Remington: The Science and Practice of Pharmacy

Volume II

19TH EDITION

Remington: Practice of

ALFONSO R GENNARO

Chairman of the Editorial Board and Editor

The Science and Pharmacy

1995

MACK PUBLISHING COMPANY
Easton, Pennsylvania 18042

Library of Congress Catalog Card No. 60-53334

ISBN 0-912734-04-3

The use of structural formulas from USAN and the USP Dictionary of Drug Names is by permission of The USP Convention. The Convention is not responsible for any inaccuracy contained herein.

NOTICE—*This text is not intended to represent, nor shall it be interpreted to be, the equivalent of or a substitute for the official United States Pharmacopeia (USP) and / or the National Formulary (NF). In the event of any difference or discrepancy between the current official USP or NF standards of strength, quality, purity, packaging and labeling for drugs and representations of them herein, the context and effect of the official compendia shall prevail.*

Printed in the United States of America by the Mack Printing Company, Easton, Pennsylvania

Table of Contents

Volume I

Part 1 Orientation

Part 2 Pharmaceutics

Part 3 Pharmaceutical Chemistry

Part 4 Pharmaceutical Testing, Analysis and Control

Part 5 Pharmacodynamics

Volume II

Part 6 Pharmaceutical and Medicinal Agents

Part 7 Industrial Pharmacy

Part 8 Pharmacy Practice

Appendix

Glossary and Index

CHAPTER 51

Medical Applications of Radioisotopes

Grafton D Chase, PhD*
Professor Emeritus of Chemistry
Philadelphia College of Pharmacy and Science
Philadelphia, PA 19104

Bernard Shapiro, MD
Chairman Emeritus
Department of Nuclear Medicine
Albert Einstein Medical Center
Philadelphia, PA 19141

Radium has the distinction of being the first radioisotope used in medicine, having been employed as early as 1901. This nuclide was the most important medical radioisotope in use up to about 1946 when artificially produced radioisotopes became available in quantity. Since that date, growth in the medical applications of radioisotopes has been very rapid as their usefulness has become more and more apparent in diagnosis, therapy and medical research and as greater numbers of physicians and other scientific personnel have been trained in their use. Current medical procedures employ more than 50 radioisotopes in a wide variety of chemical and physical forms.

Radioisotopes are used in medicine in two different ways, as radiation sources or radioactive tracers.

As *radiation sources* their principal role is in therapy. Here, the choice of the isotope for a given application is governed largely by the properties of the radiation required for treatment; the type and energy of the radiation and range in tissues are prime considerations. Except in special cases, where the radioisotope is bound to a chemical moiety or to an antibody which concentrates it in a particular tissue, the chemical properties or chemical form of a given isotope are relatively unimportant.

As a *radioactive tracer* the chemical identity and form of the nuclide are most important since, with but few exceptions, the tracer must be isotopic with the element being traced or otherwise must be capable of being incorporated as a part of a particular molecule. The nature of the radiation emitted by a tracer radioisotope is important primarily from the standpoint of its ease of detection. Radioactive tracers, available in the form of radiopharmaceuticals, are used in medicine principally for diagnostic purposes.

A radiopharmaceutical is a preparation, intended for *in vivo* use, containing a radionuclide in the form of an element, a simple salt or a complex and may exist in the form of a solid, liquid or gas.

Radiopharmaceuticals are used for diagnosis and therapy. For diagnostic applications, a radiopharmaceutical should not be pharmacologically active in that it should not produce a physiological effect. It is administered in extremely small (tracer) quantities so it does not alter that which is being measured. For therapy, the radiopharmaceutical preparation contains enough radioactivity to produce the intended specific changes in tissue.

Therapeutic Applications of Isotopes

For therapy, isotopes are used as radiation sources, not as tracers. These sources may be used either externally or internally. Their use may be summarized as

- External sources
  - Teletherapy sources—^{60}Co, ^{137}Cs, neutrons, charged particles
  - Surface sources—^{90}Sr, ^{32}P
  - Extracorporeal irradiation—^{60}Co, ^{90}Sr-^{90}Y, ^{90}Y
- Internal sources
  - Impanted sealed sources for brachytherapy
  - Locally injected radiopharmaceuticals
  - Intravenously or orally administered radiopharmaceuticals
    - Selectively absorbed or concentrated
    - Radioimmunotherapy

The therapeutic use of radioisotopes is justified basically by the fact that radioactive material, when present in a tissue or organ in sufficient quantity, will produce emanation capable of destroying existing cells and prevent the formation of new tissue. For this reason isotopic therapy generally is applied only to those diseases in which there exists extensive cellular metabolic malfunction or to those conditions in which an organ or tissue produces physiological harm through overactivity.

External Sources

Where radioisotopes are used as external sources or as sealed sources implanted in a tissue, the dose is terminated by removing the source. When they are administered internally as an unsealed source, the dose administered to the patient, either deliberately in therapy or incidentally in diagnosis, cannot be terminated at will by removing the source. In therapeutic applications the total dose must be calculated from a knowledge of the effective half-life of the isotope, the type and energy of the radiation emitted and the concentration of the isotope in the tissue.

Teletherapy sources containing kilocurie quantities of ^{60}Co or of ^{137}Cs have been used for many years for the treatment of lesions either postoperatively or where surgical removal of the lesion was not feasible. The monoenergetic nature of gamma rays provides an advantage over high-voltage X-rays which consist of a continuous spectrum of energies in addition to the characteristic energies. On the other hand, radioactive sources have the disadvantage that they cannot be turned off.

Fast neutrons, produced by neutron generators or by nuclear reactors, have received some interest for use in radiation therapy because their relative biological effectiveness surpasses that of X-rays, but their cost, and the lack of detailed knowledge concerning their effects in certain tissues and their penetrability, prevent their more widespread use. Recent research uses cyclotrons to generate high-energy, charged particles. Protons, alpha particles, heavy ions such as nitrogen, as well as pi minus mesons, are among the particles that have been considered.

Surface sources for dermatological and ophthalmological work consisting of applicators containing pure beta emitters such as ^{32}P and ^{90}Sr have been used. Bladder tumors have been treated by infiltration with ^{32}P. However, results have not created much enthusiasm for these techniques.

Extracorporeal irradiation of blood results in a depletion of lymphocytes, thereby producing an alteration in the immunological response of the individual. X-ray generators were

* Deceased.

used initially as a source of radiation; later, ^{60}Co sources were used. Attempts also have been made to prevent the rejection of grafts by the use of ^{90}Y, so placed that the blood circulating in the graft is irradiated.

Internal Sources

The use of *internal sources* for radiotherapy is confined largely to treatment with only a few different radioisotopes:

Implanted Sealed Sources—Interstitial implants of radioactive sources as seeds, ribbons or wires are used to treat tumors. They usually are put in place or the site is prepared for insertion in the operating room. Isotopes used include Cesium-137, Iridium-192, Cobalt-60, Gold-198, Iodine-125, Radium-226 and Palladium-103.

Locally Injected Radiopharmaceuticals—Phosphorus-32, as colloidal chromic phosphate, is injected intrapleurally and intraperitoneally as treatment for malignant effusions. It also may be used prophylactically in the peritoneal space following surgical removal of ovarian cancer to destroy any free-floating cells.

A number of different radionuclides have been used for radionuclide synovectomy, which is the intra-articular administration of therapeutic isotopes into a diseased joint to reduce inflamed synovium, the membrane that lines the joints. Isotopes used include colloidal Yttrium-90 and Gold-198, ferric hydroxide macroaggregates of Dysprosium-165 and Holmium-166 and microspheres of Samarium-153 and Rhenium-186.

Intravenously or Orally Administered Radiopharmaceuticals—

Selectively Absorbed or Concentrated—

Sodium Phosphate P 32 may be used in the treatment of polycythemia vera to decrease the rate of formation of the erythrocytes. Since ^{32}P is metabolized in a manner similar to naturally occurring phosphorus, the isotope is distributed readily to all tissues and is concentrated in those tissues where proliferation is most rapid. Thus, cancerous tissues concentrate the greatest amount of the isotope. A large dose of ^{32}P—1.5 to 5 mCi—will concentrate in the bone marrow but will suppress erythrogenesis only partially. In severe cases of polycythemia a phlebotomy is necessary in conjunction with ^{32}P therapy.

Sodium Iodide I 131 has several therapeutic applications. In cases of hyperthyroidism, therapeutic doses of ^{131}I will destroy thyroid tissue by means of radiation produced from within the gland. This procedure provides a more desirable mode of therapy than external roentgen-ray treatment since there is less radiation danger to the surrounding tissues. For example, in the treatment of Graves' disease, a thyroid gland that exhibits a 50% uptake at 24 hr averages 2300 to 2400 rads/mCi. The dose to be delivered generally is taken to be 5000 to 7000 rads for this malady. In the case of thyroid cancer the administration of 150 mCi of ^{131}I will deliver a tumor dose of approximately 25,000 rads, or about five times the absorbed dose that can be achieved through a typical course of external radiation therapy. This course of treatment is useful especially in cases of metastatic thyroid cancer.

Strontium Sr 89 Injection has been released for clinical use in the palliative treatment of pain from bone metastases. Strontium behaves like calcium, concentrating in active bone sites such as metastases. The diseases most often associated with bone metastases are prostate cancer and breast cancer. Pain from bone metastases can be very severe and debilitating. Eighty percent of the patients treated in one large series had significant relief. Responding patients may note relief for 1 to 15 months. Repeat treatments can be given. There are few side effects (some suppression of platelets and less likely of leukocytes). Other isotopes are being tested for the same purpose (Samarium-153 and Rhenium-186).

Radioimmunotherapy (RIT)—This is attracting interest as a potential new weapon in the arsenal for cancer therapy. In principle, monoclonal antibodies (MAbs) which have been developed against and are specific for, tumor tissue are labeled with a radionuclide. When administered intravenously the antibody seeks out the tumor and the radiation associated with the radioactive tag destroys the tumor. Among the things to be considered for a successful RIT protocol are an affinity and specificity of the antibody for the tumor, the rapidity of tumor uptake, the half-life of the antibody or nuclide in the tumor and the choice of the nuclide to maximize the radiation dose. Several achievements leading to attainment of these goals may be mentioned. High-efficiency iodination of MAbs has been achieved by using the reagent *N*-bromosuccinimide. ^{67}Cu, which is considered one of the more promising radionuclides for RIT because of its 61.5-hr half-life and abundant supply of beta particles and gamma rays, has been conjugated to antibody by using the bridging chelating agent, *p*-bromoacetamidobenzyl-tetraethylaminetetraacetic acid (TETA). ^{90}Y, which emits an energetic beta particle, also is considered a potential agent for RIT and has been coupled to antibodies by using the BCA, diethylenetriaminepentaacetic acid (DTPA). To date, however, the usefulness of labeled antibodies for RIT is still in question.

Diagnostic Applications of Isotopes

For diagnosis, isotopes are used as radioactive tracers and not as radiation sources. If results are to be meaningful the tagged substances must be handled by the body in a manner similar to that of the untagged substance.

When radioisotopes are used for diagnosis, the radiation dose delivered to the patient is maintained at as low a level as possible. This is accomplished through the judicious choice of isotope for the best combination of minimum half-life, minimum retention in the body and minimum quantity of isotope which will permit its detection and accurate measurement. Accordingly, certain isotopes, such as ^{90}Sr, ^{226}Ra and many others, are never used as unsealed internal sources or tracers. In order to reduce the radiation dose to the population there is a trend toward the use of shorter-lived isotopes, when available, for diagnostic purposes. It is for this reason that ^{57}Co and ^{58}Co often are used in place of ^{60}Co, where possible, in diagnostic procedures.

In Vitro Studies

Radioactive materials are used in performing assays on biological materials. The radioactive materials are not administered to the individual but are used as reagents in carrying out measurements of substances in biological fluids or tissues removed from the body.

Radiometric Analysis—Those radioassay methods which require the use of a standard reagent having a known relationship between chemical concentration and radiological concentration, ie, the radioactivity of a specific radioisotope per unit volume, are called radiometric analyses. For example, a sensitive method for the determination of serum calcium involves the addition of a measured excess of standard ^{14}C-oxalic acid solution to an aliquot of serum. After precipitation of calcium oxalate the radioactivity of the precipitate (or of an aliquot of the supernatant) is determined. This activity then is related to the calcium content of the serum. A variety of similar assays have been developed, including the determination of serum citric acid by the use of ^{82}Br.

Competitive Radioassay—Also known as *saturation analysis*, the basic principle of a competitive radioassay involves competitive reactions in which radioactive substrate (ligand) and nonradioactive substrate (the analyte, P) compete with each other for a binding agent Q. The *substrate* P may be a vitamin, hormone, drug or other substance the concentration of which is to be determined. To perform the assay the same substance must be available with a radioactive tag. This is P^*. ^{125}I is the most frequently used tag, with ^{3}H, ^{99m}Tc and ^{57}Co also finding limited use. A constant, known amount of tagged substrate P^* is used in all assays. The *binding agent* Q may be an ion-exchange resin, a protein, an antibody or a specific reactor for the particular substrate. The concentration of binding agent used in all assays of a series also is held constant. The independent variable is p, the concentration of nonradioactive substrate sought. Its concentration will vary. It can be seen that an increase in the concentration of P will result in an increase in the concentration of nonradioactive bound substrate, PQ, and a decrease in the concentration of radioactive bound substrate, P^*Q. The result will be an increase in free tagged substrate P^*. Therefore, the concentration of substrate P can be determined as some function of any two of the quantities B, F or T (the bound, free and total radioactivity, respectively). That is, $p = f(B, F)$, $p = f'(B, T)$ or $p = f'(F, T)$.

$$\begin{array}{ccccc} P^* & & & \rightleftarrows & PQ \\ + & & Q & & \\ + & & & \rightleftarrows & P^*Q \\ P & & & & \\ \text{FREE} & & & & \text{BOUND} \end{array}$$

If the binding between the substrate and binder is *nonspecific*, as is the case with certain protein-binding assays, it frequently is necessary to purify the substrate prior to analysis to remove interfering substances.

Alternatively, the binding agent can be made more *specific* for the particular substrate. One type of system which shows a very high degree of specificity for a particular substrate is an *immune* system. The assay is known as a *radioimmunoassay* (*RIA*) and uses an antigen-antibody reaction. If the substrate is not already antigenic it is made so by *conjugation* to a protein. Substrates requiring conjugation to a protein to produce antigenicity are known as *haptens*. Rabbits, chickens, goats and other animals then are injected with antigen to induce the production of antibodies. Usually the antigen first is mixed with an *adjuvant* in order to enhance antibody production. When the antibody level has reached a maximum level, samples of blood are removed, from time to time, to obtain serum which then must be diluted to produce a suitable antibody concentration for use in the assay. In addition, it is necessary to prepare radioactive substrate. If the substrate is a hapten which has been conjugated to a protein, tagging the compound is accomplished readily by iodination with ^{125}I. Sometimes a tritium tag is used instead.

A few specific competitive radioassays do not make use of an immune system. One typical assay is that for vitamin B_{12} in which *intrinsic factor* is used in place of an antibody as a binder. Such a binder is called a *specific reactor*.

In the simplified illustration of a RIA described, "ideal" behavior has been assumed. Most RIAs closely approach this condition. To meet the requirements of ideal behavior the following criteria should be met:

The nonradioactive and radioactive antigens, P and P^*, are indistinguishable chemically.

Both reactions go to completion. That is, the equilibrium constants not only are equal but are so great they can be considered infinite.

Antigen and antibody react in the ratio of one-to-one.

There are no cross reactions, the antibody being specific only for the single antigen indicated in the reactions.

The purpose of a RIA is to determine the concentration p of nonradioactive antigen. To conduct a RIA a standard curve first must be constructed where p is plotted as some function of radioactivity. This is known as a dose-response curve. It is constructed using data obtained by use of standard solutions as illustrated in Fig 1.

Let the concentration p^* of radioactive antigen added to each of three test tubes be 6 picomoles (p*M*)/mL. To the first tube (the blank) is added no nonradioactive antigen; to the second, 3 p*M*/mL and to the third, 12 p*M*/mL of nonradioactive antigen. Finally, equal amounts of antibody (representing 3 p*M* of antibody-binding sites/mL) are added to each of the three tubes and the content of each tube is well-mixed. The tubes then are incubated until the reactions are complete.

Bound and free antigen are now separated by some suitable means and the radioactivity B of bound antigen and the radioactivity F of free antigen are measured for each of the three standards. The total radioactivity, T $(= B + F)$, is the sum of the bound and free radioactivities. From Fig 1 it can be seen that the data tabulated in Table 1 are obtained.

The total concentration of antigen C_t $(= C_B + C_F)$ also is equal to the sum of the concentrations of radioactive and nonradioactive antigens.

$$C_t = p^* + p$$

Since radioactive and nonradioactive antigen are indistinguishable chemically, they are uniformly distributed in the system. Thus

$$\frac{C_t}{C_B} = \frac{T}{B}.$$

By combining these two relationships it follows that

$$p = -p^* + C_B\frac{T}{B}.$$

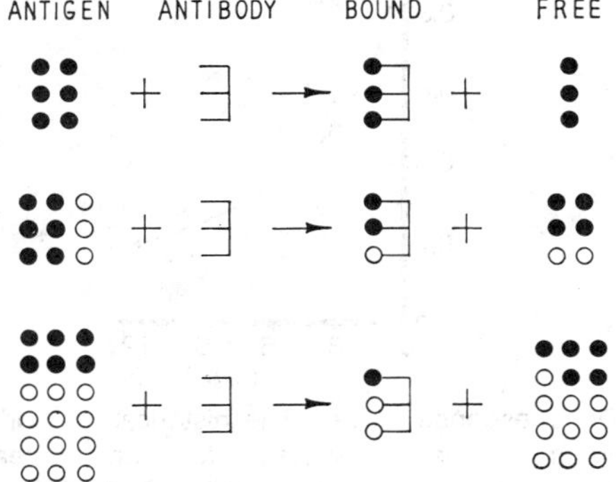

Fig 1. "Ideal" radioimmunoassay.

If q is the total concentration of antibody binding sites and q_B is the concentration of bound or occupied binding sites, then, when antigen is in excess, $q = q_B = C_B$ since the reaction is assumed to have gone to completion. Consequently

$$p = -p^* + q\frac{T}{B}.$$

By plotting the concentration p of dose antigen (nonradioactive antigen) as a function of the ratio T/B of total to bound radioactivity, a linear relationship is obtained. The y-intercept is $-p^*$ and gives the apparent concentration of radioactive antigen. The slope q gives the concentration of antibody sites. In the assay T/B is the quantity measured and p is the quantity sought. For the example cited

$$p = -6 + 3\cdot\frac{T}{B}.$$

A plot of these data is shown in Fig 2.

The usefulness of this method of data reduction lies in its clinical applicability. RIA standard curve data are essentially linearized and can be fit by a linear regression analysis. Suspect data also are recognizable readily.

In a more detailed analysis of competitive assays the equilibrium constant K must be considered. For a single species of binding site the Scatchard equation applies

$$R = \frac{B}{F} = Kq - KC_B.$$

Rearrangement shows that

$$C_B = q - \frac{R}{K}.$$

The resulting relation is

$$p = -p^* + \left(q - \frac{R}{K}\right)\frac{T}{B}.$$

Here p^* is the true concentration of radioactive antigen. The fit of experimental data is excellent and essentially linear over the clinical range of concentration.

Dose-response curves were prepared originally by plotting the ratio B/F as a function of the concentration of dose antigen p. See Fig 3. To improve linearity and to expand the graph in the region of low concentration, the ratio B/F is sometimes plotted as a function of $\log p$ as in Fig 4A. Recognizing the advantage of a linear plot of data, especially for rejection of suspect data, a *logit* plot has been used wherein logit Y is plotted as a function of $\ln p$ or $\log p$. According to one definition

$$\text{logit } Y = \ln\frac{Y'}{1 - Y'} \quad \text{where } Y' = B/B_o,$$

where B is the radioactivity of the bound antigen and B_o is the value of B for $p = 0$. For "ideal" conditions a linear plot is obtained as shown in Fig 4B. The y-intercept is $\ln p^*$ and the slope is -1 (or -2.303) depending upon whether natural or Naperian logarithms are used. This is expected since it can be shown that

$$\text{logit } Y = \ln p^* - \ln p.$$

Although the logit plot is used widely it is not recommended since it is prone to introduce plotting errors.

Immunoradiometric assays (IRMA)—These use a large excess of binder (eg, antibody) so that essentially all of the analyte becomes bound even if the binding constant is not great. In one type of IRMA a radioactively tagged antibody, Q^*, is used. Added to the analyte in large excess, analyte, P, essentially is bound completely.

$$P + Q^* \rightarrow PQ^* \; (+Q^* \text{ excess})$$

The excess of tagged antibody then is removed by using ligand (analyte) which has been immobilized by bonding to a solid phase, *P-sp*.

$$Q^* \text{ excess} + P\text{-}sp \rightarrow Q^*P\text{-}sp$$

Radioactivity remaining in solution represents radioactive antibody bound to analyte, PQ^*, and is therefore a measure of analyte concentration in the sample.

In a second, more common type of IRMA known as a "two-site sandwich" assay, analyte, P, is bound to nonradioactive antibody which is bound to a solid phase, *Q-sp*.

$$P + Q\text{-}sp \rightarrow PQ\text{-}sp \; (+Q\text{-}sp \text{ excess})$$

Table 1—Data for Simulated Standard RIA Curve

Tube no	Concentration of antigen (pM/mL)					Ratio of radioactivities		
	Radioactive p*	Nonradioactive p	Total C_t	Bound C_B	Free C_F	F/B	T/B	B/F
1	6	0	6	3	3	1	2	1
2	6	3	9	3	6	2	3	0.5
3	6	12	18	3	15	5	6	0.2

The amount of analyte bound then is determined by addition of an excess of a second radioactively tagged antibody, Q^*, to the analyte.

$$PQ\text{-}sp + Q^* \rightarrow Q^*PQ\text{-}sp$$

Bound radioactivity then is proportional to the concentration of analyte.

A modification called the "three-site sandwich" assay is similar to the two-site method except that the second antibody, specific for the analyte, is untagged. Bound analyte then is identified and quantitated by adding a third antibody, radiolabeled antigamma globulin, which binds to the second antibody. The advantage of the three-site method is that it uses the same radiolabeled Ig-G to quantify a wide variety of analytes.

Receptor Assays—Various receptor systems have been identified in body tissues and organs. These receptor systems are of physiological importance since they act as binders to specific hormones and other compounds having physiological activity. One receptor system of particular clinical importance is the estrogen receptor of breast cancers. It has been observed that breast cancers respond more dramatically to hormone treatment if they contain appreciable numbers of such estrogen receptor sites. Estrogen receptor-site assays in breast tumors, therefore, have become a routine clinical assay.

Receptors may be present either in the cell cytosol or on the cell membrane. At least certain membrane receptors have been shown to be glycoproteins and may have association constants as great as 10^9 to 10^{10} L/mole.

Receptor assays are similar to competitive binding assays, as described above, but differ in that it is the binder that is the analyte rather than the ligand. Scatchard analysis is employed most frequently to quantitate the receptor sites and to evaluate their binding constants.

In one type of receptor assay, radioactive ligand L^*, specific for the receptor in question, is added to an aliquot of tissue homogenate containing receptor R and the mixture is incubated until an equilibrium condition is achieved.

$$L^* + R \leftrightarrow LR$$

The association constant, K, is given by

$$K = (L^*R)/(L^*)(R).$$

Since the ratio of bound-to-free ligand concentration, $(L^*R)/(L^*)f$, is equal to the ratio of bound-to-free radioactivity, B/F, substitution and rearrangement yields

$$B/F = K(R).$$

The total concentration of receptor sites, r, is equal to the sum of free and bound sites, $(R) + (L^*R)$. It follows that $(R) = r - (L^*R)$ and

$$B/F = Kr - K(L^*R).$$

This is one form of the Scatchard equation. This linear form is for a single species of binding site (receptor). By repeating the measurement with a range of concentrations of radiolabeled ligand, L^*, data are obtained to plot B/F as a function of (L^*R), the bound radioactivity. The slope of the resulting curve is $-K$ and the x-intercept is r.

In practice the Scatchard plot is curved concave upward with a long tail to the right. This is due to the presence of nonspecific binding sites. It is customary to take the steepest part of the slope to represent binding to receptor. The slope at the steepest part is used for calculation of the association constant, and the intercept of the tangent with the x-axis is taken as the receptor concentration. Another complicating feature sometimes observed is a low-concentration hook resulting from positive cooperativity. The implication of such hooks is that the receptors consist of two interrelated sites, a situation often observed with antibodies.

DNA Probes—A DNA probe is a segment of a single-stranded DNA or RNA which has been tagged with a radionuclide. A probe will seek out and detect complementary sequences in the presence of a large amount of noncomplementary DNA. Since the DNA of any individual—whether human, animal, plant or microorganism is unique, except for special exceptions such as identical twins—a DNA probe is the most powerful tool for the identification of individuals. For example, through the use of DNA probes, carriers of genetic disease can be identified. Probes may be produced in several ways. They can be synthesized from the constituent nucleotides, if known, or it is possible to use an isolated and cloned segment of genomic DNA. Also, a probe can be made from messenger RNA (mRNA) using reverse transcriptase. The radioactive marker generally used for DNA probes is ^{32}P.

In Vivo Quantitative Studies

Radioactive materials are administered to the individual and then measurements are made of the distribution of the radioactive material, by detection of the radioactivity, in body fluids or tissues within the body (external counting) or after removal from the body (urine, blood, exhaled air, etc).

Thyroid Studies—Several studies of thyroid function can be carried out with the aid of radioactive ^{123}I and ^{131}I. These studies include the rate of deposition of iodine in the gland *in vivo*, the total accumulation of iodine in the gland within a specified period of time and the output of thyroid hormone into which radioactive iodine has been incorporated.

Because the thyroid has such an avidity for iodine, precautions must be taken to prevent exposure to or ingestion of even small amounts of iodine by the patient if valid results are to be obtained. Treatments to be avoided include the external application of iodine, ingestion of iodine-containing medicaments (may influence thyroid uptake for weeks), use of X-ray contrast media containing organic iodine compounds (may produce an effect on the thyroid for months) and myelography and bronchography (may have a permanent effect). The radioiodine thyroid uptake may, in addition, be lowered by such substances as thyroid preparations, antithy-

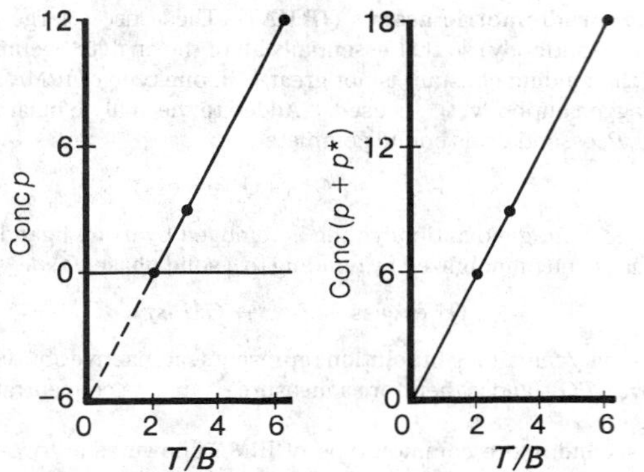

Fig 2. Dose-response curves. The linear relationship illustrated is for an elementary "ideal" radioimmunoassay and also holds for most real assays.

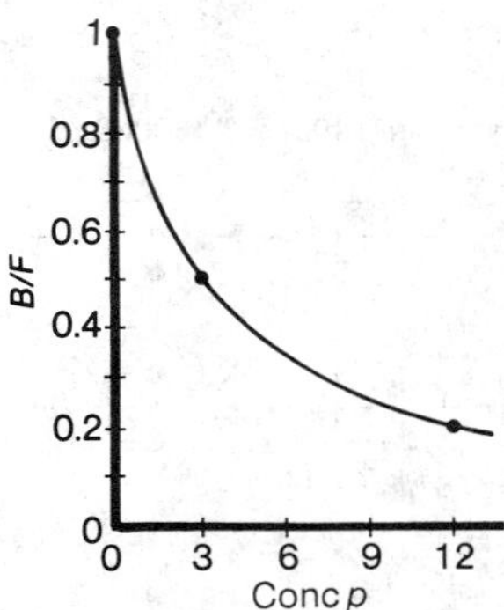

Fig 3. Dose-response curve. The historical method of plotting B/F versus p is illustrated for an "ideal" radioimmunoassay. The result is a hyperbola. The principal disadvantage of this method is the inability to recognize data which are in error.

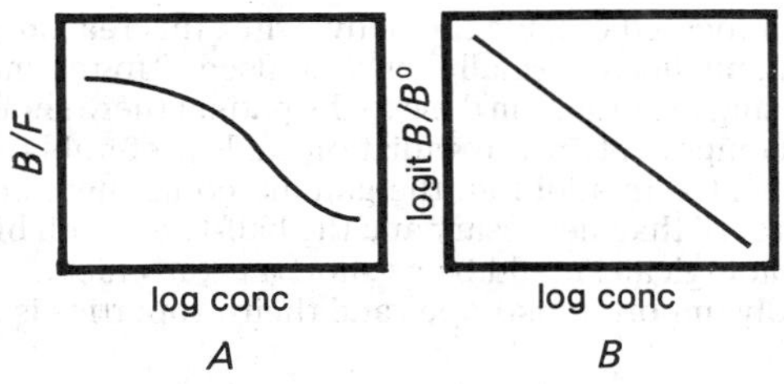

Fig 4. Dose-response curves. *A*: A semilog plot has been used in an attempt to linearize the data. This empirical approach represents an improvement over a *B/F* versus *p* plot, but falls short of being linear. *B*: A logit plot is linear for an "ideal" situation as shown here for the plot of "ideal" data. Its disadvantage is that it is empirical and does not explain readily cases which deviate from linearity. In addition, it cannot be extended to zero concentration of antigen.

roid drugs, thiocyanate perchlorate, corticotropin, corticosteroids, phenylbutazone, sulfonamides, *p*-aminosalicylic acid, arsenic, lead and mercury. Malabsorption syndromes and renal disease also will lower thyroid uptake.

The thyroid gland concentrates inorganic iodide from the blood and converts it to thyroxine, the thyroid hormone, through the action of a peroxidase enzyme. When a thyroid gland is relatively "iodine starved," ie, receiving no more iodine than is found in the normal diet, the administration of a small dose of radioactive iodine results in a portion of the dose being retained by the thyroid while the remainder of the radioactive isotope is excreted in the urine. The amount of radioactive iodine retained by the thyroid is an index of thyroid function.

For *thyroid uptake* the most commonly employed technique involves the oral administration of 50 μCi of $Na^{123}I$ or 5–10 μCi of $Na^{131}I$ followed by measurement of the radioactivity of the thyroid after the elapse of a given time. A sample of $Na^{123}I$ or $Na^{131}I$ is set aside as a standard. After the elapse of about 24 hours, the radioactivity of the thyroid is determined with a gamma-sensitive detector and pluse-height analyzer. The activity is compared to that of the standard when measured under identical conditions of geometry. A lucite neck phantom with inserted $Na^{123}I$ or $Na^{131}I$ standard are used to simulate identical geometry. See Fig 5.

The normal range for iodine uptake is about 10 to 35% in 24 hours. Uptakes from 10 to 15% and from 35 to 40% may be considered borderline. An uptake exceeding 50% may indicate hyperthyroidism while an uptake of less than 15% usually may indicate hypothyroidism.

Although the thyroid uptake is a valid measure of thyroid gland activity, blood levels of thyroid hormones, thyroxine (T-4) and triiodothyronine (T-3), and thyroid stimulating hormone (TSH) by radioimmunoassay are the primary methods currently used to assess thyroid function. However, the thyroid uptake is still important for diagnosing acute thyroiditis (where the uptake is low while the blood hormones are at hyperthyroid levels), chronic thyroiditis (where the uptake is high while the blood hormones are at hypothyroid levels) and for estimating treatment doses of Iodine-131 for hyperthyroidism.

The use of radioiodine is contraindicated during the second and third trimesters of pregnancy. The fetal thyroid gland is developed sufficiently at 12 to 14 weeks to pick up iodine from the maternal circulation. Even a tracer dose given to the mother may be sufficient to inhibit or injure the fetal thyroid.

Two mechanisms which compete for the iodine circulating in the body are uptake by the thyroid and urinary excretion. The amount of iodine excreted by the kidneys is related inversely to the amount fixed by the thyroid.

Red Blood Cell and Plasma Volume—

Isotope Dilution—The principles of isotope dilution are discussed in Chapter 25. The clinical application of this technique is illustrated by its use for the measurement of blood volume. The more popular procedure uses radioiodinated human serum albumin injected intravenously; 10 min after injection, a time sufficient to allow adequate mixing of the labeled albumin in the intravascular pool, yet not long enough for metabolic activity or seepage into extravascular pools to occur, a blood sample is withdrawn. The blood volume is calculated from the measured decrease in radioactivity of the injected sample upon its dilution by the blood. Red-blood-cell volume and plasma volume are related to the blood volume by the peripheral venous hematocrit. RBC volumes also can be determined by the use of cells labeled with ^{51}Cr in the form of sodium chromate.

Chromium-51 tagging of red blood cells is carried out by the addition of sodium chromate-Cr-51 to whole blood in ACD solution. The chromate anion diffuses rapidly into the cells where the chromate chromium is reduced to chromic chromium by the natural intracellular reducing agents. In the chromic state, chromium is rapidly bound to the globin moiety of hemoglobin where it stays permanently and provides an excellent cell label. The process provides about 90% labeling efficiency.

Radioactive hydrogen, ^{3}H, in the form of tritiated water can be used to determine total body water. Total body potassium, sodium or chloride, usually referred to as "spaces," can be determined by the use of the radioactive isotopes of these elements. In the case of chloride, ^{82}Br usually is used instead of ^{36}Cl because of the long half-life of the latter.

Red Blood Cell Survival Time—The RBC destruction mechanism and RBC half-life are measured by means of a disappearance-rate technique. If erythrocytes are labeled *in vitro* with ^{51}Cr and then reinjected, the fate of the tagged cells can be followed by assay of serial blood samples taken every 2 or 3 days for at least 2 weeks. Since the labeled cell group contains cells of all ages, only a mean survival time can be determined for them. The rate of decrease in circulating ^{51}Cr is approximately exponential and thus can be characterized by a half-clearance-time. The normal RBC half-life is about 26 days. This study is a valuable aid in the diagnosis of hemolytic anemias. See Fig 6.

Splenic Sequestration—In certain types of hemolytic anemias, red cells disappear rapidly from the blood stream, being trapped and eventually destroyed by the spleen. The extent of RBC uptake by the spleen can be determined by tagging the cells *in vitro* with ^{51}Cr, reinjecting them intravenously, counting externally over the spleen and liver and calculating the ratio of spleen/liver radioactivity. A high ratio, associated with decreased RBC survival, may indicate the need for a splenectomy.

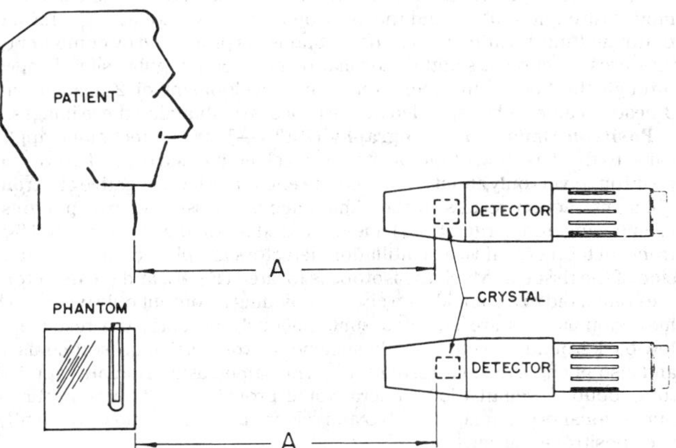

Fig 5. In practice, thyroid uptake is measured by intercomparison of the activity of the standard ^{131}I capsules (or source) in a phantom with the activity in the patient's thyroid (courtesy, Picker International).

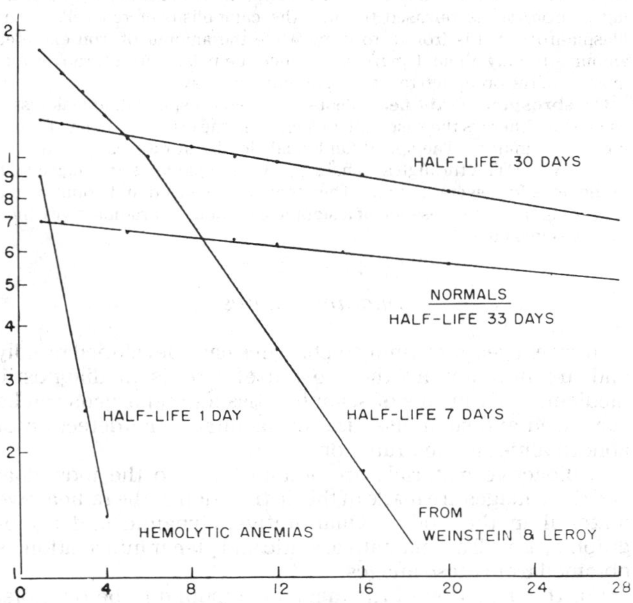

Fig 6. Red-cell tagging with ^{51}Cr permits a direct determination of erythrocyte life in anemic patients (courtesy, Picker International).

Breath Tests—*Campylobacter pylori*, an organism suspected of causing chronic gastritis and peptic ulceration, can be detected through the large amounts of urease (urea-amidohydrolase) which it produces. ^{14}C-labeled urea, administered orally, is decomposed by urease to carbon dioxide. Subsequent detection of the ^{14}C-labeled carbon dioxide in the exhaled breath is achieved by absorption in hyamine hydroxide, followed by measurement of ^{14}C in a liquid scintillation counter.

Shilling Test—The *Schilling Test* is useful for the detection of pernicious anemia and for its differentiation from other macrocytic anemias.

In a normal individual, over 50% of an oral dose of vitamin B_{12} is absorbed through the walls of the gastrointestinal tract. This absorption occurs only in the presence of the intrinsic factor of Castle with which the vitamin presumably must combine in order to pass through the intestinal walls. (The biochemical defect in pernicious anemia is the failure of the gastric mucosa to elaborate intrinsic factor.) By means of ^{60}Co-labeled vitamin B_{12} it has been shown that over half of an oral dose soon appears in the blood. Normally, only a small amount of activity appears in the urine, but if a large "flushing" dose (1000 μg) of vitamin B_{12} is given parenterally, within 1 hour after the tagged oral dose, the renal threshold is exceeded and radioactivity is observed in the urine.

In the pernicious anemia patient, there is a deficiency of intrinsic factor which causes poor absorption of the vitamin and most of the ingested B_{12} will therefore be found in the feces. The degree of absorption or of fecal excretion can be measured by the use of labeled vitamin B_{12}.

Other anemias, such as those associated with sprue and idiopathic steatorrhea, also are accompanied by a decrease in vitamin B_{12} absorption. They may be differentiated from pernicious anemia through the oral administration of intrinsic factor. A marked increase in vitamin B_{12} absorption results in the pernicious anemia patient but not in the case of sprue and other malabsorption syndromes.

In order to reduce the radiation dose received by the patient, while at the same time improving the available sensitivity of the test, ^{57}Co and ^{58}Co are used instead of ^{60}Co as the radioactive tag for vitamin B_{12} (cyanocobalamin).

If plasma iron is labeled by intravenous injection of Ferrous Citrate Fe 52, Fe 55 or Fe 59, it is possible to obtain a comprehensive evaluation of the *kinetics of iron metabolism*. Among the parameters which can be measured are

Plasma iron clearance half-time
Plasma volume
Hematocrit
Blood volume
Red-cell iron incorporation
Daily iron clearance (plasma-iron turnover; plasma-iron transport rate)
Daily hemoglobin formation
Percent daily hemoglobin replacement

The iron turnover, from the catabolism of hemoglobin, can be estimated in the following way. The average blood volume of a normal adult is about 5000 mL. The hemoglobin content is about 15 g/100 mL of blood or about 750 g/person. Iron represents 0.334% of hemoglobin. The hemoglobin-iron content per person is, therefore, about 2.6 g. If the nominal life of a red cell is 110 to 125 days, then approximately 21 to 24 mg of iron/day is released through the catabolism of red cells. The plasma-iron level is from 2 to 3 mg while the amount of iron excreted amounts to only about 1 mg/day. Hence the plasma-iron turnover rate must be of the order of 6 to 8 times, or more, per day.

Cerebrospinal Fluid Leak Test—The cerebrospinal fluid leak test is used where there is the suspicion of a crack in the cribriform plate following a head injury. The spinal fluid is labeled by intrathecal injection of Indium-111-DTPA through a spinal tap. Cotton pledgets are placed high in the nose for several hours. They then are removed and counted in a well counter. The presence of a significant amount of radioactivity indicates a spinal fluid leak.

Imaging Studies

In recent years scanning techniques have developed rapidly and are now among the most useful tools in diagnostic medicine. By means of scanning, tissues and organs can be visualized and such visualization facilitates the detection of abnormalities in their function.

Radioactive materials are administered to the individual and then images are made of the distribution of the radioactive material in the body. Quantitative, dynamic and tomographic, as well as qualitative, static and planar information, is obtained from these images.

For the detection of the tagged compound to be possible, the radiation emitted by the tagging nuclide must be sufficiently penetrating to pass through tissues so it can reach a detector located outside the body. For this reason, gamma-emitting nuclides normally must be used. In the interest of minimizing the radiation dose to the patient there should be no alpha component in the radiation and, preferably, no beta component. In addition, the gamma component should be no "harder" than necessary and the half-lives, both biological and radiological, should be as short as convenient. A list of medically important isotopes and their properties is found in Table 2.

Methodology—

Scintillation Scanning—This is a method of presenting the localization of radioactive isotope in the body by creating an image, on an oscilloscope screen and on film, wherein the variations in concentration of isotope in the body are reflected in the variations in intensity of the various points in the image. It is called scanning because the original instruments for producing the image used a scintillation probe moving back and forth over the body from the top to the bottom of the area under study registering the level of radioactivity by the frequency of dots on pressure-sensitive paper or the darkness of spots on photographic film.

At the present time these images are made by scintillation cameras. The *scintillation camera*, also known as the *radiation camera* or *gamma camera*, is a nonscanning device. Several types are available. One consists of a single sodium iodide crystal 11½ in. in diameter which is viewed by an array of 19 photomultiplier tubes. See Fig 7. Scintillations produced in the crystal are displayed on an oscilloscope as flashes of light that correspond in position with the original image in the scintillation crystal. Images are projected from the radioactive tissue onto the crystal either by pinhole collimation of the radiation or by multichannel collimation. Multichannel collimators consist of a lead block penetrated by a honeycomb-like network of holes. The image appearing on the oscilloscope screen is recorded photographically. The time required to obtain a useful image by means of the scintillation camera is only about $\frac{1}{10}$ of that required for scanning.

The scintillation camera views a large area of the body and produces an image which can be processed by computer to obtain the best possible visualization of the distribution of the radioisotope in the organ or tissue studied. The image can be analyzed quantitatively and can be dynamic as well as static. Where the radiosotope is changing in concentration in an area, this can be recorded temporally producing a motion picture which also can be analyzed quantitatively. Thus, one can visualize a beating heart or a bleeding site or passage of a radiopharmaceutical into and out of an organ or tissue. Normal versus abnormal patterns, both static and dynamic, can be correlated with normal and disease states.

A second type of scintillation camera is the *Autofluoroscope* in which, instead of one large crystal, an array of several hundred crystals is used in combination with multichannel collimation. Each crystal is coupled through light pipes to a rank-and-file system of photocells so that pulses appearing in a particular pair of photocells uniquely identify a particular crystal. Displayed on an oscilloscope, the image can be recorded photographically. Information also can be stored in a magnetic memory for future analysis to optimize contrast. Because scintillation cameras are so fast, dynamic processes can be observed. For example, serial photographs have been prepared showing heart and kidney function.

Single Photon Emission Computerized Tomography (SPECT)—This is a technique using a scintillation camera to produce sectional (slice) images of radiopharmaceutical distribution in the body. The camera is moved through 360° around the body on a fixed axis collecting information at multiple positions. The data obtained is processed by computer to give cross-sectional, sagittal, coronal or even odd angular slice images through the body. In recent years the development of 2-headed and 3-headed cameras has speeded up the process of obtaining these images.

Positron Emission Tomography (PET)—This is a technique applicable to the detection of radioisotopes which emit positrons. In tissue, a positron travels only about a 1 mm before encountering a negative electron. Their interaction results in the simultaneous emission of two photons, each having an energy of 0.51 meV, emitted at an angle of exactly 180° from each other. If two scintillation detectors are placed, one on either side of the tissue in which the isotope is located (Fig 8), and the detectors are connected to a coincidence circuit providing an output only when 0.51 meV gamma rays are detected simultaneously by both, the result is a low-background detector, highly specific for the particular isotope used and also giving excellent resolution. The same basic principles applied to a "double" scintillation camera would provide the ultimate in three-dimensional organ imaging. ^{11}C and ^{18}F are among the most frequently used positron-emitting tags.

Computerized Tomography (CT) is X-ray or gamma-ray photography of a selected plane in the body. In order to reconstruct a picture showing anatomical details clearly it is necessary to process data by a computer. CT combines an accumulation of radiation data with the advantage of its rapid analysis by computer. CT may operate on the basis of either of two fundamental concepts with regard to the source of radiation: *emission* of radiation from an internally administered radiopharmaceutical and *transmission* of radiation from an external X-ray source. Each type of CT yields distinctly different information.

Applications—

Cardiovascular Studies—

Myocardial Perfusion—The most common cardiac study performed in nuclear medicine at present is the stress test with nuclear imaging. The study involves stressing the patient with exercise on a treadmill or giving an intravenous injection of dipyridamole. An injection of Thallium-201 chloride or Technetium-99m-labeled methoxyisobutylisonitrile (MIBI) is then given and imaging is carried out preferably with tomography. Redistribution imaging at 3 to 4 hours without reinjection (for Tl-201) or on a separate day with reinjection for (Tc-99m-MIBI) are carried out for comparison.

The radioactive agents used behave like potassium in that they enter viable myocardial cells but do not enter dead cells. Myocardial cell concentration of the radioactive agents also is related to the relative perfusion of the tissue. Regions that cannot respond to stress by augmented perfusion due to coronary artery disease are relatively low in radioactivity compared to normal regions that do respond to stress with augmented perfusion. Tomographic slices are studied for localization of poorly perfused areas indicative of stenosed coronary arteries. This study helps make decisions in the management of patients with suspected cardiac disease.

Myocardial Infarction Imaging—Technetium Tc 99m Sodium Pyrophosphate Injection, while primarily a skeletal-imaging agent, has been used as a cardiac-imaging agent as an adjunct to the diagnosis of acute myocardial infarction. Deposition in the infarcted zone has been explained on the basis of increased Ca^{2+} deposition in such tissues, but pyrophosphate seems to be taken up by ischemic tissue as well.

Ventricular Function—Gated Cardiac Imaging is a technique which allows the motion of the heart to be visualized in a movie-like manner. Red blood cells can be labeled with technetium *in vivo*. The method involves the intravenous injection of the contents of a commercial vial containing 12 mg sodium pyrophosphate and 3.4 mg stannous chloride in saline. Thirty minutes later 15 to 20 mCi Tc-99m pertechnetate is injected. About 95% of the radioactivity will remain red-cell bound for 1 hour. Five percent, and sometimes more, of the activity remains free and will diffuse through the tissue and be excreted in the urine. After labeling red blood cells with technetium, sequential images of the heart are recorded with a scintillation camera. A series of 15 to 30 frames is stored in a computer. Since each frame represents only a fraction of a second it is necessary to accumulate and superimpose data for many cycles in order to obtain clear images. The synchronization of imaging cycles is made possible by use of an EKG-gating device to indicate the beginning of a heart cycle.

Left Ventricular (LV) *Function* has been evaluated using a variety of techniques. One important parameter in the evaluation of LV function is the ejection fraction (EF). It first is necessary to measure either the ventricular radioactivity or the ventricular volume during maximum contraction, ie, end-systole (ES) and during maximum volume, ie, end-diastole (ED). The value of EF then is calculated by using the relationship

$$EF = \frac{ED - ES}{ED}$$

Detection of the radiation has been by use of the standard gamma camera. Usually, the detector is synchronized to the heart beat with an EKG which identifies the times corresponding to ED and ES, as in the case of gated cardiac imaging.

Bone Imaging—This study is used widely in the diagnosis of benign and malignant, primary and metastatic bone tumors. It also is useful in the study of patients with suspected fracture, arthritis, metabolic bone disease, avascular necrosis, bone infarcts and bone healing. The major radiopharmaceutical used at present is technetium-99m-methylenediphosphonate (MDP) which is adsorbed onto the surface of hydroxapatite crystals. The images are produced by scintillation cameras taking *spot* views at various sites or whole body views with cameras that move from head to toe. Tomography of the spine is very useful in identifying the exact location of spinal abnormalities. *Triple phase* studies imaging blood flow, blood pool and delayed bone uptake are helpful in diagnosing fractures, osteomyelitis, reflex sympathetic dystrophy and septic arthritis. See Fig 9.

Renal Studies—These provide information on blood flow and function of the kidneys. They are particularly helpful in following patients with suspected kidney stones, kidney infections and with kidney transplants. There are several radiopharmaceuticals in use, technetium-99m-DTPA and iodine-131-iodohippurate being the most common. Tc-99m-DTPA is excreted entirely by glomerular filtration whereas iodohippurate-I-131 is excreted mainly (80%) by tubular secretion.

A new agent Tc-99m-mercaptoacetylglycylglycylglycine (MAG_3) is available having the advantage of a technetium tag with the pharmacokinetics of hippurate. Kidneys are imaged for 30 minutes after injection of the first two agents or the latter agent. Areas of interest over each kidney are established and time-activity curves are generated. The initial part of either Tc-99m agent curve shows the blood flow through each kidney. The rest of the curves show the concentration (rise in radioactivity) and the excretion (fall in radioactivity) for each kidney. If there is obstruction, the curve continues to rise as radioactivity continues to accumulate. Different patterns are seen with different kidney disease states.

Other renal agents, Tc-99m-glucoheptonate and Tc-99m-dimercaptosuccinic acid, are used for anatomical information because they are concentrated in the renal tubules and stay there. These agents are used for diagnosis of pyelonephritis, congenital anomalies and kidney localization.

Lung Imaging—The main purpose of lung imaging is the diagnosis of pulmonary emboli. The agent used is Tc-99m-macroaggregated albumin. After injection into an arm vein the radioactive particles lodge in the capillaries of the lung. Only 0.1% of the capillaries are blocked and only for a few hours, so the procedure is innocuous. If there is an embolus blocking the flow to the capillary bed the radioactive particles will not reach the capillaries in the segment supplied by that vessel, resulting in a defect in the image in that region. Images are obtained in multiple views to observe and localize the defect. This is known as a perfusion lung scan. It must be accompanied by a ventilation lung scan. This is carried out by having the patient breathe Xenon-133 gas and imaging the distribution of radioactive gas in the lungs after the first deep breath, after breathing Xenon-133 to equilibrium and after washing out the Xenon-133 with air. Patients with emphysema, asthma or other chronic lung disease will not ventilate certain areas of the lungs and consequently will not perfuse them. The matching perfusion defects are not necessarily pulmonary emboli. The ventilation scan is necessary to rule out false positive perfusion lung scans. See Fig 10.

Thyroid and Parathyroid Imaging—The thyroid gland was the first organ to be imaged by isotopic methods. Since iodine-131 was one of the first radioactive isotopes available for clinical use and since the thyroid gland naturally concentrates iodine, this was an excellent set of circumstances to begin nuclear imaging. Thyroid scans are obtained mainly to identify the presence of nodules and to determine whether they concentrate radioactivity (warm or hot nodule) or not (cold nodules). Cold nodules are more likely to be malignant. Thyroid scans also are used to locate the thyroid, estimate its size, determine dose of I-131 for treatment of hyperthyroidism and look for recurrent thyroid cancer and metastases. Radiopharmaceuticals used include iodine-123 and Technetium-99m-pertechnetate. The latter is concentrated in the thyroid in the same way as iodine but is not incorporated into thyroid hormones and rapidly diffuses out of the gland. See Fig 11.

Parathyroid imaging is used to look for parathyroid adenomas in patients with hyperparathyroidism. The patient receives an injection of Tc-99m-pertechnetate and Thallium-201 chloride. The Tc-99m is picked up only by the thyroid whereas the Tl-201 is picked up by both thyroid and parathyroid adenomas. The Tc-99m image is subtracted from the Tl-201 image to reveal the parathyroid adenoma.

Biliary Tract Imaging—Imaging of the biliary tract is carried out primarily to aid in the diagnosis of acute cholecystitis and to differentiate it from other causes of right-upper-quadrant abdominal pain. The radiopharmaceutical used is a Tc-99m labeled analog of iminodiacetic acid called HIDA. After the patient is injected with the agent, imaging takes place for 1 hour. In that time the hepatic and common ducts should be visualized and radioactivity should appear in the small bowel. In acute cholecystitis the cystic duct usually is blocked and the gall bladder will not be visualized by 1 hour or even in a delayed image at 4 hours. In chronic cholecystitis the gall bladder may be visualized by 4 hours. See Fig 12.

Brain Imaging—A radiopharmaceutical effective for brain imaging must be capable of crossing the blood-brain barrier. Recently, several, uncharged, lipophilic radiopharmaceuticals possessing this capability have been reported and/or are commercially available. There are two types of such radiopharmaceuticals based upon their pharmacokinetic properties. Those with a brain distribution proportional to blood flow and those whose concentration is associated with receptor binding. One of the more interesting radiopharmaceuticals for imaging cerebral perfusion is a cyclic amine, Technetium-99m-hexamethylpropylene oxime (HM-PAO), using single photon emission computed tomography (SPECT). This is a lipid-soluble neutral chelate which passes the blood-brain barrier readily, and its distribution is proportional to blood flow.

Another such agent is iodine-123-d,*l*-*N*-isopropyl-*p*-iodoamphetamine. This agent also distributes in the brain in proportion to blood flow, but it redistributes in 1 to 2 hours giving some additional information on the cerebral circulation. The major application has been to distinguish Alzheimer's disease from other dementias. Imaging must be tomographic. Some of the patterns are characteristic of some neuropsychiatric diseases.

Cisternography—This is a technique involving the intraspinal injection—usually lumbar—of a radiopharmaceutical for the purpose of observ-

Table 2—Properties of Frequently Used Medical Isotopes

Isotope	Radiological half-life	Beta energies[a] (meV)	Gamma energies (meV)
^{2}H	stable	. . .	. . .
^{3}H	12.26 yr	0.018(100%)	. . .
^{11}C	20.3 min	β+0.97(99+%)	0.51[b](200%)
^{14}C	5730 yr	0.156(100%)	. . .
^{13}N	10.0 min	β+1.20(100%)	0.51[b](200%)
^{15}O	124 sec	β+1.70(100%)	0.51(200%)
^{18}F	109.7 min	β+0.635(97%), EC(3%)	0.51[b](194%)
^{22}Na	2.60 yr	β+0.54(89%), EC(11%)	1.28(100%), 0.51[b]
^{24}Na	15.0 hr	1.39(100%)	1.37(100%), 2.75(10%)
^{32}P	14.3 days	1.71(100%)	. . .
^{35}S	88 days	0.168(100%)	. . .
^{42}K	12.4 hr	3.53(82%), 2.01(18%)	1.52(18%)
^{43}K	22.4 hr	0.82(87%), 0.46(8%)	0.373(85%), 0.619(81%), 0.59(13%)
^{45}Ca	165 days	0.25(100%)	. . .
^{47}Ca-^{47}Sc	4.53 days	0.66(83%), 1.96(17%)	1.31(16%)
(Daughter ^{47}Sc)	3.43 days	0.44(74%), 0.60(26%)	0.16(74%)
^{51}Cr	27.8 days	EC(100%)	0.32(8%)
^{52}Fe	8.2 hr	β+(56%), EC(44%)	0.165(100%), 0.511(112%)
(Daughter ^{52m}Mn)	21 min	β+	0.511(193%), 1.434(100%)
^{55}Fe	2.6 yr	EC(100%)	. . .
^{59}Fe	45 days	0.46(54%), 0.27(46%)	1.10(57%), 1.29(43%), 0.19(2.8%)
^{57}Co	270 days	EC(100%)	0.122(93%), 0.137(7%)
^{58}Co	71.3 days	β+0.48(14%), EC(86%)	0.81(100%), 0.51[b]
^{60}Co	5.26 yr	0.31(100%)	1.17(100%), 1.33(100%)
^{64}Cu	12.8 hr	EC(43%), 0.57(38%) β+0.66(19%)	 0.51[b]
^{62}Zn	9.3 hr	β+0.66(18%), EC(82%)	0.51[b]
^{65}Zn	245 days	EC(98.5%), β+0.325 (1.5%)	1.11(45%), 0.51[b]
^{69m}Zn	13.8 hr		0.439(95%)
^{67}Ga	78 hr	EC	0.093(40%), 0.184(24%), 0.296(22%), 0.388(7%)
^{68}Ga	68.3 min	β+1.90(88%), EC(12%)	0.51[b](1.76%), 1.078(3.5%)
^{74}As	17.9 days	1.36(17%), 0.69(16%), β+0.90(26%), EC(38%)	0.60(63%), 0.64(16%), 0.51[b]
^{75}Se	120.4 days	EC(100%)	0.265(71%), 0.136(24%), 0.405(14%), 0.077(14%), 0.098(6%), 0.281(5%)
^{75}Br	1.7 hr	β+(90%), 1.70(75%) EC(10%)	0.285(75%)
^{77}Br	57 hr	EC(99%), β+0.34(1%)	0.24(30%), 0.300(67%), 0.52(24%), 0.58(7%), 0.75(2%), 0.82(3%), 1.00(1.3%)
^{82}Br	35.34 hr	0.44(100%)	0.78(87%), 0.55(70%), 0.62(43%), 1.04(30%), 0.70(29%), 1.32(28%), 0.83(26%), 1.48(18%)
^{81m}Kr	13 sec	IT	0.190(65%)
^{85}Kr	10.76 yr	0.67(99+%)	0.052(0.65%)
^{81}Rb	4.7 hr	EC(87%), β+1.03(13%)	0.51[b](26%)
^{82}Rb	1.3 min	β+(96%)	0.511(192%), 0.777(9%)
^{86}Rb	18.66 days	1.77(91%), 0.7(9%)	1.08(9%)
^{85}Sr	64 days	EC(100%)	0.514(100%)
^{87m}Sr	2.8 hr	IT	0.388(80%)
^{89}Sr	50.5 days	1.47(>99%)	
^{90}Sr-^{90}Y	28.1 yr	0.54(100%)	. . .
(Daughter ^{90}Y)	64.2 hr	2.26(100%)	. . .
^{97}Ru	2.9 days	EC(100%)	0.2154(92%), 0.1091
^{99m}Tc	5.997 hr	. . .	IT0.002(98.6%), 0.140 (98.6%), 0.142(1.4%)
^{103}Pd	17.0 days	0.03975	
^{111}In	2.8 days	EC	0.173(8%), 0.247(94%)
^{113m}In	100 min		0.393(74%)
^{115m}In	4.50 hr	0.83(5%)	0.335(95%)
^{113}Sn	115 days	EC(98%)	0.08846, 0.15900
^{123m}Te	117 days		
^{123}I	13.3 hr	EC	0.159(83%)
^{125}I	60 days	EC	0.035(7%), IC(93%)
^{131}I	8.05 days	0.61(87%), 0.33(9%), 0.25(3%)	0.36(80%), 0.64(9%), 0.28(5%), 0.72(3%)

Table 2—Continued

Isotope	Radiological half-life	Beta energies[a] (meV)	Gamma energies (meV)
^{127}Xe	36.4 days	EC	0.203(65%), 0.172(22%), 0.375(20%)
^{133}Xe	5.27 days	0.346(99+%)	0.081(37%)
^{129}Cs	32 hr	EC, no β^+	0.04(2%), 0.28(3%), 0.32(4%), 0.375(48%), 0.416(25%), 0.55(5%)
^{131}Cs	9.70 days	EC, no β^+	Xe, X-rays
^{131}Ba	12 days	EC, no β^+	0.124(28%), 0.216(19%), 0.25(5%), 0.373(13%), 0.496(48%)
^{135m}Ba	28.7 hr		IT, 0.268(16%)
^{153}Sm	47 hr	. . .	0.103(28%), 0.070(5.4%)
^{157}Dy	8.1 hr	EC, no β^+	0.326(91%)
^{169}Yb	32 days	EC	0.063(45%), 0.110(18%), 0.131(11%), 0.177(22%), 0.198(35%), 0.308(10%)
^{178}Ta	2.1 hr	EC	0.328(120%), 0.427(97%), 0.214(75%), 0.093(14%)
^{182}Ta	115 days	1.71(0.3%), 0.216(29%)	0.068(42%), 0.100(14%), 0.152(7%), 0.222(8%), 1.122(34%), 1.189(16%) 1.222(27%), 1.231(13%)
^{192}Ir	74.2 days	0.67(48%), 0.53(41%), 0.26(7%), EC(3.5%)	0.296(29%), 0.31(28%), 0.60(11%), 0.61(7%), 0.48(6%), 0.59(6%)
^{195m}Au	31 sec	IT	0.0567, 0.2615, 0.318
^{198}Au	2.698 days	0.97(99%), 0.28(1%)	0.411(96%), 0.674(1%)
^{197}Hg	64.8 hr	EC(100%)	0.077(19.3%), 0.091(0.5%)
^{203}Hg	46.9 days	0.21(100%)	0.279(83%), IC(17%)
^{201}Tl	73 hr	EC(100%)	0.167(8%), 0.135(2%)
^{203}Pb	52.1 hr	EC(100%)	0.279(81%), 0.401(5%)
^{226}Ra	1602 yr	α4.78(94.3%) α4.59(5.7%)	0.187(4%)
(^{226}Ra daughters)		Many	Many

[a]Unless otherwise specified, the energies given are for negatrons.
[b]Annihilation radiation from positron emission.
Events occurring in less than 1% of the decays have been omitted.

ing the pathway of the CSF. After injection of the tracer dose, its distribution is determined periodically by scanning or imaging. Normally, the tracer moves up to the spinal subarachnoid space or into the basal cisterns, moving toward the brain. Cisternography is useful in the diagnosis of hydrocephalus, intraventricular tumor, subarachnoid hemorrhage, rhinorrhea and other pathological conditions.

Human serum albumin I 131 has been used extensively for cisternography, but human serum albumin Tc 99m is superior because it provides better photon yields. ^{99m}Tc-inulin has been used in a similar manner. The use of ^{169}Yb-DTPA offers the advantage that the longer radiological half-life of ^{169}Yb (32 days) and the stability of the ^{169}Yb-DTPA complex allow a strict quality control, a very important feature for a radiopharmaceutical intended for injection in such a critical location.

A comparison of the useful photons per rad showed ^{111}In to be superior to ^{131}I, ^{99m}Tc, ^{169}Yb and ^{203}Pb. The use of ^{111}In-transferin, ^{111}In-EDTA and ^{111}In-DTPA in cisternography has been investigated. The studies show ^{111}In-DTPA to be essentially the ideal radiopharmaceutical for cisternography.

Liver, Spleen and Bone-Marrow Imaging—These organs are readily imaged with Tc-99m-sulfur colloid. The colloid particles are concentrated in the reticuloendothelial (RE) cells by phagocytosis and remain there permanently. The liver image is used to look for liver cysts, abscesses or metastases or for cirrhosis. A separate technique using tagged red blood cells is used for diagnosis of hemangiomas of the liver. The spleen is imaged for size, accessory spleens, infarcts and metastases. Bone-marrow imaging is used to determine the distribution of active marrow in the body and to identify infarcts, metastases and osteomyelitis. Bone-marrow scanning also can be carried out using indium-111-chloride, which distributes in the body like iron. See Fig 13.

Gastrointestinal (GI) Studies—This category includes a number of different types of scans using different radiopharmaceuticals. The most common study is the measurement of gastric emptying. Tc-99m-sulfur colloid is added to eggs which then are scrambled and fed to the patient. Images of the stomach at 5 and 90 minutes are obtained, and quantitation of stomach radioactivity is carried out. Normal individuals empty 50% or more of gastric radioactivity in this interval. Patients with gastroparesis empty less.

Gastroesophageal reflux is another GI study which involves oral administration of Tc-99m-sulfur colloid in acidified orange juice to the patient. With the patient in the supine position and with a pressure cuff applied to the epigastrium, pressure is applied in 20-torr increments with imaging at each step. Normally a patient should be able to withstand 100-torr pressure on the epigastrium without the appearance of radioactivity in the esophagus. Disease of the esophagus may result in gastroesophageal reflux at much lower pressures.

Gastrointestinal bleeding can be a serious emergency. By *in vivo* labeling of red blood cells with Tc-99m and imaging over the abdomen, it may be possible to identify a bleeding site in the GI tract and direct the angiographer or surgeon to the location of the hemorrhage.

Abscess Localization—The main agents used for abscess localization are Gallium-67 citrate and radiolabeled white blood cells. Gallium is concentrated by leukocytes and therefore will appear at sites of inflammation. It is used to look for abscesses and osteomyelitis. Since it is also a bone agent and a tumor agent, it has certain limitations. The excretion of Ga-67 by the bowel makes difficult the detection of abdominal abscesses in some cases.

White blood cells can be labeled with In-111 or Tc-99m by several different methods but most require initial separation of the white cells prior to the labeling. In-111-labelled oxine and Tc-99m-hexamethylpropyleneamine oxime (HMPAO) are the radiopharmaceuticals used. Tagged white cells concentrate in the spleen, liver and in the first 24 hours in the lungs. Localization of inflammation in these areas is limited, but the method is quite sensitive for localization of abscesses in the abdomen.

Tumor Localization—The localization and treatment of tumors with radioactive isotopes always has been a highly desired goal in nuclear medicine.

Diiodofluorescein I 131 was the first radiopharmaceutical to be used for tumor localization. Since then, numerous radioactive compounds have been used for cerebral tumor detection.

The use of *gallium citrate Ga 67* to detect soft tissue tumors was first reported in 1969. Carrier-free gallium 67, a cyclotron-produced nuclide, has been useful in the differential diagnosis of liver abnormalities to detect the presence of metastases and cancerous lesions which are not visible roentgenographically. Gallium Ga 67 is useful primarily as an adjunctive

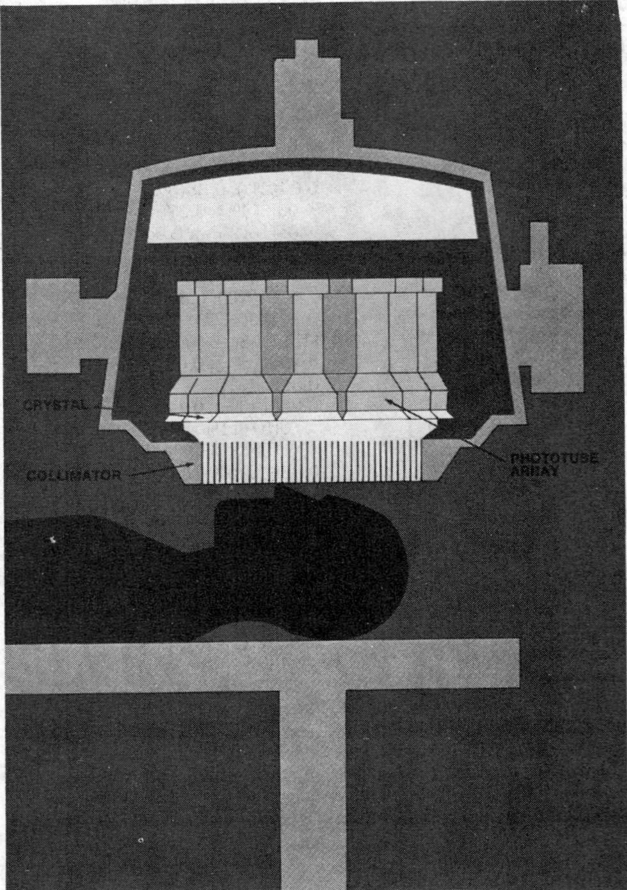

Fig 7. The Anger scintillation camera image detector with multichannel collimator (courtesy, Amersham Searle).

test in the evaluation of patients with Hodgkin's disease, histiocytic lymphoma, Burkitt's lymphoma, embryonal cell testicular tumors and in the evaluation of hepatoma, melanoma and lung carcinoma. The nonspecific accumulation of tagged macromolecules such as Iodine I 131 Albumin by tumor tissue has been used effectively for brain tumor imaging since about 1940. Success of this "nonspecific" technique depends upon the exclusion of protein from the normal surrounding brain by the blood-brain

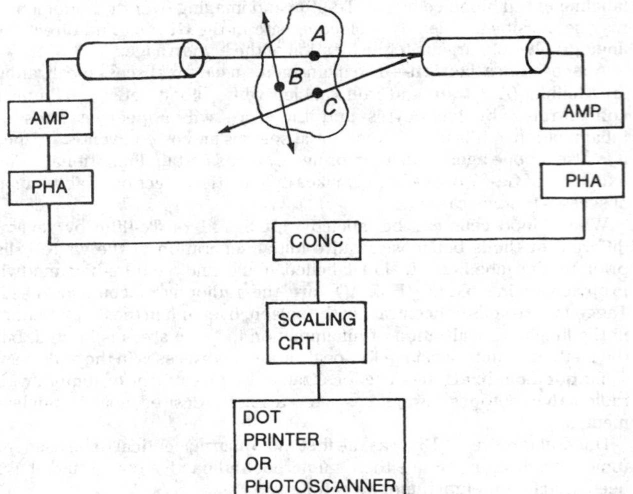

Fig 8. Principle of positron scanning. The location of the atom at *A* is recorded because both annihilation photons are detected. Atoms located at *B* or *C* are not detected since both photons are not detected.

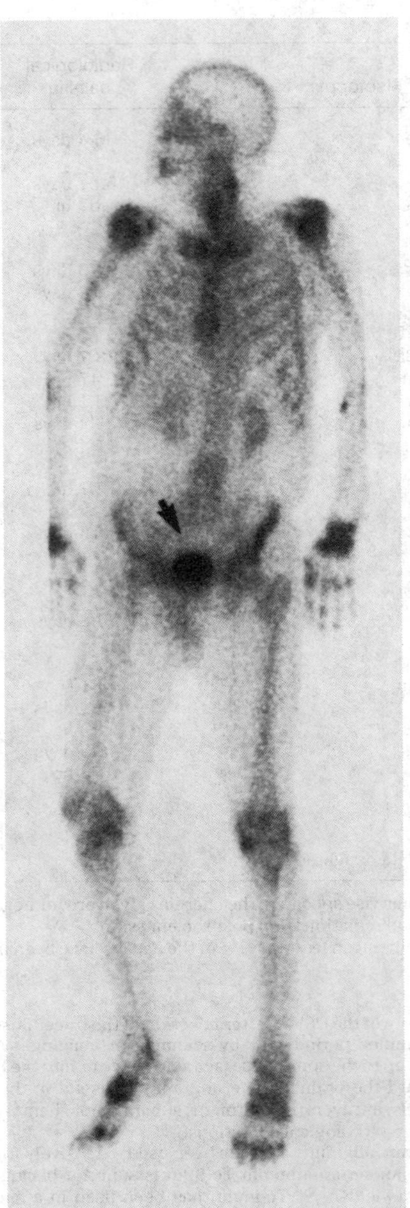

Fig 9. Bone scan, anterior view, with arrow pointing to the urinary bladder. The radiopharmaceutical is excreted by the kidneys and accumulates in the bladder until the patient urinates. The scan shows arthritis in the shoulders, wrists, knees and ankles.

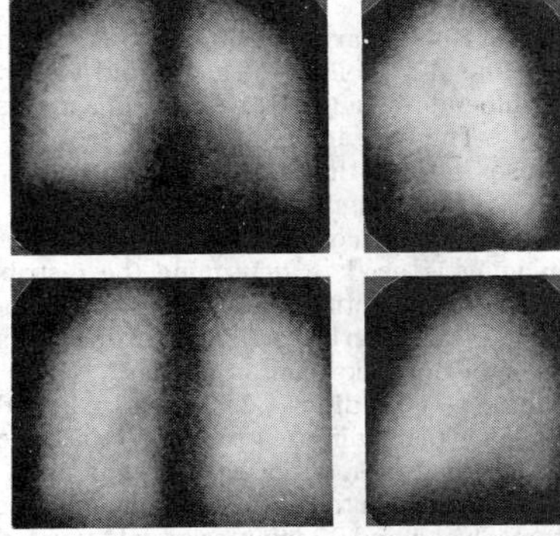

Fig 10. Perfusion lung scan in the following views: anterior (*upper left*); posterior (*lower left*); left lateral (*upper right*); right lateral (*lower right*). This is a normal scan.

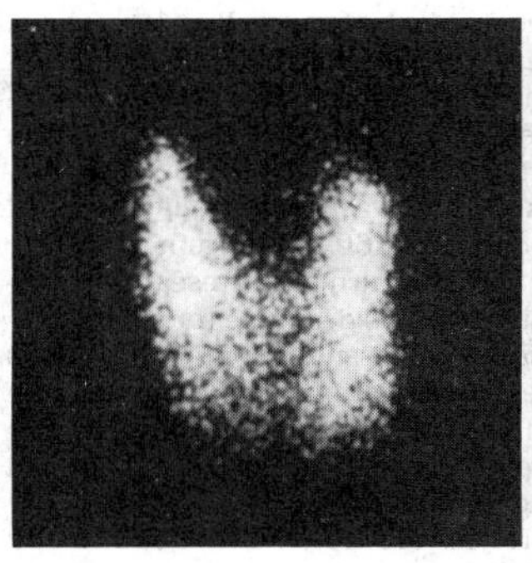
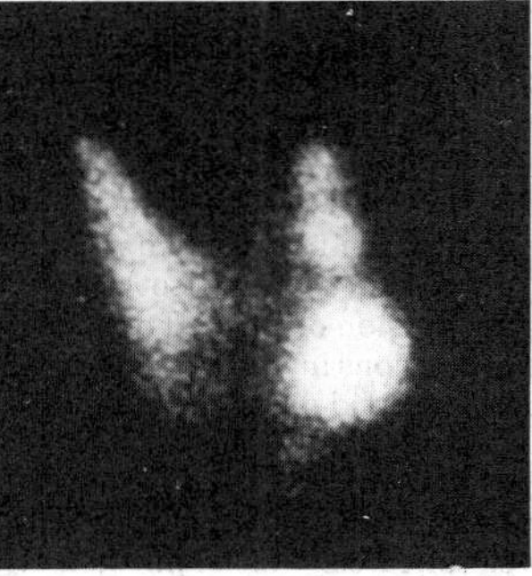

Fig 11. Thyroid scans: normal scan (*left*); scan with nodules in left lobe (*right*).

barrier (BBB) resulting in a greater accumulation in tumor tissue. Absence of a barrier, such as the BBB, in other tissues makes it difficult to identify tumors in other parts of the body by the use of nonspecific proteins. See Fig 14.

Radiolabeled polyclonal antitumor antibodies were introduced as imaging agents in order to improve the specificity of accumulation of radioactivity in the tumor. The recent availability of specific monoclonal antibodies (MAbs) has provided an alternative procedure for *in vivo* radioimmunodetection. The advantage of MAbs over polyclonal antibodies is the ability to produce them in large quantities with well-defined specificity and uniformity. In addition, the radiolabeling of MAbs with bifunctional chelating agents (BCA) such as *p*-carboxyethylphenylgloxal-di(*N*-methylthiosemicarbazone, allows the tagging of antibodies without a significant decrease in immunoactivity. Bifunctional-chelate methods use the accessible epsilon amino groups of lysine, whereas iodination methods employ the accessible tyrosines for radiolabeling.

The accumulation of a specific antibody in a tumor depends upon several factors.

Blood Flow—Antibody must be transported from the site of injection to the general site of the tumor through the circulatory system. Tumors often have a poor blood flow since tumor cells tend to outgrow their blood supply.

Permeability—To reach the tumor, the tagged antibody must cross the capillary wall and diffuse through interstitial fluid. The large size (160,000 daltons for IgG) limits the rate of diffusion. For this reason antibody fragments such as Fab and $F(ab')_2$ have been used in place of the intact antibody.

Antibody Affinity for Tumor Antigen—The greater the affinity constant of antibody for antigen, the greater the antigen concentration in the tissue and the greater the specific activity of the administered tagged antibody, the greater will be the radioactivity in the tumor and the chance for success in identifying malignant tissue.

Background resulting from nonspecific accumulation of activity in surrounding tissues often may cloud results. Background subtraction techniques often involve administration of a second nontumor-specific radiopharmaceutical to outline the blood pool or other backround area. The activity of the second radioactive material then is subtracted by a computer from the total activity. The result is an image of enhanced clarity.

Still another approach to improved imaging is the technique of antiantibody enhancement. In this technique a second antibody, also radiolabeled and specific to the first antibody, is administered. The second antibody then seeks out and attaches to the first, thus enhancing the total activity in the malignancy. The principal radionuclides which have been employed for imaging include ^{125}I, ^{131}I, ^{111}In and ^{99m}Tc.

MAbs are being used to classify malignancies (melanomas, sarcomas, lymphomas, etc) and to conduct rapid, reproducible assays for many of the proteins of the human body. The use of radiolabeled MAbs has been useful for identifying tumors of the colon, lung, heart, rectum, stomach, pancreas, ovary, testis, prostate, breast and other organs.

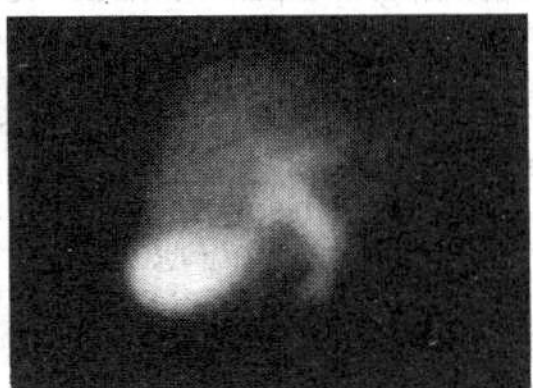

Fig 12. Biliary tract image showling hepatic ducts in liver emptying into the common duct and gall bladder (large bright oval area on left).

Establishment of a Radiopharmacy Program

Types of Programs—There are two types of clinical radioisotope programs:

Institutional programs sponsored by a medical organization or hospital and carried out under the guidance of a medical isotope committee.

Private medical practice programs.

Among the latter, a distinction may be made between private-practice programs confined primarily to the use of radioactive materials in a private office and private-practice programs where the materials are used within a medical facility. For radiological safety it is advisable that patients receiving a dose of more than 30 mCi of radioactive material be hospitalized. In most cases physicians have found it desirable to carry out their treatments within a hospital rather than in their private offices. The responsibility still remains with the individual physician, however, with the hospital merely providing the facilities.

Personnel—Radioactive compounds used in humans for therapy and diagnosis are radioactive drugs and should be treated as such. The administration of such drugs to humans must be supervised by a physician specially trained in their use. Thus, to organize a medical radioisotope program there must be at least one qualified physician. The training must be ample to satisfy the NRC that radioactive material can be used properly and safely for the particular procedure proposed. The suggested minimum experience requirements for the physician for specific diagnostic and therapeutic procedures have been published by the NRC.

The organization of an isotope committee is recommended highly. The membership on the committee may include physicians, physicists, chemists, pharmacists, business administrators or others as required for the proper functioning of the committee. One member of the isotope committee should be designated as *Radiation Safety Officer* (RSO). The specific responsibility of the RSO is to see that all radioisotopes are handled with minimum hazard to personnel and that all regulations governing the use of radioisotopes are observed.

Outlining the Program—One of the first duties of the isotope committee is to outline the radioisotope program for the institution. Although institutional programs may differ one from the other, they all have certain common problems. Some of the subjects to be considered by the committee are

Diagnostic or therapeutic procedures to be performed

Facilities and work areas required (treatment room, laboratory, counting areas, etc)

Instrumentation (selection, cost)

Licensure and reports (NRC, state, city)

Records (licenses, isotopes ordered and received, disposition of isotopes, patients' records, personnel safety records)

Isotopes (procurement, storage, waste disposal)

Facilities and Work Area—An isotope storage area, a laboratory for the manipulation of isotopes and the preparation of prescribed dosage forms, a counting area for calibration of the dose and a treatment room are among the facilities and work areas which should be considered. With the availability of precalibrated dosage forms of most radio pharmaceuticals, elaborate facilities are not required for many diagnostic procedures. An existing, standard, chemical laboratory normally will provide all necessary facilities for the preparation and handling of small amounts of radioactive drugs.

In some hospitals radiopharmaceuticals are dispensed by the hospital pharmacist. Nonradioactive pharmaceuticals have been dispensed by the pharmacist for years. Adding the property of radioactivity to these substances modifies them but does not cause them to be less of a drug than they were before. It, therefore, seems not only logical but necessary that these products be dispensed by a pharmacist who has taken the initiative to acquire the necessary knowledge and training to work with radioactive pharmaceuticals.

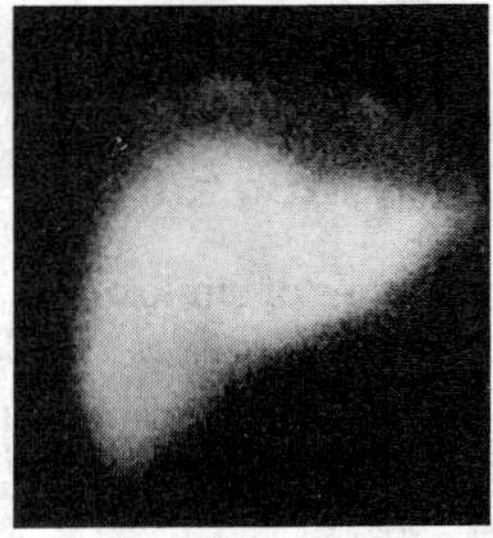
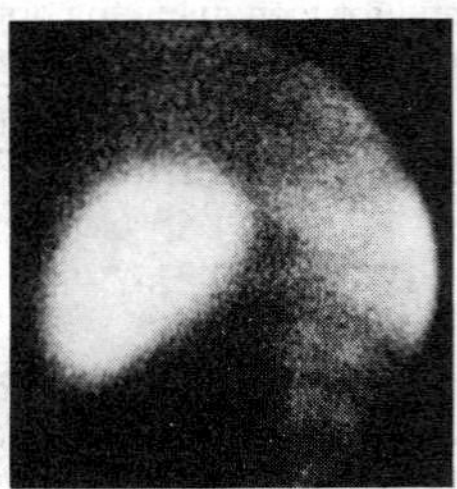

Fig 13. Liver and spleen images: normal liver scan (*left*); enlarged-spleen posterior view (*right*).

In the selection of the counting area, the location of X-ray equipment and other radiation sources must be considered lest the background in the counting area be erratic or excessively high.

Preparation of Radiopharmaceuticals—Many radiopharmaceuticals in current use require preparation. ^{99m}Tc- and ^{113m}In-cows, for example, which provide valuable, short- lived radioisotopes, complicate the procedures for the preparation of radiopharmaceuticals intended for parenteral use since on-site labeling is required. There still remains the need for a sterile, pyrogen-free product for the safety of the patient. See also Table 3.

Other factors which must be controlled are isotonicity, pH, loss of nuclide by adsorption on the walls of the container, chemical purity of reagents and radionuclidic purity and radiochemical purity of the radiopharmaceutical.

Sterility—Sterility tests must be suitable for indicating the presence of viable forms of bacteria, fungi and yeasts. Two media are used on each test: fluid thioglycollate medium and soybean-casein digest medium. After inoculation, the test samples are incubated for a minimum period of 7 to 14 days depending upon the type of sterilization adopted for the final product (7 days at 30 to 34° for autoclaved materials, 14 days at 22 to 25°C for membrane filtration). The absence of any growth in either medium during the incubation period indicates the sterile nature of the preparation.

Terminal sterilization of radiopharmaceuticals usually is preferred. This may be accomplished by steam autoclaving; when autoclaving is contraindicated, sterility can be achieved by filtration through a membrane filter, a 0.22-μm filter usually sufficing. Certain products, such as aggregated human serum albumin, cannot be sterilized terminally since the product is heat-labile, and bacterial filters will remove the aggregate. It must be prepared using aseptic techniques from sterile reactants.

Control testing for sterility should be conducted on radiopharmaeutical products prior to use, where half-life and shelf-life permit. Where such testing is not possible prior to use it should be performed after the fact.

Pyrogenicity—Pyrogens are polysaccharide or protein products that result from the growth of bacteria, viruses, yeasts or mold in any media. They are soluble, filterable and heat stable. Healthy mature rabbits are housed individually in an area of uniform temperature, and their body temperatures are recorded. A volume of test preparation equivalent to patient dosage is injected into the ear vein of each of 3 rabbits and the temperature is recorded at 1-, 2- and 3-hour postinjection. Individual rise in rectal temperature must be no more than 0.6°C in any animal, and the sum of the 3 temperature elevations must not exceed 1.4°C.

Pyrogens may contaminate parenteral radiopharmaceuticals in many ways. Obvious sources are the solvent or vehicle as well as the solutes used, especially if the solutes may have been purified by recrystallization from pyrogen-containing water. Once introduced into a product, pyrogens essentially are impossible to remove. Control of the preparation step is, therefore, of utmost importance to ensure a quality product. Glassware must be scrupulously clean. After washing it should be rinsed with pyrogen-free distilled water and heated to 160°F for 1 hour.

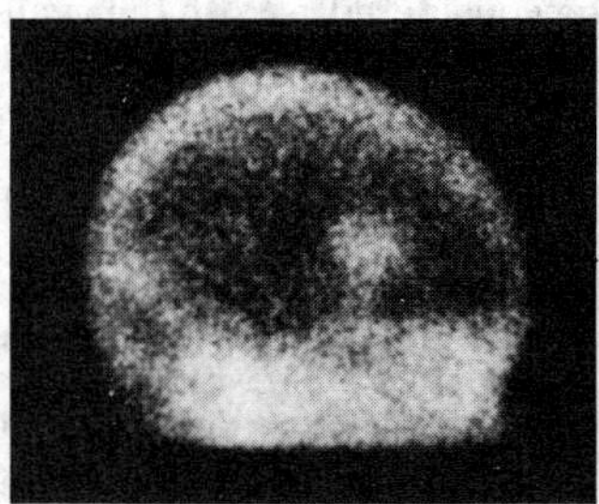
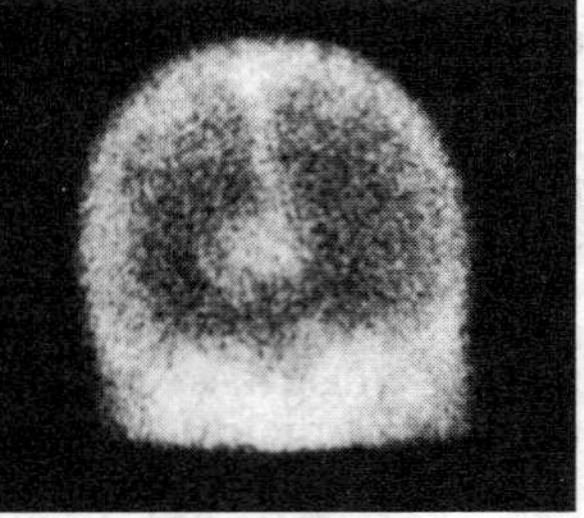

Fig 14. Brain scan, lateral and anterior views, showing pituitary tumor.

Isotonicity—Strict isotonia is only necessary in medical research involving perfusion of isolated organs. Clinically it is desirable for subcutaneous infusions in order to avoid irritation of the tissues. With intravenous use, the rapid dilution allows considerable deviations from isotonia to be tolerated without irritation of the walls of the veins, eg, 20% invert sugar (~1110 mOsm/L), 2 to 2.5% salt solutions (513 to 769 mOsm/L) and mixtures such as 10% glucose with 3 g KCl and 4 g salt (772 mOsm/L) are well tolerated. Usual infusion electrolytes are isotonic at ~310 to 330 mmol/L and glucose at ~290 mmol/L.

pH—For physiological suitability and radiochemical stability, the pH of most of the radiopharmaceutical preparations usually is adjusted in the range of 4.0 to 8.5. However, more extreme pH levels have been used without difficulty. The rapid buffering by the blood renders the extremes innocuous.

Chemicals used in the preparation of radiopharmaceuticals should be of the highest purity obtainable. Trace amounts of impurities may dilute carrier-free substances below the point of acceptability. Chemicals also should be free of pyrogens and are best procured in small bottles rather than the usually more economical large size. It also should be noted that good chemistry laboratory techniques are not always sufficient from the standpoint of radiopharmaceutical formulation.

Water and other vehicles should conform to high standards of purity with regard to pH, sterility, freedom from pyrogens and dissolved solids. The USP monograph for Water For Injection should be consulted (see Chapter 80).

Additives intended to improve or safeguard the quality of the product (antioxidants, antimicrobial agents, stabilizers, etc) must be selected carefully because one usually is dealing with an extremely dilute solution of active ingredient in a radiopharmaceutical preparation. Changes too small to be detected chemically can alter the biological behavior of the preparation.

Radionuclidic Purity—Radionuclidic purity means the proportion of the activity present as a stated nuclide. Radionuclidic purity can be measured by use of gamma-ray spectrometry, half-life measurement and other physical measurements which will detect the presence of extraneous nuclides. Often a preliminary step of chemical or chromatographic separation will be helpful.

Typical examples of the lack of radionuclidic purity are

^{198}Au contaminated with ^{199}Au
^{125}I contaminated with ^{126}I
^{197}Hg contaminated with ^{203}Hg
^{99}mTc contaminated with ^{99}Mo

Radionuclidic purity can make a big difference in absorbed radiation dose and image quality. ^{123}I is a good example of impurity effects. When produced by the ^{127}I (p, 5n) ^{123}Xe → ^{123}I reaction, the only impurity is ^{125}I (2%) at 38 hours. When produced by ^{122}Te (α, n) ^{123}I contaminants include ^{124}I, ^{126}I, ^{130}I and ^{131}I, and when produced by ^{124}Te (p, 2n) ^{123}I, there is 3.8% ^{124}I at 30 hours which increases to 12.8% at 55 hours after bombardment. Dose to the thyroid per 100 μCi ^{123}I is 1.6 rad, 2.1 rad and 2.7 rads (7.4 rads at 55 hours) for the product obtained by the three alternative production methods. Because of the absence of contaminants, using the p, 5n reaction, ^{123}I can be imaged with a low energy collimator, whereas the others require a medium energy collimator for comparable resolution. However the p, 5n reaction requires very high energy protons (over 60 meV) not available from commercial cyclotrons, (^{124}I has a $t_{1/2}$ of 4.15 days and gamma energies of .511 meV and above).

Radiochemical Purity—Radiochemical purity is a measure of the fraction of the stated radionuclide present in the stated chemical form. Chemical purity refers to a single chemical form whether radioactive or not. If there are nonradioactive contaminants, the material can be radiochemically pure but not chemically pure. If there are small amounts of a radioactive contaminant, the material can be apparently chemically pure, at least by chemical methods of testing, without being radiochemically pure. A variety of chromatographic methods are useful for purity studies. Paper and thin-layer chromatography have been used as well as gas chromatography and HPLC. In addition to impurities resulting from the manufacture and storage of the product, there is also self decomposition owing to the effects of the radiation.

Cr-51-chromic ions are formed in solutions of sodium chromate. P-32-DFP (diisopropylfluorophosphate) undergoes radiation decomposition. Rose Bengal I131 often contains a certain amount of incompletely iodinated tetrachlorofluoresceins. Iodinated triolein contains high amounts of labeled impurities in some preparations.

Where radiopharmaceuticals are prepared in the nuclear medicine de-

Table 3—Dose of Commonly Used Radiopharmaceuticals

Nuclide	Compound or form	Dose mCi per patient	Organ	Dose in rads	Purpose
^{32}P	Colloidal $CrPO_4$	10–20	Membrane	15,000	Rx malignant effusions
	Na phosphate	2.0–5.0	Bone	150	Rx polycythemian vera
^{57}Co	Vitamin B-12	0.0005	Liver	0.065	Schilling Tests
^{51}Cr	Cr-Tagged RBC	0.1–0.2	Blood	0.1–0.2	RBC volume, splenic sequestration
^{67}Ga	Gallium Citrate	5.0–10	Colon	4.5–9.0	Abscess & tumor scanning
^{99m}Tc	Pertechnetate	10.0	Stomach	2.5	Thyroid, parotid scans
	Pertechnetate	8.0	Stomach	2.0	Superior vena cava flow
	Pertechnetate	15.0	Stomach	3.75	Testicular scans
	Pertechnetate	0.1/kg	Stomach	Depends	Meckel's diverticulum scan
	Pertechnetete	25.0	Stomach	6.25	Scans for brain death
	Pertechnetate	2.5	Stomach	0.6	With ^{201}T1 parathyroid scan
	Pertechnetate	1.0	Bladder	0.03	Vesicoureteral reflux studies
	Tc-DTPA	15.0	Bladder	8.25	Renal blood flow
	Tc-gluco-heptonate	15.0	Bladder	12.0	Kidney blood flow & scan
	Tc-HIDA	6.0	Gall bladder	11.0	Biliary tract scan
	Tc-HMPAO	20.0	Lacrymal gland	5.2	Brain tomography
	Tc-MAA	5.0	Lung	1.0	Perfusing lung scans
	Tc-MDP	25.0	Bladder	5.0	Bone scans, including 3-phase
	Tc-MAG3	10.0	Kidney	0.07	Renal function & imaging
	Tc-pyrophosphate	25.0	Bladder	5.0	Acute myocardial infact scan
	Tc-S-colloid	6.0	Liver	2.0	Liver & spleen scanning
	Tc-S-colloid	0.5–1	Bowel	0.25–0.50	Gastric emptying, GE reflux
	Tc-S-colloid	1.0	Liver	0.3	LeVeen shunt patency study
	Tc-sestamibi	10–30	Bowel	3.6	Ischemic heart disease
	Tc-tagged RBCs	25.0	Heart	2.0	MUGA, GI bleed, hemangioma scans
	Tc-tagged WBCs	10.0	Spleen	8.3	Infection, inflammatory scan
^{111}In	In-DTPA	0.5–1.0	Cord	4.0	Cisternography, shunt patency
	In-tagged platelets	1.0	Spleen	33.5	Thombus & platelet study
	In-tagged WBCs	0.5	Spleen	8.6	Infection, inflammation scans
^{123}I	NaI capsules	0.200	Thyroid	1.5	Thyroid uptake, scan
	Iodoamphetamine	4.0	Retina	3.0	Brain tomography
^{125}I	I-serum albumin	0.005	Blood	0.015	Measure plasma volume
^{131}I	NaI capsules	0.01–0.02	Thyroid	8–16	Thyroid uptake
	NaI solution or capsules	5–200	Thyroid	Depends	Rx hyperthyroid thyroid CA
	Iodohippurate	0.15–0.30	Bladder	1.2–2.4	Renal & transplant scans
^{133}Xe	Xe gas	15.0	Lungs	0.25	Ventilation lung scan
^{201}Tl	Tl chloride	3.0–3.5	Kidneys	3.6–4.2	Myocardial perfusion scan
	Tl chloride	2.5	Kidneys	3.0	With ^{99m}Tc, parathyroid scan

partment, eg, using kits for making bone agent, liver agent, etc, it is necessary to check radiochemical purity. This is particularly the case with technetium compounds because of the many forms of this element. Technetium usually is obtained in the pertechnetate (TcO_4^-) state with a +7 valence. However, to bind or complex Tc, it must be reduced to Tc^{+4} (carried out with stannous ion usually). In any preparation, Tc may then exist as TcO_4^-, Tc^{4+} and Tc^{4+} complex, and the percent of forms other than the complex should be checked.

Simple, kit-formatted, miniaturized, paper chromatography solves this problem. Rapid-ascending systems with compounds either on the starting line or at the solvent front after development make it easy to do. There are kits that separate unbound or hydrolyzed Tc^{4+} from TcO^{4-} and Tc^{4+}-complex using normal saline as solvent. The former remain on the starting line, whereas the latter forms migrate with the solvent front. Other kits separate TcO^{4-} from bound and unbound Tc^{4+} using an acetone-acetic acid solvent. In this case the former form migrates with the solvent front, whereas the latter forms remain on the starting line. This is used for preparation of Tc-DTPA, Tc-pyrophosphate, Tc-polyphosphate and Tc-diphosphonate. Other kits separate TcO^{4-} from particulated Tc such as Tc-S-colloid, macroaggregated albumin and microsphere preparations. Normal saline is used as solvent and the TcO^{4-} moves with the solvent front whereas the particulated Tc remains on the starting line.

Specific Activity—Specific activity is the radioactivity per unit weight of the compound (mCi/mg). It is usually desirable to have the highest specific activity possible so that very small amounts of tracer may be used. In some cases, carrier-free material can be obtained, providing the highest possible specific activity.

In some cases, carrier must be added to provide enough of the compound to measure its physiological behavior. In the iron-absorption study, carrier iron must be added to the tracer so that the intestinal mucosa has something to work on. Otherwise, the Fe-59 gets bound to the mucosa and little absorption occurs. One of the problems with high-specific-activity radiopharmaceuticals is loss of tracer due to binding on surfaces of containers.

Concentration—Both radioactivity and chemical concentration are important. High radioactivity concentration is needed for good visualization of vessels on blood flow studies. Containers usually read

Activity: 0.100 mCi/mL
Conc: 100 mg/mL

and specific activity is calculated by

$$\text{Activity/conc} = 1\ \mu\text{Ci/mg}$$

Instrumentation—The majority of clinical studies and analyses can be performed with the aid of but a few different types of radiation-detection equipment. Of these the scintillation detector usually will be found most useful.

Instruments necessary to carry out a thyroid-uptake study may be considered essential equipment for a clinical radioisotope laboratory. The necessary components of the system are an adjustable gamma scintillation probe attached to a scaler equipped with an elapsed-time clock. With this system the uptake of gamma-emitting isotopes can be measured in any organ of the body. The uptake of ^{131}I by the thyroid and the uptake of ^{51}Cr-labeled red-blood cells by the spleen are examples of techniques possible with this basic equipment.

The use of a scintillation counter is enhanced greatly by a pulse-height analyzer. The resulting spectrometer can be "tuned" to a particular isotope. Such a system not only allows the detection of one isotope in the presence of others but also permits the use of a smaller amount of radioactive material in a diagnostic procedure because of the significant reduction in background and the improved statistics resulting therefrom. A further advantage, again resulting from the possible high selectivity or "tuning" effect, is the resulting discrimination against Compton-scattered radiation which otherwise could cause serious errors in the measurements, especially if changes in the counting geometry occur.

For the *in vitro* counting of gamma-emitting isotopes such as those above, a well-type detector will provide detection efficiencies as high as 60% or more. Accordingly, the addition of a well counter to the basic scintillation system (or, better, to a scintillation spectrometer system) will provide the necessary instrumentation for performing numerous other diagnostic procedures, including blood-volume measurements as well as other isotope-dilution techniques, RBC survival time, test of gastrointestinal bleeding, PBI conversion ratio, triiodothyronine *in vitro* uptake studies, Schilling test, fat absorption and others.

Measurements to determine the relative concentration of an isotope throughout an organ can be accomplished by means of scintillation scanning. A scintillation scanner permits accurate mapping of radioactivity uptake in such organs as the thyroid, brain, liver, kidneys, spleen and cardiac blood pool. For the optimum in organ imaging a gamma camera is recommended.

Licensure and Reports—Until recently all users of radioisotopes in the US were required to obtain a license for their use from the Atomic Energy Commission (AEC), now the Nuclear Regulatory Commission (NRC). This is still true in most states. An application for license may be made on forms AEC 313 and AEC-313A which are available from the Nuclear Regulatory Commission, Washington DC 20545.

Effective March 26, 1962, the Commonwealth of Kentucky assumed certain regulatory authority in that state. Individuals or organizations desiring to use radioisotopes in Kentucky should contact the State Commissioner of Health, Frankfort KY. Similar agreements for state regulation have been made since with a number of other states, including Alabama, Arizona, Arkansas, California, Colorado, Florida, Kansas, Louisiana, Mississippi, Nebraska, New Hampshire, Idaho, New York, North Carolina, Oregon, Tennessee, Texas and Washington.

While these state programs replace NRC regulations, some states have radiation-control programs which supplement those of the NRC. State regulations frequently require registration of radiation sources. Similar registration is desirable with the local municipality, especially with fire and police officials, even though not always required.

Radiopharmaceuticals Used in Nuclear Medicine

Iodinated I 125 Albumin Injection

Radioiodinated Serum Albumin (Human) (IHSA I-125) (*Mallinckrodt*)

A sterile, buffered, isotonic solution prepared to contain not less than 10 mg/mL of radioiodinated normal human albumin, and adjusted to provide not more than 1 mCi/mL of radioactivity. Other forms of radioactivity do not exceed 3% of the total radioactivity.

Preparation—By mild iodination of normal human albumin with ^{125}I or ^{131}I to introduce not more than 1 g-atom/g-mol (60,000 g) of albumin. Iodination usually is carried out at 10°, in a slightly alkaline medium, by dropwise addition of very dilute hypochlorite or chloramine-T to a mixture of iodide and the protein. The unbound iodide is removed by an ion-exchange column and the product is sterilized by a Seitz filtration.

Description—Clear, colorless to slightly yellow solution; upon standing, the radiation may cause both the albumin and the glass container to darken; pH 7 to 8.5.

Uses—A *diagnostic aid* in the *determination of total blood* and *plasma volumes.* There are several advantages to the use of ^{125}I as a tag over ^{131}I. The shelf-life of ^{125}I-tagged compounds is greater due to the longer radiological half-life of the isotope and, because ^{125}I emits no beta radiation and its gamma radiation is relatively "soft," the radiation dose is minimal. The resulting decrease in radioautolysis of the tracer compound further increases its shelf-life. Of even greater importance is the decrease in the dose delivered to the patient. Collimation of the radiation also is simpler so it is possible to obtain greater resolution. Shielding problems and the protection of personnel likewise are simplified.

Note—In making dosage calculations, correct for radioactive decay; for radiological constants, see Table 2.

Dose—*Intravenous,* the equivalent of **5** to **60 µCi;** *usual,* **5 µCi.**

Chromic Phosphate P 32 Injection

Chromic Phosphate P 32 Suspension; Phosphocol (*Mallinckrodt*)

A sterile suspension of $Cr^{32}PO_4$ [24381-60-0] in a suitable vehicle.

Preparation—By reacting $Na_2H^{32}PO_4$ with chromic nitrate in a saline-carboxymethylcellulose vehicle.

Description—Grayish-green to brownish-green suspension.

Uses—A *neoplastic suppressant* that has given best results for palliative treatment of pleural and peritoneal effusions. For this purpose it largely has replaced *Gold Au 198 Injection.* Because ^{32}P emits no gamma component in its radiation (other than Bremsstrahlung), the hazard to personnel is reduced greatly. In addition, the dose delivered per millicurie, during an effective half-life period, is about 10 times greater for ^{32}P than for ^{198}Au. Relatively smaller doses of ^{32}P therefore can be used. Since chromic phosphate ^{32}P remains *in situ* on interstitial injection, it may be injected directly into a malignancy. It has been investigated for use in the treatment of prostatic carcinoma, urologic tumors, liver metastases, leukemia and for lymph node irradiation.

Note—In making dosage calculations, correct for radioactive decay; for radiological constants, see Table 2.

Dose—*Intravenous, intrapleural effusion,* the equivalent of **6** to **9 mCi;** *intraperitoneal,* **10 mCi;** *ascites,* **9** to **12 mCi;** *leukemia,* **3.5** to **10 mCi.**

Cobalt Co 60 and Iridium Ir 192 Sources

^{60}Co Sources—Cobalt rods activated by neutron bombardment and ensheathed in stainless steel. Each rod may contain a radioactivity of up to several thousand curies. Sources possessing a higher activity are obtained by the use of clusters of rods in a suitable support.

^{192}Ir Sources—Generally small stainless steel ensheathed seeds measuring approximately 3 mm in length and 0.5 mm in diameter, imbedded in a nylon ribbon, the number and spacing of the seeds depending on the application.

Preparation—*^{60}Co Sources:* By the reaction $^{59}Co + n \rightarrow {}^{60}Co + \gamma$.

^{192}Ir Sources: By neutron irradiation of iridium metal by the reaction $^{191}Ir + n \rightarrow {}^{192}Ir + \gamma$. ^{194}Ir produced simultaneously due to the presence of ^{193}Ir in the target will decay largely before use due to its 17.4-hr half-life.

Uses—^{60}Co has replaced radium, which is relatively expensive, for many radiation uses of the latter element. The use of ^{60}Co in alloys rather than the pure metal has increased the physical stability, making quite feasible its incorporation in sealed cells to fit various applicators. The 1.17 and 1.3 mev gamma radiation is fully the equivalent of radium in biological effectiveness.

^{192}Ir provides a softer radiation, ie, less penetrating; the radioactive source is enclosed in nylon for interstitial use.

Note—In making dosage calculations, correct for radioactive decay; for radiological constants, see Table 2.

Dose—*^{60}Co and ^{192}Ir:* *Therapeutic,* up to **7000 rads** in a single or in several doses as an implant or external radiation source.

Cyanocobalamin Co 57 Capsules and Solution

Rubratope-57 (*Squibb*); Cyanocobalamin Co 57 Capsules (*Mallinckrodt*); Dicopac Kit (*Amersham*)

Vitamin B_{12}-^{57}Co [13115-03-2]. Cyanocobalamin (Chapter 65) in which a portion of the molecules contain radioactive ^{57}Co in the molecular structure; specific activity is not less than 0.5 μCi/μg. *Capsules* or *Solution:* Suitable for oral administration; contains a suitable antimicrobial agent.

Description—*Capsules:* May contain a small amount of solid or solids, or may appear empty. *Solution:* Clear, colorless to pink solution; pH 4 to 5.5.

Uses—A *diagnostic aid* to study the *absorption* and *deposition* of *vitamin* B_{12} in normal individuals and in patients with megaloblastic anemias. Since the normal human intestine can absorb significant amounts of the usually ingested quantities of vitamin B_{12} only in the presence of the intrinsic factor, radiocyanocobalamin solution is useful in the diagnosis of pernicious anemia, a clinical condition characterized by a marked deficiency or absence of this factor. Three different tests, using the orally administered radioactive substance, have been used for the estimation of intrinsic factor activity: (1) the estimation of the unabsorbed tracer in the stool, (2) the measurement of the radiation emanating from the liver and (3) the determination of urinary radioactivity following a large parenteral dose of nonradioactive vitamin B_{12}. The first test requires the analysis of total fecal collections for 5 to 10 days; the second necessitates repeated body surface counts using a scintillation counter and the third directly quantitates, in terms of the administered vitamin B_{12}-^{57}Co, the radioactivity in a 24-hr urine sample.

Note—In making dosage calculations, correct for radioactive decay; for radiological constants, see Table 2.

Dose—*Schilling test, usual, oral,* the equivalent of **0.5 μCi.**

Exametazime

2-Butanone, (±)-(3*RS*, 3′*RS*)-3,3′-[(2,2-dimethyltrimethylene)-diimino]di-, dioxime; Ceretec (*Amersham*)

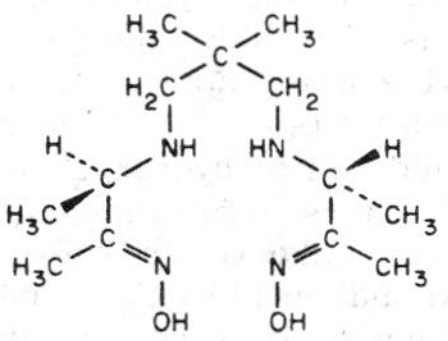

[105613-48-7] $C_{13}H_{28}N_4O_2$ (272.39)

Preparation—Incorporation of ^{99m}TcO into the exametazine molecule produces the drug as depicted below.

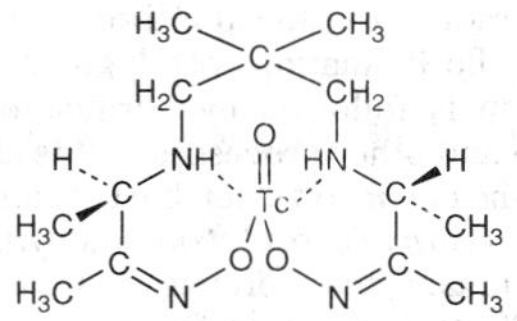

Tc = ^{99M}Tc

Uses—As an adjunct in the detection of altered regional cerebral perfusion in stroke; labeling leukocytes.

Distribution and Metabolism—Following injection HMPAO is rapidly cleared from the blood. Uptake in the brain reaches a maximum of 3.5–7.0% of the injected dose within 1 min of injection. Up to 15% of the activity is eliminated from the brain in 2 min post injection after which little activity is lost for 24 hr except for radiological decay.

The activity not in the brain is distributed throughout the body, especially in muscle and soft tissue. About 39% of the injected dose is in the GI tract immediately after injection. About 50% of this is excreted through the intestinal tract in 48 hr. About 40% of the injected dose is excreted through background.

Caution—This radiopharmaceutical cannot be used after 30 min following reconstitution due to conversion of the lipophilic complex to a secondary complex, less lipophilic, which will not cross the blood-brain barrier.

Dose—10 to **20 mCi.**

Dosage Form—Single-dose vials ready for reconstitution by adding sterile, pyrogen-free, sodium pertechnetate in isotonic solution.

Radiation Doses (rad/20 mCi)—Lacrymal glands: 5.16, gallbladder wall: 3.80, kidney: 2.60, thyroid: 2.00, upper large intestinal wall: 1.58, liver: 1.08, brain: 0.52, whole body: 0.26, eyes: 0.52.

Ferrous Citrate Fe 59 Injection

Ferrous Citrate Fe 59 (*Mallinckrodt*)

A sterile solution of radioactive iron (^{59}Fe) in the ferrous state and complexed with citrate, in Water for Injection [64521-35-3]. It may contain added sodium chloride in an amount to render the solution isotonic, and may contain bacteriostatic agents.

Preparation—By neutron bombardment of iron by the reaction $^{58}Fe(n, \gamma)^{59}Fe$. In the process, ^{55}Fe also is produced by the reaction $^{54}Fe(n, \gamma)^{55}Fe$. If enriched ^{58}Fe is bombarded the resulting ^{59}Fe will be purer.

Description—Clear, slightly yellow solution.

Uses—A *diagnostic aid* for the evaluation of the *kinetics of iron metabolism.* Among the parameters which can be measured are plasma iron clearance half-time, plasma volume, hematocrit, blood volume, red-cell incorporation (percent utilization), daily iron clearance, daily hemoglobin formation and percent daily hemoglobin replacement. Ferrous citrate is useful especially in that it may be administered directly into the blood stream, where it reacts with the metal-binding globulin normally present in excess, thus avoiding the isolation and *in vitro* tagging of that protein. The rate of disappearance of ^{59}Fe from the blood, the rate of reincorporation into red cells and the intermediate storage in the reticuloendothelial system may be followed by appropriate gamma-counting techniques.

Note—In making dosage calculations, correct for radioactive decay; for radiological constants, see Table 2.

Dose—*Intravenous,* the equivalent of **5** to **10 μCi.**

Fibrinogen I 125 Injection

Ibrin (*Amersham*)

A sterile solution of fibrinogen, suitable for intravenous administration, which has been labeled radioactively with ^{125}I. It normally is supplied as a freeze-dried preparation to be reconstituted by addition of Sterile Water for Injection.

Note: Fibrinogen is a very labile protein readily denatured by high temperature (50° or less), and by handling and labeling.

Preparation—By one of the more commonly used techniques for isolating fibrinogen, eg, that of Blombäck, which employs an alcohol and glycine fractionation of the citrated plasma. Iodination then is accomplished using a modification of one of the standard techniques in which ^{125}I is added in the form of I_2, ICl or as iodide and subsequently oxidized with chloramine-T, electrolytically or enzymatically. Unreacted iodine is reduced by addition of sodium thiosulfate, and the ^{125}I-fibrinogen immediately is separated from the reaction by-products.

Uses—In the *diagnosis* and *localization* of *deep-vein thrombosis,* the accumulation of ^{125}I-fibrinogen in clots is observable by use of a radiation detector pressed to the surface of the limb. Radiation detectors designed for maximum sensitivity to the 27–35 keV photons emitted by ^{125}I are available for this purpose. Other applications include the detection of renal transplant rejections, tumors and for the study of fibrinogen turnover.

Note—In making dosage calculations, correct for radioactive decay; for radiological constants, see Table 2.

Dose—*Usual, intravenous,* the equivalent of **100 μCi.**

Gallium Citrate Ga 67 Injection

Gallium-67 Citrate; Neoscan (*Medi-Physics*); Gallium Citrate Ga 67 (*DuPont; Mallinckrodt*)

Gallium citrate Ga 67 [41183-64-6]; a sterile, pyrogen-free, isotonic solution.

Preparation—By proton irradiation of ^{67}Zn-enriched ZnO_2. The reactions are $^{67}Zn(p, n)^{67}Ga$ and $^{68}Zn(p, 2n)^{67}Ga$. At the same time ^{66}Ga and ^{65}Ga are formed but they decay rapidly due to their short half-lives. The resulting ^{67}Ga is essentially carrier-free. The expiration date of the product is limited by the 78-hr half-life of ^{67}Ga. ^{67}Ga as the citrate has a biological half-life of 53 days and an effective half-life of 73.5 hr.

Uses—Has been shown to concentrate in tumors of soft tissue and bone. With respect to tumor-to-normal tissue concentration, it is reported to be superior to selenomethionine Se 75, chlormerodrin Hg 203 and human serum albumin I 125. It has been useful for diagnosing lesions of the lung, breast, maxillary sinuses and liver by using scanning and organ-imaging techniques. A positive ^{67}Ga uptake is a potential indicator of certain malignancies such as lymphomas, bronchogenic carcinoma and Hodgkin's disease. In addition, ^{67}Ga also is useful for the identification of certain inflammatory conditions such as pancreatitis and disc-space infection. The mechanism of ^{67}Ga uptake is unknown.

Distribution and Metabolism—Following injection, about 30% is bound to plasma proteins. Plasma clearance is slow—after 24 hr 10% still remains. One-third of the injected dose is excreted over the first week, 25% is excreted by the kidneys, predominantly in the first 24 hr. Another 10% is excreted in the stool over about 1 wk. The remaining 65% is distributed in the body, the highest concentrations appearing in the liver (5%), spleen (1%), kidney (2%) and skeleton including marrow (24%).

In the kidney, gallium is mostly in the cortex, in proximal convoluted tubules. In the spleen, gallium is in the phagocytic cells. In the liver, gallium is in both Küpffer cells and hepatocytes.

Tumor uptake is highest in osteosarcomas, lymphomas, lung cancers, melanomas and hepatomas and seminomas. Abscesses, osteomyelitis, etc, also concentrate gallium.

Note—In making dosage calculations, correct for radioactive decay; for radiological constants, see Table 2.

Dose—*Intravenous bolus,* the equivalent of **2.5 mCi;** *scanning,* the equivalent of **2** to **5 mCi.**

Indium Chlorides In 111

Indium-111 is a cyclotron-produced radioisotope that is available as a mixture of $^{111}InCl_3$ hydrates in 0.05 *N* HCl.

Indium normally exists in aqueous solution in the 3+ valence state since indium compounds of lower valencies are unstable. For example, indium monochloride and dichloride disproportionate in the presence of water.

$$3InCl \rightleftarrows 2In + InCl_3$$

$$3InCl_2 \rightleftarrows In + 2InCl_3$$

Indium (3+) ions are colorless and resemble aluminum (3+) ions in many ways. Since the solubility product constant (pK) of $In(OH)_3$ is 33.9, the hydroxide begins to precipitate when the pH is increased to about 3.6. Being amphoteric, indium hydroxide will redissolve in the presence of an excess of strong base.

In aqueous solution it is believed that indium chloride exists as a mixture of the following hydrated chlorides:

$[^{111}In(H_2O)_6]Cl_3$	Hexaaquoindium(3+)-^{111}In trichloride
$[^{111}In(H_2O)_5Cl]Cl_2$	Pentaaquochloroindium(2+)-^{111}In dichloride
$[^{111}In(H_2O)_4Cl_2]Cl$	Tetraaquodichloroindium(1+)-^{111}In chloride
$^{111}In(H_2O)_3Cl_3$	Triaquotrichloroindium-^{111}In

Preparation—By bombarding a cadmium target with 15 meV deuterons to produce ^{111}In by the reactions $^{110}Cd(d, n)^{111}In$ and $^{111}Cd(d, 2n)^{111}In$. ^{111}In then is etched from the target with HCl, carrier Fe^{3+} is added and the ^{111}In is precipitated, along with $Fe(OH)_3$, by adding NH_4OH. The precipitate is separated, dissolved in HCl and the ferric iron removed by extraction with isopropyl ether.

Uses—To tag a variety of compounds. For example, ^{111}In-transferrin, which has been used as a replacement for ^{131}I-HSA; ^{111}In-EDTA and ^{111}In-DTPA, useful for cisternography; ^{111}In-bleomycin, which has been used for tumor localization. ^{111}In-labeled platelets have been used for the noninvasive detection of coronary thrombi. ^{111}In-labeled lymphocytes are useful for monitoring cardiac antirejection therapy and ^{111}In-labeled leucocytes have been used for the diagnosis of upper-abdominal infections, inflammation and occult sepsis.

Note—In making dosage calculations, correct for radioactive decay; for radiological constants, see Table 2.

Dose—For *CSF scan (lumbar intrathecal injection),* the equivalent of **0.2** to **1 mCi** of ^{111}In.

Indium In 111 Oxyquinoline Injection

Indium Oxine; [^{111}In]oxine; Tris(8-quinolato-N^1,O^8)-Indium-111 *ln;* Indium In 111 Oxyquinoline *(Amersham)*; MPI Indium Oxine In 111 *(Medi-Physics)*

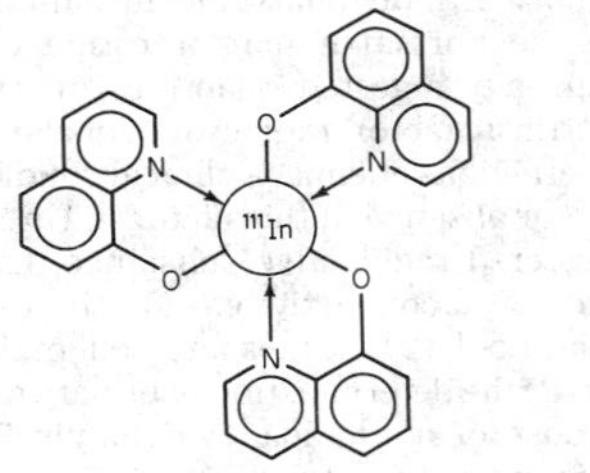

[65389-08-4]

A sterile, aqueous solution, suitable for intravenous administration, containing radioactive indium (^{111}In) oxine.

Uses—Has been used extensively to label various components of the blood. The indium-111 complex of 8-hydroxyquinoline (oxine) tightly binds to blood cells in high yield and is now used to label neutrophils, platelets and lymphocytes. Oxine is a chelating agent which forms a 3:1 complex with indium. Labeled blood platelets have been used for cardiac imaging, for the detection of thrombi and to measure platelet survival time. ^{111}In-labeled platelets largely have replaced ^{51}Cr-labeled platelets in such studies. Platelets can be labeled by preparing platelet-rich plasma (by centrifugation). Further centrifugation produces a platelet *button.* Resuspension and labeling can be done in ACD-saline using oxine sulfate. Autologous leukocytes, labeled with Indium 111 oxine have been used extensively for the detection and localization of infectious and inflammatory processes in humans. The long time (~2 hr) required to prepare ^{111}In-labeled leukocytes is a disadvantage. To label leukocytes, 50 mL of blood, anticoagulated with ACD solution, is allowed to stand so that the red cells settle out (after addition of hydroxyethyl starch, an erythrocyte agglutination agent). The plasma fraction containing suspended leukocytes is centrifuged. The leukocytes are resuspended in protein-free medium and labeled with indium-111-oxine sulfate in TRIS buffer for 20 min. Indium-11-tropolone is another complex used similarly.

Dose—*Intravenous,* the equivalent of **0.2** to **1 mCi,** as labeled blood components.

Radiation Dose (Rads/mCi)—Spleen: 23 to 30, whole body: 0.45, labelled cells: as high as 1500.

Insulin I 125 and I 131

Insulin containing a radioactive tag of ^{125}I and ^{131}I, respectively.

Preparation—By mild iodination with high-specific-activity radioactive iodine. Iodination is followed by purification of the product by dialysis, ion-exchange and other processes. It is assumed that the addition of radioactive iodine occurs on available tyrosine moieties.

Uses—For *in vitro assay of circulating insulin,* either free or bound. If prepared for use in humans, these preparations also can be used to study insulin kinetics, including plasma disappearance.

Note—In making dosage calculations, correct for radioactive decay; for radiological constants, see Table 2.

Dose—*Intravenous, Insulin ^{125}I:* the equivalent of **1** to **10 µCi.**

Iodohippurate Sodium I 123 and I 131 Injection

Glycine, *N*-[2-(iodo-^{131}*I*)benzoyl]-, monosodium salt; Hipputope-131 *(Squibb)*; Iodohippurate Sodium I 131 *(Sorin)*; Nephroflow I 123 *(Medi-Physics)*; Hippuran I 131 *(Mallinckrodt)*

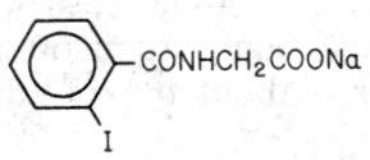

Monosodium *o*-iodo-^{131}I-hippurate [881-17-4] $C_9H_7{}^{131}INNaO_3$ or Monosodium *o*-iodo-^{123}I-hippurate [56254-07-0]. *Injection:* A sterile solution containing *o*-iodohippurate sodium in which a portion of the molecules contain radioactive ^{123}I or ^{131}I in the molecular structure. Other forms of radioactivity do not exceed 3% of the total radioactivity.

Preparation—By condensing *o*-Iodobenzoyl chloride-^{131}I with glycine with the aid of a dehydrochlorinating agent and the resulting *o*-iodohippuric acid reacted with NaOH.

Description—Clear, colorless solution; pH 7 to 8.5.

Uses—The excretion of certain compounds is almost entirely by way of the kidneys. If both kidneys are functioning properly, each should excrete approximately 50% of these compounds or any other substance with a blood concentration in excess of the renal threshold. The performance of the kidneys can be determined by injection of a radioactive compound which quickly and exclusively is excreted by the kidneys. The radioactive tag is selected from those nuclides which emit gamma radiation to permit external detection of the isotope. The relative concentration of the tagged compound in each kidney then can be measured by means of two identical crystal scintillation detectors, one being positioned over each kidney. Renal malfunction is indicated if the measured activities are unequal. The scintillation camera now is used to image and quantitate the passage of this agent through the kidneys.

Note—In making dosage calculations, correct for radioactive decay; for radiological constants, see Table 2.

Dose—*Intravenous, renogram,* the equivalent of **1** to **30 μCi;** *scanning,* **200** to **300 μCi.**

Dosage Forms—In such volumes as may be requested by the physician.

Iofetamine Hydrochloride I 123 Injection

4-(Iodo-^{123}*I*-)-α-methyl-*N*-(1-methylethyl)benzeneethaneamine hydrochloride; IMP; Spectamine (*Hoffman-La Roche*); Perfusamine (*Medi-Physics*)

p-Iodo-^{123}*I*-N-isopropyl-α-methylphenethylamine hydrochloride [85068-76-4].

A sterile, apyrogenic, aqueous sodium chloride solution for intravenous administration.

Uses—A clinical tool for assessing regional cerebral blood flow with single photon emission computerized tomography (SPECT) systems in cases of cerebrovascular disorder, epilepsy, Alzheimer's disease, multiple infarct dementia and brain tumor. It crosses the intact blood-brain barrier, concentrating in metabolically active brain cells.

Distribution and Metabolism—The compound is removed from the blood via first-pass metabolism primarily by the brain and liver; the extraction fraction in the brain is 74 to 92%. The ratio of concentration in gray to white matter is 2.4 at 15 min, 2.2 at 1 hr, 1.8 at 4 hr and 0.6 at 24 hr (primate studies). Retention in the brain is due to binding by relatively nonspecific high-capacity binding sites. The percent remaining in the brain is 5.7 at 1 hr, 4.1 at 5 hr and 2.1 at 22 hr. The liver concentrations were 12.5% at 1 hr, 14.1% at 5 hr and 5.5% at 22 hr. The lung concentration is similar.

Following injection the compound distributes rapidly in body tissues while blood concentration falls to 3 to 8.5% of the injected dose 6 to 10 min after injection and to 2.5% after 20 min. Less than 10% is bound to plasma proteins. The principal excretion is renal: 20% in 1 day and 40% in 2 days. After 24 hr, most of the activity in the plasma is in the form of metabolites with slower clearance rates. Two major metabolites are *p*-iodoamphetamine and *p*-iodobenzoic acid which are excreted as *p*-iodohippuric acid.

Note—It is desirable to decrease accumulation of radioactive iodine in the thyroid by administration of Potassium Iodide Oral Solution prior to injection of iofetamine.

Dose—*Intravenous,* the equivalent of **3** to **6 mCi.**

Radiation Doses (Rads/6mCi)—Brain: 0.66, retina: 4.7, lung: 1.6, liver: 1.4, bladder: 2.5, whole body: 0.52.

Liothyronine I 125 and I 131

Liothyronine labeled with either ^{125}I or ^{131}I by mild oxidation. For the structure of liothyronine, see Chapter 50.

Preparation—By exchange of synthetic liothyronine with ^{131}I under carefully controlled conditions. Since such reactions always result in a mixture of products, purification must be effected by column and/or paper strip chromatography.

Uses—For *in vitro* evaluation of *thyroid function.* ^{125}I-labeled T-3, added to an aliquot of the patient's serum, along with a source of secondary binding sites (Sephadex, ion-exchange resin, etc), will become bound to binding sites on thyroxine-binding proteins (TBP) not occupied by thyroxine. ^{125}I-labeled T-3 not bound to TBP becomes bound to the secondary binding sites in which form it is separated from the serum and measured, thereby providing an estimate of unoccupied binding sites on the TBP.

Note—Due to the high specific activity required, radiation damage can take place easily. This is in part prevented by the use of propylene glycol (50%) as a solvent. Packages should be refrigerated or even frozen during storage, and should not be used longer than 2 weeks.

Note—In making dosage calculations, correct for radioactive decay; for radiological constants, see Table 2.

Dose—*Not for internal use.*

Levothyroxine I 125 and I 131

L-Thyroxine ($C_{15}H_{13}I_4NO_4$), obtained by synthesis (Chapter 50), tagged with either radioactive ^{125}I [24486-40-6] or ^{131}I [20196-65-0] in the 3′-position.

Uses—To *study the metabolism of endogenous thyroxine,* supplementing other tests of thyroid function. Following administration of a tracer dose, serial blood samples are measured for radioactivity. When data are plotted on semilogarithmic paper the disappearance half-time, calculated from the curve, provides useful information on thyroid function.

Radioactively labeled thyroxine also is used to measure thyroxine-binding protein capacity. When incubated with a small amount of a patient's serum, endogenous and tagged thyroxine will exchange and equilibrate. Separated by electrophoresis, the extent of binding can be determined by measuring the radioactivity of the bound and unbound thyroxine fractions.

Note—In making dosage calculations, correct for radioactive decay; for radiological constants, see Table 2.

Dose—Primarily for *in vitro* use as with liothyronine I125 and I131.

Pentetate Indium Disodium In 111 Injection

Indate (2)-^{111}In-, [N,N-bis[2-[bis(carboxymethyl)amino]ethyl]-glycinato(5-)]-, disodium; MPI Indium DTPA In III (*Medi-Physics*)

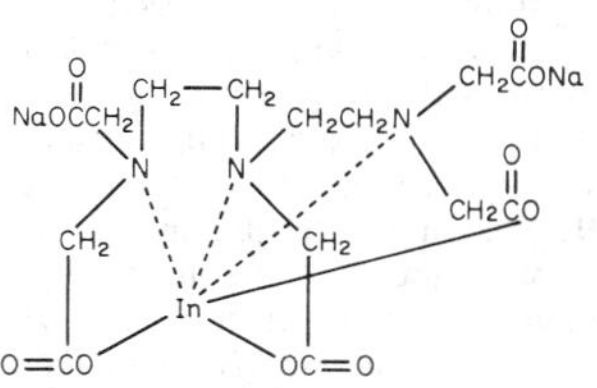

A sterile, aqueous solution of the pentetic acid (diethylenetriaminepentaacetic acid) chelate of indium 111 (^{111}In-DTPA), adjusted to a pH between 7.0 and 7.5, suitable for intravenous administration [60662-14-8]. As supplied, the radioactive concentration is 0.5 mCi/mL at the calibration time; the expiration date is established by the 67.5-hr half-life of ^{111}In.

Preparation—By mixing a solution of cyclotron-produced indium chlorides In 111 (see *Indium Chlorides In 111*), at a pH of 3.5 or less to avoid precipitation of indium hydroxide on subsequent chelation, with pentetic acid to form an indium-111 DTPA chelate. The stability of the chelate is enhanced by adjusting the pH of the solution to between 7.0 and 7.5, corresponding to formation of a trisodium salt of the complex.

Uses—A *diagnostic aid* for studies of *cardiac output,* for *cisternography,* for evaluation of *glomerular filtration* and in *renal scintigraphy.*

Dose—*Intravenous,* the equivalent of **0.2** to **1 mCi.**

Pentetate Calcium Trisodium Yb 169 Injection

Sodium salt of pentetic acid Yb 169; Diethylenetriaminepentaacetic acid chelate of ytterbium 169; Yb-169 DTPA; Ytterbium Yb-169 DTPA (*3M*)

A sterile, aqueous solution of ^{169}Yb-DTPA suitable for oral or intravenous administration.

Preparation—Usually, by adding a sterile ytterbium Yb-169 solution to buffered, lyophilized pentetic acid (DTPA) in a sterile ampul.

Uses—For *brain* and *kidney imaging,* and for *cisternographic* diagnosis of *CSF rhinorrhea.*

Note—In making dosage calculations, correct for radioactive decay; for radiological constants, see Table 2.

Dose—*Usual, intravenous,* the equivalent of **1 mCi.**

Potassium Chloride K 42 Injection

A sterile, isotonic solution of Potassium ^{42}K Chloride suitable for intravenous administration.

Preparation—By neutron bombardment of natural potassium in a nuclear reactor, whereby the ^{41}K isotope (present to the extent of 6.9% in natural potassium) undergoes the reaction $^{41}K(n, \gamma)^{42}K$.

Uses—For measuring total exchangeable potassium.

Note—In making dosage calculations, correct for radioactive decay; for radiological constants, see Table 2.

Dose—*Intravenous,* the equivalent of **50 to 100 μCi.**

Sodium Chloride Na 22 Injection

A sterile, pyrogen-free solution of sodium chloride ^{22}Na [17112-21-9] suitable for injection.

Preparation—By bombarding ^{24}Mg with deuterons in a cyclotron. The reaction is $^{24}Mg(d, \alpha)^{22}Na$.

Uses—An injection for determination of *circulation times, sodium space* and *total exchangeable sodium.* While the use of ^{24}Na has certain advantages over ^{22}Na in medicine, its half-life of only 15 hr creates problems of supply and the usual tracer dose of ^{22}Na is well within the accepted tolerance level. Because ^{22}Na emits positrons it can be detected readily by coincidence counting methods which combine the advantages of low background activity with high resolution.

Note—In making dosage calculations, correct for radioactive decay; for radiological constants, see Table 2.

Dose—*Intravenous,* the equivalent of **5** to **10 μCi.**

Sodium Chromate Cr 51 Injection

Chromic acid ($H_2{}^{51}CrO_4$), disodium salt (*Mallinckrodt*);
Chromitope Sodium (*Squibb*)

Disodium chromate ($Na_2{}^{51}CrO_4$) [10039-53-9]. *Injection:* A sterile solution of radioactive ^{51}Cr processed in the form of sodium chromate in water for injection. For uses where an isotonic solution is required, sodium chloride may be added in appropriate amounts.

The specific activity of the injection is not less than 10 mCi/mg of sodium chromate at the end of the expiration period. Other forms of radioactivity do not exceed 10% of the total radioactivity.

Preparation—By neutron bombardment of enriched ^{50}Cr.

Description—Clear, slightly yellow solution; pH 7.5 to 8.5.

Uses—A *biological tracer* to measure *circulating red-cell volume, red-cell survival time* and *whole-blood volume* (red-cell mass and plasma volume). To tag erythrocytes, a sample of the patient's blood or of donor blood is mixed with a solution of $Na_2{}^{51}CrO_4$ and allowed to remain until the isotope diffuses into cells (15 to 60 min). Once inside the cell, the hexavalent anionic chromium ($CrO_4{}^{2-}$) is reduced to the trivalent cationic chromium (Cr^{3+}), which firmly associates with the globin portion of the cell contents. The unbound chromium (in the plasma) is either reduced with ascorbic acid or removed by washing the cells. The treated blood or suspension of cells then is injected into the circulation, time allowed for complete *in vivo* mixing and samples taken for scintillation counting. Red-cell or whole-blood volume is estimated by the radioisotope dilution method. Normal mean values for whole-blood volume obtained by the isotope method are 65.6 ± 5.96 mL/kg.

Such tagged cells also provide an excellent means of studying red-cell disappearance, as in hemolytic anemias and gastrointestinal bleeding. Platelets also may be labeled, though less effectively. For such purposes, it is essential that the specific activity be high—at least 5 to 15 mCi/mg. Such a solution, prepared by the peroxide oxidation of $CrCl_3$, is essentially colorless.

For greatest tagging efficiency, sterile vials are available containing a special formula ACD solution. The blood and chromate are added directly to these vials wherein tagging takes place.

For those uses where chromic chloride is required, it easily may be secured by the addition of ascorbic acid to the above-mentioned chromate solution.

Sodium radiochromate has not been shown to produce any significant deleterious effects on normal erythrocytes.

The usual dose given below is mixed with 40 or 50 mL of whole blood withdrawn from the patient or from a compatible donor.

Note—In making dosage calculations, correct for radioactive decay; for radiological constants, see Table 2.

Dose—*Intravenous,* the equivalent of **15** to **200 μCi;** *usual,* **100** to **200 μCi.**

Sodium Iodide I 123

(*Medi-Physics; Benedict Nuclear*)

Sodium iodide ($Na^{123}I$) [41927-88-2]. Radioactive ^{123}I processed in the form of sodium iodide obtained from bombardment of enriched tellurium 124 with protons or enriched tellurium-122 with deuterons or by decay of xenon-123 in such manner that it is carrier-free. Other forms of radioactivity do not exceed 5% of the total radioactivity. *Capsules:* For oral use only. *Solution:* For oral or intravenous administration.

Preparation—By bombardment of enriched ^{124}Te with protons or enriched ^{122}Te with cyclotron-accelerated deuterons from the reaction $^{122}Te(d, n)^{123}I$. It also is produced through negatron decay of ^{123}Xe. One of the best methods for producing ^{123}Xe is by bombardment of an ^{127}I target with 50 to 60 MeV protons. The reaction is represented as $^{127}I(p, 5n)^{123}Xe$. After up to 3 hr of irradiation the iodine target is dissolved in aqueous potassium iodide and helium is flushed through the solution. Water vapor is removed from the helium stream by using a dry ice-acetone trap and the ^{123}Xe is collected in a liquid nitrogen trap. Beta decay of the ^{123}Xe yields ^{123}I. This method eliminates virtually all radioactive contaminants in the ^{123}I.

Description—*Capsules:* May contain a small amount of solid or solids, or may appear empty. *Solution:* Clear, colorless; on standing, both the solution and the glass container may darken as a result of the effects of the radiation.

Uses—For *diagnostic procedures* in *thyroid function studies* and for other studies using iodinated compounds for *organ imaging,* including the thyroid, liver, lung and brain. The half-life of 13.2 hr and the radiation characteristics result in a radiation dose far less than that delivered by other iodine isotopes.

Distribution and **Metabolism**— After oral administration, iodine is absorbed rapidly in the proximal small intestine and enters the circulation. Iodine in the circulation is concentrated rapidly by the thyroid gland which clears 50% of the iodide ions passing through and a total of 10 to 40% (average 25%) of the body pool (90 μg) in 24 hr. The biological half-life for the thyroid is 25 to 100 days. Iodide filtered by kidneys is reabsorbed in the tubules except for a small fraction. This amounts to 75% excreted in the urine in 24 hr. The biological $t_{1/2}$ for the body is 12 hr. Salivary, gastric and lactating mammary glands also concentrate and excrete iodine. Trapped iodine is organified, stored and released into the circulation and beyond. The thyroxine space is 9 L and thyroxine represents 3% of the body iodine (0.3% of dose/L). The biological $t_{1/2}$ for thyroxine is 6 days. The biological $t_{1/2}$ for triiodothyronine is 2 days and its space is 30 L.

Note—In making dosage calculations, correct for radioactive decay; for radiological constants, see Table 2.

Dose—*Oral,* the equivalent of **10** to **400 μCi;** *intravenous,* **10** to **200 μCi;** *uptake studies,* **10** to **20 μCi;** *scanning,* **100** to **400 μCi.**

Sodium Iodide I 125

Sodium iodide ($Na^{125}I$) [24359-64-6]. Radioactive ^{125}I processed in the form of sodium iodide in such manner that it is essentially carrier-free. Other forms of radioactivity do not exceed 5% of the total radioactivity. *Capsules:* For oral use only. *Solution:* For oral or intravenous administration.

Preparation—By reactor reduction by neutron bombardment of xenon gas, represented by

$$^{124}Xe(n, \gamma)^{125}Xe \xrightarrow[18\ hr]{EC} {}^{125}I$$

yields a relatively pure product in large quantities. Xenon, at pressures up to 5000 psi, is irradiated with a high neutron flux for several hours. Irradiation is terminated before large quantities of ^{125}I are produced by decay of the ^{125}Xe, otherwise the product becomes contaminated with ^{126}I produced by the reaction $^{125}I(n, \gamma)^{126}I$.

Description—*Capsules:* May contain a small amount of solid or solids, or may appear empty. *Solution:* Clear, colorless; on standing, both the solution and the glass container may darken as a result of the effects of the radiation.

Uses—A *diagnostic aid* in determining *thyroid function.* In some applications sodium iodide I 125 is superior to sodium iodide I 131 for organ imaging because the dose to the patient may be decreased and the organ is often delineated more clearly through improved resolution. Sodium iodide I 125 has been used for thyroid, liver and brain scans with good results.

Therapeutically, ^{125}I has been found useful for treatment of deep-seated tumors such as those in the chest which are not surgically resectable. In such cases, sufficient I 125 to yield a total dose of about 15,000 rads/yr has been found helpful.

Note—In making dosage calculations, correct for radioactive decay; for radiological constants, see Table 2.

Dose—*Usual, oral, diagnostic,* the equivalent of **50** to **100 μCi.**

Sodium Iodide I 131

Sodium Iodide I 131 (*Syncor; Mallinckrodt*); Iodotope (*Squibb*)

Sodium iodide ($Na^{131}I$) [7790-26-3]. Radioactive ^{131}I processed in the form of sodium iodide from products of uranium fission or neutron bombardment of tellurium in such manner that it is essentially carrier-free and contains only minute amounts of naturally occurring iodine 127. Other forms of radioactivity do not exceed 5% of the total radioactivity. *Capsules:* For oral use. *Solution:* For oral or intravenous administration.

Preparation—If prepared from the products of uranium fission it is necessary that other radioactive fission products be separated by appropriate chemical techniques. Neutron bombardment of tellurium results in production of ^{131}I by the reaction

$$^{130}Te(n, \gamma)^{131}Te \xrightarrow[24.8\ min]{\beta^-} {}^{131}I.$$

Description—*Capsules:* May contain a small amount of solid or solids, or may appear empty. *Solution:* Clear, colorless; on standing, both the solution and the glass container may darken as a result of the effects of the radiation; pH 7.5 to 9.0.

Uses—A *diagnostic aid* in determining *thyroid function* and a *neoplastic suppressant.*

Note—In making dosage calculations, correct for radioactive decay; for radiological constants, see Table 2.

Dose—*Oral* or *intravenous, thyroid function determination,* the equivalent of **5** to **15 μCi;** *usual* **5** to **10 μCi;** *thyroid inhibitor,* **2** to **10 mCi** (**2000** to **10,000 μCi**) as a single dose or in divided doses 6 to 8 weeks apart; *thyroid scanning,* **30** to **100 μCi.**

Sodium Pertechnetate Tc 99m Injection

Pertechnetic acid ($H^{99m}TcO_4$), sodium salt
Injection (*Gamma; Medi-Physics; Syncor*). Generators: Minitec (*Squibb*); Technetium Tc99m Generator (*DuPont; Medi-Physics*); Ultra-Technekow FM (*Mallinckrodt*)

Sodium pertechnetate ($Na^{99m}TcO_4$) [23288-60-0]. *Injection:* A sterile solution, suitable for intravenous or oral administration, containing radioactive ^{99m}Tc in the form of sodium pertechnetate and sodium chloride to make the solution isotonic. Technetium 99m is formed by decay of molybdenum 99, a radioactive isotope of molybdenum obtained by neutron bombardment of molybdenum 98 or as a product of uranium fission. Other forms of ^{99m}Tc do not exceed 5% of the total radioactivity.

Preparation—Commonly, by elution of a generator or "cow" containing ^{99}Mo (half-life, 67 hr). The decay of ^{99}Mo results in the buildup of its daughter, ^{99m}Tc, at a rate that permits eluting the generator about once a day.

Generators usually are sterilized by the manufacturer so a sterile, pyrogen-free solution of sodium pertechnetate ^{99m}Tc can be obtained by aseptic elution. Prior to use, the sodium pertechnetate ^{99m}Tc solution should be assayed. ^{57}Co standards usually are used for this purpose since the 123 keV and 137 keV photopeaks of ^{57}Co are of nearly the same energy as the 140 keV and 142 keV photopeaks of ^{99m}Tc.

^{99m}Tc is an almost ideal isotope for medical applications. Its half-life is long enough to allow completion of diagnostic procedures using it, yet short enough that the radiation dose to the patient is minimal. The lack of a beta component in the radiation further decreases the dose delivered to the patient. Because greater activities therefore can be used, scanning time can be reduced accordingly. The 140 keV gamma energy is weak enough that good collimation is achieved readily, yet hard enough to penetrate tissue so deep organ-scanning is possible.

The chemistry of technetium is similar to that of other members of Group VIIB, manganese and rhenium. The pertechnetate TcO_4^- resembles iodine in that it is taken up by the thyroid. To reduce thyroid uptake of ^{99m}Tc a protective dose of potassium perchlorate is often administered.

Uses—Has been used for the *detection and location of cranial lesions, thyroid and salivary gland imaging, placenta localization and blood-pool imaging.* It also has been used to tag many compounds and, in one form or other, to visualize the brain, liver, kidney, lungs, placenta and other organs and tissues. Erythrocytes also have been labeled with ^{99m}Tc.

Note—In making dosage calculations, correct for radioactive decay; for radiological constants, see Table 2.

Dose—*Usual, intravenous,* the equivalent of **1** to **5 mCi.**

Sodium Phosphate P 32 Solution

Phosphoric-^{32}P acid, disodium salt; Radioactive Phosphorus Solution; Phosphotope (*Squibb*); Sodium Phosphate P 32 Injection (*Mallinckrodt*)

Disodium phosphate-^{32}P [7635-46-3]. *Solution:* A solution, suitable for either oral or intravenous administration, containing radioactive ^{32}P processed in the form of sodium phosphate from the neutron bombardment of elemental sulfur. Inactive sodium phosphate may be added during the process. Other forms of radioactivity are absent.

Preparation—By neutron irradiation of elemental sulfur in an atomic reactor. The ^{32}P, produced by the reaction $^{32}S(n, p)^{32}P$, is leached from the melted sulfur with NaOH solution in the form $Na_3{}^{32}PO_4$. It then is purified chemically as a carrier-free solution of $Na_2H^{32}PO_4$.

Description—Clear, colorless solution; on standing, radiation may cause both the solution and the glass container to darken; pH 5.0 to 6.0.

Uses—A *neoplastic* and *polycythemic suppressant* and a *diagnostic aid* for the localization of certain ocular tumors.

Note—In making dosage calculations, correct for radioactive decay; for radiological constants, see Table 2.

Dose—*Usual, oral* or *intravenous, diagnostic,* the equivalent of **250 μCi** to **1 mCi;** *therapeutic,* **1** to **7 mCi.**

Technetium Tc 99m Albumin Aggregated Injection

Technetium (^{99m}Tc)-Labeled Macroaggregated Human Serum Albumin Injection; TechneScan MAA (*Mallinckrodt*); Macrotec (*Squibb*); Pulmolite (*DuPont*); AN-MAA (*CIS-US*); Technetium Tc 99m MAA (*Medi-Physics*); Technetium Tc 99m Albumin Aggregated Kit (*MSD*)

A sterile, aqueous suspension of human albumin that has been denatured to produce aggregates of controlled particle size that are labeled with ^{99m}Tc. It is suitable for intravenous administration. It may contain antimicrobial, reducing, chelating and stabilizing agents, buffers and non-aggregated human albumin. Other forms of radioactivity do not exceed 10% of the total radioactivity.

Preparation—By tagging human albumin, denatured by heating so as to produce aggregates of controlled particle size, with ^{99m}Tc by any of several methods which generally involve reducing systems to convert heptavalent Tc as pertechnetate (TcO_4^-) to a lower oxidation state. Albumin can be tagged by reduction of Tc (VII) with either Sn (II) or Fe (II), alone or in conjunction with ascorbic acid, at an acid pH followed by adjustment to pH 6 with NaOH. Anionic Tc is removed by use of an anion-exchange column. Only pyrogen-free water is used for reagents and the final preparation is sterilized by passage through a microbial filter.

^{99m}Tc-HSA also can be prepared by electrolytic reduction of pertechnetate 99m in the presence of albumin. Sterile ^{99m}Tc freshly eluted from a generator is added to albumin in the presence of dilute HCl and a trace of $FeCl_2$. Reduction of pertechnetate is accomplished by passing a direct current through the solution following which the pH is adjusted by adding a buffer.

Uses—For the *diagnostic study of the lungs* by isotope scanning. Its principal application is for the diagnosis of pulmonary embolism. Administered intravenously, the fragile clumps of labeled albumin become lodged in the fine pulmonary capillaries where they remain for varying periods of time (usually a few hours) depending on the particle size. Particles over 10 μm in size will lodge in the pulmonary capillaries on the first pass. All capillary beds (extremities, lung, liver and kidneys) extract spheres of 50 μm diameter with 99% efficiency; 20-μm diameter spheres may be extracted with slightly less efficiency. Microspheres are of uniform size (10 to 45 μm) and shape, whereas MAA (macroaggregated albumin) is irregular in shape and has a larger size range (50 to 150 μm). Normally fewer than 0.5% of the pulmonary capillaries become blocked so the procedure presents no hazard to the patient by impairment of ventilation. Lung clearance depends on the particle size and the number of particles. A 1% suspension containing 50 to 100 million particles/mL, 10 μm in size with few larger than 25 μm, will clear with a $t_{1/2}$ of 30 min for the first 30 min and then clearance will slow down. The biological $t_{1/2}$ for lung with a similar concentration of larger particles (10 to 70 μm) is 4 to 6 hr. Particles with a greater size range (10 to 150 μm) with a mean size of 50 μm clear with a $t_{1/2}$ of 18 to 24 hr. The effective $t_{1/2}$ of Tc microspheres in the lungs is given as 6 hr. As the aggregates disintegrate, they are carried to the liver where they are phagocytized by the Kupffer cells.

Note—In making dosage calculations, correct for radioactive decay; for radiological constants, see Table 2.

Dose—*Intravenous, lung scanning,* **5 mCi.**

Technetium Tc 99m Gluceptate Injection

Glucoscan (*DuPont*); Technescan Gluceptate (*MSD*)

A sterile, aqueous solution, suitable for intravenous administration, of sodium glucoheptonate and stannous chloride that is labeled with ^{99m}Tc; it may contain antimicrobial agents and buffers. Other forms of radioactivity do not exceed 10% of the total radioactivity.

Preparation—By lyophilizing sodium glucoheptonate in vials with stannous chloride. The addition of freshly eluted pertechnetate ^{99m}Tc, with shaking to dissolve, results in the reduction of pertechnetate to form Tc-Sn-glucoheptonate in the form of an injection ready for use. The reconstituted injection should be used within 6 to 8 hr.

Uses—A *renal imaging agent*, and possibly useful for localization of brain, lung and gallbladder lesions. Studies have shown that optimal results for both renal and brain imaging are obtained from 1 to 2 hr after administration.

Note—In making dosage calculations, correct for radioactive decay; for radiological constants, see Table 2.

Dose—*Intravenous*, the equivalent of **10** to **15 mCi.**

Technetium Tc 99m Iminodiacetic Acid (IDA) and IDA *N-* Substituted Derivatives

Etifenin, EIDA or diethyl-IDA; PIPIDA or -isopropyl-IDA; HIDA or Hepatobiliary-IDA; PBIDA or *p*-butyl-IDA; Hepatolite, Technetium Tc 99m Disofenin Injection Kit (*DuPont*); Technescan HIDA, Technetium Tc 99m Lidofenin Injection Kit (*MSD*); Choletec, Technetium Tc 99m Mebrofenin Injection Kit or 3-bromo-2,4,6-trimethylphenylcarbamoyl-IDA (*Squibb*)

HIDA

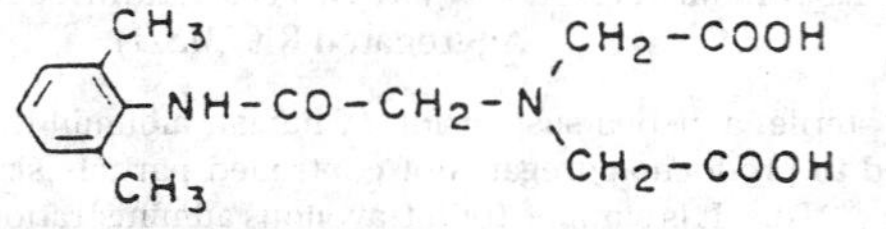

N-α-(2,6-dimethylacetanilide)iminodiacetic acid

DIETHYL

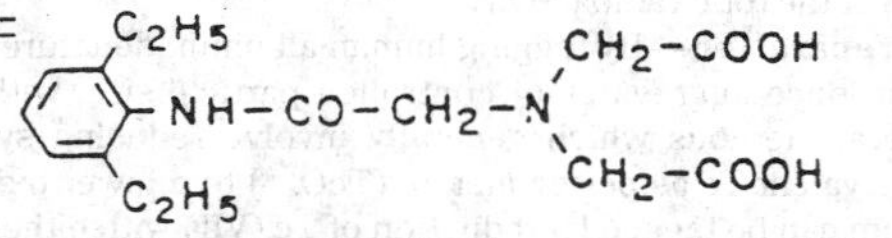

N-α-(2,6-diethylacetanilide)iminodiacetic acid

p-ETHOXY

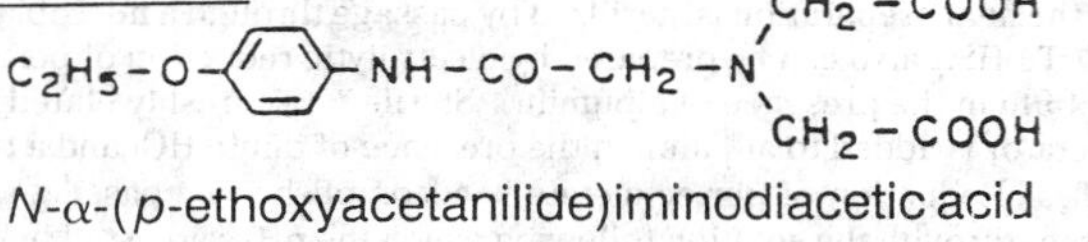

N-α-(*p*-ethoxyacetanilide)iminodiacetic acid

p-IODO

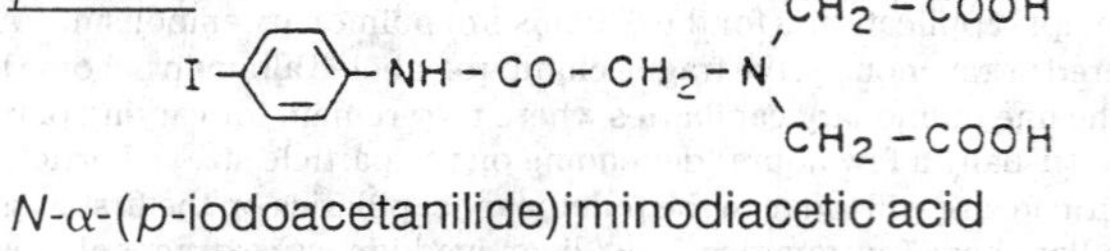

N-α-(*p*-iodoacetanilide)iminodiacetic acid

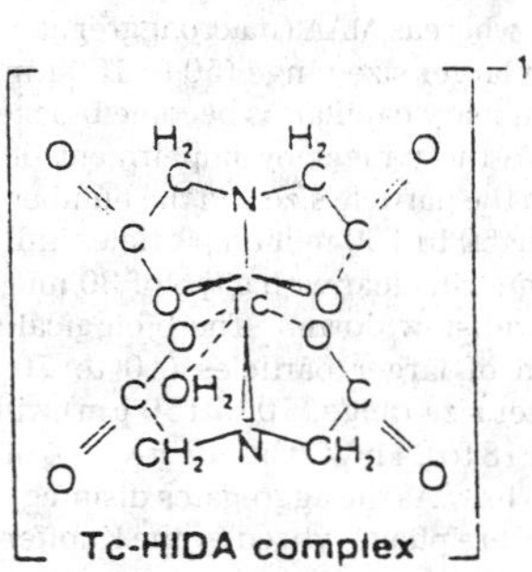

Tc-HIDA complex

Preparation—Usually, by using a commercially available kit, each vial containing the product in sterile, pyrogen-free, lyophilized form with an appropriate amount of stannous chloride. The solution is reconstituted and the substance tagged by adding sterile, pyrogen-free Sodium Pertechnetate Tc 99m.

Use—*Hepatobiliary imaging agents.*

Dose—*Intravenous: nonjaundiced patient*, **1** to **5 mCi,** *jaundiced patient*, **3** to **8 mCi.**

Technetium Tc 99m Etidronate Injection

Phosphonic acid, (1-hydroxyethylidine)bis-, sodium technetium-^{99m} salt; 1-Hydroxyethane-1,1-diphosphonate (EHDP), ^{99m}Tc-labeled; ^{99m}Tc-EHDP; Sodium Etidronate Tc 99m; Tc-99m HEDP (1-hydroxyethylidine diphosphonate); Osteoscan (*Mallinckrodt*)

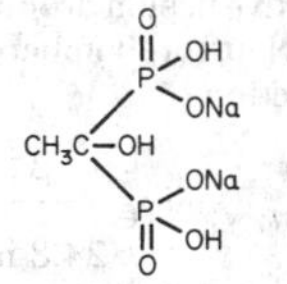

Sodium technetium-^{99m}Tc (1-hydroxyethylidine)diphosphonate [63951-52-0]. A sterile, clear, colorless solution, suitable for intravenous administration, of radioactive ^{99m}Tc in the form of a chelate of sodium hydroxyethylidinediphosphonate (etidronate sodium). Other forms of radioactivity do not exceed 10% of the total radioactivity.

Preparation—By treating acetic acid with PCl_3; the disodium salt (HEDSPA) forms when a solution of etidronic acid is adjusted to a pH of 8.5. To the solution of etidronate sodium, stannous chloride and sometimes a stabilizer such as sodium ascorbate are added, and the resulting solution is distributed into vials and lyophilized (alternatively a mixture of dry ingredients may be prepared). The labeled injection is prepared by adding a freshly eluted solution of ^{99m}Tc to a vial and mixing thoroughly.

Uses—A very useful injection for *bone imaging*, since the diphosphonate is more stable than the polyphosphate; it also has been found superior to ^{18}F bone scans and to roentgen studies; it is frequently more sensitive in detecting metastases to the bone. For this purpose it is considered to be one of the best imaging agents available.

Note—In making dosage calculations, correct for radioactive decay; for radiological constants, see Table 2.

Dose—*Intravenous*, the equivalent of **15** to **25 mCi.**

Technetium Tc 99m Mertiatide

Technatate(2-)-^{99m}Tc, (*SP*-5-25)-[*N*-[*N*-(*N*-(mercaptoacetyl)glycyl]glycyl]-glycinato(5-), *N,N',N''S*]-oxo-,disodium salt; TechneScan MAG3 (*Mallinckrodt*)

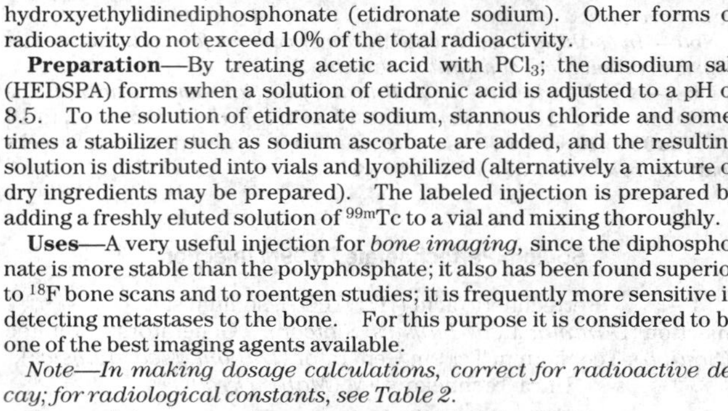

[125224-05-7] $C_8H_8N_3Na_2O_6S^{99m}Tc$.

Preparation—A kit consisting of a 10-ml vial containing 1.0 mg betiatide, 0.05 mg stannous chloride dihydrate, 40 mg sodium tartrate dihydrate and 20 mg lactose monohydrate for the production of Technetium Tc 99m Mertiatide is supplied as a lyophilized, sterile, nonpyrogenic preparation.

Caution—Betiatide is light sensitive.

Description—pH (reconstituted preparation) between 5 and 6.

Clinical Pharmacology—The appearance, concentration and excretion can be monitored to assess renal function. Technetium Tc 99m is reversibly bound to serum protein—89% in healthy subjects. It is therefore excreted rapidly by the kidneys and cleared rapidly from the blood—21.3% excreted in 3 hr.

Uses—A *renal imaging agent.* A *diagnostic aid* in providing information on renal function, split function, renal angiograms and renogram curves for whole kidney and renal cortex.

Dose—*Renal function and imaging studies*, **5** to **10 mCi.**

Radiation Dose (estimated, rads/10 mCi)—Urinary bladder wall: 4.8, large lower intestinal wall: 0.33, ovaries: 0.26, upper large intestine wall: 0.19, gallbladder wall: 0.16, small intestine: 0.16, testes: 0.16, kidneys: 0.14, red marrow: 0.048, liver: 0.036.

Dosage Form—The preparation is reconstituted with sterile Sodium Pertechnetate Tc 99m Injection.

Technetium Tc 99m Oxidronate

Hydroxymethylene Diphosphonate; HDP; Osteoscan-HDP (*Mallinckrodt*)

See the analog, *Technetium Tc 99m Etidronate Injection*

Technetium Tc 99m Pentetate Injection

Diethylenetriaminepentaacetic acid chelate of technetium 99m; Technetium-99m DTPA (Tin); ^{99m}Tc-DTPA; DTPA Technetium Tc 99m Pentetate (*Medi-Physics*); MPI DTPA—Chelate Tc 99m Pentetate (*Medi-Physics*); AN-DTPA (*Syncor*)

$$\left[Tc^{4+} \quad \begin{matrix} {}^-OOCCH_2 & CH_2COO^- & CH_2COO^- \\ | & | & | \\ NCH_2CH_2NCH_2CH_2N & & \\ | & & | \\ {}^-OOCCH_2 & & CH_2COO^- \end{matrix} \right]^- Na^+$$

A sterile, aqueous solution of the diethylenetriaminepentaacetic acid (pentetic acid; DTPA; see formula under *Pentetate Indium Trisodium In 111 Injection*) chelate of ^{99m}Tc, suitable for intravenous administration [65454-61-7].

Preparation—Usually, by adding a sterile pertechnetate ^{99m}Tc saline solution to an aliquot of buffered stock solution of DTPA at pH 7.0 containing stannous chloride as a reducing agent for pertechnetate. If sterile conditions are maintained no further purification is required. Instant DTPA ^{99m}Tc kits are commercially available which contain vials of lyophilized reagents to prolong shelf-life.

Uses—Useful for *kidney visualization*, for *vascular dynamic studies* for measurement of *glomerular filtration* and for *lung ventilation* studies (as an aerosol). Although it is thought not to be a true chelate, it does not tend to concentrate in any organ as is the case with pertechnetate 99m, which follows the pathway of iodide. DTPA ^{99m}Tc is uniformly distributed throughout the extracellular space and is cleared rapidly by the kidneys without retention.

Note—In making dosage calculations, correct for radioactive decay; for radiological constants, see Table 2.

Dose—*Intravenous*, for *kidney imaging*, the equivalent of up to **15 mCi.**

Technetium Tc 99m Pyrophosphate Injection (Tc-99m PPi)

Technescan PYP Kit (*Mallinckrodt*); AN-Pyrotec (*Cis US*); Phosphotec (*Squibb*)

A sterile, aqueous solution, suitable for intravenous administration, of pyrophosphate labeled with ^{99m}Tc. It may contain antimicrobial agents, buffers, reducing agents and stabilizers. Other forms of radioactivity do not exceed 10% of the total radioactivity.

Preparation—By using a commercially available kit of single- or multiple-dose vials, each containing sodium pyrophosphate mixed with stannous tin. Each vial contains a measured amount of pyrophosphate and stannous tin as a dry mix or as the residue of a lyophilized solution. The technetium Tc 99m pyrophosphate-tin complex is prepared by adding to the vial sodium pertechnetate Tc 99m injection.

Uses—*A skeletal imaging agent* used to demonstrate regions of altered osteogenesis. For optimal results bone imaging should be performed 2 to 4 hr following administration. As a *cardiac imaging agent* it is used as an adjunct to the diagnosis of acute myocardial infarct; imaging is recommended 45 to 60 min postinjection. Under certain conditions technetium ^{99m}Tc pyrophosphate concentrates in muscle tissue. It has been observed to concentrate in contused myocardium, with contused-to-normal ratios of 8 to 41, and in muscle following exercise in patients with McArdle syndrome.

Note—In making dosage calculations, correct for radioactive decay; for radiological constants, see Table 2.

Dose—*Intravenous*, for *bone imaging and cardiac imaging*, the equivalent of **10** to **25 mCi** administered over a 10- to 20-sec period.

Technetium Tc 99m Sestamibi

Technetium (1+)-^{99m}Tc, (*OC*-6-11)-hexakis(1-isocyano-2-methoxy-2-methylpropane)-, Cardiolite (*DuPont*)

$$^{99m}Tc\left[C{\equiv}N{-}CH_2{-}C(CH_3)_2{-}OCH_3\right]_6$$

Tc99mRP-30A [109581-73-9] $C_{36}H_{66}N_6O_6{}^{99m}Tc$.

Preparation—Usually, by using a commercial kit, each vial contains a sterile, nonpyrogenic, lyophilized mixture of Tetrakis (2-methoxyisobutylisonitrile) Copper (I) tetraborate, stannous chloride, buffers and stabilizing agents. Reconstitute with sterile, pyrogen-free, oxidant-free Sodium Pertechnetate Tc99m Injection (pH 5.0–6.0). Store at 15 to 25° before and after reconstitution.

Clinical Pharmacology—A cationic Tc99m complex which has been found to accumulate in viable myocardial tissue in a manner analogous to that of Thallous Chloride Tl-210. The major pathway for clearance is the hepatobiliary system. Activity from the gallbladder appears in the intestines within one hour of injection. Twenty-seven percent of the injected dose is excreted in the urine. Pulmonary activity is negligible, even immediately after injection. Clearance from the blood has a $t_{1/2}$ of 4.3 min (fast component) at rest. The agent is excreted without any evidence of metabolism. There is less than 1% protein binding in the serum. The biological half-life for the liver is about 30 min.

Caution—In studying patients in whom cardiac disease is known or suspected, care should be taken to assure continuous monitoring and treatment in accordance with safe, accepted clinical procedure to avoid complications usually associated with exercise stress.

Uses—*Myocardial perfusion agent* useful in the evaluation of ischemic heart disease and in distinguishing normal from abnormal myocardium and in the localization of the abnormality, in patients with suspected myocardial infarction, ischemic heart disease or coronary artery disease.

Dose—*Intravenous*, the equivalent of **10** to **30 mCi.**

Radiation Dose (Rads/30 mCi, 4-hr void)—Upper large intestinal wall: 5.4, lower large intestinal wall: 4.2, urinary bladder wall: 4.2, small intestine: 3.0, gallbladder: 2.0, kidneys: 2.0, ovaries: 1.6, thyroid: 0.7.

Technetium Tc 99m Sodium Methylene Diphosphonate Injection

Technetium Tc 99m Medronate Sodium Kit; Amerscan MDP Kit (*Amersham*); Osteolite (*DuPont*); Technetium Tc 99m MPI MDP (*Medi-Physics*); MDP-Squibb (*Squibb*); AN-MDP (*Syncor*); Technescan MDP (*MSD*)

$$NaO{-}\overset{O}{\overset{\|}{\underset{OH}{\underset{|}{P}}}}{-}CH_2{-}\overset{O}{\overset{\|}{\underset{OH}{\underset{|}{P}}}}{-}ONa$$

Sodium methylene diphosphonate (*sodium medronate*) is supplied as sterile and nonpyrogenic powder, in kits, suitable for reconstitution with sodium pertechnetate Tc 99m.

Preparation—The simple addition of pertechnetate to the reagents, supplied commercially in a reaction vial, and mixing is all that is required. Once the lyophilized reagents are dissolved, the reaction is rapid. Stannous chloride, one of the reagents, is present to reduce pertechnetate. A wait of 5 min is sufficient before use of the material. The preparation is said to be usable for 8 hr.

Uses—On *intravenous* administration, ^{99m}Tc-sodium methylene diphosphonate concentrates in areas of altered osteogenesis. It has been shown to be a superior agent for skeletal imaging, compared with other technetium complexes.

Dose—*Intravenous*, up to **5 mCi**.

Technetium Tc 99m Succimer Injection

Technetium Tc 99m meso-2,3-dimercatosuccinic acid (DMSA); MPI DMSA Kidney Reagent (*Medi-Physics*)

Preparation—Usually, by using a commercially available kit, each vial containing the product in a sterile, pyrogen-free, aqueous solution containing the appropriate amount of stannous chloride. Sterile, pyrogen-free sodium pertechnetate Tc 99min isotonic saline is added to the vial, mixed and incubated for 10 to 20 min to form the complex. The product should be used within 30 min.

Use—A *renal cortical imaging agent* to be used as an aid in the scintigraphic evaluation of parenchymal disorders.

Caution—Should be formulated within 30 min of use.

Dose—*Intravenous*, up to **10 mCi**.

Technetium Tc 99m Sulfur Colloid Injection

Kits: Technecoll (*Mallinckrodt*); AN-Sulfur Colloid (*CIS US*); Tesuloid (*Squibb*); Technetium Tc 99m TSC Kit (*Medi-Physics*); Injection; Technetium Tc 99m Sulfur Colloid (*Gamma*)

A sterile, colloidal dispersion of sulfur labeled with ^{99m}Tc, suitable for intravenous administration [7704-34-9]. It may contain chelating agents, buffers and stabilizing agents. Other forms of radioactivity do not exceed 8% of the total radioactivity.

Preparation—Pertechnetate $(TcO_4)^-$ is reduced to technetium heptasulfide, Tc_2S_7, and coprecipitated with colloidal sulfur. In practice, pertechnetate is added to a vial containing sodium thiosulfate for reduction, gelatin for stabilization, potassium phosphate and sodium edetate. Acidification is carried out, after mixing, by injection of 0.25 *N* HCl. Further shaking is followed by incubation in boiling water for 10 min. After cooling for 5 min, the solution is buffered with phosphate and sodium hydroxide at pH 5.5 to 6.0. Above this pH the heptasulfide dissolves. The preparation can be stored at room temperature but must be used within 6 hr.

Description—Slightly opalescent, colorless to light-tan colloidal dispersion, pH 4 to 7.

Uses—A *diagnostic aid* for *liver spleen and bone-marrow scanning*. Colloids are phagocytized by the liver. Plasma clearance of ^{99m}Tc sulfur colloid occurs rapidly; the average disappearance half-time is about 2.5 min. Concentration in the liver depends on careful control of the particle size. A test of biological distribution, conducted on mice, should show not less than 80% accumulation in the liver and not more than 5% in the lungs. Other potential uses include the detection of intrapulmonary bleeding and lower GI bleeding, and visualization of the lungs by inhalation of the colloid.

Note—In making dosage calculations, correct for radioactive decay; for radiological constants, see Table 2.

Dose—*Intravenous*, the equivalent of **2** to **6 mCi**.

Technetium Tc 99m Tebroxime

Technetium-^{99m}Tc, (*TPS*-7-1-232′4′54)-[bis[(1,2-cyclohexanedione dioximato)(1-)-*O*][(1,2-cyclohexanedione dioximato)-(2-)-*O*]methylborato(2-)-N,N′,N′′,N′′′,N′′′′,N′′′′′]chloro-, Cardiotec (*Bristol-Myers Squibb*)

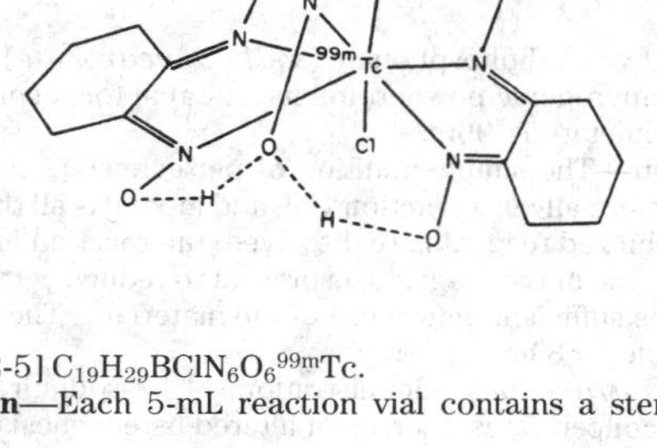

[104716-22-5] $C_{19}H_{29}BClN_6O_6{}^{99m}Tc$.

Preparation—Each 5-mL reaction vial contains a sterile, nonpyrogenic, lyophilized formulation of cyclohexanedione dioxime, methylboronic acid, pentetic acid, citric acid, sodium chloride, gamma cyclodextrin and stannous chloride. Technetium Tc99m Teboroxime is formed by the addition of sterile, pyrogen-free sodium pertechnetate and heating the mixture in the vial for 15 min at 100°: pH (reconstituted product) between range of 3.3 to 4.1.

Clinical Pharmacology—Teboroxime is a boronic acid technetium dioxime (BATO) derivative with no known pharmacological action at the recommended doses. Following intravenous administration it is rapidly cleared from the circulation with about 10% of the dose remaining after 10 min. Excretion is predominantely through the hepatobiliary system. Myocardial uptake has been detected 1 min after injection and myocardial images were seen 2 min postinjection. Substantial uptake has been observed in the liver.

Uses—A *myocardial perfusion agent* useful in distinguishing normal from abnormal myocardium in patients with suspected coronary artery disease using rest and stress techniques.

Storage—Room temperature prior to and following reconstitution. Use within 6 hr of reconstitution.

Dose—*Adult*, **15** to **50 mCi**.

Radiation Dose (rads/50 mCi)—Upper large intestine: 6.15, gallbladder wall: 4.89, lower large intestine: 4.36, liver: 3.10, ovaries: 1.81, lungs: 1.40, urinary bladder wall: 1.37, heart wall: 1.01, kidneys: 1.01, spleen: 0.75, thyroid: 0.54.

Thallium Tl 201 Chloride Injection

Thallous Chloride Tl 201 (*DuPont; Mallinckrodt; Medi-Physics*)

A sterile, isotonic, aqueous solution of ^{201}TlCl suitable for intravenous administration [55172-29-7].

Preparation—By bombarding thallium with protons to produce ^{201}Pb by the reaction ^{203}Tl(*p*, 3*n*)^{201}Pb. The lead is complexed and the undesirable thallium target material removed by ion exchange. The lead isotopes then are affixed to another column from which ^{201}Tl is eluted following its formation by decay of ^{201}Pb.

Uses—In *myocardial perfusion imaging* for diagnosing and localizing of myocardial ischemia and infarction. It is an adjunct to angiography. Thallium mimics potassium ions and is taken up by cells of the heart; a decrease in the vitality of the cells is indicated by decreased ^{201}Tl uptake. It has been reported that ^{201}Tl is also useful for thyroid imaging, in particular for the detection of marked goiter and thyroid carcinoma.

Blood disappearance is very rapid—91.5% disappears with a $t_{1/2}$ of 5 min, the rest, mostly in RBCs, with a $t_{1/2}$ of 40 hr. Only 4 to 8% is excreted by the kidneys during the first 24 hr. The effective ^{201}Tl $t_{1/2}$ is 57 hr.

The heart takes up about 1 to 2% but decreases to 0.2% in 24 hr. The lower abdomen and pelvis take up 40%, kidneys: 3 to 4% and liver (in a goat study): 11.6%, decreasing to 1.8% in 20 hr. Thyroid activity is 0.2% of the injected dose but disappears in 24 hr. The testes take up 0.15% but rate of disappearance is slower.

Dose—*Intravenous*, the equivalent of **2** to **4 mCi**.

Radiation Doses (Rads/mCi)—Whole body: 0.21, testes: 0.59, kidney: 1.17, thyroid: 1.03, large intestine: 0.90.

Water O 15

Water-^{15}O; [^{15}O]water

A sterile preparation suitable for intravenous administration [24286-21-3].

Preparation—By labeling with a cyclotron-generated radionuclide. Prepared in individual nuclear medical centers.

Uses—*Blood-flow imaging*, using PET (positron emission tomography) scanning.

Xenon Xe 127 and Xe 133 Gas

Xenon (^{127}Xe) Gas (*Mallinckrodt*)

Xenon, isotope of mass 127; a gas [13994-19-9]. As produced it contains less than 10% xenon 129m and less than 10% xenon 131m; 99% of total radioactivity is as radioxenon.

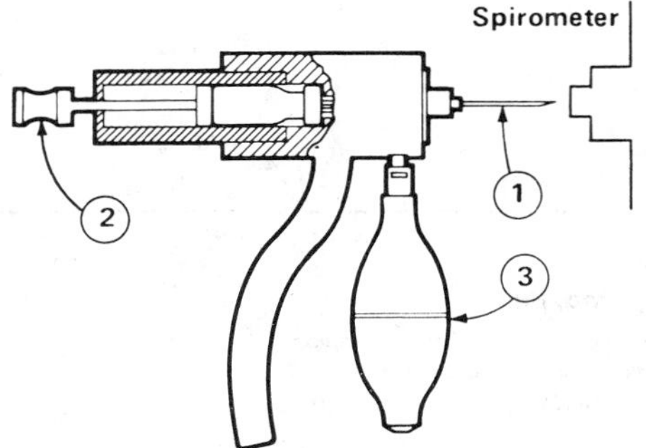

Fig 15. Using the Calidose gas dispensing system. 1: Af-fix to a spirometer or related breathing apparatus; 2: puncture septum of loaded vial by pushing plunger into dispenser and 3: immediately squeeze and hold rubber bulb for 5 sec, and then release (courtesy, New England Nuclear div, Dupont).

Preparation—By proton bombardment of cesium 133 with xenon 127.

Uses—See *Xenon Xe 133 Injection.*

Dose—*Intravenous, cerebral and pulmonary studies,* the equivalent of **0.5** to **10 mCi.**

Xenon Xe 133 Injection

Inhalation; Xenon Xe 133 (*DuPont; Mallinckrodt; Medi-Physics*); Xenon Xe 133—V.S.S. (*Medi-Physics*); Injection; Xeneisol (*Mallinckrodt*)

Xenon, isotope of mass 133; a gas [14932-42-4]. *Injection:* A sterile, isotonic solution of xenon 133 suitable for intravenous administration. Xenon 133 is a radioactive nuclide prepared from the fission of uranium 235. Other forms of radioactivity do not exceed 10% of the total radioactivity.

Preparation—A product of nuclear fission, xenon 133 also can be prepared by neutron activation according to the reaction $^{132}Xe(n, \gamma)^{133}Xe$. It is available as a gas and, being three times more soluble than oxygen, also as a solution in isotonic saline.

Uses—As a *gas,* for *lung imaging* to detect alveolar blockage. ^{133}Xe can be introduced into a spirometer or breathing apparatus by use of a special assembly illustrated in Fig 15. Its biological half-life of approximately 15 min makes it a relatively safe isotope to use. Single-photon tomography of inhaled Xe-133 has been used to map cerebral blood flow.

Dissolve in saline, as a biological tracer for regional blood-flow measurements. Injected into a tissue, the rate of clearance is a measure of the regional blood flow. Intravenously, it can be used to measure the potency of the cerebral blood supply, pulmonary functions, etc.

Note—In making dosage calculations, correct for radioactive decay; for radiological constants, see Table 2.

Dose—*Intravenous, cerebral,* and *pulmonary studies,* the equivalent of **0.5** to **10 mCi**; *inhalation,* up to **10 mCi**.

CHAPTER 52

Topical Drugs

Kristine Knutson, PhD
Associate Professor of Pharmaceutics
College of Pharmacy, University of Utah
Salt Lake City, UT 84112

Lynn K Pershing, PhD
Research Associate Professsor of Internal Medicine
School of Medicine, University of Utah
Salt Lake City, UT 84132

Chemical agents may be applied to the skin and mucous membranes for localized effects within the skin or membrane. Many of these, such as antibiotics, antiseptics, corticosteroids, anti-neoplastics and local anesthetics, belong to distinct pharmacologic classes treated elsewhere in this text, and will not be discussed specifically in this chapter. However, transdermal delivery systems for compounds whose pharmacological activity is discussed elsewhere, will be outlined briefly from the delivery viewpoint in this chapter. The heterogeneous groups of agents, which are not part of a pharmaceutical drug class, but nonetheless have effects on epithelial surfaces and are mostly nonselective in action, will be the primary focus of this chapter.

Those locally acting topical agents, which have limited chemical and pharmacological activity, generally have a *physical* basis of action. Included in this group are protectives, adsorbents, demulcents, emollients and cleansing agents. The relative inertness of many of these substances renders them of value as vehicles and excipients. Consequently, many agents in this group are also pharmaceutical necessities and may be treated in Chapter 80.

Topical agents that have general *chemical* reactivity include most astringents, irritants, rubefacients, vesicants, sclerosing agents, caustics, escharotics, many keratolytic (desquamating) agents and a miscellaneous group of dermatologicals including hypopigmenting and antipruritic agents.

Although the skin (described in further detail in Chapter 91) and other membranes (see Chapter 90 concerning the eye and Chapter 43 concerning absorption across other membranes) differ considerably in structure and function, they exhibit similar absorption profiles for some chemical agents and similar responses to certain physical and pharmacologic stimuli. Thus, many of the agents found in this chapter may be applied to other membranes. Nevertheless, it is obvious that many agents, for which there is either contraindication or no rationale for their application to the mucous membranes, may be applied only to the skin.

Protectives and Adsorbents

In its broadest pharmacological sense a protective is any agent that isolates the exposed surface (skin or other membranes) from harmful or annoying stimuli. Substances that protect by mechanical or other physical means are considered to be protectives. While the surface action of adsorbents and demulcents may impart some protection, demulcents and emollients are placed in separate categories that reflect their primarily dermatological function.

The abridged category of protectives mainly comprises the dusting powders, adsorbents, mechanical protective agents and plasters.

Dusting Powders

Certain relatively inert and insoluble substances are used to cover and protect epithelial surfaces, ulcers and wounds. Usually these substances are very finely subdivided powders. They generally absorb moisture and, therefore, also act as cutaneous desiccants. The absorption of skin moisture decreases friction and also discourages certain bacterial growth.

The water-absorbent powders should not be administered to wet, raw surfaces because of the formation of cakes and adherent crusts. Starch and other carbohydrate powders may become doughy with absorption of aqueous-based fluids, but also may ferment. Consequently, such powders often contain an antiseptic. Most impalpable powders are absorptive, to some extent. Whether absorption of substances, other than water, contributes to the protection of the skin is uncertain; however, absorption of fatty acids and perspiration constituents along with cutaneous drying, contributes to a deodorant action of such powders. It generally is held that the adsorptive capacity is important to the gastrointestinal protective action of chemically inert powders taken internally.

Chemically inert dusting powders are not entirely biologically inert, despite the name. When carried into pores or wounds or left upon skin or epithelial surfaces, certain of the dusting powders, eg, talc, may cause irritation, granulomas, fibrosis or adhesions. Even without direct irritation or obstruction of the perspiration, dust can be troublesome.

Absorbable dusting powders (Biosorb, Ezon) are available for surgical gloves. This absorbable powder is mixed with 2% magnesium oxide and contains residual amounts of sodium sulfate and sodium chloride. This mixture produces no reaction in tissues and is absorbed completely within short time periods. Starch also has drying and absorptive qualities (Fordustin powder; 90 and 24 g). These products, however, can be metabolized by *Candida* and thus can aggravate an infection.

A product containing detranomer (Debrisan) promotes debridement of secreting wounds, including venous stasis and decubitus ulcers, infected traumatic and surgical wounds, as well as infected burns. It consists of hydrophilic spherical beads (0.1 to 0.3 mm in diameter) of dextranomer. The beads are composed of a three-dimensional network of cross-linked dextran. This network selectively imbibes molecules based on molecular weight (molecules <1000 daltons are imbibed; molecules 1000 to 5000 daltons experience decreased absorption with increasing molecular weight and molecules >5000 daltons are not imbibed). Four mL of water are absorbed for each gram of dextranomer, and absorption is continuous so long as unsaturated beads are in proximity to the wound. This therapy is associated with the rapid and continuous exudate removal from wound surfaces resulting in a marked reduction in inflammation, edema and pain, as well as an increase in granuloma tissue formation and reduction in time for wound healing.

Several of the dusting powders are incorporated into ointments, creams and lotions. They also serve other functions in tablets and other pharmaceutical dosage forms.

Bentonite—page 1396.

Bismuth, Insoluble Salts—page 887.

Boric Acid—page 1407.
Calcium Carbonate, Precipitated—page 887.
Cellulose, Powdered—page 1397.
Cornstarch—page 1414.
Magnesium Stearate—page 1411.
Talc—page 1415.
Titanium Dioxide—page 884.
Zinc Oxide—page 873.

Zinc Stearate

Octadecanoic acid, zinc salt

Zinc stearate [557-05-1]. A compound of zinc with a mixture of solid organic acids obtained from fats, and consists chiefly of variable proportions of zinc stearate and zinc palmitate. It contains the equivalent of 12.5–14.0% of ZnO(81.38).

Preparation—An aqueous solution of zinc sulfate is added to a sodium stearate solution, and the precipitate is washed with water until free of sulfate and dried.

Description—Fine, white, bulky powder, free from grittiness with a faint characteristic color; neutral to moistened litmus paper.

Solubility—Insoluble in water, alcohol or ether; soluble in benzene.

Uses—In *water-repellent* ointments and as a *dusting powder* in dermatologic practice for its desiccating, astringent and *protective* effects. It has been removed from baby dusting powders, owing to accidental, fatal inhalations.

Mechanical and Chemical Protectives

Several materials may be administered to the skin to form an adherent, continuous film that may be either flexible or semirigid, depending on the materials and their formulations, as well as the manner in which they are applied. Such materials may serve several purposes including (1) to provide occlusive protection from the external environment, (2) to provide mechanical support and/or (3) to serve as vehicles for various medicaments.

The two principal classes of mechanical protectives are the collodions and plasters. Their use is decreasing with the increasing recognition of the importance of air exposure in maintaining a normally balanced cutaneous bacterial flora of low pathogenicity. Also, the mechanical protectives may be somewhat irritating due to interference with normal percutaneous water transport caused by certain oligomers, resins and other components, especially in plasters. The cerates may be employed similarly to the plasters. Bandages, dressings, new vapor-permeable polymer membranes and casts also afford mechanical protection and support (see Chapter 108 for additional information). A brief discussion of plasters is included in Chapter 90.

A number of insoluble and relatively inert powders, which remain essentially unchanged chemically in the GI tract, may possess surface properties that favor their absorption to the GI mucosa. Such materials may offer mechanical protection against abrasion and may even offer slight protection against toxins and chemical irritants. Many such protectives also are adsorbents (charcoal, bismuth compounds, kaolin) or astringents (zinc and bismuth compounds). They are discussed under those categories.

Aluminum Hydroxide Gel—page 887.

Collodion

Contains not less than 5.0%, by weight, of pyroxylin.

Pyroxylin	**40 g**
Ether	**750 mL**
Alcohol	**250 mL**
To make about	**1000 mL**

Add the alcohol and the ether to the pyroxylin contained in a suitable container, and stopper the container well. Shake the mixture occasionally until the pyroxylin is dissolved.

Description—Clear, or slightly opalescent, viscous liquid; colorless, or slightly yellowish and has the odor of ether; specific gravity between 0.765 and 0.775.

Alcohol Content—22 to 26% of C_2H_5OH.

Uses—Chiefly to seal small wounds, for the preparation of medicated collodions and to protect nonaffected areas of the skin from topically applied irritants, corrosives, etc.

Caution—Collodion is highly flammable.

Flexible Collodion [Collodion Flexile]—See *RPS 16*, page 717. See also *Salicylic Acid Collodion* (page 879).

Dimethicone

Simethicone; 360 Medical Fluid (Dow);
Sentry Dimethicone (Union Carbide)

[9006-65-9]$(C_2H_6OSi)_n$. A water-repellent silicone oil consisting essentially of dimethyl siloxane polymers (200 series of fluids; see *Silicones*, below).

Preparation—US Pat 2,441,098.

Description—Water-white, viscous, oil-like liquid.

Solubility—Immiscible with water or alcohol; miscible with chloroform or either.

Uses—Exhibits skin-adherent and water-repellent properties. It is both a *protective* and an *emollient*, for which its FDA classification is Category I. Applied to the skin, it forms a *protective* film that provides a barrier to ordinary soap and water and water-soluble irritants. The film may last several hours if the skin is exposed, mainly to aqueous media. The film provides a less effective barrier to synthetic detergents and lipid-soluble materials, such as organic solvents. It should not be applied except in contact dermatoses and dermatoses aggravated by substances that can be repelled by the silicone. It is useful in preventing irritation from ammonia produced by the urine of infants, but it may exacerbate pre-existing irritation. The occlusive protection by the silicone is detrimental to inflamed, traumatized, abraded or excoriated skin and to lesions requiring free drainage. However, applied adjacent to such lesions, it offers protection against irritating discharges and maceration. It practically is harmless, and does not sensitize skin, but it does cause temporary irritation to the eyes. It may be incorporated into creams or lotions.

Dose—Apply uniformly with rubbing as required to clean, dry skin 3 or 4 times for the first day or two, then twice daily. Allow the application area to dry before covering.

Dosage Forms—Cream: 1%; Lotion: 3%.

Petrolatum Gauze

Petrolated Gauze

Absorbent gauze saturated with white petrolatum. The weight of the petrolatum is 70 to 80% of the weight of the gauze. It is sterile.

Preparation—By adding, under aseptic conditions, molten, sterile, white petrolatum to dry, sterile, absorbent gauze, previously cut to size, in the ratio of 60 g petrolatum to each 20 g gauze.

Uses—A *protective* dressing; also as packing material for postoperative plugs, packs, rolls and tampons, and as a wick, drain or wraparound for tubing. It is claimed that there is no danger of tissue maceration and that no growth of granulation tissue through it occurs.

Gelatin Film, Absorbable—see RPS-18, page 758.
Gelatin Sponge, Absorbable—page 927.
Gelatin, Zinc—see RPS-18, page 758.
Kaolin—page 907.
Lanolin—page 1402.
Lanolin, Anhydrous—page 1401.
Mineral Oil—page 899.
Mineral Oil Emulsion—page 899.
Mineral Oil, Light—page 1411.
Olive Oil—page 1400.
Peanut Oil—page 1394.
Petrolatum—page 1400.

Silicones

Polyorganosiloxanes; Silastic; Silicone Rubber

Organosilicon polymers containing chains of alternating oxygen and silicon atoms with substituent organic groups, frequently methyl or phenyl, attached to each silicon atom.

Preparation—May be prepared synthetically by condensing alkylated or arylated *silanols*. Disubstituted *silanediols* [$R_2Si(OH)_2$] form linear polymers having the general formula:

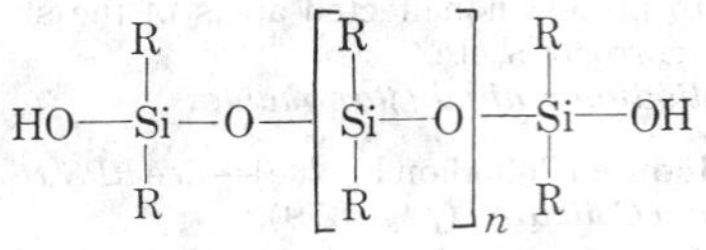

$$
\begin{array}{ccccccccc}
 & R & & & R & & & R & \\
 & | & & & | & & & | & \\
HO- & Si & -O- & \Big[& Si & -O \Big]_n & - & Si & -OH \\
 & | & & & | & & & | & \\
 & R & & & R & & & R &
\end{array}
$$

Cross-linked polymers result from condensation of mixtures of substituted silanediols and monosubstituted *silanetriols* [$RSi(OH)_3$], represented by the following partial formula where R is a hydrocarbon radical:

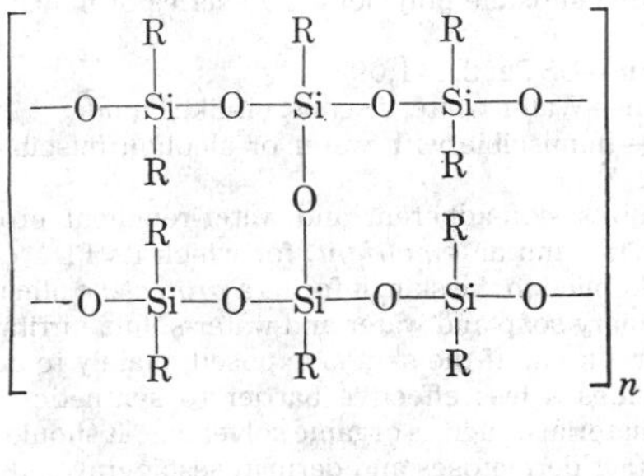

$$
\left[
\begin{array}{ccccccc}
 & R & & R & & R & \\
 & | & & | & & | & \\
-O- & Si & -O- & Si & -O- & Si & -O- \\
 & | & & | & & | & \\
 & R & & O & & R & \\
 & & & | & & & \\
 & R & & | & & R & \\
 & | & & | & & | & \\
-O- & Si & -O- & Si & -O- & Si & -O- \\
 & | & & | & & | & \\
 & R & & R & & R &
\end{array}
\right]_n
$$

One method of preparation involves interaction of silicon tetrachloride with appropriate Grignard reagents to yield alkylated or arylated dichlorosilanes. After hydrolysis to the corresponding substituted silanols, dehydration procedures are used to effect condensation polymerization. The overall reaction, as it involves a disubstituted silanediol, may be represented as:

$$SiCl_4 \xrightarrow{RMgX} R_2SiCl_2 \xrightarrow{HOH} R_2Si(OH)_2 \xrightarrow{-HOH} HO[Si(R)_2O]_nH$$

Silicon tetrachloride	Disubstituted dichlorosilane	Disubstituted silanediol	Silicone linear polymer

Description—Silicones with a wide range of properties may be produced by varying the molecular weight, tacticity, substituent R groups, R:Si ratios (whether linear, cyclic or cross-linked polymers) and the degree of cross-linking. Physically, silicones vary from mobile liquids through low-viscosity liquids and semisolids to solids. Linear silicones (liquids to semisolids) have viscosities ranging from 0.65 to 1,000,000 centistokes. Higher molecular weight, linear silicones form solids. Cross-linked silicones may exhibit gel-like to solid-like properties depending on the degree of cross-linking and chemical structure of the repeat unit. In general, silicones are odorless, tasteless, water repellent, relatively inert chemically, stable under high and low temperatures and efficient as antifoam agents.

Solubility—Unmodified silicones are generally insoluble in water, thus they frequently are termed *silicone oils*. However, a water-soluble sodium salt of a simple silicone, *sodium methyl siliconate* [$CH_3Si(OH)_2ONa$] has been marketed.

Uses—Preparations containing silicones have various dermatological uses (see *Dimethicone*) and are used as ingredients of bases for ointments and liniments. In the form of inhalation sprays, silicone preparations have been employed in the treatment of pulmonary edema involving frothing of fluid in the upper respiratory tract. They also are used orally as antiflatulent or gastric defoaming agents (see *Simethicone*, page 908). A silicone *bouncing putty* has found acceptance for use as a physical agent in treating conditions requiring finger exercise. The water-repellent properties of the silicones are employed in numerous applications where drainage of aqueous fluids from surfaces is desirable.

Silicones exhibit low irritation as a result of their surface chemical and physical, as well as bulk mechanical properties. Consequently, silicone rubbers are component materials in various indwelling catheters and tubes designed for short-time use. Solid implants that incorporate silicone into their composition include nose, chin and other types of prostheses used in plastic, reconstructive and orthopedic procedures.

In addition to uses involving antifoaming, water-repellent and nonirritating characteristics, silicone fluids also are employed to prevent adhesion between components or materials and as release agents. Examples of its usage as a release agent include release of rubber and plastics from molds, food from metal, ice from wings of aircraft and capsules and tablets from molds and dies in which they are fabricated.

Liquid silicones have been used to fill in hypoplastic body areas for cosmetic purposes, although these fluids tend to relocate due to flow under gravity and motion. While the use of silicone fluids in reconstructive breast surgery and similar applications is undergoing reassessment for safety concerns, solid materials continue to be well accepted in biomedical applications.

Higher molecular weight (solid) silicone rubbers are used to encapsulate steroid hormones and other drugs intended for chronic implantation. For example, Norplant (*Wyeth-Ayerst*) is a long-term contraceptive implant that incorporates levonorgestrel into silastic-based rods. The steroid is released slowly from the implant over an extended time period to provide approximately 5-yr continuous use.

Silicone-based materials are also an important class of contact lens materials. The silicone polymer is gas permeable, thus enabling oxygen to permeate the contact lens to the cornea. However, silicones are not hydrogels and do not absorb large amounts of water similar to hydrogel-based contact lenses. The materials exhibit minimal if any irritation as a result of surface chemical and physical properties, and are comfortable to wear due to the gas permeation and mechanical properties.

Zinc Carbonate

Smithsonite; Zincspar

[3486-35-9] CO_3Zn (125.38).

Description—White rhombohedroids.

Solubility—Soluble 10 ppm in water at 15°; soluble in dilute acids, alkalies or solutions of ammonium salts.

Uses—Both for its lubricity and as a drying agent. As a skin protectant it falls into FDA Category I. It is included in commercial topical burn and sunburn products and extemporary protectants.

Dose—*Topical*, to the *skin*, **0.2** to **2%**.

Occlusive Dressings

Occlusive dressings alter environmental aspects of certain types of wounds that may facilitate healing. While a moist wound environment may be beneficial, there are certain disadantages. Moisture has been associated with enhanced rates of reepithelialization. Brief increases in the number of inflammatory cells within the wound site may break down cellular debris. While transient increases in bacterial counts have been observed with occlusive dressings, infection usually does not occur, in part as a result of the transitory increased inflammatory cell populations. Dermal and epidermal healing also may be aided by the low-pH and low-oxygen environment. Furthermore, such dressings provide physical protection.

Gaseous permeable synthetic polymer-based dressings have been developed. These materials provide chemical and physical protection while maintaining a more acceptable micro-environment. Polyurethane-based films that are permeable to oxygen and water vapor include Op-site, Tegaderm and Bioclusive. Duo-Derm (*Conva Tec*) is a hydrophobic polymer with embedded hydroactive particles that is oxygen- and water-vapor impermeable. Application is dependent on whether the dressing is self-adherent.

Demulcents

Demulcents (L, *demulcere* = to smooth down), are protective agents that are employed primarily to alleviate irritation, particularly of mucous membranes or abraded tissues. They also often are applied to the skin. They generally are applied to the surface in viscid sticky preparations that cover the area readily. They also may be medicated. The local action of chemical, mechanical or bacterial irritants, thereby, is diminished, and pain, reflexes, spasm or catarrh are attenuated. They also prevent drying of the affected surface. The demulcents may be applied to the skin (lotions, ointments or wet dressings, GI tract (demulcent drinks or enemas), throat (lozenges or gargles) or corneal membranes (artificial tears and in wetting agents for contact lenses). When demulcents are applied as solid material (as in lozenges or powders), the liquid is provided by secreted or exuded fluids. Demulcents frequently are medicated. In such instances the demulcent may be an adjuvant, a corrective or a pharmaceutical necessity. Many of the demulcents are also laxatives (page 895) and are used as such, or they are used with laxatives or antacids for their demulcent and lubricating action.

A variety of chemical substances possess demulcent properties. Among these are the alginates, mucilages, gums, dextrins, starches, certain sugars and polymeric polyhydric glycols. Mucus, in itself, is a natural demulcent. Certain silicates that form silicic acid on exposure to air or gastric juice and glycerin, although the silicic acid has low molecular weight and relatively low binding power, frequently are placed among the demulcents. Also the colloidal hydrous oxides, hydroxides and basic salts of several metals are claimed to be demulcent, but acceptable clinical proof of the claim has not been provided.

The hydrophilic colloidal properties of most demulcents enable them to function as emulsifiers and suspending agents in water-soluble ointments and suspensions. They also retard the absorption of many injections and, thus, may be employed in various depot preparations. Many of the demulcents mask the flavor of medicaments by means of at least three physical phenomena: (1) they apparently coat the taste receptors and render them less sensitive, (2) they incorporate many organic solutes into micelles and, thereby, diminish the free concentration of such solutes and (3) they coat the surfaces of many particles in suspension. Because of the adhesiveness of the demulcents, they are employed widely as binding agents in tablets, lozenges and similar dosage forms. Consequently, certain demulcents will be discussed in Chapter 80.

Acacia—page 1395.

Agar—page 1395.

Benzoin

Gum Benjamin; Benzoe

The balsamic resin obtained from *Styrax benzoin* Dryander or *Styrax paralleloneurus* Perkins, known in commerce as Sumatra Benzoin, or from *Styrax tonkinensis* (Pierre) Craib ex Hartwich, or other species of the Section *Anthostyrax* of the genus *Styrax*, known in commerce as Siam Benzoin (Fam *Styraceae*).

Sumatra benzoin yields not less than 75.0% of alcohol-soluble extractive, and Siam benzoin yields not less than 90.0% of alcohol-soluble extractive.

Constituents—Siam benzoin contains about 68% of crystalline *coniferyl benzoate* [$C_{17}H_{16}O_4$]; up to 10% of an amorphous form of this compound is also present. Some *coniferyl alcohol* (*m-methoxy-p-hydroxycinnamyl alcohol*, mp 73–74°) occurs in the free state as well. Other compounds that have been isolated are *benzoic acid* 11.7%, *d-siaresinolic acid* 6%, *cinnamyl benzoate* 2.3% and *vanillin* 0.3%.

Sumatra benzoin has been reported to contain benzoic and cinnamic acid esters of the alcohol *benzoresinol* and probably also of coniferyl alcohol, free *benzoic* and *cinnamic acids, styrene*, 2 to 3% of *cinnamyl cinnamate* (also called *styracin*), 1% of *phenylpropyl cinnamate*, 1% of *vanillin*, a trace of *benzaldehyde*, a little *benzyl cinnamate* and the alcohol *d-sumaresinol* [$C_{30}H_{48}O_4$].

Description—*Sumatra Benzoin:* Blocks or lumps of varying size made up of compacted tears, with a reddish brown, reddish gray or grayish brown resinous mass. *Siam Benzoin:* Compressed pebble-like tears of varying size and shape. Both varieties are yellowish to rusty brown externally and milky white on fracture; hard and brittle at ordinary temperatures but softened by heat; aromatic and balsamic odor; aromatic and slightly acrid taste.

Uses—A *protective* application for irritations of the skin. When mixed with glycerin and water, the tincture may be applied locally for *cutaneous ulcers, bedsores, cracked nipples* and *fissures* of the lips and anus. For throat and bronchial inflammation, the tincture may be administered on sugar. The tincture and compound tincture sometimes are used in boiling water as steam inhalants for their *expectorant* and *soothing action* in acute laryngitis and croup. In combination with zinc oxide, it is used in baby ointments.

Dose—*Topical*, to the *skin*, as a **10%** tincture or compound tincture (below).

Compound Benzoin Tincture [Balsamum Equitis Sancti Victoris, Balsamum Commendatoris, Balsamum Catholicum, Balsamum Traumaticum, Balsamum Vulnerarium, Balsamum Persicum, Balsamum Suecium, Balsamum Friari, Balsamum Vervaini, Guttae Nader, Guttae Jesuitarium, Tinctura Balsamica, Balsam of the Holy Victorious Knight, Commander's Balsam, Friar's Balsam, Turlington's Drops, Persian Balsam, Swedish Balsam, Vervain Balsam, Turlington's Balsam of Life, Balsam de Maltha, Ward's Balsam, Jerusalem Balsam, Saint Victor's Balsam, Wade's Drops, Wound Elixir and Balsamic Tincture]—*Preparation:* With benzoin (in moderately coarse powder, 100 g), aloe (in moderately coarse powder, 20 g), storax (80 g) and tolu balsam (40 g), prepare a tincture (1000 mL) by Process M (page 1521), using alcohol as the menstruum. *Alcohol Content:* 74 to 80% of C_2H_5OH. *Uses:* Especially valuable in acute *laryngitis*, also in croup, when added to hot water and the vapor inhaled. By adding a teaspoonful of the tincture to boiling water in an inhaler, and inhaling the vapor, very effective results may be obtained. See Chapter 107. It is also administered, on sugar, for throat and bronchial inflammation and as a local application, when mixed with glycerin and water, for *ulcers, bedsores, cracked nipples* and *fissures* of the lips and anus. *Dose: Topical*, as required; *inhalation*, 1% in very hot water.

Carbomer—page 1396.

Gelatin—page 1397.

Glycerin—pages 1041 and 1405.

Glycerin Suppositories—see RPS-18, page 785.

Glycyrrhiza—page 1387.

Hydroxyethyl Cellulose—page 1397.

Hydroxypropyl Cellulose—page 1397.

Hydroxypropyl Cellulose Insert

Lacrisert (*MSD*)

Description—Sterile; translucent; rod-shaped.

Solubility—Soluble in water.

Uses—For administration into the inferior cul-de-sac of the eye. It is used when lacrimation is inadequate or to thicken tear film and prolong the tear-film breakup time, which usually is accelerated in patients with moderate to severe dry-eye states, including conjunctival hyperemia, corneal and conjunctival staining with rose bengal, exudation, itching, burning, foreign body sensation, smarting, photophobia, dryness and blurred or cloudy vision.

Dose—*Usual*, **1 insert** in each eye once a day.

Dosage Forms—Inserts: 5 mg.

Hydroxypropyl Methylcellulose—page 1397.

Hydroxypropyl Methylcellulose Ophthalmic Solution

A sterile solution of hydroxypropyl methylcellulose, of a grade containing 19.0–30.0% methoxy and 4.0–12.0% hydroxypropoxy groups; may contain antimicrobial, buffering and stabilizing agents.

Uses—A *wetting solution for contact lenses.* Its demulcent action decreases the irritant effect of the lens on the cornea. It also imparts viscous properties to the wetting solution, which assists the lens in staying in place. The demulcent effect also finds application in ophthalmic decongestants. "Artificial tear" formulations containing this drug may be used when lacrimation is inadequate. A 2.5% solution is used in gonioscopes.

Dose—*Topical*, to the *conjunctiva*, **1** to **2 drops** 3 or 4 times a day.

Dosage Forms—Solution: 0.3, 0.5 and 1%.

Methylcellulose—page 1397.

Methylcellulose Ophthalmic Solution

A sterile solution of methylcellulose; may contain antimicrobial, buffering and stabilizing agents.

Uses—For the same purposes, and in the same manner, as *Hydroxypropyl Methylcellulose Ophthalmic Solution*, above.

Dosage Forms—0.25, 0.5 and 1%.

Pectin—page 907.

Polyethylene Glycols—page 1403.

Polyvinyl Alcohol—page 1398.

Polyvinyl Alcohol Ophthalmic Solution

VasoClear A (*Cooper Vision*)

A sterile solution of polyvinyl alcohol, which may contain antimicrobial, buffering and stabilizing agents and other demulcent substances.

[9002-89-5] (Polyvinyl alcohol).

Preparation—By partial hydrolysis (*ca* 90%) of polyvinyl acetate.

Description—A white powder which is a linear polymer, —$(CH_2—CHOH)_n$—, where the value of *n* is between 500 and 5000; pH (1 in 25 aqueous solution) between 5.0 and 8.0.

Solubility—Soluble in water; insoluble in organic solvents.

Uses—A *wetting solution for contact lenses.* The polyvinyl alcohol has a demulcent action that helps protect the eye from irritation by the contact lens. It also is used in "artificial tears," employed when there is insufficient lacrimation.

Dose—*Topical*, to the *conjunctiva*, **1 or 2 drops**, 3 or 4 times a day or as needed.

Dosage Forms—Solution: 1.4 to 3.0%.

Propylene Glycol—page 1406.
Sodium Alginate—page 1396.
Tragacanth—page 1399.

Emollients

Emollients (L, *emollier* = to soften) are bland, fatty or oleaginous substances which may be applied locally, particularly to the skin, but also to other mucous membranes. Skin usually appears "dry" due to a lack of moisture. Emollients or moisturizers increase the tissue moisture content, thereby rendering the skin softer and more pliable. Increased moisture content in the skin can be achieved by preventing water loss with an occlusive water-immiscible barrier, increasing the water-holding capacity of the skin with humectants or altering the desquamation of the outermost skin layer, the strateum corneum.

The class of vehicles for emollients providing the range of the greatest moisturizing to the greatest drying effects on the skin include oleaginous bases, anhydrous absorption bases, W/O emulsions, O/W emulsions, the more-neutral, water-miscible compounds and, finally, the more-drying gel and solution bases.

Emollients have certain disadvantages. It now is recognized that retention of perspiration below the emollient and exclusion of air render conditions favorable to the growth of anaerobic bacteria. Furthermore, rubbing and massaging during application aids in the spreading of cutaneous bacteria. Consequently, the use of emollients to cover burns and abrasions is diminishing. Some emollients (eg, lanolin, both the hydroxylated and acetylated forms; isopropyl myristate and palmitate; oleyl alcohol and sodium lauryl sulfate) are comedogenic. Other liquid emollients may be used for mild catharsis (page 896) and for protection against GI corrosives; however, castor oil is hydrolyzed in the gut to the irritating ricinoleic acid and, hence, is employed as an emollient only externally. Orally administered liquid emollients may be aspirated into the trachea and lungs, especially in infants; in the debilitated, such aspiration induce "oil aspiration pneumonia." This condition also may be induced by emollient nose drops.

The chief use of emollient or moisturizing substances beyond their therapeutic actions is to provide vehicles for lipid-soluble drugs (as in ointments and liniments), hence, many of them are described among the pharmaceutical necessities (Chapter 80). It is widely, but incorrectly, held that such vehicles facilitate the transport through the skin of their active ingredients. On the contrary, when the oil:water partition coefficient is greater than 1.0, the penetration is retarded and the emollient vehicle prolongs the action of the active ingredient. Emollient substances also are employed in both cleansing and antiphlogistic creams and lotions. Compound ointment bases, creams and other medicated applications are treated in Chapter 89. Only the simple emollients and important compounded ointments that are used frequently for their emollient actions are listed below.

Animal Fats and Oils

Lanolin—page 1402.
Spermaceti—see RPS-18, page 1310.
Mineral Oil—page 899.
Mineral Oil, Light—page 1411.
Paraffin—page 1400.
Petrolatum—page 1400

Red Petrolatum

Description—UV-absorbing qualities to 340 nm. It provides a water-protective action because of its petrolatum base.

Uses—Owing to its opacity, it is used as a *sunblock* in creams, ointments and sticks. It also is used as a *sunshade* with zinc oxide in some formulations and for lip protection (20% petrolatum with 5% PABA).

Dosage Forms—*Topical:* 30 to 100%.

White Ointment—page 1400.
White Petrolatum—page 1401.
Yellow Ointment—page 1400.

Vegetable Oils

Castor Oil—page 897.
Castor Oil, Sulfated—page 1401.
Cocoa Butter—page 1409.
Coconut Oil—page 1406.
Corn Oil—page 1394.
Cottonseed Oil—page 1394.
Olive Oil—page 1400.
Peanut Oil—page 1394.
Persic Oil—page 1416.
Sesame Oil—page 1395.

Waxes

Cetyl Esters Wax—page 1400.
Cold Cream—page 1401.
Hydrophilic Ointment—page 1402.
Rose Water Ointment—page 1402.
Spermaceti—see RPS-18, page 1312.
Wax, White—see RPS-18, page 1310.
Wax, Yellow—see RPS-18, page 1311.

Other Emollients

Cetyl Alcohol—page 1401.
Glycerin—page 1405.
Petrolatum, Hydrophilic—page 1401.
Isopropyl Myristate—page 1411.

Myristyl Alcohol

Tetradecyl Alcohol

[112-72-1] $CH_3(CH_2)_{12}CH_2OH$ (214.38).

Preparation—By reduction of fatty acid esters.

Description—White, crystalline alcohol; specific gravity 0.824; melts at 30°.

Solubility—Insoluble in water; soluble in ether; slightly soluble in alcohol.

Uses—An *emollient* in cold creams.

Oleyl Alcohol—page 1398.

Shark Liver Oil

The oil extracted from the livers of the *soupfin shark, Galeorhinus zyopterus* or *Hypoprion brevirostris*, both of which are rich in vitamins A and D.

Uses—An *emollient* and *protectant* (FDA classification Category I) used in burn and sunburn ointments.

Dose—*Usual*, **3%**.

Astringents and Antiperspirants

Astringents are locally applied protein precipitants which have such a low cell penetrability that the action essentially is limited to the cell surface and the interstitial spaces. The permeability of the cell membrane is reduced, but the cells remain viable. The astringent action is accompanied by contraction and wrinkling of the tissue and by blanching. The cement substance of the capillary endothelium and the basement membrane is hardened, so that pathological transcapillary movement of plasma protein is inhibited and local edema, inflammation and exudation, thereby, are reduced. Mucus or other secretions also may be reduced, so that the affected area becomes drier.

Astringents are used therapeutically to arrest hemorrhage by coagulating the blood (*styptic* action, page 926) and to check diarrhea, reduce inflammation of mucous membranes, promote healing, toughen the skin or decrease sweating.

The principal astringents are the (1) salts of the cations aluminum, zinc, manganese, iron or bismuth, (2) certain other salts that contain these metals (such as permanganates) and (3) tannins, or related polyphenolic compounds. Zinc sulfate (0.25%) is the only nonprescription astringent recommended. Acids, alcohols, phenols and other substances that precipitate proteins may be astringent in the appropriate amount or concentration. However, such substances generally are not employed for their astringent effects, because they readily penetrate cells and promote tissue damage. Strongly hypertonic solutions dry the affected tissues and are often incorrectly called astringents, since protein precipitation also occurs. Many astringents are irritant or caustic in moderate to high concentrations. Consequently, strict attention must be paid to the appropriate concentration. Most astringents are also antiseptics and many of them are discussed in Chapter 76.

Astringents also possess some *deodorant* properties by virtue of their interaction with odorous fatty acids liberated or produced by action of bacteria on lipids in sweat, and by supressing bacterial growth, partly because of a decrease in pH. The *antiperspirant* effect is the result both of the closure of the sweat ducts by protein precipitation to form a plug and peritubular irritation that promotes an increase in inward pressure on the tubule.

Antiperspirants and deodorants can be applied as aerosols, sprays pads, sticks and roll-on liquid, creams and semisolids for the control of excessive perspiration and body odor. The general adult population secretes between 0.5 to 1.5 L of odorless perspiration a day. The unpleasant odor associated with perspiration is the result of chemical and bacterial degradation of these skin secretions. Antiperspirants are designed to decrease the flow and/or inhibit the bacterial degradation of skin secretions. Agents most commonly used as antiperspirants include aluminum chlorohydrates, aluminum chloride, buffered aluminum sulfate and zirconyl chlorohydrates. These agents reduce perspiration 20 to 40% in the general adult population.

Aluminum chlorohydrates are available in a variety of 25% (anhydrous) salt formulations that differ in the ratio of aluminum to chlorine, as well as in complexes with polyethylene glycol or polypropylene glycol. Aluminum chlorohydrates are less acidic than aluminum chloride; thus, they do not stain fabrics in contact with treated skin and maintain antiperspirant activity and antiodor activity due to inhibiting growth of gram-negative bacteria on the skin surface.

Buffered aluminum sufate (8% aluminum sulfate buffered with 8% sodium aluminum lactate) is effective and nonirritating to the skin.

Due to the sarcoid-like granulomas and allergic reactions to aluminum zirconium chlorohydrates, they are not used in aerosol-type antiperspirants. They are used topically as antihydrotics on the axillae in concentrations not exceeding 20%.

Glutaraldehyde (2 to 10% buffered solution), formaldehyde (5 to 30% solutions), methenamine (5% stick or 10% solution) and scopolamine hydrobromide (0.025% solution) also are used to treat hyperhidrosis of the planar and plantar surfaces, but not axillae surfaces. Deodorants reduce the resident bacteria flora on the skin, thereby inhibiting bacterial decomposition of perspiration.

Commonly used agents include benzalkonium chloride, methylbenzethonium chloride and neomycin sulfate. The quaternary ammonium chlorides, however, are inactivated by soaps. They can irritate skin at concentrations greater than 1%. Concurent use of antibiotics may sensitize the individual subject and or result in the production of resistant bacterial strains.

Alcohol—page 1404.

Alum

Sulfuric acid, aluminum potassium salt (2:1:1), dodecahydrate; Sulfuric acid, aluminum ammonium salt (2:1:1), dodecahydrate; Alumen; Alumen Purificatum; Purified Alum

Aluminum ammonium sulfate (1:1:2) dodecahydrate [7784-26-1]; anhydrous [7784-25-0] (237.14); or aluminum potassium sulfate (1:1:2) dodecahydrate [7784-24-9]; anhydrous [10043-67-1] (258.19).

The label of the container must indicate whether the salt is ammonium alum [$AlNH_4(SO_4)_2.12H_2O$ = 453.32] or potassium alum [$AlK(SO_4)_2.12H_2O$ = 474.38].

Preparation—Prepared from the mineral *bauxite* (a hydrated aluminum oxide) and sulfuric acid, with the addition of ammonium or potassium sulfate for the respective alums. Ammonium alum dominates the market because of its lower cost.

Description—Large, colorless crystals, crystalline fragments or a white powder; odorless and has a sweetish, strongly astringent taste; solutions are acid to litmus.

Solubility—1 g ammonium alum in 7 mL water, and 1 g potassium alum in 7.5 mL water; both are soluble in about 0.3 mL boiling water, but they are insoluble in alcohol; alum is freely but slowly soluble in glycerin.

Incompatibilities—When alum is dispensed in powders with *phenol*, *salicylates* or *tannic acid*, gray or green colors may be developed due to traces of iron in the alum. A partial liberation of its water of crystallization permits it to act as an acid toward *sodium bicarbonate*, thus liberating carbon dioxide. Ammonia is liberated simultaneously from ammonium alum. *Alkali hydroxides and carbonates*, *borax* or *lime water* precipitate aluminum hydroxide from solutions of alum. The alums possess the incompatibilities of the water-soluble sulfates.

Uses—A powerful *astringent* in acidic solutions. It is only slightly antiseptic, probably due to bacteriostasis through liberation of acid on hydrolysis. It sometimes is used as a local *styptic*, and frequently is employed in making astringent lotions and douches. It is used especially by athletes to toughen the skin. As an astringent it is used in concentrations of 0.5 to 5%. Some vulvovaginal cleansing and deodorant preparations also contain alum.

Styptic pencils are made by fusing potassium alum, usually with the addition of some potassium nitrate, and pouring it into suitable molds.

Caution—Do not confuse *styptic* pencils with *caustic* pencils (page 877); the latter contain *silver nitrate*.

Dose—*Topical*, as a **0.5 to 5%** solution.

Aluminum Acetate Topical Solution

Acetic acid, aluminum salt; Liquor Burowii; Burow's Solution

$Al(OCOCH_3)_3$

Yields, from each 100 mL, 1.20–1.45 g of aluminum oxide [Al_2O_3 = 101.96], and 4.24 to 5.12 g of acetic acid [$C_2H_4O_2$ = 60.05], corresponding to 4.8 to 5.8 g of aluminum acetate [139-12-8] $C_6H_9AlO_6$ (204.12). It may be stabilized by the addition of not more than 0.6% of boric acid.

Caution—This solution should not be confused with Aluminum Subacetate Topical Solution which is a stronger preparation.

Note—Dispense only clear Aluminum Acetate Solution.

Description—Clear, colorless liquid having a faint acetous odor, and a sweetish, astringent taste; specific gravity about 1.022; pH 3.6 to 4.4.

Uses—As an *astringent dressing* or as an *astringent mouth wash* and *gargle*. Aluminum acetate is included in preparations to treat athlete's foot, dermatidides, diaper rash, dry skin, poison ivy poisoning and inflammation of the external ear.

Dose—*Topical*, to the skin, as a wet dressing containing a **1:10** to **1:40 dilution** of the solution.

Aluminum Chloride

[7784-13-6] $AlCl_3.6H_2O$ (241.43); *anhydrous* [7446-70-0] (133.34).

Preparation—By heating aluminum in chlorine gas, then dissolving the product in water and crystallizing, or by dissolving freshly precipitated aluminum hydroxide in hydrochloric acid and concentrating to permit crystallization.

Description—White or yellowish white, crystalline powder; deliquescent; sweet, astringent taste; solutions are acid to litmus.

Solubility—1 g in about 0.9 mL water or 4 mL alcohol; soluble in glycerin.

Uses—Extensively employed on the skin as an *astringent* and *anhidrotic*; it is included in some proprietary preparations formulated for this purpose. It is used especially in the treatment of soggy athlete's foot, to promote drying and, hence, to enhance the efficacy of specific antifungal drugs. For ordinary antiperspirant use the basic salt *aluminum chlorohydroxide*, $Al_2Cl(OH)_5$, is preferable as it is less irritating and causes less deterioration of clothing than does this drug. It may have a special use in the treatment of *hyperhidrosis of the palms, soles or axillae*, for which a 20% solution in absolute alcohol is used. In the presence of water, it hydrolyzes to aluminum chlorohydroxide and hydrochloric acid, which can cause irritation, especially in fissures, discomfort and also deterioration of clothing. Concentrations below 15% cause a low incidence of irritation. Consequently, it is essential that the area to be treated is completely dry before application. To protect bedclothes, the treated area is sometimes covered with plastic wrap, but such occlusion of the axillae may result in boils or furuncles. It should not be applied to the axillae immediately after shaving or used where the skin is irritated or broken. Concentrations above 15% are used as *caustics*.

Dose—*Topical*, to the *skin*, as **6.25** to **30%** solution. The 20% alcoholic solution may be applied on 2 successive days and twice a week thereafter, except that it may be applied twice a day for athlete's foot.

Aluminum Chlorohydrates

The hydrate of aluminum chloride hydroxide [1327-41-9] Al_2- $Cl(OH)_5$].

Uses—Mainly employed in antiperspirant products, for which they have been rated safe and effective in concentrations of 25% (as anhydride) or less. Since solutions or suspensions are less acidic than those of aluminum chloride, they cause a lower incidence of irritation to the skin.

Dose—*Topical*, to the axilla, as a **2.5** to **25%** cake, ointment, solution or suspension.

Aluminum Sulfate

Sulfuric acid, aluminum salt (3:2), hydrate; Cake Alum; Patent Alum; Pearl Alum; Pickle Alum; "Papermaker's Alum"

Aluminum sulfate (2:3) hydrate [17927-65-0] $Al_2(SO_4)_3.xH_2O$; anhydrous [10043-01-3] (342.14).

Preparation—By reacting freshly precipitated aluminum hydroxide with an appropriate quantity of sulfuric acid. The resulting solution is evaporated and allowed to crystallize.

Description—White crystalline powder, shining plates or crystalline fragments; stable in air; odorless and has a sweet, mildly astringent taste; aqueous solution (1 in 20) is acid and has a pH not less than 2.9.

Solubility—1 g in about 1 mL water; insoluble in alcohol.

Uses—A powerful *astringent*, acting much like alum. It is used widely as a *local antiperspirant* and is the effective ingredient in some commercial antiperspirant products. Solutions usually are buffered with sodium aluminum lactate to make them less irritating. It is used for water purification in the "alum flocculation" process. It is a *pharmaceutical necessity* for *Aluminum Subacetate Solution*.

Dose—*Topical*, to the skin, as an **8%** solution.

Aluminum Zirconium Chlorohydrate—See RPS-18, page 763.

Bismuth Subcarbonate—see RPS-18, page 799.

Bismuth Subnitrate—page 1407.

Calamine

Iron oxide (Fe_2O_3), mixt. with zinc oxide; Prepared Calamine; Lapis Calaminaria; Artificial Calamine

Calamine [8011-96-9]; contains, after ignition, not less than 98.0% ZnO (81.38).

Preparation—By thoroughly mixing zinc oxide with sufficient ferric oxide (usually 0.5 to 1%) to obtain a product of the desired color.

It originally was obtained by roasting a native zinc carbonate, then known as *calamine*, hence, the name. This name also is applied by mineralogists to a native form of zinc silicate, which is not suitable for making medicinal calamine.

Description—Pink powder, all of which passes through a No 100 standard mesh sieve. It is odorless and almost tasteless.

Solubility—Insoluble in water; dissolves almost completely in mineral acids.

Uses—Similar to those of zinc oxide, being employed chiefly as an *astringent* and in *protective* and soothing ointments and lotions for *sunburn, ivy poisoning*, etc. It often is prescribed by dermatologists to give opacity and a flesh-like color to lotions or ointments.

Dose—*Topical*, to the skin, in various concentrations in lotions and ointments.

Calamine Lotion [Lotio Calaminae]—*Preparation:* Dilute bentonite magma (250 mL) with an equal volume of calcium hydroxide solution. Mix calamine (80 g) and zinc oxide (80 g) intimately with glycerin (20 mL) and about 100 mL of the diluted magma, triturating until a smooth, uniform paste is formed. Gradually incorporate the remainder of the diluted magma. Finally add calcium hydroxide solution (qs) to make 1000 mL, and shake well. If a more viscous consistency in the Lotion is desired, the quantity of bentonite magma may be increased to not more than 400 mL. *Note: Shake thoroughly before dispensing.*

Phenolated Calamine Lotion [Lotio Calaminae Composita; Compound Calamine Lotion]—*Preparation:* Mix liquefied phenol (10 mL) and calamine lotion (990 mL) to make 1000 mL. Commercial preparations also contain 8.4% isopropyl alcohol and have various other modifications. See *Calamine. Note: Shake thoroughly before dispensing.*

Glutaral—page 1266.

Methenamine—page 1268.

Potassium Permanganate—see RPS-18, page 1173.

Resorcinol—RPS-16, page 1107.

Silver Nitrate—page 877.

Tannic Acid

Gallotannic Acid; Tannin; Digallic Acid
Zibactin Medicated (*Zila*)

[1401-55-4]. A tannin usually obtained from nutgalls, the excrescences produced on the young twigs of *Quercus infectoria* Olivier and allied species of *Quercus* Linné (Fam *Fagaceae*).

Description—Yellowish white to light brown amorphous powder, glistening scales or spongy masses; usually odorless; strong astringent taste; gradually darkens on exposure to air and light.

Solubility—1 g in about 0.35 mL water or 1 mL warm glycerin; very soluble in alcohol; practically insoluble in chloroform or ether.

Incompatibilities—Solutions gradually darken on exposure to air and light through oxidation of phenolic groups to quinoid structures. It is incompatible with most enzymes, gums, salts of many metals and many other substances.

Uses—On an open sore or denuded surface, it forms a film of protein tannate that acts as a *mechanical protective* which excludes external irritants and infectives and, thus, provides some relief from pain. However, it is not antibacterial and not only does not inhibit the growth of bacteria entrained beneath the film but actually may create favorable conditions for the growth of certain anaerobes. For this reason, and also the fact that it is absorbed sufficiently from large denuded areas to cause liver damage, it is no longer used in the treatment of burns and should not be used on any large lesions. Nevertheless, it is incorporated in 8 to 10% concentration in several products to treat ivy or oak poisoning. As a 7% gel it is used on cold sores, fever blisters and cankers. It is included in 2.16% concentration in a hemorrhoidal preparation and in 4% concentration in a keratolytic product for removing corns, calluses and warts, these concentration probably being too low to contribute significantly to the supposed efficacies. In a 25% solution it is used to reduce inflammation and harden skin around ingrown toenails, thus increasing comfort and making nail-cutting easier.

Its content in tea accounts for the use of strong tea as an internal antidote, presumably for the dual purpose of precipitating toxic alkaloids and hardening the surface of the gastrointestinal mucosa and its mucous layer.

Dose—*Topical*, to the *skin*, 4 times a day for at least 2 days.

Dosage Forms—Gel: 7%.

White Lotion

Lotio Alba; Lotio Sulfurata

Zinc Sulfate	**40 g**
Sulfurated Potash	**40 g**
Purified Water, a sufficient quantity,	
To make	**1000 mL**

Dissolve zinc sulfate and sulfurated potash separately, each in 450 mL purified water, and filter each solution. Add slowly the sulfurated potash solution to the zinc sulfate solution with constant stirring. Then add the required amount of purified water, and mix.

Note—Prepare freshly and shake thoroughly before dispensing. For further discussion see *Sulfurated Potash* (page 1415).

Uses—An *astringent, protective* and mild *antimicrobial* preparation. The astringency is attributable to the zinc ion. The thiosulfates and polysulfides in it exert antibacterial and antifungal actions (see *Sodium Thiosulfate*, RPS-16, page 1176). White lotion is used in the treatment of acne vulgaris.

Dose—*Topical*, to the *skin*, as required.

Zinc Caprylate

Zinc Octanoate

[557-09-5] $C_{16}H_{20}O_4Zn$ (351.79).

Preparation—By the methathesis of zinc sulfate and ammonium caprylate.

Description—Lustrous scales; melts about 136°.

Solubility—Sparingly soluble in boiling water; moderately soluble in boiling alcohol.

Uses—In the treatment of *athlete's foot*. The astringency of the zinc decreases inflammation and wetness. The caprylate has a weak antifungal action.

Dose—*Topical*, to the *skin*, as a **5%** ointment.

Dosage Forms—Ointment: 5%.

Zinc Chloride

Butter of Zinc

[7646-85-7] $ZnCl_2$ (136.29).

Preparation—By reacting metallic zinc or zinc oxide with hydrochloric acid and evaporating the solution to dryness.

Description—White, or nearly white, odorless, crystalline powder, or as porcelain-like masses, or in molded pencils; very deliquescent; aqueous solution (1 in 10) acid to litmus; solution in water or alcohol usually slightly turbid, but the turbidity disappears on addition of a small quantity of hydrochloric acid.

Solubility—1 g in 0.5 mL water, about 1.5 mL alcohol or about 2 mL glycerin.

Incompatibilities—Soluble zinc salts are precipitated as zinc hydroxide by alkali hydroxides, including ammonium hydroxide; the precipitate is soluble in an excess of either the fixed or the ammonium hydroxide. *Carbonates, phosphates, oxalates, arsenates* and *tannin* cause precipitation. The precipitation with sodium borate can be prevented by addition of an amount of glycerin equal in weight to the sodium borate. In weak aqueous solutions, it has a tendency to form the insoluble basic salt by hydrolysis and about one-half its weight of ammonium chloride has been used for the purpose of stabilization. It is very *deliquescent*. It has the incompatibilities of chlorides, being precipitated by *silver* and *lead salts*.

Uses—In high concentrations it is *caustic* and has been used as a caustic agent to treat corns, calluses and warts. In the low concentrations in which it is marketed it is astringent and mildly antibacterial and probably does not contribute to keratolysis. Although it is used in mouthwashes, the contact time is too short, and only an astringent and not an antibacterial action results.

Dose—*Topical*, to the teeth, as a **10%** solution; to skin and mucous membranes for astringency and antimicrobial actions, as a **0.1** to **2%** solution.

Zinc Oxide

Flowers of Zinc; Zinc White; Pompholyx; Nihil Album; Lana Philosophica

Zinc oxide [1314-13-2] ZnO (81.38).

Preparation—By heating zinc carbonate at a low red heat until the carbon dioxide and water are expelled.

Description—Very fine, odorless, amorphous, white or yellowish white powder, free from gritty particles; gradually absorbs carbon dioxide from the air; when strongly heated it assumes a yellow color which disappears on cooling; its suspension in water is practically neutral.

Solubility—Insoluble in water or alcohol; soluble in dilute acids, solutions of the alkali hydroxides or ammonium carbonate solution.

Incompatibilities—Reacts slowly with fatty acids in *oils* and *fats* to produce lumpy masses of zinc oleate, stearate, etc. *Vanishing creams* tend to dry out and crumble. Whenever permissible, it is advisable to levigate it to a smooth paste with a little mineral oil before incorporation into an ointment.

Uses—Has a mild *astringent, protective* and *antiseptic* action. In the form of its various official ointments and pastes it is employed widely in the treatment of dry skin and such skin disorders and infections as *acne vulgaris, prickly heat, insect stings and bites, ivy poisoning, diaper rash, dandruff, seborrhea, eczema, impetigo, ringworm, psoriasis, varicose ulcers* and *pruritus*. It is contained in some sunscreens. It is included in some vulvovaginal deodorant preparations and in preparations for the treatment of hemorrhoids. It also is used in dental cements and temporary fillings. It is the essential ingredient in *Calamine* (page 872).

Dose—*Topical*, as a **5** to **25%** cream, lotion, ointment, paste, baby powder or rectal suppository.

Dosage Forms—Ointment: 20%; Paste: 25%. In numerous combinations: 2 to 15%.

Zinc Pyrithione—see RPS-18, page 1173.

Zinc Sulfate—page 1271.

Zinc Undecylenate—see RPS-18, page 1237.

Irritants, Rubefacients and Vesicants

Irritants are drugs that act locally on the skin and mucous membranes to induce, based on irritant concentration, hyperemia, inflammation and, when the action is severe, vesication. Agents that induce only hyperemia are known as *rubefacients*. Rubefaction is produced by increased circulation to the injured area and is accompanied by a feeling of comfort, warmth and, sometimes, itching and hyperesthesia. Appropriately low concentrations of directly applied or inhaled vapors of volatile aromatic irritants, such as camphor or menthol, induce a sensation of coolness rather than warmth. When the irritation is more severe, plasma escapes from the damaged capillaries and forms blisters (vesicles). Agents that induce blisters are known as *vesicants*. Most rubefacients also are vesicants in higher concentrations. Certain irritants may be relatively selective for various tissues or cell types, so that hypersecretion of the surface, seborrheic abscesses, paresthesia or other effects may be noted in the absence of appreciable hyperemia.

Irritants have been used empirically for many centuries, probably even prehistorically. They may be employed for counterirritation, the mechanism of which is poorly under stood. A moderate to severe pain may be obscured by a milder pain arising from areas of irritation appropriately placed to induce reflex stimulation of certain organs or systems, especially respiratory. Sensory and visible effects of irritation sometimes give patients the assurance that they are receiving effective medication. The rubefacient of choice is simply the applicant of heat, as drugs are much less efficient. Taken internally, many irritants exert either an emetic or laxative action. Irritant laxatives are listed on page 896. A few irritants, especially cantharides, on absorption into the blood stream, irritate the urogenital tract and, consequently, have been dangerously employed as *aphrodisiacs*. Certain irritants also possess a healing action on wounds, possibly the result of local stimulation. Many condiments are irritants. In high concentrations, many irritants even can be corrosive.

Alcohol—page 1404.

Alcohol, Rubbing—page 1264.

Ammonia Spirit, Aromatic—RPS-16, page 1452.

Anthralin

1,8,9-Anthracenetriol; Dithranol;
Dioxyanthranol; Cignolin; Anthra-Derm (*Dermik*); Lasan (*Stiefel*)

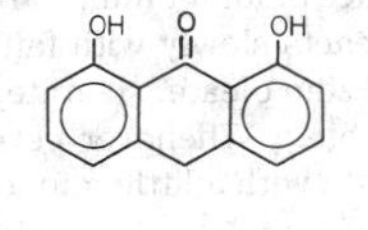

1,8-Dihydroxyanthranol [480-22-8] $C_{14}H_{10}O_3$ (226.23).

Preparation—Anthraquinone is sulfonated to the 1,8-disulfonic acid, which is isolated from the reaction mixture and then heated with a calcium hydroxide-calcium chloride mixture to form 1,8-dihydroxy-9,10-anthraquinone, which is reduced with tin and HCl to anthralin.

Description—Yellowish brown, crystalline powder; odorless and tasteless; melts between 175° and 181°.

Solubility—Insoluble in water; slightly soluble in alcohol; soluble in chloroform; slightly soluble in ether.

Uses—Although long considered to be an irritant, its principal therapeutic action is the reduction of epidermal DNA synthesis and mitotic activity. It is used in the treatment of *psoriasis, alopecia areata, eczema* and other *chronic dermatoses.* It usually is used in combination with ultraviolet light and a daily coal tar "bath." To avoid harmful irritation, medicaments containing it should not be used on the face, scalp, genitalia or intertriginous skin areas; they should not be applied to blistered, raw or oozing areas of the skin, and should be kept from the eyes, since they may cause severe conjunctivitis, keratitis or corneal opacity. Renal irritation, casts and albuminuria may result when the drug is absorbed systemically. The hands should be washed immediately after applying medication. A reversible slight discoloration of the skin may occur.

Dose—*Topical,* to the *skin,* as a **0.1** to **1%** cream or ointment, once a day with cream and once or twice a day with ointment. The concentration should be low initially and increased only as necessary.

Dosage Forms—Cream: 0.1, 0.2, 0.25, 0.4, 0.5 and 1%; Ointment: 0.1, 0.25, 0.4, 0.5, 1 and 2%.

Benzoin Tincture, Compound—page 869.

Camphor

2-Camphanone; 2-Bornanone; Gum Camphor; Laurel Camphor

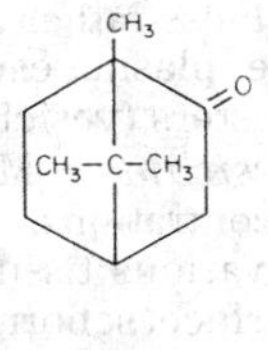

[76-22-2] $C_{10}H_{16}O$ (152.24). A ketone obtained from *Cinnamomum camphora* (Linné). Nees et Ebermaier (Fam *Lauraceae*) (Natural Camphor) or produced synthetically (Synthetic Camphor).

Preparation—Natural crude camphor may be obtained by steam distilling chips of the camphor tree; the crude camphor so obtained is purified, usually by sublimation. One method of producing synthetic camphor starts with *pinene* [$C_{10}H_{16}$], a hydrocarbon obtained from turpentine oil. The pinene is saturated with hydrogen chloride at 0° forming bornyl chloride [$C_{10}H_{17}Cl$]. On heating the bornyl chloride with sodium acetate and glacial acetic acid, it is converted into isobornyl acetate, which is subsequently hydrolyzed to isobornyl alcohol [$C_{10}H_{17}OH$] and oxidized with chromic acid to camphor. Synthetic camphor resembles natural camphor in most of its properties except that it is a racemic mixture and, therefore, lacks optical activity. When camphor is mixed in approximately molecular proportions with chloral hydrate, menthol, phenol or thymol, liquefaction ensues; such mixtures are known as *eutectic mixtures* (see page 163).

Description—Colorless or white crystals, granules or crystalline masses; or as colorless to white, translucent, tough masses; a penetrating, characteristic odor, a pungent, aromatic taste and is readily pulverizable in the presence of a little alcohol, ether or chloroform; specific gravity about 0.99; melts between 174° and 179° and slowly volatilizes at ordinary temperature and in steam.

Solubility—1 g in about 800 mL water, 1 mL alcohol, about 0.5 mL chloroform or 1 mL ether; freely soluble in carbon disulfide, solvent hexane or fixed and volatile oils.

Incompatibilites—Forms a liquid or a soft mass when rubbed with *chloral hydrate, hydroquinone, menthol, phenol, phenyl salicylate, resorcinol, salicylic acid, thymol* or other substances. It is precipitated from its alcoholic solution by the addition of water. It is precipitated from camphor water by the addition of soluble salts.

Uses—Locally, weakly *analgesic*, mildly *analgesic* (*antipruritic*) and *rubefacient* when rubbed on the skin. The spirit is applied locally to allay itching caused by insect stings. It also is used as a counterirritant in humans for *inflamed joints, sprains* and *rheumatic* and other *inflammatory* conditions such as colds in the throat and chest. Although the patient may feel improved,the inflammation is not affected. However, reflexly induced local vasoconstriction may mediate a mild nasopharyngeal decongestant effect. When taken internally in small amounts it produces a feeling of warmth and comfort in the gastrointestinal tract, and, therefore, formerly was much used as a *carminative.* Systemically, it is a reflexly active *circulatory* and *respiratory stimulant.* However, its use as a stimulant is obsolete. It also possesses a slight *expectorant* action and is included in some cough-suppressant mixtures. Concentrations above 11% are not safe. Toxicity consists of nausea and vomiting, headache, feeling of warmth, confusion, delirium, convulsions, coma or respiratory arrest. Camphor is a *pharmaceutical necessity* for *Flexible Collodion* and *Camphorated Opium Tincture.*

Dose—*Topical,* to the *skin, rectum* or *throat,* as a **0.1** to **3%** lotion, cream, spray or ointment, or **10%** tincture (spirit), no more than 3 to 4 times a day. For *topical analgesia,* concentrations of **0.1** to **3%** are used; for *counterirritation,* **3** to **11%**.

Cantharidin

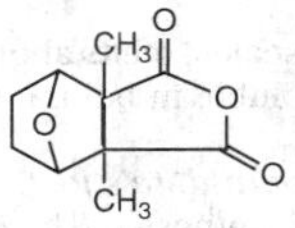

[56-25-7] $C_{10}H_{12}O_4$ (186.21). The active principle of *Cantharides.*

Preparation—*JACS, 102*: 6893, 1980.

Description—White platelets.

Solubility—1 g in 40 mL acetone, 65 mL chloroform, 560 mL ether or 150 mL ethyl acetate; soluble in oils.

Uses—An *irritant* and *vesicant* on skin. As a result of its intradermal vesiculation, it also is employed to remove benign epithelial growths such as warts (particularly the periungal type), molluscum contagiosum and thick hyperkeratotic lesions without leaving a scar. It usually is applied under occlusive bandages. The vesicle eventually breaks, becomes encrusted and falls off in 1 to 2 wk. It is not an aphrodisiac as folklore suggests.

Dose—*Topical,* to the *wart,* as a **0.7%** solution.

Dosage Forms—Solution: 0.7%.

Capsicum

The dried ripe fruit of *Capsicum frutescens* Linné, *Solonaceae,* which contains not less than 0.5% of capsaicin [(*E*)-*N*-[4-Hydroxy-3-methoxyphenyl]-8-methyl-6-nonaneamide [404-86-4] $C_{18}H_{27}NO_3$ (305.40), which is the active ingredient.

Uses—Its active ingredients are mildly irritant, causing erythema and a feeling of warmth without vesication. Its preparations are used as *counterirritants.*

Dose—The equivalent of **0.025** to **0.25%** of capsicum applied to the skin no more than 3 or 4 times a day.

Coal Tar

Pix Carbonis; Prepared Coal Tar BP; Pix Lithanthracis; Gas Tar

The tar obtained as a by-product during the destructive distillation of bituminous coal.

Description—Nearly black, viscous liquid, heavier than water, with a characteristic naphthalene-like odor and a sharp burning taste; on ignition it burns with a reddish, luminous and very sooty flame, leaving not more than 2% of residue.

Solubility—Only slightly soluble in water, to which it imparts its characteristic odor and taste and a faintly alkaline reaction; partially dissolved by alcohol, acetone, methanol, solvent hexane, carbon disulfide, chloroform or ether; to the extent of about 95% by benzene, and entirely by nitrobenzene with the exception of a small amount of suspended matter.

Uses—A *local irritant* used in the treatment of *chronic skin diseases.* Like anthralin, its primary action is to decrease the epidermal synthesis of DNA and, hence, to suppress hyperplasia. Occasionally, it may cause a rash, burning sensation or other manifestations of excessive irritation or sensitization. Since photosensitization may occur, the treated area should be protected from sunlight. It should be kept away from the eyes and from raw, weeping or blistered surfaces. Temporary discoloration of the skin may occur.

Dose—*Topical*, to the *skin*: *cleansing bar*, **2%** once or twice a day; *cream*, **1.6** to **5%** 2 or 3 times a day; *gel*, **5** to **7.5%** once or twice a day; *lotion*, **2** to **5%** 2 to 4 times a day; *ointment*, **1** to **5%** 2 or 3 times a day; *paste*, **5%** once or twice a day; *shampoo*, **0.5** to **10%** twice a wk; *solution*, **2.5** to **20% straight** or **diluted 1:3** with water 1 to 3 times a day; *suspension*, **7.5** to **33.3%** diluted in lukewarm water at intervals directed by the physician.

Dosage Forms—Cleansing Bar: 2%; Cream: 1.6 and 5%; Gel: 5 and 7.5%; Lotion: 2 and 5%; Ointment: 1 and 5%; Paste: 5%; Shampoo: 0.5, 1, 2, 3, 4.3, 5, 9 and 10%; Topical Solution: 2.5, 5 and 20%; Topical Suspension: 7.5, 30 and 33.3%.

Green Soap—see RPS-17, page 786.

Green Soap Tincture—see RPS-17, page 786.

Ichthammol

Ammonium Ichthosulfonate; Sulfonated Bitumen; Ictiol; Ichthymall (*Mallinckrodt*); Ichthyol (*Stiefel*); (*Various Mfrs*)

[8029-68-3]. It yields not less than 2.5% of ammonia and not less than 10% of total sulfur.

Preparation—By the destructive distillation of certain bituminous schists, sulfonating the distillate and neutralizing the product with ammonia.

Description—Black-brown, viscous, liquid with a coal-tar odor.

Solubility—Soluble in water, fats or oils. Partially soluble in ether or alcohol.

Constituents—It belongs to a class of preparations containing, as essential constituents, salts or compounds of a mixture of acids designated by the group name *sulfoichthyolic acid*, formed by sulfonation of the oil obtained in the destructive distillation of certain bituminous shales. Sulfoichthyolic acid is characterized by a high sulfur content, the sulfur existing largely in the form of sulfonates, sulfones and sulfides. *Description* and *Solubility:* Reddish brown to brownish black, viscous fluid, with a strong, characteristic, empyreumatic odor. Miscible with water, glycerin fixed oils or fats; partially soluble in alcohol or ether.

Incompatibilities: Becomes granular in the presence of *acids* or under the influence of *heat*. In solution, it is precipitated by acids and *acid salts* as a dark, sticky mass; *alkalies* liberate ammonia; many *metallic salts* cause precipitation.

Uses—A *mildly astringent irritant* and *local antibacterial agent* with moderate *emollient* and *demulcent* properties. It is used alone or in combination with other antiseptics for the treatment of skin disorders such as *insect stings and bites*, *erysipelas*, *psoriasis* and *lupus erythematosus* and to produce healing in *chronic inflammations*. It also is used to treat *inflammation* and *boils* in the external ear canal. Medical opinion is divided as to whether this agent is useful. In higher concentrations, irritation is frequent and rashes may develop. It should be kept away from the eyes and other sensitive surfaces. It has been reported to cause hyperepithelialization, an action that would be counterproductive in the treatment of psoriasis.

Dose—*Topical*, to the *skin* as a **10** or **20%** ointment or external ear canal as a **10%** ointment.

Juniper Tar

Cade Oil

The empyreumatic volatile oil obtained from the woody portions of *Juniperus oxycedrus* Linné (Fam *Pinaceae*).

Description—Dark-brown, clear, thick liquid; tarry odor; faintly aromatic, bitter taste.

Solubility—Very slightly soluble in water; 1 volume in 9 volumes alcohol or 3 volumes ether, leaving a slight, flocculent residue; miscible with chloroform.

Uses—A mildly irritant oil that is employed as a *topical antipruritic* in several chronic dermatological disorders, such as *psoriasis*, *atopic dermatitis*, *pruritus*, *eczema* and *seborrhea*. Since it is irritant to the conjuctiva and also may cause chemosis of the cornea, care should be taken to keep it out of the eyes. Systemic absorption may result in renal damage.

Dose—*Topical*, as **1** to **5%** ointment applied once a day; it also is used as a **4%** shampoo or **34%** bath.

Menthol

Peppermint Camphor

[1490-04-6] $C_{10}H_{20}O$ (156.27). An alcohol obtained from diverse mint oils or prepared synthetically. It may be levorotatory [(−)-Menthol] from natural or synthetic sources, or racemic [(±)-Menthol)].

Preparation—It owes its odor chiefly to menthol, which is obtained from it by fractional distillation and allowing the proper fraction to crystallize, or by chromatographic processes. Among numerous methods of synthesis of an optically inactive menthol, the most popular involves the catalytic hydrogenation of thymol (obtained from natural sources or synthesized from *m*-cresol or cresylic acid). The difficulty in the synthesis of (−)-menthol arises from the fact that menthol contains three asymmetric carbon atoms, and there are thus eight stereoisomers, designated as (−)- and (+)-menthol, (−)- and (+)-isomenthol, (−)- and (+)-neomenthol, and (−)- and (+)-neoisomenthol. To obtain a product meeting USP requirements, it is necessary to separate (−)-menthol from its stereoisomers, for which purpose fractional crystallization, distillation under reduced pressure or esterification may be used. The other stereoisomers differ from the official (−)-menthol in physical properties and possibly to some extent in pharmacological action.

Description—Colorless, hexagonal, usually needle-like crystals, or fused masses, or a crystalline powder, with a pleasant, peppermint-like odor; (−)-menthol melts between 41° and 44°; (±)-menthol congeals at 27° to 28°.

Solubility—Very soluble in alcohol, chloroform or ether; freely soluble in glacial acetic acid, mineral oil or in fixed and volatile oils; slightly soluble in water.

Identification—When mixed with about an equal weight of camphor, chloral hydrate, phenol or thymol, it forms a "eutectic" mixture liquefying at room temperature.

Incompatibilities—Produces a liquid or soft mass when triturated with *camphor*, *phenol*, *chloral hydrate*, *resorcinol*, *thymol* or numerous other substances. *Labeling:* The label on the container indicates whether it is levorotatory or racemic.

Uses—In low concentrations, it selectively stimulates the sensory nerve endings for cold and, hence, causes a *sensation of coolness*. Some *local analgesic* effects also accompany this effect. Higher concentrations not only stimulate sensory endings for heat and other pain, but also may cause some irritation. Consequently, there may first be a sensation of coolness, then a slight prickly and burning sensation. The *local analgesia* and *sensation of coolness* are employed in the treatment of insect bites and stings, itching (antipruritic effect), minor burns and sunburn, hemorrhoids, toothache, cankers, cold sores and sore throat. The local analgesic effect also is the probable basis of the *antitussive* use, although the value of the drug as an antitussive remains unproved. Care must be taken to avoid the inhalation of irritant concentrations. The contribution of a placebo effect to some of these effects cannot be discounted. It is incorporated into *irritant* products used to treat acne vulgaris, dandruff, seborrhea, calluses, corns, warts and athlete's foot and in vaginal preparations to lessen the sense of irritation. Whatever effects the rubbing of menthol-containing ointment on the chest possess to relieve pulmonary congestion in colds and allergy are attributable to *counterirritation* and placebo effects. It also is contained in counterirritants for the treatment of muscle aches.

Dose—*Topical*, to the *skin*, as **0.1** to **2%** lotion or ointment; to the throat, as a **0.08** to **0.12%** lozenge. *Inhalation*, **15mL** of **1%** liquid or **10 mL** of **2%** ointment per qt of water, to be dispensed by steam inhalation.

Methyl Salicylate—page 1387.

Peruvian Balsam

Peru Balsam; Balsam of Peru; Indian Balsam; Black Balsam

Obtained from *Myroxylon pereirae* (Royle) Klotzsch (Fam *Leguminosae*). Contains from 60 to 64% of a volatile oil termed *cinnamein* and from 20 to 28% of *resin*. Cinnamein is a mixture of compounds, among which the following have been identified: the esters *benzyl benzoate*, *benzyl cinnamate*, *cinnamyl cinnamate* (*styracin*) and the alcohol *peruviol* (considered by some to be identical with the sesquiterpene alcohol *nerolidol*, $C_{15}H_{26}O$) as ester, free *cinnamic acid:* about 0.05% of *vanillin*; and a trace of *coumarin*. The resin consists of benzoic and cinnamic acid.

Description—Dark brown, viscid liquid; transparent and appears reddish brown in thin layers; agreeable odor resembling vanilla; a bitter, acrid taste, with a persistent after-taste and free from stringiness or stickiness. It does not harden on exposure to air; specific gravity 1.150 to 1.170.

Solubility—Nearly insoluble in water; soluble in alcohol, chloroform or glacial acetic acid, with not more than an opalescence; partly soluble in ether or solvent hexane.

Uses—*A local irritant and vulnerary.* It once was used as a dressing to promote growth of epithelial cells in the treatment of *indolent ulcers, wounds* and certain *skin diseases*, eg, scabies. It presently is an ingredient in suppositories used in the treatment of hemorrhoids and anal pruritus. Allergic reactions to it occassionally occur. Ointments containing both this and sulfur present a problem in compounding, since the resinous part of the balsam tends to separate. This difficulty may be overcome by mixing the balsam with an equal amount of castor oil, prior to incorporating it into the base; or, alternatively, by mixing it with solid petroxolin—an ointment vehicle (oxygenated petroleum) consisting of liquid paraffin, oleic acid and ammoniated alcohol.

Dose—*Topical, rectal,* **1.8** to **30 mg** in suppositories.

Pine Tar

Pix Pini; Pix Liquida; Tar

The product obtained by the destructive distillation of the wood of *Pinus palustris* Miller, or of other species of *Pinus* Linné (Fam *Pinaceae*). Usually obtained as a by-product in the manufacture of charcoal or acetic acid from wood. It is a complex mixture of phenolic bodies for the most part insoluble in water. Among these are *cresol, phlorol, guaiacol, pyrocatechol, caerulignol* and *pyrogallol* ethers. Traces of *phenol* and *cresols* also are present as well as hydrocarbons of the paraffin and benzene series.

Description—Very viscid, blackish brown liquid; translucent in thin layers, but becomes granular and opaque with age; has an empyreumatic, terebinthinate odor, a sharp, empyreumatic taste and is more dense than water; solution is acid to litmus.

Solubility—Miscible with alcohol, ether, chloroform, glacial acetic acid or with fixed and volatile oils; slightly soluble in water, the solution being pale yellowish to yellowish brown.

Uses—Externally as a mild *irritant* and *local antibacterial* agent in chronic *skin diseases*, especially eczema and psoriasis. Its volatile constituents are claimed to be *expectorant* but their efficacy is unproven; its inhalations formerly were used for this purpose.

Doses—*Topical,* as a **1.8** to **30%** shampoo.

Resorcinol—see RPS-16, page 1107.
Resorcinol Ointment, Compound—see RPS-16, page 1107.
Resorcinol Monoacetate—see RPS-16, page 1107.
Storax—page 1414.
Tolu Balsam—page 1390.
Turpentine Oil, Rectified—see RPS-16, page 808.

Sclerosing Agents

A number of irritant drugs are of sufficient activity to damage cells but are not so potent as to destroy large numbers of cells at the site of application. Such agents promote fibrosis and are used to strengthen supporting structures, close inguinal rings, etc. The intimal surface of blood vessels may break down under attack by such agents and thus initiate thrombosis, which may be an undesirable side effect. This action is the basis of the use of sclerosing agents in the reduction of varicose veins and hemorrhoids. They can be harmful when used improperly and sometimes even when used with caution.

Morrhuate Sodium Injection

(*Pasadena Res*); Scleromate (*Palisades*)

A sterile solution of the sodium salts of the fatty acids of cod liver oil. It contains 50 mg of sodium morrhuate/mL. A suitable antimicrobial agent, not to exceed 0.5%, and ethyl or benzyl alcohol, not to exceed 3%, may be added.

Note—It may show a separation of solid matter on standing. Do not use the material if such solid does not dissolve completely upon warming.

Preparation—By heating cod liver oil with alcoholic sodium hydroxide until completely saponified. After dilution with water the alcohol is removed by distillation. Dilute H_2SO_4 is then added to the aqueous solution, and the liberated organic acids are separated or preferably extracted with a suitable immiscible solvent such as ether. Just-sufficient aqueous NaOH then is added to neutralize the acids. About 20 mg of benzyl alcohol/mL of the Injection usually is added to lessen the pain of injection.

Uses—Formerly, widely used as a *sclerosing* and *fibrosing agent* for obliterating *varicose veins.* Irritants of this type once were employed for closure of hernial rings, fibrosing of uncomplicated hemorrhoids, removal of condylomata acuminata and in other conditions where the ultimate objective was production of fibrous tissue.

Dose—*Intravenous,* by special injection **0.5** to **5 mL** of a **5%** injection to a localized area; *usual,* **1 mL.**

Dosage Forms—5, 10 and 30 mL.

Sodium Tetradecyl Sulfate

STS; Sotradecol (*Elkins-Sinn*)

$$CH_3(CH_2)_3CH(C_2H_5)(CH_2)_2CH(CH_2CH(CH_3)_2)OSO_2ONa$$

[139-88-8] $C_{14}H_{29}NaO_4S$ (316.43).

Preparation—One method reacts the corresponding alcohol with $ClSO_3H$ and neutralizes the resulting hydrogen sulfate ester with Na_2CO_3.

Description—White, waxy, odorless solid.

Solubility—Soluble in water, alcohol or ether.

Uses—A *sclerosing agent* similar in action to sodium morrhuate. It formerly was used widely as a buffered solution in the *obliteration of varicose veins and internal hemorrhoids.* For such purposes, the solution is injected directly into the vein. Injection outside of the vein may cause sloughing. For this reason, the substance is not used to close inguinal rings. The principal untoward effect is pain immediately upon injection, although brief; mild anaphylactoid and idiosyncratic responses rarely occur. Because the substance is an anionic surface-active agent, it also is used as a *wetting agent* to promote spreading of certain topical antiseptics.

Dose—By injection directly into the target vein, as a **1** or **3%** solution, depending on the size of the vein. The volume then to be injected as any one site varies from **0.2** to **2.0 mL,** depending on the concentration and the number of previous injections at the site, the larger volumes being given only after several previous injections. No more than 10 mL of the 3% solution or 6 mL of the 5% solution should be given at any one time. The interval between injections varies from 5 to 7 days.

Dosage Forms—Injection: 1 and 3% in 2-mL ampuls.

Caustics and Escharotics

Any topical agent that causes destruction of tissues at the site of application is a *caustic* (or corrosive).

Caustics may be used to induce desquamation of cornified epithelium ("keratolytic" action) and, therefore, are used to destroy warts, condylomata, keratoses, certain moles and hyperplastic tissues.

If the agent also precipitates the proteins of the cell and the inflammation exudate, there is formed a scab (or eschar), which later is organized into a scar; such an agent is an *escharotic* (or cauterizant). Most, but not all, caustics are also escharotic. Furthermore, certain caustics, especially the alkalies, redissolve precipitated proteins, partly by hydrolysis, so that no scab or only a soft scab forms; such agents penetrate deeply and generally are unsuitable for therapeutic use. Escharotics sometimes are employed to seal cutaneous and aphthous ulcers, wounds, etc. Since most escharotics are bactericidal, it formerly was thought that chemical cauterization effected sterilization; however, sterilization is not achieved always, especially by those agents which remain bound to the protein precipitate. The growth of certain bacteria even may be favored by the chemically induced necrosis and by the protection of the scab.

Acetic Acid, Glacial—page 1406.
Alum—page 871.
Aluminum Chloride—page 872.

Dichloroacetic Acid

Bichloracetic Acid (*Glenwood*)

$Cl_2CHCOOH$

[79-43-6] $C_2H_2Cl_2O_2$ (128.95).

Preparation—From chloral; *Chem and Ind:*718, 1960.

Description—Pungent liquid; boils about 194°.

Solubility—Miscible with water, alcohol or ether.

Uses—A *cauterizing agent.* It rapidly penetrates and cauterizes skin, keratins, etc. Its cauterizing ability compares with that of electrocautery or freezing. It is used on calluses, hard and soft corns, xanthoma palpebrarum, seborrheic keratoses, ingrown nails, cysts and benign erosion of the cervix. See also *Trichloroacetic Acid.*

Dose—The amount which is applied varies with the nature of the lesion being treated. Denser horny lesions require more than those of lower density. The number of treatments also varies with the lesion.

Dosage Forms—Liquid: 10 mL.

Nitric Acid, Concentrated

An aqueous solution containing 67–71% HNO_3.

Preparation—By oxidation of ammonia.

Description—Fuming liquid; very caustic; characteristic, highly irritating odor; boils at 120°; specific gravity about 1.41.

Solubility—Miscible with water.

Uses—A *cauterizing agent* for the immediate sterilization of dangerously infected wounds, such as the bite from a rabid animal; it does not penetrate too deeply and forms a firm eschar.

Phenol—page 1412.

Podofilox

Furo[3′,4′:6,7]naphtho[2,3-*d*]-1,3,-dixol-6(5a*H*)-one, [5*R*-(5α,5aβ,8aα,9α)]-5,8,8a,9-tetrahydro-9-hydroxy-5-(3,4,5,-trimethoxyphenyl)-,

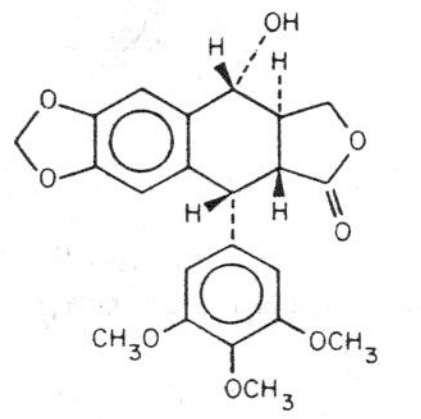

Podophyllotoxin [518-28-5] $C_{22}H_{22}O_8$ (414.41).

Found in the rhizomes of several species of plants, principally *Podophyllum peltatum* L *Berberidaceae, P emodi* and *Juniperus virginiana* L *Coniferae.*

Preparation—See *JACS 103: 6208, 1981.*

Description—Hydrated crystals; melts about 115° (dec) and about 184° after drying; a number of polymorphic forms exist.

Solubility—Very slightly soluble in water; soluble in alcohol, chloroform or acetone.

Uses—Actions, uses and adverse effects are those of *Podophyllum Resin* (below), except that the therapeutic index is greater. It is several times more potent. It is an investigational drug.

Dose—*Topical,* to the *skin, adults and children,* as a **0.5** to **1%** solution twice a day for 3 days.

Podophyllum

Mandrake; May Apple

The dried rhizome and roots of *Podophyllum peltatum* Linné (Fam *Berberidaceae*); it yields not less than 5% of podophyllum resin.

Constituents—From 3 to 6% of resin along with up to 1% of quercetin and podophyllotoxin and peltatin glucosides. At least 16 different compounds have been isolated and characterized. The aglycone *podophyllotoxin* [$C_{22}H_{22}O_8$] is the lactone of 1-hydroxy-2-(hydroxymethyl)-6,7 -methylenedioxy-4-(3′,4′,5′-trimethoxyphenyl)-1,2,3,4-tetrahydronaphthalene-3-carboxylic acid. Hydrolytic rupture of the lactone ring yields *podophyllic acid* [$C_{22}H_{24}O_9$], the 2,3-*trans* form of which is *podophyllinic acid* while the 2,3-*cis* form is *picropodophyllinic acid.*

Although podophyllotoxin has been demonstrated to possess marked caustic, cathartic and toxic properties, it is believed that not it, but an amorphous *resin,* called *podophylloresin,* is the chief cathartic principle of the drug. However, podophyllotoxin is safer and ultimately probably will replace the crude preparations.

Uses and Dose—See *Podophyllum Resin.*

Podophyllum Resin

Uses—Supersedes *Podophyllum.* Certain glycosides and polynuclear lactones in the resin interact with tubulin and, thus, interfere with cell cycling and intracellular dynamics such as to cause the eventual death of affected cells. Applied topically, it is corrosive in the region of contact. It mainly is used in the treatment of *condyloma accuminatum* but also of *juvenile papilloma of the larynx, multiple superficial epitheliomatoses* (basal cell and squamous cell carcinomas), *precancerous keratoses* (seborrheic, actinic and radiation keratoses), *verrucae fibroids* and *calluses.* Some pain usually occurs at the site of application; if it is excessive, the drug should be removed with ethyl or isopropyl alcohol. Resin on adjacent normal tissues also should be removed. Pain may be avoided somewhat by treating only a small area of surface at any one time. *It especially is irritating to the eyes and mucous membranes.* Treatment of large surfaces also may result in excessive absorption and systemic effects, such as nausea and vomiting, tachycardia, shallow respiration, leukopenia, thrombocytopenia, renal damage, paralytic ileus, lethargy, stupor, psychotic confusional states and peripheral neuropathy, including flaccid paralysis. Systemic absorption is enhanced by occlusion. The drug is contraindicated in pregnancy and lactation.

Dose—*Topical, adults* and *children,* to the skin, *condyloma accuminata,* as a **25%** solution, the resin to remain in place for 6 hr; application may be repeated weekly for up to 4 wk, if necessary; *superficial epitheliomatoses* and *precancerous keratoses,* as a **25%** solution once a day, to be continued until several days after a slough has occurred; *to laryngeal lesions, juvenile laryngeal papilloma,* as a **12.5%** solution to the papilloma, initially once a day, but progressively longer intervals may be elected as the lesions shrink (medical authorities hold that short intervals are more effective); the 12.5% solution is to be extemporized by diluting the 25% solution in 95% alcohol.

Dosage Form—Topical Solution: 25%.

Potassium Hydroxide

Caustic Potash; Lye; Potash Lye

[1310-58-3] KOH (56.11); it contains not less than 85.0% of K_2CO_3 (138.21).

Caution—Exercise great care in handling, as it rapidly destroys tissues. Do not handle it with bare hands.

Preparation—By electrolysis of a solution of potassium chloride in a diaphragm cell that does not allow liberated chlorine to react with it. It is prepared in the form of sticks, pellets, flakes or fused masses. Sticks or pellets are made by evaporating a solution of it to a fluid of oily consistency and then pouring the hot liquid into suitable molds in which it solidifies.

Description—White, or nearly white, fused masses, small pellets, flakes, sticks and other forms; hard and brittle and shows a crystalline fracture; exposed to air it rapidly absorbs carbon dioxide and moisture, and deliquesces; melts at about 360 to 380°; when dissolved in water or alcohol, or when its solution is treated with an acid, much heat is generated; solutions, even when highly diluted, are strongly alkaline.

Solubility—1 g in mL water, 3 mL alcohol or 2.5 mL glycerin at 25°; very soluble in boiling alcohol.

Incompatibilities—Bases react with *acids* to form salts, liberate alkaloids from aqueous solutions of *alkaloidal salts,* and promote various hydrolysis reactions such as the decomposition of *chloral hydrate* into chloroform and a formate or the breakdown of *salol* into phenol and a salicylate. Only the alkali hydroxides are appreciably soluble in water. Nearly all common *metals* will be precipitated as hydroxides when solutions of their salts are added to solutions of the alkali hydroxides. Certain hydroxides, however, notably those of aluminum,zinc, arsenic or lead, will dissolve in excess of sodium or potassium hydroxide.

Uses—A *caustic,* principally in veterinary practice. The end of a stick of potassium hydroxide may be inserted into a section of rubber tubing, or wrapped several times with tin foil, to avoid cauterizing the fingers of the operator. It is used also as a *pharmaceutical necessity* in several pharmacopeial preparations.

Salicylic Acid—page 879.

Silver Nitrate

Nitric acid, silver(1+) salt; Argenti Nitras

Silver(1+) nitrate [7761-88-8] $AgNO_3$ (169.87).

Preparation—By the action of nitric acid on metallic silver.

Description—Colorless or white crystals; on exposure to light in the presence of organic matter, it becomes gray or grayish black; pH of solutions about 5.5.

Solubility—1 g in 0.4 mL water, 30 mL alcohol, about 250 mL acetone, slightly more than 0.1 mL boiling water or about 6.5 mL of boiling alcohol; slightly soluble in ether.

Incompatibilities—Easily reduced to metallic silver by most *reducing agents*, including *ferrous salts, arsenites, hypophosphites, tartrates, sugars, tannins, volatile oils* and other *organic substances*. In neutral or alkaline solutions, precipitated by *chlorides, bromides, iodides, borax, hydroxides, carbonates, phosphates, sulfates, arsenites* and *arsenates*. *Potassium permanganate, tannic acid* and *soluble citrates and sulfates* may cause a precipitate if sufficiently concentrated. In acid solution, only the *chloride, bromide* and *iodide* are insoluble. *Ammonia water* dissolves many of the insoluble silver salts through formation of the silver diammine complex, $Ag(NH_3)_2{}^+$.

Uses—Silver ions combine with proteins and cause denaturation and precipitation. As a result, silver ions have *astringent, caustic, bactericidal* and *antiviral* properties. In low concentrations, silver denatured protein is confined to the interstitial spaces and the surface of denuded, weeping areas, so that only astringent and antimicrobial effects occur; with higher concentrations, cell membranes are disrupted, so that caustic effects result. The corroded site will become covered with a scab of silver protein precipitate.

It is used mainly in podiatry as a caustic to *destroy excessive granulation tissue*, such as *corns, calluses, granuloma pyogenicum* and *plantar warts, reduce neurovascular helomas, remove papillomas* and *cauterize small nerve endings* and *blood vessels*. As an astringent, it is used to treat *impetigo vulgaris* and *pruritis* as well as *indolent ulcers, wounds* and *fissures*. It also is used as a *styptic*, especially in dentistry.

As an antiseptic, it mainly is employed prophylactically against *ophthalmia neonatorum*. It formerly was applied regularly to burned surfaces because of its high efficacy against both staphylococci and pseudomonas. However, the precipitation of AgCl at the site of application and in dressing depletes plasma choride and can cause serious electrolyte disturbances; consequently, the drug seldom is used in burn therapy today. Refer to RPS-17, page 1165, for a discussion of its prior uses as an antiseptic.

Excessive corrosion at the target site and corrosion from inadvertent application or leakage away from the intended site can occur. Dental cones or pieces of toughened silver nitrate that are accidentally ingested can cause death. Elemental silver from the bioreduction of silver ion may reside permanently at the site of application and cause a bluish-to-black discoloration called argyria. Locally injected sodium thiosulfate sometimes can remove the silver. Nitrate ion absorbed from large, denuded surfaces can cause methemoglobinemia. Only concentrations 0.5% or below should be applied to raw wounds, fresh cuts or broken skin.

Dose—*Topical, antiseptic*, to the *conjunctiva*, **0.1 mL** of a **1%** solution; to the *burned skin* or *open lesion* (neither advised), **0.1** to **0.5%** solution as a wet dressing. *Astringent*, to the *affected skin*, as a **10%** solution for *impetigo vulgaris* and as a **10** or **25%** solution for *pruritis*. *Caustic*, to the *lesion* only, as a **10%** solution or ointment for *helomas* and to *cauterize small nerve endings* and *blood vessels*, as a **25** or **50%** solution for *plantar warts* and as a **50%** solution for *granulation tissue, granuloma pyogenica* and *papillomatous growths*.

Dosage Forms—Ointment: 10%; Topical Solution: 10, 25 and 50%. For *Toughened Silver Nitrate*, see RPS-17, page 784.

Trichloroacetic Acid

Tri-Chlor (*Gordon*)

[76-03-9] $C_2HCl_3O_2$ (163.39).

Preparation—Usually by oxidizing chloral hydrate with fuming nitric acid.

Description—Colorless, deliquescent crystals having a slight, characteristic odor; melts at about 58° and boils at 196 to 197°.

Solubility—1 g in about 0.1 mL water; soluble in alcohol or ether.

Uses—Precipitates proteins and used as a *caustic* on the skin or mucous membranes to destroy local lesions and for treatment of various dermatological disease. Its chief use is to destroy ordinary warts and juvenile flat warts. It is employed extensively as a *precipitant of protein* in the chemical analysis of body fluids and tissue extracts, as well as a *decalcifier* and *fixative* in microscopy.

Caution—Trichloroacetic Acid is highly corrosive to the skin.

Dose—*Topical*, to the skin, as a **15** to **100%** *w/v* solution, carefully applied with a cotton-tipped applicator or glass rod. Concentrations above 50% are not recommended.

Dosage For—Liquid: 10%.

Keratolytics (Desquamating Agents)

The epidermis consists of layers of flat cells, called *stratified squamous epithelial cells*. They are bound together by desmosomes and penetrating tonofibrils, both of which largely consist of keratin. The outer layer of the epidermis (cornified epithelium or stratum corneum) is composed of the collapsed ghosts of the squamous cells (keratinocytes or corneocytes) that are primarily tight networks of keratin and lipoprotein within a matrix of lipid multilayers. Unlike most cellular membranes, the lipids include fatty acids, neutral lipids, ceramides, etc, and are predominantly in the gel (solid-like) state. Certain fungi, especially the dermatophytes, use keratin and, therefore, reside in the stratum corneum in those places where the degree of hydration and the pH are sufficiently high. One way such mycoses may be suppressed is that of removal of the stratum corneum, a process that is called *desquamation*. Certain chemical substances, especially among phenols and sulfhydryl compounds, loosen the kera tin and, thus, facilitate desquamation. These substances are called *keratolytics*. Aqueous maceration of the stratum corneum also favors desquamation. In addition to the treatment of epidermophytosis, keratolytics are used to thin hyperkeratotic areas. Most keratolytics are irritant. Irritants also can cause desquamation by causing damage to and swelling of the basal cells.

Benzoyl Peroxide

(*Various Mfrs*)

O=C—O—O—C=O

[94-36-0] $C_{14}H_{10}O_4$ (242.23); contains 65–82% of benzoyl peroxide; also contains about 26% of water for the purpose of reducing flammability and shock sensitivity.

Preparation—Benzoyl chloride is reacted with a cold solution of sodium peroxide.

Description—White, granular powder, having a characteristic odor; melts about 104°; *may explode with heat*.

Solubility—Sparingly soluble in water or alcohol; soluble in acetone, chloroform or ether.

Caution (For the drug entity—not the dosage forms)—It may explode at temperatures higher than 60° or cause fires in the presence of reducing substances. Store it in the original container, treated to reduce static charges. Do not transfer it to metal or glass containers fitted with friction tops. Do not return unused material to its original container, but destroy it by treatment with NaOH solution (1 in 10) until addition of a crystal of KI results in no release of free iodine.

Uses—Possesses *mild antibacterial* properties, especially against anaerobic bacteria. It is also mildly irritant, and it exerts moderate keratolytic and antiseborrheic actions. Its principal use is in the treatment of mild *acne vulgaris* (in which it is comedolytic) and *acne rosaceae*, but it also is used in the treatment of decubital and stasis ulcers.

It causes stinging or burning sensations for a brief time after application; with continued use these effects mostly disappear. After 1 or 2 wk of use there may be a sudden excess dryness of the skin and peeling. The drug must be kept away from the eyes, and from inflamed, denuded or highly sensitive skin, such as the circumoral areas, neck and skin of children. It should not be used in conjunction with harsh abrasive skin cleansers. It can cause contact dermatitis. It can bleach hair and fabrics.

Dose—*Topical*, to the *skin, adults* and *children 12 yr or older*, as a **5** or **10%** cleansing bar 2 or 3 times a day, **5** to **10%** cream or gel 1 or 2 times a day, **5** to **20%** lotion 1 to 4 times a day, **5** or **10%** cleansing lotion 1 or 2 times a day, **5%** facial mask once a day, **10%** soap 1 or 2 times a day or **10%** stick 1 to 3 times a day. The 20% lotion is used only for the treatment of decubital and stasis ulcers.

Dosage Forms—Cleansing Bar: 5 and 10%; Cream: 5, 7 and 10%; Gel: 2.5, 5 and 10%; Lotion: 5, 5.5, 10 and 20%; Cleansing Lotion: 5 and 10%; Facial Mask: 5%; Stick: 10%.

Fluorouracil—page 1251.

Resorcinol—see RPS-16, page 1107.

Resorcinol Ointment, Compound—see RPS-16, page 1107.

Salicylic Acid

Benzoic acid, 2-hydroxy-, *o*-Hydroxybenzoic Acid

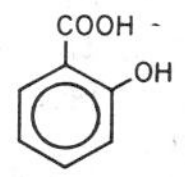

Salicylic acid [69-72-7] $C_7H_6O_3$ (138.12).

Preparation—Mostly by the Kolbe-Schmidt process in which CO_2 is reacted with sodium phenolate under pressure at about 130° to form sodium salicylate, followed by treatment with mineral acid.

Description—White, fine, needle-like crystals or as a fluffy, white, crystalline powder; the synthetic acid is white and odorless; sweetish, afterward acrid, taste; stable in the air; melts between 158° and 161°.

Solubility—1 g in 460 mL water, 3 mL alcohol, 45 mL chloroform, 3 mL ether, 135 mL benzene or about 15 mL boiling water.

Uses—Used *externally* on the skin, where it exerts a slight *antiseptic* action and considerable *keratolytic* action. The latter property makes it a beneficial agent in the local treatment of certain forms of *eczematoid dermatitis*. It also is included in products for the treatment of *psoriasis*, for which the FDA classification is Category I. Tissue cells swell, soften and ultimately desquamate. Salicylic Acid Plaster often is used for this purpose. The drug is especially useful in the treatment of *tinea pedis* (athlete's foot) and *tinea capitis* (ringworm of the scalp), since the fungus grows and thrives in the stratum corneum. Keratolysis both removes the infected horny layer and aids in penetration by antifungal drugs. It is combined with benzoic acid in an ointment long known as *Whitfield's Ointment* (see RPS-18, page 1235). It also is combined commonly with zinc oxide, sulfur or sulfur and coal tar. It is incorporated into mixtures for the treatment of acne, dandruff and seborrhea, insect bites and stings and into soaps and vaginal douches, but efficacy remains to be established. In high concentrations it is *caustic* and may be used to remove *corns, calluses, warts* and other growths.

Collodions or solutions of 17% or higher and other forms above 25% concentration should not be employed if the patient has diabetes mellitus, peripheral vascular disease or inflammation or infection at the intended site of application. Continuous application of the drug to the skin can cause dermatitis. Systemic toxicity resulting from application to large areas of the skin has been reported. It is not employed internally as an analgesic because of its local irritating effect on the gastrointestinal tract.

Dose—*Topical*, to the *skin, keratolytic*, as a **16.7** or **17%** collodion once a day, **2.5** to **10%** cream under occlusion once every 3 to 5 days, **2%** foam once or twice a day, **5** or **6%** gel under occlusion once a day, **1.8%** lotion once or twice a day, **3** to **10%** ointment once a day, **2** or **4%** shampoo once or twice a wk, **3.5%** soap once a day or **17%** solution once a day; *antipsoriatic*, as a **5** or **6%** gel under occlusion or **3** to **10%** ointment once a day; *antiseborrheic*, as a **1.8%** lotion, **3** to **10%** ointment or **2** or **4%** shampoo once a day; *antiacne*, as a **2%** foam once or twice a day, **5** or **6%** gel under occlusion once a day, **3** to **6%** ointment once a day or **3.5%** soap once a day; *caustic*, as a **25%** cream once every 3 to 5 days, **25** to **60%** ointment under occlusion every 3 to 5 days, or **40%** plaster once a day.

Dosage Forms—Flexible Collodion: 16.7 and 17%; Cream: 2.5, 10 and 25%; Gel: 5 and 6%; Lotion: 1.8%; Ointment: 25, 40 and 60% (3 to 10% ointments must be extemporized); Plaster: 40%; Shampoo: 2 and 4%; Soap: 3.5%; Topical Solution: 17%.

Sulfur, Precipitated—page 1355.

Tretinoin

Retinoic acid; Retin-A (*Ortho*)

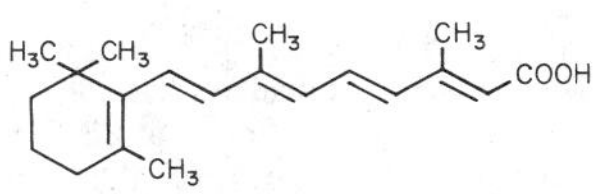

all *trans*-Retinoic acid [302-79-4] $C_{20}H_{28}O_2$ (300.44).

Preparation—By oxidation of vitamin A aldehyde which may be obtained by oxidation of vitamin A. *Biochem J 90:* 569, 1964.

Description—Yellow to light-orange crystals or crystalline powder with the odor of ensilage; should be stored in cold and protected from light and air; melts between 176 and 181°.

Solubility—Insoluble in water; slightly soluble in alcohol; slightly soluble in chloroform; 1 g in 10 mL boiling benzene.

Uses—It is retinoic acid, or so-called *vitamin A acid*, which is formed when the aldehyde group of retinene (retinal) is oxidized to a carboxyl group. It is not known whether retinoic acid has a physiological function, but some authorities consider it to be the form of vitamin A that acts in the skin. This view is supported by the fact that retinol and retinal have very little action on the skin but large systemic doses of vitamin A evoke prominent dermatologic changes.

Topically, it causes inflammation, thickening of the epidermis (acanthosis) and local intercellular edema, which leads to some separation of the epidermal cells. Follicular epithelial cells become less adhesive, the stratum corneum loosens and exfoliation may occur. High concentrations can cause vesiculation. These actions are used in the treatment of *acne vulgaris*. The loosened horny layer makes it easier for the comedo to rise up and discharge, and the inflammatory response mobilizes white cells which attack the bacteria in the follicle. In the early stages of treatment, the sudden surfacing of obscured preexisting comedones makes it appear that the acne has been exacerbated, but the new comedones do not coalesce into cysts or nodules and scarring does not occur. The exaggerated stage may last for as long as 6 wk, after which improvement comes rapidly. Shortly after discontinuation of treatment, relapses readily occur. Deep cystic nodular acne (acne conglobata) or severe cases usually are not improved by the drug.

Various hyperkeratotic conditions are reported to respond to it, responses being sometimes exceptionally dramatic. *Solar* and *follicular keratosis, lamellar ichthyosis, keratosis palmaris* and *plantaris* and other hyperplastic dermatoses have been treated successfully with the drug. It also has been used in the treatment of some skin cancers. Recent reports indicate that it may somewhat rejuvenate sun-aged skin.

It is an antioxidant and free-radical scavenger. There is some evidence not only that topical applications may provide some protection from actinic and other radiation effects on the skin, including cancer, but that internally it may be protective against carcinogenesis from radiation and carcinogens. Systemically, it does not cause the toxic effects of large doses of vitamin A.

In concentrations of 0.05 to 0.1%, it causes a transient feeling of warmth or mild stinging, and erythema follows. Peeling of the skin may occur. Irritation and peeling are marked more when the concentration exceeds 0.1%. When peeling, crusting or blistering occurs, medication should be withheld until the skin recovers, or the concentration should be reduced. The drug should not be applied around the eyes, nose or angles of the mouth, because the mucosae are much more sensitive than the skin to the irritant effects. It also may cause severe irritation on eczematous skin. It should not be applied along with, or closely following, other irritants or keratolytic drugs. Exposure to sunlight should be avoided if possible. Both hypo- and hyperpigmentation have been reported, but the conditions appear to be reversible and temporary.

Dose—*Topical, usual*, to the *skin*, **0.01** to **0.1%** once a day at bedtime.

Dosage Forms—Cream: 0.05 and 0.1%; Gel: 0.01 and 0.025%; Topical Solution: 0.05%.

Trichloroacetic Acid—page 878.

Cleansing Preparations

The skin may be cleansed with detergents, solvents or abrasives, singly or in combination. Among the detergents, the soaps have enjoyed the greatest official status, more through custom than through special merit. The nonsoap detergents became important, not only as household hand cleansers, but also in dermatological and surgical practice as well. However, because many nonsoap detergents do not decompose in sewage disposal plants, there has been a return to real soap. Some of the antiseptic "soaps" still contain synthetic detergents. Soap interferes with the action of many antiseptics, which is one reason synthetic detergents often are used in antiseptic cleansing preparations. However, synthetic detergents also interact with some antiseptics. Anionic nonsoap skin detergents rarely sensitize the skin and, thus, are prescribed when the user is allergic to soap.

Ordinary soaps tend to be alkaline, with pH ranging from 9.5 to 10.5. Superfatted soaps have a pH in the lower end of the range. Synthetic detergents usually have a pH of ≤ 5.6. Neutral toilet bars contain synthetic detergents. Anionic surfactants and cationic detergents emulsify fats with water as well as assisting in the removal of foreign particulates from the skin, scalp or hair.

Shampoos are liquid soaps or detergents used to clean the hair and scalp. Both soaps and shampoos often are used as vehicles for dermatological agents.

Many bar soaps contain either triclosan or triclocarban as antiseptics in concentrations which suppress bacterial production of body odors but which effectively are not antiseptic. A number of soaps and shampoos contain keratolytic and anti-acne ingredients. Abrasive soaps contain particles of alumina, polyethylene or sodium tetraborate decahydrate.

It commonly, but erroneously, is believed that soap has an antiseptic action. The promotion of either soap or synthetic detergents alone for the control of acne is unwarranted; antiseptic substances must be added to the cleansing material or be used separately. Quantitative studies of the cutaneous flora before and after cleansing with soap or with other anionic detergents show a negligible antiseptic effect. However, the removal of loose epidermis lessens the likelihood that cutaneous bacteria will be transferred from the skin to other structures. Certain cationic detergents employed in dermatology are antiseptic. Detergents are treated under *Surface-Active Agents* (page 239).

The choice of organic solvents to cleanse the skin depends largely upon the nature of the material to be removed. In medical practice ethanol and isopropyl alcohol are the most frequently employed organic solvents. Cleansing creams act both as solvents and as detergents. Other soapless cleansers variously contain petrolatum, vegatable oils, lanolin, high-molecular-weight alcohols, various carbohydrate derivatives, oatmeal and other ingredients.

Alcohol—page 1404.
Alcohol, Rubbing—page 1264.
Benzalkonium Chloride—page 1264.
Green Soap—see RPS-17, page 786.
Hexachlorophene Cleansing Emulsion—page 1266.
Isopropyl Rubbing Alcohol—page 1267.
Selenium Sulfide—page 1270.
Sodium Lauryl Sulfate—page 1398.

Transdermal Systems

Transdermal systems are designed to employ the skin as either a rate-controlling barrier to drug absorption or a reservoir for drug absorption. The primary compounds delivered via transdermal systems include estradiol, page 1089; nitroglycerine, page 1041; nicotine, page 1354; clonidine, page 943; fentanyl, page 1204 and scopolamine, page 905.

These drugs are discussed elsewhere since their pharmacological activity is not primarily skin-related. However, transdermal systems have been developed to deliver salicylic acid for localized therapy in the skin to remove warts (salicylic acid, page 879).

The underlying principals of percutaneous absorption is discussed in further detail in Chapter 91, while the systems are discussed in Chapter 95. However, transdermal systems may give to localized effects within skin due to increased hydration as a result of occlusion, drug metabolism or degradation within the skin, penetration enhancer-associated skin alterations, increased localized bacterial populations, etc.

Miscellaneous Dermatologics

Gargles, nasal washes, douches, enemata, etc generally contain as basic ingredients substances described under other categories in this chapter. These preparations are described under *Aqueous Solutions*, page 1497.

Antiphlogistics include alcohol and several creams and lotions that cool the skin by evaporation. Many antiphlogistic preparations also contain an astringent and a local anesthetic or camphor or menthol.

Commonly employed *antipruritics* also depend to some extent upon local anesthetics and the soothing effect of cooling, although some emollients or demulcents may be included, especially depending upon the etiology of the pruritus. The antipruritic properties of phenol preparations largely derive from superficial local anesthesia.

Vulnerary and *epithelizing* properties are attributed to numerous irritants and to several dyes; however, few reliable data exist to support most claims to vulnerary action.

Sunscreens contain aromatic compounds, like aminobenzoic acid, which efficiently absorb the harmful UV rays from the incident sunlight and transmit mainly the less harmful wavelengths, or titanium dioxide, which reflects sunlight from the surface of application. UV light in the spectral range of 290 to 320 nm causes suntan and sunburn; therefore, a sunscreen to prevent tan or burn should have a high molar absorptivity in this range. However, *photosensitization* (ie, the photoactivation of chemicals to make them toxic or allergenic) may occur with wavelengths as high as 500 nm; consequently, to protect recipients of certain drugs (tetracyclines, sulfonamides, erythromycin, promazine, chlorpromazine, promethazine, psoralens), sunscreens with a broader absorption spectrum are required. An adequate broad spectrum is usually achieved with combinations of sunscreens (eg, dioxybenzone and oxybenzone).

Melanizers are substances that promote the pigmentation of the skin. Most melanizers produce their effect by sensitizing the skin to UV light, so that the effect is principally the same as if the subject had been exposed for a long time to the sun.

This action is termed a *photodynamic action*. The term has been used loosely to include all instances of enhanced sensitivity to light, but in strict definition it is confined to photosensitization in which the participation of oxygen is required. In the photodynamic process, light of wavelengths too long to be ordinarily effective may be used, so that the activating spectrum may be shifted toward longer wavelengths.

Skin bleaches, or *demelanizers*, mostly contain hydroquinone derivatives.

Hair bleaches generally contain peroxides.

There is a large variety of *depilatories* on the market. Many of them are sulfhydryl compounds, especially thioglycollates, which reduce the disulfide bonds of keratin, thus softening the hair to the point where it can be separated easily from the epidermis. Some of the same compounds are used in lower concentrations in hairwaving preparations. There is one drug, minoxidil, an antihypertensive drug, which can *increase hair growth* and *treat baldness*.

Antiperspirants have been included among the astringents.

Allantoin

[97-59-6] $C_4H_6N_4O_3$ (158.12).

Preparation—By oxidation of uric acid.

Description—Colorless crystals; melts at 238°.

Solubility—1 g in 190 mL water or 500 mL alcohol; nearly insoluble in ether.

Uses—In World War I it was noticed that maggot-infested wounds seemed to heal better than uninfested wounds, an effect attributed to this drug produced by maggots. It is used topically as a *vulnerary* to stimulate tissue repair in suppurating wounds, resistant ulcers, acne, seborrhea, cold sores, hemorrhoids and various dermatologic infections and psoriasis. It frequently is combined with astringents, keratolytics, coal tar, antiseptics and antifungal drugs. The silver salt has been used in the topical treatment of extensive burns.

Dose—*Topical*, **0.2** to **2%** in creams, lotions or shampoos and **0.3** to **0.5%** in ointments for hemorrhoids.

Aminobenzoic Acid

Benzoic acid, 4-amino-, PABA

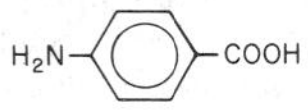

p-Aminobenzoic acid [150-13-0] $C_7H_7NO_2$ (137.14).

Preparation—*p*-Nitrotoluene is oxidized with permanganate to *p*-nitrobenzoic acid, and the nitro group is then reduced to amino with iron and hydrochloric acid.

Description—White or slightly yellow, odorless crystals or crystalline
8 powder; melts between 186° and 189°; discolors on exposure to air or light.

Solubility—Slightly soluble in water or chloroform; freely soluble in alcohol or solutions of alkali hydroxides and carbonates; sparingly soluble in ether.

Uses—A *sunscreen.* It absorbs UV light of wavelengths in the region of 260 to 313 nm; its molar absorptivity at 288.5 nm is 18,300. However, it does not absorb throughout the near UV range, so that drug-related photosensitivity and phototoxicity may not be prevented by it, but in combination with benzophenone it does protect against some drug-induced phototoxicities. Nevertheless, in the 260 to 313 nm range, it has the highest protection index of current sunscreen agents.

For animal species that do not use preformed folic acid, which contains the *p*-aminobenzoyl moiety, it is a B-vitamin. However, man does not use it, and its promotion in vitamin preparations preys on the ignorance of the consumer. It or its potassium salt is promoted as an agent that softens or regresses fibrotic tissue in Peyronie's disease, scleroderma, dermatomyositis, morphea and pemphigus. The claims for the antifibrotic actions are substantiated poorly, and the actions and uses are not mentioned in major works on pharmacology and therapeutics.

Topically, it is rarely allergenic to recipients, but phototoxicity and photoallergenicity occur. Systemic side effects include nausea, anorexia, fever and rash.

Dose—*Topical,* as a *sunscreen,* **4** to **15%** in solutions, lotions, creams and lipsticks. *Oral, adults,* **12 g** a day in 4 to 6 divided doses; *children,* **1 g/10 lb** a day in divided doses, to be diluted and taken with food.

Dosage Forms—Capsules: 500 mg; Cream: 4% (may also contain sodium PABA); Gel: 5%; Lotion: 5%; Powder: 2, 100 and 453 g; Solution: 5%; Stick: 5% (may contain red petrolatum); Tablets: 30, 100 and 500 mg.

Cetyl Alcohol—page 1401.

Cinoxate

Propenoic acid, 3-(4-methoxyphenyl)-, 2-ethoxyethyl ester

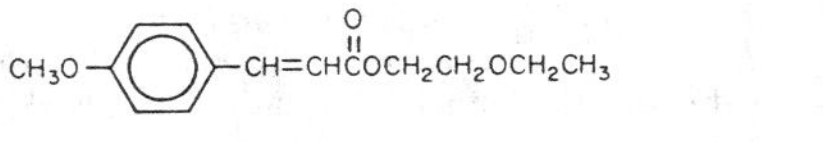

[104-28-9] $C_{14}H_{18}O_4$ (250.29).

Preparation—Brit Pat 856,411.

Description—A viscous liquid; may have a slightly yellow tinge; boils about 185°.

Solubility—Practically insoluble in water; miscible with alcohol.

Uses—A *sunscreen* that absorbs UV light at 270 to 328 nm and has a relatively high molar absorptivity (19,400 at 306 nm) but not absorbing well throughout the entire offending range of UV light. Consequently, it is used principally in preparations intended to promote tanning rather than to protect against photosensitivity and phototoxicity.

Dose—*Topical,* **1.75** to **4%** in creams, gels or lotions.

Dextranomer

Dextran Polymer; Debrisan (*J&J*)

[56087-11-7]

Preparation—By cross-linking chains of the polymer dextran to produce a three-dimensional network.

Description—Small, dry beads highly hygroscopic.

Solubility—1 g absorbs about 4 g water.

Uses—For *drying, cleansing* and *debridement* of exudative *venous stasis ulcers; infected wounds* and *burns;* it is not useful for cleansing nonexudative wounds or lesions. The beads not only absorb water but also proteins, including fibrin/fibrinogen degradation products and, thus, prevent encrustation. The beads are poured into the cleansed wound, which is circumscribed with petroleum jelly, and a compress is taped in place to retain the material. Changes may be made up to 3 or 4 times a day, as needed. The beads must be removed before skin grafting is attempted. Care must be taken to prevent cross-contamination from patient to patient. On the floor the beads are slippery and, thus, hazardous.

Dihydroxyacetone

Vitadye (*Elders*); Chromelin Complexion Blender (*Summers*)

[96-26-4] $C_3H_6O_3$ (90.08).

Preparation—By oxidation of the secondary alcohol group of glycerin.

Description—Crystalline powder; fairly hygroscopic; characteristic odor; sweet taste; melts about 77°.

Solubility—*Dimer* (normal form): slowly soluble in 1 part water or 15 parts alcohol. *Monomer* (formed in solution): very soluble in water, alcohol or ether.

Uses—Interacts with keratin in the stratum corneum to form a dark pigment that simulates the appearance of a suntan. It is incorporated in several *sunscreen* preparations. Since the sunscreen component is usually present in a concentration lower than optimal, such preparations may not provide protection to photosensitive persons. Also used to treat vitiligo.

Dosage Forms—Liquid: 5%.

Dioxybenzone

Methanone, (2-hydroxy-4-methoxyphenyl)(2-hydroxyphenyl)-, Spectra-Sorb UV 24 (*American Cyanamid*); Solaquin (*Elder*)

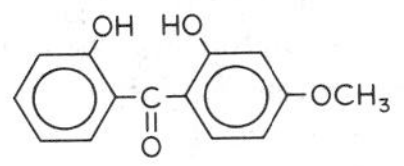

2,2′-Dihydroxy-4-methoxybenzophenone [131-53-3] $C_{14}H_{12}O_4$ (244.25).

Preparation—By a Friedel-Crafts reaction in which *o*-methoxybenzoyl chloride is added gradually to a mixture of 1,3-dimethoxybenzene, chlorobenzene and aluminum chloride. The reaction conditions are such that both methoxy groups ortho to the carbonyl bridge in the initial condensation product are demethylated. US Pat 2,853,521.

Description—Off-white to yellow powder; congeals not lower than 68°.

Solubility—Practically insoluble in water; freely soluble in alcohol or toluene.

Uses—A *sunscreen* of intermediate molar absorptivity (11,950 at 282 nm), but it absorbs throughout the UV spectrum and, hence, affords protection not only against sunburn but also against the photodynamic, photosensitizing and phototoxic effects of drugs. At present, it is marketed in combination with the closely related *Oxybenzone* (page 883).

Dose—*Topical,* as a **3%** lotion or cream.

Dosage Forms—Dioxybenzone and Oxybenzone Lotion and Cream: 3% of each ingredient.

Ethylhexyl *p*-Methoxycinnamate

Parsol MCX

Octyl methoxycinnamate [5466-77-3] $C_{18}H_{26}O_3$ (290.40).

Preparation—US Pat 4,713,473.

Description—High-boiling liquid.

Uses—A *sunscreen* with a narrow absorption band of 290 to 320 nm and a moderate molar absorptivity.

Dose—*Topical,* **2** to **7.5%** in creams, lotions and oils.

Etretinate

2,4,6,8-Nonanetetraenoic acid, 9-(4-methoxy-2,3,6-trimethylphenyl)-3,7-dimethyl-, ethyl ester (*all-E*); Tegison (*Roche*)

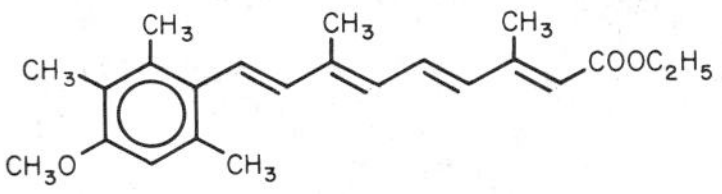

[54350-48-0] $C_{23}H_{30}O_3$ (354.49).

Preparation—One scheme involves the Wittig condensation of diphenyl 2,3,6-trimethyl-4-methoxybenzylphosphonium chloride and 8-oxo-3,7-dimethyl-2,4,6-octane-trienoic acid (*all-trans*) in the presence of butylene oxide; *Experientia 34:* 1113, 1978.

Description—Crystalline solid melting about 104°.

Solubility—Soluble in alcohol; unsoluble in water.

Uses—Although not a topical drug, it is a retinoid closely related to tretinoin and is used only for its dermatologic actions; consequently, it is included in this chapter. It is used in the treatment of recalcitrant *psoriasis*, especially the severe pustular erythrodermic type. It decreases scaling, erythema and the thickness of lesions and causes epithelial and dermal cells to redifferentiate to normal cells. Sometimes, dramatic improvement occurs within 2 wk and complete clearing in 1.5 to 4.5 mo. However, relapses are frequent once treatment is discontinued and sometimes even during chronic maintenance. It can be used alone or in low-dose combination with PUVA therapy. The mechanism of action is unknown, but it is undoubtedly like that of vitamin A. Activity resides in the acid metabolite.

Adverse effects occur in more than 75% of recipients. They include chapped lips, peeling of the palms, soles and fingertips, dryness of the mucous membranes, sore tongue, cheilitis, rhinorrhea, nosebleed, gingival bleeding, loss of hair, nail abnormalities, dry and irritated cornea, sclera and conjunctiva (50%), epidermal fragility, easy sunburning and other effects. Occasionally, pseudotumor cerebri, metastatic calcification of ligaments and tendons, and liver dysfunction or necrosis occur. In children and adolescents there may be premature closure of the epiphyses. Plasma cholesterol and triglycerides rise and high-density lipoprotein decreases. The drug is also teratogenic. Adverse effects are less with the low doses used with PUVA.

Absorption after oral administration is incomplete. It can be increased by whole milk and other lipid-containing foods. There is a rapid metabolism during which it is de-esterified to the acid metabolite. A much slower degradation and conjugation follows, the metabolites being secreted into bile and urine. Nearly all of the circulating drug is bound to plasma lipoproteins, but the active metabolite is bound to albumin. Ultimately, it is taken up into fat, where it may be found even as long as 2 yr after the last dose. The apparent elimination half-life is about 120 days. This persistence of drug in the body militates against the use of the drug in fertile women of child-bearing age, since the incidence of congenital defects is high even when conception occurs months after the drug is discontinued. The drug also is excreted into milk; effects in the nursing infant are not known.

Dose—*Oral, adult, initially* **0.25** to **1.0 mg/kg** a day in divided doses, the dose depending upon the type and seriousness of the disorder; with erythrodermic psoriasis, the initial dose is 0.25 mg/kg a day, increased weekly with increments of 0.25 mg/kg a day until a response occurs; *maintenance*, **0.5** to **0.75 mg/kg** a day. Maintenance usually is not begun until after 8 to 16 wk of treatment. The above doses are higher than those used concurrently with PUVA treatment.

Dosage Form—Capsules: 10 and 25 mg.

Homosalate

Benzoic acid, 2-hydroxy-, 3,3,5-trimethylcyclohexyl ester; Ing of Coppertone (*Plough*); Filtrosol "A" (*Norda*); Heliophan (*Greeff*)

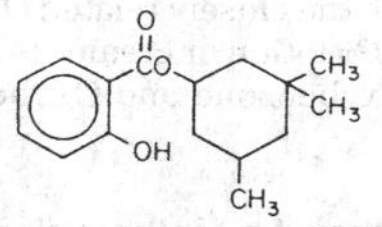

Homomenthyl salicylate [118-56-9[$C_{16}H_{22}O_3$ (262.36).

Preparation—US Pat 2,369,084.

Description—Colorless liquid boiling about 163° at 4 mm.

Uses—A liquid with relatively low molar absorptivity (6720 at 310 nm) and limited absorption in the near ultraviolet range (290 to 315 nm), so that it is used mainly to *promote tanning*. Photosensitive persons may not be protected from burns and phototoxicity.

Dose—*Topical*, **4** to **10%** in creams, lotions or oils.

Hydrogen Peroxide Solution—page 1267.

Hydroquinone

1,4-Benzenediol; *p*-Dihydroxybenzene; Hydroquinol; Quinol; Eldoquin and Eldopaque (*Elder*)

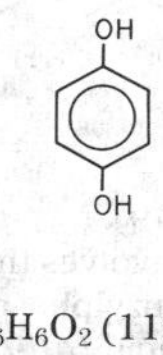

Hydroquinone [123-31-9] $C_6H_6O_2$ (110.11).

Preparation—Various processes are employed. One involves reacting a sulfuric acid solution of aniline with manganese dioxide and reducing the resulting *p*-benzoquinone with sodium bisulfite.

Description—Fine, white needles; darkens on exposure to air; melts 8 between 172 and 174°.

Solubility—1 g in about 17 mL water, 4 mL alcohol, 51 mL chloroform or 16.5 mL ether.

Uses—A *hypopigmenting* agent employed percutaneously to lighten localized areas of hyperpigmented skin, such as skin blemishes, lentigo, melasma, chloasma, freckles, etc. Its action is temporary, so that it is necessary to repeat the application at frequent intervals. It is a mild irritant, and erythema or rash may develop, which requires discontinuation of the drug. It should not be used near the eyes or in open cuts. It is contraindicated in the presence of sunburn, miliaria or irritated skin. It is not to be used in children. Ingestion of 1 g results in tinnitus, nausea, vomiting, a sense of suffocation, shortness of breath, cyanosis, convulsions, delirium and collapse. Death has occurred with ingestion of 5 g. Irritation of the GI tract occurs with oral ingestion. Dermatitis results from skin contact. Corneal staining and opacification have been noted in those exposed for prolonged periods to hydroquinone vapor at concentrations not sufficiently high for systemic effects.

Dose—*Topical*, to the *skin, adults* and *children over 12 yr*, as a **2** to **4%** cream, gel, lotion or ointment to the affected area once or twice a day.

Dosage Forms—Cream: 2 and 4%; Gel: 4%; Lotion: 2%; Ointment: 2 and 4%.

Hydroxyurea—page 1252.

Isotretinoin

13-*cis*-Retinoic Acid; Accutane (*Roche*)

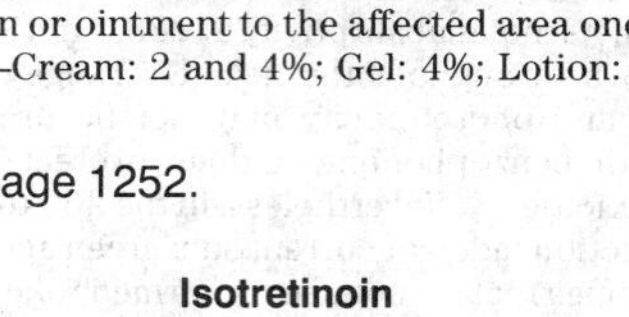

3,7-Dimethyl-9-(2,6,6-trimethyl-1-cyclohexen-1-yl)-2-*cis*-4-*trans*-6-*trans*-8-*trans*-nonatetraenoic acid [4759-48-2] $C_{20}H_{28}O_2$ (300.44). Differs from tretinoin (vitamin A) only in the configuration of the unsaturation at the α and β carbon atoms, which is *cis rather than trans.*

Uses—Although not a topical drug, it is a dermatologic agent and, hence, is described here. Its primary action is to decrease the production of sebum, which lends itself to the treatment of severe *modular* and *cystic acne* (acne conglobata). The size of the sebaceous gland is decreased and there is a change in the morphology and secretory capacity of the cells (dedifferentiation). Complete clearing of lesions is seen in about 90% of cases. A single course of treatment usually brings about long-lasting, sometimes permanent, remissions.

It also appears to diminish hyperkeratosis and has been reported to be effective in *rosacea*, gram-negative *folliculitis*, *lamellar ichthyosis*, *Darier's disease*, *pityriasis rubra pilaris* and *keratocanthoma*.

Adverse effects include facial dermatitis, fragile skin, thinning and drying of the hair, reversible cheilitis and dry skin, mouth, eyes and conjunctivitis in 25 to 80% of recipients. Peeling of the palms and soles and sensitivity to sunburn occur in about 5% of users. Urethral inflammation also occurs frequently. Joint pains and exacerbation of rheumatoid arthritis also has been reported to occur in about 16% of patients. Sedimentation rate, serum triglyceride concentration and serum levels of alanine and aspartate transaminases transiently occur in about 25% of users. Vertebral hyperostoses has been noted with the current recommended dose regimen. It was noted originally in patients receiving isotretinoin for various keratinization disorders at higher dosages and for longer periods than those recommended for acne. In spite of the relatively high incidence of side effects, treatment rarely has to be discontinued.

After oral administration, peak blood concentrations occur within 1 to 4 hr. The compound is oxidized to 4-hydroxy-13-*cis*-retinoic acid, which is then glucuronidated and is secreted into the bile. The elimination half-life is 11 to 39 (mean 20) hr. Isotretinoin should not be given during pregnancy or nursing.

Dose—*Oral, adult,* for *acne*, **0.5** to **1 mg/kg** a day in 2 divided doses for 15 to 20 wk. Although lower doses may achieve initial response rates, they are associated with higher recurrence rates on discontinuation of the drug. There appears to be no advantage to single versus divided doses, although its absorption is enhanced by taking it with meals. If the cyst count has not been reduced by more than 70%, a second course of treatment may be given after a wait of 2 mo. The skin often continues to clear after drug therapy; therefore, the waiting period is recommended. The response rate may be 90% with one to two treatment courses. Persons over 70 kg or who have severe chest and back involvement usually require doses at the high end of the range. For *severe rosacea* or gram-negative *folliculitis*, **0.25** to **0.5 mg/kg** twice a day. For *hyperkeratoses*, up to **4 mg/kg**.

Dosage Forms—Capsules: 10, 20 and 40 mg.

Lisadimate

1,2,3-Propanetriol, 1-(4-aminobenzoate) ester;
Escalol 106 (*Van Dyk*)

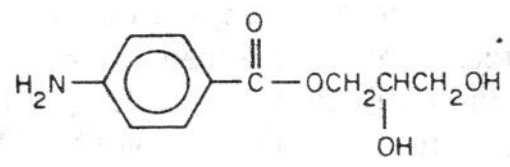

Glyceryl *p*-aminobenzoate [136-44-7] $C_{10}H_{13}NO_4$ (211.21).
Preparation—By esterification of aminobenzoic acid with glycerin.
Description—Waxy semisolid or syrup.
Solubility—Insoluble in water, oils or fats; soluble in alcohol, isopropyl alcohol or propylene glycol.
Uses—A *sunscreen* that asorbs UV light at 264 to 315 nm and which has a relatively high molar absorptivity (17,197 at 295 nm) but a limited spectrum, therefore used primarily to promote tanning rather than to protect sensitive persons.
Dose—*Topical*, **2** to **3%** in lotions.

Methoxsalen

7*H*-Furo [3,2-*g*][1]benzopyran-7-one, 9-methoxy-, Ammoidin;
9-Methoxypsoralen; Xanthotoxin; Oxsoralen (*Elder*)

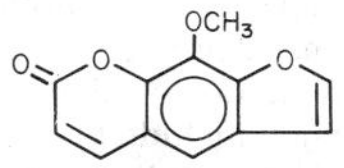

[298-81-7] $C_{12}H_8O_4$ (216.19).
Preparation—Occurs naturally in *Psorales coryfolia, Ammi majus, Ruta chalepensis* and various other plants. It may be synthesized by methods described in *JACS 79:* 3491, 1957, and in US Pat 2,889,337.
Description—White to cream-colored, odorless, fluffy, needle-like crystals; melts between 143° and 148°.
Solubility—Practically insoluble in cold water, sparingly soluble in boiling water; freely soluble in chloroform; soluble in boiling alcohol, acetone or acetic acid; soluble in aqueous alkalies with ring cleavage; reconstitution occurs on neutralization.
Uses—A *psoralen melanizer.* It increases the photodynamic pigmentation of skin; it does not induce pigmentation in the absence of UV light or melanocytes. It is used in the treatment of *vitiligo* and to *desensitize to sunlight.* Severe sunburning can occur with topical application; it is customary to protect the surrounding skin with a sunscreen. It also is used in PUVA treatment of *psoriasis, mycosis fungoides* and *cutaneous T-cell lymphoma;* in these, irradiation activates it to cross-link DNA. It may have value in the PUVA treatment of *alopecia areata, inflammatory dermatoses, eczema* and *lichen planus.* After oral administration gastrointestinal upset and central nervous system toxicities, such as vertigo and excitement, also occur. Consequently, the drug should be used orally only under medical supervision. It is additive with other photosensitizing drugs and the furocumarin pigments in carrots, celery, figs, limes, mustard, parsley and parsnips. It inhibits the metabolism of caffeine.
Dose—*Topical*, as a **1%** lotion (see the package literature for details of application and use). *Oral, adults* and *children over 12 yr*, for *vitiligo*, **30** to **40 mg** once a day 2 to 4 hr before exposure to ultraviolet light or at longer than 48-hr intervals 2 or 3 times a wk; for *psoriasis, mycosis fungoides* or *cutaneous T-cell lymphoma*, **0.6 mg/kg** 2 or 3 hr before UVA exposure (see the package literature for details).
Dosage Forms—Capsules: 10 mg; Lotion: 1%.

Methyl Anthranilate

2-Aminobenzoic acid, methyl ester

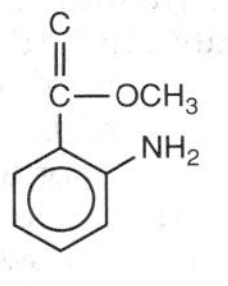

[134-20-3] $C_8H_9NO_2$ (151.16).
Preparation—A constituent of several essential oils; also, by esterification of anthranilic acid with methyl alcohol.
Description—A crystalline substance; melts at 25°.
Solubility—Slightly soluble in water; freely soluble in alcohol or ether.
Uses—A *sunscreen*, with the lowest molar absorptivity of all sunscreens (941 at 315 nm); also, it does not absorb throughout the near UV range (absorption band, 290 to 320 nm) and, therefore, is used in combination with other sunscreens or light-protectives. It also is used as a perfume in ointments and cosmetics.
Dose—*Topical*, to the *skin*, **5%** in creams, lotions or ointments.

Minoxidil—page 947.

Monobenzone

Phenol, 4-(phenylmethoxy)-, Monobenzyl Ether of Hydroquinone;
Benoquin (*Elder*)

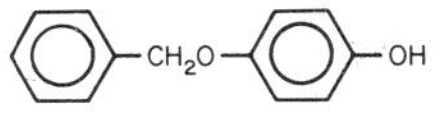

p-(Benzyloxy)phenol [103-16-2] $C_{13}H_{12}O_2$ (200.24).
Preparation—Prepared in various ways. One method involves condensing sodium *p*-nitrophenolate with benzyl chloride to produce benzyl *p*-nitrophenyl ether followed by (1) reduction of nitro to amino, (2) diazotization of amino and (3) hydrolytic decomposition of the diazonium compound to the corresponding phenol.
Description—White, odorless, crystalline powder possessing very little taste; melts between 117° and 120°.
Solubility—1 g in > 10,000 mL water, 14.5 mL alcohol, 29 mL chloroform or 14 mL ether.
Uses—A *depigmenting agent* or *demelanizer.* It acts by interfering with the formation of melanin, which is the principal cutaneous pigment. It is recommended only for the final depigmentation in *vitiligo.* It is not recommended for treatment of lentigo, severe freckling and other types of hyperpigmentation. It is not effective against pigmented moles or malignant melanoma. Its pigment-decreasing action is somewhat erratic. Irritation of varying degrees occurs in a considerable number of patients.
Dose—*Topical, adults* and *children over 12 yr*, to the *skin*, as a **20%** cream 2 or 3 times a day.
Dosage Forms—Cream: 20%.

Octyl Salicylate—See RPS-18, page 773.

Oxybenzone

Methanone, (2-hydroxy-4-methoxyphenyl)phenyl-,
(*Various Mfrs*)

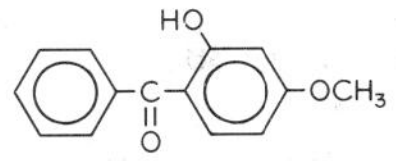

2-Hydroxy-4-methoxybenzophenone [131-57-7] $C_{14}H_{12}O_3$ (228.25).
Preparation—Benzoic acid is condensed with resorcinol monomethyl ether by heating in the presence of $ZnCl_2$ or polyphosphoric acid (103% H_3PO_4 equivalent), and PCl_3. US Pat 3,073,866.
Description—White to off-white powder; congeals not lower than 62°.
Solubility—Practically insoluble in water; freely soluble in alcohol or toluene.
Uses—A *sunscreen* with a high molar absorptivity (20,381 at 290 nm), and it absorbs in both the long and short UV spectrum 270–350 nm. Therefore, it serves not only to prevent sunburn but also to protect against the photodynamic, photosensitizing and phototoxic effects of various drugs. Contact with the eyes should be avoided. At present, it is marketed only in combination with other sunscreens.
Dose—*Topical*, as a **3** to **5%** cream, **0.5%** lipstick and **2** or **3%** lotion in combination with other sunscreens.

Padimate A

Benzoic acid, 4-(dimethylamino)-, pentyl ester
(*Various Mfrs*)

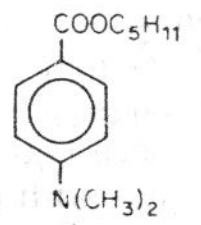

[14779-78-3] $C_{14}H_{21}NO_2$ (235.33). A mixture of pentyl, isopentyl and 2-methylbutyl esters of *p*-aminobenzoic acid.

Description—Yellow liquid; faint, aromatic odor.

Solubility—Practically insoluble in water or glycerin; soluble in alcohol, chloroform, isopropyl alcohol or mineral oil.

Uses—A *sunscreen* of moderate molar absorptivity but relatively narrow UV absorption spectrum (290 to 315 nm) characteristic of other aminobenzoic acid derivatives.

Dose—*Topical*, to the *skin*, as a **1.4** to **8%** cream, foam, lotion or stick.

Padimate O

Benzoic acid, 4-(dimethylamino)-, 2-ethylhexyl ester
(*Various Mfrs*)

$COOCH_2CH(C_2H_5)CH_2CH_2CH_2CH_3$ — benzene ring — $N(CH_3)_2$

[21245-02-3] $C_{17}H_{27}NO_2$ (277.41).

Preparation—By the esterification of p-dimethylaminobenzoic acid with 2-ethylhexanol in the presence of dry HCl. The product is liberated from the salt by neutralization with base.

Description—Light-yellow mobile liquid; faint, aromatic odor.

Solubility—Practically insoluble in water, alcohol or mineral oil.

Uses—See *Padimate A*.

Ringer's Irrigation—see RPS-16, page 762.

Roxadimate

Benzoic acid, 4-[bis-(2-hydroxypropyl)amino]-, ethyl ester
Amerscreen (*Amerchol*)

$(CH_3CH(OH)CH_2)_2N$ — benzene ring — $C(=O)-OCH_2CH_3$

[58882-17-0] $C_{15}H_{23}NO_4$ (281.35).

Uses—A *sunscreen* with a limited absorption spectrum (280 to 330 nm) characteristic of *p*-aminobenzoates but a relatively high molar absorptivity. It is used mainly in suntan products.

Dose—*Topical*, **1** to **5%**.

Sodium Bicarbonate—page 889.

Sodium Fluoride

Sodium fluoride [7681-49-4] NaF (41.99).

Preparation—By interaction of 40% HF with an equivalent quantity of NaOH or Na_2CO_3.

Description—White, odorless powder.

Solubility—1 g in 25 mL water; insoluble in alcohol.

Uses—A *dental caries prophylactic*. Fluoridation of municipal water supplies is considered a safe and practical public health measure, a concentration of about 1 ppm of fluoride in the water supply resulting in a 50 to 65% reduction in the incidence of dental caries in permanent teeth. Ingested fluoride is effective only while teeth are being formed. The fluoride is incorporated into tooth salts as fluoroapatite. Excessive intake during development of teeth may cause mottling; hence, mottling of newly erupted teeth is an indication to reduce fluoride intake. Where drinking water contains less than 0.7 ppm of fluoride, dietary supplements for children with unerupted teeth may provide some future protection.

Topical application results in changes only in the outer layers of enamel or exposed dentin. In children, repeated application of a 2% solution of the drug to cleaned teeth results in a 16 to 49% reduction of dental caries; adult teeth are protected to a lesser extent by topical application. Topical application also is used to *densensitize* teeth.

Orally administered, it produces new bone formation in some patients with osteoporosis, especially when calcium and vitamin D (and estrogens in women) are administered concomitantly to facilitate mineralization of the new bone. However, the bone may become brittle.

It removes calcium from tissues and also poisons certain enzymes. Large oral doses may cause nausea and vomiting, which usually can be prevented by taking the substance with food. Pastes, rinses, solutions and gels for topical applications should not be swallowed.

Dose (as sodium fluoride)—*Topical*, to the teeth, as a **0.02** to **2%** solution, **1.1** or **2.71%** gel (with phosphoric acid) or **0.22** to **2.3%** toothpaste. *Oral*, **1.5** to **3 ppm** (equivalent to 0.7 to 1.3 ppm of fluoride ion) in drinking water; as a supplement, when the drinking water contains less than 0.3 ppm of fluoride ion, **0.55 mg** a day for infants from 2 wk to 2 yr of age, **1.1 mg** once a day for children from 2 to 3 yr and **2.2 mg** for those from 3 to 13 yr, and when the drinking water contains 0.3 to 0.7 ppm of fluoride ion, **550 µg** once a day for children 2 to 3 yr and **1.1 mg** for those 3 to 13 yr. The fluoride ion equivalents of 550 µg, 1.1 mg, and 2.2 mg of the drug are 250 µg, 500 µg, and 1 mg, respectively. For *osteoporosis*, up to **60 mg** a day. *Caution: It is poisonous.*

Dosage Forms—Drops: 0.275, 0.55 and 1.1 mg/drop; Gel: 1.1 and 2.71%; Rinse: 0.02, 0.05, 0.2 and 0.44%; Solution: 1.1, 3.3, 5.5, and 20 mg/mL; Chewable Tablets: 0.55, 1.1 and 2.2 mg. Sodium Fluoride and Orthophosphoric Acid: Gel: 1.23% fluoride ion and 1% phosphoric acid.

Sodium Monofluorophosphate

Phosphorofluoridic acid, sodium salt

$FPO(ONa)_2$

Disodium phosphorofluoridate [10163-15-2] (143.95).

Preparation—Substantially pure drug is produced by fusing a mixture of sodium metaphosphate and sodium fluoride, in stoichiometric proportion, in a closed vessel from which moist air is excluded.

Description—White to slightly gray, odorless powder.

Solubility—Freely soluble in water.

Uses—Like *Sodium Fluoride*, above, it promotes the replacement of the hydroxyapatite by fluoroapatite in the tooth salts and, hence, is used as a *dental prophylactic* against dental caries. It has the advantage over sodium fluoride in that the teeth do not require special preparation before application, it is effective when included in dentifrices and in dentifrices there is no hazard with respect to local toxicity to the gingivae or systemic intoxication from ingestion.

Dose—*Topical*, to the *teeth*, in dentifrice containing **0.76%.**

Stannous Fluoride

Tin Difluoride; Fluoristan

Tin fluoride (SnF_2) [7783-47-3] (156.69); contains not less than 71.2% Sn^{2+} (stannous tin), and about 24% F^- (fluoride).

Preparation—Stannous oxide is dissolved in 40% HF and the solution is evaporated out of contact with air.

Description—White, crystalline powder with a bitter, salty taste; melts at about 213°.

Solubility—Freely soluble in water; practically insoluble in alcohol, ether or chloroform.

Uses—Alters the composition and crystalline structure of the hydroxyapatite-like salts that make up the bulk of enamel and dentin, so that the tooth material is more resistant to acidic erosion and dental caries (decay). The substance is applied only topically, so that the tooth substance is only affected in the superficial layers, and it must be applied periodically. It is most effective when applied to the tooth surface after the teeth have been cleaned thoroughly by a dentist. However, there is good evidence that even when incorporated into tooth pastes the drug has a retardant effect on the development of dental caries.

Dose—*Topical*, to the *teeth*, generally as **0.4%** gel or **0.1%** rinse.

Dosage Forms—Capsules (for solution): 0.4, 0.65 and 0.8 g; Concentrate: 30%; Gel: 0.4%.

Titanium Dioxide

Titanic Anhydride

Titanium oxide (TiO_2) [13463-67-7] TiO_2 (79.88).

Preparation—By adding ammonia or an alkali carbonate to a solution of titanyl sulfate ($TiOSO_4$). Titanic acid [$Ti(OH)_4$ or $TiO(OH)_2$] is precipitated and, after filtration and washing, is dried and ignited.

Description—White, amorphous, tasteless, odorless, infusible powder; density about 4; suspension in water (1 in 10) neutral to litmus.

Solubility—Insoluble in water, HCl, HNO_3 or dilute H_2SO_4.

Uses—Its powder has a very high reflectance at visible and UV wavelengths, and, hence, it serves as an excellent white pigment. In ointments or lotions it reflects a very high proportion of incident sunlight, hence, protecting the skin from sunburn and serving as a sunblock. It also is used in cosmetics and as a dusting powder. Topically, it is devoid of toxicity.

Dose—*Topical*, to the *skin*, as **2** to **25%** cream, lotion or ointment as required.

Trioxsalen

7*H*-Furo[3,2-*g*][1]benzopyran-7-one, 2,5,9-trimethyl-, 6-hydroxy-β,2,7-trimethyl-5-benzofuranacrylic acid, δ-lactone; Trisoralen (*Elder*)

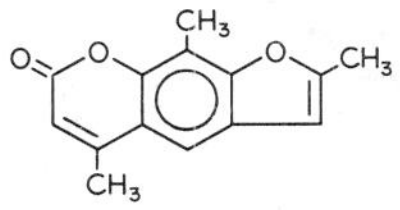

[3902-71-4] $C_{14}H_{12}O_3$ (228.25).

Caution—Avoid contact with the skin.

Preparation—2-Methylresorcinol is cyclized with ethyl acetoacetate with the aid of sulfuric acid to 7-hydroxy-4,8-dimethylcoumarin (I). Treatment with allyl bromide in the presence of potassium carbonate transforms I into the 7-allyloxy compound which, on reacting with acetic anhydride in the presence of *N,N*-diethylaniline and anhydrous sodium acetate, rearranges and esterifies to give the 7-acetoxy-6-allyl compound (II). Bromination of II followed by reaction with sodium methoxide yields trioxsalen. US Pat 3,201,421.

Description—White to off-white, odorless, tasteless crystalline solid; stable in light, air and heat; melts at about 230°.

Solubility—1 g in 1150 mL alcohol, 84 mL chloroform or 43 mL methylenedichloride; practically insoluble in water.

Uses—Although not a topical drug, it closely relates to other drugs in this section. It facilitates the action of near UV light to induce melanin (skin pigment) formation. It is used to cause repigmentation in idiopathic *vitiligo* and to enhance pigmentation to *increase tolerance to sunlight* or for *cosmetic purposes.* The increased tolerance to sunlight does not occur until enhanced pigmentation has occurred, and the patient must be cautioned that severe sunburning with less than normal exposure can occur early during the course of treatment. The increase in dermal pigment occurs gradually over a period of several days of repeated exposure. Care must be taken to protect the eyes and lips during treatment. The manufacturer's recommended schedule of exposure should be used except at high altitudes, where exposure times should be appropriately reduced.

It is contraindicated in persons with photosensitizing diseases, such as infectious leukoderma, porphyria or lupus erythematosus and when photosensitizing drugs are being given. The drug sometimes may cause gastric irritation and emesis. Children under 12 should not take it.

Dose—*Oral, adults* and *children over 12 yr*, **5** to **10 mg** 2 hr before exposure to sunlight. For the treatment of vitiligo the exposure should be repeated once a day for 4 days, and subsequent exposures should be determined according to the results of the initial 4 days. For the enhancement of pigmentation, treatment should not exceed 2 wk, and the total accumulated dose in any one treatment course should not exceed 140 mg. Persons who show side effects of the drug should take only 5 mg; the duration of use will be necessarily prolonged over that in persons taking the usual dose of 10 mg.

Dosage Forms—Tablets: 5 mg.

Urea—pages 1041 and 1416.

CHAPTER 53

Gastrointestinal and Liver Drugs

Keith G Tolman, MD
Professor of Medicine
School of Medicine
University of Utah
Salt Lake City, Utah 84132

The major categories of drugs included in this chapter are antacids, H2-receptor antagonists, H^+/K^+ ATPase inhibitors, drugs that enhance mucosal resistance, digestants including pancreatic enzymes, laxatives, antidiarrheals, emetics, antiemetics, prokinetic agents, adsorbents and miscellaneous drugs. A number of other drugs, used primarily for other indications but also used in the treatment of gastrointestinal diseases, are not included in this chapter. These include immunosuppressive drugs, anti-inflammatory drugs, immunostimulants and antibiotics.

Antacids

Antacids are drugs which react with hydrochloric acid to form salt and water. This neutralizes acid and, in so doing, raises gastric pH. The most widely used antacids are sodium bicarbonate, calcium carbonate, aluminum hydroxide and magnesium hydroxide. Refer to Chapter 23 for the chemistry of the antacids.

Antacids are used widely by the laity for the relief of heartburn and dyspepsia, as well as a large variety of nonspecific gastrointestinal symptoms. They are used by physicians for peptic ulcer disease, gastritis, reflux esophagitis, prevention of stress ulcers and gastrointestinal bleeding. Despite the widespread use of antacids, they offer little advantage, and many disadvantages over H2-receptor blockers, which have become the mainstay for the routine treatment of acid peptic disorders. The primary role of antacids in the management of acid peptic disorders is relief of pain. Antacids are marketed widely as over-the-counter (OTC) agents. For the most part, they are safe but in patients with compromised renal function, indiscriminate use can lead to alkalosis and other complications.

Antacids are used typically in combination. The differences in mixture account for the relative differences in neutralizing capacity and side effects. It is apparent that the more acid neutralized, the greater the efficacy of the antacid. For practical purposes, however, efficacy is obtained by increasing the gastric pH to 3.5-5.0. This is achieved readily with modern antacids, giving doses of 15 to 30 mL, 1 and 3 hours after meals. Such doses also heal ulcers in 4 to 8 weeks in approximately 80% of patients.

The mechanism of action of antacids is complex. A proposed mechanism is the prevention of back-diffusion of hydrogen ions across the gastrointestinal mucosa. It is not clear at what pH this action takes effect. It is readily apparent that one can neutralize 50% of the acid in a given amount of gastric juice with a pH of 1.3 by raising the pH to 1.6, 90% by raising the pH to 2.3 and 99% by raising the pH to 3.3. It generally is accepted that raising the gastric pH to approximately 4 prevents stress ulcer, which is thought to be mediated by acid back-diffusion. Another action of antacids is to prevent the conversion of gastric pepsinogen, a proenzyme, to pepsin, the active form. This is a proteolytic enzyme thought to mediate tissue injury in ulcer disease. Pepsinogens are inactivated reversibly at pH 5 and inactivated irreversibly at pH 7. It thus may be necessary to raise the pH to 5 to achieve the maximum benefit from antacids. Antacids also may enhance cytoprotection in the stomach. Finally, antacids may confer a therapeutic benefit by inactivating bile salts which are thought to reflux from the duodenum into the stomach and play some role in acid peptid disease.

There are differences in the types of antacids in terms of their cation content, neutralizing capacity, duration of action, side effects and cost. These must be considered when choosing an antacid for therapeutic use.

The Patient—Certain patients by nature of their underlying disease may be at increased risk of antacid toxicity. For example, patients with heart failure may be at risk from excess sodium intake. In terms of sodium content, antacids vary less now than in the past. Most available antacids are low in sodium and thus the presence of edema or heart failure precludes the use only of sodium bicarbonate. Patients with renal failure should not use magnesium-containing antacids because of the possibility of hypermagnesemia, or sodium bicarbonate which may cause systemic alkalosis. While patients with renal failure are sometimes given aluminum-containing antacids for their phosphate-lowering effect, there is increasing concern about aluminum neurotoxicity in such patients.

Systemic versus Nonsystemic—A systemic antacid, such as sodium bicarbonate, is soluble and readily absorbed. It can cause electrolyte disturbances and alkalosis. The so-called nonsystemic antacids, such as aluminum-, calcium- and magnesium-containing antacids, form relatively insoluble compounds in the GI tract. It is not true, however, that such compounds are not absorbed. Toxicity occurs as the result of systemic absorption of all of these antacids. Ingestion of large amounts of calcium carbonate can lead to hypercalcemia, alkalosis and renal failure with so called milk-alkali syndrome. Magnesium-containing antacids can cause both diarrhea and hypermagnesemia. Prolonged treatment with aluminum-containing antacids can cause phosphate depletion and, eventually, osteoporosis and osteomalacia as well as neurotoxicity. All of the toxicities of the nonsystemic antacid are more common and more serious in patients with renal failure.

Neutralizing Capacity—Antacids are compared quantitatively in terms of *acid-neutralizing capacity* (ANC), defined as the number of milliequivalents of hydrochloric acid required to maintain 1 mL of an antacid suspension at pH 3 for 2 hours *in vitro*. The rate of neutralization varies according to the degree of comminution, crystal form, precipitants used and presence of reactive suspending agents. Consequently, the ANC and rate of neutralization of various antacids differ enormously. For example, 5 mL of aluminum hydroxide suspension (Amphojel) will neutralize 6.5 mEq of acid in 60 minutes, whereas a similar volume of aluminum hydroxide–magnesium hydroxide suspension (Delcid) will neutralize 42 mEq in the same period of time.

Dose—It is generally agreed that 50 mEq/hr of *available* antacid is required to neutralize continuously the gastric contents of 90% of patients with duodenal ulcer. Based on the neutralizing capacity given above, this would require a dose of 6 mL of Delcid or 39 mL of Amphojel.

Dose Interval—An ideal antacid should be rapid in onset and provide a continuous buffering action. Antacids with a rapid onset include magnesium hydroxide, magnesium oxide and calcium carbonate; those with an intermediate onset, magaldrate and magnesium carbonate; and those with a slow onset, magnesium trisilicate and the aluminum compounds. The duration of buffering action is determined largely by when the antacid is administered; if administered while food is in the stomach, the buffering action will last for 2 hours. An additional dose 3 hours after meals will extend the buffering time by 1 hr. Therefore, the ideal dose interval is 1 and 3 hr *after meals and at bedtime.*

Aluminum Carbonate Gel, Basic

Basaljel (*Wyeth*)

Uses—To control gastric hyperacidity and as an adjunct in the treatment of peptic ulcer. Because it is excreted as aluminum phosphate, it also is used with a low-phosphate diet to prevent formation of phosphate urinary stones.

Dose—*Antacid,* **1000 mg** (2 capsules or tablets), **10 mL** of regular suspension (in water or fruit juice) or **5 mL** of extra-strength suspension 1 and 3 hr after meals and at bedtime; *Hyperphosphatemia*: administer 3 to 4 times a day with meals.

Other Dose Information—10 mL of the suspension or 5 mL of the extra-strength suspension will neutralize 23 mEq of acid; 2 capsules or 2 swallow tablets will neutralize 24 and 25 mEq of acid, respectively. The sodium content of each dosage form is as follows: suspension, 0.13 mEq/5mL; extra-strength suspension, 1.0 mEq/5mL; capsules and tablets, 0.12 mEq.

Dosage Forms—Capsules and Swallow Tablets, equivalent to 500 mg aluminum hydroxide; Suspension, equivalent to 400 mg aluminum hydroxide per 5 mL; Extra-strength Suspension, equivalent to 1000 mg aluminum hydroxide per 5 mL.

Aluminum Hydroxide Gel

Colloidal Aluminum Hydroxide; Amphojel (*Wyeth-Ayerst*); Alternagel (*Stuart*); (*Various mfrs*)

Aluminum Hydroxide [21645-51-2] $Al(OH)_3$ (78.00); a suspension each 100 g of which contains the equivalent of 3.6–4.4 g of aluminum oxide [Al_2O_3 = 101.96], in the form of aluminum hydroxide and hydrated oxide.

It may contain peppermint oil, glycerin, sorbitol, sucrose, saccharin or other suitable flavors, and it may contain suitable antimicrobial agents.

Preparation—One process for the preparation of this type of aluminum hydroxide is as follows:

Dissolve 1000 g of $Na_2CO_3.10H_2O$ in 400 mL of hot water and filter. Dissolve 800 g of ammonium alum in 2000 mL of hot water and filter into the carbonate solution with constant stirring. Then add 4000 mL of hot water and remove all gas. Dilute to 80,000 mL with cold water. Collect and wash the precipitate and suspend it in 2000 mL of purified water flavored with 0.01% peppermint oil and preserve with 0.1% of sodium benzoate. Homogenize the resulting gel.

The principal property desired is a very fine particle size to achieve large surface and, thus, maximum adsorption capacity.

Description—White, viscous suspension, from which small amounts of water may separate on standing; translucent in thin layers; affects both red and blue litmus paper slightly but is not reddened by phenolphthalein.

Incompatibilities—The use of Aluminum Hydroxide Gel and similar materials to reduce the gastrointestinal problem accompanying use of tetracycline antibiotics has resulted in complexation and decreased absorption of the antibiotic.

Uses—Primarily as an antacid in the management of *peptic ulcer, gastritis* and *esophagitis.* It also is used as a skin protectant and mild astringent. It is a relatively weak antacid and does not elevate gastric pH sufficiently to inhibit pepsin activity. Aluminum hydroxide does not have significant demulcent properties. Although aluminum hydroxide is a nonsystemic antacid significant amounts are absorbed in patients with renal failure. Aluminum hydroxide is excreted as the phosphate. This provides the basis not only for the occasional use of aluminum hydroxide for the treatment of *phosphate nephrolithiasis,* but also is the cause of the phosphate depletion syndrome sometimes observed after chronic administration. There is increasing concern that aluminum absorption may lead to dementation. The major advantage of aluminum hydroxide is that no systemic alkalosis is produced. Aluminum compounds decrease the absorption of certain drugs, such as tetracyclines. It also interferes with the defoaming action of simethicone. These compounds are also constipating.

Dose—*Usual, adult, oral,* **500** to **1800 mg** 3 to 6 times a day between meals and at bedtime. *Children, hyperphosphatemia,* **50** to **150 mg/kg/24 hr** in divided doses every 4 to 6 hr.

Other Dose Information—One 600-mg tablet or 10 mL of suspension will neutralize 18 and 13 mEq, respectively, of acid in 60 min.

Dosage Forms—Capsules 475 and 500 mg; Oral Suspension, 320 and 600 mg/5 mL; Dried, Tablets: 300 and 600 mg; Tablets (Chewable), 487.5 mg.

Dried Aluminum Hydroxide Gel yields not less than 50.0% of aluminum oxide [Al_2O_3 = 101.96]. *Preparation:* Aluminum hydroxide, prepared as described under *Aluminum Hydroxide Gel,* is dried at a low temperature until it has the required amount of Al_2O_3. *Description:* White, odorless, tasteless, amorphous powder. The filtrate from the aqueous suspension (1 in 25) is neutral to litmus. *Solubility:* Insoluble in water and alcohol; soluble in diluted mineral acids and solutions of fixed alkali hydroxides. *Dose:* The equivalent of 300 mg to 5 g of aluminum hydroxide daily; *usual,* the equivalent of 300 mg of aluminum hydroxide, 4 to 6 times a day.

Bismuth Subnitrate—see RPS-18, page 775.

Bismuth Subsalicylate

Basic Bismuth Salicylate; Pepto-Bismol (*Norwich Eaton*)

[14882-18-19] $C_7H_5BiO_4$ (362.11).

Solubility—Practically insoluble in water or alcohol; soluble in alkali; decomposed by hot water.

Uses—Bismuth subsalicylate is the principal ingredient in a popular OTC product employed for *indigestion, nausea* and *diarrhea.* As an antidiarrheal agent it shows good activity versus *salmonella,* but less activity versus *E Coli.* As an antiulcer drug, gastroscopic studies show little effective coating of the mucosa; nevertheless, it seems to increase the rate of healing of peptic ulcers. It also reduces active intestinal secretion induced by *E coli* and *Vibrio cholerae.* This is thought to be due to antiprostaglandin activity by the subsalicylate component. It is used sometimes as an antibiotic for the prophylaxis of traveller's diarrhea and amoebiasis. It also is used to treat the common form of gastritis and duodenal ulcer caused by *Helicobacter pylori.* In this circumstance, it usually is used in combination with an antibiotic (usually amoxicillin and/or metronidazole) and an H2-blocker, but is effective when given alone.

Bismuth subsalicylate has several properties aside from its effect on *H pylori* that may account for its efficacy in the treatment of ulcer disease. It forms a glycoprotein-bismuth complex with mucus that may create a protective barrier against acid peptic digestion. Furthermore, it may stimulate prostaglandin E2 which in turn stimulates mucus and bicarbonate secretion. Finally, it may stimulate epidermal growth factor which may enhance healing of ulcers.

The majority of ingested bismuth subsalicylate is excreted in feces as bismuth sulfide. However, small amounts are absorbed and plasma levels are detectable. Encephalopathy has been reported with other bismuth salts. Its use is not recommended in patients with renal failure. The toxicity of long-term therapy is uncertain. Since this agent is a salicylate, it may cause ringing of the ears if taken with aspirin. Bismuth subsalicylate may cause a temporary darkening of the stool and tongue. The darkening of the stool mimics melena and may mistakenly suggest GI bleeding.

Dose—*Usual, adult, oral,* **30 mL** of the liquid or **600 mg** every ½ to 1 hr as needed to a maximum of 8 doses. *Children 10 to 14 yr,* **20 mL**; *6 to 10 yr,* **2 teaspoonfuls or 1 tablet;** *3 to 6 yr,* **5 mL** or **300 mg**.

Dose—*For prophylaxis of traveler's diarrhea,* **60 mL** 4 times a day. For *H pylori gastritis of duodenal ulcer,* **600 mg** 3 times a day with meals and at bedtime.

Dosage Form—Liquid: 262 mg/15 mL (tablespoonful). Tablets: 300 mg.

Calcium Carbonate

(*Various Mfrs*)

Calcium carbonate (1:1) [471-34-1] $CaCO_3$ (100.09).

Preparation—By double decomposition of calcium chloride and sodium carbonate in aqueous solution. Its density and fineness are governed by the concentration of the solutions; heavy and light forms are available on the market.

Description—Fine, white, microcrystalline powder, without odor or taste, and stable in air; aqueous suspension is practically neutral to litmus.

Solubility—Practically insoluble in water (its solubility in water is increased by the presence of any ammonium salt and by the presence of carbon dioxide; alkali hydroxide reduces its solubility); insoluble in alcohol; dissolves with effervescence in dilute acetic, hydrochloric or nitric acids.

Uses—A rapidly acting *antacid.* Although calcium carbonate is classified as a "nonsystemic" *antacid,* long-term therapy with large doses may cause systemic alkalosis and hypercalcemia (milk-alkali syndrome) in patients with renal failure. The salt reacts with hydrochloric acid in the stomach to form calcium chloride which is largely (90%) insoluble. However, a proportion of the calcium (7 to 19%) is absorbed. Calcium is constipating. For this reason, calcium and magnesium antacids often are alternated in therapy or given in fixed combination.

Calcium-containing antacids cause "acid rebound"—an increase in acid secretion that occurs after the neutralizing effect occurs. For this reason, calcium-containing antacids are used for the prevention, not treatment, of osteoporosis. It is most effective as an antiabsorption drug. The goal of therapy is to maintain, rather than restore, bone mass. Large doses, ie, 1000 to 1500 mg, as elemental calcium daily is required.

Precipitated calcium carbonate also is employed in dentifrices and is a pharmaceutical necessity for *Aluminum Subacetate Solution* and antacid oral suspension dosage forms.

Dose—For *prevention of osteoporosis,* **1** to **1.5 g** a day and Chewable Tablets **0.5** to **1.5 g** every 2 to 4 hr.

Other Dose Information—Two 420-mg tablets or 5 mL of suspension (Titralac) will neutralize 15 and 19 mEq, respectively, of acid in 60 min.

Dosage Forms—Tablets: 350, 420, 500, 650, 750, 800 and 1000 mg.

Calcium Hydroxide Solution—page 1408.

Calcium Phosphate, Dibasic—page 929.

Calcium Phosphate, Tribasic—see RPS-16, page 774.

Clidinium Bromide—page 1023.

Dihydroxyaluminum Aminoacetate—see RPS-18, page 778.

Dihydroxyaluminum Sodium Carbonate

Aluminum, [carbonato(1-)-*O*]dihydroxy, monosodium salt; Rolaids (*Warner Lambert*)

$$\left[O{=}C\langle O,O \rangle Al(OH)_2 \right] Na^+$$

Sodium (*T*-4)-[carbonato(2-)-*O,O'*]dihydroxyaluminate (1-) [16482-55-6] $NaAl(OH)_2CO_3$ (144.00); contains the equivalent of 34.8–38.2% of Al_2O_3 (aluminum oxide).

Preparation—Aluminum isopropoxide is reacted with a basic solution of sodium bicarbonate. US Pat 2,783,179.

Description—Fine, white powder that is odorless and tasteless; stable in light, slightly hygroscopic at room temperature and dehydrates and loses CO_2 above 100°.

Solubility—Practically insoluble in water; dissolves in dilute mineral acids.

Uses—A single molecule which combines the antacid properties of aluminum hydroxide and sodium bicarbonate. Hence, it is a partial systemic *antacid.* It has a rapid onset of action as gastric acid reacts with the sodium carbonate portion of the molecule; this is followed by a sustained, but less intense, antacid action due to the generated aluminum hydroxide. It is used for symptomatic relief of heartburn and dyspepsia but is not recommended as primary therapy for ulcer disease or reflux espophagitis. Since each tablet contains 53 mg of sodium, it is contraindicated in patients on a sodium-restricted diet. This product interacts with tetracycline and should not be taken when tetracycline is being used.

Dose—*Usual,* **300** to **600 mg** as required.

Other Dose Information—Each tablet (334 mg) neutralizes approximately 7.5 mEq of acid in 60 min.

Dosage Form—Tablets (Chewable): 334 mg.

Magaldrate

Aluminum magnesium hydroxide; Riopan (*Ayerst*)

$AlMg_2(OH)_7 \cdot H_2O$

[1317-26-6] (212.66); contains the equivalent of 29–40% of MgO (magnesium oxide) and the equivalent of 18–26% of Al_2O_3 (aluminum oxide).

Preparation—By precipitation using aqueous solutions of sodium or potassium aluminate and a magnesium salt under controlled conditions of concentration and temperature. The precipitated product is collected by filtration, washed to remove soluble by-products and dried. US Pat 2,923,660. The formulas shown above have been suggested although the substance also is described as an indefinite mixture of magnesium and aluminum hydroxides.

Description—White, odorless, crystalline powder.

Solubility—Insoluble in water or alcohol; soluble in dilute solutions of mineral acids.

Uses—A chemical combination of magnesium and aluminum hydoxides. It is used as an antacid for symptomatic relief of heartburn and dyspepsia. Megaldrate has rapid and uniform buffering capability with a large neutralizing capacity. It has a low sodium content (0.1 mg sodium per teaspoonful or tablet). It often is used for treatment of peptic ulcer disease and peptic esophagitis but is not recommended as primary therapy. It is somewhat more effective as an antacid than aluminum hydroxide. Magaldrate disturbs neither electrolyte balance nor bowel function. It should not be used in patients taking any form of tetracycline. It also is available in combination with simethicone.

Dose—*Usual,* **480** to **1080 mg** as required, preferably taken between meals and at bedtime.

Other Dose Information—Each tablet (480 mg) or 5 mL of suspension (540 mg) neutralizes 13.5 and 15 mEq, respectively, of acid in 60 min and contains 0.65 mg of sodium.

Dosage Forms—Oral Suspension: 540 mg/5 mL. Chewable Tablets: 480 mg. Swallow Tablets: 480 mg.

Magnesium Carbonate—see RPS-18, page 777.

Magnesium Hydroxide

Magnesium hydroxide [1309-42-8] $Mg(OH)_2$ (58.32).

Preparation—By precipitation using aqueous solutions of magnesium chloride or sulfate and sodium hydroxide. US Pat 3,127,241. A method for preparing it in various particle sizes is described in US Pat 3,232,708.

Description—White, very fine, bulky powder; slowly absorbs carbon dioxide on exposure to air.

Solubility—Practically insoluble in water or in alcohol; dissolves in dilute acids.

Uses—As a laxative and an antacid (although at usual doses it does not have enough neutralizing capacity to be defined as an antacid). Magnesium hydroxide is a mild cathartic that usually produces bowel movements in ½ to 6 hr. It probably acts by altering intestinal motility. It should not be used in patients with vomiting or abdominal pain.

As an antacid, it is not recommended, although frequently used. As with other magnesium-containing compounds, it should not be used in patients with impaired renal function.

Dose—*Usual, adult, laxative,* **1950** to **2600 mg** or **30** to **60 mL;** *antacid,* **650** to **1300 mg** or **5** to **15 mL.**

Dosage Forms—Tablets (regular and mint-flavored): 325 mg; Liquid (regular and mint-flavored): 390 mg per 5 mL.

Magnesium Oxide

Magnesia; Light Magnesia; Calcined Magnesia; Heavy Magnesium Oxide; Heavy Magnesia; Heavy Calcined Magnesia; Magnesia Usta; Uro-Mag and Mag-Ox 400 (*Blaine*)

[1309-48-4] MgO (40.30).

Preparation—Light or heavy magnesium carbonate is exposed to red heat, whereupon, CO_2 and H_2O are expelled, and light or heavy magnesium oxide is left. The density of the oxide also is influenced by the calcining temperature, higher temperatures yielding more compact forms.

Description—Very bulky, white powder known as light magnesium oxide or as a relatively dense, white powder known as heavy magnesium oxide. Readily absorbs moisture and carbon dioxide when exposed to air.

Solubility—Practically insoluble in water to which, however, it imparts an alkaline reaction; insoluble in alcohol; soluble in dilute acids.

Uses—An effective, fairly long-acting, nonsystemic *gastric antacid.* Since in water it is converted to the hydroxide, its biological properties are the same as the hydroxide. Consequently, it does not neutralize gastric contents excessively and does not liberate carbon dioxide. It is sometimes employed as a *cathartic.*

Light magnesia is preferable to the heavy for administration in liquids because, being a finer powder, it suspends more readily.

Dose—*Capsules:* **280 mg** to **1.5 g** taken with water or milk 4 times a day. *Tablets:* **400** to **820 mg** a day.

Other Dose Information—One g has a neutralizing capacity of 50 mEq of acid; however, only 8 to 20 mEq react with gastric acid in 30 min.

Magnesium Phosphate—see RPS-18, page 777.

Magnesium Trisilicate

Hydrated Magnesium Silicate; (*Various Mfrs*)

Magnesium silicate hydrate [39365-87-2] $2MgO.3SiO_2.xH_2O$; *anhydrous* [14987-04-3] (260.86). A compound of magnesium oxide and silicon dioxide with varying proportions of water. It contains not less than 20% of magnesium oxide [MgO = 40.30] and not less than 45% of silicon dioxide [SiO_2 = 60.08].

Preparation—By precipitating a solution of sodium silicate of the proper composition [$Na_4Si_3O_8$, or having a ratio of Na_2O to SiO_2 = 1:1.5] with a solution of magnesium chloride or sulfate.

Description—Fine, white odorless, tasteless powder, free from grittiness; its suspension is neutral or only slightly alkaline to litmus.

Solubility—Insoluble in water or alcohol; readily decomposed by mineral acids with the liberation of silicic acid.

Uses—A nonsystemic *antacid* and *adsorbent*. As an antacid, it has a slow onset of action and is relatively weak; as a single entity it can not meet current pH requirements for nonprescription antacids. Approximately 5% of the magnesium and 7% of the silicate may be absorbed. Therefore, a number of cases of siliceous nephrolith have been reported following chronic use. Large doses may cause diarrhea due to the action of the soluble magnesium salts on the gastrointestinal tract. It is available only in combination with other antacids.

Dose—**1** to **16g** a day; *usual,* **1 g** 4 times a day.

Dosage Forms—Tablets 500 mg and liquid.

Milk of Bismuth—see RPS-18, page 778.

Sodium Bicarbonate

Carbonic acid monosodium salt; Baking Soda;
Sodium Acid Carbonate

Monosodium carbonate [144-55-8] $NaHCO_3$ (84.01).

Preparation—May be produced by the ammonia-soda process, or *Solvay Process*, as it is usually called. In this process, CO_2 is passed into a solution of common salt in ammonia water, sodium bicarbonate is precipitated and ammonium chloride, being much more soluble, remains in solution. The ammonium chloride solution is heated with lime, whereby, the ammonia is regenerated and returned to the process.

Description—White, crystalline powder; odorless and has a saline and slightly alkaline taste; solutions, when freshly prepared with cold water without shaking, are alkaline to litmus paper; alkalinity increases as the solutions stand, are agitated or heated; stable in dry air, but slowly decomposes in moist air.

Solubility—1 g in 12 mL water; with hot water it is converted into carbonate; insoluble in alcohol.

Uses—Widely employed as a gastric *antacid*, especially by the laity, despite its many disadvantages. Sodium bicarbonate reacts with HCl to produce CO_2, thus giving rise to epigastric distress and eructation. Although the onset of action is rapid, the duration of action is short. Sodium bicarbonate is absorbed readily. Prolonged therapy with large doses will produce systemic alkalosis. Moreover, chronic therapy along with milk or calcium may precipitate the milk-alkali syndrome in patients with renal failure. Even moderate amounts may expand plasma volume, increase blood pressure and lead to edema. Therefore, it may be hazardous in patients with renal insufficiency, hypertension or cardiac failure.

In the treatment of *systemic acidosis*, sodium bicarbonate is specific in that the salt is composed of the two ions essential to correct this condition.

Sodium bicarbonate is used locally on the skin in the form of a moist paste or a solution. In this form, it is an effective *antipruritic*. The salt also is an ingredient of many effervescent mixtures, alkaline solutions, douches, etc.

Dose—**300 mg** to **16 g** a day; *usual,* **300 mg** to **2 g** 1 to 4 times a day.

Other Dose Information—The maximum daily intake is 200 mEq of bicarbonate in patients under 60 yr and 100 mEq in those over 60. Each g will neutralize 12 mEq of gastric acid in 60 min.

Dosage Forms—Injection: 1%/20 mL, 1.4 and 5%/500 mL, 7.5%/50 mL, 8.4%/40 mL; Tablets: 325, 520 and 650 mg.

Gastric Antacid Mixtures

Antacids are used commonly in combination for three reasons: (1) to combine fast- and slow-reacting antacids in order to obtain a product with a rapid onset and relatively even, sustained action; (2) to lower the dose of each component and minimize the possibility of certain adverse effects and (3) to use one component to antagonize one or more side effects of another component (eg, laxation versus constipation). The antacid substances listed in Table 1 are employed extensively in the preparation of antacid mixtures. Indeed, they are the principal ingredients in almost 100 OTC antacid preparations, including chewable tablets, 44 suspensions and gels. For example, examination of 78 antacid mixtures reveals that 72% are composed of aluminum hydroxide and magnesium hydroxide alone or with simethicone, 12% aluminum hydroxide and either magnesium trisilicate or magnesium carbonate, 11% magnesium oxide and/or calcium carbonate with simethicone and 5% magaldrate with simethicone. Simethicone is not an antacid. It is an antiflatulent frequently used in antacid combinations to defoam gastric juice in order to decrease the incidence of gastroesophageal reflux. It does not decrease the antacid requirement.

The acid neutralizing capacity (ANC) of the suspensions closely approximates that of the tablets, but in general their neutralizing capacity tends to be greater because tablets go into solution less well. *Gaviscon* is listed in the tables although it is not used in peptic ulcer disease and the ANC of its regular preparation does not qualify it as an antacid. Its unique formulation produces a foam which floats on the stomach contents. When acid reflux occurs, the foam precedes the stomach contents into the esophagus and protects the mucosa from further irritation. Hence, it is formulated specifically for acid indigestion due to acid reflux.

H_2-Receptor Antagonists

There are three histamine receptors. The second of these receptors mediates acid secretion by the gastric parietal cells and is inhibited by the H_2-receptor blocking drugs (Black *et al*: *Nature 236*:385, 1972). The identification of this receptor and its modulation introduced an era of pharmacology and led to the awarding of the Nobel Prize to Dr Black. The H_2-receptor antagonists are histamine analogs. They consist of ring structures with side chains. While the rings in the side chains differ among compounds, they all have in common a nitrogen either in the ring or immediately adjacent to the ring and a nitrogen on the side chain that is recognized by the receptor.

Table 1—The Relative Onset and Duration of Action, Sodium Content, Acid Neutralizing Capacity (ANC) and Potential Adverse Effects of Common Single-Entity Antacids

Antacid	Onset of action	Duration of action	Sodium (mg/unit)	ANC[a]	Adverse effects[b]
Aluminum carbonate gel	Slow	Short	0.12	12	AFGI
Aluminum hydroxide gel	Slow	Prolonged	<2.5	16	AFGI
Calcium carbonate	Fast	Prolonged	<2.3	10	ABCEH
Dihydroxaluminum sodium carbonate	Fast	Moderate	53	7.5-8.0	AGI
Magaldrate	Intermediate	Prolonged	<0.1	13.5	DFI
Magnesium carbonate	Intermediate	Prolonged	—	20/g	BD
Magnesium hydroxide	Fast	Short	0.12	14	BD
Magnesium oxide	Fast	Short	—	21	BD
Sodium bicarbonate	Fast	Short	88	12/g	CEJ

[a]ANC per capsule, tablet or 5-mL suspension unless otherwise indicated.

[b]A—constipation; B—laxation; C—hypercalcemia; D—hypermagnesia; E—metabolic alkalosis; F—neurotoxicity in renal failure; G—osteomalacia and osteoporosis; H—renal calculi; I—phosphorus depletion; J—swelling of feet.

Table 2—Composition, Sodium Content and Neutralizing Capacity of Some Proprietary Antacid Suspension

Product (*Mfr*)	Content (mg/5 mL)				ANC[a] (per 5 mL)
	$Al(OH)_3$	$Mg(OH)_2$	$CaCO_3$	Na	
Aludrox (*Wyeth*)	307	103	0	2.3	12
Alternagel (*J&J-Merck*)	0	0	0	0	0
Amphojel (*Wyeth-Ayerst*)	0	0	0	0.10	10
Basaljel (*Wyeth-Ayerst*)	0	0	0	2.9	12
Camalox (*Rhone-Poulenc Rorer*)	225	200	250	1.2	18.5
Di-Gel (*Plough*)	200	200	0	<5	10.5
Gaviscon (*Marion*)	31.7	137[b]	0	13	1
Gelusil (*Parke-Davis*)	200	200	0	0.7	12
Gelusil-II	400	400	0	1.3	24
Kudrox (*Kremers-Urban*)	565	180	0	<15	25
Maalox (*Rhone-Poulenc Rorer*)	225	200	0	1.4	13.3
Maalox TC	600	300	0	0.8	28.3
Marblen (*Fleming*)	0	400[b]	520	3	18
Mylanta (*Stuart*)	200	200	0	0.68	12.7
Mylanta II	400	400	0	1.14	25.4
Nephrox (*Fleming*)	320	0	0	0.19	9
Riopan Plus (*Ayerst*)	0	540[c]	0	>0.1	15
WinGel (*Winthrop-Breon*)	180	160	0	2.5	11.6

[a]Acid-neutralizing capacity (in milliequivalents).
[b]Magnesium carbonate.
[c]Magaldrate.

The exact mechanism of gastric acid secretion has yet to be elucidated. It is known that four endogenous substances—acetyl choline, the neurotransmitter of the vagus nerve; gastrin, a systemic hormone secreted by G cells in the antrum of the stomach; histamine, a paracrine hormone secreted by enterochromasin cells in the wall of the stomach and calcium all stimulate acid secretion. There are receptors for acetylcholine (muscarinic receptor), gastrin (gastrin receptor) and histamine (H_2-receptor). Calcium may both increase gastrin and act as a second messenger for gastrin and acetylcholine. Histamine probably activates adenylate cyclase which converts cytosolic ATP to cyclic AMP which acts as a second messenger. There is some evidence that histamine may act as the common mediator of acid secretion since it augments acetylcholine and gastrin stimulated secretion, and H_2-blockers inhibit both acid and gastrin stimulated secretion. The final common pathway of acid secretion is the proton pump, Na^+/K^+ ATPase. The physiological essence of Na^+/K^+ ATPase is to exchange K^+ for H^+ and H^+ is secreted against a profound concentration gradient of 2,000,000:1 or greater. This acid secretion is stimulated by the sight, smell and ingestion of food. In addition to the stimulated acid secretion, there is a basal acid secretion that occurs independently of eating. An important feature of basal acid secretion is its diurnal variation such that acid secretion is low during the day but relatively high at night—generally peaking between 10 pm and midnight. For this reason patients tend to wake up around midnight with dyspepsia and heartburn. It is at this time that gastric pH tends to drop to 1 or 2, since acid secretion is relatively high and is not neutralized by food. During the day, the food that stimulates acid secretion also neutralizes it, keeping the gastric pH about 4 or 5. The diurnal variation in acid secretion forms the rationale for using H_2-receptor antagonists as a single evening dose in the treatment of gastric and duodenal ulcers.

In addition to a stimulatory pathway of acid secretion, there is a closely related inhibitory system. This system is activated by prostaglandin E_2. (PGE_2) which appears to act on a membrane receptor which activates an inhibitory protein (GI) which blocks the histamine activation of adenylate cyclase.

Table 3—Composition, Sodium Content and Neutralizing Capacity of Some Proprietary Antacid Chewable Tablets

Product (*Mfr*)	Content (mg/tablet)				ANC[a] (per Unit)
	$Al(OH)_3$	$Mg(OH)_2$	$CaCO_3$	Na	
Aludrox (*Wyeth*)	233	83	0	1.4	10
Camalox (*Rhone-Poulenc Rorer*)	225	200	250	1	18
Di-Gel (*Plough*)	282[b]	85	0	<5	9
Gaviscon (*Marion*)	80	20[c]	0	18.4	0.5
Gelusil (*Parke-Davis*)	200	200	0	0.8	11
Gelusil-M	300	200	0	1.3	12.5
Gelulsil-II	400	400	0	2.1	21
Maalox No 1 (*Rhone-Poulenc Rorer*)	200	200	0	0.7	8.5
Maalox No 2	400	400	0	1.4	18
Maalox Plus	200	200	0	0.8	11.4
Maalox TC	600	300	0	0.5	28
Mylanta (*Stuart*)	200	200	0	0.77	11.5
Mylanta II	400	400	0	1.3	23
Riopan Plus (*Ayerst*)	0	480[d]	0	<0.1	13.5
Tums (*Norclift Thayer*)	0	500	0	<5	20
WinGel (*Winthrop-Breon*)	180	160	0	<2.5	12.3

[a]Acid-neutralizing capacity (in milliequivalents).
[b]Magnesium carbonate.
[c]Aluminum hydroxide and magnesium carbonate.
[d]Magnesium trisilicate.
[e]Magaldrate.

Another important function of PGE_2 in the gastric mucosa is to increase bicarbonate and mucus secretion, which enhances mucosal resistance to injury. Thus, the combined effect of PGE_2 is to inhibit acid secretion and increase mucosal protection, yet another example of the adaptive or protective function of the prostaglandin. There are other inhibitors of acid secretion. Somatostatin and secretin are probably the most important under physiological conditions.

The H_2-receptor antagonists were developed as the result of the intentional modification of the histamine structure in an effort to find analogs with a higher binding infinity for the H_2-receptor. Such compounds would displace histamine and thus act as competitive inhibitors. The first such substance was burimamide, but it was only effective when given intravenously. The next substance was metiamide, effective both orally and intravenously but abandoned because it caused agranulocytosis. Finally, in 1977, cimetidine was approved by the FDA. It quickly became the number-one selling drug in the world. It contains a substituted imidazole ring, like that in histamine. Subsequently, ranitidine, a substituted furan ring and famotidine and nizatidine, substituted thiazoles, were approved.

The H_2-receptor antagonists are a remarkably safe group of drugs. The list of adverse reactions is long, but the incidence is low. Among the side effects associated with all four drugs are headache, dizziness, malaise, myalgias, nausea, diarrhea, constipation, skin rashes, pruritus and impotence. It has been said that dementation and bradycardia are more common with intravenous cimetidine (especially in elderly patients), but the evidence supporting this contention is now convincing. A mild cardiotoxicity may be more common with famotidine. Impotence is said to occur more commonly with large IV doses of cimetidine, but again, the data supporting this are less than convincing. Mild hepatotoxicity has been seen with all of the compounds, probably more commonly with ranitidine. Overall, the incidence of side effects is so low that they are of little practical importance.

Cimetidine binds to part of the cytochrome P450-dependent mixed-function oxidase system.

Cimetidine

Guanidine, *N*″-cyano-*N*-methyl-*N*′-[2-[[(5-methyl-1*H*-imidazol-4-yl)-methyl]thio]ethyl]-, Tagamet (*Smith Kline & French*)

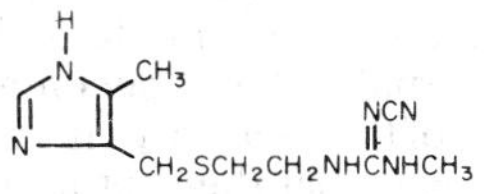

[51481-61-9] $C_{10}H_{16}N_6S$ (252.34).

Preparation—Methods of synthesis of analogs of histamine capable of functioning as H_2-receptor antagonists, of the type of cimetidine, are described in German Pats 2,344,779 and 2,344,833 (see *CA 80:* 146167h, 146168j, 1974). In one of these methods a substituted guanidine, such as $CH_3NHC(:NCN)SCH_3$, is refluxed with a histamine-related imidazole, as $NH_2CH_2CH_2SCH_2Z$ (in which Z is a methylimidazole), in methyl cyanide to produce the product N = CHNH(CH_3)C = $CHCH_2CH_2SCH_2Z$.

Description—White to off-white, crystalline powder; unpleasant odor; melts 141°–143°; pK_a 6.8.

Solubility—1 g in about 200 mL water, 18 mL alcohol, 1000 mL chloroform; insoluble in ether.

Uses—Cimetidine is used for the acute treatment of gastric ulcer, duodenal ulcer and gastroespohageal reflux. It also is used in the prophylaxis of the above conditions and the treatment of pathological hypersecretory conditions such as Zollinger-Ellison syndrome, systemic mastocytosis and multiple endocrine adenomas. Studies also suggest that cimetidine is effective in both prevention and treatment of stress ulcers.

Cimetidine competitively inhibits the action of histamine on the H_2 receptors of parietal cells, reducing gastric acid output and concentration. This reduction occurs under basal conditions as well as when gastric acid secretion is stimulated by food. The oral administration of 800 mg of cimetidine reduces nocturnal gastric acid output by 80% over an 8 hr period with no effect on daytime acid secretion in duodenal ulcer patients. The gastric pH is raised to 5 or greater for at least 2½ hr. Administered orally after a standard meal, 300 mg of cimetidine inhibited gastric secretion in duodenal ulcer patients by 50% during the first hr and by 75% during the subsequent 2 hr. Cimetidine, 800 mg at bedtime, 400 mg 2 times a day or 300 mg 4 times a day all reduce the 4-hr mean gastric pH by 50 to 60%. Nighttime dosing has the theoretical advantage of reducing nocturnal secretion while not affecting daytime secretion.

Cimetidine is absorbed rapidly, and well, after oral administration. A small portion of the drug is metabolized on its first pass through the liver; the average bioavailability is 70% when compared to intravenous injection; 19% is bound to serum proteins; volume of distribution is 1.5 L/kg; 48% is excreted unchanged; elimination half-life ranges from 2 to 3 hr; mean serum concentration is 500 ng/mL; and mean peak blood level is 1440 ng/mL.

Cimetidine has been reported to reduce hepatic metabolism of drugs that are metabolized primarily by cytochrome P-450, thereby delaying elimination and increasing blood levels of these drugs. Therefore, cimetidine should be used with caution in patients on *warfarin-type anticoagulants, phenytoin, beta-adrenergic-blocking agents, lidocaine* and *theophylline;* cimetidine reduces the hepatic metabolism of these substances, delays their elimination and increases their blood levels. The half-life of benzodiazepines is also increased in patients taking cimetidine. A *decrease* in serum digoxin may occur in patients taking both *digoxin* and cimetidine.

Adverse reactions are usually mild and transient; diarrhea, muscular pain, dizziness and rash have been reported in a few patients. A few cases of headache, ranging from mild to severe, have been reported. Reversible arthralgia, myalgia and exacerbation of joint symptoms in patients with pre-existing arthritis are observed on rare occasions. Mild gynecomastia has been reported in about 4% of patients with hypersecretory conditions; in all others the incidence was about 0.3 to 1%. A few cases of reversible confusional states in elderly or severely ill patients have been observed. Small increases in plasma creatinine and serum transaminase have been reported; all of these cleared when the drug was withdrawn. Interstitial nephritis also has been reported. The safe use of cimetidine in pregnant women or nursing mothers has not been established.

Dose—*Usual, oral, adult, duodenal ulcer,* **800 mg** in the evening. *Maintenance, healed duodenal ulcer,* **400 mg** in the evening. *Active gastric ulcer,* **800 mg** in the evening; *Gastroesophageal reflux disease,* **800 mg** 2 times a day. *Pathological hypersecretory states* (such as Zollinger-Ellison syndrome), **800 mg** 2 to 3 times a day. *Usual, adult, intravenous* (as the hydrochloride) **300 mg** administered in 20 mL of 0.9% sodium chloride solution or **300 mg** 100 mL of 5% dextrose by intermittent infusion. *Continuous infusion,* **37.5 mg/hr.** *Maintenance, duodenal ulcer,* **400 mg** at bedtime.

Dosage Forms—Tablets: 200, 300, 400 and 800 mg; Liquid (as the hydrochloride): 300 mg/5 mL; Injection (as the hydrochloride): single-dose vials, 300 mg/5 mL; multiple dose-vials, 8 mL (300 mg/2 mL); prefilled disposable syringes (300 mg/2 mL); plastic containers (300 mg/50 mL).

Cinnamon—page 1386.

Cinnamon, Ceylon—page 1391.

Cinnamon Oil—page 1391.

Coriander Oil—page 1391.

Famotidine

Propanimidamide, *N*′-(aminosulfonyl)-3-[[[2-((diaminomethylene)-amino]-4-thiazolyl]-methyl]thio-, Pepcid (*MSD*)

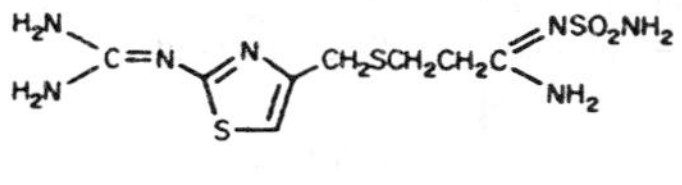

[76824-35-6] $C_8H_{15}N_7O_2S_3.HCl$ (337.43)

Preparation—Synthesized from *S*-(2-aminothiazol-4-ylmethyl)iso-thiourea, 3-chloropropionitrile and benzoylisothiocyanate in 9 steps. Belg Pat 882,071.

Description—White to pale yellow crystalline solid, melting at 163–164°.

Solubility—Freely soluble in glacial acetic acid; slightly soluble in methanol; very slightly soluble in water; practically insoluble in ethanol. At 25°, in water, pK_a is 7.1.

Uses—Famotidine, an inhibitor of H_2 receptors, is recommended for the short-term treatment of active duodenal ulcer, gastric ulcer and gastro-esophageal reflux. It also is recommended for maintenance therapy of duodenal ulcer after the active ulcer has healed and management of pathological hypersecretory conditions, such as Zollinger-Ellison Syndrome and multiple endocrine adenomas. The duration of secretion inhibition after doses of 20 and 40 mg is usually 10 to 12 hr, respectively. Famotidine is absorbed incompletely. Bioavailability of oral doses is 40 to 45%; this may be increased slightly by food or decreased slightly by antacids. After oral doses, peak plasma levels occur in 1 to 3 hr; the peak plasma level is not altered by chronic administration; and elimination half-life is 2.5 to 3.5 hr. It is eliminated largely unchanged by the renal route (65 to 70%) and the remainder (30 to 35%) by metabolic routes. The only metabolite identified is the *S*-oxide. Thus, famotidine should be used in reduced dosage and at longer time intervals in patients with severe renal insufficiency. Adverse reactions reported to occur in more than 1% of patients include headache (4.7%), dizziness (1.8%), constipation (1.2%) and diarrhea (1.7%). Other adverse reactions reported include fever, asthenia, fatigue, palpitations, nausea, vomiting and abdominal distress, anorexia, dry mouth, liver enzyme abnormalities, thrombocytopenia, orbital edema, pain, arthralgia, paresthesias, psychic disturbances (depression, anxiety, decreased libido, hallucinations, insomnia and somnolence), bronchospasm, alopecia, acne, pruritus, rash and flushing. Although reproductive studies in laboratory animals revealed no evidence of impaired fertility or harm to the fetus, safety in pregnancy or in nursing mothers has not been established.

Dose—*Usual, adult, oral, duodenal ulcer,* **40 mg** in the evening *maintenance*: **20 mg**. *Gastric ulcer,* **40 mg** in the evening. *Gastroesophageal reflux disease,* **40 mg** in the evening or **20 mg** twice a day. *Hypersecretory conditions* (such as Zollinger-Ellison Syndrome), **20 mg** every 6 hr. *Impaired renal function,* **20 mg** at bedtime or **40 mg** every 36 to 48 hr, as indicated. *Intravenous administration,* **20 mg** every 12 hr.

Dosage Forms—Tablets: 20 and 40 mg; Injection: 10 mg per mL, in 2 mL single-dose or 4 mL multidose vials (must be refrigerated); Powder for Oral Suspension: 400 mg (40 mg/5 mL when reconstituted).

Nizatidine

1,1-Ethenediamine, *N*-[2-[[[2-[(dimethylamino)methyl]-4-thiazolyl]-methyl]thio]ethyl]-*N'*-methyl-2-nitro-, Axid (*Lilly*)

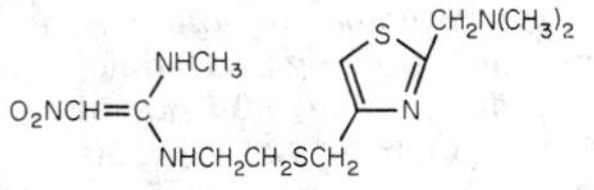

[76963-41-2] $C_{12}H_{21}N_5O_2S_2$ (331.45).

Uses—Nizatidine, a reversible inhibitor of H_2 receptors, is used in the treatment of active duodenal ulcer active, gastric ulcer, gastroesophageal reflux and maintenance of duodenal ulcer. After oral administration of 100 and 300 mg, peak plasma concentrations of 700 to 1800 μg/L and 1400 to 3600 μg/L, respectively, occur within 0.5 to 3 hr; plasma concentrations after 12 hr are less than 10 μg/L. Elimination half-life is 1 to 2 hr, plasma clearance 40 to 60 L/hr and volume distribution 0.8 to 1.5 L/kg. More than 90% of an oral dose is excreted in the urine within 12 hr; 60% as unchanged drug. Therefore, it should be used in reduced dosage in patients with severe renal insufficiency. Adverse reactions include somnolence, sweating and urticaria. Hepatocellur injury, ventricular tachycardia, decreased libido, gynecomastia and thrombocytopenia have been reported. Safety and efficacy in children has not been established.

Dose—*Usual, oral, adult, duodenal ulcer,* **300 mg** into the evening. *Maintenance of healed ulcer,* **150 mg** in the evening. *Gastric Ulcer,* **300 mg** once a day in the evening. *Gastroesophageal reflux,* **300 mg** in the evening or **150 mg** twice a day. *Impaired renal function,* **150 mg** a day or every other day.

Dosage Form—Capsules: 150 and 300 mg.

Ranitidine

1,1-Ethenediamine, *N*-[2-[[[5-[(dimethylamino)methyl]-2-furanyl]-methyl]thio]ethyl]-*N'*-methyl-2-nitro-, Zantac (*Glaxo*)

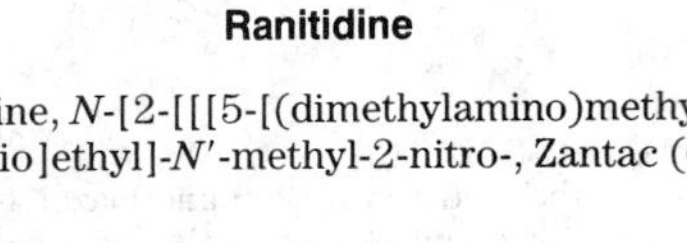

[66357-35-5] $C_{13}H_{22}N_4O_3S$ (314.40).

Preparation—See US Pat 4,128,658.

Description—White solid melting about 70°.

Uses—Ranitidine, a substituted furan derivative, is an H_2-receptor antagonist indicated for the short-term treatment of *duodenal ulcer* and the management of *hypersecretory conditions,* such as *Zollinger-Ellison Syndrome* and *systemic mastocytosis.* The pharmacokinetic profile of ranitidine is similar to that for cimetidine. Neither product is long acting and they have similar half-lives. Oral absorption appears to be variable and decreased if given concurrently with antacids; bioavailability after an oral dose of 150 mg is approximately 50% (range 40 to 88%); 15% is bound to plasma protein; volume distribution 1.4 L/kg; 30% of the administered dose is excreted unchanged; elimination half-life ranges from 2.5 to 3.0 hr; serum concentrations vary from 36 to 94 ng/mL; and mean peak blood levels are 440 to 545 ng/mL. Ranitidine is not inherently long acting and it lacks a predictable dose/response relationship. For example, 75, 100 and 150 mg of ranitidine inhibits nocturnal gastric acid output by 95, 96 and 92%, respectively. Although the limited clinical experience suggests that ranitidine may interact with only a limited number of other drugs, interactions with warfarin, benzodiazepines, fentanyl, metaprolol, nefedipine and acetaminophen have been reported. Likewise, few adverse reactions have been encountered; headache, malaise, dizziness, constipation, nausea, abdominal pain and rash have been observed most frequently. Decreased white blood cell and platelet count also have been reported. Increases (up to 5 times the upper limit of normal) in serum transaminase and gammaglutamyl transpeptidase have been noted. Rare cases of hepatitis also have been reported. In normal volunteers, SGPT were increased at least twice the pretreatment levels in 6 of 12 subjects given 100 mg 4 times a day intravenously for 7 days and in 4 of 24 subjects given 50 mg 4 times daily intravenously for 5 days. This dose-related effect suggests that ranitidine is potentially hepatotoxic. With respect to use in pregnancy and lactation, studies in rats and rabbits have revealed no evidence of impaired fertility or harm to the fetus. Nevertheless, it should not be used in pregnancy unless needed. Ranitidine is secreted in milk; therefore, it should not be used in nursing mothers unless absolutely necessary.

Dose—*Usual, adult, oral, duodenal ulcer,* **300 mg** in the evening; *maintenance, healed ulcer,* **150 mg** in the evening. *Gastric ulcer,* **200 mg** in the evening. *Gastroesophageal reflux,* **150 mg** twice a day or **200 mg** in the evening. *Hypersecretory conditions* (such as Zollinger-Ellison Syndrome): **150 mg** 2 times a day. *Impaired renal function:* **150 mg** every 12 to 24 hr.

Dosage Forms—Injection: single-dose vials 2 mL (25 mg/mL) and multi-dose vials of 10 mL (25 mg/mL); Tablets: 150 and 300 mg. All dosage forms must be refrigerated and protected from light.

Proton Pump Inhibitors

The final common pathway in gastric acid secretion is the *proton pump*—an H^+/K^+ ATPase. The physiological essence of this enzyme is the exchange of hydrogen ion for potassium ion. Thus, hydrogen is secreted by the parietal cell in exchange for potassium. In the resting state, the proton pump resides on the inner membrane of secretory vesicles within the parietal cell. When the cell is activated by eating (or by pharmacological stimulus), the inner membrane of the vesicle is externalized and becomes the outer; ie, the secretory membrane of the secretory villous. The physiological importance of this is that the proton pump inhibitors can only inhibit the H^+/K^+ ATPase when it is externalized. Thus, these drugs are more potent when taken prior to meals and when taken orally.

The proton pump inhibitors belong to a new class of antisecretory drugs called substituted benzimidazoles. The prototype, omeprazole, is an irreversible inhibitor of the proton pump. It has a plasma half life of 0.5 to 1.0 hour, but its duration of action is greater than 24 hours reflecting the time required to generate new hydrogen potassium ATPase.

The proton pump inhibitors are used for the short-term treatment of acid peptic disease, gastroesophageal reflux, gastric ulcer, duodenal ulcer and Zollinger-Ellison syndrome. The therapeutic advantages of the proton pump inhibitors over the H_2-receptor antagonists are a faster healing rate, a higher healing rate and the ability to heal patients who have not been helped by H_2-receptor antagonist therapy.

There are numerous side effects of the proton pump inhibitors, but they occur infrequently. Headache, diarrhea, abdominal pain, dizziness, rash and constipation are seen with about the same frequency as seen with H_2-blockers, ie, 1 to 5%. A major concern with the use of proton pump inhibitors is an elevation of serum gastrin. The elevations are 1.5 to 4-fold—about twice that seen with H_2-blockers. Gastrin is a trophic hormone that causes enterochromaffin cells to proliferate in rats. These cells produce histamine and are the precursor of carcinoid tumors in rats. The effect in rats is almost certainly mediated through gastrin rather than from a carcinogenic effect of the drug itself since the tumors do not occur after antrectomy—a situation that precludes an increase in serum gastrin. Human studies have shown only a slight increase in the enterochromattin cell population with chronic use of proton pump inhibitors. Carcinoid tumors have not been reported in human subjects using omeprazole. Nevertheless, there is an increased incidence of carcinoid tumors in patients with pernicious anemia, a condition that also is associated with hypergastrinemia. The FDA has warned against prolonged use of omeprazole. Long-term studies in Europe, however, support the view that omeprazole is safe and efficacious for long-term (five years plus) prophylaxis of ulcer disease.

Omeprazole

1*H*-Benzimidazole,
5-methoxy-2-[[(4-methoxy-3,5-dimethyl-2-pyridinyl)-methyl]sulfinyl]-, Prilosec (*MSD*)

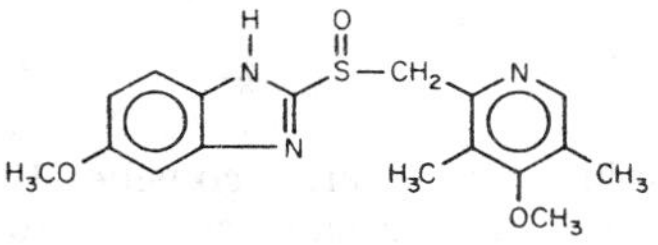

[73590-58-6] $C_{17}H_{19}N_3O_3S$ (345.42).

Preparation—US Pat 4,255,431.

Description—White crystals melting about 156°; pK_a (pyridine-N) 4.0, (imidazole-N) 8.7.

Solubility—1 g in about 8000 mL water or 25 mL alcohol.

Uses—In the treatment of acid peptic disorders. It is approved for the short-term treatment of duodenal ulcer, severe or poorly responsive gastroesophageal reflux and hypersecretory conditions such as Zollinger-Ellison syndrome, systemic mastocytosis and multiple endocrine adenomas. It is now thought that, with the exception of nonsteroidal induced and *Helicobacter pylori*-induced ulcers, the acid peptic diseases are lifelong diseases that require a lifetime of therapy. Long-term studies have demonstrated efficacy in the prevention of recurrence of reflux esophagitis and duodenal ulcer, but there is reluctance to use omeprazole long term because of the fear, probably unfounded, of carcinoid tumors. The current trend in practice is to use omeprazole for short-term healing and then switch to an H_2-receptor antagonist for maintenance. However, patients with resistant reflux esophagitis usually have already failed H_2-receptor antagonists and typically relapse rather quickly when switched back. It is becoming more common practice to continue omeprazole long term. The wisdom of this practice remains to be established.

Omeprazole, because of its acid lability, is given as a delayed-release capsule. Absorption occurs in the small bowel with peak plasma levels occurring at 0.5 to 3.5 hr. Peak plasma levels and AUC are approximately proportional to dose in the therapeutic range. Bioavailability is 30 to 40%. Plasma half-life is 0.5 to 1 hr with total body clearance 500 to 600 mL/min. Protein-binding is approximately 95%. Two plasma metabolites have been identified: hydroxyomeprazole and its corresponding carboxylic acid. The metabolites have virtually no antisecretory activity. Most of the drug is eliminated as metabolites in the urine. Dosage adjustment is not needed for patients with impaired renal function.

The antisecretory effect of omeprazole occurs within 1 hr, with maximum effect occurring within 2 hr. Inhibition of secretion remains at about 50% at 24 hr and lasts approximately 72 hr. The prolonged effect, beyond that expected for a drug with a short half-life, is due to irreversible binding to the H^+/K^+ ATPase. The effect of the treatment plateaus in 3 to 4 days and lasts for 3 to 5 days after discontinuing treatment. Omeprazole, at therapeutic doses of 20 to 40 mg causes an 80 to 95% decrease in 24-hr intragastric acidity.

Duodenal ulcer healing occurs in 80 to 95% of patients at 4 wk. Reflux esophagitis healing occurs in 8 wk in approximately 75% of patients.

Adverse reactions reported to occur in more than 1% of patients include headache (6.9%), diarrhea (3.0%), abdominal pain (2.4%), nausea (2.2%), dizziness (1.5%), vomiting (1.5%), rash (1.5%), constipation (1.1%), asthenia (1.1%) and back pain (1.1%). There continues to be concern about the development of carcinoid tumors after long-term treatment but, in fact, such tumors have not been reported.

Dose—*Usual, adult, oral, duodenal ulcer* or *gastroesophageal reflux*, **20 mg** once a day in the morning. *Hypersecretory conditions* (such as Zollinger-Ellison syndrome), dosage is adjusted to the individual needs of the patient; *usual* initially **60 mg** once a day.

Dosage Form—Delayed-Release Capsules: 20 mg.

Drugs That Enhance Mucosal Protection

Misoprostil

Prost-13-en-1-oic acid,
(11α, 13*E*)-(±)-11,16-dihydroxy-16-methyl-9-oxo-, methyl ester;
Cytotec (*Searle*)

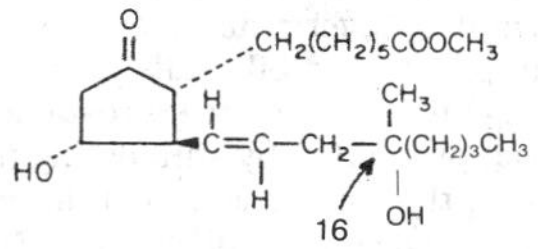

[59122-46-2]$C_{22}H_{38}O_5$(382.54).

Preparation—*J Med Chem 20:*1152, 1957.

Description—Pale yellow oil. It is a mixture of the (±)-*R* and (±)-*S* forms with reference to carbon atom no 16.

Solubility—1 g in 2500 mL of water or 100 mL of alcohol.

Uses—In the prevention of NSAIDs gastropathy. A prostaglandin E_1 analog, differs from the naturally occurring compound in that it is more water soluble and has a longer half-life. It both inhibits gastric secretion and increases mucosal resistance. Its inhibition of acid secretion, however, may not be sufficient to cause a therapeutic effect. Misoprostil probably derives its therapeutic benefit in the GI tract by increasing mucous and bicarbonate secretion by the gastric epithelium, thus enhancing mucosal protection.

Misoprostil is used for the prevention of gastric injury by NSAIDs. Controlled studies demonstrate that both the 100 μg 4 times a day and 200 μg 4 times a day dose are very effective in preventing gastric injury induced by NSAIDs. It is superior to H_2-blockers in preventing gastric ulcers, but not duodenal ulcers. It is superior to sucralfate in preventing both gastric and duodenal ulcers.

It is not yet clear which patients should receive misoprostil routinely for prophylaxis of NSAID-induced injury or under what circumstances misoprostil is cost effective. The patients at greatest risk for NSAIDs injury are patients with a previous history of ulcer disease, the elderly, patients with concomitant debilitating disease and patients on multiple drug therapy.

Misoprostil is also effective in the treatment of gastric ulcer, duodenal ulcer and stress ulcer, but is not approved for these uses, presumably because it has more side effects and no therapeutic advantage over H_2 blockers.

Side effects from misoprostil have, to some extent, limited its use. At the 200 μg 4 times a day dose, more than 30% of patients have diarrhea. This appears to be less at the 100 μg 4 times a day dose which should be the initial dose. It has no effect on gastrointestinal hormones (gastrin, motilin, somatostatin and vasoactive intestinal peptide) and no effect on gastric motility.

Misoprostil, because it causes uterine contractions, is contraindicated in pregnancy. It is rapidly (T_{max}: 12 min) and extensively absorbed. It has a terminal half-life of 20 to 40 min with 80% being recovered in the urine. Dosage adjustment is not needed in patients with renal impairment. There is no effect on hepatic mixed-function oxidase systems and no drug interactions are known. Misoprostil does not inhibit the therapeutic benefit of NSAIDs in rheumatoid arthritis.

Dose—*Usual, oral, adult,* for *prevention of NSAIDs injury*, **100 μg** 4 times a day or **200 μg** 2 times a day.

Dosage Form—Tablets: 100 and 200 μg.

Sucralfate

α-D-Glucopyranoside, β-D-fructofuranosyl-, octakis(hydrogen sulfate), aluminum complex; Carafate (*Marion Merrell Dow*)

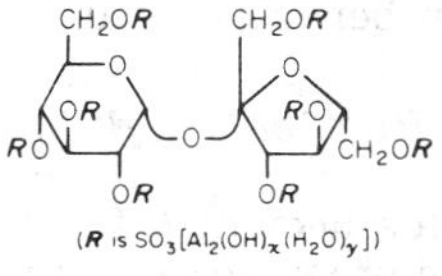

(*R* is $SO_3[Al_2(OH)_x(H_2O)_y]$)

[54182-58-0] $C_{12}H_mAl_{16}O_nS_8$ (*m* and *n* are approximately 54 and 75, respectively, giving an average molecular weight of about 2086 daltons).

Preparation—See US Pat 3,432,489.
Description—White powder; pK_a between 0.43 and 1.19.
Solubility—Practically insoluble in water; soluble in fixed alkali or acids.
Uses—Sucralfate is approved for short-term (8 wk) therapy of duodenal ulcers and, at reduced dosage, for maintenance therapy of duodenal ulcer. Clinical reports indicate that 1 g 4 times a day for 4 weeks will completely heal 73 to 92% of duodenal ulcers. Antacids may be prescribed as needed for pain relief. Sucralfate is absorbed minimally from the gastrointestinal tract. The mechanism by which sucralfate accelerates healing of duodenal ulcer remains to be defined fully. Sucralfate has negligible acid-neutralizing properties; therefore, its antiulcer effects cannot be attributed to neutralization of gastric acid. It is thought that sucralfate forms an ulcer-adherent complex with proteinaceous exudate at the ulcer site; this complex covers the ulcer site and protects it against further attack by acid, pepsin and bile salts. Animal studies, however, suggest that sucralfate may enhance local prostaglandin synthesis which would increase mucosal protection by stimulating mucous and bicarbonate secretion. Whatever the mechanism, sucralfate is effective in healing ulcers. There are no known contraindications. Nevertheless, it should not be used during pregnancy or in nursing mothers unless clearly needed. Since sucralfate is an aluminum salt of a sulfated disaccharide, it may prevent absorption of tetracycline, phenytoin, H_2 blockers, warfarin or digoxin if the drugs are given simultaneously; giving the drugs 2 hr apart minimizes these effects. Adverse effects occur in approximately 5% of patients; constipation is most common (2.2%). Other adverse effects include diarrhea, nausea, gastric discomfort, indigestion, dry mouth, rash, pruritus, back pain, dizziness, sleepiness and vertigo.
Dose—*Usual, adult, oral, for duodenal ulcer,* **1 g** 4 times a day on an empty stomach (1 hr before each meal and at bedtime); for *ulcer maintenance,* **1g** 2 times a day.
Dosage Form—Tablets: 1 g.

Digestants

Digestants are drugs which promote the process of digestion in the gastrointestinal tract. With the exception of pancreatic enzymes, they have limited usefulness in the treatment of conditions characterized by a deficiency of one or more of the specific substances essential for the digestion of foodstuffs. In a general way, they may be classified as drugs used for replacement therapy in deficiency states. The digestants commonly employed are the *choleretics* (bile, bile acids and bile salts) hydrochloric acid and pancreatic enzymes (see below).

Although bile is composed of a variety of substances, only the bile salts (salts of the native bile acids, page 782) are therapeutically important. When given by mouth the bile salts are absorbed from the intestine and re-excreted by the liver in the bile, thus, entering the same cyclic process (enterohepatic circulation) as endogenous bile salts. They are of little value in promoting the absorption of fats and fat-soluble vitamins from the intestinal tract but are useful in the dissolution of gallstones and perhaps in the symptomatic treatment of primary biliary cirrhosis and primary sclerosing cholangitis.

Hydrochloric acid exerts several physiological functions in the gastrointestinal tract. It converts pepsinogen to active pepsin, renders gastric contents relatively sterile, plays a role in the normal emptying of the stomach, aids in the secretion of intestinal and pancreatic juices, is important for the absorption of iron and plays a minor role in maintaining systemic pH homeostasis. It also may protect the GI tract from environmental carcinogens. *Achlorhydria,* a complete absence of acid secretion, frequently is associated with atrophic gastritis and pernicious anemia, both of which may predispose to adenocarcinoma of the stomach and gastric carcinoma. Despite this, there is no evidence that gastric acid replacement therapy has any beneficial effect.

Bile, Bile Acids and Bile Salts

Bile, a viscid, bitter, alkaline (pH 7.8) fluid, isotonic with serum and yellowish brown to golden yellow in color, is excreted by adults at the rate of 500 to 1100 mL per 24 hours. The principal organic constituents are bile acids (as salts), bile pigments, cholesterol, lecithin and mucin. The principal inorganic constituents are sodium, calcium, copper, iron, magnesium, potassium, bicarbonate, phosphate and sulfate.

The bile acids, present as the sodium salts of a mixture of acids, are divided into two groups: primary (derived from cholesterol) and secondary (derived from primary bile acids). The bile salts are conjugated through peptide linkages to glycine or taurine. The primary bile salts on the taurine or glycine conjugate cholic acid and chenic acid, while the secondary bile salts on the aminoacids conjugate deoxycholic and lithocholic acids.

The predominant bile acids represented in bile are cholic, chenic, deoxycholic and lithocholic. The structural relationships among these and their parent molecule, 5b-cholanic acid, are shown below. The synthetic dehydrocholic acid is included for comparison.

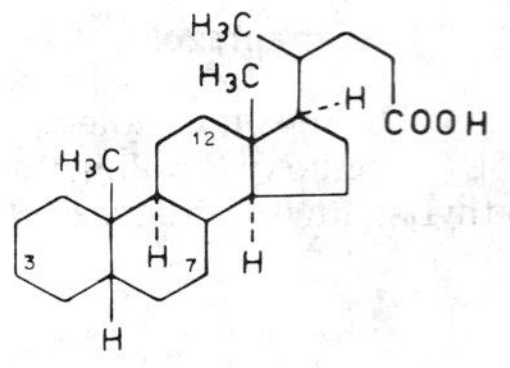

H3C H3C H COOH 12 H3C 3 H 7 H H

The composition of bile varies considerably with the species of animal. The bile salts can be isolated as stable crystals soluble in water. The free bile acids can be obtained; they are only slightly soluble in water. These acids combine with the fatty acids in the intestine as mixed micelles. In so doing, both acids are responsible for emulsifying, dispersing and, thus, promoting the absorption of fats, cholesterol and the fat-soluble vitamins. However, the primary clinical use of bile acids is the dissolution of cholesterol gallstones.

Ursodiol

Cholan-24-oic acid, (3α,5β,7β)-3,7-dihydroxy-, Ursodeoxycholic Acid; Actigall (*Summit*)

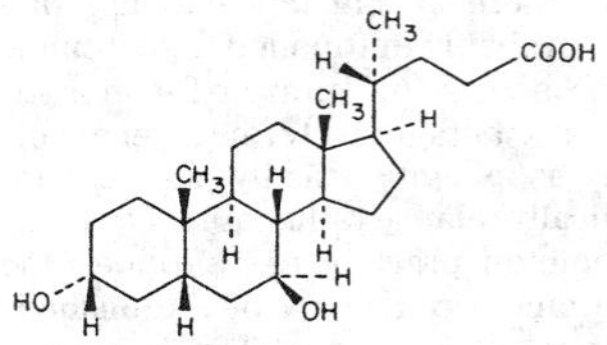

CH3 H COOH CH3 H CH3 H H H HO H H OH

[128-13-2] $C_{24}H_{40}O_4$ (392.58).
Preparation—For the isolation, see *J Biochem (Japan) 7:* 505, 1927.
Description—Platelets, melting about 203°; $pK_a \approx 5$.
Solubility—Practically insoluble in water; freely soluble in alcohol; slightly soluble in chloroform; very slightly soluble in ether.
Uses—A naturally occurring bile acid that is found in small amounts in man and in large amounts in bear (hence the name urso). It is the 7β epimer of chenodeoxycholic acid—an important primary bile acid in man. It reduces the cholesterol saturation of bile by inhibiting HMG-CoA reductase—the rate-limiting enzyme in cholesterol synthesis. It is used for the dissolution of radiolucent (ie, cholesterol) gallstones. It also has been used in the treatment of primary biliary cirrhosis, primary sclerosing cholangitis and chronic active hepatitis, but without proved therapeutic benefit. Ursodiol is 90% absorbed in the small bowel. Upon absorption, it enters the portal circulation and then is extracted by the liver, where it is conjugated with glycine or taurine and finally secreted into bile and ultimately back into the intestine. This intrahepatic recirculation of ursodiol ultimately results in some replacement of endogenous bile acids such that after about 3 wk of therapy, ursodiol makes up about 60% of the total bile acid pool. Since the total bile acid pool also is increased, cholesterol more readily can be solubilized and cholesterol gallstones are dissolved gradually. Once ursodiol is conjugated, little change occurs in the liver or intestine. Small amounts of 7-ketolithocholic acid or lithocholic acid are formed, but mostly lost in the feces. This is helpful since larger amounts of lithocholic acid are hepatotoxic. There is also some deconjugation of

ursodiol in the intestine. The resultant free ursodiol is reabsorbed and subsequently reconjugated in the liver.

Clinical trials with ursodiol demonstrate that gallstone dissolution occurs in about 30% of patients with gallstones less than 20 mm in diameter treated for up to 2 yr. Patients with larger stones or with nonvisualizing gallbladders on oral cholecystogram rarely dissolve their stones. However, patients with floating stones less than 0.5 cm in diameter have a greater than 50% chance of dissolution.

Dose—*For radiolucent gallbladder stones* **8** to **10 mg/kg/day** given in 2 or 3 divided doses.

Dosage Form—Capsules: 300 mg.

Malt Extract—page 1399.

Pancreatin—page 1138.

Resorcinol—see RPS-16, page 1107.

Pancreatic Enzymes

Pancreatic enzymes are approved for the treatment of malabsorption secondary to pancreatic insufficiency caused by chronic pancreatitis, pancreatectomy and cystic fibrosis. They also have been advocated for the treatment of chronic pancreatitis and pancreatic fistulae. Pancreatic enzyme preparations consist of mixtures of lipase, amylase and protease.

Lipase hydrolyzes dietary triglycerides at the alpha position, forming two molecules of fatty acid and a molecule of beta-monoglyceride. In so doing, the large triglyceride molecule is converted to three smaller molecules that can be incorporated in mixed micelles for solubilization and transported in the intestine.

Amylase is an alpha-1,4-glucosidase, which splits straight chain polyglucosides (the amyloses in dietary starch) into maltose and maltotriose. These subsequently are cleaved into glucose by intestinal brush-border enzymes and absorbed.

Protease is a mixture of proteolytic enzymes—trypsin, chymotrypsin and elastase—that cleaves peptide bonds in the center of proteins and polypeptides. The hydrolytic products of these enzymes are amino acids and oligopeptides. The amino acids are absorbed directly while the oligopeptides are split further by brush-border enzymes or intracellular enzymes before being transported in the portal circulation to the liver.

The treatment of malabsorption is the traditional indication for pancreatic enzymes. The major manifestation of pancreatic malabsorption is steatorrhea—a voluminous malodorous stool that is light in color and laden with the fat that is not being absorbed. Clinical steatorrhea does not occur until pancreatic lipase output is less than 10% of normal. Thus, the lipase content of the pancreatic enzyme replacement preparation is the critical factor in the treatment of steatorrhea. Only a few preparations have sufficient lipase to be effective. (see Table 4 for enzyme contents) Because lipase is inhibited irreversibly below pH 4, the enzyme preparations either have to be enteric coated or need to be given with sodium bicarbonate supplementation to avoid inactivation. The new microsphere preparations, Creon, Entolase-HP, Pancrease MT16 and Zymase, appear to have the most bioavailability. The usual dose is 3 capsules prior to each meal. When using Viokase (8 tablets), Cotazym (6 capsules) or Ilozyme (4 capsules), adjuvant therapy with 650 mg sodium bicarbonate before and after meals should be used. In general, further increasing the dose of enzymes doesn't lead to much improvement in steatorrhea and may aggravate abdominal bloating and cramping.

The treatment of abdominal pain in patients with chronic pancreatitis is complex and controversial. Many of the patients have chronic pain syndrome with narcotic addiction. An important component of pain management in these patients is withdrawal from pain medications which, in themselves, may be perpetuating the pain. Once this is done, correction of mechanical problems, ie, drainage of pseudocysts and the correction of duct stenosis, is essential. If pain persists, there is evidence that large doses of pancreatic enzymes will decrease pain in these patients. The rationale for this treatment is that "resting" the pancreas will allow it to heal. Pancreatic enzymes inhibit cholecystokinin, which stimulates pancreatic secretion when food reaches the duodenum. Putting the pancreas to rest presently eliminates the pain which occurs when the pancreas is actively secreting. The effective components of the pancreatic enzymes for relieving pain are the serine proteases (trypsin, chymotrypsin and elastase). Patients with idiopathic chronic pancreatitis appear to respond better than patients with chronic alcoholic pancreatitis. Finally, pancreatic enzymes also have been advocated for the treatment of pancreatic fistulae and for the reduction and frequency of attacks of acute recurrent pancreatitis. To date, there are no controlled studies to support this type of therapy.

Laxatives

Laxatives are drugs that either accelerate fecal passage or decrease fecal consistency. They work by promoting one or more of the mechanisms that cause diarrhea. Constipation, however, is a symptom that reflects an underlying problem. It has different meanings for different people but, in general, refers to stools that are too small, too infrequent or too difficult to expel. Patients also may describe it as a sense of incomplete evacuation. None of these definitions is easy to quantify and the normal range is wide. Normal stool weight is largely a function of diet. Thus, stools generated by the Western diet, which tends to be low in undigestible fiber, weigh 100 to 200 g a day while stools in Africa tend to weigh 400 to 500 g a day. Similarly, the frequency of stools varies greatly. Stool weight and frequency also are largely a function of the diet. It is said that normal stool frequency varies from three stools a day to three a week. There are few studies to determine what really is normal but in the Western world, it is believed that fewer than

Table 4—Pancreatic Enzymes

Name	Manufacturer	Formulation	Enzyme content[a,b]
Cotazym	Organon	Powder in capsules	L, 8000; P, 30,000; A, 30,000
Cotazym S	Organon	Enteric-coated spheres in capsules	L, 8000; P, 30,000; A, 30,000
Creon	Solvay	Enteric-coated microspheres in capsules	L, 8000; P, 13,000; A, 30,000
Creon 25	Solvay	Enteric-coated microspheres in capsules	L, 25,000; P, 62,500; A, 74,700
Entozyme	Robins	Tablets	L, 6,000; P, 7,500; A, 7,500
Pancrease	McNeil	Enteric-coated microspheres in capsules	L, 4,000; P, 25,000; A, 30,000
Pancrease MT 4	McNeil	Enteric coated microtablets in capsules	L, 4,000; P, 12,000; A, 12,000
Pancrease MT 10	McNeil	Enteric coated microtablets in capsules	L, 10,000; P, 30,000; A, 30,000
Pancrease MT 16	McNeil	Enteric coated microtablets in capsules	L, 16,000; P, 48,000; A, 48,000
Viokase	Robins	Tablets Powder (1/4 tsp.)	L, 8,000; P, 30,000; A, 30,000
Zymase	Organon	Enteric-coated spheres in capsules	L, 12,000; P, 24,000; A, 24,000

[a] L - lipase; P - protease, A - amylase.

[b] Expressed in USP units. USP units (*in vitro* test method) indicate digestive capacity such that 1000 units of lipase digests 3.5 g of fat, 1000 units of protease digests 1 g of protein and 1000 units of amylase digests 1 g of starch.

five stools a week is abnormal. Another definition may be a change to less frequency than usual for a particular individual.

Since constipation is a symptom rather than a disease, medical evaluation should be undertaken in patients who develop constipation. The wide availability and marketing of OTC laxatives has the potential to preclude appropriate diagnosis. The commonest cause is irritable bowel disease, but constipation may be associated with neurogenic diseases, systemic diseases and pharmacological causes as well as bowel disease. All of these may require primary treatment independent of symptomatic treatment with laxatives. For this reason, indiscriminate use of laxatives to relieve constipation is not recommended.

Laxatives are divided into several categories as a function of their mechanism of action.

Bulk-forming laxatives consist of polysaccharides and cellulose derivatives that are undigestible. Because they absorb water, they increase the bulk of stool and, in so doing, provide a physiological stimulus to defecation. They also may affect bile acid composition with subsequent effects on water absorption and secretion by the intestine.

Emollient laxatives, such as docusate sodium, are surfactants, which facilitate mixture of water and lipid soluble substances to soften stool. They also stimulate water secretion in the GI tract.

Lubricant laxatives, such as mineral oil, allow easier passage of a stool because of an oil coating. They may also inhibit colonic reabsorption of water.

Saline laxatives, such as magnesium citrate and sodium phosphate, exert an osmotic effect that increases the water content and volume of stool.

Stimulant laxatives, such as bisacodyl, phenolphthalein and senna, work by various mechanisms including inhibition of absorption, enhancement of secretion and effects on motility. In general, these laxatives have the most toxicity and are less physiological in their actions.

Hyperosmotic laxatives, such as lactulose, exert an osmotic effect and may have some effect on intestinal motility.

Patients who use laxatives should be reminded of the following points: laxatives are not for long-term use; if they are not effective after 1 week, a physician should be consulted. Laxative products which contain more than 15 mEq (345 mg) of sodium, more than 25 mEq (975 mg) of potassium or more than 50 mEq (600 mg) of magnesium in the maximum daily dose should not be used if kidney disease is present. Phenophthalein preparations should be discontinued if a skin rash appears. Saline laxatives should not be given orally to children under 6 or rectally to infants under 2 yr of age; mineral oil should not be given to children under 6 yr of age. To be effective, enemas and suppositories must be administered properly. *The use of laxatives to relieve gastrointestinal symptoms of unknown cause should be condemned.*

Although occasional use of a laxative is relatively harmless, depletion of fluids and electrolytes can result from their chronic use. Dioctyl sodium sulfosuccinate should not be used with mineral oil. Mineral oil should be given at bedtime in order to minimize its interference with the absorption of fat-soluble vitamins in the diet. In addition, aspiration of mineral oil may result in chronic pneumonitis; consequently, it is contraindicated in patients with disorders of gastric or esophageal emptying. Even the soft bulk-forming laxatives have been reported to cause enteric obstruction in an occasional patient with inflammatory or neoplastic strictures of the gut.

Stimulant Laxatives

The *stimulant laxatives* have multiple actions in the intestines. These include stimulation of motor activity and effects on water reabsorption and secretion. What they have in common is the ability to increase the amount of water in the stool and the ability to increase colonic motility. The more commonly employed agents are the anthraquinone laxatives, *cascara sagrada* and *senna;* the diphenylmethane derivatives, *phenolphthalein* and *bisacodyl;* and *castor oil.*

The *anthraquinone-containing laxatives,* such as cascara and senna, are used widely. The active glycosides are absorbed in the small intestine, circulated through the portal system and into the general circulation and excreted in the bile, urine, saliva, colonic mucosa and in the milk of lactating women. These glycosides stimulate Auerbach's plexus to increase peristalsis. These agents usually act within 6 to 12 hours of ingestion. The *diphenylmethane derivatives,* such as phenolphthalein and bisacodyl, have similar pharmacological actions; they stimulate sensory nerves in the colonic mucosa to initiate reflex peristalsis. Phenolphthalein is usually active within 6 to 8 hours after administration; bisacodyl results in a smooth, formed stool within 6 to 10 hours after oral administration and 15 to 60 minutes after rectal administration. *Castor oil* is classified as a stimulant laxative because lipolysis in the small intestine liberates ricinoleic acid, a short-chain fatty acid which stimulates peristalsis and inhibits the absorption of water and electrolyte from the small intestine. *Glycerin,* in the form of suppositories, promotes defecation by stimulating the rectal mucosa; it also acts to lubricate and soften inspissated fecal material. The stimulant laxatives have many characteristics in common; they increase intestinal motility leading to abdominal cramps, increase mucous secretion and increase fluidity of the stool. Intensity of effect is related to dosage, but effective doses vary markedly from one individual to another.

Aloe

The dried latex of leaves of *Aloe barbadensis* Miller (*Aloe vera* Linné), known in commerce as Curacao Aloe, or of *Aloe ferox* Miller and hybrids of this species with *Aloe africana* Miller and *Aloe spicata* Baker, known in commerce as Cape Aloe (Fam *Liliaceae*); yields not less than 50% of water-soluble extractive. The active principles are pentosides, including aloin (barbaloin, socaloin or capaloin), beta-barbaloin and iso-barbaloin.

Uses—Aloe still is employed as a cathartic in a few mixtures. The active principles are hydrolyzed in the intestine to anthraquinone derivatives that are responsible for the cathartic action. The action of aloe is accompanied by intestinal cramping and pelvic vascular congestion, the latter property having given to aloe the undeserved classification of emmenagogue. The laxative action of aloe occurs 8 to 12 hr after ingestion. Use of aloe as a cathartic has not been justified by clinical studies and should be abandoned. Aloe is also an ingredient of *Compound Benzoin Tincture,* which gives it official status as a pharmaceutic aid.

Bisacodyl

Phenol, 4,4′-(2-pyridinylmethylene)bis-, diacetate (ester); Dulcolax (*CIBA Consumer*); Fleet Bisacodyl (*Fleet*); (*Various Mfrs*)

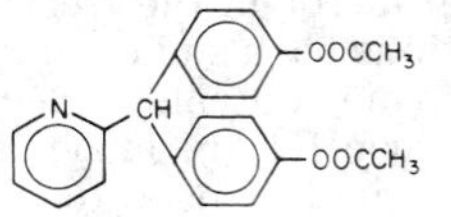

4,4′-(2-Pyridylmethylene)diphenol diacetate (ester) [603-50-9] $C_{22}H_{19}NO_4$ (361.40).

Caution—Avoid inhalation and contact with the eyes, skin and mucous membranes.

Preparation—2-Pyridinecarboxaldehyde is condensed with phenol with the aid of a suitable dehydrant such as sulfuric acid and the resulting 4,4′-(2-pyridyl)diphenol is esterified by treatment with acetic anhydride and anhydrous sodium acetate. US Pat 2,764,590.

Description—White to off-white, crystalline powder in which particles having a longest diameter smaller than 50 μm predominate; melts between 131 and 135°.

Solubility—1 g in > 10,000 mL water, 210 mL alcohol, 2.5 mL chloroform or 275 mL ether.

Uses—A stimulant laxative which acts directly on sensory nerve fibers in the colonic mucosa to increase peristalsis throughout the large intestine. It is administered either orally or rectally for constipation and for evacuation of the bowel prior to surgery, proctoscopy or radiologic examination. It is usually effective overnight or within 6 to 10 hr. Bisacodyl provides satisfactory cleansing of the bowel, obviating the need for an enema. Side effects usually are limited to abdominal cramps. Continued use of the suppository may cause rectal irritation. There are no contraindications to the use of bisacodyl, except for an acute surgical abdomen.

Dose—*Oral,* **10** to **30 mg;** *usual, oral* and *rectal,* **10 mg;** *usual, pediatric, rectal,* **8 mg/m²,** or 5 to 10 mg; *oral,* **0.3 mg/kg** or **8 mg/m².**

Other Dose Information—Do not chew or break tablet coating. Do not take within 1 hr after ingestion of antacids or milk.

Dosage Forms—Suppositories: 10 mg; Tablets, Enteric Coated: 5 mg.

Casanthrol

Peri-Colace (*Mead Johnson*); ing of Dialose Plus; ing of D-S-S Plus (*Warner-Chilcott*)

A purified mixture of the anthranol glycosides extracted from cascara sagrada.

Preparation—US Pat 2,552,896.

Uses—One of the anthraquinone-containing stimulant laxatives; reported to be 10 times as potent as cascara sagrada. In most patients a semisoft stool is produced in 8 to 12 hr. Casanthrol is an ingredient in numerous proprietary laxative preparations. Adverse reactions reported are abdominal cramping, diarrhea, nausea and rectal bleeding in patients with ulcerative colitis. It should not be used in patients with abdominal pain, nausea or vomiting. Continued use for several months may cause melanosis coli—a harmless deposition of anthraquinone pigment in the GI tract that disappears a few months after discontinuing use.

Dose—*Usual*, **30 mg** at bedtime; **60 mg** may be required in laxative-dependent patients.

Dosage Form—Capsules: 30 mg combination with 100 mg of docusate potassium.

Cascara Sagrada

Nature's Remedy (*SmithKline Beecham*); ing of Peri-Colace (*Mead Johnson*); Sacred Bark; Chittem; Dogwood; Bear-berry; Bitter Bark

The dried bark of *Rhamnus purshiana* De Candolle (Fam *Rhamnaceae).*

Constituents—The following active principles have been reported: *Aloe-emodin* (1,8-dihydroxy-3-hydroxymethylanthraquinone), *chrysophanic acid* (1,8-dihydroxy-3-methylanthraquinone), *iso-emodin* (3,5,8-trihydroxy-2-methylanthraquinone), *methylhydrocotoin* (2,4,6-trimethoxybenzophenone), and *purshianin*, a glycoside-forming red-brown crystal melting at 237°. Cascara also contains several resins, one of which is very bitter and gives a bright-red color with potassium hydroxide solution.

Uses—A widely used *cathartic.* Its precise mechanism of action is unknown. It has very little action on the small intestine but promotes peristalsis in the large intestine. The action of cascara is mild and is unaccompanied by cramping. A therapeutic dose causes a single evacuation of the bowel in approximately 8 hr. The stool may be solid or semifluid. Prolonged ingestion frequently results in melanosis coli which regresses after cascara sagrada is discontinued. It should not be given to lactating mothers, since it is excreted in breast milk.

Dose—*Usual, adult,* **650 mg** with a glass of water a day; *usual, child,* **325 mg** a day.

Dosage Form—Film-Coated Tablets; Capsules (in combination with docusate potassium).

Cascara Sagrada Extracts—See RPS-18, page 784.

Castor Oil

Emulsoil (*Paddock*); Neoloid (*Lederle*); Purge (*Fleming*).

The fixed oil obtained from the seed of *Ricinus communis* Linné (Fam *Euphorbiaceae*).

Preparation—By cold expression and subsequent clarification of the oil by heat. It consists chiefly of glycerides of ricinoleic and isoricinoleic acids. The purgative action has been attributed to hydrolysis of ricinolein in the intestine, ricinoleic acid being produced. The seeds contain two principles, *ricin*, a very poisonous albumin (150 mg toxic *per os*), and *ricinine*, a poisonous base (1,2- dihydro-4-methoxy-1-methyl-2-oxonicotinonitrile). Because of the presence of these toxic substances, the seeds are definitely poisonous.

Description—Pale yellowish or almost colorless, transparent, viscid liquid with a faint, mild odor and a bland followed by a slightly acrid and usually nauseating taste; specific gravity between 0.945 and 0.965.

Solubility—Soluble in alcohol; miscible with dehydrated alcohol, glacial acetic acid, chloroform or ether.

Uses—Externally as an *emollient*, internally as a *laxative.* The oil is bland and soothing to the skin. Castor oil is metabolized to ricinoleic acid, which stimulates water secretion in the intestine while decreasing glucose absorption. It also stimulates colonic motility. When administered orally it produces one or more copious stools within 2 to 6 hr after ingestion. It is used frequently to empty the gastrointestinal tract prior to proctoscopy or X-ray studies of the gastrointestinal tract. It should not be used in the therapy of acute constipation. Chronic use is not recommended, since absorption of nutrients may be reduced.

Dose—*Usual, adult,* **5** to **20 mL** a day; *Children 6 to 12 yr,* **5** to **10 mL** (varies with product).

Dosage Form—Oil; 60 mL.

Dehydrocholic Acid—see RPS-18, page 782.

Phenolphthalein

1(3*H*)-Isobenzofuranone, 3,3-bis(4-hydroxyphenyl)- (*Various Mfrs*)

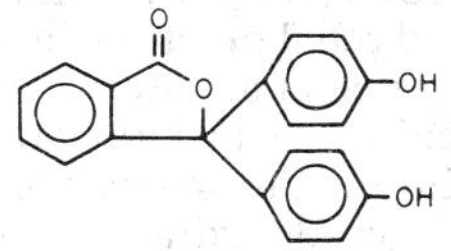

3,3-Bis(*p*-hydroxyphenyl)phthalide [77-09-8] $C_{20}H_{14}O_4$ (318.33).

Preparation—A mixture of phenol, phthalic anhydride and sulfuric acid is heated at 120° for 10 to 12 hr. The product is extracted with boiling water, the residue dissolved in dilute NaOH solution, filtered and precipitated with acid.

Description—White or faintly yellowish white, crystalline powder; odorless and stable in air; melts no lower than 258°.

Solubility—Practically insoluble in water; 1 g in about 15 mL alcohol or about 100 mL ether.

Uses—One of the most widely used of the *cathartic* drugs, being the basis of many proprietary laxatives. Classified as a stimulant cathartic, although the precise mechanism of action is unknown. It tends to act longer than other laxatives because it enters the enterohepatic circulation and is re-excreted in bile into the intestine. It acts within 4 to 8 hr after ingestion. In susceptible individuals, phenolphthalein may cause allergic reactions, including Stevens-Johnson syndrome and lupus erythematosus; the skin lesions may persist for months after discontinuing the drug. Deaths have been attributed to allergy to this drug. It also may cause a Bartter's-like syndrome with hyperaldosteronism and hypokalemia. It should be remembered that phenolphthalein colors an alkaline urine red and small portions may appear in the urine after oral ingestion. It also is used as an indicator in volumetric analysis. This reaction forms the basis of a test in which KOH is used to detect phenolphthalein in the stools of laxative abusers.

Dose—*Usual, adult, oral,* **60 mg;** *pediatric, oral,* 15 to 30 mg, preferably at bedtime.

Dosage Forms—Tablets: 60, 80, 90, 97.2 and 130 mg; Wafers: 64.8 mg; Liquid: 60 and 65 mg/5 mL.

Senna—see RPS-18, page 785.

Sennosides

Gentle Nature (*Sandoz*)

A natural complex of anthraquinone glycosides found in senna, isolated from *Cassia angustifolia* as calcium salts; contains 55–65% of the calcium salts.

Description—Brownish powder; pH (mixture, 1 g/10 mL water) between 6.3 and 7.3.

Uses—A *laxative.* Evacuation of the bowels occurs 8 to 10 hr after oral administration.

Dose—*Usual, adult,* **20** to **40 mg** a day at bedtime; *children over 6 yr,* **20 mg** a day. *Children 6 to 10 yr,* **12 mg.**

Dosage Form—Tablets: 20 mg of Sennosides A and B.

Saline (Hyperosmotic) Laxatives

A number of magnesium and sodium salts in the form of citrates, sulfates, phosphates and tartrates are used as *saline laxatives.* These cations and anions are not absorbed, or at most only slightly absorbed, from the gastrointestinal tract. Consequently, when given orally in hypertonic solutions, they draw water from the tissues into the intestine, increase peristalsis and induce a profuse, watery stool. This traditional explanation for the mechanism of action of saline laxatives has been questioned. Indeed, several studies indicate that different mechanisms, independent of osmotic effect, are responsible for the laxative properties of these salts. For example, it has been shown that magnesium stimulates release of endogenous cholecystokinin-pancreozymin, a hormone which causes the accumulation of fluid and electrolytes within the human small intestine. The laxative action of magnesium-containing salts, therefore, may result from their ability to diminish the net absorption of fluid and electrolytes.

The choice of saline laxative usually is based on cost and palatability. There are, however, situations in which the injudicious use of a saline laxative results in serious adverse effects. As much as 20% of the magnesium ion may be absorbed after oral administration of a magnesium salt. If renal function is normal, the absorbed ion is excreted so rapidly that no change in the blood level of the ion can be detected. In patients with impaired renal function, however, toxic concentrations of the ion can accumulate. Laxatives that contain sodium are contraindicated in individuals with edema and congestive heart failure. Chronic use of saline laxatives also may result in excessive dehydration. Other contraindications will be mentioned in the respective monographs.

Magnesium Carbonate—see RPS-16, page 738.

Magnesium Citrate Oral Solution—see RPS-18, page 786.

Magnesium Oxide—page 888.

Magnesium Sulfate

Sulfuric acid magnesium salt (1:1), heptahydrate; Bitter Salts; Epsom Salts (*Various Mfrs*)

Magnesium sulfate (1:1) heptahydrate [10034-99-8] $MgSO_4.7H_2O$ (246.47); *anhydrous* [7487-88-8] (120.36).

Preparation—Magnesium sulfate can be prepared by neutralizing sulfuric acid with magnesium carbonate or oxide, but it also may be obtained directly from natural sources. In the form of a double salt with alkali metals, it occurs abundantly in several mines and these comprise a large source of the salt. It also is produced in large quantities from the magnesium salts occurring in the brines used for extraction of bromine. The "liquors" after the removal of bromine are treated with calcium hydroxide, thus precipitating magnesium as the hydroxide. Sulfur dioxide and air are passed into an aqueous suspension of the magnesium hydroxide, yielding magnesium sulfate:

$$Mg(OH)_2 + SO_2 + \frac{1}{2}O_2 \rightarrow MgSO_4 + H_2O$$

Description—Small, colorless crystals, usually needlelike and has a cooling, saline and bitter taste; effloresces in warm, dry air; at 100° it loses 5 molecules of its water; aqueous solution is neutral to litmus.

Uses—An effective and widely employed *saline laxative*. The laxative action probably results from two factors: (1) magnesium sulfate is not absorbed from the intestinal tract and, thus, retains sufficient water within the lumen of the bowel to make an isotonic solution and (2) the magnesium ion stimulates the release of cholecystokinin-pancreozymin which causes an accumulation of fluid and electrolytes within the small intestine (see introduction of this section). It is the increased bulk which promotes the motor activity of the bowel. If dissolved in iced water, its nauseous taste is not so perceptible as when water at ordinary temperature is used; it may be disguised further by the use of orange juice.

A cold, wet compress of saturated magnesium sulfate solution in water has been employed in the treatment of such skin disorders as erysipelas. Hot concentrated, aqueous solutions of magnesium sulfate (about 1 lb/pint of water) are sometimes used in the treatment of deep-seated infections; cloths are saturated and applied while hot. The action is much like that of a poultice.

For parenteral anticonvulsant use see *Magnesium Sulfate Injection*, page 1175.

Dose—*Usual, adult, oral,* **10 to 15 g** in a glass of water. *Children,* **5** to **10 g** in a glass of water.

Potassium Bitartrate—see RPS-18, page 787.

Potassium Phosphate—see RPS-18, page 788.

Potassium Sodium Tartrate—see RPS-18, page 788.

Sodium Phosphate

Phosphoric acid, disodium salt, heptahydrate; Dibasic Sodium Phosphate; Disodium Orthophosphate; Disodium Hydrogen Phosphate; Secondary Sodium Phosphate Fleet Enema, Phospho-Soda (*Fleet*)

Disodium phosphate heptahydrate [7782-85-6] $Na_2HPO_4.7H_2O$ (268.07); *anhydrous* [7558-79-4] (141.96).

Preparation—From *bone phosphate* or *bone ash*, obtained by heating bones to whiteness, which consists chiefly of tribasic calcium phosphate. The mineral *phosphorite*, which is a tribasic calcium phosphate, also is used. The finely ground phosphatic material is digested with sulfuric acid, the mixture then is leached with hot water, neutralized with sodium carbonate and the sodium phosphate crystallized from the filtrate.

Description—Colorless, or white, granular salt; effloresces in warm, dry air; solutions are alkaline to litmus and phenolphthalein (pH about 9.5).

Solubility—1 g in 4 mL water; very slightly soluble in alcohol.

Uses—One of the most palatable of the *saline laxatives*. It also is used in the form of the oral solution (see below) as an *antihypercalcemic*. Its major use, however, is for diagnostic procedures such as proctoscopy, colonscopy or barium enema.

Caution—This phosphate should not be confused with tribasic sodium phosphate which is very alkaline and has a caustic action.

Dose—4 to **8 g;** *usual,* **4 g.**

Sodium Phosphate, Dried–see RPS-18, page 787.

Sodium Phosphate, Effervescent—see RPS-18, page 787.

Sodium Phosphate, Oral Solution–see RPS-18, page 787.

Sodium Phosphate and Sodium Biphosphate Enema

Sodium Phosphates Enema; Fleet Enema (*Fleet*)

Uses—A *laxative* administered as an enema primarily in preparation for surgery, endoscopy or X-ray. It should not be used in the presence of abdominal pain, nausea or vomiting.

Dose—*Usual, rectal,* **120 mL.** *Usual, pediatric, rectal,* dosage not established in children under 2 yr; over 2 yr, **60 mL.**

Dosage Forms—Enema: 6% sodium phosphate and 16% sodium biphosphate.

Sodium Phosphate and Sodium Biphosphate Oral Solution

Sodium Phosphates Oral Solution; Fleet Phospho-Soda (*Fleet*); Sodium Phosphates (*Roxane*)

Uses—An orally administered saline *laxative* used primarily in preparation for surgery, endoscopy or X-ray. It is usually effective overnight or within 1 hr if taken before meals. It should not be used in patients with abdominal pain, nausea or vomiting.

Dose—*Usual, adult, oral,* **20 to 30 mL** mixed with ½ glass water and then follow with a glass full of water; *usual, pediatric, oral,* **2.5** to **5 mL** for children 5 to 10 yr; **5** to **10 mL** for children over 10 yr.

Dosage Form—Solution: 18% sodium phosphate and 48% sodium biphosphate.

Sodium Sulfate—see RPS-18, page 787.

Potassium Bitartrate—see RPS-18, page 787.

Potassium Phosphate, Dibasic—see RPS-18, page 788.

Potassium Sodium Tartrate—see RPS-18, page 788.

Bulk-Forming Laxatives

The bulk-forming laxatives include a wide range of natural and semisynthetic polysaccharides and cellular derivatives that are only partially digested. The undigested portions are hydrophilic and swell in the presence of water to form a viscous solution or gel. The resultant changes in bowel wall tension and intraluminal pressure promote transit. Other mechanisms also may be involved. For example, bile-salt metabolism may be altered leading to a choleretic effect. The bulk-forming laxatives have become the mainstay of the management of irritable bowel syndrome. They are particularly useful in this condition because they not only relieve constipation but also, because of their hydrophilic property, decrease diarrhea. Although used widely for the treatment of irritable bowel syndrome, there is little convincing evidence of their efficacy. This may be because of the variability of this syndrome and the lack of objective parameters to measure efficacy. They also are used for symptomatic treatment of acute diarrhea and for symptomatic treatment of inflammatory bowel disease such as ulcerative colitis and Crohn's colitis. They may be useful for the continued treatment of diverticular disease or in situations where it is desirable to maintain a soft stool such as after anorectal surgery. They can ease the discomfort of bowel movements in the postoperative period.

Bulk-forming laxatives usually exert a laxative effect in 12 to 24 hr but may require as much as 3 days. Each dose of laxative should be taken with a full glass of water. These drugs interact and combine with other drugs, such as salicylates, digitalis, etc. Consequently, they should not, as a general rule, be taken with other drugs. For the most part, these drugs are safe. They are devoid of systemic side effects but may increase flatulence. Rare cases of intestinal and esophageal obstruction have been reported. It is important, therefore, to take these agents with large volumes of liquid, at least one glass with each dose. They are contraindicated in patients with known esophageal or intestinal obstruction. The dosing of these agents is highly variable and needs to be adjusted to the individual patient.

Carboxymethylcellulose Sodium—page 1396.

Methylcellulose—page 1397.

Plantago Seed

Psyllium Seed; Plantain Seed

The cleaned, dried, ripe seed of *Plantago psyllium* Linné, or of *Plantago indica* Linné ((*Plantago arenaria* Waldstein et Kitaibel), known in commerce as Spanish or French Psyllium Seed; or of *Plantago ovata* Forskal, known in commerce as Blond Psyllium or Indian Plantago Seed (Fam *Plantaginaceae*).

Uses—By virtue of its indigestibility and mucilaginous character, it acts as a mild *laxative*. It is contraindicated in patients with intestinal obstruction.

Dose—1 to **3 rounded teaspoonfuls** with a glass of liquid once or twice a day. While the manufacturer recommends teaspoon doses, it is common experience that tablespoon doses usually are required.

Polycarbophil

Acrylic Acid-Divinyl Glycol Copolymer Fiberall Chewable Tablets (*CIBA Consumer*)

Polycarbophil [9003-97-8]; polyacrylic acid cross-linked with divinyl glycol.

Preparation—Acrylic acid and divinyl glycol (1,5-hexadiene- 3,4-diol) are copolymerized in a hot salt slurry using azobis[methylpropionitrile] as the initiator. US Pat 3,202,577.

Description—White to creamy white granules, having a slight, characteristic, esterlike odor; contains a maximum of 1.5% water.

Solubility—Swells but is insoluble in water; insoluble in most organic solvents.

Uses—A pharmacologically inert substance which has the capacity to bind free fecal water. Hence, it is used in diarrheal disorders to decrease the fluidity or looseness of stools. Orally administered, polycarbophil exerts its most marked hydrosorptive action only on reaching the slightly acid or alkaline medium of the small intestine and colon. Polycarbophil also is used as a bulk-forming laxative. This hydrophilic polyacrylic resin is indigestible, nonabsorbable and binds more water than other laxatives of this type. Polycarbophil is reported to have no effect on digestive enzymes, and that it is metabolically inactive. The only adverse effect noted is a sense of fullness and bloating in some patients; this can be minimized by giving smaller doses at shorter intervals. This compound contains calcium which may interact with tetracycline. It is contraindicated in bowel obstruction or fecal impaction.

Dose—*Usual, adult, oral,* **1 g** 1 to 4 times a day. *Children 6 to 12 yr, 0.5 g* 1 to 4 times a day.

Dosage Form—Chewable tablets: 1 g.

Other Bulk-Forming Laxatives

Plantago Ovata Coating—A cream-colored to brown, granular powder; practically odorless and tasteless. It consists principally of the separated outer mucilaginous layers of plantago ovata seeds (blond psyllium). *Uses:* For correction of simple constipation of functional or nervous origin due to lack of sufficient bulk in the stool. *Dose: Oral,* **1** to **2 rounded tablespoonfuls** in a glass of liquid once or twice a day.

Psyllium Hydrophilic Muciloid [Metamucil (*P&G*) and others]—A white to cream-colored, slightly granular powder with little or no odor, and a slightly acid taste. It consists of the mucilaginous portion (outer epidermis) of blond psyllium seeds. *Uses:* A bulk-forming laxative. *Dose: Oral,* **1** to **2 rounded teaspoonfuls** in a glass of liquid, followed by another glass of liquid, once or twice a day. Common experience would suggest that tablespoon doses usually are required.

Lubricant Laxatives

The *lubricant laxatives* (mineral oil and vegetable oils) lubricate the intestinal tract, soften the fecal contents and facilitate the passage of feces. The many untoward effects induced by mineral oil, such as *lipid pneumonitis, lipoid avitaminosis A,* foreign-body reactions in the intestinal mucosa and anal leakage all argue against its use.

Cottonseed Oil—page 1394.

Mineral Oil

Liquid Paraffin; Liquid Petrolatum; White Mineral Oil; Heavy Liquid Petrolatum (*Various Mfrs*)

A mixture of aliphatic hydrocarbons obtained from petroleum. It is indigestable and thus has limited absorption.

Preparation—After removing the lighter hydrocarbons from petroleum by distillation, the residue is again subjected to distillation at a temperature between 330° and 390° and the distillate treated first with H_2SO_4, then with NaOH, and afterward decolorized by filtering through bone black, animal charcoal or fuller's earth. The purified product is again chilled, to remove paraffin, and redistilled at a temperature above 330°. In some instances the H_2SO_4 treatment is omitted.

Description—Colorless, transparent, oily liquid, free or nearly free from fluorescence; tasteless and odorless when cold and develops not more than a faint odor of petroleum when heated; specific gravity between 0.860 and 0.905; kinematic viscosity not less than 38.1 centistokes at 37.8°.

Solubility—Insoluble in water or alcohol; miscible with most fixed oils, but not with castor oil; soluble in volatile oils.

Uses—A vehicle internally as a *laxative*. It was used as a vehicle for drugs to be applied to the nasal mucous membranes. It is now recognized that neither of these procedures is as benign as once supposed. A small portion of mineral oil may be aspirated into the lungs after topical application to nasal mucous membranes and may cause "lipid" pneumonia.

When taken internally, mineral oil, by virtue of its ability to soften fecal contents and retard the absorption of water, is a mild laxative. It is probably harmless in occasional laxative doses, but if taken continuously in large amounts it may impair appetite, reduce the absorption of fat-soluble vitamins and possibly be absorbed to an extent sufficient to cause

Table 5—Composition and Dose of Some Bulk Laxatives

Product (*mfr*)	Active ingredient	Amount of fiber (g/unit dose)	Usual adult dose[a]
Citrucel Orange Flavor (*Lakeside*)	Methylcellulose	2 g	1 tbs
Effer-Syllium Natural (*Stuart*)	Psyllium	3 g	1 tsp
Fiberall Powder (*Ciba*)	Polycarbophil	2.2 g	1 tsp
Fiberall Fiber Wafers (*Ciba*)	Psyllium	2.2 g	1 wafer
FiberCon (*Lederle*)	Polycarbophil	0.5 g	2 tablets
Hydrocil Instant (*Solvay*)	Psyllium	~3.5 g	1 packet
Metamucil Regular (*Procter & Gamble*)	Psyllium	3.4 g	1 tsp
Metamucil Sugar Free Orange (*Procter & Gamble*)	Psyllium	3.4 g	1 packet
Perdiem Fiber (*Rhone-Poulenc Rorer*)	Psyllium	~4 g	1 tsp
Serutan (*SmithKline Beecham*)	Psyllium	2.5 g	1 tsp

[a]Teaspoonful and tablespoonful quantities are rounded unless otherwise stated.

recognizable changes in the liver and mesenteric lymph nodes. It should not be used when abdominal pain, nausea or vomiting is present. The adverse effects, especially lipid pneumonia, argue against its use as a laxative.

Dose—*Adult, oral,* **15** to **30 mL** at bedtime; *children over 6 yr,* **10** to **20 mL** at bedtime.

Dosage Form—Emulsified Oil (plain and flavored).

Mineral Oil, Emulsion—see RPS-18, page 788.

Light Mineral Oil—page 1411.

Olive Oil—page 1400.

Fecal Softeners

The fecal softeners represent the most recent approach to the management of constipation and fecal impaction. Substances included in this category are "surface-acting" or "wetting" agents which are nonabsorbable and relatively nontoxic. Their action is attributed to their surface-active property; by lowering surface tension they permit the intestinal fluids to penetrate the fecal mass more readily and, thus, produce soft, easily passed stools. However, agents such as dioctyl sodium sulfosuccinate have been shown to increase mucosal cAMP and alter ion transport in a manner similar to the bile acids. Thus, cAMP-mediated active anion secretion may account for the increased accumulation of luminal fluid. The relative importance of these two mechanisms remains to be determined.

Docusate Calcium

Butanedioic acid, sulfo-, 1,4-bis(2-ethylhexyl) ester, calcium salt; Bis(2-ethylhexyl) *S*-calcium sulfosuccinate; Dioctyl calcium sulfosuccinate; Surfak (*Hoechst-Roussel*)

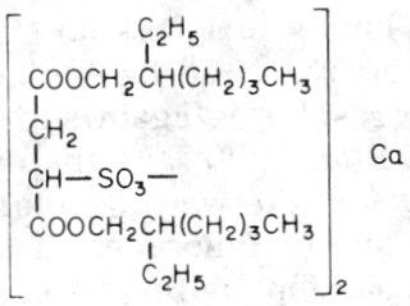

$$\left[\begin{array}{l} \quad\quad\quad C_2H_5 \\ COOCH_2CH(CH_2)_3CH_3 \\ CH_2 \\ CH-SO_3- \\ COOCH_2CH(CH_2)_3CH_3 \\ \quad\quad\quad C_2H_5 \end{array}\right]_2 Ca$$

[128-49-4] $C_{40}H_{74}CaO_{14}S_2$ (883.22).

Preparation—*Docusate Sodium* (below) is dissolved in 2-propanol and reacted with a methanolic solution of calcium chloride. US Pat 3,035,973.

Description—White, amorphous solid having the characteristic odor of octyl alcohol; free of the odor of other solvents.

Solubility—1 g in 3300 mL water, < 1 mL alcohol, < 1 mL chloroform or < 1 mL ether.

Uses—A *fecal-softening* agent useful in *preventing constipation* or in patients where laxative therapy is undesirable or contraindicated. It does not increase gastrointestinal motility and, therefore, may be used in patients in whom cathartic medication is contraindicated. Except for occasional mild, transitory, cramping pains, dioctyl calcium sulfosuccinate is free from side effects and contraindications. It is used also as an emulsifying, wetting and dispersing agent for external preparations.

Dose—*Usual, adult, oral,* **240 mg.** *Children,* and *adults with minimal needs,* **50 mg** 1 to 3 times a day.

Dosage Form—Capsules: 50 and 240 mg.

Docusate Sodium

Butanedioic acid, sulfo-, 1,4-bis(2-ethylhexyl) ester, sodium salt; Dioctyl Sodium Sulfosuccinate; Aerosol OT (*Am Cyanamid*); (*Various Mfrs*)

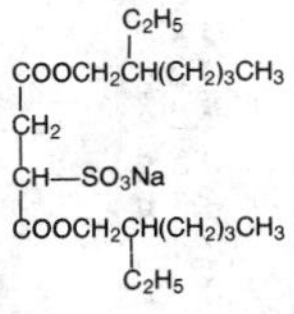

$$\begin{array}{l} \quad\quad\quad C_2H_5 \\ COOCH_2CH(CH_2)_3CH_3 \\ CH_2 \\ CH-SO_3Na \\ COOCH_2CH(CH_2)_3CH_3 \\ \quad\quad\quad C_2H_5 \end{array}$$

Sodium 1,4-bis(2-ethylhexyl) sulfosuccinate [577-11-7] $C_{20}H_{37}NaO_7S$ (444.56).

Preparation—Several patents have been issued covering the preparation of this compound. In general, maleic anhydride is treated with 2-ethylhexanol to produce dioctyl maleate which is then reacted with sodium bisulfite under conditions conducive to saturation of the olefinic bond with simultaneous rearrangement of the bisulfite to the sulfonate structure.

Description—White, wax-like, plastic solid with a characteristic odor suggestive of octyl alcohol; usually available in the form of pellets.

Solubility—1 g slowly in about 70 mL water; freely soluble in alcohol or glycerin.

Uses—A surface-active agent used in the management of constipation and painful anorectal conditions. It is not a laxative but is used to soften the stools in such conditions as anal fissures and postoperative anal pain. It is also useful for constipation in geriatric, pediatric and obstetric patients. However, 1 or 2 days of treatment may be necessary before an effect is observed. Although its action is attributed to its "detergent" or "wetting" properties, it does increase mucosal cAMP in a manner similar to bile acids. As a pharmaceutic aid, it is used as an emulsifying, wetting and dispersing agent in formulations for external use.

Dose—**50** to **500 mg** a day; *usual,* **100 mg** 2 or 3 times a day.

Other Dose Information—For infants and children the dose is 10 to 20 mg a day.

Dosage Forms—Capsules: 50, 60, 100, 240, 250 and 300 mg. Liquid: 50 mg/mL; Syrup: 20 mg/5 mL. Tablets: 50, 100, and 300 mg.

Docusate Potassium

Butanedioic acid, sulfo-, 1,4-bis(2-ethylhexyl) ester, potassium salt; Dialose or Kasof (*Stuart*)

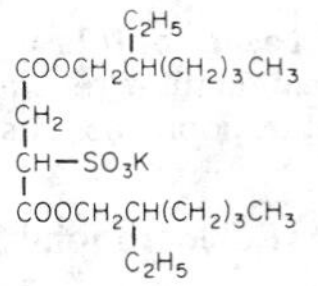

$$\begin{array}{l} \quad\quad\quad C_2H_5 \\ COOCH_2CH(CH_2)_3CH_3 \\ CH_2 \\ CH-SO_3K \\ COOCH_2CH(CH_2)_3CH_3 \\ \quad\quad\quad C_2H_5 \end{array}$$

Potassium 1,4-bis(2-ethylhexyl sulfosuccinate [7491-09-0] $C_{20}H_{37}KO_7S$ (460.67)

Preparation—See *Docusate Sodium,* above; potassium bisulfite replaces the sodium bisulfite.

Description—White amorphous solid with the odor of octyl alcohol.

Solubility—Sparingly soluble in water; soluble in alcohol or glycerol; very soluble in ligroin.

Uses—A sodium-free, nonhabit-forming stool softener. It facilitates absorption of water by the stool to form a soft, easily evacuated mass. Helps eliminate straining associated with obstetric, cardiac, surgical, anorectal or proctologic conditions. See also *Dosusate Sodium.*

Dose—*Usual, adult, oral,* **100 to 300 mg** daily until bowel move ments are normal. *Children 6 yr and older,* **100 mg** at bedtime.

Dosage Form—Capsules: 100 and 240 mg.

Laxative Combinations

There are many laxative products available to the public (OTC) that contain more than one type of laxative. For example, a product may contain both an emollient (stool softener) and a stimulant laxative. In general, combination products are more likely to cause adverse effects because of the multiple ingredients, especially when the separate ingredients are used in full dose. In addition, laxative combinations may not offer any advantage over products which contain only one type of laxative. The composition of 20 of the more commonly used laxative combinations, available in either capsule or tablet form, is shown in Table 6.

Antidiarrheals

Diarrhea is the manifestation of many illnesses. Its etiologies include infections (viral, bacterial, fungal, parasitic), irritable bowel syndrome, inflammatory bowel disease (ulcerative colitis, Crohn's disease and others), toxins (food poisoning and pseudomembranous colitis), drugs, surreptitious laxative abuse, neuroendocrine tumors, secretory tumors (villous adenoma), malabsorption syndromes (celiac sprue, lactase deficiency, etc), motility disorders, diverticular

Table 6—Composition of Some Laxative Mixtures

Product (*mfr*)	Content (mg) per capsule or tablet				Dose
	Docusate[a]	Casanthranol	Phenolphthalein	Other	
Correctol Tab (*Plough*)	100 (Na)				1–2 taps
Dialose Plus (*Stuart*)	100 (K)	30			1 cap bid
Extra Gentle Ex-Lax (*Sandoz-Cons*)	75 (Na)		65		1–2 tabs
Feen-A-Mint (*Plough*)	100 (Na)		65		1–2 tabs
Natures Remedy (*Smith Kline-Beecham*)	100 (Na)			100[b]; 150[c]	1–2 tabs
Peri-Colace (*Mead-Johnson*)	100 (Na)	30			1–2 caps
Phillips' LaxCaps (*Glenbrook*)	83 (Na)		90		1–2 caps

[a]Na = sodium; K = potassium.
[b]Aloe.
[c]Cascara sagrada.

disease and ileostomy. Treatment should be directed to the underlying cause. Nevertheless, it is occasionally necessary to use antidiarrheals for convenience or for conditions for which there is no primary treatment, eg, ileorectal anastomosis and ileoanal pull-through surgery. The most commonly used antidiarrheals are anticholinergics (page 902), opioid narcotics, meperidine congeners (diphenoxylate) and loperamide.

Diphenoxylate Hydrochloride

4-Piperidinecarboxylic acid, 1-(3-cyano-3,3-diphenylpropyl)-4-phenyl-, ethyl ester, monohydrochloride; ing of Lomotil (*Searle*)

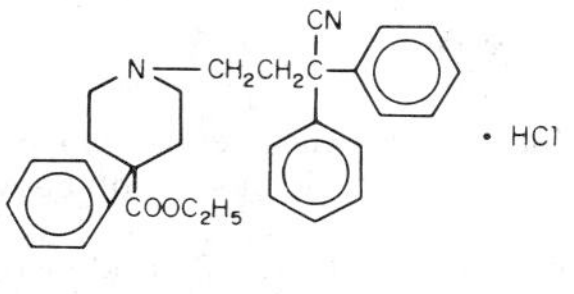

Ethyl 1-(3-cyano-3,3-diphenylpropyl)-4-phenylisonipecotate monohydrochloride [3810-80-8] $C_{30}H_{32}N_2O_2.HCl$ (489.06).

Preparation—Ethyl 4-phenylisonipecotate (prepared as described under *Meperidine Hydrochloride* (page 1204) except omitting the final step of *N*-methylation), is condensed with 2,2-diphenyl-4-bromobutyronitrile by refluxing in toluene using either an excess of the ester or another suitable dehydrobrominating agent. US Pat 2,898,340. Combined with atropine subject.

Description—White, odorless, crystalline powder; pH (saturated solution) about 3.3; melts between 220 and 226°.

Solubility—Sparingly soluble in alcohol or acetone; slightly soluble in water or isopropyl alcohol; freely soluble in chloroform; practically insoluble in ether or solvent hexane.

Uses—Diphenoxylate, a synthetic congener of meperidine, inhibits excessive gastrointestinal propulsion by slowing intestinal motility. It is *effective as adjunctive therapy* in the management of *diarrhea*, diarrhea associated with gastroenteritis, irritable bowel, acute infections, food poisoning and side effects of some drugs. Caution should be used in patients with ulcerative colitis and pseudomembranous colitis who are at increased risk of developing toxic magacolon. Also, diphenoxylate may prolong infectious diarrhea. It also is useful in the control of *intestinal transit time* in patients with and ileostomies, colostomies and ileoanal pull-through operation.

In high dosage (40 to 60 mg) diphenoxylate can produce morphine-like euphoria and prevent withdrawal symptoms in narcotic addicts, but in the recommended dosage range for antidiarrheal therapy no evidence for addiction liability has been reported. The available dosage forms contain a subtherapeutic dose of 0.025 mg of atropine sulfate and a 2.5-mg dose of diphenoxylate hydrochloride. The atropine sulfate decreases gastrointestinal motility after accumulative dosage and also discourages usage of excessive amounts, thereby minimizing abuse. The combination is listed in *Schedule V* under the *Controlled Substances Act*. *Caution:* This combination (*Lomotil*) is *not* an innocuous drug and dosage recommendations should be adhered to strictly, especially in children.

Side effects are usually minor and include nausea, sedation, vertigo, vomiting, pruritus, skin eruption, insomnia and abdominal cramps. Numbness of the extremities, headache, blurring of vision, swelling of gums and general malaise also have been reported. The drug is contraindicated in patients with cirrhosis or advanced liver disease, and in children under 2 yr. Laboratory studies demonstrate that diphenoxylate hydrochloride inhibits the hepatic microsomal enzymes. Therefore, it should be used with caution in patients on barbiturates, tranquilizers and alcohol, because the activity of these drugs may be potentiated by diphenoxylate. Concurrent use with monoamine oxidase inhibitors may, in theory, precipitate a hypertensive crisis.

Dose—**5** to **30 mg** daily; *usual, adult, oral,* **5 mg** 4 times a day. Lomotil is contraindicated in children under 2 yr; in children 2 to 12 yr, the liquid form should be used; *2 to 5 yr,* **4 mL (2 mg)** 3 times a day; *5 to 8 yr,* **4 mL (2 mg)** 4 times a day; and *8 to 12 yr,* **4 mL (2 mg)** 5 times a day.

Dosage Forms—Diphenoxylate Hydrochloride and Atropine Sulfate Solution (*Lomotil*, Searle): 2.5 mg of diphenoxylate hydrochloride and 0.025 mg (25 mg) of atropine sulfate/5 mL; Diphenoxylate Hydrochloride and Atropine Sulfate Tablets: 2.5 mg of diphenoxylate hydrochloride and 0.025 mg of atropine sulfate.

Ether—see RPS-18, page 1041.

Fennel Oil—page 1387.

Loperamide Hydrochloride

1-Piperidinebutanamide, 4-(4-chlorophenyl)-4-hydroxy-*N,N*-dimethyl-α,α-diphenyl-, monohydrochloride;
Imodium A-D (*McNeil Consumer*); Imodium (*Janssen*)

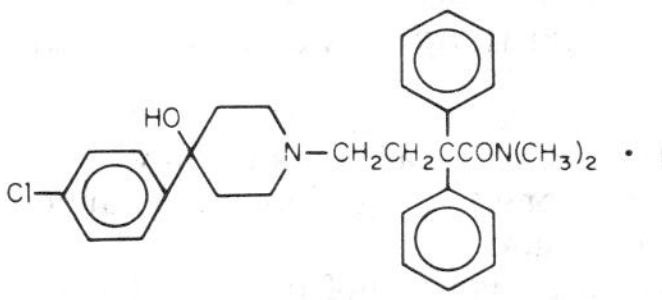

4-(*p*-Chlorophenyl) - 4 - hydroxy - *N,N*-dimethyl-α,α-diphenyl-1-piperidinebutyramide monohydrochloride [34552-83-5] $C_{29}H_{33}ClN_2O_2.HCl$ (513.51).

Preparation—4-Bromo-2,2-diphenylbutyric acid is converted in a series of reactions to dimethyl(tetrahydro-3,3-diphenyl-2-furylidene)ammonium bromide, which is reacted with *p*-chlorophenyl-4-piperidinol to produce loperamide. US Pat 3,714,159; *J Med Chem 16:* 782, 1973.

Description—White to faintly yellow, amorphous or microcrystalline powder; melts at about 222°.

Solubility—Slightly soluble in water; soluble in alcohol.

Uses—A synthetic agent used for the control and symptomatic relief of *acute nonspecific diarrhea* and *chronic diarrhea* associated with ileoanal pull-through surgery. It also is used for *reducing the volume of discharge* from ileostomies. Caution should be used in patients with ulcerative colitis and pseudomembranous colitis who are at increased risk for toxic megacolon. Also, loperamide may prolong the course of infectious diarrhea. Plasma levels are highest 5 hr after oral administration. The elimination half-life is 10.8 hr with a range of 9.1 to 14.4 hr. Unchanged drug remains below 2 ng/mL after the intake of a 2-mg capsule. Most of the drug is excreted in the feces. The safe use of this agent during pregnancy, by nursing mothers, infants and children, has not been established. Adverse effects are minimal and usually self-limiting. The following patient complaints have been reported: abdominal pain or discomfort, constipation, drowsiness, dizziness, dry mouth, nausea and vomiting and tiredness. Hypersensitivity reactions have been reported. Loperamide should be discontinued if abdominal distention occurs or if other untoward symptoms develop in patients with ulcerative colitis.

Dose—*Usual, adult, oral, initial,* **4 mg**, followed by **2 mg** after each unformed stool until diarrhea is controlled. Daily dosage should not exceed 16 mg. *Children 2 to 5 yr:* **1 mg** 3 times a day; *5 to 8 yr:* **2 mg** 2 times a day; *8 to 12 yr:* **2 mg** 3 times a day. Clinical improvement is usually observed within 48 hours.

Dosage Forms—Capsules: 2 mg. Liquid: 1 mg/5 mL.

Peppermint Spirit—see RPS-18, page 798.

Emetics

An *emetic* is a drug which induces vomiting. They may act directly by stimulation of the *chemoreceptor trigger zone* located in the area postrema of the medulla oblongata, (eg, apomorphine, morphine, hydrogenated ergot alkaloids and digitalis glycosides), or they may act reflexly by irritant action on the gastrointestinal tract (eg, copper sulfate, mustard, sodium chloride and zinc sulfate). They also may produce stimulation of the vagus (eg, veratrum). It should be remembered that the stomach tube is a safer and more efficient tool for emptying the stomach. Emetics should not be used in patients who are unconscious, semicomatose or in whom coma is expected imminently. They should not be used in patients with severe heart disease, tuberculosis, hernia or advanced pregnancy. They are contraindicated in debilitated patients and in poisoning caused by corrosive or petroleum products.

Apomorphine Hydrochloride—see RPS-18, page 790.

Emetine Hydrochloride—page 1324.

Ipecac—page 976.

Sodium Chloride—page 932.

Zinc Sulfate—page 1271.

Antiemetics

Nausea and vomiting are among the most frequent symptoms of disease. They often are induced by drugs and occur after operations and radiation therapy, during pregnancy, with gastrointestinal tumors and, as the result of certain types of motion, in sensitive persons. Of a number of drugs which block nausea, the *antiemetics (antinauseants)*, are therapeutically effective. Useful agents are found among the following six groups:

1. *Antipsychotics* (phenothiazines and butyrophenones) act at the chemoreceptor trigger zone (CTZ) to block dopaminergic emetic receptors excited by apomorphine.
2. *Antihistaminics* provide relief from motion sickness through an action on the vestibular apparatus.
3. *Anticholinergics* in combination with *d*-amphetamine and scopolamine are most effective against motion sickness (mechanism unknown).
4. *Cannabinoids* are especially useful in the emesis from cancer chemotherapy; they may cause thought disorder.
5. 5-HT_3-receptor antagonists such as ondansetron, block both peripheral and central 5-HT_3-receptors and are especially effective against the emetogenic effects of chemotherapy.
6. *Other agents,* such as trimethobenzamide and metoclopramide, block dopamine receptors in the CTZ, whereas diphenidol depresses the vestibular apparatus.

Centrally acting antiemetics, such as trimethobenzamide, the phenothiazines and similar agents, should not be used for the treatment of uncomplicated vomiting in children because the extrapyramidal symptoms which often occur with these agents may be confused with the central nervous system signs of an undiagnosed primary disease responsible for the vomiting, eg, Reye's syndrome or other encephalopathy.

The phenothiazine antiemetics are capable of potentiating central nervous system depressants (eg, anesthetics, opiates, alcohol, etc).

Adverse reactions include

Phenothiazines (aliphatic)—Drowsiness, orthostatic hypotension, ocular changes, anticholinergic effects, extrapyramidal reactions (dystonia, akathisia, parkinsonian syndrome, dysarthria), hypersensitivity reactions, amenorrhea, reversal of epinephrine pressor effect, enhancement of CNS depressant drugs, gynecomastia, lactation, hyperglycemia, hypoglycemia and glycosuria.

Antihistaminics—Drowsiness, lightheadedness, blurred vision, dryness of the mouth and urinary retention.

Anticholinergics—Glycosuria, drowsiness, excitement or hallucinations, dryness of the mouth, mydriasis, blurred vision and urinary retention.

Cannabinoids—Cardiac disorders, drug dependance, hypertension, mania or depressive states or psychoses.

5-HT_3-receptor antagonists—constipation, rash and seizures.

Since drowsiness is common to most of these agents, patients should be cautioned not to drive or operate hazardous machinery while on these drugs.

Persistent vomiting results in loss of hydrochloric acid, alkalosis and dehydration which, in turn, may precipitate further vomiting. Hence, electrolyte therapy may be necessary after vomiting has been present for some time (see pages 915 and 916).

Benzquinamide Hydrochloride

2*H*-Benzo[*a*]quinolizine-3-carboxamide, 2-(acetyloxy)-*N,N*-diethyl-1,3,4,6,7,11b-hexahydro-9,10-dimethoxy-, monohydrochloride; Emete-con (*Roerig*)

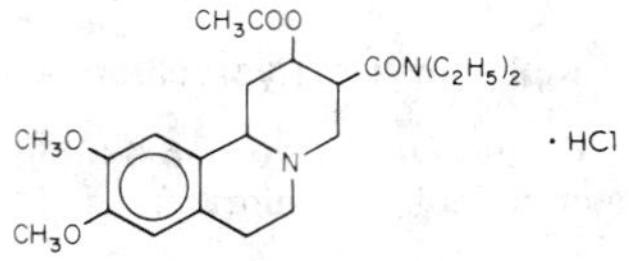

CH_3COO $CON(C_2H_5)_2$ CH_3O N   · HCl CH_3O

[30046-34-5] $C_{22}H_{32}N_2O_5$.HCl(440.97).

Preparation—See US Pat 3,053,845.

Description—White or pale yellow, crystalline powder; melts between 222 and 230°; light-sensitive; stable in solution between pH 2 and 4; pK_a 5.9.

Solubility—1 g in 12.5 mL water or 43 mL alcohol.

Uses—A benzoquinolizine derivative, chemically unrelated to the phenothiazines, with antiemetic, antihistaminic, anticholinergic and sedative properties. It is indicated for *prevention* and *treatment* of *nausea* and *vomiting* associated with anesthesia and surgery; it is contraindicated in patients with demonstrated hypersensitivity to the drug. It is not recommended for use either in pregnant women or in children. The onset of antiemetic activity occurs within 15 min; 5 to 10% of an administered dose is excreted unchanged in the urine and the remainder is metabolized by the liver. The plasma half-life is about 40 min; 58% of the drug is bound to plasma protein. Drowsiness is the most common adverse effect. Other adverse reactions reported are as follows: *autonomic nervous system*—dry mouth, shivering, sweating, hiccups, flushing, salivation, blurred vision; *cardiovascular system*—hypertension, hypotension, dizziness, atrial fibrillation, premature atrial and ventricular contractions; *central nervous system*—drowsiness, insomnia, restlessness, headache, excitement, nervousness; *gastrointestinal system*—anorexia, nausea; *musculoskeletal system*—twitching, shaking, tremors, weakness; *other systems*—fatigue, chills, increased temperature.

Dose—*Usual, intramuscular,* **50 mg** repeated in 1 hr, with subsequent doses every 3 or 4 hr as necessary. *Intravenous,* 25 mg slowly as a single dose; subsequent doses should be given intramuscularly.

Dosage Form—Injection: 50 mg, to be reconstituted with 2.2 mL sterile water.

Buclizine Hydrochloride

Piperazine, 1-[4-chlorophenylmethyl]-4-[[4-(1,1-dimethylethyl)phenyl]methyl]-, dihydrochloride; Ing of Bucladin-S, Softab (*Stuart*)

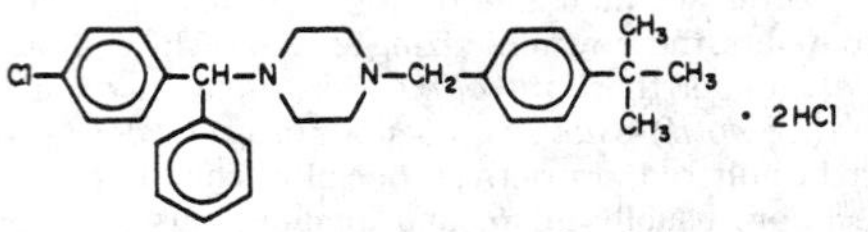

Cl   CH—N   N—CH_2 C—CH_3 CH_3 CH_3 · 2HCl

[129-74-8] $C_{28}H_{33}ClN_2$.2HCl (505.96).

Description—White, crystalline powder.

Solubility—Slightly soluble in water; insoluble in the usual organic solvents.

Uses—Buclizine hydrochloride, an agent with antihistaminic, antivertigo and CNS depressant properties, is indicated for the management of nausea, vomiting and dizziness associated with motion sickness. Adverse effects include drowsiness, blurred vision, dryness of the mouth, nose and throat, headache, nervousness, insomnia and upset stomach. It is not recommended for use during pregnancy or in breast-feeding mothers. Safety and efficacy for use in children have not been established. Drowsiness may occur and patients should be cautioned about driving or operating machinery.

Dose—*Usual, adult, oral,* **50 mg** 30 min before travel, repeated in 4 to 6 hr, if needed. *Nausea,* **50 mg,** 2 times a day; maximum dose, 150 mg a day.

Dosage Form—Tablets (Softab): 50 mg.

Chlorpromazine—page 1182.

Dimenhydrinate

1*H*-Purine-2,6-dione, 8-chloro-3,7-dihydro-1,3-dimethyl-, compd. with 2-(diphenylmethoxy)-*N*,*N*-dimethylethanamine (1:1); Dramamine (*Upjohn*); (*Various Mfrs*)

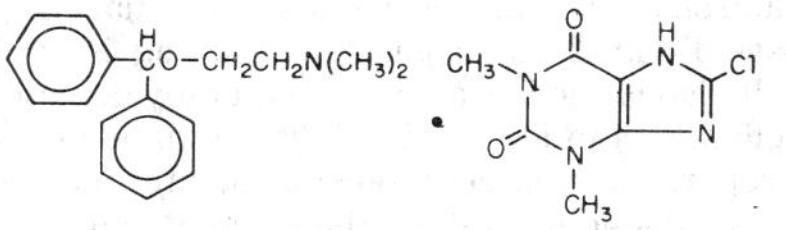

8-Chlorotheophylline, compound with 2-(diphenylmethoxy)-*N*,*N*-dimethylethylamine (1:1) [523-87-5] $C_{17}H_{21}NO.C_7H_7ClN_4O_2$ (469.97); contains 53–55.5% of diphenylhydramine ($C_{17}H_{21}NO$), and 44–47% of 8-chlorotheophylline ($C_7H_7ClN_4O_2$).

Preparation—By interaction of diphenhydramine, a base, with 8-chlorotheophylline, an acid, in isopropyl alcohol. **2**

Description—White, crystalline, odorless powder; melts between 102 and 107°.

Solubility—Slightly soluble in water; freely soluble in alcohol or chloroform; sparingly soluble in ether.

Uses—An *antihistaminic* compound which is a combination of diphenhydramine (Benadryl, *Parke-Davis)* and 8-chlorotheophyl line. The latter contributes little, if anything, to its action as an antiemetic or an antihistaminic agent. It is employed chiefly as an *antinauseant* in *motion sickness.* It also has been used with success in the management of the vertigo associated with Ménière's syndrome and radiation sickness. Mild sedation commonly attends its use. See page 902. Because of its sedating properties, patients should be cautioned about driving or operating machinery.

Dose—25 to **600 mg** daily; *usual, adult, oral,* **50** to **100 mg** every 4 hr; prophylaxis of *motion sickness*: **50 to 100 mg** 1 to 2 hr prior to exposure. *Children 8 to 12 yr, orally or rectally,* **25** to **50 mg** 2 or 3 times a day.

Dosage Forms—Injection: 50 mg/mL; Liquid: 15 mg/5 mL and 12.5 mg/4 mL; Tablets: 50 mg.

Diphenhydramine Hydrochloride—page 1225.

Diphenidol

1-Piperidinebutanol, α,α-diphenyl-, Vontrol (*SmithKline Beecham*)

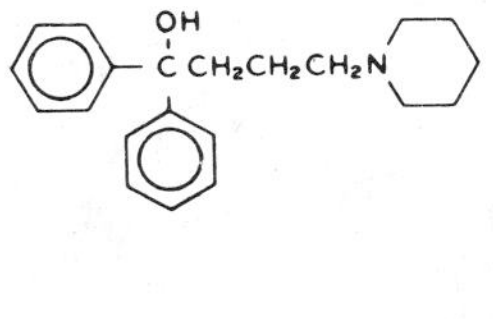

[972-02-1] $C_{21}H_{27}NO$ (309.45).

Preparation—Piperidine is reacted with 1-bromo-3-chloropropane in benzene with the aid of trimethylamine and the resulting 1-(3-chloropropyl)piperidine is converted to a Grignard reagent and reacted with benzophenone in tetrahydrofuran. Hydrolysis of the Grignard reaction complex yields crude diphenidol which may be purified by recrystallization from 2-propanol. US Pat 2,898,340.

Description—White, crystalline powder that is odorless and has a slightly bitter taste; stable in light and air; melts between 103 and 107°.

Solubility—Freely soluble in chloroform or ether; sparingly soluble in alcohol; insoluble in water.

Uses—An antiemetic agent unrelated to antihistamines or phenothiazines for the control of peripheral (labyrinthine) vertigo and associated nausea and vomiting as seen in Meniere's disease or after inner-ear surgery. It also is used to control nausea and vomiting in postoperative states and malignant neoplasms. Experimentally, it has been shown to exhibit weak parasympatholytic actions, but to lack significant sedative, tranquilizing or antihistaminic properties. Diphenidol is well absorbed after oral administration; peak concentration is reached in 1½ to 3 hr. The half-life is 4 hr with primary (90%) excretion in the urine. *Its use should be restricted to patients under close medical supervision, since auditory and visual hallucinations, disorientation and confusion have been reported.* Other untoward effects such as drowsiness, dry mouth, dizziness, skin rash, heartburn, headache, nausea, blurred vision, malaise, etc have been infrequent and minor in nature. Since diphenidol does possess parasympatholytic properties, it should not be used in patients with glaucoma, prostatic hypertrophy, peptic ulcer or gastroesophageal reflux. It is not recommended for use in the nausea and vomiting of pregnancy, since its safety has not been established.

Dose—*Usual, adult, oral,* **25** to **50 mg** every 4 hr. *Children 50 to 100 lb,* **25 mg** every 4 hr. Not recommended for use in infants under 6 months of age or 25 lb.

Dosage Form—Tablets: 25 mg.

Fluphenazine Hydrochloride—page 1184.

Dronabinol

6*H*-Dibenzo[*b*,*d*]pyran-1-ol, (6a*R*-*trans*)-6a,7,8,10a-tetrahydro-6,6,9-trimethyl-3-pentyl-, Delta-9-tetrahydrocannabinol; Marinol (*Roxane*)

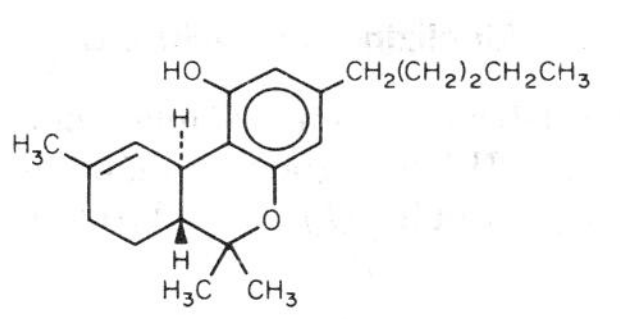

[1972-08-3] $C_{21}H_{30}O_2$ (314.47)

Preparation—The Δ^1-3,4-*trans* isomer (Δ^9-THC) is the major active component of marihuana (hashhish). For the isolation refer to *J Am Chem Soc 86:* 1646, 1964; for synthesis, *ibid 96:* 5860, 1974.

Description—Viscous, oily liquid; see *J Pharm Sci 62*: 1601, 1973 for stability under various conditions of storage.

Solubility—Insoluble in water; soluble in 1 part of alcohol or acetone, 3 parts of glycerol; soluble in fixed oils. Stability of parental solutions; *J Pharm Sci 61*: 1106, 1972.

Uses—Dronabinol, commonly known as delta 9-THC, is one of the active ingredients of marijuana. As such, it may be habit forming. It is especially useful for cancer chemotherapy-induced nausea and vomiting. It is thought to act centrally. Following oral administration dronabinol has systemic bioavailability of 10 to 20%. The drug undergoes extensive first-pass metabolism. Numerous metabolites have been identified, including 11-hydroxytetrahydrocannabinol, which appears in the plasma in about the same concentration as the parent substance. Within 72 hr after oral administration, approximately 50% of the administered dose is excreted in the feces and 15% in the urine either unchanged or as a metabolite. Patients may experience mood changes, hallucinations, mental depression, nervousness and tachycardia followed by bradycardia. Because of its effects on mental status, patients should be warned not to drive, operate machinery or make judgment decisions. Thus, strict patient compliance to dosage prescribed must be emphasized and the amount prescribed limited to that required for a single cycle of chemotherapy. Withdrawal symptoms consisting of irritability, insomnia and restlessness occur within 12 hr of abrupt withdrawal.

Dose—*Usual, adult, oral,* **5 mg** per m^2 of body surface 1 to 3 hr prior to chemotherapy, then every 2 to 4 hr after chemotherapy, for a total of 4 to 6 doses a day. *Maximum dose,* **15 mg**/m^2 of body surface per dose.

Dosage Form—Capsules: 2.5, 5 and 10 mg.

Granisetron Hydrochloride

1*H*-Indazole-3-carboxamide, endo-1-methyl-*N*-(9-methyl-9-azabicyclo[3.3.1]non-3-yl-, Kytril (*SmithKline Beecham*)

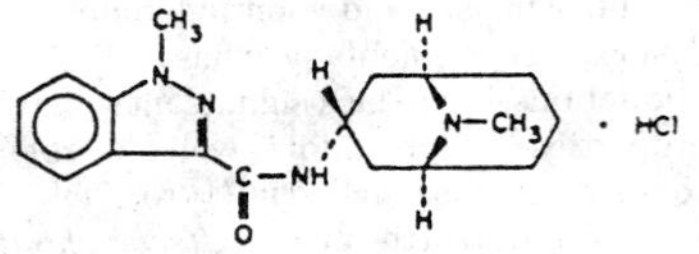

[107007-99-8] $C_{18}H_{24}N_4O.HCl$ (348.88).

Preparation—European Pat Appl. 200,444.

Description—White tufts melting about 291°.

Solubility—Very soluble in water or normal saline.

Uses—A very selective 5-hydroxytryptamine (5-HT_3) receptor antagonist with little or no affinity for other serotonin receptors (5-HT_1; 5-HT_{1A}; 5$HT_{1B/C}$; 5-HT_2; α- or β-adrenoreceptors; dopamine-D_2; histamine-H_1; benzodiazepin; picrotoxin or opioid). It is indicated to control nausea and vomiting associated with cancer chemotherapy. It is effective in preventing emesis and nausea when used with cisplatin, carboplatin and cyclophosphamide. It may also be co-administered with dexamethasone.

Principal adverse effects are headache (14%), asthenia (5%), somnolence (4%), diarrhea (4%) and constipation (3%).

Dose—*Usual, adult, intravenous,* **10 μg/Kg,** diluted in 50 mL of normal saline, infused over 5 minutes, beginning within 30 minutes before initiation of cancer chemotherapy.

Dosage Form—Injection: 1 mg/mL in normal saline in 1 mL vials.

Hydroxyzine Hydrochloride—page 1168.
Hydroxyzine Pamoate—page 1169

Meclizine Hydrochloride

Piperazine, 1-[(4-chlorophenyl)phenylmethyl]-4-[(3-methylphenyl)methyl]-, dihydrochloride, monohydrate; Antivert (*Roerig*); Bonine (*Pfizer*); (*Various Mfrs*)

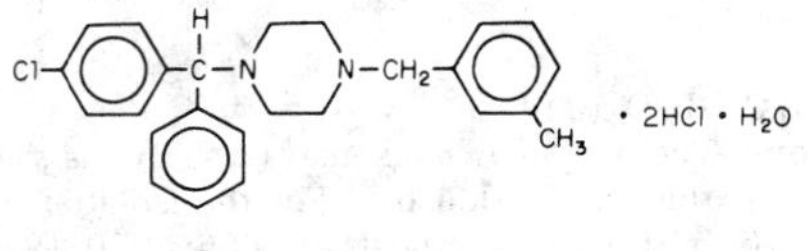

[31884-77-2] $C_{25}H_{27}ClN_2.2HCl.H_2O$ (481.89); *anhydrous* [1104-22-9] (463.88).

Preparation—Meclizine is formed by condensing *N*-(*m*-methylbenzyl) piperazine with *p*-chlorobenzhydryl chloride in the presence of triethylamine. The purified base is dissolved in a suitable solvent and converted to the dihydrochloride by a stream of hydrogen chloride.

Description—White or slightly yellowish, crystalline powder; slight odor; tasteless; melts between 217° and 224°, with decomposition.

Solubility—Practically insoluble in water and ether; freely soluble in chloroform; slightly soluble in alcohol.

Uses—Meclizine is a long-acting antihistaminic agent effective in the prevention or treatment of *nausea, vomiting* and *dizziness* associated with motion sickness. It also is used in *vertigo* associated with diseases affecting the vestibular system. The antiemetic activity starts within 60 min and lasts for 8 to 24 hr. Like other antihistamines, it may cause drowsiness and other side actions, such as blurred vision, dryness of the mouth and fatigue. Patients should be cautioned about driving and operating machinery. The action of a single dose can persist for 9 to 24 hr. Use of the drug in pregnancy or in women who may become pregnant is contraindicated. See page 790.

Dose—*Usual, adult, oral,* **25** to **50 mg** 1 hr prior to embarkation for protection against motion sickness. The dose may be repeated every 24 hr for the duration of the trip.

Dosage Forms—Tablets: 12.5, 25 and 50 mg. Chewable Tablets: 25 mg.

Metoclopramide Hydrochloride

Benzamide, 4-amino-5-chloro-*N*-[2-(diethylamino)ethyl]-2-methoxy-, monohydrochloride, monohydrate; Clopra (*Quantum*); Maxolon (*Beecham*); Reglan (*Robbins*); (*Various Mfrs*)

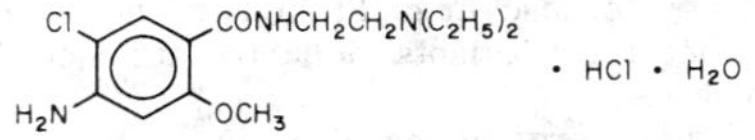

[54143-57-6] $C_{14}H_{22}ClN_3O_2.HCl.H_2O$.

Preparation—See *Arch Pharm 313:* 297, 1980.

Description—White crystals melting about 185° with decomposition.

Solubility—Soluble 1 g in about 0.7 mL of water, 3 mL of alcohol or 55 mL of chloroform. A 10% aqueous solution has a pH of about 5.5.

Uses—Metoclopramide is used for the prophylaxis of *vomiting* associated with *cisplatin* or other *cancer chemotherapeutic agents;* relief of symptoms associated with *acute* and *recurrent diabetic gastroparesis;* facilitation of *small-bowel intubation* in adults and children in whom the tube does not pass the pylorus with conventional maneuvers and the *promotion of gastric emptying and intestinal transit of barium* in cases where delayed emptying interferes with radiological examination of the stomach and small intestine. When treating diabetic gastroparesis, it should be used IV until some gastric emptying is restored to assure absorption. It also is used as adjunctive therapy in patients with gastroesophageal reflux. In addition to its ability to stimulate the gut, it also has cholinergic properties, apparently sensitizing intestinal smooth muscle to the action of acetylcholine rather than acting directly on cholinergic receptors. In addition, it is a potent dopamine antagonist. The drug is not effective in motion sickness. The use of metoclopramide is limited by two factors—a narrow therapeutic index and tachyphylaxis which usually occurs within 6 wk.

Metoclopramide is absorbed rapidly. Single oral dose peak plasma concentrations are reached within 40 to 120 min and the plasma half-life is about 4 hr. Approximately 75% of the orally administered drug is excreted in the urine. Pharmacological activity appears within 1 to 3 min following intravenous administration and 10 to 15 min following intramuscular injection; pharmacological effects persist for 1 to 2 hr. Common adverse effects include somnolence, nervousness and dystonic reactions. Parkinsonism and tardive dyskinesia also have been observed; increased pituitary prolactin release, galactorrhea and menstrual disorders have been reported. Metoclopramide should not be used in epileptics or patients receiving other drugs which are likely to cause extrapyramidal reactions, since the frequency and severity of seizure or extrapyramidal reactions may be increased.

Dose—*Prevention of cisplatin-induced emesis:* **1** or **2 mg/kg** diluted in 50 mL of a large-volume parenteral solution; infuse slowly over a period of not less than 15 min, 30 min before beginning cisplatin every 2 hr for 2 doses, then every 3 hr for 3 doses. *Diabetic gastroparesis:* **10 mg** orally, 30 min before each meal and at bed time for 2 to 8 weeks. *Direct intravenous injection: adults* **10 mg (2 mL),** *children 6 to 14 yr,* **2.5** to **5 mg,** and *under 6 yr,* **0.1 mg/kg** injected slowly over a period of 1 to 2 min.

Dosage Forms—Injection: 5 mg/mL in 2- and 10-mL ampuls. Syrup: 5 mg/5 mL. Tablets: 10 mg.

Perphenazine—page 1186.

Ondansetron Hydrochloride

4*H*-Carbazol-4-one, (±)-1,2,3,9-tetrahydro-9-methyl-3-[(2-methyl-1*H*-imidazol-1-yl)methyl]-, monohydrochloride, dihydrate; Zofran (*Glaxo*)

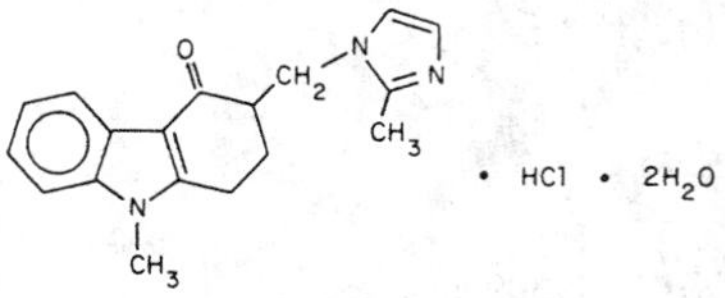

[103639-04-9] $C_{18}H_{19}N_3O.HCl.2H_2O$ (365.86).

Preparation—US Pat 4,695,578.

Description—White crystals melting about 180°; pK_a 7.4.

Solubility—1 g dissolves in 3 mL of water.

Uses—A selective 5-HT_3-receptor antagonist. Such receptors are present in vagal nerve terminals and in the chemoreceptor trigger zone of the area postrema. Ondansetron is indicated for the prevention of nausea and vomiting associated with emetogenic chemotherapy. It is not clear whether it acts peripherally, centrally or both. It appears that cytotoxic chemotherapy such as cisplatin is associated with release of serotonin from enterochromaffin cells in the small intestine. It is speculated that this serotonin triggers vomiting through 5-HT_3 vagal receptors that activate the vomiting reflex.

Ondansetron is metabolized extensively and only 5% of unchanged compound is recovered in the urine. It initially undergoes hydroxylation of the indole ring followed by glucuronidation or sulfation. The mean elimination half-life is approximately 4 to 5 hr but increases with the age of the patient. Plasma protein binding is 70 to 75%.

Ondansetron is effective in reducing emesis in both cisplatin- and cyclophosphamide-based chemotherapy. Using a visual analog scale, global satisfaction is increased from 10.5 to 96 (0 to 100) after single-day cisplatin therapy and from 52 to 100 after single-dose cyclophosphamide therapy.

The most common side effects of ondansetron are diarrhea (22%) and headache (16%). Akathisia and dystonia, seen with metoclopramide, does not occur with ondansetron. Other adverse reactions after multiple-day therapy include constipation, elevated liver enzymes, rash, bronchospasm, tachycardia, angina, hypokalemia and seizures.

Dose—*Usual, adult, intravenous* **0.15 mg/kg** diluted in 50 ml of 5% dextrose or 0.9% sodium chloride given over 15 min, 30 min prior to chemotherapy and 4 and 8 hr after chemotherapy.

Dosage Form—Injection: 2 mg/mL in 20-mL vials.

Prochlorperazine

10*H*-Phenothiazine,
2-chloro-10-[3-(4-methyl-1-piperazinyl)propyl]-,
Chlorazine (*Major*); Compazine (*SmithKline Beecham*)

[58-38-8] $C_{20}H_{24}ClN_3S$ (373.94).

Preparation—A toluene solution of 1-(3-chloropropyl)-4-methylpiperazine and 2-chlorophenothiazine is refluxed with sodamide for several hours. After filtering and distilling off the toluene, the prochlorperazine is obtained by short-path distillation under high vacuum.

Description—Clear, pale yellow, viscous liquid; sensitive to light.

Solubility—Very slightly soluble in water; freely soluble in alcohol, chloroform or ether.

Uses—A piperazine-type phenothiazine with actions, uses and limitations similar to those of *Prochlorperazine Maleate*. However, prochlorperazine, as the base, is administered rectally.

Dose—*Usual, rectal, children,* **2.5** to **10 mg** a day, according to weight, in divided doses; *adults,* **25 mg** 2 times a day.

Other Dose Information—The *child's rectal* dose should not exceed 7.5, 10 and 15 mg a day for a 20- to 29-lb, 30- to 39-lb and 40- to 58-lb child, respectively. It is not recommended for children weighing less than 20 lb.

Dosage Form—Suppositories: 2.5, 5, 10 and 25 mg.

Promethazine Hydrochloride—page 1227.

Prochlorperazine Edisylate

10*H*-Phenothiazine, 2-chloro-10-[3-(4-methyl-1-piperazinyl)propyl]-, 1,2-ethanedisulfonate (1:1); Prochlorperazine Ethanedisulfonate; Compazine (*SmithKline Beecham*)

[1257-78-9] $C_{20}H_{24}ClN_3S.C_2H_6O_6S_2$ (564.13).

For the structure of the base, see *Prochlorperazine*.

Preparation—*Prochlorperazine* is dissolved in a suitable solvent and treated with an equimolar portion of 1,2-ethanedisulfonic acid. The salt precipitates.

Description—White to very light yellow, odorless, crystalline powder; solutions are acid to litmus.

Solubility—1 g in about 2 mL water or about 1500 mL alcohol; insoluble in ether or chloroform.

Uses—Same actions and uses as prochlorperazine maleate except that it may be administered intramuscularly as well as orally. Parenteral therapy usually is reserved for the treatment of severe nausea and vomiting, for the immediate control of acutely disturbed psychotics or for patients who cannot or will not take oral medication. It should not be used in children with uncomplicated vomiting of unknown etiology. See *Prochlorperazine Maleate*.

Dose (as base equivalent)—*Adult, oral, antiemetic,* **5** to **10 mg** 3 or 4 times a day as required; *tranquilizer,* **5** to **35 mg** 3 or 4 times a day. *Usual range of oral dose,* **5** to **150 mg** a day. *Intramuscular* or *intravenous, antiemetic,* **5** to **10 mg** 6 to 8 times a day as required; *tranquilizer,* **10** to **20 mg** 4 to 6 times a day as required. *Usual range of parenteral dose,* as antiemetic, **5** to **40 mg** daily; as tranquilizer, **10** to **200 mg** a day.

Other Dose Information—No more than 40 mg of base equivalent should be injected in any 24-hr period unless the patient is hospitalized and under adequate observation. For acutely disturbed patients, the usual dose is 20 to 40 mg intramuscularly at intervals of 1 to 6 hr.

Dosage Forms (base equivalent)—Injection: 5 mg/mL; Syrup: 5 mg/5 mL; Concentrate (for institutional use): 10 mg/mL.

Prochlorperazine Maleate

10*H*-Phenothiazine, 2-chloro-10-[3-(4-methyl-1-piperazinyl)propyl]-, (*Z*)-2-butenedioate (1:2); Compazine (*SmithKline Beecham*)

[84-02-6] $C_{20}H_{24}ClN_3S.2C_4H_4O_4$ (606.09).

For the structure of the base, see *Prochlorperazine*.

Preparation—By the method described for *Prochlorperazine Edisylate* except that maleic acid is employed instead of ethanedi-sulfonic acid and it is employed in double equimolar quantity in relation to the prochlorperazine base.

Description—White or pale yellow, practically odorless, crystalline powder; saturated solution is acid to litmus.

Solubility—Practically insoluble in water or alcohol; slightly soluble in warm chloroform.

Uses—An *antiemetic, antipsychotic* and *tranquilizing agent.* It is an effective *antiemetic* in the control of mild or severe nausea and vomiting due to a variety of causes, such as early pregnancy, anesthesia, surgery and radiation therapy. Safety in pregnancy has not been established. There are reports of prolonged jaundice, extrapyramidial signs, hyperreflexia or hyporeflexia in newborns whose mothers have received phenothiazines. Nevertheless, compazine is used widely in pregnancy and has a long track record of safety. It, however, is not approved for this usage. It should not be used in children with uncomplicated vomiting of unknown etiology (*see page* 902). The drug is also an *effective antipsychotic.* Beneficial results ascribed to its action include reduction in psychomotor agitation and excitement, diminished aggressiveness and destructiveness, mitigation of hallucinations and delusions and a general calming effect. As a *tranquilizing agent,* it is possibly effective in mild mental disorders in which anxiety, tension and agitation predominate.

Adverse reactions include *drowsiness, dizziness, amenorrhea, skin reactions, hypotension, cholestatic jaundice, neuromuscular (extrapyramidal) reactions, motor restlessness, dystonias, pseudoparkinsonism, persistent tardive dyskinesia* and *contact dermatitis.* Children with acute infections (chickenpox, CNS infections, measles, gastroenteritis) or dehydration are more susceptible to neuromuscular reactions, particularly dystonias; such patients should be kept under close supervision. This agent may mask signs of overdosage of toxic drugs or obscure diagnosis of conditions such as intestinal obstruction or brain tumor. Adverse drug reactions can be minimized by periodically evaluating the dosage employed by patients on long-term therapy.

Dose (as base equivalent)—*Adult, oral, antiemetic,* **5** to **10 mg** 3 or 4 times a day as required; *tranquilizer,* **5** to **35 mg** 3 or 4 times a day, the initial low dose being increased gradually until the desired response is obtained, for which 50 to 150 mg daily usually is required.

Dosage Forms (base equivalent)—Tablets: 5, 10 and 25 mg; Sustained Release Capsules: 10, 15, 30 and 75 mg.

Scopolamine

Transderm-Scōp (*CIBA Consumer*)

Hyoscine [51-34-3] $C_{17}H_{21}NO_4$ (303.35). See *Scopolamine,* page 403 for structural formula, nomenclature and other data.

Description—Viscous liquid.

Solubility—1 g in 10 mL water; freely soluble in hot water, alcohol, ether or chloroform.

Uses—Provided as a disk for transdermal controlled release in the prevention of nausea and vomiting associated with motion sickness. It consists of a backing layer of aluminized polyester film, a drug reservoir of scopolamine, mineral oil and polyisobutylene, a microporous polypropylene membrane and an adhesive formulation of mineral oil, polyisobutylene and scopolamine. It contains 1.5 mg scopolamine and is programmed to deliver 0.5 mg per day at a constant rate over a 3-day period.

Scopolamine is a belladonna alkaloid and it is used to prevent motion sickness. Its mechanism of action is thought to be associated with inhibition of vestibular input resulting in suppression of the vomiting reflex.

The most frequent adverse reaction is dryness of the mouth and drowsiness. Transient blurred vision, disorientation, memory disturbance, restlessness, hallucinations, urinary retention, rashes and precipitation of glaucoma also have been reported. It should not be used in children, the elderly and patients on CNS depressants. Withdrawal symptoms may occur, especially if used for more than 3 days.

Dose—*usual, adult,* **one disk** applied to the hairless area behind the ear at least 4 hr prior to the desired antiemetic effect. Not recommended for children. *Note*—Hands should be washed before and after application and removal.

Dosage Form—Disks: 1.5 mg scopolamine.

Scopolamine Hydrobromide—page 1024.

Thiethylperazine Malate

10*H*-Phenothiazine, 2-(ethylthio)-10-[3-(4-methyl-1-piperazinyl)propyl]-, 2-hydroxy-1,4-butanedioate (1:2); Torecan (*Roxane*), Norzine (*Purdue Frederick*)

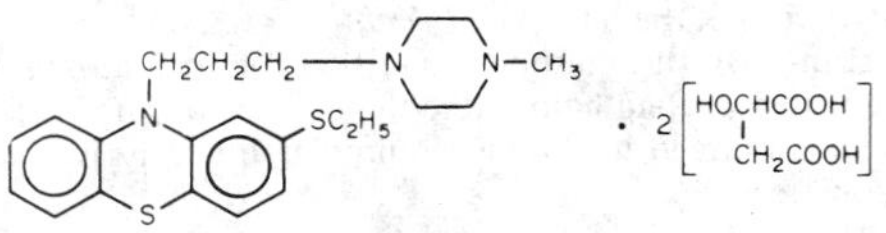

[52239-63-1] $C_{22}H_{29}N_3S_2.2C_4H_6O_5$ (533.71).

Preparation—*Thiethylperazine* is reacted with a double equimolar quantity of malic acid.

Description—White to faintly yellow crystalline powder; not more than a slight odor; pH (freshly prepared 1 in 100 solution) between 2.8 and 3.8.

Solubility—1 g in 40 mL water, 90 mL alcohol, 525 mL chloroform or 3400 mL ether.

Uses—See *Thiethylperazine Maleate.* Because of its solubility, this salt is used to prepare the injection.

Dose—*Intramuscular, usual,* **10** to **30 mg** daily.

Dosage Form—Injection: 5 mg/mL in 2 mL ampuls.

Thiethylperazine Maleate

10*H*-Phenothiazine, 2-(ethylthio)-10-[3-(4-methyl-1-piperazinyl)propyl]-, (*Z*)-1,4-butenedioate (1:2); Torecan (*Roxane*)

2-(Ethylthio)-10-[3-(4-methyl-1-piperazinyl)propyl]phenothia zine maleate (1:2) [1179-69-7] $C_{22}H_{29}N_3S_2.2C_4H_4O_4$ (631.76). For the structure of the base refer to *Thiethylpyrazine malate.*

Preparation—Thiethylperazine is prepared by reacting 2-(ethylthio) phenothiazine with 1-(3-chloropropyl)-4-methylpiperazine in the presence of sodamide or another dehydrochlorinating agent. The base is dissolved in a suitable solvent and reacted with a double molar quantity of maleic acid to produce the official salt. The starting phenothiazine compound may be prepared by condensing phenothiazine with ethanethiol and the piperazine compound similarly from methylpiperazine and trimethylene chloride. US Pat 3,336,197.

Description—Faintly yellowish, fine, crystalline, voluminous powder; odorless or has a very slight odor and is bitter to the taste; melts at about 183°, with decomposition; pH (1 in 1000 solution, warmed) between 2.8 and 3.8.

Solubility—1 g in 1700 mL water, 530 mL alcohol, >10,000 mL chlororoform or >10,000 mL ether.

Uses—A phenothiazine antiemetic *effective* in the relief of *nausea and vomiting* from various causes. It is also *possibly effective* for the management of *vertigo.* It should not be used in pregnancy or children under 12 yr. Other contraindications and side effects are the same as those for other phenothiazines (see page 1180).

Dose—*Usual, adult, oral,* **10** to **30 mg** a day.

Other Dose Information—The usual intramuscular and rectal dose is 10 to 30 mg a day.

Dosage Forms—Suppositories: 10 mg; Tablets: 10 mg.

Triflupromazine—see RPS-18, page 1090 .

Trimethobenzamide Hydrochloride

Benzamide, *N*-[[4-[2-(dimethylamino)ethoxy]phenyl]methyl]-3,4,5-trimethoxy-, monohydrochloride; Tigan (*SmithKline Beecham*)

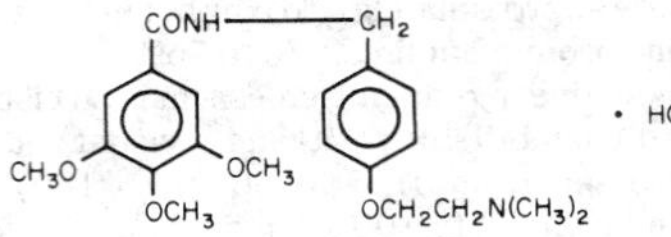

[554-92-7] $C_{21}H_{28}N_2O_5.HCl$ (424.92).

Preparation—4-[2-(Dimethylamino)ethoxy]benzylamine is condensed with 3,4,5-trimethoxybenzoyl chloride by refluxing in an inert solvent. The resulting trimethoxybenzamide may be converted to the hydrochloride by dissolving it in a suitable solvent and treating with HCl. The starting amine may be prepared in various ways, eg, by condensing sodium *p*-aminomethylphenoxide with 2- chloro-*N,N*-dimethylethylamine.

Description—White crystalline powder; slight phenolic odor; melts between 186° and 190°.

Solubility—1 g in 2 mL water, 59 mL alcohol, 67 mL chloroform or 720 mL ether.

Uses—A dimethylaminoethanol derivative indicated for the control of *nausea* and *vomiting.* Its safety in pregnancy has not been established, but trimethobenzamide frequently is used in this situation. Its antiemetic potency is about 1/10 that of chlorpromazine when given subcutaneously and 1/4 that of the latter when given orally. Minor side effects which have been reported include drowsiness, vertigo, diarrhea and local irritation. In patients with acute febrile illness, encephalitides, gastroenteritis, dehydration and electrolyte imbalance (especially in children and the elderly and debilitated), CNS reactions, such as opisthotonos, convulsions, coma and extrapyramidal symptoms, have been reported, but it is not certain that these effects were in all cases due to use of the drug. Therefore, caution should be exercised when trimethobenzamide hydrochloride is used in these conditions (*see* page 902). Drowsiness can occur and patients should be cautioned about driving and operating machinery. The use of the injectable form of the drug in children, the suppositories in premature or newborn infants and the use of the drug in patients hypersensitive to it are contraindicated. Also, suppositories should not be used in patients known to be sensitive to benzocaine or similar types of local anesthetics. Parkinson-like symptoms have been reported. Blood dyscrasias, blurred vision, coma, seizure, depression, diarrhea, drowsiness, muscle cramps and jaundice also have been reported. A blanket warning on the label, relating to Reye's Syndrome does not seem to be justified, but still should be considered.

Dose—*Usual, adult, oral,* **250 mg** 3 or 4 times a day; *rectal* or *intramuscular,* **200 mg** 3 or 4 times a day. *Children 30 to 90 lb, oral or rectal,* **100** to **200 mg** 3 or 4 times a day. *Intramuscular* not recommended for use in children.

Dosage Forms—Capsules: 100 and 250 mg; Injection: 100 mg/mL in 2-mL ampuls and 20-mL vials; Suppositories: 100 and 200 mg.

Adsorbents

Adsorbents are chemically inert powders that have the ability to adsorb gases, toxins and bacteria. The fine state of subdivision of these inert powders confers high adsorptive capacity upon them. However, in the complex milieu of the gastrointestinal secretions, physical (van der Waals) adsorbents are more likely to be selective for surface-active substances such as bile salts than for bacterial toxins and other noxious substances. Consequently, only certain materials that possess chemical adsorptive properties lend themselves effectively to gastrointestinal detoxification and to the adsorption of gases resulting from abnormal intestinal fermentation. Such substances are kaolin and activated charcoal. It is doubtful that either is an effective adsorbent in the lower gastrointestinal tract since passage through the upper tract saturates and deactivates these agents.

Many of the nonsystemic antacids may serve as internal protectives and adsorbents, especially after regeneration in the alkaline small intestine. Magnesium trisilicate is claimed to exert a protective action in the stomach by virtue of released silicic acid, which acts more as a demulcent than as a solid protective. *Antacids* commonly are combined with kaolin or other adsorbents.

Bismuth Subcarbonate—see RPS-18, page 908.

Bismuth Subnitrate—page 1407.

Activated Charcoal

Medicinal Charcoal (*Various Mfrs*)

The residue from the destructive distillation of various organic materials, treated to increase its adsorptive power.

Preparation—Formerly, a product named *Carbo Ligni* or *Wood Charcoal* was produced by burning wood out of contact with air, the residue obtained consisted of nearly pure carbon. Charcoal made by this process was variable in its adsorptive powers, frequently being entirely devoid of such properties. It was found that the adsorptive powers of charcoal could be increased tremendously by treating it with various substances such as steam, air, carbon dioxide, oxygen, zinc chloride, sulfuric acid, phosphoric acid or a combination of some of these substances, at temperatures ranging from 500° to 900°. This treatment is referred to as activation, the activating agent presumably removing substances previously adsorbed on the charcoal and, in some instances at least, breaking down the granules of carbon into smaller ones having a greater total surface area. It has been estimated that 1 mL of charcoal, finely divided, possesses a total surface of approximately 1000 m^2.

In addition to wood, many other substances are used as sources of charcoal, including sucrose, lactose, rice starch, coconut pericarp, bone, blood, various industrial wastes, etc. As many different activated charcoals are available for various purposes, one should be certain to use only the medicinal variety for medicinal purposes.

Description—Fine, black, odorless and tasteless powder, free from gritty matter.

Solubility—Insoluble in water or the other known solvents.

Uses—Activated charcoal is used for the acute treatment of poisoning—primarily as an emergency *antidote* in many forms of poisoning. Indeed, except for mineral acids, alkalies and substances insoluble in aqueous acidic solution, such as tolbutamide, it is the emergency treatment of choice for virtually all drugs and chemicals. Charcoal capsules also are used for the relief of flatulence and the discomfort of abdominal gas, but there is little evidence that it is effective for this purpose.

Industrially, it is used in large quantities in chemical and pharmaceutical manufacturing as a decolorizer. See *Clarification and Decoloration* (Chapter 37).

Dose—*Antidote*: **5** to **50 g**. *Usual, adult, oral,* **50 g;** *children, oral,* **25 g**. *Antiflatulent*: *adult,* **520** to **975 mg** after meals or at the first sign of discomfort; repeat as needed up to 4.16 daily.

Other Dose Information—Charcoal can adsorb drugs while they are in the GI tract; therefore, when used as an antiflatulent it should be taken 2 hr before or 1 hr after other oral medication. As an *antidote*, charcoal often is underutilized and given in insufficient doses; it should be given in a ratio of at least 10:1 of charcoal to estimated dose of toxin. Charcoal should not be administered simultaneously with ipecac, since it binds ipecac.

Dosage Form—Oral Solution: 20 g/150 mL, 25 g/120 mL and 50 g/240 mL.

Kaolin

Light Kaolin; White Bole; China Clay

A native hydrated aluminum silicate, powdered and freed from gritty particles by elutriation.

Preparation—Kaolin is distributed widely in nature. Most kaolin deposits, however, are contaminated with ferric oxide (hence the red color of ordinary clay) and some other impurities, such as calcium carbonate, magnesium carbonate, etc. To render kaolin suitable for pharmaceutical use, it has to be purified by treatment with hydrochloric acid or sulfuric acid, or both, then washed with water.

Kaolin of a high degree of purity, directly suitable for pharmaceutical use without acid purification, has been mined in the state of Georgia. England has large deposits of a fine grade of kaolin. The kaolin from these deposits is freed of coarse particles by elutriation or screening. Kaolin is essentially a colloid, and the *colloid kaolin* on the market differs only from ordinary kaolin in that it contains a larger percentage of fine particles and is prepared by special screening.

Description—Soft, white or yellowish white powder, or lumps; characteristic earthy or clay-like taste and, when moistened with water, becomes darker and develops a pronounced clay-like odor.

Solubility—Insoluble in water, cold diluted acids or solutions of the alkali hydroxides.

Uses—Either alone or as *Kaolin Mixture with Pectin* (see below) it is used medicinally as an *adsorbent*. It is perhaps of value in the treatment of *diarrhea* caused by agents capable of being adsorbed; for example, the diarrhea of food poisoning or dysentery. Kaolin also has been used in the treatment of chronic ulcerative colitis, but it is doubtful whether any adsorptive capacity is retained by the time the preparation reaches the colon. Externally, kaolin has some use as a poultice, dusting powder and an ingredient of toilet powders.

Dose—It usually is given suspended in water in the dose of from **50** to **100 g,** at 3-hr intervals.

Magnesium Trisilicate—page 888.

Pectin

A purified carbohydrate product obtained from the dilute acid extract of the inner portion of the rind of citrus fruits or from apple pomace. It consists chiefly of partially methoxylated polygalacturonic acids.

Pectin yields not less than 6.7% of methoxy groups and not less than 74.0% of $C_6H_{10}O_7$ (galacturonic acid), calculated on the dried basis.

Pectin may be standardized to the convenient "150 jelly grade" by addition of dextrose or other sugars, and it may contain sodium citrate or other buffer salts. Such pectin is not suitable for medicinal use.

Description—Coarse or fine powder, yellowish white in color, almost odorless, and with a mucilaginous taste.

Solubility—Almost completely soluble in 20 parts of water at 25°, forming a viscous, opalescent, colloidal solution which flows readily and is acid to litmus; insoluble in alcohol or diluted alcohol and in other organic solvents; dissolves in water more readily if first moistened with alcohol, glycerin or simple syrup, or if first mixed with 3 or more parts of sucrose.

Incompatibilities—Precipitated from solution by an excess of *alcohol*. *Metals*, particularly the heavy metals, form insoluble derivatives. In the presence of *alkalies*, pectin undergoes progressive hydrolysis resulting in a demethylation followed by a splitting of the glycosidic linkages of the galacturonic acid units. *In cold acid solution* it is more stable; prolonged heating of such a solution causes hydrolysis. Liquefaction of pectin pastes may be due to a hydrolysis which accompanies growth of certain types of *mold*.

Uses—A *protective* used in combination with kaolin for the treatment of *diarrhea* in infants and children. The unchanged molecules of the polygalacturonic acids may have an *adsorbent* action in the intestine. As a *pharmaceutic aid*, it is used as an *emulsifying* and *thickening* agent.

Dose—See *Kaolin Mixture with Pectin*.

Other Adsorbents

Kaolin Mixture with Pectin [(*Various Mfrs*)]—*Preparation:* Mix kaolin (200 g) with purified water (500 mL). Triturate pectin (10 g), powdered tragacanth (5 g) and sodium saccharin (1 g) with glycerin (20 mL) and add to this, with constant stirring, benzoic acid (2 g) dissolved in boiling purified water (300 mL). Allow the mixture to stand until it cools to room temperature and all the pectin is dissolved. Add peppermint oil (0.75 mL) and the kaolin-water mixture, mix thoroughly and finally add sufficient purified water to make 1000 mL. In order to obtain a product with suitable consistency when larger amounts are prepared, the quantity of tragacanth and, if necessary, the quantity of pectin may be altered. However, if the proportion of pectin in the form is altered by more than 10%, the pectin content of the preparation must be stated clearly on the label. This compound contains calcium which may interact with tetracycline. It is contraindicated in bowel obstruction or fecal impaction.

Uses—For the treatment of diarrhea but is only moderately effective. It can be used in children.

Dose—*Usual, adult,* **2 tablespoonfuls** and repeat every 3 to 4 hr; **4 chewable tablets** and repeat every 3 to 4 hr or **2 tablets** after initial bowel movement and each subsequent bowel movement, not to exceed 12 tablets in 24 hr. *Usual, children, 3 to 6 yr,* ¼ adult dose; *6 to 12 yr,* ½ adult dose.

Hepatic Immunostimulants

Immunostimulation is used to treat chronic hepatitis B and C. Approximately 10 to 15% of patients who become infected with the hepatitis B virus develop chronic disease, manifested by chronic hepatitis, cirrhosis or in a small number of patients, hepatocellular carcinoma. The reasons that patients develop chronic disease are uncertain. In some parts of the world, southeast Asia for example, almost 90% of infants born to hepatitis B-positive women will become chronically infected. When the disease is acquired at an older age, chronic disease is less likely to occur. Serum interferon levels are decreased in many patients with chronic hepatitis B. This may be secondary to the virus transfecting chromosome-9 at the site that codes for interferon. Interferon is antiviral because of two properties—it stimulates the synthesis of 2,5-A synthetase, which inhibits viral replication, and it induces the HLA major histocompatibility antigens on the hepatocyte surface so that they can become the target of cytotoxic T cells. The demonstration of interferon deficiency in chronic hepatitis B is the rationale for its use in that disease. It induces remission in about half the patients with a relapse rate of 2 to 3% a year. It is not known if it prevents hepatocellular carcinoma in such patients.

Approximately 70% of patients with non-A, non-B hepatitis, now largely recognized as hepatitis C, become chronically infected. Interferon trials for non-A, non-B trials were started prior to the discovery of the hepatitis C virus. It was learned subsequently that most of the patients indeed had hepatitis C and the drug-induced remission in approximately half of these patients with relapse occurring in about half of these patients by 1 year.

Interferon Alfa-2b, (Recombinant)

Interferon α2b (human leukocyte clone Hif-SN206 protein reduced); Intron A (*Schering*)

[9008-11-1] $C_{860}H_{1353}N_{229}O_{255}S_9$ (19,269.12).

Preparation—A protein chain of 165 amino acids which are naturally occuring and are derived from virus-stimulated Namawala cells or recombinant DNA-formed as a single component.

Description—White, lyophilized powder.

Uses—Interferons exert their activity by binding to specific cellular receptors and then initiating intracellular events that suppress viruses. These include induction of 2,5-A synthetase, which inhibits viral replication and HLA-1 major histocompatibility antigens which attract the cytotoxic T cells.

Interferon alfa-2b is indicated for the treatment of *chronic hepatitis C* and *chronic hepatitis B*. For chronic hepatitis C, treatment is continued for 6 mo although there is little evidence that therapy beyond 4 mo is helpful. Patients who are symptomatic with malaise, fatigue, myalgia, arthalgias and other symptoms of liver disease are candidates for treatment. Also, asymptotic patients with chronic aggressive heptitis on liver biopsy are suitable. Because of the uncertainty of the prognosis of patients with hepatitis C, some have suggested treating all patients. However, there are no data to support this approach. Therapeutic response is measured by following liver enzymes. The ALT and AST may return to normal within 2 or 3 wk, but seldom return to normal beyond 4 mo of therapy. Nevertheless, the current recommendation is to treat for 6 mo. Histological improvement is seen in 50 to 60% of patients and is characterized by a decrease in severity of necrosis. It is not known if this improves the ultimate prognosis in these patients in terms of preventing cirrhosis or hepatocellular carcinoma.

Side effects are common with interferon alfa-2b. Those seen in more than 10% of patients include fever (approximately 45%), headaches (approximately 45%), myalgias (approximately 40%), asthenia (approximately 20%), rigors (approximately 25%), fatigue (approximately 20%), arthralgias (approximately 20%), nausea (approximately 25%), diarrhea (approximately 15%) and alopecia (approximately 15%). Irritability, insomnia, depression, abdominal pain, pruritus, rash and inflammation at the injection site also are seen. Thyroid dysfunction in the form of either hyper- or hypothyroidism occurs in approximately 1% of patients and has been irreversible in some. TSH monitoring prior to therapy and at 1 mo is recommended. Anemia, leukopenia and thrombocytopenia occur in 10 to 30% of patients and may require dose modification or temporary discontinuance. CBCs are recommended at 2- to 4-wk intervals to monitor patients. Despite the long list of side effects and their rather high frequency, therapy almost always can be completed. It should not, however, be used in patients with decompensated liver disease. There is recent evidence that interferon, when given to patients with acute hepatitis C, may reduce the incidence of chronic hepatitis.

Interferon alfa-2b also is indicated for the treatment of chronic hepatitis B, which is continued for 6 mo. Because of the higher dose, therapy is difficult as the patients have more frequent and more severe side effects. There is frequently a flareup of the liver disease at 12 to 14 wk when the hepatitis e antigen converts to e antibody. This, however, generally signals the end of viral replication and a positive response to treatment. Patients with decompensated liver disease manifested by ascites, encephalopathy or coagulopathy, should not be treated except under special controlled circumstances because of the high risk of fatal side effects, especially bacterial peritonitis with sepsis.

Dose—*Usual, subcutaneous,* for *chronic hepatitis* C, **3 million units** 3 times a wk for 4-6 mo; for *chronic hepatitis B*, **5 million units** a day for 6 mo.

Dosage Form—Prefilled Syringes: 3 or 5 million units for self-administration.

Miscellaneous Gastrointestinal Drugs

Several drugs with diverse actions on the gastrointestinal tract are included in this section. They range from the empirical carminative *peppermint spirit* to the novel gallstone dissolution agent ursodiol, and the well-established *diphenoxylate hydrochloride–atropine sulfate* antidiarrheal combination. Carminatives are substances which were at one time used to relieve gaseous distention of the stomach or intestines. Many carminative volatile oils are used as flavoring agents (*see* Chapter 80 and the cross-references listed below).

Anise Oil—page 1385.
Anisotropine Methylbromide—page 1025.
Bismuth Subcarbonate—see RPS-18, page 799.
Camphor—page 874.
Camphor Spirit—see RPS-17, page 781.
Caraway—see RPS-18, page 1293.
Caraway Oil—see RPS-18, page 1293.
Cardamom Oil—page 1386.
Cardamom Seed—page 1386.
Cardamom Tincture, Compound—see RPS-18, page 1302.
Chenodiol—see RPS-18, page 797.
Chlorobutanol—page 1380.
Chloroform—page 1409.

Lactase

Lactaid (*Lactaid*)

Preparation—A β-D-galactosidase isolated from *Aspergillus oryzae* (caplets) or *Kluyveromyces lactis* (drops).

Uses—The enzyme lactase hydrolyzes lactose—the sugar found in milk—into two simple sugars: glucose and galactose. It is indicated for patients with symptomatic lactose deficiency manifested by abdominal cramps, bloating, flatuluence and diarrhea. It's only known side-effect is allergy. Diabetics should be aware that the glucose formed through degradation by lactase will be absorbed and, in effect, increase their sugar intake.

Dose—Add **5 drops** of liquid to a quart of milk, shake gently and refrigerate for 24 for 70% reduction in lactose; **10** to **15 drops** may be used for 90% or 99% reduction in lactose. *Oral,* **two caplets** with each meal; adjust for relief of symptoms, but no more than 6 caplets at a time.

Dosage Forms—Drops (each drop contains 250 neutrolactose units); Caplets (each caplet contains 3,300 Food Chemical Codex units).

Lactulose

D-Fructose, 4-*O*-β-D-galactopyranosyl-, Cephulac and Chronulac (*Marion Merrell Dow*)

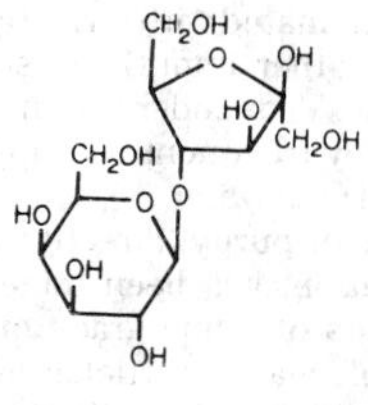

4-*O*-β-D-Galactopyranosyl-D-fructofuranose [4618-18-2] $C_{12}H_{22}O_{11}$ (342.30).

Preparation—Lactulose (a disaccharide containing 1 molecule of galactose and 1 molecule of fructose) may be prepared by epimerization of lactose (a disaccharide containing 1 molecule of galactose and 1 molecule of glucose) in a lime water medium. *J Am Chem Soc 52:* 2101, 1930.

Description—White powder; melts at about 169°; levorotatory; reduces Fehling's solution; yields galactose and fructose on acid hydrolysis. The commercially available syrup is a pale yellow to yellow, viscous, sweet liquid; each 15 mL contains 10 g of lactulose (and less than 2.2 g galactose, less than 1.2 g lactose and 1.2 g or less of other sugars).

Solubility—Very soluble in water; very slightly soluble in alcohol.

Uses—Lactulose (syrup) is used to reduce blood ammonia levels in patients with portal-systemic encephalopathy. It improves the patients' mental state and EEG patterns, but does not alter the course of the underlying liver disease. The action of lactulose, which is absorbed poorly after oral administration, depends on its breakdown by colonic bacteria to carbon dioxide, lactic acid and small amounts of acetic and formic acids, which acidify the contents of the colon. The acidic environment converts ammonia to ammonium ion (NH_4^+) which cannot be absorbed. It also favors diffusion of ammonia from blood into the colon. The osmotic laxative action of lactulose and/or its metabolites then expels the trapped ammonium ions from the colon. Therapy with lactulose is reported to reduce blood-ammonia levels by 25 to 50%, and effect a favorable clinical response in about 75% of patients. Lactulose is poorly absorbed with only 3% appearing in the urine in 24 hr.

Lactulose may produce gaseous distention with flatulence or belching and abdominal discomfort such as cramping in about 20% of patients. Excessive dosage produces diarrhea but some degree of diarrhea is needed for its maximum therapeutic effect. Nausea and vomiting have been reported infrequently.

Lactulose syrup contains some monosaccharides and should be used with caution in diabetics. Concomitant use of neomycin with lactulose may result in elimination of colonic bacteria that are essential for the required degradation of lactulose and thus prevent acidification of the colon. Other laxatives should not be used, especially during the initial phase of therapy because loose stools falsely may suggest that lactulose dosage is adequate. Lactulose does not alter the course of the underlying liver disease, for which other therapy may be required. The safety of lactulose syrup during pregnancy and the effect on the mother and fetus have not been evaluated.

Dose—*Usual, adult, oral, for portal-systemic encephalopathy,* **30** to **45 mL** of syrup (**20** to **30 g** of lactulose) 3 or 4 times a day; dosage may be adjusted every 1 or 2 days to produce 2 or 3 soft stools a day. *Usual, oral, for constipation,* **15** to **30 mL** (**10** to **20 g** of lactulose) daily (24 to 48 hr may be required for normal bowel movement). *Rectal, as retention enema,* **300 mL** of lactulose mixed with 700 mL of water or saline (retain for 30 to 60 min).

Dosage Form—Syrup, each 15 mL containing 10 g of lactulose.

Simethicone

Gas-X (*Sandoz*); Mylicon (*Stuart*); Phazyme (*Reed & Carnrick*); Silain (*Robins*); (*Various Mfrs*)

Simethicone [8050-81-5]; a mixture of fully methylated linear siloxane polymers containing repeating units of the formula $[—(CH_3)_2SiO]_n$, stabilized with trimethylsiloxy end-blocking units of the formula $[(CH_3)_3$-$SiO—]$, and silicon dioxide.

Description—Translucent, gray, viscous fluid; specific gravity between 0.964 and 0.984; refractive index between 1.400 and 1.410; viscosity (25 ± 0.1°) not less than 300 centistokes.

Uses—An agent with defoaming action which is supposed to relieve gas in the GI tract. It is used as adjunctive therapy in conditions in which gas is a problem, such as *postoperative gaseous distention, air swallowing, functional dyspepsia, irritable colon* and *diverticulosis.* It also is used in antacid combinations to defoam gastric juice, in order to decrease the tendency to gastroesophageal reflux; however, it does *not* decrease the antacid requirement. It has yet to be proved that simethicone has any therapeutic benefit. It is thought to be physiologically inert and devoid of toxicity.

Dose—*Usual, adult, oral,* Capsules: **125 mg**. Tablets: **40** to **80 mg** 4 times a day after each meal and at bedtime. Chew tablets thoroughly. Drops: **40 mg** 4 times a day after meals and at bedtime.

Dosage Forms—Drops: 40 mg/0.6 mL; Tablets: 40, 50, 60, 80 and 125 mg. Capsules: 125 mg.

CHAPTER 54

Blood, Fluids, Electrolytes and Hematologic Drugs

Karleen S Callahan, PhD
Research Assistant Professor of Pharmacology
College of Pharmacy, University of Utah
Salt Lake City, UT 84112

Blood is a unique tissue. As a tissue, it can be withdrawn from the body, and an extensive array of its parts can be separated for use in therapy. As a circulating body fluid, blood serves a vital set of physiological functions. A large number of drugs exert useful specific actions directed at maintaining or restoring these functions.

The reader is referred to Chapter 31 for a basic discussion of hematology and blood banking technology.

The responsibility for promulgating and administering federal regulations applicable to blood and blood products is that of the Food and Drug Administration (FDA), Bureau of Biologics. The applicable regulations are found in the *Code of Federal Regulations, 21 CFR 273.3.* Standards also are set by the American Association of Blood Banks and the World Health Organization (WHO).

Whole Blood and Blood Components

Blood serves many vital functions and also reflects the condition of other body tissues. Even though whole blood does not normally come into direct contact with cells other than the vascular endothelium, electrolytes and many small organic compounds found in plasma freely exchange with both the lymph and the interstitial fluid. Thus, the composition of blood is an important indicator of cellular ion and metabolic status. Plasma is the vehicle for the transport of most nutrients to, and many wastes from, the tissues. Plasma transports drugs, often in combined, or bound, form; plasma is therefore an important factor in determining the effectiveness of drugs (Chapter 41). The proteins in plasma are involved importantly in the regulation of the hydration of the tissues by virtue of osmosis resulting from the impermeability of the vascular endothelium to most of the protein. Some of the plasma proteins are involved intimately in the clotting of blood and, therefore, in its conservation.

The erythrocytes are involved especially with oxygen and carbon dioxide transport. Leukocytes play major roles in the defense against infection (see Chapter 44) and platelets exert a variety of important functions in hemostasis and response to injury.

Uses for Blood and Blood Components—The many physiological functions of blood derive from the specific roles of its many parts; in addition to the formed elements there are more than 80 discrete proteins in plasma. When whole blood has been lost, as by hemorrhage, whole blood is required for replacement. However, the use of whole blood to overcome a deficiency of a single part constitutes a dissipation of the other useful parts.

In the majority of instances, the administration of a single component in concentrated form elicits a far better response than the administration of that component as whole blood. Furthermore, by using the specific parts of the blood, the supply of blood can be used more economically; the net result is the use of the components of a single donation for several purposes.

The number of products now available is increasing but is still short of the number of known parts of blood. For example, the red cells can be made available for the treatment of anemia, albumin for the treatment of shock, immune globulins for the prophylaxis of certain infectious diseases, granulocytes for granulocytopenia and platelets for thrombocytopenia. These, and other important available blood components, are discussed in the following sections.

In the US, the collection, processing, preservation and distribution of blood and its separated components are performed by a wide variety of enterprises. For the purpose of this discussion, however, the important fact is where and how blood and its components are made available for the use of patients and the public at large. The main channels for dispensing blood services and blood products are

1. Blood centers and blood banks. These provide a wide array of services which reach the patient on prescription usually through a hospital blood bank or transfusion service. The major services include the provision of whole blood, separated red cells, platelets, granulocytes, cryoprecipitated Factor VIII, single-donor plasma and fresh frozen plasma. These usually are referred to as blood and blood components. They are distinguished by the fact that they are prepared locally in the blood center and dispensed in the form of individual units identified by the donor.
2. The pharmaceutical manufacturer and the pharmacy. This applies to the products of plasma fractionation, which are prepared by pharmaceutical manufacturers from large lots of pooled human plasma and are, therefore, subject to biological control regulations separate from those applying to simple units of blood and its components.
3. Public-health agencies and large blood centers. These may dispense directly to physicians or even to individual patients under certain circumstances.

Transmission of Infection—The use of blood and its components is accompanied by some risk of transmission of serum hepatitis cytomegalovirus, AIDS, Epstein-Barr virus, herpes simplex, infectious mononucleosis, syphillis, malaria, Chaga's disease, etc. This risk is different depending on which part of the blood is used and, also, on how it was prepared.

In the case of units of whole blood and blood components prepared and distributed by blood banks and blood centers, the degree of risk depends on the ability to detect the infectious agent in donor blood. Rapid progress is being made in this area. However, it probably will be some time, if ever, before the risk will reach zero; ie, before the absolute safety of donor blood can be assured. Still, the risk may be diminished or indeed eliminated by suitable processing treatments. Thus, immune globulin prepared by the ethanol-water fractionation procedure is free of virus even without specific viricidal treatment.

Human Albumin carries no risk of virus transmission, as a result of heating the solution to 60°C for 10 hours. Therefore, it is likely that any product which can be heated at 60°C for 10 hours will have a greatly diminished, if not zero, risk of viral transmission. Unfortunately, very few products can withstand such rigorous treatment, and other means have been sought to inactivate viruses, but with less than complete success. These include irradiation with ultraviolet light, cathode rays and chemical treatment with various substances such as β-propiolactone. None of these methods, as presently used, can be relied on to inactivate completely all viruses that might be present, although they diminish the risk associated with use of the material.

In short, except for certain products such as albumin and immune globulin which are known to be free of virus, most blood derivatives must be assumed to involve a risk of virus transmission, and this risk must be weighed against the medical consequences of withholding the product.

Whole Blood

Blood may be collected for human use only from persons who are certified by a physician as being free of transmissible disease, as far as can be determined from the donor's personal history, physical examination, etc. Unfortunately, in mass donations (eg, bloodmobiles) these examinations and certifications tend to be hasty and limited. The usual amount drawn is 500 mL. The blood is collected into an anticoagulant solution. A sample of blood is collected at the time of bleeding and subjected to serological and virological tests.

The use of the anticoagulant mixtures known as ACD and CPD (see page 921) extends the useful life of the red cells with the result that, following storage under proper conditions, the blood can be used with safety for a period of 21 days after collection. The addition of adenine to CPD solution (to make CPDA-1) increases the shelf life by another 14 days, thus enabling a useful storage time of 35 days. The use of these solutions has extended greatly the flexibility of hospital and community blood banks. However, with heparin the shelf life is much shorter, the official expiration time being 2 days.

If whole blood is used, it is handled carefully and stored in the cold without further processing or testing, except for occasional observation to detect evidence of hemolysis or contamination.

Blood Components

Blood collection agencies—blood centers and blood banks—provide an array of blood services to the areas they serve. These include providing whole blood and several blood components prepared in the center from fresh donor blood. Blood components are made from single units of blood without opening or breaking the sterility of the plastic-bag system in which the blood originally was collected. These components thus are individualized with respect to the donor; if greater amounts are required than those available from one donor, multiple units are used. In addition to whole blood, components commonly available are CPD or CPDA-1 red blood cells, frozen red blood cells, saline-washed red blood cells, leukocyte-free red blood cells, granulocyte concentrate, platelet concentrate, cryoprecipitated antihemophilic factor (page 919), fresh frozen plasma and liquid plasma.

Whole Blood

Blood that has been drawn from suitable human donors under rigid aseptic precautions. It contains citrate ion (acid citrate dextrose or citrate phosphate dextrose or citrate phosphate dextrose with adenine) or heparin as an anticoagulant. Preparations are designated ACD Whole Blood, CPD Whole Bood, CPDA-1 Whole Blood or Heparinized Whole Blood according to the anticoagulant used. Whole blood from which the antihemophilic factor has been removed is designated Modified Whole Blood (see below).

Description—Deep-red, opaque liquid from which the corpuscles readily settle, on standing for 24 to 48 hr, leaving a clear, yellowish or pinkish, supernatant layer. If the blood has been drawn soon after the donor has eaten, it may, on standing, acquire a layer of fatlike material near its surface. A deep-pink or red color in the plasma, or a purplish tint at the surface of the cell portion, usually indicates that the blood is unsatisfactory for use.

Uses—The natural replenisher for lost blood and hence is indicated when there has been hemorrhage or traumatic blood loss of over 20% of the blood volume. When the blood loss is small, it is not essential that all of the lost blood be replaced, except in persons with high oxygen demand (eg, thyrotoxicosis, beri-beri) or in anemia. Consequently, some practitioners may replace only part of the lost blood and make up the remainder of the deficit with a saline, hetastarch or dextran solution. In hemorrhagic shock, some medical opinion holds that the entire volume deficit should not be repaired by whole blood alone because of erythrocyte aggregation and sludging, and a dextran also sometimes is added concomitantly, not only to suppress erythrocyte aggregation but also platelet aggregation, since intravascular clotting sometimes is a complication. Adverse effects of whole blood include reactions from improperly matched blood, passive transfer of allergies, serum hepatitis and other infections, volume overload in improperly monitored administration and increased viscosity of the circulating blood. Stored whole blood is nearly devoid of platelets and also may be deficient in factors V and VII, so that clotting and coagulation defects may occur after massive transfusions.

Dose—*Intravenous infusion*, as needed to replenish blood volume; *usual* **1 Unit,** repeated as necessary. The dose is based on the estimated blood loss, laboratory determination of need or central venous pressure. One unit is 450 ± 45 mL of whole blood to which 63 mL of ACD, CPD or CPDA-1 solution has been added. Units must be administered through a 170-μm filter.

Dosage Form—Between 468 and 558 mL.

Whole Blood Modified

Single-donor whole blood from which antihemophilic factor (USP definition) or one or more other, nonerythrocyte components has/have been removed. Components and plasma may be removed either by sedimentation methods or by continuous separation devices; after selective separation, the plasma is reunited with the erythrocytes.

Uses—The uses are determined, in part, by the health of both the donor and recipient and the reason for removal of the component(s). If the reason for component-pheresis is to remove an adverse component, such as leukocytes in a leukemia or lymphocytes in an autoimmune disorder, the modified whole blood is returned autologously to the donor. If, instead, the donor is healthy and pheresis is conducted to provide a heterologous source of the component(s) for therapeutic purposes, the residual modified whole blood may be used for the same purposes as *Whole Blood*, provided that the volume to be transfused is small enough so as not to cause, by dilution, a clinically-significant deficit of the corresponding component(s) in the recipient.

Granulocyte Concentrate

A single-donor concentrate of leukocytes obtained either by separation from sedimented whole blood or by pheresis with a continuous- or intermittent-flow centrifuge. The granulocytes (and entrained lymphocytes) are resuspended in the plasma of the recipient. The component should be used within 24 hr of collection.

Uses—Heterologously in patients with severe leukopenia, usually that which results from cancer chemotherapy or other adverse drug reactions.

Dose—That which is necessary to bring the granulocyte count above 500/mL. A single donor usually can provide more than 10^{10} granulocytes in 2 to 3 hr. It is difficult to administer more than 10% of the normal daily output of granulocytes.

Lymphocytes Frozen

A single-donor frozen concentrate of lymphocytes obtained by differential sedimentation from whole blood or from the removal of lymph from the thoracic duct. The cells are cooled at a rate of 3.5°/min. DMSO is added to a 5% concentration when the temperature reaches 0°. Reconstitution requires careful thawing and repeated washout of DMSO. Viable cells are quantified from the uptake of radiothymidine into phytohemagglutinin-stimulated suspensions.

Uses—Investigationally in the treatment of neoplastic diseases, as exchange replacement for lymphocytes pheresed from the blood of patients afflicted with certain thymocyte-mediated autoimmune disorders, and as a diagnostic agent in specialized *in vitro* assessments of immune function.

Tumor-Infiltrating Lymphocytes—page 1262.

Single-Donor Plasma

Human Plasma

The liquid portion of a single unit of ACD, CPD- or CPDA-1-whole blood, the separation of which was accomplished within the expiration time of the whole blood. It is stored at 1 to 6°; it may be stored for 5 days beyond the dating period of the whole blood from which it was separated (26 and 40 days if from CPD- or CPDA-1-whole blood, respectively). The ABO compatibility is that of the donor whole blood. One unit is 220 to 250 mL.

Description—Straw-colored transparent fluid which may sometimes exhibit a slight opalescence.

Uses—Mostly for *volume replenishment* in the treatment of *shock*, especially after severe burns, in which plasma protein loss is considerable. It is used occasionally as a source of the stable coagulation factors II, VII, IX and X, and thus can be used to treat hemophilia B. ABO compatibility is desirable but is not a prerequisite to use.

Dose—*Intravenous infusion*, variable dose, depending upon the magnitude of the volume deficit or requirement for stable coagulation factors and upon the clinical response. When the plasma is ABO-incompatible with the blood of the recipient and a volume deficit is large, the physician may elect to repair only part of the deficit with plasma and the remainder with another plasma expander.

Single-Donor Plasma Freeze Dried

Human Plasma Freeze-Dried

Single-donor plasma that has been cryodessicated. If Fresh Frozen Plasma is the source of the cryodessicate, the plasma may be designated as an Antihemophilic Plasma. The expiration time of the reconstituted plasma is that of *Single-Donor Plasma*.

Uses and ***Dose***—If the dessicate is made from *Fresh Frozen Plasma*, see the monograph; it made from Frozen Plasma. see *Single-Donor Plasma*.

Single-Donor Plasma Fresh Frozen

Human Plasma, Fresh Frozen; Antihemophilic Plasma

Single-donor human plasma frozen within 6 hr of collection and stored at a temperature of −20° or lower (preferably below −30°). The frozen plasma shall not be stored beyond 12 mo. As a source of coagulation factors, the expiration time of thawed fresh frozen plasma is 24 hr; as a volume replenisher, the expiration time is that of Single-Donor Plasma. ABO compatibility is that of the donor whole blood. One unit is 200 to 250 mL.

Description—Light yellow to deep cream in color. When viewed microscopically, a reticulated structure without evidence of fusion may be seen.

Uses—Indicated especially for the treatment of *multiple coagulation factor deficiencies* (since the labile coagulation factors V and XIII are preserved in fresh frozen plasma), such as those which occur in cases of massive transfusion with stored blood, after heparinization in disseminated intravascular coagulation or in liver disease and for *hemophilia*. The preparation also may be used as *Single-Donor Plasma* (above), although such use is unnecessarily expensive. It is the plasma of choice in patients with thrombotic throbocytopenic purpura. It also is of value in patients with deficiencies of immunoglobulin and/or complement. Serum hepatitis virus is not killed by freezing.

Dose—*Intravenous infusion*, variable dose, depending upon the magnitude and type of coagulation factor deficit and the clinical response or upon the volume deficit and response.

Single-Donor Plasma Frozen

Human Plasma Frozen

Single-donor plasma that has been frozen within the expiration time of the liquid plasma but longer than 6 hr after removal from the donor. The expiration time of the thawed plasma is that of *Single-Donor Plasma*.

Uses and **Dose**—*See Single-Donor Plasma*.

Platelet Concentrate

Platelets taken from plasma obtained by whole-blood collection, by plasmapheresis or by plateletpheresis, from a single, suitable, human donor of whole blood; or from a plasmapheresis donor; or from a plateletpheresis donor. One unit of platelet concentrate consists of not less than 5.5×10^{10} platelets suspended in a specified volume of the original plasma. (See USP for collection procedure.)

Preserved platelets can be reinfused successfully into recipients suffering from platelet deficiency. Platelets obtained by plateletpheresis must be used within 24 hr of collection, because the open system allows bacterial contamination. Although the official expiration time is only 72 hr, it now is possible to store platelets for up to 120 hr, and it is likely methods to preserve them for a longer period will be devised in the near future.

Uses—To arrest or prevent bleeding resulting from thrombocytopenia or thrombopathia. In platelet deficiency, consequent to disseminated intravascular coagulation and thrombocytopenic purpura (in which a type of intravascular coagulation occurs), the platelets must be coadministered with heparin. When thrombocytopenia is caused by immune destruction, the administration of platelets mostly is futile because of rapid destruction of the added platelets. Likewise, in drug-induced thrombocytopenia, the effects of the platelets mostly are voided unless the drug is discontinued, preferably in advance. Platelets can be used in the priming of extracorporeal circuits, but they may be subjected to faster destruction in the circuit than endogenous platelets. The half-life of platelets is about 1 to 2 days.

Dose—*Intravenous*, usually **1 Unit**, which will increase the platelet count in an average adult by about 35,000 per μL in a 70-kg recipient without platelet antibodies, splenomegaly, sepsis or coagulopathy. Units must be administered through a 170 μm filter.

Dosage Form—1 Unit.

Red Blood Cells

Human Red Blood Cells; Red Cell Concentrate

Red cells of whole human blood, separated from plasma by centrifuging or subsidence during the dating period of the blood from which it is derived but not later than 21 days after the blood is drawn, if the anticoagulant solution is ACD or CPD solution; if acid citrate dextrose adenine solution has been used as anticoagulant, such preparation may be made within 35 days therefrom; if heparin is used, the expiration time is 48 hr. The expiration dates are valid only if the hematocrit does not exceed 80% and the seal is unbroken. Preparations are designated CPD Red Cells, CPDA-1 Red Cells or Heparinized Red Cells according to the anticoagulant used.

Description—Dark red when packed and may show a slight creamy layer on the surface and a small supernatant layer of yellow or opalescent plasma. Resuspended human blood cells is a dark-red fluid.

Uses—A *blood replenisher* in any condition in which the primary deficiency in the blood is that of the erythrocytes. Thus, they are used in the emergency treatment of a number of the anemias which formerly were treated with whole-blood transfusions. They also may be returned to the donor by autologous transfusion after plasmapheresis or apheresis of other components. Human blood cells are not suitable alone as a replacement fluid in hemorrhage, but they may be employed in cases where chronic blood loss is not too great to decrease appreciably the plasma volume and plasma protein content. Each unit of concentrate preferrably is mixed with 50 to 100 mL of 0.9% NaCl injection to decrease the viscosity. Lactated Ringer injection is contraindicated because it provides enough calcium to initiate coagulation; dextrose injection is contraindicated because it causes hemolysis. The half life is about 4 weeks, but varies considerably according to the recipient.

Dose—*Usual, intravenous infusion*, as needed to replenish red cells, prime extracorporeal circuits, etc, the equivalent of **1 Unit** (500 mL) of whole blood, repeated as necessary. One unit in a 70-kg recipient increases the hematocrit about 3%.

Dosage Form—The red-cell equivalent of 1 Unit of human blood.

Red Blood Cells Frozen

Red Blood Cells (Human) Frozen; Red Cells Fresh Frozen

A preparation in which human red cells are suspended in a glycerol solution and frozen at temperatures ranging from −80° to −120°. There are two types of preparations; one in which a low concentration of glycerol and rapid freezing are used, and the other in which a high concentration of glycerol and slow freezing are used. The expiration time is 3 yr. Before use, the suspension is thawed and the glycerol medium is replaced with a physiologic solution. At this stage the preparation is designated Deglycerolized Red Cell Concentrate. The expiration time of the thawed preparation is 24 hr.

Uses—By freezing erythrocytes immediately or shortly after withdrawal, both ATP and 2,3-diphosphoglyceric acid (2,3-DPG) are preserved better than in the classical preparation and storage methods, and frozen erythrocytes have better oxygen-transport capacity. Therefore they especially are suited for use in newborn and premature infants, and in older patients with excessive oxygen demands. Because of their single-donor origin they are used especially for autologous transfusions. They also are used when there is a rare blood requirement, in elective gynecologic and cardiac surgery, hemodialysis and kidney transplantation. They essentially are free of irregular antibodies and plasma proteins and hence are useful in patients with allergic, febrile reactions to saline-washed red cells or with nocturnal hemoglobinuria. Since there are few surviving leukocytes, the risk of graft versus host response is diminished. The freeze-thaw procedure removes senescent erythrocytes, thus leaving a younger population of cells with a longer survival time in the recipient.

The post-thaw washing procedure greatly decreases the risk of serum hepatitis and pyrogenic reactions to debris from leukocytes and platelets. Frozen red cells are very expensive.

Dose and **Dosage Form**—See the corresponding paragraphs under *Red Blood Cells* (above).

Red Blood Cells Leukocytes Removed

Red Cell Concentrate, Leukocyte-Poor

A single-donor red cell concentrate which contains less than 25% of the original leukocytes. The expiration time is that of *Red Blood Cells* and is determined by the type of anticoagulant used. The hematocrit usually ranges from 0.7 to 0.8.

Dose—See *Red Blood Cells*, page 912.

Uses—Mostly for autologous transfusion in leukemic individuals in whom a reduction in circulating leukocytes is imperative. May be used in heterologous erythrocyte replenishment if the original donor blood was normal (ie, donor blood served as a source of therapeutic leukocytes). Because the preparation has fewer pyrogenic leukocyte fragments than does Red Blood Cells, febrile reactions are less severe and less frequent. *Dose:* See *Red Blood Cells*.

Red Blood Cells Saline Washed

Red Cell Concentrate, Washed

A single-donor red-cell concentrate in which most of the plasma, leukocytes and platelets have been removed within 24 hr of transfusion by one or more washes with an isotonic saline solution. The hematocrit usually lies between 0.7 and 0.8.

Uses—Washing may be employed for five purposes: (1) to remove adverse components in specific disorders (eg, lymphocytes and/or immune globulins in certain autoimmune disorders, Rh factors in alloimmunity, anticoagulation factors in certain bleeding disorders, thyroid hormone in thyroid storm, etc; in such instances, the erythrocytes are to be reinfused into the donor; (2) to reduce the risk of blood-transmissable infections (not malaria); the erythrocytes are intended for heterologous transmission; (3) to remove citrate in citrated blood when the volume to be transfused is large and the intended recipient has a liver dysfunction in which citrate cannot be tolerated; (4) to decrease the intensity of heterologous transfusion reactions in emergency situations in which out-of-group (non-matched) blood must be used or (5) to decrease the incidence and severity of febrile transfusion reaction caused by fragments of leukocytes and platelets.

Plasma Expanders and Intravenous Fluids

Protein and Colloid Solutions

Hemorrhage and shock result in loss of blood volume, which, if carried beyond a certain critical point, leads to circulatory failure. Replacement of the plasma proteins, or injection of a substance having similar osmotic properties, will restore the blood volume at least temporarily, so that circulation of oxygen to the tissues may be maintained. Many substances have been employed for this purpose: *whole blood*, which in certain situations is ideal, but is not always immediately available; *plasma*, which is quite effective, but is unstable in the liquid form, relatively cumbersome in the dry form, involves injection of salt and water, which are in some cases undesirable and, finally, cannot readily be rendered free of pathogenic viruses; *serum albumin*, the protein in the plasma which functions to control blood volume and polysaccharides, such as *dextrans* and *hetastarch*.

Physiologically, the most clearly established role of albumin appears to be its water-retaining (osmotic) capacity. It is due chiefly to plasma albumin that the water of the plasma, instead of diffusing into the tissues, is retained in the blood stream, maintaining the volume of blood which is necessary for effective cardiac output and circulation. Albumin, although it comprises less than 60% of the plasma proteins, by virtue of having the lowest molecular weight of these proteins contributes 80% of their osmotic effect. Another highly important property of albumin is its capacity to bind various chemical substances, including certain ions, some hormones and numerous drugs.

Methods have been devised for preparing human plasma albumin more than 99% pure. Unlike most plasma proteins, it is extraordinarily stable. It does not require desiccation or continuous refrigeration and, therefore, can be kept on hand as a 25% sterile solution, ready for instant use. Separation of the albumin leaves the remaining plasma proteins as by-products. It is possible to derive many specific pharmaceutical agents from one blood donation, enabling more efficient use of a given quantity of blood.

Albumin Human

Normal Human Serum Albumin; Albuminar (*Armour*); Albutein (*Alpha*); Plasbumin (*Cutter*); Buminate (*Hyland*)

Human albumin is a sterile, nonpyrogenic preparation of serum albumin obtained by fractionating blood, plasma, serum or placentas from healthy human donors and tested for absence of hepatitis B surface antigen. It is prepared by a process ensuring safety for intravenous use. The albumin content is not less than 96% of the total protein. The solution contains 5 or 25 g of albumin, respectively, corresponding to 100 or 500 mL of normal human plasma. It may contain sodium acetyltryptophanate alone, or with sodium caprylate as a stabilizing agent. The sodium content is not less than 130 mEq/L and not more than 160 mEq/L. No antimicrobial agent is added. It meets the requirements of tests for limit of heme, heat stability and pH. Solutions are heated in final containers at 60° for 10 hr to kill any pathogenic organisms that may be present. The storage temperature is indicated on the label. The solution is not to be used if it is turbid or there is a sediment.

Description—Moderately viscous, clear, brownish fluid; practically odorless; may develop a slight granular or flaky deposit during storage. When dried, has a slight-yellow to deep-cream color.

Uses—Serves as an emergency agent for restoration of blood volume in the treatment of *shock* or *hemorrhage*. It especially is indicated when blood loss exceeds 20% of blood volume. If albumin is administered in hypertonic concentrations, it will abstract water from interstitial and intracellular fluids and increase blood volume by an amount more than the volume administered; in isotonic concentration it will expand blood volume only by an amount equal to the volume added. Each gram of albumin holds about 18 mL of water in the blood stream. Because its action depends on the availability of tissue water, hypertonic albumin should not be used in severely dehydrated patients without simultaneous administration of saline or dextrose solutions.

It has been used in protein replacement therapy where serum protein levels are low due to excessive loss, as in extensive burns and nephrosis, certain skin diseases and other conditions, or due to inadequate formation of proteins because of nutritional disturbances, cirrhosis or other causes. However, the value of albumin in the therapy of chronic nephritis or cirrhosis is less impressive than in acute hypoalbuminemia. Hyperoncotic albumin solutions may be used to cause transient diuresis in edematous patients or in those undergoing renal dialysis. It also is used in the treatment of hyperbilirubinemia and erythroblastosis fetalis to increase the binding capacity for bilirubin.

Low salt content and the high stability of the single protein component present make "salt-poor" albumin the agent of choice in certain types of protein replacement therapy, bearing in mind the following limitations: Albumin does not, in any sense, replace red cells and, therefore, should not be used in hemorrhagic shock except as an emergency remedy. It lacks the other proteins contained in plasma, hence is not an adequate agent for treatment of deficiencies of specific plasma proteins (eg, fibrinogen, prothrombin) such as occur in acute hepatitis or burns. It does not replace lost fluids, and therefore must be given with ample quantities of crystalloid solution when used in dehydrated patients, as noted above. Chills, fever, urticaria and perturbations of respiration and blood pressure sometimes occur. Albumin is contraindicated in congestive heart failure. Large doses should not be given in severe anemia, low cardiac reserve and in the absence of hypoalbuminemia.

Dose—*Intravenous, adults* and *older children*, for *replacement* or *plasma extension*, **25g,** repeated 15 to 30 min, if necessary. The total daily dose should not exceed 250 g. The 5% solution may be infused directly and the 25% solution infused as a mixture of 20 mL of 25% albumin diluted to 100 mL with an isotonic solution, the infusion rate being maintained at 2 to 4 mL/min. When the 25% solution is infused directly, the rate should not exceed 1 mL/min. In *burns*, initially **500 mL** of 5% or **100 mL** of **25%** solution along with an electrolyte solution. Children, for *hyperbilirubinemia* and *erythroblastosis* fetalis, **1 g/kg** is given with each exchange transfusion; for nonemergency use, **6.25** to **12.5 g.** 25 g is equivalent to approximately 500 mL of plasma.

Dosage Form—Injection: 5%, in 50-, 250-, 500- and 1000-mL vials; 25%, in 20-, 50- and 100-mL vials.

Antihemophilic Factor—page 918.

Plasma Protein Fraction

Human Plasma Protein Fraction; Plasmanate (*Cutter*); Plasma Plex (*Armour*); Plasmatein (*Alpha*); Protenate (*Hyland*)

A sterile solution of selected proteins derived from the blood plasma of healthy adult human donors. It contains 4.5 to 5.5 g of protein/100 mL, of which about 83 to 90% is albumin, and the remainder is alpha and beta globulins. It contains no antimicrobial agent but may contain suitable stabilizers. The expiration time is 5 yr if the storage temperature is 2 to 10°, 3 yr if 11 through 29°, the time not to include 1 yr of storage at the manufacturing plant at 5°.

Preparation—By a process similar to that by which albumin is made. The product resembles plasma from which certain unstable globulins have been removed, including gamma globulin and certain lipoproteins. The solution is treated by heating at 60° for 10 hr to reduce the risk of virus transmission. The solution is isotonic with normal plasma and is isotonic with respect to diffusible ions, the major ions being sodium and chloride.

Description—Transparent, nearly colorless or slightly brownish liquid; nearly odorless; may develop a slight, granular or flaky deposit during storage.

Uses—Indicated, like albumin, as a substitute for plasma in treating nonhemorrhagic *shock*. It also is a convenient source of protein for intravenous nutrition. Because it does not contain any clotting factors, it is not a substitute for fresh plasma in treating hemorrhagic states. The plasma half-life is about 27 days.

Untoward effects are uncommon; they include nausea, vomiting and increased salivation. Care must be exercised to prevent circulatory overload. especially in nonhypovolemic patients. Solutions of this fraction should not be mixed with other intravenous fluids, either in the bottle or in the tubing.

Dose—*Intravenous infusion, adults* and *older children, shock*, **250 mL** of **5%** solution at a rate of 5 to 8 mL/min, repeated as necessary; *burns*, initially **500 mL** to **1 L;** *hypoproteinemia*, **1** to **1.5 L/day.** *Infants* and *small children, dehydration*, **22** to **33 mL** of **5%** solution/kg of body weight at a rate not exceeding 8 mL/min.

Dosage Form—Solution: 5%, in 50-, 250- and 500-mL containers.

Plasma Extenders (Volume Expanders)

Much effort has been expended in the search for nontoxic substances, not of human origin, which might be used in an emergency to restore blood volume. It should be emphasized that these substances are in no sense substitutes for plasma; following their emergency use, plasma or blood must be replaced as rapidly as possible. Some substitutes, however, have favorable actions on the rheology of blood and on platelet adhesiveness, hence sometimes may be administered along with blood or plasma just for these effects. Furthermore, in some kinds of hypovolemic shock, the plasma actually is not lost from the vascular tree but is sequestered in various vascular beds. In these situations, it is not necessary to give plasma, because repair of the fictive volume deficit with a plasma extender will mobilize some of the plasma back into the circulation. Even plasma proteins lost into interstitial spaces return by way of the lymph. In hypovolemia, from dehydration or adrenal insufficiency, appropriate electrolyte or dextrose solutions are indicated.

Volume expansion (plasma extension) clearly is not indicated unless the pulmonary arterial wedge pressure (PAW), an approximation of the pulmonary venous pressure, is below 12 torr. It is advisable to give a test injection (about 200 mL) of isotonic saline or dextran solution. If the PAW rises only slightly but cardiac output more substantially, further plasma extension is indicated; if PAW rises sharply but cardiac output does not, plasma extension is redundant, and treatment must be directed toward improving cardiac function. In volume expansion, the end-point is usually 16 torr (rarely 18 torr), and further expansion will tend to cause pulmonary edema.

Volume expanders also are used to prime extracorporeal circuits.

Albumin—page 913.

Dextran 40

Gentran 40 (*Baxter*); 10% LMD (*Abbott*); Rheomacrodex (*Pharmacia*); Rheotran (*Pharmachem*)

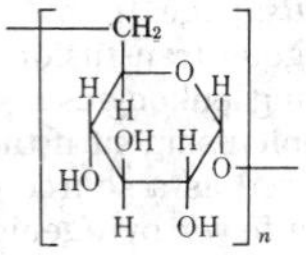

Dextran [9004-54-0] $(C_6H_{10}O_5)_n$; a polymer of glucose, with an average mol wt of about 40,000 in which the glucosidic linkages are predominantly of the $\alpha(1 \rightarrow 6)$ type.

Preparation—Sucrose is subjected to the action of the bacterium *Leuconostoc mesenteroides* B 512, and the crude, high-molecular-weight dextran thus formed is hydrolyzed and fractionated to an average molecular weight of about 40,000 as measured by light-scattering techniques. US Pat 2,644,815.

Description—White, amorphous powder that is odorless and tasteless; 10% solution in 5% dextrose in water darkens slightly over a long storage period as with other dextrose-containing solutions; darkening is accelerated by increased ambient temperatures.

Solubility—Freely soluble in water; soluble in dimethyl sulfoxide; insoluble in alcohol or ether.

Uses—As an isotonic solution to prime pumps or improve flow in surgery requiring *cardiopulmonary bypass*. It has the property of lowering the viscosity of blood and improving flow; in part the improvement in flow is the result of hemodilution. For this reason, 10% of dextran 40 in isotonic saline solution or 5% dextrose is superior to dextran 40 in whole blood. Dextrans decrease platelet adhesiveness. This property is used for *prophylaxis of thrombosis and thromboembolism during and after surgery* and occasionally to decrease coagulopathies in the shock-lung syndrome. Otherwise, it seldom is used in shock, because of the short duration in the body (2 to 4 hr) and also because of frequent adverse effects.

The size of the molecule is such that the polysaccharide is filtered in the glomeruli more rapidly than larger macromolecules, such as dextran 70 or 75. As the filtrate is concentrated in the renal tubules, it sometimes may become too viscid to flow, and renal damage can ensue. For this reason many surgeons prefer to prime their bypass with other solutions. Renal failure, severe congestive heart failure, severe coagulation disorders, hypervolemia, hypersensitivity and severe dehydration contraindicate use of this substance. It can cause allergic reactions. It interferes with the cross-matching of blood, especially when enzyme methods are used. It also interferes with some tests of renal and hepatic function and with assays for blood sugar in which acid-hydrolysis is used.

Dose—As a primer for extracorporeal circuits, **500 mL** to **1 L**, depending on volume requirement. *Intravenous infusion, adults* and *children*, for *hypovolemia*, **10 mL/kg** of **10%** solution in isotonic sodium chloride or dextrose solution, repeated as necessary, not to exceed 20 mL/kg a day on the first day and 10 mL/kg a day thereafter; for *prophylaxis* of thrombosis or thromboembolism, **10 mL/ kg** during surgery, then 500 mL a day for the next 2 or more days, according to the persistence of the risk.

Dosage Form—Injection: 10% in 5% dextrose solution, 500 mL; 10% in 0.9% sodium chloride solution, 500 mL.

Dextran 70

Hyskon, Macrodex (*Kabi Pharmacia*)

Dextran [9004-54-0] $(C_6H_{10}O_5)_n$; a polymer of glucose with an average mol wt of about 70,000, in which the glucosidic linkages are predominantly of the $\alpha(1 \rightarrow 6)$ type. For the structural formula see *Dextran 40*.

Preparation—As described for *Dextran 40* except that the hydrolysis and fractionation are adjusted to yield a product of average mol wt of about 70,000.

Description—Fine, white, amorphous powder; odorless and tasteless; stable in light and very hygroscopic; commercial grades usually contain about 5% water.

Solubility—Freely soluble in hot water or dimethyl sulfoxide; insoluble in alcohol or ether.

Uses—A plasma expander for the prevention or treatment of *hypovolemic shock*. The macromolecule is contained within the plasma and hence retains fluid in the vascular bed by osmosis. Hypertonic solutions cause the dehydration of tissues, the abstracted water being added to the plasma. For this reason it is useful in the treatment of *toxemia of pregnancy* and *nephrosis*. Although dextran 70 solution is inferior to plasma, it has the advantage that refrigeration is not required or that the solution does not have to be prepared immediately before use. Thus, it may be kept ready for use in emergency vehicles, field kits, etc. It is also less expensive than plasma. Like plasma, it is inferior to whole blood as replacement when hypovolemia is due to hemorrhage. When hypoproteinemia exists, it should not be used in place of plasma. It decreases platelet adhesiveness and hence increases clotting time. In some uses this may be a disadvantage, although hemorrhage occurs mainly in the presence of clotting disorders. In some types of shock the effect on platelet adhesiveness is an advantage, because shock-induced coagulopathies will be attenuated. Its anticoagulant effect can be useful clinically; it has been shown to be equal to dicumarol in *preventing thrombosis* after femoral neck fractures and major pelvic surgery. A solution also is used to distend the uterus for hysteroscopy and to irrigate the cavity. It also is used in artificial tears.

A small part of dextran 70, corresponding to the low-molecular-weight molecules, is excreted during the first 1 or 2 days. The remainder is taken up by the reticuloendothelial system and is metabolized later, which requires approximately 10 days.

Side effects include mainly allergic reactions (fever, hypotension, hives, angioedema, bronchospasm and anaphylaxis). The substance may interfere with cross-matching of blood, if unsuitable dilutions of erythrocytes and serum are used. The drug is contraindicated when there is hypersensitivity, severe coagulation disorders, severe congestive heart failure and hypervolemia.

Dose—*Intravenous infusion, adult,* **250** to **1500 mL,** not to exceed 20 mL/kg, in the first day; *usual,* **500** to **1000 mL** of a **6%** solution in isotonic saline, 5% dextrose or 10% invert sugar solution. The rate of infusion is usually 20 to 40 mL/min but may be accelerated if hypovolemia is severe. *Children,* proportioned to the adult dose according to body weight or surface, not to exceed 10 mg/kg/day. For *nephrosis* or *toxemia of pregnancy,* **500 mL** of a **10%** solution in 5% dextrose or 10% invert sugar may be given at a rate of about 60 mL/hr. *Intrauterine, diagnostic,* **50** to **100 mL,** to be administered by canula with a pressure of about 100 torr and maintained at a pressure of less than 150 torr during examination.

Dosage Forms—Injection: 6% in 5% dextrose solution, 500 mL; 6% in 0.9% sodium chloride solution, 500 mL; Solution: 32% in 10% dextrose solution.

Dextran 75

Gentran 75 (*Baxter*)

Chemistry, Preparation, Description, Solubility—See *Dextran 70* (above); read 75,000 in place of 70,000.

Uses and **Dose**—See *Dextran 70,* above. Dextran 75 is not used as an aid to hysteroscopy.

Dosage Form—Injection: 6% in 5% dextrose solution, 500 mL; 6% in 0.9% sodium chloride solution, 500 mL.

Hetastarch

Starch 2-hydroxyethyl ether; Hespan (*Du Pont*)

Amylose derivative:

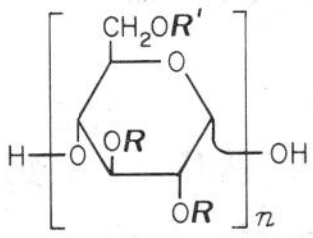

[structure: repeating glucopyranose unit with CH_2OR', O, OR, OR; H—O ... —OH; subscript n]

in which either *R* or *R'* may be either H or CH_2CH_2OH

Amylopectin derivative: Similar to the above, except that the sequence is frequently interrupted by a similar unit that differs in that *R'* is the residue of an additional *O*-hydroxyethylated α-D-glucopyranosyl moiety that constitutes the first unit in a branch or sub-branch of the polymer.

[9005-27-0]. Consists of more then 90% amylopectin which has been treated with ethylene chlorohydrin so that an average of 7 to 8 of the hydroxyl groups occurring in every 10 D-glucopyranose units of the starch polymer have been converted to 2-hydroxyethoxy groups. The molecular wt is about 450,000 daltons.

Uses—A 6% solution is osmotically equivalent to a 5% albumin solution. In the blood, it abstracts some water from interstitial and intracellular fluids, thus expanding the blood volume somewhat in excess of the volume infused. The expansion persists for 1 to 1½ days. Hetastarch is used in the prevention and treatment of *hypovolemic shock*. It also is used as a suspension medium for leukapheresis.

It does not cause the coagulation abnormalities that does dextran nor does it interfere with the cross-matching of blood. There is general but not complete agreement that it is less likely than dextran to cause anaphylaxis and other allergic manifestations (fever, chills, urticaria, pruritis). The incidence of anaphylactoid reactions is stated to be less than 0.1%.

Elimination has complex kinetics, mainly because of heterogeneity in molecular size and linkage. About 40% of molecules with molecular weights below 50,000 daltons is eliminated in the urine in 1 day, 64% in 8 days, 90% in 41 days and 100% in 48 days. Larger molecules are taken up by the reticuloendothelial system and degraded by amylase. There is a compound half-life: 90% is eliminated with a half-life of 17 days; the remainder, 48 days.

Dose—*Intravenous infusion, adults,* for *hypovolemia, intially* **500 mL** to **1 L** repeated as needed up to 3 or 4 L a day in severe hypovolemia. The rate of infusion depends upon the hemodynamic indices, but ranges up to 20 mL/kg/hr. For *leukapheresis,* **250 to 700 mL** in a 1:8 ratio with venous whole blood.

Dosage Form—Injection: 6% in 0.9% sodium chloride solution, 500 mL.

Single-Donor Plasma—page 911.

Balanced Electrolyte Solutions

Ringer's Injection

Isotonic Solution of Three Chlorides

A sterile solution of sodium chloride (8.6 g), potassium chloride (0.30 g) and calcium chloride (0.33 g) in 1 L of solution prepared with Water for Injection. It contains aproximately 147.5 mEq of sodium, 4.0 mEq of potassium, 4.5 mEq of calcium and 156 mEq of chloride ion per liter; antimicrobial agents are not present.

Description—Colorless, odorless solution having a salty taste; pH between 5.0 and 7.5.

Uses—Theoretically superior to *Sodium Chloride Injection* as a *fluid and electrolyte replenisher* in that it supplies the three important cations of the extracellular fluid. However, in actual practice, the addition of potassium and calcium increases only slightly the therapeutic value of an isotonic sodium chloride solution. Neither potassium nor calcium is present in sufficient concentration to render it useful for the repair of deficits of these ions. Further, while administration of large volumes would result in minimal distortion of the cation composition of the extracellular fluid, like *Sodium Chloride Injection,* it would alter acid–base balance. It frequently is used to prime pumps for cardiopulmonary bypass in heart surgery. It also may be applied topically for the purposes of irrigation.

Dose—*Intravenous infusion,* **500** to **1000 mL.** However, the dose may be larger or smaller, according to the size and clinical condition of the patient.

Dosage Form—Injection: 500 and 1000 mL.

Lactated Ringer's Injection

Hartmann's Solution

A sterile solution of calcium chloride, potassium chloride, sodium chloride and sodium lactate in water for injection. It contains no antimicrobial agents. The calcium, potassium and sodium contents are approximately 2.7, 4 and 130 mEq/L, respectively.

Description—pH 6.0 to 7.5.

Uses and **Dose**—See *Ringer's Injection.* Except for the concentration of lactate and absence of bicarbonate, the composition of this injection closely approximates that of the extracellular fluids. It is employed as a *fluid and electrolyte replenisher.* The lactate ultimately metabolizes to bicarbonate and thus has an alkalinizing effect in the body; in persons with normal cellular oxidative activity, this requires 1 to 2 hr to be fully effective. It is inappropriate in the treatment of lactic acidosis. The absence of bicarbonate from the solution stabilizes the calcium, which sometimes tends to precipitate as calcium carbonate from heated solutions which contain bicarbonate.

Dose—*Intravenous infusion,* **500** to **1000 mL.** However, the dose may be larger or smaller, according to the size and clinical condition of the patient. Do not administer with blood. Pediatric dosage can be determined from an analysis of the acid–base status of the young patient.

Dosage Form—Injection: 250, 500 and 1000 mL.

Miscellaneous Fluids

Sodium Chloride Injection—page 932.

Miscellaneous Parenteral Fluids—There are at least 69 commercially available parenteral fluids, some of which differ only slightly and others considerably from one or more of those described in the foregoing sections. Excellent summary tables of the composition, names, and manufacturers of these products may be found in *AMA Drug Evaluations* and *Drug Facts and Comparisons* (listed under *Intravenous Nutritional Therapy*). *AMA Drug Evaluations* also provides a useful table of peritoneal solutions.

Miscellaneous Oral Electrolyte Solutions—Oral solutions containing 2 to 2.5% dextrose, 75 to 90 mEq/L sodium and 20 mEq/L potassium have become widely used in lieu of intravenous solutions for the treatment of dehydration from diarrhea, especially in infants and children. *WHO Oral Rehydration Salts* contain 90, 20, 80 and 30 mEq/L of sodium, potassium, chloride and bicarbonate, respectively, and 20 g/L of dextrose when reconstituted. *Maintenance/prevention solutions* contain 45 to 50 mEq/L of sodium but about the same potassium, base and dextrose concentrations as the rehydration solutions.

Dextrose Injection

Injection of Glucose

A sterile solution of dextrose in water for injection. It contains 95 to 105% of the labeled amount of $C_6H_{12}O_6.H_2O$. It contains no antimicrobial agents.

Preparation—The strength of the solution may vary from 2.0, to 5, 10, 20, 25 or 50%. Quantities which are administered may vary from 100 mL to 1000 mL or more. With such large amounts being administered, a hospital will require considerable quantities of this solution daily, and many shortcuts have been developed for its manufacture. It is general practice to prepare concentrated solutions and then to dilute these with water for injection, thus saving an immense amount of labor and time, particularly in the filtration operation.

Care should be exercised in the selection of dextrose, since the sugar itself may be a source of pyrogens, and extreme care must be observed throughout the preparation of the dextrose injections to prevent contamination, for the conditions are practically ideal for the development of bacteria and, therefore, pyrogens.

Weaker solutions may be sterilized in an autoclave without producing any change in color, but with the more concentrated solutions there is greater possibility of producing a slight change in color on sterilization with high temperatures. Consequently, sterilization by filtration often is resorted to in these cases.

The pH of dextrose solutions is lowered on heating. Nevertheless, buffers seldom are added directly to the solution during its preparation since this is often the cause of discoloration and the buffer capacity diminishes after the solution stands for a period of time. Where buffers are desired, they should be dispensed separately so that the physician may add the buffer extemporaneously when the preparation is to be administered. Dextrose solutions should be tested for mold.

Note—Antimicrobial agents are prohibited since such large quantities of dextrose are administered at one time that excessive doses of the antimicrobial agent would thus be given.

Description—Clear, colorless solution having a pH of 3.5 to 6.5, determined on a portion of injection diluted with water, if necessary, to a concentration of not more than 5% of dextrose.

Uses—The most extensively used injection in hospital practice. Dextrose provides a readily metabolizable nutrient. During periods of inanition, intravenous injection of isotonic solution of dextrose *provides both fluid and carbohydrate.* Each 25 g of dextrose provides about 85 cal. A 20 to 50% solution may be infused into a high-flow vein as a source of calories in total parenteral nutrition. A 50% solution is given in insulin or suspected insulin-coma. A 20 to 50% solution, with or without insulin, is used in hyperkalemia, to move potassium intracellularly. Body protein is spared and starvation-ketosis and acidosis are prevented. It also is employed for parenteral fluid therapy when it is desired to supply water unaccompanied by electrolyte. In the body, the dextrose is converted slowly to glycogen or metabolized, thus leaving the water component of the injection without an osmotic component; the final result is the same as if water were given, but without the hemolysis that accompanies intravenous infusions of water. The injection also provides a suitable *vehicle for the slow intravenous infusion* of numerous drugs.

Dextrose usually is administered intravenously as a 5% solution which is isoosmotic with body fluids. Subcutaneous injection is less desirable since such solutions are irritating and can cause local necrosis. In addition, such solutions cause temporary sequestration of extracellular electrolyte in the subcutaneous depot, and anuria, oliguria and circulatory collapse can result. If the subcutaneous route is to be employed, *Dextrose and Sodium Chloride Injection* should be used.

When administered rapidly intravenously, hypertonic solutions of dextrose cause cellular dehydration which may be of benefit in the treatment of *cerebral edema, shock* and *circulatory collapse. However, Dextrose and Sodium Chloride Injection is preferred.* Hypertonic solutions of dextrose also are administered intravenously to initiate *osmotic diuresis.* Dextrose in the glomerular filtrate in excess of that which can be reabsorbed by the renal tubule causes excretion of an osmotic equivalent of water. Additional quantities of extracellular electrolyte also escape renal tubular reabsorption during the osmotic diuresis.

Hyperglycemia and glycosuria may result, according to the infusion rate and metabolic status. Because of both the dilution of extracellular fluid and endocellular movement of potassium during glucose uptake, hypokalemia may be a consequence. Reactive hypoglycemia may result from the abrupt termination of administration.

Dose—*Intravenous,* variable, as determined by the use, clinical condition and size of the individual. For a 5% dextrose solution, the dose frequently ranges from 500 to 1000 mL. The maximum rate of infusion that will not cause glycosuria is 0.5 g/kg/hr; about 95% is retained when the rate is 0.8 g/kg/hr. The usual diuretic dose is 50 mL of 50% solution. For emergency treatment of suspected insulin coma, 50 mL of 50% solution.

Dosage Form—Injection: 2, 2.5, 5, 10, 20, 30, 38.5, 40, 50, 60 and 70%, in various volumes. Solutions of 2.0 to 10% are for nonelectrolyte and caloric replacement; 20 to 50% are for caloric provision with minimal hydration; 50% is for use in insulin hypoglycemia; 40 to 70% solutions are for mixing with other solutions for parenteral alimentation.

Dextrose and Sodium Chloride Injection

Sodium Chloride and Dextrose Injection

A sterile solution of dextrose and sodium chloride in water for injection. It contains 95 to 105% of the labeled amount of $C_6H_{12}O_6.H_2O$ and of NaCl. It contains no antimicrobial agents.

Preparation—This title may include a highly concentrated solution for use as a sclerosing agent, or much weaker solutions to be used in a manner similar to the use of 5 or 10% dextrose solution. This may be a mixture of equal parts of isotonic sodium chloride solution and isotonic dextrose solution, or it may represent 5% of dextrose in isotonic sodium chloride solution. Both of these should be prepared according to the suggestions given for the preparation of *Dextrose Injection.*

Description—Clear, colorless solution having a pH of 3.5 to 6.5, determined on a portion of injection diluted with water, if necessary, to a concentration of not more than 5% of dextrose.

Uses—To provide dextrose as a nutrient (see above) in a medium that does not hydrate the tissues, or it may be employed as a source of isotonic sodium chloride, or both. When hypertonic solutions of dextrose are employed in cerebral edema or in hydrated states, isotonic sodium chloride in the injection prevents a delayed rebound hydration. Since dextrose, alone, cannot be given safely by the subcutaneous route (see *Dextrose Injection*), this is the preferred preparation.

Dose—*Intravenous,* variable, as determined by the use, clinical condition and size of the patient. It frequently ranges from 500 to 1000 mL.

Dosage Form—Injection: Various percentages of each ingredient, with 2.5% to 25% dextrose and 0.11% to 0.9% NaCl, in various sizes.

Fructose Injection—page 1131.

Fructose and Sodium Chloride Injection—page 1131.

Protein Hydrolysate Injection—page 1129.

Antibodies and Isoagglutinins

Human plasma contains antibodies of various types, which are concentrated almost entirely in Fractions II and III. Some of these occur naturally, others arise as a result of infection or are stimulated by artificial immunization.

The serum of all human beings contains antibodies (agglutinins or isoagglutinins) which react with those principal blood-group factors (agglutinogens) which the individual does *not* possess (see Table 1).

Thus, for example, 45% of the population of the US possesses the blood-group O factor in their red cells, and agglutinins against the A and B factors in the plasma. Should the whole blood or cells of a Group A individual be injected into a

Table 1—Blood-Group Factors

Blood groups (cells)		
Factors present	Frequency in population	Isoagglutinins (plasma)
O	45%	Anti-A and Anti-B
A	41%	Anti-B
B	10%	Anti-A
AB	4%	None

Group O patient, the anti-A agglutinins of the patient will clump the cells received, and usually will destroy (lyse) them, causing a serious reaction in many cases, even if the volume of cells injected is as little as 50 mL.

The importance of establishing the blood group of anyone either giving or receiving whole blood is therefore obvious. This is done by mixing a specimen of the cells of the subject with the serum of a selected individual whose group is known; for example, if the cells of an untyped donor are clumped by the serum of a known Group B subject, but not by the serum of a known Group A subject, the donor evidently belongs to Group A.

In practice, anti-A isoagglutinins obtained from selected group B subjects, and anti-B isoagglutinins from similarly selected Group A subjects, have for years provided highly effective reagents for identification of the blood groups. It has been demonstrated that administration of small quantities of the specific blood-group substances A or B (which can be obtained from red blood cells or, in larger quantities, from other animal tissues) to individuals having the corresponding isoagglutinins will induce a tremendous rise in titer of the agglutinin. In this fashion, extremely potent blood-grouping sera have been prepared in ample quantities. It is also possible to produce blood grouping sera as a by-product of ethanol fractionation of plasma.

In practice (see Chapter 31), it is customary not only to determine the blood group of a donor and recipient of a blood transfusion, but to "cross-match" the cells of the donor with the serum of the patient and *vice versa*, so as to detect any otherwise unpredictable incompatibility in the bloods of the two individuals. This extra precaution is invaluable, not only for the purpose indicated but also as a final check against mistaken identity of the specimens. Numerous other precautions are involved in correct blood grouping, so that it has become a highly specialized technique, which should only be performed by a qualified technician.

The Rh Factor—A much rarer antibody occurs in a small proportion of individuals as a result of injection of so-called "Rh-positive blood," or absorption of such blood across the placenta during pregnancy in gravid females. This "Rh factor" actually consists of at least nine different factors, any one or several of which may be present in the red cells of a given individual. Isoagglutinins reacting with these factors do not occur normally in humans, but appear only as a result of accidental "immunization" of an individual with a type of Rh factor which he does not possess. Actually, the blood of about 85% of Western Europeans or Americans contains one or two of the commonest of these factors, which also are the most potent as antigens. Therefore, in general practice it is customary and quite permissible to classify individuals simply as either "Rh-positive" or "Rh-negative." The technique of Rh typing is essentially like that of blood grouping.

Like anti-A and anti-B blood-grouping serum, the principal source for Rh typing serum is the blood of human donors who, by chance or intention, have become hyperimmunized to one of the Rh factors. One of the commonest sources is the blood of Rh-negative women who have borne several Rh-positive infants, absorbed their Rh factor, and thereby have become sensitized. Another source is Rh-negative individuals who have been transfused with Rh-positive blood. Injection of small amounts of Rh substance in the latter individuals will induce very high antibody titers, rendering them suitable donors of hyperimmune serum for typing purposes. The danger of mismatched transfusion in such individuals is actually decreased, since they become extremely easy to identify.

Blood-Grouping and Typing Serums

Blood-Group Specific Substances A, B and AB

A sterile, isotonic solution of the polysaccharide-amino acid complexes that are capable of reducing the titer of the anti-A and the anti-B isoagglutinins of group O blood. The blood-group specific substance A is prepared from hog gastric mucin and the blood-group specific substances B and AB are prepared from the glandular portion of horse gastric mucosa. Blood Group Specific Substances A, B and AB contains no preservative.

Description—Clear solution, which may have a slight odor due to the preservative; pH 6.0 to 6.8.

Uses—Added to group O blood as a *neutralizer of isoagglutinins* and hence it makes the blood reasonably safe for transfusions into patients whose blood is of another group. It also may be used to condition plasma. However, conditioned plasma which contains immune anti-A and anti-B agglutinins may cause reactions. Furthermore, it must not be forgotten that blood from group O donors that previously have received conditioned group O blood may contain A and B isohemagglutinins. Such blood is dangerous to use in universal donation unless it is conditioned with blood group specific substances A and B.

Dose—*Intravenous*, one transfusion unit in approximately **500 mL** of group O blood.

Anti-A Blood-Grouping Serum

Derived from high-titered serums of humans, with or without stimulation by the injection of group-specific red cells or substances. It agglutinates human red cells containing A antigens; ie, blood groups A and AB (including subgroups A_1, A_2, A_3, A_1B and A_2B). It may contain a suitable antibacterial preservative.

Description—Clear or slightly opalescent fluid unless artificially colored, when it has a blue or blue-green color. The dried product is light yellow to deep cream color, unless artificially colored as indicated for liquid serum and, microscopically, is of a honeycomb-like structure.

Use—As a diagnostic agent.

Anti-B Blood-Grouping Serum

Derived from high-titered serums of humans, with or without stimulation by the injection of group-specific red cells or substances. It agglutinates human red cells containing B antigens; ie, blood groups B and AB (including subgroups A_1B and A_2B). It may contain a suitable antibacterial preservative.

Description—Clear or slightly opalescent fluid unless artificially colored when it has a yellow color. The dried product is light yellow to deep cream color, unless artificially colored as indicated for liquid serum and, microscopically, is of a honeycomb-like structure.

Use—As a diagnostic agent.

Anti-Rh Blood-Grouping Serums

Blood Grouping Serums Anti-D, Anti-C, Anti-E, Anti-c, Anti-e

Derived from the blood of humans who have developed specific Rh antibodies. Anti-Rh Blood-Grouping Serums are free from agglutinins for A or B antigens and from alloantibodies other than those for which claims are made in the labeling. They may contain suitable antimicrobial agents.

Two varieties of Anti-Rh Grouping Serums are recognized: ie, (1) complete ("saline-agglutinating") serums, which specifically agglutinate human red blood cells in saline TS, and (2) incomplete ("blocking") serums, which agglutinate human red blood cells only in a medium containing protein or other macromolecular substances, which may be furnished in an accompanying diluent. Complete serums commonly are designated "For saline tube test," and the incomplete serums are designated "For slide or modified (rapid) tube test." In liquid form, the latter contain, as additives, the required micromolecular substances.

The left-hand column of Table 2 lists the designations of the most commonly used anti-Rh blood-grouping serums, and the right-hand column lists the blood factor(s) with which each serum specifically reacts. The designations used in an alternative system of nomenclature are indicated parenthetically.

Uses—As diagnostic agents.

Immune Globulins

Adult blood contains antibodies specific for various infectious agents to which the individual has built up a resistance.

Table 2

Serum	Antigen(s) reacting
Anti-D (Anti-Rh_0)	D (Rh_0)
Anti-C (Anti-rh')	C (rh')
Anti-E (Anti-rh")	E (rh")
Anti-CD (Anti-Rh_0')	D (Rh_0), C (rh')
Anti-DE (Anti-Rh_0")	D (Rh_0), E (rh")
Anti-CDE (Anti-Rh_0''')	D (Rh_0), C (rh'), E (rh")
Anti-c (Anti-hr')	c (hr')
Anti-e (Anti-hr")	e (hr")

In pooled normal plasma used for fractionation some of these are in high enough concentration to have a protective action. This is usually true of measles and poliomyelitis antibodies. Antibodies from adult plasma will protect against the disease if given after exposure. In certain other conditions, it is possible to select individuals with already detectable antibody levels and, by injection of an appropriate vaccine, to raise their antibody level to very high titers, much as was described for blood grouping and Rh typing sera above. This practice has been employed mainly in the production of pertussis hyperimmune globulin for the treatment or prophylaxis of whooping cough.

During the fractionation of plasma, most of the antibodies are concentrated into a single fraction (Fraction II); electrophoretically the proteins in this fraction are characterized as gamma globulins. Isolated immune globulins, dispensed as a 16% solution, represent a concentration of most antibodies approximately 25 times greater than in plasma. As a result, they have been found useful in the prophylaxis of certain infectious diseases, including measles, infectious hepatitis (not to be confused with serum hepatitis) and poliomyelitis.

The usefulness derives from the immunity conferred by the *added* antibody. However, since the added antibody is metabolized slowly and therefore disappears, the immunity is passive, and lasts only so long as the concentration of antibody is above an effective level, usually from 1 to 2 months. Thereafter, the recipient once again becomes susceptible to infection. Alternatively, and particularly when exposure to infection can be ascertained with reasonable accuracy, as in measles, a modifying dose of antibodies may be administered.

While failing to prevent active infection, the added antibody lessens the severity of the disease and the patient responds to the infection by producing antibodies of his own. This production of antibodies persists for long periods thereafter, thus conferring long-lasting immunity.

Immune globulin is administered intramuscularly; it cannot be used intravenously. Reactions are uncommon and when they do occur chiefly are local and usually mild. Another source of gamma globulin is the blood from normal human placentas. Application of the methods of processing immune globulin from human blood, however, has made possible the preparation of a similar globulin from placentas.

Immune Globulin and immune globulins for *hepatitis B, pertussis, rabies, Rh_o(D), tetanus* and *varicella-zoster* are described in Chapter 81.

Immune Sera

Various biological products obtained from the blood of humans or animals and used for their prophylactic or therapeutic effects, eg, antitoxins, immune sera and immune globulin, are discussed in Chapter 81.

Agents Affecting Blood Coagulation

The clotting of blood is a very important process (see Chapter 31). It depends on the existence of a complex system of reactions involving plasma proteins, platelets, tissue factors and calcium ion. This system normally is in a state of balance. However, if a factor is missing, as is the case in hemophilia, a hemorrhagic tendency exists which can lead to major hemorrhage under certain circumstances. In hemophilia, the defect is congenital. Other defects, often transient, may arise as the result of disease or malnutrition. Under certain circumstances, the reverse situation is encountered. Hypercoagulability—an abnormal tendency for the blood to clot—can be very serious, leading to thrombosis.

Various agents are available with which to achieve at least partial control over this system.

Blood-Clotting Proteins

Although it technically should be possible to prepare therapeutically useful concentrates of several clotting factors, only a few are marketed presently.

Antihemophilic Factor

Hemofil T (*Hyland*); Humate P, Monoclate (*Armour*); Profilate (*Alpha*)

A sterile, freeze-dried concentrate of human antihemophilic factor prepared from the Factor VIII-rich cryoprotein fraction of human venous plasma.

Preparation—Precipitated by glycine from a solution of AHF-rich first precipitate from pooled normal human plasma. After treatment to lower the content of glycine and inactive proteins, a solution of the active fraction is sterilized by filtration, aseptically filled into final containers, dried aseptically from the frozen state, stoppered under vacuum and assayed for AHF content.

Description—White or grayish, to yellow, amorphous substance dried from the frozen state; colorless or opalescent when reconstituted with the diluent provided. 1 unit is the activity in 1 mL of pooled human plasma less than 1-hr old.

Uses—The coagulation defect in classical hemophilia (hemophilia A) is predominately a deficit of the coagulation factor VIII, called antihemophilic factor (AHF). In severe hemorrhage in the patient with hemophilia A, it is used as a cryoprecipitate or concentrate, or in fresh plasma or whole blood, as required to *terminate hemorrhage* or to prevent hemorrhage in surgery or consequent to various procedures in which bleeding may occur. The concentrate generally is preferred to plasma or whole blood since the AHF titers of blood and plasma are quite variable, but in von Willebrand's disease the cryoprecipitate (below) is more effective. The preparation is poorly effective in hemophilia B. AHF has a distribution half-life of 4 to 8 hr, and an elimination half-life of 12 to 15 hr. Neither the glycine- nor cryo-precipitated preparations are entirely free of possible contamination by hepatitis B, non-A, non-B and human immunodeficiency viruses, even after heat treatment. However, monoclonal and recombinant preparations, thus far, seem to be free. Traces of ABO isohemoagglutinins are present in glycine precipitates, so that large doses may sometimes cause severe hemolysis. Mild allergic reactions are frequent. Occasionally there may be chills, fever, erythema, urticaria, bronchospasm, headache, lethargy, somnolence and backache. The concentrate is more expensive than the cryoprecipitate.

Dose—*Intravenous,* from **5 Units/kg** once a day to **25 Units/kg** every 8 to 12 hr, depending on severity of hemorrhage and its location, or whether use is for prophylaxis. To raise plasma concentration of AHF by 10% of the normal content, 4 to 5 Units/kg are usually required. The following levels of normal are desirable: for *hemarthrosis,* 20 to 30%, except 50% if severe; *mild hemorrhage,* minor episodes most often resolve with a single infusion reaching 30% or more; *moderate hemorrhage* and *minor surgery* need to reach levels of 30 to 50%; *severe hemorrhage into CNS,* or *peritoneal* or *pleural spaces* requires plasma Factor VIII levels of 80 to 100%; *major surgery* requires a level of 80 to 100% prior to procedure and a *maintenance* level of at least 30% continuing 10 to 14 days after; *general prophylaxis,* 10 to 15%. Appropriate laboratory tests are necessary to ascertain the adequacy of dosage.

Dosage Forms—Vials containing 80, 125, 250, 500, 1000 and 1500 Units; also available in many other quantities (200 to 1700 Units), the amount of which is shown on the label only.

Cryoprecipitated Antihemophilic Factor

A sterile, frozen concentrate of antihemophilic factor prepared from the Factor VIII-rich cryoprotein fraction of a single unit of human venous plasma obtained from whole blood or by plasmapheresis. It can be kept for 1 yr at −18° or below, and is thawed at a temperature not to exceed 37° just before use.

Uses and **Dose**—See *Antihemophilic Factor*. The cryoprecipitated form is used when an autologous replacement is necessary. Also, cryopreservation maintains the potency better than liquid preservation. The cryoprecipitate contains other factors, including one that improves the bleeding time in patients with von Willebrand's disease. This factor is not present in marketed preparations of antihemophilic factor, and the cryoprecipitated preparation or fresh frozen plasma should be used, instead. Since the cryoprecipitate is type-specific, it may be cross-matched to the patient's blood to avoid hemolysis.

Dosage Form—For Injection: 80 to 125 Units/15 mL.

Antithrombin III (Human)

Thrombate III (*Miles*); Kybernin (*Hoechst-Roussel*)

[52014-67-2]

Antithrombin III, is an α_2-globulin of molecular weight about 60,000 found in blood, and is a major endogenous coagulation inhibitor which inactivates various clotting cascade serine proteases including thrombin.

Preparation—Produced from pooled units of human plasma from normal donors by modifications and refinements of the cold ethanol method of Cohn (Cohn EJ *et al: J Am Chem Soc 68(3):* 459, 1946).

Description—Lyophilized powder consisitng of a glycoprotein of molecular weight 58,000 which has a pH of 6.0 to 7.5 upon reconstitution.

Uses—Administered to patients with hereditary antithrombin III deficiency prior to surgical or obstetrical procedures or when they suffer from thromboembolism. Antithrombin III (AT III) is the major plasma inhibitor of thrombin due to its covalent binding with the active residue of thrombin forming an inactive complex. Antithrombin III also inactivates other components of the coagulation cascade including Factors IXa, Xa, XIa, and XIIa. The neutralization rate of these serine proteases is relatively slow but is greatly accelerated in the presence of heparin. The hereditary deficiency of antithrombin III may result in spontaneous episodes of thrombosis and pulmonary embolism and these risks are increased with age, surgery, pregnancy or delivery. In order to either treat or prevent acute thrombotic events, the antithrombin III level should be raised to normal and maintained at this level for 2 to 8 days depending on the treatment indication as well as the patient's medical condition. In some situations such as hemorrhage or acute thrombosis, following surgery, or concommitant heparin therapy, the half-life of antithrombin III may be decreased so plasma levels should be monitored more frequently and dosage or frequency of drug administration adjusted as necessary.

Dose—*Intravenous*, administration of **1 U/kg** raises the level of antithrombin III (AT III) by 1 to 2% depending on the patient's condition. The loading dose should be determined on an individual basis based on the pretherapy antithrombin III level in order to achieve the level found in normal plasma using the following formula:

$$\text{Dosage units} = \frac{[\text{Desired AT III level (\%)} - \text{baseline AT III level (\%)}] \times \text{weight (kg)}}{1.4}$$

This formula is based on an expected incremental increase of 1.4% per IU/kg administered. As the increase varies among patients, it is essential to measure antithrombin III levels preceding and 20 min postinfusion so that subsequent doses can be adjusted if necessary based on the initial dose effect. Plasma levels of antithrombin III should be monitored initially at least twice daily until the patient is stabilized and thereafter once every 24 hr with the goal of keeping plasma antithrombin III levels above 80%. Levels should always be obtained before the next infusion of thrombate III. Plasma levels between 80 and 120% usually are maintained by dosing every 24 hr with 60% of the initial loading dose. These recommendations are a general guideline for therapy and adjustments in the maintenance dose and dosing intervals should be based on the actual antithrombin III levels achieved. The suggested rate of infusion is 50 IU/min and should not exceed 100 IU/min.

Dosage Form—Injection: Lyophilized powder in vials of 500 or 1000 IU containing 10 and 20 mL, respectively, of SterileWater for Injection as the diluent. The solution must be administered intravenously within 3 hr following reconstitution.

Anti-Inhibitor Coagulant Complex

Autoplex (*Baxter*); Feiba (*Immuno US*)

A cryodessicated complex of activated and precursor clotting factors and factors of the kinin generating system which is prepared from pooled human plasma. It is standardized by its ability to restore normal clotting time to Factor VIII-deficient plasma. One correctional unit will correct the clotting time to 35 sec in the ellagic acid-APTT test. The complex is reconstituted with Sterile Water for Injection. There should be no more than 2 Units/mL of heparin and 0.02*M* citrate after reconstitution.

Uses—As an alternative treatment for hemorrhagic diathesis in patients with titers of Factor VIII inhibitors above 5 Bethesda Units/mL only after the failure of conventional treatment. It is contraindicated when signs of fibrinolysis or disseminated intravascular coagulation are extant. It may cause transient hypofibrogenemia in children, so that fibrinogen levels should be monitored in young patients. Headache, flushing, tachycardia and hypotension may result from too-rapid infusion. It is not free of the risk of serum hepatitis.

Dose—*Intravenous, initially* **25** to **100 Units/kg**, to be adjusted according to APTT 30-min after the end of infusion. The infusion rate should not exceed 10 mL/min.

Dosage Form—Powder: in 30-mL and other vials.

Factor IX Complex

Konÿne (*Cutter*); Profilnine (*Alpha*); Proplex (*Hyland*)

A preparation of pooled human plasma protein fraction containing clotting factors II, VII, IX and X. The preparation is standardized in terms of Factor IX; the activity is not less than 0.7 and is usually 1 Unit/mg of protein.

Preparation—See US Pat 3,717,708.

Description—White powder with a slight odor; fairly stable in light and air but unstable in heat. After reconstitution, solutions are stable up to 12 hr at room temperature; they should, however, be prepared only immediately before use. 1 Unit is the activity in 1 mL of average normal fresh plasma.

Solubility—Soluble in water.

Uses—Principally, as a source of Factor IX for treatment of hemophilia B, a form of hemophilia separate and distinct from the more prevalent hemophilia A, or classic Factor VIII-deficient hemophilia. It also can be used in the treatment of congenital deficiencies of the other vitamin-K-dependent coagulation factors, namely, factors II, VII and X. Because some preparations of the product have been found to cause posttransfusion hepatitis, caution is indicated and physicians should weigh the risks against expected benefits.

Nausea, vomiting, headache, flushing, tingling, chills and fever may result shortly after administration.

Factor IX manifests two-compartment pharmacokinetics, with a distribution half-life of 3 to 6 hr, and a terminal half-life of 22 to 41 hr.

Dose—*Intravenous*, the dose is determined according to previous evaluation of the patient, the circumstances and the response. In Factor IX-deficient patients, 1 Unit/kg will cause an average increment of Factor IX of 1% of normal; in Factor VII-deficient patients, 2 Units/kg will cause an increase in Factor VII of about 4%. Presurgically, it is advisable to achieve 60% of normal initially, although a maintenance of 20% is minimally sufficient. Maintenance should continue for 8 days. Prophylactically, for ambulatory patients with a Factor IX deficiency in normal circumstances, 500 Units/wk.

Dosage Form—Vials containing approximately 500 or 1000 Factor IX Units, equivalent to Factor IX activity of 500 or 500 mL, respectively of normal plasma. The actual number of units is indicated on the label. Products differ in the volume of sterile water to be added for reconstitution.

Anticoagulants

Anticoagulants are substances or drugs which delay blood coagulation. They are of three general types.

Calcium Sequestering Agents—Calcium is essential to several steps in the clotting process; hence, its removal prevents clotting. The calcium-sequestering agents tie up calcium and other divalent cations; these agents are employed only in withdrawn blood. Thus, they find their most common use in anticoagulant solutions used by blood banks. These substances act rapidly, and their effect can be overcome rapidly by adding or otherwise restoring calcium to normal. Thus, citrate-containing blood is, in effect, recalcified on transfusion back into the bloodstream.

Heparin and Heparin Substitutes—These agents combine with antithrombin III. The complex then interacts with certain activated clotting factors, namely, Factors IX, X, XI and XII, to prevent the conversion of prothrombin to thrombin. In high concentrations the complex interacts with thrombin and inhibits its effects to promote conversion of fibrinogen to fibrin. They inhibit the aggregation of platelets. They are fast-acting drugs. Heparin has the advantage of being a naturally occurring substance.

Prothrombopenic Anticoagulants (Oral Anticoagulants)—In this group dicumarol provides the prototype of action but not necessarily of structure. Prothrombopenic anticoagulants competitively inhibit vitamin K in the hepatic production of prothrombin (Factor II), the plasma content of prothrombin thus is reduced and blood coagulation is impaired. These drugs also suppress formation of Factors VII, IX and X, although the effect on prothrombin is the predominant one. Drugs in this category are slow-acting because their effect is directed at inhibition of protein synthesis and there is a latency determined by the long half-life (about 60 hr) of prothrombin. By the same token, their action is overcome only slowly by vitamin K.

The heparin and prothrombopenic anticoagulants generally are not employed for the same purpose, since chronic medication with heparin is expensive and entails the nuisance of parenteral administration. Rather, they may be complementary, heparin being employed acutely or initially, and prothrombopenic anticoagulants being employed for longer-term therapy.

The enzymes urokinase and streptokinase are not true anticoagulants, although their effects to increase the fibrinolytic activity of blood have the effect of retarding red thrombus formation. They are described in Chapter 66.

Prothrombopenic Anticoagulants

Anisindione

Miradon (*Schering*)

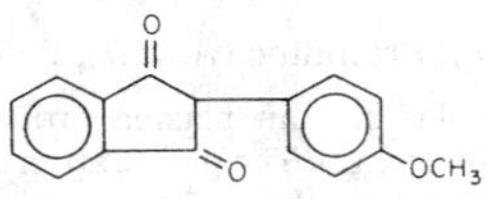

[117-37-3] $C_{16}H_{12}O_3$ (252.27).

Preparation—By rearrangement of 3-(*p*-methoxybenzylidene) phthalide. US Pat 2,899,359.

Description—White or off-white, crystalline powder.

Solubility—Practically insoluble in water.

Uses—A prothrombopenic anticoagulant with actions and uses similar to those of *Dicumarol*. Its onset of action is 24 to 72 hr, and duration of action is ordinarily 3 to 5 days. The effective dose and duration of action are affected by factors including dietary intake, bacterial synthesis of vitamin K and concurrently administered drugs that affect the hepatic microsomal drug-metabolizing system. Untoward effects include hemorrhagic diathesis resulting from overdosage and, also, dermatitis. Overdoses can be antagonized with phytonadione (vitamin K_1) but there is a long delay before prothrombin levels return to a safe range. If fever or dermatitis appear, the drug should be discontinued because of the possible danger of blood dyscrasias. It may cause some orange discoloration of urine that may obscure onset of hematuria, an important sign of impending hemorrhage; the color disappears on acidification. Hemorrhagic complications and drug interactions are as for *Dicumarol*.

Dose—Oral, adults, **300 mg** the first day, **200 mg** the second day and **100 mg** the third day; for maintenance, 25 to 250 mg a day.

Dosage Form—Tablets: 50 mg.

Dicumarol

2*H*-1-Benzopyran-2-one], 3,3′-methylenebis[4-hydroxy-,
Biscumarol; Bishydroxycoumarin; Dicoumarol; (*Abbott*)

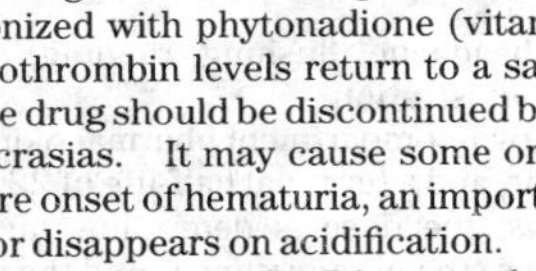

3,3′-Methylenebis[4-hydroxycoumarin] [66-76-2] $C_{19}H_{12}O_6$ (336.30).

Preparation—Methyl acetylsalicylate is stirred with sodium, thus effecting ring closure through demethanolation to form the sodium derivative of 4-hydroxycoumarin. Treatment with HCl liberates 4-hydroxycoumarin, which readily forms methylenebishydroxycoumarin on heating with formaldehyde and water.

Description—White or creamy white, crystalline powder, with a faint, pleasant odor and a slightly bitter taste; melts at about 290°.

Solubility—Practically insoluble in water, alcohol or ether; slightly soluble in chloroform; readily soluble in solutions of fixed alkali hydroxides.

Uses—A *prothrombopenic anticoagulant*. It depresses hepatic production of prothrombin, probably by competing with vitamin K, both for transportation into liver cells and at the major site of vitamin-K-dependent synthesis of clotting factors; the resultant lowering of the blood level of prothrombin renders the blood less coagulable. The plasma levels of VII, IX and X also are depressed; indeed, in some persons the major effect of dicumarol is upon these factors. Plasma levels of Factor VII are the first to fall, since it has a half-life of about 6 hr; the half-lives of Factors IX, X and II (prothrombin) are 20, 40 and 60 hr, respectively.

It has advantages over heparin (see page 922) for ambulatory and prolonged anticoagulant therapy in that it is *orally effective*, has a longer duration of action (2 to 7 days; plasma half-life, about 8.2 hr at low doses, but up to 30 hr at high doses) and is considerably less expensive. It is unsuitable for short-term or emergency therapy in that the maximal effect of a full initial dose does not occur for 48 to 96 hr after administration, which reflects both the long half-life of prothrombin and the slow onset of the steady state. During the period of onset of action, heparin may be given. This drug or one of its congeners is employed for long-term therapy to a much greater extent than heparin. However, the necessity for frequent prothrombin tests, which are more difficult to determine than clotting time, restricts its use to physicians having access to properly equipped laboratories and trained personnel. It may be used in the treatment of the following: *pulmonary embolism*, to prevent further embolism; primary acute and postoperative *thrombophlebitis* and *traumatic injuries to blood vessels*, to forestall *venous thrombosis* and to prevent *thromboemboli;* sudden *arterial occlusion from thrombosis or embolism;* prophylaxis of *postoperative venous thrombosis or embolism or vascular surgery*, and prophylaxis after mechanical prosthetic valves or tissue heart valves.

In the absence of specific contraindications, it frequently is used routinely in acute *coronary thrombosis* with myocardial infarction. It also is advocated in the treatment of chronic diseases that predispose to thrombi or emboli such as congestive heart failure, persistent phlebitis migrans, recurrent thrombophlebitis, recurrent coronary thrombosis and atrial fibrillation. However, the exact status of such long-term therapy is undetermined.

The aim of treatment is to maintain the blood prothrombin activity at a level of 15 to 25% of normal. The onset of action is 1 to 5 days; the duration is 2 to 10 days.

With the recommended dosage, the incidence of hemorrhage is 2 to 4%, and strict laboratory control is mandatory to prevent hemorrhagic diatheses. Bleeding is most common from the mucous membranes, skin, gastrointestinal tract, urogenital tract and uterus. Stools should be monitored for occult blood loss and urine for hematuria. Hemorrhage can be arrested by vitamin K (which has a latency), fresh frozen plasma, whole blood or Factor IX concentrate (which contains prothrombin along with other vitamin K-dependent coagulation factors).

Other side effects include anorexia, nausea, vomiting and diarrhea. Rarely, there may be hypersensitivity reactions, such as purpura, alopecia, urticaria, necrosis of the skin, breast and genitals and purple coloration of the toes. Tissue necrosis has been associated with protein C deficiency and may be minimized by concurrent heparin therapy for the first 5 to 7 days of treatment. Protein C, a plasma glycoprotein, is a vitamin K-dependent factor which upon activation functions as an endogenous anticoagulant.

It is sensitive to interaction with other drugs and to the nutrition and other status of the patient, all of which may lead to unpredictable results. Therefore, whenever a patient on this drug is subjected to a new drug regimen or an old drug is withdrawn, it is essential that the patient's prothrombin time be monitored and the dosage of dicumarol be adjusted if necessary.

Drug interactions occur in various ways. Mechanisms of antagonism and offending drugs are as follows (*italics* indicate the most-important clinical interactions):

Interference with absorption: *griseofulvin, cholestyramine*, clofibrate.

Stimulation of synthesis of clotting factors: *vitamin K*, glucocorticoids, estrogens.

Induction of hepatic enzymes: *barbiturates, ethchlorvynol, glutethimide, carbamazepine, griseofulvin*, meprobamate, phenytoin, *rifampin*.

Mechanisms of increasing the response to dicumarol, and the offending drugs are as follows:

Displacement from plasma protein: *chloral hydrate* (as the trichloroacetate metabolite), *clofibrate*, diazoxide, ethacrynic acid, *mefenamic acid*, nalidixic acid, *phenylbutazone* and *hydroxyphenylbutazone*, long-acting sulfonamides.

Inhibition of hepatic metabolism: *chloramphenicol, clofibrate,* oral hypoglycemics, *cimetidine, disulfiram,* allopurinol, disulfiram, mercaptopurine, methylphenidate, nortriptyline.

Decrease in availability of vitamin K: *anabolic steroids, broad-spectrum antibiotics, clofibrate, cholestyramine, mineral oil,* D-thyroxine.

Inhibition of synthesis of clotting factors: acetaminophen, *anabolic steroids, glucagon,* mercaptopurine, *quinidine, salicylates.*

Increased catabolism of clotting factors: *anabolic steroids,* D-*thyroxine.*

Increased binding affinity to receptor enzyme: D-thyroxine.

Additivity of anticoagulant effects: *heparin, salicylates,* quinidine.

A complete table of interactions may be found in *USP DI.*

The drug is contraindicated if laboratory facilities are unavailable for determining prothrombin levels, and vitamin K, fresh blood or plasma are not available. It also is contraindicated in any person with hemorrhagic tendencies, blood dyscrasias, peptic ulcer, ulcerative colitis, colitis, diverticulitis, subacute bacterial endocarditis, recent operations on the CNS, regional or lumbar block anesthesia and severe renal or liver disease. Not only is it contraindicated in threatened abortion, but it should be withheld in pregnancy, since hemorrhage in the fetus can occur, and several tetratogenic abnormalities including hydrocephaly, microcephaly, optic atrophy, other CNS defects, nasal hypoplasia and chondrodysplasia punctata have been attributed to the drug. Patients with congestive heart failure are more sensitive to dicumarol than persons with normal cardiac function.

It is metabolized by the hepatic cytochrome P450 system. The half-life is 24 to 96 hr.

Dose—*Oral, adults,* **200** to **300 mg** on the first day, for loading; *maintenance,* ranges from **25** to **200 mg** a day, according to prothrombin time.

Dosage Forms—Capsules and Tablets: 25 and 50 mg.

Warfarin Sodium

2*H*-1-Benzopyran-2-one, 4-hydroxy-3-(3-oxo-1-phenylbutyl)-, sodium salt; Coumadin (*Dupont*); Panwarfin (*Abbott*); Sofarin (*Lemmon*)

3-(α-Acetonylbenzyl)-4-hydroxycoumarin sodium salt [129-06-6] $C_{19}H_{15}NaO_4$ (330.31); an amorphous solid or a crystalline clathrate. The clathrate consists principally of sodium warfarin, isopropyl alcohol and water, the molecular proportions of which vary between 8:4:0 and 8:2:2.

Preparation—By addition of 4-hydroxycoumarin to benzalacetone under the catalytic influence of a mildly basic substance such as ammonia or piperidine. The reaction is a typical Michael "condensation." Conversion to the sodium salt is effected by reacting purified warfarin with an equimolar portion of dilute NaOH solution at room temperature.

Description—White, odorless, amorphous or crystalline powder with a slightly bitter taste; discolored by light; pH (1 in 100 solution) 7.2 to 8.3.

Solubility—Very soluble in water, freely soluble in alcohol; very slightly soluble in chloroform or ether.

Uses—The most widely used *prothrombopenic anticoagulant* (see *Dicumarol*). Although usually it is administered orally, its chief distinction from other prothrombopenic drugs is the fact that it is water-soluble and may be administered intravenously. By the intravenous route its onset of action is 12 to 18 hr and its duration is 5 to 6 days. It is metabolized by the hepatic cytochrome P450 system. The plasma half-life is 41 to 57 hr, except about 27 hr in alcoholics and probably even less in persons using phenobarbital or other hepatic microsomal enzyme inducers.

The hemorrhagic complications, precautions and drug interactions are those of *Dicumarol.* Influenza vaccine increases the response; this interaction probably occurs also with dicoumarol and anisindione.

Dose—*Oral, intramuscular,* or *intravenous, adults,* **10** to **15 mg** for 2 to 4 days, followed by a daily *maintenance* dose of **2** to **10 mg,** according to the prothrombin time. A prothrombin time 1.2 to 1.5 times the control time is effective for anticoagulation, yet is associated with an incidence of hemorrhage of only 4.3%.

Dosage Forms—for Injection: 50 mg; Tablets: 1.0, 2, 2.5, 5, 7.5 and 10 mg.

Nonprothrombopenic Anticoagulants

Anticoagulant Citrate Dextrose Solution Modified

ACD Solution Modified (*Squibb*)

Each sterile 10 mL contains 80 mg citric acid, 224 mg anhydrous sodium citrate and 120 mg anhydrous dextrose.

Uses—It is used with *Sodium Chromatic Cr 51 Injection* for the labeling of erythrocytes in *in vitro* and *in vivo* diagnostic tests.

Application—10 mL are mixed with 30 to 50 mL of whole blood and 150 μCi of sodium chromate Cr 51 and incubated for 30 to 60 min at room temperature, after which 100 mg of ascorbic acid are added. For *in vivo* use, the mixture is injected *intravenously.*

Anticoagulant Citrate Dextrose Solution

ACD Solution

A sterile solution of citric acid ($C_6H_8O_7$), sodium citrate ($C_6H_5Na_3$-O_7.$2H_2O$) and dextrose ($C_6H_{12}O_6$.H_2O) in water for injection. It contains no antimicrobial agents.

Preparation—See the USP.

Uses—The citrate chelates calcium ions and thus acts as an anticoagulant. The ratio of citric acid to sodium citrate is such that the pH is optimal for storage of whole blood. The dextrose provides a substrate for glycolysis during storage, thus extending the lifetime of the erythrocytes. The expiration time of whole blood anticoagulated with ACD solution is 21 days. The sterile solution is employed mainly for the anticoagulation and preservation of whole blood for transfusion.

Application—10 mL per 100 mL of whole blood.

Anticoagulant Citrate Phosphate Dextrose Solution

CPD Solution

A sterile solution of citric acid ($C_6H_8O_7$), sodium citrate ($C_6H_5Na_3O_7$.$2H_2O$), sodium biphosphate (NaH_2PO_4.H_2O) and dextrose ($C_6H_{12}O_6$.H_2O) in water for injection. It contains no antimicrobial agents.

Preparation—See the USP.

Description—Clear, colorless, odorless liquid; pH 5.0 to 6.0.

Uses—Citrate ion chelates calcium, thus making calcium unavailable to the coagulation system. Citric acid, sodium citrate and sodium biphosphate are in the proper proportions to buffer the solution at the optimal pH for the storage of blood and its components. Dextrose provides a substrate for glycolysis and increases both storage and posttransfusion lives of blood cells. The expiration time of whole blood with CPD solution is 21 days. The 2,3-diphosphorglycerate (2,3-DPG) content of erythrocytes stored in CPD solution is 120% of the original content at 7 and 40% at 21 days. The preservation helps keep the oxygen affinity of hemoglobin low so that it can yield its oxygen readily to the tissues. Consequently, CPD is the preferred anticoagulant for blood to be used for exchange transfusion.

The sodium concentration is 284 mEq/L, and 17.8 mEq are thus added to each unit of whole blood.

Application—In the proportion of 14 mL of solution for each 100 mL of whole blood.

Size Available—63 mL in a blood-collecting container.

Anticoagulant Sodium Citrate Solution

A sterile 4% solution of sodium citrate [$C_6H_5Na_3O_7$.$2H_2O$ (294.10)] in water for injection. It contains no antimicrobial agents.

Preparation—Dissolve 40 g sodium citrate in sufficient water for injection to make 1000 mL, and filter until clear. Place the solution in suitable containers, and sterilize.

Note—Anhydrous sodium citrate (35.1 g) may be used instead of the dihydrate.

Description—Clear, colorless solution possessing a slightly saline taste; pH 6.4 to 7.5.

Uses—Prevents clotting of blood by forming an undissociated calcium citrate chelate. The solution also prevents either crenation or swelling of the cells. The sterile solution is employed for preparation of blood for fractionation, for banked blood for transfusion and for preparation of citrated human plasma.

Application—10 mL per 100 mL of whole blood or plasma.

Edetate Disodium—page 935.

Anticoagulant Citrate Phosphate Dextrose Adenine Solution

CPDA-1 Solution; CPD-Adenine Solution (*Travenol*)

Uses—The addition of adenine to CPD solution increases the storage life of blood by 40%, that is, blood can now be stored for 35 days. However, CPDA-1 solution does not preserve 2,3-diphosphoglycerate as well as does CPD solution; there is 97% of the initial content at 7 days but only 10% at 21 days. Therefore, CPDA-1 whole blood should not be used in exchange transfusion.

Application—14 mL per 100 mL of whole blood.

Heparin Calcium

Calciparine (*Du Pont*)

[37270-89-6]. Obtained from the lungs or mucosa of cattle, sheep or pigs. Refer to *Heparin Sodium.*

Description—white to off-white powder.

Solubility—1 g in 4 to 5 mL water; pH of 1% solution, 5.0 to 7.5.

Uses abd Dose—See *Heparin Sodium.* The calcium salt is used in low doses to prevent postoperative thromboembolism. The claim that it causes fewer and less severe hemorrhagic disturbances has not been supported by controlled clinical trails. The calcium salt is indicated especially when it is desirable to restrict sodium intake.

Dosage Form—Injection: 5000, 12,500 and 20,000 Units/mL.

Heparin Low-Molecular-Weight

Enoxaparin; Lovenox (*Rorer*)

A mixture of low-molecular-weight fragments of heparin obtained by the depolymerization of the benzyl ester of porcine mucosal heparin. The molecular weights of the constituent molecules range from about 4000 to 5000 daltons. *Chem Abstr 96:* 218191s, 1982.

Uses—Standard heparin (see below) forms a ternary complex with antithrombin III and thrombin, but heparins with molecular weights below 4800 form only binary complexes with antithrombin III, thus inhibiting only Factor Xa and not thrombin. Furthermore, small heparin molecules bound to antithrombin III react only slightly with platelets. Consequently, deep-vein thrombosis can be prevented or retarded without as much risk of hemorrhage as with standard heparin. It has been used investigationally primarily as a prophylactic after elective hip surgery and other situations in which there is a high risk of deep vein thrombosis. Medical opinion about its superiority over approved medications is mixed. The elimination half-life is about 3 to 5 hr, twice as long as that of standard heparin.

Dose—Tentatively, the dose in USP units is the same as that of standard heparin, but this does not take into account the difference in half-lives; some of the differences in medical findings possibly may relate to inappropriate dosage.

Heparin Sodium

Heparin; Lipo-Hepin (*Riker*); Liquaemin Sodium (*Organon*); Panheprin (*Abbott*)

A mixture of active glycosaminoglycans, having the property of prolonging the clotting time of blood. It usually is obtained from the lungs, intestinal mucosa or other suitable tissues of domestic mammals used for food by man. Potency: not less than 120 (when derived from lungs) and not less than 140 (when derived from other tissues) USP Heparin Units/mg.

Note—USP Heparin Units consistently are established on the basis of the USP assay, independently of International Units, and the respective units are not equivalent.

Preparation—Heparin is the body's natural anticoagulant, taking part in the physiological function of maintaining the fluidity of the blood. It is produced by the mast cells of Ehrlich, which are clustered in the perivascular connective tissue of the walls of major blood vessels and capillaries. Heparin is a polysulfuric ester of mucoitin. The molecular skeleton is constructed from acetylated glucosamine and glucuronic acid. The disaccharide unit is similar to that in *mucoitin sulfuric acid* and *hyaluronic acid.* Protein-free samples of heparin contain about 10% of sulfur present as ester sulfates. Original preparations of heparin contain mixtures consisting of mucoitin disulfuric and trisulfuric acids. The anticoagulant action is greater in preparations with the highest sulfuric content. Heparin in the final, therapeutic form is supplied in a solution made from the sodium salt, but in the steps of its purification the barium salts of heparin are prepared. Heparin, being a mixture of the several sulfuric esters, is not entirely homogeneous, and there is debate as to whether a truly crystalline or homogeneous preparation has been or ever can be prepared.

Description—White or pale-colored amorphous powder: odorless, or nearly so; hygroscopic. The molecular weight may vary from 6000 to 20000 depending on the source and on the method used to determine the molecular weight. pH (1% solution) 5.0 to 7.5. It will not dialyze through a parchment membrane, and only slightly through a collodion membrane. Heparin is resistant to all kinds of chemical agents, gives an insoluble precipitate with protamine and with toluidine blue and interference with the sulfuric groups reduces its anticoagulant activity. It has a very low osmotic pressure in respect to its high degree of ionization. In contrast to the effect of oxalate, it has no osmotic influence on red blood cells. It may be stored for long periods without loss of activity.

Solubility—1 g in 20 mL of water; soluble in alcohol, acetone or glacial acetic acid.

Uses—Its anticoagulant actions are described on page 919. In addition, it releases lipoprotein lipase from the vascular endothelium, which has the effect of clearing chylomicrons and very-low-density lipoproteins from blood; only low doses are needed for this action. It has antiatherogenic activity, but only a few studies of its prophylactic efficacy have been made. It also has anti-inflammatory and antiallergy actions through its effects on the Hageman factor (XIIa), kallikreins and other enzymes that have active groups containing or act on substrates with lysine and/or arginine moieties.

It is employed clinically in conditions in which a rapid reduction in the coagulability of the blood is desired. It often is employed to initiate prolonged anticoagulant therapy in order to cover the latent period of onset of action of dicumarol-type anticoagulants. It also is used in lieu of dicumarol-type drugs in prolonged therapy when laboratory facilities are unavailable for determination of prothrombin time.

Some of the primary clinical applications are the treatment and prevention of *pulmonary embolism, prevention of mural thrombosis* after myocardial infarction, *initial treatment of deep-vein* and *proximal-vein thrombosis*, primary and postoperative *thrombophlebitis*, sudden *arterial occlusion* from thrombosis or embolism, prophylaxis of postoperative *venous thrombosis* or embolism, *prevention of cerebral thrombosis* during evolving stroke and after *vascular surgery.* For these purposes, low doses given subcutaneously are popular; however, recent reports indicate that blood levels are erratic and monitoring is advisable. It is indicated for treatment of *diffuse intravascular coagulation* (consumptive coagulopathy) in patients with acute leukemia (only) and *immune thrombocytopenia* (in which vasculitis causes coagulopathy and consumption of platelets).

It sometimes is given during and after conversion of atrial fibrillation to prevent thrombosis from emboli and mural thrombi. It is advocated by some for immediate therapy of *coronary occlusion,* but its status in that condition is still controversial after more than four decades of use. It appears to decrease mortality in women but not in men. However, it does protect against venous thrombosis resulting from stasis during coronary care.

The indications for prolonged therapy are the same as with prothrombopenic anticoagulants (see *Dicumarol*), but usually this drug is used only during the early stages of treatment when the disorder is acute, to keep blood clotting suppressed until oral anticoagulants can be given and take effect. It also has special uses, such as prevention of clotting of blood samples or whole blood for transfusion, to *prevent clotting* during *blood transfusions, extracorporeal hemodialysis* or *cardiopulmonary bypass* and for the heparin tolerance test.

It is used in low concentrations in solutions for flushing intravenous catheters for intermittent injections; the residual heparin in the catheter keeps clots from occluding the catheter orifice. It also is used to prevent pleural and peritoneal *adhesions.* Sometimes it is used as an adjuvant to antineoplastic therapy to suppress formation of a fibrin network through which the neoplasm can spread.

Constant infusion appears to be more efficacious and safer than is intermittent injection. Intramuscular injection often results in hematoma formation and should be avoided.

Hemorrhage is the principal toxic effect, usually the result of overdosage; protamine, with which it combines, may be employed for immediate control of hyperheparinemia. It must be administered cautiously when oral anticoagulants are in use or when there is thrombocytopenia because of the enhanced risk of hemorrhage; it also interferes with laboratory tests for the effect of oral anticoagulants. The risk of hemorrhage also is increased by salicylates, dipyridamole, glyceryl guaiacolate or other inhibitors of platelet adhesiveness.

Certain amine or ammonium compounds, especially bifunctional ones, interact with it directly and thus decrease the circulating levels in the blood; cimetidine, various antihistamines, quinine and quinidine are examples. Even tetracyclines supposedly interact. Polymyxins and colistins are known to interact during simultaneous infusion but have not been reported to interact when administered separately.

Hypersensitivity and other adverse side effects may occur. Manifestations include bronchospasm (dyspnea, tightness in chest, wheezing), skin rash, urticaria, pruritus, chills, fever, vasospasm (chest pain, pain in extremities, priapism), neuropathy with paresthesias and hair loss. Thrombocytopenia occurs in about 1% of cases.

It is inactive orally and must be administered parenterally. Its plasma half-life is 1.3 to 1.6 hr.

Dose—Dosage should be determined by laboratory tests of coagulability of blood during the course of therapy in each patient and not by a rigid regimen. Usually, a coagulation time 2.5 to 3, or a partial prothombin time (PPT) 1.5 to 2.5 times normal is desired. The following doses (**in USP Units**) only provide an approximate guide to dosage. *Intravenous, adults, therapeutic, initially* **10,000 Units** followed by **5000** to **10,000 Units** every 4 to 6 hr or **100 Units/kg** every 4 hr; for *heart* and *blood vessel surgery*, initially **150** to **300 Units/kg** for procedures expected to last less than 60 min and **400 Units/kg** for procedures over 60 min, maintenance doses being determined by coagulation tests; for *disseminated intravascular coagulation*, **50** to **100 Units/kg** every 4 hr, administered by bolus or constant infusion; *children, initially* **50 Units/kg** followed by **100 Units per kg** every 4 hr.

Intravenous infusion, adults, initially **35** to **70 Units/kg** or **5000 Units** followed rapidly by **20,000** to **40,000 Units** (in 1 L isotonic sodium chloride) per 24 hr; *children,* initially **50 Units/kg** followed rapidly by **100 Units/kg** every 4 hr or **20,000 Units/m^2** every 24 hr; for *heart* and *blood vessel surgery,* as for adults; for *disseminated intravascular coagulation,* one-half the adult dose.

Deep subcutaneous ("intrafat"), *adults, therapeutic, initially* (after an intravenous loading dose of 5000 USP units) **10,000 Units** followed by **8000** to **10,000 Units** every 8 hr or **15,000** to **20,000 Units** every 12 hr; for *low-dose prophylaxis,* initially **5000 Units** 2 hr prior to surgery, repeated at 8- to 12-hr intervals for 7 days or until the patient is fully ambulatory, whichever is the longer.

For *blood transfusion* or *extracorporeal circuits,* **400** to **600 Units/100 mL** of whole blood. For laboratory *blood samples,* **70** to **150 Units/10 to 20 mL.** For *filling* and *flushing intravenous catheters,* as an isotonic saline solution containing **10** or **100 Units/mL.**

Dosage Form—Injection: 10, 100, 1000, 2500, 5000, 7500, 10,000, 15,000, 20,000 and 40,000 Units/mL. It also is available in concentrations of 50 and 100 Units/mL in 5% dextrose or 0.45% sodium chloride intravenous solutions.

Heparin Sodium and Dihydroergotamine Mesylate—see RPS-18, page 814.

Potassium Oxalate

[583-52-8] $K_2C_2O_4.H_2O$ (183.23).

Description—Colorless crystals; efflorese in dry air.

Solubility—1 g in 3 mL water.

Uses—The oxalate anion of potassium oxalate combines with calcium ions to form the very insoluble calcium oxalate. Thus, when it is added to withdrawn (shed) blood it acts as an anticoagulant, for which purpose it may be employed in clinical laboratory procedures. Care must be exercised in its storage and use because it is highly toxic.

Sodium Citrate

1,2,3-Propanetricarboxylic acid, 2-hydroxy-, trisodium salt

$CH_2(COONa)C(OH)(COONa)CH_2COONa$

Trisodium citrate [68-04-2] $C_6H_5Na_3O_7$ (258.07) or trisodium citrate dihydrate [6132-04-3] (294.10).

Preparation—Usually, by adding sodium carbonate to a solution of citric acid until effervescence ceases, evaporating and granulating the product.

Description—Colorless crystals or a white, crystalline powder; cooling, saline taste; stable in air; the aqueous solution is slightly alkaline to litmus but should not be reddened by phenolphthalein.

Solubility—1 g in 1.5 mL water at 25° or in 0.6 mL boiling water; insoluble in alcohol.

Uses—The most important use is as an *anticoagulant* for blood or plasma that is to be fractionated or for blood that is to be stored. The anticoagulant effect is due to conversion of ionized calcium in the blood to a citrato-calcium chelate. It is an ingredient of *Anticoagulant Citrate Dextrose Solution, Anticoagulant Citrate Phosphate Dextrose Solution* and *Sodium Citrate and Citric Acid Solution.*

It also is used as an *expectorant* and a systemic and urine *alkalinizer.* Saline expectorants are useful especially when it is desired to liquefy thick, tenacious sputum. In the body sodium citrate is oxidized to bicarbonate and excreted in urine. Thus, when given orally it is useful in acidosis, to overcome excessive urinary acidity and to assist in the dissolution of uric acid nephroliths.

It is a chelating agent and thus increases *urinary excretion* of *calcium* and *lead.* It has been employed in hypercalcemia, urolithiasis and to facilitate elimination of lead in poisoning due to the latter. As a *pharmaceutic aid,* sodium citrate may be used to prevent darkening when iron is included in preparations containing tannin.

Dose—*Usual, expectorant,* **1** to **2 g,** well-diluted with water, every 2 hr; for *metabolic acidosis,* **1** to **4 g** 4 times a day; for *urolithiasis,* **490** or **500 mg** in combination with 334 or 640 mg of citric acid 4 times a day. Since sodium citrate is not used alone as an anticoagulant, there is no statement of application or dosage forms here.

Sodium Oxalate

[62-76-0] $Na_2C_2O_4$ (134.01). The actions and uses of sodium oxalate are virtually identical to those of *Potassium Oxalate.*

Thrombolytic Agents

The fibrinolytic system comprises a group of proteins which complexly interact to cause the lysis of thrombi and also to keep the fibrinolytic factors in check. Plasminogen plays a key role in the activation of fibrinolysis. It is a proenzyme that is converted to the active enzyme, plasmin, by interactions among circulating intrinsic factors (prekallikrein, kininogens, Factors XII, XIIIa and plasminogen proactivator and the extrinsic factor, endothelial tissue, which releases plasminogen activator [tissue plasminogen activator, TPA). Fibrinolytic activity is kept in check by the inhibitors, C1-*in*activator, alpha$_2$-macroglobulin and alpha$_2$-antiplasmin. Once formed, plasmin cleaves fibrin into its split-products. However, it also can degrade Factors V, VIII, XII and other proteins. The rates of formation and inactivation of plasmin normally are balanced, such that there is always a small amount of fibrin being formed to maintain normal vascular integrity and the remainder being lysed before clots form. Vascular injury and inflammation increase both fibrin deposition and fibrinolytic activity.

In the early 1960s, a bacterial product called streptokinase-streptodornase was discovered to activate plasminogen. Subsequently, the active component, streptokinase (SK; see page 1037), has been purified sufficiently to permit clinical use in the dissolution of thrombi. Interest has been high especially with respect to the ability to dissolve coronary thrombi and restore coronary perfusion. Timing is very critical, because once the fibrin has "aged" (greater than 4 hours), very little dissolution occurs. Consequently, for the dissolution of coronary thrombi, there is a preference for the intravenous over the intracoronary route, because it avoids the more-than-1-hr delay required to get a coronary catheter in place. However, the intravenous route carries a greater danger of hemorrhage elsewhere. SK presently still confers a considerably high risk of hypersensitivity reactions.

A natural plasminogen activator, urokinase (UK; see page 1137) was isolated and purified for the same uses as SK. It is free of allergic potential but has the slightly lesser potential for generalized fibrinolyisis and hemorrhage than SK. It is several times more expensive. More recently, several other plasminogen activators have been isolated, characterized and modified. They are anisoylated plasminogen-streptokinase activator complex (APSAC), pro-urokinase (Pro-UK) and tissue plasminogen activator (TPA). APSAC is an inactive complex of human plasminogen and streptokinase which is gradually deacylated and thus activated after injection. It has similar efficacy to intracoronary streptokinase in achieving reperfusion and may be slightly superior in preventing reocclusion. APSAC's major advantage over streptokinase is its ease of administration due to the prolonged half-life.

Both rTPA (alteplase; r denotes *recombinant*) and rPRO-UK theoretically have considerably lesser tendencies to produce hemorrhage, because they bind selectively to fibrin and not to circulating clotting factors. Thus, they are selective for the intended target, a previously formed clot. They are not free of bleeding risk, however, because they attack the many microclots that constantly are forming at the sites of endothelial breaks, and clinical opinion is divided over whether there is a significant advantage over SK and UK in this respect. In fact, target selectivity creates a bleeding problem, in that clots tend to form around the intravenous catheters used for infusion, so that heparin also is infused to prevent this effect. Furthermore, their short half-lifes favor rethrombosis unless heparin is coadministered. rTPA and rPRO-UK are more than ten times as expensive as SK.

With respect to the treatment of coronary occlusion, there is very little difference in the percentage of reopened coronary arteries and reperfusion (65 to 70%) or in the reocclusion frequencies (about 20%) if treatment is begun earlier than 4 hr after occlusion. It is thought by some that the very short lifetime of infused TPA limits the concentration at the target, a situation that might be correctable by higher rates of infusion. There appears to be some advantage with rTPA at later times, for reasons not altogether clear.

Anistreplase

Eminase (*SmithKline Beecham*)

[81669-57-0]

Preparation—By *p*-anisoylation of primary human lys-plasminogen streptokinase complex (1:1) from Group C β-hemolytic streptococci.

Description—White to off-white powder.

Uses—Indicated for *thrombolysis* in patients exhibiting symptoms consistent with acute myocardial infarction. Its comparison with streptokinase is described above. Randomized, controlled studies comparing it to either placebo- or heparin-treated patients demonstrated that anistreplase significantly reduced mortality. As with other thrombolytics, it is contraindicated in patients with active internal bleeding, a history of cerebrovascular accident, recent intraspinal or intracranial surgery or trauma, severe hypertension, arteriovenous malformation or aneurysm. Allergic-type reactions including rash, bronchospasm, fever, angiodema and anaphylaxis have been observed in patients receiving anistreplase and are similar in incidence to streptokinase. Other reported adverse effects include facial flushing, nausea, vomiting and muscle aches. The half-life of anistreplase is approximately 90 min with a fibrinolytic activity duration of from 4 to 6 hr after administration.

Dose—Intravenous, **30 units** over 2 to 5 min. Units of anistreplase are based on a reference standard specific for Eminase and are not comparable to units used for other thrombolytic agents. One unit is approximately equivalent to 1 mg. The drug is not approved currently for intracoronary administration.

Dosage Form—Injection: Lyophilized powder in 30-unit vials which is reconstituted with 5 mL of Sterile Water for Injection. It must be administered within 30 min of reconstitution.

Alteplase Recombinant

Activase (*Genentech*)

[105857-23-6] $C_{2736}H_{4174}N_{914}O_{824}S_{45}$ (59,050.00).

Purified glycoprotein of a single, continuous chain containing 527 amino acids with three carbohydrate side chains. The biological potency is determined by an *in vitro* clot lysis assay expressed in International Units as tested against a WHO standard. See Chapter 49.

Preparation—Using the complimentary DNA (cDNA) for natural human tissue-type plasminogen activator obtained from a human melanoma cell line. The enzyme alteplase is secreted into the culture medium by an established mammalian cell line (Chinese hamster ovary cells) into which the DNA for alteplase has been inserted genetically. It is harvested, purified by chromatography and lyophilized.

Description—White to off-white powder.

Uses—Its actions are described and a comparison with streptokinase is found in the general statement. It is approved for use in the attempted lysis of coronary thrombi within the critical time after coronary occlusion. Its usefulness in the management of venous thrombosis and pulmonary embolism remain to be determined. It is contraindicated if there is internal or external bleeding, arteriovenous malformation, aneurism, severe hypertension, a history of cerebrovascular accident, recent (<2 mo) trauma or intracranial or spinal surgery. Adverse effects include nausea, vomiting, mild hypersensitivity reactions, fever and bleeding. Part of the hemorrhage problem is the result of concomitant administration of heparin, which is given to prevent clots at the catheter tip and to decrease the reocclusion rate. Care must be taken if antiplatelet drugs are present. Alteplase is eliminated by the liver; the half-life is less than 5 min.

Dose—*Intravenous, adults, initially* **6** to **10 mg** as a bolus, then **50** to **54 mg/hr** by slow infusion *during the first hour* and **20 mg/hr** *for the next 2 hr*, making a total of 100 mg (34/8 million IU); for patients weighing *less than 65 kg*, **1.25 mg/kg** infused over 3 hr.

Dosage Form—for Injection: 20 and 50 mg (11.6 and 29 million IU).

Antiplatelet Drugs

Platelets play a key role in hemostasis and thrombus formation. Platelets adhere to thrombin, collagen, immunologicaly sensitized surfaces and various other substances. At the site of vascular injury, collagen is exposed, thus causing platelet adhesion and the release of ADP, prostaglandins PGG_2 and PGH_2, TXA_2 and other substances. The growing platelet aggregate becomes a "white thrombus" which may plug a small vascular break or grow sufficiently large to cause vascular occlusion. In a blood clot, adhesion to thrombin causes an aggregate known as the "white head" of a red thrombus, which by a self-regenerating process (since ADP and TXA_2 cause further aggregation) enlarges the thrombus. Serotonin, PGG_2, PGH_2, TXA_2 and platelet-derived growth factor (PDGF) cause local vasospasm, which helps arrest bleeding from ruptured capillaries.

Vascular endothelium generates prostacyclin (PGI_2) which suppresses platelet adherence and aggregation and thus is a protective substance that helps limit the progression of a white thrombus beyond the point of injury. PGI_2 is also a potent vasodilator.

Platelets adhering to the wall of a blood vessel promote atherogenesis. PDGF causes local smooth muscle cells to increase cholesterol synthesis, bind low-density lipoprotein (LDL), increase the rate of cell replication and change into the foam cells characteristic of an atheroma. Platelets also are crucial to the process of thrombotic vascular occlusion once an atheroma has ruptured. Platelets also are involved in inflammation, bronchial asthma, eosinophilia, vascular tone, microcirculatory regulation, mitogenesis and tissue growth and repair, but antiplatelet drugs have received little attention in these roles.

So-called antiplatelet drugs may suppress platelet adherence and aggregation and extend platelet viability by acting directly on mechanisms within the platelet (true antiplatelet activity) or indirectly, to decrease the availability of nonplatelet-derived agonists that promote aggregation. The greatest interest has been of inhibitors of prostaglandin and thromboxane synthesis, especially of *aspirin* (page 1209).

Aspirin irreversibly inhibits (by acetylation) the cyclooxygenase system that generates prostaglandins, prostacyclin and TXA_2. The effect of decreasing TXA_2 decreases platelet aggregation, but at first this is counterbalanced by a decrease in PGI_2. However, vascular endothelial cells continue to synthesize cyclooxygenase, whereas anuclear platelets do not. Therefore, within a few hours after the administration of aspirin, PGI_2 synthesis returns to normal but TXA_2 synthesis does not. Furthermore, oral aspirin interacts with circulating platelets during absorption but with most endothelial cells only after passing through the liver, where first-pass metabolism greatly decreases the plasma concentration, and after dilution with nonhepatic blood, consequently, platelets are the more effected, and it is possible to suppress platelet aggregation with doses that have little effect on the generation of PGI_2. In addition, aspirin probably inhibits platelet function by additional mechanism(s) unrelated to TXA_2 inhibition.

Other nonsteroidal antiinflammatory drugs (NSAID), such as other salicylates, hydroxychloroquin, indomethacin, etc are not irreversible inhibitors of cyclooxygenase and are not as effective as antiplatelet drugs. *Sulfinpyrazone* (page 1221) is a weak inhibitor of cyclooxygenase and possibly may have another mechanism of action. Aspirin also has an action to suppress secretion of ADP-containing dense granules from platelets, which also contributes to antiplatelet activity.

Ticlopidine Hydrochloride

Thieno[3,2-*e*]pyridine, 5-[(2-chlorophenyl)methyl]-4,5,6,7-tetrahydro-,hydrochloride; Ticlid Hydrochloride (*Syntex*)

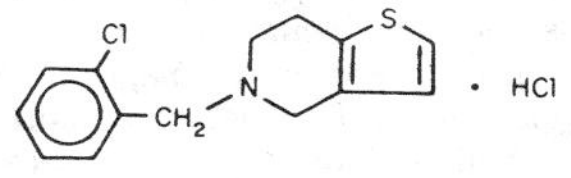

[53885-35-1] $C_{14}H_{14}ClNS.HCl$ (300.25).

Preparation—From 2-thiophenecarboxaldehyde plus 2-aminoacetaldehyde diethyl acetal to form the Schiff base, which is cyclized with acid to form pyrido[3,4-*b*]thiophene. This latter compound with α,2-dichlorotoluene yields the tertiary iminium chloride which with sodium borohydride affects reduction of the pyridine ring to yield the product. *J Med Chem* 9:483, 1974.

Description—White, crystalline solid; melts at 189°.

Solubility—Freely soluble in methanol or water to pH 3.6; sparingly soluble in methylene chloride or alcohol; slightly soluble in acetone; insoluble in a buffer solution of pH 6.3.

Uses—An orally active *platelet inhibitor* that prevents both platelet aggregation and release of granule constituents. Its mechanism of action is not completely delineated but apparently results from interference with platelet membrane function. It inhibits ADP-induced platelet-fibrinogen binding and platelet-platelet interactions but has variable effects on aggregation due to other stimuli including thrombin, platelet-activating factor, epinephrine or collagen. The inhibitory effect is irreversible and persists for the life of the platelet. After discontinuation of the drug, platelet function tests return to normal within 2 wk in most patients. Ticlopidine is indicated to reduce the risk of thrombotic stroke in patients who cannot take aspirin. In a trial comparing ticlopidine with aspirin therapy in patients experiencing stroke precursors or a minor stroke, ticlopidine significantly reduced the risk of fatal and nonfatal stroke compared to aspirin. The risk reduction by ticlopidine was similar in women and men. Side effects were more frequent with ticlopidine than with aspirin and gastrointestinal symptoms were the most common complaint. Neutropenia is the most serious adverse effect of ticlopidine and occurred in 2.4% of patients. Consequently, patients *must* have their blood tested every 2 wk for the first 3 mo of therapy. Patients also should be advised to contact their physician immediately if they experience symptoms of infection such as fever, chills or sore throat. The drug is metabolized extensively by the liver and is contraindicated in patients with severe liver impairment. In addition, it should not be given to patients who have a hematopoietic or hemostatic disorder or active pathological bleeding such as a bleeding peptic ulcer or intracranial bleeding.

Dose—*Oral, adults,* **250 mg** twice a day taken with food.

Dosage Form—Tablets: 250 mg.

Other Antiplatelet Drugs

Other drugs work in other ways.

Dipyridamole (RPS-18, page 844) inhibits platelet phosphodiesterase thus increasing cyclic AMP levels, which suppresses platelet aggregation and dense-granule secretion. It also blocks the reuptake and metabolism of adenosine, and potentiates the antiaggregating action of PGI_2.

Calcium channel blockers (page 963) decrease intraplatelet calcium concentration and, hence, also suppress dense-granule secretion.

β-*Adrenergic blockers* (page 1009) prevent β-receptor operation of calcium channels.

α-Blockers prevent α-agonist-induced dense-granule secretion.

Anagrelide (see RPS-18, page 1161) supresses platelet response to all stimuli; its mechanism may be that of inhibiting a distinct pool of cAMP phosphodiesterase.

Other inhibitors of platelet function are dextrans (page 914), glyceryl guaiacolate (very active), penicillin, tricyclic antidepressants, glucocorticoids, clofibrate, pyridinol carbamate, PGE_1, glucagon, antiserotonin drugs, certain antihistamines, caffeine, theophylline, pentoxifyllin, general anesthetics and ethanol in high concentration.

No clinical use of antiplatelet drugs is without some controversy. In general, except for dextrans 70 and 75, antiplatelet drugs have not been found effective alone in preventing or limiting venous thrombosis and pulmonary embolism, but they probably improve the response to oral anticoagulants. In such a combination, aspirin increases the incidence and severity of gastrointestinal hemorrhage whereas dipyridamole does not. This deleterious effect of combination therapy is reduced if the dose of aspirin is lowered, ie, 325 mg a day or less. In addition, it is essential that coagulation and platelet function tests are monitored routinely with anticoagulant doses adjusted accordingly.

Antiplatelet-anticoagulant drug combinations appear to be superior to oral anticoagulants alone in preventing thombosis from prosthetic heart valves and other foreign surfaces. After hip surgery, aspirin alone (in men), aspirin-dipyridamole and hydroxychloroquin have been reported to be of value in preventing venous thrombosis and pulmonary embolism. Sulfinpyrazone decreases the incidence of systemic embolism in rheumatic mitral valve stenosis.

Aspirin is approved in the US to reduce the risk of death and/or nonfatal myocardial infarction in patients with a previous infarction or unstable angina pectoris. It also is approved to reduce the risk of stroke in men experiencing transient ischemic attacks. Completed strokes are not affected. Occlusive microvascular disorders in the fingers are resolved in 2 to 3 days and further prevented after treatment with aspirin. Microvascular occlusion after organ transplants also appear to be diminished by aspirin. In general, the combination of aspirin and dipyridamole are no more effective than aspirin alone. One study did demonstrate that combination therapy was slightly more effective than aspirin alone in the prevention of aortocoronary bypass graft occlusion; however, this needs to be further confirmed.

There is much interest in the reputed ability of antiplatelet drugs to decrease the rate of myocardial infarction. There have been two randomized trials examining whether aspirin has a protective effect in the primary prevention of vascular disease with conflicting results. In a 5-year study, the US Physicians' Health Study, there was a 44% reduction (from approximately 0.4% to 0.2%/year) in the incidence of myocardial infarction in men receiving aspirin (325 mg every other day) compared to placebo. This effect was only observed in men age 50 or over. Over the 5-year period the death rate from cardiovascular processes was similar in both placebo- and aspirin-treated groups. In contrast, in the British Doctors' Trial there was no difference in the rate of myocardial infarction or cardiovascular death in the aspirin (500 mg/day) versus placebo group over a 6-year study period. In both of these studies there was a slight increase in the incidence of stroke and an increased risk of gastrointestinal hemorrhage in the aspirin-treated cohort. The US Preventive Services Task Force recommends that "low-dose aspirin therapy may be considered for men aged 40 and over who are at a significantly increased risk of myocardial infarction and who lack contraindications to the drug." Aspirin therapy should be considered an adjunct approach in the management of cardiovascular disease. Reduction of significant risk factors including hypertension, high cholesterol levels and smoking are the most effective treatment for patients at risk for myocardial infarction and stroke. Of note, current epidemiological evidence suggests that aspirin is beneficial in women as well as men, however definitive recommendations must await the results of the ongoing Women's Health Study.

Anticoagulant Antagonists

Anticoagulant therapy carries the risk of serious hemorrhage, so that there may be need to arrest the anticoagulant action. Prothrombopenic anticoagulants, as expected from their mode of action, are antagonized by vitamin K or its synthetic substitutes. Not all vitamin K preparations are equally effective, vitamin K_1 (phytonadione) being superior and menadione inferior. The efficacy of vitamin K preparations also varies according to the anticoagulant, but all agents of the dicumarol group may be antagonized by an appropriate dose of vitamin K_1. The antagonism is not manifested immediately, since normal coagulation is obtained only after the liver has had time to replenish the prothrombin and prothrombinogen.

High doses of vitamin K_1 can antagonize oral anticoagulants, despite their being continually inhibited at their site of action, because high doses can activate a second latent enzyme, not significantly productive with ordinary concentrations of vitamin K, and which enzyme is not inhibited by the anticoagulants. Heparin is antagonized by various amines, ammonium compounds and basic proteins, which precipitate the polysulfate. Circulating heparinoid substances in the blood also can be assayed with such substances.

Menadiol Sodium Diphosphate—page 1114.
Menadione—see RPS-17, page 1010.
Menadione Sodium Bisulfite—see RPS-17, page 1010.
Phytonadione—page 1115.

Protamine Sulfate

A purified mixture of simple protein principles obtained from the sperm or testes of suitable species of fish, which has the property of neutralizing heparin. Each mg neutralizes not less than 80 USP Units of heparin activity derived from lung tissue and not less than 100 USP Units of heparin activity derived from intestinal mucosa.

Preparation—Frozen, ripe, salmon testes are ground, water- washed, centrifuged and dehydrated by means of solvents and vacuum drying. The dried material then is extracted with 10% H_2SO_4 and, after filtering, a protamine sulfate-rich fraction is precipitated from the filtrate with cold alcohol. This fraction is dissolved in hot water, and the protamine sulfate separates as an oil upon cooling. This protamine-rich oil is dissolved in hot water and fractionated again with cold alcohol. The resulting fraction is dehydrated by means of solvents and vacuum dried.

Description—Fine, white or faintly colored, amorphous or crystalline, hygroscopic powder.

Solubility—Sparingly soluble in water.

Uses—A *heparin antagonist.* Because it is a strongly basic macromolecule, it combines avidly with heparin, which is a polyanionic macromolecule. It combines with heparin in an approximate 1:1 ratio by weight regardless of the source of heparin; since the potency of heparin from different sources varies, the dose of protamine based on USP unitage also varies. It is injected slowly intravenously after suitable dilution with physiological salt solution, to counteract the effect of *overmedication with heparin.* The duration of the effect is about 2 hr.

Untoward effects are uncommon. They include abrupt hypotension, dyspnea, bradycardia, flushing and a feeling of warmth. An overdose can itself exert an anticoagulant effect.

Dose—*Intravenous, adults* and *children,* **1 mg** for each 90 Units of heparin from lung or 115 units of heparin from intestinal mucosa, to be injected slowly over a span of 1 to 3 min; no more than 50 mg should be given in any 10-min period. In calculating the dose, its disappearance from the blood should be taken into account. Since the half-life is 1.3 to 1.6 hr, a dose given 1.5 hr after a single dose of heparin would be based on 50% of the dose of heparin. However, during steady-state heparin treatment, the dose of this drug required may be greater even than that estimated from the last dose of heparin, especially if the dose of this drug is administered shortly after the heparin. Therefore, laboratory checks on coagulation of blood are important in determining adequacy of dosage.

Dosage Forms—Injection: 50 mg/5 mL, 100 mg/10 mL and 250 mg/25 mL; for Injection: 50 and 250 mg.

Fibrinolysin Inhibitors

Aminocaproic Acid

"Epsilon" Aminocaproic Acid; Aminocaproic Acid (*Elkins-Sinn*)
Amicar (*Lederle*)

$$H_2C(CH_2)_3CH_2COOH$$
$$|$$
$$NH_2$$

6-Aminohexanoic acid [60-32-2] $C_6H_{13}NO_2$ (131.17).

Preparation—The lactam group of the commercially available caprolactam (hexahydro-2*H*-azepin-2-one) is cleaved at the C-N linkage by heating an aqueous solution with calcium hydroxide. The calcium aminocaproate thus formed is reacted with sulfuric acid to free the official acid and precipitate the calcium. Various other methods of preparation are also available.

Description—Fine, white, crystalline powder; odorless, or nearly so; tasteless, stable in light and air; melts at about 205°.

Solubility—1 g in 3 mL water; slightly soluble in alcohol; practically insoluble in chloroform or ether.

Uses—A competitive inhibitor of activators of profibrinolysin and, to a lesser extent, of fibrinolysin. As a consequence, it suppresses the formation of fibrinolysin, an enzyme which destroys fibrinogen, fibrin and other clotting components. For vascular integrity a low rate of fibrin deposition is normal; excessive fibrinolysis leads to hemorrhage.

It is used in the treatment of *procedures or disorders in which fibrinolysis is enhanced,* such as cardiac bypass, postcaval shunt, major thoracic surgery, prostatic postoperative hematuria and also nonsurgical hematuria, leukemia, metastatic prostatic carcinoma, cirrhosis and other hepatic diseases, eclampsia, intrauterine fetal death, amniotic fluid embolism and abruptio placentae. It also is used to correct excessive, treatment-induced fibrinolysis. It has been reported to be of use in angioedema and subarachnoid hemorrhage. The drug is of no value in hemorrhage due to thrombocytopenia, hyperheparinemia or other coagulation defects, or to vascular disruption.

It may cause itching, erythema, skin rash, diuresis, heartburn, nausea and diarrhea. It also has an antiadrenergic effect similar to guanethidine, so that nasal stuffiness, conjunctival suffusion and hypotension may occur. The drug may enhance thrombotic processes by suppression of reactive fibrinolysis, which tends to limit clot formation and favor clot resolution. Therefore, it should not be given unless there is unequivocal evidence that disseminated intravascular clotting is not the cause of elevated fibrinolytic activity. The drug is teratogenic in animals and, hence, should not be used in humans in the first two trimesters of pregnancy and in the third trimester only if its use is imperative.

It is excreted by the kidney; in the presence of renal disease the dose should be reduced.

Dose—*Intravenous infusion, adults,* for *peripheral acute hemorrhage,* **4** to **5 g** during 1 hr followed by **1 g/hr** for 8 hr or until an adequate response occurs, up to 30 g/day; *children,* **100 mg/kg** (or 3 g/m^2) in 1 hr followed by **33.3 mg/kg/hr** (or 1 g/m^2), not to exceed 18 g/m^2/day. *Intravenous infusion* or *bolus, adults,* for *subarachnoid hemorrhage,* **1** to **1.5 g/hr.** *Oral, adults,* for *peripheral acute hemorrhage, initially* **5 g** followed by **1** or **1.25 g/hr** for 8 hr or until an adequate response occurs; *children,* same as intravenous dose.

Dosage Forms—Injection: 250 mg/mL; Syrup: 250 mg/mL; Tablets: 500 mg.

Tranexamic Acid

Cyklokapron (*Kabi Pharmacia*)

COOH
CH₂NH₂

[1197-18-8] $C_8H_{15}NO_2$ (157.21).

Preparation—*J Org Chem 24:*115, 1959 and US Pat 3,499,925.

Description—White crystals; melts over 300°.

Solubility—1 g in about 6 mL water; very slightly soluble in alcohol or ether; 5% aqueous solution, pH 6.5 to 7.5.

Uses—Resembles aminocaproic acid in decreasing the activity of the fibrinolysis system, in part by inhibiting plasminogen; it is approved for use in hemophiliac patients to prevent hemorrhage and reduce the need for replacement of blood factors. Its most interesting use has been in the treatment of malignant ovarian tumors, to promote formation of a fibrin capsule to wall off and inhibit growth of the tumor. It also causes regression of ascites secondary to carcinoma. In these uses heparin was given concomitantly to prevent intravascular coagulation. It causes nausea, vomiting, diarrhea, occasional vertigo and hypotension from rapid injection. It passes through the placental barrier. It is excreted rapidly in urine.

Dose—*Oral, adult,* **25 mg/kg** 3 or 4 times a day for 1 day prior to dental extraction and 2 to 8 days after; *intravenous,* for tooth *extraction.* **10 mg/kg** immediately before extraction (along with blood factor replacement), switching to oral dosage afterward (above), unless oral medication is not possible, in which case 10 mg/kg 3 or 4 times a day is used.

Dosage Forms—Tablets: 500 mg; Injection: 100 mg/mL in 10-mL vials.

Hemostatics and Styptics

Many substances not especially related to the clotting mechanism are capable of promoting clotting. Upon contact with most surfaces, platelets adhere, aggregate and release mediators which promote fibrin deposition. Spongy and gauzy materials, which provide a large surface area, thus are used to arrest bleeding; absorbable sponges may be left permanently at the site of bleeding. Fibrin, fibrinogen and thrombin are also potent hemostatics (see page 926). Astringents (see Chapter 52) also initiate clotting by precipitating proteins and by labilizing platelets; mostly ferric salts are employed as styptics.

Alum—page 871.

Cellulose, Oxidized—page 1877.

Collagen, Microfibrillar

Avitene (*Alcon*)

A preparation of animal origin of the polypeptide substance occurring as the main constituent of skin, connective tissue and the organic substance of bones.

Uses—Platelets adhere naturally to collagen and are stimulated to release substances that promote further aggregation. Microfibrillar collagen is used to arrest bleeding, especially during surgery. It usually stops capillary bleeding in 1 min, "brisk" bleeding in 4 to 5 min and oozing from bone in 5 to 10 min. The collagen is absorbed in less than 84 days. It may cause mild, chronic inflammation at the site of application, probably as the result of slight contamination by bovine albumin. It does not interfere with regeneration of bone. It may interfere mechanically with the closure of incisions. Plugging of pores in cancellous bone diminishes the strength of methacrylate adhesives. Spillage on nonbleeding surfaces should be avoided because it may cause adhesions.

Application—1 g/50 cm² of previously dried surface. Handle with forceps, as it is adhesive.

Dosage Forms—Fibrous: 1 and 5 g: Web: 70 × 70 × 1 mm and 70 × 35 × 1 mm sterile blister packs.

Desmopressin—page 1063.

Absorbable Gelatin Powder

Gelfoam (*Upjohn*)

A fine, dry, heat-sterilized light powder prepared by milling absorbable gelatin sponge.

Uses—Sterile powder, saturated with sterile sodium chloride solution; is indicated in surgical procedures to control capillary, venous and arteriolar bleeding when conventional procedures such as pressure or ligature is ineffective.

Dose—Only the minimum amount necessary to achieve hemostasis should be used and excess material removed once hemostasis occurs. A putty-like paste is prepared from the powder by addition of 3 to 4 mL of sterile saline which is then smeared or pressed against the bleeding surface.

Dosage Form—1 g.

Absorbable Gelatin Sponge

Gelfoam (*Upjohn*)

Gelatin in the form of a sterile, absorbable, water-insoluble sponge.

Description—Light, nearly white, nonelastic, tough, porous, hydrophilic solid; 10-mm cube weighing approximately 9 mg will take up approximately 45 times its weight of well-agitated oxalated whole blood; it is stable in dry heat at 150° for 4 hr.

Solubility—Insoluble in water, but absorbable in body fluids; completely digested by a solution of pepsin.

Uses and **Application**—A *hemostatic* and *coagulant* used to control bleeding. It is moistened with sterile sodium chloride or thrombin solution and may then be left in place following closure of a surgical incision. It should not be used in the closure of skin incisions because of interference with the rejoining of edges. It is absorbed in from 4 to 6 wk.

Application Forms—Prostatectomy Cones; Dental Packs; Sterile Packs; Sterile Sponges; Sterile Compressed Sponges.

Thrombin

Thrombin, Sterile (*Upjohn*); Thrombostat (*Parke-Davis*); Thrombinair (*Armour*)

A sterile protein substance prepared from prothrombin of bovine origin through interaction with added thromboplastin in the presence of calcium. It is capable, without the addition of other substances, of causing the clotting of whole blood, plasma or a solution of fibrinogen. It may contain a suitable antibacterial agent.

Note: Solutions of thrombin should be used within a few hours after preparation, and are not to be injected.

Description—White or grayish, amorphous substance dried from the frozen state.

Uses—When concentrated, it has an extraordinarily potent hemostatic or clotting effect on blood. Its powerful coagulant action is employed in coagulating fibrinogen solution. It also is useful for local application to *cuts* or *injuries*. In surgery and in emergency, it is useful for local application in the control of minor oozing. For more extensive or inaccessible *hemorrhage*, a matrix must be applied to hold the thrombin in place and provide a structure for clot formation. Such a matrix is provided by various products, including fibrin foam, gelatin sponge, etc. It is ineffective in arterial bleeding.

Dose—*Topical*, as a powder or as a solution containing 100 to 2000 NIH units/mL in 0.9% sodium chloride solution or sterile water. For general use in *dental extractions*, *plastic surgery*, *skin grafting*, etc, solutions containing 100 units/mL are frequently used. For *profuse bleeding* such as cut surfaces of liver or spleen, concentrations as high as 2000 units/mL may be necessary. Oozing surfaces often are treated best with the dry powder.

Dosage Form—Powder: 1000, 5000, 10,000, 20,000 and 50,000 Units.

Zinc Acetate—see RPS-17, page 779.

Electrolytes and Systemic Buffers

The concentration of several of the electrolytes in plasma is critical for proper functioning of cells, especially those of the excitable tissues. The proper balance of the several ions is complex depending not only on the concentration in the extracellular fluid (of which plasma is one compartment) but also on the intracellular concentration, the ratio across the cell membrane being an essential factor as well as the ratio of one ion type to another. Thus, plasma electrolyte concentrations provide only a crude clue to the electrolyte status of the patient, and balance or other ancillary studies are often necessary to determine the true electrolyte needs. Certain electrolytes, for example calcium and phosphate, serve also as structural elements in hard tissues (bone, teeth, etc) and may be employed for that purpose.

Several of the phosphates described in this section often are used to remove calcium from blood in hypercalcemia and to prevent and even dissolve calcific kidney stones rather than to add an electrolyte.

Ammonium Chloride—page 1040.

Calcium Carbonate—page 887.

Calcium Chloride

Calcium chloride, dihydrate [10035-04-8] $CaCl_2.2H_2O$ (147.02); *anhydrous* [10043-52-4] (110.99).

Preparation—By saturating HCl with chalk or marble, then adding calcium hydroxide to alkalinity and boiling, which precipitates magnesium, iron and other metals. After filtering, the filtrate is neutralized with HCl and evaporated until it contains about 24% of water.

Description—White, hard, odorless fragments or granules; deliquescent.

Solubility—1 g in 0.7 mL of water or 4 mL of alcohol.

Uses—Provides calcium ions in the treatment of *hypocalcemic tetany*. It also relieves muscle spasms and pain from *black widow bites*. It is given during *exchange transfusions*, in order to repair the calcium deficit in citrated blood; however, calcium gluceptate is preferred for this use. It is *antispasmodic* to smooth muscle and effective in relieving the abdominal pain and diarrhea of *intestinal tuberculosis* and *lead colic;* for this purpose it is given orally, a neutral salt being preferred. It stimulates cardiac automaticity and contractility and is used in *cardiac resuscitation*. Calcium is used in the management of *hypersensitivity reactions*, especially urticaria and angioneurotic edema, and of *insect bites* and *stings*.

It is a specific antidote in cases of *magnesium poisoning*. It is used in the treatment of *hyperkalemia*, since it antagonizes the cardiac effects of potassium.

As an *electrolyte replenisher* it is a pharmaceutical necessity for *Ringer's Injection, Lactated Ringer's Injection* and *Ringer's Solution.*

Side effects result from too-rapid injection; these include vasodilation and a burning sensation in the skin. Overdosage can cause hypercalcemia, characterized by persistant nausea and vomiting, lethargy, weakness, coma and sudden death. Because of the danger of overdosage, it is contraindicated in renal insufficiency, even if hypocalcemia exists. It should be given cautiously to the digitalized patient, and the electrocardiogram should be monitored. In general, plasma electrolyte concentrations should be monitored before and during use. Extravasation and intramuscular or subcutaneous injection can cause tissue necrosis. For this reason, less irritant salts are preferred, especially in pediatrics.

Dose—*Intravenous, adults, hypocalcemia, replenishment* or *cardiotonic,* **6.8** to **13.6 mEq** (0.5 to 1 g of dihydrate or 5 to 10 mL of 10% solution) at a rate not to exceed 1.36 mEq/min (1 mL/min of 10% solution), repeated at intervals of 1 to 3 days, if necessary; *hyperkalemia,* dose to be determined by electrocardiographic response; *hypermagnesemia, initially* **6.8 mEq,** repeated if necessary; *children, hypocalcemia* or *replenishment,* **0.34 mEq/kg** (25 mg/kg) administered over a period of no less than 10 min. *Intracardiac, adults,* **2.72** to **5.48 mEq** (0.2 to 0.4 g or 2 to 4 mL of 10% solution) into the left ventricle.

Dosage Form—Injection: 13.6 mEq/10 mL (Each mL of this "10%" solution contains 1.36 mEq or 27.2 mg of Ca^{2+}, 100 mg of $CaCl_2 \cdot 2H_2O$ and 2.04 mOsm.)

Calcium Citrate

1,2,3-Propanetricarboxylic acid, 2-hydroxy-, calcium salt (2:3), tetrahydrate; Citracal *(Mission)*

```
⎡    CH2COO—  ⎤
⎢    |        ⎥
⎢ HO—C—COO—   ⎥        Ca3  •  4H2O
⎢    |        ⎥
⎣    CH2COO—  ⎦2
```

[5785-44-4] $C_{12}H_{10}Ca_3O_{14}.4H_2O$ (570.50).

Preparation—By treating citric acid obtained from citrus fruits with lime.

Description—White, odorless, crystalline powder losing all of its water of crystallization at 120°.

Solubility—1 g in 1050 mL cold water; more soluble in hot water; insoluble in alcohol.

Uses—Most calcium compounds given orally as a source of calcium are soluble in gastric acid but are converted mostly to insoluble calcium carbonate in the duodenum, so that only a fraction of the calcium is available for absorption. Calcium carbonate, especially, is dependent greatly upon gastric acid to make some of the calcium bioavailable. Persons with achlorhydria, pyloroplasty or other conditions in which a calcium compound is not in an acidic environment long enough to liberate or maintain much soluble calcium usually do not obtain adequate calcium absorption from calcium carbonate and certain other calcium compounds. In this drug, the calcium ion is chelated sufficiently firmly that a large proportion remains in the soluble form in the alkaline environment of the small intestine. In individuals with normal gastric acid secretion, 20 to 66% more calcium is bioavailable from the citrate than from the carbonate, and in persons with achlorhydria it is 100% more available. It is used to treat *hypocalcemia* and as a *supplement* to dietary calcium, especially in persons in whom there is a probability of developing or exacerbating osteoporosis.

Dose—*Oral, adults,* **10** to **20 mEq** (0.95 to 1.9 g or 200 to 400 mg of Ca) 3 or 4 times a day after meals.

Dosage Form—Tablets: 10 and 12.5 mEq (200 and 250 mg of Ca; 950 and 1188 mg).

Calcium Glubionate

Calcium, (4-*O*-β-D-galactopyranosyl-D-gluconato-*O*[1])(D-gluconato-*O*[1])-, monohydrate; Neo-Calglucon *(Sandoz)*

```
          COO—
 COO—     HCOH
 HCOH     HOCH
 HOCH     HC————————————O      Ca • H2O
 HCOH     HCOH     CH2OH
 HCOH     CH2OH  HO     O
 CH2OH             OH
                        OH
```

[12569-38-9] $C_{18}H_{32}CaO_{19}.H_2O$ (610.53).

Uses—As a source of calcium, more as a dietary supplement than for the treatment of hypocalcemia.

Dose—*Oral, adults* and *children over 4 yr* **1 tablespoonful**/3 times a day with meals; *children up to 1 yr* **1 teaspoonful** 5 times a day undiluted or mixed with formula or juice/5 times a day before meals; *1 to 4 yr,* **2 teaspoonfuls**/3 times a day before meals.

Dosage Form—Syrup: 115 mg Ca/5 mL (teaspoonful).

Calcium Gluceptate

D-*glycero*-D-*gulo*-Heptonic acid, calcium salt (2:1); Calcium Gluceptate *(Lilly; Abbott; IMS)*

```
⎡        H  H  OH H  H         ⎤
⎢        |  |  |  |  |         ⎥
⎢ HOCH2—C—C—C—C—C—COO—         ⎥   Ca
⎢        |  |  |  |  |         ⎥
⎣        OH OH H  OH OH        ⎦2
```

Calcium D-*glycero*-D-*gulo*-heptonate (1:2) [17140-60-2] $C_{14}H_{26}CaO_{16}$ (490.43); *hydrate* [56348-83-5] (508.45).

Preparation—From sodium glucoheptonate, US Pat 3,033,900.

Uses—To provide calcium ions when rapid availability is required. The clinical conditions in which calcium is required are stated under *Calcium Chloride.* This drug is even less irritating than *Calcium Gluconate,* so that it is preferred when intramuscular administration is required, as in neonatal tetany. Many authorities also prefer the gluceptate to the gluconate for intravenous injection, but, once symptoms are controlled, maintenance usually is achieved with calcium gluconate given by intravenous infusion. The duration of action after intravenous administration is 2 to 3 hr and after intramuscular injection, 1 to 4 hr.

After rapid intravenous injection there may be tingling sensations and a chalky taste. The effects of overdoses, precautions and drug interactions are those of *Calcium Chloride.* Mild local reactions may occur at the site of injection, but abscesses apparently do not occur.

Dose—*Intravenous, adults, hypocalcemia* or *replenishment,* **4.5** to **18 mEq** (1.1 to 4.4 g or 5 to 20 mL of a solution containing 0.22 g/ mL) at a rate not to exceed 1.8 mEq/min (2 mL/min); *hypermagnesemia, initially* **4.9** to **9.8 mEq** (1.2 to 2.4 g or 5.5 to 21.8 mL); *children, hypocalcemia,* **1.8** to **4.5 mEq** (0.44 to 1.1 g or 2 to 5 mL) at a rate not to exceed 0.7 mEq/min (0.75 mL/min); *exchange transfusions in neonates,* **0.45 mEq** (0.11 g or 0.5 mL) after every 100 mL of blood transfused. *Intramuscular, adults* and *children, hypocalcemia* or *replenishment,* **1.8** to **4.5 mEq** (0.44 to 1.1 g or 2 to 5 mL).

Dosage Form—Injection: 4.5 mEq/10 mL and 45 mEq/50 mL. Each mL contains 0.9 mEq or 18 mg of Ca^{2+}, 0.22 g of calcium gluceptate and 7 mOsm.

Calcium Gluconate

D-Gluconic acid, calcium salt (2:1); *(Various Mfrs)*

```
⎡        H  H  OH H          ⎤
⎢        |  |  |  |          ⎥
⎢ HOCH2—C—C—C—C—COO—         ⎥   Ca
⎢        |  |  |  |          ⎥
⎣        OH OH H  OH         ⎦2
```

Calcium gluconate (1:2) [299-28-5] $C_{12}H_{22}CaO_{14}$ (430.38).

Preparation—D-Glucose is oxidized to gluconic acid in the presence of calcium carbonate. The oxidation may be effected by certain molds, eg, *Aspergillus niger,* or by bromine.

Description—White, crystalline granules or powder, without odor or taste; stable in air and does not lose its water on drying without undergoing decomposition; solutions are neutral to litmus paper; decomposed by dilute mineral acids into gluconic acid and the calcium salt of the mineral acid used.

Solubility—1 g slowly in about 30 mL water or about 5 mL boiling water; insoluble in alcohol or many other organic solvents.

Uses—Its uses are those of *Calcium Chloride.* It is less irritating than calcium chloride and may be given orally or by intramuscular or intravenous injection. However, intramuscular injection may cause abscesses. It usually is considered to be the calcium salt of choice for intravenous use.

Dose—*Intravenous, adults, hypocalcemia* or *replenishment,* **4.5 mEq** (0.97 g or 10 mL of 10% solution) at a rate not to exceed 2.25 mEq/min (5 mL/min), repeated as necessary up to a total of 69.7 mEq (15 g)/day; *hyperkalemia* or *hypermagnesemia,* tentatively 4.65 to 9.29 mEq (1 to 2 g or 10.3 to 20.6 mL), the exact dose being determined by electrocardiographic and other responses during administration; *children, hypocalcemia,* **0.93** to **2.32 mEq** (2 to 5 mL or 0.2 to 0.5 g) at a rate not to exceed 1 mL/min. Oral, *adults, hypocalcemia,* **11 g** (51.2 mEq or 1.02 g of Ca)/**day** in divided doses *after meals; children, hypocalcemia,*

0.50 to **0.72 g** (2.32 to 3.35 mEq or 0.045 to 0.072 g of Ca)/**kg/day** in divided doses after meals.

Dosage Form—Injection: 4.51 mEq/10 mL and 9.02 mEq/20 mL. Each mL contains 0.451 mEq or 9.02 mg of Ca, 97 mg of calcium gluconate and 0.392 mOsm.); Chewable Tablets: 500, 650, 975 and 1000 mg.

Calcium Glycerophosphate

Calphosan (*Glenwood*); Neurosin; (*Various Mfrs*)

$(HOCH_2)_2CHOPO_3Ca$

[27214-00-2] $C_3H_7CaO_6P$ (210.15). A mixture of the β-calcium salt (center hydroxyl of glycerol is phosphorylated) and the α-salt (end hydroxyl is phosphorylated). Since the α-salt enjoys a chiral center, it exists as two stereoisomers of which only the racemic form is present in this salt.

Preparation—*J Chem Soc 105:* 1238, 1914.

Description—Odorless, tasteless powder; decomposes at about 170°.

Solubility—1 g in about 50 mL water at 20°; less soluble at higher temperatures.

Uses—The actions, uses and adverse effects are much like those of *Calcium Gluconate.* The effects of overdoses, drug interactions and precautions are those of *Calsum Chloride.* The salt is marketed only in combination with calcium lactate or calcium levulinate.

Dose—**6.5 mEq** of Ca^{2+} from injections containing various concentrations of calcium glycerophosphate and other calcium compounds.

Dosage Form—Injection: 10 mL ampule or 60-mL vial (Calphoson) containing 50 mg calcium glycerophosphate and 50 mg calcium lactate/10 mL in sodium chloride solution.

Calcium Lactate

Propanoic acid, 2-hydroxy-, calcium salt (2:1), hydrate (*Various Mfrs*)

$\left[CH_3\underset{OH}{CH}COO-\right]_2 Ca \cdot xH_2O$

Calcium lactate (1:2) hydrate [41372-22-9] $C_6H_{10}CaO_6.xH_2O$; *anhydrous* [814-80-2] (218.22); *pentahydrate* (308.30).

Preparation—By fermenting hydrolyzed starch with a suitable mold in the presence of calcium carbonate, and purifying until the product meets USP purity requirements. It also is obtained, now in decreasing quantities, by fermentation of the mother liquors resulting from the production of milk sugar.

Description—White, almost odorless powder or granules, somewhat efflorescent; it becomes anhydrous at 120°; aqueous solutions are prone to become moldy.

Solubility—1 g in about 20 mL of water; practically insoluble in alcohol.

Uses—An excellent source of calcium ion in the oral treatment of *calcium deficiency.* It causes less gastrointestinal irritation than does calcium chloride. It is used in the prevention and retardation of *osteoporosis.* The bioavailability of calcium is not as gastric acid-dependent as is that of $CaCO_3$; consequently, the lactate is superior in many elderly patients.

Dose (as pentahydrate)—*Oral, adults,* **50 mEq** (7.7 g) in 3 divided doses a day with meals; *children,* **2.24** to **3.24 mEq** (345 to 500 mg)/**kg** body weight a day in 3 divided doses after meals.

Dosage Form (as pentahydrate)—Tablets: 325 and 650 mg (2.11 and 4.22 mEq or 42.3 and 84.5 mg of Ca). The lactate also is available in combination with calcium glycerophosphate in injection form.

Calcium Levulinate

Pentanoic acid, 4-oxo-, calcium salt (2:1) (*Various Mfrs*)

$[CH_3COCH_2CH_2OOO—]_2Ca \cdot 2H_2O$

[5743-49-7] $C_{10}H_{14}CaO_6.2H_2O$ (306.33).

Preparation—From levulinic acid and calcium carbonate. The acid may be obtained from crude cellulose and as a by-product in the manufacture of furfural. *Ind Eng Chem 48:* 1331, 1956.

Description—White, crystalline or amorphous powder; faint odor suggestive of burnt sugar; bitter, salty taste.

Solubility—Freely soluble in water; slightly soluble in alcohol; insoluble in ether or chloroform.

Uses—Much like *Calcium Gluceptate* in that it is less irritating than calcium gluconate. The side effects also are essentially the same. The effects of overdoses, precuations and drug interactions are those of *Calcium Chloride.* The salt is marketed only in combination with calcium glycerophosphate.

Dose—(as dihydrate)—1.5 g calcium levulinate and 1 g calcium glycerophosphate/100 mL (0.19 mEq Ca^{2+}/mL) once a day.

Dosage Forms—Injection: 100 mL.

Dibasic Calcium Phosphate

Phosphoric acid, calcium salt (1:1); Dicalcium Orthophosphate (*Various Mfrs*)

Calcium phosphate (1:1) anhydrous [7757-93-9] $CaHPO_4$ (136.06); *dihydrate* [7789-77-7] (172.09).

Preparation—A phosphate mineral, eg, *apatite,* or preferably ignited animal bone, is decomposed with H_2SO_4, resulting in the production of phosphoric acid and calcium sulfate. After filtering off the calcium sulfate, the proper quantity of calcium hydroxide is added to form dibasic calcium phosphate.

It also may be prepared from animal bones as described under the preparation of *Tribasic Calcium Phosphate,* using only sufficient calcium hydroxide to form the dibasic salt.

Description—White, odorless, tasteless powder; stable in air; aqueous suspension is neutral to litmus.

Solubility—Practically insoluble in water; readily soluble in diluted hydrochloric or nitric acids; insoluble in alcohol.

Uses—An excellent *source of calcium* and *phosphorus* during pregnancy, lactation or mild-to-moderate *hypocalcemia* characterized by a low degree of tetany. Because of the phosphate content, it is contraindicated in hypoparathyroidism. If the tetany is severe, intravenous calcium medication is administered. See *Calcium Chloride, Calcium Gluconate, Calcium Gluceptate, Calcium Glycerophosphate* or *Calcium Levulinate.*

Dose (as dihydrate)—*Oral, adults,* **4.4 g** (51 mEq; 1 g of Ca^{2+}) in 3 divided doses after meals; *children,* **0.20** to **0.28 g** (3.3 mEq; 0.045 to 0.065 g of Ca^{2+})/**kg** of body weight in 3 divided doses after meals. The calcium is absorbed better if taken in small doses at frequent intervals.

Dosage Form (as dihydrate)—Tablets: 486 mg (5.65 mEq or 113 mg of Ca^{2+}).

Tribasic Calcium Phosphate

Calcium Hydroxide Phosphate

$Ca_5(OH)(PO_4)_3$

[12167-74-7] $Ca_5HP_3O_{13}$ (502.32).

Preparation—Commercially from phosphate rock; also occurs naturally.

Description—Amorphous, odorless, tasteless powder.

Solubility—Insoluble in water, alcohol or acetic acid; soluble in mineral acids.

Uses—Mainly for the prophylaxis and treatment of *hypocalcemia,* although it also serves as a source of phosphate.

Dose—*Oral, adults,* for *hypocalcemia,* **29.9 mEq** of Ca^{2+} (1.6 g of salt or 600 mg Ca^{2+}) twice a day after meals.

Dosage Form—Tablets: 14.9 and 29.9 mEq (300 and 600 mg) of Ca^{2+}.

Magnesium Sulfate Injection—page 1175.

Potassium Acetate

[127-08-2] $C_2H_3KO_2$ (98.14).

Preparation—Potassium bicarbonate or carbonate is reacted with acetic acid, previously diluted with water, and the solution is evaporated to dryness.

Description—Colorless, monoclinic crystals or a white, crystalline powder; rapidly deliquesces in moist air; saline and slightly alkaline taste; aqueous solutions are alkaline to litmus, but do not affect phenolphthalein TS.

Solubility—1 g in about 0.5 mL water or about 3 mL alcohol.

Uses—Therapeutically, as a systemic and urinary *alkalinizer,* and for the effects of the *potassium ion.* Its value in hypokalemia is limited, since the condition frequently is associated with a hypochloremic alkalosis. Consequently, potassium chloride usually is preferred in hypokalemia. Acetate anion is metabolized to bicarbonate. When used orally as an alkalinizer the salt should be diluted liberally with water or fruit juice to avoid gastric distress. Indiscriminate use of this or other potassium salts may produce toxic manifestations of hyperkalemia (see *Potassium Chloride,* page 930).

Dose—*Intravenous infusion, adults,* for *hypokalemia,* when plasma potassium is above 2.5 mEq/L, up to **200 mEq** a day, given in a concentration of no more than 40 mEq/L at a rate of no more than 10 mEq/hr; when plasma potassium is less than 2.0 mEq/L, up to 400 mEq a day at a range of no more than 40 mEq/hr; *children,* up to 3 mEq/kg (or 40 mEq/m^2) a day; the volume of fluid should be varied in proportion to body size. *Oral,* 1 **g** up to 4 times a day, in solution.

Dosage Form—Injection: 40 mEq/20 mL and 120 mEq/30 mL.

Potassium Chloride

Potassium chloride [7447-40-7] KCl (74.55).

Preparation—Occurs in sea water and in many mineral springs. Formerly it largely was imported from Germany where it is mined at Stassfurt, occurring there as *carnallite* [$KCl.MgCl_2.6H_2O$] and as *sylvite* [KCl]. It now is obtained from the Searles Lake deposit in the Mojäve Desert of southern California and from deposits of carnallite and sylvite in New Mexico and Texas. Another source is the Dead Sea, where considerable quantities are found as dissolved carnallite. This double salt, in aqueous solution, is treated with live steam, the two separate salts form, and the less-soluble salt, potassium chloride, crystallizes out as the solution cools. In the laboratory it may be prepared from potassium carbonate or bicarbonate and HCl.

Description—Colorless, elongated, prismatic or cubical crystals, or as a white granular powder; odorless, saline taste and stable in air; pH (aqueous solution) about 7.

Solubility—1 g in 2.8 mL water at 25° or about 2 mL boiling water; insoluble in alcohol.

Uses—The salt most frequently employed when the action of potassium cation is desired. It is used when *hypokalemia* or *hypochloremic alkalosis* exists, as after prolonged diarrhea or vomiting or consequent to adrenal steroid therapy or treatment with certain diuretics, especially the thiazides. It is used when it is desired to elevate normal plasma potassium levels, as in the treatment of digitalis intoxication. It may be used as a diuretic. Potassium chloride is of value for the relief of the symptoms of *hypokalemic periodic paralysis,* a rare disease characterized by recurrent attacks of muscular weakness. An increase in the daily intake of potassium decreases the risk of stroke-associated mortality; an increment of 10 mEq a day results in an average decrement in mortality of 40%. Potassium salts have been found to relieve the symptoms of *Ménière's* disease.

Potassium chloride is an ingredient of *Lactated Potassic Saline Injection, Ringer's Solution, Lactated Ringer's Injection* and *Ringer's Injection* and various other parenteral and oral electrolyte combinations.

It is irritant to the gastrointestinal tract: oral preparations may cause nausea, vomiting, epigastric distress, abdominal discomfort and diarrhea. High, local concentrations in the gastrointestinal tract can lead to ulceration. Esophageal ulceration may occur if there is dysphagia and gastric ulceration, especially if gastric emptying is delayed. Enteric coating lessens the incidence of such side effects but favors the development of small bowel lesions, especially when thiazides are used concurrently. In a wax matrix it has been promoted as a safe form, but esophageal, gastric and small bowel ulcerations nevertheless occur occasionally. It is best to avoid solid forms; if they are used, they should be taken with one or more full glasses of water. Overdoses may cause paresthesias, generalized weakness, flaccid paralysis, listlessness, vertigo, mental confusion, hypotension, cardiac arrhythmias and heart block. Death may ensue.

Signs of toxicity may occur even with apparently normal blood levels; consequently, the signs must be monitored frequently, and ambulatory patients must be apprised of premonitory symptoms. Most patients can be managed adequately and more safely with foods high in potassium and low in sodium (fruits, especially dried, and cereals).

It must be administered cautiously in the presence of heart or renal disease. It is contraindicated in untreated Addison's disease, heat cramps, adynamia episodica hereditaria, acute dehydration and hyperkalemia from any cause.

Dose—*Oral, solution, adults,* **20** to **40 mEq** (1.49 to 2.98 g) a day to *prevent depletion* and **40** to **100 mEq** (2.98 to 7.55 g) a day for *replacement,* in 3 or 4 divided doses; *children,* **1** to **3 mEq** (75 to 225 mg)/**kg** (or 15 to 40 mEq/m^2) a day in several divided doses. Doses may be higher or lower, as indicated by serum potassium levels. The oral solution should be diluted, such that each 20 mEq is contained in at least 120 mL of water or juice; *enteric-coated tablets* (not recommended), adults, 8 to 13 meq (0.6 to 1 g) 3 times/day; *extended-release capsules,* adults, *prophylactic,* **16** to **24 mEq** (1.19 to 1.79 g) a day in 2 or 3 divided doses; *replacement,* **40** to **96 mEq** (2.98 to 7.16 g) a day in 2 or 3 divided doses; *extended-release tablets, adults,* **6.7, 8, 10, 13.4, 16** or **20 mEq** *(0.5, 0.6, 0.75, 1, 1.2 or 1.5 g)* 3 times a day. Enteric-coated and wax-matrix tablets and extend- release capsules are not recommended for children; however, effervescent tablets can be used.

Intravenous infusion, adults, when plasma potassium is above 2.5 mEq/L, at a rate not to exceed **10 mEq** (750 mg)/hr and a total dose not to exceed **200 mEq** a day; when plasma potassium is less than 2 mEq/L and the clinical condition is serious, **40 mEq** (3 g)/hr may be given, up to a total daily dose of **400 mEq.** For the slower rate of infusion, a 30 mEq/L (0.25%) solution is recommended, and for the faster rate of infusion, 60 mEq/L (0.5%).

Children, **up to 3 mEq/kg** (or 40 mEq/m^2) a day; the volume of solution should be proportional to body size.

Dosage Forms—Extended-Release Capsules: 8 mEq (600 mg); Injection: 0.67, 1, 1.5, 2, 2.4, 3, and 3.2 mEq/mL; Oral Powder (for oral solution): 15, 20, and 25 mEq/packet; Oral Solution: 0.67, 1.34, 2, and 2.66 mEq/mL (5, 10, 15, and 20%, respectively); Effervescent Tablets: 20, 25, and 50 mEq; Enteric-Coated Tablets: 4, and 13.4 mEq (325, and 1000 mg, respectively); Extended-Release Tablets: 6.7, 8, 10 and 20 mEq (499, 746, 1000 and 1491 mg, respectively).

Potassium Gluconate

Kaon (*Warren-Teed*); (*Various Mfrs*)

```
         H   H   OH  H
         |   |   |   |
HOCH2 —C—C—C—C— COOK
         |   |   |   |
         OH  OH  H   OH
```

[299-27-4] $C_6H_{11}KO_7$ (234.25).

Preparation— Glucose may be oxidized to gluconic acid by various processes, eg, electrolytic oxidation of an alkaline solution, reaction with hypobromites or by fermentation using *Aspergillus niger* or other microorganisms. Neutralization with potassium hydroxide provides the salt.

Description—White to yellowish white, crystalline powder or granules; odorless; slightly bitter taste; stable in air; solutions slightly alkaline to litmus.

Solubility—1 g in 3 mL water; practically insoluble in dehydrated alcohol, ether or chloroform.

Uses—A *source of potassium* for management of *hypokalemic* states, such as occur consequent to adrenocorticosteroid therapy or use of thiazide diuretics, or for deliberate production of hyperkalemia, as for treatment of digitalis intoxication. The gluconate anion supposedly makes the compound better tolerated in the gastrointestinal tract than is potassium chloride. It also is claimed that the potassium of the gluconate is absorbed high in the gastrointestinal tract, above the location where mucosal lesions sometimes occur in combined thiazide-potassium therapy, whereas other salts are not absorbed so quickly. Such faulty suppositions and claims ignore the unavoidable chemical fact that irrespective of the salt used, potassium ion is only dissociable completely and hence is unaffected in its irritant actions and absorption by the anion in the compound.

Its sugar-coated tablets dissolve at a higher level than do enteric-coated tablets of potassium chloride but, by this very fact, are free to cause the irritation for which the chloride tablet was coated. The fact that it may cause nausea, vomiting, diarrhea and abdominal discomfort shows that the gluconate has no advantage over nonenteric-coated potassium chloride tablets. A full glass of water taken with either greatly reduces the irritant effects of either salt. Hypochloremia is a frequent accompaniment of hypokalemia; in such instances the chloride definitely is preferred. Furthermore, since gluconate metabolizes to bicarbonate, it contributes to alkalosis, which also may be present in hypokalemia. Only in a hypokalemic, hyperchloremic acidosis (as in renal failure, dehydration and occasional diabetic acidosis) is the drug rational; however, clinical experience indicates no obvious superiority over KCl. The use and toxicity of, and contraindications to, it are the same as for *Potassium Chloride.*

Dose—*Oral, adults,* **5** to **20 mEq** (2.34 to 4.68 g) 2 to 4 times a day, after meals. As the elixir, the dose should be diluted with ½ glass of water or fruit juice; *children,* **2** to **3 mEq/kg** (or 20 to 40 mEq/m^2 a day as the elixir in several divided doses well-diluted in water or juice. The tablets are not recommended.

Dosage Forms—Elixir (40 mEq of K/30 mL); Tablets: 5 mEq.

Potassium Mixtures

Potassium Mixtures—A number of potassium-containing products are mixtures of: KCl and $KHCO_3$; KCl $KHCO_3$ and K_2CO_3; KCl, $KHCO_3$ and citric acid; KCl $KHCO_3$ and potassium citrate; $KHCO_3$ and citric acid; KCl and potassium gluconate; $KHCO_3$, potassium citrate and potassium acetate; and potassium citrate and potassium gluconate. Those that combine $KHCO_3$ with citric acid are effervescent; some effervescent preparations contain betaine.HCl or lysine.HCl in lieu of, or in adition to, citric acid. Those that are not reconstituted for effervescence are intended for their alkalinizing effects in addition to their effects to repair potassium deficits. $KHCO_3$ and K_2CO_3 are directly alkalotic; potassium acetate, citrate and gluconate all metabolize to $KHCO_3$. Since hypokalemia usually is accompanied by *alkalosis*, there are few situations in which an alkalinizing source of potassium is rational. Examples in which hypokalemia and acidosis coexist are renal failure, dehydration and sometimes diabetic acidosis. Even in these, clinical experience is that KCl alone seems to be as useful as the combinations.

Dibasic Potassium Phosphate

Potassium Phosphate Dibasic; Neutra-Phos (*Baker-Norton*)

[7758-11-4] K_2HPO_4 (174.18).

Preparation—By partial neutralization of phosphoric acid with potassium hydroxide or carbonate.

Description—Granular powder; hygroscopic; pH (5% aqueous solution) about 8.5.

Solubility—Very soluble in water.

Uses—In the body, HPO_4^{2-} anion interacts with calcium ion in a way that favors the deposition of both calcium and phosphate in bone salts and in other tissues depots. Some of the phosphate also is converted to pyrophosphate, which is a chelator of calcium, the calcium-pyrophosphate complex being excreted in the urine. Furthermore, high plasma phosphate levels decrease calcitriol levels and thus decrease absorption of calcium. Thus, $KHPO_4$ causes all of redistribution from plasma to tissue, decorporation and diminished incorporation of calcium. Its principal use is in the treatment of *hypercalcemia*. It is not used alone as a source of potassium or phosphate in potassium or phosphate deficiency. It is a component of *Potassium Phosphates, Potassium and Sodium Phosphates* and *Dibasic Potassium and Sodium Phosphates*. It is also a reagent and pharmaceutical necessity for various buffers and parenteral fluids. It is no longer used as a laxative: it may cause diarrhea by the oral route. See *Monobasic Potassium Phosphate* for other adverse effects.

Dose—*Oral, adults*, for *hypercalcemia*. **8** to **16 mmol** (250 to 500 mg of P) 4 times a day, after meals and at bedtime.

Dosage Forms—Powder: 64 g/bottle, when reconstituted makes 1 gal; Packets and Capsules: 1.25–1.45 g of powder, makes 75 mL of oral solution on reconstitution.

Monobasic Potassium Phosphate

Potassium Phosphate Monobasic
K-Phos (*Beach*); Neutra-Phos (*Baker Norton*)

[7778-77-0] K_2HPO_4 (136.09).

Preparation—As for *Dibasic Potassium Phosphate*.

Description—pH (5% aqueous solution) about 5.

Solubility—1 g in about 5 mL water.

Uses—See *Dibasic Potassium Phosphate* for actions to decrease calcium absorption, depress calcium levels in plasma and enhance calcium excretion as pyrophosphate complex. The dibasic salt is likewise used to treat *hypercalcemia*. It is used to treat *nephrolithiasis* when the stones are calcific. In this, the decrease in free calcium excretion into the urine decreases stone formation and acidification of the urine (H_2PO_4- causes *acidosis*) and free pyrophosphate ion favor dissolution of stones. It is a component of *Potassium Phosphates, Monobasic Potassium and Sodium Phosphates*), and a pharmaceutical necessity for various parenteral fluids and buffers. Adverse effects are diarrhea by the oral route (it is poorly absorbed orally and acts as an osmotic cathartic), hypocalcemia (paresthesias, confusion, weakness, muscle cramps, dyspnea, irregular heartbeat), when employed vigorously in nonhypercalcemia patients and the passing of loosened kidney stones.

Dose—*Oral, adults, hypercalcemia*, **8** to **16 mmol** (250 to 500 mg of P) 4 times a day, with meals and at bedtime; for *urolithiasis*, **7.4 mmol** (1 g of salt; 228 mg of P) 4 times a day, with meals at bedtime. Because of the acidity, the dose must be diluted with 180 to 240 mL of water.

Dosage Form—Tablets: 3.7 mmol (500 mg of salt: 124 mg P).

Potassium Phosphates

A mixture of monobasic and dibasic potassium phosphate in the ratio described under each category below.

Uses—For actions, uses and adverse effects, see *Dibasic Potassium Phosphate* and *Monobasic Potassium Phosphate*. Mainly used for hypercalcemia and hypophosphatemia.

Dose—*Oral, adults*, for *hypercalcemia*, **8** to **16 mmol** (150 to 500 mg of P) 4 times a day, after meals and at bedtime; *children*, for *hypophosphatamia*, **6.4 mmol** (200 mg of P) 4 times a day, after meals and at bedtime; when capsules for oral solution are used, they must be dissolved in at least 10 mL/mmol of phosphate. *Intravenous, adults*, for *hypercalcemia*, **100 mmol** (3.1 g of P) infused over 6 to 8 hr once a day; for *hypophosphatemia*, **10 mmol** (310 mg of P) a day; *children over 4 yr*, for *hypophosphatemia*, **1.5 to 2 mmol** (46 to 62 mg of P) a day.

Dosage Forms—Injection: 3 mmol (93 mg of P, 224 mg KH_2PO_4 and 236 mg of K_2HPO_4 per mL); Capsules for Oral Solution: 8 mmol (250 mg of P); for Oral Solution: 64 g of powder to be constituted with 3.785 L of water (1 gal) to make 8 mmol (250 mg of P)/75 mL of solution.

Potassium and Sodium Phosphates

A mixture of mono- and dibasic potassium and sodium phosphates.

Uses—See *Dibasic Potassium Phosphate, Monobasic Sodium Phosphate, Dibasic Sodium Phosphate* (page 898). The mixture is advantageous in that it lessens the risk of sodium or potassium overload from a single-entity preparation. It is used mainly for *hypercalcemia* and *hypophosphatemia*.

Dose—*Oral, adults*, **8 mmol** (250 mg of P) for *hypophosphatemia* and **8** to **16 mmol** (250 to 500 mg of P) 4 times a day, after meals and at bedtime; *children, over 4 yr* for *hypophosphatemia*, **6.4 mmol** (200 mg of P) 4 times a day, after meals and at bedtime; capsules for oral solution should be dissolved in no less than 10 mL of water/1 mmol of PO_4.

Dosage Forms—Capsules for Oral Solution: 8 mmol (250 mg of P); for Oral Solution: 64 g of concentrate powder to be reconstituted in 3.875 L (1 gal) of water: each 75 mL will contain 8 mmol of PO_4 (250 mg of P).

Monobasic Potassium and Sodium Phosphates

A mixture of monobasic potassium and monobasic sodium phosphates.

Uses—See *Monobasic Potassium Phosphate* and *Monobasic Sodium Phosphate*. The combination is used to acidify the urine for the prevention and treatment of urolithiasis. The combination is advantageous in that it lessens the likelihood of excessive intake of either sodium or potassium from that of the single-entity components.

Doses—*Oral, adults*, for *urinary acidification* and *urolithiasis*, **8 mmol** (250 mg of P) dissolved in a full glass of water 4 times a day, after meals and at bedtime; for *hypophosphatemia*, **8 mmol** (150 mg of P) 4 times a day, after meals and at bedtime.

Dosage Form—Tablets for Oral Solution: 8 mmol (250 mg of P).

Ringer's Injection—page 915.

Lactated Ringer's Injection—page 915.

Sodium Acetate

Sodium Acetate Trihydrate

[6131-90-4] $C_2H_3NaO_2.3H_2O$ (136.08); anhydrous 127-09-3 (82.03).

Preparation—By neutralizing acetic acid with sodium carbonate.

Description—Colorless, transparent crystals or granular, crystalline powder; slightly bitter, saline taste; effloresces in warm, dry air; the trihydrate liquefies at about 60°.

Solubility—1 g in 0.8 mL water or 19 mL alcohol.

Uses—The acetate ion is metabolized rapidly and completely in the body; consequently administration eventually is equivalent to giving sodium bicarbonate. Solutions are stable and readily sterilized, and this salt has been used for parenteral therapy of metabolic acidosis and hypoanatremia. It also may be used to alkalinize the urine. It is a pharmaceutical necessity used in solutions for hemodialysis and peritoneal dialysis.

Dose—*Oral, adults*, **7.3** to **14.6 mEq** (1 to 2 g), but more or less may be given, depending on the size of the patient and the clinical condition.

Dosage Form—Injection: 40 mEq/20 mL.

Sodium Bicarbonate

Carbonic acid, monosodium salt; Baking Soda; Sodium Acid Carbonate

Monosodium carbonate [144-55-8] $NaHCO_3$ (84.01).

Preparation—May be produced by the ammonia-soda, or *Solvay Process*. In this process, CO_2 is passed into a solution of common salt in ammonia water, sodium bicarbonate is precipitated and ammonium chloride, being much more soluble, remains in solution. The ammonium chloride solution is heated with lime, whereby the ammonia is regenerated and returned to the process.

Description—White, crystalline powder; odorless with a saline and slightly alkaline taste; solutions, when freshly prepared with cold water without shaking, are alkaline to litmus paper; alkalinity increases as the solutions stand, are agitated or heated; stable in dry air, but slowly decomposes in moist air.

Solubility—1 g in 12 mL water; with hot water it is converted into carbonate; insoluble in alcohol.

Uses—All therapeutic uses accrue to the alkaline properties of $NaHCO_3$. Its most important uses are to *correct metabolic acidosis, alkalinize the urine* and serve as a *buffer* in various parenteral, extracorporeal and topical solutions. Examples of conditions which give rise to metabolic acidosis are uncontrolled diabetes mellitus, aspirin intoxication, ingestion of acidic or acid-forming drugs and other chemicals, hypoadrenalcorticism, renal tubular dysfunction, severe diarrhea and circulatory shock. In metabolic acidosis, cardiac arrest may occur, and *cardiac resuscitation* may be accomplished with $NaCO_3$. Its systemic alkalinizing properties also are used in the management of *sickle-cell anemia*, an elevated plasma pH suppressing the sickling of erythrocytes. Urinary alkalinization is indicated in uricosuria (to favor the formation of the more soluble sodium urate and thus prevent uric acid nephroliths), *sulfonamide treatment* (to increase the solubility of sulfonamides and their metabolites and thus prevent crystalluria and nephrolithiasis) and *intoxication with weak acids*, in which the anionic form is excreted sufficiently fast that urinary alkalinization significantly hastens elimination (eg, aspirin or certain barbiturates).

It is used widely as a *gastric antacid* in lay medicine, but such use is discouraged by gastroenterologists. This is because $NaHCO_3$ is not retained in the stomach long and the rapid evolution of CO_2 causes excessive belching, epigastric discomfort and even sometimes dangerous gastric distention. Urinary alkalinization is considerable and favors calcific nephrolithiasis, nephrocalcinosis and also the intake of sodium ion is held to be undesirable.

The effects of increased sodium intake are considered to be hypervolemia with consequent edema and hypertension. However, certain prominent medical opinion holds that it is the chloride and not the sodium ion in salt that favors hypervolemia and hypertension in persons with normal renal function. This may explain why few systemic adverse effects were found in clinical studies in which huge doses were administered chronically. This implies that systemic alkalosis, of itself, may be benign. Such studies notwithstanding, it is prudent to withhold $NaHCO_3$ from persons with congestive heart failure, edematous states, cirrhosis of the liver, hypertension or the toxemia of pregnancy. It definitely is contraindicated in renal insufficiency, hypernatremia (can cause renal damage, especially in infants younger than 2 yr) and calcific nephrolithiasis. It can promote an extracellular-to-intracellular shift of potassium, which can be especially adverse if hypokalemia and/or hypochloremia exists.

A paste or solution of $NaHCO_3$ is used topically on the skin as an antipruretic. It also is used in various effervescent mixtures as a source of carbon dioxide. Effervescence confers no therapeutic benefits except a placebo effect, but palatability is enhanced.

Dose—*Intravenous, adults* and *children*, in *systemic acidosis* and for *urinary alkalinization*, **2 to 5 mEq/kg,** infused over a period of 4 to 8 hr; *cardiac arrest* (in acidosis), *initially* **1 mEq/kg,** repeated every 10 min, if necessary. *Oral, adults, urinary alkalinization, initially* **49.8 mEq** (4 g) then **12.4** to **24.9 mEq** (1 to 2 g) every 4 hr, up to a total of 199 mEq (16 g)/day; doses should be one-half of the above in persons over 60 yr; *antacid*, **4** to **24.9 mEq** (0.325 to 2 g) 1 to 4 times a day; *children 6 to 12 yr, antacid*, **6.47 mEq** (0.52 g) repeated once in 30 min, if necessary; *all children, urinary alkalinization*, **1** to **10 mEq** (0.023 to 0.23 g)/**kg** a day in divided doses as necessary.

Dosage Forms—Injection: 0.48, 0.5, 0.595, 0.892 and 1 mEq/mL (4, 4.2, 5, 7.5 and 8.4%, respectively); Powder: 120 and 300 g and 1 lb; Effervescent Solution: To be extemporized from powder or tablets that contain $NaHCO_3$ with or without $KHCO_3$, citric acid with or without sodium citrate and other ingredients, such that the antacid strength per dose varies (14.7 mEq for Alka-Seltzer and 18.6 for Citrocarbonate); for Oral Solution: to be extemporized, 1/2 teaspoonful (20.9 mEq) to a glass of water; Tablets: 325 and 650 mg.

Sodium Chloride

Salt; Table Salt; Rock Salt; Sea Salt

Sodium chloride [7647-14-5] NaCl (58.44). It contains no added substance. (Table salt may contain added iodide and/or an anti-caking agent).

Preparation—Common salt is distributed widely over the world, and may be obtained by mining, as rock salt, by evaporating a purified solution of saline deposits or by evaporating sea water, and purifying afterward. If free from contaminating salts it is not hygroscopic.

Description—Colorless, cubic crystals or a white crystalline powder; odorless with a saline taste; the solution is practically neutral; a 23% solution in water freezes at −20°.

Solubility—1 g in 2.8 mL water, 10 mL glycerin or 2.7 mL boiling water; slightly soluble in alcohol.

Uses—Solutions of this salt more closely approximate the composition of the extracellular fluid of the body than solutions of any other single salt. For example, more than 90% of the cation of the extracellular fluid is sodium, more than 60% of the anion is chloride. Furthermore, a 0.9% solution has approximately the same osmotic pressure as body fluids, ie, is isotonic with body fluids. Thus, an isotonic solution can be injected without affecting the osmotic pressure of the body fluids and without causing any appreciable distortion in chemical composition. An isotonic solution, therefore, is the choice as a vehicle for many drugs which have to be administered parenterally. The 0.9% injection is used widely as a substitute for plasma in *volume expansion*, most practitioners preferring it to a dextran because not only is it free of allergenicity but also increases the flow of lymph. The solution has the added advantage of being nonirritating to tissue. Isotonic solutions may be used as an enema or applied topically to intact or exposed tissues for purposes of *irrigation*, to keep tissues moist or to keep a cavity flushed, as in irrigation of the urinary bladder; for this purpose 0.45 or 0.9% *Sodium Chloride Irrigation* is used. Although the *Irrigation* is sterile and meets the pyrogen requirements of the *Injection* it should not be used parenterally. Hypertonic solutions (2 or 5%) may be applied to the cornea, to diminish corneal edema in inflammation or chemosis. Hypertonic solutions also are injected into the amniotic fluid in the 16th to 24th wk of gestation to *cause abortion*. Since accidental intravenous injection can cause shock, pneumonia, fever and other adverse effects, this procedure should be performed only if an intensive care unit is available.

The injection is used as an *electrolyte replenisher* for maintenance or replacement of deficits of extracellular fluid. Since the solution potentially is capable of producing metabolic acidosis (by diluting bicarbonate ion) and does not supply all major cations of the extracellular fluid, other solutions, such as lactated Ringer's injection, may be preferred if large volumes of fluids are to be administered. Other solutions of appropriate composition also must be employed if the composition of the extracellular fluid is distorted markedly. Sterile, pyrogen-free solutions usually are administered intravenously.

In persons who are unable to take fluids by mouth, a hypotonic injection (0.45%) may be used as a source of water, but hypotonic balanced electrolyte solutions with dextrose usually are preferred. In patients in which a salt deficit exists disproportionately to dehydration, a hypertonic injection (3 or 5%) may be used, preferably in conjunction with sodium bicarbonate.

It is administered orally for the prevention of *heat cramps* (miner's cramps, low-sodium syndrome) caused by the depletion of sodium salts through copious perspiration. It is common to use tablets, but a beverage containing only 0.5% will prevent development of the symptoms. This salt is given in *adrenal cortical insufficiency* (Addison's Disease) where it decreases the requirement for adrenal cortical extract. It is used in the treatment of hypercalcemia, to increase glomerular filtration and consequent excretion of calcium.

Common salt is used as a preservative; 6% or more prevents the growth of *Cl botulinum* and other pathogens.

Overdosage may cause pulmonary edema, generalized edema, headache, tinnitus, sensation of warmth in lips, tongue and torso, hypernatremia (characterized by abdominal, back and pelvic pain, diarrhea, muscle twitching, hyperreactivity, confusion, numbness stupor, convulsions or coma) and, occasionally, cellular dehydration. It must be used cautiously in patients with cardiac or renal impairment or hypoproteinemia.

Dose—*Oral*, **8.6** to **17.1 mEq** in a full glass of water 1 to 10 times a day, not to exceed 4.8 g a day. *Intravenous infusion*, variable, according to the weight of the patient, clinical situation, the plasma electrolyte concentration and the intake-output balance, but usually about 1 L of a 0.9% injection (154 mEq), except when the plasma is hypotonic, in which case a 3 to 5% injection may be given at a rate not to exceed 100 mL/hr. *Intraamniotic*, as a **20%** sterile solution in a volume equal to that removed (usually 200 to 250 mL) given over 20 to 30 min, repeated if necessary. *Topically*, usually as **0.9%** solution, but **0.45** or **0.9%** for *bladder irrigation* and **2** or **5%** with added oncotic substances or as a **5%** ointment for corneal turgescense. *Rectal*, as *enema*, **0.9%** solution.

Dosage Forms—Injection (0.9%): 50, 100, 130, 150, 250, 500 and 1000 mL; Injection (0.45%): 100, 500 and 1000 mL; Injection (3%): 500 mL; Injection (5%), 500 mL; Injection (20%): 250 mL; Injection for Admixtures (0.9%): 50, 100, 625 mEq; Injection, Bacteriostatic: 0.9% with 0.9% benzyl alcohol; Injection for Diluents (0.9%): 5, 6, 10, 20, 30, 50 and 100 mL; Irrigation (0.9%): 250, 500, 1500, 2000 and 3000 mL; Irrigation (0.45%): 1000 and 2000 mL; Ophthalmic Ointment: 5%; Ophthalmic Solution: 2 or 5%; Tablets: 650 mg and 1 and 2.25 g; Enteric-Coated Tablets: 1 g; Sustained-Release Tablets, 600 mg; various tablets containing NaCl in combination with dextrose, $CaCO_3$, $Ca_3(PO_4)_2$, $MgCO_3$ or KCl.

Sodium Citrate and Citric Acid Solution

A solution of sodium citrate and citric acid in purified water. It contains, in each mL, 95-105 mg of sodium citrate dihydrate ($C_6H_5Na_3O_7.2H_2O$) and 57–63 mg of anhydrous citric acid ($C_6H_8O_7$). It may contain preservatives and flavoring agents.

Uses—A *systemic* and *urinary alkanizer*. In the body the citrate is metabolized to bicarbonate, so that the effect is that of a dose of bicarbonate. The citric acid is metabolized to carbon dioxide and water and, thus, has only a transient effect on the systemic acid-base status; its function is as a temporary buffer component. Citrate can mobilize calcium from the bones and increase its renal excretion; this, along with the elevated urine pH, may predispose to urolithiasis. Oral citrate also interferes with calcium absorption.

Dose—*Oral, adults, usual,* **10** to **30 mEq** as $NaHCO_3$ equivalent (10 to 30 mL) 4 times a day, but as much as 150 mEq may be given a day; *children,* **5** to **15 mEq** of Na^+ 4 times a day. Each 10 mL of solution should be diluted with a fluid ounce of water for adults and 2 fluid ounces for children. The first three doses are to be given after meals and the fourth at bedtime.

Sodium Lactate Injection

Propanoic acid, 2-hydroxy-, monosodium salt

$CH_3CH(OH)COONa$

Monosodium lactate [72-17-3] $C_3H_5NaO_3$ (112.06); a sterile solution of lactic acid ($C_3H_6O_3$) in water for injection prepared with the aid of NaOH.

Note—Sterilize sodium lactate injection preferably by steam under pressure.

Preparation—A weighed quantity of lactic acid, sufficient to yield the desired amount of sodium lactate, is diluted with water for injection. A volume of assayed concentrated NaOH solution, equivalent to the quantity of lactic acid, is added and the mixture boiled gently until all the lactic anhydride also has been converted into sodium lactate. After quickly cooling, the solution is diluted with *Water for Injection* to the proper volume, promptly filtered if necessary, ampuled and sterilized.

Description—pH, diluted if necessary to about 0.16 *M* (20 mg/mL), 6.0 to 7.3.

Uses—As a substitute for sodium bicarbonate in solutions for *parenteral fluid* and *electrolyte therapy*. Since lactate ion generally is metabolized rapidly in the body, this salt is a potential source of fixed cation for correction of *metabolic acidosis*. However, in shock, severe liver disease and various other hyperlactic acidemic states lactate oxidation is impaired, and the compound is contraindicated. In persons with normal cellular oxidative capacity, lactate will be converted to bicarbonate in 1 to 2 hr. An advantage over sodium bicarbonate is that its solutions may be sterilized by boiling. It is used to accelerate the heart in hypokalemia.

Dose—*Intravenous infusion, adults, metabolic acidosis,* **500** to **1000 mL** of **0.167 *M*** solution (equivalent to 140 to 280 mL of 5% $NaHCO_3$ solution), the dose varying according to the clinical condition of the patient, the laboratory evaluation and the response. It is given at a rate no faster than 300 mL/hr; *cardiac,* in *hypokalemia,* **20 mL** of **1 *M*** solution is given in 2 to 5 min, after which infusion is continued at a rate of 0.4 to 1 mL/min until the desired effect is achieved.

Dosage Form—0.167 *M* solution in 150-, 250-, 500- and 1000- mL containers; 5 *M* solution in 10-mL containers.

Dibasic Sodium Phosphate—page 898.

Monobasic Potassium Phosphate—page 931.

Monobasic Sodium Phosphate

Phosphoric acid, monosodium salt, monohydrate; Sodium Acid Phosphate; Sodium Dihydrogen Phosphate; Monosodium Orthophosphate; Monobasic Sodium Phosphate

Monosodium phosphate monohydrate [10049-21-5] $NaH_2PO_4.H_2O$ (137.99); *anhydrous* [7558-80-7] (119.98).

Preparation—By adding phosphoric acid to a hot concentrated solution of disodium phosphate until the liquid ceases to give a precipitate with barium chloride. The solution is then concentrated to the crystallization point.

Description—Colorless crystals or a white, crystalline powder; odorless and slightly deliquescent; solutions are acid to litmus and effervesce with sodium carbonate.

Solubility—Freely soluble in water; practically insoluble in alcohol.

Incompatibilities—Since sodium biphosphate is an acid salt, it is incompatible with *carbonate* and *alkalies* in general. In solution with *methenamine* it causes a slow evolution of formaldehyde.

Uses—A source of phosphorus in *hypophosphatemia* and *total parenteral nutrition.* Excessive plasma phosphate not only interacts with plasma calcium to transfer it to bone but also indirectly brings about a decrease in calcium absorption in the gut. Consequently, it sometimes is used to treat *hypercalcemia*. It is a pharmaceutical necessity for *Sodium Phosphates Injection.* Sodium *Phosphates Oral Solution* (page 898), *Sodium Phosphate and Sodium Biphosphate Enema* and *Oral Solution* (page 898) and *Potassium and Sodium Phosphates* (page 931), various parenteral and topical solutions and buffers. Adverse effects are diarrhea, hypertension, edema in heart failure, ascites in hepatic dysfunction, hypocalcemia, metastatic calcification and renal damage in adrenal insufficiency.

Dose—*Oral, adults, hypercalcemia,* **8** to **16 mmol** (250 to 500 mg of phosphorus) 4 times a day, after meals and at bedtime. *Intravenous, adults, hypercalcemia* and *hypophosphatemia*, dose individualized according to plasma and urine electrolyte analyses; *total parenteral nutrition,* **10** to **15 m*M*** (310 to 465 mg phosphorus/L); *infants, total parenteral nutrition,* **1.5** to **2 m*M*/kg/day.**

Dosage Forms—Injection (provides 3 mM phosphate and 4 mEq sodium per mL): 15 mL in 30-mL containers; Tablets: 250 mg.

Sodium Phosphates Injection

The usually available injection contains 276 mg (2 millimoles) of monobasic sodium phosphate ($NaH_2PO_4.H_2O$) and 142 mg (1 millimole) of dibasic sodium phosphate (Na_2HPO_4) per mL, equivalent to a total of 93 mg (3 millimoles) of phosphorus.

Uses—A source of phosphorus for *replacement* in phosphorus-depleted patients. It also can be used to treat *hypercalcemia,* since elevated plasma levels of phosphate promote deposition of calcium in bone salts and also loss in urine. The injection should be diluted before use and should be infused slowly to avoid phosphate intoxication. The patient should be monitored for serum levels of calcium, phosphorus and sodium, and for renal function at frequent intervals. Concurrent administration with thiazides may cause renal damage. Each mL of the injection described above represents 92 mg (4 mEq) of sodium, which should be taken into consideration in use of the injection in patients on sodium restriction.

Dose (phosphorus equivalent)—*Intravenous infusion, adults, usual,* for *replacement,* **10** to **15 m*M*** (310 to 465 mg of phosphorus) once a day; for *hypercalcemia,* **100 m*M*** (3.1 g of phosphorus) a day as needed; infusion should be slow, over a period of 6 to 8 hr; *children,* **1.5** to **2 m*M*** of **P/kg a day**.

Dosage Form—Injection (provides 3 m*M* phosphate and 4 mEq sodium per mL): 15 mL in 30-mL containers.

Tromethamine

1,3-Propanediol, 2-amino-2-(hydroxymethyl)-, THAM (*Abbott*)

$$HOCH_2C(CH_2OH)_2NH_2$$

2-Amino-2-(hydroxymethyl)-1,3-propanediol [77-86-1] $C_4H_{11}NO_3$ (121.14).

Preparation—Nitromethane is reacted additively with formaldehyde to yield tris(hydroxymethyl)nitromethane, and the nitro compound then is hydrogenated with the aid of Raney nickel. US Pat 2,174,242.

Description—White, crystalline powder with a slight, characteristic odor and a faint, sweet, soapy taste; stable in light and air; melts between 168 and 172°; pH (1 in 20 solution) 10.0 to 11.5.

Solubility—1 g in 1.8 mL water, 46 mL alcohol or >10,000 mL chloroform.

Uses—A weak amine base with a pK_b of 7.8 at body temperature. This is close to plasma pH (7.4), so that the compound is well-suited to the preparation of a buffer mixture for controlling extracellular pH. Furthermore, at pH 7.4 it is 30% nonionized and hence it gradually penetrates cells, where it also may buffer the intracellular contents. It can react with any proton donor, and the notion that it reacts primarily with carbonic acid or carbon dioxide is erroneous. By removing protons from hydronium ions, ionization of carbonic acid is shifted so as to decrease pCO_2 and to increase bicarbonate concentration. The excess bicarbonate then is excreted gradually in the kidney. This is an especially useful way to manage excessively high pCO_2 in *respiratory acidosis* (respiratory distress syndrome, asphyxia neonatorum, status asthmaticus, chronic respiratory insufficiency, drug intoxication, etc), in which pulmonary ventilation is inadequate. However, it equally is useful in the management of *metabolic acidosis* (drug intoxications, cardiac surgery, diabetic acidosis, etc), especially when the intracellular pH is low, since it readily penetrates cells.

It is used to prevent acidosis in cardiac bypass surgery, and it may be used in conjunction with other drugs in the treatment of cardiac arrest. The ionized drug is excreted by the kidney, so that the effect is that of excretion of hydrogen ions. Elimination of the drug from the body is entirely by renal excretion. Excretion of tromethammonium ion is accompanied by osmotic diuresis, since clinical doses of the drug add considerably to the osmolarity of the glomerular filtrate. The drug should be used cautiously in renal disease. It also is used to buffer blood for transfusions, and it may be added to ACD blood (page 921) as a buffer for storage purposes.

The principal untoward effects are related to its buffering action, namely that overdoses may cause alkalosis; respiration may be depressed because of the decrease in pCO_2 and increase in pH in plasma. Also, it is irritating locally because of its alkalinity, a slough may develop at a site of extravasation, and venospasm and thrombosis also may occur. The fact that about 70% remains in the extracellular space means that a sufficient amount of water must be given to prevent hyperosmolarity and hence to avoid tissue dehydration and the hemodynamic consequences of an increased blood volume.

Plasma hyperosmolarity, in general, causes hepatic and renal damage, and tromethamine is no exception. The hemorraghic lines necrosis seen frequently in newborn infants treated with the drug may possibly have another origin, perhaps related to the route of administration (umbilical vein). The drug also causes hyperkalemia, hypoglycemia and may depress the respiratory center, especially in neonates and premature infants.

Dose—*Intravenous,* variable, depending upon the cause of acidosis and the degree of acid-base distortion. The preferred dose is calculated by the formula; mL (of 0.3 *M*) = body weight in kg × base deficit in mEq/L × 1.1. It frequently is given in a single dose of **2.5 mEq** (300 mg)/**kg** given over a period of not less than 1 hr. Doses of up to **4.1 mEq** (500 mg)/**kg** may be required depending upon the severity and progression of the acidosis. *Intracardiac,* for *cardiac arrest in acidosis,* **16.7** to **50 mEq** (2 to 6 g in 55 to 165 mL) directly into a ventricle.

Dosage Form—Injection: 0.3 *M* solution in 500 mL (18 g) for Injection: 36 g with electrolytes such that reconstitution to 150 mL yields 300 mEq/L tromethamine, 30 mEq/L Na^+, 5 mEq/L K^+ and 35 mEq/L Cl.

Cation Complexing Agents

The introduction of the arsenical war gas, Lewisite, and the proof by Carl Voegtlin that arsenicals combine with sulfhydryl groups, led to the eventual development of dimercaprol (British antilewisite; BAL) in the 1940s. BAL has a high affinity constant because the two adjacent –SH groups enables the arsenic to attach to both sulfhydryl groups in a very stable five-membered ring structure. Such ring complexes were later called *chelates*. BAL also was shown to chelate a number of heavy metals, and it monopolized the role as a heavy metal antidote for nearly two decades.

In 1962, edetate disodium was introduced into medicine. It chelates calcium (and to a lesser extent, magnesium) in addition to various heavy metals. This led to an era in which edetate was used widely to lower plasma calcium levels and to attempt the decalcification of ateriosclerotic and calcinosed organs, and later it became an important decorporant for lead. Despite a spate of even newer chelating compounds, these early drugs are still in use.

Selectivity is a major problem in chelation therapy. Monovalent cations can not be chelated sufficiently strongly so that chelating agents can be used to decrease plasma concentrations. Certain crown ethers can sequester monovalent cations selectively, but, at present, only oral cation-exchange resins are used clinically in the decorporation of monovalent ions. With polyvalent cations, selectivity is achieved through the types of reactive groups, internal dimensions and steric relations in the reagent. Still, selectivity presently is inadequate. For example, chelating agents for calcium also decorporate zinc and other alkaline earth metals. With radionuclides, this problem is circumvented, in part, by using the zinc chelate as a reagent for the radionuclide. Development in this area has been slow, not only because of chemical limitations but also because of a small market and consequent meager investment incentives.

Cellulose Sodium Phosphate

Calcibind (*Mission*)

[68444-58-6] An insoluble, nonabsorbable ion-exchange resin with a great affinity for calcium ions.

Preparation—US Pat 2,759,924.

Description—White to cream-colored powder; must be stored in tightly closed containers to minimize hydrolysis during storage. It contains about 34% inorganic phosphate and 11% sodium. Each g exchanges approx 1.8 m*M* of Ca.

Solubility—Practically insoluble in water, dilute acids and organic solvents.

Uses—Exchanges sodium for calcium and other polyvalent cations. By the oral route it decreases the amount of calcium absorbed from the diet, supposedly without altering calcium balance. It is used to treat a type of absorptiove hypercaluria which occurs even on low-calcium diets. The effectiveness in suppressing nephrolith formation ranges from nil to much according to various reports. During treatment, hyperoxaluria and hypermagnesemia occur, both of which favor certain kinds of kidney stones. The drug is unpalatable and may cause gastrointestinal discomfort. Acute arthralgias from drug-induced hyperparathyroidism have been reported. Every 15 g contains 25 to 50 mEq of sodium.

Dose—*Oral, adults,* **5 g** 3 times a day (with meals) when urine calcium output exceeds 300 mg a day and 10 g a day in 3 divided doses when calcium falls to less than 200 mg a day.

Dosage Form—Bulk Powder: 300 g.

Deferoxamine Mesylate

Butanediamide, *N'*-[5-[[4-[[5-(acetylhydroxyamino)pentyl]amino]-1,4-dioxobutyl]hydroxyamino]pentyl]-*N*-(5-aminopentyl)-*N*-hydroxy-, monomethanesulfonate; Desferal Mesylate (*Ciba*)

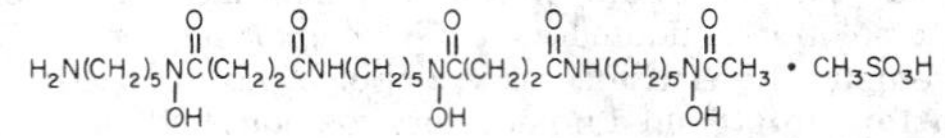

$$H_2N(CH_2)_5N(OH)C(=O)(CH_2)_2C(=O)NH(CH_2)_5N(OH)C(=O)(CH_2)_2C(=O)NH(CH_2)_5N(OH)C(=O)CH_3 \cdot CH_3SO_3H$$

[138-14-7] $C_{25}H_{48}N_6O_8CH_4O_3S$ (656.79).

Preparation—Isolated from cultures of *Streptomyces pilosus* by the method of Bickel *et al* (*Helv Chim Acta 43:* 2118, 1960) or synthesized by the method of Prelog and Walser (*Helv Chim Acta 45:* 631, 1962).

Description—White crystals; reconstituted solutions are stable for 2 wk at room temperature.

Solubility—One g in 5 mL water or 20 mL alcohol; practically insoluble in organic solvents.

Uses—A chelating agent that is selective for iron, but it does complex with aluminum. It is used for the *treatment of severe iron intoxication,* iron overload resulting from hemolysis (from drugs, thalassemia, sickle-cell anemia, frequent blood transfusions, etc.) or *iron storage disease.* It is used to treat *hemodialysis-related porphyria.* Stoichiometrically, 100 mg of deferoxamine sequesters 8.5 mg of ferric iron. Although it does not bind ferrous ion appreciably, it has, nevertheless, proved useful in the treatment of intoxication by ferrous and ferric salts, probably partly because some of the toxicity of ferrous salts is due to ferric ion resulting from oxidation of the divalent iron. Also, partly because complexation of the ferric ion favors further oxidation of ferrous ion and so promotes a diminution in the content of the divalent form. It can decorporate aluminum, and it has been used to manage aluminum accumulation in bone for patients on hemodialysis.

The drug is not absorbed orally and must be given parenterally. By intermittent or continuous subcutaneous infusion the drug is 2 to 3 times more effective than by intramuscular or intravenous injection. This can be achieved in ambulatory patients with an automatic syringe strapped to the waist. Ascorbic acid, 1 g twice a day, also greatly increases its efficacy.

Pain and induration may occur at the site of an intramuscular injection. Other untoward effects include erythema, flushing, diarrhea, blurring of vision, optic neuropathy, high-frequency hearing loss, abdominal discomfort, muscular spasms in the legs, itching, tachycardia and fever. In long-term therapy, various allergic reactions, including anaphylaxis, have been reported. It is a growth factor for many bacteria and enhances virulence; yersinia sepsis and mucormycosis have occurred in patients under treatment with the drug. Because of the side effects, it should not be used to treat mild iron intoxication. The drug is contraindicated in severe renal impairment. Long-term treatment has caused visual and hearing disturbances. The iron chelate (ferrioxamine) is excreted by the kidney and imparts a reddish color to the urine.

Dose—*Intravenous* or *intramuscular, adults,* in *acute intoxication,* initially **1 g** (500 mg twice at 4-hr intervals), then **0.5 g** every 4 to 12 hr, not to exceed 6 g a day; in *chronic iron overload,* **0.5** to **1 g** a day; in chronic iron overload, if blood is to be infused, 2 g must be administered for each unit of blood. It must be administered separately from the blood. Intravenous infusion is reserved only for iron-intoxicated patients in a state of cardiovascular collapse. The rate of intravenous infusion must not exceed 15 mg/kg/hr. *Subcutaneous*, by *infusion*, **1** to **2 g** a day, not to exceed 20 to 40 mg/kg a day; infusion should take 8 to 24 hr. *Intramuscular* or *intravenous, children*, **50 mg/kg** every 6 hr, the rate of infusion not to exceed 15 mg/kg/hr and the dose and total daily dose not to exceed 2 g and 6 g, respectively.

Dosage Form—for Injection: 500 mg to be constituted to 2 mL.

Dimercaprol

1-Propanol, 2,3-dimercapto-, British Anti-Lewisite;
BAL in Oil (*Becton Dickinson*)

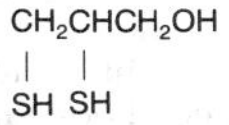

$$\begin{array}{l} CH_2CHCH_2OH \\ \;\;|\;\;\;\;\;| \\ SH\;SH \end{array}$$

[59-52-9] $C_3H_8OS_2$ (124.22) and not more than 1.5% of 1,2,3-trimercaptopropane ($C_3H_8S_3$).

Preparation—A methanol solution of NaOH is saturated with hydrogen sulfide resulting in the formation of sodium hydrogen sulfide [NaSH]. 2,3-Dibromopropanol is added and the mixture heated at 40° under pressure. 2,3-Dibromopropanol is prepared by bromination of allyl alcohol.

Description—Colorless or almost colorless liquid; offensive, mercaptan-like odor; specific gravity 1.242 to 1.244; boiling range 66 to 68° (0.2 torr).

Solubility—1 g in about 20 mL water; soluble in alcohol, benzyl benzoate or vegetable oils.

Uses—An *antidote*, in oil solution, in the treatment of *arsenic, gold* or *mercury poisoning*. The drug may be of value in the treatment of antimony, thallium or bismuth poisoning. It is used in the treatment of acute *lead encephalopathy* only in conjunction with *Edetate Calcium Disodium*. The thiol groups of dimercaprol compete with the physiologically essential–SH groups found in the tissues, and thus remove the metal ions. The combination of heavy metal and dimercaprol is a stable compound which is excreted. It particularly is useful in hemorrhage encephalitis resulting from arsenotherapy, in arsenical or gold dermatitis and, possibly, in postarsenical jaundice.

It usually causes hypertension and tachycardia, which lasts for about 2 hr. It often causes nausea, vomiting, headache, burning sensations in the mouth and throat and a feeling of pressure in the throat, chest and hands. It also may cause conjunctivitis, lacrimation, salivation and rhinorrhea, sweating and abdominal pain. Sterile abscesses often occur at the site of injection. In children, fever frequently occurs; it appears after the 3rd dose and remains throughout the course.

Dose—*Intramuscular* (deep), *adults*, and *children*, for *mild arsenic* or *gold* intoxication, **2.5 mg/kg** 4 times a day for 2 days, 2 times on the 3rd day, and then once a day for 10 days; for *severe arsenic* or *gold intoxication*, **3 mg/kg** every 4 hr for 2 days, 4 times on the 3rd day, then every 12 hr for 10 days; for *mercury intoxication, initially* **5 mg/kg** followed by **2.5 mg/kg** once or twice a day for 10 days; for *acute lead encephalopathy, initially* **4 mg/kg** then **3** to **4 mg/kg** at 4-hr intervals (in combination with calcium disodium edeate at separate sites twice a day) for 2 to 7 days.

Dosage Form—Injection (in oil): 300 mg/3 mL.

Edetate Calcium Disodium

Calciate(2-), [[*N,N'*-1,2-ethanediylbis[*N*-(carboxymethyl)-glycinato]]-(4-)-*N,N',O,O',O^NO^N'*]-, disodium, hydrate (*OC*-6-21)-, Calcium Disodium Versenate (*3M*); Versene CA (*Dow*)

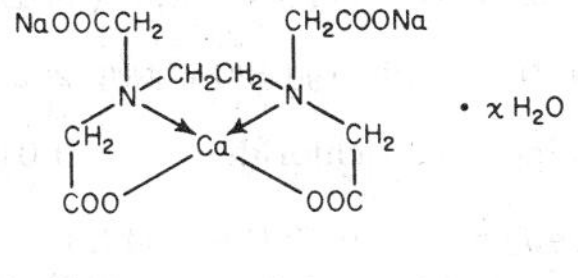

NaOOCCH₂ CH₂COONa / N–CH₂CH₂–N / CH₂ Ca CH₂ / COO OOC · x H₂O

Disodium (ethylenedinitrilo)tetraacetato]calciate(2-) hydrate; calcium disodium ethylenediaminetetraacetate hydrate [23411-34-9] $C_{10}H_{12}CaN_2Na_2O_8.xH_2O$; *anhydrous* [62-33-9] (374.27); a mixture of the dihyrate and trihydrate of calcium disodium ethylenediaminetetraacetate (predominantly the dihydrate).

Preparation—Among other ways, by boiling an aqueous solution of edetate disodium (below) with slightly more than an equimolar quantity of calcium carbonate until carbon dioxide no longer is evolved, filtering while hot and crystallizing.

Description—White, crystalline granules or white, crystalline powder; odorless, slightly hygroscopic and a faint, saline taste; stable in air.

Solubility—Freely soluble in water.

Uses—Primarily in the diagnosis and treatment of *lead poisoning*, but may be used for removing certain other heavy metals from the body. As a diagnostic agent, it causes a surge of lead into the urine, the magnitude of which reveals the extent of the body burden of lead. Treatment is usually by intravenous infusion, but in lead encephalopathy the infusion fluid exacerbates the cerebral edema, so that the drug is given, instead, by the intramuscular route in a hyperosmotic concentration. Since this agent already contains calcium it is useless as an anticoagulant or for treatment of hypercalcemia. Indeed, the purpose of calcium in the compound is to prevent the loss of calcium.

During infusion there may be transitory hypotension, inversion of the T-wave of the ECG and prolongation of prothrombin time. Fever sometimes occurs 4 to 8 hr after an infusion. It is accompanied by malaise, fatigue, thirst and chills. Myalgia, headache, vomiting and increased urinary urgency often follow. Sneezing, nasal congestion, lacrimation, glycosuria, anemia and dermatitis also occasionally occur. Edetate sometimes causes a usually reversible hydropic degeneration of the renal tubular epithelium, especially in the lower nephron. Some of the adverse effects are the result of decorporation of zinc.

It is eliminated entirely in the urine with a half-life of 1 hr, except longer in renal insufficiency.

Dose—*Intravenous infusion, adults*, **1 g** in 250 to 500 mL of isotonic solution over a period of 1 hr 2 times a day for 3 to 5 days; the total daily dose should not exceed 50 mg/kg when symptoms are only mild; for *children*, up to **35 mg/kg** (or 850 mg/m^2) as 0.2 to 0.4% solution in an isotonic injection twice a day. *Intramuscular, adults*, up to **35 mg/kg** in 0.5% procaine hydrochloride solution twice a day, not to exceed 50 mg/kg/day in mild intoxication; *children*, up to **35 mg/kg** (or 850 mg/m^2) in 0.5% procaine hydrochloride solution twice a day in divided doses at 8- to 12-hr intervals; a course may be repeated after a rest of 4 days.

Dosage Form—Injection: 1 g/5 mL.

Edetate Disodium

Glycine, *N,N'*-1,2-ethanediylbis[*N*-(carboxymethyl)-, disodium salt, dihydrate; Diso-Tate (*Forest*); Endrate (*Abbott*); Edathamil; Disodium Versenate (*Various Mfrs*)

$$(HOOCCH_2)_2NCH_2CH_2N(CH_2COONa)_2 \cdot 2H_2O$$

Disodium (ethylenedinitrilo)tetraacetate dihydrate [6381-92-6] $C_{10}H_{14}N_2Na_2O_8.2H_2O$ (372.24); *anhydrous* [139-33-3] (336.21).

Preparation—(Ethylenedinitrilo)tetraacetic acid (edetic acid, page 1410) is dissolved in a hot solution containing two equivalents of NaOH and the disodium salt is allowed to crystallize.

Description—White, crystalline powder.

Solubility—Soluble in water; pH (1 in 20 solution) 4.0 to 6.0.

Uses—To remove free calcium ions from solution, since it readily chelates calcium; thus, it may be used as an *anticoagulant* in the same manner as sodium citrate. Intravenously, it temporarily *lowers plasma calcium* concentration, but the effect is too brief to be of value in the treatment of hypercalcemia, but constant infusion can yield a more sustained effect. It is employed occasionally to *terminate* abruptly *the effects of injected calcium* and to *antagonize digitalis toxicity* or *suppress tachyarrhythmias*. The drug is not effective in the treatment of arteriosclerosis, since calcium is mobilized more easily from bone. It can dissolve precipitated calcium salts.

It may cause nausea, vomiting, diarrhea, transient circumoral paresthesias, numbness, headache and a transient hypotension. Too-rapid an injection can cause death. Fever, anemia, exfoliative dermatitis and other toxic effects on skin and mucous membranes occasionally occur. When given intravenously, it sometimes has a nephrotoxic action. Overdosage can result in damage to the reticuloendothelial system. Prolonged infusion may cause zinc and magnesium deficiencies. It is contraindicated in patients with impaired renal function with severe azotemia, and should be used cautiously in the presence of liver impairment and hypokalemia.

Dose—Depends on the use and the amount of calcium to be sequestered; 1 g chelates 0.12 g of calcium. *Usual, intravenous infusion, adults* **50 mg/kg,** up to a maximum of 3 g a day. The drug usually is employed as a 3% solution in isotonic saline or glucose. It is given by slow intravenous drip such that 3 hr or more are required to accomplish the infusion. Five consecutive daily doses may be given, after which there should be a rest of 2 days before resuming treatment; no more than a total of 15 doses should be given. For *children*, the recommended daily dose is **40 mg/kg** to be infused over a period of no less than 3 hr; the maximum daily dose is 70 mg/kg.

Dosage Form—Injection: 3 g/20 mL.

Penicillamine

D-Valine, 3-mercapto-, Cuprimine (*MSD*); Depen (*Wallace*)

$$HS-C(CH_3)_2-CH(NH_2)-COOH$$

β,β-Dimethylcysteine; D-3-Mercaptovaline [52-67-5] $C_5H_{11}NO_2S$ (149.21).

Preparation—By acid hydrolysis of penicillin. It is precipitated from the hydrolysis mixture as the mercuric salt which is then collected, suspended in water and treated with hydrogen sulfide to liberate the free acid. Purification involves only recrystallization from water. Penicillamine also is obtained by synthesis.

Description—Fine, white or practically white, crystalline powder; slight characteristic odor and a slightly bitter taste; relatively stable in both light and air; melts at about 200° with decomposition; pH (1 in 100 solution) 4.5 to 5.5.

Solubility—Freely soluble in water; slightly soluble in alcohol; insoluble in chloroform or ether.

Uses—A chelating agent useful in the treatment of *Wilson's disease* and *biliary cirrhosis* (in which the serum and liver copper concentrations, respectively, are excessively high), and *lead, gold* or *mercury poisoning.* It especially is useful in the long-term treatment of lead poisoning because of its oral efficacy, which the edetates lack. It also is useful in the treatment of *cystinuria* and *rheumatoid arthritis*; plasma cystine levels fall in the former during treatment but rise in the latter. The mechanism in rheumatoid arthritis is uncertain but has been attributed to a marked reduction in concentrations of IgM rheumatoid factor or to the scavenging of oxygen free radicals. The drug is investigational in the treatment of biliary cirrhosis.

Side effects most often appear shortly after therapy has begun. It may cause ecchymosis, hematuria dermatitis, eruptions of the mucous membranes, leukopenia, thrombocytopenia, agranulocytosis, fever, polyarthralgia, glomerulopathy, nephrosis, lymphadenopathy and optic neuritis. Anorexia, nausea, epigastric pain, diarrhea, vomiting, stomatitis, peptic ulcer and disorders of taste are also common effects. Some of these effects are the result of decorporation of zinc. Tinnitus and optic neuritis occur as the result of drug- induced pyridoxine deficiency; pyridoxine supplements are advised. Cholestatic jaundice, toxic hepatitis, lupus erythematosis, bronchiolitis, alveolitis, pemphigoid, myasthenia and pancreatitis occur rarely. Blood counts must be made every 2 wk during the first 6 mo of therapy. Once therapy has begun, treatment should be continued on a daily basis as even short interruptions have been followed by sensitivity reactions.

Dose—*Oral, adults*, as an *antidote* to heavy metals, **0.5** to **1 g** 4 times day for 1 to 2 months, the dose being adjusted according to blood and urine analyses; *antirheumatic*, initially **125 mg** once or twice a day, followed by increments of **125** to **250 mg/day** at 1- to 3- month intervals up to a maximum of **1.5 g** a day; in *cystinuria*, **0.5** to **1 g** 4 times a day; for *Wilson's disease* and *biliary cirrhosis*, **0.5** to **1 g** 4 times a day, the dose being adjusted according to blood and urine analyses. *Children*, as an antidote, **10** to **13.3 mg/kg** 3 times a day for 1 to 6 months; in *cystinuria*, **7.5 mg/kg** 4 times a day; in *Wilson's disease* and *biliary cirrhosis*, *initially* 250 mg a day in fruit juice for infants over 6 months and young children and adult dose in older children. Penicillamine should be taken on an empty stomach 30 to 60 min before meals and at bedtime.

Dosage Forms—Capsules: 125 and 250 mg; Tablets: 250 mg.

Sodium Polystyrene Sulfonate

Benzene, ethenyl-, homopolymer, sulfonated, sodium salt; Kayexalate (*Winthrop*)

Styrene polymer sulfonated, sodium salt; a cation-exchange resin prepared in the sodium form. Each g exchanges (2.8 to 3.5 mEq) of potassium.

Description—Golden brown, fine powder; odorless and tasteless.

Solubility—Insoluble in water.

Uses—An ion-exchange resin used for the treatment of hyperkalemia resulting from acute renal failure. The resin is given orally by a stomach tube or as a high-retention enema. The sodium moiety of the resin is, in part, replaced by potassium which subsequently is eliminated from the body when the resin is excreted in the feces or in the enema. The potassium-removing capacity of the resin is approximately ⅓ of that possible when measured under conditions in which potassium is the only cation present. The resin should be an adjunct to other therapeutic measures, such as restriction of electrolyte intake, control of acidosis and high-caloric diet. Untoward effects include anorexia, nausea, vomiting and constipation. Constipation and fecal impaction can be minimized by the administration of 70% sorbitol solution every 2 hr as needed to produce watery stools. Serum potassium levels should be determined daily in order to avoid hypokalemia.

The resin may cause gastric irritation, nausea, vomiting and occasional diarrhea. Especially in elderly patients, large doses may cause fecal impaction. Since the resin can sequester calcium and magnesium, hypocalcemia, hypomagnesemia or related effects may occur, and mineral metabolism should be monitored during prolonged treatment. The drug should be used with caution in patients with actual or impending cardiac failure; the absorption of the released (exchanged) sodium may be hazardous in such patients. It also may exaggerate the effects of digitalis.

Dose—*Oral, adults*, **15 g** 1 to 4 times a day; as much as 160 g/day have been administered. Each dose should be suspended in 20 to 100 mL of water or syrup. By *enema*, **25** to **100 g** in 150 to 200 mL of water, 5% dextrose solution or 2% hydroxy methylcellulose solution as a retention enema once or twice a day; a cleansing enema should follow. Duration of treatment depends on clinical condition and response, and it may be as short as 3 days; it is discontinued when plasma potassium reaches 4 to 5 mEq/L. *Oral* or *rectal, infants* and *small children*, **1 g** of resin for every mEq of potassium that is to be removed. One level teaspoonful contains approximately 3.5 g.

Dosage Forms—Suspension: 250 mg/mL in 60-, 120-, 480- and 500-mL quantities; For Suspension: 454 g (1 lb). *Note:* Each g of sodium polystyrene sulfonate contains 4.1 mEq (94 mg) of sodium.

Succimer

Butanedioic acid, (*R,S*)-2,3-dimercapto-, Chemet (*McNeil*)

$$HOOC-CH(SH)-CH(SH)-COOH$$

meso-2,3-Dimercaptosuccinic acid; DMSA; DIM-SA [304-55-2] $C_4H_6O_4S_2$ (182.21).

Preparation—*J Chem Soc 71:* 3109, 1949.

Description—White crystalline powder with an unpleasant mercaptan-like odor and taste; melts at about 193°.

Uses—Has a broader spectrum of chelating activity than does dimercaprol, owing to the presence of carboxyl groups in the molecule. However, it is selective for lead and is used in the treatment of lead intoxication. Its advantages are that it can be administered orally and that adverse effects are few and mild. Mild, transient elevation of plasma SGPT levels occurs. An increase in copper and zinc excretion have been noted, but no pathology attributed to loss of these metals has been observed. The drug probably will eventually replace dimercaprol in the treatment of lead and certain other heavy metals poisoning. ^{99}Technetium DMSA (page 864) is used for renal imaging. The compound is excreted in both the urine and bile.

Dose—*Oral*, **10 mg/kg** every 8 hr for 5 days, then every 12 hr for an additional 2 wks.

Dosage Form—Capsules, 100 mg.

Trientine Hydrochloride

1,2-Ethanediamine, *N,N'*-bis(2-aminoethyl)-, dihydrochloride; Syprine (formerly Cuprid) (*MSD*)

$$H_2N(CH_2)_2NH(CH_2)_2NH(CH_2)_2NH_2 \cdot 2HCl$$

Triethylenetetramine hydrochloride [38260-01-4] $C_6H_{18}N_4.2HCl$ (219.16).

Preparation—See *J Org Chem 9:* 125, 1944.

Description—White to pale-yellow hygroscopic crystals, melts about 117°.

Solubility—Freely soluble in water; slightly soluble in alcohol; insoluble in chloroform or ether.

Uses—A tetramine chelating agent that lacks sulfhydryl and oxygen-containing groups and hence has a low affinity for most of the transition and heavy metals, yet retains a high affinity for copper. The relative affinity for copper enables the drug to be used for the treatment of *Wilson's disease* without the side effects attributable to decorporation of zinc. It also presently does not appear to cause the hypersensitivity and immune disorders evoked by penicillamine. However, penicillamine-induced lupus erythematosis sometimes fails to remit or even recurs during treatment. It is approved only for the treatment of Wilson's disease in patients intolerant to penicillamine, but its low toxicity most certainly will result in the displacement of penicillamine in the treatment of this disease. The only significant adverse effect observed thus far is iron-deficiency anemia; that it is really the result of copper deficiency and not iron decorporation is demonstrated by the response of the anemia to copper.

Dose—*Oral, adults* and *children over 12 yr*, initially **0.75** to **1.25 g** a day in 2 to 4 divided doses, adjusted upwards to 2 g a day, if necessary; *children up to 12 yr*, **0.5** to **0.75 g** a day in 2 to 4 divided doses, adjusted upwards to 1.5 g a day, if necessary.

Dosage Form—Capsules: 250 mg.

Hematologic Drugs Affecting Blood Production

Hematopoietics

Hematopoietics are *antianemics* that aid in the production of red and white blood cells; *hematinics* are *antianemics* that increase the hemoglobin content of blood through erythropoiesis or through an increase in hemoglobin content of erythrocytes. The choice of a hematinic critically depends upon the nature of the anemia. The hypochromic anemias are nearly all iron-deficiency anemias in character and are treated with iron preparations. Occasionally, other accessory factors are indicated in the treatment of the hypochromic anemias. As long as 6 months of treatment may be required to replenish the body stores of iron and correct various anemias. For example, the anemia of nurslings may require copper to facilitate the mobilization of iron from the gut and tissues.

Ascorbic acid occasionally helps promote the antianemic action of iron. When given with iron salts, it promotes the absorption of iron, in part by reducing the less-well-absorbed ferric ion to the better-absorbed ferrous ion or maintaining the ferrous state of administered ferrous salts, and in part by forming an absorbable complex with iron. However, ascorbic acid appears to have an additional but obscure role in hematopoiesis; it is included in a number of iron-containing products.

Cobalt and molybdenum probably also play a role in hematopoiesis, but deficiency syndromes in man are unknown, and the inclusion of these metals in hematinic preparations is irrational. The use of cobalt even may be dangerous. Although copper is known to have a hematopoietic function, a deficiency in man severe enough to impair erythropoiesis has never been demonstrated (see page 1133), although trientine can cause a copper-responsive anemia.

The macrocytic anemias all respond to cyanocobalamin, but the route of administration and accessory factors are dependent critically upon the particular anemia. In tropical sprue, the absorption of folic acid is impaired to a greater extent than that of vitamin B_{12}, so that folic acid usually elicits the greater hematopoietic response. For reasons stated elsewhere (below and on page 1118), the promiscuous use of folic and folinic acids should be condemned. In pyridoxine deficiency, protoporphyrin synthesis, and hence erythropoiesis, is impaired and pyridoxine restores normal erythropoiesis.

Iron and Iron Compounds

Iron is used in medicine in the form of inorganic and simple organic ferrous compounds (ferrous sulfate, etc) and complex ferrous compounds.

Complex (nonionic) iron compounds do not respond to the ordinary tests for ferrous or ferric ions because the iron in them is part of a complex radical. The stabilities of these complex radicals differ widely. Some are converted to simple ionic iron by the action of dilute acids while others resist treatment with strong acids or with alkalies. The complex iron compounds occurring naturally in animal and vegetable tissues (termed food irons) belong generally to the more resistant class, while the complex iron compounds produced artificially are as a rule decomposed rather readily. There is, however, no sharp line of distinction between the natural complex iron compounds and those products artificially produced, nor is there any good evidence that they differ in therapeutic action.

Uses—The principal use of iron is in the treatment of *hypochromic, iron-deficiency anemias*, that is, in anemias characterized by a deficiency of hemoglobin. The two most common causes of such anemias are nutritional (deficient intake, especially in infancy, in childhood, at puberty, during pregnancy and late in menstrual life or at the menopause), and chronic blood loss (especially bleeding peptic ulcer, carcinoma of the colon or stomach, bleeding from the urinary tract or excessive loss of blood during menstruation). Iron therapy is of no particular value in other forms of anemia, such as pernicious anemia, unless the patient has entered an iron-deficiency stage of his disease.

Complex iron compounds generally are less prone to produce gastric distress than the simple ferrous compounds; they also are utilized less efficiently physiologically. Indeed, in some complexes the iron may be chelated so effectively as to escape utilization altogether.

Differences exist among the different iron preparations in their local irritant and astringent actions, which are absent in most of the complex iron compounds; for this reason the less-astringent and less-irritant ferrous salts are used rather than ferric salts. The irritation occurs mostly in the stomach and upper duodenum, where the pH is low. It can exacerbate peptic ulcer, regional enteritis, ulcerative colitis and other gastrointestinal disorders. Enteric coatings allow the preparations to pass into the more alkaline portions of the gut before release occurs. However, the absorption of iron from enteric-coated preparations is less than in uncoated ones, especially in persons with bowel hypermotility. In steatorrhea or in persons with partial gastrectomy, iron preparations often are absorbed poorly. Antacids also diminish absorption. Constipation, consequent to local actions of iron, may be countered by cathartics, properly individualized. Suitable diet (especially liver, kidney and meat) is sometimes more effective than the iron preparations, presumably by the cooperation of other factors.

All of the iron preparations are capable of causing severe intoxication in overdoses, especially in children. Iron preparations are a common cause of lethal intoxication in children.

Ascorbic Acid—pages 1116 and 1124.

Ferrous Fumarate

2-Butenedioic acid, (*E*)-, iron(2+) salt (*Various Mfrs*)

```
     HC—C=O
     ||   |
O=C—CH   O
  |      /
  O—Fe
```

Iron(2+) fumarate [141-01-5] $C_4H_2FeO_4$ (169.90).

Preparation—Ferrous sulfate and sodium fumarate are metathesized in hot aqueous solution whereupon the sparingly soluble, anhydrous ferrous fumarate precipitates.

Description—Reddish orange to red-brown, odorless powder; may contain soft lumps that produce a yellow streak when crushed.

Solubility—Slightly soluble in water; very slightly soluble in alcohol; its solubility in dilute HCl is limited by the separation of insoluble free fumaric acid.

Uses—In the clinical management of *iron-deficiency anemias*. Its efficacy is about the same as that of ferrous sulfate, but the untoward effects are somewhat less severe. The drug may sometimes be employed without difficulty in patients who cannot tolerate other preparations of iron. When side effects occur, they include anorexia, nausea, vomiting, cramping and constipation or diarrhea. Like other iron preparations, this drug may exacerbate gastrointestinal diseases, especially ulcerative ones. The effects generally subside as therapy is continued. The untoward effects are minimized if the dose is taken shortly after eating.

Dose—*Oral, adults,* **200 mg,** once a day for *prophylaxis* and 3 times a day for *treatment,* except **300 mg**/day for prophylaxis and 2 times a day for treatment with extended-release capsules; *children,* usually as the oral suspension, **3 mg/kg** once a day for prophylaxis and 3 times a day for treatment. For treatment, doses may be gradually doubled, if necessary.

Dosage Forms—Oral Suspension: 100 mg (33 mg Fe)/100 mL, 45 mg (15 mg Fe)/0.6 mL; Tablets: 63, 195, 200, 324, 325 mg (20, 64, 66, 106, 107 mg Fe, respectively); Chewable Tablets: 325 mg (106 mg Fe); Extended-Release Capsules: 325 mg (106 mg Fe).

Ferrous Gluconate

D-Gluconic acid, iron(2+) salt (2:1), dihydrate (*Various Mfrs*)

$$\left[HOCH_2-\underset{OH}{\overset{H}{C}}-\underset{OH}{\overset{H}{C}}-\underset{H}{\overset{OH}{C}}-\underset{OH}{\overset{H}{C}}-COO-\right]_2 Fe \cdot 2H_2O$$

Iron(2+) gluconate (1:2) dihydrate [12389-15-0] $C_{12}H_{22}FeO_{14}.2H_2O$ (482.17); *anhydrous* [299-29-6] (446.14).

Preparation—By metathesis between hot solutions of calcium gluconate and ferrous sulfate whereby ferrous gluconate and insoluble calcium sulfate are formed. The mixture is filtered while hot to minimize the solubility of calcium sulfate and the filtrate is evaporated to crystallization.

It also may be produced by heating freshly prepared ferrous carbonate with the proper quantity of gluconic acid in aqueous solution.

Description—Fine, yellowish gray or pale greenish yellow powder, or granules, with a slight burnt-sugar-like odor; affected by light; the ferrous iron slowly oxidizes to ferric on exposure to air; aqueous solution is acid to litmus (color of the solution depends on pH—they are light yellow at pH 2, brown at pH 4.5 and green at pH 7); the iron rapidly oxidizes at higher pH.

Solubility—1 g in about 5 mL water with slight heating; practically insoluble in alcohol; it forms supersaturated solutions which are stable for a period of time; its solubility is increased by addition of citric acid or the citrate iron.

Uses—A *hematinic,* similar to other ferrous salts. Its side effects and toxicity are those of all iron compounds; it is claimed that it causes fewer side effects than ferrous sulfate (see under *Iron and Iron Compounds*). The elixir can cause staining of the teeth if taken undiluted.

Dose—*Oral, adults,* **320** or **325 mg** once a day for *prophylaxis* and 4 times a day for *treatment*; *children, under 2 yr,* to be individualized; *2 yr and over,* **8 mg/kg** once a day for *prophylaxis* and **16 mg/kg** 3 times a day for treatment. Adult doses may be doubled gradually, if necessary.

Dosage Forms—Capsules: 86, 325 and 435 mg (10, 38 and 50 mg Fe); Elixir: 300 mg (35 mg Fe)/5 mL; Tablets: 300, 320 and 325 mg (35, 37 and 38 mg Fe).

Ferrous Sulfate

Sulfuric acid, iron(2+) salt (1:1), heptahydrate; Ferri Sulfas; Feosol (*Various Mfrs*)

Iron(2+) sulfate (1:1) heptahydrate [7782-63-0] $FeSO_4.7H_2O$ (278.01); *anhydrous* [7720-78-7] (151.90).

Note—Do not use Ferrous Sulfate that is coated with brownish yellow basic ferric sulfate.

Preparation—By dissolving iron in diluted H_2SO_4. The resulting solution is filtered and concentrated, if necessary, to the point of crystallization of ferrous sulfate. Commercially, scrap iron is used in the process.

Description—Pale, bluish green crystals or granules; odorless, has a saline, styptic taste and effloresces in dry air, becoming white; oxidizes readily in moist air to form brownish yellow basic ferric sulfate; pH (1 in 10 solution) about 3.7.

Solubility—1 g in 1.5 mL of water or 0.5 mL of boiling water; insoluble in alcohol.

Uses—One of the most commonly employed *hematinic* preparations used in iron-deficiency anemias (see under *Iron and Iron Compounds*). The drug is dispensed most commonly as capsules or tablets coated for protection from air and moisture. The salt sometimes is mixed with glucose or lactose to protect it from oxidation.

Its adverse effects are those of iron compounds in general, but they are rarely severe when the salt is taken in therapeutic doses; however, relatively small overdoses can cause serious intoxication in infants and children. The oral solution can cause staining of teeth if used undiluted.

About 20% of this drug is absorbed when taken orally. Timed- release and enteric-coated preparations tend to be absorbed more erratically and are not recommended. Magnesium and aluminum hydroxides, present in some preparations, make the iron unavailable for absorption.

Dose—*Oral, adults* **300 mg** once a day for *prophylaxis* and *initially* 2 times a day, gradually increased to 4 times a day, if necessary, for *treatment; children,* usually as liquid, **5 mg/kg** a day for *prophylaxis* and **10 mg/kg** 3 times a day for treatment.

Dosage Forms—Capsules: 190 mg (exsiccated; 60 mg Fe); Extended-Release Capsules: 150, 159 (exsiccated), 250, and 325 mg (30, 50, 50, and 65 mg of Fe, respectively); Drops: 75 mg (15 mg Fe)/ 0.6 mL and 125 mg (25 mg Fe)/mL; Elixir: 220 mg (44 mg Fe)/5 mL; Syrup: 90 mg (18 mg Fe)/5 mL; Tablets: 195, 200 (exsiccated), 300 and 325 mg (60, 39, 65, 60 and 65 mg Fe, respectively); Enteric-coated Tablets: 160 and 525 mg (50 and 105 mg Fe).

Iron Dextran Injection

InFeD (*Schein*)

A sterile, colloidal solution of ferric hydroxide in complex with partially hydrolyzed dextran of low molecular weight, in water for injection. It may contain not more than 0.5% of phenol as a preservative.

Preparation—To an aqueous solution of partially depolymerized dextran (intrinsic viscosity 0.04 to 0.07) is added a solution of alkali and a solution of a ferric salt. The mixture is heated, then cooled to room temperature, clarified by centrifugation and the solution dialyzed against running water. After concentrating to the required iron content, the solution is filtered, ampuled and sterilized by autoclaving.

Description—Dark-brown, slightly viscous liquid; pH 5.2 to 6.

Uses—Because iron is strongly chelated by dextran, it is not locally irritating on intramuscular injection. Absorption is rapid from an intramuscular site. Thus the drug is used for intramuscular injection in patients with iron-deficiency anemias in whom oral therapy cannot be tolerated or does not evoke a therapeutic response. If the drug is administered to persons not in an iron-deficiency state, hemosiderosis may occur. Absorption is very slow from a subcutaneous site and a brown stain occurs that may remain for 1 to 2 yr. Consequently, in injecting the drug, care must be taken to prevent leakage under the skin. Injections are given deeply into the upper-outer quadrant of the buttock by a special technique called a Z-track injection, which diminishes leakage to subcutaneous sites.

In the human the lymphatic system is well-developed and the dose of the complex is relatively low, so that the danger of malignancy, such as occurs in some animals, is very slight. However, it can cause fibrosis at the site of injection. Allergic reactions, even anaphylaxis, have occurred. Consequently, a test of 0.5 mL of the injection should be given prior to therapeutic administration. Headache, fever, nausea, vomiting, paresthesias and regional lymphadenopathy are relatively common side effects. Hypotension, reactivation of quiescent arthritis, leukocytosis with fever and sterile abscesses at an intramuscular injection site may occur. Phlebitis occasionally occurs after intravenous administration. The parenteral use of iron and carbohydrate has resulted in fatal anaphylactic-type reactions. Consequently, use of iron dextran should be reserved for patients with a clearly established iron deficiency state not amenable to oral iron therapy.

Dose—Intramuscular, adults, daily dose

$$\text{mg Fe} = 0.3 \times \text{wt in lb}\left(100 - \frac{\text{Hb in g/dL} \times 100}{14.8}\right)$$

To convert to mL of injection, divide by 50. The daily dose should not exceed 25 mg Fe for infants under 10 lb. 50 mg Fe for 10 to 20 lb, or 100 mg Fe for persons under 110 lb. *Intravenous,* up to **50 mg** Fe may be given slowly (less than 1 mL/min) once a day. *Intravenous infusion* (not approved in US), the calculated dose is placed in 200 to 250 mL of isotonic sodium chloride; if a test dose of 25 mg infused over 5 min evokes no adverse effect, the infusion is completed over 1 to 2 hr.

Dosage Form—Injection: 50 mg/mL in 2-, 5- and 10-mL vials.

Polyferose

β-D-Fructofuranosyl α-D-glucopyranoside deriv, polymer, iron complex; Jefron (*Marion Merrell Dow*)

[9009-29-4] A chelate of iron with a polymerized derivative of sucrose, containing about 45% Fe.

Uses—For the treatment of iron-deficiency anemias. The complex is less astringent than ferrous salts and hence is more palatable in oral suspension.

Dose—Oral, adults, **150 mg** (50 mg Fe) once a day for *prophylaxis* and twice a day, gradually doubled, if necessary, for *treatment; children*, the equivalent of 1.5 mg Fe/kg a day, for *prophylaxis* only.

Dosage Forms—Capsules: 125 mg Fe; Elixir: 100 mg Fe/5 mL; Tablets: 50 mg Fe.

Agents for Macrocytic Anemias

The macrocytic anemias are characterized by the presence of large, hypochromic erythrocytes. They include *pernicious anemia*, the *anemia* of *sprue*, *macrocytic tropical anemia*, *fish tapeworm anemia*, *achrestic anemia* and anemias resulting from gastric carcinoma and resection or disease of the intestinal tract. In all of these, insufficient intake or absorption of *cyanocobalamin* (vitamin B_{12}) is the cause of the disorder, the vitamin being essential to normal hematopoiesis and to the integrity of the central nervous system. Early work on pernicious anemia had established the need for a dietary factor, called the *extrinsic factor*, and a gastric and upper duodenal secretory factor, called the *intrinsic factor*.

It is now well-established that cyanocobalamin is the extrinsic factor; the vitamin is also the *antianemia component* of liver. The intrinsic factor is essential to the proper absorption of vitamins B_{12}. The intrinsic factor is absent in pernicious anemia; in this disease the secretion of hydrochloric acid and pepsin also is diminished or absent. Before the advent of cyanocobalamin (a vitamin B_{12}), various liver preparations were employed as sources of extrinsic factor and stomach preparations as sources of the intrinsic factor. Since orally administered liver was not reliable, because it did not provide the intrinsic factor, it was necessary to administer a stomach preparation at the same time or to administer the liver parenterally. Today, the preparation of choice is cyanocobalamin, which is cheaper and which causes less discomfort at the site of injection than liver. Oral cyanocobalamin, of course, like liver, optimally requires a source of intrinsic factor.

For the patient with uncomplicated pernicious anemia in relapse, the initial dose of cyanocobalamin is 30 μg a day, parenterally, or every other day for 5 to 10 doses, followed by 15 to 30 μg once or twice a week until the blood picture is normal. For maintenance; 40 to 60 μg every 2 weeks or 80 to 100 μg once a month is usually adequate. If there is demonstrable neurological damage, it may be necessary to administer 1000 μg a week for several months before switching to the maintenance schedule. Therapy must be maintained for life, since the basic deficiency in gastrointestinal physiology remains. Nevertheless, the patient may be kept in good health and may lead a fairly normal life.

Despite the superiority of cyanocobalamin, liver and stomach preparations still are available. The ingestion of 200 to 400 g of whole liver may be effective irregularly in inducing a remission in pernicious anemia. Concentrates for oral administration are made from such amounts of liver, but concentration results in some loss of activity. Extracts suitable for parenteral administration may be prepared from 10 to 15 g of liver. Similar effects may be produced by the ingestion of 30 to 40 g of desiccated stomach; however, the combinations of stomach and liver are required for optimal oral therapy.

Liver preparations for injection may be assayed microbiologically, employing *Lactobacillus leichmannii* ATCC 7830, the assay being expressed in terms of cyanocobalamin. However, since oral preparations rarely are effective, owing to the absence of the intrinsic factor, the assay must be made in the human pernicious anemia patient in relapse, and the assay is expressed in terms of oral units. This reflects the ridiculousness of using archaic and irregularly effective preparations when the active ingredient, cyanocobalamin, or derivatives, readily is available and is administered more easily and safely.

Megaloblastic anemia of infancy, megaloblastic anemia of pregnancy, achrestic anemia and nutritional macrocytic anemia generally respond better to liver preparations than they do to cyanocobalamin, and deficiencies in *folic* and *folinic acid* intake or metabolism are implicated; thus, either of these two acids may evoke a dramatic response in such anemias. Ascorbic acid also occasionally may confer additional benefits. The metabolic functions of folic or folinic acid and vitamin B_{12} converge in certain respects. Thus, folic or folinic acid may induce a remission in the blood pathology in pernicious anemia, but it will not revert or delay the progression of the epithelial and neurological pathology, which may develop insidiously and emerge explosively and irreversibly. Therefore, folic or folinic acid therapy of pernicious anemia is to be condemned. *Equally offensive and irresponsible is the inclusion of these acids in liver or multivitamin-hematinic preparations* because, in allaying the blood pathology of undiagnosed pernicious anemia, they prevent detection of the disease until the neurological pathology has advanced to a dangerous state. Unfortified liver preparations also may contain enough folic acid to constitute the same danger. *In general, a hematinic should be employed only upon accurate diagnosis of the anemia and upon specific indication.* Multiple preparations are to be avoided. For descriptions of cyanocobalamin, hydroxocobalamin and folic acid; see Chapter 65.

Hematopoietic Growth Factors

The hematopoietic growth factors regulate the proliferation and differentiation of progenitor stem cells found in the bone marrow. They are glycoproteins which bind to specific cell surface receptors resulting in a sequential series of events culminating in hematopoiesis. Recombinant DNA technology has allowed the manufacture of sufficient quantities of these factors thus enabling clinical trials in patients. Erythropoietin which stimulates red blood cell production was the first human hematopoietic growth factor to be isolated and studied. It improves the anemia associated with several clinical conditions. Several of the colony-stimulating factors also have been purified, molecularly cloned and expressed as recombinant proteins. Clinical trials are in progress evaluating their effectiveness in treating patients for a variety of hematological disorders (refer to Appendix A in Chapter 49). Two of the colony-stimulating factors, granulocyte colony stimulating factor (G-CSF) and granulocyte-macrophage colony stimulating factor (GM-CSF) are efficacious in the management of bone marrow hypoplasia particularly after myelosuppressive chemotherapy. They not only stimulate the progenitor cell target but also result in some functional activation of the mature cell. It is anticipated that future therapy will use additional hematopoietic growth factors in various conditions involving altered hematological status.

Epoetin Alfa

1-165-Erythropoietin (human clone λHEPOFL 13 protein moiety), glycoform α; Epogen (*Amgen*); Procrit (*Ortho*)

[113427-24-0] $C_{809}H_{1301}N_{229}O_{240}S_5$ (34,400 ± 400) A 165 amino acid glycoprotein produced by Chinese hamster ovary cells into which the human erythropoietin gene has been incorporated.

Uses—Erythropoietin, a naturally occurring glycoprotein, stimulates the division and differentiation of erythroid progenitors in the bone marrow resulting in red blood cell production. The kidney is the major source of erythropoietin in adults. Epoietin alfa stimulates erythropoiesis in chronic renal failure (CRF) patients who are anemic due to impairment of their endogenous erythropoietin production. It is effective in both patients on dialysis and those not requiring regular dialysis. As it requires several days for erythroid progenitors to mature and be released into blood, a clinically significant increase in hematocrit generally is not observed before 2 wk. The treatment goal is to increase hematocrit to 30 to 33% and eliminate the need for blood transfusions. The rate of hematocrit increase depends on several factors including availability of iron stores, baseline hematocrit, concurrent medical problems and the dose administered. For reasons discussed below, a rapid increase in hematocrit (eg, > 4 points in any 2-wk period) is undesirable. Epoetin alfa also is indicated for treatment of anemias related to zidovudine (AZT) therapy in HIV-infected patients who have endogeneous erythropoietin levels < 500 mU/mL and are receiving < 4200 mg a wk of AZT. Patients with endogenous erythropoietin levels > 500 mU/mL do not appear to have a clinically significant response with epoetin alfa.

Prior to, and during therapy, the patient's iron stores should be evaluated and transferrin saturation should be at least 20% and ferritin at least 100 ng/mL. Supplemental iron may be required to increase and maintain transferrin saturation to adequate levels. Epoetin alfa therapy has been associated with increased blood pressure in many CRF patients. Blood pressure should be controlled adequately prior to administration of the drug, and must be monitored closely and controlled during therapy. During the time when hematocrit is increasing, approximately 25% of dialysis patients require initiation of, or increases in, antihypertensive medication. The dose of drug should be decreased in patients with an excessive rate of hematocrit rise (eg, > 4 points in any 2-wk period) as this rapid increase may exacerbate the hypertensive response. Epoetin alfa is contraindicated in patients with uncontrolled hypertension or known hypersensitivity to either mammalian cell-derived products or human albumin. During hemodialysis, patients on this drug may require increased anticoagulation with heparin to prevent clotting of the artificial kidney.

Dose—In *CRF patients*, initially **50** to **100 U/kg** 3 times a wk is usually effective in increasing hematocrit and eliminating transfusion dependency. The dose should be increased if the hematocrit is not increased by 5 to 6 points after 8 wk of therapy. The dose should be reduced when the hematocrit reaches the target range or if the rate of rise is too rapid. When the hematocrit reaches 30 to 33%, the dosage should be decreased by 25 U/kg 3 times a wk with the maintenance dose individualized for each patient. In *HIV-infected patients*, initially **100 U/kg** 3 times a wk is recommended. If the response is not satisfactory in increasing hematocrit and reducing the transfusion requirements, the dose may be adjusted by 50 to 100 U/kg increments 3 times a wk. During the dose-adjustment period, the hematocrit should be monitored weekly. If the patient doesn't respond adequately to 300 U/kg 3 times a wk, higher doses are not likely to be effective. The drug is administered either as an intravenous or subcutaneous injection. In patients on dialysis, it may be administered into the venous line at the end of the dialysis procedure.

Dosage Form—Injection: Sterile solution in a single-use vial containing 2,000, 3,000, 4,000 or 10,000 U/1 mL.

Filgrastim

Colony-stimulating factor (human clone 1034), *N*-L-methionyl-, Neupogen (*Amgen*)

[121181-53-1] $C_{845}H_{1339}N_{223}O_{243}S_9$ (18,000.00). A single chain of 175 aminoacids, nonglycosylated, produced by recombinant DNA technology, expressed by *E coli*.

Uses—Granulocyte colony stimulating factor (G-CSF) is an endogenous glycoprotein which acts primarily on hematopoietic cells regulating the production of neutrophils within the bone marrow. It is effective in accelerating the recovery of neutrophil counts following a variety of chemotherapy regimens. In addition to regulating the production of neutrophils, G-CSF also enhances neutrophil functional activity including enhanced phagocytic ability, priming of the cellular metabolism associated with respiratory burst and antibody-dependent killing. It is indicated to decrease the incidence of infection in patients with nonmyeloid malignancies receiving myelosuppressive anticancer drugs. Such patients experience a significant incidence of severe neutropenia with fever. Because of the potential sensitivity of rapidly dividing myeloid cells to cytotoxic agents, it should not be used 24 hr prior to, or within 24 hr after, chemotherapy. It is essential to obtain complete blood counts and platelet counts prior to the chemotherapy, and twice a wk during treatment with filgrastim. A transient increase in the neutrophil count typically occurs within the first 1 or 2 days following administration of filgrastim; however, for a sustained therapeutic effect it should be continued until the postchemotherapy nadir count reaches 10,000/mm^3. Medullary bone pain of mild to moderate severity is the major adverse effect and occurs in approximately 24% of patients. It is most frequent in patients treated with higher doses (20 to 100 μg/kg/day) administered IV, and reported less in patients treated with lower SC doses (3 to 10 μg/kg/day). Although filgrastim is a growth factor which primarily stimulates neutrophils, it could potentially act as a growth factor for tumor cells and caution should be used if this drug is administered in any malignancy with myeloid characteristics. It is contraindicated in patients with known hypersensitivity to *E coli*-derived proteins.

Dose—*Subcutaneous* or *intravenous*, initially **5 μg/kg/day** administered as a single daily dose. It should be given daily for up to 2 wk until the absolute neutrophil count has reached 10,000/mm^3 after the expected chemotherapy-induced nadir. The duration of therapy primarily depends upon the myelosuppressive potential of the chemotherapeutic regiment administered. Doses may be increased in increments of 5 μg/kg for each chemotherapy cycle depending on the extent of neutrophil depression. It should be discontinued if the absolute neutrophil count exceeds 10,000/mm^3 after the expected chemotherapy-induced nadir.

Dosage Form—Injection: 300 μg/mL in single-dose vials of 1.0 and 1.6 mL.

Sargramostim

Colony-stimulating factor 2 (human clone pHG$_{25}$ protein moiety), 23-L-leucine-, rhu GM-CSF; Leukine (*Immunex*); Prokine (*Hoechst-Roussel*)

[123774-72-1] $C_{639}H_{1002}N_{168}O_{196}S_8$ (15,500 to 19,500). A single chain of 127 aminoacids, glycosylated, produced by recombinant DNA technology, expressed from *Saccharomyces cerevisiae*. There are three species having approx molecular weights of 19,500, 16,800 and 15,500 daltons, depending on the extent of glycosylation.

Description—White lyophilized powder.

Uses—Granulocyte-macrophage colony stimulating factor (GM-CSF) is an endogenous multipotential hematopoietic growth factor which stimulates proliferation and differentiation of both early and late progenitor cells resulting in increases in granulocytes and macrophages. It is indicated for accelerating myeloid engraftment in autologous bone marrow transplantation (BMT) in patients with non-Hodgkin's lymphoma, acute lymphoblastic leukemia and Hodgkin's disease. It is effective in decreasing median duration of antibiotic therapy, reducing duration of infectious episodes and shortening the median duration of hospitalization in these patients. It also is indicated for patients who have undergone allogeneic or autologous BMT in whom engraftment is delayed or has failed. In these patients, sargramostim is safe and effective in prolonging survival in both the presence or absence of infection. Hematological response to therapy should be assessed twice a week by CBC with differential. Sargramostim can induce WBC increases, and treatment should be interrupted or the dose reduced if excessive leukocytosis occurs (WBC > 50,000 cells/mm^3; absolute neutrophil count more than 20,000 mm^3). It is contraindicated in patients with excessive (more than 10%) leukemic myeloid blasts in the bone marrow or peripheral blood or known hypersensitivity to yeast-derived products. Adverse effects include peripheral edema and a capillary leak syndrome, and it should be used with caution in patients with pre-existing fluid retention, congestive heart failure or pulmonary infiltrates. Because of the potential for promoting tumor growth, precaution is necessary when using this drug in any malignancy with myeloid characteristics.

Dose—For *myeloid reconstitution after autologous BMT*, **250 μg/m^2/day** for 21 days as a 2-hr IV infusion starting 2 to 4 hr after the bone-marrow infusion and not less than 24 hr after the last dose of chemotherapy and 12 hr after the last dose of radiotherapy. For *bone marrow transplantation failure* or *engraftment delay*, **250 μg/m^2/day** for 14 days as a 2-hr IV infusion. The dose can be repeated after 7 days off therapy if engraftment has not occurred, which may be followed after another 7 days off therapy with a third drug course of **500 μg/m^2/day** for 14 days. If engraftment is still unsuccesful, it is unlikely that additional drug administration will be beneficial. If blast cells appear or disease progression occurs, treatment should be discontinued. If excessive leukocytosis occurs, treatment should be interrupted or the dose reduced by half.

Dosage Form—Injection: Lyophilized powder in single-use vials of 250 or 500 μg which are reconstituted with 1 mL Sterile Water for Injection.

Antihematopoietic Drugs

Polycythemia and erythrocytosis are conditions in which there is an increase in the number of circulating erythrocytes. The cause is usually the result of a deficient oxygenation of the arterial blood, and either condition may be corrected by management of the underlying primary disorder. However, in *polycythemia rubra vera* the condition is primary, and therapy thus is directed at the erythrocytes, either by their removal by venesection, their destruction by phenylhydrazines or the suppression of their formation by antihematopoietic drugs or by X-irradiation. Several of the antineoplastic drugs such as the nitrogen mustards, the antifolic acids, arsenicals or radiophosphate may be employed. The *leukemias* result from excessive leukocytic hematopoietic activity of a neoplastic nature; either the bone marrow (myelogenous or granulocytic leukemia) or lymphatic tissue (lymphocytic leukemia) may be involved. In myelogenous leukemia there may be anemia because the erythropoietic cells are crowded out by leukopoietic cells. Drugs used in the therapy of the leukemias and polycythemia are treated in Chapter 75.

Miscellaneous Drugs Affecting Blood

Hemin

Ferrate(2-), chloro[7,12-diethenyl-3,8,13,17-tetramethyl-21*H*,23*H*-porphine-2,18-dipropanoato(4-)-N^{21}, N^{22}, N^{23}, N^{24}]-, dihydrogen-, (*SP*-5-13).

Chlorohemin[16009-13-5] $C_{34}H_{32}ClFeN_4O_4$ (651.96).

Preparation—Usually from hemoglobin by treatment with a hot saline acetic acid solution. *Org Syn Coll Vol III:* 442, 1955.

Description—Polychromatic crystals (usually brownish to blue) which do not melt under 300°.

Solubility—Freely soluble in dilute base through conversion to *hematin* by replacement of the chlorine atom by hydroxyl; sparingly soluble in alcohol; insoluble in water.

Uses—Inhibits the biosynthesis of porphyrin in juvenile erythrocytes and hence also indirectly decreases the rate of formation of porphyrins. It is used to ameliorate symptoms in *intermittent porphyria, porphyria variegata* and hereditary *coproporphyria*. In some but not all patients pain, tachycardia, hypertension, mild to moderate neurological impairment and abnormal mentation are abated. Neurological improvement is sometimes delayed weeks to months after treatment. Remissions are not permanent.

It is contraindicated in hypersensitivity to itself and in porphyria cutanea tarda. Excessive doses may cause renal failure. Phlebitis may occur in the injected vein. Coagulopathy and renal failure from an overdose have been reported. It may be antagonized by barbiturates, estrogens and various steroid metabolites which induce aminolevulinate synthesis.

It is converted partially to bilirubin and partially excreted into the bile intact. Bilirubin metabolites and urobilinogen also appear in the urine.

Dose—*Intravenous infusion* into large high-flow vein, **1** to **4 mg/kg** over a 10- to 15-min period once a day for 3 to 14 days. In severe cases, the dose may be repeated at 12-hr intervals, not to exceed 6 mg/kg/day.

Dosage Form—Powder for Injection: 313 mg to be reconstituted to 43 mL with sterile water (makes 7 mg/mL).

Methylene Blue

Phenothiazin-5-ium, 3,7-bis(dimethylamino)-, chloride, trihydrate; Methylthionine Chloride; Aniline Violet

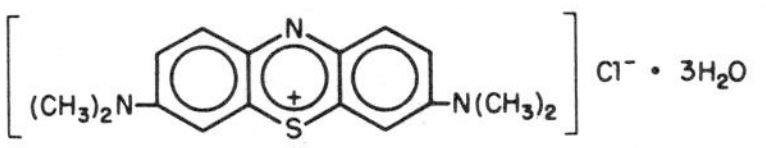

C I Basic Blue 9 trihydrate [7220-79-3] $C_{16}H_{18}ClN_3S.3H_2O$ (373.90); *anhydrous* [61-73-4] (319.85).

Preparation—By treating a solution of *N,N*-dimethyl-*p*-phenylenediamine and *N,N*-dimethylaniline hydrochlorides with H_2S and $FeCl_3$ or another suitable oxidizing agent.

Description—Dark green crystals or a crystalline powder, having a bronze-like luster; odorless or having a slight odor; stable in air; solutions have a deep-blue color.

Solubility—1 g in 25 mL water or 65 mL alcohol; soluble in chloroform.

Uses—Readily reduced to leukomethylene blue, which, in turn, is readily reoxidized to methylene blue. Thus, it is useful as a reversible *oxidation–reduction* indicator. Its principal therapeutic use, in the *treatment of methemoglobinemia*, stems from this chemical property. It acts as an electron-acceptor in the transfer of electrons from reduced pyridine nucleotides (NADPH and NATPH) to methemoglobin, thus facilitating reduction of ferric to ferrous iron. Glucose 6-phosphate dehydrogenase is required; if this enzyme is absent, as it is in certain hemolysis-prone individuals, the drug is ineffective. If the dose is high, the oxidation potential favors the formation of methemoglobin from hemoglobin. This effect is used in the *treatment of cyanide poisoning*. The methemoglobin so formed complexes cyanide, which tends to spare the cytochrome system. However, other drugs are superior.

This drug formerly was employed as a urinary antibacterial agent, but this use is now obsolete. An outgrowth of this use is the belief that the drug is effective in the treatment of urolithiasis. Although a slight effect to retard crystal formation *in vitro* has been reported, no clinical benefits have been proven, and expert opinion holds the dye to be ineffective. Its use as an analgetic, antipyretic and parasiticide has likewise been abandoned. The dye is used as a bacteriologic stain.

It colors urine and feces green and the skin blue. It may cause bladder irritation, nausea, vomiting and diarrhea. Large doses may cause vertigo, headache, confusion, sweating methemoglobinemia (paradoxical) and chest and abdominal pains. It can cause hemolysis in persons with glucose-6-phosphate dehydrogenase-deficient erythrocytes.

Dose—*Oral*, for chronic *idiopathic methemoglobinemia*, **65** to **130 mg** with a full glass of water after meals 3 times a day, in conjunction with large doses of ascorbic acid; for *urolithiasis* (but see comments above), **65 mg** 2 or 3 times a day; for *urinary antisepsis*, **55 to 130 mg** with a full glass of water 3 times a day after meals. *Intravenous*, for *drug-induced* or *toxic methemoglobinemia*, **1** to **2 mg/kg**, and for *cyanide poisoning*, **500 mg** (50 mL of 1% solution).

Dosage Forms—Injection: 10 mg/1 mL and 100 mg/10 mL; Tablets: 55 and 65 mg.

Pentoxifylline

1*H*-Purine-2,6-dione, 3,7-dihydro-3,7-dimethyl-1-(5-oxohexyl)-, Trental (*Hoechst-Roussel*)

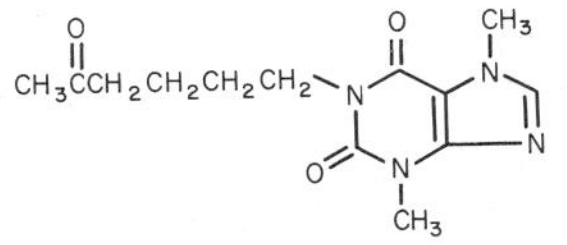

1-(5-Oxohexyl)theobromine [6493-05-6] $C_{13}H_{18}N_4O_3$ (278.31).

Preparation—Ethyl acetoacetate and 1,3-dibromopropane are reacted to form the ethyl ester of 3*H*-dihydropyran-3-carboxylic acid, which is cleaved with HBr to form 6-bromo-2-hexanone. This latter compound, with theobromine, in the presence of base yields pentoxifylline.

Description—Bitter-tasting, colorless, odorless needles; melts about 105°.

Solubility—1 g in 13 mL water at 25° or in 5.5 mL at 37°; 1 g in 9 mL benzene.

Uses—Increases the ATP content of erythrocytes, which makes them both more deformable and less likely to aggregate. Consequently, they pass through precapillary sphincters and capillaries more easily, which improves blood flow through the microcirculation. It also stimulates the synthesis of prostacyclin by endothelial cells and inhibits phosphodiesterase activity (thus increasing cyclic AMP levels) in platelets; these two actions decrease the aggregation of platelets. It increases fibrinolytic activity and thus decreases fibrinogen concentration. These effects sum to decrease the viscosity of blood, which increases blood flow and decreases myocardial work. It is approved for the treatment of *intermittent claudication*. It is also investigational in the management of cerebrovascular insufficiency, transient ischemic attacks, stroke, diabetic angiopathy, sickle cell thallasemia and leg ulcers.

Adverse effects are dyspepsia (2.8%), nausea (2.2%), vomiting (1.2%), bloating (0.6%), belching, flatus, anorexia, dry mouth, thirst, constipation and cholecystitis; dizziness (1.9%), headache (1.2%), tremor (0.3%), anxiety and confusion; anginal pain (0.3%), hypotension and edema; blurred vision, conjunctivitis and scotomata; dyspnea, flu-like symptoms, laryngitis, nasal congestion and nose- bleeds; brittle fingernails, pruritis, rash and urticaria; earache, leukopenia, malaise, sialorrhea, bad taste, sore throat and swollen neck lymph glands, and change in weight; dysrhythmias, hepatitis and jaundice, hyperfibrinogenemia, pancytopenia, purpura and thrombocytopenia are rare effects.

It is absorbed readily and first-pass metabolized by the oral route. Peak plasma levels occur in 2 to 4 hr. There are more than five metabolites, two of which probably have pharmacodynamic activity. The elimination half-life is only about 0.4 to 0.8 hr, but that of the major metabolites is 1 to 1.6 hr.

Dose—*Oral, adults,* **400 mg** 3 times a day with meals, unless there are persistent gastrointestinal side effects, in which case only twice a day.

Dosage Form—Tablets: 400 mg.

Sodium Nitrite

Sodium nitrite [7632-00-0] $NaNO_2$ (69.00).

Preparation—By various methods, as by reduction of sodium nitrate with lead, a sulfite or sulfur dioxide, or by absorption of NO obtained from catalytic oxidation of ammonia in sodium carbonate solution.

Description—White to slightly yellow, granular powder or white or nearly white, opaque, fused masses or sticks; deliquescent in air; solutions are alkaline to litmus.

Solubility—1 g in 1.5 mL water; sparingly soluble in alcohol.

Uses—Principally for treating of *cyanide poisoning,* based on its causing methemoglobin, which complexes cyanide. In cyanide poisoning, it is injected intravenously in very large doses to produce methemoglobin, which combines with the highly lethal cyanide and renders it temporarily inactive as cyanmethemoglobin. Sodium thiosulfate (RPS-16, page 1176) then is injected intravenously to form the nontoxic thiocyanate. Nitrite ion relaxes smooth muscle, so that sodium nitrite causes hypotension. Solutions are unstable and should be prepared directly before use.

Dose—*Intravenous, adults,* **10 mL** of **3%** solution, given at a rate of 2.5 to 5 mL/min; *pediatric,* **0.2 mL** of **3%** solution/**kg** (or 6 to 8 mL/m^2), not to exceed 10 mL.

CHAPTER 55

Cardiovascular Drugs

Donald N Franz, PhD
Professor of Pharmacology
University of Utah School of Medicine
Salt Lake City, UT 84132

Any drug that affects the heart or blood vessels, directly or indirectly, is a cardiovascular drug, although the term generally connotes only those drugs which are used for their cardiovascular actions. Many such drugs exist. Nearly every autonomic drug has clinically applicable cardiovascular actions.

Sympathomimetics (see Chapter 57) may be used to elevate blood pressure, stimulate the heart, slow the heart reflexly, etc, depending on the particular agents and the clinical conditions.

α-Adrenergic blocking drugs (see Chapter 59) may be used in vasospastic conditions, in the diagnosis and management of pheochromocytoma and, rarely, in malignant and toxemic hypertensive crises.

β-Adrenergic blocking drugs (Chapter 59) are employed in the treatment of essential hypertension, portal hypertension, angina pectoris and certain dysrhythmias.

The anticholinesterase, edrophonium (page 1005), is used in the diagnosis and treatment of paroxysmal atrial tachycardia.

Atropine and other *antimuscarinic drugs* (see Chapter 60) may be used to block the cardiac vagus nerve in Adams-Stokes syndrome and certain other bradycardias.

The *ganglionic blocking agents* are treated in this chapter.

A large number of drugs other than the autonomic agents have useful cardiovascular actions.

Digitalis and its allies, the *coronary* and *peripheral dilators*, and the *antidysrhythmic agents* are included below.

Parenteral fluids (see Chapter 54), which may be used in the treatment of shock, and *diuretics* (see Chapter 62), which are adjuvants in the treatment of heart failure and hypertension, are discussed elsewhere, as are numerous miscellaneous drugs.

Antihypertensive and Hypotensive Drugs

Antihypertensive drugs are used in the treatment of hypertension, although certain ones (eg, ganglionic blocking drugs) enjoy scattered uses in other therapeutic, diagnostic and surgical procedures. Some are used as hypotensive drugs in nonhypertensive patients. The predominant types of diastolic hypertension are primary (essential, idiopathic) and secondary hypertension. Malignant hypertension is a severe, progressive phase of primary hypertension. There is no universal therapy for primary hypertension, and individual cases vary widely in response to various drugs.

Evidence today suggests that there may be a sympathetic factor in some types of hypertension formerly classified as diastolic or essential hypertension. The sympathetic neural influence is exerted both directly on blood vessels and on the renin-producing system in the kidney. Irrespective of whether there is an abnormal sympathetic neural factor involved, removal of the normal sympathetic nervous support of vascular tone and cardiac output usually decreases blood pressure in the hypertensive person and favors a retardation of the progression of the disease.

The role of the renin-angiotensin system (see page 949) in the pathogenesis of essential hypertension and in the antihypertensive actions of various drugs is compelling. Clinical studies alone indicate that the renin-angiotensin system is hyperactive in less than one-third of the cases of essential hypertension, but the effects of converting-enzyme inhibitors and antagonists of angiotensin indicate that the renin-angiotensin system is involved in at least 70% of cases of essential hypertension. It is possible that the effect of sundry antihypertensive drugs to decrease plasma renin activity contributes importantly to their efficacy.

The therapy of diastolic hypertension has been improving since 1958 because of the large number of agents introduced since then. The finding that the diuretic chlorothiazide (see page 1044) not only is mildly antihypertensive but also greatly potentiates the antihypertensive effects of other drugs initiated a revolution in the medical management of hypertension. Closely following chlorothiazide came reserpine and guanethidine, (see page 1018), and later alpha-methyldopa and clonidine, β-antagonists, angiotensin converting enzyme (ACE) inhibitors and calcium channel blockers.

At the present time in the US expert opinion holds that in young persons, a diastolic blood pressure over 90 torr is an indication for treatment and in persons over 35 years of age, 95 torr. Long-term studies have proved unequivocally that treatment both decreases morbidity and prolongs life expectancy. Formerly, the first drug to be used was a thiazide diuretic, but it now appears that therapy may just as well be initiated with β-antagonists, ACE inhibitors or calcium channel blockers as single agents in early hypertension. If no single drug is effective alone, two from different classes are used in combination. In mild hypertension, the first drugs to be added to a thiazide are β-blockers, ACE inhibitors or calcium entry blockers. In moderate hypertension, hydralazine, α_1-antagonists or centrally acting drugs may be added. Since β-adrenergic blockers and converting enzyme inhibitors decrease angiotensin II levels, they are indicated whenever renin levels are high and possibly even when they are normal. β-Blockers also are combined commonly with vasodilators, such as hydralazine, to prevent reflex tachycardia and stimulation of renin secretion. Diazoxide, sodium nitroprusside, captopril or hydralazine and, to a lesser extent, trimethaphan are employed in the treatment of hypertensive crises, such as eclampsia.

It is difficult to anticipate how and when treatment of hypertension will stabilize. Currently, converting enzyme inhibitors, β-antagonists, calcium channel blockers and α_1-blockers dominate the field; the diuretics will remain essential; there has been a marked decline in use of guanethidine, reserpine, methyldopa and clonidine; hydralazine will be used mainly as a tertiary drug for resistant cases, usually with a β-antagonist and a diuretic.

Saluretics

It long has been suspected that certain hypertensive persons have abnormal salt metabolism, and epidemiological and endemiological studies have established a relationship between salt intake and blood pressure. In the essential and malignant hypertensive individual with an expanded blood volume and high sodium burden, the rationale for use of saluretic drugs is almost self-evident. However, certain saluretic drugs even have been found to lower blood pressure of persons with essential hypertension who have small extracellular fluid volumes.

It is held widely that the vascular smooth muscles in such persons have a high intracellular sodium content. When thiazide saluretics are given, the fall in blood pressure in the first week or two correlates with saluresis and the decrement in extracellular fluid volume (hence, in venous return, stroke output and systolic blood pressure). In this phase, heart rate is accelerated and peripheral resistance is increased. The antihypertensive action passes into a phase in which the extracellular volume and heart rate return toward normal and peripheral resistance falls. Not all saluretics are alike in this effect, which suggests that something more than saluresis is involved. For example, high-ceiling saluretics never lower the vascular resistance, and blood pressure is lowered only because cardiac output is decreased. Spironolactone is a useful antihypertensive agent only when aldosterone or 18-hydroxycorticosterone levels are high.

Homeostatic mechanisms increase plasma renin activity which counterproductively increase plasma levels of the potent endogenous vasoconstrictor, angiotensin II. If they were available, drugs that inhibit renin secretion would be rational agents to combine with saluretics.

At present, thiazide-like saluretics often are the first drugs to be used in the treatment of essential hypertension, customarily being used alone in mild essential hypertension; other drugs are added in moderate and severe essential hypertensions. Thiazides also are correctives for the counterproductive salt and water retention that occurs as side effects to most other antihypertensive drugs. High-ceiling diuretics are inappropriate for general use and should be used only in congestive heart failure, in renal impairment in hypertensive emergencies in which salt and water have accumulated, or in combinations with drugs in which salt and water retention are especially severe (eg, methyldopa, minoxidil, hydralazine).

For the pharmacology of specific saluretics, see Chapter 62.

Peripheral Antiadrenergic Drugs

Regardless of whether there is a sympathetic component in the perpetuation of essential or malignant hypertension, a reduction of whatever sympathetic activity exists can effect a lowering of blood pressure four ways.

A decrease in sympathetically (α_1-receptor)-mediated arteriolar constriction will decrease systemic peripheral resistance.

A decrease in sympathetically (α_1-receptor)-mediated venous tone will increase venous capacitance, decrease venous return and, hence, cardiac output. However, this effect tends not to be sustained in the long run because of compensation by fluid retention.

A decrease in sympathetically (β_1-receptor)-mediated support of cardiac contractility and heart rate will decrease cardiac output.

A decrease in sympathetically (β_1-receptor)-modulated secretion of renin by the juxtaglomerular apparatus of the kidney will decrease the plasma levels of angiotensin II, a potent vasoconstrictor and sensitizer to sympathetic nervous activity and stimulant of the secretion of aldosterone, an antisaluretic hormone.

Drugs such as reserpine and guanethidine, which act on adrenergic nerve terminals to deplete norepinephrine or prevent release of norepinephrine, potentially are antihypertensive by all four ways, although their actions are not exerted evenly throughout the sympathetic nervous system, and the heart may be affected more than the vessels, etc. α-Adrenoreceptor blocking drugs, such as phenoxybenzamine and phentolamine, have antihypertensive actions, but reflex cardiac stimulation and increased renin secretion limit their efficacy. However, both phenoxybenzamine and phentolamine are important antihypertensives in the treatment of pheochromocytoma. By a selectivity for only α_1-receptors, prazosin causes less of such counterproductive homeostatic adjustments and hence is more efficacious. β-Adrenoreceptor blocking drugs, such as propranolol, act to decrease cardiac output and renin secretion. However, they reflexly increase sympathetic activity and hence peripheral vascular resistance. Nevertheless, they not only are effective alone but also are important adjuncts to vasodilator drugs, which cause reflex sympathetic cardiac stimulation and increased renin secretion, and to diuretics, which increase renin secretion. β-Adrenoreceptor antagonists also have actions at the adrenergic nerve terminals to decrease norepinephrine release. Newer drugs, such as labetolol, with both α- and β-adrenoreceptor blocking activity possibly may change considerably the treatment of essential hypertension, since blockade of one type of receptor cannot result in counteractive reflex activation of the other.

The important antihypertensive α- and β- adrenoreceptor blocking drugs and drugs which act on the adrenergic nerve terminals are described in Chapter 59, *Adrenergic and Adrenergic Neuron Blocking Drugs:* Acebutolol, Atenolol, Guanadrel, Guanethidine, Labetelol, Nadolol, Metoprolol, Phenoxybenzamine, Phentolamine, Pindolol, Propranalol, Reserpine and Timolol.

Doxazosin Mesylate—page 1010.
Prazosin Hydrochloride—page 1010.
Terazosin Hydrochloride—page 1011.

Centrally Acting Antihypertensive Drugs

Several drugs act directly or indirectly on the vasomotor center and in the spinal cord to decrease sympathetic outflow to the blood vessels and heart. They also activate the parasympathetic (vagal) outflow to the heart. Less is known about central inhibition of outflow to the juxtaglomerular apparatus, but the clinically significant drugs of this class all decrease plasma renin activity. Only clonidine, guanabenz, guanfacine, methyldopa and methyldopate are described in this section. There is no rationale for using more than one of these drugs at a time.

The various sedative and antianxiety drugs never have been shown to have antihypertensive actions, although it might seem that a salutary effect on the progression of the reactive stage of early essential hypertension should accrue to their use. Nevertheless, the pharmaceutical industry has convinced a large proportion of the medical profession that sedatives are important adjuvants to antihypertensive treatment, and it is too common to prescribe an "antianxiety" drug (phenobarbital or a benzodiazepine) along with antihypertensive drugs.

Clonidine Hydrochloride

2-(2,6-Dichlorophenylamino)-2-imidazoline hydrochloride;
Catapres (*Boehringer Ingelheim*)

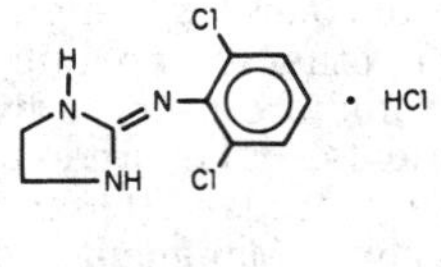

Cl
H
N
N
NH
Cl
· HCl

[4205-91-8] $C_9H_9Cl_2N_3.HCl$ (266.56).

Preparation—Ammonium thiocyanate converts 2,6-dichloroaniline to the thiourea which is treated with methyl iodide to yield the *S*-methylthiuronium salt. The latter compound, with ethylene diamine, closes the imidazoline ring to afford the product. See US Pat 3,202,660.

Description—White to off-white, odorless, bitter-tasting, crystalline powder; stable in light, air and heat; does not exhibit polymorphism; melts about 300° with decomposition; pK_a 8.2.

Solubility—1 g in about 13 mL water (20°), about 25 mL alcohol or about 5000 mL chloroform.

Uses—An antihypertensive drug used in the treatment of moderate *primary* (essential) *hypertension*. It also is used in the treatment of *postmenopausal vasomotor instability, dysmenorrhea* and in the prophylaxis of *migraine* and *cluster headaches*. It suppresses opiate, alcohol, benzodiazepine and tobacco craving and withdrawal symptoms and is an investigational drug in the management of *opiate addiction*. The antihypertensive actions are, in part, a central action. A decrease in sympathetic activity causes vasodilation, bradycardia and occasional atrioventricular block, and a decrease in renin release from the kidney; an increase in vagal activity also causes bradycardia.

The central actions, in part, appear to be the result of a stimulant action on α_2-adrenergic receptors in the vasomotor and cardioinhibitory centers, and in the spinal cord on preganglionic sympathetic neurons. It also appears to have a peripheral action to reduce release of norepinephrine from sympathetic nerves. It stimulates α_2-adrenergic receptors on the sympathetic nerve terminals, which stimulation feeds back negatively to suppress release of the mediator.

In moderate doses it causes sedation in about 65% of patients, dry mouth in about 50% and mild to moderate orthostatic hypotension in about 25%. Salt and water retention occur in the first few days of treatment but usually do not persist. Impotence, defective ejaculation, constipation, anorexia, nausea and vomiting, dry, itchy eyes, painful salivary glands, depression and nightmares also occur in less than 5% of recipients. Various side effects secondary to excessive reductions in blood pressure can occur, as with most antihypertensive drugs. Tolerance sometimes occurs, usually a result of fluid retention which can be overcome by adding a diuretic. The transdermal preparation commonly causes skin irritation; application sites should be rotated.

Serious rebound hypertension may occur if the drug is discontinued abruptly. It is somewhat fetotoxic in laboratory animals and, hence, should be avoided in pregnancy. Tricyclic antidepressants antagonize its antihypertensive actions. Clonidine increases ethanol-induced CNS depression.

It is absorbed readily by the oral route, with an absorption time of 2 to 4 hr. It is excreted mostly unchanged into the urine. The half-life is 12 to 16 hr. The duration of action is 6 to 10 hr. The transdermal patch dosage form releases drug at a constant rate for longer than a week. It provides a more stable control of blood pressure than do tablets and side effects are less severe.

Dose—For *mild* to *moderate* essential *hypertension, initially* **0.1 mg** twice a day, followed by gradual adjustments in increments of 0.1 to 0.2 mg a day until the desired effect occurs; *maintenance* doses usually range from **0.2** to **0.8 mg** a day; *severe hypertension, initially* **0.2 mg** then **0.1 mg** every hour until the blood pressure is controlled or 0.7 mg have been given; for *vasomotor instability,* **25** to **75 µg** (0.025 to 0.075 mg) twice a day; for severe *dysmenorrhea,* **25 µg** (0.025 mg) twice a day 2 wk before and during menses; for *migraine,* **25 µg** 2 to 4 times a day to **50 µg** 3 times a day. *Transdermal, adult,* **1 system/wk** which delivers 0.1, 0.2, or 0.3 mg a day; dosage adjustments are made at 1- or 2-wk intervals, if necessary, by applying larger systems.

Dosage Forms—Tablets: 0.1, 0.2 and 0.3 mg; Transdermal system: 2.5, 5 and 7.5 mg (to deliver 0.10, 0.20 and 0.30 mg/day, respectively, for 1 week).

Guanabenz Acetate

Guanidine, (2,6-dichlorobenzylidene)amino)-, acetate;
Wytensin (*Wyeth*)

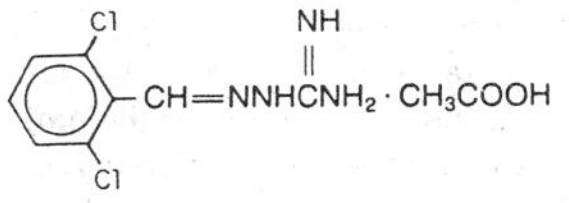

[23256-50-0] $C_8H_8Cl_2N_4.C_2H_4O_2$ (291.14).

Preparation—Brit Pat 1,019,120.

Description—White solid; melts about 193° (dec).

Solubility—1 g in 90 mL water, 20 mL alcohol or 10 mL propylene glycol

Uses—Depresses the vasomotor and cardioaccelerator centers and thus decreases the sympathetic outflow to the arterioles and heart. It acts as an α_2-adrenergic agonist at cardiovascular centers in the medulla and spinal cord as does clonidine. It is effective in mild to moderately severe essential hypertension. Although it usually is effective alone, efficacy is enhanced by saluretics. The half-life is 7 to 10 hr. It causes a mild, usually insignificant, postural or exercise hypotension. Dry mouth, sedation and constipation are common side effects. Withdrawal hypertension occurs after abrupt withdrawal from large doses. It does not cause clinically significant distortions of plasma lipoproteins.

Dose—*Oral, initially* **4 mg** twice a day, to be gradually increased at 1- or 2-wk intervals to 32 mg a day, if necessary.

Dosage Form—Tablets: 4, 8 and 16 mg.

Guanfacine Hydrochloride

Benzeneacetamide, *N*-(aminoiminomethyl)-2,6-dichloro-,
monohydrochloride; Tenex (*Robins*)

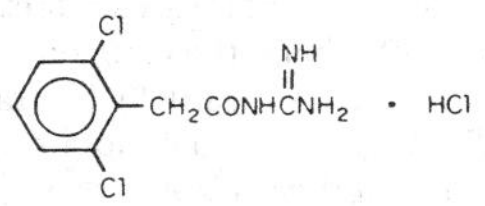

[29110-48-3] $C_9H_2Cl_2N_3O.HCl$ (282.56).

Preparation—US Pat 3,632,645

Description—White needles; melts about 215°.

Uses—An α_2-agonist which acts in the vasomotor center and the spinal cord to decrease sympathetic outflow to the blood vessels and to a lesser extent, to the heart. It is thus like clonidine and guanabenz. However, its effects last longer. It is used (usually along with a saluretic) mostly to treat *mild* to *moderate hypertension,* but it also is effective in *toxemia of pregnancy* and ultimately may prove to be useful in *hypertensive emergencies.* Tolerance is common in the absence of a saluretic. Adverse effects are mainly those of clonidine, (above), but they tend to be milder. Withdrawal hypertension may occur 2 to 7 days after discontinuation of treatment. Elimination is by both hepatic metabolism (60 to 70%) and renal excretion (30 to 40%); dosage is said not to require adjustments in renal failure. The elimination half-life is 14 to 17 hr.

Dose—*Oral, adult, initially* **1 mg** at bedtime, to be increased gradually as needed; *maintenance,* between 1 and 3 mg a day.

Dosage Forms—Tablets: 1 mg.

Methyldopa

L-Tyrosine, 3-hydroxy-α-methyl-, sesquihydrate; Alpha-methyldopa;
Aldomet (*MSD*)

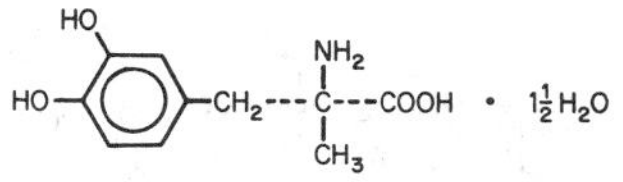

[41372-08-1] $C_{10}H_{13}NO_4.1\frac{1}{2}H_2O$ (238.24); *anhydrous* [555-30-6] (211.22).

Preparation—The product of the reaction of 3,4-dimethoxyphenylacetonitrile with sodium ethoxide is hydrolyzed with acid to give 3,4-dimethoxyphenylacetone. This is reacted with ammonium carbonate and potassium cyanide to form a substituted hydantoin intermediate which, on alkaline hydrolysis, yields racemic methyldopa. The acetylated form of this racemate is resolved using (−)-α- methylbenzylamine. The isolated acetylated (−)-methyldopate salt is deacetylated with base and treated with mineral acid to liberate (−)-methyldopa. US Pat 2,868,818.

Description—White to yellowish white, odorless, fine powder, which may contain friable lumps; almost tasteless and relatively stable in both light and air; melts above 290° with decomposition; pK_a 2.2 (COOH), 10.6 (NH_2), 9.2 and 12 (ring OH).

Solubility—Sparingly soluble in water; very soluble in diluted hydrochloric acid; slightly soluble in alcohol; practically insoluble in ether.

Uses—An *antihypertensive* in the treatment of moderate to severe essential hypertension, including malignant hypertension. It has a slight effect on cardiac output and heart rate. Renal blood flow remains nearly normal in patients without previous renal damage. The degree of orthostatic hypotension is considerably less than with guanethidine, which is an advantage. Its action is erratic, and one third of treated patients may not respond to the drug. Tolerance sometimes develops in up to a third of initially responsive patients, which is largely the result of retention of salt and water, and may be overcome by increasing the dose of concomitant diuretic drug.

In the brain, it is converted to methylnorepinephrine which displaces norepinephrine from storage sites and is released as a "false transmitter" by nervous impulses in the adrenergic nerves. The metabolite α-methylnorepinephrine has potent α_2-agonist activity and probably acts to decrease blood pressure in the same way as does clonidine. In the spinal cord and vasomotor center, the result is a decrease in sympathetic vasomotor outflow, which decreases blood pressure and lowers plasma renin activity. Its action begins in about 2 hr, becomes maximal in 6 to 8 hr and lasts 18 to 24 hr.

The most prominent side effect is somnolence. Tolerance to the sedative effects usually occurs in a few days to a few weeks. Side effects include occasional orthostatic hypotension with vertigo, nausea, weakness and headache, bradycardia, nasal stuffiness, diarrhea and impotence. Other side effects include frequent dry mouth, maculopapular skin rashes, decreased libido, defective ejaculation and impotence in males, breast enlargement and paresthesias. Like reserpine, it may cause edema and rarely psychic depression and nightmares, parkinsonism, arthralgia and myalgia. Lactation and breast engorgement occur rarely. Depression of liver function characterized by fever and malaise and occasionally jaundice may occur. The direct Coombs test may be positive in about 20% of recipients. Rarely, a lupus erythematosus-like syndrome, granulocytopenia or thrombocytopenia occurs. It is contraindicated in the presence of active liver disease and in persons known to be sensitive to the drug.

About 50% of the drug is absorbed by the oral route. Most of it is excreted unchanged, but some is conjugated to the *O*-sulfate. Sulfate-containing drugs, such as ferrous sulfate, not only decrease absorption but also increase sulfation, thereby decreasing the systemic bioavailability. Most of the drug is excreted before distribution is complete. The plasma concentration falls with an α-phase half-life of about 1.7 hr; however, in renal failure only 50% is excreted during the distribution phase ($t_{1/2}$ = 3.5 hr), and accumulation can occur.

Dose—*Oral, adult,* **250 mg** every 8 or 12 hr during the first 2 days then, if necessary, upward adjustments are made at intervals no shorter than 2 days, up to a total daily dose of 2 g; while occasional patients have responded to higher doses (maximum of 3 g daily) it is recommended that if 2 g is insufficient, another antihypertensive drug should be added to the regimen rather than to increase the dose. *Children, initially* **10 mg/kg** a day in 2 to 4 divided doses, or 100 mg/m^2 every 8 hr, to be adjusted, as necessary, at 2- to 4-day intervals; the maximum *maintenance* dose is 65 mg/kg or 2 g/m^2, up to a maximum total of 3 g a day.

Dosage Forms—Oral Suspension: 250 mg/5 mL; Tablets: 125, 250 and 500 mg.

Methyldopate Hydrochloride

L-Tyrosine, 3-hydroxy-α-methyl-, ethyl ester, hydrochloride;
Aldomet Ester Hydrochloride (*MSD*)

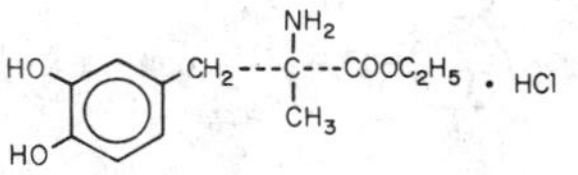

[5208-79-4] $C_{12}H_{17}NO_4$.HCl (275.73).

Preparation—By converting methyldopa to its ethyl ester and passing hydrogen chloride into a solution of the ester in a suitable organic solvent.

Description—White or practically white crystalline powder; odorless or practically odorless with a bitter taste; relatively stable both in light and air; melts at about 160°; pH (1 in 100 solution) 3.0 to 5.0.

Solubility—Freely soluble in water, alcohol or methanol; slightly soluble in chloroform; practically insoluble in ether.

Uses—The actions and uses are the same as those of *Methyldopa*. The ester is employed for intravenous use in hypertensive crises or in patients who are unable to take antihypertensive drugs by mouth. In the body the ethyl group is removed by hydrolysis to yield methyldopa. The onset of action by the intravenous route is 4 to 6 hr, whereas that by the oral route may be 1 to 2 days. The duration of action is 10 to 16 hr.

Dose—*Intravenous infusion, adult,* **250** to **500 mg** in 100 mL of 5% dextrose injection over a period of 30 to 60 min every 6 hr, if needed; single doses of as much as 3 g have been given, but syncope is more likely with such large doses, especially in arteriosclerotic patients; *children,* **5** to **10 mg/kg** (150 to 300 mg/m^2) every 6 hr if necessary.

Dosage Form—Injection: 250 mg/5 mL.

Antihypertensive Direct Vasodilators

Direct vasodilators act by several mechanisms, such as inhibition of cyclic nucleotide phosphodiesterase, adenosine mimicry, impairment of calcium and sodium influx in vascular smooth muscle, opening of potassium channels, release of nitric oxide (NO), stimulation of guanylate cyclase and unknown mechanisms. Their usefulness in the ambulatory treatment of hypertension depends a great deal on the selectivity of the drug for the resistance blood vessels, namely, the arterioles, which causes a lowering of blood pressure. If the capacitance veins also are dilated, venous return to the heart, and hence cardiovascular adjustments to posture and exercise, is impaired, and the patient may experience postural and exercise hypotensions, sometimes to the point of syncope. A slight degree of interference with venous return usually is considered to be desirable, especially in the treatment of severe hypertension, because it enables a greater lowering of blood pressure than does arteriolar dilatation alone.

Direct vasodilators invariably cause reflex palpitation and tachycardia and also increases in plasma renin activity, all of which tend to counter the hypotensive action; the cardiac effects give rise to patient discomfort. Therefore, it often is advisable to combine the vasodilators with β-adrenoreceptor antagonists to antagonize these effects.

In addition to the ultimate edema-causing sequelae to increased renin secretion, the lowering of blood pressure may decrease both pressure natriuresis and renal blood flow. This decrease promotes sodium and water retention, which, in turn, may decrease the antihypertensive effects of the drug; therefore, it is rational to use saluretics in combination with vasodilators.

Diazoxide

2*H*-1,2,4-Benzothiadiazine, 7-chloro-3-methyl-, 1,1-dioxide;
Hyperstat IV (*Schering*) (*Various Mfrs*)

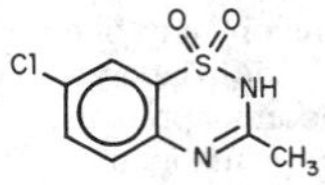

[364-98-7] $C_8H_7ClN_2O_2S$ (230.67).

Preparation—One method reacts 2,4-dichloronitrobenzene with benzyl mercaptan and KOH and the 2-(benzylthio) group thus introduced is converted to $-SO_2Cl$ with chlorine and aqueous acetic acid and thence to $-SO_2NH_2$ by reaction with NH_3. After reducing the NO_2 to NH_2 with Fe and NH_4Cl, cyclization is effected by condensation with ethyl orthoacetate. *Science 133:*2067, 1961. US Pats 2,986,573 and 3,345,365.

Description—White to cream-white crystals or crystalline powder; odorless; melts about 330°; pK_a 8.5.

Solubility—Practically insoluble to sparingly soluble in water.

Uses—Exerts prominent vasodepressor actions, especially by the intravenous route. In therapeutic doses, vasodepression is primarily the result of arteriolar dilatation, so that orthostatic hypotension is usually minimal. However, some venous dilatation does occur, which at times is sufficient to cause orthostatic hypotension. The smooth muscle-relaxing effects result from hyperpolarization of vascular smooth muscle by activating ATPase-sensitive potassium channels. It is used intravenously as a hypotensive drug in *acute hypertensive crises*. Its side effects preclude its use in the chronic management of essential hypertension, but it may be used to initiate treatment in order to control blood pressure until the oral antihypertensives can be used.

Although it is a benzothiazide, it is not a diuretic but instead actually causes salt and water retention and consequent gain in weight. This action sometimes precipitates congestive heart failure, especially if renal function is impaired. It also causes hyperglycemia by inhibiting insulin secretion from pancreatic β-cells. Occasionally, it is necessary to administer oral hypoglycemics or insulin to suppress the hyperglycemia.

Other side effects include nausea, vomiting and other gastrointestinal upsets, burning sensations along the vein of injection (because of the high pH of solutions), tachycardia, substernal pain, orthostatic hypotension, transient hyperuricemia, headache and drowsiness. Overdosage by the intravenous route can cause shock.

It is contraindicated in toxemia of pregnancy because it relaxes uterine smooth muscle and may interfere with impending delivery. It should be used in diabetics only when blood glucose is monitored closely. Blood glucose also should be determined in all persons receiving multiple injections. It should be used cautiously in persons with coronary or cerebral insufficiency and patients with impaired renal function. However, it may be safer to use in renal hypertensive crises than other antihypertensives. The drug is contraindicated if hypersensitivity to thiazides exists. Thiazide diuretics, and other antihypertensive drugs, increase the response to diazoxide, even when they fail to lower blood pressure themselves. Some authorities administer furosemide along with this drug, in order to prevent salt and water retention.

It is about 90% protein-bound, but rapid intravenous injection permits distribution to smooth muscle before it is bound to protein. Thus, a greater and longer-lasting fall in blood pressure accrues to faster rates of injection. It is of interest that the drug persists in blood longer than the hypotensive effect. The plasma half-life is 20 to 60 hr in persons with normal renal function, but the hypotensive effect lasts only 2 to 15 hr. Different populations may eliminate the drug differently, some mostly by renal tubular secretion and others mostly by biotransformation. It competes with weakly acidic drugs, such as allopurinol, aspirin, colchicine, probenecid, sulfinpyrazone and warfarin for the renal secretory system and thus increases their plasma concentrations. It also displaces several drugs from plasma proteins; in the case of warfarin, this may cause a hemorrhagic diathesis.

Dose—*Intravenous, adult,* for *hypertensive emergencies, initially* up to **150 mg** (or 1 to 3 mg/kg), repeated in 5 to 15 min, if necessary, with dose adjusted according to response, then every 4 to 24 hr until the blood pressure is under control and an oral antihypertensive drug can be substituted; *children, initially* **1** to **3 mg/kg** (or 30 to 90 mg/m^2), repeated as for adults.

Dosage Form—Injection: 300 mg/20 mL.

Hydralazine Hydrochloride

Phthalazine, 1-hydrazino-, monohydrochloride;
Apresoline (*Ciba*); (*Various Mfrs*)

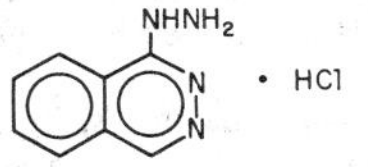

[304-20-1] $C_8H_8N_4.HCl$ (196.64).

Preparation—Phthalazone is converted to 1-chlorophthalazine by treatment with phosphorus oxychloride, condensed with hydrazine hydrate to form hydralazine and neutralized with HCl to produce the hydrochloride.

Description—White to off-white, crystalline powder; melts between 270 and 280° with decomposition; pK_a 0.5, 7.3.

Solubility—1 g in 25 mL water, 500 mL alcohol; very slightly soluble in ether.

Uses—Causes vasodilatation by stimulating guanylate cyclase in arteriolar smooth muscle; the stimulant appears to be nitric oxide (NO) from the local oxidation of the hydrazine moiety. NO is a natural, endothelial-derived relaxing factor.

It is one of the few drugs that causes substantial vasodilatation in the kidney, and it increases renal plasma flow even when the blood pressure drops considerably. Vasodilatation also is pronounced in the splanchnic, cerebral and coronary vascular beds; it exerts only slight vasodilator actions in skin and skeletal muscle. The veins participate very little in the effect, so that postural hypotension is negligible. As the result of the fall in blood pressure, reflex tachycardia, palpitations and increases in plasma renin activity occur, although the renin activity sometimes decreases in long-term treatment.

It may be used in the treatment of moderate *essential* or *early malignant hypertension* and *hypertensive emergencies,* virtually always in conjunction with other antihypertensive drugs. However, mainly because of its side effects, it generally is not used until other, safer, therapy has failed. Because it increases renal blood flow, it is often used to treat *toxemia of pregnancy.* It also sometimes is used in *acute congestive heart failure* or *after myocardial infarction* because it decreases cardiac afterload with very little effect on preload, so that cardiac output is improved.

Tolerance sometimes occurs during long-term treatment. In part, this is probably the result of depletion of tissue sulfhydryl compounds and probably is reversible with *N*-acetylcysteine. In part, it is the result of sodium retention.

Its principal serious toxic effects are syndromes resembling rheumatoid arthritis or lupus erythematosus, appearance of which necessitates withdrawal of the drug. This toxicity is more frequent in slow than in fast acetylators. Most patient complaints are of tachycardia and palpitations. These effects are counterproductive in that they tend to limit the fall in blood pressure. Furthermore, they may precipitate attacks of angina pectoris. β_1-Adrenergic blocking drugs prevent these effects and also the reflex rise in plasma renin levels and hence increase the antihypertensive response.

Other frequent side effects include dizziness, headache and cardiomegaly. Paresthesias, anxiety, nausea, vomiting, malaise, disorientation, depression, impotence, priapism edema, nasal congestion, lacrimation, red eyes, rash, giant urticaria, drug fever, agranulocytosis, leukocytosis and anemia also occasionally occur. Even when the plasma renin activity is suppressed, a counterproductive sodium and water retention occurs; saluretics suppress the effect and improve the antihypertensive effects.

It is absorbed by the oral route. With low doses, first-pass metabolism limits bioavailability to 16 to 35%; food enhances the bioavailability. Elimination is by both ring hydroxylation and *N*-acetylation, and only 10% of hydralazine is excreted unchanged. Elimination is dose-dependent, and plasma levels increase disproportionately with dose. The half-life is 1.5 to 6 hr; the difference between slow and fast acetylators is usually minor. It accumulates in fat in vascular smooth muscle, where it has a life longer than in plasma.

Dose—*Oral, adult, initially* **5** to **10 mg** 4 times a day for 2 to 4 days, then **25 mg** 4 times a day for the rest of the week; the dose may be increased to **200 mg** a day in 2 to 4 divided doses thereafter; the daily dose should not exceed 200 mg, but in preeclampsia the total daily dose may be as high as 400 mg, reached by *daily* increments of 40 to 50 mg until the desired effect is achieved; *children, initially* **0.75 mg/kg** (or 25 mg/m^2) daily, divided into 2 to 4 doses, to be adjusted upward gradually, if necessary, to no more than 7.5 mg/kg or 300 mg a day. *Intramuscular* or *intravenous, adults,* **10** to **20 mg,** increased to **40 mg** if necessary, repeated as necessary; *children,* **1.7** to **3.5 mg/kg** (or 50 to 100 mg/m^2) a day, divided into 4 to 6 doses.

Dosage Forms—Injection: 20 mg/mL; Tablets: 10, 25, 50, and 100 mg. An oral solution of 10 mg/mL may be extemporized by adding 5 mL of injection to 5 mL of 10% sorbitol solution.

Minoxidil

2,4-Pyrimidinediamine, 6-(1-piperidinyl)-, 3-oxide; Loniten;
Rogaine (*Upjohn*)

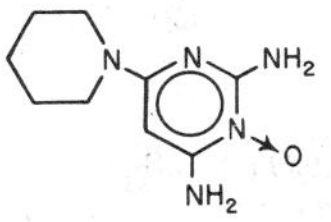

[38304-91-5] $C_9H_{15}N_5O$ (209.25).

Preparation—US Pat 3,461,461.

Description—White to off-white, crystalline powder; pK_a 4.6.

Solubility—1 g in about 500 mL water; 25 mL alcohol; practically insoluble in chloroform.

Uses—Dilates arterioles by opening potassium channels, which causes hyperpolarization and relaxation of smooth muscle. This lowers the total peripheral vascular resistance and hence the blood pressure. The maximum achievable decrease in mean blood pressure is usually at least 35 torr in most hypertensive patients. Dilatation of capacitance veins is only slight to moderate and sympathetic vascular reflexes are unimpaired, so that postural and exercise hypotensions are usually minimal.

Reflex tachycardia and palpitations occur, but they are less than that expected from the fall in blood pressure, which suggests cardioaccelerator-suppressant actions not yet elucidated. Nevertheless, a β_1-adrenoreceptor blocking drug may need to be coadministered to suppress reflex cardiac stimulation. Renal plasma flow and glomerular filtration rate are very little affected, which implies a substantial renal vasodilatation. Plasma renin activity may be elevated as the result of reflex sympathetic activity or diminished by an unknown mechanism. Irrespective of the plasma renin activity, salt and water retention occur sufficiently to cause considerable tolerance to the antihypertensive effects, and saluretics, even occasionally high-ceiling diuretics, are necessary to restore the antihypertensive effects.

In appropriate dosage, minoxidil can be used to treat all types of hypertension, although most experience has been in the treatment of *moderate* to *severe essential hypertension.* It often is effective in hypertensions refractory to all other therapy. It also is useful in *hypertensive emergencies* and for *ventricular unloading,* the effect being mainly to decrease afterload.

A side effect is excessive hair growth. Consequently, the drug is used topically to restore hair growth in *androgenetic alopecia* and *alopecia areata.* Improvement occurs in about 60% of cases but is cosmetically acceptable in only about 30%.

Adverse effects of systemic use include fluid retention, cardiac stimulation and mild postural hypotension, anginal attacks (from both cardiac stimulation and decreased coronary perfusion pressure), moderate but usually reversible hypertrichosis with increased pigmentation in about 70% of patients, and rare pulmonary hypertension (controversial), pericardial effusion and breast tenderness. A slight anemia (7% decrease in RBC, in part the result of hemodilution) and small increase in alkaline phosphatase and 6% increase in plasma creatinine and BUN transiently occur. Nausea and vomiting sometimes occur; thrombocytopenia and leukopenia, rarely. No teratogenic effects thus far have been observed, but it is wise to avoid the drug during pregnancy. It also probably should be withheld within a month after a myocardial infarction. Adverse effects usually are slight with topical administration, but some hypotension may occur with concentrations over 3%.

The drug is absorbed well by the oral route. The volume of distribution is 9 to 15 L/kg. It is concentrated in vascular tissue. Metabolism in the liver accounts for about 90% of elimination, and no modification of dose is required in renal failure or hemodialysis. The apparent half-life of about 4 hr appears to be a distribution parameter; the β-half-life is about 24 hr. The duration of action is 1 to 3 days.

Dose—*Oral, adult* and *children over 12 yr, initially* **5 mg** a day, with dose adjustments, by doubling the previous dose, at 3-day intervals, if necessary, usually up to 20 to 40 mg and no more than 100 mg a day;

children under 12 yr, initially **0.2 mg/kg** a day, to be increased gradually at 3-day intervals, usually up to 0.25 to 1 mg/kg and no more than 50 mg a day. In severe hypertension, in which a rapid reduction in blood pressure is desired, dose adjustments can be made at 6-hr intervals, if the patient is monitored carefully. *Topical,* to the *scalp,* applied thinly as a **1** to **5%** ointment or **2%** spray twice a day.

Dosage Forms—Tablets: 2.5 and 10 mg. Topical solution: 2% in 60 mL.

Pinacidil

Guanidine, (±)-*N*″-cyano-*N*-4-pyridinyl-*N*′-(1,2,2-trimethylpropyl)-, monohydrate; Pindac (*Lilly*)

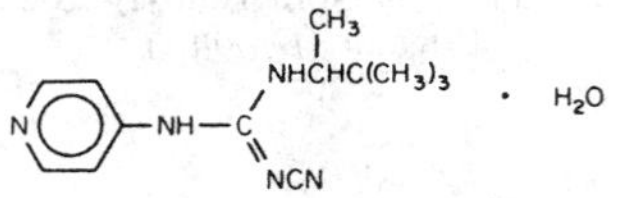

[85371-64-8] $C_{13}H_{19}N_5 \cdot H_2O$ (263.34).

Preparation—See *J Med Chem 21:* 773, 1978.

Description—White crystals melting about 165°; pK_a 6.0, 10.8.

Solubility—1 g in 7 mL alcohol.

Uses—An investigational antihypertensive drug for use in the treatment of *moderate hypertension.* It opens potassium channels in arteriolar smooth muscle, thus causing hyperpolarization and relaxation. It also decreases systolic calcium concentrations by redistributing calcium to organelles. Although it generally is considered to have a pharmacodynamic profile nearly identical to that of minoxidil (above), it seems to cause more salt and water retention, even more than hydralazine. This may be the result of an increase in plasma renin activity. However, no retention occurs when the drug is combined with either a thiazide saluretic or a β-adrenoreceptor blocking drug. Other adverse effects are usually infrequent. They include facial flushing, headache, exertional dyspnea, insomnia, fatigue, unusual dreams and postural hypotension. Palpitations and tachycardia are mild. By the oral route, pinacidil is absorbed rapidly. There is considerable first-pass metabolism into a number of metabolites; the active metabolite, pinacidil *N*-oxide, is the most important. The elimination half-like is 1.5 to 3 hr.

Dose—*Oral, adult,* **12.5** to **25 mg** twice a day.

Dosage Form—Capsules: 12.5 and 25 mg.

Sodium Nitroprusside

Ferrate(2-), pentakis(cyano-*C*)nitrosyl-, disodium, (*OC*-6-22)-dihydrate; Sodium Nitroferricyanide; (*Elkins-Sinn*); Nipride (*Roche*); Nitropress (*Abbott*)

[13755-38-9] $Na_2[Fe(CN)_5NO] \cdot 2H_2O$ (297.95); *anhydrous* [14402-89-2] (261.92).

Preparation—Potassium ferrocyanide is dissolved in 50% HNO_3 and the solution boiled for about 1 hr. After cooling and filtering to remove potassium nitrate, the solution is neutralized with Na_2CO_3 and evaporated to crystallization.

Description—Reddish brown, practically odorless, crystals or powder; freshly prepared solutions all have a faint brownish tint. Since nitroprusside ion forms colored compounds with many organic and inorganic substances, blue, green, red or any highly colored solutions should be discarded; aqueous solutions are photosensitive and should be protected from light.

Solubility—1 g in about 2.5 mL water; slightly soluble in alcohol.

Uses—A potent, directly acting peripheral vasodilator. It releases nitric oxide (NO), which is also the endogenous, endothelial-derived relaxing factor. NO activates guanylyl cyclase in vascular smooth muscle to produce vasodilation. Its actions on arterioles decrease the total systemic vascular resistance, which is the main cause of the fall in blood pressure it evokes. It has a lesser action on capacitance veins so that, with usual doses, venous return is impaired insignificantly in the recumbent position; however, in the upright position there is considerable orthostatic hypotension. Cardiac output is increased in the recumbent and decreased in the upright position. Heart rate invariably is increased reflexly. There is a variable effect on renal plasma flow and glomerular filtration rate, but it usually is increased in the recumbent position. Plasma renin activity is slightly to moderately increased.

It is given by continuous intravenous infusion for treatment of *hypertensive emergencies* and for *ventricular unloading* in acute congestive heart failure and after myocardial infarction. Its predilection for the arterioles enables it to reduce selectively the cardiac afterload. It also is used for controlled hypotension during surgery. Owing to an extremely brief duration of action, the drug must be given intravenously. Since there is a very narrow therapeutic range, the rate of infusion and the blood pressure must be monitored continuously at first and then at intervals of 5 min throughout the course of the infusion. For this reason, the drug usually is employed only in emergencies and in intensive-care units.

Discontinuation of infusion can cause rebound hypertensive instead of hypotensive effects. Other adverse effects are tachycardia (in part reflex, hence avoidable by β-blockade), nausea, retching, vomiting, transient restlessness, agitation, tremors and muscular twitching. Dyspnea, cyanosis, mydriasis and cardiovascular collapse have occurred as the result of an excessive fall in blood pressure.

Nitroprusside is broken down rapidly by reaction with hemoglobin to NO, cyanide ion, and cyanmethemoglobin with a half-life of about 2 min. Cyanide is converted to thiocyanate by the enzyme rhodanase in the liver. Infants lack this enzyme, so that the drug should not be used in neonates and probably also not in the treatment of toxemia of pregnancy. Conversion to thiocyanate requires endogenous thiosulfate, which can be depleted by high doses or prolonged administration, leading to toxic levels of cyanide. Thiocyanate is eliminated by the normal kidney with a half-life of 3 days.

Dose (as the dihydrate)—*Intravenous,* by *slow infusion, adult, initially* **0.5 μg/kg/min** (0.005 mg/kg) of a solution containing 50 mg dissolved in 500 to 1000 mL of 5% dextrose injection, adjusted in 0.5 μg-increments, as needed, up to a limit of 10 μg/kg/min or a total dose of 3.5 mg/kg in brief infusions; *children,* **1.4 μg/kg/min,** adjusted slowly, if necessary. A fresh solution should be prepared immediately before use.

Dosage Form—Sterile powder for Preparation of Injection: 50 mg in 2- and 5-mL vials.

Ganglionic Blocking Agents

The clinically available ganglionic blocking drugs compete with acetylcholine at postsynaptic nicotinic receptors. Since the ganglia of both the sympathetic and parasympathetic nervous systems are cholinergic, these drugs interrupt the outflow through both systems; thus, it is not possible to achieve a therapeutic block of autonomic outflow to a given locus without a number of undesirable but unavoidable side effects resulting from the blockade of other autonomic nerves. Blockade of sympathetic outflow to the blood vessels causes hypotension and increased blood flow (with a pink, warm skin).

Blockade of sympathetics to the heart may cause slowing, but the parasympathetic outflow also is blocked, so that acceleration can result in persons with predominantly parasympathetic tone. Orthostatic hypotension results from blockade of reflex adjustments to posture. Blockade of parasympathetic outflow results in dry mouth, mydriasis, cycloplegia (loss of ocular accommodation), diminished gastrointestinal motility and urinary retention.

The ganglionic blocking agents should be used cautiously when other hypotensive, antihypertensive or anesthetic drugs are used concomitantly, because the hypotension may be exaggerated to such an extent that blood flow through the brain, heart or kidney may be jeopardized. Overdose of the ganglionic blocking drug alone can have this effect. Because compensatory cardiovascular reflexes are suppressed by the ganglionic blocking drugs, pressor drugs given during ganglionic blockade may elicit dangerously enhanced responses.

Ganglionic blocking drugs are contraindicated when there is pyloric stenosis, cerebral arteriosclerosis, coronary insufficiency, recent myocardial infarction or glaucoma. They should be used cautiously in elderly patients and in patients with renal insufficiency or receiving neuromuscular blocking antibiotics.

Mecamylamine Hydrochloride

Bicyclo[2.2.1]heptan-2-amine, *N*,2,3,3-tetramethyl-, monohydrochloride; Inversine (*MSD*)

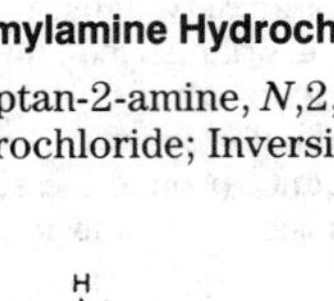

[826-39-1] $C_{11}H_{21}H \cdot HCl$ (203.75).

Preparation—From camphene; *J Am Chem Soc 78:* 1514, 1946.

Description—White, crystalline powder; melts about 245° (dec); can be sterilized by autoclaving.

Solubility—1 g in 5 mL water, 12 mL alcohol or 10 mL glycerol.

Uses—Differs from most other ganglionic blocking agents in that it is not a quaternary ammonium compound so that it is ionized poorly in the small intestine and thus is readily and completely absorbed. It is the only orally effective gnaglionic blocker available. It was used in the past to treat *essential hypertension*, but it largely has been replaced by newer drugs. Its nonionic form permits it to pass into the CNS, so that occasional bizarre central disturbances may result. It has a low renal clearance and hence a long duration of action. It will produce a variety of unpleasant, unavoidable side effects that result from the interruption of both sympathetic and parasympathetic outflow. Orthostatic hypotension, blurring of vision, dry mouth, diarrhea followed by constipation, occasional paralytic ileus, nausea and vomiting, urinary retention, fatigue, sedation and impotence are among these general side effects. Tremor and delusions or hallucinations may occur. It is absorbed readily from the gut. It penetrates the blood-brain barrier into the CNS and also into the fetus (hence, it should be avoided in pregnancy). Elimination is by renal tubular secretion. The duration of action is 6 to 12 hr.

Dose—*Oral, adult,* **2.5** to **25 mg** a day; *usual, initially* **2.5 mg** 2 times a day, increased by 2.5-mg increments at intervals of not less than 2 days as required; *maximum, maintenance,* **7.5 mg** 3 times a day.

Dosage Form—Tablets: 2.5 mg.

Trimethaphan Camsylate

Thieno[1′,2′:1,2]thienol[3,4-*d*]imidazol-5-ium, decahydro-2-oxo-1,3-bis(phenylmethyl)-, salt with (+)-7,7-dimethyl-2-oxobicyclo[2.2.1]heptane-1-methanesulfonic acid (1:1); Arfonad (*Roche*)

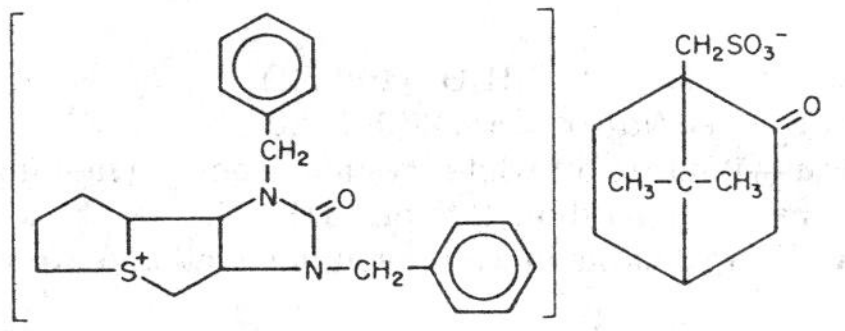

[68-91-7] $C_{32}H_{40}N_2O_5S_2$ (596.80).

Preparation—The bromide, prepared from an intermediate produced in the synthesis of biotin, is metathesized with silver *d*-camphor-10-sulfonate; the silver bromide is removed by filtration and the camsylate is obtained by evaporating the filtrate.

Description—White crystals or crystalline powder; melts between 230 and 235° with decomposition.

Solubility—Freely soluble in water, alcohol or chloroform; insoluble in ether.

Uses—Usually classified as a ganglionic blocking agent, but it only moderately blocks ganglia in the therapeutic dose range. Some of its hypotensive effects result from a direct peripheral vasodilator action. It has an extremely brief duration of action. Thus, the hypotension induced is subject to moment-to-moment control simply by varying the rate of intravenous infusion. It sometimes is used in the treatment of *hypertensive emergencies,* but other drugs usually are preferred. It occasionally is used for *induction of brief, controlled hypotension,* as for surgical procedures, to reduce an otherwise bloody field or for certain diagnostic procedures. It also is used to treat severe *autonomic dysreflexia.* Adverse effects are mostly the result of ganglionic blockade. They necessitate a reduction in dosage. They are anorexia, nausea, vomiting, constipation and possibility of paralytic ileus, mydriasis, cycloplegia and possibility of glaucomatous attack, dry mouth, anginal pain, tachycardia, postural hypotension and urinary retention. It causes release of histamine, so that it must be used with caution in allergic and asthmatic persons.

Dose—*Slow intravenous infusion, adult,* for *hypertensive emergency, initially* **0.5** to **1 mg/min** then **1** to **15 mg/min** for *maintenance,* according to blood pressure; for *controlled hypotension, initially* **3** to **4 mg/min** then **0.2** to **6 mg/min,** according to response; *children, initially* **0.1 mg/min,** adjusted according to response.

Dosage Form—Injection: 500 mg/10 mL, to be diluted to 500 mL before use.

Drugs Affecting the Renin-Angiotensin System

Renin is a protease that is released by the kidney in response to reduced renal perfusion, hyponatremia or sympathetic activity. It acts on the plasma α_2-globulin substrate, angiotensinogen, to yield the decapeptide, angiotensin I. Angiotensin I is hydrolyzed by a "*converting enzyme*" to yield the octapeptide, angiotensin II. Angiotensin II may lose one aminoacid residue to yield angiotensin III. Angiotensins II and III are destroyed by carboxypeptidases.

Angiotensin I is inactive in the cardiovascular system, although it may have some effect to contract the renal glomerular mesangium. Angiotensin II has several cardiovascular-renal actions.

It stimulates the zona glomerulosa of the adrenal cortex to secrete aldosterone. Aldosterone causes the renal retention of sodium (and hence of water) and the loss of potassium. The extracellular fluid volume and body burden of sodium are thus increased, which promotes an increase in blood pressure in many persons and edema in congestive heart failure. Angiotensin III also stimulates the adrenal secretion of aldosterone.

It is a very potent vasoconstrictor, which contributes to an elevation of blood pressure in most persons and to reduced cardiac output (from increased afterload) in congestive heart failure.

If facilitates transmission in sympathetic ganglia, increases the release of norepinephrine at adrenergic nerve terminals and increases the response of blood vessels and the heart to norepinephrine, thus amplifying sympathetic factors in the maintenance of elevated blood pressure.

It stimulates the release of ADH (vasopressin) from the neurohypophysis and thirst receptors, thus adding to volume and vasopressor factors in some conditions of hypertension and in congestive heart failure. Angiotensin II is also a putative neurotransmitter in the CNS.

The most important site of the angiotensin converting enzyme (ACE) is in the lung, but ACE also is found in the kidney, CNS and elsewhere. A form of ACE circulates in the plasma. ACE is the same enzyme as kininase II. Therefore, inhibition of ACE not only decreases the amount of the vasoconstrictor, angiotension II, but also increases the amount of the vasodilator kinins. At one time it was thought that much of the antihypertensive effects of ACE inhibitors was attributable to kinins, but careful studies have discounted this involvement. Furthermore, kinins probably do not account for rashes caused by captopril, as was commonly thought.

ACE inhibitors are used to treat *mild to moderate esential* and *renovascular hypertensions,* especially when plasma renin activity (PRA) is high, although they are effectively antihypertensive even when PRA is not elevated. They often provide effective monotherapy. They also are used in *refractory congestive heart failure,* to unload the ventricle and to suppress the renin angiotensin factor in edema formation. ACE inhibitors decrease arteriolar resistance in hypertension. They improve the cardiac work performance index and decrease ventricular enlargement in hypertension, heart failure and after myocardial infarction. They also are used to treat *diabetic proteinuria*; the action appears to be intrarenal.

Alone or in combination, ACE inhibitors are becoming the drugs of choice in the first-line treatment of essential hypertension. Many drugs that lower blood pressure homeostatically increase renin release, hence increasing angiotensin II concentrations.

Centrally acting and β-adrenoreceptor-antagonist antihypertensive drugs decrease sympathetically mediated but not hemodynamically or intrarenally mediated increases in angiotensin levels; ACE inhibitors suppress increased angiotensin levels from any cause. In combination with saluretics, they suppress the renin-angiotensin-aldosterone factor in saluretic-induced hypokalemia, thus attenuating the risk of hypokalemia. In fact, they may produce *hyper*kalemia, if there is concurrent renal failure or if potassium-sparing diuretics or potassium supplements are being taken. By preventing homeostatic rises in aldosterone levels, and even by themselves causing a decrease in extracellular fluid volume, ACE inhibitors have a greater synergism with saluretics than do other antihypertensive drugs. Lastly, ACE inhibitors are tolerated better than most other antihypertensive drugs. Patients and physicians elect to discontinue them less frequently than they do methyldopa or propranolol.

ACE inhibitors reduce lithium excretion and can produce lithium intoxication in patients taking lithium. NSAIDs tend to reduce the hypotensive effect of ACE inhibitors.

There is one available competitive antagonist of angiotension II, *saralasin,* but it has a very brief half-life and is not effective orally. Long-acting, orally effective antagonists are under investigation. There also are promising investigational inhibitors of renin. Some of these may be introduced before the next edition of this book.

Benazepril Hydrochloride

1*H*-1-Benzazepine-1-acetic acid, [*S*-(*R**,*R**)]-,3-[[1-(ethoxycarbonyl)-3-phenylpropyl]-amino]-2,3,4,5-tetrahydro-2-oxo-, monohydrochloride, Lotensin (*Ciba-Geigy*)

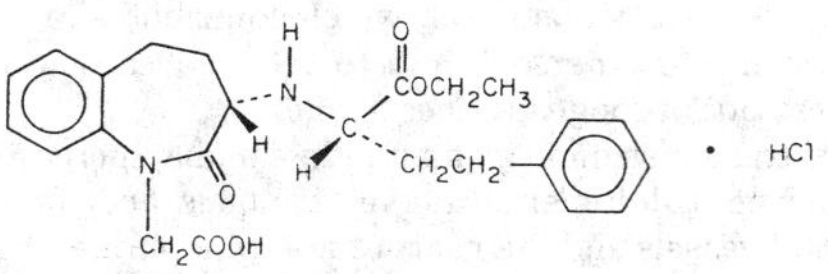

[86541-74-4] $C_{24}H_{28}N_2O_5$.HCl (490.96).

Description—White to off-white crystalline powder.

Solubility—Greater than 1 g in 10 mL of water, ethanol or methanol.

Uses—A prodrug rapidly absorbed and converted to the active ACE inhibitor, *benazerilat*, which has a half-life of 10 to 11 hr. It is approved for treating *essential hypertension* and may be effective for treating *congestive heart failure*. It produces a spectrum and incidence of side effects and drug interactions that are similar to those of enalapril; also, see the general statement.

Dose—*Oral, adult, initially* **10 mg** once a day, increasing to **20 to 40 mg** once or twice a day. *Patients taking diuretics* or with *renal impairment, initially* **5 mg** once a day.

Dosage Form—Tablets: 5, 10, 20 and 40 mg.

Captopril

L-Proline, 1-[(2*S*)-3-mercapto-2-methyl-1-oxopropyl]-, Capoten (*Squibb*)

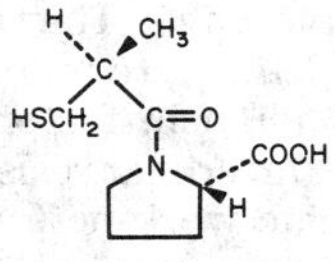

[62571-86-2] $C_9H_{15}NO_3S$ (217.28)

Preparation—See *Science 196:* 441, 1977.

Description—White crystals melting about 88° which resolidify and melt again at about 105°; $pK_1 = 3.7$, $pK_2 = 9.8$.

Solubility—Freely soluble in water, alcohol or chloroform.

Uses—The first orally effective ACE inhibitor to have been marketed. For the uses, see the general statement (above). It is especially effective in renal and malignant hypertensions. Captopril elevates mood in depressed patients, possibly by an action on converting enzyme in the brain.

Rashes (erythematous, morbilliform, macropapular, edematous, urticarial) occur during the first 4 weeks of treatment in 4 to 10% of recipients. Approximately 7 to 10% of these manifest eosinophilia and antinuclear antibody, so that the rashes may have an immune origin. Eruptions do not occur until the dose exceeds 600 mg a day; they will sometimes disappear even with continued treatment. Pruritis, flushing, swelling of the extremities, cough (all 0.5 to 2%) and angioedema (0.1%) occur; these are probably kininergic rather than immunogenic. Angioedema can be a life-threatening reaction that requires discontinuation and, if severe, emergency treatment. Approximately 1% of recipients may have chest pain, vertigo or syncope (especially in salt-depleted patients) and tachycardia and/or dysrhythmia.

Nausea, vomiting and abdominal pain occur in 0.5 to 2% of recipients. Dysgeusia occurs in 2 to 4%; zinc chelators cause the same disorder, and captopril may possibly decorporate zinc. Dizziness, fatigue, headache, insomnia and paresthesias occur in 0.5 to 2% of cases. Sore throat (with severe neutropenia) and chills and fever occur in about 0.3%. Neutropenia is "dose-related" and occurs within 10 to 30 days of treatment; it persists for about 2 weeks after discontinuation; granulocyte counts are mandatory. It increases blood urea nitrogen, creatinine and liver enzymes in some patients. It may cause false positive tests for urinary acetone. Since it decreases aldosterone levels, drugs or situations that cause hyperkalemia, hyponatremia or hypoveolemia may interact adversely.

About 50% is eliminated in the urine, the remainder being metabolized. Doses must be lowered in renal failure. The half-life is less than 2 hr.

Dose—*Oral, adult, initially* **25 mg** 2 or 3 times a day to be increased after 2 weeks to **50 mg** 2 or 3 times a day, if necessary for *hypertension* and **25 mg** 2 or 3 times a day for *ventricular unloading* in heart failure. If the patient is sodium-depleted from saluresis, the initial dose should be 6.25 mg 2 or 3 times a day; *children, initially* **300 μg** (0.30 mg)/**kg** 3 times a day, to be increased, if necessary, by 300 μg/kg at 8- to 24-hr intervals up to the optimal dose. If the child is sodium-depleted from saluresis, the initial dose should be 150 μg/kg 3 times a day.

Dosage Form—Tablets: 12.5, 25, 50 and 100 mg.

Enalapril Maleate

L-Proline, (*S*)-1-[*N*-[1-(ethoxycarbonyl)-3-phenylpropyl]-L-alanyl]-, (*Z*)-2-butenedioate (1:1); Vasotec (*MSD*)

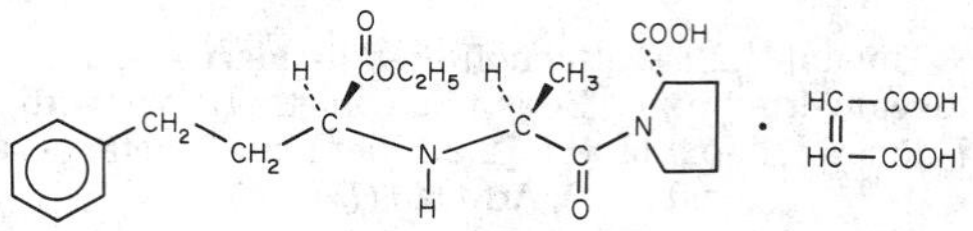

[76095-16-4] $C_{20}H_{28}N_2O_5.C_4H_4O_4$ (492.52).

Preparation—See *Nature 288*: 280, 1980.

Description—White to off-white crystalline powder melting about 143°; pH (1% aqueous solution) about 2.5; pK_a 3.0, 5.4.

Solubility—Very soluble in water; soluble in ethanol; freely soluble in methanol.

Uses—A prodrug of enaliprilat, the longer acting ACE inhibitor, used in the treatment of *renovascular, essential* and *malignant hypertensions* and for ventricular unloading in *congestive heart failure*. It can be used alone or in combination.

It lacks the sulfhydryl group of captopril and thus is less likely to cause rashes, proteinuria, leukopenia and dysgeusia. Adverse effects are excessive hypotension, especially in the elderly (0.9 to 2.3%), chest pain, palpitations (both 0.5 to 1%), nausea (1.3%), vomiting, abdominal pain (both 0.5 to 1%), diarrhea (1.6%), dysgeusia (0.5%), dyspnea, pruritis (both 0.5 to 1%), cough (1.3%), rash (1.5%), angioedema (0.2%), insomnia, paresthesias (both 0.5 to 1%), headache (4.8%), dizziness (4.6%) and fatigue (2.8%). Hyperkalemia may occur in renal failure.

About 60% is absorbed by the oral route. Peak plasma levels occur in 0.5 to 1 hr. In the body, about 40% is deesterified to enalaprilat, the active form of the drug (below). Enalaprilat and the remaining enalapril are eliminated in the urine. The half-life of enalapril is 1.3 hr but that of enalaprilat is about 11 hr, thus providing a duration of action of over a day.

Dose—*Oral, adult, initially* **2.5** to **5 mg** once a day for *hypertension* and **2.5 mg** for *heart failure*, with upward adjustments up to **10** to **40 mg** a day, divided into 1 or 2 doses, for *maintenance*; doses should be one-half the above in elderly patients or if a saluretic is also being administered.

Dosage Form—Tablets: 2.5, 5, 10 and 20 mg.

Enalaprilat

L-Proline, (*S*)-1-[*N*-[1-(carboxy)-3-phenylpropyl]-L-alanyl]-, dihydrate; Vasotec IV (*MSD*)

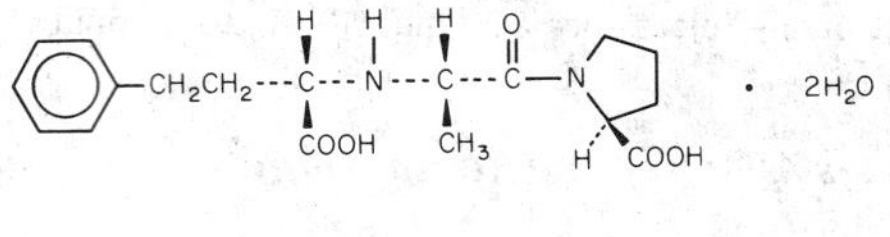

[84680-54-6] $C_{18}H_{24}N_2O_5.2H_2O$ (384.43).

Preparation—See *Enalapril Maleate*.

Description—White crystals melting about 150°.

Uses—The active form of enalapril (see above). It is water-soluble and hence is the parenteral form of enalapril. It is absorbed too slowly and erratically to be given orally.

Dose—*Intravenous, adult,* **1.25 mg** every 6 hr, except one-half that amount in elderly patients or if a saluretic also is being administered.

Dosage Form—Injection: 1.25 mg/mL in 1- and 2-mL vials.

Fosinopril Sodium

L-Proline, *trans*-4-cyclohexyl-1-[[[2-methyl-1-(1-oxopropoxy)propoxy] (4-phenylbutyl)phosphinyl]acetyl]-, sodium salt; Monopril (*Mead Johnson*)

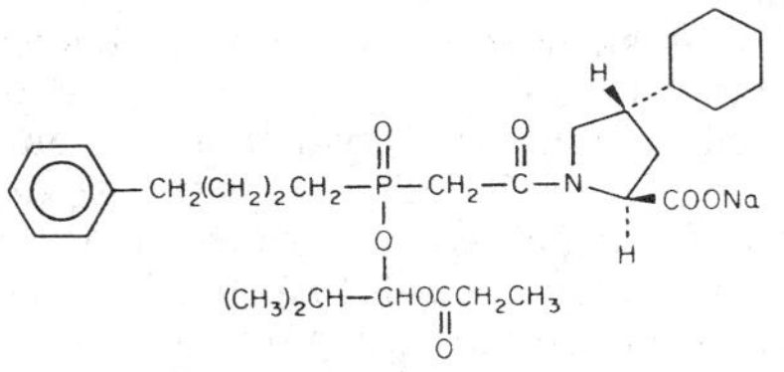

[88889-14-9] $C_{30}H_{45}NNaO_7P$ (585.65).

Preparation—See *J Med Chem 31:* 1148, 1988.

Describtion—White to off-white crystalline powder.

Solubility—1 g in 10 mL water; soluble in methanol or ethanol.

Uses—A prodrug rapidly absorbed and hydrolyzed by esterases in the intestine and liver to the active ACE inhibitor, *fosinoprilat,* which has a half-life of about 12 hr. It is approved for treating *essential hypertension.* It produces a similar spectrum and incidence of side effects and drug interactions as does enalapril; also, see the general statement. Total-body clearance is not reduced by renal impairment because it is conjugated to inactive glucuronide in the liver and excreted in the bile and urine.

Dose—*Oral, adult, initially* **10 mg** once a day, increasing to **20 to 40 mg** once or twice a day.

Dosage Form—Tablets: 10 and 20 mg.

Lisinopril

L-Proline, (*S*)-1-[N^2-[1-(carboxy)-3-phenylpropyl]-L-lysyl]-, dihydrate; Prinivil (*MSD*)

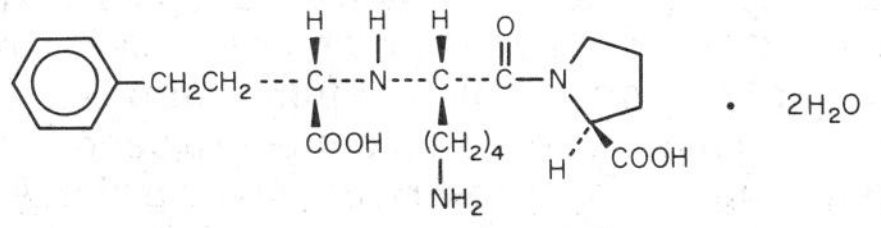

[83915-83-7] $C_{21}H_{31}N_3O_5.2H_2O$ (441.52).

Preparation—US Pat 4,555,502.

Description—White crystals; pK_a 2.5, 4.0, 6.7 and 10.1

Solubility—1 g in 10 mL water or 70 mL of methanol.

Uses—An ACE inhibitor used in the treatment of *renovascular, essential* and *malignant hypertensions* and for ventricular unloading in *congestive heart failure.* It can be used alone or in combination with other drugs.

It lacks the sulfhydryl group of captopril and thus is less likely to cause rashes, proteinuria, leukopenia and dysgeusia. Adverse effects are excessive hypotension (0.3 to 5%), chest pain (1.3%), palpitations (0.3 to 1%), nausea (2.3%), vomiting (1.3%), abdominal pain (0.3 to 1%), diarrhea (3.2%), dyspnea (1.1%), cough (2.9%), pruritis (0.3 to 1%), rash (1.5%), angioedema (0.1%), dizziness (6.3%), headache (5.3%), fatigue (3.3%), insomnia (0.3 to 1%) and paresthesias (0.8%). Hyperkalemia may occur in renal failure. There is no dysgeusia, which distinguishes this drug from captopril and enalapril.

Only about 30% is absorbed by the oral route. Peak plasma levels occur in about 7 hr. Elimination is almost entirely by renal excretion; the dose must be adjusted in renal failure. The normal half-life is about 12 hr but is longer in elderly patients.

Dose—*Oral, adult, initially* **10 mg** once a day, except **5 mg** in elderly patients or if a saluretic also is being given, adjusted upward, if necessary, to a maximum of **20** to **40 mg** once a day for *maintenance.*

Dosage Form—Tablets: 5, 10, 20 and 40 mg.

Quinapril Hydrochloride

3-Isoquinolinecarboxylic acid, [3*S*-[2[*R**(*R**)]],3*R**]-2-[2-[[1-(ethoxycarbonyl)-3-phenylpropyl]amino]-1-oxopropyl]-1,2,3,4-tetrahydro-, monohydrochloride, monohydrate; Accupril (*Parke-Davis*)

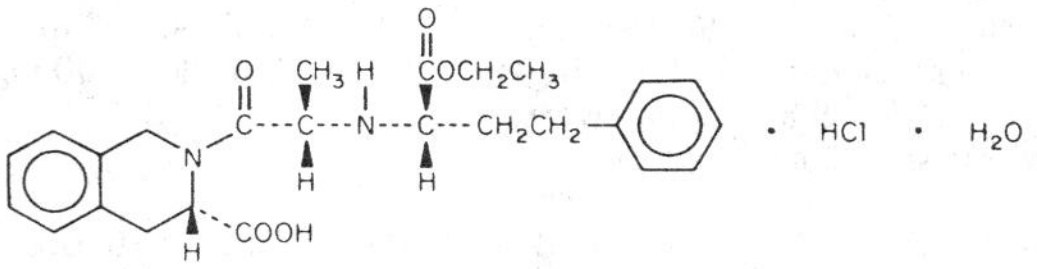

[90243-99-5] $C_{25}H_{30}N_2O_5.HCl.H_2O$ (493.00).

Preparation—*J Med Chem 29:* 1953, 1986.

Description—White crystals melting between 120 to 130° (dehydrated salt).

Uses—A prodrug rapidly absorbed and rapidly hydrolyzed to the more active ACE inhibitor, *quinaprilat,* which is active for 24 hr despite a plasma half-life of about 2 hr. It is approved for treating *essential hypertension,* and several clinical trials have shown it to be effective in treating *congestive heart failure.* Since 60% is excreted in the urine, dosage must be reduced in severe renal impairment. Its side effects and drug interactions are similar to those of other ACE inhibitors. See the general statement.

Dose—*Oral, adult, initially* **10 mg** once a day, increasing to **20 to 80 mg** a day, in one or two divided doses; *patients taking diuretics* or with *renal impairment,* initially **5 mg** once a day.

Dosage Form—Tablets: 5, 10, 20 and 40 mg.

Ramipril

Cyclopenta[*b*]pyrrole-2-carboxylic acid, [2*S*-[1[*R**(*R**)],2α,3aβ,6aβ]]-1-[2-[[1-(ethoxycarbonyl)-3-phenylpropyl]amino]-1-oxopropyl]octahydro-, Altace (*Hoechst-Roussel*)

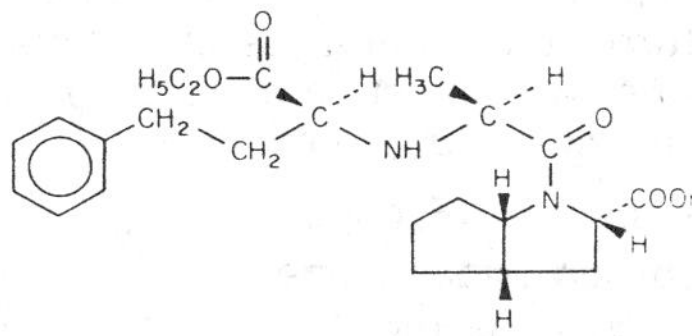

[87333-19-5] $C_{23}H_{32}N_2O_5$ (416.52).

Preparation—See *Arzneimittel-Forsch 34:* 1399, 1984.

Description—Fine needles melting about 109°; pK_a (ramiprilat) 3.1, 5.6.

Solubility—Soluble in alcohol; very slightly soluble in water.

Uses—A prodrug rapidly absorbed and converted to the highly potent, active ACE inhibitor, *ramiprilat,* which has a half-life of 13 to 17 hr. It is approved for treating *essential hypertension* and may be effective for treating *congestive heart failure.* Dosage should be reduced in renal failure because 60% is excreted in the urine. Side effects and drug interactions are similar to those of enalapril. See the general statement.

Dose—*Oral, adult, initially* **2.5 mg** once a day, increasing up to **20 mg** a day in 1 or 2 equally divided doses, as needed; *patients taking diuretics* or with *impaired renal function, initially* **1.25 mg** once a day; *maximum* in *renal impairment,* **5 mg** a day.

Dosage Form—Capsules: 1.25, 2.5, 5 and 10 mg.

Peripheral Vasodilators

Peripheral vasodilators are substances which dilate the arterioles and increase blood flow in the numerous systemic vascular beds, especially in the extremities. To the pharmacologist, the word *peripheral* may indicate that the action is directly on the arterioles, but to the clinician the word merely indicates the site of the final effect. Thus, centrally acting, reflexly acting or ganglionic blocking drugs that reduce sympathetic tone to the periphery are peripheral vasodilators, clinically speaking. Consequently, all of the hypotensives listed in the previous section may be considered to be peripheral dilators. Some sympathomimetics with prominent β_2-

Table 1—Other Peripheral Vasodilators

Drug	Description	Dosage Forms
Cyclandelate (Cyclospasmol, *Wyeth-Ayerst;* Various Mfrs)	Synthetic	Tablets: 200 and 400 mg Capsules: 200 and 400 mg
Ethaverine HCl (Ethaquin, *Ascher;* Ethatab, *Allen & Hanburys;* Various Mfrs)	Semisynthetic homolog of Papaverine	Tablets: 100 mg Capsules: 100 mg
Papaverine HCl (Various Mfrs)	Nonopioid alkaloid in crude opium	Tablets: 30, 60, 100, 150, 200 and 300 mg Timed-Release Tablets & Capsules: 200 mg Injection: 30 mg/mL

receptor stimulant actions are employed for their peripheral vasodilator effects. The adrenergic blocking drugs also are used to improve flow through specific peripheral vascular beds.

Peripheral vasodilators are employed in the treatment of vasospastic disorders such as *Raynaud's disease, causalgias* and *reflex dystrophy*, vasospasm associated with *arterial embolism* and *thrombophlebitis, immersion foot, trench foot, herpes zoster, decubitus ulcers* and degenerative arterial diseases such as *thromboangiitis obliterans, arteriosclerosis obliterans, acrocyanosis* and *diabetic gangrene*. However, there is a great deal of justifiable skepticism about the value of peripheral vasodilators in most uses, since vasospastic ischemia usually is self-limiting because of autoregulatory factors that counteract the spasms. An organic obstruction cannot be corrected for by vasodilatation, since the obstruction is the principal resistance in the line. However, vasodilatation may (or may not) improve circulation in the ischemic area through collateral vessels. Papaverine, alone or in combination with phentolamine, has been used as an intracavernous injection for impotence.

Dipyridamole—see RPS-18, page 844,

Isoxsuprine Hydrochloride—page 992.

Niacin—pages 1119 and 1126.

Nitrates and Nitrites (see **Coronary Drugs**)—page 943.

Nylidrin Hydrochloride—page 995.

Phentolamine—page 1010.

Antianginal Drugs

Drugs considered in this section are used primarily for the treatment of angina pectoris of several types: *classical* (exercise-induced or stable), *variant* (vasospastic or Prinzmetal's) and *unstable* anginas.

Two classes of drugs are the mainstays of angina therapy: the organonitrates and the calcium entry blocking drugs. Although both classes of agents dilate coronary arteries, coronary dilatation makes a minimal contribution to their antianginal effects, except in vasospastic angina, since diseased coronary arteries tend to be maximally dilated and usually are incapable of dilating further.

In the doses used for prophylaxis or relief of acute attacks of stable angina pectoris, *organonitrates* dilate the capacitance veins (which decreases ventricular-filling pressures) and the conducting arteries (which decreases arterial impedance). The former effect tends to decrease cardiac output and the latter to increase it, the net effect being a decrease in the short term but, often, an increase, when plasma levels are sustained. Both effects decrease heart size, the major determinant of myocardial oxygen demand and, hence, provide relief from anginal pain. The decrease in cardiac output lowers the blood pressure, which elicits reflex arteriolar constriction (which opposes the direct arteriolar dilating actions of the drug) and tachycardia, both of which are counterproductive.

The organonitrates are erratic in vasospastic (variant) angina. Their effect is to decrease venous return and cardiac afterload which ultimately decreases pulmonary venous pressure. The result is a decrease in pulmonary congestion and edema in left heart failure and after myocardial infarction; hence, organonitrates can be used to relieve *orthopnea* and *paroxysmal nocturnal dyspnea*. In the recumbent position, the effect to decrease venous return is less marked than in the upright position, and the effect to decrease cardiac afterload also is greater, so that cardiac output is maintained in recumbency.

Organonitrates all have a common mechanism of action briefly summarized as follows. The nitrates are denitrated *in vivo* to form nitric oxide (NO), which is also an endothelial-derived relaxing factor (EDRF) endogenously generated by the oxidation of L-arginine. In turn, NO reacts with sulfhydryl compounds in blood vessels to form adducts which stimulate guanylate cyclase, thus causing smooth muscle relaxation. Sustained use of organic nitrates depletes tissue sulfhydryl, and tolerance to the nitrates can ensue. Therefore, many experts now recommend pulse or intermittent dosing rather than continuous nitrate administration in order to reduce the likelihood of tolerance during chronic therapy. Sustained exposure to high doses of nitrates can result in a physical dependence which, upon abrupt discontinuation of drug, can be manifested as severe anginal attacks and/or myocardial infarction and sudden death.

Organonitrates are relaxants of all smooth muscle and may be employed as spasmolytics in certain instances, eg, in *biliary* and *ureteral spasms*. Since their actions are directly on the smooth muscle, they are independent of the type of innervation and cannot be prevented by any known agent.

Calcium entry blocking drugs act somewhat differently in relieving angina than do the organonitrates. Although some are extremely effective coronary and peripheral arteriolar dilators, the most important antianginal effect in exercise-induced and unstable anginas derives from the reduction in cardiac afterload. However, coronary artery dilatation is the primary cause of relief in vasospastic angina. Effects on cardiac preload are negligible. Some calcium entry antagonists directly slow the heart; this effect decreases myocardial oxygen demand as well as blunts reflex responses to arteriolar dilatation. Prevention of calcium influx into ischemic myocardial cells also may have a direct effect to decrease myocardial oxygen demand by preserving myocardial ATP. The calcium entry blocking drugs are discussed on page 952, *et seq.*

Other pharmacological approaches to the treatment of angina include the use of β-adrenoreceptor antagonists and various drugs which decrease the incidence and consequences of coronary artery disease.

Propranolol, and other β-adrenoreceptor antagonists, increase exercise tolerance in angina because they improve blood flow to the vulnerable subendocardium, mostly by slowing the heart rate and increasing diastolic time, during which subendocardial perfusion mainly occurs. Also, a decrease in heart rate decreases myocardial oxygen demand. Furthermore, β-blockade also decreases myocardial demand by decreasing calcium entry; sympathetically increased heart work has a slightly higher oxygen cost than that effected through the Starling mechanism. Therefore, β-blockade forces the heart to select the more energy-efficient mechanism to increase the work demanded by exercise. These drugs are discussed in Chapter 59. The use of drugs to decrease blood cholesterol and, hence, coronary atherosclerosis, is gaining much attention (page 966).

Antiplatelet drugs, such as aspirin and sulfinpyrazone, are under continuing investigation as prophylactics, with the rationale that thrombosis subsequent to rupture of the atheromatous plaque may be prevented and that white thrombus formation and release of a transforming factor that participates in atherogenesis is suppressed. Aspirin has been shown to decrease the incidence of myocardial reinfarction in men.

Amyl Nitrite

Mixture of nitrous acid, 2-methylbutyl ester, and nitrous acid, 3-methylbutyl ester; Vaporole (*Burroughs Wellcome*); Aspiroles (*Lilly*).

[8017-89-8] $C_5H_{11}NO_2$ (117.15).

Preparation—A good grade of commercial amyl alcohol (isoamyl alcohol) boiling above 125° is esterified with nitrous acid. The acid is generated in contact with the alcohol from sodium nitrite and dilute H_2SO_4.

Description—Clear, yellowish liquid with an ethereal, fruity odor and pungent, aromatic taste; boils at about 96° but is volatile even at low temperatures and is flammable; slowly decomposes on exposure to air and light; moisture accelerates decomposition; specific gravity 0.870 and 0.876.

Solubility—Practically insoluble in water; miscible with alcohol, chloroform or ether.

Uses—Although a *nitrite*, its actions are those of organonitrates (see the general statement). It causes more reflex arteriolar constriction than the nitrates. It is quite volatile and is inhaled to obtain a rapid effect (onset 0.5 min). In practice, however, amyl nitrite is employed rarely in the treatment of attacks of *angina pectoris* but somewhat more frequently for the relief of *biliary* or *renal colic*. An unusual, but at times life-saving, use for amyl nitrite is in the emergency treatment of *cyanide poisoning*, where nitrites are given to produce methemoglobin, which temporarily inactivates the toxic cyanide ion by combining with it to form cyanmethemoglobin. For this purpose, sodium nitrite is employed intravenously, but this drug may be inhaled while the solution of sodium nitrite is being prepared. It is administered by crushing a glass *perle of this drug* in a handkerchief and inhaling the liquid which volatilizes, or by dropping a small quantity on a handkerchief and inhaling the vapor. It has become a drug of abuse because of a "rush" (an acute vasodilatory episode) felt after inhalation. Abuse may cause methemoglobinemia, hemolytic anemia and immunological disorders.

Caution—Amyl Nitrite is very flammable. Do not use where it may be ignited.

Dose—By *inhalation*, **0.3 mL.**

Dosage Form—Volatile Inhalant: 0.3 mL.

Erythrityl Tetranitrate

(*R**,*S**)-1,2,3,4-Butanetetrol, tetranitrate; Tetranitrol; Cardilate *(Burroughs Wellcome)*

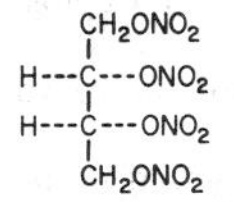

```
       CH2ONO2
        |
H---C---ONO2
        |
H---C---ONO2
        |
       CH2ONO2
```

[7297-25-8] $C_4H_6N_4O_{12}$ (302.11); a dry mixture with lactose or other suitable inert excipients, to permit safe handling and compliance with federal ICC regulations pertaining to interstate shipment.

Caution: Undiluted erythrityl tetranitrate is a powerful explosive, and proper precautions must be taken in handling. It can be exploded by percussion or by excessive heat. Only extremely small quantities should be isolated.

Preparation—Erythritol is reacted with nitric acid in the presence of sulfuric acid under controlled temperature.

Description—White powder having a slight odor of nitric oxides and a bitter taste; unstable in light or heat.

Solubility—Soluble (undiluted) in acetone or alcohol; practically insoluble in water.

Uses—See the general statement under organonitrates. By the sublingual route, it has a relatively long duration of action (about 2 hr). By the oral route, the duration is longer, but quite variable. Its principal use is in the prophylaxis of *angina pectoris* in *acute* situations in which an attack can be anticipated. Medical authorities do not consider it useful as a chronic, routine, round-the-clock prophylactic because of development of a prominent tolerance. In fact, it has been shown to be not as good as a placebo. Sensitivity can be restored by several days' rest. As with nitroglycerin and other organic nitrates, its peripheral effects to decrease venous return and arterial impedance and not coronary vasodilation account for the improved exercise tolerance in anginal patients.

Untoward effects include tachycardia, headache, flushing, dizziness, syncope and nausea; tolerance to these effects often develops. It should be given cautiously to patients with glaucoma.

The bioavailability by the oral route is unpredictable because of differences among individuals and also from time-to-time as the result of variations in hepatic metabolism during absorption. Phenobarbital increases the metabolism.

Dose—*Oral, adult, chronic therapy, initially* **10 mg** 4 times a day, gradually increased to 20 mg, if necessary, not to exceed 100 mg a day; *sublingual, adults, acute prophylaxis,* **5** or **10 mg** prior to anticipated stress; *chronic therapy,* **5** to **10 mg** 3 or 4 times a day, with adjustments as needed. The interval between increments of dosage should not be shorter than 2 days. Despite the fact that "round-the-clock" regimes are common, they run counter to authoritative medical opinion regarding the proper use of so-called long-acting organonitrates, namely, that they should be administered only in advance of anticipated situations known to cause anginal pain. Steady use causes tolerance and loss of effectiveness; to break tolerance the drug must be discontinued for more than a week, during which time other organonitrates cannot be used.

Dosage Form—Oral/Sublingual Tablets: 5 and 10 mg.

Isosorbide Dinitrate

D-Glucitol, 1,4:3,6-dianhydro-, dinitrate; Isordil *(Wyeth)*; Sorbitrate *(ICI Pharm)*; Dilatrate-SR (*Reed-Carnrick*); (*Various Mfrs*)

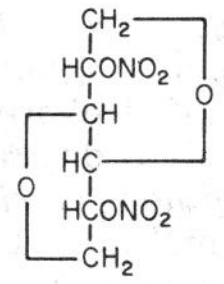

```
      CH2 ----+
       |      |
     HCONO2   |
       |      O
  +---CH      |
  |    |      |
  O   HC------+
  |    |
  |  HCONO2
  |    |
  +---CH2
```

[87-33-2] $C_6H_8N_2O_8$ (236.14).

Preparation—An aqueous syrup of 1,4:3,6-dianhydro-D-glucitol is added slowly to a cooled mixture of HNO_3 and H_2SO_4. After standing a few minutes the mixture is poured into cold water and the precipitated product is collected and recrystallized from ethanol.

Description—*Diluted* (with mannitol, lactose or other inert ingredients)*:* ivory-white, odorless powder. *Undiluted:* white, crystalline rosettes.

Solubility—*Undiluted:* very slightly soluble in water; very soluble in acetone; freely soluble in chloroform; sparingly soluble in alcohol.

Uses—The long-acting organonitrate of choice. With sublingual and chewable tablet forms, the onset of effect is 2 to 5 min (absorption from the chewable tablet is also mainly from the mouth); with oral forms, the onset is about 30 min and offset 4 to 6 hr; with sustained-release forms the offset is 8 to 12 hr. Nitroglycerin thus affords quicker relief, and isosorbide dinitrate is indicated only for the prophylaxis of attacks of angina in situations in which attacks can be anticipated. However, the dose statement includes doses for the suppression of acute attacks. Tolerance tends to limit the benefits of continuous, long-term prophylaxis. Double-blind studies show that chronic, continuously administered isosorbide dinitrate to be less effective than a placebo. The sustained-release forms have not been proved to be as effective as oral tablets for acute prophylaxis.

The most frequent complaint by users is headache. In some persons there is also a paradoxical increase in anginal pain. Mild gastrointestinal disturbances, as well as vertigo and other signs of orthostatic hypotension may occur. It should be given cautiously in patients with glaucoma.

Oral bioavailability is approximately 22% because of high first-pass metabolism. Sublingual administration is said to increase bioavailability, but there is some disagreement on this point. However, sublingual and chewable tablet dosages are predicated on bioavailabilities at least twice the bioavailability with oral administration. The metabolites of isosorbide dinitrate are the 2- and 5-monitrates, both of which have antianginal effects. The 5-mononitrate is the more active. The half-life varies with the route of administration and ranges from 20 min (IV) to 4 hr (oral), probably because there is more mononitrate formed after oral administration; mononitrate inhibits the metabolism of the parent drug. There is considerable interpatient variation. Phenobarbital, and probably other inducers of cytochrome P-450, increase the metabolism and decrease efficacy.

Dose—*Oral (capsules* or *tablets), adult, chronic prophylaxis, initially* **5** to **20 mg** in *conventional* forms or **40 mg** in *sustained-release* forms followed by *maintenance* doses of **10** to **40 mg** every 6 hr with *conventional* forms or **40** to **80 mg** every 8 to 12 hr with *sustained-release* forms. *Oropharyngeal (chewable tablets), adult, chronic prophylaxis, initially* **5** to **10 mg** every 2 to 3 hr; [*acute attack, initially* **5 mg,** to be adjusted upward at 5-min intervals until relief is obtained or adverse effects prevent further increases]. *Sublingual/buccal (sublingual tablets), adult, acute prophylaxis,* **5** to **10 mg** every 2 to 3 hr; [*acute attack, initially* **2.5** to **5 mg,** to be adjusted upward at 5-min intervals until relief is obtained or adverse effects prevent further increases]. *Topical, adult,* **100 mg a day** as an ointment (not yet available in the US).

Dosage Forms—Capsules: 40 mg; Sustained-Release Capsules: 40 mg; Tablets: 5, 10, 20, 30 and 40 mg; Chewable Tablets: 5 and 10 mg; Sustained-Release Tablets: 40 mg; Sublingual Tablets: 2.5, 5 and 10 mg.

Isosorbide Mononitrate

D-Glucitol, 1:4,3:6-dianhydro-, 5-nitrate; ISMO (*Wyeth-Ayerst*)

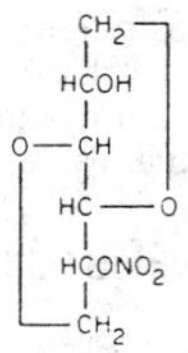

[16051-77-7] $C_6H_9NO_6$ (191.14).

Preparation—See *Acta Physiol Scand 15:* 173, 1948.

Description—White powder melting about 90°.

Solubility—About 1 g in 20 mL alcohol or water.

Uses—A metabolite of isosorbide dinitrate (above). It is effective in the treatment of all types of *angina pectoris.* Its bioavailability is about 100%. The half-life is 4 to 6 hr. Advantages over isosorbide dinitrate include no first-pass metabolism, no active metabolites and a significantly longer half-life. Interpatient variation in response is much less than with isosorbide dinitrate.

Dose—*Oral,* **20 mg** twice a day, 7 hr apart.

Dosage Form—Tablets: 20 mg.

Nitroglycerin

1,2,3-Propanetriol, trinitrate; Glyceryl Trinitrate; Glonoin; Trinitrin; (*Various Mfrs*)

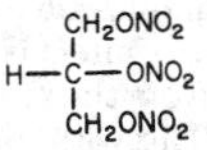

Nitroglycerin [55-63-0] $C_3H_5N_3O_9$ (227.09).

Preparation—By nitrating glycerin with a mixture of nitric and sulfuric acids called "nitration acid." This acid usually consists of 3 parts of concentrated nitric acid and 5 parts of sulfuric acid.

Description—Practically colorless, odorless liquid with a sweet taste.

Packaging—Sufficiently volatile to require packaging of tablets in glass containers with tightly fitting metal screw caps, and holding no more than 100 tablets in each container; only original unopened containers may be dispensed. Patients should keep the tablets in the original container, close it tightly after each use and avoid exposure to heat. Some manufacturers have added a "fixing" agent (polyethylene glycols) to the tablet preparation to minimize volatilization. Regardless, the unopened container *only,* should be dispensed and under no circumstance should a label, absorbent cotton or a desiccant be placed in the container.

Uses—The classical organonitrate once was long the drug of choice for the treatment of angina pectoris. See the general statement for actions and uses.

After oral administration, it is metabolized rapidly in the intestinal wall and liver, so that systemic bioavailability is rather low. Consequently, oral doses are quite high and plasma levels are erratic. Bioavailability is much greater by the buccal and sublingual routes. Medical authorities do not recommend sustained-release forms of nitroglycerin, since oral bioavailability is so poor and tolerance is favored. By the sublingual route, the vasodilator effects of the drug appear in 2 to 3 min and last about 20 min, but exercise tolerance may be increased for as long as an hour in some patients. Buccal tablets, if retained in the mouth, release nitroglycerin for 3 to 5 hr. Sustained-release oral capsules and tablets maintain plasma levels for 8 to 12 hr. A nitroglycerin ointment can provide therapeutic blood levels for 2 to 12 hr per application but is not recommended for routine use. Transdermal preparations may sustain plasma levels for 24 hr or longer.

The volume of distribution is about 3 L/kg. The distribution half-life is 1 to 4 min and the elimination half-life, about 2 hr.

Cerebral vasodilation may cause transient headaches. Paradoxical angina occurs when the dose is too large and blood pressure falls too low to sustain coronary flow. Dizziness, nausea and other symptoms of hypotension also occur. High, repetitive doses can cause methemoglobinemia.

Dose—*Buccal, adult, prophylaxis, initially* **1 mg** as a *sustained-release buccal tablet* placed between the upper lip and gingiva above the incisors every 5 hr, to be adjusted, if necessary, by changing dose or dose-interval. *Intravenous, adult,* for *angina, congestive heart failure* or *hypertension,* **0.1 mg** as a bolus or **0.005 mg/min** by slow infusion, the rate to be increased at 5-min intervals by equal increments until the response is satisfactory or the rate is 0.02 mg/min, after which increments become 0.01 mg/min, then eventually 0.02 mg/min, if necessary. *Lingual, adult, acute attack,* **0.4** or **0.8 mg** (1 or 2 metered sprays) as a *lingual aerosol* every 5 min, if necessary, not to exceed 2.4 mg in 15 min or 1.2 mg/day; *acute prophylaxis,* **0.4** or **0.8 mg** 5 to 20 min before the exertion. *Oral, adult, prophylaxis, initially* **2.5** or **2.6 mg** as an *extended-release capsule* or *extended-release tablet* 3 or 4 times a day, with adjustments, if necessary, by increasing dosage at 12-hr intervals or decreasing dose-interval to 8 hr. *Sublingual, adult, acute attack,* **0.15** to **0.6 mg,** as a *sublingual tablet* repeated every 5 min, if necessary, for 3 doses; *acute prophylaxis,* **15** to **0.6 mg,** 5 to 20 min before the exertion. *Transcutaneous, initially* **2.5** to **5 cm** of **2% ointment** (15 to 30 mg of drug) every 3 or 4 hr *or* **1 transdermal system** every 24 hr, to deliver **2.5 mg/24 hr,** with dosage adjustments by increasing the amount of ointment applied up to 12.5 cm or successively stronger transdermal systems.

Dosage Forms—Lingual Aerosol: 13.8 g, to deliver 0.4 mg/metered spray; Sustained-Release Capsules: 2.5, 6.5 and 9 mg; Injection, 0.5, 0.8 and 5 mg/mL; Ointment: 2%; Sublingual Tablets: 0.15, 0.3, 0.4 and 0.6 mg; Sustained-Release Buccal Tablets: 1, 2 and 3 mg; Sustained-Release Tablets: 2.6, 3, 5, 6.5 and 9 mg; Transdermal Systems: to deliver 2.5, 5, 7.5, 10 and 15 mg/24 hr (contents vary from 12.5 to 187.5 mg).

Pentaerythritol Tetranitrate

1,3-Propanediol, 2,2-bis[(nitrooxy)methyl]-, dinitrate, ester; Peritrate (*Parke-Davis*); (*Various Mfrs*)

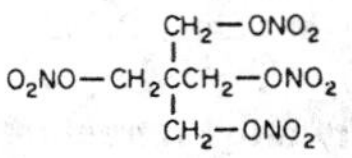

[78-11-15] $C_5H_8N_4O_{12}$ (316.14).

Description—A dry mixture of pentaerythritol tetranitrate (prepared by nitration of pentaerythritol) with lactose or other suitable inert excipient to permit safe handling of the explosive undiluted substance; melts about 140°.

Solubility—Practically insoluble in water; sparingly soluble in polar organic solvents.

Uses—A "so-called" long-acting organonitrate, the long duration of which is mainly the result of prolonged release and absorption from oral dosage forms. It is used in the prophylaxis of attacks of *angina pectoris* but not in the management of the acute attack. It is no better than a placebo as a routine chronic prophylactic in angina pectoris; tolerance develops with chronic use. Transient headache and nausea may accompany its use. It should be given cautiously to patients with glaucoma. Medical authorities state that the sustained-release forms are poorly effective. It is not absorbed sublingually. Since absorption by the oral route is erratic, efficacy is unpredictable.

Dose—*Oral, adult, usually* **10** to **20 mg** 4 times a day, increased to as much as **160 mg** a day, if necessary, administered in 4 subdivided doses as regular tablets, or **30** to **80 mg** as sustained-release tablets or capsules twice a day. For comment concerning "around-the-clock" dosage schedules, see the general statement.

Dosage Forms—Extended-Release Capsules: 30, 45 and 80 mg; Tablets: 10, 20, 40 and 80 mg; Extended-Release Tablets: 80 mg.

Vasopressor Drugs

A number of drugs of other classes treated elsewhere in this text have vasoconstrictor or cardiostimulator activity and can be used to elevate the blood pressure under appropriate conditions. The most important of these are sympathomimetics, which are treated in Chapter 57. In conditions in which the plasma volume is diminished, as in hypovolemic shock, fluid replacement tends to restore the blood pressure, but plasma extenders (Chapter 54) are not truly vasopressor, since they do not cause vasoconstriction.

The usefulness of vasoconstrictor agents in the treatment of shock has been debated intensely. In nearly every kind of shock, the body responds by reflex vasoconstriction, and it has been argued that if the arterioles and capacitance veins can respond to reflex sympathetic stimulation, vasoconstrictors are redundant. If arteriolar function has deteriorated to where it cannot respond to sympathetic impulses, it also cannot respond to vasoconstrictor drugs. Furthermore, there is much evidence that vasoconstriction increases the ischemic damage already in progress as the result of inadequate circulation. Consequently, the attention in the 1960s shifted to α-adrenergic blocking drugs and vasodilators and more recently to cardiostimulants.

Dopamine (page 988) comes close to fulfilling the requirements of an ideal vasopressor drug for supporting blood pressure in shock. In appropriate dosage it dilates blood vessels in the renal, splanchnic, cerebral and coronary beds, beds which are of vital importance, constricts in the cutaneous and skeletal muscle vascular beds, where very little flow is needed in shock, and stimulates the heart. (See also *Dobutamine*, page 988.)

Lypressin—page 1063.

Cardiac Glycosides (Digitalis)

The primary action of digitalis on the heart is a direct *cardiotonic action* on the myocardium to *increase the force of contraction*. The increased contractility results from inhibition of the membrane sodium-potassium activated ATPase, which inhibition ultimately increases the intracellular stores of calcium. In congestive heart failure, stroke volume is increased, which more effectively empties the ventricles and lowers diastolic ventricular pressures and ultimately pulmonary and central venous pressures. Congestion thus is diminished.

Increased cardiac output improves renal blood flow and glomerular filtration and decreases juxtaglomerular renin secretion, so that the renal resorption of sodium and water and, hence, of edema is diminished. Diuresis is promoted. Hepatic blood flow also is increased, which increases the clearance of aldosterone and contributes to the reduction in edema.

Slowing of the cardiac rate occurs only when the rate was originally rapid, as the result of compensatory sympathetic reflexes, consequent to failure. When the failure is abolished, there is no longer any need for the compensatory tachycardia and, consequently, the heart rate slows to normal. This slowing mistakenly has been attributed to a "vagal action" of digitalis. However, digitalis does sensitize the sinoatrial node, atrium and atrioventricular node to vagal impulses, and, in high therapeutic and toxic doses, increases vagal traffic by actions in the CNS and on the baroreceptors. High doses also may slow the ventricle by a direct action on atrioventricular conduction.

The chief therapeutic use for digitalis is in the treatment of *low-output congestive heart failure*. It is of value regardless of whether the failure is predominantly of the right or left side of the heart. There is some controversy about the benefits of extended treatment with digitalis, but the practice is exceedingly popular. Dysrhythmias and valvular defects may modify the response to digitalis, but their presence neither indicates nor contraindicates the use of the drug. However, it is generally true that the most dramatic responses are seen in patients with *both atrial fibrillation and congestive heart failure*.

Badly damaged hearts do not respond well. When the failure is due to an acute toxic or infectious process, like typhoid fever or diphtheritic myocarditis, rather than to a chronic degenerative process like arteriosclerosis or failure secondary to hypertensive heart disease, digitalis may give poor results and may even be contraindicated. High-output failure in patients with anemia, hyperthyroidism and thiamine deficiency is likewise not much benefited. Also, heart failure secondary to cardiovascular syphilis yields poorly to digitalis therapy.

Digitalis has been advocated for use in peripheral circulatory collapse, shock, etc, but it is now clear that it promotes splanchnic ischemia, which may complicate and exacerbate shock and favor small bowel ischemia.

The signs and symptoms of heart failure in persons with mild heart failure are abolished by digitalis, but bed rest, sedatives and, often, diuretics and restriction of salt intake may be required to obtain best results. Exertional and paroxysmal nocturnal dyspnea disappear; cough, cyanosis, ascites, edema and chronic passive congestion of the lungs and abdominal viscera are relieved. The enlarged diastolic size of the heart is decreased, engorged veins due to increased venous pressure are returned to normal and the diastolic rest period in each cardiac cycle is prolonged.

The action of digitalis to impair atrioventricular conduction is employed in the management of *atrial flutter*, *atrial fibrillation* and *paroxysmal supraventricular tachycardia* (PSVT). In patients with atrial fibrillation, digitalis occasionally may revert the dysrhythmia if congestive heart failure is present. Digitalis glycosides do not cure the dysrhythmia directly but by improving the condition of the heart and lessening stretch and ischemia, the fibrillation may cease in some instances. The atrial fibrillation usually persists.

The action actually sought is second-degree heart block, which will decrease the ventricular rate toward a more optimal value. The same action is sought in atrial flutter, namely a partial heart block, to decrease the number of atrial impulses that pass through to the ventricles. In an occasional case of atrial flutter, the proper use of fairly large doses of digitalis may abolish the arrhythmia. In PSVT a properly selected dose can interrupt one segment of the reentrant pathway within the AV node, thus terminating the "circus movement" yet allowing orthograde conduction of normal impulses. Cardiac glycosides commonly are used prophylactically against recurrences of PSVT.

The choice of glycoside offers considerable difficulty to many practitioners. When absorbed in adequate amounts, all the active digitalis principles produce identical effects on the myocardium, and their toxic effects are essentially the same, although there is some evidence that digitoxin gains better access to the CNS and causes more neurological side effects and CNS-initiated arrhythmias. They differ from each other largely in speed of onset of action and duration of cardiac effects and in the degree of absorption by the oral route. With some glycosides (eg, digoxin), bioavailability varies widely from product to product, which imposes strict requirements for clinical or plasma-level monitoring when unfamiliar products are employed.

Initial digitalization may be accomplished rapidly or slowly, depending on the urgency of the case. The vast majority of patients with congestive heart failure are not *in extremis* and can be digitalized without a loading dose, so that about 5 half-lives are required to achieve a maintenance steady state.

In acute heart failure or incapacitating atrial tachydysrhythmia, loading is desirable. The process of loading is known as *rapid digitalization*. It is not unusual to digitalize a patient in 12 or 24 hours by giving one-half of the calculated dose at once, and the remainder in two or three divided doses at intervals of 6 hours. This principle is applied to other cardiac glycosides and only the timing differs. No fixed formula or rule of thumb can be employed. Each case is individualized, and the physician must watch his patient constantly to observe the developing effects of the drug and to prevent unpleasant or serious toxic effects from overdosage.

Optimal effects can be obtained without toxic effects, and the optimal dose is not necessarily the largest tolerated dose. It can be found only by careful observation of the patient. When rapid digitalization is employed usually the patient should be seen immediately before an additional dose is given.

In rare cases it may be necessary to inject a parenteral preparation intravenously in order to save life. Such patients usually are *in extremis* and may die before digitalis given by mouth can exert its effect (within 2 hours) or they are patients who are unable to tolerate oral digitalis or who have gastrointestinal disorders that preclude oral dosage. Small doses are employed as a rule, and digitalization with an orally efficacious preparation then is completed by the oral route.

Cardiac glycosides have a low margin of safety. They may cause nausea, vomiting, diarrhea, abdominal pain, headache, drowsiness, fatigue, malaise, backache, decreased libido, impotence, trigeminal neuralgia, "white vision" and other visual disturbances, convulsions, mental disturbances, eosinophilia, rashes, gynecomastia and, rarely, thrombocytopenia.

Cardiac dysrhythmias of all types are relatively common as a sign of excessive plasma levels. Heart block and premature ventricular contractions (PVC) are the most frequent, ventricular tachycardia the most ominous. Toxicity is more likely in the presence of hypokalemia, a common result of concomitant diuretic therapy for the cardiac edema. Amphotericin B and mineralocorticoids also cause hypokalemia and may promote digitalis toxicity. Intravenous calcium salts also can precipitate intoxication.

Toxicity can be antagonized by Digoxin Immune Fab (page 957), edetate disodium, potassium (especially if hypokalemia exists), lidocaine, phenytoin or, to a lesser extent, propranolol, quinidine or procainamide. Toxic doses also give rise to serious ventricular dysrhythmias.

Deslanoside

Desacetyllanatoside C; Cedilanid D (*Sandoz*)

[17598-65-1] $C_{47}H_{74}O_{19}$ (943.09). Its side chain consists of 3 molecules of digitoxose and 1 molecule of glucose in glycosidic linkage.

Preparation—By deacetylating lanatoside C by treatment with alkali.

Description—Colorless or white crystals or a white, crystalline powder; odorless; hygroscopic, absorbing about 7% of moisture when exposed to air; melts indistinctly about 220°.

Solubility—Very slightly soluble in water or chloroform; 1 g in about 300 mL alcohol.

Uses—See the general statement. By the intravenous route the onset of action is about 10 to 30 min, and the peak effect occurs in about 1 to 3 hr. The duration of action is approximately 2 to 5 days. Elimination is primarily renal, and dosage adjustments may be required in renal failure. The elimination half-life is approximately 33 to 36 hr. Parenteral administration should be employed only in situations when rapid action is needed or when oral administration is not feasible.

Dose—*Intramuscular, adult, digitalization,* **800 µg** (0.8 mg) at each of 2 sites, after which an orally administered cardiac glycoside is substituted; *neonates,* **22 µg/kg** (or 300 µg/m²) divided into 2 or 3 doses given at 3- or 4-hr intervals; *infants* and *children 2 wk* to *3 yr,* **25 µg/kg** (or 750 µg/m²) divided into 2 or 3 doses given at 3- to 4-hr intervals; *children 3 or more yr,* **22.5 µg/kg** (or 750 µg/m²) divided into 2 or 3 doses given at 3- or 4-hr intervals. *Intravenous, adult, initially* **800 µg** (0.8 mg), repeated in 4 hr, after which an orally administered cardiac glycoside is substituted; *infants* and *children,* same as intramuscular dose.

Dosage Form—Injection: 0.4 mg/2 mL.

Caution—Handle with exceptional care, since it is highly potent.

Digitoxin

Card-20(22)-enolide, (3β,5β)-3-[(O-2,6-dideoxy-β-D-*ribo*-hexopyranosyl-(1 → 4)-O-2,6-dideoxy-β-D-*ribo*-hexopyranosyl-(1 → 4)-2,6-dideoxy-D-*ribo*-hexopyranosyl)oxy]-14-hydroxy-, (*Various Mfrs*)

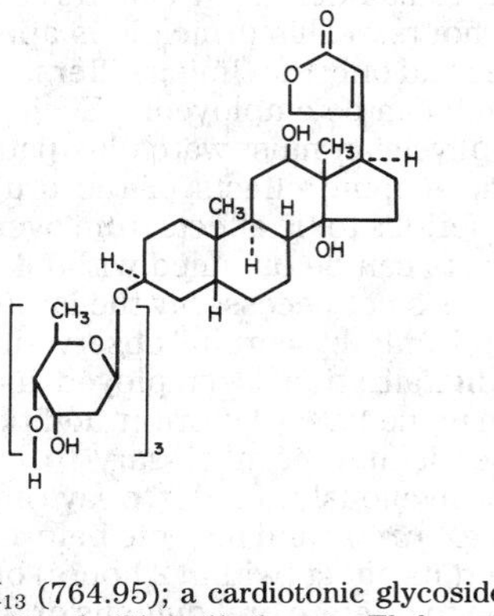

[71-63-6] $C_{41}H_{64}H_{13}$ (764.95); a cardiotonic glycoside obtained from *Digitalis purpurea* Linné, *Digitalis lanata* Ehrh and other suitable species of *Digitalis.*

The side chain consists of 3 molecules of digitoxose in glycosidic linkage. Removal of the side chain by hydrolysis yields the aglycone, digitoxigenin ($C_{23}H_{34}O_4$).

Description—White or pale buff, odorless, microcrystalline powder.

Solubility—Practically insoluble in water; 1 g in about 150 mL alcohol or 40 mL chloroform; very slightly soluble in ether.

Uses—See the general statement. It is absorbed almost completely after oral administration except when cholestyramine also is being used. Action is maximal in 4 to 12 hr. After full digitalization, the duration of action is about 14 days. In plasma, about 97% is protein-bound. The volume of distribution is about 0.6 mL/g. Plasma concentrations of 15 to 25 ng/mL are considered to be therapeutic and 35 to 40 ng/mL or more to be toxic, but plasma potassium and calcium levels and other factors cause considerable variation. Hepatic metabolism accounts for 52 to 70% of elimination. The β-half-life ranges from 2.4 to 9.6 (av 7.6) days. Phenytoin and phenobarbital can induce hepatic microsomal enzymes and shorten the half-life, hence interfering with the efficacy of the drug.

Dose—*Oral, intravenous, adult,* for *digitalization, initially* **600 µg** (0.6 mg), followed by **200** to **400** µg every 3 to 6 hr as needed, up to a total of no more than 1.6 mg in 1 or 2 days; *maintenance, usually* **50** to **300 µg** a day. In the following *pediatric* doses, only the *digitalizing* dose is stated; the *maintenance* dose is calculated as 10% of the total digitalizing dose a day: *Oral, intravenous, neonates,* **22 µg/kg** (or 300 to 350 µg/m²) divided into 3 or more doses at 6-hr intervals; *infants 2 wk to 1 yr,* **45 µg** (or 750 µg/m²) divided into 3 or more doses at 6-hr intervals; *infants 1 to 2 yr,* **40 µg/kg** (or 750 µg/m²) divided into 3 or more doses at 6-hr intervals; *children 2 yr or older,* **30 µg/kg** (or 750 µg/m²) divided into 3 or more doses at 6-hr intervals.

Loading and maintenance doses require reduction by 25 to 50% in small or elderly patients or in patients with renal, electrolyte or metabolic disorders. The above doses apply only if the patient has received no digitalis for 2 weeks.

Dosage Form—Tablets: 50, 100, 150 and 200 µg.

Caution—Handle digitoxin with exceptional care, since it is highly potent.

Digoxin

Card-20(22)-enolide, (3β,5β,12β)-3-[(O-2,6-dideoxy-β-D-*ribo*-hexopyranosyl-(1 → 4)-O-2,6-dideoxy-β-D-*ribo*-hexopyranosyl-(1 → 4)-2,6-dideoxy-β-D-*ribo*-hexopyranosyl)oxy]-12,14-dihydroxy-, Lanoxin (*Burroughs Wellcome*)

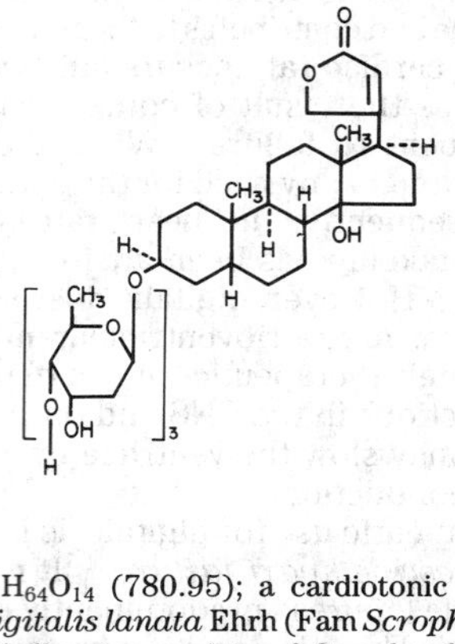

[20830-75-5] $C_{41}H_{64}O_{14}$ (780.95); a cardiotonic glycoside obtained from the leaves of *Digitalis lanata* Ehrh (Fam *Scrophulariaceae*).

The side chain of digoxin consists of 3 molecules of digitoxose in glycosidic linkage. Hydrolytic cleavage yields the aglycone, digoxigenin ($C_{23}H_{34}O_5$).

Description—Clear to white crystals or a white crystalline powder; odorless; melts with decomposition above 235°.

Solubility—Practically insoluble in water or ether; slightly soluble in diluted alcohol or chloroform.

Uses—See the general statement. Because this is a purified preparation, it frequently is used intravenously for very rapid digitalization. Intravenously, its action becomes manifest in 15 to 30 min, and the effect reaches its peak in 2 to 5 hr. Orally, its action is manifest within 1 to 2 hr and reaches a peak in 6 to 8 hr. After full digitalization, the duration of action is about 6 days. In plasma 20 to 30% is protein-bound. It has a high volume of distribution, with a v_d^{ss} of about 5.1 L/kg in normal adults and neonates and even larger in infants; in renal failure v_d^{ss} is approximately 3.3 L/kg. Extensive intracellular binding accounts for the large volume of distribution.

The therapeutic concentration in plasma is 0.5 to 2.4 ng/mL, and concentrations above 2.4 ng/mL are toxic, except that lower concentrations are toxic when hypokalemia, hypercalcemia and certain other conditions obtain. Therefore, blood-level assays have only a rough significance; they are of especial utility in determining bioavailability. In adults, renal excretion accounts for 60 to 90% of elimination; some is converted in the liver to dihydrodigoxin. Infants appear to have a greater fraction of extrarenal elimination. Biliary secretion and enterohepatic recirculation account for about 7 to 30% of the body burden. The elimination half-life is 29 to 135 (usually 36 to 41) hr in normal adults; in infants of 1 month to 2 yr, it is sufficiently shorter to require a special dose regimen. In renal failure, the β-half-life may be as long as 89 to 177 hr. Amiodarone, indomethacin, propafenone, quinidine, tiapamil and verapamil also considerably prolong the half-life.

This drug often is preferred to digitoxin because of its shorter half-life; when loading is not used, the steady state is reached earlier, and, when toxicity occurs, nontoxic levels are reached earlier after discontinuation of the drug. However, it is difficult to achieve digitalization and easier to lose control of digitalization if a dose is missed. Considerable attention to appropriate spacing of maintenance doses is required for smooth digitalization. By the oral route, about 50 to 85% is absorbed from solid dosage forms, but it is 90 to 100% from hydroalcoholic solutions in capsules. Increased gastrointestinal motility diminishes and decreased motility increases absorption.

Antacids, antineoplastic drugs, cholestyramine, dietary fiber, erythromycin, kaolin-pectate, metaclopramide, neomycin, propantheline, sulfasalazine and tetracyclines all alter its bioavailability.

Dose—[The different doses among the various dosage forms are based on assumed differences in bioavailability: *capsules* (containing hydroalcoholic solution) and *injection*, $F = 1.00$; *elixir* and *tablets*, $F = 0.80$. The higher maintenance doses with the injection are based upon more serious morbidity.] *Intravenous, adult, digitalization,* **400** to **600 μg** then **100** to **300 μg** every 4 to 8 hr as necessary or tolerated; *maintenance,* **125** to **500 μg**/day in 1 or more divided doses. *Intravenous, pediatric, digitalization, premature neonates,* **15** to **25 μg/kg;** *full-term neonates,* **20** *to* **30** μg/kg; *1 mo to 2 yr,* **30** *to* **50 μg/kg;** *2 to 5 yr,* **25** *to* **35 μg/kg;** *5 to 10 yr,* **15** to **30 μg/kg;** *10 yr and over,* **8** to **12 μg/kg;** *maintenance, premature neonates,* **20** to **30%** of the digitalizing dose/day, divided into 2 or 3 equal doses; *neonates up to 10 yr,* **25** to **35%** of the digitalizing dose/day divided into 2 or 3 equal doses; *10 yr and older,* **25** to **35%** of the total digitalizing dose once a day. *Oral, capsules, adult, rapid digitalization, initially* **400** to **600 μg**, then **100** to **300 μg** every 6 to 8 hr as necessary and tolerated; *slow digitalization, initially* **25** to **175 μg** twice a day until steady-state plasma levels are achieved (7 to 22 days); *maintenance,* **50** to **350 μg**/day in 1 or 2 divided doses; *elixir* and *tablets, adult, rapid digitalization, initially* **750** to **1250 μg** divided into 2 or more doses to be given at 6- to 8-hr intervals; *slow digitalization,* **125** to **500 μg** once a day until steady-state plasma levels are achieved; *maintenance,* **125** to **500 μg** once a day. *Capsules, pediatric: see Intravenous. Elixir* and *tablets, pediatric, digitalization, premature* and *full-term neonates up to 1 mo,* **25** to **35 μg/kg;** *1 mo to 2 yr,* **35** to **60 μg/kg;** *2 to 5 yr,* **30** to **40 μg /kg;** *5 to 10 yr,* **20** to **35 μg/kg;** *over 10 yr,* adult dose; *maintenance, all children,* **20** to **30%** of the total digitalizing dose once a day.

Dosage Forms—Capsules: 50, 100 and 200 μg; Elixir: 50 μg/mL; Tablets: 125, 250 and 500 μg; Injection: 100 and 250 μg/1 mL and 500 μg/2 mL.

Caution—Handle with exceptional care, since it is extremely poisonous.

Digoxin Immune Fab (Ovine)

F(ab); Digibind (*Burroughs Wellcome*)

Uses—The frequent toxicity and long half-life of digitalis glycosides led to the development of specific antidigoxin antibody fragments obtained from immunized sheep. The antibodies bind and inactivate molecules of digoxin or digitoxin and the resulting complex is excreted in the urine. It takes 40 mg of Fab to bind about 0.6 mg of digoxin or digitoxin. Allergic reactions are rare (0.8%), but hypokalemic reactions can develop rapidly. Measures to deal with the loss of therapeutic action of the digitalis glycoside should be available.

Dose—*Intravenous,* based on amount of drug ingested or serum digoxin concentration (see package insert).

Dosage Form—Injection (lyophilized): 40 mg/vial.

Phosphodiesterase Inhibitors

Although the cardiac glycosides have been the drugs of choice in the treatment of congestive heart failure for two centuries, they are not without serious faults. Foremost is the high incidence of adverse effects, which seems to be increasing, despite recognition of the predisposing factors and widespread attempts to educate physicians about the adverse effects and drug interactions.

As early as 1950, prominent internists sought to abandon digitalis and manage the disease with diet and saluretics alone. Later, dopamine and dobutamine were introduced for their positive inotropic actions in the management of acute, refractory, congestive heart failure. Dopamine, initially, was the focus of attention because its vasodilator actions decrease the cardiac impedence (unload the left ventricle), which increases stroke output beyond that achieved by the positive inotropic action. However, its pharmacokinetics and side effects restrict its use. In the 1980s, vasodilators became used widely, alone or as adjuncts to digitalis for the purpose of unloading the failing heart.

The discovery of amrinone in 1977 has led to renewed interest in drugs that combine positive inotropic with vasodilator actions. Such drugs are selective or nonselective phosphodiesterase inhibitors and have become known as *inodilator drugs.* They ultimately may come to displace digitalis. Amrinone and milrinone are presently the only available inodilators, but many others are in the process of development. Flosequinan has additional actions to produce similar effects.

Amrinone

[3,4′-Bipyridin]-6(1*H*)-one, 5-amino-, Inocor (*Sanofi-Winthrop*)

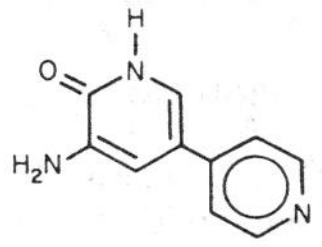

[60719-84-8] $C_{10}H_9N_3O$ (187.20).

Preparation—US Pat 4,004,012.

Description—Pale-yellow crystals; melts about 295° with decomposition.

Solubility—At pHs 4.0, 6.0 and 8.0 are 25, 0.9 and 0.7 mg/mL, respectively.

Uses—Inhibits phosphodiesterase III and thus increases intracellular cAMP and calcium. In heart muscle the result is an increase in contractility, and in vascular smooth muscle the result is relaxation. Both effects contribute to improvement in cardiac output in *congestive heart failure,* but ventricular unloading consequent to arteriolar dilatation is the more important. At present, its use should be limited to cases found to be refractory to other drugs. Only short-term treatment is advised. Adverse effects after intravenous administration include nausea (1.7%), vomiting (0.9%), anorexia (0.4%), abdominal pain (0.4%) (gastrointestinal side effects occur with an incidence of about 50% with oral administration), arrhythmia (3%), chest pain (0.2%), hypotension (1.3%), mild thrombocytopenia (2.4%, greater with oral administration), fever (0.9%) and burning at the site of injection (0.2%). Metabisulfite preservative in the preparation can cause hypersensitivity in certain individuals. Amrinone is not effective by the oral route even though it is absorbed. It has a volume of distribution of 1.2 L/kg. Over 70% is conjugated in the liver, the remainder being excreted in the urine. The half-life is about 3.6 hr in normal persons but 5 to 8 hr in subjects with heart failure. The duration of action is 30 to 120 min.

Dose—*Intravenous,* into a running dextrose infusion, *adult, initially* **0.75 mg/kg** over 2 to 3 min followed by an infusion of **5** to **10 μg/kg/min;** a second bolus of **0.75 mg/kg** may be given after 30 min, if necessary. The total daily dose should not exceed 10 mg/kg.

Dosage Form—100 mg/20 mL.

Flosequinan

4(1*H*)-Quinolone, 7-fluoro-1-methyl-3-(methylsulfinyl)-, Manoplax (*Boots*)

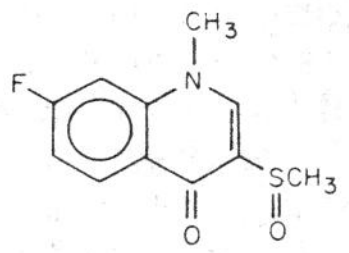

[76568-02-0] $C_{11}H_{10}FNO_2S$ (239.26).

Preparation—US Pat 4,302,460.

Description—White crystals melting about 227°.

Uses—A fluoroquinolone derivative that produces both venous and arterial vasodilatation and increases heart rate and contractility. Although its precise mechanism of action remains unknown, it appears to influence intracellular release of calcium by attenuating levels of inositol triphosphate or inhibiting protein kinase C. It is also a nonselective inhibitor of phosphodiesterases.

It is approved for treating *congestive heart failure* in patients not responding adequately to diuretics (with or without digitalis) and who either cannot tolerate ACE inhibitors or have not had an adequate response to a regimen that includes an ACE inhibitor. It increases cardiac output, stroke volume, heart rate and exercise tolerance and decreases preload and afterload by reducing peripheral resistance and blood pressure. Effects are generally additive to those of ACE inhibitors. Chief side effects are headache to which tolerance usually develops, tachycardia, hypotension and dizziness. Others are nausea and vomiting, taste disturbances and reversible increases in serum transaminase. It also has some anticoagulant activity which becomes clinically significant in patients taking anticoagulant drugs.

It is absorbed rapidly after oral administration and undergoes slow conversion to an equally active sulfone metabolite. Although the half-life of flosequinan is only about 1.7 hr, that of its active metabolite is 30 to 40 hr. Half-lives may be prolonged markedly in patients with congestive heart failure or with renal or hepatic impairment. The active and several inactive metabolites are excreted in the urine.

Dose—*Oral, adult, not taking ACE inhibitors,* **100 mg** once a day in the morning, *maximum* **150 mg** a day; *patients taking ACE inhibitors,* **50 mg** once a day in the morning, *maximum* **100 mg** a day.

Dosage Form—Tablets: 50, 75 and 100 mg.

Milrinone Lactate

[3,4′-Bipyridine]-5-carbonitrile, 1,6-dihydro-2-methyl-6-oxo-, Primacor (*Winthrop*)

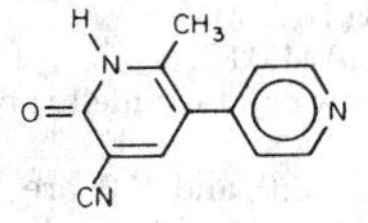

[78415-72-2] $C_{12}H_9N_3O$ (211.22).

Preparation—US Pat 4,313,951.

Description—White crystals melting over 300°.

Uses—It is 20 to 30 times more potent than amrinone as a positive inotropic agent and somewhat more potent as an arteriolar and venous dilator. It does not affect renal function significantly. In patients with congestive heart failure it improves cardiac index by 34% and decreases systemic vascular resistance 31%. It is superior to amrinone in that it is orally effective and also does not cause either thrombocytopenia or fever. However, the oral form is not yet available. The drug may be used in the long-term treatment of congestive heart failure. It has a volume of distribution of 0.4 L/kg and a mean half-life of 2.3 hr. It is excreted rapidly in the urine by active secretion.

Dose—*Intravenous,* as a *bolus,* **50 μg/kg;** *intravenous infusion,* **0.0375** to **0.75 μg/kg/min.**

Dosage Form—Injection: 1 mg/mL.

Antidysrhythmic Drugs

Cardiac dysrhythmias may result from disturbances in pacemaker function of the sinoatrial node, from alterations in conduction path and velocity so that heart block or a self-perpetuating "circus" or re-entrant rhythm occurs, or from activation of dormant pacemakers outside the sinus node. Dysrhythmias originating at the sinoatrial node may be tachycardia, bradycardia and even cardiac arrest.

Autonomic drugs often are sufficient to manage such dysrhythmias. For example, sinus tachycardia may be slowed by β_1-adrenergic blocking drugs or by reflex action resulting from the pressor effects of certain vasoconstrictors, usually sympathomimetics that lack significant direct actions on the heart (see Chapter 57), or they may be slowed directly by cholinergic drugs or by anticholinesterases. β_1-Agonists are used to revive an arrested heart and to relieve certain types of heart block. Re-entrant dysrhythmias include paroxysmal atrial tachycardia, atrial flutter and atrial fibrillation.

Circus rhythm may be terminated by

Drugs that increase atrial conduction velocity so that the circular-moving wave of excitation catches up with itself and thus dies in its own refractory zone.

Cardiac depressants that increase the refractory period of the heart muscle and decrease membrane responsiveness or change unidirectional conduction block in the re-entrant path to bidirectional block.

Drugs that improve myocardial cell responsiveness, such that unidirectional block is abolished.

Drugs that shorten the relative refractory period, so that there is less time for a premature impulse to find a relatively refractory tissue and hence aberrant conduction path.

Premature impulses from aberrant pacemakers, or ectopic foci, give rise to certain atrial tachycardias, some atrial flutters, some atrial fibrillations, nodal rhythms, ventricular tachycardias, ventricular extrasystoles and ventricular fibrillation, and they also cause reentrant dysrhythmias by discharging at a time that finds the heart muscle relatively refractory. They may be suppressed by drugs that decrease automaticity. Cardiac glycosides can be used to invoke heart block in unmanageable cases of atrial tachycardia, flutter and fibrillation, so that the ventricle is not overwhelmed with impulses of atrial origin.

Antidysrhythmic drugs are classified according to their electrophysiologic properties. The classification which follows is based on the classification of Vaughn-Williams as modified by Harrison.

Class 1 drugs have local anesthetic properties, ie, block voltage-sensitive sodium channels.

Subclass 1A drugs depress the upstroke of the action potential (Phase-0) and slow conduction moderately and they prolong membrane repolarization. Drugs discussed below, which belong to this group, are quinidine, procainamide and disopyramide.

Subclass 1B drugs have minimal effects on Phase-0 and conduction and shorten membrane repolarization. Agents in this class are lidocaine, tocainide and mexiletine.

Subclass 1C drugs depress Phase-0 and conduction but have little effect on repolarization. Flecainide and propafenone belong in this group.

Class 2 drugs have antiadrenergic properties and are β-adrenoreceptor antagonists.

Class 3 drugs prolong repolarization and increase refractoriness. Amiodarone, bretylium and sotalol comprise this group.

Class 4 drugs block slow inward calcium currents, ie, are classical calcium entry blockers, and are represented by verapamil.

For simplicity, the most prominent effects at normal doses are used to determine placement in groups, but drugs may have properties which place them in more than one group. They may act differently in different parts of the heart, and in normal and diseased hearts the effects may be modified by indirect reflex effects and the effects may be complicated by those from active metabolites.

Digitalis and Cardiac Glycosides—pages 943 to 945.

Adenosine

9*H*-Purine, 6-amino-9-β-D-ribofuranosyl-, Adenocard (*Fujisawa*)

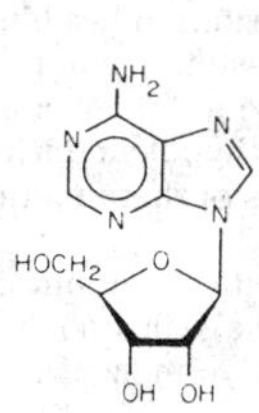

[58-61-7] $C_{10}H_{13}N_5O_4$ (267.24).

Preparation—Derived from yeast nucleic acids.

Description—White crystals melting about 235°.

Solubility—Very soluble in water; solution may be sterilized by filtration or short-term autoclaving.

Uses—A naturally occurring nucleoside formed in cells by metabolism of adenosine triphosphate (ATP). Given intravenously, it suppresses sinus node automaticity and depresses AV nodal conduction by increasing potassium conductance and reducing calcium influx. It is very effective for restoring sinus rhythm in *paroxysmal supraventricular tachycardia*, including that of *Wolff-Parkinson-White syndrome*. It is taken up rapidly by cells and has an effective half-life of about 10 sec. Adenosine frequently causes flushing, dyspnea and chest pressure; less common are headache, lighteadedness and nausea; these are generally brief due to the short half-life.

Dose—*Intravenous, initially* a **6 mg bolus** over 1 to 2 sec; if necessary, a **12-mg bolus** may be repeated, if required.

Dosage Form—Injection: 6 mg/2 mL.

Amiodarone Hydrochloride

Methanone, (2-butyl-3-benzofuranyl)[4-[2-(diethylamino)ethoxy]-3,5-diiodophenyl]-, Cordarone (*Wyeth*)

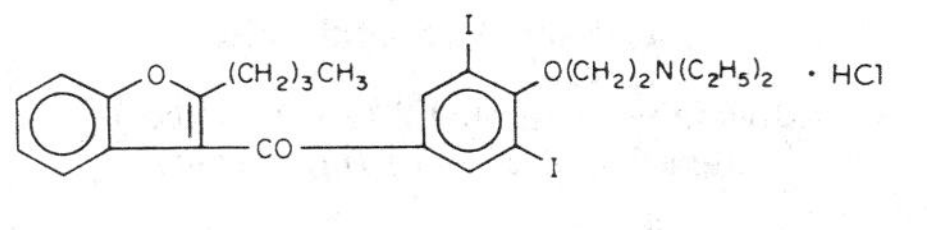

[1951-25-3] $C_{25}H_{29}I_2NO_3$ (645.32).

Preparation—US Pat 3,248,301.

Description—White to cream-colored, crystalline powder; melts about 156°; pK_a 6.56.

Solubility—Slightly soluble in water; soluble in alcohol; freely soluble in chloroform.

Uses—A Class 3 drug used only in the treatment of *documented life-threatening recurrent ventricular dysrhythmias refractory to other agents*. It prolongs the action potential and refractory period but has little direct effect on conduction. However, it also is a noncompetitive β-adrenoreceptor antagonist, and depresses depolarization by blocking sodium channels. In addition, it has been reported to block calcium channels. Therefore, it has some activity of all four classes of antidysrhythmic drugs. The drug has unusual pharmacokinetics and numerous side effects, both of which severely restrict its usefulness. It is extremely lipid-soluble and is distributed rapidly and widely in tissues (60 L/kg). Therapeutic plasma concentrations are in the range of 1.0 to 2.5 μg/mL. It is metabolized extensively to desmethylamiodarone and has a half-life of 25 to 100 days. Small amounts are excreted by lacrimal glands and in the biliary tract, but none is eliminated renally. The side effects include pulmonary fibrosis, many CNS symptoms such as ataxia, depression, nightmares and hallucinations, drug deposits in the eye and skin, hyper- and hypothyroidism, decreased libido, hematological and metabolic reactions, and photosensitivity. It increases the plasma concentrations of many drugs (eg, warfarin, digoxin, flecainide, diltiazem, phenytoin, quinidine and procainamide) by inhibition of their hepatic metabolism.

Dose—*Oral, adult, initially* **800** to **1600 mg** a day for 1 to 3 wk, decreasing gradually to 400 mg a day.

Dosage Form—Tablets: 200 mg.

Bretylium Tosylate

Benzenemethanaminium, 2-bromo-*N*-ethyl-*N,N*-dimethyl-, salt with 4-methylbenzenesulfonic acid (1:1);
Darenthin; Bretylol (*Du Pont*); (*Various Mfrs*)

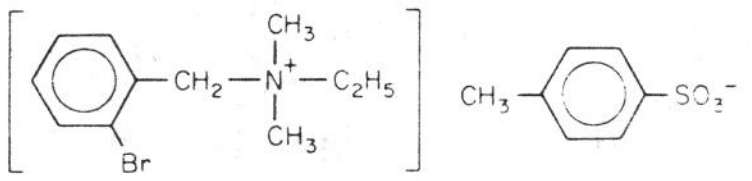

[61-75-6] $C_{18}H_{24}BrNO_3S$ (414.36).

Preparation—By interaction of *o*-bromobenzyl bromide and dimethylethylamine, the product being quaternized with *p*-toluenesulfonic acid.

Description—White, crystalline powder; melts about 98°.

Solubility—Freely soluble in water or alcohol.

Uses— A Class 3 drug presently indicated for the treatment of *life-threatening ventricular dysrhythmias that are refractory to other antidysrhythmic drugs*. It is particularly effective against ventricular tachycardia. It also is unique among antidysrhythmic drugs in the US in that it sometimes can revert a ventricular fibrillation without the use of concomitant electroversion. It is not recommended for suppression of asymptomatic premature ventricular contractions, and it has not been established that the drug has prophylactic value against ventricular dysrhythmias.

The mechanism of action is incompletely known. It depresses automaticity, increases the threshold to fibrillation-inducing electrical stimulation in both normal and infarcted myocardium and prolongs the action potential (by decreasing potassium conductance). It also has antiadrenergic effects to impair release of and partially deplete norepinephrine in adrenergic nerve terminals and also to impair norepinephrine uptake, which should assist in suppression of automaticity, once the release phase is over. However, there is no temporal correlation between the onset and duration of the antiadrenergic action with those of the antidysrhythmic action. It also increases the functional refractory period and shortens the relative refractory period, effects which discourage reentry.

Some side effects can be severe, so that the drug is held in reserve for use after other treatment fails. However, in less than 10% of patients must the drug be discontinued because of intolerance. Intravenous injection causes a high incidence of nausea and vomiting, which can be minimized by injection over a period of 10 to 30 min. Adrenergic neuron blockade by the drug causes orthostatic hypotension and severe hypotension even in the supine position in patients with inadequate heart function. During the onset of action, release of norepinephrine can cause hypertension, tachycardia, exacerbate ongoing dysrhythmias and aggravate digitalis cardiotoxicity. Therefore, careful monitoring is required until sympathetic blockade ensues. In persons with severe pulmonary hypertension or aortic stenosis, adrenergic neuron blockade removes a compensatory response system necessary to adjust to the hypotension. It sometimes causes parotid enlargement and pain. Because of blockade of the neuronal catecholamine uptake system and chemical denervation supersensitivity, directly acting sympathomimetics should be administered cautiously.

It is absorbed well from intramuscular sites. The plasma half-life averages about 10 hr but varies considerably. From excretion data, it can be surmised that it is eliminated completely by renal excretion. The dose should be adjusted in renal failure.

Dose—*Intramuscular, adult, initially* **5** to **10 mg/kg,** repeated in 1 or 2 hr, then **5** to **10 mg/kg** every 6 to 8 hr for *maintenance; intravenous, initially* **5 mg/kg,** infused over a period of no less than 8 min, followed by additional doses of 10 mg/kg every 15 to 30 min up to a total of 30 mg/kg if necessary, then **5** to **10 mg/kg** every 6 to 8 hr for *maintenance*. In *ventricular fibrillation*, the drug should be given by *rapid intravenous injection*.

Dosage Form—Injection: 500 mg/10 mL and 1 g/20 mL.

Disopyramide Phosphate

2-Pyridineacetamide, α-[2-[bis(1-methylethyl)amino]ethyl]-α-phenyl-, phosphate (1:1); Norpace (*Searle*); (*Various Mfrs*)

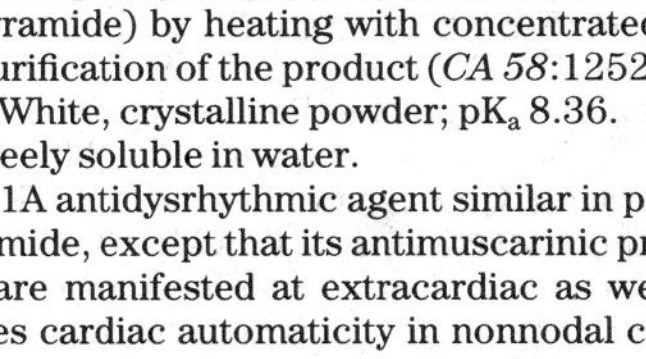

[22059-60-5] $C_{21}H_{29}N_3O.H_3PO_4$ (437.47).

Preparation—One process for one synthesis of disopyramide converts 4-diisopropylamino-2-phenyl-2-(2-pyridyl)butyronitrile to the corresponding amide (disopyramide) by heating with concentrated H_2SO_4, followed by isolation and purification of the product (*CA 58*:12522e, 1963).

Description—White, crystalline powder; pK_a 8.36.

Solubility—Freely soluble in water.

Uses—A Class 1A antidysrhythmic agent similar in properties to quinidine and procainamide, except that its antimuscarinic properties are more pronounced and are manifested at extracardiac as well as intracardiac sites. It decreases cardiac automaticity in nonnodal cells, increases the functional refractory period and shortens the relative refractory period in both atrial and ventricular cells, decreases the responsiveness of myocardial cells to electrical stimulation, decreases conduction velocity and increases the stimulus threshold. At the sinoatrial and atrioventricular nodes, its direct myocardial depressant actions are opposed by its antimuscarinic action (it has an antimuscarinic structure), so that at low to intermediate doses, especially, it may cause sinus tachycardia in some patients and decrease atrioventricular nodal capability to effect a second-degree block of high frequency atrial impulses passing through to the ventricle. For this reason, patients with supraventricular tachyarrhythmias usually are digitalized before disopyramide is administered. However, in the US, use in the treatment of supraventricular dysrhythmias is not approved. It is approved only as an oral preparation for suppression or prophylaxis of unifocal and multifocal *premature ventricular contractions, pulsus bigeminus* (coupled beats) and *ventricular tachycardia*. However, its efficacy against multifocal premature contractions and in the prevention of ventricular fibrillation as the end-sequel of ventricular dysrhythmias is in question. Given intravenously, it sometimes can arrest ventricular fibrillation, but an injection form is not marketed in the US.

It has little of the serious immunological toxicities of quinidine and procainamide and, in general, causes a lesser incidence of side effects. The most common are those reflecting its antimuscarinic properties, namely, dry mouth and skin. It also can cause blurred vision (from mydriasis and sometimes from cycloplegia), aggravation of narrow-angle glaucoma, constipation and urinary hesitancy. Nausea, vomiting, diarrhea, bloating, contractions of the pregnant uterus, urinary retention, dizziness, fatigue, headache, malaise, impotence dermatoses and nervousness also occur. Rarely, cholestasis and psychoses can occur. It has been implicated in one case of agranulocytosis. Like quinidine and procainamide, it can depress myocardial contractility and cause consequent hypotension, exacerbate heart failure and cause heart block, usually in overdoses. Disopyramide must be used cautiously in patients with heart disease and conduction disturbances. The drug increases the dose requirement for phenytoin, rifampin and warfarin by increasing hepatic metabolism.

It is absorbed almost completely by the oral route. The bioavailability is about 90%. The onset of action is 30 to 180 min. Approximately 50% is excreted unchanged in the urine with a half-life of 5 to 7 hr in persons with normal renal function and adequate cardiac output. In renal failure, congestive heart failure and shock it may be as long as 34 hr, and dose adjustments are mandatory. About 10% is secreted into bile. A substantial fraction of a dose is eliminated by *N*-monodealkylation. Therapeutic plasma levels range from 2 to 4 μg/mL, and toxic levels are approximately 9 μg/mL.

Dose—*Oral, adult, initially* **200 mg** (300 mg if loading is urgent), followed by **100** to **150 mg** every 6 hr with *conventional capsules* and **300 mg** every 12 hr with *sustained-release* capsules; *children, under 1 yr,* **10** to **30 mg/kg a day;** *1* to *4 yr,* **10** to **20 mg/kg a day;** *4* to *12 yr,* **10** to **15 mg/kg a day;** *12* to *18 yr,* **6** to **15 mg/kg a day.** Pediatric dosage has not been established.

Dosage Forms—Capsules: 100 and 150 mg; Sustained-Release Capsules: 100 and 150 mg.

β-Adrenergic Blocking Drugs—page 1009.
Calcium Entry Blockers—page 952.
Edrophonium Chloride—page 1005.
Encainide Hydrochloride—see RPS-18, page 849.
Ephedrine Sulfate—page 989.
Epinephrine—page 989.

Flecainide Acetate

Benzamide, *N*-(2-piperidinylmethyl)-2,5-bis(2,2,2-trifluorethoxy-, monoacetate; Tambocor (*Riker*)

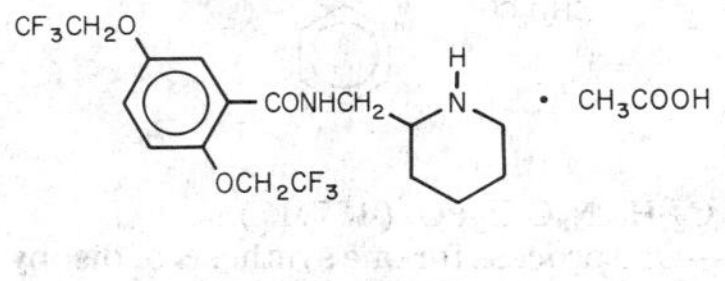

[54143-56-5] $C_{17}H_{20}F_6N_2O_3.C_2H_4O_2$ (474.40).

Preparation—See *J Med Chem 20:* 821, 1977.

Description—White crystalline solid melting about 146°; pK_a 9.3.

Solubility—1 g in about 21 mL water at 37° or 3.5 mL alcohol.

Uses—The first Class 1C agent introduced in US. It markedly inhibits Phase 0 sodium influx but differs from drugs in Class 1A and 1B in that it dissociates much more slowly from the sodium channel. It prolongs QRS duration even at normal heart rates and may cause heart block. It strongly depresses intracardiac conduction, but its effect on membrane repolarization is minimal. Conduction is particularly prolonged in the His-Purkinje system. The drug prolongs refractoriness and decreases conduction in accessory AV pathways. It strongly suppresses *ventricular dysrhythmias* but should be reserved for *documented, life-threatening ventricular dysrhythmias.*

The oral bioavailability is approximately 95%. The volume of distribution lies between 8.7 and 10 L/kg. About 32 to 47% is bound to plasma protein. Over 65% is biotransformed to two active metabolites, which, however, do not add much to the effects of the parent drug. About 27% is excreted unchanged in urine. Excretion of is by both secretion and glomerular filtration. Elevated urine pH favors tubular resorption of the unchanged drug. Plasma half-life is 18 to 27 hr in normal subjects, but the half-life may increase by 50% in patients with heart failure and may double in patients with severe renal disease. It is also longer if there is hepatic cirrhosis. Optimal therapeutic plasma concentrations have been reported to lie between 381 and 710 ng/mL.

Administration can cause dizziness and disturbances of visual accommodation. Nausea, headache and a variety of minor side effects have been associated with its use. It may further compromise left ventricular function in patients with congestive heart failure. The drug has a definite proarrhythmic potential, so that it should not be used in the treatment of nonlife-threatening dysrhythmias, particularly in patients with impaired ventricular function, coronary artery disease, myocardial infarction or heart block.

Dose—*Oral, adult,* **50** to **100 mg** twice a day, to be increased, if necessary, every 4 days by 50 mg/dose increments to a maximum of 300 mg a day.

Dosage Form—Tablets: 50, 100 and 150 mg.

Isoproterenol—page 991.
Lidocaine Hydrochloride—page 1149.
Methoxamine Hydrochloride—page 994.

Mexiletine Hydrochloride

Ethylamine, 1-methyl-2-(2,6-xylyloxy)-, Mexitil (*Boehringer Ingelheim*)

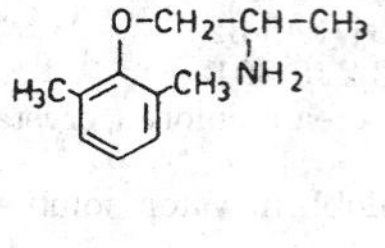

[31828-71-4] $C_{11}H_{17}NO$ (179.26).

Preparation—US Pat 3,659,019.

Description—White crystals; melts about 205°; pK_a 8.4.

Solubility—1 g in 2 mL water or 3 mL alcohol.

Uses—A Class 1B drug that resembles lidocaine in its electrophysiological effects in the heart and has the same uses and equal efficacy but is superior in that it may be used for chronic treatment. Its primary advantages are oral efficacy and relatively long half-life. Its useful actions are limited primarily to *life-threatening ventricular dysrhythmias.* It has very little effect to decrease contractility but does cause some hypotension and bradycardia. Oral bioavailability is about 88% or higher. The volume of distribution is 5.5 to 9.5 L/kg. About 70% is bound to plasma protein. Hepatic metabolism accounts for about 90% of elimination. Markedly increased half-life and volume of distribution in patients with liver dysfunction have been reported. The half-life is 10 to 12 hr. GI side effects include gastric distress, nausea and vomiting. Neurological adverse effects include lightheadedness, vertigo, tremor, nystagmus and diplopia; cardiovascular effects include bradycardia and hypotension. Decreased libido and impotence may occur. Thrombocytopenia and antinuclear factor during long-term oral treatment have been reported. Increases in SGPT and, rarely, severe liver damage have been reported.

Dose—*Oral,* for *loading,* **400 mg;** for *maintenance,* **200** to **300** mg every 8 hr.

Dosage Form—Capsules: 150, 200 and 250 mg.

Moricizine Hydrochloride

Carbamic acid, [10-[3-(4-morpholinyl)-1-oxopropyl]-10*H*-phenothiazin-2-yl]-, ethyl ester; Ethmozine (*Du Pont*)

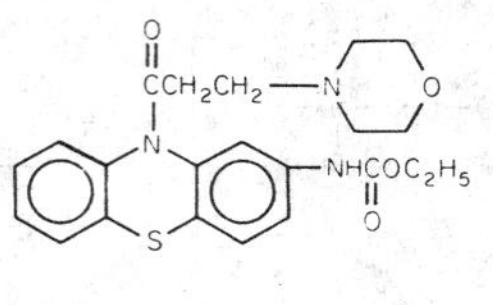

Ethyl 10-(3-morpholinopropionyl)phenothiazine-2-carbamate [31883-05-3] $C_{22}H_{25}N_3O_4S$ (427.52).

Preparation—US Pat 3,864,487.

Description—White crystals melting about 190° (dec).

Solubility—Soluble in water or alcohol.

Uses—It has some cardiac effects in common with Classes 1A, 1B and 1C antiarrhythmic drugs and is classified simply as a Class 1 drug. It prolongs AV nodal and His-Purkinje conduction times and prolongs the PR interval and QRS complex. It is used in *documented, life-threatening ventricular arrhythmias.* It exhibits proarrhythmic effects and may precipitate or worsen arrhythmias in patients with heart disease or serious arrhythmias. It is contraindicated in 2nd- or 3rd-degree AV block. It is absorbed readily from the GI tract and undergoes significant first-pass metabolism. The apparent volume of distribution is greater than 300 L, and the half-life is 1.5 to 3 hr, which may be prolonged after chronic dosing. It causes dizziness, nausea, headache, fatigue, dyspnea and palpitations in more than 5% of patients; less common are abdominal pain, vomiting, sweating, chest pain, nervousness, asthenia, paresthesias, dry mouth, sleep disorders and blurred vision. Thrombocytopenia, hepatitis, congestive heart failure and sudden cardiac death have occurred rarely.

Dose—*Oral*, **600** to **900 mg** a day in 3 divided doses.

Dosage Form—Tablets: 200, 250 and 300 mg.

Phenylephrine Hydrochloride—page 996.

Phenytoin—page 1177.

Procainamide Hydrochloride

Benzamide, 4-amino-*N*-[2-(diethylamino)ethyl]-, monohydrochloride; Procan (*Parke-Davis*); Pronestyl (*Princeton*)

$NH_2-C_6H_4-CONHCH_2CH_2N(C_2H_5)_2 \cdot HCl$

[614-39-1] $C_{13}H_{21}N_3O.HCl$ (271.79).

Preparation—Among other ways, by condensing *p*-nitrobenzoyl chloride with β-diethylaminoethylamine and then reducing the nitro group to amino by any of the usual methods. The hydrochloride forms readily when a stream of hydrogen chloride is passed into a solution of the base in an appropriate organic solvent.

Description—White to tan, crystalline powder, odorless; pH (1 in 10 solution) 5 to 6.5; melts between 165° and 169°; pK_a 9.2.

Solubility—Very soluble in water; soluble in alcohol; slightly soluble in chloroform; very slightly soluble in ether.

Uses—A Class 1A antidysrhythmic drug with properties similar to those of *Quinidine*. Myocardial automaticity and excitability are depressed, conduction is slowed and the effective refractory period, particularly that of the atrium, is increased. It is useful in suppressing *arrhythmias of ventricular origin*, including ventricular extrasystoles, and paroxysmal ventricular tachycardia. However, only treatment of documented ventricular arrhythmias is recommended because it does have proarrhythmic effects. It should not be administered to patients with heartblock, torsades de pointes or cardiomyopathy.

Many cardiologists employ this drug and quinidine interchangeably. However, either drug may be effective in an individual patient who has failed to respond to maximally tolerated doses of the other agent. It is effective immediately with intravenous injection whereas quinidine is not, so that procainamide is advantageous in arresting ventricular tachycardia.

This drug usually is well-tolerated in the short term. Gastrointestinal distress manifested by nausea, vomiting or anorexia may be noted when the drug is given orally, and hypotension, flushing and giddiness almost always occur when the intravenous route is employed. Mental depression and hallucinatory psychoses have occurred. Hypersensitivity to the drug, with fever, urticaria, angioneurotic edema, rash, hepatomegaly, leukopenia and fatal agranulocytosis occur; it is contraindicated in persons who have had these disorders. Cross-sensitivity to procaine and related drugs should be anticipated.

In the long term, the most serious side effect is a lupus-like syndrome. Ultimately, up to 30% of chronic recipients must discontinue the drug because of adverse reactions. It depresses myocardial contractility and may cause hypotension; it should be used cautiously in patients with heart failure, valvular disease or aortic stenosis. The drug has an antimuscarinic action on the atrioventricular node that may counteract its direct depressant action on that node. In patients with supraventricular tachydysrhythmias, the number of excessive impulses passing through the node may actually increase, especially at first. In addition, untoward responses may result from actions of the drug on an abnormal myocardium, such as ventricular asystole or fibrillation in patients with marked disturbances of atrioventricular conduction. It must be given cautiously if the patient is digitalized.

After oral administration, it is almost completely absorbed, and peak plasma levels are reached in 1 to 2 hr. In plasma, about 15% is protein-bound. The volume of distribution is about 2 mL/g. Renal excretion, partly by tubular secretion, accounts for 50 to 60% of elimination. From 7 to 34% is metabolized to *N*-acetylprocainamide, an active metabolite that can accumulate. The pharmacodynamic and pharmacokinetic properties differ from the parent drug and account for much of the activity during chronic administration. There are slow and fast acetylators. The β-half-life is 5 to 7 hr in patients with normal renal function but up to 25 hr in patients with renal failure, shock and congestive heart failure; doses must be adjusted in these conditions. Plasma concentrations of 4 to 10 μg/mL correct 90% of responsive ventricular tachyarrhythmias without serious adverse effects.

Dose—*Oral, adults, capsules* or *tablets, initially* **1 g** followed by **250** to **500 mg** every 3 to 6 hr; *sustained-release tablets*, **1 g** every 6 hr; *intravenous, adults*, **25** to **50 mg/min** until arrhythmia is suppressed to a *maximum* dose of **1 g**; *maintenance*, **2** to **4 mg/min.**

Dosage Forms—Capsules: 250, 375 and 500 mg; Injection: 1 g/2 mL and 1 g/10 mL; Tablets: 250, 375 and 500 mg; Sustained-Release Tablets: 250, 500, 750 and 1000 mg.

Propafenone Hydrochloride

Propiophenone, 2′-[2-hydroxy-3-(propylamino)propoxy]-3-phenyl-, hydrochloride; Rythmol (*Knoll*)

$C_6H_4(COCH_2CH_2C_6H_5)(OCH_2CH(OH)CH_2NHCH_2CH_2CH_3) \cdot HCl$

[34183-22-7] $C_{21}H_{27}NO_3.HCl$ (377.91)

Preparation—Ger pat 2,001,431.

Description—White crystals; pK_a 8.8.

Solubility—Soluble in hot water or alcohol; slightly soluble in cold water.

Uses—A Class 1C antidysrhythmic drug. Like all drugs in Class 1, it depresses the upstroke of the action potential and conduction velocity. It has only minor effects on the duration of the action potential and effective refractory period. It suppresses automaticity, elevates the threshold for ventricular fibrillation and depresses triggered ventricular activity. Ischemic cells respond better than normal cardiac cells. In high doses, it may manifest weak calcium antagonism and modest β-blocking activity. It is effective in the treatment of *life-threatening ventricular tachydysrhythmias.* It also is effective against some *supraventricular dysrhythmias*, particularly *Wolff-Parkinson-White syndrome.* After oral administration, it is 99% absorbed but undergoes extensive first-pass metabolism. Bioavailability is does-dependent; approximately 3% at low doses, but increasing to 20 to 40% after high doses of the drug. Plasma concentrations may increase 10-fold after a 3-fold increase in dose. The half-life of distribution is 4.7 min after IV administration. The volume of distribution of is 1.2 L/kg in normal subjects and 3.6 L/kg in patients with heart disease. About 90% of patients metabolize propafenone moderately rapidly to two active metabolites; 10% of patients convert the drug to the metabolizers are 2 to 10 and 10 to 52 hr, respectively. Doses of the drug require downward adjustment in patients with liver disease. Therapeutic plasma concentrations range from 60 to 3000 ng/mL. Cardiovascular side effects include exacerbation of heart failure, a proarrhythmic effect and conduction block. Noncardiovascular side effects include a bitter or metallic taste, dizziness, visual disturbances, headache, nausea and vomiting and constipation. Nausea and vomiting are a common cause of discontinuation of therapy with the drug. Drug-associated leukopenia, rash and abnormal liver tests, which disappear when the drug is stopped, have been reported rarely.

Dose—*Oral, adult*, **450** to **900 mg** a day.

Dosage Form—Tablets: 150 and 300 mg.

Quinidine Gluconate

Cinchonan-9-ol, (9*S*)-6′-methoxy-, mono-D-gluconate (salt); Quinidine Monogluconate (salt); Quinaglute (*Berlex*)

[7054-25-3] $C_{20}H_{24}N_2O_2.C_6H_{12}O_7$ (520.58); the gluconate of an alkaloid that may be obtained from various species of *Cinchona* and their hybrids, or from *Remijia pedunculata* Flückiger (Fam *Rubiaceae)*, or prepared from quinine. For the structure of quinidine, see page 402.

Description—White powder; odorless; very bitter taste.

Solubility—Freely soluble in water; slightly soluble in alcohol.

Uses—Has the same actions, uses and toxicity as *Quinidine Sulfate* (see below), but is preferred for *intramuscular* use, since it is nonirritating and stable in solution. The *intravenous* administration of quinidine only is warranted occasionally, but sometimes is a lifesaving measure in certain desperate conditions such as *ventricular tachycardia* with acute pulmonary edema or severe congestive failure. The cardiac effect may be observed in 15 to 20 min after intramuscular injection. Hypotension is frequent. It also can be used for the treatment of malaria. (See *Medical Letter Handbook of Antimicrobial Therapy* for dosage regimens.)

Dose—*Oral, adult*, as *extended-release tablets*, **324** to **972 mg,** every 8 to 12 hr; the higher doses should be used only after a trial with lower doses and clinical and laboratory re-examination and determination of plasma quinidine levels. *Intramuscular, adult, initially* **600 mg,** followed by **400 mg** at intervals as short as every 2 hr, if necessary, up to a maximum daily dose of 5 g. *Intravenous, adult,* **200** to **800 mg** in dilute solution (20 mg/mL in isotonic dextrose injection) given at a rate of no more than 1 mL/min (20 mg/min) with continuous monitoring of the electrocardiograph and blood pressure.

Dosage Forms—Injection: 800 mg/10 mL; Extended-Release Tablets: 324 mg.

Quinidine Polygalacturonate

Cardiaquin (*Purdue-Frederick*)

A compound described as a polymer of quinidine and polygalacturonic acid and assigned the molecular formula $(C_{20}H_{24}N_2O_2.C_6H_{10}O_7.H_2O)_x$ [7681-28-9].

Preparation—From quinidine and polygalacturonic acid (from pectin); described in *Am J Pharm 130:* 190, 1958, and US Pat 2,878,252.

Description—Creamy white, amorphous powder; melts about 180° with decomposition.

Solubility—Sparingly soluble in water.

Uses—The actions, uses and general toxicity are those of *Quinidine Sulfate*, except that it is not used in attempted conversion of ventricular dysrhythmias and it causes a lesser incidence and severity of gastrointestinal side effects and hence is gaining preference for oral use.

Dose—*Oral, adult, initially* **275** to **825 mg** for 3 or 4 doses at 3- to 4-hr intervals, after which upward adjustments in increments of 137.5 to 275 mg may be made on every third or fourth dose until the therapeutic endpoint is reached or toxicity supervenes, then **275 mg** 2 or 3 times a day for *maintenance*; *children,* **8** to **25 mg/kg** or **247.5 mg/m²** 3 times a day according to need and tolerance.

Dosage Form—Tablets: 275 mg, equivalent to 200 mg of quinidine sulfate.

Quinidine Sulfate

Cinchonan-9-ol, (9*S*)-6′-methoxy-, sulfate (2:1) (salt), dihydrate; (*Various Mfrs*)

[6591-63-5] $(C_{20}H_{24}N_2O_2)_2.H_2SO_4.2H_2O$ (782.95); anhydrous [50-54-4] (746.92); the sulfate of an alkaloid obtained from various species of *Cinchona* and their hybrids and from *Remijia pedunculata* Flückiger (Fam *Rubiaceae*), or prepared from quinine.

Quinidine is a stereoisomer of quinine (page 402) and occurs in cinchona bark in amounts ranging from 0.3 to over 1%, although in some barks it may be practically absent. Quinidine of commerce usually is accompanied by up to 20% of *hydroquinidine* (which is quinidine with an ethyl group replacing the vinyl) which, however, is therapeutically as potent as quinidine and no more toxic.

Preparation—By treating quinine with a metallic alkoxide [Doering WE *et al*:*J Am Chem Soc 69:*1700, (1947)] or by oxidizing quinine to quininone and then reducing the latter with sodium isopropoxide [Woodward RB *et al*:*J Am Chem Soc 67:*1428, (1945)]. It also may be obtained directly from the mother liquors remaining after removal of quinine from extracts of *Cinchona*; separation from cinchonine and other alkaloids is effected by special processes.

Description—Fine, needle-like, white crystals, frequently cohering in masses; very bitter taste; darkens on exposure to light; solutions neutral or alkaline to litmus; pK_{a1} 5.4; pK_{a2} 10.0.

Solubility—1 g in about 100 mL water, 10 mL alcohol or 15 mL chloroform; insoluble in ether.

Uses—A Class 1A antidysrhythmic drug that decreases automaticity, membrane responsiveness, excitability and conduction velocity. It prolongs the functional refractory period and shortens the relative refractory period and hence the vulnerable period for aberrant conduction. It is effective in suppressing chronic *atrial premature contractions,* and in converting and protecting against recurrences of *atrial fibrillation.* It frequently is given before attempted electroversion as a prophylactic against recurrence or new dysrhythmias. It is moderately effective against *paroxysmal atrial tachycardia, atrioventricular junctional premature systoles and tachycardia,* and *ventricular premature systoles.* It sometimes will convert atrial flutter and ventricular tachycardia. The quinidine moiety also has antimalarial actions.

It can cause dysrhythmias, in part because its effects to slow conduction favor reentrant impulses. Combined with digitalis, it may induce bizarre abnormalities of rhythm. The effect on atrioventricular conduction is erratic, especially with low doses or early in the response to high doses. This is because the drug has an antimuscarinic action on the heart to relieve vagal influences on conduction. The result is an improvement in atrioventricular conduction and an increase in the ability of the ventricle to follow atrial beats, so that during supraventricular tachyarrhythmias there may be an increase in an already excessively high ventricular rate and a consequent further impairment of ventricular filling and cardiac output. As the plasma levels increase, the ventricular rate may fall again, as a result both of control of the atrial tachyarrhythmia and a quinidine-induced AV block. Occasionally, it may cause ventricular tachycardia, fibrillation or standstill.

Orally, it commonly causes nausea, diarrhea, abdominal discomfort and, less frequently, vomiting. It decreases myocardial contractility, hence cardiac output, and can cause hypotension, sometimes severe. It also may induce cinchonism (headache, vertigo, tinnitus, nausea, vomiting, diarrhea, palpitation, syncope, photophobia, diplopia, night blindness, disturbances of color vision, scotoma and mydriasis). It also can cause hypersensitivity, characterized by various rashes, thrombocytopenia and, rarely, angioedema and anaphylaxis. In the long term, about ⅓ of all recipients discontinue the drug because of one or more of such side effects, especially thrombocytopenia. One adverse effect is the result of its therapeutic action to terminate atrial flutter, namely the dislodgement of mural thrombi with consequent embolism.

It potentiates antihypertensive drugs, other antidysrhythmic drugs in both therapeutic and cardiovascular adverse effects, and the response to prothrombopenic anticoagulants. It also increases the effects of neuromuscular paralyzants; it has a neuromuscular depressant action of its own, which has found use in testing for myasthenia gravis and treating myotonia. The drug is contraindicated when there already is heart block, thrombocytopenia or other hypersensitivity, and should be used cautiously in patients with heart failure and hypokalemia.

It is 90% absorbed by the oral route. In plasma 82% is protein-bound. The volume of distribution is 0.47 mL/g. Therapeutic plasma levels range from 3 to 6 μg/mL, and toxicity usually occurs by the time 8 μg/mL is reached. Elimination is 50 to 60% by hepatic biotransformation. The half-life ranges from 3 to 17 hr, but usually is 5 to 7 hr. An alkaline urine favors tubular resorption and, hence, prolongs the half-life and elevates plasma levels. Adjustments in dosage must be made when drugs (many antacids, carbonic anhydrase inhibitors) or diets that increase urine pH are used.

Quinidine increases the plasma levels of digoxin, making an adjustment in dosage of digoxin necessary.

Dose—*Oral, adult, conventional capsules, initially, premature atrial* and *ventricular depolarizations,* **200** to **300 mg** every 8 hr; *paroxysmal supraventricular tachycardias,* **400** to **600 mg** every 2 to 3 hr until conversion; *atrial flutter* (only after digitalization), **200 mg,** adjusted upward every 2 to 3 hr until conversion; **200 mg** every 2 to 3 hr for 5 to 8 doses; all *maintenance,* **200** to **300 mg** 3 or 4 times a day; *sustained-release tablets,* **300** to **600 mg** every 8 to 12 hr, if necessary and when tolerated; *infants* and *children,* **6 mg/kg** (or 180 mg/m²) 5 times a day. *Parenteral,* not recommended, although an injection is available.

Dosage Forms—Tablets: 100, 200 and 300 mg; Sustained-Release Tablets: 300 mg.

Sotalol Hydrochloride—page 1017.

Tocainide Hydrochloride

Propanamide, 2-amino-*N*-(2,6-dimethylphenyl)-, Tonocard (*MSD*)

$CH_3CH(NH_2)CONH$–(2,6-$(CH_3)_2C_6H_3$)

[35892-53-1] $C_{11}H_{16}N_2O.HCl$ (228.72).

Preparation—*J Med Chem 22:* 1171, 1979.

Description—White, crystalline powder; bitter taste; melts about 247°; pK_a 7.7.

Solubility—Freely soluble in water or alcohol.

Uses—A Class 1B antidysrhythmic agent with pharmacological properties similar to those of lidocaine. It is a homolog of the desethyl metabolite of lidocaine. It lacks the first-pass vulnerability of lidocaine and hence is effective orally. It resembles lidocaine in its effects on transient sodium current but differs in that it only slightly shortens action potential duration. It decreases the excitability and automaticity of Purkinje fibers. Atrioventricular conduction is not affected. Effects are most notable in patients with conduction disturbances. Effects on myocardial contractility of nonfailing hearts are negligible. Tocainide has a slight effect to increase vascular resistance. It is used to *prevent* and *suppress premature ventricular depolarizations* and *ventricular tachydysrhythmias* which are *life-threatening.*

Its effects on transient sodium currents likely accounts for such adverse CNS effects as lightheadedness, vertigo, tremor, twitching, paresthesias, sweating, hot flashes, mood alterations, blurred vision and diplopia. Gastrointestinal side effects with oral dosage include anorexia, nausea, vomiting, constipation and abdominal pain. These effects are diminished by administration with food; this delays drug absorption and decreases peak plasma concentrations but does not decrease total drug absorption. Fever, rashes and arthralgias occasionally occur. Dermatological reactions can be severe. Pulmonary fibrosis and edema, pneumonitis, hepatitis, bradycardia and antinuclear antibody have been reported. Uncommon (0.18%) but serious side effects are blood dyscrasias such as agranulocytosis and aplastic anemia.

Oral bioavailability approaches 100%. The volume of distribution is 2.5 to 3.8 mL/g. Ten to 50% is protein-bound in plasma. The distribution half-life is 5 to 15 min; the elimination half-life is 11 to 17 hr. Plasma therapeutic concentrations range from 3 to 10 μg/mL. Thirty to 40% is metabolized in the liver. Dose adjustments must be made in patients with renal disease.

Dose—*Oral, adult, initially* **400 mg** every 8 hr, subsequently adjusted as needed and tolerated, usually to a *maintenance* dose of **400** to **600 mg** every 8 hr.

Dosage Form—Tablets: 400 and 600 mg.

Verapamil—page 966.

Calcium Channel Blocking Drugs

Calcium channel blockers (CCBs) are a heterogeneous group of drugs whose main pharmacological effect is to prevent or slow the entry of calcium into cells via specialized calcium channels. Other names used for this class of drugs include calcium entry blockers, calcium antagonists and slow channel blockers, since the entry of calcium into cells is slower than sodium entry after stimulation. Nine CCBs are now available in the US (August, 1993), and others are likely to be introduced soon. Most of the CCBs are dihydropyridines.

The entry of calcium into cells is of fundamental importance for the normal functioning of the cardiovascular system. In the SA node and AV node in the heart, the slow depolarization observed in these specialized tissue cells is a consequence of the slow inward movement of calcium ions. In atrial and ventricular muscle in the myocardium, the plateau phase of the action potential (Phase 2) is the result of inward calcium movement which, in turn, couples the electrical excitation of these cells with muscle contraction. In vascular smooth muscle, calcium influx into cells is the excitation-contraction link that is necessary for smooth muscle contraction whenever smooth muscle is stimulated. Finally, inward calcium movements contribute to the resting potential and may be responsible for action potentials in some smooth muscles.

Although calcium entry into cells also is important for many tissue functions outside the cardiovascular system (eg, excitation-contraction coupling in skeletal muscle and nonvascular smooth muscle, excitation-release coupling at nerve endings, and excitation-secretion coupling in glands), the calcium channels in the cardiovascular system that are sensitive to CCBs are uniquely different. Thus, the clinical usefulness of the presently available CCBs has been their applications in the therapy of cardiovascular disease, but other potential clinical uses are being investigated.

Calcium enters cells through specialized pores in the membrane wall called calcium channels. Some channels are activated by membrane depolarization (voltage-operated) and others by activated receptors for neurotransmitters and/or sundry hormones and tissue factors (receptor-operated). CCBs decrease calcium entry in both the voltage-operated and receptor-operated channels, but the voltage-operated channel is the more sensitive to drug blockade.

Although all calcium channel blocking drugs have in common the ability to decrease calcium entry into cells, drug effects vary from site to site and from drug to drug according to the channel type, the opening frequency and the activation-inactivation kinetics.

Three different calcium channels have been characterized. L- (long opening) and T- (transient) channels have been found in neurosecretory cells and cardiac, smooth and skeletal muscle cells, and N- (neuronal) channels have been located only in neurons. Each channel type has its own characteristic activation and inactivation voltage ranges, channel conductance, sensitivity to blockade by organic and inorganic compounds, etc, such that each has a unique pharmacoresponsive profile. Also, CCBs exhibit both frequency- and voltage-dependence in their ability to block calcium movements. Verapamil, for example, binds to open channels and hence selects cells that are stimulated frequently; in contrast, dihydropyridines bind more strongly to inactivated channels and hence show little frequency-dependence. However, all CCBs are voltage-dependent in that they are much better blockers when the tissue is depolarized. None of the CCBs actually occlude the channel directly but rather act at allosteric sites on channel proteins to evoke conformational changes that cause occlusion.

CCBs have been approved for the oral treatment of *variant (vasospastic)* and chronic *stable and unstable exertional angina pectoris*. They are useful in the therapy of these diseases for three reasons: they directly dilate coronary arteries and increase myocardial blood flow, they decrease myocardial oxygen demand by peripheral arteriolar dilatation, which decreases afterload, and they exert negative chronotopic and inotropic actions which also decreases oxygen demand.

Verapamil has been approved for the intravenous therapy of *supraventricular tachyarrhythmias* because of its significant depressant effects on SA nodal automaticity and AV conduction. Oral verapamil also is approved for several chronic arrhythmias. To the extent that calcium channel activity is important for spontaneous electrical discharges in diseased myocardium, calcium channel blocking drugs also may find use in the therapy of other arrhythmias.

Seven of the nine CCBs are approved for therapy of *systemic hypertension* because they are potent arteriolar vasodilators, and they are relatively free of side effects and toxicities. CCBs provide effective monotherapy yet can be combined with other antihypertensive drugs. They do not adversely affect potassium, glucose or blood lipid metabolism, do not cause tolerance and they have appropriate pharmacokinetics. They are effective in virtually all patients and produce minimal side effects.

Other uses of CCBs include the treatment of *pulmonary hypertension, peripheral vascular disease, mild congestive heart failure* and *hypertrophic subaortic stenosis*. The role of calcium entry blockers in *protection against ischemic injury* in the heart, brain, kidneys and other tissues is under intense investigation. Presently, it appears that diltiazem decreases mortality from myocardial infarction only when there is no concomitant pulmonary congestion.

Certain CCBs have been found to be effective in central nervous system disorders such as *stroke* and *migraine*. Other investigational uses are *suppression* of *atherogenesis* and *tumor resistance to antineoplastic drugs*, treatment of *achalasia* and *esophageal spasms, bronchial asthma, premature labor* and *dysmenorrhea*, and enhancement of success in *renal transplantation*. The choice of a drug for a particular purpose depends on the pharmacological properties of the drugs (see below), the presence of other drugs and the cardiovascular status of the patient.

Untoward effects of the calcium entry blockers are consequences of calcium entry blockade and are limited primarily to the cardiovascular system. Drug-induced vasodilatation leads to hypotension and to dizziness, lightheadedness, flushing and headache. Vasodilatation may sum adversely with other vasodilators. Decreased SA automaticity causes bradycardia, and decreased AV conduction sometimes can result in heart block. Decreased myocardial contractility can result in congestive heart failure, particularly when these drugs are used with β_1-adrenergic blocking drugs. Peripheral edema caused by these drugs may be due to a combination of heart failure and peripheral vasodilatation, but direct effects to decrease sodium excretion have been noted with some CCBs. Effects of the drug outside of the cardiovascular system are minimal.

Constipation sometimes is reported and may be caused by mild excitation-contraction uncoupling in gastrointestinal smooth muscle. Excitation-secretion coupling in exocrine and endocrine glands is another important role of calcium, but the effects of calcium channel blocking drugs on glandular function have not proved to be important clinically, although nifedipine has been reported to decrease insulin secretion. In usual doses, calcium antagonists do not appear to affect norepinephrine release from sympathetic nerve endings although calcium is necessary for norepinephrine release. In sharp contrast to β_1-adrenergic blockers, calcium entry blockers do not increase airway resistance but instead appear to protect against bronchoconstriction in asthmatic patients.

Calcium channel blockers (CCBs) may enhance the neurotoxicity of lithium. Both verapamil and diltiazem slow the hepatic metabolism of carbamazepine and probably a number of other drugs. Several CCBs increase plasma digoxin concentrations when the drugs are used concurrently, probably by decreasing the renal elimination of digoxin. Verapamil has been shown also to decrease the nonrenal clearance of digoxin. Cimetidine, but not ranitidine, decreases the first-pass clearance of nifedipine by about 50% and increases bioavailability accordingly. Rifampin has been reported to decrease oral bioavailability of nifedipine by increasing hepatic cytochrome P-450 activity.

Amlodipine

3,5-Pyridinedicarboxyllic acid,(±)-2-[(2-aminoethoxy)methyl]-4-(2-chlorophenyl)-1,4-dihydro-6-methyl-, 3-ethyl 5-methyl ester, (*Z*)-2-butenedioate (1:1); Norvasc (*Pfizer*)

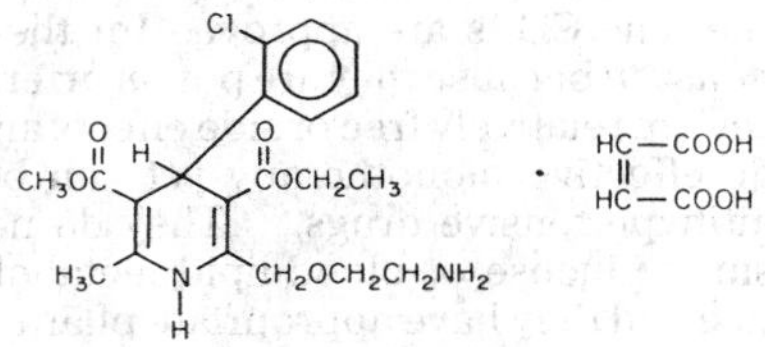

[88150-47-4] $C_{20}H_{25}ClN_2O_5.C_4H_4O_4$ (524.96).

Preparation—*J Med Chem 29:* 1696, 1986.

Description—White crystals melting about 180°; pK_a (base-NH_2) 9.0.

Uses—Like other dihydropyridines, it is more selective for arterial vascular smooth muscle than for cardiac tissue. Vasodilation is prominent and it is approved for treatment of *essential hypertension* and for *variant and stable angina.* Side effects are generally mild and typical of vasodilator CCBs. It shows some tendency to produce edema but is therapeutically compatible with thiazides as well as other classes of antihypertensive agents.

It is absorbed readily after oral administration, is 97% bound to plasma proteins, and has an apparent volume of distribution of 21 L/kg. It has a half-life of 34 h and is mostly metabolized. Patients with hepatic dysfunction should receive ½ the recommended dose.

Dose—*Oral, adult, initially* **5 mg** once a day; dosage may be increased after 2 wk to **10 mg** once a day.

Dosage Form—Tablets: 2.5, 5 and 10 mg.

Bepridil Hydrochloride

Pyrrolidineethanamine, β-[(2-methylpropoxy)methyl]-*N*-phenyl-*N*-(phenylmethyl)-, monohydrochloride, monohydrate; Vascor (*McNeil*)

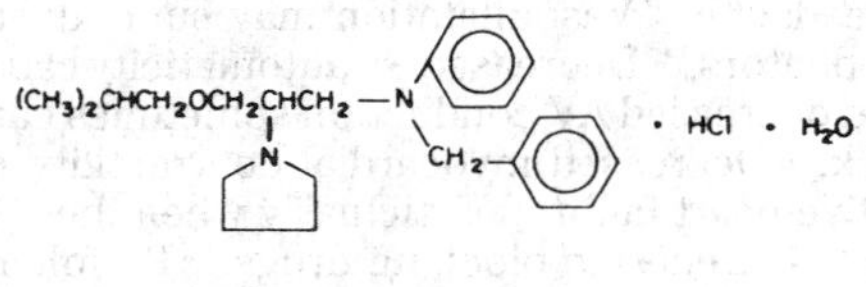

[74764-40-2] $C_{24}H_{34}N_2O.HCl.H_2O$ (421.02).

Preparation—US Pat 3,962,238.

Description—White crystals melting about 91°.

Uses—In contrast to the other CCBs, it not only blocks calcium channels but also blocks sodium channels, as do Class 1 antiarrhythmic drugs. It, therefore, significantly lengthens cardiac repolarization and depresses cardiac contraction; it is also proarrhythmogenic, which limits its usefulness. It is more selective for dilating the coronary than the peripheral vasculature.

It is approved only for treating *stable angina* in patients who do not respond to other antianginal agents. It can be given with nitrates or β-blockers. About 15% of patients discontinue use because of GI disturbances (nausea, dyspepsia, diarrhea), ventricular arrhythmias, dizziness or syncope. Torsades de pointes has been reported rarely.

It is absorbed readily with a 60% bioavailability, is 99% bound to plasma proteins and has a volume of distribution of 8L/kg. It has a half-life of 33 hr and is metabolized almost completely.

Dose—*Oral, adult, initially* **200 mg** once a day, increasing if necessary after 10 days to **300 mg** once a day; 400 mg a day is *maximal.*

Dosage Form—Tablets: 200, 300 and 400 mg.

Diltiazem Hydrochloride

Benzothiazepin-4(5*H*)-one, (+)-*cis*-3-(acetyloxy)-5-[2-(dimethylamino)ethyl]- 2,3-dihydro-2-(4-methoxyphenyl)-, monohydrochloride; Cardizem (*Marion*); Dilacor XR (*Rhone-Polenc Rorer*)

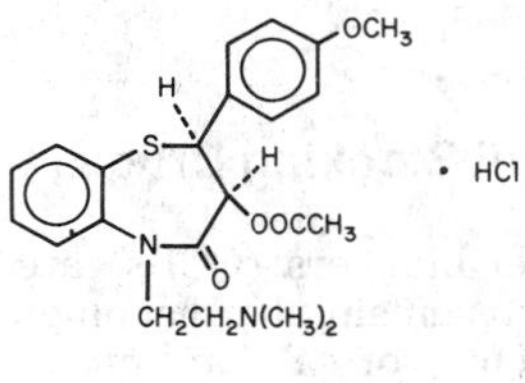

[33286-22-5] $C_{22}H_{26}N_2O_4S.HCl$ (450.98).

Preparation—*Chem Pharm Bull 19:* 595 (1971).

Description—White crystals melting about 188°; pK_a 7.7.

Solubility—Freely soluble in water, alcohol or chloroform; slightly soluble in dehydrated alcohol.

Uses—See general statement. This drug has less effect on peripheral resistance and myocardial contractility than do verapamil and nifedipine, but it is a more potent coronary vasodilator. It slows conduction in the AV node but not as much as does verapamil. Heart rate usually is decreased because of its slight effects on SA node automaticity and because its modest peripheral vasodilatory effects do not evoke powerful reflex responses.

It is approved for treating *paroxysmal supraventricular tachycardia and atrial fibrillation and flutter (IV); stable, unstable and variant angina* (regular oral); *essential hypertension* (prolonged-release) and it is used in *hypertensive emergencies* (IV).

It is 80% absorbed orally, but only 40 to 60% of an oral dose reaches the systemic circulation because of first-pass metabolism in the liver. After administration, it is 70 to 80% bound to plasma protein. Displacement from protein binding sites by other drugs does not seem to be a clinical problem. It is metabolized extensively by the liver to several metabolites, some of which have weak coronary vasodilator activity. Less than 4% of the drug appears unchanged in the urine. The plasma half-life is about 4 hr. The drug has been reported to have saturation kinetics after single doses greater than 60 mg.

Dose—*Oral, adult, tablets,* **30 mg** 4 times a day before meals and at bedtime, to be increased to 360 mg a day as necessary; *sustained-release capsules,* **60 to 120 mg** twice a day, increased to 360 mg a day, as needed; *CD or XR capsules,* **120** to **240 mg** once a day, increasing to 480 mg/day. *Intravenous, adult, arrhythmias,* **20 mg** or **0.25 mg/kg** as *bolus* over 2 min. followed by a 2nd dose, if needed/ *24-hr infusion,* **5, 10** or **15 mg/hr.**

Dosage Form—Tablets: 30, 60, 90 and 120 mg; Sustained-Release Capsules: 60, 90, 120, 180, 240 and 300 mg; Injection: 5 mg/mL.

Felodipine

3,5-Pyridine dicarboxylic acid, (±)-4-(2,3-dichlorophenyl)-1,4-dihydro-2,6-dimethyl-, ethyl methyl ester; Plendil (*MSD*)

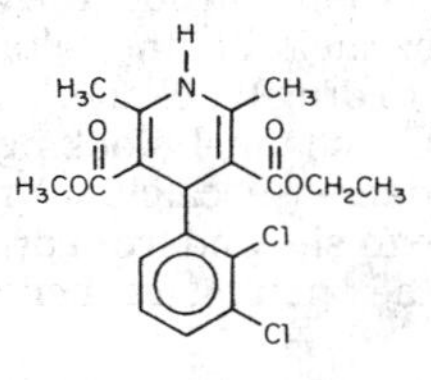

[72509-76-3] $C_{18}H_{19}Cl_2NO_4$ (384.26).

Preparation—US Pat 4,264,611.

Description—White crystals melting at 145°.

Solubility—Practically unsoluble in water, very soluble in alcohol.

Uses—A potent dihydropyridine with almost exclusive action on vascular smooth muscle, especially peripheral arterioles. It can produce some reflex tachycardia.

It is approved only for treating *essential hypertension* but may be beneficial in *renal* or *pulmonary hypertension*. It is therapeutically compatible with diuretics and other antihypertensive drugs. Common side effects include headache, dizziness, flushing and ankle edema; others include fatigue, insomnia, palpitations and dyspnea.

It is absorbed readily but undergoes extensive first-pass metabolism so that bioavailability is only 20%. It is 99% bound to plasma proteins with a V_d of only 0.6 to 1.5 L/kg. Its plasma half-life is 10 to 18 hr and it is mostly metabolized by the liver. Maximum daily dosage in the elderly and those with hepatic dysfunction is $\leq$ 10 mg once a day.

Dose—*Oral, adult, initially* **5 mg** once a day; dosage may be increased at intervals of 2 wk by 5 mg a day to a maximum of 20 mg a day.

Dosage Form—Extended-Release Tablets: 5 and 10 mg.

Isradipine

3,5-Pyridinedicarboxylic acid, (±)-4-(4-benzofurazanyl)-1,4-dihydro-2,6-dimethyl-, methyl 1-methylethyl ester; DynaCirc (*Sandoz*)

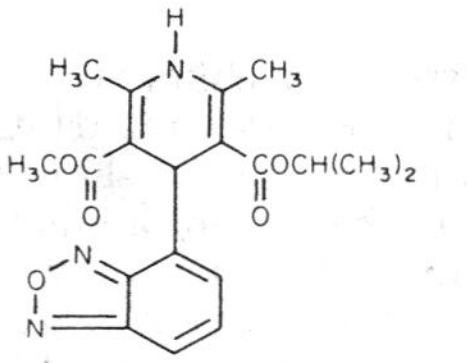

[75695-93-1] $C_{19}H_{21}N_3O_5$ (371.39)

Preparation—US Pat 4,466,972.

Description—White crystals melting about 142°.

Solubility—Practically insoluble in water; very soluble in alcohol.

Uses—A potent dihydropyridine with preferential vasodilating effects on coronary, cerebral and skeletal muscle vasculature. It has minimal depressant effects on the SA node and negligible effects on heart rate or contraction.

It is approved only for treating *essential hypertension*, but it also has been shown effective in increasing exercise tolerance in stable angina. It is undergoing a multicenter, 3-year study to determine whether it retards development of extracranial carotid artherosclerosis in hypertensive men and women. In contrast to cardiodepressant CCBs, it appears safe to use in patients with sick sinus syndrome. In general, it is tolerated well and side effects are generally extensions of dose-related vasodilation. Edema typically is common as with all potent vasodilators and is controlled readily by diuretics.

It is absorbed readily and subject to extensive first-pass metabolism providing only about 20% bioavailability. It is 97% bound to plasma proteins with a V_d of 2.9 L/kg. It has a half-life of 8 to 9 hr and is metabolized completely.

Dose—*Oral, adult, initially* **2.5 mg** twice a day for 2 to 4 wk, then increased in 5 mg a day increments every 2 to 4 wks; doses greater than 10 mg a day provide no additional benefit.

Dosage Form—Capsules: 2.5 and 5 mg.

Nicardipine Hydrochloride

3,5-Pyridinedicarboxylic acid, 1,4-dihydro-2,6-dimethyl-4-(3-nitrophenyl)-, methyl 2-[methyl(phenylmethyl)aminoethyl ester, monohydrochloride; Cardene (*Syntex*)

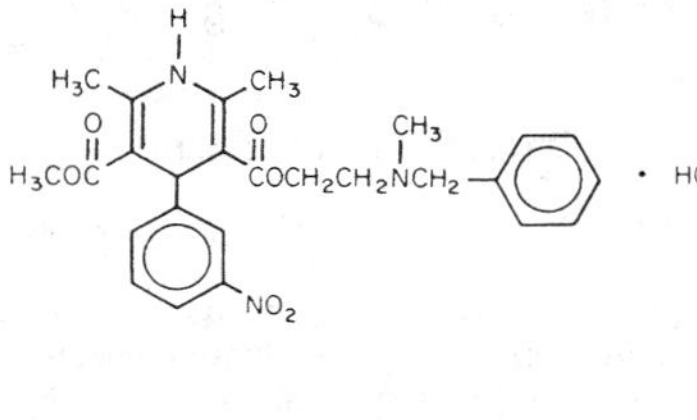

[54527-84-3] $C_{26}H_{29}N_3O_6$.HCl (515.99).

Preparation—*Chem Pharm Bull 27:* 1426, 1979.

Description—White crystals melting about 180° (α-form) or about 169° (β-form); pK_a 7.2.

Uses—A dihydropyridine with selective vasodilating actions on systemic, coronary, cerebral and renal vasculature. Reflexly increased heart rate and cardiac output reflect minimal depressant actions on the heart.

It is approved for treating *essential hypertension* and *chronic stable angina*. It produces typical vasodilator side effects. Other reactions involving the CNS, GI tract and skin are infrequent and minor.

It is absorbed readily and undergoes significant first-pass metabolism; bioavailability is 35%. It is highly protein bound and has a volume of distribution of 0.6 L/kg. It has a half-life of 3 to 4 hr and is metabolized completely.

Dose—*Oral, adult, initially* **20 mg** 3 times a day (*immediate-release*), can be increased at 3-day intervals to **40 mg** 3 times a day; for *sustained-release*, in *hypertension, initially* **30 mg** twice a day, increased in 3-day intervals to a maximum of **60 mg** twice a day.

Dosage Forms—Capsules: 20 and 30 mg; Sustained-Release Capsules: 30, 45 and 60 mg.

Nifedipine

3,5-Pyridinecarboxylic acid, 1,4-dihydro-2,6-dimethyl-4-(2-nitrophenyl)-, dimethyl ester; Adalat (*Miles*); Procardia (*Pfizer*)

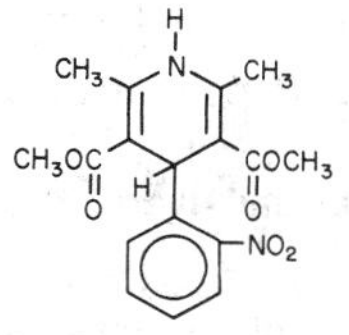

[21829-25-4] $C_{17}H_{18}N_2O_6$ (346.34).

Preparation—See US Pat 3,485,847.

Description—Yellow crystals melting about 174°.

Solubility—Practically insoluble in water; slightly soluble in alcohol; very soluble in chloroform or acetone; solutions are extremely light-sensitive.

Uses—See general statement. This drug is a potent peripheral vasodilator. This effect, coupled with its lack of significant effect to decrease SA node automaticity, causes some reflex tachycardia. Sympathetic reflex activity also tends to negate the negative intropic effects of nifedipine.

It currently is approved for treating *essential hypertension* (prolonged-release) and *vasospastic* and *stable angina*. For *hypertensive crisis*, the standard capsules are punctured and the contents are swallowed. It is also effective in treating *migraine* and *Renauds syndrome*. It is more likely to produce dizziness, nervousness and headache than verapamil. Gingival hyperplasia, gynecomastia, dermatological reactions, eye pain and neuropathies have occurred rarely.

About 90% of an oral dose is absorbed, but its bioavailability is 65 to 70%; there is significant hepatic first-pass metabolism. Greater than 90% of the drug is bound to plasma protein. It is metabolized to inactive metabolites, probably by the liver. Most (80%) of the inactive metabolites are excreted in urine; 15% are excreted in the stool. The half-life is 2 to 6 hr; sustained-release tablets provide longer effective plasma levels.

Dose—*Oral, adult, initially* **10 mg** 3 times a day, to be increased gradually to **20** to **30 mg** 3 or 4 times a day, if necessary (doses exceeding 180 mg a day are not recommended); *sustained-release, initially* **30** or **60 mg** once a day, titrate to maximum (**20 mg a day** over 7- to 14-day period).

Dosage Forms—Capsules: 10 and 20 mg; Sustained-Release Tablets: 30, 60 and 90 mg.

Nimodipine

3,5-Pyridinedicarboxylic acid, 1,4-dihydro-2,6-dimethyl-4-(3-nitrophenyl)-, 2-methoxyethyl 1-methylethyl ester; Nimotop (*Miles*)

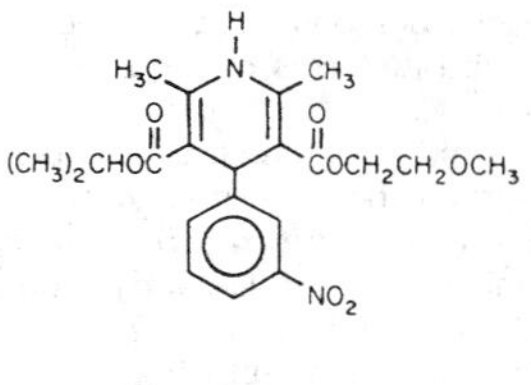

[66085-59-4] $C_{21}H_{26}N_2O_7$ (418.45).

Preparation—US Pat 3,799,934.

Description—Yellow crystals melting about 125°.

Solubility—Insoluble in water; soluble in alcohol.

Uses—A dihydropyridine that preferentially dilates the cerebral vascular and can increase cerebral blood flow without affecting systemic blood pressure or heart rate. It is the only CCB that is approved for treating *subarachnoid hemorrhage.* The aim is to improve neurological deficits due to vascular spasm following rupture of congenital intracranial aneurysms in patients who are in good neurological condition. Cerebral vasospasm is a primary cause of death or permanent disability following subarachnoid hemorrhage, but a 21-day course of nimodipine therapy initiated as soon as possible after the event has been shown to improve chances for a more favorable outcome. Side effects are minimal, the most prevalent being a dose-related reduction in systemic blood pressure.

It is absorbed rapidly after oral administration, reaching peak plasma levels within 1 hr, and it readily penetrates the brain. It undergoes extensive first-pass metabolism. Early elimination half-life is 1 to 2 hr, and terminal half-life is 8 to 9 hr. Because it is highly lipophylic, brain levels may remain higher than reflected by plasma levels. Dosage should be reduced by ½ in hepatic cirrhosis.

Dose—*Oral, adult, subarachnoid hemorrhage,* initiate therapy as soon as possible with **60 mg** every 4 hr for 21 consecutive days. If necessary, the liquid contents of the gelatin capsule can be aspirated with a syringe and administered through a nasogastric tube and flushed with 30 mL of normal saline.

Dosage Form—Gelatin capsules: 30 mg.

Nitrendipine—see RPs-18, page 855.

Verapamil Hydrochloride

Benzeneacetonitrile, α-[3-[[2-(3,4-dimethoxyphenyl)ethyl]-methylamino]propyl]-3,4-dimethoxy-α-(1-methylethyl)-, hydrochloride; Calan (*Searle*); Isoptin (*Knoll*); Veralan (*Lederle*); (*Various Mfrs*)

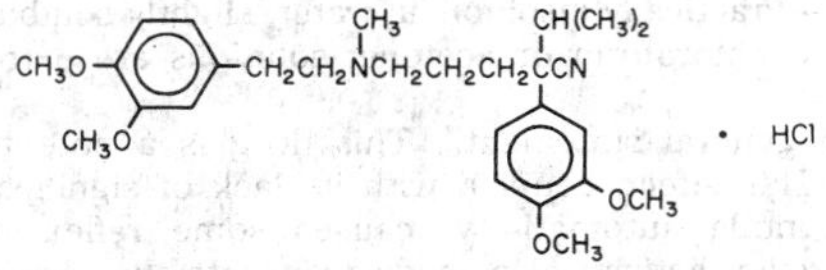

CH_3O, CH_3O — $CH_2CH_2N(CH_3)CH_2CH_2CH_2C(CH(CH_3)_2)CN$ — OCH_3, OCH_3 · HCl

[52-53-9] $C_{27}H_{38}N_2O$ (454.61).

Preparation—See *Arzneimittel-Forsch 12:* 563, 1962 and *Helv Chim Acta 58:* 2050, 1975.

Description—White to off-white crystals melting about 140°; pH (7% w/w solution) about 4.2.

Solubility—1 g dissolves in about 15 mL water, 25 mL alcohol or 2 mL chloroform; soluble in most polar organic solvents.

Uses—See general statement. Of the available calcium channel blockers, this drug has the greatest effects on the myocardium. Its effects on sinoatrial automaticity, AV conduction and myocardial contractility are greater than those of diltiazem. It dilates peripheral vascular smooth muscle more than diltiazem but not as much as does nifedipine. Effects on heart rate are variable and depend, in part, on the amount of reflex sympathetic activity evoked by peripheral dilatation.

It is approved to treat *vasospastic, stable* and *unstable angina, chronic atrial flutter and fibrillation* (combined with digitalis) and *essential hypertension.* The intravenous preparation is used to attempt *supraventricular tachyarrhymias* and to provide temporary control of rapid ventricular rate in atrial flutter or fibrillation. It is also effective prophylactically in reducing the incidence and severity of *migraine* and *cluster headaches.*

It is more than 90% absorbed, but only 20 to 35% of the dose reaches the system because of extensive hepatic first-pass metabolism. It is bound approximately 90% to plasma proteins. It is metabolized rapidly by the liver to norverapamil and traces of several other metabolites. About 70% of a dose is excreted in urine as metabolites, and 16% of a dose appears in the feces within 5 days; less than 5% is excreted unchanged. The half-life is 2 to 5 hours in normal persons but may exceed 9 hr during chronic therapy. In patients with cirrhosis of the liver, the half-life may be increased to 14 to 16 hr. The half-life is increased in patients with liver disease, due, in part, to an increased volume of distribution. Saturation kinetics have been observed after repeated doses.

Dose: *Intravenous, adult, initially* **5** to **10 mg** (0.075 to 0.15 mg/kg) over a period of 2 min (3 min in the elderly), followed by **10 mg** (0.150 mg/kg) after 30 min, if necessary; *children, up to 1 yr, initially* **0.1** to **0.2 mg/kg** over 2 min (with ECG monitoring), repeated after 30 min, if necessary; *1 to 15 yr, initially* **0.1** to **0.3 mg/kg,** not to exceed 5 mg, repeated after 30 min, if necessary. *Oral, adult,* **80 mg** 3 or 4 times a day or **240 mg** once a day in *sustained-release* form, gradually increased to as much as 480 mg a day, if necessary.

Dosage Forms—Injection: 5 mg/2 mL and 10 mg/4 mL; Tablets: 40, 80 mg and 120 mg; Sustained-Release Tablets: 120, 180 and 240 mg.

Drugs Affecting Blood Lipids

Drugs that affect blood lipids may be classified as cardiovascular drugs because of the relation of blood lipids to atherosclerosis. Atherosclerosis may be a disorder in lipid metabolism or a normal effect of a diet high in certain lipids. Since one of the major lipids in the atheroma is cholesterol, much attention has been centered upon cholesterol in the diet and blood.

There is a correlation between blood cholesterol content and the incidence of coronary occlusion, although it is far from a perfect one. Experimentally, a diet high in cholesterol can promote or exacerbate atherosclerosis in certain species. Consequently, there has been interest in drugs that affect the absorption of cholesterol from the intestine. However, cholesterol also is synthesized from fatty acids in the body, and there has been great interest in the relative abilities of different fatty acids to elevate or reduce plasma cholesterol levels.

Saturated fats, especially palmitates, induce higher blood cholesterol levels than do unsaturated fats, but it now appears that some of what was attributed to saturation was the result of cholesterol in fats derived from animals. Polyunsaturated fats have been thought to be not only the least offensive in elevating blood cholesterol but also to antagonize the cholesterologenic effects of saturated fatty acids.

The role of various fatty acids in atherogenesis now requires reevaluation. The blood β-lipoprotein and serum triglyceride levels also correlate somewhat with the incidence of coronary occlusion and with the type of fat in the diet. Since the first Framingham study, epidemiological studies and therapy have been preoccupied with the low-density (LDL) and the very-low-density (VLDL) lipoproteins and also with chylomicrons. It is now known, however, that a very important factor in atherogenesis is the plasma level of high-density lipoproteins (HDL), which serve as scavengers of cholesterol and not only protect the arteries from deposition of cholesterol but appear to be involved in the transport of cholesterol out of vessel walls. The blood lipids are only one of a number of factors that cause atherosclerosis and coronary occlusion. Thus, it should not be expected that manipulation of the blood lipids alone necessarily will bring about improvement in the disease.

In 1975 the results of a multicenter study on antilipidemic drugs was published. The essence of the report was that antihyperlipidemic drugs did not decrease the risk of coronary heart disease or lower mortality. However, many serious criticisms have been made of the study, one being that nearly one-half of the subjects in the study did not have a hyperlipidemia.

A more recent study in Sweden has indicated a remarkable decrease in coronary reinfarction rate in patients treated with a combination of clofibrate and niacin. In the US, bile acid sequestering resins have been shown to decrease the myocardial infarction rate. Furthermore, evidence continues to mount that low-fat diets in combination with antilipidemic drugs have a protective effect in coronary heart disease.

Aminosalicylic Acid—see RPS-17, page 1213.

Cholestyramine Resin

Cholybar (*Parke-Davis*); Questran (*Bristol*)

Cholestyramine [11041-12-6]; a strongly basic anion-exchange resin in the chloride form, consisting of styrene-divinylbenzene copolymer with quaternary ammonium functional groups. Each g exchanges 1.8–2.2 g of sodium glycocholate, calculated on the dried basis.

Preparation—Polystyrene trimethylbenzylammonium chloride is copolymerized through cross-linkage with divinylbenzene.

Description—White to buff-colored, hygroscopic, fine powder; odorless or has not more than a slight amine-like odor; pH between 4 and 6, in a slurry (1 in 100).

Solubility—Very slightly soluble in water or alcohol; insoluble in chloroform or ether.

Uses—Binds weak acid anions with partial hydrophobic character. It is employed to bind bile acids in the intestine and, hence, to prevent their absorption in *hypercholesterolemias*, especially the familial (Type IIa) and heterozygous (Type IIb), *cholestasis* and *bile-dependent diarrheas*. It also is used to decrease the absorption of oxalate in *hyperoxaluria*, porphyrins in *porphyria cutanea tarda* and *protoporphyria*, cardiac glycosides in *digitalis intoxication*, chlordecone in *chlordecone intoxication* and clostridial toxin in *antibiotic-associated colitis*.

The depletion of bile acids in the intestines not only decreases the absorption of dietary and enterohepatic cholesterol but also increases the synthesis of bile acids from cholesterol, which decreases the size of the systemic cholesterol pool. In familial hypercholesterolemia, the plasma concentration of low-density lipoprotein (LDL) is decreased by 20 to 30%, which upregulates LDL-receptor populations in hepatocytes and vascular myocytes and thus accelerates LDL catabolism. Atherogenesis is retarded and probably even reversed. The effect is even more pronounced in the presence of hydroxymethylglutaryl coenzyme A inhibitors (LDL is lowered by about 40%) and niacin. There now is evidence that there may be a decrease in the coronary occlusion rate.

In cholestasis, the decrease in the bile acid concentration in the skin relieves pruritus.

Side effects, attributable to depletion of intraintestinal bile acids, include constipation (20 to 50%), heartburn and dyspepsia, colic, belching, bloating, biliary stasis and lodged gallstones, steatorrhea and malapsorption syndrome (with doses $>$ 24 g/day) and consequent hypovitaminoses A, D and K. The bulkiness of the dose along with the decrease in bowel motility exacerbates constipation and favors impaction and may be the cause of nausea, vomiting and gastrointestinal bleeding from ulcers. Hypochloremic alkalosis sometimes occurs. The cause of occasional diarrhea is not known. In hypertriglyceridemias, the drug may elevate very low- and intermediate-density lipoproteins. High doses and patient age over 60 yr predispose to adverse effects. The preparation has a gritty taste. If the anhydrous bulk is ingested, accidental inhalation and pneumonitis or esophageal distress may result.

It binds numerous weakly acidic drugs and interferes with their absorption during concurrent oral administration. Prominent examples are prothrombopenic anticoagulants (warfarin, etc), saluretics, chenodiol, digitalis (especially digitoxin), penicillins, cephalosporins, tetracyclines, vancomycin, clindamycin, trimethoprim, thyroid hormones, folic acid, phenylbutazone and phenobarbital.

Dose—*Oral, adult* and *children over 12 yr, initially* **4 g** 3 times a day before meals, adjusted as necessary; *maintenance, usually* **4 g** 3 or 4 times a day before meals and at bedtime, not to exceed 32 g a day. The drug is effective even given as a single dose, but its bulkiness favors 3- or 4-doses-a-day regimens. *Children 6 to 12 yr*, **80 mg/kg** (or 2.35 g/m^2) 3 times a day before meals.

Dosage Forms—Powder (4 g of anhydrous cholestyramine/9 g of powder): 9 and 378 g. An oral suspension is prepared before use by suspending each dose in 60 of 180 mL of water or fruit juice. Bars: 4 g of resin (chewed thoroughly 1 to 6 times a day).

Clofibrate

Propanoic acid, 2-(4-chlorophenoxy)-2-methyl-, ethyl ester; Atromid-S *(Ayerst)*

CH3
CH3CCOOCH2CH3
O
Cl

Ethyl 2-(*p*-chlorophenoxy)-2-methylpropionate [637-07-0] $C_{12}H_{15}ClO_3$ (242.70), calculated on the anhydrous basis.

Preparation—By condensing phenol with ethyl 2-chloro-2-methylpropionate in the presence of a suitable dehydrochlorinating agent and then chlorinating.

Description—Stable, colorless to pale-yellow liquid with a faint, characteristic odor and a characteristic taste; boiling point 158 to 160°.

Solubility—Insoluble in water; soluble in alcohol or chloroform.

Uses—It markedly reduces the VLDL and triglyceride levels in persons with *familial dysbetalipoproteinemia* (Type III). It increases the HDL levels. In such patients, cholesterol is mobilized from xanthomata, but it has not yet been proved that it also is mobilized from atheromata.

The mechanisms of action appear to be that of suppressing release of free fatty acids from fat cells, thus decreasing precursor substrates for both triglyceride and cholesterol synthesis and of increasing the activity of lipoprotein lipase. It also decreases synthesis of glycerol and increases rate of conversion of VLDL to LDL. The principal use is in the treatment of primary dysbetalipoproteinemia (Type III) not responding to diet. It may be considered for treatment of adults with very high serum triglyceride levels (Types IV and V).

Nausea, dyspepsia, diarrhea, stomatitis and flatulence occur in about 10% of patients. Urticaria, pruritus and stomatitis occasionally occur, and alopecia areata occurs rarely. Headache, vertigo, asthenia, myalgia, dermatitis, slight weight gain, breast tenderness in males, decrease in libido, impotence, elevation in SGOT and creatine phosphokinase levels in plasma, hypouricemia and rare cardiomyopathy in the young also occur. In some women the drug causes the hair to be dry and brittle.

In the Coronary Drug Project it was found that clofibrate increased the incidence of cholesterolic gallstones twofold, presumably as the result of transferring cholesterol from tissues to bile. It also was reported that there was a small increase in thromboembolic phenomena (it is antifibrinolytic), pulmonary embolism, intermittent claudication and angina pectoris, but some of the conclusions have been challenged. There is equivocal evidence that the drug may increase the incidence of bowel cancer. It has been reported to cause cardiac dysrhythmias. It displaces weakly acidic drugs, such as thyroxine and warfarin, from plasma proteins; with warfarin the result is to increase the anticoagulant effect, and adjustments in dosage are required. It also decreases the efficacy of diuretics. It is contraindicated in pregnant women and children unless there is a history of familial hyperlipidemia.

The drug is hydrolyzed to clofibric acid during absorption and in its pass through the liver, and it is the acid to which activity is attributed. The acid is bound strongly to plasma proteins. About 60% is metabolized, mostly to a glucuronide conjugate. The rest is excreted mainly into urine; there appears to be some renal tubular secretion, and clofibric acid can compete with other anions. Some also is secreted into bile and reabsorbed. The half-life is 18 to 22 hr (av 11 hr), except over 100 hr in anuria. Patients having the slower rates of metabolism have better clinical responses.

Warning—After reviewing results of studies which raised concerns about a possible carcinogenic effect and increased incidence of gastrointestinal disease associated with its use, the FDA, in August 1979, required a boxed warning to be included in revised labeling for the drug, the warning to state, among other statements, the following: *Because of the hepatic tumorigenicity of clofibrate in rodents and the possible increased risk of malignancy associated with clofibrate in the human, as well as the increased risk of cholelithiasis, and because there is not, to date, substantial evidence of a beneficial effect on cardiovascular mortality from clofibrate, this drug should be utilized only for those patients described in the indications section* [of the labeling], *and should be discontinued if significant lipid response is not obtained.* (For the complete text of the warning see *FDA Drug Bull*, August 1979.)

Dose—*Oral, adult, antihyperlipidemic*, **500 mg** 3 times a day for persons weighing less than 120 lb, 4 times a day for those weighing 120 to 180 lb and 5 times a day for those over 180 lb. It usually takes 2 to 5 days before a discernible effect occurs and 1 to 3 mo before the full effect occurs; blood lipids return to pretreatment levels in 2 to 3 wk after treatment is interrupted.

Dosage Form—Capsules: 500 mg.

Colestipol Hydrochloride

Tetraethylenepentamine polymer with 1-chloro-2,3-epoxypropane hydrochloride; Colestid *(Upjohn)*

Copolymer of diethylenetriamine and 1-chloro-2,3-epoxypropane, hydrochloride [37296-80-3].

Preparation—Colestipol hydrochloride is a high-molecular-weight, highly cross-linked, basic anion-exchange copolymer of diethylenetriamine and 1-chloro-2,3-epoxypropane, with approximately one of five amine nitrogens protonated (chloride form). US Pat 3,692,895 and 3,803,237.

Description—White to pale-yellow beads; odorless; tasteless; hygroscopic.

Solubility—Insoluble in water, the beads swelling when placed in water or aqueous fluids.

Uses—An anion-exchange resin similar to *Cholestyramine Resin* (above) in its actions and uses, but there are differences in the anions for which it will exchange. Both resins bind and increase the fecal excretion of bile acids. The consequences and uses that derive therefrom are described under *Cholestyramine*. The adverse effects and drug interactions also are the same.

Dose—*Oral, adult, antihyperlipidemic,* **15** to **30 g** a day in 2 to 4 divided doses, each dose to be suspended in at least 90 mL water or beverage and the glass rinsed with beverage to insure ingestion of entire dose; *digitalis intoxication, initially* **10 g,** then **5 g** every 6 to 8 hr. The resin should never be ingested dry.

Dosage Form—Granules for Oral Suspension: 5 g; Bulk: 500 g.

Gemfibrozil

Pentanoic acid, 5-(2,5-dimethylphenoxy)-2,2-dimethyl-,
Lopid (*Parke-Davis*)

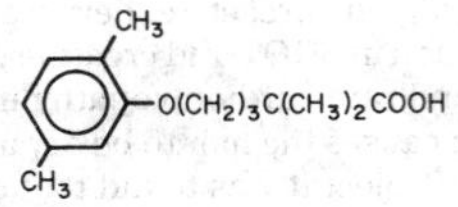

[25812-30-0] $C_{15}H_{22}O_3$ (250.34).

Preparation—See US Pat 3,674,836.

Description—White crystals melting about 61°.

Solubility—Practically insoluble in water or alcohol; slightly soluble in dilute alkali; pK_a 4.7.

Uses—Related structurally to clofibric acid. It decreases the incorporation of long-chain fatty acids into triglycerides and thus decreases the hepatic synthesis of VLDL, and it also decreases the synthesis of VLDL carrier apolipoprotein. It thus decreases VLDL and, erratically, LDL. It also increases HDL and the HDL:cholesterol ratio, more than does clofibrate. At present, it is approved for use in *Type IV hyperlipidemia* (hypertriglyceridemia) in which the patient is at risk of pancreatitis. Although 90% of patients with Types IIa and IIb hyperlipoproteinemia respond significantly, it should be considered as a last resort because of potential toxicities associated with the closely related drug, clofibrate.

The most frequent adverse effects are abdominal pain (6%), epigastric pain (5%), diarrhea (5%), nausea (4%), vomiting (1.6%) and flatulence (1%). Headache, malaise, fatigue, blurred vision, paresthesias, insomnia, dizziness, dry mouth, myalgia and arthralgia, mild hyperglycemia, rashes, dermatidides, urticaria, pruritis, leukopenia, anemia and eosinophila also occur.

It is well absorbed orally. About 30% is oxidized in the liver to two metabolites; the remaining 70% is excreted unchanged in the urine. The half-life of a single dose is 1.5 hr, but it is shortened to 1.3 hr during maintenance, which implies induction of the hepatic microsomal enzyme system.

Dose—*Oral, adult, usually* **600 mg** twice a day, before breakfast and dinner, but the dose ranges from 900 to 1500 mg a day.

Dosage Form—Capsules: 300 mg.

Neomycin—page 1301.
Niacin—pages 1119 and 1126.
Norethindrone Acetate—page 1096.
Oxandrolone—page 1103.

Lovastatin

Butanoic acid, (*S*)-2-methyl-, [1α(*R**),3α,7β,8β(2*S**,4*S**),8aβ]-1,2,3,7,8,8*a*-hexahydro-3,7-dimethyl-8-[2-(tetrahydro-4-hydroxy-6-oxo-2*H*-pyran-2-yl) ethyl]-1-naphthalenyl ester; Mevacor (*MSD*)

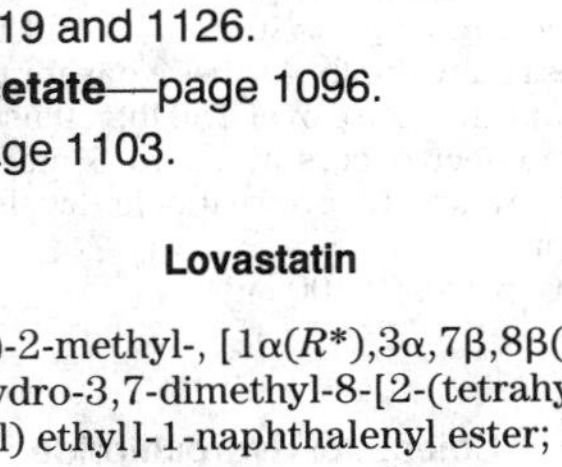

[75330-75-5] $C_{24}H_{36}O_5$ (404.55).

Description—White, nonhygroscopic, crystalline powder which is isolated from a strain of *Asperigillus terreus.* The drug is an inactive lactone which, after ingestion, is hydrolyzed to the corresponding β-hydroxy acid, the active principle.

Solubility—Insoluble in water; sparingly soluble in alcohol, methanol or acetonitrile.

Uses—An inhibitor of 3-hydroxy-3-methylglutaryl coenzyme A (HMG-CoA) reductase, which is the rate-limiting enzyme in the biosynthesis of cholesterol. The mevalonic acid moiety in lovastatin combines at the active center with an affinity over 6000 times that of the natural substrate and is itself reduced. Cholesterolgenesis is suppressed by therapeutic doses, but enough activity remains to permit sufficient cholesterol to be synthesized for body needs. Decreased intracellular concentrations of cholesterol cause upregulation of LDL receptors, so that LDL catabolism is increased and plasma LDL concentrations fall. In heterozygous familial hypercholesteremia, 80 mg a day will decrease plasma LDL levels by 35 to 40%; when combined with cholestyramine or colestipol, LDL levels may decrease by 50 to 60%. LDL is not affected in homozygous familial hypercholesterolemia. The drug is indicated for use in the treatment of *primary familial hypercholesterolemias* (heterozygous Type IIa and Type IIb). It is also effective in *dysbetalipoproteinemia* (Type III), *familial combined hyperlipidemia* (Type IV), *diabetic dyslipidemia* and *nephrotic dyslipidemia.* Combination therapy with bile-acid-binding resins is safe and effective.

Adverse effects usually are mild and transient, and side effects account for less than 2% of discontinuations of treatment. They include headache, flatus, abdominal pain/cramps, diarrhea, rash/pruritis, constipation, nausea, myalgia, dizziness, blurred vision, muscle cramps and dysgeusia.

Myopathy, occasionally leading to frank rhabdomyolysis, has been associated with therapy and may be aggravated with cyclosporin, erythromycin, niacin or gemfibrozil. Creatinine phosphokinase (CPK) levels typically are elevated mildly, but can become marked in patients with myalgias or muscle tenderness or weakness. Lovastatin is concentrated in the liver and may cause increased serum transaminases, which should be monitored during therapy; it is contraindicated in active liver disease.

By the oral route, about 40% is absorbed. In the body, the lactone ring is hydrolyzed to yield the active form of the drug. The drug also is oxidized in the liver to four metabolites. Both parent drug and metabolites are excreted mostly into the bile, but about 10% is excreted in urine.

Dose—*Oral, adult, initially* **20 mg** once a day with later adjustments at 4-wk intervals, if necessary, to up to 80 mg a day; if cholesterol levels exceed 300 mg/dL, start with 40 mg a day.

Dosage Form—Tablets: 10, 20, 40 mg.

Pravastatin Sodium

1-Naphthalene-heptanoic acid, [1*S*-[1α(β*S**,δ*S**),2α,6α,8β(*R**),8aα]]-1,2,6,7,8,8a-hexahydro-β,δ,6-trihydroxy-2-methyl-8-(2-methyl-1-oxobutoxy)-, monosodium salt; Pravachol (*Bristol-Myers Squibb*)

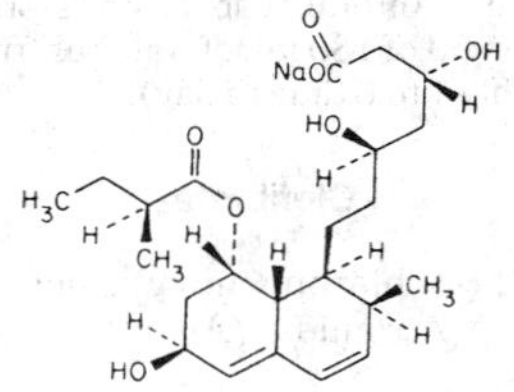

[81131-70-6] $C_{23}H_{35}NaO_7$ (446.52)

Preparation—US Pat 4,346,227; by microbial action on mevastatin.

Description—White, crystalline powder

Solubility—Very soluble in water or alcohol.

Uses—Its mechanism of action, effects, indications, side effects and precautions are essentially the same as those of *Lovastatin.* However, it is 100-fold more hydrophilic and does not cross the blood-brain barrier or enter nonhepatic cells as readily. It is absorbed more rapidly. Like lovastatin, it undergoes extensive first-pass metabolism and is concentrated in the liver, its primary site of action. It has a half-life of 77 hr and 70% of the major metabolite is excreted in the feces. Bile acid sequestrants reduce bioavailability by about 50%; it should be taken at least 1 hr before or 4 hr after the resin.

Dose—*Oral, adult,* **10 to 20 mg** once a day at bedtime, *maximum,* **40 mg** a day; *elderly,* **10 mg** once a day at bedtime, *maximum* **20 mg** a day; adjust dose at intervals of at least 4 wk.

Dosage Form—Tablets: 10 and 20 mg.

Probucol

Phenol, 4,4′-[(1-methylethylidene)bis(thio)]bis[2,6-bis(1,1-dimethylethyl)-, Lorelco (*Merrell Dow*)

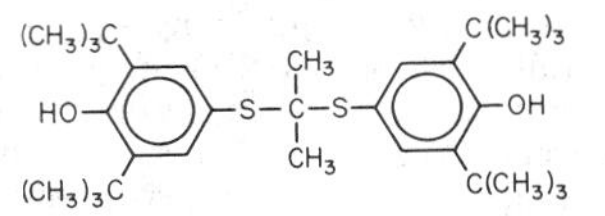

[23288-49-5] $C_{31}H_{48}O_2S_2$ (516.84).

Preparation—By acid-catalyzed condensation of 4-mercapto-2,6-di-*tert*-butylphenol with acetone (*J Med Chem 13:*722, 1970).

Description—White to yellow, crystalline powder; melts about 125°.

Solubility—Practically insoluble in water; soluble in alcohol.

Uses—Has a modest effect to lower plasma LDL (and cholesterol) levels by decreasing cholesterol synthesis at an early stage, increasing the catabolism of LDL and increasing the excretion of bile acids. In one clinical study, the plasma cholesterol content was decreased from 278 to 234 mg/dL, or 16%, after 3 months of treatment; however, after 9 months, the decrement was only 9%. It has a small and unpredictable effect on VLDL. It also tends to reduce HDL levels even more so in some patients. It is indicated for use in the treatment of *familial hypercholesterolemia* (Type IIa) and *combined hyperlipoproteinemia* (Type IIb) but not other hyperlipidemias. Although it has not been shown to reduce the atheromata or decrease coronary heart disease, it has been shown to effect the reduction or disappearance of xanthelasma and xanthomata.

Diarrhea occurs in about 10%, and transient flatulence, abdominal pain and nausea in less than 2% of patients. Hyperhidrosis, fetid sweat and vomiting occur occasionally. Dizziness, chest pain, palpitations and syncope are infrequent. Rare instances of angioneurotic edema have been reported. Other possibly drug-related but not established side effects include headache, insomnia, paresthesias, tinnitus, blurred vision, impotence, conjunctivitis and various rashes. Probucol increases the QT interval of ECG and should not be used in patients with abnormally long QT intervals or recent myocardial infarction. It also sensitizes the canine myocardium to catecholamine-induced dysrhythmias, but the effect has not been observed in other animals, so that the clinical significance is unknown. The safety of the drug in pregnancy, and in children, is not known.

About 8 to 10% of an oral dose is absorbed; absorption is increased by food. The drug accumulates in adipose tissue, and detectable amounts are found in blood for as long as 6 months after discontinuation of the drug. It mainly is eliminated in the bile.

Dose—*Oral, adult,* **500 mg** twice a day, with breakfast and evening meals.

Dosage Form—Film-Coated Tablets: 250 and 500 mg.

Simvastatin

Butanoic acid, 2,2-dimethyl-, [1*S*-[1α,3α,7β,8β-(2*S**,4*S**)8aβ]]-1,2,3,7,8,8a-hexahydro-3,7-dimethyl-8-[2-(tetrahydro-4-hydroxy-6-oxo-2*H*-pyran-2-yl)ethyl]-1-naphthalenyl ester, Zocor (*MSD*)

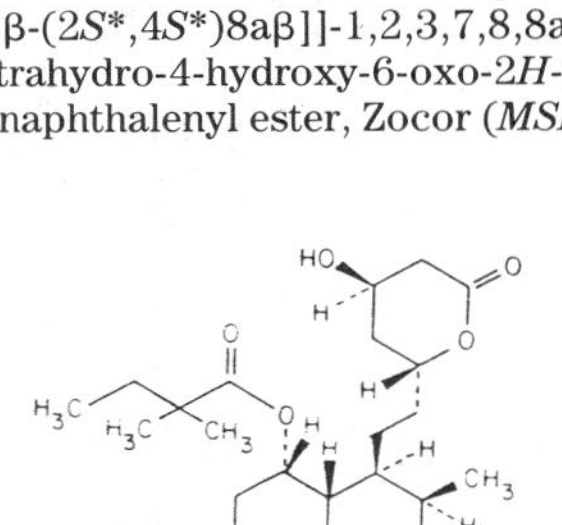

[79902-63-9] $C_{25}H_{38}O_5$ (418.57).

Preparation—*J Med Chem 29:* 849, 1986.

Description—White crystals melting about 137°; it is a derivative of lovastatin.

Solubility—Practically insoluble in water; freely soluble in alcohol.

Uses—Its mechanism of action, effects, indications, side effects and precautions are essentially the same as those of *Lovastatin*, to which it is closely related chemically. Its absorption, sequestration by the liver, metabolism and excretion are also very similar.

Dose—*Oral, adult,* **5 to 10 mg** once a day in the evening, *maximum* **40 mg** a day; *elderly,* **5 mg** once a day, *maximum* **20 mg** a day; adjust dose at intervals of at least 4 wk.

Dosage Form—Tablets: 5, 10, 20, and 40 mg.

Other Agents Affecting Blood Lipids

Dextrothyroxine Sodium

[*O*-(4-Hydroxy-3,5-diiodophenyl)-3-diiodo-, D-Tyrosine, monosodium salt hydrate; [7054-08-2] $C_{15}H_{10}I_4N\text{-}NaO_4 \cdot xH_2O$; *anhydrous* [137-53-1] (798.86); Choloxin (*Flint*)]. **Preparation**—Using D-thyroxine, the process is analogous to that described for *Levothyroxine Sodium*, page 1084. **Description and Solubility**—Light-yellow to buff-colored, odorless, tasteless powder; stable in dry air but may assume a slight, pink color on exposure to light; pH (saturated solution) about 8.9. Soluble 1 g in about 700 mL of water or about 300 mL of alcohol; insoluble in chloroform or ether. **Uses**—Thyroid hormones increase turnover of cholesterol, with catabolism increased more than biosynthesis. Furthermore they increase biliary secretion of neutral steroids and bile acids, which tends to lower plasma cholesterol levels. In addition to lowering the LDL levels, thyroid hormones lower those of the VLDL. Although some studies purport to show that the therapeutic effect is attributable to contaminating levothyroxin, general metabolic actions of this drug are less proportionately than with levothyroxine, so that it is possible to lower blood lipids with lesser increases in basal metabolic effect and other indices of thyrotoxicity. When used in combination with estrogenic substances, such as stilbestrol, the lipid-lowering effect is enhanced and the dose of this drug may be reduced, but side effects of the estrogen may make use of the combination undesirable, especially in men.

Untoward effects include increased metabolic rate, tachycardia and increased frequency of anginal attacks in persons with coronary insufficiency. Therefore the drug is not used in persons with coronary heart disease, the population that needs treatment most, and use is restricted mainly to young persons. It can elevate blood glucose levels in diabetics. It should be used cautiously in diabetics and persons with cardiac disease and in patients with hepatic or renal dysfunction. It suppresses TSH release and can, thereby, lower metabolic rate in hypothyroidism; therefore, thyroid hormones should be used first, instead of dextrothyroxine. Dextrothyroxine augments the action of anticoagulants, which requires that anticoagulant dosage be reduced appropriately. **Dose**—*Oral, adult, initially* **1** to **2 mg** a day for 1 mo, to be increased by increments of 1 to 2 mg at monthly intervals until either the desired effect is achieved or the daily dose is 8 mg. *Children, initially* **0.05 mg/kg** a day, with increments of 0.05 mg/kg a day at monthly intervals, if necessary, up to a maximum of 4 mg a day; maintenance doses are usually 0.1 mg/kg a day. **Dosage Form**—Tablets: 1, 2, 4, and 6 mg.

Fish Oils and Omega-3 Fatty Acids

Uses—Ever since Ancel Keys made worldwide epidemiological studies of the relationship of coronary heart disease (CHD) to dietary fat, the relative freedom of the eskimo from CHD posed an enigma. The eskimo has a very high fat diet which also is high in cholesterol. It was surmised that polyunsaturated fatty acids, in which fish oils and blubber are rich, protected against atherogenesis. Subsequent experimental and epidemiological studies have shown them to have protective actions alone and against saturated fat in atherogenesis. It was only in the 1980s, however, that the protective action has been attributed especially to omega-3 fatty acids, such as eicosapentaenoic and docosahexaenoic acids (which give rise to trienic prostaglandins).

Epidemiological studies reported in the mid-1980s mostly support earlier conjecture and show that substantial increases in fish and in the diet of European and sedentary people usually decrease both LDL and CHD and retard restenosis after coronary angioplasty. However, a high consumption of fish oils by persons with hypertriglyceridemia may elevate plasma LDL levels. Studies do not find that the amounts of omega-3 fatty acids contained in marketed capsules have much effect on LDL and CHD. They do, however, decrease platelet activity, prolong bleeding time and predispose to hemorrhages and stroke. They also decrease endothelial cell production of a growth factor which resembles that from platelets and suppress the production of the inflammatory mediators, interleukin-1 and tumor necrosis factor.

It has been pointed out that vegetable sources such as walnuts and walnut oil, wheat germ oil, rapeseed oil, soybean lecithin, soybeans and tofu, common beans, butternuts and seaweed all contain generous amounts of omega-3 fatty acids without either the cholesterol found in many fish oils or the expense.

Special-Use Cardiovascular Drug

Alprostadil

[(11α,13*E*,15S)-11,15-dihydroxy-9-oxoprost-13-en-1-oic acid [745-65-3] $C_{20}H_{34}O_5$ (354.49); Prostaglandin E_1; PGE_1; Prostin VR (*Upjohn*)].

Isolated from the seminal vesicle tissue of sheep. See *J Biol Chem 238:* 3555, 1963. **Preparation**—For the synthesis refer to *J Org Chem 37:* 2921, 1974. **Description**—White crystals melting about 115°; $[\alpha]_{578}$ − 61.6° (c = 0.56. THF). **Uses**—Endogenous prostaglandin E_1 helps maintain the patency of the ductus arteriosis of the fetus. After birth, prostaglandin production falls and the ductus closes. However, when there are congenital heart defects, such as the *tetralogy of Fallot, transposition of the great vessels, pulmonary atresia, pulmonary stenosis, coarctation of the aorta, tricuspid atresia* or *imperfect aortic arch*, it is necessary that the ductus remain patent until corrective surgery can be accomplished. In such instances, infusion of alprostadil (PGE) helps maintain patency pending surgery.

The following adverse effects may occur: apnea (12%), bradypnea, tachypnea, respiratory depression, bronchial wheezing (all < 1%); flushing (10%), bradycardia (7%), hypotension (4%), tachycardia (3%), cardiac arrest (1%), edema (1%), hyperemia, congestive heart failure, right ventricular spasm, second-degree heart block, supraventricular tachycardia, ventricular fibrillation, shock (all < 1%); fever (14%), convulsions (4%), opisthotomus, rigidity, hyperirritability, lethargy, hypothermia (all < 1%); diarrhea (2%), regurgitation (< 1%), hyperbilirubinemia (< 1%); intravascular coagulopathy (1%); hemorrhage, anemia, thrombocytopenia, hematuria, anuria, hypokalemia, hyperkalemia, hypoglycemia, proliferation of cortex of long bones (all < 1%) sepsis (2%) and peritonitis (< 1%).

The drug must be used cautiously when any condition preexists that may add to or exaggerate any of the above effects. There should be monitoring of arterial pressure and pulmonary status especially when pulmonary flow is already compromised). **Dose**—*Intravenous infusion, neonate, initially* **0.05** to **1.0 µg/kg/min;** after a satisfactory response is achieved, the rate is adjusted (usually lowered) to the lowest effective rate. **Dosage Form**—Injection: 500 µg/mL.

CHAPTER 56

Respiratory Drugs

Glen R Hanson, DDS, PhD
Professor of Pharmacology
College of Pharmacy and School of Medicine, University of Utah
Salt Lake City, UT 84112

The drugs discussed in this chapter are a diverse group of pharmacologic agents which can alter the function of respiratory systems and associated structures. The actions of many of these drugs are employed therapeutically to relieve respiratory disorders, but others can cause annoying respiratory effects as well as dangerous and unintended side effects. For example, alcohol, anesthetic agents, barbiturates and other hypnotic drugs and morphine and other narcotic agents compromise the respiratory system by depressing its activity. The side effects of such drugs are discussed elsewhere. The drugs used to treat respiratory disorders, which will be discussed in this chapter, include bronchodilators, corticosteroids, antitussives, expectorants, surfactant preparations, respiratory stimulants and therapeutic gases.

Bronchodilators

These drugs are used to open air passages and facilitate breathing by producing bronchodilation. They are able to diminish bronchospasms by relaxing the smooth muscles of the bronchioles, providing respiratory relief from conditions such as asthma, bronchitis, emphysema or bronchiectasis.

A number of pharmacologically different groups of drugs possess bronchodilator properties. The bronchial muscles are controlled by the autonomic nervous system with parasympathetic fibers predominating in number and effect. Stimulation of parasympathetic nerves causes calcium-dependent contraction of the bronchi and enhances the release of chemical mediators that induce bronchospasm. Consequently, *anticholinergic* drugs (eg, atropine) are useful for reducing bronchospasm.

Calcium antagonists, such as verapamil and nifedipine, selectively inhibit calcium-ion influx across the cell membrane and suppress calcium-dependent smooth muscle contraction.

Sympathomimetic drugs, such as metaproterenol, albuterol, terbutaline, bitolterol, isoetharine and pirbuterol exert a preferential effect on beta-2-adrenergic receptors and mediate relaxation of the smooth muscle of the respiratory tract.

Corticosteroids, like beclomethasone dipropionate, dexamethasone, triamcinolone acetonide and flunisolide, not only are effective anti-inflammatory agents, but also potentiate the bronchodilator effects of adrenergic drugs. These corticosteroids are not direct bronchodilators and are not effective for rapid relief of bronchospasm. Use of corticosteroid inhalers has effective anti-inflammatory activity while having minimal systemic effects. Cromolyn sodium inhibits the release of mediators of inflammation from mast cells. These mediators are induced by specific antigens, as well as non-specific mechanisms (such as exercise). It is the only antiasthmatic that blocks both early and late asthmatic responses induced by either episodic or continuous allergen inhalation or exercise. It controls the symptoms of mild to moderate chronic asthma in 60 to 70% of patients in doses that induce few, if any, adverse effects. It is not recommended for acute asthma or status asthmaticus since it has no intrinsic bronchodilator activity. Cromolyn has local effects on the lungs and consequently is administered often in aerosol forms. It frequently is used in combination with corticosteroid and/or bronchodilator treatment.

The *xanthine drugs*, especially theophylline, its soluble salts and derivatives, are thought to be the most useful bronchodilators for moderate or severe reversible bronchospasm. Moreover, they also improve respiratory exchange by increasing diaphragmatic contractility. The mechanism for the therapeutic effect of theophylline on respiratory systems is not clear; however, this drug has several notable actions, including: (1) it competitively inhibits phosphodiesterase which increases cyclic adenosine monophosphate (cAMP) and the release of endogenous epinephrine; (2) it inhibits neural transmission at certain synapses, especially in the central nervous system, where adenosine, a structural analog, may be a neurotransmitter; (3) it antagonizes the action of PGE_2 and $PGF_{2\alpha}$ and (4) it affects the mobilization of intracellular calcium. It is important to note that theophylline induces learning and behavioral problems in about 5% of school children receiving the drug.

The effectiveness of the methylxanthine preparations in the treatment of bronchial asthma depends on their hepatic conversion to theophylline, which is the active constituent. Consequently, the dosage of theophylline, its salts and dyphylline usually is expressed in terms of anhydrous theophylline base, despite the marked pharmacokinetic interpatient variability among these preparations. The approximate anhydrous theophylline content in the various theophylline derivatives is:

84 to 86% of aminophylline anhydrous
74 to 82% of aminophylline hydrous
70% of dyphylline
62 to 66% of oxytriphylline
48 to 50% of theophylline calcium salicylate
91% of theophylline monohydrate
73 to 75% of theophylline olamine
55 to 65% of theophylline sodium acetate
45 to 47% of theophylline sodium glycinate

The anticholinergic drugs are discussed in Chapter 60, beta-2 and other adrenergic drugs in Chapter 45, cromolyn sodium in Chapter 73, and corticosteroids in Chapter 64. Theophylline and its various derivatives and combinations are presented in this section.

Albuterol—page 986.

Aminophylline

1*H*-Purine-2,6-dione, 3,7-dihydro-1,3-dimethyl-, compd with 1,2-ethanediamine (2:1)

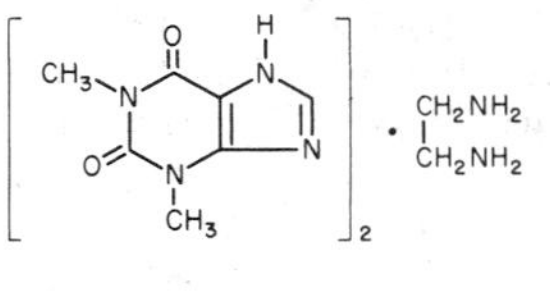

Theophylline compound with ethylenediamine [317-34-0] $C_{16}H_{24}N_{10}O_4$ (420.43); *dihydrate* [49746-06-7] (456.46).

Preparation—By adding, with vigorous stirring, a weighed quantity of theophylline to a volume of solution containing the required equivalent quantity of the diamine in anhydrous alcohol. After a few hours, the precipitate of aminophylline is filtered off, washed with cold alcohol and dried at a low temperature.

Description—White or slightly yellowish granules or powder, having a slight ammoniacal odor and a bitter taste; on exposure to air it gradually loses ethylenediamine and absorbs CO_2 with liberation of free theophylline; its solution is alkaline to litmus.

Solubility—1 g in about 5 mL water, but, owing to hydrolysis, separation of crystals of less aminated theophylline begins in a few minutes, these crystals dissolving on the addition of a small amount of ethylenediamine. When, however, 1 g is dissolved in 25 mL water, the solution remains clear; insoluble in alcohol or ether.

Incompatibilities—Aqueous solutions are alkaline and display the incompatibilities of the alkalies. *Acids* cause a precipitation of theophylline; even *carbon dioxide* of the air behaves thus.

Uses—Indicated for *bronchial asthma*, and for reversible bronchospasm associated with chronic bronchitis and emphysema. Aminophylline (injection, oral solution, enema) also is used as a respiratory stimulant in neonatal apnea and in Cheyne-Stokes respiration. It also is useful as a diuretic agent. Absorption from the gastrointestinal tract after oral or rectal administration is incomplete, slow and variable. Approximately 79% is converted to theophylline. Optimal serum therapeutic levels range from 10 to 20 μg/mL. It is most effective when given intravenously; if given slowly in dilute solution, the drug is relatively nontoxic, although nausea, vomiting and anorexia may appear in some patients. The simultaneous administration of aluminum hydroxide decreases the incidence of this side effect. See *Theophylline*.

Dose—*Usual, adult, bronchodilator, oral, loading:* Elixir, **7 mg/kg;** Tablets, **18.7 mg/kg/day** in 3 or 4 divided doses at 6- to 8-hr intervals; Enteric-Coated Tablets, see Tablets. *Intravenous, loading:* **6 mg/kg** over a period of 20 min. *Rectal, enema*, **300 mg** 3 times a day or **450 mg** 2 times a day; suppositories, **500 mg** 1 to 3 times a day. *Usual, adult, bronchodilator, oral, maintenance:* Elixir, **2.4 mg/kg** every 6 hr for 12 hr, then **2.4 mg/kg** every 12 hr; Tablets, increase 25% at 2- or 3-day intervals up to a maximum of **15.2 mg/kg/day**. *Intravenous, maintenance*, **600 μg/kg/hr** for 12 hr, then **300 μg/kg/hr**.

Pediatric, bronchodilator, rectal, enema or *suppositories*, **3** to **5 mg/kg** every 6 to 8 hr, not to exceed **20 mg/kg/day.** *Pediatric, elixir, oral solution, tablets* or *injection*, see package insert for information about the dose for a particular age group.

Dosage Forms—Enema: 60 mg/mL; Injection: 250 mg/10 mL, 500 mg/20 mL and 500/2 mL (see below); Suppositories: 250 and 500 mg; Oral Solution: 105 mg/5 mL; Tablets: 100 and 200 mg; Enteric-Coated Tablets: 100 and 200 mg; Extended-Release Tablets: 225 mg.

Aminophylline Injection [Theophylline Ethylenediamine Injection] is a sterile solution of aminophylline in water for injection, or is a sterile solution of theophylline in water for injection prepared with the aid of ethylenediamine. It contains, in each 100 mL, 2.5 g of $C_{16}H_{24}N_{10}O_4.2H_2O$. Aminophylline Injection may contain an excess of ethylenediamine, but no other substance added for the purpose of pH adjustment: it contains 131 to 152 mg of $C_2H_8N_2$ per g of $C_{16}H_{24}N_{10}O_4.2H_2O$. *Stabilization:* The aminophylline in this injection absorbs CO_2 from the air resulting in the liberation of free theophylline. The USP recognizes the difficulties experienced with the aminophylline injection and, for purposes of stabilization, permits the use of additional ethylenediamine. It appears to be advisable to prepare the solution directly from calculated quantities of theophylline and of ethylenediamine, thus entirely eliminating the possibility of previous absorption of CO_2. It has been found helpful to ampul the solution while hot, seal it at once, thus producing a slight vacuum in the ampul and then sterilize the ampul immediately by autoclaving before seed crystals can start to form. Some operators prefer to repeat the sterilization operation, believing that this also helps to prevent subsequent precipitation.

Atropine—page 1022.

Bitolterol—page 987.

Cromolyn Sodium—page 1229.

Dyphylline

1*H*-Purine-2,6-dione,
7-(2,3-dihydroxypropyl)-3,7-dihydro-1,3-dimethyl-, Dilor (*Savage*);
Lufyllin (*Wallace*); Neothylline (*Lemmon*)

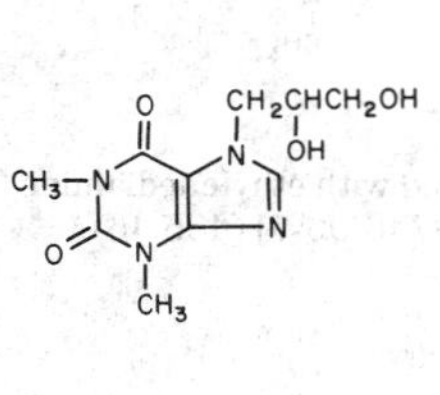

7-(2,3-Dihydroxypropyl)theophylline $C_{10}H_{14}N_4O_4$ (254.25).

Preparation—By interaction of 1-chloro-2,3-dihydroxypropane with theophylline dissolved in a sodium hydroxide or potassium hydroxide solution. US Pat 2,575,344 (see *CA 46:*1722i, 1952).

Description—White, crystalline powder; bitter taste; melts at about 158°; pH (1 in 100 solution) 6.6 to 7.3; protect aqueous solutions from light.

Solubility—1 g in 3 mL water, 50 mL alcohol or 100 mL chloroform.

Uses—Indicated for relief of *bronchial asthma* and for reversible *bronchospasm* associated with *chronic bronchitis* and *emphysema*. It exhibits peripheral vasodilator and bronchodilator actions characteristic of theophylline. It also has some diuretic and myocardial stimulant effects, and is effective orally. Dyphylline is a derivative of theophylline and is not metabolized to theophylline *in vivo*. Following oral administration, dyphylline is 68 to 82% bioavailable. Peak plasma concentrations are reached in 1 hr; its half-life is 2 hr. The minimal therapeutic concentration is 12 μg/mL; 88% is excreted unchanged in the urine. Because of its somewhat shorter half-life, other theophylline derivatives usually are preferred for chronic bronchodilator therapy. Otherwise, its pharmacological profile, effective and toxic serum levels, contraindications, precautions, adverse reactions and drug interactions are similar to those for theophylline.

Dose—*Usual, adult, oral, acute attack,* **15 mg/kg** every 6 hr, up to 4 times a day. The dosage should be individualized by titration to the condition and response of the patient. *Intramuscular, adults,* **250** to **500 mg** injected slowly. *Children,* **2** to **3 mg/lb** daily, in divided doses.

Dosage Forms—Elixir: 33.3 and 53.3 mg/5 mL; Injection: 250 mg/mL; Liquid: 100 mg/5 mL; Tablets: 200 and 400 mg.

Ephedrine—page 989.

Epinephrine—page 989.

Ethylnorepinephrine—page 990.

Isoetharine—page 991.

Isoproterenol—page 991.

Metaproterenol—page 993.

Oxtriphylline

Ethanaminium, 2-hydroxy-*N,N,N*-trimethyl-, salt with 3,7-dihydro-1,3-dimethyl-1*H*-purine-2,6-dione; Choline Theophyllinate; Choledyl (*Parke-Davis*)

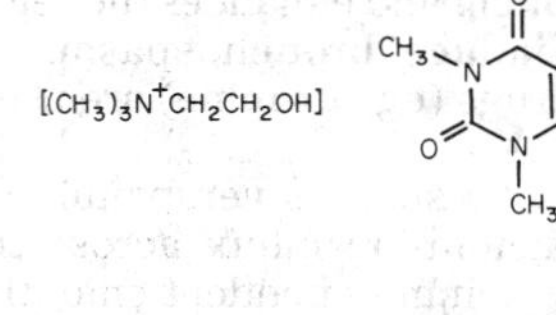

Choline salt of theophylline (1:1) [4499-40-5] $C_{12}H_{21}N_5O_3$ (283.33).

Preparation—An aqueous solution of choline bicarbonate is reacted with theophylline in 2-propanol. After concentration by vacuum distillation, the crude product is crystallized from 2-propanol–methanol solution. US Pat 2,776,287 and 2,776,288.

Description—White, crystalline powder, having an amine-like odor; pH (1 in 100 solution) about 10.3; protect aqueous solutions from light.

Solubility—1 g in 1 mL of water; freely soluble in alcohol; very slightly soluble in chloroform.

Uses—Oxtriphylline, the choline salt of theophylline, is more soluble, more stable, better absorbed from the gastrointestinal tract and produces less gastric irritation than aminophylline, but has pharmacological actions similar to other xanthine derivatives. (See *Theophylline*, page 973). Hence, it is effective orally in the management of *acute bronchial asthma* and for *reversible bronchospasm*, associated with *chronic bronchitis* and *emphysema*. Development of tolerance is infrequent; therefore, it is useful for long-term therapy. Its usefulness in premenstrual tension or in dysmenorrhea has not been established. Untoward effects include gastric distress, occasionally palpitation and central nervous system stimulation.

Dose—*Bronchodilator, usual, adult, oral,* **100** to **200 mg** every 6 hr; sustained-action, **400** to **600 mg** every 12 hr. *Pediatric*, children 2 to 12 yr, **3.7 mg/kg** every 6 hr (dosage for children under 2 yr has not been established).

Dosage Forms—Elixir: 100 mg/5 mL; Pediatric Syrup: **50 mg/5 mL;** Tablets: 100 and 200 mg. Sustained-Action Tablets: 400 and 600 mg.

Pirbuterol—page 997.

Terbutaline Sulfate—page 998.

Theophylline

1*H*-Purine-2,6-dione, 3,7-dihydro-1,3-dimethyl-, monohydrate or anhydrous; 1,3-Dimethylxanthine *(Various Mfrs)*

Theophylline monohydrate [5967-84-0] $C_7H_8N_4O_2.H_2O$ (198.18); *anhydrous* [58-55-9] (180.17); for the structural formula, see page 1232.

Preparation—Present in tea but in too small an amount to make it an economical source. It has been made from caffeine, but is produced more successfully by total synthesis. See page 1232.

Description—White, odorless, crystalline powder having a bitter taste; stable in air; melts between 270° and 274°; saturated aqueous solution is neutral or slightly acid to litmus; weaker as a base than caffeine or theobromine and scarcely forms salts even with the strong acids, but is more "acidic" than those and readily dissolves in ammonia water.

Solubility—1 g in about 120 mL water or 80 mL alcohol; more soluble in hot water; sparingly soluble in ether or chloroform; freely soluble in solutions of alkali hydroxides or ammonia.

Uses—Theophylline and its salts and derivatives are used as *bronchodilators* in the symptomatic treatment of *mild bronchial asthma* and *reversible bronchospasm* which may occur in association with *chronic bronchitis, emphysema* and *other obstructive pulmonary diseases.* It relieves the primary manifestations of asthma, including shortness of breath, wheezing and dyspnea and improves pulmonary function as measured by increased flow rates and vital capacity. The drug also suppresses exercise-induced asthma and, in doses that maintain therapeutic serum levels, prevents symptoms of chronic asthma. The bronchodilator action may be due in part to increased cAMP following inhibition of phosphodiesterase, the enzyme that degrades cAMP. Other proposed mechanisms include alteration in smooth muscle calcium ion concentration, inhibition of prostaglandins, blockade of adenosine receptors and the release of histamine and leucotrienes from mast cells. Theophylline is well absorbed after administration. Food has little effect on theophylline availability; absorption may be slower in the presence of food and more rapid in the presence of large volumes of fluid. Rectal suppositories are absorbed slowly and erratically regardless of the type of suppository base; retention enemas are absorbed more rapidly. The time required to reach peak plasma levels varies with the route and formulation used; following oral administration of liquids or uncoated tablets, peak plasma levels are reached in 2 hr. Average volume of distribution is 0.5 L/kg.

Theophylline and its derivatives frequently are combined with sympathomimetics, sedatives and expectorants for use in asthmatic patients. Many clinicians believe that theophylline doses in these combination preparations are inadequate and single-ingredient products are more effective, easier to manage and safer. There is no evidence of a therapeutic advantage with the combination products.

Theophylline plasma or serum levels of about 10 to 20 μg/mL usually are needed to produce optimum bronchodilator response. Some patients with mild pulmonary disease will experience relief of bronchospasm with theophylline plasma levels of 5 μg/mL. With plasma levels ranging from 8 to 20 μg/mL, a linear relationship exists between improvement in pulmonary function and the logarithm of theophylline plasma concentration. In premature infants, theophylline plasma levels of about 7 to 14 μg/mL may be sufficient to reverse apnea. Theophylline plasma levels of about 10 μg/mL produce a transient diuretic response. Theophylline is excreted by the kidneys. Less than 15% of the drug is excreted unchanged in the urine. Elimination kinetics vary greatly among individuals. The elimination half-life of theophylline averages about *7 to 9 hr in the adult nonsmoker* and *4 to 5 hr in the adult smoker* (one or two packs per day); *3 to 5 hr in children* and *20 to 30 hr in premature neonates.* The premature neonate excretes about 50% unchanged theophylline and may accumulate the caffeine metabolite.

Theophylline, its salts and dyphylline exert identical pharmacologic actions. Theophylline competitively inhibits phosphodiesterase, the enzyme that degrades cyclic 3′,5′-adenosine monophosphate (cAMP). Increased levels of intracellular cAMP may mediate some of the pharmacological effects of the drug.

Theophylline has less stimulatory effect on the central nervous system and skeletal muscles than caffeine but has a greater effect on coronary dilatation, smooth muscle relaxation, diuresis and cardiac stimulation than caffeine. In general, it has relatively more pharmacologic activity in all categories than theobromine.

Theophylline produces central nervous system stimulation and gastrointestinal irritation following administration by any route. Theophylline and its salts and analogs are all somewhat irritating to gastric mucosa; the significance of reported differences among the individual agents is doubtful. The most common gastrointestinal side effects (both locally and centrally mediated) include nausea, vomiting, epigastric pain, abdominal cramps, anorexia and, rarely, diarrhea. Cardiovascular side effects of theophylline include palpitation, sinus tachycardia and increased pulse rate. These side effects are usually mild and transient. Theophylline also may produce transiently increased urinary frequency, dehydration, twitching of fingers and hands and elevated SGOT levels. Hypersensitivity reactions characterized by urticaria, generalized pruritus and angioneurotic edema have been reported with theophylline administration. Drug interactions are common in patients on theophylline. Agents which *decrease* the effects of theophylline include cigarette and marijuana smoking, phenobarbital and charcoal-broiled foods. Agents which *increase* the effects of theophylline include cimetidine, erythromycin, influenza virus vaccine, troleandomycin, allopurinal and thiabendazole. Theophylline *increases* the effects of sympathomimetic drugs, digitalis and oral anticoagulants. Theophylline *decreases* the effects of phenytoin and lithium carbonate. Concomitant administration of theophylline with beta-adrenergic blocking agents may result in antagonistic effects; theophylline with reserpine or halothane may induce tachycardia or cardiac arrhythmias, respectively.

Theophylline toxicity is most likely to occur when plasma levels exceed 20 μg/mL and becomes progressively more severe at higher serum concentrations. Tachycardia, in the absence of hypoxia, fever or administration of sympathomimetic drugs, may be an indication of theophylline toxicity. Anorexia, nausea and occasional vomiting, diarrhea, insomnia, irritability, restlessness and headache commonly occur. Fatalities in adults have occurred during or following IV administration of large doses of theophylline in patients with renal, hepatic or cardiovascular complications. In other patients, the rapidity of the injection, rather than the dose used, appears to be the more important factor precipitating acute hypotension, convulsions, coma, cardiac standstill, ventricular fibrillation and death. There is no specific antidote for theophylline toxicity; therapy is usually supportive. Treatment includes stopping the drug, gastric lavage and/or emesis and administration of antacids or demulcents and oxygen. Prompt restoration of fluid and electrolyte balance is essential. Other symptomatic procedures are instituted as necessary.

Dose—All dosages should be based on lean body weight since theophylline does not distribute into fatty tissue. Moreover, all dosage should be calculated on the basis of anhydrous theophylline content, regardless of the salt used. For the rapid control of acute symptoms in patients not on theophylline, an initial loading dose is required. *Adult (nonsmoker), oral loading,* **6 mg/kg** followed by 2 doses of **3 mg/kg** every 6 hr; *maintenance dose,* **3 mg/kg** every 8 hr. *Adult (smoker),* and *children 9 to 16 yr, oral loading,* **6 mg/kg** followed by 3 doses of **3 mg/kg** every 4 hr; *maintenance dose,* 3 mg/kg every 6 hr. *Children 6 months to 9 yr, oral loading,* **6 mg/kg** followed by 3 doses of **4 mg/kg** every 4 hr; *maintenance dose,* **4 mg/kg** every 6 hr. Consult package insert for detailed dosage regimen.

Dosage Forms—Capsules: 50, 100, 200 and 250 mg; Extended-Release Capsules: 50, 60, 65, 75, 100, 125, 130, 200, 250, 260 and 300 mg; Elixir: 80, 112.5, 150 and 225 mg/5 mL; Oral Liquid: 80 mg/15 mL; Oral Suspension: 100 mg/5 mL; Tablets: 100, 125, 200, 225, 250 and 300 mg; Extended-Release Tablets: 100, 130, 200, 250, 260, 300, 400 and 500 mg.

Antiasthmatic Combinations

Some examples of antiasthmatic combinations (with content per capsule, tablet or 5 mL provided) are as follows:

Dyphylline and Guaifenesin [Dilor-G (*Savage*); Lufyllin-GG (*Wallace*); Neothyline-GG (*Lemmon*)]—200 and 200 mg, respectively.

Theophylline, Sodium Glycinate and Guaifenesin [Asbron-G (*Sandoz*)]—300 and 100 mg, respectively.

Theophylline, Ephedrine Hydrochloride and Phenobarbital [Tedral SA (*Parke-Davis*)]—130–180, 24–48 and 8–28 mg, respectively.

Theophylline, Ephedrine Sulfate and Hydroxyzine Hydrochloride [Marax (*Roerig*)]—130, 25 and 10 mg, respectively.

Theophylline Calcium Salicylate, Ephedrine Hydrochloride, Phenobarbital and Potassium Iodide [Quadrinal (*Knoll*)]—130, 24, 24, and 320 mg, respectively.

Theophylline, Ephedrine Sulfate, Guaifenesin and Phenobarbital [Bronkotabs, Bronkolixir (*Winthrop*)]—100, 24, 100 and 8 mg, respectively. Available OTC.

Theophylline, Ephedrine Hydrochloride, Potassium Iodide and Phenobarbital [Quadrinal (*Knoll*)]—65, 24, 320 and 24 mg, respectively.

Corticosteroids

In general, corticosteroids are used to treat severe asthmatic conditions when other measures, such as sympathomimetics and theophylline-like drugs do not provide adequate relief. For example, in the treatment of severe chronic asthma that is refractory to other forms of therapy, the long-term use of corticosteroids may be necessary. Adrenal insufficiency and stress management are always major concerns in patients receiving prolonged treatments with these drugs. Corticosteroid therapy for asthma is always done in combination with concurrent use of other asthma medication, such as inhaled β_2-adrenergic agonists and/or theophylline-related oral medication. Such combinations help to reduce the number of doses of corticosteroids required to provide adequate asthmatic control and decrease the chance of serious side effects. Sometimes, the use of inhaled corticosteroids as part of the therapy for bronchial asthma can reduce the need for their oral counterparts or replace them all together. If done conservatively, inhaled glucocorticoids often are effective in relieving bronchial hyperreactivity associated with moderately severe asthma without significant suppression of adrenal function. However, oral inhalation of corticosteroids such as dexamethasone should not be used for the treatment of occasional mild attacks of asthma which are controlled adequately by treatments with sympathomimetics or theophyllines.

It should be remembered that corticosteroids are not bronchodilators and will not provide rapid relief from bronchospasm and thus should not be the primary treatment for *status epilepticus* or other acute episodes of asthma. Corticosteroid therapy is most effective when used as a preventative measure. The corticosteroid agents most often used in asthma medication are dexamethasone sodium phosphate, beclomethasone dipropionate, triamcinolone acetonide and fluisolide. These drugs are discussed in greater detail in Chapter 64.

Corticosteroid Asthma Inhalants

Some examples of corticosteroid asthma inhalants are as follows:

Beclomethasone Dipropionate [Beclovent (*Allen & Hanburys*) and Vanceril (*Schering*)]—Adults: 2 inhalations, 3 or 4 times daily; Children: 1 or 2 inhalations, 3 or 4 times daily. Each actuation delivers approximately 42 μg.

Dexamethasone Sodium Phosphate [Decadron Phosphate Resphihaler (*MSD*)]—Adults: 3 inhalations, 3 or 4 times daily; Children: 2 inhalations, 3 or 4 times daily. Each actuation delivers approximately 42 μg.

Flunisolide [AeroBid (*Forest*)]—Adults: 2 inhalations, 2 times daily; Children: 2 inhalations, 2 times daily. Each actuation delivers approximately 250 μg.

Triamcinolone Acetonide [Azmacort (*Rhone-Poulenc Rorer*)—Adults: 2 inhalations, 3 to 4 times daily; Children: 1 to 2 inhalations, 3 to 4 times daily. Each actuation delivers approximately 60 μg.

Antitussives

Antitussives are substances that specifically inhibit or suppress the act of coughing. Such inhibition may be due to: (1) depression of the medullary center or associated higher centers, (2) increased threshold of the peripheral reflexogenous zones, (3) interruption of tussal impulses in the afferent limb of the cough reflex, (4) inhibition of conduction along the motor pathways and (5) removal of irritants by facilitating bronchial drainage and mucociliary activity. The first four ways of inhibiting cough are believed to characterize the "antitussive" agents, whereas the latter one is theoretically associated with "expectorant" agents.

Antitussives may be classified in various ways. For example, *centrally acting antitussives* either depress the central nervous system and inhibit the "cough center" in the medulla or raise the threshold for central noxious stimuli and diminish the cough reflex, whereas *peripherally acting antitussives* act principally within the respiratory tract. Another possible classification is to consider these drugs as "narcotic antitussives" or "nonnarcotic antitussives." This classification will not be used in this section since most of the narcotic antitussives are discussed in Chapter 72, *Analgesics and Antipyretics.* Agents that have addiction potential will be identified, however, since the addiction liability of these substances is the same regardless of therapeutic use.

Apomorphine Hydrochloride—see RPS-18, page 790.

Benzonatate

Benzoic acid, 4-(butylamino)-, 2,5,8,11,14,17,20,23,26-nonaoxaoctacosan-28-yl ester; Tessalon (*Forest*)

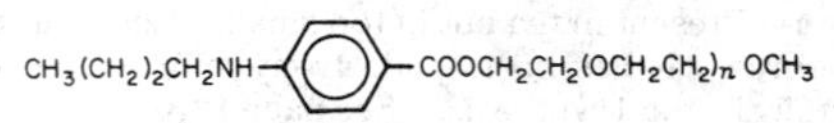

$$CH_3(CH_2)_2CH_2NH-C_6H_4-COOCH_2CH_2(OCH_2CH_2)_nOCH_3$$

Average: $n = 8$ [104-31-4] $C_{30}H_{43}NO_{11}$ (average: 603).

Benzonatate is a mixture of the *p*-butylaminobenzoate esters of the monomethyl ethers derived from a mixture of polyethylene glycols having the average composition of a nonaethylene glycol. The chemical name above is for the average compound.

Preparation—Ethyl *p*-(butylamino)benzoate is transesterified with a polyethylene glycol monomethyl ether fraction in a methanol solution of sodium methoxide. The crude ester is purified by extracting its benzene solution with sodium carbonate solution, the ester being retained in the benzene. US Pat 2,714,606.

Description—Pale yellow, clear, viscous liquid with a faint characteristic odor and a bitter taste followed by a sense of numbness.

Solubility—Freely soluble in chloroform, alcohol or benzene; miscible with water in all proportions.

Uses—An *antitussive.* It is related to tetracaine and reduces the cough reflex at its source by anesthetizing the stretch receptors in the respiratory passages, lungs and pleura. It begins to act within 15 to 20 min and its effect lasts for 3 to 8 hr. Although its antitussive potency essentially is the same as for codeine when evaluated against experimentally induced cough in animals and man, it is somewhat less effective than codeine against cough associated with clinical illness.

Benzonatate is tolerated well in therapeutic doses. Untoward effects reported to date include headache, mild dizziness, pruritus and skin eruptions, nasal congestion, constipation, nausea, gastrointestinal upset, a sensation of burning of the eyes and numbness or tightness in the chest. Hypersensitivity reactions have been reported. If the capsules are allowed to dissolve in the mouth, they exert a local anesthetic effect which is disagreeable to a few patients. Dependence, euphoria, respiratory depression or constipation have not been reported. Overdosage can lead to CNS stimulation, resulting in restlessness, tremors and, ultimately, seizures.

Dose—100 to **200 mg;** *usual,* **100 mg** 3 times a day. Capsules should not be chewed but swallowed whole.

Dosage Form—Capsules: 100 mg.

Caramiphen Edisylate—see RPS-18, page 864.
Chlophedianol—see RPS-18, page 865.
Codeine—page 1200.
Codeine Phosphate—page 1200.
Codeine Sulfate—page 1200.

Dextromethorphan Hydrobromide

(9α,13α,14α)-Morphinan, 3-methoxy-17-methyl-, hydrobromide, monohydrate (*Various Mfrs*)

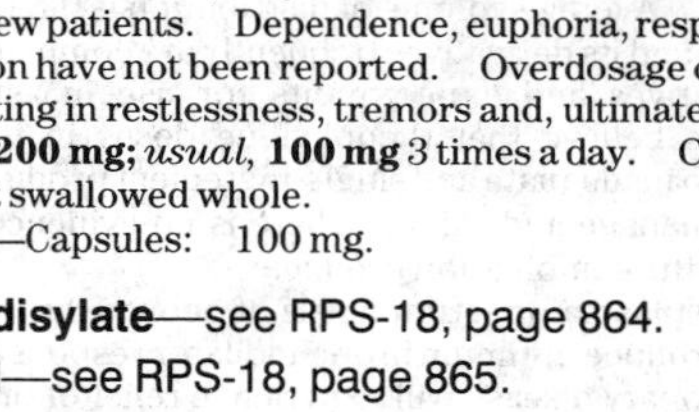

[6700-34-1] $C_{18}H_{25}NO.HBr.H_2O$ (370.33); *anhydrous* [125-69-9] (352.32).

Preparation—Dextromethorphan base (*d*-3-methoxy-*N*-methylmorphinan) is prepared from the corresponding *d*-3-hydroxy compound by methylation with phenyltrimethylammonium hydroxide. The procedure is analogous to that employed for the methylation of morphine to produce codeine. Treatment of the base with HBr yields the hydrobromide.

Description—Practically white crystals, or crystalline powder, having a faint odor; melts at about 126°, with decomposition, pH (1 in 100 solution) 5.2 to 6.5.

Solubility—1 g in about 65 mL water; freely soluble in alcohol or chloroform; insoluble in ether.

Uses—Dextromethorphan, the *d*-isomer of the codeine analog of levorphanol, is employed as an *antitussive* agent. It controls cough spasms by depressing the cough center in the medulla. Controlled studies in man indicate it has a cough suppression potency approximately one-half that of codeine. The oral administration of 30 mg to an adult provides effective antitussive activity over an 8- to 12-hr period. Unlike codeine, it is devoid of analgesic properties and produces little or no depression of the central nervous system. Addiction does not usually occur even after the administration of rather large doses for prolonged periods. However, there have been reports of abuse of OTC dextromethorphan-containing cold and cough medicines, especially by teenagers. Animal studies suggest that this drug has some effects similar to phencyclidine (PCP) which may account for its abuse. Additional data are needed to assess better the potential for dextromethorphan dependence. High doses of this drug can cause ataxia, respiratory depression and convulsions in children, while in adults high doses can alter sensory perception, and cause ataxia, slurred speech and dysphoria. The side effects include slight drowsiness and gastrointestinal upset; these are less severe and less frequent than with codeine. Accidental poisoning in children is characterized by stupor and ataxia with rapid recovery after emesis. Dextromethorphan hydrobromide should not be given to patients on monoamine oxidase inhibitors.

Dose—*Usual, Adult, oral,* **10** to **30 mg** every 4 to 8 hr; do not exceed **120 mg** in 24 hr. *Children 6 to 12,* **5** to **10 mg** every 4 hr or **15 mg** every 6 to 8 hr; do not exceed **60 mg** in 24 hr. *Children 2 to 6 yr,* Syrup and Chewy Squares: **2.5** to **7.5** mg every 4 to 8 hr; do not exceed **30 mg** in 24 hr. *Adult, controlled-release liquid,* **60 mg** twice daily; *children 6 to 12 yr,* **30 mg** 2 times a day; *children 2 to 6 yr,* **15 mg** 2 times a day.

Dosage Forms—Controlled-Release Liquid: 30 mg/5 mL; Lozenges: 5 mg; Syrup: 5, 7.5, 10 and 15 mg/5 mL. Dextromethorphan often is combined with expectorants, or other drugs in OTC cough and cold medications. The therapeutic value of these combinations is unproven.

Diphenhydramine Hydrochloride—page 1225.

Ethylmorphine Hydrochloride—see RPS-15, page 1040.

Hydrocodone Bitartrate—page 1200.

Methadone Hydrochloride—page 1205.

Morphine Sulfate—page 1199.

Antitussive Combinations

A wide array of antitussive combinations are commercially available. The combinations can consist of from two to four active ingredients and include any combination of an antitussive plus sympathomimetics, antihistamines, expectorants and/or analgesics. These cough products are very controversial and rarely offer an advantage over single ingredient cough medicines.

Some examples of antitussive combinations (with content per capsule, tablet or 5 mL provided) are as follows:

Caramiphen Edisylate and Phenylpropanolamine Hydrochloride [Tuss-Ornade (*SmithKline Beecham*)]—40 and 75 mg, respectively.

Codeine Phosphate and Pseudoephedrine Hydrochloride [Nucofed (*SmithKline Beecham*)]—20 and 60 mg, respectively.

Codeine Phosphate, Phenylpropanolamine and Brompheniramine [Dimetane-DC (*Robins*)]—10, 12.5 and 2.0 mg, respectively.

Dextromethorphan Hydrobromide and Phenylephrine Hydrochloride [Bayer Cough Syrup for Children (*Glenbrook*)]—7.5 and 9 mg/5 mL, respectively.

Dextromethorphan Hydrobromide and Doxylamine Succinate [Cough Formula (*Various Mfrs*)]—15 and 3.75/5 mL, respectively.

Dextromethorphan Hydrobromide and Chlorpheniramine Maleate [Formula 44 Cough Mixture (*Richardson-Vicks*)]—15 and 2 mg/5 mL, respectively.

Dextromethorphan, Guaifenesin and Pseudoephedrine Hydrochloride [Noratuss II Expectorant (*Vortech*)]—3.75, 50 and 15 mg/5 mL respectively.

Dextromethorphan, Acetaminophen, Doxylamine and Pseudoephedrine Hydrochloride [NyQuil Nighttime Cold Medicine (*Richardson-Vicks*)]—5, 167, 1.25, and 10 mg/5 mL, respectively.

Hydrocodone Bitartrate and Guaifenesin [Hycotuss (*Du Pont*)]—5 and 100 mg, respectively.

Hydrocodone Bitartrate and Homatropine Methylbromide [Hycodan (*Du Pont*)]—5 and 1.5 mg, respectively.

Hydrocodone Bitartrate and Chlorpheniramine [Tussionex (*Fisons*)]—10 and 8 mg, respectively.

Expectorants

Expectorants are drugs which have been proposed to be useful in loosening and liquefying mucous, in soothing irritated bronchial mucosa and in making coughs more productive. Such agents are thought to affect the respiratory tract in two ways: (1) by decreasing the viscosity of the bronchial secretions and facilitating their elimination so that local irritants are removed and ineffectual coughing is alleviated or made more productive and (2) by increasing the amounts of respiratory tract fluid a demulcent action is exerted on the dry mucosal lining, thus relieving the unproductive cough.

The FDA has proposed that orally administered expectorants available OTC be divided into three categories: (I) those generally recognized as safe and effective, (II) those not generally recognized as safe and effective and (III) those with insufficient data to classify as safe and effective. The FDA has approved only guaifenesin for classification as a Category I expectorant. Thus, it is not surprising that many of the orally administered cough and cold combinations include guaifenesin as the expectorant. Even so, there is a lack of scientific evidence to demonstrate that guaifenesin is of value in the treatment of coughing. It should be remembered, however, that humidification of room air and adequate fluid intake (six to eight glasses of water/day) can effectively liquefy respiratory mucus and are useful therapeutic procedures.

Acetylcysteine

L-Cysteine, *N*-acetyl-, Mucomyst (*Apothecon*)

$$HSCH_2-\underset{H}{\overset{NHCOCH_3}{C}}-COOH$$

N-Acetyl-L-cysteine [616-91-1] $C_5H_9NO_3S$ (163.19).

Preparation—By direct acetylation of L-cysteine.

Description—White, crystalline powder which has a very slight acetic odor and a characteristic sour taste; stable in ordinary light; nonhygroscopic (oxidizes in moist air); stable at temperatures up to 120°; melts between 104° and 110°; pK_a 3.24; pH (1 in 100) 2 to 2.75.

Solubility—1 g in 5 mL water or 4 mL alcohol; practically insoluble in chloroform or ether.

Uses—To reduce the viscosity of pulmonary secretions and facilitate their removal. Hence, it is used as adjuvant therapy in bronchopulmonary disorders when mucolysis is desirable. It is thought the sulfhydryl group in the molecule "opens" the disulfide bonds in mucus and lowers the viscosity. The mucolytic activity of acetylcysteine is related to pH; significant mucolysis occurs between pH 6 and 9. Clinical studies indicate that, after inhalation, onset of action is within 1 min and time to peak effect is 5 to 10 min. Side effects are rare. However, bronchospasm, hemoptysis and nausea and vomiting have been observed. Antimicrobial drugs, including ampicillin, tetracyclines, amphotericin B and erythromycin lactobionate, should not be administered in acetylcysteine solution since it inactivates antibiotics. Effectiveness of acetylcysteine as a mucolytic is difficult to assess and has been based on subjective observations and may not be any greater than adequate humidification.

Acetylcysteine is used orally and parenterally as an antidote to prevent or minimize hepatotoxicity in acute acetaminophen overdosage. It also has been used with some success as an ophthalmic solution for the treatment of keratoconjunctivitis sicca (dry eye) and as an enema for the management of bowel obstruction due to meconium ileus.

Dose—By *inhalation of nebulized solution,* **2** to **20 mL** of a **10%** or **1** to **10 mL** of a **20%** solution every 2 to 6 hr; by *direct instillation,* **1** to **2 mL** of a **10** or **20%** solution every 1 to 4 hr.

Dosage Form—Solution: 10 and 20% in 4-, 10- and 30-mL vials.

Ammonium Carbonate—page 978.

Ammonium Chloride—page 1040.

Antimony Potassium Tartrate—page 1338.

Calcium Iodide—see RPS-18, page 864.

Creosote—see RPS-15, page 1102.

Creosote Carbonate—see RPS-18, page 864.

Glycerin—page 1405.

Guaiacol—see RPS-18, page 864.

Guaifenesin

1,2-Propanediol, 3-(2-methoxyphenoxy)-, Glyceryl Guaiacolate
(Various Mfrs)

3-(*o*-Methoxyphenoxy)-1,2-propanediol [93-14-1] $C_{10}H_{14}O_4$ (198.22).

Preparation—Guaiacol and 3-chloro-1,2-propanediol are condensed via dehydrochlorination by warming a mixture of the reactants with a base.

Description—White to slightly gray, crystalline powder having a bitter taste; may have a slight characteristic odor; stable in light and heat and is nonhygroscopic; melts within a range of 3° between 78° and 82°; pH (1 in 100 solution) between 5.0 and 7.0.

Solubility—1 g in 60 to 70 mL water; soluble in alcohol, chloroform, glycerin or propylene glycol; insoluble in petroleum ether.

Uses—Used for the symptomatic relief of respiratory conditions characterized by a dry, nonproductive cough and in the presence of mucus in the respiratory tract. Subjective clinical studies suggest that the action of guaifenesin ameliorates dry unproductive cough by decreasing sputum viscosity and difficulty in expectoration and increasing sputum volume. However, experimentally, it only increases respiratory tract secretions, but only when given in doses larger than those used clinically. Adverse effects are infrequent and usually consist of nausea, gastric disturbance and drowsiness. Guaifenesin may produce a false positive test for 5-hydroxyindoleacetic acid. It is an ingredient in many OTC proprietary expectorant formulations.

Dose—*Usual, adult, oral,* **100** to **400 mg** every 3 to 6 hr. Maximum, **2.4 g/day.** *Usual, pediatric: children 6 to 12 yr,* **100** to **200 mg** orally every 4 to 6 hr; do not exceed **1.2 g/day;** *children 2 to 6 yr,* **50** to **100 mg** every 4 hr; do not exceed **600 mg/day.**

Dosage Forms—Capsules: 200 mg; Syrup: 67 and 100 mg/5 mL; Tablets: 100 and 200 mg; Sustained-Release Tablets: 600 mg.

Hydriodic Acid Syrup—page 1393.

Ipecac

Ipecacuanha

The dried rhizome and roots of *Cephaëlis acuminata* Karsten, known in commerce as Cartagena, Nicaragua or Panama Ipecac (Fam *Rubiaceae*). Ipecac yields not less than 2% of the total ether-soluble alkaloids of ipecac, of which not less than 90% consists of emetine ($C_{29}H_{40}N_2O_4$) and cephaeline ($C_{28}H_{38}N_2O_4$), the content of the latter varying from an amount equal to, to not more than twice, the content of emetine.

Constituents—Ipecac contains *emetine (methylcephaëline)* [$C_{29}H_{40}N_2O_4$], *cephaëline,* [$C_{28}H_{38}N_2O_4$], *psychotrine* [$C_{28}H_{36}N_2O_4$], *O-methylpsychotrine* [$C_{29}H_{38}N_2O_4$], *emetamine* [$C_{29}H_{36}N_2O_4$], *ipecamine,* also *ipecacuanhic acid,* pectin, starch, resin, sugar, etc. All of the alkaloids are interrelated and may be synthesized from each other. Brazilian roots yield as much as 2.5% of total alkaloids and Cartagena root, 2%.

Uses—Has *expectorant, emetic* and *amebicidal properties.* The syrup is preferred for use as an expectorant and emetic; it is used widely as an emetic in accidental poisoning. Emetic doses of ipecac may be used in patients with *paroxysmal atrial tachycardia,* the vagal impulses arising from the excitation of the medullary vagal vomiting mechanism acting to bring about the cessation of the arrhythmia. Ipecac has amebicidal potency by virtue of its content of emetine but is almost never used in the therapy of amebiasis.

Powdered Ipecac is ipecac reduced to a fine or a very fine powder and adjusted to a potency of 1.9–2.1% of the ether-soluble alkaloids of ipecac, by addition of exhausted marc of ipecac or of other suitable inert diluent or by addition of powdered ipecac of either a lower or a higher potency. *Description:* Pale brown, weak yellow or light olive-gray powder.

Ipecac Syrup—yields, from each 100 mL, 123–157 mg of ether-soluble alkaloids of ipecac. *Preparation:* Exhaust powdered ipecac (70 g) by percolation, using a mixture of 3 volumes of alcohol and 1 volume of water as the menstruum, macerating for 72 hr, and percolating slowly. Reduce the entire percolate to a volume of 70 mL by evaporation at a temperature not exceeding 60° and preferably in vacuum, and add water (140 mL). Allow the mixture to stand overnight, filter and wash the residue on the filter with water. Evaporate the filtrate and washings to 40 mL, and to this add hydrochloric acid (2.5 mL) and alcohol (20 mL), mix and filter. Wash the filter with a mixture of 30 volumes of alcohol, 3.5 volumes of HCl and 66.5 volumes of water, using a volume sufficient to produce 70 mL of filtrate. Add glycerin (100 mL) and syrup (qs) to make the product measure 1000 mL, and mix. *Alcohol Content:* 1 to 2.5%. *Uses:* Emetic and *nauseant expectorant.* Ipecac syrup is probably the single most important item to have in the home for the treatment of poison ingestions. It is given orally to adults and children over 1 yr in a dose of 1 tablespoonful (15 mL) followed by at least 1 glassful (250 mL) of liquid (water, juices, etc); if the victim does not vomit within 15 to 20 min, the treatment should be repeated. The dosage should be recovered by gastric lavage if emesis does not occur after the second dose. The dose in children up to 1 yr is 5 or 10 mL followed by the procedure described above. If activated charcoal is to be used, give the activated charcoal only after vomiting has been induced with ipecac syrup. Small doses of ipecac syrup (0.3 to 1 mL) also are used as an expectorant in cough preparations, but its therapeutic value has not been demonstrated. *Dose: Emetic:* 10 to 30 mL; *usual,* 15 mL. Do not use in semiconscious, unconscious or convulsing persons. Do not administer milk or carbonated beverages with this product. *Other Dose Information:* Expectorant, *oral, adults,* 0.5 to 2 mL every 6 hr.

Ipecac and Opium Powder—see RPS 13, page 561.

Potassium Iodide

Potassium iodide [7681-11-0] KI (166.00).

Preparation—Potassium iodide may be prepared by reacting iodine with a hot solution of potassium hydroxide, the iodate simultaneously formed being subsequently reduced to iodide by heating the dry reaction mixture with carbon.

Description—Hexahedral crystals, either transparent and colorless or somewhat opaque and white, or a white, granular powder; slightly hygroscopic in moist air; aqueous solution is neutral or slightly alkaline to litmus.

Solubility—1 g in 0.7 mL water, 22 mL alcohol, 2 mL glycerin, 75 mL acetone at 25° or 0.5 mL boiling water; when dissolved in water heat is absorbed; 100 mL of a saturated aqueous solution at 25° contains 100 g of KI.

Uses—An *expectorant* and when the action of iodide is desired. It is used as an expectorant to liquefy thick and tenacious sputum in chronic bronchitis, bronchiectasis, bronchial asthma and pulmonary emphysema. It also is used as adjunctive treatment in cystic fibrosis, chronic sinusitis and after surgery to prevent atelectasis. However, the therapeutic value of potassium iodide as an expectorant has not been demonstrated convincingly. Although a substantial number of patients tolerate potassium iodide well, iodide-induced goiter and hypothyroidism have been observed. Consequently, alternative drugs which are safer and more effective should be considered when an expectorant action is desired.

In regions where little iodine is obtained in the diet, iodides are completely effective in the *prevention of goiter.* Only minute doses are required and these small amounts can be administered best in the form of iodized salt (1 part of potassium iodide to 100,000 parts of salt). A saturated solution of potassium iodide also may be used with an antithyroid drug to prepare hyperthyroid patients for thyroidectomy and to treat thyrotoxic crisis or neonatal thyrotoxicosis. It also is used in place of Lugol's Solution for the treatment of *toxic goiter,* in the dose of 0.3 mL, 3 times a day. Potassium iodide also is used to treat victims of a radiation emergency in order to prevent the uptake of radioactive iodine by the thyroid gland. Administration prior to, or within 3 to 4 hr after exposure is essential. See *Strong Iodine Solution* (page 1134).

Potassium iodide solution (1 g/mL) is the drug of choice for cutaneous lymphatic sporotrichosis in patients who can tolerate the drug and do not have a history of iodism.

Mild untoward reactions occur frequently with iodide medication. The syndrome is known as iodism. The symptoms include salivation, lacrimation, coryza, soreness of the teeth and gums, eruption of the skin, headaches, swollen salivary glands and gastric irritation. The symptoms disappear when the drug is discontinued. Serious reactions occur only very rarely. Concurrent use of potassium iodide with lithium and other antithyroid drugs may potentiate the hypothyroid and goitrogenic effects of these medications. Likewise, use with other potassium-containing medications and potassium-sparing diuretics may induce hyperkalemia and cardiac arrhythmias or cardiac arrest.

Dose—*Expectorant,* **300 mg** with a glassful of water every 4 to 6 hr; *antifungal,* **600 mg** 3 times a day, gradually increased to 12 g daily if tolerated. *Preoperative preparation for thyroidectomy,* 5 drops of a saturated solution 3 times a day for 10 days.

Potassium Iodide Solution [Saturated Potassium Iodide Solution] contains, in each 100 mL, 97–103 g of KI. *Preparation:* Dissolve potassium iodide (1000 g) in hot purified water (680 mL), cool to about 25° and add sufficient purified water to make 1000 mL; filter, if necessary. *Note:* If the solution is not to be used within a short time, 500 mg of sodium thiosulfate should be added to each 1 L. *Description:* Clear, colorless and odorless solution having a characteristic, strongly salty taste; neutral or slightly alkaline to litmus paper; specific gravity about 1.700. *Uses:* Iodide supplement and expectorant; see *Potassium Iodide*. *Dose:* *Usual,* 0.3 mL, equivalent to 300 mg of potassium iodide.

Sodium Citrate—page 923.

Sodium Iodide

Sodium iodide [7681-82-5] NaI (149.89).

Preparation—From iodine and sodium hydroxide, or by metathesis between ferrosoferric iodide and sodium carbonate. See *Potassium Iodide*.

Description—Colorless, odorless crystals, or a white, crystalline powder; in moist air it cakes and then deliquesces, and frequently undergoes decomposition, developing a brown tint; its solution in water is neutral or slightly alkaline to litmus and gradually becomes yellow because of the formation of free iodine; in contrast to potassium iodide, when sodium iodide is dissolved in water heat is liberated due to the formation of the dihydrate [$NaI.2H_2O$].

Solubility—1 g in 0.6 mL water, about 2 mL alcohol or about 1 mL glycerin.

Uses—Can be used interchangeably with potassium iodide, as a therapeutic agent, except where sodium ion is contraindicated. See *Potassium Iodide*.

Dose—*Oral,* **300 mg** to **2 g** daily; *usual,* **300 mg** 2 to 4 times a day; *intravenous infusion,* **1** to **3 g** daily; *usual,* **1 g**.

Terpin Hydrate

Cyclohexanemethanol, 4-hydroxy-α,α-4-trimethyl-, monohydrate; Terpinum; Terpinol

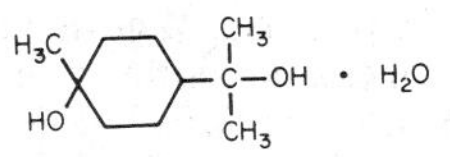

H_3C / HO — cyclohexane — $C(CH_3)_2$—OH · H_2O

p-Menthane-1,8-diol monohydrate [2451-01-6] $C_{10}H_{20}O_2.H_2O$ (190.28); *anhydrous* [80-53-5] (172.27).

Preparation—By hydration of the pinenes in turpentine oil (or pine oil) in the presence of a strong acid.

Description—Colorless, lustrous crystals, or as a white powder; slight odor, and efflorescent in dry air; a hot 1:100 aqueous solution is neutral to litmus; when dried over H_2SO_4 in a vacuum, it melts at about 103°.

Solubility—1 g in about 200 mL water, 13 mL alcohol, 140 mL chloroform or about 140 mL ether, at 25°; 1 g in about 35 mL boiling water or about 3 mL boiling alcohol.

Uses—In *bronchitis* as an *expectorant*. Terpin hydrate elixir contains too little of the compound to be effective alone and is employed mainly as a vehicle for cough mixtures such as *Terpin Hydrate and Codeine Elixir* and *Terpin Hydrate and Dextromethorphan Elixir*.

Dose—*Usual,* **125** to **300 mg** every 6 hr.

Terpin Hydrate Elixir contains, in each 100 mL, 1.53–1.87 g of $C_{10}H_{20}O_2.H_2O$. *Preparation:* Dissolve terpin hydrate (17 g) in the alcohol (430 mL); add successively sweet orange peel tincture (20 mL), benzaldehyde (0.05 mL), glycerin (400 mL), syrup (100 mL) and purified water (qs) to make the product measure 1000 mL; mix well and filter, if necessary, until the product is clear. *Note*—The sweet orange peel tincture may be replaced by 1 mL orange oil dissolved in 15 mL alcohol. *Alcohol Content:* 39 to 44%. The high alcoholic content in this elixir is required for the solution of the terpin hydrate. *Incompatibilities:* Dilution of this elixir with water or liquids of low alcohol content causes precipitation of the terpin hydrate. *Dose:* *Usual, adult, oral,* the equivalent of 85 to 170 mg 3 or 4 times a day. *Usual, pediatric, oral,* children 1 to 4 yr, 20 mg; children 5 to 9, 40 mg and children 10 to 12, 85 mg. All children's doses may be repeated 3 or 4 times a day.

Terpin Hydrate and Codeine Elixir contains, in each 100 mL, 1.53 to 1.87 g of $C_{10}H_{20}O_2.H_2O$ (terpin hydrate), and 180–220 mg of $C_{18}H_{21}NO_3.H_2O$ (codeine). *Preparation:* Dissolve codeine (2 g) in terpin hydrate elixir (qs) to make the product measure 1000 mL. *Alcohol Content:* 39 to 44%. *Uses:* This elixir is an *expectorant* and *sedative* used to allay excessive coughing. Its value resides primarily in its content of codeine. *Caution*—This elixir is sometimes used by addicts, by whom it is known as *GI Gin*, for its alcohol and codeine content. In some states pharmacists are required to register and limit its sale. Its repeated sale to an individual should be noted and stopped. *Dose:* *Usual,* 5 mL, equivalent to 10 mg of codeine and 85 mg of terpin hydrate.

Terpin Hydrate and Dextromethorphan Hydrobromide Elixir contains, in each 100 mL, 1.53–1.87 g of $C_{10}H_{20}O_2.H_2O$ (terpin hydrate), and 180–220 mg of $C_{18}H_{25}NO.HBr.H_2O$ (dextromethorphan hydrobromide). *Preparation:* Dissolve dextromethorphan hydrobromide (2 g) in terpin hydrate elixir (qs) to make the product measure 1000 mL. *Uses:* The same indications as *Terpin Hydrate and Codeine Elixir*. It is used in the control of coughs associated with the common cold, laryngitis, tracheitis and bronchitis. Dextromethorphan acts to elevate the threshold for coughing. Unlike codeine, it rarely produces drowsiness or gastrointestinal disturbances. *Dose:* *Usual,* 5 mL, equivalent to 10 mg dextromethorphan hydrobromide and 85 mg of terpin hydrate. *Other Dose Information:* The usual adult dose should not exceed 40 mL. Children, 4 to 12 yr, 2.5 to 5 mL 4 times a day; total dose should not exceed 20 mL. Children, 2 to 4 yr, 1 to 2.5 mL 1 to 4 times daily; total daily dose should not exceed 10 mL.

Tolu Balsam—page 1390.

Tolu Balsam Syrup—page 1390.

Tolu Balsam Tincture—page 1390.

Tyloxapol

Phenol, 4-(1,1,3,3-tetramethylbutyl)-, polymer with formaldehyde and oxirane (*Various Mfrs*)

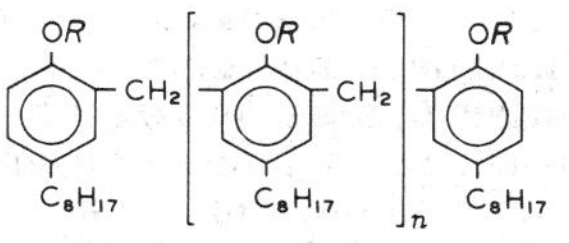

[*R* is $CH_2CH_2O(CH_2CH_2O)_mCH_2CH_2OH$; *m* is 6 to 8; *n* is not more than 5]

p-(1,1,3,3-Tetramethylbutyl)phenol polymer with ethylene oxide and formaldehyde [25301-02-4].

Preparation—*p*-(1,1,3,3-Tetramethylbutyl)phenol and formaldehyde are condensed by heating in the presence of an acidic catalyst and the polymeric phenol thus obtained is reacted with ethylene oxide at elevated temperature under pressure in the presence of NaOH. US Pat 2,454,541.

Description—Amber, viscous liquid; may show a slight turbidity; slight aromatic odor; specific gravity about 1.072; stable at sterilization temperature; stable in the presence of acids, bases or salts; oxidized by metals; pH (5% aqueous solution) between 4 and 7.

Solubility—Slowly but freely soluble in water; soluble in many organic solvents, including acetic acid, benzene, carbon tetrachloride, carbon disulfide, chloroform or toluene.

Uses—A nonionic detergent that depresses both surface tension and interfacial tension. The hydrophobic alkyl groups impart oil solubility to the molecule and the large number of hydrophilic groups impart water solubility. Hence, it may be used as an emulsifying agent for both water-in-oil and oil-in-water systems. *Note—Precaution should be exercised to prevent contact of tyloxapol with metals as this catalyzes air-oxidation and rapid discoloration.*

Tyloxapol has been used to lower surface tension and help liquefy mucus and is reported to be useful for short-term management of many inflammatory and postoperative pulmonary conditions. Some reports indicate it has value when administered intermittently in long-term management of cystic fibrosis and other chronic pulmonary diseases. Some double-blind studies, however, indicate that agents of this type are no more effective than saline aerosols. Tyloxapol also is used in contact lens cleaner formulations.

Dose—*Mucolytic, usual, adult,* **0.125%** solution administered via aerosol nebulizer with pressurized oxygen or air into a tent, face mask or by direct inhalation, as directed in package insert.

Expectorant Combinations

The most frequent expectorant combinations include an antitussive with guaifenesin. However, expectorants also are found in combination with sympathomimetics, antihistamines and analgesics in OTC cold and cough medicines. The benefit of such combinations in the treatment of coughing or other respiratory ailments is controversial.

Some examples of expectorant combinations (with content per capsule, tablet or 5 mL provided) are as follows:

Calcium Iodide and Codeine [Calcidrine Syrup (*Abbott*)]—152 and 8.4 mg, respectively.

Guaifenesin and Codeine Phosphate [Cheracol Syrup (*Upjohn*); Robitussin A-C (*Robins*)—100 and 10 mg, respectively.

Guaifenesin and Dextromethorphan Hydrobromide [Cheracol D (*Upjohn*); Naldecon Senior DX (*Apothecon*); Pertussin (*Pertussin*)]—25–200 and 3.5–15 mg. respectively.

Guaifenesin and Phenylpropanolamine Hydrochloride [Triaminic Expectorant (*Dorsey*); Triphenyl Expectorant (*Rugby*)]—100 and 12.5 mg, respectively.

Guaifenesin and Pseudoephedrine Hydrochloride [Congestac (*SmithKline Beecham*); Robitussin-PE (*Robins*)]—100–400 and 30–60 mg, respectively.

Surfactant Preparations

Surfactant preparations are used as replacement therapy for the treatment of premature infants suffering from neonatal respiratory distress syndrome (also known as hyaline membrane disease). This pulmonary condition occurs in approximately 20% of the 250,000 premature babies born in the US each year and accounts for 5000 deaths annually. A substantial deficiency in the endogenous lung surfactant (of which colfosceril palmitate is the primary phospholipid) is the principal factor contributing to the pathology of respiratory distress syndrome. The lung surfactant preparations are used in combination with supplemental oxygen and mechanical ventilation to facilitate gas exchange for either prophylactic or rescue treatment of neonatal respiratory distress syndrome. The exogenous surfactants are derived either from animals or synthesized. The efficacy of lung surfactants has been demonstrated in double-blind randomized studies in comparison to air placebo in premature infants with respiratory distress syndrome, particularly in infants with a birth weight exceeding 700 g. Studies suggest the exogenous lung surfactants are tolerated well with few direct adverse effects.

Colfosceril Palmitate

3,5,9-Trioxa-4-phosphapentacosan-1-aminium, (*R*)-4-hydroxy-*N,N,N*-trimethyl-10-oxo-7-[(1-oxohexadecyl)oxy]-, hydroxide, inner salt, 4-oxide; component of Exosurf (*Burroughs-Wellcome*)

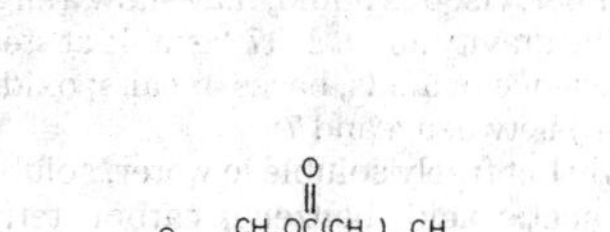

1,2-Dipalmitoyl-*sn*-glycero-3-phosphocholine [63-89-8] $C_{40}H_{80}NO_8P$ (734.05).

Beractant (*Survanta; Ross*) is a modified bovine extract consisting of phospholipids, neutral lipids, fatty acids and surfactant-associated proteins. Colfosceril palmitate, palmitic acid and tipalmitin are added to improve the surface-active properties. Mechanical ventilation must be interrupted prior to administration and such interruptions increase the risk of oxygen denaturation. It has been shown to improve the clinical outcome from respiratory distress syndrome in infants weighing between 600 and 1250 g (prophylactic therapy) and 600 and 1750 g (rescue therapy). While it appears to produce a more rapid increase in lung compliance than *Exosurf Neonatal*, it is not clear if this is a therapeutic advantage. Its use causes a significant increase in sepsis, although the increase does not appear to affect mortality. The dose is divided into four aliquots with each dose administered after a change in the infant's position. It is available as a ready-to-use suspension that requires refrigeration and protection from light. It is off-white to light brown and it should not be used if discoloration has occurred. In case of settling, gentle swirling (not shaking) should be used to resuspend the contents and it should be warmed gently before administration.

Exosurf (*Burroughs-Welcome*) is a synthetic lung surfactant composed of colfosceril palmitate, cetyl alcohol and tyloxapol. The cetyl alcohol facilitates spreading and adsorption of colfosceril palmitate at the air-alveolar interface. It is administered to premature infants suffering respiratory distress syndrome through an endotracheal tube adaptor without interfering with mechanical ventilation. The low viscosity of this product facilitates administration. It has been shown to reduce mortality in infants weighing 500 g or more at birth. For prophylactic therapy, a single 5-mL/kg dose is given immediately after birth with second and third doses administered approximately 12 and 24 hr later if the infant continues to be ventilated mechanically. Recommended treatment for rescue therapy consists of a 5-mL/kg dose given as soon as possible after diagnosis of respiratory distress syndrome and a second dose 12 hr later. It is available as a lyophilized powder to be reconstituted immediately prior to use with the accompanying preservative-free sterile water. Solutions with buffers or preservatives should not be used. The reconstituted product suspension has a milky white appearance and can be refrigerated or maintained at room temperature up to 12 hr. For administration, special endotracheal tube adaptors are included with each vital.

Respiratory Stimulants

Respiration is controlled by a respiratory center in the medulla oblongata. Drugs which act directly on the center to increase respiratory rate include atropine, caffeine, pentylenetetrazol and picrotoxin. Respiration is controlled partially by both chemical and sensory stimuli from the carotid body and carotid sinus, and drugs such as nikethamide exert at least part of their respiratory effect through this mechanism. The rate of respiration also is modified by numerous forms of sensory stimuli reaching the brain from the skin, nose, mouth, throat, etc, and drugs such as ammonia act through this mechanism. Respiration also may be modified voluntarily through the higher brain centers, and drugs which stimulate these higher centers, such as pentylenetetrazol and picrotoxin, act to increase respiration.

Drugs rarely are used to therapeutically stimulate respiration. The effectiveness of nonspecific analeptic drugs for the management of postanesthetic respiratory depression is controversial. Some clinicians believe that postanesthetic respiratory depression, irrespective of its cause, is treated most effectively with manual or mechanical methods of respiratory assistance. Others believe respiration should be stimulated pharmacologically only if a specific antidote is available; for example, narcotic antagonists for respiratory depression induced by narcotics or anticholinesterases if due to a curariform muscle relaxant. It generally is agreed that prolonged respiratory depression, such as that due to barbiturate poisoning, is treated best by methods which assure adequate ventilation and circulation and, when necessary, hemodialysis to accelerate removal of the drug. Few clinicians find nonspecific analeptics useful in the above conditions.

Aromatic Ammonia Spirit—page 873.

Ammonium Carbonate

Carbonic acid, monoammonium salt, mixt with ammonium carbamate; Ammonia Crystal; Sal Volatile; Ammonium Sesquicarbonate

Monoammonium carbonate mixture with ammonium carbamate [8000-73-5]; consists of ammonium bicarbonate [NH_4HCO_3 = 79.06] and ammonium carbamate [NH_2COONH_4 = 78.07] in varying proportions. It yields 30–34% of NH_3.

Preparation—By subliming a mixture of ammonium sulfate and calcium carbonate.

Description—White powder or hard, white or translucent masses, having a strong odor of ammonia, without empyreuma and with a sharp, ammoniacal taste; affected by light; on exposure to air, it loses ammonia and CO_2, becoming opaque, and is finally converted into friable, porous lumps or a white powder of ammonium bicarbonate; decomposed by hot water and by weak acids.

Solubility—1 g very slowly soluble in about 4 mL water; partly soluble (the carbamate portion) in alcohol; decomposed by hot water; its solution has the odor of ammonia and is alkaline to litmus. For reactions occurring in water, see *Aromatic Ammonia Spirit* (page 873).

Uses—A *pharmaceutical necessity* in the preparation of *Aromatic Ammonia Spirit* and as a source of ammonia in *smelling salts*. For the latter purpose, ¼- to 1-in. cubes generally are used. Both of these preparations are employed as *reflex respiratory stimulants* in hysterical syncope.

Dose—Up to **300 mg** in dilute solutions.

Atropine Sulfate—page 1022.

Caffeine—page 1231.

Caffeine and Sodium Benzoate—page 1233.

Camphor—page 874.

Carbon Dioxide

After-damp; Aer Fixus; Carbonic Acid Gas

Carbon dioxide [124-38-9] CO_2 (44.01).

Preparation—Various methods, eg, heating limestone, burning coke and fermentation processes.

Description—Odorless, colorless gas; 1 L at 760 mm and 0° weighs 1.977 g. Its solutions are slightly acid to litmus and have a slightly acid taste.

Solubility—1 volume in about 1 volume water at 25°; it is more soluble at lower than at higher temperatures; less soluble in alcohol or other solvents.

Uses—Has few valid therapeutic uses. Its most valuable use is with oxygen in certain types of pump oxygenators to *avoid a reduction of carbon dioxide* tension of the blood. It sometimes is used when it is of little value and possibly even harmful. Carbon dioxide is used to relieve persistent hiccups; it only occasionally produces transient relief. Its use has been suggested to *improve cerebral vascular disorders* (cerebral thrombosis), but it is of doubtful value and may be harmful because it increases intracranial pressure. Similarly, it has been used to induce deep breathing and coughing to avoid *postoperative* atelectasis, but is generally of little benefit. Carbon dioxide should not be used to resuscitate victims of carbon monoxide poisoning, drowning, electric shock or asphyxiation; the carbon dioxide content of the blood is already high and further increases may only exacerbate the respiratory depression. It should not be used to treat overdosage with central nervous system depressants; the medullary chemoreceptors are depressed and will not respond.

Carbon dioxide is administered by inhalation, most conveniently through a tight-fitting mask. The gas is administered in conjunction with oxygen. Concentrations of 5 to 7.5% are employed; 5% is the usual concentration.

Dose—By *inhalation*, up to 7% in oxygen.

Doxapram Hydrochloride

2-Pyrrolidinone, 1-ethyl-4-[2-(4-morpholinyl)ethyl]-3,3-diphenyl-, monohydrochloride, monohydrate; Dopram (*Robins*)

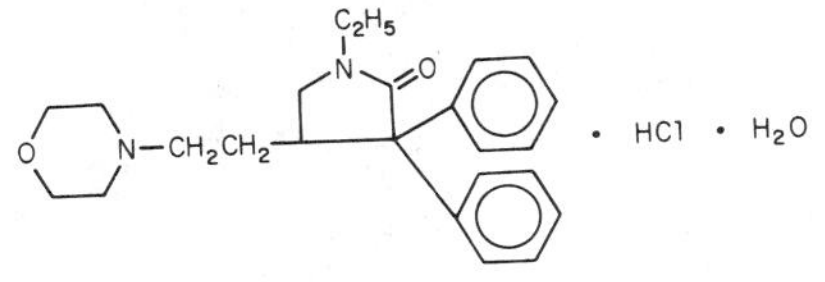

C_2H_5 N O N—CH_2CH_2 · HCl · H_2O

[7081-53-0] $C_{24}H_{30}N_2O_2.HCl.H_2O$(432.99); *anhydrous* [113-07-5] (414.97).

Preparation—1-Ethyl-3-pyrrolidinol is reacted with thionyl chloride to form the 3-chloro compound which is condensed with diphenylacetonitrile in toluene solution with the aid of sodamide. The resulting α-(1-ethyl-3-pyrrolidinyl)diphenylacetonitrile is hydrolyzed with 70% H_2SO_4 to the corresponding acid. On treatment with thionyl chloride, the acid is converted into the acid chloride which immediately isomerizes to 4-(2-chloroethyl)-3,3-diphenyl-1-ethyl-2-pyrrolidinone. Condensation of this with morpholine in a dehydrohalogenating environment yields doxapram (base) which, on reaction with HCl, gives the official salt.

Description—White to off-white, odorless, crystalline powder; stable in light and air; melts at about 220°.

Solubility—1 g in 50 mL water; soluble in chloroform; sparingly soluble in alcohol; practically insoluble in ether.

Uses—For respiratory stimulation in *postanesthesia, chronic pulmonary disease associated with acute hypercapnia* and as an adjunct to established supportive measures and resuscitative techniques in *drug-induced CNS depression*. Low doses of doxapram also have been evaluated for treatment of apnea in premature infants when methylxanthines have failed, although the presence of benzyl alcohol makes use of this drug product dangerous in newborns. The respiratory stimulation is thought to be mediated through the carotid chemoreceptors; as the dosage is increased, the respiratory centers in the medulla are stimulated with progressive stimulation in other areas of the brain and spinal cord. A pressor response, due to improved cardiac output, also may occur. An increased release of catecholamines also has been noted. The onset of respiratory stimulation after IV injection usually occurs in 20 to 40 sec with peak effect in 1 to 2 min. The effect is short and persists for only 5 to 12 min because of rapid metabolism. Doxapram is contraindicated in patients with epilepsy or other convulsive states, pulmonary disease such as pulmonary embolism, pulmonary incompetence due to muscle paresis, severe hypertension or cerebrovascular accidents and coronary artery disease. It also should be administered cautiously to patients on sympathomimetic or monoamine oxidase inhibiting drugs (addictive pressor effects) and patients given anesthetic agents (halothane, cyclopropane, enflurane) known to sensitize the myocardium to catecholamines. Adverse reactions involve the central and autonomic systems (headache, dizziness, apprehension, disorientation, convulsions and muscle spasms), respiratory system (cough, dyspnea, tachypnea, laryngospasm, etc), cardiovascular system (phlebitis, variations in heart rate, arrhythmias, chest pain, increase in blood pressure, etc), gastrointestinal tract (nausea, vomiting and diarrhea) and genitourinary system (urinary retention and spontaneous voiding). Safe use during pregnancy has not been established. Doxapram is not recommended for use in children 12 yr and younger.

Dose—Postanesthetic: *intravenous*, **0.5** to **1.0 mg/kg**, not to exceed **1.5 mg/kg** as a single injection. Drug-induced CNS depression: *intravenous*, **1.0** to **2.0 mg/kg** and repeated in 5 min; repeat same dose every 1 to 2 hr until patient awakens. Chronic obstructive pulmonary disease: *infusion*, **1** to **2 mg/min** increased to a maximum of 3 mg/min.

Dosage Form—Injection: 20 mg/mL in 20 mL vials.

Nikethamide—page 1235.

Pentylenetetrazol—page 1235.

Picrotoxin—page 1235.

Therapeutic Gases

A number of pharmacologic agents are gaseous at normal temperatures and pressures, whereas others are liquids or even solids with such high vapor pressures that they yield vapors in sufficiently high concentration to exhibit pharmacological properties. Since these gases and vapors are absorbed by way of the respiratory tract, they could be included in this section. However, only those gases which have therapeutic application are presented here. Aside from the anesthetic gases and vapors, which are discussed elsewhere (see Chapter 67), the most important therapeutic gases are carbon dioxide, oxygen and helium. Although helium is not a pharmacologically active agent, it does possess valuable therapeutic properties attributable to its unique physical properties; hence, it is included in this section.

Carbon Dioxide—page 979.

Helium

Helium [7440-59-7] He (4.003); contains not less than 99% by volume of He; the remainder consists mainly of nitrogen.

Preparation—See page 318.

Description—Colorless, odorless, tasteless, chemically inert gas; 1 L at 760 mm and 0° weighs 178–189 mg.

Solubility—Very slightly soluble in water.

Uses—A diluent for medicinal gases. Helium is inert with respect to body metabolism and has no physiologic function or pharmacologic toxicity. Its pharmacologic actions are related exclusively to its physical properties; its density is about 1/7 that of oxygen. A mixture of 80 parts helium and 20 parts oxygen is only ⅓ as heavy as air. Such mixtures are used in the treatment of *respiratory obstruction* and are of great value in relieving *status asthmaticus* and the symptoms arising from inflammatory obstructions. When administered in *asphyxia*, the light mixture penetrates the air passages more readily than mixtures of nitrogen and oxygen. Helium also may be substituted for nitrogen for divers working at high ambient pressures; the helium eliminates the possibility of nitrogen narcosis on deep dives.

Dose—By *inhalation*, **60** to **80%**, with oxygen 20 to 40%.

Oxygen

Oxygen [7782-44-7], O_2 (32.00); contains not less than 99% by volume of O_2.

Preparation—See page 329.

Description—Colorless, odorless, tasteless gas; it supports combustion more energetically than air; 1 L at 760 mm and 0° weighs 1.429 g.

Solubility—1 volume in about 32 volumes water or in about 7 volumes alcohol at 20°C and 760 mm.

Uses—Employed widely in the treatment and prevention of *hypoxia*. Hypoxia may result from an *inadequate oxygen content in inspired air* (high altitudes), *inadequate delivery of inspired air to the lungs* (asthma, obstruction of the airway, insufficiency of the respiratory muscles or respiratory depression), *inadequate oxygenation of blood due to abnormal pulmonary gas exchange* (pulmonary fibrosis, pulmonary edema, pneumonia, tachypnea, etc) and *inadequate transport of oxygen by the circulation* (carbon monoxide poisoning, cardiac decompensation, shock, coronary occlusion, cerebrovascular accidents, etc). In addition there are several miscellaneous uses, such as the treatment of abdominal distention, spontaneous pneumothorax and air embolism. Oxygen also is used by workers in pressurized spaces. Finally, in anesthesia, oxygen is a common diluent for gaseous and volatile anesthetic agents.

Oxygen, when administered by external devices, can cause significant adverse effects, which include discomfort from a dry gas mixture and hypoventilation. If oxygen is consumed in extremely high concentrations, pulmonary oxygen toxicity can result. The major target tissue of oxygen toxicity is likely the pulmonary capillary endothelium. The cellular damage may be due to the formation of the unstable superoxide free radical from the reduction of oxygen. Although often difficult to detect, oxygen toxicity can consist of tracheobronchitis, nausea, vomiting, decreases in vital capacity and tachypnea.

CAUTION: *While oxygen does not burn, it supports combustion with ease.*

Dose—By *inhalation*, as required.

CHAPTER 57

Sympathomimetic Drugs

Donald N Franz, PhD
Professor of Pharmacology
School of Medicine, University of Utah
Salt Lake City, UT 84132

The next five chapters treat specifically of autonomic drugs, and several other chapters (eg, Chapters 53, 55, 71, and 74) include descriptions of or references to a number of autonomic drugs. Consequently, it will be helpful to review briefly the autonomic nervous system and the classification of drugs that act on or simulate components of that system.

Autonomic Nervous System and Autonomic Drugs

The *autonomic (involuntary) nervous system* generally is defined as that system of motor (efferent) nerves which contains cell bodies and corresponding synapses (ie, ganglia) outside of the cerebrospinal axis. The definition includes the sensory (afferent) nerves that subserve functions mediated by the autonomic motor nerves, although a given sensory nerve also may subserve somatic motor functions. This system modulates or controls the activities of smooth (involuntary) muscles of the body, including those that control the caliber of blood vessels, the heart muscle and the digestive, salivary, sweat and some endocrine glands. Unconsciously (without conscious control), it tends to maintain a constant state (homeostasis) of the vital functions of the body, constantly adjusting one or more factors to attempt to maintain equilibrium or restore an equilibrium upset by external or internal influences; cerebral blood flow, body temperature, visual accommodation, blood sugar and body fluid composition, for example, are kept remarkably constant by means of servoadjustments mediated through the autonomic nerves. However, it should be noted that the *somatic* (voluntary) *nervous system* also unconsciously subserves vital functions such as respiration, posture, swallowing, motor reflexes, body temperature and many less vital but important unconscious modulations of skeletal muscle tone; however, the degree of conscious modulation of this control is much greater than in the autonomic nervous system. These involuntary somatic motor functions are coordinated with autonomic functions.

There are two main motor divisions to the autonomic nervous systems—the *sympathetic* (thoracolumbar) and the *parasympathetic* (craniosacral) divisions. Most organs or systems (effectors) receive innervation from both these divisions; generally, but not invariably, the two divisions qualitatively are opposed in their actions on a given effector. An abridged list of responses is presented in Table 1.

The opposition of the two divisions of the autonomic nervous system reflects the fact that the chemical substances (mediator, transmitter or neurohumor) liberated by the postganglionic nerve terminals are not the same for the two divisions. Parasympathetic postganglionic nerves liberate acetylcholine and, hence, are called *cholinergic* nerves. Most sympathetic postganglionic nerves liberate norepinephine; however, sympathetic postganglionic fibers to the sweat glands and a few fibers to the vascular beds of the mouth, face and skeletal muscles liberate acetylcholine (ie, are cholinergic). The adrenal medulla, which is innervated by sympathetic preganglionic nerves, liberates mostly epinephrine, also known as adrenaline; since adrenaline originally was thought to be the sympathetic transmitter, norepinephrine-releasing nerves are termed *adrenergic*.

At the ganglia, preganglionic nerves of either division liberate acetylcholine (ie, are cholinergic), but the character of the acetylcholine ganglionic receptors is different from those in the neuroeffectors, so that the two types of receptors are not blocked by the same drugs. Somatic motor nerves also liberate acetylcholine (ie, are cholinergic) and are similar to autonomic preganglionic nerves in this regard.

Autonomic drugs are classified according to their relation to the chemical mediator that they either mimic or block. Thus, a drug is cholinergic if it either mimics or blocks stimulation by cholinergic nerves. The terms *cholinomimetic* and *adrenomimetic* have been advanced for the appropriate mimetic agents. There also prevails an older terminology. Hence, adrenomimetics are usually called *sympathomimetics* (this chapter) and cholinomimetics are often called *parasympathomimetics* (Chapter 58); the term parasympathomimetic applies to those drugs that act upon the cholinergic neuroeffectors (ie, are muscarinic), not the ganglionic synapses. Agents that block the receptors are called *blocking agents*, according to the nature of the chemical transmitter with which they compete. Thus, there are *adrenergic blocking agents* (Chapter 59) and *antimuscarinic agents* (Chapter 60), the latter term again restricted to those drugs that block acetylcholine at the neuroeffector receptors. Those agents that block acetylcholine at the ganglionic synapses are simply called *ganglionic blocking agents* (Chapter 55); their somatic motor counterparts (generally loosely included among the autonomic drugs) are called *neuromuscular blocking agents (curarimimetics)* (Chapter 61). The suffix *lytic* sometimes is used in lieu of the word *blocking*; thus, a sympatholytic agent is an adrenergic blocking agent. Also, agents, such as the anticholinesterases, which enhance autonomic transmission by preserving the transmitter from enzymatic destruction, are endowed with no definitive designation; the *anticholinesterases* (Chapter 58) are classified awkwardly as cholinomimetics or parasympathomimetics.

An autonomic mediator not only is liberated at different sites and exerts different effects but also may act on different receptors. The actions of acetylcholine on the exocrine glands, smooth muscle and heart differ from those on autonomic ganglia and the voluntary neuromuscular junction. The former (and not the latter) effects are blocked by atropine, whereas the latter (and not the former) are blocked by tubocurarine. Since muscarine exerts the former actions (and not the latter), the corresponding receptors are called *muscarinic;* since nicotine exerts the latter reactions (and not the former), the corresponding receptors are called *nicotinic.* Three main types of muscarinic receptors are important: M_1-receptors predominate in the CNS and on gastric parietal cells where stimulation increases gastric secretion; M_2-receptors predominate in the heart and M_3-receptors are found in secretory glands and most smooth muscle.

In the adrenergic system there are also two main types of receptors: α and β. There are two types of α- adrenoreceptors: α_1 and α_2. The α_1-adrenoreceptors subserve smooth muscular stimulant functions, adrenergic sweating and adrenergic salivation. The α_2-adrenoreceptors serve to inhibit the presynaptic release of norepinephrine and other mediators and the postsynaptic activation of adenyl cyclase

Table 1—Response of Human Effector Organs to Autonomic Nerve Impulses

Effector system	Sympathetic nerve impulses	Parasympathetic nerve impulses
Systemic blood vessels	Constrict Dilate[a]	Innervate few systemic vessels, but dilate
Pulmonary blood vessels	Constrict	Dilate
Coronary blood vessels	Dilate	Dilate
Bronchioles	Dilate[b]	Constrict
Stomach motility and tone	Decrease	Increase
Gastric secretion	Little effect	Increase
Intestinal motility and tone	Decrease	Increase
Urinary bladder sphincter	Constrict	Dilate
Heart	Increase rate and strength	Decrease rate and strength, block
Pupil of eye	Dilate	Constrict
Salivary glands	Stimulate to viscid saliva	Stimulate to watery saliva
Sweat glands	Stimulate	Not innervated[c]
Lacrimal glands	Not innervated	Stimulate

[a] Constriction is produced in most vascular beds by stimulation of α-receptors. Dilation is produced primarily in skeletal muscle and the liver by stimulation of β-receptors.

[b] Adrenergic nerves do not innervate directly bronchiolar smooth muscle but instead act on cholinergic nerve terminals to decrease the release of acetylcholine.

[c] Most sweat glands *anatomically* are *sympathetic* but *functionally* are *muscarinic.*

(and hence inhibit postsynaptic responses). The β-adrenoreceptors are subdivided into β_1- and β_2-adrenoreceptors, and perhaps more. They are characterized and defined by differences in responsiveness to sympathomimetics and blocking drugs. β_1-Adrenoreceptors effect cardiac stimulation and lipolysis; β_2-adrenoreceptors subserve adrenergic smooth muscle relaxation (eg, vasodilatation, bronchodilatation and intestinal and uterine relaxation) and glycolysis. Both α-adrenoreceptors are blocked by phenoxybenzamine. α_1-Adrenoreceptors are blocked selectively by prazosin and α_2-receptors by yohimbine and rauwolscine. β-Adrenoreceptors are blocked by propranolol. β-Adrenoreceptors are blocked somewhat selectively by metoprolol and β_2-receptors somewhat selectively by butoxamine. Dopamine excites dopamine receptors that are found in kidney and mesenteric blood vessels and are blocked by haloperidol; this receptor does not appear to be activated by other adrenergic stimulants.

Sympathomimetics

The abbreviated list of functions affected by sympathetic nerves, shown in Table 1, indicates the potential complexity of the pharmacology of the sympathomimetics. It is, in fact, considerably more complex than might be surmised from the table, not only because of the several different receptors with different functions and structure-activity requirements, but also because some sympathomimetics do not even act directly upon these receptors; these act indirectly by releasing norepinephrine from adrenergic nerve terminals. Furthermore, some sympathomimetics can pass through the blood-brain barrier into the central nervous system, where they may elicit a variety of effects. Consequently, it is not possible to describe the actions, uses, adverse effects, etc of a prototype sympathomimetic that will apply to all sympathomimetics. The text below discusses prototypic actions rather than prototypic drugs, in order to explain the varied behavior among the sympathomimetics. The dependent uses, adverse effects and precautions are discussed in relation to the actions, in order that the pharmacodynamic bases of these may be comprehended better.

Peripheral Actions and Uses

Not all sympathomimetics are capable of activating all adrenergic and dopaminergic receptors; even among those which are, there is marked variation in the relative intensities of activation of the several receptor types. Thus dopamine stimulates dopaminergic receptors strongly, β_1-adrenoreceptors moderately, α-adrenoreceptors weakly and β_2-adrenoreceptors negligibly. The predominant sympathetic neurotransmitter, norepinephrine, stimulates α_1- and β_1-adrenoreceptors strongly, α_2-adrenoreceptors moderately, β_2-adrenoreceptors weakly and dopaminergic receptors negligibly. Epinephrine stimulates all of the α_1-, α_2-, β_1- and β_2-adrenoreceptors strongly and dopaminergic receptors negligibly. Obviously, then, the pharmacodynamic profiles of these three natural sympathomimetics differ considerably from one another. Several sympathomimetics act selectively on a single type of receptor.

α-Adrenoreceptor Agonists—α-Agonists cause arteriolar and venous constriction and, hence, have an action to increase blood pressure. This vasopressor action is used to *support blood pressure* in hypotensive states, such as in *orthostatic hypotension, carotid sinus syndrome, shock* and during *spinal anesthesia.* In the treatment of *hypovolemic shock,* the constriction of the capacitance vessels (ie, large veins) increases the venous return to the heart and, hence, the cardiac output, but once the blood volume is repleted, α-agonists may not be necessary. In fact, the use of α-agonists in any kind of shock (except anaphylaxis) is usually counterproductive, because there is already ischemia of certain critical organs like the kidney and bowel, and vasoconstriction exacerbates the ischemia in these two organs and contributes to irreversible damage and life-threatening complications.

The systemic vasoconstrictor effects also are employed in the management of a variety of serious allergic conditions, such as *giant urticaria, serum sickness, drug reactions, angioneurotic edema* and *anaphylaxis.* For these uses, epinephrine is the drug of choice. Also, the vasopressor effects of selective α-agonists (ie, devoid of significant β-activity) are sometimes used to elicit compensatory vagal reflexes, which slow the heart and depress atrioventricular conduction and, hence, terminate *paroxysmal supraventricular (atrial)* or *nodal tachycardia.*

The α-agonists are applied topically to induce local vasoconstriction in the nasopharyngeal, scleroconjunctival and otic blood vessels in *vasomotor rhinitis, acute rhinitis, acute coryza, nasopharyngitis, acute sinusitis, eustachian salpingitis, conjunctivitis, scleritis, hay fever, otitis media, barotitis media,* etc. This use to suppress hyperemia and the related edema is called *decongestion.* Conjunctival and scleral decongestion may relieve irritative *blepharospasm.* α-Agonists that are capable of penetrating the cornea may be used to relieve *uveal congestion.* α-Agonists also are applied topically as *styptics* to arrest superficial hemorrhage. Lastly, they may be *combined with local anesthetics;* vasoconstriction keeps the local anesthetic at the injection site for a longer time.

Topically administered α-agonists are used to stimulate the radial smooth muscle of the iris and, hence, cause *mydriasis* for ophthalmologic examination or to break *posterior synechiae* in uveitis. Their effects on the ciliary body are slight, and they do not cause significant cycloplegia or increase intraocular pressure, even in susceptible persons. However, their mydriatic effects are additive with those of antimuscarinic drugs, with which they are sometimes combined, to produce maximum mydriasis for optimal examination of the eyegrounds. In *open-angle glaucoma,* intraocular vasoconstriction causes an increase in the outflow of aqueous humor and, hence, in the intraocular pressure; they are sometimes used in combination with carbonic anhydrase inhibitors in this use.

β_1-Adrenoreceptor Agonists—The β_1-agonists increase the heart rate, enhance atrioventricular conduction and increase the strength of the heart beat (positive inotropic action).

They also induce lipolysis and, thus, increase the concentration of plasma free fatty acids. These effects are achieved, in part, through the activation of adenylyl cyclase and the synthesis of 3′,5′-cyclic adenosine monophosphate (cAMP). In the heart, especially, β_1-agonists also increase calcium influx and storage, in part the result of mediation by cAMP.

Use is made of the cardiostimulatory effects of β_1-agonists. They may be administered by intracardiac injection to restore the *heart beat* in *cardiac arrest* and *heart block with syncopal seizures* (as in Adams-Stokes syndrome) and by intravenous injection to sustain restored rhythm or to prevent a recurrence of arrests; however, β_1-agonists are not the treatment of choice, and physical and electrical measures take precedence. More often, β_1-agonists are used for their positive inotropic actions in the treatment of *acute heart failure* and in *cardiogenic* or other types of *shock*, in which contractility often is diminished. However, they are less than ideal in the treatment of shock, not only because they favor arrhythmias, which are an especial threat in cardiogenic shock, but also because they promote a metabolic acidosis through the lipolytic action.

β_2-Adrenoreceptor Agonists—The β_2-agonists relax smooth muscle and induce hepatic and muscle glycogenolysis, by activating the adenylyl cyclase system and increasing the intracellular levels of cAMP. Thus, they dilate the bronchioles, arterioles in vascular beds which are invested with β_2-receptors (such as in skeletal muscle, splanchnic and coronary but not renal or cutaneous beds) and veins, and they relax the uterus and intestines. The glycogenolytic effects in liver and muscle, respectively, result in hyperglycemia and hyperlactic acidemia. The hyperglycemic actions are sometimes used to treat *insulin overdosage*. At present, there are no "pure" β_2-agonists without some degree of β_1-agonist activity.

Most β_2-agonists are used as bronchodilators in the treatment of *bronchial asthma, emphysema, bronchitis* and *bronchiectasis*, often in combination with theophylline. They also increase ciliary activity and liquefy tenacious mucus and, so, have a mild expectorant action. These effects are usually beneficial, but they may cause mucus plugs. Tachyphylaxis to the bronchodilator effects sometimes occurs, especially if they are used continuously or in excess of recommended dosage or frequency.

Selective β_2-agonists, when administered by inhalation, may dilate bronchioles with a minimum of hypotensive side effects. However, some degree of cardiostimulation can occur with current drugs. Muscle tremor, by an action on the skeletal muscle spindles, also commonly occurs.

Certain β-agonists may be used as vasodilators in the treatment of peripheral vascular diseases. There are two preconditions for efficacy: (1) the disease process must predominantly have a vasospastic and not obliterative component and (2) the vessels involved must have an effective population of β_2-receptors. Efficacy, thus, is limited essentially to selected cases of *intermittent claudication* and *thrombophlebitis*. Some of the presumed selective β_2-agonists for peripheral vascular disease relax vascular smooth muscle partly by a direct smooth muscle depressant mechanism.

β_2-Agonists may be used to relax the uterus and delay delivery in *premature labor*. Although they do depress the premature contractions for a time, they seldom avoid subsequent premature delivery.

Dopaminergic Agonists—Dopamine is the only marketed sympathomimetic with significant dopaminergic actions in the periphery. In the periphery, dopamine receptors are prominent in the splanchnic and renal vascular beds, where they mediate vasodilatation. Dilatation in these beds is important in the treatment of *shock* and *acute heart failure*, since these beds often are constricted critically in these conditions. Dopamine is used in the management of these disorders.

Combined Agonist Activity—Most sympathomimetics act upon two or more receptor types, and the net effects are the algebraic sum of the α-, β_1- and β_2-activities. In describing the properties of a sympathomimetic, it is necessary to indicate the relative agonist activities in order to understand the overall effects.

Central Nervous System Actions and Uses

The actions of sympathomimetics in the central nervous system are exceedingly complex. Noradrenergic and dopaminergic nerves are disseminated widely throughout the central nervous system, and dopaminergic nerves are crucial to some brain functions. A limited number of epinephrine (adrenaline) nerves also are found in several areas. Not only are there α-, β-adrenergic and dopamine receptors at the synapses, but the actions subserved may be either excitatory or inhibitory at a specific structure, which structure may, in turn, have facilitatory or inhibitory influences on other structures. Furthermore, some sympathomimetics appear to activate serotoninergic and possibly histaminergic receptors in the central nervous system. Also, some centrally acting sympathomimetics appear to act as agonists at some loci and transmitter-releasing agents at other loci. One drug, thus, may display simultaneously a number of activities.

The most prominent central nervous system effects of centrally acting sympathomimetics are various manifestations of stimulation, which may give rise to nervousness, sleeplessness, hyperactivity, irritability and increased respiration. In some users they may induce anxiety and in others a kind of euphoria that gives the user a feeling of accomplishment, expectation and affectations for which some sympathomimetics may be abused widely. They allay the perception but not the reality of fatigue, and users often drive themselves to physical and emotional exhaustion (the "crash"). Large doses can cause hallucinations, and long, continued use may result in paranoia and other dangerous behavior, as well as exhaustion. Some tolerance to the euphoric and certain other central nervous system actions occurs.

The effects to promote wakefulness are used in the treatment of *narcolepsy*. They seldom are used any longer to treat central nervous system depression from overdoses of drugs, although the antagonism of respiratory depression is sometimes dramatic.

The centrally acting sympathomimetics may be beneficial in certain disorders of movement. In *parkinsonism* they often diminish rigidity, relieve oculogyric crises and improve sleep. They also may provide relief in *spasmodic torticollis*. They also have a beneficial effect on mood in depressive states, but they have been superseded by other drugs. In the *attention deficit hyperkinetic disorder* (ADHD) they have a paradoxical calming effect, but this use is controversial because of perceptions of overuse.

A very widely used and greatly abused effect is that of the *suppression of appetite* (anorexiant, anorectic or anorexigenic effect). The drugs may induce temporary weight loss in *exogenous obesity*. However, the weight loss is usually the least in those who need it most and seldom exceeds 10 lb, the effectiveness usually lasts but a few weeks (ie, tolerance develops) and there is danger of abuse; abuse potential varies among the sundry anorexiant drugs. At best, anorexiant drugs should be used only in a training program to condition the patient to new eating habits. Even so, the patient usually resumes hyperphagic behavior eventually and may even show a rebound-like gain in weight.

Centrally acting sympathomimetics may exert autonomic actions by acting both in the periphery and upon the various autonomic nervous centers in the brain. Stimulants used for their pressor effects usually act in the periphery, but central sympathoadrenal stimulation may augment such effects and may be an important factor in the cardiovascular effects of intoxication. Some centrally acting sympathomimetics are used to *support blood pressure* in the *carotid sinus syndrome* or *orthostatic hypotension;* the oral efficacy and convenient duration of action offer advantages that partially offset disadvantages accruing to central stimulation. Their effects to suppress *urinary incontinence* and *enuresis* mostly derive from their central actions to increase the genitourinary autonomic nervous outflow. They may sometimes relieve the pain of *dysmenorrhea*, probably by central nervous system and neuroendocrine mechanisms.

Indirect Sympathomimetics—Many sympathomimetics do not conform to the structural requirements for adrenergic agonist activity. The aliphatic and cycloaliphatic amine sympathomimetics, for example, deviate greatly from the prerequisite structure. These compounds derive their activity from an action to release norepinephrine from adrenergic nerve terminals, the final action, then, being mediated by norepinephrine. It might be expected that the pharmacodynamics of the indirect sympathomimetics would be identical to those of exogenously administered norepinephrine, but in some cases they are not. Firstly, the release from nerve endings may achieve high local concentrations of norepinephrine at the effector site that could not be achieved safely with injected norepinephrine. Thus, therapeutic doses of ephedrine cause substantial bronchodilatation, while those of norepinephrine do not. Secondly, release is not equal everywhere. For example, ephedrine releases norepinephrine more effectively in the bronchioles and heart than elsewhere; hence, considerable bronchodilatation and cardiostimulation often can be achieved with only mild to moderate vasoconstriction. Also, hydroxyamphetamine fails to release norepinephrine in the skin, although it does in the eye and the heart.

Disposition—Part of the norepinephrine or dopamine that is released from nerve terminals is returned to the interior of the nerve by a membrane-transport system. This provides the principal means by which the action of adrenergic neurotransmitters is terminated. Neuronal uptake also assists in the termination of the action of small doses of exogenous norepinephrine. However, the predominant route of elimination in the periphery is *O*-methylation at the ring 3-OH group by the enzyme, catechol-*O*-methyltransferase (COMT). COMT is found throughout the peripheral tissues but is quite active in the liver. Other catecholamines, and, to a lesser extent, 3-OH monophenolic amines also are *O*-methylated. Ring hydroxyl groups also are conjugated with sulfate and glycuronate in the liver. In the brain, both norepinephrine and dopamine are eliminated mostly by the mitochondrial enzyme, monoamine oxidase (MAO). In the periphery, MAO is also important to the elimination of catecholamines as well as to that of noncatecholic arylethylamines. The presence of side-chain substituents, as in ephedrine and amphetamine, renders the sympathomimetic amines resistant to oxidative deamination by MAO. Such drugs do, however, inhibit MAO.

By the oral route, a sympathomimetic must run the gamut of MAO, COMT and conjugases in the intestinal wall and liver. Sympathomimetics that are good substrates for these enzymes are ineffective or erratic orally. Most noncatecholamines also are oxidized by the cytochrome P-450 system in the liver.

Adverse Effects, Precautions and Contraindications

The multiple activities of sympathomimetics make for numerous side effects. Some of these, such as reflex homeostatic adjustments, which act to counter an effect or the elicitation of simultaneous physiologically antagonistic effects, are counterproductive but are not necessarily adverse. However, some reflex effects may be adverse, such as the prolonged reflex renal vasoconstriction that accrues to the use of isoproterenol infusion in shock. Some side effects, such as substernal pain, occur only in patients with a particular disease and indicate an adverse effect only in such patients.

The manufacturer's literature (package insert, *Physicians' Desk Reference*, etc) tends to list for each sympathomimetic drug all the collective side effects and contraindications of all sympathomimetics, without regard to the individual properties. In the discussion below, the adverse effects are enumerated according to the type of activity. For drugs with multiple activities, it will be necessary for the reader to synthesize the profile of adverse effects and contraindications from the component activities. However, certain precautions apply to all sympathomimetics, namely that elderly persons, infants and persons with thyrotoxicosis tend to be more sensitive to sympathomimetics, and that adverse effects of one kind or another are much more probable in persons with cardiovascular disease than in normal adults.

α_1-Agonists—One important adverse effect of *systemically* administered α_1-agonists is an excessive increase in blood pressure. In persons with weak or atheromatous blood vessels, a cerebrovascular accident (eg, stroke), coronary occlusion, aneurysm or other serious event may occur. The heart works harder against the increased pressure, which may induce an attack of angina pectoris or precipitate or aggravate heart failure. *Hypertensive* or *elderly persons* may show an exaggerated pressor response. Vagal reflexes to the pressor response may cause bradycardia and various degrees of atrioventricular conduction block; the disturbed electrophysiology and myocardial stretch (the heart enlarges to work against the increased pressure) favor various serious cardiac arrhythmias in persons with certain types of heart damage. Therefore, except under the most careful medical supervision, α-agonists are contraindicated in persons with *hypertension, coronary heart disease, arteriosclerosis, atherosclerosis, diabetes* (because of vascular pathology), *cardiac arrhythmias* or a history of *myocardial infarction*. They also are contraindicated in *venous thrombosis*, because venospasm not only may exacerbate the thrombosis but also may initiate thromboembolism.

The possible adverse effects of α_1-agonists in shock were mentioned under *Peripheral Actions and Uses*. Prolonged infusion of some sympathomimetics occasionally can cause shock. Extravasation of α-agonists during intravenous administration may result in a slough; sometimes phentolamine is included in the solution to antagonize the perivascular vasoconstriction. Uterine and placental vasoconstriction in *pregnancy* may harm the fetus. α_1-Agonists interfere with *lactation*. Signs and symptoms of a strong vasoconstrictor effect are bradycardia with a strong pulse, occasional tingling in the extremities, headache and sometimes anxiety, which results from the enteroceptive detection of the altered cardiovascular status and other autonomic disturbances.

Other systemic side effects of α-agonists include mydriasis and photophobia (if the drug can penetrate into the eye), sweating, piloerection and occasionally nausea and vomiting. Increased tension in the trigone muscle and urethral contraction may create a desire to urinate, but urination may be difficult; α-agonists should be used cautiously in elderly men, especially those with *prostatic hypertrophy*.

Adverse effects of α-agonists *applied topically* to the eye include photophobia (from mydriasis), browache, ocular pain, headache, aftercongestion, especially during chronic use, rebound miosis after the adrenergic effects wear off, floating opacities and scleroconjunctival and especially corneal chemosis. Prolonged use, especially of epinephrine, may cause pigmentation in the cornea, conjunctiva and lids. Intense intraocular vasoconstriction can damage the retina; special care must be exercised when there is no lens. Ophthalmologic sympathomimetics should be used cautiously when there is *retinal detachment* or before cataract surgery, because of possible rebound miosis. In *narrow-angle glaucoma*, mydriasis may close the angle sufficiently to increase the intraocular pressure. Adverse effects that may occur after topical application to the nasopharynx include aftercongestion and chemical rhinitis, with sneezing. Enough sympathomimetic may be absorbed after either conjunctival or nasopharyngeal application to cause serious hypertensive episodes in patients; *blood pressures of over 200 torr frequently are observed in infants and small children*. Therefore, the precautions and contraindications that apply to systemic use also apply to topical use.

β_1-Agonists—The side effects of β-agonists with strong β_1-activity are tachycardia and palpitation. Substernal distress may occur if there is coronary heart disease, because tachycardia and a decrease in the efficiency of oxygen utilization increase the myocardial oxygen demand. There also may be premature atrial and ventricular contractions and tachyarrhythmias. The degree of vasodepression depends upon the degree of concomitant β_2-activity; with isoproterenol, there is usually diastolic hypotension and often systolic hypertension, with a net increase or decrease in blood pressure.

Because of the cardiostimulant effects, β_1-agonists are contraindicated in *coronary heart disease* and when there are *arrhythmias*. They also are contraindicated in *thyrotoxicosis*, because the heart is hyperreactive to β-adrenergic influences and already may be in tachycardia. The potential detrimental consequences of the lipolytic effects already have been mentioned. β_1-Agonists in high concentration occasionally can cause myocardial necrosis; this warrants caution after *coronary occlusion*. Myocardial necrosis possibly may occur after inhalation of β_1-agonists. An interesting adverse effect of β_1-agonist activity in chronic *obstructive pulmonary disease* is that of an increased perfusion of the nonfunctioning portions of the lungs (consequent to the increased cardiac output), which results in a decrease in mixed pulmonary venous oxygen saturation (pO_2).

β_2-Agonists—Because some β_2-agonists decrease the blood pressure, they cause reflex tachycardia and palpitation. Consequently, they must be used cautiously in the same cardiovascular diseases as must the β_1-agonists. When β_2-agonists are administered by inhalation, especially, pulmonary vasodilatation may cause shunting of blood and uneven circulation of the lung, which may have an effect to sometimes lower the mixed pulmonary venous pO_2 similar to that of the β_1-agonists, above, despite the decrease in airway resistance. Also, pulmonary vasodilation favors peribronchiolar edema, which is counterproductive, and an α-agonist may be coadministered to antagonize the pulmonary vasodilation. Tolerance to the bronchodilator effects not only may occur, especially with high doses, but a rebound increase in airway resistance often occurs as the β_2-effects decline. Although β_2-agonists have a mild expectorant effect, they increase mucus secretion and may occasionally cause the development of mucus plugs.

When Freon-propelled inhalation aerosols of β-agonist bronchodilators were introduced, there was a sudden increase in the occurrence of both tolerance and sudden deaths. The development of metered sprays and a return to nebulization has reduced the incidence of such deaths. The deaths have been attributed to a combination of causes: a cardiotoxic effect of the propellant, an effect of the propellant (which may be regarded as a chlorocarbon) to sensitize the heart to the arrhythmiagenic effects of the component β_1-agonist activity of the bronchodilators (since the deaths mainly occurred with those agonists with combined β_1- and β_2-activity) and the ease of administration and, hence, ease of overdosing. Despite the improved safety of metered aerosols, it is important to stress the importance of waiting a few minutes between closely consecutive inhalations and not exceeding the recommended frequency of dosing.

The hyperglycemic effects of β_2-agonists impose precautions when they are used in *diabetes*, and the increased metabolic rate requires caution in *thyrotoxicosis*. The detrimental effects of lactic acidosis in shock have been mentioned under *Actions and Uses*. Local and systemic acidosis from β_2-agonists decreases the bronchodilator response. β_2-Agonists may cause tremor, vertigo and insomnia.

Both β_1- and β_2-agonists occasionally cause sweating, headache and nausea and vomiting, probably indirectly the result of other effects. They also may cause anxiety, perhaps from CNS activity. β-Agonists can cause fetal tachycardia and also inhibit uterine contractions and, thus, delay labor, so that they should be avoided, if possible, in pregnancy.

Centrally Acting Sympathomimetics—Because these drugs may act both centrally and peripherally to stimulate the heart and to cause vasoconstriction, the same precautions that apply to both systemic α- and β_1-agonists should be observed. With therapeutic doses of the amphetamines which affect the CNS, these cardiovascular side effects are often of a low order, but they may be a cause of death in intoxication. Centrally acting sympathomimetics must be used cautiously in the presence of *prostatic hypertrophy*. Other autonomic nervous system-mediated side effects include mydriasis, dry mouth, flushing, sweating, diarrhea and impotence. Because of mydriasis, these drugs are contraindicated in *narrow-angle glaucoma*. Nausea, vomiting and tremors are probably mostly of central nervous system origin. With excessive doses, there may be hyperthermia, as the result of a combination of increased metabolic rate, increased physical activity and vasoconstriction. They are contraindicated in *thyrotoxicosis*. Because of an increased sympathetic outflow to the liver, hyperglycemia occurs occasionally and this, and the increase in physical activity, may change the insulin requirement in *diabetes*.

Relatively frequent CNS side effects include restlessness, insomnia, agitation and anorexia. REM sleep is disturbed. Dysphoria occurs in some persons. There sometimes is also headache, dizziness and dyskinesias. Respiratory stimulation may result in hyperventilation; this may precipitate absence seizures in persons with *petit mal epilepsy*. There may be changes in libido as the result of changes in both endocrine and sympathetic nervous systems. When the centrally acting sympathomimetics are used chronically in children, endocrine disturbances may arrest growth, which usually rebounds after discontinuation. The anxiety and psychotic states that occur after long, continued use and the potential for drug abuse have been mentioned. These drugs are contraindicated especially when there is a *history of drug abuse*, a state of *agitation* or in *pregnancy*. They also are contraindicated in *porphyria*.

All sympathomimetics can cause allergic reactions of various types, but they are more frequent with those that have polar moieties in the structure. Contact dermatitis, especially, may occur after topical use. A history of *previous allergic reactions* to a particular or similar sympathomimetic contraindicates its use.

Drug Interactions

α-Agonists must not be given along with other *vasoconstrictor drugs*. Sympathomimetics with β_1-activity, when used in the presence of *cardiac glycosides*, may precipitate dangerous tachyarrhythmias. A hypertensive response to an α-agonist causes a vagal reflex which may combine with the action of a cardiac glycoside to increase heart block. Furthermore, cardiac glycosides themselves have vasoconstrictor actions, which not only may increase the hypertensive response to an α-agonist but the combined action also may result in bowel infarction, especially in the elderly. *Cyclopropane-* and *chlorocarbon-ether anesthetics* sensitize the heart to the arrhythmiagenic effects of β_1-agonists.

Since *reserpine* and *guanethidine*, respectively, deplete and prevent the release of norepinephrine from adrenergic nerve terminals, they tend to prevent the indirect sympathomimetics from acting. By a sort of chemical denervation supersensitivity, reserpine moderately and *guanethidine* markedly increase the responses to direct sympathomimetics, especially norepinephrine and metaraminol. Dextroamphetamine and methamphetamine, and to a lesser extent other centrally acting sympathomimetics, may hasten the offset of action of guanethidine.

Monoamine oxidase inhibitors (MAOIs) increase the peripheral effects of noncatecholamine sympathomimetics which do not have substituents in the α-position; the effect is greater with primary than with secondary amines. MAOIs also cause centrally acting sympathomimetics to evoke bizarre behavior. The use of MAOIs should be discontinued 2 weeks in advance of the use of an interacting sympathomimetic. Like guanethidine and methylphenidate, *tricyclic antidepressants* (TCAs) block the neuronal reuptake system for catecholamines and metaraminol, and they may potentiate the peripheral actions of these drugs and the central actions of some centrally acting sympathomimetics. Although only certain sympathomimetics are affected by MAOIs and TCAs, the manufacturer's and medical literature usually do not discriminate; in the absence of specific intelligence to the contrary, the reader should assume that the precautions apply to any sympathomimetic of interest.

Theophylline synergizes the β_1- and β_2- and centrally acting sympathomimetics, and should be used in combination with them only when there is a special rationale, as in asthma. Because certain *oxytocic* drugs (especially ergot alkaloids) have vasoconstrictor actions, α-agonists and oxytocics should not be given together. β_2-Agonists relax the uterus and, hence, antagonize oxytocics. Some *ganglionic blocking drugs* increase the vasoconstrictor responses to α-agonists, and α-agonists and indirect sympathomimetics should be used cautiously during ganglionic blockade. Systemic *carbonic anhydrase inhibitors* cause metabolic acidosis, which diminishes the responses to β_1- and β_2-agonists, especially. *Thyroxine, liothyronine,* etc have the same effect as thyrotoxicosis to enhance the responses to the β_1- and β_2-agonists, especially, and increase the basal metabolic effects of centrally acting sympathomimetics.

α-Adrenergic blocking agents, such as *phenoxybenzamine, prazosin* and *phentolamine,* antagonize the α-agonists; if a sympathomimetic also has β_2-activity, the usual pressor response will be reversed to a depressor response. Large doses of *chlorpromazine* have the same effect. Chlorpromazine also will suppress some of the central nervous effects of sympathomimetics. *β-Adrenoreceptor blocking drugs,* such as propranolol, will suppress the actions of both β_1- and β_2-agonists. *Haloperidol* and related drugs will antagonize the vasodilator effects of dopamine and alter the central actions of some sympathomimetics.

Albuterol

1,3-Benzenedimethanol, α[1]-[[(dimethylethyl)amino]methyl]-4-hydroxy-, Proventil (*Schering*); Ventolin (*Allen & Hanburys*)

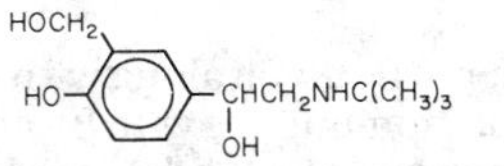

HOCH$_2$ / HO– (benzene ring) –CHCH$_2$NHC(CH$_3$)$_3$ / OH

α[1]-[(*tert*-Butylamino)methyl]-4-hydroxy-*m*-xylene-α,α′-diol, [18559-94-9] $C_{13}H_{21}NO_3$ (239.31).

Preparation—*J Med Chem 13:* 674, 1970.

Description—Off-white to white, crystalline powder; odorless; slightly bitter taste.

Solubility—1 g dissolves in 4 mL of water; slightly soluble in alcohol, chloroform or ether.

Uses—Has strong β_2- weak β_1- and no α-adrenergic agonist activity. It is used only as a *bronchodilator* in the treatment or prevention of *bronchospasm* in patients with reversible obstructive airway disease, such as bronchial asthma. Its side effects, contraindications and drug interactions are those of β_2-agonists in general (see general statement); tremor is common. The drug is teratogenic to mice and rabbits in large doses and carcinogenic in rats in huge doses; the human implications are unknown.

It lacks a 3-OH group and, hence, is not methylated by COMT; however, it is conjugated in the liver to the 4-*O*-sulfate. The half-life is about 4 hr. By inhalation, the duration of action is 3 to 6 hr. The time of peak effect is 30 to 60 min. By the oral route, the duration of action is 4 to 8 hr.

Dose—*Oral inhalation, adults* and *children over 12 yr,* **90** or **180 µg** (**1** or **2 inhalations**) every 4 to 6 hr, except **180 µg** 15 min prior to exertion, to prevent exercise-induced bronchospasm. Inhalation is not recommended for children under 12 yr.

Dosage Form—Metered Inhalation Aerosol: 17 g canister (90 µg per actuation).

Albuterol Sulfate

1,3-Benzenedimethanol, α[1]-[[(dimethylethyl)amino]methyl]-4-hydroxy-, sulfate (2:1) (salt); Proventil (*Schering*); Ventolin (*Allen & Hanburys*)

α[1]-[(*tert*-Butylamino)methyl]-4-hydroxy-*m*-xylene-α,α′-diol, sulfate (2:1) (salt) [51022-70-9] $(C_{13}H_{21}NO_3)_2.H_2SO_4$ (576.70).

Preparation—*J Med Chem 13:* 674, 1970.

Description—Off-white to white, crystalline powder; odorless; slightly bitter taste.

Solubility—One g dissolves in 4 mL of water; slightly soluble in alcohol, chloroform or ether.

Uses—See *Albuterol.*

Dose—*Oral, adults* and *children over 12 to 14 yr* or *60 lb, initially* **2** or **4 mg** 3 or 4 times a day, except only **2 mg** in elderly persons, to be cautiously increased to 8 mg a dose, if necessary, up to a total of 32 mg a day; *children 6 to 14 yr, initially* **2 mg** or 4 times a day, to be cautiously increased to no more than 24 mg a day, if necessary; *2 to 6 yr, initially* **0.1 mg/kg** 3 times a day, to be cautiously increased to no more than 0.2 mg/kg a day or 4 mg, whichever is less, if necessary. *Nebulization, adults and children over 12 yr,* **2.5 mg** inhaled 3 or 4 times a day. *Inhalation (dry powder), adults and children over 4 yr,* **200** or **400 µg** every 4 to 6 hr.

Dosage Forms—Syrup: 2 mg/5 mL; Tablets: 2 and 4 mg; Extended-Release Tablets: 4 mg. Solution for Inhalation (nebulization): 0.5% in 20 mL (to be diluted), 0.083% in 3 mL (unit dose); Capsules for Inhalation: 20 µg (administered by Rotohaler).

Amphetamine Sulfate

Benzeneethanamine, (±)-α-methyl-, sulfate, (2:1); Racemic Amphetamine Sulfate; Benzedrine Sulfate (*SmithKline Beecham*)

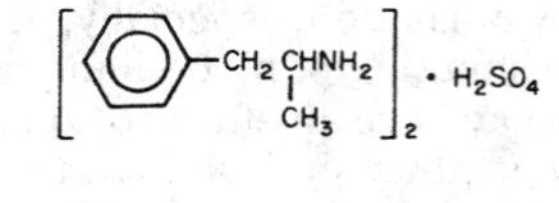

[(benzene ring)–CH$_2$CHNH$_2$ / CH$_3$]$_2$ · H$_2$SO$_4$

[60-13-9] $(C_9H_{13}N)_2.H_2SO_4$ (368.49).

α-Methylphenethylamine, sulfate (2:); For the structural formula of the (+)-form of amphetamine, see page 987.

Preparation—*J Am Chem Soc 53:* 1875, 1931.

Description—White, odorless, slightly bitter, crystalline powder; pH of 10% aqueous solution, 4.6.

Solubility—1 g in about 9 mL water or 500 mL alcohol.

Uses and **Dose**—Amphetamine has actions and uses identical to those of *Dextroamphetamine* (page 987). Although the potency is less than that of dextroamphetamine, the doses are the same.

Dosage Forms—Sustained-Release Tablets: 5, 10 and 15 mg; Tablets: 5 and 10 mg.

Apraclonidine Hydrochloride

1,4-Benzenediamine, 2,6-dichloro-*N*[1]-2-imidazolidinylidene-, monohydrochloride; Iopidine (*Alcon*)

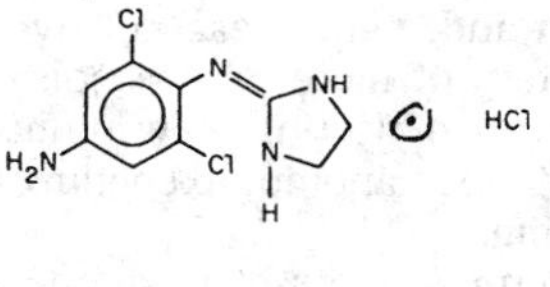

Cl / H$_2$N– (benzene ring) –N= (imidazolidine ring: NH, N–H) –Cl · HCl

[73218-79-8] $C_9H_{10}Cl_2N_4.HCl$ (281.57).

Preparation—US Pat 4,517,199.

Description—White to off-white powder.

Solubility—1 g in 34 mL water, 74 mL ethanol, 13 mL methanol; practically insoluble in chloroform or non-polar organic solvents, pH of a 1% soln about 5.5.

Uses—An aminated congener of clonidine, the α_2-adrenergic receptor agonist that acts in the CNS to lower blood pressure in hypertensive patients. Apraclonidine reduces the formation of aqueous humor and is used topically to prevent increases in intraocular pressure following eye surgery. It is used in argon laser trabeculoplasty for glaucoma, in iridotomy and capsulotomy and in cataract surgery. Its effectiveness in preventing postsurgical elevations in intraocular pressure is significantly greater than that of other topical agents that are used to treat glaucoma. Onset of action is about 1 hr, and maximal effects are attained at 3 to 5 hr. Common side effects include conjunctival blanching, upper lid retraction, mydriasis (α-adrenergic effects) and dry mouth or nose.

Dose—**1 drop** of **1% solution** instilled in the operative eye 1 hr before surgery; a second drop is instilled immediately after surgery.

Dosage Form—Sterile Solution (1%) packaged in two 0.25-mL dispensers, one for pre- and one for postsurgical use.

Benzphetamine Hydrochloride

2-Propanamine, *N*-benzyl-*N*-methyl-1-phenyl-, hydrochloride; Didrex (*Upjohn*)

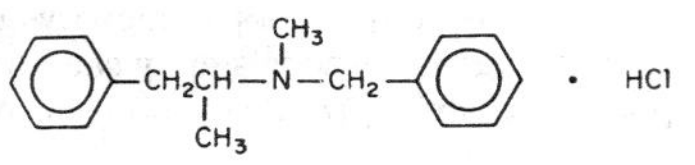

[5411-22-3] $C_{17}H_{21}N.HCl$ (275.82).

Preparation—By benzylating (+)-desoxyephedrine with benzyl chloride in the presence of sodium carbonate, the resulting benzphetamine being separated by distillation and then converted to the hydrochloride.

Description—White to off-white, crystalline powder; polymorphic, one form melting at about 130°, the other at 150°, with decomposition.

Solubility—1 g in about 1.5 mL water, 1.5 ml alcohol or 1.5 mL chloroform; slightly soluble in ether.

Uses—An indirectly acting *sympathomimetic* and central nervous system stimulant. Its only approved use is as an *anorexiant*, in which role it is about as efficacious as dextroamphetamine. Benzphetamine has euphoric action. For the limitations of anorexiant therapy and the adverse effects, precautions and drug interactions of centrally acting sympathomimetics, see the general statement. It is a Schedule III controlled substance.

Dose—*Oral, over 12 yr only, initially* **25 mg** once a day, to be increased, if necessary, to 50 mg 1 to 3 times a day.

Dosage Form—Tablets: 25 and 50 mg.

Bitolterol Mesylate

Benzoic acid, 4-methyl-, 4-[2-[(1,1-dimethylethyl)amino]-1-hydroxyethyl]-1,2-phenylene ester, methanesulfonate (salt); Tornalate *(Dura)*

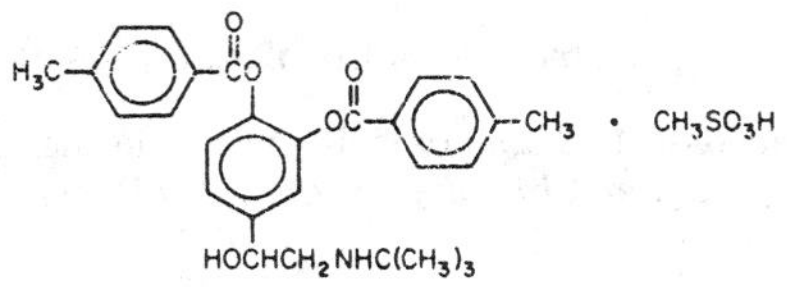

[30392-41-7] $C_{28}H_{31}NO_5.CH_4O_3S$ (557.66)

Preparation—*J Med Chem 19:* 834, 1976.

Description—Crystalline solid melting about 171°.

Uses—In the body, esterases remove the 4-methylbenzoyl groups from the prodrug, bitolterol, to generate the β-adrenoreceptor agonist, colterol (*N*-butylarterenol). Colterol is somewhat selective for β_2-adrenoreceptors, but also it causes cardiostimulatory and metabolic β_1-effects. However, when bitolterol is administered by inhalation, it is absorbed into the lung as the ester and concentrated there, at which site colterol is generated gradually. Consequently, not only is the duration of bronchodilation longer than that of any other presently available inhalant β-agonist in the US but also there is minimal cardiostimulation and vasodilatation. It is used only as a *bronchodilator*. The tissue half-life of the intact ester in the lung may be around 4 hr; the elimination half-life of colterol probably is only a fraction of 1 hr. The duration of the bronchodilator effect is from 5 to over 8 hr.

In recommended doses, it causes very little effect on the heart rate, although palpitation occurs in about 5% of recipients. There are various CNS effects, such as tremor (about 14%), nervousness (5%), vertigo (3%) and nausea (3%); these effects may be increased by concomitant administration of theophylline. There is about a 5% incidence of throat irritation and 4% of cough when the drug is inhaled.

Dose—*Oral inhalation, adults* and *children over 12 yr,* **2 inhalations (370 μg** each) every 8 hr for *prophylaxis* and *treatment*, except that for treatment, a third inhalation may be administered after 3 min, if necessary; daily dosage should not exceed 2 inhalations (740 μg) every 4 hr or 3 inhalations (1.11 mg) every 6 hr.

Dosage Form—Aerosol: 0.8% (370 μg/actuation); Inhalation Solution: 0.2%.

Bromocriptine—page 1035.

Cyclazindol—see RPS-18, page 888.

Dextroamphetamine Saccharate—see RPS-18, page 886.

Dextroamphetamine Sulfate

(*S*)-Benzeneethanamine, α-methyl-, sulfate (2:1); Dexamphetamine Sulfate; *d*-1-Phenyl-2-aminopropane Sulfate; Dexedrine Sulfate (*SmithKline Beecham*)

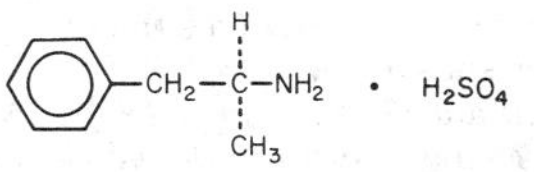

(+)-α-Methylphenethylamine sulfate (2:1) [51-63-8] $(C_9H_{13}N)_2.H_2SO_4$ (368.49).

Preparation—Racemic amphetamine may be prepared from phenylacetone by (1) catalytic reduction of the oxime or (2) heating the ketone with formamide. Resolution is affected with *d*-tartaric acid followed by treatment with 10% sulfuric acid. Also, the inefficient resolution step may be obviated by preparation from *d*-phenylalanine, with retention of conformation.

Description—White, odorless, crystalline powder; pH (1 in 20 solution) between 5 and 6; specific rotation (4% aqueous solution of a dried sample) between +20° and +23.5°.

Solubility—1 g in about 10 mL water or about 800 mL alcohol; insoluble in ether.

Uses—Amphetamine is an *indirectly acting sympathomimetic* with weak peripheral but strong central nervous system stimulant actions. As a central stimulant, the dextrorotatory isomer is approximately twice as potent as the racemic mixture (amphetamine) and 3 to 4 times as potent as the levorotatory isomer.

The approved uses are limited to the treatment of *narcolepsy*, the *attention deficit disorder* in children and *exogenous obesity*. FDA approval of use as an anorexiant in the treatment of exogenous obesity is limited to short-term use. For longer term use, clinicians generally favor anorexiants with weaker euphoria and less rapidly developing tolerance.

It is addicting and widely abused. It has been estimated that nearly one-half of that manufactured in the US is being used illegally. During chronic abuse, tolerance to the euphoric effects may be as much as 25-fold, so that enormous quantities are used. With such high doses, repetitive, nonproductive activity and hallucinatory and paranoid psychoses are common. It is classified by the DEA as a Schedule II controlled substance.

The adverse effects are those of the centrally acting sympathomimetics in general (see the general statement).

Dose—*Oral*, for *narcolepsy: adults* and *children over 12 yr, initially* **10 mg** 1 to 3 times a day (to be increased by increments of **5** to **10 mg** a day at weekly intervals up to **60 mg** a day), *except* **5** to **30 mg** once a day with *sustained-release* capsules; *children 6* to *12 yr*, **2.5 mg,** twice a day (to be increased by increments of 5 mg at weekly intervals until the desired wakefulness is achieved), *except* **5** to **15 mg** once a day with *sustained-release* capsules. For *attention deficit disorder: children 3* to *6 yr*, **2.5 mg** once a day (increased by increments of 2.5 mg at weekly intervals until the desired effect is achieved); *over 6 yr*, **5 mg** once or twice a day (increased by increments of 5 mg at weekly intervals until the desired effect is achieved), *except* **5** to **15 mg** once a day with sustained-release capsules. For *exogenous obesity, adults* and *children over 12 yr*, **5** to **10 mg** ½ to 1 hr before meals, *except* **10** to **15 mg** in the morning with sustained-release capsules.

Sustained-release capsules are not to be used to initiate treatment and should not be substituted for conventional dosage forms until the daily dose of the conventional form is equal to or exceeds the dosage provided by the sustained-release capsules.

Dosage Forms—Sustained-Release Capsules: 5, 10 and 15 mg; Elixir: 5 mg/5 mL; Tablets: 5 and 10 mg.

Diethylpropion Hydrochloride

Propanone, 2-(dimethylamino)-1-phenyl-, hydrochloride; Tenuate (*Lakeside*); Tepanil (*Riker*)

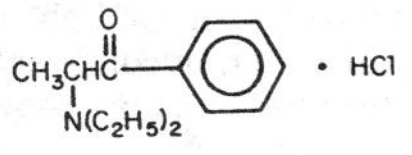

[134-80-5] $C_{13}H_{19}NO.HCl$ (241.76).

Preparation—*J Am Chem Soc 50:* 2287, 1928.

Description—White or creamy white, small crystals or crystalline powder; characteristic, mildly aromatic odor and stable in dry air; melts at about 175° with decomposition. White crystalline powder; although it has one chiral center, the dosage form is a racemic mixture.

Solubility—1 g in soluble in 0.5 mL of water or 3 mL of alcohol.

Uses—The CNS stimulatory actions of diethylpropion occur at considerably lower doses than do the cardiovascular actions. Thus, it is used only for its central effects. It is the safest anorexiant for use in hypertensive or anginal patients. Its anorexiant effects are relatively more prominent than with dextroamphetamine, so that it is used only in the treatment of *obesity*. The adverse effects and precautions are those of centrally acting sympathomimetics in general (see the general statement). It is a Schedule IV controlled substance.

Dose—*Oral, adults* and *children over 12 yr*, **25 mg** 3 times a day, 1 hr before each meal, or **75 mg** in *sustained-release* form in the morning; 25 mg may be taken midevening if insomnia is not a problem.

Dosage Forms—Extended-Release Tablets: 75 mg; Tablets: 25 mg.

Dipivefrin Hydrochloride

Propanoic Acid, (±)-2,2-dimethyl-, 4-[1-hydroxy-2-(methylamino)ethyl]-1,2-phenylene ester, hydrochloride; Propine (*Allergan*)

$(CH_3)_3CCOO$, $(CH_3)_3CCOO$–[benzene ring]–$CHCH_2NHCH_3$ (OH) · HCl

[64019-93-8] $C_{19}H_{29}NO_5$.HCl (387.90).

Preparation—By esterification of epinephrine under mildly basic conditions, with pivaloyl chloride (trimethylacetyl chloride); US Pat 4,085,270.

Description—White crystals melting about 158°.

Solubility—Soluble in water or alcohol.

Uses—Much more lipid-soluble than epinephrine; hence, it is 17 times as penetrant into the eye after topical application. Once into the eye, it is hydrolyzed to epinephrine, the active agent, which lowers intraocular pressure by increasing the outflow of aqueous humor. It is used in the treatment of *open-angle glaucoma*. After topical administration, the intraocular tension drops in about ½ hr and lasts about 12 hr.

The greater penetrance allows it to be used in a lower concentration than epinephrine. Furthermore, if it is absorbed systemically, epinephrine is generated only slowly, which greatly diminishes the peak plasma levels. Consequently, adverse effects are about 1/30 those of epinephrine. For this reason, it should become the epinephrine derivative of choice for use in the eye.

Dose—*Topical, to the conjunctiva, adults*, **1 drop** of a **0.1%** solution every 12 hr.

Dosage Form—Ophthalmic Solution: 0.1%.

Dobutamine Hydrochloride

1,2-Benzenediol, 4-[2-[[3-(4-hydroxyphenyl)-1-methylpropyl]amino]ethyl]-, hydrochloride, (±)-, Dobutrex (*Lilly*)

HO, HO–[benzene ring]–$(CH_2)_2NHCH(CH_3)(CH_2)_2$–[benzene ring]–OH · HCl

(±)-4-[2-[[3-(*p*-Hydroxyphenyl)-1-methylpropyl]amino]ethyl]pyrocatechol hydrochloride [49745-95-1] $C_{18}H_{23}NO_3$.HCl (337.85).

Preparation—For a summary of a patented process see *CA 80:* 14721z, 1974.

Description—White to off-white powder; melts at about 185°; pK_a (dobutamine) 9.4.

Solubility—Sparingly soluble in water or methanol; soluble in ethanol.

Uses—Has strong β_1- and weak β_2- and α-adrenoreceptor agonist activity. Its positive inotropic actions and effects to enhance atrioventricular and intraventricular conduction are more prominent than its positive chronotropic effects, so that with appropriately low doses (ie, less than 20 μg/kg/min) it increases cardiac output considerably but affects heart rate only slightly. Heart rate usually is increased by only 5 to 15 beats/min, and an increase of more than 30/min occurs in only 10% of patients. Therapeutic plasma concentrations lie between 40 and 190 ng/mL. Higher rates of infusion can cause substantial tachycardia. The net effect of β_2- and α-adrenergic vascular actions usually is a slight decrease in peripheral resistance. However, the increase in cardiac output compensates approximately for decreased peripheral resistance, so that blood pressure is affected mildly, tending to increase slightly with low doses and decrease slightly with high doses. In clinical use, arterial pressure usually rises only 10 to 20 torr and rises by as much as 50 torr in only 7.5% of patients. Tachyphylaxis to the actions on cardiac output usually does not occur, but there is sometimes a slight diminution in response.

The principal clinical use is in the short-term treatment of *low output acute heart failure*, such as that after myocardial infarction or after cardiopulmonary bypass surgery. In heart failure the drug increases cardiac output, decreases pulmonary artery wedge pressure and increases urine output. It more consistently lowers pulmonary artery wedge pressure than does dopamine, but it less consistently causes diuresis. It also is used to treat *hypovolemic* and *septic shock* following intravascular fluid replacement.

It is biotransformed very rapidly, mainly by catechol-*O*-methyltransferase, although some also is conjugated. The elimination half-life is only 2 min, so that the drug must be given by continuous intravenous infusion. After infusion is begun, the onset of action is 1 to 2 min; the effect requires 5 to 10 min to reach a steady state (plateau). However, in congestive cardiomyopathy the beneficial effects of a 48- to 72-hr infusion lasts from 4 to 8 wk!

It has been given safely in infusions lasting as long as 72 hr. Adverse effects other than usually mild hypertension and tachycardia (see above) occur in only 1 to 3% of patients. They include nausea, headache, palpitation, shortness of breath, anginal pain and nonspecific chest pain. Occasionally there is ectopic activity, mainly premature atrial and ventricular beats; other arrhythmias can occur. Because of facilitated AV conduction, the ventricular rate may be increased adversely in atrial fibrillation or flutter, and digitalis should be administered prior to dobutamine. The drug is contraindicated in idiopathic hypertropic subaortic stenosis. Thus far, few drug interactions are known. β-Adrenoreceptor-blocking drugs abolish the cardiac and vasodilator actions and unmask the vasoconstrictor effects. Sodium nitroprusside (and presumably any other vasodilator that decreases cardiac afterload substantially) enables a greater increase in cardiac output and decrease in pulmonary arterial wedge pressure. Neither reserpine, MAOIs nor tricyclic antidepressants affect the response to the drug. The safety of the drug in children is unknown.

Dose—*Intravenous, infusion, adult*, usually **2.5** to **10 μg/kg/min,** but occasionally as much as 40 μg/kg/min is required.

Dosage Form—For Injection: 250 mg/20 mL.

Dopamine Hydrochloride

1,2-Benzenediol, 4-(2-aminoethyl-, hydrochloride; Dopastat (*Warner-Chilcott*); Intropin (*Du Pont*)

HO, HO–[benzene ring]–$CH_2CH_2NH_2$ · HCl

3,4-Dihydroxyphenethylamine Hydrochloride [62-31-7] $C_8H_{11}NO_2$.HCl (189.64).

Preparation—Dopamine, which is 3-hydroxytyramine, may be prepared from tyramine by successive nitration to 3-nitrotyramine, reduction to 3-aminotyramine by catalytic hydrogenation and diazotization to 3-hydroxytyramine.

Description—White, crystalline powder; decomposes at about 241°; to avoid oxidation of the hydrochloride injection, the air in containers is replaced with nitrogen; yellow or brown discoloration of solutions indicates decomposition of the drug, and such solutions should not be used.

Solubility—Freely soluble in water; soluble in alcohol; practically insoluble in chloroform or ether.

Uses—The hydrochloride of a natural catecholamine formed by the decarboxylation of 3,4-dihydroxyphenylalanine (DOPA). It is a precursor to norepinephrine in noradrenergic nerves and is also itself a neurotransmitter in certain areas of the central nervous system, especially in the nigrostriatal tract. However, dopamine does not penetrate the blood-brain-barrier readily and therefore, does not produce CNS effects.

In the central nervous system and the splanchnic and renal vascular beds, it acts upon dopamine receptors that are distinct from α- and β-adrenoreceptors to cause vasodilatation. The renal vasodilatation causes diuresis. It also has moderate β_1- and weak α-agonist activities, part of which is attributable to norepinephrine released by dopamine. During a low rate of intravenous infusion, only vasodilatation in the splanchnic and renal vascular beds usually predominates, and hypotension sometimes occurs. At an intermediate rate of infusion, the heart rate and force of contraction are increased, as is cardiac output, and blood pressure may increase accordingly. At high rates of infusion (over 10 to 12 μg/kg/min), α-adrenoreceptor-mediated vasoconstriction occurs, and the blood pressure may rise substantially.

It is used in the treatment of *shock*, for which it has several advantages. Firstly, vasodilatation often can be effected in the two organs most likely to suffer ischemic damage in shock (kidney and small bowel); blood may be moved from the skeletal muscle to more vital organs, cardiac stimulation improves a usually deteriorated cardiac function and diuresis also helps to preserve the renal tubules. Although dopamine is now the vasopressor agent of choice in shock, a substantial fraction of cases, nevertheless, fail to respond. It also is used to treat *acute heart failure;* the decreased vascular resistance decreases the cardiac afterload, the cardiostimulatory actions improve cardiac output and the diuresis lessens edema.

The adverse effects, precautions and drug interactions are those expected from a β_1- and α-agonist (see the general statement). Hypotension, when it occurs, is not necessarily adverse, so long as the critical organs are perfused adequately. It usually can be counteracted by increasing the rate of infusion; if not, another pressor agent will be required. Haloperidol-like drugs suppress the vasodilator actions. It also causes nausea by a dopaminergic action at the chemoreceptor trigger zone.

The onset of action following intravenous administration occurs within 5 min, and the duration of action is less than 10 min, but in patients receiving MAOIs the duration of action may be prolonged to 1 hr. Dopamine should be used cautiously in patients taking MAOIs.

Dose—*Intravenous infusion, initially* **0.5** to **5 μg/kg/min,** to be increased at 10- to 30-min intervals until the desired blood pressure is achieved; the effective rate usually does not exceed 15 mg per kg/min, but more than 50 μg/kg/min occasionally are required; if so, urine output should be monitored. To improve response, the patient should be volume-repleted, if appropriate, to a central venous pressure of 10 to 15 cm of water or a pulmonary arterial wedge pressure of 14 to 18 torr. The safety and efficacy of this drug in children has not been established.

Dosage Forms—for Injection: 0.8, 1.6, 40, 80 and 160 mg/mL; in 5% Dextrose Injection: 200, 400 and 800 mg/250 mL and 200, 400 and 800 mg/500 mL.

Ephedrine Sulfate

Benzenemethanol, [*R*-(*R**,*S**)]-α-[1-(methylamino)ethyl]-, sulfate (2:1) (salt); (*Various Mfrs*)

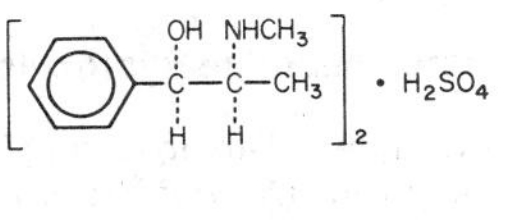

(−)-Ephedrine sulfate (2:1) (salt) [134-72-5] $(C_{10}H_{15}NO)_2.H_2SO_4$ (428.54).

Preparation—First obtained by Nagai in 1887 from a Chinese herb, *ma huang*, ephedrine is related structurally to epinephrine. Ephedrine may be obtained by alkalinizing powdered *ma huang* with milk of lime or sodium carbonate solution, and extracting the base with alcohol or benzene. It is now, however, almost exclusively produced by synthetic methods. The most economic process (Neuberg) for synthetic production commences with fermentation of a mixture of benzaldehyde and molasses to form the ketoalcohol, $C_6H_5CH(OH)COCH_3$, which is hydrogenated in a methylamine solution. The keto group is thereby reduced to —CHOH— which condenses with the methylamine.

Description—Fine, white, odorless crystals or a powder; affected by light; aqueous solution practically neutral to litmus; rotation −30.5° to −32.5°.

Solubility—1 g in about 1.3 mL water or about 90 mL alcohol; insoluble in ether.

Incompatibilities—See *Ephedrine Hydrochloride.*

Uses—In ordinary doses it acts *indirectly* through release of norepinephrine from adrenergic nerves. In higher doses it has a direct sympathomimetic action. It easily penetrates membranes and the brain, and, hence, has CNS-stimulatory actions which, however, are not as prominent as those of the amphetamines.

Although it mainly acts indirectly through the release of norepinephrine, its peripheral effects are as though it possessed weak α-agonist activity, except that it acts rather strongly on the trigone sphincter, and has moderate β_1- and β_2-agonist activity, although the β_2-activity is limited to the bronchioles. It once was used mainly as a *bronchodilator* in asthma, for which it usually is combined with theophylline; however, albuterol and other more selective, orally effective bronchodilators have made ephedrine almost obsolete in this use. It will continue to be useful in the nonemergency, outpatient treatment of Adams-Stokes syndrome. It is used occasionally to treat *enuresis.* The weak vascular α-activity actually may have some advantages in the support of blood pressure during spinal anesthesia and in other nonshock hypotensions, since the weak vasoconstrictor effects may result in less ischemic damage than with stronger α-agonists; the moderate cardiac stimulation is beneficial. The weak vasoconstrictor effects also lend themselves to the ambulatory management of various *allergic conditions*, ephedrine being safer to use than stronger α-agonists; in allergic emergencies, it is inferior to epinephrine. The only central nervous use of historic interest was in the treatment of *narcolepsy.*

It is resistant to MAO and thus is efficacious orally. By the oral route, its duration of action is 2 to 3 hr. The half-life is about 6 hr, but when the urine is alkaline, it is longer; when acidic, it is shorter. Although it is not a substrate of MAO, it is said that MAOIs may cause a hypertensive crisis in response to otherwise safe doses; therefore, caution is indicated. For other potential adverse effects and precautions, see the general statement.

As a rule, salts of ephedrine are employed instead of the free base.

Dose—*Oral, adults,* **25** to **50 mg** every 3 to 4 hr; *children,* **3 mg/kg/day** (or **100 mg/m²/day**) in 4 to 6 divided doses. *Intravenous, adults,* **5** to **25 mg** *slowly,* repeated in 5 to 10 min, if necessary, up to a limit of 150 mg a day. *Intramuscular* or *subcutaneous, adults,* **25** to **50 mg,** repeated, if necessary, up to a limit of 150 mg a day; *children,* **126** to **748 μg/kg** (or **4.2** to **25 mg/m²**) every 4 to 6 hr for no more than 3 or 4 consecutive days. *Topical, intranasal, adults* and *children over 6 yr,* **2** to **3 drops** of a **0.5** to **3%** solution or a **small amount** of **0.6%** jelly into each nostril every 4 hr.

Dosage Forms—Capsules: 25 and 50 mg; Injection: 25 and 50 mg/mL: Topical Jelly: 0.6%; Topical Solution: 0.5, 1 and 3%; Syrup: 11 and 20 mg/5 mL; Tablets: 7.5 mg (with 0.15 mg atropine sulfate).

Epinephrine

1,2-Benzenediol, (*R*)-4-[1-hydroxy-2-(methylamino)ethyl]-, Adrenaline; Suprarenalin; Nephridine; Adrenalin (*Parke-Davis*) (*Various Mfrs*)

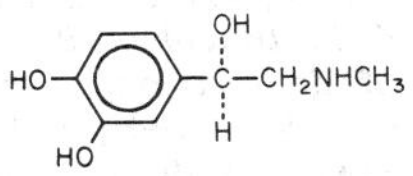

(−)-3,4-Dihydroxy-α-[(methylamino)methyl]benzyl alcohol [51- 43-4] $C_9H_{13}NO_3$ (183.21).

Preparation—By several processes, one of these starts with catechol (1,2-dihydroxybenzene), which is converted successively to (chloroacetyl)catechol with chloroacetyl chloride, then to (methyl- aminoacetyl)catechol with methylamine, and to racemic epinephrine by hydrogenation. The racemic form is resolved with D-tartaric acid.

Description—White to nearly white, microcrystalline, odorless powder, gradually darkening on exposure to light and air; combines with acids, forming salts that are readily soluble in water, and from these solutions the base may be precipitated by ammonia water or by alkali carbonates; solutions are alkaline to litmus; pK_a (apparent) 5.5.

Solubility—Very slightly soluble in water or alcohol; insoluble in ether, chloroform or fixed or volatile oils.

Incompatibilities—Solutions usually are prepared with the aid of HCl, and an acid reaction is essential to the stability of such solutions not only because of possible precipitation but also because of the possibility of rapid oxidation to inert products. Oxidation generally is evidenced by development of a pink to brown color. Air, light, heat and alkalies promote deterioration. Solutions buffered to a pH of 4.2 and containing a suitable antioxidant such as 0.1% sodium metabisulfite are stable for prolonged periods of time if protected from light, heat and undue exposure to air. *Metals,* notably *copper, iron* and *zinc,* destroy its activity.

Uses—Epinephrine is the predominant sympathomimetic in the adrenal medulla. It is liberated in conditions of stress and vigorous exertion. It possesses all of strong α_1-, α_2-, β_1- and β_2-agonist activities (see the general statement). The β-adrenoreceptors respond to lower concentrations than the α-receptors, so that with low doses or low intravenous infusion rates it is possible to stimulate the heart and relax bronchioles and at the same time decrease the diastolic blood pressure; however, the vasoconstrictor effect is stronger than the vasodilator effect, so that at higher doses there is a net increase in vascular resistance, and extreme hypertensive crises can occur with overdoses. The uses are those of α- and β_1-agonists (see the general statement). Only the outstanding uses and failures require comment here.

It is the drug of choice in the management of allergic emergencies, such as *anaphylaxis, angioneurotic edema, giant urticaria* and *serum sickness.* Despite new selective β_2-bronchodilators, epinephrine still is used in the treatment of *status asthmaticus;* the vasoconstrictor activity assists the bronchodilator actions through a reduction in bronchiolar stiffness by decreasing edema and diminishing bronchiolar secretions, and α_2-agonist activity suppresses vagal activity in the bronchioles. In chronic use as a bronchodilator, refractoriness often develops. It has a poor record in the treatment of shock (very intense splanchnic and renal vasoconstriction and metabolic acidosis), and in general should not be used to support blood pressure. As a topical decongestant it causes too much aftercongestion to be a first-choice drug. In *cardiac arrest*, epinephrine is an excellent resuscitant, but the concomitant vasoconstriction places an unwanted load on a compromised heart. It penetrates into the eye poorly from both blood stream and cornea, but high concentrations may be used to increase the outflow of the aqueous humor in *primary open-angle glaucoma;* it is used often in combination with a miotic and a carbonic anhydrase inhibitor. It is an excellent *styptic* because of both its local vasoconstrictor effects and the coagulant effects of its oxidation product, adrenochrome. It frequently is added to local anesthetic solutions to prolong their duration and to reduce their systemic toxicities. Such combinations should not be used for injections at digits, ears or penis where blood perfusion could be halted, thereby causing tissue necrosis.

The adverse effects of epinephrine are those of a strong α-, β_1- and β_2-agonist (see general statement).

Epinephrine is destroyed by MAO, catechol-*O*-methyltransferase, and is conjugated during its passage through the liver; consequently, oral dosage is ineffective. The plasma half-life of epinephrine is about 2.5 min. However, by the subcutaneous and intramuscular routes, local vasoconstriction retards absorption, so that the effects last much longer than the half-life would predict.

Note: Do not use any epinephrine preparation if it is brown or pink in color or contains a precipitate; a hallucinatory reaction may occur.

Dose—*Intravenous, adult,* **100 μg** to **250 μg** of the *diluted* injection *very slowly* for *vasopression,* repeated at 5- to 15-min intervals as needed, or **100 μg** to **1 mg** for *anaphylaxis* or *cardiac stimulation; children,* for *cardiac stimulation,* **5** to **10 μg/kg** (or **150** to **300 μg/m²**), and, for *anaphylaxis,* **300 μg** repeated at 15-min intervals for 3 or 4 doses, if necessary. *Intramuscular, adult, for anaphylaxis,* **200** to **500 μg** followed by 25 to 50 μg intravenously every 5 to 15 min, as needed, and, for *hypoglycemia* **300 μg** once; *children,* **300 μg,** repeated every 15 min for 3 or 4 doses, as needed, and for hypoglycemia, **10 μg/kg** (or 300 μg/m²) **200 μg** (0.2 mg) to **1 mg,** repeated as needed. *Subcutaneous* or *intramuscular, adult* and *children over 12 yr,* for *bronchodilatation, initially* **300** to **500 μg** of the *injection,* repeated at 20-min to 4-hour intervals, if necessary, *or initially* **500 μg** of the *Sterile Suspension (subcutaneous, only!),* repeated with doses of **up to 1.5 mg** at 4-hr intervals or longer if necessary; the duration of action of the Injection is 15 to 30 min and the Sterile Suspension up to 10 hr; *children 1 mo to 12 yr, initially* **10 μg/kg** (or **300 μg/m²**) of the injection, repeated every 20 min to 4 hr, if necessary, with up to **25 μg/kg,** except that no single dose should exceed 500 μg, or **25 μg/kg** (or **625 μg/m²**) of sterile suspension, repeated, if necessary, at intervals no less than 6 hr, no single dose to exceed 750 μg in a child weighing less than 30 kg. *Intracardiac, adult,* as the diluted *Injection,* **100 μg** to **1 mg,** repeated every 5 min, if necessary; *children under 6 yr,* **5** to **10 μg/kg** (or **300 μg/m²**), repeated every 15 min for 2 doses, then every 4 hr as needed. *Intraspinal, adults* and *children,* in combination with a local anesthetic, **200** to **400 μg,** to be added to the local anesthetic mixture. *Infiltration,* in combination with a local anesthetic, 1:100,000 to 1:20,000. *Oral Inhalation, adult* and *children over 6 yr,* as the *Inhalation Aerosol,* **200 μg** (1 metered spray), repeated in 2 or 3 min, if necessary, and not more frequently than every 4 hr, thereafter, *or,* as the *Inhalation,* **1** to **2 sprays** of a **1%** solution of the *levo* form or **1.25%** or **2.25%** of the racemic form, repeated in 1 to 2 min, if necessary, then as required thereafter; inhalation doses for children over 6 yr must be individualized. *Topical, intranasal,* as a **0.1%** solution as needed; *topical, conjunctiva, adults* and *children,* for *glaucoma,* **1 drop** of a **0.5** to **2%** solution 1 to 2 times a day, and, for *mydriasis* and *ocular hemostasis,* **1 drop** of a **1%** solution for 1 to 3 doses, as needed. For topical application in operative procedures on the nose and throat, solutions of 0.002 to 0.05% freshly prepared from the 0.1% Injection may be used.

All doses of *levo*-forms are as the equivalent of *levo*-epinephrine; the actual ingredient may be the bitartrate, hydrochloride, sulfate or other salt.

Dosage Forms—Inhalation: 1%; Inhalation Aerosol: 0.5% (200 and 270 μg per metered spray); Injection: 10 μg/mL, 100 μg/mL, 1 mg/mL; Nasal Solution: 0.1%, nonsterile; Ophthalmic Solution: 0.1, 0.25, 0.5, 1, 1.1 and 2%; Sterile Suspension: 5 mg/mL.

Epinephrine Bitartrate

1,2-Benzenediol, (*R*)-,4-[1-hydroxy-2-(methylamino)ethyl]-, [*R*-(*R**,*R*)]-2,3-dihydroxybutanedioate (1:1) (salt); Adrenaline Bitartrate BP (*Various Mfrs*)

(−)-3,4-Dihydroxy-α-[(methylamino)methyl]benzyl alcohol (+)-tartrate (1:1) salt [51-42-3] $C_9H_{13}NO_3.C_4H_6O_6$ (333.29).

For the structure of the base, see *Epinephrine.*

Preparation—By reacting epinephrine with an equimolar portion of tartaric acid and precipitating by the addition of alcohol.

Description—White, grayish white, or light brownish gray crystalline powder; odorless; slowly darkens on exposure to air and light; melting range 147° to 152° with decomposition; pH (1% solution) 3.5.

Solubility—1 g in about 3 mL water or about 500 mL alcohol; practically insoluble in chloroform or ether.

Uses—Supplied only for use in *bronchial asthma, scleroconjunctival inflammation* and *open-angle glaucoma.* For actions, uses, adverse effects, etc, see *Epinephrine.*

Dose—*Topical, adult,* to the *conjunctiva,* **1 drop** of the equivalent of a **0.25** to **2%** epinephrine (free base) solution once every 3 days to 2 times a day. *Oral inhalation, adult* and *children over 6 yr,* **160 μg** as the base equivalent (1 metered spray), to be repeated in 1 min if necessary, and at intervals no shorter than 4 hr thereafter; the dose for children under 6 yr must be individualized.

Dosage Forms—Aerosol: Inhalation Aerosol: 300 μg (equivalent to 160 μg of base) per metered spray; Ophthalmic Solution: 0.25, 0.5, 1, 1.1 and 2%, epinephrine base equivalent; for Ophthalmic Solution: 55 mg base equivalent, to be constituted to 1.1%.

Epinephryl Borate Ophthalmic Solution

1,3,2-Benzodioxaborole-5-methanol, (*R*)-2-hydroxy-α-[(methylamino)-methyl]-, Epinal (*Alcon*); Eppy/N (*Barnes-Hind*)

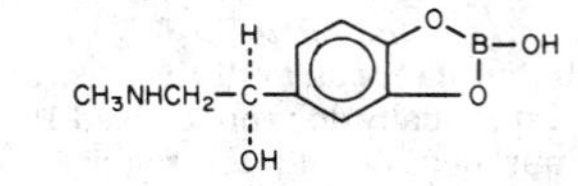

(−)-3,4-Dihydroxy-α-[(methylamino)methyl]benzyl alcohol, cyclic 3,4-ester with boric acid [5579-16-8] $C_9H_{12}BNO_4$ (209.01).

Preparation—Reported to be a 1:1 chelate formed in aqueous medium between boric acid and epinephrine (*J Pharm Sci 51:* 206, 1962). US Pat 3,149,035.

Uses—A preparation for ophthalmologic uses only. For actions, uses, adverse effects, etc, see *Epinephrine.*

Dose—*Topical,* to the *conjunctiva,* **0.1 mL** of the equivalent of a **0.25** to **2%** epinephrine solution 2 times a day.

Dosage Form—Ophthalmic Solution: 0.25, 0.5, 1 and 2%, epinephrine base equivalent.

Ethylnorepinephrine Hydrochloride

1,2-Benzenediol, 4-(2-amino-1-hydroxybutyl)-, hydrochloride; Bronkephrine (*Sanofi Winthrop*)

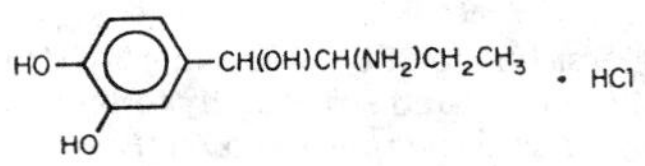

[3198-07-0] $C_{10}H_{15}NO_3.HCl$ (233.70).

Preparation—By the procedure for *epinephrine* (page 990), using ethyl amine in place of methyl amine.

Description—Crystalline substance; decompose about 200°. Darkens on exposure to light.

Solubility—Soluble in water.

Uses—Possesses moderate α-, β_1-, and β_2-agonist activities. Its only use is as a *bronchodilator,* having about one-tenth the potency of isoproterenol. The α- and β-activities often roughly balance each other with respect to blood pressure but the distribution of blood flow is altered unfavorably. For actions, uses, adverse effects, precautions and drug interactions, see the general statement.

Dose—*Subcutaneous* or *intramuscular, adults,* **0.6** to **2 mg;** *children,* **0.2** to **1 mg.** In an *emergency,* by slow *intravenous injection,* **1** to **5 mg.**

Dosage Form—Injection: 2 mg/1 mL.

Fenfluramine Hydrochloride

Benzeneethaneamine, *N*-ethyl-α-methyl-3-(trifluoromethyl)-, hydrochloride; Pondimin (*Robins*)

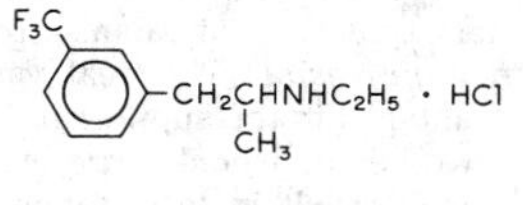

N-Ethyl-α-methyl-*m*-(trifluoromethyl)phenethylamine hydrochloride [404-82-0] $C_{12}H_{16}F_3N.HCl$ (267.12).

Preparation—From α,α,α-trifluoro-*m*-tolualdehyde, which is condensed with nitroethane; the 1-nitroethylidene group reduced to the α-aminoethyl, then acetylated to the amide and reduced to fenfluramine. French Pat M1658.

Description—White, amorphous powder with a characteristic odor; melts 165 to 170°; pK_a 9.92.

Solubility—Sparingly soluble in water.

Uses—An anorexiant that differs from most other sympathomimetic anorexiants in not stimulating the central nervous system in the majority of users; instead, it usually exerts a mild sedative action. It appears to have a low drug-abuse potential; it is a Schedule IV controlled substance. Doses of 80 to 400 mg can cause euphoria, derealization and perceptual changes in persons with a history of drug abuse. It does not affect REM sleep during use, but insomnia may occur after withdrawal. Depression of mood has been noted in some patients after discontinuation of treatment with the drug. Unlike most sympathomimetic-related anorexiants, tolerance does not appear to develop, and after 6 to 8 wk of treatment the body weight reaches a plateau that is relatively stable for at least another 16 wk. Although weight loss is sometimes dramatic, with usual dosage and without strict dietary regulation, the loss averages only about 6 lb; the most obese patients tend to be those experiencing the smallest loss. When caloric intake is restricted by a deliberate program, it enables the patient to endure the restrictions, and weight losses greater than those on an unrestricted diet can be achieved. On an unrestricted diet, the drug appears to be no more effective than dextroamphetamine in the early stages of management. It differs from dextroamphetamine in its mechanism of action since it induces a selective release and depletion of serotonin from central serotonergic neurons. With therapeutic doses, it appears to lack sympathomimetic cardiovascular actions; in fact, it appears to exert a masked inhibitory action on the sympathetic nervous system, since the drug increases the action of antihypertensive drugs.

In high doses, it can cause an increase in blood pressure, tachycardia and palpitations. It causes side effects in 2 to 20 times as many patients as does dextroamphetamine, the ratio depending on the particular effect. Drowsiness occurs in 67% of patients, gastrointestinal effects (nausea, diarrhea, constipation, abdominal discomfort, other), in about 37%, dry mouth in about 26%, insomnia in 22%, dizziness in 18%, headache in 15% and skin rashes in about 3%. In children especially, urinary frequency and incontinence also occur. It should be used cautiously when methyldopa, oral hypoglycemics or reserpine also is used.

Dose—*Oral, adults* and *children over 12 yr, initially* **20 mg** 3 times a day, 30 min to 1 hr before each meal, with increments of 20 mg a day, if necessary, up to a maximum daily dose of 40 mg. If the drug initially is tolerated poorly, one dose a day may be temporarily dropped, and the dose gradually increased thereafter.

Dosage Form—Tablets: 20 mg.

Fenoldopam—see RPS-18, page 888.

Fenoterol—see RPS-18, page 888.

Hydroxyamphetamine Hydrobromide

Phenol, 4-(2-aminopropyl)-, hydrobromide; Paredrine (*Pharmics*)

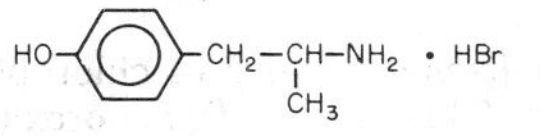

(±)-*p*-(2-Aminopropyl)phenol hydrobromide [306-21-8] C_9H_{13}-NO.HBr (232.12).

Preparation—Among other methods, by reducing *p*-methoxybenzyl methyl ketoxime followed by hydrolysis of the methoxy group with mineral acids. The free base then may be liberated with alkali, and, after extraction, converted into the salt by treatment with hydrobromic acid.

Description—White, crystalline powder; solutions are slightly acid to litmus, having a pH of about 5; melting range 189° to 192°.

Solubility—1 g in about 1 mL water or about 2.5 mL alcohol; slightly soluble in chloroform; insoluble in ether.

Uses—An indirect sympathomimetic, the actions of which are both α- and β_1-agonist in nature; it is essentially devoid of CNS activity. It is used topically as a *mydriatic*, as a *diagnostic* agent in *Horner's syndrome* and as a *provocative agent* for tests of *narrow-angle-closure glaucoma*. Mydrasis lasts several hours.

Although it shares the general properties of other sympathomimetic amines, it also presents some interesting anomalies. The drug does not cause vasoconstriction when injected intradermally; consequently, it does not prolong the duration of action of local anesthetics. In addition, its actions on the bronchi and gastrointestinal tract are of low intensity. For the adverse effects and precautions, see the general statement.

Dose—*Topical*, to the *conjunctiva*, **1** or **2 drops** of a **1%** solution, repeated as necessary.

Dosage Form—Ophthalmic Solution: 1%.

Isoetharine Hydrochloride

1,2-Benzenediol, 4-[1-hydroxy-2-[(1-methylethyl)amino]butyl]-, hydrochloride; *N*-isopropylethylnorepinephrine hydrochloride; Bronkosol (*Sanofi Winthrop*); Arm-a-Med (*Astra*)

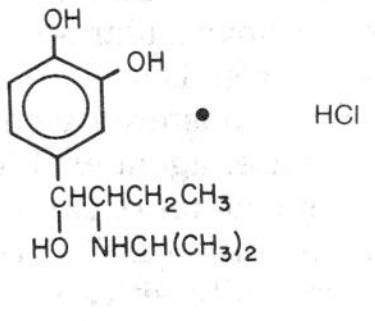

3,4-Dihydroxy-α-[1-(isopropylamino)propyl]benzyl alcohol hydrochloride $C_{13}H_{21}NO_3.HCl$ [2576-92-3] (275.77).

Preparation—Synthesis of isoetharine and other 1-(3,4-dihydroxyphenyl)-2-monoalkyl-1-butanols, starting with 3,4-dihydroxybutyrophenone, is described in German Pat 638,650 (*CA 31:* 3209[4], 1937). The base is converted to the hydrochloride or the mesylate (below).

Description—White to off-white, crystalline solid; odorless; melts between 196 and 208° with decomposition.

Solubility—Soluble in water; sparingly soluble in alcohol; practically insoluble in ether.

Uses—Possesses moderate α-, β_1- and β_2-agonist activities (see the general statement for actions, uses, adverse effects, precautions and drug interactions). It is used only as a *bronchodilator*, mainly for *intermittent bronchospasm*. The duration of action is less than 1 hr. It is administered by inhalation; abroad it also is used orally in sustained-release tablets formulated with a porous plastic base.

Dose—*Adult, inhalation*, by hand nebulizer, **3** to **7 inhalations** of a **1%** solution; by *oxygen aerosolization* (oxygen flow 4 to 6 L/min) or *intermittent positive pressure breathing* (1 ppb; inspiratory flow 15 L/min), **4 mL** of a **0.125%** solution, **2.5 mL** of a **0.2%** solution, **2 mL** of a **0.25%** solution, **0.5** to **1 mL** of a **0.5%** solution (dilute to 3 mL), and **0.25** to **0.5 mL** of a **1%** solution (dilute 1:3, ie, to 0.75 to 1.5 mL.

Dosage Form—Solution for Nebulization: 0.062, 0.08, 0.1, 0.125, 0.167, 0.17, 0.2, 0.25 and 1%.

Isoetharine Mesylate

1,2-Benzenediol, 4-[1-hydroxy-2-[(1-methylethyl)amino]butyl]-, methanesulfonate (salt); *N*-isopropylethylnorepinephrine methanesulfonate; Bronkometer (*Sanofi Winthrop*)

For the formula of isoetharine base, see *Isoetharine Hydrochloride*.

3,4-Dihydroxy-α-[1-(isopropylamino)propyl]benzyl alcohol methanesulfonate [7279-75-6] $C_{13}H_{21}NO_3.CH_4O_3S$ (335.41).

Preparation—See *Isoetharine Hydrochloride*.

Description—White to off-white, crystalline solid; odorless; slightly bitter, salty taste; melts at about 165°.

Solubility—Freely soluble in water; soluble in alcohol; very slightly soluble in ether.

Uses—See *Isoetharine Hydrochloride*.

Dose—*Oral inhalation, adults*, **340 μg** (1 metered dose), to be repeated after 1 or 2 min, if necessary.

Dosage Form—Aerosol: 0.61% (340 μg/metered dose).

Isoproterenol Hydrochloride

1,2-Benzenediol, 4-[1-hydroxy-2-[(1-methylethyl)amino]ethyl]-, hydrochloride; Isopropylarterenol Hydrochloride; (*Various Mfrs*)

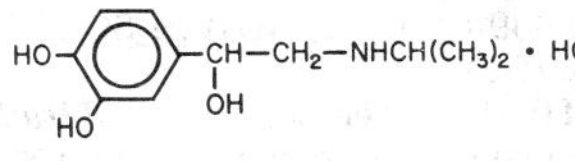

3,4-Dihydroxy-α-[(isopropylamino)methyl]benzyl alcohol hydrochloride [51-30-9] $C_{11}H_{17}NO_3.HCl$ (247.72).

Preparation—By the synthetic procedure given for *Epinephrine* (page

989), using isopropylamine in place of methylamine; the base is then converted to the hydrochloride without resolution.

Description—White to nearly white, odorless, crystalline powder, having a slightly bitter taste; gradually darkens on exposure to air and light; solutions become pink to brownish pink on standing exposed to air, and almost immediately so when rendered alkaline; pH (1% aqueous solution) about 5; melting range between 165 and 170°.

Solubility—1 g in 3 mL water or 50 mL alcohol; less soluble in dehydrated alcohol; insoluble in chloroform or ether.

Uses—A close congener of epinephrine; it has strong β_1- and β_2-agonist activities but lacks α-activity (see the general statement). Its primary use is in the treatment of *bronchial asthma,* for which it supplanted epinephrine, but it in turn is being supplanted by metaproterenol and other selective β_2-agonists. It is administered mostly by oral inhalation for this purpose, the cardiovascular side effects being much more prominent by other routes. It also is used to treat bronchospasm during anesthesia. It sometimes is administered in combination with phenylephrine, vasoconstriction by the latter agent enabling a decrease in bronchial edema and secretions. The incidence of side effects by systemic routes is over 30% but by inhalation, less than 10%. However, sudden death has occurred after inhalation, especially with aerosols. This has been attributed to the combination of a cardiotoxic action of the fluorocarbon propellant and the arrhythmiagenic action of isoproterenol, but it may also be, in part, the ease of overdosing. The incidence of sudden death has decreased dramatically after dosage metering was initiated. Chronic use occasionally results in an increase in airway resistance. Isoproterenol has been used to treat *ventricular bradycardia* and in the prophylaxis of *cardiac standstill,* but it has been displaced largely by more cardioselective sympathomimetics. In the treatment of *shock* it occasionally improves cardiovascular function, but it also sometimes worsens the condition. For the adverse effects and precautions of β-agonists, see the general statement.

Bioavailability by the oral route is poor. It is somewhat less erratic by the sublingual and rectal routes. The duration of action by the sublingual and subcutaneous routes is 1 to 2 hr; by inhalation, it is 30 to 60 min.

Note—Do not use any dosage form of isoproterenol hydrochloride if it is brown in color or contains a precipitate.

Dose—*Oral inhalation, metered aerosol, adult* and *children,* **120** or **131 μg** as a metered spray, followed by a second dose in 1 to 5 min, if necessary, and repeated up to 4 to 6 times a day (ie, no more than 6 inhalations in any 1 hr in a 24-hr period) for *asthma* or at intervals no shorter than 3 to 4 hr for *chronic obstructive pulmonary disease:* more than 3 applications a day require medical supervision. *Oral inhalation, hand nebulization, adults* and *children,* **5** to **15 sprays** of **0.5%** or **3** to **7 sprays** of **1%** solution, followed by a second dose in 5 to 10 min, if necessary, repeated up to 5 times a day; *compressed air* or *oxygen nebulization,* **2 mL** of a **0.125%** solution or **2.5 mL** of a **0.1%** solution delivered over a 15- to 20-min period up to 5 times a day. *Sublingual, adult,* for *bronchodilatation,* **10** to **15 mg** 3 to 4 times a day; for *bradydysrhythmias, initially* **10 mg,** followed by **5** to **50 mg** as necessary; for *carotid sinus syndrome,* **10** to **30 mg** 4 to 6 times a day; *children,* for *bronchodilatation,* **5** to **10 mg** 3 times a day; for *heart block, initially* **5 mg,** subsequent doses determined by response. *Intracardiac, adult,* **20 μg,** repeated as needed. *Intravenous, adult,* **20** to **60 μg,** followed by **10** to **200 μg** as necessary. *Intravenous infusion, adult,* **0.5** to **5 μg** per min, the rate adjusted to maintain the desired blood pressure (solution usually contains 2 mg/500 mL, but 1 to 10 mg in 500 mL of 5% dextrose injection). *Intramuscular, adult, initially* **200 μg** (0.2 mg), followed by **20 μg** to **1 mg,** as necessary. *Rectal,* for *bradydysrhythmias, initially* **5 mg,** repeated as necessary. *Subcutaneous, adult, initially* **200 μg,** followed by **150** to **200 μg,** as necessary. Unstated pediatric doses must be individualized.

Dosage Forms—Inhalation Aerosol: 0.25% (120 or 131 μg per metered dose); Solution for Nebulization: 0.25, 0.5 and 1%; Injection: 200 μg/mL and 1 mg/5 mL; Sublingual Tablets: 10 and 15 mg.

Isoproterenol Sulfate

1,2-Benzenediol, 4-[1-hydroxy-2-[(1-methylethyl)amino]ethyl]-, sulfate (2:1) (salt), dihydrate; Isopropylarterenol Sulfate; Medihaler-Iso (*Riker*); Norisodrine Aerotrol (*Abbott*)

3,4-Dihydroxy-α-[(isopropylamino)methyl]benzyl alcohol sulfate (2:1) (salt) dihydrate [6700-39-6] $(C_{11}H_{17}NO_3)_2.H_2SO_4.2H_2O$ (556.62); *anhydrous* [299-95-6] (520.59).

For the structure of the base, see *Isoproterenol Hydrochloride.*

Preparation—An alcoholic solution of 2-chloro-3′,4′-dihydroxyacetophenone is condensed with isopropylamine. The 3′,4′- dihydroxy-2-(isopropylamino)acetophenone formed is isolated as the sulfate and its carbonyl group is reduced to a carbinol by catalytic hydrogenation.

Description—White to nearly white, odorless, crystalline powder, having a slightly bitter taste; gradually darkens on exposure to air and light; solutions become pink to brownish pink on standing exposed to air, and almost immediately so when rendered alkaline; pH (1 in 100 solution) about 5; melting range 125° to 129°.

Solubility—1 g in 4 mL water; very slightly soluble in alcohol, benzene, or ether.

Uses—See *Isoproterenol Hydrochloride.* The sulfate is used only as a bronchodilator.

Dose—*Oral inhalation, adults* and *children,* **1 metered spray** (80 μg); a second dose may be given 2 to 5 min later, if necessary, 4 to 6 times a day; no more than 6 doses should be given in any 1 hr during a 24-hr period.

Dosage Form—Aerosol Solution: 2 mg/mL (80 μg per metered spray).

Isoxsuprine Hydrochloride

Benzenemethanol, 4-hydroxy-α-[1-[1-methyl-2-phenoxyethyl)amino)ethyl]-, hydrochloride; Vasodilan (*Mead Johnson*)

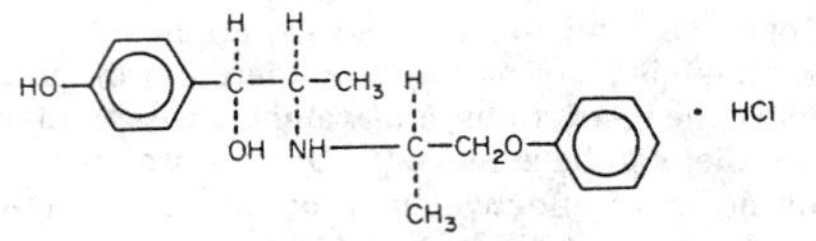

[579-56-6] $C_{18}H_{23}NO_3.HCl$ (337.85).

Preparation—Phenoxyacetone (from sodium phenoxide and chloroacetone), on reductive amination, yields 1-phenoxy-2-aminopropane (**I**). Sodium *p*-propionylphenoxide is converted to the ether with benzyl bromide, to protect the phenolic group; brominated α to the carbonyl and then condensed with **I**. The resulting secondary aminoketone is catalytically hydrogenated to remove the protective benzyl group, the carbonyl reduced to the secondary alcohol with $NaBH_4$ and the base converted to the salt. *Rec Trav Chim 75:* 1215 (1956).

Description—White, crystalline powder; odorless; bitter taste; melts with decomposition at about 200°; pH (1 in 100 solution) between 4.5 and 6.0.

Solubility—1 g in 500 mL water, 100 mL alcohol, > 10,000 mL chloroform or > 10,000 mL ether.

Uses—A β-agonist with a slight selectivity for the β_2-adrenoreceptors. However, a considerable portion of the vasodilator actions are attributable to a nonselective depression of vascular smooth muscle. It is considered to be "possibly effective" in Raynaud's disease, thromboangiitis obliterans, obliterative arteriosclerosis and cerebrovascular insufficiency. In the management of premature labor, it has been superseded by more selective β-agonists. See the general statement for the actions adverse effects and precautions of β-agonists.

Dose—*Oral, adult,* **10** to **20 mg,** 3 or 4 times a day. *Intramuscular, adult,* **5** to **10 mg** 2 to 3 times a day.

Dosage Form—Tablets: 10 and 20 mg.

Levonordefrin—see RPS-18, page 886.

Mazindol

3*H*-Imidazo[2,1-*a*]isoindol-5-ol, 5-(4-chlorophenyl-2,5-dihydro-, Mazanor (*Wyeth-Ayerst*); Sanorex (*Sandoz*)

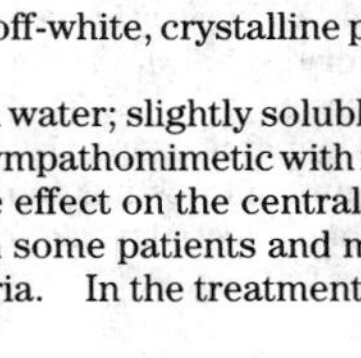

[22232-71-9] $C_{19}H_{13}ClN_2O$ (284.74).

Preparation—By catalytic condensation/addition of 2-(*p*-chlorobenzoyl)benzoic acid and ethylenediamine.

Description—White to off-white, crystalline powder; odorless or with a faint odor.

Solubility—Insoluble in water; slightly soluble in alcohol.

Uses—An *anorexiant* sympathomimetic with relatively weak cardiovascular actions and a variable effect on the central nervous system, causing signs of mild stimulation in some patients and mild depression in others. It causes little or no euphoria. In the treatment of obesity with mazindol about two-thirds of patients on a diet of 600 cal/day can adhere to the diet for over 12 wk, which appears to be a better response than with any other anorexiant. Tolerance to mazindol is of a low order, and the abuse potential appears to be less than with most centrally acting sympathomimetics. It is a Schedule IV controlled substance. The side effects, precautions and drug interactions are those of other centrally acting sympathomimetics (see general statement), but some effects, such as drowsiness (20% of patients) and moderate hypotension, differ. Reduction in blood pressure may be secondary to weight loss. Insulin requirements may change, mostly as a result of changed diet. Nausea occurs in about 10% of users.

Dose—*Oral, adults* and *children over 12 yr;* **2 mg** once a day with the first meal, or **1 mg** 3 times a day, 1 hr before each meal. Administration with food diminishes gastrointestinal intolerance.

Dosage Form—Tablets: 1 and 2 mg.

Metaproterenol Sulfate

1,3-Benzenediol, 5-[1-hydroxy-2-[(1-methylethyl)amino]ethyl]-, sulfate (2:1) salt; Orciprenaline Sulfate; Alupent (*Boehringer Ingelheim*); Metaprel (*Sandoz*)

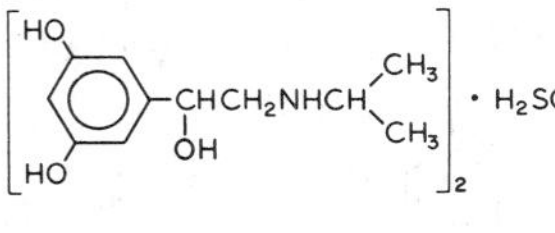

3,5-Dihydroxy-α-[(isopropylamino)methyl]benzyl alcohol sulfate (2:1) [5874-97-5] $(C_{11}H_{17}NO_3)_2.H_2SO_4$ (520.59).

Preparation—One method involves condensing 2-chloro-3′,5′-dihydroxyacetophenone with isopropylamine, reducing the CO group to CHOH and reacting the resulting metaproterenol base with H_2SO_4. US Pat 3,341,594.

Description—White to off-white, odorless, bitter, crystalline powder; photosensitive and oxidizes in air; melts at about 202°.

Solubility—Freely soluble in water or alcohol.

Uses—Possesses strong β_2-, weak β_1- and no α-agonist activity. The actions, uses, adverse effects, precautions and drug interactions of β-agonists are discussed in the general statement. Because the cardiac stimulant effects are slight, it is replacing isoproterenol and epinephrine in the management of *bronchial asthma.* It is not acted upon by catechol-*O*-methyltransferase, is only slightly degraded by MAO and is conjugated only slowly in the liver; consequently, it is effective orally. The duration of action after inhalation is about 4 hr and somewhat longer after oral administration. The duration of action, but not the maximum effect, may decrease with appropriate chronic use.

Dose—*Oral inhalation,* user *over 12 yr,* only, *metered aerosol,* **2** or **3 inhalations** (1.3 or 1.95 mg) every 3 or 4 hr, up to a limit of 7.8 mg a day; hand *nebulization,* **5** to **15 inhalations** of a **5%** solution every 3 or 4 hr for acute, and 3 or 4 times a day for chronic, bronchospasm; intermittant positive pressure breathing (IPPB), **0.2** to **0.3 mL** of a **5%** solution diluted to 2.5 mL or of a **0.6%** solution, every 3 or 4 hr for acute and 3 or 4 times a day for chronic bronchospasm. *Oral,* user *over 9 yr* (or 27 kg), **20 mg** 3 or 4 times a day; *children 6 to 9 yr,* **10 mg** 3 or 4 times a day; *children under 6 yr,* **325** to **650 μg/kg** 4 times a day (syrup only).

Dosage Forms—Inhalation Aerosol (powder): 75 and 150 mg (650 μg per metered spray); Inhalant Solution: 0.4, 0.6 and 5%; Syrup: 10 mg/5 mL; Tablets: 10 and 20 mg.

Mephentermine Sulfate

Benzeneethanamine, *N*,α,α-trimethyl-, sulfate; Wyamine Sulfate (*Wyeth-Ayerst*)

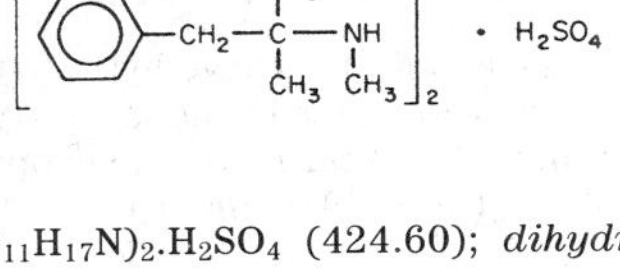

[1212-72-2] $(C_{11}H_{17}N)_2.H_2SO_4$ (424.60); *dihydrate* [6190-60-9] (460.63).

Preparation—By a seven-step synthesis starting with phenyl isopropyl ketone and conversion of the free base to the salt with sulfuric acid. US Pat 2,590,079.

Description—White, odorless crystals or a crystalline powder; solutions are acid to litmus, having a pH of about 6.

Solubility—1 g in 18 mL water, 220 mL alcohol, >1000 mL chloroform or >10,000 mL ether.

Uses—Acts both directly and by release of norepinephrine to stimulate both α- and β-receptors in the vasculature and heart. It is employed parenterally to *support blood pressure* during spinal anesthesia, or treatment with ganglionic blocking drugs or in postural hypotension. It is not recommended for routine use in the management of shock, especially hypovolemic shock, although it can be given as an interim drug while preparations are being made for fluid replacement and other measures. Parenteral injections of the drug produce a very prompt and prolonged increase in blood pressure. Tachyphylaxis occurs, so that repeated injections lose their pressor effects. The central stimulant actions are weak relative to the cardiovascular action, and it is not possible to achieve a central effect without cardiovascular side effects; nevertheless, the drug has been used to elevate mood in geriatric patients and to antagonize the central depressant effects of certain antihistamines. See the general statement for the adverse effects, precautions and drug interactions of indirect sympathomimetics and α- and β-agonists. Mephentermine is absorbed orally and excreted in the urine. An alkaline urine favors retention of the drug and tends to elevate plasma levels. The duration of action is 1 to 2 hr.

Dose—*Intramuscular, adults,* in *spinal anesthesia,* **30** to **45 mg** 10 to 20 min prior to hypotensive procedure; *children,* **400 μg/kg.** *Intravenous, adults, initially* **30** to **45 mg,** then 30 mg as needed; the dose should be half the above in cesarian section or hyperresponsive patients; *children,* **400 μg/kg.** Constant *intravenous infusion,* a **0.1% solution** infused at a rate necessary to maintain blood pressure.

Dosage Form—Injection: 15 and 30 mg/mL.

Metaraminol Bitartrate

Benzenemethanol, [*R*-(*R**,*S**)]-α-(1-aminoethyl)-3-hydroxy-, [*R*-(*R**,*R**)]-2,3-dihydroxybutanedioate (1:1) (salt) Aramine (*MSD, Bristol*); Pressonex (*Sterling*)

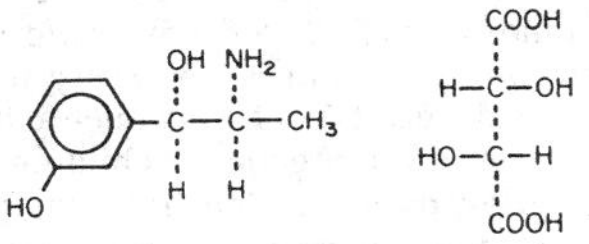

(−)-α-(1-Aminoethyl)-*m*-hydroxybenzyl alcohol, tartrate (1:1) (salt) [33402-03-8] $C_9H_{13}NO_2.C_4H_6O_6$ (317.29).

Preparation—Among other methods, by reactions using *m*-hydroxybenzaldehyde and benzylamine as the principal reactants. The base is converted to the bitartrate with an equimolar quantity of tartaric acid.

Description—White, practically odorless, crystalline powder; melts between 171 and 175°; pH (1 in 20 solution) between 3.2 and 3.5.

Solubility—Freely soluble in water; 1 g in about 100 mL alcohol; practically insoluble in chloroform or ether.

Uses—A directly acting *sympathomimetic* with strong α- and moderate β_1-agonist activity and virtually no β_2-agonist activity or actions on the central nervous system. See the general statement for actions, uses, adverse effects and precautions of α- and β_1-agonists. The drug is used mainly to support or elevate blood pressure during spinal or general anesthesia and in certain acute *hypotensive conditions,* such as anaphylactic shock (after initial management with epinephrine) or shock secondary to myocardial infarction, trauma, septicemia, gram-negative bacterial endotoxins and adverse drug reactions. It is not recommended in hypovolemic shock. In the treatment of shock, metaraminol has been superseded largely by dopamine and dobutamine. After prolonged infusion, a severe hypotensive episode often follows discontinuation, because the drug replaces norepinephrine in the adrenergic nerve terminals and becomes a false transmitter. The duration of action is about 1.5 hr after intramuscular injection.

Dose—(as the base): *Intravenous, adult,* **0.5** to **5 mg** of metaraminol; *children,* **10 μg/kg** (or **300 μg/m²**). *Intravenous infusion, adults,* **15** to **100 mg/500 mL** of 5% dextrose or dextrose-sodium chloride injection, infused at a rate adjusted to maintain systolic blood pressure at 80 to 100 torr; *children,* **400 μg/kg** (or **12 mg/m²**) in a parenteral solution such that there is 1 mg/25 mL, infused at the optimal rate. *Intramuscular adults,* **2** to **10 mg;** *children,* **100 μg/kg** (or **3 mg/m²**). *Subcutaneous* administration is not recommended because of the frequent occurrence of ischemic necrosis at the injection site; the dose is the same as for intramuscular injection.

Dosage Form—Injection: 10 mg/mL.

Methamphetamine Hydrochloride

2-Propaneamine, *N*-methyl-1-phenyl-, hydrochloride; (*Various Mfrs*)

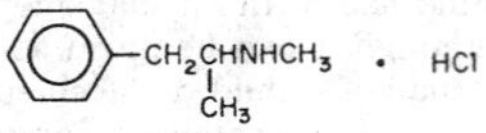

Deoxyephedrine hydrochloride, methylamphetamine hydrochloride [51-57-0] $C_{10}H_{15}N.HCl$ (185.70).

Preparation—By catalytic hydrogenation of ephedrine and subsequently converted to the hydrochloride.

Description—White crystals or a white, crystalline powder; odorless; melts between 171 and 175°.

Solubility—1 g in 2 mL water, 3 mL alcohol or 5 mL chloroform; very slightly soluble in absolute ether.

Uses—Actions are very similar to those of amphetamine, but at low doses the cardiovascular effects are less pronounced. It is mainly employed for its *central nervous system stimulant* actions in depressing appetite in the therapy of *obesity* and *abnormal behavioral states* in children. Some medical authorities do not recommend its use as an anorexiant. Tolerance to the normalizing effect in attention defective children does not occur. Because it may elevate mood, it was once used as an antidepressant. At tolerated doses, the cardiovascular effects consist mainly of cardiac stimulation, which elevates blood pressure. Vasoconstriction makes a minor contribution to the pressor effect. The cardiovascular actions are elicited principally by the levo component in a racemic mixture; they are the result of an indirect, norepinephrine-releasing action. The side effects, contraindications and drug interactions are those of centrally acting sympathomimetics (see introductory statement). Methamphetamine is abused widely for its central stimulant actions. It is the drug usually called "speed" in drug-abuse circles, although other centrally acting sympathomimetics often are given the same name. It is a Schedule II controlled substance.

Dose—*Oral, adults* and *children over 12 yr,* for *exogenous obesity initially* **2.5 mg** 3 times a day, 30 to 60 min before meals; the dose is increased as needed, but it seldom is necessary to exceed 5 mg. In *timed-release* form, the dose is **10** to **15 mg** once a day. The drug is not recommended for use as an anorectic in children under 12 yr. For *attention deficit disorder, children 6 yr and older,* **2.5** or **5 mg** 1 or 2 times a day, with 5 mg/day-adjustments at weekly intervals, if needed *or,* in *extended-release form,* **5** to **15 mg** once a day.

Dosage Forms—Tablets: 5 and 10 mg; Extended-Release Tablets: 5, 10 and 15 mg.

Methoxamine Hydrochloride

Benzenemethanol, α-(1-aminoethyl)-2,5-dimethoxy-, hydrochloride; Vasoxyl Hydrochloride (*Burroughs Wellcome*)

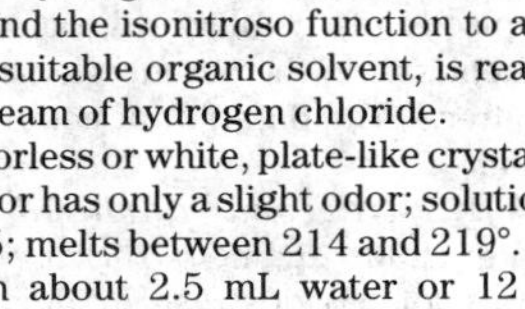

(±)-α-(1-Aminoethyl)-2,5-dimethoxybenzyl alcohol hydrochloride [61-16-5] $C_{11}H_{17}NO_3.HCl$ (247.72).

Preparation—Among other ways, from 2′,5′-dimethoxypropiophenone through reaction with nitrous acid to form the 2-isonitroso derivative followed by catalytic hydrogenation which reduces both the carbonyl function to carbinol and the isonitroso function to amino. The methoxamine, dissolved in a suitable organic solvent, is readily converted to the hydrochloride by a stream of hydrogen chloride.

Description—Colorless or white, plate-like crystals, or a white, crystalline powder; odorless or has only a slight odor; solutions are acid to litmus, having a pH of about 5; melts between 214 and 219°.

Solubility—1 g in about 2.5 mL water or 12 mL alcohol; almost insoluble in chloroform or ether.

Uses—A directly acting *sympathomimetic* amine with a prompt and prolonged pressor action which results almost exclusively from α-agonist activity to increase peripheral resistance. Not only does it not stimulate the heart but it has moderate beta-adrenergic receptor blocking properties. It actually causes bradycardia, mostly as the result of a reflex activation of the vagus nerve secondary to the increased blood pressure. It is useful for the treatment of *hypotensive states* when it is desired to raise blood pressure without cardiac stimulation. However, it has very little effect on the capacitance veins, so that its usefulness is compromised, especially in the treatment of various kinds of shock. It is used mainly to support blood pressure during anesthesia, including anesthesia by heart-sensitizing anesthetics. The reflex bradycardia is employed to terminate *paroxysmal supraventricular tachycardia.* It has no inhibitory effect on bronchial muscles, causes no central stimulation and does not increase the irritability of the anesthetic-sensitized heart. The duration of action is 60 to 90 min. For the adverse effects, precautions and contraindications of α-agonists, see the general statement.

Dose—*Intramuscular, adult, pre-* and *postoperative,* **5** to **10 mg;** with *spinal anesthesia* or *to correct hypotension,* **10** to **20 mg;** *children,* **250 μg/kg.** *Intravenous, adult,* for *hypotensive emergencies,* **3** to **5 mg** *slowly;* for *paroxysmal supraventricular tachycardia,* **10 mg** *slowly; children,* **80 μg/kg** slowly in divided doses.

Dosage Form—Injection: 20 mg/mL.

Methylphenidate Hydrochloride—page 1234.

Midodrine—see RPS-18, page 888.

Naphazoline Hydrochloride

1*H*-Imidazole, 4,5-dihydro-2-(1-naphthalenylmethyl)-, monohydrochloride; Privine Hydrochloride (*Ciba*); (*Various Mfrs*)

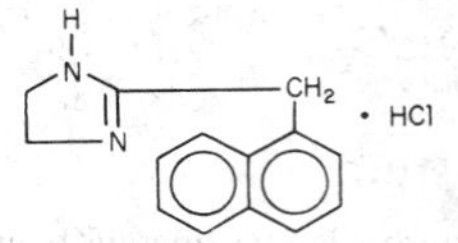

2-(1-Naphthylmethyl)-2-imidazoline monohydrochloride [550-99-2] $C_{14}H_{14}N_2.HCl$ (246.74).

Preparation—In almost quantitative yields by heating 1-naphthaleneacetonitrile with ethylenediamine monohydrochloride at 175° to 200° for 1 hr. The 1-naphthaleneacetonitrile is made from naphthalene by chloromethylation with formaldehyde and HCl followed by treatment of the resulting 1-naphthylmethyl chloride with potassium cyanide.

Description—White, crystalline, odorless, bitter powder; melting range 253 to 258°, with decomposition; pH (1 in 100 solution) between 5.0 and 6.6.

Solubility—Freely soluble in water or alcohol; very slightly soluble in chloroform; practically insoluble in ether.

Uses—Although its structure differs markedly from that of most sympathomimetic agents, it is a direct-acting *sympathomimetic* with only α-agonist activity. It is employed topically for relief of *nasal congestion.* It also may be used to relieve nasal congestion consequent to treatment with reserpine, etc, since its actions are mainly direct. Care should be exercised in its prolonged use, because naphazoline, in common with most locally applied vasoconstrictors, may cause a rebound congestion that simulates the condition for which it was employed originally; it also induces chemical rhinitis. Mere discontinuation of ill-advised vasoconstrictor therapy has been noted to produce dramatic relief of chronic nasal congestion in some cases. Naphazoline also is used as an ophthalmic solution for relief of *ocular congestion* and *blepharospasm.*

The common adverse effects include hypertension, bradycardia, sweating, sedation and, in children, occasional coma. For other potential adverse effects and precautions, see the general statement on α-agonists.

Dose—*Topical, adults,* to the *nasal mucosa,* **2 sprays** or **drops** of **0.05%** solution every 3 to 4 hr, if necessary, or as **0.05% nasal spray** no more frequently than every 3 hr; to the *conjunctiva,* **1** to **2 drops** of **0.012** to **0.1%** ophthalmic solution every 3 to 4 hr or longer, if possible. (The FDA Advisory Panel on Ophthalmologic Drugs did not endorse concentrations above 0.03%.) Use in children is not recommended.

Dosage Forms—Nasal Solution: 0.05%; Ophthalmic Solution: 0.012, 0.02, 0.025, 0.03, 0.05 and 0.1%.

Norepinephrine Bitartrate

1,2-Benzenediol, 4-(2-amino-1-hydroxyethyl)-, (*R*)-[*R*-(*R**,*R**)]-2,3-dihydroxybutanedioate (1:1) (salt), monohydrate; Levarterenol Bitartrate; Noradrenaline Acid Tartrate; Levophed Bitartrate (*Sanofi Winthrop*)

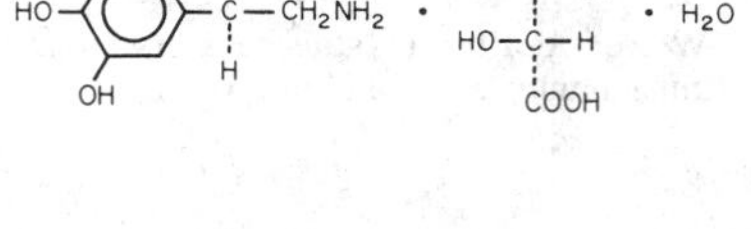

(−)-α-(Aminomethyl)-3,4-dihydroxybenzyl alcohol tartrate (1:1) (salt) monohydrate [69815-49-2] $C_8H_{11}NO_3.C_4H_6O_6.H_2O$ (337.28); *anhydrous* [51-40-1] (319.27).

Preparation—By the synthetic procedure given for *Epinephrine* (page 990), using ammonia in place of methylamine; the base is then converted to the bitartrate and resolved.

Description—White or faintly gray, crystalline powder; odorless; slowly darkens on exposure to air and light; solutions are acid to litmus, having a pH of about 3.5; melts, without previous drying, between 98° and 104° to form a turbid melt.

Solubility—1 g in about 2.5 mL water or about 300 mL alcohol; practically insoluble in chloroform or ether.

Uses—Norepinephrine is the catecholamine released at almost all adrenergic nerve terminals in the periphery and in a large proportion of adrenergic nerve terminals in the central nervous system. It constitutes 10 to 18% of the catecholamine content of the adrenal medulla and as much as 97% of that of some pheochromocytomas.

It has strong α- and β_1- but weak β_2-agonist activity. It is used only for its α-activity, but β_1-activity contributes to its systemic usefulness and adverse effects (see the general statement for actions, uses, adverse effects and precautions of α- and β_1-agonists). Its principal use is to *support blood pressure* in various acute hypotensive states, especially in myocardial *shock*. In shock, despite adequate restoration of blood pressure, failure occurs in approximately 50% of cases. Prolonged infusions sometimes themselves cause shock. Even though it possesses strong β_1-activity, an increase in heart rate often does not occur during intravenous infusion, because the vasoconstrictor actions marshal vagal reflexes that tend to slow the heart and nullify the direct effect to increase heart rate. However, the reflexes do not antagonize the effect on the strength of the heart beat, so that cardiac output usually is maintained, even though the rate is slowed. At the low blood pressures usually seen in shock, the baroreceptors are not operative, and an increase in heart rate often is seen after the administration of norepinephrine. It sometimes is used in *cardiac arrest*. Like other β_1-agonists, it is arrhythmiagenic. The β_2-activity is so weak that tolerated doses do not cause bronchodilatation or vasodilatation in muscle vascular beds; at the usual infusion rates, it also does not cause α-adrenergic bronchoconstriction.

The bitartriate is used as a vasoconstrictor in some local anesthetic solutions for dental use, usually in 0.0033% (1 in 30,000) concentration of norepinephrine.

Note—Do not use any dosage form of norepinephrine bitartrate if it is brown in color or contains a precipitate.

Dose—*Intravenous, adult*, by slow infusion, **0.03** to **0.15 μg/kg/min** (of norepinephrine base equivalent), the rate being determined by the response. An initial rate of 0.1 to 0.15 μg/kg/min often is used as a trial from which adjustments are made to achieve a systolic blood pressure of 80 to 120 torr; but many clinicians prefer to start with a low rate and increase the rate until response occurs, rather than risk a hypertensive crisis with the test rate. Especially if the patient has just had a pheochromocytoma removed, the rate may greatly exceed that given above. Average *maintenance* dose, **0.03** to **0.06 μg/kg/min**, but the infusion rate will need to be increased gradually, which is in part a sign that volume replenishment is needed. Even after the initial rate-adjusting period, vigilant monitoring (at least every 15 min) is required. *Children, initially* **2 μg/min/m²**, the rate to be adjusted according to the response. The infusion is prepared by adding 8 mg of levarterenol bitartrate (equivalent to 4 mg of levarterenol) to 1 L of 5% dextrose or dextrose-sodium chloride injection. *If extravasation occurs, the exposed tissue should be infiltrated with 5 to 10 mg of phentolamine.*

Dosage Form—Injection: 4 mg/4 mL.

Nylidrin Hydrochloride

Benzeneethanol, 4-hydroxy-α-[1-[(1-methyl-3-phenylpropyl)-amino]ethyl]-, hydrochloride; (*Various Mfrs*)

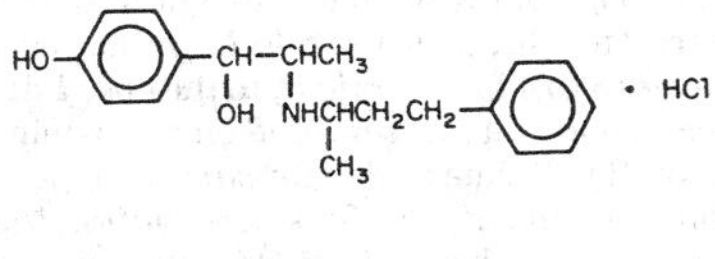

[900-01-6; 849-55-8] $C_{19}H_{25}NO_2.HCl$ (335.87).

Preparation—By reacting *p*-hydroxynorephedrine and benzylacetone in alcohol and catalytically hydrogenating the product.

Description—White, crystalline powder; odorless; practically tasteless.

Solubility—1 g in about 65 mL water or 40 mL alcohol; very slightly soluble in chloroform or ether.

Uses—Possesses β_2-agonist activity that is more selective for the skeletal muscle vasculature than the bronchioles. Some of the action appears to be a nonspecific smooth muscle relaxation. There is little effect on the cutaneous vasculature. It has mild β_1-agonist activity. See the general statement for the actions, uses, adverse effects and precautions of β_2- and β_1-agonists. In normotensive patients, the drug has little effect on blood pressure, but it is hypotensive in hypertensive patients and hypertensive in hypotensive patients. It is used in the treatment of vascular disorders of the skeletal muscle vessels, such as *intermittent claudication, thrombophlebitis* and, to a lesser extent, *diabetic vascular disease*. However, it is effective only to the extent that there may be a vasospastic component in these disorders, which are otherwise mainly occlusive. It has been advocated for use in thromboangiitis obliterans, endarteritis obliterans, Raynaud's disease and ischemic ulcers; inasmuch as the drug fails to increase significantly cutaneous blood flow, such use cannot be expected to be of benefit. It is claimed to be of benefit in *ischemic disorders* of the *inner ear*.

Dose—*Oral*, **3** to **12 mg** 3 or 4 times a day.

Dosage Form—Tablets: 6 and 12 mg.

Oxymetazoline Hydrochloride

Phenol,
3-[(4,5-dihydro-1*H*-imidazol-2-yl)methyl]-6-(1,1-dimethylethyl)-2,4-dimethyl-, monohydrochloride; (*Various Mfrs*)

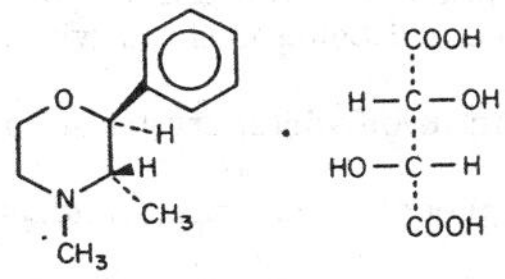

6-*tert*-Butyl-3-(2-imidazolin-2-ylmethyl)-2,4-dimethylphenol monohydrochloride [2315-02-8] $C_{16}H_{24}N_2O.HCl$ (296.84).

Preparation—2,4-Dimethyl-6-*tert*-butylphenol is converted into the benzyl cyanide intermediate, which is reacted with ethylenediamine *p*-toluenesulfonate whereby, through addition and deammoniation, the imidazoline ring is formed. The resulting oxymetazoline is converted to the salt through interaction with an equimolar quantity of hydrogen chloride. US Pat 3,147,275.

Description—White to nearly white, fine, crystalline powder; odorless; stable in light and heat, nonhygroscopic; melts at about 300° with decomposition; pH (1 in 20 solution) between 4.0 and 6.5.

Solubility—1 g in 6.7 mL water, 3.6 mL alcohol or 860 mL chloroform; practically insoluble in ether.

Uses—A *direct-acting sympathomimetic* with only α-agonist activity. It is used only topically as a *nasal* or *ophthalmic decongestant*. After-congestion is less prominent than with naphazoline, to which it is chemically related. For the action, adverse effects and precautions of α-agonists, see the general statement.

Dose—*Intranasal, adults* and *children over 6* yrs, **2** to **3 drops** or **sprays** of **0.05%** solution into each nostril every 4 to 12 hr; *children* 2 to 5 yr, **2** to **3 drops** of **0.025%** solution every 12 hr. *Ophthalmic*, **1** or **2 drops** every 6 hr.

Dosage Forms—Nasal Solution: 0.025 and 0.05%; Nasal Spray: 0.05%; Ophthalmic Solution: 0.025%.

Phendimetrazine Tartrate

Morpholine, (2*S*-*trans*)-3,4-dimethyl-2-phenyl-, [*R*-(*R**,*R**)]-2,3-dihydroxybutanedioate (1:1) (*Various Mfrs*)

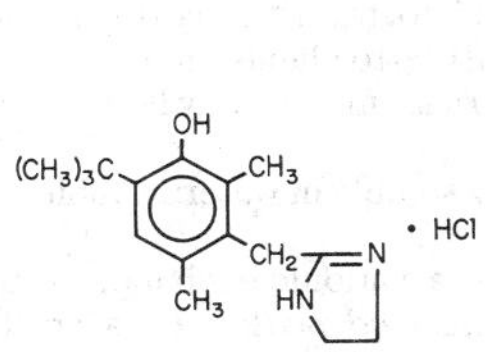

[50-58-2] $C_{12}H_{17}NO.C_4H_6O_6$ (341.35).

Preparation—The base by interaction of *l*-ephedrine and ethylene chlorohydrin.

Description—White, crystalline powder; odorless; bitter taste; melts at about 186° with decomposition; pK_a 7.2.

Solubility—Soluble in water or alcohol.

Uses—Closely related to phenmetrazine, both chemically and pharmacologically, it is an indirectly acting *sympathomimetic* with predominantly central nervous stimulant actions. It is used as an *appetite suppressant* and not as a general central stimulant or sympathomimetic. It is a Schedule II controlled substance. Except for glossitis and cystitis, the adverse effects are those of centrally acting sympathomimetics (see the general statement for actions, uses, adverse effects, etc.)

Dose—*Oral, adults* and *children over 12 yr,* **17.5** to **70 mg** 2 or 3 times a day, 1 hr before meals, or **105 mg** in *extended-release form* once a day.

Dosage Forms—Extended-Release Capsules: 105 mg; Capsules: 35 mg; Tablets: 35 mg.

Phenmetrazine Hydrochloride

Morpholine, 3-methyl-2-phenyl-, hydrochloride; Endurets, Preludin (*Boehringer Ingelheim*); Melfiat (*Solvay*)

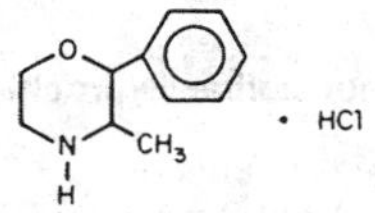

[1707-14-8] $C_{11}H_{15}NO.HCl$ (213.71).

Preparation—By an addition reaction of norephedrine and ethylene oxide, the resulting alcohol being cyclized with a suitable dehydrating agent.

Description—White to off-white, crystalline powder; melts between 172 and 182°; pK_a 7.6.

Solubility—1 g in about 0.4 mL water, 2 mL alcohol or 2 mL chloroform.

Uses—A *sympathomimetic* with CNS and weak cardiovascular activity. See the general statement for the actions, uses, adverse effects, precautions and drug interactions of centrally acting sympathomimetics. It is a little-recommended anorexiant, for which use it is about equal to dextroamphetamine. The side effects of euphoria, insomnia, headache, dizziness, nausea, urinary frequency, nervousness and hyperexcitability are claimed to be less frequent. However, some clinical studies indicate that it may have greater relative central stimulatory activity than amphetamine. Tolerance and drug dependence can occur. It is a Schedule II controlled substance. It may cause loss of antihypertensive effect of guanethidine.

Dose—*Oral, adults* and *children over 12 yr,* **25 mg** 1 to 3 times a day administered 1 hr before meals or **75 mg** a day as a single *extended-release tablet* taken 1 hr before breakfast. Not recommended for use in children under 12 yr.

Dosage Forms—Tablets: 25 mg; Extended-Release Tablets: 75 mg.

Phentermine

Benzenethanamine, α,α-dimethyl-, (*Various Mfrs*)

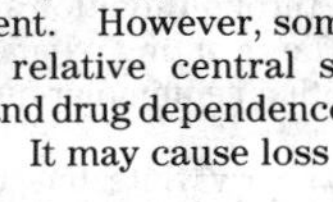

α,α-Dimethylphenethylamine [122-09-8] $C_{10}H_{15}N$ (149.23).

Preparation—By the Grignard reaction of benzylmagnesium bromide with acetone, reacting the resulting α,α-dimethylphenethyl alcohol with sodium cyanide in acid to form the corresponding 2-formamido compound, and hydrolyzing this to phentermine.

Description—Colorless, mobile, oily liquid with an odor characteristic of amines.

Solubility—Slightly soluble in water; soluble in alcohol, choroform or ether.

Phentermine Resin, a cationic-exchange resin complex of phentermine, and *Phentermine Hydrochloride,* a crystalline salt that is very soluble in water, are the two derivatives used in available dosage forms; the former is marketed under the name Ionamin (*Pennwalt*) and the latter under various names.

Uses—A centrally acting sympathomimetic with weak cardiovascular activity. It is used as an *anorexiant.* The central stimulant actions are less prominent than with the amphetamines (except that the incidence of insomnia is higher). Consequently, use of the drug is accompanied by a low incidence of side effects; however, the anorectic effects are also weaker. Clinical trials do not show unequivocal efficacy. Long-term use, particularly of doses larger than are recommended for therapy, can cause drug dependence. The adverse effects, precautions and drug interactions are those of the centrally acting sympathomimetics (see the general statement). The drug is a Schedule V controlled substance.

Dose—*Oral, adults* and *children over 12 yr, extended-release* forms, **15** to **30 mg** (as the base), to be taken on rising, or **8 mg** 3 times a day 30 min before meals or **15** to **30 mg** as a single dose before breakfast with *conventional* forms.

Dosage Forms—Phentermine Resin Capsules: 15 and 30 mg; Phentermine Hydrochloride Capsules: 15, 30 and 37.5 mg; Phentermine Hydrochloride Extended-Release Capsules: 30 mg; Tablets: 8, 15, 30 and 37.5 mg.

Phenylephrine Hydrochloride

Benzenemethanol, 3-hydroxy-α-[(methylamino)methyl]-, hydrochloride; (*Various Mfrs*)

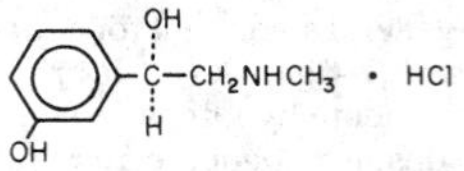

(−)-*m*-Hydroxy-α-[(methylamino)methyl]benzyl alcohol hydrochloride [61-76-7] $C_9H_{13}NO_2.HCl$ (203.67).

Preparation—*m*-Hydroxyphenacyl bromide is condensed with methylamine and the carbonyl group then is reduced to a carbinol via catalytic hydrogenation. The phenylephrine so formed is dissolved in a suitable solvent and neutralized with HCl.

Description—White or nearly white crystals; odorless; bitter taste; melts between 140 and 145°.

Solubility—Freely soluble in water or alcohol.

Uses—A *direct-acting sympathomimetic* with strong α-agonist and negligible β-agonist and CNS activity. See the general statement for the actions, uses, adverse effects, precautions and drug interactions of direct α-agonists. It is used in the treatment of *paroxysmal supraventricular tachycardia* and to support *blood pressure.* It can be used in the presence of heart-sensitizing anesthetics because of its lack of significant beta-adrenergic cardiac stimulant actions. It also is used as a nasal, scleroconjunctival and uveal *decongestant,* as a *mydriatic* and to increase aqueous humor outflow in *open-angle glaucoma.* It is included in some local anesthetic preparations to prolong local and regional anesthesia and in combination with inhaled bronchodilators.

It is absorbed orally and, since it is not attacked by MAO, it is effective by mouth for orthostatic hypotension. By the intravenous route the duration of action is about 15 to 20 min and by the intramuscular route 30 to 120 min.

Dose—*Intramuscular* or *subcutaneous, adults,* for *mild to moderate hypotension, initially* **2** to **5 mg,** repeated at intervals no less than 10 to 15 min, *or,* for *prevention of hypotension during spinal anesthesia,* **2** to **3 mg** 4 min before anesthetic; *children, to treat hypotension,* **100 μg/kg** (or **3 mg/m²**), repeated in 1 to 2 hr, as needed, *or, prior to spinal anesthesia,* **44** to **88 μg/kg.** *Intravenous injection, adults,* for *mild to moderate hypotension,* **500 μg** (*slowly!*), repeated at intervals no less than 10 to 15 min *or,* for *severe hypotension* during spinal anesthesia, *initially* **200 μg,** with subsequent increments no greater than 200 μg, up to a total of 500 μg/dose, **or** for *paroxysmal supraventricular tachycardia, initially* **up to 500/μg** given over 30 sec, with subsequent increments of 100 to 200 μg, up to a total of 1 mg/dose. *Continuous intravenous infusion, adults, initially* **100** to **180 μg/min,** usually reduced to **40** to **60 μg/min** for *maintenance.* To *prolong spinal* and *local anesthesia,* **2** to **5 mg** added to a *spinal anesthetic* solution *or* **1 mg** (as **0.005%** solution) to 20 mL of *regional anesthetic* solution. *Topical, intranasal, adults,* **2 or 3 drops** or **1 or 2 sprays** of **0.2** to **1.0%** solution, or a **small amount** of **0.5%** jelly into each nostril every 3 to 4 hr; *children, all age groups,* **2** or **3 drops** of solutions as follows: *up to 2 yr,* **0.125%** every 2 to 4 hr; *2 to 6 yr,* **0.125%** every 2 to 4 hr or **0.16%** every 4 hr; *6 to 12 yr,* **0.25%** every 2 to 4 hr; *children 6 to 12 yr* may use **1 or 2 sprays** of **0.25%** solution every 3 to 4 hr. *Topical,* to the *eye,* **1 drop** of **2.5** to **10%** solution into the conjunctival sac, repeated once in 5 min, if necessary, for *opthalmoscopy,* or, 2 to 3 times a day for *chronic mydriasis,* or, **1 drop** of **0.12%** solution 2 or 3 times a day for *scleroconjunctival decongestion* and *blepharospasm,* or, **1 drop** of a **2.5%** solution, repeated at 15-min intervals for 4 doses for *preoperative mydriasis,* or, **1 drop** of **10%** solution once a day for 3 days, to be alternated with miotics, for *post-iridectomy mydriasis,* or, **1 drop** of **10%** solution to the upper surface of the cornea for *glaucoma; children,* as adults, except 10% solution is not to be used.

Dosage Forms—Injection: 10 mg/1 mL; Ophthalmic Solution: 0.120, 2.5 and 10%; Nasal Jelly: 0.5%; Nasal Solution: 0.125, 0.160, 0.2, 0.25, 0.5 and 1%.

Phenylpropanolamine Hydrochloride

(±)-Benzenemethanol, (R^*,S^*)-α-(1-aminoethyl)-, hydrochloride; *(Various Mfrs)*

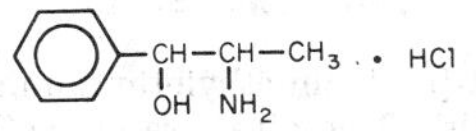

(±)-Norephedrine hydrochloride [154-41-6] $C_9H_{13}NO.HCl$ (187.67).

Preparation—By reacting benzaldehyde with nitroethane to form α-(1-nitroethyl)benzyl alcohol and then reducing this nitroalcohol to the corresponding amino compound, which is then converted to the hydrochloride. US Pat 2,151,517. For an improved industrial process, see US Pat 3,028,429.

Description—White, crystalline powder having a slight aromatic odor; affected by light; melts between 191 and 196°; pH (3 in 100 solution) between 4.2 and 5.5; pK_{a1} (0.10) 9.04; pK_{a2} (0.005) 9.06.

Solubility—1 g in 1.1 mL water, 7.4 mL alcohol or 4100 mL chloroform; insoluble in ether.

Uses—An *indirectly acting sympathomimetic* with prominent peripheral adrenergic effects and weak central stimulant actions. The principal uses of phenylpropanolamine are as a *nasopharyngeal* and *bronchial decongestant*. In cold and hay fever preparations, it often is combined with phenylephrine and codeine or hydrocodone. Promotional claims that systemic (oral) phenylpropanol-amine has a selective vasoconstrictor action in the nasopharyngeal and otic regions have not been substantiated in man; a substantial decongestant action in the above areas is accompanied by a hypertensive response. It also is used to treat *urinary incontinence*, especially in women, and *retrograde ejaculation* in men. For these purposes, it is sometimes combined with chlorpheniramine.

It has mild CNS actions and is used as a nonprescription anorexiant in the treatment of *exogenous obesity*. It is an ingredient in a number of anorexiant combinations, sometimes in insufficient dose.

The actions, adverse effects, precautions and drug interactions of indirect and centrally acting sympathomimetics may be found in the general statement. Adverse effects are most likely to occur when the dose exceeds 75 mg/day. Notable side effects include the CNS effects of nausea, dizziness, nervousness, insomnia, headache, tinnitus, fear, delusions, psychoses and convulsions and peripheral effects of palpitations, hypertension and hyperglycemia.

About 10% of the drug is metabolized to an active metabolite, the remainder being excreted unchanged with a half-life of about 6 hr.

Dose—*Oral, adults,* for *decongestion,* **25 mg** every 4 hr *or* **50 mg** every 8 hr *or* **75 mg** in extended-release form every 12 hr, not to exceed 150 mg/day: for *appetite suppression,* **25 mg** 3 times/day, ½ hr before meals, **or 75 mg** in extended-release form once a day; for *urinary incontinence,* **50** to **75 mg** 3 times a day or **75 mg** in timed-release form once a day. *Oral, children, for decongestion only, 2 to 6 yr* (not recommended), **6.25 mg** every 4 hr or **12.5 mg** every 8 hr, not to exceed 37.5 mg/day; *6 to 12 yr,* **12.5 mg** every 4 hr or **25 mg** every 8 hr, not to exceed 75 mg/day; *under 2 yr* (not recommended), dose must be individualized.

Dosage Forms—Capsules: 25, 37.5 and 50 mg; Timed-Release Capsules: 50 and 75 mg; Drops: 25 mg/5 drops; Lozenges: 25 mg; Tablets: 25 and 50 mg.

Pirbuterol Hydrochloride

2,6-Pyridinedimethanol, α^6-[[1,1-dimethylethyl)amino]methyl]-3-hydroxy-, hydrochloride Maxair *(Riker)*

[38029-10-6] $C_{12}H_{20}N_2O_3.2HCl$ (313.22); [65652-44-0 (acetate)]

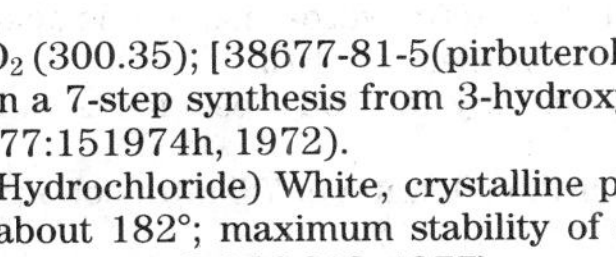

$C_{12}H_{20}N_2O_3.C_2\text{-}H_4O_2$ (300.35); [38677-81-5(pirbuterol)]

Preparation—In a 7-step synthesis from 3-hydroxypyridine; see Ger Pat 2,105,464 (CA 77:151974h, 1972).

Description—(Hydrochloride) White, crystalline powder; melts with decomposition at about 182°; maximum stability of aqueous solutions occurs at pH 1 to 2 (*J Pharm Sci 66:*819, 1977).

Solubility—Soluble in water.

Uses—A moderately selective β_2-adrenoreceptor agonist. Its approval in the US as a *bronchodilator* is imminent, to be marketed as Exirel (*Pfizer*). It also relaxes uterine and vascular smooth muscle; it has been successful in trials as an antihypertensive drug. As a bronchodilator, its efficacy is about that of albuterol (page 986), and the incidence and severity of side effects are also about the same. By the oral route, the incidence of side effects are tremor, 9%; nervousness, 7%; headache, 4.5%; tachycardia and ECG changes, 3%; dry mouth, 2%; palpitations, 2%; slight *hypo*tension is common. By inhalation, the frequency and severity are less. Its oral bioavailability is probably about 60%. Elimination occurs mainly by sulfation in the liver, only about 10% being excreted unchanged in the urine. The elimination half-life is 2 to 3 hr.

Dose—*Oral, adult,* **10** to **15 mg** 3 to 4 times a day, up to a maximum of 60 mg/day. *Inhalation aerosol, adult,* **1** to **2 inhalations** (200 to 400 μg) every 4 hr, up to 12 inhalations/day.

Dosage Forms—Syrup; 7.5 mg (as the hydrochloride)/5 mL; Inhaler: 200 μg (as the acetate) per metered dose.

Prenalterol—see RPS-18, page 888.

Procaterol—see RPS-18, page 888.

Propylhexedrine

Cyclohexaneethanamine, (±)-; *N*,α-dimethyl-, Benzedrex *(SmithKline Beecham)*; Dristan *(Whitehall)*

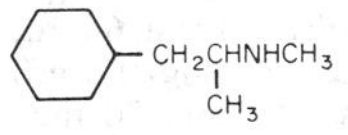

(±)-*N*-α-Dimethylcyclohexaneethylamine [101-40-6] $C_{10}H_{21}N$ (155.28).

Preparation—As described in US Pat 2,454,746, a solution of cyclohexylacetone in formic acid is reacted with *N*-methylformamide by heating for 4 hr at 160 to 180°. The resulting formyl derivative of propylhexedrine then is hydrolyzed by refluxing with 50% H_2SO_4 and the hydrolysate extracted with ether to remove acid-insoluble material. The aqueous solution then is rendered strongly alkaline with NaOH and the propylhexedrine is extracted with ether and purified by distillation under reduced pressure.

Description—Clear, colorless liquid, having a characteristic, amine-like odor; volatilizes slowly at room temperature; solutions are alkaline to litmus; absorbs CO_2 from the air; specific gravity 0.848 to 0.852; boils at about 205°.

Solubility—1 g in >500 mL water, 0.4 mL alcohol, 0.2 mL chloroform or 0.1 mL ether.

Uses—A volatile *indirect sympathomimetic* amine which, because of its lack of central excitatory effects and addiction liability, was introduced as a substitute for amphetamine for use in inhaler cartridges. One or two inhalations through each nostril produce *vasoconstriction* and a *decongestant* effect on nasal mucous membranes. Because of its wide margin of safety and relative freedom from toxic side effects, its use by inhalation is not contraindicated in patients in whom an ephedrine-like action would be undesirable. It is considered safe for self-medication by adults, but children should not have unsupervised access to an inhaler. Because the action is indirect, it will have limited efficacy in the treatment of nasal stuffiness consequent to treatment with reserpine, guanethidine and other adrenergic neuron blockers and catecholamine depletors. Untoward effects of propylhexedrine include aftercongestion, headache and, rarely, increase in blood pressure.

Dose—**1** or **2 inhalations** (approximately 350 or 700 μg), through each nostril, as required.

Dosage Form—Inhalant: 250 mg.

Pseudoephedrine Hydrochloride

Benzenemethanol, [*S*-(R^*,R^*)]-α-[1-(methylamino)ethyl]-, hydrochloride; *d*-Isoephedrine Hydrochloride; *(Various Mfrs)*

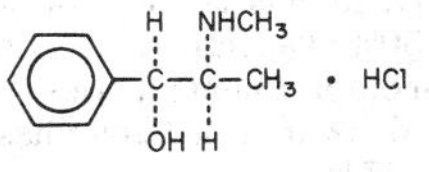

(+)-Pseudoephedrine hydrochloride [345-78-8] $C_{10}H_{15}NO.HCl$ (201.70).

Preparation—(−)-Ephedrine hydrochloride is acetylated to produce (+)-*N*-acetylpseudoephedrine hydrochloride which is then deacetylated to yield the official article. Ephedrine and pseudoephedrine are diastereoisomers, the former having the *erythro* and the latter the *threo* configuration.

Description—Fine, white to off-white crystals or powder having a faint, characteristic odor; melts between 182 and 186°; pH (1 in 20 solution) between 4.6 and 6.0.

Solubility—1 g in 0.5 mL water, 3.6 mL alcohol, 91 mL chloroform or 7000 mL ether.

Uses—Differs from ephedrine (page 989) in that it is relatively weaker in its pressor, cardiac, mydriatic and central-stimulant actions. Its nasopharyngeal vasoconstrictor and bronchodilator actions are about the same. It is used as a *nasopharyngeal* and *otic decongestant* and to treat *stress incontinence.* Promotional statements imply that systemic pseudoephedrine selectively can constrict blood vessels in the head region without generalized vasoconstriction, but most medical authorities disagree; if the dose is insufficient to raise the blood pressure, it also is insufficient to act as a decongestant. It has an anomalous action to dilate renal blood vessels and increase urine output. The adverse effects, precautions and drug interactions are those of indirect and weak centrally acting sympathomimetics (see the general statement). The drug is combined variously with phenylephrine, phenylpropanolamine and/or antihistamines in decongestant products.

Dose—*Oral,* user *over 12 yr,* **30** to **60 mg** every 6 hr, not to exceed 240 mg/day, *or,* with *extended-release* forms, **120 mg** every 12 hr. *Children,* **4 mg/kg** (or **125 mg/m²**)/day in 4 divided doses, *or by age group: 4 mo to 2 yr,* **3.75 mg** every 4 to 6 hr; *2 to 6 yr,* **15 mg** every 6 hr, not to exceed 60 mg/day; *6 to 12 yr,* **30 mg** every 6 hr, not to exceed 120 mg/day, *or,* in *extended-release* form, **60 mg** every 8 to 12 hr.

Dosage Forms—Drops: 7.5 mg/0.8 mL and 30 mg/mL; Syrup: 15 and 30 mg/5 mL; Tablets: 30 and 60 mg; Extended-Release Tablets: 120 mg.

Pseudoephedrine Sulfate—see RPS-18, page 887.

Racenephrine—see RPS-18, page 887.

Ritodrine Hydrochloride

Benzenemethanol, (*R**,*S**)-4-Hydroxy-α-[1-[[2-(4-hydroxyphenyl)-ethyl]amino]ethyl]-, hydrochloride; Yutopar (*Astra*)

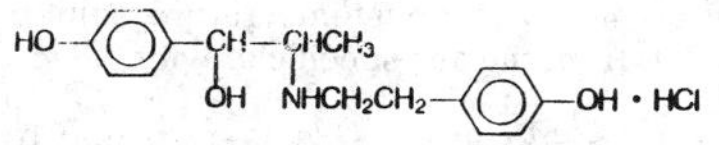

[23239-51-2] $C_{17}H_{21}NO_3.HCl$ (323.82).

Preparation—*p*-Methoxyphenethyl amine and *p*-(benzyloxy)-2-bromopropiophenone are condensed to form the corresponding secondary amine, which then successively is reduced with hydrogen, in the presence of palladium to remove the benzyl group, and HBr to cleave the methoxyl group. Reduction of the carbonyl group, using a palladium catalyst, yields the secondary alcohol, ritodrine. The base is converted to the hydrochloride in the usual fashion. US Pat 3,410,944.

Description—White, odorless crystals melting with decomposition between 196 and 205°.

Solubility—Freely soluble in water.

Uses—A β-adrenoreceptor agonist that is somewhat selective for β_2-receptors and, as such, relaxes uterine and bronchiolar smooth muscle and arterioles, especially in the skeletal muscle and splanchnic vascular beds. The heart is stimulated moderately, but blood glucose and lactate are elevated only mildly. It is used only to suppress *premature labor.*

The adverse effects are those of β-adrenergic agonists in general (see general statement). Cardiovascular effects usually are mild after oral administration, but considerable cardioacceleration and diastolic vasodepression result from intravenous infusion in both mother and fetus. Migraine headache results occasionally, presumably from cerebral vasodilatation. With concurrent administration of glucocorticoids, pulmonary edema may occur.

Its oral, systemic bioavailability is about 30%. It is conjugated in the liver, 90% of an oral and 50% of an intravenous dose being biotransformed. It appears to obey three-compartment kinetics, an early distribution phase having a half-life of 8 to 32 min; a later phase, 1.7 to 2.6 hr and an elimination phase of 7 to 27 hr.

Dose—*Intravenous infusion* (0.3 mg/mL, in 5% dextrose or other isotonic solution), *adults, initially* **0.1 mg/min,** to be adjusted at 10-min intervals by increments of 0.05 mg/min until contractions cease or excessive cardiovascular effects supravene; the effective rate usually lies between **0.15** and **0.37 mg/min**. Infusion is continued for more than 12 hr after contractions subside, after which oral dosing is substituted. *Oral, adults,* **10 mg** 30 min before termination of intravenous infusion followed by **10 mg** every 2 hr for the first 24 hr and **10** to **20 mg** every 6 hr thereafter, not to exceed 120 mg/day.

Dosage Forms—For Injection: 50 mg/5 mL and 150 mg/10 mL; Tablets: 10 mg.

Terbutaline Sulfate

1,3-Benzenediol, 5-[2-[(1,1-dimethylethyl)amino]-1-hydroxyethyl]-, sulfate (2:1) (salt); Brethaire, Brethine (*Geigy*); Bricanyl (*Merrell-Dow*)

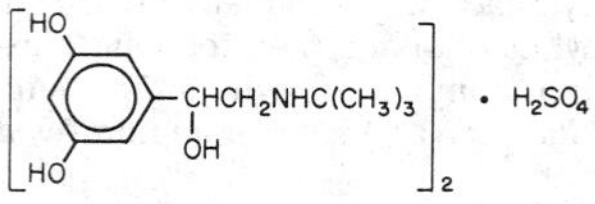

α-[(*tert*-Butylamino)methyl]-3,5-dihydroxybenzyl alcohol, sulfate (2:1) (salt) [23031-32-5] $(C_{12}H_{19}NO_3)_2.H_2SO_4$ (548.65).

Preparation—One method involves reduction of 2-(*tert*-butyl- amino)-3′,5′-dihydroxyacetophenone (I) to the carbinol by catalytic hydrogenation, followed by neutralization of the base with H_2SO_4 (Brit Pat 1,199,630). Substance I may be prepared by various routes starting with 3,5-dihydroxybenzoic acid.

Description—White to gray-white, crystalline powder; odorless or a faint odor of acetic acid; slightly bitter; unstable in light; melts at about 247°; pK_{a1} 8.8; pK_{a2} 10.1; pK_{a3} 11.2.

Solubility—1 g in 1.5 mL water or 250 mL alcohol.

Uses—Possesses strong β_2- and weak β_1- and α-agonist activities. It is used as a *bronchodilator* and *uterine relaxant* in premature labor. Of the β-agonists, it causes the greatest degree of tremor. It causes less tachycardia but more hyperglycemia than ritodrine. It is effective orally, by inhalation, and parenterally. By the subcutaneous route the onset of action is about 5 min, peak effect being reached in 30 to 60 min. The actions, uses, adverse effects, precautions, etc of the β-agonists are discussed in the general statement.

Dose—*Oral Inhalation, adult,* **2** or **3 deep inhalations** 1- to 5-min apart every 4 to 6 hr; total daily use should not exceed 16 to 20 inhalations. *Intravenous, adult, initially* **2.5 mg/min** followed by increments of 2.5 mg/min at 20-min intervals until contractions stop, the rate then being adjusted downward to the minimally effective rate. *Oral, adult,* **2.5** to **5 mg** 3 times a day at approximately 6-hr intervals during the waking hours for *bronchodilation* and **5 mg,** 30 min prior to discontinuation of intravenous infusion and every 4 hr thereafter in *premature labor; children, 12 to 15 yr,* **2.5 mg** 3 times a day; not advised for younger children. *Subcutaneous, adult,* **250 μ** to be repeated after 15 to 30 min, if necessary, and not to exceed 500 μg in any 4-hr period; not determined for children.

Dosage Forms—Inhalation Aerosol: 10.5 g (200 μg/activation.) Injection: 1 mg/mL; Scored Tablet: 2.5 and 5 mg.

Tetrahydrozoline Hydrochloride

Imidazole, 4,5-dihydro-2-(1,2,3,4-tetrahydro-l-naphthalenyl)-, monohydrochloride; Collyrium Fresh (*Wyeth-Ayerst*) Murine (*Abbott*); Soothe (*Alcon*); Tyzine (*Key*)

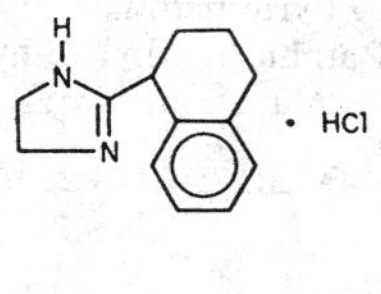

[522-48-5] $C_{13}H_{16}N_2.HCl$ (236.74).

Preparation—Ethyl phenylacetate and methyl acrylate undergo a Michael condensation and cyclization using sodium ethoxide as catalyst, followed by acidification to form 4-keto-1,2,3,4-tetrahydro-1-naphthoic acid. The keto group is reduced by catalytic hydrogenation to methylene, and the resulting 1,2,3,4-tetrahydro-1-naphthoic acid is condensed with ethylenediamine in the presence of HCl.

Description—White crystals; odorless; melts with decomposition at about 256°.

Solubility—1 g in 3.5 mL water or 7.5 mL alcohol; very slightly soluble in chloroform or ether.

Uses—Related chemically to naphazoline but differs in its actions such that in addition to topical vasoconstrictor action it has a prominent vasodilator component to its systemic effects in man. It is used only as a *nasal* and *ophthalmologic decongestant.* The local and systemic adverse effects and precautions are those of topical α-agonists. In addition, profuse sweating, sedation, severe respiratory depression, coma and shock in young children after overdosage have been reported. Overdoses in adults cause hypotension and bradycardia.

Dose—*Topical, intranasal, user over 6 yr,* **2** to **4 drops** of **0.05** or **0.1% solution** into each nostril twice a day, in the morning and in the evening; *children 2* to *6 yr,* **2** to **3 drops** of **0.05% solution** at intervals no shorter than 3 hr. *To the eye,* **1** to **2 drops** of **0.05% solution** into the conjunctival sac 2 or 3 times a day.

Dosage Form—Solution: 0.05%.

Xylometazoline Hydrochloride

1*H*-Imidazole, 2-[[4-(1,1-dimethylethyl)-2,6-dimethylphenyl]methyl]-4,5-dihydro-, monohydrochloride; Otrivin Hydrochloride (*Geigy*)

2-(4-*tert*-Butyl-2,6-dimethylbenzyl)-2-imidazoline monohydrochloride [1218-35-5] $C_{16}H_{24}N_2.HCl$ (280.84).

Preparation—Using (4-*tert*-butyl-2,6-dimethylphenyl)acetonitrile as the participating nitrile, by the method described for *Naphazoline Hydrochloride,* page 994.

Description—White, odorless crystalline powder, melts above 300° with decomposition; pH (1 in 20 solution) between 5.0 and 6.6.

Solubility—1 g in about 30 mL water; freely soluble in alcohol; sparingly soluble in chloroform; practically insoluble in benzene or ether.

Uses—A direct sympathomimetic chemically related to *Naphazoline Hydrochloride* (page 994) and *Tetrahydrozoline Hydrochloride* (page 998). It is used as a local vasoconstrictor for *nasal decongestion.* Its effects are prompt in onset and last for several hours but do not seem to be followed by as much reactive hyperemia (rebound congestion) as with naphazoline. Side effects are infrequent but are those of topical α-agonists (see the general statement for actions, uses, adverse effects, precautions and drug interactions); in addition, overdoses may cause severe central nervous depression and even coma in children.

Dose—*Intranasal, adults* and *children over 12 yr,* **2** or **3 drops** or **1** or **2 sprays** of a **0.1%** solution into each nostril every 8 to 10 hr, as needed; *children, up to 2 yr* (not recommended), **1 drop** of a **0.05%** solution every 8 to 10 hr, as needed; *2 to 12 yr,* **2** or **3 drops** of a **0.05%** solution every 8 to 10 hr, as needed.

Dosage Forms—Solution: 0.05 and 0.1%; Nasal Spray: 0.1%.

CHAPTER 58

Cholinomimetic Drugs

Donald N Franz, PhD
Professor of Pharmacology
School of Medicine, University of Utah
Salt Lake City, UT 84132

The terms *cholinomimetic* (*cholinergic*) and *parasympathomimetic* are not equivalent, but they are treated sometimes erroneously as synonyms. It will be recalled (see General Statement on *Autonomic Nervous System and Autonomic Drugs*, page 981) that acetylcholine is liberated not only at parasympathetic *post*ganglionic nerve endings but also at all autonomic *pre*ganglionic nerve endings, at somatic motor nerve endings and at certain central synapses. Thus, a cholinomimetic can be a ganglionic or neuromuscular stimulant (ie, can be *nicotinic*—see *Nicotine*, page 1002), possibly even a centrally acting drug, with or without also being a parasympathomimetic. A parasympathomimetic drug is literally an agent whose cholinomimetic action is limited to the parasympathetic neuroeffectors (ie, it is *muscarinic*). Some muscarinic substances also possess varying degrees of action on autonomic ganglia and neuromuscular junctions (ie, nicotinic actions). Even methacholine, which generally is held to be only muscarinic, exerts nicotinic actions on the neuromuscular junction in myasthenia gravis or on the adrenal medullary tumors in pheochromocytoma. There are muscarinic receptors in autonomic ganglia, but their normal function is elusive and complex. Most sweat glands are innervated by *post*ganglionic parasympathetic neurons that originate in *sympathetic* ganglia and are activated by spinal neurons that are anatomically *sympathetic*. The sweat gland receptors are therefore *muscarinic*.

Acetylcholine is hydrolyzed to choline and acetic acid by various isoenzymes called *acetylcholinesterases* at or near the site of liberation of the neurohumor. Similar specific and nonspecific esterases also are present in plasma, erythrocytes and other tissues. Drugs that inhibit these enzymes prolong the life of acetylcholine at the cholinergic neuroeffectors and synapses and thereby facilitate the normal transmission of cholinergic nervous impulses. Although this action of anticholinesterases is one of support rather than mimicry of acetylcholine, the anticholinesterases generally are classified loosely as cholinomimetics. Therefore, they also are included in this chapter. The section on *Anticholinesterases* begins on page 1003.

Cholinomimetics

Except for nicotine, therapeutic cholinomimetic drugs are used for their muscarinic actions. Muscarinic drugs dilate nearly all blood vessels, except that they constrict certain veins. Although the receptors are on the smooth myocytes, there is no direct coupling to the cell interior; rather, the receptors activate endothelial cells which, in turn, release endothelium-derived relaxing factor (EDRF) now known to be nitric oxide (NO), which elicits smooth muscle relaxation by activation of guanyl cyclase to increase cyclic GMP in smooth muscle. In high doses they may decrease heart rate and atrioventricular conduction velocity and cause varying degrees of heart block; they also may decrease the strength of atrial, but not ventricular, contractions. However, in therapeutic doses, usually only vasodilatation occurs and the heart rate and contractility actually may increase because of sympathetically mediated reflexes to the hypotension caused by vasodilatation. The muscarinic drugs stimulate gastrointestinal smooth muscle and increase peristalsis, thus decreasing bowel transit time and promoting defecation; in high doses, bowel and sphincter spasms can occur. The lower esophageal sphincter also is stimulated. There also are muscarinic actions to contract the smooth muscle of the detrusor muscle of the urinary bladder but relax that of the trigone sphincter, thus causing urination. The bronchial smooth muscle is contracted, and bronchospasm may result. Stimulation of the sphincter of the iris causes miosis (pupilloconstriction); stimulation of the ciliary muscle causes ciliary spasm and a decrease in intraocular tension in glaucoma. Miosis and ciliary spasm usually do not occur after systemic administration, since the muscarinic drugs penetrate poorly into the eye from the blood stream; topical or intraocular administration is employed to achieve therapeutic miosis. Most exocrine glands are stimulated; thus, excessive salivation, rhinorrhea, bronchorrhea (and mucous plugs), increased gastric and pancreatic secretions, and copious sweating may be elicited.

All muscarinic drugs have some degree of nicotinic activity, although some may be considered devoid of such activity for practical purposes. Even with those that have relatively strong nicotinic activity, such as acetylcholine (the natural nicotinic neurotransmitter), nicotinic effects, such as neuromuscular stimulation and paralysis and sympathoadrenal discharge, usually are manifested only in highly toxic doses; however, in therapeutic doses, carbachol appears to exert some nicotinic actions at mural ganglia in the gut and perhaps at sacral parasympathetic ganglia.

Uses—The miotic and ciliary spastic effects are used in the topical treatment of *open-angle, acute congestive* and *narrow-angle glaucoma*, prior to or *during intraocular surgery*, such as cataract surgery (after the lens is delivered), iridectomy, penetrating keratoplasty and other anterior segment surgery; they also are used in alternation with mydriatic drugs to *break adhesions between the iris and the lens*. They are used occasionally in the treatment of *accommodative strabismus*. Muscarinic drugs may be used to *antagonize mydriatics*.

In gastroenterology certain muscarinic drugs are used in the treatment of *atonic constipation, congenital megacolon* (Hirschsprung's disease), postoperative and postpartum *adynamic intestinal ileus*, and *postvagotomy gastric atony*. They also are used occasionally to stimulate pancreatic secretion in tests of pancreatic function. In genitourinary practice muscarinic drugs may be used to treat *functional urinary retention*. Their principal cardiovascular use is for the diagnosis and attempted arrest of *paroxysmal atrial tachycardia*; even though therapeutic doses usually do not depress the normal functions of the heart, they often do induce a conduction block in the aberrant conduction pathway within the atrioventricular node that permits this reentrant arrhythmia to occur. *Vasospastic peripheral vascular disorders*, such as accompany Raynaud's disease and cold exposure or frostbite, have been treated successfully with these agents, but superior drugs are available. This is also true of their use to increase cutaneous blood flow in *scleroderma*. Muscarinic drugs are not useful in the management of occlusive vascular diseases.

In pulmonary practice methacoline is used as a diagnostic agent for asthma, the asthmatic patient being ultrasensitive to the bronchoconstricting effects.

Adverse Effects—The adverse effects of muscarinic drugs are simply extensions of their pharmacodynamic actions. Thus, excessive salivary, nasopharyngeal and bronchial secretions and bronchospasm are not only uncomfortable but may be life-threatening by way of impeding the movement of air to and from the lungs. Excessive sweating may cause discomfort, affect the clothing and interfere with body temperature control. In low doses, vasodilatation mainly may be confined to the skin, causing flushing and prickly or burning sensations. Moderate to high doses may cause moderate to severe hypotension, leading to syncope and even shock. Excessive doses may cause severe bradycardia, even cardiac arrest, and atrioventricular conduction disturbances, especially heart block. Furthermore, reflex sympathoadrenal discharge coupled with direct muscarinic effects on conduction sets the stage for serious cardiac arrhythmias. Gastrointestinal adverse effects include epigastric distress, belching, diarrhea, involuntary defecation, nausea and vomiting (partly as the result of hypotension) and colic. There also may be a feeling of tightness in the urinary bladder, urinary frequency and enuresis.

Topical muscarinic drugs applied to the conjunctiva or intraocularly may interfere with near vision (accommodative myopia) and cause blurred vision, ocular pain, browache, headache, ciliary and conjunctival congestion, twitching of the eyelids and decreased vision in poor light. After conjunctival application, there may be enough local absorption and nasolacrimal drainage into the bloodstream to produce systemic side effects.

Precautions and Contraindications—Muscarinic drugs should be used cautiously in patients with hypertension, especially those under treatment with antihypertensive drugs, and when there is arteriosclerosis (since reflex adjustments to the hypotensive effects may be impaired). Systemic muscarinic drugs are contraindicated in the presence of atrioventricular conduction defects, coronary insufficiency, pheochromocytoma (catecholamine release and hypertensive crisis may be initiated), hyperthyroidism (atrial fibrillation may result), asthma and peptic ulcer. Even in ophthalmologic use, care must be exercised in these conditions. After instillation of solutions into the conjunctival sac, the nasolacrimal duct should be occluded by digital pressure to minimize drainage and oral absorption.

Atropine should be at hand, in case serious side effects occur. The muscarinic (parasympathomimetic) actions can be blocked by atropine and its congeners, which serve as antidotes to overdosage, and the ganglionic and neuromuscular (nicotinic) stimulant actions can be antagonized, respectively, by ganglionic blocking and neuromuscular blocking agents.

Acetylcholine Chloride

Ethanaminium, 2-(acetyloxy)-*N,N,N*-trimethyl-, chloride; Miochol (*CooperVision*)

$CH_3CO(CH_2)_2N^+(CH_3)_3\ \ Cl^-$

Choline chloride acetate [60-31-1] $C_7H_{16}ClNO_2$ (181.66).

Preparation—Trimethylamine is reacted with 2-chloroethyl acetate as described in *Bull Soc Chim France 15(4):* 544, 1914.

Description—Hygroscopic, crystalline powder.

Solubility—Very soluble in cold water or alcohol; decomposed by hot water or alkalies; practically insoluble in ether.

Uses—Principally a topical ophthalmological drug to *induce miosis* during certain intraocular surgical procedures, such as cataract surgery (*after* the lens is delivered), iridectomy, penetrating keratoplasty and other anterior segment surgery. It is given as an irrigant into the anterior chamber. When applied to the intact cornea, acetylcholine penetrates too poorly to be a clinically useful miotic.

Because of the rapidity by which acetylcholine is destroyed by acetylcholinesterase, it has no systemic uses; even huge doses rarely cause death. When death occurs it is usually a hypoxic death from mucous plugs in the bronchial tree or a cardiac death from fibrillation caused by the combination of cholinergic and reflex sympatho-adrenal stimulation.

Dose—*Topical,* into the anterior chamber of the eye, as a **1% solution.**

Dosage Form—for Ophthalmic Solution: 20 mg/2 mL in a 2-chamber vial.

Bethanechol Chloride

1-Propanaminium, 2-[(aminocarbonyl)oxy]-*N,N,N*-trimethyl-, chloride; Duvoid (*Norwich Eaton*); Urabeth (*Major*); Urecholine Chloride (*MSD*)

$$\left[\begin{array}{l}CH_3CHCH_2N^+(CH_3)_3\\ \quad\ \ |\\ \quad OCONH_2\end{array}\right] Cl^-$$

(2-Hydroxypropyl)trimethylammonium chloride carbamate [590-63-6] $C_7H_{17}ClN_2O_2$ (196.68).

Preparation—By treating propylene chlorohydrin with phosgene, reacting the condensation product (2-chloro-1-methylethyl chloroformate) with ammonia in ether solution and heating the resulting urethan with trimethylamine.

Description—Colorless or white crystals or a white crystalline powder, usually having a slight, amine-like odor; slightly hygroscopic; pH (1% solution) between 5.5 and 6.5; exhibits polymorphism (one form melts about 211° and the other about 219°).

Solubility—1 g in 0.6 mL water or 13 mL alcohol; less soluble in dehydrated alcohol; insoluble in chloroform or ether.

Uses—Has somewhat stronger muscarinic activity for the gastrointestinal and urinary tracts than for the cardiovascular system and hence is employed systemically only for the gastroenterological and genitourinary uses indicated in the general statement. See the general statement for ophthalmologic uses, adverse effects, precautions and contraindications. Bethanechol chloride is not hydrolyzed by the cholinesterases and it has a relatively prolonged duration of action.

Bethanechol chloride is supplied for subcutaneous and for oral administration. It should be taken on an empty stomach. It should not be administered by the intravenous or intramuscular route. Even with subcutaneous administration, adverse systemic effects may occur.

Dose—*Oral, adult, initially* **5** to **10 mg** followed by hourly increments of 5 mg until a satisfactory response is achieved, then, for *maintenance,* **5** to **50 mg** 2 to 4 times a day. *Oral, pediatric* **200 μg** (0.2 mg)/**kg** (6.7 mg/m²) 3 times a day. *Subcutaneous, adult, initially* **2.5 mg,** repeated at 15- to 30-min intervals as necessary, up to **10 mg,** to obtain a satisfactory response, then **2.5** to **10 mg** 3 or 4 times a day. *Subcutaneous, pediatric,* **150** to **200 μg** (0.15 to 0.2 mg)/**kg** (or 5 to 6.7 mg/m²) 3 times a day).

Dosage Forms—Injection: 5 mg/mL; Tablets: 5, 10, 25 and 50 mg.

Carbachol

Ethanaminium, 2-[(aminocarbonyl)oxy]-*N,N,N*-trimethyl-, chloride; Miostat (*Alcon*)

$[NH_2COOCH_2CH_2N^+(CH_3)_3]Cl^-$

Choline chloride, carbamate [51-83-2] (182.65).

Preparation—By reaction of ethylene chlorohydrin with phosgene, the resulting chloroethyl chloroformate treated with ammonia to produce chloroethyl urethan, which yields carbachol when reacted with aqueous trimethylamine.

Description—White or faintly yellow crystals or crystalline powder; odorless or with a slight amine-like odor; hygroscopic; melts between 200 and 204°; pK_a 4.8.

Solubility—1 g in about 1 mL water or 50 mL alcohol; practically insoluble in chloroform or ether.

Uses—Carbachol has a moderate degree of selectivity for the gastrointestinal and urinary tracts, hence it formerly was used widely in gastroenterology and genitourinary practice. Currently, it is used in ophthalmology, mainly for the treatment of narrow-angle glaucoma and to induce miosis prior to ocular surgery. It is not hydrolyzed by cholinesterase and hence has a longer duration of action than methacholine and acetylcholine. See the general statement for actions, adverse effects and contraindications.

Dose—*Topical, adult,* **1** to **2 drops** of **0.75** to **3% solution** instilled into the conjunctival sac 2 or 3 times a day; the nasolacrimal ducts should be occluded during application. *Intraocular, adult,* as an irrigant into the anterior chamber, **0.5 mL** of **0.01% solution.**

Dosage Forms—Ophthalmic Solution: 0.75, 1.5, 2.25 and 3%: Intraocular solution: 0.01%.

Methacholine Chloride

Propanaminium, 2-(acetyloxy)-*N*,*N*,*N*-trimethyl-, chloride; Provocholine (*Roche*)

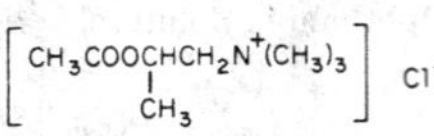

$$\left[\begin{array}{c} CH_3COOCHCH_2N^+(CH_3)_3 \\ \quad | \\ \quad CH_3 \end{array}\right] Cl^-$$

(2-Hydroxypropyl)trimethyl ammonium chloride acetate [62-51-1] $C_8H_{18}ClNO_2$ (195.69).

Preparation—From trimethylacetonylammonium chloride by reduction followed by acetylation. (US Pat 2,040,145).

Description—Highly deliquescent; faint, fishy odor; aqueous solutions are neutral and stable for only short periods even when refrigerated; alkaline excipients promote degradation.

Solubility—Freely soluble in water, alcohol or chloroform;

Uses—Methacholine is a selective muscarinic agent. However, weak nicotinic actions are manifested at the neuromuscular junction in myasthenic persons and at adrenal medullary tumors in pheochromocytoma. Presently, it is marketed only for the diagnosis of bronchial asthma. Persons with asthma are much more sensitive to the bronchoconstrictor actions than are normal persons. A positive test is a 20% or greater decrease in the forced expiratory volume. However, there is a tendency toward false positives among nonasthmatic smokers and relatives of asthmatics; there is also a small percentage of false negatives. Hypertensives are excessively sensitive to the hypotensive effects, but persons with pheochromocytoma respond with an acute hypertension. Adverse effects of the inhaled drug are syncope and cardiac arrest, for which 0.5 to 1 mg of atropine is given. There is a rare incidence of vertigo, throat irritation and itching. Methacholine is contraindicated in the presence of beta-adrenoreceptor-blocking drugs. Cromolyn may attenuate the bronchoconstrictor response.

Dose—5 breaths of a **0.025** to **25 mg/mL solution,** starting with the lowest concentration and progressing serially to the concentration that elicits a positive response.

Dosage Form—Powder: 100 mg, to be reconstituted with 4 mL of saline injection; subsequent dilutions are 10, 2.5, 0.25 and 0.025 mg/mL.

Muscarine—see RPS-18, page 891.

Nicotine

Pyridine, 3-(1-methyl-2-pyrrolidinyl-,)

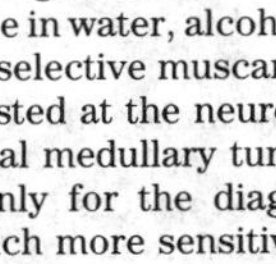

[54-11-5]$C_{11}H_{14}N_2$ (162-23). An alkaloid from *Nicotiana tabacum* or N rustica.

Preparation—Commercially, it is a byproduct of the tobacco industry where it occurs to the extent of 2 to 8%. It is extracted from waste tobacco with organic solvents and purified through the zinc chloride double salt.

Description—Poisonous, oily liquid; unpleasant tobacco-like odor; burning taste; strongly alkaline reaction; pK_1 6.16; pK_2 10.96 at 15°.

Solubility—Soluble in water, alcohol, chloroform and most common organic solvents.

Nicotine is the prototype of cholinomimetics of the so-called nicotinic type. Because it was used by early investigators to determine both cholinomimetic agonist and antagonist actions at the ganglia, at the adrenal medulla and at the neuromuscular junction the cholinergic receptors at these sites are designated as the nicotinic subtypes. The action of nicotine in the body is characterized by a primary transient stimulation followed by a persistent depression of all sympathetic and parasympathetic ganglia. The actions are explained by a common mechanism, namely, that of depolarization of the postsynaptic membrane. During the onset of depolarization, nerve action potentials are generated. Once the postsynaptic membrane becomes fully depolarized, further action potentials cannot be initiated, since they require a polarized postsynaptic membrane at their outset. Thus, a block of synaptic transmission results from the persisting depolarization induced by nicotine. Even after the membrane potential is restored, the block may persist. The synaptic stimulatory and depressant effects of nicotine cannot be overcome by atropine.

Nicotine likewise stimulates then paralyzes skeletal muscles and thus induces a succinylcholine-like action, which is the major reason for the toxic effect of the alkaloid on respiration. However, nicotine is more active on ganglia than on skeletal muscles, whereas the reverse is true of succinylcholine. In addition to the above well-established actions, nicotine also first stimulates then depresses the central nervous system.

Cardiovascular effects of nicotine are hypertension (which may tend to shift to hypotension with time), a smearing of circadian cardiovascular rhythms, tachycardia, a positive inotropic effect (only a part of which can be explained by an effect on nicotinic receptors) and, in large doses, a variety of abnormal electrocardiographic effects. The relationship of these effects to the cardiomyopathy of smoking is unknown. Nicotine does not appear to elevate blood-lipid levels, so that its relationship to smoking-aggravated coronary artery disease is unknown.

The CNS effects of nicotine probably are the most important to the initiation and maintenance of the smoking habit. Nicotine is a CNS stimulant that resembles psychomotor stimulants and it may induce subtle, complex changes in behavior. Although it is often dysphoric in the naive user, it is euphorigenic in tobacco habitues. It increases alertness and attention and, consequently, may improve memory somewhat. It decreases irritability and appetite. Deep tendon reflexes and skeletal muscle tone are diminished, which may contribute to a feeling of relaxation. However, it also may induce skeletal muscle tremor and even cause convulsions in large doses. Death may be either consequent to convulsions or respiratory arrest as the result of CNS depression and skeletal muscle paralysis. The adult lethal dose is 40 to 60 mg. Even low doses may cause nausea and vomiting by actions at the chemoreceptor trigger zone and the "vomiting center" in the medulla oblongata. The CNS actions are the result of a combination of the stimulation of nicotinic and dopaminergic receptors, blockade of some central cholinergic synapses, inhibition of choline acetylase and release of acetylcholine, dopamine, norepinephrine and serotonin. Nicotine also causes the release of several hormones, to which some effects are secondary.

Nicotine is metabolized to cotinine in the liver. The plasma half-life is about 2 hr. Nicotine, along with various other constituents of tobacco smoke, induces various hepatic microsomal enzymes in both phase 1 and phase 2 metabolism. Estrogen elimination is accelerated and may cause menopausal-like consequences. Nicotine also increases the elimination of hydrocortisone, which is counterbalanced by greater release of the hormone from the adrenal cortex because of enhanced ACTH release. The metabolism of caffeine, theophylline, imipramine, pentazocine, propranolol, propoxyphene, mexiletene and probably numerous other drugs is accelerated.

Uses—Although nicotine has never been used as a therapeutic agent, in recent years nicotine gum and transdermal nicotine patches have been introduced to suppress withdrawal symptoms in chronic tobacco users who are trying to quit. The strategy is to substitute nicotine for that previously obtained from tobacco and then to taper the dose over a period of weeks until tobacco dependency subsides.

In nicotine gum, nicotine is complexed with a polyacrylic resin. Release from the resin is slow, so that euphorigenesis is less apparent. Nevertheless, nicotine dependence is maintained. Adverse effects from the nicotine content include (in decreasing order of incidence) nausea and vomiting, eructations, vertigo, sialorrhea, headache and irritability. Effects from constant chewing are oropharyngeal soreness and jaw muscle ache. Each stick contains 2 or 4 mg of nicotine; it should be chewed for 20 to 30 min during which time about 90% of the nicotine is absorbed.

Nicotine transdermal systems are attached to hairless, clean skin once a day and deliver a rapid initial release of nicotine followed by a slow release over the next 24 hr, at which time the patch is exchanged for a new one attached to a different site. One manufacturer directs application for 16 hr/day with removal at bedtime. Daily dosage (5 to 22 mg) is regulated and tapered by using patches of differing sizes (3.5 to 30 cm^2). The most common adverse effect is a reversible erythema, pruritis or burning at the site of application. Hypersensitivity reactions occur in 2% of patients. Headache, insomnia, abnormal dreams, nervousness, insomnia and gastrointestinal complaints are relatively common. Serious toxicity can result from oral ingestion of patches or from application of multiple patches.

Dosage Forms—Nicotine Gum: 2 or 4 mg. Transdermal Systems: 5 to 22 mg delivered every 16 or 24 hr.

Pilocarpine

2(3*H*)-Furanone, (3*S*-*cis*)-3-ethyldihydro-4-[(1-methyl-1*H*-imidazol-5-yl) methyl]-, Ocusert (*Ciba-Geigy*)

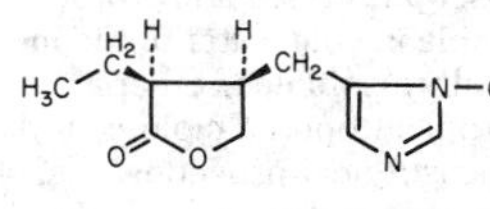

Pilocarpine monohydrochloride [92-13-7] $C_{11}H_{16}N_2O_2$ (208.25).

Preparation—The total alkaloids are extracted from the dried crushed leaves of *Pilocarpus microphyllus*, or other suitable *Pilocarpus* species, with alcohol containing a small amount of hydrochloric acid. The solvent is distilled, the aqueous residue neutralized with ammonia and allowed to stand until the resins are all deposited. It is then filtered, and the filtrate evaporated to a small bulk. Ammonia is added in excess and the free alkaloids extracted with chloroform. The solvent is removed by distillation and the residue allowed to crystallize.

Description—Colorless, translucent, odorless, faintly bitter crystals; hygroscopic and affected by light; solutions acid to litmus; melts within a range of 3° between 199 and 204°; pK_{a1} 6.8, pK_{a2} 1.3.

Solubility—Soluble in water, alcohol or chloroform; sparingly soluble in ether.

Incompatibilities—See *Alkaloids*, in Chapter 26. Since the free alkaloid is quite soluble in water, *alkalies* do not readily cause a precipitation when added to solutions of its salts. It reduces *silver nitrate*.

Uses—A muscarinic agonist that is totally devoid of nicotinic activity but is nonselective with respect to muscarinic targets. Because it is a tertiary amine, it penetrates membranes much better than do quaternary ammonium cholinomimetics. Consequently, it lends itself well to topical administration in ophthalmology (see below). Systemically, it is not selective enough to be used for gastrointestinal, genitourinary or cardiovascular purposes.

Pilocarpine is tolerated better than other miotics. It rarely causes irritation or hypersensitivity, and systemic responses following topical application are uncommon; however, absorption from solutions of high concentration may result in systemic side effects. Lens opacities may result from prolonged use. Ocular controlled- release systems may cause mechanical irritation of the conjunctiva and sometimes a slight increase in mucus secretion, which usually wanes during continued use.

The free base, pilocarpine, is employed in the ocular controlled-release system, since only the nonionized form can diffuse readily through the "hydrophobic" membrane. The hydrochloride or nitrate salt is employed to make solutions and gels; the less hygroscopic nitrate is the more convenient to handle pharmaceutically but offers no therapeutic advantage.

In narrow-angle glaucomatous patients who are responsive to pilocarpine and who can maintain the unit within the conjunctival sac, the ocular controlled-release system has the advantage of long duration, the system needing to be changed but once a week. Topically applied drops are suited better to the acute antagonism of antimuscarinic mydriatics. The salts also may be used in the management of both narrow-angle glaucoma and chronic simple glaucoma of the open-angle type.

Dose—*Topical*, as an ocular controlled-release system placed in the conjunctival sac, to release an average of **20** or **40 μg/hr** over a period of 7 days, after which time the system should be changed. Therapy usually is started with the 20 μg/hr system and switched to the 40 μg/hr system only if control with the lower-rated system is inadequate. Since pilocarpine-induced myopia may occur during the first several hours after insertion, the unit should be inserted at bedtime to allow stabilization of the myopia before arising.

Dosage Form—Controlled-Release Inserts: 5 mg (to release 20 μg/hr) and 11 mg (to release 40 μg/hr).

Pilocarpine Hydrochloride

2(3*H*)-Furanone, (3*S*-*cis*)-3-ethyldihydro-4-[(1-methyl-1*H*-imidazol-5-yl)methyl]-, monohydrochloride;
(*Various Mfrs*)

Pilocarpine monohydrochloride [54-71-7] $C_{11}H_{16}N_2O_2.HCl$ (244.72)

Description—Colorless, translucent, odorless, faintly bitter crystals; hygroscopic and affected by light; solutions acid to litmus; melts within a range of 3° between 199 and 204°; pK_{a1} 6.8, pK_{a2} 1.3.

Solubility—1 g in 0.3 mL water, 3 mL alcohol or 360 mL chloroform; insoluble in ether.

Incompatibilities—See *Alkaloids* (page 397). Since the free alkaloid is quite soluble in water, *alkalies* do not readily cause a precipitation when added to solutions of its salts. It reduces *silver nitrate*.

Uses—See *Pilocarpine*, above.

Dose—*Topical*, **1** to **2 drops** of **0.25** to **10%** solution into the conjunctival sac 1 to 6 times a day, as directed by a physician.

Dosage Forms—Ophthalmic Gel: 4%; Ophthalmic Solution: 0.25, 0.5, 1, 1.5, 2, 3, 4, 5, 6, 8 and 10%.

Pilocarpine Nitrate

2(3*H*)-Furanone, (3*S*-*cis*)-3-ethyldihydro-4-[(1-methyl-1*H*-imidazol-5-yl)methyl]-; mononitrate; P.V. Carpine Liquifilm
(*Allergan*)

Pilocarpine mononitrate [148-72-1] $C_{11}H_{16}N_2O_2.HNO_3$ (271.27).

Description—Shining, white crystals; stable in air but is affected by light; solutions are acid to litmus; melts within a range of 3° between 171 and 176°.

Solubility—1 g in 4 mL water or 75 mL alcohol; insoluble in chloroform or ether.

Incompatibilities—See *Pilocarpine Hydrochloride*.

Uses—See *Pilocarpine*, above.

Dose—*Topical*, **1** to **2 drops** of a **1** to **4%** solution into the conjunctival sac 1 to 6 times a day, as directed by a physician; the 1 and 2% solutions are the ones usually used.

Dosage Form—Ophthalmic Solution: 1, 2 and 4%.

Anticholinesterases

The term cholinesterase is a generic term that includes all enzymes capable of hydrolyzing acetylcholine. There are two main categories of cholinesterase. The term *acetylcholinesterase* is applied to any or all of a family of serine-dependent isoenzymes that very selectively hydrolyze acetylcholine and hence is called true, or specific, cholinesterase; it is not truly specific, since other choline esters may be hydrolyzed with low velocities. Acetylcholinesterase is concentrated in the region of the motor end plate, at autonomic ganglia, in cholinergic neurons in and outside the central nervous system and in erythrocytes. The term *butyrylcholinesterase* (also called cholinesterase, pseudocholinesterase or nonspecific cholinesterase) is applied to a number of enzymes that may hydrolyze acetylcholine but for which butyrylcholine, not acetylcholine, is the optimal substrate. Butyrylcholinesterase is present in glial and satellite cells in the central nervous system and autonomic ganglia, in smooth muscle, exocrine glands and various organs, such as the liver, and plasma; its concentration in cholinergic neurons is usually insignificant.

Inhibition of acetylcholinesterase and butyrylcholinesterase has various consequences depending on where the enzymes are inhibited. Neither the butyrylcholinesterase in plasma nor the acetylcholinesterase in erythrocytes have known functions, and their inhibition has no known physiological consequences, but inhibition may cause moderate increases in the plasma half-life and concentration of acetylcholine and certain other hydrolyzable choline esters. The only important effects accrue to inhibition at sites of cholinergic neuroeffector transmission. The preservation of acetylcholine at such sites prolongs and intensifies the cholinergic activity there. Thus, at the neuromuscular junction, anticholinesterases facilitate neuromuscular transmission, with an early increase in muscle strength (by recruiting subliminal junctions) and a late decrease in muscle strength, even paralysis, if many motor end plates remain depolarized by persisting levels of acetylcholine. Excessive muscular fasciculations and fibrillations also occur, which also decrease muscle strength, by causing asynchrony among motor units and fibers. At the autonomic ganglia, the predominant effect is to facilitate transmission, and the final resultant effect depends on the effector organ system innervated by the excited postganglionic nerves. In the case of the atria and the atrioventricular node, the activity in both adrenergic and cholinergic postganglionic nerves will be increased, so that the effects mediated by the parasympathetic nerves will be antagonized by those of the sympathetic nerves. However, in the parasympathetic innervation, acetylcholine is preserved by the anticholinesterase at two sites, the ganglia and the innervated heart cells, which amplifies the action, whereas, in the sympathetic innervation, transmission is facilitated only at the ganglia. Therefore, where there is dual and antagonistic innervation, as in the atria, atrioventricular node, pupil, stomach and intestines, urinary tract, etc, the parasympathetic effects predominate. Thus, bradycardia, partial heart block, miosis, increased gastric secretion and motility and tendency to urination all result from significant anticholinesterase activity. The blood pressure may be elevated, because there is little cholinergic innervation of the vascular tree and the facilitation in the sympathetic pathway is not antagonized at the vascular smooth muscle. Ciliary spasm may be intense, because there is a negligible antagonistic sympathetic innervation of the ciliary body. Facilitation in both sympathetic and parasympathetic pathways cause increased salivation and sweating (which is mostly cholinergic). Anticholinesterase action within the central nervous system may cause a bizarre mixture of stimulation and depression.

There are two main categories of cholinesterase inhibitors: those that are amine or quaternary ammonium compounds, which interact with the anionic sites of the cholinesterase as well as with the esteratic site and those that are usually organophosphates (but may contain other nucleophilic moieties) which esterify the serine hydroxyl group at the esteratic site. The amine or ammonium anticholinesterases react reversibly with the enzymes, consistent with ionic bonding; their durations of action are a few minutes to a few hours and are determined by elimination pharmacokinetics. The organophosphate-type anticholinesterases form a firmer bond, some so firm as to be essentially irreversible. With these, the duration of action is determined by the kinetics of dissociation at the esteratic site or, with essentially irreversibly acting ones (like isoflurophate), the time for resynthesis of cholinesterase (weeks to months).

The organophosphate-type anticholinesterases cannot enhance neuromuscular transmission without excessive effects on glands and smooth muscle. They are un-ionized and, hence, also readily penetrate the blood-brain barrier and cause CNS effects. They also can be absorbed through the skin. The amine and ammonium agents are more selective for acetylcholinesterase and the quaternary ammonium anticholinesterases, especially, often may enhance neuromuscular function with only minimal to moderate autonomic side effects. The amine agents, like physostigmine and tacrine, can pass the blood-brain barrier and elicit central effects, and they are employed only for their central actions, except that physostigmine also is applied topically to the eye. The quaternary ammonium compounds have a nicotinic agonist activity, which, at the ganglia and neuromuscular junction, adds to the indirect anticholinesterase effect; therefore, because of this dual effect, they are the agents chosen to enhance neuromuscular function. Because of their confinement to the periphery, the quaternary agents also are chosen for peripheral actions.

Uses—The quaternary ammonium anticholinesterases are used systemically to abolish muscular paralysis from competitive *neuromuscular blocking drugs*, to improve muscle function in *myasthenia gravis*, to treat *intestinal distention*, such as congenital *megacolon*, postoperative and postpartum *adynamic intestinal ileus*, *postvagotomy gastric atony* and *functional urinary retention*. They also have received desultory trials in the management of *gastroesophageal reflux* to increase lower esophageal pressure. They have an erratic usefulness in the treatment of *delayed menstruation*. Edrophonium is used as an antiarrhythmic drug to interrupt the reentrant conduction pathway in *paroxysmal atrial tachycardia*. Edrophonium or neostigmine are used also in the differential *diagnosis of myasthenic crisis*, in which case they will improve muscle function; *cholinergic crisis*, in which case they will worsen function; and to diagnose *myotonia congenita*. Neostigmine at one time was used in the diagnosis of early pregnancy; three successive daily doses will initiate menstruation in 72 hours unless the patient is pregnant. Anticholinesterases, especially physostigmine, are used to treat atropine or tricyclic antidepressant poisoning.

Physostigmine, a blood-brain-barrier-penetrant amine anticholinesterase, is employed to *antagonize the toxic CNS effects of antimuscarinic drugs, tricyclic antidepressants* and *H_1-antihistamines*.

The anticholinesterases are applied topically to the eye in the treatment of primary *wide-angle glaucoma, accommodative convergent strabismus, accommodative esotropia* and for the *emergency treatment of acute congestive glaucoma*. They also may be used to *treat marginal corneal ulcers*. In *myasthenia gravis* topical application may be used to improve the function of the extraocular muscles and eyelids. The reversibly acting anticholinesterases may be alternated with mydriatics to *break adhesions between lens and iris*.

Adverse Effects and Intoxication—Conjunctivally applied anticholinesterases locally may cause stinging, lacrimation, ocular pain and browache (from ciliary spasm), blurring of vision, blepharospasm, conjunctival and intraocular hyperemia, transient early rise in intraocular pressure, iridocyclitis, pigment cysts of the iris, anterior and posterior synechiae and, rarely, retinal detachment. Atropine can antagonize some of these effects. Allergies also may occur. In addition, organophosphates may cause fibrinous iritis cataracts, especially in elderly patients (in 50% of cases chronically treated), and uveitis.

Adverse systemic effects, from systemic administration or systemic absorption after topical application, include excessive salivation, sweating, tracheobronchial secretion, lacrimation, bronchoconstriction, marked miosis, blurring of vision, nausea and vomiting, diarrhea, abdominal cramps and colic, involuntary defecation, pallor, hypertension or hypotension, bradycardia and urinary frequency, urgency and enuresis. These effects can be antagonized with sufficiently large doses of atropine. Laryngospasm, tremors, muscle fasciculations and twitching, weakness (even respiratory paralysis), potentiation of succinylcholine and dizziness are nicotinic effects that cannot be antagonized with atropine. These effects usually occur only after quite large overdoses. Pralidoxime will antagonize these actions if given early enough. Acute intoxication caused by large doses of physostigmine or organophosphates also induces CNS effects, such as confusion, ataxia, loss of reflexes, slurred speech, Cheyne-Stokes respiration, convulsions, coma and respiratory and circulatory paralysis. Huge doses of atropine and pralidoxime, if used early, can suppress these effects. General supportive measures also are necessary in the management of both peripheral and central toxicity.

Some, but not all, organophosphates cause a latent demyelination and degeneration of various nerve axons.

Precautions and Contraindications—When systemic anticholinesterases are used, the margin between the first appearance of side effects and serious toxic effects is small. The first signs may be quite subtle. Furthermore, there is a wide variation among patients and in the same patient from time to time, so each patient must be approached cautiously. Therefore, careful medical supervision is mandatory. Anticholinesterases should be used cautiously, or withheld, in patients with bronchial asthma, mechanical intestinal or urinary obstruction, peptic ulcer, vagotonia, bradycardia, hypotension, recent myocardial infarction, epilepsy, parkinsonism or a known hypersensitivity to depolarizing neuromuscular blocking drugs and when cholinomimetics are to be used. Quinidine and quinine antagonize the neuromuscular effects of the anticholinesterases. They should not be applied topically to the eye when there is a history of retinal detachment, uveitis or angle-closure glaucoma. Their potential systemic effects command the same precautions as for systemic anticholinesterases. Systemic anticholinesterases will antagonize ganglionic-blocking drugs. The safety of the amine and quaternary ammonium agents in mother and fetus during pregnancy has not been established; systemic organophosphates are absolutely contraindicated.

Ambenonium Chloride

Benzenemethanaminium, *N,N'*-[(1,2-dioxo-1,2-ethanediyl)bis(imino-2,1-ethanediyl)]bis[2-chloro-*N,N*-diethyl]-, dichloride; Mysuran; Mytelase (*Winthrop*)

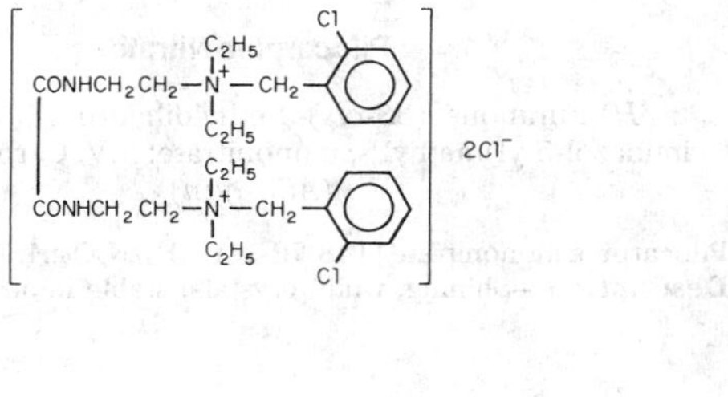

[Oxalylbis(iminoethylene)]bis[(*o*-chlorobenzyl)diethylammonium] dichloride [115-79-7] $C_{28}H_{42}Cl_4N_4O_2$ (608.48); *tetrahydrate* [52022-31-8] (680.54).

Preparation—*N,N*-Diethylethylenediamine is reacted with ethyl oxalate to give *N,N'*-bis[2-(diethylamino)ethyl]oxamide which is doubly quaternized with 2-chlorobenzyl chloride. US Pat 3,096,373.

Description—White, odorless powder melting at about 200°.

Solubility—1 g in 5 mL water, 20 mL alcohol, > 1000 mL chloroform or > 1000 mL ether.

Uses—A quaternary ammonium *anticholinesterase* drug (see general statement) with actions similar to those of *Neostigmine* (see page 1006); ambenonium chloride is 2 to 4 times more potent, and its duration of action after oral administration (4 hr) may be slightly longer. It also is claimed to have a lower incidence of side effects than neostigmine, particularly of the gastrointestinal tract. It is used in the treatment of *myasthenia gravis*. For side effects and precautions, see the general statement, above.

Dose—*Oral, adult, initially* **5 mg**, gradually increased as required up to **25 mg 3** or **4** times a day. Occasionally, as much as 75 mg per dose may be required. Doses over 200 mg a day require careful medical supervision.

Dosage Form—Scored Tablets: 10 mg.

Demecarium Bromide

Benzenaminium, 3,3'-[1,10-decanediylbis(methylimino)-carbonyloxy]bis[*N,N,N*-trimethyl-, dibromide; Humorsol (*MSD*)

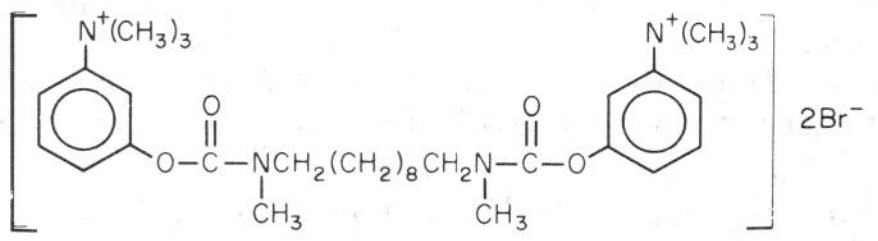

(*m*-Hydroxyphenyl)trimethylammonium bromide decamethylenebis-[methylcarbamate](2:1) [56-94-0] $C_{32}H_{52}Br_2N_4O_4$ (716.60).

Preparation—*N,N'*-Dimethyl-1,10-decamethylenediamine is added to molten 3-(dimethylamino)phenyl carbonate to produce 1,10-decamethylenebis[3-(dimethylamino)phenyl *N*-methylcarbamate]. This ester, a viscous oil, is dissolved in ethanol and doubly quaternized with an acetone solution of methyl bromide. US Pat 2,789,981.

Description—White, or slightly yellow, slightly hygroscopic, crystalline powder; melts at about 165°, with decomposition; pH (1 in 100 solution) between 5.0 and 7.0.

Solubility—Freely soluble in water or alcohol; sparingly soluble in acetone; soluble in ether; aqueous solutions are stable and may be heat-sterilized.

Uses—A quaternary ammonium *anticholinesterase* drug that has high topical penetrability into the eye. It is used topically for its ophthalmological actions (see the general statement). These actions may last an advantageous 3 to 5 days.

Dose—*Topical, adult* and *pediatric*, to the conjunctiva, **1** to **2 drops** of **0.125** to **0.25%** solution twice a wk to 1 or 2 times a day. For details of frequency and duration of application in the various uses of demecarium bromide see USP DI, vol 1, or the package literature.

Dosage Form—Ophthalmic Solution: 0.125 and 0.25% in a 5-mL ocumeter.

Echothiophate Iodide

Ethanaminium, 2-[(diethoxyphosphinyl)thio]-*N,N,N*-trimethyl-, iodide; Ecodide (*Alcon*); Phospholine Iodide (*Ayerst*)

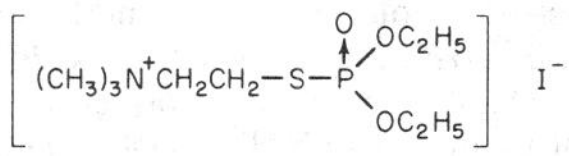

(2-Mercaptoethyl)trimethylammonium iodide *S*-ester with *O,O*-diethyl phosphorothioate [513-10-0] $C_9H_{23}INO_3PS$ (383.22).

Preparation—β-(Dimethylamino)ethanol is reacted with sodium and the resulting sodium alkoxide is condensed with *O,O*-diethyl phosphorochloridothioate [$ClP(S)(OC_2H_5)_2$] to yield *S*-[2-(dimethylamino)ethyl] *O,O*-diethyl phosphorothioate. This ester is quaternized with methyl iodide. US Pat 2,911,430.

Description—White, crystalline, hygroscopic solid having a slight mercaptan-like odor; its solutions have a pH of about 4.

Solubility—1 g in 1 mL water, 3 mL methanol or 25 mL dehydrated alcohol; practically insoluble in other organic solvents.

Uses—An *anticholinesterase* drug that is both a quaternary ammonium and organophosphate compound. It has a long duration of action. Applied topically to the eye it causes intense miosis and contraction of the ciliary body; the effects begin in 10 to 45 min and last 3 to 7 days. It is used for the treatment of *primary open-angle* and *post-cataract surgical glaucoma* and *accommodative esotropia*. It should be used only when short-acting miotics have failed. For the adverse effects and precautions, see the general statement. Echothiophate does not penetrate into the central nervous system.

Dose—*Topical, adult* and *pediatric* for *glaucoma*, **1 drop** of **0.03** to **0.25%** solution to the conjunctiva once or twice a day, in the morning and at bedtime; for *cyclostimulation*, **1 drop** of **0.03** to **0.125%** solution once or twice a day, in the morning and at bedtime; for *accommodative esotropia*, **1 drop** of **0.06** to **0.125%** solution once a day or every other day for 2 or 3 wks.

Solutions are not marketed and must be prepared from the available powder by dissolution in isotonic sodium chloride solution containing 0.5% chlorobutanol; solutions are stable for over 1 yr at 4° and for over 1 mo at room temperature.

Dosage Form—for Ophthalmic Solution: 1.5, 3, 6.25 and 12.5 mg/5 mL.

Edrophonium Chloride

Benzenaminium, *N*-ethyl-3-hydroxy-*N,N*-dimethyl-, chloride; Enlon-Plus (*Anaquest*); Tensilon (*ICN Pharm*)

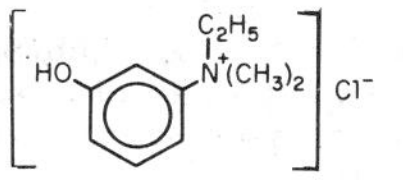

Ethyl(*m*-hydroxyphenyl)dimethylammonium chloride [116-38-1] $C_{10}H_{16}ClNO$ (201.70).

Preparation—*m*-Dimethylaminophenol is dissolved in a suitable organic solvent and quaternized with ethyl iodide. The dimethylethyl(3-hydroxyphenyl)ammonium iodide precipitates and is converted to the chloride in various ways, one of which involves treatment with moist silver oxide to form the quaternary base followed by neutralization with hydrochloric acid.

Description—White, odorless crystalline powder; 1 in 10 solution is practically colorless, pH (1 in 10 solution) between 4.0 and 5.0; melts between 165 and 170° with decomposition.

Solubility—1 g in 0.5 mL water or 5 mL alcohol; insoluble in chloroform or ether.

Uses—Inhibits cholinesterase primarily at the neuromuscular junction and very little at other sites. It also has some direct nicotinic stimulant actions at the neuromuscular junction but not at the autonomic ganglia. The duration of action of a single small dose is only about 5 min, but large doses may act for 1 to 2 hr. It is used to *abolish neuromuscular paralysis due to d-tubocurarine* or similarly acting motor end plate-stabilizing drugs. It also is used as a *diagnostic agent for myasthenia gravis* or to differentiate a myasthenic crisis from a cholinergic crisis. Edrophonium chloride may be used occasionally to treat *myasthenic crises*. It has been used for the diagnosis and attempted arrest of *paroxysmal supraventricular (atrial) tachycardia*, but calcium channel blockers or adenosine are now preferred.

Transient blurring of vision, lacrimation, perspiration and dizziness may accompany its use. It causes muscle fasciculations in the normal human. When it is used to differentiate myasthenic from cholinergic crisis, facilities for endotracheal intubation and artificial respiration must be available.

Dose—*Intravenous, adult*, for *paroxysmal atrial tachycardia, initially* **3** to **5 mg**, then **10 mg**, if necessary; for *myasthenia gravis*, as a *diagnostic agent, initially* **2 mg** injected within 15 to 30 sec, followed by **8 mg** if no response occurs within 45 sec; for *children, initially* **1 mg** if body weight is less than 34 kg, or **2 mg** if over 34 kg and, if no response occurs in 45 sec, up to a total of **5 mg** if body weight is less than 34 kg and **10 mg** if over 34 kg. The *infant* dose is **500 μg** (0.5 mg). For *myasthenic crisis*, by *intravenous drip*. To *antagonize curare-like* neuromuscular blocking drugs, initially **10 mg** repeated in 5 to 10 min as necessary; no more than a total of **40 mg** should be given. *Intramuscular, adult, diagnostic*, **10 mg;** for *children*, **2 mg** if body weight is less than 34 kg and **5 mg** if over 34 kg.

Dosage Form—Injection: 10 mg/1 mL, 100 mg/10 mL, 150 mg/15 mL.

Hexafluorenium Bromide—page 1030.

Isoflurophate

Phosphorofluoridic acid, bis(1-methylethyl) ester; DFP; Floropryl (*MSD*)

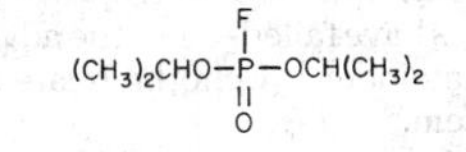

$$(CH_3)_2CHO-\underset{\underset{O}{\|}}{\overset{\overset{F}{|}}{P}}-OCH(CH_3)_2$$

Diisopropyl phosphorofluoridate [55-91-4] $C_6H_{14}FO_3P$ (184.15).

Preparation—Isopropyl alcohol is reacted with PCl_3 to form diisopropyl phosphite. Oxidation with chlorine gives diisopropyl phosphorochloridate, which metathesizes with NaF to yield the phosphorofluoridate.

Description—Clear, colorless or faintly yellow liquid; boils at 183°; specific gravity about 1.05; vapor is extremely irritating to the eye and mucous membranes; in the presence of moisture, it decomposes with formation of hydrogen fluoride.

Solubility—Sparingly soluble in water; soluble in alcohol.

Uses—An *organophosphate anticholinesterase;* consequently, it has a long duration of action. It is used topically in the treatment of *primary open-angle glaucoma,* but only when short-acting miotics have failed. It also is used in the treatment of *aphakic glaucoma* and *accommodative esotropia.* Within a day, the intraocular tension drops and it may remain depressed for as long as a week. Miosis lasts 2 to 4 wks. For the adverse effects and contraindications, see the general statement.

Caution—When handling isoflurophate in open containers, protect the eyes, nose and mouth with a suitable mask and avoid contact with the skin.

Dose—*Topical, adult,* for *glaucoma,* a strip of **0.025%** ointment approximately **0.5-cm** long every 8 to 72 hr (pediatric schedule undetermined); diagnosis of *accommodative esotropia,* once a day at bedtime for 2 wk; *uncomplicated esotropia,* once a day at bedtime, gradually decreasing to once a week for 2 mo.

Dosage Form—Ophthalmic Ointment: 0.025%.

Malathion—see RPS-18, page 897.

Neostigmine Bromide

Benzenaminium, 3-[[(dimethylamino)carbonyl]oxy]-*N,N,N*-trimethyl-, bromide; Prostigmin Bromide (*ICN Pharm*)

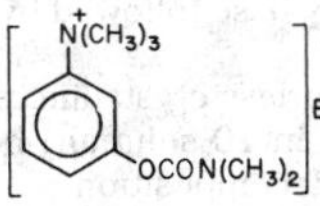

$$\left[C_6H_4\left(\overset{+}{N}(CH_3)_3\right)\left(OCON(CH_3)_2\right) \right] Br^-$$

(*m*-Hydroxyphenyl)trimethylammonium bromide dimethylcarbamate [114-80-7] $C_{12}H_{19}BrN_2O_2$ (303.20).

Preparation—It may be prepared by reacting dimethylcarbamoylchloride [$(CH_3)_2NCOCl$] with potassium *m*-(dimethylamino)-phenolate, then quaternizing with methyl bromide.

Description—White, crystalline powder; odorless and has a bitter taste; solutions are neutral to litmus; melts between 171 and 176° with decomposition.

Solubility—1 g in about 0.5 mL water; soluble in alcohol; practically insoluble in ether.

Uses—A quaternary ammonium anticholinesterase (see *Anticholinesterases,* page 1003). It acts at the esteratic site of the enzyme to form the inactive dimethylcarbamoyl enzyme. Its effects are more prominent on certain structures than on others, being particularly effective on the bowel, urinary bladder and skeletal muscle; the pupil, heart, blood pressure and secretions are affected to a much lesser extent in doses that are ordinarily effective on the structures listed above. The duration of action by the oral route is 3 to 6 hr and by the intramuscular route, 2 to 4 hr.

Neostigmine is employed for the genitourinary, gastrointestinal and neuromuscular uses indicated in the general statement. However, it is infrequently used today to antagonize curare-like drugs or in the diagnosis of myasthenia gravis because its duration of action is too long.

The adverse effects of neostigmine are those of quaternary ammonium anticholinesterases (see the general statement).

Orally, neostigmine is absorbed poorly; sometimes as little as 1%. Changes in bowel condition can alter absorption considerably, which may make management difficult. Neostigmine is administered parenterally as the methylsulfate and orally as the bromide salt.

Dose—*Oral,* for *myasthenia gravis, initially* **15 mg** 3 times a day, gradually increased to **45 mg** every 2 to 4 hr if necessary (as much as 375 mg a day may be given); for *children, initially* **7.5** to **15 mg** 3 or 4 times a day or **330 μg** (0.33 mg)/**kg** 3 to 6 times a day, gradually increasing to as much as the adult dose.

Dosage Form—Tablets: 15 mg.

Neostigmine Methylsulfate

Benzenaminium, 3-[[(dimethylamino)carbonyl]oxy]-*N,N,N*-trimethyl-,methyl sulfate; Prostigmin Methylsulfate (*ICN Pharm*)

(*m*-Hydroxyphenyl)trimethylammonium methyl sulfate dimethylcarbamate [51-60-5] $C_{13}H_{22}N_2O_6S$ (334.39).

Preparation—It is made by the method outlined under *Neostigmine Bromide,* using dimethyl sulfate in place of methyl bromide.

Description—White, crystalline powder; odorless and has a bitter taste; solutions are neutral to litmus; melts between 144 and 149°.

Solubility—Very soluble in water; soluble in alcohol.

Uses—See *Neostigmine Bromide.*

Dose—*Intramuscular, adult, diagnosis of myasthenia,* **0.022 mg/kg** (along with atropine 0.011 mg/kg) on the first test and **0.03 mg/kg** (with 0.016 mg/kg atropine) on the second, if the first is equivocal; *to control myasthenia, initially* **0.5 mg,** then up to **1** to **2 mg** (with 0.2 to 0.6 mg atropine) every 3 to 6 hr; to *prevent postsurgical bladder atony* or *intestinal paresis,* **0.25** to **0.50 mg** every 4 to 6 hr for 2 to 3 days; in *bladder* or *gastrointestinal atony,* **0.5** to **1 mg** as needed; *children, diagnosis of myasthenia,* **0.01** to **0.04 mg/kg** (with 0.01 mg/kg atropine). *Intravenous, adults,* to control *exacerbations of myasthenia,* **1** to **2 mg** (with 0.6 to 1.2 mg of atropine) every 1 to 3 hr; to *treat overdosage of nondepolarizing neuromuscular blocking drugs,* **0.5** to **2 mg** slowly; *children,* **0.07** to **0.08 mg/kg** (with 0.008 to 0.025 mg/kg atropine). *Subcutaneous, adult and children,* in *bladder* or *gastrointestinal atony or spasm* or *treatment of myasthenia,* same as intramuscular; *infants,* to treat *myasthenia gravis,* **0.1** to **0.2 mg** 1 to 4 times a day (along with 0.01 mg/kg atropine).

Dosage Form—Injection: 250 and 500 μg/mL, 5 and 10 mg/10 mL.

Physostigmine Salicylate

Pyrrolo[2,3-*b*]indol-5-ol, (3a*S*-*cis*)-1,2,3,3a,8,8a-hexahydro-1,3a,8-trimethyl-, methylcarbamate (ester); mono-(2-hydroxybenzoate); Eserine Salicylate; Isopto-Eserine (*Alcon*); Antilirium (*Forest*)

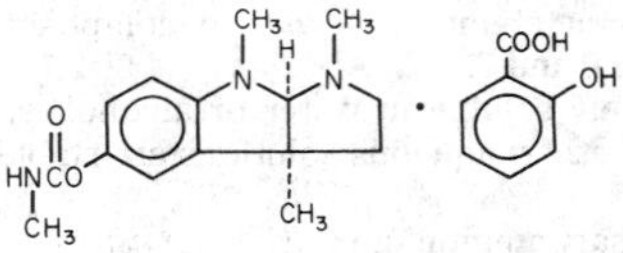

Physostigmine monosalicylate [57-64-7] $C_{15}H_{21}N_3O_2.C_7H_6O_3$ (413.47).

Preparation—By extracting powdered *Physostigma* seeds with hot alcohol. After distilling off the alcohol, the residue is mixed with sodium carbonate and extracted with ether, from which solution the physostigmine is removed with dilute sulfuric acid. The free alkaloid may be obtained by alkalinizing the acid solution. The salicylate may be made by adding 2 parts of physostigmine to a solution of 1 part of salicylic acid in 35 parts of boiling distilled water, and allowing the salt to crystallize on cooling.

Description—White or faintly yellow odorless powder or shining crystals; acquires a red tint when exposed to light and air; melts at about 184°.

Solubility—1 g in 75 mL water, 16 mL alcohol, 6 mL chloroform or about 250 mL ether.

Incompatibilities—Aqueous solutions tend to develop a red color on standing; a pink solution does not necessarily indicate complete ineffectiveness but, as the color deepens to red, the product rapidly loses its potency. Boric acid retards the change but alkalies hasten decomposition. Alkali-free glass should be used. It is precipitated by the usual alkaloidal precipitants.

Uses—The oldest of the anticholinesterases. It combines with the enzyme at the esteratic site to yield the inactive methylcarbamoyl enzyme. It shares with neostigmine marked stimulatory actions on the bowel, but causes more secretion of glands, more effect on blood pressure, more constriction of the pupil and less action on skeletal muscle. Since it is a tertiary amine, it penetrates into the nervous system and can exert central actions when given in sufficient doses. It also penetrates readily into the eye. Although its main use in medicine is topically in ophthalmology, for the purposes indicated in the general statement, there is some interest in its CNS uses. The salicylate is used for both its CNS and ophthalmologic actions; the sulfate is used only in the eye.

For adverse effects and precautions, see the general statement.

The duration of the ocular effects after topical application is 6 to 12 hr; the duration of systemic effects is less than 2 hr. The systemic bioavailability after oral administration is about 5 to 12%.

The salicylate has the advantage of being less deliquescent than the sulfate. Addition of a small amount of boric acid to a solution of the salt is said to inhibit formation of the red decomposition product produced by alkalies and which frequently occurs in solutions of physostigmine salts dispensed on prescription. A solution that has developed a red color should not be used.

Dose—*Topical, adult,* for *open-angle glaucoma* or to *antagonize antimuscarinic mydriatics,* **1** to **2 drops** of **0.25** to **0.5%** solution instilled into the conjunctival sac up to 4 times a day; for *acute-angle closure glaucoma,* **1 drop** of **0.25%** solution every 5 min for 30 min, then at 30-min intervals until the angle opens. Pediatric doses are those of the smallest adult doses. *Oral, adult,* for *CNS effects,* **1** to **2 mg** 3 times a day or **0.5 mg** every 2 hr. *Parenteral, adult,* for *drug intoxication* or *after anesthesia intramuscularly or intravenously,* **0.5** to **2 mg,** to be repeated in doses of 1 to 4 mg in life-threatening situations; *pediatric, intravenously,* **0.5 mg** very slowly over at least 1 min, to be repeated at 5- to 10-min intervals, if necessary, up to a total of 2 mg. Children should not receive the drug unless the situation is urgent.

Dosage Forms—Injection: 1 mg/1 mL and 2 mg/2 mL; Ointment 0.25%; Ophthalmic Solution: 0.25 and 0.5%.

Physostigmine Sulfate

Pyrrolo[2,3-*b*]indol-5-ol, (3a*S*-*cis*)-1,2,3,3a,8,8a-hexahydro-1,3a,8-trimethyl-, methylcarbamate (ester), sulfate (2:1);
Physostigmine Sulfate (2:1)

Physostigmine sulfate (2:1) [64-47-1] $(C_{15}H_{21}N_3O_2)_2.H_2SO_4$ (648.77).

For structure of the amine base, see *Physostigmine Salicylate.*

Description—White, odorless, microcrystalline powder; melts at about 143°; deliquescent in moist air and acquires a red tint when long exposed to heat, light, air or contact with traces of metals.

Solubility—1 g in 4 mL water, 0.4 mL alcohol or about 1200 mL ether.

Uses—See *Physostigmine Salicylate.*

Dose—*Topical, adult,* to the conjunctiva, **1 cm** of **0.25%** ointment 1 to 3 times a day. Pediatric dosage has not been established.

Dosage Form—Ophthalmic Ointment: 0.25%.

Pyridostigmine Bromide

Pyridinium, 3-[[(dimethylamino)carbonyl]oxy]-1-methyl-, bromide;
Mestinon (*Roche*); Regonal (*Organon*)

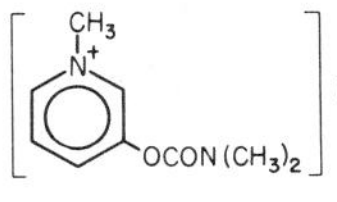

CH_3 N^+ $OCON(CH_3)_2$ Br^-

3-Hydroxy-1-methylpyridinium bromide dimethylcarbamate [101-26-8] $C_9H_{13}BrN_2O_2$ (261.12).

Preparation—3-Pyridinol is condensed with dimethylcarbamoyl chloride in the presence of a suitable basic catalyst such as dimethylaniline, magnesium oxide, etc. The resulting ester, 3-pyridyl dimethylcarbamate, is isolated, dissolved in a suitable organic solvent and quaternized with methyl bromide.

Description—White or practically white, crystalline, hygroscopic powder, having an agreeable, characteristic odor; melts between 154 and 157°.

Solubility—Freely soluble in water, alcohol or chloroform; slightly soluble in solvent hexane; practically insoluble in ether.

Uses—A quaternary ammonium anticholinesterase drug that is approximately one-fourth as potent as neostigmine at the neuromuscular junction and about one-eighth as potent on the bowel, genitourinary tract and exocrine glands. Its duration of action by the oral route usually is somewhat longer and absorption is less erratic than with neostigmine, which are advantages. Because of its relative affinity for the neuromuscular junction, its principal use is in the treatment of *myasthenia gravis,* in which use it causes fewer side effects than does neostigmine. It is also superior to neostigmine in that the patient may be carried through the night without the necessity of interrupting sleep to take medication. However, in some patients, it provides less control of muscular weakness than does neostigmine. Pyridostigmine is administered orally except when the patient is to undergo surgery or childbirth or is in myasthenic crisis. Neonates born of myasthenic mothers also may be given parenteral pyridostigmine to improve respiration, swallowing and suckling. The drug also is used to antagonize competitive neuromuscular-blocking drugs.

The adverse effects and precautions are listed in the general statement. Bromide sensitivity occasionally occurs.

Dose—*Oral, adult, initially* **60 mg** every 4 to 8 hr while the patient is awake; however, dosage usually has to be increased to **120** to **300 mg** every 4 hr. With *sustained-release tablets,* the dose is **180** to **540 mg** once or twice a day. In severe cases the dose often exceeds 1.5 g/day and as much as 6 g/day has been recorded. The *oral pediatric* dose is **1.2 mg/kg** or **33 mg/m²** every 4 hr. *Parenteral, adult, intramuscular, slow intravenous,* 1/30 of the oral dose, except to antagonize competitive neuromuscular blocking drugs, 10 to 20 mg usually is used; *pediatric, intramuscular,* **0.05** to **0.15 mg/kg.**

Dosage Forms—Injection: 10 mg/2 mL and 25 mg/5 mL; Syrup: 60 mg/5 mL; Tablets: 60 mg; Sustained-Release Tablets: 180 mg.

Tacrine Hydrochloride

Acridine, 9-amino-1,2,3,4-tetrahydro-,hydrochloride;
Cognex (*Parke-Davis*)

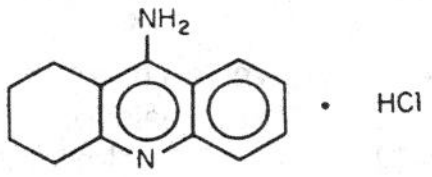

NH_2 N · HCl

[1684-40-8] $C_{13}H_{14}N_2$. HCl (234.73).

Preparation—By heating 9-chloro-1,2,3,4-tetrahydroacridine with ammonium carbonate in phenol at 130° followed by usual conversion to the hydrochloride. (See *J Soc Chem Ind 64:* 169, 1945).

Description—Yellow needles melting about 284°; Bitter taste; pH of 1.5% solution about 5.

Solubility—Soluble in water.

Uses—Possesses both an anticholinesterase action and an action to block potassium channels in cell membranes. The latter action causes prolonged action potentials, which, at cholinergic nerve endings, increases the release of acetylcholine. Thus, the two actions compliment each other. Since the drug can penetrate the blood-brain barrier readily (in the nonionized form) and gain access to the CNS, it is of special interest as an anticholinesterase for actions in the CNS. The current focus is on its effects to improve learning, memory and mood in patients with Alzheimer's type of senile dementia. Early studies reported considerable improvement, sometimes dramatic, in about 75% of recipients, especially in the early stages of the disease, but subsequent studies have been far less encouraging. At best, the drug is only palliative and does not prevent the eventual degeneration of the affected nerve tracts. Side effects occur in about 25 to 35% of recipients, but they are usually minimal and tolerated; they include belching, nausea, emesis, enuresis, abdominal discomfort, diarrhea and sweating.

Dose—The optimal dose remains to be determined. Tentatively, it is initially **25 mg/day,** increased daily by increments of **25** to **50 mg,** up to **150** to **200 mg/day.**

Related Agent

Guanidine Hydrochloride—see RPS-18, page 897.

Cholinesterase Reactivators

Several substances are capable of displacing dialkylphosphate groups (from organophosphate anticholinesterases) and methyl- or dimethylcarbamoyl groups (from physostigmine or neostigmine) from the esteratic sites of cholinesterases poisoned by the anticholinesterases. At present, all such substances of value contain oxime groups, which engage in a nucleophilic attack on the attached phosphate or carbamoyl group and rupture the bond between the inhibiting group and the esteratic site. This action especially is important in the treatment of intoxication by isopropyl and certain other organophosphate anticholinesterases, since these organophosphates have such a long duration of action. The reactivation of carbamoylated enzyme is less prominent. Unfortunately, within a period of minutes to hours after poisoning with an isopropyl organophosphate, there is a change in the phosphorylated enzyme (''aging,'' dealkylation of the alkyl phosphate moiety), so that the alkylphosphate–enzyme bond becomes too stable to be displaced by reactivators. The efficacy of any one reactivator varies according to which anticholinesterase is involved because of differences in electrophilicity of the phosphorus in the various phosphate radicals; one anticholinesterase, octamethylphosphoramide, is refractory to displacement by cholinesterase reactivators. Atropine also must be used concomitantly with reactivators for optimal therapy. The reactivators may be used prophylactically.

Pralidoxime Chloride

Pyridinium, 2-[(hydroxyimino)methyl]-1-methyl-, chloride;
2-PAM Chloride; Protopam Chloride (*Wyeth-Ayerst*)

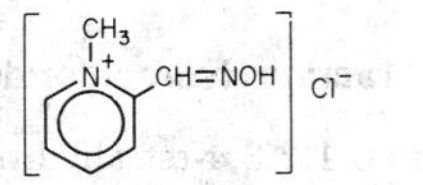

2-Formyl-1-methylpyridinium chloride oxime [51-15-0] $C_7H_9ClN_2O$ (172.61).

Preparation—Picolinal is converted to its oxime which is then quaternized with dimethyl sulfate. Metathesis of the resulting pralidoxime methosulfate with HCl yields the official chloride. US Pat 3,123, 613.

Description—White to pale-yellow, crystalline powder; odorless; stable in air; melts between 215 and 225° with decomposition.

Solubility—Freely soluble in water.

Uses—A cholinesterase reactivator. The quaternary portion of the molecule attaches to the anionic site of the cholinesterase molecule and brings the oxime into close proximity to the poisoned esteratic site. The drug is used in the treatment of poisoning by organophosphate anticholinesterases; it has questionable value in poisoning by neostigmine or physostigmine. The therapeutic effect (remission) usually occurs within 1 hr. Pralidoxime also is given prophylactically to handlers of organophosphates, but the status of this use is in dispute. Pralidoxime does not antagonize all anticholinesterase compounds; the manufacturer's package literature should be consulted to ascertain whether the drug will be effective. After a period of time, organophosphate-inhibited cholinesterase undergoes a change that makes reactivation difficult; with isoflurophate, this time is only about 1 hr.

The plasma half-life of pralidoxime is about 2.5 hr.

When pralidoxime is injected more rapidly than at the recommended rate, dizziness, nausea, headache, mild weakness, blurred vision, diplopia or tachycardia may result.

Dose—*Intravenous, adult,* for accidental intoxication, **1** to **2 g** in 100 mL of saline injection infused in a period of 15 to 30 min, to be repeated after 1 hr if muscle weakness persists. For a cholinergic crisis due to echothiophate, it is often the practice to start with 50 mg and increase the dose every 5 min until a remission occurs. For cholinergic crisis due to neostigmine, ambenonium or pyridostigmine, an initial dose of **1** to **2 g** may be followed by **250 mg** every 5 min until remission occurs. *Pediatric,* **20** to **40 mg/kg,** given in no less than 5 min. *Oral,* **1** to **3 g,** repeated in 3 hr if necessary. If signs and symptoms of cholinesterase poisoning already exist, more than two doses probably will be of little extra value. If the drug is given prophylactically after exposure, before signs of poisoning ensue, up to 5 oral doses of 1 to 3 g each may be given to protect against slowly absorbing anticholinesterase.

Dosage Forms—Injection (autoinjector): 600 mg/2 mL; Sterile: 1 g/20 mL.

CHAPTER 59

Adrenergic and Adrenergic Neuron Blocking Drugs

Donald N Franz, PhD
Professor of Pharmacology
University of Utah School of Medicine
Salt Lake City, UT 84132

The term *blockade* is used to indicate interference with a response system such that the final effect is prevented. A *blocking drug* is an agent that produces such interference. *Adrenergic* blockade indicates interference with response systems that normally involve the catecholamine neurohumoral transmitters, epinephrine (*adren*aline) and norepinephrine (nor*adren*aline, levarterenol). The term adrenergic refers to any of the cellular processes concerned with the synthesis, storage, release, transmission or activation of adrenergic receptors by catecholamines or their mimetics. Thus the locus of action of an adrenergic blocking agent might be any of these adrenergic sites.

Until the discovery of the catecholamine-depleting effects of reserpine, the only adrenergic blocking agents were those that blocked at the adrenergic neuroeffector receptor to the catecholamines or their mimetics.

Today, several drugs that block the adrenergic response system by inhibiting the synthesis, storage or release of catecholamines are used clinically. Such drugs reduce the response to stimulation of the sympathetic adrenergic nerves by reducing the delivery of catecholamines to the neuroeffector receptor; they do not reduce the actions of catecholamines or sympathomimetics on the neuroeffector receptor as do the "classical" adrenergic blocking agents.

In general, the terms *adrenergic blocking agent* or *adrenergic antagonist* usually are applied to those drugs that block adrenergic receptors, and the term *adrenergic neuron blocking agent* is applied to those drugs that reduce delivery of catecholamines to the adrenergic receptors. The adrenergic blocking agents sometimes are called *sympatholytics*, because they abolish ("lyse") the response to stimulation of the sympathetic nerves, or *adrenolytics*, because they abolish certain responses to epinephrine (adrenaline). Adrenergic neuron blocking agents are sympatholytic but not adrenolytic.

Adrenergic Blocking Agents

The classification of adrenoreceptors into α- and β-subtypes implies that two types of blocking drugs are possible, α- and β-antagonists. In fact, inasmuch as there are subcategories, α_1-, α_2-, β_1- and β_2-adrenoreceptors, there are four types of selective and three types of nonselective adrenergic antagonists. The classical adrenergic blocking drugs, ergotamine phenoxybenzamine and phenotolamine block both α_1- and α_2-adrenoreceptors. Propranolol, nadolol, timolol, pindolol and others block both β_1- and β_2-adrenoreceptors. Labetolol blocks both α- and β-receptors.

α-Adrenoreceptor Antagonists

Nonselective α-Antagonists—Only three nonselective α-adrenoreceptor antagonists, namely phenoxybenzamine, tolazoline and phentolamine, presently are marketed in the US. Other drugs, sometimes classified as α-blockers (eg, chlorpromazine), have other more prominent actions for which they are used.

Blockade of α_1-adrenoreceptors causes readily apparent effects, whereas blockade of α_2-receptors causes subtle effects. Antagonism of α_1-adrenergic impulses to the arterioles decreases vascular resistance, thus tending to lower blood pressure, cause a pink warm skin, nasal and scleroconjunctival congestion and ptosis. α_1-Antagonism at the venules (capacitance vessels) not only increases venous capacitance, which necessitates fluid loading, but also causes postural and exercise hypotension. Other obvious effects of α_1- block are mild to moderate miosis and interference with ejaculation.

α-Antagonism causes tachycardia, palpitations and increased secretion of renin. These are β_1-adrenoreceptor responses not suppressable by α-blockade. They are partially attributable to activation of baroreflexes from the hypotension produced by α_1-blockade. It now is known that there also is an increased amount of norepinephrine released from adrenergic nerve endings (transmitter "overflow") as the result of concurrent block of α_2-adrenoreceptors, which subserve a negative-feedback function to decrease the release of transmitter. Consequently, tachycardia, palpitations and elevation of plasma renin levels may occur even when blood pressure falls very little. These reflex/overflow effects are counterproductive in the major uses of nonselective α-blocking drugs.

Nonselective α-adrenoreceptor antagonists are used in the treatment of peripheral vascular disorders in which there is an adrenergically mediated vasospastic component, such as in *Raynaud's disease, acrocyanosis, frost bite, acute arterial occlusion, phlebitis, phlebothrombosis, diabetic gangrene, causalgia, shock* (to increase blood flow to intestines and kidney) and *pheochromocytoma*. In *pheochromocytoma*, the drugs may be used in advance of surgery to maintain a lower blood pressure, immediately before surgery, to prevent the occurrence of hypertensive crises caused by manipulation of the tumor, and for the long-term treatment of inoperable, metastatic pheochromocytoma.

Adverse effects of nonselective α-antagonists are postural hypotension, tachycardia, palpitations, fluid retention, nasal and ocular congestion, impotence, impaired ejaculation, priapism and aggravation of the signs and symptoms of respiratory infections.

α-Antagonists are contraindicated in severe cerebral or coronary atherosclerosis and in renal insufficiency.

Selective α-Antagonists—Highly selective antagonists for both α_1- and α_2-adrenoreceptors are known. At present, only α_1-antagonists have known clinical uses. Only *prazosin, doxazosin* and *terazosin* are available currently in the US. Theoretically, α_1-blockers should be useful for the same disorders as are the nonselective α-blockers, but α_1-antagonists are approved only for the treatment of *hypertension*. However, they enjoy a considerable use in refractory heart failure, to decrease the cardiac afterload and preload, to relieve vasospasm in Raynaud's disease and to treat benign prostatic hyperplasia.

α_1-Antagonists are advantageous in that they do not block α_2-receptors and, hence, do not cause increased release of transmitter and thus excessive tachycardia, stroke volume and plasma renin levels; in some patients, such side effects are almost absent. The most adverse side effect of α_1-blockade sometimes is severe postural hypotension and syncope, especially very early in the treatment. Impotence and priapism lead to noncompliance.

Selective α_2-antagonists include yohimbine and rauwolscine (α-yohimbine), but there are presently no approved therapeutic indications for α_2-blockade. However, yohimbine sometimes is used to treat certain types of male erectile impotence.

Doxazosin Mesylate

Piperazine, 1-(4-amino-6,7-dimethoxy-2-quinazolinyl)-4-[(2,3-dihydro-1,4-benzodioxin-2-yl)carbonyl]-, monomethanesulfonate; Cardura (*Roerig*)

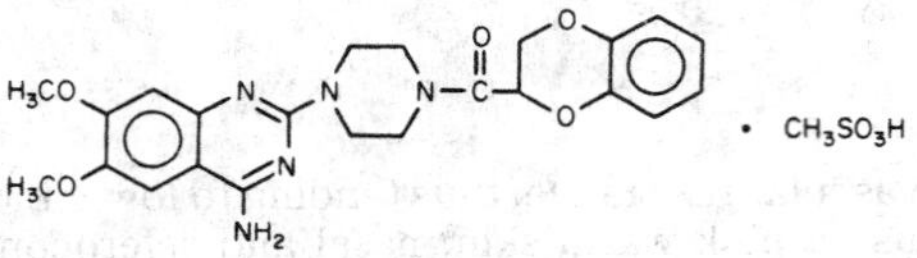

[77883-43-3] $C_{23}H_{25}N_5O_5.CH_4O_3S$ (547.58).

Preparation—See US Patent 4,188,390.

Description—Off-white powder; pK_a 6.93.

Solubility—Sparingly soluble in water and most common organic solvents.

Uses—A selective α_1-adrenorecepter blocking drug similar to *Prazosin Hydrochloride* in its pharmacological properties, clinical uses and adverse effects. It differs particularly in that the elimination half-life is about 16 to 24 hr, which enables once-a-day dosage. The volume of distribution is 3.5 L/kg.

Dose—*Oral, adult, initially* **1 mg** once a day, gradually increased, if necessary, to as much as 16 mg a day.

Dosage Form—Tablets: 1, 2, 4 and 8 mg.

Phenoxybenzamine Hydrochloride

Benzenemethanamine, *N*-(2-chloroethyl)-*N*-(1-methyl-2-phenoxyethyl)-, hydrochloride; Dibenzyline Hydrochloride (*SmithKline Beecham*)

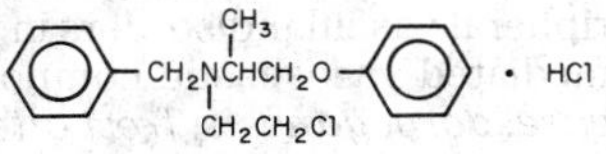

N-(2-Chloroethyl)-*N*-(1-methyl-2-phenoxyethyl)benzylamine hydrochloride [63-92-3] $C_{18}H_{22}ClNO.HCl$ (340.29).

Preparation—One method starts with phenol undergoing addition to propylene oxide to give 1-phenoxy-2-propanol, which is reacted with thionyl chloride to yield 1-phenoxy-2-chloropropane. Refluxing the latter with excess ethanolamine gives *N*-(phenoxyisopropylamino)ethanol and additional refluxing of this with benzyl chloride in the presence of $NaHCO_3$ yields 2-[*N*-benzyl-*N*-(1-methyl-2-phenoxyethyl)amino]ethanol. Treatment with thionyl chloride and HCl in $CHCl_3$ completes the synthesis. US Pat 2,599,000.

Description—White, crystalline, odorless powder; melts between 136 and 141°.

Solubility—1 g in 25 mL water, 6 mL alcohol, 3 mL chloroform or > 1000 mL ether.

Uses—A nonselective α-antagonist. It irreversibly alkylates sulfhydryl groups at the α-receptor sites. Recovery from blockade can result only from synthesis of new receptors. The duration of action may be as long as 4 to 5 days. The effects and uses are those of α-blocking drugs in general, except that this drug has too unpredictable an efficacy and causes excessive tachycardia and orthostatic hypotension in essential hypertension to be competitive with newer drugs. The long duration of action makes the drug especially useful in the management of inoperable *pheochromocytoma*, usually in combination with a β-antagonist. It also has been used to treat peripheral vascular disease and some micturition disorders characterized by urinary retention.

In addition to the side effects of α-blockade, it causes drowsiness and has a local irritancy; by the oral route it may cause nausea, vomiting and diarrhea. Contraindications are those of α-antagonists in general (see the general statement).

Dose—*Oral, adult, initially* **10 mg** a day, taken with milk, for 4 days; thereafter, the dose is increased every other day in increments of 10 mg until optimal dosage is achieved, which is usually 20 to 120 mg a day in 2 or 3 divided doses. *Children, initially* **0.2 mg/kg** or **6 mg/m²**, not to exceed 10 mg, once a day, to be increased gradually every 4 days to *maintenance*, **0.4** to **1.2 mg/kg** or **12** to **36 mg/m²** a day in 3 or 4 divided doses.

Dosage Form—Capsules: 10 mg.

Phentolamine Mesylate

Phenol, 3-[[(4,5-dihydro-1*H*-imidazol-2-yl)methyl](4-methylphenyl)-amino]-, monomethanesulfonate (salt); Regitine Mesylate (*Ciba-Geigy*)

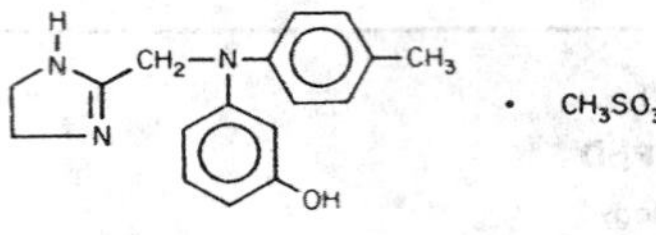

[65-28-1] $C_{17}H_{19}N_3O.CH_4O_3S$ (377.46).

Preparation—*m*-(*p*-Toluidino)phenol is refluxed with 2-chloromethylimidazoline hydrochloride and the resulting phentolamine base treated with an equimolar portion of methanesulfonic acid.

Description—White or off-white, odorless, crystalline powder; solutions are acid to litmus, having a pH of about 5, and deteriorate slowly; melts at about 178°.

Solubility—1 g in 1 mL water, 4 mL alcohol or 700 mL chloroform.

Uses—A nonselective α-adrenoreceptor antagonist. The blockade is reversible. In addition to α-blocking activity, it has mild to moderate sympathomimetic-like mydriatic and cardiostimulant (rate, force of contraction and dysrythmias) activity, weak muscarinic activity in the gastrointestinal tract and weak to mild histaminergic activity in the stomach (acid secretion) and arterioles (flushing and slight fall in blood pressure). These effects limit the dose that can be used, hence α-blockade is usually incomplete. For the effects of the α-blocking component of activity and the uses, see the general statement. Additional uses include the treatment or prevention of dermal necrosis and sloughing resulting from *extravasation of norepinephrine*, the treatment of *primary pulmonary hypertension* and the management of *hypertensive crises* caused by drug interactions with *MAO inhibitors* or the abrupt withdrawal of *clonidine*. It is used as a diagnostic agent for pheochromocytoma; a fall in diastolic blood pressure in excess of 25 torr is considered to be positive, although both false negative and positive responses occur. Analysis of urinary metanephrines is the preferred diagnostic method. It also is used during surgery for pheochromocytoma, preferably in combination with a β-antagonist. In shock, it sometimes is combined with norepinephrine to block the α-vasoconstrictor effects and permit the uncomplicated β_1-effects on the heart to prevail. Also, it has been combined with papaverine for intracavernous injection in impotence.

The adverse effects are those of α-blockade (see the general statement), in addition to which there is weakness. The contraindications are those in the general statement, with the addition that digitalis should be avoided in phentolamine-treated patients because of the danger of serious cardiac dysrhythmias.

It is metabolized in the liver. The half-life is about 19 min.

Dose—*Intramuscular, children, diagnostic* in suspected pheochromocytoma, **3 mg**; *intramuscular* or *intravenous, pheochromocytoma*, **1 mg** or **0.1 mg/kg** or **3 mg/m²** 1 to 2 hr before surgery for *prophylaxis*, repeated if necessary, and *also during surgery*, to control hypertension. *Intravenous, adult, diagnostic* in suspected *pheochromocytoma*, **2.5 mg** to be followed by 5 mg if the result of the first dose is negative; *pheochromocytoma*, **5 mg** 1 to 2 hr *before surgery* for prophylaxis, repeated if necessary, and *also during surgery*, to control hypertension; *children, diagnostic*, **1 mg** or **0.1 mg/kg** or **3 mg/m²**. *Intravenous infusion, adult*, in acute congestive *heart failure*, **0.17** to **0.4 mg/min**; *during intravenous infusion of norepinephrine*, to prevent perivascular sloughing and dermal necrosis, **10 mg/L** of norepinephrine solution. *Perivascular infiltration*, following extravasation of norepinephrine, **5** to **10 mg/10 mL**, to be given at the earliest possible time; ineffective after 10 to 12 hr.

Dosage Form: for Injection: 5 mg/1 mL.

Prazosin Hydrochloride

Piperazine, 1-(4-amino-6,7-dimethoxy-2-quinazolinyl)-4-(2-furanylcarbonyl)-, monohydrochloride; Minipress (*Pfizer*)

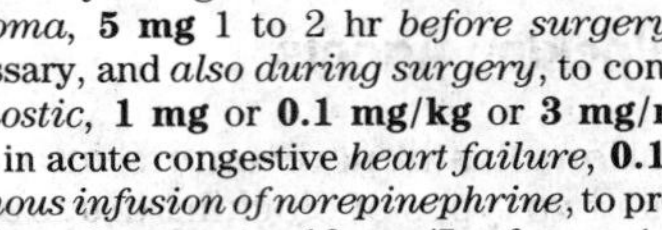

1-(4-Amino-6,7-dimethoxy-2-quinazolinyl)-4-(2-furoyl)piperazine monohydrochloride [19237-84-4] $C_{19}H_{21}N_5O_4.HCl$ (419.87).

Preparation—4,5-Dimethoxyanthranilamide is treated with sodium cyanate to form the corresponding tetrahydroquinazoline-2,4-dione. The carbonyl groups are converted to chlorine and the heterocyclic ring aromatized using $POCl_3$ plus PCl_5. Subsequent treatment with ammonia replaces the chlorine atom adjacent to the benzenoid ring with an amino function and the resulting monochloro derivative is condensed with 1-(2-furoyl)-piperazine to yield the product. See British Pat 1,156,973.

Description—White, crystalline powder; pK_a (in 1:1 water-ethanol solution) 6.5.

Solubility—Slightly soluble in water; very slightly soluble in alcohol.

Uses—Lowers blood pressure by blocking α_1-adrenoreceptors that subserve vasoconstrictor functions. It differs from nonselective α-blocking agents in that it does not block α_2-adrenoreceptors on the adrenergic nerve terminals, which receptors serve a negative feedback function to limit the release of norepinephrine. Nondiscriminatory α-blocking drugs block these receptors and thus cause an excessive continuing release of norepinephrine, which in the heart gives rise to often-intolerable tachycardia and palpitation, and in the juxtaglomerular apparatus in the kidney to elevated plasma renin activity. It is unique in avoiding this neurotransmitter overflow and, hence, causes less reflex cardiac stimulation and increased plasma renin activity than do other α-blocking drugs.

It often can be used alone in the treatment of *mild* to *moderate essential hypertension* and *with other drugs in severe hypertension.* Used alone, it is effective in 40 to 75% of patients, and, in combination, in over 80%. In combination with verapamil it is nearly 100% effective. The peripheral resistance is decreased because of α-blockade of sympathetic stimulation to the arterioles. Venous capacitance is increased, also because of α-blockade, but this plays a minor role in the antihypertensive action, except with the first few doses. It is useful in the preoperative management of *pheochromocytoma*. Because of the relative selectivity for the vascular resistance and cardiac impedance, it is useful to *decrease cardiac afterload* and, hence, increase cardiac output in severe acute congestive heart failure and cardiogenic shock. With mild to moderate doses, the slight effect on capacitance does not decrease venous return ("preload") sufficiently to compromise cardiac output, but large doses will decrease preload, even in the supine position. It relaxes spastic digital arterioles in patients with *Raynaud's phenomenon.*

The most common side effect is palpitation (15%), even though this is much less than occurs with nonselective α-adrenoreceptor blocking drugs and vasodilators. Dizziness occurs in about 10% of patients, headache in 8% of recipients; nasal stuffiness is also a frequent complaint. With small to moderate doses, postural hypotension (from α-blockade of reflex stimulation of capacitance veins) during maintenance is usually only slight to moderate, but during initiation of treatment, or when dosage is increased abruptly, a severe postural hypotension, sometimes with syncope, occurs in about 1% of patients. Therefore, treatment should begin slowly and dose increments should be made gradually; with large doses, severe postural hypotension is frequent. Diuretics increase the incidence and severity of the postural hypotension.

Other side effects include dry mouth, lassitude (7%), urinary incontinence, drowsiness (8%), nausea (5%), blurred vision, sweating, psychic depression and polyarthralgia. Fluid retenion occurs frequently but usually is limited sufficiently that the drug often can be given without the coadministration of a saluretic. Impotence and defective ejaculation occur occasionally and priapism rarely. Plasma renin levels may increase little, if at all, and do not correlate with fluid retention.

It elevates plasma norepinephrine levels by about 50%, which may account for a slight blunting of glucose regulation. Renal blood flow and filtration fraction are affected very little. Rashes and pruritus have been reported. It does not affect blood lipids adversely. Its safety in pregnancy has not been established. Saluretics favor orthostatic hypotension and syncope as do various vasodilators, such as nitroglycerin and calcium channel blockers.

It is absorbed completely by the oral route; the absorption time is 1.7 to 4.55 hr. About 97% in plasma is bound to proteins. The volume of distribution is about 0.6 L/kg. It is eliminated mainly by metabolism in the liver. The plasma half-life is 3 to 4 hr, but the antihypertensive effect outlasts the plasma levels, the duration of action being 6 to 12 hr.

Dose (base equivalent)—*Oral, adult, initially* **0.5** to **1 mg** 3 times a day, to be increased gradually in increments of only 1 mg a day to a maximum of 20 mg a day (usually 6 to 15 mg a day) in 2 or 3 divided doses; very little further effect usually is achieved above 20 mg a day, but a few patients may show increased response up to 40 mg a day. When a diuretic or another antihypertensive drug is added, the dose of prazosin should be decreased to 1 or 2 mg 3 times a day, to be followed by gradual increases in dose, if necessary. *Children, under 7 yr, initially* **0.25 mg** 2 or 3 times a day, subsequently adjusted; *7 to 12 yr, initially* **0.5 mg** 2 or 3 times a day, subsequently adjusted.

Dosage Forms (base equivalent)—Capsules: 1, 2, and 5 mg.

Terazosin Hydrochloride

Piperazine, 1-(4-Amino-6,7-dimethoxy-2-quinazolinyl-4-[(tetrahydro-2-furanyl)carbonyl], monohydrochloride, dihydrate; Hytrin (*Abbott*)

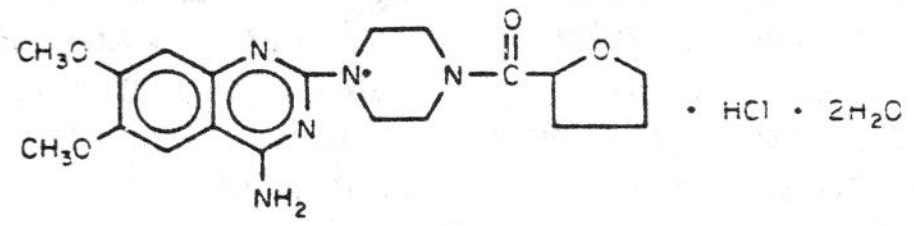

[70024-40-7] $C_{19}H_{25}N_5O_4.HCl.2H_2O$ (459.93).

Preparation—See *Prazosin Hydrochloride;* 1-(2-tetrahydrofuroyl)-piperazine is condensed with the monochloroquinazoline.

Description—White crystalline powder.

Solubility—Freely soluble in water.

Uses—A selective α_1-adrenoreceptor blocking drug with actions and uses similar to those of *Prazosin Hydrochloride.* It is advantageous in that it has a long duration of action and may be administered only once a day. In the treatment of mild to moderate hypertension, it can be used alone or in combination with other antihypertensive drugs. It is the only α_1-antagonist currently approved to treat *benign prostatic hyperplasia.* The reduction in symptoms and improvement in flow rate is due to blockade of α_1-receptors of smooth muscle in the bladder-neck and prostate.

Adverse effects are dizziness, 19%; asthenia (fatigue, lassitude, tiredness, weakness), 11%; nasal congestion, 6%; headache, 6%; peripheral edema, 5.5%; somnolence, 5.4%; nausea, 4.4%; palpitations, 4.3%; blurred vision, 1.6%. Sore throat also is frequent. Postural hypotension can occur, especially at the initiation of treatment, and syncope occasionally occurs if the regimen does not begin with the lowest dosage. It does not have an adverse effect on blood lipids. Tolerance to the antihypertensive actions has not been observed.

By the oral route, absorption is rapid and nearly complete. It manifests two-compartment kinetics, the distribution half-life being 2 to 3 hr and the elimination half life, 9 to 16 hr. It is metabolized in the liver. The metabolites are excreted mostly in the bile and, to lesser extent, in the urine.

Dose—*Oral, adult, initially* **1 mg** at bedtime with gradual upward adjustments at intervals of 2 or more days, if necessary; maintenance doses usually do not exceed 5 mg, but as much as 20 mg is needed occasionally. Once-a-day dosage is adequate.

Dosage Form—Tablets: 1, 2, 5 and 10 mg.

Tolazoline Hydrochloride

1*H*-Imidazole, 4,5-dihydro-2-(phenylmethyl)-, monohydrochloride; Priscoline (*Ciba-Geigy*)

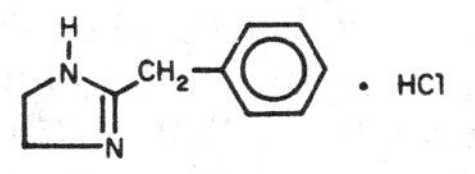

[59-97-2] $C_{10}H_{12}N_2.HCl$ (196.68).

Preparation—By heating benzyl cyanide and ethylenediamine together in the presence of carbon disulfide, whereby hydrogen sulfide and ammonia are liberated, and tolazoline is formed. After purification by distillation, the base is converted to the hydrochloride.

Description—White or creamy white, crystalline powder; solutions are slightly acid to litmus; melts between 172 and 176°.

Solubility—Freely soluble in water or alcohol.

Uses—A vasodilator with α-adrenergic blocking activity and direct vasodilator properties. It has a sympathomimetic effect to stimulate the hearts, so that blood pressure sometimes is elevated moderately, despite vasodilation. It has a histamine-like effect to stimulate gastric secretion and an acetylcholine-like effect to increase gastrointestinal motility. It also causes mydriasis by a sympathomimetic action. The only approved use is in the treatment of *persistent pulmonary hypertension in the neonate* in whom arterial oxygen cannot be maintained by oxygen or assisted ventilation. It is an effective α_2-antagonist with access to the CNS and has been used to antagonize overdoses of clonidine and other centrally acting α_2-agonists. Side effects include flushing, tingling, formication, nausea, vomiting, diarrhea, abdominal pain, gastric hyperacidity, pilomotor stimulation, palpitation, tachycardia and mydriasis. The drug is contraindicated when there is a history of angina pectoris or peptic ulcer.

Dose—*Intravenous, neonates,* **1** to **2 mg/kg/hr**, to be terminated when arterial blood gases become stable.

Dosage Form—Injection: 100 mg/4 ml.

β-Adrenoreceptor Antagonists

Nonselective β-Antagonists—Drugs such as propranolol, nadolol, pindolol and timolol suppress both β_1- and β_2-adrenoreceptor-mediated responses almost equally.

Blockade of myocardial β_1-receptors causes sinoatrial bradycardia, suppression of some ectopic pacemakers, decreased force of myocardial contraction, slowing of atrioventricular conduction and increased atrioventricular refractoriness. The effect to slow the heart rate increases the duration of diastole (that segment of the heart cycle during which most left coronary blood flow occurs) and thus increases coronary blood flow to the subendocardial region. Therefore, β-blockers are of prophylactic value in the treatment of *stable angina pectoris*. Variant (vasospastic) angina may sometimes be exacerbated. Only atenolol, metoprolol, propranolol and nadolol are approved currently in the US as antianginal drugs, but all full β-antagonists are equally effective. It is held widely that the mechanism is that of decreasing myocardial oxygen demand, especially during exercise which normally increases heart rate and contractility, thereby increasing oxygen demand and decreasing coronary blood flow. The effect to decrease sinoatrial rate also is used to *suppress tachycardia in thyrotoxicosis and pheochromocytoma*.

The effect of β-antagonists to decrease myocardial contractility is employed in *hypertrophic subaortic stenosis*, in which a reduction in the rate of development of systolic tension decreases angina, palpitations and anxiety. The effect to decrease atrioventricular nodal conduction is employed in the chronic management of *paroxysmal supraventricular* tachycardia, in which β-antagonists may block one segment of the reentrant pathway within the atrioventricular (AV) node, and in *atrial flutter* and *atrial fibrillation*, in which a drug-induced second degree AV block diminishes the number of excessive impulses from reaching the ventricles, thus increasing filling time and improving stroke output. Certain ventricular tachydysrhythmias, especially digitalis-induced, also are treated with β-blockers. Acebutolol, esmolol, propranolol and sotalol are approved antidysrhythmic drugs.

All available β-antagonists are used in the treatment of *essential hypertension*. Originally, the antihypertensive action was attributed to the decrease in cardiac output. This seems to be the mechanism of the early response, but it fails to explain the long-term effects. In the early stages of response, vascular resistance actually increases, reflexly. In a later stage, in which the greatest reduction in blood pressure occurs, the vascular resistance falls below premedication values and cardiac output returns partially toward premedication levels. β-Blockers suppress that fraction of renin release that is sustained by sympathetic activity, but this effect occurs earlier than the major fall in vascular resistance. In normal-renin and high-renin hypertensive subjects, changes in plasma renin activity correlate well with changes in blood pressure. The CNS must be ruled out as a locus of antihypertensive action, since not all effective β-blockers enter the CNS. β-Antagonists are especially useful in combination with antihypertensive vasodilators (eg, hydralazine, minoxidil) to prevent reflex tachycardia and renin release.

β-Antagonists decrease morbidity and *increase survival after myocardial infarction*. Immediately after occlusion, their effects to suppress reflex tachycardia and increase in myocardial tension decreases oxygen need. This, along with a decrease in calcium entry into the myocytes (via β-receptor-operated channels), decreases myocardial necrosis. Certain fatal tachydysrhythmias also are prevented. Continuing β-blockade decreases the incidence of sudden death from dysrhythmias and reinfarction for as long as 2 yr after an infarction. Atenolol, metoprolol, propranolol and timolol are approved for this use.

The rate of formation of intraocular fluid is decreased by β-antagonists; this is useful in the treatment of open-angle *glaucoma* and other conditions of increased intraocular pressure. Betaxolol, carteolol, levobunalol, metipranolol and timolol are applied topically in this disorder.

β-Antagonists have a varied usefulness in the prophylaxis of *migraine headache*, diminishing pain in many instances but increasing it in others. Only propranolol and timolol are approved for this purpose. The locus of action apparently is peripheral rather than central.

In the treatment of certain kinds of anxiety, such as stage fright and examination apprehension, β-antagonists are frequently effective. The efficacy is attributable to the prevention of the peripheral manifestations of sympathoadrenal discharge (eg, of tachycardia, palpitations or muscle tremor) rather than to a central action. Their value in the treatment of pathological anxiety disorders is controversial. They appear to have little effect on the underlying disorder but only to decrease certain physical manifestations.

Not all β-antagonists penetrate into the CNS, and once there, they do not all behave similarly. Propranolol, but not metroprolol or timolol, blocks certain serotonin receptors. Central actions explain the increase in slow-wave sleep, antiepileptic effects, suppression of extrapyramidal disorders such as essential tremors and tardive dyskinesias, the abolition of phantom limb sensations and possible improvement in schizophrenia after certain β-blockers. Both central and peripheral actions probably are involved in amelioration of the opiate, ethanol and amphetamine withdrawal syndromes, lessening of tremor and muscle spasms in tetanus.

Adverse effects accrue to both β_1- and β_2-antagonism. β_1-blockade in the sinoatrial node and myocardium prevents sympathetically mediated increases in cardiac output during exercise, thus forcing cardiac output to adjust purely by a Starling mechanism. Consequently, pulmonary congestion can occur during vigorous exercise, even in athletes, and pulmonary congestion limits performance. The antagonism of sympathetic nervous support to the heart also may convert a masked, compensated congestive heart failure to a frank congestive failure. However, if a tachydysrhythmia is present and the drug improves ventricular rate, congestion actually may diminish. At the AV node, β-antagonism may deepen a preexisting partial heart block and occasionally even cause ventricular asystole.

β-Antagonism in the bronchioles causes an increase in airway resistance. This can be expressed as a serious bronchospasm in bronchial asthma, bronchitis, emphysema and chronic obstructive pulmonary disease. Laryngospasm also may occur. β_2-Blockade in the liver may cause hypoglycemia in some persons. In insulin overdosage, β_2-blockade prevents the mobilization of glucose from the liver to offset hypoglycemia; furthermore, the prevention of reflex tachycardia deprives the patient of an early warning signal of impending insulin shock. β-Blockers may cause postural hypotension, with vertigo, weakness and syncope; this is more likely to occur in elderly persons or those with cerebrovascular disease or disorders of the inner ear. Prolonged use decreases renal perfusion.

Other adverse effects of β-blockade include loss of libido in both men and women, impotence, increased very low- density and decreased high-density lipoproteins, occasional nausea and vomiting, mild diarrhea or constipation, and rare allergic responses, such as rashes, fever and purpura. Centrally acting β-blockers may cause drowsiness, decreased alertness, lassitude, headache, vertigo, paresthesias, visual disturbances, insomnia, depression, mental confusion in the elderly, nightmares and hallucinations. Tolerance to these effects is frequent.

Abrupt withdrawal of β-blockers may precipitate rebound angina pectoris and/or hypertension. β-Blockers and clonidine should never be discontinued simultaneously.

Nonselective β-antagonists should be avoided, if possible, in the presence of bronchial asthma, bronchitis, emphysema, chronic obstructive pulmonary disease, sinus bradycardia, partial heart block, Raynaud's disease, diabetes, compensated and frank congestive heart failure and variant (vasospastic) angina pectoris.

β-Antagonists interact with other drugs. They usually increase the fall in blood pressure caused by other antihypertensive drugs. They increase heart block caused by digitalis and may increase the dose requirement for the inotropic actions; exacerbate the myocardial-depressant effects of halogenated general anesthetics and tricyclic antidepressants; augment the hypertensive actions of epinephrine and other α,β-adrenergic agonists; may cause MAO inhibitors to become hypertensive; prolong the action of nondepolarizing neuromuscular paralysants; increase the hypoglycemic effects of insulin and oral hypoglycemic drugs; partially antagonize indirectly the bronchodilator effects of theophylline and directly antagonize bronchodilator β_2-agonists. The effects of β-blockade are exaggerated in the presence of adrenergic neuronal blockade by reserpine, guanethidine, etc.

Selective β-Antagonists—At present there are available in the US six selective β_1-antagonists: acebutolol, atenolol, betaxolol, bisoprolol, esmolol and metoprolol. Others are practolol and tolamolol. Advantages to selective β_1-blockade are lesser effects on bronchiolar airway resistance and a diminished effect to increase insulin-induced hypoglycemia. However, β_1-block prevents the telltale reflex tachycardia that is premonitory of insulin shock. Although affinity for β_1-adrenoreceptors is many times that for β_2-receptors, care should be exercised when there is pulmonary disease or diabetes.

Selective β_1-antagonists can be used for all the purposes listed under the nonselective blockers, although they have not been approved universally for these uses.

Partial Agonist β-Antagonists—Some β-antagonists also cause some stimulation of β-adrenoreceptors (ie, have *intrinsic sympathomimetic activity, or ISA*). Of the β-antagonists presently approved in the US, only carteolol and pindolol have appreciable partial agonist properties; acebutolol and penbutolol are weak partial agonists. Some authorities hold that partial agonist activity offers no advantage over full antagonist activity. However, some advocates contend that partial agonism may be advantageous in patients prone to bradycardia or hyperlipidemia.

Acebutolol Hydrochloride

Butaneamide, ($\pm$)-*N*-[3-acetyl-4-[2-hydroxy-3-[(1-methylethyl)-amino]propoxy] phenyl-, hydrochloride; Sectral (*Wyeth*)

$CH_3CH_2CH_2CONH$ — C_6H_3(COCH$_3$) — $OCH_2CH(OH)CH_2NHCH(CH_3)_2$ · HCl

($\pm$)-3′-Acetyl-4′[2-hydroxy-3-(isopropylamino)propoxy]butyranilide, hydrochloride [34381-68-5] $C_{18}H_{28}N_2O_4$.HCl (372.93).

Preparation—S Afr Pat 68 08,345.

Description—White to slightly off-white powder melting about 142°.

Solubility—Freely soluble in water; partially soluble in alcohol.

Uses—A β_1-selective adrenoreceptor blocking agent (see the general statement) that also has weak partial agonist activity (ISA). Much of its activity is exerted by an active metabolite, diacetolol. Because of the ISA, it does not lower heart rate and increase systemic vascular resistance initially, as much as does propranolol. Although it is approved only for the treatment of *hypertension* and *tachydysrhythmias*, it is probably effective in other uses of β-blockers.

It is tolerated well. Severe bradycardia and depressed left-ventricular function are rare. Because acebutolol and diacetolol poorly penetrate the CNS, the incidence and severity of neurological side effects is low. A small proportion (0.7%) of chronic recipients develop antinuclear antibodies, but lupus-like disorders have been reported in only a few cases. Adverse effects on plasma lipids are negligible.

It undergoes first-pass intestinal and hepatic metabolism, and the oral systemic bioavailability is less than 40%. Ten to 20% is bound to plasma proteins, but there is considerable binding to erythrocytes. The steady-state volume of distribution is slightly greater than 1 L/kg, lower than any other β-blocker. Its concentration in cerebrospinal fluid is only 0.11 that in plasma and that of diacetolol is 0.04. Some of the drug is excreted into bile and feces and 30 to 40% into urine; about 70% of diacetolol is excreted in the urine. Its elimination half-life is about 3 hr but that of diacetolol is 8 to 13 hr, longer in elderly patients and persons with renal failure.

Dose—*Oral, adult,* **400 mg** a day in 2 divided doses for *dysrhythmias* and 1 or 2 divided doses for *hypertension*, to be adjusted if necessary, a daily dose of 800 mg not to be exceeded. Use one-half the above dose when creatinine clearance is 26 to 50 mL/min and one-fourth if under 25 mL/min.

Dosage Form—Capsules: 200 and 400 mg.

Atenolol

Benzeneacetamide, 4-[2-hydroxy-3-[(1-methylethyl)amino]propoxy]-, Tenormin (*Stuart*)

$OCH_2CH(OH)CH_2NHCH(CH_3)_2$ — C_6H_4 — CH_2CONH_2

2-[*p*-[2-Hydroxy-3-(isopropylamino)propoxy]phenyl]acetamide [29122-68-7] $C_{14}H_{22}N_2O_3$ (266.34).

Preparation—From *p*-hydroxyphenylacetamide, ethylene chlorohydrin and isopropylamine (US Pat 3,836,671).

Description—White crystals melting about 147°.

Uses—A selective β_1-antagonist (see the general statement) with very weak β_2-antagonist activity. It has less effect on airway resistance than metoprolol. It also has very little effect to decrease plasma renin activity.

Although it has all of the potential uses of β-antagonists, in the US it has been approved only for the treatment of hypertension, myocardial infarction and angina pectoris. Investigational data suggest an efficacy in the management of ventricular tachycardia and acute anxiety attacks.

It can cause all the adverse effects common to β-antagonists (see the general statement), but it has almost no effect on airway resistance in persons with normal lungs and has sufficiently mild effects in persons with chronic obstructive pulmonary disease that the drug can be used cautiously in such patients. It can cause bronchoconstriction and thus is contraindicated in persons with bronchial asthma. Although the brain concentration of atenolol is only one-fifth that in plasma, effects do occur in this system. Fatigue and depression are the most common noncardiovascular side effects. Allergic effects are infrequent; they include rash, fever, respiratory distress and sore throat. Agranulocytosis and both thrombocytopenic and nonthrombocytopenic purpura occasionally occur.

The oral bioavailability is 50 to 60%. Plasma protein binding is 6 to 16%. The volume of distribution is 0.7 to 1.1 L/kg. The drug is eliminated mostly unchanged in the urine and feces. The normal total body clearance is about 100 mg/min/1.73 m^2 and the half-life is 6 to 9 hr. Dose adjustments are required when the glomerular filtration rate falls below 35 mL/min/1.73 m^2.

Dose—*Oral, adult, antianginal, initially* **50 mg** once a day, to be increased after 2 wk to 100 mg once a day, if necessary. Higher doses usually produce no further therapeutic effect. If creatine clearance is 15 to 35 mL/min/1.73 m^2 (half-life, 16 to 27 hr), the maximum dose is **50 mg** a day; if it is less than 15 mL/min/1.73 m^2 (half-life, 27 hr), it is **50 mg** every second day. *Antihypertensive, initially* **25** to **50 mg** once a day, to be increased by 25 mg-increments at 2-wk intervals to as much as 100 mg a day, if necessary.

Dosage Forms—Tablets: 25, 50 and 100 mg; Injection: 5 mg/10 mL.

Betaxolol Hydrochloride

2-Propanol, 1-[4-[2-(cyclopropylmethoxy)ethyl]phenoxy]-3-[(1-methylethyl)amino]-, hydrochloride; Betoptic (*Alcon*); Kerlone (*Searle*)

$(H_3C)_2CHNHCH_2CH(OH)CH_2O$ — C_6H_4 — $CH_2CH_2OCH_2$-cyclopropyl · HCl

[63659-19-8] $C_{18}H_{29}NO_3$.HCl (343.89)

Preparation—The methyl ester of 2-(cyclopropylmethoxy)ethanesulfonic acid and *p*-benzyloxyphenol react to form 2-(cyclopropylmethoxy)-ethoxyphenyl benzyl ether, which is debenzylated to yield the free phenol, treated with epichlorhydrin to form the glycidyl ether, followed by ring opening with isopropyl amine to yield the product as the base. Treatment of the base in dry ether with HCl forms the salt. US Pat 4,252,984; *Chem Abstr*: *87*, 13454j.

Description—Crystals melting about 116°.

Uses—A selective β_1-adrenoreceptor antagonist (see the general statement). Although it is effective for the treatment of nearly all disorders for which β-blockers are used, it is approved in the US only to lower intraocular tension in *open-angle glaucoma* and certain other ocular hypertensions and in the management of essential hypertension. Because it has a low β_2-blocking activity, it does not cause the incidence and severity of pulmonary side effects of nonselective antagonists. Oral bioavailability is 90%, it has a half-life of 14 to 22 hr and most undergoes hepatic metabolism. In general, its adverse effects are those of β_1-blockers.

Dose—*Topical*, into the *conjunctival* sac, *adult*, **1 drop** of a **0.5%** (base equivalent) solution or a 0.25% suspension twice a day. *Oral, adult*, **10** to **20 mg** once a day.

Dosage Forms—Ophthalmic Solution: 0.5%; Ophthalmic Suspension: 0.25%; Tablets: 10 and 20 mg.

Bisoprolol Fumarate

2-Propanol, (±)-1-[4-[[2-(1-methylethoxy)ethoxy]methyl]-phenoxy]-3-[(1-methylethyl)amino]-, (*E*)-2-butenedioate (2:1) (salt); Zebeta (*Lederle*)

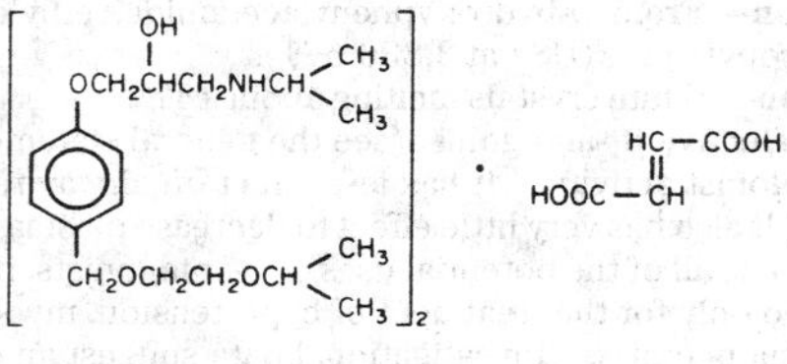

[104344-23-2] $(C_{18}H_{31}NO_4)_2 \cdot C_4H_4O_2$ (766.97).

Preparation—Cyclization of 1-(isopropylamino)-3-phenoxy-2-propanol with $COCl_2$ forms a cyclic carbamate. Treatment with paraformaldehyde and HCl yields the *p*-chloromethyl derivative which undergoes an S_N reaction with 2-isopropoxyethanol to form the ether. Aqueous base opens the protective carbamate ring yielding the product. See US Pat 4,258,062.

Description—White crystals melting about 100°; pK_a (amine) 4.8.

Solubility—Very soluble in water; 1 g dissolves in 20 mL of alcohol.

Uses—A selective β_1-antagonist with no partial agonist or local anesthetic activity. Although it is approved only for treating *essential hypertension*, it is effective for treating angina pectoris and dysrhythmias, and probably other indications for β-antagonist therapy.

It is absorbed readily after oral administration, with or without meals, with a bioavailability of 80%. Its half-life is 8 to 12 hr, and it has low lipid solubility. About 50% is excreted unchanged in urine and the rest is excreted as inactive metabolites. Dosage adjustments may be required in patients with renal impairment or severe hepatic dysfunction.

Dose—*Initially* **2.5** to **5 mg** once a day, increasing gradually to **10** or **20 mg** once a day, if necessary.

Dosage Form—Tablets: 5 to 10 mg.

Carteolol Hydrochloride

2(1*H*)-Quinolinone, 5-[3-[(1,1-dimethylethyl)amino]-2-hydroxypropoxy]-3,4-dihydro-, monohydrochloride; Cartrol (*Abbott*); Ocupress (*Otsuka America*)

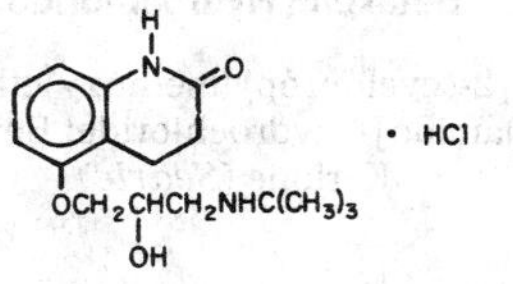

[51781-21-6] $C_{16}H_{24}N_2O_3 \cdot HCl$ (328.84).

Preparation—It is synthesized from 3,4-dihydro-5-hydroxycarbostyril and epichlorhydrin to afford the 2,3-epoxypropyl ether. Opening the epoxide with *t*-butylamine yields the base which is converted to the hydrochloride. See *J Med Chem 17*: 529, 1974.

Description—White crystals melting about 278°.

Solubility—Soluble in water; slightly soluble in alcohol.

Uses—A nonselective β-antagonist with significant partial agonist activity (ISA) and little membrane-stabilizing (local anesthetic) activity. It is approved only for treating *essential hypertension* and for lowering the intraocular pressure in *ocular hypertension* and *open-angle glaucoma*. Although it produces the typical spectrum of side effects (see the general statement, page 1012), bradycardia may be less than produced by agents without partial agonist activity, and CNS effects are less frequent due to low lipid solubility and poor brain penetration. It is as effective as other topical β-antagonists in lowering intraocular pressure, but is somewhat less potent.

Carteolol is absorbed readily providing an oral bioavailability of 85%. Since 50 to 70% is excreted unchanged, the half-life of 6 hr is increased by impaired renal function. A major metabolite, 8-hydroxycarteolol, is active with a half-life of 8 to 12 hr and represents about 5% of the administered dose excreted.

Dose—*Oral, initially* **2.5 mg** once a day, to be increased gradually to **5** or **10 mg** once a day, if necessary. Higher doses may actually decrease the response. *Topical, into the conjunctival sac,* **1 drop** of a 1% solution twice a day.

Dosage Forms—Tablets: 2.5 and 5 mg; Ophthalmic Solution: 1%.

Esmolol Hydrochloride

Benzenepropionic acid, (±)-4-[2-hydroxy-3-[(1-methylethyl)-amino]propoxy]-, methyl ester, hydrochloride; Brevibloc (*Du Pont*)

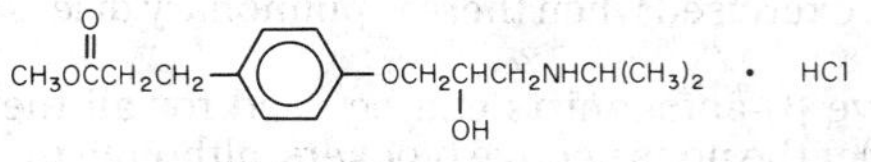

[84057-94-3] $C_{16}H_{25}NO_4.HCl$ (331.84)

Preparation—*J Med Chem 25*: 1408, 1982.

Description—White crystals melting about 85°.

Uses—A β-adrenoreceptor antagonist that is more selective for β_1 receptors than is metoprolol (see below). It has an ultrashort duration of action, which is advantageous in the treatment of supraventricular tachycardias consequent to valvular heart disease, open- heart surgery, tracheal intubation and myocardial infarction and of acute hypertension from intubation, surgery and other causes. It probably will become the β-blocker of choice for the early management of myocardial infarction. It also may be used diagnostically to assess the possible efficacy and adverse effects of β_1-adrenergic block prior to the initiation of a long-term regimen.

Its potential adverse effects are those expected from β_1-adrenergic blockade (see the general statement). Hypotension is the most frequent adverse effect. The selectivity is sufficiently high that in asthmatic patients very little change in airway resistance occurs.

It is degraded by esterases in red blood cells. The elimination half-life averages 9 min.

Dose—*Intravenous, adult, loading,* **0.5 mg/kg,** given over a period of 1 min, followed by *maintenance infusion* of **0.05 mg/kg/min,** to be adjusted by increments of 0.05 mg/kg/min at 5- to 10-min intervals, if necessary. Infusion rates rarely exceed 0.1 mg/kg/min; rates above 0.2 mg/kg/min do not achieve greater effects.

Dosage Form—Injection: 2.5 g/10 mL.

Indoramine Hydrochloride—see RPS-18, page 834.

Labetalol Hydrochloride

Benzamide, 2-hydroxy-5-[1-hydroxy-2-[(1-methyl-3-phenylpropyl)amino]ethyl]-, monohydrochloride; Normodyne (*Schering*); Trandate (*Allen & Hanburys*)

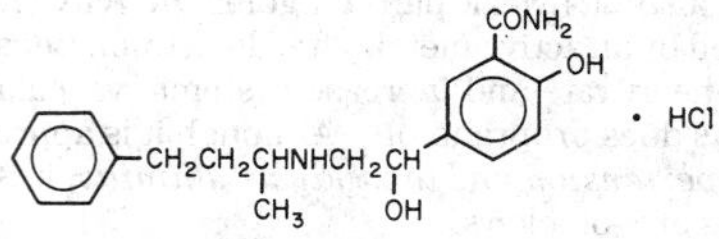

5-[1-Hydroxy-2-[(1-methyl-3-phenylpropyl)amino]ethyl]salicylamide monohydrochloride [32780-64-6] $C_{19}H_{24}N_2O_3.HCl$ (364.87).

Preparation—US Pat 4,012,444.

Description—White crystals.

Solubility—Soluble in water or ethanol; insoluble in ether or chloroform.

Uses—Combines both nonselective β- and selective α_1-antagonist activity, in a ratio of 3:1 by the oral and 7:1 by the intravenous routes. In addition, it has weak intrinsic β_2-adrenergic agonist activity, to which some investigators attribute some of its antihypertensive effects. These different actions are attributable to the different stereoisomers found in the racemate. The drug variably decreases heart rate and cardiac output, but in conventional doses has very little effect on contractility. Plasma renin activity usually is decreased. Systemic vascular resistance is decreased and venous capacitance increased. The collective effect of these actions is a reduction in blood pressure, often without much change in heart rate.

It is used in the treatment of *essential* and *renal hypertension, toxemia of pregnancy* and other *hypertensive emergencies* and *pheochromacytoma*. In essential hypertension often it is effective when other drugs have failed. It also is effective in *angina pectoris*.

The incidence of adverse effects is 6 to 25%. Effects of α-blockade include postural hypotension with accompanying dizziness, scleroconjunctival injection and irritation, nasal stuffiness and tingling of the scalp. Some tolerance to the α-blocking activity gradually occurs. Effects of β-blockade include bronchospasm (which partly is ameliorated by β_2-agonism) and occasional Raynaud's phenomenon, claudication and heart failure. Other effects include flushed, yet cold, extremities, palpitations, diarrhea, rare reversible alopecia, impotence, decreased libido, tremors, headache, lassitude, fatigue, rare myopathy, depression and abnormal dreaming. After intravenous injection there is an occasional paradoxical pressor response. Allergic and immunologic effects include rashes, pruritis, increased antinuclear antibodies and rare lupus-like syndrome.

The oral bioavailability is about 35%, because of first-pass metabolism. Food, cimetidine and liver disease increase bioavailability. In the liver, the drug mostly is conjugated to glucuronides. Oral administration selectively decreases β-blocking activity. The elimination half-life is about 6 to 8 hr.

Dose—*Oral, adult, initially* **100 mg** twice a day, to be adjusted twice a day with 100-mg increments to a *maintenance* dose of **200 mg** to **1.2 g** a day in *mild* to *moderate hypertension* and **1.2** to **2.4 g** a day in *moderately severe* hypertension. *Intravenous, adult, initially* **20 mg** slowly over a 2-min period, then **40** to **80 mg** at 10-min intervals, if necessary.

Dosage Forms—Injection: 5 mg/mL in 20, 40 and 60 mL; Tablets: 100, 200 and 300 mg.

Levobunolol Hydrochloride

1(2*H*)-Naphthalenone, (−)-5-[3-[(1,1-dimethylethyl)-amino]-2-hydroxypropoxy]-3,4-dihydro-, hydrochloride; Betagan Liquifilm (*Allergan*)

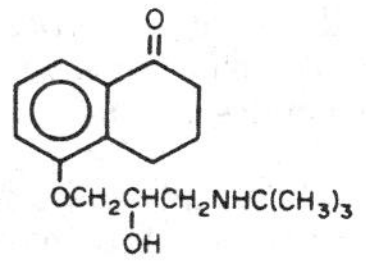

O ‖ · HCl
$OCH_2CHCH_2NHC(CH_3)_3$
OH

[27912-14-7] $C_{17}H_{25}NO_3.HCl$ (327.85).

Preparation—See *J Med Chem 13:* 684, 1970.

Description—White crystals melting about 210°.

Solubility—Soluble in water; slightly soluble in alcohol.

Uses—A nonselective β-agonist with a structure similar to that of carteolol, and its actions and averse effects are similar. It is approved in the US only for the treatment of *primary open-angle glaucoma*, and other causes of ocular hypertension.

Dose—*Topical*, into the *conjuctival* sac, *adult*, **1 drop** of **0.5% solution** 1 or 2 times a day.

Dosage Form—Ophthalmic Solution: 0.5%.

Metipranolol Hydrochloride

Phenol, (±)-4-[2-hydroxy-3-[(1-methylethyl)amino]propoxy]-2,3,6-trimethyl-, 1-acetate, hydrochloride; MPR; OptiPranolol (*Bausch & Lomb*)

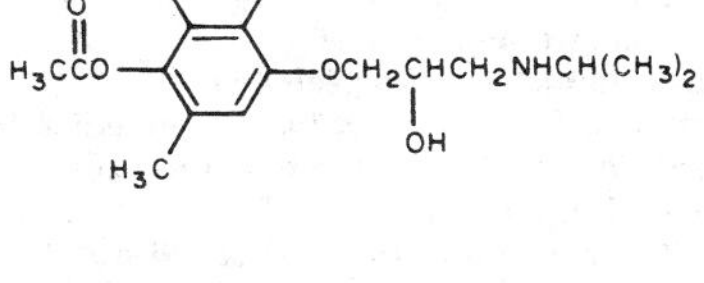

H_3C CH_3
H_3CCO (O ‖) $OCH_2CHCH_2NHCH(CH_3)_2$
H_3C OH

[22664-55-7(base)]$C_{17}H_{27}NO_4$ (345.86).

Preparation—Czech Pat 128,471.

Description—White crystals melting about 106°.

Solubility—Slightly soluble in water.

Uses—A nonselective β-antagonist with no agonist or local anesthetic activity that is approved only for topical application to reduce intraocular pressure in *open-angle glaucoma* and *ocular hypertension*. It may be more irritating than some of the other topical β-antagonists, and systemic absorption can produce typical side effects and avoidance in patients with contraindications to β-antagonists. Reduced intraocular pressure can persist for 24 hr following a single application.

Dose—*Topical*, **1 drop** into the conjunctival sac twice a day.

Dosage Form—Ophthalmic Solution: 0.3%.

Metoprolol Tartrate

2-Propanol, (±)-1-[4-(2-methoxyethyl)phenoxy]-3-[(1-methylethyl)amino]-, [*R*-(*R**,*R**)]-2,3-dihydroxybutanedioate (2:1) (salt); Lopressor (*Ciba-Geigy*); Toprol XL (*Astra*)

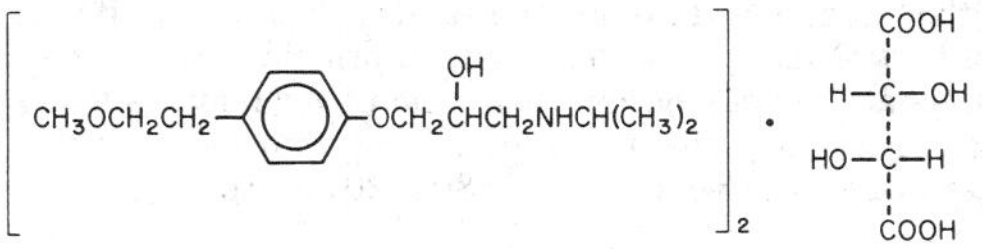

[$CH_3OCH_2CH_2$–C6H4–$OCH_2CHCH_2NHCH(CH_3)_2$ (OH)]$_2$ · COOH, H–C–OH, HO–C–H, COOH

(±)-1-(Isopropylamino)-3-[*p*-(2-methoxyethyl)phenoxy]-2-propanol, L-(+)-tartrate (2:1) (salt) [56392-17-7] $(C_{15}H_{25}NO_3)_2.C_4H_4O_6$ (684.82).

Preparation—From 4-(2-methoxyethyl)phenol, 3-chloro-1,2-propanediol and isopropylamine (Swedish Pat 368,004).

Description—White, odorless powder; bitter taste; melts about 120°.

Solubility—Very soluble in water; soluble in alcohol or chloroform; insoluble in acetone or ether.

Uses—A selective β_1-antagonist with slight β_2-antagonist activity (see general statement). Its β_2-blocking activity is sufficient that in therapeutic doses it can suppress adrenergically induced hyperglycemia and also frequently cause bronchospasm in asthmatic subjects. It only slightly increases airway resistance in normal persons and moderately in persons with obstructive airway disease.

The potential uses, adverse effects, contraindications and drug interactions are those of β-antagonists in general (see the general statement). However, it presently is approved only for the treatment of *hypertension, angina pectoris* and after *myocardial* infarction. Although it penetrates the CNS, its effects there are less intense than with propranolol. Nevertheless, about 10% of recipients will experience lassitude and dizziness. It occasionally may cause pruritis.

The oral bioavailability is about 50% for immediate-release tablets, but about 75% for extended-release tablets. The volume of distribution is 3.5 to 5 L/kg. Only 12% is protein-bound in plasma. It is hydroxylated in the liver. There are slow and fast hydroxylator subjects; the elimination half-life is about 1.7 to 4.2 hr in fast and 5 to 10 hr in slow hydroxylators.

Dose—*Oral, adult, antianginal* or *antihypertensive, initially* **100 mg** a day once or in 2 divided doses, with weekly adjustments in dosage up to a total of **450 mg** a day, if necessary; *postmyocardial infarction, initially* **50 mg** (25 mg, if tolerated poorly) every 6 hr for 48 hr, beginning 15 min after the last intravenous dose, then **100 mg** twice a day for 3 mo to 3 yr; *prophylaxis of vascular headache*, **50** to **100 mg** every 6 to 12 hr. Extended-release tablets permit once-a-day dosage in the ranges indicated above. *Intravenous, adult*, postmyocardial infarction, **5 mg** every 2 min for 3 doses, beginning at the earliest possible time. At the higher doses, β_2-antagonism may be significant.

Dosage Forms—Injection: 5 mg/5 mL; Tablets: 50 and 100 mg; Extended Release Tablets: 50, 100 and 200 mg.

Nadolol

2,3-Naphthalenediol, *cis*-5-[3-[(1,1-dimethylethyl)amino]-2-hydroxypropoxy]-1,2,3,4-tetrahydro-, Corgard (*Bristol-Myers Squibb*)

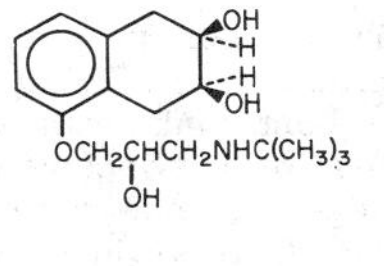

OH, H, H, OH
$OCH_2CHCH_2NHC(CH_3)_3$
OH

1-(*tert*-Butylamino)-3-[(5,6,7,8-tetrahydro-*cis*-6,7-dihydroxy-1-naphthyl)oxy]-2-propanol [42200-33-9] $C_{17}H_{27}NO_4$ (309.40).

Preparation—US Pat 3,935,267.

Description—White crystalline powder melting about 130°; pK_a 9.68.

Solubility—Freely soluble in alcohol; slightly soluble in water or chloroform; insoluble in acetone or hydrocarbon solvents.

Uses—A nonselective β-antagonist with all the actions, uses, adverse effects, contraindications and drug interactions characteristic of drugs in this class (see the general statement). However, nadolol is approved only for treatment of *hypertension* and *angina pectoris*. Its chief advantage is its long duration of action which permits once-a-day dosage. It lacks CNS actions because it fails to penetrate into the CNS.

The oral bioavailability is about 40%. Twenty to 30% is bound to plasma proteins. The volume of distribution is about 2 L/kg. Most of the drug is eliminated unchanged in the urine. Some is excreted as conjugates in the bile, which are deconjugated partially in the small intestine and reabsorbed. The normal half-life is 20 to 24 hr but it is longer in renal failure.

Dose—*Oral, adult,* for *angina pectoris, initially* **40 mg** once a day, with increments of 40 to 80 mg a day at 3- to 7-day intervals, if necessary, up to a total dose of **240 mg** a day; for *hypertension, initially* **80 mg** once a day, with increments of **80 mg** a day at weekly intervals, if necessary, up to a total of **320 mg** a day. The plateau principle establishes that dose adjustments at intervals of less than 5 half-lives may result in excessive maintenance dosage. In renal failure, dosage must be adjusted.

Dosage Form—Tablets: 20, 40, 80, 120 and 160 mg.

Penbutolol Sulfate

2-Propanol, (*S*)-1-(2-cyclopentylphenoxy)-3-[(1,1-dimethylethyl)amino]-, sulfate (2:1) (salt); Levatol (*Reed & Carnrick*)

$$\left[(CH_3)_3CNHCH_2-\overset{H}{\underset{OH}{C}}-CH_2O-C_6H_4-C_5H_9\right]_2 \cdot H_2SO_4$$

[38363-32-5] $(C_{18}H_{29}NO_2)_2 \cdot H_2SO_4$ (680.94).

Preparation—See US Pat 3,551,493.

Description—White crystals melting about 217°.

Solubility—Soluble in water; slightly soluble in alcohol.

Uses—A nonselective β-antagonist with some agonist activity but no membrane stabilizing activity and is approved only for the treatment of *essential hypertension.* Experience with other β-antagonist indications is limited. It is completely absorbed from the GI tract, highly bound to plasma proteins and completely metabolized by the liver. Despite a plasma half-life of about 5 hr, once-a-day dosage appears adequate. A lower incidence of severe bradycardia than produced by propranolol probably reflects its intrinsic agonist activity.

Dose—*Oral,* **20 mg** once a day, increased to **40 mg,** if needed.

Dosage Form—Tablets: 20 mg.

Pindolol

2-Propanol, 1-(1*H*-indol-4-yloxy)-3-[(1-methyl-ethyl)amino]-, Visken (*Sandoz*)

$$\text{Indol-4-yl}-OCH_2\underset{OH}{CH}CH_2NHCH(CH_3)_2$$

[13523-86-9] $C_{14}H_{20}N_2O$ (248.32).

Preparation—Swiss Pat 472,404.

Description—Off-white, crystalline powder; almost odorless; melts about 172°.

Solubility—Practically insoluble in water; slightly soluble in anhydrous alcohol or chloroform.

Uses—A nonselective β-antagonist with partial agonist activity (see general statement). The intrinsic sympathomimetic activity in man appears to be somewhat less than 0.5. When resting sympathoadrenal activity is low, the intrinsic activity is evident in that heart rate and force of contraction do not decrease to the extent expected from β-blockade or may actually slightly increase. When the sympathoadrenal activity is high, heart rate and force decline, as expected from β-blockade. With low doses, in hypertension, angina pectoris and ventricular tachydysrhythmias, its efficacy appears to be comparable to that of propranolol, but it is probably less effective against supraventricular tachydysrhythmias. With high doses, there may be a decrease in antihypertensive efficacy possibly because of increased renin secretion. The oral bioavailability is about 90%. In plasma, about 57% is protein-bound. The volume of distribution is about 2.9 L/kg. The effective plasma concentration is 50 to 100 ng/mL. About 60% is eliminated by hepatic metabolism and 40% by renal excretion; the (−) enantiomer is excreted faster than the (+) one. The elimination half-life is 3 to 4 hr.

Dose—*Oral, adult, initially* **10 mg** twice a day, to be adjusted at 14- to 21-day intervals up to a maximum daily dose of 30 mg; above 30 mg a day, no further reductions in blood pressure usually are achieved and adverse effects are more prominent.

Dosage Form—Tablets: 5 and 10 mg.

Propranolol Hydrochloride

2-Propanol, 1-[(1-methylethyl)amino]-3-(1-naphthalenyloxy)-, hydrochloride; Inderal (*Ayerst*); (*Various Mfrs*)

$$\text{1-Naphthyl}-OCH_2\overset{OH}{CH}CH_2NHCH(CH_3)_2 \cdot HCl$$

[318-98-9] $C_{16}H_{21}NO_2.HCl$ (295.81).

Preparation—α-Naphthol is reacted with epichlorohydrin in aqueous alkali to form 2,3-epoxypropyl α-naphthyl ether and the epoxy ring ruptured by reaction with isopropylamine. The base is converted to hydrochloride with HCl.

Description—White or almost white powder that is odorless with a bitter taste; stable to heat, unstable in light and nonhygroscopic; melts at about 161°; pK_a 9.45.

Solubility—1 g in 20 mL water or 20 mL alcohol; slightly soluble in chloroform; practically insoluble in ether.

Uses—The prototype nonselective β-antagonist, with all the actions, uses, adverse effects and contraindications characteristic of this class of drugs (see general statement), except that it is not used to treat glaucoma. Only the (−)isomer has significant β-blocking activity. It is stated frequently that the drug has quinidine-like properties to decrease myocardial sodium entry, but it appears that such actions do not occur in therapeutic concentrations and that the antidysrhythmic actions are those of β_1-blockade alone.

The drug penetrates into the CNS and causes the central effects in the general statement. It has been reported to be of value in more than 20 noncardiovascular disorders, many of which are in the CNS. It also enters adrenergic neurons, from which it can be released by nerve impulses. It decreases portal venous pressure and blood flow in the splanchnic bed and portosystemic collateral vessels; consequently, it is used to decrease the incidence of mortality of upper gastrointestinal hemorrhage in cirrhosis of the liver and esophageal varices.

It can cause an erythematous rash with fever and sore throat. It inhibits 5′-deiodination, hence, increases thyroxine and decreases liothyronine levels, thus altering thyroid physiology. It also has been reported possibly to be teratogenic.

By the oral route only 30 to 60% reaches the systemic circulation, mainly because it is metabolized actively as it passes through the liver from the gut. Most food increases the bioavailability, but high-protein meals increase hepatic clearance and lower bioavailability. Bioavailability also is lower with extended-release preparations. There are about 20 metabolites, at least one of which is also active. More metabolites appear after oral than intravenous administration. All of the drug is biotransformed in the liver. The volume of distribution is about 4 L/kg. It is 93% protein-bound. The minimal effective plasma concentration is in the range of 0.04 to 0.085 μg/mL. Plasma renin activity is suppressed at 0.10 to 0.20 μg/mL. The plasma half-life of a single dose is about 2 to 3.5 hr, but it is about 3 to 5 hr with repeated dosage and also longer in congestive heart failure. The half-life is shorter in blacks than in whites and shorter in men than women.

The oral route of administration is preferred.

Dose—*Intravenous,* for *arrhythmias* or immediately after *myocardial infarction, adult,* **1 to 3 mg** at a rate not to exceed 1 mg/min. The dose may be repeated in a few minutes if necessary. *Oral,* in *conventional form, adult,* for *arrhythmias,* **10 to 30 mg** 3 or 4 times a day, before meals and at bedtime; after *myocardial infarction,* **60 mg** 3 or 4 times a day, starting as early as possible; for *pheochromocytoma, preoperatively,* **20** to **40 mg** 3 or 4 times a day for 3 days prior to surgery but not to be given before an α-blocker has been administered first, or, for the *management* of *inoperable tumor,* **10** to **50 mg** 3 times a day; for *essential hypertension, initially* **40 mg** twice a day, increased by 20-mg increments up to **160 mg,** 4 times a day (several days to several weeks of medication may be required before a substantial effect occurs); *for angina pectoris, initially* **10** to **20 mg** 3 or 4 times a day, to be increased to as much as **80 mg,** if necessary, 3 or 4 times a day; for *hypertrophic subaortic stenosis,* **20** to **40 mg** 3 or 4 times a day; for *thyrotoxicosis,* **10** to **40 mg** 3 or 4 times a day with adjustments as necessary; for *vascular headaches,* **20 mg** 4 times a day, with upward adjustments, if necessary, up to a dose of 240 mg a day for *anxiety,* **10** to **80 mg** 30 to 90 min in advance of anxiety-inducing situations; *essential tremor, initially* **40 mg** 3 or 4 times a day, to be adjusted as needed. *Oral, children,* **500 μg** to **1 mg/kg** a day in 3 or 4 divided doses. In *sustained-release form,* the total daily dose can be taken once a day.

Dosage Forms—Sustained-Release Capsules: 60, 80, 120 and 160 mg; Injection: 1 mg/mL; Tablets: 10, 20, 40, 60, 80 and 90 mg; Oral Solution: 4, 8 and 80 mg/mL.

Terazosin Hydrochloride—page 1011.

Sotalol Hydrochloride

Methanesulfonamide, *N*-[4-[1-hydroxy-2-[(1-methylethyl)-amino]ethyl]phenyl]-, monohydrochloride; Betapace (*Berlex*)

$CH_3SO_2NH-C_6H_4-CH(OH)CH_2NHCH(CH_3)_2 \cdot HCl$

[959-24-0]$C_{12}H_{20}N_2O_3S.HCl$ (308.82).

Preparation—One method involves the reaction of methanesulfonyl chloride with *p*-aminoacetophenone to form the sulfonamide which is then brominated by a free radical procedure to yield the phenacyl bromide. A nucleophilic substitution of bromine by isopropyl amine affords the base which is converted to the salt. See *J Med Chem 10:* 462, 1967.

Description—White crystals melting about 207°; pK_1 8.3, pK_2 9.8.

Solubility—Freely soluble in water; insoluble in alcohol.

Uses—A nonselective β-antagonist with no intrinsic agonist or local anesthetic activities. It also lengthens the action potential and prolongs the refractory period in myocardial fibers by inhibiting a rapid component of the delayed rectifier potassium current. It is approved only for the treatment of *life-threatening ventricular arrhythmias.* It has been shown superior to other antiarrhythmic agents that act by blocking sodium channels in myocardial conductive tissue. It produces the typical β-antagonist side effects (see the general statement, page 1013) except that its low lipid solubility predicts a lower incidence of CNS side effects. However, its tendency to produce a serious ventricular arrhythmia, torsades de points, especially in the presence of prolonged QT intervals as determined by ECG or hypokalemia limit its recommended use to life-threatening ventricular arrhythmias, although limited trials indicate efficacy in controlling supraventricular tachycardias.

It is absorbed completely and rapidly from the GI tract and is excreted unchanged in the urine with a half-life of 12 hr. Dosing intervals require modification in the presence of renal impairment. Previous antiarrhythmic drugs should be tapered downward before starting sotalol.

Dose—*Oral, initially* **80 mg** twice a day, increasing to **240** to **320 mg** 2 or 3 times a day under close monitoring.

Dosage Form—Tablets: 80, 160 and 240 mg.

Timolol Maleate

2-Propanol, (*S*)-1-[(1,1-dimethylethyl)amino]-3-[[4-(4-morpholinyl-1,2,5-thiadiazol-3-yl]oxy-, (*Z*)-2-butenedioate (1:1) (salt); Blocadren, Timoptic (*MSD*); (*Various Mfrs*)

(–)-1-(*tert*-Butylamino)-3-[(4-morpholino-1,2,5-thiadiazol-3-yl)oxy]-2-propanol maleate (1:1) (salt) [26921-17-5] $C_{13}H_{24}N_4O_4.S.-C_4H_4O_4$ (432.49).

Preparation—*J Med Chem 15:* 651, 1972.

Description—White crystals melting about 202°; pH (5% aqueous solution) about 4; stable in aqueous solution up to about pH 12.

Solubility—Freely soluble in water; soluble in alcohol; sparingly soluble in chloroform; practically insoluble in ether.

Uses—A nonselective β-adrenoreceptor antagonist with all the potential uses, adverse effects, contraindications and drug interactions characteristic of this class of drugs (see the general statement), except that its CNS actions are very weak. Approved uses in the US include the treatment of *hypertension,* migraine prophylaxis, the prevention of reinfarction and/or sudden death *after myocardial infarction* and the treatment of most types of *glaucoma.* This was the drug used in the Norwegian studies that convincingly demonstrated the value of administering β-blockers following myocardial infarction.

As the first β-antagonist to be used in the US for treating glaucoma, it is free of intrinsic agonist and local anesthetic activities. However, systemic absorption can occur through the lacrymal ducts, and it should be used cautiously in patients with asthma, emphysema, congestive heart failure, diabetes and greater than first-degree heart block. Systemic absorption also can produce typical peripheral and CNS side effects of β-antagonists.

By the oral route the bioavailability is 60 to 75%. About 10% is bound to plasma proteins. β-Blocking concentrations are 5 to 10 ng/mL. Lipid solubility is low, so that concentrations in the CNS are low. Because of its high potency, topical efficacy in the eye is good. About 80% is eliminated by hepatic metabolism and 20% by renal excretion. The elimination half-life is about 3 to 4 hr in fast metabolizers and 7.5 hr in slow metabolizers.

Dose—*Oral, adult, initially* **10 mg** twice a day, to be maintained at that dose for prophylaxis after myocardial infarction but increased at 1-wk intervals, if necessary, up to a dose of 30 mg twice a day in angina, hypertension and vascular headache. *Topical, to the eye, initially* **1 drop** of a **0.25%** solution once or twice a day, to be increased to 0.50%, if necessary.

Dosage Forms—Ophthalmic Solution: 0.25 and 0.50%; Tablets: 5, 10 and 20 mg.

Adrenergic Neuron Blocking Drugs

The biosynthesis of the adrenergic neurohumor, norepinephrine, takes place in the postganglionic sympathetic adrenergic neuron. The substrate is 3,4-dihydroxyphenyl-alanine (DOPA), which is formed in the adrenergic neuron by the hydroxylation of tyrosine. DOPA is decarboxylated by the enzyme, dopa decarboxylase, to produce the catecholamine, dopamine (3,4-dihydroxy-β-phenylethylamine). Within the adrenergic neuron in the region of the nerve endings are granular organelles that contain the enzyme dopamine β-oxidase, which introduces the side-chain hydroxyl group onto dopamine to make norepinephrine. The norepinephrine is stored in the granular organelles. Nerve impulses cause the ingress of calcium, which releases norepinephrine from the storage granules. It also can be released by indirectly acting sympathomimetics (see Chapter 43) and drugs such as reserpine or guanethidine. After the norepinephrine is released initially from the granules by reserpine or guanethidine, newly formed or transported norepinephrine cannot be reincorporated into the depleted granules; furthermore, residual norepinephrine in the granules, of which there is considerable after treatment with guanethidine, cannot be released. The total effect is that norepinephrine is less available for delivery to the effector in response to nerve stimulation.

Drugs such as metyrosine, which suppress the biosynthesis of norepinephrine, also cause adrenergic neuronal block.

Guanadrel Sulfate

Guanidine, (1,4-dioxaspiro[4.5]dec-2-ylmethyl)-, sulfate (2:1); Hylorel (*Pennwalt*)

[22195-34-2] $(C_{10}H_{19}N_3O_2)_2.H_2SO_4$ (524.63).

Preparation—US Pat 3,547,951.

Description—White solid melting about 235° with decomposition.

Solubility—One g dissolves in about 13.5 mL water.

Uses—An adrenergic neuron blocking drug with a mechanism of action and hemodynamic properties like those of guanethidine (below), to which it is related chemically. It has a shorter duration of action and consequently causes less severe morning postural hypotension, but postural hypotension during the rest of the day is comparable to that from guanethidine. It causes somewhat less diarrhea and interferes less with ejaculation. Unlike guanethidine, it is used in the treatment of *mild* and *moderate essential hypertension.*

The drug is absorbed well orally, the bioavailability of compressed tablets being about 85%. Peak effects are reached in 30 to 120 min after oral administration, although peak plasma concentrations are not achieved until 90 to 120 min. Less than 20% of plasma guanadrel is protein-bound. The drug does not penetrate into the brain or eye. The duration of action is 4 to 14 hr. Tricyclic antidepressants, amphetamines and other drugs that inhibit the amine uptake pump into the adrenergic neuron prevent neuronal uptake of guanadrel and hence shorten the duration of action or completely "deblock" the adrenergic neuron. Elimination is about 50% by hepatic metabolism and 50% by renal excretion. The distribution and elimination half-lives are 1 to 4 hr and 5 to 45 hr, respectively.

Dose—*Oral, adult, initially* **5 mg** upon arising and again in the afternoon, to be adjusted gradually, if necessary, to a usual *maintenance* dose of **20** to **75 mg** a day; some patients may require only 1 dose a day.

Dosage Form—Scored Tablets: 10 and 25 mg.

Guanethidine Monosulfate

Guanidine, [2-(hexahydro-1(2*H*)-azocinyl)ethyl]-, sulfate (2:1); Ismelin Sulfate (*Ciba-Geigy*)

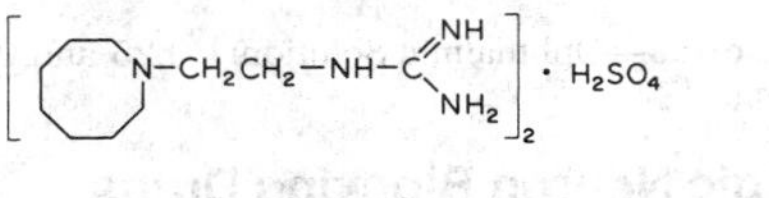

[60-02-6] $(C_{10}H_{22}N_4)_2.H_2SO_4$ (494.69).

Preparation—Cycloheptanone oxime undergoes Beckmann rearrangement to form hexahydro-2(1*H*)-azocinone [$CH_2(CH_2)_5CONH$] which is then reduced to heptamethyleneimine [$CH_2(CH_2)_6NH$]. This is condensed with chloracetonitrile and the resulting nitrile is hydrogenated to 1-(2-aminoethyl)heptamethyleneimine. Condensation with 2-methyl-2-thiopseudourea [$NH{=}C(SCH_3)NH_2$] sulfate eliminates CH_3SH to produce crude guanethidine sulfate. See *Experientia 15*: 267, 1959.

Description—White to off-white, crystalline powder.

Solubility—Sparingly soluble in water; slightly soluble in alcohol; practically insoluble in chloroform.

Uses—An antiadrenergic neuron blocking agent that partially depletes the adrenergic nerve of its norepinephrine and prevents release of that which remains after being taken up selectively by adrenergic nerve terminals. The result is vasodilatation and a decrease in plasma renin activity, both of which act to lower blood pressure. The onset of action is slow, requiring several hours to 2 or 3 days for its full effect, and its duration of action may be 4 or more days. Guanethidine lowers the blood pressure very effectively. In fact, there is danger that the blood pressure will fall to dangerously low levels in some patients. Therefore, it usually is employed in submaximal doses and is combined with thiazides or hydralazine in order to permit some adrenergic function to remain. It usually is not used to treat mild to moderate but only moderately severe to severe hypertension. In fact, it is seldom used today, having been replaced by highly effective drugs with far fewer side effects.

Its most common untoward effects are those that obligatorily accrue to the effects of sympathetic blockade. They include orthostatic hypotension with its attendant vertigo, weakness, lassitude, nausea and occasional syncope, bradycardia, nasal stuffiness, dry mouth, diarrhea, urinary incontinence, nocturia and failure of normal ejaculation. Fatigue and dyspnea from exertion also occur. Heart failure also may occur in susceptible patients. Like reserpine, the drug may cause edema and azotemia as a result of a deficient renal blood flow consequent to decreased blood pressure and cardiac output. Adrenergic neuron blockage tends to exacerbate hypoglycemia in certain patients. Other effects include fatigue, ptosis, blurred vision, parotid tenderness, angina, muscle tremor, myalgia, alopecia and mental depression.

It potentiates the pressor effects of norepinephrine, and certain other directly acting alpha sympathomimetics, by inhibiting uptake into the adrenergic nerve terminals and by causing supersensitivity of receptors. It also may cause release of catecholamines from pheochrome tumors and hence precipitate hypertensive crises. It interferes with the pressor actions of indirectly acting sympathomimetics by inhibiting both uptake of the drugs into the adrenergic neuron and release of norepinephrine, but it potentiates whatever lesser amounts of levarterenol are released. Amphetamine-type central nervous stimulants, tricyclic antidepressants levodopa, and chlorpromazine antagonize this drug. Tricyclic antidepressants and quinidine may cause cardiac arrest when given with this drug. It potentiates the hypoglycemic effects of oral hypoglycemics and insulin.

It is contraindicated in pheochromocytoma, in patients hypersensitive to the drug, and when MAO inhibitors are in use. It should be used cautiously in renal disease, cerebral vascular disease, coronary insufficiency, recent myocardial infarction, congestive heart failure, pulmonary disorders and asthma, peptic ulcer, edematous states, diabetes and anesthesia.

Only 3 to 30% is absorbed when administered orally. It is metabolized partly to two metabolites and excreted partly unchanged, (25 to 50%), mostly within a few hours; however, effective traces remain for up to 14 days. The onset of action is a few hours to a few days; the offset of action is several days.

Dose—*Oral, adult, ambulatory patients, initially* **10** or **12.5 mg** once a day, with 10- to 12.5-mg increments at 5- to 7-day intervals, if necessary to effect a therapeutic fall in blood pressure, but not to exceed 200 mg a day; **25** to **50 mg** a day is the usual *maintenance* dose. In combination with other antihypertensives the usual dose will be lower. "Minidoses" of 5 mg sometimes have been used in the treatment of moderate essential hypertension. *Hospitalized patients, initially* **25** to **50 mg,** with daily or bi-daily increments of 25 to 50 mg, if necessary. An initial large dose of 100 mg can be given without a hypertensive phase of action. *Children,* **200 μg/kg** (or 6 mg/m²), with increments of 200 μg/kg at 7- to 10-day intervals, if necessary.

Dosage Form—Scored Tablets: 10 and 25 mg.

Metyrosine

L-Tyrosine, (−)-α-methyl-, Demser (*MSD*)

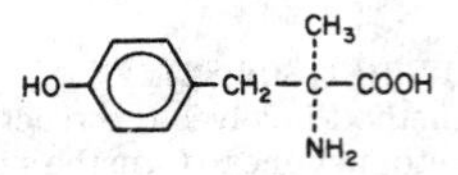

[672-87-7] $C_{10}H_{13}NO_3$ (195.22).

Preparation—*J Org Chem 32*: 4074, 1967.

Description—White, crystalline solid; melts about 310°.

Solubility—About 1 g in 1750 mL water.

Uses—Blocks tyrosine hydroxylase and thus suppresses the synthesis of catecholamines. This causes depletion of catecholamines in adrenergic neurons in both the sympathetic and central nervous systems and in the pheochrome cells in the adrenal medulla and accessory tissue. The drug is used to treat *pheochromocytoma.* It is too inconsistent in hypertension to be competitive with other drugs. Sedation is the most common side effect, but some tolerance occurs during the first week of treatment. Extrapyramidal dyskinesias occur in about 10% of recipients. Other adverse CNS effects include anxiety, confusion, depression, disorientation and hallucinations. Insomnia and hyperactivity may occur after withdrawal. Gastrointestinal side effects include diarrhea (about 10%), nausea, vomiting and abdominal pain. Nasal stuffiness, impotence and impaired ejaculation result from sympathetic adrenergic neuron blockade. Other adverse effects are dry mouth, headache, gynecomastia, galactorrhea, peripheral edema, urticaria, pharyngeal edema, eosinophilia and elevated SGOT. Crystalluria and nephrolithiasis and consequent hematuria and transient dysuria may occur. A daily urine output of over 2 L should be maintained. It potentiates the extrapyramidal effects of phenothiazines and butyrophenones. About 50 to 90% is excreted unchanged in the urine.

Dose—*Oral, adult* and *children over 12 yr, initially* **250 mg** 4 times a day with daily increments of 250 to 500 mg up to a total daily dose of 4 g, if necessary.

Dosage Form—*Capsules:* 250 mg.

Reserpine

Yohimban-16-carboxylic acid, (3β,16β,17α,18β,20α)-11,17-dimethoxy-18-[(3,4,5- trimethoxybenzoyl)oxy]-, methyl ester; (*Various Mfrs*)

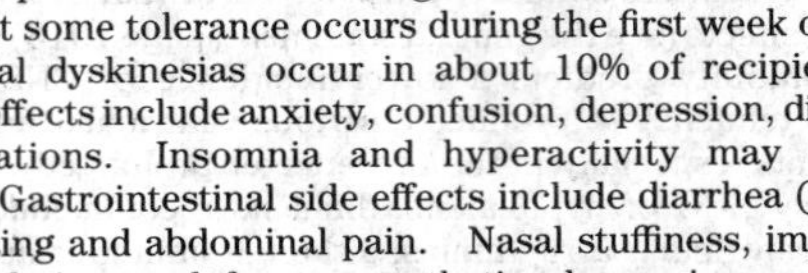

[50-55-5] $C_{33}H_{40}N_2O_9$ (608.69).

Reserpine, one of more than 20 alkaloids in *Rauwolfia serpentina,* was first isolated in pure crystalline form by Müller *et al*, (*Experientia 8*: 338, 1952). Subsequently it was found also in other species of *Rauwolfia*. A procedure for its separation is described in US Pat 2,833,771 (1958). Although it has been synthesized (Woodward *et al*, *J Am Chem Soc 78*: 2023, 1956) its production by this route is not economically feasible.

Description—White or pale-buff to slightly yellowish, odorless, crystalline powder; darkens slowly on exposure to light, but more rapidly when in solution; melts between 255 and 265° with decomposition.

Solubility—Insoluble in water; very slightly soluble in ether; 1 g in about 1800 mL alcohol or about 6 mL chloroform; slightly soluble in benzene; freely soluble in acetic acid.

Uses—The first rauwolfia alkaloid to be recognized officially, it was used first for the symptomatic management of patients with anxiety or tension psychoneuroses or chronic psychoses involving anxiety, psychomotor hyperactivity or compulsive aggressive behavior. Higher doses of the drug are required in the management of grossly disturbed psychoses than in anxiety-tension states. However, in both types of patients the drug must be administered for 1 or 2 wk before the optimal level of dosage can be determined. The tranquilizing effect of the drug makes the patient more cooperative, less destructive and more amenable to psychotherapy. Unless the dosage is adjusted carefully, the drug may induce a paradoxical form of anxiety and adverse reactive depression. In chronic psychoses, the drug does not appear to alter the basic psychopathological state. Because of the seriousness of side effects, it no longer is used much as an antianxiety or antipsychotic drug.

It still has a position in antihypertensive therapy. Because the doses used are considerably smaller than those for its tranquilizing effects, the drug may be used for its hypotensive effects with more safety than as a psychopharmacological drug. It exerts its antihypertensive effects through a partial depletion of the norepinephrine in the sympathetic postganglionic nerves. The effect is greater at the vascular smooth muscle than at the heart. Plasma renin activity is diminished. The drug is used chiefly in combination with thiazide diuretics for the management of mild *essential hypertension*. Its antihypertensive action derives from adrenergic neuronal blockade consequent to depletion of the catecholamine-containing granules of the postganglionic sympathetic neuron. The mechanism of the effects on the CNS is similar. It depletes both brain serotonin and catecholamines. It also is used to treat *Raynaud's phenomenon*.

The drug is absorbed poorly and erratically from the gastrointestinal tract, which causes considerable differences in efficacy of oral doses. It characteristically has a long latency of onset and a prolonged duration of action. For example, with daily oral administration the effects of the drug usually are not fully manifest for several days to 2 wk and may persist for as long as 4 wk after oral medication is discontinued. Tolerance to the drug does not develop with continued administration.

Nasal congestion, scleroconjunctival congestion, drowsiness, bradycardia, lacrimation, excessive salivation, nausea, vomiting, anorexia, weight gain and diarrhea are the most frequently noted side effects. Dry mouth, headache, dizziness, dysuria, myalgia and dull sensorium also occur. Suicidal depression is the most serious untoward effect. The drug may reactivate old peptic ulcers because it increases hydrochloric acid secretion by the stomach. Consequently, it should be used cautiously in patients with a history of peptic ulcer. Other serious reactions are orthostatic hypotension, fatigue, weakness, insomnia, nightmares, excitement, paradoxical anxiety, irrational behavior, parkinsonian rigidity (extrapyramidal syndrome), glaucoma, angina pectoris, dyspnea, deafness, uveitis, pruritus, rash, purpura, decreased libido, retrograde ejaculation, impotence, deafness and optic atrophy.

It is contraindicated in pregnancy and in nursing mothers because it is transmitted to the offspring. It also is contraindicated in ulcerative colitis because of the increase in bowel motility, biliary lithiasis, persons with suicidal tendencies or other mental depression and persons receiving electroconvulsive treatment. It should be used cautiously in combination with quinidine, because of the danger of heart block, cardiac arrest or arrhythmias. It may sensitize anesthetics and interfere with cardiovascular adjustments during surgery. It may decrease the response to indirect sympathomimetics.

Dose—*Oral, adult,* for *hypertension, initially* **0.05** to **0.2 mg** a day in 1 or 2 divided doses; when higher doses are used, the patient must be monitored continuously for mood depression; *children* (not recommended), for *hypertension,* **5** to **20 μg/kg** (or 150 to 600 μg/m²) a day, once or in 2 divided doses.

Dosage Forms—Tablets: 0.1, 0.25 and 1 mg.

Table 1—Other Rauwolfia Drugs

Drug	Description	Rel potency (Reserpine = 1)
Alseroxylon (Rauwiloid-*Riker*)	Fat soluble alkaloidal fraction from *R serpintina*	0.1
Deserpidine (Harmonyl-*Abbott*)	Alkaloid from *R canescens*	1.0
Rauwolfia serpentina	Dried root of *R serpentina*	0.002
Rescinnamine (Moderil-*Pfizer*)	Extracted from *R vomitoria* or synthesized from reserpine	1.0

CHAPTER 60

Antimuscarinic and Antispasmodic Drugs

Donald N Franz, PhD
Professor of Pharmacology
School of Medicine, University of Utah
Salt Lake City, UT 84132

Antimuscarinic Drugs

Cholinergic transmission occurs not only at the neuroeffectors innervated by the parasympathetic and certain sympathetic postganglionic nerves but also at all autonomic ganglia, the somatic neuromuscular junction and certain central synapses (see introductory statement, Chapter 43). *Antimuscarinic* drugs are competitive antagonists that act only on the cholinergic receptors at smooth muscle and secretory cells and certain central synapses. The term *cholinergic blocking drug* is used loosely by some as synonymous with antimuscarinic drug but it denotes any drug that can antagonize cholinergic stimuli at any cholinergic site, nicotinic or muscarinic. Other synonyms for the term antimuscarinic are *anticholinergic, cholinolytic, parasympatholytic* and *parasympathetic blocking drugs.* Since "cholinergic," ganglionic and neuromuscular blocking drugs have in common the antagonism of acetylcholine, it is to be expected that certain of these drugs may block at more than one kind of cholinergic receptor.

Actions and Selectivity—The effects of antimuscarinic drugs on the whole are predicted readily by considering the consequences of interruption of parasympathetic (and sympathetic cholinergic) nerve stimulation. Thus, the effects are decreased gastrointestinal motility, decreased gastric secretion, dry mouth, drying of the mucous membranes in general, mydriasis, loss of accommodation (with consequent tendency to increased intraocular pressure), urinary retention, decreased sweating and compensatory cutaneous flush, bronchial and biliary dilation, tachycardia (although effective block of the cardiac inhibitory nerves is difficult to achieve), etc. Some antimuscarinics have important actions in the central nervous system (see below).

There are considerable differences among the antimuscarinic drugs in the extent to which the various effects are elicited, and it now appears that there are at least three and possibly five types of muscarinic receptors, each with different structural requirements for blockade. Therefore, the selectivities (ie, profiles of activity and spectrum of efficacy) may differ considerably from drug to drug. For example, scopolamine has excellent mydriatic and cycloplegic activity yet cannot block cardiac vagal activity in nontoxic doses, whereas its derivative, methscopolamine, is the most efficacious drug for the antagonism of vagally mediated cardiac effects. Many structural features contribute to the different pharmacologic and therapeutic profiles of the antimuscarinic drugs, but the one of greatest importance is the amine function, the quaternary ammonium compounds differing in certain important respects from the secondary and tertiary amines.

Differences Between Tertiary and Quaternary Antimuscarinics—Tertiary (and secondary) amine antimuscarinic drugs can penetrate cell membranes in the nonionized form and, hence, can pass the blood-brain barrier. In the brain, they can exert both therapeutic and toxic actions. The quaternary ammonium antimuscarinic drugs do not pass the blood-brain barrier easily and, hence, usually lack prominent CNS actions. Similarly, the quaternary ammonium compounds poorly penetrate into the eye from the bloodstream or cornea and are less likely than the tertiary amine antimuscarinic drugs to cause mydriasis and cycloplegia. Most topical mydriatic antimuscarinic drugs are tertiary amines. Furthermore, the quaternary compounds usually are absorbed erratically and incompletely from the gut, in contrast to the tertiary amines.

The quaternary compounds have a greater affinity for nicotinic receptors, so that some degree of ganglionic blockade may result from therapeutic doses of some, but not all, quaternary ammonium antimuscarinic drugs. Some of the quaternary ammonium analogs also have a potential for neuromuscular paralysis, especially in drug interactions, in persons with myasthenia gravis or when taken in toxic doses.

The quaternary ammonium group seems to confer various degrees of selectivity for gastric secretory and, perhaps, other gastrointestinal functions. The extent to which ganglionic blockade may be involved is not known.

The quaternary ammonium antimuscarinic drugs are excreted mostly into the urine unchanged, whereas the secondary and tertiary members usually are biotransformed considerably in the liver.

Uses—In ophthalmology, antimuscarinic drugs are used topically to *dilate the pupil* (*cause mydriasis,* in order to facilitate visualization of the optic fundus) and to *paralyze accommodation* (*cause cycloplegia,* for refractive examination); some of these drugs (eg, eucatropine, homatropine) cannot effect a complete cycloplegia, so they are not all equivalent. Generally, short-acting topical antimuscarinic drugs (cyclopentolate, tropicamide, eucatropine, homatropine) are preferred for examination, so that interference with vision or intraocular tension will last for the shortest possible time. They are given in combination with phenylephrine to *promote maximal widening of the pupil* to allow greater surgical access and, after surgery, to *prevent adhesions* and, in alternation with miotics or with phenylephrine, to *break adhesions between the iris and lens* (synechiae). They also are used to treat *acute iritis, uveitis, iridiocyclitis* and *keratitis.* Paradoxically, these drugs may be used to treat *malignant* (ciliary block) glaucoma; in this, the rationale is that relaxation of the ciliary muscle helps to push the lens/diaphram posteriorly and reestablish an anterior direction of flow of intraocular fluid.

Antimuscarinic drugs, especially atropine, are used sometimes for *anesthetic premedication,* to *inhibit excessive salivary and bronchial* secretions and *prevent bronchospasm* and *laryngospasm.* The antisecretory effects also are sought in the treatment of *sialorrhea, acute coryza, hay fever* and *rhinitis;* proprietary "cold medicines" used to contain various belladonna alkaloids for this purpose, but the doses were mostly subliminal. The effects to antagonize parasympathetically mediated bronchospasm and bronchorrhea are employed also in the treatment of *bronchial asthma* and other chronic obstructive pulmonary diseases; given systemically, they are not as effective as certain sympathomimetic aerosols, but several antimuscarinic drugs when given as aerosols are as effective. When administered by inhalation, systemic effects are less frequent and sometimes negligible.

In cardiology and anesthesiology, antimuscarinic drugs are used to prevent or suppress *vagally mediated bradyarrhyth-*

mias (such as occur after coronary occlusion), *heart block* or *cardiac syncope* due to hyperactive carotid sinuses; in these, medical convention clings to atropine, which is less efficacious than methscopolamine (*not* scopolamine!)

In genitourinary practice, antimuscarinic drugs are used to relieve *urinary frequency and urgency*, to control *enuresis* in children and to relieve *ureteral colic* (often in combination with opiates). They also are used to control urinary incontinence.

In gastroenterology, antimuscarinic drugs are used sometimes for their gastrointestinal effects, although parasympathetic effects in the bowel are difficult to suppress completely. In the *irritable colon syndrome* ("spastic colon") they may provide some relief initially, but some refractoriness usually develops later. *Functional gastrointestinal disorders (functional diarrhea, spastic constipation, cardiospasm, pylorospasm, neurogenic colon, general hypermotility)* may respond as may mild to moderate irritative or infectious disorders, such as *mild diarrhea;* however, severe infectious dysenteries, regional enteritis and ulcerative colitis do not. *Acute enterocolitis, mucous colitis* and the *splenic flexure syndrome* may respond erratically. *Diverticulitis* sometimes may be improved. Antimuscarinic drugs may be used in combination with meperidine in the relief of *biliary dyskinesia.* In these uses, belladonna alkaloids commonly are employed; although they are less expensive than nonsolanaceous antimuscarinic drugs, they also cause more intense side effects than many synthetic, especially quaternary, ammonium, drugs. For gastrointestinal use, several antimuscarinic drugs are marketed in combination with barbiturates or other hypnotic-sedative drugs, a practice which deserves to be condemned.

Antimuscarinic drugs are used in the adjunctive *treatment of peptic ulcer.* Since they *retard gastric emptying*, the flood of acid to a duodenal ulcer is lessened, but a gastric ulcer will continue to be exposed to acid and, hence, not be benefited. However, any delay in gastric emptying will *help retain antacids* in the stomach, which should be beneficial if the appropriate regimen of antacids is used. Some gastroenterologists use antimuscarinic drugs only at bedtime, partly because nocturnal secretion presents a difficult treatment problem and partly because side effects during rest and sleep may be of less consequence to the patient than during the waking hours. With low doses of some antimuscarinic drugs side effects may be mild and tolerable even while awake.

Antimuscarinic drugs, especially those tertiary and quaternary drugs listed in Table 1, formerly were used extensively to *suppress gastric acid secretion* in peptic ulcer disease. Although the quaternary drugs were devoid of effects on the central nervous system, doses necessary to produce significant gastric acid secretion also produced significant peripheral side effects, which some patients could not tolerate and others suffered a reduced quality of life. The widespread side effects occur because these drugs not only block M_1-muscarinic receptors, which are responsible for stimulating gastric acid secretion, but they also block M_2-muscarinic receptors in the heart and some smooth muscles and M_3-muscarinic receptors in other smooth muscles (eg, sphincter muscle of the iris) and secretory glands. The relative selectivities of most antimuscarinic drugs for the receptor subtypes has not been determined. *Pirenzepine* (Gaotrozepine, *Boehringer Ingelheim*) is an antimuscarinic drug which is selective at M_1-receptors and effectively reduces acid secretion and promotes ulcer healing with a low incidence of antimuscarinic side effects. Although available in many countries, it is not yet approved in the US.

The high efficacy of the H_2-histamine antagonists such as cimetidine, which very effectively reduce gastric acid secretion with minimal side effects, has relegated the antimuscarinic drugs to adjunctive status for peptic ulcer. In addition, omeprazole (Prilosec, *MSD*), which blocks the ability of the acid secreting parietal cells in the stomach to secrete hydrogen ions, provides another highly effective treatment for gastrointestinal ulcers. Recent findings that recurrent ulcers are associated with the presence of *Helicobacter pylori* bacteria has added another strategy to prevent recurrence by appropriate antimicrobial drug therapy coadministered with an H_2-antagonist.

The secondary and tertiary amine antimuscarinic drugs may be used for their CNS actions. In the treatment of *parkinsonism,* they play a secondary role but are quite important in combinations with first-choice drugs (see page 1020). They may be of some occasional benefit in other *spastic and rigid conditions of cerebral origin.* They also are used to antidote muscarinic central nervous (and peripheral) toxicity in *anticholinesterase intoxication.* Scopolamine is highly effective against motion sickness and is sometimes used for its sedative and amnesic effects, but these effects are not typical of antimuscarinic drugs.

Other uses of antimuscarinic drugs include the treatment of *dysmenorrhea* (questionable efficacy), *hyperhidrosis* and treatment of poisoning by *Amanita muscaria.*

Adverse Effects—With nearly all antimuscarinic drugs, *dry mouth* is the first and dry skin is the second most common side effect. *Thirst* and *difficulty in swallowing* occur when the mouth and esophagus become sufficiently dry; chronic dry mouth also fosters dental *caries.* Suppression of sweating causes reflexive *flushing* and *heat intolerance* and can result in heat exhaustion or heat stroke in a hot environment; it also contributes to the hyperthermia seen in intoxication. *Mydriasis* frequently occurs, especially with secondary and tertiary compounds; *photophobia* and *blurring* of *vision* are consequences of mydriasis. With the secondary and tertiary amines, *cycloplegia* (which exacerbates blurred vision) occurs approximately concomitantly with mydriasis, but usually higher doses are required with many quaternary ammonium antimuscarinic drugs. In susceptible persons, especially the elderly, cycloplegia may contribute to an *elevation of intraocular pressure. Difficulty in urination* and *urinary retention* may occur, especially in elderly males with prostate enlargement. Tachycardia is a common side effect. *Constipation,* even *bowel stasis,* may occur. Antimuscarinic drugs relax the lower esophageal sphincter and, thus, promote gastroesophageal reflux, heartburn and reflux esophagitis. They are, therefore, contraindicated in these conditions.

In the larger therapeutic doses, the secondary and tertiary amine antimuscarinic drugs may cause *dizziness, restlessness, tremors, fatigue* and *locomotor difficulties.* Serious systemic intoxication can occur even from topical ophthalmologic application, especially in children, since both local absorption and nasolacrimal drainage into the gut can deliver considerable amounts to the circulation. In serious intoxication, *hyperpyrexia, flushing, nausea, vomiting, drowsiness, disorientation, stupor, hallucinations, leukocytosis,* nonallergic *rashes, circulatory* or *respiratory collapse* and even *death,* in addition to all aforenamed effects, may occur. Children, especially infants and children with Down's syndrome, spastic paralysis or brain damage, are more sensitive than adults to the toxic effects. Blondes and people with light irides also are reputed to be more sensitive.

When barbiturates are included in an antimuscarinic product, adverse effects of the barbiturates must be anticipated and the possibility that chronic use will lead to dependence must be considered.

The quaternary ammonium drugs mostly have a low CNS component of toxicity but instead may cause *orthostatic hypotension* (from ganglionic blockade) and *neuromuscular paralysis.*

Hypersensitivity with a variety of manifestations, usually *rash,* may follow the use of any antimuscarinic drug, but it is more common with the solanaceous alkaloids.

Drug Interactions—Other drugs, such as phenothiazines, tricyclic antidepressants, certain antihistamines, meperidine, etc, which have significant antimuscarinic activity, may intensify considerably the effects of antimuscarinic drugs. Drugs with neuromuscular paralysant activity (neuromuscular blocking drugs, aminoglycosides, polymyxin, etc) and ganglionic blocking drugs will summate with quaternary ammonium antimuscarinic drugs. Aluminum- and magnesium trisilicate-containing antacids have been shown to decrease the absorption of some antimuscarinic drugs and may possibly do so with all of them.

Precautions—If there is mydriasis and photophobia, *dark glasses* should be worn. The patient also should be warned that *driving* or *other vision-dependent capabilities* may be impaired. Appropriate dosage precautions must be taken with *infants, children* and *persons with Down's syndrome, brain damage, spasticity* or *light irides*. Elevated intraocular pressure, urinary difficulty and retention and constipation are more probable in *elderly persons*. Men with *prostatic hypertrophy*, especially, should be monitored for urinary function. Antimuscarinics should be used cautiously in *toxic megacolon*. Because of the tachycardic effects of the drugs, care must be exercised when *tachycardia*, other *tachyarrhythmias, coronary heart disease, congestive heart disease* or *hyperthyroidism* preexist. Persons with *hypertension* may experience both exaggerated orthostatic hypotension and tachycardia. Similarly, *autonomic neuropathy* requires caution. Persons with a history of *allergies* or *bronchial asthma* will show a higher than normal incidence of hypersensitivity reactions. Quaternary ammonium antimuscarinic drugs, especially, may cause neuromuscular paralysis (with fatal respiratory arrest) in persons with *myasthenia gravis*. Although these drugs sometimes are used in the treatment of *adhesions between lens and iris*, damage can occur and expert precautions must be taken. When solutions of antimuscarinic drugs are applied topically to the eye, pressure should be applied just below the internal canthus of the eye to prevent nasolacrimal drainage.

Precautions are appropriate in *ulcerative colitis*. In *hiatus hernia* or *gastroesophageal reflux*, reflux and esophagitis are exacerbated by antimuscarinic drugs, because the lower esophageal sphincter is stimulated by cholinergic nerves. In a *hot environment*, the user is more susceptible to disruption of heat regulation. *Hepatic disease* for some and *renal disease* for other antimuscarinic drugs may decrease the rate of elimination. Cognizance should be taken of possible *drug interactions*. Lastly, until proven otherwise, it must be assumed that all antimuscarinic drugs can pass the placental barrier; the threat to the fetus *in utero* is unknown, but an infant born with an effective amount of drug aboard may have gastrointestinal difficulties and problems in early nutrition.

Contraindications—An antimuscarinic drug generally is contraindicated in *narrow-angle glaucoma, pyloric* or *intestinal* obstruction, *intestinal atony* of the elderly, *paralytic ileus, achalasia of the esophagus*, frank *bladder neck obstruction* or where there is *hypersensitivity* to the drug or a closely related one. There are specific exceptions according to the route employed and the degree of selectivity (profile of activity) of the drug used.

Anisotropine Methylbromide—see Table 1.

Atropine Sulfate

Benzeneacetic acid, *endo*-(±)-α-(hydroxymethyl)-, 8-methyl-8-azabicyclo[3.2.1]-oct-3-yl ester, sulfate (2:1) (salt), monohydrate

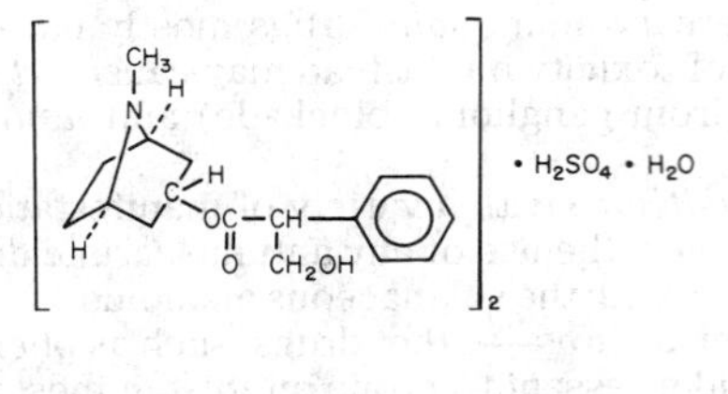

1αH,5αH-Tropan-3α-ol (±)-tropate (ester) sulfate (2:1) (salt) monohydrate [5908-99-6] $(C_{17}H_{23}NO_3)_2.H_2SO_4.H_2O$ (694.82); *anhydrous* [55-48-1] (676.82).

Caution—Atropine Sulfate is very poisonous.

Preparation—Atropine is dissolved in warm acetone, sufficient dilute sulfuric acid is added to form the 2:1 sulfate, and atropine sulfate is crystallized from the solution.

Description—Colorless crystals or a white, crystalline powder; odorless; effloresces in dry air; slowly affected by light; when previously dried at 120° for 4 hr, it melts not lower than 187°.

Solubility—1 g in 0.4 mL water, 5 mL alcohol or about 2.5 mL glycerin.

Uses—Atropine is a tertiary amine antimuscarinic drug with all of the actions, most uses and adverse effects described in the general statement at the beginning of this chapter. The antimuscarinic activity mostly resides in the *l*-isomer (*l*-hyoscyamine). By historical precedence, it has become the prototype and most widely used of antimuscarinic drugs, although in most respects it no longer deserves the special status it continues to enjoy.

Because atropine is obtained from species of *belladonna*, the word atropine often has been used as synonymous with belladonna. Actually, several genera of *Solanaceae* produce atropine and related alkaloids, so that atropine and other related natural or semisynthetic congeners are sometimes called *solanaceous* alkaloids.

Atropine is absorbed rapidly and completely from the gut and is distributed rapidly throughout the body. Following topical application it penetrates readily into the eye. It produces prolonged mydriasis and cycloplegia for more than 1 wk. It is metabolized, mainly, in the liver. The plasma half-life of *l*-hyoscyamine is less than 4 hr. The half-life in the eye is long, and effects may last for 7 to 12 days after topical application to the eye. Intraocular inflammation, however, greatly shortens the half-life in the eye.

Dose—*Oral, adult, various antimuscarinic effects*, **0.3** to **1.2 mg** every 4 to 6 hr; *antiparkinsonism*, **0.1** to **0.25 mg** 4 times a day; *preanesthetic medication*, **2 mg** 1 hr before surgery; *children, general antimuscarinic use*, **0.01 mg/kg**, not to exceed 0.4 mg, *or* **0.3 mg/m²** every 4 to 6 hr; *maintenance* in *organophosphate anticholinesterase poisoning*, **1** to **2 mg** every 4 to 6 hr. *Intramuscular, adult, antispasmodic* and *general antimuscarinic*, **0.4** to **0.6 mg** every 4 to 6 hr; *gastrointestinal radiography*, **1 mg**; *preanesthetic medication*, **0.2** to **0.6 mg** ½ to 1 hr before surgery; *muscarine (Amanita muscaria) poisoning*, **1** to **2 mg** every hr until salivation and tracheobronchial secretions abate or atropine toxicity supravenes; *moderate anticholinesterase poisoning, initially* **2** to **4 mg**, then **1** to **2 mg** every 20 to 30 min until salivation, tracheobronchial secretions and cyanosis subside or atropine toxicity supravenes, repeated as muscarinic signs reappear, finally switching to oral maintenance when the condition of the patient has stabilized (see *oral*, above); *children, organophosphate anticholinesterase poisoning, initially* **1 mg**, then **0.5** to **1 mg** every 5 to 10 min until secretions and cyanosis abate or atropine toxicity supravenes. *Intravenous, adult, various antimuscarinic uses*, **0.4** to **0.6 mg** every 4 to 6 hr; *bradydysrhythmias*, **0.4** to **1 mg** every 1 to 2 hr, as needed; *corrective to muscarinic effects of therapeutic anticholinesterases* (eg neostigmine), **0.6** to **1.2 mg** a few min before or along with the anticholinesterase (separate syringes); *muscarine (Amanita) poisoning, same as intramuscular*, above; *organophosphate anticholinesterase poisoning, initially* **2** to **4 mg** in *severe* and **1** to **2 mg** in *moderate poisoning*, then **2 mg** repeated every 5 to 10 min in *severe poisoning* and **1** to **2 mg** every 20 to 30 min in *moderate poisoning* until salivation, tracheobronchial secretions and cyanosis abate or atropine toxicity supravenes, switching to oral maintenance (see *oral*, above) when the condition stabilizes; *children, bradydysrhythmias*, **0.01** to **0.03 mg/kg**, as needed; *anticholinesterase poisoning*, same as *intramuscular*, above. *Subcutaneous, adult, various antimuscarinic uses*, **0.4** to **0.6 mg** every 4 to 6 hr; *children, various antimuscarinic uses*, **0.01 mg/kg**, not to exceed 0.4 mg, *or* **0.3 mg/m²** every 4 to 6 hr; *preanesthetic medication* or *prophylaxis of bradydysrhythmias* from succinylcholine or surgical procedures, **0.1, 0.2, 0.3, 0.4, 0.5** and **0.6 mg**, respectively, for children weighing up to 3 kg, 7 to 9 kg, 12 to 16 kg, 20 to 27 kg, 32 kg and 41 kg. *Oral inhalation*, by *nebulizer*, *prophylaxis of bronchospasm*, **0.25 mg/kg** for *adults* and **0.05 mg/kg** for *children*, diluted in 3 to 5 mL of isotonic NaCl solution, 3 or 4 times a day. *Topical*, into conjunctival sac, *adult*, for *uveitis*, **0.3** to **0.5 cm** of **1%** ointment *or* **1 drop** of **1%** solution 1 to 3 times a day; *preoperative mydriasis*, **1 drop** of **1%** solution followed by 1 drop of 2.5 or 10% solution of phenylephrine just prior to surgery; *postoperative mydriasis*, **1 drop** of **1** or **2%** solution 1 to 3 times a day; to *break posterior synechiae*, **1 drop** of **1** or **2%** solution followed in 5 min by 1 drop of 2.5 or 10% phenylephrine solution, the procedure repeated after 5 min and again for a total of 3 applications; *malignant* (ciliary block) *glaucoma, initially* **1 drop** of **1** or **2%** solution followed by 1 drop of 2.5 or 10% phenylephrine solution 3 or 4 times a day until intraocular tension falls to an acceptable value, then, for *maintenance*, **1 drop** of **1%** solution once a day or every other day; *children, cycloplegic refraction*, **0.3 cm** of **0.5%** ointment 3 times a day for 1 to 3 days before examination for *children with blue irides under 2 yr* and **2%** *for children with dark irides under 2 yr* and *all children over 2 yr or* **1 drop** of **0.125, 0.25, 0.5** or **1%**, respectively, for *infants under 1 yr, children 1 to 5 yr, over 5 yr* *and having blue irides*, and *over 5 yr and having dark irides; unveitis*, **1 drop** of **0.125** to **1%** solution 1 to 3 times a day; *postoperative mydriasis*, **1 drop** of **0.5%** solution 1 to 3 times a day or as needed; ointments are preferred for children, because intoxication is less likely than with solutions.

Dosage Forms—Inhalation Solution: 0.2 and 0.5%. Injection: 0.8 mg/0.5 mL; 0.3, 0.4, 0.5 and 1.2 mg/1 mL; 0.25, 0.5 and 2.5 mg/5 mL; 1, 4 and 10 mg/10 mL; 8 mg/20 mL; 15 mg/30 mL. Ophthalmic Ointment: 0.5 and 1%. Ophthalmic Solution: 0.5, 1, 2 and 3%. Tablets: 0.4 and 0.6 mg.

Atropine Sulfate and Diphenoxylate Hydrochloride Tablets—page 901.

Belladonna

Deadly Nightshade Leaf; Belladonna Herb; Black Cherry Leaf; Dwale; Dwayberry Leaf

The dried leaf and flowering or fruiting top of *Atropa belladonna* Linné or of its variety *acuminata* Royle ex Lindley (Fam *Solanaceae*); it yields not less than 0.35% of the alkaloids of Belladonna Leaf USP.

Uses—Its actions are those of its principal alkaloids, hyoscyamine and atropine (see the general statement). It is used to decrease gastrointestinal activity in functional bowel disorders, to delay gastric emptying, and supposedly to decrease gastric secretion, which it cannot do in tolerated doses. It also is used in the treatment of nocturnal enuresis and dysmenorrhea. In all of these uses it is among the least selective of antimuscarinic drugs, and its wide use derives from historical precedence and habit rather than from therapeutic superiority. It is included in a number of fixed-dose combinations, which may contain components of doubtful or unproven value and, in some, actually may entail hazard. Nonprescription combinations containing belladonna usually have a content too small for substantial activity. The belladonna alkaloid content of the extract and tincture are much different, and doses are expressed in mg and mL rather than as the alkaloid equivalents. One mg of extract contains 12.5 μg of alkaloids. One mL of tincture contains 0.3 mg (300 μg) of alkaloids.

Dose—Of *extract, oral, adult,* **15 mg** 3 or 4 times a day ½ to 1 hr before meals and at bedtime, with dosage adjustment as needed; 15 mg is equivalent to 0.2 mg of atropine. Of *tincture, oral, adult,* **0.6** to **1 mL** 3 or 4 times a day, ½ to 1 hr before meals and at bedtime, with dosage adjustment as needed; *children,* **0.03 mL/kg** (0.8 mL/m^2) 3 times a day.

Dosage Forms—Extract: 15 mg; Tablets: 15 mg; Tincture: 30 mg/100 mL.

Levorotatory Alkaloids of Belladonna

A synthetic mixture of the pure salts of the levorotatory alkaloids found in belladonna. The ratio of the salts is such that a single dose contains the approximate amount of each of the following: scopolamine hydrobromide, 0.006 mg; atropine sulfate, 0.02 mg and hyoscyamine sulfate, 0.1 mg.

Uses—Since the antimuscarinic activity of belladonna is only in the levorotatory isomers, the actions, uses and adverse effects of the levorotatory alkaloids are the same as those of *Belladonna*, above. Only the dose and dosage forms are different.

Dose—*Oral, adult,* **0.25** to **0.5 mg** 3 times day; *children over 6 yr,* **0.125** to **0.25 mg** 3 times a day. *Subcutaneous, adult,* **0.25** to **0.5 mg,** 1 or 2 times a day.

Dosage Forms—Tablets: 0.25 mg.

Benztropine Mesylate—page 1035.

Biperiden—page 1035.

Chlorphenoxamine Hydrochloride—see RPS-17, page 931.

Clidinium Bromide—see Table 1 and RPS-18, page 910.

Cyclopentolate Hydrochloride

Benzeneacetic acid, α-(1-hydroxycyclopentyl)-, 2-(dimethylamino)ethyl ester, hydrochloride; AK-Pentolate (*Akorn*); Cyclogyl (*Alcon*)

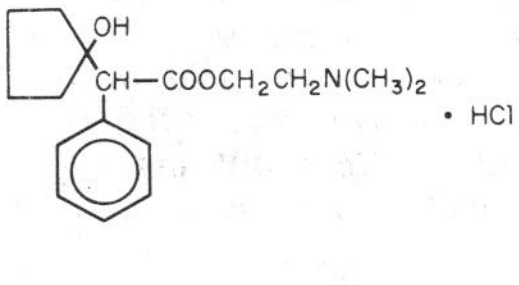

OH
CH—$COOCH_2CH_2N(CH_3)_2$ · HCl

2-(Dimethylamino)ethyl 1-hydroxy-α-phenylcyclopentaneacetate hydrochloride [5870-29-1] $C_{17}H_{25}NO_3$.HCl (327.85).

Preparation—The acid moiety of the ester, 1-hydroxy-α-phenylcyclopentaneacetic acid (I), may be prepared by adding sodium phenylacetate to an ethereal solution of isopropyl magnesium bromide; treatment of the resulting sodium phenylacetate magnesium bromide with an ethereal solution of cyclopentanone produces a Grignard addition product that on hydrolysis yields I. The ester is produced by metathesis between the sodium salt of I and 2-dimethylaminoethyl chloride in isopropyl alcohol. After crystallization from acetone, the ester is converted to the hydrochloride with HCl.

Description—White, crystalline powder, which on standing develops a characteristic odor; melts between 137 and 141°; pH (1 in 100 solution) between 4.5 and 5.5.

Solubility—Very soluble in water; freely soluble in alcohol; insoluble in ether.

Uses—An *antimuscarinic* drug used primarily for its *ophthalmologic* actions (see page 1020). After application to the cornea, cyclopegia is complete in 25 to 75 min; recovery is complete in 6 to 24 hr. The side effects and CNS toxicity are those of antimuscarinic drugs (page 1020) but the duration of the effects is very short.

Dose—*Topical, into the conjunctival sac, adult,* for *mydriatic ophthalmoscopy* or *cycloplegic refraction,* **1 drop** of a **1** or **2%** solution, repeated once in 5 min; a 2% solution is recommended when the irides are dark; for *uveitis,* **1 drop** of a **0.5** or **1%** solution 3 or 4 times a day. In *neonates* and *premature* and *small infants,* for *mydriatic ophthalmoscopy* or *cycloplegic refraction,* **1 drop** of a **0.5%** solution once only. *Older infants* and *children,* for *mydriatic ophthalmoscopy,* **1 drop** of **0.5** or **1%** solution once only; for *cycloplegic refraction,* **1 drop** of a **1** or **2%** solution, repeated in 5 min; for *uveitis,* **1 drop** of a **0.5** or **1%** solution 3 or 4 times a day. When phenylephrine is combined with cyclopentolate, a 0.2% concentration of the latter suffices for mydriatic ophthalmoscopy in all patients.

Dosage Form—Ophthalmic Solution: 0.5, 1 and 2%.

Dicyclomine Hydrochloride—see Table 1 and RPS-18, page 911.

Glycopyrrolate—see Table 1 and RPS-18, page 911.

Hexocyclium Methylsulfate—see Table 1 and RPS-18, page 914.

Homatropine Hydrobromide

Benzeneacetic acid, (±)-α-hydroxy-, endo-8-methyl-8-azabicyclo[3.2.1]oct-3-yl ester hydrobromide

1αH,5αH-Tropan-3α-ol mandelate (ester) hydrobromide [51-56-9] $C_{16}H_{21}NO_3$.HBr (356.26); the hydrobromide of tropine mandelate. For the structural formula, see page 403.

Preparation—By heating *tropine* with *mandelic acid* in the presence of hydrochloric acid; ammonia is added and the homatropine that is liberated is extracted with chloroform; the solution is evaporated, hydrobromic acid is added and the homatropine hydrobromide is crystallized.

Description—White crystals, or a white crystalline powder; affected by light; melts between 214 and 217° with slight decomposition; aqueous solution is practically neutral or only faintly acid to litmus.

Solubility—1 g in 6 mL water, 40 mL alcohol or about 420 mL chloroform; insoluble in ether.

Uses—Used only for its effects in the eye (see page 1020). It is preferred to atropine, because its effects are shorter in duration (0.5 to 2 days) and there is no protracted cycloplegia. It often is combined with sympathomimetics in ophthalmologic practice. Its systemic toxicity is considerably less than that of atropine, but rare systemic intoxication can occur from conjunctival instillation, especially in children.

Dose—*Topical,* to the conjunctiva, *adult,* for *cycloplegic refraction,* **1 drop** of a **2** or **5%** solution, repeated in 5 to 10 min, if necessary for 2 to 5 doses prior to examination; for *uveitis,* **1 drop** of a **2** or **5%** solution 2 or 3 times a day; *children* use **1** or **2%** solution in lieu of adult concentrations.

Dosage Form—Ophthalmic Solution: 2 and 5%.

Hyoscyamine Sulfate

Benzeneacetic acid, α-(hydroxymethyl)-, [3(*S*)-*endo*]-8-methyl-8-azabicyclo[3.2.1]oct-3-yl ester, sulfate (2:1), dihydrate; Cystospaz (*Alcon*); (*Various mfrs*)

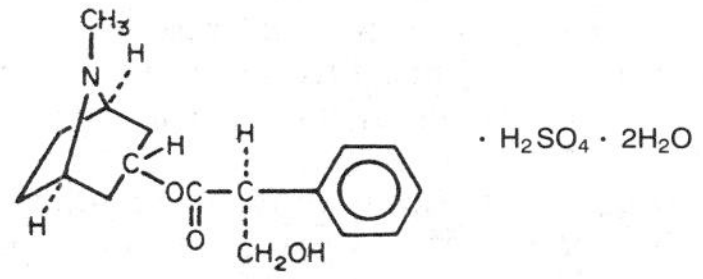

CH_3 N H H OC—C CH₂OH · H_2SO_4 · $2H_2O$

[6835-16-1] $(C_{17}H_{23}NO_3)_2.H_2SO_4.2H_2O$ (712.85); *anhydrous* [620-61-1] (676.82). The sulfate of an alkaloid usually obtained from species of *Hyoscyamus* Linné or other genera of Fam *Solanaceae*. For the structural formula of hyoscyamine, see page 403.

Caution—Hyoscyamine Sulfate is extremely poisonous.

Preparation—Isolated from the alkaloids of belladonna by resolution of atropine.

Description—White, odorless crystals or a crystalline powder; deliquescent; affected by light; when previously dried at 105° for 4 hr, does not melt below 200°; pH (1 in 100 solution) about 5.3.

Solubility—1 g in 0.5 mL water or 5 mL alcohol; practically insoluble in ether.

Uses—Hyoscyamine is the levorotatory isomer of the racemic mixture known as atropine, and therefore ½ of atropine is hyoscyamine. Since the dextrorotatory isomer is nearly inactive, the potency of hyoscyamine is approximately twice that of atropine. The actions, uses and toxicity are the same as those of antimuscarinic drugs in general (see page 1020), except that hyoscyamine has not been used for ophthalmologic purposes and is of little use to suppress gastric secretion. In fact, its use mainly has been confined to that of an *antispasmodic* although it is sometimes used in rhinitis, cystitis and parkinsonism. Hyoscyamine is marketed as the hydrobromide and sulfate salts. The hydrobromide is not marketed as a single-entity preparation but rather in a number of combinations, most of which have dubious rationales and efficacies.

Dose—*Oral, adult, general antimuscarinic effects,* in *tablet* form, **0.125** to **0.5 mg** 3 or 4 times a day before meals and at bedtime, *or,* in *oral solution* form, **0.125** to **0.25 mg** every 6 hr, *or,* in *extended-release* form, **0.375 mg** twice a day, in the morning and at bedtime; *children,* in *elixir* or *oral solution* form, **0.0125, 0.0156, 0.0188, 0.025, 0.0313, 0.063, 0.094** to **0.125** and **0.125** to **0.187 mg,** respectively, for children weighing 2.3 to 3.3, 3.4 to 4.4, 4.5 to 6.7, 6.8 to 9, 9.1 to 13.5, 13.6 to 22.6, 22.7 to 33 and 34 to 36 kg every 4 hr. *Intramuscular, intravenous* or *subcutaneous, adult, general antimuscarinic effects,* **0.25** to **0.5 mg** every 4 to 6 hr; *preanesthetic medication,* **0.005 mg/kg** *or* **0.5 mg** ½ to 1 hr before induction; *gastrointestinal radiography,* **0.25** to **0.5 mg** 5 to 10 min before radiography; *bradydysrhythmias* (intravenous only), **0.125 mg,** repeated as needed; *corrective* for muscarinic effects of anticholinesterases (intravenous only), **0.2 mg** for each mg of neostigmine equivalent; *children over 2 yr, preanesthetic medication,* **0.005 mg/kg** ½ to 1 hr before induction.

Dosage Forms—Timed-Release Capsules: 0.375 mg; Elixir: 0.125 mg/5 mL; Injection: 0.5 mg/1 mL and 5 mg/10 mL; Solution: 0.125 mg/mL. Tablets: 0.125 and 0.15 mg.

Ipratropium Bromide

(±)-(*endo, syn*)-8-Azaniabicyclo[3.2.1]octane,
3-(3-hydroxy-1-oxo-2-phenylpropoxy)-8-methyl-8-(1-methylethyl)-,
bromide monhydrate; Atrovent (*Boehringer Ingelheim*)

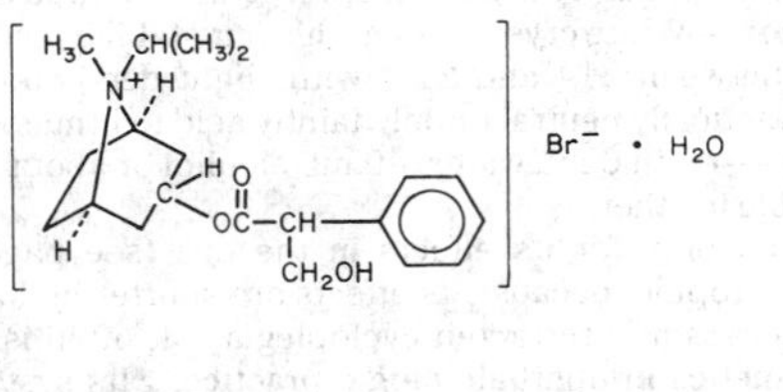

(8*r*)-3α-Hydroxy-8-isopropyl-1αH,5αH-tropanium bromide (±)-tropate monohydrate [66985-17-9]; anhydrous [22254-24-6] $C_{20}H_{30}BrNO_3.H_2O$ (430.38)].

Preparation—Atropine is quaternized with isopropyl bromide.

Description—White, crystalline substance with a bitter taste.

Solubility—Freely soluble in water or alcohol; insoluble in chloroform or ether.

Uses—A quaternary ammonium antimuscarinic drug (page 1020) used for the treatment of *bronchial asthma* and *chronic obstructive pulmonary disease,* for which it is given as an inhalant aerosol. It appears to be approximately equivalent to β_2-agonists in its efficacy against bronchial asthma, but the duration of action is longer. It appears to be more effective than β_2-agonists against chronic obstructive pulmonary disease. It seems to act mainly on the larger airways.

By inhalation, the incidence and severity of side effects is low, the most common effects being dry mouth, irritation in the throat, cough and unpleasant taste. Other effects are quite rare and include blurring of vision, drowsiness, dizziness, mild *brady*cardia and airway obstruction caused by sputum made viscous by diminished tracheobronchial secretions.

By inhalation, ipratropium causes bronchodilatation in doses 1:1000 those of oral or intravenous doses, which avoids most systemic side effects. Bronchodilatation occurs within a few minutes, peaks at 1 to 2 hr and lasts 4 to 8 hr. About half the dose is eliminated in the feces. The half-life is 3 to 4 hr.

Dose—*Inhalation, adult* and *children over 12 yr,* **1** or **2 inhalations** (0.02 or 0.04 mg) 3 or 4 times a day at intervals no shorter than 4 hr; some patients initially may require up to 0.08 mg.

Dosage Form—Metered-dose inhaler; each 14 g inhaler provides 200 doses of 18 µg of drug.

Methscopolamine Bromide—see Table 1 and RPS-18, page 912.

Isopropamide Iodide—see Table 1 and RPS-18, page 914.

Mepenzolate Bromide—see Table 1and RPS-18, page 914.

Methantheline Bromide—see Table 1 and RPS-18, page 914.

Orphenadrine Citrate—see page 1034.

Oxyphencyclimine Hydrochloride—see Table 1, page 1025 and RPS-18, page 912.

Oxyphenonium Bromide—see RPS-18, page 915.

Procyclidine Hydrochloride—page 1038.

Propantheline Bromide—see Table 1 and RPS-18, page 915.

Scopolamine Hydrobromide

Benzeneacetic acid, [7(*S*)-(1α,2β,4β,5α,7β)]-α-(hydroxymethyl)-,
9-methyl-3-oxa-9-azatricy-clo[3.3.1.0^{2,4}]non-7-yl ester,
hydrobromide, trihydrate; Transderm-Scōp (*Ciba*)

6β,7β-Epoxy-1αH,5αH-tropan-3α-ol (−)-tropate (ester) hydrobromide trihydrate [6533-68-2] $C_{17}H_{21}NO_4.HBr.3H_2O$ (438.31); *anhydrous* [114-49-8] (384.27). For the structural formula of scopolamine see page 403.

Preparation—Scopolamine, an alkaloid occurring in several solanaceous plants, may be obtained from such plants by alkaloid extraction procedures followed by fractionation of the extract to remove other alkaloids, notably hyoscyamine.

Description—Colorless or white crystals or white, granular powder; odorless; slightly efflorescent in dry air; the anhydrous salt melts between 195 and 199°; pH (1 in 10 solution) between 4.0 and 5.5.

Solubility—1 g in 1.5 mL water or 20 mL alcohol; slightly soluble in chloroform; insoluble in ether.

Uses—Differs from other antimuscarinic drugs in that in therapeutic doses it is a sedative and tranquilizing depressant to the central nervous system. In its peripheral actions, it differs from atropine in that it is a stronger blocking agent for the iris, ciliary body and salivary, bronchial and sweat glands but is weaker in its action on the heart (in which it is incapable of exerting actions in tolerated doses), the intestinal tract and bronchial musculature.

Frequently, it is given as a *preanesthetic medicament* for both its sedative-tranquilizing and antisecretory actions. It is effective as a prophylactic against *motion sickness,* for which slow-release transdermal dosage forms have been devised. It also is used sometimes in other types of *vertigo.* It occasionally is used to suppress *delirium.* It is used as an *amnesic* agent in *obstetrics* (combined with morphine it was used formerly to produce "twilight sleep"). As a *mydriatic* and *cycloplegic,* it has a somewhat shorter duration (3 to 7 days) and intraocular pressure is affected less markedly than with atropine.

Except for drowsiness, its side effects are those of tertiary amine antimuscarinic drugs (see page 1020). Occasionally, with therapeutic doses a patient may experience excitement, restlessness, hallucinations, delirium or disorientation, confusion, memory loss, stupor and, rarely, coma. Infants and young children are quite susceptible to the CNS toxicity. After a transdermal system has been in use for 3 or more days, removal sometimes causes a withdrawal syndrome consisting of dizziness, disequilibrium, nausea, vomiting and headache. Rarely there may be hypersensitivity, characterized by edema of the uvula, glottis and lips. The toxic effects of overdoses, precautions and contraindications are like those of tertiary amine antimuscarinic drugs.

Dose—*Oral, adult, motion sickness* and *vertigo,* **0.25** to **0.8 mg** 1 hr before departure, then 3 times a day or as needed or tolerated; *children,* to be determined by a physician. *Intramuscular, intravenous* or *subcutaneous, adults* and *children over 12 yr, preanesthetic medication* (usually intramuscular), **0.2** to **0.6 mg** ½ hr before induction; *sedation/hypnosis,* **0.6 mg** 3 times a day; to *cause amnesia* (in combination with an opioid), **0.32** to **0.65 mg**; *antiemetic,* **0.3** to **0.6 mg**; *children, general antimuscarinic* or *antiemetic,* **0.006 mg/kg** or **0.2 mg/m²**; *preanesthetic medication* (usually intramuscular), **0.1, 0.15, 0.2** and **0.3 mg,** respectively, for children of 4 to 7 mo, 7 mo to 3 yr, 3 to 8 yr and 8 to 12 yr. *Topical, transdermal, adult,* to the *postauricular* skin, for *motion sickness,* **1 system,** to deliver **0.5 mg over 3 days,** to be attached at least

4 hr before effect is required. *Topical*, into *conjunctival* sac, *adult*, *cycloplegic refraction*, **1** to **2 drops** of **0.25%** solution 1 hr before refraction; *mydriatic*, **1 drop** of **0.25%** as needed for diagnosis and once a day for postoperative mydriasis; *preoperative* (to prevent posterior synechiae), **1 drop** of **0.25%** solution 1 or 2 times a day as needed; to *break posterior synechiae*, **1 drop** of **0.25%** solution every min for 5 min (usually along with phenylephrine); *iridiocyclitis*, **1 drop** of **0.25%** solution 1 to 4 times a day, tapered off as inflammation abates; *uveitis*, **1 drop** of **0.25%** solution twice 1 to 3 times a day; *children, cycloplegic refraction*, **1 drop** of **0.25%** solution twice a day for 2 days before refraction; *all other ophthalmologic uses*, see adult dose, *except* that the physician should consider individualization of dose according to age, size and need.

Dosage Forms—Capsules: 0.25 mg. Injection: 0.2 and 0.43 mg/0.5 mL and 0.3, 0.4, 0.5, 0.6 and 1 mg/1 mL. Ophthalmic Solution: 0.25 and 0.3%. Transdermal Therapeutic System: 1.5 mg (delivers 0.5 mg over 3 days).

Tridihexethyl Chloride—see Table 1 and RPS-18, page 927.

Trihexyphenidyl Hydrochloride—page 1038.

Tropicamide

Benzeneacetamide, *N*-ethyl-α-(hydroxymethyl)-*N*-(4-pyridinylmethyl)-, Mydriacyl (*Alcon*)

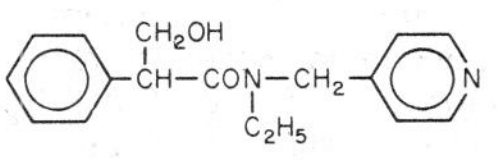

N-Ethyl-2-phenyl-*N*-(4-pyridylmethyl)hydracrylamide [1508-75-4] $C_{17}H_{20}N_2O_2$ (284.36).

Preparation—Tropic acid is esterified with acetyl chloride and the resulting tropic acid acetate is converted to the corresponding acid chloride by reaction with thionyl chloride. Condensation of the acid chloride with 4-[(ethylamino)methyl]pyridine in the presence of an appropriate dehydrochlorinating agent yields the tropicamide acetate ester which saponifies readily to tropicamide. US Pat 2,726,245.

Description—White or practically white, crystalline powder; odorless, or has not more than a slight odor; melts between 96 and 100°.

Solubility—1 g in 500 mL water or 3 mL chloroform; freely soluble in alcohol or solutions of strong acids.

Uses—An *antimuscarinic* drug that is used to induce *mydriasis* and *cycloplegia* in ophthalmologic practice. Applied topically to the eye it has short duration of action. The time to a maximal effect is usually 20 to 25 min. The duration of maximal effect is only about 15 to 20 min, but full recovery requires 5 to 6 hr. However, photophobia and other subjective indices of an effect may disappear as early as 2 hr after application. The drug, thus, has an obvious advantage over belladonna alkaloids in its shorter duration of action and, over homatropine, in its ability to induce cycloplegia. It is disadvantageous in that the ophthalmologist must time the examination to coincide with the time of maximal effect and has a brief time for examination or else it is necessary to repeat administration at 30-min intervals in order to obviate the timing problem.

Although tropicamide does not increase intraocular pressure in normal persons, it may do so in patients with glaucoma or those who have certain structural deformities of the anterior chamber of the eye. It should, thus, be used cautiously in such patients. If an antimuscarinic drug must be employed in such patients, tropicamide is indicated because of its brief duration of action.

Side effects can occur from passage of solutions through the nasolacrimal duct and subsequent absorption. Dry mouth and tachycardia have occurred. Although intoxication in children has not been reported, it must be kept in mind. Tropicamide usually stings transiently when applied.

Dose—*Topical*, to the conjunctiva, *adult*, for *cycloplegic refraction*, **1** or **2 drops** of a **0.1%** solution, repeated in 5 min; for *ophthalmoscopy*, **1** or **2 drops** of a **0.5%** solution 15 to 20 min prior to examination. *Children*, **1 drop** of a **0.5** or **1%** solution repeated in 5 min.

Dosage Form—Ophthalmic Solution: 0.5 and 1%.

Antispasmodic Drugs

Spasm may result from a local disorder, in which cellular injury initiates the contractile process, local hormones or other excitatory or irritant substances are released (or local reflexes are activated) or it may be the result of hyperactivity in efferent excitatory autonomic nerves or electrolyte disturbances that favor increased neuronal and muscular activity. Therefore, according to the locus, cause and mediators of a spastic condition, one or more of a number of classes of selective drugs may be employed, eg, neuromuscular blocking or centrally acting muscle relaxants for various spastic conditions of skeletal muscle, local anesthetics for some localized neurally mediated spasm, α-adrenoreceptor blocking drugs or β_2-adrenoreceptor agonists for vasospasm, β_2-agonists for bronchial and uterine spasms, antimuscarinic drugs for ciliary spasm or spastic bowel, calcium for hypocalcemic tetany,

Table 1—Antimuscarinic Drugs Used for Effects on the Gastrointestinal Tract [a]

Drug (trade name, mfr)	Dosage forms	Usual adult daily dosage
Quaternary amines		
Anisotropine methylbromide (Valpin, *Du Pont*)	Tablets: 50 mg	3 times a day
Clidinium bromide (Quarzan; ing of Librax, *Roche*)	Capsules: 2.5 and 5 mg	3 or 4 times a day
Glycopyrrolate (Robinul, *Robins*)	Tablets: 1 and 2 mg Injection: 0.2 mg/mL in 1, 2, 5 and 20 mL	2 or 3 times a day, preanesthetic and intraoperative
Hexocyclium methylsulfate (Tral, *Abbott*)	Tablets: 25 mg	4 times a day
Isopropamide iodide (Darbid, *SmithKline Beecham*)	Tablets: 5 mg	2 times a day
Mepenzolate bromide (Cantil, *Merrell Dow*)	Tablets: 25 mg	4 times a day
Methantheline bromide (Banthine, *Searle*)	Tablets: 50 mg	4 times a day
Methscopolamine bromide (Pamine, *Upjohn*)	Tablets: 2.5 mg	4 times a day
Propantheline bromide (Pro-Banthine, *Searle*)	Tablets: 7.5 and 15 mg	3 or 4 times a day
Tertiary amines		
Dicyclomine hydrochloride (Bentyl, *Lakeside*)	Capsules: 10 and 20 mg Tablets: 20 mg Syrup: 10 mg per 5 mL Injection: 10 mg/mL in 2 and 10 mL	3 or 4 times a day Pediatric
Oxyphencyclimine hydrochloride (Daricon, *Beecham*)	Tablets: 10 mg	2 or 3 times a day
Tridihexethyl chloride (Pathilon, *Lederle*)	Tablets: 25 mg	3 or 4 times a day

[a] For further information, see RPS-18, Chap 46, page 907.

calcium channel blockers for various smooth muscle spasms, etc. Thus, the term antispasmodic might apply to many different types of drugs. The term should be reserved, however, for those drugs that relax smooth muscle nonselectively. Only those drugs are included below which potentially influence all smooth muscle, regardless of the type of innervation and neurotransmitter affected. Calcium channel blocking drugs are discussed elsewhere. The selective antagonists are treated in the appropriate chapters. Long before the selective competitive antagonistic actions of antimuscarinic drugs were known, some antimuscarinic preparations and drugs were known to relieve certain spastic conditions of the bowel. Therefore, the term antispasmodic came to connote antimuscarinic drugs that have important gastrointestinal uses, and it has become common to include antispasmodics in chapters on antimuscarinic drugs. For want of a better alternative for this small group of agents, that tradition is maintained here.

Aminophylline—page 971.

Calcium Channel Blockers—pages 963 and 971.

Ethaverine Hydrochloride—see RPS-18, page 842.

Flavoxate Hydrochloride

4*H*-1-Benzopyran-8-carboxylic acid, 3-methyl-4-oxo-2-phenyl-, Urispas (*SmithKline Beecham*)

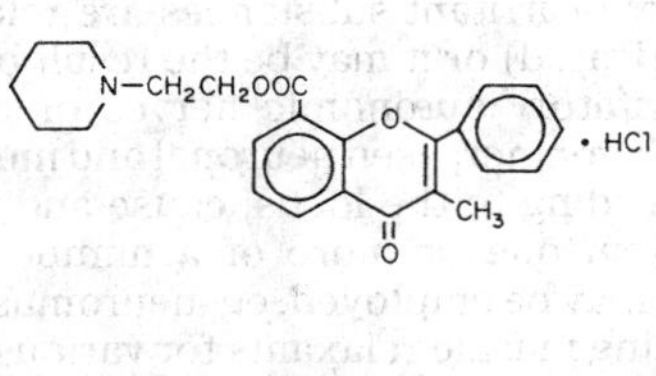

[3717-88-2] $C_{24}H_{25}NO_4$.HCl (427.93).

Preparation—*J Med Pharm Chem 2:* 263, 1960; US Pat 2,291,070.

Description—Off-white, crystalline powder; melts about 230° with decomposition.

Solubility—1 g in 6 mL water or 500 mL alcohol.

Uses—A nonspecific smooth muscle relaxant with weak antimuscarinic properties; appears to have a selectivity for the urinary tract. It is promoted for the symptomatic relief but not the definitive treatment of dysuria, urinary urgency, nocturia, suprapubic pain and urinary incontinence such as accompany urethrocystitis/urethrotrigonitis, urethritis, cystitis and prostatitis. Untoward effects include nausea and vomiting, dry mouth, blurred vision, increased intraocular tension, dysuria, tachycardia, palpitation, hyperpyrexia, headache, drowsiness, mental confusion (particularly in elderly patients), eosinophilia, leukopenia, urticaria and dermatoses. The precautions and contraindications are those of antimuscarinic drugs (page 1020). Considering that the side effects and toxicity are all antimuscarinic in character, it is interesting that the actions on the urinary smooth muscle are not held to be antimuscarinic.

Dose—*Oral, adult* or *children over 12 yr*, **100** to **200 mg** 3 or 4 times a day; not recommended for children under 12 yr.

Dosage Form—Tablets: 100 mg.

Oxybutynin Chloride

Benzeneacetic acid, α-cyclohexyl-α-hydroxy-, 4-(diethylamino)-2-butynyl ester, hydrochloride; Ditropan, Dridase (*Marion Merrell Dow*)

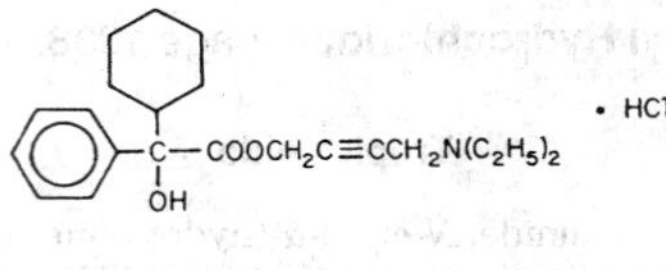

[1508-65-2] $C_{22}H_{31}NO_3$.HCl (393.95)

Preparation—By interaction of methyl phenylcyclohexaneglycolate and 4-diethylamino-2-butylnyl acetate in n-heptane solution in the presence of sodium methylate and converted to the hydrochloride by extraction with dilute hydrochloric acid. Brit Pat 940,540.

Description—White to off-white, crystalline powder; melts at about 130°; pK_a 6.96.

Solubility—Freely soluble in water or alcohol.

Uses—An antispasmodic with weak antimuscarinic activity. In patients with uninhibited neurogenic and reflex neurogenic bladder, cystometric studies have demonstrated that it increases vesical capacity, diminishes frequency of uninhibited contractions of the detrusor muscle and delays initial desire to void. It is used for relief of symptoms associated with voiding (such as urgency, urge incontinence, frequency, nocturia and incontinence) in patients confirmed by cystometry and other diagnostic procedures to have neurogenic bladder. The adverse effects, contraindications, warnings and precautions are those of antimuscarinic drugs (see the general statement), except that it also causes drowsiness. However, because of the weak antimuscarinic activity, side effects are less severe than with atropine. Safety of use in women who are, or who may become, pregnant has not been established. Safety and efficacy in children under 5 yr have not been established.

Dose—*Oral, adult*, **5 mg** 2 or 3 times a day, not exceeding 5 mg 4 times a day. *Children over 5 yr*, 5 mg 2 times a day, not exceeding 5 mg 3 times a day.

Dosage Forms—Tablets: 5 mg; Syrup: 5 mg/5 mL.

Papaverine Hydrochloride—see RPS-18, page 842.

CHAPTER 61

Skeletal Muscle Relaxants

H Steve White, PhD
Research Associate Professor of Pharmacology and Toxicology
College of Pharmacy
University of Utah
Salt Lake City, UT 84112

Skeletal muscle may be relaxed by blocking the effect of somatic motor nerve impulses, by depressing the appropriate neurons within the central nervous system so that somatic motor nerve impulses fail to be generated or by decreasing the availability of calcium ions to the myofibrillar contractile system. Interruption of certain afferent reflex pathways, as by local anesthesia, also may effect relaxation of circumscribed muscle groups; local anesthetic block of efferent somatic motor outflow also is employed sometimes to relieve localized skeletal muscle spasm. In this chapter only those drugs that act at the myoneural junction, the *neuromuscular blocking drugs* and those drugs that act upon central neurons, the *centrally acting muscle relaxants*, will be discussed.

Neuromuscular Blocking Drugs

Neuromuscular blocking drugs prevent somatic motor nerve impulses from initiating contractile responses in the effector skeletal (striated) muscles and hence cause a paralysis of the muscles. There are two categories of such drugs: the *competitive* (or *stabilizing*) paralysants and the *depolarizing* paralysants, to be discussed separately.

Uses—Competitive and depolarizing neuromuscular blocking drugs have the same major uses, in general. The pharmacokinetics and pattern of side effects, rather than their mechanism, determine the uses of any given agent. The principal use is to provide *adequate skeletal muscular relaxation* during *surgery*, *controlled respiration* and *orthopedic manipulations*. The short-acting drugs are used to relax the laryngeal muscles during *endotracheal intubation* and *bronchoscopy*. Neuromuscular paralysants may be employed to *decrease the severity of muscle contraction* during *electroconvulsive* treatment. Competitive neuromuscular paralysants have been used in the management of *tetanus* and in *various spastic disorders*, but the results usually have been disappointing. Competitive blocking drugs may be used in the *diagnosis of myasthenia gravis;* the myasthenic patient is extremely sensitive to the paralysant actions.

Competitive Neuromuscular Blocking Drugs

When impulses in the somatic motor nerves arrive in the nerve terminals in the motor end-plate region, they evoke the release of acetylcholine, which diffuses to the postsynaptic motor end plate membrane. There, acetylcholine combines with nicotinic cholinergic receptors to activate them, which leads to the opening of transmembrane ion channels, ion flow and consequent membrane depolarization. End-plate membrane depolarization is followed by depolarization of the muscle membrane and subsequent contraction. Any interruption of the above sequence of events leads to muscular paralysis.

The competitive neuromuscular blocking drugs combine with the nicotinic receptors and occupy them without activating them. Acetylcholine cannot activate the already occupied receptors, so that motor nerve impulses cannot elicit contractions, and paralysis ensues. Some of them also lodge in the receptor-operated ionophore and, thus, decrease electrical activation of the postsynaptic membrane.

Pharmacological Antagonism—The interaction of blocking drug and receptor is reversible and dynamic. Drug molecules combine, dissociate, recombine, etc, thus leaving receptor molecules transiently unoccupied. The probability that an acetylcholine molecule will find an unoccupied receptor is directly proportional to the concentration. If the concentration is elevated sufficiently, dissociated blocking drug molecules will find the receptors occupied with acetylcholine and will be prevented from recombining with the receptors to maintain blockade. Thus, a blockade can be overcome competitively. In practice, the acetylcholine concentration is raised by inhibiting acetylcholinesterase in the end plate region. Neostigmine and edrophonium are the most commonly employed anticholinesterases for antagonizing competitive neuromuscular paralysants. The anticholinesterases are discussed in Chapter 58 (page 1003).

Side Effects and Precautions—The competitive neuromuscular blocking drugs are quite selective for the nonrespiratory muscles, so that it is possible to achieve surgical relaxation of the abdominal, limb, neck or laryngeal muscles without significant loss of respiratory function. However, respiration often may be depressed to the point of danger, even apnea, so that *these drugs should be used only when facilities for prolonged respiratory assistance are at hand and the trachea is intubated,* in case respiratory assistance is needed. In hypothermic procedures such as cardiopulmonary bypass surgery, blockade is less complete, so that larger than standard doses are required; excessive paralysis may ensue subsequently when body temperature is elevated.

The two other principal side effects are the release of histamine from mast cells and ganglionic blockade. The extent to which histamine release occurs varies among the several drugs; it is greatest with tubocurarine. The histamine released may cause vasodilatation and consequent hypotension and reflex tachycardia, bronchospasm, urticaria, rash and rarely, even angioneurotic edema. *Histamine-releasing neuromuscular blocking drugs should be avoided in persons with a history of bronchial asthma, angioneurotic edema or anaphylaxis.*

Ganglionic blockade may occur, because the postsynaptic ganglionic cholinergic receptors are nicotinic. However, these receptors have somewhat different structural requirements from those at the neuromuscular junction, so that ganglionic blockade is only slight to moderate with the usual clinical doses of neuromuscular blocking drugs. The types of effects of ganglionic blockade depend upon which ganglia are blocked. Blockade of sympathetic ganglia contributes to hypotension and of vagal ganglia to tachycardia. Some curimimetics have a "vagolytic" action of unknown mechanism at cardiac muscarinic sites; this action also contributes to tachycardia. Ganglionic blockade is salutory when adverse reflexes to surgical manipulation are attenuated.

All of the marketed neuromuscular blocking drugs are quaternary ammonium compounds, hence they do not penetrate the blood-brain barrier and thus lack central nervous actions. However, some cross the placental barrier into the fetus.

Drug Interactions—Any drug with an effect to depress the excitability of the postsynaptic membrane at the motor end plate will increase the blocking effect of competitive neuromuscular blocking drugs. The anesthetic ethers, halothane, trimethaphan and propranolol, are among such drugs.

A number of antibiotics can cause neuromuscular paralysis in high doses and in therapeutic doses may increase neuromuscular blockade by the competitive blocking drugs. Some of these (gentamicin, kanamycin, neomycin, streptomycin, tobramycin, paromomycin and viomycin) apparently also act competitively on the nicotinic receptor and, hence, may be antagonized by anticholinesterases. Others (polymyxins, colistin, colistimethate, tetracyclines, lincomycin and clindamycin) have a more obscure action and are not antagonized by anticholinesterases, although anticholinesterases will antagonize the neuromuscular blocking drug and relieve the exaggerated paralysis; calcium partially antagonizes these drugs. Local anesthetics (quinine, quinidine, ganglionic blocking drugs and magnesium ion) also potentiate the neuromuscular blocking actions of the competitive blocking drugs.

Depolarizing Neuromuscular Blocking Drugs

The depolarizing neuromuscular blocking drugs are nicotinic agonists, which, like acetylcholine, interact with the postsynaptic nicotinic receptors to effect a depolarization of the membrane at the motor end plate. Unlike acetylcholine their sojourn at the end plate is long, so that the postsynaptic membrane may remain depolarized. Since the muscle membrane, and consequent contraction, can be excited only by a fresh depolarization, the muscle remains paralyzed. That is to say, the trigger for the conducted muscle impulse is the transient fall in end plate membrane potential and not the persisting depolarization.

Eventually, the motor end plate membrane repolarizes despite the continuing presence of the drug (phase two block), owing to a shift in receptor conformation. Nevertheless, despite the fact that the membrane is poised for a new depolarization, motor nerve impulses and acetylcholine fail to elicit a response, because the nicotinic receptor is not in its appropriate configuration. During this phase, the neuromuscular blockade takes on some characteristics of competitive blockade and even may be antagonized partially by anticholinesterases. This second phase is erratic in onset among the various muscles, and blockade may be of a mixed type, thus complicating the treatment of overdoses. Furthermore, not all drug recipients respond alike. Electrolyte status, muscle condition, disease, genetic factors, the presence of other drugs and temperature all affect the time of onset and extent of phase two block. Moreover, not all depolarizing drugs are identical in the pattern of blockade. Clinically, phase two is usually significant only when the drug dose is repeated or the drug is infused and blood levels sustained beyond the normal single-dose limit. Monitoring neuromuscular function by nerve stimulation to avoid overdose and/or conversion to phase two paralysis is advisable.

Side Effects and Precautions—During the onset of the drug-induced depolarization, as the membrane potential depolarizes to the critical firing potential, there may arise conducted impulses that will cause random contraction (fibrillation) of the muscle fibers. Motor nerve terminals are stimulated to generate axon reflexes that fire off entire motor units. In addition, the depolarizing neuromuscular blocking drugs stimulate both the intrafusal fibers and the muscle spindle afferent nerve endings, which results in facilitatory nerve traffic entering the spinal cord. Thus, there usually is an organized contraction pattern, namely *fasciculations* and even *twitching*. The result is muscle soreness. Fasciculations and twitching can exacerbate spasm and also cause damage in the presence of broken bones; consequently, the depolarizing drugs should be avoided in these conditions.

The muscles of respiration (intercostal and diaphragmatic) are more resistant to the paralyzing effects than are other skeletal muscles, and it usually is possible to achieve surgical relaxation of abdominal, limb, neck or laryngeal muscles without significant loss of respiratory function. Nevertheless, respiration often may be depressed, sometimes to the point of apnea. This is likely especially after prolonged use, which favors considerable loss of potassium from the motor end plate region. Consequently, *the depolarizing neuromuscular blocking drugs should be used only with tracheal intubation and when facilities for prolonged assisted respiration are at hand.* Care should be used when respiration already is depressed and also when the lithotomy or Trendelenburg positions are employed, especially in young children and the aged.

During the depolarizing phase of neuromuscular block, potassium is lost rapidly from the muscles, which may cause hyperkalemia. If a sufficient amount of the mobilized potassium is excreted, there may be a later hypokalemia. Various cardiac arrhythmias, even cardiac arrest, may result, especially if the patient is digitalized. Prolonged paralysis by these agents may lead to malignant hyperthermia.

The effects of depolarizing blocking drugs on autonomic ganglia and histamine stores are variable.

Drug Interactions—Muscle paralysis with depolarizing neuromuscular blocking drugs is increased by hypothermia, hypokalemia, hypermagnesemia, polymyxin B, colistin, colistimethate and aminoglycoside antibiotics (streptomycin, kanamycin, gentamicin, tobramycin and neomycin).

Atracurium Besylate

Isoquinolinium, 2,2′-[1,5-pentanediylbis[oxy(3-oxo-3,1-propanediyl)]]-bis[1-(3,4-dimethoxyphenyl)methyl]-1,2,3,4-tetrahydro-6,7-dimethoxy-2-methyl, dibenzenesulfonate;
Tracrium (*Burroughs-Wellcome*)

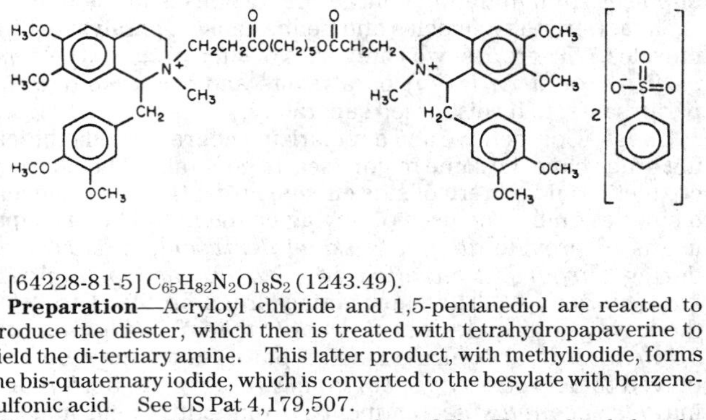

[64228-81-5] $C_{65}H_{82}N_2O_{18}S_2$ (1243.49).

Preparation—Acryloyl chloride and 1,5-pentanediol are reacted to produce the diester, which then is treated with tetrahydropapaverine to yield the di-tertiary amine. This latter product, with methyliodide, forms the bis-quaternary iodide, which is converted to the besylate with benzenesulfonic acid. See US Pat 4,179,507.

Description—Off-white powder; melts at 87°. The molecule has the potential to conform to any of 16 different isomers but, due to its symmetry, only ten exist. The drug entity consists of a mixture of several possible isomers and the synthetic procedure results in the production of a consistent ratio of isomers, but in unequal amounts. The isomer which predominates (approximately in a 3:1 ratio) is that in which the quaternary methyl group and the dimethoxybenzyl group assume a *trans* configuration about the tetrahydroisoquinoline parent.

Solubility—1 g in 20 mL water.

Uses—A competitive neuromuscular paralysant that is 2.5 times as potent as tubocurarine (see page 1031). Its effects are more predictable than are those of tubocurarine, especially with respect to repeated doses. Its duration of action is 33 to 50% of that of tubocurarine, 90% of recovery of muscle function occurring in 60 to 70 min. The drug thus lends itself to use in surgical procedures of short to intermediate duration. In therapeutic doses, side effects are minimal, but moderate degrees of histamine release and consequent sequelae occur occasionally.

Drug interactions and antagonism by anticholinesterases essentially are the same as with tubocurarine, but the potentiating effects of anesthetics are less marked.

It neither is metabolized appreciably in the liver nor excreted into the urine. Rather, the bridge between the isoquinoline moieties is ruptured spontaneously by Hoffman elimination and by hydrolysis in plasma. This unique elimination makes the effects and duration of action independent of liver and/or renal insufficiency. The elimination half-life is about 20 min.

Dose—*Intravenous, adults* and *children over 2 yr, initially* **0.4** to **0.5 mg/kg**; *supplemental* doses of **0.08** to **0.10 mg/kg** may be given in

20 to 45 min, then every 15 to 25 min, if necessary. In patients to whom histamine release might be hazardous or following succinylcholine for endotracheal intubation, the *initial* dose should be **0.3** to **0.4 mg/kg**, given singly or in divided doses over a period of 1 min. With enflurane or isoflurane anesthesia, doses should be diminished by one third; a lesser reduction is required with halothane or methoxyflurane. *Infants, 1 mo* to *2 yr*, **0.3** to **0.4 mg/ kg.**

Dosage Forms—Injection: 50 mg/5 mL and 100 mg/10 mL.

Curare

A name applied to extracts principally of the bark and other parts of plants of certain species of *Chondodendron* or *Strychnos*, especially *Chondodendron tomentosum* and *Strychnos toxiferin*, prepared by South American Indians of the Upper Amazon and Orinoco basins for use as arrow poisons. The extracts contain neuromuscular paralysant alkaloids and numerous other contaminants. The chondodendron alkaloids contain tertiary and quaternary benzylisoquinoline derivatives such as *d*-tubocurarine (see *Tubocurarine Chloride*), *curine*, and related compounds. The strychnos alkaloids contain β-carboline alkaloids such as the toxiferins and calabash *curarines*. None of the crude preparations currently is used in therapeutics. Only purified preparations or alkaloids from *Chondodendron tomentosum* are available commercially.

Dantrolene Sodium

2,4-Imidazolidinedione,
1-[[[5-(4-nitrophenyl)-2-furany]methylene]amino]-,
sodium salt, hydrate (2:7); Dantrium (*Proctor & Gamble*)

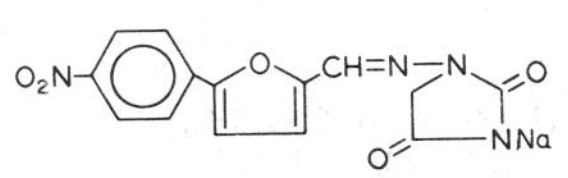

1-[[5-(*p*-Nitrophenyl)furfurylidene]amino]hydantoin sodium salt hydrate [24868-20-0] $C_{14}H_9N_4NaO_5 \cdot 3\frac{1}{2}H_2O$ (399.29).

Preparation—See *J Med Chem 10:*807, 1967 and US Pat 3,415,821.

Description—Orange powder; *free acid* melts about 280°; pK_a about 7.5.

Solubility—Slightly soluble in water; more soluble in alkali.

Uses—Differs from the classical neuromuscular blocking drugs in that its action is distal to the nicotinic receptors and neuromuscular junction. Instead, it suppresses excitation-contraction coupling by interfering with release of calcium from the sarcotubular reticulum. The muscle fibers still respond to nerve impulses, but the contractile response is lessened but not abolished. Therefore, muscle weakness, rather than paralysis, is the result. Fast muscle fibers (white) are affected more than slow muscle fibers (red). Because the contractility of the intrafusal fibers in the muscle spindles also is decreased, spinal cord-mediated stretch reflexes are attenuated, which provides the primary explanation of its ability to relieve certain types of spasm. It is used to treat *spasticity resulting from upper motor neuron* lesions, such as those in *spinal cord injury, stroke, multiple sclerosis* and *cerebral palsy* but not spasticity resulting from musculoskeletal injury, lumbago or rheumatoid disorders. It is possible that a direct effect on the motor neuron may be involved in this limited spectrum of activity, since the drug does exert some CNS-depressant actions. In fact, the drug is used to treat the *neuroleptic malignant syndrome.* Its effect on intracellular calcium also lends itself to the treatment of *malignant hyperthemia* which can be triggered by general anesthesia and neuromuscular blocking drugs.

Interference with muscle function may cause weakness and fatigue, poor posture with consequent backache and myalgia, a feeling of suffocation, difficulties in swallowing, diplopia and other visual disturbances. Effects on the CNS include drowsiness, dizziness, malaise, headache, nervousness, slurred speech, confusion, depression and, rarely, convulsions. Other adverse effects include constipation, diarrhea, abdominal cramps, gastric irritation, gastrointestinal bleeding, increased urinary frequency yet oliguria, lacrimation, sweating, disorders of taste, urticaria, acneiform rash, eczematoid dermatitis, pleural effusions and pericarditis, hepatitis, chills and fever. It is contraindicated in liver and pulmonary disease, in situations where alertness is essential and when gross postural abnormalities result from its use. It may color the urine orange to red.

Orally, it is absorbed poorly but more or less consistently, so that blood levels are proportional to the dose. It is metabolized in the liver to several products. It is stated that the plasma half-life is 5 hr by the intravenous route but 9 hr by the oral route. The former is probably an approximation of the *distribution* (α) half-life and the latter of the elimination (β) half-life.

Dose—*Oral, adult,* for *chronic spasticity, initially* **25 mg** once a day, to be increased at intervals of 4 to 7 days to as much as **100 mg** 2 to 4 times a day, if necessary; for *preoperative prophylaxis* of malignant hyperthermia, **4** to **8 mg/kg** a day in 3 or 4 divided doses 1 or 2 days before surgery, so the last dose is taken 3 to 4 hr prior to surgery; for *post-malignant hypethermia,* as for prophylaxis, for 1 to 3 days. *Children,* for *spasticity, initially* **0.5 mg/kg** 2 times a day, then gradually increasing the dose by increments of **0.5 mg/kg** a day every 4 to 7 days, up to **3 mg/kg** 2 to 4 times a day, not to exceed a total of 100 mg/day. *Intravenous, adult* and *children,* for *malignant hyperthermia, initially* **1** to **3 mg/kg** rapidly repeated in doses of 1 mg/kg, if necessary, up to total of **10 mg/kg.** Once the hyperthermia is controlled, the drug is given orally (see above).

Dosage Forms—Capsules: 25, 50 and 100 mg. Powder for Injection: 20 mg, to make 60 mL solution of 0.33 mg/mL.

Doxacurium Chloride

Isoquinolinium dichloride, 2,2′-[(1,4-dioxo-1,4-butanediyl)bis
(Oxy-3,1-propanediyl)] bis[1,2,3,4-tetrahydro-6,7,8-trimethoxy-
2-methyl-1-[(3,4,5-tri-methoxyphenyl)methyl]-, Nuromax
(*Burroughs Wellcome*)

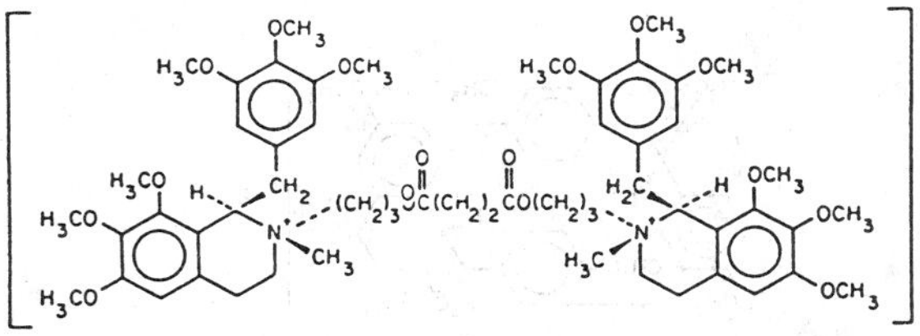

[106819-53-8], $C_{56}H_{78}Cl_2N_2O_{16}$ (1106.15).

Uses—A long-acting, nondepolarizing, competitive, neuromuscular blocking drug whose action is reversed by anticholinesterases. Doxacurium is indicated as an adjunct to general anesthesia. Its time to onset following an intravenous dose is approximately 1.5 to 2 times longer than the intermediate-acting nondepolarizing agents atracurium and vecuronium and 4 to 5 times longer than the short-acting depolarizing agent succinylcholine. Time to 25% recovery is approximately 10 to 15 times longer than succinylcholine and 2 to 3 times longer than the intermediate agents. Doxacurium does not appear to cause histamine release. The major elimination pathway for doxacurium is through excretion of unchanged drug in the urine and bile. The duration of action of doxacurium is increased in patients with end-stage kidney and hepatic disease.

Dose—*Intravenous, adults, initially* **0.05 mg/kg** will produce a clinically effective neuromuscular block for approximately 60 to 100 min. Patients undergoing surgical procedures lasting longer than 100 min will require a *maintenance* dose of **0.005** to **0.01 mg/kg** every 30 to 45 min. The *initial* dose in *children older than 2 yr* receiving halothane anesthesia is **0.03 mg/kg.** *Maintenance* doses of doxacurium generally are administered more frequently in children than in adults.

Dosage Form—Injection: 1 mg/mL.

Gallamine Triethiodide

Ethanaminium, 2,2′,2″-[1,2,3-benzentriyltris(oxy)tris]-*N,N,N*-triethyl-, triiodide; Flaxedil (*Davis & Geck*)

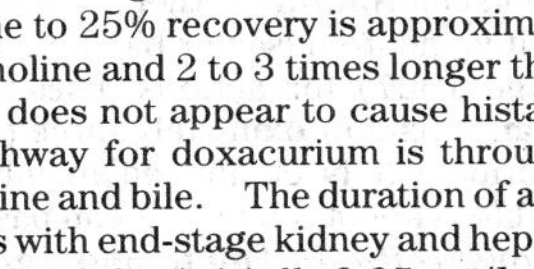

1,2,3-Tris(β-diethylaminoethoxy)benzene Triethiodide; [65-29-2] $C_{30}H_{60}I_3N_3O_3$ (891.54).

Preparation—Prepared by condensing pyrogallol with tris(2-chloroethyl)amine and quaternizing the resulting triamine with ethyl iodide in boiling acetone.

Description—White, odorless, amorphous powder; hygroscopic.

Solubility—Very soluble in water; sparingly soluble in alcohol; very slightly soluble in chloroform.

Note: It is pharmaceutically incompatible with meperidine hydrochloride (solutions must not be mixed).

Uses— A competitive neuromuscular blocking drug; see the introductory statement for actions, uses, side effects and drug interactions. It is used when an intermediate to long duration of action is desired. In general, it has very little action on autonomic ganglia, but usually blocks the cardiac vagus and hence causes tachycardia and occasionally hypertension. It releases histamine only in high doses. Hyper-sensitivity reactions occasionally occur, and severe anaphylaxis has been reported; the drug should be used cautiously in patients with a history of allergy, asthma or atopy. It should be used cautiously if tachycardia preexists. Azathioprine may antagonize gallamine. It is eliminated mainly by renal excretion, and its action may be prolonged if there is renal dysfunction. Its normal elimination half-life is about 2.5 hr.

Dose—*Intravenous adults* and *children, initially* **1 mg/kg** for *limb muscle paralysis* or **1.5 mg/kg** for *abdominal surgery,* not to exceed 100 mg, then **500 μg** to **1 mg** at 30- to 60-min intervals if necessary. Special caution must be exercized when the patient weighs less than 5 kg. The dose should be diminished if various ether anesthetics or halothane is used.

Dosage Form—Injection: 20 mg/mL.

Hexafluorenium Bromide—see RPS-18, page 918.

Metocurine Iodide

Tubocuraranium, 6,6′,7′,12′-tetramethoxy-2,2,2′,2′-tetramethyl-, diiodide; Dimethyl Tubocurarine Iodide; Metubine Iodide (*Lilly*)

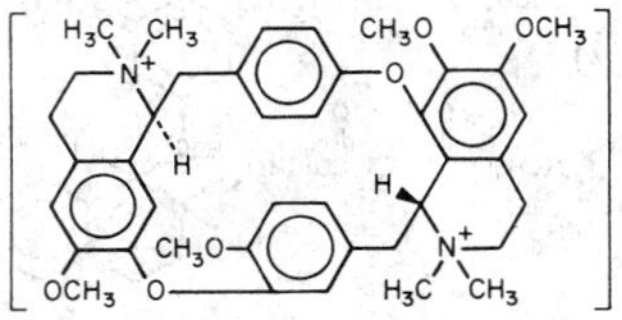

(+)-*O,O′*-Dimethylchondrocurarine diiodide [7601-55-0] $C_{40}H_{48}I_2N_2O_6$ (906.64).

Preparation—By methylation of the naturally occurring *d*-tubocurarine, with methyl iodide or dimethyl sulfate, and conversion to the diiodide.

Description—White or yellow, crystalline powder.

Solubility—1 g in 400 mL water; very slightly soluble in alcohol; practically insoluble in chloroform or ether.

Uses—A competitive neuromuscular blocking drug; see the introductory statement (page 1027) for actions, uses, side effects and drug interactions. In man, it is approximately three times more potent than *d*-tubocurarine chloride. It is eliminated mainly by renal and biliary excretions; the half-life is about 3.5 hr. It can pass the placental barrier.

Dose—*Intravenous, initially* **100** to **300 μg/kg** given over a 30- to 60-sec period. The initial dose depends on the anesthetic employed and is determined by the anesthesiologist. For limb muscle paralysis, dosage is in the lower range; for abdominal and respiratory muscle paralysis, it is at the upper end; for *endotracheal intubation,* **200** to **400 μg/kg.** *Maintenance,* **500 μg** to **1 mg** every 25 to 90 min. For *electroshock* therapy, **1.75** to **5.5 mg.**

Dosage Form—Injection: 40 mg/20 mL.

Mivacurium Chloride

Isoquinolinium, [*R*-[*R**, *R**-(*E*)]]-2,2′-[(1,8-dioxo-4-octene-1,8-diyl)bis(oxy-3,1-propanediyl)]bis-[1,2,3,4-tetrahydro-6,7-dimethoxy-2-methyl-1-[(3,4,5-trimethoxyphenyl)methyl]-, dichloride; Mivacron (*Burroughs Wellcome*)

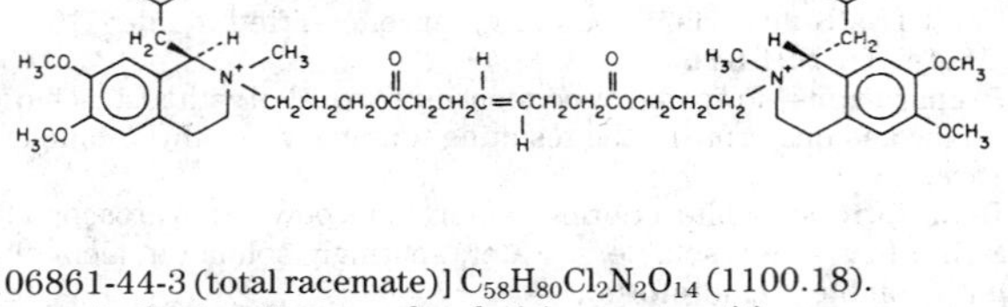

[106861-44-3 (total racemate)] $C_{58}H_{80}Cl_2N_2O_{14}$ (1100.18).

Uses—A short-acting, nondepolarizing, competitive, neuromuscular blocking drug whose action is reversed by anticholinesterases. Its time to onset following a bolus dose is equivalent to the intermediate acting nondepolarizing agents atracurium and vecuronium and 2 to 3 times longer than the short-acting depolarizing agent succinylcholine. Time to 25% recovery is approximately 2 times longer than succinylcholine (16 versus 8 min, respectively) and 2 to 3 times shorter than the intermediate agents (16 versus 25 to 45 min, respectively). For short-duration procedures not requiring rapid induction of anesthesia, mivacurium represents a viable alternative to succinylcholine. Bolus doses of mivacurium can cause histamine release which leads to cutaneous flushing of face and neck, increased heart rate and hypotension. Like succinylcholine, mivacurium is metabolized rapidly by plasma cholinesterase. The duration of action of mivacurium is increased in patients with end-stage kidney and hepatic disease and patients with a deficiency of plasma cholinesterase.

Dose—*Intravenous,* **0.15 mg/kg** over 5 to 15 sec. Administration over a 30- to 60-sec period is recommended in patients with clinically significant cardiovascular disease or in those patients who have demonstrated a greater sensitivity to histamine-releasing agents.

Dosage Form—Injection: 2 mg/mL.

Pancuronium Bromide

Piperidinium, 1,1′-[2β,3α,5α,16β,17β)-3,17-bis(acetyloxy)androstane-2,16-diyl]bis[1-methyl]-, dibromide; Pavulon (*Organon*)

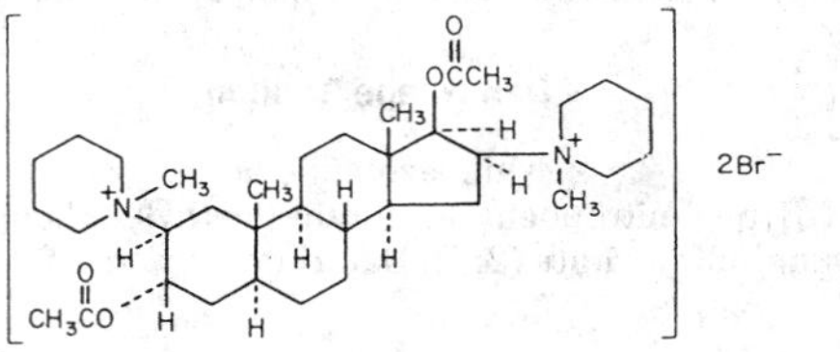

[15500-66-0] $C_{35}H_{60}Br_2N_2O_4$ (732.68).

Preparation—See US Pat 3,553,212.

Description—White, crystalline powder; hygroscopic; melts at about 215°.

Solubility—Freely soluble in water; soluble in alcohol or chloroform.

Uses—A competitive neuromuscular blocking drug; see the general statement for actions, uses, side effects and drug interactions. Its mechanism of action usually is assumed to be identical to that of tubocurarine, but the dose-response curve is steeper, which suggests a difference. It differs from tubocurarine in its side effects in that it does not block the autonomic ganglia and rarely releases histamine, so that it causes neither hypotension nor bronchospasm. In fact, it may cause a slight tachycardia and hypertension as the result of a "vagotic" action and also interference with the neuronal reuptake of norepinephrine. Also, a slight transient rash may occur occasionally. Salivary secretion during light anesthesia is common. Drug interactions are the same as with tubocurarine, except that prior treatment with succinylcholine augments the paralysis and increases the duration; also, narcotic analgesics do not seem to affect its actions. It may be used more safely in patients with cardiovascular disease or bronchial asthma than any other neuromuscular blocking drug. Indeed, it actually has been used in the *management of status asthmaticus,* to relax the muscles, thereby facilitating artificial respiration and decreasing oxygen demand. After intravenous injection, its effects become maximal in less than 4.5 min in adults and 90 sec in children. The duration of action of usual doses is generally 30 to 60 min, but it depends on various factors, such as the anesthetic, or prior dosage with succinylcholine. The plasma half-life is usually slightly less than 2 hours. It is excreted mostly unchanged into the urine, but up to one-third of a dose is deacetylated; thus, it is advisable to use the drug cautiously in the presence of either renal or liver disease.

Dose—*Intravenous, adult* and *children* over *1 mo, for surgical relaxation,* **20** to **100 μg/kg,** followed by *supplemental* doses of **10 μg/kg;** for *intubation,* **60** to **100 μg/kg.** Doses for *infants younger than 1 mo* to be determined by the physician.

Dosage Form—Injection: 1 and 2 mg/mL.

Succinylcholine Chloride

Ethanaminium, 2,2′-[(1,4-dioxo-1,4-butanediyl)bis(oxy)]bis [*N,N,N*-trimethyl-, dichloride; Suxamethonium Chloride; Anectine (*Burroughs Wellcome*); (*Organon*); Quelicin (*Abbott*); Sucostrin (*Squibb-Marsam*)

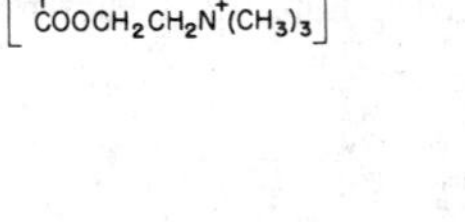

$$\left[\begin{array}{l} COOCH_2CH_2N^+(CH_3)_3 \\ (CH_2)_2 \\ COOCH_2CH_2N^+(CH_3)_3 \end{array}\right] 2Cl^-$$

Choline chloride succinate (2:1) *anhydrous* [71-27-2] $C_{14}H_{30}Cl_2N_2O_4$ (361.31); *dihydrate* [6101-15-1] (397.34); usually occurs as the dihydrate.

Preparation—It may be prepared by condensing succinyl chloride with β-dimethylaminoethanol and quaternizing the resulting ester with methyl chloride.

Description—White, odorless, crystalline powder; solutions are acid to litmus (pH of about 4); the dihydrate melts at about 160°, the anhydrous at about 190°; hygroscopic.

Solubility—1 g in about 1 mL water or about 350 mL alcohol; slightly soluble in chloroform; practically insoluble in ether.

Uses—A depolarizing neuromuscular blocking agent; see the introductory statement (page 1027) for actions, uses, side effects precautions and drug interactions. It usually has a very transient duration of action because of rapid hydrolysis of the drug by serum butyryl (pseudo) cholinesterases. The effects of a single injection usually last only a few minutes; consequently, it is of special use for muscle relaxation during brief manipulations. Prolonged muscular relaxation is achieved by continuous intravenous infusion, and the intensity of muscle paralysis is controlled readily by adjustment of the infusion rate. Alternatively, prolonged muscular relaxation may be achieved with periodic injections when the drug is given in combination with *hexafluorenium bromide* (above). Although a stabilizing phase of action can occur, its occurrence is erratic and usually results only from prolonged use.

It does not cause liberation of histamine, but hypersensitivity reactions sometimes occur. As the drug depolarizes the motor end-plate, axon reflex-conducted impulses and contractions of motor units (fasciculations) may occur. Muscle aching resulting from its transient stimulatory action is minimized by slow administration. Hyperkalemia, due to potassium loss from muscle, and myoglobinemia sometimes result from these stimulatory actions. Excessive salivation may occur; this is preventable by premedication with atropine or scopolamine. It may induce a bradycardia that can be suppressed by atropine or methscopolamine but not by scopolamine. It may cause cardiac arrhythmias in patients with myocardial damage. Among neuromuscular blocking drugs, it is unique in its effect to increase intraocular pressure; it is contraindicated in persons with glaucoma or retinal detachment and in persons with known hypersensitivity. Rarely, it may cause a severe (malignant) hyperthermia when an ether anesthetic or cyclopropane is used. No specific pharmacologic antagonist of the skeletal muscle effects is available, but dantrolene can suppress malignant hyperthermia. Calcium channel blocking drugs also are useful in this regard. Its actions may be prolonged in individuals with reduced plasma cholinesterase activity, such as results from a genetic defect or from liver disease or cachexia.

Dose—*Intravenous, adult, initially* **0.6** to **1.1 mg/kg** given over 10 to 30 sec; if paralysis is insufficient, a second dose of size to be determined according to the response to the first dose and the desired duration of effect may be given after a few minutes; for *prolonged relaxation*, repeat doses of **0.04** to **0.07 mg/kg** are administered at appropriate intervals, but intravenous infusion is preferred to repetitive dosing; in *electroshock treatment, adult,* **10** to **30 mg** total 1 min before electroshock; *older children* and *adolescents, initially* **1 mg/kg;** *infants* and *small children, initially* **2 mg/ kg.** *Intravenous infusion, adult,* **0.5** to **10 mg/ min** as a 0.1 to 0.2% solution in dextrose injection; intravenous infusion should neither exceed 1 hr nor be used in children because of the danger of malignant hyperthermia. *Intramuscular, adults* and *children,* **2.5** to **3.3 mg/kg,** not to exceed 150 mg; inaccessible or small veins are the only indication for this route.

Dosage Forms—Injection: 20, 50 and 100 mg/mL; Sterile: 500 mg and 1 g.

Tubocurarine Chloride

Tubocuraranium, (+)-7′,12′-dihydroxy-6,6′-dimethoxy-2,2′, 2′-trimethyl-, chloride, hydrochloride, pentahydrate; Tubocurarine Dichloride; *d*-Tubocurarine Chloride; (*Various Mfrs*)

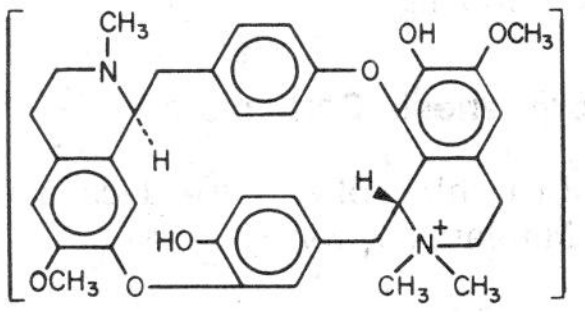

(+)-Tubocurarine chloride hydrochloride pentahydrate [6989-98-6] $C_{37}H_{41}ClN_2O_6.HCl.5H_2O$ (771.73); *anhydrous* [57-94-3] (681.65).

Preparation—Isolated from the stems and bark of the freshly gathered plant *Chondodendron tomentosum* which is extracted with small portions of water. Refer to RPS-16 for details.

Description—White or yellowish white to grayish white, odorless, crystalline powder; melts at about 270°, with decomposition.

Solubility—1 g in 20 mL water or 45 mL alcohol; insoluble in chloroform or ether.

Uses—A competitive neuromuscular blocking agent; see the introductory statement (page 1027) for the actions, uses, side effects and drug interactions.

It is not absorbed from the gut. After intravenous administration it rapidly disappears from the plasma, with a distribution half-life of about 12 min; however, its terminal plasma half-life is 1 to 3 hr. The duration of action of the first dose is 10 to 30 min, but a residual effect lasting several hours has been shown. Subsequent doses may have a longer action. It is both excreted into urine (43%) and degraded in the liver and kidneys, and either renal failure or hepatic failure can prolong the half-life.

Dose—*Intramuscular* or *intravenous,* for *paralysis of limb and back muscles* for *surgery, electroshock* or *controlled respiration, initially* **0.165 mg/kg** (6 to 9 mg) in 30 to 90 sec, followed in 5 min by **0.083 mg/kg** (3 to 4.5 mg) more if necessary, and for profound *abdominal relaxation* and *apnea,* **0.413 mg/kg** (15 to 27 mg); maintenance doses are usually about one-quarter to one-third of the initial doses, given at 45- to 60-min intervals. When the anesthetic is enflurane, isoflurane or ether, the dose should be one-third to one-half the standard dose; when it is halothane or methoxyflurane, the dose should be one-half to two-thirds the standard dose. In the diagnosis of *myasthenia gravis,* **0.007** to **0.022 mg/kg** is given. In *infants* and *children,* for *surgical relaxation, initially* **0.2** to **0.5 mg/kg,** the larger dose producing apnea; in neonates under 4 wk, supplemental doses should be one-sixth to one-fifth the initial dose. It seldom is given intramuscularly.

Dosage Form—Injection: 30 mg/10 mL and 60 mg/20 mL.

Vecuronium Bromide

Piperidinium, 1-[(2β,3α,5α,16β,17β)-3,17-bis(acetyloxy)-2-(1-piperidinyl)androstan-16-yl]-1-methyl-, bromide, diacetate; Norcuron (*Organon*)

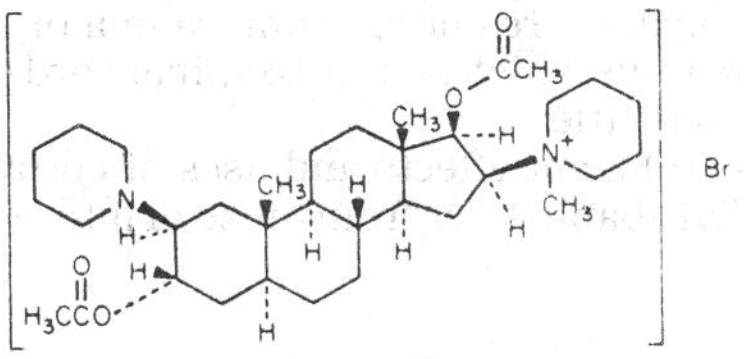

[50700-72-6] $C_{34}H_{57}BrN_2O_4$ (637.74).

Preparation—See *J Med Chem 16:*1116, 1973.

Description—White crystals; melts at about 230°.

Uses—It retains the competitive neuromuscular blocking activity of pancuronium (see page 1030 for properties of competitive blocking drugs and *Pancuronium Bromide,* this page) but is devoid of some of the side effects and, consequently, has clinical advantages over pancuronium. It does not release histamine significantly, cause ganglionic blockade or interfere with neuronal reuptake of norepinephrine, hence, has negligible cardiovascular side effects. The duration of action in adults is about 15 to 30 min for doses that cause less than 100% paralysis. Partial recovery sufficient to permit breathing may take even less time. Consequently, it may be used for relatively short surgical procedures and endotracheal intubation in adults. Recovery time is slightly longer in young children and more than twice as long in infants. When doses are repeated after only 25% of recovery of muscle function, accumulation apparently does not occur.

It is excreted mostly into the bile, and the degree of paralysis and duration of action are increased in liver failure. Ten to 25% is excreted into urine, and renal failure may prolong the duration of action by as much as 32%.

Dose—*Intravenous, adults and children 10 yr* and older, for *surgery, initially* **0.08** to **0.10 mg/kg** followed by a supplemental dose of **0.01** to **0.15 mg/kg** in 25 to 40 min and 12 to 15 min thereafter, except *after succinylcholine* (for intubation), **0.040** to **0.060 mg/kg** are given initially; in *balanced anesthesia, initially* **0.050** to **0.060 mg/kg;** *children under 10 yr,* dose must be individualized.

Dosage Form—For injection: 10 mg.

Centrally Acting Muscle Relaxants

The cell bodies of the somatic motor nerves lie within the spinal cord and, hence, within the central nervous system.

The activity of motor neurons is affected not only by facilitatory and inhibitory modulation through feedback from contralateral and ipsilateral stretch and other receptors but also from centers in the brain. Spasticity can arise from musculoskeletal injury, which may cause aberrant afferent impulse traffic into the spinal cord, from injury to or disease of the motor nerves or related interneurons within the cord, or sensory neurons in the sensory ganglia and from disorders in the brain, which alter the flow of suprasegmental impulses to the motor neurons. Involuntary movement, such as is seen in palsies, chorea or parkinsonism, mostly is the result of impairment of feedback control within the brain.

When the disorder is musculoskeletal or is within the spinal cord, the selectivity of drugs is relatively low, because the collective neurons involved in the reflex arcs are not sufficiently qualitatively different from the motor and sensory neurons in chemical sensitivity to permit a selective depression of the hyperactive influences on the motor neuron. However, some selectivity is achieved when interneurons are involved, simply because a small effect on each converging interneuron may summate to cause a moderate decrease in interneuron input to the motor neuron. Because the interneurons are involved in the fine tuning of neuronal activity, their influences are balanced critically and hence more susceptible to pharmacological action than the motor neuron itself. Consequently, most central relaxants are *interneuron depressants*, which, however, will manifest variable depressant actions throughout the central nervous system. Interestingly, many antianxiety and some sedative drugs possess muscle relaxant activity, probably because of the high sensitivity of the critically balanced interneurons to perturbation.

In tolerated doses, the centrally acting muscle relaxants are erratic, owing to their limited selectivity. Orally, they are usually ineffective (the tolerated doses being much too low); intravenously, they have some established value in treating acute muscle spasms resulting from trauma or inflammation. Motor dysfunctions which accrue to spinal cord or brain disorders are affected little.

The central relaxant effects and uses of certain benzodiazepines, like diazepam, differ from those of interneuron depressants.

Baclofen

4-Amino-3-(4-chlorophenyl)butanoic acid; Atrofen (*Athena*); Lioresal (*Ciba-Geigy*)

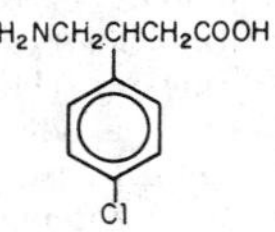

β-(Aminomethyl)-*p*-chlorohydrocinnamic acid [1134-47-0] $C_{10}H_{12}ClNO_2$ (213.67).

Preparation—Synthesis by hydrogenation of β-cyano-*p*-chlorohydrocinnamic acid, in acidified ethanol in the presence of platinic oxide catalyst, is described in Swiss Pat 449,046 (*CA 69:*106273f, 1968).

Description—Crystalline powder; melts at about 207° (190°?); pK_a 3.85, 9.25.

Solubility—Slightly soluble in water; poorly soluble in organic solvents.

Uses—Its muscle relaxant actions result from an action within the spinal cord, where both monosynaptic and polysynaptic reflexes are inhibited by the drug. It is an analog of gamma-aminobutyric acid, an inhibitory neurotransmitter, but it is not certain whether its actions are attributable entirely to a GABA-mimetic action. Its sedative and ataxic actions are consistent with such an action in the brain.

It is used in the relief of painful spasticity in *multiple sclerosis*, for which it is more effective than diazepam. Some residual ambulatory function must be present; the drug will not make nonambulatory patients ambulatory. Although spasticity may be lessened, the gait and posture of some patients may be worsened, because of the unmasking of incoordination. It also may afford some relief in patients with *spinal cord disease* and *traumatic transverse myelopathies*. It is not as effective as carbamazepine in the treatment of *neuralgias* but is an important substitute when needed. It has been reported to be of value in tardive dyskinesia. It is useful in the management of *external urinary sphincter hypertonicity* and *detrussor-external sphincter dyssynergia*. It is not indicated in musculoskeletal spastic disorders.

Sedation is the most frequent adverse effect, although it is less frequent and severe than with diazepam. Its use in combination with other CNS depressants or ethanol should be avoided, if possible. Weakness may occur, but it is less handicapping than with dantrolene. Other common side effects include dizziness, insomnia, pruritus and rashes. The drug is contraindicated when a hypersensitivity exists. Less frequent side effects include hypotension and mental confusion. Abrupt withdrawal has been reported to result in anxiety, tachycardia and even visual hallucinations; therefore, dosage must be discontinued gradually. In patients with epilepsy, it may increase the frequency of seizures. Overdoses may cause seizures, coma, loss of brain stem reflexes and respiratory depression. It is teratogenic, and this risk must be considered in pregnancy. It also has been found to cause ovarian cysts and enlarged or hemorrhagic adrenal glands in experimental animals.

It is absorbed rapidly, orally; absorption time is approximately 2 hr. More than 80% of the drug is excreted in the urine. The elimination half-life is 3 to 4 hr.

Dose—*Oral, adult, initially* **5 mg** 3 times a day, with **5 mg**- increments per dose at 4-day intervals until relief is achieved or **20 mg** (4 times a day) is reached, whichever occurs first. Neither the dose nor the efficacy in children has been established. The drug should be withdrawn slowly.

Dosage Form—Scored Tablets: 10 and 20 mg.

Carisoprodol

Soma (*Wallace*); (*Geneva, Par*)

$$(CH_3)_2CHNHCOOCH_2\underset{CH_2CH_2CH_3}{\overset{CH_3}{C}}CH_2OOCNH_2$$

N-Isopropyl-2-methyl-2-propyl-1,3-propanediol dicarbamate [78-44-4] $C_{12}H_{24}N_2O_4$ (260.33).

Preparation—Synthesis of the drug, which is an isopropyl me-probamate, is described in US Pat 2,937,119.

Description—White, crystalline powder; melts at about 93°.

Solubility—1 g in about 3300 mL water; 2.5 mL of acetone or alcohol; soluble in many common organic solvents.

Uses—A sedative drug with muscle relaxant properties that result from reticulospinal depression. It is used to treat muscle spasm of local origin, such as results from strains, sprains and lumbago. Part of its action may result from analgesia, sedation and alleviation of anxiety. Onset of relief takes about 30 min; duration of action is 4 to 6 hr.

Adverse effects of the first dose may include sedation, diplopia, extreme weakness, ataxia, transient quadriplegia, tachycardia, postural hypotension, syncope, mydriasis, temporary loss of vision, dizziness, confusion, irritability, agitation, depression, disorientation and dysarthria. Usually these subside within a few hours, but they may continue in milder form throughout treatment. Nausea and vomiting, hiccough and epigastric distress also may occur. Sedation may occur throughout treatment. The patient should be advised not to operate a motor vehicle or machinery or attempt activities requiring alertness, judgment or complex mentation. Addiction may occur; withdrawal signs and symptoms are abdominal cramps, chills, nausea, headache and insomnia. Pregnant or lactating mothers should not use the drug. Hypersensitivity occasionally occurs, in part attributable to tartrazine in some products; manifestations may be smarting of the eyes, asthmatic episodes, pruritus, rash, fixed drug eruption, eosinophilia, fever, angioneurotic edema, hypotension or anaphylaxis. It is contraindicated in acute intermittent porphyria.

The drug is metabolized mostly in the liver; the elimination half- life is usually about 8 hr.

Dose—*Oral, adult,* **350 mg** 4 times a day; *children 5 to 12 yr,* **6.25 mg/kg** 4 times a day; dose not established for younger children.

Dosage Form—Tablets: 350 mg.

Chlorphenesin Carbamate

1,2-Propanediol, 3-(4-chlorophenoxy)-, 1-carbamate; Maolate (*Upjohn*)

$$Cl-C_6H_4-OCH_2\underset{OH}{CH}CH_2OCONH_2$$

[886-74-8] $C_{10}H_{12}ClNO_4$ (245.66).

Preparation—*p*-Chlorophenol and glycidol (2,3-epoxy-1-propanol) form 3-(*p*-chlorophenoxy)-1,2-propanediol, which is esterified with carbamoyl chloride at the 1-hydroxy position. US Pats 3,161,567 and 3,214,336.

Description—White, crystalline powder; melts between 89° and 91°.

Solubility—Very sligthly soluble in water; freely soluble in alcohol; sparingly soluble in chloroform.

Uses—A centrally active skeletal muscle relaxant similar in its actions to *Methocarbamol*. It is used to diminish *skeletal muscle spasms* resulting from trauma, inflammation, vertebral disk syndrome, osteoarthritis and rheumatoid arthritis. (In the British Commonwealth, *chlorphenesin* is used topically to treat athlete's foot.) Side effects include drowsiness, dizziness, epigastric distress, nausea, skin rash, headache, insomnia, nervousness and agitation. Rarely, leukopenia, thrombocytopenia, pancytopenia or agranulocytosis may occur. Anaphylaxis and drug fever also have been reported. The various hypersensitivity effects may be caused, in part, by tartrazine in the commercial product. It probably has an addiction liability, as do other carbamates. Persons taking the drug should not drive, operate machinery or undertake activities that require alertness, judgment or mentalization. Elimination is by glucuronidation in the liver. The elimination half-life is 2.3 to 5.1 hr.

Dose—*Oral*, **400** to **800 mg** 2 to 4 times a day.

Dosage Form—Tablets: 400 mg.

Chlorzoxazone

2(3*H*)-Benzoxazolone-, 5-chloro-, Paraflex, Parafon Forte (*McNeil*); (*Various Mfrs*)

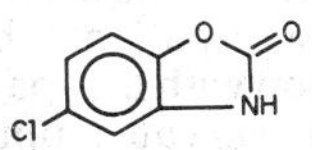

5-Chloro-2-benzoxazolol [95-25-0] $C_7H_4ClNO_2$ (169.58)

Preparation—From 2-amino-5-chlorobenzoxazole (US Pat 2,895,877).

Description—White, crystalline powder; melts about 192°.

Solubility—Sparingly soluble in water; freely soluble in aqueous solutions of alkali hydroxides or ammonia.

Uses—Inhibits polysynaptic reflexes within the spinal cord and subcortical regions of the brain. It is used to decrease muscle tone and tension and thus to relieve spasm and pain associated with musculoskeletal disorders such as fibrositis, bursitis, spondylitis, sprains and muscle injury. It is of little use in spasticity resulting from lesions involving motor neurons or in dyskinetic movement disorders. It also exerts sedative actions, which aid in providing relief.

Adverse effects are infrequent and generally mild. CNS effects include drowsiness, vertigo, lightheadedness, headache, malaise and occasional stimulation. Manifestations of hypersensitivity are rash, petechiae, ecchymosis and, rarely, angioneurotic edema or anaphylaxis. Liver damage possibly occurs, so that it is wise to avoid the drug if there is a history of liver disease. Nausea and vomiting are relatively frequent, and diarrhea and gastrointestinal bleeding also can occur, so that the drug is contraindicated in peptic ulcer. Ethanol or other CNS depressants should not be taken concomitantly.

Absorption time is 3 to 4 hr. The elimination half-life is about 60 min. More than 90% of the drug is glucuronidated in the liver.

Dose—*Oral, adult,* **250 mg** 3 or 4 times a day, except *initially* **500 mg** when pain is severe. It may be increased to **750 mg** 3 or 4 times a day, if necessary; *children,* **20 mg/kg** or **600 mg/m²** per day in 3 or 4 divided doses or 125 to 500 mg 3 or 4 times a day.

Dosage Form—Tablets: 250 and 500 mg.

Cyclobenzaprine Hydrochloride

1-Propanamine, 3-(5*H*-dibenzo[*a,d*]cyclohepten-5-ylidene)-*N,N*-dimethyl-, hydrochloride; Flexeril (*MSD*)

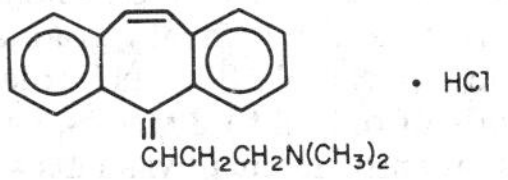

N,N-Dimethyl-5*H*-dibenzo[*a,d*]cycloheptene-$\Delta^{5,\gamma}$-propylamine hydrochloride [6302-23-9] $C_{20}H_{21}N.HCl$ (311.85).

Preparation—Cyclobenzaprine may be synthesized by Grignard addition of α-dimethylaminopropylmagnesium chloride to 10,11-dihydro-5*H*-dibenzo[*a,d*]cycloheptene-5-one, followed by elimination of water from the resulting tertiary carbinol (Villani *et al, J Med Pharm Chem 5:* 373, 1962; see also Winthrop *et al, J Org Chem 27*:230, 1962).

Description—White, crystalline powder; melts at about 217°; pK_a 8.47 (cyclobenzaprine).

Solubility—Freely soluble in water or alcohol.

Uses—Depresses suprasegmental (upper) motor neurons in the brainstem and, to some degree, spinal motor neurons to decrease reflex skeletal muscle activity and tonus. It inhibits both the alpha and gamma motor systems. It is used to diminish spasm and pain associated with *musculoskeletal disorders* and to increase the range of movement. The drug also has weak antimuscarinic activity.

Frequent side effects include sedation, dry mouth and dizziness. Weakness, fatigue, insomnia, unpleasant taste and other paresthesias, blurred vision, tachycardia, nausea and dyspepsia are less frequent. Rarely, there may be headache, nervousness, confusion, disorientation, tremors, ataxia, depression or euphoria, hallucinations, dyspnea, sweating, constipation, urinary difficulty and retention, dysarthria and various allergic reactions (eg, rash, urticaria and facial edema). The drug should be used with care in the presence of MAOIs, CNS depressants (including ethanol) and when antimuscarinic drugs also are being given. It is contraindicated in narrow-angle glaucoma, when there is prostatic hypertrophy, after myocardial infarction or during congestive heart failure, heart block, conduction disturbances, tachydysrhythmias and thyrotoxicosis.

It is absorbed erratically. The onset of action is about 1 hr. It is highly bound to plasma albumin. It is biotransformed and conjugated to glucuronides in the liver. The elimination half-life is 1 to 3 days. Very little is excreted unchanged into the urine, but some is excreted into milk.

Dose—*Oral, adult* and *children 15 yr* or older, usually **10 mg** 3 times a day, but ranges from **20** to **40 mg** a day. The duration of treatment should not exceed 2 to 3 wk.

Dosage Form—Tablets: 10 mg.

Diazepam—page 1157.

Meprobamate—page 1169.

Metaxalone

2-Oxazolidinone, 5-[(3,5-dimethylphenoxy)methyl]-, Skelaxin (*Carnrick*)

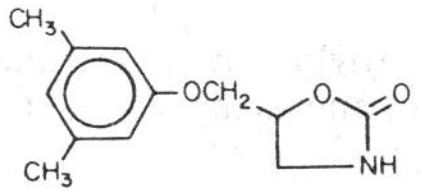

[1665-48-1] $C_{12}H_{15}NO_3$ (221.26)

Preparation—Described in *J Am Chem Soc 82:* 1166, 1960; US Pat 3,062,827.

Description—White, crystalline powder; melts at about 123°.

Solubility—Very slightly soluble in water; soluble in alcohol; freely soluble in chloroform.

Uses—Reputed to have muscle relaxant properties with a CNS focus of action. Marketed for relief of acute muscle spasm resulting from various injuries or strains, but its efficacy is in serious question, and there seems to be no reason to use the drug in lieu of drugs that obviously are more effective. Furthermore, its toxicity is greater than that of more efficacious drugs; toxic effects include anorexia, nausea, vomiting, vertigo, drowsiness, nervousness, mental confusion, dry mouth, urinary retention, pruritus, dermatitis, rarely leukopenia, anemia and jaundice, and possible pyuria, albuminuria and nephrolithiasis. It may exacerbate grand mal epilepsy. It should not be used when there is anemia, liver or renal disease or in persons with a history of such disease. Peak blood levels occur in about 2 hr; the duration of action is 4 to 6 hr. Elimination is by hepatic metabolism; the half-life is 2 to 3 hr.

Dose—*Oral, adult,* **2.4** to **3.2 g** a day in 3 or 4 divided doses for no more than 10 consecutive days. Safety and effectiveness in children 12 yr and below have not been established.

Dosage Form—Tablets: 400 mg.

Methocarbamol

1,2-Propanediol, 3-(2-methoxyphenoxy)-, 1-carbamate; Neuraxin; Robaxin (*Robins*)

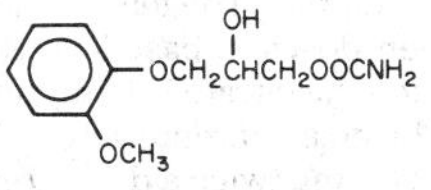

3-(*o*-Methoxyphenoxy)-1,2-propanediol 1-carbamate [532-03-6] $C_{11}H_{15}NO_5$ (241.24).

Preparation—3-(*o*-Methoxyphenoxy)-1,2-propanediol participates in a transesterification reaction with ethyl carbonate in the presence of an alkaline catalyst to eliminate ethanol and produce the cyclic carbonate of the starting diol. Subsequent treatment with ammonia ruptures the cyclic carbonate ring and forms the primary carbamate of the starting compound. US Pat 2,770,649.

Description—Fine, white powder; odorless or has a slight characteristic odor; melts between 93° and 97°.

Solubility—1 g in 40 mL water; freely soluble in alcohol; sparingly soluble in chloroform.

Uses—A *centrally acting muscle relaxant.* After parenteral administration, its action is prompt and intense enough to *facilitate orthopedic procedures.* It is used in the *treatment of muscle spasm* resulting from injury, musculoskeletal disorders, tetanus and other disorders. It has been used with limited success in the treatment of *paralysis agitans, cerebral palsy, multiple sclerosis* and *cerebrovascular accidents* (with spastic manifestations). Side effects by the oral route include drowsiness, vertigo, headache, fever, rash, itching, urticaria, gastrointestinal upsets and, rarely, syncope. After parenteral administration there also may be flushing, headache, muscular incoordination, nystagmus, diplopia, hypotension, bradycardia and metallic taste. These effects are minimized if the injection is given slowly at a rate of less than 300 mg/min and no more than 200 mg/injection. Extravasated injections are locally irritating and may cause sloughing or thrombophlebitis. The vehicle for commercial solutions, 50% polyethylene glycol 300, causes uremia in persons with renal dysfunction, and parenteral administration is contraindicated in the presence of renal disease. It should be avoided in pregnancy and in nursing mothers.

It is erratic by the oral route, probably owing to first-pass metabolism. Peak concentration occurs in about 30 min. Most of the drug is metabolized with an elimination half-life of 1 to 2 hr.

Dose—*Oral, initially* **1.5** to **2 g** 4 times a day for the first 2 or 3 days, then 2.25 to 4.5 g a day in 3 to 4 divided doses. The dose for children under 12 yr has not been established. *Intramuscular,* alternately into the gluteus maximi, **1 g** every 8 hours. *Intravenous,* **1** to **3 g** a day given at a rate not exceeding 3 mL (0.3 g)/min. It should not be given for more than 3 consecutive days; it may be resumed after a drug-free interval of 2 days.

Dosage Forms—Injection: 1 g/10 mL; Tablets: 500 and 750 mg.

Orphenadrine Citrate

N,N-Dimethyl-2-[(2-methylphenyl)phenylmethoxy]-, Ethaneamine, 2-hydroxy-1,2-3-propanetricarboxylate (1:1); Norflex (*Riker*)

$(CH_3)_2NCH_2CH_2OCH$ · $HO-C(CH_2COOH)_2-COOH$

[4682-36-4] $C_{18}H_{23}NO.C_6H_8O_7$ (461.51).

Preparation—From 2-methylbenzhydrol and 2-(dimethylamino)ethanol; the base is converted to the salt with citric acid (US Pat 2,991,225).

Description—White, crystalline powder; melts at about 136°.

Solubility—About 1 g in 70 mL water or 400 mL alcohol.

Uses— Orphenadrine, a methyl analog of the antihistamine diphenhydramine, has weak antihistaminic and mild antimuscarinic activities. The drug reduces voluntary muscle spasm by a central effect. Indications for the citrate are as an adjunct for relief of discomfort associated with acute painful musculoskeletal conditions, by a mode of action not clearly identified but that may be related to the analgesic properties of the compound. It does not directly relax tense skeletal muscles in man. It sometimes induces mild excitement and also a mild euphoria in fatigued or depressed patients. Peripheral atropine-like actions are weak, but blurred vision, dry skin and dry mouth may occur. Other side effects include nausea, vertigo, rash, headache, dizziness, drowsiness, constipation, increased intraocular pressure, weakness, mental confusion and occasional hallucinations. It is contraindicated in patients with acute-angle closure glaucoma or myasthenia gravis. It should be used cautiously in patients with gastrointestinal obstruction, urinary retention, urinary tract obstruction or tachycardia; propoxyphene appears to interact to increase mental confusion, anxiety and tremors. The manufacturer's recommendation of a longer interval between doses is based on the retarding effect of the plasticized matrix in which the citrate is compounded in the tablet dosage form. The citrate may be given parenterally.

Dose—*Oral, adult,* **100 mg** twice a day. *Intramuscular* or *intravenous,* **60 mg** every 12 hr, as necessary.

Dosage Forms—Injection: 30 mg/mL; Tablets: 100 mg.

Orphenadrine Hydrochloride—see RPS-18, page 923.

Propranolol Hydrochloride—page 1016.

Quinine Sulfate—page 1323.

Antiparkinson Drugs

Some kinds of spasticity and involuntary movement arise from disorders within discrete nervous structures which contain neurons predominately of one or two transmitter types. These disorders may be controlled more selectively by drugs directed at the particular neurotransmitters. Parkinsonism (paralysis agitans) is an example of a disorder that lends itself to such specific treatment; the antiparkinson drugs are not interneuron depressants.

The disorder in parkinsonism lies mostly within the substantia nigra and corpus striatum. The cells in the substantia nigra, which connect to the corpus striatum, are mostly dopaminergic and inhibitory; in parkinsonism, the substantia nigra is deficient in dopamine. Striatal neurons that feed back upon the nigral cells are cholinergic and excitatory. Therefore, intervention with either dopaminergic or antimuscarinic drugs is capable of enhancing nigrostriatal activity and improving the condition. Dopaminergic intervention is the more effective, especially against the rigidity. L-Dopa and amantadine exert dopaminergic influences. Used alone, the antimuscarinic drugs are second- or third-order drugs, showing efficacy in fewer than 25% of patients, but they often are used effectively in combination with L-dopa or amantadine.

The antimuscarinic drugs can suppress the extrapyramidal effects of the antipsychotic drugs (phenothiazines, reserpine, etc), but since they mask the tardive dyskinesias, they should not be used chronically with such drugs.

Amantadine Hydrochloride

Tricyclo[3.3.1.1^{3,7}]decan-1-amine, hydrochloride; Symmetrel (*Du Pont*)

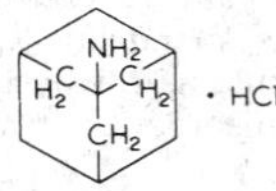

1-Adamantanamine hydrochloride [665-66-7] $C_{10}H_{17}N.HCl$ (187.71).

Preparation—Adamantane is brominated to the 1-bromo compound, which is then reacted with acetonitrile in the presence of sulfuric acid to produce *N*-(1-adamantanyl)acetamide. Alkaline hydrolysis liberates amantadine, which is reacted with hydrogen chloride in a suitable solvent to yield the official salt.

Description—White or nearly white, odorless, crystalline powder; bitter taste; stable in light, heat and air; does not melt up to 300°, but sublimes slowly; pK_a (30°) 10.36; pH (1 in 5 solution) between 3.0 and 5.5.

Solubility—1 g in 2.5 mL water, 5.1 mL alcohol, 18 mL chloroform or 70 mL polyethylene glycol 400.

Uses—Possesses both antiparkinsonism and antiviral activity, having been introduced as an antiviral agent. Its use in the *prophylaxis* of A_2 *influenza virus infection* (*Asian flu*) is less well-established and discussed in Chapter 76.

In the brain, it appears to block the reuptake of dopamine at dopaminergic nerve terminals, thus increasing the concentration of dopamine at the synapses. This facilitates the function of the remaining nigrostriatal neuronal pathways in patients with parkinsonism. It is inferior to levodopa but somewhat superior to the antimuscarinic drugs. Patients sometimes are improved dramatically, but the usual response is moderate to mediocre. Even when the response is excellent, usually after 6 to 8 weeks of continuous treatment the efficacy gradually wanes, and control may be lost between month 2 and 18. Such tolerance is minimal if the drug is used for periods of only 2 to 3 weeks, separated by intervals of several weeks. Consequently, many physicians administer the drug only for short periods, when the patient requires additional treatment. In combination with levodopa, better control is maintained than with either agent alone.

It may cause hyperexcitability, tremors, anxiety, ataxia, slurring of speech, insomnia, drowsiness, lethargy, psychic depression, vertigo and postural hypotension. Less frequently, it may induce dry mouth, constipation, abdominal pain, nausea, vomiting, headache, dizziness, dyspnea, fatigue and urinary retention. Dermatitis, pruritus and livedo reticularis occasionally occur. Edema, which may precipitate cardiac congestion, is not infrequent. Confusion and visual hallucinations are seen, especially if the recommended dose is exceeded. Alkaline phosphatase in the blood may be elevated. It exaggerates the peripheral effects of the antimuscarinic drugs used during treatment. The drug is contraindicated in epileptics. There are indications that the drug may increase the incidence of measles. Medicated persons should avoid driving or other tasks in which safety depends upon alertness.

Orally, it is absorbed rapidly and completely. Over 90% is excreted in the urine unchanged. The elimination half-life is 10 to 37 hr; the half-life is pH-dependent, being increased at higher urine pH. It also is increased in renal impairment. It crosses the placental barrier and also is excreted into milk.

Dose—*Oral, adults and children 12 yr* or older, *antidyskinetic, initially* **100 mg** 1 or 2 times a day, to be increased up to 400 mg a day if necessary; *antiviral,* **100 mg** 2 times a day or **200 mg** once a day; *children 9 to 12 yr, antiviral,* **100 mg** 2 times a day; *children 1 to 9 yr, antiviral,* **1.5** to **3.0 mg/kg** or **2.2** to **4.4 mg/m²** every 8 hr, not to exceed 200 mg a day.

Dosage Forms—Capsules: 100 mg; Syrup: 50 mg/5 mL.

Benztropine Mesylate

8-Azabicyclo[3.2.1]octane, *endo*-3-(diphenylmethoxy)-, methanesulfonate; Benztropine Methanesulfonate; Cogentin (*MSD*)

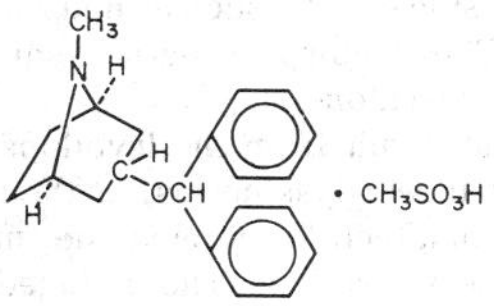

3α-(Diphenylmethoxy)-1αH,5αH-tropane methanesulfonate [132-17-2] $C_{21}H_{25}NO.CH_4O_3S$ (403.54).

Preparation—Bromodiphenylmethane, formed by bromination of diphenylmethane, is condensed with tropine, using the sodium alkoxide derivative of tropine. After purification, the benztropine base thus obtained is dissolved in a suitable organic solvent and precipitated by reaction with methanesulfonic acid.

Description—White, crystalline powder; colorless; sligtly hygroscopic melts between 141° and 145°; pK_a 10.

Solubility—Very soluble in water; freely soluble in alcohol; very slightly soluble in ether.

Uses—The structure of benztropine resembles both atropine and antihistaminics of the diphenhydramine type. It is thus an *antimuscarinic* drug of potency one-quarter that of atropine sulfate and an antihistaminic of potency equal to that of pyrilamine maleate. It also possesses local anesthetic properties. However, only its central actions to suppress tremor and rigidity are employed therapeutically. These actions are similar to those of atropine but, unlike atropine, it possesses sedative and other effects similar to those of diphenhydramine. Since some patients, particularly the elderly, often are excited by other antiparkinson drugs, the sedative property is of special value. It is used mainly in the treatment of *paralysis agitans* (parkinsonism; see general statement, above) to control tremor and rigidity and also to relieve sialorrhea, oculogyric crises, mask-like facies and pain secondary to muscle spasm. It also is used to treat extrapyramidal dyskinesia, but not tardive dyskinesia, resulting from the use of tranquilizers, such as reserpine or chlorpromazine. It may be used alone or in combination with other drugs.

Side effects include dry mouth, mydriasis, blurred vision, nausea and nervousness and, less frequently, they may include vomiting, mental confusion, ataxia, sedation or excitement, hallucinations, paralysis of some muscle groups, dysphagia, hyperpyrexia, rash and difficulty in urination. As with any antimuscarinic drug, it must be used cautiously in the presence of bladder neck obstruction or glaucoma.

Dose—*Oral, adult, idiopathic parkinsonism, initially* **0.5 mg** at bedtime, to be increased by weekly increments of 0.5 mg as needed and tolerated, usually to **1** to **2 mg** a day; *postencephalitic parkinsonism, initially* **2 mg** once a day or **1 mg** 2 times a day, to be adjusted as needed or tolerated, usually to **1** to **2 mg** a day; *drug- induced extrapyramidal dyskinesias, initially* **1** to **8 mg** a day in 1 to 3 divided doses, according to the rapidity of onset and severity of dyskinesia, the dose to be adjusted subsequently as needed or tolerated. *Intramuscular or intravenous, parkinsonism, initially* **1** to **2 mg** a day the dose subsequently being adjusted as needed up to the limit of 6 mg a day; *drug-induced extrapyramidal dyskinesias,* **1** to **4 mg** 1 or 2 times a day. *Children 3 yr* or older, dosage must be determined by the physician. Not recommended for children under 3 yr.

Dosage Forms—Injection: 2 mg/2 mL; Tablets: 500 μg and 1 and 2 mg.

Biperiden Hydrochloride

1-Piperidinepropanol, α-bicyclo[2.2.1]hept-5-en-2-yl-α-phenyl-, Hydrochloride; Akineton (*Knoll*)

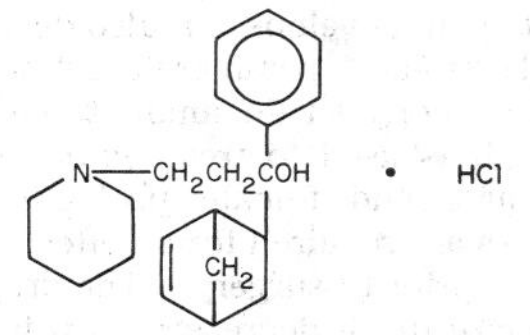

α-5-Norbornen-2-yl-α-phenyl-1-piperidinepropanol [1235-82-1] $C_{21}H_{29}NO.HCl$ (347.93).

Preparation—Acetophenone undergoes Mannich condensation with formaldehyde and piperidine hydrochloride and the resulting 3-piperidinopropiophenone is grignardized in benzene with 5-chloro-2-norbornene to yield the tertiary carbinol, biperiden, which is extracted with methanol. Saturation of the solution with dry HCl yields the salt. US Pat 2,789,110.

Description—White odorless, crystalline powder; decomposes at about 275°; somewhat light-sensitive.

Solubility—Slightly soluble in water, alcohol, chloroform or ether; sparingly soluble in methanol.

Uses—Exerts *antimuscarinic* and *antiparkinson* actions similar to those of trihexyphenidyl, of which biperiden is a congener. In the treatment of *paralysis agitans* (parkinsonism) it reduces tremor, akinesia, muscle rigidity, drooling and sweating. It may also decrease the incidence and severity of oculogyric crises. It sometimes is of value in lessening spasticity in certain disorders of the pyramidal tract, particularly drug-induced extrapyramidal dyskinesia.

Untoward effects result from the antimuscarinic properties and include dry mouth, blurring of vision, urinary retention and heat stroke in hot weather. These effects usually are of low intensity and often do not result in intolerance. Less frequently, there occur drowsiness, dizziness, headache, dysuria, gastric irritation and rash and, rarely, confusion, disorientation, hallucinations or psychotic episodes. The patient should be monitored carefully if glaucoma or urinary bladder neck obstruction exist.

Dose—*Oral, adult, parkinsonism,* **2 mg** 3 or 4 times a day, with adjustments as needed or tolerated; *drug-induced extrapyramidal dyskinesias,* **2 mg** 1 to 3 times a day, with adjustments as needed. Elderly patients are often hyperresponsive and should start with low doses.

Dosage Form—Tablets: 2 mg.

Biperiden Lactate

1-Piperidinepropanol, α-bicyclo[2.2.1]hept-5-en-2-yl-α-phenyl-, compd with 2-hydroxypropanoic acid (1:1); Akineton (*Knoll*)

α-5-Norbornen-2-yl-α-phenyl-1-piperidinepropanol lactate (salt) [7085-45-2] $C_{21}H_{29}NO.C_3H_6O_3$ (401.54). For the structure of the base, see *Biperiden Hydrochloride.*

Preparation—*Biperiden* is reacted with aqueous lactic acid.

Uses—See *Biperiden Hydrochloride.* The lactate is used only to control severe drug-induced extrapyramidal dyskinesias.

Dose—*Intravenous* (slow) or *intramuscular, adult,* **2 mg.** The dose may be repeated every ½-hr until symptoms are controlled, except that no more than four doses should be given in a 24-hr period; *children (intramuscular only), initially* **0.04 mg/kg** or **1.2 mg/m²,** to be repeated every ½ hr, if necessary, up to a total of 4 doses.

Dosage Form—Injection: 5 mg/1 mL.

Bromocriptine Mesylate

Ergotaman-3′,6′,18-trione methanesulfonate; Parlodel (*Sandoz*)

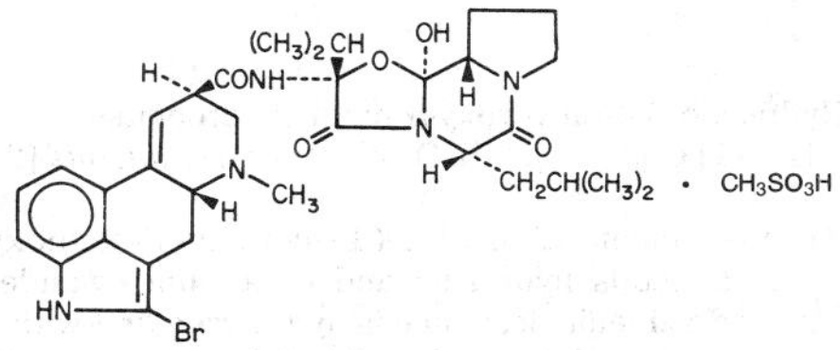

2-Bromoergocryptine monomethanesulfonate (salt) [22260-51-1] $C_{32}H_{40}BrN_5O_5.CH_3SO_3H$ (750.70).

Preparation—From N-bromosuccinimide and α-ergocryptine (US Pat 3,752,814).

Description—Yellowish-white, crystalline powder; melts about 194° with decomposition; $pK_a = 4.90$.

Solubility—Soluble in water or chloroform; very soluble in benzene or hexane; poorly soluble in most organic solvents.

Uses—Bromocriptine is the 2-bromo derivative of α-ergocryptine. Like all of the ergot alkaloids, it has dopamine-like agonist activity. In the treatment of *parkinsonism* it is used to supplement levodopa, when refractoriness to that agent develops. It also decreases the secretion of prolactin, presumably by its dopaminergic actions in the median eminence; some authorities consider dopamine to be the prolactin release-inhibiting hormone. It is used to treat *galactorrhea* and associated *amenorrhea* and male and female prolactin-induced *infertility*. Approximately 4 weeks are required for an effect to peak. It is used to *shrink prolactinomas* prior to surgery. The drug also is used to *suppress postpartum lactation*. It decreases growth hormone secretion in *acromegaly* and is used to treat that disorder, mostly as an adjunct to radiotherapy or surgery; used alone, only a low percentage of remissions occur. It also has been used in the management of senile depression and related disorders.

The incidence of adverse effects seems to differ according to the particular clinical disorder, even when the same dosage regimen is used. When it is used to treat galactorrhea/amenorrhea/female infertility, nearly 70% of recipients have adverse effects, whereas only about 23% have adverse effects when the drug is used to suppress physiological lactation. Adverse effect-related discontinuation of treatment occurs in 3 to 7% of cases. In parkinsonism, the incidence is complicated by the concomitant administration of levodopa. Nausea is the most frequent side effect (51%) in galactorrhea but occurs in only 7% in the postpartum patient. The incidences of other side effects are: headache, 10 to 18%; dizziness, 8 to 16%; postural hypotension, up to 28%; vomiting, 3 to 5%; fatigue, 1 to 7%; diarrhea, 0.4 to 3%; nasal congestion, up to 5%. Other less-frequent side effects (mostly in parkinsonism) are occasional syncope, urinary frequency and incontinence, dyskinesias, visual disturbances, paresthesias, anxiety, nightmares, anorexia, depression, convulsions, cutaneous vasoconstriction, mottling of the skin and Raynaud's phenomenon, muscle cramps, ataxia, erythromyalgia and rashes. There may be elevations in BUN, alkaline phosphatase, urate, CPK, SGOT, SGPT and GPT, which usually are transient. It is teratogenic and also may induce spontaneous abortions. The drug is contraindicated in angina pectoris, peripheral vascular disease, pregnancy and if sensitivity to ergot alkaloids exists. Since it has been reported to cause delusions and hallucinations in post-schizophrenics, it also should be withheld in patients with a history of psychoses.

Although about 28% of an oral dose is absorbed from the gut, only 6% reaches the systemic circulation, because of first-pass metabolism. One to 2 hr are required for onset of action; action persists for 6 to 14 hr.

Dose—*Oral, adult,* for *galactorrhea, postpartum suppression of lactation* or *infertility, initially* **1.5** to **2.5 mg** a day with meals, to be increased gradually over a period of a week to as much as **2.5 mg** 2 or 3 times a day. In the postpartum patient, treatment is for 2 weeks; in galactorrhea/amenorrhea, treatment is for 6 months. In female infertility, barrier contraceptives should be used until a normal cycle has occurred (to protect a possible unknown pregnancy); if menstruation does not occur within 3 days of the expected date, the drug should be discontinued and a pregnancy test given. For *pituitary prolactinoma,* **5** to **20 mg** a day in divided doses. For *parkinsonism, initially* **1.5** to **2.5 mg** a day, to be increased by increments of **2.5 mg**/day at bi- to quadra-weekly intervals, often to, and rarely exceeding, a total of 100 mg a day.

Dosage Forms—Capsules: 5 mg; Tablets: 2.5 mg.

Carbidopa

Benzenepropanoic acid, (*S*)-α-hydrazino-3,4-dihydroxy-α-methyl-, monohydrate, ing of Sinemet (*DuPont*)

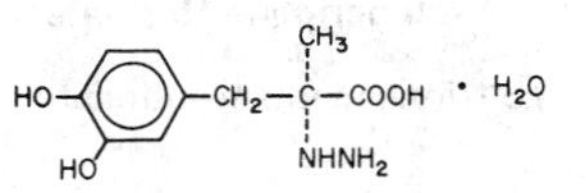

(−)-L-α-Hydrazino-3,4-dihydroxy-α-methylhydrocinnamic acid monohydrate [38821-49-7] $C_{10}H_{14}N_2O_4 \cdot H_2O$ (244.25); *anhydrous* [28860-95-9] (226.23).

Preparation—Condensation of 1-(4′-hydroxy-3′-methoxyphenyl)-2-propanone with aqueous hydrazine and potassium cyanide forms the corresponding hydrazinenitrile, which is hydrolyzed first with HCl to convert the nitrile to amide and then refluxed with HBr to convert the amide to carboxyl and the methoxy group to OH, yielding the DL-form of carbidopa (Sletzinger *et al, J Med Chem 6:* 101, 1963). To obtain the L-form, one method involves acylation of the aforementioned hydrazinenitrile and resolution with 1-menthoxyacetyl chloride, producing crystals which on hydrolysis yield the levorotatory compound (Karady *et al, J Org Chem 36:* 1946, 1949, 1971).

Description—White to creamy white powder; odorless or practically odorless, melts at about 205° with decomposition; pK_a 2.3, 7.3.

Solubility—Slightly soluble in water; practically insoluble in alcohol, chloroform or ether; freely soluble in 3*N* hydrochloric acid.

Uses—An inhibitor of L-aromatic amino acid decarboxylase, often called dopa-decarboxylase. It has no direct therapeutic actions of its own but, rather, is used only to *protect levodopa* and *L-5-hydroxytryptophan,* both of which are decarboxylated by aromatic amino acid decarboxylase. Levodopa is 95% decarboxylated in the periphery.

It does not enter the central nervous system in concentrations sufficient to inhibit aromatic amino acid decarboxylase, so that its action is limited to the periphery, which is precisely what is desired. It is essential that levodopa and 5-hydroxytryptophan be decarboxylated in the brain to their respective biogenic amine products, dopamine and serotonin (5-hydroxytryptamine), which are the active agents. But in the periphery it is not desirable that these amino acids be decarboxylated, since decarboxylation not only lowers the concentration of aromatic amino acid available to the brain but also raises the concentrations of the amine products in the periphery, which give rise to some of the untoward effects of the aromatic amino acids. When it is given concomitantly with levodopa, only about 25% as much levodopa need be given, the onset of response is more rapid, pyridoxine no longer suppresses the efficacy, dietary control no longer is necessary and certain side effects, such as nausea, vomiting and natriuresis, are diminished. The combination permits smoother control of parkinsonism than with levodopa alone.

The side effects that result from the levodopa-derived amines in the brain (psychic disturbances, dyskinesias) or the static hypotension, cardiac arrhythmias are not affected. Indeed, they may occur sooner and be more serious if the dose of levodopa is not reduced sufficiently.

In the approved doses, it does not appear to cause adverse effects, even though the production in the periphery of dopamine and serotonin, which have natural physiological roles in the periphery, may be diminished. Therefore, side effects, precautions and contraindications of a combination of levodopa and carbidopa are those of levodopa (see page 1037).

The drug may be given with levodopa from the outset of levodopa therapy or added after levodopa therapy is in progress. Since inhibition of peripheral dopa decarboxylase approximately quadruples the availability of levodopa to the brain, it is advisable to reduce ongoing levodopa dosage when adding this drug. Consequently, levodopa first should be discontinued for at least 8 hr and then begun again at 20 to 25% of the previous effective dose. Although it is available in a single-entity preparation to add to levodopa, it is simpler to employ a fixed-dose combination of the two. Fixed-dose ratios of 1/10 and 2.5/10 are available. Carbidopa saturates dopa decarboxylase in daily doses of about 70 to 100 mg. It occurs that some dosage schedules for the fixed-dose combination fail to provide a sufficient amount of this drug, and there may be persistence of some of the peripheral adverse effects of levodopa. This is especially the case when the daily dose of levodopa is less than 700 mg. Therefore, there is a place for single-entity preparation in the correction of such shortfalls of this drug. The approved dosage limit for it is 200 mg a day.

Dose (*single-entity* carbidopa)—*Oral, adult,* **12.5** to **25 mg** of carbidopa added to the first dose of levodopa each day and/or subsequent doses as appropriate to achieve a total daily dose of carbidopa of 70 to 100 mg.

Dose (as carbidopa/levodopa)—*Oral, adult, beginning levadopa therapy, initially* **10 mg** carbidopa/**100 mg** levodopa 3 times a day, to be adjusted subsequently every other day or every day by adding 10 mg carbidopa/100 mg levodopa a day until 60 mg carbidopa/600 mg levodopa a day is reached, after which further increments are achieved by substituting 25 mg carbidopa/100 mg levodopa and eventually 25 mg carbidopa/250 mg levodopa; *substitution of carbidopa/levadopa for* single-entity *levodopa* for a patient previously *having required less than 1.5 g levodopa/day, initially* **10 mg** carbidopa/**100 mg** levodopa *or* **25 mg** carbidopa/**100 mg** levodopa 3 or 4 times a day, to be adjusted every other day or every day as needed and tolerated; for a patient previously *having required over 1.5 g levodopa a day, initially* **250 mg** carbidopa/**250 mg** levodopa 3 or 4 times a day, to be adjusted every other day or every day as needed and tolerated.

Dosage Forms—Carbidopa and Levodopa Tablets: 10 mg carbidopa/100 mg levodopa, 25 mg carbidopa/100 mg levodopa and 25 mg carbidopa/250 mg levodopa. Sustained-Release Tablets: 50 mg carbidopa/200 mg levodopa.

Diphenhydramine—page 1225.

Ethopropazine Hydrochloride

Phenothiazine, 10-[2-(Diethylamino)propyl] monohydrochloride; Parsidol (*Parke-Davis*)

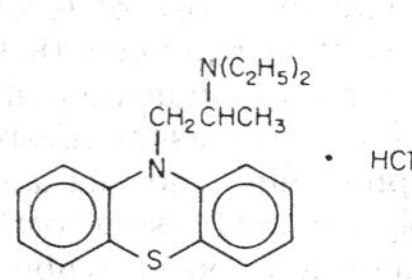

[1094-08-2] $C_{19}H_{24}N_2S.HCl$ (348.93).

Preparation—2-(Diethylamino)propyl bromide is converted to a Grignard complex and reacted with phenothiazine to give ethopropazine base. US Pat 2,607,773.

Description—A white or off-white, crystalline powder; melts at about 210° with decomposition.

Solubility—Slightly soluble in water; soluble in alcohol or chloroform.

Uses—A phenothiazine with both antimuscarinic and antihistaminic properties; used in the management of *paralysis agitans*, (parkinsonism) especially for control of rigidity. However, it also may diminish spasm, tremor and sialorrhea and prevent oculogyric crises. Except for its effects on oculogyric crises, authorities consider it to be inferior to other antimuscarinic drugs used to treat parkinsonism, and it causes as many or more side effects, including exacerbation of parkinsonism. Side effects include sedation, vertigo, lassitude, inability to concentrate, confusion, dry mouth, blurred vision and epigastric distress. Less-frequent effects are paresthesias, heavy feeling in the limbs, ataxia, muscular cramps, rash, hypotension (in large doses) and, rarely, agranulocytosis; symptoms of parkinsonism are sometimes worsened. It should be used cautiously in patients who drive, operate machinery or who have glaucoma, urinary tract obstruction or gastrointestinal obstruction. It can enhance the central depression caused by sedative-hypnotic drugs or antihistamines, and such untoward drug interactions should be avoided.

Dose—*Oral, initially* **50 mg** 1 or 2 times a day; increase gradually if necessary. Patients with mild to moderate symptoms frequently are controlled with **100** to **400 mg** a day. Severe cases may require doses gradually increased to **500** or **600 mg** or more a day.

Dosage Form—Tablets: 10 and 50 mg.

Hyoscyamine Sulfate—page 1023

Levodopa

L-Tyrosine, 3-hydroxy-, L-Dopa; Bendopa (*ICN*); Dopar (*Roberts*); Larodopa (*Roche*); ing of Sinemet (*Du Pont*)

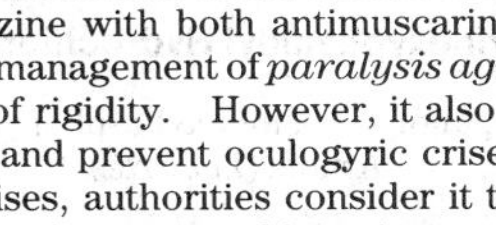

(−)-3-(3,4-Dihydroxyphenyl)-L-alanine [59-92-7] $C_9H_{11}NO_4$ (197.19).

Preparation—By indirect resolution of DL-3-(3,4-dihydroxyphenyl)alanine (DL-dopa). One method first converts this to DL-*N*- acetyl-3-methoxy-4-acetoxyphenylalanine and then resolves the latter with the aid of α-phenethylamine. Hydrolysis of the desired enantiomer with aqueous HBr yields levodopa. The starting DL- dopa may be synthesized commencing with vanillin and glycine.

Description—Fine, white to off-white, crystalline powder; oxidized by atmospheric oxygen in the presence of moisture and darkens; melts at about 280° with decomposition; pK_a 2.3, 8.7, 9.7, 13.4.

Solubility—1 g in 10 mL 0.1*N* HCl, 250 mL water, about 555 mL alcohol or 1000 mL chloroform.

Uses—The single most important drug in the treatment of incapacitating *paralysis agitans* (parkinsonism). The neurochemical basis was indicated in the introductory statement. It also is effective in nonincapacitating parkinsonism, but its cost and side effects are such that its use is not warranted in many patients. Approximately 65 to 80% of patients are improved, some quite dramatically. The greatest effects are on rigidity and hypokinesia. Sialorrhea, dysphagia, seborrhea, postural instability, speech difficulties and glabellar reflexes usually are suppressed and may be abolished. Tremor and akinesia respond only erratically and require prolonged treatment, up to 6 months, before improvement ensues. All forms of parkinsonism respond; the idiopathic form responds best, but the postencephalitic form responds to lower doses; paradoxically, the postencephalitic patient may experience more severe adverse effects, including exacerbation of oculogyric crises, than patients with idiopathic or other forms of the disease. Consequently, postencephalitic patients require a conservative dosage regimen that increases the dose quite slowly. Levodopa also is used to treat the parkinsonism-like neurological syndrome of *manganese intoxication*, in which there is also a deficiency of dopamine in the basal ganglia.

It is 40 to 70% absorbed orally. Less than 1% penetrates into the brain. There, and throughout the body, it is 99% decarboxylated to dopamine. Concurrent carbidopa (above) administration prevents peripheral decarboxylation and enhances availability to the brain. Peak concentrations of dopamine in the brain occur 1 to 2 hr after administration. The plasma half-life of levodopa alone is 0.5 to 1 hr; in combination with carbidopa it is 1.2 to 2.3 hr.

Nearly every patient experiences untoward effects, but only 5% find it desirable or necessary to discontinue medication. Nausea will occur in virtually all and anorexia, vomiting, flatulence, epigastric pain and dry mouth in the majority of patients. Peptic ulceration and gastrointestinal bleeding sometimes occur. With a slow increase in dosage, the gastrointestinal side effects are less severe, and tolerance tends to develop. If nausea and vomiting are intolerable, they may be managed with non-phenothiazine-, non-pyridoxine-containing antiemetics. The second most common type of side effect is the appearance of abnormal involuntary movements, which usually start with the face and tongue and gradually move downward to involve the arms, hands and trunk. These dyskinesias are most severe 1 to 2 hr after administration. These effects are not seen immediately but progress slowly over a year's time. Eventually, nearly 75% of patients will show some such movements; however, most patients accept such movements as the price of increased mobility. The involuntary movements can be decreased by lowering the dose or the use of haloperidol or pyridoxine, but these recourses also abolish the therapeutic response to this drug. Hypotension occurs in about 75% and orthostatic hypotension in about 30% of recipients, but vertigo and syncope are uncommon. Cardiac arrhythmias occur occasionally. After 2 or 3 mo, tolerance develops. Increased myocardial contractility, tachycardia and atrial fibrillation may occur. Behavioral changes frequently accompany treatment. Increased central nervous excitability, with nervousness, anxiety, insomnia, vivid dreams, tremor and flushing occur. Paranoid ideation, delusions, hallucinations (often olfactory), delirium and loss of judgment sometimes occur. Easy sexual arousal and loss of sexual inhibitions are common; in part this is the result of the emergence of normal desire long suppressed by physical incapacity. Serum glutamic oxaloacetate transaminase and glutamic pyruvate transaminase may be elevated somewhat early during therapy, but they usually subside later. Transient granulocytopenia may occur; agranulocytosis no longer seems to be an adverse effect since the dextro form was removed from the preparations. Dental caries is accelerated, and fillings often fall out, perhaps because the buffering effect of sialorrhea is diminished. Other miscellaneous side effects include increased pain, when pain-producing pathology or headache exists, sweating, alopecia, cough, hoarseness, urinary frequency, incontinence or retention, nocturia, mydriasis, blurred vision, Horner's syndrome, fever, hot flashes and loss or gain in weight. A mild natriuresis occurs, probably as the result of the action of dopamine formed in the kidney. Thrombocytopenia occurs rarely after long-term treatment.

Pyridoxine antagonizes levodopa, possibly by promoting premature decarboxylation (as a coenzyme to dopa decarboxylase), before levodopa has penetrated into the brain. Some antagonism occurs with even as little as a Recommended Dietary Allowance, so that patients should not take multivitamin supplements containing pyridoxine. To what extent some of the side effects of the CNS are attributable to pyridoxine deficiency is not known. Carbidopa prevents antagonism by pyridoxine. Methyldopa and reserpine, which interfere with catecholamine synthesis and storage, exacerbate the parkinson syndrome and, hence, antagonize levodopa. Tricyclic antidepressants and monoamine oxidase inhibitors given concomitantly evoke hypertensive crises and may precipitate many of the adverse side effects of the CNS, because they increase the local concentrations of dopamine formed from levodopa. Such drugs should be discontinued 2 wk prior to taking levodopa. Antacids decrease gastric emptying time and, thereby, promote absorption, thus increasing efficacy in some patients. Levodopa is synergized by antimuscarinics.

Levodopa is contraindicated when there is evidence of uncompensated endocrine, renal, hepatic, pulmonary or cardiovascular disease, narrow-angle glaucoma, blood dyscrasia or hypersensitivity to the drug. It should be used cautiously in diabetes, hyperthyroidism, wide-angle glaucoma, epilepsy, hypotension or when antihypertensives are being used. The drug should be discontinued 24 hr prior to anesthesia. Levodopa is a precursor of melanin and may activate latent malignant melanoma; it should be withheld from persons with a history of malignant melanoma or suspicious skin lesions.

Dose—*Oral, adult, initially* **100 mg** to **1 g** a day in divided doses (usually **250 mg** 4 times a day) with meals. The dose is increased gradually in increments of **100** to **750 mg** a day at 3- to 7-day intervals until intolerable side effects occur, usually abnormal movements; the *maintenance* dose is usually **2.5** to **6 g** a day and should not exceed 8 g. After a prolonged period of stabilized response, the dose sometimes can be decreased moderately without loss of control. For doses when used in combination with carbidopa, see *Carbidopa*, above.

Dosage Forms—Capsules: 100, 250 and 500 mg; Tablets: 100, 250 and 500 mg.

Pergolide Mesylate

Ergoline-, [8-(methylthio) methyl]-6-propyl-, methanesulfonate salt, Permax (*Lilly*)

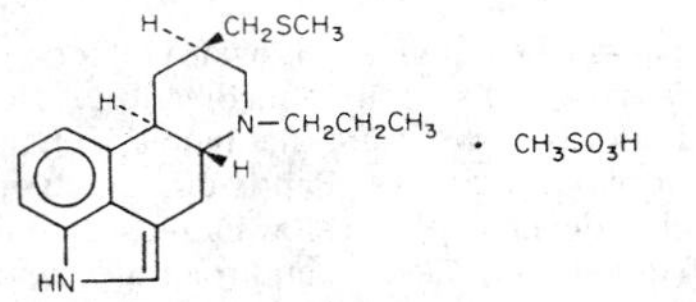

[66104-23-2] $C_{19}H_{26}N_2S.CH_4O_3S$ (410.59).

Preparation—See US Pat 4,166,182.

Description—White solid; melts at 207°.

Uses—Has actions and uses like those of bromocriptine (page 1035) and is indicated as an adjunct to levodopa/carbidopa for the management of Parkinson's disease. It has both D_1- and D_2-dopaminergic activity. Side effects include nausea and vomiting, postural hypotension, premature ventricular contractions, confusion and hallucinations, dyskinesias, elevated SGOT, sedation, hallucinations, xerostomia and, rarely, reversible pleural fibrosis. It is likely that other side effects like those of bromocriptine eventually will be reported. The duration of action exceeds 24 hr.

Dose—The optimal doses have yet to be established. *Oral, adult,* for *parkinsonism,* **0.1** to **10 mg** a day, and, for *galactorrhea/amenorrhea/female infertility,* **0.15** to **0.25** mg a day have been reported.

Dosage Form—Tablets: 0.05, 0.25 and 1 mg.

Procyclidine Hydrochloride

1-pyrrolidinepropanol, α-Cyclohexyl-α-phenyl-, hydrochloride; Kemadrin (*Burroughs Wellcome*)

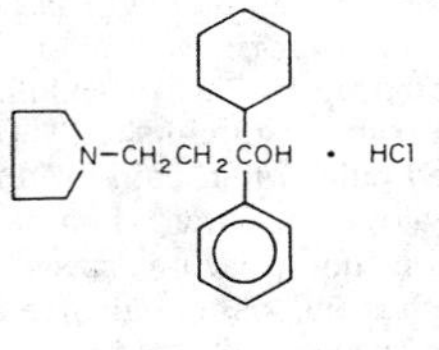

[1508-76-5] $C_{19}H_{29}NO.HCl$ (323.91)

Preparation—From the cyclohexyl Grignard reagent and 3-(1-pyrrolidinyl)propiophenone; the resulting base then converted to the hydrochloride.

Description—White, crystalline powder melts at about 226°.

Solubility—About 1 g in 33 mL water; more soluble in alcohol.

Uses—An antimuscarinic drug used mostly as a substitute for trihexyphenidyl in the treatment of parkinsonism when the latter drug fails to control symptoms. Sometimes it is used in combination with other drugs. The side effects, precautions and contraindications are those of trihexyphenidyl.

Dose—*Oral, adult, initially* **2** to **2.5 mg** 2 or 3 times a day, after meals. The dose may be increased gradually by increments of 2.5 mg a day until symptoms are controlled satisfactorily or intolerable side effects supervene; the usual *maintenance dose is* **10** to **20 mg** a day, but as much as 60 mg may be required.

Dosage Form—Tablets: 5 mg.

Selegiline Hydrochloride

Eldepryl (*Somerset*)

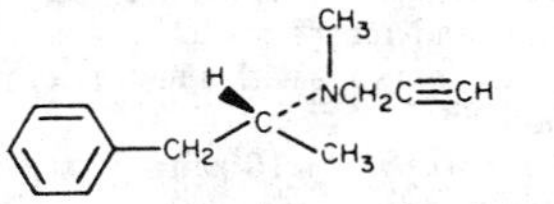

[14611-52-0] $C_{13}H_{17}N.HCl$ (223.78).

Preparation—By reacting propargyl bromide with L-(*N*,α-dimethyl)-phenethylamine and distilling the extracted oil. US Pat 3,496,195.

Description—Oil, boiling point 92 to 93° at 0.8 mm; η_D^{20} 1.518; α_D −11.2°. The HCl salt melts at 141°.

Uses—An inhibitor of monoamine oxidase B, which enzyme is selective for dopamine over norepinephrine and epinephrine. As such, selegiline is an approved adjunct to levodopa for the treatment of parkinsonism. The drug decreases the effective dose of levodopa and smoothes out dose-related fluctuations in efficacy, effects that should rouse only mild interest. However, recent reports indicate that it slows the progress of idiopathic parkinsonism and increases the lifespan of the afflicted. The drug is converted to amphetamine and methamphetamine in the body, which metabolites possibly account for some of the antiparkinson activity. Dyskinesias have been reported to occur in about one-third of users, but this high incidence of adverse effects is undoubtedly the result of failure to reduce the dose of levodopa to which the drug was added. Dry mouth, nausea and dizziness occur in 10 to 20% of cases. Side effects of low incidence are postural hypotension, unpleasant taste, circumoral paresthesias, hallucinations, depression and paranoia.

Dose—*Oral, adult, initially* **5 mg** once a day, to be increased to 10 mg a day or decreased to 5 mg every other day according to response.

Dosage Form—Tablets: 5 mg.

Trihexyphenidyl Hydrochloride

1-Piperidinepropanol, α-cyclohexyl-α-phenyl-, hydrochloride; Artane (*Lederle*)

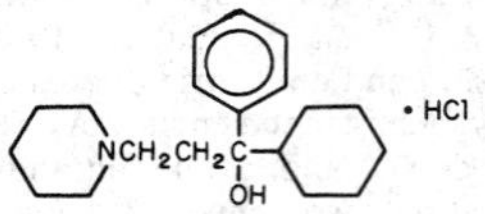

α-Cyclohexyl-α-phenyl-1-piperidinepropanol hydrochloride [52-49-3] $C_{20}H_{31}NO.HCl$ (337.93).

Preparation—From a Mannich reaction of acetophenone, piperidine and formaldehyde. The piperidinopropiophenone formed is treated as for *Procyclidine*.

Description—White or slightly off-white, crystalline powder; no more than a very faint odor; melts between 247° and 253° with slight decomposition.

Solubility—Slightly soluble in water; soluble in alcohol or chloroform.

Use—Has weak *antimuscarinic* and *antispasmodic* activity. In the treatment of parkinsonism it is preferred to levodopa in patients with mild to moderate nonincapacitating symtoms, and most neurologists prefer to begin treatment of all cases with it. It is effective in all forms of the disease, although not uniformly. It is most effective against rigidity, but it also is useful in the relief of akinesia, tremor, sialorrhea and oculogyria. Tolerance may develop, but not necessarily so. It also is useful in the treatment of *drug-induced extrapyramidal dyskinesias*.

The adverse effects mostly derive from its antimuscarinic actions, but they are much less troublesome than with atropine. The most frequent are dry mouth, blurred vision, tachycardia, constipation, dry skin, nervousness, headache, sedation and muscle weakness. Some of these effects subside after continued administration. Sometimes insomnia may occur. Urinary retention is infrequent, but it does occur. Occasionally, vomiting, severe tinnitus, vertigo, suppurative parotitis or rash occur and may require discontinuation of medication. With large doses, inability to concentrate, impaired memory, disorientation and confusion may occur, and if the dose is not reduced, they are followed by agitation, excitement, delirium, visual hallucinations and psychoses. Elderly patients or persons with arteriosclerosis especially are susceptible to the adverse central effects. It should be used cautiously in persons with cardiovascular or liver pathology, glaucoma, bladder neck obstruction, prostatitis, hyperthyroidism or arteriosclerosis and in elderly patients. Trihexyphenidyl may interact with CNS-active antihypertensive drugs, ethanol and other CNS depressants, tricyclic antidepressants, MAOIs, other antimuscarinic drugs, dopamine agonists, dopamine antagonists, phenothiazine and procainamide. When it is used in combination with levodopa, bromocryptine or amantadine, the doses of both drugs in combination may need reduction.

Dose—*Oral, adult, initially* **1 mg** on the first day, after which the dose may be increased in increments of 2 mg a day at intervals of 3 to 5 days until symptoms are controlled adequately without the supervention of serious adverse effects; the *maintenance* dose is usually **6** to **10 mg** a day in 3 to 4 divided doses, but the dose may be even larger if necessary and required, up to a limit of 20 mg. Before timed-release forms are used, the dose with the normal tablet should be established. The drug release-rate of timed-release forms is erratic.

Dosage Forms—Elixir: 2 mg/5 mL; Tablets: 2 and 5 mg; Sustained-release Capsules: 5 mg.

CHAPTER 62

Diuretic Drugs

Glen R Hansen, DDS, PhD

Professor of Pharmacology
College of Pharmacy and School of Medicine
University of Utah
Salt Lake City, UT 84112

Diuretics are drugs which reduce the volume of extracellular fluid, enhance the urinary excretion of sodium chloride and, secondarily, increase the volume of urine excreted by the kidneys. They are used primarily to prevent and alleviate edema and ascites. These conditions occur in diseases of the heart, kidneys and liver. Consequently, diuretics are used in the treatment of edema associated with chronic congestive heart failure, acute pulmonary edema, edema of pregnancy, brain edema and cirrhosis associated with ascites. They also are used in hypertension, diabetes insipidus, renal calculi, hypercalcemia, acute and chronic renal failure and the nephrotic syndrome. Some diuretics have highly *specialized* uses in glaucoma, hyperpotassemia, bromide intoxication, anginal syndrome, epilepsy, migraine and premenstrual depression, conditions in which edema is not present or at least not definitely established. In addition, diuretics sometimes are used to maintain adequate urine volume, as in the case of some severe traumatic injuries, or to reduce the concentration of a noxious agent in the urine in order to minimize renal damage.

The formation of urine from the blood, in simplest terms, consists of glomerular filtration and selective tubular reabsorption and secretion. As the glomerular filtrate passes through the tubules, substances essential to the blood and tissues—water, glucose, salts and amino acids—are reabsorbed. Other substances in the glomerular filtrate, such as urea, are not absorbed as readily by the tubules. Thus, it is thought that in the renal tubule there is a specific mechanism for the transport of each ionic species, the capacities of which are quite different. For example, the capacity of the renal tubule to reabsorb sulfate ion is limited. The tubular capacity for the reabsorption of phosphate is such that sufficient is reabsorbed to maintain the normal extracellular level and any excess is excreted. On the other hand, much larger amounts of bicarbonate ion and chloride ion can be reabsorbed.

Under normal circumstances the glomerular filtration rate is about 100 mL/min. About 99 mL of the fluid is returned to the blood and only 1 mL is excreted as urine. It follows, therefore, that drugs may increase the rate of urine formation in two ways: (1) by increasing glomerular filtration and (2) by depressing tubular reabsorption. Increasing glomerular filtration is *not* an efficient mechanism and usually causes only a moderate increase in urine formation. If, for example, the percent of fluid reabsorbed by the renal tubules is assumed to remain constant, glomerular filtration rate would have to be increased twofold in order to double the urinary output. On the other hand, a 1% decrease in the tubular reabsorption of water, induced either by the administration of excessive quantities of electrolytes or nonelectrolytes (osmotic diuretics) or by agents which alter selective reabsorption of substances in the renal tubules, would double the urinary output.

Most diuretics block sodium and/or chloride reabsorption in the renal tubules. This results in natriuresis and diuresis. However, the mechanism(s) by which diuretics block the reabsorption and the site of action varies; they may act at the proximal tubule, loop of Henle, distal tubule, collecting tubule or combinations of these sites.

Osmotic diuretics are thought to produce diuresis by multiple mechanisms. Mannitol, the most widely used osmotic diuretic, is filtered at the glomerulus and is not reabsorbed by the renal tubules. Because of its osmotic action in the proximal tubules, mannitol prevents the reabsorption of water and impairs sodium reabsorption by lowering the concentration of sodium in the tubular fluid. In the loop of Henle, mannitol reduces medullary hypertonicity by increasing medullary blood flow. In the collecting duct, it reduces sodium and water reabsorption because of papillary washout, high flow rate or some other factor.

Carbonic anhydrase inhibitors (eg, acetazolimide) act on the proximal convolution and possibly the collecting tubule, to inhibit cytoplasmic and brush border carbonic anhydrase. This enzyme catalyzes the reaction: $CO_2 + OH^- \rightleftharpoons HCO_3^-$. The overall inhibition of carbonic anhydrase decreases bicarbonate reabsorption and passive forces favoring chloride reabsorption. The excess chloride (with accompanying sodium) subsequently is reabsorbed in the loop of Henle. However, sodium bicarbonate is excreted but the total diuretic effect is minimal. Although potassium excretion is increased during initial therapy with carbonic anhydrase inhibitors, clinically significant hypokalemia is seldom a problem. After several days of continuous administration, a mild hyperchloremic acidosis develops, which decreases the diuretic effect.

Thiazide diuretics act mainly to block sodium and chloride reabsorption at the *first (thick) portion* of the *distal tubules*. They also have a *mild anti-carbonic anhydrase* effect. The resulting natriuresis is accompanied by increased excretion of potassium (particularly in short-term treatment), bicarbonate, chloride and water. However, glomerular filtration rate actually may be reduced by these drugs causing a problem in patients with diminished renal reserve. Unlike carbonic anhydrase inhibitors, thiazide diuretics are effective even though systemic acidosis or alkalosis may be present. The *antihypertensive* action of the *thiazides* may be attributable to two factors: (1) *depletion of sodium* and subsequent reduction in *plasma volume* and (2) a *decrease in peripheral resistance*. The latter is thought to be due either to the loss of sodium from the arteriolar wall or a direct action on the vascular bed. In addition, there is some *inhibition* of the *pressor activity of norepinephrine*. In contrast, the antihypertensive effect of *chlorthalidone* is thought to be due to a *decreased cardiac output*.

Potassium-sparing diuretics (*spironolactone*, *triamterene* and *amiloride*) interfere with sodium absorption in the late distal tubules and cortical collecting ducts, thereby promoting sodium excretion while conserving potassium. Spironolactone is a competitive inhibitor of aldosterone, whereas triamterene and amiloride interfere directly with electrolyte transport. These agents are not potent diuretics when used alone but, when combined with a thiazide—eg, Aldactizide (*Searle*), they reduce potassium loss, increase sodium excretion and minimize alkalosis. In addition, the onset of diuresis with combination therapy is much more rapid than with spironolactone alone (4 to 7 days).

Loop, or high-ceiling, *diuretics*, such as *furosemide*, *ethacrynic acid* and *bumetanide*, act mainly on the medullary and cortical portions of the *thick ascending loop of Henle* and cause a peak diuresis far greater than that which occurs with other diuretics. This action inhibits electrolyte reabsorption and reduces the osmotic gradient in the renal medulla which in turn impairs both the concentrating and diluting capacities of the kidney. Although initially increasing renal blood flow, the reduction in extracellular fluid volume that is caused by the diuresis can result in a decrease in renal blood flow. Since furosemide also induces significant kaluresis, supplemental administration of potassium often is necessary. Ethacrynic acid induces a greater excretion of chloride than sodium; however, it can produce systemic alkalosis. Ethacrynic acid continues to be effective in the presence of alkalosis. It also is useful in cases of edema refractory to other drugs.

Contraindications and adverse effects resulting from diuretic therapy usually are due to electrolyte imbalance induced by these agents. All commonly employed diuretics can produce acute and chronic sodium depletion, hypokalemia, hyperglycemia and hyperuricemia, as well as alterations in chloride, magnesium and calcium balance. Osmotic diuretics must be used with caution because they can produce a marked increase in extracellular fluid volume and may induce pulmonary edema. Hypersensitivity to diuretic agents frequently is encountered. Also, blood dyscrasias, pancreatitis (thiazides), decreased glucose tolerance (thiazides and ethacrynic acid) and ototoxicity (intravenous ethacrynic acid) occasionally are encountered during diuretic therapy.

Concurrent administration of diuretic agents and other drugs results in some of the most frequently encountered drug *interactions.* A common example is the prescribing of a *cardiac glycoside* and a *diuretic;* the diuretic-induced hypokalemia potentiates the cardiotoxicity of the glycoside. The adverse interaction can be minimized by either increasing potassium intake (potassium supplements, diet or potassium-sparing diuretic) or by administering the diuretic intermittently (allows homeostatic mechanisms to correct imbalance). Other examples of adverse interactions include the following:

Loss of blood sugar control in diabetic patients given thiazides, furosemide or ethacrynic acid.

More intensive skeletal muscle blockade in patients on certain muscle relaxants and hypokalemic-inducing diuretics.

Orthostatic hypotension induced by concurrent administration of methyldopa, guanethidine or a ganglionic blocking agent and a diuretic.

Increased incidence of ototoxicity when patients on aminoglycoside antibiotics (gentamicin, kanamycin, neomycin and streptomycin) are given diuretics reported to cause ototoxicity (ethacrynic acid and furosemide).

Increased incidence of nephrotoxicity when patients on cephaloridine are given diuretics which have nephrotoxic effects (ethacrynic acid and furosemide).

Hyperkalemia when potassium salts are administered with triamterene; disruption of uricosuric therapy by administration of a diuretic which increases plasma uric acid levels (thiazides).

An increased anticoagulant effect induced by displacement of warfarin from protein binding sites (thiazides).

Thoughtful management of these interactions will not only result in improved patient response, but also will spare the patient unnecessary inconvenience and expense.

Agents employed clinically as diuretics may be divided into two groups: (1) osmotic diuretics and (2) renal tubular-inhibiting diuretics. In this presentation a third category, miscellaneous renal agents, is provided for probenecid, an agent which is not a diuretic but inhibits renal tubule reabsorption of uric acid and blocks the renal excretion of a number of substances.

Osmotic Diuretics

The capacity of the renal tubule to reabsorb various electrolytes and nonelectrolytes is limited and, as previously mentioned, varies for each ionic species. If large amounts of these substances are administered to an individual, their concentration in the body fluids and, subsequently, in the glomerular filtrate exceeds the reabsorption capacity of the tubule, and the excess appears in the urine accompanied by an increased volume of water. Traditionally, substances which increase urine formation in this manner are called osmotic diuretics. It is now known, however, that osmotic diuretics, such as mannitol, have several important mechanisms of action. For example, mannitol has been shown to increase renal plasma flow and glomerular hydrostatic pressure secondary to vasodilatation of the afferent arteriole. Thus, it appears that osmotic agents have multiple sites of action; nevertheless, their major component probably is a decrease in medullary solute content resulting in less water reabsorption from the thin descending limb of Henle and collecting duct and less sodium chloride reabsorption in the ascending limb of Henle.

The *major toxic effect* of osmotic diuretics is related to the amount of solute administered and its effect on the volume and distribution of body fluids. For example, following its administration, mannitol is distributed throughout the extracellular fluid; consequently, the administration of hypertonic solutions sufficient to make a significant contribution to extracellular osmolarity will be accompanied by a significant expansion of extracellular fluid volume, largely at the expense of intracellular fluid volume. In edematous states accompanied by diminished cardiac reserve, the use of mannitol introduces a risk which far outweighs any advantages. Also, a variety of signs and symptoms suggestive of hypersensitivity reactions have accompanied the use of some osmotic diuretics.

This group of diuretics includes osmotic electrolytes (potassium and sodium salts), osmotic nonelectrolytes (urea, glycerin and mannitol) and acid-forming salts (ammonium chloride).

Acacia—page 1395.

Ammonium Chloride

Muriate of Ammonia; Sal Ammoniac

Ammonium chloride [12125-02-9] NH_4Cl (53.49).

Preparation—By the following processes: (1) the ammoniacal liquid obtained from gas works during the destructive distillation of coal is neutralized with HCl and the crude product subsequently is purified, (2) the vapors of ammonia from synthetic processes are absorbed in HCl and (3) as a by-product in the Solvay process for sodium bicarbonate.

Description—Colorless crystals, or a white, fine or coarse crystalline powder; cool, saline taste; somewhat hygroscopic; when dissolved in water the temperature of the solution is lowered; pH (1 in 20 solution) between 4.6 and 6.0.

Solubility—1 g in 3 mL water, 100 mL alcohol or 8 mL glycerin.

Uses—A *diuretic, systemic acidifier* and *expectorant.* Ammonium chloride is a combination of a labile cation and a fixed anion. When the ammonium ion is converted to urea, the liberated hydrogen ion reacts with bicarbonate and other body buffers. The end result is that chloride ion displaces bicarbonate ion; the latter is converted to CO_2. Thus, the chloride load to the kidneys is increased and an appreciable amount escapes reabsorption along with an equivalent amount of cation (predominantly sodium) and an isoosmotic quantity of water. This is the basic mechanism by which ammonium chloride brings about a net loss of extracellular fluid and promotes the mobilization of edema fluid.

Ammonium chloride has limited value when used alone for its diuretic effects. It occasionally is combined with a xanthine for short-term relief from temporary water-related weight gain, bloating or edema associated with menstrual periods.

The fact that ammonium chloride causes systemic acidosis makes the salt of some value in the treatment of alkalosis. It also renders the urine acidic and is prescribed for this purpose in conjunction with methenamine. In the rare instances when it is desired to produce an acidosis, ammonium chloride may be used. An example is in the treatment of lead poisoning where an acidosis is desired to hasten the excretion of lead or to treat alkalosis from excessive use of alkalinizing drugs.

Dose—*Adult, oral,* **2** to **12 g** daily; *usual, oral,* **500 mg** to **3 g** 4 times a day; *intravenous,* **100** to **1000 mL** of **2%** solution; *usual, intravenous,* **500 mL** of a **2%** solution is infused over a 3-hr period.

Other Dose Information—The oral dose may vary from 8 to 12 g daily in divided doses. The drug usually is taken with or after meals to avoid gastric irritation.

Dosage Forms—Injection: 2.14% (0.4 mEq/mL) in 500 mL; 26.75%

(5 mEq/mL) in 20 mL vials. Tablets: 500 mg. Enteric-Coated Tablets: 500 mg and 1 g.

Glycerin

1,2,3-Propanetriol; Glycerol; Ophthalgan (*Wyeth-Ayerst*); Osmoglyn (*Alcon*); (*Various Mfrs*)

[56-81-5] $C_3H_8O_3$ (92.09)

Preparation—Obtained in the production of soaps and fatty acids through hydrolysis or by hydration of propylene.

Description—Syrupy liquid with a sweet warm taste; hygroscopic.

Solubility—Completely miscible with water or alcohol; insoluble in most nonpolar solvents.

Uses—An *oral osmotic agent for reducing intraocular pressure*. It is used to interrupt acute attacks of glaucoma and lower intraocular pressure prior to ocular surgery. Because glycerin is rapidly metabolized, it produces little diuresis. Adverse effects include nausea, vomiting, headache, confusion and disorientation. Severe dehydration, cardiac arrhythmias and fatal hyperosmolar nonketotic coma have been reported. Therefore, oral glycerin should be used cautiously in hypervolemia, confused mental states, congestive heart disease and in elderly, senile, diabetic and severely dehydrated individuals. Safety for use in pregnancy, nursing mothers and children has not been established.

Dose—*Usual, oral,* **1** to **1.5 g/kg** 1 to 1½ hr prior to surgery. Total dose should not exceed 120 g.

Dosage Form—50%, lime flavor, in 180 mL; 75% in 120 mL.

Glucose—page 1410.

Glucose, Liquid—page 1410.

Mannitol

Mannite; Manna Sugar; Osmitrol (*Travenol*); (*Various Mfrs*)

HOCH₂–C(H)(OH)–C(H)(OH)–C(OH)(H)–C(OH)(H)–CH₂OH

D-Mannitol [69-65-8] $C_6H_{14}O_6$ (182.17).

Preparation—May be extracted from manna and other natural sources with hot alcohol or other selective solvents. Commercially, it is produced by catalytic or electrolytic reduction of certain monosaccharides such as mannose and glucose. Manufacture is somewhat complicated by the need for separation of stereoisomers.

Description—White, crystalline powder or free-flowing granules; odorless and having a sweetish taste; density about 1.52 at 20°; melts between 165° and 168°; pK_a (19°) 3.4.

Solubility—1 g in about 5.5 mL water; slightly soluble in pyridine; very slightly soluble in alcohol; soluble in alkaline solutions; practically insoluble in ether.

Uses—A *diuretic* and a *diagnostic agent for kidney function*. The intravenous administration of hypertonic solutions of mannitol is used to promote an *osmotic diuresis*. It is not absorbed significantly from the gastrointestinal tract and, if given orally, mannitol causes osmotic diarrhea. Mannitol is a useful adjunct in the treatment of acute renal failure before irreversible renal failure becomes established. However, in order to be effective, there must be sufficient renal blood flow and glomerular filtration for mannitol to reach the kidneys. It also is used to reduce intracranial pressure, treat cerebral edema by reducing brain mass, reduce intraocular pressure when elevated pressure is not amenable to other therapy and promote urinary excretion of toxic substances. When administered parenterally, mannitol is distributed in the extracellular space. Only 7 to 10% is metabolized to glycogen and the rest is excreted in the urine. Plasma half-life after a single IV dose is 15 min with normal renal function. In severe renal insufficiency, mannitol excretion is reduced greatly; retained mannitol may increase extracellular tonicity, expand extracellular fluid volume and induce hyponatremia. It is superior to dextrose in that it is metabolized only slightly in the body and is reabsorbed only slightly by the renal tubule. Although it requires a larger volume, it produces fewer side effects than urea and is equally effective. Side effects mostly are due to fluid and electrolyte imbalance. Significant accumulation of mannitol can occur, due to rapid administration of large doses or inadequate renal output, leading to an expanded extracellular fluid volume. Isolated cases of adverse reactions (such as pulmonary congestion, fluid and electrolyte imbalances, acidosis, electrolyte loss, dryness of the mouth, thirst osmotic nephrosis, marked diuresis, urinary retention, edema, headache, blurred vision, convulsions, nausea, vomiting, rhinitis, diarrhea, arm pain, thrombophlebitis, chills, dizziness, urticaria, dehydration, hypotension, hypertension and anginal-like chest pains) have been reported during or following mannitol infusion. Safe use of mannitol during pregnancy and in children under 12 yr has not been established.

Since only a negligible amount of mannitol, which appears in the glomerular filtrate, is reabsorbed by the renal tubule, it has been employed for the measurement of *glomerular filtration rate*.

Dose—*Usual, intravenous infusion,* **50** to **200 g** daily.

Other Dose Information—The usual *diuretic* dose is 50 to 100 g, administered as a 5 to 20% solution. Test dose for patients with severe oliguria or compromised renal function: infuse 0.2 g/kg over 3 to 5 min and assess urine flow.

Dosage Forms—Injection: 5 and 10% (in 500 and 1000 mL), 15% (in 150 and 500 mL), 20% (in 250 and 500 mL) and 25% (in 50 mL); Mannitol and Sodium Chloride Injection (see below): *of each ingredient*—5 and 0.3% (in 500 and 1000 mL), 10 and 0.3% (in 500 and 1000 mL), 15 and 0.45% (in 150 and 500 mL) and 20 and 0.45% (in 250 and 500 mL).

Mannitol and Sodium Chloride Injection [(*Various Mfrs*)]—A sterile solution of mannitol and sodium chloride in water for injection. It contains no bacteriostatic agents. pH between 4.5 and 7. *Uses* and *Dose:* See *Mannitol*.

Potassium Citrate—RPS-16, page 777.

Isosorbide

D-Glucitol, 1,4:3,6-dianhydro-, Ismotic (*Alcon*)

[652-67-5] $C_6H_{10}O_4$ (146.14).

Preparation—By acid dehydration of sorbitol, Brit Pat 600,870.

Description—White crystals melting at 63°; usually supplied as an aqueous solution of approximately 75% concentration.

Solubility—Completely miscible with water; insoluble in most nonpolar organic solvents.

Uses—An *osmotic diuretic* used for the *short-term reduction of intraocular pressure* prior to, and after intraocular surgery. It also is used to interrupt an acute attack of glaucoma. It is absorbed rapidly after oral administration and distributed through total body water; ocular penetration is good and time of peak effect is 1 to 1½ hr. The drug is not metabolized to any appreciable extent and is excreted unchanged in the urine. It is less likely to induce nausea and vomiting than other oral hyperosmotic agents. Other adverse effects include headache, confusion and disorientation. Very rare occurrences of hypernatremia, hyperosmolarity, rash, syncope, dizziness and lightheadedness have been reported. There is no adequate information on either the teratogenic potential or any adverse fetal effects.

Dose—*Oral* (only), *initially* **1** to **3 g/kg** 2 to 4 times a day as indicated.

Dosage Form—*Solution*: 45% (100 g/220 mL), with 4.6 mEq sodium and 0.9 mEq potassium/220 mL.

Urea

Carbonyldiamide; Ureaphil (*Abbott*)

$CO(NH_2)_2$

Carbamide [57-13-6] CH_4N_2O (60.06).

Preparation—A product of the metabolism of proteins, it is excreted in human urine in average amounts of 30 g/day. In 1828 Wöhler obtained it on evaporating a solution containing potassium cyanate and ammonium sulfate, the ammonium cyanate first produced isomerizing to urea—reputedly the first synthesis of an organic compound from inorganic material.

A large-scale process for preparing urea is by heating calcium cyanamide with water under pressure:

$$CaNCN + 3H_2O \rightarrow CO(NH_2)_2 + Ca(OH)_2$$

Description—Colorless to white, prismatic crystals or a white, crystalline powder; almost odorless with a cooling, saline taste; may gradually develop a slight odor of ammonia, especially in the presence of moisture; melts between 132° and 135°; aqueous solutions are neutral to litmus, but on standing or heating, decompose into NH_3 and CO_2; pK_a (21°) 0.1.

Solubility—1 g in 1.5 mL water, 10 mL alcohol, 20 mL anhydrous alcohol, 6 mL methanol or 2 mL glycerol; practically insoluble in chloroform or ether.

Uses—Used *intravenously* as an *osmotic diuretic* for the reduction of intracranial pressure (in the control of cerebral edema) and of intraocular pressure. It is used *topically* in the treatment of psoriasis, ichthyosis, atopic dermatitis and to remove excess keratin from dry skin. It is used by transabdominal intra-amniotic injection as an abortifacient. Urea also may have mucolytic action and help to liquify purulent or mucoid sputum. Adverse reactions include headache, nausea, vomiting, syncope, disorientation, transient confusion and electrolyte depletion (hyponatremia and hypokalemia). Extravasation at the site of injection can cause local reactions. The infusion should never be mixed with blood in a transfusion set. It is contraindicated in patients with severely impaired liver and kidney function and in patients with active intracranial bleeding.

Dose—*Usual, intravenous infusion, adult and children over 2 yr,* **500 mg** to **1.5 g/kg** as a **30%** solution in 5 or 10% dextrose injection or 10% invert sugar injection; *children less than 2 yr,* **0.1** to **1.5 g/kg** as indicated above.

Dosage Forms—Sterile: 40 g in 150 mL.

Renal Tubular-Inhibiting Diuretics

The most powerful and consistently effective diuretics are those which depress tubular mechanisms responsible for the active reabsorptive transport of certain ions. Drugs which induce diuresis in this way may be divided into five groups: carbonic anhydrase inhibitors, benzothiadiazine and related derivatives, potassium-sparing diuretics, loop diuretics and other renal tubular-inhibiting diuretics. The mechanisms, uses and limitations of these several groups of diuretics are discussed in the introductory statement to the respective section.

Carbonic Anhydrase Inhibitors

Carbonic anhydrase is an ubiquitous enzyme responsible for the catalytic reversible hydration of carbon dioxide and dehydration of carbonic acid, a process critical to the transport of carbon dioxide in the erythrocyte and its exchange in the parenchyma of the lungs. This enzyme also is found in the renal cortex, gastric mucosa, pancreas, eye and central nervous system. The renal tubular cells also contain substantial amounts of carbonic anhydrase, and the CO_2 produced metabolically in the cells of the renal tubule is converted immediately to carbonic acid by the enzyme. Urine is normally acidified by secretion of hydrogen ions derived from carbonic acid formed in the proximal tubular cells in exchange for sodium ions in the lumen of the tubule. When carbonic anhydrase is inhibited, via adenyl cyclase stimulation, pH of the urine increases because the amount of hydrogen ions available for exchange with sodium is decreased; the excess sodium ions retained in the tubule combine with bicarbonate are excreted by the kidney with an increased volume of water and a loss of potassium. The diuretic effect is self-limiting when it is administered for longer than 48 hours, since the subsequent metabolic acidosis prevents further diuretic action by the carbonic anhydrase inhibitor.

Although carbonic anhydrase inhibitors were developed originally as diuretics, their *major usefulness is in glaucoma.* Inhibition of carbonic anhydrase in the ciliary body of the eye markedly reduces secretion of aqueous humor; oral or parenteral administration of carbonic anhydrase inhibitors decreases intraocular pressure in most patients with this ocular defect. These agents also have been used in some cases of absence and generalized tonic-clonic epilepsy refractory to anticonvulsants. The anticonvulsant effects of the carbonic anhydrase inhibitors may be due to the metabolic acidosis caused by these agents.

Adverse reactions to carbonic anhydrase inhibitors are seldom serious and are reversed rapidly, since the drug is excreted rapidly. The most frequent adverse effects include paresthesia, particularly tingling in the extremities; loss of appetite; polyuria; some drowsiness and confusion. During long-term therapy, an acidotic state may supervene; this can be corrected by administration of bicarbonate. Transient myopia has been reported. Other occasional reactions include urticaria, melena, flaccid paralysis and convulsions. Drowsiness may impair ability to drive or perform other tasks requiring alertness; patients should be advised of this. Like other sulfonamide derivatives, the sulfonamide-type carbonic anhydrase agents may produce fever, rash, crystalluria, renal calculus, bone-marrow depression, thrombocytopenic purpura, hemolytic anemia, leukopenia, pancytopenia and agranulocytosis. At the first signs of such reactions the drug should be discontinued and appropriate therapy instituted.

The safe use of these agents during pregnancy has not been established. These agents are contraindicated in patients with idiopathic renal hyperchloremic acidosis, renal failure, a known depletion of sodium and/or potassium, Addison's disease and patients known to be sensitive to this class of drugs. Moreover, long-term therapy is contraindicated in patients with chronic noncongestive angle-closure glaucoma.

Acetazolamide

Acetamide, *N*-[5-(aminosulfonyl)-1,3,4-thiadiazol-2-yl]-,
Diamox (*Lederle*)

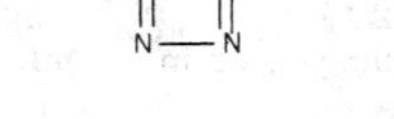

H_2NO_2S–(S, N—N thiadiazole ring)–$NHCOCH_3$

[59-66-5] $C_4H_6N_4O_3S_2$ (222.24).

Preparation—Hydrazine hydrate is reacted with a two-molar quantity of ammonium thiocyanate to produce 1,2-bis(thiocarbamoyl)hydrazine which yields, through loss of ammonia and rearrangement, 5-amino-2-mercapto-1,3,4-thiadiazole. This is acetylated and then oxidized to the 2-sulfonyl chloride with chlorine. The final step is amidation with ammonia.

Description—White to faintly yellowish white, crystalline, odorless powder; pK_a ;7.2, 9.0.

Solubility—Very slightly soluble in water; sparingly soluble in hot water (90° to 100°); slightly soluble in alcohol.

Uses—A *carbonic anhydrase inhibitor* effective for adjunctive treatment of *edema due to congestive heart failure, drug-induced edema, absence* and other *centrencephalic epilepsies,* chronic simple (open-angle) *glaucoma,* secondary glaucoma and *preoperatively in acute angle-closure glaucoma* where it is desired to lower intraocular pressure prior to surgery. It also is used in the prevention and amelioration of symptoms associated with mountain (high altitude) sickness. When used orally in tablet form to lower intraocular pressure, it has a rapid onset of action (1 to 1½ hr), reaches peak effect in 2 to 4 hr and the effect persists for 8 to 12 hr. When sustained-release capsules are employed, onset of action is approximately 2 hr, peak effect varies from 8 to 12 hr and the effects persist for 18 to 24 hr. It particularly is useful where careful following of blood electrolytes is not possible, as in outpatients. It has low toxicity. For additional information on adverse effects and precautions, see introductory statement.

Dose—*Usual, adult, oral, diuretic* or *urinary alkalizer,* **500 mg** once a day in the morning for 1 or 2 days, alternating with 1 day of rest. *Usual pediatric,* dosage not established.

Other Dose Information—In *glaucoma,* 250 mg every 4 hr; in *epilepsy,* 375 to 1 g in divided doses; when used in *combination with other anticonvulsants,* 250 mg once daily; in acute *mountain sickness,* 500 to 1000 mg daily in divided doses.

Dosage Forms—Tablets: 125 and 250 mg; Sustained-Release Capsules: 500 mg.

Sterile Acetazolamide Sodium

Acetamide, *N*-[5-(aminosulfonyl)-1,3,4-thiadiazol-2-yl]-,
monosodium salt; Diamox Sodium (*Lederle*)

[1424-27-7] $C_4H_5N_4NaO_3S_2$ (244.22); prepared from acetazolamide with the aid of NaOH. It is suitable for parenteral use. For the structure of the acidic form, see *Acetazolamide.*

Preparation—Acetazolamide is dissolved in aqueous NaOH solution containing an equimolar quantity of NaOH whereupon the acidic H of the —SO_2NH_2 group is replaced by Na. The solid sodium compound then may be produced by various drying or crystallization techniques.

Description—White solid, having the characteristic appearance of freeze-dried products; pH (freshly prepared solution, 1 in 10) between 9 and 10.

Uses—See *Acetazolamide.*

Dose—*Intravenous* or *intramuscular*, the equivalent of **250 mg** to **1 g** of acetazolamide daily; *usual*, **250 mg** 2 to 4 times a day.

Dosage Form—Sterile: 500 mg.

Dichlorphenamide

1,3-Benzenedisulfonamide, 4,5-dichloro-, Daranide (*MSD*)

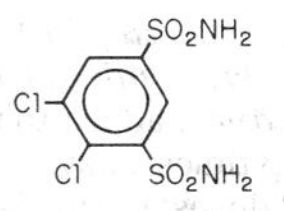

4,5-Dichloro-*m*-benzenedisulfonamide [120-97-8] $C_6H_6Cl_2N_2O_4S_2$ (305.15).

Preparation—*o*-Chlorophenol is reacted with chlorosulfonic acid to produce 5-chloro-4-hydroxy-1,3-benzenedisulfonyl chloride which is treated with PCl_5 to replace the 4-hydroxy with chlorine. Ammonolysis of the sulfonyl chloride yields the disulfonamide.

Description—White or nearly white, crystalline powder having not more than a slight characteristic odor; melts between 236.5° and 240°.

Solubility—Very slightly soluble in water; freely soluble in 1 *N* NaOH; soluble in alcohol; slightly soluble in ether.

Uses—A *carbonic anhydrase inhibitor* used in the treatment of *primary glaucoma*, the acute phase of *secondary glaucoma* and in the preoperative control of intraocular tension. The drug lowers intraocular pressure by reducing the rate of secretion of aqueous humor. After oral administration, the effect on intraocular pressure is observed within 1 hr, reaches a peak in 2 to 4 hr and persists for 6 to 12 hr. Although it has diuretic properties, it is not advocated for this purpose. Side effects and precautions are the same as other carbonic anhydrase inhibitors (see page 1042).

Dose—*Initial, adult, oral, antiglaucoma,* **100** to **200 mg** followed by **100 mg** every 12 hr until desired response is obtained; *maintenance,* **25** to **50 mg** 1 to 3 times a day. *Urinary alkalizer or diuretic, oral,* **100** to **200 mg** once a day in the morning for 1 to 2 days, alternating with 1 day of rest.

Dosage Form—Tablets: 50 mg.

Methazolamide

Acetamide, *N*-[5-(aminosulfonyl)-3-methyl-1,3,4-thiadiazol-2(3*H*)-ylidene]-, Neptazane (*Lederle*)

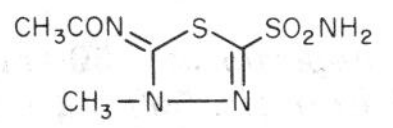

N-(4-Methyl-2-sulfamoyl-Δ^2-1,3,4-thiadiazolin-5-ylidene)acetamide [554-57-4] $C_5H_8N_4O_3S_2$ (236.26).

Preparation—2-Acetamido-5-mercapto-1,3,4-thiadiazole, prepared as described under *Acetazolamide,* is treated with *p*-chlorobenzyl chloride to produce the *p*-chlorobenzylmercapto derivative which, on treatment with methyl bromide in the presence of sodium methylate, undergoes methylation and rearrangement to yield the acetylimino thiadiazoline derivative. This is oxidized with chlorine water to the 2-sulfonyl chloride which yields methazolamide on amidation with ammonia.

Description—White or faintly yellow, crystalline powder having a slight odor; melts at about 213°; pK_a 7.30.

Solubility—Very slightly soluble in water or alcohol; soluble in dimethylformamide; slightly soluble in acetone.

Uses—A *carbonic anhydrase inhibitor* chemically related to acetazolamide and used as *adjunctive treatment* of chronic simple glaucoma, secondary glaucoma and preoperatively in acute angle-closure glaucoma where delay of surgery is desired to lower intraocular pressure. It is of doubtful value in glaucoma due to severe peripheral anterior synechiae or hemorrhage. Significant reduction in intraocular pressure occurs in 2 to 4 hr, reaches a peak in 6 to 8 hr and persists for 10 to 18 hr. It is indicated in patients who do not respond to acetazolamide or in those who are intolerant to it. The contraindications, precautions and adverse reactions are similar to those observed with acetazolamide and other carbonic anhydrase inhibitors (see page 1042).

Dose—*Usual, adult, oral, glaucoma,* **50** to **100 mg** 2 or 3 times a day. *Urinary alkalizer,* **50** to **100 mg** once a day in the morning for 1 or 2 days, alternating with 1 day of rest.

Dosage Form—Tablets: 50 mg.

Mersalyl with Theophylline—RPS-18, page 933.

Benzothiadiazine and Related Diuretics

The benzothiadiazine diuretics resulted from efforts to develop more potent carbonic anhydrase inhibitors. Some very potent disulfonamides (see *Dichlorphenamide,* this page) were synthesized but were no more useful as diuretics than other members of the group, until a compound with ring closure of one of the sulfonamide groups was accomplished. This resulted in the introduction of the prototype thiazide, chlorothiazide, in 1958, a widely used, reliable, well-tolerated, orally effective diuretic. The thiazide diuretics increase urinary excretion of sodium and water by inhibiting sodium reabsorption in the cortical (thick) portion of the ascending limb of Henle's loop and in the early distal tubules. They also increase excretion of chloride, potassium and, to a lesser extent, bicarbonate ions. The latter effect is due to their slight carbonic anhydrase-inhibitory action, although this action is usually of minor diuretic consequence . Because of their site of action, they interfere with the dilution but not the concentration of urine. The thiazide drugs also decrease the glomerular filtration rate. This effect does not appear to contribute to the diuretic action of these drugs and may explain their diminished efficacy in the presence of impaired kidney function.

The thiazide drugs are among the most widely used prescription drugs. They are often the first drug to be employed in the treatment of *hypertension* and can add to the effectiveness of other antihypertensive drugs and reverse the fluid retention caused by some of these agents. Although the precise mechanism of their antihypertensive action is unknown, it may be due to an altered sodium balance. Since the thiazides induce only a limited (10%) reduction in blood pressure, they are useful either in mild cases of hypertension or as adjunctive therapy to other drugs. The thiazide diuretics are *effective* as adjunctive therapy in *edema* associated with *congestive heart failure, hepatic cirrhosis* and *corticosteroid* and *estrogen therapy,* as well as edema due to *various forms* of *renal dysfunction (nephrotic syndrome, acute glomerulonephritis* and *chronic renal failure).* Thiazide diuretics also have been used successfully (alone or in combination with amiloride and/or allopurinol) to prevent the formation and recurrence of calcium stones in *hypercalciuric* and *normal calciuric patients.*

Thiazide diuretics are contraindicated in anuria, patients hypersensitive to these and other sulfonamide drugs and in otherwise healthy pregnant women with or without mild edema. Diuretics can decrease placental perfusion. Thiazides are excreted into breast milk; therefore, use by nursing mothers is not recommended. These drugs should be used with caution in patients with renal disease, since they may precipitate azotemia. They also should be used with caution in patients with impaired liver function, diabetes, gout or a history of lupus erythematosus.

Adverse effects have been observed as follows: *gastrointestinal* (anorexia, gastric irritation, nausea, vomiting, cramping, diarrhea, constipation, jaundice, pancreatitis, sialadenitis), *central nervous system* (dizziness, vertigo, paresthesias, headache, xanthopsia), *hematologic* (leukopenia, agranulocytosis, thrombocytopenia, aplastic anemia), *cardiovascular* (orthostatic hypotension), *hypersensitivity* (purpura, photosensitivity, rash, urticaria, necrotizing angiitis, fever, respiratory distress, anaphylactic reactions) and *other* (hyperglycemia, glycosuria, hyperuricemia, muscle spasm, weakness, restlessness, transient blurred vision). Periodic serum electrolyte determinations should be done on *all* patients in order to detect electrolyte imbalance such as hyponatremia, hypochloremic alkalosis and hypokalemia.

Thiazides are involved in several clinically important drug interactions. They interact with adrenal corticosteroids to enhance hypokalemia, with vitamin D and calcium to induce hypercalcemia, with diazoxide to cause hyperglycemia and with indomethacin to decrease the natriuretic and/or antihypertensive effect and with digitalis glycosides to produce digitalis toxicity. Moreover, the thiazides *increase* lithium levels and the neuromuscular blocking effect of tubocurarine, but decrease the anticoagulant effect of the oral anticoagulants.

Four agents included in this section—chlorthalidone, indapamide, metolazone and quinethazone—are nonthiazide sulfonamide derivatives. Their mechanisms of action and therapeutic indications are similar to the benzothiadiazines. Demonstrable differences between these agents and the thiazide diuretics are largely due to dosage and duration of action, although indapamide and metazolone may be effective in patients with compromised kidney function when thiazides are not. Because of their similarities, these drugs will be discussed with the thiazide diuretics.

Bendroflumethiazide

2*H*-1,2,4-Benzothiadiazine-7-sulfonamide, 3,4-dihydro-3-(phenylmethyl)-6-(trifluoromethyl)-, 1,1-dioxide; Naturetin (*Princeton*)

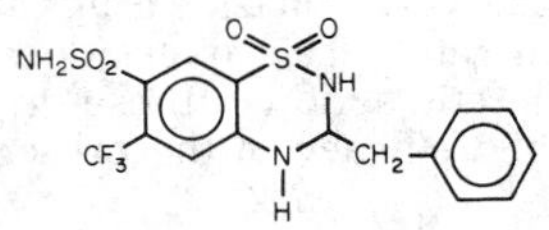

[73-48-3] $C_{15}H_{14}F_3N_3O_4S_2$ (421.41).

Preparation—One method consists of cyclization of 4-amino-6-trifluoromethyl-*m*-benzenedisulfonamide through condensation with phenylacetaldehyde (*J Am Chem Soc 81:* 4807, 1959).

Description—White to cream-colored, finely divided, crystalline powder which is odorless or has a slight, characteristic floral odor; melts about 220°. pK_a 8.5.

Solubility—1 g in 23 mL alcohol or 200 mL ether; practically insoluble in water chloroform or benzene.

Uses—A potent, orally effective thiazide *diuretic* and *antihypertensive* agent. It is indicated as adjunctive therapy in *edema, congestive heart failure, nephrosis* and *nephritis, cirrhosis* and *ascites* and other *edematous states.* It is also of value in *hypertension,* alone or when combined with other antihypertensive drugs—eg, *Rauwolfia serpentina* (Rauzide, *Apothecon*) or nadolol (Corzide, *Bristol*). Diuresis occurs within 2 hr and lasts 6 to 12 hr. After 10 mg orally, peak plasma levels (86 ng/mL) are reached in 2 hr; the mean half-life is 3 hr and the apparent volume of distribution averages 1.48 L/kg. The major part of the drug is eliminated unchanged in urine. Urinary recovery of the thiazide averages 30%. Side effects and contraindications are similar to those reviewed above.

Dose—*Usual, adult, oral, diuretic, initially* **5** to **20 mg** daily; *maintenance,* **2.5** to **5 mg** daily. *Antihypertensive, initially* **5** to **20 mg** daily; *maintenance,* **2.5** to **15 mg** daily. *Children, oral, initially* up to **0.4 mg/kg** daily in 2 divided doses; *maintenance,* **0.05** to **0.1 mg/kg** daily in a single dose.

Dosage Form—Tablets: 2.5, 5 and 10 mg.

Benzthiazide

2*H*-1,2,4-Benzothiadiazine-7-sulfonamide, 6-chloro-3-[[(phenylmethyl)thio]methyl]-, 1,1-dioxide; Aquatag, Proaqua (*Reid-Rowell*); Exna (*Robins*); Hydrex (*Trimen*); Marazide (*Vortech*); Urazide (*Hauck*)

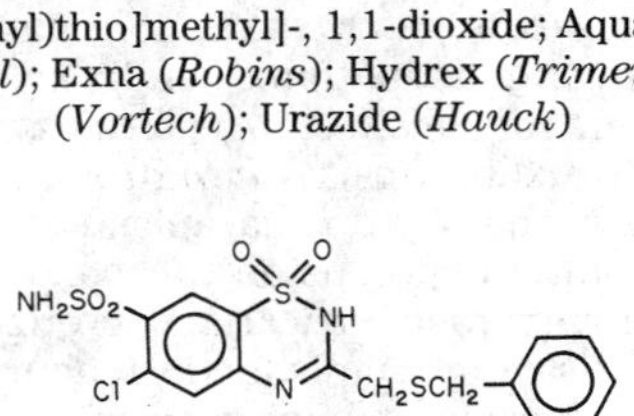

3-[(Benzylthio)methyl]-6-chloro-2*H*-1,2,4-benzothiadiazine-7- sulfonamide 1,1-dioxide [91-33-8] $C_{15}H_{14}ClN_3O_4S_3$ (431.93).

Preparation—4-Amino-6-chloro-*m*-benzenedisulfonamide is reacted with chloroacetic anhydride to give 2,3′-dichloro-4′,6′-disulfamoylacetanilide which is then condensed and cyclized with benzyl mercaptan in the presence of sodium hydroxide. US Pat 3,111,517.

Description—Fine, white, crystalline powder having both a characteristic odor and taste; stable in both light and air; melts about 240°.

Solubility—1 g in 41,000 mL water, 480 mL alcohol, 24,000 mL chloroform or 2900 mL ether; soluble in alkaline solutions.

Uses—A *diuretic* and *antihypertensive* agent with pharmacologic characteristics and uses similar to the thiazides. Diuresis occurs within 2 hr, reaches peak activity in 4 to 6 hr and lasts 12 to 18 hr. It is about 10 times as potent on a milligram basis as chlorothiazide. For a discussion of the action, precautions, side effects and possible drug interactions see pages 1039, 1040 and 1042.

Dose—*Usual, adult, oral, diuretic, initially* **50** to **200 mg** daily; *maintenance,* **50** to **150 mg** daily; *usual, antihypertensive, initially* **25** to **50 mg** twice daily; *maintenance,* adjust to the response of the patient with a maximal dose of **50 mg** 3 times a day. *Children, oral, initially* **1** to **4 mg/kg** daily divided into 3 doses; *maintenance,* reduce as needed.

Dosage Form—Tablets: 50 mg.

Chlorothiazide

2*H*-1,2,4-Benzothiadiazine-7-sulfonamide, 6-chloro-, 1,1-dioxide; Diachlor (*Major*); Diuril (*MSD*); (*Various Mfrs*)

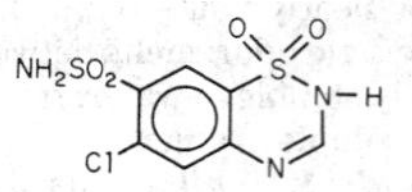

[58-94-6] $C_7H_6ClN_3O_4S_2$ (295.72).

Preparation—3-Chloroaniline is acylated with chlorosulfonic acid to produce the 4,6-disulfonyl chloride which is amidated with ammonia to give the 4,6-disulfonamide. Heating the latter with formic acid results in cyclization through double condensation.

Description—White or practically white, odorless, crystalline powder; melts at about 340°, with decomposition. pK_a 6.7, 9.5.

Solubility—Very slightly soluble in water (0.4 g per L at pH4, 0.65 g per L at pH 7) ; freely soluble in dimethylformamide or dimethyl sulfoxide; slightly soluble in methanol or pyridine; practically insoluble in ether, benzene or chloroform. Soluble in alkaline solutions but decompose on heating or standing.

Uses—The prototype benzothiadiazine diuretic having the therapeutic indications, warnings, precautions, drug interactions and adverse reactions described on pages 1039–1043. Diuretic effects are apparent within 2 hr after oral administration, reach peak activity in 4 hr and persist for about 6 to 12 hr; after intravenous administration, effects are apparent in 15 min, reach a peak in 30 min and persist for about 2 hr. Refractoriness to the drug is relatively uncommon even after prolonged periods of continuous administration. For information on drug interactions of benzothiazides, see page 1043.

Dose—*Adult, oral, antihypertensive,* **500 mg** or **1 g** given as a single or 2 divided doses; *usual, diuretic,* **500 mg** 1 or 2 times a day; *Adult, intravenous,* **500 mg** 2 times a day. *Children, oral,* **22 mg/kg** a day in 2 divided doses; *infants,* under 6 mo, up to **33 mg/kg** a day in 2 divided doses.

Other Dose Information—Dosage must be individualized according to the response of the particular patient and the severity of the condition under treatment.

Dosage Forms—Oral Suspension: 250 mg/5 mL; Tablets: 250 and 500 mg; Chlorothiazide Sodium for Injection: 500 mg.

Chlorthalidone

Benzenesulfonamide, 2-chloro-5-(2,3-dihydro-1-hydroxy-3-oxo-1*H*-isoindol-1-yl)-, Hygroton (*Rhone-Poulenc Rorer*); Hylidone (*Major*); Combipres (*Boehringer-Ingelheim*)

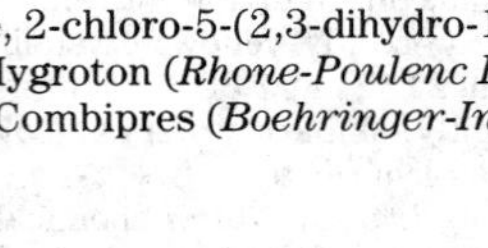

2-Chloro-5-(1-hydroxy-3-oxo-1-isoindolinyl)benzenesulfonamide [77-36-1] $C_{14}H_{11}ClN_2O_4S$ (338.76).

Preparation—3-Amino-4-chlorobenzophenone-2-carboxylic acid is diazotized and the resulting diazonium chloride is reacted in the cold with sulfur dioxide in the presence of cupric chloride to form 4-chloro-2′-carboxybenzophenone-3-sulfonyl chloride (I). Heating I with thionyl chloride yields 3-chloro-3-(3′-chlorosulfonyl-4′-chlorophenyl)phthalide which is reacted with ammonia. Removal of the solvent and treatment of the residue with HCl yields chlorthalidone. US Pat 3,055,904.

Description—White to yellowish white, crystalline powder; melts with decomposition above 215°; pK_a 9.4.

Solubility—Practically insoluble in water (12 mg/100 mL at 20°), chloroform or ether; slightly soluble in alcohol; soluble in methanol. Soluble in alkali carbonates or basic solutions.

Uses—An orally effective nonthiazide *diuretic* useful in the treatment of edema associated with *congestive heart failure, renal disease, hepatic cirrhosis, obesity* and the *premenstrual syndrome.* The diuretic effects start within 2 hr after administration, reach a peak in 2 to 6 hr, and persist for 24 to 72 hr. Therefore, the drug usually is given only every other day. Biochemical studies suggest that the prolonged duration of action is due to slow gastrointestinal absorption, enterohepatic recirculation and binding to red blood cells in the body. Approximately 30 to 60% of this drug is excreted unchanged by the kidney. It also exerts an antihypertensive effect and may be administered with other agents, such as reserpine, ganglionic blocking agents, hydralazine and guanethidine. Since it contains a sulfonamide group, its pharmacological actions and many of its untoward effects are similar to those of the other orally administered diuretics. See page 1039. It is contraindicated in patients with severe renal or hepatic disease. Patients on this drug should be watched closely for symptoms of renal damage or of electrolyte disturbance.

Dose—*Adult, oral, diuretic,* **50** to **100 mg** a day or **100 mg** on alternate days or 3 times a wk. Some patients may require 150 to 200 mg at these intervals.

Other Dose Information—Initial antihypertensive, 25 mg/day increased to 50 mg/day if necessary; maximum, 100 mg/day; *maintenance,* adjusted individually.

Dosage Form—Tablets: 25, 50 and 100 mg.

Cyclothiazide

2*H*-1,2,4-Benzothiadiazine-7-sulfonamide, 3-bicyclo[2.2.1]hept-5-en-2-yl-6-chloro-3,4-dihydro-, 1,1-dioxide; Anhydron (*Lilly*)

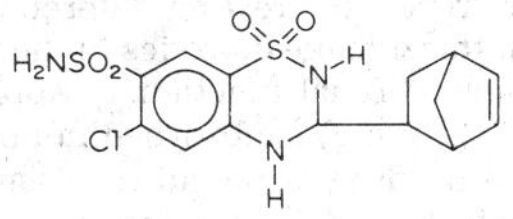

6-Chloro-3,4-dihydro-3-(5-norbornen-2-yl)-2*H*-1,2,4-benzothiadiazine-7-sulfonamide 1,1-dioxide [2259-96-3] $C_{14}H_{16}ClN_3O_4S_2$ (389.87).

Preparation—The process is analogous to that for *Chlorothiazide,* except that 5-norbornene-2-carboxaldehyde is employed in the cyclization step instead of formic acid. US Pat 3,275,625.

Description—White to nearly white, practically odorless powder; melts within a range of 4° between 217° and 225°.

Solubility—1 g in 70 mL alcohol or 30 mL methanol; practically insoluble in water, chloroform or ether.

Uses—An orally effective *diuretic* and *antihypertensive* agent. Diuresis occurs within 6 hr, reaches a peak in 7 to 12 hr and lasts 18 to 24 hr. Its site and mechanism of action, pattern of electrolyte excretion, untoward effects and clinical applications are similar to those of other thiazides. See page 1039. Like other agents of this type, it may be used as an adjunct to other antihypertensive agents, such as reserpine and the ganglionic blocking agents.

Dose—*Usual, adult, oral, diuretic, initially* **1** to **2 mg** a day; *maintenance,* **1** to **2 mg** every other day or 2 or 3 times a week; *usual, antihypertensive,* **2 mg** 1 to 3 times a day. *Children, initially* **0.02** to **0.04 mg/kg** a day; *maintenance,* dose reduced as needed.

Dosage Form—Tablets: 2 mg.

Flumethiazide—see RP5-18, page 935.

Hydrochlorothiazide

2*H*-1,2,4-Benzothiadiazine-7-sulfonamide, 6-chloro-3,4-dihydro-, 1,1-dioxide; HydroDiuril (*MSD*); (*Various Mfrs*)

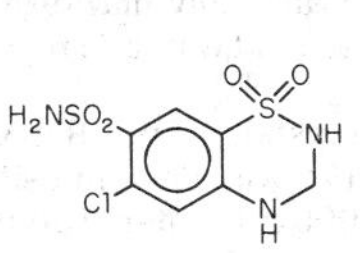

[58-93-5] $C_7H_8ClN_3O_4S_2$ (297.73).

Preparation—The process is identical with that for *Chlorothiazide,* except that formaldehyde is employed in the final cyclization step instead of formic acid.

Description—White, or practically white, odorless, crystalline powder; melts about 268° with decomposition; pK_{a1} 7.9; pK_{a2} 9.2.

Solubility—Slightly soluble in water; freely soluble in sodium hydroxide solution or dimethylformamide; sparingly soluble in methanol; insoluble in ether or chloroform.

Uses—Effective *diuresis,* comparable to that produced by 500 mg of chlorothiazide twice daily, is induced with 50 mg of this drug twice daily; diuresis occurs within 2 hr, reaches a peak in 4 hr, and lasts 6 to 12 hr. Otherwise, the pharmacologic actions, clinical uses, drug interactions and untoward effects are the same as for chlorothiazide. See pages 1043, 1044 and 1051. It also is used in combination with potassium-conserving agents such as triamterene (Dyazide, *SmithKline Beecham*) or amiloride (Moduretic, *MSD*).

Dose—*Adult, oral, antihypertensive, initially* **50** or **100 mg** a day as a single or divided dose; increased or decreased according to response, some patients requiring up to 200 mg a day in divided doses. *Adult, diuretic,* **25** to **100 mg** once or twice a day, or on alternate days. *Children, oral,* **2 mg/kg** a day, divided into 2 doses; *infants under 6 months,* up to **3 mg/kg** a day, in 2 doses.

Dosage Form—Tablets: 25, 50 and 100 mg.

Hydroflumethiazide

2*H*-1,2,4-Benzothiadiazine-7-sulfonamide, 3,4-dihydro, 6-(trifluoromethyl)-, 1,1-dioxide; Diucardin (*Wyeth-Ayerst*); Saluron (*Apothecon*)

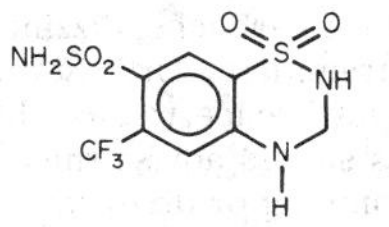

[135-09-1] $C_8H_8F_3N_3O_4S_2$ (331.28).

Preparation—4-Amino-6-(trifluoromethyl)-*m*-benzenedisulfonamide is heated with formaldehyde in a sulfuric acid environment thus effecting concomitant condensation and cyclization to hydroflumethiazide. US Pat 3,254,076.

Description—White to cream-colored, finely divided, crystalline powder; odorless; melts between 270° and 275°; pH (1 in 100 dispersion in water) between 4.5 to 7.5; pK_1 8.9, pK_2 10.7.

Solubility—1 g in > 5000 mL water, 39 mL alcohol, > 5000 mL chloroform or 2500 mL ether.

Uses—A potent, orally administered thiazide *diuretic* useful in the management of edema associated with *cardiac failure, hepatic cirrhosis, premenstrual tension* and *steroid administration.* It also is recommended for the treatment of mild to moderate *hypertension,* either alone or in combination with other antihypertensive agents. Diuresis occurs within 2 hr, reaches a peak in 4 hr, and lasts 6 to 12 hr. Since it potentiates the actions of other antihypertensive agents, the dose of other agents may need to be reduced when this drug is added to the regimen. Except for the fact that a smaller dosage is required for it, there is no convincing evidence of significant differences in therapeutic, metabolic or toxic or sensitization in edematous or hypertensive patients over that of the parent compound, flumethiazide or the prototype chlorothiazide. See page 1044.

Dose—*Adult, oral,* **25** to **200 mg;** *usual,* **50** to **100 mg** a day. *Children, initially* **1 mg/kg**; *maintenance,* adjusted as needed.

Other Dose Information—Refractory cases may require as much as 200 mg a day in divided doses. Dosage should be adjusted to provide the minimum effective dose for the individual patient.

Dosage Form—Tablets: 50 mg.

Indapamide

Benzamide, 3-(aminosulfonyl)-4-chloro-*N*-(2,3-dihydro-2-methyl-1*H*-indol-1-yl)-, Lozol (*Rhone Poulenc Rorer*)

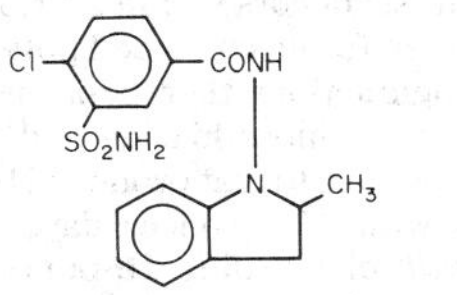

4-Chloro-*N*-(2-methyl-1-indolinyl)-3-sulfamoylbenzamide [26807-65-8] $C_{16}H_{16}ClN_3O_3S$ (365.83).

Preparation—*p*-Chlorotoluene is sulfonated and converted to the sulfonamide yielding 3-chloro-4-sulfamoylbenzoic acid. This acid is reacted with thionyl chloride to form the carbonyl chloride and treated with 2-methylindole (skatole) to give the product. See US Pat 3.565.911.

Description—White to yellow orthogonal crystals melting about 161°; weak acid, pKa = 8.8

Solubility—Soluble in aqueous solutions of strong bases.

Uses—An orally effective diuretic acid and antihypertensive agent related chemically to the indolines. It is used for the management of *edema* associated with *congestive heart failure* and, alone or in combination with other agents, in the treatment of *hypertension*. Its diuretic effect is similar to that induced by hydrochlorothiazide. Diuresis occurs within 1 to 2 hr, reaches a peak within 2 hr and lasts as long as 36 hr. Its antihypertensive effect results from decreased peripheral resistance, perhaps due to an alteration of transmembrane calcium events. Chronic administration does not tend to reduce glomerular filtration rate or renal blood flow; thus, its use may be preferred in patients with renal insufficiency who require diuretic treatment. With multiple-dose therapy, antihypertensive action usually appears within 1 to 2 wk and reaches a peak in 8 to 12 wk.

It is taken up preferentially and reversibly by erythrocytes in peripheral blood. The whole blood/plasma ratio is about 6:1 at the time of peak concentration and decreases to 3.5:1 at 8 hr. From 71 to 79% of the drug is bound to plasma proteins. It is metabolized extensively; only 7% of the unchanged drug is excreted by the kidneys. Few drug interactions have been reported; it reduces the renal clearance of lithium and tends to decrease arterial responsiveness to norepinephrine.

Adverse effects are usually mild and transient. Like the thiazide diuretics, indapamide-induced diuresis can cause hypokalemia, hypochloremic alkalosis, dilutional hyponatremia and hyperuricemia. Other side effects commonly observed include headache, dizziness, fatigue, muscle cramps or numbness of the extremities. Orthostatic hypotension, premature ventricular contractions, impotence, reduced libido and hypokalemia have been reported. Patients should advise their physician if muscle weakness, cramps, nausea, vomiting or dizziness occur. The safe use in the pregnant or nursing mother has not been established.

Dose—*Usual, hypertension* and *edema of congestive heart failure*, **2.5 mg** as a single daily dose taken in the morning; if the response is not satisfactory after 1 (edema) to 4 (hypertension) wk, the dose is increased to **5 mg** once daily. The dose of other agents should be reduced by 50% when used in combination with indapamide.

Dosage Form—Tablets: 2.5 mg.

Methyclothiazide

2*H*-1,2,4-Benzothiadiazine-7-sulfonamide,
6-chloro-3-(chloromethyl)- 3,4-dihydro-2-methyl-, 1,1-dioxide;
Aquatensen (*Wallace*); Enduron (*Abbott*); Methyclodine (*Rugby*)

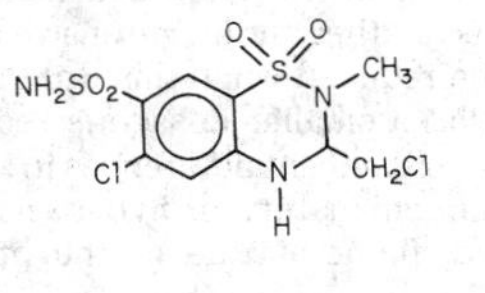

[135-07-9] $C_9H_{11}Cl_2N_3O_4S_2$ (360.23).

Preparation—By a process analogous to that for *Chlorothiazide*, 4-amino-6-chloro-N^3-methyl-*m*-benzenedisulfonamide is cyclized through condensation with monochloroacetaldehyde or an acetal thereof. US Pat 3,163,644.

Description—White or practically white, crystalline powder; odorless or has a slight odor and is tasteless; chars slightly below 220° and decomposes at 220°; pK_a (extrapolated from water-acetone) 9.4.

Solubility—1 g in > 10,000 mL water, 92.5 mL alcohol, > 10,000 mL chloroform or 2700 mL ether; freely soluble in acetone.

Uses—An orally effective *diuretic* and *antihypertensive* agent of the thiazide group. Diuresis occurs within 2 hr, reaches a peak within 6 hr and lasts 24 hr. Except for its enhanced potency and longer duration of action, its pharmacologic actions, therapeutic uses, side effects and contra-indications are similar to chlorothiazide and related agents. See page 1043. Diuresis comparable to that produced by 500 mg of chlorothiazide twice a day is induced with 2.5 mg once a day. See page 1044.

Dose—*Usual, adult, oral,* **2.5** to **10 mg** once daily, 10 mg being the maximum single effective dose. *Usual maintenance* and *antihypertensive*, 2.5 to 5 mg once daily. *Children*, **0.05** to **0.2 mg/kg** daily.

Dosage Form—Tablets: 2.5 and 5 mg.

Metolazone

6-Quinazolinesulfonamide,
7-chloro-1,2,3,4-tetrahydro-2-methyl-3-(2- methylphenyl)-4-oxo-,
Diulo (*Searle*); Mykrox, Zaroxolyn (*Fisons*)

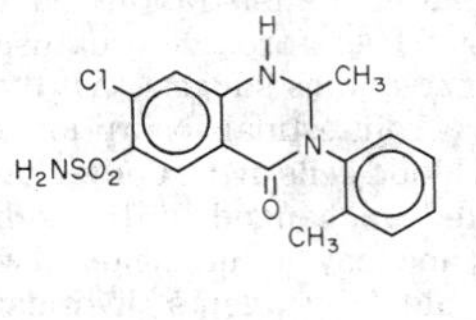

[17560-51-9] $C_{16}H_{16}ClN_3O_3S$ (365.83).

Preparation—5-Chloro-*o*-toluidine is converted through a series of reactions into *N*-(*o*-tolyl)-2-amino-4-chloro-5-sulfamoylbenzamide, which undergoes ring closure through reaction with acetaldehyde. US Pat 3,360,518; J Med Chem *13*:886, 1970.

Description—Colorless, odorless, tasteless, crystalline powder; light-sensitive; pK_a 9.72; melts between 253 to 259°.

Solubility—Sparingly soluble in water or alcohol.

Uses—A quinazoline-derived nonthiazide *diuretic* and *antihypertensive* drug. It acts primarily to inhibit sodium reabsorption at the cortical diluting site and in the proximal convoluted tubule. Sodium and chloride ions are excreted in approximately equal amounts; increased potassium excretion also may occur. Diuresis usually begins within 1 hr, reaches a peak in 2 hr and persists for 12 to 24 hr. This long duration of action is attributed to protein binding and enterohepatic recycling. It is indicated for *hypertension, edema* accompanying *congestive heart failure, renal diseases* including the *nephrotic syndrome* and other *conditions of diminished renal function.*

Clinical pharmacokinetic studies in normal patients and in patients with cardiac or renal failure reveal interesting differences. Metolazone may be more effective than thiazidelike diuretics in the treatment of edema in patients with compromised renal function. Approximately 65% of an administered oral dose (2.5 mg) is absorbed in normal control subjects. About 95% of the plasma drug is bound to plasma proteins in normal controls; about 90% is bound in patients with severe renal failure. Clearance of the drug is approximately equal to creatinine clearance and ranges from 110 mL/min in normal controls to 20 mL/min in patients with severe renal failure. Metolazone undergoes some enterohepatic recycling; consequently, in normal subjects about 10% of the administered dose is excreted in the bile. It is contraindicated in anuria, hepatic coma, known allergy or hypersensitivity, pregnancy and nursing mothers. Besides the adverse reactions reported for thiazide agents metolazone also may cause abdominal bleeding, palpitations, chest pains and chills.

Dose—*Usual, adult, oral, edema of cardiac failure,* **5** to **10 mg** once daily; *edema of renal disease,* **5** to **20 mg** once daily; *mild essential hypertension,* **2.5** to **5 mg** once daily.

Dosage Form—Tablets: 0.5, 2.5, 5 and 10 mg.

Polythiazide

2*H*-1,2,4-Benzothiadiazine-7-sulfonamide, 6-chloro-3,4-dihydro-2-
methyl-3-[[(2,2,2-trifluoroethyl)thio]methyl]-, 1,1-dioxide;
Renese (*Pfizer*)

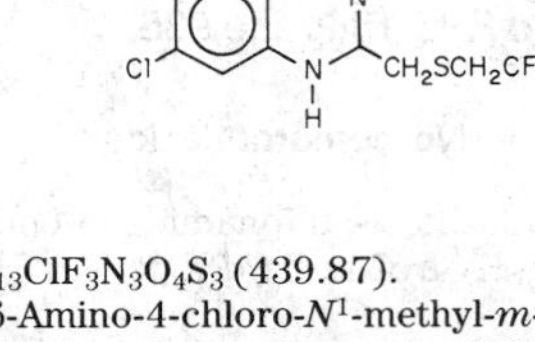

[346-18-9] $C_{11}H_{13}ClF_3N_3O_4S_3$ (439.87).

Preparation—6-Amino-4-chloro-N^1-methyl-*m*-benzenedisulfonamide is condensed with the dimethyl acetal of 2,2,2-trifluoroethylmercaptoacetaldehyde. The crude polythiazide, which precipitates when the reaction mixture is added to cold water, is recrystallized from 2-propanol. US Pat 3,009,911.

Description—White, crystalline powder with a characteristic odor; melts between 207° and 217°, with decomposition; pK_a 9.1.

Solubility—1 g in > 1000 mL water, 150 mL alcohol, 175 mL chloroform or >1000 mL ether; soluble in acetone; soluble in aqueous alkali carbonates or hydroxides with increasing decomposition as pH increases.

Uses—An orally effective long-acting *diuretic* and *antihypertensive agent* of the thiazide class. Diuresis occurs within 2 hr, reaches a peak in 6 hr and lasts 24 to 48 hr. Studies in 18 normal subjects receiving single 1-mg oral doses of this drug indicate a maximum plasma level of 3.22 ng/mL were reached 5 hr after its administration. The mean plasma half-lives for absorption and elimination were 1.2 and 25.7 hr, respectively. The latter is consistent with its extended duration of action. Approximately 20% of the drug was excreted unchanged in the urine. Its clinical effectiveness, untoward reactions and contraindications are similar to those of other benzothiadiazine diuretics. When compared on a milligram basis, 2 mg has approximately the same diuretic activity as 500 mg of chlorothiazide. See pages 1045 and 1043.

Dose—*Usual, adult, oral,* **1** to **4 mg** daily; *maintenance,* **0.5** to **8 mg** daily, adjusted to optimal response. *Children, oral, initially* **0.02** to **0.08 mg/kg** daily; *maintenance,* adjusted to need.

Other Dose Information—Antihypertensive, 2 to 4 mg daily, adjusted to achieve desired results.

Dosage Form—Tablets: 1, 2 and 4 mg.

Quinethazone

6-Quinazolinesulfonamide, 7-chloro-2-ethyl-1,2,3,4-tetrahydro-4-oxo-, Hydromox (*Lederle*)

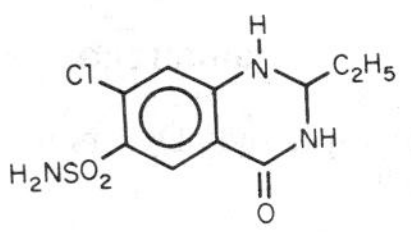

[73-49-4] $C_{10}H_{12}ClN_3O_3S$ (289.74).

Preparation—4′-Chloro-*o*-acetotoluidide is subjected to chlorosulfonation and subsequent amination to form 2-amino-4-chloro-5-sulfamoylbenzamide. Refluxing with an acidulated alcoholic solution of the diethylacetal of propionaldehyde effects the required condensation cyclization to yield quinethazone. US Pat 2,976,289; also J Amer Chem Soc *82:*2731, 1960.

Description—White to yellowish white, odorless, crystalline powder with a bitter taste; discolors in the presence of strong light and alkaline materials; melts between 250° and 252°.

Solubility—1 g in 500 mL alcohol; freely soluble in solutions of alkali hydroxides and carbonates; very slightly soluble in water.

Uses—A quinazoline derivative with *diuretic* and *antihypertensive* action similar to the thiazides. It differs chemically from the benzothiazide type only in the replacement of a sulfur atom by a carbon. Diuresis occurs within 2 hr, reaches a peak in 6 hr and lasts from 18 to 24 hr. Available clinical evidence indicates that its site, mechanism of action, electrolyte excretion pattern, therapeutic actions and untoward effects are similar to those of chlorothiazide and related agents. See pages 1045 and 1049.

Dose—*Adult, oral,* **50** to **200 mg** daily; *usual,* **50** to **100 mg** once a day.

Dosage Form—Tablets: 50 mg.

Trichlormethiazide

2*H*-1,2,4-Benzothiadiazine-7-sulfonamide, 6-chloro-3-(dichloromethyl)-3,4-dihydro-, 1,1-dioxide; Metahydrin (*Marion Merrell Dow*); Naqua (*Schering*) (*Various Mfrs*)

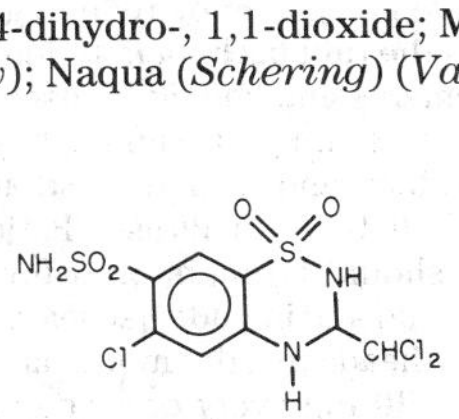

[133-67-5] $C_8H_8Cl_3N_3O_4S_2$ (380.65).

Preparation—By reacting 4-amino-6-chloro-*m*-benzenedisulfonamide with dichloroacetaldehyde, or an acetal thereof, in a suitable condensation environment. US Pats 3,163,645 and 3,264,292.

Description—White, crystalline powder that is odorless or has a slight characteristic odor; light-sensitive, but stable in air and heat; melts at about 274° with decomposition.

Solubility—1 g in 1100 mL water, 48 mL alcohol, 5000 mL chloroform or 1400 mL ether.

Uses—An orally effective and long-acting *diuretic* and *antihypertensive* of the thiazide class. Diuresis occurs within 2 hr, reaches a peak in 6 hr and lasts 24 hr. As an antihypertensive, it also is used in combination with reserpine. Pharmacologic actions, therapeutic uses, untoward effects and contraindications are similar to those of the parent substance, chlorothiazide. See pages 1039 and 1049. On a milligram basis, it is approximately 250 times more active than chlorothiazide.

Dose—*Usual, adult, oral,* **2** to **4 mg** daily, then 1 to 2 mg once daily. *Children,* **0.07mg/kg** daily in single or divided doses.

Dosage Form—Tablets: 2 and 4 mg.

Potassium-Sparing Diuretics

The potassium-sparing diuretics include *spironolactone, triamterene* and *amiloride.* The effects of these agents on urinary electrolyte composition are similar in that they cause a mild natriuresis and decrease potassium and hydrogen-ion excretion. Despite this similarity, these agents actually compose two groups with respect to mechanism of action.

Spironolactone, the prototype agent of the so-called "aldosterone antagonists," is a specific competitive inhibitor of aldosterone at the receptor site level; hence, it is *effective only* when aldosterone is present. The other two potassium-sparing diuretics, triamterene and amiloride, exert their effect independent of the presence or absence of aldosterone. Triamterene, on the peritubular side, inhibits the potential in the collecting duct and not on the distal tubule. Amiloride, on the other hand, inhibits the potential in both the collecting duct and the distal tubule. In addition, amiloride also decreases sodium transport in the proximal tubule. The potassium-sparing action common to all three of these agents is due to alteration of passive forces controlling movement of these ions.

The potassium-sparing agents are used in the management of *edema* associated with *congestive heart failure, hepatic cirrhosis with ascites, the nephrotic syndrome* and *idiopathic edema.* Because these diuretics have little antihypertensive action of their own they are used mainly in combination with other drugs in the management of hypertension and to correct hypokalemia often caused by other diuretic agents. Spironolactone also is used in *primary hyperaldosteronism.*

Potassium-sparing diuretics are contraindicated in patients with anuria, acute renal insufficiency, impaired renal function or hyperkalemia. Adverse reactions include diarrhea, nausea, vomiting, weakness, headache, erythematous rash and urticaria. Gynecomastia and carcinoma of the breast have been reported after spironolactone; however, no causal relationship between the latter and the drug has been established. These drugs can cause life-threatening hyperkalemia in patients using potassium-containing "salt substitutes" or in those with renal impairment. Serum potassium levels should be monitored in diabetics, the elderly and patients with renal failure.

Amiloride Hydrochloride

Pyrazinecarboxamide, 3,5-diamino-*N*-(aminoiminomethyl)-6-chloro-, monohydrochloride, dihydrate; Midamor (*MSD*)

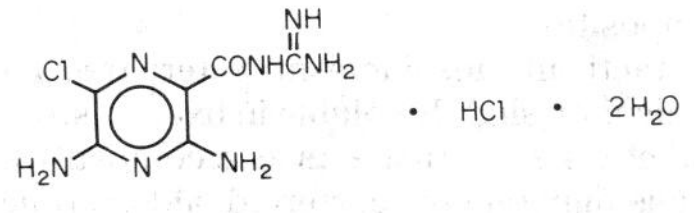

N-Amidino-3,5-diamino-6-chloropyrazinecarboxamide hydrochloride, dihydrate [2016-88-8] $C_6H_8ClN_7O.HCl.2H_2O$ (302.12).

Preparation—Pyrazine-2,3-dicarboxamide is converted to 3-amino-2-carboxamide through a Hoffman degradation using one equivalent of NaOBr; the carboxamide forming the ethyl ester by ethanolysis followed by reaction with sulfuryl chloride. This latter treatment forms the 5,6-dichloro derivative. As the 5-chloro is activated by the *p*-carboxyl it is readily converted to the amine with ammonia. Finally, the ester group is condensed with guanidine to yield the product. See Belg Pat 639,386 [CA 62:14698f,1965].

Description—Odorless, pale yellowish-green powder melting about 240°; pK_a 8.7.

Solubility—Soluble 1 g in 200 mL water or 350 mL alcohol; practically insoluble in chloroform or ether.

Uses—A potassium-conserving drug with natriuretic, diuretic and antihypertensive activity. It is approved only for concurrent use with other thiazide diuretics or other saliuretic-diuretic agents in the management of congestive heart failure or hypertension. It is used to restore normal serum potassium levels in patients who develop hypokalemia and in patients who would be exposed to a particular risk if hypokalemia were to develop. Its effect on electrolyte excretion is first observed 2 hr after drug administration, reaches a peak between 6 and 10 hr and lasts about 24 hr. Peak plasma levels are reached in 3 to 4 hr and plasma half-life varies from 6 to 9 hr. The drug is not metabolized by the liver and is excreted unchanged in the urine. It is contraindicated in patients with hyperkalemia or those taking potassium supplements or other potassium-sparing drugs. It should be used with extreme care in patients with diabetes or impaired renal function.

Amiloride usually is well tolerated and serious side effects are infrequent, although minor adverse effects occur in 20% of the users. Adverse effects include headache, nausea, anorexia, diarrhea and vomiting (3 to 8%). Other adverse effects such as dizziness, encephalopathy, abdominal pain, constipation, weakness, muscle cramps, decreased libido, cough and impotence occur less frequently. Amiloride alone has little effect on electrolytes, other than potassium; however, electrolyte disturbances may occur when combined with other diuretics. Serum potassium levels should be monitored.

Dose—*Single drug therapy:* **5** to **10 mg** daily; if persistent hypokalemia is documented with **10 mg/kg,** the dose can be increased to **15** and then **20 mg** daily with careful electrolyte monitoring.

Dosage Form—Tablets: 5 mg.

Dose—*Multiple drug therapy:* Amiloride and Hydrochlorthiazide (*Moduretic*, MSD), **1 tablet** daily. The dosage may be increased to **2 tablets** daily if necessary.

Dosage Form—Tablets: Amiloride hydrochloride, 5 mg, and hydrochlorthiazide, 50 mg.

Spironolactone

(7α,17α)- Pregn-4-ene-21-carboxylic acid, 7-(acetylthio)-17-hydroxy-3-oxo-, γ-lactone, Aldactone (*Searle*)

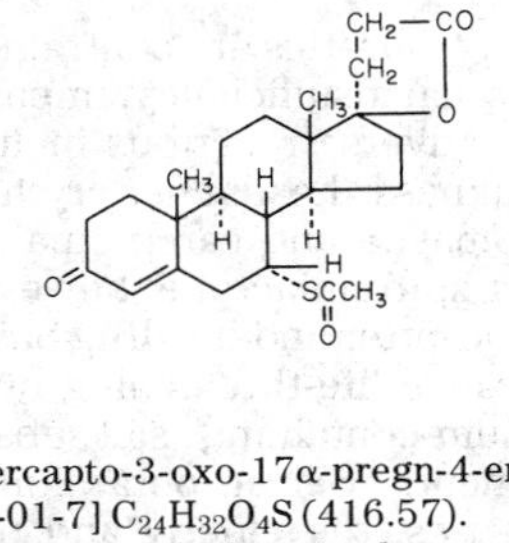

17-Hydroxy-7α-mercapto-3-oxo-17α-pregn-4-ene-21-carboxylic acid γ-lactone acetate [52-01-7] $C_{24}H_{32}O_4S$ (416.57).

Preparation—By treating dehydroepiandrosterone (prepared from cholesterol or sitosterol) with acetylene to form the 17α-ethynyl-17β-hydroxy derivative which is carbonated to the 17α-propiolic acid. Reduction of the unsaturated acid in alkaline solution yields the saturated acid which cyclizes to the lactone on acidification. Bromination to the 5,6-dibromo compound, followed by oxidation of the 3-hydroxyl group to the ketone, then dehydrobromination to the 7α-hydroxyl derivative, produces spironolactone when esterified with thiolacetic acid.

Description—Light, cream-colored to light tan, crystalline powder; faint to mild mercaptan-like odor; stable in air; melts between 198° and 207°, with decomposition.

Solubility—Practically insoluble in water; freely soluble in chloroform; soluble in alcohol; slightly soluble in fixed oils.

Uses—A synthetic steroid that acts as a competitive antagonist of the potent endogenous mineral-corticosteroid, aldosterone. It has a slower onset of action than triamterene or amiloride, but its natriuretic effect is slightly greater during long-term therapy. It is indicated in the treatment of *essential hypertension, edema* associated with *congestive heart failure, hepatic cirrhosis* with ascites, the *nephrotic syndrome, idiopathic edema* and in the diagnosis of primary aldosteronism. By blocking the sodium-retaining effects of aldosterone on the distal convoluted tubule, it corrects one of the most important mechanisms responsible for the production of edema but spironolactone is effective only in the presence of aldosterone. Its onset of diuretic action is gradual (24 to 48 hr), reaches a peak in 48 to 72 hr and lasts for 48 to 72 hr. It is a relatively weak diuretic and usually is employed as an adjunct to other diuretics, such as the thiazides. When used in this combined manner, it enhances the excretion of sodium and decreases the excretion of potassium. Further increase in diuresis may be obtained by the use of a glucocorticoid with this drug in combination with another diuretic. It is metabolized rapidly after oral administration. The metabolites are excreted largely in the urine, but also in bile. The primary metabolite, canrenone, reaches peak plasma levels 2 to 4 hr after oral administration of the drug. The half-life of canrenone, following multiple doses of the drug, is 13 to 24 hr. Both this drug and canrenone are more than 90% bound to plasma proteins. It has been shown to be a tumorigen in chronic toxicity studies in rats; 500 mg/kg induced hepatocytomegaly hyperplastic liver nodules and hepatocellular carcinoma.

It is contraindicated in acute renal insufficiency, anuria and hyperkalemia. It also is contraindicated in patients on digoxin; concurrent use elevates digoxin plasma levels and may induce digoxin toxicity. Similarly, concurrent use with lithium increases the risk of lithium toxicity. Side effects include hyponatremia, hyperkalemia and drowsiness. Other adverse effects include headache, diarrhea, skin rashes and urticaria, mental confusion, drug fever, ataxia, gynecomastia, decreased libido in the male and mild androgenic effects, such as hirsutism, irregular menses and deepening of the voice in the female.

Dose—*Usual, adult, oral,* **25 mg** 4 times a day; range, **25** to **200 mg** a day. *Children,* **3.3 mg/kg** a day in divided doses.

Other Dose Information—If satisfactory diuretic effect is not achieved in 5 days, a thiazide diuretic should be added to the regimen.

Dosage Form—Tablets: 25, 50 and 100 mg.

Triamterene

2,4,7-Pteridinetriamine, 6-phenyl-, Dyrenium (*SmithKline Beecham*)

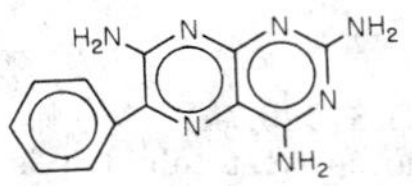

2,4,7-Triamino-6-phenylpteridine [396-01-0] $C_{12}H_{11}N_7$ (253.27).

Preparation—5-Nitroso-2,4,6-triaminopyrimidine is refluxed with phenylacetonitrile in the presence of sodium methoxide. US Pat 3,081,230; J Org Chem 28:1191, 1963.

Description—Yellow, odorless, crystalline powder; stable to temperature and light; pK_a 6.2.

Solubility—Practically insoluble in water, chloroform or ether; very slightly soluble in alcohol.

Uses—Inhibits reabsorption of sodium ions in exchange for potassium and hydrogen ions at that segment of the distal tubule under the control of adrenal mineralocorticoids. The effect is unrelated to the level of aldosterone secretion. After oral administration, 30 to 70% is absorbed and 50 to 67% is bound to plasma protein. Diuresis appears within 2 hr after administration, reaches a peak in 6 to 8 hr and lasts for 12 to 16 hr. It is metabolized primarily by the liver (hydroxytriamterene sulfate, an active metabolite) and about 3 to 5% is excreted unchanged in the urine. It also is used in combination with hydrochlorothiazide (Dyazide, *SmithKline Beecham*) in the treatment of edema associated with *congestive heart failure, cirrhosis* and the *nephrotic syndrome.* It also is indicated in steroid-induced edema, idiopathic edema, edema due to secondary hyperaldosteronism and in edematous patients unresponsive to other therapy. It directly inhibits the reabsorption of sodium and chloride independent of aldosterone. Although it promotes the excretion of sodium and chloride, it is believed to conserve potassium by reducing the transport of this ion from the tubular cell to the tubular lumen. Hence, it should not be used with potassium supplements and should be used with caution in patients with preexisting elevated serum potassium. It also is contraindicated in patients with severe kidney and liver disease and should be used with caution in patients with diabetes mellitus. Patients receiving long-term triamterene treatment should be monitored for electrolyte imbalances. Side effects are usually mild and include nausea, vomiting, gastrointestinal disturbances, weakness, headache, dry mouth and rash.

Dose—*Adult, oral,* **100 mg** every other day to **300 mg** daily; *usual,* **100 mg** twice a day.

Other Dose Information—The usual dose should be taken after meals. For *maintenance,* 100 mg daily or every other day. The total dose should not exceed 300 mg daily.

Dosage Form—Capsules: 50 and 100 mg.

Loop Diuretics

The loop, or high-ceiling, diuretics, ethacrynic acid (Edecrin, *MSD*), furosemide (Lasix, *Hoechst-Roussell*) and bumetanide (Bumex, *Roche*), are the most potent currently available diuretic agents. Although differences do exist between these agents, they are similar in that their most important action is in the medullary and cortical (thick) ascending limb of the loop of Henle. Loop diuretics inhibit active chloride, and possibly sodium, transport in the ascending thick limb of Henle. The loop diuretics have a much greater diuretic effect than the thiazides and are effective even in the presence of electrolyte and acid-base disturbances. Excess amounts of the potent diuretics can lead to serious water and electrolyte depletion; thus, careful medical monitoring is required. The time of onset and duration of action of the loop diuretics are shorter than those with the thiazides. These potent agents usually are reserved for patients with impaired renal function, acute pulmonary edema or hypertensive crises.

Despite their similar actions, there are some essential differences between the loop diuretics. Furosemide usually is preferred to ethacrynic acid for a number of reasons: (1) it has a broader dose-response curve, (2) it is less ototoxic, (3) it causes fewer gastrointestinal side effects, (4) it is more convenient for intravenous use and (5) it may be less likely to cause alkalosis.

Considerable controversy persists relative to their antihypertensive effectiveness as compared to the thiazides. Studies have suggested that the loop diuretics are not more effective than the thiazides in the management of uncomplicated mild to moderate hypertension in most patients. There is little controversy relative to the superiority of the loop diuretics in hypertension associated with renal insufficiency. Moreover, the loop diuretics *increase* renal blood flow, whereas the thiazides tend to *decrease* renal blood flow and further compromise renal function.

Many of the adverse effects are similar for both the thiazides and loop diuretics, and the management of these effects are the same. However, because of the much greater potency of the loop diuretics as compared to the thiazides, close monitoring is warranted to avoid severe electrolyte imbalances.

Bumetanide

Benzoic acid, 3-(aminosulfonyl)-5-(butylamino)-4-phenoxy-, Bumex (*Roche*)

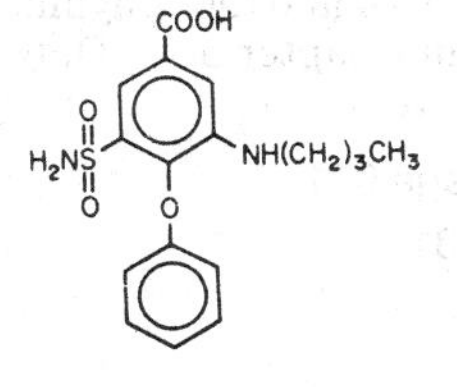

3-(Butylamino)-4-phenoxy-5-sulfamoylbenzoic acid [28395-03-1] $C_{17}H_{20}N_2O_5S$ (364.42).

Preparation—3-Chloro-5-(chlorosulfonyl)benzoic acid is nitrated in the 3-position with nitric/sulfuric acid, treated with ammonia to form the sulfonamide, then with sodium phenoxide to form the phenyl ether (replacing the active ring halogen), the nitro group reduced with acid bisulfite to the amine and a butylamino group generated by reductive coupling of the ring amino group with butyraldehyde in the presence of Pd and H_2. This latter step also produces the butyl ester of the carboxylic acid function, which subsequently is saponified with base and the free acid generated with HCl. See *J Med Chem 14*: 432, 1971.

Description—White crystals melting about 230°; pK_{a_1} 0.3; pK_{a_2} 4.0; pK_{a_3} 10.

Solubility—1 gm in 30 mL alcohol or 10,000 mL water.

Uses—A metanilamide derivative that is a potent *loop diuretic* with efficacy and biochemical effects similar to those of furosemide. Orally, it is effective in patients with *chronic congestive heart failure, chronic renal failure, cirrhosis with ascites* and the *nephrotic syndrome*. It also is useful when given intravenously in *acute pulmonary edema*. Orally, 1 mg is equivalent to 40 mg of furosemide. It is 95% protein bound and the volume of distribution is 12 to 35 L. Approximately 45% of an oral dose is excreted unchanged. The half-life is 1 to 1.5 hr and is prolonged in patients with renal failure. Onset of diuresis is observed within 30 to 60 min, reaches a peak in 1 to 2 hr and persists for 3 to 6 hr. It inhibits both chloride and sodium reabsorption in the ascending limb of the loop of Henle; it is somewhat more chloruretic than natriuretic. Bumetanide causes dilation of renal vasculature and increases renal blood flow. Since fluid and electrolyte changes are similar to those for furosemide, the same precautions apply (see page 1050). It also may cause azotemia, hyperuricemia and, rarely, impaired glucose tolerance. Nausea, vomiting, musculoskeletal pain, abdominal pain, rashes and Stevens-Johnson syndrome have been reported. Blood dyscrasias have occurred rarely. Reported drug interactions are similar to those for furosemide.

Dose—*Usual, adult, oral edema,* **0.5** to **2 mg** daily; *initially* **1 mg** in the morning, repeated 6 to 8 hr later if necessary. Patients with severe renal failure may require up to 15 mg. *Usual, adult, intravenous, pulmonary edema, initially* **0.5** to **1 mg;** repeat if necessary after 20 min.

Dosage Forms—Tablets: 0.5, 1 and 2 mg; Injection: 0.25 mg/mL in 2 mL ampuls.

Ethacrynic Acid

Acetic acid, [2,3-dichloro-4-(2-methylene-1-oxobutyl)phenoxy]-, Edecrin (*MSD*)

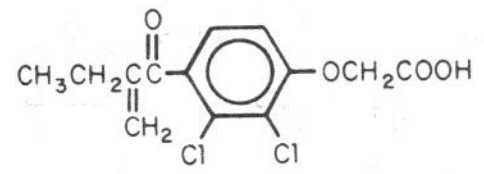

[2,3-Dichloro-4-(2-methylenebutyryl)phenoxy]acetic acid [58-54-8] $C_{13}H_{12}Cl_2O_4$ (303.14).

Caution—Use care in handling, since it irritates the skin, eyes and mucous membranes.

Preparation—2,3-Dichlorophenoxyacetic acid is subjected to a Friedel-Crafts reaction with butyryl chloride to form the 4-butyryl derivative. This undergoes a Mannich reaction with formaldehyde and dimethylamine, the product decomposing thermally to introduce the methylene group; *J Med Pharm Chem 5*: 660, 1962.

Description—White or practically white, crystalline powder that is odorless or practically odorless and has a bitter taste; relatively stable in light and at room temperature; nonhygroscopic; melts between 121° and 125°; pK_a 3.5.

Solubility—1 g in 1.6 mL alcohol, 3.5 mL ether or 6 mL chloroform; very slightly soluble in water.

Uses—An aryloxyacetic acid derivative that is a potent, short-acting diuretic. Maximum water and sodium diuresis is similar to that with furosemide, but greatly exceeds that with the thiazides. It is useful especially in patients who require an agent with greater diuretic potential than those commonly employed. It is used in the treatment of *fluid retentive states* caused by *congestive heart failure, cirrhosis of the liver* and *renal disease*, including the nephrotic syndrome. It also is recommended for the short-term management of ascites due to malignancy, idiopathic edema and lymphedema. In addition, it is useful for the short-term management of hospitalized pediatric patients with congenital heart disease or the nephrotic syndrome. It exerts its action on the cortical ascending (thick) loop of Henle and on the proximal and distal tubule, where it affects both the concentrating and diluting mechanisms of the kidney. It causes the excretion of virtually an isoosmotic urine by preventing sodium reabsorption from the loop of Henle; chloride excretion is even greater than sodium. After oral administration, diuresis begins within ½ hr, reaches a peak in 2 hr and persists for 6 to 8 hr. After intravenous administration, diuresis begins within 5 min, reaches a peak in 15 to 30 min and lasts about 2 hr. Approximately 95% of the drug is bound to plasma proteins. Plasma half-life is about 1 hr. It can be used with additive effect with diuretics having different sites of action. Adverse reactions include: *gastrointestinal* (anorexia, abdominal discomfort, dysphagia, nausea, vomiting and diarrhea; gastrointestinal bleeding and pancreatitis also have occurred); *renal* (hyperuricemia, acute gout and acute hypoglycemia with convulsions in uremic patients); *carbohydrate metabolism* (hyperglycemia in a few patients); *hemopoietic* (agranulocytosis or severe neutropenia; thrombocytopenia has been observed only rarely); *hepatic* (jaundice and abnormal liver function) and *miscellaneous* (vertigo, deafness and tinnitus with a sense of fullness in the ears; infrequently, skin rash, headache, fever, chills, hematuria, blurred vision, fatigue, apprehension and confusion). Patients should have determinations of blood urea nitrogen, serum carbon dioxide and electrolytes and white blood cell counts made frequently.

Dose—*Adult, oral,* **50** to **400 mg** daily; *usual,* **50 mg** 2 times a day or 2 times every other day. *Children, initially* **25 mg;** increase by **25 mg** until desired effect obtained. Dose for infants has not been established.

Other Dose Information—Dosage must be regulated carefully to prevent excessive fluid and electrolyte loss.
Dosage Forms—Tablets: 25 and 50 mg.

Ethacrynate Sodium for Injection

Acetic acid, [2,3-dichloro-4-(2-methylene-1-oxobutyl)phenoxy]-, sodium salt; Edecrin Sodium (*MSD*)

Sodium [2,3-dichloro-4-(2-methylenebutyryl)phenoxy]acetate [6500-81-8] $C_{13}H_{11}Cl_2NaO_4$ (325.12).
Preparation—A sterile, cryodesiccated powder prepared by the neutralization of ethacrynic acid with NaOH.
Uses—See *Ethacrynic Acid.*
Dose—*Intravenous*, the equivalent of **50** to **100 mg** of ethacrynic acid; *usual*, the equivalent of **50 mg** of ethacrynic acid.
Dosage Form—Vials: the equivalent of 50 mg of ethacrynic acid.

Furosemide

Benzoic acid, 5-(aminosulfonyl)-4-chloro-2-[(2-furanylmethyl)amino]-, Lasix (*Hoechst-Roussel*); (*Various Mfrs*)

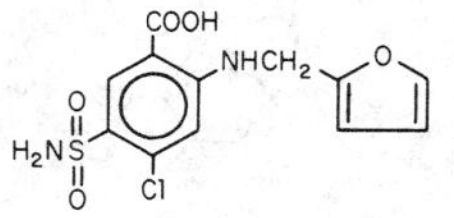

4-Chloro-*N*-furfuryl-5-sulfamoylanthranilic acid [54-31-9] $C_{12}H_{11}ClN_2O_5S$ (330.74).
Preparation—2,4-Dichlorobenzoic acid is heated with chlorosulfonic acid and the resulting 5-chlorosulfonyl derivative is reacted with concentrated ammonia to convert it to the 5-sulfamoyl analogue (I). Refluxing I with furfurylamine in large excess or in the presence of sodium bicarbonate yields crude furosemide which is recrystallized from aqueous ethanol. US Pat 3,058,882.
Description—Fine, white to slightly yellow, crystalline powder; odorless and practically tasteless; unstable in light but stable in air; melts between 203° and 205° with decomposition; pK_a 3.9 (acid).
Solubility—Practically insoluble in water; freely soluble in acetone, or solutions of alkali hydroxides; sparingly soluble in alcohol; slightly soluble in ether; very slightly soluble in chloroform.
Uses—A *diuretic* chemically related to the sulfonamide diuretics. It is characterized by high efficacy, rapid onset of action, comparatively short duration of action and a tenfold ratio between minimum and maximum diuretic dose. Moreover, it is slightly more potent than the organomercurial agents, orally effective and its diuretic action is independent of alterations in body acid-base balance. It acts not only on the proximal and distal tubules but also on the ascending limb of the loop of Henle.
It is indicated for the treatment of *edema* associated with *congestive heart failure, cirrhosis of the liver* and *renal disease,* including the *nephrotic syndrome.* It is indicated particularly when a greater diuretic potential is needed than that produced by commonly employed diuretic agents. It is also useful in the management of selected patients with *hypertension.* It is thought to decrease peripheral resistance in hypertensive patients and dilate the veins in patients with congestive heart failure (*TIPS 8*:254, 1987). It is given by both oral and parenteral routes of administration; parenteral administration should be reserved for those cases where oral therapy is not practical. Orally, the diuretic effect begins within 1 hr, reaches a peak in 1 or 2 hr and persists for 6 to 8 hr. Administered intravenously, the diuretic effect begins within 5 min, reaches a peak in 30 min and persists for 2 hr.
Clinical pharmacokinetic studies carried out after a single intravenous dose of 0.5, 1.0 or 1.5 mg/kg indicate that peak diuresis occurs between 20 and 60 min after injection. Apparent volume of distribution of the drug averages 11.4% of the body weight and is independent of the dose. Mean plasma half-life in these studies was 29.5 min with a clearance rate of 162 mL/min. Renal excretion was found to be the main route of elimination and averaged 92% of the administered dose with a mean renal clearance of 149 mL/min. Since this exceeds the glomerular filtration rate, it is thought that tubular secretion of this drug occurs, despite the fact that 95% of it is bound to plasma protein.
Like the other diuretics, furosemide is known to be involved in a number of drug interactions. It increases the toxicity of lithium, digitalis and theophylline. It decreases the arterial responsiveness of norepinephrine and antagonizes the skeletal muscle relaxant effects of tubocurarine and may potentiate the action of succinylcholine. Concomitant administration of indomethacin may reduce the natriuretic and antihypertensive effects of the drug. This effect also may occur with other nonsteroidal anti-inflammatory drugs such as ibuprofen or naproxen. Metolazone acts synergistically with this to stimulate profound diuresis in patients resistant to it.
It is contraindicated in anuria, hepatic coma and in patients known to be sensitive to the drug. Adverse effects which may result from therapy include reduction of renal, cerebral and cardiac blood flow, potassium loss with resultant cardiac and neuromuscular abnormalities, elevation of blood uric acid and blood sugar levels, allergic reactions, rare cases of exfoliative dermatitis, pruritus and blood dyscrasias (thrombocytopenia and leukopenia). Paresthesia, blurring of vision, postural hypotension, nausea, vomiting or diarrhea may occur. In addition, cases of reversible deafness and tinnitus have been reported. Diuresis induced by the drug also has been accompanied by weakness, fatigue, light-headedness or dizziness, muscle cramps, thirst and urinary frequency. Excessive therapy can lead to profound diuresis with water and electrolyte depletion. Patients on this drug should be tested at frequent intervals for blood urea nitrogen, sodium, potassium, chloride and carbon dioxide concentrations. The drug should not be used in cirrhotic patients, unless they do not respond to other therapy. It is contraindicated in women with child-bearing potential.
Dose—*Adult, oral,* **20** to **80 mg** daily; *usual,* **40** to **80 mg** once a day; *intramuscular or intravenous,* **20** to **40 mg,** after not less than 2 hr increased by 20 mg to desired effect. *Usual, pediatric,* **2 mg/kg** as a single dose. If response is not adequate, increase by **1** or **2 mg/kg** after 6 to 8 hr; do not exceed **6 mg/kg.**
Dosage Forms—Injection: 10 mg/mL; Oral Solution: 8 and 10 mg/mL; Tablets: 20, 40 and 80 mg.

Other Renal Tubular-Inhibiting Diuretics

All of the xanthines (caffeine, theophylline and theobromine) appear to induce diuresis by a direct action on the renal tubule. The increased urinary output involves an increase in the rate of sodium and chloride excretion, with no significant effect on urinary acidification. Although diuretic action is altered only slightly by changes in acid-base balance, it is potentiated by the coadministration of carbonic anhydrase inhibitors. In clinical practice, the xanthines are considered obsolete as diuretics and seldom used for three reasons: (1) they lack the efficacy of the newer agents, (2) their continued use leads to decreased effectiveness and (3) they cause some gastric irritation. Therefore, caffeine, a CNS stimulant, is presented in Chapter 74 and theophylline, a useful bronchodilator, is discussed in Chapter 56. Only theobromine will be presented in this section.

Aminophylline—page 971.
Caffeine—page 1231.

Theobromine

1*H*-Purine-2,6-dione, 3,7-dihydro-3,7-dimethyl-,

3,7-Dimethylxanthine [83-67-0] $C_7H_8N_4O_2$ (180.17).
Preparation—An alkaloid prepared from the dried ripe seed of *Theobroma cacao* Linné(Fam *Sterculiaceae*), or made synthetically. For the structural formula, see page 404.
Description—White, crystalline powder with a bitter taste; sublimes at about 290°.
Solubility—1 g in 1800 mL water, 2400 mL alcohol or 6000 mL chloroform; soluble in solutions of fixed alkali hydroxides; insoluble in ether.
Uses—It shares with other methylxanthines an ability to produce diuresis, relax smooth muscle (ie, bronchial muscle), stimulate the central nervous system and cardiac muscle. Because of the low pharmacological potency of theobromine, it rarely is used therapeutically and no longer is included as an active ingredient in prescription or OTC medications. Even so, theobromine frequently is consumed because of its presence in chocolate-related products and rarely causes significant adverse effects.

Theophylline—page 973.
Theophylline Sodium Acetate—RPS-17, page 875.

Miscellaneous Renal Agent

Probenecid

Benzoic acid, 4-[(dipropylamino)sulfonyl]-, Benemid (*MSD*); (*Various Mfrs*)

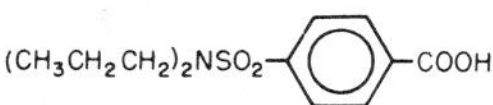

[57-66-9] $C_{13}H_{19}NO_4S$ (285.36).

Preparation—Oxidation of the methyl group of *p*-toluenesulfonyl chloride produces *p*-carboxybenzenesulfonic acid. This acid is then converted into the corresponding sulfonyl chloride by treatment with chlorosulfonic acid, which is condensed with di-*n*-propylamine (US Pat 2,608,507).

Description—White or nearly white, fine, crystalline powder; practically odorless; melts between 198° and 200°; pK_a 5.8.

Solubility—Soluble in alcohol, chloroform or acetone; practically insoluble in water. Soluble in dilute aqueous alkali.

Uses—An agent which blocks both renal and CSF transport of weak acids. With respect to the inward renal transport, it is an effective *uricosuric* agent for the treatment of gout and gouty arthritis. It inhibits tubular reabsorption of urate at the proximal convoluted tubule, thus increasing urinary excretion of uric acid and decreasing serum uric acid levels. With regard to outward renal transport probenecid blocks secretion of weak organic acids at the proximal and distal tubules and is effective as an adjuvant therapy with penicillin G, O or V, or with ampicillin, methicillin, oxacillin, cloxacillin or nafcillin, for elevation and prolongation of penicillin plasma levels by whatever route the antibiotic is given. It inhibits the renal excretion and may increase the plasma levels of methotrexate, sulfonamides, sulfonylureas, naproxen, indomethacin, rifampin, aminosalicylic acid, dapsone, clofibrate or pantothenic acid. Patients concurrently taking any of these agents should be monitored closely and the dosage regimen adjusted appropriately.

It is absorbed rapidly and completely after oral administration. Plasma levels of 100 to 200 μg/mL are necessary for an adequate uricosuric effect, whereas plasma levels of only 40 to 60 μg/mL produce maximal inhibition of penicillin excretion. Plasma levels of 25 μg/mL are reached 30 min after a single 1-g oral dose; plasma levels reach a peak in 2 to 4 hr and remain above 30 μg/mL for 8 hr. Following a single 2-g oral dose, peak plasma levels of 150 to 200 μg/mL are reached in 4 hr and levels of 50 μg/mL are sustained for 8 hr; the plasma half-life ranges from 4 to 17 hr. At a plasma concentration of 14 μg/mL, about 17% of the drug is bound to plasma protein.

It is contraindicated in hypersensitive individuals, children under 2 yr and persons with known blood dyscrasias or uric acid stones. Therapy should not be started until an acute gouty attack has subsided. Exacerbation of gout following therapy may occur; in such cases, colchicine or other appropriate therapy is advisable. The drug should not be given with methotrexate, since plasma levels of the latter agent have been reported to be increased. Use of salicylates also is contraindicated because these substances antagonize the drug's uricosuric action. Patients who require a mild analgesic should be advised to use acetaminophen rather than salicylates. Probenecid is devoid of analgesic activity.

It is tolerated well but an occasional patient may experience headache, anorexia, nausea, vomiting, urinary frequency, hypersensitivity reactions, sore gums, flushing, dizziness and anemia. In gouty patients, exacerbation of gout and uric acid stones with or without hematuria, renal colic and costovertebral pain have been observed. Nephrotic syndrome, hepatic necrosis and aplastic anemia occur rarely. Hemolytic anemia, which in some cases could be related to genetic deficiencies of red blood cell glucose 6-phosphate dehydrogenase, has been reported.

Dose—*Adult, oral,* **500 mg** to **2 g** daily; *usual,* **250 mg** twice a day for 1 week, then **500 mg** twice a day thereafter.

Dosage Form—Tablets: 500 mg.

Diuretic Combinations

Some examples of diuretic combinations (with content per capsule, tablet or 5 mL provided) are as follows:

Amiloride Hydrochloride and Hydrochlorathiazide [Moduretic (*MSD*)]—5 and 50 mg, respectively.

Hydrochlorothiazide and Deserpidine [Oreticyl 25, Oreticyl 50 and Oreticyl Forte (*Abbott*)]—25–50 and 0.125–0.25 mg, respectively.

Methylclothiazide and Deserpidine [Enduronyl and Enduronyl Forte (*Abbott*)]—5 and 0.25–0.5 mg, respectively.

Quinethazone and Reserpine [Hydromox R (*Lederle*)]—50 and 0.125 mg, respectively.

Rauwolfia Serpentina (powdered whole root) and Bendroflumethiazide [Rauzide (*Princeton*)]—50 and 4 mg, respectively.

Spironolactone and Hydrochlorothiazide [Aldactazide (*Searle*)] — 25–50 and 25–50 mg, respectively.

Triamterene and Hydrochlorothiazide [Dyazide (*SmithKline Beecham*); Maxzide (*Lederle*)]—50–75 and 25–50 mg, respectively.

CHAPTER 63

Uterine and Antimigraine Drugs

Glen R Hanson, DDS, PhD
Professor of Pharmacology
College of Pharmacy and School of Medicine, University of Utah
Salt Lake City, UT 84132

Drugs that stimulate the smooth muscle of the uterus are known as *oxytocics*. Three chemical types of oxytocics are used clinically: (1) the oxytocic fraction (oxytocin) of the posterior pituitary extract, (2) certain ergot alkaloids and (3) certain prostaglandins. However, a number of other agents possess mild to intense oxytocic actions. Some of these, eg, hydrastis and quinine, have been used formerly but are now archaic. The lay public, and sometimes also the physician, employ cathartics and abdominal congestants such as castor oil to induce reflex uterine movement, but it is doubtful whether such agents are effective until the uterus is prepared to present the fetus normally.

The response of the uterus to oxytocics depends on estrogenic and progestational hormonal influences. Progesterone hyperpolarizes the uterine smooth muscle and, thus, diminishes its responsiveness and coordination, while estrogen increases myometrial excitability. Consequently, and fortunately, during the first two terms of pregnancy, oxytocics generally are incapable of inducing labor. Late in the third term, as the progesterone levels decline and the estrogen influence increases, uterine responsiveness rises sharply in advance of pelvic relaxation, cervical dilatation and the coordination of uterine contractions necessary for proper delivery of the fetus. The premature induction of labor by oxytocics can result in harm to both mother and infant and may result in stillbirth if premature separation of the placenta, placental vasoconstriction or umbilical strangulation occur. Therefore, only under rare circumstances should oxytocics be used to induce labor; indeed, they generally are withheld *during* labor until the cervix is dilated and presentation of the fetus has occurred (ie, until the third stage of labor). The oxytocic then is given to hasten the delivery of the placenta and to diminish uterine bleeding by contractile compression of the blood sinuses and vasoconstriction. Oxytocics also may be employed during the puerperium to aid in the involution of the uterus to normal. Oxytocin promotes and facilitates the normal phasic contractions which are characteristic of normal delivery. The ergot alkaloids induce prolonged contractions or contracture, which may be detrimental to safe delivery and, hence, they are employed mainly in the third stage of labor to diminish bleeding. Prostaglandins, notably PGE_2 and PGF_2, promote normal-type phasic contractions. However, the effects of the prostaglandins are not so dependent on the estrogen-progesterone balance as those of oxytocin, so that prostaglandins can induce labor considerably in advance of term and, hence, can be used to induce abortion.

Nonoxytocic ergot alkaloids are listed in this section because of their relationship to the oxytocic prototypes.

The so-called uterine sedatives comprise an ill-defined class of drugs that diminish, or supposedly diminish, uterine activity. They are employed to interrupt premature labor, diminish pain in dysmenorrhea and diminish premenstrual discomfort. Some of these agents, such as central nervous system sedatives like ethanol, have questionable effects on uterine activity at all. Uterine activity and premature labor may be decreased after opiates have been administered. Ammonium chloride and other diuretics may give relief in dysmenorrhea, not by their effects on uterine activity, but by the relief of pelvic congestion and edema. Both estrogens and progestational hormones (see Chapter 64) have been employed in the treatment of dysmenorrhea. Though the estrogens may suppress uterine motility under certain circumstances, the prophylactic action in this instance is through the prevention of ovulation. Progestational hormones alone may decrease uterine motility in appropriate circumstances, but the mechanism of their action in dysmenorrhea is undetermined, except that it is not a proliferative effect. Usually, however, the progestins are used in combination with estrogens to normalize a menstrual cycle and, hence, diminish dysmenorrhea. The balance between estrogens and progestational hormones may be more important to uterine activity than either type of hormone alone. Nonsteroidal anti-inflammatory drugs, which inhibit the synthesis of prostaglandins (see page 410), play a major role in the management of dysmenorrhea. β_2-Agonists, especially ritodrine, are used widely to treat premature labor. Miscellaneous "uterine sedatives" may be no more than placebos.

Most of the oxytocic ergot alkaloids also cause cerebral vasoconstriction. Since the painful phase of a migraine attack appears to be due to cerebral vasodilatation, a vasoconstrictor often will provide relief; this is thought to be the basis of the use of vasocontrictor ergot alkaloids in the treatment of migraine headache. However, the migraine headache is preceded by vasoconstriction, which appears to be associated with subsequent vasodilatation. This prodromal vasoconstriction has been thought to be the result of excessive release (probably from platelets) of serotonin in the region of the vessels, and serotonin antagonists are effective in preventing not only the aura (vasoconstrictor phase) but also the subsequent headache.

Carboprost Tromethamine

Prosta-5,13-dien-1-oic acid, (5*Z*,9α,11α,13*E*,15*S*)-9,11,15-trihydroxy-15-methyl-, compound with 2-amino-2-(hydroxymethyl)-1,3-propanediol (1:1); Hemabate (*Upjohn*)

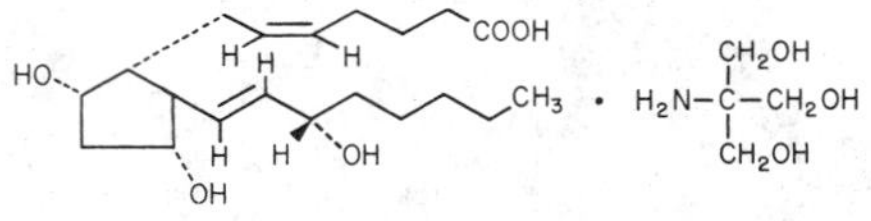

(15*S*)-15-Methylprostaglandin F_α tromethamine [58551-69-2] $C_{21}H_{36}O_5 \cdot C_4H_{11}NO_3$ (489.65)

Preparation—By a series of complex alterations on a prostaglandin precursor. See US Pat 3,728,382.

Uses—A modification of the prostaglandin, $PGF_{2\alpha}$ (see *Dinoprostone*, below) which occurs during normal term labor. It is used to *induce abortion* in weeks 13 to 20 of gestation or to help expulse a fetus in combination with another abortion method. Successful induction is achieved in about 96% of trials, 78% being complete. It may be used during the second trimester to complete failed spontaneous or drug-induced abortions or to *initiate delivery* after fetal death or/premature rupture of the membranes. Although it is not approved for these uses, it is employed postpartum to diminish blood loss when conventional therapy is precluded or ineffective, in hydatiform mole and to ripen the cervix preparatory to curettage. Advantages over dinoprost are a longer duration of action and the consequent intramuscular, rather than intra- or extra-amniotic, route of administration.

Vomiting and diarrhea occur in about 67% of cases and nausea in 33%. Pretreatment or concurrent administration of antiemetic and antidiarrheal drugs decrease the GI effects and are recommended strongly. Fever (to be differentiated from that of endometritis) occurs in about 12%. Flushing and hot flashes, chills and/or shivering, hiccough, uterine pain, muscular pain, backache, eye pain, breast tenderness, pain at the injection site, paresthesias and alteration of taste, tinnitus, vertigo, faintness, syncope, drowsiness, dry mouth and throat, thirst, respiratory distress and hyperventilation, coughing, weakness, hematemesis, chest pain or tightness, wheezing, sweating, blepharospasm, thyroid storm, tachycardia, palpitations, hypertension and uterine rupture also may occur sometimes. Incomplete abortion is also adverse and requires dilatation and curettage or suction. It is contraindicated in patients with a history of asthma, cardiovascular or renal disease, hypertension, diabetes, liver disease, jaundice, epilepsy, anemia or uterine surgery. It must not be given simultaneously with other oxytocics lest uterine hypercontractility and rupture occur.

Dose—*Intramuscular* (deep), *initially* **250 μg** (0.25 mg) to be repeated at 1½ to 3½-hr intervals, or an optional test dose of **100 μg** (0.1 mg) initially, followed by **250 μg** (0.25 mg) at 1½-hr intervals. Maintenance doses may be increased to 500 μg (0.5 mg), after several unsuccessful smaller doses. The total cumulative dose should not exceed 12 mg; the average dose is 2.6 mg. Continuous administration should not be longer than 2 days; the mean time to abortion is 16 hr.

Dosage Form—Injection: 250 μg of carboprost/1 mL.

Cyproheptadine—page 1230.

Dihydroergotamine Mesylate

Ergotaman-3′,6′,18-trione, 9,10-dihydro-12′-hydroxy-2′-methyl-5′-(phenylmethyl)-, (5′α)-, monomethanesulfonate (salt); DHE 45 (*Sandoz*)

Dihydroergotamine monomethanesulfonate [6190-39-2] $C_{33}H_{37}N_5O_5 \cdot CH_4O_3S$ (679.79).

For the structural formula of dihydroergotamine, see page 405.

Preparation—Dihydroergotamine, prepared by catalytic hydrogenation of ergotamine, is reacted with an equimolar portion of methanesulfonic acid in a suitable solvent.

Description—White, yellowish, or faintly red powder; pH (1 in 1000 solution) between 4.4 and 5.4.

Solubility—1 g in 125 mL water, 90 mL alcohol, 175 mL chloroform or 2600 mL ether.

Uses—A smooth muscle stimulant with somewhat weaker actions than those of ergotamine (see *Ergotamine Tartrate*, below). It causes peripheral vasoconstriction in the presence of low vascular tone because of the stimulation of α-adrenergic receptors. However, in high doses, it has some α-adrenergic antagonist effects. Its actions are erratic, and it is the least effective of the vasoactive drugs used in the treatment of *migraine* and *cluster headaches*. However, when it does abolish headache, it usually does so without producing nausea and vomiting. Its greatest disadvantage is that it must be given parenterally. It has oxytocic activity and it has been used in the third stage of labor, but it is inferior to other ergot alkaloids used for this purpose. It depresses the vasomotor center more than does ergotamine and constricts the arterioles less, and its net effect is one of moderate hypotension. However, in hypertension it is not useful because of its other side effects. Paradoxically, it increases blood pressure in hypotensive persons and is used in the treatment of *postural* (orthostatic) *hypotension*. Because it constricts large veins, the velocity of blood in the veins is increased; this effect is used in the treatment of *deep vein thrombosis* and for *prophylaxis against thrombosis* after major abdominal surgery or hip replacement, the agent being combined with heparin. It is an antagonist of serotonin (5- hydroxytryptamine), but it is doubtful that this activity contributes to the therapeutic effect against migraine, in the doses used.

Dihydroergotamine is most effective against vascular headaches when administered immediately after the first symptoms. The onset of action is 15 to 30 min; the duration of action is 3 to 4 hr.

Adverse effects include occasional nausea and vomiting, precordial "pressure" and pain (from coronary vasoconstriction), tachycardia or bradycardia, hypotension, muscle pain in the limbs, weakness in the legs, numbness and tingling in the digits, localized edema and itching. Gangrene, especially of the extremities, can occur with chronic use or after a large overdose. It is contraindicated when there is peripheral vascular disease, coronary insufficiency, hypertension, renal impairment, hepatic dysfunction, sepsis, pregnancy or hypersensitivity.

Dose—*Intramuscular, adult, vascular headaches,* **1 mg** at the first sign of impending headache, then **1 mg** at the end of the first hour, if necessary, and *again* at the end of the second hour, making a total of 3 mg; once the accumulative minimal effective dose is determined, it may be given as a single dose at the onset of an attack; *postural hypotension,* **1 mg** once a day. *Intravenous, adult,* **1 mg,** to be repeated after 1 hr, if necessary. *Subcutaneous, adult, antithrombotic,* **0.5 mg,** in combination with heparin and lidocaine. No more than a total of 6 mg by any route should be given per week.

Dosage Form—Injection: 1 mg/mL.

Dinoprost Tromethamine—see RPS-18, page 944.

Dinoprostone

Prosta-5,13-dien-1-oic acid, (5*Z*,11α,13*E*,15*S*)-11,15-dihydroxy-9-oxo-, PGE_2; Prostin E_2 (*Upjohn*)

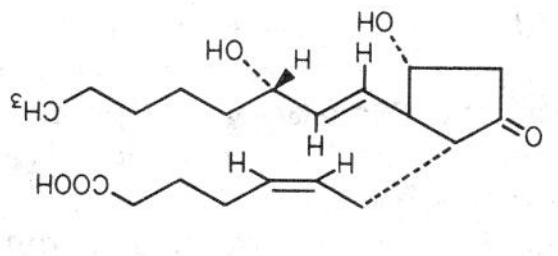

Prostaglandin E_2 [363-24-6] $C_{20}H_{32}O_5$ (352.47).

Preparation—The limited availability of the prostaglandins (page 410) from natural sources has spurred efforts to synthesize them, and total synthesis of prostaglandins F_2 (dinoprost) and E_2 (dinoprostone) has been achieved. The complex syntheses are described in articles in *J Am Chem Soc 91:* 5675, 1969; *92:* 397, 1586, 1970; *94:* 2123, 4342, 1972.

Description—Colorless crystals or white to off-white crystalline solid; melts between 66° and 68°.

Solubility—1 g in about 1000 mL water; soluble in alcohol.

Uses—It is one of a family of over 30 natural, partially cyclic alkenoic acids, called *prostaglandins,* derived from arachidonic acid (see page 410). They are involved in the regulation of endocrine, reproductive, secretory, digestive, nervous, cardiovascular, respiratory, renal and hemostatic systems. Certain prostaglandins are involved in the cyclical changes in uterine tone and activity and the changes consequent to pregnancy. Furthermore, prostaglandins in semen (whence the name prostaglandin) stimulate the myometrium and fallopian tubes in a way that facilitates the transport of sperm to the ovum. Not all prostaglandins have the same actions, some being vasodilator and others vasoconstrictor, etc. Some prostaglandins, eg, prostaglandins E_2 (PGE_2, dinoprostone), are oxytocic and also induce cervical softening. Unlike oxytocin, they are oxytocic even in the second trimester of pregnancy and, hence, can be used as an early abortifacient. Dinoprostone is used to *terminate pregnancy* from the 12th week through the second trimester (80 to 90% effective), to *evacuate the uterus* in intrauterine fetal death or missed abortion up to 28 weeks after conception and to *manage benign hydatidiform mole.* It also is used to induce labor in midtrimester and later, contract the postpartum uterus and, hence, decrease hemorrhage, and ripen the cervix prior to curettage or abortion procedures.

Endovaginally, it may be absorbed sufficiently into the bloodstream to cause systemic side effects; some of the effects attributed to the drug possibly may be the result of hormonal changes and of release of substances from the fetoplacental unit or hydatidiform mole consequent to sloughing and movement or to movement itself. Adverse effects include the following: nausea and vomiting (67%), transient fever (50%; PGE_2 is the mediator of pyrogens), diarrhea (40%), headache (10%), chills and shivering (10%), hypotension (10%), backache, arthralgia, flushing, vertigo, vaginal pain, chest pain, dyspnea, endometritis, faintness, syncope, vulvovaginitis, asthenia, muscle cramps and myalgia, tightness in the chest, breast tenderness, blurred vision, cough, rash, stiff neck, dehydration, tremor, paresthesias, impaired hearing, urinary retention, pharyngitis, laryngitis, sweating, wheezing, tachycardia, skin discoloration, vaginismus, tension and convulsions (rare). Also, it is not fetotoxic, and near the end of the second trimester a live fetus may be presented. Caution should be exercised when there is asthma or chronic obstructive pulmonary disease, hypotension, hypertension, other cardiovascular disease, renal or hepatic disease, anemia, jaundice, diabetes, a past history of epilepsy, endocervical disease, vaginitis or cervicitis. It is contraindicated in acute pelvic inflammatory disease and when there is hypersensitivity to the drug.

Dose—*Intrauterine, abortifacient,* high in the uterus, **20 mg,** to be repeated at 3- to 5-hour intervals until delivery of the fetus, not to exceed 240 mg; *induction of labor* at term or *cervical ripening,* **0.2** to **5mg.**

Dosage Form—Vaginal Suppository: 20 mg.

Ergoloid Mesylates—page 1183.

Ergonovine Maleate

Ergoline-8-carboxamide, [8β(*S*)]-9,10-didehydro-*N*-(2-hydroxy-1-methyl-ethyl)-6-methyl-, (*Z*)-2-butenedioate (1:1) (salt); Ergometrine Maleate; Ergotrate Maleate (*Lilly*)

9,10-Didehydro-*N*-[(*S*)-2-hydroxy-1-methylethyl)-6-methyl-ergoline-8β-carboxamine maleate (1:1) (salt) [129-51-1] $C_{19}H_{23}N_3O_2.C_4H_4O_4$ (441.48).

For the structural formula of ergonovine, see page 405.

Preparation—May be prepared from the natural alkaloid ergonovine by dissolving the latter in a suitable solvent and reacting it with an equimolar portion of maleic acid.

Ergonovine alkaloid also is prepared synthetically from isolysergic acid obtained by alkaline hydrolysis of ergot alkaloids. One of the methods of synthesis involves the following steps: (1) conversion of the acid to its methyl ester by reaction with diazomethane; (2) hydrazinolysis of the ester to lysergic acid hydrazide; (3) condensation of the hydrazide with nitrous acid to form the azide; (4) metathesis of the azide with D-2-amino-1-propanol to form the amide and (5) isomerization of the amide to the normal form by treatment with acetic or phosphoric acid.

Description—White to grayish white or faintly yellow, odorless, microcrystalline powder; affected by light.

Solubility—1 g in about 36 mL water or about 120 mL alcohol; insoluble in ether or chloroform.

Uses—Ergonovine is the most valued of the ergot alkaloids for obstetrical use. It is a powerful *uterine stimulant* and is active after both oral or parenteral administration. It is less toxic than the other natural alkaloids of ergot (see *Ergot*, page 405) and is much less prone to cause gangrene. The maleate is given after the delivery of the placenta for the purpose of inducing prolonged, nonphasic contractions of the uterus in order to *reduce postpartum bleeding*. It also may be administered during the puerperium to *promote involution of the uterus*. In incomplete abortion, it may be used to accelerate the expulsion of the uterine contents. It constricts the cerebral vessels and, hence, is used in the treatment of migraine headache, but it is inferior for this purpose and not recommended. It constricts coronary arteries; in variant angina pectoris the arteries respond to otherwise ineffective doses, so that low doses may be used in the *diagnosis of variant angina pectoris*.

It may cause nausea and vomiting, especially when given intravenously. Like other oxytocics, occasionally it evokes severe hypertensive episodes, especially in hypertensive or toxemic patients or when regional anesthetics containing vasoconstrictors have been used. Such hypertensive episodes can be suppressed by chlorpromazine. Hypersensitivity, including anaphylactic shock, has been reported.

It is contraindicated before the fetus has been presented and should not be used to induce or augment labor. In addition, ergonovine should not be used in persons with known allergy to ergot alkaloids, in uterine sepsis, toxemia of pregnancy, peripheral vascular disease, coronary insufficiency, kidney or liver disease. It should be used cautiously if there is cardiac disease or hypertension. The actions are antagonized by hypocalcemia, and calcium gluconate can be used judiciously to improve the response.

When used properly, there is little problem with adverse side effects; however, high doses administered by the IV route can cause nausea and vomiting, headaches, tinnitus, dyspnea, muscle cramps, nasal congestion, diarrhea and a foul taste.

Dose—*Oxytocic, intramuscular,* **200 μg,** to be repeated in 2 to 4 hr, up to 5 times, if needed; *intravenous,* **200 μg,** only in emergency when there is uncontrolled severe bleeding; *oral,* **200** to **400 μg** 2 to 4 times a day, usually for 2 days postpartum but longer if necessary. *Diagnosis of variant angina pectoris, intravenous,* **50 μg** every 5 min until anginal pain occurs or 400 μg have been given.

Dosage Forms—Injection: 200 μg/1 mL; Tablets: 200 μg.

Ergot Alkaloids

Over 20 have been isolated, and a number of semisynthetic compounds have been made. Sources and a brief chemistry are discussed in Chapter 26.

Uses—The pharmacology is quite complex. Although there are similarities among them, each possesses distinct properties. Natural alkaloids of the peptide type (ergotamine, ergosine, ergocornine, ergocryptine and ergocristine; see Chapter 26) are potent vasoconstrictors and oxytocics of unknown mechanism and also weak α-adrenoreceptor blocking agents. They also possess weak dopaminergic activity, except bromocriptine, which has strong dopaminergic activity.

Hydrogenation at the 9,10-positions considerably diminishes the vasoconstrictor activity, especially in the ergotoxine group (ergocornine, ergocryptine and ergocristine) and moderately diminishes the oxytocic activity, but the α-blocking activity is increased; vasodepression, mostly due to a central action, obscures the residual vasoconstrictor action.

Both the parent and dihydro alkaloids possess serotonin-antagonist activity, but there is also partial serotonin-agonist activity with some. They also increase phosphodiesterase activity, and some derivatives appear to block cAMP, which gives some members the appearance of having β-adrenoreceptor blocking activity.

The so-called amine alkaloids (which are actually alkanolamides), such as ergonovine and methylergonovine (see page 1054), possess only slight vasoconstrictor activity but retain oxytocic activity, for which they mainly are used; they are nearly devoid of adrenergic or serotonin-blocking, serotonin-agonist or dopaminergic activity, except that methysergide is an effective serotonin antagonist.

The ergoline derivatives (LSD, lergotrile, lisuride, etc) lack significant peripheral actions but have complex central actions. LSD is a partial serotonin agonist, acting like serotonin at some loci and as antagonist at others, and it possesses dopaminergic activity as well; the hallucinogenic properties have been attributed to its serotoninergic activity. Other ergolines and some clavines have weak serotoninergic activity and lack hallucinogenic activity but have strong dopaminergic activity in some central loci and dopamine-antagonist activity in others.

Emetic actions probably are attributable to dopaminergic activity at the chemoreceptor trigger zone on the floor of the fourth ventricle, and the hypotensive activity of the dihydrogenated ergot alkaloids possibly is attributable to dopaminergic and/or α-adrenergic activity in the vasomotor center. The effects of bromocriptine and lergotrile to diminish some senile dementia also may result from a dopaminergic action.

Ergotamine Tartrate

Ergotaman-3′,6′,18-trione, 12′-hydroxy-2′-methyl-5′-(phenylmethyl)-, (5′α)-[*R*-(*R**,*R**)]-2,3-dihydroxybutanedioate (2:1) (salt); Ergomar (*Fisons*); Ergostat (*Parke-Davis*); Medihaler Ergotamine (*3M*); Wigraine (*Organon*)

Ergotamine tartrate (2:1) (salt) [379-79-3] $(C_{33}H_{35}N_5O_5)_2.C_4H_6O_6$ (1313.43).

For the structural formula of ergotamine, see page 405.

Description—Colorless crystals or a white to yellowish white, crystalline powder, usually containing solvent of crystallization; these crystals lose the solvent of crystallization in a high vacuum; melts at about 180° with decomposition.

Solubility—1 g in about 500 mL water or about 500 mL alcohol; slightly more soluble in the presence of a slight excess of tartaric acid.

Uses—Possesses the characteristic actions of *Ergot Alkaloids* (page 405). It is the drug of choice in the treatment of *migraine, cluster* and other *vascular headaches*, and it affords relief in about 90% of cases. It contracts the painfully dilated cerebral vessels in these disorders. The drug is most effective if given early in the course of the attack. It usually is administered sublingually or by oral inhalation. When combined with caffeine, ergotamine is given orally or rectally. Ergotamine also exerts oxytocic actions, but stimulates uterine contractions much less effectively than ergonovine. There is no acceptable evidence that ergotamine is of benefit in menopausal disorders. The use of ergotamine to treat cardiovascular disorders could be dangerous.

Many of the ergotamine-containing products are combinations. Caffeine (100 mg) frequently is included in these combination products and may enhance the relief of vascular headaches by ergotamine by increasing its GI absorption or by causing cerebral vasconstriction of its own.

Some products contain belladonna alkaloids in marginally effective amounts, with the unsupported rationale that the alkaloids correct some hypothetical autonomic imbalance. Products containing pentobarbital also are promoted with faulty rationale; if an antianxiety drug is justified, a benzodiazepine should be used.

Peak plasma levels after oral administration occur within 0.5–3 hours, but the pharmacokinetics after sublingual, oral inhalation or rectal applications are not well studied.

Adverse effects are most common after large doses or accumulation of small doses. They include nausea, vomiting, epigastric distress, diarrhea, muscle weakness, precordial distress and pain (indicative of coronary spasm), coldness of the skin (from vasoconstriction), bradycardia or tachycardia, paresthesias in the extremities, myalgia (especially in the thigh and neck muscles), localized edema (mostly in the face and extremities), itching and dermatitis. Occasionally, hypertensive episodes occur. With continued administration, severe vasoconstriction, endarteritis and gangrene may result. With combinations, the potential adverse effects of the other components also must be kept in mind. It is contraindicated in pregnancy, peripheral vascular disease, coronary insufficiency or angina pectoris, thrombophlebitis, peptic ulcer, kidney disease, liver disease, sepsis, malnutrition and when there is a history of hypersensitivity to ergot alkaloids.

Dose—Doses should be titrated for each patient during several attacks and the minimum dose used. *Oral, adult,* **1 to 2 mg;** this dose may be repeated in 30 min and again in 1 hr. In subsequent attacks up to 3 or 4 mg may be taken, but no more than 6 mg should be taken in any 1 day. No more than 10 mg should be taken per week. *Sublingual, adult,* **1 mg;** this dose may be repeated after 30 to 60 min; at the *next attack,* the dose is **2 mg,** and 1 or 2 mg may be given in 30 to 60 min, if needed. In this way the initial dose with each attack may be increased to 5 mg. No more than 10 mg should be taken per week. *Inhalation, adult,* **360 μg;** this dose may be repeated at intervals no shorter than 30 min up to a total of 2.16 mg (6 inhalations) per day but no more than 5.4 mg (15 inhalations) per week. *Rectal, adult,* **2 mg** with 100 mg of caffeine; this dose may be repeated once only in 1 hour if necessary. No more than 5 suppositories (10 mg of ergotamine) should be taken per week.

Dosage Forms—Inhalation: 9 mg/mL; Suppositories: 2 mg (with 100 mg of caffeine); Tablets: 1 mg (with 100 mg of caffeine); Sublingual Tablets: 2 mg.

Methylergonovine Maleate

Ergoline-8-carboxamide, 9,10-didehydro-*N*-[1-(hydroxymethyl)propyl]-6-methyl-, [8β(*S*)]-, (*Z*)-2-butenedioate (1:1) (salt); Methergine (*Sandoz*)

9,10-Didehydro-*N*-[(*S*)-1-(hydroxymethyl)propyl]-6-methyl- ergoline-8β-carboxamide maleate (1:1) (salt) [7054-07-1] [57432-61-8] $C_{20}H_{25}N_3O_2.C_4H_4O_4$ (455.51).

For the structural formula of methylergonovine, see page 405.

Preparation—Synthesized by the method described above for ergonovine except that in step (4), D-2-amino-1-butanol is employed. The base, dissolved in a suitable solvent, yields the maleate by reaction with an equimolar quantity of maleic acid.

Description—White to pinkish tan, microcrystalline powder; odorless and a bitter taste; must be protected from light and heat; pH (1 in 5000 solution) between 4.4 and 5.2.

Solubility—1 g in 100 mL water, 175 mL alcohol, 1900 mL chloroform or 8400 mL ether.

Uses—Similar in its actions to ergonovine, and it shares the same uses as an *oxytocic* drug (see *Ergonovine Maleate*). It may induce uterine contractions upon either oral or parenteral administration. The intensity and duration of its oxytocic action is greater than that of ergonovine but less than that of ergotamine. Despite a lesser incidence of side effects compared to other drugs used to treat migraine, authorities do not recommend this use because the efficacy is less.

The side effects are the same as those of *Ergonovine Maleate*, but they are of a lesser intensity. The precautions and contraindications are also the same.

Dose—*Oxytocic, oral, adult,* **200** to **400 μg** 2 to 4 times a day, usually for 2 days postpartum and no longer than 1 week. *Intramuscular* or *intravenous,* **200 μg,** to be repeated in 2 to 4 hr if necessary.

Dosage Forms—Injection: 200 μg/mL; Tablets: 200 μg.

Methysergide Maleate

Ergoline-8-carboxamide, 9,10-didehydro-*N*-[1-(hydroxymethyl)propyl]-1,6-dimethyl-, (8β)-, (*Z*)-2-butenedioate (1:1) (salt); Sansert (*Sandoz*)

9,10-Didehydro-*N*-[1-(hydroxymethyl)propyl]-1,6-dimethyl-ergoline-8β-carboxamide maleate (1:1) (salt) [129-49-7] $C_{21}H_{27}N_3O_2.C_4H_4O_4$ (469.5⁄).

For the structural formula of methysergide, see page 405.

Preparation—Methylergonovine (base) (see *Methylergonovine Maleate*) is methylated at the indole nitrogen with methyl iodide and the resulting methysergide (base) is dissolved in a suitable solvent and reacted with an equimolar portion of maleic acid. US Pat 3,113,133.

Description—White to yellowish white or reddish white crystalline powder; melting point uncharacteristic showing decomposition above approximately 165°; odorless or not more than a slight odor.

Solubility—1 g in 200 mL water, 165 mL alcohol or 3400 mL chloroform; practically insoluble in ether.

Uses—Methysergide is the *N*-methyl derivative of methylergonovine. However, its oxytocic activity is much weaker, and it is not employed as an oxytocic. Its principal therapeutic use is in the *treatment and prophylaxis of migraine* and *cluster headaches,* for which the drug is quite effective, but it is of very little use during an acute attack. Since it has only weak vasoconstrictor activity, cerebral vasoconstriction has been discounted as the mechanism of action against migraine; thus, its action likely differs from that of ergotamine (see *Ergotamine Tartrate,* page 1054). It is a potent serotonin antagonist, and it has been suggested that its usefulness against migraine is based on this action; various facts contradict this suggestion. The drug is not effective in tension and other types of headache.

Side effects occur in more than a third of patients, but they usually are mild and of brief duration. They are severe enough in 20% of users to require discontinuation of the drug. The most common adverse effects are nausea, abdominal cramps, leg cramps, vertigo, restlessness, insomnia, drowsiness, confusion, epigastric pain (with increased secretion of gastric acid), feelings of depersonalization and mental disturbances. Less-frequent effects include vomiting, diarrhea, constipation, muscle weakness, myalgia, arthralgia, paresthesias in the extremities, ataxia, facial flush, skin rash, telangiectasis, edema and weight gain, weakness, tachycardia, postural hypotension, coronary and peripheral arterial insufficiency, alopecia and induction of premature labor. Neutropenia and eosinophilia are rare. Prolonged therapy has been known to cause retroperitoneal fibrosis. Patients should be instructed in the signs and symptoms of the syndrome, and a urogram should be taken at 6-month intervals during chronic use. It also causes pleuropulmonary, myocardial and aortic fibrosis, the last-named to the point of obstruction. It suppresses sleep-related prolactin secretion and increases growth hormone secretion during sleep, effects that may be adverse or beneficial, depending on circumstances. Many of the side effects diminish after continued administration of the drug. It is contraindicated during pregnancy, in patients with peripheral vascular disease, valvular heart disease, coronary artery disease, thrombophlebitis, severe hypertension, renal, hepatic or pulmonary disorders, rheumatoid arthritis or other collagen diseases or any condition which may cause fibrosis.

Dose—*Oral, adult,* **2 mg** 2 to 3 times a day, *preferably with meals.* It should not be used continuously for a period longer than 6 months without a 1- to 2-month drug-free interval. When discontinuing use, the dose must be reduced gradually to avoid rebound headache.

Dosage Form—Tablets: 2 mg.

Oxytocin

Alpha-Hypophamine; Pitocin (*Parke-Davis*); Syntocinon (*Sandoz*); (*Invenex, Wyeth*)

H-Cys-Tyr-Ile-Glu(NH2)-Asp(NH2)-Cys-Pro-Leu-Gly-NH2
1 2 3 4 5 6 7 8 9

[50-56-6] $C_{43}H_{66}N_{12}O_{12}S_2$ (1007.19).

Preparation—Obtained from the posterior lobe of the pituitary of healthy hogs or cattle; from either source it has the same amino-acid composition. Synthesis was achieved by du Vigneaud and is beyond the scope of this text (see *J Am Chem Soc 76:* 3107, 1954). Commercial preparation is described in US Pat 3,076,797.

Description—White powder; $[\alpha]_D^{22}$ − 26.2° (c = 0.53).

Solubility—Soluble in water, 1-butanol or 2-butanol.

Uses—See *Posterior Pituitary,* page 1062. Natural, endogenous oxytocin is involved in normal parturition. The hormone stimulates guanyl cyclase in myometrial tissue, which promotes inward movement of sodium ion and the consequent increase in both the frequency and strength of contractions. The contractions that are induced are normal phasic contractions. It does not appear to initiate activity not already latent. Hence, the drug is not very active until close to term, and it is less likely than ergonovine to cause harm to the fetus and mother. Nevertheless, unless the cervix is dilated, oxytocin can cause injury. Oxytocin is used antepartum when an early vaginal delivery is desired. It is the drug of choice for the *induction* and *maintenance of labor* once the pregnancy is at term. It is used more frequently when there is prolonged *uterine inertia* than when labor is only somewhat sluggish. It may be used to *assist an ongoing abortion.* It cannot induce an abortion except in high doses (20 to 30 units) and usually not until after the 20th week of pregnancy. It may be used to *control postpartum hemorrhage* and *promote uterine involution,* but the appropriate ergot alkaloids are preferred. It induces contraction of the myoepithelial cells around the breast alveoli, thus squeezing milk into the larger ducts and increasing flow through the nipple, and it is used occasionally in the treatment of *breast engorgement* or to *increase milk flow* to the infant.

It has a weak antidiuretic hormone-like activity, and during prolonged infusion it can cause water intoxication with convulsions and coma, especially in patients with toxemia of pregnancy. For infusion, saline, rather than dextrose, lessens this danger. The drug also occasionally induces a hypertensive episode, which may cause subarachnoid hemorrhage or fetal death. Pelvic hematomas and allergic reactions may occur in the mother and cardiac arrhythmias and jaundice in the fetus. The drug is contraindicated in toxemia, abruptio placentae, undilated cervix, over-distended uterus, abnormal presentation and renal or cardiovascular disease. Extreme care must be used when combining it with another oxytocic drug.

Dose—*Intramuscular,* to *control postpartum bleeding,* **3** to **10 Units** after the delivery of the placenta. *Intravenous infusion,* for *induction and/or maintenance of labor, initially* **1** to **2 mUnits/min** then gradually increasing the rate by increments of 1 to 2 mUnits/min at 15- to 30-min intervals until a near-normal contraction pattern has been achieved or a rate of 20 mUnits/min has been established; to *control postpartum uterine bleeding,* **10 Units** in 1000 mL of isotonic sodium chloride solution with or without 5% dextrose infused at a *rate* **20** to **40 mUnits/min,** except up to 100 mUnits/min following abortion; to *manage incomplete or impending abortion,* **10 Units** at a rate of **20** to **40 mUnits/min.** *Intranasal,* to *stimulate milk flow,* **one spray** or **3 drops into one or both nostrils** of a solution containing 40 Units/mL, to be administered 2 to 3 min prior to nursing or breast pumping.

Dosage Forms—Injection: 10 Units/mL; Nasal spray: 40 Units/mL.

Sodium Chloride—page 932.

Sumatriptan Succinate

1*H*-Indole-5-methanesulfonamide, 3-[2-(dimethylamino)ethyl]-*N*-methyl-, butamedioate; Imitrex (*Glaxo*)

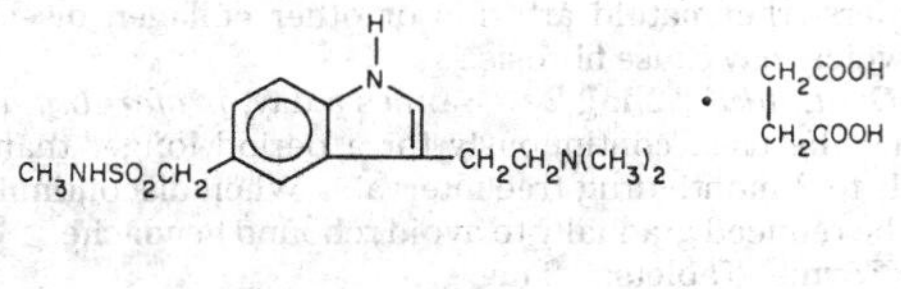

[103628-8-4] $C_{14}H_{21}N_3O_2S.C_4H_6O_4$ (413.49).

Preparation—Ger Pat 3,320,521.

Description—White crystalline powder; melts about 165°.

Uses—A serotonin agonist used for treatment of migraine headaches. It is thought to relieve migraines by selectively constricting the large intracranial blood vessels of the carotid circulation. This action is thought to be therapeutically advantageous because it helps to relieve the inflammation around sensory nerves caused by vasodilation of intracranial vessels during migraine episodes (*Med Lett 34 Oct 2*): 91, 1992). Sumatriptan does not cross the blood-brain barrier; also, it neither decreases cerebral blood flow nor has any direct analgesic action. Sumatriptan is administered subcutaneously and, due to rapid absorption, reaches peak concentrations in 5 to 20 min. The drug is inactivated by hepatic metabolism and following oral administration only 15% reaches systemic circulation due to first-pass clearance by the liver. The mean $t_{1/2}$ after subcutaneous administration is approximately 2 hr.

Sumatriptan is not recommended for prophylatic use. In clinical trials, 70% of the patients receiving this drug reported relief from migraine headache pain compared to 22% receiving placebo. In addition, 33% of the patients treated with sumatriptan remained pain-free for 24 hr compared to 11% of the patients receiving placebo (Cady RK *et al: JAMA 265:* 2831, 1991). In another trial it was observed that 30 min after subcutaneous injection of 6 mg of sumatriptan, 50% of the patients received relief from migraine pain, and within 2 hr of treatment, 90% of the migraine suffers experienced diminished pain (Study Group, *N Engl J Med 325:* 316, 1991). This serotonin agonist also is more effective than placebo in relieving migraine-associated nausea, vomiting, phonophobia and photophobia. In addition, sumatriptan has been reported to relieve pain associated with cluster headaches within 15 min of a subcutaneous administration in 70% of the patients.

In general, sumatriptan appears to be more effective than previously available drugs for treatment of acute attacks of migraine and cluster headaches, although additional confirming studies are needed. The auto-injected, subcutaneous formulation appears to be faster acting and more effective than tablets; however, neither form is recommended for prophylactic use.

The long-term safety of sumatriptan has not been established. If given intravenously it can cause a transient increase in blood pressure and occasionally constriction of coronary arteries. Angina has been reported in patients with coronary artery disease or Prinzmetal's angina after use of sumatriptan; thus, this drug is contraindicated in these patients. Subcutaneous injection of sumatriptan can cause localized pain and redness. Other side effects of injected sumatriptan include tingling, flushing, burning of the skin, nausea, a sense of tightness and thoracic pressure. The most frequent complaints with oral sumatriptan are nausea and vomiting. Sumatriptan should not be used until 24 hr after administering an ergotamine, and ergotamine preparations should not be used until 6 hr after sumatriptan.

Dose—*Oral, for relief of migraine,* **100 mg** with maximum of 300 mg in 24 hr. *Subcutaneous, for relief of migraine,* **6 mg** with maximum of 12 mg in 24 hr. The injection should be administered in the lateral thigh using an autoinjector supplied with the drug. A second dose is not effective if pain does not respond to the first dose.

Dosage Forms—Tablet: 100 mg; Injection: 12 mg/mL (comes with autoinjector).

Urea—page 1041.

CHAPTER 64

Hormones

William K Nichols, PhD
Associate Professor of Pharmacology
College of Pharmacy
University of Utah
Salt Lake City, UT 84112

Hormones are substances secreted by the endocrine, or ductless, glands and nonglandular tissues which serve to integrate metabolic processes. The regulatory function of the hormones differs from other regulatory mechanisms (such as the nervous system and other glandular secretions) in that the hormones are transported to the affected tissues by the blood. Some of the hormones affect nearly all the tissues of the body; the action of others is restricted to but a few tissues or organs.

Chemically, the hormones represent a very diverse group of compounds. Some, like epinephrine and thyroxine, are relatively simple amino acid derivatives. Several groups of hormones, such as those produced by the adrenal cortex and the gonads, are steroids, while the pituitary, parathyroid and pancreatic hormones are polypeptides or proteins; the molecular weights of the latter range from about 1000 to 30,000 or more. The gastrointestinal, thymic, renal, atrial natriuretic, adrenal medullary and neural (other than hypothalamic) hormones and colony-stimulating factor, interleukins, interferons, various growth factors and platelet-activating factor (which plays a role in ovulation) are not discussed in this chapter.

In most instances, the existence of a trophic hormone was usually first recognized when degeneration or destruction of a gland by disease or accident in humans or its experimental removal from animals was found to result in unfavorable physiological consequences. (The hypothalamic releasing and inhibitory hormones were anticipated on theoretical grounds and discovered as the result of theory-directed research.) Attempts then were made to reverse such untoward effects by implanting tissues from healthy animals (frequently at other sites) or by supplying extracts prepared from them. Once the type of physiological activity attributable to any one gland has been recognized and a biologically effective extract has been produced, the way is opened for the development of an assay method by means of which the hormone content of various preparations can be compared. The ultimate goal with each extract is to obtain a demonstrably pure active substance, to establish its chemical structure and to develop either a method of synthesis or a convenient method of preparation from natural sources so as to make it available for therapeutic or experimental use. Frequently, the successful conclusion of attempts to isolate, purify and identify a hormone also has permitted the development of chemical methods for its determination—for example, in body fluids. However, for some of the hormones, available chemical methods for identification and quantitative determination are still inferior to biological methods as regards specificity and sensitivity.

Standardization—Many of the hormones, or substances which possess nearly identical biological properties, have been prepared in chemically pure (usually crystalline) form, either from natural sources, or by synthesis. For such materials, the standard practice is to specify a dose in terms of weight. With others, especially some of the polypeptide or protein hormones, potency is expressed in terms of biological activity. In such instances, a unit of biological activity is established as the amount necessary to produce a predetermined response in a test animal, or by comparison with an arbitrarily accepted standard preparation. For some preparations, eg, insulin and the posterior lobe hormones, the custom of designating dosage in terms of biological "units" has persisted even after the substance has become available in chemically pure form. The use of units is important especially when hormones of different sources differ in chemical composition and activity. In any event, no hormone preparation should be used therapeutically unless it is a pure substance or its activity can be precisely assayed biologically.

Administration—A few of the hormones can be administered *orally* with full effect, eg, thyroid and certain steroid hormones. There is usually some loss due to destruction of the hormone in the digestive tract, its elimination from the circulation or inactivation while it is in transit through the liver immediately after absorption. Some hormones must be administered by injection, either *subcutaneously* or *intramuscularly*, because they are inactivated in the digestive tract. The intramuscular injection usually is chosen, and it gives rapid absorption if the hormone is in aqueous solution, or slower absorption if the hormone is in oil. This use of oil is not ideal, for oil is not readily removed from the site of injection, and oils are difficult to free from allergens. Suspensions of crystals of differing size also have variable repository actions. Another technique is the *implantation* of compressed pellets of those hormones which are only slightly soluble in tissue fluid; these pellets are placed in the subcutaneous tissues and are absorbed during a period of a few months. This technique has the disadvantage of requiring a careful surgical procedure, and, even with good technique, certain pellets may be extruded due to infection, or they may be of no value because of fibrous tissue barriers which develop about the pellets in some cases. Hormones entrained in degradable polymers, or even in silicones, can be used for slow-release forms. Still another form is the buccal tablet of very highly compressed steroid hormone which is held in the buccal area (usually anteriorly between the upper lip and gingiva) for up to 45 minutes. During this time there is absorption through the buccal mucous membrane, providing direct access of the steroid to the systemic circulation. This avoids the disadvantage of the oral route, by which steroids must pass through the liver where they are largely inactivated. Some of the synthetic or semisynthetic hormones are structured so as to greatly diminish enzymatic destruction in the liver and hence are effective orally. Notable among these are the oral contraceptives. Some drugs, particularly insulin, may be delivered subcutaneously through a permanently implanted canula, the injection powered by a tiny attached pump; considerable progress has been made toward demand-actuated pumps.

The Pituitary Hormones

The pituitary body (hypophysis) comprises anterior, intermediate and posterior portions or lobes, which have distinguishing structures and functions. Active principles have been discovered in extracts prepared in various ways from all three portions of the pituitary, and these will be listed and discussed separately.

The Anterior Pituitary

The pituitary body is known as the "master gland" because it has so many important actions in the body and it regulates the function of several of the other glands. Without the anterior portion of the pituitary gland, the sex functions and growth cease, and the functions of the adrenal cortex, the thyroid and the parathyroids decrease markedly. The anterior lobe of the pituitary has at least *six* separate hormones. Some of the anterior pituitary hormones also are produced outside of the adenohypophysis and extrapituitary production plays a role in physiological functions of certain pituitary hormones. For example, a growth lactogenic hormone and ACTH elaborated by the placenta, undoubtedly are important during pregnancy. Growth hormone also is produced by monocytes.

1. Somatropin (*Growth Hormone, GH, Somatotropin, STH;* The recombinant methionine derivative is known as *Somatrem.*)—This hormone causes an increase in weight and length of the body. The increase in length is especially prominent, due to the bone growth, but its effect is manifested in nearly all the tissues of the body. Human GH also possesses most of the activities of lactogenic hormone. For maximum action of growth hormone, all the essential and quasiessential amino acids must be present in abundance. Some, perhaps all, of the effects of GH are mediated by several *somatomedins,* two of which are called *insulin-like growth factors* (I and II) and at least one of which is the *sulfation factor.*

Human GH contains 191 amino acid residues and has a molecular weight of 22,000 daltons. It also is found in a much larger molecule which is probably an association of the primary molecule with another protein. The biological properties of GH can be assayed by observing the growth of hypophysectomized young rats in response to injections of the hormone, or by measuring the extent of bone growth (tibia) adjacent to the epiphyseal line. In humans, the protein anabolic action of GH is most readily measured by its nitrogen-retaining effect. Other assay methods involve the effect on the plasma sulfation factor, plasma phosphate, insulin tolerance and especially radioimmunoassay.

In addition to effects upon protein metabolism, GH affects the metabolism of carbohydrates, fats and steroids. These effects include (a) maintenance of a normal amount of muscle glycogen in hypophysectomized animals, (b) decreased responsiveness to insulin, (c) increased concentration of nonesterified fatty acids in plasma and promotion of steroid-metabolizing cytochrome P450s that differ in males and females. In turn, sex hormones regulate GH secretion. Human GH also exerts prominent effects on the kidney and electrolyte metabolism.

Unlike corticotropin, insulin and some of the other protein hormones, a considerable species difference has been observed in response to GH administration. Thus, GH active in fishes can be isolated from fish pituitaries, but this substance is inactive in mammals. Bovine GH is active in fishes, rats, dogs (and presumably in cattle) but is inactive in monkeys and men, whereas GH prepared from simian or human pituitaries is active in both primate species, as well as in nearly all lower orders of animals in which it has been tested. These differences appear to be reflections of significant variations in the chemical composition of the hormones from various sources. For example, the molecular weight of primate GH is much smaller than that of the bovine variety (29,000 versus 46,000).

These facts explain why attempts to demonstrate beneficial effects when GH preparations from domestic animals are used clinically have been disappointing. Human GH is used successfully in stimulating growth (height and weight increase) in hypopituitary dwarfs. It also is used to treat other forms of retarded growth. An interesting diagnostic application of human GH is based upon its ability to increase the concentration of free fatty acids in the blood. Patients suffering from acromegaly (a disease caused by excessive secretion of GH) are sometimes treated by radiation therapy. In order to assess the effects of the treatment, GH is administered and its effects upon plasma free fatty acid is determined. If the treatment is successful, production of endogenous GH diminishes or ceases; subsequent injection of growth hormone will cause an increase in free fatty acids in the plasma. The effect to increase blood glucose concentration has been used in the treatment of hypoglycemia (especially that which is lysine- sensitive) in children. The nitrogen-sparing anabolic effect has been employed to suppress catabolism from burns and other severe trauma. Potential uses include the stimulation of hematopoiesis and postmenopausal and other bone mineralization, the treatment of renal failure, obesity, hyperlipidemia immune disorders, aging and hypothalamic hypofunction.

2. The Gonadotropic Hormones—Two separate gonadotropins are secreted by the anterior pituitary. They act both in concert and sequentially to control the sexual (estrous) cycle in lower animals and the menstrual cycle in primates.

a. Follicle-stimulating Hormone (FSH)—Human FSH is a two-subunit glycoprotein with a molecular weight of 32,000. The carbohydrate content is 18%. It promotes maturation of the primordial follicle and in combination with small amounts of LH (see below) stimulates secretion of estrogen by the developing follicle. During the first 7 days of the estrous cycle, estrogens suppress the release of FSH, as a result of negative feedback actions on both the anterior pituitary and hypothalamus. In days 9 to 18, estrogens have a positive feedback effect to increase FSH secretion; progesterone blocks the positive but not the negative feedback effect.

b. Luteinizing Hormone (LH)—Human LH is also a two-subunit glycoprotein with a molecular weight of 32,000 and a carbohydrate content of 18%. The secretion of LH increases near the middle of the cycle. As noted above, small amounts of LH, acting with FSH, stimulate the secretion of estrogen by the ovarian follicle. As the amount of LH increases, ovulation occurs, and the corpus luteum begins to form.

LH also acts upon the male gonads, specifically upon the interstitial cells of the testis, to produce testosterone. Because of this property, LH is also sometimes referred to as interstitial cell-stimulating hormone (ICSH).

As with FSH, estrogens have a suppressant effect on LH secretion early and an augmenting effect later in the estrous cycle, but the time course of sensitivity is somewhat different from that with FSH. Progesterone similarly blocks the positive feedback effect. Androgens also suppress the secretion of LH.

Other Gonadotropic Substances—In addition to the anterior pituitary glands, three other sources of gonadotropic activity are known. Two are produced by the chorionic cells of the placenta of women and mares, respectively. The third is a gonadotropin (*urofollitropin*; human menopausal gonadotropin or HMG) present in the serum of postmenopausal women and is a mixture of FSH:LH in approximately a 1:1 ratio. Human chorionic gonadotropin (HCG) is secreted into the maternal blood and is excreted in the urine, where it may be detected within 48 hr after the ovum is implanted. The biological properties of HCG approximate most closely those of LH and prolactin (Prl) in combination, although it differs substantially from either in chemical properties. Thus, like Prl, HCG maintains the secretion of the corpus luteum, enabling pregnancy to continue. Like LH, it will act upon gonadal interstitial cells. Unlike FSH, it will not act upon the ovary of the hypophysectomized rat, although it will exert a marked synergism with FSH in this respect.

Human chorionic gonadotropin is a glycoprotein of molecular weight 35,000; the carbohydrate content is about 28%. The molecule has α and β subunits, the β-subunit conferring the special activity. There is about an 80% homology in structure and aminoacid sequence to HLH-β. HCG-α is nearly identical to FSH-α, except for the terminal three amino acids.

The international unit of HCG is defined as the activity of 0.1 mg of the international standard. Purified HCG contains approximately 12,000 IU/mg.

Uses of Gonadotropic Hormones—Although many attempts have been made to demonstrate in humans an effect of pituitary gonadotropins from domestic animals, the evidence obtained so far has been equivocal or frankly negative. This may be due to a species specificity of the kind already noted in connection with growth hormone preparations. Preparations of FSH from human pituitaries or menotropins from the serum of postmenopausal women, administered in conjunction with LH or HCG, have been found to induce ovulation in women suffering from diminished gonadotropin secretion. However, evidence of superovulation (production of more than one ovum) sometimes is obtained following administration of FSH or menotropins of human origin. Human chorionic gonadotropin also is used for stimulation of androgen secretion by testicular interstitial cells, and for expediting the descent of the testes in boys and young men with cryptorchidism. It also has been found to be effective in prolonging luteal function and in inducing ovulatory cycles in anovulatory women with metropathia hemorrhagica. However, HCG appears to induce ovulation only when a mature ovarian follicle is present. Unfortunately, a mature follicle is not common in anovulatory women. HCG is not effective in the treatment of obesity.

3. Prolactin (Prl; lactogenic hormone, mammotropin)—It is a protein of MW 20,000, which is derived from a prohormone of MW 50,000. In the last 50 *N*-terminal aminoacids of prolactin there is 24% identity with growth hormone in the aminoacids and sequence. Human placental lactogen has an identity of 76%, which accounts for the greater growth hormone-like properties of the placental lactogen. Both prolactin and growth hormone have "big" and "little" circulating forms, the release of which appears to be under separate controls. A related hormone, placental lactogen (PL; chorionic somatomammotropin) is produced by the placenta.

It now is recognized that Prl is a hormone with many different actions, perhaps more so than growth hormone, of which primitive prolactin appears to be the phylogenetic precursor. By itself, Prl does not cause breast development, but in concert with estrogens, progesterone and permissive actions of hydrocortisone and insulin it is mammotropic. It widely is thought to be a cocarcinogen for breast cancer, but the evidence is not conclusive. In the human, it also stimulates milk secretion by the mammary glands, but only after suitable priming by estrogens and progesterone. Other effects in humans include lipolysis, luteotropism and luteolysis, promotion of growth and secretion, increase in testicular steroidogenesis and development of the male accessory sex organs and involvement in the regulation of gonadotropin release.

4. Thyrotropic Hormone (*Thyrotropin, TSH*)—The most potent TSH preparations which have been obtained thus far are still impure. TSH obtained from beef pituitaries is a glycoprotein of molecular weight of about 28,000. The sugars are mannose, fucose, galactose and *N*-acetylglucosamine. Human TSH contains sialic acid. There are two subunits. The β subunit contains the specific activity; it has 113 amino acid residues, without carbohydrate moieties. The α subunit has 96 residues and the carbohydrate moieties. The α unit is functionally interchangeable with the α unit of LH or HCG, and the α units are nearly identical.

Thyrotropin sustains the activity of the thyroid gland, promoting increased uptake of inorganic iodine and release of organically bound iodine. In the absence of TSH, the thyroid gland atrophies, producing only small amounts of thyroid hormone. An excess of TSH causes hypertrophy and hyperplasia of the thyroid, and a clinical picture resembling Graves' disease.

In Graves' disease an abnormal thyrotropic substance is present in the blood. Because of its long duration of action it is called long-acting thyroid stimulator (LATS). It is a 7S globulin of the immunoglobulin G (IgG) class. It may be an autoantibody to TSH which is capable of mimicking its antigen. It differs from TSH in that it crosses the placental barrier, and its production is not suppressed by thyroid hormone; the nonsuppressibility is the basis of a diagnostic test for borderline hyperthyroidism.

5. Adrenal Corticotropic Hormone (*Corticotropin, ACTH*)—It is a polypeptide containing 39 amino acid residues with a molecular weight of 4566. ACTH is produced not only by the adenohypophysis but also by the placenta. The hormones from pituitaries of various species of animals differ with respect to the sequence of amino acids 25 to 32, but these differences do not affect their biological actions. When corticotropin is treated briefly with pepsin, 11 amino acid residues at the *C*- terminal end are removed. The product (β-corticotropin) retains full biological activity. In contrast, even slight alteration of the *N*-terminal end of the molecule results in substantial inactivation. A synthetic polypeptide containing the first 23 amino acid residues of naturally occurring corticotropin has essentially all of the biological and clinical properties of corticotropin. Several peptides have been synthesized which are more potent than natural ACTH.

Physiological Effects—ACTH maintains and controls the functions of the adrenal cortex and thus indirectly affects carbohydrate, protein and mineral metabolism. Since the known physiological actions of corticotropin are mediated through the adrenal cortex, its effects are similar to those of the adrenal cortical hormones, especially the glucocorticoids (see *Adrenal Hormones*, page 1064). ACTH also slightly enhances the adrenal cortical output of aldosterone and hence has a minor action on mineral metabolism. However, aldosterone secretion is mostly under the control of the renin-angiotensin system (see page 949).

Since the first 13 amino acids of ACTH are identical in sequence to those of α-MSH (melanocyte-stimulating hormone), ACTH causes some hyperpigmentation of the skin. ACTH also causes ketosis, fat mobilization (adipokinesis), hypoglycemia and insulin resistance in high doses. There is evidence that both ACTH and α-melanotropin are contained in cerebral neurons and function as neurotransmitters and/or neuromodulators.

6. Other Pituitary Principles—From time to time the existence of anterior pituitary hormones other than those listed above has been postulated. Generally, the effects attributed to them have been shown to be referable to one or more of the known pituitary hormones. Thus, for example, the diabetogenic effect of anterior pituitary extracts has been shown to be due to the action of somatotropin under conditions of limited insulin supply. Several of the anterior lobe hormones possess adipokinetic properties as well as melanocyte-stimulating and adrenocorticotrophic activity. The adenohypophysis also contains some β-lipotropin and β-endorphin.

Hypothalamic Regulation of Anterior Pituitary Secretion: Releasing and Inhibiting Factors (*Hypothalamic Hormones*)—The secretion of an anterior pituitary hormone is not constant but rather undergoes intrinsic cyclical variations and additionally is affected by noncyclical factors, such as stress and input from sensory nerves. The intrinsic cycles are determined mostly by what are called *negative feedback loops*, that is to say that a hormone eventually suppresses its own release indirectly by suppressing the secretion of a hormone from the tuberoinfundibular neuron system of the median eminence of the hypothalamus, which hormone stimulates the release of the anterior pituitary hormone. Such a hypothalamic hormone is called a *hypothalamic releasing factor* if its structure is unknown and as a *hormone* if its structure is known. For each anterior pituitary hormone there is one such factor (except that LH and FSH share the same factor); the designation RF (releasing factor) or RH (releasing hormone) is applied to each factor, CRH designating that for corticotropin, TRH for thyrotropin, LH-RH/FSH-RH (LRH/FRH; LRH, GnRH) for luteinizing and follicle-stimulating hormones, GH-RF for growth hormone, MRF for melanocyte-releasing hormone and PRF for prolactin-releasing factor. For growth hormone, prolactin and melanocyte-stimulating hormones there are also respective release inhibitory factors (GH-RIH, PIF and MIF, respectively). These factors are secreted into the bloodstream of the pituitary portal system, by which route they reach the anterior hypophysis, where they evoke burst electrical activity. To be effective, releasing factors must be released in pulses. Sustained-release and long-acting congeners (eg, leuprolide) down-regulate receptors and thus have inhibitory actions. GH-RIH, LHRH and TRH are distributed widely in the brain and probably are also neurotransmitters; CRF also is produced in the periphery and is released during stress; GH-RIH (*somatostatin*) also is produced in the pancreas. There is also a pro GH-RIH which is a stronger inhibitor of insulin release but weaker inhibitor of glucagon release than is GH-RIH. PIF is released from the same cells as LRH.

The negative feedback loop that goes from the anterior hypophysis to the hypothalamus is called the *short negative feedback loop*. There is also a *long negative feedback loop* that involves the appropriate target-gland hormone (cortisol for ACTH, thyroid hormone for TSH, estrogen for FSH, etc). The target hormone not only feeds back negatively on the hypothalamus but also directly on the anterior hypophysis, which appears to be the main locus of feedback for some target-cell hormones. Negative feedback to the hypothalamus apparently elicits both a decrease in secretion of a releasing factor and an increase in the secretion of the inhibitory factor. There is also a nonestrogen-mediated long negative feedback on FSH secretion; the factors involved are called *inhibins*. In the case of LH there is a *long positive feedback* loop in which secretion of estrogens favors secretion of LRH. The noncyclical perturbations in anterior pituitary hormone output are also effected through the hypothalamic releasing and inhibiting factors. PIF is thought to be two factors, namely, dopamine and gamma-aminobutyric acid (GABA).

The hypothalamic releasing factors are relatively small polypeptides with molecular weights ranging up to 8000 daltons. In man, the prolactin-releasing factor may be both norepinephrine and vasoactive intestinal polypeptide (VIP). The simplest releasing factor is TRH, the structure of which is *pyro*Glu-His-Pro-NH_2. *Pyro* means the glutamic acid is internally cyclized; this unit is common to several of the releasing factors. Some releasing factors appear to function as neurotransmitters or neuromodulators elsewhere in the CNS and autonomic nervous system.

The natural and synthetic hypothalamic releasing factors lend themselves to diagnostic as well as therapeutic uses. For example, if a hypothyroid patient responds to TRH with an increase in TSH, then the hypothyroidism may be a lesion in the hypothalamus or pituitary portal system rather than in the anterior hypophysis; this appears to be the situation in cretinism, and treatment with TRH rather than TSH or thyroid hormone may be indicated, because some releasing factors appear to have beneficial actions beyond that of releasing its pituitary hormone. If there is a limited pituitary response to TRH, even in large doses, then the pituitary reserve of TSH is limited. In thyrotoxicosis, TRH fails to affect plasma TSH or thyroid hormone concentrations, so that TRH may distinguish between thyrotoxicosis and apparent hyperthyroid states. LRH/FRH can distinguish between hypothalamic and pituitary defects in hypogonadotropic hypogonadism in men but is not reliable in women. However, it does reveal the existence of primary gonadal failure and hypernormal negative feedback systems in amenorrheic women. LRH/FRH can be used to treat infertility if the defect is in the hypothalamus; even when the defect appears to be at the anterior pituitary level, after a course of treatment anovulatory women frequently go on to secrete normal amounts of LH. GH-RH is used to accelerate growth in growth-retarded children. GH-RIH may be used to treat acromegaly, gigantism and diabetes mellitus associated with excess GH secretion. Structural analogues of the releasing factors are under investigation as agonists and antagonists. An antagonist of LRH would have a considerable potential as a contraceptive. Leuprolide (page 1253), an analog of LRH, presently is available for treating prostatic cancer. The Nle^{27} analog of the first 29 amino acid-segment of GH-RH has been shown clinically to be an effective growth promoter.

The releasing and inhibiting factors are not only under the control of the various peripheral hormones but the brain as well, and the secretion of some has been demonstrated to be affected by neuropharmacological drugs. Thus drugs such as reserpine and methyldopa that decrease the release of dopamine and/or norepinephrine increase the output of lactogenic and growth hormones. *Bromocriptine, lergotrile* and *pergolide,* potent dopaminergic agonists, suppress the output of these two hormones and consequently have been tried, successfully, in the treatment of galactorrhea, prolactin-secreting tumors with hypogonadism in men, hyperprolactinemia-associated infertility in women and acromegaly.

Arginine Hydrochloride—page 1130.

Bromocriptine Mesylate—page 1035.

Buserelin—see RPS-18, page 952.

Chorionic Gonadotropin

Human Chorionic Gonadotropin; HCG (*Various Mfrs*)

A gonad-stimulating polypeptide hormone obtained from the urine of pregnant women. Its potency is not less than 1500 USP Chorionic Gonadotropin Units in each mg.

Description—White or practically white, amorphous powder.

Solubility—Freely soluble in water.

Uses—See *Uses of Gonadotropic Hormones* (page 1058). This drug alone rarely induces ovulation in anovulatory women. In sequence with *Menotropins* (this page), which favors the maturation of ovarian follicles, or after clomiphene, ovulation may be effected in women with low gonadotropin secretion. There have been claims that the hormone may be effective in the treatment of *female infertility* from luteal hypofunction. There is some evidence of a usefulness of the drug in the treatment of *male sterility.* The hormone stimulates testosterone secretion in the male, and some authorities consider it to be superior to either oral or parenteral androgens for replacement therapy in androgenic insufficiency, but the necessity for the injection of it is disadvantageous and such therapy is expensive.

To achieve full spermatogenesis in *hypogonadotropic eunuchoidism,* the hormone is used in combination with menotropins or clomiphene. However, the spermatic tubules may be damaged by prolonged treatment. In *cryptorchidism,* chorionic gonadotropin usually promotes descent of the testicles if the testes are retractile. It seldom causes descent in true cryptorchidism. HCG is used as a *diagnostic* tool to assess the cause of delayed puberty in males, to test the responsiveness of the testes to gonadotropins, and to identify the source of androgens in hirsute females, for which HCG is unreliable.

It may cause virilization and precocious puberty in prepuberal males, and such an effect is an indication to stop treatment. Ovarian hyperstimulation with abdominal bloating and pelvic pain occurs in about 7% of women given combined chorionic gonadotropin and menotropins. It may favor arterial thromboembolism and rupture of ovarian cysts. There are also frequent multiple births. In boys, it may cause acne, growth of pubic hair and rapid increase in height. In men, there may be edema from increased secretion of testosterone. It also may cause gynecomastia, headache, restlessness, irritability, depression, asthenia, edema of the lower limbs and pain at the injection site. HCG has not been demonstrated to be effective in the treatment of obesity.

Dose—*Intramuscular,* for *cryptorchidism in boys,* one of **4000 USP Units** 3 times a week for 3 wk, **5000 USP Units** every other day for 4 injections, 15 injections of **500** to **1000 USP Units** over a period of 6 wk, or **500 USP Units** 3 times a week for 4 to 6 wk; for *hypogonadism in men,* one of **500** to **1000 USP Units** for 3 wk, then twice a week for 3 wk, **1000** to **2000 USP Units** 3 times a week for several weeks to months, or **4000 USP Units** 3 times a week for 6 to 9 mo then **2000 USP Units** 3 times a week for 3 mo; in *diagnosis of male hypogonadism,* **2000 USP Units** a day for 3 days; to *induce ovulation,* in combination with menotropins or clomiphene, **5000** to **10,000 USP Units** once following the last dose of menotropins or 5 to 7 days after the last dose of clomiphene; to *induce spermatogenesis* (in combination with menotropins), **5000 USP Units** 3 times a week for 4 to 6 mo.

Dosage Form—For Injection: 2000, 5000, 10,000 and 20,000 Units.

Corticotropin

ACTH; Adrenocorticotropin; (*Various Mfrs*)

The polypeptide hormone derived from the anterior lobe of the pituitary of mammals used for food by man, which increases rate of secretion of adrenal corticosteroids.

Preparation—Most commercial preparations of *corticotropin* are obtained from either hog or sheep pituitary glands, although beef and whale glands also have been used. Isolation of the hormonal principle(s) from swine and sheep pituitaries was reported in 1943 by Sayers *et al: J Biol Chem 149:*425, 1943, and by Li *et al: Ibid:*413, 1943. A process of purification of the hormonal substance is described in US Pat 3,124,509. For other information see *Adrenal Corticotropic Hormone,* page 1059.

Two types of preparations are available: short- and long-acting. The short-acting preparations consist of a lyophilized powder or a stable aqueous solution containing 1% phenol. The powder is dissolved in physiological saline or other suitable medium before injection. Short-acting preparations are administered either intramuscularly or intravenously.

Long-acting preparations (repository and gel) contain *the drug* incorporated in a gelatin menstruum designed to delay the rate of absorption and increase the period of effectiveness. Combination with zinc hydroxide suspension also delays the rate of absorption. These are injected intramuscularly.

It is standardized by the Sayers assay. The clinical effectiveness, however, varies with the mode of administration. The difference is evident particularly in comparisons of short-acting preparations injected intramuscularly with long-acting preparations similarly administered. For this reason, gel preparations are labeled in terms of "clinical units" to conform more nearly to their expected physiological potency. Fourteen USP Units in gelatin medium possess the approximate clinical efficacy of 40 USP Units of aqueous solution by intermittent intramuscular injection.

Description—White or practically white, soluble, amorphous solid having the characteristic appearance of substances prepared by freeze-drying; pH (of the liquid form or after reconstitution from the solid state) between 3 and 7.

Uses—Stimulates the adrenal gland to produce hydrocortisone, desoxycorticosterone and androgens. It is used as a *diagnostic* drug to assess the functional capacity of the adrenal gland. After injection, a rise in plasma cortisol or urinary 17-hydroxycorticosterone indicates a functional gland. This is at present the most important clinical use of this agent. However, *cosyntropin is preferred* because it is less allergenic. This drug has been promoted as a therapeutic agent in a wide variety of glucocorticoid-responsive disorders (see page 1067). In general, with the exception of primary adrenal insufficiency, it is effective in all of the conditions for which glucocorticoids are found useful, but it is ineffective when applied locally. Except for *infantile myoclonus,* there is no evidence that it can achieve any therapeutic effect that cannot be achieved by appropriate doses of a glucocorticoid and its cost and allergenicity are definite disadvantages. However, some clinicians consider it to be somewhat superior to glucocorticoids in the management of *acute exacerbations of multiple sclerosis* and *inflammatory bowel disease* and as an antiemetic during cancer chemotherapy.

The fact that corticotropin has a trophic action at the neuromuscular jucntion leads to an interesting use in which the peptide hormone may be superior to glucocorticoids is in the management of severe myasthenia gravis. The hormone is given for 10 to 20 days, during which time muscle strength actually deteriorates to the extent that assisted respiration may be required. After treatment stops, the muscle strength returns to normal in 2 to 7 days and then increases above the pretreatment level for several months. Glucocorticoids cause less deterioration during administration but also bring about less improvement afterward. The margin between optimum clinical effectiveness and undesirable side effects is frequently narrow.

The continued administration of large amounts of the hormone may result in one or more of the manifestations of Cushing's syndrome, may exacerbate the symptoms of latent or frank diabetes, and, because of its anti-inflammatory action, may mask symptoms of infection. The need for adequate medical supervision during its use, therefore, cannot be over-emphasized. Various side effects mediated by the glucocorticoids released from the adrenal gland are listed on page 1066. They occur frequently when the dosage exceeds 40 Units a day.

Abrupt cessation of corticotropin injections may be followed by withdrawal effects which take the form of symptoms of adrenal insufficiency. These result from pituitary inhibition which occurs during treatment with corticotropin and may be minimized or eliminated by gradually reducing the amount injected. Corticotropin causes some side effects not caused by glucocorticoids, namely, hypersensitivity, salt and water retention and androgenic effects (acne, hirsutism and amenorrhea) in women. It is contraindicated if there is osteoporosis, systemic mycosis, corneal herpes or scleroderma.

Dose—*Intramuscular, repository, adult,* **40 USP Units** every 12 to 24 hr; *infants,* for *myoclonic seizures, regular* or *repository,* **4** to **8 USP Units** a day; *intramuscular* (or subcutaneous; intramuscular preferred), *adult, hypoadrenal corticism, regular,* **40** to **80 USP Units** a day, variously divided; *repository,* **40** to **80 USP Units** every 24 to 72 hr; *acute multiple sclerosis, regular* or *repository,* **80** to **120 USP Units** a day, variously divided, for 2 to 3 wk; *intramuscular* or *intravenous, children, regular,* **1.6 USP Units/kg** or **50 USP Units/m^2** a day in 3 or 4 divided doses; *intravenous infusion, adult, diagnostic, regular* (only!), **10** to **25 USP Units** in 500 mL of 5% dextrose solution infused over 8 hr; *subcutaneous, children, respository,* **0.8 USP Units/kg** or **25 USP Units/m^2** a day in 1 or 2 divided doses. Corticotropin zinc hydroxide injection should be injected deep into the gluteal muscle.

Dosage Forms—Injection: 25 and 40 Units; Repository Injection: 40 and 80 Units/1 mL, 200 and 400 Units/5 mL; Sterile Zinc Hydroxide Suspension: 200 Units/5 mL.

Cosyntropin

Cortrosyn (*Organon*)

Ser-Tyr-Ser-Met-Glu-His-Phe-Arg-Trp-Gly-Lys-Pro-Val-Gly-Lys-Lys-Arg-Arg-Pro-Val-Lys-Val-Tyr-Pro
1 2 3 4 5 6 7 8 9 10 11 12 13 14 15 16 17 18 19 20 21 22 23 24

α^{1-24}-Corticotropin [16960-16-0] $C_{136}H_{210}N_{40}O_{31}S$ (2933.46).

Preparation—This synthetic polypeptide is identical with the moiety of corticotropin containing the first 24 of its 36 amino acids. For detailed information concerning the synthesis see *Helv Chim Acta 44:* 1136, 1961; *46:*1550, 1963.

Description—A white to off-white lyophilized mixture with 40 parts of mannitol.

Solubility—Soluble in water.

Uses—The full adrenocorticotropic activity of corticotropin resides in the first 23 amino acids, whereas the allergenicity resides in the segment 22 to the C-terminal end. Thus, this drug has full corticotropic activity but negligible antigenicity. Consequently, it is preferred for *diagnostic tests of adrenal function.* Repository preparations are unavailable, so that it usually is not used therapeutically.

Dose—*Intramuscular* or *intravenous, adults and children over 2 yr,* **250 μg**; *children under 2 yr,* **125 μg;** intravenous injection should take at least 2 min or be infused at a rate of **40 μg/ hr** for 6 hr. If the increase in plasma cortisol is at least 7 μg/100 mL and the absolute level is at least 18 μg/100 mL 30 to 60 min after injection, no further tests are made, the patient having normal adrenocortical function. If the response is subnormal, 250 μg is given as a 4- to 8-hr infusion (or corticotropin by the schedule under *Corticotropin Injection)* to distinguish between hypopituitarism, in which an adequate plasma cortisol or urinary 17-hydroxysterol response occurs, and Addison's disease, in which little response occurs.

Dosage Form—for Injection: 0.25 mg in 1-mL vials.

Gonadorelin Acetate

Luteinizing hormone-releasing factor acetate (salt) hydrate; LH-RH; Lutrepulse (*Ferring*)

5-oxoPro-His-Trp-Ser-Tyr-Gly-Leu-Arg-Pro-Gly-NH_2 • $xC_2H_4O_2$ • yH_2O
1 2 3 4 5 6 7 8 9 10

[52699-48-6] $C_{55}H_{75}N_{17}O_{13}$. $xC_2H_4O_2 \cdot yH_2O$

Preparation—By synthesis or from the hypothalamus, *Science 179:* 341, 1973.

Description—Faint-yellow powder.

Solubility—1 g in 25 mL water, 50 mL methanol or 25 mL 1% acetic acid.

Uses—Identical to natural GnRH. Gonadorelin is used in the treatment of primary hypothalmic amenorrhea. Gonadorelin hydrochloride (Factel, *Ayerst*) is a related preparation and is used as a diagnostic agent to determine whether hypogonadism is the result of a defect in anterior pituitary release of LH or in hypothalamic release of LH-RH. If gonadorelin evokes a rise in LH levels, the disturbance is in the hypothalamus; if it does not, the disturbance is in the anterior pituitary. Administered in pulsatile fashion, it evokes secretion of both FSH and LH. However, if plasma levels remain high for periods longer than a few hours, preceptor down regulation occurs. LH receptors are affected more than FSH receptors. By careful selection of dose-regimen it is thus possible to increase or decrease male or female fertility, in the latter instance without marked changes in estrogen secretion.

Gondorelin is used as an investigational drug to treat infertility, prostatic carcinoma, induction of puberty in hypogonadal males, precocious puberty, metastatic breast cancer in premenopausal women, cryptorchidism, premenstrual syndrome, and endometriosis and as a male contraceptive agent. Local swelling, itching or pain and occasional rash at the injection site may occur after subcutaneous injection. Headache, nausea, lightheadedness, abdominal discomfort and rare flushing may occur. It does not cause multiple births.

Dose—*Intravenous* or *subcutaneous, adults* and *children over 12 yr,* **5 μg,** every 90 min (range 1 to 20 μg) usual interval is for 21 days.

Dosage Form—Injection: Powder, 0.8 mg or 3.2 mg/10 mL for reconstitution.

Lergotrile Mesylate—see RPS-18, page 953.

Leuprolide—page 1253

Menotropins

Pergonal (*Serono*)

Menotropins [9002-68-0]; an extract of postmenopausal urine containing the follicle-stimulating hormone (FSH) and luteinizing hormone (LH) in a 1:1 ratio.

Uses—Has the gonadotropic activities of FSH and LH (see page 1060). It is used to *induce ovulation* in women with infertility consequent to insufficient endogenous production of gonadotropins. Clinical experience is that about 75% of anovulatory women ovulate after treatment and 25% become pregnant after 2 courses of treatment. Multiple gestation occurs in about 15 to 30% of completed pregnancies. The hyperstimulation syndrome occurs in 1 to 2% of cases. If urinary estrogen excretion is used to guide treatment with large doses and the need for concomitant chorionic gonadotropin, the ovulatory rate can be increased to 98% and the percentage of live births is improved, but multiple gestation is increased and hyperstimulation is more common. It sometimes is used to treat hypogonadotropic male infertility.

Side effects include ovarian enlargement, flatulence, abdominal discomfort, oliguria, weight gain, ascites, pleural effusion, hypotension and hypercoagulability; these are all evidence of hyperstimulation. Other adverse reactions include arterial thromboembolism, hypersensitivity and febrile reactions. Birth defects occurred in 5 of 287 pregnancies. Occasionally, ovarian rupture and intraperitoneal hemorrhage occur, and surgery is required.

Dose—*Intramuscular,* in *females, induction of ovulation initially* **75 IU** of each component/day for 9 to 12 days, followed by **10,000 IU** of chorionic gonadotropin 1 day after the course of menotropins is stopped. If estrogen levels rise to normal but no ovulation occurs, the same course is repeated twice more. If there is no pregnancy, the dose is increased to **150 IU/day** for 9 to 12 days, followed by **10,000 IU** HCG 1 day after last dose of menotropins. Two such courses may be repeated, if necessary. Some clinicians stop the administration of menotropins when estrogen secretion reaches 50 to 100 μg/day and give 10,000 IU of chorionic gonadotropin 1 day later; others wait until the estrogen secretion is 100 to 150 μg/day. If the estrogen excretion is higher than 150 μg/day, chorionic gonadotropin is withheld, to minimize hyperstimulation. In *male hypogonadism,* **75 IU** of each component 3 times a wk for 4 mo; pretreatment and concomitant treatment with HCG 2000 IU twice a wk.

Dosage Form—for Injection: 75 and 150 IU of each component.

Nafarelin Acetate

Lutenizing hormone-releasing factor (pig), 6-[3-(2-naphthadenyl)-D- alanine, acetate (salt), hydrate; Synarel (*Syntex*)

H-5-oxo-L-Pro-L-His-L-Trp-L-Ser-L-Tyr—N(H)---C(H)(CH_2-naphthyl)---C(=O)—
L-Leu-L-Arg-L-Pro-Gly—NH_2 • xCH_3COOH • yH_2O

[86620-42-0] $C_{66}H_{83}N_{17}O_{13}$. $xC_2H_4O_2$. yH_2O.

Preparation—US Pat 4,234,571.

Uses—An agonist for LH-RH receptors. However, the duration of action is too long for pulsatile dosing, so that the effect of repetitive administration is that of down-regulation of LH-RH receptors. It has been found to be effective in the treatment of *endometriosis* and *central precocious puberty.* It probably will prove to be effective also on the treatment of premenstrual syndrome, metastatic breast cancer, prostatic cancer and as a male contraceptive agent. In women, adverse effects are those of hypoestrogenemia, namely, hot flashes, vaginal dryness, decreased libidio and a moderate decrease in trabecular bone mineralization in the spine in about 67% of patients. In men, weight gain, hot flashes, decreased libidio and decreased drive and initiative occur. These effects disappear after discontinuation of the drug. It is absorbed rapidly by the intranasal but not sublingual route. Intranasal bioavailability is about 21%. The drug is metabolized to at least six metabolites. The half-life is about 2 hr. **Dose**—For *endometriosis, intranasal, adult,* **200** to **400 μg** twice a day starting between days 2 and 4 of the menstrual cycle; for *central precocious puberty,* **1600 μg/day.**

Dosage Form—Nasal Solution: 2 mg/mL.

Octreotide

L-Cysteinamide, [*R*-(*R**,*R**)]-D-phenylalanyl-L-cysteinyl-L-phenylalanyl-D-tryptophyl-L-lysyl-L-threonyl-*N*-[2-hydroxy-1-(hydroxymethyl)propyl]-, cyclic (2 → 7)-disulfide, Sandostatin (*Sandoz*)

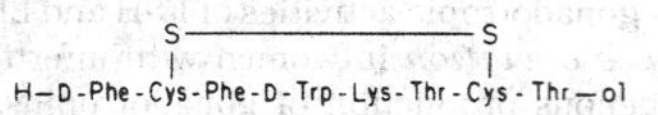

H—D-Phe-Cys-Phe-D-Trp-Lys-Thr-Cys-Thr—ol (S—S bridge between the two Cys)

[83150-76-9] $C_{49}H_{66}N_{10}O_{10}S_2$ (1019.24).

Preparation—US Pat 4,395,403.

Uses—An analog of somatostatin (see page 1078) which differs in that it inhibits growth hormone secretion in lower doses than affect insulin secretion, it is long acting (2-hr half-life), there is no rebound hypersecretion after discontinuation and it is orally effective. It is approved for *symptomatic treatment of carcinoid tumors and profuse diarrhea associated with vasoactive intestinal peptide tumors* (lipomas). The drug is tolerated well. During the first few days of treatment there are flatulence, loose stools, diarrhea and abdominal pains. A mild steatorrhea occurs in some patients and may persist during treatment or disappear in a few days. Malabsorption does not occur. There may be a moderate decrease in postprandial glucose tolerance, but no complications have been recorded.

Dose—*Subcutaneous, adult,* **100** to **600 μg** a day, in 2 to 4 divided doses.

Dosage Form—Injection: 50, 100 and 500 μg/mL.

Pergolide Mesylate

Permax (*Lilly*)

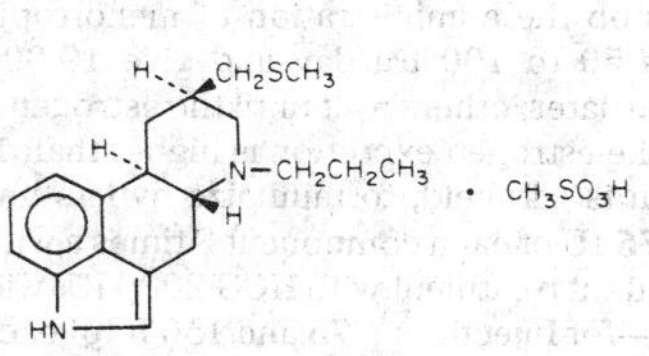

[66104-22-1] $C_{19}H_{26}N_2S.CH_4O_3S$ (410.59).

Preparation—A derivative of the ergot alkaloid, ergoline. US Pat 4,166,182.

Description—Off-white crystals; melt about 225°.

Uses—Has all of the actions and uses of *Bromocriptine* (page 1035). Its advantage is a longer duration of action, namely, over 24 hr.

Dose—*Oral, adults, initially* **50 μg,** on the first day to be adjusted subsequently according to plasma prolactin levels.

Dosage Forms—Tablets; 50, 250 and 1000 μg (0.05, 0.25 and 1.0 mg), as the base.

Protirelin—see RPS-18, page 953.

Somatrem and Somatropin
Somatrem

N-L-Methionylsomatotropin (human) Protropin (*Genentech*)

[82030-87-3] $C_{995}H_{1537}N_{263}O_{301}S_8$ (22,256.21)

Somatropin

Humatrope (*Lilly*)

Growth hormone, human; somatotropin (human) [12629-01-5] $C_{990}H_{1528}N_{262}O_{300}S_7$ (21,500.00)

Preparation—A single polypeptide chain of 191 aminoacids once obtained from the anterior lobe of the human pituitary gland. See US Pat 3,118,815.

Uses—Both somatrem and somatropin products are from recombinant DNA-directed syntheses. *Humatrope* is identical to human pituitary-derived somatropin. Somatrem (*Protropin*) is identical to natural growth hormone except it contains an additional methionine on the *N*-terminus of the molecule. However, the effects and potencies are identical; therefore, both peptides are considered together. Somatropin from pituitary extracts was discontinued because of reports that its use was sometimes the cause of Creutzfeldt-Jakob disease. For description, actions and uses see *Growth Hormone* (page 1058).

Intramuscular administration of the hormone is preferred to subcutaneous injection because the hormone causes lipodystrophy or lipoatrophy at the cutaneous injection site. Pain and swelling usually occur on injection, so that sites should be rotated. Hypercalciuria occurs frequently but usually regresses in 2 to 3 mo. Hyperglycemia and frank diabetes mellitus due to insulin resistance may occur. Myalgia and early morning headaches are relatively frequent. Antibodies to the hormone may be found in 30 to 40% of recipients given somatren, but patients rarely fail to respond to therapy. Approximately 2% of patients receiving somatropin developed antibodies, but growth responses have not been limited in such patients. Occasionally, somatotropin causes hypothyroidism. If the epiphyses are closed, the hormone should not be used because continued stimulation of growth of the phalanges and jawbone, but not other bones, can cause abnormal body proportions. Available products are exceedingly expensive.

Dose—*Intramuscular or subcutaneous,* individualize dosage; up to **0.26 IU/kg** for somatrem or up to **0.16 IU/kg** for somatropin 3 times a wk is recommended.

Dosage Forms—Somatrem for Injection: 13 IU (5 mg); Somatropin for Injection: 13 IU (5 mg).

Thyrotropin—see RPS-18, page 953.

Urofollitropin—see RPS-18, page 954.

The Intermediate Lobe

The intermediate lobe of the pituitary produces a substance, *intermedin,* or *melanocyte-stimulating hormone* (MSH), which disperses the pigment granules in the melanophores and other chromatophores in some amphibians and fishes. The biological assay of MSH depends upon its capacity for darkening the skin of frogs either *in vivo* or *in vitro.*

Extracts of mammalian pituitaries contain two substances with MSH activity: α- and β-MSH. These are polypeptides containing 13 and 18 amino acids, respectively; the amino acid sequences in both are known. Although MSH has no known physiological role in mammals, alkali-treated MSH (which has a more prolonged action than the native material) will cause some darkening of the skin in man. Purified ACTH possesses intrinsic MSH activity, probably due to similarity of structure between ACTH and α-MSH. It has been suggested that the hyperpigmentation of Addison's disease is due to excessive ACTH secretion.

The hypothalamus produces both an MSH-releasing factor (MRF) and MSH-inhibitory factor (MIF).

The Posterior Pituitary (Neurohypophysis)

The posterior pituitary contains two peptide hormones, *oxytocin* and *vasopressin.* Neither is made in the posterior pituitary, but rather they are synthesized in neurons in the hypothalamus. Oxytocin is synthesized in the paraventricular nucleus and vasopressin the supraoptic nucleus. The axons of the hormone-secreting nerve cells pass from the hypothalamus to the internal infundibular zone of the posterior pituitary (hence the name neurohypophysis). The hormones flow down the axons as granules or vesicles composed of a hormone and a carrier protein called *neurophysin.* Their release at the nerve terminals is effected by nerve impulses. Thus, the control of release is actually in the appropriate hypothalamic nuclei.

Human and most mammalian vasopressin is Cys-Tyr-Phe-Gln-Asn-Cys-Pro-Arg-GlyNH_2, called *arginine* vasopressin. Oddly, *USAN* has not assigned a special name to arginine vasopressin as it has to lysine vasopressin (*lypressin*), obtained from the pig. The USAN name, *vasopressin,* applies to either peptide. The two do not have identical activities. Vasopressin is usually called *antidiuretic hormone* (ADH) by physiologists and biochemists, because it decreases urine flow by increasing the resorption of water from the distal convoluted tubules and collecting ducts of the kidney. Not only does it promote water retention but under certain circumstances it increases the excretion of sodium and chloride. The effect is a decrease in the osmolarity of the extracellular fluid. When ADH secretion is suppressed (as from various physiological stimuli or ethanol) a watery diuresis ensues. When there is a defect in the hypothalamicopituitary secretion of ADH, *diabetes insipidus* results. Vasopressin is used mainly for its antidiuretic effects in this disease rather than for its vasoconstrictor actions, from which the name vasopressin is derived. However, not only does vasopressin stimulate vascular smooth muscle, but also it increases bowel motility and it has been used to treat bowel stasis and to expel gas postsurgically; however, cholinergic drugs are considered to be superior for this purpose. The vasoconstrictor and bowel spastic actions have special usefulness in arresting hemorrhage from peptic ulcers. The smooth muscle stimulant effects occur with higher doses than are necessary to affect renal function. Vasopressin also causes the release of ACTH much like the hypothalamic releasing hormone, CRF. Consequently, vasopressin sometimes is used diagnostically to assess the pituitary reserve of ACTH. Vasopressin also has weak oxytocic activity. Vasopressin has a brief half-life (less than 20 minutes). Lypressin has much weaker smooth-muscle stimulant activity than vasopressin, the ratio of antidiuretic to pressor activity being about 1000:1.

Oxytocin stimulates the contraction of smooth muscle in the uterus and alveoli of the lactating breast. At coitus, uterine stimulation by oxytocin causes peristaltic activity that assists the migration of spermatozoa. During parturition, the hormone enhances the uterine contractions. The uses of oxytocin in labor and breast engorgement are described in Chapter 63.

Neither vasopressin nor oxytocin survives the acid and enzymes of the gastrointestinal tract, so they must be given parenterally or intranasally.

Each of the octapeptides has been synthesized. Oxytocin has the structure

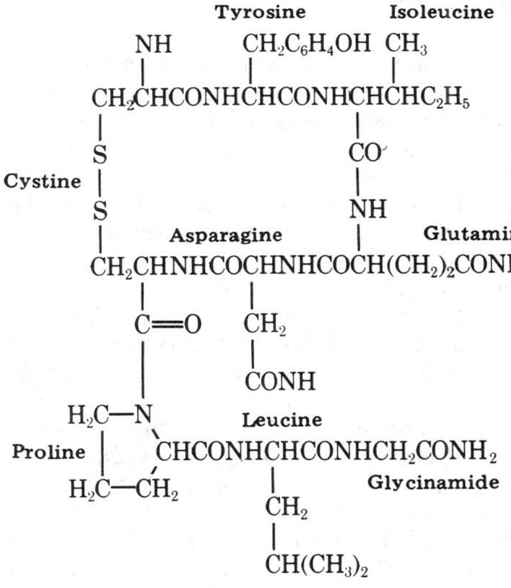

```
                    Tyrosine         Isoleucine
          NH       CH2C6H4OH  CH3
          |        |          |
        CH2CHCONHCHCONHCHCHC2H5
        |                 |
        S                 CO
Cystine |                 |
        S                 NH
        |    Asparagine   |     Glutamine
        CH2CHNHCOCHNHCOCH(CH2)2CONH2
          |       |
          C=O     CH2
          |       |
          |       CONH
          |
    H2C—N         Leucine
Proline |  CHCONHCHCONHCH2CONH2
    H2C—CH2       |        Glycinamide
                  CH2
                  |
                  CH(CH3)2
```

Oxytocin

The *structure of vasopressin* from human, monkey, dog, cat, ox, camel, rabbit and rat pituitaries *is identical with that of oxytocin, except* that the isoleucine and leucine residues are replaced by residues of phenylalanine and arginine, respectively. Vasopressin prepared from pig pituitaries (lypressin) contains lysine instead of arginine.

The synthesis of oxytocin by du Vigneaud *et al* in 1953 represented the first synthesis of a peptide hormone. The synthetic product is qualitatively and quantitatively identical in biological properties with the purified natural hormone. Purified oxytocin contains 500 to 600 USP Units/mg.

The successful synthesis of the naturally occurring posterior lobe hormones has provided the impetus for the synthesis of a number of analogues of both oxytocin and vasopressin. Thus, substances in which one or more of the amino acids of the native hormones have been replaced by others, or containing fewer or additional amino acid residues, have been prepared and their pharmacological properties explored. One of these was the compound vasotocin, containing the pentapeptide ring of oxytocin and the tripeptide side chain of vasopressin. This substance possesses the biological properties of both neurohypophyseal hormones, although in lesser degree. Subsequently, it was shown that vasotocin is, in fact, the naturally occurring neurohypophyseal hormone of birds and amphibians.

It has become rather common practice to name those synthetic analogues of oxytocin and the two vasopressins in which one or more of the amino acids of the native hormones have been replaced by others by the simple expedient of assigning consecutive numbers to the amino acid residues in the native hormone and using these numbers to denote the alterations represented in the synthetic. The numbering system can be seen with the structures for *Lypressin* and *Vasopressin* (see below). A synthetic vasopressin in which the moiety at position 8 is arginine is named simply 8-arginine vasopressin; if it is lysine, the peptide is 8-lysine vasopressin.

Desmopressin Acetate

Vasopresssin, 1-(3-mercaptopropionic acid)-8-D-arginine, monoacetate (salt), trihydrate; DDVAP (*Rhone-Poulenc Rorer*); Concentraid (*Ferring*)

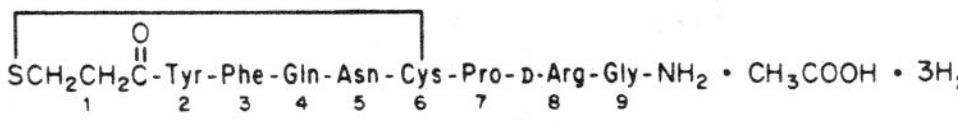

```
┌───────────────────────────────┐
|           O                   |
|           ||                  |
SCH2CH2C-Tyr-Phe-Gln-Asn-Cys-Pro-D-Arg-Gly-NH2 • CH3COOH • 3H2O
    1      2   3   4   5   6   7    8    9
```

[62357-86-2] $C_{48}H_{68}N_{14}O_{14}S_2.3H_2O$ (1183.22).

Preparation—A synthetic analog of 8-arginine vasopressin in which the amino group has been removed from the *N*-terminus cysteine and L-arginine at position 8 has been replaced by the D-enantiomer. *Helv Chim Acta 49:*695, 1966.

Description—White fluffy powder; pK_a (gly-NH_2) 4.8.

Solubility—Soluble in alcohol or water.

Uses—In the treatment of *central* ("neurogenic") *diabetes insipidus*. It also is used to test the ability of the kidney to concentrate urine. Since the hormone can raise the plasma levels of factor VIII (antihemophilic factor), it is sometimes used to treat Factor VIII *bleeding disorders* and to increase Factor VIII levels prior to surgery. It may be used alone or as an adjunct for some refractory cases of primary nocturnal enuresis. Headache, mild hypertension, nasal congestion, mild abdominal cramping, water intoxication and vulval pain sometimes occur. Chlorpropamide and clofibrate potentiate, and glyburide inhibits, antidiuretic action.

Dose—For *diabetes insipidus, intransal, adult* **10** to **40 μg** a day in 1 to 3 divided doses; *children*, **5** to **30 μg** a day. For *primary nocturnal enuresis, intranasally*, **20** to **40 μg** at bedtime. *Subcutaneous* or *intravenous, adult*, **2** to **4** μg.

Dosage Forms—Nasal Solution: 0.1 mg/mL; for Injection: 4 μg/mL.

Lypressin

Vasopressin, 8-L-lysine-, Diapid (*Sandoz*)

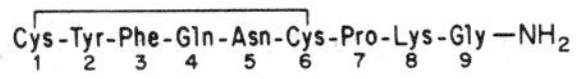

```
┌────────────────────┐
Cys-Tyr-Phe-Gln-Asn-Cys-Pro-Lys-Gly—NH2
 1   2   3   4   5   6   7   8   9
```

[50-57-7] $C_{46}H_{65}N_{13}O_{12}S_2$ (1056.22).

Preparation—Isolated from hog pituitaries and prepared synthetically (*J Biol Chem 222:* 951, 1956; *J Am Chem Soc 82:* 3195, 1960). One commercial synthetic method concludes by reacting the protected tripeptide, *N*-tosyl-*S*-benzyl-L-cysteinyl-L-tyrosyl-L-phenylalanylhydrazide, with the protected hexapeptide, L-glutaminyl-L-asparaginyl-*S*-benzyl-L-cysteinyl-L-prolyl- *N*-tosyl-L-lysyl-glycinamide, and then splits off the protecting groups with metallic sodium.

One mg of lypressin is stated to be equivalent to 270 USP Posterior Pituitary Units (1 Unit is equivalent to 3.7 μg).

Uses—Has strong antidiuretic but weak pressor activity. It is used only in the control or prevention of mild to moderate neurogenic *diabetes insipidus*. When the condition is severe, it does not give sufficient control because of its brief duration of action; even in moderate diabetes insipidus, control is only periodic, in accordance with the dosage regimen. In the severe condition, vasopressin tannate is used, although this hormone may be used as an adjunct between injections of the tannate. Diabetes insipidus from renal disorders is not affected. After nasal application, antidiuresis peaks within ½ to 2 hr and lasts 3 to 8 hr. The half-life is about 15 min.

When used as recommended, its untoward effects are infrequent and mild; they include nasal irritation and congestion, rhinorrhea, nasal pruritus, nasal ulceration, conjunctivitis and headache. Overdosage may cause heartburn from postnasal drip, abdominal cramps, bowel hypermotility and fluid retention. Inhalation of the spray can result in asthma-like tightness in the chest, dyspnea and coughing. Thus far, allergic responses have not been reported. Because the marketed substance is synthetic and thus free of traces of foreign proteins, it may possibly lack allergenicity, even though its composition differs slightly from the human hormone.

Dose—*Intranasal, usually* **1** or **2 sprays** (about 7 to 14 μg) into each nostril 4 times a day or whenever urinary frequency or substantial thirst indicates a need. The average interval is 6 hr. Increases in dosage should be achieved by more frequent administration rather than by increased number of sprays per application.

Dosage Form—Nasal Spray: 185 μg/mL in 8 mL (185 μg = 50 posterior pituitary units).

Posterior Pituitary—see RPS-18, page 955.

Vasopressin

Lys—Tyr—Phe—Glu—Asp—Cys—Pro—Arg*—Gly—NH_2
1 2 3 4 5 6 7 8 9

(*in pig vasopressin, Arg is Lys)

Beta-Hypophamine; Pitressin (*Parke-Davis*)

8-L-Lysine (or arginine) vasopressin: Lysine form-[50-57-7] $C_{46}H_{65}N_{13}O_{12}S_2$ (1056.22); Arginine form-[113-79-1] $C_{46}H_{65}N_{15}O_{12}S_2$ (1084.23).

Uses—Its actions are discussed on page 1062. It is employed for its *antidiuretic* effect in central diabetes insipidus and to dispel gas shadows in bowel roentgenography and pyelography. It should not be used as a pressor agent.

Untoward effects related to overdosage include water intoxication (with headache, nausea and vomiting, confusion, lethargy, coma and convulsions), especially when patients drink excessive amounts of water or are given intravenous fluids, and stimulation of vascular, uterine and intestinal smooth muscle, which may result in pallor, hypertension, coronary constriction (with anginal chest pain, electrocardiographic changes and occasional myocardial infarction), uterine cramps, menorrhagia, and nausea, vomiting, diarrhea and abdominal cramps. Hypersensitivity occasionally occurs; manifestations include urticaria, neurodermatitis, flushing, fever, wheezing, dyspnea and rare anaphylactic shock. Large doses are oxytocic and also cause milk ejection. Alcohol, heparin, demeclocycline, lithium and large doses of epinephrine antagonize it; carbamazepine, chlorpropamide, clofibrate, glucocorticoids and urea potentiate it.

The plasma half-life is 10 to 20 min. However, the effect of an intramuscular injection lasts from 2 to 8 hr. From 10 to 15% is excreted unchanged. Vasopressin tannate is also available as a longer acting preparation.

Dose—*Intramuscular* or *subcutaneous*, for *central diabetes insipidus*, **5** to **10 USP Units** (0.25 to 0.5 mL) 2 to 3 times a day; for *children, reduce dose proportionately. May also be given intranasally* on cotton pledgets, with a dropper, or as a spray, at intervals determined by return of polyuria or thirst. For *hypotonic bowel, initially* **5 Units,** increased to 10 Units, if necessary, repeated at 3- to 4-hr intervals, as needed; for *bowel roentgenography,* **10 Units** 2 hr and ½ hr before the procedure.

Dosage Form—Injection: 20 Units/0.5 and 1 mL; Injection (Tannate, in oil): 5 Units/mL.

The Adrenal Hormones

The adrenal hormones include both the adrenocorticoids from the adrenal cortex and epinephrine and norepinephrine from the adrenal medulla. The discussion below will deal only with the adrenocorticoids. Epinephrine and norepinephrine are treated in Chapter 57.

The cortex, or outer portion, of the adrenal gland is one of the endocrine structures most vitally necessary for normal metabolic function. While it is possible for life to continue in the complete absence of adrenal cortical function, serious metabolic derangements ensue, and the capacity of the organism to respond to physiological or environmental stress is lost completely. The vital role of the adrenal cortex is due to its production of a group of hormones, all *steroid* in nature.

Physiology—Four general patterns of adrenal cortical hormone action have been described.

1. Retention of sodium ions in extracellular fluid and potassium ions within cells, thus maintaining the normal distribution of water and chloride ion and resulting maintenance of blood volume and blood pressure.
2. Maintenance of normal blood glucose levels and facilitation of liver glycogen deposition.
3. Enhanced mobilization of tissue protein and gluconeogenesis from protein.
4. Androgenic effects (see page 1101) from androgenic steroids, mainly dehydroepiandrosterone, produced in the adrenal cortex.

Steroids that affect the electrolyte metabolism as in (1) are called *mineralocorticoids;* those that affect carbohydrate and protein metabolism as in (2) and (3) and which favor lipolysis are called *glucocorticoids.* Glucocorticoids exert a regulatory influence upon lymphocytes, erythrocytes and eosinophils of the blood, and upon the structure and function of lymphoid tissue. They also function in the regulation of cerebrospinal fluid composition and secretion and serve as modulators of nerve transmission. There is evidence for locally synthesized glucocorticoids, the *neurocorticoids,* in the CNS. The relative or complete absence of adrenocortical function, known as *Addison's disease,* is accompanied by loss of sodium chloride and water, retention of potassium, lowering of blood-glucose and liver-glycogen levels, increased sensitivity to insulin, nitrogen retention and lymphocytosis. The disturbances in electrolyte metabolism are the cause of morbidity and mortality in most cases of severe adrenal insufficiency. All of these disorders may be corrected by administration of adrenal cortical extract or the pure adrenal cortical steroids now available.

In its biosynthesis of the steroid hormones, the adrenal cortex uses cholesterol, which is present in large amounts in the gland; during periods of secretory activity it also consumes large quantities of ascorbic acid, which is likewise present in high concentration.

The synthesis and secretion of the glucocorticoids (essentially hydrocortisone) takes place in the *zona fasciculata.* Corticotropin (ACTH) is the primary stimulus to hydrocortisone secretion. ACTH is released in response to the hypothalamic hormone, CRH (see page 1059). Glucocorticoid secretion, then, is regulated through suprahypothalamic and hypothalamic nuclei, which integrate responses to sensory, emotional and chemical inputs, including the glucocorticoids themselves, and the basophilic cells of the adenohypophysis, release from which is suppressed by circulating glucorticoids. Physical (injury, surgery, etc) and emotional stress and hypoglycemia increase secretion. Synthesis in the zona fasciculata can be altered by drugs which inhibit specific enzymes involved. CRH, ACTH and glucocorticoid release follows a circadian rhythm such that blood concentrations of hydrocortisone are highest between 6 and 8 am and lowest around midnight.

The synthesis and release of the mineralocorticoid, aldosterone, takes place in the *zona glomerulosa.* ACTH has only a slight effect on secretion. Rather, angiotensins II and III are the primary stimulants, although hyperkalemia is also an important stimulus. The production of the angiotensins is under renal and central and sympathetic nervous system control.

In the kidney, the macula densa around the juxtaglomerular distal tubules monitors Na^+ and Cl^- concentrations and luminal osmolarity. Low [Na^+] and osmolarity or high [Cl^-] cause signals to be sent to the juxtaglomerular (JG) cells in the afferent arterioles, which then release renin. Renin secretion also is increased by low blood pressure at the JG cells and by sympathetic impulses, which work through β_1-adrenoreceptors. Renin then cleaves angiotensin I from angiotensinogen, both locally and in the blood. Angiotensin I is converted to angiotensin II by a converting enzyme (CE or kininase II), mainly in the lung. (Angiotensin III is a metabolite of II.) Thus, a variety of electrolyte, emotional, cardiovascular and drug factors can affect aldosterone secretion indirectly.

Structure-Activity Relationship—Over 50 steroids have been shown to be present in the adrenal cortex. Only seven of these, however, have been shown to exert a significant biological effect related to gluco- and mineralo-corticoid function. All of the adrenal cortical steroids, except the androgens, contain 21 carbon atoms, an α,β-unsaturated ketone in Ring A and an α-ketol chain (—$COCH_2OH$) attached to Ring D. They differ in extent of oxygenation or hydroxylation at carbons 11, 17 or 19.

In general, clinical experience has indicated that the anti-inflammatory activity of adrenal cortical steroids in man correlates well with their glucocorticoid activity. The undesirable side effects of sodium retention and edema are associated with mineralocorticoid activity. Synthetic steroids possessing higher glucocorticoid and lower mineralocorticoid activity than cortisone or cortisol have been prepared and marketed. All adrenal corticoids require the 3-keto group and 4–5 unsaturation. Additional unsaturation in Ring A enhances the anti-inflammatory and antirheumatic properties while at the same time reduces the sodium-retaining effect. Thus, prednisolone has 4 times the anti-inflammatory activity of cortisol and yet has only 0.8 of the mineralocorticoid activity. The presence of oxygen at position 11 is necessary for significant glucocorticoid activity but not for mineralocorticoid activity; the 11β-hydroxy group is more potent than the 11-keto group; the 11-keto group is converted to the active β-hydroxy group in the body. The 17α-hydroxy group also is important to glucocorticoid activity. The 21-hydroxy group is essential to mineralocorticoid activity; it favors, but is not required for, glucocorticoid activity. Introduction of either a methyl or hydroxyl group at position 16 markedly reduces mineralocorticoid activity but only slightly decreases glucocorticoid and anti-inflammatory activity. Thus, paramethasone (16α-methyl), betamethasone (16β-methyl), dexamethasone (16α-methyl) and triamcinolone (16α-hydroxy) have no significant mineralocorticoid activity; 6α-methylation has unpredictable effects as it enhances the mineralocorticoid activity of cortisol but virtually abolishes that of prednisolone. The 9α-fluoro group enhances both glucocorticoid and mineralocorticoid activities, but the effects of substituents at the 6 and 16 positions override this effect. Further examples will become apparent from the discussions provided in the following individual monographs.

Biological Activity—The glucocorticoids appear to affect all cells, although not all in the same way. Clinical interest primarily focuses on their anti-inflammatory and immunosuppressant effects. They prevent release of various lytic enzymes that not only extend tissue damage during inflammation but also generate leukotactic substances. Directly and indirectly, glucocorticoids decrease phagocytosis by macrophages and also the disruption of macrophages by ingested materials. Anti-inflammatory effects include the retardation of the migration of polymorphonuclear leukocytes, suppression of repair and granulation, reduction in the erythrocyte sedimentation rate, decreased fibrinogenesis and diminished elaboration of C-reactive protein. Glucocorticoids do not affect antigen-antibody interaction or the release of the mediators of immediate hypersensitivity. The immunosuppressant effects may be partly the result of the suppression of phagocytosis and immunoinformation processing and a decrease in the number of eosinophils and lymphocytes, suppression of delayed hypersensitivity reactions, decrease in tissue reaction to antigen-antibody interactions (but not in the interaction itself) and reduction in plasma immunoglobulins. Effects on carbohydrate, fat and protein metabolism are responsible for both beneficial and untoward effects. These hormones increase gluconeogenesis and glycogen deposition, both lipolysis and lipogenesis (but increase fat deposition at only a few specialized sites), and protein catabolism in various tissues.

In addition to the above-mentioned changes brought about by glucocorticoids are the so-called *permissive* effects. In these, the steroids do not themselves cause change but physiological amounts are required for certain organs or structures to respond to stimuli. For example, neither the kidney can respond to a water load nor the arterioles to epinephrine in the absence of adequate levels of glucocorticoids.

Once a steroid hormone has permeated a cell membrane, it combines with a cytosolic protein called a receptor, or aporeceptor. The steroid-protein complex is altered and then translocated to the cell nucleus, where it attaches to chromatin. The result is an enhancement or reduction of the transcription of both messenger RNA and ribosomal RNA, which, in turn, leads to an increased or decreased synthesis of certain proteins. Other transcription factors also interact at the same DNA binding sites. The protein produced probably is determined, in part, by the aporeceptor, of which there is more than one kind within the cell. However, tissue selectivity seems to be considerably determined by steroid- metabolizing enzymes that differentially alter intracellular steroids.

In renal tubular cells, mineralocorticoids appear mainly to induce the synthesis of a protein that decreases intracellular sodium content; it is not clear whether this protein acts directly to increase the activity of membrane [Na^+-K^+]-activated ATPase or indirectly to increase the mitochondrial production of ATP for the ATPase or whether it decreases sodium permease activity. Because of the manifold actions of the glucocorticoids, it is to be expected that many intracellular proteins would be induced, but this has been difficult to verify. Inhibitors of protein- and RNA-synthesis prevent the effects of glucocorticoids, and the cellular content of some enzymes is affected, but with a number of membrane-bound enzymes, only the activities, and not the content, are affected.

The activities of some enzymes are increased and others decreased. These are enzymes that have phospholipid adjuvants. Since the glucocorticoids alter the phospholipid composition of a number of cell membranes, it is likely that the enzyme activities are altered through the phospholipid composition, possibly through the induction of phospholipid-synthesizing and/or lytic enzymes. Alterations in membrane composition may possibly explain the membrane-stabilizing effects. Some, but not all, lysosomal membranes are stabilized.

Glucocorticoids also inhibit membrane lipid peroxidation, which possibly contributes to the salutary effects in brain edema; the effect appears to be one of decreasing the activity of membrane-bound, superoxide radical-generating mixed-function enzymes. Possibly related is an action to block phospholipase-A_2, which prevents the release of arachidonic acid from membrane phospholipids and its subsequent conversion to eicosanoids. This inhibitory effect results from the production of an inhibitory protein, lipocortin, in leucocytes. Alterations in the prostaglandin system change the cyclic nucleotide balance, often in favor of cyclic guanosyl phosphate. In the proliferative skin diseases, glucocorticoids decrease the markedly elevated arachidonic acid and cyclic-AMP levels.

Effects on the prostaglandin and cyclic nucleotide systems undoubtedly are involved in the anti-inflammatory response, as is also membrane stabilization. They also induce the production of an antileukokinetic (antichemotactic) peptide. This peptide may prevent the proper assembly of the microtubules, an effect that also would explain the antimitotic effect seen with lymphoblasts and certain other proliferating cells and hence explain certain immunosuppressant and antineoplastic activity and the effect to retard growth. The sundry anabolic (eg, gluconeogenic) and catabolic (eg, proteolytic) effects of the glucocorticoids also are probably indirect.

The primary effects of mineralocorticoids are on cortical collecting tubule cells in the kidney to increase sodium reabsorption and potassium secretion. Thus, elevated aldosterone titers cause sodium retention and potassium depletion with accompanying volume expansion and weight gain, hypertension and metabolic alkalosis. There are effects on electrolyte transport in other tissues (eg, salivary glands, choroid plexus or intestines), but they are not clinically important.

Side Effects—Certain side effects may appear during the first week of treatment with glucocorticoids; they include euphoria and a rare paradoxical suicidal depression, psychoses (especially with high doses), rare hypertension, anorexia, occasional hyperglycemia, rare colonic ulceration (even though the drugs are used to treat ulcerative colitis), increased susceptibility to infections (especially vaccinial, herpetic, varicellar and other viral infections, fungal infections, tuberculosis) and acne. They also mask some of the signs of infections, thus causing a postponement of appropriate anti-infective treatment. Glucocorticoids appear to increase peptic ulceration, especially of the stomach. After 2 to 3 days of treatment, the pituitary release of ACTH is suppressed, and the adrenal secretion of cortisol is inadequate once glucocorticoid administration ceases; this condition is temporary after short-term treatment. In the case of a medical emergency, the depressed pituitary-adrenal response may make the patient unable to respond to stress. Additional exogenous corticosteroid is given in a dosage and for a duration appropriate for the severity of the stress. Consequently, patients on high-dose or long-term treatment should carry identification stating that they are under treatment with corticosteroids. Withdrawal of corticosteroids should be slow.

From the first week through the first year of therapy, additional side effects may appear, namely, fat redistribution to the nape of the neck ("buffalo hump") and lower abdomen, diabetes mellitus and hyperglycemia, "moon face" and other edematous states and renal potassium loss (from mineralocorticoid activity), alkalosis, additional infections (including tuberculosis), papilledema, glaucoma, posterior subcapsular cataracts, diplopia, 6th nerve palsies, osteoporosis, myopathy, ecchymoses and purpura and cutaneous striae.

Because of the long-loop negative feedback suppression of ACTH output, the normal adrenal production of corticosteroids from cholesterol is decreased considerably, and hypercholesterolemia results; some of the excess cholesterol is diverted to increase the production of adrenal and testicular androgens, so that masculinization of the female or virilization of the young male and premature cessation of growth may occur. After prolonged suppression of the anterior pituitary secretion of ACTH, there may be a permanent defect in pituitary-adrenal function. Continuous or repetitive use of glucocorticoids may cause painless joint destruction, especially if the drug is given intra-articularly.

After prolonged glucocorticoid therapy, additional untoward effects include bone fractures and vertebral collapse (from marked osteoporosis), hyperlipidemia and possible premature atherosclerosis. Patients also become physically and psychically dependent upon glucocorticoids, pressure the physician to continue prescriptions and engage in drug-seeking behavior characteristic of addicts.

Adverse effects of glucocorticoids applied to the skin include stinging or burning sensations, itching, irritation, dryness, scaliness, vasoconstriction, folliculitis, acne, bacterial or yeast infections, hypopigmentation, atrophy and striae. Systemic effects also can occur, especially if occlusive dressings are used. Topical ophthalmologic glucocorticoids not only may cause serious exacerbations of viral, fungal and bacterial infections of the eye but also glaucoma; examinations for intraocular tension and corneal integrity should be made every 4 to 6 weeks. From all of the above, it can be seen that glucocorticoids are dangerous drugs.

Because the mineralocorticoids are used mainly in physiological doses for replacement therapy, untoward effects are usually infrequent and mild. Sodium and water retention (with "moon face"), potassium loss, alkalosis and hypertension can occur with excessive doses.

Drug Interactions—Glucocorticoids decrease the hypoglycemic activity of insulin and oral hypoglycemics, so that a change in dose of the antidiabetic drugs may be necessitated. In high doses, glucocorticoids also decrease the response to somatotropin. The usual doses of mineralocorticoids and large doses of some glucocorticoids cause hypokalemia and may exaggerate the hypokalemic effects of thiazide and high-ceiling diuretics. In combination with amphotericin B they also may cause hypokalemia. Glucocorticoids appear to enhance the ulcerogenic effects of nonsteroidal anti-inflammatory drugs. They decrease the plasma levels of salicylates, and salicylism may occur on discontinuing steroids. Glucocorticoids may increase or decrease the effects of prothrombopenic anticoagulants. Estrogens, phenobarbital, phenytoin and rifampin increase the metabolic clearance of adrenal steroids and hence necessitate dose adjustments.

Other Precautions and Contraindications—Both glucocorticoids and mineralocorticoids must be used cautiously in congestive heart failure, hypertension, liver failure, renal failure or nephrolithiasis. When glucocorticoids are used in persons with emotional instability or psychotic tendencies, hyperlipidemia, diabetes mellitus, hypothyroidism, myasthenia gravis, osteoporosis, peptic ulcer, ulcerative colitis, chronic infections (especially tuberculosis or a positive test) or a history of herpetic infections, patients should be monitored frequently for untoward effects. Topical application to the eye is absolutely contraindicated in the presence of ophthalmological infections.

Pharmacokinetics—All corticosteroids are absorbed rapidly and completely from the gastrointestinal tract. Some, however, particularly the natural ones, are destroyed so rapidly as they pass through the liver that they are poorly effective by the oral route, hence must be given parenterally for systemic effects. Esterification with large hydrophobic organic acids decreases solubility and therefore slows systemic absorption from sites of injection. Esterification with water-soluble acids, such as phosphoric or succinic, increases the rate of absorption from injection sites and even may permit intravenous administration. All of the glucocorticoids are absorbed from the skin, but some slowly enough that metabolic destruction can limit systemic accumulation.

Many glucocorticoids also are metabolized in the skin. Fluorination at the 9-position and various substituents at the 17-position make glucocorticoids resistant to local destruction and hence make these derivatives more likely to cause systemic effects. For this reason, topical use usually is avoided in children. In the liver, the carbonyl groups at positions 3, 11, 17 and 20 are reduced to hydroxyl, and the resulting compounds may be conjugated with sulfate or glucuronic acid. Double bonds in the A ring also are reduced. Less than 1% of unchanged steroid is excreted.

In the plasma, corticosteroids are bound to both corticosteroid-binding globulin (CBG, transcortin, α_1-macroglobulin) and albumin, which serve as transport vehicles. The extent of binding varies among the steroids. Various drugs and diseases can affect the concentration of transport proteins and their capacities.

Corticoids cross the placental barrier and may cause congenital malformations. They also appear in breast milk and may suppress growth of the infant.

The action of a steroid-receptor complex at the genes long outlasts significant plasma concentrations of the steroid, so that the plasma half-life has little relevance to a dosage regimen. Instead, a parameter known as the biological half-life is the primary determinant of dosage-intervals.

Therapeutic Uses—The adrenal corticosteroids are used for replacement therapy in *adrenal insufficiency* (eg, *Addison's disease* and *congenital adrenal hyperplasia).* In this use, toxic effects are infrequent, since the aim is to approximate the equivalent of physiological body concentrations. Both mineralocorticoids and glucocorticoids may be required; sometimes adrenocortical extracts, which contain both, are used. Glucocorticoids additionally are used to treat rheumatic, inflammatory, allergic, neoplastic and other disorders; the effects are palliative only and do not eradicate the underlying disorders. It is necessary to use supraphysiological doses, so that some untoward effects are unavoidable.

The anti-inflammatory actions of the glucocorticoids are employed in the treatment of *noninfectious acute ocular inflammation* (*allergic blepharitis, iritis, uveitis, choroiditis, conjunctivitis, sympathetic ophthalmia*) and certain infectious inflammations, especially in combination with antibiotics. Glucocorticoids are of value, in decreasing some *cerebral edemas*, eg, vasogenic, but are of dubious value in cerebral edema from other causes except that their value in the treatment of *bacterial meningitis* probably accrues to decreased permeability of the blood-brain barrier and the suppression of cerebral edema plus inhibition of cytokine production, especially tumor necrosis factor (TNF).

In *infantile massive spasms* (minor motor epilepsy) glucocorticoids may be of benefit, but it is not clear how this derives from anti-inflammatory activity. In serious *acute allergic disorders*, glucocorticoids may be indicated; they should not be used chronically in allergic disorders, except in acute flareups. (However, they are approved for intranasal application for chronic noninfectious rhinitis.) Similarly, *acute bronchial asthma, status asthmaticus* and some chronic *obstructive pulmonary disease* may require glucocorticoids, but they should be avoided, if possible, in chronic asthma because of the implications for lifetime medication. These drugs suppress allergic and inflammatory manifestations of *trichinosis*.

Topical or systemic glucocorticoids often markedly improve certain skin diseases, such as *pruritus, psoriasis, dermatitis herpetiformis* and *eczema; pemphigus, erythema multiforme, exfoliative dermatitis* and *mycosis fungoides* usually require systemic treatment, which may be life-saving.

Probably the most widely known application of the anti-inflammatory actions of the glucocorticoids is in the treatment of the arthritic and rheumatic disorders. Immunosuppressant actions also may play a role in the treatment of such disorders. These disorders are *systemic lupus erythematosus, polyarteritis nodosa, temporal arteritis, Wegener's granulomatosis, polymyositis* and *polymyalgia rheumatica*. Glucocorticoids may be indicated in severe cases of *rheumatoid arthritis* unresponsive to other treatment, *Still's disease, mixed connective tissue disease, drug-induced lupoid syndromes* and *psoriatic arthropathy*.

Rheumatic or arthritic conditions in which glucocorticoids may or may not provide temporary relief but are not justified chronically because of a high toxicity/benefit ratio are osteoarthritis, systemic ankylosing spondylitis, gout fibrositis and Reiter's syndrome. Even though the *nephrotic syndrome* is not inflammatory, it may respond to treatment, perhaps as the result of immunosuppression. *Ulcerative colitis* sometimes may respond dramatically. The beneficial effects in *myasthenia gravis* are probably immunosuppressant. Chronic *multiple sclerosis* does not respond but acute relapses may.

The incidence and severity of the *respiratory distress syndrome* in premature infants can be decreased by glucocorticoid treatment.

Glucocorticoids may be palliative in *acute leukemia* and also in *chronic lymphocytic leukemia*, and they are components of certain curative antineoplastic combinations. They suppress the associated autoimmune hemolytic anemia and the nonhemolytic anemia, granulocytopenia and thrombocytopenia that result from encroachment on the bone marrow, and also the cachexia and fever. The effects are only temporary, and the patient eventually becomes refractory to steroid therapy. *Hodgkin's disease, lymphosarcoma* and *multiple myeloma* also may be suppressed temporarily, though most frequently only the pain is diminished. The mechanism of the palliative effects on these neoplasms is unknown.

In the treatment of *endotoxin shock*, massive doses of glucocorticoids suppress the vasculotoxic effects of the toxin. In all kinds of *shock*, massive doses decrease peripheral resistance, stimulate the heart and decrease the amount of circulating myocardial depressant factor. To be optimally effective they must be given as boluses.

Modalities and Regimens of Corticosteroid Therapy—*Replacement Therapy*—Treatment of primary and secondary adrenal insufficiency requires replacement of both glucocorticoids and mineralocorticoids in sufficient doses to relieve the signs and symptoms of insufficiency. However, when the patient experiences an additional stress, supplements of glucocorticoids may be required. The dose and dose-interval vary from patient to patient, but the doses are small and complications are infrequent and minimal; the most difficult challenge is in the adjustment of dosage in response to changes in stress.

Chronic Low-Dose Systemic Therapy of Disease—In mild inflammatory or collagen disorders, low doses of glucocorticoids often are sufficient to be palliative, and low-dose regimens are preferable, since adverse effects usually are of low intensity, provided that the therapeutic end point is only an amelioration and not elimination of the morbidity. Although low-dose therapy may cause some suppression of pituitary-adrenal function, the suppression is readily reversible, and some reserve in the system is extant. However, abrupt withdrawal of the drug not only may be followed by a return to the previous condition but an acute exacerbation of the disease. Pituitary-adrenal suppression and consequent acute flare-up after withdrawal may be lessened by avoiding round-the-clock administration and, instead, giving the drug between 6 and 9 am, in order that plasma levels and, hence, pituitary-adrenal suppression be at a minimum during the early morning sleeping hours, when pituitary adrenal function is at its diurnal peak. Moreover, the selection of a steroid with a short biological half-life allows for some drug- free time during the day, during which pituitary-adrenal recovery can occur.

Chronic High-Dose Systemic Therapy—In serious chronic inflammatory or immunologic disorders or in glucocorticoid-responsive neoplasia, large doses of glucocorticoids may be given for long periods of time. Consequently, side effects are frequent, and pituitary-adrenal suppression may be severe. The suppression may continue for weeks to months after cessation of treatment, so that withdrawal must be tapered off slowly to allow the pituitary-adrenal system to recover. Abrupt withdrawal will result in adrenal insufficiency, which may be life-threatening, as well as an acute recrudescence of the original disorder. Pituitary-adrenal suppression and systemic side effects may be less severe if the dose is given in the morning, so that nocturnal pituitary-adrenal activity is less inhibited. Another device to minimize such adverse systemic effects is that of *alternate-day therapy*. Thus, twice the usual daily dose is given but only every other day, which permits the hypothalamico-pituitary segment of the pituitary-adrenal negative feedback system, and various undiseased target organs, time to recover partially between doses. Only glucocorticoids with an intermediate duration of action (12 to 36 hours) should be used for alternate-drug therapy.

Intensive Short-Term Systemic Therapy—Massive doses of glucocorticoids may be required in certain acute conditions, such as bacteremic shock or status asthmaticus. The short duration of such treatment, sometimes no longer than 48 hours, is not enough to give rise to pituitary-adrenal suppression, serious immunosuppression or opportunistic infections, although in septic shock, suprainfections may occur. Psychosis, gastrointestinal bleeding and hyperosmolar diabetic coma can occur in such short-term use.

Local Treatment (Topical Application)—Topical efficacy depends on the inherent glucocorticoid activity (or potency) of the steroid, the concentration in the preparation, permeability coefficient, the vehicle and excipients and local metabolic processes. Except for serious conditions, low-potency glucocorticoids are preferred by many authorities, because adverse effects on the skin appear to be less severe than with high-potency agents, even if the latter are used at appropriately lower concentrations. Only hydrocortisone and its acetate are available for nonprescription topical use.

Drugs with a high lipid-water distribution coefficient penetrate well from absorbable or nonoleaginous vehicles and tend to remain longer in the skin than water-soluble agents, exerting a more extended local action but lesser systemic side effects, especially if the drug is metabolized rapidly systemically. However, it is desirable that the agents be metabolized in the skin, so that less is delivered to the systemic circulation. Steroids that have the 17-OH group substituted and/or which are fluorinated are metabolized poorly locally and hence may have a significant potential for systemic effects; for this reason, especial caution is urged when such compounds are used in children.

Occlusive dressings may be used, especially for low-potency, poorly penetrant steroids. The stratum corneum under the dressing becomes macerated and more permeable. However, such dressings increase absorption into the blood stream and hence favor systemic effects.

Local Treatment (Local Injection)—In order to achieve high, rapidly acting local concentrations of a glucocorticoid, it sometimes is injected as a very soluble derivative which rapidly generates the parent steroid. However, such soluble forms also rapidly leave the region of injection. For this reason, insoluble derivatives may be included or injected alone,

Table 1—Potency Ranking of Some Commonly Used Topical Corticosteroids[a]

Super-Potent	
I.	Clobetasol propionate ointment 0.05%
	Betamethasone dipropionate ointment 0.05%
	Diflorasone diacetate ointment 0.05%
	Clobetasol priopionate cream 0.05%
	Betamethasone dipropionate cream 0.05%
Potent	
II.	Amcinonide ointment 0.1%
	Betamethasone dipropionate ointment 0.05%
	Desoximetasone cream, gel, ointment 0.25%
	Diflorasone diacetate ointment 0.05%
	Fluocinonide cream, gel, ointment 0.05%
	Halcinonide cream 0.1%
III.	Betamethasone dipropionate cream 0.05%
	Betamethasone valerate ointment 0.1%
	Diflorasone diacetate cream 0.05%
	Mometasone furoate cream, ointment 0.1%
	Triamcinolone acetonide cream, ointment 0.5
Mid-Strength	
IV.	Betamethasone benzoate ointment 0.025%
	Clocortolone pivalate cream 0.1%
	Desoximetasone cream 0.05%
	Fluocinolone acetonide cream 0.2%
	Fluocinolone acetonide ointment 0.025%
	Flurandrenolide ointment 0.055
	Hydrocortisone valerat ointment 0.2%
	Triamcinolone acetonide cream, ointment 0.1%
V.	Betamethasone benzoate cream 0.025%
	Betamethasone diproprionate lotion 0.02%
	Betamethasone valerate cream 0.1%
	Fluocinolone acetonide cream 0.025%
	Flurandrenolide cream 0.05%
	Hydrocortisone butyrate cream 0.1%
	Hydrocortisone valerate cream 0.2%
	Triamcinolone acetonide lotion 0.1%
Mild	
VI.	Alclometasone dipropionate cream, ointment 0.05%
	Betamethasone valerate lotion 0.1%
	Desonide cream 0.05%
	Fluocinolone acetonide solution 0.01%
VII.	Hydrocortisone, dexamethasone, flumethasone, prednisolone and methylprednisolone

[a] Summarized from "*Drug Evaluations Annual 1992*," American Medical Association, Chicago, 1099.

so that a sustained action in parallel with slow dissolution may be effected.

Inhibitors of Biosynthesis—Several drugs that interfere with the biosynthesis of adrenocorticoids are used clinically as "antiadrenal" drugs. Their mechanisms of action vary. *Mitotane* causes adrenocortical atrophy and a consequent decrease in the biosynthesis of all products of adrenocortical cells. *Aminoglutethimide* blocks the conversion of cholesterol to pregnenolone, and *trilostane* the dehydrogenation of the 3β-hydroxyl group of pregnenolone; hence, they both interrupt the biosynthesis of *all active* adrenal-derived steroids, including androgens and estrogens.

Mitotane blocks 11β-hydroxylation and hence the biosynthesis of aldosterone, cortisone and hydroxycortisone. Mitotane and aminoglutethimide, especially, are used in the treatment of adrenal tumors and aminoglutethimide also to suppress the production of androgens and estrogens in carcinoma of the breast. These two drugs are discussed in Chapter 75. Since blocking 11-hydroxylation leads to the homeostatic overflow of ACTH and the 11-deoxy precursors of cortisone and hydrocortisone, *metyrapone* is used diagnostically to ascertain the source of excess hydrocortisone in suspected adrenal carcinoma or autonomous adenoma by monitoring plasma ACTH and 11-deoxycorticods. Metyrapone and trilostane are used in the management of Cushing's syndrome.

Beclomethasone Dipropionate

Pregna-1,4-diene-3,20-dione, (11β,16β)-9-chloro-11-hydroxy-16-methyl-17,21-bis(1-oxopropoxy)-, Beclovent; Beconase (*Glaxo*); Vanceril, Vancenase (*Schering*)

[5534-09-8] $C_{26}H_{37}ClO_7$ (521.05).

Preparation—Synthesis of beclomethasone, a 9-chloro-16β-methyl derivative of prednisolone, and esters of beclomethasone, from steroid intermediates is described in British Pats 901,093 and 912,378 (*CA 58:* 3488e, 1963; *59:*14082b, 1963).

Description—White to cream-white powder; odorless.

Solubility—Very slightly soluble in water; very soluble in chloroform; freely soluble in alcohol or acetone.

Uses—Has 500 times the topical anti-inflammatory activity of dexamethasone but is less active as a systemic glucocorticoid and is almost inactive by the oral route. The low systemic activity is the result of rapid deesterification and further metabolism in the liver. Also, it has a high lipid, but low water, solubility, so that it not only is absorbed well topically but also tends to remain at the site of application. Thus, it may be administered by oral inhalation with usually negligible systemic side effects. It is indicated only in the treatment of *bronchial asthma* in which bronchodilators and cromolyn sodium are ineffective. As long as 2 to 4 weeks may be required for the onset of a beneficial effect. It alsois employed in the treatment of *noninfectious rhinitis*.

The most-common side effects of the inhaled drug are dry mouth, hoarseness, sore throat, and pharyngeal or tracheal candidiasis. Usually, the effects on pituitary-adrenal function are negligible, but suppression of plasma cortisol levels occurs in a few percent of adult patients who receive 1600 μg a day and in all who receive 4000 μg a day. In children, doses of 400 to 800 μg a day have effects on adrenal function comparable to alternate-day therapy with prednisone. Patients who switch from continuous oral glucocorticoids to aerosols of this drug often show signs and symptoms of systemic glucocorticoid deficiency, and deaths from adrenal insufficiency have been reported. Adverse effects of intranasal administration include epistaxis, nasal irritation, sneezing and nasopharyngeal candidiasis. Hypersensitivity or other adverse effects to the propellants (CHF_3 and CH_2F_2) and oleic acid (a dispersing agent) may occur; hypersensitivity absolutely contraindicates use of the aerosol. Its effects on the fetus *in utero* and the extent of secretion into milk are not yet known.

The plasma half-life is about 15 hr. The drug is 60% bound to plasma albumin but is not bound to transcortin.

Dose—*Oral inhalation (aerosol), adults* and *children over 12 yr, initially* **84 μg** (2 metered inhalations) 3 or 4 times a day, to be adjusted later to the minimal number of daily inhalations that will control symptoms; in *severe asthma*, the initial dose is **504** to **672 μg** (12 to 16 metered sprays) a day in divided doses, to be subsequently adjusted as needed, usually to a lower dose but occasionally to doses as high as 840 μg a day or more; *children 6 to 12 yr*, **42** to **84 μg** (1 to 2 metered sprays) 3 or 4 times a day, not to exceed 420 μg a day. [*Oral inhalation* (capsules; in *Canada*), *adult*, 200 μg 3 or 4 times a day, to be adjusted subsequently to the minimal effective dose; *children*, 100 μg 2 or 3 times a day, adjusted subsequently to a dose not to exceed 500 μg a day.] The mouth and throat should be rinsed after each oral or intranasal insufflation. *Topical*, to the *skin*, as a **0.025%** cream, lotion or ointment applied thinly once or twice a day.

Dosage Forms—Aerosol: 16.8 g/canister; each metered spray releases approximately 42 μg; Capsules, for Inhalation (Canada): 100 and 200 μg.

Betamethasone

Pregna-1,4-diene-3,20-dione, (11β,16β)-
9-fluoro-11,17,21-trihydroxy-16-methyl-, Celestone (*Schering*)

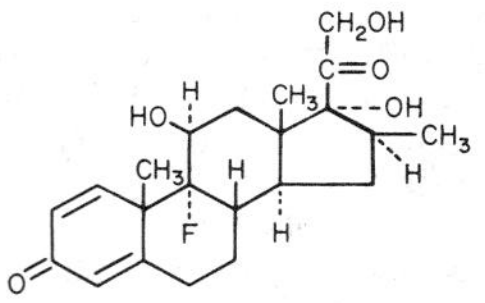

[378-44-9] $C_{22}H_{29}FO_5$ (392.47).

Preparation—Betamethasone is prepared from 16-dehydropregnenolone (see *Progesterone*, page □□□) by treatment with methyl magnesium iodide to insert the 16β-methyl group, catalytic reduction of the remaining double bond, enol acylation at position 20 and reaction with peracetic acid followed by hydrolysis to the 16β-methyl-17α-hydroxy compound. Bromination and acetoxylation gives the 3β-hydroxy-21-acetoxy derivative which is oxidized to the 3-oxo compound with chromic acid. Dibromination at positions 1 and 4 followed by dehydrobromination with dimethylformamide to the 1,4-diene, then incubation with *Pestalotia foedans* (or a similar organism) results in the 11α-hydroxy derivative. Esterification at the 11-position with ethyl chloroformate, elimination of the ester function with acetic acid to form the 1,4,9(11)-triene, treatment with *N*-bromoacetamide and perchloric acid gives the 9α-bromo-11β-hydroxy compound. Abstraction of HBr with potassium acetate affords the 9β,11β-epoxy derivative which by treatment with HF in a halogenated hydrocarbon yields the 9α-fluoro-11β- hydroxy analog, betamethasone.

Description—White to practically white, odorless, crystalline powder; melts at about 240° with some decomposition.

Solubility—1 g in 5300 mL water, 65 mL alcohol or 325 mL chloroform; very slightly soluble in ether.

Uses—An extremely potent glucocorticoid with actions, uses and side effects typical of this class of steroids (see the introduction to this section). Its activity is 20 to 30 times that of cortisol. However, it only rarely induces sodium and water retention and potassium loss such as accompany treatment with cortisone and many other adrenal corticoids; on occasion, it even may increase sodium excretion and induce diuresis. In the usual doses, the incidence of characteristic adrenal corticoid untoward effects such as anorexia, protracted weight loss, vertigo, headache and muscle weakness is quite low. The plasma half-life is about 6.5 hr and the biological half-life 36 to 54 hr. The volume of distribution is 1.8 L/kg.

Dose—*Oral, adult, initially* **0.6** to **7.2 mg** (usually **2.4** to **4.8 mg**) daily in single or divided doses; *maintenance*, usually **0.6** to **1.2 mg** a day or on alternate days; *children, replacement*, **17.5 μg/kg** or **500 μg/m²** a day in 3 divided doses, and, for *disease*, **62.5** to **250 μg/kg** or **1.88** to **7.5 mg/m²** in 3 or 4 divided doses. [With extended-release tablets (Canada), the adult dose is initially 2 to 6 mg a day.] *Topical*, as **0.2%** cream applied to skin 2 or 3 times a day in adults and once a day in children.

Dosage Forms—Cream: 0.2%; Syrup: 0.6 mg/5 mL; Tablets: 0.6 mg.

Betamethasone Acetate

Pregna-1,4-diene-3,20-dione, (11β,16β)-
9-fluoro-11,17-dihydroxy-16-methyl-21-(acetyloxy)-,

Betamethasone 21-Acetate [987-24-6] $C_{24}H_{31}FO_6$ (434.50).

For the structure of the parent, see *Betamethasone*.

Preparation—*Betamethasone* is acetylated with acetic anhydride in the presence of pyridine. US Pat 3,164,618.

Description—White to creamy white, odorless powder; sinters and resolidifies at about 165° and remelts with decomposition between 200° and 220°.

Solubility—1 g in 2000 mL water, 9 mL alcohol or 16 mL chloroform.

Uses—The actions are the same as those of the parent compound, *Betamethasone*. However, at present, the acetate is marketed only in combination with the sodium phosphate. The acetate is less soluble than the sodium phosphate, so that it provides a sustained action after intramuscular or intra-articular injection.

Betamethasone Benzoate

Pregna-1,4-diene-3,20-dione, (11β,16β)-17-(benzoyloxy)-9-fluoro-
11,21-dihydroxy-16-methyl-, Uticort (*Park-Davis*)

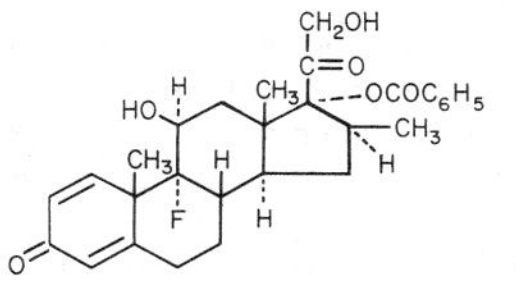

[22298-29-9] $C_{29}H_{33}FO_6$ (496.57).

Preparation—See *J Med Chem 15*:783, 1972.

Description—White crystals melting about 226°.

Solubility—Practically insoluble in water; soluble in ethanol, methanol or chloroform.

Uses—See the general statement and *Betamethasone*. The benzoate has a low aqueous solubility and high lipid/water distribution coefficient, hence the drug has potent topical glucocorticoid activity and persistence in the skin.

Dose—*Topical*, to the skin, as a **0.025%** cream, gel, lotion or ointment, applied 2 to 4 times a day on adults and once a day in children.

Dosage Forms—Cream, Gel, Lotion or Ointment: 0.025%.

Betamethasone Sodium Phosphate

Pregna-1,4-diene-3,20-dione, (11β,16β)- 9-fluoro-11,17-dihydroxy-
16-methyl-21- (phosphonooxy)-, disodium salt, Betamethasone 21-
(Disodium Phosphate); (*Various Mfrs*)

[151-73-5] $C_{22}H_{28}FNa_2O_8P$ (516.41).

For the structure of the parent, see *Betamethasone*.

Preparation—Starting with *Betamethasone*, by the method described for *Dexamethasone Sodium Phosphate*, page 1070. US Pat 3,164,618.

Description—White to practically white, odorless powder; hygroscopic.

Solubility—1 g in 2 mL water, 470 mL alcohol, >10,000 mL chloroform or >10,000 mL ether.

Uses—A soluble derivative of *Betamethasone*, to which it is converted in the body. Following injection, the plasma or synovial fluid levels rise at a rapid rate to high levels, which effects a prompt response. This parenteral form is employed when oral glucocorticoids cannot be used or when it is desirable to inject the drug directly into the affected structure. It is employed singly or in combination with *Betamethasone Acetate*.

Dose—The following doses are stated in terms of the *betamethasone equivalents*, but the content of ampules and vials is stated for betamethasone sodium phosphate itself. *To convert*, 4 mg of the sodium phosphate derivative is equivalent to 3 mg of betamethasone. *Intramuscular* or *intravenous, adult, initially* up to **9 mg**/day, to be repeated and adjusted as necessary; *intra-articular, intralesional* or into *soft tissue*, up to **9 mg**/day as needed. *Children, intramuscular*, for *replacement*, **17.5 μg/kg** or **500 μg/m²** every third day *or* **5.8** to **8.75 μg/kg** or **166** to **250 μg** once a day; for *disease*, **20.8** to **125 μg/kg or 625 μg** to **3.75 mg/m²** once or twice a day.

Dosage Forms—Injection: 20 mg/5 mL, equivalent to 3 mg/mL of betamethasone. Pellets for the local treatment of aphthous ulcers, an enema and effervescent tablets are available abroad.

Betamethasone Valerate

Pregna-1,4-diene-3,20-dione, (11β,16β)-
9-fluoro-11,21-dihydroxy-16-methyl-17-[(1-oxopentyl)oxy]-,
Bethamethasone 17-Valerate; Valisone (*Various Mfrs*)

[2152-44-5] $C_{27}H_{37}FO_6$ (476.58).
For the structure of the parent, see *Betamethasone*.

Preparation—A solution of *Bethamethasone* in an organic solvent is treated with a lower alkyl orthovalerate such as trimethyl orthovalerate [$C_4H_9C(OCH_3)_3$] to produce betamethasone-17,21-ylene alkyl orthovalerate. This is then hydrolyzed with dilute acid and the resulting crude betamethasone 17-valerate is extracted and crystallized from a suitable organic solvent. US Pat 3,312,590.

Description—White to practically white, odorless, crystalline powder; melts about 190°, with decomposition.

Solubility—1 g in 10,000 mL water, 16 mL alcohol, <10 mL chloroform or 400 mL ether.

Uses—The actions are the same as those of the parent compound, *Betamethasone*. However, the physicochemical properties of the compound favor penetration into the skin. It is thus employed for treatment of inflammatory and allergic dermatoses and dermatitides (see the introduction to this section).

Unless extensive areas of the skin are dressed with betamethasone valerate cream under occlusion, systemic effects are unlikely to occur. However, prolonged topical use may cause cutaneous and subcutaneous atrophy and consequent striae. Irritation, folliculitis and sensitization are rare.

Dose—*Topical, adult,* as a cream, lotion, or ointment containing the equivalent of **0.01** or **0.1%** of betamethasone to the affected area 1 to 3 times a day. *Children,* as a **0.01%** cream 1 or 2 times a day or as a **0.1%** cream, lotion, or ointment once a day.

Dosage Forms (betamethasone equivalent)—Cream: 0.01 and 0.1%; Lotion: 0.1%; Ointment: 0.1%.

Cortisone Acetate

Pregn-4-ene-3,11,20-trione, 21-(acetyloxy)-17-hydroxy-, Kendall's Compound E Acetate; Wintersteiner's Compound F Acetate; Reichstein's Substance Fa Acetate; Cortone Acetate (*MSD*)

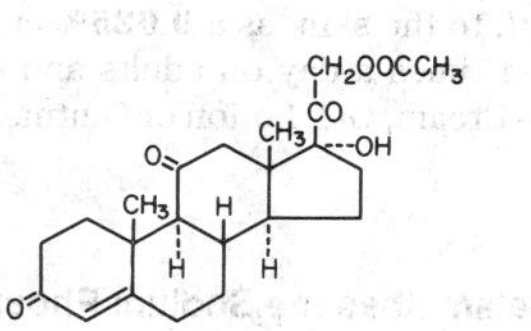

[50-04-4] $C_{23}H_{30}O_6$ (402.49).

Preparation—By a variety of methods using easily obtainable starting materials such as ergosterol, diosgenin or hecogenin from plant materials and cholesterol or desoxycholic acid from animal sources. The cortisone is esterified with acetic anhydride to give the acetate.

Description—White or practically white, odorless, crystalline powder; stable in air; melts about 240° with some decomposition.

Solubility—Insoluble in water; 1 g in about 350 mL alcohol, 4 mL chloroform, 30 mL dioxane or 75 mL acetone.

Uses—Cortisone is a natural glucocorticoid with a slight degree of mineralocorticoid activity; it has 0.8 the glucocorticoid activity of cortisol. The acetate is used specifically, in combination with desoxycorticosterone acetate, in *adrenal cortical insufficiency*. It also may be used for the numerous purposes described in the introduction to this section, where its untoward effects also are described. Although this drug is applied locally in some conditions, it requires conversion to cortisol to be substantially effective, and there is little to justify topical use. The plasma half-life of cortisone is about 30 min, which is shorter than the half-time for absorption of the acetate and conversion to cortisone. The plasma half-time for hydrocortisone, the active form of cortisone, is 1½ to 2 hr and the biological half-life is 8 to 12 hr.

Dose—*Oral, adult,* for *replacement therapy,* **20** to **70 mg** a day, ⅔ taken in the morning and ⅓ in the afternoon, and, for *anti-inflammatory effects,* **25** to **50 mg** a day in mild chronic disorders and **75** to **300 mg** in acute and severe chronic disorders; *children, replacement,* **700 µg/kg** (or **20** to **25 mg per m²**) a day in divided doses once a day; for *anti-inflammatory effects,* **2.5** to **10 mg/kg** (or **75** to **300 mg/m²**) a day in single or divided doses. *Intramuscular, adult,* **20** to **300 mg** a day for serious chronic disorders; absorption is too slow and erratic by this route to lend itself to treatment of acute disorders; *children, replacement,* **700 µg/kg** or **37.5 mg/m²** a day every 3rd day; *anti-inflammatory,* **833 µg** to **5 mg/kg** or **25** to **150 mg/m²** every 12 to 24 hr. Once a satisfactory initial response has been obtained, the dose gradually is lowered to the satisfactory maintenance minimum.

Dosage Forms—Sterile Suspension: 250 and 500 mg/10 mL and 500 mg/20 mL; Tablets: 5, 10 and 25 mg.

Dexamethasone

(11β,16α)-Pregna-1,4-diene-3,20-dione, 9-fluoro-
11,17,21-trihydroxy-16-methyl-, (*Various Mfrs*)

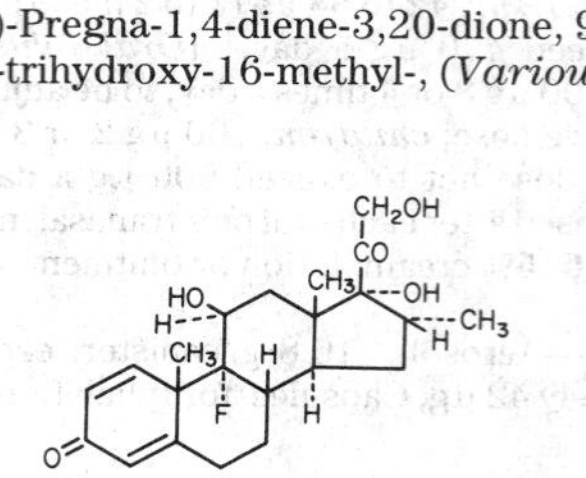

[50-02-2] $C_{22}H_{29}FO_5$ (392.47).

Preparation—In a manner quite similar to that for *Betamethasone*, the difference being that the 16-methyl group is inserted in the α-configuration.

Description—White to practically white, odorless, crystalline powder; stable in air; melts about 250° with some decomposition.

Solubility—1 g in 42 mL alcohol or 165 mL chloroform; sparingly soluble in acetone, dioxane or methanol; very slightly soluble in ether; practically insoluble in water.

Uses—Possesses glucocorticoid activity, for which it is used clinically (see the introduction to this section). It especially is used as an anti-inflammatory and antiallergic drug. Topically, it is employed in the treatment of glucocorticoid-responsive dermatoses. Systemically, it decreases the incidence and severity of hearing loss consequent to bacterial meningitis. Its systemic glucocorticoid potency is about 25 times that of cortisone. It is capable of inducing all the usual side effects of adrenal corticoids, except that the mineralocorticoid-like side effects are less pronounced than with cortisone acetate.

Its effect to suppress pituitary-adrenocortical function is used for differential diagnostic purposes in Cushing's syndrome. In the *rapid overnight test,* 1 mg given at 11 or 12 pm will have a marked suppressant effect on plasma cortisol levels at 8 am in persons who do not have Cushing's syndrome but little effect on those who do. In the *low-dose 2-day test,* 0.5 mg every 6 hr for 2 days will fail to suppress 24-hr urinary output of 17-hydroxysteroids in patients with bilateral adrenal hyperplasia and autonomous adenomas but not in others. In the *high-dose 2-day test,* 2 mg every 6 hr for 2 days will suppress urinary 17-hydroxysteroids in adrenal hyperplasia (except multinodular hyperplasia) and most ACTH-responsive adrenal adenomas. Some multinodular hyperplasias and ACTH-responsive adrenal adenomas will not show suppression until the dose of the drug is increased to 4 to 8 mg every 6 hr. When adrenal hyperplasia is secondary to an ACTH-producing tumor, no suppression will occur in any of these tests.

The plasma half-life is 3 to 4 hr and the biological half-life is 36 to 54 hr. The volume of distribution is 0.75 L/kg. It binds linearly to albumin but does not bind to transcortin.

Dose—*Oral, adult, initially* **500 µg** to **9 mg** a day in single or divided doses, and usually less for *maintenance;* for *multiple sclerosis* (after initial therapy with prednisolone acetate), **8 mg** every other day for 1 mo; for *cerebral edema,* **2 mg** 2 or 3 times a day for *maintenance* only after initial control with parenteral dexamethasone sodium phosphate; for *diagnostic doses,* see *Uses,* above; *children,* for *replacement,* **23 µg/kg** (or **670 µg/m²**) a day, and, for *disease,* **83** to **333 µg/kg** (or **2.5** to **10 mg/m²**) a day in 3 or 4 divided doses. *Topical,* to the *skin,* as **0.01** or **0.04%** aerosol 2 to 4 times a day or **0.1%** gel 3 or 4 times a day, except only 1 or 2 times a day with any preparation in children. *Topical,* to the *conjunctiva,* **1 drop** of **0.1%** suspension 3 or 4 times a day.

Dosage Forms—Topical Aerosol: 0.01 and 0.04%; Elixir: 0.5 mg/5 mL; Gel: 0.1%; Ophthalmic Suspension: 0.1%; Tablets: 0.25, 0.5, 0.75, 1, 1.5, 2, 4 and 6 mg.

Dexamethasone Sodium Phosphate

Pregn-4-ene-3,20-dione, (11β,16α)- 9-fluoro-11,17-dihydroxy-16-methyl-21-(phosphonooxy)-, disodium salt, Dexamethasone 21-(Disodium Phosphate); Decadron (*MSD*); Dalalone (*Forest*)

[2392-39-4] $C_{22}H_{28}FNa_2O_8P$ (516.41).
For the structure of the parent, see *Dexamethasone*.

Preparation—Dexamethasone is esterified with methanesulfonyl chloride at the 21-position, and the ester is refluxed with sodium iodide in ethanol to form the 21-iodo derivative. This is treated with silver dihydrogen phosphate and the resulting 21-(dihydrogen phosphate) is neutralized with sodium hydroxide.

Description—White, or slightly yellow, crystalline powder; odorless or has a slight odor of alcohol; very hygroscopic; pH (1 in 100 solution) between 7.5 and 10.5.

Solubility—1 g in about 2 mL water; slightly soluble in ether or chloroform.

Uses—The same actions as *Dexamethasone*. It is one of the most soluble adrenocortical compounds. Thus, it lends itself well to intravenous administration, local injection and inhalation, and to solutions and water-based ointments for topical application, especially for ophthalmological use. The inhalation aerosol is used in the management of bronchial asthma. Although it may be given intra-articularly, it usually is not recommended by this route because of the danger of painless joint destruction. The adverse effects and contraindications are those of other glucocorticoids (see the introduction to this section).

Dose (dexamethasone equivalents)—*Intravenous* or *intramuscular, adult,* **420 μg** to **7.5 mg** a day, the dosage being decreased when a response occurs. *Intra-articular, intralesional* or *soft-tissue injection,* **170 μg** to **5 mg.** *Intramuscular, children, replacement,* **19.6 μg/kg** or **563 μg/m²** every 3rd day *or* **6.52** to **9.79 μg/kg** or **196** to **281 μg/m²** once a day; for *disease,* **23** to **140 μg/kg** or **700 μg** to **4.2 mg/m²** once or twice a day. *Oral inhalation,* **3 metered sprays (252 μg)** in *adults,* maximum of 12 inhalations a day, and **2 metered sprays (168 μg)** in *children,* 3 or 4 times a day, maximum of 8 inhalations a day. *Intranasal, adult,* **2 metered sprays (168 μg)** into each nostril 2 or 3 times a day up to 1008 mg, maximum of 8 sprays (672 μg) a day; *children over 6 yr,* **1** or **2 metered sprays** into each nostril twice a day. *Topical,* to the *skin,* as **0.1%** cream, 3 or 4 times a day for *adults* or once a day for *children;* to the *conjunctiva* as **0.05%** ointment 3 or 4 times a day or 1 drop of **0.05%** solution 4 to 6 times a day or **1 drop** of **0.1%** suspension 3 or 4 times a day; *otic,* **3** or **4 drops** of **0.1%** ophthalmic solution into the ear canal 2 or 3 times a day.

Dosage Forms—(dexamethasone equivalents) Inhalation Aerosol: 84 μg/metered spray 170 doses; Nasal Aerosol: 84 μg/metered spray 170 doses; Cream: 0.1%; Injection: 3.3, 8.33, 16.66 and 20 mg/mL; Ophthalmic Ointment: 0.05%; Ophthalmic Solution: 0.1%; Opthalmic Suspension: 0.1%.

Fludrocortisone Acetate

(11β)-Pregn-4-ene-3,20-dione, 21-(acetyloxy)-9-fluoro-11,17-dihydroxy-, Florinef Acetate (*Squibb*)

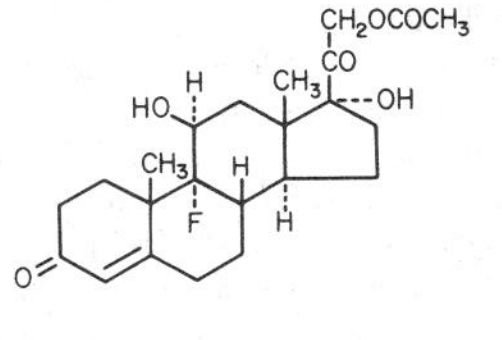

[514-36-3] $C_{23}H_{31}FO_6$ (422.49).

Preparation—One method starts with *Hydrocortisone Acetate* which is first dehydrated to the 4,9-diene. The 9α-fluoro and 11β-hydroxy groups are inserted by a method similar to that used for *Betamethasone.*

Description—Fine, white to pale-yellow powder that is odorless or practically odorless; hygroscopic; melts at about 225° with some decomposition.

Solubility—Insoluble in water; soluble 1 g in 50 mL alcohol, 50 mL chloroform or 250 mL ether.

Uses—A potent mineralocorticoid with considerable glucocorticoid activity. Its uses and side effects are those of mineralocorticoids (see page 1064), except that when used for replacement therapy in adrenal insufficiency it may not always be necessary to use a glucocorticoid concurrently, although usually hydrocortisone or cortisone are administered also. With the doses used for replacement therapy, glucocorticoid side effects of the drug alone are mild and infrequent. The plasma half-life is about 3.5 hr and the biological half-life is 18 to 36 hr.

Dose—*Oral, adult,* for *chronic adrenal insufficiency,* **100 μg** a day; for *congenital adrenogenital syndromes,* **0.1** to **0.2 mg** a day; *children,* **50** to **100 μg** a day. In both of the above, a glucocorticoid usually is administered concomitantly.

Dosage Form—Tablets: 0.1 mg.

Flunisolide

Pregna-1,4-diene-3,20-dione, (6α,11β,16α)-6-fluoro-11,21-dihydroxy- 16,17-[(1-methylethylidene)bis(oxy)]-, hemihydrate; Aerobid, Nasalide (*Syntex*)

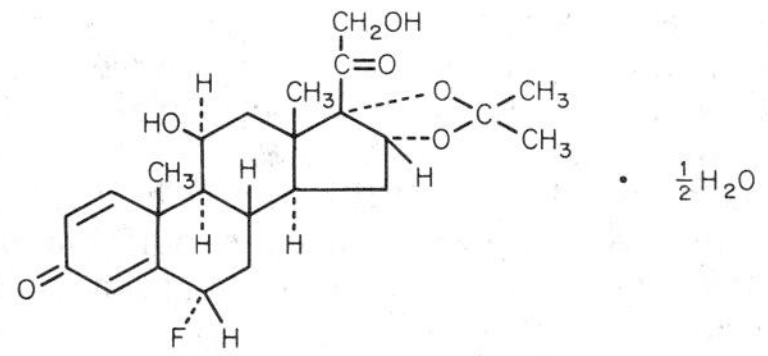

[77326-96-6] $C_{24}H_{31}FO_6 \cdot \frac{1}{2}H_2O$ (443.51).

Preparation—See US Pat 3,124,571.

Description—White to creamy white crystalline powder melting about 245°.

Solubility—Soluble in acetone; sparingly soluble in chloroform; slightly soluble in methanol; practically insoluble in water.

Uses—A topical glucocorticoid for the treatment of *noninfectious rhinitis* and *bronchial asthma.* It has a high lipid/water-distribution coefficient, which favors both absorption into nasal and pulmonary tissue and retention at the site of application. By inhalation, about 40% is absorbed, which is considerably more than is absorbed of beclomethasone. The plasma half-life is about 1.8 hr, so that absorbed steroid is destroyed rapidly enough so that pituitary-adrenocortical suppression does not occur with recommended doses. Dry mouth, hoarseness, sore throat and pharyngeal, laryngeal or tracheal candidiasis sometimes occurs after continuous use. Occasional coughing, wheezing and chest tightness are attributable to the vehicle and/or propellant.

Dose—*Intranasal, age 14 yr or over, initially* **50 μg** (2 metered sprays) into each nostril 2 (preferably) or 3 times a day, maximum of 8 sprays in each nostril (400 μg a day), then **25 μg** once a day for *maintenance; children 6* to *14 yr, initially* **25 μg** (1 metered spray) into each nostril 3 times a day *or* **50 μg** (2 metered sprays) twice a day, maximum of 4 sprays in each nostril (200 μg a day), then **25 μg** (1 metered spray) into each nostril once a day for *maintenance. Oral inhalation, age 15 yr or over, usually* **500 μg** (2 metered sprays) twice a day (morning and evening), not to exceed 2 mg a day.

Dosage Forms—Metered Aerosol: 250 μg/actuation, 100 doses; Metered Nasal Spray: 25 μg/actuation, 200 doses.

Fluocinolone Acetonide

(6α,11β,16α)-Pregna-1,4-diene-3,20-dione, 6,9-difluoro-11,21-dihydroxy-16,17-[(1- methylethylidene)bis(oxy)]-, (*Various Mfrs*)

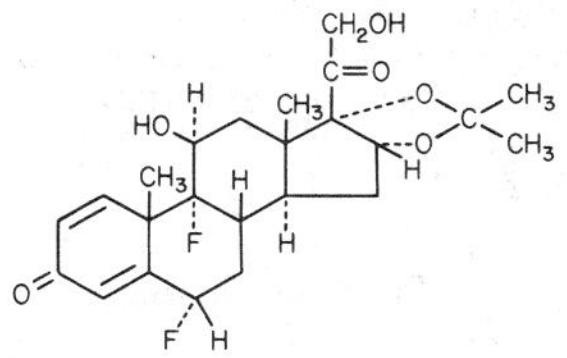

6α,9-Difluoro-11β,16α,17,21-tetrahydroxypregna-1,4-diene-3,20-dione, cyclic 16,17-acetal with acetone [67-73-2] $C_{24}H_{30}F_2O_6$ (452.50).

Preparation—From the 21-acetate of 16α,17α-epoxy-3β,21-dihydroxypregn-5-en-20-one (available by synthesis from naturally occurring sapogenins such as diosgenin). Treatment of this pregnene with HF and *N*-bromoacetamide, followed by chromic acid oxidation and then treatment with HBr in acetic acid gives the Δ^4- 16β-bromo-6α-fluoro derivative. This latter compound on refluxing with potassium acetate in acetic acid and then saponifying with sodium carbonate yields the 6α-fluoro-16α,17α-dihydroxy compound which when incubated with minced, defatted bovine adrenals adds an 11β-hydroxyl group. From the 16,21-diacetate, with dimethylformamide and methanesulfonyl chloride, the 4,9-diene is synthesized, which is converted to the 9β,11β-epoxide and then to the 9α-fluoro-11β-hydroxy compound in a manner similar to that for *Betamethasone.* Oxidation of this product with selenium dioxide yields the 1,4-diene (fluocinolone) which on reaction with acetone and perchloric acid yields the acetonide.

Description—White, crystalline powder that is odorless; stable in light; melts about 270°, with decomposition.

Solubility—1 g in > 1000 mL water, 45 mL alcohol, 25 mL chloroform or 350 mL ether.

Uses—A glucocorticoid with potent anti-inflammatory and metabolic actions and negligible mineralocorticoid actions (see page 1064). It is employed topically in the treatment of various *dermatoses.* In resistant nummular dermatitis, psoriasis or chronic neurodermatitis it usually is used under occlusive dressings. Even in instances in which nearly the whole body has been covered by a cream containing the corticoid, evidences of systemic side effects are rare. However, folliculitis or striae is a frequent complication, especially if occlusive dressings are used. Topically, it is contraindicated in the presence of tuberculosis, fungal infections and most viral lesions of the skin (vaccinia, varicella, herpes simplex, etc). Neomycin often is included in topical preparations of the glucocorticoid to suppress infections secondary to the inflammatory process or which result from its use.

Dose—Topical, to the *skin, adult,* as **0.01** to **0.2%** cream, **0.025%** ointment or **0.01%** solution, applied 2 to 4 times a day or under an occlusive dressing; *children,* as **0.01%** cream or solution once or twice a day or as **0.025** to **0.2%** cream or **0.025%** ointment once a day.

Dosage Forms—Cream: 0.01, 0.025 and 0.2%; Ointment: 0.025%; Topical Solution: 0.01%.

Fluocinonide

(6α,11β,16α)-Pregna-1,4-diene-3,20-dione, 21-(acetyloxy)-6, 9-difluoro-11-hydroxy- 16,17-[(1-methylethylidene)bis(oxy)]-, Fluocinolide; Lidex, Topsyn (*Syntex*); Lionide (*Syosset*)

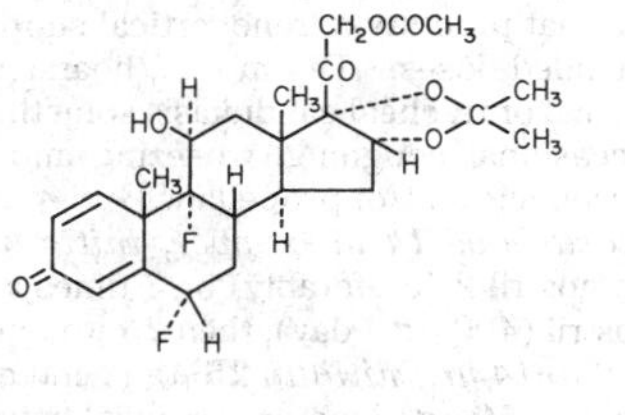

6α,9-Difluoro-11β,16α,17,21-tetrahydroxypregna-1,4-diene-3,20-dione, cyclic 16,17-acetal with acetone, 21-acetate [356-12-7] $C_{26}H_{32}F_2O_7$ (494.53).

Preparation—*Fluocinolone Acetonide* is esterified with acetic anhydride in the presence of pyridine. US Pat 3,126,375 and 3,592,930.

Description—White to creamy white, odorless, crystalline powder; stable in light, air and at room temperature; melts, within a range of 3°, at about 300°, with decomposition.

Solubility—Insoluble in water; 1 g in 70 mL of alcohol, 10 mL of acetone or 10 mL of chloroform.

Uses—A glucocorticoid used only topically for its anti-inflammatory effects in glucocorticoid-responsive *dermatoses* (see the introduction to this section). Systemic side effects are infrequent, but the local side effects are those of other glucocorticoids.

Dose—*Topical,* as **0.05%** cream, gel, ointment or solution applied 2 to 4 times a day for *adults* or once a day for *children.*

Dosage Forms—Cream: 0.05%; Gel: 0.05%; Ointment: 0.05%; Topical Solution: 0.05%.

Flurandrenolide

(6α,11β,16α-)-Pregn-4-ene-3,20-dione, 6-fluoro-11,21-dihydroxy-16,17-[(1-methylethylidene)bis(oxy)]-, Flurandrenolone; Cordran (*Oclassen*)

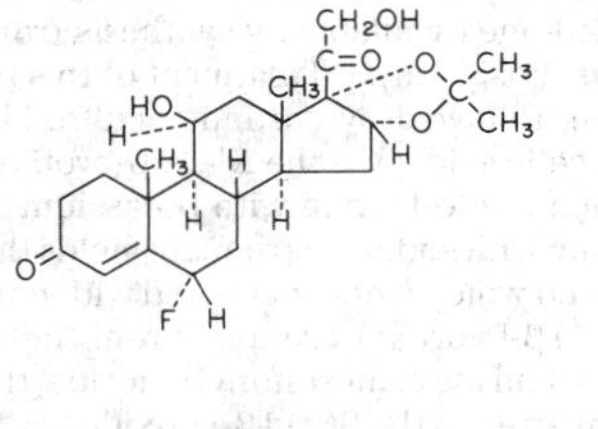

6α-Fluoro-11β,16α,17,21-tetrahydroxypregn-4-ene-3,20-dione, cyclic 16,17-acetal with acetone [1524-88-5] $C_{24}H_{33}FO_6$ (436.52).

Preparation—Flurandrenolone (6α-fluoro-16α-hydroxycortisol) is condensed with acetone by treating its solution in acetone with 70% perchloric acid. US Pat 3,126,375.

Description—White to off-white, fluffy, odorless, crystalline powder.

Solubility—1 g in 72 mL alcohol or 10 mL chloroform; practically insoluble in water or ether.

Uses—A glucocorticoid with a high potency topically but low potency systemically because of rapid destruction in the liver. Consequently, its use is limited to the topical management of *glucocorticoid-responsive dermatological disorders.* Under occlusive dressings it is used especially to treat nummular dermatitis, psoriasis and chronic neurodermatitis. Local side effects are uncommon but are typical of drugs of this class (see the introduction to this section). Neomycin is included in some topical preparations of this drug to suppress infections secondary to the inflammatory process or to the use of the glucocorticoid.

Dose—*Topical,* to the *skin, adult,* as **0.025** or **0.05%** cream or ointment or **0.05%** lotion 2 or 3 times a day or as a tape (plaster) containing **4 μg/cm²** 1 or 2 times a day. *Children,* as **0.025%** cream or ointment 1 or 2 times a day or as **0.05%** cream, lotion or ointment, or as tape containing **4 μg/cm²** once a day.

Dosage Forms—Cream: 0.025 and 0.05%; Lotion: 0.05%; Ointment: 0.025 and 0.05%; Tape: 4 μg/cm².

Hydrocortisone

(11β)-Pregn-4-ene-3,20-dione, 11,17,21-trihydroxy-, Compound F; Reichstein's "Substance M"; (*Various Mfrs*)

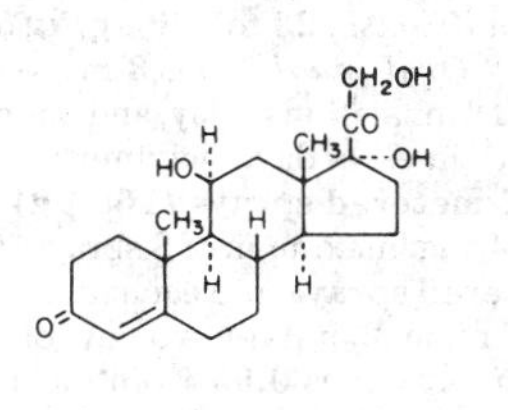

Cortisol [50-23-7] $C_{21}H_{30}O_5$ (362.47).

Preparation—The most attractive commercial synthesis involves the oxidation of 17α,21-dihydroxypregn-4-ene-3,20-dione, which is readily obtainable from diosgenin. Microbiological hydroxylation at the 11β-position is affected on the diacetate of the above compound employing organisms of the *Rhizopus, Aspergillus* or *Streptomyces* species. Saponification then yields hydrocortisone.

Description—White to practically white, odorless, crystalline powder; melts about 215°, with decomposition.

Solubility—1 g in 40 mL alcohol; very slightly soluble in water or ether; slightly soluble in chloroform.

Uses—The principal natural glucocorticoid in man and thus the prototype of all glucocorticoids (for actions, uses and side effects of glucocorticoids, see the introduction to this section). Systemic side effects can result from topical application. Allergic bronchospasm after use in asthmatics has been reported. The plasma half-life is 1½ to 3 hr and the biological half-life is 8 to 12 hr. The volume of distribution is 0.3 to 0.5 L/kg, varying with the dose.

Some topical preparations include neomycin and/or other antibiotics to suppress the emergence of infections.

Dose—*Enema,* **100 mg** once a day. *Intramuscular, adult,* for *replacement,* **560 μg/kg** (or **30** to **37.5 mg/m²**) once a day; for *disease,* **15** to **240 mg** a day; *children,* for *disease,* **666 μg** to **4 mg/kg** (or **20** to **120 mg/m²**) once or twice a day. *Oral, adult,* for *replacement,* **25** to **50 mg**/day, ⅔ of which is to be taken in the morning and ⅓ in the afternoon; for *disease,* **15** to **240 mg**/day in 3 or 4 divided doses; *children,* for *replacement,* **0.56 mg/kg** (or **15** to **20 mg/m²**) once a day; for *disease,* **2** to **8 mg/kg** (or **60** to **240 mg/m²**) once a day. *Rectal,* as **1%** cream or **0.5%** ointment 3 or 4 times a day; *Topical, adult,* to the *skin,* as **0.125** to **2.5%** cream, as **1%** gel, **0.5%** spray solution or **0.125%** to **2.5%** lotion 3 or 4 times a day; *children,* as **0.125** to **1%** cream or lotion or **1%** gel or ointment 1 or 2 times a day or **2.5%** cream or ointment once a day.

Dosage Forms—Cream: 0.5, 1 and 2.5%; Rectal Cream: Retention Enema: 100 mg/60 mL; Gel: 1%; Lotion: 0.25, 0.5, 1, and 2.5%; Ointment: 0.5, 1 and 2.5%; Rectal Ointment: 0.5%; Sterile Suspension: 25 and 50 mg/mL; Suppositories: 10 and 25 mg; Tablets: 5, 10 and 20 mg; Topical Spray Solution: 0.5%; Topical Solution: 1%.

Hydrocortisone Acetate

(11β)-Pregn-4-ene-3,20-dione, 21-(acetyloxy)-11,17-dihydroxy-, Hydrocortisone 21-Acetate; (*Various Mfrs*)

Cortisol 21-acetate [50-03-3] $C_{23}H_{32}O_6$ (404.50).

Preparation—Hydrocortisone is esterified with acetic anhydride to give the 21-acetate.

Description—White to practically white, odorless, crystalline powder; melts about 220° with decomposition.

Solubility—Insoluble in water; 1 g in 230 mL alcohol or 200 mL chloroform.

Uses—Actions of *Hydrocortisone,* to which it is converted in the body.

However, it is not used for systemic therapy. It is used topically in the treatment of glucocorticoid-sensitive dermatoses, anorectal inflammations, inflammatory conditions of the eye and intra-articularly in the treatment of arthritides. Systemic effects can result from local application.

The inclusion of neomycin or antifungal drugs in lotions and creams containing this drug is for the purpose of protecting against bacterial or fungal infections that might be favored by the suppression of the inflammatory response and of clearing up infections secondary to the inflammatory condition.

Dose—*Intra-articular, intralesional* or *soft-tissue injection, adult,* **5** to **75 mg** repeated at 2 or 3-wk intervals, if necessary. *Topical, to the skin, adult,* as **0.5%** cream or lotion 3 or 4 times a day or **0.5** or **1%** ointment 1 to 4 times a day; *children,* as **0.5%** cream or lotion or **0.5** or **1%** ointment 1 or 2 times a day or as a **2.5%** ointment once a day. *Topical,* to the conjunctiva, *adults* and *children,* as a 0.5 or 1% cream (which also contains antibiotics); 3 or 4 times a day. *Rectal, adult* as **1.0%** aerosol foam (90 mg per application) or **0.5%** cream 1 or 2 times a day for 3 wk, after which dosage is diminished every other day, or as suppository **10** to **50 mg** twice a day for 2 wk.

Dosage Forms—Aerosol Foam: 1%; Rectal Aerosol Foam: 1%; Dermatological and Rectal Creams: 0.5%; Ophthalmological Cream (containing antibiotics): 0.5 and 1%; Dental Paste: 0.5%; Lotion: 0.5%; Ointment: 1; Sterile Suspension: 25 and 50 mg/mL; Suppositories: 10 and 25 mg.

Hydrocortisone Cypionate

(11β)-Pregn-4-ene-3,20-dione, 21-(3-cyclopentyl-1-oxopropoxy)-11,17-dihydroxy-, Cortisol Cypionate; Cortef (*Upjohn*)

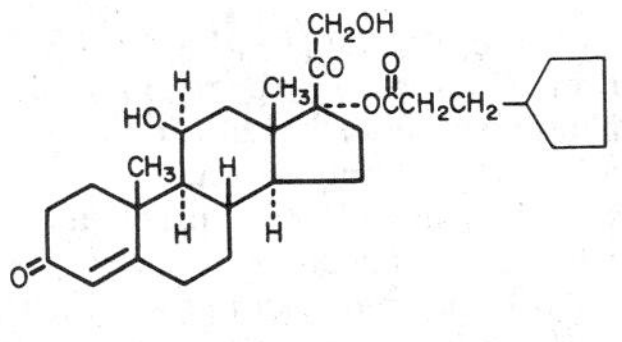

Cortisol 21-cyclopentanepropionate [508-99-6] $C_{29}H_{42}O_6$ (486.65).

Preparation—*Hydrocortisone* is esterified by treatment with cyclopentanepropionyl chloride in the presence of pyridine.

Description—White to practically white, crystalline powder; odorless or has a slight odor.

Solubility—Insoluble in water; slightly soluble in ether; soluble in alcohol; very soluble in chloroform.

Uses—Actions and systemic uses of *Hydrocortisone,* to which it is converted in the body. Because of its low solubility, its absorption from the gastrointestinal tract is slower than that of hydrocortisone; also, its taste is more pleasant than that of hydrocortisone, so that it is used for oral therapy.

Dose—*Oral, adult,* the equivalent of **20** to **240 mg** of hydrocortisone daily, as a single dose or in divided doses; *children,* for *replacement,* the equivalent of **0.56 mg/kg** (or 15 to 20 mg/m^2) of hydrocortisone a day, or, for *anti-inflammatory* use, the equivalent of **2** to **8 mg/kg** (or 60 to 240 mg) a day.

Dosage Form—Oral Suspension: the equivalent of 10 mg of hydrocortisone/5 mL.

Hydrocortisone Sodium Phosphate

(11β)-Pregn-4-ene-3,20-dione, 11,17-dihydroxy-21-(phosphonooxy)-, disodium salt; Cortisol Sodium Phosphate; Hydrocortone Phosphate (*MSD*); Corphos (*Cooper*)

Cortisol 21-(disodium phosphate) [6000-74-4] $C_{21}H_{29}Na_2O_8P$ (486.41).

For the structure of the parent, see *Hydrocortisone.*

Preparation—From hydrocortisone by a method similar to that used for *Dexamethasone Sodium Phosphate.* US Pat 2,870,177.

Description—White to light-yellow, odorless or practically odorless, bitter-tasting powder; relatively stable in light and heat and very hygroscopic; pH (1% solution) 7.5 to 8.5.

Solubility—1 g in about 1.5 mL water; slightly soluble in alcohol; practically insoluble in chloroform, dioxane or ether.

Uses—Actions and uses of *Hydrocortisone,* to which it is converted in the body. However, the phosphate is quite soluble and hence has special usefulness as a parenteral form of cortisol in emergency situations in which a rapid response is essential or when oral medication cannot be tolerated.

Dose (hydrocortisone equivalents)—*Intramuscular, intravenous,* or *subcutaneous, adult,* **15** to **240 mg** a day in 2 or 3 divided doses until the condition responds, after which the dosage is gradually decreased; in *acute adrenal insufficiency,* **100 mg** is given *intravenously* followed by **100 mg** every 8 hr until the patient is out of danger. *Intramuscular, children,* for *replacement,* **186** to **280 μg**/kg or **10** to **12 mg/m²** a day in 3 divided doses; for *disease,* **660 μg** to **4 mg/kg** or **20** to **120 mg/m²** every 12 to 24 hr. *Intravenous,* for *acute adrenal insufficiency, infants,* **1** to **2 mg/kg** followed by **25** to **150 μg/kg**/day and *older children,* **1** to **2 mg/kg** followed by **150** to **250 μg/kg**/day in divided doses.

Dosage Form—Injection: the equivalent of 50 mg of hydrocortisone/mL.

Hydrocortisone Sodium Succinate

(11β)-Pregn-4-ene-3,20-dione, 21-(3-carboxy-1-oxopropoxy)-11,17- dihydroxy-, monosodium salt, A-hydroCort (*Abbott*); SoluCortef (*Upjohn*)

Cortisol 21-(sodium succinate) [125-04-2] $C_{25}H_{33}NaO_8$ (484.52).

Preparation—Hydroxycortisone 21-(hydrogen succinate) is first prepared by reacting hydrocortisone with succinic anhydride dissolved in pyridine. When the reaction is complete, the mixture is added to cold, dilute HCl whereupon the acid ester precipitates. It is collected, washed with water, dried and purified by recrystallizing from acetone. The sodium salt is then prepared by neutralizing the acid with dilute NaOH solution followed by drying the solution from the frozen state.

Description—White or nearly white, odorless, hygroscopic, amorphous solid.

Solubility—Very soluble in water or alcohol; insoluble in chloroform; very slightly soluble in acetone.

Uses—Actions and uses of *Hydrocortisone,* to which it is converted in the body. However the sodium succinate derivative is highly soluble and hence is a desirable form for infusion concentrates and for intravenous or intramuscular administration when intense rapid action is desired. It is intended only for systemic short-term emergency therapy.

Dose—*Intramuscular* or *intravenous, initially* **100** to **500 mg** and may be repeated at 2-, 4- or 6-hr intervals depending on patient response and clinical condition.

Dosage Form—For Injection: the equivalent of 100, 250 and 500 mg and 1 g of hydrocortisone.

Methylprednisolone

(6α,11β)-Pregna-1,4-diene-3,20-dione, 11,17,21-trihydroxy-6-methyl-, Medrol (*Upjohn*); Meprolone (*Major*)

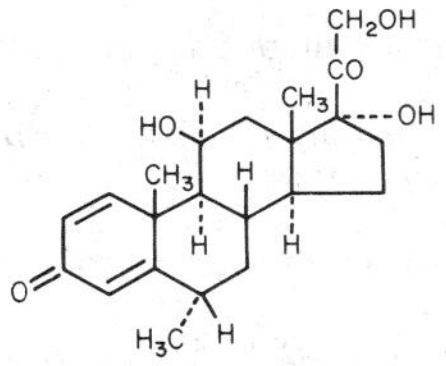

[83-43-2] $C_{22}H_{30}O_5$ (374.48).

Preparation—*Progesterone* (page 1097) is converted to the 6α-methyl derivative in the same manner as indicated in the synthesis of *Medroxyprogesterone Acetate* (page 1095). Incubation of the 6α-methyl compound with an Ascomycete, such as *Pestalotia,* forms the 11α-hydroxy derivative which is oxidized to the 3,11-diketo compound with chromic acid. Further treatment with ethyl oxalate followed by bromination, rearrangement with sodium methoxide and debromination with zinc dust gives the methyl ester of the 4,17(20)-diene-21-carboxylate. With pyrrolidine, lithium aluminum hydride reduction and treatment with alkali, the 11β,21-dihydroxy-4,17(20)-diene is formed which is converted to the 21-acetate and then oxidatively hydroxylated to 6α-methylhydrocortisone acetate. Saponification, followed by dehydrogenation with *Septomyxa affinis* gives the 1,4,17(20)-triene, which is again converted to the 21-acetate, oxidatively hydroxylated to yield the 17α-hydroxy derivative and saponified to give methylprednisolone.

Description—White to practically white, odorless, crystalline powder; melts about 240° with some decomposition.

Solubility—1 g in 10,000 mL water, 100 mL alcohol, 800 mL chloroform or 800 mL ether.

Uses—A glucocorticoid with actions, uses and side effects typical of drugs of this class (see the introduction to this section). It induces considerably less retention of sodium and water than the parent prednisolone. Because it possesses only weak mineralocorticoid activity, it is not employed in the management of acute adrenal insufficiency. The plasma half-life is 3 to 4 hr and the biological half-life is 18 to 36 hr. The volume of distribution is 0.7 L/kg. The drug does not bind to transcortin.

Dose—*Oral, adult,* **4** to **48 mg** a day; *children,* for *replacement,* **117 μg/kg** (or **3.3 mg/m²**) a day; for *disease,* **417** μg to **1.67 mg/kg** (or **12.5** to **50 mg/m²**) a day in 3 or 4 divided doses.

Dosage Form—Tablets: 2, 4, 8, 16, 24 and 32 mg.

Methylprednisolone Acetate

(6α,11β)-Pregna-1,4-diene-3,20-dione, 21-(acetyloxy)-11,17-dihydroxy-6-methyl-, Medralone (*Keene*); Medrone (*Kay*); Depo-Medrol and Medrol Acetate; (*Upjohn*)

Methylprednisolone 21-acetate [53-36-1] $C_{24}H_{32}O_6$ (416.51).

For the structure of the parent, see *Methylprednisolone.*

Preparation—The 21-acetate compound obtained in the synthesis of *Methylprednisolone,* just prior to the final saponification.

Description—White or practically white, odorless, crystalline powder; melts at about 225° with some decomposition.

Solubility—1 g in 1500 mL water, 400 mL alcohol, 250 mL chloroform or 1500 mL ether.

Uses—Converted in the body to *Methylprednisolone,* over which it has no advantage in systemic therapy; thus, the acetate is employed principally for local therapy. As a suspension it may be given intra-articularly or topically. Topical uses and adverse effects are discussed in the introduction to this section. It is combined with neomycin in some topical preparations.

Dose—*Intramuscular, adult, initially* **40** to **120 mg** repeated at 1-day to 2-wk intervals, if necessary; *children,* for *replacement,* **117 μg/kg** (or **3.33 mg/m²**) in 3 divided doses in one day, repeated every 3rd day, *or* **39** to **58 μg/kg** (or **1.11** to **1.66 mg/m²**) once a day; for *disease,* **139** to **835 μg/kg** (or **4.16** to **25 mg/m²** every 12 to 24 hr. *Intra-articular, intralesional* or into *soft tissue, adult,* **4** to **80 mg,** repeated at 1- to 5-wk intervals if necessary. *Topical,* as **0.25%** or **1%** ointment, applied 1 to 4 times a day on *adults* and 1 or 2 times a day on *children. Rectal, adult,* **40 mg** as retention enema 3 to 7 times a week for 2 or more weeks; *children,* **500 μg** to **1 mg/kg** (or **15** to **30 mg/m²**) every 1 or 2 days for 2 or more weeks.

Dosage Forms—for Enema: 40 mg; Ointment: 0.25 and 1%; Sterile Suspension: 20, 40 mg/1 mL, 100, 200 and 400 mg/5 mL, and 200 and 400 mg/10 mL.

Methylprednisolone Sodium Succinate

Pregna-1,4-diene-3,20-dione, 21-(3-carboxy-1-oxopropoxy)-11,17-dihydroxy-6-methyl-, monosodium salt, (6α,11β)-, Solu-Medrol (*Upjohn*); A-methaPred (*Abbott*)

Methylprednisolone 21-(Sodium Succinate); [2375-03-3] $C_{26}H_{33}NaO_8$ (496.53).

For the structure of the parent, see *Methylprednisolone.*

Preparation—*Methylprednisolone* is treated with succinic anhydride in pyridine and added to dilute HCl to precipitate the hemisuccinate which is neutralized with NaOH in aqueous acetone solution and the solvent removed by lyophilization.

Description—White, or nearly white, odorless, hygroscopic, amorphous solid.

Solubility—1 g in 1.5 mL water, 12 mL alcohol or >10,000 mL chloroform or ether.

Uses—Actions of *Methylprednisolone,* to which it is converted in the body; for actions, uses and adverse effects of glucocorticoids see the introduction to this section. The solubility of this drug makes its use advantageous for parenteral and intra-articular administration when rapid and intense action is desired. It is used systemically only for short-term treatment.

Dose (methylprednisolone equivalent)—*Intravenous* or *intramuscular, adult,* **10** to **40 mg** as needed, except **5 mg/kg** as a *bolus* every 4 hr in *shock. Intramuscular, children,* for *replacement* and *disease* therapy, see *Methylprednisolone Acetate. Intra-articular* or *intralesional,* **4** to **80 mg,** as needed.

Dosage Form—For Injection: 40, 125 and 500 mg, and 1 and 2 g (methylprednisolone equivalent).

Prednisolone

(11β)-Pregna-1,4-diene-3,20-dione, 11,17,21-trihydroxy-, (*Various Mfrs*)

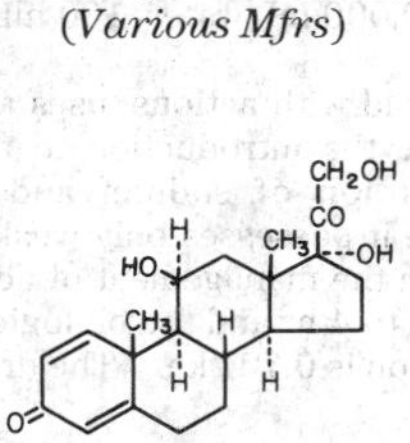

[50-24-8] $C_{21}H_{28}O_5$ (360.45); *sesquihydrate* [52438-85-4] (387.47); anhydrous or contains one and one-half molecules of water of hydration.

Preparation—From hydrocortisone by a microbiological process using *Corynebacterium simplex* which selectively dehydrogenates cortisol at the 1 and 2 positions.

Description—White to practically white, odorless, crystalline powder; melts about 235° with some decomposition.

Solubility—1 g in 30 mL alcohol or 180 mL chloroform; very slightly soluble in water.

Uses—A glucocorticoid with the actions, uses and side effects typical of drugs of this class (see the introduction to this section). It is 4 times as potent as, but relatively somewhat weaker than, hydrocortisone as a mineralocorticoid although sodium retention and potassium depletion can occur. The plasma half-life is said to be about 3 hr and the biological half-life is 18 to 36 hr. However, the pharmacokinetics are dose-dependent because of nonlinear protein binding. With high doses the plasma half-life may approach 1.7 hr. Except for its higher solubility, it may be considered equivalent to prednisone; it is the biologically active metabolite of prednisone.

Dose—*Oral, adult, initially* usually **5** to **60 mg** but may be as high as **250 mg** a day until a response occurs, when the dose gradually is diminished to the smallest effective maintenance dose; *children,* for *replacement,* **140 μg/kg** (or **4 mg/m²**) a day in 3 divided doses, or, for *disease,* **500 μg** to **2 mg/kg** (or **15** to **60 mg/m²**) a day in 3 or 4 divided doses.

Dosage Forms—Syrup: 15 mg/5 mL; Tablets: 5 mg.

Prednisolone Acetate

(11β)-Pregna-1,4-diene-3,20-dione, 21-(acetyloxy)-11, 17-dihydroxy-, (*Various Mfrs*)

Prednisolone 21-Acetate[52-21-1] $C_{23}H_{30}O_6$ (402.49).

Preparation—From *Prednisolone* by reaction with acetic anhydride.

Description—White to practically white, odorless, crystalline powder; melts about 235° with some decomposition.

Solubility—1 g in 120 mL alcohol; practically insoluble in water; slightly soluble in chloroform or acetone.

Uses—Actions and uses of *Prednisolone,* to which it is converted in the body. The acetate is relatively nonirritating to the tissues and hence is suitable for intramuscular or local injection; esterification also prolongs absorption. It may be used particularly in those situations in which oral prednisolone is not feasible, but there are no contraindications to substitution of the parenteral acetate for oral prednisolone for any purpose. It is used in combination with prednisolone sodium phosphate; because of its low solubility, it confers a sustained action upon the mixture.

Dose—*Intramuscular, adult, initially* **4** to **60 mg** a day in 4 divided doses until a satisfactory response occurs, then a gradual reduction to a minimal *maintenance* dose, which usually is in the range of **5** to **20 mg** a day; *multiple sclerosis, initially* **200 mg** a day for 1 wk, then **80 mg** every other day (or switch to dexamethasone) for 1 mo; *children,* for *replacement,* **140 μg/kg** (or **4 mg/m²**) every 3rd day or **46** to **70 μg/kg** (or **1.33** to **2 mg/m²**) once a day; for *disease,* **166 μg** to **1 mg/kg** (or **5** to **30 mg/m²**) every 12 to 24 hr. *Intra-articular, intralesional* or *soft-tissue injection,* **4** to **100 mg** as needed. *Topical,* to the *eyes,* **1** or **2 drops** of a **0.12** to **1%** ophthalmic suspension; to the *skin,* as **0.5%** ointment (containing 0.5% neomycin).

Dosage Forms—Ointment: 0.6% (with 0.3% gentamicin); Ophthalmic Suspension: 0.12, 0.125, 0.5 (in combination with neomycin and polymyxin B), and 1%; Sterile Suspension: 250, 500 and 1000 mg/10 mL and 750 mg/30 mL.

Prednisolone Sodium Phosphate

11β-Pregna-1,4-diene-3,20-dione, 11,17-dihydroxy-21-(phosphonooxy)-, disodium salt; (*Various Mfrs*)

Prednisolone 21-(Disodium Phosphate); [125-02-0] $C_{21}H_{27}Na_2O_8P$ (484.39).

Preparation—From *Prednisolone* by a method similar to that used for *Dexamethasone Sodium Phosphate.*

Description—White or slightly yellow, friable granules or powder; odorless or has a slight odor; slightly hygroscopic.

Solubility—1 g in 4 mL water or 13 mL methanol; slightly soluble in alcohol or chloroform; very slightly soluble in acetone or dioxane.

Uses—A soluble form of *Prednisolone,* to which it is converted in the body. It is employed parenterally in emergency situations in which an intense glucocorticoid action is required. Since absorption by the intramuscular route is quite rapid, the intravenous route is employed infrequently. The high solubility of the drug also lends itself well to intrasynovial injection in the treatment of arthritides and bursitides and to local injection for inflammatory cysts and soft-tissue inflammations; it is often combined with prednisolone acetate in these uses. It also is employed in the local treatment of a number of inflammatory eye diseases and for inflammatory and pruritic dermatoses, bites and burns.

Dose (prednisolone phosphate equivalents)—*Intravenous* or *intramuscular, adult,* **4** to **60 mg** a day. *Intramuscular, children,* for *replacement,* **140 μg/kg** (or **4 mg/m²**) in 1 day in 3 divided doses every 3rd day, *or* **46** to **70 μg/kg** (or **1.33** to **2 mg/m²**) per day; for *disease,* **166 μg/kg** to **1 mg** (or **5** to **30 mg/m²**) every 12 to 24 hr. *Intra-articular, intralesional* or *soft-tissue injection,* **2** to **30 mg** every 3 to 5 days to 2 to 3 wk. *Oral, adult,* **5** to **60 mg** a day. *Topical,* to the *conjunctiva,* **1** or **2 drops** of **0.113** to **0.9%** ophthalmic solution 4 to 6 times a day: to the *ear* canal **3** or **4 drops** of a **0.5%** solution 2 or 3 times a day.

Dosage Forms (prednisolone phosphate equivalent)—Injection: 40 mg/2 mL, 100 mg/5 mL and 200 mg/10 mL; Ophthalmic Solution: 0.125, and 1%; Ophthalmic/Otic Solution: 0.5%; Oral Solution: 5 mg/5 mL.

Prednisolone Tebutate

(11β)-Pregna-1,4-diene-3,20-dione, 11,17-dihydroxy-21-[(3,3-dimethyl-1- oxobutyl)oxy]-, Hydeltra T.B.A. (*MSD*); Prednalone T.B.A. (*Forest*)

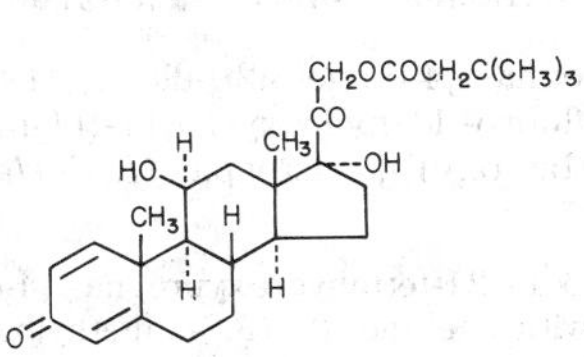

Prednisolone *tert*-butylacetate; [7681-14-3] $C_{27}H_{38}O_6$ (458.59); *monohydrate* (476.61).

Preparation—From *Prednisolone* by esterification of the 21-hydroxyl group with 3,3-dimethylbutyryl chloride.

Description—White to slightly yellow powder; odorless or has not more than a moderate, characteristic odor; melts between 240 and 250°.

Solubility—Very slightly soluble in water; freely soluble in chloroform; soluble in acetone; sparingly soluble in alcohol.

Uses—Converted in the body to *Prednisolone.* At present, its use is confined to local injection into inflamed joints, tendons and bursae, or into soft-tissue lesions. Its low solubility results in a repository action, with an onset of action of 1 to 2 days and a duration of 2 to 3 wk. Temporary local discomfort may follow injection.

Dose—*Intra-articular, intralesional* or *soft-tissue injection,* **4** to **40 mg** once every 2 or 3 wk.

Dosage Form—Sterile Suspension: 20 mg/1 mL, 100 mg/5 mL and 200 mg/10 mL.

Prednisone

Pregna-1,4-diene-3,11,20-trione, 17,21-dihydroxy-, (*Various Mfrs*)

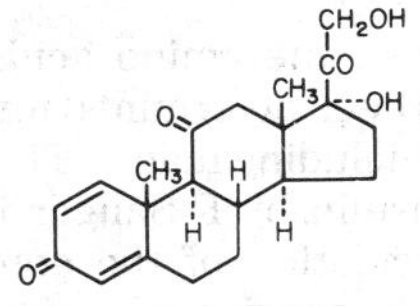

[53-03-2] $C_{21}H_{26}O_5$ (358.43).

Preparation—As described for *Prednisolone* except that cortisone is used instead of hydrocortisone.

Description—White to practically white, odorless, crystalline powder; melts about 230°, with some decomposition.

Solubility—1 g in 150 mL alcohol or 200 mL chloroform; very slightly soluble in water.

Uses—A dehydrogenated derivative of cortisone with actions, uses and side effects typical of glucocorticoids (see the introduction to this section). The active form of the drug is its metabolite, prednisolone. It has 3 to 5 times the glucocorticoid activity of hydrocortisone but somewhat less of mineralocorticoid activity, although sodium retention and potassium depletion may occur. It cannot be used alone for replacement therapy in adrenal insufficiency. It is the glucocorticoid predominantly used in *cancer chemotherapy,* always in combination with other drugs. In pediatrics it is used widely to treat *nephrosis, rheumatic carditis, leukemias, other tumors* and *tuberculosis.* The plasma half-life is 3 to 5 hr, but the biological half-life is 12 to 36 hr.

Dose—*Oral, adult, initially* usually **5** to **60 mg** a day but may be as high as **250 mg** a day until a satisfactory response occurs, when the dose is gradually diminished to the smallest effective *maintenance* dose, usually **10** to **20 mg** a day; *children,* **35** to **500 μg/kg** (or **1** to **15 mg/m²**) 4 times a day. However, dose regimens vary greatly with the use; for the details, see the *USP DI, AMA Drug Evaluations, Physicians Desk Reference* or the package literature.

Dosage Forms—Oral Solution: 5 mg/5 mL and 5 mg/mL (oral concentrate); Tablets: 1, 2.5, 5, 10, 20, 25 and 50 mg.

Triamcinolone

(11β,16α)-Pregna-1,4-diene-3,20-dione, 9-fluoro-11,16,17, 21-tetrahydroxy-, Aristocort (*Lederle*); Kenacort (*Squibb*)

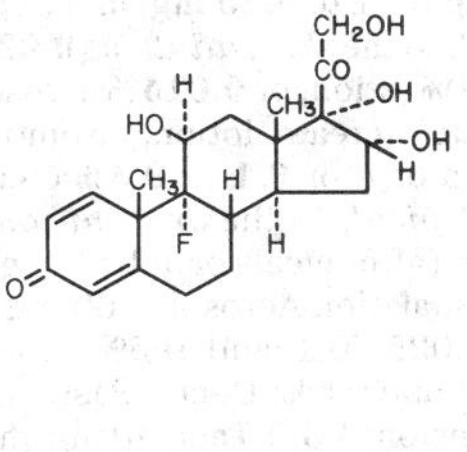

[124-94-7] $C_{21}H_{27}FO_6$ (394.44).

Preparation—From hydrocortisone acetate via the 3,20-bisketal by treatment with thionyl chloride, refluxing with potassium hydroxide and acetylation to give 21-acetoxy-4,9,11(16)-pregnatriene-3,20-dione. Oxidation with osmium tetroxide to the 16α,17α-dihydroxy derivative and subsequent insertion of the 9α-fluoro and 11β-hydroxy groups as indicated for *Betamethasone* (page 1069), gives a product lacking only a double bond at the 1-position. This latter step is accomplished by incubation with *Nocardia corallina,* followed by saponification of the acetate to yield triamcinolone. Alternatively, the compound can be made from *Fludrocortisone* by enzymatically inserting the 16α-hydroxyl group and dehydrogenating as above at the 1,2-position.

Description—Fine, white or practically white, crystalline powder having not more than a slight odor; its polymorphic forms and/or solvates melt between 248 and 250°, 260° and 263° or 269° and 271°.

Solubility—1 g in about 5000 mL water, 70 mL propylene glycol or less than 20 mL dimethyl sulfoxide; slightly soluble in alcohol or chloroform.

Uses—A glucocorticoid with actions, uses and side effects typical of drugs of this class (see the introduction to this section). It is 7 to 13 times more potent than hydrocortisone. It has been claimed that therapeutic doses of this drug are nearly devoid of mineralocorticoid and other side effects of hydrocortisone but the mineralocorticoid actions vary from patient to patient. It appears that the drug may induce naturesis, negative sodium balance with weight loss in most patients (along with headache, dizziness and fatigue) and sodium retention with weight gain, moon face, etc in others. Nearly every side effect seen with hydrocortisone has been observed with this drug, but the relative frequencies are less; however, it does not increase appetite and thus differs from other glucocorticoids. By the oral route, more of it survives the first pass through the liver than does hydrocortisone, and blood levels are somewhat more predictable. The plasma half-life is about 5 hr and the biological half-life is 18 to 36 hr. The volume of distribution is 1.4 to 2.1 L/kg, depending upon the dose.

Dose—*Oral, adult,* in *adrenal insufficiency,* **4** to **12 mg** a day in single or divided doses (along with a mineralocorticoid); in *disease,* **4** to **60 mg** a day. *Children,* in *adrenal insufficiency,* **117 μg/kg** (or **3.3 mg/m²**) a day; in *disease,* **416 μg** to **1.7 mg/kg** (or **12.5** to **50 mg/m²**) a day.

Dosage Form—Tablets: 1, 2, 4 and 8 mg.

Triamcinolone Acetonide

(11β,16α)-Pregna-1,4-diene-3,20-dione, 9-fluoro-11,21-dihydroxy-16,17- [(1-methylethylidene)bis(oxy)]-, (*Various Mfrs*)

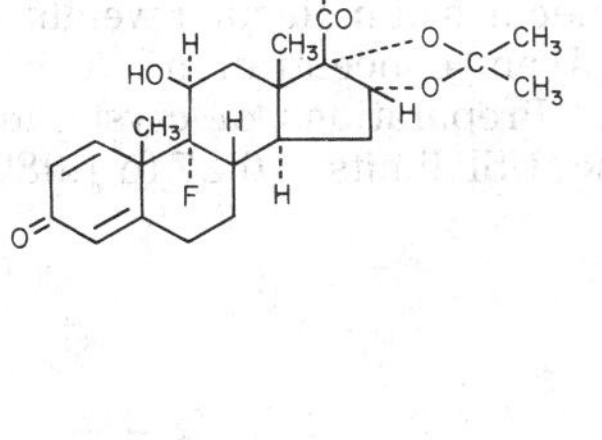

Triamcinolone 16,17-cyclic acetal with acetone; [76-25-5] $C_{24}H_{31}FO_6$ (434.50).

Preparation—*Triamcinolone* is treated with acetone and perchloric acid followed by neutralization and vacuum concentration.

Description—White to cream-colored, crystalline powder having not more than a slight odor; melts between 290 and 294°.

Solubility—Practically insoluble in water; very soluble in dehydrated alcohol, chloroform or methanol; sparingly soluble in acetone or ethyl acetate; slightly soluble in alcohol.

Uses—A high-potency glucocorticoid with the actions, uses and side effects typical of that class of drugs (see the introduction to this section). It has a higher lipid-water distribution coefficient than triamcinolone and is thus more suitable for topical use.

Dose—*Inhalation,* **2 inhalations (200 μg**) 3 or 4 times a day; *children 6 to 12 yr,* **1 or 2 inhalations** (100 to 200 μg) 3 or 4 times a day. *Intraarticular, intrabursal* or into the *tendon sheath, adults* and *children,* **2.5** to **15 mg** at weekly intervals or more frequently. *Intradermal* or *intralesional, adults,* up to **1 mg** at intervals up to 1 wk. *Intramuscular,* **40** to **80 mg,** repeated at 4-wk intervals, in *adults,* and **40 mg** or **30** to **200 μg/kg** (or **1** to **6.25 mg/m²**), repeated at 7-day intervals, in *children. Topical,* to the *skin, adult,* as **0.025, 0.1,** or **0.5%** cream or ointment, **0.025** or **0.1%** lotion, or **0.015%** aerosol solution, 2 to 4 times a day; *children,* as **0.025%** cream, lotion, or ointment, or **0.015%** aerosol solution 1 or 2 times a day, or **0.1** or **0.5%** cream or ointment or **0.1%** lotion once a day. *Topical,* to the *oral mucous membranes,* as **0.1%** paste 1 to 3 times a day (after meals or at bedtime).

Dosage Forms—Inhalation Aerosol: 60 mg (each actuation delivers 100 μg); Cream: 0.025, 0.1 and 0.5%; Lotion: 0.025 and 0.1%; Ointment: 0.025, 0.1 and 0.5%; Dental Paste: 0.1%; Aerosol Solution: 0.015%; Sterile Suspension: 3, 10 and 40 mg/mL.

Triamcinolone Diacetate

(11β,16α)-Pregna-1,4-diene-3,20-dione, 16,21-bis(acetyloxy)-9-fluoro-11,17- dihydroxy-, (*Various Mfrs*)

Triamcinolone 16,21-Diacetate; [67-78-7] $C_{25}H_{31}FO_8$ (478.51).

For the structure of the parent, see *Triamcinolone.*

Preparation—By direct acetylation of triamcinolone. Among other ways, it has also been prepared from 11β,16α,17,21-tetrahydroxypregn-4-en-3,20-dione (16α-hydroxycortisone) through the following sequence of reactions: (a) microbiological oxidation with *Nocardia corallina* or *Corynebacterium simplex* to the pregna-1,4-diene analog, (b) acetylation yielding the 16α,21-diacetate, (c) selective dehydration involving the 11-hydroxy with thionyl chloride to form the 1,4,9(11)-pregnatriene compound, (d) addition of hypobromous acid to the 9,11-double bond followed by treatment with potassium acetate in ethanol to form the 9,11-epoxy compound, and (e) rupturing of the epoxy ring with hydrogen fluoride to introduce the 9α-fluorine.

Description—Fine, white or slightly off-white crystals that have not more than a slight odor and a slight, bitter taste; prolonged heating above 100° will convert the hydrate to the anhydrous form.

Solubility—1 g in 13 mL alcohol or 80 mL chloroform; practically insoluble in water; slightly soluble in ether.

Uses—Actions and uses identical to *Triamcinolone.* However, its slight solubility is such that on injection it has reasonably prompt onset of action yet a duration of action longer than that of more soluble preparations. It also has a more agreeable taste than triamcinolone and can thus be given in liquid oral preparations.

Dose (triamcinolone equivalent)—*Intra-articular, intrasynovial intralesional* or into *soft tissue, adult,* **5** to **48 mg.** *Intramuscular, adult* and *children* over *6 yr,* **40 mg** once a week. *Oral, adult,* for *replacement,* **4** to **12 mg** per day (along with a mineralocorticoid) and, for *anti-inflammatory* use, **8** to **48 mg** a day; *children,* for *replacement,* **117 μg/kg** (or **3.3 mg/m²**) a day (with a mineralocorticoid) and, for *anti-inflammatory* use, **416 μg** to **1.7 mg/kg** (or **12.5** to **50 mg/m²**) a day.

Dosage Forms—Sterile Suspension: 40 mg/1 mL and 125 and 200 mg/5 mL; Syrup: 2 and 4 mg/5 mL.

Triamcinolone Hexacetonide

(11β,16α)-,Pregna-1,4-diene-3,20-dione, 21-(3,3-dimethyl-1-oxobutoxy)-9-fluoro- 11-hydroxy-16,17-[(1-methylethylidene) bis(oxy)]-, Aristospan (*Lederle*)

9-Fluoro-11β,16α,17,21-tetrahydroxypregna-1,4-diene-3,20- dione cyclic 16,17-acetal with acetone, 21-(3,3-dimethylbutyrate) [5611-51-8] $C_{30}H_{41}FO_7$ (532.65).

For the structure of the parent, see *Triamcinolone.*

Preparation—*Triamcinolone Acetonide* is 21-esterified by reaction with 3,3-dimethylbutyryl chloride in the presence of pyridine.

Description—White to cream-colored, crystalline powder; odorless and tasteless to slightly bitter tasting; relatively stable to light, heat and air; decomposes at about 295°; no polymorphs have been reported.

Solubility—1 g in 167 mL methanol or less than 20 mL chloroform; practically insoluble in water.

Uses—Gradually converted to *Triamcinolone* in the body and hence has the same potential actions, uses and side effects. At present, it is used only for injection into inflamed joints and soft- tissue lesions. It is quite insoluble and hence has a repository action.

Dose—*Intra-articular* or *intrasynovial, adult,* **2** to **20 mg,** repeated at 3- or 4-wk intervals, if necessary. *Intralesional* or *sublesional, adult,* up to **0.5 mg/in²** of diseased skin.

Dosage Forms—Sterile Suspension: 20 mg/1 mL and 25 and 100 mg/5 mL.

The Pancreatic Hormones

The larger portion of the pancreas consists of glandular tissue which secretes digestive enzymes, but there also are isolated groups of cells, called *Islets of Langerhans,* the beta cells of which produce a hormone known as *insulin* and the alpha cells, one known as *glucagon.*

Insulin—

Chemistry—Insulin is obtained by extraction of beef, sheep, swine or whale pancreas; human insulin now is produced by chemical conversion from porcine insulin and by *E coli* into which the human genes for insulin have been inserted. The recombinant product has the same physiological properties as insulin from beef or pork but is much less likely to cause allergic reactions and refractoriness. Insulin was one of the first proteins obtained in crystalline form. Insulin (monomer) is a polypeptide of molecular weight 6000; it consists of two peptide chains containing 21 and 30 amino acids, respectively, the two chains being held together by disulfide (—S—S—) bonds of cystine.

In aqueous solution, the insulin monomer polymerizes to form macromolecules of molecular weight 12,000 or 36,000, depending on pH and concentration. The isoelectric point of insulin is 5.3. Preparations of crystalline insulin contain about 0.5% zinc (USP limits: 0.27 to 1.08%), the function of which is unknown. The potency of crystalline insulin, calculated on the anhydrous basis, is not less than 26 USP Insulin Units in each mg.

The arrangement of the amino acids in each of the two chains of insulin has been determined for insulins from several species of animals, including man. The determination of the structure of beef insulin by F Sanger in 1954 was the first example of the elucidation of the complete structure of a protein. Although the species differences are relatively small, involving mainly substitutions among amino acids 8–10 of the shorter (A) chain, antibodies to insulin can be prepared in some animals.

Successful syntheses of both chains of bovine insulin has been achieved.

In patients with insuloma, an insulin of molecular weight 100,000 can be found in the plasma. It is much larger than proinsulin, and it probably is a form of preproinsulin.

Physiology and Actions—Insulin is the hormone which facilitates the uptake of glucose into all cells. It also decreases hepatic gluconeogenesis and increases glycogenesis. When the supply of or response to insulin is inadequate, a disease known as *diabetes mellitus* occurs (see page 681). In this disorder, glucose accumulates rapidly in the body fluids, and as the blood glucose concentration increases beyond a certain point it is excreted by the kidneys. The amount of sugar in the urine is a rough index of the severity of the diabetes and may be used to approximate the amount of insulin necessary for treatment. Diabetic acidosis requires larger doses of insulin than does simple hyperglycemia. When there is diabetic coma, heroic doses are required. Although attention focuses on the intervention of insulin in glucose metabolism, it also has independent actions to stimulate lipogenesis and promote the synthesis of many proteins but suppress the synthesis of some.

Diabetes mellitus is classified as insulin-dependent diabetes mellitus (IDDM, Type I); noninsulin-dependent diabetes mellitus (NIDDM, Type II); diabetes mellitus associated with other conditions (eg, pancreatic disease, hormonal imbalances, drugs), formerly known as secondary diabetes, or gestational diabetes (impaired glucose tolerance during pregnancy).

Once IDDM was termed juvenile-onset diabetes (because the age of onset is predominantly before adulthood) or ketosis-prone diabetes. Patients with IDDM require insulin to prevent ketosis and to sustain life. Islet cell antibodies and autoantibodies against endogenous insulin commonly occur early in the disease. The onset of this type of diabetes occasionally follows viral infection. A strong, positive correlation exists between IDDM and the presence of HLA antigens DR3 and/or DR4.

The condition, NIDDM, previously was identified as maturity-onset diabetes (MOD), adult-onset or ketosis-resistant diabetes. It is further subdivided into nonobese and obese types; the latter is more common (incidence, approximately 80% of NIDDM patients). Although insulin may be necessary to control hypoglycemia, patients with NIDDM are not prone to ketosis and have either relatively low insulin levels or normal to high insulin levels associated with peripheral tissue resistance to the hormone. With NIDDM, antagonism to insulin occurs at a postreceptor site. Hepatic glucose output is elevated because of insulin insensitivity, and insulin secretion in response to appropriate stimuli is impaired. Diet therapy and exercise alone, or in conjugation with oral hypoglycemic agents or insulin, are appropriate to treat this form of diabetes.

When there is an excess of insulin, serious or dangerous symptoms from hypoglycemia may result. There may be sweating, hunger, incoherence, tachycardia and palpitations, convulsions, coma and death. Glucose administration relieves the symptoms of overdosage, and the diabetic patient often carries some source of glucose to alleviate hypoglycemia. Glucagon may be administered when hypoglycemia is severe.

Insulin binds to the α-subunit of the insulin receptors. This evokes tyrosine kinase activity in the β-subunit and autophosphorylation of the receptor and also the translocation of glucose transporters to the plasma membrane. Phosphatidylinositol system coupling also occurs; inositol phosphates mediate recruitment of intracellular calcium and inositol phosphate glycans and diacylglycerol mediate the activation of receptor-contained threonine and serine kinases and gene transcription. Furthermore, phosphodiesterase activity is increased, which decreases cAMP, and guanylate cyclase activity is increased. Inward potassium and magnesium transports are stimulated. Intracellular enzyme activities are altered variously by phoshorylation, dephosphorylation and changes in protein synthesis. Overall, protein, lipid and DNA syntheses are increased and cell growth is promoted. Down-regulation of the insulin receptors begins within minutes of receptor activation and becomes maximal within a few hours.

Insulin is absorbed rapidly and exerts its maximum action within three hours. The plasma half-life is only 9 minutes. In severe diabetes, injections must be spaced throughout the day, usually being given before meals. During the night, when no insulin is available, the blood sugar rises and is usually at its highest point before the morning dose. This erratic behavior on the level of blood sugar can be controlled more adequately by the use of insoluble insulins, which are absorbed more slowly and thus can exert a continuous even action over a period as long as 24 hours (see below). Continuous infusion pumps for insulin also are available. Pumps that deliver insulin on demand are in development, as are other delivery systems. Sustained blood levels have the disadvantage of suppressing glucagon-mediated homeostasis, thus favoring prolonged hypoglycemic episodes and encephalopathy.

Insulin is degraded locally, so that sometimes subcutaneous insulin has a low efficacy.

Preparations—

Crystalline Zinc Insulin—By addition of appropriate amounts of zinc salts, insulin may be crystallized. This achieves a superior degree of purification, which is of advantage when treating diabetics who demonstrate an allergic sensitivity to Insulin Injection, the earlier and more commonly used, but less highly purified, type. The speed and duration of action of the zinc insulins depends on the crystal size. The microcrystalline form (regular insulin or crystalline zinc insulin) dissolves promptly and hence, by the intramuscular route, has an onset of action of 0.5 to 1 hour and duration of 5 to 7 hours, and duration of action (8 hours) nearly the same as that of zinc-free insulin (prompt zinc insulin or semilente insulin; duration 6 hours), and they may be used interchangeably. Either form meets USP standards. The Reference Standard of the USP consists of dried Zinc-Insulin Crystals and is defined as containing 22 USP Units/mg. Zinc insulins of larger crystals size have slow-release properties that depend on crystal size. Thus Prompt Insulin Zinc Suspension, Insulin Zinc Suspension (Lente) and Extended Insulin Zinc Suspension, with durations of action of 14, 24 and 36 hours, respectively, represent increasing crystal sizes.

Insoluble Insulins—Insulin or zinc insulin may be combined with globin or protamine to yield complexes of larger molecular weight, and the complexes may be mixed in various proportions. The isoelectric point of globin zinc insulin, isophane insulin or protamine zinc insulin is near pH 7.3. This means that at the pH of body fluids they are very insoluble. Crystalline zinc insulin has a higher solubility than the protein complexes but goes into solution at a very slow rate. Protamine zinc insulin (PZI) is injected as a suspension. It goes into solution only slowly and this limits the rate of absorption. It has a duration of action of about 36 hours. By the use of protamine zinc insulin the number of injections required to control the level of blood sugar often can be reduced to one a day. What is more important, wide fluctuations in the level of blood sugar are less likely to occur. In certain cases combinations of protamine zinc insulin and regular insulin may be employed.

Distinguishing Characteristics—FDA regulations require that the labels of various insulin preparations shall have distinctive colors.

The onsets and durations of action, purity and animal sources of the various commercial products vary, even among those of supposedly identical constitution. For details of the differences, see *AMA Drug Evaluations* (Annual), Chap 48, Table 2, 941–942, 1992.

Proinsulin—This is the single-chain protein precursor of insulin. The removal of the C-peptide moiety leaves insulin. When administered exogenously, its metabolic effects differ somewhat from those of insulin in that it mostly suppresses hepatic glucose output and has only a slight action to stimulate peripheral glucose uptake. Therefore, it has a much lesser probability of causing severe hypoglycemia. The locus of action especially lends itself to the treatment of *noninsulin-dependent diabetes mellitus*. The pharmacokinetics permit once-a-day dosage. A recombinant human product is undergoing clinical trials.

Glucagon (*Hyperglycemic Factor; HGF*)—In addition to insulin, the pancreas also produces a substance which exerts an effect on blood sugar opposite to that of insulin. This HGF, or glucagon, is produced by the alpha cells of the Islets of Langerhans. It plays an important role in the physiological regulation of blood sugar, and defects in the control of glucagon secretion are a factor in certain types of diabetes mellitus. Contamination of an insulin preparation by glucagon is manifested by a transitory *increase* in blood glucose following insulin injection. Some insulins, eg, recombinant human insulin and the Danish *Novo* insulins, do not contain this HGF.

Somatostatin (*GH-RIF*)—Somatostatin (see page 1077) also is produced in the pancreas, where it inhibits release of both insulin and glucagon; it is involved in the physiologic regulation of the secretion of these hormones. In diabetes mellitus, the persistence of glucagon output contributes to hyperglycemia and ketoacidosis; administration of somatostatin improves the metabolic condition by suppressing glucagon blood levels. Unfortunately, the half-life of somatostatin is very short, so that longer-lived congeners with separate activities to treat diabetes, acromegaly, peptic ulcer and other disorders are being developed.

Glucagon

Glucagon (pig); (*Lilly*)

H-His-Ser-Glu(NH$_2$)-Gly-Thr-Phe-Thr-Ser-Asp-Tyr-Ser-Lys-Tyr-Leu-Asp-Ser-
1 2 3 4 5 6 7 8 9 10 11 12 13 14 15 16

Arg-Arg-Ala-Glu(NH$_2$)-Asp-Phe-Val-Glu(NH$_2$)-Trp-Leu-Met-Asp(NH$_2$)-Thr-OH
17 18 19 20 21 22 23 24 25 26 27 28 29

Glucagon [16941-32-5] $C_{153}H_{225}N_{43}O_{49}S$ (3482.78); a polypeptide occurring in the pancreas glands of domestic mammals used for food by man, which has the property of increasing the blood glucose concentration. It is employed as the hydrochloride.

Description—Fine, white or faintly colored, crystalline powder; practically odorless and tasteless.

Solubility—Soluble in dilute alkali or acid solutions; insoluble in most organic solvents.

Uses—Stimulates the hepatic adenylate cyclase system and hence promotes the breakdown of liver glycogen. The end result is the release of glucose and an elevation of blood glucose. Stimulation of adenylate cyclase in the heart causes positive inotropy and in intestinal muscle, relaxation. After parenteral injection the glucose response is quite prompt. The action lasts but 45 to 90 min. It is used primarily to *terminate hypoglycemic coma*, such as may occur from an overdose of insulin. It is dubious that it offers any compelling advantage over intravenous dextrose for this purpose, except when it is difficult to give an intravenous infusion. Its value in idiopathic hypoglycemia, islet cell carcinoma, and glycogen storage disease has not yet been determined fully. However, it can be used to *diagnose glycogen storage disease* and *to determine pancreatic β-cell secretory reserve*; in the latter test, the amount of C-peptide that appears in the plasma quantifies the reserve. It must be used cautiously in islet cell carcinoma, because it stimulates the release of insulin and may cause hypoglycemia. Even in the diabetic patient it may cause rebound hypoglycemia, mostly, however, because of the persistence of insulin levels from the overdose for which glucagon was administered. It is used as an adjunct in hypotonic *radiography of the gastrointestinal tract*, to relax the smooth muscle. Side effects include dizziness, nausea, vomiting, hypotension and rebound hypoglycemia, especially after intravenous administration. Occasional allergy causes dyspnea or rash.

Dose—*Subcutaneous, intramuscular or intravenous, adult,* for *hypoglycemia,* **0.5** to **1 mg** (Unit) repeated in 20 min if necessary; if there is no response within 20 min intravenous dextrose is mandatory; for *diagnostic use,* **0.25 mg IV** or **2 mg IM**; *children,* **0.025 mg/kg**, repeated in 20 min, if necessary.

Dosage Form—For Injection: 1 and 10 mg (1 and 10 Units).

Insulin Injection

Regular Insulin; Crystalline Zinc Insulin; (*Various Mfrs*)

A sterile, acidified or neutral solution of insulin. The solution has a potency of 40, 80, 100, or 500 USP Insulin Units in each mL.

Description—When containing in each mL not more than 100 USP Units, it is a colorless or almost colorless liquid; that containing 500 Units may be straw-colored; substantially free from turbidity and from insoluble matter; contains from 0.1 to 0.25% (*w/v*) of either phenol or cresol and 1.4 to 1.8% (*w/v*) of glycerin; pH, determined potentiometrically, between 2.5 and 3.5 for acidified injection, and 7.0 and 7.8 for neutral injection.

Uses—For the actions and uses, see the introduction to this section. In diabetes mellitus, the dosage varies with the individual case. Insulin must be given by hypodermic injection, the hormone being destroyed in the gastrointestinal tract. Diabetic individuals are trained to inject themselves. For this purpose a special syringe measuring the dosage of insulin directly in units is employed.

Regular insulin is a *rapid acting* insulin. The time interval from a hypodermic injection of regular insulin until its action can be demonstrated is ½ to 1 hr. The duration of action is relatively short but longer than the plasma half-life, which is approximately 9 min. The duration of action is not linearly proportional to the size of the dose, but it is a simple function of the logarithm of the dose; if 1 Unit will last 4 hr, 10 Units will last 8 hr. Since the usual duration is from 5 to 8 hr after subcutaneous injection, the insulin injection usually is planned in 2 to 4 daily doses for proper control of severe diabetes. This is ordinarily timed a few minutes before the ingestion of food, in order to avoid an unpleasant reduction of the blood-glucose level.

A large number of drugs interact with insulin; they are listed in USP DI.

Dose—There is no standard dosage; each case must be studied individually and monitored closely. The amount given is based on the amount of glucose the patient uses from the diet, the response to treatment and whether insulin injection is used in combination with longer-acting insulins.

Subcutaneous, for a patient with *newly diagnosed mild diabetes,* to be individualized, but usually *initially* **5** to **10 USP Units** 15 to 30 min before each meal. After the period of stabilization of dose, the dose is usually **10** to **20 Units** 3 or 4 times a day, but as much as **40 Units** is occasionally required. A general guideline is 0.5 to 1 Units/kg/day with slightly higher doses of 0.8 to 1.20/kg/day for adolescents during the growth spurt. As an adjunct to intermediate-acting insulins, **5** to **10 Units** given in the same syringe, except with protamine zinc insulin. *Intravenous infusion, adults* and *children,* in coma or severe acidosis, **0.1 Units/kg/hr.** *Intramuscular,* for diabetic ketoacidosis when facilities for intravenous infusion are inadequate, **5** to **10 Units/hr** following an *intravenous bolus* of **10** to **20 Units.** Blood glucose must be titrated to avoid hypoglycemia.

The dosage of insulin should always be expressed in Units rather than in cubic centimeters or minims.

Dosage Form—Injection, Beef: 1000 Units/10 mL; Beef *and* Pork: 400 and 1000 Units/10 mL; Pork: 1000 Units/10 mL and 10,000 Units/20 mL; Human (Recombinant): 1000 Units/10 mL; Human (Semisynthetic); 150 Units/1.5 mL and 1000 Units/10 mL.

Isophane Insulin Suspension

Isophane Insulin; Isophane Insulin Injection; NPH Insulin (*Squibb*); NPH Iletin (*Lilly*)

A sterile suspension of zinc-insulin crystals and protamine sulfate in buffered water for injection, combined in a manner such that the solid phase of the suspension consists of crystals composed of insulin, protamine, and zinc. The protamine sulfate is prepared from the sperm or from the mature testes of fish belonging to the genus *Oncorhynchus* Suckley, or *Salmo* Linné (Fam *Salmonidae*).

Each mL is prepared from sufficient insulin to provide either 40, 80, or 100 USP Insulin Units of insulin activity.

Description—White suspension of rod-shaped crystals approximately 30 μm in length and free from large aggregates of crystals following moderate agitation; contains either (1) 1.4 to 1.8% (*w/v*) of glycerin, 0.15 to 0.17% (*w/v*) of metacresol and 0.06 to 0.07% (*w/v*) of phenol or (2) 1.4 to 1.8% (*w/v*) of glycerin and 0.20 to 0.25% (*w/v*) of phenol; contains 0.15 to 0.25% (*w/v*) of dibasic sodium phosphate; contains also 0.01 to 0.04 mg of zinc and 0.3 to 0.6 mg of protamine for each 100 USP Insulin Units; when examined microscopically, the insoluble matter in the suspension is crystalline, and contains not more than traces of amorphous material; pH between 7.1 and 7.4, determined potentiometrically.

Uses—An insoluble, repository form of insulin (see the introduction to this section). It is an *intermediate-acting* insulin. The action begins in 1 to 2 hr, reaches a peak in 6 to 10 hr, and lasts 18 to 28 hr, except that human isophane insulin has a somewhat shorter duration of action. There may be occasional hypersensitivity to the protamine. *It is never given intravenously.*

Dose—*Subcutaneous,* to be individualized, but the *adult* dose is usually *initially,* **10** to **20 Units** ½ to 1 hr before breakfast; sometimes as much as **80 Units** a day may be required.

Note—It differs in its actions from that of other insulin injections in the USP in both time of onset and duration. To secure accuracy of dosage, the preparation must be brought into uniform suspension by careful shaking before use.

Dosage Form—Injection, Beef, Beef *and* Pork, Pork or Human (Recombinant or Semisynthetic): 1000 Units/10 mL.

Insulin Zinc Suspension

Lente Insulin (*Various Mfrs*)

A sterile suspension of insulin in buffered water for injection, modified by the addition of zinc chloride in a manner such that the solid phase of the suspension consists of a mixture of crystalline and amorphous insulin in a ratio of approximately 7 parts of crystals to 3 parts of amorphous material. Each mL is prepared from sufficient insulin to provide either 40, 80 or 100 USP Insulin Units of insulin activity.

Description—Almost colorless suspension of a mixture of characteristic crystals predominantly 10 to 40 μm in maximum dimension and many particles which have no uniform shape and do not exceed 2 μm in maximum dimensions; contains 0.15 to 0.17% (*w/v*) of sodium acetate, 0.65 to 0.75% (*w/v*) of sodium chloride and 0.09 to 0.11% (*w/v*) of methylparaben; contains also, for each 100 USP Insulin Units, 0.12 to 0.25 mg of zinc of which 20 to 65% is in the supernatant liquid; pH between 7.2 and 7.5.

Uses—The "amorphous" zinc insulin component has a duration of action of about 6 to 8 hr and the crystalline zinc insulin component a duration of longer than 36 hr, owing to the slowness with which the larger crystals dissolve. An appropriate dose of the 3:7 mixture used has an onset of action of 1½ to 4 hr and an *intermediate* duration of action which is very close to that of isophane insulin suspension (18 to 28 hr), with which preparation it may be used interchangeably. The advantage of zinc insulin is its freedom from foreign proteins, such as globin or protamine, to which certain patients are sensitive. For the actions and uses, see the introduction to this section.

Dose—*Subcutaneous*, to be individualized, but the *adult* dose is usually *initially* **10** to **20** but sometimes as much as **80 USP Units** a day; the dose may be initially 10 Units a day with adjustments for newly developed moderate cases or 80% of an established dose of unmodified insulin (eg, *Insulin Injection*) or protamine zinc insulin for cases of longer standing. *It must never be given intravenously!*

Dosage Form—Injection, Beef, Pork or Human (Recombinant or Semisynthetic): 1000 Units/10 mL; Beef *and* Pork: 400 and 1000 Units/10 mL.

Extended Insulin Zinc Suspension

Ultra-Lente Iletin (*Lilly*); Ultralente Insulin/Ultratard (*Squibb-Novo*)

A sterile suspension of insulin in buffered water for injection, modified by the addition of zinc chloride in a manner such that the solid phase of the suspension is predominantly crystalline. In its preparation, sufficient insulin is used to provide either 40, 80 or 100 USP Insulin Units for each mL of the suspension.

Description—Almost colorless suspension of a mixture of characteristic crystals the maximum dimension of which is predominantly 10 to 40 μm; contains, for each 100 USP Units of insulin, 0.12 to 0.25 mg of zinc (of which 20 to 65% is in the supernatant liquid) and not more than 0.70 mg of nitrogen; contains also 0.15 to 0.17% (*w/v*) of sodium acetate, 0.65 to 0.75% (*w/v*) of sodium chloride and 0.09 to 0.11% (*w/v*) of methylparaben; pH, between 7.2 and 7.5.

Uses—For the actions and uses of the insulins, see the introduction to this section. The crystals in this form are of sufficient size to have a slow rate of dissolution. It is a *long-acting* insulin with an onset of action of 4 to 6 hr, a peak at 10 to 14 hr, and duration usually in excess of 36 hr, which is slightly longer than that of *Protamine Zinc Insulin*. Since it is free of protamine and other foreign proteins, the incidence of allergic reactions is minimized. The dose needs to be individualized to the patient on the basis of a study of responses of blood and urine glucose to trial doses of the drug.

Dose—*Subcutaneous* (deep), to be individualized, but *adult* dose is usually **7** to **20** but sometimes as much as **80 USP Units** a day. *It must never be given intravenously!*

Dosage Form—Injection, Beef: 1000 Units/10 mL; Beef *and* Pork: 400 and 1000 Units/10 mL; Human: 1000 Units/10 mL.

Prompt Insulin Zinc Suspension

Semi-Lente Iletin (*Lilly*); Semitard (*Squibb-Novo*)

A sterile suspension of insulin in buffered water for injection, modified by the addition of zinc chloride in a manner such that the solid phase of the suspension is amorphous. In its preparation, sufficient insulin is used to provide either 40, 80 or 100 USP Insulin Units for each mL of the suspension.

Description—Almost colorless suspension of particles that have no uniform shape and the maximum dimension of which does not exceed 2 μm; contains, for each 100 USP Units of insulin, 0.12 to 0.25 mg of zinc (of which 20 to 65% is in the supernatant liquid) and not more than 0.70 mg of nitrogen; contains also 0.15 to 0.17% (*w/v*) of sodium acetate, 0.65 to 0.75% (*w/v*) of sodium chloride and 0.09 to 0.11% (*w/v*) of methylparaben; pH between 7.2 and 7.5.

Uses—For the actions and uses of the insulins, see the introduction to this section. The zinc insulin in this form is a mixture of amorphous and extremely fine crystalline materials. Consequently, it is a *rapid-acting* insulin with an onset of ½ to 3 hr, a peak of 4 to 6 hr and a duration of 12 to 16 hr. Because this form is essentially free of foreign proteins, the incidence of allergic reactions is extremely low.

Dose—*Subcutaneous* (deep), to be individualized, but *adult* dose is usually **10** to **20** but sometimes as much as **80 USP Units** a day. *It should never be given intravenously!*

Dosage Form—Injection, Beef: 1000 Units/10 mL; Beef *and* Pork: 400 and 1000 Units/10 mL.

Protamine Zinc Insulin Suspension

Protamine Zinc Insulin; Protamine Zinc Insulin Injection (*Squibb*); Protamine Zinc and Iletin (*Lilly*)

A sterile suspension of insulin in buffered water for injection, modified by the addition of zinc chloride and protamine sulfate. The protamine sulfate is prepared from the sperm or from the mature testes of fish belonging to the genus *Oncorhynchus* Suckley, or *Salmo* Linné (Fam *Salmonidae*). In the preparation, the amount of insulin used is sufficient to provide either 40, 80 or 100 USP Insulin Units for each mL of the suspension.

Description—White, or almost white, suspension, free from large particles following moderate agitation; must contain from 1.4 to 1.8% (*w/v*) of glycerin, and either from 0.18 to 0.22% (*w/v*) of cresol or from 0.22 to 0.28% (*w/v*) of phenol; contains from 0.15 to 0.25% (*w/v*) of Na_2HPO_4; must contain from 0.15 to 0.25 mg of zinc and from 1 to 1.5 mg of protamine for each 100 USP Insulin Units; pH, determined potentiometrically, between 7.1 and 7.4.

Uses—For the actions and uses of the insulins, see the introduction to this section. This is a *long-acting* insulin with an onset of action of 4 to 6 hr, a peak at 10 to 12 hr, and a duration of about 36 hr. Consequently, it need not be given with any definite time relation to food intake, and it must not be depended upon when very prompt action is needed, as in diabetic acidosis and coma. Also, due to the prolonged action, it need not be given more often than once a day, but this should be done at a fairly uniform, scheduled time. Since subliminal levels persist for 3 or 4 days, the dose should be adjusted at intervals of not less than 3 days.

This and the more rapidly acting insulins have been mixed in various proportions and in different ways. Such variations produce mixtures that give intermediate patterns of speed and duration of physiological activity. This method, however, makes it possible through the long-acting insulin to take care of the sugar requirements during the night, while short-acting insulin causes full utilization of food taken during the day. It thus permits one to avoid large doses of the long-acting insulin such as might cause hypoglycemia in the early morning hours. However, the need to individualize the insulin schedule makes commercial fixed mixtures impractical and places the responsibility for the preparation in the hands of the physician. Except for the inconvenience of an extra injection, the short-acting insulin can just as well be administered by separate injection.

It is administered by injection usually into the loose subcutaneous tissue. *It must never be given intravenously!*

Dose—*Subcutaneous*, to be individualized, but the *adult* dose is usually **7** to **20** but sometimes as much as **80 USP Units** a day.

Note—It differs in its action from that of other insulin injections in the USP in both time of onset and duration. To secure accuracy of dosage, the preparation must be brought into uniform suspension by careful shaking before use.

Dosage Form—Injection, Beef or Pork: 1000 Units/10 mL; Beef *and* Pork: 400 and 1000 Units/10 mL.

Secretin—page 1374.

Oral Hypoglycemic and Hyperglycemic Drugs

Compounds from several different chemical classes are capable of lowering blood sugar. The best known of these compounds are benzenesulfonylurea derivatives of the type $R_1C_6H_4SO_2NHCONHR_2$. Certain biguanides (formamidinyliminoureas) also cause the same effect, but are no longer used in the US.

Oral hypoglycemics were received enthusiastically by the medical profession. However, the sulfonylureas especially have proved to be efficacious only in certain types of diabetes, primarily in noninsulin-dependent Type II diabetes mellitus. Limitations to the usefulness of oral hypoglycemics most certainly are connected with the mechanism of their hypoglycemic action and with the nature of the metabolic deficiency in each of the various types of diabetes. The principal action of the sulfonylureas seems to be to increase secretion of insulin by increasing the number of potassium channels that close in response to glucose. Some functional β-cells must be present for an effect on blood glucose. In addition, hepatic glucogenesis is decreased, and also the number of insulin receptors per cell appears to be increased by certain agents. During chronic treatment tolerance may occur (except with glipizide), so that neither insulin nor glucose blood levels may be much affected.

In 1970 the results of a collaborative study among a number of university medical centers were reported (University Group Diabetes Program, UGDP). The findings were that life expectancy with diet, plus tolbutamide or phenformin, was no greater than with diet alone, thus raising serious doubts about the advisability of using oral hypoglycemic agents at all. Furthermore, cardiovascular complications appeared to be higher when these drugs were used than in their absence, although the findings were by no means conclusive. Critics have pointed out serious defects in the design and execution of the study, and the American Diabetes Association no longer endorses the report. Consequently, the status of these drugs is uncertain. The usual advice is that the use of oral hypoglycemics should be limited to the management of noninsulin-dependent diabetes *which does not respond to diet* and in which the patient will not or can not tolerate insulin. Glipizide has been shown to reverse the thickening of the vascular basement membrane in diabetics.

Oral hypoglycemic drugs interact with over 50 different drugs. A list can be found in *Drug Facts and Comparisons*.

Acetohexamide

Benzenesulfonamide, 4-acetyl-*N*-[[cyclohexylamino]carbonyl]-, Dymelor (*Lilly*); (*Various Mfrs*)

$CH_3CO-C_6H_4-SO_2NHCONH-C_6H_{11}$

1-[(*p*-Acetylphenyl)sulfonyl]-3-cyclohexylurea [968-81-0] $C_{15}H_{20}$- N_2O_4S (324.39), calculated on the dried basis.

Preparation—*p*-Acetylbenzenesulfonamide is treated with anhydrous potassium carbonate and the resulting potassium salt of the sulfonamide is reacted with cyclohexyl isocyanate. After removal of acetone, the residue (potassium salt of acetohexamide) is dissolved in water and acidified with hydrochloric acid to precipitate acetohexamide. Purification is by recrystallization from aqueous ethanol. US Pat 3,320,312.

Description—White, practically odorless, crystalline powder; melts between 182.5 and 187°.

Solubility—1 g in 230 mL alcohol or 210 mL chloroform; practically insoluble in water or ether.

Uses—A sulfonylurea oral hypoglycemic drug with actions and uses similar to those of *Tolbutamide*. Thus, it is used in the treatment of mild to moderately severe *diabetes mellitus* of the *noninsulin-dependent* type in patients in whom diet alone cannot control glycosuria. It is ineffective in *insulin-dependent* diabetes and is contraindicated in diabetes complicated by acidosis, ketosis, severe infections, coma, severe trauma or major surgery.

The side effects are similar to those of other sulfonylureas (see *Tolbutamide*). The incidence of adverse effects is low, and such effects are reversible. Contraindications and drug interactions are similar.

It is metabolized in the liver to a metabolite that has 2.5 times the activity of the parent compound. The metabolite is excreted in the urine; consequently, care must be exercised in renal failure. The plasma half-life of the parent drug is 6 to 8 hr, and the duration of action is 8 to 12 hr.

Dose—*Oral, adult, initially* **250 mg** once a day, with upward adjustments, if necessary, to a total of 1.5 g a day. Doses of 1 g or above should be divided into two separate doses.

Dosage Form—Tablets: 250 and 500 mg.

Chlorpropamide

Benzenesulfonamide, 4-chloro-*N*-[(propylamino)carbonyl]-, Diabinese (*Pfizer*); (*Various Mfrs*)

$Cl-C_6H_4-SO_2-NH-C(=O)-NH-CH_2CH_2CH_3$

1-[(*p*-Chlorophenyl)sulfonyl]-3-propylurea [94-20-2] $C_{10}H_{13}Cl$-N_2O_3S (276.74).

Preparation—*p*-Chlorobenzenesulfonamide undergoes addition to propyl isocyanate by warming a solution of equimolar quantities of the two reactants.

Description—White, crystalline powder, having a slight odor; melts between 125 and 129°.

Solubility—Practically insoluble in water; soluble in alcohol; sparingly soluble in chloroform.

Uses—An oral hypoglycemic agent with actions and uses essentially the same as those of *Tolbutamide*. As with tolbutamide, its use is limited to patients with stable, mild to moderately severe diabetes mellitus who still have some residual pancreatic beta-cell function. A patient who requires more than 40 Units of insulin/day, usually will not respond to this drug. Refractoriness sometimes develops. Elimination is about 80% hepatic. The half-life (25 to 60 hr) and duration of action (about 24 to 48 hr) are much longer than those of tolbutamide. The side effects are of the same type as with tolbutamide but have a somewhat higher incidence, namely, about 6%, half of which are cutaneous. Severe, refractory hypoglycemic coma occurs more often with chlorpropamide than with other oral hypoglycemic drugs. It increases the endogenous release of vasopressin (ADH) and thus causes water retention with resultant hyponatremia and hypo-osmolality. This action is used in the treatment of central *diabetes insipidus*. Patients under treatment with this drug have a disulfiram-like intolerance to alcohol. It is contraindicated in the presence of *renal* glycosuria because of the possibility of fatal hypoglycemia.

Dose—*Oral, adult, diabetes mellitus initially* **250 mg** in *middle-aged patients* and **100** to **125 mg** in *elderly patients*, given once a day, with breakfast. After 5 to 7 days, when the blood glucose response becomes constant, the dosage may be increased or decreased by 50 to 125 mg at weekly intervals; the *usual maintenance* dose is **100** to **500 mg** a day. Doses above 500 mg do not usually increase the response; the dose should not exceed 750 mg a day. *Diabetes insipidus*, initially **100** to **200 mg** once a day, with upward adjustments of 50 to 125 mg at 2- to 3-day intervals, if necessary and tolerated, to as much as 750 mg a day.

Dosage Form—Tablets: 100 and 250 mg.

Glipizide

Pyrazinecarboxamide, *N*-[2-[4-[[[(cyclohexylamino)carbonyl]amino]sulfonyl]phenyl]ethyl]-5-methyl-, Glucotrol (*Roerig*)

(5-methylpyrazinyl)$-CONHCH_2CH_2-C_6H_4-SO_2NHCONH-C_6H_{11}$

[29094-61-9] $C_{21}H_{27}N_5O_4S$ (445.54).

Preparation—By the condensation of 4-[2-(5-methyl-2-pyrazinecarboxamido)ethyl]benzenesulfonamide and cyclohexyl isocyanate; *Arzneimittel Forsch 21:* 200, 1971.

Description—White, odorless powder; pK_a 5.9; melts about 205°.

Solubility—Insoluble in water or polar solvents; freely soluble in dimethylformamide or fixed alkalies.

Uses—A sulfonylurea 100 times more potent than tolbutamide in evoking pancreatic secretion of insulin. It differs from other oral hypoglycemic drugs in that tolerance to this action apparently does not occur. It also upregulates insulin receptors in the periphery, which seems to be the primary action. It is thought not to have a direct effect on glucagon secretion. It is mildly diuretic. It has a special status in the treatment of *noninsulin-dependent diabetes mellitus* because it is effective in many cases which are resistent to all other oral hypoglycemic drugs. It differs from other oral hypoglycemic drugs in that it is more effective during eating than during fasting. It has been shown to be superior to tolbutamide and at least as effective as chlorpropamide. It was the first oral hypoglycemic drug shown to thin a diabetes-thickened endothelial basement membrane and, hence, to reverse diabetic angiopathy.

Adverse effects have been reported to occur in as few as 3% and as many as 12% and may cause discontinuation in 0.3 to 3% of cases. Gastrointestinal effects, such as nausea, heartburn, diarrhea, constipation, vomiting and colic, are the most common and occur with a frequency of 1.7 to 3.7%. Rashes occur in 0.5 to 1.5%. Mild headache, drowsiness, asthenia, and dizziness occasionally occur. Although minor episodes of hypoglycemia can occur, no instance of severe hypoglycemia has been observed except where there were complications of age, hypocaloric diet, other drugs or liver disease.

Peroral absorption is almost complete. It is rapid (about 30 min) if the stomach is empty, but 1.2 to 3.5 hr is required in the presence of food. About 98% is bound to plasma albumin by nonionic forces. The volume of distribution is about 0.16 L/kg. About 90% is metabolized in the liver to several inactive metabolites. The half-life is about 2 to 4 hr. The duration of action is 10 to 16 hr.

Dose—*Oral, adult, initially* **5 mg** 30 min before breakfast, to be adjusted subsequently, if necessary, in increments of 2.5 to 5 mg, at intervals of several days to a *usual maintenance dose* of **15 mg** once a day. Daily doses should not exceed 40 mg. Doses above 15 mg a day should be divided.

Dosage Form—Tablets: 5 and 10 mg.

Glyburide

Benzamide, 5-chloro-*N*-[2-[4-[[[(cyclohexylamino)carbonyl]amino]sulfonyl]phenyl]ethyl]-2-methoxy-, DiaBeta (*Hoechst-Roussel*); Glynase Pres Tab, Micronase (*Upjohn*)

Cl

CONHCH₂CH₂—SO₂NHCONH—

OCH₃

Glybenclamide [10238-21-8] $C_{23}H_{28}ClN_3O_5S$ (494.00).

Preparation—See *Arzneimittel Forsch 16:* 640, 1966; *CA 66:* 65289h.

Description—White to off-white crystalline powder; melts about 170°; pK_a 5.3.

Solubility—Sparingly soluble in water or ether; 1 g dissolves in 330 mL of alcohol or 36 mL of chloroform.

Uses—A sulfonylurea hypoglycemic drug 200 times as potent as *Tolbutamide* in evoking the release of insulin from the pancreatic islets. It is more effective in suppressing fasting than postprandial hyperglycemia. Like glipizide, it is mildly diuretic. After its introduction it quickly became the most widely prescribed oral hypoglycemic drug in the world, because it is as effective as tolbutamide but has a lower incidence of adverse effects than chlorpropamide. However, side effects are less frequent and severe with glipizide.

The incidence of adverse effects is reported to be 3.6%. Gastrointestinal side effects, such as nausea, anorexia, vomiting, heartburn, diarrhea, constipation and abdominal pain, occur with a frequency of about 2%. Pruritus and rashes may occur. Cholestatic jaundice and eosinophilia have been reported. Transient leucopenia sometimes occurs. A disulfiram-like reaction to alcohol may occur. Hypoglycemic episodes sometimes are prolonged and severe, and deaths have resulted.

About 90% of oral drug is absorbed from an empty stomach. The absorption time is 1.5 to 2 hr. Food decreases absorption, some fibers decreasing it by as much as 50%. About 97% is bound to plasma albumin as a weak-acid anion and, hence, is susceptible to displacement by many weak acid drugs. The volume of distribution is about 0.16 L/kg. Elimination is by hepatic metabolism. The 50% biliary elimination stated in promotional literature is as a metabolite, and this drug has no clinical advantage over other sulfonylureas in either renal or hepatic failure. The half-life is 1.5 to 5 hr. The duration of action is 24 hr. The micronized tablets are not strictly bioequivalent to nonmicronized tablets in their onset of action or half-life. See product information if patient changes products.

Dose—*Oral, adult, initially* **1.25** to **5 mg** with breakfast, to be adjusted, if necessary, at weakly intervals with 2.5-mg increments to no more than 20 mg a day.

Dosage Forms—Tablets: 1.25, 2.5 and 5 mg. Micronized Tablets: 1.5 and 3 mg.

Linogliride—see RPS-18, page 976.

Tolazamide

Benzenesulfonamide, *N*-[[(hexahydro-1*H*-azepin-1-yl)amino]-carbonyl]-4-methyl-; Tolinase (*Upjohn*); (*Various Mfrs*)

CH₃—SO₂NHCONH—N

1-(Hexahydro-1*H*-azepin-1-yl)-3-(*p*-tolylsulfonyl)urea [1156-19-0] $C_{14}H_{21}N_3O_3S$ (311.40).

Preparation—Methyl *p*-tolylsulfonylcarbamate undergoes an ammonolysis type of reaction with 1-aminohexamethyleneimine. US Pat 3,063,903.

Description—White to off-white, crystalline powder that is odorless or has a slight odor; melts between 161 and 169° with decomposition; pK_a (25°) 3.6; (37.5°) 5.68.

Solubility—Very slightly soluble in water; freely soluble in chloroform; soluble in acetone; slightly soluble in alcohol.

Uses—A sulfonylurea oral hypoglycemic drug with actions and uses similar to *Tolbutamide*. Thus, it is used in the treatment of mild to moderately severe *diabetes mellitus* of the maturity-onset, nonketotic type in patients in whom glycosuria cannot be controlled by diet alone. It is ineffective in *insulin-dependent* diabetes and is contraindicated in diabetes complicated by acidosis, ketosis, severe infections, coma, severe trauma or major surgery. After oral administration the plasma levels reach a peak in 4 to 8 hr. The plasma half-life is about 7 hr and the duration of action is 12 to 24 hr.

The total incidence of side effects is about 5%; about 2% of patients find it necessary to discontinue the drug. The side effects are the same types as those of *Tolbutamide*. Korsakoff-Wernicke encephalopathy has been reported; hypoglycemic episodes increase the need for thiamin.

Dose—*Oral, adult, initially* **100** to **250 mg** once a day taken with breakfast; the dose is then adjusted every 4 to 6 days until a satisfactory response is achieved or toxicity requires discontinuation. Doses larger than 1.5 g/day will usually not increase the response. If the daily dose exceeds 500 mg, it should be given in 2 divided doses.

Dosage Form—Tablets: 100, 250 and 500 mg.

Tolbutamide

Benzenesulfonamide, *N*-[(butylamino)carbonyl]-4-methyl-, Orinase (*Upjohn*); (*Various Mfrs*)

CH₃—SO₂—NHCONH(CH₂)₃CH₃

1-Butyl-3-(*p*-tolylsulfonyl)urea [64-77-7] $C_{12}H_{18}N_2O_3S$ (270.35).

Preparation—Toluene is treated with chlorosulfonic acid and the resulting *p*-toluenesulfonyl chloride is converted into *p*-toluenesulfonamide by interaction with ammonia. Condensation of the sulfonamide with ethyl chloroformate in the presence of pyridine or another suitable basic catalyst produces ethyl *N*-*p*-toluenesulfonylcarbamate. Aminolysis with butylamine in ethylene glycol monomethyl ether solutions yields tolbutamide.

Description—White, or practically white, crystalline powder; slightly bitter and practically odorless; melting range 126 to 132°.

Solubility—Practically insoluble in water, soluble in alcohol or chloroform.

Uses—An oral hypoglycemic drug. It is useful in the treatment of selected cases of *noninsulin-dependent diabetes mellitus*. In order to respond, patients must have some remaining functional islet beta cells which can be stimulated by the drug. If the patient requires more than 40 Units of insulin/day, he generally will not respond to this drug. In diabetic patients the peak effect is reached in 5 to 8 hr. The duration of action is usually 6 to 12 hr (average plasma half-life 5.6 hr but longer in elderly patients; dose-dependent kinetics occur with high doses), so that two daily doses are required in most patients. The hypoglycemia induced by even high doses of the drug is generally not as severe as can be induced by insulin; hence, the incidence of acute hypoglycemic reactions is lower with tolbutamide; however, severe, refractory hypoglycemia sometimes does occur. Refractoriness to it sometimes develops. See also page 1079 for the findings of the UGDP.

Toxic effects include diarrhea, nausea, vomiting, abdominal cramps, weakness, headache, tinnitus, paresthesias, allergic reactions (pruritus, erythema multiforme, maculopapular rash, all usually transient), photosensitivity and alcohol intolerance. Water retention and hyponatremia may result from enhancement of ADH (vasopressin) release. Cholestatic jaundice may occur (rarely), and the drug is contraindicated in the presence of liver damage. Rare leukopenia, thrombocytopenia, pancytopenia and agranulocytosis occur. Furthermore, because the hypoglycemic action of the drug is mild, the patient is more susceptible to loss of control of the blood sugar through dietary indulgence or infections. Hypoglycemic reactions are rare. It is contraindicated in nondiabetic patients with renal glycosuria and liver disease.

The sulfonylureas interact with a number of drugs. The following substances increase the hypoglycemic activity of sulfonylureas:

dicumarol, phenylbutazone, oxyphenbutazone, several sulfonamides, chloramphenicol, large doses of salicylates, monoamine oxidase inhibitors, clofibrate, anabolic steroids, fenfluramine, guanethidine, β-adrenoreceptor blocking drugs and alcohol.

Dose—*Oral, adult, initially* **500 mg** once or twice a day. The dose is individualized and adjusted gradually to the minimal *maintenance* dose that satisfactorily controls the hyperglycemia and glycosuria. Doses greater than 3 g are usually no more effective than smaller doses and greatly increase the likelihood of toxicity.

Dosage Form—Tablets: 250 and 500 mg.

The Parathyroid Hormone

Spontaneous atrophy, or injury (as at thyroidectomy), of the parathyroid glands is followed by a decrease in the concentration of serum calcium and an increase in serum phosphorus. These changes can be reversed by the parenteral administration of suitably prepared extracts of the parathyroids of domestic animals. The active principle of the parathyroid gland is a protein of molecular weight 9500. Active amino terminal and carboxyl terminal fragments of lower molecular weight (3800 and 6900, respectively) are found in plasma. These products possess ¼ to ½ the specific calcium-mobilizing activity of parathormone (PTH).

Various cancers produce an active peptide homologous to the amino end of PTH, which peptide (called parathyroid hormone-like peptide or PTH-LH) causes hypercalcemia, bone destruction and pain. PTH-LH also is found in lactating mammary tissue and plays a role in the mobilization of calcium to milk.

Secretion of PTH is stimulated by a fall in the free Ca^{2+} concentration of the plasma. The hormone then acts to restore Ca^{2+} concentration by (1) increasing reabsorption of calcium and the excretion of phosphate and decreasing the absorption of bicarbonate by the kidney, (2) increasing resorption of bone, with release of Ca^{2+} and (3) increasing absorption of calcium and phosphate from the gastrointestinal tract. The gastrointestinal effects are mediated by 1α,25-dihydroxycholecalciferol, a metabolite of vitamin D_3 that may be considered a hormone; PTH is a trophin for renal synthesis of the metabolite. The metabolite also promotes the action of vitamin D_3 on bone. Vitamin D_2 (calciferol) and dihydrotachysterol can simulate the hypercalcemic effect of PTH; these compounds, moreover, are active orally. Overdosage with any of these compounds can lead to dangerously high calcium concentrations in the blood, with attendant complications, such as calcification of kidneys and blood vessels. Their use, therefore, should have careful medical supervision and be controlled by frequent determinations of blood calcium.

The thyroid gland produces a hormone, *thyrocalcitonin* (see page 1083), that reduces serum calcium concentration. A small amount of calcitonin also is produced in the parathyroid gland as well as the thymus, but the main source is the thyroid gland. The biological function of calcitonin is to prevent excessive hypercalcemia from parathyroid hormone activity.

Calcitriol—page 1116.

Dihydrotachysterol

9,10-Secoergosta-5,7,22-trien-3-ol, (3β,5*E*,7*E*,10α,22*E*)-, Dihydrotachysterol; DHT (*Roxane*)

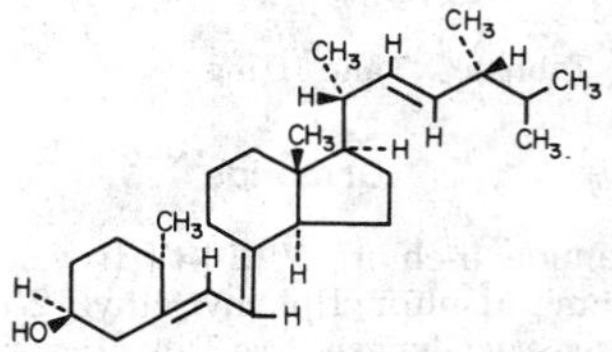

9,10-Secoergosta-5,7,22-trien-3β-ol [67-96-9] $C_{28}H_{46}O$ (398.67).

Preparation—Calciferol (activated ergosterol) is dissolved in a suitable organic solvent and subjected to catalytic hydrogenation until the proper amount of hydrogen has reacted.

Description—Colorless or white crystals, or a white, crystalline powder; odorless; melts between 123.5 and 129° for one form, or about 113° for the other form.

Solubility—Practically insoluble in water; soluble in alcohol; freely soluble in ether or chloroform; sparingly soluble in vegetable oils.

Uses—Chemically closely related to vitamin D_2 (calciferol) and consequently is classified frequently as a D vitamin. However, it possesses very weak antirachitic activity, being only about ¹⁄₄₀₀ as potent as calciferol in this respect, mainly because its effects on calcium absorption from the intestine are quite weak. But it has potent calcemic activity (ie, raises plasma calcium concentration) and is similar to parathyroid hormone in this action. Consequently, it long has been used in lieu of parathyroid hormone in the treatment of *idiopathic* and *postoperative tetanies, hypocalcemia* and *hypoparathyroidism*. The drug should not be used in the presence of renal insufficiency or hyperphosphatemia. Extreme care must be used to prevent overdosage.

Adverse effects result mainly from hypercalcemia. They include anorexia, nausea, vomiting, diarrhea, languor, osteoporosis, weight loss, metastatic calcification, renal damage, anemia, band keratitis and convulsions. In severe hypercalcemia there may be headache, vertigo, innitus, abdominal cramps, polyuria, thirst, ataxia, albuminuria and xanthemia.

Dose—*Oral, adult, initially* **0.8** to **2.4 mg** a day for several days, after which adjustments are made according to plasma calcium concentrations; *maintenance, usual,* **0.2** to **1 mg** a day.

Dosage Forms—Capsules: 0.125 mg; Oral Solution: 0.2 and 0.25 mg/mL; Tablets: 0.125, 0.2 and 0.4 mg.

The Thyroid Hormones

The thyroid gland modulates the energy metabolism and certain nonenergetic metabolic functions of the body. In the absence of the thyroid gland the basal metabolic rate is less than 55% of normal, and growth and development are impaired. In the presence of a hyperactive gland the metabolic rate may be up to 160% of normal; the excitability of irritable tissues is increased, and tachycardia, nervousness, etc result. Thyroid "hormone" is used clinically mainly to replenish the corporal hormone supply in conditions of thyroid insufficiency (hypothyroidism), such as may result from a natural thyroid or pituitary pathology or from thyroid surgery. The "hormone" rarely is administered to increase the metabolic rate and organic activity above normal, and such iatrogenic hyperthyroidism may indeed be dangerous.

The mediator by which the thyroid gland stimulates the tissues to a higher activity and rate of metabolism is called the *thyroid hormone*, but there are actually four active substances, all iodinated thyronines, released by the gland. Thyroxine (L-3,5,3′,5′-tetraiodothyronine or T-4) is found in the greatest amount in blood (about 75% of the thyroid hormone content of the plasma), and the moderately less- active L-3,3′-*diiodothyronine* is present in the next greatest amount (25%). L-3,5,3′-*Triiodothyronine* (liothyronine or T-3), which is 3 to 10 times as active as thyroxine, and L- 3,3′,5′-*triiodo-thyronine* comprise less than 3% of the plasma thyroid hormone content. But since the triiodothyronines disappear more rapidly from blood than thyroxine, they probably comprise a somewhat larger proportion of the glandular secretion; in the thyroid gland they account for about ⅕ of the hormone content and as much as 40% of its hormone activity. Furthermore, in the tissues, some thyroxine is converted to liothyronine and perhaps as much as ½ to ⅔ of the body liothyronine is derived from thyroxine. Liothyronine regulates TRH release in the hypothalamus and is probably the principal hormone involved in the long negative feedback loop regulation of TSH (thyroid-stimulating hormone, or thyrotropin) release.

The thyroid gland concentrates iodide ion from the plasma and converts it to free iodine, which then reacts with tyrosine moieties within the substance of the gland eventually to produce the thyroid hormones. The glandular accumulation of iodine and the conversion to the intermediate, 3,5-diiodotyrosine, are under the control of the thyrotropic hormone (see page 1059). Iodine deficiency results in a compensatory increase in the size of the thyroid gland in a usually fruitless homeostatic attempt to manufacture more hormone. Iodine administration corrects this type of goiter and permits the normal production of the thyroid hormones. The incorporation of sodium iodide into table salt helps protect against iodine-deficiency thyroid disorders. In children under 14 years, iodine supplementation corrects endemic cretinism.

In the colloid of the thyroid gland these thyronine derivatives are bound to a globulin, *thyroglobulin*, which formerly was thought to be the thyroid hormone. About 90% of the thyroid hormone content of the gland is in the thyroglobulin complex. The molecular weight of thyroglobulin is 650,000 daltons. Before thyroxine and liothyronine can be released into the bloodstream, the thyroglobulin must be assimilated by the thyroid follicular cells, within which the globulin is split by proteases to release the hormones. In the blood, the hormones are bound mainly to an albumin; the complex is dissociable, so that the hormones are free to pass into the body cells.

The thyroid hormones interact with nuclear receptors to increase RNA polymerase and also to increase the number of initiation sites for the polymerase. The result is an increase in transcription for a number of proteins, and the synthesis thereof is increased. Thyroid hormone also has a regulatory action on t-RNA. The synthesized proteins in turn regulate various enzymes and enzyme complexes, so that oxidative phosphorylation in the mitochondria may become partially uncoupled, membrane ATPase activity is increased, adenylate cyclase activity is enhanced, etc. There also are some direct actions on cellular functions, such as stimulation of autocrine growth factors and amino acid transport systems, and inhibition of some zinc-dependent dehydrogenases, prostaglandin dehydrogenases, etc.

The uses and adverse effects of the thyroid hormones are indicated in the monograph on *Thyroid* (page 1086). Thyroid hormones lower plasma lipid concentrations. However, because of their effect to increase the metabolic rate, they are not used clinically to lower blood lipids. The lipid-lowering action is possessed also by the dextro isomers of thyroid hormones, but the dextro forms have only a very weak effect on the metabolic rate. Consequently, dextrothyroxine is employed to lower blood lipids.

Calcitonin—Thyrocalcitonin also is a thyroid hormone, but its effects are to decrease plasma calcium concentration rather than to affect energy and lipid metabolism. It has an effect to decrease osteoclastic activity, thus inhibiting the movement of bone salts from bone to the blood. It decreases the renal tubular secretion of calcium and probably inhibits calcium pumping in many types of cells. It also increases renal excretion of phosphate. It has very little effect on the absorption of calcium from the intestine. It plays a role in the homeostasis of blood calcium. When plasma calcium levels are elevated, thyrocalcitonin is released in increased quantities. Thus it tends to oppose parathyroid hormone but at different cell targets. The molecular weight of monomeric thyrocalcitonin is 3500 daltons. It is a polypeptide of 32 amino acid units. Despite only a 50% homology between human and salmon calcitonins, their biochemical actions are the same. However, salmon calcitonin is allergenic.

Calcitonin

Calcitonin (Human) [Cibacalcin (*Ciba*); Calcitonin (Salmon) [Calcimar (*Rhone-Poulenc Rorer*); Miacalcin (*Sandoz*)]

Cys-Ser-Asn-Leu-Ser-Thr-Cys-Val-Leu-Gly-Lys-Leu-Ser-Gln-Glu-Leu-His-
1 2 3 4 5 6 7 8 9 10 11 12 13 14 15 16 17

Lys-Leu-Gln-Thr-Tyr-Pro-Arg-Thr-Asn-Thr-Gly-Ser-Gly-Thr-Pro—NH_2
18 19 20 21 22 23 24 25 26 27 28 29 30 31 32

[47931-85-1] $C_{145}H_{240}O_{48}S_2$ (3431.88).

A polypeptide hormone secreted by the parafollicular cells of the thyroid gland in mammals and by the ultimobranchial gland of birds and fish, isolated from various of these sources, all apparently containing 32 amino acid residues but differing in the linear sequence. Human and salmon calcitonin differ at 18 positions. Both human and salmon calcitonins are available as synthetic products. The source of the product is indicated in the labeling.

Description—White, fluffy powder; lyophilized.

Solubility—Very soluble in water; slightly soluble in alcohol; insoluble in chloroform or ether.

Uses—The actions are described in the introductory section. The hormone does not have much effect on normal plasma calcium, and patients with calcitonin-producing tumors of the thyroid medulla often do not manifest disturbances of calcium metabolism. It appears to act only in *hypercalcemia*, such as that caused by hyperparathyroidism, various carcinomas and multiple myeloma. It normalizes plasma calcium and causes a favorable change in bone structure in *Paget's disease*; 3 to 12 mo of treatment may be required to restore plasma electrolyte, alkaline phosphatase and hydroxyproline to normal. Human calcitonin is less potent than salmon calcitonin because it is the more rapidly degraded. Used alone against osteoporosis the hormone has a variable effect, and there have been several reports that bone pain was alleviated. Since few studies have been conducted with human calcitonin, no final judgment is yet possible. In combination with calcitriol and calcium it may be effective against senile and *postmenopausal osteoporosis*.

Side effects are mild nausea, vomiting, diarrhea, facial flushing and malaise. Rashes may occur with salmon calcitonin. Inflammation and pain at the injection site sometimes occur. Diuresis at the onset of treatment often occurs.

The half-life of human calcitonin is about 1 hr; that of salmon calcitonin is considerably longer, but the exact figure is unknown. The duration of action is 6 to 8 hr.

Dose—*Intramuscular* or *subcutaneous, adult,* for *hypercalcemia* (approved for salmon calcitonin only), *initially* **4 IU/kg** every 12 hr, to be increased as needed up to no more than **8 IU/kg** every 6 hr; for *Paget's disease* with serious osseous deformities, *initially* **100 IU** once a day, then **50 IU** (salmon calcitonin) every other day or 3 times a wk; **0.5 mg** (human calcitonin) 2 to 3 times a wk; for *postmenopausal osteoporosis* (approved for salmon calcitonin, only), **100 IU** once a day, every other day or 3 times a wk.

Dosage Form—Injection (salmon calcitonin): 100 and 400 USP Units/2 mL. One USP Unit is equal to 1 MRC Unit Injection (human calcitonin): 0.5 mg/vial.

Dextrothyroxin—page 969.

Etidronate Disodium

Phosphonic acid, (1-hydroxyethylidene)bis-, disodium salt; Didronel (*Norwich-Eaton*)

$C_2H_6Na_2O_7P_2$ (249.99).

Preparation—Etidronic acid may be prepared in various ways, as by passing gaseous phosphorus trichloride into acetic acid at about 75°, by reaction of the same substances in a lower aliphatic tertiary amine such as tributylamine, or by reaction of an anhydrous mixture of phosphorous acid, acetic anhydride and acetic acid.

Description—White powder.

Solubility—Very soluble in water.

Uses—The actions are unique, and there is no separate category in this volume into which the drug logically can be placed. Since it resembles calcitonin in its uses, it is placed here, but the drug is neither a hormone nor is its mechanism of action that of calcitonin. It is adsorbed onto hydroxyapatite (bone crystal), where it interferes with resorption of the crystals in osteoclasia and, in higher concentration, with osteoblastosis. In *Paget's disease* (osteitis deformans), for which it mainly is used, it slows the rate of turnover of bone, decreases excessive osteoclastic and osteoblastic cellular activities, and diminishes hydroxyproline levels in blood and urine and brings the elevated serum alkaline phosphate down toward normal. With appropriate (low) doses, bone pain is decreased, and mobility is increased. Where there is impairment of hearing or high-output heart failure, these also are improved. Deformity and fracturing are not prevented. Usually several months of treatment are required to effect a considerable improvement. Sometimes after a single course of treatment remission may be sustained for several years before another course becomes necessary. Etidronate is advantageous, relative to calcitonin, in not requiring parenteral administration, in freedom from antibody formation, and in cost. It also is used in the *prophylaxis* or *slowing of heterotopic ossification* (eg, after hip replacement or vertebral injury) and to suppress *hypercalcemia of malignancy*.

In high doses (above 20 mg/kg and possible above 10 mg/kg) or after prolonged use, increased bone pain, decreased mineralization and increased bone fractures may occur as the result of inhibition of osteoid formation. It sometimes is used deliberately to suppress heterotropic ossification after injury or bone surgery. Even with the usual dosage, there may be occasional nausea, vomiting, diarrhea and abdominal cramps, which can be lessened by dividing the dose into two or more portions. It should not be used if there is enterocolitis. The drug increases plasma levels of phosphate by an effect that increases renal resorption (probably indirectly through hormonal homeostasis), but no adverse effects have thus far been attributable to this effect. The drug does not appear to be teratogenic, but it increases the number of still-born fetuses in experimental animals, and it may also impair bone formation. Therefore, the drug should not be used during pregnancy, except in unusual circumstances.

It is 50% absorbed by the oral route. Various constituents in food and antacids, especially calcium, impair absorption. The distribution half-life is 5 to 7 hr; the elimination half-life is about 24 hr. The drug is eliminated entirely by renal excretion. Therefore, it should be used cautiously in renal failure. Urine hydroxyproline levels and serum alkaline phosphatase activity should be monitored periodically during treatment.

Dose—*Intravenous infusion, adult,* for *hypercalcemia, initially* **7.5 mg/kg** over a period of no less than 2 hr once a day for 3 days. *Oral, adults,* for *Paget's disease, initially* **5** to **10 mg/kg** a day, usually as a single dose, to be taken 2 hr before eating; when there is *accelerated disease* or *high cardiac output,* **10** to **20 mg/kg** a day may be given, but for no longer than 3 mo; *heterotopic ossification,* **20 mg/kg** a day for 1 mo prior to *surgery* and 3 mo afterwards or *initially* **20 mg/kg** a day for 2 wk then **10 mg/kg** a day for 10 wk after *spinal injury*; for *hypercalcemia,* **20 mg/kg** a day for 30 to 90 days.

Dosage Forms—Injection: 300 mg/6 mL; Tablets: 200 and 400 mg.

Gallium Nitrate

Nitric acid, gallium salt, nonahydrate: Ganite (*Fujisawa*)
$Ga(NO_3).9H_2O$

[135886-70-3] $GaN_3O_9.9H_2O$ (417.87)

Preparation—By dissolution of gallium metal or gallium oxide in nitric acid.

Description—White, deliquescent crystals; decomposes about 110°; forms Ga_2O_3 at 200°.

Solubility—Very soluble in water; soluble in anhydrous alcohol.

Uses—To treat cancer-related hypercalcemia unresponsive to adequate hydration. It inhibits calcium resorption from bone, possibly by reducing increased bone turnover. The precise mechanism has not been determined. The plasma half-life is 72 to 115 hr with a prolonged intravenous infusion and the major route of elimination is renal excretion.

Adverse effects include nephrotoxicity, transient hypophosphatemia, anemia and leukopenia. It should not be used with other nephrotoxic drugs.

Dose—*Intravenous infusion,* **100** to **200 mg/m²** over 24 hr for 5 days.

Dosage Form—Injection: 500 mg/20 mL.

Levothyroxine Sodium

l-Tyrosine, *O*-(4-hydroxy-3,5-diiodophenyl)-3,5-diiodo-, monosodium salt, hydrate; Levothroid (*USV*); Levoxine (*Daniels*) Synthroid (*Boots*); Synthrox (*Vortech*); Syroxine (*Major*); (*Various Mfrs*)

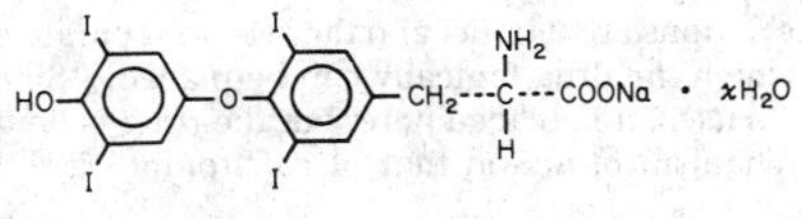

Monosodium L-thyroxine hydrate [25416-65-3] $C_{15}H_{10}I_4NNaO_4.xH_2O$; *anhydrous* [55-03-8] (798.86); the sodium salt of the levo isomer of thyroxine, an active physiological principle obtained from the thyroid gland of domesticated animals used for food by man, or prepared synthetically. It contains 61.6–65.5% of iodine, corresponding to 97–103% of levothyroxine sodium.

Preparation—L-Thyroxine is dissolved in dilute NaOH solution and the resulting sodium salt is precipitated by saturating the solution with NaCl.

Thyroxine may be prepared from thyroid glands or by synthesis. Preparation from the glands (fresh or desiccated) involves extraction with dilute sodium hydroxide followed by acidification with hydrochloric acid whereupon a very crude form of thyroxine is precipitated. Purification involves repeated solubilization by means of sodium hydroxide and reprecipitation with acid, these operations being conducted under increasingly refined conditions and with the aid of auxiliary operations designed to enhance the purity of the final precipitate of thyroxine.

The key compound in the synthesis of thyroxine is 3,5-diiodo-4-(*p*-methoxyphenoxy)nitrobenzene (I) which is readily formed by condensing *p*-methoxyphenol with 3,4,5-triiodonitrobenzene under the influence of anhydrous potassium carbonate. A series of subsequent operations involves (*a*) reduction of nitro to amino; (*b*) replacement of amino by cyano by treatment with cuprous cyanide and butyl nitrite; (*c*) hydration of cyano to carboxyl and (*d*) reduction of carboxyl to formyl. The resulting aldehyde may be converted into thyroxine in various ways. One involves condensation with 2-phenyl-2-oxazolin-5-one to produce II which is then simultaneously hydrogenated, demethylated and reductively cleaved by hydrogen iodide in the presence of phosphorus and acetic anhydride to give the DL-form of 3-[4-(4-hydroxyphenoxy)-3,5-diiodophenyl]alanine (III), which is resolved and the isolated L-enantiomorph is iodinated with ammoniacal potassium triiodide solution at the 3,5-positions on the phenoxy ring to give levothyroxine. Neutralization of this acid with NaOH yields the salt.

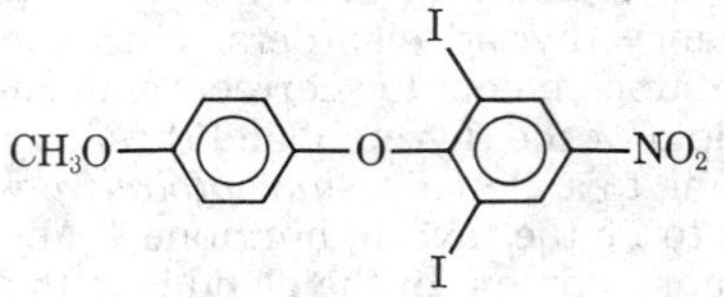

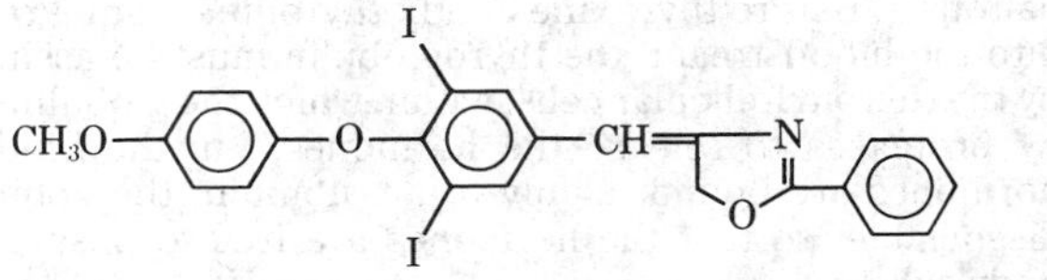

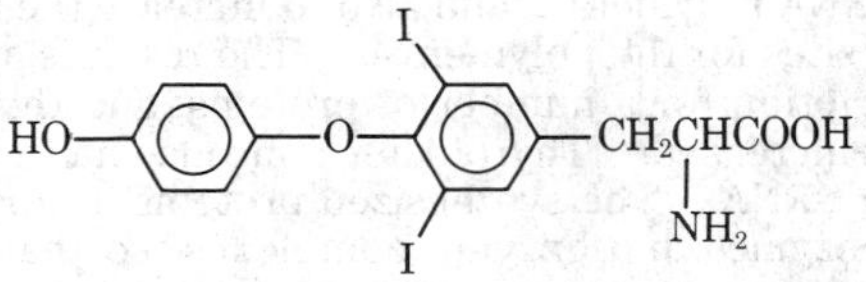

Description—Light yellow to buff-colored, odorless, tasteless, hygroscopic powder; stable in dry air but may assume a slight pink color upon exposure to light; pH (saturated solution) about 8.9.

Solubility—1 g in about 700 mL water or about 300 mL alcohol; insoluble in acetone, chloroform or ether; soluble in solutions of alkali hydroxides.

Uses—Has the actions, uses, side effects and limitations of *Thyroid.* The sodium salt lends itself to intravenous administration in the treatment of myxedemic coma, although the more rapidly acting liothyronine is preferred. Approximately 50% of an oral dose is absorbed. The plasma half-life is about 9 to 10 days in hypothyroid, 6 to 7 days in euthyroid and 3 to 4 days in hyperthyroid persons, but the time for the intensity of its effect to fall to ½ of its initial value is 9 to 12 days, and some residual effects may be apparent for several weeks after the last dose. Although the L-form is twice as active as the racemic mixture, it offers no particular therapeutic advantage over the DL-form, and it has the disadvantage of being more expensive.

Dose—*Intravenous,* for *myxedemic coma* or *stupor, initially* **400 μg** on the first day, to which 100 to 200 μg more may be added on day 2, after which the daily dose is decreased and finally converted to oral medication when the patient can tolerate it. *Intravenous* or *intramuscu-*

lar, adults, **50** to **100 μg** as a single dose; *children* **75%** of the appropriate **oral dose.** *Oral,* for *mild hypothyroidism* in *young* and *middle-aged adults, initially* **50 μg** a day, then adjusted by increments of 25 to 50 μg every 3 or 4 wk until a satisfactory response occurs; in *severe* hypothyroidism the *initial* dose **12.5** to **25 μg** a day and increments are 25 μg until a total daily dose of 100 μg is reached, after which the schedule for mild hypothyroidism is used; in *elderly adults, initially* **12.5** to **25 μg** a day for the first 6 wk, after which the dose is doubled every 6 to 8 wk until the desirable response is achieved; adult *maintenance* doses range from **100** to **200 μg** a day or **2** to **3 μg** a day up to 175 to 250 μg a day; *children under 6 mo,* **5** to **6 μg/kg** or **25** to **50 μg** a day; *6 to 12 mo,* **5** to **6 μg/kg** or **50** to **75 μg** a day; *1 to 5 yr,* **3** to **5 μg/kg** or **75** to **100 μg** a day; *6 to 12 yr,* **4** to **5 μg/kg** or **100** to **150 μg** a day; *over 12 yr,* **2** to **3 μg/kg** a day, not to exceed adult dose or 200 μg a day; *premature infants,* **25 μg** a day for 4 to 6 wk, then **50 μg** a day.

Dosage Forms—Injection: 200 and 500 μg/6 and 10 mL; Tablets: 25, 50, 75, 88, 100, 112, 125, 150, 175, 200 and 300 μg.

Liothyronine Sodium

L-Tyrosine, *O*-(4-hydroxy-3-iodophenyl)-3,5-diiodo-, monosodium salt; Cytomel (*SmithKline Beecham*); Liothyronine Sodium (*Various Mfrs*)

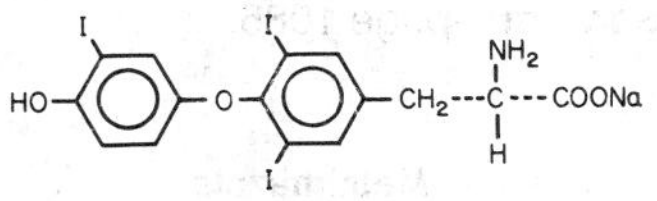

Monosodium L-3-[4-(4-hydroxy-3-iodophenoxy)-3,5-diiodophenyl]alanine [55-06-1] $C_{15}H_{11}I_3NNaO_4$ (672.96).

Preparation—3,5-Diiodo-L-thyronine, the L-enantiomorph of compound (III) in the thyroxine synthesis described under *Levothyroxine Sodium,* is dissolved in methanol and iodinated only at the 3-position by treatment with ammonia and iodine at room temperature. The liothyronine (acid) is then liberated by acidifying the reaction mixture. It is purified and neutralized with NaOH to give the salt.

Description—Light-tan, odorless, crystalline powder.

Solubility—Very slightly soluble in water; slightly soluble in alcohol; practically insoluble in most other organic solvents.

Uses—Three to ten times more potent than *Levothyroxine Sodium.* The actions and uses are those of *Thyroid* and *Levothyroxine Sodium,* except that it is considered to be more suitable for treatment of a vague syndrome known as *metabolic insufficiency,* which perhaps is due to a deficiency in tissue utilization of thyroxine, and experimentally for treatment of *male infertility* and certain *menstrual disorders* associated with hypothyroidism. It also has been used to *reduce goiter,* but it is less effective than Levothyroxine in suppressing TSH release. Because of the lesser pituitary suppression and the wide fluctuation in plasma levels, which negate monitoring, it is not the agent of choice for maintenance, especially after ablative radioiodine treatment. It is the treatment of choice to treat *myxedemic coma,* because of the rapid onset of action. It may be used to *suppress goiter* preparatory to surgery.

It has a rapid onset of action. The peak effect occurs in 1 to 3 days, and the offset of action is about 3 days. The prompt onset and rapid offset (compared to levothyroxine) are considered to be an advantage over thyroid or levothyroxine. The time for the intensity of its effect to fall to ½ of its initial value is 4 to 10 days. Liothyronine is erratically absorbed from the gastrointestinal tract, and 30 to 40% may be recovered from the stools. Liothyronine is only loosely bound to plasma proteins and hence does not elevate the plasma protein-bound iodine (PBI) significantly. It crosses the blood-brain barrier and hence is not recommended for use in children.

Dose—*Oral,* for *mild hypothyroidism* in *young* and *middle-aged adults, initially* **5 μg** a day with increments of 5 to 10 μg a day every 1 to 2 wk until 25 μg a day is reached, after which the daily dose is increased by 12.5 to 25 μg at intervals of 1 to 3 wk until the desired response is achieved (usually 50 to 100 μg); for *severe hypothyroidism, initially* **2.5** to **5 μg** a day for 1 to 3 wk, then increased by 5- to 10- μg increments to a *maintenance* dose of **25** to **50 μg** a day; in *older adults* and in patients with cardiovascular disease, *initially* **5 μg** a day for 3 to 6 wk, after which the dose is doubled every 6 wk until the desired response is obtained; in *simple nontoxic goiter,* initially **5 μg** a day, then increased by 5 to 10 μg a day at 1- to 2-wk intervals up to 25 μg a day, then by 12.5 to 25 μg a day every week to a *maintenance* dose of **50** to **100 μg** a day.

Dosage Form—Tablets: 5, 25 and 50 μg; Injection: 10 μg/mL.

Liotrix

Euthroid (*Warner-Chilcott*); Thyrolar (*Armour*)

A uniform mixture of synthetic levothyroxine sodium (T-4) and liothyronine sodium (T-3) in a 4:1 ratio by weight.

Uses—Since the endogenous thyroid hormone is actually not a single hormone but rather levothyroxine and liothyronine, some medical opinion holds that the 4:1 mixture in liotrix more closely approximates the normal physiological thyroid hormone in activity than either of the separate hormones. Furthermore, the effect on the protein-bound iodine more nearly correlates with the clinical response than that of either of the separate hormones, since the amount of iodine in equieffective doses of the two separate hormones differs by a factor of about 6 to 10.

Dose—*Oral, adult,* in *mild hypothyroidism, initially* **30 μg** of levothyroxine and **7.5 μg** of liothyronine a day, with equal increments at 2 wk intervals until the desired effect is achieved; in *myxedema* or patients with *cardiovascular disease,* **12.5 μg** of levothyroxine and **3.1 μg** of liothyronine a day, with equal increments at 2- to 3-wk intervals until the desired effect is achieved; for *maintenance* in both of the above, **60** to **120 μg** of levothyroxine and **15** to **30 μg** of liothyronine a day.

Dosage Form—Tablets: (T-4:T-3)—12.5 μg:3.1 μg, 25 μg:6.25 μg, 30 μg:7.5 μg, 50 μg:12.5 μg, 60 μg:15 μg, 100 μg:25 μg, 120 μg:30 μg, 150 μg:37.5 μg, and 180 μg:45 μg.

Pamidronate Disodium

Phosphonic acid, (3-amino-1-hydroxypropyl-idene)bis-, disodium salt, pentahydrate; Aredia (*Ciba*)

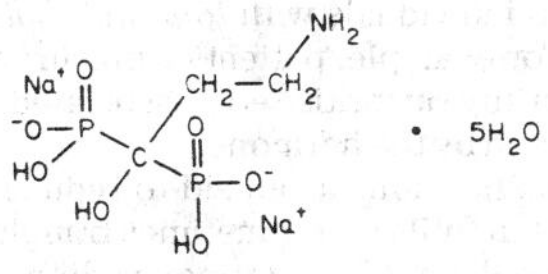

[109552-15-0]$C_3H_9NNa_2O_7P_2.5H_2O$ (369.11).

Preparation—US Pat 4,327,039.

Uses—Acts similarly to *Etidronate Disodium* and is used to inhibit bone resorption in treating hypercalcemia of malignancy. It differs from etidronate in that it does not inhibit bone formation. Its body retention is 49% of intravenous dose over a 72-hr period with a distribution half-life of 1.6 hr and plasma half-life of 27.2 hr. Bone uptake occurs preferentially in areas of high bone turnover. The rate of elimination from bone has not been determined.

Adverse effects include transient fever, infusion site reactions, fluid overload, generalized pain, hypertension, urinary infection and bone pain. Nausea and vomiting occur with doses of 90 mg.

Dose—*Intravenous infusion,* **60** to **90 mg** over 24 hr.

Dosage Form—Injection: 30 mg.

Thyroglobulin

Proloid (*Parke-Davis*)

A substance obtained by the fractionation of thyroid glands from the hog, *Sus scrofa* Linné var *domesticus* Gray (Fam *Suidae*). It contains not less than 0.7% of organically bound iodine (I) [9010-34-8].

Preparation—Hog thyroid glands are grouped and extracted with dilute aqueous sodium chloride solution. Adjusting the pH to the isoelectric point with acetic acid and heating precipitates the crude product which is then defatted with an appropriate solvent, dried, milled and blended.

Description—Cream- to tan-colored free-flowing powder that has a characteristic odor and taste; stable in air, heat and light, although it may deteriorate on prolonged exposure to strong light.

Solubility—Insoluble in water, alcohol or other common organic solvents.

Uses—A glycoprotein in the thyroid follicular lumen and epithelial cells that contains the iodinated thyroid hormones (see page 1082). The actions and uses of thyroglobulin are the same as for *Thyroid.* However, it is less likely to cause hypersensitivity, although it is not completely free of contaminating proteins; to this extent it may have some advantage over thyroid, but it is difficult to see any advantage over levothyroxine sodium or liothyronine sodium. It is twice as expensive as *Thyroid.*

Dose—*Oral, adult,* in *mild hypothyroidism, initially* **30 mg** a day with equal increments of 15 mg at 2- or 3-wk intervals until the desired effect is achieved; *maintenance,* usually **60** to **120 mg** a day; in *myxedema* or with *cardiovascular disease, initially* **15** to **30 mg** a day with equal increments at 2-wk intervals until the desired effect is achieved; for *maintenance,* in both of the above, **60** to **180 mg** a day. For *children,* for *cretinism* use the adult dose for myxedema; otherwise use the appropriate adult dose.

Dosage Form—Tablets: 30, 60, 90, 120 and 180 mg.

Thyroid

Desiccated Thyroid; Thyroid Extract; Thyroid Gland; (*Various Mfrs*)

The cleaned, dried and powdered thyroid gland previously deprived of connective tissue and fat. It is obtained from domesticated animals that are used for food by man.

Thyroid contains 0.17–0.23% of iodine (I) in thyroid combination, and is free from iodine in inorganic or any form of combination other than that peculiar to the thyroid gland. A desiccated thyroid of a higher iodine content may be brought to this standard by admixture with a desiccated thyroid of a lower iodine content or with lactose, sodium chloride, starch, sucrose or dextrose.

Description—Yellowish to buff-colored, amorphous powder, having a slight characteristic, meat-like odor and a saline taste.

Uses—Essential for normal metabolism and development. The congenital absence of thyroid hormone results in a condition known as *cretinism.* In childhood or adult life, absence of thyroid hormone causes *myxedema.* These conditions are characterized by an abnormally low basal metabolic rate. The primary therapeutic use is in their treatment.

These preparations may be used to *suppress the secretion of thyrotropin* in simple *nonendemic goiter* (hence decreases thyroid size) and chronic lymphocytic thyroiditis (Hashimoto's disease). These hormones do not decrease hyperthyroid exophthalamus. The use of them in the *diagnosis* of hyperthyroidism is outlined under *Liothyronine Sodium.*

It is often given to individuals with *low metabolic rates* unassociated with myxedema. For example, patients with chronic constipation, menstrual disorders, sterility, arthritis, etc, associated with a low metabolic rate, are often benefited by the hormone.

Employment of the hormone as an aid to reduce excessive weight is a frequent practice, often futile and sometimes fraught with danger. In the absence of hypothyroidism, these hormones do not improve skin conditions, mental depression, fatigue, lethargy, irritability, nervousness, menstrual irregularities and other endocrine and reproductive disorders, and there is danger that untoward effects may be produced.

Untoward effects of overdoses of these hormones include tachycardia, arrhythmias, angina pectoris, hypertension, insomnia, nervousness, hyperkinesis, tremors, diaphoresis, hot skin, gastrointestinal disturbances and hypoadrenocorticism. Even with physiological doses, it may be advisable to administer glucocorticoids concurrently. It may cause allergic reactions.

It has a very slow onset of action. A given dose does not exert its maximum effect for several days and will continue to have some degree of action for 2 to 3 mo. Therefore, caution must be exercised in judging the dose in that cumulative effects must be anticipated.

Dose—*Oral, adult,* for *mild hypothyroidism, initially usually* **30 mg** a day with increments of 15 mg every 2 to 3 wk until the desired effect is achieved: for *myxedema* or with *cardiovascular disease, initially* **15 mg** a day for 2 wk, 30 mg a day for 2 wk, 60 mg a day for 2 wk, then, if necessary, 120 mg a day for 2 mo, then even 180 mg a day; *maintenance,* for both of the above, usually **60** to **120 mg** a day, but failure to respond to 180-mg doses suggests a lack of compliance or malabsorption; in the *elderly, initially* **7.5** to **15 mg** a day, doubling every 6 to 8 wk, if necessary; *children,* for *cretinism,* adult dose for myxedema; otherwise use the appropriate adult dose. Doses of *Thyroid Strong* should be ⅓ less, since the preparation is 50% stronger than Thyroid.

Dosage Form—Tablets: 15, 30, 60, 90, 120, 180, 240 and 300 mg; Thyroid Strong Tablets: 30, 60, 120 and 180 mg.

Teriparatide Acetate—see RPS-18, page 981.

Antithyroid Drugs

A number of linear and heterocyclic derivatives of thiourea inhibit the production of thyroid hormone by the thyroid gland. The mechanism of action is that of preventing iodination of tyrosine and the coupling between iodotyrosines. They also inhibit the conversion of thyroxine to liothyronine in the periphery. The decline in thyroid hormone output and the resultant lowering of plasma levels of the thyroid hormones is sensed in the hypothalamus, which through the long-loop feedback and intermediation of the thyrotropin-releasing factor stimulates the adenohypophysis to produce more thyrotropic hormone. Consequently, the thyroid gland is stimulated to enlarge, even though the enlarged gland cannot produce more thyroid hormone.

Because of the thyroid enlargement consequent to the use of the thiourea class of antithyroid compounds, such compounds are called goitrogens. The goitrogens are employed in the control of *hyperthyroidism.* An enlarged thyroid gland is very vascular and friable, which makes surgery difficult. Therefore, iodine (or a thyroid hormone), which reduces the size of the gland, is added to the regimen preparatory to thyroid surgery.

Antithyroid drugs also decrease T-lymphocyte cytotoxicity and restore normal suppressor-cell activity and are thought thus to decrease thyroid autoimmunity in Grave's disease.

Several other classes of compounds also are antithyroid agents. Compounds such as thiocyanates and perchlorates competitively inhibit the iodine uptake mechanism. Large doses of iodine inhibit the enzyme tyrosine iodinase and thus interfere with the production of thyroid hormone. Therefore, iodine also may be used in the treatment of hyperthyroidism. Curiously, this action of iodine is not goitrogenic; in fact, iodine opposes the goitrogenic effects of certain antithyroid drugs. Radioiodine (^{131}I) is antithyroid by virtue of tissue destruction caused by radiation. Thyroid hormones are antigoitrogenic by the long-loop homeostatic feedback mechanism to reduce the hypothalamic release of thyrotropin-releasing factor.

Liothyronine Sodium—page 1085.

Methimazole

2*H*-Imidazole-2-thione, 1,3-dihydro-1-methyl-, Tapazole (*Lilly*)

1-Methylimidazole-2-thiol [60-56-0] $C_4H_6N_2S$ (114.16).

Preparation—One method consists of cyclizing (methylamino)acetaldehyde diethyl acetal with thiocyanic acid via de-ethanolation. Details are provided in *J Am Chem Soc 71:* 4000, 1949.

Description—White to pale buff, crystalline powder, having a faint characteristic odor; solutions are practically neutral to litmus; melting range 144 to 147°.

Solubility—1 g in 5 mL water, 5 mL alcohol, 4.5 mL chloroform or 125 mL ether.

Uses—An antithyroid drug for the preparation of the hyperthyroid patient for surgery and for the total treatment of *hyperthyroidism.* It is approximately 10 times as potent as *Propylthiouracil* and is more prompt in eliciting an antithyroid response. The drug also exhibits a more prolonged action than propylthiouracil; a single dose of 5 mg may inhibit the synthesis of thyroid hormone for 24 hr. The plasma half-life is 6 to 8.5 hr in hyperthyroid but 8 to 18 hr in hypothyroid patients; therefore, as the drug lowers the metabolic rate, its own metabolism is slowed, and accumulation will occur unless the dose is adjusted.

The toxic side effects are similar to those of *Propylthiouracil.* Approximately 6% of patients taking the drug experience some untoward effect. Thus, the incidence of untoward reactions is somewhat higher than with propylthiouracil, but considerably lower than with other antithyroid drugs. Cross-sensitization to other thiouracils can occur. Three times as much of this drug crosses the placental barrier as propylthiouracil, so that the former is the more likely to cause aplasiacutis.

Dose—*Oral, adult, initially* **15 mg** a day for *mild hyperthyroidism,* **30** to **40 mg** for *moderately severe hyperthyroidism* and **60 mg** or more for *severe hyperthyroidism,* given in 3 divided doses; once the patient is euthyroid (may require up to 2 mo!), the dose is diminished to **5** to **15 mg** a day for *maintenance.* In *children, initially* **400 µg/kg** a day in 3 divided doses 8 hr apart and, for *maintenance,* ⅓ to ⅔ of initial dose beginning when patient is euthyroid. For preparation *prior to thyroid surgery,* as above, except that when the patient becomes euthyroid **6 mg** a day of *iodine* for 10 days is added to the regimen. In *thyrotoxic crisis,* **15** to **20 mg** every 4 hr for the first day, followed by downward adjustments according to the response.

Dosage Form—Scored Tablets: 5 and 10 mg.

Potassium Iodide—page 976.

Propylthiouracil

4(1*H*)-Pyrimidinone, 2,3-dihydro-6-propyl-2-thioxo-, Propacil; (*Various Mfrs*)

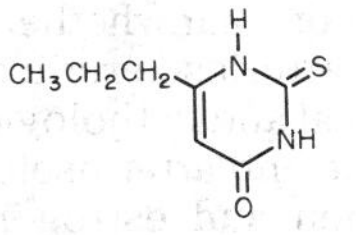

6-Propyl-2-thiouracil [51-52-5] $C_7H_{10}N_2OS$ (170.23).

Preparation—By condensation of ethyl 3-oxocaproate with thiourea (*J Am Chem Soc 67:* 2197, 1945).

Description—White, powdery, crystalline substance; starch-like in appearance and to the touch; bitter taste; melts about 220°.

Solubility—Slightly soluble in water; sparingly soluble in alcohol; slightly soluble in chloroform or ether; soluble in ammonia or alkali hydroxides.

Uses—See the introduction to this section. Since the drug does not interfere with the release or use of stored thyroid hormone, the period which elapses between the beginning of medication and the manifestations of its antithyroid action is dependent upon the quantity of thyroid hormone stored in the gland. The marked hyperplasia of the thyroid gland which follows its administration is a result of a compensatory increase of thyrotropin release consequent to a reduction in the thyroid hormone titer of the blood. In the *preparation of the hyperthyroid patient for surgery*, when treatment with the drug has brought the basal metabolic rate to normal (euthyroidism) or nearly so, iodine is administered to reduce the marked vascularity and friability of the gland. In the total (medical) *treatment of hyperthyroidism*, the duration of treatment usually ranges from 6 mo to 3 yr, after which time thyroid function may remain normal. However, at least half the patients so treated may be expected to have a recurrence 6 to 12 mo after cessation of medication. It also decreases mortality in *alcoholic liver disease*.

It exerts toxic actions in a small but significant number of patients. The most serious of these toxic actions are granulocytopenia, leukopenia, drug fever and dermatitis. Joint pains and urticaria may occur. Cross-sensitivity to other thiouracils may occur. A small percentage of patients experience nausea, abdominal discomfort, headache, drowsiness, vertigo, paresthesias and loss of taste sense. The overall incidence of untoward reactions to propylthiouracil is approximately 4%; the incidence of agranulocytosis approaches 0.5%. Therefore, the patient who receives chronic medication with this drug should be kept under close surveillance. The drug passes the placental barrier and may affect the fetus, so that during pregnancy the lowest possible dose should be used. It also is secreted into milk, and the drug should be withheld from nursing mothers.

Only about 75% is absorbed by the oral route. There is considerable confusion about the elimination half-life, probably because redistribution has been confused with elimination and because of analytical difficulties. The elimination half-life is probably about 3 to 5 hr in hyperthyroid, 6 to 8 hr in euthyroid and 24 to 34 hr in hypothyroid persons, so that as the drug decreases the metabolic rate, the dose should be adjusted accordingly, to avoid accumulation.

Dose—*Oral, adult,* for *hyperthyroidism, initially* **300** to **900 mg** a day in 3 or 4 divided doses at equal intervals, until the patient becomes euthyroid; *maintenance,* **50** to **600 mg** a day in 2 to 4 divided doses. *Neonates,* **10 mg/kg** a day in divided doses; *children 6 to 10 yr,* **50** to **150 mg** a day in 2 or 3 divided doses; *children 10 yr or older,* **150** to **300 mg** a day in 3 divided doses at 8-hr intervals. For *preparation* prior to *thyroid surgery,* as above, except that when the patient becomes euthyroid **6 mg** a day of *iodine* for 10 days is added to the regimen. In *thyrotoxic crises,* **200** every 4 to 6 hr during the 1st day, followed by downward adjustments according to the response.

Dosage Form—Tablets: 50 mg.

Sodium Iodide—page 977.

Sodium Iodide I 131—pages 844 and 861.

The Sex Hormones

The sex hormones, like the hormones of the adrenal cortex, are steroids. They may be classified into the following groups, according to chemical structure and physiological activity:

1. Estrogenic hormones (female).
2. Progestational hormone (female).
3. Androgenic hormones (male).

Groups (1) and (2) are known collectively as the *ovarian hormones.* They include synthetic as well as natural products.

Structure—The natural estrogens are all steroids (see Chapter 26) containing 18 carbon atoms, oxygenated at carbons 3 and 17. Ring A of all the estrogens is aromatic; some estrogenic hormones found in the urine of *Equidae* possess further unsaturation in Ring B.

Progesterone, the hormone of the corpus luteum, is a 21-carbon-atom steroid, possessing, like adrenal cortical steroids, an α,β-unsaturated ketone component in Ring A. It differs from the latter in that its C_{17} does not carry hydroxyl.

The natural androgenic steroids are 19-carbon-atom compounds. They are characterized by a partly or completely saturated ring A, and by either a hydroxyl or a keto group at C_3 and C_{17}.

As with all other classes of steroids, stereoisomerism is of fundamental importance with the sex hormones; and the α- and β-configuration conventions are applied in drawing the structural formulas.

The Ovarian Hormones

The ovaries serve the dual purpose of secreting the female hormones and producing the ova which, after the menarche, are liberated normally at the rate of one every 4 weeks. The ovaries secrete two principal types of hormones which are related intimately to the entire process of sex development and function. The first category of these hormones is the group of steroids named *estrogens.* The second category of ovarian steroidal hormone is the *luteal* or *progestational hormone* named *progesterone.* The ovaries also secrete small amounts of androgens, adrenal steroids and the nonsteroidal hormone relaxin (see below).

The ovarian production of hormones is regulated by the gonadotropic hormones of the anterior pituitary (see page 1058). However, the control of pituitary gonadotropin production is, in turn, modulated by the estrogens and progesterone, which in low plasma concentrations appear to stimulate and at high concentrations inhibit the production of FSH, LH and LRH. Thus, a complex positive and negative feedback system subserves the cyclic phenomena of ovulation and menstruation. The exact details in this concert are not known completely for humans. It is known that in women ovulation can be prevented by estrogens as the result of suppression of FSH production. However, estrogen alone is not satisfactory for oral contraception, owing to what is termed "breakthrough" bleeding, except when dangerously high doses of estrogen are used. In impractically large doses, progesterone also inhibits ovulation, presumably because of suppression of the production of the hypothalamic luteinizing hormone-releasing factor; furthermore, it can favor infertility by a second mechanism, namely, that of maintaining the endometrium in a hypoproliferative and hyposecretory state which is unfavorable to implantation of the fertilized ovum. It now is known that some progestins have an antifertility effect at doses well below those necessary to suppress endometrial proliferation and secretion.

Interest in oral contraceptives originally started with progestins. However, intermenstrual bleeding occurs during continuous treatment with many progestins, and it was found desirable to add estrogens, which, although they favor endometrial proliferation, have a hemostatic effect on uterine bleeding. Furthermore, the 19-norprogestogens originally were synthesized by a route that contaminated the intended product with an estrogen. It was accepted gradually that the estrogen not only helped normalize cyclic bleeding but also contributed to the contraceptive effect. In fact, some authorities argued that the estrogen alone was responsible for the antifertility effect and that the progestin was only promoting a normal mense. Now it is appreciated that progestins alone can be contraceptive in low doses which do not disturb the menses of many users.

Progestins alone avoid the drawbacks of estrogens, namely nausea, vomiting, headache, a tendency to venous thrombosis and other untoward effects, but they are less effective contraceptives than are the estrogens. The progestins have been combined with estrogens in oral contraceptives in a way such that anovulatory doses of estrogen are followed in sequence by a progestin, in order to simulate the sequence of hormone dominance during the estrous cycle and hence to allow a near-normal mense, but such sequential contraceptives are no longer available in the US.

The luteinized granulosa cells of the corpus luteum also produce *relaxin*, a peptide with a tertiary structure similar to insulin and some growth factors. There are two chains linked through disulfide bonds. The molecular weight is about 6000 daltons. It relaxes the estrogen-primed symphysis pubis and increases the viscous pliability of the cervix, thus assisting the birth canal to prepare for parturition. It also increases glycogen synthesis and water uptake by the myometrium and decreases uterine contractility, which suggests a role during gestation. During the menstrual cycle, blood levels are high just following the LH surge and during menstruation. Much of its physiology remains to be learned. Relaxin also is found in the placenta and uterus.

Another relaxing peptide, *lututrin*, is produced in the ovary. Very little is known of its physiological functions.

Relaxin and lututrin have been used to treat dysmenorrhea, premature labor, cervical dystocia and scleroderma, but efficacy never has been proved.

Natural Estrogenic Hormones and Congeners

Natural estrogenic hormones are secreted by the ovarian follicles. They stimulate or regulate the growth and development of the uterus, the vaginal mucous membrane and also other structures such as mammary glands, subcutaneous fat, axillary and pubic hair and certain elements in the skin. These latter comprise the secondary female sex characteristics. Therefore the estrogens also are called *female sex hormones*. Of the estrogens the most potent occurring naturally is β-*estradiol*, and its two principal metabolic products, *estrone* and *estriol*, which also are estrogenic. Several other products of metabolic change occur in smaller amounts, but these are not offered as single substances for therapy. Estrogens are secreted throughout the period of activity of the ovaries, but at varying rates at different times of the menstrual cycle.

The naturally occurring estrogens can be prepared synthetically, but at greater cost than by extraction from natural materials or by simple chemical processing of natural estrogens as they occur in urine. An interesting improvement of the natural estrogen has been the synthetic modification of β-estradiol, the most potent of natural estrogens, by the addition of a side chain, producing *ethinyl estradiol*. This has a very high activity when administered orally. All present-day estrogens are available in crystalline form, hence doses are expressed in terms of weight. Biological units still sometimes are referred to; biological assay is by the rapid cornification of the vaginal mucosae of spayed female rats.

Uses—Estrogens are used as *substitution therapy* when menopausal symptoms occur after cessation of ovarian function, following ovariectomy or X-ray or radium therapy, or in the natural menopause (also called the climacteric). The purpose of the treatment is to afford relief from any of a long list of complaints which are recognized widely as characteristic of the menopause. However, the use of estrogens for this purpose is not accepted universally. There is evidence that estrogens have clinically useful effects. There is general agreement that low-dose estrogen treatment will ameliorate the symptoms of vasomotor instability (hot flashes), prevent or reverse urogenital atrophy in menopausal women and slow or prevent postmenopausal osteoporosis, especially when given with calcium supplements, calcitriol and fluoride.

The beneficial effects of estrogen therapy on irritability, depression, anxiety, memory and insomnia are more unpredictable. It is not clear whether or not estrogen administration can prevent arteriosclerotic cardiovascular disease. Several epidemiological and pathological studies suggest that coronary heart disease and arteriosclerosis are less severe in premenopausal women and estrogen-treated men than in women without ovarian function or normal men. However, other influences among the various treatment groups such as the presence or absence of hypertension have been invoked to explain these data.

High-density lipoproteins are elevated by these drugs, but there is no evidence that changes in lipoprotein patterns decrease atherogenesis. However, any potential benefits of estrogen replacement therapy must be weighed against serious risk (see *Side Effects*, below).

A reasonable position at present regarding estrogen therapy in postmenopausal women seems to be an optimistic one. There is no compelling reason to withhold treatment from women suffering with debilitating vasomotor instability or in whom osteoporosis can be delayed. Whether or not cyclic or sequential use of estrogens or use of different preparations will decrease side effects significantly remains to be established, but sequential combinations with progestins appear to diminish adverse effects. It is clear that even very low doses of estrogens are effective against menopausal symptoms and have low toxicity. However, such low doses do not provide optimal prophylaxis against osteoporosis. Careful monitoring for untoward effects is mandatory with estrogen use.

Estrogens are used in young women in whom there is *failure of steroidogenesis;* treatment brings about acceleration of delayed development of the uterus, the appearance of secondary sex characteristics and subtle biochemical and behavioral changes. Applied locally, the estrogens are useful in the treatment of *atrophic* or *senile vaginitis, vulvovaginitis* or *cervicitis* resulting from hypoestrogenesis but not from other causes.

A number of menstrual irregularities may be treated with estrogens. Some of these, such as *amenorrhea*, may be the result of steroid agenesis. Some have various causes, among them an asynchrony in the release of hypothalamic release factors and pituitary gonadotropin release. Estrogens used cyclically may regularize some of these conditions; *secondary amenorrhea* is such a condition. They are of value in decreasing electrolyte imbalance, headache, tension, breast engorgement and nipple tenderness in *premenstrual tension*, but they are of dubious value in relieving neurological and mood changes in that disorder. In *dysmenorrhea* their efficacy is unproven, but if they are of value, it is in cyclic therapy. In *endometriosis*, estrogens are effective for only a short time, endometrial hyperplasia eventually resulting. In *dysfunctional uterine bleeding*, combined treatment with estrogens and progestogens is used, and normal withdrawal bleeding may follow the abrupt cessation of treatment.

Since estrogens suppress gonadotropin (FSH) release and also inhibit blastocyst implantation, they are used as *contraceptives* (see page 1058). A contrasting use is to assist reproduction as an adjunct in the *prevention of habitual abortion*. They may be used in the *induction of parturition* and in the postpartum period to reduce *breast engorgement*.

Estrogens decrease plasma cholesterol and hence have been used as *hypocholesteremic* drugs, but side effects are usually unacceptable to the male recipient. Estrogens also are used to treat *acne vulgaris* and *hirsutism*. They also are used to inhibit the growth of *prostatic cancer* of men and *carcinoma of the breast* or carcinoma elsewhere in the reproductive tract of women who are more than 4 years beyond the menopause (see Chapter 75, page 1236).

There is a choice of compounds for estrogenic therapy. Estrone is employed commonly by intramuscular injection.

Considerable activity is lost if the oral route is used. Ethinyl estradiol is the most active of all oral estrogens, and its oral activity is nearly equal to its parenteral activity. On a weight basis, estradiol benzoate is more powerful in action than estrone. Its action also is more sustained. It commonly is given by intramuscular injection. Estriol is considerably less active than estrone given hypodermically, and its activity following oral administration is probably too low to make it important. Conjugated estrogens (see page 986) retain much of their activity on oral administration and are used extensively by this route. Estrogens also can be given by inunction or with transdermal systems. In addition, various concentrates of estrogenic hormones are available.

Synthetic estrogens (see below), of which the best known is diethylstilbestrol, possess most of the therapeutic and untoward actions of the natural estrogenic hormones and are often cheaper. Since they lose little activity after oral administration, they have advantages over the natural estrogens, but the comparative toxicities are not clear.

Side Effects—Nausea and vomiting are frequent side effects of estrogens; these are claimed to be more frequent and intense with diethylstilbestrol (see *Synthetic Estrogens*, below). These effects appear to be mainly of central nervous system origin. Anorexia also is frequent. Although estrogens may decrease salt and water accumulation in premenstrual tension, they also may cause such retention. This retention may be one factor in the breast tenderness caused by estrogens. They also may cause breast engorgement, in part by promoting the proliferation of the secretory acini and ducts. High doses of estrogens often cause dizziness. Headache is more frequent with high doses but does occur even with low doses. Malaise, irritability and depression occasionally occur with small doses and frequently with large doses. The effect on libido is erratic, being increased in some and decreased in others.

Estrogens effect changes in the concentration of some of the clotting factors in blood, and there is considerable evidence that therapeutic doses of semisynthetic and synthetic estrogens increase the incidence of thrombophlebitis and thromboembolism in both the superficial and deep veins. These disorders are favored additionally by venodilation caused by the drugs. Pulmonary embolism, cerebral embolism with stroke and mesenteric vascular occlusion occur. Coronary thrombosis also seems to be increased among users of estrogens. The incidence of these pathologies is low but definite. Women over 35 years and having blood type O are most susceptible. Evidence that replacement doses of natural estrogens favor thromboembolic disorders is not at hand.

Estrogens alter hepatic function, which may alter various tests of liver function as well as various synthetic and biotransformation processes. There may be a decrease in glucose tolerance, and diabetes mellitus may be exacerbated. Serum triglycerides rise, and dangerous hyperlipidemia may occur in persons who already have a Type-4 hyperlipidemia. 17-"Alkyl" derivatives, especially, occasionally cause cholestatic jaundice. Estrogens sometimes favor hepatic adenomas.

The composition of the bile is altered, and there is a slightly increased incidence of gallstones after long-term use. Although rare, porphyria may be provoked. Changes in the concentration of blood proteins may occur; thyroxine- and glucocorticoid-binding proteins are increased, which may alter endocrine relationships. Aldosterone secretion is increased, which not only accounts for sodium retention but also for an abnormal incidence of hypertension among users of estrogens. Estrogen-induced hypertension is reversible.

Estrogens may induce changes in the skin, such as itching, increased pigmentation (in combination with progestins, causes chloasma), a tendency to candidiasis (also in the vagina) and spider angiomas. Pigmentation caused by diethylstilbestrol is marked especially in the nipples and facies. Photosensitization may occur, and protective measures are advisable. Although estrogens may improve acne, they only do so after a temporary worsening of the condition. Estrogens may cause a loss of scalp hair in some users and hypertrichosis in others. Allergic reactions include rashes, erythema multiforme, erythema nodosum and cholestatic jaundice.

It has long been held that estrogens increase the incidence of breast cancer in premenopausal women. However, the incidence is not increased among users of oral contraceptives, so that this belief is nonsupportable at present.

Estrogens increase the risk of cervical and endometrial carcinoma, and periodic examinations are advisable. When diethylstilbestrol is taken during pregnancy, there is an increased likelihood of vaginal adenocarcinoma in the daughter after maturity; whether natural and semisynthetic estrogens are similarly fetotoxic is not known. There also is an increased likelihood of functional abnormalities in the reproductive tracts in both female and male offspring.

It has long been stated that estrogens cause premature arrest of growth and epiphyseal closure in girls, but the subject requires greater study. Neuroophthalmic lesions during estrogen treatment have been described. Hypercalcemia may occur, especially in men taking large doses for prostatic carcinoma.

In women, chronic use may cause spotting or breakthrough vaginal bleeding; after discontinuation, withdrawal bleeding usually occurs.

For a discussion of the role of estrogens in the adverse effects of oral contraceptives, see under *Oral Contraceptives. Adverse Effects*.

Pharmacokinetics—Naturally occurring estrogens are not effective orally because they are destroyed almost totally in a single pass through the liver (first-pass effect). Oral effectiveness can be improved by administration of conjugated or esterified estrogens, by use of synthetic estrogens that are metabolized more slowly, or, in the case of estradiol, by preparation of the drug in a micronized form that is absorbed into the thoracic duct rather than into the portal circulation. Estrogens are absorbed rapidly from intramuscular sites, mucous membranes, skin and other sites of therapeutic application. The half-life of estradiol is 40 to 50 minutes, but other estrogens persist much longer.

Estrogens circulate in both free and conjugated forms. These are bound in varying amounts to albumin and to a specific sex hormone binding globulin (SSHBG).

Estrogens are excreted primarily in the conjugated form in urine. Some free estrogen is secreted in bile from which some is excreted in feces and most return to the systemic circulation by the enterhepatic route. Estrogens are excreted in breast milk, so their use in nursing mothers is not recommended.

Drug Interactions—Drugs that induce the hepatic microsomal mixed oxygenase system (eg, phenobarbital, phenytoin, rifampin, etc) will accelerate estrogen metabolism. Estrogens antagonize oral anticoagulants and also interfere with tests of coagulation. They also interfere with tests of thyroid function. By an unknown mechanism, estrogens increase the effects of tricyclic antidepressants.

Estradiol

(17β)-Estra-1,3,5(10)-triene-3,17-diol; 17-Beta-estradiol; (*Various Mfrs*)

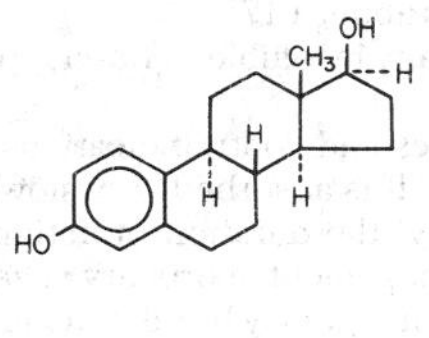

Dihydrotheelin; [50-28-2] $C_{18}H_{24}O_2$ (272.39).

Preparation—Has been isolated from ovarian follicular fluid and from placental tissue, and is the most potent of the natural estrogens. It is usually prepared through reduction of the 17-keto group of *Estrone*.

It is curious that the urine of stallions and of the males of other *Equidae* contains 3 to 5 times as much estradiol as that of the female of the species.

Description—White or creamy white, small crystals or a crystalline powder; odorless and stable in air; hygroscopic; melts about 175°.

Solubility—1 g in 28 mL alcohol, 435 mL chloroform or 150 mL ether; practically insoluble in water.

Uses—A natural estrogen used for *replacement* mainly in the postmenopause but also in ovarian hypofunction and after ovarectomy. It has a high, presystemic elimination rate, hence a low bioavailability by the oral route. However, a micronized preparation (*Estrace*) is absorbed rapidly enough to flood the pertinent liver enzyme sufficiently that oral administration is feasible. Transdermal systems also are used effectively for replacement. Intravaginal estradiol works topically in *atrophic vaginitis*, but the action to correct *kraurosis vulvae* is probably partly systemic. Estradiol is considerably converted to estrone in the body. The half-life is about 1 hr.

Dose—*Intravaginal, adult,* **200** to **400 μg** as a **0.01%** cream (2 to 4 g of cream) a day for 1 to 2 wk, then **100 μg** 1 to 3 times a wk until a normal vaginal mucosa is achieved. *Oral, adults,* for *replacement* therapy, **1** to **2 mg** a day for 21 days, to be repeated cyclically every 28 days; for *breast cancer,* **10 mg** 3 times a day for at least 3 mo; *prostatic cancer,* **1** to **2 mg** 3 times a day; for *osteoporosis prevention,* **0.5 mg** a day cyclically (3 wk on, 1 wk off). *Transdermal,* for *replacement,* **1 system,** to deliver **50** or **100 μg** a day, twice a week for 3 wk, then a 1-wk rest, each month.

Dosage Forms—Vaginal Cream: 0.01%; Scored Tablets: 1 and 2 mg; Transdermal System: to deliver 50 or 100 μg a day.

Estradiol Cypionate

(17β)-Estra-1,3,5(10)-triene-3,17-diol, 17-cyclopentanepropanoate; Estradiol Cyclopentylpropionate NF XI; (*Various Mfrs*)

Estradiol 17-cyclopentanepropionate [313-06-4] $C_{26}H_{36}O_3$ (396.57).

For the structure of the parent, see *Estradiol.*

Preparation—Estradiol is esterified at both the 3- and 17-positions by treatment with cyclopentylpropionyl chloride in pyridine, the diester being recovered in the usual way by pouring the reaction mixture into an excess of cold, dilute hydrochloric acid. The solid 3,17-diester is collected and treated with potassium carbonate in aqueous methanol whereby saponification is effected only at the 3-position. Water is then added, and the crude 17-ester which precipitates is collected and crystallized from 80% methanol.

Description—White to practically white, odorless, crystalline powder; melting range 149 to 153°.

Solubility—1 g in > 10,000 mL water, 40 mL alcohol, 7 mL chloroform or 2800 mL ether.

Uses—The same actions and uses as *Estradiol* and its other esters (see *Estradiol Valerate*). However, intramuscularly injected vegetable oil solutions of the cypionate have a more-prolonged action than do those of the benzoate or valerate. The average duration of action is 3 to 8 wk.

Dose—*Intramuscular, adults,* for female *hypogonadism,* **1.5** to **2 mg** once a mo; *postmenopausal,* for vasomotor instability, **1** to **5 mg** every 3 or 4 wk.

Dosage Form—Injection (in oil): 10 and 50 mg/10 mL and 25 mg/5 mL.

Estradiol Valerate

(17β)-Estra-1,3,5(10)-triene-3,17-diol, 17-pentanoate; Delestrogen (*Squibb*); (*Various Mfrs*)

Estradiol 17-valerate [979-32-8] $C_{23}H_{32}O_3$ (356.50).

For the structure of the parent, see *Estradiol.*

Preparation—By the method described above for the cypionate, using valeryl chloride as the esterificant.

Description—White, crystalline powder; usually odorless but may have a faint, fatty odor; melts about 147°.

Solubility—Practically insoluble in water; sparingly soluble in sesame oil and peanut oil.

Uses—Its action, uses and contraindications are those of other estrogens (see page 1087). It is absorbed very slowly from an oil suspension injected intramuscularly; the duration of action of suspensions in oil is about 3 wk. In the management of primary or secondary amenorrhea and functional uterine bleeding, it may be administered along with the progestational agent employed.

Dose—*Intramuscular,* for *replacement,* **10** to **20 mg** every 4 wk; for *postpartum breast engorgement* and to *suppress lactation,* **10** to **25 mg,** at the end of the 1st stage of labor; for *prostatic carcinoma, initially* **30 mg** every 1 or 2 wk, to be adjusted as necessary.

Dosage Form—Injection (in oil): 50, 100 and 200 mg/5 mL and 100, 200 and 400 mg/10 mL.

Conjugated Estrogens

Premarin (*Wyeth-Ayerst*); Progens (*Major*)

A mixture containing the sodium salts of the sulfate esters of the estrogenic substances, principally estrone and equilin, that are of the type excreted by pregnant mares. Conjugated estrogens contains 50–65% of sodium estrone sulfate, and 20–35% of sodium equilin sulfate, calculated on the basis of the total estrogens content.

Preparation—The urine of pregnant mares is subjected to a solvent extraction process. US Pat 2,565,115 and 2,720,483.

Description—Buff-colored powder; odorless or with a slight, characteristic odor.

Solubility—Soluble in water.

Uses—See *Estrone.* Estrone sulfate, the principal constituent of these substances, retains a greater potency by the oral route than does estrone, so that it is superior for oral administration. Some clinical opinion holds that this mixture causes fewer and milder gastrointestinal side effects than other estrogens.

It has been advocated for rapid control of spontaneous "capillary bleeding" and to reduce "capillary bleeding" in surgery. However, in controlled studies no short-term hemostatic effect has been found, although such effects may result from chronic use.

Dose—*Intramuscular* or *intravenous,* in *dysfunctional uterine bleeding,* **25 mg,** repeated in 6 to 12 hr, if necessary. *Intravaginal,* for *atrophic vaginitis* and *kraurosis vulvae,* **2** to **4 g** of a **0.0625%** cream a day for 3 wk of each month. *Oral,* in *menopause, postmenopause, primary ovarian failure,* or *postovariectomy,* **0.625** to **1.25 mg** a day for 21 days, to be repeated cyclically every 28 days; *osteoporosis,* **0.625 mg** a day cyclically; in *hypogonadism* (hypoestrogenesis) and *amenorrhea,* **2.5** to **7.5 mg** a day for 20 days followed by a rest for 10 days, to be repeated cyclically until menstruation occurs (a progestin may be added during days 16 to 20); for *postcoital contraception,* **10 mg** 3 times a day for 5 days; for *prostatic carcinoma* **1.25** to **2.5 mg** 3 times a day; in *carcinoma* of the *breast,* **10 mg** 3 times a day for at least 3 mo.

Dosage Forms—Cream: 0.0625%, for Injection: 25 mg; Tablets: 0.3, 0.625, 0.9, 1.25 and 2.5 mg.

Esterified Estrogens

Estratab (*Solvay*); Menest (*Beecham*)

A mixture of the sodium salts of the sulfate esters of the estrogenic substances, principally estrone, that are of the type excreted by pregnant mares. Esterified estrogens contains 75–85% of sodium estrone sulfate, and 6–15% of sodium equilin sulfate, calculated on the basis of the total esterified estrogens content.

Description—White or buff-colored, amorphous powder; odorless or has a slight characteristic odor.

Uses and **Dose**—See *Conjugated Estrogens, oral administration only.*

Dosage Form—Tablets: 0.3, 0.625, 1.25 and 2.5 mg.

Estrone

Estra-1,3,5(10)-trien-17-one, 3-hydroxy-, Theelin (*Parke-Davis*); *Various Mfrs*

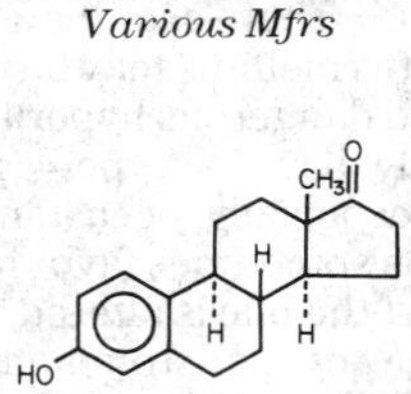

Folliculin; [53-16-7] $C_{18}H_{22}O_2$ (270.37).

Preparation—The first sex hormone isolated in pure form (Doisy and Allen in 1929). It is present, along with traces of other estrogens, in the urine of pregnant mares to the extent of about 10 mg/L and was formerly obtained exclusively from this source. It has also been prepared "synthetically" from stigmasterol, a phytosterol found in soya bean oil. Urinary estrone is regarded as resulting from the metabolic oxidation of the 17-hydroxy group of estradiol to a ketone group.

Estrone may be prepared from the Mexican yam (*Dioscorea*) via 16-dehydropregnenolone acetate as outlined in the synthesis of *Progesterone* (page 1097). The side chain at position-17 is degraded by first forming the 20-oxime and then effecting a Beckmann rearrangement with *p*-acetamidobenzenesulfonyl chloride to the 17-acetamido derivative, which on treatment with dilute sulfuric acid forms the enamine acetate and is hydrolyzed to the 17-keto compound, estrone.

Note—The estrogenic activity of 0.1 μg of crystalline estrone constitutes the International Unit of estrogenic activity.

Description—Small, white crystals, or a white to creamy white, crystalline powder; odorless and stable in air; melts at about 260°.

Solubility—1 g in 250 mL alcohol (15°) or 110 mL chloroform (15°); practically insoluble in water; soluble in vegetable oils.

Uses—See the introduction to this section.

Dose—*Intramuscular,* in *female hypogonadism, primary ovarian failure,* or *postovariectomy, initially* **0.1** to **2 mg** a wk in 1 to 3 divided doses for 3 wk of each month; for *kraurosis vulvae, atrophic vaginitis* or *vasomotor instability,* **0.1** to **0.5 mg** 2 or 3 times a wk for 3 wk of each month; for *abnormal uterine bleeding,* **2** to **5 mg** a day for several days; for *carcinoma of the prostate,* **2** to **4 mg** 2 or 3 times a wk.

Dosage Form—Aqueous Suspension: 20 and 50 mg/10 mL, 60 mg/30 mL. In several products, estrone potassium sulfate is included for a prompt action.

Estropipate

Estra-1,3,5(10)-trien-17-one, 3-(sulfooxy)-, compound with piperazine (1:1); Ogen (*Abbott*)

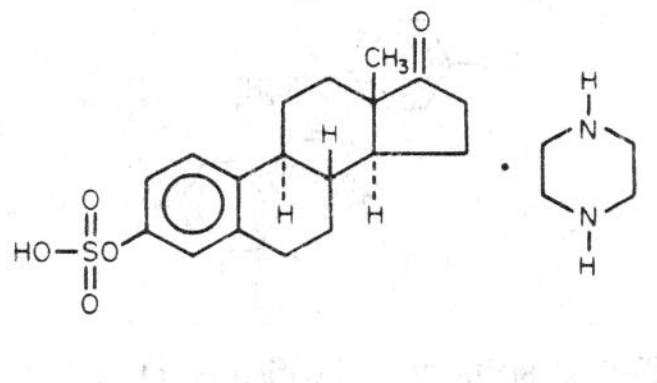

Piperazine estrone sulfate (1:1) [7280-37-7] $C_{18}H_{22}O_5S.C_4H_{10}N_2$ (436.56).

Preparation—Estrone is reacted with SO_3 in *N,N*-dimethylformamide and piperazine is then added in excess whereby the product precipitates. US Pat 3,525,738.

Description—White to yellowish white, fine, crystalline powder; odorless or may have a slight odor; melts about 190° to a light-brown viscous liquid which solidifies on further heating, and finally melts about 245° with decomposition.

Solubility—1 g in 2000 mL water, alcohol, chloroform or ether.

Uses—Has the same actions and limitations as *Estrene.* The cream is used in the treatment of atrophic vaginitis and kraurosis vulvae.

Dose—*Oral, adults,* for *menopause, postmenopause,* or *postovariectomy,* **0.625** to **7.5 mg** a day for 3 wk of each month; for, *osteoporosis prevention,* **0.625 mg** a day for 25 days of a 31-day cycle per month. *Intravaginal,* **2** to **4 g** of a **0.15%** cream daily for 3 of every 4 wk.

Dosage Forms—Tablets: 0.625, 1.25, 2.5 and 5 mg (of estrone sodium sulfate equivalent); Vaginal Cream: 0.15%.

Ethinyl Estradiol

(17α)-19-Norpregna-1,3,5(10)-trien-20-yne-3,17-diol, 17- Ethynylestradiol; (*Various Mfrs*)

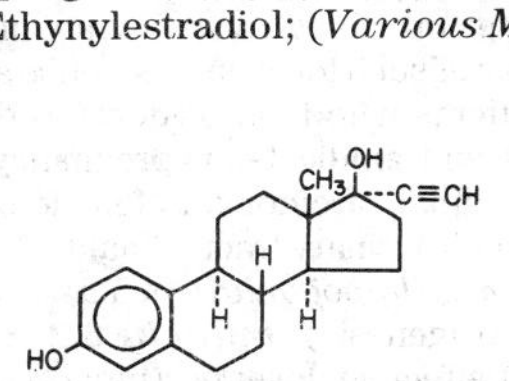

[57-63-6] $C_{20}H_{24}O_2$ (296.41).

Preparation—By the Nef reaction, or a modification thereof, whereby estrone is caused to react with sodium acetylide in liquid ammonia. Hydrolysis of the sodoxy addition complex yields the desired carbinol. It also may be prepared by a typical Grignard reaction from estrone and ethynyl magnesium bromide.

Description—White to creamy white, odorless, crystalline powder; melting range 180 to 186°; also exists in a polymorphic modification melting between 142 and 146°.

Solubility—Insoluble in water; soluble in alcohol, chloroform or ether.

Uses—Has the actions, uses and limitations of the other estrogens (see page 1087). It has an anovulatory effect at relatively low doses; it is the most widely used estrogen in oral contraceptive combinations. The ethinyl radical delays the decomposition of the estradiol molecule that occurs during absorption by the oral route. It is one of the most potent oral estrogens known.

Dose—*Oral,* for *postmenopausal vasomotor instability,* **20** to **50 μg** a day for 21 days, to be repeated cyclically every 28 days; for *female hypogonadism,* **50 μg** 1 to 3 times a day for 14 days each month with progestin during the last 2 wk to be repeated cyclically; for *secondary amenorrhea,* as above, except cycling is stopped after 3 to 6 cycles to see if normal cycling will take over; for inoperable *prostatic cancer,* **150 μg** to **2 mg** a day; for inoperable *breast cancer* in postmenopausal women, *initially* **1 mg** 3 times a day.

Dosage Form—Tablets: 20, 50 and 500 μg.

Ethinyl Estradiol and Ethynodiol Diacetate Tablets—page 1099.

Ethinyl Estradiol and Levonorgestrel Tablets—page 1099.

Ethinyl Estradiol and Norethindrone Acetate Tablets—page 1099.

Ethinyl Estradiol and Norgestrel Tablets—page 1100.

Quinestrol

(17α)-19-Norpregna-1,3,5(10)-trien-20-yn-17-ol, 3-(cyclopentyloxy)-, Estrovis (*Parke-Davis*)

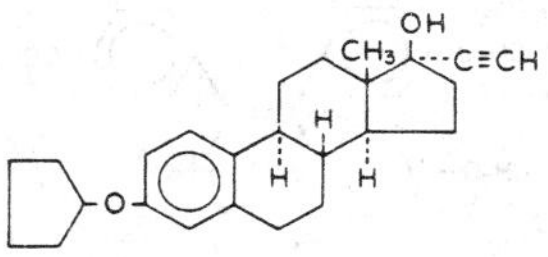

[152-43-2] $C_{25}H_{32}O_2$ (364.53).

Preparation—US Pat 3,231,567.

Description—White powder; melts about 108°.

Solubility—Practically insoluble in water; soluble in alcohol, chloroform or ether.

Uses—For estrogen replacement therapy, primarily for relief of vasomotor symptoms. This cyclopentyl ether of ethinyl estradiol is stored in adipose tissue after oral absorption. It is released slowly and metabolized to the parent compound. Side effects occur infrequently and are similar to other estrogens.

Dose—*Oral, initially* **100 μg** a day for 7 days, followed by a maintenance dose of 100 to 200 μg per week. Cyclic therapy should be considered as a regimen more in keeping with the principles of estrogen treatment.

Dosage Form—Tablets: 100 μg.

Synthetic Estrogens

The exciting discovery by Dodds *et al* in 1938 that diethylstilbestrol and other relatively simple nonsteroidal organic compounds possess estrogenic activity gave considerable impetus to research in this field during the next decade. This research was designed to discover compounds that had more favorable therapeutic indices because of either greater potency or lesser toxicity. Hundreds of compounds were synthesized and tested and numerous methods for the synthesis of these compounds starting with readily available materials have been devised.

Attempts to explain why such nonsteroidal compounds are estrogenically potent have been intriguing. Dodds pointed out that when the formulas are written appropriately there is a spatial resemblance between them and the true hormone estradiol. Others have focused attention on the closeness of the dimensions of the synthetics (especially length, width and distance between OH groups) with those of estradiol. The synthetic estrogens combine with the same cytoplasmic receptors as natural estrogens and presumably also with the same nuclear receptor. The configuration of methallenestril does not conform to the hypothetical dimensions prerequisite to estrogenic activity.

Synthetic estrogens are less expensive than natural ones, and they have a greater bioavailability. Regarding the latter it must be recalled that the oral doses of natural estrogens, with the possible exception of ethinyl estradiol (a derivative of a natural estrogen), may have to be five or more times that of the parenteral doses to secure similar results. This is the result of first-pass metabolism, excretion into bile and destruction in the intestines. One disadvantage of some synthetic estrogenic compounds is that nausea follows the use of even the minimum effective dose in some women, but probably not over 20% of those who use the materials carefully. It is most distressing in the first 2 weeks of use, after which tolerance develops. In such women the synthetic materials must be replaced by natural products. One other slight difference, which is possibly debatable, is the general impression that the natural estrogens give the patient a greater feeling of well-being than do the synthetics. Whether the synthetic estrogens are more toxic than natural estrogens is not established unequivocally, but diethylstilbestrol differs significantly from natural compounds (see the introduction and *Diethylstilbestrol*).

Chlorotrianisene

Benzene, 1,1′,1″-(1-chloro-1-ethenyl-2-ylidene)tris [4-methoxy]-, TACE (*Marion Merrell Dow*)

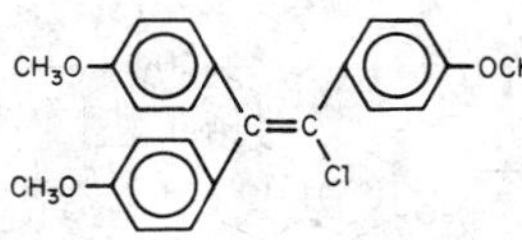

Chlorotris(*p*-methoxyphenyl)ethylene, [569-57-3] $C_{23}H_{21}ClO_3$ (380.87).

Preparation—An alcoholic solution of anisaldehyde is refluxed with potassium cyanide to yield anisoin which may be converted to deoxyanisoin (I) by reduction with zinc and hydrochloric acid. Performing a Grignard reaction on I with *p*-methoxyphenylmagnesium bromide yields 1,1,2-tri-*p*-anisylethanol (II). Dehydration of II by treatment with phosphoric acid produces 1,1,2-tri-*p*-anisylethene which is chlorinated directly in carbon tetrachloride solution. The resulting crude chlorotrianisene is purified by recrystallization from an acetone-alcohol mixture.

Description—Small white crystals, or as a crystalline powder; odorless and stable in air; exhibits polymorphism, one form melting about 116° and the other at about 118°.

Solubility—1 g in about 4200 mL water, 360 mL ethanol, 28 mL ether or 1.5 mL chloroform.

Uses—An estrogen with most of the actions, uses and limitations of the other estrogens. See page 1087. However, it is unique in that its potency is greater by the oral than by any other route, because drug is converted in the liver to a more active form. Also, it apparently induces less anterior pituitary and adrenal hyperplasia than other estrogens. In fact, it appears to be *anti*estrogenic at the hypothalamic locus that regulates adenohypophyseal gonadotropin release. Furthermore, it causes a lesser incidence of withdrawal bleeding. It is stored in the fat, from which it is released slowly to give a sustained action. The consequent long duration of action makes this drug unsuitable for the treatment of menstrual disorders or other conditions in which cyclic therapy is desired.

Dose—*Oral, adults,* for *postmenopause, postovariectomy* or *prostatic carcinoma,* **12** to **25 mg** a day; in *female hypogonadism* (hypoestrogenesis), **12** to **25 mg** a day for 21 days (with a progestogen on days 17 to 21), the cycle to be repeated after the 5th day of induced menstruation; for *senile vaginitis* or *kraurosis vulvae,* **12** to **25 mg** a day cyclically for 1 or 2 cycles; to *prevent postpartum breast engorgement,* **12 mg** 4 times a day for 7 days or **50 mg** every 6 hr for 6 doses, the first dose to be given within 8 hr of delivery for an immediate postpartum effect; for *prostatic carcinoma,* **12** to **25 mg** a day.

Dosage Form—Capsules: 12 and 25 mg.

Dienestrol

Phenol, (*E, E*)-4,4′-(1,2-diethylidene-1,2-ethanediyl)bis-, Dienoestrol (*Ortho*); DV (*Marion Merrell Dow*)

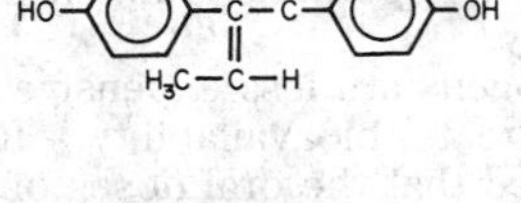

4,4′-(Diethylideneethylene)diphenol [84-17-3] $C_{18}H_{18}O_2$ (266.34).

Preparation—Among other methods, from diethylstilbestrol diacetate. Saturation of the olefinic bond with bromine yields the dibromo derivative which is then dehydrobrominated by refluxing with pyridine to yield dienestrol diacetate. Saponification then yields dienestrol.

Description—Colorless or white, or practically white, odorless needle-like crystals, or a white, crystalline powder; melts within a range of 3° between 227 and 234°.

Solubility—Practically insoluble in water; soluble in alcohol or ether; slightly soluble in chloroform.

Uses—A potent estrogen, now used only topically, for the treatment of *atrophic vaginitis* and *kraurosis vulvae.* It should not be used in patients with known or suspected cancer of the breast, known or suspected estrogen-dependent neoplasia, undiagnosed abnormal genital bleeding, active thrombophlebitis or thromboembolic disorders or a past history of such conditions, hypersensitivity to the ingredients of the cream or suppositories of dienestrol or during pregnancy.

Dose—*Intravaginal,* as **0.01%** cream 1 or 2 times a day for 7 to 14 days, the frequency afterward gradually reduced to 1 to 3 times a week.

Dosage Form—Cream: 0.01%

Diethylstilbestrol

Phenol, (*E*)-4,4′-(1,2-diethyl-1,2-ethenediyl)bis-, DES; (*Various Mfrs*)

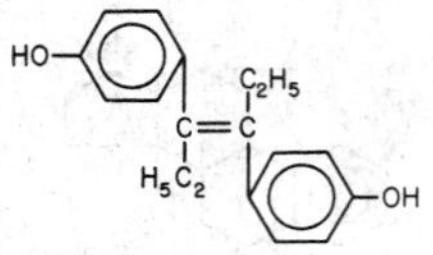

α,α′-Diethyl-(*E*)-4,4′-stilbenediol [56-53-1] $C_{18}H_{20}O_2$ (268.35).

Preparation—A synthetic estrogen first synthesized by Dodds *et al* in 1938. As to be expected, the compound exists in 2 geometric isomeric forms. The *cis*-isomer(*Z*), which has less than one-tenth the activity of the *trans*(*E*) and does not form readily, is unstable and tends to revert to the *trans*-isomer; hence the official product is *trans*-diethylstilbestrol.

Several methods of synthesis have been devised. That of Kharasch and Kleiman (*Medicinal Chemistry,* vol II, Wiley, New York, 1956) uses anethole hydrobromide as the starting material and is most convenient.

Description—White, odorless, crystalline powder; melts within a range of 4° between 169 and 175°.

Solubility—Practically insoluble in water; soluble in alcohol, ether, chloroform, fatty oils or dilute alkali hydroxides.

Uses—For the same conditions for which natural estrogens are employed; see page 1087 for uses, contraindications and side effects. It is advantageous because it is absorbed well orally. Because the rate of inactivation is slow, it can be administered orally in single daily doses even with large doses.

In large doses it is used as an emergency postcoital contraceptive; it is not to be used routinely but only after rape or in other emergencies, because the total amount given is equivalent to a several-months' estrogen requirement. Success is 100% if the drug is used within 72 hr of insemination.

Nausea and vomiting appear to be caused, in part, by local actions of the drug. Enteric coatings on tablets slow the rate of release and lessen the incidence and intensity of such local effects. It is advised to start with the smaller doses for patients who tend to develop disagreeable symptoms such as nausea. It is contraindicated in pregnancy because of the danger of inducing a latent vaginal carcinoma in female offspring and structural abnormalities in the genitourinary tract in male offspring.

Dose—*Oral,* in *female hypogonadism, castration* or *primary ovarian failure,* (hypoestrogenesis), *initially* **0.2** to **0.5 mg** a day, to be adjusted to the lowest effective dose; *postmenopausal vasomotor instability, atrophic vaginitis* or *pruritus vulvae,* **1** and occasionally **2 mg** a day until a response occurs; *postmenopausal* or *postovariectomy,* **0.2** to **0.5 mg** a day; for *prostatic carcinoma, initially* **1** to **3 mg** a day; for *breast carcinoma* in postmenopausal women, *initially* **15 mg** a day, then gradually adjusted upward to the limit of tolerance; for *postcoital emergency contraception (use not currently included in labeling approved by FDA),* **25 mg** twice a day for 5 days, starting within 72 hr of insemination.

Dosage Forms—Tablets: 1, 2.5 and 5 mg.

Diethylstilbestrol Diphosphate

Phenol, (*E*)-4,4′-(1,2-diethyl-1,2-ethenediyl)bis-, bis(dihydrogen phosphate), Stilphostrol (*Miles*)

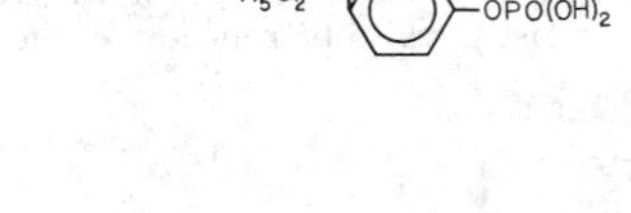

α,α′-Diethyl-(*E*)-4,4′-stilbenediol bis(dihydrogen phosphate) [13425-53-1] $C_{18}H_{22}O_8P_2$ (428.31).

Preparation—*Diethylstilbestrol* is reacted with phosphorus oxychloride in the presence of pyridine.

Description—White, crystalline powder; decomposes between 204 and 206°; stable solutions at pH 10.

Solubility—Sparingly soluble in water (the disodium salt is soluble in water).

Uses—Indicated only for the treatment of *prostatic carcinoma,* in which it is claimed that it is more efficacious than other estrogens, and it has proven effective after tolerance to other estrogens has occurred. Whether it has a unique cytotoxic action on the cancer cells is not clear. It has been hypothesized that the drug enters the cell as the diphosphate and is hydrolyzed therein by the acid phosphatase that is in such high concentrations in prostatic carcinomatous cells, thereby precipitating diethylstilbestrol intracellularly. Present indications are that untoward effects are less frequent and less severe than with any other estrogen. Even with very large doses gynecomastia has been infrequent. Nausea, vomiting, dizziness, pain in the perineum and transient pain at the sites of metastases are the most common side effects.

Dose—*Oral, initially* **50 mg** 3 times a day, gradually increased to as much as **200 mg** 3 times a day; *intravenous infusion, initially* **500 mg** in 300 mL of isotonic parenteral fluid over a 20- to 30-min period on the 1st day and **1 g** over a period of 1 hr on the next 5 days, then **250** to **500 mg** once or twice a wk for maintenance.

Dosage Forms—Injection: 250 mg/5 mL (as the disodium salt); Tablets: 50 mg.

Mestranol

(17α)-19-Norpregna-1,3,5(10)-trien-20-yn-17-ol, 3-methoxy-,

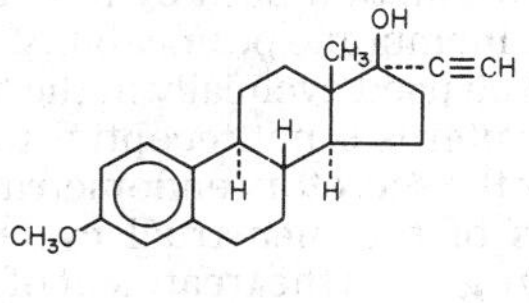

OH CH3 C≡CH H H H CH3O

[72-33-3] $C_{21}H_{26}O_2$ (310.44).

Preparation—Estrone is converted to its 3-methoxy analog by reaction with methyl sulfate. The ethynyl group may then be introduced at position 17 either through reaction with sodium acetylide in liquid ammonia followed by hydrolysis of the sodoxy compound, or through grignardization with ethynyl bromide. US Pat 2,666,769.

Description—White to creamy white, odorless, crystalline powder; melts within a range of 4° between 146 and 154°.

Solubility—Freely soluble in chloroform; sparingly soluble in ether; slightly soluble in alcohol; insoluble in water.

Uses—A contaminant in early preparations of norethynodrel. Such impure preparations were superior to pure norethynodrel for oral contraception. Therefore, this drug was incorporated with norethynodrel in the historically famous oral contraceptive, *Norethynodrel with Mestranol* (page 1100), and it is now combined with several progestins in oral contraceptives. When suppression of the pituitary release of gonadotropins occurs with these preparations, it is likely that inhibition is more attributable to this drug than to the progestin. However, oral contraceptive preparations containing mestranol do not suppress ovulation in a large fraction of users, and the oral contraceptive effect cannot thus be correctly attributed to an anovulatory effect of the estrogen. It is an effective estrogen for the usual uses of estrogens, but it is not marketed as a single entity.

Dose and **Dosage Forms**—see *Hormonal Contraceptives* (page 1097).

Ethynodiol Diacetate and Mestranol Tablets—see RPS-18, page 995.

Norethindrone and Mestranol Tablets—page 1100.

Norethynodrel and Mestranol Tablets—page 1100.

Antiestrogens and Aromatase Inhibitors

In a broad sense, antiestrogens are substances which suppress the effects of estrogens, regardless of mechanism. Androgens and progestins would thus qualify as incomplete antiestrogens, since they are antagonists to estrogens in some of their effects. With the advent of competitive antagonists of estrogens, the term antiestrogen has become restricted in use to apply only to such drugs. A number of estrogens have been found which reduce the intensity of response to other estrogens, behaving as partial agonists, as it were. Some, such as tamoxifen, are complete antagonists; tamoxifen has been effective in the treatment of breast cancer in premenopausal women. Some substances appear to exert antiestrogenic effects only on some but not all target organs; for example, chlorotrianisene is estrogenic in the periphery but antiestrogenic in the hypothalamus, so that it interrupts the normal negative feedback system that modulates anterior pituitary gonadotropin release.

A closely related compound, clomiphene, has even a stronger antiestrogenic action in the hypothalamus but is sufficiently weak in the periphery so as not to interfere with the peripheral effects of endogenously released estrogens. By blocking the effects of endogenous estrogen to suppress adenohypophyseal release of gonadotropins, antiestrogens allow the anterior pituitary to produce more gonadotropins than normally. The ovaries are thus stimulated to a greater extent and follicular development and maturation are enhanced. In cases of infertility resulting from failure to ovulate this effect may result in ovulation and the development of fertility.

Another approach to suppress the effects of endogenous estrogens is to decrease their synthesis. The most promising drugs for this purpose are the *aromatase* inhibitors. Aromatase is an enzyme complex which converts androgen precursors into estrogens. Inhibition of this enzyme complex would thus decrease estrogen synthesis; synthesis of adrenal steroids would not be compromised since they are formed earlier in the steroid synthetic pathway.

The most potent and selective inhibitor now available is *4-hydroxyandrostenedione (4-OHA),* a competitive inhibitor of the enzyme complex. *Aminoglutethimide* (page 1241) also inhibits the aromatase complex, but it is not as selective or as potent as is 4-OHA. The inhibition of steroid hydroxylases by aminoglutethimide decreases the synthesis of adrenal steroids, a side effect which severely limits its clinical usefulness. 4-OHA has been shown to be effective in patients with breast cancer who were resistant to, or had relapsed from, tamoxifen (see below). It has not been established that 4-OHA is more effective than tamoxifen. Several steroidal active site-directed inhibitors, which are more selective for aromatase complex and which inhibit the complex irreversibly, and a nonsteroidal inhibitor more selective for aromatase than aminoglutethimide, show promise.

Clomiphene Citrate

Ethanamine, 2-[4-(2-chloro-1,2-diphenylethenyl)phenoxy]-*N,N*-diethyl-, 2-hydroxy-1,2,3-propanetricarboxylate (1:1); Clomid (*Marion Merrell Dow*); Milophene (*Milex*); Serophene (*Serono*)

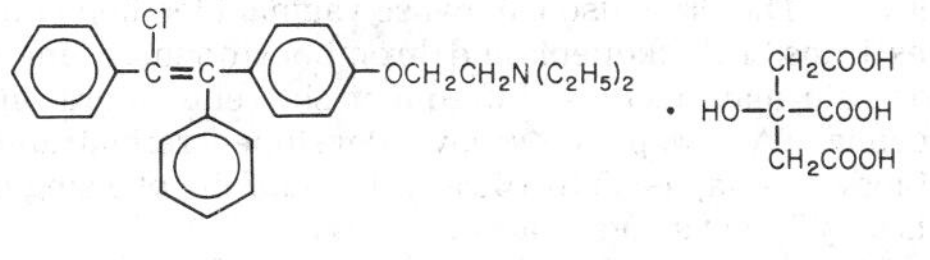

Cl C=C OCH2CH2N(C2H5)2 · CH2COOH HO—C—COOH CH2COOH

2-[*p*-(2-Chloro-1,2-diphenylvinyl)phenoxy]triethylamine citrate (1:1) [50-41-9] $C_{26}H_{28}ClNO.C_6H_8O_7$ (598.09).

Preparation—4-Hydroxybenzophenone is condensed with 2-(diethylamino)ethyl chloride in toluene in the presence of alkali. The 4-[2-(diethylamino)ethoxy]benzophenone thus formed is grignardized with benzyl chloride and the tertiary carbinol thus produced is dehydrated to give 2-[*p*-(1,2-diphenylvinyl)phenoxy]triethylamine. This compound is chlorinated to yield clomiphene and then reacted with an equimolar quantity of citric acid. Clomiphene citrate is a mixture of (*E*)- and (*Z*)-geometric isomers containing 30.0–50.0% of the latter isomer.

Description—White to pale yellow powder, essentially odorless; not appreciably hygroscopic; melts about 118° with decomposition.

Solubility—Sparingly soluble in alcohol; slightly soluble in water or chloroform; insoluble in ether.

Uses—An antiestrogenic drug that blocks the negative feedback action of endogenous estrogens by blocking cytosolic estrogen receptors in the hypothalamus and diminishing their number. The result is an increase in the secretion of LH-RH/FSH-RH and, hence, in gonadotropins. However, its effect is uneven, since it seems to be most effective in the late follicular and not in the luteal phase of the estrous cycle. The elevated LH levels bring about ovulation; sometimes more than one ovum is released, which may result in multiple pregnancies. It is used to *induce ovulation* (increase fertility) in anovulatory and oligoovulatory women who have adequate endogenous estrogens and in whom the hypothalamic-anterior pituitary has a latent capacity to function. In properly selected patients, 80% may be induced to ovulate, and successful pregnancy is achieved in 30 to 40%. The probability of multiple pregnancy is increased to 8 times normal. This is about the same order of success as with human chorionic gonadotropin (HCG); HCG plus clomiphene does not increase efficacy. It also is under investigation as an agent to increase sperm production in oligospermic males.

In addition to multiple pregnancy, the major side effect is cystic enlargement of the ovaries. Increased cyclic ovarian pain, breast enlargement and hot flashes which resemble those of the menopause also occur. Nausea is frequent. Blurred vision and scintillating scotoma may occur, and they require discontinuation of the treatment. Sulfobromophthalein retention may be increased. Desmosterol levels are elevated by high doses. All side effects are reversible, except pregnancy itself.

Dose—*Oral, initially* **50 mg** a day for 5 days, starting on the 5th day of the menstrual cycle or at any time in the amenorrheic patient. If ovulation occurs, the same dosage is continued cyclically until conception is achieved or 3 to 4 cycles have passed. If ovulation does not occur, the cycle is repeated with 100 mg a day.

Dosage Form—Tablets: 50 mg.

Tamoxifen Citrate

Ethanamine,
(*Z*)-2-[4-(1,2-diphenyl-1-butenyl)phenoxy]-*N,N*-dimethyl-,
Nolvadex (*Zeneca*)

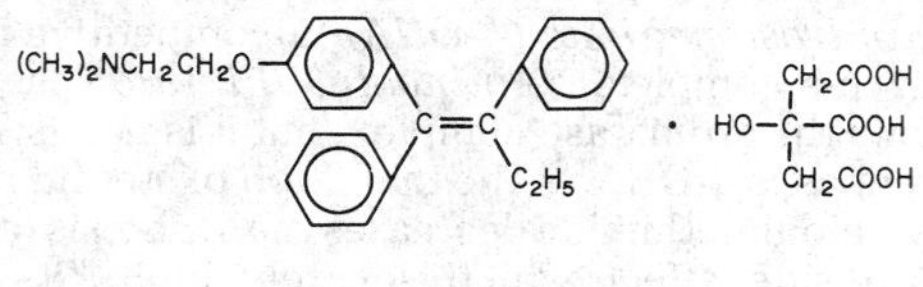

(*Z*)-2-[*p*-(1,2-Diphenyl-1-butenyl)phenoxy]-*N,N*-dimethylethylamine citrate (1:1) [54965-24-1] $C_{26}H_{29}NO.C_6H_8O_7$ (563.65).

Preparation—4-β-Dimethylaminoethoxy-α-ethyldesoxybenzoin by reaction with phenylmagnesium bromide or phenyl lithium is converted to 1-(4-β-dimethylaminoethoxyphenyl)-1,2-diphenyl butanol, which on dehydration yields a mixture of tamoxifen and its *cis*-isomer that may be separated with petroleum ether; tamoxifen is converted to the 1:1 citrate for dispensing use. See *Nature 212:* 733, 1966; *CA 67:* 90515g, 1967.

Description—White, crystalline powder; melts at about 140°.

Uses—A nonsteroidal antiestrogen for palliative *therapy of breast cancer in postmenopausal women*. The drug competes with estrogens for cytosol estrogen receptors and thus blocks estrogen effects in the target tissue. Tumors with negative receptor assays do not respond to it. The drug has been used investigationally to treat *female infertility*, the mechanism being that described for *Clomiphene*. Unapproved uses include the reduction of breast size in gynecomastia and the relief of mastalgia. Adverse effects frequently reported are hot flashes, nausea and vomiting. The drug also can cause vaginal bleeding and discharge, skin rashes, transient leukopenia and thrombocytopenia. Increased bone and tumor pain may occur. Infrequent side effects are anorexia and hypercalcemia. A few patients have developed retinal abnormalities. The oral bioavailability is 25 to 100%. The half-life of a single dose is 18 hr, but it is only 7 hr at steady state.

Dose—*Oral, adult* for *breast cancer*, **10** or **20 mg**, twice a day; for *stimulating ovulation (use not currently included in labeling approved by FDA)*, **5** to **40 mg** twice a day for 4 days.

Dosage Form—Tablets: 10 mg.

Testolactone—page 1104.

Progestins (Progestogens) and Antagonists

The second type of hormone produced in the ovaries is *progesterone*, which is excreted in the form of pregnanediol glucuronide. Although it originates in cells which also may produce estrogen and although it has a molecular structure very similar to that of the estrogens, progesterone has a unique physiological action. Under its influence the numerous minute glands which line the uterine cavity are transformed into secreting glands. This alteration is part of the change which is essential to provide for the implantation of a fertilized ovum and for the continuing development of the placenta. This endometrial alteration requires the cooperation of an estrogen; in the absence of an estrogen, a progestin that is devoid of estrogenic activity will exert an atrophic effect on the endometrium.

Progestins also cause a change in the cervical secretions to suppress "ferning," a dendritic crystallization of cervical mucopolysaccharides. When the cervical mucus is not dendritic, it forms a tight net of fibers, through which it is believed sperm cannot pass. The antifertility effect of some progestins possibly may be due in part to the suppression of ferning. Progestins in high doses suppress the pituitary release of luteinizing hormone and the hypothalmic release of the LH-releasing factor (LRF), thus preventing ovulation. Progestins also decrease uterine motility, which may contribute to a contraceptive effect. In addition, they antagonize the endometrial actions of estrogens, especially the natural estrogens. Progestins have the ability to stimulate development of the glandular portions of the mammae. They also exert some effects upon the capacity of tissues to retain water in the intercellular spaces. They also have a thermogenic action.

Progesterone is biotransformed *in vivo*, beginning with 5-alpha and 5-beta reductions, to several active metabolites which affect the central nervous system in multiple ways and which may be responsible for some of the effects of progesterone described above. The metabolites decrease brain electrical activity, inhibit calcium ingress into nerve terminals and norepinephrine release and modify behavior. They also participate in the control of gonadotropin secretion. The metabolites appear to function both by modifying gene expression or by altering membrane permeability.

Progestins may be used cyclically in the treatment of *infertility* in which the uterus is not receptive to implantation; the progestin sustains the secretory endometrium during the third and fourth weeks of the menstrual cycle. They are used cyclically with estrogens in the treatment of *secondary amenorrhea* and *dysfunctional uterine bleeding*. They also may be used to lessen *premenstrual tension*, although they cause salt and water retention, which is a factor in this disorder. The effect to suppress the release of LH and LRF is used to prevent ovulation, not only with some oral *contraceptives* but also in the treatment of *primary dysmenorrhea* and *endometriosis*. In *sexual infantilism* in the female, progestins may be combined with estrogens to bring about genital development and maturation. Progestins may decrease breast size in *mastodynia*.

In *preeclampsia* and *toxemia* of pregnancy due to hormonal imbalance, progestins plus estrogens may improve the condition, even though both types of hormone can cause salt and water retention and estrogens can cause hypertension. They may be used in huge doses as adjunctive treatment in *endometrial carcinoma*. They have been used in the past to prevent habitual abortion or treat threatened abortion. An intriguing use of progestins is to stimulate respiration in the *Pickwickian syndrome*.

The use of these agents during the first 4 months of pregnancy is not recommended because there is no evidence that the treatment is effective and there is evidence that the fetus may be harmed. In fact, the FDA now requires that women taking progestins must be informed that the use of these drugs during the first 4 months of pregnancy may increase the risk of heart defects and deformed arms and legs in their children.

Untoward effects of progestins include nausea, vomiting, diarrhea, edema and weight gain, headache, fatigue, hirsutism, urticaria, ulcerative stomatitis, pruritus vulvae and a tendency to galactorrhea and vaginal candidal infections. Some are locally irritating. Some have mild androgenic activity that may result in masculinization, especially in the female fetus. Others have a weak estrogenic component of activity. Some have both estrogenic and androgenic actions. Progestins increase the cutaneous pigmenting effect of estrogens, thus favoring cloasma (melasma) when used in combination. It is probable that they increase the intensity of adverse effects of estrogens, especially headache and hypertension. There may be breakthrough bleeding when continuous high doses are used which suppress menstruation, yet there also may be decreased menstrual flow in many patients.

Most oral contraceptives contain both an estrogen and a progestogen. Certain progestins may be used alone. The oral contraceptives are discussed on page 1098.

Progesterone Antagonists—In addition to the widespread use of progestins in oral contraceptive agents, drugs which are classified as progesterone antagonists are receiving considerable attention in reproductive pharmacology. Since progesterone is essential for nidation and maintenance of early pregnancy, blockade of progesterone receptors or interference with progesterone synthesis prevents pregnancy and/or causes abortion early in gestation. Two such agents, dubbed *abortion pills* by the lay press, have been studied in some detail in experimental animals and humans.

Mifepristone (RU486) combines with progesterone receptors and acts as a progestrone antagonist. The drug is an abortifacient and acts as a contraceptive.

Epostane inhibits 3-beta-hydroxysteroid dehydrogenase, the enzyme which converts pregnenelone to progesterone. Thus, progesterone synthesis is decreased and the effects of progesterone are negated. Epostane causes abortion in the first 8 weeks of pregnancy and appears to be reasonably safe for this use.

The exact clinical status of mifepristone and epostane as abortifacients remains to be established, but the potential availability of methods to produce safe, noninvasive abortions raises significant medical, social and legal questions.

Ethynodiol Diacetate

(3β,17α)-19-Norpregn-4-en-20-yne-3,17-diol, diacetate

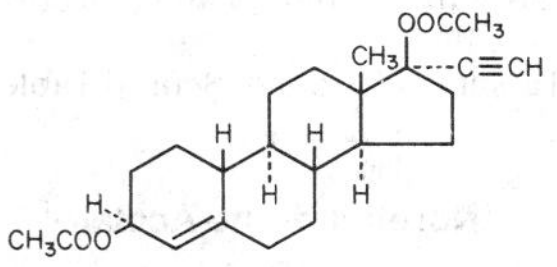

[297-76-7] $C_{24}H_{32}O_4$ (384.51).

Preparation—From *Norethindrone* by reducing the keto group to the carbinol state and then esterifying the 3- and 17-hydroxyls with acetyl chloride in the presence of pyridine.

Description—White, odorless, crystalline powder; stable in air; melts about 129°.

Solubility—Insoluble in water; very soluble in chloroform; freely soluble in ether; soluble in alcohol; sparingly soluble in fixed oils.

Uses—A *progestin* with actions and uses similar to *Norethindrone*, to which it is closely related chemically. However, because of the hydroxyl rather than keto character of the 3-position of the A ring, it has a stronger estrogenic activity and is essentially devoid of androgenic activity. It is useful in the treatment of all conditions in which progestins are indicated (see page 1094). The drug is promoted as an *oral contraceptive*, for which purpose it is combined with an estrogen (mestranol or ethinyl estradiol) in 6 of 49 products; however, because of its inherent estrogenic activity, it probably could be used alone. It suppresses the midcycle elevation of luteotropin that is the immediate stimulus to ovulation.

Dose and **Dosage Form**—See *Ethynodiol Diacetate and Ethinyl Estradiol Tablets*, page 1099.

Hydroxyprogesterone Caproate

Pregn-4-ene-3,20-dione, 17-[(1-oxohexyl)oxy]-, Delalutin (*Squibb*); Hy-Gestrone (*Pasadena Research*); (*Various Mfrs*)

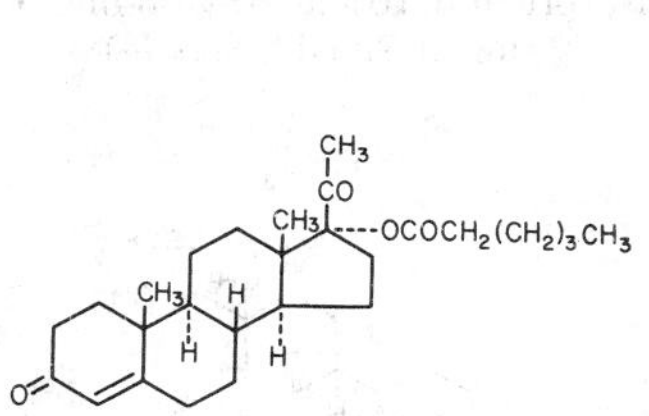

17-Hydroxypregn-4-ene-3,20-dione hexanoate [630-56-8] $C_{27}H_{40}O_4$ (428.61).

Preparation—Hydroxyprogesterone is esterified by heating with caproic anhydride in the presence of *p*-toluenesulfonic acid under an atmosphere of nitrogen. US Pat 2,753,360.

Description—White or creamy white, crystalline powder which is odorless or has a slight odor; melts between 120 and 124°.

Solubility—Insoluble in water; 1 g in about 20 mL ether or 800 mL benzene.

Uses—Actions and uses of the progestins (see page 1094), except that it does not prevent ovulation. It is several times more potent than progesterone, and its duration of action is longer, but its onset of action is also slower. A single injection of a solution of hydroxyprogesterone caproate in oil will exert progestational effects for 1 to 2 wk. It is not converted to progesterone or hydroxyprogesterone in the body. When used to regulate an irregular estrous cycle, it usually is combined with an estrogen.

In addition to a potential to cause the usual side effects of progestins, this drug occasionally causes hypersensitivity, coughing or dyspnea. In rare instances it may cause virilization of the female fetus.

Dose—*Intramuscular*, cyclically (with estradiol valerate), for *amenorrhea*, **375 mg** every 4 wk for 4 cycles and, to *induce a secretory endometrium* and *desquamation*, **375 mg** every 4 wk; for *uterine carcinoma*, **1 g** once a day to once a wk (1 to 7 g/wk).

Dosage Form—Injection: 125 and 250 mg/mL.

Levonorgestrel

(17α)-(−)-18,19-Dinorpregn-4-en-20-yn-3-one, 13-ethyl-17-hydroxy-, Norplant (*Wyeth-Ayerst*)

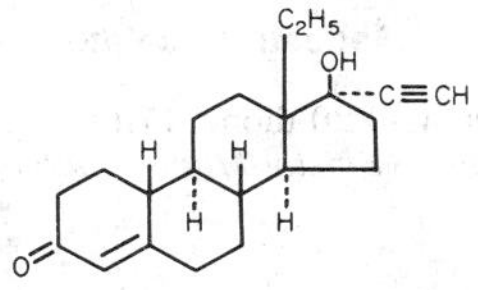

[797-63-7] $C_{21}H_{28}O_2$ (312.45). This compound is the (−)-isomer of norgestrel, but the D-configurational isomer. A former designation as the d-enantiomer is incorrect.

Preparation—Refer to *Experientia 19:* 394, 1963 for the (±)-form and US Pat 3,413,314 for both enantiomers.

Description—White crystals melting about 240°.

Solubility—Practically insoluble in water; soluble in chloroform; slightly soluble in ether or dioxane; sparingly soluble in ether.

Uses—The (−)-isomer of norgestrel (page 1097). It is the active form of norgestrel, hence it is twice as potent on a weight basis as is norgestrel. Otherwise, the pharmacological properties of norgestrel and this drug are the same. It is used alone in subdermal implants and in combinations with ethinyl estradiol as an oral contraceptive.

Dose and **Dosage Form**—See *Levonorgestrol and Ethinyl Estradiol Tablets*, page 1099. Implants: Set of 6 capsules, 36 mg each (effective as a contraceptive for 5 yr after implantation).

Medroxyprogesterone Acetate

(6α)-Pregn-4-ene-3,20-dione, 17-(acetyloxy)-6-methyl-, Provera, Depo-Provera (*Upjohn*); Curretab (*Solvay*); Cycrin (*Wyeth-Ayerst*)

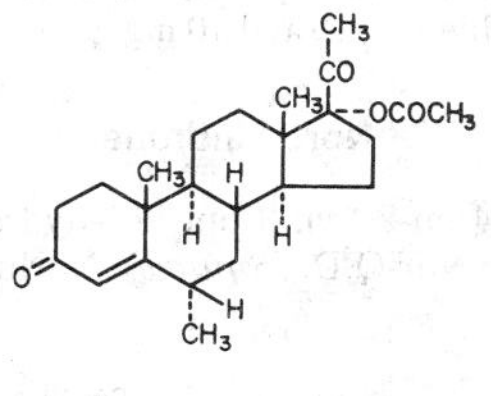

17-Hydroxy-6α-methylpregn-4-ene-3,20-dione acetate [71-58-9] $C_{24}H_{34}O_4$ (386.53).

Preparation—From 17α-hydroxyprogesterone by first forming the 3,21-bisethylene acetal with ethylene glycol, then treating with peracetic acid to give a mixture of the 5α,6α- and 5β,6β-epoxides. With methyl magnesium iodide the α-epoxide isomer yields the 5α-hydroxy-6β-methyl derivative which dehydrates and epimerizes with hydrogen chloride in chloroform to the Δ^4-6α-methyl compound, medroxyprogesterone. Acylation with acetic anhydride and *p*-toluenesulfonic acid in acetic acid gives medroxyprogesterone acetate.

Description—White to off-white, odorless, crystalline powder; melts about 205°; stable in air.

Solubility—Insoluble in water; freely soluble in chloroform; soluble in acetone or dioxane; sparingly soluble in alcohol or methanol; slightly soluble in ether.

Uses—Actions, uses and side effects of the progestins in general (see page 1094). Its oral efficacy is an advantage over progesterone. There is no clinical evidence to date confirming the supposed efficacy in threatened or habitual abortion. Furthermore, the drug is teratogenic during the first 4 mo of pregnancy and hence should not be used for threatened abortion. The long duration of action of intramuscular drug makes it popular in some countries. It is effective as a contraceptive when given IM at the recommended dose to women every 3 mo. Gonadotropin secretion is inhibited, which prevents follicular maturation and ovulation and results in endometrial thinning. It has been found to be beneficial in some cases of *sleep apnea*. Aqueous suspensions administered intramuscularly have a duration of action of weeks to months.

Dose—*Oral,* for *secondary amenorrhea* and *functional uterine bleeding,* **5** to **10 mg** a day for 5 to 10 days, starting on the assumed 16th to 21st day of the cycle, to be continued for 2 cycles in the case of bleeding; for *endometriosis,* **30 mg** a day; as an *adjunct to cyclical therapy with estrogen,* **10** to **20 mg** a day for the last 7 to 10 days of each cycle. *Intramuscular,* for *endometriosis,* **150 mg** every 3 mo; in *endometrial carcinoma, initially* **400 mg** to **1 g** a week, adjusted eventually to 400 mg a week, as an adjunct to other treatment. *Deep intramuscular* for *contraception,* **150 mg** every 3 mo.

Dosage Forms—Sterile Suspension: 100, 150 and 400 mg/mL; Tablets: 2.5, 5 and 10 mg.

Megestrol Acetate

Pregna-4,6-diene-3,20-dione, 17-(acetyloxy)-6-methyl-, Megace (*Bristol-Myers Oncology*)

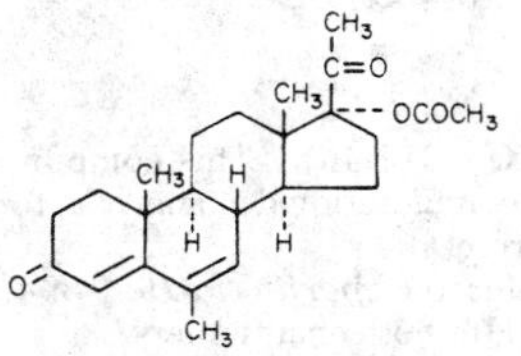

[595-33-5] $C_{24}H_{32}O_4$ (384.51).

Preparation—See RPS-15, page 925.

Description—White or almost white, crystalline powder; odorless; tasteless; melts about 215°.

Solubility—Insoluble in water; sparingly soluble in alcohol; slightly soluble in ether; very soluble in chloroform.

Uses—See the introduction to this section for actions, uses and side effects. It is very potent in inhibiting ovulation, and is employed outside the US as an oral contraceptive. For such use it is supplemented by an estrogen, generally ethinyl estradiol. In the US it is used for palliative treatment of inoperable advanced carcinoma of the breast or endometrium, as an adjunct to other therapy. It has no estrogenic or androgenic properties of its own. Side effects include nausea and vomiting, headache, tiredness, breast discomfort and weight gain.

Dose—For *endometrial carcinoma,* **40** to **320 mg** a day in divided doses; for *breast cancer,* **160 mg** a day, divided into 4 doses. An adequate trial of the potential efficacy is at least 2 mo.

Dosage Form—Tablets: 20 and 40 mg.

Norethindrone

(17α)-19-Norpregn-4-en-20-yn-3-one, 17-hydroxy-, Norethisterone; Micronor (*Ortho*); Nor-Q.D. (*Syntex*); Norlutin (*Parke-Davis*)

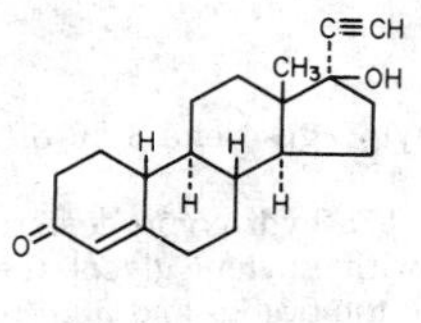

[68-22-4] $C_{20}H_{26}O_2$ (298.42).

Preparation—The methyl ether of estrone is reacted with lithium metal in liquid ammonia to reduce ring A to the 4-ene state and the reduced compound is oxidized with chromic acid in aqueous acetic acid to form estr-4-ene-3,17-dione (I). In order to prevent the 3-keto group from participating in the ensuing ethynylation reaction, I is reacted with ethyl orthoformate in the presence of pyridine hydrochloride to form the 3-ethoxy-3,5-diene compound (II). Acetylene is passed into a solution of II in toluene, previously admixed with a solution of sodium in *tert*-amyl alcohol, to form the 17-ethynyl-17-hydroxy compound. Hydrolysis at the 3-ethoxy linkage by heating with dilute HCl is accompanied by rearrangement of the 3-hydroxy-3,5-diene compound to the 3-oxo-4-ene state. US Pat 2,744,122.

Description—White to creamy white, odorless, crystalline powder; melts about 205°; stable in air.

Solubility—Practically insoluble in water; sparingly soluble in alcohol; soluble in chloroform or dioxane; slightly soluble in ether.

Uses—For the actions and uses, see page 1094. In addition to its progestational actions, it has weak estrogenic actions, owing to biotransformation to an estrogenic metabolite. Among the progestational drugs, it ranks high in ability to postpone menstruation, and it is used for this purpose for both medical and social reasons. In high doses it prevents ovulation by suppressing pituitary gonadotropin output. In lower doses it suppresses the endometrium and decreases the fluidity of the cervical mucus. Consequently, the steroid is an important *oral contraceptive.* As an oral contraceptive, it is used alone or combined with an estrogen, especially *Mestranol* and *Ethinyl Estradiol;* when used alone, the pregnancy rate is about 3 times that when used in combination with an estrogen.

In some women with Type V hyperlipoproteinemia, it markedly decreases the concentrations of VLDL and chylomicrons; however, it also lowers HDL and hence is used only when the condition is refractory to other drugs. The drug has weak androgenic properties and may cause deepening of the voice, hirsutism and acne and it may cause masculinization of the fetus.

Dose—For *amenorrhea, dysfunctional uterine bleeding, premenstrual tension* or *dysmenorrhea, cyclically* **5** to **20 mg** a day for 21 days, starting on the 5th and ending on the 25th day of the menstrual cycle; for *endometriosis, initially* **10 mg** a day for 2 wk, after which the dose is increased in increments of **5 mg** every 2 wk until a *maintenance* dose of **30 mg** a day is reached; for *contraception,* **0.35 mg** (350 μg) a day continuously, starting on the 1st day of menstruation. See also *Norethindrone and Ethinyl Estradiol Tablets* and *Norethindrone and Mestranol Tablets.*

Dosage Form—Tablets: 0.35 mg; Scored Tablets: 5 mg.

Norethindrone Acetate

(17α)-19-Norpregn-4-en-20-yn-3-one, 17-(acetyloxy)-, Aygestin (*Ayerst*) Norlutate (*Parke-Davis*)

17-Hydroxy-19-nor-17α-pregn-4-en-20-yn-3-one acetate [51-98-9] $C_{22}H_{28}O_3$ (340.46).

For the structure of the parent, see *Norethindrone.*

Preparation—*Norethindrone* is acetylated by treatment with acetic anhydride in the presence of pyridine.

Description—White to creamy white, odorless, crystalline powder.

Solubility—1 g in > 10,000 mL water, 10 mL alcohol, < 1 mL chloroform, 18 mL ether or 2 mL dioxane.

Uses—For the actions, uses and side effects, see *Norethindrone.* However, it is 2 to 3 times as potent as the parent steroid. Although it may be employed alone as a progestin, it is used most commonly in combination with an estrogen (ethinyl estradiol) for oral contraception or cyclic therapy.

Dose—For *amenorrhea, dysfunctional uterine bleeding, premenstrual tension* or *dysmenorrhea, cyclically* **2.5** to **10 mg** a day for 21 days, starting on the 5th and ending on the 25th day of the menstrual cycle; for *endometriosis, initially,* **5 mg** a day for 2 wk, with increments of 2.5 mg a day every 2 wk until a *maintenance* dose of **15 mg** a day is reached. See also *Norethindrone Acetate and Ethinyl Estradiol Tablets,* page 1100.

Dosage Form—Scored Tablets: 5 mg.

Norethynodrel

(17α)-19-Norpregn-5(10)-en-20-yn-3-one, 17-hydroxy-, ing of Enovid (*Searle*)

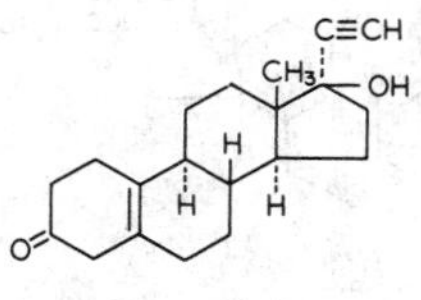

[68-23-5] $C_{20}H_{26}O_2$ (298.42).

Preparation—Dehydroepiandrosterone acetate is simultaneously saponified and oxidized by a series of reactions to 19-hydroxyandrost-6(6)-ene-3,17-dione. The hydroxymethyl group at the 10-position is then oxidized to carboxyl. The resulting acid is decarboxylated with simultaneous shifting of the double bond to give estr-5(10)-ene-3,17-dione. Selective addition of acetylene at the expense of the 17-one group yields norethynodrel. US Pat 2,725,389.

Description—White or nearly white, odorless, crystalline powder; stable in air; melts within a range of 3°, between 174 and 184°.

Solubility—Freely soluble in chloroform; sparingly soluble in alcohol or ether; very slightly soluble in water or solvent hexane.

Uses—A *progestin* which is isomeric with *Norethindrone*. However, the shift of the double bond in the A ring abolishes the weak androgenic properties found in norethindrone. In fact, norethynodrel exerts weak estrogenic actions because it is biotransformed to an estrogenic metabolite. Nevertheless, for progestational therapy or for oral contraception it is usual to supplement norethynodrel with an estrogen, both to prevent withdrawal bleeding and to favor an anovulatory effect. The prevention of ovulation is the result of suppression of pituitary gonadotropin release. However, contraception results from other mechanisms. The drug is the primary ingredient of the oral contraceptive *Norethynodrel and Mestranol* (page 1100). It is not advocated for infertility and maintenance of pregnancy, since it appears not to promote an endometrium which is favorable to nidation and support of the fetus. Furthermore, it causes some masculinization of the fetus, even though it otherwise lacks androgenic properties. This androgenic activity is somewhat antagonized by the estrogenic actions of mestranol and other estrogens. The drug is not used separately from its estrogenic adjuvant even in general progestational therapy.

Dose and **Dosage Form**—see *Norethynodrel and Mestranol Tablets*, page 1100.

Norgestrel

(17α)-(±)-18,19-Dinorpregn-4-en-20-yn-3-one, 13-ethyl-17-hydroxy-, Ovrette, (*Wyeth-Ayerst*)

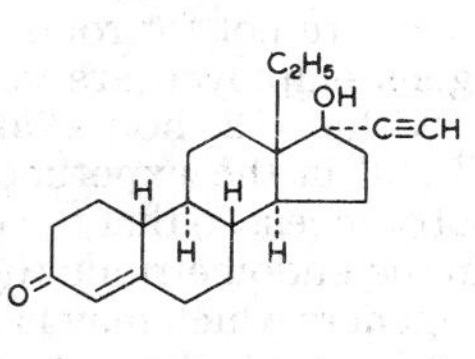

[6533-00-2] $C_{21}H_{28}O_2$ (312.45).

Preparation—Described by the manufacturer as a total, stereoselective chemical synthesis. 6-Methoxy-α-tetralone is reacted with vinylmagnesium bromide and the resulting 1,2,3,4-tetrahydro-6-methoxy-1-vinyl-1-naphthol is condensed with 2-ethyl-1,3-cyclopentanedione to obtain initially a tricyclic intermediate (secosteroid) containing all of the gonane skeleton carbon atoms. Cyclization of the secosteroid via dehydration yields a 13-ethylgona-1,3,5(10),-8,14-pentaene structure which is then successively reduced and ethynylated.

Description—White or nearly white, practically odorless, crystalline powder; melts within a range of 4° between 205 and 212°.

Solubility—Insoluble in water; sparingly soluble in alcohol; freely soluble in chloroform.

Uses—Although a progestin with potentially all the actions, uses and side effects of drugs of this class (see page 1094), it is marketed only as an *oral contraceptive*, both as a single entity product and in combination with ethinyl estradiol. Its action is to make the endometrium unreceptive to implantation. It is free from estrogenic activity. Although it has been demonstrated to have an androgenic effect in animals, such effects have not been reported in the human with the doses used.

Dose—*Oral*, as a single agent for *contraception*, **75 μg** a day, continuously, starting on the 1st day of menstruation. See also *Norgestrel and Ethinyl Estradiol Tablets*, page 1100.

Dosage Form—Tablets: 75 μg.

Progesterone

Pregn-4-ene-3,20-dione; (*Various Mfrs*)

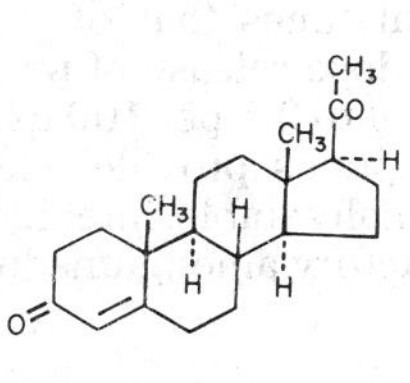

Progesterone [57-83-0] $C_{21}H_{30}O_2$ (314.47).

Preparation—From animal ovaries, synthesized from stigmasterol, or better from diosgenin (extracted from *Dioscorea mexicana*, a Mexican yam). The latter synthesis involves acetolysis, chromic acid oxidation, cleavage of the ketoester diacetate with boiling acetic acid to 16-dehydropregnenolone acetate, which on catalytic reduction yields pregnenolone acetate. Saponification of the acetate ester to the 3β-alcohol followed by Oppenauer oxidation affords progesterone. Progesterone in pure form was first isolated, from corpus luteum, in 1934 by Butenandt.

Description—White or creamy white, crystalline powder; odorless and stable in air; melts 128°; a polymorphic modification melts about 121°.

Solubility—Practically insoluble in water; soluble in alcohol, acetone or dioxane; sparingly soluble in vegetable oils.

Uses—The natural endogenous progestin; its actions, uses and side effects are described on page 1094. However, its plasma half-life is only about 5 min, so that it is extremely difficult to achieve effective blood levels with any convenient dosage schedules. Authorities doubt its usefulness in the treatment of habitual or threatened abortion. However, some consider it to be the drug of choice in luteal phase dysfunction, a disorder that causes infertility or repeated early abortion. It is not effective orally and is of limited and erratic efficacy buccally; consequently it is given intramuscularly as a suspension or solution in oil. The steroid is irritant, more so in aqueous suspension than in oil solution.

One intrauterine contraceptive device (Progestasert, *Alza*) contains 38 mg of progesterone in silicone oil. The hormone is said to enhance the contraceptive effectiveness of the device by a local effect on the endometrium and by effects on sperm motility, capacitation and metabolism. Progesterone is released at an average rate of 65 μg daily for 1 yr, at which time the device is replaced. The device increases the risk of pelvic inflammation and actinomycotic infections.

Dose—*Intramuscular*, for *primary* and *secondary amenorrhea*, **5** to **10 mg** a day for 6 to 8 days; in combination with an estrogen for *functional uterine bleeding* and *menorrhagia*, **5** to **10 mg** a day for the last 6 days of the cycle. *Intrauterine contraceptive system*, **38 mg** in silicone oil, once a yr.

Dosage Forms— Injection (in oil): 500 mg/10 mL 750 and 1500 mg/30 mL; Intrauterine Contraceptive System: 38 mg in silicone oil.

Hormonal Contraceptives

Mechanisms—The various mechanisms whereby hormonal contraceptives can prevent conception are complex. Knowledge in this field is still incomplete, but some mechanisms are understood relatively well. The mechanisms involved vary with the particular agent(s) in a preparation, the dose(s) and whether a cyclic or continuous schedule is used. It is probable that several mechanisms operate simultaneously with some preparations.

Suppression of Gonadotropic Output—During the menstrual cycle, there are two periods of elevated FSH secretion, a sharp peak just preceding ovulation and a long wave beginning just before menstruation. In sufficient doses, *estrogens* can suppress both phases by feedback actions on both the hypothalamus and the anterior hypophysis; FSH-LH output is desynchronized at the early peak, ovulation may be prevented and the estrogen-progestin priming of the uterus is defective. Estrogens also suppress the hypophyseal output of LH. *Progestins* also can suppress the LH peak (by an action at the hypothalamus, only), but their action is weak, owing to their antiestrogenic effects, which oppose the suppressant actions of endogenous and exogenous estrogen. Very high doses of progestins are necessary to suppress LH output, unless the progestin is combined with an estrogen. A progestin alone desynchronizes the FSH and LH output, thus sometimes preventing ovulation; long-term use of a combination of progestin and estrogen depresses the output of both gonadotropins and more consistently prevents ovulation.

Ovarian Effects—Estrogens and progestins decrease the ovarian response to their respective gonadotropins, a short-loop target-hormone negative feedback, so to speak. The result may be a failure to ovulate, or, if ovulation does occur, a smaller, hyposecreting corpus luteum, the latter especially when a progestin is in the contraceptive preparation. This latter effect has been demonstrated with chlormadinone and megestrol.

Tubal Effects—In some species progestins and in others estrogens accelerate the ciliary and peristaltic egg transport in the fallopian tubes and increase secretions. Consequently, the ovum arrives in the uterus before the endometrium is prepared for nidation. The tubal effects of these hormones in man are unknown, but it is thought that the contraceptive effects of large postcoital doses of estrogens (see *Diethylstilbestrol*, page 1092) may involve a tubal action.

Effects on the Endometrium—Long-acting injectable progestins (see *Medroxyprogesterone*, page 1095) in appropriate doses cause endometrial atrophy. Oral preparations vary according to the drug and the dose, some permitting a normal endometrium and others causing regression. In combination with estrogens, progestins effect a decrease in tortuosity and secretion of the endometrial glands and sometimes a regression to a stage of secretory exhaustion, with thinning of the endometrium after several cycles of use. With some combinations, the effect may be mainly an asynchrony in the development of the stroma and glands.

Effects on the Cervix—Estrogens favor ferning (the parallel alignment of pinnate-structured mucoid cervical secretions), which creates open channels through which spermatozoa may pass. Progestins inhibit ferning and favor an impenetrable mucoid network. In the combination contraceptives, the progestins predominate.

Effects on Capacitance—Capacitance is the ability of the sperm to penetrate into the ovum. Progestins are thought to decrease capacitance, by an unknown mechanism, probably involving prostaglandins. It is speculated that the low-dose, continuously administered progestin contraceptives are effective by the anticapacitant action.

Types of Preparations—The first oral contraceptives to be marketed were *progestin-estrogen combinations*, and the majority of currently marketed products are of this type. In some preparations, called *monophasic* combinations, the progestin and estrogen are present in fixed amounts, so that blood levels rise and fall together, in contrast to the levels in the normal menstrual cycle, in which one estrogen peak appears 11 days in advance of the combined estrogen-progesterone peak. With the combined preparations, an artificial menstrual cycle is induced by using the contraceptive for only 20 to 21 days out of every 28; if they were to be used continuously, instead, no regular mense would occur, but breakthrough bleeding would occur eventually.

The artificial mense caused by the cyclic use of combination contraceptives usually is not normal but oligemic. During the 7 to 8 days in which no hormones are taken, some products provide placebo or iron tablets in lieu of the combination; in these products, the pills are packaged to be taken serially by number to save the user the nuisance of keeping track of her pill consumption and of coordinating her consumption with her menstrual cycle. Over the years since combinations appeared on the market, the estrogen content has been decreased considerably in several products, because of the possible adverse effects of the estrogen component.

To provide a more normal mense and also possibly to decrease the incidence of adverse effects, *sequential* products were introduced. The estrogen was given alone during the first 14 to 16 days then combined with a progestin in the same pill for the next 5 to 7 days, thus covering 20 to 23 days of the cycle. These preparations have been removed from the market in the US because they were not acceptably effective as contraceptives and because their use was associated with elevated risk of adenocarcinoma and thromboembolic disease. Continued stimulation by estrogens unopposed by progestins during half of the cycle probably accounted for the increased risks associated with these drugs. Attempts to develop more nearly physiological regimens have led to the so-called *biphasic* and *triphasic* combinations. In the former, the progestin dose is increased during the last 11 days of the medication cycle; in the latter, the progestin/estrogen ratio is changed 3 times during the cycle by altering the doses of either progestin or estrogen or both.

Continuous progestin-only oral products do not contain any estrogen and furthermore contain the progestin in amounts smaller (the so-called "mini-pill") than those used in combination or sequential products. The dose is small enough not to prevent ovulation and menstruation in most users, yet to act sufficiently on the uterus, cervix or capacitance to prevent conception. However, the efficacy is less than with combination or sequential products. A progesterone containing IUD and *continuous-progestin injectable* products, repository forms of progestins, also are available.

An *implanted progestin system* has been approved for use as contraceptive therapy by the FDA. The levonorgestrol contraceptive implant system consists of six elongated silastic capsules that are all implanted subdermally in the upper arm. Levonorgestrol is metabolized in the liver at a much slower rate than endogenous progestins. The amount of progestin initially released daily from implants is more than double the daily amount released after 1 year; however, the daily amount after 1 year is similar to the amount contained in oral progestin-only contraceptives. Plasma concentrations vary widely, presumably due to individual differences in metabolism and body weight. Most patients have irregular menstruation during the first year and some women experience progestin-associated side effects, especially headaches and acne, that make implants unacceptable (see general comments on *Progestins*, page 1094). The levels of exogenous progestin released from implants decrease secretion of gonadotropins FSH and LH, and ovulation is suppressed in some patients. When ovulation does occur, a thick scanty mucus is induced that prevents sperm migration and endometrial development is suppressed by the constant low levels of progestin. The continuous low-dose release of progestin has a duration of action of up to 5 years.

Postcoital oral contraceptives (so-called "morning-after pills") have been used for a long time in emergencies, such as rape, and they now are used somewhat more widely, as in student health services, to prevent pregnancy in girls or women who are caught without contraceptive preparation; these preparations, however, are not for routine use, inasmuch as the doses of estrogens employed are very high. They are effective if taken within 72 hours after coitus. *Postconception* "pills," still in the experimental stage, contain various antiluteal substances, so that the embryo is unable to remain implanted in the endometrium; there is great interest in prostaglandin congeners which may have antiluteal effects but minor gastrointestinal and other activity.

Antagonist analogs of the gonadotropins and gonadotropin-releasing hormones provide the impetus for a way to prevent ovulation without the side effects of the steroid hormones. Oral contraception in the male has been approached experimentally by the use of drugs that inhibit sperm production, maturation or transport. No safe drugs have been found yet. An interesting nonpharmacological development is immunization against the sperm or certain of its enzymes; in the female there seem to be few complications to such immunization, but there are in the male.

Efficacy and Failures—The efficacy of an oral contraceptive depends on the type and the dose of hormonal ingredients. The combined type, which contains relatively high doses of estrogens, is nearly 100% effective when taken correctly; failures probably can be attributed to the negligence of the user. There appears to be a finite, though small, probability of ovulation and hence of later conception if a single pill is missed, because of the rebound oversecretion of the gonadotropins. If one pill is skipped, the user should take it immediately upon discovery of the skip and take the rest on their schedule; if two or more are missed, she should additionally use other methods of contraception until her next cycle. Lowering the estrogen content in combination preparations decreases the side effects but increases the risk of pregnancy. The long-acting combinations have a relatively high failure rate. The continuous low-dose oral progestin products have a failure rate several times that of combination products. The continuous low-dose release of progestin from implants has a failure rate of 0.4 to 0.5 per 100 users per year.

The oral contraceptives provide excellent contraception when used by emotionally stable, intelligent, educated women, but are not as satisfactory among uneducated or emotionally labile women. This is because the demanding uninterrupted use requires understanding of the importance of the schedule as well as the consequences of pregnancy and consistent determination. In underdeveloped countries, intrauterine devices or surgical sterilization are much more practical.

Adverse Effects—The medical and lay literature, alike, have been filled with accounts of adverse effects of the oral contraceptives, and many previous or potential users have been frightened away from these drugs. The adverse effects vary in incidence and severity according to the type of preparation. Most side effects are from the estrogens (see page 1088) in combination contraceptives, but progestins also cause adverse effects. The estrogen-progestin ratio is important to the type and incidence of side effects.

Some side effects are of little consequence to the health of the user and present difficulties only as the user or physician reacts to them. Oligomenorrhea occurs in 20 to 80% of users of combination and some continuous progestin contraceptives, and amenorrhea occurs in some. The greatest offenders are the 19-nortestosterone derivatives. Some users consider oligomenorrhea a boon, yet others are emotionally disturbed by this innocuous effect. Spotting and breakthrough bleeding is more annoying, since its irregularity and unpredictability are inconvenient; sometimes such bleeding is more voluminous than in regular menstruation.

Side effects such as tiredness, weakness, malaise, changes in libido, dizziness, nonspecific headaches and psychiatric symptoms often are the result of suggestion and conditioning and occur frequently when placebos are used, so it is difficult to state to what degree such effects are attributable to the oral contraceptives. An increase in the incidence of migraine headaches, however, is indisputable; the estrogen component appears to be responsible. Weight gain occurs with some but not all preparations; salt and water retention is caused mostly by estrogen components, whereas anabolic effects are caused by higher doses of the 19-nortestosterone-derived progestins (not the 17α-hydroxyprogesterones).

Chloasma occurs in about 4% of users of combination contraceptives during the 1st year and 37% by the 5th year; it is attributable to the combined action of the two active components. Milk flow in lactating women may be decreased by an average of 50% when combination preparations are used. Changes in the color and secretions of the cervix may be misinterpreted as infection or carcinoma by the uninformed physician. Bacteriuria and urinary tract infections are more common in users than in nonusers. Estrogen-containing contraceptives also cause an uncommon choreiform movement.

Serious side effects of oral contraceptives are multiple. A reversible hypertension is observed in approximately 15% of users of estrogen-containing contraceptives; this is more than the incidence when estrogens are used alone for noncontraceptive purposes and suggests modulation by progestins. The prevalence of hypertension increases with duration of use and is greater in older women. Incidence of thromboembolic disorders, including stroke and myocardial infarction, is higher in women using oral contraceptives; the relative risk may be several times greater in users as compared to control populations. Further, the risk increases sharply in women over 35 years.

Contraceptive use also has been associated with increased evidence of benign liver tumors. The relative risk of liver tumors appears to rise with duration of use of the drugs. In one study, mestranol-containing preparations were implicated almost exclusively, thus indicating that the type of synthetic estrogen might be important. The risk of gallbladder disease is increased twofold in contraceptive users. Fetal abnormalities may result if the mother continues to take the pill after becoming pregnant. Neuroocular lesions have been associated with use of oral contraceptives. Some other possible complications of contraceptive use include breast cancer (pill use actually protects against the development of benign breast lesions), and cancer of the uterus, cervix and vagina. Any of the other side effects of estrogens or progestins given above also may be caused by these drugs. Irregular bleeding is initially a problem for some women with progestin implants and depot progestin administration. However, after 1 year most women are completely amenorrheic. Patients taking oral contraceptives must be informed of their effectiveness and risks.

Perspectives—Oral contraceptives are potent drugs that are remarkably effective in the prevention of pregnancy. They are not benign drugs and have many recognized and potential side effects. However, pregnancy itself is not without hazard, and it can be argued that risks of death and serious illness are less with oral contraceptives than with pregnancy in most women. The risks of serious complications with oral contraceptive use increase as the dose, duration of therapy and age of the patient increase, and as other risk factors, such as smoking, increase. The long-term safety of both depot progestin and progestin implants has not been established. Therefore, a prudent attitude toward oral contraceptives as a birth-control method would be as follows:

> There are relatively few contraindications to their use in young, healthy, sexually active women who seek careful control of family size and spacing. The risks associated with the low-dose combinations are less than with high-dose preparations. Once reproduction is completed or as a female approaches middle age, it probably would be wise to seek other methods of contraception.

Conjugated Estrogens—page 1090.

Diethylstilbestrol—page 1092.

Estrone—page 1090.

Ethinyl Estradiol—page 1091.

Ethynodiol Diacetate and Ethinyl Estradiol Tablets

Demulen (*Searle*)

Uses—For *combination oral contraception* (see page 1097). For the actions of the separate components, see *Ethynodiol Diacetate* (page 1095) and *Ethinyl Estradiol* (page 1091). The adverse effects are mainly those of the ethinyl estradiol (page 1091); see also above for adverse effects of combinations).

Dose—**1 mg** of ethynodiol diacetate and either **35** or **50 μg** of ethinyl estradiol a day for 21 days, starting on the 5th day after the beginning of menstruation. One commercial product provides 7 placebo pills for the other 7 days of the cycle, in order to avoid interruption of the daily routine of pilltaking.

Dosage Form—Tablets: Ethynodiol Diacetate/Ethinyl Estradiol, 1 mg/35 or 50 μg.

Norethindrone—page 1096.

Levonorgestrol and Ethinyl Estradiol Tablets

Tri-Levlen (*Berlex*); Triphasil (*Wyeth-Ayerst*)

Uses—For *combination oral contraception* (see page 1097). For the actions of separate components, see *Levonorgestrol* (page 1095) and *Ethinyl Estradiol* (page 1091).

Dose—*Combinations levonorgestrol:ethinyl estradiol: Oral, monophasic,* **0.15 mg:30 μg** once a day for 21 days, starting on the 5th day after menstruation begins; *triphasic,* **0.05 mg:30 μg** once a day for 6 days, followed by **0.075 mg:40 μg** for 5 days, followed by **0.125 mg:30 μg** once a day for 10 days. Products are available in both the monophasic and triphasic forms which provide 7 inert tablets to be taken during days 22 through 28, to simplify the dose schedule for the patient.

Dosage Form—Tablets: Levonorgestrol/Ethinyl Estradiol, Monophasic, 0.15/30 mg/μg; Triphasic, 0.05/30, 0.075/40 and 0.125/30 mg/μg.

Norethindrone and Ethinyl Estradiol Tablets

Ortho-Novum (*Ortho*)

Uses—For *combination oral contraception* (see page 1097). For the action of the separate components, see *Norethindrone* (page 1096) and *Ethinyl Estradiol* (page 1091).

Dose—*Combinations (norethindrone:ethinyl estradiol): Oral, monophasic,* **1 mg:50 μg** or **1 mg:35 μg** or **0.5 mg:35 μg** or **0.4 mg:35 μg**

a day for 21 days, starting on the 5th day after beginning of menstruation; *biphasic* **0.5 mg:35 μg** a day for the first 10 days, starting on the 5th day after the beginning of menstruation, followed by **1 mg:35 μg** a day for 11 days; *triphasic*, **0.5 mg:35 μg** a day for the first 10 days, starting on the 5th day after the beginning of menstruation, followed by **0.75** or **1 mg:35 μg** a day for 7 days, then **0.5** or **1 mg:35 μg** a day for 7 days. Several preparations are available in a 28-day pack in which 7 inert tablets are supplied for the other 7 days of the cycle so that the daily routine of pilltaking is not altered.

Dosage Form—Tablets: Norethindrone/Ethinyl Estradiol, monophasic, 1 mg/50 μg, 1 mg/35 μg, 0.5 mg/35 μg, 0.4 mg/35 μg; Biphasic, 0.5 mg/35 μg (x10) and 1 mg/35 μg (x11); Triphasic, 0.5 mg/35 μg (x7), 1 mg/35 μg (x7) and 0.5 μg/35 μg (x7) or 0.5 mg/35 μg (x7), 0.75 mg/35 μg (x7) and 1 mg/35 μg (x7).

Norethindrone and Mestranol Tablets

(*Various Mfrs*)

Uses—For *combination oral contraception* (see page 1097). For the actions and uses of the separate components, see *Norethindrone* (page 1096) and *Mestranol* (page 1093). In the higher dose forms, at least, suppression of gonadotropin release by both components probably occurs, but in the products with low doses of norethindrone, the mestranol is the primary anovulatory agent. In addition to its role in the anovulatory effect, mestranol antagonizes some of the androgenic actions of norethindrone. The combination has been used in nearly all conditions in which progestins are indicated (see page 1094), particularly in those situations where anovulation is desirable. It has also been used to regularize uterine bleeding.

For the side effects, see pages 1087, 1094 and 1099.

Dose—*Combinations (norethindrone:mestranol)*: *Oral*, for *contraception, monophasic*, **1 mg:50 μg** a day for 20 or 21 days starting on the 5th day after the beginning of menstruation.

Dosage Form—Tablets: Norethindrone/Mestranol, *monophasic*, 1 mg/50 μg.

Norethindrone Acetate and Ethinyl Estradiol Tablets

(*Various Mfrs*)

Uses—For *combination oral contraception* (see page 1097). Some products are quite low in estrogen content. For the actions of the separate components, see *Norethindrone Acetate* (page 1096) and *Ethinyl Estradiol* (page 1091). The antifertility effect appears to be due more to the progestogen than the estrogen. Adverse effects are essentially the same as those of the separate components (pages 1091 and 1096) and of combination preparations in general (page 1098).

Dose—*Combinations (norethindrone acetate: ethinyl estradiol)* are used: **2.5 mg:50 μg, 1.5 mg:30 μg, 1 mg:50 μg**, and **1 mg:20 μg**. All are taken for 21 days, starting with the 5th day of menstruation, except for the 2.5 mg:50 μg combination which can be taken for only 21 days, if desired. Each of these combinations is available in a product which provides 7 iron ("brown") tablets, to be taken on days 27 through 4, during which no hormones are given.

Dosage Form—Tablets: Norethindrone Acetate/Ethinyl Estradiol, 1/20, 1.5/30, 1/50 and 2.5/50 mg/μg.

Norethynodrel and Mestranol Tablets

Enovid (*Searle*)

Uses—This combination became famous the world over as an oral contraceptive and has been dubbed "The Pill." See page 1093. For the effects of the separate components, see *Norethynodrel* (page 1096) and *Mestranol* (page 1093). The contraceptive action is not entirely the result of prevention of ovulation; the endometrium is rendered inhospitable to the fertilized ovum, so that nidation cannot take place. In addition to oral contraceptive use, preparations containing 5 mg or more of norethynodrel may be used in the treatment of *dysmenorrhea* and *menorrhagia* and to produce cyclic withdrawal bleeding.

The side effects are those of the separate components as well as of combination contraceptives (page 1099). The most frequent effects are bleeding irregularities, nausea, and vomiting in about ¼ of all users, breast fullness, chloasma, headache, weakness, dizziness and diarrhea. The effects diminish with continual use. Sometimes fluid retention and acne occur. Cholestatic jaundice occurs rarely.

Dose—For *contraception*, *norethynodrel* (**2.5** or **5 mg**) plus *mestranol* (**100** or **75 μg**, respectively) daily for 20 or 21 days, starting on the 5th day after menstruation begins. For *cyclic therapy* in dysmenorrhea, functional uterine bleeding (once it is controlled), premenstrual tension, amenorrhea (once a menses has been accomplished) or idiopathic infertility, one 5:75 or 9.85:150 tablet a day for 20 days of each cycle, beginning on the 5th day after menstruation begins; for emergency control of *dysfunctional uterine bleeding*, one 9.85:150 (so-called 10-mg) tablet 2 or 3 times a day until bleeding is arrested, then once a day through the 24th day after menstruation began; for *endometriosis*, one 5:75 or 9.85:150 tablet a day for 2 wk, beginning on the 5th day after menstruation begins, increasing in dosage every 2 wk until 20 mg of norethynodrel a day is being given, to be continued for 6 to 9 mo; to *delay menstruation*, one to two 9.85:150 tablets a day, beginning at least 1 wk in advance of the expected menstruation; to *advance menstruation*, one 5:75 or 9.85:150 tablet for 10 days, beginning on the 5th day after the start of menstruation.

Dosage Form—Tablets: Norethynodrel:Mestranol, 5:75 and 9.85:150 mg:μg.

Norgestrel—page 1097.

Norgestrel and Ethinyl Estradiol Tablets

Ovral (*Wyeth*)

Uses—For *combination oral contraception* (see page 1099). For the actions of the separate components see *Norgestrel* (page 1097) and *Ethinyl Estradiol* (page 1091). The adverse effects are those of the estrogens (page 1091), progestins (page 1096), and combinations (page 1098).

Dose—*Oral, adult*, for *contraception*, **500 μg** of *norgestrel* plus **50 μg** of *ethinyl estradiol* or **300 μg** of *norgestrel* plus **30 μg** of *ethinyl estradiol* a day for 21 days, starting on the 5th day of the menstrual cycle; for *postcoital contraception*, **1 mg** of *norgestrel* plus **100 μg** of *ethinyl estradiol* twice at 12-hr intervals.

Dosage Form—Tablets: Norgestrel : Mestranol, 500:50 and 300:30 μg:μg.

Norethindrone—page 1096.

Norgestrel—page 1097.

Progesterone—page 1097.

Male Contraceptives

Since 1980 there has been considerable effort to develop male contraceptives. In China, *gossypol*, a polyphenolaldehyde isolated from cottonseed oil, has been under investigation since the mid-1950s. It is an inhibitor of human sperm acrosin and an LDD isoenzyme known as LDH-C. It also interferes with epididymal function and elicits structural alterations. A clinical trial in over 4000 healthy men found gossypol to be 99.9% effective as a contraceptive. However, it causes hypokalemia and other untoward effects and has a narrow margin of safety. Its effects are irreversible in 10 to 20% of users. Investigations of related compounds are in progress.

The inhibitory effect of *testosterone* and other androgens on hypothalamic release factor signalling and anterior pituitary secretion of gonadotropins results in a decreased spermatogenesis, and aspermia may result from prolonged, vigorous use. Because of the adverse effects, however, (see the introduction under *The Testicular Hormones*), this approach has limited promise. Low dose androgen-progestin combinations, which suppress anterior pituitary release of LH/FSH with less intense androgenic side effects, are being investigated also.

A more encouraging approach is the use of analogs of LH-RH/FRH-RH, such as *nafarelin* (see page 1061), which causes a down-regulation of pituitary release hormone receptors during nonpulsatile administration, or various antagonists of the releasing factor. Both steroidogenisis and spermatogenesis are diminished reversibly. Decreased libido occurs, so that, to be acceptable to many men, use must be supplemented with androgens.

The Sertoli cell peptide, *inhibin*, and related proteins, which inhibit the anterior pituitary release of FSH, are under active investigation, but are not ready for clinical trials. They, too, probably will decrease libido and hence may not be acceptable to a large percentage of potential users.

Perhaps the most promising but nascent developments are vaccines against one or more of spermatic proteins. The sperm lactic dehydrogenase, LDH-C_4, and possibly various protamines are presently investigational targets for monoclonal and other antibodies. The first vaccines for human use are likely to be against LDH-C_4. The effects of vaccines, are not likely to be readily reversible, although some memory immune cells have relatively short lifetimes. The approach has great promise for undeveloped nations.

The Testicular Hormone

The testis has a dual function, to produce the germ cell (the *sperm*) and supply the male hormone (*testosterone*). Two clearly defined groups of cells are found in the testes; the one group in the tubules produces the sperm, while the other, clustered in between the tubules, consists of interstitial cells (Leydig cells). The spermatogenic tissue produces an exocrine secretion and probably also androgens needed for spermatogenesis.

The interstitial cells are the seat of production of a steroid hormone, testosterone. However, it is mainly the metabolite, dihydrotestosterone, which stimulates and maintains the secondary sex organs; these are the penis, prostate gland, seminal vesicles, vas deferens and scrotum. It also exerts sustaining effects on the spermatogenic cells, and it stimulates the development of bone, muscle, nerves, skin and hair growth, and emotional responses to produce the characteristic adult masculine traits. Testosterone, itself, regulates the hypophyseal release of LH. This group of combined actions of this hormone is termed *androgenic actions*. Testosterone also antagonizes a number of the effects of estrogens, and sometimes is employed clinically for this purpose. This is especially important in the suppression of metastatic carcinoma of the breast. Since it promotes development of the clitoris, which is an anatomic homolog of the penis, androgens may increase the libido of women.

The naturally occurring androgens (androsterone, testosterone) are derivatives of androstane. Testosterone and its esters (testosterone propionate) and derivatives (methyltestosterone) are the most commonly used androgenic steroids. In addition to their androgenic properties, however, these compounds exert widespread anabolic effects and promote the retention of calcium. In attempts to dissociate the virilizing and anabolic properties (for use in women) a number of compounds with high anabolic:androgenic ratios have been prepared. However, it has not been possible yet to abolish completely the androgenic effects.

Uses—For *replacement therapy* in men who have climacteric symptoms, or in men or youths with *hypogonadism* (eunuchism, Klinefelter's syndrome). They have been employed to facilitate development of adult masculine characteristics when the adolescent process has been delayed. In *cryptorchidism* they may be used adjunctively with gonadotropins. They also are very useful in therapy of patients with *hypopituitarism* and with *Addison's disease*. They are of value in the treatment of *frigidity* and occasionally in *impotence*. The use of androgens for relief of impotence not associated with evidence of testicular underactivity (psychic causes) is known to be futile in most cases. Low doses of androgens have been used in pituitary dwarfism to *accelerate growth*, but care must be exercised not to arrest growth by epiphyseal closure. They also are used sometimes to *promote hematopoiesis*. In large, supratherapeutic doses, anabolic steroids increase athletic performance and aggressiveness. Their use has been condemned by the American College of Sports Medicine. Female performance is improved, but at the expense of virilization and acne vulgaris. Their use subjects the athlete to disqualification for official competition.

With estrogens, androgen therapy may be efficacious in the treatment of the *menopause*. The anabolic effects are possibly of some benefit in the postclimacteric person, and they may retard *osteoporosis*, although many authorities do not believe that any lasting benefit is achieved. They also help *relieve vasomotor instability* in postmenopausal women in whom estrogens alone do not relieve symptoms. In functional *dysmenorrhea* androgens may give relief through an antiestrogenic action, although they also are combined often with estrogens to treat this disorder. They may be used to treat *endometriosis*. They also may be used in the treatment of *postpartum breast engorgement* and for *suppression of lactation*.

Testosterone and related compounds find widespread application in the palliative treatment of *cancer of the breast* in women. Its use in men with prostatic cancer, however, is contraindicated.

Side Effects—Androgens cause hirsutism, deepening or hoarseness of the voice, precocious puberty and epiphyseal closure in immature males, increased libido (in both male and female!), priapism, oligospermia and testicular atrophy (from negative feedback on LH and FSH production), enlargement of the clitoris in the female, flushing, decreased ejaculatory volume and sperm population, gynecomastia (from conversion to estrogens), hypersensitivity, acne, weight gain, edema and hypercalcemia. Prolonged use increases aggressiveness, sometimes enormously, and many assaults are stated to be attributable to androgen abuse. Paranoia-like and other psychotic behavior has been reported. Biliary stasis and jaundice occur. There have been a few cases reported of hepatoma following long-term therapy. The 17α-methylated androgens are more prone to disturb liver function than are the nonsubstituted drugs. Hypercalcemia requires discontinuation of therapy, and edema requires diuretic therapy. Except in the treatment of breast cancer, a reduction in dosage is indicated upon virilization in women.

The administration of androgens to patients on anticoagulant therapy may increase the effect of anticoagulants and, thus, may require an adjustment of the dose of the latter. Likewise, dosage of insulin or oral hypoglycemic agents may require adjustment when anabolic androgens are administered to diabetic patients.

Cyproterone Acetate

3′*H*-Cyclopropa[1,2]pregna-1,4,6-triene-3,20-dione, (1β,2β)-17-(acetyloxy)-6-chloro-1,2-dihydro-, ing of Androcur (*Berlex*); (*Various Mfrs*)

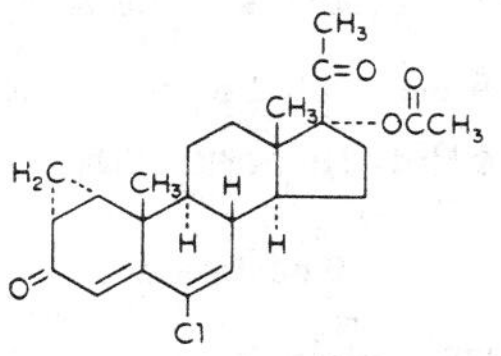

[427-51-0] $C_{24}H_{29}ClO_4$ (416.94).

Preparation—US Pat 3,234,093.

Description—White crystals; melts about 200°.

Solubility—Soluble in water; slightly soluble in alcohol.

Uses—An androgen antagonist orphan drug. It also has strong progestin activity that suppresses the otherwise expected increase in LH/FSH secretion consequent to attenuated androgen activity. It is used to treat *severe hirsutism in women* (used in sequence with estrogens), *excessive sexual drive in men* and *precocious puberty*. Adverse effects include oligospermia, decreased volume of ejaculate, loss of libido in both men and women, gynecomastia in men, galactorrhea and glandular enlargement, mastodynia, alterations in hair pattern, skin reactions, weight changes, anemia, vasomotor instability in both men and women, irregular menses in women, headache and depression.

Dose—*Intramuscular, adult, excessive sexual drive*, **300 mg** once a wk, decreased to once every other wk after orchiectomy. *Oral, adult, excessive sexual drive*, **50** to **100 mg** a day; *hirsutism* in women, **100 mg** a day for 10 days each mo, beginning on the 5th day of the mense; *boys, precocious puberty*, **70** to **150 mg/m²** for 6 to 40 mo. *Intramuscular or subcutaneous*, **107** to **230 mg/m²** every 2 to 4 wk.

Dosage Form—Tablets: 50 mg.

Danazol

(17α)-Pregna-2,4-dien-20-yno[2,3-*d*]isoxazol-17-ol, Chronogyn; Danocrine (*Winthrop*)

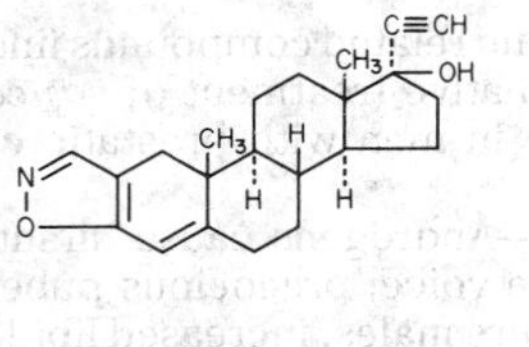

[17230-88-5] $C_{22}H_{27}NO_2$ (337.46).

Preparation—Danazol is a derivative of ethisterone (17α-ethynyltestosterone) in which an isoxazole ring is fused to the 2,3-position of the steroid nucleus. Methods for preparing such steroidal heterocycles have been described by Manson *et al*, *J Med Chem 6*:1, 1963; also in US Pat 3,135,743.

Description—Pale yellow, crystalline powder; melts about 225°.

Solubility—Practically insoluble in water; sparingly soluble in alcohol.

Uses—An "impeded" androgen (ie, weak androgenic activity). It binds to androgen, glucocorticoid and progesterone receptors, but it evokes no glucocorticoid, progestational or estrogenic effects except that it suppresses the release of LH and FSH, even in women. It suppresses ovarian steroidogenesis, induces the hepatic metabolism of progesterone and binds to α_1-macroglobulin, causing partial displacement of other steroids. It is used in the treatment of *endometriosis* in patients who do not respond to or cannot tolerate other drug therapy and in the management of *fibrocystic breast disease* and *periareolar abscesses.* It may prevent attacks of *hereditary angioedema.* It increases platelet populations in *idiopathic* and *immune thrombocytopenias.* However, it also can cause thrombocytopenia. It relieves *migraine* in some persons.

Androgenic side effects include deepening of the voice in women, acne, edema, mild hirsutism, decrease in breast size, oiliness of the skin and hair, weight gain and clitoral hypertrophy. Hypoestrogenic manifestations include amenorrhea, vasomotor instability, vaginitis with itching, burning and vaginal bleeding and emotional lability. It also may cause muscle cramps, asthenia, rhabdomyolysis, testicular atrophy and rare hematuria. It has an adverse effect on plasma lipids. In doses over 400 mg a day, it may cause hepatic injury, including carcinoma. It has been reported to lower serum levothyroxine levels.

Dose—*Oral, adult,* for *mild endometriosis,* **100** to **200 mg** twice a day for at least 3 to 6, and as long as 9 mo; for *moderate* to *severe endometriosis,* **400 mg** twice a day for at least 3 and as long as 9 mo; for *fibrocystic breast* disease **50** to **200 mg** twice a day, preferably beginning during the mense; for *angioedoma, initially* **200 mg** 2 or 3 times a day then, once the effect has been achieved, decrements of no more than 50%, according to the frequency of attacks. During an attack, the dose may be increased by 200 mg.

Dosage Form—Capsules: 50, 100 and 200 mg.

Ethylestrenol—see RPS-18, page 1001.

Finasteride

4-Azaandrost-1-ene-17-carboxamide, (5α,17β)-*N*-(1,1-dimethylethyl)-3-oxo-, Proscar (*MSD*)

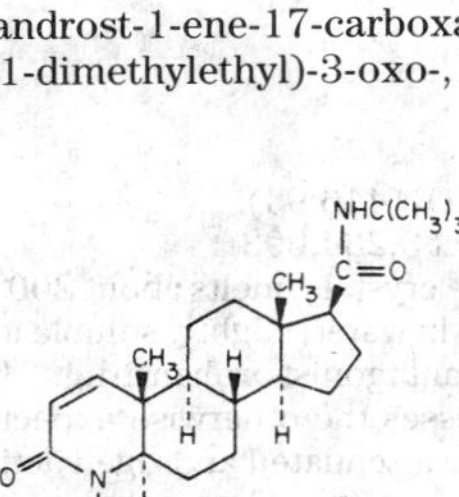

[98319-26-7] $C_{23}H_{36}N_2O_2$ (372.55).

Preparation—*J Am Chem Soc 110*:3319, 1988.

Description—White to off-white crystals; melts about 257°.

Solubility—Very slightly soluble in water or dilute acid or base; freely soluble in alcohol or chloroform.

Uses—An androgen hormone inhibitor that acts by competitive inhibition of steroid 5-reductase which converts testosterone to potent 5-dihydrotestosterone (DHT) in the prostate gland, liver and skin. DHT induces its effects by binding to androgen receptors in cell nuclei of organs containing this enzyme. It is used to treat *symptomatic benign prostatic hyperplasia.* Oral bioavailability is 63% and its mean plasma half-life is 6 hr. About 39% of the drug is eliminated in the urine as metabolites and 57% is excreted in feces. The drug generally is tolerated well with reports of impotence (3.7%), decreased libido (3.3%) and decreased volume of ejaculation (2.8%).

Dose—*Oral,* **5 mg** once a day.

Dosage Form—Tablets: 5 mg.

Fluoxymesterone

(11β,17β)-Androst-4-en-3-one, 9-fluoro-11,17-dihydroxy-17-methyl-, Halotestin (*Upjohn*)

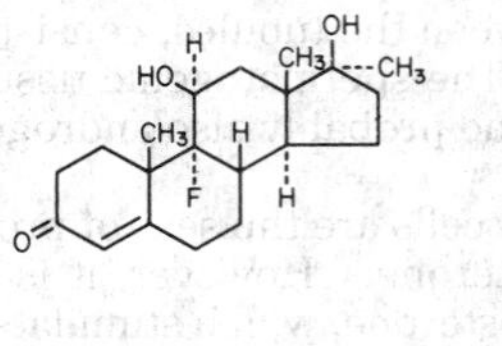

[76-43-7] $C_{20}H_{29}FO_3$ (336.45).

Preparation—From 17-methyltestosterone first by introduction of a hydroxyl group at position 11 through oxidation with a microorganism (such as *Pestalotia* or *Aspergillus*), followed by dehydration, epoxidation and treatment with HF, as for *Betamethasone* (page 1069).

Description—White or practically white, odorless, crystalline powder; melts about 240° with some decomposition.

Solubility—Practically insoluble in water; sparingly soluble in alcohol; slightly soluble in chloroform.

Uses—The same actions, uses and limitations as the androgens (page 1101). It is approximately five times more potent than testosterone, and is orally effective. Nevertheless, it is less effective than testosterone in hypogonadism and is seldom used to initiate treatment but rather for maintenance. In addition to the side effects of testosterone, this drug may cause occasional cholestatic jaundice, gynecomastia, oligospermia after prolonged use and hypersensitivity. It sometimes is combined with an estrogen for treatment of postmenopausal osteoporosis. The half-life is about 10 hr.

Dose—*Oral, adult, replacement therapy,* **5 mg** 1 to 4 times a day; *adolescent boys,* for *delayed puberty, initially* **2.5 mg** a day followed by gradual increments, if necessary to as much as 20 mg a day for 4 to 6 mo; *inoperable breast carcinoma in women,* **10** to **40 mg** a day in divided doses; in *hypoplastic* or *aplastic anemia,* **10** to **20 mg** twice a day; for *postpartum breast engorgement, initially* **2.5** to **5 mg** just after delivery, then **5** to **10 mg** a day in divided doses for 4 or 5 days postpartum.

Dosage Form—Tablets: 2, 5 and 10 mg.

Methyltestosterone

(17β)-Androst-4-en-3-one, 17-hydroxy-17-methyl-, (*Various Mfrs*)

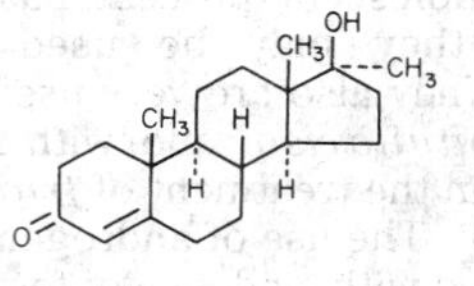

[58-18-4] $C_{20}H_{30}O_2$ (302.46).

Preparation—From dehydroepiandrosterone (prepared from cholesterol) by subjecting it to a Grignard reaction with CH_3MgI followed by an Oppenauer oxidation. The first reaction creates the tertiary carbinol structure at C_{17}, while the second oxidizes the secondary carbinol group at position 3 to carbonyl and causes a rearrangement of the double bond from the 5,6- to the 4,5-position.

Description—White or creamy white crystals or a crystalline powder; odorless; stable in air, but slightly hygroscopic; affected by light; melts about 165°.

Solubility—Practically insoluble in water; soluble in alcohol, methanol, ether or other organic solvents; sparingly soluble in vegetable oils.

Uses—The same actions, uses and limitations as the androgens (page 1101). It is effective orally. It also is combined with various estrogens for treatment of menorrhagia, menopausal symptoms, dysmenorrhea, osteoporosis, malnutrition and to suppress postpartum lactation. In addition to the side effects caused by testosterone, it may cause oligospermia, hypersensitivity with dermatologic manifestations, and a rare type of cholestatic jaundice. It often is stated that virilization in women does not occur unless the dose exceeds 300 mg a mo, but virilization can occur with doses considerably less than this.

It is metabolized rapidly by the liver and undergoes first-pass metabolism. By the buccal route, potency is twice that by the oral route. The half-life is about 2.5 hr.

Dose—*Buccal, adult, replacement,* **5** to **25 mg** a day; *postpubertal cryptorchidism,* **5 mg** 3 times a day; *inoperable breast cancer* in women, **2.5** to **12.5 mg** 1 to 4 times a day. *Oral (conventional tablet) adult, replacement,* **10** to **50 mg** a day; *postpubertal cryptorchidism,* **10 mg** 3 times a day; *postpartum breast engorgement,* **20 mg** 4 times a day for 3 to 5 days; *inoperable breast cancer* in women, **50 mg** 1 to 4 times a day.

Dosage Forms—Capsules: 10 mg; Tablets: 10 and 25 mg; Buccal Tablets: 10 mg.

Nandrolone Decanoate

(17β)- Estr-4-en-3-one, 17-[(1-oxodecyl)oxy]-, (*Various Mfrs*)

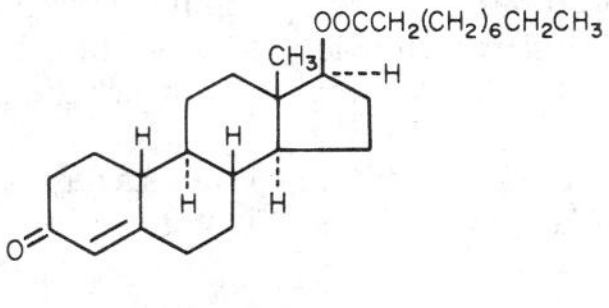

17β-Hydroxyestr-4-en-3-one decanoate [360-70-3] $C_{28}H_{44}O_3$ (428.65).

Preparation—A dry benzene solution of 17β-hydroxy-estr-4-en- 3-one (19-nortestosterone) and pyridine is mixed with a dry benzene solution of decanoyl chloride and the esterification is allowed to proceed overnight in an atmosphere of nitrogen. After washing successively with acid, alkali and water, the solvent is evaporated and the crude ester is recrystallized from petroleum ether or some other suitable solvent. US Pat 2,998,423.

Description—Fine, white to creamy white, crystalline powder; odorless or may have a slight odor; melts about 34°.

Solubility—Soluble in chloroform, alcohol, acetone or vegetable oils; practically insoluble in water.

Uses—The *management of the anemia of renal insufficiency.* Oil solutions of the decanoate have a duration of action 3 to 4 times longer than that of the phenpropionate.

Dose—*Intramuscular, adult* and *children over 14 yr, anabolic* or for *osteoporosis, males,* **100** to **200 mg** and *females,* **50** to **100 mg** once a wk; *metastatic breast carcinoma* or *refractory anemias,* **100** to **200 mg** a wk; *children 2* to *13 yr, anabolic,* **25** to **50 mg** every 3 to 4 wk; other pediatric doses not determined.

Dosage Form—Injection: 50 mg/1 mL, 100 mg/2 mL, 200 mg/1 mL, 200 mg/2 mL.

Nandrolone Phenpropionate

(17β)- Estr-4-en-3-one, 17-(1-oxo-3-phenylpropoxy)-, Durabolin (*Organon*); Nandrobolic (*Forest*) (*Various Mfrs*)

17β-Hydroxyestr-4-en-3-one hydrocinnamate [62-90-8] $C_{27}H_{34}O_3$ (406.56).

For the structure of the steroid moiety, see *Nandrolone Decanoate.*

Preparation—19-Nortestosterone is esterified with hydrocinnamoyl chloride by the method described for *Nandrolone Decanoate.*

Description—Fine, white to creamy white, crystalline powder having a slight characteristic odor; melts about 97°.

Solubility—Practically insoluble in water; soluble in alcohol (1 g in 2 mL), chloroform, dioxane or vegetable oils.

Uses—A synthetic androgen with actions more prolonged than those of *Testosterone.* Although it is less androgenic than testosterone in doses which exert anabolic actions, virilization may occur after high doses or during chronic administration. Indeed, the androgenic virilizing actions are sought in the treatment with this agent of *inoperable breast cancer* in women. It is used mainly in the treatment of *chronic wasting diseases, conditions in which negative nitrogen balance exists* and *osteoporosis.* Low doses may *accelerate the growth of children* with retarded growth without excessively accelerating bone age; higher doses accelerate bone maturation more than body growth. The phenylpropionate ester moiety confers a long duration of action to suspensions in oil injected intramuscularly. The potential side effects are those of testosterone. The drug does not appear to cause cholestatic jaundice, probably because it lacks an alkyl group on carbon 17.

Dose—*Intramuscular, adults,* **50** to **100 mg** once a wk; *children,* use the decanoate.

Dosage Form—Injection (in oil): 100 mg/2 mL, 125 mg/5 mL.

Oxandrolone

(5α,17β)-2-Oxaandrostan-3-one, 17-hydroxy-17-methyl-, Oxandrin (*Gynex*)

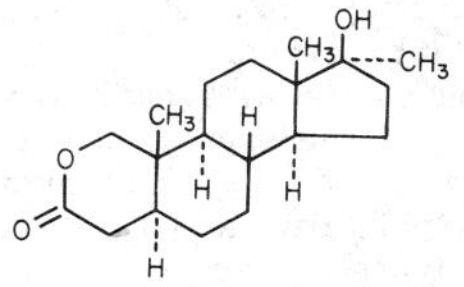

17β-Hydroxy-17-methyl-2-oxa-5α-androstan-3-one [53-39-4] $C_{19}H_{30}O_3$ (306.44).

Preparation—Methyldihydrotesterone is converted into the corresponding 1,2-dehydro compound by bromination followed by dehydrobromination. Ring A is then ruptured through ozonization and subsequent hydrolysis to yield the aldehyde-acid (I). Reduction of the formyl group in I yields the expected hydroxy acid implied in the partial structure (II) which is lactonized to oxandrolone.

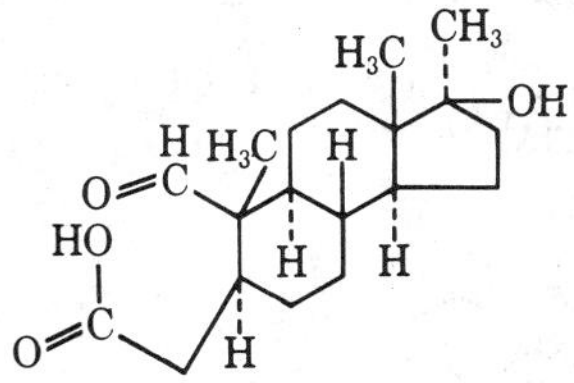

(I) 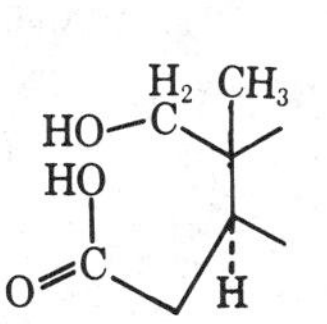 (II)

Description—White, odorless, crystalline powder; stable in air but darkens when exposed to light; melts about 225°.

Solubility—1 g in 5200 mL water, 57 mL alcohol, <5 mL chloroform, 860 mL ether or 69 mL acetone.

Uses—Although strictly speaking not a steroid, its configuration is that of a 17-methyl androgenic steroid. Its anabolic actions are strong relative to its androgenic actions. Consequently, it is used in the treatment of *chronic wasting diseases,* conditions in which *negative nitrogen balance* exists and *osteoporosis,* especially that caused by glucocorticoids. The drug may cause virilization in children or women, especially if the recommended doses are exceeded. The potential toxicity is that of the androgens but the incidence and severity are less than with testosterone. It may affect liver function tests adversely, and the possibility of cholestatic jaundice must be kept in mind. Leukopenia also has been reported. It is contraindicated in prostatic cancer, breast cancer in some women, pregnancy, nephrosis, and premature and newborn infants. It is also available as an IND for treatment of constitutional delay of growth and puberty.

Dose—*Oral, adults, initially* **2.5 mg** 2 to 4 times a day, then **2.5** to **20 mg** a day for *maintenance,* not to be taken for more than 3 mo in any one course; for *children,* **250 μg/kg** a day, repeated as indicated.

Dosage Form—Tablets: 2.5 mg.

Oxymetholone

(5α,17β)-Androstan-3-one, 17-hydroxy-2-(hydroxymethylene)-17-methyl-, Anadrol (*Syntex*)

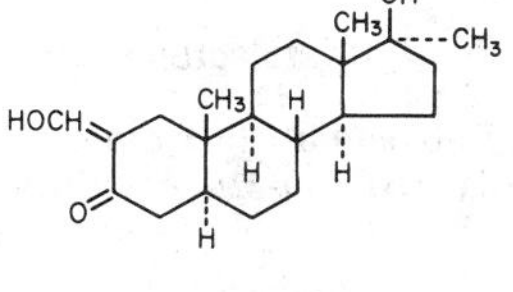

[434-07-1] $C_{21}H_{32}O_3$ (332.48).

Preparation—17β-Hydroxy-17-methylandrostan-3-one (17-methyldihydrotestosterone) is reacted with ethyl formate and sodium hydroxide by stirring the mixture under nitrogen for several hours thus forming the 2-(sodoxymethylene) derivative. Treatment of the washed sodium compound with cold dilute hydrochloric acid liberates the oxymetholone which may be purified by recrystallization from ethyl acetate. *J Am Chem Soc 81:*427, 1959.

Description—White to creamy white crystals or crystalline powder; odorless and stable in air; tautomeric in nature and can exist as either tautomer or as a mixture of both, the exact composition depending on solvent and rate of crystallization; melts about 175°.

Solubility—1 g in >10,000 mL water, 40 mL alcohol, 5 mL chloroform, 82 mL ether or 14 mL dioxane.

Uses—An androgenic steroid with relatively greater anabolic activity than androgenic activity. Consequently, it is employed mainly to *promote nitrogen anabolism* and weight gain in cachexia and debilitating diseases and after serious infections, burns, trauma or surgery. It may relieve pain in certain types of *osteoporosis,* and it promotes calcium retention, so that the condition of the bone may improve. It may be used for its erythropoietic effects in the treatment of *hypoplastic* and *aplastic anemias.* Side effects include nausea, vomiting, anorexia, burning of the tongue, increased or decreased libido, acne, suppression of gonadotropin secretion, virilization (especially in women and children), gynecomastia in males, oligospermia, sodium retention and edema, abnormal liver function tests, cholestatic jaundice, decrease in several clotting factors and hemorrhagic diathesis in the presence of anticoagulants.

Dose—*Oral, adults, children and infants,* **1** to **5 mg/kg** a day given for a trial of 3 to 6 mo.

Dosage Form—Tablets: 50 mg.

Stanozolol

(5α,17β)-2′*H*-Androst-2-eno[3,2-*c*]pyrazol-17-ol, 17-methyl-, Winstrol (*Winthrop*)

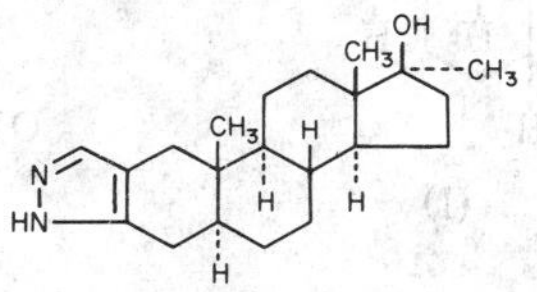

[10418-03-8] $C_{21}H_{32}N_2O$ (328.50).

Preparation—17-Methyl-5α-androstan-17β-ol-3-one is converted into its 2-formyl derivative which is then condensed with hydrazine hydrate. US Pat 3,030,358.

Description—Nearly colorless, odorless, crystalline powder; exists in two forms: *needles,* melting about 155°, and *prisms,* melting about 235°.

Solubility—1 g in >1000 mL water, 41 mL alcohol, 74 mL chloroform or 370 mL ether.

Uses—An *androgen* with relatively strong anabolic and weak androgenic activity. Consequently, it is employed mainly to *promote nitrogen anabolism* and weight gain in cachexia and debilitating diseases and after serious infections, burns, trauma or surgery. Although it may relieve pain in certain types of *osteoporosis,* it apparently does not affect bone density. It may have an erythropoietic effect in *hypoplastic* and *aplastic anemias.* It also is used in the *prophylaxis* of *heretitary angioedema,* which is now the only approved use.

Side effects include increased or decreased libido, virilization (especially in women and children), sodium retention and edema, hypercalcemia, insomnia, restlessness, chills, hemorrhage in patients on anticoagulants, acne and hepatic dysfunction. Potentially, any of the side effects of *Testosterone* may occur. However, these rarely occur during the usual 5-day course.

Dose—*Oral, adults, initially* **2 mg** 3 times a day to **4 mg** 4 times a day for 5 days, except twice a day in women who are virilized easily by the usual dose; *children under 6 yr,* **1 mg** twice a day, to be administered only during an acute attack of angioedema; *children 6 to 12 yr,* up to 2 mg 3 times a day, to be administered only during an acute attack.

Dosage Form—Scored Tablets: 2 mg.

Testolactone

D-Homo-17a-oxaandrosta-1,4-diene-3,17-dione; Teslac (*Bristol-Myers Oncology*)

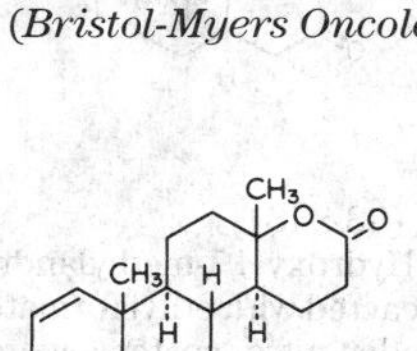

13-Hydroxy-3-oxo-13,17-secoandrosta-1,4-dien-17-oic acid δ-lactone [968-93-4] $C_{19}H_{24}O_3$ (300.40).

Preparation—By microbial transformation of progesterone, testosterone, and various other steroidal substances. US Pat 2,744,120; *J Org Chem 30:*760, 1965.

Description—White to off-white, practically odorless, crystalline powder; stable in light, air and normal temperatures; melts about 218°.

Solubility—Slightly soluble in water or benzyl alcohol; soluble in alcohol or chloroform; insoluble in ether or solvent hexane.

Uses—An aromatase inhibitor that prevents the synthesis of estrogens. Although structurally related to the androgens, it is essentially devoid of androgenic activity in therapeutic doses. It is used in the adjunctive and palliative treatment of inoperable *breast cancer* in women. When the tumor cells possess estrogen receptors and lesions are nonosseus, about 50% of cases will show some improvement. Remissions occur in approximately 15% of cases.

Except possibly for hypercalcemia, the side effects are not those of the androgens. There may be mild pain, irritation and inflammation at the site of injection. Other reported side effects are anorexia, nausea, vomiting, diarrhea, aches, myalgia, arthralgia, edema of the extremities, swelling of the tongue, peripheral neuritis (tingling of the face and extremities), maculopapular rash and hypertension; these all subside without discontinuation of the drug, and it is not always clear to what extent the drug or the disease is responsible.

Dose—*Usual, oral, adult,* **250 mg** 4 times a day.

Dosage Form—Tablets: 50 and 250 mg.

Testosterone

(17β)-Androst-4-en-3-one, 17-hydroxy, (*Various Mfrs*)

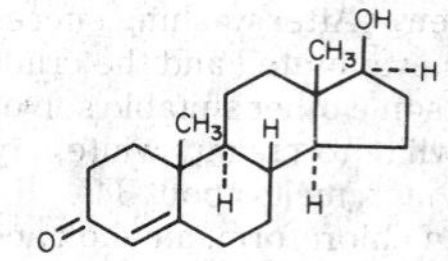

17β-Hydroxyandrost-4-en-3-one [58-22-0] $C_{19}H_{28}O_2$ (288.43).

Preparation—First isolated in crystalline form by Laquer in 1935 who obtained it from animal testes. Although small amounts of testosterone may be extracted from testicular material, the synthetic commercial supply is derived from cholesterol. The key intermediate in the synthesis is dehydroepiandrosterone which can be treated further, by either chemical or microbiological processes, to yield testosterone. US Pat 2,236,574.

Description—White or slightly creamy white crystals or crystalline powder; odorless; stable in air; melts about 155°.

Solubility—Practically insoluble in water; 1 g in about 6 mL of dehydrated alcohol, 1 mL chloroform or 100 mL ether; soluble in vegetable oils.

Uses—See the introduction to this section, page 1101. It is not effective orally because it is destroyed in the liver on absorption. Its plasma half-life is 10 to 20 min.

Dose—*Intramuscular, replacement therapy,* **25** to **50 mg** 2 or 3 times a wk; *delayed puberty* or *postpubertal cryptorchidism,* **12.5** to **25 mg** 2 or 3 times a wk; to *prevent postpartum breast engorgement,* **25 mg** once or twice a day for 3 or 4 days; in *metastatic breast cancer,* **50** to **100 mg** 3 times a wk.

Dosage Form—Sterile Suspension: 25, 50 and 100 mg/mL.

Testosterone Cypionate

(17β)-Androst-4-en-3-one, 17-(3-cyclopentyl-1-oxopropoxy)-, (*Various Mfrs*)

Testosterone cyclopentanepropionate [58-20-8] $C_{27}H_{40}O_3$ (412.61).

For the structure of the base, see *Testosterone.*

Preparation—Testosterone is esterified by interaction with 3-cyclopentylpropionyl chloride [$C_5H_{11}CH_2CH_2COCl$] in the presence of pyridine.

Description—White or creamy white, crystalline powder which is odorless or has a slight odor and is stable in air; melts about 100°.

Solubility—Insoluble in water; freely soluble in alcohol, chloroform, dioxane or ether; soluble in vegetable oils.

Uses—The same actions, uses and limitations as the androgens (see the introduction to this section) but the cypionate has a much longer duration of action (3 to 4 wk) than testosterone when administered intramuscularly in oil.

Dose—*Intramuscular, replacement* in various *male hypogonadal states* and *impotence*, **50** to **400 mg** every 2 to 4 wk; for *delayed puberty*, **25** to **200 mg** every 2 to 4 wk, usually for no longer than 6 mo; *metastatic breast cancer* in women, **200** to **400 mg** every 2 to 4 wk.

Dosage Form—Injection (in oil): 100 and 200 mg/mL

Testosterone Enanthate

(17β)-Androst-4-en-3-one, 17-[(1-oxoheptyl)oxy]-, (*Various Mfrs*)

Testosterone heptanoate [315-37-7] $C_{26}H_{40}O_3$ (400.60).

For the structure of the parent, see *Testosterone*.

Preparation—A solution of enanthic acid in benzene is refluxed for about one hour after which it is allowed to cool, testosterone is added and the mixture is refluxed for about 21 hr. The resulting light brown solution is cooled, extracted with a sodium hydroxide solution to remove surplus enanthic acid, washed with water and dried over magnesium sulfate. After removal of solvent, the crude ester is purified by molecular distillation.

Description—White or creamy white, crystalline powder; odorless or has a faint odor characteristic of enanthic acid; melts about 36°, the initial temperature of the bath not exceeding 20°.

Solubility—Insoluble in water; 1 g in about 0.3 mL ether; soluble in vegetable oils.

Uses—The same actions, uses and limitations as *Testosterone Cypionate*, except that the enanthate also is used for the treatment of osteoporosis. The effects of a single intramuscular injection may last 3 to 4 wk.

Dose—*Intramuscular*, for *replacement* in *male hypogonadal states* and for *impotence*, **50** to **400 mg** every 2 to 4 wk; treatment of *anemia*, *initially* **400 mg** a day for 7 days, then once or twice in the next week, and **200** to **400 mg** every 4 wk for *maintenance*; for *metastatic breast cancer* in women, **200** to **400 mg** every 2 to 4 wk.

Dosage Form—Injection (in oil): 100 and 200 mg/mL.

Testosterone Propionate

(17β)-Androst-4-en-3-one, 17-(1-oxopropoxy)-, (*Various Mfrs*)

17β-Hydroxyandrost-4-en-3-one propionate [57-85-2] $C_{22}H_{32}O_3$ (344.49).

For the structure of the parent, see *Testosterone*.

Preparation—From testosterone by refluxing with propionic anhydride.

Description—White or creamy white crystals or crystalline powder; odorless and stable in air; melts about 120°.

Solubility—Insoluble in water; freely soluble in alcohol, dioxane, ether or other organic solvents; soluble in vegetable oils.

Uses—See the introduction to this section. Intramuscular injection of the propionate provides a somewhat more intense action than with testosterone, but the duration of action is somewhat shorter, even though the half-life is about 4 hr. The parenteral route is not suited to long-term treatment. The other esters of testosterone and synthetic congeners have considerably diminished the importance of the propionate.

Dose—*Intramuscular, adult, replacement* in various *male hypogonadal states*, **25** to **50 mg** 2 or 3 times a wk; *adolescent boys*, for *delayed puberty*, **12.5** to **25 mg** 2 or 3 times a wk for up to 6 mo; for *metastatic breast cancer* in women, **50** to **100 mg** 3 times a wk. For *postpartum breast engorgement*, **25** to **50 mg** a day for 3 or 4 days.

Dosage Form—Injection (in oil): 50 and 100 mg/mL

CHAPTER 65

Vitamins and Other Nutrients

Ernestine Vanderveen, PhD
National Institute on Alcohol Abuse and Alcoholism
NIH
Rockville, MD 20857

John E Vanderveen, PhD
Center for Food Safety and Applied Nutrition
Food and Drug Administration
Washington, DC 20204

Man consumes food to provide him with energy for growth, maintenance of normal body functions, and work. Energy is made available through conversion of carbohydrate, fat, and protein, which yield 4, 9 and 4 kilocalories per gram of the nutrient, respectively, when completely metabolized. The proportion or each of these nutrient sources in the human diet varies with environment, food availability, culture, and personal food behavior of the individual.

In the US the percent of total calories provided by carbohydrate, fat, and protein in most diets is approximately 50, 38 and 12%, respectively. There is growing evidence that the amount and form of carbohydrates and fats have a profound effect on the development of degenerative diseases.

Metabolism, growth and tissue repair require adequate ingestion of protein, minerals, vitamins, water, and oxygen. The latter two generally are not classed as nutrients in the usual sense but are substances that must be supplied on a continuing basis and in sufficient amount to sustain life. Current recommendations are that diets should not contain more than 30% of total calories from fat, of which not more than ⅓ should be from saturated fat and not more than ⅓ from polyunsaturated fat. The remainder of the fat will be monounsaturated. Olive oil is a good source of monounsaturated fatty acids.

Mineral elements present in organic compounds serve structural, catalytic and modulator roles in the metabolic processes. Minerals are present as free ions in body fluids, where they act osmotically as electrolytes. The solid structure of the body, which is primarily bone tissue, contains mineral compounds. Vitamins are a heterogeneous group of organic compounds that participate in metabolic processes in minute amounts compared to other nutrients. The combination of complex processes through which living animal organisms obtain and utilize these materials is nutrition. The various disciplines of study aimed at elucidating those processes are collectively termed nutritional science.

Understanding of the significance of nutrients in human physiology has evolved largely from research studies on lower forms of life, mainly bacteria and animals, such as the chicken, rat, guniea pig, mouse, dog, pig and monkey. These studies have been substantiated and enlarged by clinical observations on human populations in healthy states and various conditions of disease, in malnutrition and by some experimental studies conducted with human subjects.

Misinformation About Food—A vast amount of confusion and nonscientific information surrounds that relationship of foods, as specially formulated food products, to health and preventing or cure of various disease conditions. The consumption of appropriate amounts of food selected from a variety of plant and animal sources will, over a period of time, furnish adequate to abundant amounts of all known essential nutritients for virtually the entire population.

A very few individuals with inborn errors of metabolism, or who have injury or diseases of the GI tract or are exposed to substances which decrease absorption or alter metabolism of certain nutrients, may need supplements or special foods to meet their needs. However, food behaviors of increasing numbers of people are influenced by misrepresentations and false claims made for "health" foods, fad diets and miracle cures by individuals and groups who profit from sale of such foods or ideas. Often these purveyors are convincing in their approach, claiming to have experienced a "cure" or presenting evidence of their product's success in curing people of a variety of real or imagined illnesses. When the unwary consumer uncritically accepts the advice of the purveyors of falsely labeled products in place of needed medical treatment, serious consequences can result. Risks incurred through following bizarre diet schemes for weight loss can be equally serious. Deaths have occurred from causes directly or indirectly associated with fad diets and other forms of self diagnosis and treatment.

The FDA has the responsibility and authority to control interstate traffic of products which are falsely promoted. This includes authority to regulate nutritional supplements for safety; insure that labeling is informative, accurate and does not contain false or misleading statements; and that supplements for infants, children under 12 years, pregnant women and lactating women have appropriate potency. Compliance with regulations that pertain to safety, label requirements and promotion is accomplished through nationwide monitoring of labeling as well as of composition of the enormous number and variety of packaged foods in the market. Pharmacists and others who are informed in the sciences that make up nutritional science should report instances of false and misleading claims in labeling to the FDA.

Particularly in the field of nutrition, where misinformation may endanger the health of individuals, the consumer must be provided opportunity to learn to make sound decisions regarding his health and nutritional status. Effective nutrition education programs are perceived to be essential if consumers are to make decisions in their own best interest when faced with the complexities of the modern marketplace.

Pharmacists, because of their day-to-day contact with the public most directly concerned, have a responsibility to be well-informed to allay the fears that are created by pseudoscientific writings of sensationalists, and to protect the health as well as the pocketbooks of patrons.

Nutrient Requirements and Dietary Standards—The determination of quantitative human requirements for nutrients could be made if it were possible to correlate known nutrient intake with specific biological responses in precisely controlled studies. Although that is not possible, there are three kinds of studies which do yield information that can be used to closely estimate requirements.

Balance studies, which employ a method of comparing nutrient intake and output and therefore measure body gain or loss of a stable component.

Biochemical measurements of a nutrient, nutrient metabolites or related functional and structural components in a body fluid, compartment, tissue or excreta.

Clinical evaluation and performance tests on subjects maintained on carefully controlled nutrient intakes to determine dietary levels that maintain health and will prevent deterioration of physiological and cognitive functions.

Ideally, data from all three enable the investigator to determine the smallest amount of a nutrient that will prevent deficiency symptoms or support a well-defined physiological or biochemical response, eg, the maintenance of serum ferritin levels in women of childbearing ages. An *average* requirement, however, is derived most often from such data to denote the amount of a nutrient that will support health in most persons of a given population group. It implies that the *true* requirement for *individuals* may be either above or below the average for the group. Obviously, neither the perfect tool for determining human requirements nor the perfect criterion of physiological and cognitive responses have yet been devised or ascertained.

To use the knowledge about nutrient requirements in a practical way, ie, to develop dietary standards as goals for food selection, it is necessary to add amounts above estimated requirements as "safety factors" to cover both variation among individuals and the lack of precision inherent in the estimated requirement. The resulting values are called *allowances*, and the dietary standards used in the US are the Recommended Dietary Allowances (RDA) developed by the Food and Nutrition Board of the National Academy of the Sciences-National Research Council (NAS-NRC) (Table 1). The Food and Nutrition Board also published Estimated Safe and Adequate Daily Dietary Intakes for 12 nutrients for which less information existed than was necessary to establish allowances (Table 2).

In 1940 the FDA independently established a set of dietary standards called Minimum Daily Requirements (MDR), which were used in labeling to help consumers relate the nutrient content claimed for certain foods to their own nutrient needs. In 1974 these were replaced by the FDA with a new set of labeling standards, the US Recommended Daily Allowances (US RDA), which include values for more nutrients and which were adapted and condensed from the Food and Nutrition Board's RDA. To reduce confusion the FDA has renamed these labeling standards as Reference Daily Intakes (RDI). See Table 3. Federal regulations require that manufacturers who make nutritional claims on the label of foods, including dietary supplements, must include a statement of the percentages of the RDIs of the vitamins, minerals and protein supplied by an amount of the food usually consumed or recommended for consumption in 1 day.

Dietary standards are necessary and useful tools and are a means through which the findings in nutritional science can be applied for the improvement and maintenance of human health. They are assessed periodically and revised as new data become available.

Therapeutic Nutrition—Any interference with the body's ability to use the nutrients present in available food or, for that matter, its inability to obtain enough nutrients from the available food, calls for the intervention by professionals who are able to diagnose and treat the condition. The treatment or therapy, may involve a range of actions from simple adjustment of nutrient intake to the intravenous feeding of special nutrient formulas. Diet therapy is practiced when a change in nutrition status of a patient can be effected gradually. This would be in cases where it is important to maintain optimal nutritional status during prolonged periods of physical stress, to bring about changes in body weight, and to adjust food intake (both qualitatively and quantitatively) when the body is functioning abnormally or when surgery or trauma have depleted the body's reserves. Specific kinds of diet therapy are also needed for long periods, often for life, to compensate for inborn errors of metabolism.

Radical means of therapy in both the management and treatment of certain conditions is often necessary. For example, in correcting a nutritional deficiency such as pernicious anemia and preventing its recurrence in a susceptible individual, large doses of the missing nutrient are administratered parenterally. Feeding by nasogastric tube or by gastrostomy or jejunostomy, is instituted when it is not possible for a patient to take food by mouth. Patients with extensive burns present nutritional problems much more far-reaching than those who have undergone major surgery or sustained severe hemorrhage. The first need for those individuals is for fluid and electrolyte replacement followed as quickly as possible by a diet or intravenous solution markedly increased in protein, calories, and vitamins. The focus in all these cases is on restoration of nutrient supply commensurate with the specific need as soon as possible.

An understanding of the necessity for nutrient therapy is aided by recognizing the following factors which can affect nutrient needs:

Interference with food consumption (eg, impaired appetite, gastrointestinal disease, traumatic neurological disorders interfering with self-feeding, neuropsychiatric disorders, disease of soft or hard oral tissue, alcoholism, pregnancy anorexia and vomiting, food allergy and disease requiring a restricted diet).

Interference with absorption (eg, abscence of normal digestive secretions, intestinal hypermotility, reduction of effective absorbing surface, impairment of intrinsic mechanism of absorption and drugs preventing absorption.)

Interference with utilization or storage (eg, impaired liver function, hypothyroidism, neoplasm of gastrointestinal tract and drug therapy or radiation).

Increased destruction of tissues and/or function (eg, severe trauma, achlorhydria in the gastrointestinal tract, heavy metals and other metabolic antagonists).

Increased excretion or loss of nutrients (eg, lactation, burns, glycosuria and albuminuria and acute of chronic blood loss).

Increased nutrient requirements (eg, increased physical activity, periods of rapid growth, pregnancy and lactation, dever, hyperthyroidism and drug therapy).

Vitamins

Vitamins are organic compounds required for normal growth and maintenance of life by animals, including man. As a rule, animals are unable to synthesize these compounds by anabolic processes that are independent of environment other than air. These compounds are effective in small amounts, do not furnish energy and are not used as building units for the structure of the organism, but are essential for transformation of energy and for regulation of the metabolism of structural units. They or their precursors are found in plants and, so far as is known, have specific metabolic functions to perform in plant cells. Plant tissues are sources for the animal kingdom of these protective nutritional factors. In addition to carbohydrates, fats, proteins, mineral salts and water, it is essential that the food of main and animals contain small amounts of these organic substances called vitamins. If any one of at least 13 of these compounds is lacking in the diet, this breakdown results in a reduced rate or complete lack of growth in children and in symptoms of malnutrition that are known as deficiency diseases.

Vitamins are unlike each other in chemical composition and function. They are alike only in that they cannot be synthesized at all or at least not at an adequate rate in the tissues of animals or humans. The functions they serve fall into two categories, the maintenance of normal structure and of normal metabolic functions. For example, vitamin A is essential for the maintenance of normal epithelial tissue; vitamin D functions in the absorption of normal bone salts for the formation and growth of bone and other tissue. Certain vitamins of the water-soluble group, among them thiamin, riboflavin, pantothenic acid and niacin, are known to be essential constituents of the respiratory enzymes that are required in the use of energy from oxidative catabolism of sugars and fats.

It is convenient in a discussion of this subject to divide these nutritional substances into two groups, the *fat-soluble* and the

Table 1—Food and Nutrition Board, NAS—NRC[a] Recommended Dietary Allowances,[b] Revised 1989

Designed for the maintenance of good nutrition of practically all healthy people in the US

							Fat-soluble vitamins				Water-soluble vitamins							Minerals						
Category	Age (yr) or condition	Weight[c] (kg)	Weight[c] (lb)	Height[c] (cm)	Height[c] (in)	Protein (g)	Vitamin A (μg RE)[d]	Vitamin D (μg)[e]	Vitamin E (mg α-TE)[f]	Vitamin K (μg)	Vitamin C (mg)	Thiamin (mg)	Riboflavin (mg)	Niacin (mg NE)[g]	Vitamin B_6 (mg)	Folate (μg)	Vitamin B_{12} (μg)	Calcium (mg)	Phosphorus (mg)	Magnesium (mg)	Iron (mg)	Zinc (mg)	Iodine (μg)	Selenium (μg)
Infants	0.0–0.5	6	13	60	24	13	375	7.5	3	5	30	0.3	0.4	5	0.3	25	0.3	400	300	40	6	5	40	10
	0.5–1.0	9	20	71	28	14	375	10	4	10	35	0.4	0.5	6	0.6	35	0.5	600	500	60	10	5	50	15
Children	1–3	13	29	90	35	16	400	10	6	15	40	0.7	0.8	9	1.0	50	0.7	800	800	80	10	10	70	20
	4–6	20	44	112	44	24	500	10	7	20	45	0.9	1.1	12	1.1	75	1.0	800	800	120	10	10	90	20
	7–10	28	62	132	52	28	700	10	7	30	45	1.0	1.2	13	1.4	100	1.4	800	800	170	10	10	120	30
Males	11–14	45	99	157	62	45	1,000	10	10	45	50	1.3	1.5	17	1.7	150	2.0	1,200	1,200	270	12	15	150	40
	15–18	66	145	176	69	59	1,000	10	10	65	60	1.5	1.8	20	2.0	200	2.0	1,200	1,200	400	12	15	150	50
	19–24	72	160	177	70	58	1,000	10	10	70	60	1.5	1.7	19	2.0	200	2.0	1,200	1,200	350	10	15	150	70
	25–50	79	174	176	70	63	1,000	5	10	80	60	1.5	1.7	19	2.0	200	2.0	800	800	350	10	15	150	70
	51+	77	170	173	68	63	1,000	5	10	80	60	1.2	1.4	15	2.0	200	2.0	800	800	350	10	15	150	70
Females	11–14	46	101	157	62	46	800	10	8	45	50	1.1	1.3	15	1.4	150	2.0	1,200	1,200	280	15	12	150	45
	15–18	55	120	163	64	44	800	10	8	55	60	1.1	1.3	15	1.5	180	2.0	1,200	1,200	300	15	12	150	50
	19–24	58	128	164	65	46	800	10	8	60	60	1.1	1.3	15	1.6	180	2.0	1,200	1,200	280	15	12	150	55
	25–50	63	138	163	64	50	800	5	8	65	60	1.1	1.3	15	1.6	180	2.0	800	800	280	15	12	150	55
	51+	65	143	160	63	50	800	5	8	65	60	1.0	1.2	13	1.6	180	2.0	800	800	280	10	12	150	55
Pregnant						60	800	10	10	65	70	1.5	1.6	17	2.2	400	2.2	1,200	1,200	320	30	15	175	65
Lactating	1st 6 mo					65	1,300	10	12	65	95	1.6	1.8	20	2.1	280	2.6	1,200	1,200	355	15	19	200	75
	2nd 6 mo					62	1,200	10	11	65	90	1.6	1.7	20	2.1	260	2.6	1,200	1,200	340	15	16	200	75

[a] Reproduced from Recommended Dietary Allowances, 10th ed NAS, Washington, DC, 1989.

[b] The allowances, expressed as average daily intakes over time, are intended to provide for individual variations among most normal persons as they live in the US under usual environmental stresses. Diets should be based on a variety of common foods in order to provide other nutrients for which human requirements have been less well defined. See text for detailed discussion of allowances and of nutrients not tabulated.

[c] Weights and heights of Reference Adults are actual medians for the US population of the designated age, as reported by NHANES II. The median weights and heights of those under 19 years of age were taken from Hamill *et al*: *Am J Clin Nutr 32*:607, 1979. The use of these figures does not imply that the height-to-weight ratios are ideal.

[d] Retinol equivalents. 1 retinol equivalent = 1 μg retinol or 6 μg β-carotene. See test for calculation of vitamin A activity of diets as retinol equivalents.

[e] As cholecalciferol. 10 μg cholecalciferol = 400 IU of vitamin D.

[f] α-Tocopherol equivalents. 1 mg d-α tocopherol = 1 α-TE. See text for variation in allowances and calculation of vitamin E activity of the diet as α-tocopherol equivalents.

[g] 1 NE (niacin equivalent) is equal to 1 mg of niacin or 60 mg of dietary tryptophan.

Table 2—Summary Table: Estimated Safe and Adequate Daily Dietary Intakes of Selected Vitamins and Minerals [a,b]

Category	Age (yr)	Vitamins: Biotin (μg)	Vitamins: Pantothenic acid (mg)	Age (yr)	Trace Elements[c]: Copper (mg)	Manganese (mg)	Fluoride (mg)	Chromium (μg)	Molybdenum (μg)
Infants	0–0.5	10	2	0–0.5	0.4–0.6	0.3–0.6	0.1–0.5	10–40	15–30
	0.5–1	15	3	0.5–1	0.6–0.7	0.6–1.0	0.2–1.0	20–60	20–40
Children and adolescents	1–3	20	3	1–3	0.7–1.0	1.0–1.5	0.5–1.5	20–80	25–50
	4–6	25	3–4	4–6	1.0–1.5	1.5–2.0	1.0–2.5	30–120	30–75
	7–10	30	4–5	7–10	1.0–2.0	2.0–3.0	1.5–2.5	50–200	50–150
	11 +	30–100	4–7	11 +	1.5–2.5	2.0–5.0	1.5–2.5	50–200	75–250
Adults		30–100	4–7		1.5–3.0	2.0–5.0	1.5–4.0	50–200	75–250

[a] Reproduced from Recommended Dietary Allowances, 10th ed NAS, Washington, DC, 1989.
[b] Because there is less information on which to base allowances, these figures are not given in the main table of RDA and are provided here in the form of ranges of recommended intakes.
[c] Since the toxic levels for many trace elements may be only several times usual intakes, the upper levels for the trace elements given in this table should not be habitually exceeded.

water-soluble factors. Vitamins A, D, E and K fall into the fat-soluble group, since they can be extracted with fat solvents and are found in the fat fractions of animal tissues. The water-soluble vitamins include ascorbic acid and the B group of vitamins, which consists of some ten or more well-defined compounds. Additional vitamin nomenclature can be found in Table 4. The characterization of vitamins as essential metabolic factors with discrete chemical structures required their isolation in pure form from natural sources and subsequent laboratory synthesis. Commercial chemical or microbiological syntheses, some from relatively simple compounds, are the source of most of the vitamins now used in pharmaceutical preparations, dietary supplements, and fortified foods.

Standardization—Vitamin activity or potency is measured by three principal types of methods:

Biological, in which rats, mice, guinea pigs and chickens serve as the assay animals.

Microbiological, which employ bacteria that require certain of the water-soluble vitamins, are rapid, specific and precise. Such methods are used for manufacturing and laboratory control of the production of some vitamins.

Chemical, using a characteristic color or a sensitive reaction specific for the compounds, are available for most vitamins in uncomplicated mixtures. Chromatographic separations followed by a variety of detection techniques provide alternative means of quantification.

The status of vitamin methods of assay is now such that manufacturers of vitamin preparations find it possible to state with precision the potency of their products, and tables of vitamin content of foods are, for most vitamins, quite complete. Methods of assay are described briefly in the individual vitamin sections.

In the interest of improvement and uniformity of expressing the results of such assays, the World Health Organization

Table 3—Reference Daily Intakes (RDI) for Labeling Purposes

	Units	Infants	Children under 4 yr of age	Adults and children 4 or more yr of age	Pregnant or lactating women
Vitamin A	IU	1500	2500	5000	8000
Vitamin D	IU	400	400	400	400
Vitamin E	IU	5	10	30	30
Vitamin C	mg	35	40	60	60
Folacin	mg	0.1	0.2	0.4	0.8
Thiamin	mg	0.5	0.7	1.5	1.7
Riboflavin	mg	0.6	0.8	1.7	2.0
Niacin	mg	8	9	20	20
Vitamin B_6	mg	0.4	0.7	2	2.5
Vitamin B_{12}	μg	2	3	6	8
Biotin	mg	0.05	0.15	0.3	0.3
Pantothenic Acid	mg	3	5	10	10
Calcium	g	0.6	0.8	1.0	1.3
Phosphorus	g	0.5	0.8	1.0	1.3
Iodine	μg	45	70	150	150
Iron	mg	15	10	18	18
Magnesium	mg	70	200	400	450
Copper	mg	0.6	1.0	2.0	2.0
Zinc	mg	5	8	15	15
Protein	g	14[a]	16[a]	50[b]	60, 65[b]

[a] Quality measured by Protein Efficiency Ratio (PER).
[b] Value for protein in adults and children 4 or more years of age is referred as a *daily reference value* and quality is measured by a scoring process based on amino acid content.

Table 4—Vitamin Nomenclature

Vitamin	Synonym or descriptive terms
A group	Antixerophthalmic vitamin
A_1	Retinol
A_2	Dehydroretinol
A acid	Retinoic acid (Tretinoin)
Provitamin A Carotenoids	Carotene (α & β, cryptoxanthin (hydroxy β-carotene)
B group	Formerly vitamin B complex
Thiamin	Vitamin B_1, aneurin, antiberiberi vitamin
Riboflavin	Vitamin B_2, lactoflavin
Niacin	Nicotinic acid and nicotinamide, pellagra-preventive factor
Pantothenic acid	Formerly vitamin B_3
B_6	Pyridoxine, pyridoxal, pyridoxamine
Biotin	Coenzyme R
Folacin	Folic acid (pteroylmonoglutamic acid, PGA) and folic acid polyglutamates, tetrahydrofolic acid, formyl tetrahydrofolic acid (formerly citrovorum factor, folinic acid)
B_{12}	Antipernicious anemia vitamin, cyanocobalamin, hydroxocobalamin (formerly vitamin B_{12b}), nitritocobalamin (formerly vitamin B_{12c})
C	L-Ascorbic acid, antiscorbutic vitamin
D group	Antirachitic vitamin
D_2	Ergocalciferol (formerly calciferol), activated ergosterol
D_3	Cholecalciferol, activated 7-dehydrocholesterol
E group: alpha-, beta-, gamma-, delta- tocopherols & tocotrienols	Possess vitamin E activity in varying degrees. Occur as fatty acid esters
K group	Antihemorrhagic vitamin
K_1	Phylloquinone (naturally occurring)
K_2	Farnoquinone (naturally occurring)
K_3	Menadione, menaquinone
K_{4-7}	Biologically active analogues of menadione (synthetic)

(WHO) of the United Nations has sponsored the preparation and distribution of Standards. As a rule, an International Standard is no longer provided once the substance responsible for its characteristic activity has been isolated, identified, and made readily available. The USP has set up comparable Reference Standards in this country, and the biological potency of vitamins A and D is expressed in USP Units that are equal to International Units (IU). However, availability of the vitamins in pure form encourages transition from the use of units to the use of weight in expressing amounts present in vitamin products.

The Fat-Soluble Vitamins

Vitamin A and Carotene

Vitamin A was the first fat-soluble vitamin discovered. Animal nutritionists observed growth failures in calves born of cows maintained on wheat or oats alone, whereas whole cornplants supported growth and development of the animals. The vitamin was found to be related to chlorophyll and carotenoid-containing plants. Later study revealed that the vitamin is essential for the maintenance of normal tissue structure and for other important physiological functions such as vision and reproduction.

Chemistry and Assay—Vitamin A is represented primarily by the cyclic polyene alcohol vitamin A_1 (retinol) with an empirical formula of $C_{20}H_{30}O$ and whose four conjugated double bonds in the side chain are in the *trans* arrangement.

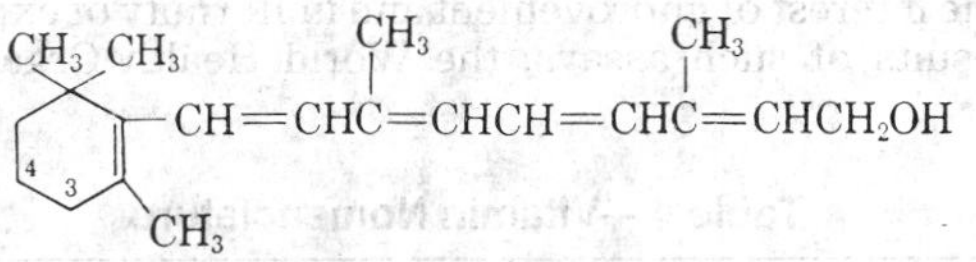

CH_3 CH_3 CH_3 CH_3
$-CH{=}CHC{=}CHCH{=}CHC{=}CHCH_2OH$
4 3
CH_3

Vitamin A (Retinol) (Vitamin A₁)

Another representative of vitamin A occuring in nature is vitamin A_2, which has an additional double bond in the ring at the 3–4 position. It has only about ¼ to ½ the biological activity of vitamin A_1 for the rat and has no commerical significance. A third such representative is neovitamin A-a in which the terminal double bond in the side chain of vitamin A_1 is *cis*. It has low biological activity.

Vitamin A_1 is a pale yellow crystalline compound, is soluble in lipid solvents, and has a UV absorption maximum at 328 nm. The vitamin is not readily destroyed by heat but is oxidized easily and is less stable in acid than in alkaline solution. The esters of vitamin A_1 with the fatty acids, acetic and palmitic, are commercially important since they are considerably more stable than the alcohol.

The source of most of the vitamin A in animals, birds and fish is the carotenoid pigments, the yellow-colored compounds in all chlorophyll-containing plants. At least ten different carotenoids exhibit provitamin A activity, but only α- and β-carotene and cryptoxanthin (founded in yellow corn) are important in animal nutrition, β-carotene being the most impor tant.

Theoretically one molecule of β-carotene should yield two molecules of vitamin A_1; however, the availability of carotene in foods as sources of vitamin A for humans is low and extremely variable. Often, factors of ½, ⅓, ¼ or less are used arbitrarily to compensate for this. This utilization efficiency of carotene is generally considered to be ⅙ for humans; that is, 1 μg of β-carotene would have the same biological activity as 0.167 μg of retinol. This conservatively takes into account the decremental effects on carotene utilization of absorption, transport and tissue conversion to

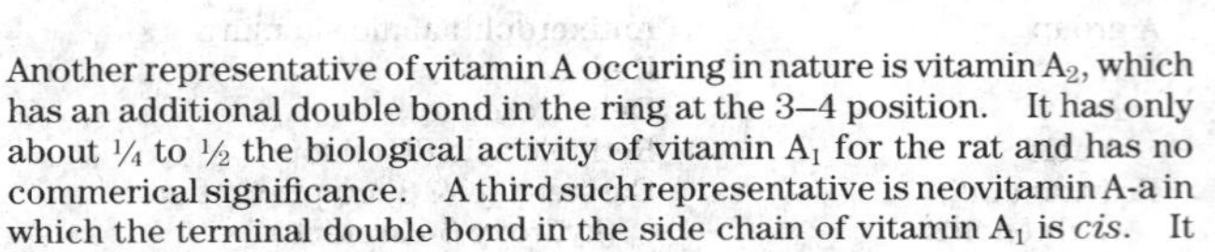

CH_3 CH_3 CH_3 CH_3 CH_3 CH_3
$(CH{=}CHC{=}CH)_2CH{=}CH(CH{=}CCH{=}CH)_2$
CH_3 CH_3

β-Carotene

the active vitamin. The conversion of the provitamin to vitamin A occurs primarily in the walls of the small intestine and perhaps to a lesser degree in the liver; conversion is linked to body stores of vitamin A. Like vitamin A_1, the carotenes are soluble in fat solvents, in crystalline form appear deep orange or copper-colored, and have characteristic absorption spectra.

Total synthesis of vitamin A_1 and β-carotene is achieved commercially, vitamin A usually being prepared as the acetate. Concentration of vitamin A from animal fats and fish liver oil is still important. The principal steps in the process are molecular distillation, saponification, and crystallization of the distillate and acylation to the desired ester.

The USP Unit for vitamin A is identical to the International Unit. The USP Reference Standard for vitamin A is a solution of crystalline vitamin A acetate in cottonseed oil such that there is contained 1 USP Unit (0.344 μg)/0.1 mg of solution. Although there is no USP Unit for carotene, there is an International Unit (IU); the relation between carotene and vitamin A is 6 to 3.44 by weight of the respective pure compounds.

Vitamin A can be assayed by direct measurement of its ultraviolet absorption by photometric evaluation of the color reaction with antimony trichloride in chloroform (the Carr-Price rection), by high-pressure liquid chromatographic separation and ultraviolet and visable spectrometry or by a biological method based on the resumption of growth of rats when the vitamin activity is added to a vitamin A-deficient diet. The chemical or physicochemical determination of β-carotene depends on measurement of the yellow color of its solutions in organic solvents. Chromatographic separation of associated carotenoids is usually necessary before an accurate analysis of the biologically active compounds can be made.

Carotenoids are photo-degradable and deficiency resulting from excessive exposure of the human to UV light has been reported.

Metabolic Functions—Of the known functions of vitamin A in the body, its role in the visual process is established best. The retina of man contains two distinct photoreceptor systems. The rods, which are the structural components of one system, are especially sensitive to light of low intensity. A specific vitamin A aldehyde is essential for the formation of rhodopsin (the high-molecular-weight glycoprotein part of the visual pigment within the rods) and the normal functioning of the retina. By virtue of this relation to the visual process, vitamin A alcohol has been named retinol and the aldehyde form named retinal. A vitamin A-deficient person has an impaired dark adaptation ("night-blindness").

Vitamin A also participates in the maintenance of the integrity of the epithelial membranes such that normal structures may be substituted by stratified keratinizing epithelium in the eyes and paraocular glands, respiratory, alimentary and genitourinary tracts under the stresses of a deficiency. The basal cells do not lose their function under such conditions, however, and are able to be restored to normal when sufficient vitamin A is absorbed. Abnormalities of nerve and connective tissue and of bones are further consequences of a dietary deficiency of the vitamin. In severe deficiency the affected epithelial and connective tissue may become the site of infections due to the cells' reduced resistance to bacterial invasion. This gave rise to the notion that administration of vitamin A was useful in the treatment of skin infections. Both topical and oral vitamin A, and especially vitamin A acid (trans-retinoic acid, tretinoin), are prescribed by some physicians to treat acne vulgaris; however, *trans*-retinoic acid has been shown to be equally effective with less harmful side effects than with oral isotretinoin (*cis*-retinoic acid).

There is a growing body of epidemiological data which suggest that foods which are a good source of vitamin A and carotenoids are protective against a variety of epithelial cancers. This association simply may be a result of a chronic vitamin A deficiency, since vitamin A is required for normal cell differentiation of stem cells in epithelial tissue. Also, there is the possibility that the observed protective effect could have been due to other undetected carotenoids, other vitamins, indoles or unknown compounds present in these foods. Some, but not all, animal studies show a positive effect for vitamin A and synthetic retinoids against epithelial cancers of the skin, lung, bladder and breast. Clinical studies are now in progress to assess the potential for these compounds to reduce the risk of recurrence of some forms of epithelial cancer in humans, but data from these studies will not be available until 1995.

The common severe deficiency symptoms are increased susceptibility to microbial infections, xerophthalmia and other eye disorders, loss of appetite and weight, and sterility, conditions which require a long time for their development. Although the recommended dietary allowance is no more than 6000 IU/day, in a deficiency much greater amounts are indicated. For example, the usual therapeutic oral dose range is from 10,000 to 20,000 IU daily for 7 to 10 days for infants and growing children and 25,000 to 100,000 IU daily for 7 to 10 days for older children and adults.

If large doses of vitamin A are ingested for long periods of time, manifestations of toxicity develop. In the absence of a deficiency, chronic administration of vitamin A of 25,000 to 50,000 IU daily induces pathologic changes in bone and periosteal tissues, skin and mucous membranes, liver, and changes in behavior. Doses as low as 18,500 IU of a water-dispersed vitamin A preparation daily for 1 to 3 months are reported to be toxic for infants 3 to 6 months of age. Vitamin A toxicity has occurred in infants who were given liver daily for a period of 3 months. Animal studies show that levels as low as four times the requirements increase the incidence of birth defects. Epidemiological studies in humans have indicated that levels as low as 15,000 IU during the first trimester of pregnancy may increase the risk of birth defects in humans.

Dietary Requirement and Food Sources—According to the National Research Council's "Recommended Dietary Allowances," the requirement for vitamin A appears to be proportional to body weight. The recommended allowances for the maintenance of good nutrition of healthy adults in the US is 1000 Retinolequivalents (RE) for males and 800 RE for females per day (1000 RE is equivalent to 5000 IU), although the adult requirement for maintenance of normalcy in important vitamin A functions is about ½ this value. Somewhat more vitamin A than the allowance should be provided during the latter ⅔ of pregnancy and even more during lactation. These increments would assure the nutritional well-being of the rapdily growing fetus and nursing infant, who are dependent on the mother's vitamin A intake.

About ½ of the vitamin A activity in the average American diet comes from β-carotene and related compounds. The other ½ is provided by the vitamin itself present in foods of animal origin. Not all of the carotene present in the food eaten is converted into vitamin A. Some passes through the digestive tract and is excreted as such. Of that absorbed, only the amounts necessary to meet requirements are converted to vitamin A. The rest is stored in the body or excreted. Intake of large amounts of carotene frequently causes a yellow orange color to the skin which is considered to be harmless. The richest sources of carotene are yellow and green (leafy) vegetables and yellow fruits. Preformed vitamin A_1 is supplied primarily from the fat of dairy products and egg-yolk, but other important sources in some diets are liver, kidney and fish. Federal regulations provide for the optional addition of 15,000 IU of vitamin A/lb of margarine. Almost all margarine is so fortified. There are also provisions for marketing vitamins A & D-fortified nonfat dry milk containing 500 IU vitamin A and 100 IU vitamin D/8 fl oz reconstituted.

Vitamin D

Vitamin D is the antirachitic vitamin effective in promoting calcification of the bony structures of man and animals. It sometimes is known popularly as the "sunshine" vitamin because it is formed by the action of the sun's ultraviolet rays on precursor sterols in the skin. Exposure to sunlight, therefore, has a powerful antirachitic effect. The term rachitic denotes the condition of a person or animal affected with the deficiency disease rickets, where bone is poorly mineralized and unable to support the weight of the body.

Chemistry and Assay—The two immediate biological precursors (provitamins) to the vitamins D are the steroid alcohols ergosterol (egosta-5,7,22*E*-trien-3β-ol) and 7-dehydrocholesterol (cholesta-5,7-dien-3β-ol). Under the influence of UV light, each undergoes scission of the 9(10) bond of the steroid nucleus with the simultaneous creation of a 10(19) double bond yielding, respectively vitamin D_2 (ergocalciferol) and vitamin D_3 (cholecalciferol).

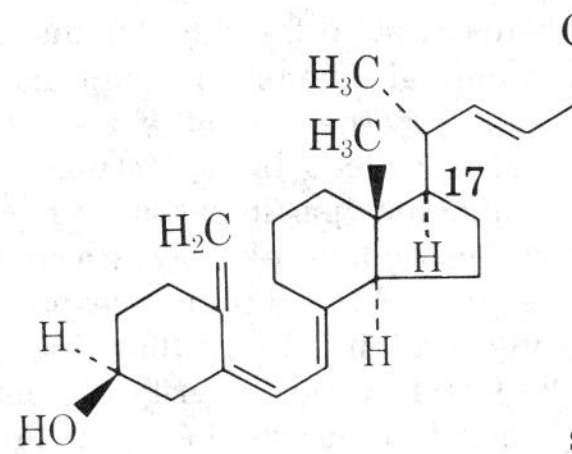

Vitamin D_2 (Ergocalciferol)
Vitamin D_3 (Cholecalciferol): same except C_{17} side chain is

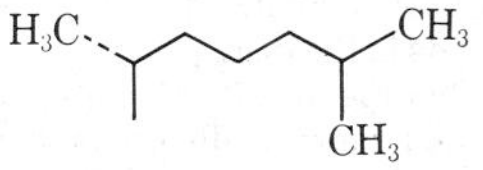

Pure vitamins D_2 and D_3 are white, odorless crystals that are soluble in fat solvents such as either, alcohol or chloroform, but insoluble in water. The compounds have characteristic absorption spectra, which property is useful in their identification. Both forms of the vitamin are stable to oxidation by air and to moderate heat in neutral and alkaline solutions. Upon alkaline saponification of fats, the vitamin appears in the nonsaponifiable fraction. It withstands autoclaving temperatures of 120° in the absence of air, but at this temperature is subject to oxidation, and it is destroyed completely by heating at 170°. Vitamin D is stable over long periods of storage in oil solution but is quite unstable in the presence of mineral salts, such as tricalcium phosphate, when compounded in tablet form. It may be stabilized by dispersion in gelatin or a similar protective coating.

The international standard for vitamin D is a crystalline preparation of pure vitamin D_3 assigned a potency of 40 million units/g. The USP adopted an equivalent standard of vitamin D_3 with the same assigned potency, distributed in the form of a cottonseed oil solution. The USP unit for vitamin D, therefore, is equivalent to the IU.

The provitamins D are found in both plant and animal tissue; 7-dehydrocholesterol is found principally in animal skin and ergosterol in relatively large amounts in yeasts, although it was first isolated from ergot. The vitamin D which is absorbed thrugh the intestinal wall from dietary sources or which is formed in the skin from 7-dehydrocholesterol enters the circulatory system, and excesses are stored. Like vitamin A, vitamin D is stored in animal body fats, principally in the liver. The liver oils, particularly of fish, are the most potent natural sources of the vitamin. The vitamin D of commerce now is synthesized principally from readily available structurally related compounds, such as cholesterol, which are often obtained as packinghouse by-products.

There are three methods for quantitative physiochemical assay of vitamin D. For years, the biological assay based on the curative effects of the vitamin on experimental rickets in young rats has been used to measure the total biological activity of the vitamin in complex materials of low potency. Minimal amounts of the vitamin are needed by the rat; therefore, the rachitic condition is produced by using an extremely low-calcium, low-phosphorus diet. Now the prefered method for minimal amounts is high-pressure liquid chromatography for separation and UV spectrometry. For relatively concentrated solutions of vitamin D in alcohol (but not in oil), UV spectrometric determination is made at the wavelength of maximum absorption. Antimony trichloride reacts with various vitamins D in a Carr-Price reaction to yield a yellow color whose intensity is proportional to the vitamin D present. The reaction is satisfactory only for concentrated preparations; cholesterol and vitamin A interfere only when present in amounts in excess of certain limits.

Metabolic Functions—Both vitamin D_2 and vitamin D_3 are biologically inactive molecules. After absorption, they are converted, primarily in the liver, to 25-hydrocholecalciferol D_2 and D_3 (25-HCCD_2 and 25-HCCD_3 calciferol), respectively, and are the most predominant forms found in the blood. Both of these compounds appear to facilitate phosphate resorption in the renal tubule; however, their most important functions is a precursor of 1,25-dihydroxycholecalciferol (1,25-DHCC calciferol), which is formed in the kidney. This compound is a true hormone and is extreted in response to specific stimuli from an organ distal to its target organ. Calcitriol is transported in the blood bound to a protein. There is a rapid turnover of 1,25-DHCC, which depends on vitamin D status (greater turnover if bodystores and plasma levels are low). Normal plasma values range from 18 to 60 pg/mL in children and 15 to 45 pg/mL in adults. Vitamin D, therefore, is a precursor of a true hormone, 1,25-DHCC, which is secreted by an organ and performs a vital function. It is likely that some forms of vitamin D-resistant rickets can be explained by possible genetic inability of the body to produce adequate amounts of either 25-HCC or 1,25-DHCC. Conversely, some children may have an enhanced capacity to convert vitamin D to the more active metabolites and, thereby, manifest a hyperreactivity to amounts of the ingested vitamin very slightly in excess of recommended dietary allowances.

Vitamin D, through the action of these active metabolites, aids in the absorption of calcium from the intestinal tract and the resorption of phosphate in the renal tubule. Vitamin D is necessary for normal growth in children, probably having a direct effect on the osteoblast cells which influence calcification of cartilage in the growing areas of bone. 1,25-DHCC also plays an essential management role in the regulation of various genes important to cell proliferation and lymphokine expression in systems not involved in mineral homeostasis.

A deficiency of vitamin D leads to inadequate absorption of calcium and phosphorus from the intestinal tract and retention of these minerals in the kidney and thence to faulty mineralization of bone structures. The inability of the soft bones to withstand the stress of weight results in skeletal malformations. Early rickets is difficult to diagnose, but fully developed cases in infants and children present characteristic signs. These include delayed closure of the fontanelles and softening of the skull, soft fragile bones with bowing of the legs and spinal curvature, enlargement of wrist, knee and ankle joints, poorly developed muscles, restlessness and nervous irritability. A form of "adult rickets" called osteomalacia similarly may occur. It, too, represents a failure of the process of calcification caused by simple vitamin D lack and calcium or phosphorus inadequancy.

With adequate calcium-phosphorus intake, adult osteomalacia and uncomplicated rickets can be cured by the ordinary daily intake of 400 IU of vitamin D. Larger doses (about 1600 IU or more daily) are more rapidly effective, the first evidence of improvement—a rise in serum phosphorus—occurring in about 10 days.

Vitamin D has a serious toxic potential. There is a wide range of susceptibility to the toxic effects of vitamin D. Most adults will require more than 50,000 units of vitamin D/day to produce intoxication. However, levels as low as 15,000 IU/kg for 2 weeks have produced acute toxicity in adults. Long-term consumption of levels as low as 1000 IU/kg may lead to hypercalcemia and attendant complications, such as metastatic calcification and renal calculi in adults, provided there are high levels of cacium in the diet. As little as 2000 IU can inhibit linear growth of normal children. In advanced stages, demineralization of bones occurs, and multiple fractions may result from very slight trauma. Chronic excessive intake will result in liver accumulation and detoxification will take several months. Classic features of vitamin D intoxication are hyperclacemea and hyperphosphatemia, and impaired renal function. Painful joints and muscle weakness also may occur, which impairs mobility.

Dietary Requirement and Food Sources—Requirements for vitamin D vary with the amount of exposure to ultraviolet light. Some individuals can obtain their entire requirements by skin irridiation, but age, skin pigment and other conditions can effect the need for dietary supplies.

There are few reliable data concerning minimum vitamin D requirements, except for infants. For most healthy individual 400 IU/day is sufficient to meet requirements without exposure to sun. However, recent studies on older individuals indicate that higher levels may be desirable. In normal full-term infants, intakes of as little as 100 IU/day have prevented rickets. There is no evidence that diets need supply more than 400 IU/day for normal growth of infants and children.

Vitamin D is not found naturally in many food sources. Egg yolks, which are the best food source, vary in content from winter to summer depending most upon the content of the vitamin in the hen's diet. Unfortified dairy products contain some vitamin D, but again the potency varies with the season. Varities of fish, whose muscle tissues contain substantial quantities of oil and fat, may supply an appreciable part of the dietary requirement. The livers of a number of fish, or the oils extracted from the livers, are extremely rich in vitamin D. Addition of vitamin D to appropriate foods has been an important factor in the prevention of any significant incidence of rickets in this country.

The major sources of Vitamin D in the diets of most Americans are those foods which have been fortified. Vitamin D-fortified whole milk, nonfat dry milk and evaporated milk containing 400 IU/qt (or reconstituted quart in the case of nonfat dry milk and evaporated milk) are particularly effective because of their use in infant feeding during the stage of growth most susceptible to rachitic changes. Fortification is accomplished by addition of vitamin D concentrates, mainly in the form of vitamin D_3. Fortification of other foods, such as processed cereals and margarine, is practiced to a limited degree.

Vitamin E

Vitamin E designates the group of compounds (tocol and tocotrienol derivatives) which exhibit qualitatively the biological activity of α-tocopherol. Studies which led to its discovery as an essential factor in animal metabolism showed that it was, among other things, necessary for reproduction in rats. It often is called the antisterility vitamin, an inappropriate term, since it is not known to specifically function in this capacity in humans.

Chemistry and Assay—As with several of the other vitamins, there are a series of closely related compounds, tocopherols, known to occur in nature. Biological activity associated with the vitamin nature of the group is exhibited by four major compounds: α-, β-, γ- and δ-tocopherol, each of which can exist in various stereoisomeric forms. These are all methyl-substituted tocols; α tocopherol, the most important member of the series because of its activity and occurrence, is 5,7,8-trimethyltocol, ie, 2,5,7,8-tetramethyl-2-(4,8,12-trimethyltridecyl)-6-chromanol.

α-Tocopherol

The tocopherols are oily liquids at room temperature. High temperatures and acids do not affect the stability of vitamin E, but oxidation does take place readily in the presence of iron salts or in rancid fats. The tocopherols themselves act as antioxidants, the δ-tocopherol having the greatest antioxidant power. Decomposition also occurs in UV light. Tocopherols are isolated on a commercial scale from vegetable oils, usually by molecular distillation, extraction with organic solvents or by absorption chromatography, α-tocopherol is usually the most important homolog isolated from these sources; it also can be prepared synthetically and made available as the acetate and acid succinate esters.

The international standard for vitamin E used as a reference in all assays for this vitamin is a solution of *dl*-α-tocopheryl acetate in coconut oil. Each 0.1 g of this solution contains 1 mg of the acetate. Results of an assay are expressed in terms of mg of the vitamin. The following relationship exists between IUs (or the equivalent USP Units) of the vitamin and the respective weights of the common forms:

1 USP or IU = 1 mg *dl*-alpha tocopheryl acetate = 0.91 mg *dl*-alpha tocopherol = 0.735 mg *d*-alpha tocopheryl acetate (the ester of the natural form) = 0.671 mg *d*-alpha tocopherol (the natural form)

The IU represents biological activity as determined by the rat antisterility test.

The usual methods for quantitative assay of vitamin E depend either directly or indirectly upon the ease with which free α-tocopherol is oxidized. The esters, which are almost exclusively used in pharmaceuticals, must first by hydrolyzed. The free alcohol, then, because of its instability, must be handled with care in all other analytical operations. The physiocochemical methods generally applied employ either of two oxidation-reduction reactions: (1) the formation of a red orthoquinone by treatment of the tocopherol with concentrated nitric acid and (2) the reduction of ferric chloride in the presence of α,α′-dipyridyl which forms a red-colored complex with ferrous ions. Both methods are relatively nonspecific and are suitable only when combined with adequate separation procedures. A gas-liquid chromatographic procedure coupled with a visable-light detector and a high-pressure liquid chromagraphic procedure using a UV detector provide highly specific determinations.

The classic biological method is the rat assay in which female rats are depleted of vitamin E and mated with normal males. The dose of the material to be tested and of the standard is administered over a period of several days after conception. On the 20th day of pregnancy the female rates are killed and the numbers of living and dead fetuses, and resorption sites, are recorded. Another more simple bioassay is based on the dialuric acid hemolysis test in which the red-blood-cell fragility is measured as a criterion of vitamin E status in the rat.

Metabolic Functions, Dietary Requirement and Food Sources—The exact biochemical mechanism whereby vitamin E functions in the body is still unknown; however, its most critical function occurs in the membranous parts of cells. Here, it interdigitates with phospholipids, cholesterol and triglycerides, the three main structural elements of membranes. Since vitamin E is an antioxidant, a favored reaction at this site is with very reactive and usually destructive compounds called free radicals. These are products of oxidative deterioration of such substances as polyunsaturated fat. Vitamin E converts the free radical into a less reactive and nonharmful form. In its role as a protector against oxidation, vitamin E shows nutritional interactions with a wide variety of nutrients: vitamin A, the trace element selenium, the sulfur amino acids methionine and cysteine/cystine, polyunsaturated fatty acids, and, to a lesser extent, vitamin C. Interestingly enough, the order of antioxidant power among the tocopherols, as measured by their effect on the rate of peroxide formation in fats, is the reverse of the order of biological potencies. Other physiological functions probably includes participation in nucleic acid metabolism, and it appears also that the tocopherols may be a component of the cytochrome reductase segment of the terminal respiratory chain in intermediary metabolism. In general, it appears that vitamin E plays an important role in insuring the stability and integrity of cellular membranes; thus far in man, the only such demonstrated effect is on the red blood cell. The effect is also modified by the level of polyunsaturated fatty acids in the diet.

The therapeutic effectiveness of vitamin E in the prevention of abortion, in certain menstrual disorders, in the improvement of lactation, in muscular dystrophy or in cardiovascular diseases has not been substantiated, and the promotion of vitamin E for such purposes is fraudulent. One use that is established and sound is in hemolytic anemia in premature infants. Vitamin E also generally is considered to provide protection against pulmonary oxygen poisoning. Essentially all other examples of clinical indications of need for vitamin E at nutritional levels are related to malnourishment or malabsorption problems. The latter are found in humans with cystic fibrosis, liver cirrhosis, postgastrectomy, obstructive jaundice, pancreatic insufficiency and sprue.

There are some data which suggest that vitamin E may be useful in protecting the epithelial tissue of the lungs from free radical damage associated with air pollution, but more research is needed to achieve a consensus of medical opinion. Similarly, more data are required to substantiate claims that vitamin E promotes rapid healing of tissue damaged by severe burns or other skin injuries. Studies which suggest the vitamin E is useful for preventing some forms of cancer and preventing and treating coronary heart disease have been supported by epidemiological data, but replication of finding is still needed using human subjects.

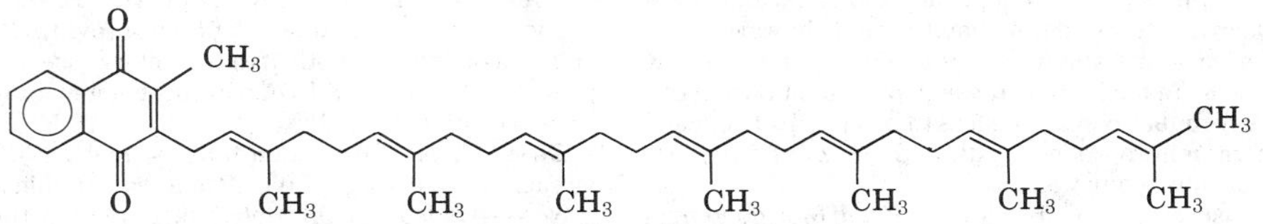

A clearly defined uncomplicated vitamin E-deficiency disease has not been recognized as a public health problem. A deficiency state with respect to vitamin E has been demonstrated in human subjects, especially in premature and newborn infants and in infants with steatorrhea. The evidence rests mainly on determination of *in vitro* hemolysis and blood tocopherol level. However, peripheral neuropathy and vitamin E-deficient nerves in deficient patients has been reported. Vitamin E requirement apparently is not related to body weight directly or to a caloric intake, but seems to be related to body weight in kilograms to the three-quarter power, sometimes designated as physiological or metabolic size. Requirements of Vitamin E are known to increase with high-intakes of polyunsaturated fatty acids and in selenium deficiency.

Vitamin E is ubiquitous in its distribution and is found particularly in vegetable fats and oils, dairy products and meat, eggs, cereals, nuts, and leafy green and yellow vegetables. *Vitamin E is distributed so widely in nature that it is difficult to prepare a diet which does not meet NAS RDAs for all sex and age groups. However, attainment of levels expected to be needed for lowering the risk of cancer and heart disease likely will require supplimentation.* In direct contrast to the more rapid turnover of some of the water-soluble vitamins, vitamin E is stored in fatty tissue and is removed from it only when the fat is mobiized. This means that many months of deprivation would have to pass in order to deplete the body stores.

Vitamin K

Vitamin K refers to a group of substances, widespread in nature, having similar biological activity; one form was isolated first from alfalfa and the other from putrefied fish meal. The primary activity which makes the vitamin essential in humans is its function in post-translation of γ-carboxylation of glutamate in a number of proteins associated with blood clotting.

Chemistry and Assay—The parent structure of the K family of vitamins is 2-methyl-1,4-naphthoquinone. The various forms of vitamin K differ by the hydrophobic substituent at 3-position. This fat-soluble compound and several water-soluble derivatives such as the sodium bisulfite and diphosphoric acid ester are the common commercial forms used in medical practice. Vitamin K_1 (isolated from plants) is 2-methyl-3-phytyl-1,4-naphthoquinone.

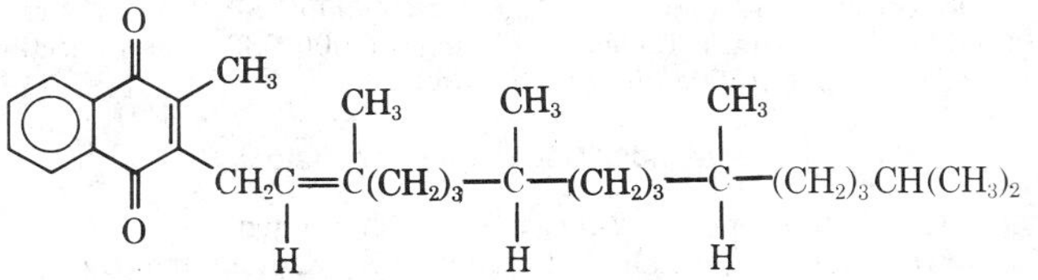

Vitamin K_1—phylloquinone; phytonadione

Vitamin K_2 exists as a chemical series which, instead of the phytyl side chain in the 3-position, have side chains of varying number of unhydrogenated isoprene units depending on the bacterial source. The vitamin K_2 having a 35-carbon side-chain and originally isolated from the putrefied fish meal is 2-methyl-3-*all-trans*-farnesylgeranylgeranyl-1,4-naphthoquinone. The synthetic compound, menadione, lacks a hydrophobic group at position 3 but can be alkylated in mammalian liver. The synthetic form is used as a source of vitamin K in most commercial animal feeds.

The naturally occurring substances in pure form are light-yellow solids or oils, insoluble in water but soluble in fat solvents. Transparent colloidal solutions of vitamin K_1 can be prepared by means of nonionic surfactants. Although menadione, too, is fat-soluble, it is easily soluble in boiling water and it is also slightly volatile at room temperature. Vitamins K_1 and K_2 as well as menadione are redox substance stable in the quinone form. In this respect there is a structural analogy between the vitamins K and E and a series of naturally occurring quinones called *ubiquinones*. The latter do not possess any demonstrable vitamin activity. Vitamins K have characteristic absorption spectra in the UV range and are sensitive to alkali, light and ionizing radiation.

Vitamin $K_{2(35)}$ (farnoquinone)

There is neither an international nor USP standard (or Unit) for vitamin K. There is, however, a USP Reference Standard of menadione. The activity of test materials is generally measured in terms of biological equivalency to milligrams of micrograms of meandione in a chick-feeding test.

After extraction and separation from interfering substances, the vitamins K can be determined by their UV spectra or by color reactions. They react with sodium ethylate to give a blue color, which changes to brown. A more sensitive reaction occurs with sodium diethyldithiocarbamate to give a transient blue color. A method for assay of menadione in injections is the photometric assay of Menotti, in which 2,4-dinitrophenylhydrazine in ethanol is heated with meandione in the presence of HCl. The vitamin thus is converted to the hydrazone, which when treated with ammonia yields a blue-green color. Vitamin K also can be assayed by the use of high performance liquid chromatography (HPLC) coupled with UV detection. Vitamin K_1 content of food homogenates and plasma are analyzed using reverse-phase HPLC with postcolumn solid phase-reduction of vitamin K_1 to its hydroquinone form, followed by fluorometric detection.

The chick is suited particularly for the biological assay of vitamin K because of the ease in producing a dietary vitamin deficiency and the high requirement, and the criterion of activity (blood "prothrombin time") is readily measurable but species differences in biological activity are known to occur.

Metabolic Functions, Dietary Requirement and Food Sources—Vitamin K is necessary for the formation of prothrombinogen and other blood-clotting factors in the liver. During clotting, circulating prothrombin is required for the production of thrombin; in turn, the thrombin converts fibrinogen to fibrin, the network of which constitutes the clot. It is obvious from this description that interference with formation of prothrombin will reduce the clotting tendency of the blood. In a severe deficiency of the vitamin, a condition of hypoprothrombinemia occurs, and blood-clotting time may be prolonged greatly, or even indefinitely. Internal or external hemorrhages may ensue either spontaneously or following injury or surgery. Other vitamin K-dependent proteins, including osteocalcin and matrix gla protein, have been identified in bone.

A group of substances termed vitamin K antagonists are characterized by their property to decrease plasma prothrombin levels and their usefulness in medicine as anticoagulants (see page 919). Representative of this group is dicumarol, originally isolated from spoiled sweet clover hay, in which it is formed by bacterial action on coumarin. An important use of vitamin K is in the treatment of hypoprothrombinemia consequent to prothrombopenic anticoagulant therapy. Vitamin K_1 is the preferred form. Large doses of salicylates also antagonize vitamin K.

A few chemically related derivatives of dicumarole are commercially used as rodenticides. Another compound with similar antagonist activity is sulfaquinoxaline, a sulfonamide drug used in veterinary medicine for treatment of various infectious intestinal diseases. It increases the animal's requirement for vitamin K in some undetermined manner, probably by eliminating vitamin K-synthesizing enteric bacteria, upon which the animal depends, in part, for a source of the vitamin. Extended treatment with antibacterial drugs than alter the enteric flora also increases the dietary vitamin K requirement in man.

Optimal absorption of vitamins K requires the presence of bile or bile salts in the intestine. Menadione, the synthetic water soluble analog, is absorbed easily in the absence of bile. The average diet apparently contains adequate amounts of vitamin K_1 since few if any malnourished humans have presented findings of dietary lack of vitamin K uncomplicated by intestinal disease, which prevents absorption. In 1989 the NAS established RDA's for Vitamin K_1 at 80 μg/day for men and 65 μg/day for women.

The premature infant appears to be particularly sensitive to a lack of the vitamin, and to an excess in the case of menadione. Because of this potential toxicity, the inclusion of menadione in OTC dietary supplements for the pregnant women is prohibited. Vitamin K_1 does not ehxibit this toxicity and is the preferred form. For newborn infants and especially those born prematurely (and anoxic), a single dose of 1 mg of vitamin K_1, immediately after birth, is often a routine measure to prevent hemorrhagic disease. Vitamin K_1 may be administered to the mother 12 to 24 hours prior to the expected delivery, or at the first sign of labor, especially if the mother has been receiving prothrombopenic anticoagulants. Requirements normally decrease after the neonatal period; however, it is important to ensure that adequate amounts of vitamin K_1 are present in infant formulas, since these are likely to be the sole nutriment during this period. Milk-substitute formulas containing less than 4 μg/100 kilocalories is required to have vitamin K_1 added to attain the level of 4 μg/100 Kcal required by infant formula regulations.

Although extensive measurements of dietary intakes and food content of the vitamins K_1 have not been made, primarily because suitable analytical methods have not been developed, most diets contain sufficient amounts as evident by adequate body stores for a very high proportion of the population. The green, leafy vegetables, tomatoes, cauliflower, egg yolk, soybean oil and liver of all kinds are good sources. Since it is insoluble in water, there is no loss in ordinary cooking. The human also uses vitamin K synthesized by certain enteric bacteria.

Fat-Soluble Vitamin Preparations

Cholecalciferol

(3β)-9,10-Secocholesta-5,7,10(19)-trien-3-ol, Vitamin D_3; Activated 7-Dehydrocholesterol

9,10-Secocholesta-5,7,10(19)-trien-3β-ol [67-97-0] $C_{27}H_{44}O$ (384.64); an antirachitic vitamin obtained from natural sources or prepared synthetically. See page 1111.

Description—White, odorless crystals; affected by air and light; melts between 84 and 88°.

Description—Insoluble in water; soluble in alcohol, chloroform or fatty oils.

Uses—The only valid therapeutic (as opposed to dietary) uses are in the *treatment* of vitamin D *deficiency* or in the *prophylaxis* of deficiency in persons with a known deficiency, a high requirement or an absorption defect. However, the substance may be employed to treat *hypocalcemic tetany* and *hypoparathyroidism.* Also, there is a growing medical opinion that it facilitates the prophylaxis of osteoporosis by calcium in postmenopausal women. It should not be employed in the presence of renal insufficiency or hyperphosphatemia.

Dose—The same as for *Ergocalciferol.*

Cod Liver Oil

Oleum Morrhuae; Oleum Jecoris Aselli; Oleum Gadi

The partially destearinated fixed oil obtained from fresh livers of *Gadus morrhua* Linné and other species of the Family *Gadidae;* contains in each g, not less than 255 μg (850 USP Units) of vitamin A and not less than 2.125 μg (85 USP Units) of vitamin D.

It may be flavored by the addition of not more than 1% of a suitable flavoring substance or a mixture of such substances.

Preparation—The highest grade of this medicinal oil is manufactured from fresh cod livers of healthy fish, removed from the fish within a few hours after they are caught. The oil is separated from the livers by heating with low-pressure steam. When livers of high quality are used and the manufacturing procedure is carried out under carefully controlled sanitary conditions the resulting crude oil is of a light yellow color, and of good flavor and odor. Such an oil requires no purification or chemical refining.

Due, however, to long-established trade demands, it is necessary to remove the code liver stearin so that the oil will remain clear at temperatures above freezing. To accomplish this, the oil is chilled to precipitate the stearin, which is removed by pressure filtration. To preserve the natural vitamin content of the oil it should be stored out of contact with air and light, preferably in a cold place.

Constituents—Consists chiefly of unsatured glycerides but contains *palmitin* and *stearin*, as well as traces of *chlorine, bromine, phosphorus* and *sulfur*. American cod liver oils may contain as much as 3 ppm of arsenic, but there is little evidence as to how completely it may be assimilated. American cod liver oils are rich in *iodine*—one sample was found to contain nearly 15,000 parts of iodine/billion parts of oil.

The vitamins of this oil occur in the unsaponifiable fraction. Since some persons object to taking oils, tablets and capsules containing the unsaponifiable fraction of the oil are manufactured. In general the procedure consists of saponifying the oil, separating the unsaponifiable portion, and extracting it with suitable solvents. The extract is diluted with corn oil and filled with capsules or mixed with solid materials and manufactured into tablets. The vitamin potency of these preparations can be adjusted to the patient's requirements but oviously they do not supply the constituents present in the saponifiable portion of the oil from which they were prepared.

Description—Thin, oily liquid, with a characteristic, slightly fishy, but not rancid, odor and a fishy taste; specific gravity 0.918 to 0.927.

Solubility—Slightly soluble in alcohol; freely soluble in either, chloroform, carbon disulfide or ethyl acetate.

Uses—A source of vitamins A and D. The vitamins are present in such proportion that an oral dose of 5 mL provides the daily requirements for children or adults of both of these dietary essentials. However, it may not provide 100% of a US RDA. It has been employed in the prophylaxis of rickets in infants.

Dose—5 mL, to contain no less than **1170 μg** (3900 USP units) of vitamin A and **9.7 μg** (386 USP units) of vitamin D.

Note—Code Liver Oil containing more than the minimum requirements for both vitamin A and vitamin D may be administered in proportionally smaller doses. The concentrate contains 10,000 Units of vitamin A and 400 Units of vitamin D per capsule or 4000 and 200 Units, respectively, per tablet.

Dihydrotachysterol—page 1082.

Ergocalciferol

(3b,5*Z*,7*E*,22*E*)-9,10-Secoergosta-5,7,10(19),22-tetraen-3-ol, Calciferol; Vitamin D_2; (*Various Mfrs*)

See page 1111 for the structure.

[50-14-6] $C_{28}H_{44}O$ (396.65). It is obtained by exposing ergosterol to ultraviolet light for the proper length of time. Insufficient irradiation results in the production of products with little or no antirachitic activity and prolonged exposure causes the production of toxic products. See page 1111.

Note—In stating the potency and dosage of vitamin D (cholecalciferol, ergocalciferol) dosage forms it is customary to use either the International Unit (IU) or the equivalent USP Unit. One USP Unit (or International Unit) of vitamin D (cholecalciferol or ergocalciferol) is defined as the specific biologic activity of 0.025 μg of the crystalline international standard or pure vitamin D_3.

Description—White, odorless crystals; affected by light and air; melting range 115 to 118°.

Solubility—Insoluble in water; soluble in alcohol, chloroform, ether or fatty oils.

Uses—Like other forms of vitamin D, it exhibits both antirachitic and calcemic effects. It has a relatively high potency and is thus especially useful for the treatment of severe or refractory *rickets.* It also may be used in the management of *hypocalcemia* and *hypoparathyroidism.* Care must be exercised to prevent overdosage. It should not be employed when renal insufficiency or hyperphosphatemia prevails. The serious toxic effects that may be caused by vitamin D are summarized in the general statement on *Vitamin D* under *Metabolic Functions.*

Dose—*Prophylactic, to prevent rickets,* **10 μg** (400 USP Units) a day (see Tables 1 and 2); in the *treatment of vitamin D-resistant rickets (refractory rickets),* **300 μg** to **12.5 mg** (12,000 to 500,000 Units) a day; in *hypoparathyroidism,* **1.25** to **5 mg** (50,000 to 200,000 Units) a day, plus 4 g of calcium lactate administered 6 times a day. *Caution: Pediatric dosage must be individualized under close medical supervision; the range between therapeutic and toxic doses is narrow.*

Dosage Forms—Capsules: 1.25 mg (50,000 USP Units); Solution (8000 USP Units/mL); Tablets: 1.25 mg (50,000 USP Units); Injection (in oil): 12.5 mg (500,000 USP Units)/mL.

Menadiol Sodium Diphosphate

1,4-Naphthalenediol, 2-methyl-, bis(dihydrogen phosphate), tetrasodium salt, hexahydrate; Vitamin K_4; Kappadione (*Lilly*); Synkavite (*Roche*)

2-Methyl-1,4-naphthalenediol bis(dihydrogen phosphate) tetrasodium salt, hexahydrate [6700-42-1] $C_{11}H_8Na_4O_8P_2.6H_2O$ (530.18); *anhydrous* [131-13-5] (422.09).

Preparation—Reduction of menadione to the diol compound by treatment with zinc in the presence of acid followed by double esterification with HI, metathesis of the resulting 1,4-diiodo compound with AgH_2PO_4, and neutralization of the bis(dihydrogen phosphate) ester thus formed with NaOH.

Description—White to pink powder, having a characteristic odor; hygroscopic; solutions are neutral or slightly alkaline to litmus, pH about 8.

Solubility—Very soluble in water; insoluble in alcohol.

Uses—See *Menadione* and *Phytonadione*. In the body it is converted to menadione and, consequently, it has the same uses and limitations, except that it is water-soluble and does not require the presence of bile salts for its absorption; therefore, it is especially useful in the presence of biliary obstruction.

Dose—*Adult, oral, subcutaneous, intramuscular,* or *intravenous, usual,* for *hypoprothrombinemia,* **5** to **15 mg** daily: *children,* **5** to **10 mg**; *intramuscular* or *subcutaneous,* to *antagonize prothrombopenic anticoagulants,* up to **75 mg,** to be repeated as needed; to *antagonize the prothrombopenic actions of salicylates,* **10** to **25 mg** daily, in 3 divided doses; for *liver function test,* **75 mg** IV.

Dosage Forms—Injection: 5 to 10 mg/mL, 75 mg/2 mL; Tablets: 5 mg.

Phytonadione

1,4-Naphthalenedione, *R*-[R^*, $R^*(E)$]]-, 2-methyl-3-(3,7,11,15-tetramethyl-2-hexadecenyl)-, 2-Methyl-3-phytyl-1,4-naphthoquinone; Vitamin K_1; Mephyton (*MSD*)

Phylloquinone [84-80-0] $C_{31}H_{46}O_2$ (450.70). It is a mixture of *cis-* and *trans*-isomers; it contains not more than 20.0% of the *cis*-isomer. See page 1113.

Description—Clear, yellow to amber, very viscous, odorless or nearly odorless liquid; specific gravity about 0.967; stable in air but decomposes on exposure to sunlight; solution (1 in 20) in alcohol is neutral to litmus; refractive index 1.523 to 1.526 at 25°.

Solubility—Insoluble in water; soluble in dehydrated alcohol, benzene, chloroform, ether or vegetable oils.

Uses—The natural product, vitamin K_1. For the metabolic functions of vitamin K, see the general statement.

It has a more prompt and prolonged action than menadiol and other synthetic analogs of vitamin K, and it is the more reliable in restoring prothrombin to the blood in conditions of *hypoprothrombinemia. Hypoprothrombinemia in the newborn* may be prevented or treated by the administration of phytonadione to the mother shortly before parturition or by giving the infant a single dose shortly after birth. In *hypoprothrombinemia consequent to prothrombopenic anticoagulant therapy,* an adequate intravenous injection will usually stop hemorrhage within 3 to 4 hr and restore the plasma prothrombin level to normal in 12 to 24 hr. In hypoprothrombinemia resulting from liver disease it may have limited value, especially if the disease is hepatocellular; in *biliary obstruction or fistula,* in which only the absorption of vitamin K is impaired, hypoprothrombinemia responds promptly to parenteral phytonadione. In other enteric diseases in which absorption is defective—as in *sprue, regional enteritis, enterocolitis, ulcerative colitis, dysentery* and *extensive bowel resection*—it will correct hypoprothrombinemia if given parenterally.

It must be emphasized that it cannot be used to check bleeding irrespective of its origin. It is of no benefit in diseases of the blood-forming organs, thrombocytopenic purpura, hemophilia, etc.

Excessive doses occasionally may cause hyperprothrombinemia and a tendency toward thrombosis.

Dose—*Oral,* for *hypoprothrombinemia,* **2.5** to **10 mg** or up to **25 mg** (rarely **50 mg**), repeated in 12 to 48 hr if necessary; *subcutaneous* or *intramuscular* (*intravenous* if unavoidable, at rate of 1 mg/min), **2.5** to **10 mg** or up to **25 mg** (rarely **50 mg**), repeated in 6 to 8 hr if necessary. For prophylaxis of hemorrhagic disease of the newborn, a single *intramuscular* dose of **0.5** to **1 mg;** less desirably, **1** to **5 mg** to mother 12 to 24 hr before delivery. For treatment of hemorrhagic disease of the newborn, **0.5** to **1 mg** *subcutaneously* or *intramuscularly* (higher doses if mother has been receiving oral anticoagulants).

Dosage Forms—Injection: 1 mg/0.5 mL, 10 mg/mL, 25 mg/2.5 mL, 50 mg/5 mL; Tablets: 5 mg.

Tretinoin—page 879.

Vitamin A

Contains a suitable form of retinol ($C_{20}H_{30}O$; vitamin A alcohol). It may consist of retinol or esters of retinol formed from edible fatty acids, principally acetic and palmitic acids. It may be diluted with edible oils, or it may be incorporated in solid, edible carriers or excipients, and it may contain suitable antimicrobial agents, dispersants, and antioxidants. See page 1110.

Note—In stating the potency and dosage of vitamin A dosage forms it is customary to use either the International Unit (IU) or the equivalent USP Unit. One USP Unit (or International Unit) of vitamin A is defined as the specific biological activity of 0.3 μg of the all-*trans* isomer of retinol.

Description—Yellow to red, oily liquid that may solidify upon refrigeration; in solid form, it has the appearance of any diluent that has been added; may be nearly odorless or may have a fish odor, but has no rancid odor or taste; unstable to air and light.

Solubility—In liquid form, insoluble in water or glycerin; soluble in absolute alcohol or vegetable oils; very soluble in ether or chloroform. In solid form, may be dispersible in water.

Uses—The only valid therapeutic uses are in the treatment of vitamin A *deficiency* or in the *prophylaxis* of deficiency in persons with a known dietary deficiency, a high requirement or an absorption defect. Large doses produce toxicity (see the general statement), symptoms of which may not be evident for 6 mo or longer. Daily doses larger than 25,000 USP Units should not be prescribed unless severe deficiency exists.

Dose—*Deficiency, adults and children over 8 yr,* **10,000 to 25,000 Units** a day for 1 or 2 wk; Refer to Tables 1 and 2 for dosage variations with different age groups; for *xerophthalamia,* initially **25,000 to 50,000 Units** a day for 5 days; *Intramuscular,* 50,000 to 100,000 Units a day for 10 days, followed by **50,000 Units** a day for 10 days; *children* (IM), **5000 to 15,000 Units** a day for 10 days; *pediatric, deficiency,* initially **5000 Units/kg.**

Dosage Forms—Capsules: 1.5, 3, 7.5 and 15 mg (5000, 10,000, 25,000 and 50,000 USP Units); Drops: 15 mg (50,000 USP Units)/mL; Tablets: 15 mg (50,000 USP Units); Injection: 15 mg (50,000 USP Units)/mL.

Vitamin E

A form of alpha tocopherol [$C_{29}H_{50}O_2$ = 430.71]. See page 1112. It includes the following: *d-* or *dl*-alpha tocopherol ($C_{29}H_{50}O_2$); *d-* or *dl*-alpha tocopheryl acetate [$C_{31}H_{52}O_3$ = 472.75]; *d-* or *dl*-alpha tocopheryl acid succinate [$C_{33}H_{54}O_5$ = 530.79].

The generic title *Vitamin E Preparation* is officially recognized for any single form of the vitamin with one or more inert substances. The product may be in liquid or solid form, and it must contain not less than 95.0% and not more than 120.0% of the labeled amount of the vitamin. For a preparation labeled to contain a *dl*-form of the vitamin allowance is made for it to contain a small amount of a *d*-form occurring as a minor constituent of an added substance.

Alpha tocopherol (also written α-tocopherol) is a trivial generic name (which embraces all stereoisomeric forms of 2,5,7,8-tetra-methyl-2-(4,8,12-trimethyltridecyl)-6-chromanol. The term *d*-alpha tocopherol is employed in the pharmaceutical field to designate that form of the compound which (1) occurs naturally and (2) is dextrorotatory. The term *dl*-alpha tocopherol designates the mixture of stereoisomers prepared synthetically, commonly from racemic isophytol.

The phenolic hydroxyl is readily susceptible to acylation and the resulting esters, eg, the acetate and acid succinate, are much more resistant to oxidation and discoloration on exposure to air and light than the phenolic form.

Description—Little or no odor or taste. *The alpha tocopherols and alpha tocopheryl acetates:* clear, yellow, viscous oils. *d-Alpha tocopheryl acetate:* may solidify in the cold. *Alpha tocopheryl acid succinate:* white powder; the *d*-isomer melts at about 75°, and the *dl*-form melts at about 70°. *The esters:* stable to air and to light but are unstable to alkali; *the acid succinate:* also unstable when held molten.

Solubility—*Alpha tocopheryl acid succinate:* insoluble in water; slightly soluble in alkaline solutions; soluble in alcohol, ether, acetone or vegetable oils; very soluble in chloroform. *Other forms of vitamin E:* insoluble in water; soluble in alcohol; miscible with ether, acetone, vegetable oils or chloroform.

Uses—The only valid therapeutic use is as a supplement to the diet of the newborn infant, especially if premature, or in the treatment of the infant with steatorrhea, in which the gastrointestinal absorption of it is impaired. No need for administration to children or adults has been demonstrated. For additional information see the general statement.

Dose—*Usual, prophylactic,* from **5** to **30** USP Units of vitamin E. 30 IU corresponds to the US RDA (see Tables 1 and 2); only persons on diets high in polyunsaturated fatty acids or who have previously been on such diets for a long period of time actually require this daily intake. *Therapeutic,* **4 to 5 times** the RDA or **1 Unit** per kg of body weight a day.

Dosage Form—Capsules: 30, 37.5, 50, 75, 100, 200, 400, 500, 600, and 1000 IU.

Other Fat-Soluble Vitamins

Calcifediol [(3β,5*Z*,7*Z*)-9,10-Secocholesta-5,7,10(19)-triene-3,25-diol monohydrate $C_{27}H_{44}O_2.H_2O$ (418.66) Palderol (*Organon*)]—The form of vitamin D_3 found in the circulation; differs from calcitriol (below) in that hydroxylation in the liver occurs only at C-25. Produced synthetically; see *Am J Clin Nutr 22:* 412, 1969. A white powder practically insoluble in water. *Uses:* In the treatment and management of metabolic bone disease or hypocalcemia associated with chronic renal failure. It should not be given to patients with hypercalcemia or evidencing toxicity to vitamin D. *Dose: Usual adult, oral,* initially 300 to 500 μg/wk administered daily or on an alternate-day schedule; the dosage may be increased, if necessary, at 4-wk intervals; *pediatric, oral, children up to 2 yr,* 20 to 50 μg a day; *children,* 2 to 10 yr, *oral,* 50 μg a day; *children,* over 10 yr, use adult dose. *Dosage Forms:* Capsules, 20 and 50 μg.

Calcitriol [9,10-Seco(5*Z*,7*E*)-5,7,10(19)-cholestatriene-1α,3β,25-triol; 1,25-dihydroxycholecalciferol; 1,25-hydroxyvitamin D_3; 1,25-DHCC; $C_{27}H_{44}O_3$ (416.65); Rocaltrol (*Roche*)]—The biologically active form of vitamin D_3 (see page 1111) resulting from sequential hydroxylation of the vitamin at C-25 in the liver and at C-1 in the kidney; produced also synthetically. A colorless, crystalline compound. *Uses:* The form of vitamin D_3 that stimulates intestinal calcium transport. Based on the observation that in acutely uremic rats, it stimulates intestinal calcium absorption it has been suggested that a vitamin D-resistant state exists in uremic patients because of failure of the kidney to convert precursors to calcitriol, hence the indication for use of the latter compound in the management of hypocalciuria in patients undergoing chronic renal dialysis. Its efficacy in reversing not only the calcium metabolic disorder but also of reducing elevated parathyroid hormone levels in some patients has been demonstrated. *Dose:* Optimal daily dose, administered *orally*, must be determined for each patient. The recommended initial dose is 0.25 μg/day; most patients undergoing hemodialysis respond to doses between 0.5 and 1 μg/day but dosages up to 2 μg/day have been reported. *Dosage Form:* Soft gelatin capsules containing 0.25 μg.

Vitamin A Acetate [Retinol Acetate; $C_{22}H_{32}O_2$]—Light-yellow to red oil with a slight fishy odor; light and oxygen cause deterioration; tasteless. Soluble in lipid solvents; insoluble in water. *Uses:* A form of vitamin A; 0.344 μg is equivalent to 1 USP unit or to 0.6 μg of β-carotene. *Dose:* See *Vitamin A* (page 1110).

Vitamin A Palmitate [Retinol Palmitate; $C_{36}H_{60}O_2$]—Light-yellow to red oil; odorless in the pure state but otherwise has a slight fishy odor; unstable in light and air. Soluble in oils and lipid solvents; insoluble in water. *Uses:* A form of vitamin A. *Dose:* See *Vitamin A* (page 1110); by weight, the palmitate is approximately half as potent as vitamin A.

The Water-Soluble Vitamins

Except for ascorbic acid, all the vitamins in this water-soluble category belong to the B-group of vitamins. Some still retain their original individual designations, such as B_1, B_6 and B_{12}, whereas comparable names for other vitamins have become obsolete.

In 1930, when it was clear that vitamin B was of multiple nature, the term vitamin B complex was coined to refer to the group of water-soluble animal growth factors found in relatively high concentrations in such products as liver, yeast and rice bran. This was a convenient term to use in the early scientific literature, but it was not intended to be a specific name for pharmaceutical preparations that contain varying proportions of the B vitamins. The term was intended to apply to a group of vitamins whose identity was being sought, rather than to a group of compounds whose identity had been established. Since the nature of the "complex" has been characterized, the term vitamin B com plex is no longer appropriate.

Ascorbic Acid (Vitamin C)

Vitamin C, or ascorbic acid (antiscorbutic vitamin), is necessary for the prevention and cure of the deficiency disease scurvy.

Scurvy has been recognized since the Middle Ages and was found widespread in northern Europe and among the crews of sailing ships. During the 18th century it was learned that when fresh fruit was made available aboard sailing vessels, scurvy was avoided. In 1907 Holst and Frolich observed a scurvy-like syndrome in guinea pigs that was similar to human scurvy and cured it by feeding citrus juices. This gave an experimental means for the rapid development of our knowledge of vitamin C, to which many workers have contributed.

Chemistry and Assay—Ascorbic acid is a white, crystalline compound structurally related to the monosaccharides. It exists in nature in both a reduced and the oxidized form, dehydroascorbic acid. These substances are in a state of reversible equilibrium in biological systems, and both have the same biological activity.

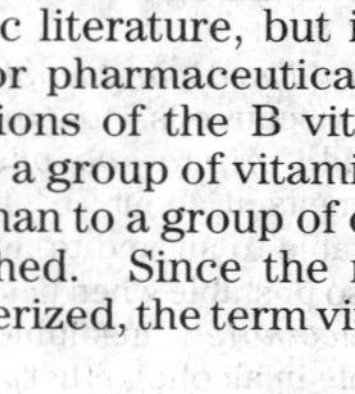

L-Ascorbic Acid 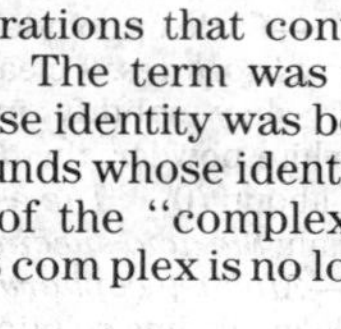 **Dehydroascorbic Acid**

Ascorbic acid is stable in the dry state but is easily oxidized in aqueous solution in the presence of air. Oxidation is accelerated by heat, light, alkalies, oxidative enzymes and traces of copper and iron. Because of its relative instability, ascorbic acid is readily lost during cooking if simple precautions to avoid aeration are not taken. Also, because of its high aqueous solubility, the vitamin is lost to a considerable extent when large amounts of cooking water are discarded. Progressive loss of vitamin C in fresh fruits and vegetables occurs during storage.

Solutions of ascorbic acid are strongly reducing, and the vitamin is oxidized easily. In animal tissues the greater part of the vitamin is in the reduced form, but, as scurvy develops, the ratio of oxidized to reduced form rises. This property of reversible oxidation–reduction is the most likely basis for the role of the vitamin in biochemical reactions.

The article of commerce is produced exclusively by synthesis. Sorbitol, a hexose occurring in several fruits but commercially obtained by hydrogenating dextrose, is the raw material for production of ascorbic acid. Amounts of ascorbic acid are expressed in terms of weight, as milligrams. The USP provides a Reference Standard of L-ascorbic acid for assay purposes. The practical methods of ascorbic acid assay are based on its powerful reducing properties which enable determination by oximetric titration. The three most-used reagents for this titration are chloramine-T, 2,6-dichlorophenolindophenol, and iodine. Another practical assay is based on the conversion of ascorbic acid to oxalic acid 2-nitrophenylhydrazide by treatment with diazotized 2-nitroaniline. This yields a colored compound which is measured photometrically. Still another is the photometric assay of total ascorbic acid (ascorbic acid plus dehydroascorbic acid) by conversion of the vitamin to its 2,4-dinitrophenylhydrazone.

Metabolic Function, Dietary Requirement and Food Sources—Vitamin C is known to be essential for the formation of intercellular collagen. In scorbutic tissues the amorphous ground substance, and the fibroblasts in the area between the cells appear normal but without the matrix of collagen fibers. These bundles of collagenous material appear within a few hours after the administration of ascorbic acid. This points to the relationship of the vitamin in maintenance of tooth structures, matrix of bone and the walls of capillaries. In scurvy, these are the tissues found to be faulty.

The picture of clinical scurvy in humans is one that can be related to the general breakdown of intercellular collagen substance. Bleeding is common, particularly at sites of pressure. The occurrence of petechiae, pinpoint hemorrhages that occur in the skin under reduced pressure, has been used as a diagnosis of scurvy. This is an indication of weakness or fragility of the walls of capillaries. Bones become brittle and cease to grow, and normal structures are replaced by connective tissue that contains calcified cartilage. Anemia is a common occurrence in scurvy, caused by an impairment of hematopoiesis. Also, vitamin C has been shown to change iron absorption. Tooth enamel, cementum and particularly dentin, change in structure, and the gums about the teeth become spongy and bleed easily. Keratoconjunctivitis sicca, xerostomia, salivary gland enlargement, xerosis, hyperpigmentation, ichthyosis, neuropathies and mental depression may occur, even when the full-blown picture of scurvy is absent.

Vitamin C is essential for the healing of bone fractures. Such fractures heal slowly in a patient deficient in vitamin C. Wound-healing also is impaired.

There is evidence to indicate that the vitamin functions in the metabolism of tyrosine. There is an abnormal excretion of homogentisic, *p*-hydroxyphenylpyruvic and *p*-hydroxyphenyllactic acids in scorbutic guinea pigs following administration of tyrosine, which, of course, is corrected with ascorbic acid. The excretion of "tyrosyl" derivatives in humans on a vitamin C-low diet given 20 g of tyrosine daily is also affected by ascorbic acid administration. In some newborn, the occurrence of tyrosinemia possibly accruing to high protein intakes suggests that this relationship be taken into consideration in evaluating the ascorbic acid requirement for the infant.

An intake of 10 to 20 mg a day of ascorbic acid is sufficient to protect an adult from classical scurvy and 45 mg a day will maintain an adequate body pool of 1500 mg. Except for pregnant and lactating women, 60 mg is the recommended dietary allowance (Table 1) for both men and women over 11 years. For infants, 35 mg of ascorbic acid provides about the same amount as supplied daily by 850 mL of milk from mothers living in the US. The vitamin C requirements are increased following trauma, during infections, and during periods of vigorous physical activity; in such circumstances the requirement may be 100 to 200 mg a day.

The regular ingestion of from 1 to 4 g of ascorbic acid a day has been suggested as a means of shortening the illness period and alleviating the symptoms of the "common cold." A few clinical studies offer some support for this hypothesis, but other studies have failed to replicate these results. Definitive long-term studies with large populations which might confirm the practice as a reliable public health measure have not been done.

A number of epidemiological studies show a protective association between the consumption of foods which contain vitamin C and cancers of the esophagus, stomach and cervix. Animal studies testing precursors of known carcinogens show a reduced number of tumors when the animals were given vitamin C. Biochemical studies suggest that vitamin C blocks the formation of active carcinogenics from precursors. There is also the hypothesis that vitamin C has an effect as a free radial scavenger. Although vitamin C in large amounts may have some pharmacological effects, these are not related to the normal functioning of the vitamin at nutritional levels. There is no evidence that levels in excess of few times the RDA has any additional benefit and contrary to those who advocate the use of megadose quantities (gram quanities); such practices can be harmful to some individuals.

The prolonged ingestion of supplements of ascorbic acid in excess of about 3 g a day is not without potential danger. Gastrointestinal disturbances (nausea followed by diarrhea), kidney or bladder stone formation (resulting from an increased excretion of oxalate, urate, and calcium), prenatal conditioning of the fetus to deficiency symptoms, interference with simple tests for glycosuria and interference with the anticoagulant effect of heparin are clinical problems which may occur.

For therapeutic purposes in treatment of adult scurvy, 1000 mg of ascorbic acid a day, in divided doses, for 1 week is recommended, then 500 mg until all signs disappear. It also is used in the treatment of idiopathic methemoglobinemia to reduce the ferric iron in heme to the ferrous state.

Ascorbic acid facilitates the absorption of iron by keeping the iron in the reduced form. A few microcytic anemias respond to ascorbic acid treatment, which may be in part due to improved absorption of iron.

Vitamin C is found in all living plant cells, is synthesized during the germination of seeds, and is concentrated relatively in the rapidly growing parts of the plant. It is present in all animal tissues as well, but only guinea pigs, primates, a few exotic animal species and man are unable to meet body needs by synthesis, and must rely upon a dietary source.

Although vitamin C appears to be present in all living tissues, our best sources of supply are fresh fruits such as citrus fruits, strawberries, melons and green vegetables such as lettuce and cabbage. An average serving of potatoes contains enough vitamin C when first harvested to meet the adult male RDA, but contains only half that amount by the following spring. It is a common practice, and a sound one, to rely to a large extent on citrus fruits and juices as important vitamin C carriers, particularly in infant feeding. An ounce of orange or lemon juice a day is sufficient to prevent scurvy in humans on an otherwise vitamin C-low diet.

It is fairly common practice to add ascorbic acid to foods for technical purposes; eg, as an antioxidant to protect natural flavors and colors.

The B Vitamins

The "water-soluble B" of McCollum, or the "antiberiberi vita mine" of Funk, has now been differentiated into at least eleven separate and distinct chemical entities. It has been established that eight of these are required in human nutrition. They are *thiamin, riboflavin, niacin, folic acid, pyridoxine, biotin, pantothenic acid and vitamin B_{12}*. Para-aminobenzoic acid, choline, and inositol have an essential part in cellular metabolism in plants and animals, but this alone does not constitute presumptive evidence of their importance in human nutrition. When the dietary intake of methionine is adequate, choline can be synthesized endogenously; therefore, the human requirement is relative to the methionine intake, similar to the relationship between niacin and tryptophan. It can be stated categorically that the human does not require either an exogenous or endogenous source of para-aminobenzoic acid. Although inositol deficiency has not been demonstrated in humans, it may be an important nutrient in infant nutrition. Mammalian milk contains inositol and, since milk is the sole item of the diet of infants during this critical growth period, is appropriate to include it in nonmilk-based formulas, a practice which has existed since the early 1960s.

There is no one natural source of the B vitamins as a group that is necessarily superior to another source. No natural source contains all the water-soluble factors in the proportions that are needed in human nutrition, and the therapeutic value of any vitamin-containing material depends on the needs of the individual to whom it is being administered. Nevertheless, multiple deficiencies of B vitamins often coexist. Furthermore, the repair of one B-vitamin deficiency may increase the need for another; thus, the administration of thiamin in clinical or subclinical beriberi increases the need for riboflavin. Consequently, there is some justification for multivitamin therapy with those five B vitamins for which *clinical* deficiencies occur (thiamin, niacin, riboflavin, folic acid and vitamin B_{12}). Human deficiencies in biotin and pantothenic acid have only been produced experimentally, and pyridoxine deficiency has occurred in infants fed an unfortified formula.

Biotin

cis-Hexahydro-2-oxothieno[3,4-*d*]imidazole-4-valeric acid

Before this nutritional factor was identified as a discrete chemical substance, it variously was called vitamin H, anti-egg-white injury factor, coenzyme R, Bios II and others. Its discovery was an outgrowth of studies on the "toxicity" of large amounts of unheated egg white as the sole source of protein for rats.

Chemistry and Assay—Biotin is a colorless, crystalline monocarboxylic acid, only slightly soluble in water or alcohol (its salts are quite soluble). Water solutions are stable at 100°, and the dry substance is both thermostable and photostable. Biotin is unstable, however, in strong acids and alkaline solutions and in oxidizing agents. The vitamin is optically active and the natural isomer, which alone possesses biological activity, is the D-form (rings are *cis*-fused and the isomer is designated (+)-biotin).

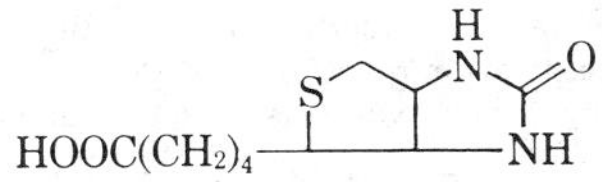

H
S N O
$HOOC(CH_2)_4$ NH

Biotin

Although biotin with the above structure is the compound present in food sources, the sulfur atom can be replaced with an oxygen atom without reduction of its metabolic activity. Biotin occurs in animal and plant tissues primarily in combined forms which are liberated by enzymatic hydrolysis during digestion. One of the simplest such complexes is biocytin, ε-*N*-biotinyl-L-lysine. The amount of the vitamin in a product is expressed solely in terms of the weight of the chemically pure substance, the free monocarboxylic acid.

Only microbiological methods are feasible for the quantitative assay of biotin because of their sensitivity to the low concentrations usually encountered. After simple aqueous or acid extraction combined with heating, a microbiological assay using growth of the test organisms *Allescheria boydii* or *Lactobacillus arabinosus* as the criterion is carried out.

Metabolic Functions, Dietary Requirement and Food Sources—Attempts to induce deficiency in man by inclusion of large amounts (200 g) of dried unheated egg white for several days in the diet have resulted in the appearance of vague symptoms such as change in skin color and dermatoses, slight change in lingual papillae of the tongue, muscle pains, loss of appetite, sleeplessness and extreme lassitude. Raw egg white contains a protein, avidin, which combines with biotin and prevents absorption of the vitamin from the intestine. Rapid relief from such symptoms was observed with administration of biotin. This condition is difficult to produce in human subjects and, since a frank and specific deficiency disease is not discernible, there is uncertainty as to the exact nature of the deficiency syndrome as well as the need for a dietary source of biotin in human nutrition. Intestinal synthesis is undoubtedly the important factor in the supply of biotin to the body.

Biotin functions in carbon dioxide fixation reactions in intermediary metabolism, transferring the carboxyl group to acceptor molecules. It similarly acts also in decarboxylation reactions. For its part in these vital enzymatic steps, in catalyzing deamination of amino acids, and in oleic acid synthesis, biotin is essential in human metabolism and presumed to be a dietary essential in the absence of adequate microbial synthesis in the intestine.

Diets providing a daily intake of 150 to 300 μg of biotin are considered adequate. And these amounts are readily met and exceeded when milk, meat, and eggs are frequent items of the diet.

Choline

The propriety of classifying choline as a vitamin and a member of the B group is questionable because it is synthesized in the human body, and there is no evidence that a lack of choline has a disturbing effect on human metabolism. Nevertheless, choline plays an important role both as a structural component of tissues and in biological methylation reactions. Dietary deficiency of it leads to gross pathology in several species of animals.

Chemistry—Choline is (β-hydroxyethyl)trimethylammonium hydroxide. Since it is completely dissociated, it is comparable to alkali hydroxides as a base. Consequently, it does not exist as a base at body pH but rather as a salt, the anion is that present in its immediate biological environment. The β-(hydroxyethyl)trimethylammonium cation is the biologically important moiety. The cation is incorporated into phospholipids, such as lecithin and sphingomyelin, and acetylcholine, a substance released at cholinergic nerve junctions during transmission of nerve impulses. Acid hydrolysis of phospholipids yields the free choline salt which is very soluble in water, and to a lesser extent in ethanol. Assay for choline is accomplished with a microbiological method using a mutant strain of *Neurospora*.

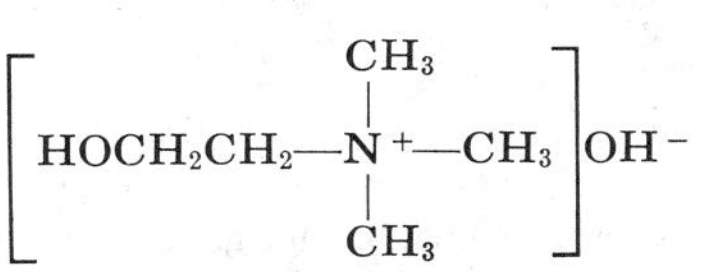

$$\left[HOCH_2CH_2—\overset{\displaystyle CH_3}{\underset{\displaystyle CH_3}{N^{+}}}—CH_3 \right] OH^-$$

Choline

Metabolic Functions, Dietary Requirement and Food Sources—Besides its vital function as a precursor of acetylcholine, which is important in the sequence of nerve-muscle stimulations, choline is an important contributor of methyl groups needed for the *in vivo* synthesis of metabolites and perhaps some hormones. The biogenesis of choline appears to be universal in nature, and is the result of the three-step transfer of methyl groups to an acceptor, which may be either free aminoethanol or phosphatidyl aminoethanol. Such transfers require methionine as a methyl donor (actually, *S*-adenosylmethionine). Choline is indirectly a source of methyl groups; it is first oxidized to betaine, which then may transfer a methyl group to homocysteine to form methionine. By thus regenerating methionine lost in transmethylation reactions, exogenous choline can spare the amino acid for use in protein synthesis. Methionine is an essential amino acid.

Choline has the property of preventing the deposition of excess fat, or of causing the removal of excess fat from the liver of experimental animals fed high-fat diets and, because of this, is often classified as a "lipotropic agent." The lipotropic action probably relates to the incorporation of choline into phosphatidyl choline (lecithin), which, in turn, is incorporated into phospholipids and lipoproteins. The lipotropic action is independent of the function of choline as a reservoir of methyl groups.

There is presumptive evidence from nutritional and metabolic studies and teleological considerations that choline is important, if not essential, for the infant. It is appropriate to ensure, therefore, that choline is present in infant formulas at least to the level found in human milk. This is about 90 mg/L. Most infant formulas contain about 1½ times this amount. It is equally appropriate to include choline in chemically defined diets to be used as the sole source of nutrients for critically ill patients. An average mixed diet consumed by man in the US has been estimated to contain 500 to 900 mg choline a day, an amount known to be adequate when compared with animal requirements. Foods that supply large amounts of choline are liver, kidney, brain, muscle meats, fish, nuts, beans, peas and eggs. Moderate amounts exist in cereals, milk and a number of vegetables.

Folic Acid (Folacin)

The vitamin derives its name from the Latin word *folium*, leaf. It was first isolated from spinach leaves where it is now known to occur in relatively minute amounts, compared to other food sources. Several apparently unrelated factors had been isolated in various laboratories before realization that they had in common the same parent compound, pteroyl-L-glutamic acid: Factor U (a chick growth factor), vitamin M (a factor for monkeys), vitamin B_c (a chick anti-anemia factor), liver and yeast *L casei* factors (bacterial growth factors) and others. In 1972 the International Union of Nutritional Sciences Committee on Nomenclature decided that the term folacin should be used as the generic descriptor for folic acid pteroylmono-L-glutamic acid. However, the USP continues to call pteroylglutamic acid by the descriptor, folic acid, and medical and biochemical practice usually does the same.

Chemistry and Assay—Pteroylglutamic acid crystallizes from cold water, in which it is only slightly soluble, as yellow spear-shaped platelets. It is readily destroyed by boiling in acid solution and its solutions will deteriorate in sunlight. It is insoluble in alcohol or the usual organic solvents but readily dissolves in dilute solutions of alkali hydroxides and carbonates. The characteristic UV absorption spectrum of pteroylglutamic acid in dilute NaOH is used to aid in identification and measurement of the compound.

A series of compounds with several molecules of glutamic acid attached to the first glutamic acid radical in peptide linkage have been synthesized. Compounds with one, two, three and seven glutamic acid groups have been isolated. The latter three are known as conjugates. Some animals and man can utilize them as a source of pteroylglutamic acid, presumably because appropriate digestive enzymes can hydrolyze them. Microorganisms can use them to only a variable and limited extent, unless they are first hydrolyzed to the free form with liver, kidney or pancreatic enzymes, called conjugases.

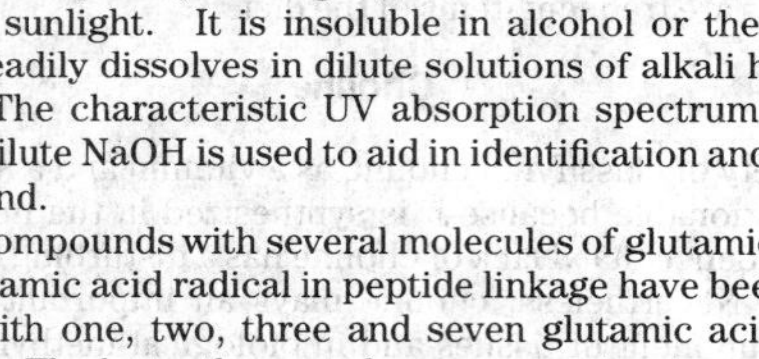

The functional form of this vitamin group is basically the 5,6,7,8-tetrahydrofolic acid in which a formyl group (—CHO), when present, is attached at either or both the N^5 or N^{10} positions. The hydrogenated N^5-formyl compound, formerly called *folinic acid*, or leucovorin, is available, as is the monosodium salt of folic acid, as a discrete pharmaceutical preparation. It properly is termed 5-formyltetrahydrofolic acid. These compounds similarly serve as standards during assay of the vitamin. A USP Reference Standard Folic Acid is available. Separately, the three moieties which make up the folic acid molecule (pteroic acid, *p*-aminobenzoic acid and glutamic acid) have no vitamin activity.

The quantitative assay of folacin in natural products is mainly by biological or microbiological methods. In the chick assay, the birds are placed on a folic acid-free diet until they became anemic, after which folic acid supplements and the test material are administered. The degree of recovery is related to the quantity of reference folic acid fed. The two organisms most used in the microbiological method are *Lactobacillus casei* and *Streptococcus faecalis*. The method is based on the fact that pteroylglutamic acid is a required growth factor for each; however, the assay is complicated when biological material is analyzed, because naturally occurring folic acid derivatives do not all have the same biological activity for the two organisms.

Folic acid can be determined by either of two physicochemical methods, provided the compound is present in relatively pure form. One method is the spectrophotometric measurement of the extinction maxima of the UV absorption curve; the other is the spectrometric measurement after oxidative fission of folic acid to 4-aminobenzoylglutamic acid followed by diazotization and coupling to give an azo dye. Folic acid also can be determined with high-pressure liquid chromatography.

Metabolic Functions—Folic acid is one of the important hematopoietic agents necessary for proper regeneration of the blood-forming elements and their functioning. Although the mechanism whereby folic acid performs this vital role is not understood, much is known about the involvement of folic acid as a coenzyme in intermediary metabolic reactions in which one-carbon units are transferred. These reactions are important in interconversions of various amino acids and in purine and pyrimidine synthesis. This role is in contrast to that of choline in furnishing and transferring so-called labile methyl groups in transmethylation reactions. The biosynthesis of purines and pyrimidines is linked ultimately with that of nucleotides and ribo- and deoxyribo-nucleic acids, functional elements of all cells.

The concept of antivitamins or vitamin antagonists is exemplified in a particular aspect of folic acid metabolism. By virtue of its structural similarity, sulfanilamide competes with *p*-aminobenzoic acid in the biological synthesis of folic acid. The organism is thus deprived of needed folic acid. Sulfonamides act, therefore, as growth inhibitors of certain pathogenic organisms, a competitive antagonism which is responsible for the antibacterial action of sulfa drugs. Since mammals use preformed folic acid, sulfonamides do not disrupt the host metabolism.

Numerous analogs of pteroylglutamic acid have been prepared which exhibit potent antifolic acid activity. Several compounds, notably aminopterin (4-aminopteroylglutamic acid) and methotrexate (4-amino-N^{10}-methylpteroylglutamic acid), compete with folic acid in nucleic acid synthesis and have been used in the treatment of various cancers, psoriasis and certain immune disorders. The antimicrobial drugs, trimethoprim and pyrimethamine, are also antifolate drugs.

Dietary Requirement and Food Sources—Folic acid deficiency results in megaloblastic anemia, glossitis, diarrhea and weight loss. A deficiency is best diagnosed by the demonstration of low levels of the vitamin in serum or blood by microbiological assay or by the hematological response to a physiological dose of folic acid, 50 to 200 μg intramuscularly a day for 10 days. The condition of megaloblastic anemia arising as a result of dietary deficiency of folacin occurs most frequently after the age of 65, in persons suffering from malabsorption syndromes, in women during the last trimester of pregnancy and in infants receiving unfortified proprietary formulas or goat's milk. In the treatment of megaloblastic or macrocytic anemia, folic acid should be administered as the sole therapeusis *only* when the possibility of pernicious anemia and other primary diseases of the small bowel has been excluded absolutely, a restriction necessitated because of the vitamin's ability to mask other diagnostic signs of these conditions.

In recent years folic acid has been linked as a possible agent in lowering the risk of rare but serious defects in fetal development of the brain and spinal cord, including spina bifida and anencephaly. These conditions generally are referred to as neural tube defects (NTDs). In some intervention and observational studies in which women of child-bearing age were given folic acid supplements, lower levels of NTDs were observed compared with placebo controls. It should be noted that these studies were accomplished in areas where the pretreatment rates of NTDs were near or above 2 per 1000 live births and supplemental levels of folic acid were between 0.4 and 4 mg/day. Also, data obtained for populations where folic acid intakes were exceedingly low show no relationship with the rates of NTDs and, therefore, the condition does not appear to be caused by classic folic acid deficiency. Furthermore, research with animals has not shown any increase in NTDs with folic acid deficient diets.

No mechanism for the observed relationship of folic acid consumption and NTD rates in humans has been proposed. The US Public Health Service has recommended that all women who are capable of becoming pregnant should consume 0.4 mg of folic acid per day throughout their child-bearing years for the purpose of reducing their risk of an NTD pregnancy.

This recommendation was made after the 1989 revision of the RDAs was released by the Food and Nutrition Board of the NAS. The 1989 RDAs are 0.2, 0.18 and 0.4 mg for men, women and pregnant women, respectively.

A balanced American diet for adults contains approximately 0.2 to 0.6 mg of total folic acid activity, and the intestinal microflora also provide some absorbable amounts of the vitamin. The best food sources of folic acid are liver, kidney, dry beans, asparagus, mushrooms, broccoli and collards. Other good sources include spinach, peanuts, lima beans, cabbage, sweet corn, chard, turnip greens, lettuce, milk and whole wheat products.

Inositol

Inositol is hexahydroxycyclohexane (1,2,3,4,5,6-cyclohexanhexol; *i*-inositol; *myo*-inositol; *meso*-inositol). Actually, there are nine stereoisomeric cyclohexanols, all of which now are referred to commonly as inositols. Several occur in nature; the isomer described above is by far the most prevalent and is the only one that is biologically active.

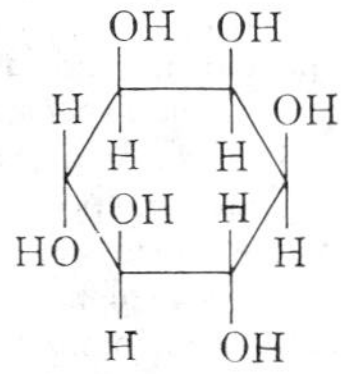

Inositol

Inositol occurs normally in nearly all plant and animal cells, either free or combined, suggesting that it is an essential cell constituent. In animal tissues it occurs as a constituent of phospholipids. In plants it usually is found as *phytic acid*, the hexaphosphate ester of inositol. There has as yet been no demonstration of need for inositol in human nutrition. In fact, large amounts of phytic acid in the diet interfere with the absorption of minerals, especially calcium, zinc and iron.

Although inositol possesses weak lipotropic activity, it is not as effective as methionine or choline. There is no valid therapeutic use of the compound. It may, however, be important to ensure its presence, at levels customarily found in human milk, in foods which are fed to infants and critically ill patients as the sole item of the diet. Inositol is measured by a microbiological assay.

Niacin (Nicotinic Acid and Nicotinamide)

Nicotinic acid (niacin) and nicotinamide (niacinamide) have identical properties as vitamins. Both compounds had been known for approximately 20 years before their biological significance was realized. In 1867 nicotinic acid was synthesized by the oxidation of nicotine with nitric acid. But it was not until 1937 that it was isolated from biological sources and found to be effective in the cure of black tongue in dogs and, later, pellagra in humans. The vitamin has none of the pharmacological properties of nicotine, however. In the 1940s the term "niacin" was adopted as a synonym for food labeling purposes to avoid association with the nicotine of tobacco. The term "niacin" is used generically to include both nicotinic acid and nicotinamide.

Chemistry and Assay—Nicotinic acid is pyridine-3-carboxylic acid. The structures of nicotinic acid and nicotinamide are shown below.

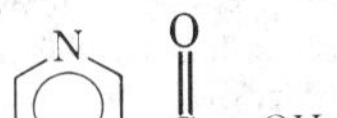

Nicotinic Acid 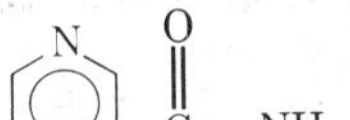 **Nicotinamide**

Niacin, the most stable of the vitamins, is not destroyed by heating in acid or alkaline solution. It withstands mild oxidation, and retains its biological activity during the processing of food and the preparation and storage of pharmaceuticals. It is readily soluble in water or alcohol but insoluble in ether or chloroform. Niacinamide, on the other hand, may be extracted from water solution with ether. The amide is hydrolyzed readily to the free acid by heating in acid or alkaline solution.

The usual commercial synthesis of nicotinic acid used in foods and drugs is by the oxidation of quinoline with potassium permanganate or manganese dioxide, and monodecarboxylation of the purified quinolinic acid with controlled heating. Nicotinamide usually is prepared by esterifying nicotinic acid with methanol followed by ammonolysis.

The activity of both forms of the vitamin is expressed in milligrams of the chemically pure substance. Because they have identical biological activity and their molecular weights are nearly identical, they are equivalent on a weight basis. Reference Standard Niacin and also Niacinamide Reference Standard are available from the USP.

Niacin may be determined in food, drugs, and biological materials by microbiological assay or by chemical methods. No animal biological method exists. The chemical determination involves reaction of the pyridine ring with cyanogen bromide and coupling of the fission product with an aromatic amine. The yellow polymethine dye which is formed is measured in a spectrometer at 436 nm. In natural products niacin occurs mainly in combined form as a coenzyme and must be liberated by acid hydrolysis before assay.

The microbiological assays employs *Lactobacillus arabinosus* as the test organism. A quantitative discrimination between nicotinic acid and nicotinamide in a sample is possible by assaying with both this organism, which uses both forms, and *Leuconostoc mesenteroides*, which can use only nicotinic acid.

Metabolic Functions—In the body niacin is converted to niacinamide, which is an essential constituent of coenzymes I and II that occur in a wide variety of enzyme systems involved in the anaerobic oxidation of carbohydrates. The coenzyme serves as a hydrogen acceptor in the oxidation of the substrate. These enzymes are present in all living cells and take part in many reactions of biological oxidation.

Nicotinamide-adenine dinucleotide (NAD) is the inner salt of the 5′-ester of 3-carbamoyl-1-D-ribofuranosylpyridinium hydroxide with adenosine 5′-pyrophosphate, and has the structure shown below. Nicotinamide-adenine dinucleotide phosphate (NADP) differs only in that the adenosine moiety is esterified at its 2′-position with phosphoric acid.

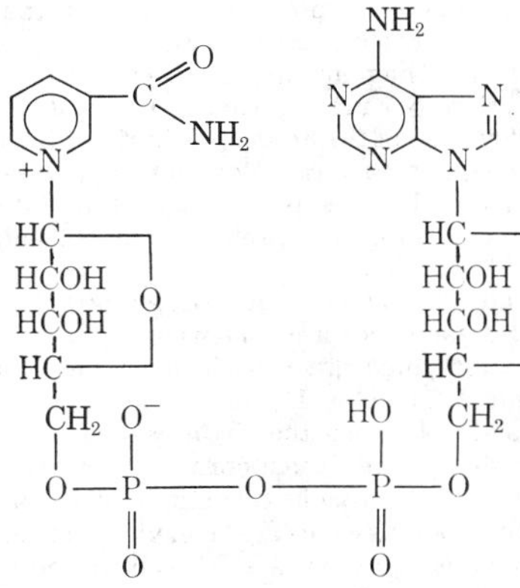

NAD

These coenzymes are synthesized in the body and take part in the metabolism of all living cells. Since they are of such widespread and vital importance, it is not difficult to see why serious disturbance of metabolic processes occurs when the supply of niacin to the cell is interrupted.

The observations of numerous nutritionists that the daily requirement for niacin is influenced by the amount and kind of dietary protein led to the discovery that the amino acid tryptophan functions as a potential precursor of niacin. The efficiency of the conversion indicates that 60 mg of dietary tryptophan is equivalent to 1 mg of niacin. This relationship has given rise to the use of the term "niacin equivalent," which is defined for the purpose of estimating the adequacy of diets in this vitamin as 1 mg of niacin or 60 mg of dietary tryptophan.

Niacin is absorbed readily from the intestinal tract, and large doses may be given orally or parenterally, with equal effect. Niacin, as nicotinic acid, is prescribed widely by physicians in gram amounts for the purpose of lowering blood cholesterol levels. The mechanism for this action is not fully understood; however, the effect is known to occur as a result of decreased cholesterol synthesis in the liver. Only the nicotinic acid form of the vitamin provides the effects. The use of such high doses of nicotinic acid can have serious side effects, including impairment of liver function. Nicotinic acid at these levels should only be used in conjunction with appropriate monitoring of normal liver function.

The principal excretory product of niacin in the urine is *N*-methylnicotinamide, a fluorescent compound formed in the liver. On a normal diet approximately one-fourth of the niacinamide ingested is excreted as

N-methylnicotinamide. With increased levels of niacin intake the percentage of ingested niacin excreted as the fluorescent substance is decreased.

Dietary Requirement and Food Sources—Pellagra, which means rough skin, is the primary deficiency disease due to lack of sufficient niacin in the diet, and it appears only after months of dietary deprivation. The condition involves the gastrointestinal tract, the skin, and the nervous system. Loss of weight, anorexia, weakness, insomnia, headache and diarrhea are common and appear without obvious cause. Other early symptoms may include abdominal pain, nervousness and mental confusion.

Typical manifestations of pellagra in a well-advanced stage are diarrhea, dermatitis and dementia. Gastrointestinal difficulties vary in severity, and absence of gastric secretion is a common finding. In the more advanced state, diarrhea is severe. Dermatitis has a characteristic appearance and occurs at those sites subject to exposure or irritation. The skin lesions are usually bilaterally symmetrical and appear first as erythematous patches, changing to brown pigmented areas, followed by desquamation and thickening. Glossitis is common; it is characterized by swelling and redness at the margins and tip of the tongue. Because of inflammation and superficial desquamation, the tongue, gums and lips appear scarlet and smooth. Mental symptoms vary in occurrence and intensity; they include irritability, mental depression and emotional instability. A confused mental state with hallucinations, mania, and delirium is seen in advanced stages of the disease. Pellagra is a complex deficiency, and symptoms of riboflavin, thiamin and folacin deficiency frequently complicate the clinical picture.

Treatment of the disease requires immediate change to a nutritionally adequate diet and the administration of niacin or niacinamide. Where neurological symptoms are present, use of thiamin and riboflavin may be necessary as well. Recovery from the acute condition is dramatic in most instances, and occurs within 24 to 48 hours. Small doses given frequently during the day have been found to be more effective than a single large daily dose. Niacinamide is preferable to niacin because it does not produce vasodilation in the skin with sensations of itching, burning, or tingling. With severe nausea and diarrhea, intravenous injection of niacinamide is of additional advantage.

In considering dietary requirement and the foods which contribute to it, one must consider the content of preformed niacin and the niacin available by conversion from tryptophan, an essential amino acid present in all good-quality proteins. The minimum requirement to prevent pellagra is the equivalent of about 4.4 mg of niacin/1000 kcal/day. The recommended dietary allowance of the Food and Nutrition Board is 6.6 mg per 1000 kcal and not less than 13 mg at caloric intakes of less than 2000 kcal. Most diets consumed in the US supply from 500 to 1000 mg or more of tryptophan a day and 8 to 17 mg of preformed niacin, equivalent to 16 to 33 mg of niacin.

Poultry, meats and fish constitute the most important single food group source of niacin. Organ meats are somewhat superior to muscle tissue. Potatoes, legumes and some green leafy vegetables contain moderate amounts of preformed niacin, as do whole grains. An important public health nutrition practice, begun in the 1940s, is the nutrient enrichment of cereal products: wheat flour, farina, corn products, rice, macaroni and noodle products and bread. Niacin, thiamin, riboflavin and iron are mandatory ingredients in products which are labeled "enriched." The level of enrichment for niacin is such that a significant proportion of the daily requirement is obtainable from a generous serving of these foods.

Pantothenic Acid

Knowledge of the identity and importance of pantothenic acid grew principally from experimental studies on microorganisms and chicks. Because of its wide distribution in nature it was named "pantothenic" (Greek, *pantothen*, from all sides). The terms vitamin B_3 and chick antidermatitis factor once were applied to variously purified concentrates of the factor, but they are now obsolete. No known therapeutic value exists for pantothenic acid, except perhaps in the treatment of frank or suspected cases of combined nutritional deficiencies.

Chemistry and Assay—Pantothenic acid is optically active (chiral). Maximum vitamin activity resides only in the D-form, and it is readily available as either the sodium or calcium salts which are crystalline substances. Another commercially available form used in liquid preparations is D-pantothenyl alcohol (panthenol). Chemically, pantothenic acid is a composite structure of β-alanine and 2,4-dihydroxy-3,3-dimethylbutyric acid γ-lactone, connected in peptide linkage.

$$HOCH_2-\underset{CH_3}{\overset{CH_3}{C}}-\underset{H}{\overset{OH}{C}}-\overset{O}{\overset{\|}{C}}-NHCH_2CH_2COOH$$

D-Pantothenic Acid

The free acid is fairly stable in neutral solution but sensitive to acids, bases and heat. The salts are somewhat more stable, but even these are destroyed by autoclaving.

Pantothenic acid, its salts and alcohol, can be assayed by both chemical and microbiological methods. A chick growth method has been used but it is time-consuming and has been replaced since suitable methods are available for releasing the bound vitamin (a protein enzyme) from its firm combination in plant and animal tissue. The first step in chemical assay is acid or alkaline hydrolysis. This cleaves the molecule at the peptide linkage into an alanine part and a pantoic acid part. These fission products can then be determined photometrically by suitable color reactions. In addition both gas-liquid chromatography and high-pressure liquid chromatographic methods now exist. *Saccharomyces carlsbergensis* and *Lactobacillus plantarum* are used for the microbiological assay of pantothenic acid and its salts. There is available a USP Reference Standard Calcium Pantothenate.

Metabolic Functions, Dietary Requirement and Food Sources—Pantothenic acid is of the highest biological importance because of its incorporation into coenzyme A (CoA), which is involved in many vital enzymatic reactions transferring a two-carbon compound (the acetyl group) in intermediary metabolism. It is involved in the release of energy from carbohydrate, in the degradation and metabolism of fatty acids, and in the synthesis of such compounds as sterols and steroid hormones, porphyrins, and acetylcholine. CoA is composed of one mole each of adenine, ribose and β-mercaptoethylamine and three moles of phosphate for each mole of pantothenate.

Many microorganisms depend on the same metabolic pathways for their growth and reproduction as do animal species and humans and thus also require pantothenic acid. Some have the ability to synthesize pantothenic acid at a life-sustaining rate from proper precursors. Synthesis by the bacterial flora of the intestine in man appears to be an important source of the vitamin and is the probable explanation, in part, that pantothenic acid deficiency in man is seldom encountered. A deficiency syndrome has been experimentally induced in human volunteers by the oral administration of a pantothenic acid antagonist, ω-methylpantothenic acid, imposed on a pantothenic acid-deficient diet. It has been impossible so far to induce an isolated deficiency of the vitamin in less than at least 9 months on anything resembling a natural diet alone because of the occurrence of significant amounts of pantothenic acid in such a wide variety of foods.

The symptoms which appear to be specific for a lack of available pantothenic acid from the studies using the antivitamin are neuromuscular disorders (paresthesias of the hands and feet and cramping of the legs and impairment of motor coordination), loss of normal eosinopenic response to adrenal corticotrophic hormone (ACTH), heightened sensitivity to a test dose of insulin and, in concert with pyridoxine, a loss of antibody production. Fatigue, malaise, headache, sleep disturbances, nausea, abdominal cramps, epigastric distress, occasional vomiting and an increase in flatus were subjective observations of the pantothenic acid-deficient human volunteers.

Usual diets of adult Americans furnish about 10 to 15 mg of pantothenic acid a day, with a probable range of 6 to 20 mg. A daily intake of 5 to 10 mg is probably adequate for children and adults, and there is no evidence for or against a greater requirement during pregnancy or lactation. Human milk contains about 2 mg/L; cow's milk, about 3.5 mg/L. Liver and other organ meats and eggs are particularly good sources. Broccoli, cauliflower, white and sweet potatoes, tomatoes and molasses are quite high in pantothenic acid. Muscle tissue of beef, pork, lamb and chicken are also good sources.

Pyridoxine (Vitamin B_6)

Vitamin B_6 does not denote a single substance but is rather a collective term for a group of naturally occurring pyridines that are metabolically and functionally interrelated; namely, pyridoxine, pyridoxal, and pyridoxamine. They are interconvertible *in vivo* in their phosphorylated form. There is no information on the relative biologic activity of the three compounds in humans, and since pyridoxine is the most stable, it probably contributes the most vitamin activity to the diet.

Chemistry and Assay—Pyridoxine as the free base has a bitter taste and is readily soluble in water, alcohol or acetone. It crystallizes as the hydrochloride and is prepared in this form for commercial use. Pyridoxine is one of the more stable vitamins and in the alcohol form withstands heating in acid or alkaline solution. Pyridoxal and pyridoxamine are less stable, however, and are known to undergo destruction in the more severe heat treatments sometimes used in food processing. Under most conditions of processing and storage of foods and pharmaceutical preparations, the vitamin is retained well.

The structures of the three active forms of the vitamin and the phosphorylated form of one of them, pyridoxal phosphate, are shown below.

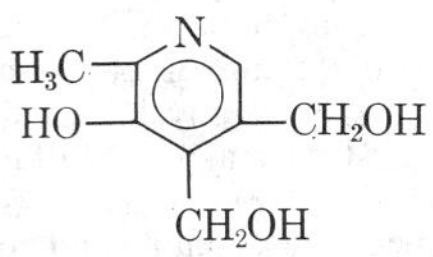

Pyridoxine 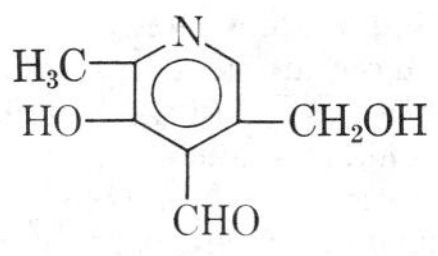 **Pyridoxal**

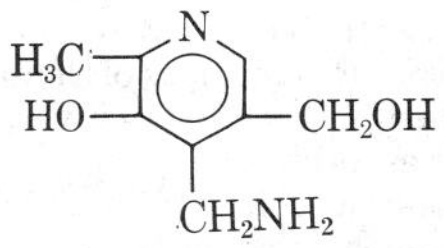

Pyridoxamine

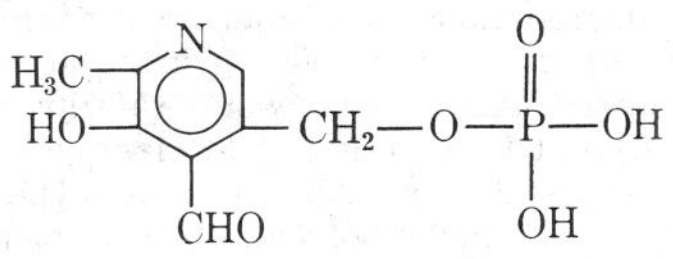

Pyridoxal Phosphate

The biological activity of the vitamin is expressed in milligrams of the chemically pure substance, usually pyridoxine hydrochloride, for which a USP Reference Standard is available. Chicks and rats have been used for the biologic assay of vitamin B_6 by placing the animals on a deficient basal diet which, when supplemented with known amounts of the test vitamin, supports a degree of growth related to the amount present. It is necessary to measure the three forms of vitamin B_6 to determine accurately the total biological activity. This can be accomplished with a high-pressure liquid chromatographic method. Microbiological assays, can also discriminate between the individual vitamin B_6 components. A very useful technique employed in this type of assay is the preliminary separation of the different vitamin forms by a column chromatographic procedure using an ion exchanger. The column eluates then are analyzed by procedures suited to the vitamin form present in the eluates. The organisms most commonly used are *Saccharomyces carlsbergensis*, *Lactobacillus casei* and *Streptococcus faecalis*.

Metabolic Functions, Dietary Requirement and Food Source—Vitamin B_6 in the form of pyridoxal phosphate or pyridoxamine phosphate functions in carbohydrate, fat and protein metabolism; its major functions are most closely related to protein and amino acid metabolism. The vitamin is a part of the molecular configuration of many enzymes (a coenzyme), notably glycogen phosphorylase, various transaminases, decarboxylases and deaminases. The latter three are essential for the anabolism and catabolism of proteins.

The biological activity of vitamin B_6 seems to be a function of the molecule as a whole, since small changes in structure render it inactive. Deoxypyridoxine, a derivative of the vitamin in which one of the methanol groups is reduced to a methyl group, has potent antivitamin activity, but it is of limited experimental use in man because of its toxicity. The antivitamin isonicotinic acid hydrazide (isoniazid) has been used widely in the treatment of tuberculosis. It is chemically related to pyridoxine and acts also as an antagonist, thus requiring the physician to be alert to the pyridoxine nutriture of his patients so treated. A similar antagonism is possible during treatment of hypertension with the drug hydralazine.

No classic syndrome of pyridoxine deficiency exists, probably because it is distributed widely in nature and unique or unusual dietary habits have not so far produced an uncomplicated deficiency. That it is essential for the growth of animals and human infants is well-established. Other manifestations of deficiency in humans are probably an acrodynia-like syndrome characterized by edema and loss of hair, nerve degeneration resulting in behavioral changes and, in infants, convulsive seizures. The latter symptom was shown to result when infants were fed a proprietary milk-based formula, unsupplemented with pyridoxine, in which the natural vitamin content was destroyed inadvertently during sterilization. Clearly, in this instance, marked changes in electroencephalogram patterns of the infants were produced; and they returned to normal minutes after pyridoxine administration.

In infants, although daily requirements of the vitamin are met by consumption of adequate quantities of normal breast milk, the protein-vitamin B_6 relationship is critical. General experience with proprietary formulas suggests that metabolic requirements are satisfied if the vitamin is present in amounts of 0.015 mg/g of protein, or 0.04 mg/100 kcal. The recommended dietary allowances of the Food and Nutrition Board for adolescents and adults, including conditions of pregnancy and lactation, range from 2.3 to 2.6 mg a day.

The best food sources of vitamin B_6 are muscle meats, liver, green vegetables and whole-grain cereals. The bran from the cereal grains has especially large amounts. Nuts, corn, eggs and milk are also good sources.

If large doses of vitamin B_6 are ingested for long periods of time, peripheral neuropathies develop. In most observations involving levels in excess of 500 mg a day; however, one case as low as 250 mg a day has been reported.

Riboflavin

Riboflavin was formerly known as vitamin B_2 or G and lactoflavin. It owes its discovery as one of the components of the B vitamin group to its characteristic fluorescence and pigmenting quality in such common foods as milk and egg yolk. Isolation and characterization of the yellow protein enzyme originally from yeast led to studies on the essential nature of the flavin pigment part of the enzyme in human metabolism, growth, and health.

Chemistry and Assay—Riboflavin is a yellow to orange-yellow, crystalline powder having a slight odor. When dry, it is not appreciably affected by diffused light.

In alkaline solution it is readily soluble but quite unstable to heat and to light, forming lumiflavin, a fluorescent degradation product that is without biological activity. Riboflavin is more stable to heat in acid solution, particularly from pH 1 to 6.5, but upon irradiation forms lumichrome, also biologically inactive. Photodegradation occurs in the skin, and infants with kernicterus who are treated with UV light may become riboflavin-deficient. Riboflavin is adsorbed readily from acid or neutral solution on such agents as frankonite, fuller's earth and certain zeolites, and eluted with acetone or pyridine solutions. Adsorbates have been used in pharmaceutical preparations, but from some of these the vitamin has been found to be unavailable to the human because of difficulty of elution in the intestinal tract.

Solutions of riboflavin have a characteristic yellow-green fluorescence that has a maximum absorption at 565 nm in the acid pH range. This property is made use of in the chemical determination of riboflavin. It is reduced rapidly by hydrosulfite, or by hydrogen in the presence of zinc in acid solution, to the leuco form which is colorless and nonfluorescent. The leucoriboflavin is reoxidized easily by shaking in air. This oxidation–reduction property (see below) is the probable basis for the biological importance of riboflavin in the respiratory enzyme systems.

One gram dissolves in from 3000 to about 20,000 mL of water, the variations in the solubility being due to differences in the internal crystalline structure of the riboflavin; it is more soluble in isotonic sodium chloride or alkaline solution than in water, and less soluble in alcohol. It is insoluble in most lipid solvents. Derivatives such as the phosphate or acetate have been prepared for use in pharmaceutical preparations when higher concentrations are desired.

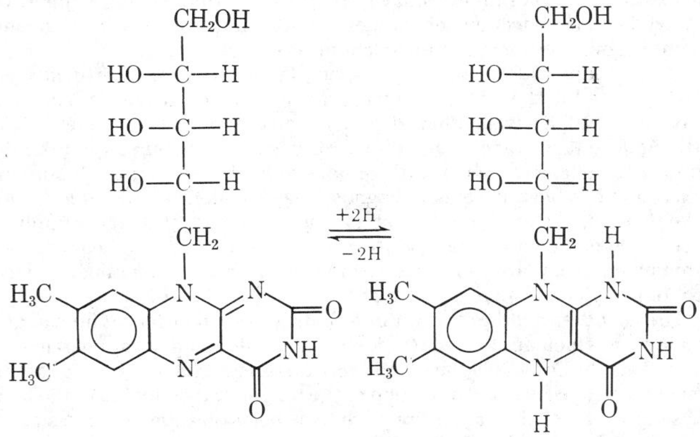

$$\text{Riboflavin} \underset{-2H}{\overset{+2H}{\rightleftharpoons}} \text{Leucoriboflavin}$$

Riboflavin **Leucoriboflavin**

The activity of riboflavin is expressed in milligrams of the chemically pure substance, and a USP Reference Standard Riboflavin is available for assay purposes. In early work, the riboflavin content of substances was measured by a rat growth bioassay method, but this has been replaced by both physicochemical and microbiological methods.

Chemical determinations are based on colorimetric and fluorometric procedures. Straightforward measurement of the intrinsic yellow color of riboflavin is often sufficient for assaying pharmaceutical preparations. The fluorometric method is more sensitive and free of interferences and is therefore more suited to the assay of the vitamin in foods. It depends upon the extraction of the vitamin with dilute acid, filtration, treatment of the filtrate with permanganate and hydrogen peroxide to destroy interfering pigments and measurement of the fluorescence. Assays also can be accomplished using high-pressure liquid chromatography and a fluorometric detector.

Lactobacillus casei is used as the test organism for microbiological assay of riboflavin. It is determined by measurement of the growth stimulation of the organism or by alkaline titration of the acid produced during incubation.

Metabolic Functions—Riboflavin plays its physiological role as the prosthetic group of a number of enzyme systems that are involved in the oxidation of carbohydrates and amino acids. It functions in combination with a specific protein either as a mononucleotide containing phosphoric acid (FMN), or as a dinucleotide combined through phosphoric acid with adenine (FAD).

Flavin-adenine dinucleotide (FAD)

The specificity of each of the enzymes is determined by the protein in the complex. By a process of oxidation–reduction, riboflavin in the system either gains or loses hydrogen. The substrate, either carbohydrate or amino acid, may be oxidized by a removal of hydrogen. The first hydrogen acceptor in the chain of events is NAD or NADP, the di- or trinucleotide containing nicotinic acid and adenine. The oxidized riboflavin system then serves as hydrogen acceptor for the coenzyme system and in turn is oxidized by the cytochrome system. The hydrogen finally is passed on to the oxygen to complete the oxidative cycle. A number of flavoprotein enzymes have been identified, each of which is specific for a given substrate.

There is evidence now that some of the flavin enzymes contain metallic constituents. These metalloflavoproteins may contain iron, copper, or molybdenum. Succinic dehydrogenase, for example, contains iron, and xanthine oxidase contains molybdenum, as well as iron.

Riboflavin is absorbed after phosphorylation from the intestinal tract, and excreted in the urine. A human adult on an ordinary diet excretes from 0.5 to 1.5 mg in 24 hours, depending on the content of the diet. Of a 10-mg dose taken by mouth, 50 to 70% is excreted within 24 hours. In riboflavin deficiency there is little or none found in the urine. Measure of excretion has been used as a diagnostic sign of deficiency. Riboflavin, like thiamin, is stored to a limited extent, and constant dietary supply is needed to maintain normal body levels. Liver, kidney, and heart tissues contain relatively large amounts of riboflavin because of their high enzyme content.

Dietary Requirement and Food Sources—Symptoms of human ariboflavinosis include cheilosis (reddening of the lips and the appearance of fissures at the corners of the mouth), characteristic changes in color of the mucous membranes, inflammation of the tongue and denuding of the lips. Lesions of a seborrheic nature have also been observed as a result of riboflavin deficiency. Ocular manifestations that appear in man and animals are characterized chiefly by corneal vascularization, in which the cornea is extensively invaded by small capillaries. This usually is accompanied by sensations of itching, burning, and roughness of the eyelid, lacrimation, photophobia and visual fatigue. Some of these conditions may, of course, arise from other causes and are not necessarily indicative of riboflavin deficiency.

Riboflavin deficiency in humans has not been found to be widespread in any part of the world, but is undoubtedly a complicating factor in other deficiency diseases such as pellagra. For therapeutic purposes, doses of 1 to 10 mg a day have been given. Rapid disappearance of symptoms of ariboflavinosis occurs with 10-mg doses, and there is some question of the need for administering amounts larger than this.

Studies dealing with the quantitative riboflavin requirement of the human indicate that it is related to body size, metabolic rate and rate of growth. And the parameter used to express these most closely is metabolic body size, represented as kilograms of body weight taken to the ¾ power. The recommended daily dietary allowance of the Food and Nutrition Board for riboflavin is 0.4 to 0.6 mg for infants, 0.8 to 1.2 mg for children up to 10 years, 1.0 to 1.7 mg for adolescents and adults and slightly higher for women during pregnancy and lactation. In general, the minimum requirement for riboflavin is about 0.3 mg for adults and 0.8 mg for infants on a 1000-kcal-intake basis. From a physiological point of view, an intake of more than 0.5 to 0.6 mg/1000 kcal may be of little extra value in normal adult persons.

Riboflavin is widely distributed in nature, in both plants and animals, as an essential constituent of all living cells, and therefore is found widely distributed in small amounts in foods. It is quite stable during the processing of food, except where there is excessive exposure to light. Because of its water solubility, there is moderate loss of riboflavin in cooking when the cooking water is discarded. This loss, however, is generally smaller than that of thiamin, niacin or ascorbic acid.

Foods that make important contributions of riboflavin to the diet are liver and other organ tissues, milk and eggs. Vegetables and fruits furnish a small but constant supply.

Many species of microorganisms are capable of synthesizing riboflavin, and because of the extensive bacterial growth in the human intestinal tract, this may form an important and constant source of supply of riboflavin and may account for the limited occurrence of deficiency in humans.

When it was recognized that cereal products would be a good vehicle to use to improve the content of riboflavin in many diets, its mandatory addition as an enriching ingredient was adopted. In concert with thiamin, niacin and iron, riboflavin is present in nutritionally significant amounts in enriched wheat flour, farina, corn products, bread, macaroni and noodle products. Because of certain cooking habits and the apparent unacceptability of the unnatural yellow color, the enrichment of rice with riboflavin has been resisted.

Thiamine

Concentrates of thiamine, often termed vitamin B_1, were given the latter name by early workers in this country who recognized that at least two accessory dietary factors were needed for normal growth of laboratory rats, one in butter fat and the other in "milk sugar." The names they suggested for these factors were fat-soluble vitamin A and water-soluble vitamin B. It was shown subsequently by a number of investigators that the latter consisted of a group of substances rather than a single compound, but vitamin B_1 was finally the first pure compound of the group to be laboriously isolated from rice polishings. In the pioneer studies on this substance it was found that a thiamine concentrate prevented polyneuritis in chickens, which later was found to be caused by the absence of thiamine in their diet. Deriving from this observation, an early name for the factor is aneurin (from antineuritic), which has persisted in some countries.

Chemistry and Assay—Thiamine is a generic term applied to all substances possessing vitamin B_1 activity, regardless of the anion attached to the molecule. The cationic portion of the molecule, which is the part that may properly be called "thiamine," is made up of a substituted pyrimidine ring connected by a methylene bridge to the nitrogen of a substituted thiazole ring. A general structural formula is where *A* is any appropriate anion but usually chloride (see structure below). In addition, ammonium salts may be formed with the amine substituent on the pyrimidine ring. The common nomenclature is confusing, but, in general, the term mono, as in thiamine mononitrate or thiamine monophosphate, designates the thiazolium type salt. Thiamine chloride hydrochloride is the ammonium salt formed by reacting thiamine chloride with hydrochloric acid (see page ☐).

Thiamine compounds are usually readily soluble in water or in alcohol but insoluble in fat solvents. They are stable in acid solution, and may be heated without decomposition, but unstable in neutral or alkaline solution. At neutral or alkaline pH splitting occurs at the methylene bridge upon heating in the presence of moisture. Splitting of the molecule takes place quantitatively in the presence of bisulfite ions, a reaction that is made use of in preparing dietary constituents free of thiamine for bioassay purposes.

Thiamine is oxidized in alkaline solution to thiochrome, a biologically inactive, highly fluorescent substance. This reaction is the basis for the chemical method of estimating thiamine. The pure vitamin is not readily oxidized in air.

An alternate commercial form of vitamin B_1 widely used because of its greater stability than the hydrochloride is the mononitrate.

The activity of the vitamin is expressed in milligrams of the chemically pure substance and a USP Reference Standard Thiamine Hydrochloride is available.

The determination of thiamine in food, biological materials and pharmaceutical products is done almost exclusively by the thiochrome fluorometric method. On oxidation with ferricyanide in alkaline solution, thiamine is transformed into thiochrome which has a strong blue fluorescence. It is a very sensitive method and correlates well with bioassay results. The sequence in the determination involves extraction of the vitamin, enzyme hydrolysis, adsorption, elution and oxidation to thiochrome which is extracted with isobutanol and determined fluorometrically.

Before the development of suitable physicochemical methods, thiamine was determined in a typical rat-growth assay which is based on the growth response of young thiamine-depleted rats to supplemental doses of a reference standard and to the test material either fed in or separate from the diet or injected parenterally.

Metabolic Functions—In a phosphorylated form, thiamine (thiamine pyrophosphate; cocarboxylase) serves as the prosthetic group of enzyme systems that are concerned with the decarboxylation of α-ketoacids. For example, pyruvic acid is decarboxylated to form a two-carbon residue. This process of decarboxylation is catalyzed by the pyruvic acid decarboxylase enzyme system which consists of a specific protein, manganese ions, and diphosphothiamin. An α-hydroxyethyl group (the "acetaldehyde" residue of the decarboxylated pyruvic acid) attaches to the 2-carbon of the thiazole ring. The hydroxyethyl group (active "acetate," active "acetaldehyde," or two-carbon fragment) attaches to one of the sulfur atoms of lipoamide, from which it is removed by coenzyme A. Pyrophosphorylated thiamine is effective in the decarboxylation of other α-ketoacids as well. Some decarboxylation processes are reversible, so that synthesis (condensation) may be achieved; thus, thiamine is also important to the biosynthesis of keto-acids. It is involved in transketolase reactions.

Thiamine is absorbed readily in aqueous solution from both the small and large intestine, and then is carried to the liver by the portal circulation. In the liver, as well as in all living cells, it normally combines with phosphate to form cocarboxylase. It may be stored in the liver in this form or it may combine further with manganese and specific proteins to become active enzymes known as carboxylases.

Thiamine is excreted in the urine in amounts that reflect the amount taken in and the amounts stored in the tissues. Measurement of the urinary excretion of thiamine after giving a small dose of thiamine is useful in determining whether body stores are adequate or deficient.

Dietary Requirement and Food Sources—Polyneuritis (dysfunctioning of the nervous system) or beriberi is the frank disease associated with thiamine deficiency in man. Peripheral neuritis is a pathological condition of the nerves of the extremities; usually both legs are affected and sometimes the arms as well. The symptoms include loss of sensation, muscle weakness and paralysis. In beriberi this condition is also associated with edema and abnormal electrocardiogram patterns.

Severe cases of beriberi are commonly found in the Orient among people whose diets consist principally of milled or polished rice, from which the vitamin, contained in the bran and germ of the cereal, is largely removed during the milling process. American dietaries generally furnish sufficient thiamine to meet requirements, and with the use of a varied diet, including whole grain cereals or enriched bread or flour, the adequacy of thiamine in most instances is beyond question. Symptoms of thiamine deficiency have been observed among chronic alcoholics, who use alcohol in place of food as a source of energy. Deficiency also occurs in cases of chronic diarrhea, in which absorption is interfered with over a period of time and during pregnancy complicated with anorexia and nausea.

In the diagnosis of thiamine deficiency, symptoms to be noted in particular are anorexia, fatigue, loss of weight, sensation of burning in the soles of the feet, tenderness in calf muscles, muscle cramps and general muscular weakness. Such signs are not in themselves specific, however, without supplementary laboratory findings that indicate a reduced thiamine content of blood and urine.

For treatment of beriberi or thiamine deficiency in humans, the first requisite is a nutritionally complete, well-balanced diet. Good diet is essential, because beriberi in most instances results from a complex or multiple deficiency, and administration of thiamine alone may precipitate a condition resulting from a lack of other water-soluble factors. Doses of 10 to 100 mg of thiamine have been used in severe cases to bring about a cure, but evidence of superiority of the larger doses is lacking. As size of the dose is increased, the proportion of thiamine retained rapidly decreases, the excess being excreted rapidly in the urine. Frequent small doses are to be preferred to a single large daily dose. Only in the most severe cases, or in patients with impaired intestinal absorption, does parenteral administration appear advantageous. Pharmaceutical preparations of many types and potencies are available commercially.

It is generally assumed that thiamine need is related to calorie need, particularly to those calories derived from carbohydrate. The Food and Nutrition Board considers that 0.5 mg/1000 kcal will maintain satisfactory thiamine nutriture under normal conditions in the US. As the caloric allowance varies with age, so does the recommended daily dietary allowance for thiamine; for infants, 0.3 to 0.5 mg; for children up to 12 years, 0.7 to 1.4 mg; for adolescents and adults, 1.0 to 1.5 mg, the highest allowance being for boys and men 15 to 22 years. The literature on thiamine needs in maternal and child nutrition suggests an increased need for thiamine during pregnancy, and an additional 0.3 mg a day is recommended, in accordance with the increased calorie recommendation.

Thiamine is found widely distributed in foods. Thiamine is found in all plants, and is synthesized by some microorganisms, particularly yeasts. No one food can be considered of particular importance above all others, although the cereal grains, milk, legumes, nuts, eggs and pork probably furnish the larger proportion of thiamine in diets used in this country. Sophistication and processing of foods generally tend to reduce the thiamine supply. For example, in the preparation of wheat flour, separation of the bran coat and germ removes ¾ or more of the thiamine present in the whole wheat. This is true for other cereal grains as well. Much of the white flour, corn grits and rice used in this country is enriched to approximately the whole grain level. Because of the lability of thiamine to heat, cooking and baking processes reduce the raw food content of the vitamin.

The loss of thiamine in home cooking is not considered excessive, except with foods cooked in large amounts of water that then is discarded. Because of its solubility, the thiamine content of the cooking water is always appreciable.

Vitamin B_{12}

Vitamin B_{12}, the most recently discovered of the B group, was isolated from liver fractions in crystalline form in 1948 and was soon after shown to be specific for the treatment of Addisonian pernicious anemia. It was established that vitamin B_{12} is the active principle in extracts of liver, employed for more than 30 years in the control of pernicious anemia. Liver continues to be an important dietary source of the vitamin, but liver injection is no longer used in the treatment of pernicious anemia, because of the ready availability of crystalline forms of the vitamin.

Chemistry and Assay—Vitamin B_{12} is a complex water-soluble compound which crystallizes as small red needles that have a specific rotation in dilute aqueous solution of −59°. Characteristic absorption maxima occur at 278, 361 and 550 nm. The crystalline substance blackens without melting at 300°. The compound is a cobalt coordination complex, in which the cobalt is trivalent and has a coordination number of six. The complex is neutral. Vitamin B_{12} is composed of two heterocyclic systems, a benzimidazole and a modified porphyrin nucleus, with the following structure:

Cyanocobalamin

Actually, the cyanide group coordinated to the cobalt is not a part of the true vitamin but rather is an artifact caused by isolation of the vitamin on charcoal; in the liver the ligand is 5′-deoxyadenosyl anion. Nevertheless, by strict organic chemical definition, by virtue of the fact that the cyanide was the first form of the vitamin to be isolated, cyanocobalamin *is* vitamin B_{12}. When the ligand is hydroxide instead of cyanide, the compound is *vitamin* B_{12a} (hydroxocobalamin); when it is water, the substance is *vitamin* B_{12b} (aquocobalamin); when it is nitro, the compound is *vitamin* B_{12c}; *the 5′-deoxyadenosyl form is coenzyme* B_{12}; if the ligand is methyl, the compound is *methyl* B_{12}. Sulfito- and thiocyanatocobalamins also are known. In practice, all of these compounds are vitamin B_{12}. A similar situation obtains with respect to the name *cobalamin*, which strictly is synonymous with cyanocobalamin but in loose practice applies to any active compound containing the α-(5,6-dimethylbenzimidazoyl)corrin nucleus. *Cobamides* is a generic term which has been used for these compounds.

Vitamin B_{12} (cyanocobalamin) in an atmosphere of hydrogen with a platinum catalyst is reduced to a red crystalline compound with slightly changed UV-absorption maxima, and a reduced stability to heat. Vitamin B_{12a} results from such reduction. Vitamin B_{12b}, another reduced form, occurs in natural sources.

Commercially, vitamin B_{12} is obtained from the fermentation of *Streptomyces griseus*. The vitamin is precipitated from aqueous solutions saturated with ammonium sulfate by 1-butanol. Purification is achieved by chromatography, using bentonite or aluminum silicate as the adsorbent.

Sharply defined red bands are formed during the development of the chromatograms indicating the location of the vitamin. The red band is separated mechanically and eluted with water. The concentrated water solution on addition of acetone gives the crystalline vitamin which can be further purified by recrystallization from aqueous acetone.

The USP provides a Reference Standard Cyanocobalamin for use in assay of the vitamin. A physicochemical method for determining vitamin B_{12} involves measurement of light absorbance at certain specific wavelengths characteristic for cyanocobalamin. This method is only applicable to relatively concentrated solutions of the compound, such as in pharmaceutical preparations. Vitamin B_{12} also can be determined with high performance liquid chromatography.

Vitamin B_{12} is one of the most active biological factors known; its activity for bacteria is measured in terms of millimicrograms. Because of this sensitivity of some bacteria to such low levels of the vitamin and the fact that foods contain exceptionally low concentrations of the vitamin, microbiological methods are widely used. The following three organisms, which require vitamin B_{12} for growth, are used: *Lactobacillus leichmannii, Ochromonas malhamensis* and *Euglenia gracilis.*

Metabolic Functions, Dietary Requirement and Food Sources—The vitamin is essential for the normal functioning of all cells, but particularly for cells of the bone marrow, the nervous system and the gastrointestinal tract. It appears to facilitate reduction reactions and participate in the transfer of methyl groups. Evidence exists that vitamin B_{12} is involved in protein, carbohydrate and fat metabolism, but its chief importance in mammalian tissues seems to be, together with folic acid, in the anabolism of deoxyribonucleic acid in all cells. Coenzyme forms of vitamin B_{12}, in which the vitamin is linked to adenine and a sugar, which catalyze specific reactions in intermediary metabolism have been isolated from bacterial cultures and probably have similar vitamin roles in mammalian cells.

The biochemical fault in pernicious anemia, a condition caused by a prolonged deficiency of vitamin B_{12}, is a failure of elaboration of the intrinsic factor, normally secreted by the parietal cells of the stomach mucosa. This intrinsic factor, which is essential for the absorption of the vitamin through the intestinal wall, forms a complex with vitamin B_{12}. Intrinsic factor is a glycoprotein of 45,000 daltons.

Vitamin B_{12} is a requisite for normal blood formation, and certain macrocytic anemias respond to its administration. In pernicious anemia, unless accompanied by intrinsic factor, the vitamin is not absorbed orally in effective amounts and must be administered parenterally in microgram quantities. Preparations containing vitamin B_{12} and intrinsic factor concentrate are now available for oral use, and have been shown for short-term use at least to be equivalent in value to the injections. Clinical studies indicate that if milligram amounts of the vitamin are administered orally, in the absence of intrinsic factor, enough of the vitamin passes through the intestinal wall to be effective in maintaining the pernicious anemia patient. However, the injectable form of vitamin B_{12} continues to be the drug of choice because of the desirability of regular attention of a physician to the condition of the patient.

The evidence indicating that vitamin B_{12} is the antipernicious anemia factor is complete. In treating pernicious anemia, vitamin B_{12} administered intramuscularly produces a maximal reticulocyte response in 4 to 9 days, and a restoration of red- and white-cell count in 4 to 6 weeks. The change in bone marrow, from a megaloblastic to a normoblastic state, is dramatic and occurs within a few hours after the injection of as little as 1 μg of the vitamin. Vitamin B_{12} is considered to be the extrinsic factor of Castle, the absorption of which from the intestinal tract is facilitated by the intrinsic factor present in normal gastric juice. The biochemical defect in pernicious anemia, then, is a failure of elaboration of the intrinsic factor. Because of this relationship, vitamin B_{12} given orally is much less effective in the pernicious anemia patient, and entirely ineffective if there is complete absence of intrinsic factor.

The vitamin is effective in preventing the occurrence of neurological changes common to pernicious anemia. These symptoms are observed more frequently among the elderly because absorption of vitamin B_{12} has been shown to decrease among this population. However, it is not uncommon to identify women with neurological changes caused by vitamin B_{12} deficiency in their mid to late thirties. Acute symptoms of combined system disease have been found to disappear rather promptly after B_{12} administration, but recovery appears to depend more on the chronicity of the disease than on the extent of neurological involvement, and conditions of long standing are less apt to show recovery.

Osteoblast activity probably also depends upon vitamin B_{12}.

A simple nutritional concept of pernicious anemia which seems valid is that of essentially an uncomplicated deficiency of vitamin B_{12} conditioned by the lack of intrinsic factor and, hence, the inability to absorb the vitamin from ingested food. This validation rests on several types of evidence, of which particularly convincing is the comparison of the clinical development of vitamin B_{12} deficiency in vegans, in patients following total gastrectomy (resulting in removal of intrinsic factor and interference with absorption of the vitamin) and the relapse following withholding of therapy from previously adequately treated patients with pernicious anemia. Simple experimental dietary deficiency of vitamin B_{12} has not yet been produced in the adult human under conditions of careful continuous observation. It seems probable that the requirements of parenterally administered (or absorbed) vitamin B_{12} by the patient with pernicious anemia or gastrectomy is similar to the requirements of the normal subject.

The recommended daily dietary allowance of the Food and Nutrition Board for vitamin B_{12} ranges from 0.5 to 3 μg; the lower value is for infants, and the higher value is for women during pregnancy.

Vitamin B_{12} occurs in meat and dairy products but is not present to any measurable extent in plants or cereal grains. It is probable that indigenous bacteria in plant foods synthesize sufficient vitamin B_{12} to meet the requirement of those individuals whose dietary habits preclude the use of animal food sources.

Water-Soluble Vitamin Preparations

Aminobenzoic Acid—page 881.

Ascorbic Acid

(Various Mfrs)

L-Ascorbic acid [50-81-7] $C_6H_8O_6$ (176.13). See page 1116.

Preparation—The article in commerce is produced exclusively by synthesis. Sorbitol, a hexose sugar, occurring in several fruits but commercially obtained by hydrogenating dextrose in the presence of a Cu–Cr catalyst, is the raw material for the production of ascorbic acid. The D-sorbitol in aqueous solution is converted by the action of the organism *Acetobacter suboxydans* to L-sorbose, which is a ketose. The L-sorbose is then condensed with acetone by means of sulfuric acid to form diacetone sorbose. The object of the acetonation is to protect the hydroxyl group from oxidation in the subsequent steps. The diacetone sorbose, after suitable purification, is oxidized by potassium permanganate and then hydrolyzed forming 2 keto-L-gulonic acid. This acid is esterified with methanol and an intermediate sodio compound is formed with sodium methoxide. Hydrolysis with aqueous HCl removes the methyl group and sodium and lactonizes it to form ascorbic acid. The process is illustrated as follows.

CHO–HCOH–HOCH–HCOH–HCOH–CH_2OH (**D-Glucose**) $\xrightarrow{H_2}$ CH_2OH–HCOH–HOCH–HCOH–HCOH–CH_2OH (**D-Sorbitol**) $\xrightarrow{A\ Suboxydans}$ CH_2OH–C=O–HOCH–HCOH–HOCH–CH_2OH (**L-Sorbose**)

$\xrightarrow{(CH_3)_2CO}$ **Diacetone L-Sorbose** $\xrightarrow{KMnO_4}$ (diacetone derivative with COOH) $\xrightarrow{H_2O}$

COOH–C=O–HOCH–HCOH–HOCH–CH_2OH (**2-Keto-L-gulonic Acid**) $\xrightarrow[\text{then } CH_3ONa]{CH_3OH\ +\ HCl}$ [$COOCH_3$–HOC=NaOC–HCOH–HOCH–CH_2OH] $\xrightarrow{HCl}$ **L-Ascorbic Acid**

Description—White or slightly yellow crystals or powder; odorless and on exposure to light gradually darkens; in the dry state, reasonably stable in air, but in solution rapidly deteriorates in the presence of air; melts at about 190°; specific rotation (1 in 10 aqueous solution) between +20.5 and +21.5°; aqueous solution has the acidic properties of a monobasic acid and it forms salts with metallic ions. pK_a 4.2 and 11.6.

Solubility—1 g in about 3 mL water or 40 mL alcohol; insoluble in chloroform, ether or benzene.

Incompatibilities—Stable in the dry state but in solution oxidizes rapidly in the presence of air. The reaction is accelerated by *alkalies and certain metals*, especially *copper*; it is retarded by acids. Aqueous solutions are strongly acidic, having a pH of 2 to 3.

Uses—In addition to the uses described on page 1013, it is sometimes given with iron salts in the treatment of iron-deficiency anemia; it functions to keep the iron in the ferrous state and hence to improve absorption. Apart from coadministration of vitamin C and iron preparations, a few cases of hypochromic anemia improve upon increasing the intake of vitamin. For additional information, see the general statement on *Ascorbic Acid*.

It is also used as a urinary-acidifier to enhance the effectiveness of methenamide by lowering the pH of the urine and thus aiding in the formation of formaldehyde.

The effect of megadoses (10 to 15 times the RDA) has not been proved and large overdosing should be discouraged.

Numerous, unapproved uses for ascorbic acid have been claimed, such as in the prevention and treatment of cancer, for infections of the gingiva, hemorrhagic states, mental depression, dental caries, acne, collagen disorders, ulcers of the skin, hay fever and the common cold.

No more than the recommended daily allowance should be given to the pregnant woman; the metabolism of the fetus adapts to high levels of the vitamin, and scurvy may develop after birth when the intake drops to normal levels.

Dose—*Nutritional supplement, oral,* **50 to 100 mg** a day; *treatment of deficiency,* **100 to 250 mg** a day; *urinary acidification, oral,* **4 to 12 g** a day in divided doses; *methemoglobinemia, oral,* **300 to 600 mg** a day in divided doses; *pediatric; solution oral* (nutritional supplement), **20 to 50 mg** a day; *therapeutic,* **100 to 300 mg** a day in divided doses.

Dosage Forms—Extended Release Capsules: 250 and 500 mg; Solution: 35 mg/0.6 mL and 100 mg/mL: Syrup; 20 and 100 mg/mL; Tablets: 25, 50, 100, 250, 500 and 1000 mg; Injection: 50, 100, 200, 250, and 500 mg/mL. It is also available in chewable, effervescent and other extended-release forms.

Sodium Ascorbate

L-Ascorbic acid, monosodium salt; Cevalin (*Lilly*)

Monosodium L-ascorbate [134-03-2] $C_6H_7NaO_6$ (198.11).

Description—White or very faintly yellow crystals, or crystalline powder; odorless or practically odorless; relatively stable in air; on exposure to light it gradually darkens; pH (1 in 10 solution) between 7.5 and 8.

Solubility—1 g in 1.3 mL of water; very slightly soluble in alcohol; insoluble in chloroform or ether.

Uses—A pharmaceutical necessity for *Decavitamin Capsules and Decavitamin Tablets.* It also is used as an antioxidant in fruit and vegetable canning, and in the processing of meat.

Dose—See *Ascorbic Acid.*

Calcium Pantothenate

β-Alanine, (*R*)-*N*-(2,4-dihydroxy-3,3-dimethyl-1-oxobutyl)-, calcium salt (2:1); Dextro Calcium Pantothenate; Pantholin (*Lilly*)

$$\left[HOCH_2C(CH_3)_2-\overset{OH}{\underset{H}{C}}-CONH(CH_2)_2COO- \right]_2 Ca$$

Calcium D-pantothenate (1:2) [137-08-6] $C_{18}H_{32}CaN_2O_{10}$ (476.54); the calcium salt of tne dextrorotatory isomer of pantothenic acid.

Preparation—Several syntheses are available. In one, isobutyraldehyde is converted to the lactone of 2,4-dihydroxy-3,3-dimethylbutyric acid, the D-enantiomer of which obtained by resolution is combined with β-alanine to form D-pantothenic acid and then converted to the calcium salt.

Description—Slightly hygroscopic, white powder; odorless, has a bitter taste, and is stable in air; unstable to heat both in the dry state and in acid or alkaline solution; most stable at pH 5.5 to 6.5 and its solutions may be autoclaved at this pH for a short time without appreciable loss; solutions are neutral or slightly alkaline to litmus, having a pH of 7 to 9; specific rotation (calculated on the dried basis and in a 5% solution) +25 to +27.5°.

Solubility—1 g in about 3 mL water; soluble in glycerin; practically insoluble in alcohol, chloroform or ether.

Uses—See the general statement on *Pantothenic Acid.* Since a deficiency of pantothenic acid, alone, is virtually unknown, the primary indication for use is a general nutritional deficiency. Clinical cases have been too few to supply creditable data on dosage; consequently, the dose that follows is more customary than meaningful.

Dose—*Oral, adults* and *children,* **5** to **10 mg** once a day.

Dosage Form—Tablets: 10 and 30 mg.

Cyanocobalamin

α-5,6-Dimethylbenzimidazolylcobamide cyanide; Vitamin B_{12}

Vitamin B_{12} [68-19-9] $C_{63}H_{88}CoN_{14}O_{14}P$ (1355.38). 1123.

Preparation—Vitamin B_{12} can be isolated from aqueous liver extracts and from *Streptomyces griseus* fermentation. Commercially, it is obtained from the latter source (see page 1123).

Description—Dark red, hygroscopic crystals or amorphous or crystalline powder; when the anhydrous compound is exposed to air it may absorb about 12% of water.

Solubility—1 g in 80 mL water; soluble in alcohol; insoluble in acetone, chloroform or ether.

Uses—This and other forms of vitamin B_{12} are used to treat various megaloblastic anemias, especially *pernicious anemia* and other anemias in which the secretion of the intrinsic factor is impaired, as in *gastric cancer, gastric atrophy, total* or even *subtotal gastrectomy.* It also may be used to treat the megaloblastic anemias of *tropical sprue, idiopathic steatorrhea, gluten-induced enteropathy, regional ileitis, ileal resection, malignancies, granulomas, strictures or other structural disorders of the ileum* in which vitamin B_{12} absorption is impaired; in most of these folic acid deficiency is even more severe, and combined therapy is indicated. Its deficiencies untreated for periods of more than 3 months may result in permanent degenerative spinal cord lesions. The megaloblastic anemia associated with *fish tapeworm infestation* also responds to the vitamin. The megaloblastic anemias of pregnancy, infancy, alcoholism, and poverty are usually due to folic acid deficiency and only infrequently respond to it. The vitamin is *not useful* in the treatment of infectious hepatitis, multiple sclerosis, trigeminal neuralgia, anorexia, miscellaneous neuropathies, thyrotoxicosis, retarded growth, aging and various psychiatric disorders, and claims to the contrary and promotion therefore represent an abuse. It should not be administered intravenously and is contraindicated in patients who are sensitive to it or cobalt. Patients with Leber's disease have been found to suffer severe and rapid opticatrophy when treated with it. Either cyanocobalamin or hydroxocobalamin may be used for a loading dose in the Schilling test for malabsorption of the vitamin in diseases which affect the lower bowel, such as *sprue.*

A nasal spray has been developed recently which is said to provide significant absorption in the nasal mucosa and may supplant the parenteral dosage forms.

In addition to intrinsic factor, gastrointestinal absorption requires an alkaline pH. In the presence of pancreatic disease it may be necessary to administer the oral vitamin with bicarbonate or give the vitamin parenterally.

For additional information about cyanocobalamin see the general statement on *Vitamin B_{12}.*

Dose—Tablets: *nutritional supplement, adult, oral,* **1 μg** a day up to **25 μg** when indicated; *children* (up to 1 yr), *oral,* **0.3 μg** a day; (over 1 yr), **1 μg** a day; Injection (IM): *deficiency,* **100 μg** a day for 6 to 7 days, followed by **100 μg** every 3rd or 4th day for 2 or 3 wk; *Maintenance,* **100 to 200 μg** once a month; *diagnostic aid,* **1 μg** a day for 10 days; *Schilling test* (loading dose), **1000 μg** IM; *children, deficiency, initially* **30 to 50 μg** a day for 2 or more weeks with a total dose of 1 to 5 mg; *maintenance,* **100 μg** once a month as needed.

Dosage Forms—Injection: 100 μg and 1 mg/mL; Tablets: 10, 25, 50, 100, 250 and 1000 μg; Soluble Tablets; 25, 50, 100 and 200 μg.

Hydroxocobalamin

Cobinamide, dihydroxide, dihydrogen phosphate (ester), mono(inner salt), 3′-ester with 5,6-dimethyl-1-α-D-ribofuranosyl-1*H*-benzimidazole; Vitamin B_{12a}

Cobinamide dihydroxide dihydrogen phosphate (ester), mono(inner salt), 3′-ester with 5,6-dimethyl-1-α-D-ribofuranosylbenzimidazole [13422-

51-0] $C_{62}H_{89}CoN_{13}O_{15}P$ (1346.37); an analog of *Cyanocobalamin* in which a hydroxyl radical has replaced the cyano radical.

Preparation—Cyanocobalamin in solution is hydrogenated at room temperature with the aid of Raney nickel. The solution is then exposed to air and diluted with acetone. Oxidation takes place and, upon standing, the hydroxocobalamin crystallizes.

Description—Dark red crystals or red crystalline powder; odorless or has not more than a slight acetone odor; anhydrous form is very hygroscopic; pH (2 in 100 solution) between 8 and 10.

Solubility—1 g in 50 mL water, 100 mL alcohol, 10,000 mL chloroform or 10,000 mL ether. It is preferable to make aqueous solutions in acetate buffer at a pH between 3.5 and 4.5 in which 1 g dissolves in about 100 mL water.

Use and Dose—See *Cyanocobalamin.*

Nutritional supplement efficiency, initial, **30 to 50 μg** a day for 5 to 10 days; *megoblastic anemia (severe),* **100 μg** a day for 5 to 10 days; *maintenance,* **100 to 200 μg** a month. Although the indications for cyanocobalamin and hydroxocobalamin are the same, the latter may be preferred for the treatment of deficiency since cyanocobalamine may cause degeneration of optic neuropathies. Some patients may develop antibodies to the hydroxocobalamin-transcobalamin-II complex.

Dosage Form—Injection: 1 mg/mL, 10 mg/10 mL.

Folic Acid

L-Glutamic acid, *N*-[4-[[(2-amino-1,4-dihydro-4-oxo-6-pteridinyl)-methyl]amino]benzoyl]-, PGA; Folacin; Pteroylglutamic Acid; Folvite (*Lederle*)

N-[*p*-[[(2-Amino-4-hydroxy-6-pteridinyl)methyl]amino]benzoyl]-L-glutamic acid [59-30-3] $C_{19}H_{19}N_7O_6$ (441.40). See page 1118.

Preparation—Commercial syntheses use different processes. In one of these 2,3-dibromopropionaldehyde, dissolved in a water-miscible organic solvent (alcohol, dioxane), is added to a solution of equal molecular quantities of 2,4,5-triamino-6-hydroxypyrimidine and *p*-aminobenzoylglutamic acid, maintaining a pH of about 4 by the controlled action of alkali as the reaction progresses. The scheme of the reaction is analogous to that described for *Methotrexate* (1256), the only difference being in the starting pyrimidine compound.

Description—Yellow or yellowish orange, odorless, crystalline powder.

Solubility—Very slightly soluble in water; insoluble in alcohol, chloroform or ether; readily dissolves in dilute solutions of alkali hydroxides or carbonates, and is soluble in hot diluted hydrochloric or sulfuric acid, forming very pale yellow solutions.

Uses—The only valid therapeutic use is in the treatment of a deficiency of the vitamin or prophylactically in instances in which the folacin requirement is increased, as in the third trimester of pregnancy. *Megaloblastic anemias* in which folic acid deficiency occurs may result from malabsorption syndromes, such as *sprue, idiopathic steatorrhea, celiac disease, intestinal reticulosis, regional jejunitis, jejunal diverticulosis, blind loop syndrome and gastroenterostomy* and from antacid use in the elderly. Megaloblastic anemia of infancy is generally the result of generalized malnutrition, as is nutritional megaloblastic anemia. In all of the above-named megaloblastic anemias vitamin B_{12} deficiency often coexists, and folic acid, alone, may be inadequate. Pernicious anemia should be ruled out, lest the vitamin mask the disease (see below). In the megaloblastic anemias of deficiency, a low serum folic acid level will obtain. However, in megaloblastic anemias consequent to treatment with pyrimethamine, phenytoin, and related substances, or methotrexate, the serum folic acid levels may be normal; the signs of deficiency result from the antimetabolite effects of the drugs, and they may be overcome competitively by increasing its intake. It is not effective in the treatment of aplastic anemia, leukemia, anemias of infection and nephritis, and general reduction in bone marrow activity of unknown origin.

The vitamin is usually absorbed readily from the gastrointestinal tract and from parenteral sites of administration. The portion of administered folic acid which is excreted in the urine varies directly with the dose; only a small fraction appears in the urine following the oral ingestion of 0.1 mg, but up to 90% may be excreted by the kidney when a single dose of 15 mg is ingested. The fate of the unrecovered vitamin is unknown. The indications for parenteral use are rare. A solution in water for injection, prepared with the aid of sodium hydroxide or sodium carbonate, is the preferred form for injection.

It is capable of bringing about an incomplete and temporary hematopoietic response in pernicious anemia, which may cause the physician to overlook the basic disorder. But it does not affect the progressive neurological lesions of the disease, which may appear explosively and in an irreversible stage. Doses which will correct a deficiency but which will not generally cause a remission in pernicious anemia are on the order of 0.1 to 0.4 mg.

Infants fed on a goat milk formula should have a 50 μg a day supplement of folic acid.

For additional information concerning folic acid see the general statement on *Folic Acid.*

Dose—*Usual, maintenance, oral, intramuscular, intravenous* or *subcutaneous (deep)* **0.1** to **0.25 mg** (100 to 250 μg) once a day; *therapeutic, oral* or *parenteral,* **0.25 mg** (250 μg) to **1 mg** once a day; diagnostic aid (folate deficiency), **100 to 200 μg** a day for 10 days; *pediatric, supplement,* **100 μg** a day and may require increasing to 500 or 1000 μg a day; *deficiency,* **250 to 1000 μg** a day; *maintenance, infants,* **100 μg a day**; *children up to 4 yr,* up to **300 μg**; *over 4 yr,* **400 μg** a day.

Dosage Forms—Injection: 15 mg/mL, 150 mg/10 mL; Tablets: 100, 250, 400 and 800 μg and 1 and 5 mg.

Leucovorin Calcium

L-Glutamic acid, *N*-[[(2-amino-5-formyl-1,4,5,6,7,8-hexahydro-4-oxo-6-pteridinyl)methyl]amino]benzoyl]-, calcium salt (1:1), pentahydrate; Folmic Acid; Citrovorum Factor; (*Various Mfrs*)

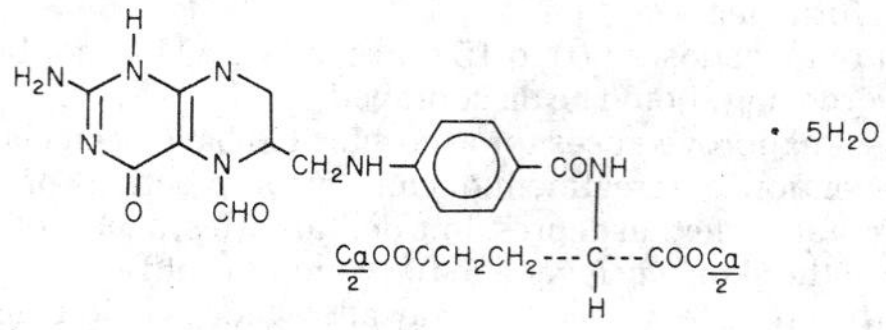

Calcium *N*-[*p*-[[(2-amino-5-formyl-5,6,7,8-tetrahydro-4-hydroxy-6- pteridinyl)methyl]amino]benzoyl]-L-glutamate (1:1) pentahydrate [6035-45-6] $C_{20}H_{21}CaN_7O_7.5H_2O$ (601.58); *anhydrous* [1492-18-8] (511.51).

Preparation—Folic acid simultaneously is hydrogenated and formylated in 90 to 100% formic acid under the influence of platinum oxide catalyst at low temperature and atmospheric pressure to yield leucovorin. Conversion to the calcium salt may be accomplished by dissolving the leucovorin in NaOH solution, treating with $CaCl_2$, and precipitating with ethanol.

Description—Yellowish white or yellow, odorless powder. pK_a 3.8, 4.8 and 10.4.

Solubility—Very soluble in water; practically insoluble in alcohol.

Uses—Leucovorin is folinic acid (see *Folic Acid,* page 1118). The calcium salt is a convenient pharmaceutical form that is preferred for intramuscular injection. Consequently, its uses and limitations in the *treatment of the megaloblastic anemias* are the same as for folic acid. However, it is superior to folic acid in *counteracting the excessive effects of the folic acid antagonists* (methotrexate, etc; see page 1256), since the antagonists competitively antagonize the conversion of folic acid to leucovorin and not the leucovorin itself, and also since leucovorin is an excellent competitor for the inward transport system.

Dose—*Intramuscular, adults* and *children* in *folate-deficiency anemia,* the equivalent of **1 mg** of leucovorin once daily; *folic acid antagonist antidote,* administer an amount of leucovorin sufficient to produce blood levels equal to, or greater than the antagonist, as soon as possible.

Dosage Forms—Injection: 3 and 5 mg (base)/mL; Oral Solution: 60 mg (base) to be reconstituted to 60 mL with Aromatic Elixir NF; Tablets: 5, 15 and 25 mg (base).

Niacin

3-Pyridinecarboxylic acid; Nicotinic Acid

Nicotinic acid [59-67-6] $C_6H_5NO_2$ (123.11). See page 1119.

Preparation—Niacin may be variously prepared, as by oxidation of nicotine with nitric acid or potassium permanganate, by oxidation of quinoline, or synthesis from pyridine.

Description—White crystals or crystalline powder; odorless or has a slight odor; melts at about 235°; pK_a 4.85.

Solubility—1 g in about 60 mL water; freely soluble in boiling water, boiling alcohol or also solutions of alkali hydroxides or carbonates; practically insoluble in ether.

Uses—Chiefly in the treatment of pellagra, a disease common among the poor in subtropical countries due to diet deficiency. It also has been found useful in conjunction with vitamin B_1 and riboflavin in the treatment of nutritional deficiency in chronic alcoholism.

In doses of 20 mg or more in humans, niacin elicits a vasodilator effect that occurs a few minutes after oral ingestion, or immediately after intravenous injection, and lasts for a few minutes to an hour. Symptoms of flushing, itching, burning, or tingling occur, along with an increased skin temperature and increased motility and gastric secretion. Nicotinyl alcohol also shares this vasodilator property, and at one time both nicotinic acid and the alcohol popularly were used in the treatment of peripheral vascular disease and senility (as a cerebral vasodilator). These uses are obsolete and now are but an annoying side effect of large doses. The vasodilator effect of the oral drug is less if it is given with a meal.

Larger doses lower blood cholesterol, phospholipids, triglycerides and free fatty acids, and the drug is used in the treatment of hypercholesterolemia mostly in combination with cholestyramine, colestipol or clofibrate. Nicotinamide does not possess the hypolipemic or the vasodilator property.

Large doses, especially those over 3 g a day, cause abnormalities in liver function, including jaundice.

Niacin is absorbed well orally, and the oral and parenteral doses are the same. With large doses, a considerable amount is excreted into the urine, so that it is advisable to give several small doses during the day rather than one large one.

For additional information see the general statement on *Niacin*.

Dose—*Oral, pellegra,* **50 mg**, 3 to 10 times a day; *dietary supplement,* **10 to 20 mg** a day; *Hartnup disease,* **50 to 200 mg** a day; *antihyperlipidemic, initial,* **100 mg** 3 times a day, increased in increments of **300 mg** a day every 4 to 7 days, as needed; *parenteral (IM),* **50 to 100 mg**, 5 or more times a day; *(IV) slow,* **25 to 100 mg**, 2 or more times a day; *pediatric, IV, slow,* less than oral dose.

Dosage Forms—Injection: 50 and 100 mg/mL; Tablets: 25, 25, 50, 100, 250 and 500 mg; (Extended release): 150 and 300 mg; Capsules (extended release): 125, 200, 250, 300, 400 and 500 mg; Oral Solution: 50 mg/5 mL.

Niacinamide

3-Pyridinecarboxamide; Nicotinamide; Nicotinic Acid Amide

Nicotinamide [98-92-0] $C_6H_6N_2O$ (122.13). See page 1119.

Preparation—From niacin by various methods, as by reaction with thionyl chloride followed by treatment with ammonia, or by interaction of ammonia gas with molten niacin.

Description—White, crystalline powder; odorless or nearly so, and has a bitter taste; solutions are neutral to litmus paper; melts between 128 and 131°

Solubility—1 g in 1.5 mL water, 5.5 mL alcohol or 10 mL glycerin.

Uses—See page 1119 and *Niacin*. This drug lacks the vasodilator, gastrointestinal, hepatic and hypolipemic actions of niacin. Consequently, it is preferred to niacin in the treatment of deficiency.

Dose—*Usual, oral, pellegra,* **50 mg**, 3 to 10 times a day; *supplement,* **10 to 20 mg** a day; *Hartnup disease,* **50 to 200 mg** a day; *pediatric, pellegra,* **100 to 300 mg** a day in divided doses; *supplement,* **50 to 200 mg** a day; *intramuscular, adult, pellegra,* **50 to 100 mg**, 5 or more times a day; *intravenous, slow,* **25 to 100 mg**, 2 or more times a day; *pediatric, intravenous, slow,* less than oral dose.

Dosage Forms—Injection: 100 mg/2 mL, 500 mg/5 mL, 1 g/10 mL, 3 and 6 g/30 mL; Tablets: 25, 50, and 100 mg.

Pyridoxine Hydrochloride

3,4-Pyridinedimethanol, 5-hydroxy-6-methyl-, hydrochloride; Vitamin B_6 Hydrochloride (*Various Mfrs*)

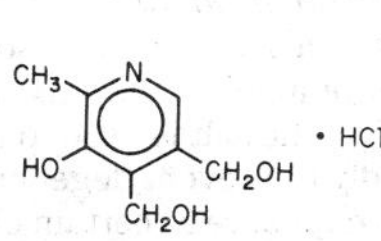

Pyridoxol hydrochloride [58-56-0] $C_8H_{11}NO_3.HCl$ (205.64).

Preparation—Several processes are available. One may be viewed as a cyclizing dehydration of ethyl glycinate (I), ethyl pyruvate (II), and 1,4-diethoxy-2-butanone (III) followed by saponification and decarboxylation at position 2 and cleavage of the three ethoxy groups with HI or another suitable reagent. Reaction of the base with HCl yields the hydrochloride. US Pats 2,904,551, 3,024,244, and 3,024,245.

Description—Colorless or white crystals or a white, crystalline powder; stable in air and slowly affected by sunlight; solutions are acid to litmus, having a pH of about 3; melting range 202 to 206° with some decomposition.

Solubility—1 g in 5 mL water or 115 mL alcohol; insoluble in chloroform or ether.

Uses—Deficiency in adults is extremely difficult to induce, and the therapeutic need for this vitamin, alone, in the adult is of rare occurrence. However, it is justified to give it along with other B vitamins when there is evidence of a *multiple B-vitamin deficiency*. It may be used prophylactically to prevent, or to treat, peripheral neuritis in *patients treated with isoniazid*. It has been claimed that the vitamin controls the *nausea and vomiting of pregnancy* or of *radiation sickness*, but unequivocal proof has never been presented. In infants with *convulsive seizures due to pyridoxine dependency*, administration of the vitamin promptly corrects the condition (see the general statement on *Pyridoxine*). It has been claimed to be medically effective in treating the carpal-tunnel syndrome; however, more data are required to substantiate this claim. Extremely high doses (600 to 3000 mg per day) have been administered to schizophrenics, autistic children and children shown hyperkinesis. However, clear evidence of benefit has not been established. Caution needs to be exercised with these levels of administration because of reports of severe sensory-nervous-system dysfunction after daily consumption of 2 to 5 g. It may be effective in correcting hypochromic or megaloblastic anemia in patients with adequate levels of iron who have not responded to other hematopoietic agents. Since it antagonizes levodopa, patients with Parkinson's disease treated with the latter drug should not take multivitamin supplements containing pyridoxine (see *Levodopa*, page 1037).

Dose—*Usual, adult, oral, supplement,* initially **10 to 20 mg** a day for 3 wk, followed by **2 to 5 mg** a day for several weeks; *Pyridoxine dependency syndrome,* initially **30 to 600 mg** a day, *maintenance,* **50 mg** a day for life; *deficiency, prevention,* **10 to 300 mg** a day; *treatment,* **50 to 200 mg** a day for 3 wk followed by **25 to 100 mg** a day as needed; *Alcoholism,* **50 mg** a day for 2 to 4 wk; *hereditary sideroblastic anemia,* **200 to 600 mg** a day for 1 or 2 mo, followed by **30 to 50 mg** a day for life; *pediatric, oral, pyridoxine dependency,* **2 to 10 mg** a day for life; *dietary supplement,* **2.5 to 10 mg** a day for 3 wk followed by **2 to 5 mg** a day for several weeks.

Dosage Forms—Injection: 50 and 100 mg/mL; Tablets: 5, 10, 25, 50, 100, 200, 250 and 500 mg; Extended-Release Capsules: 5, 10, 25, 50, 100, 200, 250 and 500 mg.

Riboflavin

Lactoflavin; Vitamin B_2; (*Various Mfrs*)

Riboflavine [83-88-5] $C_{17}H_{20}N_4O_6$ (376.37). See page 1121.

Preparation—Mostly by synthesis. In one method, 1-(6-amino-3,4-xylidino)-1-deoxy-D-ribitol (I) is condensed with alloxan (II) in acetic acid with boric acid as a catalyst. Among other ways, I may be prepared by condensing D-ribitol with 4,5-dimethylphenylenediamine. US Pat 2,807,611.

Description—Yellow to orange-yellow, crystalline powder having a slight odor; melts at about 280°; saturated solution is neutral to litmus; when dry not appreciably affected by diffused light, but when in solution, light induces quite rapid deterioration especially in the presence of alkalies.

Solubility—Very slightly soluble in water, alcohol or isotonic sodium chloride solution; very soluble in dilute solutions of alkalies; insoluble in ether or chloroform.

Uses—To treat ariboflavinosis (riboflavin deficiency) and also to supplement other B vitamins in the treatment of pellagra and beriberi (see the general statement on *Riboflavin*).

Dose—*Adult, deficiency, oral,* **5 to 30 mg** a day in divided doses for several days; *Supplement,* **1 to 4 mg** a day; *Children, over 12 yr,* **3 to 10 mg** a day; *Supplement,* **600 μg** a day for each 1000 calories ingested.

Dosage Form—Tablets: 5, 10, 25, 50, 60 and 100 mg.

Thiamine Hydrochloride

Thiazolium, 3-[(4-amino-2-methyl-5-pyrimidinyl)methyl]-5-(2-hydroxyethyl)-4-methyl-, chloride, monohydrochloride; Vitamin B_1 Hydrochloride; Aneurine Hydrochloride; (*Various Mfrs*)

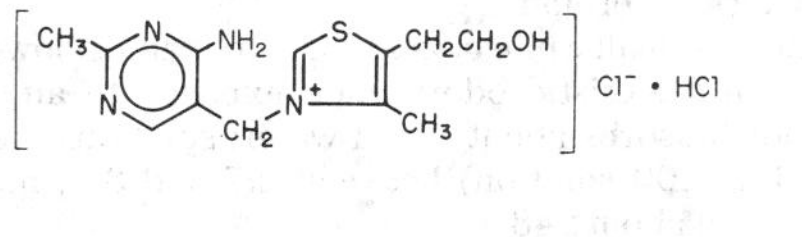

[67-03-8] $C_{12}H_{17}ClN_4OS.HCl$ (337.27).

Preparation—This vitamin consists of two ring systems, a pyrimidine portion and a thiazole portion joined by a methylene bridge.

The *pyrimidine* may be prepared by several processes, one of which is as follows: Ethyl acrylate [$CH_2{=}CHCOOC_2H_5$] is heated with ethyl alcohol forming β-ethoxypropionic ester [$C_2H_5OCH_2CH_2COOC_2H_5$] which is condensed in the presence of sodium metal with formic acid to form ethyl sodioformyl-β-ethoxypropionate **I**. This is then condensed with acetamidine yielding 2-methyl-5-ethoxymethyl-5-hydroxypyrimidine, **II**. This compound is treated with phosphorus oxychloride thereby replacing the OH on carbon 6 with Cl, and by reacting the resulting chloro derivative with ammonia, the Cl is replaced by NH_2. Finally, on treating the latter product with HBr, 2-methyl-5-bromomethyl-6-aminopyrimidine hydrobromide, **III**, is produced.

The *thiazole* portion of the thiamine molecule may be built up in the following matter: Ethyl acetoacetate **IV** is treated with ethylene oxide [C_2H_4O] and the resulting acetyl-butyryl lactone, when reacted with sulfuryl chloride, yields chloroacetyl butyrolactone. This compound is decarboxylated when heated with HCl, splitting off CO_2 and forming 3-chloro-5-hydroxy-2-pentanone, **V**. The latter, when condensed with thioformamide yields the thiazole, 4-methyl-5-hydroxyethylthiazole, **VI**.

$CH_3C(=NH)NH_2$ + $NaOCH=C(CH_2OC_2H_5)C(=O)OC_2H_5$ $\xrightarrow[C_2H_5OH]{Na}$

Acetamidine **Enol form of Ethyl Sodioformyl-β-ethoxypropionate**

I

$C_2H_5OCH_2$-pyrimidine(CH_3, OH) **II** $\xrightarrow[\text{then HBr}]{POCl_3\text{, then }NH_3}$ $BrCH_2$-pyrimidine(CH_3, $NH_2 \cdot HBr$) **III**

$O{=}CCH_3$ / $CH_2COOC_2H_5$ **IV** $\xrightarrow{C_2H_4O}$ $O{=}CCH_3$ / $CHC(=O)O$ / CH_2CH_2 $\xrightarrow[\text{then }CO_2]{SO_2Cl_2}$

$ClCHCH_2CH_2OH$ / $O{=}CCH_3$ **V** + $S{=}CH$ / NH_2 $\longrightarrow$ $HOCH_2CH_2$-thiazole(CH_3) **VI**

III + VI $\xrightarrow[\text{then AgCl}]{\text{Condense}}$ Product

The final step of this process is the combination of the pyrimidine and the thiazole to form a thiazolium halide. Since this is a simple addition of an alkyl halide, the (bromomethyl) pyrimidine to a tertiary amine, the thiazole, it is readily effected by bringing the two components together in a suitable solvent. The vitamin- bromohydrobromide so obtained is transformed into the corresponding chlorine compound, thiamine, with freshly precipitated silver chloride. The silver combines with the bromine to form the less soluble silver bromide and the chloride from the silver chloride replaces the bromine.

Description—Small white crystals or a crystalline powder usually having a slight, characteristic odor; when exposed to air, the anhydrous product rapidly absorbs about 4% of water; solutions are acid to litmus paper; pH (1 in 100 solution) between 2.7 and 3.4; melts, with some decomposition, at about 248°.

Solubility—1 g in about 1 mL water or about 170 mL alcohol; soluble in glycerin; insoluble in ether or benzene.

Incompatibilities—In the dry state, it is stable. Acidic solutions having a pH below 5.5, preferably from 5.0 to 3.5, are also relatively stable. *Alkalies* destroy it. It is precipitated from solution by several of the *alkaloidal reagents* such as *mercuric chloride, iodine, picric acid, tannin,* and *Mayer's reagent*. It is sensitive to both *oxidizing* and *reducing agents*.

Elixirs of thiamine hydrochloride are necessarily acid in reaction and are, therefore, incompatible with any acid-neutralizing substance. *Phenobarbital sodium* has been an occasional offender in this respect, the result frequently being such as to cause precipitation of the phenobarbital as well as a partial lowering of the acidity of the mixture with consequent deterioration of the vitamin. Phenobarbital, not the sodium derivative, may be dispensed in such an instance provided that sufficient alcohol is present to keep it in solution. If a part of the elixir is replaced with alcohol for this purpose, an amount of thiamine hydrochloride equivalent to that contained in the volume so replaced must be added to the product.

Uses—To treat *beriberi* and also *general B-vitamin deficiency*. The fact that it cures the neuropathologies of beriberi has given rise to a widespread use of the vitamin in nearly any type of neuropathology. Although such indiscriminate use can do no organic harm to the patient, it constitutes an unnecessary expense; the promotion of the vitamin for such promiscuous use constitutes an abuse. For additional information see the general statement on *Thiamine*.

Dose—*Oral, adult, nutritional supplement* or *deficiency, beriberi,* **5 to 10 mg**, 3 times a day; *alcohol-induced deficiency,* **40 mg** a day; *dietary supplement,* **1 to 2 mg** a day; *genetic enzyme deficiency,* **10 to 20 mg** a day (single dose); *pediatric, beri-beri,* **10 mg** a day; *deficiency,* **10 to 50 mg** a day in divided doses; *dietary supplement, infants,* **300 to 500 μg** a day; *children,* **500 μg to 1 mg** a day; *adult, parenteral, nutritional supplement, intramuscular* or *slow intravenous,* **5 to 100 mg**, 3 times a day followed by oral maintenance; *pediatric IM or slow IV,* **10 to 25 mg.**

Dosage Forms—Injection: 100 and 200 mg/mL; Tablets: 5, 10, 25, 50, 100, 250 and 500 mg.

Other Water-Soluble Vitamin Preparations

Carnitine [L-(3-Carboxy-2-hydroxypropyl)trimethylammonium hydroxide inner salt; [461-06-3] Vitamin B_T; $C_7H_{15}NO_3$ (161.20) (*Tyson*); Carnitor (*Sigma-Tau*)]—*Preparation:* See Wolf G, ed: *Monograph: Recent Research on Carnitine*, MIT Press, Cambridge MA, 1965. It may be isolated from meat extracts or prepared synthetically. *Description and Solubility:* White, very hygroscopic solid melting about 197°. Readily soluble in water or hot alcohol; practically insoluble in most organic solvents. *Uses:* Required in mammalian energy metabolism and has been shown to facilitate long-chain fatty acid entry into cellular mitochondria, therefore providing the substrate for β-oxidation and subsequent production of energy. It is synthesized in the liver from lysine. Deficiency may occur from impaired hepatic synthesis or transport from liver to muscle. Carnitine deficiency may lead to elevated triglyceride and free fatty acid concentrations, diminished ketogenesis and lipid infiltration of muscle and liver. *Dose: Usual, adult, oral* or *enteral,* initially 1 g, 1 to three times a day with meals; *pediatric,* initially 50 mg/kg a day with food, increased as needed to a maximum of 3 g a day. *Dosage Forms:* Oral Solution: 100 mg/mL; Tablets: 330 mg.

Choline Bitartrate [(2-Hydroxyethyl)trimethylammonium Bitartrate; $C_9H_{19}NO_7$ (253.25)]—*Preparation:* See *Choline Chloride*, below. *Description and Solubility:* A white, hygroscopic, crystalline powder with an acidic taste; odorless or may have a faint trimethylamine-like odor. Freely soluble in water, slightly soluble in alcohol and insoluble in benzene, chloroform or ether. *Uses:* As a nutrient or dietary supplement.

Choline Chloride [(2-Hydroxyethyl)trimethylammonium chloride; [67-48-1] $C_5H_{14}ClNO$ (139.62)]—*Preparation:* For the preparation of choline, see *Choline Dihydrogen Citrate. Description and Solubility:* White, deliquescent crystals; a 10% aqueous solution has a pH of about 4.7. Very soluble in water or alcohol. *Uses:* For the metabolic effects of *Choline*, see page 1117. The salt is used to reduce fatty infiltration of the liver and thus supposedly to prevent degeneration and cirrhosis. Such infiltration may occur after exposure to certain chemical intoxicants, such as carbon tetrachloride, chloroform and various other halogenated hydrocarbons (including several general anesthetics), divinyl ether, etc. Moderate to severe ethanol intoxication and habitual ingestion of ethanol also predispose to fatty infiltration of the liver. Patients who are acutely ill and cannot eat or persons on a high-fat diet frequently develop fatty livers, for which this vitamin may be given. In none of these conditions has there been clearly demonstrable efficacy. Furthermore, a high-protein diet, especially one that includes eggs, meat, liver and milk, not only provides some of this vitamin but also methionine, which promotes the endogenous synthesis of *Choline* (see page 1117). Once cirrhosis occurs, it is probably too late for any possible benefits. There is no evidence that it is helpful in infectious hepatitis. For the above reasons, there is no longer any official preparation of it. Since the anion is irrelevant to the metabolic effects, the chloride is neither superior nor inferior to other salts.

Choline Dihydrogen Citrate [(2-Hydroxyethyl)trimethylammonium Dihydrogen Citrate; $C_{11}H_{21}NO_8$ (295.29)]—*Preparation:* By treating aqueous trimethylamine with ethylene oxide. Conversion to the dihydrogen citrate is conveniently effected by dissolving the base in a suitable solvent such as ethanol and treating with an equimolar portion of citric acid. *Description and Solubility:* Colorless, translucent crystals, or a white, granular to fine, crystalline powder; odorless or may have a faint trimethylamine odor and has an acidic taste; hygroscopic when exposed to air; melts between 103 and 107.5°. 1 g dissolves in 1 mL water or 42 mL alcohol; very slightly soluble in ether, chloroform or benzene. *Uses:* See *Choline Chloride*, above.

Sodium Folate [Monosodium Folate [6484-89-5] $C_{19}H_{18}N_7NaO_6$ (463.38); Folvite Sodium (*Lederle*)]—For the structure of the acid, see page 1118. *Preparation: Folic Acid* is reacted with $NaHCO_3$. *Description* and *Solubility:* Clear, mobile liquid having a yellow or orange-yellow color; pH between 8.5 and 11. *Uses:* Has the actions of *Folic Acid* (page 1118). However, the salt is preferred for parenteral use. *Dose:* Parenteral, 5 to 15 mg daily.

Thiamine Mononitrate [Thiazolium, 3-[(4-amino-2-methyl-5-pyrimidinyl)methyl]-5-(2-hydroxyethyl)-4-methyl-, nitrate (salt); Thiamine Nitrate; Vitamin B_1 Mononitrate; Thiamine nitrate [532-43-4] $C_{12}H_{17}N_5O_4S$ (327.36)]—*Preparation:* In one method thiamine hydrochloride is reacted with sufficient NaOH to remove the HCl and replace the chloride ion by OH, and the resulting thiamine hydroxide is neutralized with nitric acid. *Description:* White crystals or crystalline powder, usually having a slight, characteristic odor; pH (1 in 50 solution) 6 to 7.5. *Solubility:* 1 g in about 44 mL water; slightly soluble in alcohol or chloroform. *Uses:* More stable than the hydrochloride; solutions of the nitrate are practically neutral, while those of the hydrochloride are acid. Its vitaminergic actions and uses are identical to those of the hydrochloride. See *Thiamine Hydrochloride.*

Multivitamin Preparations

In the preceding text and in various monographs, attention was called in several instances to the fact that it is desirable at times to administer more than one vitamin for what appear to be the symptoms of a single deficiency. The quotation "In the shadow of pellagra walks beriberi" has considerable substance in fact. Diets deficient in niacin are frequently also deficient in thiamin and certain other B vitamins of similar dietary source. The same relationship holds frequently for folacin and vitamin B_{12}. Malabsorption syndromes affect the assimilation of several vitamins. Furthermore, the repair of a deficiency of one vitamin may increase the requirement of another; for example, repletion of thiamin increases the need for riboflavin. Diseases in which there is increased metabolism, such as thyrotoxicosis, increase the need for more of the vitamins, as do periods of hard physical work, stress, pregnancy and lactation. Therefore, multivitamin therapy is often rational. Multivitamin therapy also is recommended for individuals, who on restricted diets for weight control or lacks verity, those who are debilitated, and those working in hazardous environments. Use of multivitamin supplements for infants and preschool children should be done on the advice of a pediatrician.

Other Nutrients

Amino Acids and Proteins

Nutritional Role—Protein hydrolysates, in which proteins have been reduced to short-chain peptides and amino acids, long have been used orally or in relatively dilute solutions intravenously as supplementary nutrients for patients unable to metabolize intact protein adequately. More recently, patients in whom oral or tube feeding is contraindicated or inadequate, good nutrition may be achieved and maintained, for several months if necessary, by the procedure of intravenous feeding known as *total parenteral nutrition (TPN)*, sometimes called *intravenous* or *parenteral hyperalimentation.* Such feeding provides essential nutrients in a sufficiently concentrated form that does not exceed normal daily fluid requirements; this necessitates formulation of markedly hypertonic solutions (2000 mOsm/L and higher). Such solutions must be infused, at a constant rate throughout the entire day, into a large-diameter *central* vein where rapid dilution by high blood-flow minimizes vascular damage and the risk of phlebitis or thrombosis that is likely to occur on injection into a peripheral vein. The infusion route is generally through a surgically placed subclavian catheter into the superior vena cava, but in infants and small children it may be through a catheter in the jugular vein.

The most critical component in TPN is a nitrogen source available for repletion and/or maintenance of lean body mass and proteins essential for wound healing, tissue repair, and growth. Protein hydrolysate injections, sometimes supplemented with amino acids, are used as nitrogen sources, but in most hospitals solutions of mixed crystalline L-amino acids have replaced the former. Crystalline L-amino acids appear to be more efficiently metabolized and better tolerated in the body than are the peptides of protein hydrolysates. Also, individual acids may be readily and reproducibly formulated to meet specific requirements of patients, such as those with renal failure and infants that are premature.

So that amino acids may be used for protein synthesis and to achieve positive nitrogen balance and weight gain in debilitated patients it is necessary to provide the equivalent of at least 150 nonprotein calories per gram of nitrogen administered. When relying on total parenteral nutrition it is preferable to use intravenous fat emulsion to provide energy needs* (see *Fats and Oils*, below). If an intravenous emulsion is not used then large amounts of dextrose are required to achieve caloric balance, and to avoid the fluid overload that would result from use of weaker solutions, markedly hypertonic concentrations of dextrose (25%—five times the isotonic concentration—or higher) must be supplied. As solutions so concentrated are prone to produce thrombosis when injected into a peripheral vein, they must be infused into a central vein, as described above.

In addition to dextrose and amino acids, TPN solutions may contain vitamins and electrolytes (often added to meet individual patient requirements). Various solutions for TPN use are commercially available, as are kits that include, for example, a 1-L bottle containing 500 mL of 50% dextrose solution under vacuum, a 500-mL bottle of 8.5% solution of a crystalline amino acid mixture composed of 8 essential and 7 nonessential amino acids in biologically usable proportion (FreAmine III,† *McGaw*), and a transfer set and additive cap

* A 10% soybean oil emulsion (Intralipid), developed and used in Europe since 1961, that has an osmolarity of 280 mOsm/L (essentially isotonic with blood) and can be administered through peripheral veins. The fat particles of this egg-yolk phospholipid emulsion are less than 0.5 μm in diameter, similar in size to naturally occurring chylomicrons. The emulsion is a useful source of calories and will also prevent and correct essential fatty acid deficiencies that may develop during long-term parenteral nutrition using nonlipid calorie sources.

† The composition of FreAmine III, in g/100 mL is: *Essential Amino Acids:* L-isoleucine 0.59; L-leucine 0.77; L-lysine acetate 0.87; L-methionine 0.45; L-phenylalanine 0.48; l-threonine 0.34; L-tryptophan 0.13; L-valine 0.56. Nonessential Amino Acids: L-alanine 0.60; L-arginine 0.81; L-histidine 0.24; L-proline 0.95; L-serine 0.50; aminoacetic acid 1.19; L-cysteine HCl <0.02. The calculated osmolarity of the solution is approximately 850 mOsm/L. Aminosyn (*Abbott*), a preparation of crystalline amino acids containing a somewhat different proportion of the same essential acids, and with the exception of L-tyrosine replacing L-cysteine the same nonessential amino acids, is supplied in concentrations of 5%, 7%, and 10% of the total acids, with calculated osmolarities of approximately 500, 700, and 1000 mOsm/L, respectively.

for aseptic preparation of the final solution. Total parenteral nutrition solutions, which often require extemporaneous addition of compatible vitamins and/or electrolytes to solutions such as described above, should be prepared by a pharmacist experienced in parenterals production, using aseptic techniques performed under a laminar-flow, filtered-air hood (see Chapter 85, on *Intravenous Admixtures*).

In recent years certain free amino acids have been prescribed for a variety of medical conditions for which neither drug nor food approval have been obtained. Regulations on the food-additive use is limited to providing protein requirements. Therefore, these uses of single amino acids are without approved status. Consumption of high levels of single amino acids have been associated with severe metabolic and medical consequences.

Chemistry—The USP has provided monographs of standards and tests for each of the crystalline amino acids used in amino acid dosage forms. For comparative purposes the formulas and chemical names of the L-amino acids are given in Chapter 26, page 393, and other chemical data are provided in Table 5.

Each of the amino acids is synthesized readily, by a variety of methods, but always as a DL-mixture. While resolution to obtain the L-form can in some cases be conveniently accomplished, often it is easier and more economical to isolate individual acids from the mixed amino acids obtained by hydrolysis of selected proteins. Chromatographic fractionation of amino acids in such hydrolysates has generally replaced the tedious fractional precipitation and derivative distillation methods formerly employed.

The articles that follow describe certain amino acids which are used for certain nonnutritional purposes as well as components of nutritional formulations; also included are brief articles on Protein Hydrolysate Injection and on Oral Protein Hydrolysates.

Arginine Hydrochloride

R-Gene 10 (*KabiVitrium*)

L-Arginine monohydrochloride [1119-34-2] $C_6H_{14}N_4O_2.HCl$ (210.66). For the structural formula of arginine, see page 393.

Preparation—Arginine is present in the hydrolysis products of many proteins; for a method of separating it from gelatin hydrolysate see *J Biol Chem 132:* 325, 1940. It is converted to the hydrochloride by reaction with HCl.

Description—White crystals or crystalline powder; practically odorless.

Solubility—Soluble in water; slightly soluble in hot alcohol.

Uses—Arginine has been variously used in clinical practice. Intravenous administration in the symptomatic management of severe encephalopathies associated with ammoniacal azotemia, on the theory that arginine combines with ammonia to form asparagine, has not been of value in significantly reducing blood ammonia levels or in improving the clinical status of patients, and use of the amino acid for this purpose is no longer approved by the FDA. Oral administration to patients with cystic fibrosis to correct malabsorption and steatorrhea, and by inhalation as a mucolytic, have not been effective. It is used as a nutritional supplement in conditions in which its dibasic amino character or possible blood ammonia reducing power is useful has been reported.

It stimulates pituitary release of growth hormone and prolactin, and pancreatic release of glucagon and insulin, and arginine hydrochloride is used diagnostically to evaluate pituitary growth hormone reserve and detect deficiency of the hormone in various conditions. It is administered by intravenous infusion and blood samples are taken at 30-min intervals after beginning infusion for 2.5 hr; the plasma growth hormone levels in these samples and in others taken 30 min before and at the start of infusion are determined and diagnostically evaluated.

Dose—*Intravenous infusion,* for *pituitary function test,* **30 g** of arginine hydrochloride, in 10% solution, infused at a constant rate over 30 min, preferably with the aid of an infusion pump; in *children* a dose of **500 mg/kg** of body weight is infused.

Dosage Form—Injection: 10% solution, 300 mL.

Glutamic Acid Hydrochloride—see RPS-18, page 782.

Table 5—L-Amino Acids

Amino acid[a]	Molecular formula	Molecular weight	Solubility in water	pK values
L-Alanine 56-41-7	$C_3H_7NO_2$	89.09	1 g in 6 mL	pK_1 3.34 pK_2 8.17
L-Arginine 74-79-3	$C_6H_{14}N_4O_2$	174.20	1 g in 5 mL	pK_1 2.18 pK_2 9.09 pK_3 13.2
L-Aspartic Acid 56-84-8	$C_4H_7NO_4$	133.10	1 g in 200 mL	pK_1' 1.88 pK_2' 3.65 pK_3' 9.60
L-Cysteine 52-90-4	$C_3H_7NO_2S$	121.16	Freely soluble	pK_1 1.71 pK_2 8.33 pK_3 10.78
L-Cystine 56-89-3	$C_6H_{12}N_2O_4S_2$	240.30	1 g in 9000 mL	pK_1 1 pK_2 2.1 pK_3 8.02 pK_4 8.71
L-Glutamic Acid 56-86-0	$C_5H_9NO_4$	147.13	1 g in 115 mL	pK_1 2.19 pK_2 4.25 pK_3 9.67
L-Histidine 71-00-1	$C_6H_9N_3O_2$	155.16	1 g in 24 mL	pK_1 1.78 pK_2 5.97 pK_3 8.97
L-Hydroxy-proline	$C_5H_9NO_3$	131.13	1 g in 3 mL (α-form)	pK_1 1.82 pK_2 9.65
L-Isoleucine[b] 73-32-5	$C_6H_{13}NO_2$	131.17	1 g in 25 mL	pK_1 2.36 pK_2 9.68
L-Leucine[b] 61-90-5	$C_6H_{13}NO_2$	131.17	1 g in 42 mL	K_a 2.5 × 10^{-10} K_b 2.3 × 10^{-2}
L-Lysine[b] 56-87-1	$C_6H_{14}N_2O_2$	146.19	Freely soluble	pK_1 2.20 pK_2 8.90 pK_3 10.28
L-Methionine[b] 63-68-3	$C_5H_{11}NO_2S$	149.21	Soluble	pK_1 2.12 pK_2 9.28
L-Phenylalanine[b] 63-91-2	$C_9H_{11}NO_2$	165.19	1 g in 34 mL	pK_1 2.16 pK_2 9.18
L-Proline 147-85-3	$C_5H_9NO_2$	115.13	1 g in 0.7 mL	pK_1 1.99 pK_2 10.60
L-Serine 56-45-1	$C_3H_7NO_3$	105.09	1 g in 20 mL	pK_1 2.19 pK_2 9.21
L-Taurine 107-35-7	$C_2H_7NO_3S$	125.14	1 g in 16 mL	pK_1 1.50 pK_2 8.74
L-Threonine[b] 72-19-5	$C_4H_9NO_3$	119.12	Freely soluble	pK_1 2.15 pK_2 9.12
L-Tryptophan[b] 73-22-3	$C_{11}H_{12}N_2O_2$	204.22	1 g in 88 mL	pK_1 2.38 pK_2 9.39
L-Tyrosine 60-18-4	$C_9H_{11}NO_3$	181.19	1 g in 2200 mL	pK_1 2.20 pK_1 9.11 pK_2 10.07
L-Valine[b] 72-18-4	$C_5H_{11}NO_2$	117.15	1 g in 12 mL	pK_1 2.32 pK_2 9.62

[a] The number below the name of each amino acid is its Chemical Abstracts Service (CAS) Registry Number. For structures and nomenclature see Chapter 26.

[b] Essential amino acids.

Glycine

Aminoacetic Acid; Glycocoll

NH_2CH_2COOH

[56-40-6] $C_2H_5NO_2$ (75.07).

Preparation—Aminoacetic acid is a constituent of many proteins. It may be synthesized by many processes; industrially it is prepared by interaction of ammonia with chloroacetic acid.

Description—White, odorless, crystalline powder, having a sweetish taste; solution is acid to litmus; pK_a 9.78.

Solubility—1 g in 4 mL water or 1254 mL alcohol; very slightly soluble in ether.

Uses—As an irrigating fluid in transurethral resection of the prostate. The acid is also used in an antacid preparation, as a complex salt. However, its limited buffering capacity does not warrant the expense of such a preparation. It is used primarily in admixture with other amino acids in TPN formulations.

Dose—*Usual*, **30 g** daily, in divided doses; *application*, irrigating solution as a **1.5%** solution.

Dosage Form—Irrigation: 1.5%/1500, 2000 and 3000 mL, 15% (concentrate)/1000 mL.

Sugars

Sugars are carbohydrates that are sweet to the taste and highly soluble in water. They may be either monosaccharides or disaccharides. The chemistry of the sugars is discussed in Chapter 26. In the section below are listed only those sugars that are used in medicine as aliments. Some of the sugars also have important uses as pharmaceutical necessities, in parenteral fluids, as diuretics, as osmotic "stuffing" for injection of other drugs, etc; consequently, the monographs of certain nutrient sugars may be found elsewhere in this volume.

Dextrose—page 1409.

Dextrose Injection—page 916.

Dextrose and Sodium Chloride Injection—page 916.

Fructose

D(−)-Fructose; Levulose

β-D-Fructopyranose

D-Fructose [57-48-7] $C_6H_{12}O_6$ (180.16); a sugar usually obtained by the inversion of aqueous solutions of sucrose and subsequent separation of fructose from glucose.

Preparation—Sucrose is inverted by treatment with dilute acid at moderate temperature, and the fructose is separated by precipitation of the lime-fructose complex. Fructose is released from the complex with carbon dioxide, which precipitates the calcium as carbonate. After filtering, the fructose solution is purified with activated carbon and ion-exchange resins and evaporated to dryness.

Description—Colorless crystals or as a white, crystalline or granular powder, which is odorless and has a sweet taste; specific rotation −89 to −91°.

Solubility—1 g in about 15 mL alcohol or about 14 mL methanol; freely soluble in water.

Uses—A ketohexose used parenterally as a carbohydrate nutrient. It is converted to liver glycogen and metabolized more rapidly than dextrose, without requiring insulin, and thus may be used in diabetic patients. It is indicated in patients requiring fluid replacement and caloric feeding but contraindicated in hypoglycemia, for which dextrose should be used. It also is contraindicated in patients with hereditary fructose intolerance.

Dose—*Intravenous* as required.

Dosage Forms—Injection: 100 g/1000 mL; Fructose and Sodium Chloride Injection: 100 g of fructose and 9 g of sodium chloride/1000 mL. 1 L contains 555 mosm and supplies 375 cal.

Lactose—page 1411.

Liquid Glucose—page 1410.

Sucrose—page 1390.

Syrup—page 1393.

Other Sugars

Invert Sugar [8013-17-0]—An equimolar mixture of glucose and fructose produced by hydrolysis of sucrose. Forms clear, colorless solutions having a pH of 3.5 to 6. *Uses:* Instead of dextrose, for parenteral administration of carbohydrate. While it has the same caloric value as dextrose (4 kcal/g), invert sugar is utilized more rapidly and may be administered intravenously twice as fast as dextrose. *Dose:* 1 L of a 5 or 10% solution in either water or isotonic sodium chloride solution.

Fats and Oils

The role of fat in the nutritional physiology of man is both complex and contradictory. The unique and essential part it plays in metabolic processes and in the palatability of food points out its importance. Stored fat (adipose tissue) as well as dietary fat are concentrated sources of energy which the body can use efficiently for physical activity and in times of physical stress. Fat when oxidized to carbon dioxide and water yields 9 kcal/g, whereas protein and carbohydrates both yield approximately 4 kcal/g. Energy consumed in excess to metabolic needs is stored in the body as fat and represents the major body reserve of energy during periods of low calorie intake. Certain components of fat, called polyunsaturated fatty acids, are essential dietary components for tissue biosynthesis of prostaglandins, which perform vital hormone-like activities in the transmission of genetic information in all cells. Food fats are carriers, to varying degrees, of fat-soluble vitamins (A, D, E and K). Also, a diet too restricted in fats lacks flavor and satiety value.

That fats also are involved or indicated in such significant pathologies as obesity and atherosclerosis or the syndrome called coronary heart disease (CHD) well is known. Epidemiological, experimental and clinical investigations have identified a number of "risk factors" associated with susceptibility to CHD that may be controlled. These include an elevation in plasma lipids, especially plasma cholesterol, high blood pressure (hypertension), heavy cigarette smoking, obesity and physical inactivity. Persons falling into "risk categories" on the basis of their plasma lipid levels can be made aware of this during a physician's examination and appropriate professional dietary advice then can be followed. For such persons it is important, in addition to maintaining a desirable body weight, to decrease substantially the intake of total fat, saturated fat, and to lower cholesterol consumption. Recent studies not yet conclusive indicate that so-called ω-3-fatty acids contained in oils obtained from fish harvested in cold-water regions and also found in lesser amounts in soybeans and rapeseed oils may have beneficial effects in lowering plasma low-density lipoprotein (and cholesterol) triglycerides and lowering the tendency for platelet aggregation.

There are many abnormal conditions in which faulty digestion and absorption of fat occur and excessive amounts of fat are present in the feces. When these conditions exist, there is fecal fat loss, poor absorption of other nutrients and diarrhea. As a result, there may be substantial weight loss and general malnutrition.

In recent years, it has been shown that the digestion and absorption of short- and medium-chain triglycerides (MCT's) are different from those of the long-chain triglycerides which are characteristic of most food fat. The hydrolysis and absorption of MCTs are faster than of long-chain triglycerides and it is possible for MCTs to be absorbed directly into the intestinal mucosa without first being hydrolyzed, making it possible to absorb MCTs in the absence of pancreatic juice and bile. Coconut oil contains more medium-chain fatty acids than other fats and oils and is used as a source for fractionation and preparation of MCTs. MCTs are commercially available as relatively pure 8-carbon or 10-carbon triglycerides and as a 4:1 mixture.

MCTs have been found to be useful in conjunction with the usual therapy in the treatment of such diseases as pancreatic insufficiency, cancer of the pancreas, cystic fibrosis of the pancreas, obstruction of the bile duct, certain abnormalities in the lymphatic system, regional enteritis and in postoperative cases involving the removal of much of the stomach or small intestine. The most consistent beneficial effects reported from the use of MCTs are a decrease in the fecal loss of fat and less diarrhea. In recent years fat emulsions have gained wide use in providing the energy needs of critically ill patients, particularly those with severe burns or those who must rely on TPN for long periods of time. These intravenous fat emulsions were developed in the early 1960s, in Europe, and typically contain soybean oil, egg yolk phospholipids, glycerin and water for injection. The fat particles are less than 0.5 μm in diameter, similar in size to naturally occurring chylomicrons. These emulsions are available in 10 and 20% suspensions and provide the essential fatty acids. The levels of use have been shown to be safe up to 35 to 40% of calorific needs.

Other Fats

Intravenous Fat Emulsion [Liposyn (*Abbott*); Intralipid (*KabiVitrum*); Soyacal (*Alpha Therapeutic*)]—*Description*: Water emulsions of 10 and 20%; osmolarity, approximately 300 to 350 mOsm/kg of water, 260 to 268 mOsm/kg emulsion; particle size less than 0.5 μm in diameter. *Use*: As source of calories and essential fatty acids, usually for patients requiring parenteral nutrition for more than 5 days. *Dose*: Up to 500 mL, 10% solution over 4-hr period, not more than 40% of total caloric administration. Up to 500 mL, 20% solution over 8-hr period, not more than 40% of total caloric administration.

Corn Oil—page 1394.
Olive Oil—page 1400.
Peanut Oil—page 1394.
Safflower Oil—see RPS-16, page 803.

Trace Elements

The trace elements are those inorganic nutrients that are required in small or "trace" amounts, a few micrograms to a few milligrams per day for man or per kilogram of diet for an experimental animal. The essentiality of several trace elements was established for animals and man during the 1930s. A resurgence of interest in this area has occurred due to technological advancements in analytical methodology and development of highly purified diets and "clean" environments for experimental animals.

Fourteen elements now are thought to be essential; however, evidence to support required functions in animals and man is still incomplete for nickel, silicon, tin and vanadium. It is expected that all 14 of these, and possibly others, will be shown to be required by human beings. There is also evidence that boron may be essential. Some pertinent chemical and biological information on these elements is shown in Table 6. Some elements, notably manganese and chromium, can exist in several oxidation states; however, only one or two are compatible with a biological environment and function.

The amount of each element in a normal 70-kg adult man may vary considerably, depending on requirement and whether or not the element can be stored in certain tissues. Daily requirements ("allowances") have been established for a few of the trace elements (Table 3). Ranges of typical daily intakes of the other elements by healthy individuals provide a very rough guide to maximal needs. These values are based on limited data.

Information on trace-element distribution in foods is presented in Table 7. This is an attempt to indicate important sources of the elements or the level, particularly if low, in important foods. This table is of rather limited usefulness because it is based on so little information. At present, too little is known about the effect of agricultural practices and manufacturing processes on trace-element content.

Table 6—Biological Data for the Essential Trace Elements

Element	Amount in 70-kg human, mg	Daily human intake range,[a] mg
Chromium	6.6	0.06–0.36
Cobalt	1.1	0.015–0.160
Copper	75–150	0.75–1.2
Fluorine	2600	0.5–1.7[b]
Iodine	10–20	0.3–0.7
Iron	4000–5000	10–17
Manganese	12–20	1.5–3.0
Molybdenum	9.3	0.1–0.2
Nickel	10	0.10–0.15
Selenium	. . .	0.6–1.0
Silicon	18,000	. . .
Tin	17	1.5–3.5
Vanadium	10–25	0.01–0.02
Zinc	1400–2300	8–16

[a] Values from FDA total diet study.
[b] Excludes high-fluoride areas.

Our understanding of trace-element function in man is less complete than that for vitamins. Study of a deficiency syndrome in animals often precedes recognition of deficiency or metabolic problems in man, particularly as related to a disease. For this reason, deficiency syndromes in animals are described for each element known to be essential.

Similarly, our knowledge of trace-element toxicity in man is limited and we must rely on animal data. Two problems must be considered. One is the effect of long-term supplementation with a "moderate" excess above requirement. For children and adults the FDA regulations on dietary supplements for each of four trace elements permit an excess of 50% above the US RDA (see Table 3). It is important to consider not only the amount of a single trace element, but also the balance among all required elements. This area requires periodic review as knowledge increases. The other toxicity problem relates to short-term intake of multiple recommended doses, either accidentally or purposefully. This must be regarded as undesirable, depending on the excess intake level. It is known well to be very serious in the case of infants swallowing capsules containing ferrous sulfate.

Inorganic elements are very different from the various organic nutrients in that they cannot be destroyed or converted into another substance by the metabolic processes in the animal. In most cases the trace elements are bound to an organic ligand. This is the means for effecting elemental transport and function and minimizing toxicity. The binding may be very loose or very firm. Many of the elements are part of metalloenzymes. Nucleic acids also bind metal ions in a consistent pattern; however, the significance of this is not established. Other mechanisms of function are described for individual elements below.

Many pairs or larger groups of essential elements may have chemical properties that are closely similar. This can result in competition for binding sites that may alter transport, storage, excretion and function.

There are many elements in biological systems that have no known essential function but which have some chemical properties similar to those of required elements. These elements can become a health threat when they are present in sufficient quantity to replace a required element or to bind excessively to some organic ligand and cause a physiological aberration. Modern industrial technology has effected translocation of large quantities of many minerals from their native stores in the ground to the air, water and ultimately to the food supply. Three elements that have caused concern and some isolated severe problems for man are mercury, cadmium and lead. The nutritional status of an exposed person can modify the severity of adverse response to a toxic level of an element. A deficiency of certain nutrients can result in a more severe adverse effect while a moderate excess of other nutrients can afford some protection. The possibility must be kept in mind that elements now regarded only as toxic may have an essential function at a very low level of intake.

Analysis of trace elements can be accomplished by both chemical and physical techniques. Modern advances such as induction coupled plasma, atomic absorption spectrometry and neutron activation analysis provide rapid, accurate and low-cost measurements.

Chromium

Deficiency Syndrome and Function—The principal defect in chromium deficiency is an impairment of glucose utilization; however, disturbances in protein and lipid metabolism have also been observed. In the young animal, growth rate may be reduced. Corneal lesions have been observed in rats deficient in both chromium and protein; no lesions have been seen with either single deficiency.

Impaired glucose utilization occurs in many middle-aged and elderly human beings. In experimental studies, significant numbers of such persons have shown improvement in their glucose utilization after treatment with chromium. There have also been improvements in diabetic children and infants with kwashiorkor.

For biological activity, chromium must be trivalent. The most active form of chromium is that which is incorporated into a low-molecular-

Table 7—Distribution of Essential Trace Elements in Foods[a]

Element	Food source content: Average to high	Low
Chromium	Dried brewers' yeast, bran and germ of cereal grains, molasses, liver	Refined cereals, refined sugar
Cobalt	Leafy vegetables	Milk, refined cereals
Copper	Liver, kidney, shellfish, nuts, dry legumes, whole grain cereals	Milk, muscle meat, eggs, fruit, vegetables
Fluorine[b]	Seafish, red meat, eggs, tea	Milk
Iodine[b]	Seafish, shellfish, iodized salt, milk	
Iron	Liver, kidney, shellfish, muscle meats, poultry, heart, egg yolk, dried legumes, cane molasses, nuts	Milk, refined sugar
Manganese	Whole grain cereals, dried legumes, tubers, fruits, nonleafy vegetables	Milk, poultry, fish
Molybdenum	Liver, kidney, dried legumes, whole grain cereals, leafy vegetables	Fruits, root and stem vegetables, muscle meats, milk
Nickel	Whole grain cereals, vegetables	Muscle meats, fats, eggs, milk
Selenium	Liver, kidney	
Silicon	Whole grain cereals, chicken skin, beer	Animal foods
Tin[d]	Cereals, muscle meats	Milk
Vanadium[b]	Liver, muscle meats, fish, bread, some cereal grains, nuts, a few root vegetables, oils from corn and soybeans	Milk, most vegetables
Zinc	Meat, egg yolk, whole grain cereals, oysters, fowl, milk	Fruits, fish, vegetables

[a] Bioavailability is not taken into consideration; see text of individual elements.
[b] Most foods are highly variable.
[c] Selenium content is markedly affected by available selenium during growth of the plant or animal food. Cooking losses can occur.
[d] The tin content is markedly increased by exposure to tin-plated containers.

weight organic molecule that occurs in many foods. Its structure is not known yet. This compound has been designated GTF (glucose tolerance factor). From a variety of biochemical studies, it appears that the presence of insulin is required for all functions of chromium. GTF is the only one of many compounds tested that passed the rat placenta into the fetus.

Metabolism and Bioavailability—Chromium is transported by transferrin in the plasma and competes with iron for binding sites. The main excretory route is through the urine; however, some chromium is excreted in the bile and by the small intestine. The newborn animal has large stores of chromium that decline with age.

Toxicity—In animals, a wide margin of safety separates toxicity from the nutritional requirement of chromium (III).

Cobalt

Deficiency Syndrome, Function, and Metabolism—The only known essential function of cobalt is as a component of vitamin B_{12} (see page 1123).

Cobalt salts are absorbed poorly. Excretion is via the bile and through the intestinal wall. Cobalt is widely distributed in the body, with the highest concentrations in the liver, kidney and bone.

Toxicity—High levels of cobalt can produce a polycythemia in many species, an effect that is unrelated to vitamin B_{12}. Cobalt usually is considered relatively nontoxic; however, severe cardiac failure and some deaths in man have resulted from consumption of large amounts of beer containing 1.2 to 1.5 ppm of cobalt. The element was added to the beer to promote optimal foam stabilization.

Copper

Deficiency Syndrome and Function—The most common defect observed in copper-deficient animals is anemia. Other abnormalities include growth depression, skeletal defects, demyelination and degeneration of the nervous system, ataxia, defects in pigmentation and structure of hair or wool, reproductive failure and cardiovascular lesions, including dissecting aneurysms. Copper deficiency occurs very infrequently in human beings. A deficiency has been observed in some South American infants and a few in the US receiving an artificial formula diet deficient in copper.

Several copper-containing metalloproteins have been isolated from animal tissues, including tyrosinase, ascorbic acid oxidase, laccase, cytochrome oxidase, uricase, monoamine oxidase, delta-aminolevulinic acid dehydrase and dopamine-β-hydroxylase. Copper functions in the absorption and utilization of iron, electron transport, connective tissue metabolism, phospholipid formation, purine metabolism and development of the nervous system. Ferroxidase I (ceruloplasmin), a copper-containing enzyme, effects the oxidation of Fe (II) to Fe (III), a required step for mobilization of stored iron. There is evidence that a copper-containing enzyme is responsible for the oxidative deamination of the epsilon amino group of lysine to produce desmosine and isodesmosine, the cross-links of elastin. In copper-deficient animals the arterial elastin is weaker and dissecting aneurysms may occur.

Metabolism and Bioavailability—Copper is absorbed from the small intestine. Most of the copper in the plasma is in ceruloplasmin; however, significant amounts are loosely bound to albumin, the fraction important in transport. The plasma copper level increases in acute infections, pregnancy and in women taking birth-control pills. Small amounts of copper are excreted in the urine, but the major excretory pathway is via bile and feces.

Copper is present in high concentrations in the brain, liver, heart and kidney, with the highest levels occurring at birth. It is important that pregnant women receive adequate copper during pregnancy, so that the infant will have adequate stores of copper at birth.

A variety of salts of copper have been found to be available to experimental and domestic animals. These include the sulfate, nitrate, chloride, carbonate, oxide, hydroxide, iodide, glutamate, glycerophosphate, aspartate, citrate, nucleinate and pyrophosphate. Elemental copper and copper sulfide are utilized poorly. The chemical form of copper in food is largely unknown. The absorption of copper can be decreased by large amounts of phytic acid, ascorbic acid, calcium and zinc.

Toxicity—Wilson's disease, a genetic disease in man, leads to excess copper accumulation in the brain, liver and kidney, which results in mental and neurological abnormalities. The disease is treated by administration of a chelating agent, penicillamine (β,β-dimethylcysteine), which removes excess copper from the tissues and results in its excretion.

Fluorine

Deficiency Syndrome and Function—The most important relationship of fluoride to health is that of preventing dental caries. Fluoride has been shown to enter the hydroxyapatite of teeth to form a more perfect crystal, which resists acid attack more effectively. (See *Sodium Fluoride*, page 884.) In areas where the fluoride content of the drinking water is unusually high, osteoporosis and calcification of the aorta of elderly persons are less than in control population groups not receiving high fluoride. In these areas the effective fluoride concentration is high enough to cause mottling of the tooth enamel in young children.

Metabolism and Bioavailability—The absorption of fluoride from the gastrointestinal tract is rapid and complete. Even the water-insoluble forms are absorbed fairly well. Fluoride can cross membranes easily, and it passes readily from the plasma into the tissues; however, the mammary gland and the placenta offer some resistance to transport. Excess fluoride is excreted in the urine.

Bones typically have high concentrations of fluoride, which gradually increase throughout life to about age 55 years. Fluoride supplementation increases bone density but is reported to increase brittleness. Of the soft tissues, the kidney is highest in fluoride. Calcium and aluminum can decrease the absorption of fluoride and sodium chloride can depress the skeletal uptake of fluoride.

Toxicity—Toxic doses of fluoride cause loss of appetite and body weight, muscular weakness, clonic convulsions, pulmonary congestion and respiratory and cardiac failure.

Chronic exposure to fluoride most often comes through consumption of drinking water, usually from deep wells drilled through or near fluoride-containing rocks. Levels of fluoride around 2 ppm or higher produce a permanent brownish mottling of tooth enamel when the exposure is during the time of tooth formation.

Iodine

Deficiency Syndrome, Function and Metabolism—The iodine-deficiency disease is goiter (see *The Thyroid Hormones*, page 1082). In iodine-deficient young, growth is depressed and sexual development is delayed, the skin and hair are typically rough and the hair becomes thin. Cretinism, feeble-mindedness and deaf-mutism occur in a severe deficiency. There is reproductive failure in the female and decreased fertility in the male.

Goiter has been observed in human beings in many areas of the world, with incidence in women and children usually higher than in the adult male. As a public-health measure, use of iodized salt has markedly reduced the incidence of goiter. Goitrogens also can cause goiter (see *Antithyroid Compounds*, page 1086).

The only known function of iodine is for the production of the thyroid hormones, which regulate cellular oxidation.

The absorption of iodide can occur at all levels of the gastrointestinal tract. Iodinated amino acids can be absorbed as such, but less efficiently than iodide. Excretion of iodine is primarily via the urine, and the amount is a reasonably good indicator of thyroid status. Iodine in saliva is reabsorbed.

Iron

Deficiency Syndrome and Function—Hypochromic microcytic anemia is the characteristic result of iron deficiency. Depending on the severity, the anemia is accompanied by listlessness and tiredness, palpitation on exertion, sore tongue, angular stomatitis, dysphagia and koilonychia.

Iron is an essential component of several important metalloproteins. These include hemoglobin, myoglobin and many oxidation-reduction enzymes. In iron deficiency, there may be reduced concentrations of some of the iron-containing enzymes, such as cytochrome c in liver, kidney and skeletal muscle and succinic dehydrogenase in the kidney and heart.

Metabolism—Iron is absorbed from the small intestine; however, the exact mechanism regulating the amount absorbed is still a matter of controversy. The proportion of dietary iron absorbed is greater in iron-deficient anemic individuals. Iron is transported via the blood, in which it is bound to transferrin, a β_1-globulin.

The iron from deteriorated red blood cells is reutilized. Under normal circumstances, the loss of iron from the body is very small, about 1 mg a day for men and an additional average daily loss of 0.5 mg a day by menstruating women. Iron is stored in the bone marrow, intestinal wall, liver and spleen, with the latter organs containing the largest amounts.

Bioavailability—The recognition of anemia as a major public-health problem for menstruating women and young children throughout the world has focused on the need for more extensive and better fortification of foods. This has stimulated a great deal of research on the availability of iron from foods and inorganic sources. Iron compounds that are utilized readily by experimental animals and man are ferric ammonium citrate, ferrous sulfate, ferrous gluconate, ferrous fumarate and ferrous ammonium sulfate. Average to poor sources of iron are reduced iron, ferric chloride and ferric pyrophosphate, whereas very poor sources are ferric oxide, ferrous carbonate, sodium iron pyrophosphate and ferric orthophosphate. The availability of iron from foods can vary also.

Several dietary components can affect the availability of iron from many sources. Phytic acid and antacids can decrease iron absorption. The availability of iron is increased by a variety of reducing compounds such as ascorbic acid and molecules with sulfhydryl groups, as well as histidine and lysine. The smaller the particle size of elemental iron, the greater is the intestinal absorption and utilization. Heme iron is absorbed as such. Very high intakes of zinc, copper, manganese and cadmium can decrease the absorption of iron. Many additional studies are needed to evaluate adequately the availability of iron as influenced by composition of the diet and method of food preparation.

Toxicity—Because iron absorption is regulated by the body, moderate excess above the RDA was considered harmless. Recent epidemiological data suggest that continued high intake of iron may raise the risk for chronic disease occurrence, particularly those which are increased with free radical formations such as cancer. Deaths have occurred, however, in children who swallowed capsules or tablets containing a readily available source of iron, such as ferrous sulfate. Acute effects include vomiting, hematemesis, hepatic damage, tachycardia and peripheral vascular collapse.

Some individuals have a metabolic defect so that their iron absorption is not carefully controlled, and even a normal iron intake can lead to excess tissue accumulation. A disease known as hemochromatosis results. It usually can be controlled by phlebotomy at periodic intervals; however death can result if the disease is not treated.

Manganese

Deficiency Syndrome and Function—Manganese deficiency has been produced experimentally in many animals. Characteristics of the deficiency include growth depressions of the young animal, skeletal abnormalities (ranging from mild rarefaction to crippling deformities), mortality of the young, perosis (slipping of the Achilles tendon and accompanying joint deformity) in birds, depressed reproduction of both males and females, nutritional chondrodystrophy of the chick embryo and ataxia in newborn mammals with head retraction, tremor, abnormal otoliths and semicircular canals in the ears. Newborn manganese-deficient guinea pigs have aplasia or marked hypoplasia of the pancreas. Manganese deficiency never has been recognized in man.

Manganese is required for the synthesis of mucopolysaccharides of cartilage and for the conversion of mevalonic acid to squalene. Glucose utilization is impaired in manganese deficiency. Pyruvate carboxylase is a manganese metalloenzyme.

Metabolism and Bioavailability—The homeostatic mechanism for regulating the concentration of manganese in the body is very precise. Manganese is absorbed from the small intestine and is then transported via the blood in the trivalent form bound to a β_1-globulin, transmanganin. Manganese is excreted in the bile and through the intestinal wall. The latter constitutes the principal mechanism for regulating the amounts of manganese in the tissues. With a high manganese intake, the element is also excreted in the pancreatic juice. The amount excreted in the urine is very small.

High levels of manganese occur in bone, liver, kidney, pancreas and the pituitary, whereas the concentration in the skeletal muscle is very low. The manganese in bone cannot be mobilized to meet a need. The stores of manganese, in the order of their importance, are found in the liver, skin and skeletal muscle. There is not a special store in the newborn.

In chick studies it was found that manganese was equally available from the oxide, carbonate, sulfate and chloride. High dietary intakes of calcium and phosphorus can decrease manganese absorption.

Toxicity—Miners exposed to manganese oxide dust for long periods of time develop psychiatric abnormalities that resemble schizophrenia. This is followed by crippling neurological disorders similar to those found in Parkinson's disease. Most young animals are unaffected by 1000 ppm of manganese in the diet.

Molybdenum

Deficiency Syndrome, Function and Metabolism—Adverse effects due to simple deficiency of molybdenum in man and in experimental animals have never been observed. Xanthine oxidase is an important molybdenum-containing enzyme. Due to a variety of indirect evidence and the importance of xanthine oxidase, molybdenum is considered to be an essential trace mineral for man, probably required in very small amounts. No RDA has been established.

Molybdenum supplied by water-soluble salts is absorbed readily. The element crosses the mammary gland easily. Excretion is into both urine and feces. The liver and kidney have the highest soft-tissue concentrations of molybdenum. Changes in level of dietary intake can be reflected in the concentrations in liver, kidney, skin, bones and hair. The newborn does not have special stores of the element. Sulfate can affect the absorption, tissue distribution and excretion of molybdenum. The content of molybdenum in erythrocytes decreases in many types of anemia.

Toxicity—The tolerance of animals to high intakes of molybdenum varies with species, age and the level of numerous other dietary components. The toxicity is decreased by copper, inorganic sulfate and the sulfur amino acids.

Nickel

Evidence that nickel is an essential element is based on abnormalities produced in chicks and rats fed diets containing 3 to 4 ppb of nickel. Lipid metabolism was affected. Rats maintained through successive generations on the nickel-deficient diet had increased fetal mortality.

Absorption of nickel is small from ordinary diets. Excretion is primarily through the feces; however, significant amounts can be lost in sweat. Phytate can form a very stable complex with nickel so it is possible that phytate may decrease absorption of nickel. Further studies are required to establish clearly the essentiality of nickel and its significance to human health.

A low level of toxicity has been established for nickel in rats, mice, monkeys and chicks.

Selenium

Deficiency Syndrome and Function—Depending on species, age and specific diet composition, a deficiency of selenium can lead to one or more of the following abnormalities: growth depression, muscular dystrophy, degeneration of the myocardium, neurological lesions, liver necrosis, pancreatic fibrosis, exudative diathesis, ceroid-pigment deposition in adipose tissue and death. Deficiency occurs in domestic animals with intakes below 0.02 to 0.05 ppm. Deficiency in man has only been demonstrated in China where extremely low intake causes a cardiomyopathy in children (Keshan disease). The NAS safe and adequate daily dietary intake of selenium are 10 to 80 μg for children and 50 to 200 μg for adults.

Most deficiency syndromes responsive to selenium also respond favorably to vitamin E. An exception is pancreatic fibrosis, which occurs only in selenium deficiency. Selenium is an essential component of the enzyme glutathione peroxidase. This provides a link between the antioxidant properties of vitamin E and the biological function of selenium in preventing most of the same selenium-deficiency problems. Animal studies have indicated that selenium may be useful as a chemoprevention agent but studies in man have not been accomplished. Experimentally, selenium has been shown to provide protection to pulmonary oxygen toxicity similar to that observed for vitamin E.

Metabolism—Selenium is absorbed from the duodenum. It can be metabolized to a variety of compounds and lost from the body via the bile, pancreatic and intestinal secretions, and ultimately through the feces, urine and expired air. Selenium can replace sulfur in the normal sulfur amino acids and selenite can also bind to sulfur amino acids. It also is incorporated into selenonucleosides and may be involved in genetic translation. The highest tissue concentrations of selenium occur in the kidney, pancreas, pituitary and liver.

Toxicity—Acute selenium toxicity is characterized by abdominal pain, excess salivation, grating of the teeth, paralysis and blindness. Eventually disturbed respiration leads to death.

Selenium is one of the most toxic of the essential nutrients and the quantitative separation of required and chronic toxic levels is not very large. The source of selenium has a significant impact on the level which will cause toxicity to develop. Organic compounds containing selenium enhance absorption and, therefore, are toxic at lower levels. For domestic animals, the requirement is about 0.1 to 0.2 ppm, and 3 to 4 ppm in the diet are beginning levels for chronic toxicity. Intakes above 500 μg for long periods of time are considered to present a risk of toxicity in man. A reported carcinogenicity for selenium is an elusive association that has not been clarified finally.

Silicon

With highly purified diets it has been possible to produce a deficiency of silicon in chicks and rats. The deficiency affected growth rate, bones and integumental tissues. The primary biochemical lesion in the deficient animals was an effect on the cartilage matrix.

Silicon (as silicates) is absorbed easily from the intestinal tract and excreted readily in the urine, in part as SiO_2. Silicon is distributed widely in soil, plants and animal tissues. It is relatively nontoxic; however, siliceous kidney stones have been reported in persons who live in regions with water high in silicate concentration or who chronically ingest magnesium trisilicate antacids.

Tin

Through rigid exclusion of environmental and dietary tin, it has been possible to produce growth retardation responsive to this element in rats. A maximal growth effect was obtained with 1 ppm of tin in the diet, a level similar to that found in many foods.

Tin is absorbed poorly and most of that in the diet is excreted in the feces. Tin has a low order of toxicity.

Vanadium

Chicks and rats fed a diet containing less than 10 ppb vanadium had slow growth, defective bones and altered lipid metabolism. Vanadium is a rather toxic element. The addition of 25 to 50 ppm vanadium to the diet of rats causes diarrhea and mortality.

Zinc

Deficiency Syndrome and Function—Zinc is required for growth of every animal species studied; therefore, growth depression of young animals is invariably observed if the zinc deprivation is severe enough. Other characteristics of deficiency include skin lesions, alopecia, abnormal feathering in birds, deformed and poorly mineralized bones, hyperkeratinization of the esophagus, reduced numbers of circulating lymphocytes, impaired reproduction in males and females, fetal abnormalities and decreased learning ability. Persons with impaired taste acuity and discrimination and delayed healing of wounds and burns have responded favorably to therapeutic doses of zinc in some cases.

Nutritional dwarfism has been studied extensively in the Middle East. The syndrome includes delayed sexual development, reduced height and weight, hepatosplenomegaly, spoon nails and usually anemia. Although the subjects were deficient to some degree in several nutrients, zinc was required for correcting the hypogonadism and growth depression. The syndrome occurs in both males and females. Indolent ulcers and delayed wound healing in patients with low plasma zinc levels has been reported, and both systemic and topical administration of zinc compounds is followed by accelerated healing. There is limited evidence that some young children and elderly persons in the US do not receive adequate zinc.

Zinc is known to occur in many important metalloenzymes. These include carbonic anhydrase, carboxypeptidases A and B, alcohol dehydrogenase, glutamic dehydrogenase, D-glyceraldehyde-3-phosphate dehydrogenase, lactic dehydrogenase, malic dehydrogenase, alkaline phosphatase, aldolase and others. Impaired synthesis of nucleic acids and proteins has been observed in zinc deficiency. There is some evidence that zinc may be involved in the secretion of insulin and in the function of the hormone. It appears to be a modulator of neurohumoral transmission.

Metabolism and Bioavailability—Zinc can bind readily to sulfhydryl groups, amino groups and imidazole groups of proteins, amino acids and other organic molecules.

Zinc is absorbed primarily from the duodenum. It binds to all proteins of the plasma; however, it is bound most loosely to albumin and this may be important for transport to and from tissues. The concentration of zinc in plasma decreases rapidly when a low-zinc diet is fed, and it is reduced in pregnancy and in women taking birth control pills. The principal route of excretion is via the feces. Small amounts of zinc are excreted daily in the urine; these increase when there is tissue catabolism such as occurs in burns and in fasting. Significant losses of zinc also can occur in the sweat.

Zinc is present in all tissues, with very high concentrations in the prostate and choroid of the eye. Generally, tissue concentrations are not affected greatly by zinc deficiency. The stores of zinc in the body are thought to be small.

Zinc is equally available to normal animals from a wide variety of inorganic salts as well as metallic zinc. Phytic acid markedly can decrease absorption of zinc, particularly in the presence of large amounts of calcium. Consumption of whole wheat bread, which contains phytic acid, has been shown to be primarily responsible for the zinc-deficiency dwarfism observed in the Middle East. The toxic effects of cadmium are probably partially related to interference with the normal physiological pathways and functions of zinc.

Toxicity—The taste threshold for a soluble salt of zinc in water is 15 ppm of zinc, whereas 40 ppm have a very definite taste. A dose of 225 to 450 mg of zinc has an emetic effect in an adult man. Acute toxicity of zinc is characterized by dehydration, electrolytic imbalance, stomach pain, lethargy, dizziness, muscular incoordination and renal failure. High zinc intakes are known to lower copper absorption and therefore consumption of zinc supplements should be done only with adequate intakes of copper. Zinc has been used successfully to treat Wilson's disease.

Zinc Sulfate—page 1271.

Bibliography

Beaton GH, McHenry EW, eds: *Nutrition: A Comprehensive Treatise*, 3 vols, Academic, New York, 1964 (1st & 2nd vols), 1966 (3rd vol).

Beeson PB, McDermott W, Wyngaarden JB, eds: *Textbook of Medicine*, 15th ed, Saunders, Philadelphia, 1979.

Chaney MS, Ross ML: *Nutrition*, 8th ed, Houghton-Mifflin, Boston, 1971.

Davidson S *et al*: *Human Nutrition and Dietetics*, 6th ed, Longman, London, 1975.

Fomon SJ: *Nutrition of The Normal Infant*, Mosby, St. Louis, 1993.

Shils ME, ed: *Modern Nutrition in Health and Disease*, 8th ed, Lea & Febiger, Philadelphia, 1993.

Mitchell HS *et al*: *Cooper's Nutrition in Health and Disease*, 15th ed, Lippincott, Philadelphia, 1968.

Pike RL, Brown ML: *Nutrition: An Integrated Approach*, Wiley, New York, 1975.

Robinson CH: *Normal and Therapeutic Nutrition*, 14th ed, Macmillan, New York, 1972.

Scott JM *et al.* *In, Olson RE, Bier DM, McCormick DB, eds: The Role of Nutrition in Neural Tube Defects*, Annual Review of Nutrition, Palo Alto, CA, 277, 1990.

Stanbury JB *et al:* *The Metabolic Basis of Inherited Disease*, 5th ed, McGraw-Hill, New York, 1983.

Underwood EJ: *Trace Elements in Human and Animal Nutrition*, 4th ed, Academic, New York, 1977.

Diet and Health: Implications for Reducing Chronic Disease Risk, NAS-NRC National Academy Press Washington, DC, 1989.

Recommended Dietary Allowances, NAS-NRC, Washington, DC, 1989.

The Surgeon General's Report on Nutrition and Health, US Dept of Health and Human Services, Public Health Service, DHHS (PHS) Publ No 88-50210, Washington DC, 1988.

Assay

Freed M, ed: *Methods of Vitamin Assay*, 3rd ed, Interscience, New York, 1966.

Joslyn MA, ed: *Methods in Food Analysis: Physical, Chemical and Instrumental Methods*, 2nd ed, Academic, New York, 1970.

Official Methods of Analysis, 15th ed, Assoc Off Anal Chem, Washington DC, 1990.

The United States Pharmacopeia, XXIInd rev, Mack, Easton PA, 1990.

Food Composition

Composition of Foods Raw-Processed-Prepared, USDA Handbook 8, Washington DC, 1976-1993; available from the USGPO.

Nutritive Value of Foods, Handbook 456, USDA, Washington DC, 1975; available from the USGPO.

Pennington JAT: Bowes & Church's: *Food Values of Portions Commonly Used*, 16th ed, Lippincott, Philadelphia, 1993.

CHAPTER 66

Enzymes

Michael R Franklin, PhD

Professor of Pharmacology
College of Pharmacy and School of Medicine
University of Utah
Salt Lake City, UT 84112

The functions of all living organisms depend on chemical reactions. For example, conversion of sugar to carbon dioxide and water with the release of energy proceeds through a series of chemical reactions, each of which requires a biological catalyst for the reaction to occur. Enzymes are proteins that serve as biological catalysts. Without these enzymes conditions for reaction would be required which would be incompatible with the life of the cell. Thus, enzymes play a vital role in the function of the normal cell.

The importance of enzymes in normal body function is illustrated dramatically in conditions where an enzyme is nonfunctional as a result of a disease state or a congenital abnormality. Patients with these "inborn errors of metabolism" are strikingly abnormal. Phenylketonuric infants who are born without the enzyme phenylalanine hydroxylase (which is responsible for the conversion of phenylalanine to tyrosine) develop motor disturbances, light coloration of the skin, hair and eyes and, and in early childhood (if not in infancy), remain mentally retarded.

Since most chemical reactions in the body require the action of an enzyme, these biological catalysts often serve as the focal point for the regulation of body function. Increased enzyme activity accelerates the formation of a given product that may be essential for a particular function. The synthesis of norepinephrine illustrates this principle well. Heart rate will increase when norepinephrine is released from the sympathetic nerves. Norepinephrine is synthesized through a series of enzymatic reactions of which the rate-limiting and, therefore the most important, regulating enzyme is tyrosine hydroxylase. Increased tyrosine hydroxylase activity brings about conversion of more tyrosine to dihydroxyphenylalanine (DOPA), which is converted by dopa decarboxylase to dopamine. Dopamine is converted to norepinephrine by the enzymatic activity of dopamine-β-hydroxylase. The formation of norepinephrine can be regulated by a number of factors, including a feedback mechanism. Increased levels of norepinephrine inhibit the enzyme tyrosine hydroxylase so that less norepinephrine is synthesized. Thus, levels of norepinephrine can control the amount of norepinephrine synthesized.

The actions of a considerable number of drugs representing a wide variety of pharmacological agents depend on an enzyme-drug interaction. Notable examples demonstrating this diversity are:

The hydrolysis of acetylcholine by cholinesterase is blocked in a competitive manner by physostigmine, and in a noncompetitive manner by diisopropyl fluorophosphate, organophosphate insecticides and several chemical warfare agents.

The oxidation of norepinephrine and serotonin by monoamine oxidase is inhibited by the antidepressant, phenelzine.

The oxidation of acetaldehyde to acetate by aldehyde dehydrogenase is inhibited by disulfiram.

The oxidation of arachidonic acid to prostaglandins by cyclooxygenase is inhibited by and is the common mode of action of nonsteroidal antiinflammatory drugs such as aspirin and indomethacin.

The hydrolysis of one of the cellular mediators of hormonal action, cyclic 3′,5′-adenosine monophosphate, by phosphodiesterase is inhibited by methylated xanthines, such as caffeine and theophylline.

The 11β-hydroxylation reaction in the synthesis of cortisol, corticosterone and aldosterone is inhibited by metyrapone.

The thyroid peroxidase responsible for the synthesis of thyroxine is inhibited by propylthiouracil and methimazole.

The conversion of xanthine to uric acid by xanthine oxidase is inhibited by allopurinol, which is used therefore in the treatment of gout.

The bacterial synthesis of the essential vitamin folic acid is competitively inhibited by the sulfonamide antibiotics.

The cancer chemotherapeutic agent fluorouracil is converted to a compound which inhibits the enzyme thymidylate synthetase which is needed for DNA synthesis.

These examples illustrate the importance of drug-enzyme interactions in the pharmacological actions of therapeutic agents. The actions of drugs of the future also undoubtedly will depend on drug-enzyme interaction. Indeed, the pharmacological action of many drugs currently being prescribed by the physician probably will be found to involve such interplay. Since enzymes are involved so intricately in regulation of function, it is only logical to suppose that drugs may increase or decrease function by stimulating or depressing enzyme activity, respectively. A knowledge of enzymes and their properties, therefore, becomes increasingly important to the pharmacist in order to understand the action of drugs.

In addition to the action, the pharmacokinetics, drug interactions and toxicities of many drugs depend on enzyme activity. The enzymes responsible for these phenomena are those generally termed drug-metabolizing enzymes and are located predominately in the liver. Contrary to most others, these enzymes typified by cytochrome P-450 and UDP-glucuronosyl transferase exhibit broad substrate specificity. The ability to metabolize a wide variety of drugs to more readily excretable products carries with it the potential for mutual competition when several drugs are administered simultaneously, thus altering the pharmacokinetics from that seen if a single drug is given. Toxicities arise from the two-phase nature of drug metabolism, the introduction of a reactive site suitable for conjugation and masking of that site with an endogenous polar molecule to form an excretable water-soluble conjugate. Failure to mask a reactive site allows it to interact with cell macromolecules (proteins, DNA, membranes) to produce cell damage, carcinogenesis or cell death.

Properties—Four properties of enzymes make them specialized catalysts.

1. Most enzymes will catalyze only a specific range of reactions and in many cases only one reaction will be catalyzed by a given enzyme. Some enzymes have a low degree of specificity; eg, pepsin hydrolyzes almost all soluble native proteins but the hydrolysis is limited to certain very specific peptide linkages. On the other hand, urease is a highly specific enzyme; its only known substrate is urea. Almost all enzymes show a high degree of spatial specificity. Arginase acts only on L-arginine; it does not attack D-arginine. The specificity of enzymes is one of their most fundamental and important properties.

2. Enzymes are exceedingly efficient. Most enzymatic reactions, under optimal conditions, proceed 10^8 to 10^{11} times more rapidly than the corresponding nonenzymatic reactions.

3. Enzymes as a group are exceptionally versatile catalysts. For example, they effectively catalyze hydrolytic reactions, dehydrations, acyl transfer reactions, oxidation–reduction reactions, polymerizations, aldol condensations and free-radical reactions.

4. Enzymes are subject to a variety of cellular controls. Their final concentration and rate of synthesis are under genetic control. In addition, enzymes can be present in the cell in both inactive as well as active forms. The rate of conversion from inactive to active form is influenced by environmental changes; eg, phosphorylase *b* is converted to phosphorylase *a* very rapidly through a series of reactions which are triggered by the release of catecholamines.

Nomenclature—Enzymes usually are named in terms of the reactions that are catalyzed. Usually, the suffix "-ase" is added to the name of the substrate upon which the enzyme acts, ie, the enzyme which attacks urea is urease, and arginine is acted upon by arginase. Enzymes also are classified according to the reaction they catalyze, eg, reductases and dehydrogenases. Some older names, which are unrelated to the function of the enzyme, remain in usage, eg, rennin, trypsin and pepsin.

The Commission on Enzymes of the International Union of Biochemistry has established a complete but rather complex system of classification and nomenclature. According to this classification enzymes are divided into six general groups:

1. *Oxidoreductases*—catalyzing oxidation–reduction reactions.
2. *Transferases*—catalyzing transfer of a chemical group from one molecule to another.
3. *Hydrolases*—catalyzing hydrolytic reactions.
4. *Lyases*—catalyzing the addition of groups to double bonds or *vice versa.*
5. *Isomerases*—catalyzing intramolecular rearrangements.
6. *Ligases* (also known as synthetases)—catalyzing the condensation of two molecules coupled with the cleavage of a pyrophosphate bond of ATP or similar triphosphate.

In this system every enzyme is coded in a four-number system according to the type of reaction catalyzed, type of isomerization, type of bond hydrolyzed, etc.

Many enzymes possess nonprotein chemical groups. Thus, an enzyme often can be dissociated into a protein component, an *apoenzyme* and a nonprotein component, a *prosthetic group.* Prosthetic groups also are referred to as coenzymes or cofactors. Vitamins and certain metals are examples of these prosthetic groups.

Despite the ubiquity of enzymes in normal physiology, and as the basis of many drug effects and drug interactions, the use of enzymes as drugs is extremely limited. Being proteinaceous they can be inactivated by conditions and enzymes present in the GI lumen if given orally and, if given parenterally, can elicit immune responses. Most of the enzymes currently available on the market are hydrolases (Group 3 above). These enzyme preparations are of limited use in: (1) debridement, ie, as aids in resolving and removing blood clots or fibrinous or purulent accumulations and (2) replacement therapy to correct certain gastrointestinal deficiencies.

Alteplase—page 924.

Asparaginase—page 1242.

Collagenase

Santyl (*Knoll*)

A product of *Clostridium histolyticum,* which breaks down native and denatured collagen in necrotic (not in healthy) tissue at physiological pH and temperature. It is a fermentation-produced enzyme complex.

Description—Fine, brown, amorphous powder; heat-labile.

Solubility—Soluble in water or alcohol.

Uses—Collagen comprises about 75% of the dry weight of the skin and is the main constituent of necrotic debris and of the eschar which covers the surface of an ulcer; hence, collagenase is indicated for debridement of severely burned areas and dermal ulcers. Its effectiveness in the treatment of other necrotic skin lesions requires further investigation. The enzyme is compatible with antibiotics such as polymyxin B sulfate, neomycin or bacitracin. It is adversely affected by heavy metal antiseptics, detergents and hexachlorophene so that these agents must be removed before using the enzyme.

Dose—The ointment (250 units/g) is applied daily (hospital) or every other day (outpatient) to the lesions and covered with sterile dressings.

Dosage Form—Ointment: 250 units/g White Petrolatum USP in 15- and 30-g tubes.

Hyaluronidase for Injection

Wydase (*Wyeth-Ayerst*)

A sterile, dry, soluble, enzyme product prepared from mammalian (bovine) testes and capable of hydrolyzing mucopolysaccharides of the hyaluronic acid type; its potency is not less than the labeled potency in Hyaluronidase Units and it contains not more than 0.25 μg of tyrosine for each Hyaluronidase Unit. It may contain a suitable stabilizer.

Description—White, odorless amorphous solid or a nearly colorless glass-like solid; it is destroyed by heat; its solutions are colorless.

Uses—Intercellular cement, which binds together the parenchymal cells of organs; appears to be a gel of highly polymerized polysaccharide, hyaluronic acid. The latter is present in all organs but is most abundant in tissues of mesenchymal origin (eg, connective tissue and blood vessels); the testis is the richest source of hyaluronidase in mammals. Hyaluronidase hydrolyzes hyaluronic acid by splitting the glucosaminidic bond between carbon-1 of the glucosamine moiety and carbon-4 of glucuronic acid. Hyaluronidase accelerates the subcutaneous spread of both particulate matter and solutions by depolymerizing the hyaluronic acid. This results in a larger area of distribution of drugs in the tissue spaces and facilitates their absorption.

The chief clinical use of hyaluronidase is to facilitate administration of fluids by hypodermoclysis. It has been used as an adjunct in subcutaneous urography for improving resorption of radiopaque agents and to enhance absorption of drugs in tissue spaces, transudates and various edemas. Its use with local anesthetics is not recommended. Hyaluronidase should not be used in infected areas because of the danger of spreading the infection.

Dose—*Usual, hypodermoclysis,* **150 units.**

Other Dose Information—A dose of 150 units is dissolved in 1 mL of isotonic NaCl solution and either added to 1000 mL of hypodermoclysis fluid or injected at the proposed site of infusion. In order to avoid overhydration the rate of administration should not exceed that employed for intravenous infusion.

Dosage Forms—for Injection: 150 and 1500 units; Injection: 150 units/mL.

Lactase

Lactaid (*Lactaid*); (*Various Mfrs*)

A β-D-galactosidase derived from *Kluyveromyces lactis* yeast.

Uses—Added to, or ingested with, milk to convert the disaccharide lactose into glucose and galactose for patients suffering from lactase insufficiency.

Dosage Forms—Drops, for addition to milk; Caplets, for swallowing with meals containing dairy products.

Malt Extract—page 1399.

Pancreatic Enzymes

A substance containing enzymes, principally amylase, protease and lipase, obtained from the pancreas of the hog, *Sus scrofa* Linné var. *domesticus* Gray (Fam *Suidae*) or of the ox, *Bos taurus* Linné (Fam *Bovidae*).

Pancreatin contains, in each mg, not less than 2 Units of lipase activity, not less than 25 Units of amylase activity and not less than 25 Units of protease activity. Pancreatin of a higher digestive power may be labeled as a whole-number multiple of the three minimum activities or may be diluted by admixture with lactose, or with sucrose containing not more than 3.25% of starch, or with pancreatin of lower digestive power.

Pancrelipase contains, in each mg, not less than 24 Units of lipase activity, not less than 100 Units of amylase activity and not less than 100 Units of protease activity.

Description—Cream-colored, amorphous powders, having a faint, characteristic, but not offensive, odor. They hydrolyze fats to glycerol and fatty acids, change protein into proteoses and derived substances and convert starch into dextrins and sugars. Their greatest activities are in neutral or slightly alkaline media; more than traces of mineral acids or large amounts of alkali hydroxides render them inert. An excess of alkali carbonate also inhibits their action.

Solubility—Slowly and incompletely soluble in water; insoluble in alcohol.

Incompatibilities—*Mineral acids* or excess *alkali hydroxides* or carbonates render it inert. They are precipitated by *strong alcoholic solutions* and by many *metallic salts.*

Uses—In the treatment of patients with cystic fibrosis (mucoviscidosis), chronic pancreatitis, partial or complete surgical pancreatectomy, and other conditions associated with exocrine pancreatic insufficiency. The administration of pancreatin decreases the nitrogen and fat content of

Table 1—Pancreatic Enzymes: Dose and Dosage Forms

Trade name (*Mfr*)	Lipase[a]	Protease[a]	Amylase[a]	Dose
Pancrease-MT (*McNeil*)				
Capsules				In units of lipase activity: *children, 6 mo to 1 yr,* 2000 Units/meal; *1 to 6 yr,* 4000 to 8000 Units/meal; *7 to 12 yr,* 4000 to 12,000 Units/meal; *adults,* 4000 to 16,000 Units/meal.
MT4	4	12	12	
MT10	10	30	30	
MT16	16	48	48	
MT25	25	75	75	
Cotazym-S (*Organon*)	8	30	30	1 to 3 capsules prior to each meal or snack.
8X Pancreatin (*Vitaline*)				
Tablets	22.5	180	180	1 or 2 tablets with each meal; 1 tablet with a snack.
Creon (*Solvay*)				
Capsules	8	13	30	Same as above.
Ku-Zyme-HP (*Schwarz*)				
Capsules	8	30	30	1 to 3 capsules with each meal.
VioKase (*Robins*)				
Tablets	8	30	30	Same as above.
Powder	16.8	70	70	For *cystic fibrosis,* ¼ tsp (0.7 g) with meals.
Zymase (*Organon*)				
Capsules	12	24	24	1 or 2 capsules with each meal.

[a] In thousands of USP Units/dosage unit.

the stool. The use of pancreatin except in pancreatic insufficiency is of no known value. The efficacy of pancreatin in the treatment of gaseous distention has not been demonstrated. When treating pancreatic insufficiency, a high-caloric diet which is high in protein and low in fat is recommended. A significant amount of the enzyme activity can be lost by peptic digestion during passage through the stomach. The efficacy of pancreatin is enhanced by simultaneous administration of cimetidine which increases intragastric pH. Dietary and enzyme regimens are best based on repeated clinical evaluation and, in hospitalized patients, periodic measurements of fecal fat and nitrogen loss. Since the underlying pancreatic deficiency is unchanged, replacement pancreatin therapy is permanent. At high doses, pancreatin can cause nausea, abdominal cramps and diarrhea. The enzyme dust is irritating to the nasal membrane so inhalation should be avoided.

Dose—See Table 1.

Dosage Forms—See Table 1.

Papain

Panafil (*Rystan*)

A proteolytic enzyme from the fruit of the tropical melon tree, *Carica papaya.* It exhibits broad-spectrum specificity over a wide pH range, including peptides, amides, esters and thioesters, all being susceptible to papain-catalyzed hydrolysis. Nonviable protein is susceptible, but it is harmless to viable tissue.

Uses—In the debridement of necrotic tissue.

Dosage Forms—Ointment (10%) combined with the urea (which denatures nonviable protein matter present in lesions and also releases papain activators). Also available as a 0.5% copper-chlorophyll complex.

Sutilains

Travase (*Boots*)

A substance, containing proteolytic enzymes, derived from the bacterium *Bacillus subtilis.* Elaborated by fermentation with *B subtilis* and purified by filtration, salt and solvent precipitation, and lyophilization. Potency: not less than 2,500,000 Casein Units of proteolytic activity/g.

Description—Cream-colored odorless powder; *do not taste* (irritating to oral membranes); stable in light, hygroscopic and decomposes in solvents.

Solubility—1 g in 100 mL of water; insoluble in alcohol or other organic solvents.

Uses—An adjunct to established methods of wound care for biochemical debridement of the following lesions: 2nd- and 3rd-degree burns, decubitus ulcers, incisional, traumatic and pyrogenic wounds, and ulcers secondary to peripheral vascular disease. The enzyme digests denatured proteins found in necrotic tissues and a moist environment is essential to optimal enzyme activity. Detergents and antiseptics may render the substrate refractory, and heavy-metal antibacterials may denature the enzyme. It is contraindicated for wounds communicating with body cavities or those containing exposed nerves or nervous tissue, for fungating neoplastic ulcers and in wounds in women of childbearing potential. It should not be allowed to come in contact with the eyes. If this should occur inadvertently, the eyes should be rinsed immediately with copious amounts of water (preferably sterile water).

Dose—*Topical,* to the cleansed and moist wound, 3 to 4 times a day.

Dosage Form—Ointment: 82,000 Casein Units of proteolytic activity/g in 95% mineral oil and 5% polyethylene.

Crystallized Trypsin

Granulex (*Hickam*)

A proteolytic enzyme crystallized from an extract of the pancreas of the ox, *Bos taurus* Linné (Fam *Bovidae*); its potency is not less than 25,000 Trypsin Units/mg.

Description—White to yellowish white, odorless or amorphous powder.

Solubility—An amount equivalent to 500,000 Units Soluble in 10 mL water or saline TS; pH (1% soln) 3.0 to 5.5; max activity at pH 8.

Uses—Promotes proteolysis of a variety of protein substrates, including clotted blood, purulent exudates (pus) and necrotic tissue, but not living tissue. Especially in the presence of blood its duration of action is limited, because of the presence of inhibiting substrates. Solutions also have been inhaled to liquefy viscous sputum.

Dosage Form—Aerosol: 0.12 mg Trypsin/mL together with Peru Balsam and castor oil for debridement of eschar and other necrotic tissue.

Other Enzymes

Fibrinolysin and Desoxyribonuclease [Elase (*Parke-Davis*)]—A mixture of fibrinolysin of bovine plasma and desoxyribonuclease obtained from bovine pancreas. These two enzymes function together when used topically to lyse fibrin and liquefy pus, thus aiding in the removal of necrotic material both from the skin and certain body cavities. It is used as a debriding agent in surgical wounds, ulcerative lesions and 2nd and 3rd degree burns, and is used intravaginally in severe cervicitis and vaginitis. It is not suitable for parenteral use and is not to be used in thromboembolic diseases. The commercial product named above is supplied as a lyophilized powder (25 units of fibrinolysin and 15,000 units of deoxyribonuclease), from which a solution for topical use may be prepared, and in ointment form (30 units of fibrinolysin and 20,000 units of deoxyribonuclease). It also is available combined with 1% chloramphenicol.

Digestive Aids

Numerous preparations, both prescription and OTC, are available as aids for digestion, particularly for conditions where deficiencies of natural digestive enzymes exist. They contain some or all of the following categories of enzymes: amylolytic, proteolytic, cellulytic and lipolytic. In addition, the preparations often include bile salts or bile extracts.

CHAPTER 67

General Anesthetic Drugs

Michael A Ashburn, MD
Associate Professor of Anesthesiology
University of Utah Health Sciences Center
Sale Lake City, UT 84132

Anesthetics are drugs which produce anesthesia, a condition of partial or complete loss of sensation. Two types of anesthesia are usually recognized: local anesthesia and general anesthesia. In *local anesthesia*, the anesthesia is confined to a portion of the body and the patient is usually conscious (see Chapter 68). General anesthetics induce unconsciousness and loss of sensation. This type of anesthesia is employed for most surgical operations and is the subject of this chapter.

The general anesthetic drugs may, for convenience in presentation, be divided into two groups: inhalation anesthetics and intravenous anesthetics. The first group includes the volatile liquids and gases and the second group, the rapidly acting barbiturates and nonbarbiturates.

An ideal general anesthetic would be an agent with rapid onset of effect as well as rapid recovery when the drug is discontinued. In addition, the drug would lead to analgesia, muscle relaxation, amnesia, be physically stable, nonflammable, nonarrhythomogenic, resistant to biodegradation and nontoxic. Unfortunately, no such drug exists. The extent to which existing anesthetics can exert the desired effects is variable. Since no single anesthetic agent meets all objectives, the practice of anesthesia involves the use of multiple agents. Each agent is selected to obtain a desired effect while decreasing the incidence and severity of undesired effects. This technique is referred to as balanced anesthesia.

This chapter will review the agents commonly used to provide general anesthesia. Other agents used during the conduct of anesthesia, such as opioids, benzodiazepines and muscle relaxants, are discussed elsewhere.

Inhalation Anesthetics

Inhaled anesthetics remain the most frequently used agents for the maintenance of anesthesia. Intravenous agents are used most frequently to induce anesthesia, but inhaled anesthetics also are used for this purpose, especially in children. Three expressions are used commonly to characterize the properties of inhaled anesthetics. (1) Vapor pressure (vp), in torr (1/760 of atmosphere) at 20°, is used as a measure of volatility; (2) the blood-gas partition coefficient at 37° (blood/gas) is used to describe the rate at which the partial pressure of an inhalation anesthetic in the arterial blood approaches that in the alveoli. When solubility is low, equilibrium is approached rapidly and (3) clinical potency is defined in terms of the minimal alveolar concentration (MAC) necessary to prevent movement in 50% of individuals subjected to a painful stimulus, such as skin incision. Values for these expressions are shown in the respective monographs.

The administration of an anesthetic results in progressive depression of the central nervous system, which may be preceded by varying degrees of excitation. These drugs first depress the cerebral cortex and then the basal ganglia and cerebellum. This is followed first by sensory and then motor paralysis of the functions of the spinal cord from below, upward. If the administration of the anesthetic is increased to high levels, the medullary centers become affected and death may result from paralysis of the respiratory and vasomotor centers.

Chloroform—page 1409.

Cyclopropane—see RPS-18, page 1043.

Desflurane

Ethane, (±)-2-(difluoromethoxy)-1,1,2,2-tetra-fluoro-,
Suprane (*Anaquest*)

```
    F  H     F
    |  |     |
F — C — C — O — C — H
    |  |     |
    F  F     F
```

[57041-67-5]$C_3H_2F_6O$(168.04)

Description—Extremely volatile; non-flammable and not explosive at clinical concentrations.

Solubility—Insoluble in water; soluble in organic solvents.

Uses—Desflurane (vp-644 torr, blood/gas-0.42, MAC-7.3%) is the most recent inhaled anesthetic to be introduced into clinical use in the US. Desflurane has a very rapid onset, much more rapid than seen with isoflurane or halothane. Recovery from anesthesia also is more rapid than with other available inhaled anesthetics. The recovery from anesthesia with desflurane is comparable to that seen with propofol and alfentanil.

Desflurane is very resistant to metabolism. It is stable in soda lime, even at elevated temperatures. In man, desflurane undergoes little or no metabolism, even after hepatic stimulation with barbiturates or ethanol. Serum fluoride levels are very low, several times lower than that seen with isofluorane. Hepatotoxicity or nephrotoxicity rarely, if ever, occur.

Desflurane has a vapor pressure of approximately 1 atmosphere at room temperature (644 torr at 20°), and requires the use of new vaporizer technology.

It leads to dose-related decreases in blood pressure and cardiac output similar to that seen with isoflurane. While increases in heart rate are small with low concentrations of desflurane, concentrations higher than 1 MAC can lead to tachycardia. Induction with desflurane can lead to transient tachycardia and hypertension. As with isoflurane, desflurane has minimal arrhythomogenic potential.

It can be very irritating to the airway. Induction with desflurane can provoke coughing or breath-holding at concentrations greater than 7%. Inhalation induction is not recommended for children. As opposed to isoflurane, a slow induction with desflurane increases rather than decreases signs of airway irritability.

Desflurane depresses respiration; $PaCO_2$ is increased and the response to increases in $PaCO_2$ is depressed. Concentrations higher than 1.5 MAC may produce apnea.

Desflurane has potent muscle relaxant properties and endotracheal intubation often can be completed without the use of additional muscle relaxants. The depression of neuromuscular function is dose related.

Dose—*Induction:* adults, induction can be begun with **3%** desflurane, and then increased in **0.5** to **1.0%** increments every 2 to 3 breaths. End-tidal concentrations of 4 to 11% desflurane, with and without nitrous oxide, produces anesthesia within 2 to 4 min. *Maintenance, surgical levels of anesthesia in adults* may be maintained with concentrations of **2.5** to **8.5%** desflurane, with or without nitrous oxide. *Children, surgical levels of anesthesia* may be maintained with concentrations of **5.2** to **10%** desflurane, with or without nitrous oxide.

Dosage Form—Liquid: 240 mL.

Enflurane

Ethane, 2-chloro-1-(difluoromethoxy)-1,1,2-trifluoro-, Ethrane (*Anaquest*)

```
    F     F  F
    |     |  |
H—C—O—C—C—H
    |     |  |
    F     F  Cl
```

2-Chloro-1,1,2-trifluoroethyl difluoromethyl ether [13838-16-9] $C_3H_2ClF_5O$ (184.49).

Preparation—May be synthesized by a series of reactions starting with trifluorochloroethylene. US Pats 3,469,011 and 3,527,813.

Description—Clear, colorless, volatile liquid; pleasant hydrocarbon-like odor; boils at 56.6°; nonflammable.

Solubility—Soluble in water to the extent of 0.275%, and water-soluble in enflurane to the extent of 0.13%; miscible with organic solvents.

Uses—Enflurane (vp-172 torr, blood/gas-2.11, MAC-1.68%) is a methyl ethyl ether derivative which was introduced for clinical use in 1973. Enflurane has intermediate solubility in blood and is very potent, thus causing rapid onset and recovery from anesthesia. It can be used alone, or in combination with other anesthetics, frequently nitrous oxide.

It does not require a preservative, such as thymol; it is resistant to metabolism and unlikely to lead to hepatotoxicity. About 2.4% of the absorbed dose is metabolized; the most important metabolite is fluoride. High concentrations of fluoride is associated with high output renal failure. This occurs with fluoride levels of 50 μm/L or greater, which can be seen with enflurane use at 1 MAC for 9.6 hr. An increase in enflurane metabolism is seen in patients receiving isoniazid and in obese patients.

Enflurane, like halothane, is a myocardial depressant. Cardiac output is decreased to 70% of normal at 1 MAC and 65% of normal at 2 MAC. Enflurane can cause a dose-dependent increase in heart rate, up to a 40% increase at 2 MAC. Enflurane does not enhance the arrhythmogenecity of epinephrine.

Dose—*Induction,* **2.0** to **4.5%** in oxygen alone or with oxygen-nitrous oxide mixtures. Induction usually requires 7 to 10 min. Maintenance usually is accomplished with 0.5 to 3% concentrations.

Dosage Form—Liquid: 125 and 250 mL.

Ether—see RPS-18, page 1041.

Ethyl Chloride—see RPS-18, page 1043.

Ethylene—see RPS-18, page 1044.

Fluoroxene—see RPS-18, page 1043.

Halothane

Ethane, 2-bromo-2-chloro-1,1,1-trifluoro-, Fluothane (*Wyeth-Ayerst*)

```
     Br  F
     |   |
H—C—C—F
     |   |
     Cl  F
```

2-Bromo-2-chloro-1,1,1-trifluoroethane [151-67-7] $C_2HBrClF_3$ (197.38); contains 0.008–0.012% of thymol, by weight, as a stabilizer.

Preparation—Commercially available 2-chloro-1,1,1-trifluoroethane is subjected to direct bromination and halothane is isolated from the reaction product by fractional distillation.

Description—Colorless, mobile, nonflammable, heavy liquid; characteristic odor resembling that of chloroform; sweet taste and produces a burning sensation; distils between 49 and 51°; specific gravity between 1.872 and 1.877 at 20°.

Solubility—Slightly soluble in water; miscible with alcohol, chloroform, ether or and fixed oils.

Uses—Halothane (vp-243 torr, blood/gas-2.3, MAC-0.77%) was synthesized in 1951 and introduced into clinical practice in 1956 and is the most frequently used anesthetic for inhalation induction. Halothane has an intermediate solubility in blood and a high potency, which allows for rapid onset and recovery from anesthesia. It can be used alone or in combination with other anesthetics, frequently nitrous oxide.

Halothane is susceptible to decomposition to many compounds, including hydrochloric acid, hydrobromic acid, chloride, bromide and phosgene. Because of this, halothane is stored in amber-colored bottles and thymol is added to prevent spontaneous oxidative deocmposition. Thymol remains in vaporizers following the administration of halothane, and can cause malfunction of some of the vaporizer components.

Halothane is a myocardial depressant. Cardiac output is decreased to 80% of normal at 1 MAC, 70% of normal at 2 MAC, and 45% of normal at 2.5 MAC. Halothane sensitizes the myocardium to the action of epinephrine and norepinephrine; injection of these drugs during halothane anesthesia may induce ventricular arrhythmias. In patients who are breathing spontaneously, halothane leads to CO_2 retention. In addition, halothane may decrease the ventilatory response to hypoxemia.

Halothane undergoes both oxidative and reductive metabolism. Up to 20% of the absorbed agent undergoes oxidative metabolism, producing trifluoracetic acid, chloride and bromide. Rarely, bromide toxicity can occur when bromide levels are 6 meq/L or higher, leading to somnolence and mental confusion. Reductive metabolism is more likely to occur during hepatocyte hypoxemia or as a result of stimulation of hepatocyte activity by certain drugs. Reductive metabolism results in reactive metabolites and fluoride ion. The reactive metabolites appear to cause direct damage to the hepatocyte and can lead to hypersensitivity. Very rarely, patients who become hypersensitive may experience increased hepatocyte destruction after a second exposure to halothane and significant liver damage can occur. Presence of fluoride after halothane administration may be indicative of reductive metabolism.

Dose—By *inhalation* as required.

Other Dose Information—For *induction,* **1** to **4%** vaporized by a flow of oxygen or nitrous oxide-oxygen mixture. For *maintenance,* **0.5** to **1.5%.**

Dosage Form—Liquid: 125 and 250 mL.

Isoflurane

Ethane, 2-chloro-2-(difluoromethoxy)-1,1,1-trifluor-, Forane, AErrane [Veterinary] (*Anaquest)*

```
  F
  |
HC—O—CHCF3
  |     |
  F     Cl
```

1-Chloro-2,2,2-trifluoroethyl difluoromethyl ether [26675-46-7] $C_3H_2ClF_5O$ (184.49).

Preparation—Trifluoroethanol is methylated with dimethyl sulfate to form the methyl ether which is then chlorinated to the dichloromethyl ether, $CF_3CHClOCHCl_2$. This latter compound, on treatment with HF/$SbCl_5$ forms the product. See *J Med Chem 14:* 517, 1971.

Description—Low-boiling liquid (48.5°) with a slight odor; nonflammable.

Solubility—Miscible with most organic solvents including fats or oils; practically insoluble in water.

Uses—Isoflurane (vp-240 torr, blood/gas-1.46, MAC-1.2%), is an isomer of enflurane and was introduced into clinical practice in 1981. Isoflurane has an intermediate solubility an a high potency, which allows for rapid onset and recovery from anesthesia. However, its pungency limits the rate of induction—too rapid an increase in the inspired concentration can lead to breath holding, coughing or laryngospasm.

Isoflurane is very stable and undergoes no detectable deterioration during 5 yr of storage or with exposure to soda lime or sunlight. Therefore, it contains no preservatives. In man, isoflurane is resistant to metabolism. Only 0.2% of the absorbed drug is metabolized. The most important metabolite is fluoride, but fluoride levels are clinically unimportant, and isoflurane has little or no renal or hepatic toxicity.

Isoflurane can cause up to a 20% non-dose-dependent increase in heart rate. Isoflurane has minimal effect on myocardial contractility at clinical doses. Cardiac output is not affected at 1 MAC, and is decreased to 90% of normal at 2 MAC. Cardiac output is maintained because isoflurane can cause up to a 50% decrease in systemic vascular resistance. It is probably a mild beta-agonist, and has been implicated in the coronary steal phenomenon in animal models. However, the clinical significance of this in man is debatable.

Halothane, enflurane and isoflurane all cause some bronchodilation in lungs with bronchospasm, but isoflurane is the most bronchodilating of the three agents. Isoflurane has significant muscle relaxant properties and often causes sufficient muscle relaxation for many operations.

Dose—*Induction:* Inspired concentrations of **1.5** to **3.0%** usually produce surgical anesthesia in 7 to 10 min. *Maintenance:* Surgical levels of anesthesia can be sustained with **1.0** to **2.5%** concentrations when nitrous oxide is used concomitantly. An additional 0.5 to 1.0% may be required when isoflurane is used with oxygen alone.

Dosage Form—Liquid: 100 mL.

Methoxyflurane—see RPS-18, page 1042.

Nitrous Oxide

Dinitrogen Monoxide; Laughing Gas

Nitrogen oxide (N_2O) [10024-97-2]; contains not less than 99.0%, by volume, of N_2O (44.01). The remainder is chiefly nitrogen.

Preparation—Usually by heating ammonium nitrate to about 170° to produce nitrous oxide and water.

Nitrous oxide is furnished in compressed form in metallic cylinders.

Description—Colorless gas, without appreciable odor or taste; specific gravity 1.53; 1 L, at a pressure of 760 mm at 0°, weighs about 1.97 g.

Solubility—1 volume dissolves in about 1.4 volumes of water at 20° under normal pressure; freely soluble in alcohol; soluble in ether or oils.

Uses—Nitrous oxide (blood/gas-0.47, MAC-101%) is a low molecular weight, odorless inhaled anesthetic of weak to moderate potency. It is considered to be nonflammable, but will support combustion. Nitrous oxide is not very soluble in blood, which leads to rapid onset of effect as well as rapid rapid recovery when the drug is discontinued. Because of its relatively low potency, nitrous oxide cannot be used as the sole agent to achieve general anesthesia. However, it often is used in combination with one of the other more potent inhaled anesthetics, thus decreasing the necessary concentration of both. Animal studies have shown nitrous oxide to be teratogenic; however, studies in man are inconclusive. The FDA advises health professionals who are or may become pregnant that chronic occupational exposure to nitrous oxide may pose a risk to the fetus.

Dose—By *inhalation, sedation,* **25%;** *analgesia,* **25** to **50%;** *maintenance,* **30** to **70%**. Administered with at least 25 to 30% oxygen.

Dosage Form—Supplied in blue metallic cylinders.

Sevoflurane

Propane, 1,1,1,3,3,3-hexafluoro-2-(fluoro-methoxy)-,

CF_3CHCF_3 with OCH_2F on the central carbon

[28523-86-6] $C_4H_3F_7O$ (200.06)

Description—Non-flammable, highly volatile.

Solubility—Insoluble in water.

Uses—Sevoflurane (vp-160 torr, blood/gas-0.6, MAC-1.71%) is a new inhaled anesthetic expected to be available soon in the US. Sevoflurane is half as soluble in blood than isoflurane, and induction of anesthesia is achieved rapidly and easily. In addition, recovery is more rapid than seen with isoflurane, enflurane and halothane.

Sevoflurane is not stable and it undergoes decomposition in soda lime, producing at least one alkylating agent. In man, sevoflurane is metabolized extensively, producing inorganic fluoride. Plasma fluoride concentrations average 22 μM/L after 1 hr of administration, and prolonged exposure can produce levels in excess of 50 μM/L. Metabolism of sevoflurane is increased by pretreatment with compounds that induce hepatic enzymes, such as phenobarbital or ethanol. However, sevoflurane has been used extensively in Japan with few reports of hepatotoxicity or nephrotoxicity associated with its use.

As with other inhaled anesthetics, sevoflurane is a cardiorespiratory depressant. Heart rate is not effected by sevoflurane as it is with isoflurane. This probably is due to depression of sympathetic activity without alteration of parasympathetic activity. Sevoflurane is not arrhythomogenic.

Dose—*Induction, inspired concentrations* of **2** to **3.5%** produce rapid onset of general anesthesia. *Maintenance, surgical levels of anesthesia* can be sustained with **1.5** to **2.5%** concentrations. MAC is decreased to 0.66% with the addition of 63% nitrous oxide.

Dosage Forms—Sevoflurane currently is not available in the US.

Intravenous Anesthetics

Intravenous anesthetics differ from inhalation anesthetics in that, once injected, there is practically nothing that can be done to facilitate their removal or alter the course of effects. The time course of effects from induction and rapidly deepening anesthesia to gradual emergence depends almost entirely on progressive redistribution of these drugs within the body. Understanding the pharmacokinetics of the intravenous anesthetics is important to their sound, safe and practical use. Pharmacokinetics allows predictions about drug concentrations in the body as related to dosage, time and physiological and pathological alteration in biological functions. It also may provide preliminary indications of the likelihood and types of drug interactions that may be encountered.

Historically, barbiturates have been used to induce general anesthesia. However, since barbiturates are poor analgesics and have relatively long elimination half-lives, they seldom are used alone to maintain general anesthesia. Barbiturates and nonbarbiturate anesthetics have been used mainly for induction of anesthesia and for short operative procedures. However, with the introduction of newer agents, such as propofol, intravenous anesthetics are being used for maintenance of anesthesia, particularly for outpatient procedures.

The general principles which apply to the use of intravenous anesthetics are the same as those that govern the use of other general anesthetic agents.

Adverse reactions commonly encountered may include the following:

Induction Complications—Excitatory phenomena (eg, tremors and involuntary muscle movements mostly involving the limbs); respiratory upset (eg, cough, hiccup, laryngospasm); respiratory depression; cardiovascular changes.

Tissue Irritation and Damage (drug and solvent)—Pain on injection and venous complications; effects of accidental arterial injection.

Recovery Reactions—Psychic phenomena (eg, dreaming, hallucinations, dissociative phenomena, delirium, anxiety and agitation, emotional reactions, long-term effects of frequent repeated administrations); motor phenomena (eg, increased tone, tremors and convulsions); effects on pain; nausea and vomiting.

Hypersensitivity or Idiosyncratic Reactions—True allergy–immune-based anaphylaxis; idiosyncratic–anaphylactoid reactions.

The most frequently encountered adverse reactions will be described in each monograph.

Alfentanil Hydrochloride—page 1203.

Droperidol—page 1183.

Etomidate

1*H*-Imidazole-5-carboxylic acid, 1-(1-phenylethyl)-, ethyl ester, (+)-, Amidate (*Abbott*)

CH_3CH_2OOC–imidazole–N–$CH(CH_3)$–phenyl

(+)-Ethyl 1-(α-methylbenzyl)imidazole-5-carboxylate [33125-97-2] $C_{14}H_{16}N_2O_2$ (244.99).

Preparation—From a-methylbenzyl amine and ethyl chloroacetate in 8 steps.

Description—White or yellow crystals or amorphous; melts about 67°.

Solubility—Insoluble in water; soluble in common polar organic solvents.

Uses—Etomidate, a nonbarbiturate hypnotic without analgesic activity, is injected intravenously for *induction* of general anesthesia. It also is indicated for *supplementation* of less-potent anesthetic agents, such as nitrous oxide in oxygen, during maintenance of anesthesia for short operative procedures (dilation and curettage or cervical conization). Intravenous etomidate produces a rapid induction of anesthesia with minimal cardiovascular and respiratory changes. Intravenously administered etomidate produces rapid induction of anesthesia with minimal cardiovascular and respiratory changes. Onset of unconsciousness occurs within one arm-to-brain circulation time. Awakening following a single intravenous dose is more rapid than seen with barbiturates. However, recovery of psychomotor function is intermediate between methohexital and thiopental.

Etomidate is associated with cardiovascular stability following intravenous administration. Administration of 0.3 mg/kg intravenously leads to minimal changes in heart rate, stroke volume or cardiac output. Blood pressure may decrease only up to 15% as a result of an increase in systemic vascular resistance. The use of etomidate may lead to apnea following rapid intravenous injection, but appears to cause less respiratory depression than barbiturates. The effects on ventilation following a single intravenous injection last only 3 to 5 min. It is a weak base (pK_a 4.24) with moderate lipophilic properties. Etomidate is metabolized rapidly by the liver. Approximately 75% of the dose is excreted in the urine as an inactive metabolite, 10% in the bile and 13% in feces. Adverse reactions include transient venous pain on injection and transient skeletal muscle movements, including myoclonus. Myoclonus occurs in about ⅓ of patients and is not associated with central seizure activity.

Etomidate causes adrenocortical suppression which lasts 4 to 8 hr after an induction dose. The clinical importance of this effect is controversial.

Etomidate, as with all intravenous anesthetics, should be administered only by persons trained in the use of intravenous anesthetics. Appropriate resuscitative equipment for prevention and treatment of anesthetic emergencies should be available. Available data are not sufficient to justify its use in pregnancy, obstetrics, nursing mothers or children under 10 yr of age.

Dose—*Intravenous*, **0.2** to **0.6 mg/kg**; *usual intravenous*, **0.3 mg/kg** over a period of 30 to 60 sec.

Dosage Form—Ampuls: 10 and 20 mL, containing 2 mg/mL; Abbojet syringes, 20 mL.

Fentanyl Citrate—page 1204.

Fentanyl Citrate and Droperidol Injection—see RPS-18, page 1045.

Hexobarbital—see RPS-17, page 1069.

Ketamine Hydrochloride

Cyclohexanone, 2-(2-chlorophenyl)-2-(methylamino)-, hydrochloride; Ketaject (*Bristol*); Ketalar (*Parke-Davis*)

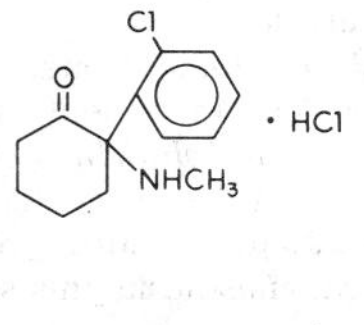

(±)-2-(*o*-Chlorophenyl)-2-(methylamino)cyclohexanone hydrochloride [1867-66-9] Base [6740-88-1] $C_{13}H_{16}ClNO.HCl$ (274.19).

Preparation—The product resulting from a Grignard reaction involving *o*-chlorobenzonitrile and bromocyclopentane is treated in the presence of strong alkali to form the epoxy compound (I). Reaction of this with methylamine yields the imine (II) which rearranges on heating in the presence of hydrochloric acid. Belgian Pat 634,208

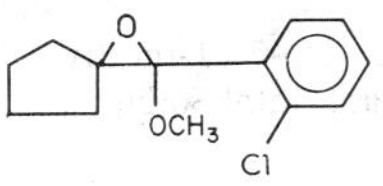

Description—White, crystalline powder with a characteristic odor; solutions are acid to litmus; melts between 258 and 261° with decomposition; pH (1 in 10 solution) between 3.5 and 4.1.

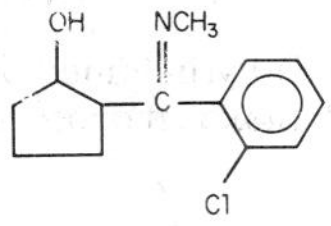

Solubility—1 g in 5 mL water, 14 mL alcohol, 60 mL chloroform or 60 mL absolute alcohol.

Uses—A rapidly acting nonbarbiturate anesthetic that produces anesthesia and profound analgesia. The anesthetic state produced by ketamine is described as *dissociative anesthesia* since the patient may appear awake but is dissociated from the environment and does not respond to pain. The patient is noncommunicative, but may appear to be awake. Analgesia is intense and the patient is amnestic.

Ketamine is useful as an intravenous or intramuscular induction agent before the use of other anesthetics and as the primary anesthetic for short operative procedures requiring intense analgesia, such as wound care. Intravenous induction doses (2 mg/kg) produce surgical anesthesia within 30 sec and lasts about 10 min. Intramuscular induction doses (9 to 13 mg/kg) produce surgical anesthesia in 3 to 4 min and last 12 to 25 min. The anesthetic action of ketamine is terminated by redistribution from the central nervous system and by hepatic biotransformation. Ketamine is metabolized extensively in the liver by the cytochrome P-450 system.

Ketamine is associated with normal to hyperactive pharyngeal-laryngeal reflexes. However, protection of the airway is not assured with ketamine-induced general anesthesia. Respiratory depression, apnea and laryngospasm can occur with rapid intravenous administration.

Ketamine produces cardiovascular stimulation. Heart rate, arterial blood pressure and cardiac output usually are increased 2 to 4 min after intravenous injection and return to normal levels in 15 min. Ketamine is thought to have its effect by sympathetic nervous system outflow stimulation from the central nervous system. Patients who are critically ill may experience hypotension and decreased cardiac output, probably as a result of depletion of catecholamine stores and the inability of the sympathetic nervous system to compensate, leading to an unmasking of a direct myocardial effect.

Adverse reactions include elevated blood pressure and pulse rate. Occasionally hypotension, bradycardia and arrhythmia can occur. Diplopia, nystagmus and slight elevation of intraocular pressure also can occur. Ketamine can lead to enhanced skeletal muscle tone, including tonic and clonic movements. Other adverse effects include anorexia, nausea and vomiting, local pain at the injection site and transient erythema and/or morbilliform rash.

Ketamine may interact with thyroid medication to produce severe hypertension and tachycardia. Ketamine also potentates the neuromuscular blocking effects of tubocurarine but not of succinylcholine.

Low doses of ketamine (0.2 mg/kg) appear to be safe for obstetrical anesthesia, but larger doses have been associated with fetal depression.

Special Note: Emergence reactions have occurred in approximately 1% of patients. The psychological manifestations vary in severity between pleasant dream-like states, vivid imagery, hallucinations and emergence delirium. In some cases these states have been accompanied by confusion, excitement and irrational behavior which a few patients recall as an unpleasant experience. The duration ordinarily lasts no more than a few hours; in a few cases, however, recurrences have taken place up to 24 hr postoperatively. No residual psychological effects are known to have resulted from use of ketamine. The incidence of these emergence phenomena is least in the young (15 yr of age or less) and elderly (over 65 yr of age) patient; also, they are less frequent when the drug is given intramuscularly. These reactions may be reduced if verbal, tactile and visual stimulation of the patient is minimized during the recovery period. This does not preclude the monitoring of vital signs. In addition, the use of a small hypnotic dose of a short-acting or ultrashort-acting barbiturate or other agent such as diazepam may be required to terminate a severe emergence reaction. Certain drugs, such as droperidol or diazepam intramuscularly, also have been used in an attempt to reduce the incidence of emergence reactions. The incidence of emergence reactions is reduced as experience with the drug is gained. When ketamine is used on an outpatient basis, the patient should not be released until recovery from anesthesia is complete and then should be accompanied by a responsible adult.

Some reports indicate that ketamine hydrochloride may interact with thyroid medication to produce severe hypertension and tachycardia. It also potentiates the neuromuscular-blocking effects of tubocurarine but not of succinylcholine. Large doses (over 2 mg/kg body wt) are likely to cause fetal depression. Although lower doses appear safe, it is not the preferred drug for obstetrical anesthesia.

Ketamine, as with all intravenous anesthetics, should be administered only by persons trained in the use of intravenous anesthetics. Appropriate resuscitative equipment for prevention and treatment of anesthetic emergencies should be available.

Dose—*Induction, intravenous*, **1** to **2 mg/kg,** intramuscular, **5** to **10 mg/kg.** A dose of 10 mg/kg usually produces 12 to 25 min of surgical anesthesia. *Maintenance*, ½ of the full induction dose repeated as necessary for maintenance of the desired level of anesthesia.

Dosage Form—Injection: 10 mg/mL in 20-, 25- and 50-mL vials; 50 mg/mL in 10-mL vials; 100 mg/mL in 5-mL vials.

Methohexital Sodium

2,4,6(1*H*,3*H*,5*H*)-Pyrimidinetrione, (±)-1-methyl-5-(1-methyl-2-pentynyl)-5-(2-propenyl)-, monosodium salt; Brevital Sodium (*Lilly*)

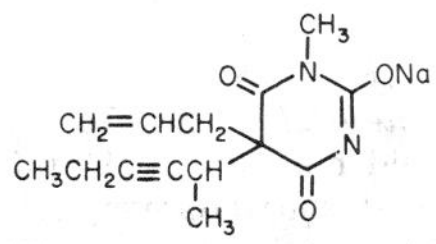

Sodium 5-allyl-1-methyl-5-(1-methyl-2-pentynyl)barbiturate [309-36-4] $C_{14}H_{17}N_2NaO_3$ (284.29).

Preparation—1-Butynyl magnesium bromide is treated with acetaldehyde and the resulting alcohol is treated with PCl_5 to produce 2-chloro-3-pentyne. Condensation with ethyl cyanoacetate in the presence of sodium ethylate yields ethyl 1-methyl-2-pentynylcyanoacetate which, on similar further condensation with allyl bromide, yields ethyl (1-methyl-2-pentynyl)allylcyanoacetate. Reaction with *N*-methylurea yields the iminobarbituric acid which, on acid-catalyzed hydrolysis, forms methohexital. Neutralization with sodium hydroxide produces the sodium salt.

The two diastereoisomers of the barbituric acid have been designated as α- and β-forms in the literature. The α-form is the one used medicinally (the β-form causes undesirable side effects) and is formed almost exclusively by the above process. The malonic ester synthesis described under *Barbital* is not used because it yields mainly the unwanted β-form.

Description—White to off-white hygroscopic powder; essentially odorless solutions are alkaline to litmus.

Solubility—Soluble in water.

Uses—The principal use of methohexital is for the induction of general anesthesia and the maintenance of anesthesia for very short procedures. Induction doses of methohexital (1 mg/kg) leads to unconsciousness within 30 sec. Although methohexital is less ionized than is thiopental (24% vs 39% at pH 7.4), its plasma protein binding is essentially the same (72 to 86%). It is thought the pattern of distribution of the two drugs immediately after injection and recovery following a single dose is due to the same mechanism, namely, redistribution of the drug from the brain into the muscle mass. Induction of anesthesia is about as rapid as with thiopental sodium, but recovery is more rapid. This is reflected in the short elimination half-life (70 to 125 min); this is a result of a high plasma clearance rate (657 to 999 mL plasma/min). Methohexital is metabolized extensively and rapidly in the liver. While metabolism may have little effect on early awakening, it is important in complete psychomotor recovery.

Methohexital is useful for very brief procedures, such as reduction of fractures, gynecological examinations and electroconvulsive therapy. The principal disadvantage of methohexital as compared to thiopental is the increased incidence of excitatory phenomena, such as muscle twitching and hiccups. Other adverse reactions include thrombophlebitis, pain at the injection site, respiratory depression, laryngospasm, bronchospasm, salivation, delirium, headache, nausea and emesis. Histamine release can occur following intravenous injection, but is rarely of clinical significance. Induction doses of methohexital leads to cardiovascular effects similar to that seen with thiopental.

Methohexital is contraindicated in patients with latent or manifest porphyria or in patients with a known hypersensitivity to barbiturates. As with thiopental, methohexital should be administered only by persons trained in the use of intravenous anesthetics, in an environment where appropriate resuscitative equipment is readily available.

Solutions of methohexital sodium are incompatible with silicone and should not be allowed to come in contact with rubber stoppers or parts of disposable syringes that have come in contact with silicone.

Dose—For *induction of general anesthesia, adults, intravenous* **1 mg/kg,** titrated to desired effect. The dose of methohexital required to induce anesthesia appears to decrease with age. *Rectal, children,* **20** to **30 mg/kg** has been advocated to induce anesthesia.

Dosage Form—Liquid: 1%.

Midazolam—page 1159.

Paraldehyde—page 1169.

Pentobarbital Sodium—page 1164.

Phencyclidine—see RPS-17, page 1047.

Propofol

Phenol, 2,6-diisopropyl-, Diprivan (*Stuart*)

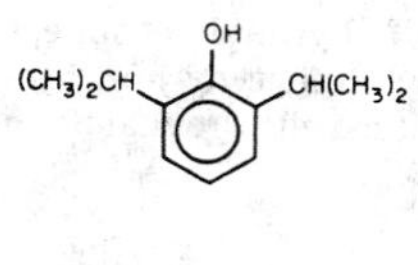

OH
$(CH_3)_2CH$ $CH(CH_3)_2$

[2078-54-8] $C_{12}H_{18}O$ (178.27)

Preparation—*J Org Chem 21:* 712, 1956.

Description—Oily liquid; melts about 19°, pK_a 11.

Solubility—Slightly soluble in water; very soluble in alcohol.

Uses—Indicated for the induction and maintenance of anesthesia, especially for short procedures or outpatient surgery. Intravenous injection of propofol produces hypnosis rapidly (one arm-brain circulation time). Propofol can be used as the sole anesthetic, or as an adjuvant to other inhaled or injected anesthetics and analgesics.

The termination of the effects of propofol after a single intravenous dose or a maintenance infusion is rapid. Following induction and maintenance of anesthesia for periods up to 2 hr, most patients are responsive to verbal commands and are oriented within 8 min. This is due to extensive redistribution from the CNS to other tissues. In addition, propofol undergoes high metabolic clearance (1.6 to 3.4 L/min).

Propofol solution contains no preservatives. The vehicle is capable of supporting rapid growth of microorganisms, and strict aseptic technique must be maintained during handling and administration.

Induction doses of propofol can lead to decreases in blood pressure greater than that seen with comparable doses of thiopental. These changes are associated with little or no change in heart rate or cardiac output. The effects of propofol on blood pressure may be exaggerated in hypovolemic or elderly patients, or in patients with pre-existing cardiac disease. The most frequent respiratory complications are cough, upper airway obstruction, apnea, hypoventilation and dyspnea.

Frequently, propofol leads to local pain during intravenous injection, which may be reduced by prior injection of IV lidocaine or adding lidocaine to the propofol solution.

Propofol is not recommended for obstetrics, including cesarean section deliveries. Propofol crosses the placenta and, as with other general anesthetic agents, the administration of propofol may be associated with neonatal depression.

Perioperative myoclonia, rarely including convulsions and opisthotonus, has been associated with propofol use. Propofol injection decreases cerebral blood flow, cerebral metabolic oxygen consumption and intracranial pressure and increases cerebrovascular resistance. However, propofol is not recommended for use in patients with increased intracranial pressure or impaired cerebral circulation because it may cause substantial decreases in mean arterial pressure, and consequently, substantial decreases in cerebral perfusion pressure.

Propofol, as with all intravenous anesthetics, should be administered only by persons trained in the use of intravenous anesthetics. Appropriate resuscitative equipment for prevention and treatment of anesthetic emergencies should be available.

Dose—*Induction, healthy adults,* titrated to effect, but usually **2.0** to **2.5 mg/kg.** The dose is less in patients who have received other sedatives/hypnotics. *Induction, elderly, usually,* **1.0** to **1.5 mg/kg.** *Maintenance, healthy adults* (also receiving 60 to 70%, nitrous oxide plus oxygen), *usual,* **100–200 μg/kg/min.** *Sedation,* for *minor surgical procedures* (under local anesthesia plus sedation), *usual, infusion,* **25** to **50 μg/kg/min.**

Dosage Form—Injection (10 mg/mL): 20-mL ampules and 50-mL infusion vials.

Secobarbital Sodium—page 1165.

Sufentanil Citrate—page 1207.

Thiamylal Sodium

4,6-(1*H*,5*H*)-Pyrimidinedione, dihydro-5-(1-methylbutyl)-5-(2-propenyl)-2-thioxo-, monosodium salt; Surital Sodium (*Parke-Davis*)

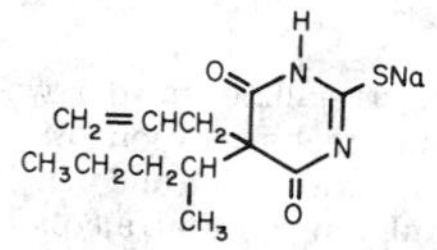

H
O N SNa
$CH_2{=}CHCH_2$
$CH_3CH_2CH_2CH$ N
CH_3 O

Sodium 5-allyl-5-(1-methylbutyl)-2-thiobarbiturate [337-47-3] $C_{12}H_{17}N_2NaO_2S$ (276.33), with anhydrous sodium carbonate as a buffer.

Preparation—The thiobarbituric acid, thiamylal, may be prepared by the general process described under *Amobarbital,* page 1163, except using allyl bromide and 1-methylbutyl bromide as the alkylating agents instead of ethyl bromide, and condensing the resulting allyl 1-methylbutyl malonic ester with thiourea instead of urea. The free acid is neutralized with sodium hydroxide to form the sodium salt.

Description—Pale yellow, hygroscopic powder; disagreeable odor.

Solubility—Soluble in water; pH (5% solution) approx 11.

Uses—A rapidly acting barbiturate indicated for *induction of anesthesia.* Its anesthetic potency, profile of action and untoward effects are similar to those of thiopental.

Dose—For *induction of general anesthesia, intravenous, adults,* **2.2** to **4.5 mg/kg,** titrated to desired effect. The dose required to induce anesthesia appears to decrease with age.

Dosage Form—Injection: 2.5% solution.

Thiopental Sodium

4,6-(1*H*,5*H*)-Pyrimidinedione, 5-ethyldihydro-5-(1-methylbutyl)-2-thioxo-, monosodium salt; Thiopentone Sodium; Pentothal Sodium (*Abbott*)

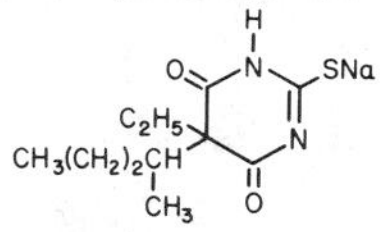

Sodium 5-ethyl-5-(1-methylbutyl)-2-thiobarbiturate [71-73-8] $C_{11}H_{17}N_2NaO_2S$ (264.32).

Preparation—In the same manner as *Thiamylal* (above), using 2-bromopentane as the alkyl halide and the ethyl 1-methylbutylmalonate is condensed with thiourea [$CS(NH_2)_2$].

Description—White to off-white, crystalline powder or a yellowish white to pale greenish yellow hygroscopic powder; may have a disagreeable odor; aqueous solution is alkaline to litmus; solutions decompose on standing and, on boiling, precipitation occurs. Carbon dioxide also causes precipitation in the solution.

Solubility—Soluble in water or alcohol; insoluble in absolute ether, benzene or solvent hexane.

Incompatibilities—Thiopental precipitates in acid solutions.

Uses—The most commonly employed rapidly acting depressant of the central nervous system which induces *hypnosis* and *anesthesia*, but not analgesia. It produces anesthesia within 30 to 40 sec after intravenous injection. Recovery after single doses is rapid, due to redistribution of the drug away from the central nervous system to inactive tissues. Thiopental may produce some retrograde amnesia, and patients are frequently somnolent following awakening. Thiopental is used widely to induce general anesthesia. It is not used frequently as the primary anesthetic for short procedures because other intravenous anesthetics, such as methohexital and propofol, are associated with more rapid recovery.

Thiopental is metabolized almost completely (99%) by the liver. Its half-life is 11.5 hr, the volume of distribution at the steady state is 1.4 L/kg and clearance is 150 mL/min. These values are increased markedly during pregnancy and in obese individuals. The elimination half-life in pediatric patients is one-half that in adults, whereas, the clearance value in children is approximately double that in adults.

Adverse reactions include excitatory phenomena, such as muscle twitching or hiccups, thrombophlebitis, pain at the injection site, respiratory depression, laryngospasm, bronchospasm, salivation, delirium, headache, nausea and emesis. Histamine release can occur following intravenous injection, but is rarely of clinical significance. Thiopental is contraindicated in patients with latent or manifest porphyria or in patients with a known hypersensitivity to barbiturates.

The hemodynamic effects of equivalent induction doses of thiopental and methohexital are similar. Thiopental, 5 mg/kg, IV, produces a transient 10 to 20 torr decrease in blood pressure. In addition, a 15 to 20 beats/min compensatory increase in heart rate occurs. These hemodynamic changes are due principally to peripheral vasodilatation and not direct myocardial depression. The hemodynamic changes may be exaggerated in patients with limited cardiac reserve and hypovolemic patients. Signs of clinically important direct myocardial depression can be seen with high doses of all the barbiturates.

Thiopental, as with all intravenous anesthetics, should be administered only by persons trained in the use of intravenous anesthetics. Appropriate resuscitative equipment for prevention and treatment of anesthetic emergencies should be available.

Dose—For *induction of general anesthesia, adults, intravenous,* **2.5** to **5 mg/kg** titrated to desired effect. The dose required to induce anesthesia appears to decrease with age.

Dosage Form—Injection: 2.5% solution.

Bibliography

Bahlman SH, Eger EI, Halsey MJ *et al:* The cardiovascular effects of halothane in man during spontaneous ventilation. *Anesthesiology 36:* 494, 1972.

Becker KE, Tonnesen AS: Cardiovascular effects of plasma levels of thiopental necessary for anesthesia. *Ibid. 49:*197, 1978.

Bentley JB *et al:* Serum inorganic fluoride levels in obese patients during and after enflurane anesthesia. *Anesth Analg 58:* 409, 1979.

Berthoud MC, Reilly CS: Adverse effects of general anaesthetics. *Drug Safety 7:* 434, 1992.

Calverley RK *et al:* Ventilatory and cardiovascular effects of enflurane anesthesia during spontaneous ventilation in man. *Anesth Analg 57:* 610, 1978.

Carpender RL *et al:* The extent of metabolism of inhaled anesthetics in humans. *Anesthesiology 65:* 201, 1986.

Choi SD *et al:* Comparison of the ventilatory effects of etomidate and methohexital. *Ibid 62:* 442, 1985.

Clarke RSJ: Adverse effects of intravenously administered drugs in anaesthetic practice. *Drugs 22:* 26, 1981.

Duthie DJR, Fraser R, Nimmo WS: Effect of induction of anaesthesia with etomidate on corticosteroid synthesis in man. *Br J Anaesth 57:* 156, 1985.

Eger, EI: Current status of sevoflurane and desflurane. *Anesth Analg (suppl)* 81, 1992.

Eger EI: *Isoflurane (Forane). A Compendium and Reference,* Ohio Medical Products, Madison, WI, 1981.

Giovannitte JA, Trapp LD: Adult sedation: oral, rectal, IM, IV. *Anesth Progr 38:* 154, 1991.

Hudson RJ, Stanski DR, Burch PG: Pharmacokinetics of methohexital and thiopental in surgical patients. *Anesthesiology 59:* 215, 1983.

Janeczko GF, El-Etr AA, Younes S: Low dose ketamine anesthesia for obstetrical delivery. *Anesth Analg 53:* 828, 1974.

Jastak JT, Donaldson D: Nitrous oxide. *Anesth Progr 38:* 142, 1991.

Jones RM: Desflurane and sevoflurane: Inhalation anaesthetics for this decade? *Br J Anaesth 65:* 527, 1990.

Owen H, Spence AA: Etomidate. *Ibid 56:* 555, 1984.

Pace NA, Victory RA, White PF: Anesthetic infusion techniques—how to do it. *J Clin Anesth 4:* 45S, 1992.

Pocock G, Richards CD: Cellular mechanisms in general anaesthesia. *Br J Anaesth 66:* 116, 1991.

Ray DC, Drummond GB: Halothane hepatitis. *Ibid 67:* 84, 1991.

Rosenberg M, Weaver J: General anesthesia. *Anesth Progr 38:* 172, 1991.

Sear JW: Practical treatment recommendations for the safe use of anaesthetics. *Drugs 43:* 54, 1992.

Shafer A *et al:* Pharmacokinetics and pharmacodynamics of propofol infusions during general anesthesia. *Anesthesiology 69:* 348, 1988.

Stanley TH: Intravenous anesthesia of the future. *J Clin Anesth 4:* 53S, 1992.

Stoelting RK, Miller RD: *Basics of Anesthesia,* Churchill Livingstone, New York, 1984.

Stoelting RK, ed: *Pharmacology and Physiology in Anesthetic Practice,* 2nd ed, Lippincott, Philadelphia, 1991.

White PF, Way WL, Trevor AJ: Ketamine: its pharmacology and therapeutic uses. *Anesthesiology 56:* 119, 1982.

Whitwam JG: Methohexitone. *Br J Anaesth 48:* 617, 1976.

CHAPTER 68

Local Anesthetics

Glen R Hanson, DDS, PhD

Professor of Pharmacology
College of Pharmacy and School of Medicine
University of Utah
Salt Lake City UT 84112

Local anesthetics reversibly block impulse conduction in any part of the nervous system and in all nerves, including sensory, motor and autonomic types. They often are used to produce a transient loss of sensation in a circumscribed area of the body without causing a general loss of consciousness. This action can be used to block pain sensation—or sympathetic vasoconstrictor impulses—to specific areas of the body. Hence, local anesthetics are used to prevent pain in surgical procedures, dental manipulations, injury and disease. The synthetic local anesthetic agents may be divided into two groups: the slightly soluble compounds and the soluble compounds. The *slightly soluble* local anesthetics are used only for surface (topical) application, since their slow absorption renders them safe for use on ulcers, wounds and mucous surfaces. The anesthesia which they induce is not as complete as that induced by soluble compounds, but the duration is longer. Many soluble anesthetics also may be used for topical anesthesia. On the other hand, only *soluble* local anesthetics of relatively low toxicity should be injected.

Local anesthesia induced by injectable agents is designated according to the technique or anatomic site of the injection. *Infiltration anesthesia* refers to injection directly into the area that is painful or to be subjected to surgical trauma. *Field block* is accomplished by administering the local anesthetic to a region of the nerve proximal to the site to be anesthetized. *Peripheral nerve block*, commonly called *regional anesthesia*, places the anesthetic agent in direct contact with the nerve or nerve plexus. *Paravertebral nerve block* places the anesthetic agent in direct contact with the nerve as it exits the intervertebral foramina. *Epidural* and *caudal blocks* are similar; caudal block is an epidural block in the caudal region. *Subarachnoid block*, commonly called *spinal anesthesia*, but more correctly *spinal analgesia*, requires that the anesthetic be placed within the subarachnoid space so that the anesthetic agent mixes with spinal fluid. The use of a hyperbaric (heavy) solution or hypobaric (light) solution and proper positioning of the patient on the operating table permits manipulation of anesthesia for various body areas.

Local anesthetics prevent both the generation and the conduction of the nerve impulse. The excitable membrane of nerve axons maintains a transmembrane potential of −90 to −60 mV. During excitation, the sodium channels open and a fast inward sodium current quickly depolarizes the membrane toward the sodium equilibrium potential (+40 mV). As a result of depolarization, the sodium channels close (inactivate) and potassium channels open. The outward flow of potassium repolarizes the membrane toward the potassium equilibrium potential (−95 mV); repolarization returns the sodium channels to the rested state. The transmembrane ionic gradients are maintained by the sodium pump.

When increasing concentrations of a local anesthetic are applied to a nerve fiber, the threshold for excitation increases, the impulse conduction slows, the rate of rise of the action potential declines, the action potential amplitude decreases and, finally, the ability to generate an action potential is abolished. All these effects result from the binding of the local anesthetic to sodium channels which in turn blocks the transient permeability to sodium. If the sodium current is blocked over a critical portion of nerve, propagation of an impulse over the blocked area is no longer possible.

When infiltration, conduction or regional techniques are employed, both nerve fibers and nerve endings are anesthetized. The ease with which a nerve fiber may be anesthetized is related to its type and size. Although there are exceptions, large myelinated nerves usually require a greater concentration of anesthetic solution and more time to be blocked than do small nonmyelinated fibers. Accordingly, small nerve fibers concerned with vascoconstriction, temperature and surface pain are anesthetized most easily, whereas large fibers associated with the sensation of touch, pressure, deep pain and the sensations from joints and tendons are anesthetized with more difficulty. In spinal anesthesia, it is probable that both sensory and motor nerve fibers are anesthetized. In surface (topical) anesthesia, the sensory nerve endings are the chief nerve structures affected.

The nerve-blocking action of the local anesthetics is pH sensitive. Because these drugs generally are marketed as water-soluble salts, the injected solutions are mildly acidic. In order to block nerve activity, the local anesthetic must become deprotonated and diffuse through cellular membranes to reach its intracellular site of action. However, because the cationic species is the form of the local anesthetic which interacts preferentially with the sodium channels, molecules which have crossed the membranes must be protonated again to be effective. Changes in extracellular pH can disrupt the balance between protonated and deprotonated forms and interfere with local anesthetic activity. This can occur in areas of tissue damage or inflammation or following multiple administrations of the acidic local anesthetic solutions.

The duration of action of a local anesthetic is proportional to the time during which it is in actual contact with nervous tissues. Consequently, procedures that help localize the drug at the nerve prolong anesthesia. Cocaine itself constricts blood vessels, prevents its own absorption and has a duration of action longer than most local anesthetics. A vasoconstrictor drug, such as epinephrine, norepinephrine, levonordefrin, is included frequently in local anesthetic solutions. The presence of one of these drugs in the local anesthetic solution retards absorption of the local anesthetic solution, thereby reducing its systemic toxicity, increasing its duration of action and increasing its efficiency by decreasing the volume of solution required. The pressor potency relative to epinephrine (shown in parentheses), maximal total dose and usual concentration are as follows: epinephrine (1), 0.2 mg, 1:50,000 to 1:200,000; norepinephrine (0.6), 0.34 mg, 1:30,000 and levonordefrin (0.5), 1 mg, 1:20,000. While vasoconstriction helps prolong the effects of the local anesthetics, it can be problematic in areas with restricted blood supply. Consequently, it is inadvisable to inject local anesthetics with vasoconstrictors around the base of fingers, toes or the penis. Some of the vasoconstrictor may be absorbed systemically causing adverse effects associated with their sympathomimetic actions. Such side effects can be particularly dangerous in the presence of cardiovascular disease or concurrent use of other drugs which enhance sympathetic nervous activity such as MAO inhibitors or tricyclic antidepressants. In addition, injection of these vasoconstrictor additives into damaged tissue may result in delayed healing.

A number of precautions should be observed when injection anesthesia is contemplated.

Resuscitation equipment and appropriate drugs should be immediately available.

The safe use of these agents in pregnancy, with respect to adverse effects on fetal development, has not been established.

Local anesthetic procedures should be used with caution when there is inflammation and/or sepsis in the region of the proposed injection.

Local anesthetics containing epinephrine should be used with *extreme caution* in patients on MAO inhibitors, tricyclic antidepressants, phenothiazines, etc, as either severe hypertension or hypotension may occur.

Vasopressor agents used in caudal or other epidural blocks should be used with *extreme caution* in patients on oxytocic drugs, since the resulting interaction may produce severe persistent hypertension and/or rupture of cerebral blood vessels.

Serious dose-related cardiac arrhythmias may occur if local anesthetics containing a vasoconstrictor such as epinephrine are employed in patients during or following the administration of chloroform, halothane, cyclopropane, trichloroethylene or other inhalation anesthetics.

Factors that must be given careful consideration prior to concurrent use of general and local anesthetics include the effect of both agents on the myocardium, the concentration and volume of the vasoconstrictor and the elapsed time since injection.

Adverse reactions to local anesthetics may be divided into two groups: systemic and local adverse reactions. In general, these reactions are qualitatively similar for all local anesthetic agents.

Systemic adverse reactions usually are associated with high blood levels of the drug and result from over-dosage, rapid systemic absorption or inadvertent intravenous injection. Because local anesthetics can affect all excitable membranes, the reactions usually involve the central nervous and cardiovascular systems.

The initial *central nervous system reactions* are excitatory and/or depressant, and may be characterized by nervousness, agitation, dizziness, blurred vision and tremors, followed by drowsiness, convulsions, unconsciousness and possibly respiratory arrest. Other systemic effects may include nausea, vomiting, chills, pupil contraction or tinnitus. The excitatory reactions may be very brief or absent, in which case the first manifestation of toxicity may be drowsiness, merging into unconsciousness and respiratory arrest.

Cardiovascular reactions usually require high systemic concentrations, are depressant and may be characterized by hypotension, cardiovascular collapse, bradycardia and, possibly, cardiac arrest. Treatment of a patient with toxic manifestations includes reassurance, maintaining a patent airway and supporting ventilation using oxygen and assisted or controlled respiration. Should circulatory depression occur, vasopressors such as ephedrine or metaraminol, and IV fluids may be used. Should a convulsion persist despite oxygen therapy, diazepam given IV is usually the treatment of choice.

Allergic reactions are characterized by cutaneous lesions, urticaria, edema or anaphylactoid reactions. Untoward reactions from overdosage with epinephrine and other vasoconstrictor agents added to local anesthetics are relatively common. Anxiety, palpitation, dizziness, headaches, restlessness, tremors, tachycardia, anginal pain and hypertension are observed frequently. These reactions may be differentiated from those caused by local anesthetics in that epinephrine does not produce convulsions and causes tachycardia rather than bradycardia. Reactions of this kind respond to sedatives and oxygen.

Local adverse reactions to these anesthetic drugs, although infrequent, are either cytotoxic or allergic and are manifested by skin discoloration, pain, edema, slough, neuritis or neurolysis. Eczematoid dermatitis, characterized by erythema and pruritus which proceeds to inflammation, swelling, vesiculation and oozing, is the predominant local reaction. *The aminobenzoic acid* derivatives are by far the most likely to cause allergic sensitivity reactions; cross-sensitivity between members of this group often is reported. If a patient is allergic or does not tolerate a particular local anesthetic, it is advisable to use a drug from a different chemical family. Unfortunately, tests for sensitivity such as skin, conjunctival and patch tests are not reliable for predicting the possibility of allergic reactions.

All local anesthetics are toxic, and the tolerance of patients varies. Safe dosage, therefore, is limited for each drug and must be individualized. The choice of drug, concentration, rate and site of injection, age and emotional and physical status of the patient represent a few factors which must be considered. In general, the smallest amount of the least toxic drug that will serve the purpose should be used, if reactions are to be avoided. In some patients, premedication with diazepam may be advisable to minimize the incidence of toxic reactions. Many local anesthetics occasionally give rise to dermatitis. When this is severe, the use of the anesthetic should be discontinued.

The interested reader is referred to the following reviews on the subject: Courtney KR: Structural elements which determine local anesthetics activity. In, Local anesthetics. (Strichartz, GR, ed) *Handbook of Experimental Pharmacology*, vol 81 Springer-Verlag, Berlin, 1987, 53–94 and McLeskey CH: Rational use of local anesthetics. *NC Med J 43:* 496–500, 1982.

Injection Anesthetics

Injectable local anesthetic drugs can be divided conveniently into two groups: esters and nonesters. The esters are primarily of the para-aminobenzoic acid type and include chlorpromazine, procaine, propoxycaine and tetracaine. The nonesters are anilides (amides or nonesters) which include lidocaine, mepivacaine, bupivacaine, etidocaine and prilocaine. This classification is particularly important from the point of view of possible allergic reactions as well as biotransformation. Thus, local anesthetics with an *ester linkage* (aromatic acid + amino alcohol) such as procaine and those with an *amide linkage* (aromatic amine + amino acid) such as lidocaine, differ significantly in hypersensitivity, metabolism and duration of action. Hypersensitivity seems to occur most prominently in response to local anesthetics of the *ester-type* and frequently extends to chemically related compounds. Allergic reactions to the amide type are extremely rare, and substitution of such extremely rare, compounds to avoid allergic responses is usually possible.

The *metabolic fate* of local anesthetics is of great practical importance because their toxicity depends largely on the balance between their rate of absorption and their rate of destruction. The *ester-type* local anesthetic appears to be hydrolyzed by both liver esterase and plasma esterase. Metabolic degradation by plasma esterase is particularly important in man; human plasma esterase can hydrolyze local anesthetics 4 to 20 times faster than can animal plasma esterases. Consequently, very little of the *ester-type* agent is available for hydrolysis by liver esterase. Spinal fluid contains little or no esterase; hence, anesthesia produced by intrathecal injection of an ester-type local anesthetic will persist until the local anesthetic agent is absorbed into the blood.

On the other hand, *amide-type* local anesthetics are degraded by hepatic microsomes; the initial reactions involve *N*-dealkylation and subsequent hydrolysis. Consequently, the *amide-type* local anesthetics usually have a longer duration of action than the ester type.

Considerable pharmacokinetic data have been accumulated on the amide-type local anesthetics, particularly lidocaine, mepivacaine, bupivacaine and etidocaine (the data will be presented in the respective monographs). Comparatively little such information is available on the older ester-type agents; for the most part their rapid metabolism has hindered most attempts to measure their blood concentrations after less than heroic doses in man. Consequently, most studies with the latter agents deal with potency, toxicity, time for onset and duration of action. The descriptive phrase short-acting suggests a duration of 45 to 75 minutes, medium-acting, 90 to 150 min and long-acting, 180 minutes or longer.

With the exception of solutions for use in spinal anesthesia, local anesthetic solutions should be isotonic to avoid edema, local irritation and inflammation at the site of injection. Solutions for spinal anesthesia may be either isobaric, hypobaric or hyperbaric, depending on the desired level of anesthesia. The total maximal dosages employed with injection anesthetics vary markedly, depending on the technique used and the patient's age, weight and physical condition. In general, the physician should administer the least volume of the most dilute solution that is effective. For adverse effects and special warnings in the use of these agents, refer to the introductory statement.

Bupivacaine Hydrochloride

2-Piperidinecarboxamide, 1-butyl-*N*-(2,6-dimethylphenyl)-, hydrochloride; Marcaine Hydrochloride (*Winthrop*); Sensorcaine (*Astra*); (*Various Mfrs*)

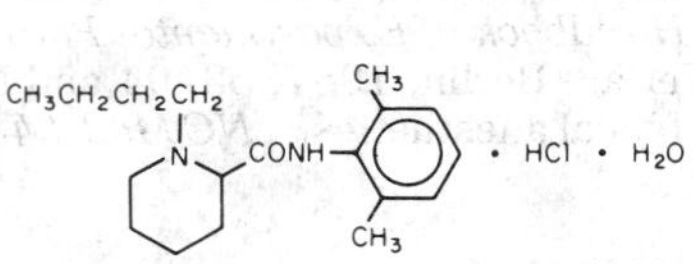

1-Butyl-2′,6′-pipecoloxylidide monohydrochloride [14252-80-3] $C_{18}H_{28}N_2O.HCl.H_2O$ (342.91).

Preparation—Similar to that of *Mepivacaine Hydrochloride*, except that butyl bromide instead of dimethyl sulfate is used for alkylation. *J Med Chem 14:* 891, 1971.

Description—White, crystalline powder; odorless; melts with decomposition about 250°. pK_a 8.05.

Solubility—1 g in 25 mL water or 8 mL alcohol; slightly soluble in chloroform.

Uses—For *local infiltration* (0.25% sol), *lumbar epidural* (0.25%, 0.5% and 0.75% sol), *caudal block* (0.25% and 0.5%), *peripheral nerve block* (0.25% and 0.5% sol), *retrobulbar block* (0.75% sol), *sympathetic block* (0.25% sol) and dental block (0.5% sol). It is *not* used for obstetric paracervical block or topical anesthesia. The onset of action after local injection is rapid (5 min); onset may be delayed as long as 20 min when used for brachial plexus or peridural anesthesia. The duration of peripheral nerve blocks produced may last up to 7 hr, whereas the duration of peridural anesthesia is about 4 hr. Epidural block with 0.75% solution induces complete motor block; hence, abdominal operations requiring complete muscle relaxation may be done. It also has been noted that a period of analgesia persists after the return of sensation; during this time the need for analgesics is reduced. It has a $t_{1/2}$ of 2.7 hrs, V_d of 1.04, a partition coefficient of 130, and 84 to 95% of the drug is bound to plasma protein. Consequently, it has a low degree of placental transmission of parenteral local anesthetic and may cause the least fetal depression. After injection for caudal, epidural or peripheral nerve block in humans, peak blood levels of approximately 1.2 μg/mL are reached in 30 to 45 min, followed by a decline to insignificant levels within 3 to 6 hr. Like other local anesthetics with an amide structure, it is not detoxified by plasma esterases but is detoxified in the liver, via conjugation with glucuronic acid.

Contraindications, general warnings, precautions and adverse reactions are similar to those of other amide-type local anesthetics (see *Lidocaine*, page 1153). It is not recommended for children under 12 yr and the solution for spinal anesthesia should *not* be used in children under 18 yr. The safe use in pregnancy, with respect to adverse effects on fetal development, has not been established.

Dose—*Infiltration*, a **0.25** or **0.5%** solution, with or without epinephrine. *Caudal block*, **15** to **30 ml** of a **0.25** or **0.5%** solution (37.5 to 150 mg). *Epidural block*, **10** to **20 mL** of a **0.25** or **0.5%** solution (25 to 100 mg); obstetrics incremental doses of **3** to **5 mL** of a **0.5%** solution (50 to 100 mg); *single-dose epidural*, **10** to **20 mL** of a **0.75%** solution (75 to 150 mg). *Peripheral nerve block*, **5 mL** of a **0.25** or **0.5%** solution (12.5 to 25 mg) with or without epinephrine up to 400 mg a day. *Sympathetic nerve block*, **20** to **50 mL** of a **0.25%** solution (50 to 150 mg). *Retrobulbar anesthesia*, **2** to **4 mL** of a **0.75%** solution (15 to 30 mg). *Maxillary and mandibular anesthesia*, **1.8 mL** of a **0.5%** solution (9 mg) with epinephrine. *Spinal anesthesia, lower extremity*, **1 mL** of a **0.75%** solution (7.5 mg) with 8.25% dextrose; *lower abdominal procedures*, **1.6 mL** (12 mg); *obstetrical*, **0.8 mL** (6 mg); *cesarean section*, **1** to **1.4 mL** (7.5 to 10.5 mg).

Dosage Forms—Ampuls or Vials: 20-, 30- and 50-mL, 0.25%, with or without epinephrine 1:200,000; 20-, 30- or 50-mL, 0.5%, with or without epinephrine 1:200,000; Ampuls, 20- or 30-mL, 0.75% with or without epinephrine 1:200,000; 0.5% with 1:200,000 epinephrine in 1.8-mL dental cartridges.

Chloroprocaine Hydrochloride

Benzoic acid, 4-amino-2-chloro-, 2-(diethylamino)ethyl ester, monohydrochloride; Nesacaine, Nesacaine-MPF (*Astra*)

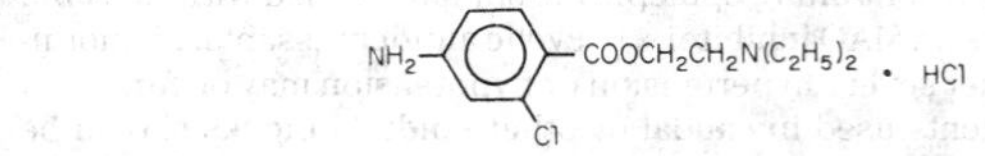

2-(Diethylamino)ethyl 4-amino-2-chlorobenzoate monohydrochloride [3858-89-7] $C_{13}H_{19}ClN_2O_2.HCl$ (307.22).

Preparation—2-Chloro-4-nitrobenzoic acid is reacted with thionyl chloride and the resulting acid chloride is condensed with 2-(diethylamino)ethanol. Reduction of the nitro ester with iron and acidulated water yields chloroprocaine base which may be converted into the hydrochloride by dissolving in a suitable solvent and introducing hydrogen chloride.

Description—White, crystalline powder; odorless and stable in air; solutions acid to litmus; exhibits local anesthetic properties when placed on the tongue; melts about 175°.

Solubility—1 g in about 20 mL water or about 100 mL alcohol; very slightly soluble in chloroform; practically insoluble in ether. Aqueous solutions are acid to litmus and if discolored, should not be used.

Uses—*Infiltration* and *nerve block* (mandibular, infraorbital or brachial plexus anesthesia, 2% solution; digital, 1%; pudendal, 2% and paracervical block, 1% solution). Caudal and epidural block, 2 or 3% solution. It is not effective topically. Its onset of action is about 6 to 12 min and anesthesia lasts from 30 to 60 min; with the addition of epinephrine 1:200,000, duration is increased to 60 to 90 min. For adverse reactions see the introductory statement.

Dose: *Maximum* **0.8 g** without epinephrine, **1.0 g** with epinephrine (1:200,000) as a **1** to **3%** solution. Repeated doses of up to 300 mg without epinephrine and 600 mg with epinephrine (1:200,000) may be given at 50-min intervals. *Usual, infiltration*, without epinephrine, up to **60 mL** of a **1%** solution depending on the site of injection; with epinephrine (1:200,000), up to **80 mL** of a **1%** solution. *Peripheral nerve block*, **1** or **2%** with or without epinephrine. *Caudal*, **15** to **25 mL** of a **2** or **3%** (Nesacaine-CE) solution, repeated at 40- to 60-min intervals as required. *Epidural*, **15** to **25 mL** (2 to 2.5 mL per nerve segment to be blocked) of a **2** or **3%** (Nesacaine-CE) solution; supplemental doses of 10 to 20 mL may be given at 40- to 50-min intervals; *peripheral nerve block*, **50 mL** of **1%** solution.

Dosage Form—Injection: 1 and 2% in 30 mL (not for caudal or epidural anesthesia); 2 and 3% in 30 mL (for caudal and epidural).

Dibucaine Hydrochloride—see RPS-18, page 1050.

Etidocaine Hydrochloride

Butanamide, (±)-*N*-(2,6-dimethylphenyl)-2-(ethylpropylamino)-, monohydrochloride; Duranest Hydrochloride (*Astra*)

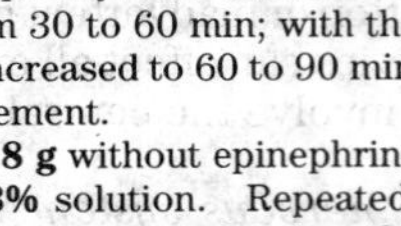

(±)-2-(Ethylpropylamino)-2′,6′-butyroxylidide monohydrochloride [3667-18-0 (free base)] $C_{17}H_{28}N_2O.HCl$ (312.88).

Preparation—Etidocaine is synthesized by the interaction of 2,6-xylidine, 2-bromobutyric acid, and ethyl *n*-propylamine. German Pat 2,162,744 (*CA 77:* 101244c, 1972).

Description—White, crystalline powder; pK_a 7.74 (etidocaine).

Solubility—Soluble in water; freely soluble in alcohol.

Uses—It has a rapid onset (3 to 5 min) and a prolonged duration of action (5 to 10 hr). The duration of sensory analgesia is 1.5 to 2 times longer than that for lidocaine; duration in excess of 9 hr is not infrequent in peripheral nerve blocks. It also produces a significant degree of motor blockade and abdominal muscle relaxation when used for peridural analgesia. Because of its tendency to block voluntary expulsive muscles, etidocaine should not be used in vaginal deliveries. This drug also should not be used for spinal anesthesia.

Contraindications, warnings for use, precautions and adverse reactions are similar to those for lidocaine. Its safe use in pregnancy, with respect to adverse effects of fetal development, has not been established. The use of this agent in children under 14 yr has not been investigated.

Dose—*Peripheral nerve, central neural* and *lumbar peridural block,* **5** to **40 mL** of a **1%** solution (50 to 400 mg); *Intraabdominal* or *pelvic surgery,* **10** to **30 mL** of **1%** solution (100 to 300 mg); *Caesarean section,* **10** to **20 mL** of a **1.5%** solution (150 to 300 mg); *dental,* **1** to **5 mL** of **1.5%** solution (15 to 75 mg). All of the above doses with epinephrine.

Dosage Forms—1.0% with or without epinephrine 1:200,000, 30-mL single-dose vials; 1.5% with epinephrine 1:200,000, 20-mL ampul.

Lidocaine—page 1153.

Lidocaine Hydrochloride

Acetamide, 2-(diethylamino)-*N*-(2,6-dimethylphenyl)-, monohydrochloride, monohydrate; Lignocaine; (*Various Mfrs*)

2-(Diethylamino)-2′,6′-acetoxylidide monohydrochloride [6108-05-0] $C_{14}H_{22}N_2O.HCl.H_2O$ (288.82); *anhydrous* [73-78-9] $C_{14}H_{22}N_2O.HCl$ (270.80).

For the structure and preparation of the base, see *Lidocaine*, page 1153.

Description—White, odorless, crystalline powder; slightly bitter taste; melts about 76°. pK_a 7.86 (base).

Solubility—1 g in 0.7 mL water or 1.5 mL alcohol; pH (0.5% soln), 5.0 to 7.0; solutions may be sterilized by autoclaving.

Uses—A widely employed amide-type *local anesthetic* and *antiarrhythmic* drug. As a local anesthetic, it is employed for *infiltration* and *field block anesthesia* in a concentration of 0.5%; for *peripheral nerve block* in a concentration of 0.5 and 1%; for *paravertebral nerve block* in a concentration of 0.5 to 1.5%; for *epidural or caudal anesthesia* in a concentration of 1.5% with 7.5% dextrose; and in *subarachnoid block (spinal analgesia)* in a concentration of 5% made hyperbaric with 7.5% dextrose. It also is used topically on mucous membranes as a 1 to 4% aqueous solution, 2% jelly, 2.5% and 5% ointment, and 2.0% viscous. It is also used in the form of suppositories for temporary relief of pain associated with inoperative, irritated or inflamed anorectal conditions.

Some of its injections contain epinephrine to delay absorption, prolong its action and reduce its toxic effects. Because it is also effective without a vasoconstrictor, it appears to be the anesthetic of choice for use in those individuals who are sensitive to epinephrine and its congeners. In addition, it is so dissimilar in chemical structure to procaine and related anesthetics that it is the agent of choice in individuals sensitive to procaine.

Its local anesthetic action is more rapid in onset, more intense and of longer duration than that of procaine. It also is more potent than procaine. Because of its local vasodilating action, epinephrine often is combined with lidocaine. When used alone, anesthesia after perineural injection lasts 60 to 75 min; with epinephrine, anesthesia lasts 2 hr or more. This drug and procaine are approximately equally toxic when administered extravascularly in 0.5% solutions; when higher concentrations are used, this is 1½ times as toxic as procaine. By the intravenous route, it is twice as toxic as procaine.

As an *antiarrhythmic agent* it is administered intravenously for the management of ventricular arrhythmias occurring during cardiac manipulation such as cardiac surgery, and life-threatening arrhythmias which are ventricular in origin, such as occur during acute myocardial infarction. For this purpose it usually is given in a dose of 50 to 100 mg intravenously at a rate of 25 to 50 mg/min. If the initial injection does not produce the desired clinical response, a second dose (⅓ to ½ the initial dose) may be given after 5 min.

No more than 200 to 300 mg of lidocaine should be administered during a 1-hr period. Smaller doses should be used in cardiac failure, a reduced cardiac output from any cause and in patients over 60 yr. It exhibits a biphasic half-life. The distribution phase ($t_{1/2}$: 7 to 8 min) accounts for the short duration of action after intravenous administration (10 to 20 min). The terminal elimination half-life is 1 to 2 hr.

Therapeutic antiarrhythmic plasma levels range from 1.5 to 5.5 μg/mL; subjective toxic effect levels range from 3 to 5 μg/mL; and objective adverse manifestations such as muscular irritability, convulsions and coma appear at plasma levels of 6 to 10 μg/mL. Thus, there is considerable overlap between therapeutic levels and subjective toxic effect levels. Moreover, toxicity may be significantly altered by the coadministration of other drugs. For example, coadministration with propranolol impairs the clearance of lidocaine and enhances toxicity, concomitant intravenous administration of phenytoin and lidocaine may induce excessive cardiac depression and additive neurological effects may be produced during concurrent administration of procainamide and lidocaine.

It should be emphasized that after administration as a local anesthetic agent, systemic absorption may result in blood concentrations in the usual therapeutic antiarrhythmic or even toxic ranges. Plasma levels vary according to the site at which the local anesthetic is injected: subcutaneous, 1.2 μg/mL/100 mg; epidural, 1.1 μg/mL/100 mg and subcutaneous (abdominal), 0.5 μg/mL/100 mg. Thus, the epidural injection of 25 mL of a 1.5% solution (375 mg) has the potential for producing a plasma level of 4.13 μg/mL, a value well within the range which induces subjective toxic effects (3 to 5 μg/mL) and approaching that which results in objective adverse manifestations (6 to 10 μg/mL).

After absorption, it partitions extensively into body tissues. Studies in monkeys indicate that it has a high affinity for spleen (tissue to plasma coefficient 3.5), lung (3.1), kidney (2.8), adipose tissue (2.0), brain (1.2), heart (0.96) and musculoskeletal tissues (0.6). Because of the avidity with which tissues take up the drug, only about 6% of a given dose is found in the blood at steady state. It then redistributes to muscle and adipose tissue; these tissues then become the major storage reservoirs. For more detailed pharmacokinetic data, the interested reader is referred to the excellent review by Benowitz and Meister (*Clin Pharmacokinet 3:* 177, 1978).

This drug is a weak base with a pK_a of 7.86, $t_{1/2}$ of 1.6 hr, V_d of 1.3 L/kg and 60 to 80% is bound to plasma protein. Maximal excretion in an acid urine is only 10%. The major portion of this agent is metabolized by the liver microsomal system. Two major metabolites have been identified: monoethylglycinexylidide and glycinexylidide. Animal experiments indicate both metabolites have antiarrhythmic and convulsant activities; the former has potency similar to this drug itself while the latter is only 10 to 26% as potent. Both metabolites, after further biotransformation in the liver, are excreted in the urine.

Some adverse central nervous system effects frequently are observed during therapy. These commonly include drowsiness, dizziness, paresthesia and euphoria. Typical symptoms with higher doses include confusion, agitation, dysarthria, vertigo, visual disturbances, tinnitus and nausea. Sweating, muscle tremor or fasciculations also may occur. Manifestations of severe toxicity include psychosis, seizures, respiratory depression and coma. Seizures which persist after the administration of oxygen may be controlled by intravenous administration of 2.5-mg increments of diazepam. Caution must be exercised since overdosage may occur if sufficient time is not allowed for the anticonvulsant action of the individual doses to become apparent. Diazepam has been recommended for prophylaxis of convulsions during local anesthetic therapy.

Dose—*Infiltration and nerve block,* up to **4.5 mg/kg** of **0.5** to **1.0%** solution without epinephrine. When used with epinephrine, up to **6.0 mg/kg.** *Spinal,* up to **100 mg.** *Caudal block,* **15** to **20 mL** of a **1.5%** solution. *Topical,* up to **250 mg** as a **2** to **4%** solution or as a **2%** jelly, to mucous membranes.

Dosage Forms—*Injection:* 0.5% in 50-mL single- and multiple-dose vials; 1% in 2- and 5-mL ampules and 2-, -30- and 50-mL vials, and 5-, 10-, 20- and 30-mL dispensing syringes; 1.5% in 20-mL single-dose ampules or vials; 2% in 2-, 5-, 10-, 20-, 30- and 50-mL vials, 2- and 10-mL ampules, and 5- and 10-mL dispensing syringes and 1.8-mL dental cartridges; 4% in 5-mL ampules and dispensing syringes. *Injection with epinephrine:* 0.5% with 1:200,000 epinephrine in 50-mL vials; 1.0% with 1:100,000 epinephrine in 20-, and 50-mL vials; 1% or 1.5% with 1:200,000 epinephrine in 5- and 30-mL ampules; 2% with 1:50,000 epinephrine in 1.8-mL dental cartridges; 2% with 1:100,000 epinephrine in 20-, and 50-mL vials and 1.8-mL dental cartridges; 2% with 1:200,000 epinephrine in 20-mL ampules or single-dose vials. *Injection with dextrose:* 1.5 and 5% with 7.5% dextrose in 2-mL ampules. *Topical:* 2.5 and 5% ointment and 0.5% cream.

Mepivacaine Hydrochloride

2-Piperidinecarboxamide, *N*-(2,6-dimethylphenyl)-1-methyl-, monohydrochloride; Carbocaine (*Winthrop*); Cavacaine (*Graham*); Polocaine (*Astra*)

1-Methyl-2′,6′-pipecoloxylidide monohydrochloride [1722-62-9] $C_{15}H_{22}N_2O.HCl$ (282.81).

Preparation—Picolinic acid (2-pyridinecarboxylic acid) is condensed with 2,6-xylidine to 2′,6′-picolinoxylidide which is reacted with dimethyl sulfate in xylene solution. Reduction of the pyridine ring followed by treatment with HCl yields the product. *Acta Chem Scand 11:* 1183, 1957

Description—White, odorless, crystalline solid; melts with decomposition about 258°; pH (1 in 50 solution) about 4.5; pK_a 7.73 ± 0.08.

Solubility—Freely soluble in water or methanol; very slightly soluble in chloroform; practically insoluble in ether.

Uses—An amide anesthetic employed for *nerve block* (1 or 2% sol), *paracervical block* in obstetrics (1% sol), *caudal* and *epidural block* (1, 1.5 or 2% sol), *infiltration* (1% sol), *therapeutic block* (1 or 2% sol) and *dental procedures* (1, 2 or 3% sol). It is not effective topically, except in large doses; therefore it should not be used for this purpose. It has a $t_{1/2}$ of 1.9 hr, V_d of 1.2 L/kg, and a partition coefficient of 12.1. Approximately 60 to 80% of that in blood is bound to serum proteins. When used in obstetrics, maternal plasma concentrations vary from 2.9 to 6.9 μg/mL, whereas the umbilical vein concentration varies from 1.9 to 4.9 μg/mL; thus, the fetus is exposed to only 60 to 70% of that in maternal plasma. It has an action similar to that of lidocaine hydrochloride; however, its onset is faster and its duration of action is somewhat longer.

Anesthesia develops in 3 to 5 min and lasts 2 to 2½ hr. It may be used for many purposes without epinephrine. Thus, it particularly is indicated in circumstances in which epinephrine is contraindicated. The systemic effects are similar to those produced by other local anesthetics. For additional information, see the introductory statement.

Dose—*Injection, adults, maximum single dose,* **7 mg/kg** but not to exceed **550 mg;** total dose should not exceed **1 g** in any 24-hr period. *Children* tolerate the local anesthetic as well as adults; however, the dose should be carefully measured as a percentage of adult dose based on weight (5 to 6 mg/kg). *Usual dose, therapeutic block,* **1** to **5 mL** of **1** or **2%** solution; *infiltration,* up to **40 mL** of **1%** solution; *caudal* and *epidural,* **15** to **30 mL** of **1%** solution, **10** to **25 mL** of **1.5%** solution, or **10** to **20 mL** of **2%** solution; *paracervical block,* up to **10 mL** of **1%** solution; *nerve block,* **5** to **20 mL** of **1** or **2%** solution.

Dosage Forms—1% in 30- and 50-mL vials; 1.5% in 30-mL vial; 2% in 20- and 50-mL vials; 2% with 1:20,000 levonordefrin and 3% in 1.8-mL dental cartridges.

Prilocaine Hydrochloride

Propanamide, *N*-(2-methylphenyl)-2-(propylamino)-, monohydrochloride; Citanest (*Astra*)

$$CH_3C_6H_4\text{–}NHCOCHCH_3(NHCH_2CH_2CH_3) \cdot HCl$$

2-(Propylamino)-*o*-propionotoluidide monohydrochloride [1786-81-8] $C_{13}H_{20}N_2O.HCl$ (256.77).

Preparation—*o*-Toluidine is condensed with 2-bromopropionyl bromide and the resulting 2-bromo-*o*-propionotoluidide is condensed with propylamine to yield prilocaine (base). An acetone solution of the base treated with hydrogen chloride yields the official salt. Brit Pat 839,943.

Description—White, odorless, crystalline powder; initially an acid and then bitter taste, stable in light and air; melts about 167°; pK_a 7.89.

Solubility—1 g in 3.5 mL water, 4.2 mL alcohol or 175 mL chloroform; practically insoluble in ether.

Uses—An amide-type local anesthetic chemically related to lidocaine and mepivacaine. For the most part, its use is confined to dental procedures administered either by infiltration or nerve block. An initial dose of 40 to 80 mg (1 to 2 mL of a 4% solution) is usually sufficient, with a maximum dose of 600 mg (8 mg/kg). Onset of action after infiltration averages 1 or 2 min; duration of action is 60 min or longer. For major nerve blocks (epidural), the onset of analgesia is approximately 2 min longer than that for lidocaine; whereas the duration of action is 30 to 60 min longer. Approximately 55% is bound to plasma protein. After 600 mg of the drug, peak plasma levels are reached in 20 min, at which time plasma levels average 4 μg/mL; the same dose with epinephrine also peaks at 20 min, but the plasma level is only 2 μg/mL. Consequently, this drug generally is used without epinephrine. Hence, this local anesthetic is particularly useful for patients who cannot tolerate vasopressor agents, eg, patients with hypertension, diabetes, thyrotoxicosis or other cardiovascular disorders.

Like other amide-type local anesthetics, prilocaine is not metabolized by plasma esterases; it is metabolized by both the liver and the kidney and excreted by the kidney. One of its metabolites is *o*-toluidine, a substance known to induce methemoglobinemia. Methemoglobin levels up to 15% and cyanosis have been reported following doses of 600 mg or more. Other clinical symptoms of methemoglobinemia, such as tachycardia, fatigue, headache, lightheadedness and dizziness may occur at higher doses. Except for methemoglobinemia, its side effects are similar to those observed with other local anesthetics. When methemoglobinemia occurs, it can be reversed by intravenous injection of methylene blue, 1 to 2 mg/kg of a 1% solution administered over a 5-min period. As with other local anesthetics, prilocaine is contraindicated in the presence of shock, severe cardiovascular disease or heart block. For other adverse effects, see the introductory statement.

Dose—*Usual, infiltration* and *nerve block in dentistry,* **1** to **2 mL** of a **4%** solution.

Dosage Form—Injection: 4%/1.8 mL or 4% with epinephrine 1:200,000/1.8 mL.

Procaine Hydrochloride

Benzoic acid, 4-amino-, 2-(dimethylamino)ethyl ester, monohydrochloride; Novocain (*Winthrop*); (*Various Mfrs*)

$$NH_2\text{–}C_6H_4\text{–}COOCH_2CH_2N(C_2H_5)_2 \cdot HCl$$

2-(Diethylamino)ethyl *p*-aminobenzoate monohydrochloride [51-05-8] $C_{13}H_{20}N_2O_2.HCl$ (272.77).

Preparation—2-(Diethylamino)ethanol is made by reacting ethylene chlorohydrin or bromohydrin with diethylamine. The diethylaminoethanol is then heated with *p*-nitrobenzoyl chloride, forming diethylaminoethyl *p*-nitrobenzoate. The NO_2 group is reduced with iron or tin and HCl. US Pat 812,554.

Description—Small, white, odorless crystals or a white crystalline powder; melts about 157°; pK_a 8.7 (base).

Solubility—1 g in 1 mL of water or 15 mL of alcohol; slightly soluble in chloroform; practically insoluble in ether.

Uses—An ester-type local anesthetic. It is used for *infiltration* (0.25 to 0.5% sol), *peripheral nerve block* (0.5 to 2% sol) and *spinal anesthesia* (10% sol). It is ineffective when applied topically. The drug has a slower onset of action than lidocaine or prilocaine; its duration of action is short, about 1 hr.

It produces vasodilation and therefore vasoconstrictor drugs such as norepinephrine or levonordefrin may be required to retard absorption, prolong duration of action and maintain homeostasis. Following absorption, it is hydrolyzed rapidly by esterases in both the plasma and liver (see the introductory statement). Since spinal fluid contains little or no esterase, when given by this route of administration it remains active until it is absorbed into the general circulation.

The products of metabolic degradation include *para*-aminobenzoic acid and diethylaminoethanol; the former inhibits the action of sulfonamides. Therefore, it and other ester-type local anesthetics should not be used in any condition in which therapy with sulfonamide is being employed. This drug and its congeners also interfere with the laboratory determination of sulfonamide concentration in biological fluids. Local anesthetics other than derivatives of *para*-aminobenzoic acid should be used in all circumstances where sulfonamide therapy has been instituted. The IV use of procaine is contraindicated in patients receiving digitalis, anticholinesterase drugs or succinyl choline. For adverse effects, see the introductory statement.

Dose—*Infiltration,* maximum of **350** to **600 mg** as a **0.25** or **0.5%** solution. *Peripheral nerve block,* up to **200 mL** of a **0.5%** solution, **100 mL** of a **1.0%** solution, or **50 mL** of a **2%** solution. The initial dose should not exceed 1000 mg. *Subarachnoid block,* **0.5** to **2.0 mL** of a **10%** solution.

Dosage Forms—1% in 2- and 6-mL ampules and 30- and 100-mL vials; 2% in 30-, and 100-mL vials; 10% in 2-mL ampules.

Propoxycaine Hydrochloride

Benzoic acid, 4-amino-2-propoxy-, 2-(diethylamino)ethyl ester, monohydrochloride; ing of Blockain Hydrochloride (*Winthrop*); Ravocaine Hydrochloride (*Cook-Waite*)

$$NH_2\text{–}C_6H_3(OCH_2CH_2CH_3)\text{–}COOCH_2CH_2N(C_2H_5)_2 \cdot HCl$$

[550-83-4] $C_{16}H_{26}N_2O_3.HCl$ (330.85).

Preparation—In the same manner as procaine hydrochloride (above), except 2-propoxy-4-nitrobenzoic acid is condensed with diethylaminoethanol. US Pat 2,689,248.

Description—White, odorless crystals which discolor on exposure to light and air; pH (2% *w/v*) about 5.4; pK_a 8.6; melts between 146° and 151°.

Solubility—1 g in 2 mL water, 10 mL alcohol or 80 mL ether; insoluble in acetone and chloroform.

Uses—An ester-type local anesthetic with an intermediate duration of action. When used as a *nerve block*, a 0.5% solution induces anesthesia which persists for about 2 hr. Hence, its duration of action is longer than that of procaine. Like other ester-type agents it is hydrolyzed primarily by plasma pseudocholinesterases and excreted by the kidneys. It is used primarily for dental procedures and given as infiltration or block anesthesia. It is combined with procaine and either norepinephrine or levonordefrin. Since it shares the toxic potentials of other local anesthetics, it should be used with similar precautions. See the introductory statement.

Dose—*Usual*, **7.2 mg** with 36 mg procaine.

Dosage Forms—Injection: Propoxycaine and Procaine Hydrochlorides and Norepinephrine Bitartrate Injection: 0.4% to 2% and 1:30,000/1.8 mL cartridge or Propoxycaine and Procaine Hydrochloride and Levonordefrin Injection: 0.4% to 2% and 1:20,000/1.8 mL cartridge.

Tetracaine—See page 1153.

Tetracaine Hydrochloride

Benzoic acid, 4-(butylamino)-, 2-(dimethylamino)ethyl ester, monohydrochloride; Amethocaine Hydrochloride; Pontocaine Hydrochloride (*Winthrop*)

2-(Dimethylamino)ethyl *p*-(butylamino)benzoate monohydrochloride [136-47-0] $C_{15}H_{24}N_2O_2.HCl$ (300.83).

For the structure of the base see page 1153.

Preparation—By dissolving tetracaine (base) in a solvent such as benzene and passing hydrogen chloride into the solution whereupon the salt precipitates. For the preparation of the base, see *Tetracaine*.

Description—Fine, white, crystalline, odorless powder; slightly bitter taste followed by a sense of numbness; solutions neutral to litmus; melts about 148°; two polymorphic modifications melt about 134° and 139°, respectively; mixtures of these may melt between 134° and 147°; pK_a 8.39. Protect solutions from light.

Solubility—Very soluble in water; soluble in alcohol; insoluble in ether or benzene.

Uses—An ester-type local anesthetic used topically on the eye, in the nose or throat and by *infiltration* for *subarachnoid block* (*spinal analgesia*). When used in the eye, it does not dilate the pupil, paralyze accommodation or increase intraocular pressure. It is particularly suitable for *spinal anesthesia*, especially for surgical procedures requiring 2 to 3 hr. Although it is an ester-type local anesthetic, it is only slowly hydrolyzed by plasma and liver esterases. It has a delayed onset of action, often as long as 15 min, but a long duration of action; spinal anesthesia may last as long as 3 hr. Since its *para*-aminobenzoic acid metabolite may antagonize the activity of aminosalicylic acid and sulfonamides, it should not be used in patients receiving these drugs. For information on cautions, contraindications and adverse effects, see the introductory statement.

Dose—*Subarachnoid block* (*spinal analgesia*), **0.2** to **1.0%** solution; *Niphanoid* (instantly soluble), perineum **5 mg**, perineum and lower extremeties **10 mg**, and up to costal margin **15 mg**. *Ophthalmic solution*, instil **1** or **2** drops.

Dosage Forms—Injection: 0.2 and 1.0% in 2-mL ampules, 0.3% in 5-mL ampuls, and *Niphanoid* (instantly soluble) 20-mg ampules; Ophthalmic Solution: 0.5%; Cream: 1%; Ointment: 0.5%; Topical Solution: 2%.

Injection Anesthetic Combinations

Some examples of injection anesthetic combinations (with %, or mg/unit provided) are as follows:

Propoxycaine Hydrochloride and Procaine Hydrochloride with Levonordefrin [Ravocaine and Novocain with Neo-Cobefrin (*Cook-Waite*)]—7.2, 36 and 0.09 mg/1.8 mL, respectively.

Propoxycaine Hydrochloride and Procaine Hydrochloride with Norepinephrine [Ravocaine and Novocaine with Levophed (*Cook-Waite*)]—7.2, 36 and 0.6 mg/1.8 mL, respectively.

Topical Anesthetics

The salts and base forms of the esters and amides included in this section are used to produce topical (surface) anesthesia. The salts do not penetrate intact skin, but both forms penetrate abraded or raw granulated skin surfaces. The base forms relieve pruritus, burning and surface pain on intact skin, but penetrate only to a limited degree. Wounds, ulcers and burns preferably are treated with preparations that are relatively insoluble in tissue fluids. Mucous membranes of the nose, mouth, pharynx, larynx, trachea, bronchi and urethra are anesthetized readily by both salt and base forms. Consequently, these agents are used prior to inserting intratracheal catheters, pharyngeal and nasal airways, nasogastric and endoscopic tubes, urinary catheters, laryngoscopes, proctoscopes, sigmoidoscopes and vaginal specula. Many of these agents also are used in the eye for such procedures as tonometry, gonioscopy and for removal of foreign bodies from the cornea, or for short operative procedures on the cornea or conjunctiva. For precautions, warnings and adverse effects, see the introductory statement.

Benoxinate Hydrochloride—see RPS-18, page 1056.

Benzocaine

Benzoic acid, 4-amino-, ethyl ester; Benzocaine; Anesthesin; (*Various Mfrs*)

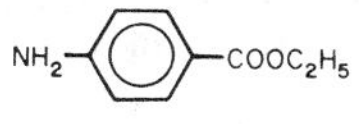

$NH_2-C_6H_4-COOC_2H_5$

Ethyl *p*-aminobenzoate [94-09-7] $C_9H_{11}NO_2$ (165.19).

Preparation—*p*-Nitrobenzoic acid, obtained by nitration of toluene and oxidation of the resulting *p*-nitrotoluene, is converted into the ethyl ester by heating with alcohol and sulfuric acid. The resulting ethyl *p*-nitrobenzoate is reduced with tin and hydrochloric acid.

Description—Small, white, odorless crystals or as a white crystalline powder; melts within a 2° range between 88 and 92°. pK_a 2.5.

Solubility—1 g in about 2500 mL water, 5 mL alcohol, 2 mL chloroform, 4 mL ether or 30 to 50 mL expressed almond oil or olive oil; soluble in dilute mineral acids.

Uses—An insoluble *local anesthetic*. It usually is employed as an ointment to relieve pain associated with *ulcers*, *wounds* and mucous surfaces. It also is used as a lubricant and anesthetic on intratracheal catheters, pharyngeal and nasal airways, nasogastric and endoscopic tubes, etc. It is included in proprietary creams, lozenges, ointments, powders, sprays and suppositories to relieve pain of damaged skin surfaces and inflamed mucous membranes, particularly those in the anorectal area. It also is used as an otic preparation for the temporary relief of ear pain. Benzocaine commonly is combined with antitussives, such as dextromethorphan, in cold medications. It acts only as long as it is in contact with the skin or mucosal surface. Peak effect occurs within 1 min after application and lasts for 36 to 60 min. For adverse reactions, see the introductory statement in this chapter.

Dose—*Topical*, as a **1** to **20%** aerosol, cream or ointment to the skin.

Dosage Forms—Aerosol: 5 and 20%; Cream: 1 and 5%; Solution: 2.5 to 20%; Gel or Paste: 6.3 to 20%; Spray: 5 to 20%; Oral Lozenges: 5 to 10 mg.

Benzyl Alcohol—see RPS-18, page 1056.

Butacaine—see RPS-18, page 1056.

Butamben Picrate—see RPS-18, page 1056.

Clove Oil—see RPS-18, page 1056.

Chlorobutanol—page 1380.

Cocaine

8-Azabicyclo[3.2.1]octane-2-carboxylic acid, [1*R*-(*exo*,*exo*)]-3-(benzoyloxy)-8-methyl-, methyl ester;

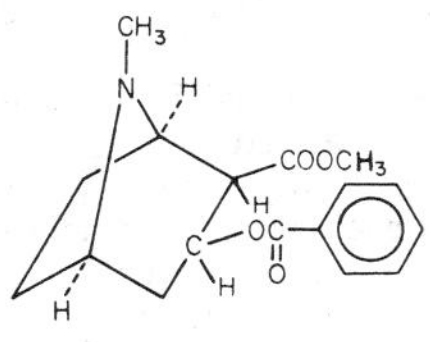

Methyl 3β-hydroxy-1αH,5αH-tropane-2β-carboxylate benzoate (ester) [50-36-2] $C_{17}H_{21}NO_4$ (303.36); an alkaloid obtained from the leaves of

Erythroxylon coca Lamarck and other species of *Erythroxylon* Linné (Fam *Erythroxylaceae*), or by synthesis from ecgonine or its derivatives.

History—Isolated by Gaedken in 1844 from Brazilian coca leaves, which for many years was the only source of cocaine. At present the alkaloid is obtained principally from Java coca leaves. Brazilian coca leaves contain from 0.5 to 1% of methylbenzoylecgonine or cocaine, whereas the Java leaves contain very little cocaine as such. However, there are present in the latter such derivatives as benzoylecgonine, cinnamoylecgonine, methylecgonine, etc, to the extent of 1.5 to 2%, all of which are converted to cocaine in the manufacturing process. For the structural relationships among the ecgonine derivatives, see page 404.

Preparation—By moistening ground coca leaves with sodium carbonate solution, percolating with benzene or other solvents such as petroleum benzin, shaking the liquid with diluted sulfuric acid and adding to the separated acid solution an excess of sodium carbonate. The precipitated alkaloids are removed with ether and, after drying with sodium carbonate, the solution is filtered and the ether distilled off. The residue is dissolved in methyl alcohol and the solution heated with sulfuric acid or with alcoholic hydrogen chloride. This treatment splits off any acids from ecgonine and esterifies the carboxyl group. After dilution with water, the organic acids which have been liberated are removed with chloroform. The aqueous solution is concentrated, neutralized and cooled with ice, whereupon methylecgonine sulfate crystallizes. This is benzoylated by heating with benzoyl chloride or benzoic anhydride at about 150°. On adding water and sodium hydroxide, methylbenzoylecgonine or cocaine is precipitated. The cocaine is extracted with ether and the solution concentrated to crystallization. For the purification of cocaine, recrystallization from a mixture of acetone and benzene generally is preferred.

Total synthesis of cocaine was achieved by Willstäter *et al*, *Ann 434:* 111, 1923.

Description—Colorless to white crystals, or a white, crystalline powder; odorless; melts about 97°; solution (in diluted HCl) levorotatory; saturated solution alkaline to litmus.

Solubility—1 g in about 600 mL water, 7 mL alcohol, 1 mL chloroform, 3.5 mL ether, about 12 mL olive oil or from 80 to 100 mL liquid petrolatum; very soluble in warm alcohol.

Uses—The first local anesthetic to be discovered. While it is considered too toxic for any anesthetic procedure requiring injection, it is still employed topically in a 1 or 2% solution for anesthesia of the ear, nose, throat, rectum and vagina because of its intense vasoconstrictive action. Besides its local anesthetic properties, cocaine enhances catecholamine systems by interfering with uptake of their transmitters into neuronal terminals. Peak effect is reached within 2 to 5 min and lasts from ½ to 2 hr. Toxic symptoms occur frequently because it is absorbed readily and dosage often is not monitored carefully. CNS effects include euphoria and cortical stimulation manifested by excitement and restlessness. Stimulation of the lower motor centers causes hypertension, tachycardia and tachypnea. Repeated use results in psychic dependence and tolerance, the euphoric effects of which are almost indistinguishable from those induced by amphetamines. Indeed, knowledgeable human subjects cannot distinguish between the subjective effects induced by the intravenous injection of 8 to 10 mg of the drug and those induced by 10 mg of dextroamphetamine. The drug is abused by intranasal, parenteral or inhalation administration because of its CNS-stimulating effects. It is listed under *Schedule II* of the *Controlled Substances Act.* Severe toxic effects have been reported with doses as low as 20 mg, while the fatal dose is approximately 1.2 g. For adverse reactions, see the introductory statement.

Dose—See *Cocaine Hydrochloride.*

Dosage Forms—See *Cocaine Hydrochloride.*

Cocaine Hydrochloride

8-Azabicyclo[3.2.1]octane-2-carboxylic acid, 3-(benzoyloxy)-8-methyl-, methyl ester, hydrochloride, [1*R*-(*exo,exo*)]-, Neurocaine Hydrochloride

Methyl 3β-hydroxy-1αH,5αH-tropan-2β-carboxylate, benzoate (ester) hydrochloride [53-21-4] $C_{17}H_{21}NO_4.HCl$ (339.82).

Preparation—By adding cocaine to an alcoholic solution of hydrochloric acid and crystallizing.

Description—Colorless crystals or a white crystalline powder. pK_a 5.59 (amine).

Solubility—1 g in 0.5 mL water, 3.5 mL alcohol or 15 mL chloroform; soluble in glycerin or insoluble in ether.

Uses—A *local anesthetic* (in solution) for mucous membranes. For topical application (ear, nose, throat or bronchoscopy) concentrations of 4 to 10%. Concentrations greater than 4% are not advisable. For adverse effects, see the introductory statement in this chapter.

Dose—*Topical,* as a **4** to **10%** solution, to mucous membranes.

Dosage Forms—Soluble Tablets: 135 mg with lactose (in 100s); Topical Solution: 40 mg/mL in 10 mL and unit dose 4 mL; 100 mg/mL in 10 ml and unit dose 4 mL; Powder: In 5 and 25 g.

Dibucaine

4-Quinolinecarboxamide, 2-butoxy-*N*-[2-(diethylamino)ethyl]-, Nupercainal (*Ciba*); (*Various Mfrs*)

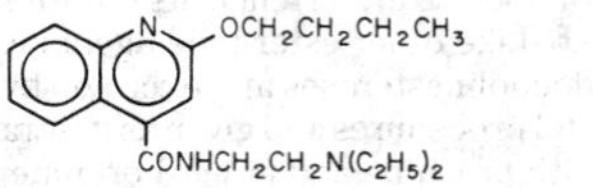

2-Butoxy-*N*-[2-(diethylamino)ethyl]cinchoninamide [85-79-0] $C_{20}H_{29}N_3O_2$ (343.47).

Preparation—May be synthesized by the following sequence of reactions: (1) Acetylation of isatin (obtained by oxidation of indigo) to *N*-acetylisatin, (2) rearrangement of 2-hydroxycinchoninic acid by treatment with alkali, (3) formation of 2-chlorocinchoninoyl chloride by reaction with phosphorus pentachloride, (4) conversion to 2-chloro-*N*-[2-(diethylamino)ethyl]cinchoninamide with *asym*-diethylethylenediamine and (5) heating with sodium butoxide. US Pat 1,825,623.

Description—White to off-white powder; slightly characteristic odor; somewhat hygroscopic; darkens on exposure to light; melts about 63°.

Solubility—1 g is soluble in 4600 mL water, less than 1 mL of alcohol or chloroform or in 1.4 mL ether.

Uses—Topically, for the temporary relief of pain and itching associated with burns, sunburn, insect bites or minor skin irritation. Ointment or suppositories are used topically for the relief of the pain and itching of hemorrhoids. Its toxicity caused it to be removed from the U.S. market as an injectable local anesthetic.

Dose—*Topical,* as a **0.5%** cream or a **1%** ointment several times a day.

Dosage Forms—Cream: 0.5%; Ointment: 1%.

Dyclonine Hydrochloride

1-Propanone, 1-(4-butoxyphenyl)-3-(1-piperidinyl)-, Dyclone (*Astra*)

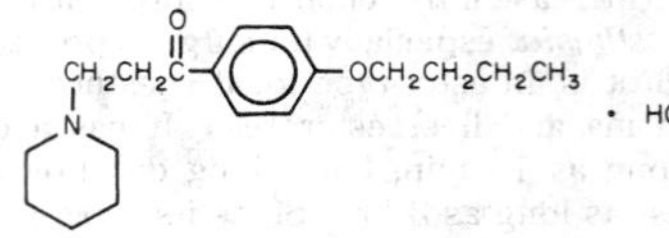

4′-Butoxy-3-piperidinopropiophenone hydrochloride [536-43-6] $C_{18}H_{27}NO_2.HCl$ (325.88).

Preparation—*p*-Hydroxyacetophenone is reacted with butyl bromide in a basic environment to produce the butoxy compound, which is reacted with piperidine hydrochloride and formaldehyde in an organic solvent under acidic conditions. US Pat 2,771,391 and 2,868,689.

Description—White crystals or white, crystalline powder; may have a slight odor; melts about 175°; pH (1 in 100 solution) 4.0 to 7.0.

Solubility—1 g in 60 mL water, 24 mL alcohol or 2.3 mL chloroform. Insoluble in ether or hexane.

Uses—To anesthetize accessible mucous membranes (eg, the mouth, pharynx, larynx, trachea, esophagus and urethra) prior to various endoscopic procedures. The 0.5% solution also may be used to block the gag reflex and to relieve pain associated with oral or anogenital lesions. Dyclonine-containing lozenges are used to relieve minor sore throat or mouth discomfort. It is contraindicated in cystoscopic procedures following intravenous pyelography; the drug precipitates iodine and interferes with visualization. When instilled into the conjunctival sac, it induces anesthesia without miosis or mydriasis. It also has antimicrobial properties. The clinical significance of this property has not been determined. Because of irritating properties, dyclonine should not be injected. For adverse effects, see the introductory statement.

Dose—*Topical,* as a **0.1**, **0.5** or **1%** solution, to the mucous membranes.

Dosage Forms—Oral Lozenges: 1, 2 and 3 mg; Solution: 0.5 and 1%.

Ethyl Chloride—page 1141.

Eugenol—see RPS-18, page 1056.

Lidocaine

Acetamide, 2-(diethylamino)-*N*-(2,6-dimethylphenyl)-, Xylocaine (*Astra*)

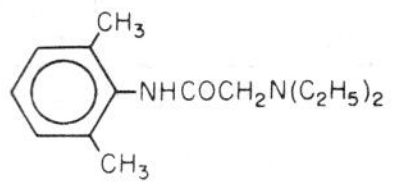

2-(Diethylamino)-2′,6′-acetoxylidide [137-58-6] $C_{14}H_{22}N_2O$ (234.34).

Preparation—By chloroacetylation of 2,6-xylidine and condensation of the resulting chloroacetoxylidide and diethylamine.

Description—White or slightly yellow, crystalline powder; characteristic odor; stable in air; melts about 67°; pK_a 7.86.

Solubility—Very soluble in alcohol or chloroform; freely soluble in benzene or ether; practically insoluble in water; dissolves in oils.

Uses—A *local anesthetic* used as an ointment topically on mucous membranes on minor burns, abrasions and anorectal lesions; also used as an anesthetic lubricant for endotracheal intubation. See *Lidocaine Hydrochloride.*

Dose—*Topical,* as a **2.5** to **5%** ointment, **0.5%** cream or **10%** oral spray.

Dosage Forms—Cream: 0.5%; Ointment: 2.5 and 5%; Oral Spray: 10%.

Lidocaine Hydrochloride—page 1149.

Pramoxine Hydrochloride

Morpholine, 4-[3-(4-butoxyphenoxy)propyl]-, hydrochloride; Tronothane (*Abbott*); Proctofoam (*Reed-Carnrick*); Prax (*Ferndale*)

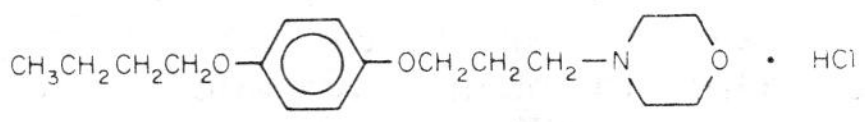

4-[3-(*p*-Butoxyphenoxy)propyl]morpholine hydrochloride [637-58-1] $C_{17}H_{27}NO_3.HCl$ (329.87).

Preparation—An aqueous mixture of 4-(3-chloropropyl)morpholine and *p*-butoxyphenol is refluxed until condensation is complete. The reaction mixture is cooled and the base is extracted with benzene. After evaporation of the benzene, the purified base is converted to the hydrochloride with HCl. *J Amer Chem Soc 73:* 2281, 1951

Description—White to nearly white, crystalline powder; numbing taste; may have a slight aromatic odor; pH (1 in 100 solution) about 4.5; melts about 182°.

Solubility—1 g in about 35 mL chloroform; freely soluble in alcohol and water; very slightly soluble in ether.

Uses—A surface anesthetic which has low indices of sensitization and toxicity, and is unrelated structurally to either ester- or amide-type agents. Consequently, it may be useful in patients sensitive to these classes of drugs. Local anesthesia develops in 3 to 5 min; its potency is comparable to that of benzocaine and is not sufficient to abolish the gag reflex. It is applied locally in a 1% concentration for the relief from discomfort and pain in hemorrhoids and rectal surgery, episiotomies, anogenital pruritus, itching dermatoses and minor burns. It is too irritating to be used in the eye. For adverse effects, see the introductory statement.

Dose—*Topical,* as a **1%** cream or aerosol every 3 to 4 hr.

Dosage Forms—Cream: 1%; Aerosol: 1%.

Proparacaine Hydrochloride

Benzoic acid, 3-amino-4-propoxy-, 2-(diethylamino)ethyl ester, monohydrochloride; Alcaine (*Alcon*); Ophthaine (*Squibb*); Ophthetic (*Allergan*)

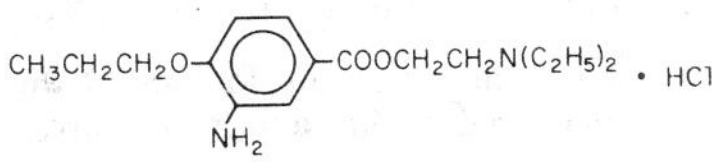

2-(Diethylamino)ethyl 3-amino-4-propoxybenzoate monohydrochloride [5875-06-9] $C_{16}H_{26}N_2O_3.HCl$ (330.85).

Preparation—*p*-Hydroxybenzoic acid is reacted with *n*-propyl chloride in alkaline solution and the resulting *p*-propoxybenzoic acid is nitrated to the 3-nitro compound. Treatment with thionyl chloride yields the acid chloride, which is coupled with 2-(diethylamino)ethanol. The resulting nitro ester is reduced to the base, which reacts with an equimolar quantity of HCl to form the hydrochloride. *J Amer Chem Soc 74:* 592, 1952.

Description—White to off-white, or faintly buff-colored, crystalline powder; odorless; on heating or exposure to air the compound tends to discolor; solutions exposed to air slowly discolor and finally become dark, with some loss of potency; crystals melt within a 2° range between 178 and 185°. pK_a 3.2.

Solubility—1 g in about 30 mL water or 30 mL warm alcohol or methanol; insoluble in ether or benzene. Solutions are neutral to litimus.

Uses—An effective ester-type surface anesthetic with a potency about equal to that of tetracaine. It is a useful anesthetic in ophthalmology and induces little or no initial irritation. Its onset of action is rapid; surface anesthesia of sufficient intensity to permit tonometry can generally be obtained within about 20 sec after the instillation of 1 or 2 drops of a 0.5% solution. The duration of such anesthesia is about 15 min. It is useful for most ocular procedures that require topical anesthesia such as, cataract extraction, tonometry, removal of foreign bodies and sutures, gonioscopy, conjunctival scraping for diagnosis and short operative procedures involving the cornea and conjunctiva. Although it is too toxic for use as an injection anesthetic, its ophthalmic use has been relatively free from side effects of untoward reactions. For adverse effects, see the introductory statement.

Dose—*Topically, cataract extraction,* **1 drop** in the eye every 5 to 10 min for 5 to 7 doses; *removal of sutures,* **1** or **2 drops** instilled 2 or 3 min before removal of sutures; *removal of foreign objects,* instill **1** or **2 drops** prior to operating; *tonometry,* **1** or **2 drops** immediately before measurement.

Dosage Form—Ophthalmic Solution: 0.5%.

Tetracaine

Benzoic acid, 4-(butylamino)-, 2-(dimethylamino)ethyl ester; Pontocaine (*Winthrop*)

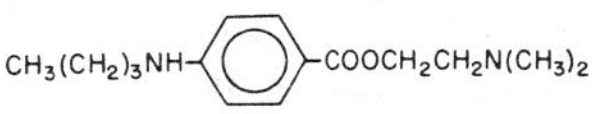

2-(Dimethylamino)ethyl *p*-(butylamino)benzoate [94-24-6] $C_{15}H_{24}N_2O_2$ (264.37).

Preparation—Ethyl *p*-aminobenzoate is butylated by refluxing with *n*-butyl bromide and ethanol in the presence of sodium carbonate. The resulting ethyl *p*-butylaminobenzoate is transesterified by heating with 2-(dimethylamino)ethanol in the presence of sodium ethoxide such that the liberated ethanol is distilled continuously from the reaction mixture. US Pat 1,889,645.

Description—White, or light yellow, waxy solid; melts about 43°.

Solubility—1 g in 1000 mL water, 5 mL alcohol, 2 mL chloroform or 2 mL ether.

Uses—See *Tetracaine Hydrochloride.*

Dose—*Topical,* as a **0.5%** ointment, apply ¼ to 1 inch to lower conjunctival fornix. Prolonged use is not recommended.

Dosage Forms—Ointment: 0.5%; Ophthalmic Ointment: 0.5%.

Tetracaine Hydrochloride—page 1151.

Other Topical Anesthetics

Other anesthetic agents used for topical applications include *benoxinate hydrochloride,* a benzoic acid ester related to procaine, for ophthalmic, surface anesthesia; *butamben picrate,* for temporary relief of pain due to minor burns; *clove oil* and *eugenol,* extracted from the volatile oil distilled from the dried flower buds of *Eugenia caryophyllus* for their germicide and counterirritant properties as a dental obtundent to alleviate toothache and treat root canals.

Topical Anesthetic Combinations

Some examples of topical anesthetic combinations (with %, or ng/unit provided) are as follows:

Benzocaine, Butamben and Tetracaine Hydrochloride [Cetacaine (*Cetylite*)]—14%, 2.0% and 2%, respectively.

Benzalkonium Chloride and Lidocaine Hydrochloride [Bactine (*Miles*)]—0.13% and 2.5%, respectively.

CHAPTER 69

Sedative and Hypnotic Drugs

Glen R Hanson, DDS, PhD
Professor of Pharmacology
College of Pharmacy and School of Medicine
University of Utah
Salt Lake City, UT 84112

The term *sedative* refers to a quieting effect accompanied by relaxation and rest, but not necessarily sleep. Sedative drugs are used to allay excitement and anxiety without inducing sleep. The term *hypnotic* refers to the production of sleep. Hence, hypnotic drugs are used to induce drowsiness and help the onset and maintenance of sleep. With most of the current drugs both sedative and hypnotic actions occur; a small dose of a drug may act as a sedative, whereas a large dose of the same drug may act as a hypnotic. However, it appears that a drug can have an anxiolytic effect without the sedative actions associated with most of the currently used medications. For example, the drug buspirone represents a new generation of anxioselective agents which do not impair psychomotor function significantly and are devoid of abuse potential.

Agents used as sedatives and hypnotics include a large number of compounds of diverse chemical structure and pharmacological properties which, with the exception of the benzodiazepines (e.g., diazepam) and buspirone, have in common the ability to induce a nonselective, reversible depression of the central nervous system. Thus, inorganic salts (bromide), chloral derivatives (chloral hydrate), acetylenic alcohols (ethchlorvynol), cyclic ethers (paraldehyde), carbamic acid esters of alcohols (ethinamate), carbamic acid esters of glycols (meprobamate), diureides (barbiturates), piperidinedione derivatives (glutethimide), disubstituted quinazolones (methaqualone) and some miscellaneous aromatic tertiary alkylamines, such as antihistaminics (diphenhydramine), and parasympatholytics (scopolamine) all exhibit pronounced sedative and hypnotic effects.

Some of these agents, such as buclizine, diphenhydramine, methotrimeprazine and scopolamine, exhibit primary pharmacological actions which dictate they should be classified in other sections of this text. On the other hand, agents such as diazepam, flurazepam, pentobarbital, meprobamate and related agents exhibit primary pharmacological actions which characterize them as sedative and hypnotic agents. For convenience, the sedatives and hypnotics presented herein will be divided into three groups: benzodiazepines, barbiturates and miscellaneous sedative and hypnotic agents.

In addition to their use as *sedatives* and *hypnotics*, the drugs discussed in this chapter also are administered as *muscle relaxants, anticonvulsants, preanesthetic medication* and *diagnostic* and *therapeutic aids* in psychiatry.

As *sedatives*, they are used in the management of neuroses and to allay anxiety, apprehension and panic episodes. Anxiety is perceived as a pervasive feeling of apprehension about some unspecified future threat to self esteem. This threat is assumed to arise within the person, perhaps based on a memory of a past threat triggered by some unrecognized present situation. The memory may signal the emotions and the somatic responses of the past fearful state. A unique form of anxiety is the panic attack. This disorder is characterized by periods of intense fear or discomfort which can last from minutes and occasionally to hours. These attacks are characterized by a sudden onset of severe anxiety or terror, often with a feeling of impending doom. Panic attacks can be spontaneous or situational.

The somatic manifestations of anxiety include fatigue, dizziness, palpitations, indigestion, bowel disturbances, headaches, muscle aches, insomnia, excessive perspiration, tremulousness of the hands or voice and other signs of nervous tension. Anxiety may be a primary symptom associated with emotional disorders or a secondary symptom of physical illness. In either case, it can be extremely disabling and worthy of careful diagnosis and treatment. Symptoms of related panic disorder include faintness, tachycardia, trembling, chest pain, fear of dying or going crazy and a general sense of losing control.

To induce sleep, hypnotic agents are selected based on the characteristics of the insomnia. Some patients have difficulty only in falling asleep and, once asleep, need no drug assistance; a rapidly acting hypnotic drug with a short duration of action will suffice for these patients. Other patients fall asleep readily, but experience one or more periods of wakefulness during the night; a hypnotic drug with a longer duration of action usually is indicated in such cases. Still other patients have trouble falling and in staying asleep; a rapidly acting hypnotic drug which exerts an effect throughout part or most of the night is required for such patients.

In all cases, however, consideration should be given to what the patient does on the day following a night of drug-induced sleep. Persons who must be alert the following day usually will object to drugs which leave residual sedation, whereas hospitalized patients, or individuals with no place to go and nothing to do, actually may benefit from the sedative after effects the next day.

It should be remembered that not all patients with insomnia require hypnotic drug therapy. Often, in cases when the insomnia is spontaneous, chronic and with no apparent cause, long-term use of a hypnotic is undesirable and the patient likely is served better with behavior-modification techniques and counseling. Moreover, there are many instances where nonhypnotic drugs are superior to hypnotic drugs. For example, methylphenidate may improve sleep in some hyperkinetic patients, phenytoin in patients with insomnia due to paroxysmal nightmares, analgesics when sleep is impaired by pain, antithyroid drugs or beta-blockers when sleep is difficult due to hyperthyroidism, bethanechol or similar drugs in nocturnal gastroesophageal reflux, cimetidine in peptic ulcers and others. Nonspecific hypnotic therapy should be employed only in those cases where specific causes of the insomnia *cannot* be identified and eliminated.

A number of the sedative-hypnotic drugs have *anticonvulsant* properties. Several benzodiazepines have excellent anticonvulsant actions and some are used to treat epilepsy.

Clonazepam is used alone or as an adjunct in the management of absence (petit mal), petit mal variant and, especially, akinetic and myoclonic seizures.

Diazepam is used as adjunctive therapy in status epilepticus and severe recurrent seizures as well as treatment for acute seizures resulting from drug overdoses or exposure to toxins.

All barbiturates exhibit anticonvulsant activity, but only phenobarbital, mephobarbital and metharbital are sufficiently selective to be clinically useful *antiepileptics*. Phenobarbital is useful in the management of generalized tonic-clonic seizures and as adjunctive therapy in complex partial (temporal lobe) seizures.

Sedative and hypnotic agents frequently are used as *preanesthetic medication* and as *adjunctive therapy* in psychiatry. Benzodiazepines and barbiturates are used commonly to allay anxiety and apprehension prior to surgery or other medical and dental procedures. In psychiatry, barbiturates with a short half-life have been used in *narcoanalysis* and *narcotherapy*. Sedative and hypnotic drugs also are employed in the treatment of dependence on CNS depressants. For example, diazepam often is used to manage symptoms associated with acute alcohol withdrawal.

A number of the sedative-hypnotic drugs cross the placental barrier. Consequently, their chronic use during pregnancy may cause withdrawal effects in the newborn infant. Moreover, many of these substances are excreted in breast milk. Their chronic use during breast feeding may cause sedation in the nursing infant.

Drowsiness is a side effect common to sedative-hypnotic agents. Patients taking such substances should be cautioned about operating hazardous machinery or operating a motor vehicle while taking such medication. Concurrent use of sedative-hypnotic drugs with alcohol, other CNS depressants, MAO inhibitors or tricyclic antidepressants should be avoided. More-detailed information with respect to adverse effects and drug interactions is provided in the introductory statement to each section and in the individual monographs.

Prolonged overdosage with most of these drugs can result in habituation and dependence liability. However, the "dependence risk" varies markedly among the various agents.

For example, the dependence risk with benzodiazepines is very low and has been estimated to be as few as one case per 5 million patient-months "at risk" for all recorded cases and one case per 50 million months in therapeutic use. Even though it is likely that in the past problems with benzodiazepines have been underestimated, there is no question that these agents are considerably safer than most other sedative and hynotic drugs, such as barbiturates. Accordingly, flurazepam, chlordiazepoxide, diazepam and other benzodiazepines are listed in *Schedule IV* under the *Controlled Substances Act*.

On the other hand, the dependence risk with methaqualone, amobarbital, pentobarbital and related substances is very high, with severe abuse potential. Consequently, these agents are listed in *Schedule II* under the *Controlled Substances Act*. It should be emphasized that with usual hypnotic doses and close medical supervision, the problem of dependence with these agents can be minimized. Nevertheless, they should be used with extreme caution, if at all, in patients with a history of previous drug dependence.

Finally, the marketing of buspirone as an anxiolytic provides another therapeutic option for treatment of anxiety in patients with a high risk dependence. Because of its lack of sedative and amnesic effects, buspirone lacks significant abuse potential.

Benzodiazepines

This group includes the most frequently prescribed sedative-hypnotic agents. In 1990 diazepam and lorazepam were the only sedative-hypnotic agents in the top 20 most frequently prescribed generic drugs and Xanax (alprazolam) and Halcion (triazolam) were the only sedative-hypnotic agents in the top 25 most prescribed brand-name drugs. These findings demonstrate the great popularity enjoyed by the benzodiazepines.

The benzodiazepines are not general depressants of the CNS like the barbiturates, ethanol, various other sedative-hypnotic agents and general anesthetics. There are marked differences among the various agents in selectivity, pharmacological profile, clinical usefulness and pharmacokinetic properties (see Table **1**). Moreover, they do not induce a true "anesthetic effect," since awareness is still present and total muscular relaxation is not obtained even after large doses.

Table 1—Elimination of benzodiazepines

Drug	Half-life ($t_{1/2}$) (hr)	Active metabolites
Alprazolam	12–15	None
Chlordiazepoxide	5–30	Four
Clonazepam	18–50	None
Clorazepate	–	Two
Diazepam	20–50	Three
Estazolam	10–24	None
Flurazepam	–	Two
Halazepam	14	One
Lorazepam	10–20	None
Midazolam	1–12.3	One
Oxazepam	3–21	None
Prazepam	–	Two
Quazepam	25–41	Two
Temazepam	10–20	None
Triazolam	1.6–5.4	None

Retrograde amnesia may take place and this creates the illusion that anesthesia has occurred. True surgical anesthesia can be obtained only when benzodiazepines are combined with other drugs which depress the CNS.

Gamma-aminobutyric acid (GABA) is a major inhibitory neurotransmitter in the mammalian CNS. It is believed that the benzodiazepines exert at least some of their actions via the inhibitory neurotransmitter GABA. The benzodiazepines potentiate GABA-mediated inhibitory neurotransmission and antagonize seizures caused by GABA depletion. *In vitro* binding studies support a GABA-benzodiazepine interaction. GABA stimulates [^{3}H]diazepam binding to synaptosomal membranes. The neurophysiological and biochemical evidence indicates that a GABA-benzodiazepine-chloride ionophore comprises a supramolecular structure. Therefore, an interaction between a benzodiazepine and its receptors stimulates GABA receptors, activates chloride channels and increases inhibition. The cellular mechanisms, pharmacokinetics, basic pharmacology and clinical pharmacology of the benzodiazepines have been reviewed by Lader (*Ann Rev Med 38:* 19, 1987).

The benzodiazepines are used in the symptomatic relief of anxiety and tension states resulting from a stressful environment or emotional factors. They also are useful in psychoneurotic states characterized by tension, anxiety, apprehension, fatigue, depression symptoms or agitation and the benzodiazepine, alprazolam, has been approved for treatment of panic attacks. Certain benzodiazepines (chlordiazepoxide and diazepam) also are useful in acute alcohol withdrawal to provide symptomatic relief from acute agitation, tremors and impending delirium tremens and hallucinosis.

Clonazepam is useful alone or as an adjunct in the management of several types of epileptic seizures. Diazepam is used as an adjunct therapy to endoscopic procedures, to the management of acute skeletal muscle spasm, and, by parenteral injection, to status epilepticus, to control convulsions resulting from overdosage with local anesthetics and other severe recurrent convulsive seizures. The benzodiazepines also are useful adjunct therapy in the management of apprehension and anxiety which precedes or accompanies surgical procedures and disease states.

Benzodiazepines markedly influence CNS activity of humans in both the awake and sleep state. In the waking human EEG, alpha activity is decreased, fast activity (primarily beta) is increased and the energy content of the EEG is decreased.

With respect to sleep, the benzodiazepines decrease sleep latency and decrease the number of awakenings and the time spent in Stage 0 (wakefulness). They also increase the awakening threshold. The time spent in Stage 1 (descending drowsiness) is decreased by flurazepam, lorazepam and nitrazepam, but increased by chlordiazepoxide, diazepam and oxazepam. The time spent in Stage 2 (major fraction of non-REM sleep) is increased by all benzodiazepines. The time spent in Stages 3 and 4 (slow wave sleep) usually is decreased; however, a few agents may increase these stages. Because of suppression of Stage 4 sleep, diazepam has been used to prevent night terrors in adults.

The benzodiazepines increase the latency to REM sleep, decrease REM sleep time and increase the number of REM cycles. Total sleep time is increased by the benzodiazepines. The greatest increase is observed in subjects with the shortest base-line sleep time. In such individuals, total sleep time may increase threefold.

After oral administration, the benzodiazepines are absorbed in from 1 to 6 hours, depending on the formulation given. Binding to serum albumin varies widely; after oral administration of flurazepam only a few percent is bound, whereas after nitrazepam 87% is in bound form. The extent to which benzodiazepines interact with other protein-bound drugs is not known; the absence of reports of such adverse interactions suggest that such competition is not of clinical significance.

Biotransformation takes place in the liver by the microsomal drug metabolizing system. Clorazepate, chlordiazepoxide, diazepam, halazepam, flurazepam and prazepam are transformed to active metabolites, primarily to *N*-demethylated products with a longer half-life than the parent drug. This metabolite may be particularly significant in the elderly, newborn or those with severe liver disease. Only lorazepam, oxazepam, temazepam and triazolam do not form long-acting active metabolites; thus, their action is not prolonged significantly in the elderly and liver-diseased patient. Benzodiazepines cross the placental barrier and are excreted in human milk.

Patients on these drugs should be warned about potential effects induced by the concomitant use of alcohol or other CNS depressants such as other antianxiety and hypnotic drugs, tricyclic antidepressants, opiate analgesics, antipsychotics, antihistamines, including nonprescription sleep aids and cold remedies. They also should be warned not to operate a motor vehicle or hazardous machinery while on these drugs.

Side effects most commonly reported after benzodiazepines include drowsiness, fatigue, confusion, dizziness, weakness, ataxia and syncope; venous thrombosis and phlebitis at the site of the injection. Other less-frequent side effects include anterograde amnesia, blurred vision, diplopia and nystagmus; urticaria and skin rash; hiccups, changes in salivation, constipation, changes in appetite, bizarre behavior, antisocial acts, neutropenia and jaundice. Paradoxical reactions such as acute hyperexcited states, anxiety, hallucinations, increased muscle spasticity, insomnia, rage and sleep disturbances also have been reported; should these occur the drug should be discontinued. Since significant amounts of benzodiazepines are found in maternal and cord blood, these agents are not recommended for obstetrical use. The safe use of benzodiazepines in children under 12 years has not been established.

Physical and *psychological* dependence may occur, especially following prolonged use, although dependence also can occur with short-term high-dose treatment. Symptoms of a benzodiazepine dependence can resemble those associated with barbiturate or alcohol dependence and include slurred speech, ataxia and drowsiness. Abrupt discontinuation of long-term benzodiazepine treatment can result in severe withdrawal symptoms like other CNS depressants. To prevent such consequences, these drugs should be withdrawn gradually. Individuals known to be addictive-prone, or those whose history suggests they modify drug dosage on their own initiative, should not be given the drug. Withdrawal symptoms resemble those resulting from barbiturate withdrawal. The benzodiazepines are listed in *Schedule IV* under the *Controlled Substances Act*.

Alprazolam

4H-[1,2,4]Triazolo [4,3-*a*][1,4] benzodiazepine, 8-chloro-1-methyl-6-phenyl-, Xanax (*Upjohn*)

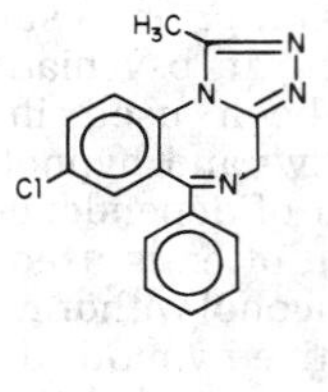

[28981-97-7] $C_{17}H_{13}ClN_4$ (308.77).

Preparation—See *J Med Chem 20*:1694, 1977.

Description—White crystals; melts about 228°.

Solubility—Practically insoluble in water; soluble in methanol or ethanol.

Uses—For the management of anxiety disorders or the short-term relief of the symptoms of anxiety. It also is indicated for the adjunctive treatment of anxiety associated with mental depression. Alprazolam also has been found to be effective in the short-term (4- to 10-wk) treatment of panic disorder with or without agoraphobia. Although not evaluated in well-controlled studies, the drug has been used effectively for 8 months or longer. In many patients, discontinuation of alprazolam results in a relapse of panic attacks and anxiety. After oral administration peak plasma levels are reached in 1 to 2 hr and half-life is 12 to 15 hr. Thus, it has a short to medium half-life when compared with other benzodiazepines. Accumulation is minimal during multiple dosage and steady-state plasma concentration usually is attained within 2 to 3 days. Elimination is rapid following discontinuation of therapy. Therefore, chronic therapy should not be terminated abruptly. Medical problems and adverse effects are similar to those for other benzodiazepines. See the introductory statement.

Dose—*Usual anxiety disorders, adult, oral,* **0.25** to **0.5 mg** 3 times a day; the dosage adjusted to the needs of the patient (maximum, 4 mg/day). *Geriatric* or *debilitated patients, oral,* **0.25 mg** 2 or 3 times a day. *Children up to 18 yr,* dosage not established. *Usual panic disorders,* **0.5 mg** 3 times a day initially; increase dose up to **1 mg/day** if needed for a response. Effective doses range from 1 to 10 mg/day.

Dosage Form—Tablets: 0.25, 0.5 and 1 mg.

Chlordiazepoxide

3H-1,4-Benzodiazepin-2-amine, 7-chloro-*N*-methyl-5-phenyl-, 4-oxide; Libritabs; Menrium (*Roche*); A-poxide (*Abbott*); Brigen-G (*Grafton*)

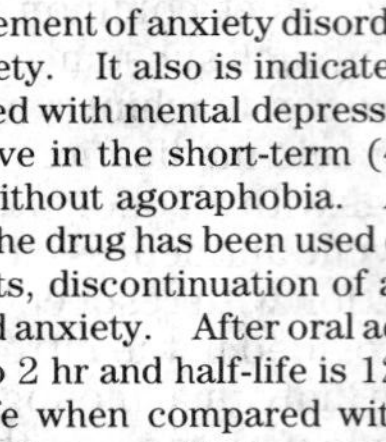

7-Chloro-2-(methylamino)-5-phenyl-*3H*-1,4-benzodiazepine 4-oxide [58-25-3] $C_{16}H_{14}ClN_3O$ (299.76).

Preparation—For the preparation of chlordiazepoxide, see *Chlordiazepoxide Hydrochloride*, below.

Description—Yellow, practically odorless, crystalline powder; sensitive to sunlight; melts about 242° pK_a 4.6.

Solubility—1 g in > 10,000 mL water, 50 mL alcohol, 6250 mL chloroform or 130 mL ether.

Uses—See *Chlordiazepoxide Hydrochloride*.

Dose—See *Chlordiazepoxide Hydrochloride*.

Dosage Form—Tablets: 5, 10 and 25 mg.

Chlordiazepoxide Hydrochloride

3H-1,4-Benzodiazepin-2-amine, 7-chloro-*N*-methyl-5-phenyl-, 4-oxide, monohydrochloride; Librium (*Roche*); Lipoxide (*Major*); Reposans-10 (*Wesley*); (*Various Mfrs*)

[438-41-5] $C_{16}H_{14}ClN_3O.HCl$ (336.22).

For the structure of the base, see above.

Preparation—By condensation cyclization of 2-amino-5-chlorobenzophenone oxime with chloroacetyl chloride to form 6-chloro-2-chloromethyl-4-phenylquinazoline 3-oxide, which subsequently is reacted with methylamine in methanol solution. US Pat 2,893,992.

Description—White or nearly white, crystalline powder; odorless; sensitive to sunlight; melts about 215°, with decomposition.

Solubility—1 g in 10 mL water or 40 mL alcohol.

Uses—Indicated for the relief of anxiety and tension, withdrawal symptoms of acute alcoholism, preoperative apprehension and anxiety, and adjunct therapy in various disease states in which anxiety and tension are prominent features. Its efficacy for long-term use (ie, for longer than 4 mo) has not been established; therefore, the need for continued therapy with the drug should be reevaluated periodically. It has a pK_a of 4.6 and a half-life of 8 to 20 hr. During chronic administration, accumulation occurs, not only of the parent substance but also of three active metabolites (desmethylchlordiazepoxide, demoxepam and desoxydemoxepam). Demoxepam has a half-life of 37 (range 28 to 63) hr and desoxydemoxepam of 44 (range 39 to 61) hr. These metabolites probably contribute to the overall activity of this drug, since they are pharmacologically active in animals. Steady-state plasma levels of chlordiazepoxide, desmethylchlordiazepoxide and demoxepam average 0.75, 0.54 and 0.36 μmg/mL, respectively. It is excreted in the urine; 1 to 2% is excreted unchanged and 3 to 6% as a conjugate.

As with other benzodiazepines, this drug requires the same warnings and precautions regarding its use in patients with known hypersensitivity, elderly and excessively depressed individuals, pregnant and lactating mothers, patients with known renal and hepatic impairment, patients on other CNS-depressant drugs and in patients with either a history of drug addiction or of indiscriminate alteration of drug dosage (page 1155).

Chlordiazepoxide is also available commercially in anxiolytic products combined with estrogens, anticholinergic (clidinium) and antidepressant (amitriptyline) agents. The therapeutic value of these fixed combinations has not been established.

Adverse reactions include drowsiness, ataxia, confusion, skin eruptions, edema, menstrual irregularities, nausea and constipation, extrapyramidal symptoms and decreased libido in some patients; blood dyscrasias (agranulocytosis), jaundice and hepatic dysfunction have occasionally been reported. Paradoxical reactions of rage, excitement, stimulation, hostility and depersonalization have sometimes followed administration to severely disturbed patients. Skin rashes, nausea, headache and decreased tolerance to alcohol also have been reported. The chronic administration of large doses of chlordiazepoxide hydrochloride may result in the development of tolerance and physical dependence.

Dose—*Anxiety, mild to moderate, oral,* **5** to **10 mg** 3 or 4 times a day; *severe,* **20** or **25 mg** 3 or 4 times a day. *Acute alcohol withdrawal oral* or *intravenous,* **50** to **100 mg**, repeated as necessary. *Preoperatively, intramuscular,* **50** to **100 mg** 1 hr prior to surgery. *Geriatric patients, debilitated patients* or *children over 6 yr,* **5** to **10 mg** 2 or 3 times a day.

Dosage Forms—Capsules: 5, 10 and 25 mg; Sterile Powder: 100 mg/ampule; Tablets: 5, 10 and 25 mg.

Chlormezanone—page 1167.
Clobazam—see RPS-18 page 1080.
Clonazepam—page 1173.

Clorazepate Dipotassium

1*H*-1,4-Benzodiazepine-3-carboxylic acid, 7-chloro-2,3-dihydro-2-oxo-5-phenyl-, potassium salt compd with potassium hydroxide (1:1); Tranxene (*Abbott*)

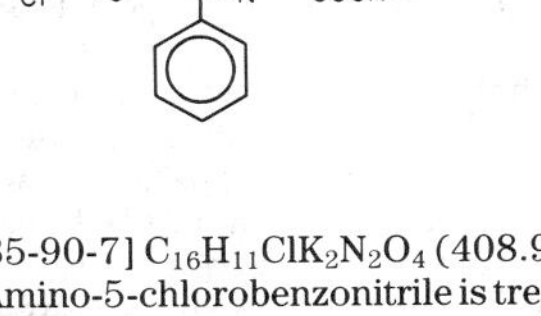

[57109-90-7; 15585-90-7] $C_{16}H_{11}ClK_2N_2O_4$ (408.92).

Preparation—2-Amino-5-chlorobenzonitrile is treated with phenylmagnesium bromide and the resulting ketimine is condensed via deamination with diethyl aminomalonate. The diester is then saponified with KOH in aqueous methanol and the resulting dipotassium dicarboxylate cyclizes via isomerization. US Pat 3,516,988.

Description—Fine, light-yellow, practically odorless, crystalline powder; slightly burning taste; sensitive to light, moisture and excessive heat; aqueous solutions are unstable (clear, light-yellow and alkaline to litmus).

Solubility—Very soluble in water; very slightly soluble in alcohol; insoluble in chloroform, ether, benzene or acetone.

Uses—For the symptomatic relief of anxiety associated with neurosis, psychoneuroses with symptoms of anxiety, acute alcohol withdrawal, other conditions in which anxiety is a prominent feature and as adjunctive therapy in the management of partial seizures. This substance is hydrolyzed in the stomach to desmethyldiazepam, a metabolic precursor of oxazepam and also a metabolite of both chlordiazepoxide and diazepam. The metabolite is absorbed rapidly (1 to 2 hr); the volume of distribution is 0.93 to 1.47 L/kg and the half-life ranges from 50 to 100 hr. Desmethyldiazepam accumulates for about 7 days, and then reaches a steady state. Consequently, clorazepate can be given once a day as well as in divided doses.

It requires the same warnings and precautions regarding use with other drugs, in hypersensitive individuals, during pregnancy and in young children, in elderly and excessively depressed patients, in patients with impaired renal or hepatic function and in patients with a history of drug addiction as with other benzodiazepines (see page 1155). Drowsiness is the most common adverse effect. Less-common untoward reactions include dizziness, various gastrointestinal complaints, nervousness, blurred vision, dry mouth, headache and mental confusion. Other adverse reactions include insomnia, transient skin rashes, fatigue, ataxia, genitourinary complaints, irritability, diplopia, depression and slurred speech. Hypotension, decreased hematocrit and abnormal liver and kidney function also have been reported.

Dose—*Adult, oral,* **15** to **60 mg** a day; *usual,* **30 mg** a day in divided doses or 22.5 mg as a single-dose tablet every 24 hr. Elderly or debilitated patients, 7.5 to 15 mg a day. See also package insert.

Dosage Forms—Capsules: 3.75, 7.5 and 15 mg; Single-Dose Tablets: 3.75, 7.5, 15 and 22.5 mg. Half-Strength Tablets, 11.25 mg.

Diazepam

2*H*-1,4-Benzodiazepin-2-one, 7-chloro-1,3-dihydro-1-methyl-5-phenyl-, Valium (*Roche*); Vazepam (*Major*); Zetran (*Hauck*); Diazepam Solution (*Roxane*)

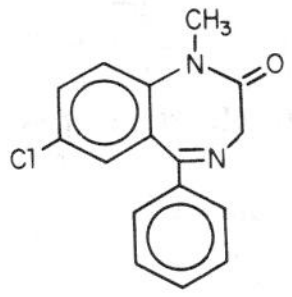

[439-14-5] $C_{16}H_{13}ClN_2O$ (284.74).

Preparation—2-(Methylamino)-5-chlorobenzophenone in ethereal solution is reacted with bromoacetyl bromide to form 2-(2-bromo-*N*-methylacetamido)-5-chlorobenzophenone. The latter is then reacted with ammonia in methanol solution whereby the bromine is replaced by amino followed by cyclization through a dehydration involving the hydrogens of the amino group and the oxygen of the starting phenone. The crude diazepam may be purified by recrystallization from ether. US Pat 3,136,815.

Description—Off-white to yellow, practically odorless, crystalline powder; stable in the air; melts about 133°; pK_a 3.7, 3.2.

Solubility—1 g in 333 mL water, 16 mL alcohol, 2 mL chloroform or 39 mL ether.

Uses—A benzodiazepine indicated for the symptomatic relief of tension and anxiety, acute alcohol withdrawal, adjunct therapy in skeletal muscle spasms and preferred by many clinicians for the management of status epilepticus. It is used preoperatively due to its ability to relieve anxiety, sedate and cause light anesthesia and anterograde amnesia. It is absorbed well after single oral doses (pK_a 3.3), leading to rapid onset of clinical effects. Initially these effects may be transient, due to extensive distribution to body tissues.

After distribution is complete, elimination is slow, with a half-life of 20 to 50 hr. Effective plasma levels vary from 0.2 to 0.5 μg/mL. With chronic administration, the drug and its major active metabolite, desmethyldiazepam, accumulate and reach a steady state in about 7 days. Consequently, it may take this long to achieve maximal sedative and antianxiety effects, at which time the patient can usually be maintained by giving the drug once or twice a day.

More details of its clinical uses as well as warnings, precautions, contraindications, addiction liability and a detailed enumeration of its adverse reactions and side effects are given on page 1155. Patients on the drug should be cautioned not to drive an automobile or to operate dangerous machinery until a few days after it has been stopped.

Dose—*Adult, oral,* **2** to **10 mg** 2 to 4 times a day; *intramuscular* or *intravenous,* **2** to **15 mg,** repeated in 3 to 4 hr, if necessary, but no more than **30 mg** should be given in an 8-hr period. *Pediatric, oral,* over 6 mo, **1** to **2.5 mg** 3 or 4 times a day.

Dosage Forms—Injection: 5 mg/mL; Tablets: 2, 5 and 10 mg; Sustained-Release Capsules: 15 mg; Solution: 1 and 5 mg/mL.

Droperidol—page 1183.

Estazolam

4H-[1,2,4]Triazolo [4,3-*a*][1,4]benzodiazepine, 8-chloro-6-phenyl-, ProSom (*Abbott*)

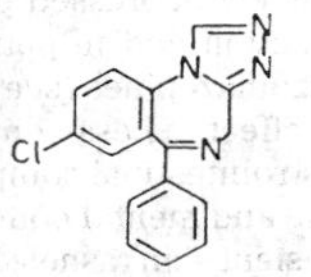

[29975-16-4] $C_{16}H_{11}ClN_4$ (294.74).

Preparation—From 7-chloro-1,3-dihydro-5-phenyl-*2H*-benzo-[1,4]-diazepin-2-thione and formylhydrazine in boiling *n*-butyl alcohol; see *J Org Chem 29:*231, 1964 and *J Med Chem 14:*1078, 1971.

Description—White crystals; melts about 230°.

Uses—A triazolobenzodiazepine derivative which structurally resembles alprazolam and triazolam. Estazolam has an intermediate half-life: the peak plasma concentration is reached 1.5–2 hr after oral administration, it undergoes hepatic microsomal oxidation, and has an elimination half-life of 10–24 hr. Some clinicians believe that triazolobenzodiazepines, such as estazolam, cause more serious toxicity and withdrawal reactions than other benzodiazepines. The adverse effects of estazolam are like other benzodiazepines and include sedation, drowsiness, dizziness, incoordination and possible recall impairment. Sudden discontinuation can cause significant transient rebound insomnia. Because use of benzodiazepines during pregnancy can result in fetal damage, estazolam should not be administered to pregnant women. Since the elimination of this drug may be slowed in geriatric patients, the doses of estazolam should be individualized carefully for this age group.

Dose—*Adult, oral,* **1** to **2 mg** at bedtime. *Geriatric, oral,* **0.5** to **1 mg** at bedtime.

Dosage Form—*Tablets:* 1 mg.

Fentanyl Citrate—page 1204.

Flurazepam Hydrochloride

2H-1,4-Benzodiazepin-2-one, 7-chloro-1-[2-(diethylamino)ethyl]-5-(2-fluorophenyl)-1,3-dihydro-, dihydrochloride; Dalmane (*Roche*); Durapam (*Major*)

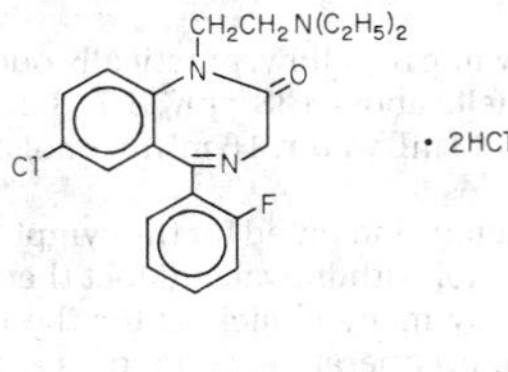

[1172-18-5] $C_{21}H_{23}ClFN_3O.2HCl$ (460.81).

Preparation—Aqueous CrO_3 is added dropwise to an acetic acid solution of 2-aminomethyl-5-chloro-1-[2-(diethylamino)ethyl]-3-(*o*-fluorophenyl)indole dihydrochloride and the mixture is stirred overnight.

Description—Off-white to yellow, crystalline powder; slight odor to odorless; melts with decomposition about 212°; moderately hygroscopic pK_a 1.9, 8.2.

Solubility—1 g in 2 mL water; ΔmL alcohol; slightly soluble in chloroform.

Uses—A benzodiazepine widely used in short-term treatment (up to 4 wk) of all types of insomnia such as difficulty in falling asleep, frequent nocturnal awakenings and/or early morning awakening. It also is used in acute and chronic medical situations in which restful sleep is desirable. It is absorbed rapidly from the GI tract and rapidly metabolized by the liver. Following a single oral dose, peak plasma concentrations ranging from 0.5 to 4.0 ng/mL are reached in 30 to 60 min. The major metabolite, N^1-desalkylflurazepam, reaches steady-state levels after 7 to 10 days of treatment of 5- to 6-fold higher than the 24-hr levels observed on day 1. The parent compound disappears rapidly from the blood; *N*-desalkylflurazepam remains active and has a half-life that ranges from 47 to 100 hr. The major urinary metabolite is conjugated N^1-hydroxyethylflurazepam and accounts for 22 to 55% of the dose.

This drug is excreted primarily in the urine. Less than 1% is excreted in the urine as N^1-desalkylflurazepam. The onset of sleep ranges from 15 to 45 min. Maximum effectiveness may not be achieved for 3 or 4 nights. Thus, the metabolite is responsible for the clinical effect as well as the residual effects which persist after the drug is discontinued. It requires the same warnings and precautions regarding use with other drug therapy, in hypersensitive individuals, during pregnancy, in children under 12 yr, in elderly and excessively depressed patients, in patients with impaired renal or hepatic function and in patients with a history of drug addiction as with other benzodiazepines (see page 1155).

Adverse reactions include dizziness, drowsiness, light-headedness, ataxia and falling (especially in elderly or debilitated persons) and severe sedation. The last usually is due to drug intolerance or overdosage. Other reported side effects include headache, heartburn, upset stomach, nausea, vomiting, diarrhea, constipation, gastrointestinal pain, nervousness, talkativeness, apprehension, irritability, weakness, palpitation, chest pains, body and joint pain and genitourinary complaints. Less frequently, sweating, flushes, blurred vision, difficulty in focusing, burning eyes, faintness, hypotension, shortness of breath, pruritus, skin rash, dry mouth, bitter taste, excessive salivation, anorexia, euphoria, depression, slurred speech, confusion, restlessness, hallucinations and paradoxical reactions (excitement, stimulation and hyperactivity) have been observed.

Dose—*Usual, adult,* **15** to **30 mg** before retiring. *Elderly* and/or *debilitated patients, initially* **15 mg** until individual response is determined. The drug is not recommended for use in children under 15 yr.

Dosage Form—Capsules: 15 and 30 mg.

Halazepam

2H-1,4-Benzodiazepin-2-one, 7-chloro-1,3-dihydro-5-phenyl-1-(2,2,2-trifluoroethyl)-, Paxipam (*Schering*)

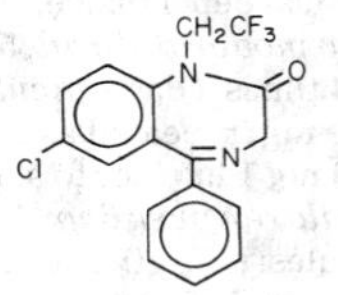

[23092-17-3] $C_{17}H_{12}ClF_3N_2O$ (352.74).

Preparation—The synthesis is similar to that for diazepam, page 1157. See *J Med Chem 66:*1354, 1973.

Description—A white crystalline solid; melts about 165°; its physical properties are similar to diazepam.

Uses—Indicated primarily for *anxiety* disorders or for the short-term relief of *symptoms of anxiety* not controlled by other more specific medication. It is absorbed rapidly and well after oral administration and excreted primarily in the urine. At least 90% of the absorbed drug is bound to plasma proteins. Maximum plasma concentration is achieved within 1 to 3 hr after oral administration; half-life following a 40-mg oral dose is approximately 14 hr. The major active metabolite of halazepam is *N*-desmethyldiazepam; maximum plasma concentrations of this metabolite occur in 3 to 6 hr and has a half-life of elimination of approximately 50 to 100 hr. Less than 1% of the parent substance is excreted in the urine as unchanged drug.

Common adverse effects include drowsiness, headache, apathy, psychomotor retardation, disorientation, confusion, euphoria, dysarthria, depression and syncope. Ataxia, fatigue and paradoxical agitation or rage also have been reported. No adverse drug interactions peculiar to this drug have been reported. However, additive sedation with alcohol and other CNS-depressant drugs would be anticipated, as well as those common to benzodiazepines (see page 1058). It should be used with caution in patients required to perform hazardous tasks and those with a history of drug abuse.

Dose—*Usual, adult, oral,* **20** to **40 mg** 3 or 4 times a day. *Elderly* or *sensitive patients,* **20 mg** once or twice a day. Information is inadequate to establish a dose for patients under 18 yr.

Dosage Form—Tablets: 20 and 40 mg.

Lorazepam

2*H*-1,4-Benzodiazepin-2-one,
7-chloro-5-(2-chlorophenyl)-1,3-dihydro-3-hydroxy-,
Ativan (*Wyeth-Ayerst*); Alzapam (*Major*); Loraz (*Quantum*)

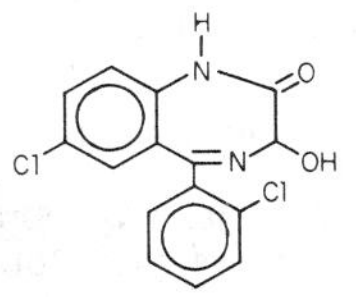

[846-49-1] $C_{15}H_{10}Cl_2N_2O_2$ (321.16).

Preparation—Syntheses of a number of substituted 1,4-benzodiazepin-2-ones, including lorazepam, have been described by Bell *et al* (J Med Chem 11:457, 1968; see also *J Org Chem 27*:1691, 1962). It differs from oxazepam in having a 5-*o*-chlorophenyl substituent in place of the 5-phenyl.

Description—White to off-white powder; no characteristic odor; melts about 173°, with decomposition pK_a 1.3, 11.5.

Solubility—Practically insoluble in water; slightly soluble in alcohol or chloroform.

Uses—A benzodiazepine used orally for anxiety and transient situational stress. Its effectiveness for long-term use (more than 4 mo) has not been assessed. It is used parenterally for *preanesthetic medication*, producing sedation and decreased ability to recall events related to the surgery. It is absorbed rapidly after oral administration; peak plasma levels after a 2-mg dose are about 20 ng/mL and maximal clinical effects occur within 2 hr after administration. Its mean plasma half-life is about 12 hr, whereas that of its conjugated metabolite, lorazepam glucuronide, is about 18 hr. Approximately 85% is bound to plasma proteins. There is no evidence of its accumulation on administration for up to 6 mo.

Adverse reactions, if they occur, usually appear at the beginning of therapy and disappear on continued medication or on decreasing the dose. Sedation is the most frequent adverse reaction (15.9%) and may persist up to 6–8 hours following an injection. Other common side effects include dizziness (6.9%), weakness (4.2%) and unsteadiness (3.4%). Less-frequent adverse effects are disorientation, depression, nausea, headache, sleep disturbance, agitation, dermatological symptoms, eye function disturbance, gastrointestinal symptoms and autonomic manifestations. The incidence of sedation and unsteadiness usually increases with age.

It requires the same warnings and precautions regarding use with other drugs, in hypersensitive individuals, during pregnancy and in young children, in elderly and excessively depressed patients, in patients with impaired renal or hepatic function and in patients with a history of drug addiction as with other benzodiazepines (see page 1155).

Dose—*Adult, oral,* **1** to **10 mg** a day, according to patient response; *usual,* **2** to **6 mg** in divided doses. In *anxiety,* **2** to **3 mg,** 2 or 3 times a day; *insomnia caused by anxiety,* **2** to **4 mg** at bedtime. A divided daily dose of **1** to **2 mg** initially is advised for elderly or debilitated patients. *Preoperative sedation, adults, deep intramuscular,* 0.05 mg/kg 2 hr prior to surgery or *intravenous,* 0.04 mg/kg 15 to 20 min prior to surgery. Dosage in children up to 12 yr has not been established.

Dosage Forms—Tablets: 0.5, 1 and 2 mg; Solution: 2 mg/mL; Injection: 2 and 4 mg/mL in 1 and 10 mL vials and 1 mL fill in 2 mL Tubex.

Midazolam Hydrochloride

4*H*-Imidazo[1,5-*a*][1,4]benzodiazepine, 8-chloro-6-(2-fluorophenyl)-1-methyl-, monohydrochloride; Versed (*Roche*)

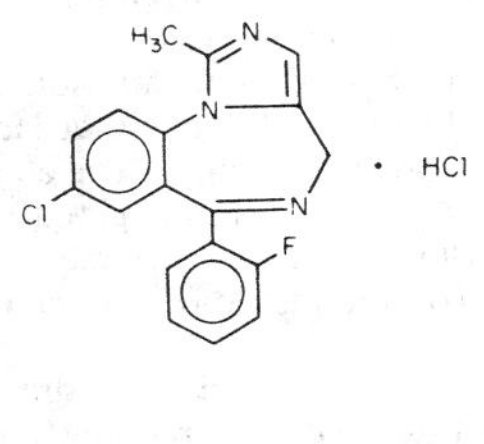

[59467-96-8]$C_{18}H_{13}ClF_3N.HCl$ (362.23); [59467-70-8] (335.76) (base).

Preparation—One method starts with 2-amino-4-chloro-2′-fluorobenzophenone in eight steps. See J Org Chem 43:936 and 4480, 1978

Description—Colorless crystals melting about 159°; pK_a 6.2.

Uses—An imidazobenzodiazepine, short-acting CNS depressant. The sedative potency of midazolam is likely 2 to 4 times that of diazepam. It is administered intramuscularly for preoperative sedation and perioperative amnesia. Because of its relatively rapid onset and short duration, it is considered by some clinicians to be the best benzodiazepine for preoperative use with short surgical procedures. Midazolam also is administered by the intravenous route, often combined with a narcotic, for conscious sedation associated with minor surgical or dental procedures or for short diagnostic or endoscopic procedures. It has been used IV as part of balanced anesthesia (eg, nitrous oxide and oxygen). It also has been administered orally for preoperative sedation and short-term management of insomnia. Midazolam is absorbed rapidly from IM injection sites, and pharmacological effects are apparent within 5 to 15 min and maximal 20 to 60 min. The duration of action of this drug is 1 to 6 hr. Following IV injection, onset of sedation and amnesic effect is usually within 1 to 5 min. After oral dosing, midazolam is absorbed rapidly from the GI tract and achieves maximum plasma concentration within 1 hr; however, up to 60% is altered with first-pass hepatic metabolism to 1-hydroxymethylmidazolam or 4-hydroxymidazolam. Approximately 95% of midazolam is bound to plasma proteins, and it is excreted principally as a conjugated metabolite in the urine.

Midazolam can cause serious respiratory depression or arrest, especially with high doses, when given IV for conscious sedation. Consequently, it should only be given IV in hospital or ambulatory-care facilities which are equipped to provide respiratory and cardiac monitoring and render resuscitative care if necessary. Patients with COPD are particularly sensitive to midazolam-induced respiratory depression. There also have been rare reports of hypotensive responses to this drug which required treatment, although changes in blood pressure and heart rate frequently occur after parenteral administration of midazolam. Adverse responses to this drug, which are similar to the side effects of other benzodiazenines, include excessive sedation, drowsiness, prolonged emergence from anesthesia, euphoria, dysphoria, confusion, agitation, sleep disturbance, weakness, lethargy, slurred speech, nausea and vomiting, blurred vision and visual disturbances. Some local tenderness following parenteral administration of midazolam has been reported, but this appears to be less than with other benzodiazepines.

Similar cautions should be used for midazolam as for other benzodiazepines. Midazolam is a potent drug and dosing should be individualized for the patient. It should not be administered during pregnancy nor to children younger than 18 yr. Midazolam will potentiate the action of other CNS depressants.

Dose—*Preoperative sedation, adults, deep intramuscular,* **70** to **80 μg/kg** administered 30 to 60 min prior to surgery. *Conscious sedation, adults, intravenous,* administer slowly prior to procedure, initial dose not to exceed **2.5 mg,** wait for 2 minutes to evaluate effect and then titrate to desired level of sedation. *Induction of anesthesia, adults,* administer **300** to **350 μg/kg** intravenously over 20 to 30 min prior to other anesthetic agents, wait 2 min to assess effect, supplemental doses may be necessary to complete induction.

Dosage Form—Injection: 1 or 5 mg/mL. The base is used to prepare the injection and the pH is adjusted to about 3, using HCl. Therefore, the solution is the salt form.

Oxazepam

2*H*-1,4-Benzodiazepin-2-one, 7-chloro-1,3-dihydro-3-hydroxy-5-phenyl-, Serax (*Wyeth-Ayerst*)

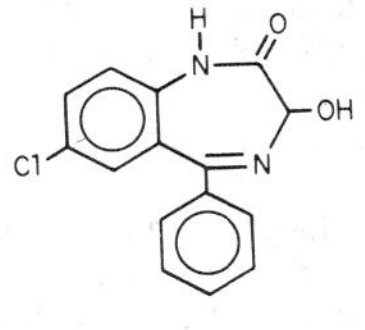

[604-75-1] $C_{15}H_{11}ClN_2O_2$ (286.72).

Preparation—2-Amino-5-chlorobenzophenone is acylated with chloroacetyl chloride and the product is refluxed with sodium iodide to form the iodoacetamido compound (I). Reaction of I with hydroxylamine effects dehydration and dehydrohalogenation to form the benzodiazepine derivative (II). Treatment of II with acetic anhydride causes rearrangement to oxazepam which is simultaneously esterified to acetate. Saponification liberates oxazepam.

Description—Creamy white to pale-yellow powder; practically odorless; bitter taste; stable in light and nonhygroscopic; melting point indefinite; pH (1 in 50 suspension) 4.8 to 7.0.

Solubility—1 g in > 10,000 mL water, 220 mL alcohol, 270 mL chloroform or 2200 mL ether.

Uses—A congener of chlordiazepoxide and diazepam; it is a mild sedative useful in the management and control of anxiety, tension, agitation, irritability and related symptoms, particularly in elderly patients. Also, it is useful for the control of acute tremulousness, inebriation or anxiety associated with alcohol withdrawal. Unlike diazepam, this drug is absorbed slowly after oral administration (1 to 4 hr) and has a simple, one-step elimination pathway without active intermediate metabolites. Its half-life is short (5 to 15 hr), there is little accumulation and full therapeutic effect can be expected with the first few doses. However, several daily doses may be necessary to reach a clinical steady state. Excessive and prolonged use may result in the development of physical dependence on the drug. Withdrawal symptoms following abrupt discontinuance of oxazepam are similar to those seen with barbiturates.

As with other sedative agents, patients on this drug should be cautioned against driving automobiles or operating dangerous machinery. Other warnings, contraindications and precautions are similar to those for other benzodiazepines (see page 1155). Untoward effects include transient mild drowsiness, dizziness, vertigo, headache and, rarely, syncope. Mild paradoxical reactions such as excitement and excessive stimulation also have been recorded.

Other side effects which have been observed include skin rashes, nausea, lethargy, edema, slurred speech, tremor and altered libido. More severe reactions include leukopenia and jaundice. Fortunately, the latter reactions only occasionally are observed. Patients on the drug should be observed carefully for the appearance of other untoward effects characteristic of benzodiazepine drugs.

Dose—**10** to **30 mg**; *usual, adult, oral,* **10** to **15 mg** 3 or 4 times a day; severe anxiety and alcoholic patients with marked withdrawal effects, **15** to **30 mg** 3 or 4 times a day. *Geriatric patients:* **10 mg** 3 times a day and increased to 15 mg 3 or 4 times a day, if necessary. Dosage for children 6 to 12 yr has not been established.

Dosage Forms—Capsules: 10, 15 and 30 mg; Tablets: 15 mg.

Prazepam

2*H*-1,4-Benzodiazepin-2-one, 7-chloro-1-(cyclopropylmethyl)-1,3-dihydro-5-phenyl-, Centrax (*Parke-Davis*)

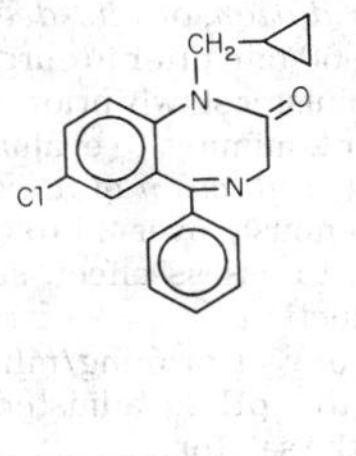

[2955-38-6] $C_{19}H_{17}ClN_2O$ (324.81).

Preparation—In one process 2-amino-5-chlorobenzophenone is acylated with cyclopropanecarbonyl chloride using triethylamine as an acid-receptor, reduced with lithium aluminum hydride to give 2-cyclopropylmethylamino-5-chlorobenzhydrol, and then oxidized with MnO_2 to the corresponding benzophenone. This is acylated with phthalimidoacetyl chloride and cyclized with hydrazine hydrate to produce prazepam. US Pats 3,192,199 and 3,192,200.

Description—Colorless, crystalline powder; melts about 145°.

Solubility—Practically insoluble in water; soluble in alcohol or chloroform.

Uses—For the management of *anxiety disorders* or for the short-term relief of the *symptoms of anxiety.* Prazepam is absorbed slowly after oral administration. Like diazepam and clorazepate, it is converted primarily to desmethyldiazepam, which appears to be the principal active metabolite. This conversion occurs slowly in the liver and peak levels of this metabolite are observed approximately 6 hr after oral administration. A mean half-life of desmethyldiazepam, measured in subjects given 10 mg 3 times a day for 1 week, was 60 hr before and 70 hr after multiple dosing. It is excreted largely as metabolites. It is contraindicated in patients with known sensitivity to the drug and those with acute narrow-angle glaucoma. The warnings, precautions, drug interactions and addiction liability for benzodiazepines are stated on page 1155.

Adverse reactions most frequently encountered are fatigue, dizziness, weakness, drowsiness, lightheadedness and ataxia. Of lesser frequency are headache, confusion, tremor, vivid dreams, slurred speech, palpitations, stimulation, dry mouth, diaphoresis and various gastrointestinal complaints; also pruritus, skin rashes, swelling of the feet, joint pains, genitourinary complaints, blurred vision and syncope have been reported. The safety and effectiveness of the drug in patients under the age of 18 have not been established.

Dose—*Adult, usual, oral,* **30 mg** a day in divided doses, adjusted gradually within the range of **20** to **60 mg** a day, depending on patient response. Alternatively, it may be given as a single dose at bedtime, starting at **20 mg,** with a usual range of **20** to **40 mg.** A divided daily dose of **10** to **15 mg** initially is advised for elderly or debilitated patients.

Dosage Forms—Capsules: 5, 10 and 20 mg; Tablets: 10 mg.

Quazepam

2*H*-1,4-Benzodiazepine-2-thione, 7-chloro-5-(2-fluorophenyl)-1,3-dihydro-1-(2,2,2-trifluorethyl)-, Doral (*Baker Cummins*)

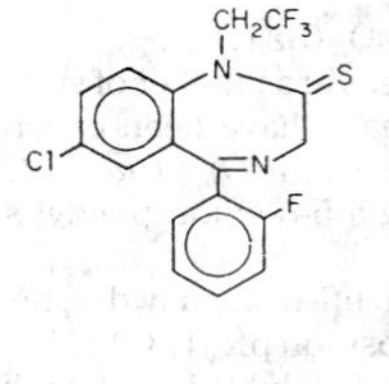

[36735-22-5] $C_{17}H_{11}ClF_4N_2S$ (386.79)

Preparation—It is synthesized in a manner similar to midazolam (page 1159); *J Med* Chem *16:*1354, 1974.

Uses—A benzodiazepine with a relatively long elimination half-life (39.3 hr). It is used for the short-term (up to 4 wk) management of insomnia. Its two principal metabolites (2-oxoquazepam and *N*-desalkylflurazepam) are pharmacologically active with long elmination ($t_{1/2s}$, 40.2 and 69.5 hr). These long half-lives likely account for the drowsiness and hangover effects which persist for 2 to 3 days following discontinuation of therapy. However, because of its slow elimination, this drug is unlikely to cause significant withdrawal, like hyperexcitability or rebound insomnia. Adverse effects, drug interactions and precautions aqppear to be similar to other benzodiazepines.

Doses—*Usual, adult, oral,* **7.5** to **15 mg** at bedtime. *Geriatric or debilitated patients,* a range of **7.5** to **15 mg** generally is used.

Dosage Form—Tablets: 7.5 and 15 mg.

Temazepam

2*H*-1,4-Benzodiazepin-2-one, 7-chloro-1,3-dihydro-3-hydroxy-1-methyl-5-phenyl-, Restoril (*Sandoz*); Razepam (*Major*); Temaz (*Quantum*); (*Various Mfrs*)

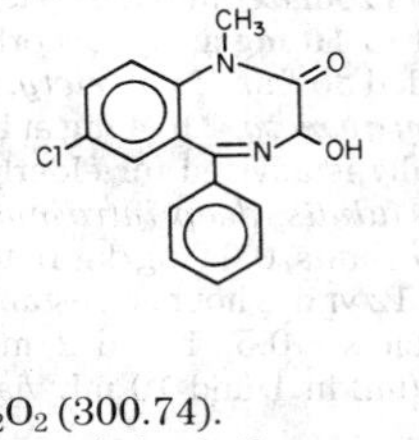

[846-50-4] $C_{16}H_{13}ClN_2O_2$ (300.74).

Preparation—The synthesis is similar to oxazepam using 2-(methylamino)-5-chlorobenzhydrol as the starting material. See *J Org Chem 27:* 1691, 1962.

Description—White crystals melting about 120°.

Solubility—Very slightly soluble in water; sparingly soluble in alcohol; pK_a 1.6.

Uses—A hypnotic drug indicated for the short-term (up to 5 wk) relief of *insomnia* associated with difficulty in falling asleep, frequent nocturnal awakenings and/or early morning awakenings. Oral bioavailability is relatively slow (mean times to peak concentration, 2 to 3 hr); 96% is bound to plasma proteins. Volume distribution ranges from 1.4 to 1.5 L/kg and clearance from 1.10 to 1.36 mL/kg/min. The elimination half-life varies from 3 to 38 hr (mean, 14.7 hr). It is conjugated with glucuronic acid and excreted in the urine. Since metabolic enzyme induction does not appear to occur after 5 to 7 days of administration, tolerance to repeated use is not troublesome.

Adverse effects are usually mild and diminish with continued administration. Those observed most frequently include morning drowsiness, dizziness, lethargy, confusion and gastrointestinal disturbances (anorexia, diarrhea). Other less-frequent adverse effects include vertigo, dryness of the mouth, paresthesias, tachycardia, panic reactions, nystagmus, paradoxical excitement and hallucinations. Precautions and possible drug interactions are the same as those for other benzodiazepines (see page 1155). Dysmorphogenic changes in rib formation have been observed in two animal species given 50 to 100 times the human therapeutic dose. Use during pregnancy should be avoided if possible.

Dose—*Usual, adult, hypnotic,* **15** to **30 mg** at bedtime. *Elderly* or *sensitive patients,* **15 mg.** Dosage in patients under 18 yr has not been established.

Dosage Form—Capsules: 15 and 30 mg.

Triazolam

4H-1,2,4-Triazolo[4,3-*a*][1,4]benzodiazepine, 8-chloro-6-(2-chlorophenyl)-1-methyl-, Halcion (*Upjohn*)

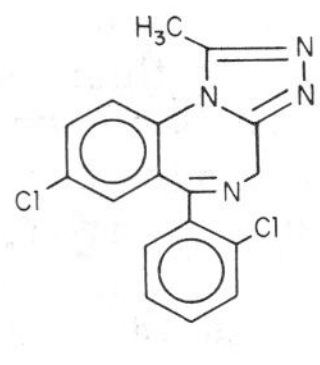

[28911-01-5] $C_{17}H_{12}Cl_2N_4$ (343.21).

Preparation—Ethyl α-aminoacetate and 2-amino-2′,4-dichlorobenzophenone are reacted in pyridine which, upon elimination of the elements of water and ethanol, yields 7-chloro-5-(2-chlorophenyl)benzodiazepin-2-one. The latter, with P_2S_5 forms the 2-thiono derivative, which, when treated with acetyl hydrazide gives the 2-acetamidoimino compound (I). Upon heating I over 200°, water is eliminated to form the triazole ring of triazolam. See Ger Pat 2,533,924.

Description—Tan crystals from isopropyl alcohol; melts about 235°.

Solubility—Very slightly soluble in water; slightly soluble in alcohol.

Uses—In the short-term management (up to 6 wk) of insomnia characterized by difficulty in falling asleep, frequent nocturnal awakenings and/or early morning awakenings. It is absorbed rapidly after oral administration; approximately 90% is bound to plasma proteins. Time to peak concentration is 1.25 hr. Volume distribution ranges from 0.8 to 1.3 L/kg. The elimination half-life is 2.6 (1.7 to 5.2) hr. The metabolites have little if any hypnotic activity. Common adverse effects include drowsiness, dizziness and headache. Hallucinations and marked confusion also have been reported. Some reports suggest that anterograde amnesia and other side effects, such as confusion, bizarre behavior, agitation and hallucinations may occur more often with triazolam than with most of the other benzodiazepines. Thus, patients using this drug should be monitored and treatment discontinued if such symptoms appear. Prescribers should be alert to the usual drug interactions common to benzodiazepines (see page 1155). The safe use of this drug during pregnancy or lactation has not been established.

Dose—*Usual, adult, oral,* **0.125** to **0.5 mg** at bedtime; elderly or sensitive patients, **0.125** to **0.25 mg.** The dose for children under 18 yr has not been established.

Dosage Form—Tablets: 0.125 and 0.25 mg.

Benzodiazepine Combinations

Some examples of benzodiazepine combinations (with mg/unit provided) are as follows:

Chlordiazepoxide with Amitryptyline Hydrochloride [Limbritol, Limbritol DS (*Roche*)]—5 or 10 mg with 12.5 or 25 mg, respectively.

Chlordiazepoxide Hydrochloride with Clidinium Bromide [Clindex (*Rugby*); Librax (*Roche*); Lidox (*Major*)]—5 mg with 2.5 mg, respectively.

Chlordiazepoxide with Esterified Estrogens [Menrium 5-2; Menrium 5-4; Menrium 10-4 (*Roche*)]—5, 5 or 10 mg with 0.2, 0.4 or 0.4 mg, respectively.

Benzodiazepine Antagonist

Because of the widespread use and the growing abuse of the benzodiazepines, attempts have been made to develop selective benzodiazepine antagonists to treat suspected benzodiazepine overdoses. These efforts have met with some success and the FDA has approved the use of flumazenil (Mazicon) as an adjunct to conventional therapy for overdosing with the benzodiazepines.

Flumazenil

4H-Imidazo[1,5-*a*][1,4]benzodiazepine-3-carboxylic acid, 8-fluoro-5,6-dihydro-5-methyl-6-oxo-, ethyl ester; Mazicon (*Roche*)

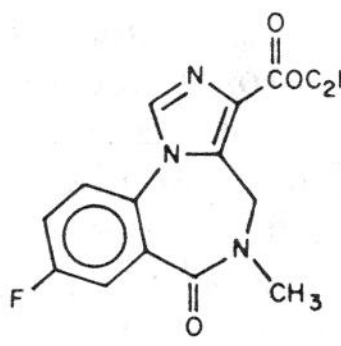

[78755-81-4] $C_{15}H_{14}FN_3O_3$ (303.29).

Preparation—Sarcosine and 6-fluorisatoic anhydride are condensed to 7-fluoro-5-methylbenzo[1,4] diazepin-2,5-dione. The dione, with ethyl α-isonitriloacetate forms a Schiff base, through nucleophilic reaction with the amido hydrogen atom. A Claisen condensation closes the imidazole ring between positions 1 and 2 on the diazepine ring to yield the product. US Pat 4,316,839.

Description—White crystals melting about 202°.

Uses—An imidazobenzodiazepine that binds directly to the benzodiazepine (BDZ) recognition site on the GABA/BDZ receptor complex. It acts as a selective competitive antagonist to block the CNS actions of the benzodiazepines. Flumazenil only blocks the psychomotor, cognitive and memory impairment caused by the benzodiazepines and has no effect on the actions of other CNS depressants (eg, ethanol, barbiturates or general anesthetics). The effects are dose-dependent with approximately 0.1 to 0.2 mg of flumazenil causing partial antagonism and 0.4 to 1.0 mg producing complete blockade of benzodiazepine effects. After IV administration, the reversal of BDZ effects occurs within 1 to 2 min with peak inhibition at 6 to 10 min. However, because of extensive first-pass elimination, oral administration results in low plasma drug concentration and is not recommended. Extensive and rapid ($t_{1/2}$ = 0.7 to 1.3 hr) hepatic metabolism results in no active metabolites. Despite a rapid clearance (31 to 78 L/hr), flumazenil can block benzodiazepine effects up to 6 hr. This drug was found to improve psychomotor performance, coordination, short-term memory loss and subjective feelings of pain and drowsiness within 30 min of administration to patients pretreated with midazolam.

Flumazenil is to be used as an adjunct to, not a substitute for, proper airway and circulatory management in the case of BDZ overdosing. Although large IV doses produce no serious side effects in healthy volunteers, in BDZ-dependent patients this BDZ antagonist can provoke severe withdrawal effects such as anxiety, panic attacks, hot flashes, tremors and seizures. Consequently, flumazenil generally is not to be used in patients with BDZ-dependence. Deaths have resulted from using this drug in patients with serious underlying diseases or in patients who overdosed on benzodiazepines in combination with large amounts of nonbezodiazepine drugs (eg, tricyclic antidepressants). In such cases, the flumazenil blocks the protective action of the benzodiazepines and unmasks the toxic effects of the other drugs. In the absence of benzodiazepines, it causes no serious adverse effects.

Besides the treatment of benzodiazepine overdoses, flumazenil has been used to reverse the sedative effects of BDZ used for general anesthesia. It has been suggested that this drug is able to reverse hepatic encephalopathy in some patients with acute and chronic liver failure. However, its effects are short-lasting.

Flumazenil should be titrated to the desired pharmacological effect by administering a series of small infusion (not a single large bolus) through a freely flowing IV in a large vein.

Doses—*Reversal of benzodiazepine sedation, intravenous,* **0.2 mg** (2 mL) over 15 sec, may repeat at 60-sec intervals to maximum dose of **10 mg;** *known or suspected benzodiazepine overdose: intravenous,* **0.2 mg** over 30 sec, may give additional doses of **0.5 mg** over 30 sec. at 1-min intervals to a maximum cumulative dose of **3.0 mg.**

Dosage Form—*Injection:* 0.1 mg/mL in 5- and 10-mL vials.

Barbiturates

The introduction of barbital in 1903 and phenobarbital in 1912 initiated the barbiturate era. For a period of over half a century they reigned as the preeminent sedative-hypnotic agents. Although several so-called nonbarbiturates attempted to displace the barbiturates from time to time, it was not until chlordiazepoxide was marketed in 1961 that their position was challenged seriously. During the ensuing quarter century the benzodiazepines displaced the barbiturates as the sedative-hypnotics of choice. Indeed, a careful comparison of the barbiturates and the benzodiazepines reveals the following cogent reasons for this obsolescence: dependence liability, potential for suicide, quality of sleep, antianxiety selectivity, propensity for tolerance and for drug interactions, safety and side effects. Nevertheless, the barbiturates continue to be prescribed by a number of physicians and are preferred for a few specialized uses.

The development of clinical pharmacokinetic data on hypnotic drugs revealed that the traditional classification of barbiturates into long-, intermediate- and short-acting compounds bears little relation to the rate of elimination of these agents in man. Moreover, these data indicate that onset (rate of absorption) and duration of action (rate of elimination) are essential factors to be considered in their use. In general, barbiturate salts are absorbed rapidly, in contrast to the free acids. Liver disease tends to decrease the elimination rate of these substances, whereas renal insufficiency may give rise to accumulation of polar metabolites. For these reasons and for ready reference, the elimination half-lives, apparent volumes of distribution and clearance values of barbiturates are summarized in each monograph.

Although traditionally used as nonspecific CNS depressants for daytime sedation and short-term treatment of insomnia, the barbiturates generally have been replaced by the benzodiazepines for these purposes. However, they are still given for preoperative medication to allay anxiety and facilitate induction of anesthesia. The anticonvulsant barbiturates, such as phenobarbital, mephobarbital and metharbital, are still useful alternatives for the long-term management of generalized tonic-clonic and cortical focal seizures and given intravenously for the management of acute convulsive episodes, such as status epilepticus, eclampsia, meningitis, tetanus and toxic reactions to strychnine or local anesthetics. The barbiturates also are administered rectally in infants and children when oral or parenteral therapy may be undesirable.

Elixirs of certain barbiturates are still available for use as somnifacients and sedatives for children, despite the availability of more effective agents. They also are used in the relief of colic, excitation and restlessness due to illness. Sedative doses may be administered as frequently as 3 to 4 times a day in cases of pylorospasm, whooping cough, nausea and vomiting of functional origin, etc.

Barbiturates are contraindicated in patients with a history of porphyria. They should be used with caution in patients with impaired hepatic or renal function, and in debilitated patients with depressed respiration. They also are contraindicated in persons with known previous addiction to the sedative/hypnotic drugs. Moreover, they should not be used in women of childbearing age, since their safe use in pregnancy has not been established. Patients on barbiturates should avoid alcoholic beverages as well as other CNS depressants and refrain from driving an automobile or operating hazardous machinery while receiving such drugs.

Drug interactions are relatively common in patients taking barbiturates in combination with other drugs. For this reason patients on these drugs should be monitored closely. The most common problems relate to the ability of barbiturates (especially phenobarbital) to induce the hepatic microsomal enzyme system and increase the rate of metabolism of coumarin anticoagulants, tricyclic antidepressants, oral contraceptives, corticosteroids, digitoxin, phenytoin, phenothiazines, doxycycline and other agents. Accordingly, the effectiveness of these agents may be decreased when given to a patient already on a barbiturate and, contrariwise, patients on both a barbiturate and one of these agents may experience adverse effects if the barbiturate is discontinued during chronic therapy, *ie* a patient on coumarin may hemorrhage if the barbiturate is stopped and anticoagulant dosage is not readjusted.

Barbiturates (especially phenobarbital) may competitively inhibit the metabolism of some drugs, such as phenytoin. Barbiturates have been shown to decrease the gastrointestinal absorption of dicumarol and griseofulvin. Some barbiturates potentiate the adverse effects of tricyclic antidepressants by competing for the same hydroxylating enzymes. Monoamine oxidase inhibitors, valproic acid, chloramphenicol and acute alcoholic intoxication inhibit the metabolism of barbiturates. Chronic alcoholic intoxication, on the other hand, increases the metabolism of barbiturates. Concomitant use of ether or curare-like drugs may produce additive respiratory depression. It also has been suggested that sulfisoxazole competes with thiopental for plasma-protein binding sites and decreases the amount of the latter necessary for anesthesia. Finally, additive depressant effects may occur with concomitant use of barbiturates and other CNS-depressant drugs.

Adverse reactions to barbiturates include

CNS: somnolence, agitation, confusion, hyperkinesia, ataxia, nightmares, lethargy, paradoxical excitement, nervousness, hallucinations, insomnia, anxiety and dizziness.

Respiratory: apnea, hypoventilation, respiratory depression, bronchospasm and circulatory collapse.

Cardiovascular: bradycardia, hypotension and syncope.

Hypersensitivity: skin rashes, angioneurotic edema, fever, serum sickness, morbiliform rash, urticaria, exfoliative dermatitis and Steven-Johnson syndrome.

Other: physical and psychological dependence, headache, blood dyscrasias, myalgia, neuralgia and arthritic pain.

For these and other reasons mentioned in this section, their indiscriminate use should be avoided.

Accidental and suicidal deaths from acute barbiturate poisoning are encountered frequently although the incidence has decreased with their diminished use. Treatment varies with the degree of intoxication. In general, emergency measures in *acute* poisoning are directed toward maintenance of respiration and cardiac function, followed by gastric decontamination. The latter is accomplished by gastric lavage, administration of activated charcoal (20 to 25 g in a child, 50 g in an adult) by gastric lavage tube and a saline cathartic to clear the gut. In severe intoxication, measures to enhance elimination of absorbed barbiturate may be necessary, such as diuresis, urine alkalinization, dialysis and hemoperfusion. The prognosis in barbiturate poisoning, with adequate medical care, is very good; mortality is less than 1%.

Continual use of barbiturates can result in tolerance which encourages an increase in dosages. Tolerance to the effects of barbiturates on mood, sedation and hypnosis is greater than tolerance to respiratory depression; consequently, with tolerance comes a decrease in the therapeutic index.

Chronic barbiturate poisoning involves a large number of individuals in this country. Some authorities consider the problem of chronic barbiturate poisoning as serious as morphine addiction. Consequently, three barbiturates (*amobarbital*, *pentobarbital* and *secobarbital*), either alone or in combination, have been placed under *Schedule II* of the *Controlled Substances Act*. Serious withdrawal symptoms, including convulsions and psychoses, may occur when a barbiturate is withheld from dependent patients. In some chronically intoxicated individuals, even though they have no previous history of epilepsy, major convulsive seizures follow the sudden withdrawal of barbiturate. It is advisable to reduce the dose of barbiturate gradually in both epileptic and nonepileptic patients when cessation of chronic barbiturate medication is contemplated. It also should be emphasized that barbiturate therapy is contraindicated in patients with a history of drug addiction.

Amobarbital

2,4,6(1*H*,3*H*,5*H*)-Pyrimidinetrione, 5-ethyl-5-(3-methylbutyl)-, Amylobarbitone; Amytal (*Lilly*); (*Various Mfrs*)

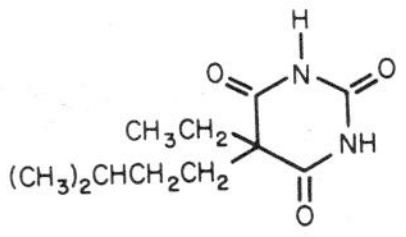

5-Ethyl-5-isopentylbarbituric acid [57-43-2] $C_{11}H_{18}N_2O_3$ (226.27).

Preparation—A typical method starts with monochloroacetic acid, which is treated with sodium cyanide to form cyanoacetic acid; the latter is reacted with hydrochloric acid in the presence of alcohol, yielding the diethyl ester of malonic acid. This ester, in absolute alcohol solution, is treated with the theoretical quantity of metallic sodium to replace one hydrogen of the CH_2 group, then a slight excess of the theoretical amount of an ethylating agent, such as ethyl bromide, is added. The second hydrogen is replaced similarly using isopentyl bromide as the alkylating agent. The diethyl ester of ethyl isopentyl malonic acid thus obtained is heated in an alcoholic solution, in the presence of sodium, with urea. Sodium amobarbital is formed, from which amobarbital is liberated with HCl. The alkylation of the CH_2 group of the malonic ester, whether the alkyls are both the same as in barbital or different, as in amobarbital, may be done in two stages, introducing one alkyl group at a time.

Description—White, crystalline, odorless, bitter powder; pH (saturated solution) about 5.6; melts within a 3° range between 156 and 161°.

Solubility—1 g in about 1300 mL of water, 5 mL of alcohol, about 17 mL of chloroform or 6 mL of ether; soluble in solutions of fixed alkali hydroxides and carbonates.

Uses—A *sedative* and *hypnotic*. It may be used in any condition that requires sedation ranging from relief of anxiety and tension to hypnotic doses for preanesthetic medication. Because of tolerance, its use as a hypnotic is limited to 2 wk. See the introductory statement on *Barbiturates*. It is a *Schedule II* drug under the *Controlled Substances Act*.

Dose—*Adult, usual: oral, sedative,* **30** to **50 mg** 2 or 3 times a day; *hypnotic,* **100** to **200 mg.** *Pediatric, usual: oral, sedative,* **2 mg/kg** or **60 mg/m²** 3 times a day.

Dosage Form—Tablets: 30, 50 and 100 mg.

Amobarbital Sodium

2,4,6(1*H*,3*H*,5*H*)-Pyrimidinetrione, 5-ethyl-5-(3-methylbutyl)-, monosodium salt; Amylobarbitone Sodium; Amytal Sodium (*Lilly*); (*Various Mfrs*)

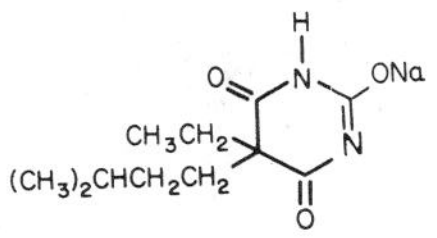

Sodium 5-ethyl-5-isopentylbarbiturate [64-43-7] $C_{11}H_{17}N_2NaO_3$ (248.26).

Preparation—By reacting amobarbital with a solution containing a chemically equivalent quantity of sodium hydroxide or sodium carbonate, evaporating to dryness and crystallizing the residue from a solution in a suitable solvent such as alcohol.

Description—White, friable, hygroscopic, odorless, granular powder with a bitter taste; pH (1 in 20 solution) 9.6 to 10.4.

Solubility—Very soluble in water; soluble in alcohol; practically insoluble in ether or chloroform.

Uses—A *hypnotic* and *sedative*. It is indicated for sedation and relief of anxiety, preanesthetic medication and the control of acute convulsive disorders. The onset of action varies from 45 to 60 min, half-life is approximately 25 hr and duration of action is 6 to 8 hr. See the introductory statement on *Barbiturates*. It is a *Schedule II* drug under the *Controlled Substances Act*.

Dose—*Adult, usual: oral, sedative,* during *labor,* **200** to **400 mg** every 1 to 3 hr up to a total of 1 g, *preoperative,* **200 mg** 1 or 2 hr before surgery; *hypnotic,* **65** to **200 mg** on retiring. *Intramuscular or intravenous, sedative,* **30** to **50 mg** 2 or 3 times a day; *intravenous, anticonvulsant* or *hypnotic,* **65** to **500 mg;** *intramuscular, hypnotic,* **65** to **500 mg.** *Pediatric, usual: oral, sedative,* **2 mg/kg** or **60 mg/m²** 3 times a day; *hypnotic,* dosage not established; *intramuscular* or *intravenous, anticonvulsant,* **3** to **5 mg/kg** or **125 mg/m²** per dose; *intramuscular, hypnotic,* **3** to **5 mg/kg** or **125 mg/m²**; dosage as *sedative* to be individualized by physician.

Dosage Forms—Capsules: 65 and 200 mg; Sterile Powder: 15- and 30-g vials.

Aprobarbital

Barbituric acid, 5-allyl-5-isopropyl-; Alurate (*Roche*)

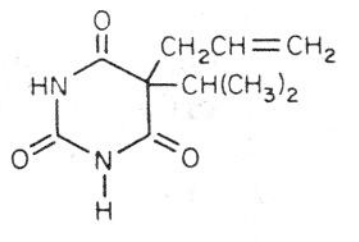

[77-02-1] $C_{10}H_{14}N_2O_3$ (210.23).

Preparation—By a method similar to that described for *Amobarbital*, this page, using allyl and isopropyl bromides as the alkylating agents.

Description—White, crystalline powder; odorless; slightly bitter taste; melts about 141°.

Solubility—Slightly soluble in cold water; soluble in alcohol, chloroform or ether.

Uses—A *sedative* and *hypnotic* used in the short-term (up to 2 wk) management of insomnia. Following oral administration, peak plasma levels are reached within 3 to 4 hr. Plasma concentrations of 2 to 3 μg/mL induce sedation; those of 25 μg/mL, sleep, and those greater than 30 μg/mL, coma. Elimination half-life ranges from 16 to 40 hr. See the introductory statement on *Barbiturates*.

Dose—*Usual, oral, sedative,* **40 mg** 3 times a day; *hypnotic,* **40** to **160 mg** on retiring.

Dosage Form—Elixir: 40 mg/5 mL.

Butabarbital Sodium

2,4,6(1*H*,3*H*,5*H*)-Pyrimidinetrione, 5-ethyl-5-(1-methylpropyl)-, monosodium salt; Butisol Sodium (*Carter-Wallace*);(*Various Mfrs*)

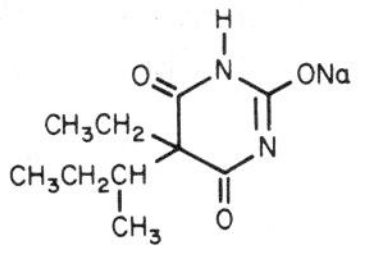

Sodium 5-*sec*-butyl-5-ethylbarbiturate [143-81-7] $C_{10}H_{15}N_2NaO_3$ (234.23).

Preparation—By preparing butarbital using a method similar to that for *Amobarbital* using ethyl bromide and *sec*-butyl bromide as the alkylating agents. Then treating an alcoholic solution of butabarbital with an equimolar quantity of NaOH and removing the solvent by evaporation.

Description—White, bitter powder; pH (1 in 10 solution) 9.5 to 10.2.

Solubility—1 g in 2 mL of water, 7 mL of alcohol, 7000 mL of chloroform or > 10,000 mL of ether.

Uses—A *sedative* and *hypnotic*. Used for short-term treatment of insomnia. Because of tolerance, barbiturates lose efficacy after 2 wk of use. See the introductory statement on *Barbiturates*. It is a *Schedule III* drug under the *Controlled Substances Act*.

Dose—*Adult, usual: oral, sedative, daytime,* **15** to **30 mg** 3 or 4 times a day; *preoperative,* **50** to **100 mg;** *hypnotic,* **50** to **100 mg** on retiring. *Pediatric, usual: oral, sedative,* **7.5** to **30 mg**, depending on age, weight and sedation desired; *preoperative,* **2** to **6 mg/kg**, maximum 100 mg; *hypnotic,* dosage based on age and weight.

Dosage Forms—Capsules: 15 and 30 mg; Elixir: 30 and 33.3 mg/5 mL; Tablets: 15, 30, 50 and 100 mg.

Hexobarbital Sodium—RPS-15, page 983.

Mephobarbital

2,4,6(1*H*,3*H*,5*H*)-Pyrimidinetrione, 5-ethyl-1-methyl-5-phenyl-, Prominal; Phemitone; Mebaral (*Winthrop*)

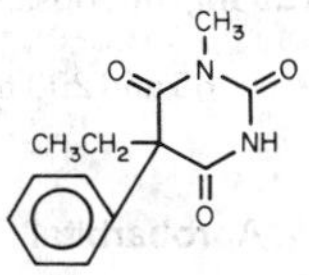

5-Ethyl-1-methyl-5-phenylbarbituric acid [115-38-8] $C_{13}H_{14}N_2O_3$ (246.27).

Preparation—The diethyl ester of ethylphenylmalonic acid is prepared by the general method described under *Amobarbital*, and is then condensed with *N*-methylurea in the presence of sodium ethylate. The resulting sodium mephobarbital is treated with HCl, whereupon mephobarbital crystallizes.

The *N*-methylurea is prepared as follows. Methylamine is passed into a mixture of sulfuric acid and absolute alcohol until the mixture is alkaline. Potassium cyanate then is added and the mixture is refluxed overnight whereupon the monomethyl ammonium cyanate produced initially by metathesis rearranges (Wöhler) to *N*-methylurea.

Description—White, crystalline powder; odorless; bitter taste; saturated solution acid to litmus; melts about 178°; pK_a 8.8.

Solubility—1 g in > 1000 mL water, > 1000 mL alcohol, 50 mL chloroform or > 1000 mL ether; soluble in solutions of fixed alkali hydroxides or carbonates.

Uses—A barbiturate with strong *sedative* and *anticonvulsant* actions but a relatively mild *hypnotic* action. Hence, it is used for relief of anxiety, tension and apprehension, and as an antiepileptic in the management of generalized tonic-clonic (grand mal) and absence (petit mal) seizures. See also the introductory statement on *Barbiturates*.

Dose—*Adult, usual, oral, anticonvulsant,* **400** to **600 mg** a day; *sedative,* **32** to **100 mg** 3 or 4 times a day; *delirium tremens,* **200 mg** 3 times a day. *Pediatric, usual, oral, anticonvulsant, up to 5 yr,* **16** to **32 mg** 3 or 4 times a day; *over 5 yr,* **32** to **64 mg** 3 or 4 times a day.

Dosage Form—Tablets: 32, 50 and 100 mg.

Metharbital—page 1176.

Methohexital Sodium for Injection—page 1143.

Pentobarbital

2,4,6(1*H*,3*H*,5*H*)-Pyrimidinetrione, 5-ethyl-5-(1-methylbutyl)-, Dorsital (*Dorsey*); Nembutal (*Abbott*); (*Various Mfrs*)

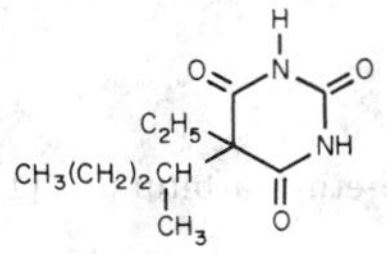

5-Ethyl-5-(1-methylbutyl)barbituric acid [76-74-4] $C_{11}H_{18}N_2O_3$ (226.27).

Preparation—By the general method described under *Amobarbital* (page 1163) using ethyl bromide and 1-methylbutyl bromide as alkylating agents.

Description—White to practically white, fine powder; practically odorless; melts about 130°.

Solubility—1 g in > 2000 mL water, 4.5 mL alcohol, 4 mL chloroform or 10 mL ether.

Uses—See *Pentobarbital Sodium.* It is a *Schedule II* drug under the *Controlled Substances Act.*

Dose—*Adult, usual: oral, sedative,* equivalent of **20 mg** of pentobarbital sodium 3 or 4 times a day; *hypnotic,* equivalent of **100 mg** of pentobarbital sodium on retiring. *Pediatric, usual: oral, sedative, equivalent of* **2** to **6 mg/kg** of pentobarbital sodium 3 times a day; *hypnotic,* as individualized by physician.

Dosage Form—Elixir: 18.2 mg/5 mL (equivalent to 20 mg/5 mL of pentobarbital sodium).

Pentobarbital Sodium

2,4,6(1*H*,3*H*,5*H*)-Pyrimidinetrione, 5-ethyl-5-(1-methylbutyl)-, monosodium salt; Pentobarbitone Sodium; Soluble Pentobarbital; Nembutal Sodium (*Abbott*); (*Various Mfrs*)

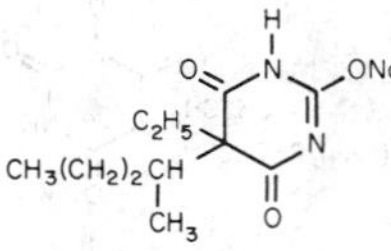

Sodium 5-ethyl-5-(1-methylbutyl)barbiturate [57-33-0] $C_{11}H_{17}N_2NaO_3$ (248.26).

Preparation—By the process given for *Amobarbital* (page 1163), using 2-bromopentane instead of ethyl bromide to react with one of the hydrogens in the CH_2 of the malonyl group. It then is converted into the soluble sodium salt by the addition of the required amount of NaOH.

Description—White, odorless, crystalline granules or a white powder with a slightly bitter taste; pH (1 in 10 solution) 10.0 to 10.5 when used in parenterals; otherwise, 9.7 to 10.2; solutions decompose on standing, heat accelerating the decomposition; pK_{a1} 8.17; pK_{a2} 12.67.

Solubility—Very soluble in water; freely soluble in alcohol; practically insoluble in ether.

Uses—Widely used as a *sedative* or *hypnotic* for the short-term (up to 2 wk) management of insomnia and as preanesthetic medication. It also is indicated, in anesthetic doses administered intravenously, for control of certain convulsive syndromes. This barbiturate is thought to reduce cerebral blood flow and thereby decrease edema and/or intracranial pressure. See also the introductory statement on *Barbiturates.* It is a *Schedule II* drug under the *Controlled Substances Act.*

Dose—*Oral, adult,* daytime *sedation,* **20 mg** 3 or 4 times a day; *hypnotic:* **100 mg** at bedtime. *Oral, children, preoperative sedation,* **2** to **6 mg/kg/day;** maximum, 100 mg. *Rectal, adults,* **120** to **200 mg;** *children 12 to 14 yr,* **60** to **120 mg;** *5 to 12 yr,* **60 mg;** *1 to 4 yr,* **30** to **60 mg;** *2 mo to 1 yr,* **30 mg.** *Parenteral, adult, intravenous, initially* **100 mg,** followed with **200** to **500 mg** as indicated by patient response; *intramuscular, adult,* based on age, weight and condition, **150** to **200 mg;** *usual, children,* **25** to **80 mg** or **2** to **6 mg/kg** as a single injection.

Dosage Forms—Capsules: 50 and 100 mg; Injection: 50 mg/mL, in 1-, 2-, 20- and 50-mL containers; Suppositories: 30, 60, 120 and 200 mg.

Phenobarbital

2,4,6(1*H*,3*H*,5*H*)-Pyrimidinetrione, 5-ethyl-5-phenyl-, Phenylethylmalonylurea; Phenobarbitone; Gardinal; Luminal; (*Various Mfrs*)

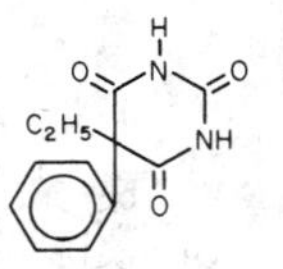

5-Ethyl-5-phenylbarbituric acid [50-06-6] $C_{12}H_{12}N_2O_3$ (232.24).

Preparation—Benzyl chloride is converted into phenylacetic ester (ethyl phenylacetate) by treating with sodium cyanide and then hydrolyzing with acid in the presence of alcohol. The ester is condensed in the presence of alcohol and metallic sodium with ethyl oxalate, forming diethyl sodium phenyloxaloacetate. HCl is added to liberate diethyl phenyloxaloacetate which, on being distilled at about 180°, splits off carbon monoxide and forms phenylmalonic ester [$C_6H_5CH(COOC_2H_5)_2$]. The hydrogen of the CH in the phenylmalonic ester is then ethylated and the resulting ethylphenylmalonic ester condensed with urea as described under *Amobarbital* (page 1163).

Description—White, odorless, glistening, small crystals or a white crystalline powder, which may exhibit polymorphism; stable in air; pH (saturated solution) about 5; melts about 176°; pK_a 7.6.

Solubility—1 g in about 1000 mL water, 10 mL alcohol, about 40 mL chloroform or 15 mL ether.

Uses—This classical barbiturate is a *sedative, hypnotic* and *antiepileptic* drug. In appropriate doses it is used in neuroses and related tension states when mild, prolonged sedation is indicated, as in hypertension, coronary artery disease, functional gastrointestinal disorders and preoperative apprehension. In addition, it has specific usefulness in the symptomatic therapy of *epilepsy.* It is especially useful in patients with generalized tonic-clonic seizures (grand mal) and complex partial (psychomotor) seizures. Effective doses usually produce a degree of drowsiness or sluggishness. Phenobarbital also has been found to be effective in the treatment and prevention of hyperbilirubenemia in neonates. Approximately 80% of an oral dose is absorbed and peak plasma levels are reached in 16 to 18 hr. Because of its slow onset of action, phenobarbital generally is not used orally to treate insomnia, but is used to help withdraw people who are physically dependent on other CNS depressants. The apparent volume of distribution is 0.7 to 1 L/kg. Therapeutic plasma levels range from 10 to 30 μg/mL. About 45 to 50% of the drug is bound to plasma protein. Apparent plasma half-life varies from 50 to 120 hr in adults and 40 to 70 hr in children. Approximately 65% of the drug is metabolized (largely to the inactive *p*-hydroxyphenyl derivative) and 35% is excreted by the kidney unchanged. Plasma clearance is slow and approximates 0.004 L/kg/hr. With the exception of metharbital and mephobarbital, this is the only barbiturate effective in epilepsy. See the introductory statement on *Barbiturates*.

Dose—*Adult, usual: oral, sedative,* **30** to **120 mg** in 2 or 3 divided doses; *hypnotic,* **100** to **320 mg;** *anticonvulsant,* **50** to **100 mg** 2 or 3 times a day. *Usual range of dose,* **30** to **600 mg** a day. *Pediatric, usual: oral, sedative,* **2 mg/kg** or **60 mg/m²** 3 times a day; *hypnotic,* individualized by physician; *anticonvulsant* or *antidyskinetic,* **3** to **5 mg/kg** or **125 mg/m²** a day until a blood level of 10 to 15 μg/mL is attained.

Dosage Forms—Elixir: 15 or 20 mg/5 mL; Capsules: 16 mg; Tablets: 8, 16, 32, 65 and 100 mg.

Phenobarbital Sodium

2,4,6(1*H*,3*H*,5*H*)-Pyrimidinetrione, 5-ethyl-5-phenyl-, monosodium salt; Sodium Phenobarbital; Soluble Phenobarbital; Phenobarbitone Sodium; Luminal Sodium (*Winthrop*); (*Various Mfrs*)

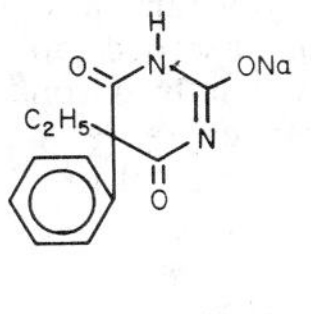

Sodium 5-ethyl-5-phenylbarbiturate [57-30-7] $C_{12}H_{11}N_2NaO_3$ (254.22).

Preparation—By dissolving phenobarbital in an alcohol solution of an equivalent quantity of NaOH and evaporating at low temperature.

Description—Flaky crystals or white, crystalline granules, or white powder; odorless; bitter taste; hygroscopic; solutions alkaline to phenolphthalein, and decompose on standing; pH (1 in 10 solution) 9.2 to 10.2.

Solubility—Very soluble in water; soluble in alcohol; practically insoluble in ether or chloroform.

Uses—Because it is soluble in water, it may be administered parenterally. It is given by slow intravenous injection for control of acute convulsive syndromes. For additional information see *Phenobarbital*, and the introductory statement on *Barbiturates*.

Dose—*Adult, usual: oral,* as for phenobarbital. *Intramuscular or intravenous, sedative,* **100** to **130 mg;** *anticonvulsant,* **200** to **300 mg** repeated in 6 hr if necessary; *preoperative medication,* **130** to **200 mg** every 6 hr; *postoperative sedation,* **32** to **100 mg.** *Pediatric, usual, intramuscular,* **60 mg/m²** 3 times a day; *anticonvulsant,* **125 mg/m²**/dose; *preoperative medication,* **16** to **100 mg;** *postoperative sedation,* **8** to **30 mg.**

Note: Doses should be reduced significantly in elderly or debilitated patients. No barbiturate should be given parenterally without full knowledge of its particular characteristics, dosage and recommended rate of administration. Because of potentially severe respiratory depression, phenobarbital sodium should not be administered at a rate that exceeds 60 mg/min.

Dosage Forms—Injection: 30, 60, 65 and 130 mg/mL; Sterile Powder, 120-mg ampuls.

Secobarbital

2,4,6(1*H*,3*H*,5*H*)-Pyrimidinetrione, 5-(1-methylbutyl)-5-(2-propenyl)-, Seconal (*Lilly*); (*Various Mfrs*)

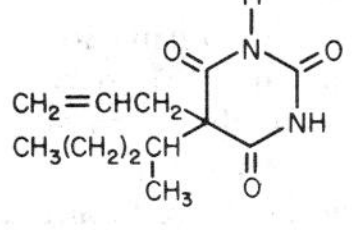

5-Allyl-5-(1-methylbutyl)barbituric acid [76-73-3] $C_{12}H_{18}N_2O_3$ (238.29).

Preparation—By the general method described under *Amobarbital* (page 1163) using allyl bromide and 1-methylbutyl bromide as alkylating agents at the 5-position.

Description—White, amorphous or crystalline, odorless powder; slightly bitter taste; pH (saturated solution) about 5.6; melts about 98°.

Solubility—Very slightly soluble in water; freely soluble in alcohol, ether or solutions of alkali hydroxides; soluble in chloroform.

Uses—A *sedative* and *hypnotic.* See also *Secobarbital Sodium* and the introductory statement on *Barbiturates.* It is a *Schedule II* drug under the *Controlled Substances Act.*

Dose—See *Secobarbital Sodium.*

Dosage Forms—See *Secobarbital Sodium.*

Secobarbital Sodium

2,4,6(1*H*,3*H*,5*H*)-Pyrimidinetrione, 5-(1-methylbutyl)-5-(2-propenyl)-, monosodium salt; Quinalbarbitone Sodium; Seconal Sodium (*Lilly*); (*Various Mfrs*)

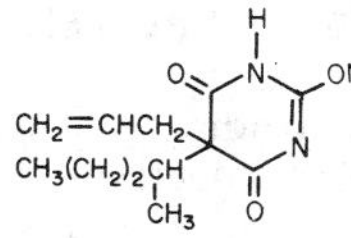

Sodium 5-allyl-5-(1-methylbutyl)barbiturate [309-43-3] $C_{12}H_{17}N_2NaO_3$ (260.27).

Preparation—By treatment of secobarbital with a chemically equivalent portion of NaOH as described under *Phenobarbital Sodium.*

Description—White, odorless, hygroscopic powder; bitter taste; pH (1 in 20 solution) 9.7 to 10.5; solutions decompose on standing, heat accelerating the decomposition.

Solubility—Very soluble in water; soluble in alcohol; practically insoluble in ether.

Uses—A short-acting barbiturate widely used *sedative* and *hypnotic.* The drug also is used, in anesthetic doses intravenously, for the control of certain acute convulsive conditions, such as those associated with tetanus, status epilepticus and toxic reactions to strychnine and local anesthetics. Within 2 hr after oral administration, 90% is absorbed from the GI tract. The effect after a hypnotic dose occurs in 15 to 30 min with oral or rectal administration and persists for 1 to 4 hr. The elimination half-life is about 30 hr. Secobarbital has been used rectally in children to induce anesthesia. See the introductory statement on *Barbiturates.* It is a *Schedule II* drug under the *Controlled Substances Act.*

Dose—*Adult, usual: oral, sedative,* **30** to **50 mg;** *hypnotic,* **100 mg** at bedtime; *preoperative sedation,* **200** to **300 mg** 1 to 2 hr before surgery. *Intramuscular, hypnotic,* **100** to **200 mg;** *rectal, hypnotic,* **120** to **200 mg.** *Pediatric, usual, oral, sedation,* **6 mg/kg** a day in 3 divided doses; *intramuscular,* **3** to **5 mg/kg** (maximum, **100 mg**); *rectal,* **6 mg/kg** daily in 3 divided doses.

Note: Doses should be reduced significantly in elderly or debilitated patients. No barbiturate should be given parenterally without full knowledge of its particular characteristics, dosage and recommended rate of administration.

Dosage Forms—Capsules: 50 and 100 mg; Injection: 50 mg/mL; Rectal Injection: 50 mg/mL.

Talbutal

2,4,6(1*H*,3*H*,5*H*)-Pyrimidinetrione, 5-(1-methylpropyl)-5-(2-propenyl)-, Lotusate (*Winthrop*)

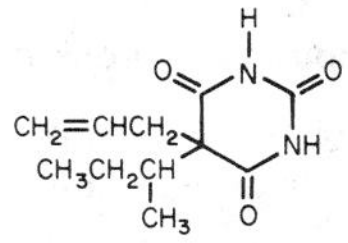

5-Allyl-5-*sec*-butylbarbituric acid [115-44-6] $C_{11}H_{16}N_2O_3$ (224.26).

Preparation—By the general method described under *Amobarbital,* page 1163, using allyl bromide and *sec*-butyl bromide as alkylating agents.

Description—White, crystalline powder; may have a slight odor of caramel; melts about 108°, or may occur in a polymorphic form which melts about 111°.

Solubility—1 g in 500 mL of water, 1 mL of alcohol, 2 mL of chloroform or 40 mL of ether.

Uses—A *hypnotic* which, in appropriate dose, induces sleep in 15 to 30 min that lasts 6 to 8 hr. See the introductory statement on *Barbiturates*.

Dose—*Adult, usual, oral, hypnotic,* **120 mg** 15 to 30 min before retiring; *sedative,* **30** to **60 mg** 2 or 3 times a day. *Pediatric,* dosage not established.

Dosage Form—Tablets: 120 mg.

Thiamyl Sodium—page 1144.

Thiopental Sodium—page 1145.

Barbiturate Combinations

Some examples of barbiturate combinations (with mg/unit provided) are as follows:

Butalbital, Acetaminophen and Caffeine [Fioricet (*Sandoz*)]—50, 325 and 40 mg, respectively.

Butalbarbital, Aspirin and Caffeine [Fiorinal (*Sandoz*)]—50, 325 and 40 mg, respectively.

Miscellaneous Sedatives and Hypnotics

In addition to the benzodiazepines and barbiturates discussed in the previous two sections, there are a number of other agents which possess useful sedative and hypnotic properties. These are derived from several heterogeneous structures, including alcohols (ethchlorvynol), carbamates (ethinamate, meprobamate), chloral hydrate and related drugs (triclofos), cyclic ether (paraldehyde), piperidine-diones (glutethimide, methyprylon) and quinazolinone (methaqualone). In addition to sedative-hypnotic properties, several of these substances possess anticonvulsant, antispasmodic, local anesthetic and weak antihistaminic properties. In general, the effective hypnotic dose of these substances is larger than that for either the benzodiazepines or barbiturates. Nevertheless, they do not differ qualitatively from the barbiturates in their desirable and undesirable effects. Hence, patients should be cautioned about concomitant use of alcohol or other CNS depressants and warned about operating a motor vehicle or hazardous machinery while on such drugs. It should be remembered that safe and effective use of many of these agents during pregnancy and in pediatric patients has not been established. Also, many of these agents will produce physical dependence and habituation when taken chronically in excessive doses. For this reason methaqualone is listed in *Schedule II* and glutethimide in *Schedule III* under the *Controlled Substances Act*. Other substances in this section have lower abuse potential and are listed in *Schedule IV*. Nevertheless, they all should be used with caution in patients with a previous history of drug dependence.

An anxiolytic drug that is structurally and pharmacologically distinct from the benzodiazepines and barbiturates is the arylpiperazine derivative, buspirone. This drug is distinguished from the other sedatives because it relieves anxiety without causing drowsiness, impairing psychomotor function and appears to lack abuse potential.

Disulfiram (Antabuse), an antioxidant agent devoid of sedative and hypnotic properties, is included in this section because of its use as an adjunct in the management of alcoholism.

Buclizine Hydrochloride—page 902.

Buspirone Hydrochloride

Azaspiro [4,5]decane-7,9-dione, 8-[4-[4-(2-pyrimidinyl)-1-piperazinyl]butyl]-, monohydrochloride; BuSpar (*Mead-Johnson*)

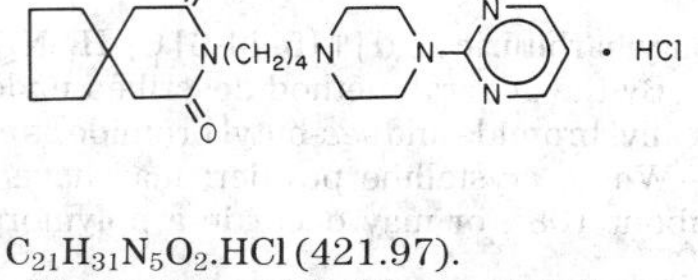

N(CH2)4 · HCl

[33386-08-2] $C_{21}H_{31}N_5O_2.HCl$ (421.97).

Preparation—Piperazine and 2-chloropyrimidine are reacted to form 2-(1-piperazinyl)pyrimidine(I). Treatment of **I** with γ-chlorobutyronitrile *N*-alkylates the free piperazinyl nitrogen atom to yield **II**. With spirocyclopentane-1, 3′-glutaric anhydride (**III**), the free base of buspirone is produced, which is then converted to the hydrochloride; *J Med Chem 12:*876, 1969 and *Ibid*, 15; 477, 1972.

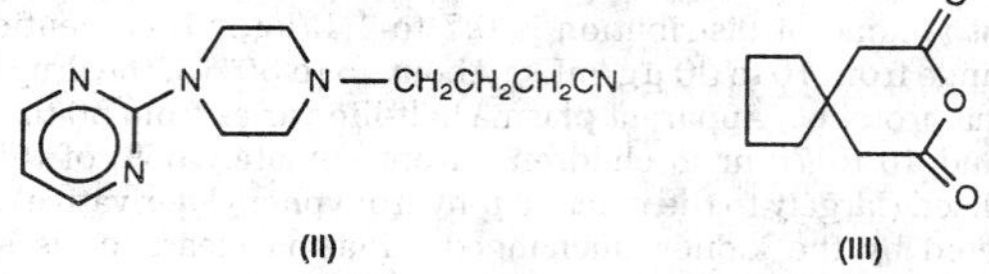

$N—CH_2CH_2CH_2CN$

(II) (III)

Description—White, crystalline solid melting at 200°; pK_a 1.22 and 7.32.

Solubility—1 g in 1 mL water, 50 mL alcohol.

Uses—An antianxiety agent unrelated either chemically or pharmacologically to the benzodiazepines, barbiturates or other sedative/anxiolytic drugs. It is used in the management of anxiety disorders, the short-term relief of the symptoms of anxiety or phobic neurosis. Although its long-term effectiveness as an anxiolytic has not been proven, there are reports of use in patients 6 to 12 mo without apparent loss of clinical benefit. The antianxiety effects of buspirone in general have been found to be comparable to that of the benzodiazepines, with some exceptions, while causing fewer adverse CNS side effects, such as sedation, psychomotor impairment or dependence. Buspirone has been used successfully as an anxiolytic in patients who experience disinhibition or aggressive behavior when taking benzodiazepines. The mechanism of its anxiolytic effect is not known, but appears to be different from the benzodiazepines and barbiturates and likely involves multiple transmitter systems, particularly those of a serotonergic nature. It is absorbed rapidly and undergoes extensive first-pass metabolism. However, buspirone tends to have a slow onset of antianxiety action which can cause patients to be discouraged during initial therapy. Peak plasma levels of 1 to 6 mg/mL usually occur within 40 to 90 min; approximately 95% is bound to plasma protein; 29 to 63% is excreted in the urine and 18 to 38% in the feces. Elimination half-life of the unchanged drug is about 2 to 3 hr.

Even though it appears that this drug has no abuse potential and does not induce either tolerance or psychological dependence, patients on the drug should be monitored closely. Although animal studies suggest the drug does not cause fetal damage, use during pregnancy should be limited to those clearly in need of the medication. Since it is excreted in breast milk, administration to nursing women is not recommended. Safety and efficacy in children under 18 yr has not been established.

Common adverse effects include dizziness, nausea, headache, nervousness, drowsiness, light-headedness, excitement and mood changes. Chest pain, tachycardia, syncopy, hypo- and hypertension, sore throat, blurred vision, skin rashes, leukopenia and shortness of breath also have been observed. Patients should notify their physician if any abnormal chronic muscle movements occur. Although buspirone generally does not impair psychomotor function at usual therapeutic doses, there is enough individual variation that patients should be warned that their ability to perform mental or motor tasks may be impaired.

Dose—Adult, oral, initially **5 mg** 3 times a day; this may be increased 5 mg every 2 or 3 days until the optimal therapeutic response is achieved. Daily dosage should not exceed 60 mg.

Dosage Form—Tablets: 5 and 10 mg.

Chloral Hydrate

1,1-Ethanediol, 2,2,2-trichloro-, Chloral; (*Various Mfrs*)

$CCl_3CH(OH)_2$

Chloral hydrate [302-17-0] $C_2H_3Cl_3O_2$ (165.40).

Preparation—By hydration of trichloroacetaldehyde (chloral) obtained by action of chlorine on alcohol.

Description—Colorless, transparent or white crystals; aromatic, penetrating and slightly acrid odor; slightly bitter, caustic taste. Melts about 55°; slowly volatilizes in air.

Solubility—1 g in 0.25 mL water, 1.3 mL alcohol, 2 mL chloroform or 1.5 mL ether; very soluble in olive oil.

Uses—Principally for the short-term (2-wk) treatment of insomnia. It is used preoperatively to allay anxiety and to induce sedation and/or sleep. It is used postoperatively as an adjunct to opiates and other analgesics to control pain. It also has been used to produce sleep prior to EEG evaluations. It is also effective in reducing anxiety associated with the withdrawal of alcohol and other drugs such as opiates and barbiturates.

Following oral administration, chloral hydrate is converted rapidly to trichloroethanol (TCE), which is largely responsible for its hypnotic action. Other metabolites are trichloroacetic acid (TCA) and trichloroethanolglucuronide (TCEG). Peak plasma levels of TCE and TCEG are reached in 20 to 60 min; plasma half-lives are 8.0 (7.0 to 9.5) hr and 6.7 (6.0 to 8.0) hr for TCE and TCEG, respectively. The half-life for TCA is 4 days. These data suggest that this drug has desirable properties, since the half-life of its active metabolite is short. The formation of TCA is a matter of concern, since its effect on the patient is unknown. It must be used with caution in patients receiving oral anticoagulants because TCA displaces warfarin from plasma protein binding sites; it is likely that dicumarol is affected similarly. Also, concomitant administration of alcohol and chloral hydrate should be avoided; significant potentiation may occur.

Gastric irritation occurs in some patients. Paradoxical excitement is observed rarely. The continued use of large doses causes peripheral vasodilation, hypotension, ventilatory depression, arrhythmias and myocardial depression. Overdosage produces symptoms similar to those caused by barbiturate overdosages and may result in coma. Patients with serious heart, kidney or liver disease should not be given this drug. If gastritis is present, the drug may be administered by rectum in olive oil as a retention enema. The acute toxic oral dose for adults is approximately 10 g; death has been reported after as little as 4 g and individuals have survived after ingesting 30 g.

For oral use, it is sometimes given in a flavored syrup. As alkali causes decomposition of chloral hydrate, it is important that the vehicle not be alkaline.

Dose—*Adult, oral or rectal, usual, sedative,* **250 mg** 3 times a day; *hypnotic,* **500 mg** to **1 g**, on retiring. *Usual range,* **250 mg** to **2 g** a day. *Pediatric, usual, oral, hypnotic,* **50 mg/kg** or at the rate of **1.5 g/m²**, up to **1 g** per single dose, at bedtime; *sedative,* **8 mg/kg** or **250 mg/m²**, up to **500 mg** per dose, 3 times a day.

Dosage Forms—Capsules: 250 and 500 mg; Suppositories: 325, 500 and 650 mg; Syrup: 250 and 500 mg/5 mL.

Chlormezanone—see RPS-18, page 1071.

Disulfiram

Thioperoxydicarbonic diamide, tetraethyl-, Tetraethylthiuram Disulfide; Antabuse (*Wyeth-Ayerst*)

$$(C_2H_5)_2NC(=S)-S-S-C(=S)N(C_2H_5)_2$$

Bis(diethylthiocarbamoyl) disulfide [97-77-8] $C_{10}H_{20}N_2S_4$ (296.52).

Preparation—A cold solution of diethylamine and carbon disulfide in alcohol is treated with an alcoholic solution of iodine. Ice water may be added to hasten separation of the disulfiram. *Ind Eng Chem 20:*1173, 1928. US Pat 1,796,977.

Description—White to off-white, odorless, crystalline powder; melts about 70°.

Solubility—1 g in >5000 mL water, 30 mL alcohol or 15 mL ether; soluble in chloroform.

Uses—An adjunct in the treatment of selected chronic alcoholic patients who *want* to remain in a state of enforced sobriety. It is not a cure for alcoholism, when used alone without supportive therapy. It blocks the oxidation of alcohol at the acetaldehyde stage, which then accumulates in the body and produces unpleasant symptoms characterized by flushing, palpitation, dyspnea and hyperventilation, increased pulse rate, nausea and vomiting, cyanosis and decreased blood pressure and, occasionally, profound collapse. These symptoms usually are followed by drowsiness and sleep, after which the patient fully recovers. The duration of the reaction varies from 30 to 60 min to several hours in the more severe cases, or as long as there is alcohol in the blood.

The drug should not be used without the patient's consent and only after the patient has been made fully aware of risks associated with the treatment. Extreme caution is necessary during its use because severe and alarming reactions (and some deaths) have been reported. These include cardiovascular complications involving unusual fall in blood pressure, cardiac arrhythmia and electrocardiographic evidence of myocardial ischemia and even myocardial infarction. Some patients complain of mild drowsiness, fatigability, impotence, headache or peripheral neuritis and, occasionally, skin rashes.

Patients on this drug should avoid contact with all alcohol, even that in a partially disguised form such as cough syrup or other medicinals and alcoholic lotions applied to the skin. In addition to alcohol-induced reactions, physicians should be alert to drug-induced psychotic episodes that may occur during therapy. It should not be used in patients recently treated with paraldehyde, and paraldehyde should not be given to patients receiving this drug. It appears to decrease the rate at which certain drugs are metabolized and so may increase the blood levels and, thus, the clinical toxicity of drugs given concomitantly.

It should be given with caution in patients receiving phenytoin, oral anticoagulant drugs, metronidazole and isoniazid. Because of the possibility of an accidental disulfiram-alcohol reaction, it should be used with extreme caution in patients with diabetes mellitus, hypothyroidism, epilepsy, cerebral damage, chronic and acute nephritis and hepatic cirrhosis or insufficiency and is contraindicated in patients with alcohol intoxication, cardiovascular disease or psychosis. Patients should be informed of the reactions and cautions stated above. Disulfiram itself can cause adverse effects such as drowsiness, fatigue, headache and skin reactions.

Dose—*Usual, oral, initially* up to **500 mg** a day for the first 2 or 3 wk; *usual, maintenance,* **250 mg** a day.

Dosage Form—Tablets: 250 and 500 mg.

Doxepin Hydrochloride—page 1190.
Droperidol—page 1183.

Ethchlorvynol

1-Penten-4-yn-3-ol, 1-chloro-3-ethyl-, Placidyl (*Abbott*)

$$HC{\equiv}C-C(OH)(CH_2CH_3)-CH{=}CHCl$$

[113-18-8] C_7H_9ClO (144.60).

Preparation—By reacting ethyl chlorovinyl ketone (I) with lithium acetylide under Grignard reaction conditions. The alkoxide addition complex reacts readily with dilute acid to form crude ethchlorvynol which is extracted with a suitable, water-immiscible organic solvent such as ether and is subsequently purified by distillation. Compound I may be prepared in good yield by addition of propionyl chloride to acetylene at a temperature of about 40° in the presence of zinc chloride.

Description—Colorless to yellow liquid possessing a characteristic pungent odor; darkens on exposure to light and air; specific gravity 1.068 to 1.071; refractive index 1.476 to 1.480.

Solubility—Immiscible with water; miscible with most organic solvents.

Uses—A mild hypnotic that induces sleep within 15 min to 1 hr and has duration of action of approximately 5 hr. Elimination half-life varies from 10 to 25 hr. Its effect is less profound and not as predictable as that obtained with benzodiazepines. It is indicated as short-term (up to 1 wk) hypnotic therapy in insomnia. This drug is thought to have little effect on REM sleep; hence, REM rebound is not a major problem. It has been reported to increase the metabolism of coumarin anticoagulants by enzyme induction; patients on oral anticoagulants should be monitored closely when this drug is started or stopped. It is contraindicated in patients with porphyria and those with known hypersensitivity to the drug.

Patients should be cautioned about concomitant use of alcohol, barbiturates, other CNS depressants or MAO inhibitors, since such combinations may produce exaggerated depressant effects. Also, they should be warned against operating a motor vehicle or hazardous machinery while on the drug. The excessive chronic use of large doses has been reported to cause psychic and physical dependence, tolerance and withdrawal symptoms much like that caused by chronic use of barbiturates or alcohol and can include severe convulsions, when the drug is discontinued. It should not be used in patients with a history of drug abuse, mental depression or suicide tendencies, and the drug should be withdrawn gradually from patients taking excessive quantities. The drug is metabolized primarily by the liver, although the kidneys appear to contribute also.

Side effects, such as nausea, mental confusion, headache, and dermatitis, have been observed in some patients. In addition, hypotension, blurring of vision, dizziness, facial numbness and allergic reactions have been reported. There have been rare reports of cholestatic jaundice and a few instances of thrombocytopenia. The safe and effective use of this agent during pregnancy and in pediatric-age patients has not been established.

Dose—*Hypnotic, adult,* **500 mg** at bedtime; **750 mg** may be used in patients whose sleep response to 500 mg is inadequate; maximum, **1000 mg.** An additional 100 to 200 mg may be given to reinstitute sleep in patients who awaken after the usual 500 to 750 mg.

Dosage Form—Capsules: 200, 500 and 750 mg.

Ethinamate

Cyclohexanol, 1-ethynyl-, carbamate; Valmid (*Dista*)

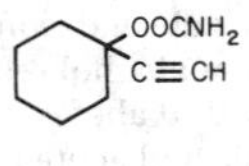

[126-52-3] $C_9H_{13}NO_2$ (167.21).

Preparation—By condensing 1-ethynylcyclohexanol with carbamoyl chloride in the presence of pyridine. The crude ester is obtained by treating the reaction mixture with dilute hydrochloric acid. The 1-ethynylcyclohexanol may be synthesized by a typical Grignard reaction using cyclohexanone and ethynylmagnesium bromide.

Description—White, essentially odorless powder; melts 94 to 98°; pH (saturated solution) about 6.5.

Solubility—1 g in 400 mL water or 2.9 mL alcohol; freely soluble in chloroform or ether.

Uses—A mild hypnotic useful for the induction of sleep in simple insomnia. For the most part, it has been replaced by more effective and safer hypnotic agents. It is contraindicated in patients hypersensitive to the drug. It is absorbed rapidly after oral administration, inactivated by the liver and excreted in the urine. Following a single dose of 1 g, peak plasma levels are reached in 36 min and decline to negligible values within 8 hr. Approximately 36% of the dose appears in the urine within 24 hr. Onset of action is 20 to 30 min. Therefore, it is more effective in inducing sleep than in maintaining sleep. When taken in high doses, physical and psychological dependence can occur; thus, abrupt abstinence may cause typical withdrawal symptoms, including seizures. Rare cases of thrombocytopenic purpura and drug idiosyncrasy with fever have been reported. Paradoxical excitement in children, mild gastrointestinal disorders and skin rashes also have been observed. Although no maternal or fetal adverse effects have been reported, sufficient laboratory work has not been done in this area to warrant its use in pregnant and lactating women.

It should not be taken concurrently with alcohol or other CNS depressants and patients on this drug should be warned against operating a motor vehicle or operating hazardous machinery for at least 4 or 5 hr after taking the drug. It has not been studied in children; hence, it is not recommended for pediatric use. Habituation and physical dependence may result from excessive use of the drug. The abstinence syndrome is similar to that of the barbiturates. It should be used with caution in patients with a history of drug abuse.

Dose—*Adult, oral, usual,* **500 mg** to **1 g** 20 min before bedtime. *Geriatric or debilitated patients,* **500 mg;** the risk of oversedation, dizziness, confusion and/or ataxia is increased substantially with higher doses; this dose may be increased when the potential benefits justify the risks. Dosage in children not established.

Dosage Form—Capsules: 500 mg.

Glutethimide

2,6-Piperidinedione, 3-ethyl-3-phenyl-, Dorimide (*Cenci*); Rolathimide (*Robinson*); Doriden (*USV*)

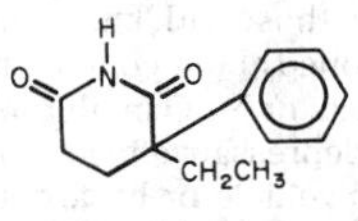

2-Ethyl-2-phenylglutarimide [77-21-4] $C_{13}H_{15}NO_2$ (217.27).

Preparation—Benzyl cyanide in toluene solution is treated with ethyl chloride in the presence of sodamide to yield α-ethylbenzyl cyanide. This is then caused to undergo addition (Michael condensation) to methyl acrylate under the catalytic influence of piperidine, thus forming methyl 4-cyano-4-phenylhexanoate (I). After purifying by low-pressure distillation, I is cyclized in acid medium. The cyclization may be represented as involving hydration of the cyanide group to amide and saponification of the ester, followed by dehydration between the amide and carboxyl groups.

Description—White, crystalline powder; saturated solution slightly acid; melts about 88°.

Solubility—Freely soluble in ethyl acetate, acetone, ether or chloroform; soluble in alcohol or methanol; practically insoluble in water.

Uses—A hypnotic used to induce sleep in all types of insomnia. Overdosage is less likely to depress respiration, but more likely to cause hypotension, than most barbiturates. The onset of action begins about 30 min after the administration of a hypnotic dose and generally lasts from 4 to 8 hr. Oral absorption is variable with peak plasma level times between 1 and 6 hr. Elimination half-life varies from 5 to 22 hr, with an average value of 11.6 hr. It is contraindicated in hypersensitive patients and patients should be warned about the concomitant use of alcohol and other CNS-depressant drugs. Patients also should be cautioned about engaging in activities which require alertness until 4 or 5 hr have elapsed following ingestion of the drug. It induces liver microsomal enzymes; therefore, therapy in patients on coumarin anticoagulants may require adjustment of the coumarin dose during and upon cessation of such therapy.

Adverse reactions include a generalized skin rash (in this case the drug should be withdrawn); occasionally, a purpuric or urticarial rash; exfoliative dermatitis has been observed rarely; nausea, hangover, paradoxical excitation and blurred vision have occurred. Some of these side effects may be due to the anticholinergic activity of this drug. Porphyria or blood dyscrasias (thrombocytopenic purpura, aplastic anemia or leukopenia) also have been reported. Habituation and physical dependence, like that which occurs with the barbiturates, may result from the prolonged administration of excessive doses. It is currently a Schedule II drug under the *Controlled Substances Act.* The drug should be used with caution in patients with a history of drug abuse.

Dose—*Usual, hypnotic,* **250** to **500 mg** at bedtime; *Elderly and debilitated patients,* a maximum of **500 mg.** Not recommended in children under 12 yr.

Dosage Form—Tablets: 250 and 500 mg.

Hydroxyzine Hydrochloride

Ethanol, 2-[2-[4-[(4-chlorophenyl)phenylmethyl]-1-piperazinyl-]ethoxy]-, dihydrochloride; Atarax (*Roerig*); (*Various Mfrs*)

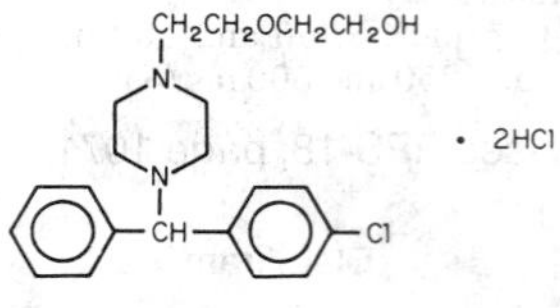

[2192-20-3] $C_{21}H_{27}ClN_2O_2.2HCl$ (447.83).

Preparation—By condensing *p*-chlorobenzhydryl chloride (**I**) with *N*-[2-(2-hydroxyethoxy)ethyl]piperazine (**II**). Conversion to the hydrochloride may be effected by dissolving the base in a double molar quantity of hydrochloric acid and evaporating the solution to dryness.

I may be synthesized by treating benzaldehyde with *p*-chlorophenylmagnesium bromide and reacting the resulting *p*-chlorobenzhydrol with a suitable halogenating agent. **II** may be synthesized by interaction of piperazine and ethylene oxide.

Description—White, odorless powder; melts with decomposition about 200°.

Solubility—1 g in 1 mL of water, 4.5 mL of alcohol, 13 mL of chloroform or > 1000 mL of ether.

Uses—A piperazine-derivative used for the management of neuroses and emotional disturbances characterized by anxiety, tension, agitation, apprehension or confusion. This includes its use in anxiety and apprehension associated with organic diseases, alcoholism, allergic conditions, pre- and postoperative conditions and cardiac conditions. Hydroxyzine also is used to control motion sickness, nausea and vomiting of various etiologies. It is contraindicated in early pregnancy and in patients who have shown a previous hypersensitivity to it. Like most other sedatives it should be used with caution and proper dose adjustment in patients on other CNS-depressant drugs. Therefore, when used as preanesthetic medication with other agents, such as meperidine and a barbiturate, the dosage should be adjusted on an individual basis. Because of its anticholinergic action, the effects of hydroxyzine may be additive with atropine and other belladonna alkaloids. Since the drug may cause drowsiness, the patient should be warned not to drive a car or operate hazardous machinery while on the drug.

Adverse reactions are relatively mild and include drowsiness and dryness of the mouth. Less frequent side effects are dizziness, ataxia, agitation and anxiety. Involuntary motor activity, including rare instances of tremor and convulsions have been reported. Because of marked local irritation and possible tissue necrosis, hydroxyzine should not be administered by subcutaneous, intra-arterial or IV injection. Clinical studies substantiate the absence of toxic effects on the liver or blood. *The potentiating effect of this drug must be taken into consideration when it is used in conjunction with CNS-depressants such as narcotics and barbiturates.*

Dose—*Adult, oral, range,* **25** to **100 mg;** *usual,* **25 mg** 3 or 4 times a day, not to exceed 400 mg in a day. *Intramuscular, usual,* **25** to **100 mg** every 4 to 6 hr. *Pediatric, oral, usual, under 6 yr,* **50 mg** a day in divided doses; *over 6 yr,* **50** to **100 mg** a day in divided doses.

Dosage Forms—Injection: 25 and 50 mg/mL; Syrup: 10 mg/5 mL; Tablets: 10, 25, 50 and 100 mg.

Hydroxyzine Pamoate

Ethanol, 2-[2-[4-[(4-chlorophenyl)phenylmethyl]-1-piperazinyl]ethoxy]-, compd with 4,4′-methylenebis[3-hydroxy-2-naphthalenecarboxylic acid] (1:1); Vistaril (*Pfizer*); Vamate (*Major*); Vistacon (*Hauck*); (*Various Mfrs*)

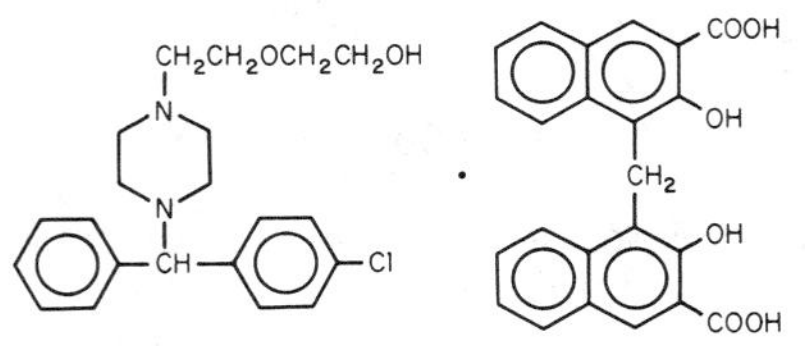

[10246-75-0] $C_{21}H_{27}ClN_2O_2.C_{23}H_{16}O_6$ (763.29).

Preparation—Hydroxyzine, prepared as described under *Hydroxyzine Hydrochloride*, is reacted with an equimolar portion of 4,4′-methylenebis[3-hydroxy-2-naphthoic acid].

Description—Light-yellow, practically odorless, powder.

Solubility—1 g in >1000 mL water, 700 mL alcohol, >1000 mL chloroform, >1000 mL ether or 10 mL dimethylformamide.

Uses and Dose—See *Hydroxyzine Hydrochloride*.

Dosage Forms—Capsules: 25, 50 and 100 mg; Oral Suspension: 25 mg/5 mL.

Magnesium Sulfate Injection—page 1175.

Meprobamate

1,3-Propanediol, 2-methyl-2-propyl-, dicarbamate; (*Various Mfrs*)

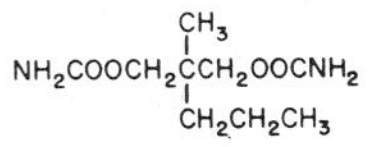

[57-53-4] $C_9H_{18}N_2O_4$ (218.25).

Preparation—2-Methyl-2-*n*-propyl-1,3-propanediol, in toluene solution, is condensed at about 0° with phosgene in the presence of dimethylaniline to yield the chloroformate diester, which is then subjected to ammonolysis to form the dicarbamate ester.

Description—White powder; characteristic odor and a bitter taste; melts within a range of 2° between 103 and 107°.

Solubility—Slightly soluble in water; freely soluble in alcohol or acetone; sparingly soluble in ether.

Uses—A propanediol derivative chemically related to mephenesin indicated for the management of *anxiety disorders* or for the short-term relief of the *symptoms of anxiety*. Anxiety or tension associated with the stress of everyday life usually do not require treatment with an anxiolytic. It is contraindicated in patients with acute intermittent porphyria and in patients allergic to meprobamate or related agents, such as carisoprodol, mebutamate or carbromal. Much like the barbiturates, physical and psychological dependence are known to occur after chronic use of high doses. Sudden withdrawal of the drug after prolonged, excessive use should be avoided in order to minimize withdrawal effects. Withdrawal symptoms usually appear 12 to 48 hr after discontinuation of meprobamate and usually cease within the next 12 to 48 hr. The drug should not be prescribed for patients with a history of drug abuse or those known to increase the dose of drugs on their own initiative. Patients should be warned not to attempt potentially hazardous tasks or take other CNS-depressant drugs while on this drug. The drug should be used with caution in elderly or debilitated patients, epileptic patients, patients with compromised hepatic or renal function and patients with suicidal tendencies. It is capable of producing a variety of side effects and untoward reactions. Briefly, these include *CNS:* drowsiness, ataxia, dizziness, slurred speech, headache, vertigo, weakness, paresthesias, impaired visual accommodation, euphoria, overstimulation and paradoxical excitement; *gastrointestinal:* nausea, vomiting and diarrhea; *cardiovascular:* palpitation, arrhythmias, syncope and hypotensive crises; *allergic or idiosyncratic:* a variety of reactions including various skin, blood and hypersensitivity reactions (also, Stevens-Johnson syndrome and bullous dermatitis) have been observed: *hematological:* agranulocytosis, aplastic anemia and rare cases of thrombocytopenic purpura have been reported. Exacerbation of porphyric symptoms also has been observed. Plasma half-life ranges from 6 to 17 hr (average 10 hr). Therapeutic blood levels range from 0.5 to 2.0 mg%; levels of 3 to 10 mg% usually correlate with mild to moderate symptoms of overdosage, ie, stupor or slight coma; and levels of 10 to 20 mg% with deeper coma requiring intensive therapy, with some fatalities occurring. At levels above 20 mg% more fatalities than survivors can be expected. It is evident, therefore, that the drug should be employed with the same discretion as other CNS-depressant agents and with due cognizance of the possibility of untoward effects.

Dose—*Adult, oral,* **1.2** to **1.6 g/day** in 3 to 4 divided doses; do not exceed 2.4 g/day. *Sustained release;* **400** to **800 mg** in the morning and at bedtime. *Pediatric, under 6 yr,* use not recommended; *6 to 12 yr,* **100** to **200 mg** 2 or 3 times a day. *Sustained release,* **200 mg** in the morning and at bedtime.

Dosage Forms—Sustained-Release Capsules: 200 and 400 mg; Tablets: 200, 400 and 600 mg.

Methapyrilene Hydrochloride—RPS-16, page 1070.

Methotrimeprazine Hydrochloride—page 1220.

Methyprylon

2,4-Piperidinedione, 3,3-diethyl-5-methyl-, Noludar (*Roche*)

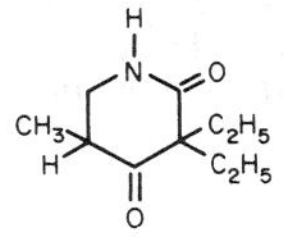

[125-64-4] $C_{10}H_{17}NO_2$ (183.25).

Preparation—3,3-Diethyl-2,4(1*H*,3*H*)-pyridinedione is hydroxymethylated at the 5-position by treatment with formaldehyde in the presence of an alkaline catalyst. The resulting methylol derivative is hydrogenated catalytically, whereupon the ring is saturated and the hydroxymethyl group deoxygenated.

Description—White, or nearly white, crystalline powder; slight, characteristic odor; melts about 76° pK_a 12.0.

Solubility—1 g in 11 mL water, 2 mL alcohol, 2 mL chloroform or 2 mL ether.

Uses—A hypnotic used in the management of insomnia of varied etiology although generally replaced by safer and more effective drugs. It usually induces sleep within 45 min; it provides sleep for 5 to 8 hr. Mean plasma levels in patients following a single 650-mg dose peak 1 or 2 hr postadministration at approximately 7.8 to 10 μg/mL; the levels decline to 3.3 to 7.8 μg/mL after 4 hr. Physical and psychological dependence can occur causing barbiturate-like withdrawal when abruptly discontinued. There have been cases of morning drowsiness, dizziness, mild to moderate gastric upset (diarrhea, esophagitis, nausea and vomiting), headache, paradoxical excitement and skin rash. A few isolated cases of neutropenia and thrombocytopenia have been reported. Patients should be warned against the concomitant use of this drug and alcohol or other CNS depressants. It is a *Schedule III* drug under the *Controlled Substances Act*. Its safe use during pregnancy and in children under 3 yr has not been established.

Dose—*Adult, oral, hypnotic,* **200** to **400 mg** before retiring, individualized for maximum beneficial effect. *Children,* the effective dose varies greatly and should be individualized; *initially* **50 mg** may be given, increased up to **200 mg,** if required, at bedtime. Should not be given to children under 12 yr.

Dosage Forms—Capsules: 300 mg; Tablets: 200 mg.

Paraldehyde

1,3,5-Trioxane, 2,4,6-trimethyl-, Paracetaldehyde; Paral (*Forest*)

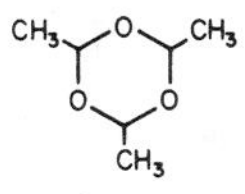

2,4,6-Trimethyl-*s*-trioxane [123-63-7] $C_6H_{12}O_3$ (132.16); a trimer of acetaldehyde.

Caution—*It is subject to oxidation to form acetic acid. It may contain a suitable stabilizer.*

Preparation—By treating acetaldehyde with small quantities of sulfur dioxide, hydrochloric acid, carbonyl chloride or zinc chloride; almost complete conversion occurs, and by freezing the liquid and then distilling the crystallized material, if necessary, the pure compound is produced.

Description—Colorless, transparent liquid; a disagreeable taste and a strong, characteristic, but not unpleasant or pungent odor; specific gravity about 0.99; congeals not below 11° and distils 120 to 126°; in contact with air it slowly oxidizes to acetic acid.

Solubility—1 mL in about 10 mL water or about 17 mL boiling water; miscible with alcohol, chloroform, ether or volatile oils.

Incompatibilities—*Acids* convert it into acetaldehyde, which is prone to oxidation.

Uses—One of the oldest *sedatives* and *hypnotics*. It is absorbed rapidly after oral administration and produces sleep within 10 to 15 min after a 4- to 8-mL dose. It is detoxified by the liver (70 to 80%) and 11 to 28% is excreted by the lungs. A negligible amount is excreted in the urine. Its chief disadvantage is that, being in part excreted through the lungs, it imparts an odor to the exhaled air, causes irritation and, thus, should not be used in patients with asthma or other pulmonary diseases. Also, it has an unpleasant taste and may irritate the throat and gastric mucosa unless dispensed in suitable vehicles and should not be used in patients with gastroenteritis. It is poorly soluble in water; hence, it usually is prescribed in combination with alcoholic liquors, elixirs, etc. The drug also can be taken in milk, fruit juices, iced tea or with cracked ice. Finally, it can be administered as a rectal retention enema in olive oil. It is effective in status epilepticus, but should be reserved for patients who do not respond to phenobarbital. It occasionally is employed as an *obstetrical analgetic*, in which case large doses are administered, usually by rectum. The drug also is used frequently in *delirium tremens* and in patients undergoing *withdrawal therapy for alcoholism*.

Dose—*Adult, oral: hypnotic,* **4** to **8 mL** in milk or iced fruit juice; *delerium tremens,* **10** to **35 mL.** *Rectal,* **10** to **20 mL** with 1 or 2 parts of olive oil. *Children, sedative,* **0.15 mL/kg** IM.

Dosage Forms—Oral and Rectal Liquids: 1 g/mL in 30 mL.

Promethazine Hydrochloride—page 1227.

Propiomazine Hydrochloride—see RPS-18, page 1071.

Propranolol Hydrochloride—page 1016.

Pyrilamine Maleate—page 1227.

Scopolamine Hydrobromide—page 1024.

Tybamate—see RPS-18, page 1071.

Sedative Combinations

Some examples of sedative combinations (with mg/unit provided) are as follows:

Meprobamate with Aspirin [Equagesic (*Wyeth*); Equazine-M (*Rugby*)]—200 and 325 mg, respectively.

Meprobamate with Conjugated Estrogens [Milprem-200 or -400 (*Wallace*); PMB-200 or -400 (*Ayerst*)]—200 or 400 and 0.45 mg, respectively.

Meprobamate with Trihexethyl Chloride [Pathibamate-200 or -400 (*Lederle*)]—200 or 400 and 25 mg, respectively.

Meprobamate with Benactyzine Hydrochloride [Deprol (*Wallace*)]—400 and 1 mg, respectively.

CHAPTER 70

Antiepileptic Drugs

H Steve White, PhD
Research Associate Professor of Pharmacology and Toxicology
College of Pharmacy
University of Utah
Salt Lake City, UT 84112

Epilepsy may be defined as a paroxysmal, self-sustaining and self-limiting cerebral dysrhythmia characterized by an abnormal and excessive EEG discharge and a loss of consciousness. It may or may not be associated with body movements or hyperactivity of the autonomic nervous system. The epileptic attack is initiated by an abnormal focus of electric discharge, originating either in the grey matter or other part of the brain. The discharge spreads to other parts of the central nervous system and results in convulsions and other manifestations of the disorder.

There are many conditions which result in seizures. These include the entire range of neurological diseases from infection to neoplasm to head injuries. Contrary to popular opinion, hereditary factors are involved in only a few subtypes of seizures. The antiepileptic drugs described in this chapter also are used in patients with febrile seizures or with seizures as a result of an acute illness such as meningitis, even though the term epilepsy is not applied to such patients unless they later develop chronic seizures. Seizures also may result from an acute toxic or metabolic disorder; in such cases appropriate therapy is directed to the specific abnormality, such as hypocalcemia. In most cases of epilepsy, the choice of medication is dictated by the seizure classification.

Based on a modification of the International Classification (Epilepsia 22:489, 1981), epileptic seizures may be divided into two groups:

I. *Partial Seizures* (Focal Seizures).

A. Partial seizures with elementary symptomatology (cortical focal). Generally without impairment of consciousness. Includes seizures confined to a single limb or muscle group (Jacksonian motor epilepsy), those with sensory or somatosensory symptoms (Jacksonian sensory epilepsy) and those with other limited symptoms depending upon the particular cortical area involved.

B. Partial seizures with complex symptomatology (temporal lobe; psychomotor seizures). Generally with impairment of consciousness. Attacks of confused behavior with a wide variety of clinical manifestations, associated with bizarre generalized EEG activity during the seizure and temporal lobe abnormalities during the interseizure period.

C. Partial seizures secondarily generalized.

II. *Generalized Seizures* (bilaterally, symmetrical seizures). Includes *absences* (petit mal), characterized by brief, abrupt loss of consciousness associated with synchronous, 3-per-second spike-and-wave pattern in the EEG, usually with symmetrical clonic motor activity (eyelid blinking or jerking of entire body). *Bilateral massive epileptic myoclonus*, isolated clonic jerks with brief burst of multiple spikes in EEG; *infantile spasms*, motor spasms with bizarre diffuse changes in the interseizure EEG, ie, hypsarrhythmia and progressive mental retardation; *clonic seizures*, rhythmic clonic contraction of all muscles, loss of consciousness and autonomic manifestations; *tonic seizures*, opisthotonous, loss of consciousness and autonomic manifestations; *tonic-clonic seizures* (grand mal), characterized by a sequence of maximal tonic spasms of all body musculature followed by synchronous clonic jerking and profound depression of all central functions; *atonic seizures*, loss of postural tone with sagging of the head or falling; *akinetic seizures*, impaired consciousness and complete muscle relaxation, secondary to excessive inhibitory discharge.

The limitation of this type of description is that it is confined to describing individual seizure types and does not take into account a description of the numerous epileptic syndromes which continue to be described. To satisfy the need for a more accurate description of a seizure disorder, the International Classification of Epilepsies and Epileptic Syndromes was proposed to supplement the above classification. An epileptic syndrome is characterized by a variety of signs and symptoms. A particular syndrome will attempt to incorporate a number of items including type of seizure, etiology, anatomy, precipitating factors, age of onset, severity, chronicity, diurnal and circadian cycling and often prognosis (*Epilepsia 30(4)*: 389, 1989).

A number of specific childhood epileptic syndromes have been recognized and classified by age. The notable examples include Early Myoclonic Encephalopathy; Lennox-Gastaut Syndrome; Absence Epilepsy Syndromes such as typical absence, juvenile absence and juvenile myoclonic epilepsy; and Progressive Myoclonic Epilepsy. One major advantage of this classification is that it recognizes that a simple partial seizure can progress to a complex partial seizure, and then to a secondary generalized seizure. In so doing, this classification does not require that a seizure be classified into one specific seizure category (*Univ Rep Epilepsy 1(1)*, 1, 1992.

One approach to the treatment of seizure disorders employs the use of antiepileptic drugs. The many medical therapies of antiquity have been replaced by a rational therapeutic approach which had its origin in the beginning of the 19th century. It has progressed from the use of bromides in 1857 and phenobarbital in 1912 to the modern era marked by introduction of dipenylhydantoin (phenytoin) in 1938. The clinical efficacy of the latter established the fact that chemicals effective in epilepsy need not by hypnotics and stimulated the laboratory search for other effective anticonvulsant agents. As a result, a number of anticonvulsant barbiturates, benzoidiazepines, deoxybarbiturates, dipropylacetic acid derivatives, hydantoins, oxazolidinediones and succinimides have been introduced in the last 50 years. Felbamate is the newest anticonvulsant approved in the US and is the first new drug introduced in 15 years. As a result of these advances in drug therapy, it generally is stated that 50% of all individuals with epileptic disorders can be satisfactorily controlled with available drugs and that the incidence of seizures can be reduced in another 25% of epileptic persons.

Knowledge of the underlying causes of various types of seizure disorders is still incomplete. Nevertheless, most experimental models of epilepsy are designed to simulate, either in isolated animal brain tissues (*in vitro*) or in the intact laboratory animal (*in vivo*), various chemical, electrical or overt manifestations of the disorder.

Because of the variety of clinical types of epilepsy and their differences in response to drugs, a battery of tests usually is employed for the laboratory study of candidate anticonvulsant drugs in animals. In general, these tests measure the ability of drugs to elevate the *threshold* for minimal seizures induced in laboratory animals by chemical stimulation (metrazol, bicuculline and picrotoxin; sc Met, sc Bic and sc Pic tests, respectively) and to *modify the pattern* of maximal seizures induced by electrical stimulation (MES test). The laboratory profile of anticonvulsant action provides the first insight as to the possible clinical usefulness of a drug. For example, the drugs of choice for generalized tonic-clonic and complex seizures (phenytoin, carbamazepine) are effective against MES seizures but ineffective against sc Met seizures, block repetitive firing and decrease $Na^+$and Ca^{2+} influx. The drug of choice for generalized absence seizures (ethosuximide) is ineffective against MES seizures but effective against sc Met seizures and reduces the current through a specific type of voltage-sensitive calcium channel called the low-threshold T-type calcium channel (*Epilepsia 34* (*5*): 1, 1993). It has been suggested that the T-channel plays an important role in the abnormal thalamocortical rhythmicity that underlies the characteristic spike and wave discharge. The finding that ethosuximide and dimethadione inhibit this current at clinically relevant concentrations support this hypothesis. The drug of choice for myclonic, generalized absence, generalized tonic-clonic and partial seizures (valproic acid) is effective against MES, sc Bic, sc Pic and sc Met seizures, blocks repetitive firing and, in larger doses, may enhance GABA-mediated transmission and reduce T-channel calcium currents.

The mechanisms of action of currently marketed anticonvulsant drugs are not understood fully. Although numerous molecular targets exist wherein anticonvulsants may exert an effect, the final common pathway appears to be through modulation of voltage-gated and/or neurotransmitter-gated ion channels. Most of the prototype anticonvulsants presently are thought to exert their primary action by

Reducing sustained, high-frequency, repetitive firing of action potentials by modulating voltage-dependent sodium channels (phenytoin, carbamazepine and valproate.

Enhancing GABA-mediated inhibitory neurotransmission via a receptor-gated chloride channel (benzodiazepines).

Modulating neurotransmitter release and neuronal bursting through an effect on voltage-gated and receptor-gated calcium channels (ethosuximide, dimethadione and valproate (*Epilepsia 30* (*4*): 389, 1989).

In addition, newer anticonvulsant substances still under preclinical development have been found to open potassium channels (Brain Res *495*: 189, 1989; *Eur J Pharmaco 167*: 181, 1989). Another promising area currently being pursued involves identifying novel therapies which are aimed at either reducing excitation by blocking specific excitatory amino acid receptors and those aimed at enhancing inhibition by blocking high-affinity uptake of neuronally released GABA. It is anticipated that our increased appreciation of the processes underlying the initiation, propagation and amelioration of seizure activity will lead to the introduction of mechanistically novel drugs in the not-too-distant future.

No one anticonvulsant drug is equally effective in all types of epilepsy. Hence, antiepileptic therapy must be individualized and drug therapy selected on the basis of seizure type, epileptic syndrome and patient response. In generalized tonic-clonic seizures (grand mal) and simple and complex partial (focal, psychomotor), the drugs of choice are phenytoin, carbamazepine or valproate; in generalized absence seizures (petit mal), ethosuximide and valproate with clonazepam as an alternate; for myclonic epilepsy, valproate. It should be noted that valproate is effective in all of the above.

Status epilepticus, a succession of tonic-clonic seizures without intervening return of consciousness, requires prompt intravenous medication. The objective of treatment is suppression of the seizures, but all of the drugs used to treat this medical emergency can be lethal if they are given too rapidly or in overdosage. Intravenous diazepam is preferred by many clinicians but since it is short-acting, maintenance must be started promptly. Some clinicians prefer intravenous phenytoin, especially in patients already on this drug. Phenobarbital is an effective alternative for the management of this disorder. If these drugs do not suppress the continuous seizure activity, general anesthesia may be used as an emergency treatment.

Until the 1970s, antiepileptic polytherapy was the most widely accepted practice in the treatment of epilepsy. Now, monotherapy is considered the superior therapeutic practice in the management of this disorder. This change was encouraged by refinements in diagnosis and the availability of broad-spectrum antiepileptics such as valproic acid. Successful monotherapy involves three basic principles.

Careful diagnosis of the specific type of seizures.

Accurate selection of the most suitable antiepileptic drug for the patient's seizures.

Appropriate drug use and monitoring.

Monotherapy has been shown to improve seizure control and reduce the risk of idiosyncratic reactions, dose-related adverse effects and complex drug interactions. Monotherapy also encourages better patient compliance and is cost effective.

The monitoring of plasma levels of these drugs is now considered part of the routine management of patients with epilepsy. These drugs exert their action after forming reversible bonds with brain-tissue molecules (receptors). Consequently, their intensity of action tends to be proportional to the drug concentration in the biophase in the vicinity of the receptors. Antiepileptic drug molecules in cerebral extracellular water are in dynamic equilibrium with drug molecules in plasma water. Therefore, the antiepileptic drug concentration in plasma water is a measure of the drug concentration in brain and, hence provides a measure of antiepileptic effect. The clinician needs to know the latter in order to manage his epileptic patients.

When should plasma antiepileptic drug levels be measured? Ideally, plasma levels should be measured in the steady state at fixed times in relation to the drug dosage interval. For most drugs which are eliminated according to processes which follow monoexponential kinetics, virtually steady-state plasma levels are achieved after approximately five drug-elimination half-lives. In the case of antiepileptics, their elimination half-lives are so long in relation to dosage regimens that the change in plasma level over a dosage interval is likely to be within the experimental error in an individual drug concentration measurement. Therefore, unless the dosage is changed or other drug therapy added, the time of measurement of antiepileptic drug levels does not present too much of a problem.

From a clinical standpoint antiepileptic drug levels should be monitored at the outset of therapy, to see if a satisfactory plasma level has been obtained and during the course of therapy. The latter is especially important if the seizures are not controlled, intercurrent illness develops, antiepileptic drug dosage is changed, dosage of any other drug is changed or symptoms occur which appear to be due to the drug. It also is important to monitor the epileptic patient during pregnancy, since antiepileptic drug levels tend to fall during pregnancy and rise again during puerperium. Such monitoring increases the changes of controlling epilepsy in patients and decreases the risk of their being overdosed in the process.

Behavioral disturbances and cognitive effects have been observed in patients on antiepileptic drug therapy (*Pediatrics 76*:644, 1985). Phenobarbital is associated with hyperactivity, fussiness, lethargy, disobedience and stubbornness; phenytoin with unsteadiness, involuntary movements, tiredness and alterations of emotional state; carbamazepine with sleep disorders, agitation, irritability and emotional liability; clonazepam with irritability, aggression, hyperactivity, disobedience and antisocial activities; and valproic acid with drowsiness. In addition, some have been shown to induce deficits in neuropsychological tests and impair attention and short-term memory. Physicians and parents should be alert for such behavioral and cognitive changes.

Antiepileptic drugs may add to or potentiate the action of other central nervous system depressants, including other anticonvulsants and alcohol. A number of drugs, when concurrently administered with various antiepileptic agents, have been reported to alter the patient's response either to the antiepileptics or the other drugs (see Chapter 105 for additional information concerning specific drug interactions). Whether or not the effects are clinically significant cannot be stated categorically; they must be evaluated by careful observation of the individual patients, with monitoring of blood plasma levels of the concurrently administered drugs after which dosage adjustments of the interacting drugs may be necessary. For these reasons patients on antiepileptic medication should not take other drugs, either OTC or prescription, without the knowledge and approval of the physician responsible for their seizure therapy.

As tricyclic antidepressants may precipitate seizures, patients being treated with anticonvulsants should be observed closely for decreased seizure control if tricyclic antidepressant therapy is commenced; if necessary, the dosage of the anticonvulsant should be adjusted.

Children of epileptic mothers who receive anticonvulsant medication during the early months of pregnancy have an increased incidence of birth defects. The risk is about 7% as compared to 2 or 3% in the general population. Data are more extensive with respect to phenytoin, phenobarbital and trimethadione. More recent observations indicate that valproate may be associated with spinal defects in the fetus. Although systematic or anecdotal reports suggest a possible similar association with the use of all known anticonvulsant drugs, therapeutic abortion should be considered when trimethadione has been used during pregnancy. The great majority of mothers on anticonvulsant medication, however, deliver normal infants. It also is important to note that anticonvulsant drugs should not be discontinued in patients in whom the drug is administered to prevent generalized tonic-clonic seizures because of the strong possibilty of precipitating status epilepticus with an attendant hypoxia and threat to life. In individual cases where the severity and frequency of the seizure disorder are such that the removal of medication does not pose a serious threat to the patient, discontinuation of the drug may be considered prior to and during pregnancy, although it cannot be said with any confidence that even seizures do not pose some hazard to the developing embryo or fetus. The prescribing physician will wish to weigh the risk/benefit of these considerations in treating or counseling epileptic women of child-bearing age.

Antiepileptic agents have several uses in the nonepileptic patient. They have been used to soften the seizures in patients undergoing electroshock therapy, control convulsions occuring in dementia paralytica and tetanus and lessen muscular rigidity in certain cases of cerebral palsy. Phenytoin administered intravenously has been reported to be effective in suppressing recurrent cardiac arrhythmias. In addition, phenytoin, trimethadione and phenacemide have been employed for the treatment of disturbed nonepileptic psychotic patients, particularly in catatonic excitement states, and in the management of children with behavioral disorders. The latter use is especially intriguing and warrants careful clinical study.

Acetazolamide—page 1042.

Carbamazepine

5H-Dibenz[*b*, *f*]azepine-5-carboxamide (*Rugby*); Tegretol (*Ciba-Geigy*)

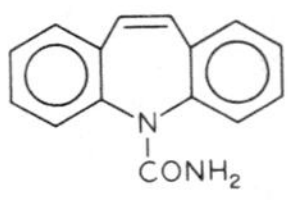

[298-46-4] $C_{15}H_{12}N_2O$ (236.27).

Preparation—5*H*-Dibenz[*b*, *f*]azepine, which may be prepared by thermal deammoniation of 2-(*o*-aminostyryl) aniline hydrochloride, is condensed with carbamoyl chloride by refluxing in an inert solvent in the presence of sodamide. US Pat 2,948,718.

Description—White to off-white powder; melts within a range of 3° between 187 and 193°.

Solubility—Practically insoluble in water; soluble in alcohol or acetone.

Uses—Considered the drug of choice for complex partial seizures (temporal lobe, psychotomotor). It is preferred by many physicians for *generalized tonic-clonic seizures* (grand mal) and simple partial (focal, Jacksonian) seizures, particularly in patients who have not responded to other less-toxic anticonvulsants. It sometimes is effective in patients with mixed seizure patterns which include the above, or other partial or generalized seizures. It is also useful in treatment of pain associated with true trigeminal neuralgia. Beneficial results also have been reported in glosspharyngeal neuralgia. Carbamazepine also has been used with some benefit for the management of acute mania, maintenance therapy of bipolar affective disorder and for the management of aggression and alcohol withdrawal syndrome (*Am Pharm NS33*(*2*): 47, 1993). The drug has a neutral pK_a; from 60 to 73% of the drug is bound to plasma protein, volume distribution usually is between 0.8 to 1.4L/kg; and half-life varies from 10 to 25 hr in adults and 8.5 to 19 hr in children. Therapeutic plasma levels range from 4 to 12 μg/mL. It should not be used in combination with other drugs; for example, troleandomycin, erythomycin, cimetidine, isoniazid and propoxyphene inhibit the metabolism of carbamazepine and elevates the plasma concentration of this agent. The steady-state plasma concentration of carbamazepine is reduced by the concomitant administration of felbamate (see below). In contrast, felbamate increases the concentration of carbamazepines-active metabolites. On the other hand, carbamazepine decreases the plasma levels of clonazepam, diazepam, ethosuximide, phenytoin, phenobarbital, primidone and valproic acid.

To minimize adverse effects, initial dosage and daily increments should be limited to 200 mg. Adverse are encountered in approximately 50% of patients with serum levels from 8.5 to 10 μg/mL, but few occur with concentrations below 5 μg/mL. Diplopia, dizziness, drowsiness and ataxia occur above 6 μg/mL; nystagmus may occur at serum levels below the therapeutic range. Other reactions include anorexia and nausea, rash (including the Stevens-Johnson syndrome) and edema. More-serious adverse effects include aplastic anemia, agranulocytosis, thrombocytopenia and transient leukopenia. Therefore, all patients should be subjected to a complete blood test before being placed on the drug; additional blood tests should be done at weekly intervals during the first month of therapy, every 2 weeks during the 2nd and 3rd month, and at monthly intervals as long as the patient is on the drug. Patients should be made aware of the early toxic signs and symptoms of hematological problems such as fever, sore throat, ulcers in the mouth, easy bruising and petechial or purpuric hemorrhage. If any blood abnormality is observed, the drug should either not be used or stopped if the patient is already on the drug. If adverse effects are of such severity that the drug must be withdrawn, the physician must be aware that abrupt discontinuation of any anticonvulsant drug in a responsive patient may lead to increased seizure incidence or even status epileptics.

The drug's safe use in pregnancy, lactation and in women of child-bearing age has not been established. See the introductory statement.

Dose—*Range*, **200** to **1200 mg.** *Usual, oral, anticonvulsant, adults and children over 12 yr*—**200 mg** twice a day (tablets) or **100 mg** 4 times a day (oral suspension); increase gradually by **200 mg/day** in divided doses until desired response is obtained. Do not exceed **1200 mg** a day in patients over 15 yr or **1000 mg** a day in children 12 to 15 yr. *Maintenance*—usually **800** to **1200 mg** a day. *Usual, oral, trigeminal neuralgia*, **100 mg** twice the first day (tablets) or **50 mg** 4 times a day (oral suspension), increased by **100 mg** twice a day until desired response obtained; *maintenance, oral*, **400** to **800 mg** twice a day as needed. *Usual, pediatric*, dose has not been established. *Maximum daily oral dose, children 12 to 15 yr*, 1000 mg.

Dosage Forms—Oral Suspension: 100 mg/5mL; Tablets: 200 mg; Chewable Tablets 100 mg.

Chloropromazine Hydrochloride—see RPS-18, page 1084.

Clonazepam

2*H*-1,4-Benzodiazepin-2-one, 5-(2-chlorophenyl)-1,3-dihydro-7-nitro-, Klonopin (*Roche*)

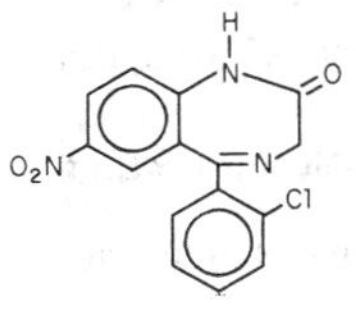

[1622-61-3] $C_{15}H_{10}ClN_3O_3$(315.72).

Preparation—*o*-Chlorobenzoyl chloride is reacted with *p*-nitroaniline to form 2-amino-5-nitro-2′-chlorozophenone, and this is condensed with bromacetyl to form 2-bromoacetamido-5-nitro-2′-chlorobenzophenone, then with ammonia to form the corresponding acetamido compound. The acetamido compound is converted to its hydrochloride with anhydrous HCl in methanol, dissolved in boiling methanol and cyclized to clonazepam using pyridine as the catalyst.

Description—Light-yellow, crystalline powder; faint odor; melts at about 238°; pK_a 1.5 (deprotonation fo nitrogen in 4 position), 10.5 (deprotonation of nitrogen in 1 position).

Solubility—Practically insoluble in water; slightly soluble in alcohol; sparingly soluble in chloroform; very slightly soluble in ether.

Uses—One of the drugs of choice for the management of myoclonic epilepsy. It also is useful alone or as an adjunct in the management of several types of generalized seizures such as absence (petit mal) attacks not responsible to either valproate or ethosuximide, the Lennox-Gestaut syndrome (petit mal variant) and akinetic seizures. About 87% of the drug is bound to plasma protein; volume distribution is 3.2 L/kg and a half-life varies from 19 to 46 hr in adults and 13 to 33 hr in children. Therapeutic plasma levels range from 20 to 80 ng/mL.

Like with diazepam, which it resembles, tolerance develops in approximately 30% of patients as shown by a loss of anticonvulsant activity; adjustment of dosage may reestablish efficacy. Consequently, the drug should be withdrawn gradually during simultaneous substitution of another anticonvulsant. When used in patients with mixed seizure types, it may increase the incidence or precipitate the onset of generalized tonic-clonic seizures (grand mal). This may require the use of either increased dosage or addition of other antiepileptic medication. Like other benzodiazepines, it is characterized in laboratory animals by its remarkable ability to antagonize pentylenetetrazol-induced seizures; it also has a taming effect in aggressive primates and induces muscle weakness and hypnosis.

Its depressant effects may be potentiated by alcohol, narcotics, barbiturates, nonbarbiturate hypnotics, antianxiety agents, the phenothiazines, thioxanthene and butyrophenone classes of antipsychotic agents, monoamine oxidase inhibitors and the tricyclic antidepressants, as well as by other anticonvulsant drugs. Phenobarbital or phenytoin may decrease steady state plasma levels of this drug by enzyme induction. Its concomitant use with valproate may produce absence status.

The most frequently occurring side effects are referable to CNS depression; drowsiness occurs in approximately 50% of patients and ataxia in approximately 30%. Other adverse reactions, listed by systems are: *Neurological:* abnormal eye movements, aphonia, choreiform movements, coma, diplopia, dysarthria, dysdiadochokinesis, "glassy-eyed" appearance, headache, hemiparesis, hypotonia, nystagmus, respiratory depression, slurred speech, tremor and vertigo. *Psychiatric:* confusion, depression, forgetfulness, hallucinations, hysteria, increased libido, insomnia, psychosis and suicidal tendencies. *Respiratory:* chest congestion, rhinorrhea, shortness of breath and hypersecretion in upper respiratory passages. *Cardiovascular:* palpitations. *Dermatologic al:* hair loss, hirsutism, skin rash and ankle and facial edema. *Gastrointestinal:* anorexia, coated tongue, constipation, diarrhea, dry mouth, encopresis, gastritis, hepatomegaly, increased appetite, nausea and sore gums. *Genitourinary:* dysuria, enuresis, nocturia and urinary retention. *Musculoskeletal:* muscle weakness and pains. *Miscellaneous:* dehydration, general deterioration, fever, lymphadenopathy and weight loss or gain. *Hematopoietic:* anemia, leukopenia, thrombocytopenia and eosinophilia.

Its safe use in pregnancy, lactation and in women of child-bearing age has not been established. See the introductory statement.

Dose—*Adults,* **1.5 mg** in 3 divided doses; dosage may be increased **0.5** to **1.0 mg** every 3 days until seizures are controlled or side effects preclude further increase. Maximum daily dose is **20 mg.** *Infants and children under 10 yr,* **0.01** to **0.03 mg/kg/day** , but not to exceed **0.05 mg/kg/day** given in 3 divided doses. Dosage may be increased by **0.25** to **0.5 mg** every 3rd day until a maintenance dose of **0.1** to **0.2 mg/kg** has been reached.

Dosage Form—Tablets: 0.5, 1.0, and 2.0 mg.

Clorazepate Dipotassium—page 1157.

Dextroamphetamine Sulfate—see RPS-18, page 876.

Diazepam—page 1157.

Dimenhydrinate—see RPS-18, page 792.

Diphenhydramine Hydrochloride—see RPS-18, page 1126.

Ephedrine Sulfate—see RPS-18, page 878.

Divalproex Sodium

Pentanoic acid, 2-propyl-, sodium salt (2:1); Depakote (*Abbott*)

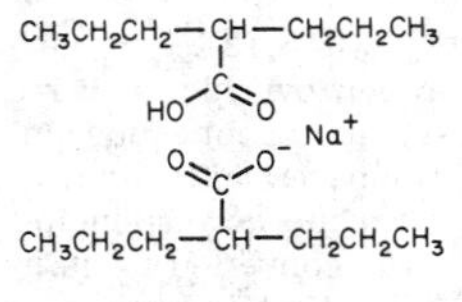

$CH_3CH_2CH_2-CH-CH_2CH_2CH_3$ (HO–C=O) ; Na^+ ; $O=C-O^-$; $CH_3CH_2CH_2-CH-CH_2CH_2CH_3$

Sodium hydrogen bis(2-propylvalerate) [76584-70-8] $C_{16}H_{31}NaO_4$ (310.41).

Preparation—Neutralization of a solution of valproic acid (page 1179) with ½ equivalent of sodium hydroxide and the solvent removed yields the product.

Uses—An antiepileptic agent that dissociates in the gastrointestinal tract into two mols of valproate. Hence, it has the same indications, adverse reactions and contraindications as valproate. It differs from *Valproate*, however, in that it is available in tablet form. See *Valproate Sodium*, page 1179.

Dose—**15** to **60 mg/kg/day.** *Usual,* **15 mg/kg/day,** increasing at weekly intervals by **5** to **10 mg/kg/day** until seizures are controlled. A twice-a-day dosage is suggested wherever feasible.

Dosage Forms—Capsules; 125 mg; Enteric-Coated Tablets; 125, 250 and 500 mg.

Ethosuximide

2,5-Pyrrolidinedione, 3-ethyl-3-methyl-, Zarontin (*Parke-Davis*)

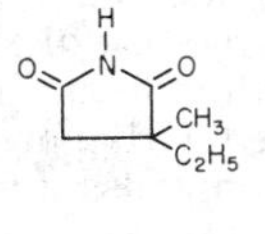

2-Ethyl-2-methylsuccinimide [77-67-8]$C_7H_{11}NO_2$ (141.17).

Preparation—Methyl ethyl ketone is condensed with ethyl cyanoacetate to yield ethyl 2-cyano-3-methyl-2-pentenoate which, in ethanolic solution, adds hydrogen cyanide to form ethyl 2,3-dicyano-3-methylpentanoate. Proton-catalyzed saponification of the latter ester is accompanied by decarboxylation to produce 2-methyl-2-ethylsuccinonitrile. This, on heating with aqueous ammonia, cyclizes to ethosuximide. US Pat 2,993,835.

Description—White to off-white crystalline powder or waxy solid; characteristic odor; stable in light, air and heat at 37°; melts about 50°; pK_a 9.5.

Solubility—Very soluble in alcohol or ether; freely soluble in water or chloroform; very slightly soluble in solvent hexane.

Uses—The drug of choice for control of uncomplicated absence seizures (petit mal). It suppresses the paroxysmal three-cycle-per-second spike and wave activity associated with lapses of consciousness characteristic of this disorder. It should not be used alone in mixed seizure types since it may increase the incidence of generalized tonic-clonic seizures in such patients. It is absorbed completely after oral administration. The drug is not bound to plasma protein; volume distribution is 0.7 L/kg; and half-life is about 60 hr in adults and 30 hr in children. It is excreted slowly in the urine; about 20% is excreted unchanged and up to 50% as the hydroxylated metabolite and/or its glucuronide. Therapeutic plasma levels range from 40 to 100 μg/mL. Maximal serum concentrations are usually achieved within 5 days after beginning oral therapy.

Adverse effects involve the gastrointestinal, hemopoietic, nervous and integumentary systems. Gastrointestinal symptoms occur frequently and include anorexia, nausea, vomiting, cramps, epigastric distress and abdominal pain; blood disturbances such as leukopenia, agranulocytosis, pancytopenia, aplastic anemia and eosinophilia have occurred; neurologic and sensory reactions observed include drowsiness, headache, dizziness, euphoria, hyperactivity and ataxia; skin manifestations include urticaria, Stevens-Johnson syndrome, lupus erythematosus and pruritic erythematous rashes; other reactions reported include myopia, vaginal bleeding, gum hypertrophy and hirsutism. Periodic blood and urine tests should be made on patients on the drug. It should be administered with extreme caution in patients with known liver or renal disease. Its safe use in pregnancy, lactation and women of child-bearing age has not been established. See the introductory statement.

Dose—*Adults and children over 6 yr, oral* **250 mg** twice a day, increased **250 mg** every 4 to 7 day until seizures are controlled or untoward effects develop; *Children under 6 yr,* **250 mg** once a day. *Usual range of dose,* **500 mg** to 1.5 **g** a day.

Dosage Forms—Capsules: 250 mg; Syrup: 250 mg/5 mL.

Ethotoin BP

Imidazolidin-2,4-dione, 3-ethyl-5-phenyl-, Peganone (*Abbott*)

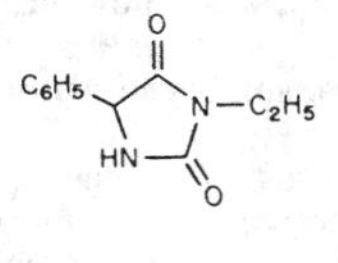

[86-35-1] $C_{11}H_{12}N_2O_2$ (204.23).

Preparation—From mandelonitrile and urea to form *N*-(α-cyanobenzyl) urea which cyclizes with HCl to yield the imino derivative of hydantoin. Hydrolysis of the imine followed by ethylation with C_2H_5I forms ethotoin. See *Ber, 21:* 2320, 1888.

Description—White, crystalline powder; melts about 94°.

Solubility—Sparingly soluble in water; freely soluble in alcohol.

Uses—Management of grand mal and psychomotor seizures. With plasma levels below 8 μg/mL, the half-life ranges from 3 to 9 hr. Therapeutic plasma levels range from 15 to 50 μg/mL. Contraindicated in patients with hepatic and hematological disorders. Should be used with extreme caution in combination with phenacemide, as paranoid symptoms have been reported with such use. Untoward effects include nausea, vomiting, fatigue, dizziness, headache, diplopia, nystagmus, skin rash, numbness, fever, diarrhea and chest pain. Ataxia and gum hyperplasia have occurred rarely; lymphadenopathy has been reported in some patients. See the introductory statment on the use of antiepileptics during pregnancy.

Dose—*Initial, oral, adult,* **1 g** a day taken in 4 to 6 divided doses, after food; *usual, adult, maintenance,* **2** to **3 g** a day. *Pediatric, initially* **not over 750 mg** a day, according to age and weight; *usual, maintenance,* **500 mg** to **1 g** a day although occasionally **2** or (rarely) **3 g** a day may be necessary.

Dosage Forms—Tablets: 250 and 500 mg.

Felbamate

1, 3-Propanediol, 2-phenyl-, bis(carbamate) ester;
Felbamyl (*Carter-Wallace*)

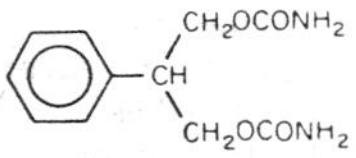

[25451-15-4] $C_{11}H_{14}N_2O_4$ (238.24).

Uses—The first new drug approved for the management of epilepsy since 1978. It represents the first new chemical entitiy to emerge from the National Institute for Neurological Disorders and Stroke's comprehensive Anticonvulsant Drug Development Program. Felbamate is approved for the treatment of partial seizures in patients 14 yr and older either as monotherapy or as adjunctive therapy. It also has been approved for the adjunctive therapy of partial and generalized seizures associated with Lennox-Gastaut syndrome, which is characterized by a mixture of several seizure types and usually is uncontrolled with other available anticonvulsants.

In laboratory animal models of epilepsy, it is effective against seizures induced by maximal electroshock, pentylenetetrazol or picrotoxin. This unique profile is broader than that of phenytoin, carbamazepine or ethosuximide, and slightly narrower than that of valproate; this suggests that felbamate has the ability to limit the spread of seizure activity and to raise seizure threshold. Its mechanism of action has yet to be clearly established. However, felbamate has been shown to inhibit high frequency repetitive firing of spinal cord neurons and to modulate the strychnine-insensitive glycine recognition site of the NMDA receptor-ionophore complex. Felbamate is a weak inhibitor at the benzodiazepine recognition site of the $GABA_A$ receptor and the $GABA_A$-receptor. It is devoid of any activity at the MK- 801 binding site of the NMDA-preferring receptor.

Felbamate is well absorbed after oral administration. Absorption of the tablet formulation does not appear to be affected by food. About 40 to 50% of the absorbed dose is excreted in the urine unchanged. An additional 40% appears as unidentified metabolites and conjugates. It is approximately 22 to 25% bound to protein and displays a terminal half-life of 20 to 23 hr. The C_{max} and AUC are proportional to dose after single and multiple doses over a range of 100 to 800 mg and single doses of 1200 to 3600 mg.

Felbamate is reported to produce only mild side effects. The most common adverse reactions seen in adults receiving felbamate monotherapy include anorexia, vomiting, insomnia, nausea and headache. The most commonly reported side effects in pediatric patients during adjunctive therapy are anorexia, vomiting, headache and somnolence.

The addition of felbamate to other anticonvulsant drugs affects the steady-state plasma concentrations of the coadministered drug. It has been shown in clinical trials to increase the plasma concentration of phenytoin or valproate, decrease the plasma concentration of carbamazepine and increasing the concentration of the active metabolite of carbamazepine. Phenytoin and carbamazepine have been shown to increase the clearance of felbamate and to reduce its steady-state concentration. The available data suggest that there is no significant effect of valproate on the clearance of felbamate. These interactions necessitate the careful titration of felbamate and scheduled dosage reduction of concomitant anticonvulsants when it is administered concurrently with other antiseizure drugs. The safety and efficacy of felbamate during pregnancy has not been established and the drug should only be used during pregnancy if clearly needed.

Dose—*Adults, 14 yr. and older,* monotherapy range, **1200** to **3600 mg** a day in 3 or 4 divided doses (the manufacturer recommends initiating monotherapy at 1200 mg a day in 3 or 4 divided doses). The dose can be increased in 600-mg increments every 2 wk to 2400 mg a day and thereafter to 3600 mg a day if clinically indicated. *Conversion to monotherapy, initially* **1200 mg** a day in 3 to 4 divided doses while reducing the dosage of concomitant anticonvulsant by one-third; at week 2, increase the felbamate dose to 2400 mg a day and reduce the dosage of other anticonvulsant up to an additional one-third; at week 3, increase the felbamate dose to 3600 mg a day and continue to reduce the dose of the other anticonvulsant as clinically indicated. *Adjunctive therapy, initially* **1200 mg** a day in 3 to 4 divided doses and reduce the dosage of concomitant anticonvulsant by 20%. The dose of felbamate can be increased at weekly intervals to 3600 mg a day in 3 to 4 divided doses; the dosage of the other anticonvulsant may need to be reduced further to minimize side effects due to drug interactions.

Children, 2 to 14 yr, adjunctive therapy, felbamate can be added to existing therapy at **15 mg/kg** a day in 3 to 4 divided doses while reducing the concomitant anticonvulsant by 20% in order to control plasma levels of phenytoin, valproate, carbamazepine and its metabolite. The dosage of felbamate can be increased by 15 mg/kg a day increments at weekly intervals up to 45 mg/kg a day, further reductions in the other anticonvulsant may be necessary to minimize side effects due to drug interactions. The majority of side effects observed during adjunctive therapy decrease as the dosage of concomitant drug is reduced.

Dosage Forms—Tablets: 400 and 600 mg; Oral Suspension: 600 mg/5 mL.

Magnesium Sulfate—page 898.

Magnesium Sulfate Injection

Sulfuric acid, magnesium salt (1:1), heptahydrate; Magnesium Sulfate Ampuls

A sterile solution of magnesium sulfate in water for injection. Magnesium sulfate (1:1) heptahydrate [10034-99-8] $MgSO_4 7H_2O$ (246.47); *anhydrous* [7487-88-9] (120.36).

Preparation—The magnesium sulfate is dissolved in water for injection, and the solution, suitably filtered until free from suspended matter, is placed in cleansed and sterile ampuls. These are sealed and sterilized suitably.

Since the water of hydration content of the salt may vary sufficiently to be troublesome in making solutions of required concentration, some operators have found it advisable to prepare solutions slightly stronger than required and to have these assayed promptly, thereafter making up to final volume of the exact strength desired according to the assay results. The stock solution, in the meantime, is kept under refrigeration to protect it.

Uses—For replacement therapy in *acute hypomagnesia* accompanied by signs of *tetany;* to control *hypertension, encephalopathy* and *convulsions* associated with acute nephritis in children; and to prevent or control convulsions in patients with preeclampsia and eclampsia. It acts at the myoneural junction to prevent the presynaptic release of acetylcholine and to decrease the motor endplate potential. Uterine contractions are inhibited and uterine blood flow enhanced. Since its action on the cardiovascular system is unpredictable, it usually is used concomitantly with an antihypertensive drug.

Principal adverse reactions are related to the high plasma levels of magnesium and include flushing, sweating, hypotension, circulatory collapse and cardiac and CNS depression. Respiratory depression is the most life-threatening effect. The magnesium ion rapidly crosses the placenta but rarely causes symptoms of toxicity in the neonate. Toxicity in the mother is indicated by loss of the pateller reflex; this occurs with magnesium plasma concentrations of 7 to 10 mEq/L. Plasma concentrations greater than 10 mEq/L affect the respiratory muscles. A salt of calcium, such as the gluconate, should be readily available for use as an antidote. The intravenous administration of 5 to 10 mEq of calcium (10 to 20 mL of 10% calcium gluconate) is usually adequate to reverse heart block or respiratory depression. In extreme cases peritoneal dialysis or hemodialysis may be necessary. It should be administered parenterally to patients with heart block or myocardial damage. It should be used with caution in patients with impaired renal function. Magnesium sulfate will enhance the CNS depressant effects of barbiturates, opiates, general anesthetics and other CNS depressants. It also enhances the effect of neuromuscular blockers and cardiac glycosides, and should be used with caution in patients receiving treatment with either of these pharmacological classes.

It also is used as an electrolyte replenisher for the treatment of magnesium deficiency.

Dose—*Magnesium deficiency, adult,* **1 g**, equivalent to 8.12 mEq of magnesium (2 mL of a 50% sol) injected *intramuscularly* every 6 hr for 4 doses. In *nephritic seizures, children,* **20** to **40 mg** (0.1 to 0.2 mL of a 20% solut)/**kg** *intramuscularly* as needed. *Preeclampsia or eclampsia, adult, intravenous infusion,* **4** to **5 g** in 250 mL of 5% dextrose solution or 0.9% sodium chloride solution. Simultaneously, *Intramuscular* doses of **up to 10 g** (10 mL of the undiluted 50% sol in each buttock) are given. Subsequently, **4** to **5 g** (8 to 10 mL of the 50% sol) are injected *intramuscularly* into alternate buttocks every 4 hr, depending upon the presence of the pateller reflex respiratory function. Therapy should be continued until paroxysms cease.

Dosage Forms—Injection: 10% (*w*/*v*), 12.5% (*w*/*v*) and 50% (*w*/*v*) in containers of various sizes; Intravenous Injection: 4% (*w*/*v*) and 8% (*w*/*v*), and 1% and 2% in 5% dextrose.

Mephenytoin

2,4-Imidazolidinedione, 5-ethyl-3-methyl-5-phenyl-, Mesantoin (*Sandoz*)

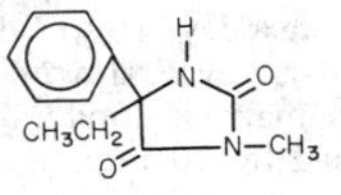

5-Ethyl-3-methyl-5-phenylhydantoin [50-12-4] $C_{12}H_{14}N_2O_2$ (218.25).

Preparation—5-Ethyl-5-phenylhydantoin, which may be prepared by condensing ethyl α-ethylmandelate with urea in the presence of sodium alcoholate, is monoethylated through reaction with dimethyl sulfate.

Description—White, crystalline powder; melts about 137°. pH (dissolve 500 mg in 10 mL alcohol, add 10 mL water, mix and determine pH without delay) 7.5 to 8.5.

Solubility—1 g in 1400 mL water, 15 mL alcohol, 3 mL chloroform or 90 mL ether.

Uses—An anticonvulsant with a spectrum of clinical activity similar to phenytoin. It may be useful in generalized tonic-clonic seizures (grand mal), complex partial seizures (temporal; psychomotor) and focal seizures (Jacksonian) and grand mal-type status epilepsy, particularly in those patients who have become refractory to or do not respond to less-toxic anticonvulsants. It is demethylated to nirvanol, an anticonvulsant employed clinically in 1920 but abandoned because of a high incidence of serious toxicity. Approximately 8% of the total plasma level (this drug and nirvanol) is this drug, but this can vary widely. Approximately 40% of this drug and 30% of nirvanol is bound to plasma protein and half-life varies from 18 to 34 hr. Therapeutic plasma levels range from 5 to 16 μg/mL for this drug and 25 to 40 μ/mL for nirvanol. Drug interactions which may occur are similar to those for phenytoin sodium (see page 1177).

The major side effects are blood dyscrasias such as leukopenia, neutropenia, agranulocytosis, thrombocytopenia and pancytopenia. Eosinophilia, monocytosis and leukocytosis have been reported. Various kinds of anemia, including aplastic anemia, have occurred, but are uncommon. Severe skin manifestations, including maculopapular, morbilliform, scarlatiniform, urticarial, purpuric and nonspecific skin rashes have been observed. Exfoliative dermatitis, Stevens-Johnson syndrome, toxic epidermal necrolysis and fatal dermatitides have been described as rare occurrences. Central effects such as ataxia, diplopia, nystagmus, dysarthria, fatigue, irritability, choreiform movements, depression and tremor also have ocurred. Hepatitis, jaundice and nephrosis have been reported, but not convincingly related to the drug. Polyarthropathy, pulmonary fibrosis, lupus erythematosus syndrome and lymphadenopathy are extremely rare.

Its safe use in pregnancy, lactation and women of child-bearing age has not been established. See the introductory statement.

Dose—*Oral*, **50** to **100 mg** a day and increasing the dose by **50** to **100 mg** a day at weekly intervals in accordance with the patient's need; the maximum daily dose **800 mg.** Children usually require **100** to **450 mg** orally in 3 divided doses a day, according to the nature of the seizure and the age and weight of the patient.

Dosage Form—Tablets: 100 mg.

Mephobarbital—page 1164.

Meprobamate—page 1169.

Metharbital—see RPS-18, page 1076.

Methsuximide

2,5-Pyrrolidinedione, 1,3-dimethyl-3-phenyl, Celontin (*Parke-Davis*)

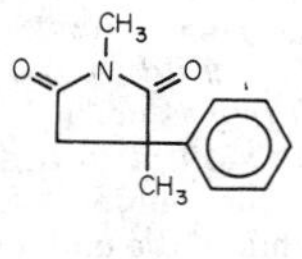

N,2-Dimethyl-2-phenylsuccinimide [77-41-8] $C_{12}H_{13}NO_2$ (203.24).

Preparation—2-Methyl-2-phenylsuccinic acid is dissolved in excess 40% methylamine. The water and excess amine are distilled off and the residue of the di(methylamine) salt of the acid is pyrolyzed at about 250° until no more distillate is formed. The residue of crude methsuximide may be purified by vacuum distillation. US Pat. 2,643,257.

Description—White to grayish white, crystalline powder; odorless or not more than a slight odor; melts about 53°.

Solubility—1 g in 350 mL water, 3 mL alcohol, < 1 mL chloroform or 2 mL ether.

Uses—An antiepileptic agent indicated for the control of absence seizures (petit mal) that are refractory to other drugs. Unlike ethosuximide and phensuximide, it usually does not unmask or increase the incidence of tonic-clonic (grand mal) seizures and may be useful in combination with other anticonvulsants such as phenytoin or phenobarbital in the treatment of mixed-seizure types. This drug, like ethosuximide, is not bound to plasma protein; volume distribution in dogs ranges from 13.5 to 22.5 L/kg; plasma half-life varies from 1.2 to 1.6 hr for methsuximide and from 28 to 36 hr for the *N*-desmethylmethsuximide metabolite. In view of its longer half-life, the desmethyl metabolite probably exerts the major antiepileptic effects.

Adverse effects are similar to those of ethosuximide. Gastrointestinal disturbances, such as nausea, vomiting, anorexia, diarrhea, weight-loss, epigastric and abdominal pain and constipation occur frequently. Hemopoietic complications including eosinophilia, leukopenia, monocytosis and pancytopenia have been reported. Neurologic and sensory reactions observed include drowsiness, ataxia, irritability and insomnia. Dermatological disturbances include urticaria, Stevens-Johnson syndrome and pruritic erythematous rashes. Periorbital edema and hyperemia also have been reported. Except for the skin and periorbital hypermia, most untoward effects disappear when the dose of drug is reduced. Patients on this therapy should be examined periodically for evidence of blood dyscrasias and liver and kidney function.

Its safe use in pregnancy, lactation and women of child-bearing age has not been established. See introductory statement.

Dose—*Usual, initially* **300 mg** a day; *maintenance,* **300 mg** to **1.2 g** a day. Optimum dosage must be determined by trial; a suggested schedule is 300 mg a day for the first week, increased 300 mg a day at weekly intervals until a daily dosage of 1.2 g is reached.

Dosage Form—Capsules: 150 and 300 mg.

Oxazepam—page 1159.

Paraldehyde—page 1169.

Paramethadione

2,4-Oxazolidinedione, 5-ethyl-3,5-dimethyl-, Paradione (*Abbott*)

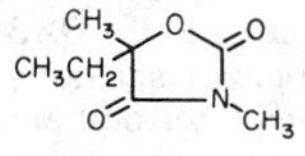

[115-67-3] $C_7H_{11}NO_3$ (157.17).

Preparation—Ethyl α-hydroxy-α-methylbutyrate and urea are refluxed for 24 hours in the presence of sodium methoxide, resulting in condensation cyclization with formation of the sodium derivative of 5-ethyl-5-methyl-2,4-oxazolidinedione. After distilling off the alcohol, dimethyl sulfate is slowly added to effect *N*-methylation.

Description—Clear, colorless liquid; may have an aromatic odor; pH (1 in 40 solution) about 6; refractive index 1.449 to 1.501.

Solubility—Sparingly soluble in water; freely soluble in alcohol, benzene, chloroform or ether.

Uses—For the control of absence seizures (petit mal) in patients refractory to other drugs. It is ineffective against other types of epilepsy. Its pharmacological properties, therapeutic uses, dosage and toxicity are similar to those of trimethadione. However, the incidence of serious adverse effects may be less for this drug. More importantly, individuals who cannot tolerate one of the oxazolidinediones may tolerate the other. See *Trimethadione*, page 1178.

Dose—**300 mg** to **2.4 g** a day; *usual,* **300 mg** 3 or 4 times a day. It is generally advisable to start therapy at a dosage of **900 mg** a day and increase this by **300 mg** at weekly intervals until therapeutic effects are seen or until toxic. The *initial* dose for *children under 2 yr* is 300 mg in 24 hr; *2 to 6 yr*, 600 mg in 24 hr; *over 6 yr*, 900 mg in 24 hr.

Dosage Forms—Capsules: 150 and 300 mg.

Phenacemide

Benzeneacetamide, *N*-(aminocarbonyl)-, Phenurone (*Abbott*)

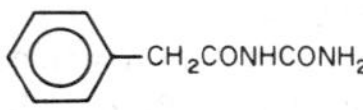

(Phenylacetyl)urea [63-98-9] $C_9H_{10}N_2O_2$ (178.19).

Preparation—Urea is reacted with phenylacetyl chloride. *J Am Chem Soc 70:* 4189,1948.

Description—White to practically white, fine, crystalline powder; odorless, or practically so; melts about 213°.

Solubility—1 g in >2000 mL water, alcohol, chloroform or ether, 500 mL of warm alcohol or 300 mL of methanol.

Uses—In severe forms of epilepsy, particularly mixed forms of complex partial seizures (psychomotor), refractory to other drugs. It can produce serious side effects as well as direct organ toxicity. Its use, therefore entails the assumption of certain risks which must be evaluated against the potential benefit to the patient. This drug should be used *only* in those cases which do not respond to other anticonvulsant medication. Extreme caution must be exercised in treating patients who have previously shown personality disorders, liver dysfunction or a history of allergy. Concurrent use with ethotoin is not recommended since paranoid symptoms have been reported.

The untoward effects which may occur include the following: gastrointestinal disturbances, anorexia and weight loss, headache, drowsiness, insomnia, paresthesias, psychic changes, hepatitis, blood dyscrasias, skin rash and nephritis. Its safe use in pregnancy, lactation or women of child-bearing age has not been established. See introductory statement. Liver function tests should be performed before and during therapy.

Dose—*Oral*, **0.5 g** 3 times a day with meals. After the 1st week, if seizures are not controlled and the drug is tolerated well, an additional 0.5 g may be taken on arising. In the 3rd week, if necessary, the dosage may be further increased by 0.5 g at bedtime. The usual total adult dose ranges from 2 to 3 g a day, although some patients may require about ½ the adult dose and others have required as much as 5 g a day. The usual initial dose for children 5 to 10 yr is 250 mg 3 times a day the 1st week, an additional 250 mg on arising the 2nd week a final 250 mg at bedtime may be added the 3rd week.

Dosage Form—Tablets: 500 mg.

Phenobarbital Sodium—page 1165.

Phensuximide

2,5-Pyrrolidinedione, 1-methyl-3-phenyl-, Milontin (*Parke-Davis*)

N-Methyl-2-phenylsuccinimide [86-34-0] $C_{11}H_{11}NO_2$ (189.21).

Preparation—By the method described above for *Methsuximide* using phenylsuccinic acid as the starting compound. US Pat 2,643,258.

Description—White to off-white, crystalline powder; odorless or not more than a slight odor; melts about 71°.

Solubility—1 g in 210 mL water, 11 mL alcohol, <1 mL chloroform or 19 mL ether.

Uses—The first succinimide introduced for the therapy of absence seizures (petit mal), it is now relegated to secondary status. It generally is not effective in the management of partial seizures with complex symptomatology and tonic-clonic (grand mal) seizures. It contrast, it may increase the frequency of tonic clonic seizures when used in patients with mixed epilepsy. Its lesser effect is thought to be due to the fact that its desmethyl metabolite does not accumulate in the body. The drug, although relatively free from serious toxic effects, may reproduce such side reactions as nausea, vomiting, anorexia, muscular weakness, drowsiness, ataxia, lethargy and occasional skin disorders such as pruritus, skin eruptions, erythema multiforme and erythematous rashes. Increased urinary frequency, renal damage, hematuria, granulocytopenia, transient leukopenia and pancytopenia have been reported. Therefore, periodic urinalysis, hepatic function tests and blood studies are advisable in patients taking the drug for prolonged periods.

Its safe use in pregnancy, lactation and women of child-bearing age has not been established. See the introductory statement.

Dose—*Usual*, **500 mg** to **1 g** 2 times or 3 times a day, irrespective of age. As with other anticonvulsant medication, the dose should be adjusted to the individual patient.

Dosage Forms—Capsules: 500 mg.

Phenytoin

2,4-Imidazolidinedione, 5,5-diphenyl-, Diphenylhydantoin; Dilantin Infatabs, Dilantin-30 Pediatric and Dilantin-125 (*Parke-Davis*)

5,5-Diphenylhydantoin [57-41-0] $C_{15}H_{12}N_2O_2$ (252.27). See *Phenytoin Sodium* for the formula.

Preparation—Phenytoin sodium, prepared as described below yields the base on acidification of its aqueous solution.

Description—White powder, odorless; melts about 295°.

Solubility—Practically insoluble in water; slightly soluble in cold alcohol, chloroform or ether.

Uses—See *Phenytoin Sodium*.

Dose—*Range, oral,* **300** to **600 mg** a day; *usual, adult,* **100 mg** 3 times a day; the dose then is individualized. *Usual, pediatric, initially* **5 mg/kg/day** in 2 or 3 equally divided doses; the dose then is individualized to a maximum of 300 mg/day. *Maintenance,* **4** to **8 mg/kg.** *Children over 6 yr* may require the minimum adult dose (300 mg/day).

Dosage Forms—Chewable Tablets: 50 mg. Oral Suspension: 30 mg/5 mL and 125 mg/5 mL.

Phenytoin Sodium

2,4-Imidazolidinedione, 5,5-diphenyl-, monosodium salt; Diphenylhydantoin Sodium Salt; Diphenylhydantoin Sodium; Soluble Phenytoin; Alepsin; Epanutin; Eptoin; Dilantin Sodium (*Parke-Davis*)

5,5-Diphenylhydantoin sodium salt [630-93-3] $C_{15}H_{11}N_2NaO_2$ (274.25).

Preparation—By treating benzaldehyde with a solution of sodium cyanide, 2 moles of benzaldehyde are condensed (benzoin condensation) into one mole of benzoin, which is oxidized to benzil with nitric acid or cupric sulfate. The benzil is then heated with urea in the presence of sodium ethoxide or isopropoxide, forming phenytoin sodium.

Description—White, odorless powder; somewhat hygroscopic and on exposure to air gradually absorbs carbon dioxide with the liberation of the base.

Solubility—Freely soluble in water, the solution usually being somewhat turbid due to partial hydrolysis and absorption of carbon dioxide; soluble in alcohol; practically insoluble in ether or chloroform.

Uses—One of the drugs of choice for the management of generalized tonic-clonic (grand mal) seizures, complex partial (temporal lobe; psychomotor) seizures and simple partial (focal, Jacksonian) seizures. It is not recommended for the management of pure absence (petit mal) epilepsy. Parenterally, it is used for the control of status epilepticus of the generalized tonic-clonic (grand mal) type and in the management of seizures occurring during neurosurgery. Intravenous phenytoin sodium may be useful in the treatment of paroxysmal atrial tachycardia, ventricular tachycardia and digitalis-induced cardiac arrhythmias. Oral phenytoin sodium also may afford benefit in the treatment of behavioral disorders and, in large doses, the management of trigeminal neuralgia. It is much less effective in the latter than carbamazepine (see page 1173). This drug has $pK_a$of 8.31 to 8.33, 87 to 93% of the drug is bound to plasma protein, volume distribution ranges from 0.5 to 0.8 L/kg and half-life is about 22 hr in adults and 18 to 22 hr in children. Therapeutic plasma levels range from 10 to 20 μg/mL in adults and 5 to 20 μg/mL in children. Toxic levels range from 30 to 50 μg/mL and lethal levels approximate 100 μg/mL.

It acts on the motor cortex where it stabilizes the neuronal membrane and inhibits the spread of the seizure discharge. Present evidence suggests that it limits sustained high-frequency repetitive firing by blocking Na^+-channels in a use- and frequency-dependent manner. It also enhances calcium binding to phospholipids in neuronal membranes. These effects result in a more stable membrane configuration.

These observations are in harmony with the fact that its most easily demonstrated properties are its ability to limit the development of maximal seizure activity and to reduce the spread of the seizure process from the active focus. Both features are undoubtedly related to its clinical usefulness.

There are two distinct forms of Phenytoin Sodium Capsules: the rapid-release type (Prompt Phenytoin Sodium Capsules) and the slow-dissolution type (Extended Phenytoin Sodium Capsules). The former have a dissolution rate of not less than 85% in 30 min and are used for 3 or 4 times a day dosing, whereas the latter have a slow dissolution rate of 15 to 35% in 30 min, 45 to 65% in 1 hr and not less than 85% in 2 hr and may be used for once-a-day dosing. Studies comparing doses of 100 mg three times a day of Prompt Phenytoin Sodium Capsules with a single, daily dose of 300 mg of Extended Phenytoin Sodium Capsules (Dilantin Kapseals, *Parke-Davis*) indicate that absorption, peak plasma levels, biological half-life, difference between peak and minimum values and urinary recovery are equivalent. Because of the differences in dissolution rates among various brands, *physicians should be cautioned to keep patients on one manufacturer's product.*

Its metabolism may be altered significantly by concomitant use of other drugs. Drugs which *increase* its serum levels include chloramphenicol, dicumarol, tolbutamide, isoniazid, phenylbutazone, acute alcohol intake, salicylates, chlordiazepoxide, phenthiazines, felbamate, diazepam, estrogens, ethosuximide, halothane, methylphenidate, sulfonamides, cimetidine and trazodone. Drugs which *decrease* its serum levels include carbamazepine, chronic alcohol abuse, reserpine and preparations containing calcium. Drugs which *either increase or decrease* its serum levels include phenobarbital, valproic acid and valproate sodium.

This is a relatively safe anticonvulsant, although many adverse effects have been observed. Nystagmus may appear with serum concentrations of 8 to 20 μg/mL and is nearly always present at higher levels. At concentrations greater than 30 μg/mL, ataxia and dysarthria commonly occur. Gingival hyperplasia and hirsutism are often intolerable, particularly in the young. A morbilliform rash may occur, usually in the first 10 days of treatment, and rarely progresses to exfoliate dermatitis or the Stevens-Johnson syndrome; the drug should be stopped if a rash appears. There also are reports of peripheral neuropathy, a lupus erythematous syndrome, hepatitis, lymphadenopathy, megaloblastic anemia and rickets and osteomalacia due to interference with vitamin D metabolism. Serum folic acid and vitamin K levels also may be depressed, and bleeding disorders have been reported in infants born to mothers taking the drug. Overdosage causes an acute cerebellar syndrome, delirium and, rarely, coma.

It is contraindicated in patients with a history of sensitivity to hydantoins. Abrupt withdrawal of this medication may precipitate status epilepticus; when the dosage needs to be reduced or substitution of another antiepileptic appears desirable, such alteration in therapy should be done gradually. Recent reports suggest an association between the use of anticonvulsant drugs by women with epilepsy and an increased incidence of birth defects in children born to these women. The prescribing physician should weigh the benefit/risk potential of antiepileptic agents when treating or counseling epileptic women of child-bearing age. See the introductory statement.

Dose—*Range, oral,* **200** to **600 mg** a day; *usual, oral,* **100 mg** up to 4 times a day; *usual, intravenous,* **150** to **250 mg,** followed, if necessary, by **100** to **150 mg** 30 min later (intravenous administration should not exceed 50 mg/min); *usual, intramuscular,* **100** to **200 mg** every 6 to 8 hr for a total of 3 or 4 injections. *Usual, pediatric, anticonvulsant,* **1.5** to **4 mg/kg** or 125 mg two times a day, not to exceed 300 mg a day administered orally, intravenously or less preferably, intramuscularly. See package insert for detailed information concerning dosage for all patients. *Note*—If seizure control in *adults* is established with 100-mg capsules administered 3 times a day, once-a-day dosage with 300-mg Phenytoin Sodium Capsules SD (Dilantin Kapseals, *Parke-Davis*) may be considered as an alternative, but patients should be cautioned not to miss a dose inadvertently or to use another manufacturer's product (see under *Uses*).

Dosage Forms—Capsules: 100 mg (with phenobarbital 0.16 or 0.32 mg); Prompt Capsules: 30 and 100 mg; Extended (once-a-day dosing) Capsules: 30 and 100 mg.

Primidone

4,6-(1*H*,5*H*)-Pyrimidinedione, 5-ethyldihydro-5-phenyl-, Mysoline (*Wyeth-Ayerst*)

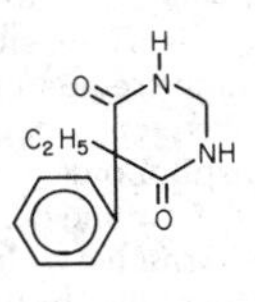

[125-33-7] $C_{12}H_{14}N_2O_2$ (218.25).

Preparation—A solution of ethylphenylmalonamide (I) in a large molar excess of formamide (II) is refluxed for 2 hours. The cyclization may be looked upon as being brought about by a Cannizzaro type of disproportionation of II followed by a deammoniation and a dehydration between I and the highly reactive methanolamine resulting from the disproportionation.

Description—White, odorless; crystalline powder; slightly bitter taste; melts about 281°.

Solubility—1 g in 2000 mL water or 200 mL alcohol; very slightly soluble in most organic solvents.

Uses—Either alone or in combination with other antiepileptics, used as alternate therapy in the control of generalized tonic-clonic seizures (grand mal), complex partial seizures (temporal lobe; psychomotor) and focal epileptic seizures. It is metabolized to phenylethylmalonamide (PEMA) and phenobarbital. Phenobarbital formation ranges form 15 to 25%. The plasma half-life of PEMA is 24 to 48 hr, whereas that of phenobarbital is 48 to 120 hr. Both substances tend to accumulate during chronic medication.

PEMA is an active antiepileptic but is less potent and less toxic than phenobarbital. From 0 to 30% of this drug is bound to plasma protein, volume distribution averages 0.6 L/kg and plasma half-life in adults range from 9 hr in combination therapy to 15 hr in monotherapy; in children, half-life varies from 6 to 8 hr. Therapeutic plasma concentrations range from 6 to 12 μg/mL for this drug and from 15 to 45 μg/mL for phenobarbital. Few interactions with other drugs have been reported, but those for phenobarbital also apply. The ratio of phenobarbital to this unmetabolized drug in serum is significantly higher in epileptic patients treated with a combination of this drug and phenytoin than in patients on this drug alone. It decreases the prothrombin response to dicumarol and warfarin. Also, concurrent treatment with valproate increases the plasma level of phenobarbital in patients on this drug.

The most frequent side effects include ataxia and vertigo; these tend to disappear with continued or reduced therapy. Occasionally, nausea, anorexia, vomiting, fatigue, irritability, emotional disturbances, diplopia, nystagmus, drowsiness and morbilliform rashes occur. Megaloblastic anemia may occur as a rare idiosyncrasy; this anemia responds to folic acid, 15 mg a day, without discontinuing the medication.

Dose—**125 mg** to **2 g** a day; *usual,* **250 mg** daily, at bedtime, the 1st week. The dose is increased in increments of 250 mg at weekly intervals to tolerance or therapeutic effectiveness; a total daily dose of 2 g should not be exceeded. For children under 8 yr, ½ the adult dosage is given on a similar schedule.

Dosage Forms—Oral Suspension: 250 mg/5 mL; Tablets: 50 and 250 mg.

Sodium Bromide—see RPS-16, page 1019.

Trimethadione

2,4-Oxazolidinedione, 3,5,5,-trimethyl-, Tridione (*Abbott*)

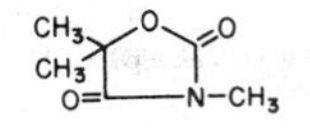

[127-48-0] $C_6H_9NO_3$ (143.14).

Preparation—By a series of reactions beginning with acetone and involving the following steps: conversion with HCN to acetone cyanhydrin, hydrolysis and esterification with alcohol to ethyl dimethylglycolate, condensation with urea to 5,5-dimethyloxazolidine-2,4-dione and methylation with dimethyl sulfate to trimethadione.

Description—White, crystalline granules; slight, camphor-like odor; melts about 46°.

Solubility—Soluble in water; freely soluble in alcohol, ether or chloroform.

Uses—An alternative drug for absence seizures (petit mal), not used widely because of its toxicity and the fact that reliable tests for plasma concentrations are generally not available. A frequent troublesome effect is hemeralopia, a peculiar glare effect or photophobia; hemeralopia is managed by having the patient wear tinted glasses. It is demethylated to an active more potent metabolite, dimethadione; dimethadione is not further metabolized, but is excreted unchanged in the urine. Dimethadione has a pK_a of 6.15; neither dimethadione nor this drug is bound to plasma protein and the half-life is 240 hr for dimethadione and 16 to 20 hr for this drug. Therapeutic plasma levels are >700 μg/mL for dimethadione and 20 μg/mL for this drug.

Clinically significant drug interactions have not been reported. Nevertheless, concurrent administration of drugs that produce similar adverse effects should be avoided.

Serious untoward effects may be associated with therapeutic doses. Gastrointestinal effects reported include hiccups, nausea, vomiting, abdominal pain and gastric distress. Anorexia and weight loss have been reported. CNS disturbances such as photophobia, diplopia, hemeralopia, drowsiness, fatigue, malaise, insomnia, vertigo, headache, paresthesia, precipitation of grand mal seizures, increased irritability and personality changes. Drowsiness appears to subside as therapy is continued.

Skin rashes, bleeding gums, epistaxis, retinal and petechial hemorrhages, vaginal bleeding and blood dyscrasias including leukopenia, neutropenia, thrombocytopenia, pancytopenia, agranulocytosis and hypoplastic anemia, and fatal aplastic anemia have been reported.

A lupus erythematosus-like syndrome also has been reported. In addition a syndrome simulating malignant lymphoma has been noted. Lymphadenopathy with hepatosplenomegaly associated with pruitus in hypersensitive individuals also has been observed. If lupus-like manifestations or lymph node enlargement should appear, therapy should be discontiued and the patient observed for a reversal of these symptoms before therapy is instituted for lupus erythematous or lymphoma.

Other reactions observed include changes in blood pressure, albuminura, nephrosis, hepatitis and precipitation of grand mal seizures. Since certain anticonvulsant drugs, including this drug and paramethadione, have been reported to be associated with an increased incidence of congenital malformations, the use of these drugs in pregnant women or women of child-bearing age requires careful evaluation of the risks and benefits. See introductory statement.

Dose—*Range*, **900 mg** to **2.4 g** a day; *usual*, **300** to **600 mg** 3 or 4 times a day.

Other Dose Information—The adult dose for the treatment of epilepsy is 900 mg to 2.4 g a day, in divided amounts. Therapy is usually started at 900 mg a day and increased by 300 mg a day at weekly intervals until the desired therapeutic results are achieved or toxic symptoms appear. For infants and children the dose ranges from 300 to 900 mg a day, depending on the age and weight of the patient, in 3 or 4 equally divided doses. The usual maintenance dosage for children is 40 mg/kg a day or 1 g/m^2 a day.

Dosage Forms—Capsules: 300 mg; Oral Solution: 40 mg/mL; Chewable Tablets: 150 mg.

Valproate Sodium

Pentanoic acid, 2-propyl-, sodium salt; Depakene (*Abbott*)

$$CH_3CH_2CH_2\underset{\displaystyle |\atop \displaystyle CH_3CH_2CH_2}{C}HCOONa$$

Sodium 2-propylpentanoate; sodium 2-propylvalerate [1069-66-5] $C_8H_{15}NaO_2$ (166.20).

Preparation—Valproic acid may be synthesized from 4-heptanol by successive conversions to 4-bromoheptane with HBr, to 4-cyanoheptane with HCN, and to 2-propylpentanoic (valproic) acid by alkaline hydrolysis of the 4-cyanoheptane.

Description—White, crystalline powder; odorless; saline taste; pK_a 4.95.

Solubility—Soluble in water or alcohol.

Uses—An 8-carbon branched-chain fatty (carboxylic) acid, unique both in its experimental an clinical profile of anticonvulsant action. It is effective in nontoxic doses against tonic seizures induced by either electroshock or strychnine, as well as against minimal-threshold seizures induced by either pentylenetetrazol, bicuculline or picrotoxin. Clinical efficacy confirms this broad-spectrum of antiepileptic activity. It is one of the drugs of choice in the management of simple absence seizures. Similarly, atypical absence seizures and myoclonic epilepsies respond well and, since there has never been an entirely satisfactory drug for these types of childhood epilepsy, this is an important advance. It also is effective in generalized tonic-clonic. In some refractory patients it has been used effectively in the management of partial seizures with complex symptomatology (psychomotor or temporal lobe seizures) or myoclonic and akinetic seizures. Like carbamazepine, valproate, has been used with some success in the management of bipolar disorder and in the treatment of aggression or violence (*Am Pharm NS33* (*2*): 47, 1993).

It has a pK_a, of 4.5, 90 to 95% is bound to plasma protein, volume distribution ranges from 0.1 to 0.5 L/kg (mean 0.2 L/kg) and half-life varies from 6 to 17 hr in adults and 4 to 14 hr in children. Therapeutic plasma levels range from 50 to 100 μg/mL; levels above 100 μg/mL are potentially toxic. More than ten metabolites have been identified in human blood and urine. Only 0.5 to 20% is excreted unchanged in the urine. Of the several metabolites, only 2-propyl-2-pentenoic acid (2-en-VPA) has been shown to accumulate in the brain. The 2-en-VPA metabolite is about 1.3 times more potent than the parent drug and may contribute significantly to the anticonvulsant effect of chronically administered valproate.

The precise mechanism of its anticonvulsant action is still unknown. It has been postulated that its administration inhibits GABA-transaminase, and thus, increases the concentration of cerebral GABA. However, other saturated straight-chain fatty acids (propionic, butyric and pentanoic) which lack anticonvulsant properties are more potent inhibitors of GABA-transaminase than is valproic acid. It also has been reported that there is a strong correlation between the anticonvulsant potency of valproate and other branched-chain fatty acids and their ability to reduce the concentration of cerebral aspartate.

It may decrease binding to serum proteins or block hepatic metabolism of phenobarbital. Administration of the drug to patients in a steady state while on phenobarbital (or primidone, which is metabolized to phenobarbital) can increase the plasma levels of phenobarbital from 35 to 200%, causing excessive somnolence. Present evidence indicates this is due to an immediate decrease in the rate of elimination of phenobarbital. This drug interacts unpredictably with phenytoin; it has been associated not only with lowered serum phenytoin levels and increased seizure frequency, but also with increased free phenytoin levels and phenytoin toxicity. Valproate also has been found to significantly increase the clearness of felbamate and correspondingly to reduce its plasma concentration. Conversely, phenobarbital, primidone, phenytoin and other drugs may induce enzymes that metabolize this drug and reduce its half-life. In contrast, felbamate has been shown to increase the plasma concentration of valproate when the two drugs are administered concurrently.

Over 40 cases of fatal hepatic failure have been reported in patients on this therapy. The risk of hepatic failure is dramatically less in patients on monotherapy (*ca* 1/37,000) as compared to those on polytherapy (*ca* 1/6500). Moreover, the incidence is much greater in children under 2 yr and on polytherapy (monotherapy, 1.42/10,000; polytherapy, *ca* 1/500).

The most commonly observed side effects in patients on monotherapy (valproate) are weight gain (11%), sedation (10%), nausea (6%), headache (3%), tremor (3%), hair loss (1%) and dizziness (1%). Other rarely observed untoward effects include skin rashes, enuresis, insomnia, anxiety, fatigue and paresthesias. Teratogenic effects have been reported in animals. Moreover, its use by women with epilepsy during the first trimester (3 months) of pregnancy has been reported by the Centers for Disease Control, USPHS, to be associated with increased risk (1.2%) of spina bifida in their infants (*MMWR 31:* Oct 28, 1982). Although the majority of women with epilepsy taking this drug will give birth to nonaffected babies, it is recommended that they consider prenatal testing for neural tube defects.

Dose (valproic acid equivalent)—*Adult* and *pediatric*, *initially* **15 mg/kg/day;** increase at 1-wk intervals by **5** to **10 mg/kg/day;** maximum daily dose, **30 mg/kg** (some patients may require up to **60 mg/kg/day**). If the daily dose exceeds 250 mg, it should be given in divided doses.

Dosage Forms—Capsules: 250 mg; Syrup: 250 mg in 5 mL.

CHAPTER 71

Psychopharmacologic Agents

Lane J Wallace, PhD

Associate Professor
College of Pharmacy, Ohio State University
Columbus OH 43210

Drugs that alter the mind and behavior have attracted the attention of man since the beginning of recorded history. Without the benefits of science and medicine, mankind has sought emotional comfort or novelty through the use of drugs for a venerable period of time. To cite two examples, alcohol and opium have been used for this purpose since antiquity. However, it was the inadvertent discovery of the unusual psychotomimetic properties of lysergic acid diethylamide in 1943 and the subsequent demonstration that these effects were similar to those induced by mescaline which marked the beginning of psychopharmacology.

Additional interest in this new science was created with the introduction of chlorpromazine for the empiric treatment of mental disorders; the successful clinical use of this agent not only led to the realization that behavior can be studied objectively in laboratory animals, but also resulted in the discovery of a host of new drugs which stimulate, sedate or otherwise change behavior.

Indeed, over 1500 compounds classified as *psychoactive* or *psychotropic* drugs have been described, and approximately 20% of all prescriptions written in the US are for medications intended to alter mental processes and behavior. Moreover, a large number of drugs prescribed for other purposes also modify thought, mood and emotion. However, the primary characteristic of psychopharmacological drugs, in contrast to the many other drugs that act on the central nervous system, is that they alter the mental state and behavior in a predictable way.

While pharmacotherapy does not cure mental disorders in the same sense that antibiotics cure infectious diseases, the available drugs do control most symptomatic manifestations and behavioral deviances, facilitate the patient's tendency toward remission and improve his or her capacity for social, occupational and familial adjustment. For example, the treatment of schizophrenic symptoms such as anxiety, delusions, hallucinations, paranoid states, catatonia, social withdrawal and autonomic nervous system dysfunctions has been changed markedly by pharmacotherapy.

The widespread use of these relatively safe compounds has reduced greatly the number of chronic patients residing in public mental hospitals, shortened the duration of hospitalization for acute episodes and shifted the focus of treatment of mental disorders from institutional care to community based ambulatory treatment programs. Moreover, the advent of effective pharmacotherapy also has influenced research methodology and theory. Indeed, the important information gathered on the mechanism of action of psychoactive drugs has generated new hypotheses about the pathogenesis of these disorders.

Drugs used in the treatment of behavioral disorders and those which are known to mimic certain of these disorders in man have been classified in various ways. For the purpose of this presentation, the psychopharmacological drugs (psychoactive drugs) are divided into antipsychotic, antianxiety, antidepressant and psychogenic agents.

Antipsychotic Agents

The several classes of drugs described in this section are used in the symptomatic treatment of psychosis, which may be operationally defined as the inability to function in society because of loss of reality recognition, affective disorder or orientation. Psychoses include schizophrenia, organic psychoses and the manic phase of manic-depressive illness. Drugs in this group act primarily on the lower brain areas to produce emotional calmness and relaxation without significant sedation, hypnosis, motor impairment or euphoria. Structurally the antipsychotic drugs can be divided into six groups:

1. *Phenothiazines* (chlorpromazine, etc).
2. *Thioxanthenes* (chlorprothixene and thiothixene).
3. *Butyrophenones* (haloperidol).
4. *Dihydroindolone* derivatives (molindone).
5. *Dibenzoxazepines* (loxapine).
6. *Dibenzodiazepine* (clozapine).

The numerous *phenothiazines* and related congeners have qualitatively similar effects, but their potency and side effects are influenced markedly by their chemical structure. For example, congeners with an aliphatic side chain, such as chlorpromazine, are relatively low in potency and high in sedative effects. Conversely, congeners with a piperazine constituent are more potent and have less sedative effects but more prominent extrapyramidal toxicity.

The mechanism of action of the antipsychotic agents is obviously complex, and many details remain to be established. Nevertheless, all antipsychotic agents currently employed clinically block postsynaptic dopaminergic receptors (in the basal ganglia, hypothalamus, limbic system, brain stem and medulla) and act as competitive antagonists of dopamine centrally and peripherally. However, the effective drugs vary markedly in selectivity and potency for the five known subtypes of dopaminergic receptor, and all to some degree are competitive antagonists of other neurotransmitters. It is likely that a combination of interference with some subset of dopaminergic and serotonergic neurotransmission is required for clinical effectiveness. The desired antipsychotic and antiemetic effects and the undesired extrapyramidal effects are related, at least in part, to dopaminergic blockade. Extrapyramidal toxicity also is related inversely to the central anticholinergic properties of these agents. Many of the various peripheral effects, including the cardiovascular effects of some of these agents, are attributable to anticholinergic properties and peripheral alpha-adrenergic blockade.

Experimentally, the *phenothiazines* suppress or abolish conditioned reflexes in trained rats, prevent morphine-induced mania in cats and reduce the toxicity of amphetamine in aggregated mice. Many of these compounds also suppress vomiting from apomorphine, irradiation and motion sickness but, in laboratory animals, do not affect the emesis from morphine, veratrum alkaloids, digitalis and copper sulfate. In addition, they decrease spontaneous motor activity, lower electroshock seizure threshold and cause skeletal muscle relaxation. The phenothiazines also exhibit weak adrenolytic, hypotensive, antispasmodic, hypothermic and antihistaminic effects and potentiate the action of many pharmacological agents.

Antipsychotic drugs are usually highly lipid-soluble and protein-bound (92 to 99%). They tend to have large volumes of distribution (usually more than 7 L/kg); bioavailability after oral administration is variable and quite low (25–35%). Plasma half-life tends to be short, ranging from 10 to 20 hr, but the duration of the antipsychotic action is much longer. Metabolites may be found in the urine weeks after the last dose of drug. This suggests that large amounts of the drug are sequestered in the tissues.

A *thioxanthene* is a phenothiazine in which the nitrogen at the 10-position is replaced by a carbon atom with a double bond to the side chain. The thioxanthene *chlorprothixene* has high sedative and adrenergic-blocking properties and a low to moderate tendency to induce extrapyramidal reactions. In contrast, *thiothixene* has low sedative and adrenergic-blocking properties and a high tendency to induce extrapyramidal reactions. Moreover, the former has a milligram for milligram potency somewhat less than most phenothiazines, whereas the latter has a potency essentially the same as the most potent phenothiazines.

The *butyrophenone haloperidol* is less sedative than the phenothiazines, but extrapyramidal symptoms occur even more frequently with this agent. It also is one of the most potent antipsychotic agents.

The *phenothiazines* are indicated for the management of *psychotic disorders*, control of *nausea and vomiting*, control of *manic depression*, relief of *intractable hiccups*, relief of *restlessness and apprehension* prior to surgery, *acute intermittent porphyria* and as an adjunct in the treatment of *tetanus*. The thioxanthenes (chlorprothixene and thiothixene) are used for the management of the symptoms of *psychotic disorders*. The *butyrophenone* (haloperidol) also is employed for the management of symptoms of *psychoses*, including *schizophrenia*, the manic type of *manic depressive* illness or *psychotic reactions* associated with organic brain syndrome or mental retardation. The dibenzoxazepine (loxapine succinate) is indicated for the management of *schizophrenia*.

The *dibenzodiazepine* (clozapine) is an "atypical" antipsycotic agent which is reserved for the treatment of patients refractory to other antipsychotic agents.

Although lithium carbonate is quite different from other antipsychotic drugs, it is included in this chapter because of its clinical use in treatment of a subset of psychotic illnesses. Lithium carbonate is indicated for treatment of bipolar (manic/depressant) affective disorder. It also is used sometimes as an adjunct with antipsychotic drugs in treatment of other psychotic disorders. Although the mechanism of action of lithium is not established, its known biochemical actions suggest suppression of inositol phosphate second-messenger systems as a possibility.

Contraindications—Many of the contraindications to the use of these drugs are similar. For example, they are contraindicated in comatose patients who have received large amounts of CNS-depressant drugs (alcohol, barbiturates, narcotics, etc), in patients with Parkinson's disease and in patients with a known history of hypersensitivity to these agents. It is not known whether there is cross-sensitivity between the phenothiazines and the thioxanthenes, but this possibility should be kept in mind.

Warnings—The safe use of these agents during pregnancy has not been established with respect to possible adverse effects on fetal development. The safe use of butyrophenones and thioxanthenes in children has not been established. It is recommended that these agents not be used in children under 12 years of age. Geriatric or debilitated patients usually require a lower initial dose of these agents; the dose then is increased as needed and tolerated. Both phenothiazines and thioxanthenes have an anticholinergic effect; hence, they should be used with extreme caution in patients with a history of glaucoma or prostatic hypertrophy. All agents in these groups tend to impair mental and physical ability required to operate a motor vehicle or complex hazardous machinery. Patients should be warned accordingly.

Precautions—Phenothiazines and thioxanthenes may significantly affect the actions of other drugs (see Chapter 105 for additional information concerning specific drug interactions). They may increase, prolong or intensify the action of CNS depressants (anesthetics, alcohol, barbiturates, narcotics, etc); therefore, appropriate adjustments in dosage of narcotics and barbiturates should be made when such agents are to be administered concomitantly. These agents also lower convulsive threshold; hence, they should be used with extreme caution in patients with a history of epilepsy. They also should be used cautiously in patients receiving atropine and related drugs, because of the possible additive anticholinergic effect. Since these agents have antiemetic properties, they may mask signs of drug overdosage and obscure symptoms of brain tumor or intestinal obstruction. These agents also should be used with extreme caution in patients with cardiovascular disease, chronic respiratory disorders, impaired liver function or a history of gastric ulcer; the aggravation of a preexisting ulcer has been reported.

Adverse Reactions—Although not all the adverse reactions listed herein have occurred following administration of either phenothiazines or thioxanthenes, the chemical and pharmacological similarities of the two groups suggest that *all* of the known side effects and toxicities associated with such therapy should be kept in mind. *CNS effects: drowsiness*, particularly during the 1st or 2nd week of therapy; *extrapyramidal reactions* may be fairly common, usually three types: (1) parkinsonian-like syndrome, (2) dystonia and dyskinesia, including torticollis, tics and other involuntary muscle movements and (3) akathisia, shown by restlessness and an urge to move about; *hyperreflexia*, reported in the newborn when phenothiazines are used during pregnancy; *grand mal seizures, catatonic-like states, psychotic symptoms* and *cerebral edema* also have been reported. *Cardiovascular effects:* postural hypotension, tachycardia, bradycardia, faintness, dizziness and cardiac arrest. *Hematological effects:* agranulocytosis, eosinophilia, leukopenia, hemolytic anemia, thrombocytopenic purpura and pancytopenia have been reported. *Liver:* jaundice has been observed but is usually reversible. *Allergic reactions:* urticaria or dermatitis in about 5% of patients. Three types have been identified: hypersensitivity reactions, contact dermatitis and photosensitivity resembling sunburn. *Endocrine effects:* these agents block ovulation, suppress the menstrual cycle, cause infertility and pseudopregnancy, lactation and breast engorgement in females. They reduce urinary levels of gonadotropins, estrogens and progestins. In males, gynecomastia or change in libido have been observed. Cholesterol levels also are increased significantly. *Other reported reactions:* these include dry mouth, nasal congestion, constipation, myosis, mydriasis, urinary retention, increased appetite, weight gain, peripheral edema, fever and suppression of cough reflex. The last may enhance the potential of aspiration and/or asphyxia. *Long-term effects:* prolonged therapy with high doses may cause pigmentation of exposed skin areas, ocular changes consisting of lenticular and corneal opacities, epithelial keratopathies and pigmentary retinopathy; vision may be impaired. See also Chapter 45.

Acetophenazine Maleate

Ethanone, 1-[10-[3-[4-(2-hydroxyethyl)-1-piperazinyl]propyl]-10*H*-phenothiazin-2-yl]-, (*Z*)-2 butenedioate (1:2) (salt);
Tindal (*Schering*)

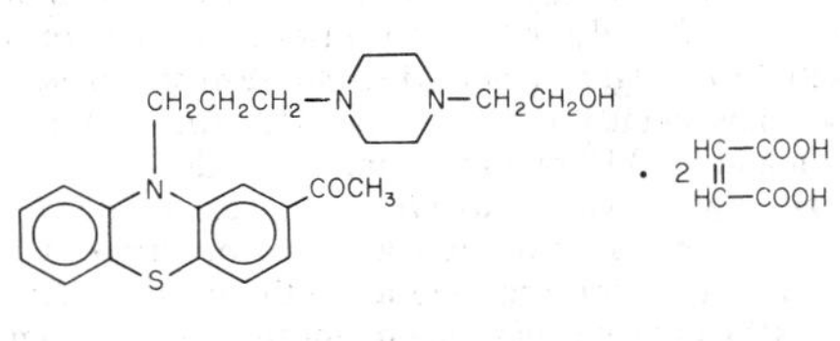

$CH_2CH_2CH_2$—N(piperazine)N—CH_2CH_2OH ; phenothiazine ring with $COCH_3$ · 2 HC—COOH ‖ HC—COOH

[5714-00-1] $C_{23}H_{29}N_3O_2S.2C_4H_4O_4$ (643.71).

Preparation—Piperazineethanol is condensed with 10-(3-chloropropyl)phenothiazin-2-yl methyl ketone (I) in the presence of a dehydrochlorinating agent such as sodamide. The resulting acetophenazine (base) is reacted with a double equimolar portion of maleic acid. I is prepared from phenothiazine through: (a) acetylation with acetic anhydride and aluminum chloride to the 2,10-diacetyl compound, (b) deacetylation at the 10-position with alkali, and (c) condensation of 2-acetylphenothiazine with 1-bromo-3- chloropropane. US Pat 2,985,654.

Description—A fine, yellow, powder that is odorless and has a bitter taste; sensitive to light and reasonably stable in dry air; melts about 165° with decomposition.

Solubility—1 g in 10 mL water, 260 mL alcohol, 2850 mL chloroform, 6000 mL ether, 370 mL acetone or 11 mL propylene glycol.

Uses—A piperazine-substituted phenothiazine for the management of the manifestations of *psychotic disorders* and the short-term treatment of anxiety, nausea and vomiting. Contraindications, warnings, precautions and adverse effects are similar to those for other phenothiazines, except extrapyramidal symptoms occur more frequently after administration of piperazine-substituted phenothiazines. See page 1181.

Dose—*Usual, adult, oral,* **20 mg** 3 times a day; range of total daily dose, **40** to **80 mg.** For hospitalized patients the optimum daily dosage ranges from **80** to **120 mg,** in divided doses, but patients with severe schizophrenia have received 400 to 600 mg a day. Not recommended for pediatric age group since safety and effectiveness in children have not been established.

Dosage Form—Tablets: 20 mg.

Chlorpromazine

10*H*-Phenothiazine-10-propanamine, 2-chloro-*N,N*-dimethyl-, Thorazine (*SmithKline Beecham*)

$CH_2CH_2CH_2N(CH_3)_2$ N Cl S

2-Chloro-10-[3-(dimethylamino)propyl]phenothiazine [50-53-3] $C_{17}H_{19}ClN_2S$ (318.86).

Preparation—The base is prepared from 2-chlorophenothiazine and (3-chloropropyl)dimethylamine in the presence of sodamide, then filtering and distilling off the toluene.

Description—White, crystalline solid; amine-like odor; darkens on prolonged exposure to light; melts about 60°.

Solubility—1 g in 3 mL alcohol, 2 mL chloroform or 3 mL ether; practically insoluble in water.

Uses—See *Chlorpromazine Hydrochloride.*

Dose—*Antiemetic, rectal,* **50** to **100 mg** every 6 to 8 hr. *Dose range,* **50** to **400 mg**. *Pediatric, antiemetic, children 6 mo and older,* **1 mg per kg** or ½ of a 25 mg suppository 3 or 4 times a day as necessary; *children under 6 mo* not recommended.

Dosage Form—Suppositories: 25 and 100 mg.

Chlorpromazine Hydrochloride

10*H*-Phenothiazine-10-propanamine, 2-chloro-*N,N*-dimethyl-, mono- hydrochloride; (*Various Mfrs*)

2-Chloro-10-[3-(dimethylamino)propyl]phenothiazine monohydrochloride [69-09-0] $C_{17}H_{19}ClN_2S.HCl$ (355.32).

See *Chlorpromazine* for the structure of the base.

Description—White or slightly creamy white, odorless, crystalline powder; darkens on prolonged exposure to light; melts about 196°.

Solubility—1 g in 1 mL water, 1.5 mL alcohol or 1.5 mL chloroform; insoluble in ether or benzene.

Uses—The first *tranquilizer* of the phenothiazine group of compounds. It is *effective* in the management of manifestations of *psychotic disorders, nausea and vomiting,* manifestations of *manic depressive illness* (manic phase), *intractable hiccups, apprehension and anxiety* prior to surgery, *acute intermittent porphyria* and as an adjunct in the treatment of *tetanus.* It is *probably effective* for control of symptoms in mild *alcohol withdrawal,* and for the control of *moderate to severe agitation,* hyperactivity or aggressiveness in *disturbed children.* The volume of distribution has been reported to be 21.8 L/kg after intramuscular administration and 80.6 L/kg after a single oral dose. This 4-fold difference reflects the low bioavailability *via* the oral route (32%). At least 100 metabolites of chlorpromazine appear in man. Two of these, 11-hydroxy- and 7-hydroxychlorpromazine, are active in man. Effective plasma levels in acute schizophrenia have been reported to vary from 30 ng/mL to 300 ng/mL; plasma levels ranging from 750 to 1000 ng/mL usually are accompanied by neurotoxicity, manifest by tremors and convulsions. Because of great interindividual differences, plasma levels for this agent are largely of research interest. A detailed listing of contraindications, warnings, precautions and adverse effects is given on page 1181.

Dosage is extremely variable and requires strict individualization. Administration is oral, intramuscular or intravenous. Parenteral administration should be reserved for bedfast or hospitalized patients. If used in ambulatory patients, the patient must remain in a supine position for at least 1 hr after the injection. Alarming reactions with failure to respond to pressor agents have been reported from even small intravenous doses. Epinephrine should never be used in treating these cases since the adrenolytic action of this drug may cause epinephrine reversal. Phenylephrine or levarterenol may be used to control the hypotension.

Dose—*Antiemetic, adults, oral,* **10** to **25 mg** every 4 to 6 hr; *intramuscular,* **25** to **50 mg** every 3 or 4 hr until vomiting ceases. *Children, oral,* **0.5 mg/kg** every 4 to 6 hr; *intramuscular,* **0.5 mg/kg** every 6 to 8 hr as required. *Tranquilizer, adults, oral, usual,* **10** to **50 mg** 2 or 3 times a day to a total dose of **1 g** a day when indicated; *intramuscular,* **25** to **50 mg,** repeated in 1 hr if necessary to a total dose of **1 g** a day when indicated. *Children, oral,* **0.5 mg/kg** every 4 to 6 hr; *intramuscular,* **0.5 mg/kg** every 6 to 8 hr as required. Consult the package literature for more specific information.

Dosage Forms—Injection: 25 mg/mL in 1, 2 and 10 mL; Timed-Release Capsules: 30, 75, 150, 200 and 300 mg; Syrup: 2 mg/mL; Concentrate: 30 and 100 mg/mL; Tablets: 10, 25, 50, 100 and 200 mg.

Chlorprothixene

1-Propanamine, 3-(2-chloro-9*H*-thioxanthen-9-ylidene)-*N,N*-dimethyl-, (*Z*)-, Taractan (*Roche*)

$H-C-CH_2CH_2N(CH_3)_2$ Cl S

(*Z*)-2-Chloro-*N,N*-dimethylthioxanthene-$\Delta^{9,\gamma}$-propylamine [113-59-7] $C_{18}H_{18}ClNS$ (315.86).

Preparation—One method cyclizes 5-chloro-2-(phenylthio)benzoic acid with the aid of polyphosphoric acid to 2-chlorothioxanthen-9-one, followed by reaction with [3-(dimethylamino)propylidene]triphenylphosphorane to introduce the 9-substituent. US Pat 3,115,502 describes a process for converting the *cis* form of the compound to the therapeutically active *trans* form by heating in the presence of a strongly basic agent.

Description—Yellow, crystalline powder; slight amine-like odor; unstable when exposed to light and air; melts about 99°.

Solubility—1 g in 1700 mL water, 29 mL alcohol, 2 mL of chloroform, 14 mL of ether or 18 mL of acetone.

Uses—A thioxanthene derivative chemically and pharmacologically related to chlorpromazine. In place of the nitrogen in the phenothiazine ring, it has a carbon atom with a double bond to the dimethylaminopropyl side chain. This structural difference is not associated with any striking pharmacological difference. It induces less sedation, adrenergic blockade and extrapyramidal reactions than does chlorpromazine. It is indicated for the management of the manifestations of *psychotic disorders.* Thus, it has been used in the treatment of acute and chronic schizophrenia and in psychotic and other conditions in which anxiety, agitation and tension predominate. Because of its structural similarity to the phenothiazines, all the known contraindications, warnings, precautions and serious side effects associated with phenothiazine therapy should be borne in mind (see page 1181).

Dose—*Usual, adult, oral* or *intramuscular,* **25** to **50 mg** 3 or 4 times a day; maximum, up to 600 mg a day. For *elderly or debilitated patients,* **10** to **25 mg** 3 or 4 times a day. *Usual, pediatric, oral, children 6 to 12 yr,* **10** to **25 mg** 3 or 4 times a day; *children under 6 yr,* dosage not established. *Intramuscular,* not to be used in children under 12 yr.

Dosage Forms—Injection: 25 mg (as hydrochloride)/2 mL; Oral Suspension: 100 mg (as lactate and hydrochloride)/5 mL; Tablets: 10, 25, 50 and 100 mg.

Clozapine

5*H*-Dibenzo[*b,e*][1,4]diazepine, 8-chloro-11-(4-methyl-1-piperazinyl)-, Clozaril (*Sandoz*)

N NCH_3 Cl N N H

[5786-21-0] $C_{18}H_{19}ClN_4$ (326.83).

Preparation—Clozapine may be prepared by intramolecular condensation of 2-amino-4-chlorodiphenylamine-2′-carboxylic acid 4-methylpiperazide in the presence of phosphoroxychloride and *N,N*-dimethylformamide. The desired product is extracted with benzene, extracted from the organic solution with dilute acetic acid, and then precipitated by addition of concentrated ammonia water. Neth Pat Appl 293,201.

Description—Yellow, tasteless crystals; melts between 183 and 184°.

Solubility—Slightly soluble in water, soluble in ether.

Uses—A dibenzodiazepine-derived atypical antipsychotic agent. It is effective and relatively rapid-acting in the treatment of schizophrenia. Many of its CNS effects differ from other antipsychotic drugs. It is likely that the antipsychotic effects of clozapine are more complex than other antipsychotic agents, and besides blocking dopamine D-2 and 0-1 receptors in mesolimbic and mesocortical brain regions, they also may involve cholinergic, serotonergic and noradrenergic systems.

Unlike the typical antipsychotic drugs, clozapine has regional specific antidopaminergic activity with relatively weak antagonism on extrapyramidal dopaminergic action; this may account for its low propensity to cause extrapyramidal side effects such as tardive dyskinesia and dystonias. In addition, compared to typical antipsychotic agents, clozapine produces greater blockade of dopamine D-1 receptors, although it is not clear if such action contributes to its antipsychotic effects. It is used to treat schizophrenia-related symptoms in severely ill patients who are not managed adequately by other antipsychotic therapy or in whom such therapy causes intolerable adverse side effects.

In comparative studies, clozapine was found to be more effective than chlorpromazine, haloperidol, perphenazine or trifluoperazine in patients with relatively severe disease, although rebound psychosis from discontinuance of drug therapy was observed to be more severe in patients receiving clozapine.

While clozapine lacks most of the extrapyramidal side effects associated with the traditional antipsychotic agents, it is more likely to cause agranulocytosis (1 to 2%) or seizures (3 to 5%). Because of these potentially serious adverse responses to clozapine, this drug should be reserved for those patients who are not controlled satisfactorily by standard antipsychotic agents. Those who do receive clozapine should be monitored closely with periodic (every 2 to 4 weeks) white blood cell (WBC) assessments.

Other potential side effects for clozapine include drowsiness, headaches, disturbed sleep, dizziness, fever (5%), changes in blood pressure (less than 10%), tachycardia (25%), cardiac arrhythmias, dry mouth or hypersalivation (50 to 80%), nasal congestion, pallor, bowel irregularities, nausea/vomiting, respiratory irregularities and rash (2%). Clozapine is absorbed rapidly from the GI tract and extensively metabolized during first pass through the liver. Peak plasma levels occur about 1.5 hr after a single oral dose. There is sixfold interindividual variability in steady-state plasma levels in patients using high doses of this drug. Pharmacological effects are apparent within 15 min after administration and the duration of action is 4 to 12 hr after a single dose. Elimination is biphasic and after a low dose averages 8 hr. Clozapine and its metabolites are excreted primarily in the urine.

Dose—*Usual, adult, oral, initially,* **25 mg** 1 or 2 times a day. If this is well tolerated, the dose is increased by **25 to 50 mg** a day until the target of **300 to 450 mg** a day is reached.

Dosage Form—Tablets: 25 and 100 mg.

Droperidol

2*H*-Benzimidazol 2 one, 1- [1-[4-(4-fluorophenyl)-4-oxobutyl]-1,2,3,6-tetrahydro-4-pyridinyl]-1,3-dihydro-,
Inapsine, ing of Innovar (*Janssen*)

1-[1-[3-(*p*-Fluorobenzoyl)propyl]-1,2,3,6-tetrahydro-4-pyridyl]-2-benzimidazolinone [548-73-2] $C_{22}H_{22}FN_3O_2$ (379.43).

Preparation—4-Chloro-4′-fluorobutyrophenone is prepared from γ-butyrolactone and reacted with 1-(1,2,3,6 tetrahydro-4-pyridyl)-2-benzimidazolinone in the presence of a suitable condensing agent. US Pat 3,161,645.

Description—White to light tan, amorphous or microcrystalline powder; odorless and tasteless (*Note:* because this compound is extremely potent, no taste test is recommended); sensitive to light, air and heat; hygroscopic; melts about 146° after drying in vacuum at 70° for 4 hr, pK_a 7.6.

Solubility—1g in 10,000 mL water, 140 mL alcohol, 4 mL chloroform or 500 mL ether.

Uses—A butyrophenone derivative, it is a *neuroleptic* used as an adjunct to anesthesia to produce sedation and reduce incidence of nausea and vomiting. It often is used in combination with the analgesic fentanyl citrate (for uses, see *Fentanyl Citrate and Droperidol Injection,* page 1143. It has been used as an intravenous antiemetic in cancer chemotherapy. Following intravenous or intramuscular administration, onset of action occurs in 3 to 10 min and full effect in 30 min. Duration is generally 2 to 4 hr, but may persist for as long as 12 hr. Terminal half-life averages 2.2 hr. Safety and use during pregnancy, labor and delivery and lactation has not been established.

Dose—*Premedication, intravenous* or *intramuscular,* **2.5** to **10 mg** 30 to 60 min before induction; *induction,* usually *intravenous,* **2.5 mg/20** to **25 lb;** *maintenance,* usually *intravenous,* **1.25** to **2.5 mg.** *Use alone in diagnostic procedures, intramuscular* **2.5** to **10 mg** 30 to 60 min prior to the procedure; *additional doses,* intravenous, **1.25** to **2.5 mg** as needed.

Dosage Form—Injection: droperidol lactate equivalent to 2.5 mg of droperidol/mL in 2- and 5-mL ampuls and 2-, 5- and 10-mL vials.

Ergoloid Mesylates

Hydergine (*Sandoz*); (*Various mfrs*)

	R
Dihydroergocornine	$-CH(CH_3)_2$
Dihydroergocristine	$-CH_2C_6H_5$
Dihydro-α-ergocryptine	$-CH_2CH(CH_3)_2$
Dihydro-β-ergocryptine	$-CH(CH_3)CH_2CH_3$

A mixture of equal amounts of the methanesulfonate (mesylate) salts of dihydroergocornine, dihydroergocristine and α- and β-dihydroergocryptine. [8067-24-0] [11032-41-0].

Preparation—By catalytic by hydrogenation of the several alkaloids isolated from ergot, *Claviceps purpurea* (Fries), a parasite on the rye plant. The salt mixture is prepared by reaction with methanesulfonic acid.

Description—White, to off-white powder.

Solubility—1 g in 50 mL of water, 30 mL alcohol or 100 mL of chloroform; sparingly soluble in acetone.

Uses—For individuals over 60 who manifest signs and symptoms of an *idiopathic decline in mental capacity, ie, cognitive* and *interpersonal skills, mood, self-care* and *motivation.* Pharmacokinetic studies in man indicate about 25% oral absorption; peak plasma levels of 0.5 ng Eq/mL/mg are achieved in 1.5 to 3 hr; elimination is apparently biphasic with half-lives of 4 and 13 hr. It is contraindicated in individuals who have previously shown hypersensitivity to the drug. The drug may cause sublingual irritation, nasal stuffiness, nausea, vomiting and sinus bradycardia; orthostatic hypotension sometimes occurs.

Dose—*Sublingual* or *oral,* **1 mg** 3 times a day. Alleviation of symptoms is gradual and may not be apparent for 3 or 4 wk.

Dosage Forms—Liquid: 1 mg/mL; Tablets: 1 mg; Sublingual Tablets: 0.5 and 1 mg.

Fluphenazine Decanoate

1-Piperazineethanol, 4-[3-[2-(trifluoromethyl)-10*H*-phenothiazin-10-yl]-propyl]-, decanoate (ester);
Prolixin Decanoate (*Princeton*)

[30909-31-4] $C_{32}H_{44}F_3N_3O_2S$ (591.77).

Preparation—Fluphenazine (see *Fluphenazine Hydrochloride*) is esterified with decanoyl chloride in the presence of pyridine. US Pats 3,194,733 and 3,394,131.

Description—Pale-yellow to yellowish orange viscous liquid with a characteristic odor; light-sensitive; melts about 31°.

Solubility—Insoluble in water; soluble in alcohol, acetone, benzene or ether.

Uses—A trifluoromethyl phenothiazine derivative indicated for the management of patients requiring prolonged parenteral neuroleptic therapy (eg, chronic schizophrenics). Peak plasma level usually is achieved in 1 to 2 days; half-life (after a single dose) is 6.8 to 9.6 days, onset of action is 1 to 3 days and duration of action is about 4 wk.

Dose—*Intramuscular* or *subcutaneous*, **12.5 to 100 mg;** *usual*, **12.5** to **25 mg;** subsequent injections and dosage interval are based with patient response. The safety and efficacy of this drug in children have not been established.

Dosage Forms—Injection: 25 mg/mL in 5-mL vials and 1-mL single dose syringes.

Fluphenazine Enanthate

Prolixin Enanthate (*Princeton*)

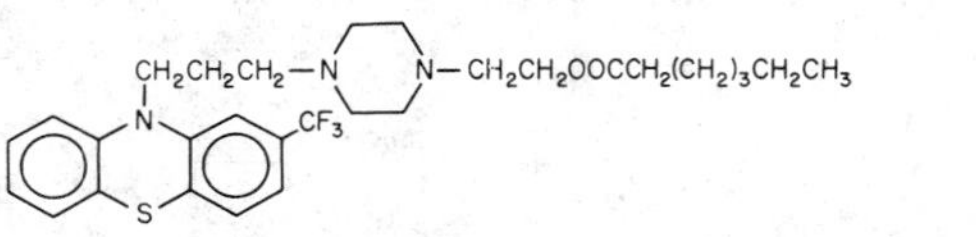

[2746-81-8] $C_{29}H_{38}F_3N_3O_2S$ (549.69).

Preparation—Fluphenazine is esterified through reaction with enanthoyl chloride in the presence of pyridine. For the preparation of fluphenazine, see *Fluphenazine Hydrochloride*. US Pat 3,058,979.

Description—Pale-yellow to yellow-orange, clear to slightly turbid, viscous liquid with a characteristic odor; *not recommended to be tasted;* unstable in strong light, but stable in air at room temperature.

Solubility—1 g in < 1 mL of alcohol, < 1 mL chloroform or 2 mL ether; insoluble in water.

Uses—Except for duration of action, it has actions, uses, contraindications and untoward effects similar to those of the hydrochloride. The esterification of fluphenazine with the enanthate moiety markedly prolongs the drug's duration of action without unduly attenuating its beneficial effects. The onset of action generally appears between 24 to 72 hr after injection and the effects of the drug on psychotic symptoms become significant within 48 to 96 hr. Amelioration of symptoms continues for 1 to 3 wk or longer, with an average duration of effect of about 2 wk. It is especially useful when the patient or his family can not be relied upon to insure that an oral antischizophrenic drug will be given every day. See *Fluphenazine Hydrochloride*.

Dose—*Intramuscular* or *subcutaneous*, **12.5** to **100 mg** every 1 to 3 wk; *usual*, **12.5** to **25 mg;** subsequent injections and dosage interval are based on patient response. The safety and efficacy of this drug in children have not been established.

Dosage Form—Injection: 25 mg/mL in 5-mL vials.

Fluphenazine Hydrochloride

Permitil (*Schering*); Prolixin (*Squibb*)

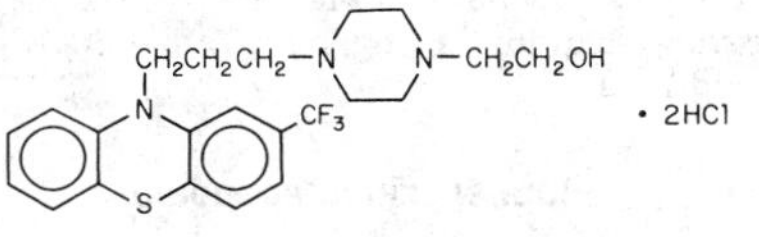

[146-56-5] $C_{22}H_{26}F_3N_3OS.2HCl$ (510.44).

Preparation—Fluphenazine may be prepared by condensing 2-(trifluoromethyl)-10-(3-chloropropyl)phenothiazine with 1-piperazineethanol in toluene with the aid of sodamide. Reaction of the purified base with a double molar quantity of hydrogen chloride yields the official salt. The starting phenothiazine compound may be prepared by heating 3-(trifluoromethyl)diphenylamine with sulfur and condensing the resulting 2-(trifluoromethyl)phenothiazine with 1-bromo-3-chloropropane. US Pat 3,058,979.

Description—White or nearly white, odorless, crystalline powder; melts within a 5° range above 225°.

Solubility—1 g in 1.4 mL water or 6.7 mL alcohol; slightly soluble in chloroform; practically insoluble in ether.

Uses—A trifluoromethyl phenothiazine derivative intended for the management of manifestations of *psychotic disorders*. Although the pharmacological effects are, in general, similar to those of other phenothiazines, laboratory and clinical studies indicate that this drug exhibits several important differences. The drug is more potent, exhibits a more prolonged duration of action, is less likely to induce hypotension, is less sedative and does not potentiate CNS depressants and anesthetics to the same degree as other phenothiazines.

It is absorbed rapidly after oral or intramuscular administration, onset of action occurs within 1 hr, peak plasma levels in 1.5 to 2 hr and duration of action is 6 hr. The intramuscular or subcutaneous administration of the enanthate salt has an average duration of 2 wk. Therefore, it is useful in those patients who refuse to take the oral preparation. It appears to be particularly effective in modifying psychotic behavior patterns and ameliorating such symptoms as agitation, delusions and hallucinations. The principal disadvantage of therapy with the decanoate or enanthate is the inability to terminate their action when severe adverse effects occur. Like other phenothiazines, it should not be used in patients receiving large doses of hypnotics, and should be used with caution in patients with a history of convulsive disorders.

Side effects induced by this drug are similar to those encountered with other phenothiazines. Those most frequently encountered include reversible extrapyramidal symptoms (approximately 60% of patients) including parkinsonism, dystonia, dyskinesia, akathisia, oculogyric crises, opisthotonos and hyperreflexia; liver damage manifest by jaundice or biliary stasis; blood dyscrasias, including leukopenia, agranulocytosis, thrombocytopenic purpura, eosinophilia and pancytopenia; skin disorders such as itching, erythema, urticaria and even exfoliative dermatitis; peripheral edema, endocrine disturbances and autonomic reactions. Hypotension rarely has been a problem with the drug. Patients should be under medical supervision and observed carefully for other untoward effects characteristic of phenothiazine agents (see page 1181).

Dose—*Usual, adult, oral, initially* **0.5** to **10 mg** a day in divided doses; *maintenance*, **1** to **5 mg** as a single dose a day. *Intramuscular*, **1.25** to **10 mg** a day divided into 4 doses. Daily dosages exceeding 20 mg orally or 10 mg intramuscularly should be used with caution. Safety and efficacy of this drug in children have not been established.

Dosage Forms—Elixir: 1 mg/2 mL; Concentrate: 5 mg/mL; Injection: 25 mg/10 mL; Tablets: 1, 2.5, 5 and 10 mg.

Haloperidol

1-Butanone, 4-[4-(4-chlorophenyl)-4-hydroxy-1-piperidinyl]-1-(4-fluorophenyl)-, Haldol (*McNeil*)

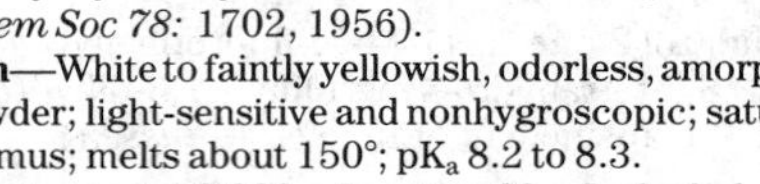

4-[4-(*p*-Chlorophenyl)-4-hydroxypiperidino]-4′-fluorobutyrophenone [52-86-8] $C_{21}H_{23}ClFNO_2$ (375.87).

Preparation—4-(*p*-Chlorophenyl)-4-piperidinol is condensed with 4-chloro-4′-fluorobutyrophenone in a toluene solution. The haloperidol thus formed is isolated and recrystallized from a solvent such as diisopropyl ether. The starting substituted piperidinol may be prepared from *p*-chloro-α-methylstyrene by the method described by Schmidle and Mansfield (*J Am Chem Soc 78:* 1702, 1956).

Description—White to faintly yellowish, odorless, amorphous or microcrystalline powder; light-sensitive and nonhygroscopic; saturated solution is neutral to litmus; melts about 150°; pK_a 8.2 to 8.3.

Solubility—1 g in > 10,000 mL water, 60 mL alcohol, 15 mL chloroform or 200 mL ether.

Uses—A butyrophenone derivative that is an antipsychotic agent useful in the management of such symptoms as moderate to severe *agitation, anxiety* and *tension, assaultiveness, delusions, hallucinations, hostility* and *hyperactivity*, when they are *manifestations of psychoses* including *schizophrenia*, the manic type of *manic depressive illness* or *psychotic reactions* associated with organic brain syndromes or mental retardation. It has been reported to be useful in *Gilles de la Tourette's disease* (motor tics, unusual barking and hissing sounds). The bioavailability of this drug has been reported to be approximately 60% *via* the oral route. The half-life of elimination ranges from 10 to 19 hours after intravenous administration and 12 to 38 hours *via* the oral route. Therapeutic plasma levels range from 3 to 10 ng/mL, but some patients require significantly higher levels before adequate antipsychotic effects are observed. It has the same contraindications, warnings and precautions as other drugs in this category (see page 1181).

Like the phenothiazines, it frequently produces extrapyramidal reactions such as parkinsonism, dystonia, dyskinesia, oculogyric crises and akathisia. Occasional adverse effects include blood dyscrasia, postural hypotension and tachycardia. Rarely, cholestatic jaundice, photosensitivity reactions and allergic skin reactions may occur. Care should be exercised when antihypertensive agents, general anesthetics, hypnotics, alcohol, analgesics and other CNS depressants are used concomitantly with this drug, since it may potentiate their actions. See 1181 for a more detailed listing of potential adverse effects.

Dose—*Usual, adult, oral,* **0.5** to **5 mg** 2 to 3 times a day; maximum, **100 mg** a day. *Note: geriatric* or debilitated patients, *oral,* **0.5** to **2 mg** 2 or 3 times a day, increased gradually as needed and tolerated. *Intramuscular,* **2** to **5 mg** initially, repeat at hourly intervals if necessary, or at 4- to 8-hr intervals if symptoms are controlled; doses above 15 mg a day are seldom required. *Hyperkinesia* with mental retardation, *intramuscular,* **5 mg** 4 times a day initially, increased gradually to 60 mg a day if necessary. Not recommended for pediatric age group since safety and effectiveness in children have not been established.

Dosage Forms—Concentrate: 2 mg/mL; Solution: 2 mg/mL; Tablets: 0.5, 1, 2, 5, 10 and 20 mg; Injection: 5 mg/mL.

Lithium Carbonate

Carbonic acid, dilithium salt; (*Various Mfrs*)

Dilithium carbonate [554-13-2] Li_2CO_3 (73.89).

Preparation—Lithium chloride is metathesized with sodium carbonate in aqueous solution.

Description—White, light, granular powder; melts at 618°.

Solubility—1 g in 78 mL cold water or 140 mL boiling water; very slightly soluble in alcohol; dissolved by dilute acids.

Uses—For the treatment of the manic phase of *manic-depressive psychoses.* Maintenance therapy prevents or diminishes the intensity of subsequent episodes in those manic-depressive patients with a history of mania. Other psychiatric conditions which may be benefited include recurrent severe depressions without manic episodes, schizo-affective psychosis, episodic alcoholism and periodic antisocial behavior and periodic schizophrenic illness; its value in these conditions awaits further research. It is water-soluble and absorbed and excreted rather rapidly; consequently, it must be taken in divided doses over the day to maintain relatively constant plasma concentrations. It has been used investigationally to improve the neutrophil count in patients with cancer-chemotherapy-induced neutropenia and in AIDS patients receiving zidovudine. Lithium alters sodium transport in nerve and muscle cells and effects a shift toward interneuronal metabolism of catecholamine.

This salt is absorbed completely 6 to 8 hours following oral administration. Its plasma half-life is about 24 hours. It is excreted by the kidneys; about 80% of filtered lithium is reabsorbed. The lithium ion is distributed in total body water, but is concentrated in various tissues to different degrees. After a steady state has been reached, about 40% is contained in cerebrospinal fluid and renal clearance is relatively constant. Serum levels should be maintained between 0.7 and 1.3 mEq/L. Adverse effects are noted at levels above 1.5 mEq/L and serious toxicity is common when concentrations exceed 2.0 mEq/L. Since toxicity develops at serum levels little higher than effective therapeutic levels frequent monitoring and dosage adjustments are mandatory for successful therapy.

Nausea, vomiting and diarrhea are presumptive evidence of toxicity and indicate the dose should be reduced. The most-common untoward effects are slight tremor and polyuria; these ordinarily do not require a reduction in dosages. CNS effects, such as slurred speech, blurred vision, confusion and lethargy, require immediate withdrawal of the drug and the administration of sodium chloride (at least 4 g extra/day) to facilitate the excretion of lithium.

Adverse cardiovascular effects include arrhythmias and hypotension. Goiter, hypothyroidism and diabetes insipidus also have been observed. It should not be used in patients with cardiovascular or renal disease. The safe use of the drug during pregnancy has not been established; it can cause cardiac and other birth defects. The drug should not be used in children under 12 yr.

Dose—*Usual, initially* **600 mg** 3 times a day; *maintenance,* **300 mg** 3 times a day, to maintain a serum lithium level of 0.6 to 1.2 mEq/L 8 to 12 hr following administration; *usual range of dose,* **900 mg** to **1.8 g** a day. Dosage for children under 12 yr has not been established.

Warning, toxicity can occur at doses close to therapeutic levels.

Dosage Forms—Capsules: 150, 300 and 600 mg; Tablets: 300 mg; Slow-Release Tablets: 300 and 450 mg.

Loxapine Succinate

Butanedioic acid, compd with 2-chloro-11-(4-methyl-1-piperazinyl)-dibenz[*b, f*][1,4]oxazepine (1:1); Loxitane (*Lederle*)

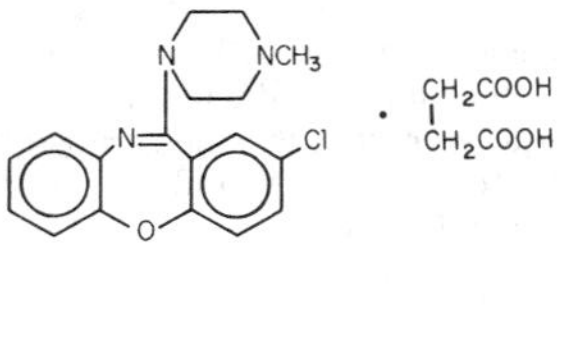

2-Chloro-11-(4-methyl-1-piperazinyl)dibenz[*b, f*][1,4]oxazepine succinate (1:1) [27833-64-3], $C_{18}H_{18}ClN_3O.C_4H_6O_4$ (445.90).

Preparation—A method of synthesis of loxapine starting with xanthone oxime is described in US Pat 3,412,193. Other procedures are summarized in *CA 63:* 11592h, 1965.

Description—White to off-white, crystalline powder; pK_a 6.6 (loxapine).

Solubility—Slightly soluble in water or alcohol.

Uses—A dibenzoxazepine antipsychotic agent indicated for symptomatic control of schizophrenia; the mode of action has not been established. It is contraindicated in comatose or severe drug- induced depressed states and also in individuals with known hypersensitivity to the drug. Absorption following oral administration is virtually complete; after distribution to tissues it is metabolized and excreted in the urine and feces, mainly in the first 24 hr. In normal human volunteers, signs of sedation were seen within 20 to 30 min after administration, were most pronounced within 1.5 to 3 hr and lasted through 12 hr.

Adverse reactions include drowsiness, dizziness, faintness, staggering gait, muscle twitching, weakness, confusional states, extrapyramidal symptoms, tardive dyskinesia, tachycardia, hypotension, hypertension, lightheadedness and syncope, dermatitis, edema, pruritus, seborrhea and skin rashes, dry mouth, nasal congestion, constipation, blurred vision, nausea, vomiting, weight gain or loss, dyspnea, ptosis, hyperpyrexia, flushed facies, headache, paresthesia and polydipsia.

It should be used with extreme caution in patients with a history of convulsive disorders since it lowers the convulsive threshold; seizures have been reported in epileptic patients receiving it, even with maintenance of anticonvulsant therapy. As an antiemetic effect may occur in man, this drug may mask signs of overdosage of toxic drugs and may obscure conditions such as intestinal obstruction and brain tumor. It should be used with caution in patients with cardiovascular disease. Increased pulse rates have been reported in most patients receiving antipsychotic doses; transient hypotension has been reported. In the presence of severe hypotension that requires vasopressor therapy, norepinephrine or angiotensin is preferred over epinephrine, which may be ineffective because of inhibition of its vasopressor effect by the drug. Since the possibility of ocular toxicity from loxapine exists, careful observation for pigmentary retinopathy and lenticular pigmentation should be made. Because of possible anticholinergic action, it should be used cautiously in patients with glaucoma or a tendency to urinary retention. Safe use during pregnancy or lactation has not been established; as studies have not been performed in children, use in children below the age of 16 is not recommended.

Dose—*Usual, adult, oral,* the equivalent of **10 mg** of loxapine 2 times a day; *maintenance, oral,* the equivalent of **15** to **25 mg** 2 to 4 times a day. Note: *Geriatric* or *debilitated patients,* the equivalent of **5 mg** of loxapine 2 times a day. *Maximum dose, adult, oral,* the equivalent of **250 mg** of loxapine a day. Not recommended for use in children below the age of 16.

Dosage Forms—Capsules: 5, 10, 25 and 50 mg of loxapine (as the succinate); Oral Concentrate: 25 mg (as the hydrochloride)/mL; Injection: 50 mg (as the hydrochloride)/mL.

Mesoridazine Besylate

10*H*-Phenothiazine, 10-[2-(1-methyl-2-piperidinyl)ethyl]-2-(methylsulfinyl)-, monobenzenesulfonate; Serentil (*Boehringer-Ingelheim*)

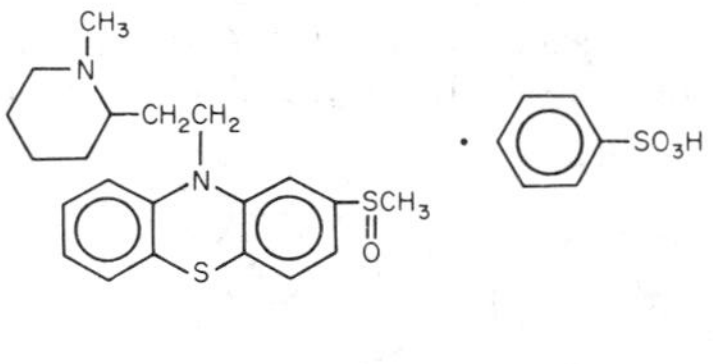

[32672-69-8] $C_{21}H_{26}N_2OS_2.C_6H_6O_3S$ (544.74).

Preparation—Nitrophenide [bis(3-nitrophenyl)disulfide)] is converted by a series of reactions into 2-(methylthio)phenothiazine. Oxidation with H_2O_2 yields the corresponding sulfinyl compound which is reacted with 1-methyl-2-(2-chloroethyl)piperidine in the presence of a suitable condensing agent and the mesoridazine thus formed is converted, with benzenesulfonic acid, to the besylate salt. US Pat 3,084,161.

Description—White to pale-yellow, crystalline powder with a faint odor; melts about 178° with decomposition.

Solubility—1 g in 1 mL water, 11 mL alcohol, 3 mL chloroform or 6300 mL ether.

Uses—The salt of a metabolite of thioridazine, a phenothiazine derivative, indicated for the management of *schizophrenia, organic brain disorders,* symptoms of *alcohol withdrawal* and *psychoneuroses.* It has pharmacological properties similar to thioridazine, except that antiemetic activity and pigmentary retinopathy has not yet been associated with its use. Otherwise, it has the warnings, precautions, contraindications and adverse effects similar to those for other phenothiazines (see page 1181).

Dose—*Usual, adult, oral,* **50** to **400 mg** a day; *initially* **50 mg** 3 times a day. *Intramuscular, usual,* **25** to **200 mg** a day; *initially* **25 mg;** repeat in 30 to 60 min if necessary. Use in children under 12 yr is not recommended because safe conditions for its use have not been established.

Dosage Forms—Concentrate: 25 mg/mL; Injection: 25 mg/mL; Tablets: 10, 25, 50 and 100 mg.

Molindone Hydrochloride

4*H*-Indol-4-one, 3-ethyl-1,5,6,7-tetrahydro-2-methyl-5-(4-morpholinylmethyl)-, monohydrochloride; Moban (*DuPont*)

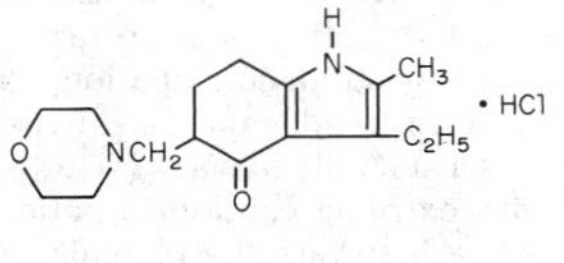

[15622-68-8] $C_{16}H_{24}N_2O_2$.HCl (312.84).

Preparation—From 4-(morpholinyl)-1,3-cyclohexanedione and 2-oximino-3-pentanone in acetic acid by refluxing with powdered zinc yields the base which may be converted to the hydrochloride by usual procedures. See Belg Pat 670,798; *CA: 65,* 7148f, 1966.

Description—White crystals; melts about 180°.

Solubility—Freely soluble in water or alcohol.

Uses—A dihydroindolone derivative effective in patients with chronic schizophrenia and in acute schizophrenic reactions. It may control symptoms of schizophrenia such as disorientation, conceptual disorganization, perceptual distortion, hallucinations, grandiosity, emotional withdrawal and tension. It is absorbed rapidly from the gastrointestinal tract; peak blood concentrations occur within 1 hr; plasma half-life is 1.5 hr and duration of action following a single dose is 36 hr. It is metabolized rapidly by the liver; 36 inactive metabolites have been identified in the urine and feces. More than 90% of a single dose is excreted in feces and urine within 24 hr. A small amount is excreted via the lungs as carbon dioxide.

Adverse effects include drowsiness (notify physician if this occurs), dryness of the mouth, tremors, involuntary muscle twitching or impaired vision. It is contraindicated in comatose patients and patients with severe CNS depression or known hypersensitivity to the drug. It is not recommended for use in children under 12 yr.

Dose—*Oral, initially* **50** to **75 mg** a day, increased to **100 mg** a day in 3 or 4 days. Patients with severe symptoms may require up to 225 mg/day. *Elderly* and *debilitated patients,* start on lower dosage. *Maintenance therapy, mild,* **5** to **15 mg** 3 or 4 times a day; *moderate,* **10** to **25 mg** 3 or 4 times a day; *severe,* **225 mg** a day may be required.

Dosage Forms—Tablets: 5, 10, 25, 50 and 100 mg; Concentrate: 20 mg/mL.

Perphenazine

1-Piperazineethanol, 4-[3-(2-chloro-10*H*-phenothiazin-10-yl)propyl]-, Trilafon (*Schering*)

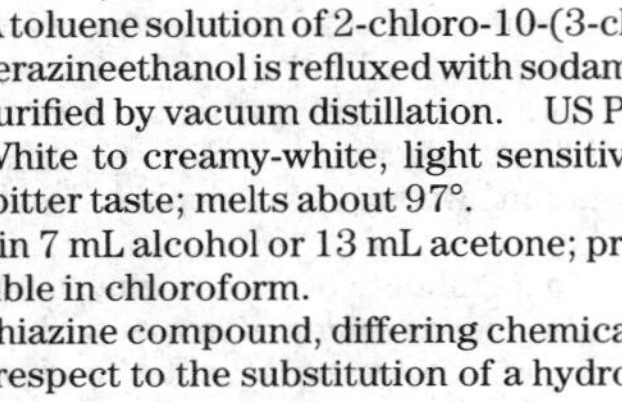

$C_{21}H_{26}ClN_3OS$ (403.97).

Preparation—A toluene solution of 2-chloro-10-(3-chloropropyl)phenothiazine and 1-piperazineethanol is refluxed with sodamide and the resulting perphenazine purified by vacuum distillation. US Pat 2,766,235.

Description—White to creamy-white, light sensitive powder; almost odorless and has a bitter taste; melts about 97°.

Solubility—1 g in 7 mL alcohol or 13 mL acetone; practically insoluble in water; freely soluble in chloroform.

Uses—A phenothiazine compound, differing chemically from prochlorperazine only with respect to the substitution of a hydroxyethyl group for the methyl group of the latter drug. It is indicated for the management of *psychotic disorders,* for the control of severe *nausea* and *vomiting* and intractable hiccoughs in adults. Since it is a phenothiazine, it is subject to similar contraindications, warnings and precautions as other members of this chemical class. Likewise, it should be considered capable of inducing similar adverse reactions. See page 1181 and *Chlorpromazine Hydrochloride.*

Dose—*Usual, oral, nonhospitalized patients,* **2** to **8 mg** 3 times a day; *hospitalized patients,* **8** to **16 mg** 2 to 4 times a day; *intramuscular,* **5** to **10 mg** *initially,* followed by **5 mg** in 6 hr. Severe *nausea* and *vomiting, adults, oral,* **8** to **16 mg** a day in divided doses or one repeat-action tablet twice a day. Not recommended for children under 12 yr.

Dosage Forms—Injection: 5 mg/mL; Solution: 16 mg/5 mL; Tablets: 2, 4, 8 and 16 mg; Repeat-Action Tablets: 8 mg.

Pimozide

2*H*-Benzimidazol-2-one, 1-[1-[4,4-bis(4-fluorophenyl)butyl]-4-piperidinyl]-1,3-dihydro-, Orap (*McNeil*)

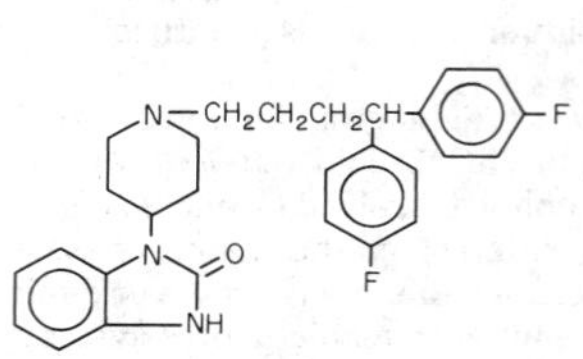

[2062-78-4] $C_{28}H_{29}F_2N_3O$ (461.55).

Preparation—The ethyl ester of 1-benzyl-4-oxo-3-piperidinecarboxylic acid and *o*-phenylenediamine are condensed, with the loss of the elements of water and ethanol, to yield I. With hydrogen and Pd catalyst the benzyl group is removed from I and the unsaturation reduced to give II, 1(2*H*)-(4-piperidinyl)benzimidazol-2-one. The other necessary intermediate is formed from a Grignard reaction between *p*-fluorophenylmagnesium bromide and ethyl cyclohexylpropanecarboxylate to give 4,4′-difluoro-α-cyclopropylbenzhydrol. Then, treatment with $SOCl_2$ opens the cyclopropane ring by a homoallylic rearrangement to produce 1,1-bis(4-fluorophenyl)-4-chloro-1-butene. Catalytic reduction of the double bond followed by condensation with II in the presence of Na_2CO_3 yields pimozide.

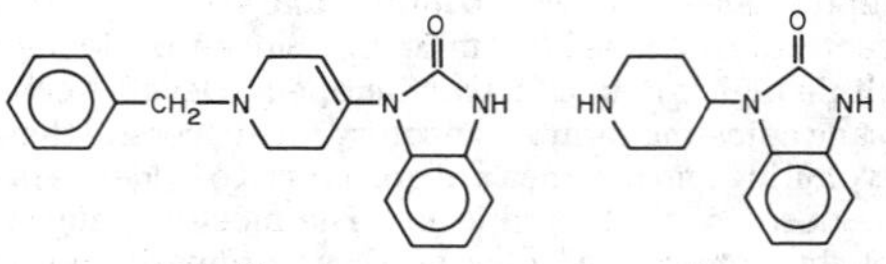

(I) (II)

Description—Crystals; melts about 216°; pK_a, 7.32.

Solubility—Practically soluble in water; 1 g in 140 mL alcohol; 5 mL chloroform or 500 mL ether; very slightly soluble in dilute aqueous acid solution.

Uses—A drug structurally similar to haloperidol for the suppression of motor and vocal tics of Tourette's disorder in children and adults. It also has been used for the symptomatic management of a variety of psychiatric illnesses, principally chronic schizophrenia, but other agents generally are preferred. It should *not* be used in schizophrenic patients whose main manifestations include excitement, agitation or hyperactivity, since the efficacy of the drug in these conditions has not been established. It is thought to block CNS dopaminergic receptors. It has no effect on norepinephrine receptors. Its ability to block motor and phonic tics in Tourette's Disorder is thought to be a function of its dopaminergic blocking activity. After oral administration approximately 50% is absorbed. Peak serum levels occur in 6 to 8 hr. It is metabolized extensively by the liver; two metabolites with undetermined neuroleptic activity have been identified. Its mean elimination half-life is approximately 55 hr. The major route of elimination is the kidney; 38 to 45% of an oral dose is excreted in the urine, mostly as metabolites. Although it is considered nonsedating, common adverse effects include sedation, lethargy and/or drowsiness. Hypotension, orthostatic hypotension, tachycardia and palpitations also have been observed. In addition, amenorrhea, dysmenorrhea, salivation, nausea, vomiting, diarrhea, constipation and abdominal cramps have been reported. Its safety and effectiveness in children under 12 yr has not been evaluated fully.

Dose—*Initial, oral,* **1** to **2 mg** a day in divided doses; if necessary, increase the dose every other day; *maintenance,* **0.2 mg/kg** or **10 mg** a day, whichever is less. Do not exceed 10 mg a day.

Dosage Form—Tablets: 2 mg.

Prochlorperazine and Its Salts—page 905.

Promazine Hydrochloride

10*H*-Phenothiazine-10-propanamine, *N,N*-dimethyl-, monohydrochloride; Sparine (*Wyeth-Ayerst*); Prozine (*Hauck*)

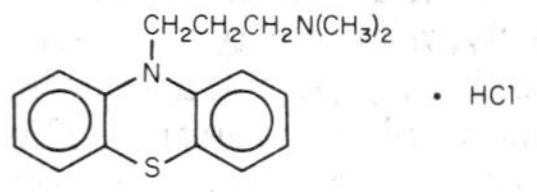

10-[3-(Dimethylamino)propyl]phenothiazine monohydrochloride [53-60-1] $C_{17}H_{20}N_2S.HCl$ (320.88).

Preparation—Phenothiazine is dissolved in an inert solvent and condensed with 3-chloro-*N,N*-dimethylpropylamine in the presence of sodium hydride to yield promazine. After purification, it is dissolved in an organic solvent and reacted with an equimolar quantity of HCl.

Description—White to slightly yellow, practically odorless, crystalline powder; oxidizes upon prolonged exposure to air, and acquires a blue or pink color; melts within a 3° range between 172 and 182°; pH (1 in 20 solution) between 4.2 and 5.2.

Solubility—1 g in 3 mL water; freely soluble in chloroform.

Uses—An aliphatic phenothiazine used in the management of the manifestations of *psychotic disorders.* It is *probably effective* for the control of *nausea and vomiting,* for the relief of *apprehension prior to surgery* and for *reducing agitation and tension associated with mild alcohol withdrawal* under supervision. It has the same contraindications, warnings and precautions as other phenothiazines. Because of the close pharmacological similarities among the various phenothiazines, each agent must be considered capable of inducing any untoward reaction common to this group of agents (see page 1181).

It has the same therapeutic applications and limitations as chlorpromazine. Although some of the more serious toxic effects of chlorpromazine have not been encountered with this drug, it should be used with the same degree of caution. See *Chlorpromazine Hydrochloride.*

Dose—*Usual, adult, oral, intramuscular* and *intravenous,* **10** to **200 mg** every 4 to 6 hr. To avoid enhancing the CNS-depressant effect of alcohol the initial dose for the inebriate should not exceed 50 mg. *Usual, pediatric, oral, children 12 yr and older,* **10** to **25 mg** every 4 to 6 hr; *under 12 yr,* dosage not established.

Other Dose Information—Total daily dose ranges from 25 to 300 mg to a maximum of 1 g a day.

Dosage Forms—Injection: 25 and 50 mg/mL; Tablets: 25, 50 and 100 mg.

Promethazine—page 1227.

Rauwolfia Serpentina—page 1018.

Rescinnamine—page 406.

Reserpine—page 1018.

Syrosingopine—RPS-16, page 849.

Thioridazine

10*H*-Phenothiazine, 10-[2-(1-methyl-2-piperidinyl)ethyl]-2-(methylthio)-, Mellaril-S (*Sandoz*); Millazine (*Major*)

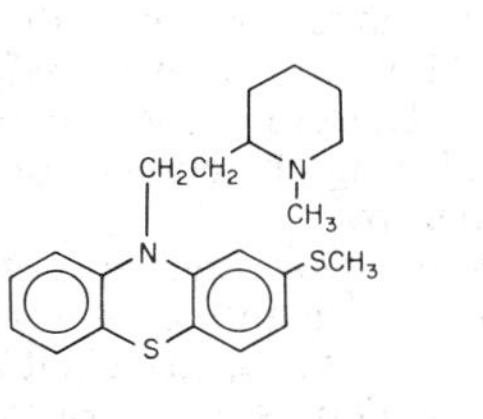

[50-52-2] $C_{21}H_{26}N_2S_2$ (370.57).

Preparation—2-(Methylthio)phenothiazine, which may be prepared by reacting 2-chlorophenothiazine with (methylthio)sodium, is condensed with 2-(1-methyl-1-piperidyl)ethyl chloride with the aid of a dehydrochlorinating agent such as sodamide. US Pat 3,239,514.

Description—Crystals; melts about 73°; pK_a 9.5 (methylamino group).

Solubility—1 g in 6 ml alcohol; practically insoluble in water.

Uses and Dose—See *Thioridazine Hydrochloride.*

Thioridazine Hydrochloride

10*H*-Phenothiazine, 10-[2-(1-methyl-2-piperidinyl)ethyl]-2-(methylthio)-, monohydrochloride; Mellaril (*Sandoz*); Intensol (*Roxane*)

[130-61-0] $C_{21}H_{26}N_2S_2.HCl$ (407.03).

For the structure and preparation of the base, see *Thioridazine.*

Description—White to slightly yellow, granular powder with a faint odor and a very bitter taste; stable in moderate heat, nonhygroscopic and darkens on exposure to light; melts within a range of 3° between 157 and 163°; pH (1 in 100 solution) between 4.2 and 5.2.

Solubility—1 g in 9 ml alcohol or 10 mL of water; freely soluble in chloroform or methanol; slightly soluble in benzene; insoluble in ether.

Uses—A piperidyl-type phenothiazine tranquilizer with central sedative and behavioral effects similar to those of chlorpromazine. It has minimal antiemetic action and produces minimal extrapyramidal stimulation. Sedation and drowsiness are less intense with this drug than with chlorpromazine and related compounds. It is *effective* in the management of manifestations of *psychotic disorders,* for relief of symptoms of *neurotic depressive reactions,* control of moderate to severe *agitation, hyperactivity* or *aggressiveness in disturbed children,* and *possibly effective* in *alcohol withdrawal* syndrome, *intractable pain, psychoneuroses* and *senility.* Half-life appears to be multiphasic with an early phase of 4 to 10 hr and a late phase of 26 to 36 hr; 96 to 99% is bound to plasma protein. The effective plasma level and the relation to clinical improvement remain to be established. The drug is sulfoxidized to mesoridazine and small amounts of sulforidazine; both are pharmacologically active.

Contraindications, warnings and precautions are similar to those for other phenothiazines. Untoward effects, such as extrapyramidal reactions, sedation and drowsiness are less intense and occur less frequently with this drug than with any other phenothiazine. Serious pigmentary retinopathy (decreased visual acuity, brownish color of vision and impaired night vision), a complication attributed only to this drug, may occur with doses in excess of 800 mg a day. Other untoward effects are potentially the same as those for other agents in this chemical class. See page 1181.

Dose—*Adult, usual, initially* **25** to **100 mg** 3 times a day; *maintenance,* **10** to **200 mg** 2 to 4 times a day. For the management of agitation, anxiety, depressed mood, tension, sleep disturbances and fears in *geriatric patients, usual, oral* **25 mg** 3 times a day. Total daily dose ranges from 200 to 800 mg, divided into two to four doses. *Usual, pediatric, children 2 to 12 yr,* **0.5** to a maximum of **3.0 mg/ kg/day,** dosage increased daily until optimum therapeutic effect obtained or the maximum dose reached; *children under 2 yr,* not recommended.

Dosage Forms—Concentrate: 30 and 100 mg/mL; Suspension: 25 and 100 mg/5 mL; Tablets: 10, 15, 25, 50, 100, 150 and 200 mg.

Thiothixene

(*Z*)-9*H*-Thioxanthene-2-sulfonamide, *N,N*-dimethyl-9-[3-(4-methyl-1- piperazinyl)propylidene]-, Navane (*Roerig*)

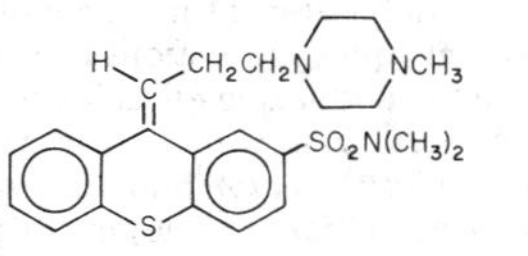

[5591-45-7 and 3313-26-6(*Z*)] $C_{23}H_{29}N_3O_2S_2$ (443.62).

Preparation—2-Chlorobenzoic acid is converted into its 5-dimethylsulfamoyl derivative by successive reaction with chlorosulfonic acid and dimethylamine. The chlorine is then replaced by the phenylthio group by treatment with benzenethiol in the presence of alkali and the resulting 2-phenylthio derivative is cyclized with polyphosphoric acid to form *N,N*-dimethyl-9-oxothioxanthene-2-sulfonamide. Reaction of this compound with [3-(4-methyl-1-piperidyl)propylidene]triphenylphosphorane replaces the oxo oxygen by the appropriately substituted propylidene group to yield thiothixene. US Pat 3,310,553.

Description—White to tan, crystalline powder; practically odorless; very bitter taste; unstable in light; melts about 150° (*cis* or *Z* isomer).

Solubility—Practically insoluble in water; 1 g in 110 of anhydrous alcohol, 2 mL of chloroform or 120 mL of ether; slightly soluble in methanol or acetone.

Uses—A thioxanthene derivative used as an antipsychotic agent in the treatment of *psychotic disorders.* It is also helpful in the management of secondary symptoms of schizophrenia, such as, hallucinations, tension and suspiciousness. Since it is related chemically to the phenothiazines closely, its contraindications, warnings, precautions and adverse reactions are similar to the latter agents. See page 1181 for a detailed discussion of these factors.

Dose—*Usual, adult, oral,* **2** to **5 mg** 2 or 3 times a day; maximum 60 mg a day. Use in children under 12 yr is not recommended because safe conditions for its use have not been established.

Dosage Form—Capsules: 1, 2, 5, 10 and 20 mg.

Thiothixene Hydrochloride

(*Z*)-9*H*-Thioxanthene-2-sulfonamide, *N,N*-dimethyl-9-[3-(4-methyl-1- piperazinyl)propylidene]-, dihydrochloride, dihydrate, Navane Hydrochloride (*Roerig*)

[22189-31-7 and 49746-09-0(*Z*)] $C_{23}H_{29}N_3O_2S_2.2HCl.2H_2O$ (552.57); *anhydrous* [49746-04-5] (516.54). For the structure of the base, see *Thiothixene.*

Preparation—*Thiothixene* is reacted with aqueous HCl and the hydrochloride is crystallized therefrom.

Description—White, or nearly white, crystalline powder; slight odor; affected by light.

Solubility—1 g in 8 mL water, 270 mL anhydrous alcohol, or 280 mL of chloroform, practically insoluble in benzene, acetone or ether.

Uses—See *Thiothixene.*

Dose—*Usual, adult, oral,* **2** to **5 mg** 2 or 3 times a day; *intramuscular,* **4 mg** 2 to 4 times a day; *daily range,* **16** to **30 mg.** Use in children under 12 yr is not recommended because safe conditions for its use have not been established.

Dosage Forms—Injection: 2 mg/1 mL; Oral Solution: 5 mg/mL; Powder for Injection: 5 mg in 2-mL vials.

Trifluoperazine Hydrochloride

10*H*-Phenothiazine, 10-[3-(4-methyl-1-piperazinyl)propyl]-2-(trifluoromethyl)-, dihydrochloride; Stelazine (*SmithKline Beecham*); Suprazine (as the base) (*Major*)

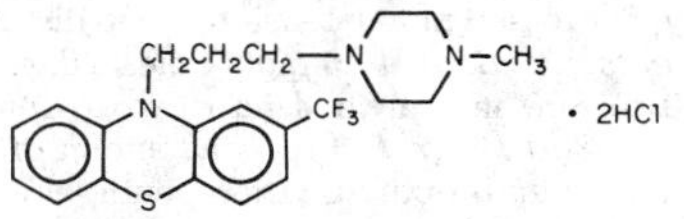

[440-17-5] $C_{21}H_{24}F_3N_3S.2HCl$ (480.42).

Preparation—By the process described for *Triflupromazine Hydrochloride* except that 1-(3-chloropropyl)-4-methylpiperazine is used as the condensing amine in place of (3-chloropropyl)dimethylamine. US Pat 2,921,069.

Description—White to pale-yellow, crystalline powder; practically odorless; bitter taste; melts at about 242° with decomposition. pK_a 8.1 (piperazine).

Solubility—1 g in 3.5 mL water, 11 mL alcohol or 100 mL chloroform; insoluble in ether; protect aqueous solutions from light.

Uses—A piperazine phenothiazine *effective* in the management of the manifestations of *psychotic disorders.* It is possibly effective for the control of *excessive anxiety, tension* and *agitation* seen in *neurosis* or associated with *somatic conditions.* The general profile of pharmacological action is similar to other phenothiazine derivatives. Bioavailability, time to peak effect, metabolism and elimination half-life resemble those for chlorpromazine. Untoward effects such as hypotension, blurred vision and other manifestations of autonomic blockade appear to be less troublesome than with other phenothiazines. Drowsiness is the most common minor untoward effect. Extrapyramidal symptoms occur much more frequently with it than with the dimethylaminopropyl-type phenothiazines. Other warnings, contraindications, precautions and potential adverse effects have been reviewed in detail (see page 1181).

Dose—*Usual, oral, nonhospitalized patients,* **1** to **2 mg** 2 times a day; *hospitalized patients,* **2** to **5 mg** 2 times a day initially, gradually increasing to the optimum level of **15** to **20 mg** a day, although a few patients may require **40 mg** a day or more; *intramuscular,* **1** to **2 mg** every 4 to 6 hr as required. *Elderly patients,* lower doses are usually sufficient; the elderly are more susceptible to hypotension and neuromuscular reactions, observe closely and increase dosage gradually. *Nonpsychotic anxiety,* **1** to **2 mg** 2 times a day; maximum, **6 mg** a day, not to exceed 12 wk. (Doses stated in base equivalents.) *Usual, pediatric, oral, hospitalized children 6 to 12 yr,* **1 mg** 1 or 2 times a day, dosage gradually increased until symptoms controlled; maximum, 15 mg a day.

Dosage Forms (base equivalent)—Injection: 20 mg/10 mL; Concentrate: 10 mg/mL; Tablets: 1, 2, 5 and 10 mg.

Triflupromazine Hydrochloride—see RPS-18, page 1090.

Antianxiety Agents

Antianxiety agents, or more precisely sedative-antianxiety drugs, now have surpassed antibiotics in sales and are the most widely prescribed drugs in the US. Pharmacologically they are sedative-hypnotic in type. Anxiety is a universal human experience; it may permeate one's existence or be an intermittent transient phenomenon. The kinds of internal and external stimuli that can produce anxiety include most events in life. A wide range of sedative-antianxiety drugs is available. For example, certain antihistaminics (diphenhydramine), acetylenic carbinols (ethchlorvynol), monoureides (carbromal), barbiturates (phenobarbital), piperidinediones (methyprylon), propyl alcohol derivatives (meprobamate), benzodiazepines (chlordiazepoxide), etc, have in common the ability to induce various levels of sedation. All antianxiety agents produce mild sedation in doses unlikely to affect adversely the clarity of consciousness and the quality of psychomotor performance. Likewise, many of these drugs exhibit other pharmacological properties, such as hypnotic, muscle relaxant and anticonvulsant actions. For these reasons the antianxiety agents are discussed in Chapter 69 with the conventional sedative and hypnotic agents. They are mentioned here only to recognize their wide use in anxiety and neuroses.

Antidepressants

Antidepressants are drugs which relieve the symptoms of major depressive disorders and may result in an increased output of behavior. For many years, all of the available antidepressants could be divided into two groups on the basis of their pharmacological properties: *tricyclic antidepressants* (imipramine hydrochloride, imipramine pamoate, amitriptyline hydrochloride, amoxapine, desipramine hydrochloride, doxepin, protriptyline hydrochloride and trimipramine) and *monoamine oxidase inhibitors* (MAOIs) (isocarboxazid, phenelzine sulfate and tranylcypromine sulfate). During the past several years, newer agents have become available that do not fit into these groups. Such antidepressants, which are sometimes classified as *second-generation* drugs, include amoxapine, maprotaline, trazodone, fluoxetine and buproprion.

The *tricyclic antidepressant* compounds are more effective, and generally safer, than the monoamine oxidase inhibitors in moderate and severe depression, especially the endogenous type. They also have antianxiety and sedative properties, which make them useful in the treatment of mild depression. In addition, some tricyclic antidepressants (imipramine and to a lesser extent amitriptyline and nortriptyline) are helpful in alleviating enuresis in children and adolescents.

The *MAOIs* are used for symptomatic relief of severe reactive or endogenous depression in hospitalized or closely supervised patients who have not responded to other antidepressant therapy. They are more toxic than the tricyclic antidepressants. Therefore, the tricyclic compounds generally are the initial drugs of choice for patients who require antidepressant therapy.

The *second-generation* antidepressants appear to be as effective as the *tricyclic* antidepressants in the treatment of depression. Also, these agents elicit fewer adverse effects than the *tricyclic* antidepressants. Because of the combination of efficacy with minimum adverse effects, *second-generation* agents are now often the drug of choice for treating depression.

Both tricyclic compounds and MAOIs potentiate central noradrenergic and serotonergic function, although they act through different mechanisms. Tricyclic compounds inhibit the reuptake of norepinephrine and serotonin by neuron terminals. MAOIs block intracellular metabolism of biogenic amines; this results in increased amine concentrations in the neuron terminals.

Several of the *second-generation* compounds have a primary effect to augment serotonin neurotransmission. Although all effective antidepressants acutely enhance central norepinephrine and/or serotonin neurotransmission, such effects occur immediately, whereas clinical improvement requires 2 or more wk of continued therapy. Recent research shows a delayed down regulation of the number of β-adrenergic receptors and decreased ability to increase levels of cAMP by activation of β-adrenergic receptors as well as increased response to α-adrenergic and serotonergic stimulation. Such observations suggest that clinical effectiveness may be produced through adaptations in second-messenger systems.

The antidepressant drugs induce a wide variety of *adverse effects*. The most common of these induced by *tricyclic compounds* include dryness of the mouth, excessive perspiration, constipation, blurred vision, hypotension, drowsiness and weight gain; occasionally, manic episodes, tremors, heart block, tachycardia and other arrhythmias, rashes and facial sweating; rarely, cholestatic jaundice, bone-marrow depression, epileptiform seizures, peripheral neuropathy and photosensitization. Urinary retention, especially in men, also has been reported.

The untoward reactions produced by MAOIs include paradoxical hypertension. This hypertensive crisis is characterized by headache, palpitation, nausea and vomiting and, occasionally, subarachnoid or intracranial hemorrhage. This reaction may be induced by the ingestion of certain kinds of sharp cheese, yeast extracts, broad beans, chicken livers, pickled herring and chocolate. Other adverse reactions include hypotension, restlessness, insomnia, dry mouth, nausea, dizziness, constipation and anorexia; occasionally, flushing, urinary retention, tremors, impotence and paresthesias; rarely, skin rash, hepatitis, tinnitus, muscle spasms and mania.

A uniform spectrum of adverse effects is not seen when comparing all of the agents in the *second-generation* group. However, the subset classified as selective serotonin reuptake inhibitors (fluoxetine hydrochloride and sertraline hydrochloride) show fewer untoward reactions than other antidepressants. The adverse effects of these drugs are mainly gastrointestinal disturbances that manifest as nausea, loose stools or diarrhea.

Special *precautions* should be taken when antidepressants are used with other medications. Patients should avoid all other medications including OTC preparations, unless specifically approved by their physician. They should be advised not to use alcoholic beverages and to limit the amount of caffeine-containing beverages while on these medications.

The *tricyclic* compounds may decrease the effect of anticonvulsant medication, necessitating dosage adjustment. They potentiate the effects of antihistaminics, antimuscarinics and other CNS depressants; they block the antihypertensive effects of clonidine and guanethidine; they alter blood-glucose levels and decrease the effectiveness of hypoglycemic medication. Their effectiveness is reduced by concurrent use of estrogens; their concurrent use with MAOIs should be avoided as a hyperpyretic crisis, severe convulsions and death may occur, and a minimum of 14 days should elapse between the discontinuance of MAOIs and the initiation of tricyclic antidepressant therapy and vice versa. Likewise, their concurrent use with sympathomimetics may result in severe hypertension or hyperpyrexia; and these agents may enhance the possibility of cardiac arrhythmias in patients on thyroid medication. The tricyclic compounds are contraindicated in patients with congestive heart failure, angina pectoris and paroxysmal tachycardia; also, they should be used with caution in patients with urinary retention, glaucoma, diabetes, impaired liver function, asthma and a history of convulsive seizures.

MAOIs potentiate a number of other drugs (barbiturates, insulin, procaine, adrenergic agents, methyldopa, thiazide diuretics, antiparkinson agents, phenothiazines and morphine analgesics); thus, reduced dosage of each agent is necessary if the drugs are used concomitantly. The MAOIs should not be administered with or immediately following other MAOIs or other antidepressants, such as dibenzazepines and phenothiazines. Such combinations can produce a hypertensive crisis, fever, marked sweating, excitation, delirium, tremor, twitching, convulsions, chorea and circulatory collapse. At least 14 days should elapse between discontinuing an MAOI and the institution of another antidepressant or MAOI. A similar period of time should elapse before patients on MAOIs undergo elective surgery. The MAOIs should not be used in patients with cerebrovascular defects or in patients with cardiovascular disease, hypertension or pheochromocytoma.

The safe use of tricyclic compounds or MAOIs during pregnancy or lactation has not been established. These agents should not be used in children under 12 years for the same reason. Also, geriatric, adolescent and black patients on tricyclic compounds usually require reduced dosage; this is thought to be related to slower drug metabolism. Antidepressant drugs are toxic agents and should be employed only with a full knowledge of their precautions and potential adverse effects.

Amitriptyline Hydrochloride

1-Propanamine, 3-(10,11-dihydro-5*H*-dibenzo[*a*,*d*]cyclohepten-5-ylidene)-*N*,*N*-dimethyl-, hydrochloride; Elavil (*MSD*); Amitril (*Parke-Davis*); Emitrip (*Major*); Endep (*Roche*)

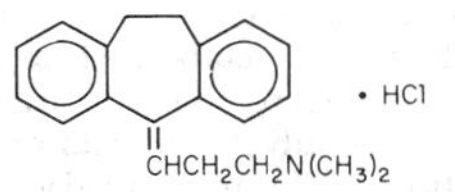

• HCl

$CHCH_2CH_2N(CH_3)_2$

[549-18-8] $C_{20}H_{23}N.HCl$ (313.87).

Preparation—Phthalic anhydride is reacted with phenylacetic acid to form 3-benzylidenephthalide, which is hydrogenated to 2-phenethylbenzoic acid. Conversion to the acid chloride followed by intramolecular dehydrochlorination yields the ketone (5*H*-dibenzo[*a*,*d*]cyclohepten-5-one), which is grignardized with 3-(dimethylamino)propyl chloride. Dehydration of the resulting tertiary carbinol gives amitriptyline which is dissolved in a suitable solvent and converted to the hydrochloride by a stream of HCl. US Pat 3,205,264.

Description—White or practically white, odorless or practically odorless, crystalline powder or small crystals; melts about 197°; pH (1 in 100 solution) 5 to 6; pK_a 9.4.

Solubility—1 g in 1 mL water, 1.5 mL alcohol, 1.2 mL chloroform or 1 mL methanol; insoluble in ether.

Uses—A tricyclic antidepressant chemically and pharmacologically related to imipramine hydrochloride used for the relief of symptoms of *depression*. Endogenous depression is more amenable to therapy than other depressive states. It is useful in the management of depression accompanied by anxiety. It is also useful in temporarily alleviating enuresis in children and adolescents.

It is absorbed rapidly after either oral or parenteral administration; (31 to 61% is bioavailable); peak plasma levels occur within 2 to 12 hr; 96% is bound to plasma proteins. The plasma half-life ranges from 31 to 46 hr; volume distribution is 5 to 10 L/kg; therapeutic plasma levels range from 80 to 200 ng/mL. It is metabolized via the same pathways as other tricyclic antidepressants. At least one active metabolite, nortriptyline, has been identified. Approximately 25 to 50% is excreted in the urine as inactive metabolites within 24 hr; small amounts are excreted in the feces *via* the bile.

Although the incidence of adverse effects appears to be less with this than with other effective antidepressants, drowsiness, xerostomia, tremor, fatigue, weakness, blurring of vision, constipation, urinary retention, edema, tachycardia, orthostatic hypotension, etc, have been observed. Most untoward effects can be controlled by a reduction in dosage. Patients taking large doses over an extended period of time should be watched closely for possible changes in liver and hematopoietic functions. See also page 1188.

Dose—*Usual, adult, oral, initially* **75 mg** a day in divided doses, or **50** to **100 mg** once a day at bedtime; if necessary, the dose may be increased gradually to a total of **150 mg** a day; *adolescent, elderly* or *black patients* may require only **10 mg** 3 times a day and **20 mg** at bedtime; *hospitalized patients* may require 100 mg a day initially, increased gradually to 200 mg a day if necessary, and to as much as 300 mg a day in some patients. *Usual, maintenance,* **50** to **100 mg** a day. *Usual, intramuscular,* **20** to **30 mg** 4 times a day initially. Not recommended for patients under 12 yr.

Dosage Forms—Injection: 10 mg/mL; Tablets: 10, 25, 50, 75, 100 and 150 mg.

Amoxapine

Dibenz[*b, f*][1,4]oxazepine, 2-chloro-11-(1-piperazinyl)-, Asendin (*Lederle*)

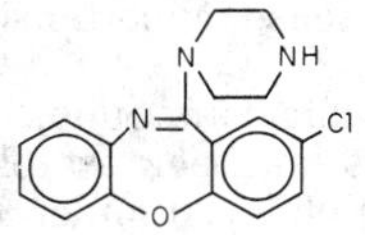

[14028-44-5] $C_{17}H_{16}ClN_3O$ (313.79).

Preparation—See *Helv Chim Acta 50:*245, 1967.

Description—White crystals; melts about 175°.

Solubility—Practically insoluble in water, freely soluble in chloroform; sparingly soluble in acetone or methanol.

Uses—An antidepressant with a mild sedative component. It is used for the relief of *depression* in patients with *neurotic and reactive depressive* disorders as well as *endogenous* and *psychotic depressions.* It also is used for *depression* accompanied by *anxiety and agitation.* The mechanism of its clinical action in man is not understood well. In animals, it reduces the uptake of norepinephrine and serotonin and blocks the response of dopamine receptors to dopamine. It is absorbed rapidly and reaches peak plasma levels in about 90 min. Approximately 90% is bound to plasma proteins; half-life is about 8 hr and it is metabolized almost completely. The major metabolite is active and has a half-life of 30 hr. The metabolites are excreted in the urine as glucuronides. The most frequently encountered adverse effects are drowsiness (14%), dry mouth (14%), constipation (12%) and blurred vision (7%). Renal impairment may develop 3 to 5 days after substantial overdosage. Treatment is the same as that for nondrug renal impairment. Safety and effectiveness in children below the age of 16 have not been established.

Dose—*Adult, oral, initially* **50 mg,** 2 or 3 times a day. Depending upon tolerance, increase dosage by the end of the 1st week (initial 300 mg a day may cause sedation the first few days). Increase above 300 mg/day dose only if it is ineffective for at least 2 wk. *Elderly patients,* **25 mg** 2 or 3 times a day; if not adequate, carefully increase but don't exceed 300 mg/day. *Maintenance,* lowest dose that will maintain remission.

Dosage Form—Tablets: 25, 50, 100 and 150 mg.

Clorazepate Dipotassium—page 1157.

Bupropion Hydrochloride

1-Propanone, 1-(3-chlorophenyl)-2-[(1,1-di-methylethyl)amino]-, hydrochloride; Wellbutrin (*Burroughs Wellcome*)

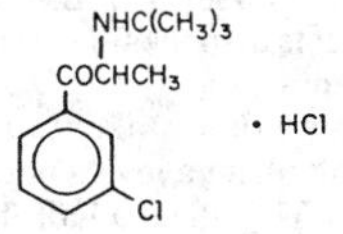

(±) - 2 - (*tert*-butylamino) - 3′ - chloropropiophenone [31677-93-7] $C_{13}H_{18}ClNO.HCl$ (276.22)

Preparation—*m*-Chlorobenzonitirile is reacted with ethyl Grignard reagent in ether to produce *m*-chlorobenzyl ethyl ketone, which is brominated in dichloromethane. The product is reacted with tertiary butyl amine in acetonitrile to yield bupropion base. Treatment of an ethereal solution of the base with dry HCl yields the salt. Ger Offen 2,059,618.

Description—White solid; melts between 233 and 234°.

Solubility—1 g in 3.5 mL water or 5 mL ethanol.

Uses—Related to the phenylethylamines, but chemically unrelated to the other currently used antidepressant agents. Its antidepressant mechanism of action is unknown: it is a relatively weak blocker of monoamine uptake carriers. Bupropion does cause dose-related CNS stimulation. It is indicated for the treatment of major depression and has been used to treat obsessive/compulsive disorder. More than any of the other antidepressant agents, bupropion has been associated with seizures. Approximately 0.4% of patients treated at doses up to 450 mg/day experience seizure episodes. Because of this serious side effect, use of bupropion is contraindicated in patients with seizure disorders, a current or prior diagnosis of bulimia or anorexia nervosa and should be used with extreme caution in patients with other predisposing conditions for seizures, such as a history of head trauma, CNS tumors or concomitant medications which lower seizure threshold. Other significant side effects include, agitation, dizziness, insomnia, psychosis, confusion, constipation, dry mouth and sweating. Peak plasma levels occur within 2 hr of oral administration. The plasma concentrations are approximately 30% of the peak concentration, 6 hr after a single dose. Bupropion is metabolized into several active metabolites and principally excreted in the urine.

Dose—*Usual adult,oral, initially* **200 mg** a day, taken as **100 mg** 2 times a day. If needed, after 3 days the dose can be increased to **300 mg** a day, taken as **100 mg** 3 times a day; maximum, 450 mg a day. As higher doses are associated with risk of seizures, no more than **150 mg** should be taken at one time.

Dosage Form—Tablets: 75 and 100 mg.

Desipramine Hydrochloride

5*H*-Dibenz[*b, f*]azepine-5-propanamine, 10,11-dihydro-*N*-methyl-, monohydrochloride; Norpramin (*Merrell Dow*); Pertofrane (*USV*)

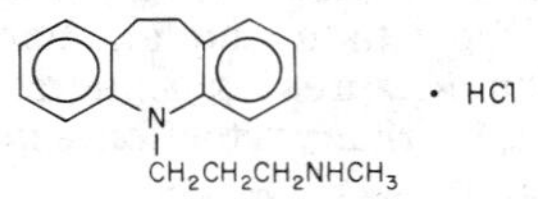

[58-28-6] $C_{18}H_{22}N_2.HCl$ (302.85).

Preparation—Pyrolysis of the methanesulfonate of 4,4′-diaminobibenzyl results in cyclization with formation of 10,11-dihydro-5*H*-dibenz [*b, f*]azepine. This is condensed with *N*-(3-chloropropyl)-*N*-methylbenzylamine in the presence of alkali to form *N*-benzylated desipramine which, following debenzylation through reductive cleavage, is reacted with an equimolar quantity of HCl. Brit Pat 908,788; US Pat 3,454,698.

Description—White to off-white, crystalline powder; odorless; bitter taste; unstable after long exposure to light, heat and air; melts within a 5° range between 208° and 218°; pK_a 10.2 (methylamino).

Solubility—1 g in 12 mL water, 14 mL alcohol, 3.5 mL chloroform or >10,000 mL ether.

Uses—A primary metabolite of imipramine used in the management of *depressive states.* It has pK_as of 1.5 and 10.2. It is absorbed well after oral administration; 69 to 76% is bound to plasma protein. Approximately 60 to 70% is bioavailable. Therapeutic plasma concentrations average 145 ng/mL. The plasma half-life ranges from 14 to 25 hr. Metabolism is *via* the same pathways as other tricyclic compounds. Desipramine is reported to be of benefit in endogenous *depressions* such as *manic depressive reactions,* and *reactive depressions.*

It is contraindicated in patients on MAOI therapy. Since the drug possesses anticholinergic and epinephrine-potentiating properties, it should not be given to patients with glaucoma, urethral or ureteral spasm or those who have had a myocardial infarction within 3 wk. It is also contraindicated in patients with severe coronary heart diseases or with active epilepsy. See page 1188 for a more complete listing of precautions and adverse effects. Although not all those mentioned have been reported for this drug, its pharmacological and chemical similarities suggest it should be suspect.

Dose—*Usual, adult, oral, initially* **75** to **200 mg** a day in divided doses or as a single dose at bedtime; if necessary dose may be increased to a total of 300 mg a day; *adolescent, elderly* or *black patients* may require only **25** to **100 mg** a day in divided doses, to a maximum, if necessary, of 150 mg a day. Not recommended for patients under 12 yr.

Dosage Forms—Capsules: 25 and 50 mg; Tablets: 10, 25, 50, 75, 100 and 150 mg.

Doxepin Hydrochloride

1-Propanamine, 3-(dibenz[*b,e*]oxepin-11(6*H*)-ylidene)-*N,N*-dimethyl-, hydrochloride; Adapin (*Pennwalt*); Sinequan (*Roerig*)

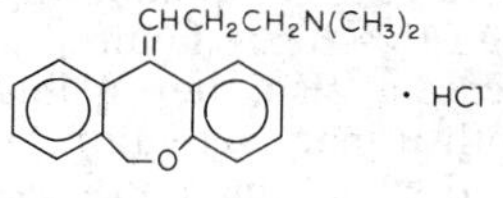

[1229-29-4; 4698-39-9(*E*); 25127-31-5(*Z*)] $C_{19}H_{21}NO.HCl$ (315.84). Doxepin hydrochloride, an (*E*) and (*Z*) geometric isomer mixture, contains the equivalent of not less than 85.0% and not more than 92.0% of $C_{19}H_{21}NO$ (doxepin), calculated on the dried basis. It contains not less than 12.0% and not more than 16.0% of the (*Z*)-isomer, and not less than 72.0% and not more than 78.0% of the (*E*)-isomer.

Preparation—6,11-Dihydrodibenz[*b,e*]oxepin-11-one is prepared from ethyl 2-(bromomethyl)benzoate and phenol to produce 2-(phenoxymethyl)-benzoic acid which is converted to 6,11-dihydrobenzo[*b,e*]oxepin-11-one by cyclization with polyphosphoric acid. This latter compound is transformed to 11-[3-(dimethylamino)propyl]-6*H*-dibenz[*b,e*]oxepin-11-ol through Grignard reaction with 3-(dimethylamino)propyl chloride. Dehydration of the alcohol with mineral acid yields the base which is reacted with HCl.

Description—White, odorless, bitter, crystalline substance; decomposes slowly in light, nonhygroscopic up to 75% RH, and relatively stable in heat; melts about 188°; pK_a 8.

Solubility—1 g in 1 mL water, 2 mL alcohol or 10 mL chloroform.

Uses—A dibenzoxepin derivative that is a psychotherapeutic agent with antianxiety and antidepressant properties. It is recommended for the management of anxiety and/or depressive states associated with psychoneurosis, psychosis, alcoholism and organic disease. It apparently is absorbed well from the gastrointestinal tract, but only 13 to 45% is bioavailable; volume distribution approximates 9 to 33 L/kg; therapeutic plasma levels range from 30 to 150 ng/mL. The plasma half-life is 8 to 24 hr. Metabolism appears to be *via* the same pathways as other tricyclic antidepressants; its *N*-demethylated metabolite is pharmacologically active.

Adverse reactions, such as dry mouth, blurred vision, constipation, tachycardia, hypotension and drowsiness, are usually mild and tend to subside as therapy is continued. Other side effects infrequently encountered include extrapyramidal symptoms, gastrointestinal disturbances, increased sweating, weakness, dizziness, fatigue, edema, paresthesia, flushing, chills, tinnitus, photophobia, decreased libido, rash and pruritus. It is contraindicated in patients with glaucoma or a tendency to urinary retention. The drug should not be administered to patients either on MAOIs or who have been on such agents within the prior 2 wk. The drug also may potentiate the depressant effect of alcohol. Its use in the pregnant patient or in children under 12 yr is not recommended, because safe conditions for its use have not been established.

Dose—*Usual, adult, oral,* **25 mg** 3 times a day; or up to **150 mg** once a day at bedtime; maximum, up to 300 mg a day. Dosage as low as **25** to **50 mg** a day suffices for some patients. Dilute oral concentrate with 120 ml water, milk or fruit juice prior to administration. Not recommended for patients under 12 yr.

Dosage Forms (base equivalent)—Capsules: 10, 25, 50, 75, 100 and 150 mg; Oral Concentrate: 10 mg/mL.

Fluoxetine Hydrochloride

(±)-3-(p-trifluoromethylphenoxy)-*N*-methyl-3-phenylpropylamine; Prozac *(Dista)*

F_3C–C_6H_4–O–$CHCH_2CH_2NHCH_3$ (with C_6H_5 on CH)

[56296-78-7] $C_{17}H_{18}F_3NO.HCl$ (345.79)

Preparation—β-(Dimethylamino)propiophenone is reduced by diborane to the corresponding secondary alcohol. The hydroxyl group is substituted by cholorine using hydrochloric acid in chloroform. The product is reacted with sodium 4-trifluoromethylphenoxide in a Williamson synthesis to produce the dimethyl analog of the desired compound. Mono-demethylation is accomplished by successive reaction with BrCN and KOH. German patent 2,500,110.

Description—Off-white crystalline solid.

Solubility—1 g in 70 mL water.

Uses—A phenylpropylamine-derived antidepressant agent. Although in some ways its pharmacology resembles that of other antidepressants which enhance serotonergic activity (eg, clomipramine, trazodone), fluoxetine is somewhat unique because it is a highly selective presynaptic serotonin uptake blocker which has little or no effects on other neurotransmitters. Although its effects on serotonin have not been proved to be responsible for its antidepressant activity, it almost certainly is involved. Fluoxetine is used as treatment for major depression. There is some evidence to suggest that patients with atypical depression, a history of poor response to prior antidepressant treatment, chronic depression or a younger age of depression onset are more likely to respond to fluoxetine than to tricyclic antidepressants. However, these findings need to be confirmed. The lack of anticholinergic activity associated with fluoxetine use is an important advantage over the tricyclic antidepressants, as such activity often causes very annoying side effects. Fluoxetine also suppresses appetite which may be useful in the treatment of obese patients with affective disorders. Besides its use in the treatment of major depression, fluoxetine also has been used in patients with bipolar disorder, obesity, eating disorders (eg, anorexia nervousa, bulimia nervosa), obsessive compulsive disorder and panic attacks. Although fluoxetine has a wide margin of safety and lacks most of the adverse effects of the other antidepressants, it can have undesirable actions on nervous and GI systems that cause discontinuance in 15% of patients. These effects include anxiety, nervousness, insomnia, dizziness, headaches and nausea. It is well absorbed from the GI tract (60 to 80%) and peak plasma levels occur 4 to 8 hours after administration. The elimination half-life of fluoxetine is approximately 2 to 3 days (range of 1 to 9 days) and the half-live of its active metabolite, norfluoxetine, is 7 to 9 days (range of 3 to 15 days); thus, adverse effects may disappear slowly after discontinuing the drug. Fluoxetine is metabolized principally in the liver and excreted in the urine.

Dose—*Usual, initially* **20 mg** a day taken in the morning. If increased dose is necessary, the medication should be taken 2 times a day, once in the morning and once at noon; maximum should not exceed **80 mg** a day.

Dosage Forms—Capsules: 20 mg; Liquid: 20 mg/5mL.

Imipramine Hydrochloride

5*H*-Dibenz[*b, f*]azepine-5-propanamine, 10,11-dihydro-*N,N*-dimethyl-, monohydrochloride; Tofranil *(Geigy)*; Janimine *(Abbott)*; SK-Pramine *(SmithKline)*; Tipramine (as the base) *(Major)*; *(Various Mfrs)*

(tricyclic ring; N–$CH_2CH_2CH_2N(CH_3)_2$ · HCl)

5-[3-(Dimethylamino)propyl]-10,11-dihydro-5*H*-dibenz[*b, f*]azepine monohydrochloride [113-52-0] $C_{19}H_{24}N_2.HCl$ (316.87).

Preparation—Dimerization of *o*-nitrotoluene is affected with sodium ethoxide and an oxidizing agent to produce 1,2-bis(*o*-nitrophenyl)ethane. This compound is reduced to the corresponding diamine, 2-(*o*-aminophenethyl)aniline hydrochloride, which is heated to yield 10,11-dihydro-5*H*-dibenz[*b, f*]azepine, which is condensed with 3-chloro-*N,N*-dimethylpropylamine by refluxing in benzene solution with the aid of sodamide. The basic constituents are then extracted with aqueous HCl and the extract is rendered alkaline and extracted with ether. After drying, the solvent is evaporated and the residue is vacuum-distilled to yield the base. Treatment with alcoholic HCl produces the hydrochloride. US Pat 2,554,736.

Description—White to off-white, odorless crystalline powder; melts about 172°; pK_a 9.4.

Solubility—1 g in about 5 mL water, about 10 mL alcohol or about 15 mL acetone; insoluble in ether or benzene.

Uses—A dibenzazepine-derivative tricyclic antidepressant effective in depressive syndromes, particularly those associated with *manic-depressive* and *involutional psychoses*, and to a lesser degree, with *reactive depressions*. It may be useful as temporary adjunctive therapy in *reducing enuresis* (bed wetting) in children aged 6 yr and older, after excluding possible organic causes. It has a pK_a of 9.5. It is absorbed completely from the gastrointestinal tract. Peak plasma levels occur within 1 to 2 hr after oral administration and 30 min after intramuscular administration. Approximately 90% is bound to plasma proteins. Plasma half-life ranges from 8 to 16 hr. It is metabolized *via* the same pathways as other tricyclic compounds; desipramine, its *N*-monodemethylated metabolite, is pharmacologically active. About 40% is excreted in the urine as inactive metabolites within 24 hr and 70% within 72 hr; small amounts are excreted in the feces *via* the bile.

Side effects are common, especially in patients over 65 yr. Most of these occur in patients receiving more than 200 mg a day and include hypotension, seizures, tremors, diplopia, involuntary staring, visual hallucinations and agitation. Because of possible congenital malformations associated with the use of this drug, it should not be used during the first trimester of pregnancy. It should not be used in patients on MAOIs. For more detailed information on precautions and adverse effects, see page 1188.

Dose—*Usual, adult, oral, initially* **75 mg** a day in divided doses, if necessary increased to a total of 150 mg a day (dosages over 200 mg a day are not recommended for outpatients); *adolescent, elderly* or *black patients* may require only **30** to **40 mg** a day initially and generally not over 100 mg a day; *hospitalized patients* may require 100 mg a day initially, increased gradually to 200 mg a day if necessary, and to as much as 250 to

300 mg a day if no response occurs after 2 wk. *Usual maintenance* dose, for *outpatients*, **50 to 150 mg** a day. *Intramuscular, initially* up to **100 mg** a day, in divided doses. Not recommended for children under 6 yr. In *childhood enuresis*, an oral dose of **25 mg,** once a day 1 hr before bedtime, may be tried in children 6 yr and older; after 1 wk the dose may be increased, if necessary, to 50 mg nightly in children under 12 yr and to 75 mg in children over 12 yr.

Dosage Forms—Injection: 25 mg/2 mL; Tablets: 10, 25 and 50 mg.

Imipramine Pamoate

Tofranil-PM (*Geigy*)

5-[3-4(Dimethylamino)propyl]-10,11-dihydro-*dH*-dibenz[*b, f*]-azepine compound (2:1) with 4,4-methylene-bis[3-hydroxy-2-naphthoic acid] [10075-24-8] $(C_{19}H_{24}N_2)_2.C_{23}H_{16}O_6$ (949.20).

Description—Yellow powder; tasteless; odorless.

Solubility—Insoluble in water; soluble in alcohol, ether or chloroform.

Uses—For relief of symptoms of depression. See *Imipramine Hydrochloride.*

Dose—*Usual, adult, oral, initially* the equivalent of **75 mg** of the hydrochloride a day; optimum response usually is obtained with the equivalent of **150 mg** of the hydrochloride daily, usually given at bedtime. Maximum dose, the equivalent of 200 mg of the hydrochloride a day. Should not be used in children of any age because of the increased potential for acute overdosage due to the high potency of the capsule dosage forms.

Dosage Form (hydrochloride equivalent)—Capsules: 75, 100, 125 and 150 mg.

Isocarboxazid

3-Isoxazolecarboxylic acid, 5-methyl-, 2-(phenylmethyl)hydrazide; Marplan (*Roche*)

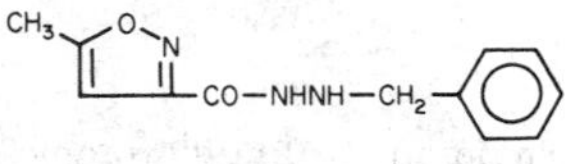

[59-63-2] $C_{12}H_{13}N_3O_2$ (231.25).

Preparation—Acetonylacetone is reacted with nitric acid to form 5-methyl-3-isoxazolecarboxylic acid which is converted to its ethyl ester. The ester is reacted with hydrazine hydrate to form the acid hydrazide which is condensed with benzaldehyde to yield the 2-benzylidenehydrazide. This is reduced in anhydrous ether with lithium aluminum hydride to isocarboxazid. US Pat 2,908,688.

Description—White or nearly white, crystalline powder; slight, characteristic odor; stable in dry air; melts about 107°; pK_a 10.4.

Solubility—1 g in 2000 mL water, 83 mL alcohol, 2 mL chloroform or 58 mL ether.

Uses—A MAOI recommended only for *depressed* patients who are refractory to tricyclic antidepressants or electroconvulsive therapy and depressed patients in whom tricyclic antidepressants are contraindicated. As with other MAOIs, patients treated with this drug should be kept under close medical supervision. Untoward effects are those characteristic of MAOIs in general. See page 1188 for additional information on adverse reactions, precautions and a discussion on the use of this with other drugs. It should be discontinued at the first sign of jaundice or impaired liver function. It is contraindicated in patients with a history of liver disease or impaired liver function.

Dose—*Usual, initially* **30 mg** a day as a single dose or in divided doses; *maintenance*, **10** to **20 mg** a day. If a favorable response is not obtained in 3 or 4 wk, continued administration is unlikely to be beneficial. Use in patients under 16 yr is not recommended since safety or efficacy in this group has not been established.

Dosage Form—Tablets: 10 mg.

Methylphenidate—page 1234.

Maprotiline Hydrochloride

9,10-Ethanoanthracene-9(10*H*)-propanamine, *N*-methyl-, hydrochloride; Ludiomil (*Ciba*)

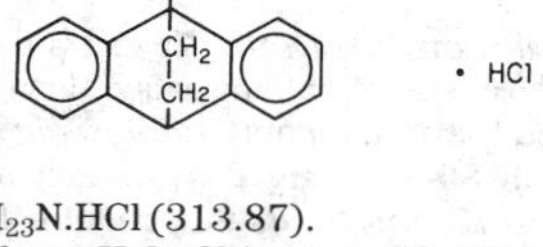

[10347-81-6] $C_{20}H_{23}N.HCl$ (313.87).

Preparation—Refer to *Helv Chim Acta 52:* 1385, 1969.

Description—White crystals; melts about 230°; pK_a 10.5.

Uses—For the treatment of patients with *depressive neurosis (dysthymic disorder)* and *manic-depressive* illness, depressed type (major depressive disorder). It is also effective for the relief of *anxiety associated with depression.* It belongs to the chemical series, dibenzobicyclo-octadienes. It has been postulated that it acts by potentiation of central adrenergic synapses by blocking reuptake of norepinephrine at nerve endings. This action is thought to account for its antidepressant action. The mean time to peak effect is 12 hr; half-life of elimination averages 51 hr; and steady state levels induced by 50 mg 3 times a day averages 238 ng/mL. Adverse reactions are similar to those observed with tricyclic antidepressants (see page 1188). Safety and effectiveness in children under the age of 18 have not been established.

Dose—*Adult, oral, mild to moderate depression,* **75 to 150 mg** a day; elderly, **25 mg** a day; maximum, **225 mg** a day. *Severe depression,* **100 to 150 mg** a day; maximum, **300 mg** a day.

Dosage Form—Tablets: 25, 50 and 75 mg.

Nortriptyline Hydrochloride

1-Propanamine, 3-(10,11-dihydro-5*H*-dibenzo[*a,d*]cyclohepten-5-ylidene)-*N*-methyl-, hydrochloride; Aventyl Hydrochloride (*Lilly*); Pamelor (*Sandoz*)

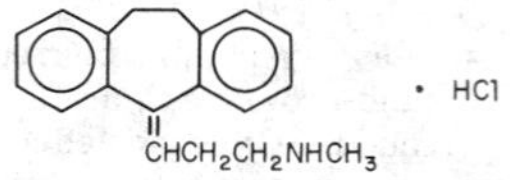

[894-71-3] $C_{19}H_{21}N.HCl$ (299.84).

Preparation—10,11-Dihydro-5*H*-dibenzo[*a,d*]cyclohepten-5-one, which may be prepared as described under *Cyproheptadine Hydrochloride* (page 1229), is reacted with an alkali metal derivative of *N*-methyl-2-propynylamine and the product hydrolyzed to form the carbinol. The acetylenic bond is then saturated by hydrogenation and the resulting carbinol dehydrated to yield nortriptyline (base). Reaction of the base with hydrogen chloride produces the hydrochloride.

Description—White to off-white powder; slight, characteristic odor; melts within a range of 3° between 215° and 220°. pK_a is 9.73.

Solubility—1 g in 90 mL water, 30 mL alcohol, 20 mL chloroform or 10 mL methanol.

Uses—A dibenzocycloheptene-derivative tricyclic antidepressant drug which is the active metabolite of amitriptyline. It is more likely to be effective in endogenous depressions than in other depressive states. Peak plasma levels occur within 7 to 18.5 hr after oral administration; about 90% is bound to plasma protein. Therapeutic plasma levels range from 50 to 150 ng/mL. Plasma half-life ranges from 18 to 35 hr after oral administration. Approximately 30% is excreted in the urine in 24 hr, and small amounts are excreted in the feces *via* the bile. Pharmacological studies indicate it inhibits the activity of such diverse agents as histamine, 5-hydroxytryptamine and acetylcholine. It also increases the pressor effect of norepinephrine but blocks the pressor response of phenethylamine. Studies suggest that the drug interferes with the transport, release and storage of catecholamines. Pharmacological studies further show that it has a combination of stimulant and depressant properties. In some clinical studies, the drug appeared to cause excitement or increased agitation in some patients and to have sedative effects in others. Similar effects have been observed with other drugs of this general type.

Untoward side effects include dryness of the mouth, drowsiness and a confusional state. Tremulousness and orthostatic hypotension also have been reported. Since drugs of this type can produce a sinus tachycardia and a first-degree heart block, they should be used with great caution in patients with vascular disease. The drug should not be used in combination with a MAOI. The potentiation of adverse effects can be serious, even fatal. It is advisable to discontinue the MAOI for at least 10 to 21 days before starting treatment with this drug. It should be used with caution in patients with glaucoma or urinary retention. Epileptiform seizures may be associated with its use. Therefore, patients on this drug should be supervised closely during the initial phase of treatment. See page 1188 for additional information on the adverse reactions and precautions for tricyclic antidepressants.

Dose—*Usual, adult, oral,* **25 mg** 3 or 4 times a day (doses above 150 mg a day are not recommended); *adolescent, elderly* or *black patients,* **30** to **50 mg** a day, in divided doses. Not recommended for children since safety and effectiveness in pediatric age group have not been determined.

Dosage Forms (base equivalent)—Capsules: 10, 25, 50 and 75 mg; Solution: 10 mg/5 mL.

Pemoline—page 1234.

Phenelzine Sulfate

Hydrazine, (2-phenylethyl)-, sulfate (1:1); Nardil (*Parke-Davis*)

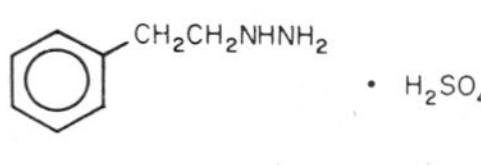

Phenethylhydrazine sulfate (1:1) [156-51-4] $C_8H_{12}N_2.H_2SO_4$ (234.27).

Preparation—Phenethyl alcohol is reacted with thionyl chloride to give phenethyl chloride which is then added to hydrazine hydrate to yield phenethylhydrazine hydrochloride. Reaction with sodium hydroxide liberates the base which is then reacted with sulfuric acid to form the sulfate. US Pat 3,314,855.

Description—White to yellowish white powder; characteristic odor; subject to oxidation and must be protected from heat and light; melts about 166°; pH (1 in 100 solution) 1.4 to 1.9.

Solubility—1 g in about 7 mL water; practically insoluble in alcohol, chloroform or ether.

Uses—A MAOI effective in depressed patients clinically characterized as "atypical," "nonendogenous" or "neurotic." Such patients often have mixed anxiety and depression and phobic or hypochondriacal features. Its use in endogenous depression is less convincing. It rarely should be the first drug used; it should be used in patients who fail to respond to the more commonly used antidepressant drugs. Maximal effects appear only after 1 to 2 wk of therapy.

It is contraindicated in elderly, debilitated patients, or in patients with a cerebrovascular defect, cardiovascular disease, hypertension, history of headache, pheochromocytoma or a history of liver disease. It is a potent MAOI. Since this enzyme is distributed widely throughout the body, diverse adverse effects can be expected. These are summarized in the introductory statement (page 1188). Physicians should know and be alert for the more serious toxic effects which can be induced by these agents.

Dose—*Usual, adult, oral, initially* **15 mg** 3 times a day, increased with patient tolerance to **60 mg** a day and, if necessary, to **90 mg** a day; *maintenance,* **15 mg** a day or every 2nd day. Not recommended for patients under 16 yr since safety and effectiveness in this age group have not been established.

Dosage Form—Tablets: 15 mg.

Protriptyline Hydrochloride

5*H*-Dibenzo[*a,d*]cycloheptene-5-propanamine, *N*-methyl-, hydrochloride; Vivactil (*MSD*)

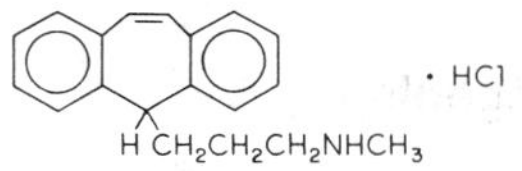

[1225-55-4] $C_{19}H_{21}N.HCl$ (299.84).

Preparation—5*H*-Dibenzo[*a,d*]cyclohepten-5-one, prepared as described under *Cyproheptadine Hydrochloride* (page 1229), is reduced to the corresponding carbinol which is then converted to the 5-chloromethyl compound (I). Reaction with the Grignard reagent of (3-chloropropyl)dimethylamine converts I into the 5-(3-dimethylamino)propyl compound which, on monodemethylation with cyanogen bromide and hydrolysis, yields protriptyline. Reaction with HCl gives the hydrochloride.

Description—White to yellowish powder; odorless or has not more than a slight odor; a bitter taste; reasonably stable in light, air and heat under the usual prevailing temperature conditions; melts about 168°; pH (1 in 100 solution) 5.0 to 6.5.

Solubility—1 g in 2 mL water, 4 mL alcohol, 2.3 mL chloroform or 2 mL methanol; practically insoluble in ether.

Uses—A tricyclic (dibenzocycloheptene) antidepressant drug useful in the management of mental *depression* in patients under close medical supervision. It also increases psychomotor activity; this property enhances its use in withdrawn and anergic patients. It is absorbed completely from the gastrointestinal tract. Peak plasma levels occur within 24 to 30 hr. About 92% is bound to plasma proteins. Therapeutic plasma levels range from 70 to 170 ng/mL. Metabolism and excretion are by the same pathways as other tricyclic antidepressants. The drug is eliminated slowly; 50% is excreted in the urine as metabolites within 16 days. Very little is excreted in the feces. It also possesses anticholinergic properties and, hence, should not be used in patients with pyloric obstruction, glaucoma or urinary retention.

Tachycardia and postural hypotension occur more frequently with it than with other antidepressant drugs; hence, patients with cardiovascular disorders and elderly patients should be observed closely for these untoward effects. This agent also is contraindicated in patients taking any of the MAOI antidepressants, such as nialamide, isocarboxazid, tranylcypromine or phenelzine. Antidepressants of this type reverse the effects of antihypertensive drugs such as guanethidine and should not be used concurrently with them. Adverse reactions attributable to antidepressant drugs are numerous and varied. The similar pharmacological properties of these agents suggest that each of these reactions should be considered when therapy with these agents is contemplated. See page 1188 for additional information on precautions and adverse reactions for this group of agents.

Dose—*Usual, adult, oral,* **15** to **40 mg** a day divided into 3 or 4 doses, increased to **60 mg** a day if necessary; *adolescent, elderly* or *black patients,* **5 mg** 3 times a day, increased gradually if necessary but in elderly patients the cardiovascular response should be closely monitored if the daily dose exceeds 20 mg. Not recommended for use in children because safety and effectiveness in this age group have not been established.

Dosage Form—Tablets: 5 and 10 mg.

Sertraline Hydrochloride

Naphthalenamine, (1*S-cis*)- 4-(3,4-dichlorophenyl)-1,2,3,4-tetrahydro-*N*-methyl-, hydrochloride Zoloft (*Roerig*)

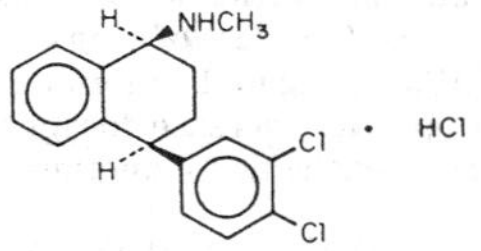

[79559-97-0] $C_{17}H_{17}Cl_2N.HCl$ (342.70)

Preparation—4-(3,4-Dichlorophenyl)-3,4-dihydro-1(2*H*)-naphthalenone, methylamine, and titanium tetrachloride are reacted to form a Schiff base, which then is reduced with sodium borohydride to produce a mixture of geometric isomers. The *cis* and *trans* isomers are separated via chromatography on silica gel. The purified base is dissolved in ether and converted to the salt with HCl gas in ether. *J Med Chem 27:*1508, 1984.

Uses—Chemically unrelated to other antidepressants although it has a three-ring structure. Like fluoxetine, its ability to block CNS neuronal uptake of serotonin likely is responsible for its therapeutic activity. Sertraline is relatively selective for the serotonin uptake carrier and has only very weak effects on norepinephrine and dopamine uptake. The lack of anticholinergic activity usually makes sertraline better tolerated than the tricyclic antidepressants. It has been approved for treatment of depression with an unlabeled use in the treatment of obsessive-compulsive disorder. Due to potentially fatal interactions, it should not be used with MAOIs. Although generally better tolerated than the MAOIs and tricyclic antidepressants, sertraline can cause nausea, diarrhea/loose stools, dyspepsia, tremor, dizziness,insomnia, anorexia, sweating, dry mouth and male sexual dysfunction. Approximately 15% patients given sertraline will discontinue treatment due to adverse effects. The peak plasma concentrations occur 4.5 to 8.4 hr after a single dose of sertraline. The elimination half-life is about 26 hr. Sertraline undergoes extensive first-pass metabolism and is metabolized principally to *N*-desmethyl-sertraline.

Dose—*Usual, adult, oral, initially* **50 mg** once a day. If needed, dosage can be increased to **200 mg** a day taken once a day.

Dosage Form—Tablets: 50 and 100 mg.

Tranylcypromine Sulfate

Cyclopropanamine, *trans*-(±)-2-phenyl-, sulfate (2:1); Parnate (*SmithKline Beecham*)

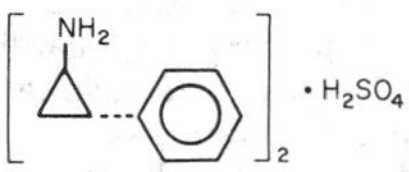

[13492-01-8] $(C_9H_{11}N)_2.H_2SO_4$ (364.46).

Preparation—Styrene is reacted with ethyl diazoacetate to form ethyl 2-phenylcyclopropanecarboxylate. Saponification of this ester with sodium hydroxide and subsequent acidification yields a mixture of the *cis* and *trans* forms of the corresponding acid and the *trans* form is isolated by fractional crystallization from water. The *trans* acid is then subjected to the Curtius reaction whereby carboxyl is transformed successively through the acyl chloride, acyl azide, and isocyanate states to yield finally the base. Reaction with a ½ equimolar quantity of H_2SO_4 gives the sulfate. US Pat 2,997,422.

Description—White, crystalline powder; either odorless or a faint, cinnamaldehyde-like odor; slightly acid taste; stable in light, heat and air; melts with decomposition at 218°; pK_a 8.2.

Solubility—1 g in 25 mL water; very slightly soluble in alcohol or ether; practically insoluble in chloroform.

Uses—A nonhydrazine MAOI used in the treatment of depression. It is probably effective for the symptomatic relief of severe reactive or endogenous depression in hospitalized or closely supervised patients who have not responded to other antidepressant therapy. It is contraindicated in any patient over 60 yr or in patients with confirmed or suspected cerebrovascular defects, cardiovascular disorders or pheochromocytoma; it should not be used concomitantly with other MAOIs or sympathomimetic agents. In addition, patients on this drug should not eat cheese or other foods with a high tyramine content.

Adverse effects most commonly observed include postural hypotension, dizziness, restlessness, insomnia, weakness, drowsiness, anxiety, agitation, manic symptoms, nausea, vomiting, diarrhea, abdominal pain, constipation, anorexia, dryness of the mouth, blurred vision, chills, tachycardia, edema, palpitation, impotence and headaches not associated with a rise in blood pressure. A number of deaths have resulted in patients on this drug; death usually is attributed to intracranial hemorrhage. Severe reactions may appear without warning and develop rapidly. This drug, like other antidepressants, should be used only under close medical supervision. See page 1090 for additional information on precautions, warnings and adverse reactions induced by this class of drugs.

Dose—*Usual, initially* **10 mg** in the morning and afternoon each day for 2 wk; if no response appears, increase dosage to **20 mg** in the morning and **10 mg** in the afternoon each day for another week; *maintenance,* **10** to **20 mg** a day.

Dosage Form (base equivalent)—Tablets: 10 mg.

Trazodone Hydrochloride

1,2,4-Triazolo[4,3-*a*]pyridin-3(2*H*)-one, 2-[3-[4- (3-chlorophenyl)-1-piperazinyl]propyl]-, monohydrochloride; Desyrel (*Mead Johnson*)

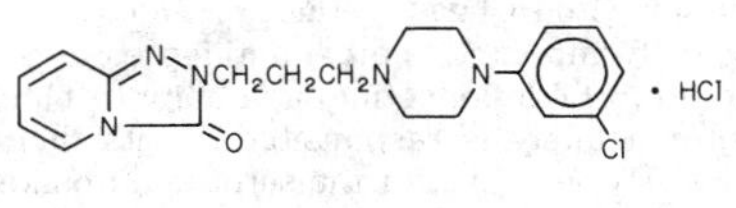

[25332-39-2] $C_{19}H_{22}ClN_5O.HCl$ (408.33).

Preparation—Semicarbazide and 2-chloropyridine are condensed with loss of water and ammonia to form 1,2,4-triazolo[4,3-*a*]pyridin-3(2*H*)-one, which on treatment with 1-(3-chlorophenyl)-4-(3-chloropropyl)piperazine (I) and sodamide, yields trazodone. I is prepared from 1-(3-chlorophenyl)piperazine with 1-bromo-3-chloropropane. See US Pat 3,381,009.

Description—White crystals; melts about 90°; pK_a (in 50% ethanol) 6.14.

Solubility—Sparingly soluble in water or alcohol; soluble in chloroform.

Uses—A triazolopyridine derivative for the treatment of *depression.* The mechanism responsible for its antidepressant action in man is not fully understood. In animals, it selectively inhibits serotonin uptake by brain synaptosomes and potentiates the behavioral changes induced by 5-hydroxytryptophan. The drug is absorbed well after oral administration without selective localization in any tissue. Peak plasma levels occur in 1 hr when taken on an empty stomach and 2 hr when taken with meals. Elimination is biphasic; initial phase, half-life, 3 to 6 hr is followed by a slower phase, half-life, 5 to 9 hr. Clearance from the body is variable in some patients; the drug may accumulate in plasma. It may be arrhythmogenic in some patients. Consequently, it is not recommended for use during the initial recovery phase of myocardial infarction. The most frequently encountered adverse effects include blurred vision, dry mouth, dizziness/light-headedness, drowsiness, nausea/vomiting, fatigue and headache. Various endocrine disturbances, such as decreased or increased libido, impotence, priapism, retrograde ejaculation, early menses and missed periods also have been reported. Safety and effectiveness in children below the age of 18 have not been established.

Dose—*Adults, oral, initially* **150 mg a day,** increased by **50 mg a day** every 3 or 5 days. *Maximum, outpatients,* **400 mg a day;** *inpatients,* **600 mg a day** in divided doses.

Dosage Form—Tablets: 50, 100, 150 and 300 mg.

Trimipramine Maleate

5*H*-Dibenz[*b,f*]azepine-5-propanamine, 10,11-dihydro-*N,N*,β-trimethyl-, (*Z*)-2-butenedioate (1:1); Surmontil (*Wyeth*)

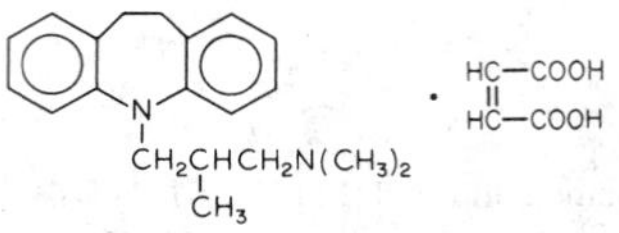

[521-78-8] $C_{20}H_{26}N_2.C_4H_4O_6$ (410.51).

Preparation—As per imipramine, page 1191, except that the side chain is attached using 3-dimethylamino-2-methylpropylchloride. See *Compt Rend 252:* 2117, 1961.

Description—White crystals; bitter taste; slight numbing characteristic; melts about 143°; pK_a 7.72 (dimethylamino).

Solubility—Slightly soluble in water or alcohol; freely soluble in chloroform.

Uses—To relieve the symptoms of *depression. Endogenous depression* is more likely to be alleviated than other depressive states. Clinical studies suggest that it is about equally as effective as amitriptyline in mild depression and less effective than amitriptyline in severely depressed patients. It has a pK_a of 8.0; peak plasma concentrations occur 2 hr after a single oral dose; 95% is bound to plasma protein; half-life is about 23 hr. In view of the pharmacological similarities among tricyclic antidepressants, adverse effects may be similar to those listed on page 1188. The drug is not recommended for use in children, since the safety and effectiveness have not been established.

Dose—*Adult, outpatient, oral, initially* **75 mg a day** in divided doses, increased to **150 mg a day.** Dosages over 200 mg are not recommended. *Adult, hospitalized patients, oral, initially* **100 mg a day** in divided doses; this may be increased to **200 mg a day.** *Maximum,* **250 to 300 mg a day.** *Adolescent* and *elderly patients: initially* **50 mg a day** with gradual increments up to **100 mg a day.** *Maintenance,* lowest dose that will maintain remission, usually **50** to **150 mg a day.**

Dosage Form—Capsules: 25, 50 and 100 mg.

Psychotherapeutic Combinations

Some examples of psychotherapeutic combinations (with mg/unit provided) are as follows:

Meprobamate and Benactyzine Hydrochloride [Deprol (*Wallace*)]—400 and 1 mg, respectively.

Perphenazine and Amitriptyline Hydrochloride [Etrafon (*Schering*); Triavil (*MSD*); Talazil (*Major*)]—2 or 4 and 10, 25 and 50 mg, respectively.

Psychogenic Agents

Psychogenic agents are drugs that consistently induce temporary abnormalities of the mental state of human subjects or the behavior of animals. This definition serves to separate the psychogenic agents from the many drugs which may produce similar effects when taken in excessive amounts or when given to susceptible individuals. Psychogenic drugs produce major disturbances of sensory perception and alter the ability of the subject to organize perceptions and thoughts for the purpose of adaptative behavior. In so doing they produce subjective effects, such as hallucinations and alterations in gross behavior, which bear some similarity to certain features of the major psychoses. For example, marihuana usually only produces mood changes, but in high doses it produces psychological syndromes that can be characterized as psychoses. Intensive investigation is directed toward elucidating those features which are common to both "clinical" and "experimental" psychoses. There are no recognized therapeutic applications for these agents. Consequently, they are listed in Schedule I of the Controlled Substances Act and are not available for prescription use. Nevertheless, they can be obtained for clinical and experimental research purposes. These agents are subjected to intensive abuse, a practice which only can be condemned. For a detailed discussion of the abuse potential of these agents see Chapter 47.

Cannabis [Marihuana]—The dried flowering tops of the pistillate plants of *Cannabis sativa* (Fam *Moraceae*). Uses: No rational or indispensable therapeutic use in modern medicine. Formerly used in migraine, insomnia, neuralgia and other syndromes. Currently, the active principles of the drug are under investigation for use as antiepileptic, anticancer and immunosuppressive agents. The use of this drug as an intoxicant and euphoric agent has increased sharply in recent years. It frequently is smoked in the form of cigarettes. It produces aggressive tendencies in some individuals and stimulates the senses so that external stimuli are magnified and distorted. Cannabis causes habituation but, unlike morphine, not true addiction.

Lysergic Acid Diethylamide [*d-N,N*-Diethyllysergamide; LSD-25; LSD [50-37-3] $C_{20}H_{25}N_3O$ (323.42).—Closely related structurally (page 405) to ergonovine, one of the principal alkaloids of ergot, but it is distinctly different in its physiological actions. It is an extremely potent agent; as little as 1 μg per kg will induce a hallucinogenic effect. Persons who have taken the drug experience a mental intoxication which has many of the features common with the perceptual disturbances of some cases of schizophrenia. Persons under the influence of LSD experience ataxia, tremors, auditory and visual hallucinations, depersonalization and disturbances in space, olfactory and taste perception, but retain the knowledge that these unusual effects are induced by the drug. Contact with reality is not lost, except after massive doses. Repeated administration of the drug produces serious mental disturbances in some individuals.

The first effects from an oral dose appear within ½ hr, reach a peak intensity in 1½ hr and disappear within 8 hr. Recovery is usually complete, except for some residual depression which may persist for as long as 24 hr after taking the drug. Tolerance to the drug develops within 3 to 7 days after repeated administration. When tolerance has developed a 4-fold dosage increase fails to evoke the hallucinatory syndrome.

LSD should be considered, at least for the present, a tool for the study of "experimental psychoses." The indiscriminate use of the agent cannot be condemned too severely.

Mescaline [3.4.5-Trimethoxyphenethylamine [54-04-6] $C_{11}H_{17}NO_3$ (211.25).—Knowledge of this drug psychosis dates back to antiquity, since, as the principal alkaloid of peyote, the dried flowering tops of the cactus *Lophophora Williamsii* Coulter, it has been used by various American Indian tribes for religious purposes. Interest in the drug stems from its use as an experimental tool for the investigation of schizophrenia and other psychotic states, and for the study of visual hallucinations. It also has been used as an adjunct to psychotherapy in depth interviews.

When it is given orally or intravenously to normal subjects in doses of 5.0 to 7.0 mg/kg, it causes unusual psychic effects and visual hallucinations. Diffuse anxiety is one of the early symptoms. Other symptoms include sympathomimetic autonomic effects, hyperreflexia of the limbs, static tremors and vivid hallucinations which are usually visual and consist of brightly colored lights, geometric designs, animals and, occasionally, human images; color and space perception is often impaired but, otherwise, the sensorium is normal and insight is retained. An extreme anxiety state may develop in some schizophrenic patients given this drug, and the hallucinations in others may be sexual in character. The effects induced by a single full dose appear within 1 hr and persist for about 12 hr. In some respects, the psychic changes are similar to those caused by LSD. Psychoses induced by this drug are of academic interest only and the drug has no therapeutic application.

Bibliography

Antipsychotics

Deutch AY, Moghaddam B, Innis RB *et al:* Mechanisms of action of atypical antipsychotic drugs. Implications for novel therapeutic strategies for schizophrenia. *Schizophrenia Res 42:* 121, 1991.

Ereshefsky L, Tran-Johnson TK, Watanabe MD: Pathophysiologic basis for schizophrenia and the efficacy of antipsychotics. *Clin Pharm 9:* 682, 1990.

Levinson DF: Pharmacologic treatment of schizophrenia. *Clin Ther 13:* 326, 1991.

Reynolds GP: Developments in the drug treatment of schizophrenia. *Trends Pharmacol Sci 13:* 118, 1992.

Ryan PM: Epidemiology, etiology, diagnosis, and treatment of schizophrenia. *Am J Hosp Pharm 48:* 1271, 1991.

Antidepressants

Caldecott-Hazard S, Schneider LS: Clinical and biochemical aspects of depressive disorders: III. Treatment and controversies. *Synapse 10:* 141, 1992.

de Jonghe F, Swinkels JA: The safety of antidepressants. *Drugs 43(suppl 2):* 40, 1992.

Kasper S, Fuger J, Moller JJ: Comparative efficacy of antidepressants. *Drugs 43(suppl 2):* 11, 1992.

Nutt DJ, Glue P: Clinical pharmacology of anxiolytics and antidepressants: A psychopharmacological perspective. *Pharm Ther 44:* 309, 1989.

Schatzberg AF: Recent developments in the acute somatic treatment of major depression. *J Clin Psychiatry 53(3, suppl):* 20, 1992.

CHAPTER 72

Analgesic, Antipyretic and Anti-inflammatory Drugs

Glen R Hanson, DDS, PhD

Professor of Pharmacology
College of Pharmacy and School of Medicine, University of Utah
Salt Lake City, UT 84112

Analgesics are agents which relieve pain by elevating the pain threshold without disturbing consciousness or altering other sensory modalities. Antipyretics are drugs which reduce elevated body temperature. Certain analgesics, aminopyrine and phenylbutazone, also possess antirheumatic and anti-inflammatory properties; such substances, as well as gold compounds, are used in the treatment of arthritis and other inflammatory conditions. Drugs which exhibit one or more of these actions are considered in this chapter.

Despite the fact that pain is a universal experience of all mankind and everybody appreciates its aversive properties, attempts to define this term have not proved entirely satisfactory. Pain has been defined in psychological language as a particular type of sensory experience distinguished by nerve tissue from sensations such as touch, pressure, heat and cold. Since there are several types of pain (bright, dull, aching, pricking, cutting, burning, etc) and many causes (injury, body derangements or disease), it is apparent that this definition is incomplete. Furthermore, it now is agreed generally that pain involves a large psychological component that depends on perception. Thus, it must be concluded that pain cannot be defined, except as one defines it introspectively.

All persons in good health have the ability to perceive pain. The point at which sensory stimuli are perceived as being noxious and unpleasant is referred to as the "pain threshold." If it is raised, more stimuli are required before pain is experienced, if it is lowered, less stimuli induce the pain experience. Many factors such as sex, circulatory change, skin temperature, sweating, carbon dioxide tension, anxiety, fear, emotion, etc, alter the pain threshold. Consequently, it is not the same for everyone and can even vary in the same individual. Thus, data obtained from laboratory and clinical studies on the effect of drugs on pain threshold are difficult to interpret.

A mechanism by which some analgesic drugs obtund pain (raise the threshold) has been based on the discovery of opiate receptors in selected portions of the central nervous system (Pert CB, Snyder SH: *Science 179:* 1011, 1973) and the subsequent identification of an endogenous substance from brain with properties similar to morphine (Hughes J: *Brain Res 88:* 295, 1975). Drugs which activate certain opiate receptors can be very potent analgesics.

Opiate receptors are located (1) in the *medial thalamus* which processes deep, chronic, burning pain that is most susceptible to relief by narcotic analgesics, (2) in the brain stem's *vagus nuclei* where coughing is triggered and (3) in *Layers I and II* of the spinal cord at the point where the afferent nerves which carry pain perception first synapse. Interestingly, the greatest concentration of opiate receptors is found in the *amygdala*, that part of the limbic system which plays a major role in regulating emotions. These receptors bind morphine and related narcotic analgesic drugs, as well as the narcotic antagonist naloxone, and account for the pharmacological profile of action of these drugs.

Based on the assumption that there is no reason why the body would have receptors for narcotic drugs unless it produces some narcotic-like substance of its own, pharmacologists John Hughes and Hans W Kosterlitz at the University of Aberdeen in Scotland isolated (from pig brain) and identified such material (*Nature 258:* 577, 1975), which they called *enkephalins.* Two of the identified brain peptides differed only in the *N*-terminal amino acid, one peptide being methionine and the other leucine. The methionine-enkephalin is tyrosine-glycine-glycine-phenylalanine-methionine, while leucine-enkephalin is tyrosine-glycine-glycine-phenylalanine-leucine.

Endorphins (a generic name contracted from endogenous and morphine, and used for all native brain peptides with opiate-like activity) probably diminish pain intensity by modulating the so-called pain threshold, the point at which one begins to perceive a stimulus as painful. Naloxone, an opiate antagonist on the other hand, tends to increase one's sensitivity to pain. These observations have not only markedly increased understanding of the mechanism by which narcotic analgesics obtund pain, but also have provided an explanation for the antitussive and euphoric action of these drugs as well as an insight into how tolerance and addiction develops. More importantly, perhaps, this research has resulted in the development of a number of opioid analgesics with diverse pharmacological actions.

The available opioid analgesics are derivatives of five chemical groups (phenanthrenes, phenylheptylamines, phenylpiperidines, morphinans and benzomorphans). Pharmacologically, these opiates and nonopiates differ significantly in activity. Some are strong agonists (morphine); others are moderate to mild agonists (codeine). In contrast, some opiate derivatives exhibit mixed agonist- antagonist activity (nalbuphine), whereas others are opiate antagonists (naloxone). Table **1** classifies selected opiate and nonopiate analgesics and antagonists based on their agonist, agonist-antagonist or antagonist properties.

Many drugs used to relieve pain are not analgesics. The general anesthetics obtund pain by interfering with consciousness, the local anesthetics prevent pain by blocking peripheral nerve fibers, the antispasmodics relieve certain kinds of pain by relaxing smooth muscle and the adrenal corticoids relieve pain associated with rheumatoid arthritis by an anti-inflammatory action. These drugs are considered elsewhere.

Many of the drugs described in this section come under the control of the *Comprehensive Drug Abuse Prevention and Control Act of 1970.* This law, commonly referred to as the "*Controlled Substances Act,*" is designed to regulate the distribution of all drugs with abuse potential as designated by the Drug Enforcement Administration, Department of Justice (Chapter 110).

Morphine is the prototype of the opioid analgesics, all of which have similar actions on the central nervous system (CNS). Moreover, they have overlapping clinical usefulness. They are indicated in the management of *acute pain, chronic pain, severe pain of acute myocardial infarction, obstetric analgesia, preanesthetic medication, pulmonary edema, cough* (see Chapter 56), *gastrointestinal* and *urinary tract disorders* (see Chapter 53).

Agents used principally for symptomatic relief of pain may for convenience in presentation be divided into four groups: opiate analgesics, analgesics which also have antipyretic and/or antiinflammatory action, gold compounds (to treat pain associated with arthritis) and "other drugs" used to treat pains associated with a variety of unrelated medical conditions.

Table 1—Chemical and Pharmacological Classification of Selected Opiate and Nonopiate Analgesics and Antagonists

Chemical group	Strong agonists	Mild to moderate agonists	Mixed agonist-antagonist	Antagonists
Phenanthrene	Morphine	Codeine	Nalbuphine (Nubain)	Nalorphine[a] (Nalline)
	Hydromorphone (Dilauded)	Oxycodone (Percodan)		
	Oxymorphone (Numorphan)	Hydrocodon (Hycodan)		Naloxone (Narcan)
Phenyl heptylamines	Methadone (Dolophine)	Propoxyphene (Darvon)		
Phenylpiperidines	Meperidine (Demerol)			
	Fentanyl (Sublimaze)			
Morphinans	Levorphanol (Levo-Dromoran)		Butorphanol (Stadol)	Levallorphan[a] (Lorfan)
Benzomorphans			Pentazocine (Talwin)	

[a] Not a pure antagonist.

The drugs considered in this section are classified according to this scheme.

Opiate Analgesics

The opium group of narcotic drugs are among the most powerfully acting and clinically useful drugs producing depression of the CNS. Drugs of this group are used principally as analgesics, but possess numerous other useful properties. Morphine, for example, is used to induce sleep in the presence of pain, check diarrhea, suppress cough, ease dyspnea and facilitate anesthesia.

Unfortunately, morphine also depresses respiration. In addition, it can increase nonpropulsive intestinal spasms but decreases the propulsive motility of the small and large intestines and diminishes biliary, pancreatic and intestinal secretions. The consequences of these actions is a period of relative atony causing a delay in the passage of bowel contents and an increase in stool viscosity. Also, it causes nausea and vomiting in some individuals and may induce cutaneous pruritus. These and other actions of morphine and related compounds tend to limit their usefulness. If these agents are given over a long period of time, tolerance to the analgesic effect develops so that the dose must be increased periodically to obtain equivalent pain relief.

Tolerance and physical dependence develop, which, combined with euphoria, results in excessive use and addiction by those patients who are susceptible. For these reasons, it is important that morphine and its derivatives be taken only as directed by the physician (never in greater dose, more often or longer than prescribed) and never used for pain when some other type of analgesic is satisfactory. Since drowsiness and decreased alertness are not uncommon, the patient taking any of these drugs usually should avoid tasks that require intact reflexes, coordination and mental alertness.

The opiate analgesics generally are *contraindicated* in patients with myxedema, Addison's disease and hepatic cirrhosis. Such patients are especially sensitive to these agents. Consequently, respiratory depression, stupor and even coma may result from relatively small doses of the narcotics. Since opiates decrease ventilation, which causes hypercapnia and progresses to cerebrovascular dilatation and increased intracranial pressure, they should be used with caution in head injuries, cerebral edema and delirium tremens. These agents also should be used with caution in patients with cardiac arrhythmias, chronic ulcerative colitis and impaired kidney function. Moreover, narcotic analgesics cross the placental barrier; hence, newborn infants whose mothers have been administered such analgesics during labor should be observed closely for signs of respiratory depression and treated for narcotic overdosage if necessary. Individuals sensitive to a particular narcotic agent, or group of agents, should avoid these drugs.

The analgesic and depressant effects of these agents provide the basis for a number of *interactions* with other drugs. Alcohol, antihistamines, muscle relaxants, antipsychotics, tricyclic antidepressants or sedative-hypnotics may interact with opiates to intensify their overlapping actions, such as respiratory depression and anticholinergic effects. Particular caution is necessary if monoamine oxidase inhibitors (MAOIs) are administered concurrently with narcotic analgesics because of intensification of action (use of meperidine in patients treated with MAOIs has produced severe and occasionally fatal reactions). Doses of the opiate analgesics should be adjusted to avoid these enhanced reactions.

The combined use of propoxyphene and orphenadrine has been reported to cause mental confusion, anxiety and tremors. Although clinical impressions regarding the seriousness of this problem differ widely, the problem can be avoided by using alternative analgesic and anticholinergic drugs. Further, anticholinergics, such as atropine, can reverse partially the biliary spasms induced by opiates, but add to the gastrointestinal and urinary tract effects of opiates. Consequently, severe constipation and urinary retention can occur during intensive anticholinergic-analgesic therapy.

The preparations of opium and its alkaloids are numerous and for convenience are divided into three groups: opium preparations, opium alkaloids and semisynthetic opium alkaloids.

Opium and its preparations exhibit analgesic and narcotic effects which directly are proportional to their morphine content. Traditionally, opium is employed more frequently in the form of tinctures for diarrhea and dysenteries.

Diacetylmorphine—see RPS-18, page 1101.

Diacetylmorphine Hydrochloride—see RPS-18, page 1101.

Opium

Gum Opium; Crude Opium; Raw Opium; Thebaicum; Meconium

The air-dried milky exudate obtained by incising unripe capsules of *Papaver somniferum* Linné or its variety *album* De Candolle (Fam *Papaveraceae*). It yields not less than 9.5% of anhydrous morphine.

History—As a medicinal drug it has been known and cultivated for many centuries, but it was not until the investigations of Sertüner, published in 1817, that it was known that the drug contained certain definite principles now called *alkaloids*.

Dioscorides, in the 2nd century, was the first writer to discuss opium and its uses at length. He gave the recipe for a preparation called *diacodion*, which is the prototype of the formerly official syrup of poppies. Paracelsus used opium extensively in the 15th century and referred to it as the "stone of immortality." Van Helmont, early in the 17th century, used opium so freely that he was referred to as Doctor Opiatus. Sydenham, a little later in the same century, praised opium as the most valuable gift of God to man.

The principal opium exporting countries have been: Turkey, Iran, Yugoslavia and India. The Turkish and Yugoslavian products are nearly alike in their physical properties: color, odor and consistency. Iranian and Indian opiums, while closely resembling each other, differ from the former in physical properties—they are darker and have a somewhat different odor and consistency. There also is a marked difference between the two groups in the amounts of the principal opium alkaloids as shown in Table **2**.

Constituents—It owes its activity to the narcotic alkaloids; 25 have been found in the various kinds of opiums, and several more have been suspected but their existence has not been confirmed. Three acids occur combined with the alkaloids—*viz*, meconic, lactic and sulfuric acids. Also present are *meconin* [$C_{10}H_{10}O_4$], pectin, glucose, mucilage,

Table 2—Alkaloidal Content of Opiums[a]

Exporting country	% morphine	% narcotine	% codeine	% papaverine	% thebaine
Turkey	11–12	3–4	0.8–1.4	1–1.5	1.0–1.5
Yugoslavia	13–15	3	1.1–1.5	1–1.5	0.8–1.2
Iran	9.5–10.5	5–6	2.5–4	2–2.5	3–4
India	10–11	···	2.5–3.5	0.8	0.5–1

[a] *Note*—For medicinal preparations only Turkish or Yugoslav opium is used.

caoutchouc, wax and odorous, fatty and coloring matters. The known alkaloids are tabulated and classified on pages 400 to 406.

Description—More or less rounded, oval, brick-shaped or elongated, somewhat flattened masses, usually about 8 to 15 cm in diameter and weighing about 300 g to 2 kg each. Externally, it is pale olive-brown or olive-gray having a coarse surface and covered with a thin coating consisting of fragments of poppy leaves and, at times, with fruits of a species of *Rumex* adhering from the packing. It is more or less plastic when fresh, becoming hard or tough on storage. Internally, it is reddish brown and coarsely granular. It has a very characteristic odor and a very bitter taste.

Uses—It owes its chief pharmacological effects to its morphine content, other alkaloids not being present in sufficient amount to modify significantly the morphine type of action. Thus, it has many of the same uses as morphine, but the latter drug nearly always is preferred, inasmuch as it can be administered in a variety of ways. The average adult dose of opium is 60 mg, taken orally. This is the equivalent of 6 mg of morphine. Like morphine, this drug has *analgetic* and *narcotic* effects. It acts as an *antiperistaltic* agent by causing spasm of the bowel musculature and preventing propulsive movements. Traditionally, it is used for *diarrheas* and *dysenteries* rather than morphine. It produces *sedation* and *sleep*. It also controls *cough* and *dyspnea*. Thus, it has a variety of therapeutic uses in medicine and surgery.

Caution—Opium, and all opium derivatives and related synthetic compounds, are listed in *Schedule II* of the *Controlled Substances Act* (Chapter 110). It should not be dispensed except upon the presentation of a physician's prescription. See *Morphine*.

Powdered Opium is opium dried at a temperature not exceeding 70° and reduced to a very fine powder; yields 10.0 to 10.5% of anhydrous morphine. It may contain any of the diluents, with the exception of starch, permitted for powdered extracts under *Extracts* (page 1543). *Description:* Light brown to moderate yellowish brown, consisting chiefly of yellowish brown to yellow, more or less irregular and granular fragments of latex, varying from 15 to 150 μm in diameter; a few fragments of strongly lignified, thick-walled, 4- to 5-sided or narrowly elongated, epidermal cells of the poppy capsule; very few fragments of tissues of poppy leaves, poppy capsules and, occasionally, *Rumex* fruits. In addition there will be the microscopic characteristics of the diluent if any has been used in the preparation of the powder. *Uses:* A pharmaceutical necessity for *Paregoric*. See *Opium* and *Morphine*.

Paregoric [Camphorated Opium Tincture USP XVI; Paregoric Elixir; Tinctura Opii Benzoica; Tinctura Thebaica Benzoica] yields, from each 100 mL, 35 to 45 mg of anhydrous morphine. *Preparation:* Macerate powdered opium (4.3 g), anise oil (3.8 mL), benzoic acid (3.8 g), and camphor (3.8 g) for 5 days, with occasional agitation, in a mixture of diluted alcohol (900 mL) and glycerin (38 mL). Then filter, and pass enough diluted alcohol through the filter to obtain 950 mL of total filtrate. Assay a portion of this filtrate as directed in the USP, and dilute the remainder with a sufficient quantity of diluted alcohol containing, in each 100 mL, 0.4 mL of anise oil, 400 mg of benzoic acid, 400 mg of camphor and 4 mL of glycerin, to produce a solution containing, in each 100 mL, 40 mg of anhydrous morphine. *History:* This preparation was originated by Professor LeMort of the University of Leyden about 1715. It was official in the 1721 edition of the London Pharmacopaeia as *Elixir Asthmaticum*, which was changed to *Elixir Paregoricum*, meaning soothing elixir, in 1746. It also has been known as *Tinctura Camphorae Composita* and *Tinctura Opii Benzoica*, and the formula has changed in minor details many times since its introduction into medicine. *Alcohol Content:* 44 to 46%. *Uses:* An *antidiarrheal agent* and mild *anodyne* in *cough, nausea* and *abdominal pains*. It should never be used to quiet restless infants, as a habit may be induced. It contains 0.4% of opium. Paregoric is listed in *Schedule III* of the *Controlled Substances Act;* hence, it only can be obtained on a prescription order (either oral or written) of a licensed practitioner. *Dose: Usual, adult, oral,* 5 to 10 mL 1 to 4 times a day; *children,* 0.25 to 0.5 mL/kg 1 to 4 times a day.

Opium Alkaloids

The pharmaceutically important opium alkaloids commonly are subdivided into two chemical groups: the isoquinoline derivatives which are, as a general rule, antispasmodic drugs, such as papaverine and narcotine (see RPS-18, page 842) and the phenanthrene derivatives described in this section, such as morphine and codeine, which are analgesic and narcotic. (For a more detailed classification of the opium alkaloids, see page 400.) The Narcotic Act of 1956 required that all heroin in the hands of pharmacists, physicians, veterinarians, hospitals, etc, be surrendered to the federal government. Presently, heroin is under *Schedule I* of the *Controlled Substances Act*.

Morphine

History—Morphine was the first alkaloid discovered. In the 17th and 18th centuries many attempts were made to separate from opium the active ingredient. Preparations thought to represent these active principles, but were really extracts, were employed in medicine under the name of *Magisterium Opii*. Bucholz was the first to endeavor to obtain a crystalline product from opium. About 1800 a number of learned apothecaries of the time devoted their attention to the separation of the suspected active drug. One of these apothecaries, Derosne, succeeded in isolating narcotine in 1803, and the following year Seguin read a paper to the Institute of France describing the isolation of a substance which is now recognized as morphine. He did not publish his paper however, until 1814 and in 1806, Friedrich William Adam Sertüner, an apothecary of Einbeck, Germany, announced the separation of a basic crystalline substance which existed in opium in combination with a special acid. He later published, in 1817, the results of further investigation in which he named the substance *morphium* and described it as a *vegetable alkali*. Liebig, in 1831, assigned to it the formula $C_{34}H_{36}N_2O_6$, which was later modified by Laurent to the present formula, $C_{17}H_{19}NO_3$ (285.33).

It was only after almost 100 years of intensive research by many able chemists that the correct structural formula (page 401), which adequately explains the chemical transformations of morphine, could be proposed. Final confirmation of this structure came with the successful total synthesis of morphine in 1952.

Preparation—Several processes are in use. In all or nearly all of them the morphine and most of the other opium alkaloids are extracted from the opium with water alone or with slightly acidulated water. In one of the processes, the extract, after concentration, is neutralized, a solution of calcium chloride added and the mixture filtered and further concentrated. Crude morphine hydrochloride crystallizes and is purified by precipitation with ammonia and recrystallized as the sulfate or hydrochloride. In another process the concentrated water extract is mixed with alcohol and made alkaline with ammonia. The morphine, being but slightly soluble in dilute alcohol, separates while the greater part of the other alkaloids remain in solution. The crude morphine so obtained is purified by repeated crystallization as the sulfate or hydrochloride and reprecipitation if necessary in the presence of alcohol.

Description—*Monohydrate:* colorless or white, shining, rhombic prisms, fine needles or a crystalline powder; darkens on exposure to air; a saturated aqueous solution is alkaline to litmus; melts with decomposition about 255°.

Solubility—*Monohydrate:* 1 g in about 5000 mL water (1100 mL boiling water), 210 mL alcohol (98 mL boiling alcohol), 1220 mL chloroform, about 6500 mL ether or 100 mL lime water; insoluble in benzene; readily soluble in solutions of fixed alkali or alkaline earth hydroxides from which it is reprecipitated by ammonium chloride or sulfate.

Uses—An *analgesic, adjunct to anesthesia, antitussive* and *nonspecific antidiarrheal* agent. It is a strong analgesic, alters the psychological response to pain and suppresses anxiety and apprehension. It is the drug of choice for the treatment of pain associated with myocardial infarction and for dyspnea associated with acute left ventricular failure and pulmonary edema. It is used in small to moderate doses to relieve constant dull pain, and in moderate to large doses to alleviate intermittent, sharp pain of traumatic or visceral origin. Although effects may begin earlier, maximal analgesic effect occurs about 20 min after intravenous injection, 50 to 90 min after subcutaneous injection and 30 to 60 min after intramuscular injection. Analgesia persists for approximately 4 hr but, in some patients, it may be as short as 2.5 hr or as long as 7 hr.

Although it has played a dominant and controversial role in *preanesthetic* medication, it generally is agreed that it is of particular value when pain is present preoperatively, in selected types of cardiac surgery and in poor-risk patients in general. It is an effective antitussive agent, but because of its erratic absorption after oral administration and its dependence liability, it should be used as an *antitussive* agent only when cough is associated with severe pain and cannot be controlled by antitussives having less potential for abuse. This drug and other opiates, such as paregoric, are the most effective and prompt-acting *nonspecific antidiarrheal* agents. They act by enhancing tone in long segments of the longitudinal muscle and inhibiting propulsive contraction of both circular and longitudinal muscle. They are used to treat acute, self-limited diarrhea.

When administered orally, it is absorbed rapidly but incompletely and metabolized equally rapidly to the glucuronide. Thus, the plasma levels after this route are usually only 1/5 to 1/3 those obtained after parenteral injection. The half-life of morphine in plasma or serum during the first 6 hr is between 2 and 3 hr; the serum half-life, between 6 and 48 hr after intravenous administration, ranges from 10 to 44 hr. Approximately 35% of the drug is bound, primarily to the albumin fraction. After parenteral administration 70 to 80% is excreted during the first 48 hr with 60% as conjugated morphine. Following oral administration, only about 60% of a given dose is excreted; this probably reflects the incomplete absorption from the gastrointestinal tract.

For a review of untoward effects, contraindications, interactions with other drugs and precautions see introductory statement.

Overt symptoms of *overdosage* include coma, pinpoint pupils and depressed respiration. Shock, decreased body temperature and pulmonary edema may occur. Treatment includes establishing a patent airway and ventilating the patient. If significant respiratory depression occurs, a suitable narcotic antagonist, such as naloxone, should be administered. Other supportive measures should be applied as indicated.

Morphine is a *Schedule II* drug under the *Controlled Substances Act.*

Dose—See *Morphine Sulfate* below.

Morphine Hydrochloride—see RPS-18, page 1101.

Morphine Sulfate

Morphinan-3,6-diol, 7,8-didehydro-4,5-epoxy-17-methyl-, (5α,6α)-, sulfate (2:1) (salt), pentahydrate; (*Various Mfrs*)

[6211-15-0] $(C_{17}H_{19}NO_3)_2.H_2SO_4.5H_2O$ (758.83); *anhydrous* [64-31-3] (668.76).

For the structural formula of morphine, see page 401.

Description—White, feathery, silky crystals, as cubical masses of crystals, or as a white crystalline powder; odorless and when exposed to air gradually loses water of hydration; darkens on prolonged exposure to light.

Solubility—1 g in 16 mL of water, 570 mL of alcohol, 1 mL of water at 80° or about 240 mL of alcohol at 60°; insoluble in chloroform or ether.

Uses—See *Morphine* and *Morphine Sulfate Injection.*

Dose—*Usual, adult, oral,* **10** to **30** mg every 4 hr or as directed by a physician. *Extended-release:* **15** or **30 mg** every 8 to 12 hr. *Adults, rectal,* **10** to **20 mg** every 4 hr.

Dosage Forms—Oral Solution: 10, 20, and 100 mg/5 mL; Rectal Suppositories: 5, 10, 20, and 30 mg; Extended-Release Tablets: 30 mg; Soluble Tablets: 10, 15 and 30 mg.

Morphine Sulfate Injection

A sterile solution of morphine sulfate in water for injection. It may contain suitable antimicrobial agents.

Preparation—Solutions of morphine sulfate at a pH above 7 decompose quickly even at room temperature. At a pH of less than 5.5 no change is reported in a 1% solution heated for 1 hr. The pH should be between 2.5 and 6.0. Sterilization should be conducted with a minimum of heat.

Uses—Indicated for the relief of severe pain. It is effective in the control of postoperative pain as well as for relieving preoperative apprehension. Its most important actions are on the brain, especially its higher functions. An initial transitory stimulation is followed by depression of the brain, its higher functions and medullary centers. The reflexes and spinal functions usually are stimulated. It affects perception in such a way that the patient is more tolerant to discomfort and pain. In addition it appears to interfere with pain conduction. It depresses the respiratory center, stimulates the vomiting center, depresses the cough reflex, constricts the pupils, increases the tone of the gastrointestinal and genitourinary tracts and produces mild vasodilation.

It is contraindicated in bronchial asthma, respiratory depression or idiosyncrasy to the drug. Overdoses may cause respiratory depression, coma and death. The drug should be used with caution in extreme ages (infants and elderly) as well as in the debilitated patient, or in patients with increased intracranial pressure, toxic psychoses, myxedema or prostatic hypertrophy. Untoward reactions may include allergic reactions, nausea, vomiting, constipation, urinary retention, depression, delirium and convulsions. Morphine Sulfate Injection is a *Schedule II* drug under the *Controlled Substances Act.*

Dose—*Usual, adult, subcutaneous* or *intramuscular,* **5** to **20 mg/70 kg;** *children,* **0.1** to **0.2 mg/kg**. *Intravenous,* **4** to **10 mg** administered very slowly. Morphine should not be administered intravenously unless a narcotic antagonist is available immediately. *Epidural,* **5 mg** in the lumbar region may provide adequate pain relief for 24 hr; if adequate pain relief is not achieved within 1 hr, further doses of 1 to 2 mg may be given; do not exceed 10 mg in 24 hr.

Dosage Form—Injection: 1, 2, 4, 5, 8, 10 and 15 mg/mL.

Morphine Tartrate—see RPS-18, page 1101.

Codeine

Morphinan-6-ol, (5α,6α)-7,8-didehydro-4,5-epoxy-3-methoxy-17-methyl-, monohydrate, Methylmorphine

[6059-47-8] $C_{18}H_{21}NO_3.H_2O$ (317.38); *anhydrous* [76-57-3] (299.37).

For the structural formula, see page 401.

History—Isolated from opium by the French chemist Robiquet in 1832, and the name given it by the discoverer is derived from the Greek word meaning poppy capsules.

Preparation—While some codeine is obtained from opium directly the quantity is not sufficient to meet the extensive use of this alkaloid as a very valuable medicinal agent. Much more codeine is used than morphine. This need is met by making it by partial synthesis from morphine. The process involves methylating the phenolic OH of the latter with phenyltrimethylammonium hydroxide. Dry morphine is dissolved in a solution of potassium hydroxide in absolute alcohol, the methylating agent added and the solution heated. After cooling, water is added, the solution acidified with sulfuric acid, the dimethylaniline product separated and the alcohol removed by distillation. Treatment with caustic soda solution precipitates the codeine, while any unreacted morphine is held in solution by the sodium hydroxide. The crude codeine is purified by crystallization as the sulfate.

Description—Colorless or white crystals, or a white, crystalline powder; effloresces slowly in dry air and is affected by light; when rendered anhydrous by drying at 80° it melts within a 2°-range between 154 and 158°; sublimes (anhydrous) under reduced pressure; pH (saturated aqueous solution) about 9.8.

Solubility—1 g in 120 mL water, 2 mL alcohol, about 0.5 mL chloroform, 50 mL ether or about 20 mL benzene. When heated in an amount of water insufficient for complete solution, it melts to oily drops which crystallize on cooling.

Incompatibilities—Precipitated from its aqueous solution by most *alkaloidal precipitants* but not by sodium, potassium or ammonium carbonate or sodium bicarbonate. Aqueous solutions are sufficiently alkaline to precipitate other less soluble alkaloids from solutions of their salts. Ammonia may be liberated from *ammonium salts.* See also page 399.

Uses—May be viewed as a weakened morphine, which fails to produce proportionately greater narcotic effects as the dose is increased. Indeed, large amounts of codeine may cause excitement. Average doses are *sedative, analgetic* and *antitussive.* When administered by the oral route 30 to 60 mg is equivalent in analgesic effectiveness to approximately 650 mg of aspirin; subcutaneously, 60 mg is somewhat less effective than 10 mg of morphine. Because of different mechanisms of action, codeine plus salicylates or acetaminophen produces additive analgesic action. Codeine is useful for inducing sleep in the presence of mild pain. It is absorbed rapidly following either oral or parenteral administration; onset of action occurs in 15 to 30 min and analgesia is maintained for 4 to 6 hr. Codeine is metabolized mainly in the liver where it undergoes *O*-demethylation, *N*-demethylation and partial conjugation with glycuronic acid. The drug is excreted largely in the urine as narcodeine and free and conjugated morphine. Like morphine, this drug also produces cortical and respiratory depression, but serious degrees of either are practically unknown. It is less apt than morphine to cause nausea, vomiting, constipation and miosis. Both tolerance and *addiction* occur, however, and the same precautions should be observed in its use as for morphine. *Naloxone* is a specific antagonist in cases of acute intoxication.

This drug, like morphine, is employed as an *analgetic, sedative, hypnotic, antiperistaltic* and *antitussive* agent. It commonly is given in combination with aspirin, acetaminophen or other agents. Administered alone, codeine is a *Schedule II* drug under the *Controlled Substances Act. In combination with aspirin-like drugs it is classified as Schedule III.*

Dose—*Analgesic,* **15** to **60 mg;** *usual, adult, oral, analgesic* **30 mg** every 4 hr; *usual, antitussive,* **5** to **10 mg** every 4 hr. *Usual, pediatric, oral,* **500 μg** (0.5 mg)/**kg** (or 16.7 mg/m^2) every 4 hr.

Other Dose Information—The dose varies from 15 to 60 mg, and the drug may be taken orally or injected parenterally as a solution of one of its water-soluble salts, such as the phosphate or sulfate.

Codeine Phosphate

Morphinan-6-ol, (5α,6α)-7,8-didehydro-4,5-epoxy-3-methoxy-17-methyl-, phosphate (1:1) (salt), hemihydrate

[41444-62-6] $C_{18}H_{21}NO_3.H_3PO_4.½H_2O$ (406.37); *anhydrous* [52-28-8] (397.36).

Preparation—By dissolving codeine in an equimolecular quantity of aqueous phosphoric acid, adding alcohol and allowing the salt to crystallize from solution.

Description—Fine, white, needle-shaped crystals or a white, crystalline powder; odorless; readily loses water of hydration on exposure to air and is affected by light; solutions are acid to litmus and levorotatory.

Solubility—1 g in 2.5 mL water, 325 mL alcohol, 0.5 mL water at 80° or 125 mL boiling alcohol.

Uses—See *Codeine, Morphine* and *general statement*. Being more soluble than codeine sulfate, the phosphate is preferred to the sulfate.

Dose—*Analgesic,* **15** to **300 mg** a day; *usual, adult, analgesic, oral* or *parenteral,* **30 mg** 4 to 6 times a day; *usual, antitussive, oral,* **10 mg** 6 to 8 times a day as necessary. *Usual, pediatric, oral,* **500 μg** (0.5 mg)/**kg** (or 16.7 mg/m²) every 4 hr.

Dosage Forms—Injection: 15, 30 and 60 mg/mL, 600 mg and 1.2 g/20 mL; Soluble Tablets: 15, 30 and 60 mg.

Codeine Sulfate

Morphinan-6-ol, (5α,6α)-7,8-didehydro-4,5-epoxy-3-methoxy-17-methyl-, sulfate (2:1) (salt), trihydrate

[6854-40-6] $(C_{18}H_{21}NO_3)_2.H_2SO_4.3H_2O$ (750.86); *anhydrous* [1420-53-7] (698.81).

Preparation—By crystallization from a solution of codeine in diluted H_2SO_4.

Description—White crystals, usually needle-like or a white, crystalline powder; effloresces in dry air and is affected by light; aqueous solution is practically neutral or only slightly acid to litmus.

Solubility—1 g in 30 mL water, 1300 mL alcohol or about 6.5 mL water at 80°; insoluble in chloroform or ether.

Incompatibilities—See *Alkaloids* (page 399). It reacts with *phenobarbital sodium* to produce the free alkaloid and phenobarbital, both of which may precipitate unless the vehicle contains a moderate proportion of alcohol.

Uses—See *Codeine, Morphine* and the introductory statement.

Dose—*Usual, analgesic, adult, oral, intramuscular, intravenous or subcutaneous,* **15** to **60 mg** every 4 to 6 hr. Do not exceed **120 mg** in 24 hr; *children* (≥ 1 yr) **0.5 mg/kg** every 4 to 6 hr. *Antitussive, adult,* **10** to **20 mg** every 4 to 6 hr; do not exceed **120 mg** in 24 hr. *Children, oral* (6 to 12 yr), **5** to **10 mg** every 4 to 6 hr; do not exceed **60 mg** in 24 hr. *Children, oral* (2 to 6 yr), **2.5** to **5 mg** every 4 to 6 hr; do not exceed **30 mg** in 24 hr.

Dosage Forms—Tablets: 15, 30 and 60 mg. Soluble Tablets: 15, 30 and 60 mg.

Diacetylmorphine—see RPS-18, page 1101.

Diacetylmorphine Hydrochloride—see RPS-18, page 1101.

Morphine Hydrochloride—see RPS-18, page 1101.

Morphine Tartrate—see RPS-18, page 1101.

Semisynthetic Opiate Analgesics

In the effort to obtain an agent with the advantages of morphine or codeine without their disadvantages, chemists have modified the structure of these natural alkaloids of opium. Some of these modifications, eg, hydrocodone, hydromorphone, ethylmorphine or nalorphine result from making minor chemical alterations in the natural alkaloids, the characteristic nucleus (see page 401) remaining intact. Others, eg, dextromethorphan, levorphanol levallorphan are truly synthetic compounds constructed around the non-opiate morphinan nucleus (see page 401) which readily is synthesizable from coal-tar derivatives. For pharmacological convenience, all of these agents are classified here as semi-synthetic opium alkaloids. In general, the pharmacological properties exhibited by these agents differ quantitatively from those of the parent substance, but qualitatively they are similar. The several semisynthetic agents employed clinically are described below.

Dextromethorphan Hydrobromide—page 974.

Hydrocodone Bitartrate

Morphinan-6-one, (5α)-4,5-epoxy-3-methoxy-17-methyl-, [*R*-(*R*,**R**)]- 2,3-dihydroxybutanedioate (1:1), hydrate (2:5); Dihydrocodeinone Bitartrate USP XVI; (*Various Mfrs*)

[34195-34-1] [6190-38-1] $C_{18}H_{21}NO_3.C_4H_6O_6.2½H_2O$ (494.50); *anhydrous* [143-71-5] (449.46).

For the structure of hydrocodone, see page 401.

Preparation—This synthetic alkaloid, 7,8-dihydrocodeinone, is prepared either by catalytic rearrangement of codeine or by controlled hydrolysis and oxidation of dihydrothebaine.

Description—Fine white crystals or a fine white crystalline powder; affected by light; pH (1 in 50 solution) 3.2 to 3.8.

Solubility—1 g in 16 mL water; slightly soluble in alcohol; insoluble in ether or chloroform.

Uses—For the relief of moderate to severe pain and for the symptomatic relief of cough. It is a narcotic which is somewhat more sedating and addictive than codeine, and is a *Schedule III* drug under the *Controlled Substances Act. It frequently is combined with other drugs such as aspirin-like analgesics, antihistamines, expectorants and sympathomimetics.*

Dose—**5** to **50 mg** a day; *usual, adult, oral,* **5** to **10 mg** 3 to 4 times a day. *Usual, pediatric,* adequate dosing information is not available.

Dosage Forms—Capsules: 5 mg; Solutions: 1.66 to 5 mg/mL. Tablets: 5 mg.

Hydromorphone Hydrochloride

Morphinan-6-one-, (5α)-4,5-epoxy-3-hydroxy-17-methyl-, hydrochloride, Dihydromorphinone Hydrochloride; Dilaudid Hydrochloride (*Knoll*)

[71-68-1] $C_{17}H_{19}NO_3.HCl$ (321.80).

Hydromorphone hydrochloride is 7,8-dihydromorphinone hydrochloride; for the structure, see page 401.

Preparation—By electrolytic reduction of morphine or by oxidation of dihydromorphine and then reacting with HCl. US Pat 2,649,454.

Description—Fine, white, odorless, crystalline powder, affected by light; aqueous solution is practically neutral or only slightly acid to litmus.

Solubility—1 g in about 3 mL water; sparingly soluble in alcohol; practically insoluble in ether.

Incompatibilities—Reactions characteristic of alkaloids are generally applicable to this substance.

Uses—A semisynthetic *analgetic,* chemically and pharmacologically similar to morphine, indicated for the relief of moderate to severe pain of myocardial infarction, cancer, trauma (soft tissue and bone), biliary and renal colic, burns and postoperative pain. (See introductory statement). It also is used occasionally for its antitussive effects. It is one-fifth as potent orally as intramuscularly; the peak effect occurs later and the duration of analgesia is longer after oral administration. After *parenteral* administration, analgesic action is apparent within 15 to 30 min and lasts for 4 to 5 hr. After *oral* administration, onset of analgesia is about 30 min. Slower absorption and, hence, longer relief from pain can be obtained from its use in suppository form. It has less tendency to cause sleep than morphine when given in equivalent analgetic doses, and thus relief from pain can be obtained without sleep or stupefaction. It is contraindicated in bronchial asthma, respiratory depression or idiosyncrasy to the drug. It is claimed that the drug causes less constipation and vomiting than morphine; also, it produces less euphoria. However, *tolerance* and *addiction* do occur with the drug and it must be used with the same precautions as for morphine. It can be given by mouth, by rectum in suppository form or injected subcutaneously or intravenously (in emergency). The high-dose injection (10 mg/mL) should be used only in patients who are tolerant to the narcotics and require large doses of these drugs for relief.

Caution—This drug, being a morphine derivative, is a *Schedule II* drug under the *Controlled Substances Act. Naloxone* (page 1103) is a specific antagonist in cases of acute intoxication.

Dose—*Oral* and *subcutaneous,* **1** to **4 mg;** *usual,* **2 mg** every 4 hr as necessary. The dose for children has not been established.

Dosage Forms—Injection: 1, 2, 3, 4 and 10 mg/mL; Suppositories: 3 mg; Solution: 1 mg/5 mL. Tablets: 1, 2, 3 and 4 mg.

Levallorphan Tartrate—see RPS-18, page 1103.

Levorphanol Tartrate

Morphinan-3-ol, 17-methyl-, [*R*-(*R**,*R**)]-2,3-dihydroxybutanedioate (1:1) (salt), dihydrate; Levo-Dromoran (*Roche*)

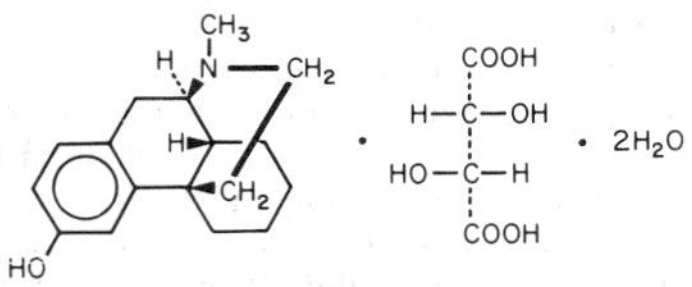

17-Methylmorphinan-3-ol tartrate (1:1) (salt) dihydrate [5985- 38-6] $C_{17}H_{23}NO.C_4H_6O_6.2H_2O$ (443.49); *anhydrous* [125-72-4] (407.46).

Preparation—5,6,7,8-Tetrahydro-2-methylisoquinolinium bromide (I) is metathesized with *p*-methoxybenzyl magnesium bromide (II), and the product rearranges at the expense of the 1,2-double bond to form 1-(*p*-methoxybenzyl)-2-methyl-1,2,5,6,7,8-hexahydroisoquinoline (III). III may be redrawn as shown below to display the ensuing reactions more clearly. A solution of the hydrochloride of III is then hydrogenated at the 3,4-positions with the aid of platinized charcoal, and subsequent treatment with ammonia liberates the *dl*-1,2,3,4,5,6,7,8-octahydro compound (IV), which may be resolved into its (+)- and (−)-enantiomorphs by the usual procedures. The final step in the preparation of the base involves heating the (−)-enantiomorph with phosphoric acid at 150° whereby cyclization between the isoquinoline residue and the benzene ring occurs at the expense of the remaining double bond of the isoquinoline. During the treatment with phosphoric acid, the methoxy group simultaneously is converted to hydroxy, thus producing levorphanol (V).

The tartrate may be produced by dissolving the base in aqueous tartaric acid solution and crystallizing.

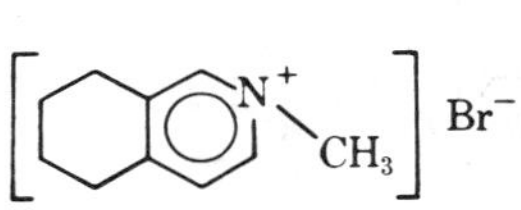

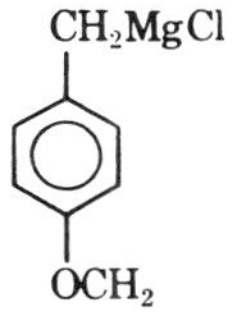

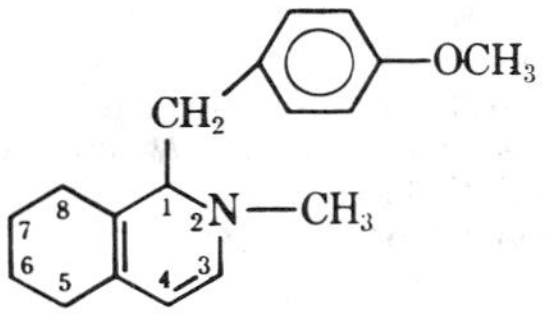

Description—Practically white, odorless, crystalline powder; melts about 115° (anhydrous, about 207°).

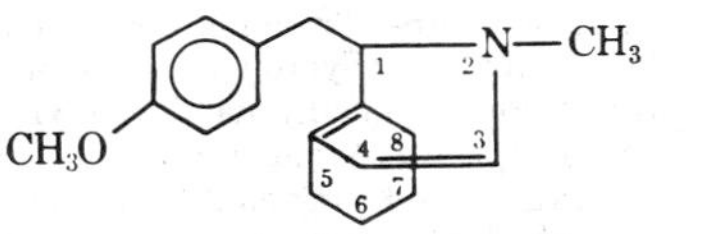

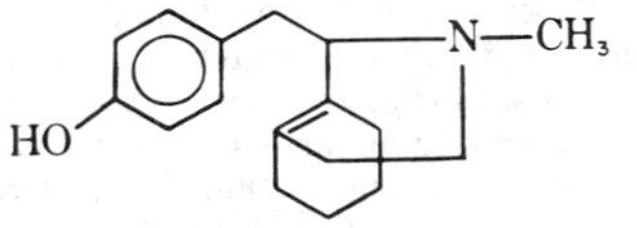

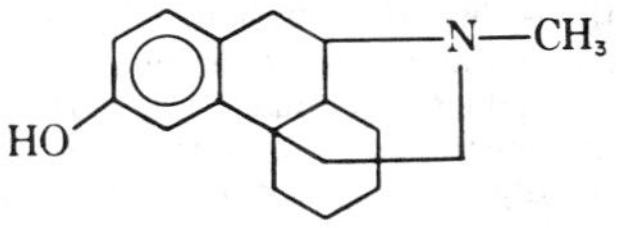

Solubility—1 g in 50 mL water or 120 mL alcohol; insoluble in chloroform and ether.

Uses—A potent synthetic analgesic related chemically and pharmacologically to morphine (see *morphine*, page 1198 and introductory statement). It produces analgesia at least equal to that of morphine and greater than that of meperidine with much smaller doses than either. It also is longer-acting than either of the above; from 6 to 8 hr of pain relief can be achieved after either oral or parenteral administration. Its margin of safety is essentially the same as morphine, but it is less likely to produce nausea, vomiting and constipation. It is indicated whenever a narcotic analgesic is required; it is effective for moderate to severe pain and is used parenterally for preoperative sedation as well as an adjunct to nitrous oxide-oxygen anesthesia. The drug is contraindicated in acute alcoholism, bronchial asthma, increased intracranial pressure, respiratory depression and anoxia. Other precautions and adverse reactions are similar to those induced by other narcotic analgesics. It is a narcotic with addiction liability similar to that of morphine; therefore, the same precautions should be observed when prescribing this drug as for morphine. The drug is a *Schedule II* drug under the *Controlled Substances Act*.

Dose—*Oral* and *subcutaneous*, **1** to **3 mg;** *usual*, **2 mg.**

Dosage Forms—Injection: 2 mg/mL and 20 mg/10 mL; Tablets: 2 mg.

Oxycodone Hydrochloride

4,5-Epoxy-14-hydroxy-3-methoxy-17-methylmorphinan-6-one Hydrochloride; Dihydrodihydroxycodeinone Hydrochloride; (*Various Mfrs*)

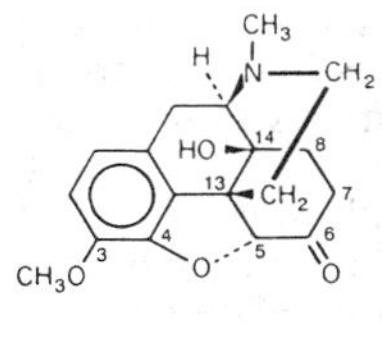

[124-90-3] $C_{18}H_{21}NO_4.HCl$ (351.83).

Preparation—From thebaine, also obtained from opium. Thebaine is the 3,6-dimethoxy-$\Delta^{6,8}$-diene which on oxidation with H_2O_2 inserts an OH at position 14 and a hemiacetal at 6. Hydrolysis of the hemiacetal forms the ketone at position 6; see Manske, *Chemistry of the Morphine Alkaloids*, Oxford Press, 1954. The hydrochloride is prepared from the base by the usual means.

Description—Odorless, white, crystalline powder; saline, bitter taste; melts with decomposition between 274° and 278°.

Solubility—1 g in 10 mL water or 60 mL alcohol.

Uses—For the relief of moderate to moderately severe pain. Like codeine and methadone, it retains one-half of its analgesic activity after oral administration. It often is used to relieve postoperative, postextractional and postpartum pain. Although oxycodone has less analgesic capability than morphine, it possesses comparable addiction potential and is a *Schedule II* drug under the *Controlled Substances Act*. *It frequently is used in combination with aspirin or acetaminophen.*

Dose—Usual, adult, oral, **5 mg** every 6 hr as needed for pain.

Dosage Forms—Solution: 5 mg/5 mL and 20mg/mL; Tablets: 5 mg (scored).

Oxymorphone Hydrochloride

(5α)-Morphinan-6-one, 4,5-epoxy-3,14-dihydroxy-17-methyl-, hydrochloride; Numorphan (*Du Pont*)

[357-07-3] $C_{17}H_{19}NO_4.HCl$ (337.80).

For the structure, see page 401.

Preparation—Thebaine is dissolved in aqueous formic acid and treated with 30% hydrogen peroxide, after which neutralization with aqueous ammonia yields 14-hydroxycodeinone. This then is dissolved in acetic acid and hydrogenated with the aid of palladium-charcoal catalyst to form 14-hydroxy-7,8-dihydrocodeinone (oxycodone). In the form of its hydrochloride, this compound is demethylated by heating with pyridine hydrochloride to yield crude oxymorphone hydrochloride, which then is purified. US Pat 2,806,033.

Description—White, acicular crystals or as a white or slightly off-white powder; odorless; darkens on prolonged exposure to light; pH (aqueous solutions) about 5.

Solubility—1 g in 4 mL water, 100 mL alcohol, > 1000 mL chloroform or > 1000 mL ether.

Uses—A semisynthetic narcotic analgesic with actions, uses and side effects similar to those of hydromorphone and morphine, except it possesses no significant antitussive activity. After parenteral administration, 1 mg of this drug is approximately equivalent in analgesic activity to 10 mg of morphine. Onset of action is rapid; initial effects usually are seen within 5 to 10 min, duration of action is approximately 3 to 6 hr. It satisfactorily controls postoperative pain, the more severe pain of advanced neoplastic diseases and other types of pain that ordinarily can be controlled by morphine. It is also used parenterally for preoperative medication as well as a supplement to anesthesia. Except that it is somewhat less constipating, the overall incidence and severity of side effects are similar to those of morphine. Its addiction liability is about the same as morphine. It is a *Schedule II* drug under the *Controlled Substances Act.*

Dose—*Usual, adult, oral, subcutaneous* and *intramuscular,* **1.0** to **1.5 mg** every 4 to 6 hr as needed; *intravenous,* **0.5 mg** *initially,* repeated in 4 to 6 hr if necessary; *suppository,* 5 mg every 4 to 6 hr as needed. Dosage in children has not been established.

Dosage Forms—Injection: 1 and 1.5 mg/mL; Suppositories: 5 mg.

Opiate Antagonists

Although *N*-allylnorcodeine was observed in 1915 to prevent or abolish morphine- and heroin-induced respiratory depression, more than 25 years elapsed before it was demonstrated that *N*-allylnormorphine (nalorphine; no longer available in the US) had even more pronounced morphine-antagonizing properties. Even then the clinical significance of this antagonizing effect was not explored until 1951. Two years later it was shown that nalorphine would precipitate acute abstinence syndromes in postaddicts who had been given morphine, methadone or heroin for brief periods. It also was shown that nonaddicted subjects given large doses of nalorphine exhibited dysphoria and anxiety rather than euphoria. Subsequently, it was noted that, although nalorphine antagonized the analgesic effects of morphine, it was a potent analgesic when given to patients with postoperative pain.

Except for meperidine, the substitution of an allyl group for the *N*-methyl group in most of the narcotics—eg, morphine, levorphanol, methadone, oxymorphone and phenazocine—results in drugs with varying levels of narcotic antagonistic effect. It should be emphasized that this is not restricted to allyl substitution, since the substitution of other groups (methallyl, propyl, isobutyl, propargyl or cyclopropargylmethyl) for the *N*-methyl group of narcotic analgesics also produces substances that are antagonists.

The term *antagonist,* as used in this section, includes naloxone and naltrexone which are antagonists with little or no agonist actions. These competitive narcotic antagonists are effective in the management of *severe respiratory depression* induced by narcotic drugs, *asphyxia neonatorum* caused by administration of these drugs to the expectant mother and for the *diagnosis or treatment of narcotic addiction.*

Nalorphine Hydrochloride—see RPS-18, page 1104.

Naloxone Hydrochloride

(5α)-Morphinan-6-one, 4,5-epoxy-3,14-dihydroxy-17-(2-propenyl)-, hydrochloride, Narcan (*Du Pont*)

[357-08-4] $C_{19}H_{21}NO_4$.HCl (363.84); *dihydrate* [51481-60-8] (399.87).

For the structure, see page 401.

Preparation—*Oxymorphone* (page 1201) is demethylated and the resulting 4,5α-epoxy-3,14-dihydroxymorphinan-6-one is *N*-allylated by reaction in ethanol with allyl bromide in the presence of $NaHCO_3$. The resulting naloxone is reacted with ethanolic HCl. US Pat 3,254,088.

Description—White to slightly off-white powder; aqueous solutions are acidic; melts about 203°.

Solubility—Soluble in water; slightly soluble in alcohol; practically insoluble in chloroform or ether.

Incompatibilities—Long-chain or high-molecular-weight anions (forms relatively insoluble salts) and with alkaline solutions (base precipitates if concentration is high enough); however, the injection is compatible with bulk IV solutions that are slightly alkaline. Also, oxygen, oxidizing agents, bisulfites or metabisulfites.

Uses—A synthetic narcotic antagonist essentially devoid of narcotic agonist properties. Hence, it does not possess morphine-like properties, such as respiratory depression, psychotomimetic effects and pupillary constriction, characteristic of other narcotic antagonists. Available evidence suggests that it antagonizes these opioid effects by competing for the same receptor sites. It is the drug of choice for management of respiratory depression induced by natural and synthetic narcotic analgesics, including depression induced by the partial agonist pentazocine. It also is indicated for diagnosis of acute narcotic overdosage. It is not effective against nonnarcotic respiratory depression. Naloxone has been used to detect opiate abuse and can precipitate severe opioid withdrawal symptoms in physically dependent patients. The use of this drug may diminish opiate-dependent euphoria and help reduce the desire for these drugs.

The drug rapidly disappears from serum in man. Following an intravenous dose naloxone is distributed rapidly in the body. The onset of activity generally is apparent within 2 to 5 min; the onset of action is only slightly less rapid when administered by the subcutaneous or intramuscular routes. The mean half-life in adults ranges from 30 to 81 min (mean 64 ± 12 min); the mean half-life in neonates is 3.1 ± 0.5 hr. It is metabolized in the liver, primarily by glucuronide conjugation, and excreted in the urine. This short duration of action necessitates multiple dosing and severely limits its value. Hence, considerable research effort has been directed toward the development of antagonists with a much longer duration of action (*see Naltrexone* and *Nalbuphine,* following). Safe and effective use in children under 12 yr and in pregnant women has not been established. Adverse effects are said to be rare and usually consist of nausea and vomiting. It is *unscheduled* under the *Controlled Substances Act.*

Dose—*Usual, parenteral,* **0.4** to **2 mg** (1 mL); if the desired level of response is not attained immediately, the same dose may be repeated at 2- or 3-min intervals. Lack of response after 2 or 3 injections suggests conditions may be due to other disease processes or nonnarcotic drugs. For postoperative respiratory depression caused by narcotic overdosage, *adult, intravenous,* **0.1** to **0.2 mg** at 2- or 3-minute intervals until the desired effect is achieved. This dose may be repeated at 1- or 2-hr intervals as necessary. *Pediatric, intravenous, initially* **0.01 mg per kg,** repeated at 2- or 3-min intervals as necessary. To reverse narcotic-induced respiratory depression in *newborn infants,* same as *pediatric, intravenous,* above.

Dosage Form—Injection: 0.4 and 1 mg/mL; Neonatal Injection: 0.02 mg/mL.

Naltrexone Hydrochloride

Morphinan-6-one, (5α)-17-(cyclopropylmethyl)-4,5-epoxy-3,14-dihydroxy-, Trexan (*Du Pont*)

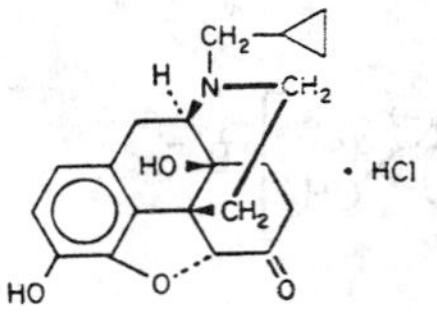

[16676-29-2] $C_{19}H_{21}NO_4$.HCl (377.87).

Preparation—From normorphine by oxidation at the allylic positions tions C6 and C14; hydrogenation of the C7-8 double bond and *N*-alkylation with cyclopropylmethyl halide. US Pat 3,332,950.

Description—White crystals; melts about 275°.

Solubility—1 g in about 1 mL water.

Uses—Naltrexone generally has little or no agonist activity. Its opiate antagonist activity is reported to be 2 to 9 times that of naloxone and 17 times that of nalorphan. Consequently, it is used as an adjunct to the maintenance of the opioid-free state in detoxified, formerly opioid-dependent, individuals. It also has been used in the treatment of postconcussional syndrome unresponsive to other treatments. It is absorbed rapidly and almost completely following oral administration, but undergoes extensive first-pass metabolism in the liver. Only 5 to 20% of an orally administered dose reaches systemic circulation unchanged. The major metabolite is 6β-naltrexol; this also is a pure antagonist and may contribute to the opioid receptor blockade. Mean elimination half-lives for naltrexone and 6β-naltrexol are 3.9 and 12.9 hr, respectively; pharmacological effects are apparent for 24 and 72 hr and appear to be independent of dose. The drug does not accumulate after chronic administration, but is excreted primarily in the urine. Adverse effects most frequently observed (10%) include anxiety, nervousness, headache, low energy, abdominal cramps, nausea, vomiting and joint and muscle pain. Liver test abnormalities and lymphocytosis have been reported. Patients should wear some identification indicating they are taking this drug.

Dose—*Usual,* treatment should not be initiated until naloxone challenge is negative and the patient has remained opioid-free for 7 to 10 days. Two or three dosage regimens have been suggested: **50 mg** every 24 hr; **50 mg** every weekday with **100 mg** on Saturday or **100 mg** Monday, **100 mg** Wednesday and **150 mg** Friday.

Dosage Form—Tablets: 50 mg.

Synthetic Opiate Agonist/Antagonist

The many undesirable side actions of morphine and the dependence on the Mediterranean and Near East countries for opium stimulated the search for synthetic drugs as analgesic as morphine, but with fewer side actions and less addiction liability. An ideal analgesic drug is theoretically possible and conceivably could make morphine and other opium derivatives obsolete as analgesics.

It generally is agreed that an ideal analgesic drug should

Not become ineffective through the development of tolerance.
Not be habit-forming or addicting.
Have a wide margin of safety.
Be effective against all types of pain.
Possess a short latent period and a long duration of action.
Not alter sensory modalities.
Not depress respiration or the cardiovascular system.
Not affect the gastrointestinal tract.
Be effective both orally and parenterally.
Be relatively inexpensive.

Since all the potent synthetic opiate analgesics developed for clinical use are addicting, mimic some of the pharmacological properties of morphine and are antagonized to some extent by nalorphine, it is obvious that the ideal analgesic agent has yet to be developed. Nevertheless, currently available synthetic agents have valuable analgesic and pharmacological properties which are described in this section.

Alfentanil Hydrochloride

Propanamide, *N*-[1-[2-(4-ethyl-4,5-dihydro-5-oxo-1*H*-tetrazol-1-yl)ethyl]-4-(methoxymethyl)-4-piperidinyl]-*N*-phenyl-, monohydrochloride, monohydrate; Alfenta (*Janssen*)

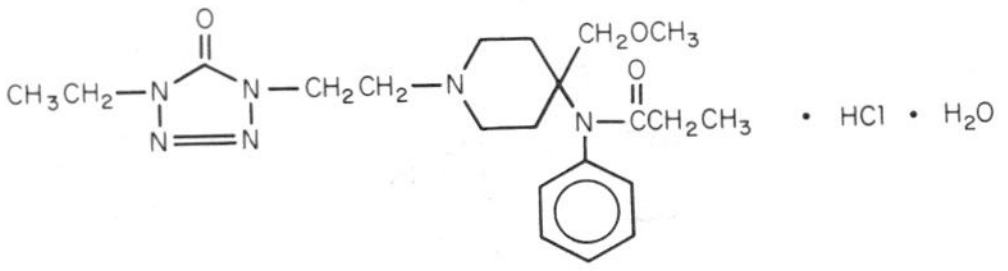

[70879-28-6] $C_{21}H_{32}N_6O_3.HCl$ (471.00).

Preparation—See *J Med Chem 29:* 2290, 1986.

Description—White crystals; melts at 138°.

Uses—A potent synthetic opioid analgesic related to fentanyl but with a more rapid onset of action and shorter duration of narcotic effects. The brief duration (30 to 60 min following 50 μg/kg IV) is advantageous for short surgical procedures but requires frequent injection or continuous infusion for longer operations. Because it is less lipid soluble then fentanyl, it is less likely to accumulate with prolonged or repeated administration.

Adverse effects include muscular rigidity (chest wall, trunk and extremities), hypotension and bradycardia, respiratory depression, nausea, vomiting and dizziness. Large doses over a long period of time also may prolong postoperative awakening and respiratory depression. Fentanyl and sufentanil frequently have been abused; this drug also is likely to be abused.

Dose—*Incremental injection, 30-min anesthesia, induction,* **8** to **20 μg/kg;** *maintenance,* **3** to **5 μg/kg/min;** *30 to 60 min anesthesia, induction,* **20** to **50 μg/kg;** *maintenance,* **5** to **15 μg/kg.** *Anesthetic induction,* **130** to **245 μg/kg/;** *maintenance,* **0.5** to **1.5 μg/kg/min.** *Continuous infusion, induction,* **50** to **75 μg/kg;** *maintenance,* **0.5** to **3 μg/kg/min.**

Dosage Form—Injection 500 μg of the base (as the HCl)/mL.

Buprenorphine Hydrochloride

6,14-Ethenomorphinan-7-methanol, 17-(cyclopropylmethy)-α-(1,1-dimethylethyl)-4,5-epoxy-18,19-dihydro-3-hydroxy-6-methoxy-α-methyl-, hydrochloride; Buprenex (*Reckitt & Coleman*)

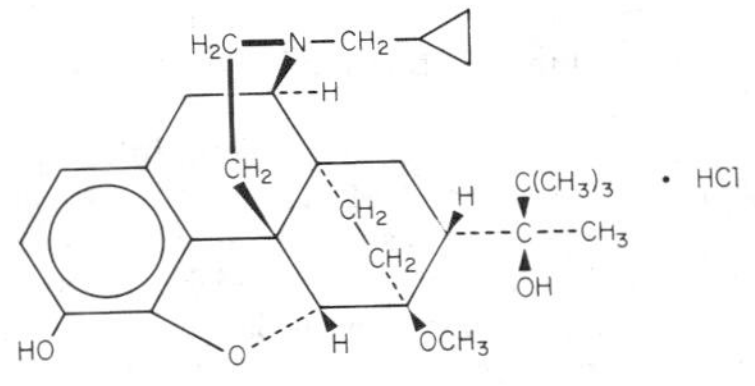

[53152-21-9] $C_{29}H_{41}NO_4.HCl$ (504.11).

Preparation—From thebaine; US Pat 3,433,791.

Description—White crystalline powder; aqueous solutions are weakly acidic.

Solubility—Slightly soluble in water.

Uses—A semisynthetic centrally acting opioid analgesic derived from thebaine, it is used for the relief of moderate to severe pain particularly associated with postoperative discomfort. It is approximately 30 times as potent as morphine and exerts its analgesic effect by binding to CNS opiate receptors. It is classified as a partial agonist and exhibits antagonist effects in higher doses. Onset of analgesia occurs within 15 min after IM injection, peaks at 1 hr and persists for up to 6 hr. Approximately 96% is bound to plasma protein and metabolized by the liver. Terminal half-life is 2 to 3 hr. The drug is excreted in the feces as free buprenorphine. Chronic use may produce psychological dependence and infrequently produce limited physical dependence. Adverse effects related to the *CNS* include sedation (66%), dizziness (5 to 10%), headache (1 to 5%), confusion, slurred speech, depression and hallucinations; *cardiovascular:* hypo- or hypertension, tachycardia or bradycardia; *gastrointestinal:* nausea/vomiting, dry mouth, dyspepsia or flatulence; *respiratory:* hypoventilation, dyspnea or cyanosis; *ophthalmological:* miosis, blurred vision, diplopia or conjunctivitis; other adverse effects include pruritus, urinary retention, flushing, chills/cold and tinnitus. Safety and efficacy in children has not been established.

Dose—*Usual, adult, intramuscular* or *intravenous,* patients 13 yr and older: **0.3 mg** every 6 hr. Maximum **0.6 mg.**

Dosage Form—Injection: 0.3 mg/mL.

Butorphanol Tartrate

(−)-Morphinan-3,14-diol, 17-(cyclobutylmethyl)-, [*R*(*R**,*R**)]-2,3-dihydroxybutanedioate (1:1) salt; Stadol (*Bristol*)

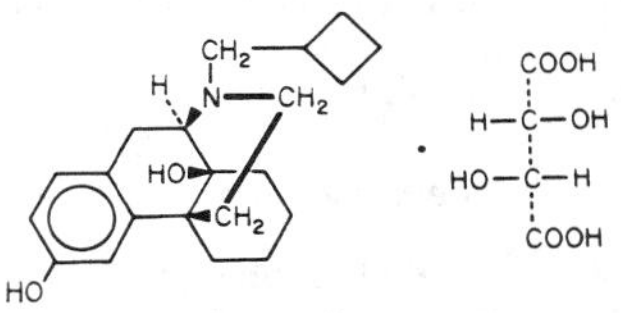

(−)-17-(Cyclobutylmethyl)morphinan-3,14-diol tartrate (1:1) salt [58786-99-5] $C_{21}H_{29}NO_2.C_4H_6O_6$ (477.55).

Preparation—Total synthesis of *N*-substituted 3,14-dihydroxymorphinans, including butorphanol, from 7-methoxy-1-tetralone, has been reported by Monković *et al* (J Am Chem Soc 95: 7910, 1973).

Description—White, crystalline powder; melts about 219°.

Solubility—Soluble in water.

Uses—A potent analgesic with both narcotic agonist and antagonist effects. Analgesic potency is 3.5 to 7 times that of morphine, 30 to 40 times that of meperidine, 15 to 20 times that of pentazocine and 1/40 the antagonist potency of naloxone. It is indicated for moderate to severe postsurgical pain to supplement balanced anesthesia and to relieve postpartum pain. After intramuscular injection, analgesia begins within 10 min, reaches peak activity in 30 to 60 min and persists for 3 to 4 hr. After intravenous administration, peak activity is reached within a few minutes. A 2-mg intramuscular dose is equivalent in analgesic effect to 10 mg of morphine. Although completely absorbed from the GI tract after oral administration, it undergoes approximately 80% first-pass metabolism. Adverse effects observed are similar to those observed after morphine, including dizziness, lightheadedness and nausea. Transient but disturbing psychotomimetic reactions have been reported after doses of 2 to 4 mg. Two mg depresses the respiration to the same extent as 10 mg of morphine; slow, shallow respiration has been reported in patients taking recommended doses of the drug. The respiratory depression and other effects can be reversed by naloxone. Like pentazocine, the drug increases arterial resistance and the work of the heart; consequently, it is contraindicated in patients with acute myocardial infarction. It is known to cause euphoria, and tolerance to the analgesic effect has been reported in animals. It also can precipitate withdrawal in opioid-dependent patients. It is an *unscheduled drug* under the *Controlled Substances Act.*

Dose—*Usual, adult, intramuscular,* **2 mg** every 3 to 4 hr; *usual, dose range,* **1** to **4 mg.** *Usual intravenous,* **1 mg** every 3 or 4 hr; *usual dose range,* **0.5** to **2 mg** every 3 or 4 hr.

Dosage Form—Injection: 1 or 2 mg/mL.

Dezocine

(−)(5α,11α,13s)-5,11-Methanobenzocyclodecen-3-ol, 13-amino-5,6,7,8,9,10,11,12-octahydro-5-methyl-, Dalgan (*Astra*)

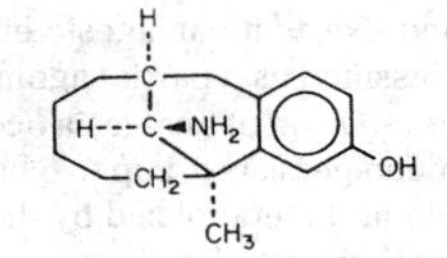

[53648-55-8] $C_{16}H_{23}NO$ (245.36).

Preparation—1-Methyl-7-methoxy-2-tetralone is treated with $Br(CH_2)_5Br$ and NaH to insert a pentamethylene bridge between positions 1 and 3 of the tetralone. Reductive amination of the carbonyl group with NH_2OH and Ni/H_2 followed by demethylation of the 7-methoxy group with HBr affords the product; *J Med Chem 16:* 595, 1973.

Uses—A synthetic opioid agonist/antagonist structurally similar to pentazocine. Its analgesic and pharmacokinetic properties are similar to morphine. Its adverse effects are like those of other opioid analgesics and include nausea, vomiting, sedation and respiratory depression. Dizziness, anxiety, disorientation, hallucinations and sweating also have been reported. Dezocine is not recommended for use in patients physically dependent on narcotics. Extreme caution should be exercised if dezocine is used in combination with other CNS-depressant drugs due to an increased risk to the patient. Although it is likely that because of its opioid agonist/antagonist properties, dezocine has less abuse potential than some of the other opioid analgesics, it probably does have some potential for dependence, particularly in patients with a history of opioid drug abuse. Dezocine is metabolized extensively in the liver by glucuronide conjugation and excreted in the urine.

Dose—*Usual, adult, intramuscular,* **5** to **20 mg;** repeat in 3 to 6 hr as necessary. Maximum, **120 mg/day.** *Usual, intravenous,* **2.5** to **10 mg** repeated every 2 to 4 hr as needed. Not recommended for children less than 18 yr.

Dosage Form—Injection: 5, 10 or 15 mg/mL.

Fentanyl Citrate

Propanamide, *N*-phenyl-*N*-[1-(2-phenylethyl)-4-piperidinyl]-, 2-hydroxy-1,2,3-propanetricarboxylate (1:1); Sublimaze; ing of Innovar (*Janssen*)

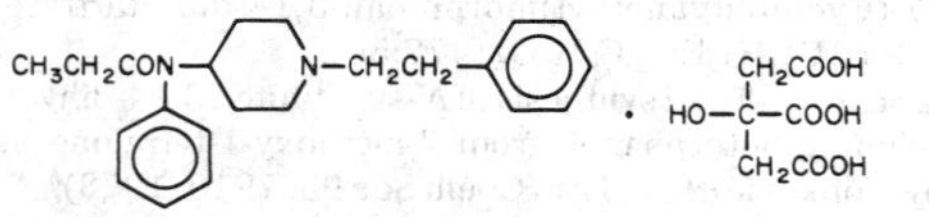

N-(1-Phenethyl-4-piperidyl)propionanilide citrate (1:1) [990-73-8] $C_{22}H_{28}N_2O.C_6H_8O_7$ (528.60).

Preparation—One method consists of condensing propionyl chloride with *N*-(4-piperidyl)aniline, then treating the resulting *N*-(4-piperidyl)propionanilide with phenethyl chloride, aiding each condensation by the presence of a suitable dehydrochlorinating agent. Reaction of the base with an equimolar portion of citric acid yields the (1:1) citrate. US Pat 3,164,600.

Description—White, crystalline powder or glistening crystals; odorless and tasteless (*Note:* because this compound is extremely potent, no taste test is recommended); stable in air; melts 147 to 152°; pK_a 8.3.

Solubility—1 g in about 40 mL of water, 140 mL of alcohol or 350 mL of chloroform.

Uses—A potent narcotic analgesic with rapid onset and short duration of action when administered parenterally. Administration of the base via a transdermal patch has a much slower onset (8 to 12 hr) and longer duration of action (greater than 72 hr) and often is used to manage chronic pain that requires an opiate analgesic. It has a profile of pharmacological action similar to morphine, except that it does not cause emesis or release histamine. Equianalgesia can be obtained with a dose 1/150 that of morphine. After intravenous injection, peak analgesia appears within 3 to 5 min and lasts 30 to 60 min. Fentanyl produces signs and symptoms typical of narcotic analgesics, such as miosis, euphoria and respiratory depression. It is used primarily as an analgesic for the control of pain associated with all types of surgery. It also can be used as a supplement to all agents commonly employed for general and regional anesthesia. It also is an ingredient in *Fentanyl Citrate and Droperidol Injection,* page 1143.

It is contraindicated in children 2 yr and younger, in asthmatic patients and in patients with a history of myasthenia gravis. Other depressant drugs, such as barbiturates, major tranquilizers, tricyclic antidepressants, narcotics and general anesthetics have an additive or potentiating effect on the drug. Its safe use in pregnancy has not been established. It crosses the placental barrier; use during labor may lead to respiratory depression in the newborn infant. It should be used with caution in patients with liver and kidney disease. Adverse reactions include respiratory depression, apnea, muscular rigidity and hypotension. Less frequently, nausea and vomiting may occur. Infrequently, dizziness, visual disturbance, itching, euphoria and spasms of the sphincter of Oddi have been observed. It is a *Schedule II* drug under the *Controlled Substances Act.*

Dose—*Usual, intramuscular,* as part of preoperative medication, **0.05** to **0.1 mg** 30 to 60 min prior to operation. For prompt analgesia during induction, *intravenous,* **0.05** to **0.1 mg,** repeated at 2- to 3-min intervals until desired effect is achieved; dosage reduced to **0.025** to **0.05 mg** in poor-risk and in very young and very old patients. For maintenance of analgesia during anesthesia, *intravenous,* **0.025** to **0.05 mg.** For control of postoperative pain, restlessness and tachypnea, *intramuscular,* **0.05** to **0.1 mg;** repeated in 1 to 2 hr as needed. Children (2 to 12 yr), *induction and maintenance* **1.7** to **3.3 μg/kg;** safety in children under 2 yr has not been established. *Transdermal patch,* **25 μg/hr;** higher doses (50, 75 and 100 μg/hr) in patients who are opiate tolerant.

Dosage Forms—Injection: 0.05 mg/mL; Transdermal system: 20, 50, 75 and 100 μg/hr.

Meperidine Hydrochloride

4-Piperidinecarboxylic acid, 1-methyl-4-phenyl-, ethyl ester, hydrochloride; Pethidine Hydrochloride; Dolantin, Dolantol, Eudolat, Isonipecaine; Demerol Hydrochloride (*Sanofi-Winthrop*)

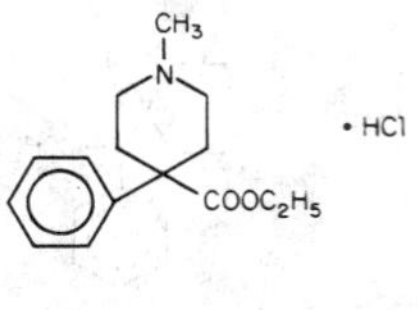

Ethyl 1-methyl-4-phenylisonipecotate hydrochloride [50-13-5] $C_{15}H_{21}NO_2.HCl$ (283.80).

Preparation—One of several methods utilizes benzyl chloride, diethanolamine and benzyl cyanide in the following principal steps:

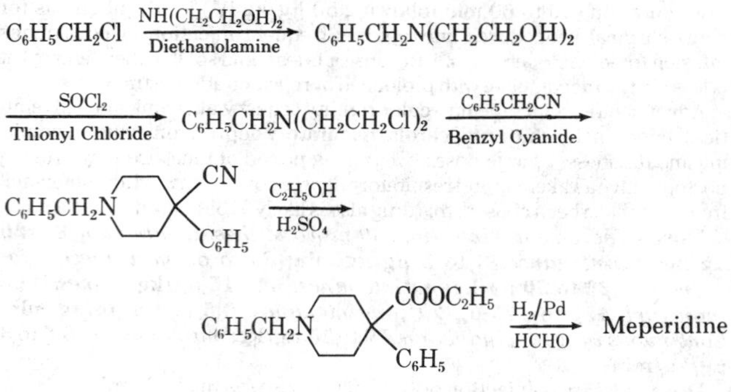

$$C_6H_5CH_2Cl \xrightarrow[\text{Diethanolamine}]{NH(CH_2CH_2OH)_2} C_6H_5CH_2N(CH_2CH_2OH)_2$$

$$\xrightarrow[\text{Thionyl Chloride}]{SOCl_2} C_6H_5CH_2N(CH_2CH_2Cl)_2 \xrightarrow[\text{Benzyl Cyanide}]{C_6H_5CH_2CN}$$

$$C_6H_5CH_2N\langle\rangle(CN)(C_6H_5) \xrightarrow[H_2SO_4]{C_2H_5OH}$$

$$C_6H_5CH_2N\langle\rangle(COOC_2H_5)(C_6H_5) \xrightarrow[HCHO]{H_2/Pd} \text{Meperidine}$$

Removal of the *N*-benzyl group is accomplished by catalytic hydrogenation in acetic acid solution using a palladium catalyst. The addition of formaldehyde to the reduction mixture followed by further catalytic hydrogenation leads to meperidine. The free base is converted to the hydrochloride by neutralization with HCl.

Description—Fine, white, crystalline, odorless powder; stable in air at ordinary temperatures; pH (1 in 20 solution) about 5; melts 186 to 189°; pK_a 7.7 to 8.15.

Solubility—Very soluble in water; soluble in alcohol; sparingly soluble in ether.

Uses—A synthetic narcotic analgesic with multiple actions qualitatively similar to those of morphine; the most prominent of these actions are on the CNS and on organs composed of smooth muscle. It acts principally to induce analgesia and sedation. It is indicated for preoperative use, relief of moderate to severe pain, support anesthesia and for obstetrical analgesia. It crosses the placental barrier; use during labor may lead to respiratory depression in the newborn infant. Available evidence suggests it produces less smooth muscle spasm, constipation and depression of cough reflex than equianalgesic doses of morphine. In a 60- to 80-mg parenteral dose, it essentially is equal in analgesic effectiveness to 10 mg of morphine; the onset of action is slightly more rapid and the duration of action somewhat shorter than morphine.

It is significantly less effective by the oral than by the parenteral route. Following intravenous administration of meperidine in healthy adults, the volume distribution at steady state was 269 L; plasma clearance was 1.06 L/min and elimination half-life was 3.6 hr. There is evidence that the disposition of meperidine varies between day and night, with elimination half-life shorter and plasma clearance greater at night. It is contraindicated in patients on MAO inhibitors; it inconsistently has precipitated severe, and occasionally fatal, reactions in patients who have received such medication within 14 days. The drug should be used with caution and in reduced dosage in patients on other narcotic analgesics, general anesthetics, phenothiazines, sedatives, tricyclic antidepressants and other CNS depressants. Major adverse reactions include respiratory depression, circulatory depression, respiratory arrest, shock and cardiac arrest. The most frequent untoward effects include dizziness, sedation, nausea, vomiting and sweating. Other adverse reactions include euphoria, weakness, headache, agitation, tremor, seizures, transient hallucinations and disorientation. Some of the CNS toxicity may be due to the neurotoxic metabolite, normeperidine. Because of concern about the incidence and severity of the CNS adverse effects, many clinicians recommend its short-term use only in otherwise healthy adults who are unable to receive either morphine or hydromorphone. Other effects involving the gastrointestinal tract, cardiovascular system and genitourinary tract are similar to morphine. Analgesia is possible with doses which do not cause stupefaction, a decided advantage over morphine. Pain usually is relieved within 20 min to 1 hr, analgesia lasting from 2 to 5 hr.

Naloxone is a specific antagonist in cases of acute intoxication.

It is a *Schedule II* drug under the *Controlled Substances Act.*

Dose—*Usual, adult, oral and parenteral,* **50** to **150 mg** every 3 or 4 hr as necessary; *usual range,* **50 mg** to **1.2 g** a day. *Children, oral,* **1** to **1.8 mg/kg,** not to exceed adult dose, 6 to 8 times a day as necessary.

Dosage Forms—Injection: 25, 50, 75 and 100 mg/mL. Syrup: 50 mg/5 mL; Tablets: 50 and 100 mg.

Methadone Hydrochloride

3-Heptanone, 6-(dimethylamino)-4,4-diphenyl-, hydrochloride; (*Roxane*) Dolophine Hydrochloride (*Lilly*);

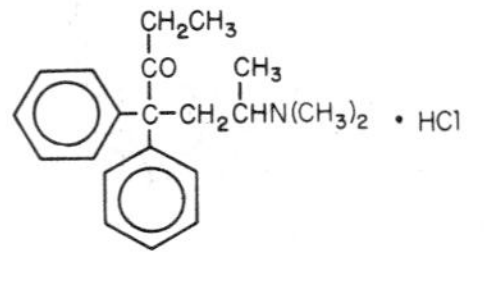

$$(C_6H_5)_2C(COCH_2CH_3)CH_2CH(CH_3)N(CH_3)_2 \cdot HCl$$

Amidone Hydrochloride; [1095-90-5] $C_{21}H_{27}NO.HCl$ (345.91).

Preparation—Diphenylacetonitrile is condensed with 2-chloro-1-dimethylaminopropane in the presence of sodamide, yielding 4-(dimethylamino)-2,2-diphenylvaleronitrile and an unwanted isomeric nitrile in approximately equal amounts. The isomers are separated and the former is subjected to Grignard addition with ethyl magnesium bromide. Subsequent hydrolysis in the presence of hydrochloric acid yields methadone hydrochloride.

Cyclized form of 2-chloro-1-dimethylaminopropane $[CH_3CH—CH_2 (N^+)(CH_3)_2]Cl^-$ $\xrightarrow[\text{NaNH}_2\text{ sodamide}]{(C_6H_5)_2CHCN\text{ diphenylacetonitrile}}$ $(C_6H_5)_2C(CN)CH_2CH(CH_3)N(CH_3)_2$ 4-(dimethylamino)-2,2-diphenylvaleronitrile

$\xrightarrow{C_2H_5MgBr}$ $(C_6H_5)_2C(CH_2CH(CH_3)N(CH_3)_2)—C(C_2H_5)=N—MgBr$ $\xrightarrow[\text{(HCl)}]{\text{Hydrolysis}}$ Methadone Hydrochloride

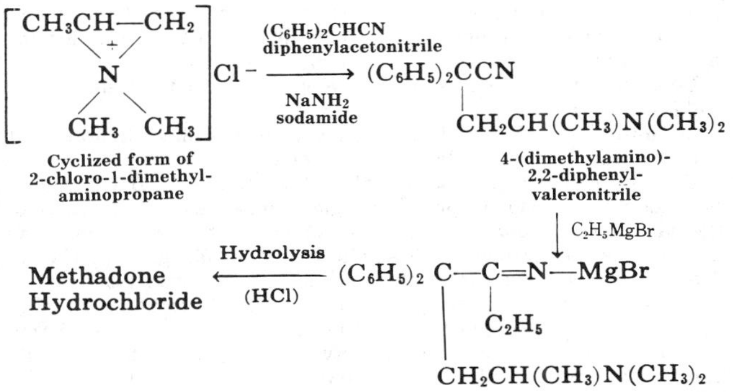

Description—Colorless crystals or a white, crystalline, odorless powder; pH (1 in 100 solution) 4.5 to 6.5; optically inactive (the official salt is a racemic mixture of which only the levo form has analgetic activity).

Solubility—1 g in 13 mL water, 8 mL alcohol or 3 mL chloroform; practically insoluble in ether or glycerin.

Uses—A synthetic *narcotic analgesic* with multiple actions quantitatively similar to morphine, the most prominent of which involve the CNS and organs composed of smooth muscle. The principal actions of therapeutic value are those of *analgesia, sedation* and *detoxification* or *temporary maintenance* in narcotic addiction. It also has significant *antitussive* properties but is no longer approved for this use in the US. It is rapidly but probably incompletely absorbed after oral administration, since only 52% of a given dose appears in the urine. Mean plasma levels of 182 and 420 ng/mL have been reported in patients maintained on a daily oral dose of 40 and 80 mg, respectively, 71 to 87% of which is in bound form. The half-life is approximately 25 hr, with a range of 13 to 47 hr. A parenteral dose of 8 to 10 mg is approximately equivalent in analgesic effectiveness to 10 mg of morphine; onset and duration of action of the two drugs are similar.

It is approximately ½ as potent orally as parenterally. It is indicated for the relief of moderate to severe pain, for detoxification treatment of narcotic addiction and for temporary maintenance treatment of narcotic addiction. If it is administered for heroin treatment for more than 3 weeks, the procedure passes from treatment of the acute withdrawal syndrome (detoxification) to maintenance therapy; the latter use can be undertaken *only* in approved programs, unless the addict is hospitalized for conditions other than addiction. Its abstinence syndrome qualitatively is similar to that of morphine; however, the onset is slower, the course is more prolonged and the symptoms less severe. It can produce drug dependence of the morphine type; therefore, it should be prescribed and administered with the same degree of caution as morphine.

It is contraindicated in patients known to be sensitive to it. The drug should be used with caution and in reduced dosage in patients on other narcotic analgesics, general anesthetics, phenothiazine and other tranquilizers, sedative-hypnotics, tricyclic antidepressants, monoamine oxidase inhibitors and CNS depressants as respiratory depression, hypotension, profound sedation or coma may result. Patients on a maintenance program are given methadone only as an oral liquid form and should not be given pentazocine or rifampin since these drugs may induce withdrawal symptoms. The safe use of the drug in pregnancy has not been established. It is not recommended for obstetrical analgesia, because its long duration may induce respiratory depression in the newborn. Adverse reactions are similar to those for other narcotic analgesics (see especially *Meperidine*).

It is employed widely in the withdrawal management of patients addicted to morphine, heroin and related narcotic drugs.

Naloxone is an effective antagonist in cases of acute intoxication. It is a *Schedule II* drug under the *Controlled Substances Act.*

Dose—*Analgesic: oral, adult, intramuscular* or *subcutaneous,* **2.5** to **10 mg** 6 to 8 times a day as necessary; *usual range,* **15** to **80 mg** a day. *Narcotic withdrawal management: adult, oral, detoxification,* 15 to 40 mg once a day, the dosage being decreased according to patient response; *maintenance,* **40** to **120 mg** once a day.

Dosage Forms—Injection: 10 mg/mL; Oral Solution: 1 or 2 mg/mL; Tablets: 5 and 10 mg; Dispersible Tablets.

Nalbuphine Hydrochloride

(5α,6α)-Morphinan-3,6,14-triol, 17-(cyclobutylmethyl)-4,5-epoxy-, hydrochloride, Nubain (*Du Pont*)

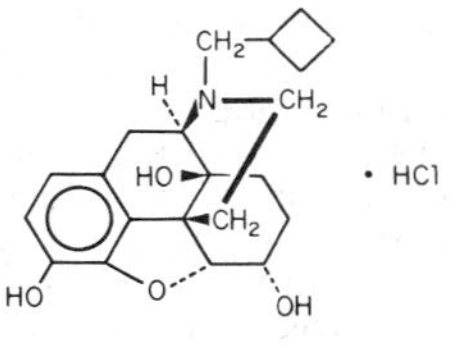

[23277-43-2] $C_{21}H_{27}NO_4.HCl$ (393.91)

Preparation—Refer to US Pat 3,393,197.

Description—*Base:* white crystals; melts about 230°.

Uses—For the relief of moderate to severe pain. It also may be used for preoperative analgesia, as a supplement to surgical anesthesia and for obstetrical analgesia during labor. It is related chemically to oxymorphone and the opiod antagonist, naloxone. It possesses both agonist and antagonist properties. Thus, it resembles pentazocine pharmacologically. Its analgesic potency, when administered parenterally on a milligram basis, is approximately the same as that of morphine and about 3 to 4 times greater than that for pentazocine; its antagonistic potency is about ten times greater than that of pentazocine. The onset of action occurs within 2 to 3 min after intravenous administration and within 15 min after intramuscular or subcutaneous administration; it is metabolized in the liver; its plasma half-life is 5 hr and the duration of effect is 3 to 6 hr. Adverse reactions are the same as those for morphine and other potent analgesics (see page 1196). Those most frequently observed include sedation (36%), sweaty/clammy (9%), nausea and vomiting (6%), dizziness and vertigo (5%), dry mouth (4%) and headache (3%). Respiratory depression may occur with usual doses of nalbuphine, but is not dose-related; however, it plateaus with a cumulative IV dose of approximately 30 mg. The abrupt withdrawal following prolonged administration causes opiate-like abstinence symptoms which are milder than those of morphine but more intense than those of pentazocine. Although it possesses narcotic antagonist activity, there is evidence that in *nondependent* patients it will not antagonize a narcotic analgesic administered just before, concurrently with or just after an injection of the drug. Therefore, patients receiving narcotic analgesics, general anesthetics, phenothiazines, other sedatives, hypnotics or CNS depressants concomitantly may exhibit additive effects. Thus, the dose of one or both agents should be reduced. Clinical experience to support use in children under 18 yr is not presently available.

Dose—*Usual, adult, parenteral* (all routes), **10 mg/70 kg,** repeated every 3 to 6 hr as necessary. Dosage should be adjusted according to the severity of the pain, physical status of the patient and other medications the patient may be receiving.

Dosage Form—Injection: 10 or 20 mg/mL.

Pentazocine

2,6-Methano-3-benzazocin-8-ol, (2α,6α,11*R**)-1,2,3,4,5,6- hexahydro-6,11-dimethyl-3-(3-methyl-2-butenyl)-, Talwin (*Sanofi-Winthrop*)

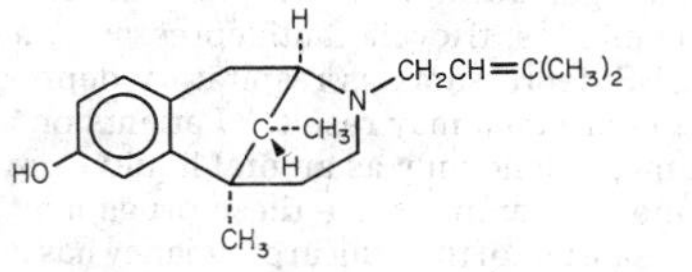

[359-83-1] $C_{19}H_{27}NO$ (285.43).

Preparation—1,2,3,4,5,6-Hexahydro-6,11-dimethyl-2,6-methano-3-benzazocin-8-ol (I) is condensed with 1-bromo-3-methyl-2-butene by refluxing in *N,N*-dimethylformamide in the presence of sodium bicarbonate. The reaction mixture is filtered and the crude pentazocine is isolated by means of a suitable solvent extraction process and finally crystallized from aqueous methanol. US Pat 3,250,678.

Compound I may be prepared by the following sequence of reactions: 3,4-dimethylpyridine methiodide is converted to 1,3,4-trimethyl-2-(*p*-methoxybenzyl)-1,2-dihydropyridine with *p*-methoxybenzylmagnesium chloride, reduced to 1,3,4-trimethyl-2-(*p*-methoxybenzyl)-1,2,5,6-tetrahydropyridine with sodium borohydride, cyclized (with H_3PO_4 or HBr) to 1,2,3,4,5,6-hexahydro-3,6,11-trimethyl-2,6-methano-3-benzazocin-8-ol, esterified with acetic anhydride and reacted with cyanogen bromide to form 3-cyano-1,2,3,4,5,6-hexahydro-6,11-dimethyl-2,6-methano-3-benzazocin-8-ol acetate, and hydrolyzed with dilute HCl to compound I.

Description—White to very pale tan, crystalline powder; odorless; slightly bitter taste; stable in light, heat (ambient room temperature), and air; melts between 147 and 158°; pK_a about 8.95.

Solubility—1 g in > 1000 mL water, 11 mL alcohol, 2 mL chloroform or 42 mL ether.

Uses—A synthetic *analgesic* agent. When administered orally in a 50-mg dose it appears to be equivalent in analgesic effectiveness to 60 mg of codeine. When given in usual parenteral doses, it is as effective in relieving moderate to severe pain as usual parenteral doses of morphine, meperidine, butorphanol or nalbuphine. Significant analgesia occurs within 15 to 30 min after oral administration, 15 to 20 min after intramuscular injection and 2 to 3 min after intravenous administration. Duration of action is usually 3 hr or longer. Half-life after intramuscular administration is 2.1 hr. Onset, duration of action and degree of pain relief are related both to dose and the severity of pain. It weakly (about 1/50 that of nalorphine) antagonizes the analgesic effect of morphine and meperidine. It also produces incomplete reversal of the cardiovascular, respiratory and behavioral depression induced by morphine and meperidine. It also has some sedative properties. It is indicated for the control of moderate to severe pain. It is contraindicated in patients hypersensitive to it. It should be used with caution in patients with head injuries and increased intracranial pressure. Except during labor, its use during pregnancy has not been established. Because of limited experience in children under 12 yr, its use in this age group is not recommended. Patients on the drug should be warned not to drive an automobile, operate machinery or expose themselves to hazards. While some patients on therapeutic doses exhibit acute CNS manifestations (hallucinations, disorientation and confusion), such instances are rare and usually clear spontaneously.

Adverse effects reported include gastrointestinal (nausea, vomiting, diarrhea, infrequent constipation and abdominal distress); CNS (dizziness, light-headedness, sedation, euphoria, headache, disturbed dreams, insomnia, syncope, visual blurring and hallucinations); autonomic (sweating, flushing and chills); allergic (rash, urticaria and edema of the face); cardiovascular (hypotension and tachycardia); respiratory depression.

It has been reported to cause psychological and physical dependence after both oral and parenteral use. This is more common in patients with a history of drug abuse. It has been abused in combination with the antihistamine, tripelennamine, by parenteral injection. This combination is reported to cause effects similar to those of heroin. It is a *Schedule IV* drug under the *Controlled Substances Act.*

Dose—*Parenteral,* **20** to **60 mg** (as the lactate); *usual,* **30 mg** every 3 to 4 hr. Maximum daily dose, **360 mg.**

Dosage Form—Lactate Injection: 30 mg (of base)/mL.

Pentazocine Hydrochloride

2,6-Methano-3-benzazocin-8-ol, (2α,6α, 11*R**)-1,2,3,4,5,6-hexahydro-6,11-dimethyl-3-(3-methyl-2-butenyl)-, hydrochloride; Talwin Hydrochloride (*Sanofi-Winthrop*)

[64024-15-3] $C_{19}H_{27}NO.HCl$ (321.89).

For the structure of the base, see *Pentazocine.*

Preparation—*Pentazocine* is reacted with HCl.

Description—White, crystalline powder; exhibits polymorphism, one form melts about 254° and the other about 218°.

Solubility—1 g in 30 mL water, 7 mL alcohol, > 10,000 mL chloroform or 3 mL ether.

Uses—See *Pentazocine.*

Dose (base equivalent)—*Usual,* **50 mg** every 3 to 4 hr; may be increased to **100 mg** when needed. Total daily dose should not exceed **600 mg.**

Dosage Form—Tablets: 50 mg. *Warning:* for oral use only; severe potentially lethal reactions may result from misuse by injection.

Propoxyphene Hydrochloride

Benzeneethanol,
[*S*-(*R**,*S**)]-α-[2-(dimethylamino)-1-methylethyl]-α-phenyl-, propanoate (ester), hydrochloride; Darvon (*Lilly*); (*Various Mfrs*)

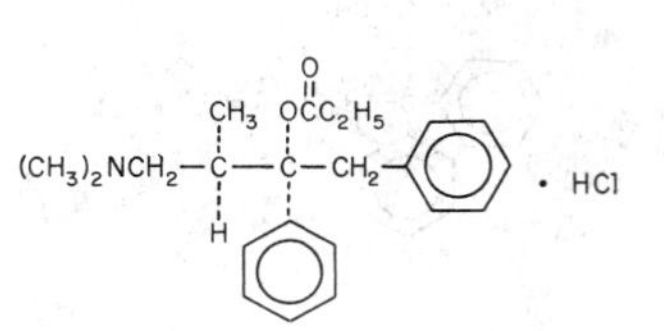

[1639-60-7] $C_{22}H_{29}NO_2.HCl$ (375.94).

Preparation—The Mannich base formed by condensing propiophenone and dimethylamine with formaldehyde is grignardized with benzyl magnesium chloride to produce a mixture of the racemates of the two diastereoisomers (designated commercially as α and β) of the alcohol. The desired α-*dl* form is isolated by fractional crystallization and resolved by means of *d*-camphorsulfonic acid. The desired α-*d* enantiomorph is propionylated with propionic acid in the presence of trimethylamine to form propoxyphene which adds an equivalent of HCl in forming the hydrochloride.

Description—White, crystalline powder; oderless; bitter taste: melts within a 3° range between 163.5° and 168.5°.

Solubility—Freely soluble in water; soluble in alcohol, chloroform or acetone; practically insoluble in benzene or ether.

Uses—A mild analgesic structurally related to the narcotic analgesic methadone. Although its pharmacological properties resemble those of the narcotics as a group, it does not compare with them in analgesic potency. Well-controlled studies indicate that the milligram potency of propoxyphene is about 1/2 to 2/3 that of codeine. It appears that its effectiveness in a dose of 32 mg is questionable and in a dose of 65 mg it is not more, and usually less, effective than the same dose of codeine or 650 mg of aspirin. It has no anti-inflammatory or antipyretic action and little antitussive activity, despite the fact its levo isomer is used for this purpose. It is indicated for the control of *mild to moderate pain.* It is absorbed completely after oral administration; however, first-pass elimination of 30 to 70% markedly reduces its bioavailability. The apparent volume of distribution is 700 to 800 L, oral clearance is 1.3 to 3.6 L/min and half-life is 6 to 12 hr. The major metabolite, norpropoxyphene, has a half-life of

30 to 36 hr. It is contraindicated in patients hypersensitive to it and to aspirin, phenacetin or caffeine. The drug should not be used during pregnancy unless, in the physician's judgment, the potential benefits exceed the potential hazards. The most frequent adverse effects are dizziness, sedation, nausea and vomiting. Other adverse reactions include constipation, abdominal pain, skin rashes, light-headedness, headache, weakness, euphoria, dysphoria and minor visual disturbances. The chronic ingestion of 800 mg/day has caused toxic psychoses and convulsions. The depressant effects of propoxyphene may be additive with those of other depressant drugs, such as alcohol, tranquilizers and sedative-hypnotics. Moreover, a number of deaths have been reported in patients on excessive doses, either alone or in combination with other CNS depressant drugs. Since both psychological and physical dependence have been induced with this agent, it should be prescribed with the same degree of caution as codeine.

Drowsiness or dizziness may occur which may impair ability to drive or perform other tasks requiring alertness. It is not recommended for children.

Dose—32 to **390 mg** a day; *usual*, **65 mg** 6 times a day as necessary.

Dosage Form—Capsules: 32 and 65 mg.

Propoxyphene Napsylate

Benzeneethanol, [*S*-(*R**, *S**)]-α-[2-(dimethylamino)-1-methylethyl]-α-phenyl-, propanoate (ester), compound with 2-naphthalenesulfonic acid (1:1) monohydrate; Darvon-N (*Lilly*)

[26570-10-5] $C_{22}H_{29}NO_2.C_{10}H_8O_3S.H_2O$ (565.72); *anhydrous* [17140-78-2] (547.71).

For the structure of the base, see *Propoxyphene Hydrochloride*.

Preparation—*Propoxyphene* is reacted with an equimolar quantity of aqueous 2-naphthalenesulfonic acid and the salt is crystallized therefrom.

Description—White, bitter, crystalline powder; essentially no odor; melts in a 4° range between 158° and 165°.

Solubility—1 g in 10,000 mL of water, 15 mL of alcohol or 10 mL of chloroform; soluble in ether.

Uses—Actions, uses and precautions are the same as *Propoxyphene Hydrochloride*, except that, because of its larger molecular weight, a dose of 100 mg is required instead of the 65 mg dose of the hydrochloride. This compound permits more stable liquid and tablet dosage forms because of its very slight solubility in water.

Dose—*Usual*, **100 mg** every 4 hr as needed for pain. Do not exceed 600 mg per day.

Dosage Forms—Oral Suspension: 10 mg/mL; Tablets: 100 mg.

Sufentanil Citrate

Propanamide, *N*-[4-(methoxymethyl)-1-[2-(thienyl)ethyl]-4-piperidinyl]-*N*-phenyl-, 2-hydroxy-1,2,3-propanetricarboxylate (1:1); Sufenta (*Janssen*)

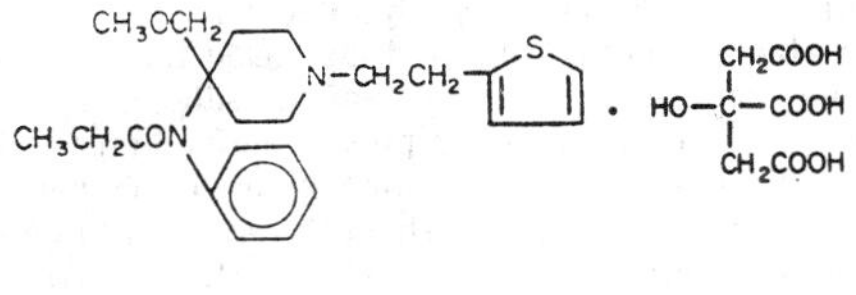

[60561-17-3] $C_{22}H_{30}N_2O_2S.C_6H_8O_7$ (578.68).

Preparation—*Arzneimittel-Forsch 26:* 1521, 1976.

Description—White crystals; melts about 97°.

Uses—A strong opioid analgesic. Its analgesic potency is 5 to 12 times that of fentanyl on a weight basis. High doses can cause amnesia and a loss of consciousness. It is used for balanced anesthesia in general surgery as an adjunct to nitrous oxide and oxygen. It also may be used for induction of surgical anesthesia and as the sole anesthetic agent with a muscle relaxant and oxygen for cardiovascular and neurosurgical procedures. Given intravenously it is metabolized rapidly (elimination half-life, 2.4 hr). The volume of distribution is 2.5 L/kg; 92.5% is bound to plasma protein; plasma clearance is 0.8 L/min. The most common adverse effects include respiratory depression and skeletal muscle rigidity. The rapid intravenous administration of sufentanil may induce a general increase in muscle tone, including chest-wall spasm. Other adverse effects include bradycardia, hypotension and hypertension. After low doses recovery time is about the same as that for fentanyl. Sufentanil is a *Schedule II* drug under the *Federal Controlled Substances Act*.

Dose—*Adult, intravenous, general surgery:* **1 to 2 μg/kg** with nitrous oxide/oxygen; *maintenance*, **10 to 25 μg** as needed. *Cardiovascular or neurological surgery*: **2** to **8 μg/kg** or more with oxygen and a nondepolarizing (curariform) muscle relaxant; *maintenance*, 25 to 50 μg as needed. *Children 2 to 12 yr, cardiovascular surgery*: 10 μg/kg or more with oxygen only. *Children under 2 yr:* no dose has been established.

Dosage Form—Solution: 50 μg/mL in 2, 5, 10, 20 and 50 mL.

Narcotic Analgesic Combinations

Some examples of narcotic analgesic combinations (with mg/unit provided) as as follows:

Codeine Phosphate and Acetaminophen [Tylenol with Codeine #1 (*McNeil*); Tylenol with Codeine Elixir (*McNeil*); Tylenol with Codeine #2 (*McNeil*); Phenaphen with Codeine #2 (*Robins*); Papadeine #3 (*Vangard*); Tylenol with Codeine #3 (*McNeil*); Phenaphen with Codeine #3 (*Robins*); Phenaphen 650 with Codeine (*Robins*); Papadeine #4 (*Vangard*); Tylenol with Codeine #4 (*McNeil*); Phenaphen with Codeine #4 (*Robins*)]—7.5 and 300; 12 and 120; 15 and 300; 15 and 325; 30 and 300; 30 and 325; 30 and 650; 32 and 325; 60 and 300; 60 and 325 mg, respectively.

Codeine Phosphate and Aspirin [Empirin with Codeine #2 (*Burroughs Wellcome*); Empirin with Codeine #3 (*Burroughs Wellcome*); Empirin with Codeine #4 (*Burroughs Wellcome*)]—15 and 325; 30 and 325; 60 and 325 mg, respectively.

Codeine Phosphate, Acetaminophen and Caffeine [Codalan #1, 2 and 3 (*Lannett*)]—8, 500 and 300; 15, 500 and 30; 30, 500 and 30 mg, respectively.

Codeine Phosphate, Aspirin, Caffeine and Butalbital [Fiorinal with Codeine (*Sandoz*)]—30, 325, 40 and 50 mg, respectively.

Dihydrocodeine Bitartrate, Aspirin and Caffeine [Synalgos-DC (*Wyeth*)]—16, 365.4 and 30 mg, respectively.

Hydrocodone and Acetaminophen [Amacodone (*Trimen*); Dolacet (*Hauck*); Hydrocet (*Carnrick*); Vicodin (*Knoll*); Zydone (*Dupont*)]—5 and 500 mg, respectively.

Meperidine Hydrochloride and Acetaminophen [Demerol APAP (*Winthrop-Breon*)]—50 and 300 mg, respectively.

Meperidine Hydrochloride and Promethazine Hydrochloride [Mepergan (*Wyeth*); Mepergan Fortes (*Wyeth*)]—25 and 25; 25 and 50 mg, respectively.

Morphine Sulfate and Atropine Sulfate [Morphine and Atropine Injection (*Beecham*)]—16 and 0.4 mg/mL, respectively.

Oxycodone Hydrochloride and Acetaminophen [Percocet (*Dupont*); Tylox (*McNeil*)]—5 and 325; 5 and 500 mg, respectively.

Propoxyphene Hydrochloride and Acetaminophen [Dolene AP-65 (*Lederle*); Wygesic (*Wyeth*)]—65 and 650 mg, respectively.

Propoxyphene and Aspirin [Darvon with ASA (*Lilly*)]—65 and 325 mg, respectively.

Propoxyphene Hydrochloride, Aspirin and Caffeine [Darvon Compound-65 (*Lilly*)]—65, 389 and 32.4 mg, respectively.

Propoxyphene Napsylate and Acetaminophen [Darvocet-N 50 (*Lilly*); Darvon-N 100 (*Lilly*); Doxapap-N (*Major*); Propacet (*Lemmon*)]—50 amd 325; 100 and 650 mg, respectively.

Propoxyphene Napsylate and Aspirin [Darvon-N with ASA (*Lilly*)]—100 and 325 mg, respectively.

Analgesics, Antipyretics and Anti-Inflammatories

The analgesic, antipyretic and antiinflammatory drugs include a small, heterogeneous group of compounds which, unlike those presented in the two preceding sections, are without significant addiction liability and, therefore, are not subject to regulation under the *Controlled Substances Act*. Many of these agents affect pain, fever and inflammation and are referred to as the nonsteroidal antiinflammatory drugs (NSAIDs). Consequently, they are used widely for minor aches and pains, headaches and the general feeling of malaise that accompanies febrile illnesses, and to alleviate symptoms of rheumatic fever, arthritis, gout and other musculoskeletal disturbances. Several agents (allopurinol, colchicine, probenecid, etc) do have pain-relieving properties in various conditions (gout, arthritis, etc), but since they are of no value in other types of pain, they cannot be classed as true analgesic drugs and will be discussed in a separate section.

Nonsteroidal Anti-inflammatory Drugs (NSAIDs)

The number of NSAIDs continues to increase. In addition to aspirin-like drugs, the NSAIDs available in this country include meclofenamate sodium, phenylbutazone, indomethacin, piroxicam, sulindac and tolmetin for the treatment of arthritis; mefenamic acid for analgesia; and ibuprofen, fenoprofen flurbiprofen, diclofenac, etodolac, ketorolac and naproxen for both analgesia and arthritis. Ibuprofen, mefenamic acid and naproxen are used also for the management of dysmenorrhea. For the most part, the newer nonsalicylate NSAIDs have similar pharmacological properties with some differences in their pharmacokinetic properties (see Table 3). The principal mechanism of action for all NSAIDs appears to be inhibition of prostaglandin synthesis by blocking the activity of the precursor enzyme, cyclooxygenase. Their actions on prostaglandins likely account for many of the side effects of the NSAIDs. Although, in general, there is little difference between the efficacy of different NSAIDs, some patients may respond to one agent better than another. This is difficult to predict and often requires trial and error to find the most suitable drug.

The clinical usefulness of NSAIDs is restricted by a number of adverse effects. Phenylbutazone has been implicated in hepatic necrosis and granulomatous hepatitis; and sulindac, indomethacin, ibuprofen and naproxen with hepatitis and cholestatic hepatitis. Transient increases in serum aminotransferases, especially alanine aminotransferase, have been reported. All of these drugs, including aspirin, because of their inhibition of prostaglandins, can interfere with regulation of glomerular filtration and renal sodium and water excretion. Thus, the NSAIDs can cause fluid retention and decrease sodium excretion, followed by hyperkalemia, oliguria and anuria. Moreover, all of these drugs can adversely affect the stomach and even cause peptic ulceration. Other side effects include diarrhea with meclofenamate; tinnitis with aspirin; headache with indomethacin and upper abdominal pain with ketoprofen, meclofenamate and tolmetin. The ranking of NSAIDs according to toxicity shows indomethacin, tolmetin, melofenamate and ketoprofen to be the most toxic with coated or buffered aspirin and ibuprofen the least.

Blood dyscrasias associated with NSAIDs are rare, but death has been attributed to the use of these drugs. All of them can interfere with platelet function and may cause bleeding in patients taking anticoagulants. In addition, agranulocytosis or aplastic anemia have been reported in patients on indomethacin, ibuprofen, fenoprofen, naproxen, tolmetin and piroxicam. Phenylbutazone has caused agranulocytosis and aplastic anemia, especially in the elderly, and may cause leukemia.

Other adverse effects attributed to these drugs include dermatitis and allergic reactions as well as CNS effects, such as sedation, agitation, headaches and tinnitis. Patients taking these drugs for long periods of time should have periodic white cell counts and determinations of serum creatinine levels and hepatic enzyme activities.

Table 3—Properties of Nonsalicylate NSAIDs

Nonsalicylate NSAIDs ($t_{1/2}$ hr)	Uses: Analgesic Onset (hr)	Analgesic Duration (hr)	Antiinflammatory Onset (days)
Propionic acids			
Fenoprofen (2–3)	—	—	2
Flurbiprofen(3–9)	—	—	NAv[a]
Ibuprofen (1.8–2.5)	0.5	4–6	≤7
Ketoprofen (2–4)	NAv[a]	NAv[a]	NAv[a]
Naproxen (12–15)	1	≤7	≤7
Acetic acids			
Diclofenac (1–2)	—	—	NAv[a]
Etodolac (~7)	0.5	4–12	—
Indomethacin (4.5)	0.5	4–6	≤7
Ketorolac (2.4–8.6)	0.15	≤6	—
Sulindac (7.8)	—	—	≤7
Tolmetin (1–2)	—	—	≤7
Fenamates			
Meclofenamate (2)	NAv[a]	NAv[a]	several days
Mefenamic acid (2–4)	NAv[a]	NAv[a]	—
Oxicam			
Piroxicam (30–86)	1	48–72	7–12
Others			
Nabumetone (22–30)	—	—	NAv[a]

[a] NAv—information not available.

Amodiaquine—RPS-17, page 1217.

Salicylate-Like NSAIDs

The salicylate group of analgesics and antipyretics are by far the most commonly employed. Indeed, these are consumed at a rate in excess of 10,000 tons annually. In general, salicylates are *contraindicated* in hypersensitive individuals and in those with gastrointestinal disturbances, particularly hemorrhaging ulcers. They also should be used with caution in patients on anticoagulant therapy and avoided in patients on uricosurics. The *salicylates interact* with a wide variety of agents, some of which are important clinically while others are largely of theoretical interest. Nevertheless, the well-informed pharmacist will acquaint himself with the potential interactions between salicylate drugs and;

Antidiabetic agents (increased hypoglycemia).
Oral anticoagulants (displacement of anticoagulants from protein binding sites, increased anticoagulant effect).
Uricosuric agents (relative effect of large and small doses of salicylates).
Antiarthritic drugs (may lower plasma concentrations of these agents).
Alcohol (which enhances gastrointestinal bleeding).
Tetracycline (may complex with buffering agent in some aspirin products).
Other drugs (see Chapter 105).

Acetaminophen

Acetamide, *N*-(4-hydroxyphenyl)-, *N*-Acetyl-*p*-aminophenol; *p*-Acetamidophenol; (*Various Mfrs*)

4′-Hydroxyacetanilide [103-90-2] $C_8H_9NO_2$ (151.16).

Preparation—*p*-Nitrophenol is reduced and the resulting *p*-aminophenol is acetylated by heating with a mixture of acetic anhydride and glacial acetic acid. The crude product may be purified by recrystallization from an ethanol–water mixture.

Description—White, odorless, crystalline powder; slightly bitter taste; melts about 170°; pH (saturated solution) 5.3 to 6.5; pK_a 9.51.

Solubility—1 g in 70 mL water, 20 mL boiling water, 10 mL alcohol, 50 mL chloroform, 40 mL glycerin; slightly soluble in ether.

Uses—An effective antipyretic and analgesic that exerts its clinical effects by a mechanism similar to that of the salicylates. It is a major metabolite of phenacetin, a *p*-aminophenol-derived analgesic no longer available in the US due to its association with analgesic nephropathy. It produces antipyresis by acting on the hypothalamic heat-regulating center and analgesia by elevating the pain threshold. It is effective in the treatment of a wide variety of arthritic and rheumatic conditions involving musculoskeletal pain as well as the pain of headache, dysmenorrhea, myalgias and neuralgias. It also is useful in diseases accompanied by pain, discomfort and fever, such as the common cold and other viral infections. It is useful particularly as an analgesic-antipyretic in patients who experience untoward reactions to aspirin. It rarely induces untoward effects in therapeutic doses and usually is well-tolerated by aspirin-sensitive patients. Rarely, a sensitivity reaction may occur; in this case the drug should be stopped. Acetaminophen frequently is combined with other drugs, such as caffeine and aspirin. The value of such combinations is questionable. However, acetaminophen combined with opiates, such as codeine and oxycodone does enhance analgesic potency. It lacks the anti-inflammatory action of the salicylates; hence, it is of only limited usefulness in inflammatory rheumatic disorders and often is not considered an NSAID agent. It does not produce the methemoglobinemia, agranulocytosis and anemia which sometimes result from long-continued use of acetanilid and phenacetin. Unlike aspirin, acetaminophen does not antagonize the effects of uricosuric agents. Although large doses have been reported to potentiate anticoagulants, therapeutic doses have no effect on prothrombin time.

Absorption of the drug after oral administration is rapid and peak plasma levels are reached in 30 to 120 min. The therapeutic half-life is approximately 3 hr. Approximately 2% is excreted unchanged in the urine; the glucuronide and sulfate conjugates are nontoxic and account for about 95% of the drug. A much smaller amount, estimated to be 3%, is oxidized via the hepatic cytochrome P-450 system to a chemically reactive intermediate which combines with liver glutathione to form a nontoxic substance. However, after massive single doses of the drug the supply of liver glutathione is exhausted and the excess reactive arylating intermediate covalently binds to vital hepatocellular macromolecules, leading to necrosis. Hepatic necrosis and death have been observed following overdosage; hepatic damage is likely if an adult takes more than 10 to 15 g in a single dose or if a 2-yr-old child takes more than 3 g. Young children are less likely to develop hepatotoxicity than adults.

Both *in vivo* and *in vitro* studies have shown that agents which stimulate metabolism, such as phenobarbital and phenytoin, potentiate acetaminophen-induced hepatotoxicity. The best indicator of potential liver injury is the half-life of its elimination. A half-life greater than 4 hr is associated uniformly with liver injury. Also, plasma levels greater than 300 μg/mL at 4 hr post-ingestion are consistent with liver injury, whereas levels less than 120 μg/mL at 4 hr post-ingestion usually are not. Treatment of overdosage includes administration of acetylcysteine to help conjugate the hepatotoxic metabolite plus symptomatic and supportive care.

The label on its dosage forms carries the following (or equivalent) statement: *Warning—Do not use more than 10 days unless directed by a physician. Keep this medication out of reach of children.*

Dose—*Usual, adult, oral,* **300 mg** to **1 g** 3 or 4 times a day. *Usual, pediatric, oral,* **175 mg/m²** 4 times a day; or **60 mg** 3 or 4 times a day for children under 1 yr, **60** to **120 mg** 3 or 4 times a day for children 1 to 2 yr, **120 mg** 3 or 4 times a day for children 3 to 5 yr, 150 to **325 mg** 3 or 4 times a day for children 6 to 12 yr.

Dosage Forms—Capsules: 500 mg; Drops: 100 mg/mL and 120 mg/2.5 mL; Elixir: 120, 160, and 325 mg/5 mL; Liquid: 160 mg/5 mL and 500 mg/15 mL. Suppositories: 120, 125, 325, and 650 mg; Tablets: 160, 325, 500, and 650 mg; Chewable Tablets: 80 mg.

Antipyrine—See RPS-18, page 1114.

Aspirin

Benzoic acid, 2-(acetyloxy)-,

COOH
$OCOCH_3$

Acetylsalicylic acid [50-78-2] $C_9H_8O_4$ (180.16).

Preparation—Salicylic acid is acetylated directly with acetic anhydride and the crude material purified by recrystallization from benzene or various other nonaqueous solvents. A granulated form of aspirin, either white or colored, also is available commercially for compression into tablets.

Description—White crystals, commonly tabular or needle-like, or a white, crystalline powder; odorless or a faint odor; stable in dry air (in moist air it gradually hydrolyzes into salicylic and acetic acids, the odor of the latter becoming noticeable); melts about 135°, but the exact melting temperature varies with the conditions of the test; an alcoholic solution is not colored violet by ferric chloride (distinction from salicylic acid).

Solubility—1 g in about 300 mL water, 5 mL alcohol, 17 mL chloroform or about 10 to 15 mL of ether; less soluble in absolute ether; dissolves with decomposition in aqueous solutions of alkali hydroxides or carbonates.

Incompatibilities—Can form a damp to pasty mass when triturated with *acetanilid, acetophenetidin, antipyrine, aminopyrine, methenamine, phenol* or *salol.* Powders containing aspirin with an alkali salt such as *sodium bicarbonate* may become gummy on contact with atmospheric moisture due to a partial solution and subsequent hydrolysis of the aspirin. Hydrolysis likewise occurs in admixture with salts containing water of crystallization. Solutions of alkali acetates and citrates, as well as alkalies themselves, dissolve this drug, but the resulting solutions hydrolyze rapidly to form salts of acetic and salicylic acids. Sugar and glycerin have been shown to hinder the decomposition. It very slowly liberates hydriodic acid from *potassium* or *sodium iodide.* Subsequent oxidation by the air produces free iodine.

Uses—Employed, as well as the salts of salicylic acid (eg, sodium, choline and magnesium salicylate) as an *antipyretic* and *analgetic* in a variety of conditions. It is indicated for the relief of pain from simple headache, discomfort and fever associated with the common cold and minor muscular aches and pains. When drug therapy is indicated for the reduction of a fever, it is one of the most effective and safest drugs.

Epidemiological evidence has suggested the possibility of an association between the use of aspirin in the treatment of fever in children with varicella (chickenpox), a common cold or influenza virus infections and the subsequent development of Reyes syndrome. The current opinion is that aspirin should not be prescribed under usual circumstances for children with upper respiratory, viral infections. If control of fever, aches and pains are necessary alternative measures should be employed. Because the drug inhibits platelet function, it prophylactically reduces the incidence of *myocardial infarction* and *transcient ischemic attacks* in men and to a lesser extent in women.

In *gout* and in *acute rheumatic fever,* the salicylates, including aspirin, have a fairly specific action. In gout, large doses must be given often, and the results obtained are somewhat less dramatic than with phenylbutazone or allopurinol. In acute rheumatic fever, full doses are given every hour until salicylism occurs (ringing in ears, dizziness), and then every 4 hr for days or weeks. In neither of the above-mentioned conditions are the salicylates a cure, and other forms of treatment are employed simultaneously. Following oral administration, peak plasma levels are reached within 1 to 2 hr, and fairly constant levels are maintained for 4 to 6 hr.

Plasma half-life following oral administration of one gram of aspirin ranges from 4.7 to 9 hr, with an average of 6 hr. With toxic doses (10 to 20 g) the half-life may be increased to 22 hr. A direct correlation between plasma levels and clinical effectiveness has not been established, but analgesia usually is achieved at plasma levels of 15 to 30 mg/100 mL, anti-inflammatory activity at 20 to 40 mg/100 mL and some symptoms of salicylism at 35 mg/100 mL. It is bound poorly to plasma protein; nevertheless, with therapeutic doses, from 50 to 80% is bound to plasma proteins.

Adverse effects from usual doses of the drug are infrequent; most common are gastrointestinal disturbances (dyspepsia, nausea, vomiting and occult bleeding). Prolonged administration of large doses (3.6 g a day) results in occult bleeding and may result in anemia. Massive gastrointestinal hemorrhage occurs rarely and, although its relationship to peptic ulcer is uncertain, a nonsalicylate analgesic may be preferred in high-risk patients.

As evidenced by substantial fecal blood loss, alcohol increases the gastric bleeding caused by aspirin in many patients. Concomitant use of the drug and corticosteroids or pyrazolone derivatives (phenylbutazone) may increase the risk of gastrointestinal ulceration. Its use with fenoprofen, ibuprofen, indomethacin or naproxen may cause lowering of plasma concentrations and thus reduce the effectiveness of the latter drugs. It displaces highly bound coumarin-type anticoagulants from protein-binding sites and thus increases the concentrations and effects of the anticoagulants.

The hypoglycemic action of oral sulfonylureas may be increased by concurrent administration of the drug. The uricosuric activity of probenecid and sulfinpyrazone are inhibited when either drug is administered simultaneously with the drug. Buffered aspirin formulations that contain calcium, magnesium or aluminum may form complexes with tetracycline from which absorption of the antibiotic is impaired.

Salicylates account for many accidental poisonings, and may result from promiscuous use of large doses of these agents by the laity. To avoid accidental poisoning of children, this drug and other salicylate drugs should be kept out of their reach; also, caution in use of these drugs in children with fever and dehydration is necessary because they are particularly prone to intoxication from relatively small doses of the drugs. In addition, some few people manifest idiosyncrasy in the form of an allergic sensitivity to salicylates, especially this drug, and may suffer from serious, if not fatal, asthma after ingestion of a single 300-mg dose. Consequently, it should be used with great care in patients with asthma, nasal polyps or allergies.

It crosses the placental barrier, and is excreted into breast milk. As use of aspirin prior to delivery may have inhibited platelet aggregation and diminished factor XII plasma levels in newborn infants, it has been suggested that no salicylate be ingested during the last month of pregnancy. Chronic high-dose therapy has been reported to increase the length of gestation and to prolong labor.

Dose—*Usual, adult, minor aches* and *pain:* **325** to **650 mg** every 4 hr as needed; *arthritis* and *rheumatic conditions,* **3.6** to **5.4 g** a day in divided doses; acute *rheumatic fever* **5** to **8 g** a day initially; *myocardial infarction* **300** to **325 mg** a day. Juvenile *rheumatoid arthritis,* **90** to **130 mg/kg** every 24 hr; *pediatric analgesic,* not to exceed 3.6 g a day.

Dosage Forms—Enteric-Coated Capsules: 325 and 500 mg; Suppositories: 60, 120, 125, 130, 195, 200, 300, 325, 600 and 650 mg and 1.2 g; Tablets: 65, 81, 325 and 500 mg; Enteric-Coated Tablets:

325, 600, 650 and 975 mg; Timed-Release Tablets: 650 and 800 mg; Gum Tablets: 227.5 mg.

Carprofen—see RPS-18, page 1111.

Choline Salicylate

(2-Hydroxyethyl)trimethylammonium salicylate; (*Various Mfrs*)

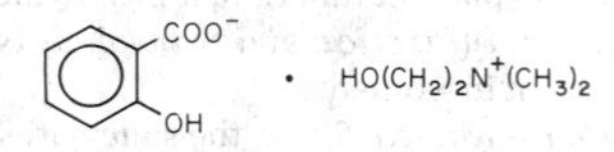

[2016-36-6] $C_{12}N_{19}NO_4$ (241.29).

Preparation—By mixing stoichiometric quantities of choline chloride and sodium salicylate in acetone, filtering the insoluble sodium chloride which is formed and precipitating the salicylate salt with petroleum ether. US Pat 3,069,321.

Description—White, hygroscopic solid; melts about 50°; pH (10% aqueous solution) 6.5.

Solubility—Freely soluble in water; soluble in most hydrophilic solvents; insoluble in organic solvents.

Uses—A salt of salicylic acid. It is a nonsteroidal anti-inflammatory agent used in the management of pain, rheumatoid arthritis and osteoarthritis. Each gram of choline salicylate contains 568 mg of salicylate (equivalent to 760 mg of aspirin). There is no evidence that one salicylate salt is superior therapeutically to another; nevertheless, sodium or magnesium salts should be avoided in patients in whom excessive amounts of these electrolytes might be harmful. Moreover, this drug has fewer gastrointestinal side effects than aspirin. Adverse effects, precautions and contraindications are the same as those for other salicylate salts. The safe use of this drug during pregnancy or lactation has not been established.

Dose—*Usual, adults* and *children (over 12 yr)*: **80 mg** (5 mL) every 3 or 4 hr; maximum, 6 times a day. Rheumatoid arthritis patient may start with 5 to 10 mL; up to 4 times a day.

Dosage Form—Mint-Flavored Liquid: 870 mg/5 mL, in 240 and 480 mL.

Magnesium Salicylate

Magnesium, bis(2-hydroxybenzoato-O^1,O^2)-, Amamate (*Winston*); Magan (*Adria*)

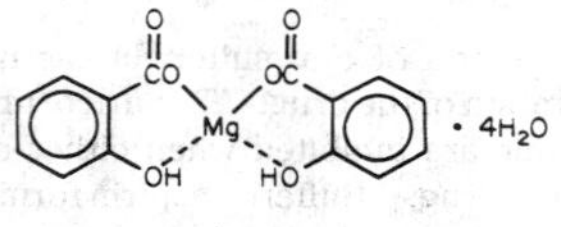

Magnesium salicylate [18917-95-8] $C_{14}H_{10}MgO_6 \cdot 4H_2O$ (370.60); *anhydrous* [34200-52-7] (298.53).

Preparation—Salicyclic acid is reacted with a sufficient quantity of magnesium oxide in a hot mixture of 2-propanol and water, and the hydrated salt crystallizes on cooling.

Description—White to slightly pink, free-flowing crystalline powder; odorless or has a faint characteristic odor; aqueous solution is acid to litmus.

Solubility—1 g in 13 mL water; soluble in alcohol.

Uses—Although it has analgesic, antipyretic and anti-inflammatory effects similar to those of aspirin and other salicylates, it is indicated only for symptomatic relief of signs and symptoms of rheumatoid arthritis, osteoarthritis, bursitis and other *musculoskeletal* disorders. Salicylates inhibit the synthesis of prostaglandins; the importance of this mechanism in analgesia and anti-inflammatory effect has not been fully elucidated. Following ingestion of 524 mg of magnesium salicylate, a peak concentration of 3.6 mg salicyclic acid/dL is reached in 1½ hr with a half-life of 2 hr. Except for the danger of hypermagnesemia in advanced chronic renal disease and the fact that safe use of this agent in children under 12 yr has not been established, the contraindications, warnings, precautions, drug interactions and treatment of overdosage are the same as for *Aspirin* (page 1110) and *Sodium Salicylate* (page 1114).

Dose—*Usual, adult, oral*, **600 mg** 3 or 4 times a day. It may be increased to **3.6 to 4.8 g** a day in divided doses at intervals of 3 to 6 hr. In rheumatic fever, as much as **9.6 g** a day may be required.

Dosage Form—Tablets: 325, 545 and 600 mg.

Phenacetin—see RPS-18, page 1114.

Salicylamide

Benzamide, 2-hydroxy-, (*Various Mfrs*)

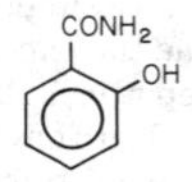

[65-45-2] $C_7H_7NO_2$ (137.14).

Preparation—From methyl benzoate by ammonolysis with ammonia at room temperature.

Description—White to faint-pink crystals; bitter taste and imparts a warm sensation to the tongue; melts about 140°; pH (saturated aqueous solution) almost 5.

Solubility—(g/100 mL)—Water: 0.2 g in 500 mL water at 30° or 167 mL at 47°; 1 g in 20 mL glycerin at 39°; soluble in hot water, alcohol or chloroform.

Uses—Has analgesic and antipyretic properties similar to the salicylates; however, anti-inflammatory action has not been demonstrated. However, the drug is *not* hydrolyzed to salicylic acid; therefore, it is not considered a true salilcylate. It is absorbed rapidly and completely after oral administration; it is metabolized almost completely to inactive metabolites during absorption and first pass through the liver and has an elimination half-life of 1.2 hr. Only trace amounts of unchanged drug are detected in plasma. It is 40 to 55% bound to serum proteins at concentrations of 20 to 500 μg/mL. In patients with normal hepatic function, 90 to 100% of a single dose is excreted in the urine within 24 hr. Adverse reactions such as gastrointestinal irritation, dizziness or headache are common; hemorrhagic lesions, leukopenia and thrombocytopenia have been reported. It is generally available in combination preparations.

Dose—*Usual, adult, oral, minor aches and pains*, **325** to **667 mg** 3 or 4 times a day. *Children under 12 yr*, consult physician.

Dosage Form—Tablets in combination with other drugs: 65 to 162 mg.

Salsalate

Benzoic acid, 2-hydroxy-, 2-carboxyphenyl ester; Disalcid (*3M*); Mono-Gesic (*Central*); Salflex (*Carnrick*)

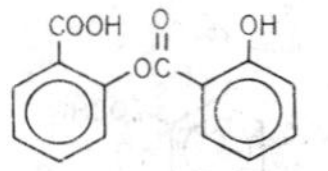

Preparation—By condensation of 2 moles of salicylic acid in the presence of thionyl chloride. See Ger Pat 214,044.

Description—A crystalline solid; melts about 148°.

Solubility—Slightly soluble in water but hydrolyzes slowly into two molecules of salicylic acid; soluble in alcohol or ether; sparingly soluble in benzene; insoluble in dilute acids.

Uses—For the relief of the signs and symptoms of rheumatoid arthritis, osteoarthritis and related rheumatic disorders. The drug, also known as salicylsalicylic acid, is a dimer of salicylic acid. It is insoluble in gastric juice, but soluble in the small intestine where it is hydrolyzed partially to two molecules of salicylic acid and absorbed. On a molar basis, the amount of salicylic acid available from the drug is about 15% less than that from aspirin. Biotransformation of the drug is saturated at anti-inflammatory doses; hence, the half-life of salicylic acid is increased from 3.5 to more than 16 hr. Thus, twice a day dosing will maintain blood levels within the desired therapeutic range (10 to 30 mg/100 mL) throughout 12-hr intervals. Therapeutic blood levels continue for up to 16 hr after the last dose. The mechanism of anti-inflammatory action of this and other anti-inflammatory drugs remains unclear. In contrast to aspirin, it does not cause gastrointestinal blood loss and can be given to aspirin-sensitive patients. Otherwise, precautions and adverse effects resemble those of the salicylates (see page 1209).

Dose—*Usual, adult, oral*, **325** to **1000** mg 2 or 3 times a day. If necessary, adjust frequency of dosage based on response.

Dosage Forms—Capsules: 500 mg; Tablets 500 and 750 mg.

Sodium Salicylate

(*Various Mfrs*)

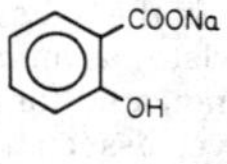

Monosodium salicylate [54-21-7] $C_7H_5NaO_3$ (160.10).

Preparation—Salicylic acid is mixed with sufficient distilled water to form a paste, then sufficient pure sodium carbonate is added in small portions to neutralize all but a small fraction of the salicylic acid. The resulting solution is filtered through a filter free from iron, as even slight contact with iron will discolor the product. The filtered solution is evaporated at a low temperature to dryness, preferably in a vacuum.

Description—Amorphous or microcrystalline powder or scales; colorless or has not more than a faint, pink tinge; odorless, or has a faint, characteristic odor, and a sweet, saline taste; affected by light; aqueous solution is neutral or acid to litmus.

Solubility—1 g in 1 mL water, 10 mL alcohol or about 4 mL glycerin; very soluble in boiling water or boiling alcohol.

Incompatibilities—Solutions of salicylates slowly darken in color due to an *oxidation reaction* influenced by the presence of *alkalies* or *iron* and leading to a quinoid structure. The reaction is retarded by the presence of more easily oxidized substances such as sodium bisulfite, sodium hypophosphite or sodium thiosulfate.

Uses—The analgetic, antipyretic actions and limitations of the salicylates are presented in detail under *Aspirin* (page 1209). Like the latter compound, this drug is employed for the *relief of pain* and the *reduction of fever*. It also is useful in the symptomatic therapy of *gout* and in acute *rheumatic fever*. It is about 1/3 less potent, on a weight basis, than aspirin, and therefore the equivalent analgetic dose is somewhat higher. The sodium salt tends to cause gastric irritation due to the liberation of free salicylic acid by the acid gastric juice. For this reason, an equivalent amount of sodium bicarbonate usually is employed along with this drug. It does not affect platelet function but, like aspirin, does increase prothrombin time. It should not be used by patients on a low-sodium diet.

Dose—**300 mg** to **4 g** a day; *usual, adult, oral*, **300** to **650 mg** every 4 to 8 hr as needed.

Dosage Forms—Tablets: 325 and 650 mg; Enteric-Coated Tablets: 324, 325 and 650 mg; Injection: 1 g/10 mL.

Sodium Thiosulfate—see RPS-16, page 1176.

Sodium Thiosalicylate

(Various Mfrs)

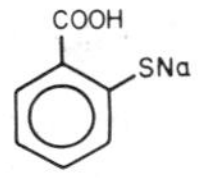

[147-93-3; free acid] $C_7H_5NaO_2S$ (176.16).

Preparation—From *o*-halobenzoic acids heated with NaSH in alkali or reduction of *O,O'*-dithiodibenzoic acid produced by treating the diazonium salt, prepared from anthranilic acid, with a solution of sulfur in sodium sulfide. *Org Syn Coll Vol II:* 580, 1943.

Description—Off-white crystals.

Solubility—Soluble in water.

Uses—An investigational drug which may be useful in the symptomatic treatment of osteoarthritis, rheumatic fever, muscular pain, musculoskeletal disorders and acute gout. The drug is absorbed rapidly and detectable in the blood 1.5 hr following intramuscular administration. It appears to share the same adverse effects, precautions and contraindications as other salicylates. The safe use of it during pregnancy and lactation has not been established.

Dose—*Usual, adult, intramuscular, acute gout:* **100 mg** every 3 or 4 hr for 2 days, then **100 mg** a day; *muscular pain:* **50** to **100 mg** a day or on alternate days; *rheumatic fever:* **100** to **150 mg** every 4 to 6 hr for 3 days, then reduce to **100 mg** twice a day. Continue until the patient is asymptomatic.

Dosage Form—Injection: 50 mg/mL.

Analgesic Combinations with Salicylate-Like NSAIDs

Some examples of analgesic combinations with salicylate-like NSAIDs (with mg/unit provided) are as follows:

Acetaminophen and Diphenhydramine Citrate [Excedrin P.M. (*Bristol Myers*)]—500 and 38 mg, respectively.

Acetaminophen, Aspirin and Caffeine [Trigesic (*Squibb*); Excedrin (*Bristol Myers*)]—125, 230 and 30 mg; 250, 250 and 65 mg, respectively.

Acetaminophen, Pambrom and Pyrilamine Maleate [Midol PMS (*Glenbrook*); Pamprin (*Chattem*)]—500, 25 and 15 mg, respectively.

Aspirin, Acetaminophen and Caffeine [Trigesic (*Squibb*); Excedrin (*Bristol Myers*)]—230, 125 and 30; 250, 250 and 65 mg, respectively.

Aspirin and Caffeine [Anacin (*Whitehall*); APAC Improved (*Vortech*); PAC (*Upjohn*); Midol Caplets (*Glenbrook*); Anacin Maximum Strength (*Whitehall*)]—400 and 32; 454 and 32.4; 500 and 32 mg, respectively.

Aspirin and Meprobamate [Epromate (*Major*); Equagesic (*Wyeth*); Equazine (*Rugby*); Micrainin (*Wallace*)]—325 and 200 mg, respectively.

Nonsalicylate NSAIDs

This group of NSAIDs include derivatives from propionic, acetic and anthranilic acids, as well as oxicam. There is little to distinguish these NSAIDs, as discussed above, although there certainly will be new drugs from these groups marketed in the future.

Diclofenac Sodium

Benzeneacetic acid, 2-[(2,6-dichlorophenyl)amino]-, monosodium salt; Voltaren (*Geigy*)

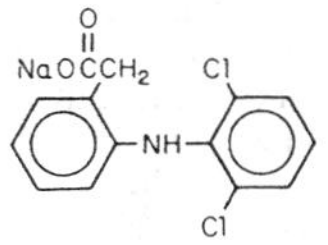

[15307-79-6] (salt); [15307-86-5] (free acid) $C_{14}H_{10}Cl_2NN_aO_2$ (318.13).

Preparation—Oxalyl chloride and 2,6-dichlorodiphenylamine are condensed to form the N,N-diphenyloxanilyl chloride which cyclizes under Friedel-Crafts conditions to yield 1-(2,6-diphenyl)isatin. Wolff-Kishner reduction of the 3-oxo group gives the lactam, which on hydrolysis affords the free acid. Neutralization with NaOH produces the salt; US Pat 3,558,690.

Description—White crystals; melts about 284°; pK_a 4.0.

Solubility—Soluble in water; insoluble in organic solvents.

Uses—A pharmacological activity much like the other NSAIDs. As with other drugs in this group, diclofenac is thought to exert many of its effects as a result of its ability to inhibit prostaglandin synthesis. Diclofenac is used as an anti-inflammatory, analgesic and occasionally an antipyretic. Its anti-inflammatory action is similar to other NSAIDs with a potency, on weight basis, that is approximately 2.5 times that of indomethacin. On a weight basis, its analgesic potency is 8 to 16 times that of ibuprofen. It is used in the symptomatic relief of acute and chronic rheumatoid arthritis, osteoarthritis and ankylosing spondylitis. It also has been used to relieve mild-to-moderate postoperative pain associated with dental, orthopedic or postpartum procedures. It is also effective in relieving some cancer-related visceral pains. Diclofenac doses of 75 to 100 mg a day are equally effective in relieving pain as 0.9 to 2.7 g of aspirin or 1.2 g of ibuprofen. It is also effective in relieving some of the discomforts associated with dysmenorrhea.

Most of the adverse effects of diclofenac are similar to those of other NSAIDs and occur in several systems. The GI effects can include irritation, bleeding, ulceration and eventually wall perforation: such effects usually are associated with chronic, high-dose treatments. However, with usual therapeutic doses, diclofenac is less likely to cause serious GI problems than aspirin or naproxen. Diclofenac can cause headaches in 3 to 9% of the patients and dizziness in 1 to 3%. Use of this drug has been associated with renal impairment in less than 1% of the patients. Severe hepatic reactions occur rarely, while 1 to 3% of the patients may experience a rash or pruritus when using the drug. Tinnitus has been reported in 1 to 3% of the patients using this drug and fluid retention occurs in 3 to 9%. Diclofenac should be used with caution in patients who would be put at risk by prolonging bleeding time because of its anticlotting actions.

Dose—*Usual, adult, mild-to-moderate pain,* **75 to 100 mg** a day. *Anti-inflammatory, adult,* **150 to 200 mg** a day, given at **75 mg** 2 times a day or **50 mg** 3 or 4 times a day.

Dosage Forms—Ophthalmic Solution: 0.1% in 2.5 and 5 mL. Enteric-Coated Tablets: 25, 50 and 75 mg.

Diflunisal

[1,1'-Biphenyl]-3-carboxylic acid, 2',4'-difluoro-4-hydroxy-, Dolobid (*MSD*)

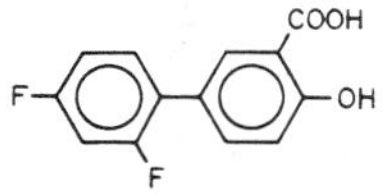

[22494-42-4] $C_{13}H_8F_2O_3$ (250.20).

Preparation—Refer to US Pat 3,714,226.

Description—White crystals; melts about 210°.

Solubility—Sparingly soluble in water; soluble in most organic solvents or dilute aqueous bases.

Uses—A prostaglandin inhibitor, nonsteroidal analgesic and anti-inflammatory drug used in the management of *mild* to *moderate* pain and osteoarthritis. It also has measurable, but not clinically useful, antipyretic activity. Double-blind studies indicate that a 500 mg dose of the drug is more effective in the control of postoperative episiotomy pain than 600 mg of aspirin, in postoperative oral surgery 500 to 1000 mg of the drug was more potent than 600 mg of acetaminophen alone and comparable to 600 mg of acetaminophen with 60 mg of codeine, and more effective than 100 mg of propoxyphene napsylate. Moreover, it had a longer duration of action. Following oral administration, peak plasma levels occur within 2 to 3 hr. Approximately 99% is bound to plasma proteins. Plasma half-life is 8 to 12 hr. About 90% of the drug is excreted in the urine as two soluble glucuronide conjugates. Although it is a derivative of salicylic acid it is not metabolized to salicylic acid.

The drug is contraindicated in patients in whom acute asthmatic attacks, urticaria or rhinitis are precipitated by aspirin. It prolongs the clotting time in patients on anticoagulant therapy, significantly increases plasma levels of hydrochlorathiazide and acetaminophen, decreases the hyperuricemic effect of furosemide and significantly decreases the urinary excretion of naproxen and its glucuronide metabolite. The most prominent side effects include nausea, dyspepsia, gastrointestinal pain and diarrhea; dizziness, headache and rash also have been reported in 3 to 9% of patients. It appears to cause less gastrointestinal bleeding than aspirin. Do not take aspirin or acetaminophen with this drug, except on professional advice.

Dose—*Usual, adult, oral, mild to moderate pain, initially* **1000 mg** followed by **500 mg** every 12 hr. *Osteoarthritis,* **500 to 1000 mg** daily in two divided doses; *maintenance,* maximum of **1500 mg** a day. Take with water, milk or meals.

Dosage Form—Film-Coated Tablets: 250 and 500 mg.

Etodolac

Pyrano[3,4-*b*]indole-1-acetic acid, 1,8-diethyl-1,3,4,9-tetrahydro-, Lodine (*Wyeth-Ayerst*)

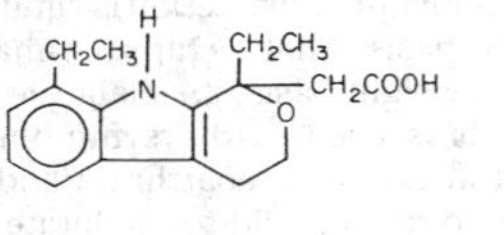

[41340-25-4] $C_{17}H_{21}NO_3$(287.36).

Preparation—See *J Med Chem 19:* 391, 1976.

Description—White crystals; melts about 147°; pK_a 4.65.

Solubility—1 g in 10 mL water or 4 mL alcohol.

Uses—Its structural uniqueness (a pyrancarboxylic acid) does not appear to distinguish it pharmacologically from the other NSAIDs. It is well absorbed from the gut and serum concentrations are maximum 1 to 2 hours after ingestion. Etodolac is converted by the liver to inactive metabolites which are excreted in the urine. Its elimination half-life is 6 to 7 hours. It is likely that the general analgesic and anti-inflammatory actions of etodolac are like those of aspirin, and it is used to treat osteoarthritis and as a general-purpose analgesic. Although it likely has many of the common side effects related to NSAIDs use, it is possible that etodolac causes fewer gastrointestinal problems than most other drugs in this group.

Dose—*Osteoarthritis, initially* **800** to **1200 mg** a day in divided doses, do not exceed a daily intake of **1200 mg** or **20 mg/kg;** acute pain, **200** to **400 mg** every 6 to 8 hr, not to exceed **1200 mg** a day.

Dosage Form—Capsules: 200 and 300 mg.

Fenoprofen Calcium

Benzeneacetic acid, (±)-α-methyl-3-phenoxy-, calcium salt (2:1), dihydrate; Nalfon (*Dista*)

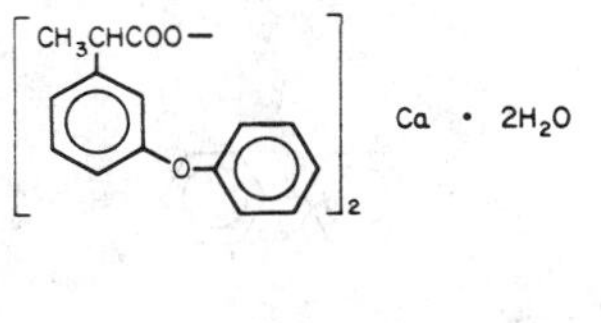

(±)-Calcium *m*-phenoxyhydratropate dihydrate [53746-45-5] $C_{30}H_{26}CaO_6.2H_2O$ (558.64); *anhydrous* [34597-40-5] (522.61).

Preparation—From *p*-phenoxyacetophenone by reducing the phenone carbonyl group to the secondary alcohol; replacing the OH with Br, using PBr_3; nucleophilic substitution of Br by CN followed by hydrolysis to one acid which is converted to the calcium salt. *J Med Chem 19:* 391, 1976.

Description—White, crystalline powder; pK_a 4.5 (fenoprofen).

Solubility—Slightly soluble in water; sparingly soluble in alcohol.

Uses—A nonsteroidal compound that has *anti-inflammatory* (antiarthritic) and *analgesic* properties. It is a propionic acid derivative related to ibuprofen and naproxen. Its mechanism of action likely relates to its inhibition of prostaglandin synthesis. It is used for the relief of the signs and symptoms of rheumatoid arthritis and osteoarthritis (acute flares and long-term management) and the relief of mild to moderate pain.

It is absorbed rapidly after oral administration. Peak plasma levels (of about 50 μg/mL) are reached within 2 hr after oral administration of a 600-mg dose. The plasma half-life is approximately 3 hr. It is highly bound (99%) to albumin. About 90% of a single oral dose is eliminated within 24 hr as fenoprofen glucuronide and 4′-hydroxyfenoprofen glucuronide, the major urinary metabolites of the agent.

It is contraindicated in patients sensitive to aspirin and other nonsteroidal anti-inflammatory drugs. The safety of this drug in pregnancy and lactation has not been established. Likewise, the safety and effectiveness in children are unknown. It interacts with a number of drugs. Patients receiving hydantoins, sulfonamides or sulfonylureas should be observed for signs of toxicity to these drugs. It prolongs prothrombin time in patients receiving coumarin-type anticoagulants. Peripheral edema, platelet aggregation and prolonged bleeding time have been observed.

Adverse reactions most commonly encountered are similar to other NSAIDs and include dyspepsia, constipation, nausea, vomiting, abdominal pain, anorexia, occult blood in the stool, diarrhea, flatulence and dry mouth. Other adverse effects are *skin:* pruritus, rash, increased sweating and urticaria; *CNS:* somnolence, dizziness, tremor, confusion and insomnia; *cardiovascular:* palpitations, tachycardia and occasionally anemia.

Dose (fenoprofen equivalent)—*Usual, adult, oral, rheumatoid arthritis* and *osteoarthritis,* **300** to **600 mg** 3 to 4 times a day; the dosage to be adjusted in accordance with the patient's age, condition and changes in disease activity. *Maximum daily dosage,* not to exceed 3200 mg. *Mild to moderate pain,* **200 mg** every 4 to 6 hr as needed.

Dosage Forms (fenoprofen equivalent)—Capsules: 200 and 300 mg; Tablets: 600 mg; Film-Coated, Tablets: 600 mg.

Flurbiprofen

(±)-[1,1′-Biphenyl]-4-acetic acid, 2-fluoro-α-methyl-, Ansaid (*Upjohn*)

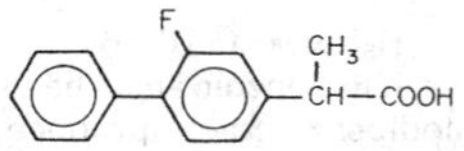

[5104-49-4] $C_{15}H_{13}FO_2$ (255.26)

Preparation—The Willgerodt reaction on 3-fluoro-4-phenylacetophenone yields the corresponding phenylacetic acid ester which, with $NaOC_2H_5$ and ethyl carbonate forms the substituted malonic ester. The ester is methylated by the classical method, hydrolyzed and decarboxylated to the product; US Pat 3,755,427.

Description—White to slightly yellow powder; melts at 110°.

Solubility—Slightly soluble in water; soluble in dilute alkali; freely soluble in alcohol.

Uses—A propionic acid derivative structurally and pharmacologically related to fenoprofen, ibuprofen and ketoprofen. Flurbiprofen has actions similar to other NSAIDs; ie, it possesses anti-inflammatory, analgesic and antipyretic properties. Flurbiprofen is used for its ocular effects and is administered topically to the eye prior to some ocular surgeries (eg, cataract extraction) in order to prevent intraoperative miosis. The value of flurbiprofen for the prevention and management of postoperative ocular inflammation remains to be established. In general, flurbiprofen sodium ophthalmic solution is well tolerated when used on the eye. No significant systemic side effects have been associated with use of the ophthalmic solution; however, with significant systemic absorption, the possibility of NSAID-type side effects does exist.

Flurbiprofen also is used systemically for the acute or long-term treatment of the signs and symptoms of rheumatoid arthritis and osteoarthritis. Adverse effects seen in more than 1% of the users include dyspepsia, diarrhea, nausea, abdominal pain, GI bleeding, flatulence, vomiting, headaches, CNS stimulation, rhinitis, rash, dizziness, tinnitus and edema.

Dose—*Inhibition of intraoperative miosis,* 1 drop of 0.03% solution beginning 2 hr prior to surgery and repeated at 30-min intervals for a total of 4 drops per eye. *Rheumatoid arthritis and osteoarthritis*, **200** to **300 mg** total daily administered 2, 3 or 4 times a day. The largest recommended single dose in a multiple-dose daily regimen is 100 mg.

Dosage Forms—Ophthalmic Solution: 0.03% (as the sodium salt); Tablets: 50 and 100 mg.

Hydroxychloroquine Sulfate—RPS-18 page 1227.

Ibuprofen

Benzeneacetic acid, (±)-α-methyl-4-(2-methylpropyl)-, Rufen (*Boots*); Nuprin (*Bristol-Myers*); Advil (*Whitehall*); Haltran, Motrin (*Upjohn*); Medipren (*McNeil*)

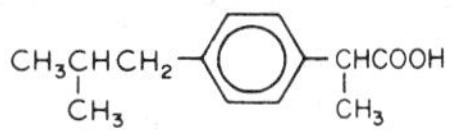

$CH_3CH(CH_3)CH_2$–C_6H_4–$CH(CH_3)COOH$

(±)-*p*-Isobutylhydratropic acid; (±)-2-(*p*-isobutylphenyl)propionic acid [15687-27-1] $C_{13}H_{18}O_2$ (206.28).

Preparation—Isobutylbenzene is acetylated in the *para* position by a Friedel-Crafts procedure to the acetophenone, which is treated with HCN to yield the cyanohydrin. Heating with HI and red P hydrolyzes the nitrile to the acid and simultaneously reduces the hydroxyl group; *J Org Chem 43:* 2936, 1978.

Description—White to off-white, crystalline powder; slight characteristic odor and taste; melts about 75°; apparent pK_a 5.2.

Solubility—Very slightly soluble in water; very soluble in alcohol or other organic solvents.

Uses—A nonsteroidal *anti-inflammatory agent* that possesses *analgesic* and *antipyretic* activities. In mild to moderate pain, 200 mg appears to be as effective as 650 mg of aspirin. When used to relieve dysmenorrhea, it is as effective as mefenamic acid and more effective than aspirin or propoxyphene. Like other nonsteroidal anti-inflammatory agents its mechanism of action likely relates to its inhibition of prostaglandin synthesis. Evidence that it does have a salutary effect in the treatment of chronic rheumatoid arthritis and osteoarthritis is shown by a reduction of joint swelling, decrease in pain, decrease in duration of morning stiffness and improved functional capacity as indicated by an increase in grip strength, a delay in the time to onset of fatigue and a decrease in the time to walk 50 ft.

The drug is absorbed rapidly after oral administration and peak plasma serum levels generally are attained within 1 to 2 hr after oral administration. With single doses from 200 mg to 800 mg, a dose-response relationship exists between the amount of drug administered and the integrated area under the serum drug concentration vs time curve. It is metabolized rapidly and eliminated in the urine; excretion virtually is complete 24 hr after the last dose of drug. The serum half-life is 1.8 to 2.0 hr.

It is indicated for relief of symptoms of *rheumatoid arthritis* and *osteoarthritis*. It also is indicated for the relief of mild to moderate pain, the treatment of primary dysmenorrhea, and as an antipyretic. It is contraindicated in individuals sensitive to the drug or in individuals with the syndrome of nasal polyps, angioedema and bronchospastic reactivity to aspirin or other nonsteroidal anti-inflammatory agents. Peptic ulceration and gastrointestinal bleeding have been reported. Consequently, it should be given under close supervision to patients with a history of upper gastrointestinal tract disease. Blurred and/or diminished vision, scotomata and other changes in color vision have been noted; the drug should be discontinued and the patient given an ophthalmological examination. Patients should be cautioned to report to their physicians signs or symptoms of gastrointestinal ulceration or bleeding, blurred vision or other eye symptoms, skin rash, weight gain or edema.

This drug, like aspirin and other NSAIDs, can inhibit platelet function and prolong bleeding time, but the effects are reversible and not as long lasting as those of aspirin. Nevertheless, it should be administered with caution to patients on anticoagulants. It is not recommended for use during pregnancy or in nursing mothers.

Adverse reactions with an incidence greater than 1% may be categorized as: *gastrointestinal:* (4 to 16%), nausea, epigastric pain, heartburn, diarrhea, abdominal distress, nausea and vomiting, indigestion, constipation and abdominal cramps or pain; *CNS:* dizziness (3 to 9%), headache, nervousness and tinnitus; *dermatologic:* rash (3 to 9%) and pruritus; *metabolic:* decreased appetite, edema and fluid retention.

Adverse effects with an incidence of less than 1% include : *gastrointestinal:* gastric or duodenal ulcer with bleeding and/or perforation; *dermatologic:* vesiculobullous eruptions, urticaria, erythema multiforme; *CNS:* depression, insomnia; *special senses:* amblyopia (blurred and/or diminished vision, scotomata and/or other changes in vision); *hematologic:* leukopenia and decreases in hemoglobin and hematocrit; *cardiovascular:* congestive heart failure in patients with marginal cardiac function and elevated blood pressure. Other reactions have been reported but under circumstances where a causal relationship could not be established.

Dose—*Usual, adult, oral, analgesia* (dysmenorrhea), **200** to **400 mg** every 4 to 6 hr as needed; *rheumatoid arthritis* and *osteoarthritis*, including flareups of chronic disease, **300** or **400 mg** 3 or 4 times a day, adjusted to meet the need of the patient. *Maximum total daily dosage*, 3200 mg.

Dosage Forms—Oral Suspension: 100 mg/5 mL. Tablets: 200, 300, 400, 600 and 800 mg.

Indomethacin

1*H*-Indole-3-acetic acid, 1-(4-chlorobenzoyl)-5-methoxy-2-methyl-, Indocin, Indocin SR (*MSD*); (*Various Mfrs*)

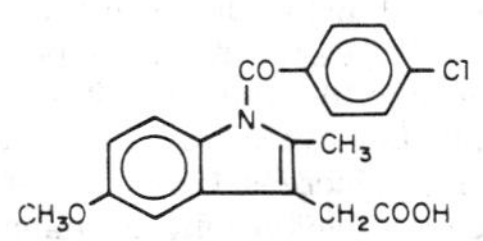

[Structure: indole ring with CH_3O at 5, N–CO–C_6H_4–Cl, CH_3 at 2, CH_2COOH at 3]

[53-86-1] $C_{19}H_{16}ClNO_4$ (357.79).

Preparation—*p*-Anisidine is diazotized and the diazonium compound reduced with sodium sulfite. The resulting *p*-methoxyphenylhydrazine undergoes the Fisher indole synthesis with methyl levulinate. The steps involved include formation of the hydrazone (I), rearrangement of I to the enamine compound II, and cyclization of II through loss of ammonia to form III. III is then hydrolyzed to the acid which is re-esterified via the anhydride to give the *tert*-butyl ester. Acylation with *p*-chlorobenzoyl chloride followed by debutylation yields indomethacin. US Pat 3,161,654.

Description—Pale-yellow to yellow-tan, crystalline powder; odorless

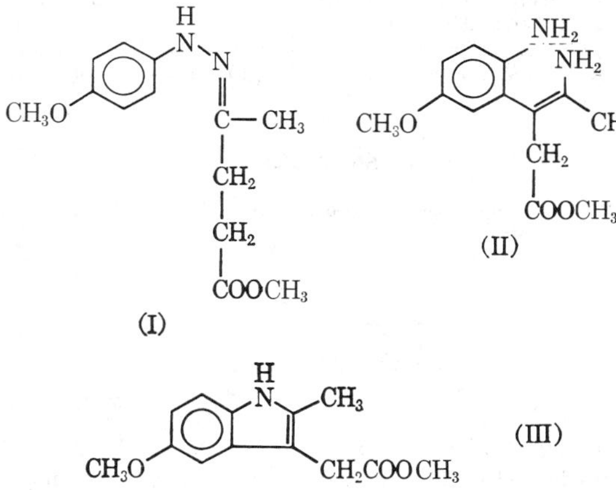

(I) CH_3O–C_6H_4–NH–N=C(CH_3)–CH_2–CH_2–$COOCH_3$

(II) CH_3O–$C_6H_3(NH_2)$–C(CH_2COOCH_3)=C(NH_2)–CH_3

(III) 5-CH_3O-2-CH_3-indole-3-CH_2COOCH_3

or a slight odor; slightly bitter taste; light-sensitive, stable in air and stable in heat under the usual prevailing temperature conditions; one polymorphic form melts about 155°, the other about 162°.

Solubility—1 g in 50 mL alcohol, 30 mL chloroform or 40 mL ether; practically insoluble in water.

Uses—A nonsteroidal drug with anti-inflammatory, antipyretic and analgesic properties. *It is not a simple analgesic and, because of its potential serious untoward effects, should not be used for trivial or minor problems.* It is indicated for the treatment of *rheumatoid arthritis, ankylosing (rheumatoid) spondylitis, osteoarthritis bursitis, tendinitis, gouty arthritis and patent ductus arteriosus in premature neonates.* The drug is absorbed rapidly after oral administration; peak plasma levels are reached in 2 hr: 97% of the drug is protein-bound. It has a half-life of 2.6 to 11.2 hr; 10 to 20% of the drug is excreted unchanged in the urine. Since it is a potent drug and has a potential to cause severe adverse effects, it should be considered carefully for an active disease unresponsive to adequate trial with salicylates and other established measures, such as appropriate rest. The drug is contraindicated in children, pregnant women and nursing mothers, patients with gastrointestinal problems and in patients allergic to aspirin.

The incidence of untoward effects has been reported to vary from a few percent to 75% of patients. Most frequent untoward actions include *gastrointestinal:* single or multiple ulcerations, hemorrhage, gastrointestinal bleeding, increased pain in ulcerative colitis, gastritis, nausea, vomiting, epigastric distress; *eye reactions:* corneal deposits and retinal disturbances, and blurring of vision; *hepatic:* toxic hepatitis, jaundice, some fatalities have been reported; *hematologic:* aplastic anemia, hemolytic anemia, depression of the bone marrow, agranulocytosis, leukopenia and thrombocytopenia purpura; *hypersensitivity:* acute respiratory including asthma and dyspnea, angiitis, pruritus, urticaria, skin rashes, etc; *ear:* deafness rarely, tinnitus; *CNS:* psychotic disturbances, depersonalization, depression, mental confusion, coma, convulsions, peripheral neuropathy, drowsiness, light-headedness, dizziness and headache; *cardiovascular-renal:* edema, hypertension, hematuria; *dermatologic:* loss of hair, erythema nodosum; *miscellaneous:* vaginal bleeding, hyperglycemia, glycosuria, ulcerative stomatitis and epistaxis. Both the incidence and severity of side effects appear to be dose-related.

The high potential for dose-related adverse reactions (see above) makes it imperative that the smallest effective dosage be determined for each patient. Gastrointestinal reactions may be reduced by giving the drug with food, immediately after meals or with antacids. The occurrence of ocular and/or hematological disturbances in some patients on prolonged therapy with the drug indicates the need for periodic ophthalmological examination and appropriate blood tests. Whether or not the drug has any effect on anticoagulants is uncertain, but concurrent administration may be hazardous because of increased risk of gastrointestinal bleeding.

It may aggravate psychiatric disturbances, epilepsy and parkinsonism; it should be used with considerable caution in patients with these conditions. Patients should be warned that ability to drive or perform other activities requiring alertness may be affected adversely. The drug should be discontinued if any of the untoward effects listed above occurs, pending consultation with the physician.

Dose—*Usual, adult, oral, gout, initially* **100 mg,** then **50 mg** 3 times a day until pain is relieved, then dosage is rapidly reduced until discontinued. *Antirheumatic, oral,* **50 mg** 2 or 3 times a day; if well-tolerated, increase by 25 mg weekly until satisfactory response is obtained or until a total daily dose of 150 to 200 mg is reached. *Acute bursitis or tendinitis, oral,* **75** to **100 mg** a day in 3 or 4 divided doses. Discontinue after inflammation has been controlled for several days.

Other Dose Information—The dose is increased gradually until optimum control is achieved. A dose of 200 mg a day should not be exceeded because of the high incidence of adverse effects. It should not be administered to children under 14 yr.

Dosage Forms—Capsules: 25, 50 and 75 mg; Sustained-Release Capsules: 75 mg; Suppositories: 50 mg; Oral suspension: 25 mg/5 mL.

Ketoprofen

Benzeneacetic acid, 3-benzoyl-α-methyl-, Orudis (*Wyeth-Ayerst*)

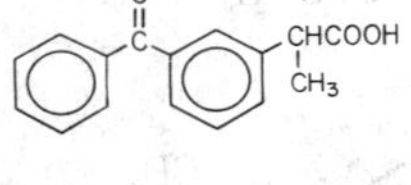

[22071-15-4] $C_{16}H_{14}O_3$ (254.28).

Preparation—The diazonium salt prepared from 2-(*p*-aminophenyl)-propionic acid is converted to the mercaptan (**I**) with potassium ethyl xanthate followed by hydrolysis. **I,** with *o*-iodobenzoic acid yields the corresponding diphenyl sulfide. The carboxyl group *ortho* to the sulfur atom cyclizes with the adjacent ring to form a thioxanthone configuration followed by desulfurization to reopen the ring and reform the benzophenone product; *Farmaco Ed Sci 35:* 684, 1980.

Description—White to off-white, odorless, crystalline, nonhygroscopic powder; melts about 95°.

Solubility—Practically insoluble in water; soluble in fixed bases; freely soluble in alcohol, chloroform, acetone or ether.

Uses—Indicated for the acute and long-term management of rheumatoid arthritis and osteoarthritis as well as mild to moderate pain and dysmenorrhea. It is absorbed rapidly and completely after oral administration; peak plasma levels are reached in 0.5 to 2 hr; 99% of the drug is bound to plasma protein; mean plasma elimination half-life is 2 to 4 hr; approximately 60% of the administered dose is excreted in the urine primarily as the glucuronide metabolite; the remaining 40% is thought to undergo enterohepatic recirculation. Adverse effects are similar to those induced with other NSAIDs and include

Digestive: dyspepsia, nausea, vomiting and diarrhea. Causes fewer GI problems than usual anti-inflammatory doses of aspirin.

Central nervous system: headache, dizziness, malaise, depression, insomnia, etc.

Urogenital: renal irritation and impairment.

Other: tinnitus, visual disturbances and skin rash. It should not be given to patients sensitive to other NSAIDs.

Dose—*Usual, adult, oral, rheumatoid arthritis,* **150** to **300 mg** divided into 3 or 4 doses. Starting dose—**75 mg** 3 times a day or **50 mg** 4 times a day. Do not exceed **300 mg a day.** *Mild to moderate pain and primary dysmenorrhea,* **25** to **50 mg** every 6 to 8 hr as needed.

Dosage Form—Capsules: 25, 50 and 75 mg.

Ketorolac Tromethamine

(±)-1*H*-Pyrrolizine-1-carboxylic acid, 5-benzoyl-2,3-dihydro-, compd with 2-amino-2-(hydroxymethyl)-1,3-propanediol (1:1); Acular (*Allergans*) (*Fisons*): Toradol (*Syntex*)

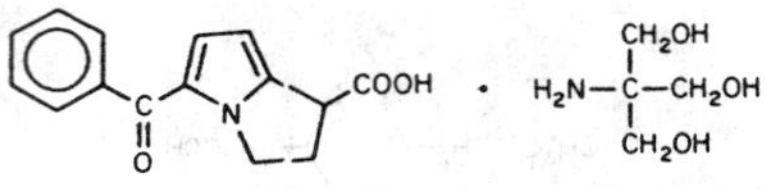

[74103-07-4] $C_{19}H_{24}N_2O_6$ (376.41).

Preparation—In seven steps from pyrrole; see US Pat 4,089,969 and *J Med Chem 29:* 589, 1986.

Description—white crystals; melts about 160°.

Uses—An NSAID which is structurally and pharmacologically related to tolmetin and indomethacin. Its anti-inflammatory, analgesic and antipyretic effects are likely due to its inhibition of prostaglandin synthesis. It is used for the short-term management of pain. Specifically, it provides symptomatic relief from moderate to severe pain associated with orthopedic, gynecological, oral or urological surgical procedures. It also has been found to be effective in the treatment of trauma-related pain as well as pain associated with cancer. Approximately 10 mg of ketorolac administered IM is equivalent to a 6 mg IM dose of morphine sulphate. Long-term oral doses (10 mg given 4 times a day for 1 yr) have been used to relieve chronic pain associated with osteoarthritis, fibromyalgias or tension headaches and found to be more effective than comparably administered aspirin (650 mg/dose).

Ketorolac has the toxic potential of other NSAIDs. Usually, adverse effects are minor and occur in approximately 40% of patients. Adverse GI effects occur in 13% of the patients and include dyspepsia, nausea and other forms of GI discomfort. Adverse CNS effects include drowsiness, headache, dizziness, depression, euphoria, nervousness and insomnia and occur in about 23% of those that use ketorolac. Less frequently, impairment of renal and hepatic functions have been reported with ketorolac use. In general, the incidence and severity of side effects are less with ketorolac than aspirin. Other possible side effects include problems with prolonged bleeding, visual disturbances, dyspnea, myalgia and edema. The safety of ketoraolac has not yet been established in children under 18 yr.

Dose—*Usual, short-term pain relief, initial loading dose,* **30** to **60 mg** IM, then maintenance with **15** to **30 mg** every 6 hours. Dosage should not exceed 150 mg the first day and 120 mg each day thereafter. *Oral, management of moderate-to-severe pain,* **5** to **10 mg** up to 4 times a day.

Dosage Forms—Injection: 15 and 30 mg/mL; Tablets: 10 mg.

Meclofenamate Sodium

Benzoic acid, 2-[(2,6-dichloro-3-methylphenyl)amino]-, monosodium salt, monohydrate; (*Various Mfrs*)

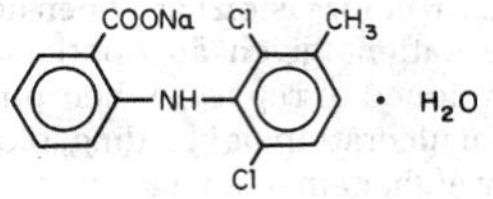

Monosodium *N*-(2,6-dichloro-*m*-tolyl)anthranilate monohydrate [6385-02-0] $C_{14}H_{10}Cl_2NNaO_2.H_2O$ (336.15).

Preparation—By the Ullman condensation of *o*-iodobenzoic acid and 2,6-dichloro-*m*-toluidine in the presence of copper-bronze, *J Med Chem 11:* 1009, 1968.

Description—White crystals; melts about 290°; a saturated solution in water (1 g in 65 mL) is slightly turbid; pH about 7.5.

Uses—Related to mefenamic acid and used for the treatment of *acute* and *chronic rheumatoid arthritis* and *osteoarthritis* as well as mild-to-moderate pain. Its pharmacological actions and adverse side effects are similar to other NSAIDs. Following oral administration, peak plasma levels are reached in 30 min to 1 hr. Plasma half-life after 4 days chronic dosing is 3.3 hr. The drug does not accumulate in the body; it is metabolized to an active hydroxymethyl derivative (25%) and an inactive carboxy derivative (6%); both metabolites are excreted as glucuronides. Approximately two-thirds of the dose is excreted in the urine and one-third in the feces. It is not recommended as the initial drug because of gastrointestinal side effects which are sometimes severe and often include diarrhea (see page 1207). Other potential adverse effects include drowsiness, dizziness, blurred vision, renal impairment (especially in the elderly) and skin eruptions. It is not recommended for use in children less than 14 yr. Patient selection should be based on a careful assessment of the benefit/risk ratio.

Dose—*Usual, oral,* **200 to 400 mg** a day in 3 or 4 equal doses. After satisfactory response has been obtained, adjust dosage as required. May be taken with meals or milk. Terminate therapy if any severe adverse reactions occur.

Dosage Forms—Capsules: 50 and 100 mg; Tablets: 50 and 100 mg.

Mefenamic Acid

Benzoic acid, 2-[(2,3-dimethylphenyl)amino]-,
Ponstel (*Parke-Davis*)

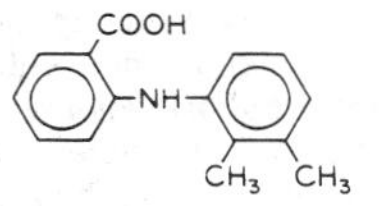

N-(2,3-Xylyl)anthranilic acid [61-68-7] $C_{15}H_{15}NO_2$ (241.29).

Preparation—*o*-Chlorobenzoic acid is condensed with 2,3-xylidine with the aid of potassium carbonate and the resulting potassium salt is treated with mineral acid to liberate the desired acid. *J Med Chem 11:* 111, 1968.

Description—White to off-white, crystalline powder; odorless; very little initial taste, but a bitter aftertaste; darkens on prolonged exposure to light, nonhygroscopic; stable up to 45°; decarboxylates at temperatures above its melting point (at 300°, 100% is decarboxylated in 3 min); melts about 230°.

Solubility—1 g in 220 mL alcohol; insoluble in water; sparingly soluble in chloroform or ether.

Uses—An analgesic drug used for the relief of moderately severe pain when *therapy will not exceed 1 wk* and for the treatment of *primary dysmenorrhea.* It also is indicated for the relief of pain resulting from postoperative pain. It is contraindicated in patients with ulceration of the upper or lower intestinal tract, children under 14 yr, women during pregnancy or patients known to be hypersensitive to the drug. Untoward effects include diarrhea which may be severe and indicates the drug should be stopped, autoimmune hemolytic anemia, thrombocytopenic purpura, leukopenia, pancytopenia, agranulocytosis and bone-marrow hypoplasia.

Minor reactions include drowsiness, gastrointestinal discomfort, dizziness, headache, vomiting, urticaria, rash, eosinophilia, blurred vision, insomnia and perspiration. Rarely, palpitations, facial edema, dyspnea, eye pain, ear pain, dysuria, hematuria, reversible loss of color vision and increased insulin need in diabetic patients. Mild renal and hepatic toxicity also have been reported (see page 1207). Since this drug is useful in moderate pain, physicians would be well-advised to consider its use only in cases which either can not tolerate or do not respond to less-toxic agents.

Dose—*Usual, adults* and *children over 14 yr, oral,* **500 mg,** followed by **250 mg** every 6 hr, as needed. Take with food.

Caution: Do not use for more than 7 days.

Dosage Form—Capsules: 250 mg.

Nabumetone

2-Butanone, 4-(6-methoxy-2-naphthalenyl)-, Relafen
(*SmithKline Beecham*)

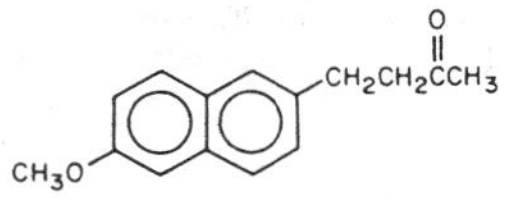

4-(6-Methoxy-2-naphthyl)-2-butanone; [42924-53-8] $C_{15}H_{16}O_2$ (228.29).

Preparation—Acetone and 6-methoxynaphthalenecarboxaldehyde are reacted in aldol fashion to form 4-(6-methoxy-2-naphthyl)-3-buten-2-one which is reduced catalytically to nabumetone. See *J Med Chem 21:* 1260, 1978.

Description—White crystals; melts about 80°

Solubility—Practically insoluble in water; sparingly soluble in alcohol.

Uses—In contrast to other NSAIDs, it is a weak inhibitor of cyclooxygenase, a prostaglandin-synthesizing enzyme, but nabumetone is metabolized to 6-methoxy-2-naphthaleneacetic acid, a strong cyclo-oxygenase inhibitor. Thus, it is likely the metabolite helps to relieve the signs and symptoms of rheumatoid arthritis and osteroarthritis as well as mild-to-moderate pain and the discomforts associated with primary dysmenorrhea. The active metabolite has a serum half-life of approximately 24 hr and is degraded to inactive metabolites in the liver and eliminated mainly by the kidney. The adverse side effects appear to be similar to other NSAIDs, with the most common problems occurring in the GI system: these include diarrhea, abdominal pain, dyspepsia and nausea. Other less frequent side effects are photosensitivity, headache, dizziness, rash, edema and nightmares.

Dose—*Usual, adult, oral, initially* **1000 mg** a day and increase as necessary to a maximum of **2000 mg** a day. Lower initial doses are used in geriatric patients, or others with a high risk of GI bleeding.

Dosage Form—Tablets: 500 and 750 mg.

Naproxen

2-Naphthaleneacetic acid, (+)-6-methoxy-α-methyl-, Equiproxen
(Veterinary); Naprosyn (*Syntex*)

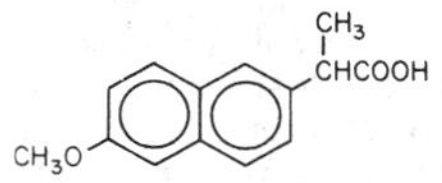

[22204-53-1] $C_{14}H_{14}O_3$ (230.26).

Preparation—6-Methoxynaphthalene is acetylated in the 2-position and the acetyl group is then converted to —$CH(CH_3)COOH$ by a sequence of reactions—Willgerodt-Kindler, esterification, alkylation and hydrolysis—yielding DL-naproxen (*CA 71:* 91162j, 1969). Resolution of the racemate may be effected through precipitation of the more potent D-enantiomer as the cinchonidine salt (*J Med Chem 13:* 203, 1970).

Description—White to off-white, crystalline powder; bitter taste; melts about 155°; apparent pK_a 4.15.

Solubility—Practically insoluble in water at pH 2; freely soluble in water at pH 8 or above; sparingly soluble in alcohol.

Uses—A propionic acid derivative that has anti-inflammatory, analgesic and antipyretic activities. It is commercially available both as the acid and the sodium salt. It is indicated for relief of symptoms of rheumatoid arthritis, both of acute flares and long-term management of the disease. Symptomatic improvement, where use of the drug is indicated, usually begins within 2 weeks but a longer trial period may be necessary. It is comparable to aspirin in controlling disease symptoms, but with lesser frequency and severity of nervous system and milder gastrointestinal adverse effects. It is used to relieve mild to moderate postoperative pain as well as postpartum pain, primary dysmenorrhea, orthopedic pain, headache and visceral pain associated with cancer. Its analgesic effects are comparable to those of aspirin or indomethacin with usual doses.

It appears to be absorbed completely from the gastrointestinal tract after oral administration. Peak plasma levels (about 55 μg/mL) are reached in 2 to 4 hr after a 500-mg dose, and steady-state levels are attained after 4 or 5 doses at 12-hr intervals. More than 99% is bound to serum albumin. The mean plasma half-life is about 13 hr. Approximately 95% of a dose is excreted in the urine, principally as conjugates of naproxen and its inactive metabolite 6-demethylnaproxen.

The adverse effects, precautions, contraindications and drug interactions are essentially the same as for *Fenoprofen Calcium* (page 1115).

Dose—*Adult, rheumatoid arthritis, osteoarthritis, ankylosing spondylitis, initially* **250 to 500 mg** twice a day (morning and evening), increased or decreased according to response of patient. Daily dosage in excess of 1000 mg is not recommended. *Juvenile arthritis,* **10 mg/kg** a day in 2 divided doses. *Acute gout,* **750 mg** followed by **250 mg** every 8 hr until relieved.

Dosage Forms—Oral Suspension: 125 mg/5 mL; Tablets: 250, 375 and 500 mg.

Naproxen Sodium

2-Naphthaleneacetic acid, 6-methoxy-α-methyl-, sodium salt
Anaprox (*Syntex*)

[26159-34-2] $C_{14}H_{13}NaO_3$ (252.24).

Uses—See *Naproxen.*

Dose—*Adult, rheumatoid arthritis, osteoarthritis, ankylosing spondylitis, initially* **275 mg** twice daily (morning and evening). Adjust dose according to clinical response. Daily doses in excess of 1000 mg have not been studied. *Acute gout, initially* **825 mg** followed by 275 mg every 8 hr until the attack has subsided.

Dosage Form—Tablets: 275 and 550 mg.

Oxyphenbutazone

3,5-Pyrazolidinedione, 4-butyl-1-(4-hydroxyphenyl)-2-phenyl-, monohydrate; (*Various Mfrs*)

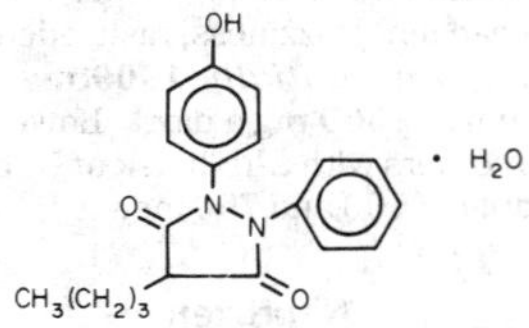

4-Butyl-1-(*p*-hydroxyphenyl)-2-phenyl-3,5-pyrazolidinedione monohydrate [7081-38-1] $C_{19}H_{20}N_2O_3.H_2O$ (342.39); *anhydrous* [129-20-4] (324.38).

Preparation—Diethyl butylmalonate is condensed with *p*-benzyloxyhydrazobenzene, with the aid of a solution of sodium ethoxide in anhydrous ethanol, to form 1-(*p*-benzyloxy)-2-phenyl-4-butyl-3,5-pyrazolidinedione (I). Completion of the reaction is effected by adding xylene and heating the mixture to about 140° for several hours, thus removing the alcohol released by the cyclizing condensation. Debenzylation of I is effected by Raney nickel hydrogenation at ambient temperature and pressure. Recrystallization of the initial product is from ether/petroleum ether. US Pat 2,745,783.

Description—White to yellowish white, odorless, crystalline powder; melts over a wide range between about 85° and 100°.

Solubility—1 g in >10,000 mL water, 1.5 mL alcohol, 4 mL chloroform 15 mL ether.

Uses—A derivative of phenylbutazone which exhibits the same analgesic, antipyretic, anti-inflammatory and mild uricosuric properties as the parent drug. Because of the increased risk of agranulocytosis and aplastic anemia, neither oxyphenbutazone nor phenylbutazone should be used as initial therapy. It is absorbed rapidly and completely after oral administration. Protein binding *is high;* time to peak serum concentration is 6 hr and peak serum concentration after 300 mg is 35 μg/mL; elimination half-life is 72 hr; and excretion is primarily by the kidneys. Except that it causes less gastrointestinal distress, its effectiveness, indications, contraindications and adverse reactions are the same as those for *Phenylbutazone*, below.

Dose—*Usual, adult, oral, antirheumatic,* **100** or **200 mg** 3 times a day. *Maintenance,* **100 mg** 1 to 4 times a day; *antigout, initially* **400 mg** as a single dose, then **100 mg** every 4 hr or until desired response is obtained.

Other Dose Information—It always should be taken immediately after meals or with a full glass of milk, to minimize gastric irritation. It should not be used in children under 14 yr.

Dosage Form—Tablets: 100 mg.

Penicillamine—page 936.

Phenylbutazone

3,5-Pyrazolidinedione, 4-butyl-1,2-diphenyl-, Butazolidin (*Geigy*); (*Various Mfrs*)

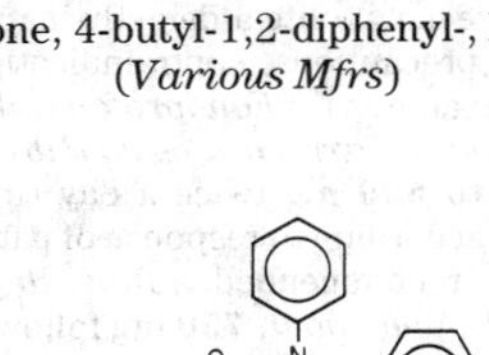

[50-33-9] $C_{19}H_{20}N_2O_2$ (308.38).

Preparation—Butylmalonyl chloride is condensed with hydrazobenzene in ether solution at 0° with the aid of pyridine. After extracting the pyridine with aqueous HCl, the phenylbutazone is extracted with aqueous Na_2CO_3 and then precipitated by addition of HCl. US Pat 2,562,830.

Description—White to off-white, odorless, crystalline powder; melts about 105°.

Solubility—1 g in about 20 mL of alcohol; very slightly soluble in water; freely soluble in acetone or ether.

Uses—A synthetic pyrazolone derivative chemically related to aminopyrine which has anti-inflammatory, antipyretic, analgesic and mild uricosuric properties. Like other NSAIDs, these pharmacological effects likely relate to inhibition of prostaglandin synthesis caused by this drug. It is indicated for the symptomatic relief of *gout, rheumatoid arthritis, rheumatoid spondylitis, osteoarthritis, psoriatic arthritis, acute superficial thrombophlebitis* and *painful shoulder.* Its anti-inflammatory and analgesic actions are comparable to that of usual doses of indomethacin, ibuprofen or tolmetin. Because of the risk of agranulocytosis and aplastic anemia, it should be used *only* after other nonsteroidal and anti-inflammatory drugs have proved unsatisfactory and is not recommended for use as a simple analgesic or antipyretic.

Therapy should not be started until the patient has been subjected to a complete physical and laboratory examination, including a hemogram and urinalysis and adequately warned of potential adverse effects. In particular, it is contraindicated in patients with severe renal, hepatic or cardiac disease and should not be prescribed for those not available for frequent observation. Patients should be warned not to exceed the recommended dosage and immediately to report any fever, sore throat or lesions in the mouth (symptoms of blood dyscrasia), dyspepsia, epigastric pain, symptoms of anemia, unusual bleeding, bruising, black or tarry stools (symptoms of intestinal lesions) and significant weight gain or anemia.

The goal of therapy should be *short-term* relief of *severe* symptoms to a level tolerable with the *smallest* possible drug dosage. If a favorable response is not observed within 1 week, the drug should be discontinued. The drug is contraindicated in patients with gastrointestinal problems, a history of drug allery and in children under 14 yr. It also is contraindicated in patients on other concurrent therapy, such as potent chemotherapeutic drugs and anticoagulant medication.

It is absorbed rapidly after oral administration and very highly bound to plasma protein. Time to peak serum concentration approximately 2.5 hr; however, the usual time for onset of antigout activity varies from 1 to 4 days and that for antirheumatic activity 3 to 7 days. Therapeutic serum concentrations average about 43 mg/mL; elimination half-life is about 84 hr. The drug (1%) and its major metabolite (oxyphenbutazone, 2%) are excreted by the kidneys.

It produces untoward effects in about 40% of patients; approximately 15% have to discontinue the drug because of toxic effects. Consequently, the drug should be employed only in those patients who fail to respond adequately to less hazardous substances. The most frequently encountered untoward effects are water retention, nausea, rash, epigastric pain, vertigo and stomatitis. Other less frequent but more severe effects include hepatitis, hypertension, transient psychosis, moderate leukopenia, agranulocytosis and thrombocytopenia. CNS stimulation, visual symptoms, anemia, lethargy, constipation, diarrhea, gastrointestinal hemorrhage, fever and cardiac arrhythmias also have been observed.

Numerous drug interactions have been reported. Some of these interactions may be due to microsomal induction caused by phenylbutazone and its metabolite, oxyphenylbutazone. In general, it should not be administered to patients taking anticoagulants, anti-inflammatory agents, bone-marrow depressants, digitoxin, hypoglycemics, methotrexate, phenytoin or sulfonamides.

Since it is a potent drug and misuse can lead to serious results, physicians are well advised to familiarize themselves with its gastrointestinal, acid-base balance, hepatic, dermatological, allergic, renal, cardiovascular, ocular, metabolic and endocrine effects before prescribing this drug. It should be used with caution in pregnant women, nursing mothers, elderly patients and patients known to have other illnesses.

This drug should be taken with milk or with meals to minimize gastric irritation.

Dose—**100 to 600 mg** a day; *usual, antirheumatic, initially* **100 mg** 3 to 6 times a day; *maintenance,* **100 mg** 1 to 4 times a day. *Antigout,* **400 mg** as a single dose, then **100 mg** ever 4 hr for approximately 4 days or until desired response is obtained, with duration not exceeding 1 week.

Dosage Forms—Capsules: 100 mg; Tablets: 100 mg.

Piroxicam

2*H*-1,2-Benzothiazine-3-carboxamide, 4-hydroxy-2-methyl-*N*-pyridinyl-, 1,1-dioxide; (*Pratt*); Feldene (*Pfizer*)

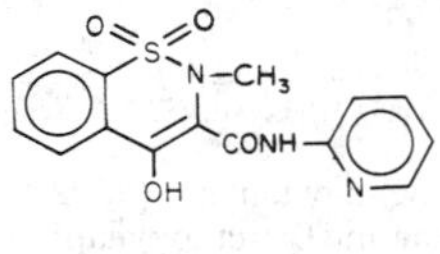

[36322-90-4] $C_{15}H_{13}N_3O_4S$ (331.35).

Preparation—See *J Med Chem 14;* 1171, 1971 and *15:* 848, 1972.

Description—White crystals; melts about 200° a saturated solution in dioxane: water (2:1) has a pK_a of about 6.3.

Solubility—Very slightly soluble in water.

Uses—An oxicam derivative which is structurally unrelated to other NSAIDs. It most frequently is used for acute or long-term use in the relief of signs and symptoms of *osteoarthritis* and *rheumatoid arthritis*. It also is used for symptomatic relief of pain associated with surgical procedures. In patients with osteoarthritis, piroxicam 20 mg/day was as effective against pain and improving joint movement as aspirin 3.9 g/day or indomethacin 75 mg/day. Like other nonsteroidal anti-inflammatory drugs, it inhibits prostaglandin synthesis chemotaxis and release of liposomal enzymes. It is absorbed rapidly after oral administration; peak plasma levels occur within 3 to 5 hr. Chronic administration with 20 mg a day produces steady state plasma levels of 3 to 5 μg/mL in 7 to 12 days. Volume distribution approximates 0.12 to 0.14 L/kg; mean half-life is about 50 hr (range, 30 to 86 hr). It is metabolized primarily by hydroxylation and excreted in the urine.

Adverse GI effects occur in approximately 20% of patients. For other adverse effects and precautions, see the general discussion for NSAIDs. Safety and efficacy in children has not been established although it is occasionally used to treat juvenile rheumatoid arthritis.

Dose—*Usual, adult, oral,* **20 mg a day.** Because of its long half-life, the effect of therapy should not be assessed for 2 wk.

Dosage Form—Capsules: 10 and 20 mg.

Sulindac

1*H*-Indene-3-acetic acid, (*Z*)-5-fluoro-2-methyl-1-[[4- (methylsulfinyl)-phenyl] methylene]-, Clinoril (*MSD*); (*Various Mfrs*)

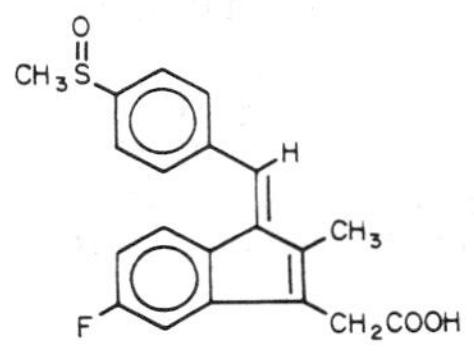

[38194-50-2] $C_{20}H_{17}FO_3S$ (356.41).

Preparation—The reaction of *p*-fluorobenzyl chloride with methylmalonic ester in the classic malonic ester synthetic route yields 3-(*p*-fluorophenyl)-2-methylpropanoic acid. Cyclization with polyphosphoric acid gives 6-fluoro-2-methylindanone which is reduced via a Reformatsky reaction to the alcohol, dehydrated to the indene, condensed with *p*-(methylthio)benzaldehyde to the 3-benzylidene derivative, the ester hydrolyzed and the thio group oxidized to the sulfoxide; *J Org Chem 42:* 1914, 1977.

Description—Yellow crystals; melts about 183° with decomposition; pK_a 4.5.

Solubility—Practically insoluble in water; sparingly soluble in alcohol.

Uses—An indene-type anti-inflammatory agent structurally and pharmacologically related to indomethacin and indicated for acute and long-term relief of signs and symptoms of *osteoarthritis, rheumatoid arthritis, ankylosing spondylitis, acute painful shoulder* and *acute gouty arthritis.* It also possesses analgesic and antipyretic properties. Its precise mechanism of action is unknown; however, it is thought the sulfide metabolite may inhibit prostaglandin synthesis. It is absorbed approximately 90% after oral administration. Peak plasma levels are achieved in about 2 hr in the fasting patient and 3 to 4 hr when administered with food. The mean half-life of sulindac is 7.8 hr; the mean half-life of the sulfide metabolite is 16.4 hr. It is contraindicated in Functional Class IV arthritis (incapacitated, largely or wholly bedridden, or confined to a wheelchair; little or no self-care), patients in whom acute asthmatic attacks, urticaria or rhinitis are precipitated by aspirin or other nonsteroidal anti-inflammatory agents and in patients sensitive to the drug.

Adverse reactions include gastrointestinal pain (10%); dyspepsia, nausea with or without vomiting, diarrhea, constipation, rash, dizziness, headache (3 to 9%), flatulence, anorexia, gastrointestinal cramps, pruritus, nervousness, tinnitus, edema (1 to 3%), gastritis or gastroenteritis, peptic ulcer, gastrointestinal bleeding, liver function abnormalities associated with jaundice, stomatitis, sore or dry mucous membranes, vertigo, hypersensitivity (including fever which may be accompanied by chills, skin rash, leukopenia or eosinophilia) (in less than 1% of patients). Other rare adverse reactions reported include congestive heart failure, Stevens-Johnson syndrome, toxic epidermal necrolysis, bone-marrow depression, thrombocytopenia, leukopenia, gastrointestinal perforation, nephropathy, pancreatitis, adverse ocular effects including diplopia, cloudy vision, eyeball swelling, noninflammatory ulceration of the cornea, retinal hemorrhage, blurred vision and spots before the eyes.

Although it has less effect on platelet function and bleeding time than aspirin, it should be used with caution in patients who may be affected adversely by this action. It also should be used with caution in patients with impaired liver and kidney function. Its safe use during pregnancy and in nursing mothers has not been established.

Dose—*Usual, adult, oral, osteoarthritis, rheumatoid arthritis and ankylosing spondylitis,* **150 mg** twice a day with food. *Usual, maximum dose,* **400 mg** a day; *acute gouty arthritis* and *painful shoulder,* **200 mg** twice a day. *Pediatric* indications and dosage have not been established.

Dosage Form: Tablets: 150 and 200 mg.

Tolmetin Sodium

1*H*-Pyrrole-2-acetic acid, 1-methyl-5-(4-methylbenzoyl)-, sodium salt, dihydrate; (*USV*) (*Mylan*); Tolectin, Tolectin DS (*McNeil*)

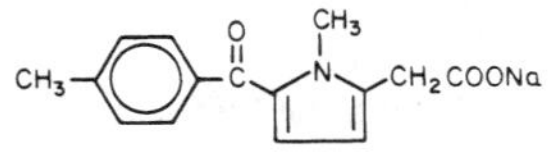

[64490-92-2] $C_{15}H_{14}NNaO_3.2H_2O$ (315.31).

Preparation—The corresponding acetonitrile is obtained by a Friedel-Crafts reaction between 1-methylpyrrole-2-acetonitrile and *p*-methylbenzoyl chloride; after separation from the 4-aroyl isomer, produced simultaneously, by fractional crystallization and/or adsorption chromatography, the acetonitrile is converted to tolmetin by saponification and subsequently to its sodium salt (*J Med Chem 14:* 646, 1971).

Description—Light yellow, crystalline powder; pK_a 3.5 (free acid).

Solubility—Freely soluble in water; slightly soluble in alcohol.

Uses—A nonsteroidal compound that has anti-inflammatory, analgesic and antipyretic activities. Its mode of action is unknown, although inhibition of prostaglandin synthesis likely contributes to its anti-inflammatory action. In patients with rheumatoid arthritis various manifestations of its anti-inflammatory and analgesic actions are observed, but there is no evidence of alteration of the progressive course of the underlying disease.

The drug is absorbed rapidly and almost completely with peak plasma levels being reached within 30 to 60 min after an oral therapeutic dose (40 μg/mL after a 400-mg dose). It is bound approximately 99% to plasma proteins; the mean plasma half-life is about 1 hr. Essentially all of a dose is excreted in the urine within 24 hr, either as an inactive oxidative metabolite or as conjugates of tolmetin.

The drug is indicated for the relief of signs and symptoms of rheumatoid arthritis, both of acute flares and long-term management of the disease. Safety and effectiveness in patients who are incapacitated, largely or wholly bedridden or confined to a wheelchair, with little capacity for self-care (Functional Class IV rheumatoid arthritis) have not been established. The drug is comparable to aspirin and to indomethacin in controlling disease activity but the frequency of the milder gastrointestinal adverse effects is reported to be less than in aspirin-treated patients and the incidence of CNS adverse effects less than in indomethacin-treated patients. Concomitant administration of this drug and aspirin is not recommended since there does not appear to be any greater benefit from the combination over that achieved with aspirin alone and the potential for adverse reactions is increased.

It is contraindicated in patients demonstrated to be hypersensitive to the drug, and also in those in whom aspirin and other nonsteroidal anti-inflammatory drugs induce symptoms of asthma, rhinitis or urticaria. In patients with active rheumatoid arthritis who also have an active peptic ulcer, treatment with nonulcerogenic drugs should be attempted; if it must be given, the patient should be observed closely for signs of ulcer perforation or severe gastrointestinal bleeding. As it is eliminated primarily by the kidneys, patients with impaired renal function should be monitored closely and dosage reduced or discontinued if necessary. As it prolongs bleeding time, patients who may be affected adversely should be observed carefully when treated with the drug. Patients with compromised cardiac function should be treated with caution because the drug causes some retention of water and sodium, with a resultant mild peripheral edema.

The most frequent adverse reactions are gastrointestinal and include, in descending order of frequency, epigastric or abdominal pain or discomfort (about 1 of 6 patients), nausea, vomiting, indigestion, heartburn, constipation and dyspepsia. The most common nervous system reactions are headache (1 of 15 patients), followed by dizziness and lightheadedness, tension and nervousness and drowsiness. Tinnitus occurs in 1 of 40 patients. Mild edema is observed in about 1 of 50 patients. Rash, including maculopapular eruptions or urticaria, develops in 1 of 30 patients; pruritus in about 1 of 50 patients. Small and transient decreases in hemoglobin and hematocrit, not associated with gastrointestinal bleeding, occur infrequently as well as a few cases of granulocytopenia. Also, see page 1207.

Safe use in children under 2 yr has not been established although the drug has been used safely and effectively in children over 2 yr. Use of the drug in pregnancy is not recommended and since it is secreted in human milk, its use by nursing mothers also is not recommended.

Dose (tolmetin equivalent)—*Adult, initially* **400 mg** 3 times a day, subsequently adjusted to patient's response. Symptom control is usually achieved with a daily dosage of **600** to **1800 mg,** given in 3 or 4 divided doses. Daily dosage exceeding **2000 mg** for adults with rheumatoid arthritis or **1600 mg** for adults with osteoarthritis has not been studied and therefore are not recommended. For the symptomatic treatment of juvenile rheumatoid arthritis, the initial dose for children 2 yr and older is **20 mg/kg** a day in 3 or 4 divided doses. Therapeutic response can be expected in a few days to a week, with progressive improvement in succeeding weeks of therapy. If gastrointestinal symptoms occur, the drug should be given with meals, milk or antacids other than sodium bicarbonate.

Dosage Form—(tolmetin equivalent)—Capsules: 400 mg; Tablets: 200 mg; Film-Coated Tablets: 600 mg. *Note:* Each dosage form contains sodium as follows: capsules (36 mg); tablets (18 mg); film-coated tablets (54 mg).

Dimethyl Sulfoxide

Methane, sulfinylbis-, Rimso-50 (*Research Industries*)

$(CH_3)_2S{=}O$

Methyl Sulfoxide; [67-68-5] C_2H_6OS (78.13).

Preparation—Obtained as a by-product in the manufacture of wood-pulp

Description—Hygroscopic liquid; bitter-sweet taste; boils about 190°

Solubility—Soluble in water and most organic solvents

Uses:—An aprotic solvent with remarkable properties to enhance penetrance of many locally applied drugs. During the course of its agricultural use as a solvent it was discovered to relieve arthritic pain, and it soon became used rather widely and promiscuously in the topical treatment of various collagen diseases. The discovery of DMSO-induced lens opacities in animals resulted in termination of these uses. At present it is approved only for the treatment of *interstitial cystitis.* Unlabeled uses of DMSO include treatment of scleroderma, arthritis, tendinitis and renal amyloidosis, although therapeutic value in these conditions has lnot been demonstrated clearly. Locally applied DMSO, in concentrations above 50%, breaks down collagen, and has anti-inflammatory and local anesthetic effects, all of which probably contribute to relief of pain and improvement in bladder function and mucosal cytology. DMSO is converted to dimethyl sulfide, which imparts to the skin and breath a foul odor described as "garlic-like," but more offensive. No other side effects of intravesical instillation of 50% solutions have been reported but transient disturbances of color vision, photophobia, headache, nausea, diarrhea, urethral burning sensation on urination and allergies have occurred from topical application to the skin.

Dosage Form—Aqueous Solution: 50%/50mL.

Gold Compounds

Most authorities prefer the gold compounds over the adre nal steroids or nonsteroidal anti-inflammatory drugs for the adjunctive treatment of selected cases of active rheumatoid arthritis. Gold compounds suppress or prevent, but do not cure, arthritis and synovitis in the rapidly progressive forms of the diseases. Although their exact mechanism is not known, localized high concentrations of gold are found in Kupffer cells and synoviocyte liposomes; this suggests that gold therapy may inhibit liposomal enzyme activity in macrophages and decrease macrophage phagocytic activity. Some of the cellular effects of these compounds may be due to the strong affinity of gold for sulfur which causes inhibition of sulfhydral systems. Accumulation occurs with repeated administration and levels persist for many years in subsynovial tissues and in macrophages of many tissues. Macrophages are thought to be involved in the antigen process and in the interaction of helper T lymphocytes with antibody forming B lymphocytes. Whether or not this action is responsible for the effectiveness of gold compounds in arthritis is unknown.

The *oral* gold compound available (auranofin) contains 29% gold by weight, whereas the *parenteral* preparations (aurothioglucose; gold sodium thiomolate) contain 50% gold by weight. Before gold therapy is initiated, the patient's hemoglobin, erythrocyte, leukocyte, differential and platelet counts should be determined and a urinalysis done to serve as a basic reference. Urine should be analyzed for protein and sediment changes, and a complete blood count should be done prior to every administration or injection throughout the course of treatment.

Adverse reactions to gold therapy may occur at any time during treatment or many months after therapy has been discontinued. Common adverse reactions include *cutaneous:* dermatitis, pruritic eruptions, erythema, vesicular and exfoliative dermatitis, alopecia, loss of nails; *mucous membranes:* stomatitis, buccal ulcers, glossitis or gingivitis; *pulmonary:* interstitial pneumonitis, fibrosis, fever, rash, cough, shortness of breath, etc; *renal:* nephrotic syndrome, glomerulitis with hematuria and, rarely, renal failure; *hematologic:* granulocytopenia, thrombocytopenia, leukopenia, eosinophilia, hemorrhagic diathesis, hypoplastic and aplastic anemia; and *miscellaneous:* flushing, dizziness, sweating, nausea, vomiting and malaise. It is important to note that, except for diarrhea, serious toxicity occurs most frequently when parenteral therapy is used. The overall incidence and frequency of termination of therapy due to adverse effects from oral and injectable gold are shown in Table 4.

If toxicity develops, gold therapy should be discontinued immediately. Treatment includes topical or systemic corticosteroids, as appropriate, and the chelating agent dimercaprol (BAL) to increase the excretion of gold.

Auranofin

Gold, (2,3,4,6-tetra-*O*-acetyl-1-thio-β-D-glucopyranato-*S*)-(triethylphosphine)-, Ridaura (*SmithKline Beecham*)

[34031-32-8] $C_{20}H_{34}AuO_9PS$ (678.48).

Preparation—By condensation of the tetraacetate ester of aurothioglucose with triethylphosphine to form the coordination complex. US Pat 3,635,945.

Description—Colorless crystals; melts about 110°; contains about 29% by weight of gold.

Uses— It is used in the treatment of rheumatoid arthritis. Although auranofin does not have analgesic activity, it may slow the progress of this inflammatory disease. The therapeutic benefits usually are not apparent until after 3 to 4 months of use. The value of gold salts in rheumatoid arthritis is well-established; except for this drug, all available gold preparations must be administered intramuscularly. Although it is administered orally, it appears to retain the efficacy of the parenteral gold substances albeit with fewer major side effects and perhaps with slightly less efficacy. Approximately 25% of the gold in the drug is absorbed. The mean terminal body half-life is 21 and 31 days (range 42 to 128); approximately 60% of the absorbed gold is excreted in the urine; the remainder is excreted in the feces. Patients on 6 mg/day display a mean steady state of blood-gold concentrations of 0.68 ± 0.45 mg/mL. Approximately 40% of its gold is associated with red blood cells and 60% with serum proteins. The mechanism by which auranofin exerts its therapeutic effect in rheumatoid arthritis is unknown, although the drug does affect numerous cellular processes associated with inflammation. In contrast to parenteral gold preparations, it is not a potent inhibitor of sulfhydryl group reactivity. Adverse effects include diarrhea (46.6%) and microscopic hematuria (14%); skin reactions (pruritus, rash, 24%) were mild and occurred in about 30% of the patients; and mucosal ulcerations in approximately 10%; proteinuria was observed in 4% and was serious enough in 0.7% of patients to discontinue therapy. Liver function test abnormalities occurred in 0.4% of patients. Its contraindications are the same as those for parenteral gold compounds. Auranofin should be administered only to carefully selected patients who can be monitored closely during therapy.

Table 4—Overall Incidence and Frequency of Terminations Due to Adverse Effects from Oral and Injectable Gold

	Oral gold (n = 527)		Injectable gold (n = 526)	
Adverse effect	Reported[a]	Withdrawn[a]	Reported[a]	Withdrawn[a]
Diarrhea	44 (230)[b]	4.6 (24)[b]	13 (69)	1.3 (7)
Rash	32 (168)	5.7 (30)	41 (213)[b]	15.2 (80)[b]
Stomatitis	15 (78)	2.7 (14)	18 (95)	5.3 (28)[b]
Anemia	5.7 (30)	0.6 (3)	4.9 (26)	0.4 (2)
Thrombocytopenia	1.9 (10)	0.2 (1)	1.9 (10)	1.7 (9)[b]
Leukopenia	1.5 (8)	0.9 (5)	2.9 (15)	1.3 (7)
Proteinuria	7 (39)	1.7 (9)	12 (64)	4.9 (26)[b]
Liver enzymes > twice normal	4 (21)	1.1 (6)	4 (22)	1.5 (8)

[a] % (number).
[b] Significant increase.

Dose—*Usual, adult, oral,* **6 mg** a day. If response is inadequate after 6 mo, increase to **9 mg** a day; if response is inadequate after 3 mo, discontinue the drug.

Dosage Form—Capsules: 3 mg.

Aurothioglucose

Gold, (1-thio-D-glucopyranosato)-, Gold Thioglucose; Solganal (*Schering*)

[12192-57-3] $C_6H_{11}AuO_5S$ (392.18). It is stabilized by the addition of not more than 5% of sodium acetate.

Preparation—By refluxing an aqueous solution of thioglucose with gold tribromide in the presence of sulfur dioxide. The compound is thus precipitated, and is purified by dissolving in water after which it is reprecipitated by the addition of alcohol.

Description—Yellow powder; odorless or nearly so; stable in air; pH (1 in 100 solution) about 6.3; aqueous solutions are unstable on long standing.

Solubility—Freely soluble in water; practically insoluble in acetone, alcohol, chloroform or ether.

Uses—It is an *antirheumatic* used for treatment of active and progressing *rheumatoid arthritis* and nondisseminated *lupus erythematosus.* The adrenal steroids once largely displaced gold compounds from the therapeutic armamentarium, but recognition of the dangers of steroid therapy and the potential curative properties has restored the use of gold. No other antirheumatic drug is capable of arresting the progression of the disease, as gold can do in some cases. However, the gold compounds do not permanently arrest or reverse the associated disease process. The best therapy usually occurs when it is used in the early active stages of the disease and is based on the daily excretion rate of gold in the individual patient. It contains 50% gold; time to peak effect is 4 to 6 hr; 95 to 99% is bound to plasma protein; plasma half-life after a single dose varies from 3 to 27 days; 70% is excreted in the urine and 30% in the feces.

Parenterally administered gold compounds tend to cause more adverse effects than auranofin and should only be given to carefully selected patients by experienced physicians. Pruritus is generally the first sign of toxicity. Other toxic manifestations are listed in the introduction to this section and include mucocutaneous, hematological, renal, hepatic, GI and ocular effects. Although side effects can occur after the first dose, severe side effects do not usually occur until at least 300 to 500 mg has been administered; sometimes they do not occur until several months after treatment has been discontinued. Glucocorticoids increase toxicity yet protect against serious consequences such as nephrosis. Dimercaprol and penicillamine increase the excretion of gold.

Dose—*Intramuscular, adult, weekly injections, 1st dose,* **10 mg;** *2nd* and *3rd dose,* **25 mg;** *4th* and *subsequent doses,* **50 mg.** Continue the 50-mg dose at weekly intervals until **0.8 to 1 g** has been given. If the patient has improved and shows no signs of toxicity, continue the 50-mg dose many months or longer, at 3- to 4-week intervals. If no improvement is observed after a total administration of 1 g, reevaluate the necessity of gold therapy. *Children,* 6 to 12 yr, **2.5 mg** the 1st week, **6.25 mg** the 2nd and 3rd weeks, and **12.5 mg** a week until **200** to **250 mg** has been given, after which **6.25** to **12.5 mg** every 3 to 4 weeks is used for maintenance. A relapse during the lengthening intervals requires a shortening of the intervals. Toxicity requires discontinuation.

Dosage Form—Suspension: 50 mg/mL.

Gold Sodium Thiomalate

Butanedioic acid, mercapto-, monogold(1+) sodium salt; mercaptosuccinic acid, monogold(1+) sodium salt; Myochrysine (*MSD*)

A mixture of mono- and di-sodium salts of gold thiomalic acid, $C_4H_4AuNaO_4S$ (368.09) and $C_4H_3AuNa_2O_4S$ (390.07).

Preparation—Sodium thiomalate is reacted with gold chloride. US Pat 1,994,213.

Description—White to yellowish white, odorless, fine powder; affected by light; pH (1 in 10 solution) 5.8 to 6.5.

Solubility—Very soluble in water; insoluble in alcohol or ether.

Uses—It is an *antirheumatic* with the same gold content, pharmacokinetic properties, uses and toxicity as *Aurothioglucose,* except for reported nitritoid reactions with gold sodium thiomalate. It is given intramuscularly only.

Dose—*Usual, adult, weekly injections—1st dose,* **10 mg;** *2nd dose,* **25 mg;** *3rd* and *subsequent doses,* **25** to **50** mg until major clinical improvement or toxicity occurs, or until the cumulative dose reaches **1 g.** *Maintenance*—**25** to **50 mg** every other week for 2 to 20 weeks. If clinical condition remains stable, give **25** to **50 mg** every 3rd or 4th week indefinitely. *Children,* up to 12 yr, **1 mg/kg,** not to exceed **50 mg** for a single injection. Otherwise, adult guidelines apply.

Dosage Form—Injection: 50 mg/mL.

Other Drugs to Relieve Pain

This section includes discussions of unrelated drugs with distinct mechanisms of action. Although, technically some of these drugs are not analgesics because they do not directly affect the nociceptive system, they do relieve pain by altering the underlying cause of a medical condition. For example, some drugs are discussed here which are used to relieve gouty pain because they block the formation, or enhance the excretion, of uric acid. In addition, methysergide is listed here because it is used to relieve the pain of migraine headaches due to its blockade of serotonin receptors and its vasoconstriction properties.

Allopurinol

4*H*-Pyrazolo[3,4-*d*]pyrimidin-4-one, 1,5-dihydro-, Zyloprim (*Burroughs Wellcome*); (*Various Mfrs*)

[315-30-0] $C_5H_4N_4O$ (136.11).

Preparation—(Ethoxymethylene)malononitrile is reacted with hydrazine hydrate via deethanolation and addition thus cyclizing to form 3-aminopyrazole-4-carbonitrile. Controlled hydration of the nitrile forms the corresponding carboxamide which, on condensation with formamide, yields allopurinol. US Pat 2,868,803.

Description—Fluffy white to off-white powder; slight odor; tasteless; stable in light and air; melts about 300° with decomposition.

Solubility—Very slightly soluble in water or alcohol; soluble in solutions of fixed alkali hydroxides; practically insoluble in chloroform or ether.

Uses—A structural analogue of hypoxanthine used in the *treatment of gout,* primary or secondary *uric acid nephropathy, uric acid stone formation* and to prevent urate deposition, renal calculi or uric acid nephropathy in patients with leukemias, lymphomas and malignancies who are receiving cancer chemotherapy with its resultant effect of increasing serum uric acid levels. It is not an analgesic *per se;* relief from pain is secondary to the reduction in blood uric acid levels. It is not uricosuric; it inhibits the production of uric acid by blocking the biochemical reactions immediately preceding uric acid formation. Thus, it inhibits xanthine oxidase, the enzyme responsible for the conversion of hypoxanthine to xanthine and of xanthine to uric acid.

In addition, the drug inhibits *de novo* purine synthesis by a feedback mechanism, which provides another benefit to the patient. It is metabolized by xanthine oxidase to oxypurinol, which also inhibits xanthine oxidase. Oxypurinol has a much longer half-clearance time from plasma than allopurinol (18 to 30 hr and less than 2 hr, respectively). This accounts for its long duration of action and permits use of a single daily dose. It is contraindicated in children (except those with hyperuricemia secondary to malignancy) and in nursing mothers; also contraindicated in patients who develop a severe reaction to the drug.

A few cases of reversible hepatotoxicity have been observed; hence, periodic liver function studies should be done during the early stages of therapy. It should not be given concomitantly with iron salts, since laboratory studies suggest increased hepatic iron concentration may occur. Moreover, it increases the effect of the oral anticoagulants and enhances the toxicity of azathioprine, cyclophosphamide and mercaptopurine by decreasing the rate at which these agents are metabolized. It particularly is useful in patients who are resistant to or cannot tolerate uricosuric drugs and in patients with renal function so reduced as to not respond to conventional drugs. It precipitates acute gouty arthritis in early therapy more frequently than uricosuric drugs. This can be minimized by giving maintenance doses of colchicine and by starting therapy on a small dose and increasing the dose gradually.

Untoward effects include a rash, usually maculopapular; less frequently exfoliative, urticarial or purpuric; the rash may be accompanied by fever, leukopenia, arthralgias or other symptoms of hypersensitivity. Diarrhea is frequently observed. Isolated cases of peripheral neuritis, depression of the bone marrow, cataracts and reversible hepatic damage have been reported.

Dose—100 to **800 mg** a day; *usual, adult, oral, antigout,* **100** to **200 mg** 1 to 3 times a day; *oral, antiurolithic,* **200 mg** 1 to 4 times a day. *Pediatric, secondary hyperuricemia* associated with malignancies, children under 5 yr, *oral,* **50 mg** 3 times a day; 6 to 10 yr, *oral,* **100 mg** 3 times a day.

Dosage Form—Tablets: 100 and 300 mg.

Colchicine

Acetamide, (*S*)-*N*-(5,6,7,9-tetrahydro-1,2-3,10-tetramethoxy-9-oxobenzo[*a*]heptalen-7-yl)-,

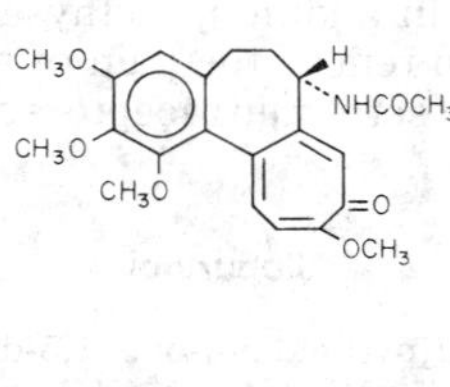

Colchicine [64-86-8] $C_{22}H_{25}NO_6$ (399.44); an alkaloid obtained from various species of *Colchicum.*

Caution—*Colchicine is extremely poisonous.*

Preparation—By extracting the corm or seed of the plant with alcohol. After distilling off the alcohol, the syrupy residue is diluted with water to precipitate fats and resins and filtered. The filtrate is digested with some lead carbonate, refiltered, evaporated to a small volume and the colchicine extracted with chloroform.

Description—Pale yellow to pale greenish yellow, amorphous scales, or powder or crystalline powder; odorless or nearly so; darkens on exposure to light; melts about 145°; pK_a 12.35.

Solubility—1 g in 25 mL water or about 220 mL ether; freely soluble in alcohol or chloroform.

Uses—The agent of choice in the symptomatic treatment of *acute* attacks of *gouty arthritis* and sometimes used for long-term prophylactic treatment of gouty arthritis. When properly administered, it will usually terminate an attack in 24 to 48 hr. It also is used in combination with either phenylbutazone or allopurinol in the management of acute gout. Colchicine is not an analgesic and the precise mechanism of action is unknown, although it is thought to decrease leukocyte motility, phagocytosis and lactic acid production, thereby decreasing the deposition of urate crystals and the inflammatory response. These effects may relate to the interference by colchine on cellular mitotic spindles. The drug is well-absorbed after oral administration; 31% is bound to plasma protein. It often is combined with probenecid to improve prophylactic therapy of chronic gouty arthritis. It is eliminated by both urinary and fecal routes. It is practically useless in chronic gout but its routine administration does lessen the frequency and severity of acute attacks.

It is very toxic, and it should be discontinued at the first evidence of toxicity, namely, diarrhea, nausea, vomiting and abdominal pain. Patients taking the drug for long periods are under some risk of occurrence of agranulocytosis, aplastic anemia, myopathy and alopecia, hence should have periodic examinations for possible blood dyscrasias or other adverse effects. Caution should be exercised in prescribing the drug for aged and debilitated patients, and for those with cardiac, renal, hepatic, gastrointestinal or hematological disease.

Dose—*Usual, adult, prophylactic, mild gout,* **0.5** to **0.6 mg** once a day for 1 to 4 days each week; *moderate to severe gout,* **0.3** to **0.6 mg** 1 to 3 times a day. *Therapeutic, oral,* **0.5** to **1.2 mg** initially, followed by **0.5** to **1.2 mg** every 2 hr until pain is relieved or until nausea, vomiting or diarrhea occurs. Total accumulative dose ranges from 4 to 8 mg. Pediatric dosage has not been established. *Intravenous, acute attacks of gout, initially* **2 mg,** followed by **0.5 mg** every 6 hr until a satisfactory response is achieved. The total intravenous dose for one course of treatment generally should not exceed 4 mg; subcutaneous extravasation may be painful.

Dosage Forms—Injection: 1 mg/2 mL; Tablets: 0.5 and 0.6 mg.

Dihydroergotamine Mesylate—page 1053.
Ergotamine Tartrate—page 1054.

Methotrimeprazine

10*H*-Phenothiazine-10-propanamine,
(−)-2-methoxy-*N*,*N*,β-trimethyl-, Levoprome (*Immunex*)

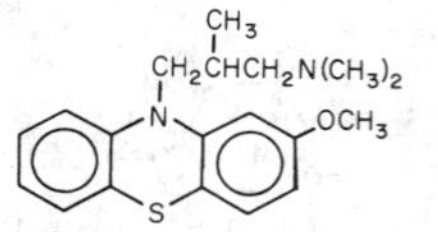

(−)-10-[3-(Dimethylamino)-2-methylpropyl]-2-methoxyphenothiazine [60-99-1] $C_{19}H_{24}N_2OS$ (328.47).

Preparation—By (1) condensation of *o*-chlorobenzoic acid with *m*-anisidine via dehydrochlorination with potassium carbonate and a copper catalyst to form 2-(*m*-anisidino)benzoic acid; (2) decarboxylation of the acid via pyrolysis to form 3-methoxydiphenylamine; (3) cyclization of the amine by heating with sulfur to form 2-methoxyphenothiazine; and (4) condensation of the 2-methoxyphenothiazine with 2-methyl-3-(dimethylamino)propyl chloride via dehydrochlorination with sodamide.

Description—Fine, white, practically odorless, crystalline powder; unstable in light and nonhygroscopic; melts about 126°.

Solubility—Practically insoluble in water; sparingly soluble in methanol; freely soluble in chloroform or ether; sparingly soluble in alcohol at 25° but freely soluble in boiling alcohol.

Uses—A phenothiazine derivative which depresses subcortical regions of the brain causing a decrease in sensory impulses, reduction of motor activity, sedation, and some amnesia. It is reported that 15 mg of the drug has the analgesic equivalence of 10 mg morphine sulfate. Methotrimeprazine also has antihistaminic, anticholinergic and antiadrenergic effects. It is available only in a form for intramuscular administration. It is indicated for the relief of pain of moderate to marked degree of severity in nonambulatory patients. It also is indicated for obstetrical analgesia and sedation where respiratory depression is to be avoided. It also can be used as preanesthetic medication for producing sedation, and for relieving anxiety and apprehension.

The drug is contraindicated for use with an unusually large number of other drugs: anesthetics, aspirin, CNS depressants, reserpine or tricyclic antidepressants (may potentiate the effects of either these medications or methotrimeprazine; dosage adjustments may be necessary); anticholinergics (may produce paralytic ileus); antihypertensive or MAO inhibitors (concurrent use is not recommended); atropine, scopolamine or succinylcholine (may produce tachycardia and hypotension, and aggravate other CNS effects such as stimulation, delirium and extrapyramidal symptoms) and epinephrine (may produce paradoxical hypotension).

The potential usefulness of methotrimeprazine must be weighed against its major adverse reactions, *orthostatic hypotension and sedation;* the former may last from 12 to 16 hr after drug administration. Because of the orthostatic hypotension patients receiving the drug should remain in bed for at least 6 to 12 hr after each of the first several doses. In addition, its use in geriatric or debilitated patients with heart disease must be done with great caution. Other untoward effects include dizziness, disorientation, amnesia, slurred speech, blurred vision, light-headedness, nausea, vomiting, dry mouth, nasal congestion, pain at site of injection, difficulty in urination, chills and uterine inertia. Leukopenia, agranulocytosis, jaundice and extrapyramidal symptoms also have been reported. Since this is a phenothiazine, the physician should be alert for other untoward effects characteristic of these agents.

Dose—*Intramuscular*, **5** to **40 mg;** *usual, initially* **10 mg** followed by **10** to **20 mg** every 4 to 6 hr. *Ambulation should be avoided or carefully supervised for at least 6 to 12 hr following the initial dose.*

Other Dose Information—For preanesthetic medication, intramuscular, 10 to 20 mg.

Dosage Form—Injection: 20 mg/mL (as the hydrochloride).

Methysergide Maleate

Ergoline-8-carboxamide, (8β)-9,10-didehydro-*N*-[1-hydroxymethyl)-propyl]-1,6-dimethyl-, (*Z*)-2-butenedioate (1:1) (salt); Sansert (*Sandoz*)

[129-49-7] $C_{21}H_{27}N_3O_2.C_4H_4O_4$ (469.54).

Preparation—See US Pat 3,218,324.

Description—Off-white to pinkish white crystals; melts with decomposition above 165°; pH (0.2% aqueous solution) about 4.

Solubility—1 g in about 500 mL water, 125 mL methanol, 165 mL ethanol or 10,000 chloroform.

Uses—A semisynthetic ergot alkaloid used for the *prevention* or *reduction of intensity* and *frequency* of vascular headaches in patients suffering from one or more severe vascular headaches per week. It also is indicated in patients suffering from vascular headaches that either are uncontrollable or so severe that preventive therapy is indicated regardless of the frequency of the attack. It may prove beneficial in the prophylaxis of migraine or cluster headaches.

Warning: Retroperitoneal fibrosis, pleuropulmonary fibrosis and fibrotic thickening of cardiac valves may occur in patients receiving long-term methysergide maleate therapy. Therefore, this preparation should be reserved for prophylaxis in patients whose vascular headaches are frequent and/or severe and uncontrollable and who are under close medical supervision.

Its use is contraindicated in patients with peripheral vascular disease, severe hypertension, coronary artery disease, pulmonary disease or collagen disease. Other adverse effects include *vasoconstrictor effects* (angina-like pain, vascular insufficiency), *central nervous system effects* (insomnia, nervousness, euphoria, dizziness, ataxia, hallucinations, drowsiness, mental depression, etc), *gastrointestinal reactions* (nausea, vomiting, diarrhea, abdominal pain) and *miscellaneous reactions* (dermatitis, alopecia, edema, weight gain, arthralgia and myalgia).

It should not be used for more than 6 months without imposing a 3- or 4-week drug-free period (the dosage should be reduced gradually 2 or 3 weeks before discontinuation of the drug to prevent rebound headaches).

Dose—*Usual, adult, oral,* **4 to 8 mg** a day in divided doses taken with food. It should not be used in children or during pregnancy.

Dosage Form—Tablets: 2 mg.

Penicillamine—page 936.

Probenecid—page 1051.

Sulfinpyrazone

3,5-Pyrazolidinedione, 1,2-diphenyl-4-[2-(phenylsulfinyl)ethyl]-, (*Par*); Anturane (*Ciba*)

[57-96-5] $C_{23}H_{20}N_2O_3S$ (404.48).

Preparation—[2-(Phenylsulfinyl)ethyl]malonic acid diethyl ester is condensed with hydrazobenzene using sodium ethoxide in absolute ethanol. The reaction is completed by adding xylene and heating at about 130° whereby the residual ethanol and that liberated during the condensation is removed. The sulfinpyrazone is isolated by a solvent extraction process and recrystallized from ethanol. US Pat 2,700,671.

Description—White to off-white powder; melts about 132°.

Solubility—Practically insoluble in water or solvent hexane; soluble in alcohol or acetone; sparingly soluble in dilute alkali.

Uses—A pyrazolone derivative with potent uricosuric activity and some antithrombotic and platelet inhibitory activity. It has no anti-inflammatory or analgesic properties. It is used to lower serum urate concentration for chronic and intermittent gouty arthritis. It is well-absorbed after oral administration; 98 to 99% is bound to plasma protein; plasma half-life is about 2.2 to 3 hr, about 50% of the administered dose is excreted unchanged in the urine.

The drug is contraindicated in patients with active peptic ulcer, renal impairment or a history of renal calculi, especially uric acid stones, because of the possibility of aggravating these conditions. Its uricosuric action is mutually antagonistic with that of salicylates. It should be used with caution in patients on sulfa drugs, sulfonylurea hypoglycemic agents and insulin since it may potentiate these agents. Side effects include upper gastrointestinal disturbances, rash (reported in about 3% of patients), and, rarely, anemia, leukopenia, agranulocytosis and thrombocytopenia.

Dose—**200** to **800 mg** a day; *usual, initially,* **100** to **200 mg** 1 or 2 times a day; *maintenance,* **100** to **400 mg** 2 times a day, with meals or milk.

Dosage Forms—Capsules: 200 mg; Tablets: 100 mg.

CHAPTER 73

Histamine and Antihistaminic Drugs

H Steve White, PhD
Research Associate Professor of Pharmacology and Toxicology
College of Pharmacy
University of Utah
Salt Lake City, UT 84112

Histamine is a physiologically active, endogenous substance (autocoid) that is produced within the body by the decarboxylation of the amino acid, histidine, and then stored in mast cells and basophils where it is protected from ubiquitous destructive enzymes, such as histaminase. It binds to and activates histamine H_1- and H_2-receptors in various sites in the body. H_3-receptors, which may be involved in the control of histamine synthesis, also have been described. The action of histamine on the cells depends to some extent upon the function of the cell as well as upon the ratio of its H_1- and H_2-receptors. The cardiovascular effects of histamine include direct and indirect microvascular dilation (involving H_1- and H_2-receptors) and increased vascular permeability (probably involving H_1-receptors); as a result, intracutaneous injection of histamine produces a "triple response" characterized by local reddening, a bright halo or flare and wheal formation. Histamine also binds to and activates specific receptors in the nose, eyes, respiratory tract and skin, causing characteristic allergic signs and symptoms. Activation of H_1-receptors (H_1-antagonists) block these actions.

Historically, the term *antihistamine* has been used to describe drugs that act as H_1-receptor antagonists. Activation of H_2-receptors stimulates gastric acid secretion; drugs which antagonize H_2-receptors (eg, cimetidine/nizatidine, ranitidine or famotidine) are referred to as H_2-receptors antagonists (see Chapter 53). The H_2-antagonists inhibit gastric secretion stimulated not only by histamine, but also by insulin, pentagastrin, food or physiological vagal reflex.

Another amine, 5-hydroxytryptamine, also is widely distributed in animals and is present in some plants. This substance, discovered independently by three groups of workers, also is known as *enteramine* and *serotonin*. It is found in largest amounts in the brain, blood, spleen, stomach, intestine, lungs and skin. It has been suggested that 5-hydroxytryptamine may be involved in the regulation of vascular tone, motor and secretory activity of the gastrointestinal tract and kidney function. It has been postulated, also, that 5-hydroxytryptamine serves as a neurotransmitter in the brain and that it may be involved in mental function. These observations, and the demonstration that tumors of the argentaffin cells of the intestinal mucosa (argentaffinomas or carcinoids) secrete large amounts of 5-hydroxytryptamine, have stimulated the search for 5-hydroxytryptamine antagonists. A number of substances, including ergot alkaloids and derivatives, indole derivatives, adrenergic blocking agents, anticholinergic drugs, morphine-like analgesics and some phenothiazines have been shown to possess this property. In addition, at least two agents that exhibit both antihistaminic and anti-5-hydroxytryptamine properties are available to clinicians, and more selective 5-hydroxytryptamine antagonists are under clinical investigation. Therefore, they also are included in this chapter.

Histamine Phosphate

1*H*-Imidazole-4-ethanamine, phosphate (1:2); Histamine Phosphate; Histatrol (*Center*)

HN N · $2H_3PO_4$
$CH_2CH_2NH_2$

4-(2-Aminoethyl)imidazole phosphate (1:2) [51-74-1] $C_5H_9N_3.2H_3PO_4$ (307.14).

Preparation—Histamine occurs in very small amounts in ergot. It is among the products of bacterial decomposition of histidine, and this constitutes one of the methods for its production. It also is produced synthetically from imidazolylpropionic acid by several methods.

Description—Long prismatic crystals; colorless; odorless stable in air but affected by light; aqueous solutions are acid to litmus; when dried at 105° for 2 hr, melts at about 140°; pH (4.1% aq soln, iso-osmotic with serum) about 5.

Solubility—1 g in about 4 mL water; slightly soluble in alcohol.

Pharmacology—Although many tissues contain a lethal amount of histamine in a bound or inactive form, no effect is produced until it is released in free form into body fluids as a result of certain stimuli. Since it is destroyed in the intestinal tract by the enzyme histaminase, it is ineffective when taken orally. After injection, it constricts certain smooth muscles such as the bronchi, uterus and intestines and dilates the capillary bed. Characteristically, increased capillary permeability accompanies the dilation, and there is a seepage of fluid, plasma proteins and even some cellular elements of the blood into extracellular spaces. Dilation of the capillaries and arterioles produces flushing of the face, fall in blood pressure and increase in skin temperature.

It stimulates all types of glandular secretions—gastric, duodenal, salivary and lacrimal. An important effect in man is the stimulation of the gastric glands, which increases the hydrochloric acid of the stomach. This effect of histamine was the basis of a diagnostic test which had been used in the past to differentiate between nonspecific hypochlorhydria and that caused by pernicious anemia (see page 690). The preferred agent for this purpose is pentagastrin (see page 1370, Chapter 79).

One highly characteristic effect of this agent is the "triple response" induced by the intracutaneous injection of small amounts of this agent. It consists of (1) local reddening at the site of the injection, (2) a wheal or patch of localized edema which obscures the original red spot and (3) the scarlet flare that surrounds the wheal. The initial red spot is due mostly to local capillary dilatation, and the wheal develops from arteriolar dilation and increased capillary permeability. The flare is a local phenomenon produced by an axon reflex involving peripheral sensory nerves. Since the flare does not appear in the presence of atrophy or degeneration of the nerve, this reaction has been used as a diagnostic test to distinguish between real and pseudoanesthesia.

When injected intravenously, it provokes an increased output of epinephrine from the adrenal medulla as indicated by a secondary rise in blood pressure. In the past, clinical use was made of this action on the adrenals by employing it as a test agent in the diagnosis of pheochromocytoma. This test is now considered obsolete because of its hazardous nature and because chemical assays are now available for detecting and quantitating the levels of catecholamines and their metabolites in patients suspected of having pheochromocytoma.

Uses—Histamine is used primarily as a positive control in evaluation of allergenic skin testing. It has a few other minor diagnostic applications. Since the "flare" that results from intracutaneous injection of this agent is mediated by an axon reflex, this approach has been used as a test for the integrity of sensory nerves; the wheal that results has been used as a test for circulatory competency.

Adverse reactions are observed even after small doses, such as employed in gastric analysis (0.01 mg/kg subcutaneously). These include flushing, dizziness, headache, bronchial constriction, dyspnea, visual disturbances, faintness, syncope, urticaria, asthma, marked hypertension or hypotension, palpitation, tachycardia, nervousness, abdominal cramps, diarrhea, vomiting, metallic taste, allergic manifestations or collapse with convulsions. The hypotension usually is postural and requires no treatment other than assuming a recumbent position. If treatment is required, epinephrine (0.3 mg SC) is an effective physiological antagonist.

Dose—*Percutaneus testing*, a **small drop** of histamine base (1 mg/mL) is placed on an abraded skin site no closer than 4 to 5 cm from an adjacent skin site. *Intradermal testing*, **0.01** or **0.02 mL** of histamine base (0.1 mg/mL) is injected intracutaneously into and slightly under the skin to form a small bleb 3 to 5 mm in diameter.

Dosage Form—Injection: 1 and 0.1 mg/mL of histamine base containing 2.75 and 0.275 mg/mL of histamine phosphate, respectively.

Pentagastrin—page 1370.

Antihistamines

All clinically available antihistamines antagonize histamine to approximately the same extent, regardless of their chemical class (ethanolamines, ethylenediamines, alkylamines, phenothiazines or piperidines). Except for phenindamine, they all induce some sedation and anticholinergic activity. Phenindamine may induce some stimulation. Only the ethanolamines and phenothiazines possess antiemetic properties. The clinical and pharmacological differences, therefore, are related chiefly to variations in adverse effects and to nonhistamine antagonizing actions, such as their atropine-like effects, central nervous system effects (depression, stimulation, antiemetic, antitremor and motion sickness) and local anesthetic properties. A knowledge of these factors is essential for proper drug selection.

All presently available antihistamines (H_1-receptor antagonists) act by competitively antagonizing the effects of histamine at receptor sites; they do not block the release of histamine and, hence, offer only palliative relief of allergic symptoms. After oral administration, effects are apparent within 15 to 30 min, are maximal within 1 hr and persist for 4 to 6 hr. The liver is the principal site of metabolism; the agents are excreted in urine as unidentified metabolites.

Clinically, indications for the use of the various antihistaminic drugs vary considerably. The majority of these agents are *effective* in *perennial* and *seasonal allergic rhinitis, vasomotor rhinitis, allergic conjunctivitis, urticaria and angioedema, allergic reactions to blood and plasma, dermographism* and as adjuncts to conventional therapy in *anaphylactic reactions*. A few antihistamines probably are effective in mild, local *allergic reactions to insect bites, physical allergy* and minor *drug* and *serum* reactions characterized by *pruritus*. Selected antihistamines (eg, diphenhydramine hydrochloride) reduce rigidity and tremors in *paralysis agitans* (Parkinson's disease) and in *drug-induced extrapyramidal symptoms*. Some antihistamines (eg, buclizine, cyclizine, dimenhydrinate, diphenhydramine, meclizine and others) also are effective in the *active and prophylactic* management of *motion sickness*. The more sedative agents (eg, diphenhydramine, doxylamine, promethazine and others) sometimes are used in *insomnia* and *insomnia* predominant in certain medical disorders. Certain antihistamines, such as chlorpheniramine, doxylamine succinate and pyrilamine maleate, are used in proprietary medication advertised as daytime sedatives and sleep aids. Methapyrilene, formerly used in virtually all nonprescription sleep aids in the US, was removed from these products in 1979 because of its possible carcinogenic properties.

The phenothiazine antihistamines possess other useful clinical properties not shared by conventional antihistamines. For example, promethazine hydrochloride is useful for *preoperative, postoperative* and *obstetric sedation*, prevention and control of *nausea* and *vomiting* associated with certain types of anesthesia and surgery and as *adjunctive therapy* to meperidine or other analgesics for the *control of postoperative pain*.

The usefulness of antihistamines in various other clinical conditions, such as bronchial asthma, atopic dermatitis, neurodermatitis, allergic eczema, various contact and chemotoxic dermatitides, generalized pruritus, and for cardiac arrhythmias, spasmolysis in gastrointestinal allergies, prophylaxis of drug reactions, etc, must await further clinical investigation before a final assessment can be made.

It is agreed generally that *most* antihistamines are *ineffective* in migraine and histamine headache, prevention or reduction of the sequelae of pain, edema and hemorrhage in oral surgery, potentiation of narcotic analgesic drugs, as antiemetics in postoperative patients, as antitussives or for treatment of nocturnal leg cramps, leg cramps of pregnancy and functional dysmenorrhea.

The most common side effect of antihistamines is sedation, evidenced principally by drowsiness, plus a diminished alertness and ability to concentrate. Less-common effects—unless large doses are used—include dryness of the mouth, blurred vision, vertigo and gastrointestinal distress (see also above). The sedative effect may be so intense as to impair driving ability and performance of duties requiring mental alertness. Other side effects elicited by these drugs include nausea, headache and restiveness. Dermatologic complications and skin eruptions have followed local application or oral administration of antihistamines. In a few individuals, certain antihistamines produce signs of central excitation such as insomnia and nervousness. Since the depressant effects of alcoholic beverages and other drugs that depress the central nervous system (tranquilizers, hypnotics, sedatives, antianxiety agents, depressants, analgesics, etc) are increased by antihistamines, the physician may forbid concurrent use or modify the conditions of such use. Patients being treated with MAO inhibitors, or who have been treated with such drugs within the preceding 2 weeks, should not be given antihistamines.

Because of their drying effect on mucous membranes, antihistamines may exacerbate wheezing and therefore should not be used during an asthmatic attack. Because of the anticholinergic action of antihistamines, their use in the following diseases may be contraindicated or subject to great caution: narrow-angle glaucoma, prostatic hypertrophy, stenosing peptic ulcer, pyloroduodenal obstruction, bladder-neck obstruction, increased intraocular pressure, history of bronchial asthma, hyperthyroidism, cardiovascular disease or hypertension. Antihistamines should not be given to premature or newborn infants, and may be denied by the physician for patients breast-feeding infants.

These brief observations call attention to the enormous number of clinical conditions for which antihistaminic drugs have been suggested. They also point up the fact that these drugs vary from *effective* to *ineffective* in these conditions.

When considering the multiplicity of available antihistamines, their numerous untoward reactions and their propensity to induce sedation of variable intensity, one can appreciate the complex therapeutic problem that confronts the thoughtful physician in the selection of an antihistamine for a particular patient with a histamine-related clinical condition.

Astemizole

1*H*-benzimidazol-2-amine, 1-[(4-fluorophenyl)methyl]-*N*-[1-[2-4-methoxyphenyl)ethyl]-4-piperidinyl]-, Hismanal (*Janssen*).

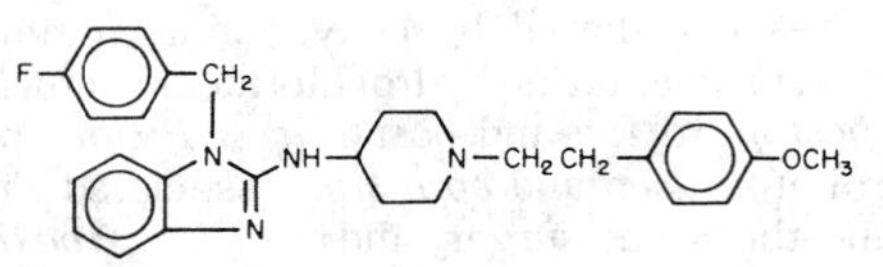

[68844-77-9] $C_{28}H_{31}FN_4O$ (458.58).

Preparation—The ethyl ester of 4-thiocyanato-1-piperidine carboxylic acid is treated with *o*-phenylenediamine to form the monourea. The unreacted primary arylamine is alkylated with *p*-fluorobenzyl bromide and the urea is then cyclized to the benzimidazole. Removal of the carbethoxy group (a carbamate) with base liberates the free piperidine nitrogen atom, which *N*-alkylated with *p*-methoxyphenethyl bromide to form the product. See US Pat 4,219,599.

Description—Melts about 150°, pK_a 8.35.

Solubility—Insoluble in water; 1 g in 30 mL alcohol.

Uses—A long-acting, peripherally selective nonsedating H_1 antagonist. It is indicated for the relief of symptoms associated with seasonal allergic rhinitis and chronic idiopathic urticaria. It is absorbed rapidly from the gastrointestinal tract. Peak plasma levels are reached within 1 hr; however, because of extensive first-pass effect and significant tissue distribution, plasma levels are low. Astemizole is metabolized extensively in the liver and excreted in the urine and feces. Elimination of astemizole plus its hydroxylated metabolites, which are considered active, occurs in a biphasic manner; distribution half-life of 20 hr and elimination half-life of 7 to 11 days. Adverse effects include drowsiness, headache, fatigue, increased appetite and weight gain, nervousness, dry mouth and, in rare cases, cholestatic jaundice. Concomitant administration of astemizole with erythromycin, ketoconazole or itraconazole is contraindicated because these drugs inhibit the cytochrome P450 enzyme system which metabolizes astemizole, and their concurrent use may lead to elevated plasma concentrations of astemizole. High concentrations of astemizole can lead to serious and potentially life-threatening cardiac arrhythmia's which require hospitalization (see also Terfenadine, page 1227). Astemizole should only be used in pregnancy and in lactation when the potential benefit justifies the potential risk to the fetus or infant.

Dose—*Usual, adults* and *children over 12 yr, oral,* **10 mg** once a day. Patients should be cautioned not to exceed the recommended dose in an attempt to accelerate the onset of action.

Dosage Form—Tablets: 10 mg.

Brompheniramine Maleate

2-Pyridinepropanamine, γ-(4-bromophenyl)-*N,N*-dimethyl-, (*Z*)-butenedioate (1:1); Dimetane (*Robins*); Rolabromophen (*Robinson*); (*Various Mfrs*)

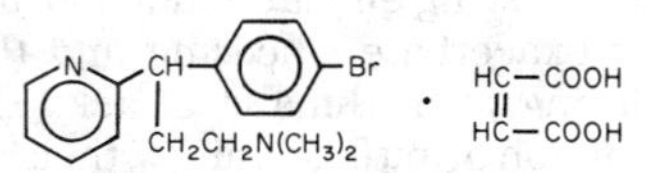

2-[*p*-Bromo-α-[2-(dimethylamino)ethyl]benzyl]pyridine maleate (1:1) [980-71-2] $C_{16}H_{19}BrN_2.C_4H_4O_4$ (435.32).

Preparation—α-(*p*-Bromophenyl)-2-pyridineacetonitrile is converted to its sodium derivative with sodium amide and condensed with 2-chloro-*N,N*-dimethylethylamine. The resulting nitrile is hydrolyzed to the corresponding acid, which is decarboxylated by treatment with H_2SO_4. The base, obtained on alkalinization, is solvent-extracted and reacted with maleic acid.

Description—White, crystalline powder; odorless; melts 130 to 135°; pH (1 in 100 solution) 4.0 to 5.0; pK_a 3.9, 9.1.

Solubility—1 g in 5 mL water, 15 mL alcohol or 15 mL chloroform; slightly soluble in ether or benzene.

Uses—The bromine analog of chlorpheniramine; an antihistamine with anticholinergic (drying) and sedative side effects. It is *probably effective* for temporary relief of hay fever and upper respiratory allergy symptoms, such as itchy, watery eyes, sneezing, itching nose or throat and for amelioration and prevention of allergic reactions to blood or plasma in patients with a known history of such reactions. It appears to be well-absorbed after oral administration; peak serum concentrations of 7.7 and 15.7 ng/mL occur within 2 to 5 hr after a dose of 0.13 mg/kg; the antihistaminic effect appears maximal within 3 to 9 hr and antipruritic effect maximal within 9 to 12 hr. See also the general statement.

Dose—*Usual, adult, oral,* **4 mg** every 4 to 6 hr; extended-release tablets, **8** or **12 mg** every 12 hr. Do not exceed 24 mg in 24 hr. *Parenteral, intramuscular, intravenous,* or *subcutaneous,* **10 mg** 2 times a day; maximum, 40 mg. *Pediatric, children* under 5 yr, *oral,* **125 µg/kg** or **3.75 mg/m²** every 6 hr or as directed by a physician; *children* over 6 yr, *oral,* **2** to **4 mg** 3 or 4 times a day or **8** to **12 mg** as extended-release tablet every 12 hr; *parenteral, children* 11 yr and under, **125 µg/kg** or **3.75 mg/ m²** every 6 hr; contraindicated for premature and full-term neonates.

Dosage Forms—Elixir: 2 mg/5 mL; Injection: 10 mg/mL. Tablets: 4 mg; Extended-Release Tablets: 8 and 12 mg.

Buclizine—page 902.

Carbinoxamine Maleate

Ethanamine, 2-[(4-chlorophenyl)-2-pyridinylmethoxy]-*N,N*-dimethyl-, (*Z*)-2-butenedioate (1:1); ing of Rondec (*Ross*)

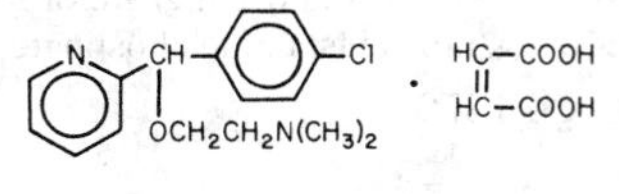

2-[*p*-Chloro-α-[2-(dimethylamino)ethoxy]benzyl]pyridine maleate (1:1) [3505-38-2] $C_{16}H_{19}ClN_2O.C_4H_4O_4$ (406.87).

Preparation—Picolinaldehyde and *p*-chlorophenylmagnesium bromide undergo a Grignard reaction to produce *p*-chloro-α-(2-pyridyl)benzyl alcohol. This is converted into its sodium alkoxide derivative with sodamide; β-Dimethylaminoethyl chloride is added to form carbinoxamine and the base converted into the maleate by reaction with maleic acid.

Description—White, crystalline powder; odorless melts 116 to 121°; pH (1 in 100 solution) 4.6 to 5.1; pK_a 8.7.

Solubility—1 g in < 1 mL water, 1.5 mL alcohol, 1.5 mL chloroform or 8300 mL ether.

Uses—An antihistamine with anticholinergic and antiemetic activity similar to other ethanolamines. It is *probably effective* in allergic rhinitis, vasomotor rhinitis, allergic conjunctivitis, mild uncomplicated allergic skin manifestation of urticaria and angioedema. Adverse reactions are relatively mild and rarely occur; dizziness, drowsiness, nausea and dryness of the mouth have been observed. Other precautions and contraindications are the same as those for other antihistamines (see the introductory statement).

Dose—*Adult, oral,* **4 mg** 3 or 4 times a day or **8 mg** (as timed-release) 2 times a day. *Children 12 and older, oral,* **8 mg** (as timed-release) 2 times a day. *Children 6 yr to 12 yr, oral,* **4 mg** 3 or 4 times a day. *Children 18 mo to 6 yr, oral syrup,* **2 mg** 3 or 4 times a day. *Pediatric children, 9 to 18 mo, oral drops,* **2 mg** 3 or 4 times a day; *6 to 9 mo, oral drops,* **1.5 mg** 3 or 4 times a day; *3 to 6 mo, oral drops,* 1 mg 3 to 4 times a day; *1 to 3 mo* **0.5 mg** 3 or 4 times a day. Contraindicated for premature and full-term neonates.

Dosage Forms—Tablets: 4 mg timed release tablets: 8 mg; syrup: 4 mg/5 mL; oral drops: 2 mg/mL.

Chlorpheniramine Maleate

2-Pyridinepropanamine, γ-(4-chlorophenyl)-*N,N*-dimethyl-, (*Z*)-2-butenedioate (1:1); Chlor-Trimeton (*Schering-Plough*); (*Various Mfrs*)

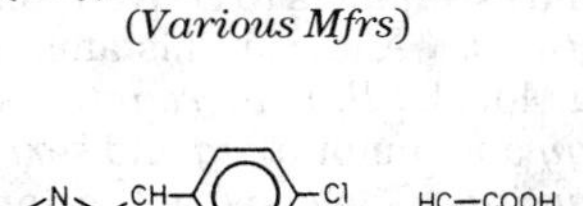

2-[*p*-Chloro-α-[2-(dimethylamino)ethyl]benzyl]pyridine maleate (1:1) [113-92-8] $C_{16}H_{19}ClN_2.C_4H_4O_4$ (390.87).

Preparation—By condensing 2-[*p*-chloro-α-(2-chloroethyl)benzyl-]pyridine with dimethylamine in the presence of sodamide. Treatment of the base with an equimolar portion of maleic acid results in the formation of the maleate.

Description—White, crystalline powder; odorless; solutions are acid to litmus (pH 4 to 5); melts 130 to 135°; pK_a 9.2.

Solubility—1 g in 4 mL water, 10 mL alcohol or 10 mL chloroform; slightly soluble in ether or benzene.

Uses—An *antihistamine* which is *probably effective* in allergic and vasomotor rhinitis, allergic conjunctivitis, mild urticaria and angioedema, allergic reactions to blood and plasma in sensitive patients, dermographism and as adjunct therapy in anaphylactic shock. It is used widely as an ingredient in proprietary antitussive formulations. It undergoes significant first-pass metabolism (40 to 55%). Peak plasma levels of 5.9 and 11 ng/mL are achieved in 2 to 6 hr. It has a low incidence of side effects, which are similar to those induced by other antihistamines. See the introductory statement.

Dose—*Usual, adult, oral,* **4 mg** 4 to 6 times a day; extended- release capsules or tablets, **8** to **12 mg** every 8 to 12 hr; not to exceed 24 mg in 24-hr period. *Children 6 to 12 yr,* **2 mg** every 4 to 6 hr, or **8 mg** extended-release once a day not to exceed 12 mg in 24 hr; *2 to 6 yr,* **1 mg** every 4 to 6 hr; *parenteral,* **5** to **20 mg** as a single dose, with a maximum of 40 mg in 24 hr. Extended-release forms not recommended for children under 6 yr.

Dosage Forms—Extended-Release Capsules: 6, 8 and 12 mg; Injection: 10 and 100 mg/mL; Solution: 1 and 2 mg/5 mL; Tablets: 4 mg; Chewable Tablets: 2 mg; Extended-Release Tablets: 8 and 12 mg.

Clemastine Fumarate

Pyrrolidine, [*R*-(*R**,*R**)]-2-[2-[1-(2-[2-[1-(4-chlorophenyl)-1-phenylethoxy]ethyl]-1-methyl-, (*E*)-2-butenedioate (1:1); Tavist (*Sandoz*)

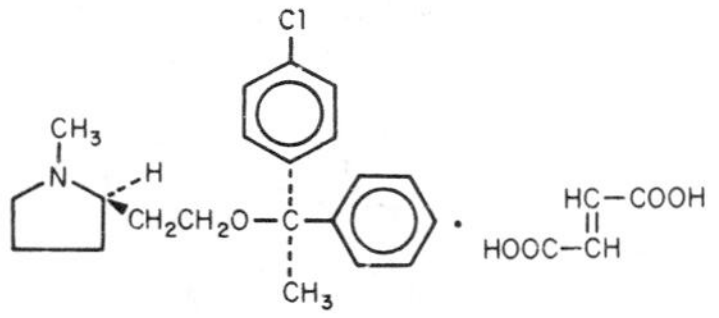

(+)-(2*R*)-2-[2-[(*R*)-*p*-Chloro-α-methyl-α-phenylbenzyl)oxy]-ethyl]-1-methylpyrrolidine fumarate (1:1) [14976-57-9] $C_{21}H_{26}ClNO.C_4H_4O_4$ (459.97).

Preparation—Various benzhydryl ethers that have histamine-inhibiting action, of which clemastine is one, may be prepared by heating a mixture of the appropriate benzhydryl bromide and *N*-methyl-2-piperidylethanol in the presence of sodium carbonate. Details of the process, as well as of an alternate synthesis, are described in British Pat 942,152 (see *CA 60*: 9250g, 1964).

Description—White to faintly yellow, crystalline powder; practically odorless; melts 176 to 181° with decomposition.

Solubility—Very slightly soluble in water, chloroform or ether; slightly soluble in alcohol.

Uses—A long-acting *antihistamine* with anticholinergic (drying) and sedative side effects. It is indicated for relief of symptoms associated with seasonal allergic rhinitis and mild uncomplicated allergic skin manifestations of urticaria and angioedema. The drug rapidly and almost completely is absorbed after oral administration; peak plasma concentrations are attained within 2 to 5 hr; it is metabolized extensively and excreted principally in the urine. Side effects and contraindications are similar to those of other agents in this group (see the general statement).

Dose—*Usual, adult, oral,* **1.34 mg** twice a day to **2.68 mg** 3 times a day; may be repeated as required but not to exceed **8.04 mg** a day. *Children 6 to 12 yr, oral,* **0.67 mg** twice a day to **1.34 mg** twice a day, not to exceed 4.02 mg daily. Not recommended for children under 6.

Dosage Form—Syrup, 0.67 mg/5 mL; Tablets: 1.34 and 2.68 mg of clemastine fumarate (equivalent to 1 and 2 mg of clemastine base).

Cyproheptadine Hydrochloride—page 1229.

Cyclizine—RPS-18, page 791.

Dexbrompheniramine Maleate

2-Pyridinepropanamine,(*S*)-γ-(4-bromophenyl)-*N*,*N*-dimethyl-, (*Z*)-2-butanedioate (1:1); ing of Disophrol, Drixoral (*Schering*)

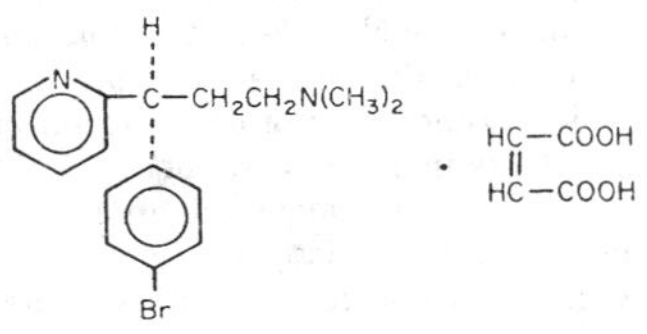

(+)-2[*p*-Bromo-α-[2-dimethylamino)ethyl]benzyl]pyridine maleate (1:1). [2391-03-9] $C_{16}H_{19}BrN_2.C_4H_4O_4$ (435.32).

Preparation—As for *chlorpheniramide*, using the *p*-bromo derivative, rather than chloro. The racemic mixture produced is resolved to yield the product. See US Pats 2,676,964 and 3,061,517.

Description—White, crystalline powder; odorless; pH (1 in 100 solution) about 5; melts 103 to 113°.

Solubility—1 g in 1.2 mL water, 2.5 mL alcohol, 2 mL alcohol, 2 mL chloroform or 3000 mL ether.

Uses—The dextro-isomer of brompheniramine maleate. The major portion of the antihistaminic activity is said to reside in the dextro-isomer; the levo form is relatively inactive. It has actions, untoward effects and therapeutic applications similar to brompheniramine maleate. See *Brompheniramine Maleate* (page 1224) and also *Antihistamine Combinations* (page 1230).

Dexchlorpheniramine Maleate

2-Pyridinepropanamine, (*S*)-γ-(4-chlorophenyl)-*N*,*N*-dimethyl-, (*Z*)-2-butenedioate (1:1); Polaramine (*Schering)*

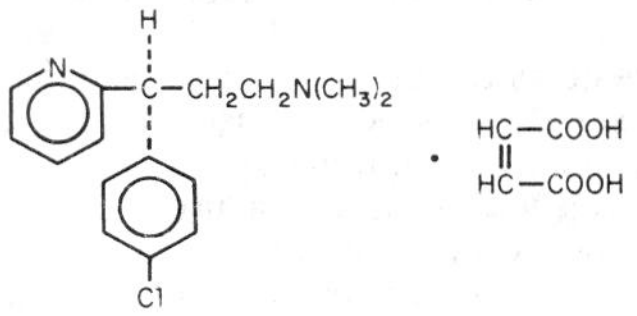

(+)-2-[*p*-Chloro-α-[2-(dimethylamino)ethyl]benzyl]pyridine maleate (1:1) [2438-32-6] $C_{16}H_{19}ClN_2.C_4H_4O_4$ (390.87).

Preparation—Racemic chlorpheniramine (see *Chlorpheniramine Maleate*) is resolved with the aid of (+)-phenylsuccinic acid. The (+)-enantiomorph of the base then is liberated from its (+)-phenylsuccinate salt by treatment with sodium hydroxide and reacted with an equimolar portion of maleic acid.

Description—White, crystalline powder; odorless; melts 110 to 115°; pH (1 in 100 solution) 4.0 to 5.0.

Solubility—1 g in 1.1 mL water, 2 mL alcohol, 1.7 mL chloroform or 2500 mL ether.

Uses—The dextro-isomer of chlorpheniramine; an antihistamine which has about twice the potency of chlorpheniramine and a wide margin of safety. Its uses and limitations are similar to those for *Chlorpheniramine Maleate*. See also the general statement.

Dose—*Usual, adult* and *children 12 yr and older, oral,* **2 mg** every 4 to 6 hr, or **4** to **6 mg** as repeat-action tablets every 8 to 12 hr, not to exceed 12 mg in 24 hr. *Pediatric, infants, oral,* **500 μg** (0.5 mg) every 4 to 6 hr; *children* 6 to 12 yr, **1 mg** every 4 to 6 hr, not to exceed 6 mg in 24 hr, or a **4 mg** repeat-action tablet once a day at bedtime; *children* 2 to 5 yr, **500 μg** (0.5 mg) every 4 to 6 hr, not to exceed 3 mg in 24 hr. Do not use repeat-action form; contraindicated for premature and full-term neonates.

Dosage Forms—Syrup: 2 mg/5 mL; Tablets: 2 mg; Repeat-Action Tablets: 4 and 6 mg.

Dimenhydrinate—page 903.

Diphenhydramine Hydrochloride

Ethanamine, 2-(diphenylmethoxy)-*N*,*N*-dimethyl-, hydrochloride; Benadryl Hydrochloride (*Parke-Davis)*; (*Various Mfrs*)

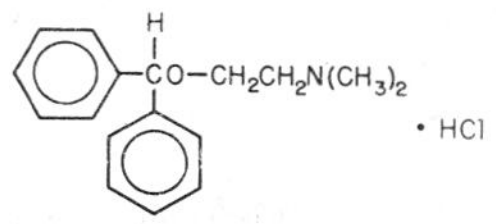

2-(Diphenylmethoxy)-*N*,*N*-dimethylethylamine hydrochloride [147-24-0] $C_{17}H_{21}NO.HCl$ (291.82).

Preparation—By heating diphenylbromomethane, β-dimethylaminoethanol and sodium carbonate in toluene. After distilling off the toluene, the purified diphenhydramine is converted to the hydrochloride with hydrogen chloride.

Description—White, crystalline powder; slowly darkens on exposure to light; solutions are practically neutral to litmus; melts 167 to 172°.

Solubility—1 g in 1 mL water, 2 mL alcohol, 2 mL chloroform or 50 mL acetone; very slightly soluble in benzene or ether.

Uses—A potent antihistamine that possesses anticholinergic (drying), antitussive, antiemetic and sedative effects. It is *effective* for use in perennial and seasonal allergic rhinitis; vasomotor rhinitis; allergic conjunctivitis due to inhalant allergens and foods; mild, uncomplicated allergic skin manifestations of urticaria and angioedema; amelioration and prevention of allergic reactions to blood or plasma in patients with a known history of such reactions; dermographism; therapy for anaphylactic reactions adjunctive to epinephrine and other standard measures after the acute manifestations have been controlled; parkinsonism (including drug-induced) in the elderly unable to tolerate more potent agents; mild cases of parkinsonism (including drug-induced) in other age groups; other cases of parkinsonism (including drug-induced) in combination with centrally acting anticholinergic agents and active and prophylactic treatment of motion sickness. It also has significant antitussive activity; the syrup is used as a cough suppressant for the control of cough due to colds or allergy.

It is *probably effective* for use in mild, local allergic reactions to insect bites; physical allergy; minor drug and serum reactions characterized by pruritus; and intractable insomnia and insomnia dominant in certain medical disorders. Other suggested uses require further investigation.

Although it is well-absorbed after oral administration, first-pass metabolism is so extensive that only 40 to 60% reaches systemic circulation unchanged. Peak plasma concentrations are attained in 1 to 4 hr, 80 to 85% is bound to plasma protein and elimination half- life ranges from 2.4 to 9.3 hr.

Numerous side effects are observed by patients on this drug, such as drowsiness, confusion, restlessness, nausea, vomiting, diarrhea, blurring of vision, diplopia, difficulty in urination, constipation, nasal stuffiness, vertigo, palpitation, headache, insomnia, urticaria, drug rash, photosensitivity, hemolytic anemia, hypotension, epigastric distress, anaphylactic shock, tightness of the chest and wheezing, thickening of bronchial secretions, dryness of the mouth, nose and throat and tingling, heaviness, and weakness of the hands.

Dimenhydrinate (Dramamine) contains approximately 50% diphenhydramine. The former agent is capable of masking symptoms of ototoxicity; therefore, dimenhydrinate and diphenhydramine should be used with caution in patients receiving aminoglycoside antibiotics (streptomycin, neomycin or kanamycin) or other ototoxic drugs.

Since it has an atropine-like action, it should be used with caution in patients with asthma. Likewise, patients should be cautioned about taking this drug with other depressant substances, because of the additive effect. Persons also should be advised not to operate a motor vehicle, fly an airplane or operate hazardous machinery while on this drug. The incidence of side effects is about 30 to 60%.

Dose—*Usual, adult, oral,* **25** to **50 mg** 3 or 4 times a day, with maximum of 300 mg a day; *intravenous* or deep *intramuscular,* **10** to **50 mg**, with maximum of 400 mg a day; *topical,* to skin, **1** and **2%** cream 3 or 4 times a day. *Pediatric, children, oral, intravenous* or deep *intramuscular,* **1.25 mg/kg** or **37.5 mg/m²** 4 times a day not to exceed 300 mg a day; *topical,* to skin, same as adult; contraindicated for neonates.

Dosage Forms—Capsules: 25 and 50 mg; Elixir: 12.5 mg/5 mL; Injection: 10 and 50 mg/mL; Syrup: 12.5 mg/5 mL; Tablets: 25 and 50 mg. Topical Cream: 1 and 2%.

Diphenylpyraline Hydrochloride—see RPS-18, page 1126.

Doxylamine Succinate

Ethanamine, *N,N*-dimethyl-2-[1-phenyl-1-(2-pyridinyl)ethoxy]-, butanedioate (1:1); Decapryn Succinate (*Merrell-Dow*); Unisom Night-time Sleep Aid (*Leeming*)

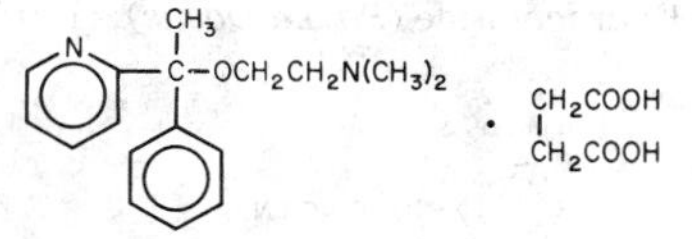

2-[α-[2-(Dimethylamino)ethoxy]-α-methylbenzyl]pyridine succinate (1:1) [562-10-7] $C_{17}H_{22}N_2O.C_4H_6O_4$ (388.46).

Preparation—Methylphenyl-2-pyridylcarbinol is converted into its sodium alcoholate and refluxed in toluene with 2-(dimethylamino)ethyl chloride. The doxylamine thus formed is reacted with an equimolar quantity of succinic acid in warm acetone.

Description—White or creamy white powder; characteristic odor; melts within a range of 3° between 103 and 108°.

Solubility—Very soluble in water or alcohol; freely soluble in chloroform; very slightly soluble in ether or benzene.

Uses—Shares the actions and uses of other antihistamines. Because of its sedative effect, it is used as a sleep aid. It also is used in combination with antitussives and decongestants for the temporary relief of cough and cold symptoms. Following oral administration (single 25-mg dose) mean plasma concentrations reach about 100 μg/mL within 2 to 3 hr; its elimination half-life is about 10 hr. Untoward effects and contraindications are similar to those for other members of this group of drugs. See the general statement.

Dose—*Usual, adult* and *children 12 yr and older, oral,* **7.5** to **12.5 mg** every 4 to 6 hours, not to exceed 75 mg in 24 hr. Under the direction of a physician, these patients may receive up to **25 mg** every 4 to 6 hr, not to exceed 150 mg in 24 hr. *Pediatric, children 6 to 12 yr, oral,* **3.75** to **6.25 mg** every 4 to 6 hrs, not to exceed 37.5 mg in 24 hr. Under the direction of a physician, pediatric patients may receive up to **12.5 mg** every 4 to 6 hr, not to exceed 75 mg in 24 hr; contraindicated for premature and full-term neonates.

Dosage Form—Tablets: 25 mg. Also available in combination with antitussives and decongestants.

Hydroxyzine Hydrochloride—page 1168.

Meclizine—page 904.

Methdilazine

10*H*-Phenothiazine, 10-[(1-methyl-3-pyrrolidinyl)methyl]-, Tacaryl (*Westwood*)

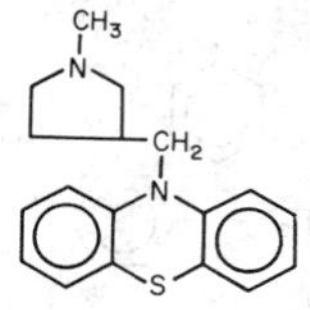

10-[(1-Methyl-3-pyrrolidinyl)methyl]phenothiazine [1982-37-2] $C_{18}H_{20}N_2S$ (296.43).

Preparation—By condensation of phenothiazine with 1-methyl- 3-pyrrolidinylmethyl chloride. US Pat 2,945,855.

Description—Light-tan, crystalline powder; characteristic odor; melts within a range of 2° between 83 and 88°; pK_a 7.45.

Solubility—1 g in > 10,000 mL water, 2 mL alcohol, 1 mL chloroform or 8 mL ether.

Uses—See *Methdilazine Hydrochloride.*

Dose—*Usual, adult, oral,* **7.2 mg** (equivalent to 8 mg of methdilazine hydrochloride) 2 to 4 times a day. *Pediatric, children over 3 yr,* **3.6 mg** 2 to 4 times a day.

Dosage Form—Chewable Tablets: 3.6 mg.

Methdilazine Hydrochloride

10*H*-Phenothiazine, 10-[(1-methyl-3-pyrrolidinyl)methyl]-, monohydrochloride; Tacaryl Hydrochloride (*Westwood*)

10-[(1-Methyl-3-pyrrolidinyl)methyl]phenothiazine monohydrochloride [1229-35-2] $C_{18}H_{20}N_2S.HCl$ (322.89). For the structure of the base, see *Methdilazine.*

Preparation—Methdilazine is reacted with an equimolar quantity of hydrogen chloride in a nonaqueous solvent.

Description—Light-tan, crystalline powder; slight characteristic odor; bitter anesthetic taste; melts 184 to 190°; pH (1 in 100 solution) 4.8 and 6.0.

Solubility—1 g in 2 mL water, 2 mL alcohol, 6 mL chloroform or > 10,000 mL ether.

Uses—A phenothiazine antihistamine *effective* for the symptomatic relief of urticaria. It also has been used for the therapy of migraine headache. It is contraindicated in asthma, narrow-angle glaucoma, prostatic hypertrophy, peptic ulcer, pyloroduodenal obstruction and newborn infants; it also is used in acutely ill or dehydrated children, because of the greater susceptibility of dystonias with phenothiazines. It should not be given concomitantly with other phenothiazines, antihistamines or MAO inhibitors. Adverse effects include drowsiness, dizziness, gastrointestinal disturbances, dryness of the mucous membranes, headache and skin rash. Extrapyramidal symptoms also have been reported. Other untoward reactions may include those for phenothiazines in general (see the general statement).

Dose—*Usual, adult, oral,* **8 mg** 2 to 4 times a day. *Children over 3 yr,* **4 mg** 2 to 4 times a day.

Dosage Forms—Syrup: 4 mg/5 mL; Tablets: 8 mg.

Phenindamine Tartrate

1*H*-Indeno[2,1-*c*]pyridine, 2,3,4,9-tetrahydro-2-methyl-9-phenyl-, Nolahist mixture (*Carnrick*)

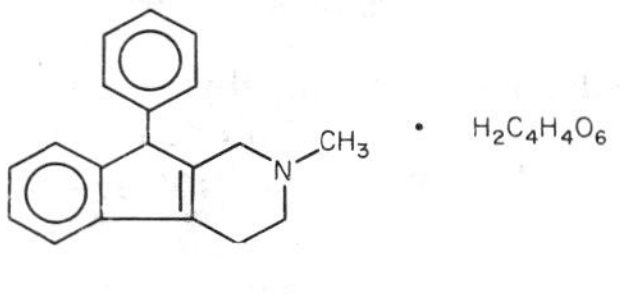

[569-59-5] $C_{19}H_{19}N.C_4H_4O_6$ (411.45).

Preparation—An aqueous solution of methylamine hydrochloride is reacted with molar quantities of acetophenone and paraformaldehyde by refluxing in alcohol. The 3,3′-methyliminobis(propiophenone) hydrochloride so obtained is refluxed with hydrobromic acid to form 2,3-dihydro-1-methyl-9-phenyl-1*H*-indeno[2,1-*c*]pyridine hydrobromide, which is then hydrogenated catalytically until an equimolar portion of hydrogen is taken up, after which treatment with alkali yields the base. Treatment with an equimolar portion of tartaric acid produces the official tartrate.

Description—Creamy white powder; usually a very faint odor; its solutions are acid to litmus; melts 160 to 162°; on continued slow heating, resolidifies at about 163°, and melts again with decomposition, at about 168°.

Solubility—1 g in about 40 mL water or about 350 mL of alcohol; practically insoluble in chloroform, ether or benzene.

Uses—For the temporary relief of running nose, sneezing, itching of the nose and throat and itchy, watery eyes due to hay fever or other upper respiratory allergies or allergic rhinitis. Also, it temporarily relieves running nose and sneezing associated with the common cold. It is contraindicated in asthma, glaucoma, emphysema, chronic pulmonary disease and shortness of breath unless directed by a physician. It may cause excitability (especially in children), nervousness and insomnia. It should be used with caution in patients with hypertension, cardiovascular disease, diabetes or hyperthyroidism. Use with caution in patients with prostatic hypertrophy or glaucoma.

Dose—*Usual, adult oral,* **25 mg** every 4 to 6 hr; do not exceed **150 mg** in 24 hr. *Children 6 to 12 yr,* **12.5 mg** every 4 to 6 hr; not to exceed 75 mg in 24 hr. *Children under 2 yr,* as directed by physician.

Dosage Form—Tablets, 25 mg. Also, available in combination with chlorpheneramine maleate and phenylpropanolamine as Nolamine (*Carnick*).

Promethazine Hydrochloride

10*H*-Phenothiazine-10-ethanamine, *N,N,α*-trimethyl-, monohydrochloride; Mepergan; Phenergan (*Wyeth-Ayerst*); (*Various Mfrs*)

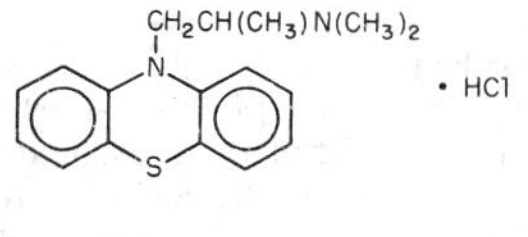

10-[2-(Dimethylamino)propyl]phenothiazine monohydrochloride [58-33-3] $C_{17}H_{20}N_2S.HCl$ (320.88).

Preparation—By reacting phenothiazine with 1-chloro-2-(dimethylamino)propane hydrochloride in the presence of sodamide and sodium hydroxide in xylene. The base is extracted, purified and converted to the hydrochloride.

Description—White to faint yellow, crystalline powder; practically odorless; slowly oxidized, particularly when moistened, on prolonged exposure to air, becoming blue in color; pH (1 in 20 solution) 4.0 to 5.0; melts within a 3° range between 215 and 225°; pK_a 9.1.

Solubility—Very soluble in water, hot dehydrated alcohol or chloroform; practically insoluble in ether, acetone or ethyl acetate.

Uses—A phenothiazine antihistamine of marked potency and prolonged duration of action. It is *effective* for use in perennial and seasonal allergic rhinitis; vasomotor rhinitis; allergic conjunctivitis due to inhalant allergens and foods; mild, uncomplicated allergic skin manifestations of urticaria and angioedema; amelioration and prevention of allergic reactions to blood or plasma in patients with a known history of such reactions; dermographism; therapy for anaphylactic reactions adjunctive to epinephrine and other standard measures after the acute manifestations have been controlled; preoperative, postoperative or obstetric sedation; prevention and control of nausea and vomiting associated with certain types of anesthesia and surgery; therapy adjunctive to meperidine or other analgesics for control of postoperative pain; sedation in both children and adults as well as relief of apprehension and production of light sleep from which the patient easily can be aroused; active and prophylactic treatment of motion sickness and antiemetic action in postoperative patients.

It is well-absorbed and peak effects occur within 20 min following oral, rectal or IM administration; 76 to 80% is bound to plasma proteins; the duration of antihistaminic effect may persist for 12 hr or more. The drug is excreted slowly in the urine and feces, primarily as inactive sulfoxides and glucuronides.

Untoward reactions include dryness of the mouth, blurring of vision and, rarely, dizziness. Rare cases of leukopenia and one case of agranulocytosis have been reported. Minor increases in blood pressure and occasional mild hypotension have been documented. The appearance of photosensitivity may contraindicate further treatment. Excessive doses in adults have resulted in deep coma, sedation and, rarely, convulsions; in children, hyperexcitability and nightmares. See the general statement.

Dose—*Antihistaminic: adults, oral, parenteral,* or *rectal,* **25 mg** before retiring or **12.5 mg** before meals and before retiring. *Pediatric, oral, parenteral,* or *rectal,* **6.25** to **12.5 mg** 3 times a day or **25 mg** once a day at bedtime; contraindicated in premature and full-term neonates. *Sedative: adults, oral, parenteral,* or *rectal,* **25** to **50 mg** at bedtime. *Pediatric, oral, parenteral, rectal,* **12.5** to **25 mg** at bedtime. *Antiemetic: adults, parenteral,* **12.5** to **25 mg** 4 to 6 times a day as needed. *Pediatric, oral, parenteral, rectal,* **0.5** to **1.0 mg/kg** or **7.5** to **15 mg/m²** 4 to 6 times a day as needed. *Preoperative: adults, oral,* **50 mg** given the night before surgery. *Pediatric,* **12.5** to **25 mg** the night before surgery. *Postoperative sedation and adjunctive use with analgesics: adults,* **25** to **50 mg;** *children,* **12.5** to **25 mg.**

Dosage Forms—Injection: 25 and 50 mg/mL; Suppositories: 12.5, 25 and 50 mg; Syrup: 6.25 and 25 mg/5 mL; Tablets: 12.5, 25 and 50 mg. Also available in combination with meperidine (Mepergan Fortis; *Wyeth-Ayerst*) and with phenylephrine Phenergan VC (*Wyeth-Ayerst*).

Pyrilamine Maleate

1,2-Ethanediamine, *N*-[(4-methoxyphenyl)methyl]-*N′,N′*-dimethyl-*N*-2-pyridinyl-, (*Z*)-2-butenedioate (1:1); Antallergan Maleate; Anthisan Maleate; Pyranisamine Maleate; (*Various Mfrs*)

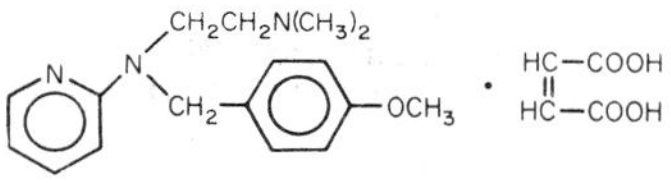

2-[[2-(Dimethylamino)ethyl](*p*-methoxybenzyl)amino]pyridinemaleate (1:1) [59-33-6] $C_{17}H_{23}N_3O.C_4H_4O_4$ (401.46).

Preparation—By condensing 2-[[2-(dimethylamino)ethyl] amino]pyridine with *p*-methoxybenzyl chloride in the presence of sodamide. Treatment of the base with maleic acid yields the maleate.

Description—White, crystalline powder; usually having a faint odor; solutions are acid to litmus, melts 99 to 103°.

Solubility—1 g in 0.5 mL water, 3 mL alcohol or 2 mL chloroform; slightly soluble in ether or benzene.

Uses—An antihistamine with a low incidence of sedative effects. The effectiveness and clinical applications are essentially the same as those for diphenhydramine, except it is not recommended for use in the management of parkinsonism or drug-induced extrapyramidal symptoms. It also is employed in a number of proprietary antitussive formulations. See *Diphenhydramine* and the general statement.

Dose—*Adults, oral,* **25** to **50 mg** 3 or 4 times a day. *Pediatric 6 yr and older,* **12.5** to **25 mg** 3 to 4 times a day.

Dosage Form—Tablets: 25 mg.

Terfenadine

1-Piperidinebutanol, α-[4-(1,1-dimethylethyl)phenyl]-4-(hydroxydiphenylmethyl)-, Seldane (*Marion Merrell Dow*)

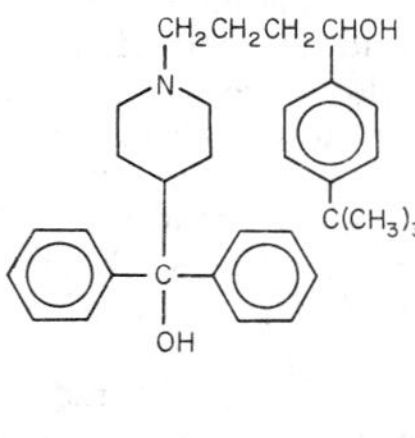

[50679-08-8] $C_{32}H_{41}NO_2$ (471.68).

Preparation—Azacyclonol (see RPS-14, page 1091) is reacted with 4-(*tert*-butyl-4′-chlorobutyrophenone) in the presence of $KHCO_3$ and KI in toluene to yield the carbonyl analog of the drug. This material is converted to hydrochloride for purification, the free base regenerated with KOH in methanol and reduced to the secondary alcohol with KBH_4. See *Arzneim Forsch 32*; 1153, 1982.

Description—White to off-white crystalline powder; melts at about 147°; pK_a 8.58.

Solubility—Freely soluble in chloroform; soluble in ethanol; very slightly soluble in water.

Uses—A peripheral distinct H_1-receptor antagonist, although chemically and pharmacologically distinct from other antihistamines. Terfenadine alone or in combination with pseudoephedrine is indicated for the relief of symptoms associated with seasonal allergic rhinitis such as sneezing, rhinorrhea, pruritus and lacrimation. It is absorbed rapidly and almost completely after oral administration; because of extensive first-pass metabolism, less than 1% reaches the systemic circulation unchanged and 97% of this is bound to plasma protein. Peak effect is observed within 1 to 2 hr; peak plasma levels range from 1.5 to 4.5 ng/mL. Plasma concentrations decline in a biphasic manner; distribution half-life is 3.5 hr and terminal elimination half-life is 16 to 23 hr. Adverse effects include headache, drowsiness, fatigue, sore throat, nausea, nasal stuffiness and cough. Rare cases of serious cardiovascular adverse events, including cardiac arrest, torsades de pointes, ventricular arrhythmias and even death have been observed in certain clinical settings. Terfenadine is contraindicated in patients taking ketoconazole, itraconazole or erythromycin, and in those patients with significant hepatic impairment. Concomitant administration of terfenadine with drugs which inhibit a specific isozyme of P450 may lead to elevated plasma terfenadine concentrations which have been shown to produce a prolongation in the QT interval and serious cardiovascular adverse effects. Physicians are advised to question patients about pregnancy or lactation before starting therapy, since the drug should be used in pregnancy and lactation only if the potential benefit justifies the potential risk to the fetus or infant.

Dose—*Usual, adults and children over 12 yr, oral,* **60 mg** twice a day.

Dosage Form—Tablets: 60 mg.

Trimeprazine Tartrate

10*H*-Phenothiazine-10-propanamine, *N,N,*β-trimethyl-, [*R*(*R**,*R**)]-2,3-dihydroxybutanedioate (2:1); Temaril (*Allergan Herbert*)

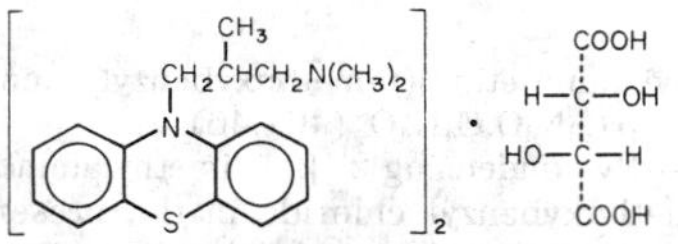

10-[3-(Dimethylamino)-2-methylpropyl]phenothiazine tartrate (2:1) [41375-66-0 (replaced); 4330-99-8] $(C_{18}H_{22}N_2S)_2.C_4H_6O_6$ (746.98).

Preparation—A xylene solution of phenothiazine is refluxed with sodamide and then with (3-chloro-2-methylpropyl)dimethylamine. The trimeprazine thus formed is extracted with aqueous acid, liberated with alkali and extracted with ether. After removal of the ether, the base is distilled under reduced pressure and reacted with tartaric acid. US Pat 2,837,518.

Description—White to off-white, crystalline powder; odorless; darkens on exposure to light; melts 160 to 164°; pK_a 9.2.

Solubility—1 g in 2 mL water, 20 mL alcohol, 5 mL chloroform or 1800 mL ether.

Uses—A phenothiazine compound more active than promethazine and less active than chlorpromazine in histamine-induced bronchospasm in guinea pigs. Its tranquilizing properties are of a low order and its chief use is as an antipruritic drug. It is considered *effective* for use in the treatment of pruritic symptoms due to urticaria and *possibly effective* for prolonged relief of pruritic symptoms in a variety of allergic and nonallergic conditions, including neurodermatitis, allergic dermatitis, contact dermatitis, pityriasis rosea, eczematous dermatitis, poison ivy dermatitis, drug rash, pruritus ani and vulvae. Side effects may mimic both phenothiazines and antihistamines; drowsiness, dryness of mucous membranes and gastrointestinal disturbances are observed commonly. Patients on therapy lasting over 1 mo should be monitored for possible agranulocytosis, hypotension or parkinson-like symptoms. MAO inhibitors and thiazide diuretics intensify these symptoms. For a more detailed description of untoward reactions see *Chlorpromazine Hydrochloride* (see pages 1181 and 1182).

Dose (base)—*Usual, adult, oral,* **2.5 mg** 4 times a day or **5 mg** as extended-release capsules every 12 hr. *Pediatric, oral, 6 mo to 3 yr,* **1.25 mg** at bedtime or **1.25 mg** 3 times a day if needed. *Children over 3 yr,* **2.5 mg** at bedtime or **2.5 mg** 3 times a day if needed. Alternatively, *children over 6 yr,* **5 mg** as extended-release capsule once a day.

Dosage Forms (base)—Extended-Release Capsules: 5 mg; Syrup: 2.5 mg/5 mL; Tablets: 2.5 mg.

Tripelennamine Citrate

1,2-Ethanediamine, *N,N*-dimethyl-*N*′-(phenylmethyl)-*N*′-2-pyridinyl-, 2-hydroxy-1,2,3-propanetricarboxylate (1:1); Pyribenzamine (*Geigy*)

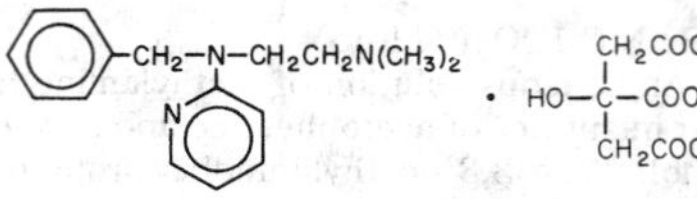

2-[Benzyl[2-(dimethylamino)ethyl]amino]pyridine citrate (1:1) [6138-56-3] $C_{16}H_{21}N_3.C_6H_8O_7$ (447.49).

Preparation—Tripelennamine is reacted with an equimolar portion of citric acid in a suitable volatile solvent. For the preparation of the base, see *Tripelennamine Hydrochloride*.

Description—White, crystalline powder; solutions are acid to litmus; melts at about 107°.

Solubility—1 g in about 1 mL water; freely soluble in alcohol; very slightly soluble in ether; practically insoluble in chloroform or benzene.

Uses—An antihistamine said to be more palatable by the oral route of administration than the hydrochloride. Otherwise, its actions and uses are the same. See *Tripelennamine Hydrochloride*.

Dose (tripelennamine hydrochloride equivalent)—*Usual, adult, oral,* **25** to **50 mg** every 4 to 6 hr, up to 600 mg a day. *Pediatric, oral,* equivalent of **1.25 mg/kg** or **37.5 mg/m²** every 6 hr, not to exceed 300 mg a day.

Dosage Form (tripelennamine hydrochloride equivalent)—Elixir: 25 mg/5 mL.

Tripelennamine Hydrochloride

1,2-Ethanediamine, *N,N*-dimethyl-*N*′-(phenylmethyl)-*N*′-(2-pyridinyl)-, monohydrochloride; (*Danbury*); Pyribenzamine (*Geigy*); Ro-Hist (*Robinson*)

2-[Benzyl[2-(dimethylamino)ethyl]amino]pyridine monohydrochloride [154-69-8] $C_{16}H_{21}N_3.HCl$ (291.82). For the structure of the base, see *Tripelennamine Citrate*.

Preparation—As follows: 2-aminopyridine, prepared by the action of sodamide on pyridine, is reacted with β-dimethylaminoethyl chloride in the presence of sodamide, and the resulting 2-[2-(dimethylamino)ethylamino]pyridine is condensed with benzyl bromide in the presence of sodamide. The hydrochloride is formed from the base by treatment with hydrogen chloride in an organic solvent.

Description—White, crystalline powder; slowly darkens on exposure to light; solutions practically neutral to litmus; melts 188 to 192°.

Solubility—1 g in 1 mL water, 6 mL alcohol, 6 mL chloroform or about 350 mL acetone; insoluble in benzene, ether or ethyl acetate.

Uses—An antihistamine *effective* in perennial and seasonal allergic rhinitis, vasomotor rhinitis, allergic conjunctivitis due to inhalant allergens and foods, mild, uncomplicated allergic skin manifestations of urticaria and angioedema, amelioration and prevention of allergic reactions to blood or blood plasma in patients with known history of such reactions, dermographism, anaphylactic actions adjunctive to epinephrine and other standard measures after the acute manifestations have been controlled.

This drug (and its citrate) are well-absorbed after oral administration. After a 100-mg dose, mean peak plasma levels of 0.06 μg/ mL are achieved within 2 to 3 hr. It appears to be metabolized completely to quaternary ammonium *N*-glucuronide or *O*-glucuronides of hydroxylated metabolites. The drug also undergoes aromatic ring hydroxylation, *N*-oxidation and *N*-demethylation. All but the *N*-oxide appear to conjugate with glucuronic acid. Therefore, the drug is excreted in the urine principally as metabolites.

It has a low incidence (20 to 35%) of side effects; gastrointestinal irritation is common, but not severe; sedation is moderate and central nervous system stimulation occurs occasionally. See the general statement.

Dose—*Usual, adult, oral,* **25** to **50 mg** every 4 to 6 hr or **100 mg** as extended-release tablet every 8 to 12 hr; range **25** to **600 mg** a day. *Pediatric, oral, children,* **1.25 mg/kg** or **37.5 mg/m²** every 6 hr, not to exceed 300 mg a day. The 100-mg extended-release tablet should not be used in children.

Dosage Forms—Tablets: 25 and 50 mg. Extended-Release Tablets: 100 mg.

Triprolidine Hydrochloride

Pyridine, *E*-2-[1-(4-methylphenyl)-3-(1-pyrrolidinyl)-1-propenyl]-, monohydrochloride, monohydrate, Actidil(*Burroughs Wellcome*)

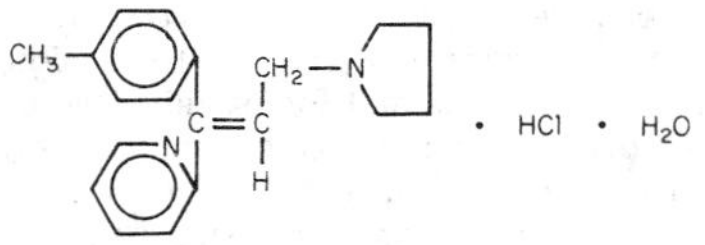

[6138-79-0] $C_{19}H_{22}N_2.HCl.H_2O$ (332.87); *anhydrous* [550-70-9] (314.86).

Preparation—4′-Methylacetophenone is reacted with formaldehyde and pyrrolidine to form 3-(1-pyrrolidinyl)-4′-methylpropiophenone. Reaction with 2-pyridylsodium and subsequent hydrolysis produces the tertiary carbinol, α-[2-(1-pyrrolidinyl)-ethyl]-α-*p*-tolyl-2-pyridinemethanol, which is dehydrated with sulfuric acid to introduce the propenyl double bond. Alkalinization liberates triprolidine, which is purified and reacted with an equimolar portion of HCl. US Pats 2,712,020 and 2,712,023.

Description—White, crystalline powder; no more than a slight, but unpleasant, odor; bitter taste; solutions are alkaline to litmus; melts at about 115°; light-sensitive; nonhygroscopic; stable to reasonable heat; pK_a 3.6, 9.3.

Solubility—1 g in 2.1 mL water, 1.8 mL alcohol, 1 mL chloroform or 2000 mL ether.

Uses—An unusually potent antihistamine with a rapid onset and long duration of action. The maximum effect occurs in about 3½ hr; the duration of effect is about 12 hr. The actions, uses and incidence of side effects are comparable to those of *Doxylamine Succinate*.

Dose—*Usual, adults* and *children over 12 yr, oral,* **2.5 mg** 4 to 6 times a day, *children 6 to 12 yr,* **1.25 mg** 4 to 6 times a day, not to exceed 5 mg in 24 hr. *Under direction of a physician, children 4 to 6 yr,* **0.9 mg** (syrup) 4 to 6 times a day, not to exceed 3.7 mg in 24 hr. *Children 2 to 4 yr,* **0.6 mg** (syrup) every 4 to 6 hr, not to exceed 2.5 mg in 24 hr. *Children 4 mo to 2 yr,* **0.3 mg** (syrup) every 4 to 6 hr, not to exceed 1.25 mg in 24 hr.

Dosage Forms—Syrup: 1.25 mg/5 mL; Tablets: 2.5 mg.

Inhibitors of Histamine Release

The antihistamines described in the previous section antagonize in varying degree most but not all pharmacological effects of histamine. They appear to accomplish this by occupying the "receptor sites" on the effector cell to the exclusion of the agonist, histamine, without initiating a response. Typically, they are competitive antagonists and do not prevent the release of histamine in response to injury, drugs or antigens. However, a more recently developed drug, cromolyn sodium, can prevent the release of histamine from mast cells which have been sensitized by specific antigens.

Cromolyn Sodium

4*H*-1-Benzopyran-2-carboxylic acid, 5,5′-[(2-hydroxy-1,3-propanediyl)- bis[4-oxo-, disodium salt; DSCG; Sodium Chromoglycate; Gastrocrom, Intal, Nasalcrom, Opticrom (*Fisons*)

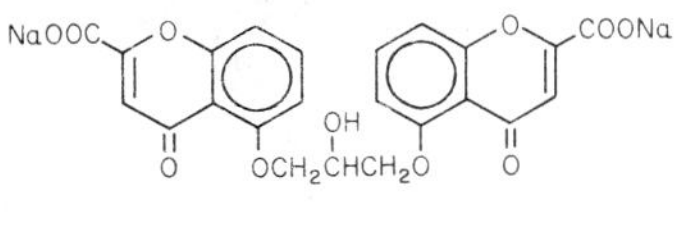

[15826-37-6] $C_{23}H_{14}Na_2O_{11}$ (512.34).

Preparation—2,6-Dihydroxyacetophenone is reacted with epichlorohydrin in the presence of a basic catalyst to yield the diether, 2′,2‴-[(2-hydroxytrimethylene)dioxy]bis[6′-hydroxyacetophenone]. Reaction with diethyl oxalate effects dehydration and deethanolation of each hydroxyacetophenone portion, thus introducing the fused oxopyrancarboxylate groups as ethyl esters. This diester is then saponified with NaOH. US Pat 3,419,578.

Description—White, crystalline powder; odorless; tasteless but with a slightly bitter aftertaste; hygroscopic; pK_a believed by analogy with similar monochromes to be about 1.5 to 2; melts at about 261°; does not exhibit polymorphism.

Solubility—1 g in 20 mL water; insoluble in alcohol or chloroform.

Uses—An antiasthmatic, antiallergic and mast cell stabilizer used in the management of severe bronchial asthma, the prevention of exercise-induced and acute bronchospasm and allergic rhinitis, the treatment of allergic ocular disorders, such as vernal keratoconjunctivitis, vernal conjunctivitis, giant papillary conjunctivitis, vernal keratitis and allergic keratoconjunctivitis and in the management of mastocytosis.

Animal studies show that it inhibits the degranulation of sensitized mast cells which occurs after exposure to specific antigens. Thus, it inhibits the release of histamine and SRS-A (slow-reacting substance of anaphylaxis) from the mast cell. It has no vasoconstrictor, antihistaminic or anti-inflammatory activity.

It is absorbed poorly from the gastrointestinal tract, lung (7 to 8%) or eye (0.03%). The systemically absorbed drug is excreted unchanged in the bile and urine. Adverse reactions from the use of *capsule and aerosol preparations* include lacrimation, swollen parotid glands, nausea, dysuria, dizziness, headache, rash, urticaria, angioedema, joint swelling and pain; from *nebulizer or nasal solutions:* cough, nasal congestion, sneezing, nasal itching, epistaxis, postnasal drip, headache and abdominal pain and from *ocular solutions:* stinging or burning on instillation, puffy eyes, irritation and styes. It is contraindicated in patients hypersensitive to cromolyn or any component of the product.

Dose—*Nebulizer Solution and Capsules*: *Adults* and *children* (>5 yr for capsules; >2 yr for nebulizer), **20 mg** inhaled 4 times a day at regular intervals. *Nasal Solution*: **One spray** in each nostril 3 to 6 times a day at regular intervals. *Allergic Ocular Disorders: Adults and children,* **1** to **2 drops** in each eye 4 to 6 times a day at regular intervals. For the management of mastocytosis. *Adults* and *children over 12 yr,* **200 mg** 4 times a day. *Children 2 to 12 yr,* **100 mg** 4 times a day. *Full-term infants to 2 yr,* **20 mg/kg** a day in 4 divided doses.

Dosage Forms—Aerosol Spray (each activation delivers 800 mcg); Capsules (for inhalation), 20 mg; Nasal Solution (each activation delivers 5.2 mg); Ophthalmic Solution, 40 mg/mL. Solution (for nebulizer), 20 mg/2 mL. Capsules (for oral administration): 100 mg.

5-Hydroxytryptamine (Serotonin) Antagonists

The pharmacological actions of 5-hydroxytryptamine are varied and complex. Liberation of excessive amounts in man, as in argentaffin cell tumors, produces episodic flushing, tachycardia and hypertension followed by cyanosis, diarrhea, asthma and pulmonary stenosis. 5-Hydroxytryptamine antagonists have been employed in the management of this malignancy, as well as certain skin diseases and psychoses. The most likely effective clinical application of these antagonists, however, is in the treatment of malignant carcinoid.

In addition to the agents described below, methysergide maleate exhibits 5-hydroxytryptamine antagonist properties. It also has other more prominent actions and uses; consequently, it is described in Chapter 63.

Azatadine Maleate

5*H*-Benzo[5,6]cyclohepta[1,2-*b*]pyridine, 6,11-dihydro-11-(1-methyl-4-piperidinylidene)-, (*Z*)-2-butenedioate (1:2); Trinalin (*Key*)

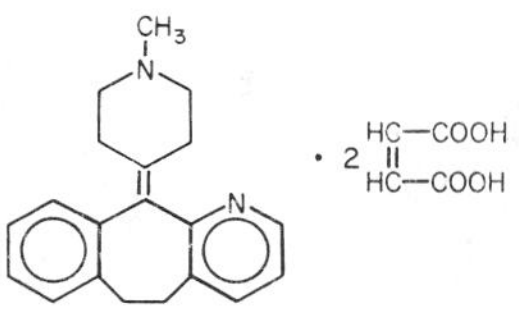

6,11-Dihydro-11-(1-methyl-4-piperidylidene)-5*H*-benzo[5,6]-cyclohepta[1,2-*b*]pyridine maleate (1:2) [3978-86-7] $C_{20}H_{22}N_2.2C_4H_4O_4$ (522.55).

Preparation—Azatadine is a chemical relative of cyproheptadine, differing from the latter in that a pyridine ring replaces one of the benzene rings of cyproheptadine and in the saturation of the cycloheptane ring of the latter compound. It may be prepared by dehydrating the condensation product formed in the presence of sodium and liquid ammonia, from 4-chloro-*N*-methylpiperidine and 5,6-dihydro-11*H*-benzo-[5,6]cyclohepta[1,2-*b*]pyridine-11-one. Treatment of the base with a bimolar quantity of maleic acid forms the maleate salt. US Pat 3,326,924.

Description—White to off-white powder; nonhygroscopic; melts about 153°; pK_a 8.4.

Solubility—1 g in 30 mL water or 30 mL alcohol.

Uses—Like its prototype cyproheptadine, an antihistamine with antiserotonin, anticholinergic and sedative effects. Stated indications for the drug are treatment of perennial and seasonal allergic rhinitis, and chronic urticaria. In general, the same contraindications, warnings and precautions apply to this drug as to the antihistamines (see the general statement). It is absorbed readily after oral administration; peak plasma concentrations are reached in about 4 hr after a single oral dose; it is bound minimally to plasma protein and elimination half-life ranges from 9 to 12 hr. The most frequent adverse reactions are sedation, sleepiness, dizziness, disturbed coordination, epigastric distress and thickening of bronchial secretions. Some reactions of lesser occurrence are anaphylactic shock, hypotension, hemolytic anemia, fatigue, blurred vision, wheezing and nasal stuffiness. It should be used with caution in patients with stenosing peptic ulcer, pyloroduodenal obstruction, urinary bladder obstruction and those patients with hypertension, ischemic heart disease or increased intraoccular pressure. Its use in pregnancy is inadequate to determine because of possible harmful effects.

Dose—*Usual, adult, oral,* **1 mg** twice a day. Not intended for use in children under 12 yr.

Dosage Form—Repeat-Action Tablets: 1 mg azatadine maleate in combination wtih 120 mg pseudoephedrine sulfate (see page 997 for uses and contraindications).

Cyproheptadine Hydrochloride

Piperidine, 4-(5*H*-dibenzo[*a,d*]cyclohepten-5-ylidene)-1-methyl-, hydrochloride, sesquihydrate; Periactin Hydrochloride (*MSD*)

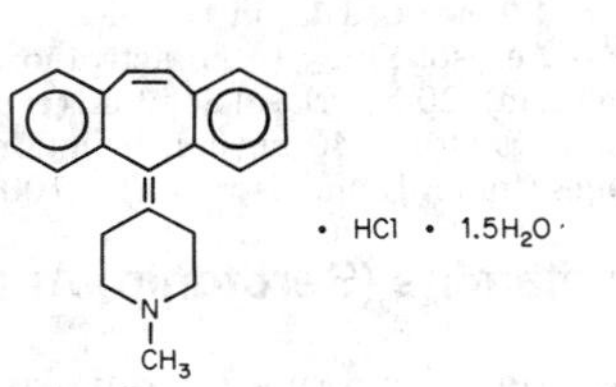

N, CH_3 · HCl · 1.5H_2O ·

4-(5*H*-Dibenzo[*a,d*]cyclohepten-5-ylidene)-1-methylpiperidine hydrochloride sesquihydrate [41354-29-4] $C_{21}H_{21}N.HCl.1\frac{1}{2}H_2O$ (350.89); *anhydrous* [969-33-5] (323.86).

Preparation—Phthalic anhydride is reacted with phenylacetic acid to form 3-benzylidenephthalide which, on isomerization and hydrogenation, gives 2-phenethylbenzoic acid. This is converted to its acid chloride, which then undergoes condensation to close the 7-membered ring and give 10,11-dihydro-5*H*-dibenzo[*a,d*]cyclohepten-5-one. Bromination at the 10 position followed by dehydrobromination introduces the 10,11 double bond. Grignardization of this ketone with 4-chloro-1-methylpiperidine followed by dehydration of the resulting carbinol yields cyproheptadine (base) which, on reacting with an equimolar quantity of hydrogen chloride, forms the hydrochloride. US Pat 3,014,911.

Description—White to slightly yellow, crystalline powder; odorless or practically odorless; slightly bitter taste; relatively stable in light, stable at room temperature; nonhygroscopic; sesquihydrate is stable in air; anhydrous form melts at about 250° and sesquihydrate melts at about 162°.

Solubility—1 g in 275 mL water, 35 mL alcohol or 26 mL chloroform; practically insoluble in ether.

Uses—An antihistamine with antiserotonin, anticholinergic, antialdosterone and sedative effects. It is *effective* for the treatment of perennial and seasonal allergic rhinitis, vasomotor rhinitis, allergic conjunctivitis due to inhalant allergens and foods, mild uncomplicated allergic skin manifestations of urticaria and angioedema, amelioration and prevention of reactions to blood or plasma in patients with a known history of such reactions, cold urticaria, dermographism, and as therapy for anaphylactic reactions adjunctive to epinephrine and other standard measures after the acute manifestations have been controlled. It is *probably effective* in mild, local allergic reactions to insect bites, physical allergy and minor drug and serum reactions characterized by pruritus. It is *possibly effective* in pruritus of allergic dermatoses including contact dermatitis and pruritus of chicken pox. In general the same contraindications, warnings and precautions apply to this drug as do to the antihistamines (see the general statement). Untoward effects which appear frequently include drowsiness, and somnolence. Dry mouth, dizziness, jitteriness, faintness, dryness of the mucous membranes, headache, nausea and allergic skin manifestations also have been reported to occur in low incidence. Rarely, central nervous system stimulation may appear.

Dose—*Usual, adult, oral,* **4 mg** 3 or 4 times a day, with a maximum of **500 µg** (0.5 mg)/**kg** a day. *Pediatric, children 2 to 6 yr, oral,* **2 mg** 2 or 3 times a day, with a maximum of **12 mg** a day; *7 to 14 yr, oral,* **4 mg** 2 or 3 times a day, with a maximum of **16 mg** a day; contraindicated for premature and full-term neonates.

Dosage Forms—Syrup: 2 mg/5 mL; Tablets: 4 mg.

Granisetron Hydrochloride—see page 904.

Methysergide Maleate—pages 1055 and 1221.

Ondansetron Hydrochloride—see page 904.

Antihistamine Combinations

Typically, most antihistamine combinations include an antihistamine, a decongestant (eg, phenylephrine, phenylpropanolamine or pseudoephadrine), a cough suppressant (eg, dextromethorphan, codeine or hydrocodone) and an analgesic (eg, acetaminophen or aspirin). Because there are literally dozens of OTC and prescription antihistamine combinations available, it is recommended that the reader refer to a current *Facts and Comparisons Drug Information* or *Physicians' Desk Reference* (for both prescription and nonprescription drugs) for a listing of the available products, dosage and suppliers.

CHAPTER 74

Central Nervous System Stimulants

Patricia K Sonsalla, PhD
Assistant Professor of Neurology
University of Medicine and Dentistry of New Jersey
Robert Wood Johnson Medical School
Piscataway, NJ 08854

Central nervous system (CNS) stimulants are substances which increase excitability within various regions of the brain or spinal cord. The prominent effects produced by many of these drugs are arousal and increased motor function which result in subjective feelings of increased mental alertness, decreased fatigue, improved concentration, increased energy and motivation and an elevation in mood. Excessive excitation can lead to convulsions, and most, if not all, of these drugs produce seizures in a dose-dependent manner.

Excitability of the CNS reflects an intricate balance between excitatory and inhibitory activity within the brain. Stimulants of the CNS directly or indirectly enhance excitatory activity or block inhibitory components. The excitatory transmitters, glutamate and aspartate, are important neurotransmitters at excitatory synapses where their actions are mediated through *N*-methyl-D-aspartate (NMDA) or non-NMDA (kainate or AMPA/quisqualate) receptors. In contrast, gamma-aminobutyric acid (GABA) and glycine are prominent inhibitory neurotransmitters. The neuromodulator, adenosine, also plays an important role in CNS excitation in that it can exert a depressant action, most likely on the basis of its ability to decrease impulse-generated transmitter release and to limit excitation of postsynaptic elements by direct hyperpolarization. Many CNS stimulants produce excitation through their antagonism at GABA, glycine or adenosine receptors whereas others, the indirect-acting sympathomimetics, produce pronounced CNS stimulation by enhancing the actions of endogeneous catecholamines due to their ability to increase release and/or prevent the uptake of endogenous catecholamines (see Table 1).

The CNS stimulants are much less imporant therapeutically than the CNS depressants, but they can produce dramatic pharmacological effects and some frequently are abused. For example, CNS stimulants (eg, methylphenidate) are among the most commonly prescribed drugs for *attention deficit disorders* in children. The amphetamines or their analogs are used in narcolepsy, as adjunct therapy in *attention deficit disorders* and as *appetite suppressants* in *obesity*. The mild CNS stimulants, such as caffeine, are used in drug-induced *respiratory* and/or *circulatory depression* and *vascular headaches;* caffeine also is used in a number of analgesic combinations. The strong CNS stimulants, such as pentylenetetrazol and picrotoxin, have no established therapeutic use since the therapeutic dose is very close to the convulsant dose.

A number of CNS stimulants have therapeutically useful actions on other parts of the body, and a number of drugs not included in this chapter stimulate the CNS when administered in toxic doses. For example, caffeine, a classical central nervous system stimulant, has clinically useful actions on the heart, blood vessels and kidneys. On the other hand, atropine and ephedrine, drugs with primary actions on the peripheral autonomic nervous system, stimulate the CNS.

Only those drugs which have central stimulation as a predominant action are listed in this section. Those agents whose central stimulant properties are secondary (atropine, many sympathomimetic amines, nicotine, lobeline, carbon dioxide, cyanide, apomorphine and emetine) and those whose central stimulant properties are induced only with toxic doses (phenol, salicylates, local anesthetics, ergot alkaloids, etc) are listed in other chapters. For convenience, the drugs described are divided into three groups: xanthine derivatives, psychostimulants and miscellaneous CNS stimulants.

Xanthine Derivatives

Stimulation of the CNS can be produced in man and animals by a large number of natural and synthetic substances. None, however, occupy as prominent a place in the environment of man as do the xanthine derivatives. The most popular sources of these substances are the xanthine beverages, which include coffee, tea, cocoa and cola-flavored drinks. Coffee and tea contain caffeine, whereas cocoa contains theobromine. The caffeine content of tea leaves (2 to 3%) is higher than that of coffee beans (0.7 to 2.0%) but the beverages as finally prepared contain about equal amounts of this stimulant. Caffeine is present in amounts of about 100 to 150 mg/180 mL of brewed coffee; 60 to 80 mg/180 mL of instant coffee; 40 to 100 mg/180 mL of tea and 17 to 55 mg/180 mL of cola beverage. There is little doubt that the popularity of these beverages depends on their stimulant action, although most people are unaware of any stimulation.

Xanthine derivatives include caffeine, theobromine, theophylline and a number of related synthetic derivatives, all of which have similar pharmacological properties that differ markedly in the intensity of their actions in various structures. For example, the stimulant effects of caffeine and theophylline on the CNS and on skeletal muscle are much greater than those of theobromine. Furthermore, theophylline surpasses caffeine in its diuretic, cardiac and smooth muscular actions. Therefore, in the therapeutic application of these drugs for a specific effect, side effects can be minimized and the desired effect intensified by careful selection of the xanthine employed.

The principal therapeutic application of caffeine is as a CNS stimulant. Therefore, caffeine and its congeners which possess this effect will be discussed in this section. The principal therapeutic use of theophylline and related compounds is as a bronchodilator in the management of asthma. For this reason theophylline derivatives are discussed in Chapter 56, *Respiratory Drugs*.

Aminophylline—page 971.

Caffeine

1*H*-Purine-2,6-dione, 3.7-dihydro-1,3,7-trimethyl-, Theine: Nō Dōz (*Bristol-Myers*); Tirend (*Norcliff Thayer*); Vivarin (*Beecham*); Dexitac (*Republic*); Quick Pep (*Thompson*)

1,3,7-Trimethylxanthine [58-08-2] $C_8H_{10}N_4O_2$ (194.19); *monohydrate* [5743-12-4] (212.21).

For the structural formula, see page 404.

Preparation—Caffeine may be isolated from tea or coffee by boiling with water in the presence of lime or magnesium oxide, which serves to precipitate the tannins and some of the coloring matter. After filtration, the crude caffeine that separates is recrystallized from hot water after

Table 1—Various Classes of CNS Stimulants and Representative Compounds

Class	Compound	Mechanism
Xanthines	Caffeine	Adenosine antagonist
	Theophylline	Adenosine antagonist
Psychostimulants	Amphetamines	Enhance actions of endogenous catecholamines
	Methylphenidate	
	Cocaine	
	Mazindol	
	Pemoline	
	Diethylpropion	
Miscellaneous stimulants	Bicuculline	Competitive GABA antagonist
	Picrotoxin	Non-competitive GABA antagonist
	Pentylenetetrazol	Non-competitive GABA antagonist
	Strychnine	Competitive antagonist at non-NMDA glycine receptor
	Doxapram	Unknown

treatment with decolorizing charcoal. A source of the commercial supply is tea dust or sweepings. Increasing quantities of caffeine are now obtained as a by-product in the manufacture of "decaffeinized coffee." It is also produced by methylation of theobromine (partial synthesis) and by total synthesis from urea or dimethylurea by variations of Traube's classic process (*Ber 33:* 3052, 1900). The essential steps of a synthesis of theophylline and caffeine from urea are shown below:

NH_2–C(=O)–NH_2 (**Urea**) —CH_3NH_2→ CH_3NH–C(=O)–$NH CH_3$ (**1,3-Dimethylurea**) —$NCCH_2COOH$→ CH_3N–CO–CH_2–CN / C=O / CH_3NH —Alkali→ CH_3–N ... NH —HNO_2→ CH_3–N ... NO_2 ... NH —reduction→ CH_3–N ... NH_2, NH_2 —HCOOH→ CH_3–N ... NH_2, NHCHO —Alkali→ CH_3–N ... NH, =CH (**Theophylline**) —methylation→ Caffeine

Description—White powder or white, glistening needles, usually matted; odorless and has a bitter taste; pH (1% solution) 6.9; the hydrate is efflorescent in air and loses all its moisture at 80°; when rendered anhydrous by drying, melts between 235° and 237.5°; pK_a 13.9.

Solubility—1 g of anhydrous caffeine dissolves in about 50 mL water, 6 mL water at 80°, 75 mL alcohol, about 25 mL alcohol at 60°, about 6 mL chloroform or 600 mL ether. Being a weak base, caffeine does not form stable salts, and even its salts of strong acids, such as the hydrochloride or hydrobromide, are hydrolyzed readily by water. The solubility of caffeine in water is increased by the presence of organic acids or their alkali salts, eg, benzoates, salicylates, cinnamates or citrates and this is the reason for the use of several such preparations.

Uses—Used orally as a mild *CNS stimulant* to aid in staying awake and to restore mental alertness in fatigued patients. In combination with ergotamine tartrate it is used to abort *vascular headaches* such as migraine and cluster headaches. It often is used in combination with analgesics (acetaminophen, aspirin, etc) for the treatment of mild pain. Since its analgesic activity is suspect, such use is controversial. It is used in combination with anthihistamines and other sedative agents to overcome the sedative properties of such drugs; however, effective dosage for this purpose has not been established adequately. It is used parenterally in the form of caffeine and sodium benzoate for the treatment of *respiratory depression* associated with overdosage of CNS depressant drugs (narcotic analgesics, alcohol, etc). Because of the questionable benefit of such use and its transient action, most authorities believe caffeine and other analeptics should not be used in these conditions and recommend other supportive therapy. Finally, caffeine is used orally either alone or in combination with other drugs (analgesics, diuretics, etc) to relieve tension and fluid retention associated with menstruation. In view of its minimal diuretic action, its usefulness in this condition is questionable.

Caffeine and citrated caffeine are absorbed well following oral administration. Absorption by the oral route is more rapid than that after intramuscular injection. Absorption from suppositories following rectal administration is slow and erratic. Following the oral administration of 100 mg of caffeine (as in coffee), peak plasma levels of about 1.5 to 1.8 μg/mL are reached after 50 to 75 min. Following oral administration of 250 mg to "caffeine-naive" subjects, peak plasma levels of 4.2 to 26 μg/mL are reached in a mean time of 60 min. Therapeutic plasma concentrations range from 6 to 13 μg/mL; concentrations >20 μg/mL commonly produce adverse reactions. The lethal concentration is >100 μg/mL. It is distributed rapidly throughout all body tissues, readily crossing the placenta and blood-brain barrier. Approximately 17% of the drug is bound to plasma proteins. Plasma half-life is 3 to 4 hours in adults. Plasma half-life in neonates born of women given caffeine prior to delivery has been estimated to be about 80 hr. The drug is metabolized rapidly by the liver to 1-methyluric acid, 1-methylxanthine and 7-methylxanthine. About 10% is excreted unchanged by the kidneys.

For many years it was thought that the stimulant actions of caffeine were due to its inhibition of the enzyme phosphodiesterase in the brain and the resulting accumulation and actions of cyclic 3′,5′-adenosine monophosphate (c-AMP). However, several compounds which are more potent than caffeine in inhibiting phosphodiesterase activity lack CNS stimulant actions. Moreover, the concentration of caffeine needed to inhibit phosphodiesterase activity is 100 times greater than blood levels achieved after caffeine consumption. Rather, substantial evidence indicates that the stimulant actions of caffeine are due to its blockade of adenosine receptors. Adenosine exerts prominent presynaptic and postsynaptic inhibition of neuronal activity. Blockade of this inhibition by caffeine likely is responsible for its stimulant effects.

In one double-blind clinical study, oral administration of 250 mg of the drug to nine healthy young non-coffee drinkers who had no coffee, tea or cola in the previous 3 wk *increased plasma renin* activity 57%, plasma *norepinephrine* 75% and plasma *epinephrine* by 207%; urinary *normetanephrine* and *metanephrine* were *increased* 52 and 100%, respectively; mean *blood pressure increased* 14/10 torr within 1 hr; *heart rate* first *decreased* and then *increased;* and *respiratory rate increased* 20%.

Caffeine stimulates all levels of the CNS. In oral doses of 100 to 200 mg, it stimulates the cerebral cortex producing a more rapid and clear flow of thought, wakefulness or arousal in fatigued patients and improved psychomotor coordination. Its cortical effects are milder and of shorter duration than those of the amphetamines. In slightly larger doses, caffeine stimulates medullary vagal, vasomotor and respiratory centers, inducing bradycardia, vasoconstriction and an increased respiratory rate.

The drug exerts multiple effects on the heart. It has a positive inotropic effect on the myocardium and a positive chronotropic effect on the sinoatrial node, causing a transient increase in heart rate, force of contraction, cardiac output and work of the heart. In doses in excess of 250 mg, the centrally mediated vagal effects of caffeine may be masked by increased sinus rates; tachycardia, extrasystoles or other ventricular arrhythmias may result.

Caffeine, in normally ingested amounts, produces vasoconstriction of blood vessels, presumably by blocking adenosine receptors located in the smooth muscle of the vasculature. It is thought that the vasoconstriction of the cerebral blood vessels by caffeine contributes to its ability to relieve headaches. In the peripheral vasculature, caffeine ingestion results in increased vascular resistance and a slight increase in blood pressure, probably due to the action of caffeine on both the smooth muscle of the vessels and on catecholamine release.

Other pharmacological effects of caffeine include the following: it stimulates voluntary skeletal muscle, increasing the force of muscle contraction and decreasing muscular fatigue; it stimulates parietal cells, increasing gastric acid secretion; it induces a mild diuresis by increasing renal blood flow and glomerular filtration rate and decreasing proximal tubular reabsorption of sodium and water; and it stimulates glycogenolysis and lipolysis, but the increases in blood glucose and plasma lipids usually are not significant in normal patients. Repeated use of this substance may result in the development of tolerance to its diuretic, cardiovascular and central nervous system effects.

This drug and other xanthines may enhance the cardiac inotropic effects of beta-adrenergic stimulating agents and decrease the effect of benzodiazepines. Because caffeine ingestion results in reduced liver blood flow, the metabolism and elimination of drugs which are eliminated primarily by hepatic metabolism may be slowed. The ingestion of caffeine can cause a slight increase in urine levels of vanillylmandelic acid, catecholamines and 5-hydroxyindoleacetic acid. Since high urine levels of vanillylmandelic acid or catecholamines may result in a false-positive diagnosis of pheochromocytoma or neuroblastoma, caffeine intake should be avoided during these tests.

Acute toxicity involving caffeine has been reported only rarely. Overdosage usually is associated with gastrointestinal pain, mild delirium, insomnia, diuresis, dehydration and fever. More serious symptoms include cardiac arrhythmias and convulsions. The acute lethal dose of caffeine in adults appears to be about 5 to 10 g either intravenously or orally. Death has occurred in a child following oral ingestion of 3 g.

Prolonged, high intake may produce tolerance, habituation and psychological dependence. Abrupt discontinuation of the stimulant may result in headache, irritation, nervousness, anxiety and dizziness.

The ingestion of large amounts of combinations containing aspirin and caffeine has been associated with analgesic nephropathy, characterized by sterile pyuria, asymptomatic bacteruria, pyelonephritis, papillary necrosis, interstitial fibrosis and nephritis. The role of caffeine in the etiology of this condition has not been established conclusively. For an indepth review of "The Health Consequences of Caffeine" the interested reader is referred to the interesting article by Sawynok and Yaksh (*Pharmacol Rev 45:* 43, 1992).

Dose—100 to **500 mg;** *usual,* **200 mg** as necessary.

Dosage Forms—Extended-Release Capsules: 200 and 250 mg; Tablets: 100, 150 and 200 mg.

Citrated Caffeine

Caffeine citrate (1:1) [69-22-7]; a mixture of caffeine and citric acid containing 50% $C_8H_{10}N_4O_2$ (anhydrous caffeine) and 50% $C_6H_8O_7$ (anhydrous citric acid).

Preparation—The formula of USP IX was

Caffeine	50 g
Citric Acid	50 g
Distilled Water, hot	100 mL

Dissolve the citric acid in the hot distilled water, add the caffeine, and evaporate the resulting solution to dryness on a water bath, constantly stirring towards the end of the operation. Reduce the product to a fine powder and transfer it to well-closed containers. It is, however, usually prepared by mixing equal proportions of finely powdered anhydrous caffeine and anhydrous citric acid.

Description—White, odorless powder; slightly bitter, acid taste; acid reaction.

Solubility—1 g in about 4 mL warm water, the caffeine gradually precipitating on diluting the solution with an equal volume of water but redissolving on further dilution with sufficient water.

Incompatibilities—Neutralization of the citric acid by *alkalies* or *alkaline salts* will cause precipitation of caffeine if in sufficient concentration. The alkali salts of organic acids may release either caffeine or the free organic acid. In general it displays the incompatibilities of the citric acid which it contains.

Uses—See *Caffeine.*

Dose—100 to **500 mg;** *usual,* **300 mg** as necessary.

Dosage Forms—Tablets: 65 mg.

Caffeine and Sodium Benzoate Injection

A sterile solution of caffeine and sodium benzoate in water for injection; contains an amount of anhydrous caffeine ($C_8H_{10}N_4O_2$) equivalent to 45 to 52%, and an amount of sodium benzoate ($C_7H_5NaO_2$) equivalent to 47.5 to 55.5%, of the labeled amounts of caffeine and sodium benzoate.

Description—pH between 6.5 and 8.5.

Use—See *Caffeine,* page 1231.

Dose—*Parenteral,* **200 mg** to **1 g;** *usual,* **500 mg,** repeated as necessary.

Dosage Form—Injection: 250 mg (Caffeine Anhydrous 125 mg and Sodium Benzoate 125 mg) per mL.

Dyphylline—page 972.

Oxtriphylline—page 972.

Theophylline—page 973.

Theophylline Calcium Salicylate—see RPS-17, page 875.

Theophylline, Ephedrine Hydrochloride and Phenobarbital—page 973.

Theophylline Olamine—see RPS-18, page 868.

Theophylline Sodium Acetate—see RPS-17, page 875.

Theophylline Sodium Glycinate—see RPS-17, page 874.

Psychostimulants

Most of the compounds included under this heading are indirect-acting sympathomimetic drugs and are more potent central stimulants than the xanthine derivatives. These compounds (amphetamine and several of its analogs, cocaine, mazindol, methylphenidate; see Table 1) do not stimulate monoaminergic receptors directly, but rather increase the actions of endogenous catecholamines. This is due to their ability to inhibit the uptake of the catecholamine from the synaptic cleft after release or to cause catecholamine release. Because of their propensity to produce euphoria, many of these drugs are widely abused and are controlled substances. The approved use for most of these drugs is as anorectic agents, although several are used in the treatment of attention deficit disorders (methylphenidate, pemoline, amphetamine) or narcolepsy (amphetamine). Given the abuse liability and dependence potential of many of these compounds, the therapeutic use of these drugs should be monitored closely.

A number of drugs that stimulate the central nervous system are promoted for treatment of hyperactive behavior in children. A degree of hyperactivity which is not acceptable, either at home or at school, often is accompanied by difficulty in learning and sometimes by other neurological signs, such as "clumsiness." Although the usefulness of psychostimulant drugs in treatment of "hyperactivity" has been controversial, there is a patient group with severe, persistent hyperactivity and a short attention span that is likely to benefit from treatment with these agents. The psychostimulants most frequently used for this purpose include *methylphenidate* and *pemoline.*

Amphetamine and methamphetamine are two of the most potent sympathomimetic drugs with regard to CNS stimulation. They can improve psychomotor performance and enhance wakefulness, although it is questionable whether concentration in complex learning situations or judgement is improved. The effects of these amphetamines are thought to be mediated through cortical stimulation and possibly through stimulation of the reticular activating system. The (S), or (+), isomer of amphetamine is three to four times more potent than the (R), or (−), isomer in elicitation of CNS responses (only the *d* isomer of methamphetamine is available clinically). The alerting effect of the amphetamines, their anorectic effect and some component of their locomotor-stimulating action are likely mediated by norepinephrine release. Some aspects of locomotor activity, as well as euphoria, are due to dopamine release within the basal ganglia and the limbic system.

That the CNS stimulating effects of these compounds are mediated through the catecholamines is suggested by findings in animal studies that inhibition of catecholamine synthesis prevents the behavioral activation produced by the drugs. In humans, acute toxicity produces restlessness, dizziness, tremor, hyperactive reflexes, talkativeness, irritability, weakness, insomnia and fever. Larger doses can produce confusion, increased libido, anxiety, panic states, hallucinations and psychotic behavior. Some of these effects may be due to the release of 5-hydroxytryptamine (5-HT) from serotonergic neurons. In addition, there may be pronounced cardiovascular and gastrointestinal effects. Excessive toxicity results in convulsions, coma and cerebral hemorrhages. See Chapter 57 for more discussion on the amphetamines.

Cocaine is also a potent sympathomimetic CNS stimulant with actions very similar to those of the amphetamines but with a much shorter duration of action. Cocaine has local anesthetic actions; however, its use for this purpose is limited, having been replaced by synthetic local anesthetics which have little CNS stimulation. The importance of cocaine lies in its abuse potential; it is currently one of the most widely abused drugs in the US. See also Chapters 47 and 68.

Amphetamine Sulfate—page 986.
Benzphetamine Hydrochloride—page 987.
Cocaine—page 1151.
Deanol Acetaminobenzoate—see RPS-18, page 1136.
Dextroamphetamine Phosphate—see RPS-16, page 820.
Dextroamphetamine Sulfate—page 987.
Diethylpropion—page 987.
Mazindol—page 992.
Methamphetamine—page 994.

Methylphenidate Hydrochloride

2-Piperidineacetic acid, (R^*, R^*)-(±)-α-phenyl-, methyl ester, hydrochloride, Ritalin (*Ciba*)

[298-59-9] $C_{14}H_{19}NO_2$,HCl (269.77).

Preparation—2-Chloropyridine is condensed with phenylacetonitrile and the resulting α-phenyl-2-pyridineacetonitrile is hydrated to its corresponding amide. The pyridine ring then is hydrogenated catalytically and the amide converted to its corresponding carboxylic acid. Esterification with methanol, with the aid of HCl, yields the final product.

Description—White, odorless, fine, crystalline powder; melts about 75°; solutions are acid to litmus, pK_a 8.9.

Solubility—Freely soluble in water or methanol; soluble in alcohol; slightly soluble in chloroform or acetone.

Uses—A mild *CNS stimulant* with a potency intermediate to caffeine and amphetamine. Its pharmacological properties are essentially the same as those of the amphetamines. It also shares the abuse potential of the amphetamines. It is *effective* as adjunctive therapy to other remedial measures (psychological, educational and social) in the management of *attention deficit disorders*. Double blind studies with placebo control demonstrate that methylphenidate can improve behavior, concentration and learning ability in 70 to 80% of children with this disorder. Drug treatment is not indicated for all children with this disorder; stimulants are not intended in the child who exhibits symptoms secondary to environmental factors or primary psychiatric disorders. Consequently, these should be ruled out and available psychological, educational and social resources should be used before drug therapy is instituted. It also is *effective* in *narcolepsy* and *possibly effective* in *mild depression*, as well as *apathetic* or *withdrawn senile behavior*.

It appears to be absorbed well from the gastrointestinal tract. Peak blood levels are reached in 1 to 3 hr and the plasma half-life ranges from 1 to 3 hr. The pharmacological effects persist from 4 to 6 hr. Approximately 80% of an oral dose is metabolized to ritalinic acid and excreted in the urine. The mechanism of action has not been determined. It is thought to act on the cerebral cortex and subcortical structures, including the thalamus; stimulation by this drug causes an increase in motor activity, mental alertness, diminished sense of fatigue, brighter spirits and mild euphoria. It also produces an anorexigenic effect.

The drug is contraindicated in patients with anxiety, tension and agitation or those known to be sensitive to the drug. The safe use in children under 6 yr of age has not been established. It also is contraindicated in patients with a prior history of epilepsy or those with EEG abnormalities in absence of seizures and in patients with glaucoma, motor tics or with a family history or diagnosis of *Tourette's syndrome*. It may decrease the hypotensive effect of guanethidine. It should be used with caution in patients on pressor agents or MAO inhibitors. Human pharmacological studies indicate the drug may inhibit metabolism of coumarin anticoagulants, anticonvulsants and tricyclic antidepressants. Dosage of these agents may require downward adjustment when given concomitantly with this drug.

Adverse reactions include nervousness, insomnia, hypersensitivity reactions (including various skin manifestations), anorexia, nausea, dizziness, palpitations, headache, dyskinesia, blood pressure and pulse changes, tachycardia, angina, cardiac arrhythmias, abdominal pain and weight loss. Toxic psychoses, leukopenia, anemia and a few cases of scalp hair loss have been reported. Tolerance, psychic dependence and abnormal behavior have been reported in patients who have abused this drug. Consequently, it should be administered cautiously, if at all, in emotionally unstable patients, those with a history of drug dependency and those known to alter drug dosage on their own initiative.

Dose—*Oral*, **10** to **60 mg** a day; *usual*, **10 mg** 2 or 3 times a day. Sustained-release tablets have an 8-hr duration of action; these may be used when the dose of slow-release (SR) tablets correspond to the 8-hr dose of the drug. Symptoms of overdose may include vomiting, agitation, tremors, hyperreflexia, muscle twitching, convulsions (may be followed by coma), euphoria, confusion, hallucinations, delirium, sweating, hyperpyrexia, tachycardia, palpitations, cardiac arrhythmias, hypertension, mydriasis and dryness of the mucous membranes.

Dosage Forms—Tablets: 5, 10 and 20 mg. Sustained-Release Tablets: 20 mg.

Pemoline

4(5*H*)-Oxazolone, 2-amino-5-phenyl-, Cylert (*Abbott*)

[2152-34-3] $C_9H_8N_2O_2$ (176.17).

Preparation—Ethyl mandelate $C_6H_5CH(OH)COOC_2H_5$, is reacted with guanidine, $HN{=}C(NH_2)_2$, in boiling alcohol solution, US Pat 2,892,753.

Description—White, crystalline powder; odorless and tasteless; melts at about 256° with decomposition.

Solubility—Practically insoluble in water, chloroform, dilute HCl or ether; slightly soluble in alcohol or propylene glycol.

Uses—A *CNS stimulant* which is structurally dissimilar to the amphetamines and methylphenidate. Although laboratory studies indicate that pemoline may act through dopaminergic mechanisms, the mechanism and site of action in man are not known. Indicated as adjunctive therapy in children with *attention deficit disorder*. It also has been used in the treatment of fatigue, mental depression, chronic schizophrenia and as a mild stimulant in geriatric patients; however, clinical benefits from such use are minimal. It should *not* be used for the prevention or treatment of normal fatigue. Peak serum levels of the drug are reached 2 to 4 hr after ingestion of a single oral dose; the serum half-life is approximately 12 hr, and a steady state level is reached in 2 to 3 days of multiple dosage. About 50% of the drug is bound to serum proteins. Approximately 75% of an oral dose is excreted in the urine within 24 hr, about 43% unchanged and 22% as pemoline conjugates.

Insomnia, usually transient, is the principal adverse effect. Anorexia with weight loss may occur during early weeks of therapy; weight gain usually resumes within 3 to 6 mo. Stomachache, skin rashes, increased irritability, mild depression, nausea, dizziness, headache, drowsiness and hallucinations have been reported. Other adverse effects reported include seizures; dyskinetic movements of the tongue, lips, face and extremities; abnormal aculogyric function (nystagmus and oculogyric crises) and symptoms of *Tourette's syndrome*.

It is contraindicated in patients with hypersensitivity or idiosyncrasy to the drug. It is not recommended for children less than 6 yr of age since safety and efficacy in this age group have not been established. Sufficient data on safety and efficacy of long-term use in children are not yet available. Safety for use during pregnancy and lactation has not been established.

Dose—*Oral, initial*, **37.5 mg** given as a single dose each morning; may be increased by **18.75 mg** a day at weekly intervals until the desired clinical response is obtained. The effective dose for most patients is **56.25** to **75 mg** a day; the maximum recommended dose is **112.5 mg** a day. Significant benefit from the drug may not be evident until the 3rd or 4th wk of treatment.

Dosage Forms—Tablets: 18.75, 37.5 and 75 mg. Chewable Tablets: 37.5 mg.

Phendimetrazine Tartrate—page 995.
Phenmetrazine Hydrochloride—page 996.
Phentermine—page 996.

Miscellaneous Central Nervous System Stimulants

Included in this category are strychnine and compounds which formerly were referred to as analeptic drugs. The analeptics are substances which stimulate various regions of the brain. Excessive doses may cause the stimulation to spread to motor areas and precipitate convulsions. Analeptics formerly were used in an attempt to counteract severe intoxication by general depressants. However, none of the compounds is a safe and selective respiratory stimulant, although doxapram is still available for use in certain circumstances. Moreover, depressant drug intoxications can be managed effectively with more conservative measures that stress intensive supportive care. Hence, the airway is kept clear by suction or by endotracheal tube, the patient is turned regularly and oxygen is administered as needed. Shock is overcome by the use of blood or plasma expanders and vasopressors. Where available, dialysis is used to remove the drug.

Although most of the formerly classified analeptics are not used therapeutically nor are available clinically, several have become important research tools for evaluating the efficacy and mechanism of action of various drugs, particularly of anticonvulsants, because the mechanism by which these convulsants exert their actions is well characterized. It is known that strychnine is a glycine antagonist with actions primarily in the spinal cord, whereas bicuculline, picrotoxin and pentylenetetrazol are GABA antagonists which act within various regions of the brain. Strychnine is used as a pesticide for destroying rodents and other predatory animals and thus is encountered frequently as a cause of poisoning in man.

Doxapram Hydrochloride—page 979.

Nikethamide—see RPS18, page 1134.

Pentylenetetrazol—see RPS-18, page 1134.

Picrotoxin—see RPS-18, page 1135.

Pipradrol Hydrochloride—see RPS-15, page 1034.

Racephedrine Hydrochloride—see RPS-17, page 893.

Strychnine—see RPS-18, page 1136.

Theobromine—see RPS-18, page 941.

Theobromine Salts—see RPS-15, page 1070.

CHAPTER 75

Antineoplastic and Immunoactive Drugs

Louis R Barrows
Professor of Pharmacology and Toxicology
College of Pharmacy, University of Utah
Salt Lake City, UT 84132

Formerly, nearly all the drugs used to intervene in the immune system were antineoplastic drugs. Indeed, the leukemias and lymphomas, which were the first major neoplastic diseases to be treated successfully with chemotherapeutic agents, may be thought of as disorders of the immune system. Until recently and except for the use of gold, progress in the suppression of autoimmune disorders was achieved mainly with antineoplastic drugs or congeners. Therefore, in previous editions of this textbook, immunosuppressive drugs were described in the chapter on antineoplastics. For want of a better place, the sole immunostimulatory drug, levamisol, was included. With this edition, there is a greatly enlarged armamentarium of immunoactive drugs owing to dramatic developments in immunology. Nevertheless, the present focus with most of these new agents pertains to their usefulness in cancer chemotherapeutic regimens or organ transplantation. Consequently, it is still appropriate to treat antineoplastic and immunoactive drugs together, even though some agents may seem out of place.

Antineoplastic Drugs

Prior to the 1940s the principal nonsurgical treatment of neoplasms was X-ray and radium therapy, although certain arsenicals and urethane were also in use. During the 1940s there were three main developments: radioisotopes, nitrogen mustards and antifolic acid agents. The use of sex hormones for the treatment of certain types of neoplasms and of adrenal corticoids and ACTH for the treatment of leukemia also developed considerably during these years.

Much excitement was generated by these early developments in antineoplastic therapy, but it was tempered later by the realization that not only were the drugs not curative but also that, for the most part, life-expectancy was negligibly increased, the drugs being mainly palliative. Subsequently, there has been a great proliferation in both the number and classes of anticancer drugs and in the theory of cell kinetics and cell-population statistics, so that with the consequently improved armamentarium and regimens, long-term disease-free remissions are achievable with several neoplasms, and even a few carcinomata can be cured.

Tumor Growth and Kinetics

The principal difference between mature normal tissues and tumors is not in the rate of cell replication but that in most normal tissues the rate of proliferation equals the rate of cell death, whereas in neoplasms proliferation exceeds the death rate. Proliferation in normal tissue responds to subtle signals that indicate when proliferation is needed for repair, regeneration or growth and development. Neoplasms seem to lack such an autoregulation of proliferation, and the rate of cell-replication appears to depend mostly on an intrinsic rate modulated by the adequacy of the vascular supply.

Exponential Growth and Doubling Times—In the early stages, the growth of a tumor is approximately constant. The doubling time is the mean ("average") interval between successive mitoses. It is characteristic of the particular type of tumor cell. Doubling time varies markedly among various kinds of tumors. In Burkitt's tumor, it is approximately 24 hours; in acute leukemia, 2 weeks; in breast cancer, 3 months; and in multiple myeloma, 6 to 12 months. Contrary to common belief, these doubling times are within the range of those for normal tissues. For example, white-cell precursors divide approximately every 12 hours and mucosal cells of the rectum every 24 hours.

A tumor becomes detectable when the number of cells reaches about 10^9 to 10^{10} cells. This requires 30 to 33 doubling times. The neoplasm becomes lethal when the population reaches about 5×10^{11} to 5×10^{12} cells, after 39 to 42 doubling times.

Phases of the Cell Cycle—Some drugs can exert a lethal action only when a cell is in a particular stage of activity and growth. Therefore, a resumé of cell kinetics will be useful. After mitosis and cell division, the new daughter cells are in a resting state, terms phase G_0 (G for gap). The length of time spent in G_0 depends on both the type of cell and the autoregulatory factors. In some tissues, such as bone marrow, gastrointestinal mucosae and skin, G_0 is prolonged only moderately during maturation and aging, whereas with others, such as nerve and skeletal muscle cells, G_0 becomes essentially infinitely long well in advance of maturity.

In solid tumors, G_0 is longer when the cell mass is large than when small, because the vascular supply cannot keep pace with the rate of growth. Ultimately, the cell enters a postresting phase, called G_1. In this phase, metabolism appears to be normal, but the cell is committed to divide. After a latency, the cell enters the S-phase, in which DNA synthesis is activated, in preparation for mitosis. The cell then enters another phase, G_2, the premitotic phase, in which DNA synthesis is essentially at rest but protein synthesis and other metabolic activities are increased and the cell volume grows. Finally, the cell undergoes mitosis (phase M) and cellular fission.

The cell cycle can be thought of as existing in two super-stages: G_0 as one, and all of $G_1 + S + G_2 + M$ as the other, the latter comprising all phases committed to cellular division. The entity $(G_1 + S + G_2 + M)/(G_0 + G_1 + S + G_2 + M)$ is known as the *growth fraction*. In tumors, it usually lies between 0.2 to 0.7. The growth fraction tends to be greater in the more rapidly proliferating tissues and tumors, but not always.

Chemotherapeutic Intervention

Phase Specificity—Antineoplastic drugs are of two general categories: (1) those that can act upon the cell throughout its cycle; such drugs are said to be *phase-non-specific* and (2) those that act preferentially during one or more of the nonresting phases; these drugs tend to be ineffective if delivered to the cell during the wrong phase. Even phase-nonspecific drugs have greater activity during the growth phases. The particular phase during which a drug acts depends on the lethal mechanism. Those that combine irreversibly with DNA can do so at any time and hence are phase-nonspecific. However, more DNA is exposed during the growth phases than during G_0, so that even these drugs have some phase selectivity. Drugs that interfere with DNA synthesis will be specific to the S-phase, those that block protein synthesis mainly to phases S and G_2, and those that inhibit microtubule assembly mainly to M.

Tumor Selectivity and Response—Especially for phase-specific drugs, the probability of a lethal action on a tumor cell (or normal cell) is directly proportional to the percent of time spent in the vulnerable phase. It follows that the percent of time spent in the vulnerable phase will be an important determinant of the susceptibility of tumors of different cell types. Even without reference to any particular growth phase, the generality that *those tumors with a large growth fraction are more susceptible to chemotherapy than those with a low fraction* is an important precept. Examples of tumors with high growth fractions that respond well to chemotherapy are acute leukemia in children, Burkitt's lymphoma, choriocarcinoma, chronic myelogenous leukemia (these last three now are considered to be curable), lymphocytic leukemia, Hodgkin's disease, Wilms' tumor and breast cancer. Examples of neoplasms that respond poorly are malignant melanoma, carcinoma of the gastrointestinal tract, bronchogenic carcinoma and tumors of the uterus and cervix.

Since growth fractions are higher in small, recent tumors, it follows that efficacy is enhanced by early treatment.

Different cell types spend different proportions of time in one as opposed to another phase (ie, more in G_2 than S, etc). Therefore, the most effective drug would be expected to be of a type that is specific to the phase of longest duration. In part, this may account for the differences in efficacy among drugs of different mechanisms and phase specificity.

There has been interest in and investigation of the possibility of *synchronizing* tumor cells so that all cells are in the same phase of the cycle. If the cells were synchronized and the host cells were not, then the tumor could be made more vulnerable to appropriate drugs given at the proper time and the therapeutic index could be increased. Synchronization is attempted by a holding "pulse" of a mitostatic or some other drug that holds the cells in a given phase until the out-of-phase cells also come into that phase. Discontinuation of the synchronizing drug simultaneously releases the cells to resume their cycle, all starting from the same phase. In combination chemotherapy, drugs often are administered in sequence, rather than simultaneously; the first-given drug sometimes serves as a synchronizing drug.

Determinants of Sensitivity and Selectivity—In addition to the growth fraction or vulnerable phase time of a tumor, other factors also determine the selectivity of drugs for certain cell types. The demand for nutrients varies among tumor types but also differs between tumor cells and normal cells. For example, many tumors require more asparagine than normal cells, so that if the plasma asparagine is destroyed enzymatically (see *Asparaginase*, page 1242), the tumor cells are selectively "starved" to death.

Some drugs are metabolized in the peripheral cells as well as in the liver, and the different cell types differ in their ability to metabolize these drugs. For example, with bleomycin there is evidence to suggest that the drug is metabolized less in susceptible tumor cells than in other cells, thus permitting higher local concentrations. Several drugs are converted to active metabolites by the target cells ("lethal synthesis"), and differences in the rates of conversion may contribute to selectivity.

Differences in penetrance account for some differences among drugs; lipid-soluble antineoplastic drugs are more effective than water-soluble ones for neoplasms in the central nervous system. With some drugs, active transport into tumor cells is greater than into normal cells; with other drugs, there are differences in outward transport. An unassessed factor in selectivity is that of effects on the immune system. There are not only tumor-cell-attacking "killer" T cells but also suppressor T cells and blocking factors from B cells which protect certain neoplastic cells from immune attack. According to which immune cells are the most suppressed, some antineoplastic drugs might antagonize the immune response to neoplastic cells and other drugs augment it.

Requirements for "Kill"—A remission usually can be achieved with a kill of 90 to 99% of the neoplastic cells. A kill of 99% would leave at least 10^7 to 10^8 surviving cells to carry on tumor growth, and the remission would last only 3 to 4 doubling times. With those neoplasms against which the immune system is ineffective, a 100% kill is necessary to effect a true cure, since it has been shown experimentally that a single implanted neoplastic cell can develop into a tumor. However, a true cure may not always be necessary. For example, with a tumor the doubling time of which is 12 months, a kill of 99.99% (which would leave perhaps 10^6 surviving cells) would require about 13 years for the tumor cell population to recover to the number extant at the time of treatment.

A second course of an appropriate chemotherapy might add another 13 years which, with middle-aged or elderly patients, might be beyond the normal life-expectancy. However, with a rapidly doubling tumor like Burkitt's tumor, the survival time in the untreated patient is measured in days, not years; even if all but a single cell were killed by an antineoplastic drug, survival would be prolonged less than two months; therefore, either a complete kill or sustained or frequently repeated courses are imperative. Fortunately, 50 to 60% of Burkitt's tumor cells are in the S-phase and are thus highly susceptible to drugs that are S-phase-specific.

Combination Chemotherapy—One way of increasing the percent of kill is to combine two or more antineoplastic drugs. Radiation also is a modality that often can be combined effectively with drugs. There are four criteria to optimize such combinations:

1. Each component drug must have some efficacy by itself.
2. Each component drug should have a different mechanism of cytotoxic activity and, preferably, phase-specificity.
3. Each component drug should have a different spectrum of toxicity than the other components, in order to avoid overwhelming toxicity of a given type.
4. The mechanism of resistance to each component should be different to that of the other components.

Log Cell-Kill Principle—Antineoplastic drugs may be characterized by their *log cell-kill index*, that is, by the negative log of the fraction of the tumor cell population that survives a single course of treatment. Thus a drug that kills 99.9% of the tumor cell population, ie, leaves 0.0001 (or $1/10^4$) of the population, is known as a 4-log drug; a second drug that kills 99.9% is known as a 3-log drug. The log cell-kill index is a tenuous number, but it serves a usefulness in predicting the effects of combinations that meet criteria 1 and 2. The predicted effect of a combination is obtained by adding the indices of the component drugs. Theoretically, a 4-log drug plus a 3-log drug should provide a 7-log combination, that is, kill 99.99999% or leave $1/10^7$ of the population. A third drug that kills 99% (2-log drug) would further reduce the remaining population to $1/10^9$, which comes close to complete eradication of a tumor caught early.

Drug Resistance—Some tumor populations appear to be heterogeneous by the time the tumor is discovered, some of the cells being resistant to certain drugs at the outset of treatment. This is well established for adrenal, colon, jejunal, kidney and liver carcinomas. As many as four different cancer cell types have been identified in a single tumor. Differences among some of these cell types do not represent different genes necessarily but rather, sometimes, differences in the number of copies of a single gene. Some resistance seems to be acquired in much the same way as microbial resistance, a resistance-conferring genetic change occurring during treatment; the resistant daughter cells then can proliferate in the environment of the drug. Whatever the cause, resistance often terminates the usefulness of an antineoplastic drug.

Nine mechanisms of resistance have been identified:

1. Loss of a transport system essential for the permeation of the drug into the tumor cell, as happens with methotrexate.

2. Disappearance of the enzyme necessary for the intratumor "lethal synthesis" of an essential active metabolite.
3. An increase in the production of the target enzyme, as sometimes happens with methotrexate.
4. A decrease in the affinity for or amount of the target enzyme, as sometimes happens with methotrexate and fluorouracil or topoisomerase inhibitors.
5. An increase in outward active transport of the drug, so that effective intracellular concentrations cannot be achieved or maintained (so-called pleiotropic drug-resistance functions by this mechanism).
6. Overexpression of metallothionine in resistance to platinum-containing and certain alkylating antineoplastics.
7. Antibody formation (eg, interferons).
8. Membrane changes that confer resistance to natural killer cells.
9. Increase glutathione synthesis in cancer cells treated with anthracyclinedione cells.

Lipophilic anticancer drugs such as the vinca alkaloids, certain alkylaminoanthraquinones actinomycin-D, colchicine, verapamil and probably other drugs are transported outwardly by an ATP-dependent pump, known as *P*-glycoprotein. This is produced excessively by some tumor cells, which accounts for multiple drug resistance. Verapamil competes for this pump; it is this property, and not its calcium channel blocking activity, that accounts for the ability of verapamil to restore the sensitivity of some tumors to formerly efficacious drugs. Other mechanisms are easy to conceive and undoubtedly will be observed.

Toxicity—Neoplastic cells have compositions and activities very much like those of the host cells. This has made it impossible thus far to design antineoplastic drugs which also will not attack normal cells. Every antineoplastic drug has a therapeutic index less than 1.0. The principles which apply to antitumor efficacy also apply to the toxicity. Thus the tissues most affected are those with high growth fractions, and the integrity of the highly proliferative tissues can be disturbed considerably. Consequently, the bone marrow, lymphoblasts, mucous membranes, skin and gonads are affected to a greater extent than other cells. Since the myelogenous leukocyte turnover is faster and the growth fraction is greater than those of erythrocytes, *bone-marrow depression* usually causes a more severe neutropenia and thrombocytopenia than anemia. Bone-marrow depression is a major adverse effect of antineoplastic drugs reviewed.

Suppression of proliferation of mucosal cells causes *mucositis,* characterized by aphthous and gastrointestinal ulceration. Fifteen of the 36 drugs reviewed prominently cause mucositis. Arrest of the proliferation of the cutaneous epithelial cells may cause *alopecia* (18 of 36 drugs), scaliness of the skin and sometimes even desquamation. Some drugs which lack significant dermatological actions may nevertheless recall cutaneous toxicities induced by previous drugs or radiation.

Aspermia may result from actions on the seminiferous tubules and amenorrhea from actions on the ovaries (where the growth fraction but not the turnover rate is high). The immune cells have a rapid turnover and are highly susceptible to certain cytotoxic agents. *Immunosuppression* makes the patient more vulnerable to *infection;* it is noteworthy that 50% of cancer patients die of intercurrent infections rather than from the terminal phases of the neoplastic disease.

Immunosuppression probably enhances the growth of certain neoplasms. Since they interfere with genetic mechanisms, certain antineoplastic drugs are mutagenic and carcinogenic, and the patient is subjected to the risk of future neoplasia. The incidences of acute leukemia and bone sarcoma are considerably higher in persons who have been treated with antineoplastic drugs than in the general population. Theoretical considerations predict that all neoplastic drugs are teratogenic, and teratogenic activity has been shown with some.

There are also other toxicities related to antineoplastic actions. For example, massive cell destruction results in the release of large quantities of purine bases from the nucleic acids of the dead cells, which purine bases are metabolized to uric acid. Hyperuricemia, renal damage consequent to hyperuricuria and also some neurological damage may result. Hence, it is common to give allopurinol along with antineoplastic drugs. Massive destruction of certain leukemic cells also may cause an acute hypotensive crisis which sometimes is called "anaphylaxis," although it is not a true allergic response. For reasons not understood, treatment of breast cancer is thrombogenic in about 7% cases, irrespective of the drug used.

Some of the local adverse effects also are related to the antineoplastic mechanisms. Extravasation, or accidental contamination of the skin or lungs, may present very high concentrations to the cells in the local area, such that the cells will be killed by the cytotoxic actions, leading to vesication, ulceration, sloughing, bronchitis, etc. With the nitrogen mustards, the drugs need not interact with DNA to be caustic, since the nitrogen mustards readily alkylate crystal chemical groups in the cell membranes and in the cytoplasm. Local toxicity in the gastrointestinal tract prevents certain antineoplastic drugs from being administered orally. Local gastrointestinal toxicity may cause nausea, vomiting, diarrhea, cramping, etc, but these are also acute side-effects of many antineoplastic drugs administered intravenously, and it is not always clear whether they relate to the antineoplastic actions.

With good nutrition, toxicity is less severe. Total parenteral nutrition is advised when nutrition is otherwise difficult to manage.

Precautions and Contraindications—With all drugs that cause bone-marrow depression, it is essential to monitor the blood cell count, which may serve both as a guide to adequate dosage and as a precaution against overdoses. The minimum advisable leukocyte and platelet count varies somewhat among the drugs but is usually 3000 to 4000 leukocytes and 20,000 to 100,000 platelets. When the count falls below these limits, the drug dosage should be reduced or the drug discontinued until there is recovery. It usually is not advisable to begin treatment with a bone-marrow depressant drug within 4 weeks of the administration of another bone-marrow depressant drug or radiation therapy. When two bone-marrow depressant drugs are used in combination, it is necessary to reduce the dose and to monitor more frequently.

Other toxicities with notable exceptions, usually are not as life-threatening as bone-marrow depression, but analogous precautions should be observed, even though monitoring cannot be as quantitative as cell counts. However, aphthous ulcers can be visualized and monitored. With patients in poor condition, it is imperative to proceed cautiously and to monitor more closely than with patients in good condition. Not only may elderly patients be more susceptible to the adverse actions of antineoplastic drugs but toxicity will be more incapacitating and life-threating, so that therapy should be undertaken most cautiously. Antineoplastic drugs should not be used during pregnancy unless alternatives are exhausted. There is even evidence that anticancer drugs are fetotoxic in pregnant nurses that handle such drugs. Since most antineoplastic drugs can be found in breast milk, infants must not be nursed during antineoplastic therapy.

Classes and Mechanisms of Drugs—Antineoplastic drugs may be grouped into seven categories. Some of the categories are based on chemical and mechanistic properties and others on the origins of natural products.

Alkylating Agents—There are five subgroups of the alkylating agents: nitrogen mustards, nitrosoureas, methylhydrazines, ethylenimines and alkylsulfonates. The nitrogen mustards are all bis(β-chloroethyl)amines. The mustards are important drugs in treatment regimens; cyclophosphamide, the most useful alkylating agent, is a member of this class. The ethylenimines contain three ethylenimine groups per molecule, and the alkylsulfonates are bismethylsulfonates. Thus these compounds are all polyfunctional alkylating agents, a fact that relates importantly to the mechanism of action. The alkylating groups react with nucleophilic centers in many different kinds of molecules; guanine in DNA is the most reactive target. However, their bi- or tri-functional character allows them to cross-link double-stranded DNA, thus preventing the strands from separating for replication.

Nitrosoureas—These usually are classified as alkylating agents. Carmustine is bifunctional and may be able to cross-link double-stranded DNA. Lomustine and semustine each contain a single β-chloroethyl group, but can cross-link DNA by using the nitroso group as a second electrophilic group. Streptozocin lacks an alkylating moiety. Carbamoylation of the nucleoside bases in nucleic acids has been suggested as a possible mechanism of action. However, the nitroso group is also a free radical and ion generator, which could confer radiomimetic properties.

Methylhydrazines—Procarbazine and dacarbazine sometimes are classified as alkylating agents, because an "alkylating" moiety supposedly is liberated within the target cell. However, like other hydrazines, they generate free hydroxyl radicals and ions and thus also are considered to be radiomimetic.

Antimetabolites—There are three subcategories of antimetabolites: purine analogs, pyrimidine analogs and folinic acid analogues. The purine analogues are incorporated into DNA as the deoxyribotides and into RNA as the ribotides, where they interfere with coding and replication. They also act like the natural purine bases in inhibiting synthesis of purine bases by acting through the allosteric feedback systems (pseudo-feedback). The pyrimidine analogues inhibit enzymes in the biosynthetic pathways for pyrimidine ribotides and deoxyribotides; thymidylate synthetase, orotic acid decarboxylase, aspartate carbamoyltransferase and dihydroorotase are inhibited. Methotrexate and trimetrexate are the only folinic acid analogues in use; they bind very tightly to dihydrofolate reductase and thereby prevent the conversion of dihydrofolate (folinate) to tetrahydrofolate.

Antibiotics—This is a miscellaneous group of drugs with respect to mechanism of action. Mitomycin appears to be an alkylating agent, the anthracyclines and epipodophyllotoxins act therapeutically by inhibiting topoisomerase II and the *Vinca* alkaloids and taxol interfere with microspindle function. Dactinomycin binds to DNA and inhibit DNA synthesis, and mithramycin inhibits DNA-dependent RNA polymerase. Bleomycin acts both as an antimetabolite of thymidine and causes fragmentation of DNA.

Steroid Hormones—The steroid hormones are transported to the cell nucleus, where they attach to chromatin and usually stimualte transcription and, hence, protein synthesis. However, the glucocortoids suppress mitosis in lymphocytes and fibroblasts and appear to inhibit transcription. This so-called lympholytic effect is employed in the chemotherapy of the lymphocytic leukemias and in immunosuppression.

The estrogens, progestins and androgens probably also inhibit transcription and prevent mitosis in those cell types which are derived from normal cells that are suppressed by these hormones in the natural hormonal physiology. Thus, the normal prostate gland is suppressed by estrogens, apparently by a comparative antagonism of androgens, and estrogens are used to treat cancer of the prostate gland, etc. Similarly, androgens exert an antiestrogen effect on certain breast tumors; only tumors of a cell type that contain estrogen receptors are responsive. Antiestrogens also are used to suppress such tumors. Estrogens also suppress the growth of some breast tumors, but the mechanism of the effect is understood poorly. Progestins behave as antiestrogens in the endometrium and, hence, may be employed in the chemotherapy of endometrial carcinoma.

Tetrahydrodesoxycorticosterone suppresses tumor angiogensis without exerting glucocorticoid or mineralocorticoid activity.

The hormones are described in Chapter 64. Drugs that induce local inflammation and fibrosis may suppress effusions secondary to various neoplasms. Thus, quinacrine may be given into the pleural and peritoneal cavities to control such effusions. Since the neoplastic process is unaffected, quinacrine is not truly antineoplastic.

Cytokines and Growth Factors—Cytokines formerly were called lymphokines, but the finding that some not only are elaborated by, but also act upon, nonlymphoid cells brought about the change in name. Research on these factors is extremely active and productive, and a number of exciting discoveries have been made. Most of the current cytokines act as modulators of the immune system such that killer and natural killer cells are stimulated to increased activity against cancer cells. However, recent research indicates that some cytokines may act upon cancer cells directly to cause differentiation or even cell death. Others may act upon endothelial cells to alter invasiveness. Colony-stimulating growth factors are becoming an important part of dose-intensified regimens, by allowing reimplantation of extracorporeally amplified bone marrow, or the stimulation of severely suppressed bone marrow *in situ*. Erythropoetin, likewise, can counteract some myelosuppressive effects. Interleukins and interleukin-activated lymphocytes, interferons, macrophage-stimulating factor, granulocyte colony-stimulating factors pentostatin, thymopentin, transfer factor, transforming growth factor-beta$_2$ and tumor necrosis factor either are available or are in therapeutic trials.

Antitumor Antibodies—There are presently a number of antitumor antibodies that have been produced for clinical trials. Success has been erratic thus far. Upon FDA approval, one manufacturer is prepared to custom-produce antibodies.

Kinetics and Regimens—With drugs with phase-specific actions, the temporal window of vulnerability is the duration of the vulnerable phase of the cell cycle. With rapidly proliferating cells, this may be only a few hours for any given cell. If the cell cycles are synchronized, only a brief exposure to the drug may be required to accomplish a high degree of cell kill; the optimal drug would be one with a half-life such that it does not persist in the body beyond the time necessary to act upon the tumor cells, so that there would be the least necessary exposure of normal cells to the drug. However, the synchronization of cell cycles is yet in its infancy, and most regimens attack a tumor cell population that randomly is in various phases of the cell cycle. In this case, it is optimal to keep the drug in the body for slightly longer than the duration of the entire cell cycle.

In the case of Burkitt's lymphoma, with a doubling time of 24 hours, exposure to drug should be about a day to effect the greatest tumor cell kill. Unfortunately, white-cell stem cells have a doubling time of only 12 hours and gastrointestinal cells about 24 hours, so that it is not possible to expose Burkitt's lymphoma cells for the duration of an entire cell cycle without causing a life-threatening kill of certain kinds of normal cells. The clinical problem, then, is to devise a regimen that is more sparing of normal cells yet causes an adequate remission, though not complete elimination of the tumor. This is possible, despite the shorter cell cycles of certain normal cells, because the normal cells spend more time in G_0 than do Burkitt's lymphoma cells. Problems of this kind usually are resolved by repeating courses of submaximal tumor-killing doses.

It is much more difficult to devise an effective yet safe regimen for the treatment of tumors with long doubling times, since the tumor doubling time may be many times longer than the hematopoietic stem, immune and mucosal cells. Long, multicourse combination treatments are the rule. Most are quite empirical with respect to kinetic considerations. In these, since the duration of a course is inevitably longer than the elimination lifetime of the drugs in use, a regimen requires maintenance dosing or constant infusion. It might be expected that constant infusion would be more effective than intermittent dosing. This has proven to be the case with breast carcinoma. It also has proved to be less toxic.

Site-directed administration of antineoplastic drugs by intra-arterial infusion is advantageous to intravenous administration only if the concentration of drug in the blood in systemic circulation is substantially lower than that infused into the artery. This was thought to obtain when there is a high rate of systemic clearance of the drug, so that toxic amounts of the drug do not accumulate systematically. However, experience with intra-arterial fluorouracil, a drug with a half-life on less than 20 minutes, has been disappointing. It has been explained that the local extraction ratio of fluorouracil during prolonged intra-arterial infusion is sufficiently low that there is not a sufficiently selective uptake into the target to gain much advantage by local infusion.

In contrast, the nitrosourea, BCNU, has a high extraction ratio by the intracarotid arterial route and, consequently, is advantageous by this route (for CNS tumors), even though there is considerable local toxicity. Similarly, diaziquone has a high local extraction ratio and is advantageous by the intra-arterial route. The local clearance of an intra-arterially infused drug of low extraction ratio may be increased by decreasing the rate of blood flow with a vasoconstrictor.

Although most regimens are largely empirical, improvisation, or failure to follow the regimen as recommended, is a common cause of early relapse, especially in pediatrics.

Not only are there circadian rhythms in the metabolism of many drugs but also in the susceptibility of the patient to the toxic effects of antineoplastic drugs. In the future, circadian kinetics may be incorporated into anticancer regimens.

As among drugs in general, various antineoplastic drugs are involved in pharmacokinetic drug interactions. For example, cisplatin and daunorubicin induce the hepatic enzymes for the metabolism of carbamazepine, phenytoin and valproate. Verapamil competes for the active transport of lipophilic anticancer drugs out of cells. Any drug that causes mucositis will interfere with the peroral absorption of other drugs.

Immunoactive Drugs

The immune system is quite complex. Several types of cells are involved. These are cells, the ancestral line of which has derived from bone marrow stem cells. Some of the descendants of the stem cells migrate to sites elsewhere in the body, where they become small lymphocytes. There are two general types of small lymphocytes involved in the immune responses: the B cells and the T cells. The B lymphocytes get the designation B from the fact that in birds they derive from stem cell clones in the bursa of Fabricus; in man, the location of analogous clones may be in the intestinal mucosal Peyer's patches. The T cells get their designation from the fact that they are derived from stem cells cloned in the thymus gland. Undifferentiated small lymphocytes take up residence in lymph tissue in the spleen, tonsils, intestines and other sites.

B and T cells respond to antigen by cellular transformation, proliferation and differentiation. Proliferation increases the population of immunocompetent cells and differentiation creates cells with various roles to play in the immune response. Both B and T cells differentiate into what broadly may be termed effector cells and memory cells. The memory cells revert to an inactive state (G_0) but respond to later immune challenge by accelerated proliferation, differentiation and activity. During their residence in the bursa equivalent, the future effector B cells become programmed to respond to an antigen by transformation into plasma cells, which produce antibodies (immunoglobulins I_A, I_D, I_E, I_G and I_M), the role of which is to combine with circulating antigens. The immunity conferred by B cells is known as *humoral immunity*.

Hypersensitivity mediated through the humoral immune system is called immediate hypersensitivity, since the response is rapid. T cells become programmed in the thymus to respond in various ways to antigen that has become fixed to cell surfaces or engulfed by macrophages. The cytotoxic T cell (effector cell, "killer" cell), with the aid of complement, attacks and lyses those cells to which the offending antigen is attached. There are different cytotoxic T cells for different antigens. There are also helper T cells, which promote B cell activity, and suppressor T cells, which restrain both the cytotoxic T cells and the B cells. Helper and suppressor B cells also exist. T cell-mediated immunity is known as cell-mediated immunity. This is the immune response involved in graft-rejection, autoimmunity and delayed hypersensitivity.

The priming of lymphocytes in response to antigen is known as the primary response. The final effector response is known as the secondary, or efferent, response.

There are other bone-marrow stem-cell-derived cells, such as macrophages and K cells, that participate in the immune response. In the primary response, the macrophages phagocytose antigens, process them and present the processed antigen to helper T lymphocytes, which initiate the recruitment of other lymphocytes. Thus the macrophages are an integral part of the afferent limb of the primary response. They also appear to be involved in the efferent response; they fix and alter antigen prior to its recognition by the T cells. Details of the immune system may be found in Chapter 44.

Immunosuppressives—An immunosuppressive drug is one that can attenuate the expression of at least one type of immune response. The numerous cell types involved in the immune system afford an equal number of places of immunosuppressive drugs to intervene. It is conceivable that a T cell responsive to one antigen may be affected more than is another T cell specific to another antigen, or that suppressor T cells might be affected more than cytoxic or helper T cells. In general, information on drug selectivity is lacking. However, the increase in the incidence of lymphomas in persons with a past history of immunosuppression lends credence to the hypothesis of a selectivity for suppressor T cells. The ability of indomethacin to delay graft rejection also suggests a selective action on suppressor cell function, since prostaglandins are suppressor mediators. In general, though, cells involved in the primary response seem to be more susceptible to immunosuppressive treatment than those in the secondary response. The overall effect of an immunosuppressive drug probably depends on its phase specificity and the differences and similarities of the cell cycle phasing among the various cell types.

The immunosuppressive drugs comprise a number of classes of drugs, not all of which are antineoplastic drugs. For example, the antimalarial drug, pyrimethamine, and the antibacterial drug, trimethopterin, have immunosuppressant properties and have been used clinically as immunosuppressants. Also penicillamine and gold salts are employed as immunosuppresants in the treatment of rheumatoid arthritis, as have cytotoxic agents like methotrexate and cyclophosphamide. Biological agents, such as lymphocyte immune globulin and antimacrophage serum are actively under investigation. Physical interventions, such as radiation, desenstization and surgery still are used in the management of certain immune diseases, which testifies to the present limitations of the drugs.

The alkylating agents mainly affect the short-lived and not the long-lived small lymphocytes. They also suppress proliferation of macrophages but do not interfere with phagocytosis. Therefore, the primary immune response mainly is affected, although cyclophosphamide acts on both afferent and efferent limbs in certain immune disorders. The antipurines, 6-mercaptopurine and azathioprine, have a strong effect on cellular immunity and act mainly on the efferent limb (according to their program of use), although they also have suppressant effects on macrophage proliferation and display afferent activity in certain circumstances. The antipyrimidines mainly behave as efferent suppressants. Experimentally, methotrexate has mixed properties, but in man it behaves mostly as an afferent suppressant. Adrenalcorticoids both suppress macrophage activity and decrease the population of small lymphocytes. Clinically, they behave mostly as afferent suppressants, but they are adjuvant to efferent and mixed suppressants.

The adverse effects and precautions of the primary immunosuppressant drugs are those of the antineoplastic drugs.

The isolation of various cytokines and other growth factors, elucidation of their roles in immune responses and sequencing of the peptides has opened up a class of immunosuppressives that are more selective for the immune system than are the antineoplastic drugs used for immune suppression. This new class is made up of synthetic or recombinantly engineered competitive analogs of the cytokines that block the actions of cytokines on the target immune cells. Also under investigation are other ligands of the cytokine receptors.

A great deal of publicity has been given the use of immunosuppressive drugs to prevent rejection of organ and bone-marrow transplants. However, they have a greater potential usefulness in the management of the autoimmune diseases.

Diseases in which they are of established benefit include systemic lupus erythematosus, rheumatoid arthritis, nonglomerular nephrosis, psoriasis and chronic active hepatitis. Diseases for which these drugs unequivocally have not been proved to be sufficiently efficacious for general use include ulcerative colitis, Crohn's disease, Behçet's disease, chronic glomerulonephritis (membranous), chronic thrombocytopenic purpura and autoimmune hemolytic anemia.

Other Immunomodulators—Since immunosuppression is a common adverse effect of antineoplastic drugs and also since many immunosuppressive drugs have come from among the antineoplastics, it is common to believe that antineoplastic cytotoxicity automatically suppresses the immune system. However, the immune system has helper, suppressor and killer components, so that the net effect depends upon which components are affected most. Indeed, there is thought to be immunostimulatory components to the actions of some antineoplastic drugs. Nevertheless, no antineoplastic drug is used for immune stimulation.

Conversely, the situation is analogous with the so-called immunostimulants, because the net effect on any given immune response depends upon which of the sundry participating cells are stimulated most. For example, levamisole is called an immunostimulant, but it either can augment or suppress an immune response depending upon factors such the type of response, dose and timing. T lymphocyte function is augmented more than B lymphocyte function. The drug tends to normalize a disturbed immune system. A similar bifunctionalism exists among the various cytokines. Interferons, for example, stimulate some immune cells and suppress others. Diethyl dithiocarbamate, however, is nearly a pure immunostimulant; it induces the recruitment of T lymphocytes and promotes cytotoxicity. Every vaccine is an immunostimulant, often quite selective. However, some, such as staphage lysate, cause rather general immunostimulation and may be used to confer varying degrees of immunity to various nonbacterial invaders.

It is now known that certain autonomic and CNS transmitters and neuromodulators also have influences on the immune system. Enkephalins and endorphins stimulate B-lymphocyte proliferation and antibody production and promote T lymphocyte and natural killer cell cytotoxicity. Opioid drugs mimic some of the immunomodulatory actions of the peptides. It is believed that these peptides are part of a neuroendocrine-immune system loop. Histamine stimulates suppressor T lymphocytes and thus tends to limit immune responses. The action is mediated through H_2-receptors. Consequently, H_2-antagonists, such as cimetidine and ranitidine, tend to augment the efferent immune response. Various immune cells also possess alpha- and beta-adrenoreceptors, through which immune functions can be affected by circulating epinephrine and sympathetically released norepinephrine and their antagonists. The overall effect of alpha-agonism is immunosuppression but that of beta-agonism varies according to the immune status under various conditions.

Antineoplastic and Immunoactive Drugs

Aldesleukin

Interleukin-2 Recombinant; Proleukin (*Chiron/Cetus*)

2-133-Interleukin 2 (human reduced) [110942-02-4] $C_{690}H_{1115}N_{177}O_{203}S_6$ (15,600.00)

Preparation—A continuous chain of 133 amino acid residues; a product of recombinant DNA technology using genetically engineered *E Coli* strains containing an analog of the human interleukin-2 gene.

Uses—Identical to a cytokine, IL-2, secreted by activated hleper T lymphocytes that is a colony-stimulating factor for active T lymphocytes, immature thymocytes, natural killer (NK) cells, antigen-activated B lymphocytes and probably other cells of the immune system. The ability to stimulate proliferation of cytotoxic T lymphocytes and NK cells has led to clinical trials against several kinds of cancer. It is approved for *metastatic renal cancer*. Treatment consists in the admistration of IL-2 alone or prior to, and along with, autologous lymphokine-activated killer (LAK) cells; the IL-2 for the purpose of encouraging the proliferation of LAK cells. At present, the combination has been found effective in some cases of *metastatic renal carcinoma, melanoma, colorectal carcinoma* and *Hodgkin's disease*, but treatment of other cancers is under active investigation. It is also under investigation as an anti-infective agent; it is in Phase II trials for use in AIDS.

Common adverse effects attributable to IL-2 are nausea, vomiting, diarrhea, fever, malaise, pruritus, severe anemia, hyperbilirubinemia and elevated plasma creatinine. Less-common effects are elevated capillary permeability with pulmonary edema, fluid retention, hypotension, cardiac dysrhythmias, thrombocytopenia and disorientation, even coma. About 20% of patients treated with IL-2 and LAK cells develop hyothyroidism. Treatment is prohibitively expensive. The peptide nature of IL-2 requires parenteral administration. The half-life is less than 1 hr, so that constant intravenous infusion is the optimal mode of administration.

Dose (tentative)—*Intravenous, adult* **30,000** to **300,000 units** (Cetus)/kg/day for 5 days, as a continuous infusion or divided into 3 doses/day at 8-hr intervals. In regimens in which LAK cells are a activated *in vivo* and administered, leukopheresis is conducted on days 7 to 12, each day's collection being cultured with IL-2 for 5 days then infused into the patient concomitantly with IL-2. When IL-2 is given alone, 2 or 3 courses may be given, each after a rest of 1 wk. IL-2 also has been administered intraperitoneally.

Dosage Forms—Ampules: to be reconstituted with normal saline. Stable for no more than a few hours in aqueous solution. Vials: containing 22 × 10^6 IU; must be stored between 2° to 8°C; reconstituted solutions are stable up to 48 hr when stored at 2° to 25°.

Altretamine

1,3,5-Triazine-2,4,6-triamine, *N,N,N′,N′,N″,N″*-hexamethyl-, Hexamethylmelamine; Hexalen (*UAD Labs*)

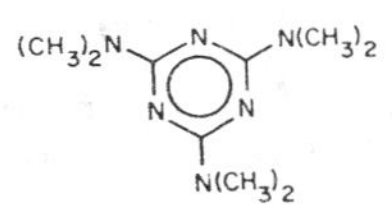

[645-05-6] $C_9H_{18}N_6$ (210.28).

Preparation—*J Am Chem Soc 73:*2984, 1951.

Description—White needles; melts about 173°.

Solubility—Practically insoluble in water; increasingly soluble below pH 3.

Uses—A Group C alkylating agent related to triethylenemelamine, an early alkylating agent. It is one of several secondary drugs for treatment of *ovarian tumors*. It is approved as a single agent for *refractory ovarian cancer*. It also has proven useful in the treatment of both *Hodgkin's* and *non-Hodgkin's lymphomas, oat-cell bronchogenic carcinoma* and *breast tumor*. Nausea and vomiting are the main acute adverse effects. Delayed toxicity includes bone-marrow depression, CNS depression, peripheral neuritis, ataxia, hallucinations, psychoses, pruritus and dermatitis. The drug is metabolized in the liver. The terminal half-life is 4.7 to 10.2 hr.

Dose—*Oral*, **240** to **320 mg/m²**/day in 4 divided doses for 21 days.

Dosage Forms—Capsules: 50 mg.

Aminoglutethimide

2,6-Piperidinedione, 3-(4-aminophenyl)-3-ethyl-, Cytadren (*Ciba-Geigy*)

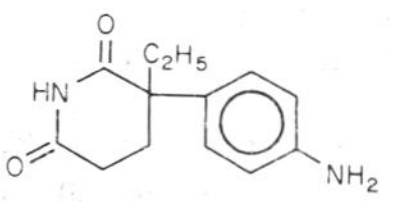

2-(*p*-Aminophenyl)-2-ethylglutaramide [125-84-8] $C_{13}H_{16}N_2O_2$ (232.28).

Preparation—By a procedure similar to gluthethamide (page 1168) with nitration of the α-ethylbenzyl cyanide to the *p*-nitro derivative. This is then reduced to the amine after ring closure. US Pat 2,848,455.

Description—White crystals; melts about 150°.

Solubility—Very slightly soluble in water; freely soluble in many organic solvents.

Uses—Inhibits the first step in adrenalcorticoid biosynthesis by inhibiting the conversion of cholesterol to Δ^5-pregrenolone. It also inhibits the aromatase that converts androstenedione to estrone and estradiol, thus eliminating the adrenal source, the only source of estrogens in postmenopausal and oophorectomized women. It is approved for *suppression of adrenalcorticoid production* in selected Cushing's syndrome patients. Treatment with aminoglutethimide is preferred to adrenalectomy in postmenopausal women with *estrogen receptor-positive breast carcinoma.* Hydrocortisone is administered concomitantly to suppress the counterproductive, counter-regulatory increase in ACTH release that accrues to the drug-induced lowering of plasma hydrocortisone. The regimen, however, causes more adverse effects than does tamoxifen and hence is a second-choice treatment. It also is useful in the management of certain cases of *Cushing's syndrome.*

Early adverse effects include lethargy (in 40% of recipients), ataxia (in 10%), nausea, vomiting and anorexia, to all of which tolerance develops in 1 to 6 weeks, and morbilliform rash. Delayed adverse effects mostly relate to mineralocorticoid insufficiency and include orthostatic hypotension (in 10%; symptoms are dizziness and weakness) so that mineralocorticoids may require supplementation. Occasional adverse effects include pruritis, myalgia, headache, masculinization and hirsuitism in women, precocious sexual development in boys, hypothyroidism with goiters after long-term use, leucopenia, thrombocytopenia, granulocytopenia and pancytopenia. Alkaline phosphatase and SGOT activities in serum frequently occur, and cholestatic jaundice occurs rarely. Aminoglutethimide induces the metabolism of dexamethasone, thus that particular glucocorticoid should not be used concomitantly. It also increases the metabolism of digitoxin and theophyllin.

Aminoglutethimide is well-absorbed orally. Initially, about 50% is excreted in the urine unchanged, but induction of liver metabolism diminishes the importance of renal elimination. The elimination half-life is initially about 13 hr but decreases to about 7 hr after 1 to 2 wk.

Dose—*Oral, adult, initially* **250 mg,** 3 times a day for 2 wk and every 6 hr thereafter for *maintenance* but may be increased up to 2 g/day in Cushing's syndrome. In breast cancer, 40 mg/day of hydrocortisone is administered concurrently in 2 divided doses at 5 am and at bedtime.

Dosage Form—Tablets: 250 mg.

Amsacrine

Methanesufonamide, *N*-[4-(acridinylamino)-3-methoxyphenyl]-, Amsidyl (*Parke-Davis*); (*Bristol*)

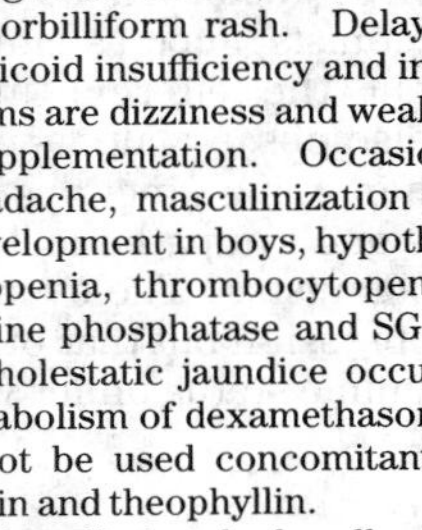

OCH_3 CH_3SO_2NH NH N

[51264-14-3] $C_{21}H_{19}N_3O_3S$ (393.46).

Preparation—From 2′-methoxy-4′-nitrobutyranilide. The nitro group is reduced to the amine, converted to the methanesulfonamide, and the resulting free amino group reacted with 9-acridinyl chloride to yield the product. *J Med Chem,* 18:1110, 1975.

Description—Reacts with some plastics and should be given in glass syringes.

Solubility—Reported to be incompatible in solutions of ionic chloride, causing precipitation; stable in dilute lactic acid or 5% dextrose solutions.

Uses—Intercalates into DNA and inhibits topoisomerase II. Phases S and G_2 of the cell cycle are the most sensitive. It is currently the primary drug for the treatment of *refractory acute myelocytic leukemia* of adults; complete remissions are achieved in 10 to 20% of such patients. It also is effective in refractory *diffuse histiocytic lymphoma,* the *acute* phase of *chronic myelocytic leukemia* and *non-Hodgkin's lymphomas.* Immediate toxicity includes nausea, vomiting, local irritation at the injection site, acute cardiotoxicity and occasional convulsions. Delayed toxicity includes leukopenia in almost all recipients, mucositis and delayed cardiotoxocity. The drug is not absorbed effectively by the oral route. It is metabolized in the liver and secreted into the bile. The elimination half-life is 7 to 17 hr.

Dose—*Intravenous,* for induction of remission in acute myelocytic leukemia, **120** to **200 mg/m²** a day for 5 days, to be repeated every 4 wk.

Dosage Form—Formulated as two sterile liquids in separate 2 mL ampules; one containing 75 mg of drug in 1.5 mL of *N,N*-dimethylacetamide, the other 13.5 mL of 0.0353 *M* lactic acid. On mixing aseptically the resulting solution contains 5 mg/mL of drug.

Asparaginase

L-Asparagine amidohydrolase; E.C. 3.5.1.1.; Elspar (*MSD*)

L-Asparaginase [9015-68-3], an enzyme of molecular weight 133,000 ± 5000, believed to consist of four equivalent subunits.

Preparation—L-Asparaginase, an enzyme that catalyzes hydrolysis of L-asparagine to L-aspartate and ammonia, occurs in many species. Isolated in pure form from several sources, it usually is obtained from *Escherichia coli* or *Erwinia caratovora* which produces also an asparaginase devoid of antileukemic activity, that is removed on purification of the enzyme. See Mashburn and Wriston, *Arch Biochem Biophys 105:* 450, 1964.

Description—White, crystalline powder.

Solubility—Freely soluble in water; practically insoluble in chloroform or methanol.

Uses—Protein synthesis in several normal as well as malignant cell types is dependent partly upon exogenous asparagine, and, in a few cells, such as lymphoblasts and certain other leukemic cells, essentially is dependent totally. The enzymatic destruction of asparagine by asparaginase injected into plasma deprives the dependent cells of the essential asparagine and, thus, not only arrests their growth but may even result in some cell death and tumor regression. It is approved for use in *acute lymphocytic leukemia.*

At present, it is used mainly in chemotherapy of *acute lymphocytic leukemia,* and T-cell leukemias and lymphomas in sequential combinations with other drugs. When it is administered immediately after a course of vincristine and a glucocorticoid (usually prednisone or dexamethasone) for the induction of the first remission in children, the median duration of remission is more than doubled. Addition of doxorubicin and intrathecal cytarabine further prolongs survival. Some studies indicate a small increase in the incidence of complete remissions. The enzyme also is useful for induction of remission in children with relapse of acute lymphocytic leukemia. It is not recommended for maintenance. Asparaginase protects some tissues and cancers froms ome antimetabolities (eg, methotrexate, ara-c), probably by preventing DNA synthesis. Such interactions, especially with methotrexate, should be anticipated. Erwinia asparaginase is an orphan drug that is reserved for use in patients allergic to asparaginase from *E coli.*

Sixty to 90% of recipients of asparaginase will show laboratory evidence of an impairment of liver function, such that plasma fibrinogen and other clotting factors may be diminished and most patients will have a considerable elevation of blood ammonia. Effects on the pancreas also are common; insulin production is diminished and there may be hyperglycemia, serum amylase activity may increase and acute pancreatitis, sometimes hemorrhagic, may occur in as many as 5% of the recipients. There also are actions on the central nervous system to cause impairment of the sensorium, mental depression and rare coma. Nausea, vomiting, chills and fever also occur frequently. Hypersensitivity reactions, ranging from mild rash to anaphylaxis and death, occur in 5 to 20% of recipients, so that sensitivity testing before administration is necesssry and desensitization may be required before a second course is administered. *Erwina* (Porton) asparaginase is less sensitizing than that from *E. coli.* Both enzymes also have immunosuppressant activity.

It must be administered parenterally. The rate of clearance varies considerably between preparations. Its half-life is about 16 hr.

Dose—*Intravenous, adults* and *children,* **200 IU/kg/day** for 10 days. *Intramuscular, children,* **6000 IU/m²** at 3-day intervals for a total of 9 doses.

Dosage Form—Injection: 10,000 units vial.

Azacitidine

1,3,5-Triazin-2(1*H*)-one, 4-amino-1-β-D-ribo-furanosyl-, Mylosar (*Upjohn*)

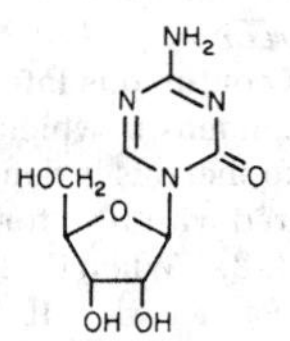

NH_2 N N $HOCH_2$ N O O OH OH

[320-67-2] $C_8H_{12}N_4O_5$ (244.20).

Preparation—A ring analog of cytidine, obtained by synthesis or produced microbiologically. US Pat 3,350,388.

Description—White powder melting about 229°.

Solubility—1 g in 25 mL water or 1000 mL alcohol. Reconstituted IV solutions are not stable for more than a few hours.

Uses—An antimetabolite used investigationally to treat refractory *acute myelocytic leukemias* and the *acute phase of chronic myelocytic leukemias*. It has been reported to arrest the progress of *AIDS* in 84% of cases. Acutely it causes nausea, vomiting, diarrhea and fever. Delayed toxicity includes prolonged leukopenia, thrombocytopenia and hepatotoxicity, not dose-related. The mortality rate has been reported to be about 6%.

Dose—*Intravenous,* **50** to **400 mg/m²/day** for 5 days, repeated at intervals of 2 to 3 wk, the length of the interval being determined by the time required for the white blood-cell count to pass its nadir. The least amount of nausea and vomiting occurs when the drug is given by continuous infusion over the entire 5-day period, but if each daily dose is infused over 18 hr, the acute toxicity is increased negligibly. If the daily dose is given in 15 to 30 min, the acute toxicity is enhanced greatly and will result in a substantial proportion of patients refusing treatment.

Dosage Form—Injection: lyophilized powder in a 30 mL vial containing 100 mg azacitidine and 100 mg mannitol. Reconstitute with 20 mL of water and dilute with normal saline or lactated Ringer's. *Note*—Investigational drug only available through NIH.

Azathioprine

1*H*-Purine, 6-[(1-methyl-4-nitro-1*H*-imidazol-5-yl)thio]-, Imuran (*Burroughs Wellcome*)

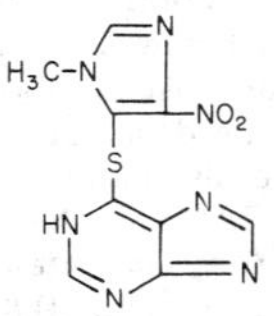

6-[(1-Methyl-4-nitroimidazol-5-yl)thio]purine [446-86-6] $C_9H_7N_7O_2S$ (277.26).

Preparation—*N,N'*-Dimethyloxaldiamide is reacted with phosphorus pentachloride to give 5-chloro-1-methylimidazole. This is nitrated and the resulting 5-chloro-1-methyl-4-nitroimidazole condensed with purine-6-thiol (mercaptopurine) in an appropriate dehydrohalogenating environment. US Pat 3,056,785.

Description—Yellow, matted powder that is odorless and has a slightly bitter taste; light-sensitive, nonhygroscopic and stable to reasonable temperatures; decomposes about 245°.

Solubility—Insoluble in water; very slightly soluble in alcohol or chloroform; soluble in dilute solutions of alkali hydroxides (unstable); sparingly soluble in dilute mineral acids.

Uses—Approved for prevention of renal transplant rejection. It is a derivative of *Mercaptopurine* into which it largely is converted in the body, but not all of its actions are those of mercaptopurine. It is used only as an *immunosuppressive* drug. It suppresses T-lymphocyte and monocyte (hence macrophage) production more than B-lymphocyte production. It probably has been used more than any other immunosuppressive drug in *kidney transplantations.* At present, about one-half of kidney transplants survive for longer than 3 yr when azathioprine is used, but other measures also contribute to this rate of success. It also is used in other organ transplantations.

Azathioprine works in the afferent and not the efferent immune phase and hence does not suppress ongoing graft rejection. It appears to bring about a satisfactory response in a high percentage of patients with *ulcerative colitis, regional enteritis, polymyositis* or *refractory idiopathic thrombocytopenic purpura* but induces considerable toxicity. In *rheumatoid arthritis,* it is used when conventional therapy fails. It is about as effective as gold, penicillamine or cyclophosphamide and less toxic than penicillamine or cyclophosphamide. It may improve metabolic control in *recent-onset diabetes* mellitus. It is usually of little benefit in *systemic lupus erythematosus.*

Nausea and vomiting is quite frequent. Other toxicity or intercurrent infection (see introduction) occurs in about one-third of patients under immunosuppressive treatment with the drug. Bone-marrow depression is the most frequent, occurring in about 11% of patients; leukopenia (28 to over 50%, as much as 16% serious), thrombocytopenia and, to a lesser extent, anemia or panctyopenia are manifested.

In antiarthritic doses, infections are not increased, and other adverse effects are less frequent and less severe. Pancreatitis, alopecia, arthralgia, skin rashes, serum sickness, stomatitis, esophagitis, steatorrhea, retinopathy, peritoneal hemorrhage and pulmonary edema also may occur in a small percentage of cases. Occasionally, hepatic damage, with elevation of the plasma content of liver enzymes and jaundice, is seen, but damage seems to be slight and to disappear during the course of treatment. However, in the presence of liver dysfunction the drug should be withheld. Although the incidence is rare, an increase in reticulum cell sarcoma and lymphoma has been noted in transplant patients receiving azathioprine; it is not clear whether this is from immunosuppression or from the successfully sustained transplant. However, the drug is carcinogenic in experimental animals.

Although it is degraded rapidly in the liver, the kidney importantly regulates the plasma concentration of the effective metabolites, so that toxicity is greatly increased in the presence of allopurinol or renal impairment, unless the dosage is properly adjusted. It should not be used during pregnancy if possible.

It is metabolized rapidly to 6-mercaptopurine (6-MP), so that its useful half-life is that of 6-MP (page 1255). Since allopurinol inhibits the metabolism of 6-MP, the dosage of this drug must be reduced to about ⅓ of the usual dose when allopurinol is used concurrently. Hepatic insufficiency diminishes efficacy.

Dose—*Oral* or *intravenous, immunosuppressive,* if treatment is begun at the time of transplantation, *initially,* **3** to **5 mg/kg/day,** after which adjustments are made to attempt to maintain the homograft without toxicity; the *maintenance dose* may be as low as **1 mg/kg** but usually is **2** to **3 mg/kg/day**. Treatment must be started within 24 hr of transplantation. When treatment is started 1 to 5 days before transplantation, **1** to **5 mg/kg/day.** In the presence of renal damage or allopurinol the dose should be reduced to ¼ to ⅓ of the above. Reduce dose or stop treatment at the first sign of bone-marrow depression. For *rheumatoid arthritis, initially* **1.0 mg/kg** as a single or twice daily dose to be increased by 0.5 mg/kg/day after 6 to 8 wk and thereafter at 4-wk intervals, if necessary, to a total of 2.5 mg/kg/day or the supravention of severe toxicity; once an effect is established, downward adjustments to a minimal effective dose should be made.

Dosage Forms—For Injection (as sodium salt): 100 mg of azathioprine equivalent; Scored Tablets: 50 mg.

Bacterial Antigen Made from Staphylococcus

Staphage Lysate (SPL) (*Delmont Labs*)

A sterile preparation of lysed cultures of *Staphylococcus aureus,* Cowan Serologic Types I & III.

Uses—Approved for staphylococcus infections. Types I & II staphylococci have broad antigenicity. *In vitro,* they have been shown to stimulate lymphoproliferative responses in certain subpopulations of both B cells and T cells. A controlled study in laboratory animals has shown elevated immunoglobulin levels. The preparation appears to induce cell-mediated immunity not only to sundry staphylococcal infections but also to aphthous ulcers (cankers) and herpes viral infections. Vaccine-type reactions (eg, malaise, fever or chills) may occur. Since there is the possibility not only of promoting allergies to staphylococcal components but also to various media components, it must be used judiciously in subjects with histories of allergies. An intracutaneous skin test is recommended.

Dose—*Intranasal, oral, subcutaneous* or *topical.* Dose regimens depend upon the type and chronicity of the disorder, age and condition of the patient and whether there is a history of allergies. For details see *Drug Facts and Comparisons* or the *Physicians' Desk Reference.*

Dosage Forms—Injection: 1 mL; Intranasal, Oral or Topical: 10 mL.

Bleomycin Sulfate

Blenoxane (*Bristol*)

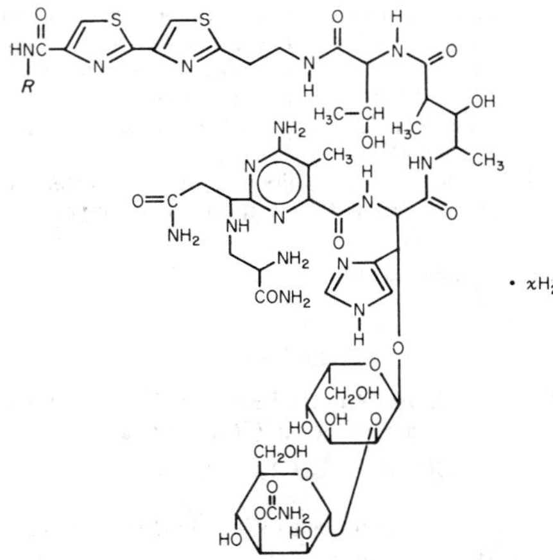

(Main component: Bleomycin A_2, in which *R* is $(CH_3)_2S^+CH_2CH_2CH_2—$)

Bleomycin Sulfate (salt) [9041-93-4]

A mixture of the sulfate salts of a group of related basic glycopeptide antibiotics, notably bleomycin A_2 and bleomycin B_2, obtained from cultures of *Streptomyces verticillus;* bleomycin A_2 is the main component of the bleomycin used clinically.

Preparation—For the purification and separation of the bleomycins see Umezawa *et al., J Antibiot 19:*200, 210, 1966, also Takita *et al, ibid. 71:*79, 1968 and *22:*237, 1969.

Description—Cream-colored, hygroscopic powder.

Solubility—Very soluble in water; sparingly soluble in alcohol.

Uses—Causes fragmentation of DNA and also inhibits incorporation of thymidine into DNA. It stops the progression of cells through the G_2 and M phases of the cell cycle. In spite of these actions, it has very little effect on bone marrow, a circumstance that gives it a special usefulness in drug combinations. Its selectivity appears to be related to distribution. It is approved as palliative treatment of *lymphomas, testicular carcinoma* and *squamous cell carcinoma.* It is a component of all three preferred combinations for the treatment of *testicular carcinoma* and of both for cervical cancer. It is included in one of two preferred combinations to treat *squamous cell carcinoma of the head and neck.* It also has been used successfully in the treatment of squamous cell carcinomas of the skin, penis and vulva. It is in two of five preferred for *Hodgkin's disease.* It is a component of four of seven preferred combinations to treat diffuse lymphocytic lymphoma. It has shown efficacy against reticulum cell sarcoma, lymphosarcoma, chloriocarcinoma and teratocarcinoma. It is also effective against *common warts.*

It is very toxic, and 10 to 40% of patients develop a pneumonitis which progresses to pulmonary fibrosis: 1% of bleomycin-treated patients die of pulmonary complications. The effect is most likely to occur in elderly patients or those who have received a total of 400 Units. The drug must be used extremely cautiously in the presence of pulmonary disease. Acute hyperpyrexia and cardiorespiratory collapse also occur, especially in patients with lymphomas; for this reason, patients with lymphomas are given two test doses of 5 units or less and are observed for a day before treatment is begun. Anticalmodulin drugs (eg, trifluperazine) enhance lethal toxicity. Bleomycin commonly causes nausea, vomiting, chills and fever, and in half of the patients it causes erythema and hyperkeratosis, which sometimes progresses to vesication. Other occasional adverse effects are cutaneous desquamation, hyperesthesia, confusion, vertigo, pruritus, tenderness, alopecia and aphthous ulcers. Cutaneous toxicity is most likely to occur when the total cumulative dose exceeds 150 Units.

It is absorbed poorly orally and also is inactivated in the gut and liver. Consequently, it must be administered parenterally. Higher concentrations are reached in certain neoplasms (carcinomas more than sarcomas), lungs and skin than in other tissues, which accounts for the selectivity and the loci of toxicities. In the tissues, the drug appears to be deaminated and, possibly, also hydrolyzed by peptidases. The enzymatic destruction is less in those tissues in which the higher concentrations are reached. Sixty to 70% is excreted in the urine. In patients with normal renal function, the elimination half-life is about 2 hr; in renal failure the half-life may be as long as 21 hr. Care must be exercised in the presence of renal impairment.

Dose (base equivalent)—*Intralesional, adults* and *children,* for *warts,* **0.2** to **0.8 Units** in a concentration of 3 to 15 Units/mL in water or sodium chloride injection, to be given one or more times at 2- to 4-wk intervals up to a total dose of 2 Units. *Intramuscular, intravenous* or *subcutaneous, adults and children,* for *Hodgkin's disease, squamous-cell carcinoma, lymphosarcoma, reticulum cell carcinoma* or *testicular carcinoma, initially* **0.25** to **0.50 Units/kg** *or* **10** to **20 Units/m²** once or twice a week; in *Hodgkin's disease,* for *maintenance, intramuscular* or *intravenous,* **1 Unit/day** *or* **5 Units/week.** *Intrapleural, adults and children,* for *malignant effusions* in Hodgkin's disease, **15** to **120 Units** in 100 mL of sodium chloride injection, to be removed after 24 hr. *Intraperitoneal, adults and children,* for *malignant effusions* in Hodgkin's disease, **60** to **100 Units** in 100 mL of sodium chloride injection, to be removed after 24 hr. *Regional arterial infusion, adults and children,* for *squamous-cell carcinoma* of the *head, neck* or *cervix,* **30** to **60 Units/day** for 1 hr to 1 day.

Dosage Form—Injection: 15 Units (1 unit is equivalent to the activity, microbiologically determined, of 1 mg of a bleomycin A_2 reference standard).

Bromocriptine—page 1035.

Busulfan

1,4-Butanediol, dimethanesulfonate; Tetramethylene Dimethanesulfonate; Myleran (*Burroughs Wellcome*)

$CH_3SO_2O(CH_2)_4OSO_2CH_3$

1,5-Butanediol dimethanesulfonate [55-98-1] $C_6H_{14}O_6S_2$ (246.29).

Caution—It is very poisonous. Great care should be taken to prevent inhaling its particles and exposing the skin to it.

Preparation—By esterifying 1,4-butanediol with methanesulfonyl chloride in the presence of pyridine.

Description—White, crystalline powder; melts about 116°.

Solubility—Very slightly soluble in water; slightly soluble in alcohol; 1 g in about 45 mL of acetone.

Uses—An alkylating agent which is efficacious as an *antineoplastic* drug in certain cases. It is phase nonspecific. Its principal distinction is that in the usual doses it exerts very little action on rapidly proliferative tissues other than bone marrow. With low doses, granulocytopoiesis can be suppressed selectively without affecting erythropoiesis. Thus, it is approved for the palliative treatment of *chronic granulocytic* (myelogenous, myeloid, myelocytic) *leukemia,* for which it is one of two drugs of choice. It is not to be used in terminal or acute phases of the disease. It is also quite effective in the treatment of *polycythemia vera* and *primary thrombocytosis.* Since it has little effect on lymphopoiesis, it is of no value in lymphocytic leukemia, Hodgkin's disease or malignant lymphoma. It is useless against solid tumors.

Its principal toxicity is pancytopenia and long-lasting thrombocytopenia. Lymphocytopenia is uncommon. A complete differential blood count (including thrombocytes) once a week is mandatory. Nausea, vomiting, diarrhea, impotence, amenorrhea, sterility and fetal malformation occasionally occur. Granulocyte destruction results in a high rate of excretion of urates, the precipitation of which may cause renal damage; cotreatment with *Allopurinol* (page 1110) may avoid such damage. It also sometimes causes cheilosis, glossitis, interstitial pulmonary fibrosis, anhidrosis, skin pigmentation (which may be the result of adrenalcortical hypofunction), alopecia and gynecomastia.

It is not immunosuppressive.

The elimination half-life is 2 to 3 hr.

Dose—*Adult, oral,* for *chronic intermittent therapy,* **0.065** to **0.1 mg/kg** *or* **3 mg/m²** (usually 4 to 8 mg)/**day** in two divided doses until leukocyte count drops below 15,000 cells/mm³; for *chronic continuous therapy, initially* as above but with dose reduction to maintain the leukocyte count at 15,000/mm³ (usually about 2 mg/day), keep leukocyte count in the normal range, the dose varying from **2 mg/wk** to **2** to **4 mg/day.** The drug must be discontinued if there is a precipitous decrease in leukocyte count. The *pediatric dose initially* is **60** to **120 µg/kg** or **1.8** to **4.6 mg/m²/day;** *maintenance,* the dose necessary to maintain the leukocyte count at about 20,000/mm³.

Dosage Form—Tablets: 2 mg.

Calusterone—see RPS-17, page 1001.

Carboplatin

Platinum, diammine [1,1-cyclobutanedicarboxylato(2-)-*O,O'*]-, Paraplatin (*Bristol-Myers Oncology*)

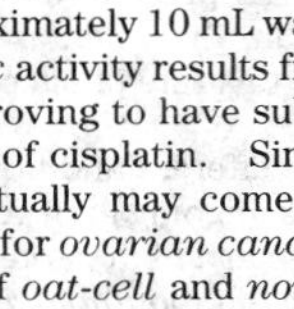

[41575-94-4] $C_6H_{12}N_2O_4Pt$ (371.25).

Preparation—Silver sulfate is reacted with *cis*-diammine platinum diiodide to yield the diaquodiammine platinum sulfate. Interaction with barium 1,1-tyclobutanedicarboxylate precipitates $BaSO_4$ and forms the product. *Inorg Chem Acta, 46:*L15, 1980.

Description—White crystals.

Solubility—1 g in approximately 10 mL water or 1000 mL alcohol.

Uses—Its *antineoplastic* activity results from the same mechanism as that of cisplatin, and it is proving to have substantially the same clinical antitumor spectrum as that of cisplatin. Since this drug is less nephrotoxic and ototoxic, it eventually may come to replace cisplatin. It is approved as palliative relief for *ovarian cancer.* It is presently an alternative drug for treatment of *oat-cell* and *non-small cell bronchogenic, ovarian* and *testicular carcinomas.* Immediate adverse effects are nausea and vomiting. Delayed toxicity includes myelosuppression with sometimes pronounced thrombocytopenia and renal and otic toxicities. The drug is not effective orally. In plasma, less than 10% is protein-bound. The elimination half-life is 3 to 7 hr.

Dose—*Intravenous, adult,* **440 mg/m²** every 28 days.

Dosage Forms—Vials (injection): 50 mg/5 mL, 150 mg/15 mL, 450 mg/45 mL. Reconstitute with water, 5% dextrose on normal saline.

Carmustine

Urea, *N,N'*-bis(2-chloroethyl)-*N*-nitroso-, BiCNU (*Bristol-Myers Oncology*)

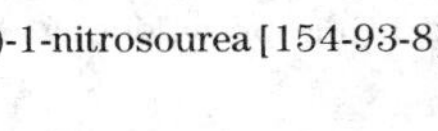

1,3-Bis(2-chloroethyl)-1-nitrosourea [154-93-8] $C_5H_9Cl_2N_3O_2$ (214.05).

Preparation—Like other cytotoxic nitrosoureas, it may be synthesized by nitrosation with sodium nitrite of the appropriate substituted urea—in this case 1,3-bis(2-chloroethyl)urea—in a cold, acid medium (eg, formic acid). Methods of synthesis of nitrosoureas have been published by Johnston *et al: J Med Chem 6:* 669, 1963.

Description—White or light yellow powder; melts, with decomposition, to an oily liquid at about 30°.

Solubility—Slightly soluble in water; freely soluble in alcohol; highly soluble in lipids; decomposes rapidly in acid or aqueous solutions above pH 7.

Uses—Although this is an alkylating drug, it also carbamoylates amino and other groups. Its cytotoxic effect is likely due to its ability to cross-link cellular DNA. Synthesis of DNA and RNA is inhibited. It is phase nonspecific. Carmustine is approved for use in *brain tumors, multiple myeloma, Hogdkin's disease* and *non-Hodgkin's lymphomas.* The drug is used mainly in the treatment of *brain glioblastoma* (for which it shares drug-of-choice status with its congener lomustine), *Hodgkin's disease* and other *lymphomas;* it is a component of a first-choice combination for *myeloma.* It has been reported to have a high efficacy against *Burkitt's tumor.* Although it has activity against various other carcinomas, including melanoma and renal cell carcinoma, it is not among the usual choices for such diseases. It usually is given in combination with radiotherapy in the treatment of brain tumors and with vincristine, procarbazine and glucocorticoids (eg, prednisone) in the treatment of the various lymphomas and multiple myeloma.

Within 2 hr after administration and lasting for 4 to 6 hr, nausea and vomiting occur frequently and usually severely. Rapid intravenous infusion causes intense flushing and conjunctival suffusion with a similar time-course. There may be a burning sensation but rarely thrombosis at the site of injection. Delayed bone-marrow toxicity occurs; also, thrombocytopenia that reaches a nadir in about 4 wk and a less severe leukepenia in about 6 wk, each lasting 2 to 7 wk; mild anemia may occur. With repeated doses, bone-marrow depression is cumulative. Leukocyte and platelet counts and signs of intercurrent infections should be monitored carefully throughout treatment. Severe dyspnea and a sometimes fatal interstitial pulmonary fibrosis occasionally occur. There also may be a mild, reversible hepatotoxicity in about 25% of recipients. Other adverse effects include slight nephrotoxocity (with a transient elevation of BUN) to severe nephrotoxicity and renal failure, with large cumulative doses, vertigo and ataxia. There is an increased risk of nonlymphocytic leukemia.

By the oral route, it is metabolized almost completely as it passes through the liver; consequently, it must be given intravenously. After intravenous administration, its plasma half-life is short, reported variously as from 3 to 30 min. Because the drug is highly lipid-soluble, it readily passes the blood-brain barrier, and concentrations of metabolites in the cerebrospinal fluid range from approximately 50 to 115% of those in plasma.

Dose—*Intravenous, adults* and *children, initially* **200 mg/m²** in a single dose every 6 or 8 wk *or* **75** to **100 mg/m²** on each of 2 *or* **40 mg/m²** an each of 5 successive days once every 6 wk. Subsequent adjustments of dosage are determined according to the therapeutic and toxic response (see the manufacturer's literature, *Drug Facts and Comparisons or USP DI*). A preexisting bone-marrow depression or concomitant use of other myelosuppressive drugs requires that lower doses be used.

Other Dose Information—Into each vial is injected 3 mL of sterile absolute ethanol and 27 mL of sterile water, to yield a solution containing 3.3 mg/mL. This solution then is added to an injection of isotonic sodium chloride or dextrose solution.

Dosage Form—Injection, 100 mg.

Chlorambucil

Benzenebutanoic acid, 4-[bis(2-chloroethyl)amino]-, Leukeran (*Burroughs Wellcome*)

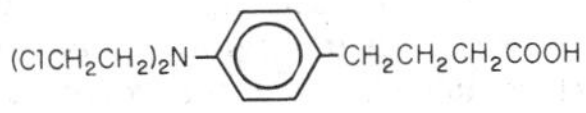

$(ClCH_2CH_2)_2N-C_6H_4-CH_2CH_2CH_2COOH$

4-[*p*-[Bis(2-chloroethyl)amino]phenyl]butyric acid [305-03-3] $C_{14}H_{19}Cl_2NO_2$ (304.22).

Caution—It is very poisonous. Great care should be taken to prevent inhaling its particles and exposing the skin to it.

Preparation—4-Phenylbutyric acid is nitrated and the resulting *p*-nitric acid is esterified with isopropyl alcohol. The nitro ester is then hydrogenated to the aminoester. Reaction with ethylene oxide converts the $—NH_2$ into $—N(CH_2CH_2OH)_2$ which is then converted into $—N(CH_2CH_2Cl)_2$ by treatment with $POCl_3$. Hydrolysis of the ester yields the acid, chlorambucil.

Description—Off-white, slightly granular powder.

Solubility—Very slightly soluble in water; soluble in dilute alkali; 1 g in 2 mL of acetone.

Uses—An alkylating agent effective by the oral route. It is approved for and is the agent of choice in the treatment of *chronic lymphocytic leukemia.* It also is effective in the treatment of Waldenstrom's *macroglobulinemia, multiple myeloma, lymphosarcoma, giant cell follicular lymphoma* and, to a lesser degree, in choriocarcinoma, Hogdkin's disease and ovarian and testicular tumors. As an immunosuppressant it is considered to be of value in the treatment of the *nephrotic syndrome* and *vasculitis* associated with *systemic lupus erythematosus, Wegner's granulomatosis, idiopathic membranous nephropathy* and *Behçet's disease.*

It is the slowest-acting and least toxic of currently used nitrogen mustards. Its toxicity is manifested mainly as bone-marrow depression, although in therapeutic doses it generally is moderate and reversible. Most patients will have some neutropenia after the third week of treatment until about 10 days after discontinuation of treatment. Slowly progressing lymphopenia also occurs, but it repairs itself quickly after treatment. Thrombocytopenia and anemia also occur sometimes. When the total accumulated dose exceeds 6.5 mg/kg the incidence of severe bone-marrow damage becomes high, and even irreversible toxicity may occur. It is mandatory that hemoglobin, leukocyte and platelet counts be monitored closely. It is contraindicated for four weeks after radiotherapy or other drugs that depress bone marrow. If possible, it should be avoided during the first trimester of pregnancy.

It is adsorbed well by the oral route. It is degraded extensively in the body. The elimination half-life is about 1.5 hr.

Dose—*Oral, adult, antineoplastic,* **0.1** to **0.2 mg/kg** *or* **3** to **6 mg/m²** a day once or in divided doses; *alternatively, initially* **0.4 mg/kg** or **12 mg/m²** a day, to be increased by 0.1 mg/kg or 3 mg/m² at biweekly intervals until either a therapeutic response or toxicity supravenes, after which the dosage is adjusted as needed; *immunosuppressant* in *nephrosis,* **0.1** to **0.2 mg/kg** once a day for 8 to 12 wk, not to exceed a total dose of 14 mg; *children, antineoplastic,* **0.1** to **0.2 mg/kg** or **4.5 mg/m²** a day once or in divided doses.

Dosage Form—Tablets: 2 mg.

Chloroquine Hydrochloride and Phosphate—page 1321.
Chromic Phosphate P32—page 856.

Cisplatin

Platinum, diamminedichloro-, (*SP*-4-2), Platinol (*Bristol*)

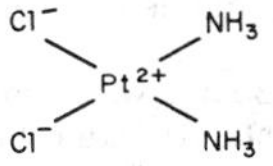

Cl^-, NH_3, Pt^{2+}, Cl^-, NH_3

cis-Diamminedichloroplatinum [15663-27-1] $Cl_2H_6N_2Pt$ (300.06).

Preparation—A solution of potassium tetrachloroplatinate(II), which is prepared by reduction of the hexachloroplatinate(II) salt with hydrazine, is neutralized with ammonium chloride and ammonium hydroxide. The *cis*-isomer precipitates (*Inorg Synth 7:*239, 1963).

Description—White, lyophylized powder; melts about 207°.

Solubility—1 g in about 1000 mL water or normal saline; 1 g in about 42 mL of dimethylformamide.

Uses—Cross-links DNA and hence acts like alkylating *antineoplastic* agents. It is approved as palliative relief for *metastatic testicular* and *ovarian tumors,* and *advanced bladder cancer.* It is used in various first-choice combinations for the treatment of *metastatic carcinomas of the testes, ovary, prostate, cervix* and *squamous cell carcinoma of the head and neck, small oat cell* and *non-small cell cancer of the lung, advanced cancer of the bladder, medulloblastoma* and *retinoblastoma* that has proved refractory to surgery and/or radiation. It also is used alone in the treatment of bladder cancer.

Acute toxicity includes severe nausea, vomiting and anorexia, occurs in almost all recipients but can be controlled largely with antiemetics. Occasional anaphylactoid reactions occur. Delayed toxicity includes ototoxicity (tinnitus and/or hearing loss in about 30% of patients), which requires audiometric monitoring: Fosfomycin has been reported to attenuate this side effect. Nephrotoxicity, which requires monitoring of serum creatinine, urate and of BUN and avoidance of other nephrotoxic drugs is a serious side effect in all patients and is controlled by forced diuresis (administration of drug in mannitol and saline) and hydration prior to administration. Bone marrow depression (in 25 to 30% of recipients), which requires leukocyte and platelet counts; occasional peripheral neuropathies, loss of taste and convulsions. Electrolyte deficits, perhaps from hemodilution by fluids, have been reported. It combines tightly with various proteins, which stimulates the immune system to produce various antibodies; the adverse effect of such immune stimulation are not known.

It is not absorbed orally and must be given intravenously. About 90% is bound to plasma proteins. It does not cross the blood-brain barrier. Elimination is mainly renal, partly by tubular secretion; excretion is nonlinear. The distribution half-life of the unbound drug is 25 to 49 min and the elimination half-life of total platinum is normally 58 to 73 hr but may be as long as 240 hr in anuria. However, platinum can be identified in tissues, especially liver, kidney, testes and intestine, for prolonged periods of time. Sodium thiosulfate decomposes the drug and complexes platinum and thus protects against renal damage and certain other toxicity.

Dose—*Intravenous,* for *metastatic testicular tumors* (in combination with bleomycin and vinblastine), **20 mg/m²** for 5 days every 3 wk for three courses; then, *maintenance* is accomplished with vinblastine alone; for *metastatic ovarian tumor* (in combination with doxorubicin); **50 mg/m²** every 3 wk or, *as a single agent,* **100 mg/m²** every 4 wk; for *bladder cancer,* **50** to **70 mg/m²** every 3 or 4 wk. All regimens are subject to modification according to hematologic, nephrologic, audiometric and other indices of toxicity. Intraperitoneal regimens for ovarian cancer and mesothelioma are more effective and less toxic than intravenous ones but presently are investigational.

Dosage Form—Injection: 10 and 50 mg. *Note*—Do not use aluminum-containing needles.

Cyclophosphamide

2*H*-1,3,2-Oxazaphosphorin-2-amine, *N,N*-bis(2-chloroethyl)tetrahydro-, 2-oxide, monohydrate; Cytoxan (*Bristol*); Neosar (*Adria*)

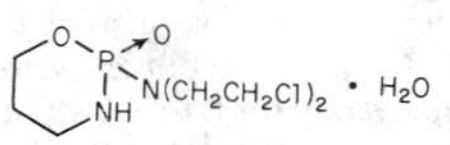

[6055-19-2] $C_7H_{15}Cl_2N_2O_2P.H_2O$ (279.10); anhydrous [50-18-0] (261.09)

Caution: Great care should be taken to prevent inhaling its particles and exposing the skin to it.

Preparation—3-Amino-1-propanol is condensed with *N,N*-bis(2-chloroethyl)phosphoramidic dichloride [$(ClCH_2CH_2)_2N$—$POCl_2$] in dioxane solution under the catalytic influence of triethylamine. The condensation is double, involving both the hydroxyl and the amino groups, thus effecting the cyclization.

Description—White, crystalline powder; liquefies on loss of its water of crystallization.

Solubility—1 g in about 25 mL water; soluble in alcohol.

Uses—An alkylating agent. Unlike other β-chloroethylamino alkylators, it does not cyclize readily to the active ethyleneimonium form until activated by hepatic enzymes. The liver is protected by the further metabolism of activated metabolites to inactive end products. Thus, the substance is stable in the gastrointestinal tract, tolerated well and effective by the oral and parenteral routes and does not cause local vesication, necrosis, phlebitis or even pain.

Cyclophosphamide is approved for *Stage III and IV, malignant lymphomas, multiple myeloma, leukemias, mycosis fungoides, neuroblastoma, retinoblastoma* and *carcinoma of the breast.* Alone or in combination, it is the drug of choice for treatment of *Burkitt's* and *non-Hodgkin's lymphomas.* It is a component of various first-choice combinations for treatment of *Hodgkin's disease, follicular lymphoma, diffuse histiocytic lymphoma, multiple myeloma, squamous cell* and *large-cell anaplastic carcinomas,* and *adenocarcinoma of the lung, small (oat) cell lung cancer, soft tissue sarcomas, embryonal rhabdomyosarcoma, osteogenic sarcoma, retinoblastoma, neuroblastoma, pediatric solid tumors, Ewing's sarcoma, breast tumor, ovarian tumors* and *testicular tumors.* In combination, it shares alternative drug status with various other drugs for chemotherapy of *acute lymphocytic leukemia, testicular cancer, Wilm's tumor, glioblastoma, cervical cancer, head and neck squamous cell carcinoma, islet cell carcinoma, Kaposi's sarcoma* and *chronic lymphocytic leukemia.* Active metabolites appear in CSF but in insufficient quantities to treat meningeal leukemia.

It is an *immunosuppressive drug.* It has been shown to be of value in the treatment of *rheumatoid arthritis, Wegner's granulomatosis, hemophilia A with factor VIII destruction, idiopathic thrombocytopenic purpura* (alone or in combination), *erythroid aplasia, childhood nephrotic syndrome, pemphigus vulgaris* and *dermatomyositis* (in combination). It appears to be erratic against *systemic lupus erythematosus.* It possibly may be efficacious in the management of *uveitis.* In combination with radiation treatment, it improves the survival of *bone marrow* and probably of *heart transplants.* The long-term toxicities of cyclophosphamide should be weighed if the drug is to be used as other than a cancer chemotherapeutic agent.

Alopecia occurs in about 50% of patients receiving maximal prolonged treatment. Leukopenia is the inevitable side effect and is used as an index of dosage. Other side effects include sterile hemorrhagic cystitis in 20% of those receiving treatment, anorexia, nausea and vomiting (regardless of route of administration), anaphylactoid reactions, fever, hemolytic-uremic reaction, pulmonary infiltrates and fibrosis, mucosal ulcerations, dizziness, occasional thrombocytopenia, hypoprothrombinemia, nail ridging, cutaneous pigmentation, water intoxication, aspermia in males (3 to 6 months or longer in onset), anovulation in 30 to 50% of females and occasional hepatic dysfunction. Bladder telangiectasis and abnormal urinary cytology occur; in long-term use, bladder fibrosis and transitional cell carcinoma occasionally occur. 2-Mercaptoethanesulfonate (Mesna) protects the bladder from this acrolein metabolite. The blood count should be monitored closely during induction and at least weekly thereafter. Cyclophosphamide is relatively platelet sparing; cyclophosphamide is carcinogenic.

It is absorbed orally. It is distributed to the tissues with a volume of distribution greater than the total body water. The drug is metabolized by the hepatic microsomal system to alkylating metabolites which, in turn, are converted to phosphoramide mustard and acrolein. High doses rapidly induce the metabolism of the drug. The plasma half-life is 4 to 6 hr.

Dose—*Oral, adult antineoplastic,* **1** to **5 mg/kg/day** (usually in combination), depending upon gastrointestinal tolerance; *rheumatoid arthritis, initially* **1.5** to **2 mg/kg/day,** to be increased to no more than 3 mg/kg/day; *Wegener's granulomatosis,* **1** to **2 mg/kg/day** (in combination with prednisone); *children, antineoplastic, initially* **2** to **8 mg/kg/day** *or* **60** to **250 mg/m²/day** in divided doses for 6 or more days then, for *maintenance,* **2** to **5 mg/kg** *or* **50** to **150 mg/m²** twice a week. *Intravenous, adult, antineoplastic, initially* **40** to **50 mg/kg** in divided doses over a period of 2 to 5 days then, for *maintenance,* **10** to **15 mg/kg** every 7 to 10 days *or* **3** to **5 mg/kg** twice a week *or* **1.5** to **3 mg/kg/day;** *children, antineoplastic, initially* **2** to **8 mg/kg/day** *or* **250 mg/kg/m²/day** for 6 or more days then, for *maintenance,* **10** to **15 mg/kg** every 7 to 10 days or every 3 to 4 wk, depending upon when hematopoiesis recovers. Because of gastrointestinal adverse effects, the intravenous route is preferred for loading. During maintenance, a leukocyte count of 3000 to 4000/mm³ usually is desired. The drug also sometimes is administered intramuscularly, by infiltration or into body cavities.

Dosage Forms—Injection: 100, 200 and 500 mg; Tablets: 25 and 50 mg.

Cyclosporine

Sandimmune (*Sandoz*)

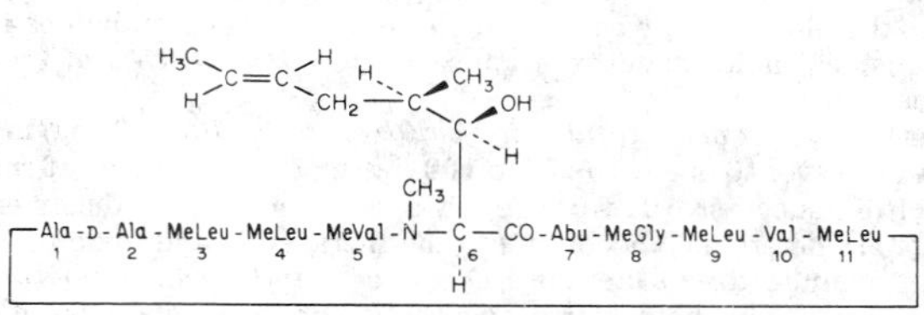

Cyclosporin A [59865-13-3] $C_{62}H_{111}N_{11}O_{12}$ (1202.63).

Preparation—A metabolite of *Cylindrocarpon lucidum* and *Trichoderma polysporum.*

Solubility—Practically insoluble in water; soluble in ethanol or fixed oils.

Uses—Suppresses helper T lymphocytes without significantly affecting suppressor T or B lymphocytes. Thus, it is a selective immunosuppressive drug without the cytotoxicity characteristic of most other immunosuppressive drugs. Since it works only in the primary (afferent) immune phase, it must be administered before exposure to the attacking antigen. It has a modest effect to suppress some humoral immunity.

It is the most efficacious *immunosuppressive* and is approved for prevention of graft rejection in *allogenic transplantation of kidney, liver* or *heart.* It is less successful in *pancreatic, lung* or *bone-marrow transplantation.* It also is used in the management of severe aplastic anemia, some cases of myasthenia gravis, childhood diabetes (Type I) of recent onset, Graves' disease, Crohn's disease, multiple sclerosis, pemphigus and pemphigoid, dermatomyositis, polymyositis, atopic dermatitis, severe psoriasis, Bechçet's disease, uveitis, biliary cirrhosis and pulmonary sarcoidosis. It usually is employed in combination with a glucocorticoid. Although combination with other immunosuppressives usually is avoided, in bone-marrow transplantation it commonly is combined with methotrexate.

Nephrotoxicity is a common, serious adverse effect, occurring with an incidence of about 25% in renal and 40% in heart transplantations. In renal transplantation, nephrotoxicity is difficult to distinguish from graft rejection. NSAIDs, aminoglycosides, trimethoprim and/or sulfamethoxozole favor nephrotoxicity. Hepatotoxicity occurs in 4 to 7% of cases.

Hypertension occurs in about 26% of cases. Benign breast tumors and lymphoproliferative disorders may occur; the latter usually remit after the drug is discontinued.

CNS toxicity includes headache, parethesias (50%), lethargy, weakness, loquaciousness, sleep disorders, confusion, depression, blurred vision, tremors (12%), ataxia, quadraplegia, coma, hallucinations, mania and convulsions. Severe CNS effects have been associated with low plasma cholesterol, hypomagnesemia, hypokalemia, high-dose methylprednisolone, aluminum overload (from dialysis) and hypertension.

Hirsutism occurs with an incidence of 21% and acne with 6%. Gum hyperplasia and diarrhea occur in 3 to 4% of cases. Leucopenia, anemia and thromboembolism occur rarely. Insulin-dependent diabetes may result from cyclosporine-glucocorticoid combination. Rare anaphylactoid reactions occur during intravenous infusion; polyoxyethylated castor oil in the injection is the usual culprit. There is a danger of severe infection, especially when other immunosuppressives or verapamil are used concurrently. It is teratogenic. It also is exceedingly expensive, which leads some authorities to doubt the cost-effectiveness of the drug.

The systemic bioavailability by the oral route averages 27% but varies greatly; the intravenous dose is about ⅓ the oral dose. Plasma levels peak in about 3.5 hr. In plasma, about 90% is protein-bound. The pharmacokinetics are multicompartmental. The volume of distribution is 1 to 13 (av 4) L/kg; it is concentration-dependent. Nearly all of the drug is metabolized by cytochrome P450 III in the liver; 94% of the metabolites are excreted into the bile and 6% into the urine. The elimination half-life is 10 to 27 hr; there is a circadian periodicity to the elimination rate, the rate being faster in the morning. In infants and children, the volume of distribution and clearance are greater than in adults. Androgens, cimetidine, danazol, erythromycin, ketoconazole and miconazole each slows the elimination rate and increases plasma levels. Trough plasma levels should be monitored daily as should be renal function since many treatment failures result from low concentrations.

Dose—*Intravenous infusion, adults and children,* **2** to **6 mg/kg/day,** starting 4 to 12 hr before transplantation and continuing until oral dosage can be tolerated. (The IV route is to be used only when the oral route is precluded.) *Oral, adults and children, initially* **12** to **15 mg/kg/day** starting 4 to 12 hr before transplantation or after IV infusion and continuing for 1 to 2 wk, after which the dose is diminished by 5% wk to a *maintenance* dose of **5** to **10 mg/kg/day.**

Dosage Forms—Injection: 250 mg/5 mL; Oral Solution: 5 g/100 mL.

Cytarabine

2(1*H*)-Pyrimidinone,4-amino-1-β-D-arabinofuranosyl-, Cytosine Arabinoside; Cytarabine (*Quad*) Cytosar-U (*Upjohn*)

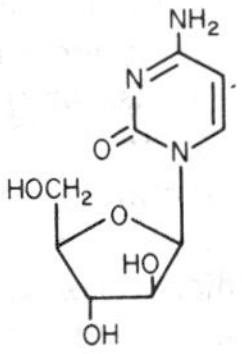

1-β-D-Arabinofuranosylcytosine [147-94-4] $C_9H_{13}N_3O_5$ (243.22).

Preparation—Cytidine is reacted with fuming HNO_3 and the resulting cytidine 2′,3′,5′-trinitrate is boiled in alcohol containing dilute alkali hydroxide to form the inverted 2′-hydroxy compound. Remaining nitrate groups are removed via saponification. *CA 75:*130077q, 1971.

Description—White to off-white, odorless, crystalline powder; nonhygroscopic and stable at 40°; melts about 216°.

Solubility—1 g in 5 mL water, 500 mL alcohol, 1000 mL chloroform or 300 mL methanol.

Uses—A pyrimidine nucleoside antimetabolite that is cytotoxic to a number of cell types. Incorporation of the nucleotidase into DNA inhibits polymerization by termination of strand synthesis. It is S-phase specific. It is approved for use in *acute lymphocytic leukemia.* It is a component of first-choice combinations to treat both *acute* and *chronic myeloblastic leukemias* and *non-Hodgkin's* and *Burkitt's lymphomas.* By the intraventricular route, it is the first alternate to methotrexate to treat *leukemic metastases in the CNS* and also other meningeal soft-tissue metastases. With other drugs it shares alternative-drug status for treatment of *acute lymphocytic leukemia* and *diffuse histiocytic lymphoma.* There does not appear to be cross-refractoriness to mercaptopurine, methotrexate or prednisone. By constant intravenous infusion, or with frequent low doses, it is also effective in the treatment of *preleukemic syndromes.*

As an immunosuppressant, it suppresses primary (afferent) responses in doses that cause little or no other toxicity. It is under active clinical investigation.

This drug is not absorbed sufficiently orally to be maximally effective by this route. Oral bioavailability is less than 0.2. However, it does penetrate into the cerebrospinal fluid and reaches a concentration up to 40% of that in plasma. Conversely, intrathecal administration can result in systemic toxicity. In the body, 90% is destroyed by deamination; the plasma elimination half-life is 1 to 3 hr. The elimination half-life in cerebral spinal fluid is about 3.5 hr. Since detoxification takes place throughout the body, the drug may be given in the presence of renal impairment, but the dose should be reduced in hepatic failure.

The primary adverse effects are leukopenia (66%), thrombocytopenia (62%) and, less frequently, anemia and megaloblastosis, which are actually closely related to the therapeutic response and, hence, are essentially unavoidable. Bone-marrow depression is more severe when the drug is given in high-dose regimens (15 times the usual dose) and by continuous intravenous infusion than by single injection. However, there are indications that with low rates of infusion an antineoplastic effect can be achieved without serious immunosuppression.

Other side effects are nausea, vomiting (especially after intravenous administration), diarrhea, aphthous ulceration, abdominal pain and bowel-necrosis, esophagitis, chest pain, thrombophlebitis at the site of injection, neuritis, arthalgias, flushing, rash, alopecia, sepsis and teratogenicity. Liver damage may occur. It should be given cautiously and in reduced doses to patients with liver impairment or bone-marrow depression. It must not be given in combination with methotrexate. Leukocyte and platelet counts should be made daily during the initial course of treatment and at regular intervals during maintenance. High-dose treatment may cause serious neurotoxicity (in peripheral nerves, mood, ideation, memory, cerebellum and seizures) and skin and ocular toxicities.

Dose—*Adult and children, rapid intravenous injection, initially* **200 mg/m²/day** *or* **3 mg/kg/day** in divided doses for 7 days; causes are repeated at intervals of about 2 wk; once an antileukemic response (neutrophils less than 1000/mm³) or hematologic toxicity (platelets less than 50,000/mm³) has occurred, the dose-interval is increased or subcutaneous maintenance is instituted; *preleukemic syndrome,* **10 mg/m²** twice a day for 21 days. *Constant intravenous infusion, initially* **200 mg/m²/day** or **3 mg/kg/day** for 7 days; courses are repeated and maintenance conducted as above; in combination with other antineoplastics, **100 mg/kg/day** for 7 to 10 days per course; constant infusion is preferred to rapid injection. *Subcutaneous, for maintenance,* **1 mg/kg/day** or semiweekly. *Intrathecally,* for acute CNS leukemia, **5** to **75 mg/m²** once a day for 4 days to once every 4 days; 30 mg/m² is the usual dose.

Dosage Form—Injection: 100, 500 mg, and 2g (vials).

Dacarbazine

1*H*-Imidazole-4-carboxamide,5-(3,3-dimethyl-l-triazenyl)-, DIC; DTIC-Dome (*Miles*)

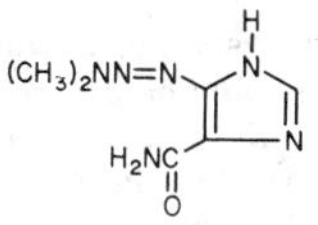

5-(3,3-Dimethyl-l-triazeno)imidazole-4-carboxamide [4342-03-4] $C_6H_{10}N_6O$(182.18).

Preparation—5-Diazoimidazole-4-carboxamide, obtained by reaction between 5-aminoimidazole-4-carboxamide and sodium nitrite in acid solution, is reacted with an anhydrous solution of dimethylamine in methanol at 5° to produce dacarbazine (Shealy *et al, J Org Chem 17:* 2150, 1962).

Description—Colorless to ivory-colored microcrystalline powder; sensitive to light and heat; reported to melt at 205° and decompose explosively at 250 to 255°; pK_a 4.42.

Solubility—Slightly soluble in water or alcohol.

Uses—It is converted in the body to an alkylating metabolite that primarily impairs DNA. It is approved for and shares a first-choice status with semustine in the treatment of *metastatic malignant melanoma.* The objective response rate is only about 20%. It is also a component of first-choice combinations for *Hodgkin's disease* (ABVD), and is useful in some adult soft tissue tumors. With several drugs it shares alternative status for *islet-cell carcinoma* and *neuroblastoma.*

The most serious adverse effect is bone-marrow depression, which occasionally is fatal; the myelogenous leukocytes and platelets are the most affected, anemia being mild, when it occurs. Careful monitoring of leukocytes, platelets and erythrocytes is required. If there is preexisting bone-marrow depression, or if another bone-marrow suppressant drug is in use or has been used within 4 wk, the dose must be reduced. Anorexia, nausea and vomiting lasting 1 to 12 hr occur in over 90% of recipients of the drug; tolerance occurs after the first few doses; phenobarbital or prochlorperazine occasionally will arrest the vomiting. Diarrhea occurs rarely; food and fluid intake usually are restricted. An influenza-like syndrome accompanied by fever up to 39°, myalgia and malaise, sometimes occurs approximately 1 week after large doses and may continue for 1 to 3 wk. Facial flushing, facial paresthesias and alopecia also have been observed. Abnormalities in liver or renal function have been reported, and the drug should be used cautiously in patients with liver or renal damage. Extravasation of dacarbazine may cause pain and local necrosis. The drug is fetotoxic and teratogenic.

It is eliminated with a terminal half-life of 5 hr. Approximately 50% of an intravenous dose is metabolized in the liver; by the oral route, very little remains unchanged, thus making the intravenous route necessary. About 40% of the drug appears unchanged in the urine within 6 hr. The unmetabolized drug is excreted in the urine by tubular secretion. The volume of distribution is larger than total body water.

Dose—*Intravenous, adult,* **2** to **4.5 mg/kg/day** for 10 days; the higher doses do not appear to be more efficacious than the lower ones. The course is repeated at 4-wk intervals. Alternative regimens are **150 mg/m²/day** for 5 days, repeated every 3 wk.

Other Dose Information—100 mg and 200 mg are reconstituted with 9.9 and 19.7 mL of sterile water, respectively. The duration of injection should be no less than 1 min.

Dosage Form—Injection: 100/10 mL and 200 mg/20 mL.

Dactinomycin

Dactinomycin; Meractinomycin; Cosmegen (*MSD*)

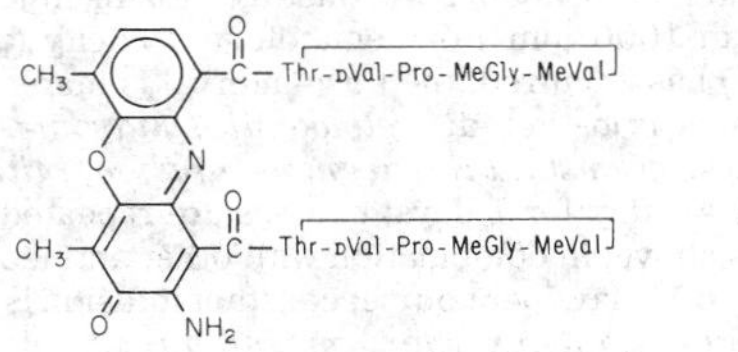

Actinomycin D [50-76-0]; $C_{62}H_{86}N_{12}O_{16}$ (1255.43).

Caution—Handle it with exceptional care, to prevent inhaling particles of it and exposing the skin to it.

Preparation—Elaborated during the culture of *Streptomyces parvulus.* After extracting from the fermentation broth, it is purified through chromatographic and crystallization processes. US Pat 2,378,876.

Description—Bright-red crystalline powder; light-sensitive and should be protected appropriately; should be protected from excessive heat and moisture; melts about 246° with the decomposition; contains in each mg an amount of antibiotic activity of not less than 900 μg of dactinomycin.

Solubility—1 g in about 8 mL alcohol, 25 mL water (at 10°), 1000 mL water (at 37°) or about 1666 mL ether.

Uses—An antineoplastic drug that inhibits DNA-dependent RNA polymerase, approved for use in *Wilm's tumor, rhabdomyosarcoma* and *carcinoma of the testis and uterus.* It is a component of first-choice combinations for treatment of *choriocarcinoma, embryonal rhabdomyosarcoma* and *Wilm's tumor.* It no longer has alternative drug status for any purpose, although it is still approved for use against Ewing's sarcoma, testicular carcinoma and sarcoma botyroides. Tumors which fail to respond to systemic treatment sometimes respond to local perfusion. Dactinomycin potentiates radiotherapy ("radiation recall"). It is a secondary (efferent) immunosuppressive.

Nausea and vomiting are usual and occur within the first few hours after administration of dactinomycin. Anorexia, abdominal pain, diarrhea, proctitis and gastrointestinal ulceration follow. The patient also may experience malaise, fatigue, lethargy, myalgia and fever. Cheilitis, ulcerative stomatitis, pharyngitis, esophagitis and proctitis are common. Because agranulocytosis, leukopenia, pancytopenia, thrombocytopenia and anemia frequently occur, *the blood picture must be monitored daily.* Cutaneous eruptions, alopecia, hyperpigmentation and erythema also occur. Anaphylaxis has been reported. Side effects appear to be reversible. The drug is toxic locally, and phlebitis and cellulitis may occur at the site of injection; extravasation may cause serious local tissue damage. Venous thrombosis also may result from local effects.

Half of the dose is excreted intact into the bile and 10% into the urine; the half-life is about 36 hr. The drug does not pass the blood-brain barrier.

Dose—*Intraarterial tumor perfusion, adults* and *children, lower extremity* or *pelvis,* **0.05 mg/kg;** *upper extremity,* **0.035 mg/kg.** *Intravenous, adult,* **0.01 to 0.015 mg/kg** for no more than 5 days every 4 to 6 wk *or* **0.5 mg/m²**, not to exceed 2 mg, once a week for 3 wk; *children,* **0.01 to 0.015 mg/kg** for no more than 5 days *or* **2.4 mg/m²** divided over 7 days, to be followed in 4 to 6 wk by a second course if toxicity has abated.

Dosage Form—Injection: 0.5 mg (500 μg).

Diethylstilbestrol Diphosphate—page 1092.

Daunorubicin Hydrochloride

5,12-Naphthacenedione, (8*S*-cis)-8-acetyl-10-[(3-amino-2,3,6-trideoxy-α-L-*lyxo*-hexanopyranosyl)oxy]-7,8,9,10-tetrahydro-6,8,11-trihydroxy-10-methoxy-, hydrochloride; Cerubidine (*Wyeth*).

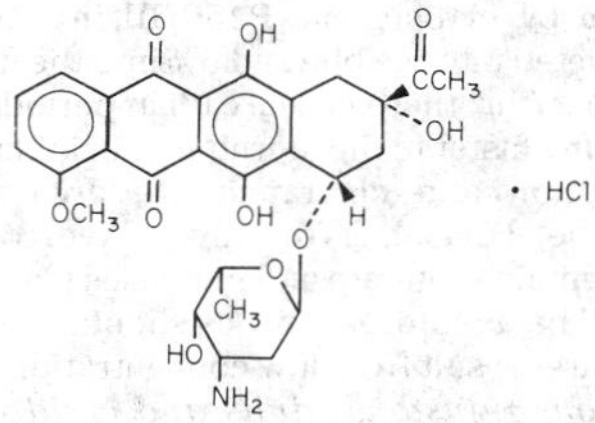

[23541-50-6] $C_{27}H_{29}NO_{10}.HCl$ (563.99).

Preparation—An antibiotic produced by *S peuceticus* or *S coeruleorubidus.*

Description—Red needles decomposing about 190°; pH (aqueous solution containing 5 mg per mL) 4.5 to 6.5

Solubility—Soluble in water, methanol or ethanol; insoluble in ether or chloroform.

Uses—Intercalates into DNA, inhibits topoisomerase II, and produces oxygen radicals and inhibits DNA synthesis. It can prevent cell division in doses that do not interfere with nucleic acid synthesis.

It is approved for use in *acute nonlymphocytic leukemia* in adults and for *acute lymphocytic leukemia* in adults and children. In combination with other drugs it is included in the first-choice chemotherapy of *acute myelocytic leukemia* in adults (for induction of remission), *acute lymphocytic leukemia* and the *acute phase of chronic myelocytic leukemia.* The drug is not given as a single agent.

Acutely, it causes nausea, vomiting, fever and rarely convulsions, cardiac dysrhythmias and S-T depression and pulmonary edema, occasionally fatal. Phlebitis at the site of injection or a slough from extravasation may occur. It also colors the urine red. Delayed toxicity includes frequent bone-marrow depression (with leukopenia and thrombocytopenia), which may be severe, and a dose-limiting congestive heart failure. Other toxicities include stomatitis and aphthous ulceration, anorexia, hemorrhagic mucositis enterocolitis, abdominal pain, fever, rashes, usually reversible alopecia (in 80% of recipients), renal tubular damage and hematuria. Cardiotoxicity also may be delayed. Rhythm disturbances are not related to cumulative dose, but a late congestive heart failure is frequent when the cumulative dose exceeds 550 mg/m². The onset of failure may occur as long as 1 to 6 mo after discontinuation of treatment. Daunorubicin is teratogenic, mutagenic and carcinogenic. Monitoring of blood-cell counts, renal function and ECG is required.

Oral absorption is poor, and it must be given intravenously. The half-life of distribution is 45 min and of elimination, about 19 hr. The half-life of its active metabolite, daunorubicinol, is about 27 hr. Daunorubicin is metabolized mostly in the liver and also secreted into the bile (*ca* 40%). Dosage must be reduced in liver or renal insufficiencies.

Dose (base equivalent)—*Intravenous adult, younger than 60 yr* **45 mg/m²/day** (30 mg/m² for patients older than 60 yr) for 1, 2 or 3 days every 3 or 4 wk or **0.8 mg/kg/day** for 3 to 6 days every 3 or 4 wk; no more than 550 mg/m² should be given in a lifetime, except only 450 mg/m² if there has been chest irradiation; *children,* **25 mg/m²** once a week unless the age is less than 2 yr or the body surface less than 0.5 m, in which case the weight-based adult schedule is used.

Dosage Form (base equivalent)—Injection: 20 mg (as the base equivalent to 21.4 mg of the hydrochloride).

Doxorubicin Hydrochloride

5,12-Naphthacenedione, (8*S-cis*)-10-[(3-amino-2,3,6-trideoxy-α-L-*lyxo*-hexopyransoyl)oxy]-7,8,9,10-tetrahydro-6,8,11-trihydroxy-8-(hydroxyacetyl)-1-methoxy-, hydrochloride; Hydroxydaunorubicin Hydrochloride; Adriamycin (*Adria*)
Rubex (*Bristol*); Doxorubicin (*Cetus*)

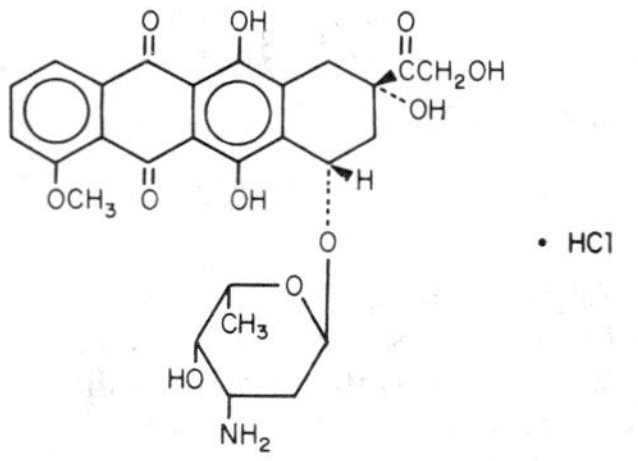

14-Hydroxydaunorubicin hydrochloride [25316-40-9] $C_{27}H_{29}NO_{11}$.HCl (579.99).

Preparation—An anthracycline antibiotic isolated from cultures of *Streptomyces peucetius* var *caesius* (US Pat 3,590,028). It differs from *Daunorubicin* only in having a hydroxyacetyl group in place of the acetyl group in daunorubicin, in postion 8.

Description—Red-orange, crystalline powder; almost odorless; hygroscopic; melts about 205° with decomposition; pK_a 8.22.

Solubility—1 g dissolves in about 10 mL water or about 2000 mL alcohol.

Uses—Approved for use in *acute lymphoblastic* and *myeloblastic leukemias, Hodgkin's* and *non-Hodgkin's lymphomas, Wilm's tumor, neuroblastoma, sarcomas* and *breast, ovarian, transitional cell, bronchogenic, gastric* and *thyroid carcinomas.* Has the widest antineoplastic spectrum and usefulness of the antineoplastic drugs. It binds to DNA and inhibits nucleic acid synthesis, inhibits topoisomerase II and produces oxygen radicals. Administered alone, it is the drug of first choice for the treatment of *thyroid adenoma* and *primary hepatocellular carcinoma.* It is a component of 31 first-choice combinations for the treatment of *ovarian, endometrial* and *breast tumors, bronchogenic oat-cell carcinoma, non-small cell lung carcinoma, gastric adenocarcinoma, retinoblastoma, neuroblastoma, mycosis fungoides, pancreatic carcinoma, prostatic carcinoma, bladder carcinoma, myeloma, diffuse histiocytic lymphoma, Wilms' tumor, Hodgkin's disease, adrenal tumors, osteogenic sarcoma, soft tissue sarcoma, Ewing's sarcoma, rhabdomyosarcoma* and *acute lymhocytic leukemia.* It is an alternative drug for the treatment of *islet cell, cervical, testicular* and *adrenocortical* cancer. It is also an immunosuppressant, but its status remains to be determined. Tumor resistance to this drug may be suppressed by verapamil.

There is a high incidence of bone-marrow depression, which manifests itself mainly as a neutropenia that is most severe 10 to 14 days after treatment and lasts about 7 days; a white-cell count as low as 1000/mm^3 is to be expected. Monitoring of leukocytes and erythrocytes and signs of intercurrent infection is mandatory. Other frequent adverse effects are nausea and vomiting and reversible alopecia. Stomatitis and esophagitis may occur 5 to 10 days after treatment. Anorexia and diarrhea occur occasionally. Rarely, there may be hypersensitivity (fever, chills, urticaria), hyperpigmentation of the nails, lacrimation, conjunctivitis and recurrence of skin reactions caused by prior radiotherapy. Hyperuricemia from rapid lysis of neoplastic cells may occur.

A serious toxicity is acute left-ventricular cardiomyopathy, which is refractory to digitalis. An early change in ECG patterns is not prodromal of the more serious congestive heart failure. This cardiotoxicity is most likely to occur with patients in whom the cumulated dose is 550 mg/m^2. Prior radiotherapy to the chest, concomitant cyclophasphamide therapy or hyperthermia may cause the cardiomyopathy to occur with a total dose as low as 400 mg/m^2. Antineoplastic activity has been dissociated from cardiotoxicity in certain chemical congeners which may eventually replace this drug. Toxicity appears to result from oxidant and free-radical metabolites. Certain antioxidants, especially bispiperazinedione (ICRF-187) and α-tocopherol protect against cardiotoxicity without affecting the antineoplastic properties.

It is locally toxic and causes venous streaking, and extravasation results in pain, cellulitis and sloughing. Its natural color may cause the urine to be red. It may potentiate hemorrhagic cystitis caused by cyclophosphamide, mucositis by radiotherapy, hepatotoxicity by 6-mercaptopurine and the bone-marrow depressant actions of other antineoplastic drugs.

It is absorbed poorly and must be administered intravenously. The pharmacokinetics are multicompartmental. Distribution phases have half-lives of 12 min and 3.3 hr. The elimination half-life is about 30 hr. Forty to 50% is secreted into the bile. Most of the remainder is metabolized in the liver, partly to an active metabolite (doxorubicinol), but a few percent is excreted into the urine. In the presence of liver impairment, the dose should be reduced.

Dose—*Intravenous, adult,* **60** to **75 mg/m²** at 21-day intervals or **25** to **30 mg/m²** on each of 2 or 3 successive days repeated at 3- or 4-wk intervals *or* **20 mg/m²** once a wk. The lowest dose should be used in elderly patients, when there is prior bone-marrow depression caused by prior chemotherapy or neoplastic marrow invasion, or when the drug is combined with other myelopoietic suppressant drugs. The dose should be reduced by 50% if the serum bilirubin lies between 1.2 and 3 mg/dL and by 75% if above 3 mg/dL. The lifetime total dose should not exceed 550 mg/m^2 in patients with normal heart function and 400 mg/m^2 in persons having received mediastinal irradiation. Children, **30 mg/m²** on each of 3 consecutive days, repeated every 4 wk. Prescribing limits are as with adults.

It has been reported that a 96-hr continuous infusion is as effective as and much less toxic than the same dose given by bolus injections by decreasing peak blood level.

Other Dose Information—The contents of the vial should be reconstituted to a final concentration of 2 mg/mL. The solution then should be injected into a freely running intravenous infusion of sodium chloride injection or 5% dextrose injection at a rate such that the dose not be administered in less than 5 min.

Dosage Form—Injection: 10 and 50 mg.

Dromostanolone Propionate—see RPS-17, page 998.

Estramustine Phosphate Sodium

Estra-1,3,5(10)-triene-3,17-diol(17β)-, 3-[bis (2-chloroethyl)carbamate] 17-(dihydrogen phosphate), disodium salt; Emcyt (*Roche*)

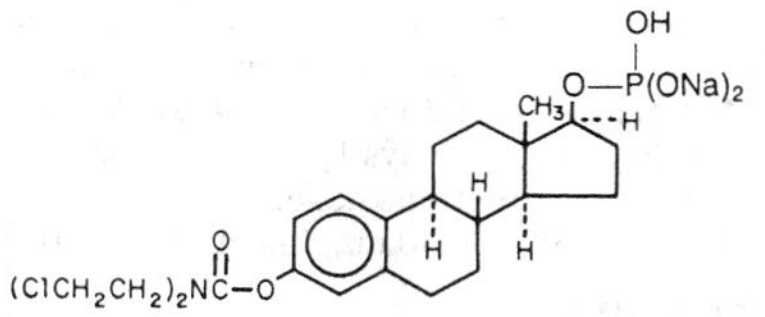

[52205-73-9] $C_{23}H_{30}Cl_2NNa_2O_6P$ (564.35).

Preparation—A compound of estradiol with a nitrogen mustard moiety.

Description—Off-white powder.

Solubility—Freely soluble in water or methanol; very slightly soluble in chloroform or anhydrous ethanol; pH of 0.5% solution; 8.5 to 10.0.

Uses—An alkylating agent that is among several aternative drugs for treatment of *cancer of the prostate* gland. It is approved for *metastatic cancer of the prostate.* It causes nausea and vomiting, delayed bone-marrow depression, mild gynecomastia, perianal anesthesia, thrombophlebitis, occasional myocardial infarction, hypertension, hypoglycemia and hepatotoxicity. It is carcinogenic in animals.

Dose—*Oral.* **600 mg/m²/day** (10 to 16 mg/kg/day) in 3 or 4 divided doses; treatment has been continued for as long as 3 yr. In combinations, the dose may be the same, but when combined with other bone-marrow depressant drugs it may have to be reduced.

Dosage Form—Capsules: equivalent to 140 mg of estramustine phosphate.

Ethinyl Estradiol—page 1091.

Etoposide

Vepesid (*Bristol*)

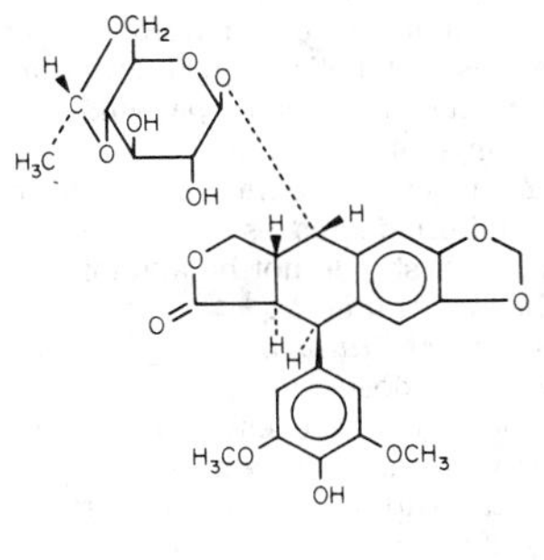

9-[(4,6-*O*-Ethylidene-β-D-glucopyranosyl)oxy]-5,8,8a,9-tetrahydro-5-(4-hydroxy-3,5-dimethoxyphenyl)furo[3′,4′:6,7]-naphtho[2,3-*d*]-1,3-dioxol-6(5a*H*)-one [33419-42-0] $C_{29}H_{32}O_{13}$ (588.56).

Preparation—A semisynthetic derivative of podophyllotoxin. See *J Med Chem 14:* 936, 1971.

Description—White to yellow-brown powder; melts about 221°.

Solubility—Very soluble in methanol or chloroform; slightly soluble in ethanol; sparingly soluble in water or ether.

Uses—Damages DNA, most likely via topoisomerase II cleavage, and arrests the cell cycle primarily in Phase G_2, although it has some action in late S and M. It is approved for *refractory testicular tumors* and *small cell lung cancer*. Alone, it is one of two drugs of choice for the treatmentof *Kaposi's sarcoma* and one of three for *non-Hodgkin's lymphoma*. It also is a component of first-choice combinations to treat *oat-cell bronchogenic carcinoma* and *refractory disseminated germ-cell tumors*. It is an alternative drug for use against *acute lymphocytic leukemia, acute myelocytic leukemia, Hodgkin's disease, Wilm's tumor, choriocarcinoma, diffuse histiocytic lymphoma, Ewing's sarcoma, hepatocellular carcinoma, neuroblastoma, non-Hodgkin's lymphoma* and *non-small cell bronchogenic carcinoma*.

Acute adverse effects are mild nausea and vomiting, chills and fever; postural hypotension, tachycardia, palpitations and bronchospasm occur during and after rapid intravenous infusion. Delayed toxicity includes leukopenia (in 60 to 90% of recipients), thrombocytopenia (in 28 to 41%), anemia (in ≤33%), diarrhea, fever, alopecia, rash, stomatitis, Stevens-Johnson syndrome, various other allergic responses, hepatotoxicity (in 3%) and peripheral neuropathy. It increases the hypoprothrombopenic affects of warfarin.

Peroral absorption is 25 to 75%. In plasma, about 94% is protein-bound, and the concentration in the cerebral spinal fluid is less than 10% of that in plasma. Distribution is slow, the initial half-life being about 1.5 hr. About 35% is excreted unchanged in the urine and about 6% into bile. A hydroxyacid metabolite is excreted in the bile, and the sulfate and glucuronide metabolites are excreted in urine. The elimination half-life is 4 to 11 hr.

Dose—*Intravenous, adult, small cell lung carcinoma,* **35** to **50 mg/m²/day** for 4 or 5 days, repeated every 3 or 4 wk; *testicular carcinoma,* **50** to **100 mg/m²/day** (infused over 30 to 60 min) for 5 days every 3 or 4 wk *or* **100 mg/m²/day** on days 1, 3 and 5, repeated every 3 or 4 wk. *Oral, adult,* **twice** the **intravenous** dose.

Dosage Forms—Capsules: 50 mg; Injection: 100 mg/5 mL.

Etretinate—page 881.

Filgrastim

Granulocyte-Colony-Stimulating Factor Recombinant; Neupogen (*Amgen*)

See also *Filgrastim,* Chapter 54, page 940.

Uses—A single-chain polypeptide containing 175 amino acids. Filgrastim is produced by *E coli,* and therefore has an *N*-terminal methionine. Unlike the human protein, the recombinant form is not glycosylated. The drug is purified from bacterial cultures primarily by chromatographic means. Neupogen is approved for use in patients with nonmyeloid malignancies, suffering neutropenia receiving myelosuppressive anticancer agents. Endogenous G-CSF is produced by monocytes, fibroblasts and other cells, and acts on neutrophil-granulocyte progenitor cells by binding to specific G-CSF receptors. G-CSF is relatively cell line specific, acting to stimulate neutrophil-committed stem cell proliferation, differentiation and activation. It also appears to stimulate mature neutrophil chemotaxis and phagocytosis, among other functions. Eosinophils, basophils and erythrocytes do not appear to be affected by filgrastim.

It generally is tolerated well; bone pain is the most common adverse effect. Adverse dermatological effects may be due to increased neutrophils. Such reactions include acute febrile neutrophilic dermatosis, leukoblastic vasculitis and exacerbated psoriasis. Splenomegaly also has been documented, possibly due to extramedullary myelopoiesis. Drug should be discontinued at blood white cell counts >10,000/µl. Clinical studies have thus far failed to detect development of antibodies to *E coli* or *filgrastim* in filgrastim-treated patients. Use of filgrastim may promote the growth of myeloid leukemic blasts.

The half-life of filgastrim is approximately 1.3 hr, but may be longer at higher doses. Renal failure decreases clearance. It is absorbed rapidly following SC injection. It should not be administered within 24 hr of a myelosuppressive chemotherapeutic.

Dose—*Subcutaneous, initially* **5 µg/kg**/day, given for up to 2 wk after chemotherapy. The dose may be increased in increments of 5 µg/kg/day on subsequent cycles; doses of 20 and 60 µg/kg/day have been used after bone-marrow transplantation, and patients have received as much as 115 µg/kg/day without adverse effects. A 2-week supply of filgrastim costs over $2000.

Dosage Form—Injection: 1 mL (contains 300 µg filgrastim, 0.59 mg acetate, 50 mg mannitol, and 0.004% Tween.

Floxuridine

Uridine, 2′-deoxy-5-fluoro-, FUDR (*Roche*)

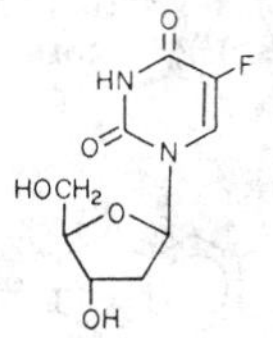

[50-91-9] $C_9H_{11}FN_2O_5$ (246.19).

Preparation—*J Am Chem Soc, 81:*4112, 1959.

Description—White to off-white, odorless solid; melts about 151°.

Solubility—1 g in 3 mL water, 12 mL alcohol or more than 10,000 mL chloroform or ether; pH of 2% solution, 4.0 to 5.5.

Uses—In the body it is converted into a false nucleotide which interferes with the synthesis of DNA. It also is converted to fluorouracil, so that it potentially has all the actions and uses of *Fluorouracil* (page 1251). It is approved for *GI adenocarcinoma with metastasis to the liver*. However, at present its use is restricted to regional intraarterial infusion of carcinomata which are judged incurable by surgery or other chemotherapy, mainly *colorectal cancer metastatic to the liver* and *hepatocellular carcinoma*. In these uses, it does not appear to be superior to fluorouracil.

The most frequent adverse effects are nausea, vomiting, diarrhea, enteritis, localized erythema along the course of infused artery, leukopenia and elevation in serum transaminase, alkaline phosphatase, bilirubin and lactic dehydrogenase. Other effects are abdominal cramps, anorexia, duodenal ulcer, duodenitis, gastroenteritis, pharyngitis, glossitis, gastritis, alopecia, dermititis, hyperpigmentation, edema, peeling of the skin, pruritus, various rashes and skin ulceration, abscesses, ataxia, blurred vision, convulsions, depression, hemiplegia, hiccoughs, lethargy, nystagmus, malaise, pain, vertigo, asthenia, dysuria, fever, hypoadrenalism, thrombocytopenia, prothrombinopenia, hypoproteinemia and aberrations in the sedimentation rate and BSP test.

It is contraindicated in patients with cachexia, potentially serious infections or bone-marrow depression. The drug is metabolized mainly in the body, but some is excreted unchanged in the urine.

Dose—*Continuous arterial infusion,* **0.1** to **0.6 mg** (100 to 600 µg)/kg/day. The higher end of the dose range (0.4 to 0.6 mg/kg/day) is reserved for hepatic artery infusion, since the liver metabolizes the drug and so decreases systemic toxicity.

Dosage Forms—Injection: 500 mg to be reconstituted with 5 mL of Water for Injection.

Fludarabine Phosphate

9*H*-Purin-6-amine, 2-fluoro-9-(5-*O*-phosphono-β-D-arabinofuranosyl)-, Fludara (*Berlex*)

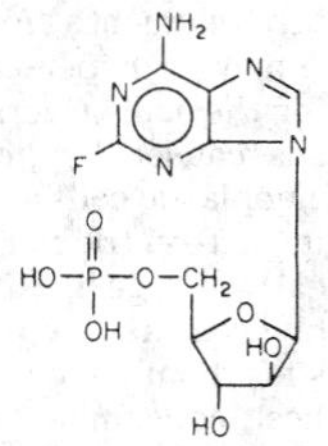

[75607-67-9] $C_{10}H_{13}FN_5O_7P$ (365.21).

Preparation—US Pat 4,357,324.

Description—White powder.

Solubility—Soluble in water.

Uses—Supplied as the monophosphate but is rapidly dephosphorylated *in vivo* to yield the free nucleoside which is actively transported into susceptible cells. Once rephosphorylated and part of the nucleotide pool of the cell fludarabine is a potent inhibitor of DNA and RNA synthesis, by inhibiting many enzymes involved in nucleic acid synthesis. The synthesis of DNA appears to be inhibited at lower intracellular concentrations of fludarabine nucleotides. Fludarabine is approved for use in *chronic lymphocytic leukemia* that has proven refractory to at least one alkylating agent. It also has activity against *Hodgkin's* and *non-Hodgkin's* *lymphomas, mycosis fungoides* and *macroglobulinemia.* Fludarabine, administered IV, has a short initial half-life of approximately 80 min. The most severe adverse effects involve a CNS syndrome, and suppression of the hematopoietic system. The CNS syndrome includes a delayed blindness, coma and death which appear at high doses. This syndrome is rare in patients receiving the recommended dose for chronic lymphocytic leukemia. Severe bone-marrow suppression results in decreased neutrophil counts ($<500/\mu l$ in 59% of patients), decreased hematocrit and platelet counts in 50 to 60% of patients. The myelosuppression may be cumulative. It also is reported to cause pulmonary disfunction.

Dose—25 mg/m²/day for 5 days, repeated every 28 days as permitted by toxicities.

Dosage Form—Injection: 50 mg/6 mL vials.

Fluorouracil

2,4(1*H*,3*H*)-Pyrimidinedione, 5-fluoro-, 5-FU; Adrucil (*Adria*); Efudex (*Roche*); Fluoroplex (*Herbert*)

5-Fluorouracil [51-21-8] $C_4H_3FN_2O_2$ (130.08).

Caution—Great care should be taken to prevent inhaling its particles and exposing the skin to it.

Preparation—Potassium fluoroacetate is reacted with methyl bromide to form methyl fluoroacetate which is then subjected to a Claisen condensation with methyl formate and sodium ethoxide to produce the potassium enolate of the methyl ester of α-fluoromalonaldehydic acid (I). Cyclization of I is affected through condensation under anhydrous conditions with *S*-benzylisothiourea. The resulting 2-(benzylthio) compound is hydrolyzed readily in the presence of acid to form fluorouracil. US Pat 2,802,005.

Description—White to practically white, practically odorless, crystalline powder; stable when exposed to air; decomposes about 282°.

Solubility—1 g in 80 mL water, 170 mL alcohol or 55 mL methanol; practically insoluble in chloroform, ether or benzene; solubility in aqueous solutions increases with increasing pH.

Uses—A congener of uracil that acts both as a surrogate and as an antimetabolite of that nucleotide. Its metabolite, 5-fluorodeoxyuridine-5′-monophosphate (FUMP), blocks the synthesis of thymidylic acid and hence of deoxyribonucleic acid; it also is incorporated into ribonucleic acid. Uracil is used preferentially by neoplastic tissue; thus the antimetabolite has some degree of selectivity for the neoplasm. It is approved for palliative treatment of *cancer of the colon, rectum, stomach, breast* and *pancreas.* It is not curative, but it may bring about regression of a number of neoplasms. It is the antineoplastic of choice of the treatment of *colorectal cancer.*

In combination with other drugs it provides chemotherapy of first choice in the treatment of *breast cancer, islet cell tumors, squamous cell carcinoma* of the *head* and *neck, non-small cell carcinoma* of the *lung, pancreatic* and *gastric carcinomas, primary hepatocellular carcinoma, testicular* and *prostatic carcinomas* and *bladder tumors.* It shares alternative-drug status for the treatment of *endometrial carcinoma, squamous cell tumors of the head, neck and cervix* and *ovarian tumors.* It may be useful in the treatment of *neoplasms of the gallbladder* and, to a lesser extent, those of the esophagus, larynx, thyroid and pharynx. Remissions of as long as 4 yr have been noted in a few instances, although the average is a few months.

The drug also is used topically in the treatment of precancerous dermatoses, especially *actinic keratosis*, for which it is the treatment of choice if the lesions are multiple. Even lesions which are not clinically discernible respond. For this reason, the drug is applied to the entire affected area. Healing continues for one to two months after treatment. The drug does not affect nonkeratotic lesions. It is a secondary (efferent) immunosuppressive agent and therefore has not been used in organ transplantation.

The drug is quite toxic, about two-thirds of patients showing signs of toxicity; the mortality rate is about 3% when treatment is initiated by daily doses. When the drug is administered by intravenous bolus, leukopenia is the principal adverse effect, usually occurring between the 7th and 14th day, with a nadir at 21 to 25 days. Leucocytes readily recover if the dose is lowered promptly. Thrombocytopenia is less frequent; the nadir occurs between the 7th and 17th day. Aphthous ulceration may occur or the appearance of diarrhea are signs tha therapy should be discontinued temporarily. Other toxic effects include vomiting, nausea, gastrointestinal ulceration (the dose-limiting effect of constant infusion), alopecia, dermatitis, hyperpigmentation, pharyngitis, esophagitis, cerebellar ataxia (sometimes irreversible) and epistaxis. Lassitude and asthenia, lasting from 12 to 35 hr after an injection, may occur; severe CNS depression may occur in patients with familial pyrimidinemia. When this drug causes death, it is usually from septicemia, so that concomitant antibiotic therapy is advisable. Topically, it may induce photosensitization and always erythema, scaling, fissuring, tenderness and usually erosion, ulceration, necrosis and re-epithelialization as the result of the therapeutic action, although some persons appear to be resistant to this effect.

By the oral route, there is poor absorption and variable first-pass elimination of the drug by the gut and liver, so that intravenous administration is required. At least 60% is metabolized to CO_2, but over 15% is excreted into the urine. The drug enters the cerebrospinal fluid and effusions. The plasma half-life is about 10 min, but the active metabolite, FUMP, may be detectable for days.

Dose—*Intravenous, adults* and *children, initial* course, **12 mg/kg** a day (not to exceed 800 mg) for 5 days. If toxicity has not occurred, **6 mg/kg** a day on days 7, 9, 11 and 13; poor-risk patients should receive **6 mg/kg** a day for 3 days and, if no toxicity, **3 mg/kg** a day on days 5, 7 and 9. When used with leucovorin for metastatic GI cancer, a dose of 370 mg/m² a day is used. For *maintenance*, if toxicity to the first course was minimal, either repeat the course every 30 days or give **10** to **15 mg/kg** (not to exceed 1 g) once a wk, after recovery from the initial toxicity is complete. Levamisole increases objective response rate when used in combination with 5FU for colon cancer and as an adjunctive therapy to colon surgery. The FDA-approved dosages above differ somewhat from those in the *USP DI.* When it is used in combination with nitrosoureas, only 75% of the full dose should be used; the dose should also be reduced when it is used in other combinations. It sometimes is given intraperitoneally to suppesss hepatic metastases from carcinomas in the abdominal cavity; constant infusion with implantable pumps is more effective and less toxic than periodic bolus injections. *Topical*, to the *skin, actinic keratosis*, as a **1% cream** or **1** or **2% solution**, applied once or twice a day to the entire affected area until necrosis, erosion and ulceration occur, except 5% concentration may be required on the hands; *basal cell carcinoma*, as a **5% cream** or **solution** twice a day for 3 to 12 wk.

Dosage Forms—Cream: 1 and 5%; Injection: 500 mg/10 mL; Topical Solution: 1, 2 and 5%.

Fluoxymesterone—page 1102.

Flutamide

Propaneamide, 2-methyl-*N*-[4-fluoro-3-(trifluoromethyl)phenyl]-, Eulexin (*Schering*)

[13311-84-7] $C_{11}H_{11}F_3N_2O_3$ (276.21).

Preparation—See *J Med Chem 10:*93, 1967.

Description—Yellow crystals melting about 110°.

Solubility—Practically insoluble in water.

Uses—This drug and its primary hydroxy metabolite are nonsteroidal *antiandrogens.* They not only block androgens at the target cells in the secondary sex organs but also decrease the metabolism of C-19 steroids by the cytochrome P-450 system. This drug is approved for use in combination with leuprolide (see below) in the treatment of *prostatic carcinoma* to prevent the temporary exacerbations of the cancer resulting from enhancement of gonadotrophin release during the first few weeks of treatment. It not only suppresses the early flare-ups but also increases the number of complete responders 6-fold and diminishes the number of nonresponders by 75%. It also is used in effective combination with aminoglutethamide to increase the percentage of responders. It is not useful alone because alone it results in increased plasma testosterone levels.

It is metabolized in the liver primarily to the 5-hydroxy derivative.

It is not yet available in the US but is in Canada.

Dose—*Oral, adult,* **250 mg** 3 times a day, starting 1 day before leuprolide is begun or concurrently with aminoglutehamide.

Dosage Form—Tablets: 250 mg.

Gold Au 198—page 255.

Goserelin Acetate

Luteinizing hormone-releasing factor (pig)
6-[*O*-(1,1-dimethylethyl)-D-serine]-10-deglycinamide-,
2-(aminocarbonyl)hydrazide, acetate salt; Zoladex (*ICI*)

H—5-oxoPro-His-Trp-Ser-Tyr-D-Ser(*t*-Bu)-Leu-Arg-Pro-NH—NH—C(=O)—$NH_2 \cdot CH_3COOH$
1 2 3 4 5 6 7 8 9

[65807-02-5 (goserelin)] $C_{59}H_{84}N_{18}O_{14} \cdot C_2H_4O_2$ (1329.48).

Preparation—*J Med Chem, 21,* 1018, 1978.

Description—White to off-white powder.

Solubility—Soluble in water, dilute acids or bases; aqueous solution pH approx 6.0.

Uses—A synthetic LHRH (GnRH) analog that acts as a potent inhibitor of pituitary gonadotropin secretion. Proliferation of prostatic cells and usually prostatic neoplastic cells are simulated by dihydortestosterone generated locally from circulating testosterone (80%); hence, it is directly under the control of LH-RH/FSH/RH. Like the natural releasing hormone, treatment with this drug initially causes an acceleration of the growth of prostatic tumors; however, it later causes a decline in tumor growth rate, as a result of down-regulation (densensitization) of LH-RH/FSH-Rh receptors in the anterior hypophysis and androgen receptors in prostatic tumor cells. It is approved for palliative treatment of *prostatic carcinoma;* however, it is active against *estrogen receptor positive breast cancer.*

Recipients often experience an exacerbation of the cancer during the first few weeks of treatment. This will result in temporarily increased bone destruction and pain in about 8% of cases; hypercalcemia, renal insufficiency and urinary obstruction may occur. The concurrent use of the antiandrogen, flutamide, prevents these flareups. As down-regulation develops and androgen/estrogen blood levels decline to castration levels, about 60% of the patients have hot flashes which gradually recede. In male patients loss of libido and sexual disfunction are common. Plasma levels of phosphatase and appropriate sex hormone should be monitored; hormone levels reach castration values in about 2 wk, and phosphatase returns to baseline levels in 4 wk.

Dose—*Subcutaneous, installation,* **3.6 mg** every 28 days.

Dosage Form—Preloaded syringes, supplied in a biodegradable lactic and glycollic acid copolymer matrix loaded with the acetate equivalent to 3.6 mg of the base. As the implanted matrix degrades the drug in released slowly over 28 days.

Hydroxyprogesterone Caproate—page 1095.

Hydroxyurea

Hydroxycarbamide; Hydrea (*Bristol-Myers Squibb*)

$H_2NCONHOH$

[127-07-1] $CH_4N_2O_2$ (76.05).

Preparation—By interaction of hydroxylamine hydrochloride and potassium cyanide.

Description—White powder; odorless; essentially tasteless; melts about 135°.

Solubility—Freely soluble in water.

Uses—Inhibits synthesis of DNA but not of RNA. It is lethal to cells in the S-phase and also holds cells in the G_1-phase, in which they are more sensitive to irradiation. It shares first-choice status with busulfan for the treatment of the *chronic phase* of *chronic myelocytic leukemia.* The value of either drug as a backup drug for the other may be limited by cross-resistance. It sometimes is combined with radiation to treat squamous-cell carcinoma of the head and neck, or used alone to treat inoperable ovarian carcinoma, in which it has erratic palliative actions; superior chemotherapy is retiring it from such uses.

As an *immunosuppressant,* it may be used in the treatment of *psoriasis.* It appears to improve the condition of the patient in a high percentage of cases, but the quality of the response may not be as good as with some other drugs. Thus it has an unsettled status.

Its most serious side effect is bone-marrow depression, in which the neutrophils are most affected: the leukocyte count drops about 50% in 2 to 4 days but recovers within a week. Thrombocytopenia and anemia are uncommon. Megaloblastosis may occur. Aphthous ulceration, nausea, vomiting, diarrhea, headache, vertigo, disorientation, hallucinations, convulsions, minor rashes and pruritus also may occur. Elevated BUN and hyperuricemia and urate nephrolithiasis have been reported. It is eliminated mainly by renal excretion. The drug is contraindicated in renal failure and when there is prior bone-marrow depression. The blood-cell population, and kidney and liver functions must be monitored weekly.

Dose—*Oral,* for *chronic myelocytic leukemia* or *continuous therapy of solid tumors,* **20** to **30 mg/kg/day** in 1 or 2 divided doses; for *intermittent therapy of solid tumors* or *combined with radiation therapy for carcinoma of the head and neck,* **60** to **80 mg/kg** (or 2000 to 3000 mg/m^2) every third day.

Idoxuridine—see RPS-17, page 1232.

Ifosfamide

2*H*-1,3,2-Oxazaphosphorin-2-amine,
N,3-bis(2-chloroethyl)tetrahydro-, 2-oxide; Ifex (*Mead Johnson*)

[3778-73-2] $C_7H_{15}Cl_2N_2O_2P$ (261.09).

Preparation—Reaction of 3-(chloromethylamino)-1-propanol with $POCl_3$ yields the *N*-(2-chloroethyl)-*P*-chlorooxaphosphorane oxide, which with 2-chloroethylamine yields the product. US Pat 3,732,340.

Description—White crystals; melts about 40°.

Solubility—Soluble in water.

Uses—An investigational alkylating agent isomeric with cyclophosphamide. It is a component of a first-choice combination for the treatment of adult soft-tissue sarcomas and *testicular cancer.* It is an alternative drug for the treatment of *acute lymphocytic leukemia, acute myelocytic leukemia, breast carcinoma, Burkitt's lymphoma, colorectal carcinoma, diffuse histiocytic lymphoma, Ewing's sarcoma, melanoma, non-small cell lung carcinoma, oat-cell carcinoma, pancreatic carcinoma, testicular carcinoma, ovarian carcinoma* and *Wilm's tumor.* Nausea and vomiting occur acutely. Delayed toxicity includes bone-marrow depression, hemorrhagic cystitis, alopecia and a usually temporary sterility. It is converted slowly to an active metabolite, the half-life being approximately 15 hr. The active metabolites are rapidly bound to proteins. The volume of distribution is larger than that of total body water.

Dose—**1-2 g/m²** once a day for 5 days: courses are repeated at approximately 3-wk intervals, depending on whether the blood cell count has passed its nadir. The drug is always given concurrently with forced hydration to reduce the risk of urothelial and renal toxicity.

Dosage Form—Injection: 1 g or 3 g single dose vials.

Interferon Alfa-2a, Recombinant

H—Cys-Asp-Leu-Pro-Gln-Thr-His-Ser-Leu-Gly-Ser-Arg-Arg-Thr-Leu-Met-Leu-Leu-Ala-Gln-
1 2 3 4 5 6 7 8 9 10 11 12 13 14 15 16 17 18 19 20
Met-Arg-Lys-Ile-Ser-Leu-Phe-Ser-Cys-Leu-Lys-Asp-Arg-His-Asp-Phe-Gly-Phe-Pro-Gln-
21 22 23 24 25 26 27 28 29 30 31 32 33 34 35 36 37 38 39 40
Glu-Glu-Phe-Gly-Asn-Gln-Phe-Gln-Lys-Ala-Glu-Thr-Ile-Pro-Val-Leu-His-Glu-Met-Ile-
41 42 43 44 45 46 47 48 49 50 51 52 53 54 55 56 57 58 59 60
Gln-Gln-Ile-Phe-Asn-Leu-Phe-Ser-Thr-Lys-Asp-Ser-Ser-Ala-Ala-Trp-Asp-Glu-Thr-Leu-
61 62 63 64 65 66 67 68 69 70 71 72 73 74 75 76 77 78 79 80
Leu-Asp-Lys-Phe-Tyr-Thr-Glu-Leu-Tyr-Gln-Gln-Leu-Asn-Asp-Leu-Glu-Ala-Cys-Val-Ile-
81 82 83 84 85 86 87 88 89 90 91 92 93 94 95 96 97 98 99 100
Gln-Gly-Val-Gly-Val-Thr-Glu-Thr-Pro-Leu-Met-Lys-Glu-Asp-Ser-Ile-Leu-Ala-Val-Arg-
101 102 103 104 105 106 107 108 109 110 111 112 113 114 115 116 117 118 119 120
Lys-Tyr-Phe-Gln-Arg-Ile-Thr-Leu-Tyr-Leu-Lys-Glu-Lys-Lys-Tyr-Ser-Pro-Cys-Ala-Trp-
121 122 123 124 125 126 127 128 129 130 131 132 133 134 135 136 137 138 139 140
Glu-Val-Val-Arg-Ala-Glu-Ile-Met-Arg-Ser-Phe-Ser-Leu-Ser-Thr-Asn-Leu-Gln-Glu-Ser-
141 142 143 144 145 146 147 148 149 150 151 152 153 154 155 156 157 158 159 160
Leu-Arg-Ser-Lys-Glu—OH
161 162 163 164 165

Interferon αA (human leukocyte protein moiety reduced); rIFN-αA [76543-88-9] $C_{860}H_{1353}N_{227}O_{255}S_9$ (19,241.11).

Uses—Identical to one of the human alpha-interferons. Interferons and other cytokines are discussed in Chapter 44. It increases class I histocompatibility molecules on lymphocytes, enhances the production of interleukins-1 and -2 (which mediate much of the toxic and therapeutic effects), modulates antibody responses and enhances natural killer (NK) cell activity. It also inhibits tumor cell growth by its ability to inhibit protein synthesis. It also is antiproliferative and thus can be immunosuppressive. The action on NK cells is the most important for its *antineoplastic* action. It is approved for use in *hairy cell leukemia* and *AIDS-related Kaposi's sarcoma.* It shares first choice status for the treatment of *hairy-cell leukemia* and *Kaposi's sarcoma* and is the drug of choice for treatment of *renal cell carcinoma*. It also is an alternative drug for use against *chronic myelocytic leukemia multiple myeloma* (21% respond), *melanoma* (13 to 23% respond) and *advanced cutaneous T-cell lymphomas*. Preliminary trials also show promising efficacy against ovarian carcinoma, non-Hodgkin's lymphoma and metastatic carcinoid tumor.

It has *antiviral* activity, especially against RNA viruses. It has been shown to be effective in the treatment of varicella in immunocompromised children, non-A and non-B hepatides, genital warts and lymphoproliferative disorders caused by Epstein-Barr virus, the prevention of cytomegalovirus, rhinoviral colds, and even possibly opportunistic bacterial infections in renal and other transplant recipients. Other investigations are in progress.

It enhances the targeting of monoclonal antibody-tethered cytotoxic drugs to cancer cells.

Toxicity varies directly with the dose and the rate of absorption. Antiviral effects, without toxicity, can be achieved with 3×10^5 IU. No adverse effects accrue to intranasal doses of 2.5×10^7 IU.

Antibodies to rIFN-αA develop, which may cause refractoriness to occur.

The following adverse effects with antineoplastic doses have incidences of 75 through 98% (in order of decreasing incidence): fever (interleukin-1-mediated), fatigue, elevated SGOT, myalgias; 50 through 74%: headache, leukopenia, chills, neutropenia, hypocalcemia; 25 through 49%: proteinuria, elevated alkaline phosphatase, anorexia, thrombocytopenia, nausea, hyperglycemia, hyperbilirubinemia, diarrhea, proteinuria; 10 through 24%: dizziness, rash, hyperphosphatemia, oropharyngeal inflammation, hyperuricemia, weight loss, pruritis, dry skin, azotemia; 5 through 9%: anemia, emesis, confusion, arthralgia, sweating, alopecia, paresthesias, numbness, lethargy, hypotension; below 5%: lethargy, nervousness, night sweats, conjunctivitis, sleep disturbances, edema, dysrhythmias and chest pain, decreased libido, impotence, etc. Interstitial nephritis and renal failure rarely occur. Many of the adverse effects diminish after several days of continued treatment. Interferons are expensive.

It is not absorbed perorally. By the intravenous route, it entirely disappears within 4 hr, but by the intramuscular or subcutaneous route disappearance takes 6 to 7 hr.

Dose—*Intralesional*, for *genital warts*, **10^6 IU** 3 times a week for 3 wk. *Intramuscular or subcutaneous, adult, antineoplastic, initially* **3×10^6 IU** a day for 16 to 24 wk; *maintenance*, **3×10^6 IU** 3 times a wk, except diminished by half if severe adverse effects occur. For Kaposi's sarcoma, 36×10^6 IU daily. *Intranasal*, for *rhinoviral prophylaxis*, **1.25×10^5 IU** into each nostril twice a day for 7 days. *Intravenous*, for *rhinoviral prophylaxis*, **10^6 IU** a day for 7 days.

Dosage Form—Injection: 3 and 18 million IU/vial.

Interferon Alfa-2b, Recombinant

Alferon (*Interferon Sciences*); Intron-A (*Schering*)

Alferon (*Interferon Sciences*); Intron-A (*Schering*)

H—Cys-Asp-Leu-Pro-Gln-Thr-His-Ser-Leu-Gly-Ser-Arg-Arg-Thr-Leu-Met-Leu-Leu-Ala-Gln-
1 2 3 4 5 6 7 8 9 10 11 12 13 14 15 16 17 18 19 20

Met-Arg-Arg-Ile-Ser-Leu-Phe-Ser-Cys-Leu-Lys-Asp-Arg-His-Asp-Phe-Gly-Phe-Pro-Gln-
21 22 23 24 25 26 27 28 29 30 31 32 33 34 35 36 37 38 39 40

Glu-Glu-Phe-Gly-Asn-Gln-Phe-Gln-Lys-Ala-Glu-Thr-Ile-Pro-Val-Leu-His-Glu-Met-Ile-
41 42 43 44 45 46 47 48 49 50 51 52 53 54 55 56 57 58 59 60

Gln-Gln-Ile-Phe-Asn-Leu-Phe-Ser-Thr-Lys-Asp-Ser-Ser-Ala-Ala-Trp-Asp-Glu-Thr-Leu-
61 62 63 64 65 66 67 68 69 70 71 72 73 74 75 76 77 78 79 80

Leu-Asp-Lys-Phe-Tyr-Thr-Glu-Leu-Tyr-Gln-Gln-Leu-Asn-Asp-Leu-Glu-Ala-Cys-Val-Ile-
81 82 83 84 85 86 87 88 89 90 91 92 93 94 95 96 97 98 99 100

Gln-Gly-Val-Gly-Val-Thr-Glu-Thr-Pro-Leu-Met-Lys-Glu-Asp-Ser-Ile-Leu-Ala-Val-Arg-
101 102 103 104 105 106 107 108 109 110 111 112 113 114 115 116 117 118 119 120

Lys-Tyr-Phe-Gln-Arg-Ile-Thr-Leu-Tyr-Leu-Lys-Glu-Lys-Lys-Tyr-Ser-Pro-Cys-Ala-Trp-
121 122 123 124 125 126 127 128 129 130 131 132 133 134 135 136 137 138 139 140

Glu-Val-Val-Arg-Ala-Glu-Ile-Met-Arg-Ser-Phe-Ser-Leu-Ser-Thr-Asn-Leu-Gln-Glu-Ser-
141 142 143 144 145 146 147 148 149 150 151 152 153 154 155 156 157 158 159 160

Leu-Arg-Ser-Lys-Glu—OH
161 162 163 164 165

Interferon α2b (human leukocyte clone Hif-SN206 protein moiety reduced) [99210-65-8] $C_{860}H_{1353}N_{229}O_{255}S_9$ (19,269.12). The structure of the alfa-2b compound differs from the alfa-2a in that the twenty-third amino acid in the sequence is *arginine* rather than *lysine*.

Uses—It is approved for use in *hairy cell leukemia*, *AIDS-related Kaposi's sarcoma*, *condylomata acuminata* and *chronic hepatitis*. Its actions very nearly are those of rIFN-αA, and the uses are presently the same, except that it appears to be somewhat less effective against melanoma, and antibody formation is less Neither alpha interferon has been studied in a sufficient number of cases to ascertain whether adverse effects differ substantially; they seem to be qualitatively the same but perhaps of slightly lower incidence and severity with rIFN-α-2.

Dose—*Intramuscular* or *subcutaneous, adult, antineoplastic*, **2 million IU/m²** 3 times a wk, except only half this does if severe adverse effects occur.

Dosage Form—Injection: 3, 5, 10 and 25 million IU/vial.

Leucovorin Calcium—page 1126.

Leuprolide Acetate

6-D-Leucine-9-(*N*-ethyl-L-prolinamide)-10-deglycinamide-, monoacetate salt; Lupron (*TAP*)

H—5-oxoPro-His-Trp-Ser-Tyr-D-Leu-Leu-Arg-Pro—NHEt · CH_3COOH
1 2 3 4 5 6 7 8 9

Leuprorelin; Lutenizing hormone releasing factor (pig). [74381-53-6] $C_{59}H_{84}N_{16}O_{12}.C_2H_4O_2$ (1269.47).

Uses—An analog of the gonadotropin-releasing hormone, LH-RH/FSH-RH. Proliferation of prostatic and usually of prostatic neoplastic cells is stimulated by dihydrotestosterone generated locally from circulating testosterone (80%): hence it is indirectly under the control of LH-RH/FSH/RH. Like the natural releasing hormone, treatment with this drug initially causes an acceleration of the growth of prostatic tumors, but, however, later causes a decline in tumor growth rate, as the result of down-regulation (densensitization) of LH-RH/FSH-RH receptors in the anterior hypophysis and androgen receptors in prostatic tumor cells. It is approved only for use for palliative treatment of *prostatic carcinoma* when orchiectomy or estrogen therapy is rejected by the patient; however, it is analogously active against estrogen receptor-positive breast cancer.

Recipients often experience an exacerbation of the cancer during the first few weeks of treatment. This will result in temporarily increased bone destruction and pain in 3 to 10% of cases, and hypercalcemia and urinary obstruction may occur. The concurrent use of the antiandrogen, flutamide, prevents these flareups. As down-regulation develops and androgen/estrogen blood levels decline to castration levels, about half of the patients have hot flashes which gradually recede. In male patients there is commonly loss of libido, impotence and gynecomastia. Nausea and vomiting, edema, changes in bone density and thrombophlebitis are uncommon complications. Plasma levels of phosphatase and appropriate sex hormone should be monitored; hormone levels reach castration values in about 2 wk and phosphatase to baseline levels in 4 wk.

Dose—*Subcutaneous, adult*, **1 mg/day.**

Dosage Form—Injection: 5 mg/mL (in 2.8-mL vials); Depot Suspension: 3.75 mg/mL or 7.5 mg/mL (single dose vials with diluent).

Levamisole Hydrochloride

Imidazo[2,1-*b*]thiazole, (*S*)-2,3,5,6-tetrahydro-6-phenyl-, monohydrochloride; Ergamisol (*Janssen*)

[16595-80-5] $C_{11}H_{12}N_2S.HCl$ (240.75).

Preparation—US Pat 3,274,209 or 3,579,530.

Description—White to cream-colored crystals.

Solubility—1 g in 2 mL water or 5 mL methanol; practically insoluble in ether.

Uses—A drug that predominantly stimulates, but also suppresses, immune responses to a variety of antigens, depending upon dose and timing of administration. It acts upon T lymphocytes, B lymphocytes, monocytes, macrophages and neutrophils to modify their proliferation, mobility and factor-release. It does not act on killer or natural killer cells. An increase in monocyte chemotaxis is thought to be the most important action. Its effects on T lymphocytes are more pronounced than those on B-lymphocytes. Clinical interest focuses on the immune stimulatory effects, especially in the treatment of cancer. It is approved for use *after surgical resection of colon cancer* and for *coadministration with 5 FU*. It is mostly ineffective in the induction of tumor regression, although it may be occasionally effective against breast carcinoma, ovarian carcinoma and acute myelocytic leukemia. It is most useful for the *stabilization of remission* in *breast carcinoma, bronchogenic carcinomas, squamous-cell sarcomas of the head and neck, gastric carcinoma, leukemias* and *myeloma*. It has been reported to be effective in the management of certain immune disorders, namely, erythema multiforme, lupus erythematosis and *rheumatoid arthritis*, against which it seems to be as effective as penicillamine. There also are reports of anti-infectious activity against aphthous stomatitis, chronic brucellosis, leprosy and staphylococcal infections. Adverse effects are usually mild and infrequent. They include vertigo (especially with ethanol), nausea, vomiting, headache, fever, dermatitis and granulocytopenia. It readily is absorbed orally. It is metabolized nearly entirely in the liver. The elimination half-life is about 4 hr.

Dose—*Oral*, to be individualized: a common regimen is **150 mg/a day** for 4 days each wk or every other wk.

Dosage Form—Tablets: 50 mg (base).

Lomustine

Urea, *N*-(2-chloroethyl)-*N'*-cyclohexyl-*N*-nitroso-, CCNU; CeeNU (*Bristol*)

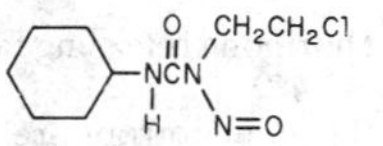

1-(2-Chloroethyl)-3-cyclohexyl-1-nitrosourea [13010-47-4] $C_9H_{16}ClN_3O_2$ (233.70).

Preparation—This drug, a cytotoxic nitrosourea, may be prepared by nitrosation of its substituted urea moiety (see preparation of *Carmustine*), page 1244.

Description—Yellow powder.

Solubility—Practically insoluble in water, soluble in alcohol; highly soluble in lipids.

Uses—It has been approved for use in *brain cancer* and *Hodgkin's disease*. A chemical congener of *Carmustine* (page 1244) and has similar mechanisms of action and shares some of the same uses. Like carmustine, it reaches high concentrations in the cerebrospinal fluid and hence shares with carmustine a first-choice status for the treatment of *glioblastoma*. It has alternative drug status for treatment of *Hodgkin's* and *diffuse histiocytic lymphomas, multiple myeloma, non-small cell lung cancer* and *renal carcinoma*. It also is used in *bone marrow transplantation* in Hodgkin's disease.

The adverse effects are similar to those of carmustine except that there may be rare interstitial pulmonary fibrosis. Nausea and vomiting occur later (3 to 6 hr) and last longer (24 hr). Thrombocytopenia and leukokpenia reach nadirs in 4 and 6 weeks, respectively, and last 1 to 2 wk. Stomatitis, alopecia, anemia and mild, transient hepatotoxicity occasionally occur. Dysarthria, ataxia, lethargy and disorientation have been reported. Monitoring of leukocyte counts is required. When other myelosuppressive drugs are in use or have been used within the prior 4 wk, the dose of lomustine should be reduced.

Lomustine is absorbed well orally and survives the first pass through the liver to be effective by the oral route. It is distributed among the tissues with a volume of distribution greater than total body water. In the cerebrospinal fluid, the concentration of metabolites reaches 150% of that in plasma. Biotransformation occurs throughout the body; the half-life is about 15 min; the half lives of metabolites are 48 hr.

Dose—*Oral, adult* and *pediatric*, **130 mg/m²** every 6 wk, except 100 mg/m² if bone-marrow function is depressed. Repeat courses should not be given until the platelet count has returned to 100,000/mm³ and the leukocyte count to 4,000/mm³, and they should never be given at intervals less than 6 wk.

Dosage Form—Capsules: 10, 40 and 100 mg.

Lymphocyte Immune Anti-thymocyte Globulin (Equine);

Atgam (Upjohn)

A preparation of equine immunoglobulin containing antibodies (primarily IgG) prepared from the hyperimmune serum of horses immunized with human thymus lymphocytes.

Description—Transparent to slightly opalescent (pink) aqueous solution of the protein.

Uses—Attacks T lymphocytes but not B lymphocytes. Its approved use is the *prevention* of *allograft rejection* in renal transplantation. Efficacy is enhanced and adverse effects are attenuated when the globulin is used in combination with other immunosuppressive agents. The globulin also has been reported to be of value in the treatment of T-cell leukemias, graft-versus-host disease and selected cases of aplastic anemia. Frequent adverse effects include chills, fever, urticaria, pruritis, generalized rashes, leukopenia and thrombocytopenia. Less frequently experienced adverse effects are nausea, vomiting, stomatitis, diarrhea, hypotension, chest pain, back pain, night sweats, pain at the injection site and peripheral thrombophlebitis. Rarely there may be tachycardia, myalgias, pulmonary edema, serum sickness, anaphylaxis, laryngospasm, local and systemic infections and activation of herpes simplex infections. Prior to use, a skin test for sensitivity to horse serum is advisable. The half-life 3 to 9 days.

Dose—*Slow intravenous infusion, adults*, to *delay rejection*. **15 mg/kg/day** for 14 days, then every other day for 14 days: the first dose should be within 24 hr before or after transplantation; *treatment of ongoing rejection*, **10** to **15 mg/kg/day** for 14 days, then every other day for 14 days, if necessary: *children*, **5** to **25 mg/kg/day.**

Dosage Form—Injection: 5 mL; 50 mg of horse gamma globulin/mL.

Lymphocyte-Activated Killer Cells—see RPS-18, page 1159.

Mechlorethamine Hydrochloride

Ethanamine, 2-chloro-*N*-(2-chloroethyl)-*N*-methyl, hydrochloride; Nitrogen Mustard; HN2; Mustargen (*MSD*)

$CH_3N(CH_2CH_2Cl)_2 \cdot HCl$

2,2'-Dichloro-*N*-methyldiethylamine hydrochloride [55-86-7] $C_5H_{11}Cl_2N.HCl$ (192.52).

Caution—This is a vesicant, and the powder or its solution is irritating to the respiratory tract.

History—The medical uses for nitrogen mustards were discovered as a result of chemical warfare research on vesicant agents during World War II. After noting that these agents brought about dissolution of lymphoid tissue, L Goodman, A Gilman and T Dougherty were prompted to study the effect of nitrogen mustards on transplanted lymphosarcoma in mice. The first clinical trial with these agents was conducted in 1942.

Preparation—Among other ways, the base may be synthesized by reacting methylamine with a double equimolar portion of ethylene oxide to produce *N*-methyldiethanolamine, which is then reacted with thionyl chloride. After purification, the base then may be converted conveniently to the hydrochloride by dissolving it in a suitable organic solvent and passing HCl into the solution.

Description—White, crystalline, hygroscopic powder; melts about 109°; pH (1:500 aqueous solution) 3 to 5.

Solubility—Very soluble in water, soluble in alcohol.

Uses—The prototype of a series of alkylating agents called the nitrogen mustards. The β-chloroethyl groups lose chloride ions to generate carbonium and azaridium (ethylenimonium) ions, which are very reactive and alkylate many biologically important chemical groups. In DNA they alkylate guanine groups; if one "arm" alkylates one guanine moiety and the second arm another guanine on the opposing strand of double-stranded DNA, the DNA becomes irreversibly cross-linked. This inhibits mitosis and may also cause chromosomal breakage. Relatively undifferentiated germinal cells are nonproliferative and hypertrophied during exposure to the drug, but the more differentiated germinal cells disintegrate. Certain neoplastic growths, particularly of the lymph nodes and bone marrow, are somewhat more sensitive to the drug than are the normal more slowly proliferative tissues. It is approved for use in *Hodgkin's disease, lymphosarcoma, chronic lymphocytic* and *myelocytic leukemia, polycythemia vera, mycosis fungoides* and *bronchogenic carcinoma.*

Although this was the drug that ushered in the era of cancer chemotherapy, it is still used today. The combinations known as MOPP (mechlorethamine, vincristine, procarbazine, prednisone) and MOP (MOPP without prednisone) offer two first-choice treatments for *Hodgkin's disease*. It is also a component of first-choice combinations to treat *medulloblastoma* and *diffuse histiocytic lymphoma*. Mechlorethamine's only other therapeutic status of note is as the drug of choice in the topical treatment of *mycosis fungoides* and plural or intraperitoneal effusions. In *polycythemia vera*, remissions of several months to 2 yr have been achieved. All of the above diseases eventually develop resistance to nitrogen mustards.

It is an immunosuppressive drug, but the requirement for intravenous administration and its high toxicity have discouraged its use. In the treatment of "*malignant*" *rheumatoid arthritis* it effects a good initial response in nearly all patients; maintenance is carried on with cyclophosphamide or other immunosuppressive drugs. It also has been reported to improve the condition of a high percentage of patients with *ulcerative colitis*.

Nausea and vomiting commonly occur within 30 to 180 min after administration, but sedative and antiemetic agents greatly diminish the incidence of such untoward actions originating centrally. Diarrhea also occurs frequently. Bone-marrow depression may result in lymphocytopenia followed by leukopenia and occasionally thrombocytopenia and thus in bleeding tendencies; hyperheparinemia also may rarely lead to hemorrhagic complications. Serious and potentially lethal hematological responses mainly occur when the total accumulated dose in a course of therapy exceeds 0.4 mg (400 μg)/kg. Skin eruptions are noted rarely, but herpes zoster (shingles) commonly occurs, especially in the treatment of malignant lymphoma. Sometimes temporary menstrual irregularities occur in females. In patients with large tumor masses which involute rapidly with treatment, there may be hyperuricemia, and adequate fluid intake and allopurinol are required to prevent crystalluria and kidney damage. Alopecia, metallic taste, headache, drowsiness, asthenia, tinnitus and deafness sometimes occur.

It is teratogenic and carcinogenic and should not be used during the first trimester of pregnancy. Several local reactions to mechlorethamine, as well as rapid chemical breakdown of the drug, require that therapy be limited to the intravenous route; even so, extravasation may cause tender local induration and sloughs, and irritation from within the lumen of the vessel may cause phlebothrombosis or thrombophlebitis, especially if the infusion rate is too rapid or the concentration of solution is too high. Extravasation should be followed with 1/6 *M* sodium thiosulfate solution.

Dose—*Intravenous, adult* and *pediatric,* **0.4 mg** (400 μg)/**kg** per course, as a single dose or divided into 2 doses given on 2 separate days or 4 doses on 4 consecutive days; after prior radiation or chemotherapy, the dose should be 0.2 mg (200 μg) to 0.3 mg (300 μg)/kg; as much as 0.8 mg/kg can be tolerated by some patients. The single dose is preferable, since it spares the patient the unnecessary repetition of bouts of nausea and vomiting. MOPP regimen is 6 mg/m² IV on days 1, 8 and 28 of treatment cycle. Patients with normal bone-marrow function can sometimes tolerate up to twice the usual dose, although serious bone-marrow depression will result at the higher doses. Courses may be repeated only when bone-marrow function has recovered, as indicated by the cellular composition of the peripheral blood; the required wait is usually not less than 6 wk. The drug is best injected (as a 1 mg/mL solution) into intravenous tubing which is rapidly conducting some isotonic fluid; the injection should be made slowly but completed within a few minutes.

Intracavity, **0.4 mg/kg** in an isotonic solution to which is added a 1 mg/mL solution of the drug; accumulated fluids are removed, and the solution instilled, after which the position of the patient is changed every minute for several minutes, to spread the solution around.

Topical, to the *skin, initially* as a **0.01** to **0.04%** ointment or **0.02%** solution to the entire skin usually once a day until 6 to 12 mo after remission, then, for *maintenance* 1 to several times a week until 3 yr have elapsed since remission.

Dosage Form—For Injection: 10 mg. Topical dosage forms must be extemporized.

Medroxyprogesterone Acetate—page 1095.
Megestrol Acetate—page 1096.

Melphalan

L-Phenylalanine, 4-[bis(2-chloroethyl)amino]-,
Alkeran (*Burroughs Wellcome*)

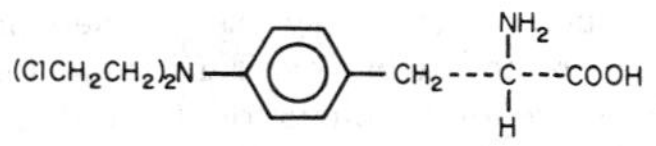

$(ClCH_2CH_2)_2N-C_6H_4-CH_2-CH(NH_2)-COOH$

[148-82-3] $C_{13}H_{18}Cl_2N_2O_2$ (305.20).

Caution—Do not inhale.

Preparation—L-3-Phenylalanine is nitrated and the *p*-nitro compound is reduced to L-3-(*p*-aminophenyl)alanine. This is reacted with ethylene oxide to form the corresponding bis(2-hydroxy-ethyl)-amino compound which is then treated with phosphoryl chloride to yield the drug.

Description—Off-white to buff powder having a faint odor; sensitive to light, heat and moisture; melts about 180° with decomposition.

Solubility—Practically insoluble in water, chloroform or ether; slightly soluble in alcohol; soluble in dilute mineral acids.

Uses—An alkylating agent of the nitrogen-mustard type. It is approved for use in *multiple myeloma* and *nonresectable epithelial carcinoma of the ovary.* In combination with prednisone either it or cyclophosphamide is the drug of choice for treatment of *multiple myeloma.* Seventy to 80% of patients show subjective improvement and 33 to 50% show objective improvement for periods from 6 mo to 2 yr, and life expectancy may be increased even when no objective signs of improvement are obtained. It is a component of the combination of choice against *ovarian carcinoma.* It is used occasionally in the treatment of *tumors of the testis, osteogenic sarcoma* and *chronic granulocytic leukemia.*

It is a primary (afferent) immunosuppresive drug.

Adverse effects include mild nausea and vomiting after large doses, bone-marrow depression with anemia, neutropenia, thrombocytopenia and occasional azotemia. Aphthous ulceration, gastrointestinal hemorrhage, skin eruptions and bronchopulmonary dyplasia also occur occasionally. Regular blood-cell counts are required. It should be given cautiously if the patient has been receiving radiation or other cancer chemotherapy. It is contraindicated in thrombocytopenia, anemia, leukopenia and during the first trimester of pregnancy. In the presence of impaired renal function the drug should be used cautiously.

It is absorbed well by the oral route, being as efficacious as by the intravenous route. It is transformed into active metabolites in probably all tissues. The elimination half-life is about 1 to 3 hr.

Dose—*Oral, myeloma, daily schedule, initially* **0.1** to **0.15 mg/kg/day** for 7 to 10 days followed by a rest until the leukocyte count begins to rise again (2 to 6 wk); *maintenance,* **0.05 mg/kg/day,** to be subsequently adjusted to 1 to 3 mg per day, according to hematological toxicity; *intermittent schedule, initially* **0.25 mg** (250 μg)/**kg/day** for 4 days; every 6 wk the course is repeated, except that the dose is adjusted according to the leukocyte and platelet count; it is desired to keep the leukocyte count slightly below 3500 cells/mm³ and the platelet count below 100,000/mm³. Various other regimens can be found in the package literature and *Drug Facts and Comparisons. Ovarian cancer,* **0.2 mg/kg/day** for 5 days, repeated every 4 to 5 wk according to hematological findings.

Dosage Form—Scored Tablets: 2 mg.

Mercaptopurine

6*H*-Purine-6-thione, 1,7-dihydro-, monohydrate;
Purinethol (*Burroughs Wellcome*)

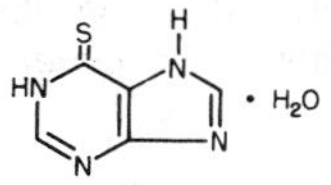

[Structure: mercaptopurine · H_2O]

Purine-6-thiol monohydrate (tautomer) [6112-76-1] $C_5H_4N_4S.H_2O$ (170.19); *anhydrous* [50-44-2] (152.17).

Preparation—Thiourea and ethyl cyanoacetate are reacted in the presence of sodium methylate to give 2-thiol-4-amino-6-hydroxypyrimidine (I) which is then converted to the 5-nitroso derivative (II) by treating with sodium nitrite and acetic acid. Reduction of II with sodium hydrosulfite yields the corresponding diamino compound (III) which is then desulfurized by hydrogenolysis in the presence of Raney nickel to yield 4,5-diamino-6-hydroxypyrimidine (IV). The imidazole ring closure is then effected by double condensation of IV with formic acid (V), and the resulting hypoxanthine is thiolated with P_2S_5.

Description—Yellow, crystalline powder; odorless or practically odorless; melts with decomposition above 308°.

Solubility—Insoluble in water, acetone or ether; soluble in hot alcohol or dilute aqueous alkali; slightly soluble in diluted H_2SO_4.

Uses—It is converted to 6-thioinosinic acid, which acts as an antimetabolite to inhibit synthesis of adenine and guanine and also to prevent conversion of purine bases into nucleotides. It also mimics inosinic acid in exerting a negative feedback suppression of the synthesis of inosinic acid. Some mercaptopurine also is converted to thioguanine, which is incorporated into DNA and RNA to generate defective nucleic acids. Thus nucleic acid synthesis and functions are impaired several ways. Cell mitosis is inhibited.

In combination with methotrexate it provides a combination of first choice in the *maintenance chemotherapy of acute lymphocytic leukemia* (this is its approved use). It is an alternative drug for the treatment of stable *chronic myelocytic leukemia;* the remission rate is about 80% if the disease is caught early, but cures are not achieved. Induction sometimes is accomplished with busulfan and maintenance with mercaptopurine. There is no cross-resistance between this drug and nonpurine antineoplastic drugs.

It is mostly a secondary (efferent) *immunosuppressive* drug that is capable of eliciting a high percentage of favorable responses in *ulcerative colitis* and *psoriatic arthritis.* It also is moderately effective in the treatment of *systemic lupus erythematosus, dermatomyositis* and *polymyositis.* However, it probably will not become the drug of choice for any of these disorders. Immunosuppression predisposes to intercurrent infections.

Bone-marrow depression occurs during treatment. Leukopenia and thrombocytopenia (with hemorrhage) are common and may be severe, but anemia is rare. Frequent monitoring of the blood-cell population is mandatory. Nausea, vomiting and anorexia may occur; they signal onset of gastrointestinal toxicity, which may take the form of mucositis and ulceration. Oral, pharyngeal and esophageal mucositis may also occur, with thrush-like stomatitis or aphthous ulceration. Diarrhea and sprue-like symptoms occasionally occur. There also may be jaundice in 10 to 40% of patients with acute leukemia. In patients with high white-cell counts or massive disease, cellular destruction leads to hyperuricemia and sometimes to tubular clogging with urate crystals and consequent oliguria, thus necessitating use of allopurinol.

The systemic bioavailability by the oral route ranges from 5 to 37%, owing to first-pass metabolism in the intestinal mucosa and liver. Both oxidation by xanthine oxidase and *S*-methylation occur. The xanthine oxidase inhibitor, allopurinol, considerably increases plasma levels from oral, but not from intravenous, drug, so that only about one-third of the usual oral dose should be given in the presence of allopurinol. Approximately 20% of the drug in plasma is protein-bound, and the volume of distribution is larger than the extracellular space; however, the access to cerebrospinal fluid is slight. The half-life averages 47 min in adults and 21 min in children.

Dose—*Oral, adult antineoplastic,* **2.5 mg/kg/day** *or* **80** to **100 mg/m²/day** in one or more divided doses, to be increased at the end of 4 wk, if necessary, to 5 mg/kg/day; for antineoplastic *maintenance,* **1.5** to **2.5 mg/kg/day** *or* **50** to **100 mg/m²/day;** *immunosuppressive,* **1.5 mg/kg/day,** adjusted upward at the end of 3 mo, if necessary, to 2.5 mg/kg/day; *children* 5 yr or older, **2.5 mg/kg/day** *or* **75 mg/kg/day** in one or more divided doses.

Dosage Form—Scored Tablets: 50 mg.

Methotrexate

L-Glutamic acid, *N*-[4-[[(2.4-diamino-6-pteridinyl)methyl]methylamino]benzoyl], benzoyl-,
Folex (*Adria*); Methotrexate (*Lederle*); Mexate (*Bristol*)

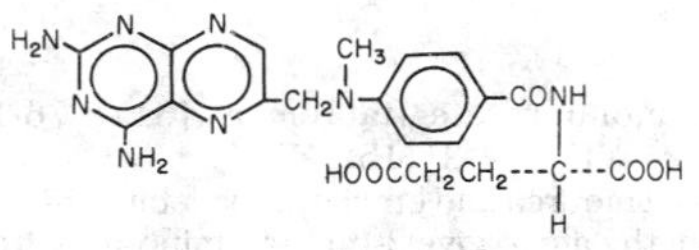

4-Amino-10-methylfolic acid; [59-05-2]; a mixture of 4-amino-10-methylfolic acid and closely related compounds and contains not less than 85.0% of $C_{20}H_{22}N_8O_5$ (454.44).

Caution—It is extremely poisonous.

Preparation—2,3-Dibromopropionaldehyde (I) is condensed in an aqueous medium with 2,4,5,6-tetraminopyrimidine (II). The condensation is multiple, consisting of: (*a*) dehydrobromination, involving a hydrogen of the 5-amino group and the 2-bromine; (*b*) dehydration, involving two hydrogens of the 6-amino group and the oxygen in II; and (*c*) dehydrogenation, involving the remaining hydrogen of the 5-amino group and the 2-hydrogen of II. The dehydrogenation in step (*c*) is brought about by another molecule of II which, by effecting the dehydrogenation, is reduced to 2,3-dibromo-1-propanol. The overall effect of these condensations is the cyclization of I with II to produce 6-bromomethyl-2,4-diaminopteridine (III). Further condensation (dehydrobromination involving the bromine in III and the hydrogen of the methylamino group in *N*-[*p*-(methylamino)benzoyl]glutamic acid) yields the crude drug, which is purified.

Description—Orange-brown, crystalline powder.

Solubility—Practically insoluble in water, alcohol, chloroform or ether; freely soluble in dilute solutions of alkali hydroxides or carbonates; slightly soluble in dilute hydrochloric acid.

Uses—Inhibits dihydrofolate reductase, and thus prevents conversion of deoxyuridylate to thymidylate and blocks the synthesis of new DNA needed for cellular replication. Methotrexate is approved for use, and is the drug of choice, in *trophoblastic tumors* such as choriocarcinoma, *hydatidiform mole* and *chorioadenoma destruens.* It also is approved for *prophylaxis of and treatment of meningeal leukemias* and for *breast cancer* and *nonmetastatic osteosarcoma.* It sometimes is combined with dactinomycin in these uses. It is the drug of choice for *CNS prophylaxis* in *acute lymphocytic leukemia.* In combination with other drugs it provides the therapy of choice. It is a component of first-choice combinations for induction and maintenance in *acute lymphocytic leukemia, diffuse histiocytic leukemia, cervical cancer, medulloblastoma, osteogenic sarcoma, breast cancer, non-Hodgkin's lymphomas, Burkitt's lymphoma, bladder carcinoma, squamous-cell carcinoma of the head and neck, oat-cell* and *non-small cell lung cancers.* It is an alternative drug for treatment of *adult soft-tissue sarcoma, follicular lymphoma, embryonal rhabdomyosarcoma,* and *colorectal carcinoma.* It also is used sequentially with fluorouracil in the treatment of node-negative breast cancer.

It may be given by intra-arterial infusion into the affected region in the treatment of a variety of carcinomata of the head, neck, pelvis and limbs; the local concentrations achieved may be high enough to be effective and yet low enough in the rest of the body not to be toxic. The endocellular transport competitor, folinic acid (leucovorin), is also often given systematically to prevent generalized toxicity.

It is a secondary (efferent) immunosuppressive drug. It is one of a few drugs used to treat *Reiter's syndrome,* although results range from poor to good. It is employed to treat *psoriasis* refractory to other drugs; with methotrexate about 50% of affected joints and 65% of skin lesions improve. It is used successfully to treat severe, progressive, refractory *rheumatoid arthritis* and glucocorticoid-dependent *asthma.* It has provided improvement in *dermatomyositis* and *polymyositis* (40 to 100% improvement), *Wegner's granulomatosis, pemphigus vulgaris, pityriasis rubra pilaris, bullous pemphigoid* and *thrombocytopenic purpura,* but other drugs appear to be equal or superior.

The toxic effects are extensions of its antimetabolite effects; sometimes toxicity occurs first. They include bone-marrow hypoplasia with leukopenia, thrombocytopenia (with hemorrhage) and anemia. Depression of cellular proliferation along the gastrointestinal tract results in diarrhea, ulcerative stomatitis, hemorrhagic enteritis and perforation. Alopecia also may occur. Dosage schedules in which methotrexate is given chronically daily may cause liver damage. The drug must not be used when there is preexisting liver damage or bone-marrow depression, or during pregnancy. Daily blood counts and triweekly creatinine determinations are mandatory. The toxicity and therapeutic effects may be antagonized by leucovorin (leucovorin or thymidine "rescue"); if the leucovorin is given after an appropriate delay, it can prevent the toxic but not the therapeutic effect on certain tumors or the immune system. The drug is concentrated in the urine, and precipitation may cause renal failure; alkalinazation and high water intake help protect the kidneys. Nitrous oxide, often used in pediatric oncology units, increases its cytotoxicity and probably its efficacy.

In doses below 30 mg/m², it is absorbed well by the oral route, but about ⅓ of an oral dose is metabolized by intestinal bacteria, and antibiotics affect the amount absorbed. In doses above 80 mg/m², the amount absorbed is reduced further by 30 to 50%. Only about 50% of the drug is bound to plasma protein, but it does not gain much access to the cerebrospinal fluid because it is strongly ionized and outwardly transported at the choroid plexus; consequently, it must be administered intrathecally for use in the CNS. In the usual doses, it actively is transported into all tissues, but it is transported preferentially into responsive neoplastic cells. Intensification of therapy, alternating with or followed by leucovorin rescue, may achieve sufficient plasma levels (1 μM) to effect meningeal leukemias and lymphomas without intrathecal administration. Plasma clearance is triexponential, with a distribution half-life of about 45 min, a second phase of about 3.5 hr (possibly an enterohepatic component, since 10% of the drug is secreted into bile), and an elimination half-life of 6 to 69 hr. Renal tubular secretion accounts for about 80% of elimination, and probenecid, salicylate and other NSAIDs, etc, interfere with excretion. The dose must be adjusted in renal failure.

Dose—(Free acid-equivalent),—*intramuscular* or *intravenous adult, antineoplastic,* **15** to **50 mg/m²** once or twice a wk, the dose varying according to the type of neoplasia, the condition of the patient and concomitant drugs employed; *mycosis fungoides* (intramuscular only), **up to 50 mg/70 kg** once a wk *or* **25 mg/70 kg** twice a wk; *psoriasis,* usually **10** to **25 mg/70 kg,** but up to 50 mg/70 kg, one a wk; *children, antineoplastic,* **25** to **30 mg/m²** once a wk. *Oral, adult, antineoplastic,* **15** to **50 mg/m²** once or twice a wk according to circumstances; *mycosis fungoides,* **2.5** to **5 mg/70 kg/day;** *psoriasis,* **10** to **25 mg/70 kg,** not to exceed 50 mg, a week *or* **2.5** to **5 mg/70 kg** every 12 hr for 3 doses or every 8 hr for 4 doses, not to exceed 30 mg/wk, *or* **2.5 mg/70 kg** once a day, not to exceed 6.25 mg/day, for 5 days, after which drug is discontinued for 2 days before continuing with each similar course; *psoriatic* or *rheumatoic arthritis,* **2.5** to **25** (usually 7.5) **mg/70 kg/wk;** *children, antineoplastic,* **20** to **30 mg/m²** once a wk.

Dosage Forms—Tablets: 2.5 mg; Methotrexate Sodium for Injection (methotrexate equivalent): 5 mg/2 mL, 50 mg/2 mL, 100 mg/4 mL and 200 mg/8 mL. Methotrexate Sodium Poweder for Injection: 20, 50, 100 and 250 mg.

Mitobronitol—see RPS-18, page 1159.

Mitomycin

Azirino[2′,3′:3,4]pyrrolo[1,2-*a*]indole-4,7-dione, [1a*R*-(1aα,8β,8aα,8bα)]-6-amino-8-[[(aminocarbonyl) oxy]methyl]-1,1a,2,8,8a,8b-hexahydro-8a-methoxy-5-methyl-, Mitocin-C; Mutamycin (*Bristol*)

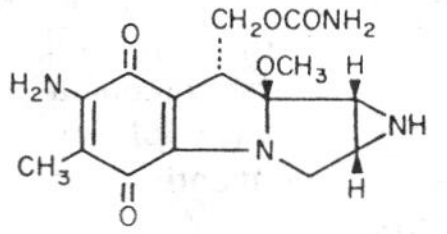

Mitomycin C [50-07-7] $C_{15}H_{18}N_4O_5$ (334.33).

Preparation—One of three closely related entities isolated from the antibiotic complex produced by *Streptomyces caespitosus*, an organism from Japanese soil.

Description—Blue-violet, crystalline powder.

Solubility—Soluble in water and common organic solvents.

Uses—Inhibits DNA synthesis by cross-linking double-stranded DNA through guanine and cytosine. It is approved for palliative treatment of *disseminated adenocarcinoma of the stomach and pancreas that have failed other treatments*. It is a component of second-line combinations for the treatment of *cervical, gastric* and *pancreatic carcinomas* and *non-small cell bronchogenic carcinoma*. It is instilled into the bladder in *papilloma*. It is an alternative drug for use against *head* and *neck squamous cell carcinoma, bladder carcinoma* and *osteogenic sarcoma*. Acute adverse effects occur in about 14% of patients: they include nausea, vomiting, anorexia, fever and local irritation and cellulitis from extravasation at the site of injection. Delayed toxicity includes cumulative, frequently irreversible, bone-marrow depression (in 64% of recipients), stomatitis, alopecia and renal impairment (in 20% of recipients).

Dose—*Intravenous, adults* and children either **10** to **20 mg/m²** as a single dose or **2 mg/m²/day** for 5 days, an interval of 2 days, then again 2 mg/m²/day for 5 days. The course is repeated at 6- to 8-wk intervals, recovery of the blood picture permitting; treatment should be resumed until the platelets recover to 75,000/mm³ and the leukocytes to 3000/mm³.

Dosage Form—Injection: 5 mg, 20 mg or 40 mg/vial.

Mitoguazone—see RPS-18, page 1160.

Mitotane

Benzene, 1-chloro-2 [2,2-dichloro-1-(4-chlorohenyl)ethyl]-, *o, p′*-DDD; Lysodren (*Bristol*)

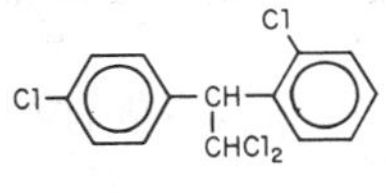

1,1-Dichloro-2-(*o*-chlorophenyl)-2-(*p*-chlorophenyl)ethane [53-19-0] $C_{14}H_{10}Cl_4$ (320.05).

Preparation—Chlorobenzene is condensed with 2,2-dichloro-1-(*o*-chlorophenyl)ethanol with the aid of H_2SO_4.

Description—White, tasteless, crystalline powder; slight aromatic odor; stable in light, air and heat; melts about 78°.

Solubility—Practically insoluble in water; soluble in alcohol, ether, solvent hexane or fixed oils or fats.

Uses—Since it is toxic to the adrenal cortex, it is approved for the treatment of *inoperable adrenal cortical carcinoma*. Nearly 50% of patients will respond to treatment. It also is used to treat *Cushing's syndrome*. Adverse effects adrenal insufficiency may require adrenal steroid replacement, include anorexia, nausea, vomiting (in 80%), diarrhea, lethargy, somnolence (25%), dizziness (15%), headache, confusion, asthenia, tremors, ataxia, speech difficulties, neuropathies, dermatitis (15%), hypersensitivity, flushing, hyperpyrexia, postural hypotension, alopecia, pigmentation, leukopenia, thrombocytopenia, hyperbilirubinemia, albuminuria, hemorrhageic cystitis, elevated serum transaminase, blurred vision, diplopia, lens opacities and retinopathy. The drug should be used with caution in the presence of liver damage, bone-marrow depression, dermatitis or neuropathy. It is metabolized in the liver.

Dose—*Oral, adult, antineoplastic, initially* **2** increased to a maximum of no more than **16** (usually 8 to 10) **g/day** in 3 or 4 divided doses, to be increased gradually until toxicity occurs; for *Cushing's syndrome, initially* **3** to **6 g/day** in 3 or 4 divided doses, continued until a remission occurs; maintenance, **0.5 mg** twice a week to **2 g/day;** *children, antineoplastic, initially* **1** to **2 g/day** in divided doses, to be increased gradually to **5** to **7 g/day** for *maintenance*.

Dosage Form—Tablets: 500 mg.

Mitoxantrone Hydrochloride

9,10-Anthracenedione, 1,4-dihydroxy-5,8-bis-[[2-[(2-hydroxyethyl)-amino]ethyl]amino]-, dihydrochloride; Novantrone (*Lederle*)

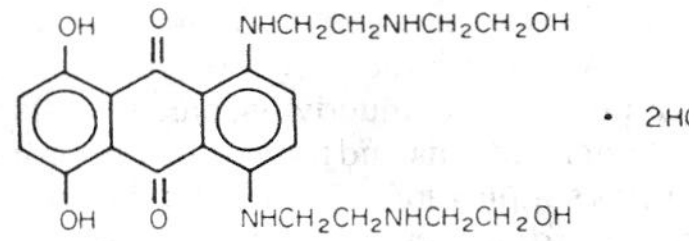

Mitozantrone [70476-82-3] $C_{22}H_{28}N_4O_6.2HCl$ (517.41).

Preparation—*J Med Chem 21*:291, 1978.

Description—Blue-black solid; hygroscopic; melts about 161°; pK_a 5.99, 8.13.

Solubility—Sparingly soluble in water; slightly soluble in methanol.

Uses—An alkylaminoanthraquinone antineoplastic drug related to doxorubicin. In the US it is approved for the treatment of *acute nonlymphocytic leukemia*, for which it is combined with cytarabine; the remission rate is about 63%. It is an alternative drug for the treatment of *acute lymphocytic* and *breast carcinoma*. It possibly may come to replace both daunarubicin and doxorubicin in some uses. Immediate adverse effects include nausea, vomiting and phlebitis. Tissue necrosis and sloughing result from extravasation. Delayed adverse effects include myelosuppression, and cardiac, renal and hepatic toxicities. The *N*-substitution on the aminosugar decreases the cardiotoxicity. The drug is not absorbed perorally. It is eliminated mostly in the bile with a half-life of 20 to 36 hr.

Dose—*Intravenous, adult,* **14 mg/m²** every 3 wk.

Dosage Form—Injection: 10 mL, 12.5 mL and 15 mL equiv to 2 mg/mL of the base.

Muromonab CD3

Orthodone OKT3 (*Ortho*)

A murine monoclonal antibody (anti CD3), $IgG_{2\alpha}$, of two chains having molecular weights of approx 50,000 and 25,000 daltons.

Preparation—Mouse myeloma is fused into lymphocytes from immunized animals producing a hybridoma which then secretes antigen-specific antibodies to the T3 antigen of T-lymphocytes.

Uses—Anti-CD3 blocks cell signals that induce proliferation of cytotoxic lymphocytes and also causes the removal of T lymphocytes from the circulation. This causes reversal of acute allograft rejection of renal and certain other transplants. In renal graft rejections, the success rate has been reported to be as high as 94%. Most adverse effects persist only during the first two days of treatment. They include fever (90%), chills (59%), dyspnea consequent to pulmonary edema (21%), nausea (19%), vomiting (19%), chest pain (14%), diarrhea (14%), wheezing (13%), tremor (13%), headache (11%) and tachycardia (10%). The antibody is antigenic and has caused occasional serum sickness and one case of anaphylaxis. Various opportunistic infections have occurred, herpes simplex and cytomegalovirus infections being the most common.

Dose—*Intravenous, adult,* **5 mg/day** it should be administered by bolus. It is advisable to premedicate the patient with methylprednisolone sodium succinate and postmedicate with hydrocortisone sodium succinate.

Dosage Form—Injection: 1 mg/mL in 5 mL ampule.

Penicillamine—page 936.

Pentostatin

Imidazo[4,5-*d*][1,3]diazepin-8-ol, (*R*)-3-(2-deoxy-β-D-*erythro*-pentofuranosyl)-3,6,7,8-tetrahydro-, Nipent (*Parke-Davis*)

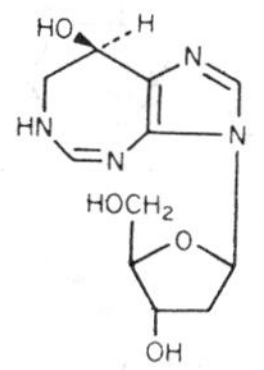

[63677-95-2] $C_{11}H_{16}N_4O_4$ (268.27).

Preparation—*J Org Chem 47*, 3457, 1982. Usually isolated from *Streptomyces antibioticus*.

Description—White crystals; melts about 223°; pK_a 5.2.

Uses—Inhibits adenosine deaminase, thus leading to an accumulation of 2′-deoxyATP. Inhibition of cell proliferation results. Lymphocytes are especially sensitive to this drug. It is approved for use in *α-interferon refractory hairy cell leukemia.* Presently it shares drug-of-choice status with interferon alpha-2 for the treatment of *hairy cell leukemia,* and it is an alternative drug for use against *chronic lymphocytic leukemia* and *mycosis fungoides.* Adverse effects include myelosuppression sometimes with severe lymphopenia, conjuctivitis, panserositis, lethargy, coma, pulmonary toxicity, hyperuricemia and immunosuppression; various infections may occur, herpes simplex infections being the most common.

Dose—*Intravenous, adult,* **5 mg/m²** for 3 days every 4 wk.

Dosage Form—Injection: 10 mg.

PGE-Adenosine Deaminase—see RPS-18, page 1038.

Pipobroman

Piperazine, 1,4-bis(3-bromo-1-oxopropyl)-, Vercyte (*Abbott*)

$$BrCH_2CH_2\overset{O}{\overset{\|}{C}}-N\langle\rangle N-\overset{O}{\overset{\|}{C}}CH_2CH_2Br$$

[54-91-1] $C_{10}H_{16}Br_2N_2O_2$ (356.06).

Preparation—By condensation of piperazine with 3-bromopropionyl chloride.

Description—White or practically white, crystalline powder; melts about 103°.

Solubility—1 g in 230 mL water, 35 mL alcohol or 5 mL chloroform.

Uses—An antineoplastic drug of the alkylating type. Its use is limited mainly to treatment of *polycythemia vera* and *chronic granulocytic leukemia.* Even in these disorders, however, it generally is not as effective as older modes of treatment. Consequently, it is held in reserve for use in patients who have become refractory to X-irradiation and busulfan in the case of leukemia and phlebotomy and radiophosphate in the case of polycythemia vera.

Adverse effects include severe anemia, in part of a hemolytic nature, and reticulocytosis. Leukopenia and thrombocytopenia are the result of the intended action of the drug, but the leukocyte count should be kept above 3000/mm³ and the platelet count above 100,000/mm³. Transient nausea, vomiting, abdominal cramps and diarrhea sometimes occur. There is an occasional rash. The drug is contraindicated in patients whose bone-marrow function remains depressed from radiation or previous chemotherapy. It should not be used in pregnancy.

Dose—*Oral,* for *polyerythemia vera,* initially **1 mg/kg/day** for at least 30 days, after which the dose may be increased to 1.5 to 3 mg/kg if there was no previous response; once the hematocrit has been reduced by 50%; *maintenance,* begun at **0.1** to **0.2 mg** (100 to 200 μg)/**kg/day.** For *chronic myelocytic leukemia, initially* **1.5** to **2.5 mg/kg/day** until the optimal therapeutic response of serious untoward effects occur; *maintenance* doses range from **7** to **175 mg/day;** maintenance is withheld until the leukocyte count rises again to 10,000 cells/mm³.

Plicamycin

Aureolic acid; Mithramycin; Mithracin (*Miles*)

[18378-89-7] $C_{52}H_{76}O_{24}$ (1085.16).

Preparation—Produced by cultures of *Streptomyces argillaceus, S plicatus* and *S tanashiensis.*

Description—Yellow, crystalline powder; odorless; hygroscopic; melts about 182°.

Solubility—Slightly soluble in water; very slightly soluble in alcohol; freely soluble in ethyl acetate.

Uses—An antibiotic elaborated during culture of certain strains of *Streptomyces.* A yellow, crystalline powder; odorless; hygroscopic; slightly soluble in water; very slightly soluble in alcohol. *Uses:* Binds to guanine-rich DNA and thus inhibits DNA-dependent RNA polymerase. It acts mainly during the S-phase. It is approved for and used to treat *carcinoma* of the *testes.* It also is an alternative drug for *acute phase* of *chronic myelocytic leukemia,* especially in combination with hydroxyurea. Because it suppresses osteoclast activity, it often is used to treat *malignant hypercalcemia* (neoplasms that cause dissolution of bone salts) not responsive to conventional treatment and other severe, refractory *hypercalcemias.*

It is quite toxic, and drug-induced mortality ranges from 0.09 to 0.7%, depending on dose. Death results from hemorrhagic diatheses resulting from prothrombinopenia, thrombocytopenia, increased clotting and bleeding times and abnormal clot retraction. The hemorrhagic episode usually begins with nosebleed, but may begin with hematemesis. The most common untoward effects are nausea, vomiting, diarrhea, anorexia and stomatitis. Less frequently there occur fever, facial flushing, rash, phlebitis, malaise, headache, drowsiness, asthenia, lethargy, depression, hepatic dysfunction, renal insufficiency, hypocalciuria, hypopotassemia, hypophosphatemia and leukopenia. The hemorrhagic syndrome occurs in about 5% of patients who receive no more than 30 μg/kg/day for no more than 10 doses, whereas it is about 12% for higher doses. It is locally toxic and can cause necrosis and sloughing if extravasated.

Dose—*Intravenous infusion,* for *testicular tumors,* **0.025** to **0.03 mg** (25 to 30 μg)/**kg** in 1 L of 5% dextrose injection, infused over a 6-hr period, once a day for 8 to 10 days or **0.025** to **0.050 mg** (25 to 50 μg)/**kg** every other day for 8 doses, unless toxicity supervenes; additional courses of treatment are given at monthly intervals until the tumor completely regresses or begins to regrow. For *hypercalcemia* and *hypercalciuria,* **0.015** to **0.025 mg** (15 to 25 μg)/**kg**/day for 3 or 4 days; additional courses or 2 to 4 doses/wk may be given, if necessary.

Podophyllum Resin—page 887.

Podophyllotoxin—see RPS-18, page 767.

Polyestradiol Phosphate—see RPS-18, page 987.

Prednisone—page 1075.

Procarbazine Hydrochloride

Benzamide, *N*-(1-methylethyl)-4-[(2-methylhydrazino)methyl]-, monohydrochloride; Matulane (*Roche*)

$$(CH_3)_2CHNH\overset{O}{\overset{\|}{C}}-C_6H_4-CH_2NHNHCH_3 \cdot HCl$$

N-Isopropyl-α-(2-methylhydrazino)-*p*-toluamide monohydrochloride [366-70-1] $C_{12}H_{19}N_3O.HCl$ (257.76).

Preparation—1,2-Bis(carbobenzoxy)-1-methylhydrazine is reacted with 4-(bromoethyl)benzoic acid methyl ester utlimately to yield 4-[[2-methyl-1,2-di(carbobenzoxy)hydrazino]methyl]benzoic acid. Thionyl chloride is used to obtain the acid chloride which is reacted with isopropylamine to give the *N*-isopropylamide compound. Treatment with 33% HBr in glacial acetic acid removes the protecting carbobenzoxy groups and the resulting hydrobromide may be converted to the hydrochloride by the usual process. US Pat 3,520,926.

Description—White to pale yellow, crystalline powder; slight odor and a bitter taste; solutions are acid to litmus; stable in light, slowly oxidized in air and stable at room temperature (in the presence of oxygen, oxidation is accelerated by increased temperature); melts about 223° with decomposition; pK_a (at room temperature) 6.8.

Solubility—1 g in 7 mL water or 100 mL alcohol; slightly soluble in chloroform; insoluble in ether.

Uses—Unstable in aqueous solutions, it breaks down to form the methylazoxy derivative, the active form of the drug. It generates hydrogen peroxide, hydroxyl and methyl-free radicals, the latter being thought to alkylate DNA resulting in degradation and chromosomal breaks; DNA synthesis, and hence protein synthesis, is impaired. It is approved as part of a combination therapy for *Hodgkin's disease.* The most important use of procarbazine is as a component of several combinations of choice for *Hodgkin's disease, histiocytic lymphoma* and *medulloblastoma.* It is an alternative drug to treat non-small cell *bronchogenic carcinoma;* it is rarely used alone. Cross-resistance with other agents or radiation apparently does not occur.

Untoward reactions include frequent leukopenia, thrombocytopenia, anemia, less frequent nausea, vomiting and, rarely, anorexia, dry mouth, stomatitis, dysphagia, diarrhea, constipation, myalgia and arthralgia, chills and fever, sweating, fatigue, asthenia, lethargy and drowsiness. Ascites, edema, effusions, cough, intercurrent infections, epistaxis, hemorrhaging, melena, pruritis, allergic dermatitis, allergic pneumonitis, flushing, alopecia, pigmentation, herpes, jaundice, headache, vertigo, depression, paresthesias, neuropathies, insomnia, nightmares, ataxia, confusion, coma, tremors and convulsions may occur. Rarely, there may be hoarseness, hypotension, tachycardia, syncope, hemolysis, nystagmus, photophobia, photosensitivity, retinal hemorrhage, diplopia, papilledema, impaired hearing and slurred speech. It is mutagenic, teratogenic and carcinogenic in experimental animals. Thus, it must be regarded as a dangerous drug.

Central nervous system depressants should not be given at the same time except under supervision. Since the drug is a monoamine oxidase inhibitor, tricyclic antidepressants, various sympathomimetics and tyramine-containing foods should be avoided. Since it has disulfiram-like activity, patients should be warned against ingestion of alcoholic beverages. Caution must be exercised in the presence of liver damage, respiratory disorders, renal impairment or bone-marrow depression.

It is absorbed almost completely by the oral route. It penetrates readily into the cerebrospinal fluid. Peak plasma and CSF levels occur about 60 min after an oral dose. It is metabolized rapidly and auto-oxidized, with an elimination half-life of only about 7 min. Almost none is excreted unchanged.

Dose—*Adult, oral, initially* **2** to **4 mg/kg/day** of procarbazine equivalent, in divided doses if desired, for 1 wk, then 4 to 6 mg/kg/day until the leukocyte count falls below 4000/mm^3 or the platelet count falls below 100,000 mm^3 or a remission occurs. In MOPP combination for Hodgkin's disease, **100 mg/m^2**/day for 2 wk, per course. If hematological toxicity occurs, treatment is suspended until the blood picture is normal, then resumed at 1 to 2 **mg/kg/day.** Once remission has occurred, the dose is maintained at 1 to 2 mg/kg/day. The *pediatric* dose is **50 mg** once a day for 1 wk, then 100 **mg/m^2/day** until the response reaches its maximum, and **50 mg** once a day thereafter.

Dosage Form—Capsules: containing the equivalent of 50 mg of procarbazine.

Semustine—see RPS-18, page 1160.

Sodium Iodide I 131—pages 844 and 861.

Sodium Phosphate P 32—pages 844 and 861.

Sargramostim

Granulocyte-Macrophage Colony-Stimulating Factor Recombinant; Prokine (*Hoechst-Roussel*); Leukine (*Immunex*)

See also *Sargramostim*, Chapter 54.

Uses—A single-chain glycopeptide containing 127 amino acids with a substitution of leucine at position 23. Sargramostim is produced by yeast. The drug is purified from yeast cultures primarily by chromatographic means. Sargramostim is approved for acceleration of bone-marrow recovery in all Hodgkin's, non-Hodgkin's disease and acute lymphocytic leukemia patients undergoing autologous bone-marrow transplantations, and for use in all patients undergoing allogenic or autologous bone-marrow transplants in whom engraftment has failed or is delayed. GM-CSF stimulates relatively uncommitted progenitor cells to produce eosinophils, monocytes, macrophages and neutrophils. It also prolongs WBC survival, and increases phagocytosis, chemotaxis and cell-mediated cytotoxicity.

It generally is tolerated well; bone pain is the most common adverse effect. Adverse dermatological effects may be due to increased neutrophils. Such reactions include acute febrile neutrophilic dermatosis, leukoblastic vasculitis and exacerbated psoriasis. Splenomegaly also has been documented, possibly due to extramedullary myelopoiesis. Rare effects of pericarditis, eosinophilic pulmonary infiltrates and capillary leak syndrome and inflammation at injection site have been reported. Clinical studies have identified anti-sargramostim antibodies in some patients, which may speed clearance of the drug. Its half-life is approximately 2 hr. It usually is administered by IV infusion over 2 hr, but may be administered SC. It should not be administered within 24 hr of a myelosuppressive chemotherapeutic.

Dose—*Intravenous* or *subcutaneous*, **250 µg/m^2** a day for 21 days, beginning 2 to 4 hr after bone-marrow instillation; higher doses may not be well tolerated. Twenty one days worth of sargramostim costs over $3000.

Dosage Form—Injection: 250 or 500 µg sargramostim (with 40 mg mannitol, 10 mg sucrose and 1.2 mg tromethamine).

Streptozocin

D-Glucopyranose, 2-deoxy-2-[[(methylnitrosoamino)-carbonyl]amino]-, Streptozocin; Zanosar (*Upjohn*)

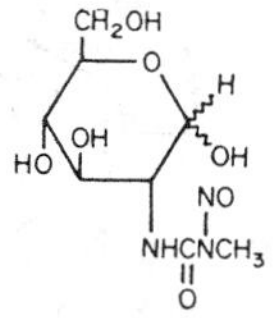

[18883-66-4] $C_8H_{15}N_3O_7$ (265.22).

Preparation—A nitrosourea antiobiotic isolated from *Streptomyces achromogenes* fermentation broth; also synthesized; *J Am Chem Soc 52*, 2555, 1969.

Description—Plates or prisms; melts about 115° with decomp.

Solubility—Very soluble in water; soluble in alcohol.

Uses—It is approved for and has become the drug of first choice (in combination with fluorouracil) for treatment of *islet cell carcinoma.* It also is used with fluorouracil and mitomycin for *pancreatic carcinoma.* It is an alternative drug for use against *malignant carcinoid tumor* and *Hodgkin's disease.* Acute adverse effects include nausea and vomiting, local pain at the site of administration and chills. Renal damage is the principal delayed toxicity but hepatotoxicity also occurs. Bone-marrow depression occurs in about 20% of recipients. The drug is mainly metabolized; its half-life is about 15 min.

Dose—*Intravenous* or *intra-arterial*, **0.5g/m^2** day for 5 days every 4 to 6 wk or **1 g/m^2** once a wk for 2 wk, then adjusted up to maximum of **1.5 g/m^2.**

Dosage Form—Powder for Injection: 1g/vial, reconstitute to 100 mg/mL.

Tamoxifen—page 1094.

Taxol

Paclitaxal; (*Bristol-Myers Oncology*)

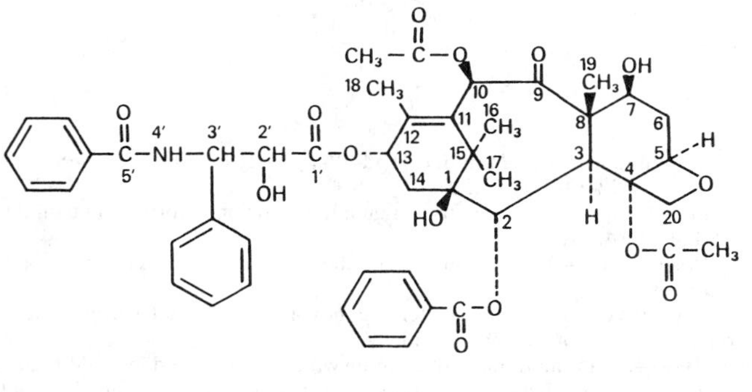

[33069-62-4] $C_{47}H_{51}NO_{14}$ (853.92)

Preparation—Extracted from the bark of the Pacific yew tree (*Taxus brevifolia*, Taxaceae).

Description—White needles; melts about 215° with decomp.

Uses—Inhibits mitosis by stabilizing mitotic spindles and promoting their formation, apparently inappropriately. Taxol is approved for use in *ovarian cancer;* it also has significant activity against breast cancer. Dose-limiting toxicity appears to be neutropenia, which reaches a nadir during the second week after therapy. This appears to be attenuated by G-CSF.

Dose—*Intravenous infusion, initially* (over 24 hr) **250 mg/m^2.** Doses may require reductions in subsequent cycles due to WBC suppression.

Dosage Form—Injection: 30 mg in 5-mL ampuls.

Teniposide

Furo[3′,4′:6,7]naphtho[2,3-*d*]-1,3-dioxol-6(5a*H*)-one, [5*R*-[5α,5aβ,8aα,9β(*R**)]]-5,8,8a,9-tetrahydro-5-(4-hydroxy-3,5-dimethoxyphenyl)-9-[[4,6-*O*-(2-thienylmethylene)-β-D-glucopyranosyl]oxy]-, Vee M-26 (*Bristol-Myers Oncology*)

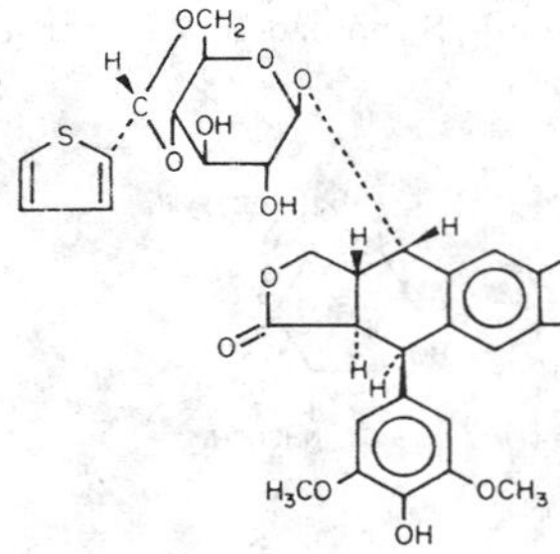

[29767-20-2] $C_{32}H_{32}O_{13}S$ (656.66).

Preparation—A semi-synthetic derivative of podophyllotoxin.

Description—White crystals; melts about 245°.

Uses—A drug related to podophyllotoxin and similar to etoposide in antieoplastic activity. It arrests the cell cycle in late S and G_2 phases. It is approved for use in *refractory acute lymphocytic leukemia*. It is an alternative drug for the treatment of *diffuse histiocytic lymphoma, Hodgkin's disease, non-Hodgkin's lymphoma, acute lymphocytic leukemia, acute myelocytic leukemia, breast cancer* and *neuroblastoma*. The principal adverse effects (leukopenia, thrombocytopenia, etc) result from myelosuppression, but hypotension, thrombophlebitis and anaphylaxis also occur. The drug is not absorbed orally. In plasma it is almost completely protein-bound. It is eliminated mainly by hepatic metabolism, with a half-life of 8 to 24 hr.

Dose—*Slow intravenous*, **50 mg/m²** for 5 days every 4 wk.

Dosage Form—Injection: 50 mg in 5-mL ampuls.

Testolactone—page 1104.

Testosterone Propionate—page 1105.

Thioguanine

6*H*-Purine-6-thione, 2-amino-1,7-dihydro-, Tabloid (*Burroughs Wellcome*)

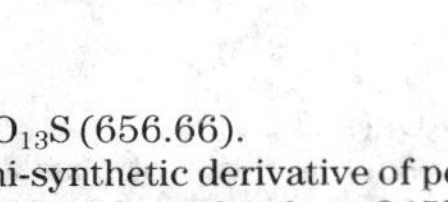

2-Aminopurine-6(1*H*)-thione [154-42-7] $C_5H_5N_5S$ (167.19); *hemihydrate* [50322-14-0] (176.20).

Preparation—By thionation of guanine with phosphorus pentasulfide. US Pat 2,884,667.

Description—Pale yellow, crystalline powder; odorless or practically odorless.

Solubility—Insoluble in water, alcohol or chloroform; freely soluble in dilute solutions of alkali hydroxides.

Uses—An antimetabolite of guanine which is converted into 6-thioguanine-ribose-phosphate; this not only is incorporated into DNA and RNA but also interferes with guanine synthesis. It acts mainly in the S-phase of the cell cycle, but cell replication ultimately is prevented. It also promotes differentiation of some cancer cells. Although its actions are very similar to those of mercaptopurine, some of which is converted to thioguanine, and cross-resistance occurs between the two drugs, so that the actions and uses are not identical. It is approved for *acute nonlymphocytic leukemia*. With other drugs, thioguanine is a component of combinations that are treatments of choice for *acute myelocytic leukemias* and the *acute* phase of *chronic granulocytic leukemia*. It is an alternative drug for use against *acute lymphocytic leukemia*. It sometimes is used in the stable phase of *chronic myelocytic leukemia*. It also is a potent *immunosuppressive drug*, but its status has yet to be settled. It has been used especially in the treatment of *nephrosis* and *collagen-vascular disorders*.

Its adverse effects are virtually the same as those for mercaptopurine (see page 1255), except that the incidence of gastrointestinal toxicity is less and there is no adverse interaction with allopurinol.

It is metabolized nearly completely in the body; the 6-thiol group is methylated and the 8-amino group removed to yield 6-methylmercaptopurine. Xanthine oxidase is not involved.

Dose—*Oral, adult* and *pediatric, initially* **2 mg/kg** a day (to the nearest 20 mg) *or* **75** to **100 mg/m²** a day for 4 wk, after which the dose may be cautiously advanced to as much as **3 mg/kg** a day *or* 100 **mg/m²** a day if the response has been inadequate; if response is still inadequate, treatment is stopped and another drug tried. In combination with daunorubicin and vincristine for induction of remission of *acute myelocytic leukemia*, **100 mg/m²** twice a day for 7 days, to be repeated every 28 days.

Dosage Form—Tablets: 40 mg.

Triethylenethiophosphoramide

Aziridine, 1,1′,1″-phosphinothioylidynetris-, Thiotepa (*Lederle*)

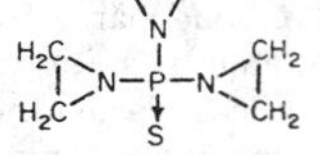

[52-24-4] $C_6H_{12}N_3PS$ (189.2).

Caution—It is extremely poisonous.

Preparation—By condensing ethylenimine with thiophosphorylchloride ($PSCl_3$) in the presence of triethylamine as the acid receptor.

Description—Fine, white, crystalline flakes; faint odor; melts about 54°.

Solubility—1 g in 13 mL water, 8.3 mL alcohol, 1.9 mL chloroform or 4.1 mL ether.

Uses—It is an alkylating agent. However, it has a much lower chemical reactivity than the β-chloroethylamines, hence, has a low degree of local irritancy and lacks the vesicant properties. For this reason it presently is used mainly for local application, where appropriate. It is approved for use in *adenocarcinoma of the breast and ovary*. Local instillation into the urinary bladder for *papillary carcinoma* is sometimes quite effective. It also may be instilled into other cavities to control serous infusions consequent to certain neoplasms. It occasionally may be infiltered directly into tumors, especially obstructive lesions. Given systemically, its bone-marrow toxicity is quite unpredictable, so that such use is dangerous; consequently, it is nearing obsolescence for systemic treatment. The neoplasm for which it is still a possible desperation choice is *embryonal rhabdomyosarcoma*.

Local adverse effects include local pain, weeping and occasional perforation through the lesion. The most serious systemic adverse effect is bone-marrow depression, characterized by neutropenia, thrombocytopenia and usually low-grade anemia. It is mandatory to monitor the blood cell counts. The effects may not appear for 5 to 30 days, which complicates management. Anorexia, nausea and vomiting are not as common as with other alkylating agents. Headache, dizziness, fever and tightness in the throat may occur. Hyperuricemia may result from massive cell destruction, and crystalluria and oliguria are possible. Hypersensitivity is uncommon, but hives, skin rash and even anaphylaxis can occur. Depression of spermatogenesis and ovarian function have been reported. Systemic side effects from local instillation can occur. Thiotepa is excreted mostly unchanged, so that the dose should be reduced in renal failure. It is contraindicated if there is prior bone-marrow depression or pregnancy.

Dose—*Parenteral*, **0.3** to **0.4 mg/kg** at intervals of 1 to 4 wk. *Intrapleural, intraperitoneal, intrapericardial* or *intratumor*, **0.6** to **0.8 mg/kg** once a wk; if the leukocyte count is below 3000 cells/mm³, treatment is discontinued until the count rises above that value (preferably until about 10,000 cells/mm³). For *maintenance*, **0.07** to **0.08 mg/kg** every 1 to 4 wk. In malignant ascites the *intraperitoneal* dose is **10** to **15 mg** once a wk as long as leukocyte and paltelet counts are sufficient. For instillation into the *bladder*, **60 mg** in 30 to 60 mL of distilled water once a wk for 4 wk: the solution should be retained inthe bladder for 2 hr at each instillation. Solutions for topical application can be mixed with 2% procaine and/or 1:1000 epinephrine.

Dosage Forms—Injection: 15 mg/vial.

Uracil Mustard

2,4(1*H*, 3*H*)-Pyrimidinedione, 5-[bis(2-chloroethyl)amino-, Uramustine; Uracil Mustard (*Upjohn*)

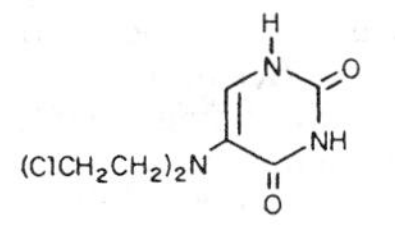

5-[Bis(2-chlorethyl)amino]uracil [66-75-1] $C_8H_{11}Cl_2N_3O_2$ (252.10).

Preparation—Using 5-aminouracil, ethylene oxide and thionyl chloride as reactants.

Description—Off-white, crystalline powder; odorless; melts about 200° with decomposition. Unstable in high humidity or aqueous vehicles.

Solubility—1 g in more than 1000 mL water or 150 mL alcohol.

Uses—An alkylating agent of the nitrogen mustard type. It is essentially an obsolete drug, having been displaced by the more efficacious and less toxic chlorambucil. However, this drug still may have a special use in the treatment of *primary thrombocytosis*. Other neoplasms for which the drug is used occasionally are non-Hodgkin's lymphomas, chronic lymphocytic leukemia, chronic myelocytic leukemia, mycosis fungoides and polycythemia vera. The most common untoward effects are nausea, vomiting and diarrhea. Pruritus, dermatitis and partial alopecia do occur, but less frequently than with cyclophosphamide. Nervousness, irritability, depression, amenorrhea and oligospermia occur infrequently. Bone-marrow depression with leukopenia, thrombocytopenia and even anemia may occur, and the blood picture must be monitored twice a week during the first month of treatment. The bone-marrow damage may become irreversible when the cumulative dose approaches 1 mg/kg. Rapid involution of tumors may cause hyperuricemia and consequent nephropathy and renal failure, so that plasma uric acid levels should be determined regularly and the patients should drink much water.

Dose—*Oral, adults and children, Schedule A, initially* **1** to **2 mg/day** until a therapeutic response or hematopoietic toxicity occurs. The drug then is withdrawn until adverse effects subside or the clinical condition deteriorates. The *maintenance* dose is **1 mg/day** for 3 wk out of each 4-wk period. *Schedule B, initially* **3** to **5 mg/day** for 1 wk; the total dosage not to exceed 0.5 mg/kg. The *maintenance* dose is **1 mg/day** for 3 wk out of each 4-wk period. Critical bone-marrow toxicity is indicated by a leukocyte count below 1500 cells/mm^3, platelet count below 50,000/mm^3 or a hemoglobin concentration less than 70% of pretreatment values.

Dosage Forms—Capsules: 1 mg.

Vinblastine Sulfate

Vincaleukoblastine, sulfate (1:1) (salt); Velban (*Lilly*)

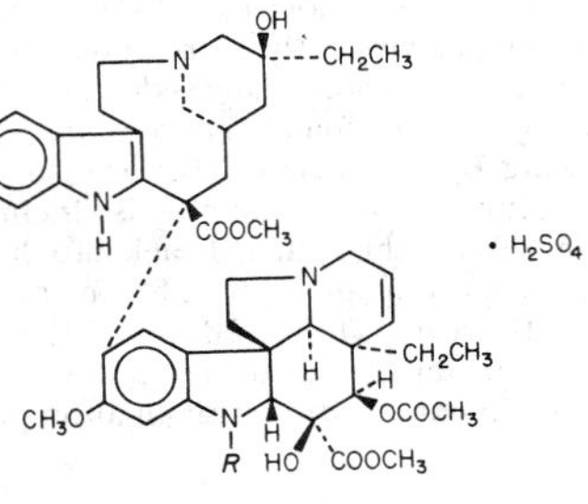

(*R* is CH_3)

[143-67-9] $C_{46}H_{58}N_4O_9.H_2SO_4$ (909.06).

Preparation—By extracting the leaves, bark or stems of *Vinca rosea* with aqueous or aqueous-alcoholic sulfuric acid, isolating the alkaloid from the extract by the usual precipitation and solvent techniques and purifying by chromatography on aluminum oxide. Conversion to the (1:1) sulfate may be effected by dissolving the alkaloid in an equimolar quantity of dilute H_2SO_4 and either evaporating to dryness or precipitating with a suitable organic solvent. US Pat 3,097,137.

Description—White to slightly yellow, amorphous or crystalline powder; odorless; hygroscopic.

Solubility—Freely soluble in water.

Uses—Interferes with the assembly of the microtubules, by combining with tubulin: the result is mitotic arrest in metaphase. However, there is also evidence that vinblastine exerts its antineoplastic effect by interfering with glutamate and aspartate metabolism. The antineoplastic spectrum and toxicity are much different than for vincristine, which also interacts with tubulin. It is approved for use in *advanced Hodgkin's disease, lymphocytic* and *histiocytic lymphoma, mycosis fungoides, testicular cancer* and *Kaposi's sarcoma.* This drug is a component of first-choice combinations for the treatment of *testicular carcinoma, Hodgkin's disease* and *bladder cancer.* It is an alternative drug for *choriocarcinoma, squamous cell carcinoma* of the head and neck, *renal-cell carcinoma, neuroblastoma, breast tumors, cervical carcinoma, Kaposi's sarcoma, melanoma* and *mycosis fungoides.* It also has been used to treat lymphosarcoma, lymphocytic lymphoma, reticulum-cell sarcoma and Letterer-Siwe's disease. This drug is subject to pleiotropic drug resistance.

It is a secondary (efferent) immunosuppressive drug, but it has not been exploited for this purpose.

Nausea, vomiting, headache and paresthesias occur within 4 to 6 hr and last from 2 to 10 hr. Severe bronchospasm may occur, especially if mitomycin has been given. Diarrhea, constipation, adynamic ileus, anorexia and stomatitis also may occur and are premonitory of neurotoxic effects, such as severe headache, malaise, mental depression, paresthesias and loss of deep tendon reflexes. Neurotoxicity occurs in 5 to 20% of cases, more frequently at higher doses. Central nervous system damage occasionally is permanent when excessive doses have been used. Blindness and death have been reported. Alopecia occurs in about 30 to 60% of users, but it generally is reversible. Mild bone-marrow depression with leukopenia occurs in a high percentage of patients and may require discontinuation of the drug. The thrombocytes are less affected, unless other thrombocytogenic drugs are also being given or have recently been given. Anemia is rare. The blood-cell count must be determined each week. The drug is toxic locally, and extravasation should be avoided. It may cause phlebitis at the site of injection. Inappropriate secretion of ADH may occur. It is teratogenic in animals, and probably should not be used during the first trimester of pregnancy.

In plasma it is about 75% protein-bound. It manifests three-compartment kinetics, the second phase having a half-life of 1 to 1½ hr and the elimination half-life 18 to 40 hr. It is metabolized largely by the liver and doses should be reduced by 50% in patients with impaired liver function.

Dose—*Adult, intravenous, initially* **0.1 mg** (100 μg/**kg** *or* **3.7 mg/m²**; 7 days later and each week thereafter the dose is increased by 0.05 mg (50 μg)/kg *or* 1.8 to 1.9 mg/m^2 until the leukocyte count falls to 3000 cells/mm^3, the tumor regresses, or a maximal dose of 0.5 mg (500 μg)/kg or 18.5 mg/m^2 is reached (usually 0.15 to 0.2 mg/kg). Thereafter the dose is *maintained* at a level one increment smaller than the last dose, given at intervals of 1 to 2 wk. Some authorities use a maintenance dose of 10 mg once or twice a month. *Pediatric, intravenous, initially* **2.5 mg/m²** for the first dose; thereafter, weekly doses are increased by 1.25 mg/m^2 until the leukocyte count falls to 3000 cells/mm^2, the tumor regresses or a maximal dose of 7.5 mg/m^2 is reached; *maintenance* is with the aforementioned dose at weekly to biweekly intervals.

Dosage Forms—Injection: 10 mg/10 mL ampul; Sterile Powder: 10 mg.

Vincristine Sulfate

Vincaleukoblastine, 22-oxo-, sulfate (1:1) (salt); Oncovin (*Lilly*); Vincasar PFS (*Adria*)

Leurocristine sulfate (1:1) (salt) [2068-78-2] $C_{46}H_{56}N_4O_{10}.H_2SO_4$ (923.04).

The structure is the same as for *Vinblastine Sulfate,* except that *R* is CHO, an aldehyde.

Preparation—Using suitable modifications in the chromatographic part of the process, vincristine sulfate may be prepared as described above for *Vinblastine Sulfate.* US Pat 3,205,220.

Description—White to slightly yellow, amorphous or crystalline powder: odorless; hygroscopic.

Solubility—Freely soluble in water.

Uses—Combines with the protein tubulin and prevents assembly of microtubules, thus disrupting various cellular processes, including spindle-formation and mitosis. Synthesis of RNA and proteins also is suppressed. It is approved for use in *Hodgkin's lymphomas, rhabdomyocsarcoma, neuroblastoma* and *Wilm's tumor.* The alkaloid is the second most widely used of the antineoplastic drugs. It is especially useful in the treatment of hematological malignancies. It is a component in 27 first-choice combinations for the treatment of *acute lymphocytic leukemia,* the *acute phase* of *chronic myelocytic leukemia, Hodgkin's disease, non-Hodgkin's lymphoma, Burkitt's lymphoma, diffuse histiocytic lymphoma, follicular lymphoma, cervical carcinoma, oat-cell bronchogenic carcinoma, Wilms' tumor, medulloblastoma, soft tissue sarcomas, Ewing's sarcoma* and *embryonal rhabdomyosarcoma.* It is an alternative drug for treatment of *breast carcinoma, cervical carcinoma, testicular carcinoma, glioblastoma, neuroblastoma* and *chronic lymphocytic leukemia.* Some authorities prefer to use this drug only to induce remissions and not for maintenance, because chronic use favors neurotoxicity. Cross-resistance to other drugs occurs via pleiotropic drug resistance.

It differs from most other antineoplastics in that bone-marrow depression frequently does not occur; this is one reason why vincristine is used in combinations. However, leukopenia can occur, and white-cell counts should be made before each dose. Treatment usually is limited by the neurotoxic effects. Adverse effects usually begin with nausea, vomiting, constipation, abdominal cramps and weight loss; these effects readily are reversible. Severe bronchospasm may occur, especially if mitomycin has been given. The drug also may cause slowly reversible reactions, such as alopecia and peripheral neuropathy. Serious neuropathic effects may occur; they include loss of deep tendon reflexes, neuritic pain, numbness of extremities, headache, ataxia and visual defects; paresis or paralysis and atrophy of certain extensor muscles may occur late; paralysis of cranial nerves 2, 3, 6 and 7 may occur. Neuropathies may persist for several months. Severe hypertension, agitation or mental depression also may occur transiently. The drug is toxic locally, and extravasation should be avoided. It is best given into the tubing for a running intravenous solution.

It is cleared rapidly from the blood. It manifests 3-compartment kinetics, with half-lives of 0.08, 2.3 and 85 hr. Seventy percent is secreted into the bile. In obstructive jaundice or impaired liver function the toxicity is greater, and the dose should be reduced by 50%. About 12% is excreted in urine. It does not penetrate into the brain, hence it cannot be used for CNS leukemias.

Dose—*Intravenous, adult,* **0.01** to **0.03 mg/kg** *or* **0.4** to **1.4 mg/m²** as a bolus once a week; *children,* **1.5** to **2 mg/m²** once a week, *except* **0.05 mg/kg** once a week if the weight is 10 kg or less or the surface area less than 1 m². Constant intravenous infusion of 0.25 mg/m²/day for 5 days is proving to be more efficacious and perhaps less toxic than is bolus administration.

Dosage Form—Injection: 1 mg/1 mL, 2 mg/2 mL and 5 mg/5 mL.

Vindesine Sulfate

Eldisine (*Lilly*)

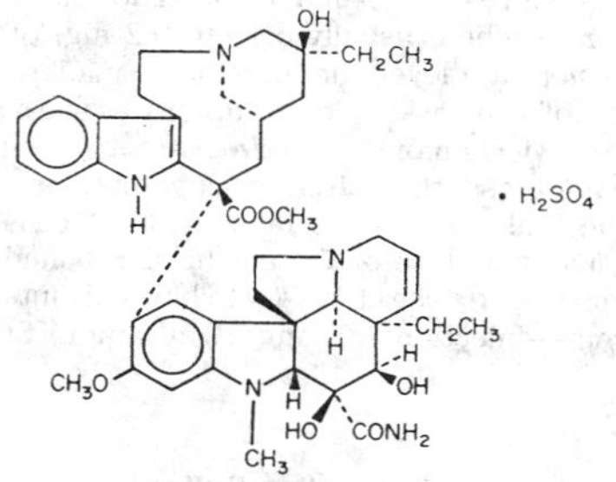

[59917-39-4] $C_{43}H_{55}N_5O_7.H_2SO_4$ (852.01).

Preparation—A semi-synthetic derivative of vinblastine obtained from *Catharanthus.* *J Med Chem 21:*88, 1978.

Description—White crystals melting about 230° (base).

Solubility—pH (reconstituted solution for injection) 4.2 to 4.5; above pH 6 the free base precipitates.

Uses—An investigational drug that combines the therapeutic and toxic properties of vincristine and vinblastine. It is active agianst *vinca-resistant acute lymphocytic leukemia,* the *blast crisis* of *chronic myelocytic leukemia, melanoma, Hodgkin's* and *non-Hodgkin's lymphomas* and *breast carcinoma.* In combination with cisplatin it especially is effective against *non-small cell bronchogenic carcinoma.* Toxicity includes occasional nausea and vomiting, severe bronchospasm, especially in the presence of mitomycin, common but moderate myelosuppression (especially leukopenia, alopecia, constipation, ileus, muscle aches, paresthesias, weakness, occasional chills and fever, phlebitis and rare confusion and lassitude. Vindesine is absorbed poorly orally. It manifests 3-compartment pharmacokinetics, with half-lives of 2 min, 1 hr and 24 hr.

Dose—*Intravenous,* into the tubing of a free-flowing IV line, either **3** or **4 mg/m²** wk for induction and every 2 wk for maintenance, or **1.2** to **2 mg/m²** on days 1, 3 and 5 every 3 wk.

Dosage Form—Injection: 5 mg.

Investigational and Orphan Briefs

BCG Vaccine (*Antigen International*) acts to stimulate the reticuloendothelial system, activates natural killer cells and increases proliferation of hematopoietic stem cells. Trials of systemically-administered vaccine are equivocal, but intralesional injection in melanoma and intravesicular installation in papilloma of bladder are effective. It can stimulate the growth of some types of cancer.

4′-Deoxydoxorubicin has antineoplastic activity similar to doxorubicin but has less cardiotoxicity.

Diethyldithiocarbamate [Imuthiol, (*Merieux Institute*)] is an orphan immunomodulator that is reported to stimulate T-lymphocyte activity in persons with AIDS.

Interferon Alpha-nl [Wellferon (*Burroughs Wellcome*)] is an orphan drug for the treatment of Kaposi's sarcoma in AIDS patients. Its properties are similar to the other alpha interferons. It is approved for use in *Chondylomata acuminata.*

Interferon, Gamma, Human, Recombinant (*Genentech*) induces Class I and II and other cell surface antigens, activates macrophages and endothelial cells, enhances natural killer cell activity, modulates various cytokines and has antiviral activity. It is in trials for the treatment of AIDS. Its ability to inhibit the development of exoerythrocytic forms of malarial parasites is of interest in tropical medicine. It is approved for use in *chronic granulomatosis disease.*

Trimetrexate [Glucuronate (*Parke-Davis*)] is an analog of methotrexate and trimethoprim that has a broader antineoplastic spectrum than does methotrexate, owing, in part, to not being as actively transported out of cells. Consequently, it is effective against methotrexate-resistant cancers of the transport type but not those with resistant dihydrofolate reductase. It is a stronger inhibitor of dihydrofolate reductase than is trimethoprim. With leucovorin rescue, it is safer than methotrexate. It is effective agianst *Pneumocystis carinii.* It is being investigated for activity against AIDS.

Tumor Necrosis Factor [TNF; Cachectin] is a glycoprotein that kills some kinds of cancer cells, activates cytokine production, activates macrophages and endothelial cells, promotes the production of collagen and collagenases, is an inflammatory mediator and also a mediator of septic shock, and promotes catabolism, fever and sleep. Some infectious agents cause tumor regression through the stimulation of TNF production. TNF can be quite toxic when used alone in effective doses, so that the optimal regimens probably will use it in lower doses in combination with other drugs. Its immunosuppressive actions are potentiated by gamma-interferon, so that the combination potentially is dangerous. A hybrid of TNF and interferon-αA also has been found to possess anticancer activity.

Tumor-Infiltrating Lymphocytes [TIL] are isolated from a human tumor and are cultured. Interleukin-2 is included to stimulate proliferation. The cells are then infused back into the patient along with interleukin-2 in the same way as are lymphokine-activated killer (LAK) cells (page 1159). However, TIL are 50 to 100 times as cytotoxic than LAK cells. In experimental animals the antitumor efficacy is most effective when TIL is used in combination with an appropriate antineoplastic drug.

CHAPTER 76

Anti-Infectives

William K Nichols, PhD
Associate Professor of Pharmacology
College of Pharmacy, University of Utah
Salt Lake City, UT 84112

The antimicrobial drugs occupy a unique niche in the history of medicine. The germ theory of disease was the vehicle of a dramatic revolution in medicine, and aseptic procedures and antiseptic drugs were its agents. During the entire preceding history of medicine, fewer than a handful of drugs had a known locus of action, and even fewer had been submitted to systematic laboratory investigation. The first systemic antimicrobial drugs revolutionized the treatment of certain protozoal infections, especially syphilis, but the second major revolution in medicine in which the antimicrobial drugs played a major role awaited the appearance of sulfanilamide and penicillin; the exponential development in the antibiotic and systemic antibacterial field is the inevitable result of the momentum created by those two agents.

The term *microbe* sometimes is applied only to the unicellular microphytes. However, in its broader sense it includes not only the multicellular microphytes but the microzoa as well. Therefore, this chapter includes the antifungal and antiprotozoal agents as well as the antibacterial agents.

The uses of the drugs in this chapter are extracted from a world literature, and, since this book is not addressed specifically to any particular national readership, uses may be listed that are not approved by the US FDA. In the US, the package literature should be used as the guide to approved uses. However, the approved indications are often vague, such as "infections caused by susceptible organisms," and the susceptibility of microorganisms change with time. Although the monographs may give some indication as to the probable susceptibility of various infectious organisms, it is incumbent upon the user to apply standard sensitivity tests and clinical acumen, rather than the monographs, to define the suitability of an antimicrobial drug in a given clinical case.

Antiseptics, Disinfectants and Spermicides

The words *antiseptic, disinfectant* and *germicide* all connote an agent which kills microbes upon contact, although certain denotations are more rigid and discriminatory. Drugs in this category are applied locally, although a few may be applied systemically as well. Thousands of chemical compounds have germicidal properties, and hundreds are now available. Unfortunately, many of these are poorly effective in the presence of serum or other organic media, or else they are excessively damaging to the tissues. Tissue damage, of course, is not of concern when such agents are employed for the disinfection of inanimate objects; on the other hand, corrosiveness, staining and other effects then become important considerations. The best and most effective antiseptics are iodine and chlorhexidine in combination with alcohol. Notable problems of commonly used preparations are listed in each monograph. Cationic detergents are very poor antiseptics or disinfectants due to their inactivation by soap and organic tissue components.

It commonly is believed that antiseptics are nonselective and that they have a continuous spectrum of activity. Although this is essentially true, certain significant absolute exceptions exist, and the relative susceptibilities of the numerous microorganisms must be considered in antiseptic use. For example, hexachlorophene is effective primarily against gram-positive organisms, and cationic antiseptics are not effective against sporulating organisms. Certain bacteria are even capable of growing in 70% ethanol. But bichloride of mercury and iodine have very broad and therapeutically complete spectra of efficacy against bacteria, fungi and viruses.

No really satisfactory classification of antiseptics exists. The most widely used scheme is the chemical classification. Nevertheless, the drugs listed below are not arranged according to chemical type. However, it will be noted that the major chemical categories represented are oxidizing agents (including the halogens and halogen-releasing compounds), phenols and related compounds, compounds of heavy metals (especially of mercury), surface-active agents (especially the cationic detergents) and scattered representatives from the alcohols and glycols, aldehydes and acids. Locally effective antibiotics are discussed with the antibiotics. A summary of some common antiseptics available in various preparations are included in Table 1.

It should be kept in mind that systemic antimicrobial drugs are often superior to topical ones. This is because topical agents usually do not penetrate into infected sites as well as systemic agents do. Nevertheless, topical drugs are often efficacious, simply by limiting surface infections so that tissue defenses can clean up below without continual reinfection from superficial foci. Furthermore, some superficial disorders do not seem to respond to safe systemic agents, or, if they do, there may be cogent reasons for with holding systemic drugs, for example, to avoid sensitizing the patient or creating resistant microorganisms. Therefore, there is still an important place for topical antiseptics. However, topical antiseptics can damage tissue defenses, so that sometimes they may exacerbate lesions. Such occasions are not always predictable, and they evidently depend in part on the condition of the patient and the activity of the immunological response to infection.

Many antiseptics have spermicidal activity, although not all of these can be safely administered into the vagina. There are only two spermicides that are not used also as antiseptics, too few a number to warrant a separate chapter or section. Consequently, spermicides are included here.

Acetic Acid, Diluted—page 1406.

Acetic Acid Irrigation

A sterile solution of glacial acetic acid in water for injection. It contains, in each 100 mL, 237.5–262.5 mg of $C_2H_4O_2$.

Description—pH between 2.8 and 3.4.

Uses—Microorganisms will not proliferate at low pH, and all acids are bacteriostatic at low concentrations and bactericidal at high concentrations. However, the small, lipid-soluble, weak acids penetrate intracellularly and

Table 1—Classes of Antiseptic Agents

Class and agent	Concentration (%)	Uses
Acids		
Acetic acid	0.1-5	Irrigant
Boric acid	2.17, 5 and 10	Irrigant
Alcohols		
Ethyl alcohol	70, 91 and 100	Antiseptic
Isopropyl alcohol	70	Antiseptic, rubefacient
Aldehydes		
Formaldehyde	37	Disinfectant
Glutaraldehyde	2-3.2	Disinfectant
Biguanide		
Chlorhexidine gluconate	0.12-4	Antiseptic, mouthwash
Carbanilide		
Triclocarban	1.5	Antiseptic soap
Chlorine Compounds		
Sodium hypochlorite	0.1-0.2	Wound irrigant
Oxychlorosene	0.1-0.5	Irrigant
Iodine Compounds		
Iodine	2	Antiseptic
Povidone-Iodine	0.5-10	Antiseptic
Metals		
Organic Mercurial Compounds		
Phenylmercuric acetate	0.02-0.2	Irrigant, antiseptic, preservative
Phenylmercuric nitrate	0.0025-0.004	Irrigant, antiseptic, preservative
Thimerosal	0.1	Irrigant, antiseptic
Silver Compounds		
Mild silver protein	10	Antiseptic
Oxidizing Agents		
Hydrogen peroxide	1.5-3	Wound cleanser, irrigant
Potassium permanganate	0.0025-0.007	Antiseptic, disinfectant
Phenols		
Hexylresorcinol	0.1	Mouthwash, wound cleanser
Hexachlorophene	3	Soap, shampoo
Menthol	0.5	Irrigant, antiseptic
Parachlorometaxylenol	0.5-2.0	Handwashes, shampoo
Phenol	1	Irrigant, antiseptic
Thymol	0.5-1.0	Irrigant, antiseptic
Triclocarban	0.5-1.5	Antiseptic soap
Triclosan	0.1-2.0	Antiseptic soap
Parabens	0.05-0.25	Preservative
Quaternary Ammonium Compounds		
Benzalkonium choice	0.01-0.5	Mouthwash, irrigant
Cetylpyridinum chloride	0.05-0.5	Mouthwash, irrigant
Benzethonium chloride	0.01-0.3	Mouthwash, irrigant

will exert a greater antimicrobial effect at a given pH than will a mineral acid. This is used to discourage bacterial infections in surgical wounds, to suppress growth by *Pseudomonas aeruginosa* in extensive burns of the skin, as a component of a number of dermatological lotions. It is used to treat external otitis caused by *Pseudomonas, Candida* and *Aspergillus* and vaginal infections caused by *Candida, Trichomonas* or *Hemophilus vaginalis.* Acetic acid has a long history of lay use as a spermicide. The 0.25% solution is used for bladder irrigation, especially during catheterization. It also is used in mouthwashes/gargles, but the contact time is much too short for the acid to have an effect.

It can cause irritation and inflammation, especially in the vagina.

Dose—*Topical,* as a **1%** surgical dressing, **5%** solution in burn therapy, **0.1%** dermatological lotion, **1** to **5%** solution for otitis and **0.25%** for irrigation.

Acrisorcin—see RPS-17, page 1226.

Alcohol—page 1404.

Rubbing Alcohol

Rubbing alcohol, and all preparations coming under the classification of *Rubbing Alcohols,* must be manufactured in accordance with the requirements of the US Treasury Department, Bureau of Alcohol, Tobacco and Firearms, using *Formula 23-H* (8 parts by volume of acetone, 1.5 parts by volume of methyl isobutyl ketone and 100 parts by volume of ethyl alcohol). It contains 68.5–71.5% by volume of absolute ethyl alcohol, the remainder consisting of water and the denaturants, with or without color additives, and perfume oils. Rubbing Alcohol contains in each 100 mL not less than 355 mg of sucrose octaäcetate or not less than 1.40 mg of denatonium benzoate. The preparation may be colored with one or more color additives, listed by the FDA for use in drugs. A suitable stabilizer also may be added. Rubbing Alcohol complies with the requirements of the Bureau of Alcohol, Tobacco, and Firearms, of the US Treasury Department.

Note—Rubbing Alcohol must be packaged, labeled, and sold in accordance with the regulations issued by the US Treasury Department, Bureau of Alcohol, Tobacco, and Firearms.

Description—Transparent, colorless or colored as desired, mobile, volatile liquid; extremely bitter taste; in the absence of added odorous substances, a characteristic odor; flammable; specific gravity of *Formula 23-H* is between 0.8691 and 0.8771 at 15.56°.

Uses—Applied externally as a *cooling, soothing* application for bedridden patients and athletes. It also is used widely for cleansing the surgeon's hands and instruments and for disinfection of the skin prior to penetration of the skin by a hypodermic needle. As an *antiseptic* it is good against vegetative bacteria and fair against fungi and viruses. It is ineffective against spores. It is believed widely that 70% ethanol provides the greatest reduction in bacterial count; however, this is in error. Other concentrations may be more effective, but their rate of kill is slower. In order to reduce the skin bacterial count to 5% of normal, 70% ethanol must be left on the skin for at least 2 min. It is also a feeble *anesthetic* and a mild *counterirritant.* See *Alcohol* (page 1404). *It is not potable.*

Aluminum Acetate Solution—page 871.

Aluminum Subacetate Solution—see RPS-17, page 778.

Aminacrine Hydrochloride—see RPS-18, page 1170.

Bacitracin—page 1305.

Benzalkonium Chloride

Ammonium, alkyldimethyl(phenylmethyl)-, chloride; Zephiran Chloride (*Winthrop*); *(Various Mfrs)*

Alkylbenzyldimethylammonium chloride [8001-54-5]; a mixture of alkylbenzyldimethylammonium chlorides of the general formula $[C_6H_5CH_2N(CH_3)_2R]Cl$, in which *R* represents a mixture of alkyls, including all or some of the group beginning with n-C_8H_{17} and extending through higher homologs, with n-$C_{12}H_{25}$, n-$C_{14}H_{29}$ and n-$C_{16}H_{33}$ comprising the major portion. On the anhydrous basis, the content of n-$C_{12}H_{25}$ homolog is not less than 40%, and the content of the n-$C_{14}H_{29}$ homolog is not less than 20%, of the total alkylbenzyldimethylammonium chloride content. The amounts of the n-$C_{12}H_{25}$ and n-$C_{14}H_{29}$ homolog components comprise together not less than 70% of the total alkylbenzyldimethylammonium chloride content.

Preparation—By treating a solution of *N*-alkyl-*N*-methylbenzylamine in a suitable organic solvent with methyl chloride, the solvent being so chosen that the quaternary compound precipitates as it is formed.

Description—White or yellowish white, thick gel or gelatinous pieces; aromatic odor and a very bitter taste; solutions are alkaline to litmus and foam strongly when shaken.

Solubility—Very soluble in water and alcohol; 1 g of the anhydrous form dissolves in about 6 mL benzene and in about 100 mL ether.

Incompatibilities—Like other cationic surface-active agents, benzalkonium chloride is incompatible with *soap* and other *anionic agents.* The large organic ions of the two agents are oppositely charged and, in sufficient concentration, can precipitate from solution. *Nitric acid* and *nitrates* cause precipitation.

Uses—A bacteriostatic in low and bactericidal in high concentrations. Gram-positive bacteria are more sensitive than gram-negative bacteria. Indeed, some gram-negative bacteria, especially *Pseudomonas cepacia,* have been known to grow in solutions of this drug and thus to cause epidemics of hospital infections. *Mycobacterium tuberculosis* is also relatively resistant. The antiseptic has a slow action. It requires 7 min for the bacterial count on the skin to be decreased by a mere 50%, while only 36 sec is required by 70% ethanol; to effect a 90% reduction, 25 min is required for this compared to 2 min for the 70% ethanol. Some gram-negative bacteria require hours of exposure to be killed. Tinctures are more rapidly acting and effective.

It is used for application to skin and mucous membranes. It is used widely in OTC ophthalmic solutions and as applications to contact lenses. It also is used for the sterilization of inanimate articles, such as surgical instruments. Its solutions have low surface tension and possess detergent and emulsifying actions. It is also a mild astringent and is used as such. It has relatively low systemic toxicity, but poisoning from oral ingestion has been reported. After repetitive use it sometimes may cause dermatitides. Like other cationic surface-active agents, it has certain limitations. It does not destroy bacterial spores, it is ineffective against some viruses, it is inactivated by soap and other anionic surface-active agents and, when applied to the skin, it has a tendency to form a film under which bacteria remain viable. Organic matter from tissue inactivates the drug, so that it has limited efficacy in the disinfection of wounds. It is adsorbed by various organic substances, so that the concentration in a sterilizing solution may drop below the antibacterial level, and the sterilization of surgical gloves, sponges, etc. may be erratic. The drug can cause irritation and damage the epidermis, and it also can cause allergies. In view of the availability of more reliable and more rapidly acting antiseptics, there is little to commend its continued use.

Dose—*Topical*, **0.02** to **0.5%** solution; to the *conjunctiva*, 0.1 mL of 0.01% aqueous solution. For *preoperative disinfection* of unbroken skin or treatment of superficial injuries or fungus infections, 1:750 aqueous solution or tincture. For *preoperative disinfection* of mucous membranes and denuded skin, 1:10,000 to 1:2000; for instillation or irrigation of the *vagina*, 1:5000 to 1:2000 aqueous solution; for irrigation of widely *denuded surfaces*, 1:10,000 or 1:5000; for irrigation of the *eye*, 1:10,000 to 1:5000 aqueous solution; for irrigation of the *urinary bladder* and *urethra*, 1:20,000 to 1:5000; for retention lavage of the bladder, 1:20,000 to 1:40,000; for disinfection of *deep lacerations*, 1:1000; for irrigation of *deep wounds*, 1:20,000 to 1:3000; for treatment of infected denuded areas with wet dressings, 1:5000; as a detergent solubilizer of water-insoluble drugs, up to 0.5%; for sterile storage of *metallic instruments* and *rubber articles*, 1:1000 to 1:750; for sterilization of catheters and other adsorbent articles, 1:500. When the drug is used for sterile storage of metal instruments, sodium nitrite (0.5%) is added to the solution to prevent corrosion of metal.

Dosage Forms—Vaginal Gel: 0.05%; Solution: 0.1 (1 in 1000), 0.133% (1 in 750) and 50%; Tincture: 0.133%; Tincture Spray: 0.133%; Concentrates: 12.8, 17, 17.5 and 50% aqueous, and 17% tincture.

Benzethonium Chloride

Benzenemethanaminium, *N,N*-dimethyl-N-[2-[2[4-(1,1,3,3-tetramethylbutyl)phenoxy]ethoxy]ethyl]-, chloride; (*Various Mfrs*)

Benzyldimethyl[2-[2-[*p*-(1,1,3,3-tetramethylbutyl)phenoxy]-ethoxy]ethyl]ammonium chloride. [121-54-0] $C_{27}H_{42}ClNO_2$ (448.09).

Preparation—From *p*-diisobutylphenol with dichlorodiethyl ether, dimethylamine and benzyl chloride.

Description—White crystals; mild odor; very bitter taste; melts at about 160°; aqueous solution (1%) slightly alkaline and foams strongly when shaken.

Solubility—1 g in 0.6 mL water, 0.6 mL alcohol, 1 ml chloroform or 6000 mL ether.

Uses—A *quaternary ammonium detergent antiseptic* and *spermicide* once used widely. It has the same limitations and erratic behavior that characterize *Benzalkonium Chloride* (page 1264). Its present uses are as as a preservative in ophthalmic preparations, vaginal contraceptive foams and nursing lubricants.

Dose—To the *vagina*, as a **3.17%** solution of the monohydrate; as a *preservative*, **0.01%**.

Dosage Form—Solution: 0.01 and 3.17%.

Benzoic Acid—see RPS-18, page 1235.

Benzyl Alcohol—page 1151.

Bismuth Tribromophenate—see RPS-18, page 1170.

Boric Acid—page 1407.

Butylparaben—see RPS-18, page 1170.

***p*-tert-Butylphenol**—see RPS-18, page 1170.

Carbamide Peroxide

Urea Peroxide; (*Various Mfrs*)

Urea, compound with hydrogen peroxide (1:1); [124-43-6] $CH_6N_2O_3$ (94.07); contains about 35% H_2O_2.

Description—White crystals or crystalline powder; decomposes in air to urea, oxygen and water.

Solubility—1 g in 2.5 mL water; incompatible with alcohol or ether, which cause partial decomposition.

Uses—An *oxidant* much like hydrogen peroxide. Peroxide ion in sufficient concentration is bactericidal to most bacteria; low concentrations are lethal to anaerobes and microaerophiles. It is used to relieve minor irritation of the gingivae and oral mucosae. The action may be, in part, an antibacterial action against organisms that produce irritating substances, but relief of irritation also may be attributed partly to the high glycerin content of the gel. There may be some efficacy against cankers.

Dose—*Topical, to the gums and oral mucosae*, as a **11%** gel in a water-free gel base, or as a **10%** solution in anhydrous glycerol.

Dosage Forms—Gel: 11%; Solution: 10%.

Cetyldimethylethylammonium Bromide—see RPS-18, page 1170.

Cetylpyridinium Chloride—see RPS-18, page 1171.

Chlorhexidine Gluconate

D-Gluconic acid, compd with *N,N″*-bis(4-chlorophenyl)-3,12-diimino-2,4,11,13-tetraazatetradecanediimidamide (2:1); Hibiclens, Hibistat (*Stuart*)

1,1′-Hexamethylenebis[5-(*p*-chlorophenyl)biguanide] di-D-gluconate [18472-51-0] $C_{22}H_{30}Cl_2N_{10}.2C_6H_{12}O_7$ (897.77).

Preparation—Chlorhexidine base may be prepared by refluxing a mixture of hexamethylenebis[dicyandiamide], [NCNHC(:NH)-NH-$(CH_2)_3]_2$, and *p*-chloroaniline hydrochloride in 2-ethoxyethanol at 130°–140° for two hours (Rose and Swain, *CA 50:* 1082h, 1956). The digluconate, diacetate, and dihydrochloride salts may be obtained by neutralizing the base with the respective acids.

Description—Colorless to pale-yellow solution. Usually available in 5 or 20% aqueous solution. pH (5% aqueous solution) 5.5 to 7.0.

Solubility—Very soluble in water; 1 g in 5 mL alcohol or 3 mL acetone.

Uses—Bactericidal to both gram-positive and gram-negative bacteria, although it is not as potent against the latter. It disrupts the plasma membrane of the bacterial cell, and cellular contents are lost.

In a 4% aqueous solution as a surgical scrub, it decreases the cutaneous bacterial population more than either hexachlorophene or povidone-iodine. It is slightly less effective than povidone-iodine if the skin is contaminated with certain gram-negative bacteria. A 1% aqueous solution has erratic antiseptic effects, but a 0.5% solution in 95% ethanol is more effective than a 4% aqueous solution. Chlorhexidine solutions leave a residue on the skin which gives a persistent antibacterial effect lasting 1 or 2 days. Its actions are not affected by blood, pus or soaps.

It is used for the preoperative preparation of both surgeon and patient, for the treatment of *superficial skin infections, burns, acne vulgaris* and the *irrigation of wounds* and *surgical infections*. It can be used in the hospital nursery to bathe neonates for prophylaxis against staphylococcal and streptococcal infections. Abroad, it is used as a mouthwash for *oral hygiene* and *oropharyngeal infections*, especially *aphthous ulcers*. It is absorbed onto tooth enamel, where it exerts a persisting action to *decrease the growth of dental plaque*.

It is absorbed negligibly from the skin and mucous membranes; it has low systemic toxicity. Thus, it would not be expected to cause systemic intoxication from topical application. However, serious injury may occur when it enters open wounds of the eye and deafness may occur if it enters the middle ear through a perforated eardrum. A few cases of sensitization have been reported. Bacterial resistance to the drug has not been reported, but overgrowth (superinfection) by naturally resistant gram-negative bacteria may sometimes occur. Instances of hospital epidemics caused by *Pseudomonas maltophilia* actually growing in its aqueous solutions have been reported. The substance is considerably adsorbed by new glass, and the concentration of weak solutions may thus be lowered; it is not adsorbed by polyethylene.

Dose—*Topical*, as a **4%** cleanser or sponge or **0.5%** tincture.

Dosage Forms—Aqueous Emulsion: 4%; Tincture Rinse: 0.5%.

Chlorothymol—see RPS-18, page 1171.

Cloflucarban—see RPS-18, page 1171.

Clorophene—see RPS-18, page 1171.

Cloroxine—see RPS-18, page 1171.

Ethylene Oxide

Oxirane

Oxirane

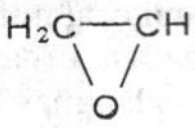

$H_2C—CH_2$ (O bridge)

Ethylene oxide [75-21-8] C_2H_4O (44.05).

Preparation—Ethylene is catalytically oxidized with air at high temperature.

Description—Colorless, flammable gas; liquid below 12°.

Solubility—Soluble in water, alcohol or ether.

Uses—An alkylating agent that has a very broad germicidal spectrum, including spores and viruses. Since it is reactive at room temperature, it may be used for the disinfection and sterilization of heat-labile objects, such as certain catheters and endoscopes in the hospital and various materials in the pharmaceutical and other industries. Because it is applied as a gas, it is advantageous for the sterilization of objects that would be harmed by immersion in aqueous or other media.

Because of the high chemical reactivity of ethylene oxide, it reacts with many pharmaceutical substances and with vitamins, amino acids and other food constituents, so that its use needs to be carefully limited. It is no longer legal to treat fruit with this gas because it reacts with tissue constituents and renders them toxic. Inhalation of the gas causes nausea, vomiting and neurological disorders, and severe exposures can cause death. Consequently, sterilization must be done only in appropriate chambers or rooms. Chemical burns can result from the wearing of ethylene oxide-sterilized clothing, shoes or gloves that have been aired inadequately after sterilization; thrombophlebitis or hemolysis can result from the use of catheters, and tracheitis from endotracheal tubes which have retained a residue of the gas. Polyvinyl tubing, bags and ware are especially dangerous because of the formation of chlorohydrin. Therefore, after exposure, such items should be aired for 5 days at room temperature or 8 hours at 120°. The gas also is used as a fumigant.

The gas is highly explosive at concentrations above 3%, so that it needs to be mixed with CO_2 or fluorocarbons before use.

The gas kills vegetative bacteria very rapidly, but desiccated microorganisms and spores are killed only slowly, so that a 3-hr exposure at 30° is advised. The optimal humidity for action is 30 to 40%.

The gas also is discussed on page 1474.

Application—120 mg/L to **100%** ethylene oxide, depending upon the use, temperature, humidity and gaseous diluents.

Ethylparaben—see RPS-18, page 1171.

Formaldehyde Solution—see RPS-18, page 1171.

Gentian Violet—see RPS-18, page 1171.

Glutaral

Pentanedial; Glutaraldehyde; Glutaric Dialdehyde;
Cidex (*Surgikos*)

$OCH(CH_2)_3CHO$

[111-30-8] $C_5H_8O_2$ (100.12).

Preparation—The 1:1 Diels-Alder adduct of acrolein and a vinyl alkyl ether is hydrolyzed, forming glutaral and an alkanol.

Description—Colorless liquid; pungent odor; boils about 188° with decomposition; stable in light; oxidizes in air; polymerizes on heating. *Glutaral Concentrate* is a 50% (*w/w*) solution in water.

Solubility—Soluble in water and in alcohol.

Uses—A *disinfectant* superior to formaldehyde. It is microbicidal against all microorganisms, including spores and viruses. Of low volatility, it does not release odorous and irritant vapor as does formaldehyde solution, and it is much more rapidly acting than the latter. It is used to sterilize endoscopes, plastic and rubber respiratory equipment, surgical and dental instruments and thermometers. A 2% alkaline solution in 70% isopropanol kills dried spores in 10 hr, but an acid-stabilized solution kills them in 20 min. Solutions can be aerosolized to kill bacteria in the air and also on surfaces (tables, floors, walls, etc.). Because it is astringent, it is used as an anhidrotic on the palms and soles but not elsewhere. It also is employed as a tissue fixative for optical and electron microscopy; being bifunctional, glutaral cross-links proteins in tissue and thus limits movement during staining and handling.

Alkaline and neutral solutions polymerize and have shelf-lives of less than 2 wk. Acid-stabilized solutions have a somewhat longer shelf-life. When poloxamers or polyethylene glycols are used to stabilize solutions, the shelf-life is increased to as long as several months, and antimicrobial activity also is enhanced.

Application—As a **2** and **3.2%** solution, applied directly or aerosolized.

Halazone

Benzoic acid, 4-[(dichloroamino)sulfonyl]-,

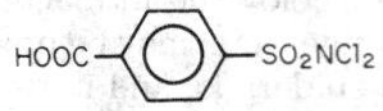

HOOC–C_6H_4–SO_2NCl_2

p-Dichlorosulfamoyl)benzoic acid [80-13-7] $C_7H_5Cl_2NO_4S$ (270.09).

Preparation—*p*-Toluenesulfonylchloride obtained by the reaction of toluene and chlorosulfonic acid is converted to the amide, which is treated with hypochlorite to form *p*-toluenesulfondichloramide. The methyl group is then oxidized with dichromate or permanganate to form halazone.

Description—White, crystalline powder; a chlorine-like odor; melts about 194° with decomposition; affected by light.

Solubility—1 g in >1000 mL water, 140 mL alcohol, >1000 mL chloroform, >2000 mL ether; soluble in solutions of alkali hydroxides or carbonates, forming the corresponding salts; soluble in glacial acetic acid.

Uses—For the extemporaneous *disinfection of drinking water*, as tablets. The chemical hydrolyzes to yield HClO and Cl_2. Organic matter in the water competes with microorganisms for the active molecules, so that dirty water requires more of it than clear water. It is poorly effective against *Giardia*.

Application—2 to **10 ppm** (0.0002 to 0.001%), in drinking water. Tablets for Solution: 4 mg. One 4-mg tablet to 1 pt of water theoretically yields 8 ppm. For polluted water, use 2 or 3 tablets. A 30-min wait is required before the water may be considered potable. The HClO and Cl_2 can be removed with sodium thiosulfate to remove the odor and improve the taste.

Hexachlorophene

Phenol, 2,2′-methylenebis[3,4,6-trichloro-, G-11; AT-7;
(*Various Mfrs*)

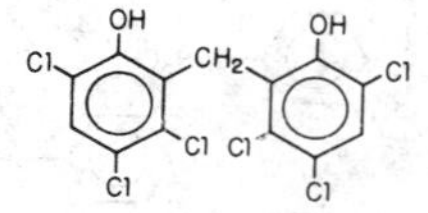

[70-30-4] $C_{13}H_6Cl_6O_2$ (406.91).

Preparation—By the Baeyer condensation reaction involving two molecules of 2,4,5-trichlorophenol, and one molecule of formaldehyde. Sulfuric acid is employed as the dehydrant.

Description—White to light tan, crystalline powder; odorless or only slightly phenolic odor; melting range 161 to 167°; incompatible with benzalkonium chloride; pK_a 5.7.

Solubility—Insoluble in water; freely soluble in acetone, alcohol and ether; soluble in chloroform and dilute solutions of fixed alkali hydroxides.

Uses—An effective bacteriostatic *antiseptic* against gram-positive bacteria but it has low activity against gram-negative organisms; *in vitro* a 3% solution will kill *Staphylococcus aureus* in 15 to 30 sec, but as long as 24 hr may be required to kill some gram-negative organisms. On the skin the bacterial population initially will decrease by only 30 to 50% but within 1 hr the decrease will exceed 90%. When washes are repeated 2 or more times a day, the decrease will reach an asymptote of 95 to 99% in 3 or 4 days from a persisting residuum of the drug in the skin. This reservoir can be removed by ethanol, isopropyl alcohol and soap and water washes or other detergents. The drug is effective whether applied as a tincture, detergent emulsion or soap; the tincture is the most effective and a 0.23% tincture foam has been reported to be more effective than a 3% soap. In soaps, one hydroxyl group is neutralized, which moderately decreases activity.

Preparations containing this are used widely as *antiseptic scrubs* by physicians, dentists, food handlers and others. The incidence and severity of *pyogenic skin infections* are reduced by routine use. Such preparations, however, are not available OTC because of concern over potential toxicity.

In infants, it can cause myelinopathy and spongiform encephalomalacia following topical application; for this reason, it is no longer used in hospital nurseries to bathe infants. Avoid contact with eyes and do not use on burns or mucous membranes. By the oral route it can cause nausea, vomiting and abdominal cramps with associated water and electrolyte derangements. Topically, the drug can cause dermatitis and sensitization. It is teratogenic. Hospital epidemics have resulted from resistant gram-negative bacteria actually growing in its nonalcoholic preparations. Superinfections caused by gram-negative bacteria or *Candida* sometimes result from repetitive applications.

Dose—*Topical,* to the *skin,* as a **0.25** or **3%** emulsion, **0.25** or **3%** solution, **0.23%** foam tincture or **3%** sponge. Aqueous preparations containing less than 2% have low efficacy. Two or more applications a day are required. As a disinfectant of inanimate objects, 3%.

Dosage Forms—Cleansing Emulsion: 0.25 and 3%; Foam: 0.23%; Sponge: 3%. Some products also contain parachlorometaxylenol to prevent contamination by gram-negative bacteria and to broaden the antibacterial spectrum.

Hexylresorcinol—see RPS-18, page 1171.

Hydrogen Peroxide Solution

Hydrogen Dioxide; (*Various Mfrs*)

[7722-84-1] H_2O_2 (34.01).

Preparation—*Hydrogen peroxide:* by many methods, one of the most important ones involving electrolysis of sulfuric acid in a solution containing sulfate, whereby persulfate is formed, which is hydrolyzed to hydrogen peroxide. Solutions containing up to about 90% H_2O_2 in each 100 mL.

Description—Clear liquid; colorless; odorless or having an odor resembling that of ozone; usually deteriorates on standing or on protracted agitation; decomposes rapidly when in contact with many oxidizing or reducing substances; when rapidly heated, it may decompose suddenly.

Uses—A *germicide* active by virtue of the release of nascent oxygen; it is short acting because the release occurs rapidly. It is the substance released by activated neutrophils, and it is an effective *microbicide* when applied in close contact with most microorganisms. However, the ubiquitous enzyme catalase often destroys it before it reaches organisms in wounds. Effervescence helps cleanse wounds mechanically. It is somewhat effective as a *mouthwash* in the treatment of Vincent's stomatitis; continued use for this purpose may lead to the condition known as "hairy tongue." The solution may be employed in the treatment of *Trichomonas viginalis vaginitis* and of *balanitis,* but is much inferior to metronidazole. It also is used popularly as a *hair bleach.*

Dose—*Topical,* for *cleansing wounds,* **1.5** to **3%** solution; as a *mouthwash,* **3%** solution; for *intravaginal use,* **2% solution.**

Dosage Forms—Concentrate; Solution: 30%; Topical Solution: 3%.

8-Hydroxyquinoline—see RPS-18, page 1171.

Iodine

Iodine [7553-56-2] I (126.90).

Preparation—From the iodide in the ashes of seaweed by chlorination, from the iodate in chile saltpeter by reduction with sulfite ion, or from the iodide in oil well brines by oxidation with chlorine or nitrite ion.

Description—Heavy, grayish black plates or granules, a metallic luster; characteristic odor; specific gravity about 4.9; melts at about 114° but volatilizes even at room temperature.

Solubility—1 g in 3000 mL water, 13 mL alcohol, 80 mL glycerin; freely soluble in chloroform, carbon tetrachloride, ether, and glacial acetic acid; soluble in solutions of iodides by the formation of I_3^-.

Incompatibilities—Oxidizes *hypophosphites, sulfites,* the lower valence forms of some *metals* and *other reducing agents,* the iodine being reduced to an iodide. *Thiosulfates* (hyposulfites) also react with free iodine. It reacts with *fixed oils* to form addition compounds, and with *volatile oils* to form various derivatives. The reaction with *turpentine oil* is violent. An explosive iodide of nitrogen may be formed with *ammonia water* or *ammoniated mercury. Alkali hydroxides* and *carbonates* react with iodine to form iodides and iodates. Many *alkaloids* are precipitated from aqueous solutions of their salts. In *alcoholic solution* iodine slowly forms hydrogen iodide if alkali iodide is absent.

Uses—One of the best all-around antiseptics. It is active against bacteria, fungi, spores, yeasts, protozoa and viruses. Although it is available in high concentration in various complexonates (with iodide ion, poloxamer, povidone, etc, called iodophores) or tinctures, its solubility in water is only 0.033% (1:3,000). Therefore, in tissue, plasma, serum or only water, no preparation or dosage form can present a higher concentration of HIO (the active form of I_2 in water) to the microbe than saturated iodine solution, alone. The advantage of iodophores or concentrates is that they provide a reservoir (called *available iodine*) from which to replenish iodine that is depleted in combining with microbial components and organic materials in the area of application and thus to permit a sustained action. Iodine in the sundry preparations can complex loosely with amino and heterocyclic groups in tissues constituents, the complexes serving as repository iodine. Only on dry surfaces, such as intact skin, instruments, containers, etc, can a tincture present a concentration of iodine to the microorganism higher than 0.033%. Ethanol and other organic solvents in tinctures act superadditively with free iodine.

Most bacteria are killed within 10 sec by a 1% solution, 1 min by 1:20,000 (0.05%) and 10 min by 1:500,000 (0.0002%). A 0.15% solution may kill wet bacterial spores, amebic cysts and enteric viruses in about 15 min, but dry spores may require hours, even with 1:3000. On the skin, a 1% tincture will kill 90% of the bacteria in 90 sec.

Its tinctures and solutions are used widely by the lay public for the *disinfection of cuts and abrasions.* The 2% solution is the best-available OTC preparation for this purpose because it lacks the irritancy of tinctures and hypertonicity of the strong solution. Solutions are effective even in strengths as low as 0.1%, which is sometimes used for wound irrigation. A 2% solution in glycerin is the preparation of choice for *application to mucous membranes.* The tincture is the best preparation for *presurgical preparation of the intact skin.* Under the surgeon's gloves, action begins to diminish in about 15 min but will persist for several hours. It may be used to "purify" drinking water. However, *Giardia* is less sensitive than bacteria and amebae, and requires higher concentrations and longer incubations. The strong solution is sometimes used orally as a source of iodide ion to *suppress thyroid function.* It is also keratolytic and is used to treat *keratoscleritis.*

It has a high therapeutic index among antiseptics. The 2% solution is nearly isotonic and does not sting in open wounds. Nevertheless, there is evidence that tissue defenses may be compromised. The hypertonicity and potassium ion in the strong solution causes some stinging and local damage. Tinctures sting and also cause local damage. The strong tincture, especially, can cause burns, even on intact skin; it was this toxicity that gave iodine a bad reputation.

Dose—*Oral, usually* **0.1** to **0.3 mL** of a **5%** (or strong) **solution** a day, not to exceed 3 mL a day. *Topical,* to the *intact skin,* for *disinfection,* as a **2% solution** or **tincture;** for *keratolysis,* as a **5%** (or strong) **solution;** to *abraded surfaces* or *open wounds,* as a **2% solution;** for *wound irrigation,* as a **0.1** to **1% solution.** For *purification of water,* **5** to **10 drops** of a **2% tincture**/qt, to stand for at least 15 min, except 30 min or more for *Giardia.*

Dosage Forms—Solution: 2% (with 2.4% KI); Strong Solution: 5% (with 10% KI); Tincture: 2% (with 2.5% KI); Strong Tincture: 7% (with 5% KI).

Iodoform—see RPS-18, page 1172.

Isopropyl Alcohol

2-Propanol

$CH_3CH(OH)CH_3$

[67-63-0] C_3H_8O (60.10).

Preparation—Most of the isopropyl alcohol prepared commercially is obtained by treating propylene with H_2SO_4 followed by hydrolysis. The olefin is obtained in the cracking of petroleum.

Some of the alcohol also is obtained by the reduction of acetone through high-pressure hydrogenation.

Description—Transparent, colorless, mobile, volatile liquid; characteristic odor; slightly bitter taste; specific gravity 0.783 to 0.787; distilling range 81° to 83°; refractive index 1.376 to 1.378 at 20°.

Solubility—Miscible with water, alcohol, ether and chloroform.

Uses—For the disinfection of hypodermic syringes and needles and, as the rubbing alcohol, as a skin antiseptic. It is superior to ethyl alcohol in regard to its *antiseptic* properties. All concentrations greater than 70% are effective skin disinfectants. The 91% concentration does not appear to affect the potency of subcutaneous insulin and hence may be used to prepare the skin for injection. It does promote bleeding at an injection site, which may make reading of allergic tests difficult. It can not be relied on to destroy the spores of organisms such as *Clostridium tetani, Clostridium welchii or Bacillus anthracis.* It has a greater effect than ethanol to dry and irritate the skin. *It is not potable* and should not be given by mouth. It also is used in hair and scalp preparations, hand and face lotions, aftershave lotions, liniments, various antiseptic and antifungal mixtures, cleansers and in the *Isopropyl Rubbing Alcohol* described below. It is recognized as a rubefacient, although it is used more widely as an antiseptic.

Dose—As an antiseptic it is applied to the skin in concentrations greater than 70% *v/v.* It should be left on the skin for at least 2 min.

Dosage Forms—Isopropyl Rubbing Alcohol: 70%; Isopropyl Alcohol: 91% and 100%.

Lactic Acid—page 1411.

Lime, Chlorinated—see RPS-18, page 1172.

Mafenide Acetate

Benzenesulfonamide, 4-(aminoethyl)-, monoacetate;
Sulfamylon (*Winthrop*)

α-Amino-*p*-toluenesulfonamide monoacetate [13009-99-9] $C_7H_{10}N_2O_2S.C_2H_4O_2$(246.28).

Preparation—*p*-Cyanobenzenesulfonamide is dissolved in ethanolic HCl and hydrogenated using Pd-charcoal catalyst (*J Am Chem Soc 62:* 2099, 1940) yielding the hydrochloride; ammonia is added to an aqueous solution of the hydrochloride and the base thus liberated is collected and reacted with acetic acid.

Description—White, crystalline powder; melts at about 167°; pH (1 in 10 solution) between 6.4 and 6.8.

Solubility—Freely soluble in water.

Uses—Has an irregular antibacterial spectrum that includes both gram-positive and gram-negative microorganisms. Although it is generally more active against the gram-positive organisms, a higher percentage of strains of *Pseudomonas aeruginosa* respond than of staphylococci and streptococci. Since *Ps aeruginosa* is the most-common pathogenic invader in burned surfaces, this drug is especially useful in the adjunctive therapy of the burned patient. Staphylococci and streptococci are also common invaders in burned tissue, but many of the strains do not respond to mafenide, so that combination treatment is generally necessary. It is also quite effective against anaerobes, such as the clostridia.

Although it is a sulfonamide, the para-substituent differs from the sulfa drugs, and its mechanism of action is much different. Thus there is no correlation between bacterial sensitivities to this and those to sulfa drugs. It is only bacteriostatic, not bactericidal, so that at best it only holds the growth of the sensitive bacteria in check to allow the body defenses a chance to recover. The drug is more effective if it is applied early, before bacterial colonization has become extensive. The *p*-NH_2CH_2— group is oxidized to —CO_2H, and the metabolite is excreted in the urine.

It is applied topically. It penetrates tissues well without loss of potency, so that it reaches most of the infected sites.

Mafenide and its metabolite inhibit carbonic anhydrase. Consequently, the treated burn patient with a large burn surface (usually over 30%) may suffer from systemic hyperchloremic acidosis with an alkaline urine and hyperventilation. Since burn patients often get pneumonia or renal complications, the metabolic acidosis action can be serious. Recovery follows removal of the drug by bathing; it should not be reapplied for several days. Other untoward effects frequently include pain at the site of application, which lasts for 20 to 30 min, and occasional allergic reactions, which usually appear as some form of dermatitis, but agranulocytosis has been reported. Also, certain fungi tend to grow beneath the cream.

Dose—*Topical*, as **8.5%** cream, to be applied in a layer approximately 2-mm thick, once or twice a day. Recovery is facilitated if the old layer is washed away, to aid debridement and the removal of microorganisms, before each reapplication. Also, whenever the cream is wiped away prematurely, as by patient movement, it should be reapplied.

Dosage Form—Cream: The equivalent of 8.5% of free base.

Merbromin—see RPS-18, page 1172.

Yellow Mercuric Oxide—see RPS-18, page 1172.

Ammoniated Mercury—see RPS-18, page 1172.

Methenamine

1,3,5,7-Tetraazatricyclo[3.3.1.1^{3,7}]decane; Aminoform; Cystamin; Cystogen; Hexamine; Uritone; Urised (*Webcon*)

Hexamethylenetetramine [100-97-0] $C_6H_{12}N_4$ (140.19).

Although a cyclic tetramine, the therapeutic action of this compound depends exclusively on its ability to liberate formaldehyde under suitable environmental conditions.

Preparation—By adding a moderate excess of ammonia water to formaldehyde solution, and evaporating to dryness.

Description—Colorless, lustrous crystals or a white crystalline powder; practically odorless; aqueous solution is alkaline to litmus; sublimes about 260°; when ignited it burns with a smokeless flame.

Solubility—1 g in 1.5 mL water, 12.5 mL alcohol, 10 mL chloroform or 320 mL ether.

Incompatibilities—Alkaline in reaction and forms salts with weak acids. *Strong acids* and concentrated solutions of organic acids decompose it with liberation of formaldehyde. With prolonged contact, weak acids also decompose it, as do acidic vehicles.

It liquefies, in some cases with decomposition, when rubbed with *aspirin, antipyrine, benzoic acid, lithium carbonate, menthol, phenol, potassium acetate, sodium benzoate, sodium salicylate,* etc. *Ammonium salts* and *alkalies* darken it. In capsules, it may combine slowly with the gelatin, rendering it insoluble.

Uses—A *urinary tract anti-infective,* provided it is acting in an acid medium. It is excreted rapidly and thus reaches effective antiseptic concentrations in the urine. The drug depends for its action on the liberation of free formaldehyde. This occurs to the extent of 20% of theoretical at pH 5, 6% at pH 6 and almost not at all at pH 7.6. Consequently, precaution must be taken to maintain an acid urine (pH 6 or below) during medication with it. This usually is accomplished by administration of sodium biphosphate, mandelic acid, hippuric acid, ascorbic acid or cranberry juice. Ammonium chloride should not be used, since NH_4^+ drives the equilibrium to the left. At a pH of 6, a daily dose of 2 g will yield an average 24-hr urine concentration of about 18 to 60 μg/mL, which is about 40 times the minimum to inhibit the growth of most bacteria that cause urinary tract infections. However, it will not prevent growth of *Candida albicans.* It is improbable that products which provide only 40.8 to 81.6 mg/dose can provide a high enough concentration of formaldehyde, since the urine contains substances that bind some of the formaldehyde.

It is of particular value in the treatment of *E coli* infections of the urinary tract. It also is especially useful in patients with renal insufficiency. Because of its low systemic toxicity, failure to excrete the drug causes no harmful consequences, unless renal insufficiency is severe.

Approximately 10 to 30% is converted to formaldehyde in the acid stomach contents unless enteric capsules are employed. Even with enteric coatings, nausea, vomiting, diarrhea and other gastrointestinal distress often occur when the dose exceeds 500 mg 4 times a day. Take with food to minimize GI upset. Formaldehyde liberated from the compound presumably is the cause of the distress. Other untoward effects are occasional pruritis and skin rashes and bladder irritation, painful and frequent urination, and hematuria in persons who have taken the drug longer than 3 to 4 wk. Dyspnea, lipoid pneumonitis and headache occur rarely. In persons with acidosis or renal failure, the acid salts usually given concomitantly may be detrimental. The drug should not be used if hepatic insufficiency exists.

Dose—*Oral, adults,* **300 mg** to **1.5 g;** *usual,* **900 mg** 4 times a day. *Children, 6* to *12 yr,* **300** or **600 mg** 4 times a day; *under 6 yr,* **18.3 mg/kg** 4 times a day; oddly, the convenient elixir form is no longer available, so that the mandelate is the preferred pediatric preparation. If therapy has begun with a high dose, it should be reduced for long-term treatment, once the urine is bacteriologically clear. When methenamine and sodium biphosphate tablets are administered the usual dose is 500 mg. Products which contain as little as 40.8 mg/tablet contain other antiseptics in addition to the drug. The doses of the drug as the mandelate and hippurate are given in the separate monographs.

Dosage Forms—Tablets Methenamine and Sodium Biphosphate, 300 mg/500 mg; also 40.8 mg in combination with benzoic acid, phenylsalicylate and belladonna alkaloids.

Methenamine Hippurate—see RPS-18, page 1172.

Methenamine Mandelate

Benzeneacetic acid, α-hydroxy-, compd with 1,3,5,7-tetraazatricyclo[3.3.1.1.^{3,7}]decane (1:1); Mandelic Acid Hexamethylenetetramine Compound (1:1); Mandelamine (*Parke-Davis*)

Hexamethylenetetramine monomandelate [587-23-5] C_6-H_{12}-N_4.-$C_8H_8O_3$ (292.34); contains not less than 95.5% of $C_6H_{12}N_4.C_8H_8O_3$ and not less than 50% of mandelic acid [$C_8H_8O_3$ = 152.15].

For the structure of the base, see *Methenamine.*

Preparation—By reacting equimolar quantities of methenamine and mandelic acid in water or alcohol and concentrating until crystallization occurs.

Description—White, crystalline powder, practically odorless; sour taste; melts about 127° with decomposition; pH (solution) about 4.

Solubility—Very soluble in water; 1 g in about 10 mL alcohol, 20 mL chloroform or 350 mL ether.

Uses—See *Methenamine*. Mandelic acid alone also possesses antiseptic activity at a pH below 5.5, which synergizes the action of the formaldehyde released from methenamine. Furthermore, mandelic acid itself tends to decrease urine pH and aid the action of both components. Because mandelic acid is excreted into urine, this salt is contraindicated in renal insufficiency, though methenamine alone is not.

Dose—*Oral, adults,* **1 g** 4 times a day; *children 6 to 12 yr,* **0.5 g** 4 times a day; *under 6 yr,* **18.3 mg/kg** 4 times a day.

Dosage Forms—Granules (for reconstitution): 1 g; Oral Suspension: 250 and 500 mg/5 mL; Tablets: 500 mg and 1 g; Enteric-Coated Tablets: 500 mg and 1 g.

Methylbenzethonium Chloride

Benzenemethanaminium, *N,N*-dimethyl-*N*-[2-[2-[methyl-4-(1,1,3,3-tetramethylbutyl)phenoxy]ethyl]-, chloride, monohydrate; (*Various Mfrs*)

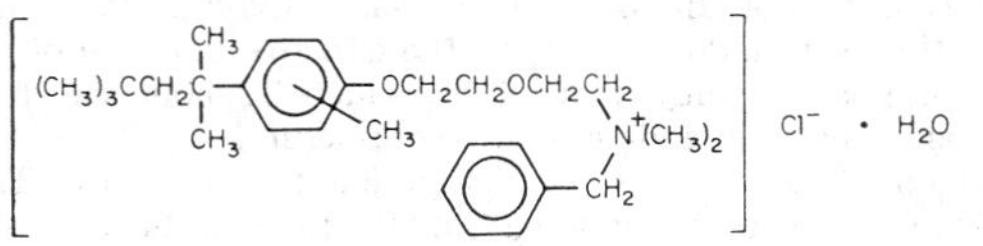

Benzyldimethyl[2-[2-[[4-(1,1,3,3-tetramethylbutyl)tolyl]oxy]ethoxy]-ethyl]ammonium chloride monohydrate. [1320-44-1] $C_{28}H_{44}ClNO_2 \cdot H_2O$ (480.13); *anhydrous* [25155-18-4] (462.11).

Preparation—By the method described for *Benzethonium Chloride* (page 1265), except that cresol is employed instead of phenol. Inasmuch as the starting cresol contains both *o*- and *m*-isomers, the corresponding isomers of the quaternary are both present in the final product.

Description—White crystals; hygroscopic; mild odor; very bitter taste; solutions are neutral or slightly alkaline to litmus; melts between 159 and 163°.

Solubility—1 g in 0.5 mL water, 0.9 mL alcohol, 0.7 mL ether or 10,000 mL chloroform.

Uses—A *quaternary ammonium antiseptic* with actions and limitations like those of *Benzalkonium Chloride* (page 1264). It is ineffective against sporulating organisms. At present, its primary use is in the treatment of *ammonia dermatitis* (diaper rash), by application both to the skin and to diapers, undergarments and bed linens. It is included in some *burn/sunburn* and *personal-care products*. Like other quaternary detergent antiseptics, it is inactivated by soap and inhibited by organic matter. Quaternary ammonium antiseptics can cause sensitization, usually manifested as rashes.

Dose—*Topical,* as a **0.1** or **0.2%** cream or **0.067, 0.1** or **0.13%** ointment and as a powder in combination with various other ingredients.

Dosage Forms—Cream: 0.1 and 0.2%; Ointment: 0.067, 0.1 or 0.13%; Powder.

Methylene Blue—page 941.

Methylparaben—see RPS-18, page 1172.

Mupirocin—see RPS-18, page 1220.

Nitrofurazone

Hydrazinecarboxamide, 2-[(5-nitro-2-furanyl)methylene]-, Furacin (*Norwich/Eaton*); Amifur (*SmithKline*)

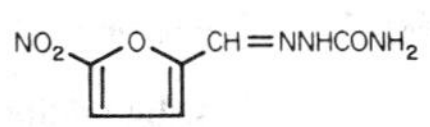

5-Nitro-2-furaldehyde semicarbazone [59-87-0] $C_6H_6N_4O_4$ (198.14).

Preparation—By condensing 5-nitro-2-furaldehyde with semicarbazide hydrochloride in the presence of sodium acetate.

Description—Odorless, lemon-yellow, crystalline powder; nearly tasteless, but develops a bitter aftertaste; darkens slowly on exposure to light; melts about 236° with decomposition; pH (saturated solution) 5 to 7.5.

Solubility—1 g in 4200 mL water, 590 mL alcohol, 350 mL propylene glycol, and polyethylene glycol mixtures up to about 1%; practically insoluble in chloroform and ether.

Uses—A local antibacterial agent with a broad spectrum of activity. Most bacteria of surface infections of the skin or mucosal surfaces are sensitive to the drug. It is applied topically in the treatment of mixed, superficial infections of the skin. It finds use, especially, in the treatment of 2nd- and 3rd-degree burns and in skin grafting in which there are complications from bacterial infections that are refractory to the usual drugs of choice but in which bacterial sensitivity to the drug is demonstrable. It has not yet been shown to be useful in the treatment of minor burns, wounds or cutaneous ulcers which are infected. It retains its antibacterial activity in blood, serum and pus; phagocytosis is not inhibited and nitrofurazone does not interfere with healing. However, it is a slowly acting drug, and at least 24 hr are required for it to take effect properly. Therefore, no treatment should be less than 2 or 3 days in duration.

Approximately 1% of patients become sensitized to the drug, sometimes within 5 days of initiation of treatment. The systemic toxicity is low.

Dose—*Topical,* **0.2%.** The dosage interval and duration of treatment vary with the particular use and dosage form. Five days is the usual duration, except for severe burns. Except in burn therapy, a duration of less than 1 wk is usually desirable, to avoid sensitization.

Dosage Forms—Cream, Soluble Dressing or Topical Solution: 0.2%.

Caution (for all dosage forms)—Avoid exposure at all times to direct sunlight, strong fluorescent light, excessive heat or alkaline materials.

Nonoxynol 9

α-(*p*-Nonylphenyl)-ω-hydroxytetra(oxyethylene); Igepal CO-630 (GAF); (*Various Mfrs*)

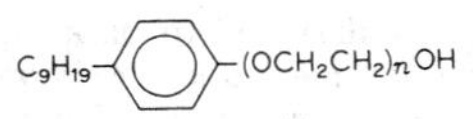

(n = approx 9)

[26027-38-3] $C_{15}H_{24}O(C_2H_4O)_n$.

Preparation—By reacting nonylphenol and ethylene oxide.

Description—Almost colorless liquid.

Solubility—Soluble in water, alcohol, polar or chlorinated organic solvents, xylene or corn oil; insoluble in aliphatic hydrocarbons (kerosene).

Uses—The most widely used spermicide in the US. It is 100% effective *in vitro*, but the failure rate in practice in the US probably lies between 1 and 8%, depending on the dosage form, concentration, user care in application and compliance. Failure rates as high as 40%, mainly with creams and gels alone (no condoms or diaphrams) have been reported. It also is an ingredient in some products for feminine hygiene.

Dose—*Topical,* high in the vaginal vault, as a **2** to **5%** cream, **8** or 12.5% foam, **1** to **5%** gel, or **100 mg** as a vaginal suppository.

Dosage Forms—Cream: 2, 4, and 5%; Foam: 8 and 12.5%; Gel: 1, 2, 3, 4 or 5%; Vaginal suppositories: 100 mg.

Octoxynol 9

Poly(oxy-1,2-ethanediyl, α-[4-(1,1,3,3-tetramethylbutyl)phenyl]-ω-hydroxy-, Octylphenoxy Polyethoxyethanol NF XII; Koromex (*Holland-Rantos*); Ortho-Gynol (*Ortho*)

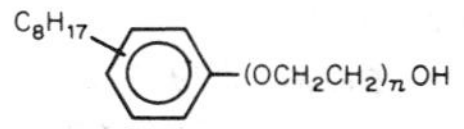

Polyethylene glycol mono[*p*-(1,1,3,3-tetramethylbutyl)phenyl]-ether [9002-93-1]; an anhydrous liquid mixture of mono-*p*-(1,1,3,3-tetramethylbutyl)phenyl ethers of polyethylene glycols in which n varies from 5 to 15, and which has an average molecular weight of 647, corresponding to the formula $C_{34}H_{62}O_{11}$.

Preparation—By reacting *p*-(1,1,3,3-tetramethylbutyl)phenol with ethylene oxide at elevated temperature under pressure in the presence of NaOH.

Description—Clear, pale yellow, viscous liquid; a faint odor; bitter taste; specific gravity between 1.059 and 1.068; pH (1 in 100 aqueous solution) between 6 to 8.

Solubility—Miscible with water, alcohol or acetone; soluble in benzene or toluene; insoluble in solvent hexane.

Uses—A nonirritating spermicide that is used widely in vaginal creams and jellies. It is highly spermicidal in vitro, but the exact failure rate in practice remains to be determined accurately. It is probably about 2 to 8% with creams or gels alone but 1 to 4% when used with condoms, rates that reflect differences in dispersion, concentration and user practice in application.

It is a nonionic detergent, emulsifier and dispersing agent that is a pharmaceutical necessity for *Nitrofurazone Solution.*

Dose—*Topical,* high in the vaginal vault, as **3%** cream or **1%** gel.
Dosage Forms—Cream: 3%; Gel: 1 and 2%.

Oxychlorosene Sodium—see RPS-18, page 1172.
Parachlorometaxylenol—see RPS-18, page 1172.
Parachlorophenol—see RPS-18, page 1172.
***p*-tert-Pentylphenol**—see RPS-18, page 1172.

Phenazopyridine Hydrochloride

2,6-Pyridinediamine, 3-(phenylazo)-, monohydrochloride; Pyridium *(Parke-Davis)*

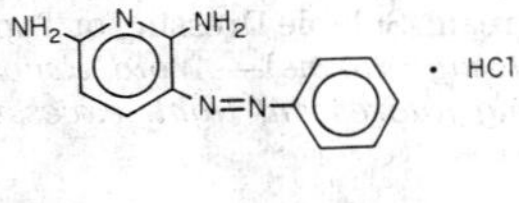

2,6-Diamino-3-(phenylazo)pyridine monohydrochloride [136-40-3] $C_{11}H_{11}N_5.HCl$ (249.70).

Preparation—Aniline is diazotized with sodium nitrite and excess HCl, and the resulting benzenediazonium chloride is coupled with 2,6-diaminopyridine.

Description—Light or dark red to dark violet, crystalline powder; odorless or has a slight odor; melts about 235° with decomposition.

Solubility—1 g in < 10 mL water, 59 mL alcohol, 331 mL chloroform, > 5000 mL ether or 100 mL glycerin.

Uses—A drug used for symptomatic relief of pain, burning, urgency, frequency and other discomforts arising from irritation of lower urinary tract mucosa caused by infection, trauma, surgery, endoscopic procedures or passage of catheters. When taken systemically it is excreted quickly into the urine, so that a high local concentration is reached. Thus, the drug either may be administered orally or instilled locally. However, a considerable proportion of the drug is converted metabolically to an inactive form, so that large oral doses are required to exert a therapeutic effect. The relief of discomfort is attributable mostly to a local anesthetic action rather than to an antibacterial action. Treatment should not continue beyond two days because there is no evidence it provides greater benefit than sulfonamides alone. When instilled locally in cystitis, the anesthetic effect may allow other therapeutic measures to be executed with a minimum of pain. It occasionally may cause gastrointestinal irritation. Jaundice, hemolytic anemia and methemoglobinemia have been reported. After oral administration the color of the urine may be orange red to dark red, if the urine is acidic. Large doses and prolonged treatment can give rise to renal stones of the drug. It is contraindicated in renal insufficiency, severe hepatitis and pyelonephritis of pregnancy, and it should be used cautiously in the presence of gastrointestinal disturbances. It often is combined with sulfonamides or methenamine salts.

Dose—*Oral, adult,* **200 mg** 3 times a day after meals; *children 6 to 12 yr,* **4 mg/kg** 3 times a day after meals.
Dosage Form—Tablets: 100 and 200 mg.

Phenol—page 1412.
Phenylethyl Alcohol—page 1389.
Phenylmercuric Acetate—see RPS-18, page 1172.
Phenylmercuric Nitrate—see RPS-18, page 1172.
Pine Tar—page 876.
Polymyxin B Sulfate—page 1307.
Potassium Permanganate—see RPS-18, page 1173.

Povidone-Iodine

2-Pyrrolidinone, 1-ethenyl-, homopolymer, compd with iodine; *(Various Mfrs)*

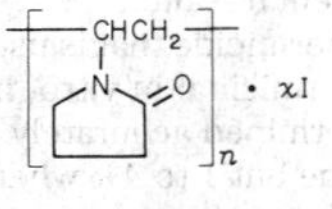

1-Vinyl-2-pyrrolidinone polymer compd with iodine [25655-41-8]; contains 9–12% of available iodine.

Preparation—Povidone having an average molecular weight of 40,000 is heated with elemental iodine in the presence of a little water whereby a small amount of the iodine enters into loose organic union with the polymer to form a compound which contains approximately 10% of available iodine.

Description—Yellowish-brown, amorphous powder; slight, characteristic odor; aqueous solution is acid to litmus.

Solubility—Soluble in water or alcohol; practically insoluble in chloroform, carbon tetrachloride, ether, solvent hexane or acetone.

Uses—Kills both gram-positive and gram-negative bacteria, fungi, viruses, protozoa and yeasts. The povidone component serves the functions of iodide in iodine solution and tincture, namely, to increase the solubility of iodine and to provide a slow-release form of iodine. The affinity of povidone for iodine is greater than that of iodide, so that the concentration of free iodine is less than 1 ppm. Consequently the immediate bactericidal action of povidone-iodine is only moderate compared to that of iodine solutions. A 10% povidone-iodine solution (1% of available iodine) kills only about 85% of cutaneous bacteria, much less than with iodine solutions or tinctures of comparable iodine content. Although it takes 6 to 8 hr for the skin bacterial population to return to normal, which is longer than with iodine solutions, the effective duration of action for surgical purposes is only about 1 hr, which is about the duration of effective antisepsis with iodine solution or tincture.

It is claimed that it stings less than iodine preparations. This is not true; it is iodine tincture that stings, and tinctures of this drug also sting. Iodine solutions are more effective in wound irrigation. It stains the skin and clothing less than iodine solutions and is also less of an irritant under occlusive dressings, which simply reflect that there is less free iodine. It is absorbed sufficiently from the skin to cause hypothyroidism in infants. It is mutagenic in the Ames test. Therefore, there is no clear advantage of povidone-iodine over iodine solutions or tinctures. Use with caution during pregnancy, lactation and in infants.

Its antiseptic preparations are indicated clinically for the prevention and treatment of surface infections as well as to degerm the skin prior to injection and hyperalimentation procedures; for seborrhea; for disinfection of wounds, burns, lacerations and abrasions; for preoperative and postoperative scrubbing and washing of hospital operating-room personnel and for preoperative skin preparation of patients.

Dose—*Topical,* **0.5** to **10%** (0.05 to 1% available iodine equivalent). To the skin, 4.7 to 10%, in various liquid forms, as ointment or as aerosol; to the mouth and pharynx, 0.5 to 1% solution; to the vaginal mucosa as 0.5 to 1% solution or gel; for baths, from 30 to 50 ppm. Available iodine equivalents can be calculated by dividing the povidone-iodine concentration by 10; actual free-iodine concentrations are less than available iodine concentrations.

Dosage Forms—Aerosol: 5%; Solution: 5, 7.5, 10, and 30% (some are diluted before use). Also available as Foam, Gauze, Mouthwash-Gargle (0.5%), Ointment (4.7 and 10%), Shampoo (7.5%), Surgical Scrub/Skin Cleanser (7.5%), Scrub Applicator (2%), Scrub Solution (2%), Swab (10%), Vaginal Douche (10%), Vaginal Gel (10%), Perineal Wash (10%), Vaginal Suppositories (10%), and Whirlpool Concentrate, for bathing patients (10%).

Propylene Oxide—see RPS-18, page 1173.
Propylparaben—see RPS-18, page 1173.
Pyrithione Zinc—see RPS-18, page 1173.
Salicylic Acid—page 879.

Selenium Sulfide

Selenium Disulfide; Selsun *(Abbott)*; Exsel *(Herbert)*; Selsun Blue *(Ross)*

Selenium sulfide (SeS_2) [7488-56-4] SeS_2 (143.08); contains 52.0 to 55.5% of selenium.

Preparation—Among other ways, by adding an aqueous solution of selenious acid to an aqueous solution containing a stoichiometric excess of hydrogen sulfide.

Description—Reddish brown to bright-orange powder; not more than a faint odor.

Solubility—Practically insoluble in water or organic solvents.

Uses—An *antibacterial, antifungal* and *mildly keratolytic* agent used in the local treatment of seborrheic dermatitis of the scalp. It is effective in the treatment of *tinea versicolor.* It is also useful in the management of *acne vulgaris* and *juvenilis* and *atopic eczema,* but it has not been approved for these uses. Some authorities attribute its antiseborrheic efficacy to cytostatic actions. It induces inflammation of the mucous membranes and exposed tissues, so that care should be exercised in the application of the compound. It also causes "rebound" oiliness of the scalp. It should not be allowed to get into the eyes. Occasionally it causes loss of hair. Although it has considerably lower toxicity than selenites and some other selenium compounds and is available OTC, care nevertheless should be taken to keep preparations away from the mouth.

Dose—*Topical*, to the scalp, **5** or **10 mL** of **1** to **2.5%** lotion and massage, after 2- or 3-min rinse thoroughly and repeat application and rinsing. The 1% cream or lotion is applied in sufficient amount to lather, afterward rinsed, and the treatment repeated.

Dosage Form—Lotion Shampoo: 1 and 2.5%.

Silver Nitrate—page 877.

Silver Protein, Mild—see RPS-18, page 1173.

Silver Sulfadiazine

Benzenesulfonamide, 4-amino-*N*-2-pyrimidinyl-, monosilver (1+) salt; Silvadene (*Marion*); SSD (*Boots*)

N^1-2-Pyrimidinylsulfanilamide monosilver(1+) salt [22199-08-2] $C_{10}H_9AgN_4O_2S$ (357.13).

Description—A white powder.

Solubility—Practically insoluble in water.

Uses—Combines in one compound the *antibacterial* properties of silver ion and sulfadiazine; it is especially effective against *Pseudomonas aeruginosa*. It is indicated for topical use as an adjunct for prevention and treatment of wound sepsis in patients with second- and third-degree burns. Its solubility product is lower than that of silver chloride, thus insoluble silver chloride is not formed when the drug comes in contact with body fluids and, also, the electrolyte disorders that result from use of silver nitrate in the topical treatment of burns are avoided. It can penetrate the eschar. Although some sulfadiazine is absorbed, it is rarely sufficient to cause crystalluria. However, bacterial resistance to sulfonamides can occur. The drug does not cause pain at the site of application. Hypersensitivity may occur. Silver inactivates proteolytic enzymes used for debridement.

Dose—*Topical*, to the affected skin, as **1%** cream, applied once or twice a day with sterile, gloved hand.

Dosage Form—Cream (water-miscible): 1%.

Sodium Benzoate—see RPS-18, page 1173.

Sodium Hypochlorite Solution

Antiformin; Dakin's Solution; Hyclorite; (*Century Pharm*)

An aqueous solution containing 4.0 to 6.0% *w/w* of sodium hypochlorite [7681-52-9] NaClO (74.44).

Preparation—By electrolysis of a solution of sodium chloride in a cell permitting reaction of chlorine with sodium hydroxide; an equivalent quantity of sodium chloride is produced simultaneously.

Description—Clear, pale greenish yellow liquid; slight odor of chlorine; affected by light.

Uses—A powerful *disinfectant* and *deodorant*, and also a *bleaching agent*. Not only is it effective against vegetative bacteria, but also against viruses and to some degree against spores and fungi. It is used for disinfecting utensils and apparatus. The 0.5% solution usually is not used on or in the human, although it is sometimes used in root canal therapy and is considered by some authorities to be much better than parachlorophenol for this puspose. For therapeutic uses it is diluted 10 to 30 times. The diluted solution is employed in full strength, as a freshly prepared solution. It is used in the treatment of suppurating wounds, often by continuous irrigation (Carrell technique). Not only does the solution exert a *germicidal action* but it also dissolves *necrotic tissue*. The disadvantages are that its solutions dissolve blood clots, delay clotting and are irritating to the skin. For prophylaxis of *epidermophytosis*, the diluted solution is employed sometimes as a foot bath. The solution is also a deodorant.

Dose—*Topical*, as a solution containing 0.15 to 0.5% of NaClO.

Dosage Form—Solution: 0.25, 0.5 and 5%.

Thimerosal—see RPS-18, page 1173.

Thymol—see RPS-18, page 1173.

Triclocarban—see RPS-18, page 1173.

Triclosan—see RPS-18, page 1173.

Zinc Sulfate

Sulfuric acid, zinc salt (1:1), heptahydrate; White Vitriol; Zinc Vitriol

Zinc sulfate (1:1) heptahydrate [7446-20-0] $ZnSO_4.7H_2O$ (287.54); *anhydrous* [7733-02-0] (161.44); contains 55.6–61% of $ZnSO_4$, corresponding to 99–108.7% of the hydrated salt.

Preparation—By reacting metallic zinc or zinc oxide with diluted sulfuric acid. It also is prepared by roasting zinc sulfide in a limited supply of oxygen and extracting the sulfate with water.

Description—Colorless, transparent prisms or small needles, or a granular, crystalline powder; odorless; astringent metallic taste; efflorescent in dry air; solutions are acid to litmus.

Solubility—1 g in 0.6 mL water or about 2.5 mL glycerin; insoluble in alcohol.

Incompatibilities—See *Zinc Chloride* (page 873). Combinations of zinc sulfate and *sodium borate* with or without *boric acid* to be used as collyria are frequently troublesome due to precipitation of zinc borate. A quantity of glycerin, equal in weight to the borate, suffices to maintain a clear solution. There is also a tendency for solutions of zinc sulfate to form a slight cloudiness due to the separation of a basic salt formed through partial hydrolysis.

Insoluble sulfates are formed with *lead, barium, strontium* and *calcium salts*. *Silver* and *mercury* form slightly soluble salts. Zinc sulfate has a dehydrating action on *methylcellulose* suspensions which leads to precipitation of the latter. *Acacia, proteins* and *tannins* also may be precipitated.

Uses—An *astringent, emetic* and weak *antiseptic*. Its antiseptic and astringent properties make it a valuable agent for use as an eyewash (aqueous solution) for temporary relief of minor eye irritation. Antibiotics largely have replaced it in general ophthalmic antiseptics. It may also be applied to the skin as a solution or as *White Lotion* (see page 873) for the treatment of *acne, dandruff, ivy poisoning, lupus erythematosus* and *impetigo*. It is the principal ingredient in some deodorant anhidrotics. It is included in some *vulvovaginal deodorants*. Large (but subemetic) doses of zinc accelerate the healing of chronic lesions or wounds, especially in patients with low serum-zinc concentrations. Topical zinc preparations also seem to accelerate the heating of chronic ulcers of the skin. Other disorders reported to respond to oral use are *rheumatoid arthritis* and *acrodermatitis enteropathica*.

Dose—*Topical, ophthalmic*, **0.1 mL** of **0.05, 0.217** or **0.25%** aqueous solution to the *conjunctiva* 3 or 4 times a day; *dermatologic*, as an *astringent*, **0.5%**, or *antiseptic*, **1%**. As a *deodorant*, **7.5%**. *Oral, adult*, for daily *dietary allowance*, **66 mg** a day; for *treatment*, initially **110** to **220 mg** 1 to 3 times a day; *infants*, **50 mg** twice a day. It is a prompt emetic in doses of 0.6 to 2 g. *Intravenous, adults*, and *children over 5 yr*, **2.5** to **4 mg** a day; *full-term infants* and *children up to 5 yr*, **100 µg/kg** a day; *premature infants*, **300 µg/kg** a day.

Dosage Forms—Injection: 1 and 5 mg/mL; Ophthalmic Solution: 0.217%, in combination with other antiseptics and/or ocular decongestants; Tablets: 66, 110, 200 and 220 mg (15, 25, 45 and 50 mg, respectively, of zinc; 1 mg contains 0.23 mg of zinc).

Systemic Antibacterial Drugs

During the early part of this century, giant strides were made in the systemic treatment of certain microzoal infections. Nevertheless, these advances did not affect, either greatly or directly, the overall practice of medicine. The advent of sulfanilamide in 1935 marked the beginning of a major revolution in the practice of medicine. The subsequent profusion of antibacterial agents overwhelmed the physician with golden tools. Several leading causes of death were deposed to a minor status and some to a mere nuisance. The consequent lengthening of the life span turned medicine toward the degenerative diseases and the problems of aging.

The social, economic and political consequences of these effects will reverberate for generations. Meanwhile, certain of the arts of "nondrug" management of infection nearly have been forgotten, and carelessness has been fostered by the glitter and security of the "wonder drugs." The realization that certain microorganisms are successfully resisting the "wonder drugs" not only impels a ceaseless search for new systemic antibacterial agents but also forces a sober return to certain ancillary arts of the medical and surgical management of infectious disease.

Although some of the drugs listed in this section are used only for their local actions, their obvious relationship to parent systemic agents warrants their inclusion.

In the dose statements under the various drugs, the permissible range of doses is indicated usually. The reader can assume the low dose is for use in mild infections or in patients with abnormally low rates of elimination and that the high dose is for use in serious or very serious infections or in patients with abnormally high rates of elimination. With many drugs, oral medication should never be used in serious infections, either because of intolerance to appropriately high doses or to erratic or limited absorption; thus, parenteral administration may be obligatory. Serious untoward effects are much more likely to occur with parenteral, especially intravenous, administration, so that for most drugs intravenous use should be replaced by oral or intramuscular use at the earliest possible time that the patient's condition permits.

Treatment should always extend at least 2 or 3 days after signs of infection have cleared, and in some types of infections for weeks or months. There are rare exceptions, such as the single-dose treatment of acute gonorrhea and urinary tract infections. These details are not given in the monographs, but they usually are found in the package inserts or other descriptive literature.

Sulfonamides

History—The compound *p*-aminobenzenesulfonamide, now known as *sulfanilamide,* was first synthesized in 1908, but it was many years before its therapeutic value was discovered. In 1932 a German firm prepared a red dye, 4-(4′-sulfamylphenylazo)-*m*-phenylenediamine or, *p*′-sulfamylchrysoidine, and in 1935 Domagk reported remarkable curative effects of this compound and named it *Prontosil.* In the same year, a group of French investigators found that the antibacterial property of the drug resided in the *p*-aminobenzenesulfonamide portion of the molecule. In 1937 Ewins and Phillips of England synthesized sulfapyridine, which was the first sulfonamide used with great success in combating pneumonia. Then followed sulfathiazole, sulfadiazine and a large number of other sulfonamides. Over 3300 sulfonamides have been prepared since, but only a few have been accepted for medicinal use.

All the official, and generally all the therapeutically useful, antimicrobial sulfonamides are characterized by the structure

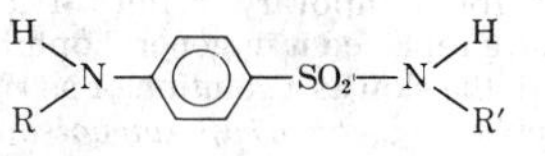

$$(H)(R)N-C_6H_4-SO_2-N(H)(R')$$

Preparation—*p*-Acetamidobenzenesulfonyl chloride, made by treating acetanilide with chlorosulfonic acid, is the basic intermediate of all the sulfonamides. This is treated with the desired amine in the presence of a weak base such as pyridine, and the resulting acetyl compound is deacetylated via proton- or hydroxyl-catalyzed hydrolysis. The reactions taking place in the synthesis of sulfadiazine are illustrated in the following:

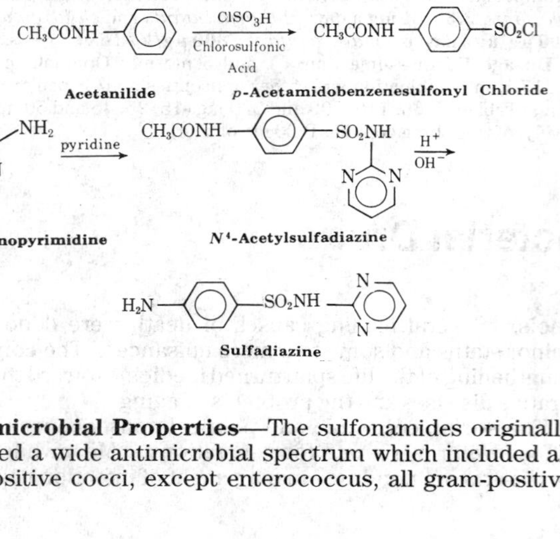

$CH_3CONH-C_6H_5$ (**Acetanilide**) $\xrightarrow{ClSO_3H \text{ (Chlorosulfonic Acid)}}$ $CH_3CONH-C_6H_4-SO_2Cl$ (***p*-Acetamidobenzenesulfonyl Chloride**)

2-Aminopyrimidine $\xrightarrow{\text{pyridine}}$ $CH_3CONH-C_6H_4-SO_2NH$-pyrimidinyl (***N*⁴-Acetylsulfadiazine**) $\xrightarrow{H^+ / OH^-}$

$H_2N-C_6H_4-SO_2NH$-pyrimidinyl (**Sulfadiazine**)

Antimicrobial Properties—The sulfonamides originally possessed a wide antimicrobial spectrum which included all gram-positive cocci, except enterococcus, all gram-positive bacilli, nearly all *Enterobacteriaceae* and gram-negative cocci, *H influenzae*, *B pertussis*, *Pasteurella*, some *Pseudomonas*, *Chlamydia* (psittacosis, *Trachoma*, *Lymphogranuloma venereum*), *Actinomycetes*, *Nocardia* and some *Toxoplasma* and malaria. However, resistance to the drugs has limited the spectrum greatly. The extent of acquired resistance to sulfonamides varies among communities, so that sensitivity testing is essential to the optimal use of these drugs.

In most circumstances, these agents exert only a bacteriostatic action, and ultimate elimination of the invading microorganisms depends upon the cellular and humoral defense mechanisms of the host, which are neither enhanced nor inhibited by the sulfonamides. However, bactericidal concentrations of these agents sometimes are attained in the urinary and intestinal tracts, where the concentration of drug may be quite high.

The mechanism of the antimicrobial action of the sulfonamides has been analyzed extensively. The sulfonamides compete with *p*-aminobenzoic acid and prevent its normal cellular use, particularly its incorporation into folic acid (pteroylglutamic acid, PGA). Thus, sulfonamide-sensitive organisms are primarily those which synthesize their own folic acid. Organisms able to use preformed folic or tetrahydrofolic acid or the tetrahydrofolate-dependent pyrimidines and thymidine are not affected by these agents generally. This mechanism is of importance as an example of the general concepts of *biological antagonism* and *antimetabolites.* The efficacy of sulfonamides generally is enhanced when the drugs are used in combination with the folic acid antagonist trimethoprim.

Microorganisms initially sensitive to the sulfonamides may become resistant to these drugs. The clinical importance of such acquired bacterial resistance is attested by the fact that the majority of the strains of *Neisseria gonorrhoeae* now isolated from patients with gonococcal urethritis are resistant to these agents, whereas the sulfonamides were once the agents of choice against such organisms. *Enterobacteriaceae,* especially, have become resistant. Numerous other examples could be cited, including the occurrence of epidemics among military populations caused by sulfonamide-resistant microorganisms after mass oral prophylactic use of these drugs. While such epidemics fortunately have not yet been of importance in civilian medicine, they do emphasize the necessity for proper precautions to minimize the development of acquired bacterial resistance. The sulfonamides should be employed only when specific indications exist for such medication. Further, when these agents are employed, they should be administered in adequate dosage as early as possible in the course of the infection.

Certain combinations of the sulfonamides with various antibiotics minimize the development of bacterial resistance and achieve chemotherapeutic results not attainable with either agent alone. However, not all combinations of chemotherapeutic agents have a rational basis. The microbe must be sensitive to both drugs used in combination. Occasionally, antibacterial drugs in combination are antagonistic. Specific examples of valid combinations of the sulfonamides with other chemotherapeutic agents are indicated below.

Absorption, Distribution and Fate—Sulfonamides in which the para-amino group is free are absorbed readily into the blood stream, mostly via the small intestine. Although only a small amount may remain unabsorbed, the local concentration in the bowel may be high enough to exert a prominent antibacterial action on some of the bowel flora. Absorption from the skin and vagina is erratic. Once into the bloodstream, sulfonamides bind to serum albumin to varying degrees, ranging from less than 10 to over 90%, depending on the particular drug. Protein binding limits penetrance into the tissues and glomerular filtration is a determinant of the rate of excretion.

Concentrations in tissue fluids usually range from about 50 to 80% of those in the plasma. Highly polar sulfonamides do not penetrate tissues well, but they are excreted rapidly. Thus, sulfisoxazole is mainly extracellular in distribution and is of limited usefulness in systemic infections; because it is filtered rapidly in the renal glomerulus and resorbed poorly by the renal tubules (being lipid-insoluble), high concentrations are reached in the urine, which makes it effective in the treatment of urinary tract infections. Nevertheless, when the urinary tract infection is extraluminal, more widely distributed sulfonamides, such as sulfadiazine, may be more effective.

Sulfonamides are acetylated in the liver to an extent of 30 to 85% depending on the sulfonamide and the patient. The fraction of the acetylate conjugate in the urine varies accordingly. Crystallization of sulfonamide, conjugate or both may occur in the urine, depending on the solubility properties of each form of the drug at the pH of the urine and on the volume of urine. In general, both parent and acetylated sulfonamides are more soluble in alkaline than acid urine.

Toxicity—Untoward effects during therapy with sulfonamides represent the major limitation to their clinical use. The most frequently observed side effects are crystalluria and related renal damage, hematuria being noted in approximately 2% of patients receiving sulfadiazine or other pyrimidine congeners.

Gastrointestinal side effects include nausea, vomiting, abdominal pain, diarrhea, anorexia, stomatitis and rare pancreatitis. Of the neurological effects, headache, vertigo and insomnia are the most frequent, but tinnitus, psychic depression, ataxia, hallucinations, peripheral and optic neuritis, acute myopia and convulsions occasionally occur. This incidence is less when adjuvant alkali and fluid therapy is instituted or when sulfonamide mixtures or the more soluble congeners are employed.

Hypersensitivity reactions, such as drug fever, dermatitis, hepatitis, polyarteritis nodosa, lupoid syndrome, pulmonary eosinophilia and rare myocarditis, occur in about 2% of patients receiving most present-day sulfonamides. The incidence of hypersensitivity reactions is higher in patients receiving sulfapyridine. Agranulocytosis, aplastic anemia, leukopenia and thrombocytopenia have been noted during sulfonamide therapy, but the incidence is low when sulfadiazine and the other newer congeners are employed.

Hemolytic anemia may occur; persons whose erythrocytes are deficient in glucose 6-phosphate dehydrogenase (G6PD) are especially susceptible. Sulfonamide-induced hepatocellular jaundice is now rare. Long-acting sulfonamides which may cause exudative erythema multiforme (Stevens-Johnson syndrome), are no longer available in the US.

Central nervous system effects are observed infrequently during current sulfonamide therapy, and cyanosis, acid-base disturbances and other miscellaneous toxic effects, formerly common during therapy with sulfanilamide, sulfathiazole or sulfapyridine, are observed only rarely during the administration of sulfadiazine.

Sulfonamides displace bilirubin from plasma proteins and hence can cause kernicterus in the newborn. It is not recommended that sulfonamides be administered to infants younger than 2 months. Consequently, sulfonamides should be avoided in pregnant women near term and in newborn or premature infants. Some sulfonamides have been shown to be teratogenic in rats. If at all possible, then, sulfonamides should be avoided in pregnancy.

Because the sulfonamides may cause serious untoward effects, they should be administered only when bacteriological diagnosis indicates that these agents can be expected to be superior to drugs of other classes. Constant medical surveillance, preferably daily, is necessary, and periodic blood counts and urinalysis are mandatory.

Uses—In spite of the dominance of antibiotics, sulfonamides still retain a minor place in the chemotherapy of infectious diseases. In only one infection, does a sulfonamide remain the agent of choice. In several infections, a sulfonamide-containing combination is the treatment of choice. In some serious infections, a sulfonamide is employed occasionally in combination with an appropriate antibiotic. In addition, sulfonamides have certain important prophylactic uses. Major advantages of sulfonamides are their low cost and ease of administration; major disadvantages are their untoward effects and limited efficacy.—Sulfonamides are the drugs of choice only for the treatment of *nocardiosis*. The combination, trimethoprim-sulfamethoxazole is the treatment of choice for infections caused by *Shigella*, *Ps maltophila*, *Ps cepacia*, *Yersinia enterocolitica*, *Aeromonas hydrophila* and *Pneumocystis carinii*. Sulfonamides share alternate-drug status with other drugs in the treatment of infections caused by *H influenzae* (if not life-threatening), *Mycobacterium fortuitum*, *Chlamydia trachomatis*, *lymphogranuloma venereum* and *meningococcal meningitis*, for which trisulfapyrimidines is indicated. Trimethoprim-sulfamethoxazole is an alternative treatment for infections caused by methicillin-resistant *Staph aureus* and *epidermidis*, *Enterobacter*, *E coli*, *Pr mirabilis* and *vulgaris*, *Morganella morganii*, *Providencia stuartii*, *Salmonella typhii*, *Klebsiella*, *Serratia*, *Acinetobacter*, *Brucella*, *H influenzae* and *ducreyi*, *Vibrio cholerae (cholera)*, *Listeria monocytogenes*, *Bordetella pertussis*, *Legionella midadei* and *pneumoniae*, *Branhamella* (Neisseria) *catarrhalis*, *Neisseria gonorrhoeae* and *meningitidis*, *Mycobacterium marinum*, *Chlamydia trachomatis* and *Nocardia*.

Sulfonamides sometimes are combined with penicillin in the treatment of otitis, with streptomycin in meningitis caused by *H influenzae* and may be combined with pyrimethamine in toxoplasmosis. Many strains of *meningococcus* are more sensitive to sulfonamides, but the occurrence of resistant strains has made penicillin G the drug of first choice. They are of use in some urinary tract infections caused by *E coli*, *Salmonella*, *Shigella*, *Staphylococcus*, *Klebsiella-Enterobacter*, *Pr mirabilis* and *Pr vulgaris*.

Sulfonamides are given with pyrimethamine to treat *toxoplasmosis* in immunosuppressed patients. Sulfonamides may be combined with penicillin in certain *selected* cases of *subacute bacterial endocarditis* not responsive to antibiotics alone. In regions in which there is a problem of resistance of malarial parasites to the usual antimalarials, sulfonamides may be given in combination with trimethoprim, quinine, pyrimethamine or other antimalarials. Prolonged treatment with sulfapyridine, but not other sulfonamides, is often useful in the treatment of *dermatitis herpetiformis;* the mechanism is unknown. Similarly, the beneficial effect of sulfasalazine in *ulcerative colitis* is understood poorly.

Important prophylactic uses of sulfonamides include their employment to reduce the *meningococcal* carrier rate and thus decrease the spread of meningococcal infections in congested populations, and for mass chemoprophylaxis during outbreaks of *bacillary dysentery*. They offer an alternative to penicillin in the prevention of recrudescences of rheumatic fever.

Types and Choice of Preparations—The antimicrobial spectrum of all sulfonamides is essentially the same. However, on the basis of solubility and degree of absorption from the gastrointestinal tract, the sulfonamides can be divided into two broad classes, namely, those employed for systemic chemotherapy and those intended only for intestinal chemotherapy.

Sulfonamides employed for their systemic actions include sulfacytine, sulfadiazine, sulfadoxine (in combination, only), sulfamerazine, sulfamethazine, sulfamethizole, sulfamethoxazole, sulfisoxazole, sulfapyridine and the sulfonamide mixtures (see below). These agents are absorbed readily from the gastrointestinal tract and adequate blood concentrations are maintained easily. All of these agents yield sufficiently high concentrations in urine to be useful against some urinary tract infections, but the more rapidly excreted ones yield higher concentrations and generally are preferred, except where tissue penetrance also is important.

Differences exist among these sulfonamides regarding distribution among the tissues and especially penetration into the cerebrospinal fluid. Differences in distribution have not been formulated well into guidelines for clinical choice. This is partly because differences resulting from protein binding are irrelevant to defining the penetrance of the free, or active, form of the drug, and not enough is yet known about the complete distribution of the free form of most of the sulfonamides.

Plasma half-lives have some bearing on choice, other than the simple matter of the convenience to the patient of the dose-interval. The relevance of rapid excretion has been noted. Very-long-acting sulfonamides bind strongly to proteins, which favors allergic responses.

Systemic sulfonamides and their conjugates differ in solubility in urine, and sulfonamide mixtures, particularly certain congeners, cause a lower incidence of crystalluria and related renal toxicity than do the other sulfonamides.

Oral administration of the sulfonamides is preferred. However, when medication cannot be taken by mouth, the soluble sodium or diolamine salts may be given parenterally.

Topical chemotherapy rarely is effective, except in the most superficial infections, and may be dangerous because of sensitization and the development of acquired bacterial resistance. Thus, topical administration of the sulfonamides, with the possible exception of sulfacetamide sodium, is not recommended and is discouraged strongly, except in trachoma and inclusion conjunctivitis, for which both topical and systemic treatment are used.

An important consideration in the choice of sulfonamide should be the cost to the patient.

Mixtures—Sulfonamide mixtures are designed to minimize the incidence of crystalluria and related renal injury associated with systemic use of sulfonamides. Since the solubility of a particular sulfonamide is not influenced by the presence of others in the same solution, a higher total concentration of sulfonamide can be attained in the urine without precipitation after administration of a mixture than is possible if a single sulfonamide is given.

There is no clinical necessity for less soluble triple sulfonamides because preparations which are more water-soluble are available. Presently marketed mixtures contain equal weights of sulfadiazine, sulfamerazine and sulfamethazine. Sulfonamide mixtures are available only for oral administration, but mixtures of parenteral preparations have been prepared extemporaneously and employed to advantage.

The antimicrobial potencies of the components of a mixture are additive, and the spectrum and therapeutic uses of sulfonamide mixtures are the same as those of the individual components. The incidence of renal toxicity is reduced, even without concomitant administration of alkalinizing salts. It can be reduced further if adjuvant urine alkalinization is employed. The incidence of hypersensitivity reactions is not enhanced and may be reduced. Precautions for the use of sulfonamide mixtures are the same as those for use of the individual congeners. Adequate 24-hour urine volume should be assured by fluid therapy if necessary. The dosage for the sulfonamide mixtures is essentially the same as that for the components.

Incompatibilities—The sodium derivatives are soluble in water, invariably imparting to the solution a marked alkalinity. Hence, such solutions are incompatible with all acidic substances and with precipitable amines.

Local anesthetics related to para-aminobenzoic acid antagonize the action of the sulfonamides. *Ethyl aminobenzoate, procaine, isocaine, butacaine* and *tetracaine* are related in this way.

Sulfabenzamide

Benzamide, *N*-[(4-aminophenyl)sulfonyl]-, ing of Sultrin (*Ortho*), Trysul (*Savage*)

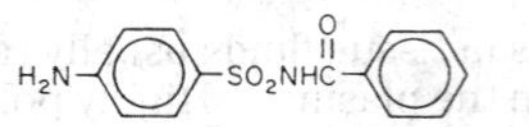

N-Sulfanilylbenzamide [127-71-9] $C_{13}H_{12}N_2O_3S$ (276.31).

Preparation—*J Am Chem Soc 61:* 2950, 1939.

Description—Crystalline powder; melts about 182°; pK_a 4.57.

Solubility—1 g in 3225 mL water, 33 mL alcohol or 9 mL acetone. Soluble in fixed alkalies.

Uses—A sulfonamide employed topically, in combination with other sulfonamides, for treatment of *Gardnerella (Hemophilus) vaginalis* vaginitis. It can cause sensitization and development of drug resistance that may compromise future systemic therapy with other sulfonamides.

Dosage Forms—Include a "triple-sulfa" cream containing as one of the ingredients 3.7% of sulfabenzamide and a vaginal tablet containing 184 mg of sulfabenzamide and other sulfonamides.

Sulfacetamide

N^1-Sulfanilylacetamide; ing of Sultrin (*Ortho*), Trysul (*Savage*)

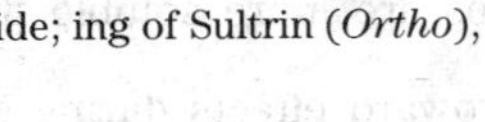

[144-80-9] $C_8H_{10}N_2O_3S$ (214.24).

Preparation—By reacting sulfanilamide with acetic anhydride, followed by controlled alkaline hydrolysis to remove the N^1-acetyl group and subsequent acidification to a pH of about 4.

Description—White, crystalline powder; melts about 183°; pK_a 1.78.

Solubility—1 g in about 140 mL water; soluble in alcohol; insoluble in ether.

Uses—Employed topically in combination with sulfabenzamide and sulfathiazole for the treatment of vaginitis caused by *Gardnerella (Hemophilus) vaginalis.*

Dose—*Topical,* as vaginal cream containing 2.86% sulfacetamide (with other sulfonamides) twice a day for 4 to 6 days or as a vaginal tablet containing 144 mg of sulfacetamide (with other sulfonamides) twice a day for 10 days.

Sulfacetamide Sodium

Acetamide, *N*-[(4-aminophenyl)sulfonyl]-, monosodium salt, monohydrate; Soluble Sulfacetamide; (*Various Mfrs*)

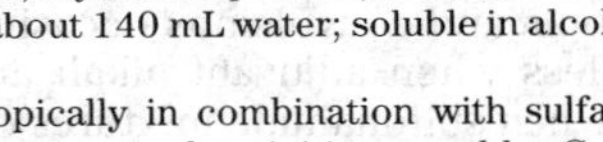

N-Sulfanilylacetamide monosodium salt monohydrate [6209-17-2] $C_8H_9N_2NaO_3S.H_2O$ (254.24); *anhydrous* [127-56-0] (236.22).

Preparation—By reacting sulfanilamide with acetic anhydride, followed by controlled alkaline hydrolysis to remove the N^1-acetyl group and subsequent acidification to a pH of about 4 to form sulfacetamide which is dissolved in the required quantity of NaOH solution and the solution is evaporated to dryness or precipitated with alcohol.

Description—White, crystalline powder; odorless; bitter taste; pH (1 in 20 solution) between 8 and 9.5.

Solubility—1 g in 2.5 mL water; sparingly soluble in alcohol; practically insoluble in benzene, chloroform or ether.

Uses—Its *antibacterial* spectrum is similar to that of the other sulfonamides, but it is less potent, owing to poor penetration into both tissues and bacteria. Employed in high concentration by local application, it is of benefit in various *ophthalmologic infections*, especially those caused by pyogenic cocci, gonococcus, *E coli* and Koch-Weeks' bacillus. *Trachoma* also may respond well sometimes. Since the drug is nonirritating even in high concentration, it can be employed in sufficient concentration to achieve penetration of the ocular tissues. Although the high local concentrations thus attained obviate certain of the undesirable aspects of local chemotherapy, the usual limitations and dangers of such therapy are not completely eliminated.

It is used also in the topical treatment of *acne vulgaris, seborrheic dermatitis* and various bacterial infections of the skin caused by susceptible organisms. It is a component of mixtures for the treatment of vaginal infections caused by *Candida, Trichomonas* and *Gardnerella*, but there is no clinical evidence that proves its efficacy for this purpose. In many infections, systemic chemotherapy also may be necessary. It is contraindicated if sensitivity to any sulfonamide exists. It is capable of causing hypersensitivity.

Dose—*Topical*, as **10%** ointment to the *conjunctiva* and lash margins 5 times a day or **1** to **3 drops** of a 10 to 30% solution every 2 to 3 hr during the day and less frequently at night; to the *skin*, as **10%** lotion.

Dosage Forms—Lotion: 10%; Ophthalmic Ointment: 10%; Ophthalmic Solution: 10, 15 and 30%.

Sulfacytine—see RPS-18, page 1177.

Sulfadiazine

Benzenesulfonamide, 4-amino-*N*-2-pyrimidinyl-, (*Various Mfrs*)

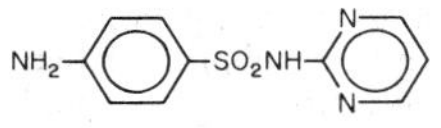

N^1-2-Pyrimidinylsulfanilamide [68-35-9] $C_{10}H_{10}N_4O_2S$ (250.27).

Preparation—By combining *p*-acetamidobenzenesulfonyl chloride (see page 1272) with 2-aminopyrimidine in the presence of a mild alkaline agent, then splitting off the acetyl group by hydrolyzing with acid or alkali.

Description—White or slightly yellow powder; odorless or nearly so; stable in air, but slowly darkens on exposure to light; melts between 251° and 254°.

Solubility—1 g in about 13,000 mL water; sparingly soluble in alcohol and acetone; 1 g in about 620 mL human serum at 37°; freely soluble in dilute mineral acids, solutions of potassium and sodium hydroxides or ammonia TS.

Uses—The therapeutic uses have been described in the general statement. Minimal therapeutic blood levels of the drug are in the range of 100 to 150 μg/mL.

Sulfadiazine is bound to plasma proteins to the extent of 40 to 50%, and concentrations of the drug in the cerebrospinal fluid vary from 50 to 80% of those in the plasma; this is a good tissue concentration, as antibacterial agents go. A dose of about 60 mg/kg will provide a therapeutic concentration in cerebrospinal fluid. Higher concentrations are attained when the meninges are inflamed, and intrathecal administration of the drug is usually not necessary. Thus, it is the sulfonamide of choice for CNS infections susceptible to sulfonamides and for which superior agents are not available; nocardiosis is an example, as is antibiotic-resistant meningococcal meningitis. It readily enters cells, and the volume of distribution is slightly greater than total body water. The tissue-penetrating properties have proven to be of importance in combatting urinary tract infections, so that in some such infections it may be superior to the more soluble sulfonamides.

Sulfadiazine is acetylated in the liver to the extent of 15 to 40%; both the free and acetylated forms are excreted in the urine. The elimination half-life is about 12 to 17 hr but varies considerably.

Untoward effects occur in approximately 6 to 8% of patients receiving therapy. Crystalluria and related renal damage can be minimized by administration of adjuvant alkalinizing salts and by maintenance of an adequate 24-hr urine volume. Urinary volume in the adult should be maintained at more than 1500 mL/24 hr. If adjuvant alkali therapy is employed, an initial dose of 4 g of sodium bicarbonate and subsequent doses of 2 g at intervals of 4 hr are necessary to achieve adequate alkalinization of the urine. To minimize crystalluria, the drug also is combined with other sulfapyrimidines. Hypersensitivity reactions are observed in 1 to 2% of patients, but agranulocytosis and other serious blood dyscrasias have been reported only rarely.

Dose—*Oral, adult, initially* **2** to **4 g** and, for *maintenance*, **4** to **8 g** a day in 4 to 6 divided doses; *infants older than 2 mo* and *children*, initially **75 mg/kg** (or **2 g/m²**) a day, followed by **150mg/kg** a day divided into 4 or 6 even doses, up to a maximum of 6 g a day. For the *prophylaxis* of rheumatic fever, **0.5 g** for persons weighing less than 30 kg, and **1 g** for persons weighing more than 30 kg, once a day. In severe infections, the initial oral dose for adults of 100 mg/kg is followed by 1 to 1.5 g every 4 hr day and night until the temperature has been normal for 5 to 7 days. In severe infections in children, the initial dose is 100 to 150 mg/kg. Subsequent doses of ¼ the initial dose are administered every 6 hr. In moderate or mild infections in both adults and children, an initial dose of 50 mg/kg and maintenance dose ⅓ of the initial dose at intervals of 4 to 6 hr are adequate.

Dosage Form—Tablets: 500 mg.

Sulfadoxine

N^1-(5,6-Dimethoxy-4-pyrimidinyl) sulfanilamide; Fanasil; Fanzil (*Roche*)

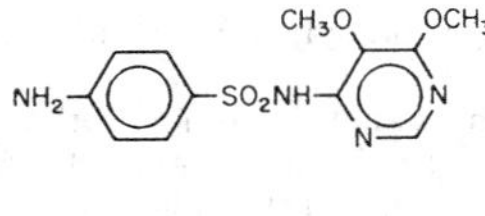

[2447-57-6] $C_{12}H_{14}N_4O_4S$ (310.34).

Preparation—By the general method for N^1-substituted sulfanilamides described on page 1272 using 4-amino- 5,6-dimethoxypyrimidine for the condensation with the sulfonyl chloride.

Description—White, to creamy white, crystalline powder; melts about 192°.

Solubility—Very slightly soluble in water; slightly soluble in alcohol.

Uses—Has antimicrobial activity similar to that of *Sulfadiazine*. Its principal use, however, is in the prophylaxis or suppression of malaria caused by chloroquine-resistant *P falciparum*. It is used only in combination with pyrimethamine, in a fixed-dose formulation.

Dose—Oral, for *acute attack, adult*, 2 to 3 tablets, alone or in sequence with primaquine or quinine. *Children 9 through 14 yr*, 2 tablets; *4 through 8 yr*, 1 tablet; *under 4 yr*, ½ tablet. *Prophylaxis, adult*, 1 tablet a week or 2 tablets every other week. *Children, 9 through 14 yr*, ¾ tablet for each tablet used by adult; *4 through 8 yr*, ½ tablet for each tablet used by adult; *under 4 yr*, ¼ tablet for each used by adult. Each scored tablet contains 500 mg of sulfadoxine and 25 mg of pyrimethamine.

Sulfamerazine

Benzenesulfonamide, 4-amino-*N*-(4-methyl-2-pyrimidinyl)-, Sulfamethyldiazine; (*Various Mfrs*)

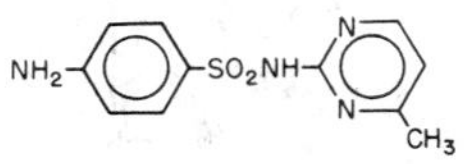

N^1-(4-Methyl-2-pyrimidinyl)sulfanilamide [127-79-7] $C_{11}H_{12}N_4O_2S$ (264.30).

Preparation—By the method described for *Sulfadiazine*, using 4-methyl-2-aminopyrimidine instead of 2-aminopyrimidine.

Description—White or faintly yellowish white crystals or powder; slightly bitter taste; odorless or nearly so; stable in air, but slowly darkens on exposure to light; melts between 234 and 239°.

Solubility—1 g in about 6250 mL water; readily soluble in dilute mineral acids or solutions of potassium, ammonium or sodium hydroxides; slightly soluble in alcohol; very slightly soluble in ether or chloroform.

Uses—Closely resembles sulfadiazine in its *antibacterial* properties, toxicity and therapeutic uses. It has a minimal effective concentration of 3 to 20 μg/mL. It is employed widely in sulfonamide mixtures in those infections in which the systemic antimicrobial actions of the sulfonamides are indicated (see the general statement and also *Sulfadiazine*).

It is absorbed more completely from the gut and excreted more slowly by the kidneys than is sulfadiazine. Hence doses required to maintain effective blood levels are smaller and are administered at slightly greater intervals than are those of sulfadiazine. About 75% is bound to plasma proteins, which is a greater extent than with sulfadiazine, and its concentration in the cerebrospinal fluid is only about 25% of that in plasma. Consequently, it is necessary to maintain a higher blood level with this drug in order to achieve efficacy equal to that of sulfadiazine. The elimination half-life is about 24 hr. Approximately 35 to 60% of the drug in the urine is in the inactive acetylated form. Both the free and acetylated forms are less soluble than those of sulfadiazine, so that crystalluria may occur, even despite a lower rate of excretion than with sulfadiazine. Consequently, it presently is used only in combination with other sulfapyrimidines.

Dose—There is no single-entity dosage form of sulfamerazine, and it is used only in combinations.

Sulfamethazine

Benzenesulfonamide, 4-amino-*N*-(4,6-dimethyl-2-pyrimidinyl)-, Sulphadimidine; Neotrizine (*Lilly*)

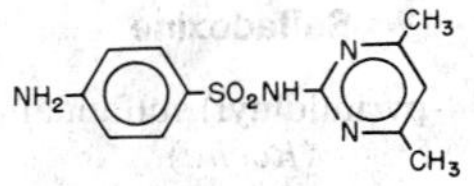

N^1-(4,6-Dimethyl-2-pyrimidinyl)sulfanilamide [57-68-1] $C_{12}H_{14}N_4O_2S$ (278.33).

Preparation—By the general method for N^1-substituted sulfanilamides described on page 1272 using 2-amino-4,6-dimethylpyrimidine for the condensation with the sulfonyl chloride.

Description—White or yellowish white powder which may darken on exposure to light; slightly bitter taste; melts between 197° and 200°.

Solubility—Very slightly soluble in water or ether; slightly soluble in alcohol; soluble in acetone.

Uses—Closely resembles *Sulfamerazine* in its antimicrobial properties, toxicity and therapeutic uses. It has a minimal effective concentration of 10 to 100 μg/mL. It is employed as a component of sulfonamide mixtures in those infections in which the systemic antimicrobial actions of sulfonamides are indicated (see the general statement, and also *Sulfamerazine*).

Like sulfamerazine, it usually is considered to be excreted more slowly by the kidney than is sulfadiazine, yet its half-life is reported to be only 7 hr. A longer half-life is consistent with the fact that doses required to maintain effective blood levels are smaller and are administered at slightly longer intervals than are those of sulfadiazine. The drug is 70 to 90% acetylated in the liver. About 80% is bound to plasma proteins.

Dose—There is no single-entity dosage form of sulfamethazine and it is used only in combinations.

Sulfamethizole

Benzenesulfonamide, 4-amino-*N*-(5-methyl-1,3,4-thiadiazol-2-yl)-, (*Various Mfrs*)

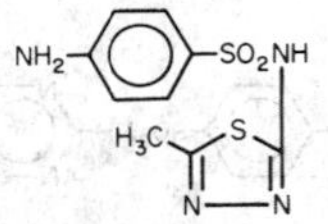

N^1-(5-Methyl-1,3,4-thiadiazol-2-yl)sulfanilamide [144-82-1] $C_9H_{10}N_4O_2S_2$ (270.32).

Preparation—By the general method for N^1-substituted sulfanilamides described on page 1272 using 5-methyl-2-amino-1,3,4-thiadiazole for the condensation with the sulfonyl chloride.

Description—White crystals or powder; slightly bitter taste; almost odorless; it has no odor of hydrogen sulfide; melting range 208° to 212°; pK_a 5.45.

Solubility—1 g in 2000 mL water, 38 mL alcohol, 1900 mL chloroform or 1900 mL ether; freely soluble in solutions of ammonium, potassium or sodium hydroxides; soluble in dilute mineral acids.

Uses—The bacterial actions and toxicity are those of other sulfonamides (see the general statement). The degree of protein binding in plasma is very low, so that the drug is filtered rapidly in the glomerulus and excreted; the rate of excretion is only 10 to 20% slower than that of creatinine. About 90% is excreted unmetabolized. The half-life is about 4 hr. The rapid rate of excretion (and consequent high concentrations in urine) and high solubility (hence low incidence of crystalluria) make the drug useful in the treatment of urinary tract infections caused by sulfonamide-susceptible organisms. It is excreted too rapidly to be of use in systemic infections. There is very little cross-sensitization between this and other sulfonamides, so that it often may be used when sensitivity exists to other sulfonamides. The drug has been reported to inhibit the metabolism of phenytoin, warfarin and tolbutamide.

Dose—*Oral, adult, usual,* **0.5** to **1 g** 3 or 4 times a day; *children and infants (over 2 mo),* **30** to **45 mg**/kg/24 hr, divided into 4 doses.

Dosage Form—Tablets: 500 mg.

Sulfamethoxazole

Benzenesulfonamide, 4-amino-*N*-(5-methyl-3-isoxazolyl)-, Gantanol (*Roche*)

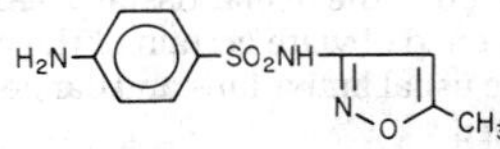

N^1-(5-Methyl-3-isoxazolyl)sulfanilamide [723-46-6] $C_{10}H_{11}N_3O_3S$ (253.28).

Preparation—By the general method for N^1-substituted sulfanilamides (page 1272) using 3-amino-5-methylisoxazole as the coupling amine. The latter may be prepared by heating ethyl 5-methylisoxazole-3-carbamate with aqueous sodium hydroxide. US Pat 2,888,455.

Description—White to off-white, crystalline powder; practically odorless; stable in air; melts 172°.

Solubility—1 g in 3400 mL water, 50 mL alcohol, 1000 mL chloroform or 1000 mL ether.

Uses—Chemically, closely related to *Sulfisoxazole;* has high aqueous solubility and low tissue penetrance, with the volume of distribution being considerably less than the extracellular space. It is bound to plasma proteins to the extent of about 68%. Thus, it is best suited to treatment of *urinary tract infections* caused by susceptible organisms. It is not rational to use it for systemic infections when there are other sulfonamides with more-favorable distribution, although it has been used successfully against gonorrhea, meningitis and serious respiratory-tract infections, and prophylactically against susceptible meningococci. Despite its unfavorable pattern of distribution, it is the sulfonamide most used around the world in combination with trimethoprim or pyrimethamine for the treatment of various systemic infections. The combination with trimethoprim is discussed in the following monograph, *Sulfamethoxazole and Trimethoprim.* (The main use, however, is for the treatment of urinary tract infections.) With pyrimethamine it is used in the treatment of chloroquine-resistant falciparum malaria. It is absorbed slowly and incompletely and is excreted more slowly than is sulfisoxazole, so that its duration of action is longer. Conjugation in the liver to the *N*-acetyl metabolite accounts for about 70% of elimination. The plasma half-life is 9 to 12 hr. The minimal effective concentration is 0.2 to 50 μg/mL. The toxicity is typical of sulfonamides, including crystalluria.

Dose—*Oral, adult, initially* **2 g,** followed by **1 g** 2 times a day. *Infants over 1 mo* and *children, initially* **50** to **60 mg/kg,** followed by **25** to **30 mg/kg** every 12 hr. Do not exceed **75 mg/kg** a day.

Dosage Forms—Oral Suspension: 500 mg/5 mL; Tablets: 500 mg and 1 g.

Sulfamethoxazole and Trimethoprim

Co-Trimoxazole; TMP-SMZ; Bactrim (*Roche*); Septra (*Burroughs Wellcome*); (*Various Mfrs*)

Uses—Sulfamethoxazole and trimethoprim inhibit sequential steps in the formation of tetrahydrofolic acid, the sulfonamide inhibits formation of dihydrofolic acid, and trimethoprim inhibits conversion of dihydrofolate to tetrahydrofolic acid and thence to folinic acid. Thus, the inhibition is magnified by the independent actions at two consecutive metabolic steps, and bacteriostasis may be altered to that of bactericidal. The minimal inhibitory concentration of the sulfamethoxazole is decreased to ½ to 1/15 that of sulfamethoxazole alone, depending on the microorganism. Moreover, even if resistance develops to the action at one step, inhibition at the other step helps to maintain the antibacterial action; incidence of resistance is low but has been increasing with widespread use of the drug.

The double blockade also widens the antibacterial spectrum from that of either agent alone. Thus, some strains of sulfonamide-insensitive *Pseudomonas aeruginosa* may become sensitive to the combination. All strains of *Streptococcus pneumoniae, Neisseria meningitidis* and *Corynebacterium diphtheriae* are sensitive to the combination. Also, 50 to 95% of strains of *Staphylococcus aureus and epidermidis; Streptococcus pyogenes, fecalis* and *viridans; Hemophilus ducreyi; Proteus mirabilis, vulgaris, morganii* and *rettgeri; Pseudomonas cepaciae* and *pseudomallei; Salmonella; Shigella; Enterobacter; Serratia* and *Alcaligenes* are inhibited. Other microorganisms that show a considerable incidence of sensitivity are *Brucella abortus, Isospora belli, Pasteurella haemolytica*, various *Klebsiella, Nocardia asteroides, Pneumocystis carinii* and some species of *Yersinia*. The frequent sensitivity of methicillin-resistant *Staph aureus* is noteworthy.

The predominant use is in the treatment of *urinary tract infections*, especially recurrent, chronic or complicated infections not considered controllable by single drugs. With these limitations of use, the rate of development of resistant strains in a community can be retarded. Urinary tract infections caused by *E coli, Klebsiella-Enterobacter* and *Proteus* species are the ones mostly treated. The combination provides the treatment or prophylaxis of choice for *pneumonitis* caused by *Pneumocystis carinii* and enterocolitis caused by *Isospora* in immunocompromised patients; it also affords successful chemoprophylaxis, even in intermittent dosage (3 days a wk). However, tissue distribution of sulfamethoxazole is poor, and the pharmacokinetics of the mixture is not optimal for treatment of systemic infections. Nevertheless, the combination has been successfully used to treat the infections noted in the general statement.

Trimethoprim is absorbed in about 2 hr and sulfamethoxazole in about 4 hr. During maintenance at steady state, 400 mg of sulfamethoxazole and 80 mg of trimethoprim (5:1 ratio) yield plasma levels (C^{ss}_{min}) of about 20 and 1 μg/mL of unbound drug, respectively. Trimethoprim enters the cerebrospinal fluid and tissues more readily than does sulfamethoxazole, so that the ratio is less than 20:1 at these sites.

In the presence of the sulfonamide, trimethoprim is bound poorly by plasma proteins, so that it filters rapidly into the urine, and less than 40% is metabolized. Consequently, the urine concentration may be 100 times that in plasma, whereas the sulfamethoxazole concentration may be only 3 times higher, thus departing from the supposedly optimal 20:1 ratio. The half-life of trimethoprim is about 9 hr. Impairment of renal function increases the half-life of each drug, the greater effect being on that of sulfamethoxazole.

The adverse effects of recommended doses are those of short-acting sulfonamides (page 1273), except that crystalluria is rare. Nausea, vomiting, glossitis and stomatitis also occur and are probably attributable to trimethoprim. In persons with subclinical folate deficiency, trimethoprim may precipitate megaloblastic anemia and leukopenia and exaggerate the probability of thrombocytopenia. Headache, peripheral neuritis, depression, convulsions, ataxia, hallucinations, fatigue and muscle weakness may occur. An increased incidence of rash and fever is observed in AIDS patients. The combination increases the effects of the coumarin anticoagulants, sulfonylurea oral hypoglycemics, phenytoin and methotrexate. Diuretics increase the risk of thrombocytopenia, especially in elderly patients with heart failure. Alkalinization of the urine decreases elimination of trimethoprim.

Dose—*Intravenous infusion, adults* and *children over 2 mo, against bacteria,* **15** to **20 mg/kg** of sulfamethoxazole and **3** to **4 mg/kg** of trimethoprim every 6 hr *or* **13.3** to **16.7 mg/kg** of sulfamethoxazole and **2.7** to **3.3 mg/kg** of trimethoprim every 8 hr *or* **20** to **25 mg/kg** of sulfamethoxazole and **4** to **5 mg/kg** of trimethoprim every 12 hr; against *Pneumocystis,* **25 mg/kg** of sulfamethoxazole and **5 mg/kg** of trimethoprim every 6 hr *or* **33.3 mg/kg** of sulfamethoxazole and **6.7 mg/kg** of trimethoprim every 8 hr. *Oral, adults and children over 40 kg against bacteria,* **800 mg** of sulfamethoxazole and **160 mg** of trimethoprim every 12 hr for 10 to 14 days; *adults* and *children over 32 kg,* against *Pneumocystis,* **25 mg/ kg** of sulfamethoxazole and **5 mg/kg** of trimethoprim every 6 hr; *children under 40 kg,* for *urinary tract infections,* **20 mg/kg** of sulfamethoxazole and **4 mg/kg** of trimethoprim every 12 hr; *children under 32 kg,* against *Pneumocystis,* **25 mg/kg** of sulfamethoxazole and **5 mg/kg** of trimethoprim every 6 hr.

Dosage Forms—Infusion: 400 mg sulfamethoxazole and 80 mg trimethoprim/5 mL; Oral Suspension: 200 mg sulfamethoxazole and 40 mg trimethoprim/5 mL; Tablets: 400 mg sulfamethoxazole and 80 mg of trimethoprim, and 800 mg sulfamethoxazole and 160 mg trimethoprim.

Sulfanilamide—see RPS-18, page 1180.

Sulfapyridine—see RPS-18, page 1180.

Sulfasalazine

Benzoic acid, 2-hydroxy-5-[[4-[(2-pyridinylamino)sulfonyl]-phenyl]azo]-, Salicylazosulfapyridine; Azulfidine (*Pharmacia*); (*Various Mfrs*)

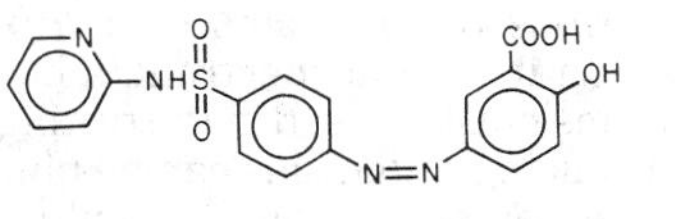

[599-79-1] $C_{18}H_{14}N_4O_5S$ (398.39).

Preparation—N^1-2-Pyridylsulfanilamide is diazotized and coupled with salicylic acid.

Description—Light brownish yellow to bright yellow, fine powder; practically tasteless and odorless; melts about 255° with decomposition.

Solubility—1 g in > 10,000 mL water, 2900 mL alcohol, > 10,000 mL chloroform or > 10,000 mL ether.

Uses—Poorly absorbed from the small intestine, so that the major portion of drug passes into the colon where bacterial enzymes release both 5-aminosalicylic acid and sulfapyridine from the drug. It has a suppressive effect on *ulcerative colitis*, that is not defined precisely. The local antibacterial effect of sulfapyridine in decreasing anaerobic bacteria may not be significant due to systemic absorption. The 5-aminosalicylate inhibits arachidonic acid cascade, both cyclooxygenase and lipoxygenase pathways. Most important may be the inhibition of leukotriene B_4 production by PMNs.

Since some sulfapyridine is absorbed from the colon, this drug has the toxic potential of *Sulfapyridine* (see under *Other Sulfonamides*). Adverse effects mostly occur when plasma levels exceed 50 μg/mL of sulfapyridine. Heinz-body and acute hemolytic anemias occur, so that the hematological status of the patient must be monitored regularly. Folic acid absorption also is impaired by the drug. Toxic epidermal necrolysis has been reported. If the initial dose does not exceed 2 g/day, the toxic potential is said to be minimized without seriously compromising therapeutic action. It imparts a yellow color to alkaline urine. Iron compounds decrease its absorption, the therapeutic significance of which is unknown. There have been a few instances in which sulfasalazine exacerbated ulcerative colitis. Desensitization has been used when reinstitution is required in patients with hypersensitivity.

Relapses occur in about 33% of cases, so that continuous prophylactic use often is advocated. However, after a year of continuous successful suppression, the relapse rate is about the same as when no prophylaxis is used.

Dose—*Oral, adult, initially* **3** to **4 g** a day in evenly divided doses; however, *initial doses* of **1** to **2 g** a day may lessen adverse GI effects, then 2 g/day for maintenance. *Children 2 yr or over, initially* **40** to **60 mg/kg** every 4 to 6 divided doses, then **20** to **30 mg/kg** a day for maintenance. Occasionally, initial doses of up to 150 mg/kg/day are required to achieve control.

Dosage Forms—Oral Suspension: 250 mg/5 mL; Enteric-Coated Tablets: 500 mg; Tablets: 500 mg.

Sulfathiazole—see RPS-18, page 1181.

Sulfisoxazole

Benzenesulfonamide, 4-amino-*N*-(3,4-dimethyl-5-isoxazolyl)-, Gantrisin (*Roche*); (*Various Mfrs*)

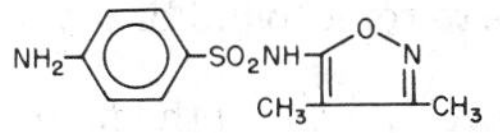

N^1-(3,4-Dimethyl-5-isoxazolyl)sulfanilamide [127-69-5] $C_{11}H_{13}N_3O_3S$ (267.30).

Preparation—By the general method for N^1-substituted sulfanilamides described on page 1272 using 3,4-dimethyl-5-aminoisoxazole for the condensation with the sulfonyl chloride.

Description—White to slightly yellowish crystalline powder; odorless; melts 199°.

Solubility—1 g in about 6700 mL water; soluble in diluted hydrochloric acid.

Uses—The *antibacterial* properties and therapeutic uses resemble those of sulfadiazine. The minimum inhibitory concentrations for bacteria to be treated in urinary tract infections are 1 to 20 μg/mL. However, it does not penetrate cells and pass barriers as well as most sulfonamides; the volume of distribution is only 0.16 mL/g. Consequently, it is not always effective against systemic infections which are sensitive to other sulfonamides. Urinary tract infections caused by sulfonamide-susceptible bacteria respond favorably, and the drug is useful in the treatment of many such infections. However, in genitourinary tract infections in which penetration into the involved tissues is required, it may not be as effective as sulfadiazine. It is secreted into prostatic fluid, but it is not known whether it is secreted into other genitourinary fluids. The extent of protein binding in plasma is 86%. It is metabolized primarily by acetylation and oxidation in the liver. Both it and the conjugate are excreted rapidly by the kidney and reach high concentrations in the urine. The half-life is about 6 hr. Since both the free and acetylated forms are highly soluble, even in acidic urine, adjuvant alkali therapy is not necessary and fluids need not be forced. The incidence of renal toxicity is lower than that caused by sulfadiazine or sulfonamide mixtures. With this exception, untoward effects during its therapy are similar to those caused by other sulfonamides (see the general statement). Topical use may compromise subsequent use of sulfonamides by causing occasional sensitization or bacterial resistance.

Dose—*Oral, adult, initially* **2** to **4 g**, followed by **4** to **8 g** a day in 4 to 6 divided doses, not to exceed 12 g a day; *infants over 2 mo* and *children, initially* **75 mg/kg** (or **2 g/m²**), followed by **150 mg/kg** a day in 4 to 6 divided doses, not to exceed 6 g a day.

Dosage Forms—Tablets: 500 mg. Vaginal Cream: 10% in combination with aminacrin and allantoin.

Sulfisoxazole Acetyl

Acetamide, *N*-[(4-aminophenyl)sulfonyl-*N*-(3,4-dimethyl-5-isoxazolyl)-, Acetyl Gantrisin, Lipo Gantrisin (*Roche*); ing of Pediazole (*Ross*)

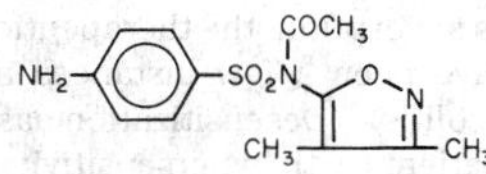

[80-74-0] $C_{13}H_{15}N_3O_4S$ (309.34).

Preparation—Sulfisoxazole is selectively acetylated at the *N*-position by converting it into its sodium salt which may then be metathesized with an equimolar quantity of acetyl chloride.

Description—White or slightly yellow, crystalline powder; melting range 192° to 195°.

Solubility—Practically insoluble in water; 1 g in 176 mL alcohol, 35 mL chloroform or 1064 mL ether.

Uses—Converted to sulfisoxazole in the gastrointestinal tract, which slows the rate of absorption. Thus, its actions and toxicity are identical to those of *Sulfisoxazole*. It is tasteless, hence is more suitable for liquid oral preparations used for children. The half-life is about 10 hr. When it is incorporated into a vegetable oil suspension, oral absorption is slowed, and the duration of action is prolonged.

Dose (base equivalent)—With the Oral Suspension and the Syrup, the dose is the same as that of *Sulfisoxazole*. With the Extended-Release (delayed absorption) Oral Suspension, the *adult* dose is **4** to **5 g** every 12 hr, and the *pediatric* dose (*children over 1 mo*) is **60** to **75 mg/kg** every 12 hr, not to exceed 6 g a day.

Dosage Forms (base equivalent)—Oral Suspension: 500 mg/5 mL; Extended-Release Oral Suspension: 1 g/5 mL; Syrup: 500 mg/5 mL.

Sulfisoxazole Diolamine

Benzenesulfonamide, 4-amino-*N*-(3,4-dimethyl-5-isoxazolyl)-, compd with 2,2′-iminobis[ethanol] (1:1); Gantrisin (*Roche*)

N^1-(3,4-Dimethyl-5-isoxazolyl)sulfanilamide compound with 2,2′-iminodiethanol (1:1) [4299-60-9] $C_{11}H_{13}N_3O_3S.C_4H_{11}NO_2$ (372.44).

Preparation—Sulfisoxazole is dissolved in an aqueous solution containing an equimolar portion of diethanolamine [$HN(CH_2CH_2OH)_2$] and the solution is evaporated to dryness.

Description—White to off-white, fine, crystalline powder; odorless; melts between 119° and 124°.

Solubility—1 g in 2 mL water, 16 mL alcohol, 1000 mL chloroform or >10,000 mL ether.

Uses—Actions and uses are the same as those of *Sulfisoxazole*, except that the diolamine salt is more soluble and hence is suitable for injection and for ophthalmic application. The ophthalmic preparations are employed in the treatment of corneal ulcers, conjunctivitis and other superficial ocular infections caused by sensitive organisms and as an adjunct in the treatment of trachoma.

Dose (base equivalent)—The *initial* dose for patients *over 1 mo*, **50 mg/kg** (or **1.125 g/m²**), is the same for all parenteral routes. *Maintenance* doses are as follows: *intramuscular*, **33 mg/kg** (or 750 mg/m²) every 8 hr *or* **50 mg/kg** (or **1.125 g/m²**) every 12 hr; *intravenous*, **25 mg/kg** (or **562.5 mg/m²**) every 6 hr; *subcutaneous*, **33 mg/kg** (or **750 mg/m²**) every 8 hr. The injection must be diluted 1 to 6 to make a 5% solution for subcutaneous or intravenous administration. Intravenous administration should be by slow infusion. *Topical*, to the conjunctiva and lid margin, **1.25** to **2.5 cm** of **4%** ointment or **1 drop** of **4%** solution every 8 hr or more frequently with solution.

Dosage Forms (sulfisoxazole equivalent)—Injection: 400 mg/mL in 5 mL; Ophthalmic Ointment: 4%; Ophthalmic Solution: 4%.

Antibiotics

Antibiotic substances are chemical compounds produced by living cells and which inhibit, in very low concentrations, the growth of microorganisms. While antibiotics have been isolated from tissues of higher plants and animals, the term generally has come to refer to inhibitory substances of microbial origin.

The historical development of the field of antibiotics began with the discovery by Chain, Florey and associates at Oxford University who discovered the favorable therapeutic and pharmacological properties of extracts of cultures of the mold *Penicillium notatum*, found to produce *penicillin* by Fleming in 1929.

As a result of these studies, and particularly because of the demands due to World War II, a remarkable impetus was imparted to the search for new antibiotics. During the decade 1940 to 1950 a large number were described, and in the following 9 years still more were reported and research in this field continues unabated. More than 4000 are known today.

The increased use of antibiotics in man and animals and the extension of uses to areas other than the treatment and prophylaxis of disease have created serious problems. More and more strains of organisms have become resistant to the available antibiotics. The staphylococci have created the greatest problem, and in "closed populations," such as hospitals, frequently more than 90% of the strains isolated are resistant to penicillin G. In most communities, the incidence of resistance is about 70%. Therefore, hospital controls are required to discourage the unnecessary use of antibiotics, so that the incidence of resistant strains in the hospitals can return toward that in the surrounding communities. The incidence in the community also could be lowered by a more selective, less frequent use.

The wide use of antibiotics in animal nutrition and disease has resulted in the sensitization of a relatively large number of the susceptible people, many of whom have serious reactions upon contact with these drugs. Such agricultural use also contributes to the pool of antibiotic-resistant bacteria in a community.

In this chapter penicillin is considered in detail since it is the historical prototype. It was the first antibiotic to be produced commercially and still assumes a position of major importance in this field.

Detection and Isolation of Antibiotic-Producing Organisms

The detection of productive organisms is based on the ability of cultures of the candidate organism to inhibit certain concomitantly cultured test bacteria under controlled conditions *in vitro*. A number of different test organisms are used, because no one organism is representative of the antibiotic susceptibilities or organisms in general. Thus, the use of a certain strain of *S aureus* as the test organism will detect all antibiotics inhibitory to that organism, but the antibiotic may or may not also be effective against *E coli*, for example, or even against various other strains of *S aureus*. To insure securing a valid antibacterial spectrum, a number of species and types of strains must be used in the testing.

Antibiotic-producing organisms can be obtained by testing pure cultures of organisms available in culture collections or isolated from natural sources, and "screening," or selection through suitable techniques from the vast heterogeneous mixed population of the soil or other natural habitations of microorganisms. In the first case, the practice consists simply of adding to broth or agar cultures, seeded with the test organism, suitable quantities or culture filtrates of the cultures being examined, incubating and inspecting for inhibition of the test organism. The screening method involves plating out in serial dilution an aqueous extract of soil or other natural substrate using a medium, usually agar, previously seeded with the test organism. During incubation the various organisms of the soil population develop, and those forming antibiotic substances are distinguished by a clear zone or halo around the colony, indicative of inhibition of the test organism which, in the region beyond the clear zone, grows abundantly in the form of a marked turbidity throughout the agar.

Many modifications of this principle are employed. Thus, the use of different media, pH, temperature and substrates will expose, for screening, different types of soil organisms. These conditions must be compatible with the growth of the particular test organism employed. Theoretically, the best chance for detecting the largest possible number of antagonists lies in the preincubation of the agar cultures containing the soil dilutions, but without the test bacteria. This is followed by a secondary incubation after the test organism is applied to the plate by streaking or spraying. In this manner slow-growing soil organisms are given the opportunity to develop and manifest antibiotic-producing ability.

Once detected, the antagonist is isolated in pure culture and identified, and the optimal conditions for production of the antibiotic substance produced by it are investigated. The composition of the medium is important. Different organic and inorganic nitrogenous substances are tested, with and without various carbohydrates, minerals, heavy metals, etc.

Once a favorable medium is established, other known strains of the antagonist, obtained either from stock-culture collections or isolated from nature, are compared for the character and amount of the antibiotic produced, and the highest yielding strain selected for further work. The antibacterial spectrum is obtained, ie, the relative effectiveness of the antibiotic in inhibiting the growth of a large variety of gram-positive and gram-negative bacteria, rickettsiae, viruses and fungi, especially those which are pathogenic. This indicates those infections in which it may be useful chemotherapeutically.

Several concentrates or isolates of the antibiotic, not necessarily pure, then are examined for toxicity in mice. Only low-toxicity preparations and, in particular, those in which toxicity is inversely proportional to the antibacterial potency are of interest. Toxicity and pharmacological data are obtained in animals and, if favorable, in clinical trials on human beings. If the clinical trials show the antibiotic to be a promising therapeutic agent, attention is turned to large-scale manufacture. Chemical studies of the structure of the pure compound will indicate the feasibility of chemical synthesis. Generally, antibiotics are complex substances whose synthesis may be extremely difficult, or at least uneconomical, compared to microbiologic production. This is the case now with most of the successful antibiotics, such as penicillin, streptomycin or chlortetracycline.

The gradual increase in numbers of strains of microorganisms resistant to antibiotics, especially the staphylococci, and the numbers of individuals developing sensitivity to them make it extremely desirable that screening programs for the isolation and development of new agents be continued.

Production

The development and operation of the large-scale commercial production of antibiotic substances may be exemplified by a description of the manufacture of penicillin. In general, the approach and methods employed are typical. Two types of processes for the microbiological production of antibiotics are:

The surface process, in which the antibiotic-producing organism grows in the form of a pad on the surface of a liquid medium in trays or bottles, or on the surface of a finely divided moist solid substrate such as wood shavings or wheat bran.

The submerged process, in which the organism develops in a liquid medium, maintained continuously under mechanical agitation and aeration, so that the organism develops uniformly and homogeneously in the form of a suspension of single cells, or small aggregates or colonies, throughout all portions of the culture liquid.

The penicillin is excreted into the culture fluid. The molds used industrially today are derived from *Penicillium chrysogenum.*

In the submerged process, growth is accelerated greatly and the handling of large quantities greatly facilitated. It is considerably more efficient than the surface processes, and hence is the only feasible method for large-scale commercial production. Stationary, closed tanks, known as fermenters, of 5000- to 30,000-gal capacity, are used in penicillin manufacture. Most of these are equipped with vertical single-shaft propeller or turbine-type agitators and with a mechanical means of comminuting and distributing sterile air, introduced for maximum dispersal effect in the region of the agitator. The tanks have a detachable manhole on the top, sight glasses and outlets to valve-closed sampling lines and accessory feed chambers, enabling inoculation by hand if necessary, particularly in small seed tanks, and the addition whenever necessary of other (sterile) materials, such as antifoam agents, during the fermentation. All outlets from the tank are exposed continuously to flowing steam to minimize chances of contamination. The culture medium is sterilized by high-pressure steam and subsequently cooled. Temperature control during growth of the mold is maintained automatically at 23° to 25°. The compressed air, which is introduced into the fermenters, is sterilized by filtration through steam-sterilized cartridges of suitable size and filled, for example, with glass wool.

Inoculum for large tanks is obtained by building up the amount of growth successively through a series of seed tanks, from tank to tank, and transferring under air pressure through sterile pipe lines. Generally, this massive inoculum amounts to 5 to 10% of the main batch and, consequently, seed tanks are about 1/10 the volume of the next larger tank. The first and smallest seed tank is inoculated with a laboratory-prepared culture, consisting either of spores or of a small flask of submerged growth obtained on a laboratory-, rotary- or reciprocal-type shaking machine.

The stock or master culture of the penicillin-producing mold is dry and cold-preserved in the form of spores. Continuous vegetative transfer of the mold on artificial media leads to loss of penicillin-producing power (physiological degeneration). Hence, the number of intermediate transfers between master culture and the final batch is kept at a minimum.

A Typical Production Medium

Corn-steep liquor (solids)	2 to 5%
Crude lactose	2 to 3%
Calcium carbonate	0.5 to 1%

The culture medium used for commercial production of penicillin generally contains natural nitrogenous material, nitrate, α-aminoadipic acid, cottonseed meal or corn-steep liquor, which is a by-product of the corn-milling industry, lactose, side-chain precursor, surface-active agent and mineral salts (including sulfate). The penicillin potency is followed by assay every 3 to 6 hours and, at the time when the potency stops rising, the batch is harvested. Maximum activity generally is reached in 50 to 90 hours. Due to the instability of penicillin at ordinary temperatures, the batch is cooled to 5° and the mycelium filtered off by pressure filtration.

The penicillin is extracted and concentrated by charcoal adsorption or solvent extraction.

Improvements in Production—The greatest advancements in the production of penicillin have been the use of the submerged or tank method of production, the use of corn-steep liquor and the progressive improvement in the penicillin- producing capacity of the mold.

The earliest widely used strain in tank production was *Penicillium notatum*, No 832, which yielded 50 to 60 units/ mL. Later, a strain of *Penicillium chrysogenum*, No 1951B25, with maximum yields of 250 units/mL, was discovered. Spores of this organism, exposed to X-ray irradiation and tested from single spore isolates, led to selection of a mutant strain X1612 producing approximately 500 units/mL. Strain X1612 was subjected to ultraviolet irradiation and strain Q176, yielding penicillin potencies of more than double that of X1612, was obtained. This strain has been used widely in commercial production, but industry has even improved on it. Some variant strains produce several thousand units per mL. The improvement in strains suitable for the surface production of penicillin followed a similar path although these were obtained by testing single spore isolates from parent cultures. A strain excellent in submerged culture is not necessarily good for surface culture, and *vice versa*. Surface culture methods are no longer used for commercial production of any of the presently useful antibiotics.

A large number of different fungi are now known to produce penicillin. Over 20 different species of *Aspergillus* and *Penicillia* produce penicillin, as do the dermatophyte *Trichophyton mentagrophytes* and a thermophilic fungus, *Malbranchea pulchella*.

Control

Federal control of antibiotics dates back to an amendment of the 1938 Food, Drug and Cosmetic Act (Section 507) under which the FDA was required to pretest all forms of penicillin and its preparations before releasing them for sale. This certification covered potency, demonstration of nontoxicity and moisture content (the presence of excess moisture makes penicillin less stable). When intended for parenteral use, it also was tested for freedom from pyrogens, for sterility, clarity and pH of its solutions.

This amendment included the provision that when it was found by the Federal Security Administrator (now Secretary HHS) that the pretesting of penicillin or its preparations was no longer necessary to insure safety and efficacy of such drugs, they could be exempted from the pretesting requirement.

Under this provision of the Act the Federal Security Agency, FDA Division, finding that certain new, highly purified forms of penicillin no longer required pretesting, issued a notice in the *Federal Register* of April 13, 1949, exempting Crystalline Penicillin G Potassium and Crystalline Penicillin G Sodium from this provision.

In March, 1947, the Congress of the US placed streptomycin under the certification system and in July of 1949 included chlortetracycline, chloramphenicol and bacitracin. Since these amendments include all derivatives as well, both dihydrostreptomycin and tetracycline, as well as pyrrolidinomethyl tetracycline and demeclocycline, were certifiable drugs.

In May, 1963, the Drug Amendments passed by Congress in 1962 became effective and superseded all previous rulings. These now provide that *all* antibiotics used in humans are subject to certification. Furthermore, those certifiable prior to passage of these latest amendments, ie, chlortetracycline, bacitracin, streptomycin, penicillin and chloramphenicol, also must be certified for veterinary use.

Classes and Agents

Antibiotics are classified by various schemes, the two most important being according to mechanism of action and according to chemical relationship. The antibiotic monographs that follow will be arranged according to chemical relationships.

Beta-Lactam Antibiotics

Penicillins

History—During an inspection of some culture plates in the laboratory of St Mary's Hospital London, in 1928, Professor Alexander Fleming observed the lysis of staphylococcus organisms by a contaminating mold. Upon subculturing the mold he found in the broth a powerful, but nontoxic, antibacterial substance. He gave it the name "penicillin" from the organism *Penicillium notatum* which caused the generation of the antibiotic.

Chemistry—The name "penicillin" now designates a number of antibiotic substances produced by the growth of various *Penicillium* species or by other means. The better known natural penicillins are listed in Table 2. Penicillins F, G and X were referred to formerly as I, II and III, respectively.

The parent compound is (2*S*-*cis*)-4-thia-1-azabicyclo-[3.2.0]hepatane-2-carboxylic acid (I). The 3,3-dimethyl-7-oxo derivative of I is known commonly by the trivial name penicillanic acid (II) and the penicillins are α-carboxamido derivatives of it (III):

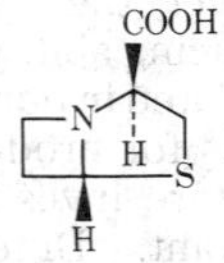

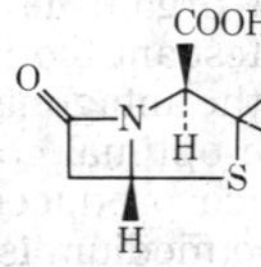

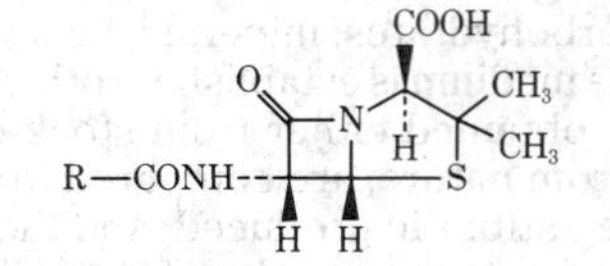

Penicillins are named variously in the literature as derivatives of I, II or III above. Nomenclature by I is purely systematic, whereas that by II or III is trivial. As derivatives of II, it is merely necessary to identify the specific 6α- carboxyamido group; as derivatives of III, only the R of the 6α-carboxamido group is identified.

The introduction of various acids, amines or amides into the medium in which the mold is developing leads to the production of biosynthetic penicillins which differ only in R. Dozens of biosynthetic *penicillins* have been prepared in this manner in an attempt to obtain compounds superior to penicillin G with respect to various physical, microbiological or pharmacological properties. In 1958 methods were devised for preparing the penicillin nucleus, thus making it possible to biosynthesize penicillins that could not be formed in a more normal medium. The resulting compounds were often more acid-stable, more penicillinase-resistant or had a wider antibacterial spectrum.

Table 2—Some Natural Penicillins

Natural penicillin	Radical (R)
Penicillin G	benzyl
Penicillin F	2-pentenyl
Penicillin dihydro-F	*n*-pentyl
Penicillin K	*n*-heptyl
Penicillin O	(allylthio)methyl
Penicillin V	phenoxymethyl
Penicillin X	*p*-hydroxybenzyl
Penicillin N	D-4-amino-4-carboxybutyl
Penicillin S	γ-chlorocrotylmercaptomethyl
Penicillin BT	butylmercaptomethyl

Much of the penicillin of commerce is pure crystalline G. It occurs in fermentation liquors together with variable amounts of K and F penicillins and smaller amounts of others, and is separated from the other penicillins during purification. Commercial practice suppresses, to a certain extent, the natural tendency of the mold to form penicillins other than the desired G by the incorporation of a precursor of G, namely phenylacetic acid, phenylacetamide, phenylethylamine or other substance containing the phenylacetyl radical, which is built directly into the penicillin G molecule. Penicillin G has the additional advantage of being much easier to crystallize than K or F.

As seen in figures I, II and III, penicillins are acids. The potassium salt predominates in use, with the sodium salt next. These salts are very soluble in water. The acid moiety can be used to combine penicillins with various bases, such as procaine or benzathine, to create insoluble salts, for repository use, or for the purpose of decreasing solubility so as to make the compound more resistant to gastric acid.

Penicillin in solution is very unstable at pH 5 or less and at 8 or above. Solutions of penicillin begin to deteriorate upon standing a few days, even in the cold. Certain penicillins are more resistant to acid hydrolysis and thus lend themselves better to oral administration.

Classification and Spectrum—Penicillins formerly were classified according to pseudohistorical divisions, by "generation", similar to the classification of the cephalosporins. However, it is more useful to classify them according to a mixture of chemical and antimicrobial designations. The categories are *penicillin G, acid-stable penicillins, penicillinase-resistant penicillins, aminopenicillins, extended-spectrum penicillins* and *amdinopenicillins.* There is a great deal of overlap in the properties among the cateogies. For example, two of the penicillinase-resistant, all of the aminopenicillins and one extended-spectrum penicillin are sufficiently acid-stable to be orally effective; aminopenicillins, extended-spectrum penicillins and amdinocillin are all resistant to certain β-lactamases (which often are called penicillinases indiscriminately) and variably resistant to Class II β-lactamases, to which the term, penicillinase, is becoming restricted. All penicillins are bacteriostatic at low and bactericidal at high concentrations. Their antimicrobial spectra differ according to the pattern of β-lactamase resistance, the ability to penetrate the outer membrane of gram-negative bacteria and selectivities for the various bacterial transpeptidases (penicillin binding proteins; PBPs).

Although penicillin G is destroyed largely by gastric acid, its low oral bioavailability can be compensated by increased dosage. Penicillin V is the only marketed member of the acid-stable class. These two drugs/classes have nearly identical antimicrobial spectra, except that sensitivities to penicillin-V are not high enough for a number of gram-negative infections to be treated by the oral route. The spectrum is *narrow* and mostly limited to gram-positive bacteria, gram-negative cocci and a few miscellaneous bacteria. They are especially active against gram-positive bacteria, particularly *Strep pyogenes*, most *pneumococci, Cl tetani* and *perfringens, Coryn diphtheriae, B anthracis, Bacteroides, Eubacterium, Fusobacterium, Listeria monocytogenes, Peptococcus and Peptostreptococcus.*

Although *Staph aureus* and *epidermidis* were originally mostly sensitive, they are now over 90% resistant in hospital populations and 50% in the community. *Strep viridans* is variably sensitive. *Strep faecalis* (enterococcus) is usually resistant. The gram-negative cocci, *N meningitidis* and *N gonorrhoeae*, are mostly sensitive, although resistance is increasing rapidly. Activity against the gram-negative bacilli is usually too low to be of clinical significance, but over 80% of strains of *E coli, Enterobacter*, most *Prot mirabilis* and some *Salmonella* and *Shigella* are sufficiently sensitive to respond in the urinary tract, where drug concentrations are high. Concentrations are also high in the bile, and these penicillins may be used to treat biliary tract infections caused by some enterobacteria and enterococci. These drugs are also active against *Actinomycetes, Leptospira, Providencia, Spirillum minus, Streptobacillus moniliformis* and *Treponema pallidum.*

Table 3—Members of Penicillin Classes

Class and Generic Name	Trade Name	Routes	Penicillinase-Resistant
Natural penicillins			
Penicillin G	Many	IM, IV, oral	No
Penicillin V	Many	IM, IV, oral	No
Penicillinase-resistant			
Cloxacillin	Cloxapen, Tegopen	oral	Yes
Dicloxacillin	Dycill, Dyanpen, Pathocil	oral	Yes
Methicillin	Staphcillin	IM, IV	Yes
Nafcillin	Nafcil, Unipen, Nallpen	IM, IV, oral	Yes
Oxacillin	Bactocill, Prostaphlin	IM, IV, oral	Yes
Aminopenicillins			
Amoxacillin	Amoxil, Larotid, Polymox, Trimox	oral	No
Amoxacillin-clavulanate	Augmentin	oral	Yes
Ampicillin	Many	IM, IV, oral	No
Ampicillin-sulbactam	Unasyn	IM, IV	Yes
Bacampicillin	Spectrobid	oral	No
Cyclacillin	Cyclapen	oral	No
Extended-spectrum (antipseudomonal) penicillins			
Carbenicillin	Geopen	IM, IV	No
Indanyl-carbenicillin	Geocillin	oral	No
Mezlocillin	Mezlin	IM, IV	No
Piperacillin	Pipracil	IM, IV	No
Ticarcillin	Ticar	IM, IV	No
Ticarcillin-clavulanate	Timentin	IV	Yes

Resistance of gram-positive and a number of gram-negative bacteria to penicillins G and V results from the bacterial elaboration of so-called penicillinase. This kind of resistance was obviated by the development of penicillins which penicillinase cannot destroy. The first member of the penicillinase-resistant class was *methicillin*, to which *cloxacillin, dicloxacillin, nafcillin* and *oxacillin* were added. These drugs have about the same spectrum of activity as the former two drugs, except increased activity against most staphylococci (especially), enterococci, gonococci and meningococci.

The *aminopenicillins* include *ampicillin, amoxacillin, becampicillin, cyclicillin* and *epicillin.* Each has an amino group adjacent to the carbonyl of the *N*-acyl substituent. Efficacy is increased against enterococcus, meningococcus and several gram-negative bacilli, such as community-acquired *E coli, H influenzae, Pr mirabilis*, various *Salmonella and Shigella.* However, there is less activity against most gram-positive bacteria, *N gonorrhoeae, B anthracis, Bacteroides, Clostridium, Corynebacterium, Enterobacter, Eubacterium, Listeria, Peptococcus, Peptostreptococcus, Providencia, Streptobaccillus, Actinomyses* and *Treponema;* consequently, this group also has been called *shifted-spectrum penicillins.* There are important differences among the spectra of the various members, ampicillin having the broadest spectrum but amoxacillin being the only one to be effective against *Strep viridans.* Only ampicillin has clinically significant activity against *Salmonella* and *Shigella.*

The *extended-spectrum* (antipseudomonal) *penicillins* include *azlocillin, carbenicillin, indanylcarbenicillin, mezlocillin, piperacillin* and *ticarcillin.* There is increased activity against *Acinetobacter, Citrobacter, E coli, Enterobacter, H influenzae, Klebsiella, Morganella morganii, Pr mirabilis* and *vulgaris, Providencia rettgeri* and *stuartii, Ps aeruginosa, Bacteroides, Clostridium, Eubacterium,*

Fusobacterium, Peptococcus, Peptostreptococcus and *Veillonella*. They are even less active than aminopenicillins against most gram-positive bacteria, *Actinomycetes* and *Treponema*, and they are not used to treat infections by these pathogens. There are considerable differences among the members. Neither azlocillin nor mezlocillin is active against staphylococci; azlocillin is inactive against *Pseudomonas* or *Neisseria* and *carbenicillin* is inactive against *Eubacterium*. Only piperacillin is active against *Strep viridans* and azlocillin and mezlocillin against *Providencia stuartii*.

Amdinocillin is the only marketed member of the class by the same name. It has a very limited spectrum. No infections by gram-positive or anaerobic bacteria are treatable. Among the gram-negative bacteria only *Citrobacter, Enterobacter, E coli, Klebsiella, Salmonella, Serratia* and *Shigella* are sensitive enough so that this drug is used alone to treat infections by them. In combination with other β-lactams, it may be used against *Prot mirabilis, Morganella morganni* and *Providencia*.

Resistance—The penicillin resistance of many gram-positive and gram-negative bacteria is due to their elaboration of penicillin-destroying enzymes called *beta-lactamases*. They are produced by large numbers of bacteria and actinomycetes and convert penicillin into inactive *penicilloic acid* by liberation of a second carboxyl group. The enzymes from staphylococci, enterococci, meningococci, gonococci and various other bacteria were the first-known beta-lactamases and were called *penicillinases*. Penicillinases are Group II beta-lactamases, acidic proteins which are resistant to mercuricions. Although they are inducible, the capacity for induction is determined by a plasmid-located gene.

Resistance of bacteria to penicillin cannot be explained entirely on penicillinase production because many resistant organisms produce little or no penicillinase. Nonpenicillinase-mediated resistance is called *methicillin resistance*. It is caused by an alteration in the target transpeptidase (penicillin- binding protein I). With some bacteria, eg, *Staph aureus*, resistance develops very fast clinically, but some microorganisms, eg, *T pallidum*, never become resistant. Resistance by staphylococci currently is a major hospital problem.

More resistant bacteria dwell in hospital personnel than in the community at large, because such personnel are close to patients under treatment. Acquired resistance is the result of the selection of natural penicillin-resistant strains that ordinarily are held in check by the sensitive parent strain. Resistant genes may be acquired by mutation, transduction by viruses, transformation and conjugative transfer of resistant-gene-containing plasmids.

Mechanism—Penicillin is known to interfere with the synthesis of peptidoglycans, which are part of the cell-wall material. Consequently, the growing protoplast cannot form a protective cell wall. Several wall enzymes are reversibly inhibited, the most important being a D, D-carboxypeptidase which also functions as a transpeptidase. Conditions favoring rapid growth of bacteria are best for the inhibitory action of penicillin, owing to the fact that the cell must be producing cell wall-lysing enzymes during the time transpeptidases are inhibited in order for cell-wall lysis to occur. Under favorable conditions, penicillin exerts a direct bactericidal action, and successful penicillin therapy may be relatively independent of immunity mechanisms of the host.

Potency—The potency of penicillin is expressed in units per mg. *One International Unit is equivalent to the activity of* 0.6 μg *of pure crystalline sodium penicillin G* to which, by international conference, a potency of 1667 *units/mg* has been assigned. See Table 4. Because of the large doses now used, it is common to speak in terms of megaunits, ie, 1 megaunit equals 10^6 Units.

Assay—See *Biological Testing* (page 491).

Uses—Although penicillin G is the original penicillin, it remains the drug of choice for the treatment of almost all infections caused by nonpenicillinase-producing, nonmethicillin-resistant gram-positive bacteria, the integrity of which depends upon cell walls. Thus, it is the drug of choice against infections by gram-positive, nonpenicillinase-producing cocci, such as *Staph aureus* or *epidermidis, Strep bovis*, Group B, *pyogenes, viridans, faecalis* (enterococcus; in combination with gentamycin, for serious infections, only) or *pneumoniae* (pneumococcus), *Peptococcus* or *Peptostreptococcus* and gram-positive bacilli, such as *B anthracis* or *Cl perfringens* or *tetani*. It is thus also the drug of choice against infections by nonpenicillinase-producing strains of the gram-negative coccus, *N meningitidis*, the gram-negative bacillus *Bacteroides fragilis* (especially oropharyngeal strains), *Fusobacterium, Leptotrichia buccalis, Pasteurella multicida, Spirillum minus* or *Streptobacillus moniliformis*, the actinomycete, *Actinomyes israelii*, or the spirochete, *Leptospira* or *Treponema pallidum*.

Table 4—Potencies of Some Penicillin Products

Drug	MW	Units/mg
Penicillin G benzathine	981.2	1211
Penicillin G potassium	372.5	1595
Penicillin G procaine	588.7	1009
Penicillin G sodium reference standard	356.4	1667
Penicillin V reference standard	350.4	1695

It is an alternative drug to treat infections by *Coryn. diptheriae, Vibrio vulnificus* or *Borrelia burgdorferi*. Penicillin V shares with penicillin G first choice status in the treatment of lesser staphylococcal infections and streptococcal (pneumococcal) pneumonia.

Penicillinase-resistant penicillins are drugs of choice only for the treatment of infections by penicillinase-producing staphylococci. They also can be used as penicillinase inhibitors, to combine with penicillin G; however, clavulanate and sulbactam are preempting that use.

An aminopenicillin is the drug of choice for the treatment of infections by *Strep* Group B (ampicillin; shares status with penicillin G), *Branhamella* catarrhalis (amoxacillin), E coli (ampicillin, combined with an aminoglycoside), *Prot mirabilis, Salmonella* (except *typhi*), *Eikenella corrodens* (with or without clavulanate or sulbactam), mild-to-moderate infections by *H influenzae* (with or without clavulanate or sulbactam) or *Listeria monocytogenes* (with or without gentamycin).

It is an alternate drug for the treatment of infections by penicillinase-producing *Staphylococcus* (with clavulanate), *Bordetella pertussis, E coli* (with clavulanate or sulbactam), *Gardnerella vaginalis, H influenzae* (serious infections; initially in combination with chloramphenicol), *Kl pneumoniae* (with clavulanate or sulbactam), *Morganella morganii, Prot vulgaris* (with clavulanate or sulbactam), *Pasteurella multicida* (with clavulanate or sulbactam), *Salmonella typhi* or *Shigella*.

An extended-spectrum (antipseudomonal) penicillin is the drug of choice only for the treatment of infections by sensitive *Ps aeruginosa*. It is an alternate drug for the treatment of infections by penicillinase-producing *Staphylococcus, Acenetobacter, Bacteroides fragilis* (gastrointestinal strains), *Enterobacter, Kl pneumoniae* (with clavulanate or sulbactam), *Morganella morganii* (with clavulanate or sulbactam), *Prot mirabilis* or *vulgaris* (with clavulanate or sulbactam), *Providencia rettgeri* or *stuartii* (with clavulanate or sulbactam), *Ps aeruginosa* (urinary tract infections) or *Serratia*.

A penicillin is employed sometimes in *combination* with other agents. The results of such therapy are often, but not invariably, superior to those obtainable with a penicillin alone. When it is administered with the tetracyclines, chloramphenicol or the sulfonamides, antagonism may be noted if the microorganism is highly susceptible to a penicillin when it is administered alone. Nevertheless, it often is used in combination with chloramphenicol in the treatment of bacterial meningitis caused by *H influenzae*.

The number of bacteria and the quantity of pus appear to have only a minor influence upon the antibacterial action of penicillin, except when the organism produces an appropri ate β-lactamase.

Adverse Effects—Penicillin is practically nontoxic. However, hypersensitivity reactions occur in several percent of patients, depending on the type of preparation employed and the route of administration. The most-common manifestation of this allergic response is a skin rash. Nondermatological manifestations of allergy include serum sickness, angioedema, nephropathy, rare hemolytic anemia, Arthus reaction, rare pericarditis, enteropathy, hepatotoxicity and anaphylaxis. Neutropenia, which occasionally results from high-dose therapy, does not appear to involve an immune process.

Side effects of oral administration of penicillins are nausea, vomiting, epigastric distress, diarrhea and black "hairy" tongue.

Like other antibiotics, penicillin markedly can alter the normal bacterial flora of man. As a result, superimposed infection by a penicillin-resistant microorganism may develop during the course of treatment, and appropriate chemotherapy should be instituted as soon as possible. Overgrowth (suprainfection) even occurs in the bowel, because penicillin is secreted into the bile, which keeps the intestinal levels high. Coagulation disorders also may occur as the result of the suppression of enteric bacteria which synthesize vitamin K.

Very high concentrations of penicillin are neurotoxic, and nerve damage has resulted from intramuscular administration. Crystalline penicillin has an irritating effect when applied directly to the central nervous system. Symptoms following intrathecal administration include listlessness, headache, nausea, vomiting, respiratory difficulty, cyanosis, fall in blood pressure, thready pulse, muscular twitching and convulsions. These are reduced or eliminated by lowering dosage.

With sodium and potassium salts, the effect of the cation load must be considered. Lastly, untoward effects sometimes result from the rapid bactericidal effects, because of the release of endotoxins and other bacterial cell components.

Absorption, Distribution and Excretion—Penicillin G in the form of its sodium or potassium salt is absorbed rapidly from subcutaneous and intramuscular sites. The intramuscular route is preferred. Penicillin G is given intravenously by continuous infusion only when it is imperative to maintain very high blood concentrations such as in the treatment of subacute *bacterial endocarditis*. The rate of absorption from intramuscular sites of injection may be slowed markedly by the use of repository (depot) preparations consisting of relatively insoluble salts of penicillin in a suitable vehicle. For example, therapeutic blood levels (for some purposes) persist 12 to 24 hours after a single 300,000-unit dose of *Procaine Penicillin in Aqueous Suspension*, 24 to 48 hours after *Procaine Penicillin in Oil* and 1 wk or more after 1.2 million units of *Benzathine Penicillin G*. However, the slower the absorption, the lower the peak plasma level, and some uses are precluded.

The absorption of penicillin G from the gastrointestinal tract is incomplete and irregular, but some acid-stable penicillins are absorbed well. To obtain the same blood concentrations as by the intramuscular route, 3 to 5 times the parenteral dose of penicillin G must be employed. Penicillin G should be ingested when the stomach is empty because penicillin binds to food substances. Although hydrochloric acid in the gastric juice destroys penicillin G, buffer agents have not proved to be necessary for successful oral medication, since the dose can be raised to compensate. Oral penicillin G therapy should never be relied upon alone in severe infections.

Penicillins are distributed in the extracellular water, but they penetrate cells poorly. Tissue concentrations are about ¼ the plasma concentration *at equilibrium*. Plasma levels fall so fast that there is not enough time for the build-up of high concentrations in many tissues. Diffusion of penicillins into CSF is minimal unless the meninges are inflamed. The preferred route of administration for treatment of bacterial meningitis is IV supplemented by IM injection. It usually is not recommended to use intrathecal administration of penicillins because of the irritative effect of even low doses of penicillin on the CNS. Local instillation may be used in various body cavities to supplement systemic administration.

Penicillins are secreted mostly into the urine, partly by glomerular filtration but mostly by tubular secretion (80%). Substances which interfere with renal tubular excretion of penicillin (see *Probenecid*, page 1051) serve to enhance and prolong the effective blood levels of the antibiotic. Probenecid can block completely the renal tubular secretion of penicillin, which slows excretion; it also decreases removal from the CSF. Phenylbutazone also interferes with excretion to a degree comparable to probenecid; sulfinpyrazone, aspirin, indomethacin and some sulfonamides also moderately interfere with the excretion of penicillin. The normal plasma half-time of penicillin G is about 45 minutes, but in persons over 65 years it is up to twice as long. In oliguria, it may be 7 to 10 hours.

Amoxicillin

[2*S*-[2α,5α,6β(*S**)]]-4-Thia-1-azabicyclo[3.2.0]heptane-2-carboxylic acid, 6-[[amino(4-hydroxyphenyl)acetyl]amino]-3,3-dimethyl-7-oxo-, trihydrate; (*Various Mfrs*)

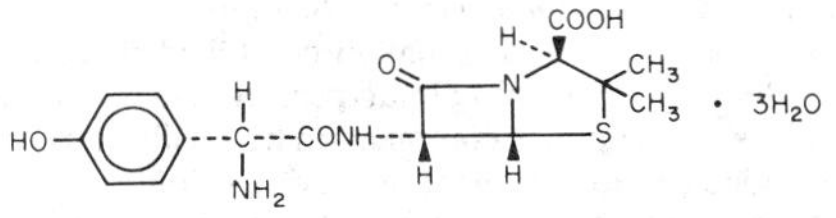

D(−)-α-Amino-*p*-hydroxybenzylpenicillin; [61336-70-7] $C_{16}H_{19}N_3O_5S.3H_2O$ (419.45); *anhydrous* [26787-78-0] (365.30).

Preparation—By acylation of 6-aminopenicillanic acid with D-(−)-2-(*p*-hydroxyphenyl)glycine.

Description—Fine, white to off-white, crystalline powder; bitter taste; high humidity and temperature over 37° adversely affect stability.

Solubility—1 g in 370 mL water or 2000 mL alcohol.

Uses—Amoxicillin, chemically *p*-hydroxyampicillin, has an antibacterial spectrum similar to that of *Ampicillin*, except that it is less active against *Streptococcus*, *N meningitidis*, *Clostridium*, *Salmonella* and *Shigella*. Like ampicillin, it is destroyed by β-lactamases and hence cannot be used to treat infections caused by resistant strains of bacteria of the β-lactamase-producing type. However, it is more acid-stable than ampicillin and absorption is not affected appreciably by food; it cannot be given parenterally. It is the drug of choice for infections caused by *Strep faecalis*, *Branhammella catarrhalis* or *Bacteroides fragilis* (mild to moderate infections). It is an alternate drug for infections by penicillinase-producing *Staphylococcus* (combined with clavulanate), *N gonorrhoeae* (with probenecid), *E coli* (with clavulanate) or *Pasteurella multicida* (with clavulanate). It cannot be given parenterally for severe infections. The toxicity is that of ampicillin, but there is less diarrhea and rash.

By the oral route, 75 to 90% is absorbed. An oral dose of 250 mg will provide a peak plasma concentration of about 4 μg/mL. In plasma, it is 17% protein-bound. The volume of distribution is 0.31 mL/g. From 50 to 72% is eliminated by renal tubular secretion. The half-life is about 1 hr when renal function is normal and 8 to 16 hr in renal failure.

Dose (trihydrate equivalent)—*Oral, adult,* and *children 20 kg or more*, **250** to **500 mg** every 8 hr, but as much as **4.5 g** a day may be given, if necessary; for *gonorrhea* **3 g** is given as a single dose along with 1 g of probenecid. *Infants less than 6 kg*, **25** to **50 mg** every 8 hr; *infants 6 to 8 kg*, **50** to **100 mg** every 8 hr; *infants 8 to 20 kg*, **6.7** to **13.3 mg/kg** every 8 hr. When it is used in combination with clavulanate, the *adult dose* is **500 mg** with 125 mg of clavulanate potassium for *serious infections* and **250 mg** with 125 mg of clavulanate for *lesser infections*; for *children under 40 kg*, **40 mg/kg** every 8 hr for serious infections and **20 mg/kg** every 8 hr for lesser infections.

Dosage Forms (trihydrate equivalent)—Capsules: 250 and 500 mg; for Oral Suspension: 50 mg/mL, and 125 and 250 mg/5 mL; Chewable Tablets: 125 and 150 mg. See also *combinations*, page 1290.

Ampicillin

[2S-[2α,5α,6β(S*)]]-4-Thia-1-azabicyclo[3.2.0]heptane-2-carboxylic acid, 6-[(aminophenylacetyl)amino]-3,3-dimethyl-7-oxo-, (*Various Mfrs*)

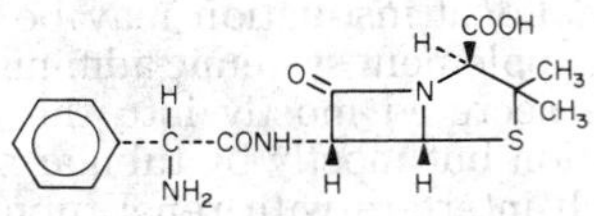

[69-53-4] $C_{16}H_{19}N_3O_4S$ (349.40); *trihydrate* [7177-48-2] (403.45). Potency: 900 to 1050 μg of $C_{16}H_{19}N_3O_4S$/mg, calculated on the anhydrous basis.

Preparation—6-Aminopenicillanic acid is acylated with D-glycine. US Pat 2,985,648.

Description—White, crystalline powder; practically odorless; occurs as the trihydrate, which is stable at room temperature.

Solubility—1 g in about 90 mL water or 250 mL absolute alcohol; practically insoluble in ether or chloroform.

Uses—The first aminopenicillin (see the statement). Its *in vitro* spectrum against gram-positive cocci is similar to but generally somewhat less effective than that of penicillin G, except that it is somewhat more effective against *Strep faecalis (enterococcus)*. It is ½ as effective against *Staph aureus* and 1/20 against *Strep pyogenes*.

It is poorly effective against penicillinase-producing organisms. It is the drug of choice for treatment of infections due to sensitive strains of *Strep* Group B, *Strep faecalis* (combined with gentamycin), *Listeria monocytogenes* (with or without gentamycin), *E coli* (with or without gentamycin) and *Prot mirabilis, Eikenella corrodens* and *Salmonella* (not typhi). It is an alternative drug against *Kl pneumoniae* (with sulbactam), indole-positive *Proteus* (*M morganii, Pr vulgaris* and *Prov rettgeri;* with sulbactam), *Salmonella typhi, Shigella, Gardnerella vaginalis, H influenzae* (serious infections; initially combined with chloramphenicol) or *Nocardia*. Some of these readily acquire resistance by elaboration of penicillinase, so it is given often in combination with sulbactam.

It causes allergic reactions typical of other penicillins. It is 5 times as allergenic as phenoxymethyl penicillin. The incidence of rashes is about 7%, but most of these are not allergenic; they are especially prevalent in patients with infectious mononucleosis. Patients allergic to penicillin G are often also allergic to ampicillin. The drug also may cause nausea and vomiting, diarrhea, glossitis and stomatitis.

It is acid-resistant and is 30 to 50% absorbed by the oral route. Bioavailability is dose-dependent. It is bound to plasma proteins to the extent of 8 to 20%. The volume of distribution is 0.26 to 0.31 mL/g. About 45% is excreted unchanged in the urine. Its half-life in plasma is about 1 to 1.5 hr, but it maybe 10 to 15 hr in renal failure.

It may be used in the anhydrous form or as the trihydrate.

Dose (anhydrous or trihydrate)—*Oral, adult* and *children 20 kg or more,* **250** to **500 mg** every 6 hr; as much as 4 g/day may be given, if necessary; for *gonorrhea,* a single dose of **3.5 g,** with 1 g of probenecid. *Infants* and *children up to 20 kg,* **50 mg/kg** a day every 6 to 8 hr in divided doses.

Dosage Forms (anhydrous or trihydrate)—Capsules: 250 and 500 mg; for Oral Suspension: 100 mg/mL and 125, 250 and 500 mg/5 mL on reconstitution. See also *Combinations,* page 1290.

Ampicillin Sodium

[2S-[2α,5α,6β(S*)]]-4-Thia-1-azabicyclo[3.2.0]heptane-2-carboxylic acid, 6-[(aminophenylacetyl)amino]-3,3-dimethyl-7-oxo-, monosodium salt; (*Various Mfrs*)

[69-52-3] $C_{16}H_{18}N_3NaO_4S$ (371.39). Potency: not less than 845 μg of ampicillin/mg, on the anhydrous basis.

Preparation—*Ampicillin* is dissolved in a suitable organic solvent and precipitated as the sodium salt by the addition of sodium acetate.

Description—White to off-white, crystalline powder; hygroscopic; pK_{a1} 2.66; pK_{a2} 7.24.

Solubility—Very soluble in water, isotonic NaCl or dextrose solutions.

Uses—Has the actions and uses of *Ampicillin,* and is the form in which ampicillin is employed for intramuscular and intravenous administration.

Dose (anhydrous ampicillin equivalent)—*Intramuscular* or *intravenous, adult* and *children 20 kg or more,* **250** to **500 mg** every 6 hr; for bacterial *meningitis* or *septicemia,* **1** to **2 g** every 3 or 4 hr *or* **18.8** to **25 mg/kg** every 3 hr *or* **25** to **33 mg/kg** every 4 hr; for *gonorrhea* **500 mg** repeated in 8 to 12 hr; daily limit is 300 mg/kg (or 16 g) a day; *infants* and *children less than 20 kg,* usually **6.25** to **25 mg/kg** every 6 hr, *or* **8.3** to **33.3 mg/kg** every 8 hr; for *meningitis* or *septicemia,* use the **adult dose.**

Dosage Forms (anhydrous ampicillin equivalent)—Sterile: 125, 250 and 500 mg, and 1, 2 and 10 g. Each g contains 3 mEq of sodium.

Azlocillin Sodium—see RPS-18, page 1187.

Bacampicillin Hydrochloride

4-Thia-1-azabicyclo[3.2.0]heptane-2-carboxylic acid, [2S-[2α,5α,6β(S*)]]-6-[(aminophenylacetyl)amino]-3,3-dimethyl-7-oxo-, 1-[(ethoxycarbonyl)oxy]ethyl] ester, monohydrochloride; Spectrobid (*Roerig*)

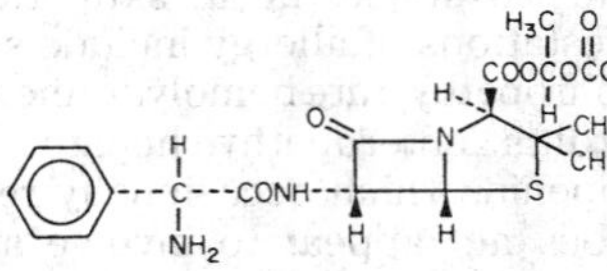

[37661-08-8] $C_{21}H_{27}N_4O_7S.HCl$ (501.98).

Preparation—US Pat 3,939,270.

Description—White crystals; melts about 175°; pH (2% aqueous solution) 3.0 to 4.5.

Solubility—1 g in about 15 mL water, 7 mL alcohol or 10 mL chloroform.

Uses— Converted in the body to ampicillin, so that its antibacterial efficacy, uses and adverse effects are those of ampicillin. By the oral route, it is absorbed almost 100%, so that an oral dose equal (mole for mole) to that of ampicillin or amoxicillin will yield a plasma concentration of ampicillin nearly 200% higher than will ampicillin itself and about 30% higher than that of amoxicillin. After 4 hr there are no significant differences in levels. The drug is administered in a "pulsed" (twice-a-day) dosing regimen (plasma levels return nearly to zero between doses). In such a regimen, bacampicillin has an efficacy equal to that of oral ampicillin or amoxicillin at 6- or 8-hr intervals; it has not been shown whether ampicillin or amoxicillin in pulsed regimens also would not be equally efficacious, especially if doses were used to achieve equivalent plasma levels. The greater bioavailability results in a lower incidence of diarrhea. It costs two to four times as much as a molar equivalent dose of ampicillin and more than twice as much as a bioequivalent dose; it is two to three times as expensive as a bioequivalent dose of amoxicillin. Medical authority does not hold it to offer any advantages over amoxicillin. Other than the differences in absorption and systemic bioavailability, the pharmacokinetics should be that of ampicillin.

Dose—*Oral, adult* and *children over 25 kg,* for *lower respiratory tract infections,* **800** mg every 12 hr; for *skin, soft-tissue urinary tract* and *upper respiratory tract infections,* **400** mg every 12 hr; for *uncomplicated gonorrhea,* **1.6** g (and 1 g of probenecid) as a single dose; *infants* and *children* weighing *up to 25 kg,* for *lower respiratory tract* infections, **25** mg/kg every 12 hr; for *skin, soft-tissue,* and *upper respiratory tract infections,* **25** mg/kg every 12 hr. Dosage adjustments are required in renal failure.

Dosage Forms—Tablets: 400 mg (equivalent to 280 mg ampicillin); Powder (for Oral/Suspension): 125 mg/5 mL (equivalent to 87.5 mg ampicillin/5 mL).

Carbenicillin Disodium

[2S-(2α,5α,6β)]-4-Thia-1-azabicyclo[3.2.0]heptane-2-carboxylic acid, 6- [(carboxyphenylacetyl)amino]-3,3-dimethyl-7-oxo-, disodium salt; (α-Carboxybenzyl)penicillin Disodium; Geopen (*Roerig*); Pyopen (*Beecham*)

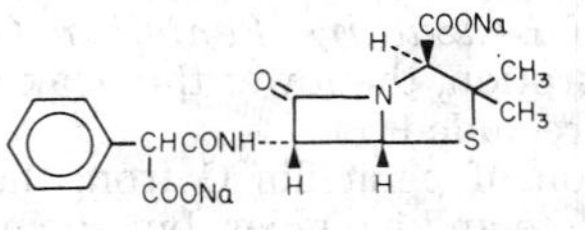

[4800-94-6] $C_{17}H_{16}N_2Na_2O_6S$ (422.36). Potency: the equivalent of not less than 770 μg of carbenicillin/mg, calculated on the anhydrous basis.

Preparation—One method consists of hydrolyzing esters of the type

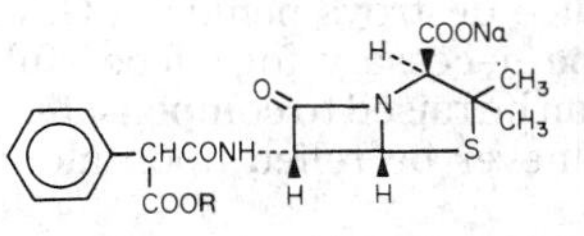

(R = alkyl, aryl, or benzyl) with the aid of a suitable esterase, such as α-chymotrypsin or pancreatin, and extracting the acid and reacting it with

aqueous $NaHCO_3$. *Chem Abstr 72:* 41674a, 1970. The starting esters may be prepared by acylating 6-aminopenicillanic acid with monoesters of phenylmalonic acid. US Pats 3,282,926 and 3,492,291.

Description—White to off-white, crystalline powder; bitter taste; hygroscopic; odorless, pH (1% solution, *w/v*) 8.0. pK_{a1} 2.76; pK_{a2} 3.5.

Solubility—1 g in 1.2 mL water or 25 mL alcohol; practically insoluble in chloroform or ether.

Uses—An extended-spectrum penicillin (see the statement). Penicillin G-resistant species and strains are also resistant to carbenicillin. Since both penicillin G and ampicillin are more potent and effective against the gram-positive bacteria, this drug is not for use in the treatment of infections caused by them. Against the gram-negative bacteria, its spectrum of activity differs not only from penicillin G but also from ampicillin in being moderately effective in high doses against most strains of *Ps aeruginosa;* however, these bacteria rapidly acquire resistance to the drug. Nevertheless, its use in the treatment of pseudomonas infections is what primarily distinguishes this drug and ticarcillin among the penicillins. It shares with ticarcillin drug-of-choice status in treating urinary tract infections caused by this bacterium. It is seldom used alone, but rather in combination with an aminoglycoside, against systemic pseudomonal infections. It is an alternative drug for use against infections caused by *Acinetobacter, Enterobacter, E coli, Morganella morganii, Prot vulgaris, Prov rettgeri* or *Serratia.* Although it is approved for use against a number of other infections, better, or less-expensive, drugs are recommended. It is inactivated by various β-lactamases and resistance rapidly develops when used alone against *Ps aeruginosa.*

Adverse effects are those of penicillins in general. The rare penicillin-type coagulopathy has been reported. Reversible elevated serum SGOT levels occasionally occur. It can prolong bleeding time. Cation toxicity can occur. Intramuscular injections cause pain; intravenous injections occasionally cause thrombophlebitis. Suprainfections caused by *Klebsiella* may occur. It can cause hypokalemic alkalosis. In persons with a low sodium tolerance, the sodium content must be taken into account. It is expensive.

The drug is entirely destroyed in gastric acid and hence is not suited for oral administration. An indanyl ester (see below) is more stable and is used for oral therapy. The volume of distribution is 0.18 mL/g. About 60 to 90% is secreted into the urine, but it also is destroyed partly in the liver and also excreted into the bile. The normal half-life is 1 to 1.5 hr, but in severe renal insufficiency it may be as long as 13 to 16 hr. If liver failure simultaneously exists, the half-life may be as long as 23 hr.

Dose (carbenicillin equivalent)—*Intramuscular* or *intravenous, adults,* for *urinary tract infections,* up to **50 mg/kg** or **1** to **2 g** every 6 hr; for *respiratory tract* and *soft-tissue infections, septicemia* and *meningitis,* **50** to **83.3 mg/kg** every 4 hr; for *gonorrhea,* **4 g** divided between two intramuscular sites and with 1 g of probenecid. The maximum daily dose recommended is 42 g. If the creatinine clearance is less than 5 mL/min, the dose should be 2 g intravenously every 8 to 12 hr; if both renal and hepatic failure exist, it is 2 g intravenously every 24 hr. *Older infants* and *children,* for *urinary tract infections,* **12.5** to **50 mg/kg** every 6 hr (or **8** to **33 mg/kg** every 4 hr); for *respiratory tract* and *soft-tissue infections, septicemia* and *meningitis,* use the adult dose. Some infants and children may require as much as 600 mg/kg/day (in divided doses), and as much as 800 mg/kg/day has been given. *Neonates over 2 kg,* for *respiratory tract* and *soft-tissue infections, septicemia,* and *meningitis,* initially **100 mg/kg,** followed by **75 mg/kg** every 6 hr during the first 3 days of life and **100 mg/kg** every 6 hr thereafter; *neonates up to 2 kg,* same as larger neonates except every 8 hr during the first week.

Dosage Form (carbenicillin equivalent)—Powder for Injection: 1, 2, 5, 10, 20 and 30 g. Each g contains 4.7 to 5.3 mEq of sodium.

Carbenicillin Indanyl Sodium

[2*S*-(2α,5α,6β)]-4-Thia-1-azabicyclo[3.2.0]heptane-2-carboxylic acid, 6-[[3-[(2,3-dihydro-1*H*-inden-5-yl)oxy]-1,3-dioxo-1-phenylpropyl]amino]-3,3-dimethyl-7-oxo-, monosodium salt; Geocillin (*Roerig*)

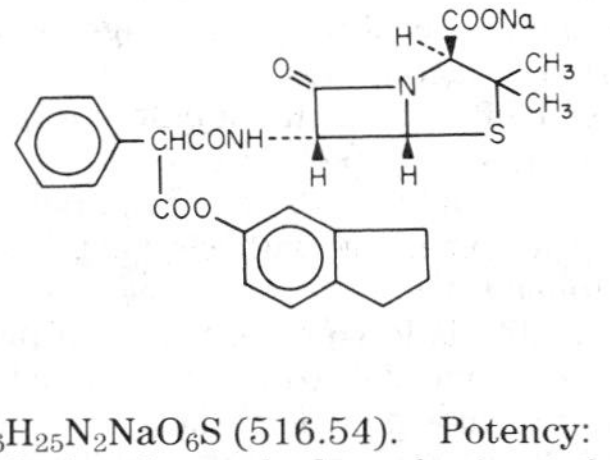

[26605-69-6] $C_{26}H_{25}N_2NaO_6S$ (516.54). Potency: 659 to 769 μg of carbenicillin/mg, calculated on anhydrous basis, at time of certification, and not less than 630 μg at any time during expiration period.

Preparation—6-Aminopenicillanic acid is coupled with 5-indanyl α-chloroformylphenylacetate (prepared from phenylmalonic acid), producing carbenicillin indanyl, which is neutralized with NaOH.

Description—White, or nearly white, powder; hygroscopic; bitter taste.

Solubility—Soluble in water; insoluble in chloroform or ether.

Uses—Converted to carbenicillin in the body, so that its actions and adverse effects are those of *Carbenicillin.* However, the indanyl derivative is stable in gastric juice and can be administered orally. Its uses are limited to treatment of uncomplicated *urinary tract infections* caused by carbenicillin-sensitive organisms. The oral bioavailability is 30 to 50%. Oral doses of 500 mg and 1 g give rise to peak plasma concentrations of about 2 and 6 μg/mL, respectively, of carbenicillin. The amount of unchanged carbenicillin secreted into urine is 35 to 40%, which is inconsistent with the belief that all of the indanyl derivative is converted to carbenicillin during its rapid absorption.

Dose—*Oral, adult,* **382** to **764 mg** every 6 hr. Pediatric dosage has not been established.

Dosage Form—Tablets: 382 mg.

Cloxacillin Sodium

[2*S*-(2α,5α,6β)]-4-Thia-1-azabicyclo[3.2.0]heptane-2-carboxylic acid, 6-[[[3-(2-chlorophenyl)-5-methyl-4-isoxazolyl]carbonyl]-amino]-3,3-dimethyl-7-oxo-, monosodium salt, monohydrate; Cloxacillin Sodium Monohydrate; Tegopen (*Apothecon*); Cloxapen (*Beecham*)

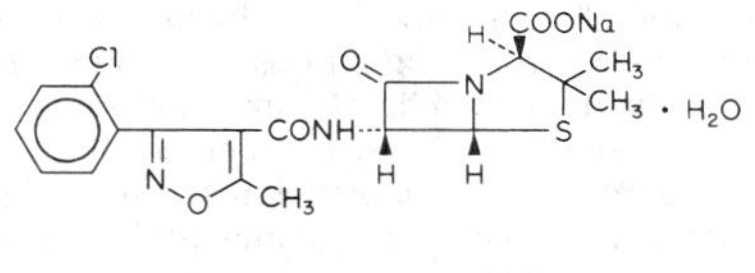

[7081-44-9] $C_{19}H_{17}ClN_3NaO_5S.H_2O$ (475.88); *anhydrous* [642-78-4] (457.86). Potency: the equivalent of not less than 825 μg of cloxacillin/mg.

Preparation—6-Aminopenicillanic acid is acylated with 3-(*o*-chlorophenyl)-5-methyl-4-isoxazolecarboxylic acid and the resulting cloxacillin is purified by recrystallization and converted to the sodium salt.

Description—White, odorless, crystalline powder having a bitter taste; stable in light and only slightly hygroscopic; decomposes 173°; pH (1 in 100 solution) 7.5; pK_a (COOH) 2.7.

Solubility—Freely soluble in water; soluble in alcohol; slightly soluble in chloroform.

Uses—An oral penicillinase-resistant penicillin (see statement). The drug shares a first-choice status with other penicillinase-resistant penicillins in the treatment of staphylococcal infections caused by penicillin G-resistant strains. However, it is less active than penicillin G against nonpenicillinase-producing bacteria, especially streptococci. It is not effective against gram-negative organisms. Consequently, its use should be limited to treating infections caused by penicillinase-producing susceptible microorganisms which are resistant to penicillin G. A parenteral penicillinase-resistant penicillin should be used initially for serious staphylococcal infections.

The adverse effects are virtually identical to those caused by other penicillins (see statement). Rash and urticaria are the principal allergic manifestations. Not all patients allergic to penicillin G are sensitive to this drug, but cross-sensitization is usual. It also may cause occasional nausea, vomiting, abdominal discomfort, epigastric fullness or diarrhea. Suprainfections occasionally occur. In persons with a low sodium tolerance, the sodium content must be taken into account.

The drug is relatively stable in gastric acid. Its absorption by the oral route is about 50%, which is better than that of nafcillin, but it is nevertheless erratic; the recommended dose is high enough to compensate for irregularity in the affected blood levels. Food in the stomach interferes with absorption. About 90% is bound to plasma proteins. The volume of distribution is 0.18 mL/g. Only 30 to 45% is excreted unchanged in the urine. The half-life is 0.8 to 1 hr in persons with normal renal function.

Dose (cloxacillin equivalent)—*Oral, adult* and *children 20 kg or more,* **250** to **500 mg** every 6 hr; *infants* and *children less than 20 kg,* 50 to 100 mg/kg every 6 hr. Adults may be given up to 6 g a day, if necessary.

Dosage Forms (cloxacillin equivalent)—Capsules: 250 and 500 mg; for Oral Solution: 125 mg/5 mL (reconstituted).

Cyclacillin—see RPS-18, page 1193.

Dicloxacillin Sodium

[2*S*-(2α,5α,6β)]-4-Thia-1-azabicyclo[3.2.0]heptane-2-carboxylic acid, 6- [[[3-(2,6-dichlorophenyl)-5-methyl-4-isoxazolyl]-carbonyl]amino]-3,3-dimethyl-7-oxo-, monosodium salt, monohydrate; Dynapen (*Apothecon*); Pathocil (*Wyeth-Ayerst*); Dycill (*Beecham*)

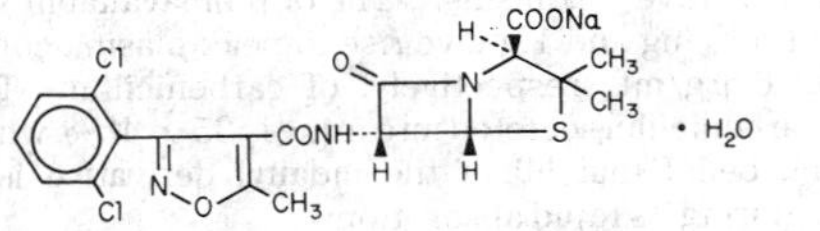

[13412-64-1] $C_{19}H_{16}Cl_2N_3NaO_5S.H_2O$ (510.32); *anhydrous* [343-55-5] (492.31). Potency: the equivalent of not less than 850 μg of dicloxacillin/mg.

Preparation—6-Aminopenicillanic acid is acylated with 3-(2,6-dichlorophenyl)-5-methyl-4-isoxazolecarboxylic acid and the resulting dicloxacillin (acid) is purified by recrystallization and converted to the sodium salt.

Description—White to off-white, crystalline powder; faint, characteristic odor; melts 225° with decomposition; pK_a 2.67.

Solubility—Freely soluble in water; soluble in alcohol.

Uses—A penicillinase-resistant penicillin (see the general statement). As with all penicillinase-resistant penicillins, it is not as effective as penicillin except against those organisms whose resistance depends on penicillinase production. Therefore, its use should be limited to the treatment of susceptible penicillinase-producing strains, mostly of *Staph aureus* or *epidermidis* resistant to penicillin G, for which it shares first-choice status with the other penicillinase-resistant penicillins.

The toxicity is the same as that of penicillins in general (see the general statement). Many patients allergic to penicillin G are not allergic to this drug, but others are, so that appropriate precautions must be taken. Nausea and diarrhea sometimes occur, but they usually do not necessitate discontinuation of the drug. Elevated serum SGOT is seen in some patients, as with other penicillins, but the significance is not clear; rare hepatotoxicity has been observed. In persons with a low sodium tolerance, the sodium content must be taken into account.

By the oral route the amount absorbed is 37 to 50%. It is bound to plasma proteins to the extent of 90 to 97%, the highest among the penicillins. The volume of distribution is only 0.1 mL/g. About 60% is excreted into the urine. Its half-life in plasma is 0.5 to 1.5 hr in normal patients but is 1 to 3 hr in renal insufficiency.

Dose (dicloxacillin equivalent)—*Oral, adult* and *children 40 kg or more,* usually **125** to **250 mg** every 6 hr, but may be taken up to **6 g** a day, if necessary; *infants* and *children under 40 kg,* **12.5** to **25 mg/kg** every 6 hr. Dosage for neonates has not been established.

Dosage Forms (dicloxacillin equivalent)—Capsules: 125, 250 and 500 mg; for Oral Suspension: 62.5 mg/5 mL (reconstituted).

Floxacillin Sodium—see RPS-18, page 1193.

Methicillin Sodium

4-Thia-l-azabicyclo[3.2.0]heptane-2-carboxylic acid, [2*S*-(2α,5α,6β)]-6-[(2,6-dimethoxybenzoyl)amino]-3,3-dimethyl-7-oxo-, monosodium salt, monohydrate, (*Various Mfrs*)

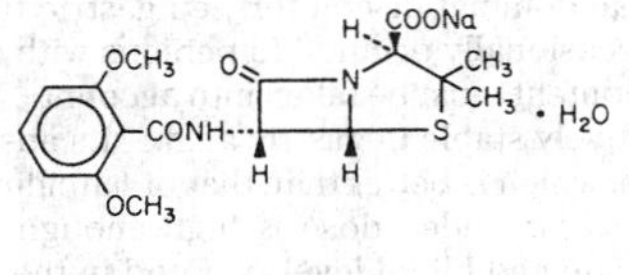

[7246-14-2] $C_{17}H_{19}N_2NaO_6S.H_2O$ [132-92-3](anhydrous),[61-32-5](methicillin, acid)(420.41).

Preparation—Fermentation-produced 6-aminopenicillanic acid is condensed with 2,6-dimethoxybenzoyl chloride in a suitable organic solvent and the resulting methicillin is precipitated as the sodium salt by the addition of sodium acetate.

Description—Fine, white, crystalline powder; odorless, or a slight odor.

Solubility—Freely soluble in water; slightly soluble in chloroform; insoluble in other.

Uses—A penicillinase-resistant penicillin. It is about 1/20 as potent as penicillin G against nonpenicillinase-producing but 10 times as potent as penicillinase-producing gram-positive cocci. Its use is limited to treatment of infections caused by penicillinase-producing cocci. It is destroyed by gastric acid and must be given parenterally. About 40% is bound to plasma proteins. The volume of distribution is 0.31 mL/g. Approximately 67% is eliminated by renal tubular secretion; the half-life is about 1.1 hr. There is more pain after its intramuscular injection than after similar injections of other penicillins. It can cause the well-known allergic reactions typical of all penicillins. However, many patients allergic to penicillin G are not sensitive to it, but the drug should be used cautiously if penicillin sensitivity exists. It occasionally causes depression of red bone-marrow functions, resulting in anemia, neutropenia or granulocytopenia. These symptoms are reversible after prompt termination of therapy. Allergic hemolytic anemia also can occur. Allergic nephropathy, which includes acute interstitial nephritis, has been reported more frequently with IV methicillin than other penicillinase-resistant penicillins. When used in persons with low sodium tolerance the sodium content must be taken into account. Because of the side effects, need for frequent injections and lower potency than nafcillin, it is not the anti-staphylococcal penicillin of choice.

Dose—(methicillin equivalent)—*Intramuscular, adult, usually* **1 g** every 4 to 6 hr; *infants* and *children,* **25 mg/kg** every 6 hr. *Intravenous, adult, usually* **1** to **2 g** every 4 hr, but in severe infections the dose can be increased to as much as 24 g/day; *infants* and *children,* **16.7** to **33.3 mg/kg** every 4 hr *or* **25** to **50 mg/kg** every 6 hr, but in severe infections the dose may be as high as 300 mg/kg/day.

Dosage Form—for Injection: 1, 4, 6 and 10 g.

Mezlocillin Sodium

[2*S*[2α,5α,6β(*S**)]]-4-Thia-1-azabicyclo[3.2.0]heptane-2-carboxylic acid, 3,3-dimethyl-6-[[[[[3-(methylsulfonyl)-2-oxo-1-imidazolidinyl]carbonyl]amino]phenylacetyl]amino]-7-oxo-, monosodium salt; Mezlin (*Miles*)

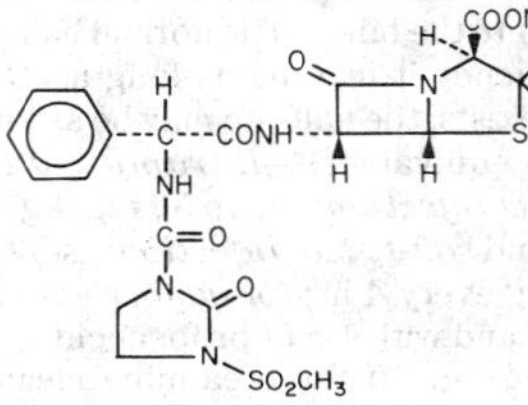

[51841-65-3] $C_{21}H_{24}NaN_5O_8S_2$ (561.56).

Preparation—Ger Pat 2,318,955.

Description—Yellowish-white powder; pK_a 2.7.

Solubility—Very soluble in water; soluble in DMF or methanol; very slightly soluble in alcohol or acetone.

Uses—An extended-spectrum penicillin (see the general statement). It has greater activity than either ampicillin or carbenicillin against *Acinetobacter, B fragilis, Citrobacter, Enterobacter, E coli, Klebsiella, Ps aeruginosa* and *Serratia.* Its activity against entercocci is comparable to that of ampicillin. Against *Ps aeruginosa* its activity is equal to that of ticarcillin but less than that of piperacillin, and it shares antipseudomonal drug of choice with those drugs except for the treatment of urinary tract infections. It is recommended for use against systemic pseudomonal infections only in combination with an aminoglycoside. It is an alternative drug against infections caused by *Enterobacter, E coli, Kl pneumoniae, Morganella morganii, Prot vulgaris* and *Prov rettgeri* or *stuartii, Serratia* or *Ps aeruginosa.* Although mezlocillin is approved for use against other infections, the drug has not been proven to have a clear-cut advantage over any other appropriate drug. For this and the reason that resistance of *Pseudomonas* and some other *Entero bacteriaceae* develops rapidly, it probably should be held in reserve for infections sensitive to this drug but insensitive to the longer-established antibiotics. It is sensitive to various β-lactamases.

It causes no adverse effects which are different from other penicillins. The overall incidence is about 10%, local reactions accounting for about 3% and skin reactions about 2%. Pseudomembranous colitis, interstitial nephritis, hepatitis and bleeding diathesis have not been reported, although thrombocytopenia has.

The oral bioavailability is low and erratic. In plasma, 16 to 42% is protein-bound. The volume of distribution is about 0.1 mL/g. The drug penetrates into cerebrospinal fluid, especially in meningitis. Urinary excretion eliminates 55 to 60% of the drug and biliary excretion 5 to 25%. The remainder is metabolized; this fraction of elimination is dose dependent. The half-life is 0.8 to 1.5 hr, except longer in either impaired renal or hepatic function.

Dose (mezlocillin equivalent)—*Intramuscular* or *intravenous, adult,* for *uncomplicated gonorrheal urethritis,* **1** or **2 g** as a single dose 0.5 hr after 1 g of probenecid; for *uncomplicated urinary tract infections,* **25** to **31.3 mg/kg** or **1.5** to **2 g** every 6 hr; *other infections,* **33.3** to **58.3 mg/kg** every 4 hr, **50** to **87.5 mg/kg** every 6 hr, or **3** to **4 g** every 4 to 6 hr; *infants over 1 mo* and *children up to 12 yr,* **50 mg/kg** every 4 hr; *younger infants,* **75 mg/kg** every 6 to 8 hr for infants up to 8 days of age and every 12 hr for infants younger than 8 days. *Intravenous, adults,* for *complicated urinary tract infections,* **37.5** to **50 mg/kg** or **3 g** every 6 hr. Dosage adjustments are required in renal failure.

Dosage Form (mezlocillin equivalent)—Powder for injection: 1, 2, 3 and 4 g. Each g contains 1.85 mEq of sodium.

Nafcillin Sodium

[2*S*-(2α,5α,6β)]-4-Thia-1-azabicyclo[3.2.0]heptane-2-carboxylic acid, 6- [[(2-ethoxy-1-naphthalenyl)carbonyl]amino]-3,3-dimethyl-7-oxo-, monosodium salt, monohydrate; Unipen (*Wyeth-Ayerst*); Nafcil (*Apothecon*); Nallpen (*Beecham*)

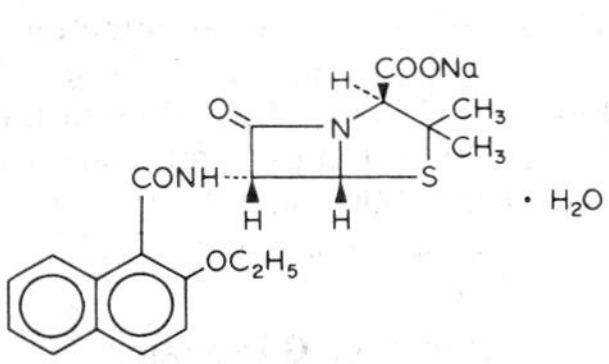

[7177-50-6] $C_{21}H_{21}N_2NaO_5S.H_2O$ (454.47); *anhydrous* [985-16-0] (436.46). Potency: equivalent to not less than 820 μg of nafcillin/mg.

Preparation—6-Aminopenicillanic acid is acylated by treatment with 2-ethoxy-1-naphthoyl chloride in an anhydrous organic solvent containing triethylamine. An aqueous extract of this product is admixed with a water-immiscible solvent and nafcillin is precipitated by the addition of sulfuric acid. Nafcillin sodium is precipitated by mixing ethanolic solutions of the acid and sodium ethylhexanoate. US Pat 3,157,639.

Description—White to yellowish white powder; not more than a slight characteristic odor.

Solubility—Freely soluble in water or chloroform; soluble in alcohol.

Uses—A penicillinase-resistant penicillin, the use of which is restricted to the treatment of infections caused by penicillinase-producing cocci (mostly staphylococci). After oral administration serum levels are low and unpredictable, therefore the oral route is not recommended.

It is destroyed partly by gastric acid, and about 36% is absorbed from the gut, somewhat erratically. For serious infections, initial therapy should be by parenteral administration. About 90% is bound to protein in plasma. The volume of distribution is 0.26 to 0.44 mL/g. Only about 10 to 30% is eliminated unchanged in the urine. Nafcillin is excreted primarily by the liver with 60% of dose metabolized and 10% secreted unchanged in the bile. The half-life is 0.5 to 1 hr, except 1.2 to 1.5 hr in renal failure.

Untoward reactions are similar to those shown by other penicillins. It causes occasional nausea and diarrhea. It is irritating and may cause pain and an increase in serum transaminase activity after intramuscular injection. Thrombophlebitis can occur with intravenous injection. Cross-sensitivity between it and other penicillins may occur, but penicillin-sensitive patients often can tolerate this drug. It is preferred in adults because of the association of interstitial nephritis with methicillin. The sodium content must be considered when the drug is used in persons with a low sodium tolerance.

Dose (nafcillin equivalent)—*Oral, adult,* **250 mg** to **1 g** every 4 to 6 hr; *older infants* and *children,* **6.25** to **12.5 mg/kg** every 6 hr, except **250 mg** every 8 hr in *streptococcal pharyngitis; neonates,* **10 mg/kg** every 6 to 8 hr. *Intramuscular, adult,* usually **500 mg** every 4 to 6 hr, but as much as 12 g/day may be given; *older infants* and *children,* usually **25 mg/kg** every 12 hr; *neonates,* usually **10** to **20 mg/kg** every 12 hr. *Intravenous, adults,* usually **500 mg** to **1.5 g** every 4 to 6 hr, but as much as 20 g/day may be given; *neonates, older infants* and *children,* usually **10** to **20 mg/kg** every 4 hr *or* **20** to **40 mg/kg** every 8 hr, but up to 225 mg/kg/day may be given.

Dosage Forms (nafcillin equivalent)—Capsules: 250 mg; for Oral Solution: 250 mg/5 mL; for Injection: 500 mg and 1 and 10 g; Tablets: 500 mg. Each g contains 2.9 mEq of sodium.

Oxacillin Sodium

[2*S*-(2α,5α,6β)]-4-Thia-1-azabicyclo[3.2.0]heptane-2-carboxylic acid, 3,3-dimethyl-6-[[(5-methyl-3-phenyl-4-isoxazolyl)carbonyl]-amino]-7-oxo-, monosodium salt, monohydrate; Bactocill (*Beecham*); Prostaphlin (*Apothecon*); (*Various Mfrs*)

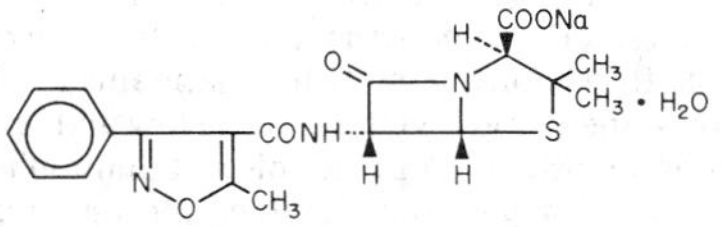

[7240-38-2] $C_{19}H_{18}N_3NaO_5S.H_2O$ (441.43); *anhydrous* [1173-88-2] (423.42). Potency: equivalent to 815 to 950 μg of oxacillin ($C_{19}H_{19}N_3O_5S$)/mg.

Preparation—Fermentation-produced 6-aminopenicillanic acid is condensed with 5-methyl-3-phenyl-4-isoxazolyl chloride in a suitable organic solvent and the resulting oxacillin is precipitated as the sodium salt by the addition of sodium acetate.

Description—Fine, white, crystalline powder; odorless or a slight odor.

Solubility—Freely soluble in water; slightly soluble in absolute alcohol, chloroform; insoluble in ether.

Uses—A penicillinase-resistant penicillin (see the general statement). Its actions and uses are nearly identical to those of *Nafcillin Sodium.* Its absorption is nearly equal to that of nafcillin but less than that of *Dicloxacillin.* Like methicillin, dicloxacillin and nafcillin, it should be restricted to treatment of penicillin G-resistant *staphylococci* infections, to minimize the development of resistant strains. Because of its variation in absorption after oral administration, oral oxacillin is not the antistaphylococcal penicillin of choice for most serious infections such as bacteremia and osteomyelitis, but the drug may be given parenterally. It may be given orally after the infection is under control.

Oral bioavailability is 30 to 33%. The presence of food in the stomach interferes with absorption. About 93% of oxacillin in plasma is bound to protein. The volume of distribution is 0.19 mL/g. About 30 to 50% of oxacillin is excreted in the urine, the remainder is secreted into the bile and metabolized, so its half-life is less affected by decreased renal function. Its half-life is 0.5 to 1 hr, except in oliguria it is 1 to 3 hr.

Allergenic effects are similar to those of other penicillins, although cross-reactions do not always occur. It also may cause nausea, vomiting, diarrhea, fever, eosinophilia, hairy tongue and, rarely, moniliasis. Because an increased plasma concentration of SGOT occasionally occurs it is suggested that special attention be paid to its use in newborn infants and in patients with hepatic dysfunction. The sodium content of the drug must be considered when the drug is to be used in persons with a low sodium tolerance.

Dose (oxacillin equivalent)—*Oral, adult* and *children more than 20 kg,* usually **500 mg** to **1 g** every 4 to 6 hr, but up to 6 g a day may be given; *infants* and *children less than 20 kg,* **12.5** to **25 mg/kg** every 6 hr. *Intramuscular or intravenous, adult* and *children over 40 kg,* usually **1 g** every 4 to 6 hr, but up to **12 g** a day may be given; *infants* and *children less than 40 kg,* **12.5** to **25 mg/kg** every 6 hr *or* **16.7 mg/kg** every 4 hr; *neonates* **25 mg/kg** every 6 hr if *over 2 kg* and 15 to 30 days of age, every 8 hr if under 2 kg and 15 to 30 days of age, and every 12 hr if under 2 kg and 1 to 14 days of age.

Dosage Forms (oxacillin equivalent)—Capsules: 250 and 500 mg; for Injection: 250 and 500 mg, and 1, 2, 4 and 10 g; for Oral Solution: 250 mg/5 mL. Each g contains 2.8 mEq of sodium.

Penicillin G Benzathine

[2*S*-(2α,5α,6β)]-4-Thia-1-azabicyclo[3.2.0]heptane-2-carboxylic acid, 3,3-dimethyl-7-oxo-6-[(phenylacetyl)amino]-, compd with *N,N′*-bis-(phenylmethyl)-1,2-ethanediamine (2:1), tetrahydrate; Bicillin (*Wyeth-Ayerst*; Permapen (*Roerig*)

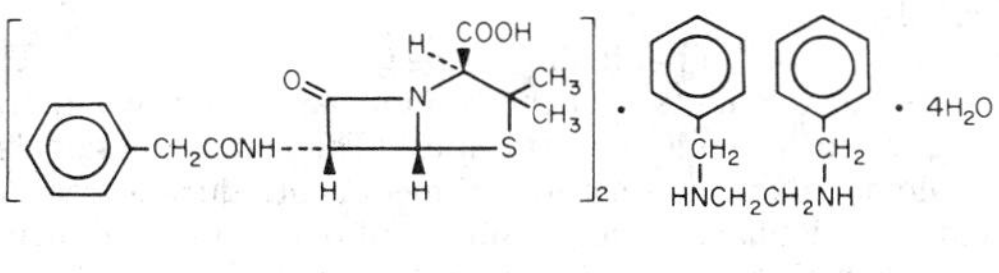

[41372-02-5] $C_{16}H_{20}N_2.2C_{16}H_{18}N_2O_4S.4H_2O$ (981.19); *anhydrous* [1538-09-6] (909.13). Potency: 1090 to 1272 penicillin Units/mg. One mg of penicillin G benzathine represents 1211 penicillin G units.

Preparation—Precipitates on mixing aqueous solutions containing *N,N*-dibenzylethylenediamine diacetate and sodium penicillin G in the required molar proportion.

Description—White, odorless, crystalline powder; pH (saturated solution) 5 to 7.5.

Solubility—1 g in about 5000 mL water and about 65 mL alcohol.

Uses—Low water-solubility; hence, on intramuscular injection, it is released slowly and yields prolonged blood levels of penicillin, generally for 1 to 4 wk. Its antibacterial activity is that of the penicillin G moiety (see the general statement), except that its long duration of action makes it especially suitable for prophylaxis of rheumatic fever. However, by the intramuscular route the blood levels are quite low and are not suitable for most of the uses of the drug. For example, 1.2 million units will yield an average plasma level of only 0.15 unit/mL on the 1st day, and by the 14th day it will have fallen to 0.03 unit/mL. Cerebrospinal fluid concentrations are negligible. With concurrent probenecid the levels will be somewhat higher. Consequently, it is indicated *only* for the *prophylaxis* and *treatment* of *infections* caused by highly susceptible *group A streptococcus, syphilis, yaws, bejel* and *pinta.*

Dose (penicillin G equivalent)—*Intramuscular, adult,* **1,200,000 units** as a single dose for upper *respiratory tract streptococcal infections;* **2,400,000 units** for *primary, secondary* and *latent syphilis,* as a single dose, and **2,400,000 units** once a week for 3 wk for *late syphilis,* but as much as 2,400,000 units a day can be given, if necessary; for *continuous prophylaxis* against streptococcal infections, **1,200,000 units** once a month or **600,000 units** every 2 wk. *Children more than 27.3 kg* (60 lb), for upper *respiratory tract streptococcal infections,* **900,000 to 1,200,000 units** as a single dose; *infants* and *children less than 27.3 kg,* for upper *respiratory tract infections,* **300,000** to **600,000 units** as a single dose; *infants* and *children up to 2 yr,* for *congenital syphilis,* **50,000 units/kg** as a single dose; *children 2 to 12 yr* with *congenital syphilis,* the adult dose diminished according to relative body weight. *Oral, adults* and *children over 12 yr,* for *prophylaxis* of streptococcal infections usually **400,000** to **600,000 units** every 4 to 6 hr, but as much as 12,000,000 units a day may be given, if necessary for *prophylaxis* of streptococcal infections, **200,000 units** every 12 hr; *infants* and *children up to 12 yr,* **4167** to **15,000 units/kg** every 4 hr or **6250** to **22,500 units/kg** every 6 hr or **8333** to **30,000 units/kg** every 8 hr.

Dosage Form (penicillin G equivalent)—Sterile Suspension: 600,000 units/1 mL, 1,200,000 units/2 mL, 2,400,000 units/4 mL, 3,000,000 units/10 mL.

Penicillin G Potassium

[2*S*-(2α,5α,6β)]-4-Thia-1-azabicyclo[3.2.0]heptane-2-carboxylic acid, 3,3-dimethyl-7-oxo-6-[(phenylacetyl)amino]-, monopotassium salt; Benzylpenicillin Potassium; *(Various Mfrs)*

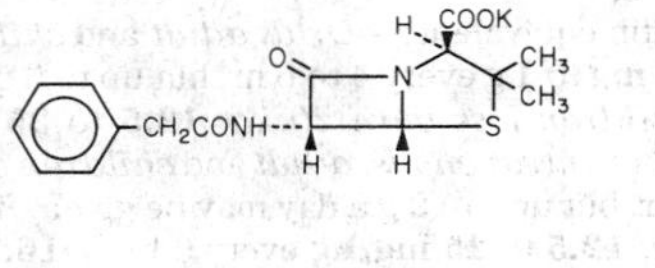

[113-98-4] $C_{16}H_{17}KN_2O_4S$ (372.48). Penicillin G Potassium has a potency of not less than 1440 and not more than 1680 Penicillin G Units per mg.

Preparation—From 6-aminopenicillanic acid and phenylacetyl chloride in an inert organic solvent; the sodium salt is precipitated with sodium acetate.

Description—Colorless or white crystals, or a white, crystalline powder; odorless or practically so; moderately hygroscopic; decomposed by prolonged exposure to temperatures of about 100°, moisture accelerating decomposition; not appreciably affected by air or light; solutions deteriorate at room temperature, but solutions stored below 15° remain stable for several days; rapidly inactivated by acids and alkalies, and also by oxidizing agents; pH (aqueous solution, 30 mg/mL) 5 and 7.5; pK_a (acid) 2.8.

Solubility—Very soluble in water, saline TS or dextrose solutions; soluble in alcohol (but is inactivated by this solvent), glycerin or many other alcohols.

Uses—See the uses of penicillins in the general statement. The potassium salt has no advantage over the sodium salt except when high doses are used in patients on sodium restriction. The potassium salt also avoids the hypokalemic alkalosis that sometimes occurs during treatment with high doses of penicillins. The possibility of potassium intoxication from massive doses in oliguric patients should be kept in mind. The bioavailability by the oral route is 15 to 33%. In plasma 50 to 65% is protein-bound. The volume of distribution is 0.47 mL/g. Renal elimination is 60 to 90% of the total, the remainder being mostly biliary. The half-life is 0.5 to 0.7 hr, except 2.5 to 10 hr in renal failure or after probenecid.

Dose (penicillin G equivalent)—*Oral, adult* and *children 12 yr or older, for treatment of infections,* usually **200,000** to **500,000** units every 6 to 8 hr, for *prophylaxis* of streptococcal infections, **200,000** to **250,000 units** every 12 hr; *infants* and *children under 12 yr,* **4167** to **15,000 units/kg** of body weight every 4 hr, *or* **6250** to **22,500 units/kg** every 6 hr, *or* **8333** to **30,000 units/kg** every 8 hr; for *prophylaxis of rheumatic fever* and/or *chorea,* **adult dose**. The drug should be taken with a full glass of water on an empty stomach. *Intramuscular* or *intravenous, adult,* usually **1,000,000** to **5,000,000 units** every 4 to 6 hr; *neonates* and *premature infants, usually* **30,000 units/kg** of body weight every 12 hr, except 500,000 to 1,000,000 units/day for neonates with *Listeria infections; older infants* and *children,* usually **4167** to **16,667 units/kg** every 4 hr, or **6250** to **25,000 units/kg** every 6 hr, except up to 400,000 units/kg/day for life-threatening infections. *Intravenous infusion, adults, for actinomycosis, fusospirochetosis (gingivostomatitis), rat-bite fever, erysipeloid endocarditis, gonorrheal endocarditis* and *arthritis,* and *Pasteurella bacteremia* and *meningitis,* **10,000,000** to **20,000,000 units a day;** for *clostridial infections,* **20,000,000 units a day;** for *Listeria endocarditis* and *meningitis,* **15,000,000** to **20,000,000 units a day;** for *meningococcal meningitis,* **20,000,000** to **30,000,000 units a day** or **1,000,000** to **2,000,000 units** every 2 hr. Such high daily doses or rapid intravenous injection of doses of 5,000,000 units or higher may occasionally cause convulsive seizures. A few doses are smaller than the above. Consult the package literature or USP DI for details of dosage in various other infections.

Dosage Forms (penicillin G equivalent)—for Injection: 500,000, 1,000,000, 5,000,000, 10,000,000 and 20,000,000 units; for Oral Solution: 200,000, 250,000, and 400,000 units/5 mL (reconstituted); Tablets for Oral Solution: 200,000, 250,000 and 400,000 units; Tablets: 200,000, 250,000, 400,000, 500,000 and 800,000 units.

Penicillin G Procaine

[2*S*-(2α,5α,6β)]-4-Thia-1-azabicyclo[3.2.0]heptane-2-carboxylic acid, 3,3-dimethyl-7-oxo-6-[(phenylacetyl)amino]-, compd with 2-(diethylamino)ethyl 4-aminobenzoate (1:1) monohydrate; *(Various Mfrs)*

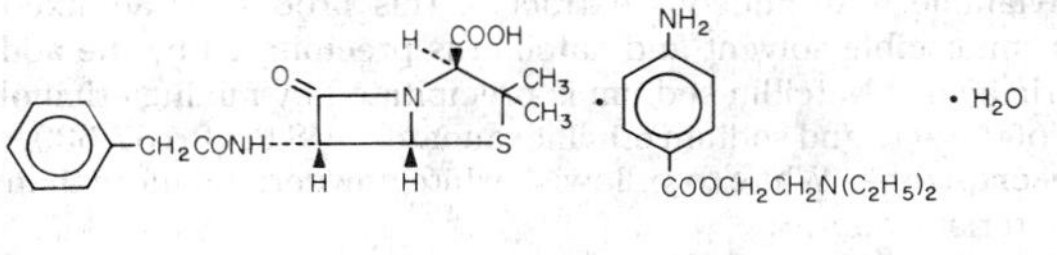

[6130-64-9] $C_{16}H_{18}N_2O_4S.C_{13}H_{20}N_2O_2.H_2O$ (588.72); *anhydrous* [54-35-3] (570.70). Potency: 900 to 1050 Penicillin Units/mg. One mg represents 1009 Penicillin G units.

Preparation—An aqueous solution of sodium (or potassium) penicillin G undergoes metathesis with an equimolar quantity of procaine hydrochloride.

Description—White, fine crystals or a white, very fine, microcrystalline powder; odorless or practically so; not appreciably affected by air or light; pH (saturated solution) 7.5; rapidly inactivated by acids and by alkali hydroxides, also by oxidizing agents.

Solubility—1 g in 250 mL water, about 30 mL alcohol or about 60 mL chloroform.

Uses—Upon intramuscular injection it slowly releases the penicillin G and provides prolonged duration of effective blood levels. An intramuscular dose of 300,000 units yields a peak plasma concentration of 1.5 units/mL at 1 to 3 hr, and the level is about 0.2 unit/mL at 24 hr and 0.05 unit/mL at 48 hr. Because of the relatively low peak blood levels, the drug is indicated only for mild to moderately severe infections by very susceptible organisms. For its uses and toxicity see the general statement. Allergies can occur due to the procaine component but other toxic effects of procaine are very rare. Intravenous injection will cause embolism.

Dose (penicillin G equivalent)—*Intramuscular, adult* and *children over 12 yr,* usually **600,000** to **1,200,000** units once a day, but up to 4,800,000 units a day may be given; for *diphtheria,* **300,000** to **600,000** units a day (with antitoxin); in *gonorrhea,* **4,800,000 units** in a single dose divided between 2 sites plus 1 g of probenecid given 30 min before injection; for *syphilis,* **600,000 units** a day for 8 days when early, secondary or latent or 10 to 15 days when tertiary or neurosyphilis; *infants* and *children up to 32 kg,* for *congenital syphilis,* **50,000 units/kg** a day for 10 days; for some infections the pediatric dose may be as much as 100,000 units/kg a day. Consult the package literature for dosage for specific infections. For most mild to moderately severe infections, 600,000 to

1,200,000 units a day suffices. Severe infections should be treated with parenteral penicillin G potassium.

Dosage Form (penicillin G equivalent)—Sterile Suspension: 300,000, 600,000, 1,200,000 and 2,400,000 units/mL.

Penicillin G Sodium

[2*S*-(2α,5α,6β)]-4-Thia-1-azabicyclo[3.2.0]heptane-2-carboxylic acid, 3,3-dimethyl-7-oxo-6-[(phenylacetyl)amino]-, monosodium salt; Benzylpenicillin Sodium;

[69-57-8] $C_{16}H_{17}N_2NaO_4S$ (356.37). Penicillin G Sodium has a potency of not less than 1500 and not more than 1750 Penicillin Units per mg.

The structure is analogous to that for *Penicillin G Potassium.*

Preparation—Refer to *Penicillin G Potassium,* using potassium acetate in place of the sodium salt.

Description—Colorless or white crystals, or as a white to slightly yellow, crystalline powder; odorless or practically so; moderately hygroscopic; relatively stable in air, but is inactivated by prolonged heating at about 100°, especially in the presence of moisture; solutions lose potency fairly rapidly at room temperature, but retain substantially full potency for several days at temperatures below 15° and at pH 5.5 to 6; solutions are rapidly inactivated by acids, alkali hydroxides, oxidizing agents and penicillinase; $pK_a = 2.76$.

Solubility—1 g in 40 mL water. Soluble in *normal* saline and glucose solutions; soluble in alcohols and glycerol. Practically insoluble in acetone, ether or chloroform.

Uses—See the uses of penicillins in the general statement. When massive doses of this drug are used, a considerable sodium load is introduced, which expands the extracellular space and may cause edema in patients with heart failure. Massive doses also can cause hypokalemic alkalosis.

Dose (penicillin G equivalent)—*Intramuscular* and *intravenous,* identical to those of *Penicillin G Potassium* (1 mg represents 1667 units).

Dosage Form (penicillin G equivalent)—for Injection: 5,000,000 units. Each 1,000,000 units contains 1.69 mEq of sodium.

Penicillin V Potassium

[2*S*-(2α,5α,6β)]-4-Thia-1-azabicyclo[3.2.0]heptane-2-carboxylic acid, 3,3-dimethyl-7-oxo-6-[(phenoxyacetyl)amino]-, monopotassium salt; Penicillin Potassium Phenoxymethyl; (*Various Mfrs*)

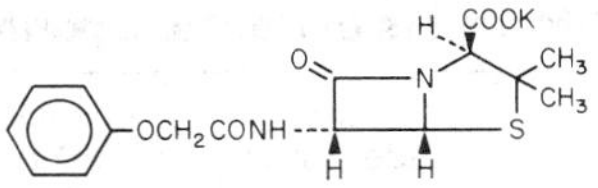

[132-98-9] $C_{16}H_{17}KN_2O_5S$ (388.48). Penicillin V Potassium has a potency of not less than 1380 and not more than 1610 Penicillin V units per mg.

Preparation—As for *Penicillin G,* using phenoxyacetyl chloride.

Description—White, odorless, crystalline powder; pH (aqueous solution, 30 mg/mL) 7.5; pK_a 2.73.

Solubility—Very soluble in water; 1 g in about 150 mL alcohol.

Uses—The antibacterial spectrum is essentially that of penicillin G against gram-positive bacteria but this is less potent and effective against gram-negative bacteria. Consequently, it shares the same uses (see the general statement), except that in severe acute infections parenteral penicillin G is mandatory. It is inactivated less by gastric juice than is penicillin G. Penicillin V is the preferred oral penicillin for less serious infections because serum levels are 2 to 5 times higher than comparable doses of penicillin G and there is less individual variability in absorption. Like penicillin G, it may cause allergic reactions, and it frequently shows cross-sensitivity to the other penicillins. However, allergic reactions are much less common with administration of oral penicillin than with intramuscular forms. Its other toxicities are also those of penicillin G. The oral bioavailability is about 60% at best. Plasma levels are two to five times higher than observed with penicillin G potassium. A dose of 1,000,000 units of the potassium salt will provide levels of 4.5 to 9 μg/mL. It is 75 to 80% bound to plasma proteins. The volume of distribution is 0.73 mL/g, which is considerably larger than that of penicillin G. Only 20 to 40% is excreted unchanged in the urine. The half-life is about 0.5 to 1 hr.

Dose (penicillin V equivalent)—*Oral, adult* and *children 12 yr or older,* usually **125** to **500 mg** (200,000 to 800,000 units) every 6 to 8 hr, except **125** to **250 units** every 12 hr for prophylaxis of rheumatic fever. Up to 7.2 g (11,520,000 units) a day may be given. *Children under 12 yr,* **2.5** to **9.3 mg/kg** every 4 hr *or* **3.75** to **14 mg/kg** every 6 hr *or* **5** to **18.7 mg/kg** every 8 hr.

Dosage Forms (penicillin V equivalent)—for Oral Solution: 125 and 250 mg/5 mL (reconstituted); Tablets: 250 and 500 mg.

Piperacillin Sodium

[2*S*-[2α,5α,6β(*S**)]]-4-Thia-1-azabicyclo[3.2.0]heptane-2-carboxylic acid, 6-[[[[(4-ethyl-2,3-dioxo-1-piperazinyl)carbonyl]amino]-phenylacetyl]amino]-3,3-dimethyl-7-oxo-, monosodium salt; Pipracil (*Lederle*)

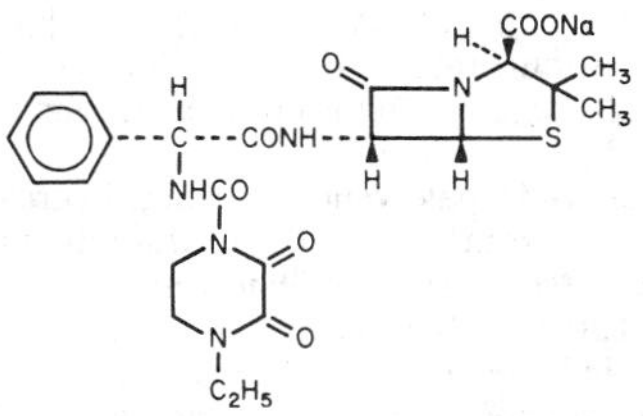

[59703-84-3] $C_{23}H_{26}N_5NaO_7S$ (539.54). Potency: the equivalent of not less than 863 μg piperacillin/mg.

Preparation—US Pat 4,087,424.

Description—White crystals.

Solubility—1 g in about 1.5 mL water or methanol; 5 mL of ethyl alcohol.

Uses—An extended-spectrum penicillin with antibacterial activities characteristic of its class (see the general statement). It is the most active penicillin against *Ps aeruginosa,* with a potency nearly that of gentamicin. It is one of five drugs of choice for use against infections caused by *Ps aeruginosa.* It is more potent against *Klebsiella* and several other enteric bacilli than is carbenicillin or ticarcillin. It is an alternative drug for use against infections by *Acinetobacter, Bacteroides fragilis* (gastrointestinal strains), *Enterobacter, E coli, Kl pneumoniae, Morganella morganii, Prot mirabilis* or *vulgaris, Prov rettgeri or stuartii, Ps aeruginosa* (urinary tract infections) or *Serratia.* It has a low efficacy against penicillinase- and other β-lactamase-producing bacteria. Resistance can develop rapidly to piperacillin during use, so that it should be administered only in combination with an aminoglycoside or penicillinase inhibitor when used against *Ps aeruginosa* and other hard-to-suppress bacilli. Present authoritative medical opinion holds that it should be reserved for use against various pseudomonal and severe enteric bacillary infections. Although it is approved for use in gonorrhea, ceftriaxone is a superior choice. This drug causes no unique adverse effects. It is expensive.

The oral bioavailability is too low and erratic to be of use. In plasma, 16 to 22% is protein-bound. The volume of distribution is about 0.18 to 0.30 mL/g. Renal excretion accounts for 60 to 80% of elimination. The half-life is 0.5 hr, except 0.6 to 1.2 hr in renal failure.

Dose (piperacillin equivalent)—*Intramuscular, adult* and *children 12 yr* or *older,* for *gonorrhea,* **2 g** as a single dose (after 1 g of probenecid. *Intramuscular* or *intravenous, uncomplicated urinary tract infections,* **1.5** to **2 g** (or **25** to **31.3 mg/kg**) every 6 hr *or* **3** to **4 g** (or **50** to **62.5 mg/kg**) every 12 hr. *Intravenous infusion adult,* for *gynecological, intra-abdominal, skin* and *soft-tissue infections,* hospital-acquired *pneumonia* and *septicemia,* **2** to **3 g** (or **31.3** to **50 mg/kg**) every 4 hr *or* **3** to **4 g** (or **50** to **75, mg/kg**) every 6 hr; for *complicated urinary tract infections,* **3** to **4 g** or **31.3** to **50 mg/kg,** every 6 to 8 hr or **41.7** to **66.7 mg/kg** every 8 hr; for *perioperative prophylaxis, abdominal hysterectomy,* **2g** 0.5 to 1 hr before surgery, upon entering the recovery room and again after 6 hr; for *vaginal hysterectomy,* **2g** ½ to 1 hr before surgery and at 6 and 12 hr after the first dose; for *intra-abdominal surgery,* **2g** 0.5 to 1 hr before surgery, once during, and every 6 hr for 24 hr; for *cesarian section,* **2g** when the umbilical cord is clamped and at 4 and 8 hr after. Dosage adjustments are required in renal failure.

Dosage Form (piperacillin equivalent)—Powder for Injection: 2, 3, 4 and 40 g. Each g contains 1.85 mEq of sodium.

Pivampicillin Hydrochloride—see RPS-18, page 1193.

Ticarcillin Disodium

[2*S*-[2α,5α,6β(*S**)]]-4-Thia-1-azabicyclo[3.2.0]heptane-2-carboxylic acid, 6-[(carboxy-3-thienylacetyl)amino]-3,3-dimethyl-7-oxo-, disodium salt; Ticar (*SmithKline Beecham*)

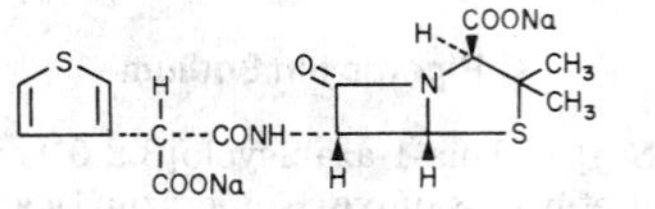

[4697-14-7] $C_{15}H_{14}N_2Na_2O_6S_2$ (428.38). Potency: equivalent to not less than 800 μg of ticarcillin ($C_{15}H_{16}N_2O_6S_2$)/mg, calculated on the anhydrous basis.

Preparation—Belgian Pat 646, 991. 2-(3-Thienyl)malonic acid, monobenzyl ester is converted to the acid chloride which is condensed with 6-aminopenicillanic acid, followed by hydrogenation to convert the ester to the free acid.

Description—White to pale-yellow powder; hygroscopic; unstable in acid medium; pK_a (acid form) 2.44, 3.64; acid solutions are unstable.

Solubility—1 g in 10 mL water or 66 mL ethanol; pH of a concentrated solution (> 100 g/100 mL) about 7.0.

Uses—An extended-spectrum penicillin almost identical to carbenicillin in its antibacterial spectrum and potency, except that it is twice as active against *Ps aeruginosa.* However, resistance to carbenicillin automatically confers resistance to this and *vice versa.* Resistance develops rapidly. With many infections, resistance is obviated by adding clavulanate. Also, for gram-negative infections, it is often combined with gentamicin or tobramycin to enhance activity and delay resistance. With carbenicillin it shares penicillin of first-choice status for the treatment of urinary tract infections caused by *Ps aeruginosa,* and in combination with gentamicin or tobramycin the treatment of all other infections caused by the bacterium. It is an alternative drug as follows, (clavulanate unnecessary): *Acinetobacter, Enterobacter* and *Serratia;* (clavulanate optional): *Bacteroides fragilis* (gastrointestinal strains), *E coli, Prot mirabilis* or *vulgaris, Morganella morganii* and *Prov rettgeri* or *stuartii;* (clavulanate *mandatory*): *Kl pneumoniae* and *Staph aureus* or *epidermidis.*

The adverse effects are those of penicillins in general (see the general statement), and cross-sensitivity to penicillin occurs. Sodium overload and hypokalemia can occur, especially with high doses. In renal failure, high doses may inhibit platelet aggregation, and hemorrhagic phenomena may result. It is expensive, but less so than carbenicillin.

It is not absorbed orally. An intravenous dose of 3 g provides a serum concentration of 260 μg/mL. In plasma, 55 to 65% is protein-bound. The volume of distribution is 0.22 mL/g. It is 86% eliminated by renal excretion. The half-life is 0.5 to 1 hr, except 15 hr in renal failure.

Dose (ticarcillin equivalent)—*Intramuscular* or *intravenous, adult* and *children 40 kg or over,* for *uncomplicated urinary tract infections,* **1 g** every 4 to 6 hr; *children up to 40 kg,* for *uncomplicated urinary tract infections,* **12.5** to **25 mg/kg** every 6 hr *or* **16.7** to **33.3 mg/kg** every 8 hr; *neonates,* for *all infections, initially* **100 mg/kg,** then **75 mg/kg** every 4 to 6 hr for 1 wk *if under 2 kg* and 2 wk if *2 kg or over,* then **100 mg/kg** every 4 hr. *Intravenous infusion, adults,* and *children 40 kg* or *over, for intra-abdominal genitourinary, pneumonia, septicemia, skin and soft-tissue infections,* **3 g** every 3 to 6 hr *or* **25** to **37.5 mg/kg** every 3 hr *or* **33.3** to **37.5 mg/kg** every 4 hr *or* **50 to 75 mg/kg** every 6 hr; for *complicated urinary tract infections,* **3 g** every 4 to 6 hr *or* **25** to **33.3 mg/kg** every 4 hr *or* **37.5** to **50 mg/kg** every 6 hr; *children up to 40 kg,* for *intra-abdominal, genitourinary, pneumonia, septicemia, skin and soft-tissue infections,* **33.3** to **50 mg/kg** every 4 hr or **50** to **75 mg/kg** every 6 hr; for *complicated urinary tract infections,* **25** to **33.3 mg/kg** every 4 hr *or* **37.5** to **50 mg/kg** every 6 hr. *In combination with clavulanate* (100 mg/3 g of ticarcillin) *adults 60 kg or over, for all infections,* **33.3** to **50 mg/kg** every 4 hr *or* **50** to **75 mg/kg** every 6 hr; *under 60 kg,* **3 g** every 4 to 6 hr.

Dosage Form (ticarcillin equivalent)—Sterile Powder: 1, 3, 6, 20 and 30 g. Each g contains 5.2 to 6.5 mEq of sodium.

Penicillin-Containing Combinations

Some examples of penicillin-containing combinations (with content per capsule, tablet or 5 mL provided) are as follows:

Amoxicillin and Clavulanate Potassium [Augmentin (*SmithKline Beecham*)—125 mg:25 mg and 250 mg:62.5 mg, tablets, chewable; 250 mg:125 mg and 500 mg:125 mg, tablets; 125 mg:25 mg and 250 mg:62.5 mg, for oral suspension.

Ampicillin—Probenicid [Polycillin-PRB (*SmithKline*); Probampacin (*Various Mfrs*)]—3.5 g:1 g, for oral suspension.

Ampicillin—Sulbactam Sodium [Unasyn (*Roerig*)]—1.5 g:0.5 g and 3 g:1 g, for injection.

Ticarcillin—Clavulanate Potassium [Timentin (*Apothecon, Beecham*)]—3 g:0.1 g, for injection.

Cephalosporins

The cephalosporins are a group of antibiotics closely related to the penicillins. The cephalosporanic acid moiety characteristic of cephalosporins is an analog of the penicillanic acid moiety characteristic of penicillins; cephalosporanic acid contains a dihydrometathiazine ring, while penicillanic acid contains a tetrahydrothiazole (thiazolidine) ring. Both have a β-lactam ring. The 7-Aminocephalosporanic acid derivatives are much more acid-stable than the corresponding 6-aminopenicillanic acid compounds. Moxalactam has a dihydrometaoxazine ring in lieu of the thiazine ring. Cephamycins are cephalosporins which possess a 7-methoxy group which enhances β-lactamase resistance. Cephamycins may induce β-lactamase production.

Antibacterial Actions—The cephalosporins have a mechanism of action very similar to that of the penicillins, namely, they bind to one or more penicillin-binding proteins (PBPs) which are transpeptidases and inhibit the cross-linking of the peptidoglycan units in the bacterial cell wall by occupying the D-alanyl-D-alanine substrate site of the transpeptidase. The intrinsic activity of acephalosporin depends in part on resistance to β-lactamases, affinity to PBPs and their ability to reach these targets which are extracellular for gram-positive bacteria and periplasmic for gram-negative bacteria. Because of the similar mechanisms, it is to be expected that the antibacterial spectra would be very similar, as they are. Cephalosporins presently are classified as first-, second- and third-generation cephalosporins.

The first-generation drugs have the highest activity against gram-positive and the lowest against gram-negative bacteria. Thus, they are active against most staphylococci (even penicillinase-producers, but not methicillin-resistant staphylococci). They also are active against most streptococci, including *S pyogenes, viridans* and *pneumoniae.* They

Table 5—Members of Cephalosporin Classes

Class and generic name	Trade names	Administration Route	Half-life (hrs)
First generation			
Cefadroxil	Duricef, Ultracef	Oral	1.4
Cefazolin	Ancef, Kefzol	IM, IV	1.8
Cephalexin	Keflex, Keftab	Oral	0.9
Cephalothin	Keflin	IM, IV	0.5-0.9
Cephapirin	Cefadyl	IM, IV	0.6-0.8
Cephradine	Anspor, Velosef	IM, IV, oral	0.8
Second generation			
Cefaclor	Ceclor	Oral	0.6-0.9
Cefamandole	Mandol	IM, IV	0.6-1
Cefmetazole	Zefazone	IV	1.2
Cefonicid	Monocid	IM, IV	3.4-4.5
Ceforanid	Precef	IM, IV	2.7-3
Cefotetan	Cefotan	IM, IV	3-4.6
Cefoxitin	Mefoxin	IM, IV	0.7-1
Cefpodoxime	Vantin	Oral	1.9-2.8
Cefprozil	Cefzil	Oral	1.3
Cefuroxime	Zinacef, Kefurox	IM, IV, oral	1.3-1.7
Loracef	Lorabid	Oral	1
Third generation			
Cefixime	Suprax	Oral	3-4
Cefoperazone	Cefobid	IM, IV	1.9-2.1
Cefotaxime	Claforan	IM, IV	1-1.1
Ceftazidime	Fortaz, Tazicef, Tazidime	IM, IV	1.9
Ceftizoxime	Cefizox	IM, IV	1.4-1.8
Ceftriaxone	Rocephin	IM, IV	6-9
Moxalactam	Moxam	IM, IV	2-2.3

are not active against *S faecalis*. Other susceptible gram-positive bacteria are *Cl perfringens*, *Listeria* and *Corynebacterium*. First-generation cephalosporins also are moderately active against certain gram-negative bacteria, such as *Neisseria gonorrheae* and *meningitidis*, many *E coli*, some *H influenzae*, and nonhospital-acquired *Klebsiella* and *Pr mirabilis* and some *Salmonella* and *Shigella*.

The second-generation cephalosporins are more active against gram-negative and less active against gram-positive bacteria than are first-generation members. Notable of the increased activity against gram-negative organisms is greater efficacy against most *H influenzae*, the efficacy of cefoxitin against *B fragilis* and indole-positive *Proteus* and the activity of cephamandole against *Enterobacter* and indole-positive *Proteus*. Like the first-generation, members of this group are inactive against *Ps aeruginosa*.

The third-generation cephalosporins are considerably less active than first-generation drugs against gram-positive but have a much expanded spectrum of activity against gram-negative organisms and have more resistance to β-lactamases. They are quite active against gram-negative anaerobes, and, except for cefsulodin, are frequently active against *Enterobacteriaceae* (*E coli*, *Enterobacter*, *Klebsiella pneumoniae*). Of special interest is the activity against *Ps aeruginosa*, although ceftazidime and cefoperazone have high activity. These drugs are inactive against *Acinetobacter*.

Resistance—As with the penicillins one common mechanism of resistance is that of elaboration of a β-lactamase. Although some cephalosporins are inactivated by penicillinase-types of β-lactamase, some are not, but are affected by cephalosporinase types. Therefore, there may be cross-resistance between penicillins and cephalosporins, but not necessarily so. In addition to β-lactamase-related resistance, other types of resistance, analogous to methicillin resistance, occur.

Indications

The cephalosporins are effective in a wide variety of infections because they have a broad spectrum and high therapeutic/toxic ratio. The first- and second-generation cephalosporins are used frequently for prophylaxis during certain surgical procedures to reduce the risk of postoperative wound infections. Cefazolin is preferred over other first-generation analogs because it has a higher serum concentration and longer elimination half-life; also it is less painful upon intramuscular administration. Cefoxitin, cefotefan, cefmetazole and moxalactam are cephamycins that are preferred for intra-abdominal surgery because of their β-lactamase resistance and activity against *Bacteroides fragilis*. A number of second- and third-generation cephalosporins are effective alternatives as prophylactic agents for various surgical procedures.

Cephalosporins are generally not the first drug of choice for any bacterial infections because of the availability of equally effective and less expensive alternatives. First-generation cephalosporins are preferred alternatives to antistaphylococcal penicillins or penicillin G for serious staphylococcal and/or streptococcal infection except enterococcal infections or meningitis. The non-cephamycin second-generation cephalosporins such as cefamandole, cefuroxime, ceforanide and cefonicid have similar antimicrobial spectra and may be used as alternatives to treat most serious infections caused by staphylococci and aerobic gram-negative bacilli. Only the third-generation cephalosporins are approved for treatment of meningitis caused by enteric gram-negative bacilli. Cefuroxime may be used to treat meningitis caused by *Haemophilus influenzae*, although a third-generation cephalosporin is still the preferred choice.

Cefotaxime, ceftizoxime, ceftriaxone and moxalactam are third-generation cephalosporins that are effective against serious hospital-acquired infections caused by enteric gram-negative bacili, such as *Enterobacter*, indole-positive *Proteus*, *Providencia stuartii* and *Serratia*. Against *H influenzae*, cefotaxime and ceftriaxone are preferred for parenteral therapy, although cefuroxine is an alternative. Ceftriaxone is the drug of choice for treatment of gonorrhea, and any cephalosporin may be preferred over an extended-spectrum penicillin against *Klebsiella pneumoniae*. The cephalosporins are also alternatives to penicillins to treat infections caused by *Moxarella (Branhamella) catarrhalis* and less serious infections of streptococci, staphylococci, *H influenzae*, *Neisseria menningitidis* and *E Coli*.

Several oral cephalosporins have increased activity against *H influenzae* including cefaclor, cefuroxime axetil, cefixime, cefprozil and cefpodoxime proxetil. Ceftazidime and cefoperazone are preferred in the treatment of infections caused by *Pseudomonas aeruginosa*, *P cepacia* or *P maltophilia*. Third-generation cephalosporins such as cefatoxime and ceftizoxime are expensive alternatives against indole-positive *Proteus*, *Providencia* and *nontyphoid Salmonella*.

Adverse Effects—Hypersensitivity occurs in about 5 to 10% of recipients of cephalosporins; manifestations are eosinophilia, drug fever, maculopapular rash, urticaria, serum sickness, angioneurotic edema, anaphylaxis, positive Coombs test associated with rare hemolytic anemia and infrequent transient hepatic abnormalities (increased SGOT, SGPT and total bilirubin), thrombocytopenia, neutropenia and interstitial nephritis. There is an appreciable incidence of cross-sensitization with penicillin; when previously manifested, penicillin sensitivity has not been serious, a cephalosporin, especially cefazolin, may be administered cautiously after sensitivity testing, but *only if necessary;* skin tests often give false negatives. If the previous reaction to penicillin was severe, such as with anaphylaxis or angioneurotic edema, or if the patient reacts to penicillin minor determinants, a cephalosporin usually is discouraged.

Other adverse effects of cephalosporins include pain, induration, sterile abscess and sloughing at the site of intramuscular injection, thrombophlebitis after intravenous administration, nausea, vomiting, glossitis, diarrhea, loose stools, abdominal pain and heartburn, especially with oral administration, sodium load and water retention with sodium salts, antibiotic-associated colitis (especially with poorly absorbed members) and a false-positive urine test for glucose (Benedict, Fehling and Clinitest, but not Tes-Tape). Present cephalosporins are not significantly nephrotoxic alone but may increase considerably the nephrotoxicity of an aminoglycoside. Cephalosporins should not be used in combination with other antibiotics that cause nephrotoxicity or ototoxicity. High-ceiling diuretics (eg, furosemide and ethacrynic acid) also enhance nephrotoxicity and make certain cephalosporins ototoxic. The acquisition costs of some cephalosporins is very high. Suprainfections by gram-negative bacteria and *Candida* may occur. There may be occasional hypoprothrombinemia and disulfiram-like reaction with alcohol; those drugs with *N*-methylthiotetrazole side chains seem to be the serious offenders which includes cefamandole, cefoperazone, moxalactam, cefotetan and cefmetazole.

Pharmacokinetics—Cephalosporins vary considerably in their peroral bioavailability (15 to 86%), protein binding (14 to 96%) and half-lives (0.5 to 6.5 hr). Elimination is mainly by glomerular filtration and tubular secretion (except for cefoperazone) and some biliary secretion (and reabsorption), except that most of cephaloglycin and some of cefotaxime, cephalothin, cephapirin and cephacetrile are deacetylated and subsequently further transformed; consequently, renal failure may greatly increase the half-lives of most cephalosporins. Cephalosporins vary in their penetrance into tissues. Only cefuroxime and third-generation cephalosporins achieve therapeutic concentrations in cerebrospinal fluid, and then only in inflammation of the meninges. The first- and second-generation cephalosporins should not be used for meningitis. Cephalosporins cross the placental barrier and reach plasma concentration in the fetus in about 10% of maternal concentrations; effects on the fetus are unknown, but it is advisable to avoid treatment of pregnant women with cephalosporins if possible.

Cefaclor

5-Thia-1-azabicyclo[4.2.0]oct-2-ene-2-carboxylic acid, [6*R*-[6α,7β(*R**)]]-7- [(aminophenylacetyl)amino]-3-chloro-8-oxo-, monohydrate; Ceclor (*Lilly*)

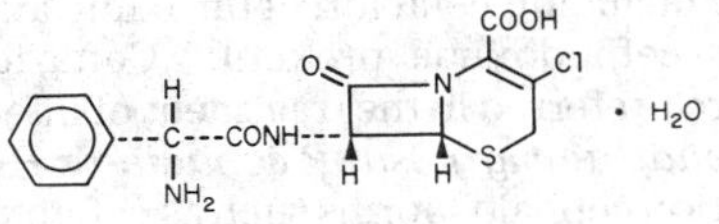

[70356-03-05] $C_{15}H_{14}ClN_3O_4S.H_2O$ (385.82)]. Cefaclor is a semi-synthetic cephalosporin related to cephalexin.

Preparation—See *J Med Chem 18:* 403, 1975.

Description—White crystalline solid; aqueous solutions are most stable at pH of about 3.5, which is the pH of a 2% solution.

Solubility—Soluble in water (1 in 100); practically insoluble in most organic solvents.

Uses—A second-generation cephalosporin with typical antibacterial activities and adverse effects (see the general statement). It was the first *orally* efficaceous member of its group. It is approved for use in the treatment of *upper respiratory tract infections, pharyngitis* and *tonsillitis* caused by *Str pyogenes; lower respiratory tract infections* caused by *Str pneumoniae, pyogenes* and *H influenzae; otitis media* caused by *Str pneumoniae, Str pyogenes,* staphylococci and *H influenzae; cutaneous infections* caused by *Staph aureus* and *Str pyrogenes;* and *urinary tract infections* caused by *E coli, Pr mirabilis, Klebsiella* spp and coagulase-negative staphylococci. A 250-mg dose causes a peak plasma concentration of about 7 μg/mL. In plasma, 25% is bound to protein. The volume of distribution is 0.24 to 0.36 mL/g. About 60 to 85% is excreted unchanged into the urine. The half-life is 0.6 to 0.9 hr, except longer in renal failure.

Dose (as the anhydride)—*Oral, adult,* **250** to **500 mg** every 8 hr; *infants 1 mo* and *older* and *children,* **6.7** to **13.4 mg/kg** every 8 hr. In uncomplicated urinary tract infections, a single 2-g dose may be given to adults.

Dosage Forms—Capsules: 250 and 500 mg; for *oral* suspension: 125, 187, 250 and 375 mg/5 mL (reconstituted).

Cefamandole Naftate

5-Thia-1-azabicyclo[4.2.0]oct-2-ene-2-carboxylic acid, [6*R*-[6α,7β(*R**)]]-7-[[(formyloxy) phenylacetyl]amino]-3-[[(1-methyl-1*H*-tetrazol-5-yl)-thio]methyl]-8-oxo-, monosodium salt, Mandol (*Lilly*)

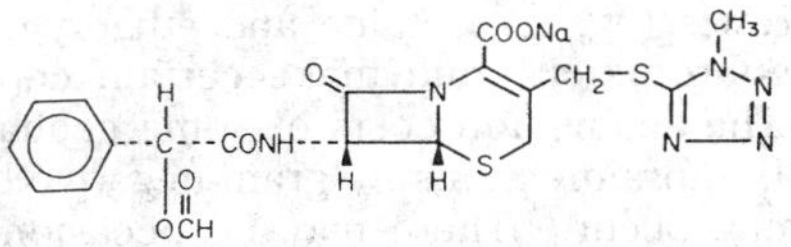

[42540-40-9] [34444-01-4(acid)] $C_{19}H_{17}N_6NaO_6S_2$ (512.49).

Preparation—US Pat 3,641,021.

Description—White crystals; melts about 190° with decomposition; pK_a 2.8.

Solubility—Soluble in water or methanol; insoluble in nonpolar solvents.

Uses—A cephalosporin (see the general statement). It is active against 80 to 90% of indole-positive strains of *Proteus* and is also active against *H influenzae, E coli, Klebsiella, Enterobacter, Serratia* and *Providencia.* However, it is not as effective as amikacin, gentamicin or tobramycin. Most *B fragilis* are resistant. There is no cross-resistance to ampicillin. In general, indications for use are those of the cephalosporins as a group (see the general statement). The adverse effects are those of other cephalosporins (see the general statement), but hypoprothrombinemia and a disulfiram-like reaction may occur. Its sodium content and that of the sodium carbonate added to it, amounts to a total of approximately 77 mg of sodium/g of its activity, should be taken into account when the drug is used in persons with low sodium tolerance. It is not absorbed when administered orally. It is 67 to 80% bound to plasma proteins and has a volume of distribution of 0.16 mL/g. An intramuscular dose of 500 mg yields a peak plasma concentration of 12 to 15 μg/mL in 0.5 to 1 hr. About 65 to 85% is secreted in to the urine; the half-life is 0.75 to 1 hr.

Dose—(cefamandole equivalent): *Intramuscular* or *intravenous, adult,* for *various infections,* **0.5** to **2 g** every 4 to 6 hr; for *pneumonia* and *skin infections,* **0.5 g** every 6 hr; for *urinary tract infections,* **0.5** to **1g** every 8 hr: for *surgical prophylaxis* **1** to **2g** 0.5 to 1 hr before and every 6 hr for 1 day after surgery; *infants 1 mo or older* and *children, for all infections,* **8.3** to **16.7** mg/kg every 4 hr *or* **12.5** to **25 mg/kg** every 6 hr *or* **16.7** to **33.3 mg/kg** every 8 hr; for *surgical prophylaxis,* **12.5** to **25 mg/kg** 0.5 to 1 hr before and every 6 hr for 1 day after surgery.

Dosage Form—Injection: 0.5 and 1 g/10 mL; 2 g/20 mL; 1, 2 and 10 g/100 mL. There are 3.3 mEq of sodium per g.

Cefazolin Sodium

5-Thia-1-azabicyclo[4.2.0]oct-2-ene-2-carboxylic acid, 3-[[(5-methyl-(6*R-trans*)- 1,3,4-thiadiazol-2-yl)thio]methyl]-8-oxo-7-[[(1*H*-tetrazol-1-yl)acetyl]-amino]-, monosodium salt; Ancef (*SmithKline Beecham*); Kefzol (*Lilly*); (*Squibb*)

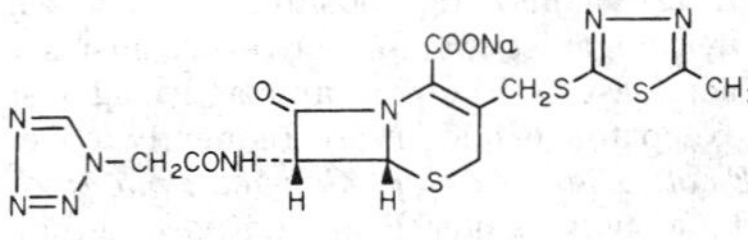

[27164-46-1] $C_{14}H_{13}N_8NaO_4S_3$ (476.48). Potency: Not less than 850 μg and not more than 1050 μg of cefazolin ($C_{14}H_{14}N_8O_4S_3$) per mg, calculated on the anhydrous basis.

Preparation—The sodium salt of 7-aminocephalosporanic acid is acylated with 1*H*-tetrazole-1-acetyl chloride and the acetoxy group is then displaced by reaction with 5-methyl-1,3,4-thiadiazole-2-thiol; the resulting cefazolin is converted to the sodium salt.

Description—White to off-white, crystalline powder.

Solubility—Freely soluble in water, saline TS or dextrose solutions; very slightly soluble in alcohol; practically insoluble in chloroform or ether.

Uses—Those of first-generation cephalosporins (see the general statement). Some gram-negative organisms and penicillinase-producing staphylococci resistant to both penicillin G and ampicillin are sensitive to cefazolin. Gram-negative activity essentially limited to *E coli, Klebsiella* and *Proteus mirabilis.*

The drug can be used to treat *infections of the respiratory tract, skin, soft tissues, bones, joints* and *urinary tract* and *endocarditis* and *septicemia* caused by susceptible organisms. Among urinary tract infections, cystitis responds much better than pyelonephritis. It is the preferred cephalosporin for most surgical prophylaxis, because of its (relatively) long half-life.

The adverse effects are those of cephalosporins in general (see the general statement). It causes some pain at the site of injection and occasional phlebitis. Oral, genital and vaginal candidiasis and anal pruritus occur. It causes a transient increase in blood urea nitrogen yet seems to have negligible nephrotoxicity.

It is not absorbed orally. It is bound to the extent of 70 to 85% by plasma proteins and has a low volume of distribution of only 0.10 to 0.14 mL/g. An intramuscular dose of 500 mg will yield a peak plasma concentration of 37 μg/mL at 1 hr; intravenously 500 mg will yield a concentration of >94 μg/mL. From 95% is excreted into urine. The half-life is 1.5 to 2 hr in normal persons but 3 to 42 hr in renal failure.

Dose (cefazolin equivalent)—*Intramuscular* or *intravenous, adult,* for *most infections,* **0.25** to **1 g** every 6 to 8 hr; for *pneumococcal pneumonia,* **0.5 g** every 12 hr; for *urinary tract infections,* **1 g** every 12 hr; for surgical *prophylaxis,* **1 g** 0.5 to 1 hr before, **0.5** to **1 g** during and every 6 hr for 1 day after surgery; *infants over 1 mo* and *children, for all infections,* **6.25** to **25 mg/kg** every 6 hr *or* **8.3** to **33.3 mg/kg** every 8 hr.

Dosage Forms (cefazolin equivalent)—Injection: 500 mg and 1 g/50 mL; Sterile Powder: 250 and 500 mg, and 1 and 10 and 20 g.

Cefixime

5-Thia-1-azabicyclo[4.2.0]oct-2-ene-2-carboxylic acid, [6*R*-[6α,7β(*Z*)]]-7-[[(2-amino-4-thiazolyl)[(carboxymethoxy)imino]acetyl]amino]-3-ethenyl-8-oxo-, Suprax (*Lederle*)

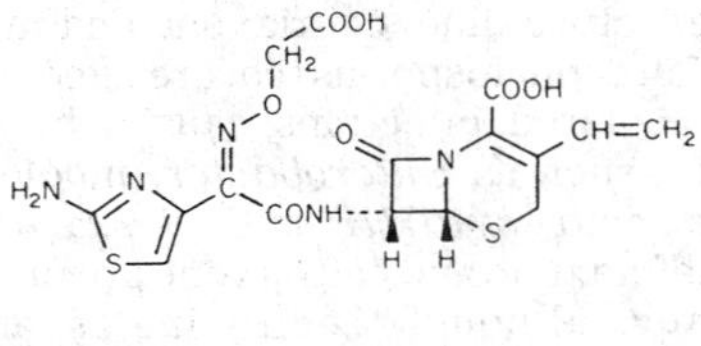

[79350-37-1] $C_{16}H_{15}N_5O_7S_2$ (453.44).

Preparation—US Pat 4,098,888.

Description—Off-white crystals; melts over 250°; distinguished from the *E*-trihydrate which melts about 220° with decomposition; pK_a (acid) 2.5.

Solubility—1 g in 125 mL water or 2000 mL alcohol.

Uses—An oral third-generation cephalosporin with excellent activity against most *E coli and Klebsiella, Haemophilus influenzae, Moraxella catarrhalis, Neisseria gonorrhea* and *Neisseria meningitidis*, including β-lactamase-producing strains. It is active against common streptococci but staphylococci are resistant. It is used for respiratory infections, otitis media and uncomplicated urinary tract infections, but its therapeutic role remains to be defined.

It is absorbed slowly and incompletely from the gastrointestinal tract and has a bioavailability of 40 to 50%. The oral suspension produces peak concentrations that are 25 to 50% higher than equivalent doses of tablet formulations. Food does not affect the amount of cefixime absorbed but delays absorption. Approximately 65 to 70% is bound to plasma protein. Renal excretion is the main route of elimination although biliary excretion is greater than 10%. The serum half-life is 3 to 4 hr but is prolonged with renal impairment.

The most common adverse reactions are gastrointestinal, primarily diarrhea. Other GI side effects may occur such as nausea, dyspepsia and flatulence. Dizziness, headache, genital pruritis and hypersensitivity reactions may occur.

Dose—*Adult, oral,* **400 mg** once a day or **200 mg** every 12 hr; *Children 6 mo to 12 yr,* **8 mg/kg** once a day or **4 mg/kg** of suspension every 12 hr. Efficacy and safety has not been established for infants less than 6 months.

Dosage Forms—Tablets: 200 and 400 mg; Oral Suspension: 100 mg/5 mL in 50 and 100 mL.

Cefmetazole Sodium

5-Thia-1-azabicyclo[4.2.0]oct-2-ene-2-carboxylic acid, (6*R*-*cis*)-7-[[[(cyanomethyl)thio]acetyl]amino]-7-methoxy-3-[[(1-methyl-1*H*-tetrazol-5-yl)thio]methyl]-8-oxo-, monosodium salt, Zefazone (*Upjohn*)

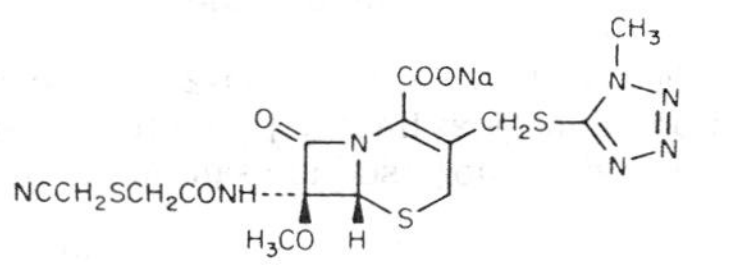

[56796-39-5], [5796-20-4 (acid)] $C_{15}H_{16}N_7NaO_5S_3$ (493.51).

Preparation—*J Antibiot 29:* 554, 1976.

Description—White solid.

Solubility—Very soluble in water or methanol; soluble in acetone.

Uses—A second-generation cephalosporin that is similar to other cephamycins such as cefoxitin and cefotetan. It has good antibacterial activity against gram-positive cocci and gram-negative bacilli as well as anaerobes such as *Bacteroides fragilis* and is very stable to gram-negative β-lactamases. It is more active that other cephamycins against *Streptococcus pneumoniae* and *Staphylococcus aureus.*

It is 85% bound to serum proteins. It has a half-life of 1.3 hr and depends primarily upon renal excretion for elimination. It also contains a *N*-methylthiotetrazole side chain which is associated with hypoprothrombinemia and can induce a disulfiram-like reaction with alcohol.

Dose—*Intravenous, adult,* **2 g** every 6 to 12 hr, for *surgical prophylaxis,* **2 g** administered 30 to 90 min before surgery and repeated 8 and 16 hr later; for *cesaerean section,* **2 g** administered after clamping cord or **1-g** doses after clamping cord and repeated 8 and 16 hr later.

Dosage Form—Powder for Injection: 1 and 2 g.

Cefonicid Sodium

5-Thia-1-azabicyclo[4.2.0]oct-2-ene-2-carboxylic acid, [6*R*-[6α,-7β(*R**)]-7-[(hydroxyphenylacetyl)amino]-8-oxo-3-[[[1-(sulfomethyl)-1*H*-tetrazol-5-yl]thio]methyl]-, disodium salt, Monocid (*SmithKline Beecham*)

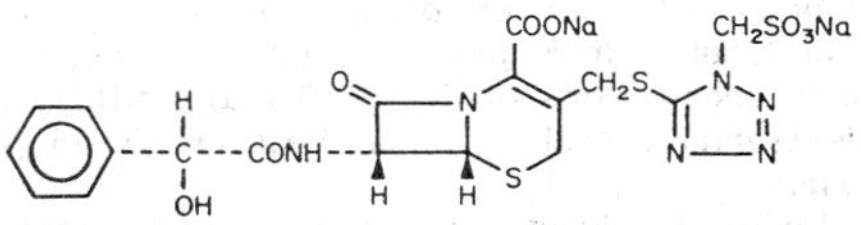

[61270-78-8] $C_{18}H_{16}N_6Na_2O_8S_3$ (586.52).

Preparation—Ger Pat 2,611,270; *CA 86:* 2985t, 1977.

Description—pH (5% solution) 3.5 to 6.5.

Uses—A second-generation cephalosporin (see the general statement). It is approved for use in the treatment of *bone* and *joint* infections caused by *Staph aureus; lower respiratory tract* infections by *E coli, H influenzae, K pneumoniae* or *Strep pneumoniae; septicemia* by *E coli* or *Strep pneumoniae; skin* infections by *Staph aureus* or *epidermidis,* or *Strep pyogenes* or *agalactiae;* and *urinary tract* infections by *E coli, K pneumoniae* or *Prot mirabilis* and for *perioperative prophylaxis.* It is absorbed poorly by the oral route. Intramuscular and intravenous doses of 1 g yield peak plasma concentrations of 99 and 220 μg/mL, respectively. Elimination is almost entirely by renal excretion. The half-life is 3.5 to 4.5 hr, except 17 to 56 hr in renal failure.

Dose—*Intramuscular* or *intravenous, adults,* **0.5** to **2 g** every 24 hr; for *perioperative prophylaxis,* **1 g** 1 hr before surgery or at the time the umbilical cord is clamped in Cesarean section.

Dosage Forms—Injection: 0.5, 1 and 10 g. Each g contains 3.7 mEq of sodium.

Cefoperazone Sodium

5-Thia-1-azabicyclo[4.2.0]oct-2-ene-2-carboxylic acid, [6*R*[6α,-7β(*R**)]]- 7-[[[[(4-ethyl-2,3-dioxo-1-piperazinyl)carbonyl]amino]-(4-hydroxyphenyl)acetyl]amino]-3-[[(1-methyl-1*H*-tetrazol-5-yl)-thio]methyl]-8-oxo, monosodium salt, Cefobid (*Roerig*)

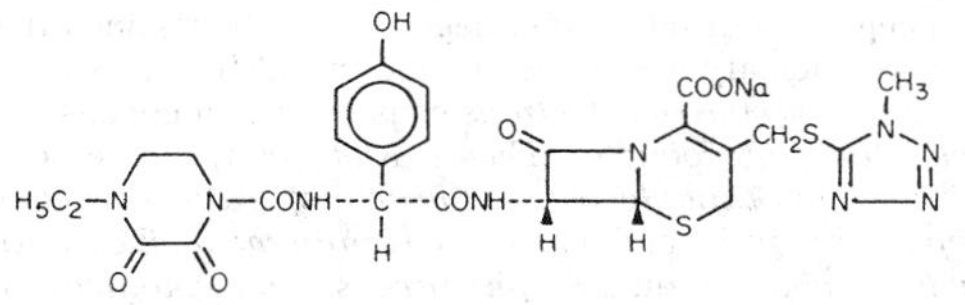

[62893-20-3] $C_{25}H_{26}N_9NaO_8S_2$ (667.65).

Preparation—See Belg Pat 837,682; *CA 87:* 6002v, 1977.

Description—White powder; melts about 170°; pH (25% aqueous solution), 4.5 to 6.5; unstable in alkaline solution.

Uses—A third-generation cephalosporin with antibacterial activities typical of that class (see the general statement). It is more active than other third-generation cepohalosporins except ceftazidime against *Ps aeruginosa* but is not active against β-lactamase-producing *B fragilis.* It is less active than cefotaxime or moxalactam against most gram-negative enteric bacteria but is more active against *Ps aeruginosa.* It is unique among cephalosporins in that dosage adjustments are not required in renal failure. It is approved for use in *urinary tract infections* caused by *Enterobacter, Ps aeruginosa* and anaerobic cocci and bacilli; *respiratory tract infections* caused by *Enterobacter, E coli, H influenzae, K pneumoniae,* pneumococci, *Proteus, Ps aeruginosa, Staph aureus* and *Strep pyogenes; cutaneous infections* by *Ps aeruginosa, Staph aureus* and *Strep pyogenes; gynecological infections* by *Bacterioides, Clostridia,* anaerobic cocci, *E coli,* gonococcus, *Staph aureus* and *epidermidis* and *Strep agalactiae; bone* and *joint infections* by *Enterobacter, E coli, Klebsiella, Proteus, Pseudomonas* and *Staph aureus;* and *septicemina* by anaerobic gram-positive cocci, *Clostridium, E coli, H influenzae, Klebsiella,* pneumonococcus, *Ps aeruginosa*), *Staph aureus* and *Strep agalactiae* and *pyogenes.* In serious infections by gram-negative bacilli, it is customary to combine it with an aminoglycoside. The adverse effects are those of cephalosporins in general (see the general statement), but the incidence is low. There is a tendency towards hypoprothrombinemia. It causes a disulfiram-like reaction to ethanol.

Orally, it is absorbed poorly. An intravenous infusion of 1 g yields a peak plasma concentration of 153 μg/mL depending on the rate of delivery, an intramuscular dose 65 to 74 μg/mL. In plasma, 82 to 93% is protein-bound. The volume of distribution 0.13 to 0.20 mL/g in adults but 0.5 mL/g in neonates. Biliary secretion eliminates 70% and urinary excretion 30% of the drug. Serum half-life is 1.9 to 2.1 hr. Dose adjustments are needed in hepatic but not in renal failure.

Dose—(cefoperazone equivalent): *Intramuscular* or *intravenous infusion, adults,* for *mild infections,* **1** to **2 g** every 12 hr and, for *severe infections,* **1.5** to **3 g** every 6 hr, **2** to **4 g** every 8 hr *or* **3** to **6 g** every 12 hr. Pediatric dosage has not been determined.

Dosage Forms—(cefoperazone equivalent): Powder for Injection: 1 and 2 g. Injection: 1 and 5 g/50 mL. Each g contains 1.5 mEq of sodium.

Ceforanide—see RPS-18, page 1199.

Cefotaxime Sodium

5-Thia-1-azabicyclo[4.2.0]oct-2-ene-2-carboxylic acid, [6R-[6α,7β(Z)]]-3-[(acetyloxy)methyl]-7-[[(2-amino-4-thiazolyl)-(methoxyimino)acetyl]amino]-8-oxo-, monosodium salt, Claforan (*Hoechst-Roussel*)

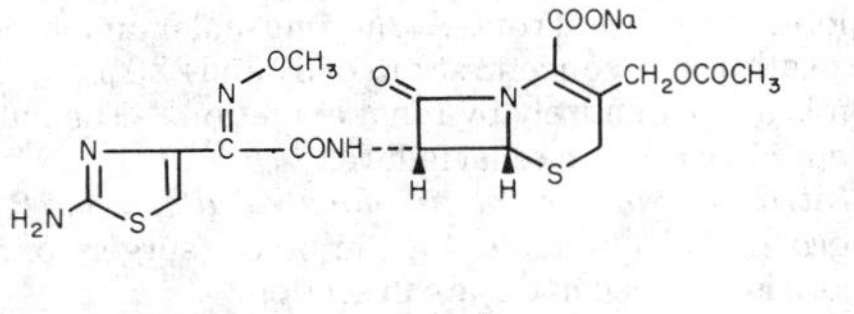

[64485-93-4] $C_{16}H_{16}N_5NaO_7S_2$ (477.44).

Preparation—*Chem Pharm Bull 28:* 2629, 1980.

Description—White to off-white solid; pH (10% solution) about 5.5; pK_a (acid) 3.75.

Solubility—Freely soluble in water; practically insoluble in most organic solvents.

Uses—A third-generation cephalosporin with an antibacterial spectrum characteristic of its class (see the general statement). Against many gram-negative bacilli it is equal to the aminoglycosides, except against *Ps aeruginosa, Acinetobactor* and some *Enterobacter.* It is more active against multiple-drug-resistant gram-negative bacilli than are moxalactam ceftazidime and cefoperazone. It is more resistant to β-lactamases than are earlier generation drugs. Against *Staph aureus,* it is less active than first- or second-generation cephalosporins. It is a preferred third-generation cephalosporin for gram-negative meningitis and other serious gram-negative bacillary infections outside the CNS. It is approved for use against *genitourinary infections* caused by gonococcus, *Enterococcus, Atrobacter, Enterobacter, E coli, Klebsiella,* indole-positive *Proteus, Serrata* and *Staphylococcus; lower respiratory tract infections* from *Strep pneumoniae* and *pyogenes, H influenzae, E coli, Klebsiella, Serratia Enterobacter* and *Staph aureus; gynecological infections* caused by *E coli, Enterococcus, Klebsiella, Pr mirabilis, Bacterioides, Clostridium,* anaerobic cocci and *Staph epidermidis; cutaneous infections* caused by *Staph aureus* and *epidermidis, Strep pyogenes, Enterococcus, Enterobacter, E coli, Klebsiella, Serratia, Pr mirabilis,* indole-positive *Proteus, Pseudomonas, Bacterioides* and anaerobic streptococci; *intra-abdominal infections* from *Bacterioides, E coli, Klebsiella* and anaerobic streptococci; *bone* and *joint* infections from *Staph aureus; CNS infections* caused by meningococcus, *H influenzae, K pneumoniae, Strep pneumoniae* and *E coli;* and *septicemia* caused by *E coli, Klebsiella* and *Serratia.* It is used for surgical prophylaxis. When appropriate, it may be combined with an aminoglycoside. It has no unique toxicity (see the general statement). It is very expensive.

The drug is absorbed poorly by the oral route. A plasma level of 80 to 90 μg/mL results from 2 g intravenously. In plasma, 38% is protein-bound. The volume of distribution is 0.25 to 0.39 mL/g. It penetrates into the cerebrospinal fluid. About 85% is eliminated in the urine and 8% in the feces. The half-life is 1 to 1.2 hr, except 3 to 12 hr in renal failure. It is 30 to 50% metabolized to an active β-lactamase-stable metabolite.

Dose (cefotaxime equivalent)—*Intramuscular, adult* and *children over 50 kg,* for *gonorrhea,* **1 g** as a single dose; *Intramuscular* or *intravenous* for *various serious infections,* **1** to **2 g** every 4 to 8 hr, except **1 g** every 12 hr for *uncomplicated infections; surgical prophylaxis* in *cesarian section,* **1 g** intravenously when the umbilical cord is clamped then **1 g** intramuscularly or intravenously at 6 and 12 hr; *other surgical prophylaxis,* **1 g** 0.5 to 1 hr before, once during, and every 6 to 8 hr after, surgery; *infants* and *children 4 wk to 50 kg,* **8.3** to **30 mg/kg** every 4 hr *or* **12.5** to **45 mg/kg** every 6 hr. *Intravenous, neonates up to 4 wk,* **50 mg/kg** every 8 hr.

Dosage Form (cefotaxime equivalent)—Powder for injection: 0.5, 1, 2 and 10 g. Each g contains 2.2 mEq of sodium.

Cefotetan Disodium

5-Thia-1-azabicyclo[4.2.0]oct-2-ene-2-carboxylic acid, [6R-6α,7α)]-7-[[[4-(2-amino-1-carboxy-2-oxoethylidene)-1,3-dithietan-2- yl]-carbonyl]amino]-7-methoxy-3-[[(1-methyl-1H-tetrazol-5- yl)-thio]methyl]-8-oxo-, disodium salt; Cefotan (*Stuart*)

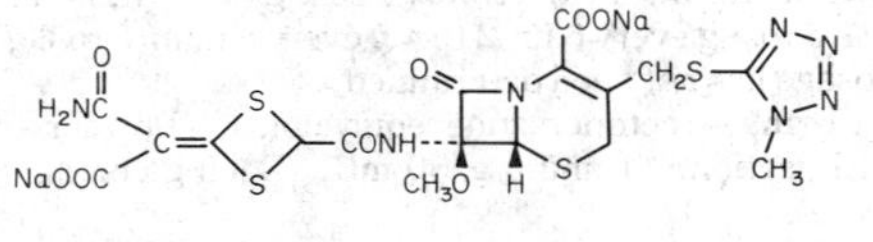

[74356-00-6] $C_{17}H_{15}N_7Na_2O_8S_4$ (619.57).

Preparation—See *Chem Pharm Bull 28:* 2629, 1980.

Description—White to pale yellow powder; pH (freshly reconstituted solution) about 5.5; pK_a 2.1, 3.3.

Solubility—Very soluble in water (the color varies from colorless to yellow depending on the concentration).

Uses—Generally classified as a second-generation cephalosporin that is actually a cephamycin similar to cefoxitin. It is very resistant to β-lactamases and has increased potency plus a broader spectrum against gram-negative bacteria than other second-generation cephalosporins. It is approved for bone and joint infections caused by *Staph aureus;* gynecologic infections by *Bacteroides* (except *B distasonis, ovatus* or *thetaiotamicron), E coli, N gonorrhoeae, Fusobacterium, Peptococcus, Peptostreptococcus* or other gram-positive anaerobic cocci, *Prot mirabilis, Staph aureus* or *epidermidis* and *Streptococcus* (except enterococci); intra-abdominal infections by *Bacteroides* (except *B distasonis, ovatus* or *thetaiotamicron), E coli, Klebsiella* spp and *Streptococci* (except enterococci); lower respiratory tract infections by *E coli, H influenzae, Klebsiella, Staph aureus* or *Strep pneumoniae,* skin infections by *E coli, Staph aureus* or *epidermidis* or *Streptococcus* (except enterococci); and *urinary tract infections* by *E coli, Klebsiella* spp, *Proteus* spp, *Providencia rettgeri* or *Morganella morgani.* It also is used in perioperative prophylaxis.

It has a methylthiotetrazole side chain that is associated with hypoprothrombinemia and bleeding (see the general statement for effects caused by cephalosporins). It is less costly than cefoxitin.

It is 88% protein-bound. Fifty one to 81% is excreted in the urine. The half-life is 3 to 4.5 hr, except 13 to 35 hr in renal failure. A 1-g intravenous dose provides a peak plasma concentration of 150 μg/mL. One g contains 3.5 mg of sodium.

Dose (acid equivalent)—*Intramuscular of intravenous, adult, for mild to moderate systemic infections,* **1** to **2 g** every 12 hr for 5 to 10 days; *for urinary tract infections,* **0.5** to **2 g** every 12 hr *or* **1** to **2 g** every 24 hr; *Intravenous, adult, for severe infections,* **2 g** every 12 hr; *for life-threatening infections,* **3 g** every 12 hr; *for perioperative prophylaxis,* **1** to **2 g** ½-hr prior to surgery except at the time the ubilical cord is clamped in caeserian section.

Dosage Form—For Injection: 1, 2 and 10 g.

Cefoxitin Sodium

(6R-cis)-5-Thia-1-azabicyclo[4.2.0]oct-2-ene-2-carboxylic acid, 3- [[(aminocarbonyl)oxy]methyl]-7-methoxy-8-oxo-7-[(2-thienylacetyl)amino]-, sodium salt; Mefoxin (*MSD*)

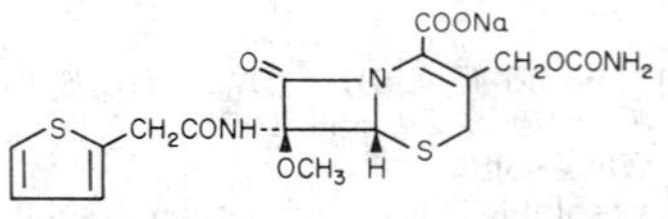

[33564-30-6] $C_{16}H_{16}N_3NaO_7S_2$ (449.43).

Preparation—A semi-synthetic, broad spectrum cepha antibiotic derived from cephamycin C, which is produced by *S lactamdurans.* See *J Amer Chem Soc 94:* 1410, 1972.

Description—Crystals melting about 150°; pK_a 2.2 (acid).

Solubility—Very soluble in water; soluble in methanol; sparing soluble in ethanol or acetone.

Uses—A second-generation cephalosporin. It is not the drug of choice for any infection, but it is an alternative drug for intra-abdominal infections, colorectal surgery or appendectomy and ruptured viscus. It is approved for use in the treatment of *bone* and *joint* infections caused by *Staph aureus, gynecological* infections by *Bacterioides* spp, *Clostridium* spp, *E coli, N gonorrhoeae, Peptococcus* spp, *Peptostreptococcus* spp or *Streptococcus* Group B, *intra-abdominal* infections by *Bacteroides* spp, *Clostridium* spp, *E coli* or *Klebsiella* spp, *lower respiratory tract* infections by *Bacteroides* spp, *E coli, H influenzae, Klebsiella* spp, *Staph aureus* or *Streptococcus* spp (except enterococci), *septicemia* by *Bacteroides* spp, *E coli, Klebsiella* spp, *Staph aureus* or *Strep pneumoniae, skin* infections by *Bacteroides* spp, *Clostridium* spp, *E coli, Klebsiella* spp, *Peptococcus* spp, *Peptostreptococcus* spp, *Prot mirabilis, Staph aureus* or *epidermidis* or *Streptococcus* spp (except enterococci) or *urinary tract* infections by *E coli, Klebsiella* spp or indole-positive *Proteus,* and for *perioperative prophylaxis.* It is absorbed poorly by the oral route. Intramuscularly or intravenously, a 1-g dose will yield plasma concentrations of 24 or 110 μg/ mL, respectively. Elimination is essentially renal. The half-life is 40 to 60 min, except 13 to 22 hr in renal failure.

Dose—(cefoxitin equivalent) *Intravenous, adult,* for *infections,* **1** or **2 g** every 4 to 8 hr; for *perioperative prophylaxis,* **2 g** ½ to 1 hr before surgery, then every 6 hr for 24 hr, except started at the time the umbilical cord is clamped in cesarean section or **1 g** just prior to *transurethral surgery* and every 8 hr for up to 5 days; *infants over 3 mo* and *children,*

13.3 to **26.7 mg/kg** every 4 hr *or* **20** to **40 mg/kg** every 6 hr, except, for *perioperative prophylaxis,* **30** to **40 mg/kg** 1 hr before surgery and then every 6 hr for up to 5 days.

Dosage Forms—Powder for injection: 1, 2 and 10 g; Solution: 1 and 2 g/50 mL. Each g contains 2.3 mEq of sodium.

Cefpodoxime Proxetil

5-Thia-1-azabicyclo[4.2.0]oct-2-ene-2-carboxylic acid, [6*R*-[6α,-7β(*Z*)]]- 7-[[(2-amino-4-thiazolyl)(methoxyimino)acetyl]amino]-3-(methoxymethyl)-8-oxo-, 1-[[(1-methylethoxy)-carbonyl]oxy]ethyl ester, Vantin (*Upjohn*)

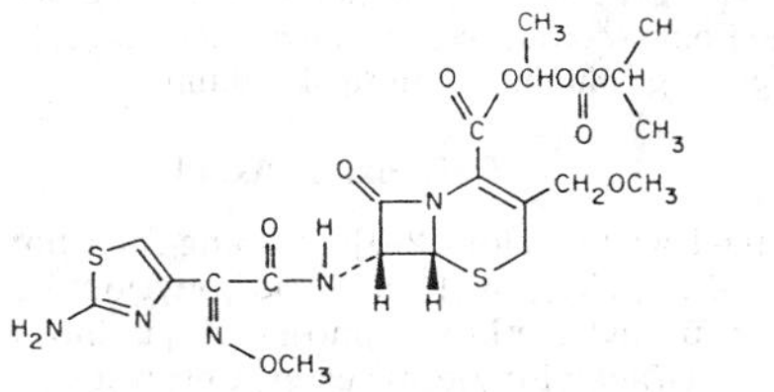

[87239-81-4], [80210-62-4 (acid)] $C_{21}H_{27}N_5O_9S_2$ (557.59).

Preparation—*J Antibiot 40:* 370, 1987. The ester is the prodrug of the metabolite, cefpodoxime, with the free carboxyl group at position 4 of the thiazine ring.

Uses—A newer oral third-generation cephalosporin with good β-lactamase resistance and an antibacterial spectrum similar to cefixime. It is active against gram-positive pathogens of the respiratory tract including *Streptococcus pneumonia, Haemophilus influenzae* and *Moraxella catarrhalis.* Limited clinical experience has indicated it has good activity against β-lactamase-producing *Nesseria gonorrhea* and has better *in vitro* activity than some second-generation cephalosporins against *Staphylococci* and gram-negative bacilli.

It is an ester prodrug that is hydrolyzed during passage through the intestinal wall and only free drug appears in the blood. Oral absorption is increased by concomitant administration of food but is decreased by antacids and H_2-antihistamine receptor antagonists. Serum protein binding is 18 to 23%. It is eliminated primarily by renal excretion and has a serum half-life of about 2.5 hr and impaired renal function increases the half-life. The most common adverse effect reported is diarrhea, but nausea, vomiting and vaginal candidiasis may occur. Patients allergic to penicillin may have allergic reactions to cefpodoxime.

Dose—Oral, *adult and children* ≥ *13 yr,* **100** to **400 mg** every 12 hr; *Children 6 mo to 12 yr,* **10 mg/kg** a day every 12 hr for a maximum of **200 mg** a day for pharyngitis and **400 mg** a day for acute otitis media.

Dosage Forms—Tablets: 100 and 200 mg; Oral Suspension: 50 and 100 mg/5 mL.

Cefprozil

5-Thia-1-azabicyclo[4.2.0]oct-2-ene-2-carboxylic acid, [6*R*-[6α,-7β(*R**)]]- 7-[[amino(4-hydroxyphenyl)acetyl]amino]-8-oxo-3-(1-propenyl)-, Cefzil (*Bristol-Myers Squibb*)

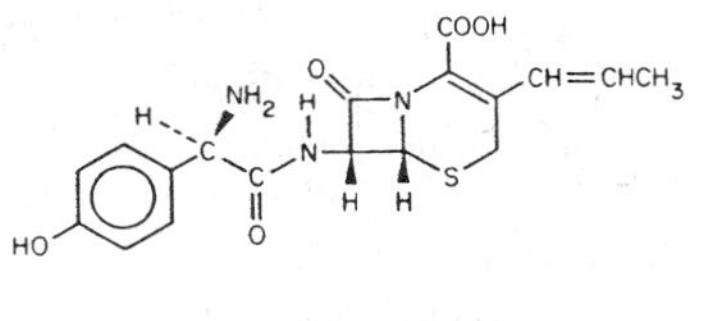

[92665-29-7] $C_{18}H_{19}N_3O_5S$ (389.43).

Uses—A newer oral, second-generation cephalosporin with good resistance to β-lactamases and an antibacterial spectrum similar to cefaclor and cefuroxime axetil. It is as effective as other agents used for upper respiratory tract infections (pharyngitis, otitis media and acute bronchitis) common in children caused by β-hemolytic *Streptococcus, Streptococcus pneumonnia, Haemophilus influenzae* and *Moxarella catarrhalis* including β-lactamase-producing strains.

It is 95% absorbed from gastrointestinal tract and is unaffected by the presence of food. It is excreted mainly by the kidney and has a serum half-life of about 1.3 hr that is prolonged with impaired renal function.

It has some gastrointestinal side effects of nausea, vomiting and diarrhea that tend to be less than those observed with other cephalosporins, erythromycin and amoxacillin-clavulanic acid.

Dose—*Oral, adult and children* ≥ *13 yr,* **500 mg** every 12–24 hr; *infants and children 6 mo to 12 yr,* **15 mg/kg** every 12 hr.

Dosage Forms—Tablets: 250 and 500 mg; Oral Suspension: 125 and 250 mg/5 mL.

Ceftazidime

Pyridinium, [6*R*-[6α,7β(*Z*)]]-1-[[-7-[[(2-amino-4-thiazolyl)-[(1-carboxy- 1-methylethoxy)imino]acetyl]amino]-2-carboxy-8-oxo-5-thia-1- azabicyclo[4.2.0]oct-2-ene-3-yl]-methyl]-, hydroxide, inner salt; Fortaz (*Glaxo*); Tazidime (*Lilly*); Tazicef (*SmithKline Beecham*)

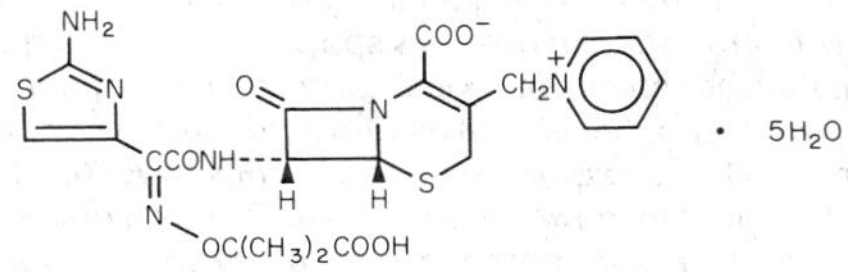

[78439-06-2] $C_{22}H_{22}N_6O_7S_2.5H_2O$ (636.65).

Preparation—See Ger Pat 2,921,316; *CA 92:* 198413c, 1980.

Description—Ivory-colored powder; pK_a 1.8, 2.7, 4.1.

Uses—A third-generation cephalosporin (see the general statement). It is a broad-spectrum antibiotic. It is of special interest because of its high activity against *Pseudomonas* and *Enterobacteriaceae.* It is stated to be as effective as aminoglycosides against most gram-negative bacteria. The drug is more effective than azlocillin against both gram-positive and gram-negative organisms. It is resistant to penicillinases. It is an alternative drug for the treatment of hospital-acquired gram-negative infections. It may be combined with amikacin in the treatment of infections in immunocompromised patients when *Ps aeruginosa* is a potential causative organism.

It is approved for use in the treatment of *bone* and *joint infections* caused by *Enterobacter, Klebsiella, Ps aeruginosa* or *Staph aureus; CNS infections* by *H influenzae, N meningitidis, Ps aeruginosa* or *Strep pneumoniae; gynecological infections* by *E coli; intra-abdominal infections* by sensitive *Bacteroides, Klebsiella, Staph aureus* or *mixed infections; lower respiratory tract infections* by *Citrobacter, Enterobacter, E coli, H influenzae, Klebsiella, Prot mirabilis, Pseudomonas, Serratia, Staph aureus* or *Strep pneumoniae; septicemia* by *E coli, H influenzae, Klebsiella, Ps aeruginosa, Serratia, Staph aureus* or *Strep pneumoniae; skin infections* by *Enterobacter, E coli, Klebsiella* spp, *Proteus, Ps aeruginosa, Serratia, Staph aureus* or *Strep pyogenes* or other Group A hemolytic streptococci; and *urinary tract infections* by *Enterobacter, E coli, Klebsiella, Proteus* or *Ps aeruginosa.*

The adverse effects are those of the cephalosporins in general.

It is absorbed poorly by the oral route. After 1-g intramuscular and intravenous doses, the plasma concentrations are 40 and 70 μg/ mL, respectively. It is 80 to 90% eliminated in the urine. The half-life in normal persons is about 2 hr but longer in renal failure.

Dose—*Intramuscular, intravenous* or *intravenous infusion, adult* for *most infections,* **1** to **2 g** every 8 to 12 hr; for *urinary tract infections,* **0.25 g** every 12 hr for *uncomplicated* and **0.5 g** every 8 to 12 hr for *complicated* infections; *infants* and *children 1 mo* to *12 yr* (intravenous only), **30** to **50 mg/kg** every 8 hr; *neonates up to 1 mo* (intravenous only), **30 mg/kg** every 12 hr.

Dosage Form—Powder for Injection: 0.5, 1, 2 and 6 g.

Ceftizoxime Sodium

[6*R*-[6α,7β,(*Z*)]]-5-Thia-1-azabicyclo[4.2.0]-oct-2-ene-2-carboxylic acid, 7-[[(2,3-dihydro-2-imino-4-thiazolyl)-(methoxyimino)acetyl]amino]-8- oxo-, monosodium salt; Cefizox (*Fujisawa*)

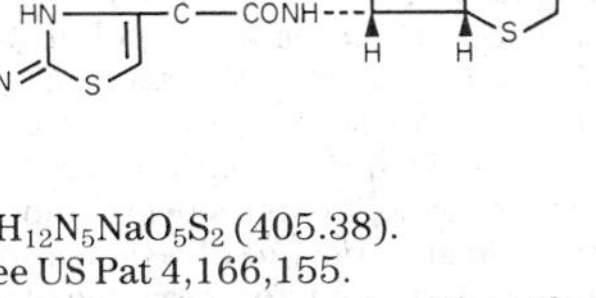

[68401-82-1] $C_{13}H_{12}N_5NaO_5S_2$ (405.38).

Preparation—See US Pat 4,166,155.

Uses—A third-generation cephalosporin with antibacterial activity typical of this class (see the general statement). It is about as active as cefotaxime or moxalactam and more active than cefoperazone against gram-negative enteric bacilli but is less active than cefoperazone against *Ps aeruginosa*. It has unreliable activity against anaerobes. It is not active against enterococci. It is approved for the treatment of *bone* and *joint infections* caused by *Bacteroides* spp, *Peptococcus* spp, *Peptostreptococcus* spp or other anaerobic cocci, *Prot mirabilis, Staph aureus* or *Streptococcus* (except enterococci); *gonorrhea; intra-abdominal infections* by *Bacteroides* spp, *Peptococcus* spp, *Peptostreptococococcus* spp or other anaerobic cocci, *Enterobacter* spp, *E coli, Klebsiella* spp, *Staph epidermidis* or *Streptococcus* (except enterococci); *lower respiratory tract infections* by *Bacteroides* spp, *E coli, H influenzae, Klebsiella* spp, *Prot mirabilis, Serratia* spp, *Staph aureus* or *Streptococcus* spp (except enterococci); *meningitis* by *H influenzae* or *Strep pneumoniae; septicemia* by *Bacteroides* spp, *E coli, Klebsiella spp, Serratia* spp, *Staph aureus* or *Streptococcus* (including pneumococcus but not enterococci); *skin infections* by *Bacteroides* spp, *Peptococcus* spp, *Peptostreptococcus* spp or other anaerobic cocci, *Enterobacter* spp, *E coli, Klebsiella* spp, *Serratia* spp, *Staph aureus* or *epidermidis* or *Streptococcus* (except enerococci); or *urinary tract infections* by *Enterobacter* spp, *E coli, Klebsiella* spp, *Morganella morganii, Prot mirabilis* or *vulgaris, Providencia rettgeri, Pseudomonas* spp or *Staph aureus*. In serious infections caused by gram-negative bacilli, it usually is combined with an aminoglycoside.

Its adverse effects are those of cephalosporins in general.

The drug is not effective orally. Intramuscular and intravenous doses of 1 g yield respective concentrations of 36 and 80 to 90 μg/ mL 30 min after administration. Only 30% is protein-bound in plasma. About 80% is eliminated in the urine. The half-life is about 1.7 hr but much longer in renal failure.

Dose (ceftizoxime equivalent)—*Intramuscular, adult,* for *gonorrhea,* **1 g** as a single dose. *Intramuscular* or *intravenous, adults,* **1** to **4 g** every 8 to 12 hr, except **0.5 g** every 12 hr for *urinary tract infections; infants over 6 mo* and *children,* **50 mg/kg** every 6 to 8 hr.

Dosage Forms (ceftizoxime equivalent)—Injection: 1 and 2 g; Powder for Injection: 1, 2 and 10 g.

Ceftriaxone Sodium

[6*R*-[6α,7β(*Z*)]]-5-Thia-1-azabicyclo[4.2.0]-oct-2-ene-2-carboxylic acid, 7-[[(2-amino-4-thiazolyl)(methoxyimino)-acetyl]amino]-8-oxo-3-[[(1,2,5,6-tetrahydro-2-methyl-5,6-dioxo-1-2,4-triazin-3-yl)-thio]methyl]-, disodium salt; Rocephin (*Roche*)

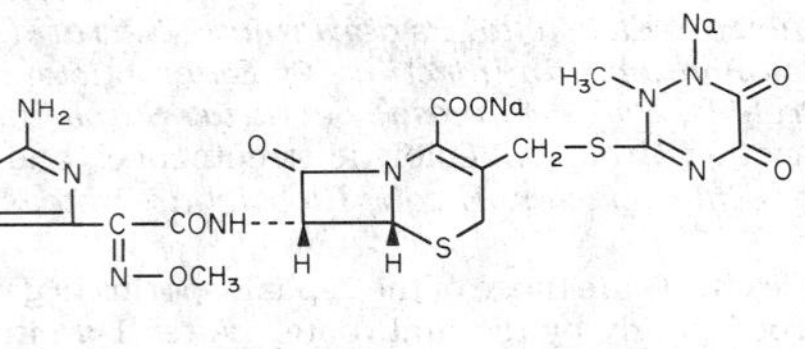

[74578-69-1] $C_{18}H_{16}N_8Na_2O_7S_3$ (598.53).

Preparation—See Brit Pat 2,022,090; *CA 93:* 95289h, 1980.

Description—White to yellowish orange crystalline powder (hemiheptahydrate); melts over 155° with decomposition; $pK_a \approx 3$ (COOH); 3.2 (NH_3^+); 4.1 (enolic OH); solution color varies from light yellow to amber depending on concentration and length of storage; pH (1% solution) about 6.7).

Solubility—Readily soluble in water (about 40g/100 mL at 25°); sparingly soluble in methanol; very slightly soluble in alcohol.

Uses—A third-generation cephalosporin that is the drug of choice for *uncomplicated* and *disseminated gonococcal infections*. It is an effective alternative for meningitis in infants caused by *H influenzae, N meningitidis* and *Strep pneumoniae*. It is effective against gram-negative bacillary meningitis and other serious gram-negative infections, including complications associated with Lyme disease. It is approved for the treatment of *bone* and *joint infections* caused by *Enterobacter* spp, *E coli, Kl pneumoniae, Prot mirabilis, Staph aureus or* various *Streptococcus*, including *pneumoniae* but excluding enterococci, *intra-abdominal infections* by *E coli* or *Kl pneumoniae; lower respiratory tract infections* by *Enterobacter aerogenes, E coli, H influenzae* or *parainfluenzae, Klebsiella* spp, *Prot mirabilis, Serratia marcescens, Staph aureus, Strep pneumoniae* or *Strep spp; meningitis* by *H influenzae, N meningitidis* or *Strep pneumoniae; pelvic infections* by *N gonorrhoeae; septicemia* by *E coli, H influenzae, Kl pneumoniae, Staph aureus* or *Strep pneumoniae; skin infections* by *Enterobacter cloacae, Klebsiella* spp, *Prot mirabilis, Ps aeruginosa, Staph aureus* or *epidermidis* or *Streptococcus* (except enterococci); and *urinary tract infections* by *E coli, Klebsiella* spp, *Morganella morganii* and *Prot mirabilis* or *vulgaris*. It also is indicated for *perioperative prophylaxis*, for which it is as effective as cefazolin.

The side effects are those of the cephalosporins. Some patients show symptoms of cholecystitis.

It is not orally effective. An intravenous dose of 1 g yields a plasma level of about 151 μg/mL after redistribution. Redistribution time is about 2 hr. In plasma, 83 to 96% is protein-bound. Elimination is 40 to 65% renal. The elimination half-life is 6 to 9 hr, except up to 34 hr in renal failure; the long half-life is an important advantage of the drug that permits a single daily administration.

Dose (ceftriaxone equivalent)—*Intramuscular, adult, gonorrhea* (uncomplicated), **0.25 g** as a single dose. *Intramuscular* or *intravenous, adults,* **1** to **2 g** every 24 hr or **0.5** to **1 g** every 12 hr, not to exceed 4 g a day; *children,* **25** to **37.5 mg/kg** every 12 hr, not to exceed 2 g a day. *Intravenous, adults,* for *perioperative prophylaxis,* **1 g** ½ to 2 hr prior to surgery; *children,* for *meningitis, initially* (optional) **75 mg/kg** followed by **50 mg/kg** every 12 hr, not to exceed 4 g a day.

Dosage Form (cefratriaxone equivalent)—for Injection: 0.25, 0.5, 1, 2 and 10 g. 1 g contains 3.6 mEq of sodium.

Cefuroxime Axetil

5-Thia-1-azabicyclo[4.2.0]oct-2-ene-2-carboxylic acid, [6*R*-[6α,7β(*Z*)]]- 3-[[(aminocarbonyl)oxy]methyl]-7-[[2-furanyl(methoxyimino)acetyl]amino]-8-oxo-, 1-(acetyloxy)ethyl ester, Ceftin (*Glaxo*)

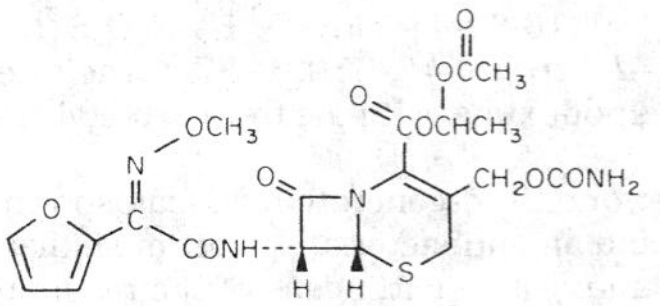

[64544-07-6] $C_{20}H_{22}N_4O_{10}S$ (510.48).

Preparation—US Pat 3,974,153.

Uses—See *Cefuroxime Sodium* for general uses and pharmacokinetics. The axetil amide is more lipid-soluble than the sodium salt, so that it is better absorbed by the oral route. Oral bioavailability without food is 36% compared to 50% fasting. It is approved for the treatment of *otitis media* caused by *B catarrhalis, H influenzae* and *Strep pneumoniae* or *pyogenes; pharyngitis* and *tonsilitis* by *Strep pyogenes; lower respiratory tract infections* by *H influenzae* or *parainfluenzae* and *Strep pneumoniae; skin infections* by *Staph aureus* and *Strep pyogenes;* and *urinary tract infections* by *E coli* and *Kl pneumoniae.*

Dose—*Oral, adults and children over 12 yr,* **250** to **500 mg** every 12 hr, except **125** to **250 mg** every 12 hr for *urinary tract infections; up to 12 yr,* **125 mg** every 12 hr, except **250 mg** every 12 hr for *otitis media* in children *2 to 12 yr.*

Dosage Form—Tablets: 125, 250 and 500 mg.

Cefuroxime Sodium

5-Thia-1-azabicyclo[4.2.0]oct-2-ene-2-carboxylic acid, (6*R*,7*R*)-7-[2-(2-furyl)glyoxylamido]-3-(hydroxymethyl)-8-oxo-, (*Z*)-mono(*O*- methyloxime) carbamate (ester); Kefurox (*Lilly*); Zinacef (*Glaxo*)

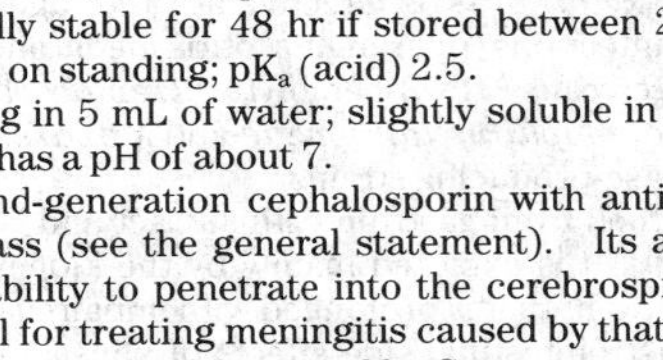

[56238-63-2] $C_{16}H_{15}N_4NaO_8S$ (446.37).

Preparation—See US Pat 3,974,153.

Description—Off-white to white powder; unbuffered aqueous solutions are stable for about 12 hr at room temperature; about 15% decomposition occurs after 24 hr. Suspensions for IM use and solutions for IV infusion are usually stable for 48 hr if stored between 2° and 10°. May become yellowish on standing; pK_a (acid) 2.5.

Solubility—1 g in 5 mL of water; slightly soluble in alcohol. A 10% aqueous solution has a pH of about 7.

Uses—A second-generation cephalosporin with antibacterial activity typical of that class (see the general statement). Its activity against *H influenzae* and ability to penetrate into the cerebrospinal fluid make it particularly useful for treating meningitis caused by that organism; it also is approved to treat *meningitis* caused by *Strep pneumoniae, N meningitidis* and *Staph aureus*. It has excellent activity against all gonococci, hence is used to treat *gonorrhea*. It may be used to treat lower *respiratory tract infections* caused by *H influenzae*, *H parainfluenzae*, *Klebsiella* spp, *E coli*, *Strep pneumoniae* and *pyogenes* and *Staph aureus*. It is approved for use against *urinary tract infections* caused by *E coli* and *Klebsiella*, a more limited approval than for other second-generation drugs. It may be used against *cutaneous infections* caused by *Enterobacter* spp, *E coli*, *Klebsiella* spp, *Staph aureus* and *Strep pyogenes*. *Bone* and *joint infections* caused by *Staph aureus* respond. *Septicemias* that may be treated with cefuroxime are those caused by *E coli*, *H influenzae*, *Klebsiella* and *Staph aureus*. It is approved for surgical prophylaxis. The adverse effects are those of cephalosporins in general (see the general statement). Pain at the injection site is usually slight. However, suprainfections caused by *Pseudomonas* and *Candida* may occur more frequently than with first- and other second-generation cephalosporins.

It is absorbed poorly by the oral route. An intravenous dose of 1.5 g will yield over 100 μg/mL. In plasma, 33% is protein-bound. The volume of distribution is 0.19 mL/g. It penetrates into cerebrospinal fluid. More than 85% is eliminated in the urine; the half-life is 1.3 to 1.7 hr but may be as much as 24 hr in renal failure.

Dose (cefuroxime equivalent)—*Intramuscular* or *intravenous, adults*, for *cutaneous, disseminated gonococcal* and *urinary tract infections* and *pneumonia*, **0.75** to **1.5 g** every 8 hr for 5 to 10 days; for uncomplicated *gonorrhea*, **1.5 g** (intramuscularly) as a single dose; for *serious infections* or those from *less-sensitive organisms*, **1.5 g** every 6 hr; for *meningitis*, **≤3 g** every 6 hr; for *perioperative prophylaxis*, **1.5 g** intravenously 0.5 to 1 hr before and **0.75 g** every 8 hr for 24 hr, if a prolonged procedure; for open heart surgery a total of 6 g, begin when anesthesia is induced and continue every 12 hr for 1 day. *Infants over 3 mo* and *children*, **12.5** to **25 mg/kg** every 8 hr or **16.7** to **33.3 mg/kg** every 12 hr except in *meningitis*, *initially* **200** to **240 mg/kg** a day iv in divided doses every 6 to 8 hr.

Dosage Form (cefuroxime equivalent)—Powder for injection: 0.75 and 1.5 g. Each g contains 2.4 mEq of sodium.

Cephalexin

5-Thia-1-azabicyclo[4.2.0]-oct-2-ene-2-carboxylic acid, [6*R*-[6α,7β(*R**)]]- 7-[(aminophenylacetyl)amino]-3-methyl-8-oxo-, monohydrate Keflex (*Dista*); (*Various Mfrs*)

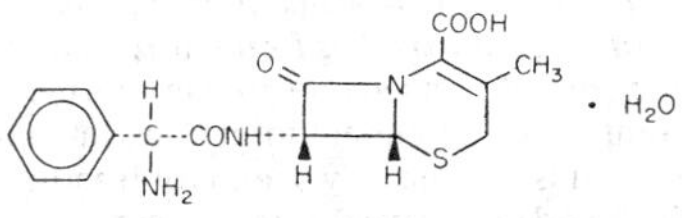

[23325-78-2] $C_{16}H_{17}N_3O_4S.H_2O$ (365.40).

Preparation—*J Med Chem 12:* 310, 1969.

Description—White crystals; pK_a 5.2, 7.3; pH (0.5% solution) about 4.5.

Solubility—1 g in 100 mL water; soluble in dilute aqueous alkaline solutions; very slightly soluble to practically insoluble in organic solvents.

Uses—A first-generation cephalosporin with antimicrobial activity and adverse effects characteristic of that class (see the general statement). It is approved for use against *respiratory infections* by pneumococcus and Group A beta-hemolytic streptococci; *otitis media* by *H influenzae*, *N catarrhalis*, pneumococcus, staphylococci and streptococci; *bone and joint infections* by *Pr mirabilis* and *staphylococci; skin and soft tissue infections* by staphylococci and streptococci; and *urinary tract infections* by *E coli*, *Klebsiella* and *Pr mirabilis*. It is effective orally. Elimination is by renal excretion with a half-life of 0.9 hr, except 5 to 30 hr in renal failure.

Dose—*Oral, adult*, **250** to **1000 mg** every 6 hr, except **500 mg** every 12 hr for *skin* and *soft-tissue infections; children*, for *otitis media*, **18.8** to **25 mg/kg** every 6 hr; for *skin* and *soft-tissue infections*, **12.5** to **50 mg/kg;** and for *other infections*, **6.25** to **25 mg/kg** every 6 hr.

Dosage Forms—Capsules: 250 and 500 mg; Oral Suspension: 100 mg/mL and 125 and 250 mg/5 mL; Tablets: 250 and 500 mg and 1 g.

Cephalothin Sodium

5-Thia-1-azabicyclo[4.2.0]oct-2-ene-2-carboxylic acid, (6*R-trans*)-3-[(acetyloxy)methyl]-8-oxo-7-[(2-thienylacetyl)amino]-, monosodium salt, Keflin, Leutral (*Lilly*); (*Various Mfrs*)

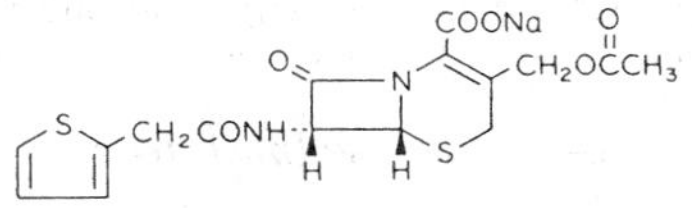

[58-71-9] $C_{16}H_{15}N_2NaO_6S_2$ (418.41).

Preparation—7-Aminocephalosporanic acid is *N*-acetylated with 2-thiopheneacetyl chloride in a dehydrochlorinating environment. The starting acid may be prepared from the natural antibiotic, cephalosporin C, by either proton-catalyzed or enzymatic hydrolysis. The cephalothin thus prepared may be converted into its sodium salt by interaction with sodium acetate in a suitable organic solvent.

Description—White to off-white, crystalline powder; practically odorless; moderately hygroscopic; decomposes on heating; pK_a 2.2.

Solubility—Freely soluble in water, normal saline or dextrose solution; slightly soluble in alcohol; insoluble in most organic solvents.

Uses—Actions, uses and toxicity primarily those of first-generation cephalosporins (see the general statement). It is not the drug of choice or alternate drug for any infection. It is approved for the treatment of *bone* and *joint infections* caused by *Staphylococcus* spp, *gastrointestinal* infections by *Salmonella* and *Shigella* spp; *genitourinary infections* by *E coli*, Klebsiella spp and *Prot mirabilis; meningitis* by *Staphylococcus* sp and *Strep* Group A and *viridans; septicemia* by *E coli*, *Klebsiella* spp *Prot mirabilis*, *Staphylococcus* spp and *Streptococcus* Group A, *pneumoniae* and *viridans; respiratory tract infections* by *H influenzae*, *Klebsiella* spp, *Staphylococcus* spp and *Streptococcus* Group A and *pneumoniae; skin and soft-tissue* infections by *E coli*, *Klebsiella* spp, *Prot mirabilis*, *Staphylococcus* spp and *Streptococcus* Group A; and for *perioperative prophylaxis*. It may cause occasional urticaria, rash, eosinophilia or fever; leukopenia or neutropenia are rare. Superinfections (overgrowth) may occur, especially with *Pseudomonas*. The drug is irritating and may cause pain, induration, sterile abscesses or thrombophlebitis. Acute tubular necrosis is rare, but granular casts in the urine are common after large doses. The sodium can cause adverse effects in persons with congestive heart failure or renal failure. High plasma levels interfere with the determination of creatinine. It is destroyed in the gastrointestinal tract and must be given parenterally. It is bound by plasma proteins to the extent of 70%. The volume of distribution is 0.26 mL/g. An intravenous dose of 1 g will effect a concentration in normal cerebrospinal fluid of 0.4 to 1.4 μg/mL and up to 5.6 μg/mL when the meninges are inflamed. Plasma half-life is 0.5 to 1 hr; it may be as long as 3 to 8 hr in severe renal failure.

Dose—(cephalothin equivalent): *Intramuscular* or *intravenous, adult*, **0.5** to **1 g** every 4 to 6 hr; *perioperative prophylaxis* (*intravenous only*), **1** to **2 g** 0.5 to 1 hr before, during, and every 6 hr after surgery for 24 hr; *children*, **20** to **40 mg/kg** every 4 to 6 hr. See the package literature for other doses and for dose adjustments in renal faiure.

Dosage Forms—Injection: 1 and 2 g; Powder for Injection: 1, 2, and 10 g. Each g contains 2.8 mEq of sodium.

Loracarbef

1-Azabicyclo[4.2.0]oct-2-ene-2-carboxylic acid, [6*R*-[6α,7β(*R**)]]-7-[(aminophenylacetyl)amino]-3-chloro-8-oxo-, monohydrate, Lorabid (*Lilly*)

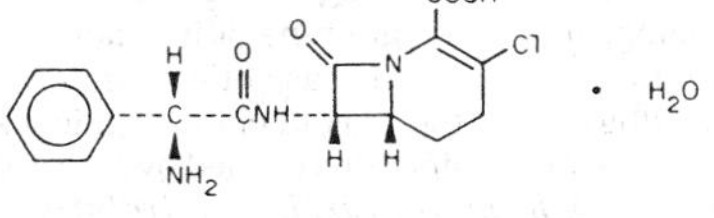

[124750-99-8] $C_{16}H_{16}ClN_3O_4.H_2O$ (367.79).

Uses—A new oral second-generation cephalosporin with good β-lactamase resistance. It is actually a carbacephem that has an antibacterial spectrum similar to cefaclor, cefprozil or cefuroxime axetil. It is an alternative agent for upper and lower respiratory tract infections due to *Streptococcus pneumoniae*, *Haemophilus influenzae* or *Moraxella catarrhalis*. It also may be used for uncomplicated urinary tract infections caused by *E coli* or *Staph saprophyticus*.

It has a serum half-life of 1 hr and is eliminated almost entirely by renal excretion. Protein binding is 25%. The most common adverse effect is diarrhea, but limited experience with this β-lactam antibiotic suggests that one consider its potential for allergic reactions including anaphylaxis. Patients allergic to penicillin may also be allergic to loracarbef.

Dose—**200** to **400 mg** every 12 hr; *infants and children 6 mo to 12 yr*, **15** to **30 mg/kg** a day in divided doses every 12 hr.

Dosage Forms—Capsules: 200 mg; Oral Suspension: 160 mg/mL.

Moxalactam Disodium—see RPS-18, page 1198.

Carbapenems and Monobactams

Carbapenems are penicillin-related antibiotics in which the sulfur atom in the A ring of penicillanic acid has been replaced by carbon. A double bond in the A ring helps the planarity of the ring to approximate that of penicillanic acid. The carbapenems bind to penicillin-binding proteins 1 and 2 and thus have antibacterial actions similar to those of the penicillins. However, they also bind to binding-protein 7, which enables them to kill nongrowing bacteria, a property that undoubtedly will be found to be important in the treatment of infections with large populations of dormant cells (endocarditis, meningitis, ophthalmitis, osteomyelitis, etc). Carbapenems induce β-lactamases but are resistant to them, which resistance accounts for their efficacy against more than 90% of gram-negative species of bacteria.

Monobactams are natural or synthetic analogs of a monocyclic β-lactam antibiotic isolated from certain soil bacteria. The structure is the B ring of penicillin, to which 1-sulfonic acid and various other activating substituents are attached. They bind only to penicillin-binding protein 3, so that their activity is limited to aerobic gram-negative organisms; gram-positive and anaerobic organisms are insensitive. β-4-Alkyl groups confer resistance to most β-lactamases. Monobactams do not induce β-lactamases.

Aztreonam

Propanoic acid, [2-*S*-[2α,3β(*Z*)]]- 2-[[[1-(2-amino-4-thiazolyl)-2-[(2-methyl-4-oxo-1-sulfo-3-azetidinyl)amino]-2-oxoethylidene]amino]-oxy]- 2-methyl-, Azactam (*Squibb*)

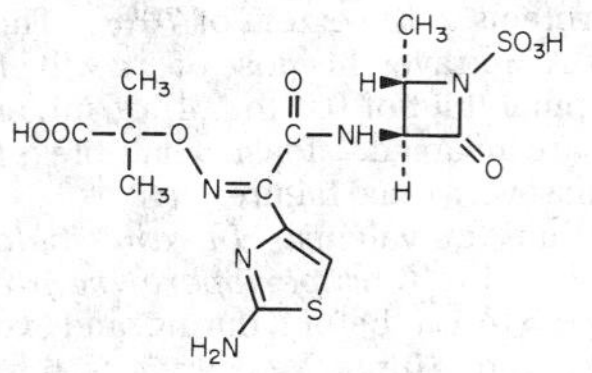

[78110-38-0] $C_{13}H_{17}N_5O_8S_2$ (435.43).

Preparation—Neth Pat Appl 81 00571; *CA 96:* 181062x, 1982.

Description—White powder; decomposes about 227°; pK_a −0.5, 2.6, 3.7.

Solubility—Very soluble in water; slightly soluble in methanol; soluble in DMF; practically insoluble in nonpolar solvents.

Uses—A monobactam with antibacterial activity against most *Enterobacteriaceae* comparable to that of the extended-spectrum penicillins or third-generation cephalosporins. However, it is not active against *Acinetobacter* and is variably active against *Ps aeruginosa.* Against β-lactamase-producing, nonenteric gram-negative bacilli, such as *H influenzae* and *N. gonorrhoeae*, it is as effective as third-generation cephalosporins. It is not yet the drug of choice against any infection. It is an alternative drug against infections caused by *Enterobacter, E coli, Kl pneumoniae, Morganella morganii, Prot mirabilis* or *vulgaris, Prov rettgeri* or *Ps aeruginosa.* This drug and aminoglycosides mutually enhance antibacterial efficacy, and they are combined frequently in serious gram-negative infections. However, in many serious (except urinary tract) infections it often is combined with clindamycin or metronidazole (for anaerobes) or antistaphylococcal penicillin or vancomycin (for gram-positive cocci). Medical opinion holds that, in general, suprainfections are less likely if such combinations are avoided. In bacteremias, intra-abdominal infections, pneumonias, skin and soft-tissue infections and urinary tract infections, efficacy ranges from 80 to 90%. The combination aztreonam-clindamycin is as effective as tobramycin-clindamycin in the treatment of gram-negative pneumonias or intra-abdominal infections.

It causes the adverse effects characteristic of penicillins and cephalosporins except that coagulation defects do not occur. However, it does not cause cross-sensitization with penicillins or cephalosporins.

Oral bioavailability is low. Parenteral doses of 1 and 2 g every 8 hr produce mean steady state plasma levels of 125 or 240 μg/mL, respectively. In plasma, 56% is protein-bound. The volume of distribution is 0.18 mL/kg. The drug crosses the placental barrier and also is excreted in milk. Renal tubular secretion accounts for about 67% of elimination; 7% is converted to a metabolite and excreted and over 1% is secreted into bile. The half-life is 1.7 hr in healthy adults but longer in renal failure or if given with probenecid.

Dose—*Intramuscular* or *intravenous, adult,* for *moderately serious systemic infections,* **1** to **2 g** every 8 to 12 hr; for *serious systemic infections,* **2 g** every 6 to 8 hr; for *urinary tract infections,* **0.5** to **1 g** every 8 to 12 hr.

Dosage Form—Powder for Injection: 0.5, 1 and 2 g. (Contains about 780 mg of arginine per g of aztreonam.)

Imipenem

1-Azabicyclo[3.2.0]hept-2-ene-2- carboxylic acid, [5*R*-[5α,6α(*R**)]]- 6-(1-hydroxyethyl)-3-[[2-[(iminomethyl)amino]-ethyl]thio]-7-oxo-, monohydrate; ing of Primaxin (*MSD*)

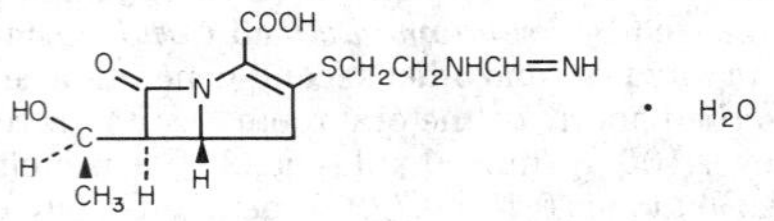

Imipemide[74431-23-5] $C_{12}H_{17}N_3O_4S.H_2O$ (317.36).

Preparation—*J Med Chem 22*:1435, 1979. A crystalline derivative of thienamycin, produced by *S cuttleya.*

Description—White solid; nonhygroscopic; pKa 3.2, 9.9.

Solubility—1g in 1000 mL water or 2000 mL methanol; practically insoluble in ethanol, DMF or DMSO.

Uses—A carbapenem. It binds to bacterial penicillin-binding proteins 1 and 2 and thus interferes with cell-wall synthesis, so that elongation and lysis occur. It is not destroyed by β-lactamases except those from *Ps maltophila* and occasional strains of *Bacteroides fragilis.* It has a broader antibacterial spectrum than any other β-lactam. It includes all cocci (except methicillin-resistant staphylococci and enterococci), *Enterobacteriaciae, Haemophilus, Ps aeruginosa* and most anaerobes, including *Bacteroides fragilis.* It surpasses cephalosporins against staphylococci, equals penicillin G against streptococci, equals third-generation cephalosporins against most aerobic gram-negative bacilli and is comparable to ceftazidime against *Ps aeruginosa.* It is comparable to clindamycin or metronidazole against anaerobes. In the short time since its release it already has become a notable alternate drug for the treatment of infections caused by *Aeromonas hydrophila, B fragilis, E coli, Kl pneumoniae, Morganella morganii, Mycobact avium, Prot mirabilis* or *vulgaris, Prov rettgeri* or *stuartii* or *Ps aeruginosa* or *cepacia.* Some opinion holds that it should be used only for serious nosocomial infections or community-acquired pseudomonal infections in which multiple resistance has occurred. It is particularly useful for treatment of mixed bacterial infections. It should not be used alone for serious infections due to *Ps aeruginosa* because resistance may occur.

The adverse effects are those of other β-lactams. Nausea and vomiting occur with an incidence of 4%, diarrhea 3% and hypersensitivity 3%. A reported incidence of seizures in 1.5% of recipients of imipenem-cilastatin requires confirmation; high doses, neurological disorders and renal failure are said to contribute. The incidence of suprainfections is about 4%. The induction of β-lactamases jeopardizes other β-lactam therapy. There is acquired resistance in up to 60% of strains of *Pseudomonas.*

The oral bioavailability is low. Intravenous doses of 0.5 and 1 g every 6 to 8 hr yield plasma levels of 35 and 70 μg/mL, respectively. Inflamed meninges are penetrated by the drug. Elimination is primarily renal, but the renal tubular cells inactivate the drug. The dehydropeptidase inhibitor, cilastatin, prevents inactivation and enables tubular reabsorption; when it is coadministered, renal excretion of it is about 70%. It is marketed only in combination with cilastatin. Elimination half-life of both imipenem and cilastatin is 1 hr but is increased with decreased renal function.

Dose (anhydrous equivalent)—*Intravenous, adult* and *children 12 yr or older,* for *mild infections,* **0.25** to **0.5 g** every 6 to 8 hr; for *moderate infections,* **0.5 g** every 6 hr to **1 g** every 8 hr; for *severe, life-threatening infections,* **0.5 g** every 6 hr to **1 g** every 8 hr. The dose should not exceed 4 g or 50 mg/kg. The dose of cilastatin is identical to that of imipenem.

Dosage Forms—See *Carbapenim-Containing Combination,* below.

Carbapenem-Containing Combination

An example of a carbapenem-containing combination is as follows:

Impenem and Cilastin [Primaxin (*MSD*)]—250, 500 or 750 mg of each (anhydrous equivalent), powder for injection.

β-Lactamase Inhibitors

Enzymes that open the β-lactam rings of penicillins, cephalosporins and related compounds at the β-lactam bond are known as β-lactamases. There are several classes; classification is based upon general substrate selectivity and inhibition, the acidity or basicity of the enzyme protein and the intra- and extracellular location of the enzyme. Those that are excreted mainly from the bacterium and the genes for which are located on plasmids are called penicillinases. They are Type II β-lactamases. They are mainly responsible for the penicillin-resistance of gram-positive bacteria, gram-negative cocci and a number of gram-negative bacilli.

Penicillinase-resistant penicillins bind to the penicillinases but dissociation of the drug-enzyme complex is relatively rapid. They have been supplanted by clavulanate and sulbactam. These newer inhibitors are β-lactams which acylate the enzyme by forming a double bond and consequently dissociate very slowly. They greatly increase the potency of the penicillins against certain bacteria and thus enhance efficacy.

Clavulanate Potassium

[2*R*-(2α,3*Z*,5α)]-4-Oxa-1-azabicyclo[3.2.0]heptane-2-carboxylic acid, 3- (2-hydroxyethylidene)-7-oxo-, monopotassium salt; ing of Augmentum and Timentin (*SmithKline Beecham*)

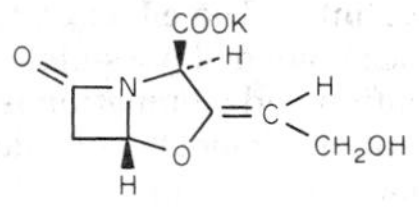

[61177-45-5] $C_8H_8KNO_5$ (237.25).

Preparation—A β-lactamase inhibitor, produced by *S clavuligerus*. It is the first reported naturally occurring fused β-lactam containing oxygen. *J Antibiot 29*:668, 1976.

Description—White powder; bitter-tasting.

Solubility—1 g in 2.5 mL alcohol or in less than 1 mL water.

Uses—The sulfur at Position 1 of the β-lactam ring has been replaced by oxygen and there is an ethylidene moiety at Position 2, which greatly enhances reactivity with the classic exopenicillinases of *Staph aureus* and *epidermidis* and the gram-negative β-lactamases of the Richmond Types II and III (*Haemophilus, Niesseria, E coli, Salmonella* and *Shigella*), IV (*Bacteroides, Klebsiella* and *Legionella*) and V. These are all plasmid-mediated enzymes; chromosomally mediated enzymes are not inhibited. It reacts irreversibly with some but not all β-lactamases. It is not presently available in a single-entity product but is marketed only in combination with amoxicillin and ticarcillin. (See the separate monographs for use in particular infections.)

It is absorbed well by the oral route but is also suitable for parenteral administration. In plasma, about 30% is protein-bound. About 25 to 50% is eliminated by renal tubular secretion, which is inhibited by probenecid; some is metabolized. The half-life is about 1 hr.

Dose—See *Amoxicillin* and *Ticarcillin*.

Dosage Forms—See *Common or Important Penicillin-Containing Combinations*, page 1290.

Sulbactam Sodium

(2*S*-*cis*)-4-Thia-1-azabicyclo[3.2.0]heptane-2-carboxylic acid, 3,3-dimethyl-7-oxo-4,4-dioxide, sodium salt; ing of Unasyn (*Roerig*)

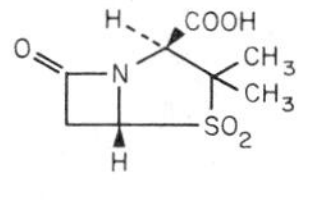

[69388-84-7] $C_8H_{10}NNaO_5S$ (255.22)

Preparation—6-aminopenicillanic is diazotized to form the unstable diazo derivative, which is immediately converted to the 6,6-dibromo compound if the reaction is carried out in the presence of bromine. Catalytic hydrogenolysis of the bromine atoms forms the product. *J Org Chem 47*:3344, 1982.

Uses—A greater activity against Type I β-lactamases than clavulanate, but does not penetrate the cell walls of gram-negative bacteria as well. It extends the antibacterial spectrum of ampicillin to include β-lactamase-producing strains of *Acinetobacter, Bacteroides* and other anaerobes, *Branhamella, Enterobacter, E coli, Klebsiella, Neisseria, Proteus* and *Staphylococcus*. It has weak antibacterial activity of its own.

It is absorbed by the oral route but is also suitable for parenteral administration. The volume of distribution is about 0.27 mL/g. Elimination is mostly by renal tubular secretion; however, it does not interfere significantly with the elimination of ampicillin, the only β-lactam antibiotics with which it is combined. It also is secreted into milk. The plasma half-life is about 1 hr. It is not currently available in a single-entity product.

Dose—See *Ampicillin*.

Dosage Forms—See *Common or Important Penicillin-Containing Combinations*, page 1290.

Aminoglycosides

The aminoglycosides each contain one or more aminosugars, such as glucosamine or neosamine, linked by glycoside linkages to a basic (amino or guanidino) 6-membered carbon ring, eg, streptidine or streptamine.

Antibacterial Spectrum—The major spectrum of activity of aminoglycosides include aerobic gram-negative bacilli and *Staphylococcus aureus*. Only gentamicin, tobramycin, amikacin and netilmicin are reliable against most hospital-acquired infections due to aerobic gram-negative bacteria. Other aminoglycosides have distinct limitations and disadvantages that restrict their uses. For example, gentamicin will inhibit over 90% of strains of *Pseudomonas aeruginosa* but kanamycin will inhibit almost none; similarly, *Actinobacillus mallei* is among the bacteria most predictably sensitive to streptomycin and least to gentamicin. It is easier to state what organisms are not affected: anaerobes (*Bacteroides, Clostridium, Entameba histolytica, Trichomonas vaginalis*), *Rickettsia*, fungi, *Trypanosoma* and viruses. The important antibacterial activities will be described for each agent in its monograph.

Mechanism—The aminoglycosides combine with bacterial (not mammalian) ribosomes to arrest protein synthesis. The initiation complex can be formed, but cannot pass into, subsequent stages of protein synthesis. The binding is quite firm, so that inhibition is severe enough that a bactericidal effect can result. The drugs also appear to interfere with the binding of aminoacetyl-t-RNA, which prevents chain elongation. They further appear to cause misreading of some RNA codons, such that inappropriate proteins can be formed when protein synthesis is not prevented completely. Toxicity in the human is unrelated, and, instead, results from blockade of N-type calcium channels and inhibition of lysosomal phospholipase and sphingomyelinase.

Resistance—Resistance to aminoglycosides develops very rapidly with some bacteria, sometimes as a single-step high resistance. With meningococcus, *Hemophilus* and some other bacteria, even dependence on the drug can occur. Although resistance to one aminoglycoside often confers resistance to others, there are important exceptions that may determine the choice of aminoglycoside for the treatment of certain infections. Both acquired and natural resistance often resulting from bacterial elaboration of aminoglycoside-destructive enzymes; nine such enzymes have been identified. Because of the rapid acquisition of resistance, it is common to employ aminoglycosides only in combination with other antibacterial drugs when the organism is one that rapidly develops high resistance.

Uses—Aminoglycosides have been a very important class of antibiotics because of a former lack of safe drugs to treat infections caused by gram-negative bacilli. Although they still largely are considered to be the cornerstone of antibiotic treatment of nosocomial gram-negative bacillary infections advances in other drug classes threaten to replace aminoglycosides as drugs of choice. Presently, some uses are common to all members of the group, but there are also considerable differences; consequently the uses will be described for each drug.

Toxicity—Most of the toxic actions are common among all aminoglycosides, although there are important quantitative differences in incidence and severity. Hypersensitivity, mostly manifested as rashes but sometimes as drug fever and blood dyscrasias, occurs in 5 to 10% of recipients. Eosinophilia is relatively common. A history of sensitization contra-indicates use. Cross-sensitization occurs. Vestibular and auditory function may be impaired; in the early stages it may be reversible, but often it becomes irreversible if medication is not stopped. Headaches, dizziness and nausea and vomiting during movement are early signs of impairment of vestibular function. Loss of auditory perception of high-frequency sound signals onset of auditory toxicity. Aminoglycosides vary with respect to whether auditory or vestibular function is most affected. High-ceiling diuretics increase risk of ototoxicity.

Nephrotoxicity, manifested by albuminuria, hematuria, cylindruria, azotemia, tubular necrosis and renal failure, is common to all aminoglycosides, although there are marked differences in incidence and severity. Aminoglycosides should not be used in combination with other nephrotoxic substances. Neuromuscular blockade also occurs with high doses, as the result of both postjunctional and prejunctional inhibitory actions, probably because of interference with movement of calcium into nerve terminals and motor endplate. Low plasma-calcium predisposes to the blockade. Aminoglycosides greatly will increase neuromuscular paralysis induced by curarizing drugs and ether anesthetics. Suprainfections ("overgrowth"), most often candidal, may occur during prolonged use, as the result of interference with the normal microbial flora. They favor hypomagnesemia.

The seriousness of toxicity mandates that signs, symptoms and plasma levels be monitored (see in Chapter 37).

Pharmacokinetics—At the pH of the lower small bowel, aminoglycosides are polycationic and, hence, are absorbed poorly from the gut. For the same reason, they are confined mostly to the extracellular space and penetrate cells poorly. The distribution coefficients (Δ') range from 0.19 to 0.28 mL/g. Aminoglycosides penetrate the blood-brain barrier only slightly, unless the meninges are inflamed. Binding to plasma protein is low and ranges from 0 to 34%. The drugs are excreted mostly into urine, the amount ranging from 60 to 100%. The average clinically significant half-lives are about 2 to 3 hr, but there is a much slower phase of elimination that relates to the gradual release of tissue-bound drug; there is greater variation among recipients than there is among the drugs. Renal failure greatly prolongs the half-life. Half-lives in the inner ear are 4 to 5 times those in plasma; the half-lives in the renal cortex range from 25 to 700 hr. These facts help explain the predisposition to vestibular, auditory and renal toxicities.

Amikacin Sulfate

D-Streptamine, *O*-3-amino-3-deoxy-α-D-glucopyranosyl-(1→6)-*O*-[6-amino-6-deoxy-α-D-glucopyranosyl-(1→4)]-N^1-(4-amino-2-hydroxy-1- oxobutyl)-2-deoxy-, (*S*)-sulfate (1:2) salt; (*Elkins-Sinn*); Amikin (*Apothecon*)

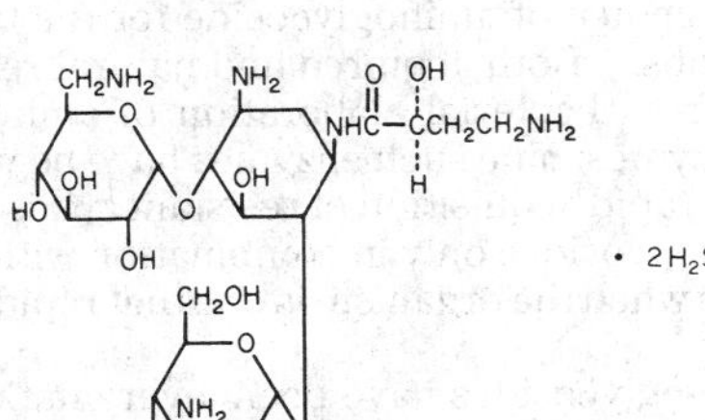

$\cdot\ 2H_2SO_4$

[39831-55-5] $C_{22}H_{43}N_5O_{23}.2H_2SO_4$ (781.78).

Preparation—Amikacin, the 1-L-(−)-4-amino-2-hydroxybutyryl derivative of kanamycin, is obtained by acylation of the C-1 amino group of the 2-deoxystreptamine moiety of kanamycin with L-(−)-4-amino-2-hydroxybutyric acid. German Pat 2,234,315, corresponding to US Pat 3,781,268 (*CA 78:* 136615x, 1973).

Description—Amikacin base: white to off-white flocculent powder, which is converted to the sulfate salt in preparing injection dosage forms; melts (base) at about 203°, (sulfate) at about 225° with decomp; pK_a (base) 8.1.

Solubility—Amikacin base: freely soluble in water; insoluble in alcohol.

Uses—The *N*-(4-amino-2-hydroxy-1-oxobutyl) group protects the aminoglycoside from all but one of the nine aminoglycoside-inactivating enzymes and acetyltransferase. In one study, more than 80% of strains of bacteria resistant to one or more aminoglycosides were sensitive *in vitro* to this drug. The greatest differences are shown with *Ps aeruginosa* and to a lesser extent with various *Enterobacteriaceae*. Most streptococci and a number of strains of otherwise sensitive gram-negative organisms are naturally resistant to the drug by virtue of mechanisms other than drug-destructive enzymes.

The most important bacterial species that are usually sensitive are *E coli, Ps aeruginosa, Proteus spp* (regardless of indole character), *Klebsiella pneumoniae, Serratia marcescens, Providencia stuartii, Citrobacter freundii* and *Acinetobacter spp*. Various staphylococci are also susceptible, irrespective of penicillinase production. The minimum effective concentration is 2 to 4 µg/mL for 90% of "sensitive" bacteria.

Amikacin is considered the drug of choice for empirical therapy of infections caused by gram-negative bacilli in hospitals where bacterial strains are common that are resistant to gentamicin or tobramycin. Development of resistance to amikacin has not occurred where hospitals have used it as the primary aminoglycoside. Septicemia, and serious infections of burns, urinary tract, respiratory tract and various soft tissues, meningitis, peritonitis, osteomyelitis, omphalitis in neonates and serious surgical infections are indications for use, provided the criteria of bacterial sensitivity to amikacin and insensitivity to both less toxic drugs and other aminoglycosides are met.

The toxicity is that of the aminoglycosides in general (see the general statement). Tremors, paresthesias, arthralgia and hypotension also occur. Plasma levels should be monitored where possible, and auditory tests and examination of the urine are mandatory. It is desirable to keep the plasma levels below 35 µg/mL. The effect on the fetus is unknown, and use in pregnancy should be avoided, if possible.

The absorption, distribution and elimination is that of aminoglycosides in general (see the general statement). Intramuscular injection of 7.5 mg/kg will yield a peak plasma concentration of 17 to 25 µg/mL within 1 hr, and intravenous infusion of 500 mg in 30 min yields a mean level of 38 µg/mL. The drug is eliminated totally unchanged in the urine. The half-life is 2 to 3 hr in adults with normal renal function but up to 30 hr in renal failure; in neonates it is 4 to 8 hr. Because of the short half-life, it has been suggested that the usual dose interval of 8 to 12 hr may be too long, but the effect on bacterial protein synthesis outlasts the time above the minimum inhibitory concentration.

Dose—*Intramuscular or intravenous, adult, children* and *older infants*, (use ideal body weight for patients in calculating dose) **15 mg/kg** a day divided into 2 or 3 equal doses for 7 to 10 days, not to exceed 1.5 g a day, except in *urinary tract infections*, in which case the dose is 250 mg every 12 hr; in *neonates, initially* **10 mg/kg** followed with **7.5 mg/kg** every 12 hr, not to exceed 15 mg/ kg/day. In renal failure, the dose is based on creatinine clearance, assuming 100% renal elimination (or see package literature). For intravenous administration, 5% dextrose or physiological saline is used. The duration of infusion should be 30 to 60 min, except 1 to 2 hr in infants.

Dosage Form—Injection: 100 and 500 mg/2 mL, and 1 g/4 mL.

Gentamicin Sulfate

Gentamicin, sulfate; (*Various Mfrs*)

Gentamycins sulfate [1405-41-0]; the sulfate salt of the antibiotic substances produced by the growth of *Micromonospora purpurea*. Potency: not less than 590 µg of gentamicin/mg, on the anhydrous basis.

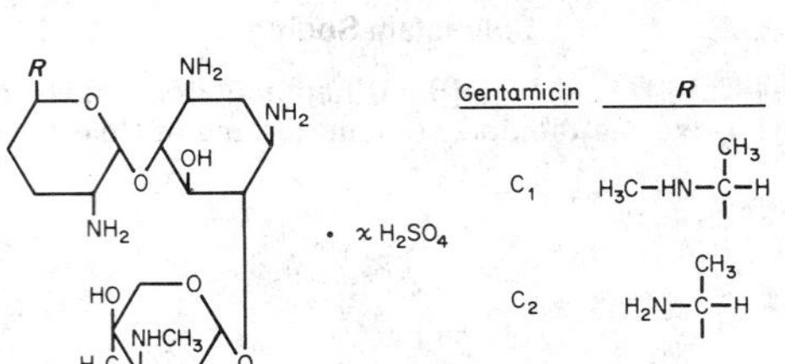

$\cdot\ x\ H_2SO_4$

Gentamicin	R
C_1	$H_3C-HN-C(CH_3)-H$
C_2	$H_2N-C(CH_3)-H$
C_{1A}	CH_2NH_2

Gentamicin is a mixture of gentamicin C_1, gentamicin C_2 and gentamicin C_{1A}. Gentamicin C_{1A} is *O*-3-deoxy-4-*C*-methyl-3-(methylamino)-β-L-arabinopyronosyl-(1→6)-*O*-[2,6-diamino-2,3,4,6-tetradeoxy-α-D-*erythro*-hexopyranosyl-(1→4)-2-deoxy-D-streptamine.

Preparation—Recovered from a fermentation broth produced when submerged cultures of two subspecies of *Micromonospora purpurea* are grown in a yeast extract-cerelose medium. US Pat 3,136,704.

Description—White to buff powder; odorless; stable in light, air and heat; melts with decomposition between 220 and 240°.

Solubility—Soluble in water; insoluble in alcohol, acetone or benzene.

Uses—Currently the most important aminoglycoside for use in the treatment of infections caused by gram-negative bacteria. It has broad-spectrum antibacterial activity. It will inhibit many strains of *Staph aureus* most indole-negative and some indole-positive *Proteus*, nonpigmented *Serratia*, all penicillin-resistant and some methicillin-resistant *Staph aureus* and *Ps aeruginosa*. *Enterobacter-Klebsiella* and *E coli* are also usually highly sensitive. *Citrobacter, Pr inconstans, Salmonella, Shigella, Listeria* and *Brucella* have variable sensitivities. *Neisseria, Clostridia, Corynebacterium Streptococci* and *Ps pseudomallei* are relatively resistant. For most infections, plasma levels of 4 to 8 μg/mL should be achieved.

The action against *Pseudomonas* is of especial interest, since species of that genus resistant to other antibiotics have become an important cause of surgical infections. They also almost always invade burned skin and, furthermore, cause some serious urinary tract infections. However, because of systemic toxicity, present systemic use is limited mainly to life-threatening infections caused by *Pseudomonas, Klebsiella-Enterobacter-Serratia, Citrobacter* and *Proteus*. In these infections it may be combined with an appropriate cephalosporin or penicillin; carbenicillin in high doses can *inhibit* its action. The promiscuous use in the treatment of urinary tract infections amenable to other agents must be condemned.

It is used topically in the treatment of *impetigo*, infected *bed sores, burns* and nasal *staphylococcal carrier state, pyodermata* and in infections of the external eye and adnexa. Its use in minor infections is an abuse. This also applies to its use in preoperative bowel sterilization in most instances.

The toxicity and precautions are those of the aminoglycosides in general (see the general statement). The peak serum concentration should be kept below 12 μg/mL. Cutaneous sensitizing potential is low, but allergic skin reactions and photosensitivity have been reported. Systemic toxicity includes auditory and vestibular impairment (2.3%), nephrotoxicity (2%; if the kidneys are previously normal, nephrotoxicity occurs only with high dose) and neuromuscular blockade, which may interact with neuromuscular blocking drugs.

The absorption, distribution and elimination are those of aminoglycosides in general (see the general statement).

Dose (base equivalent)—*Intravenous, adult*, **3 mg/kg** a day in 3 equal doses every 8 hr for 7 to 10 days; for *life-threatening infections*, up to **5 mg/kg** a day in 3 or 4 equal doses; *neonates older than 7 days, infants and children*, **2.5 mg/kg** every 8 hr; *premature infants* and *neonates less than 7 days old*, **2 to 2.5 mg/kg** every 12 hr. In renal failure, dosage is adjusted according to the creatinine clearance, based on the assumption of 100% excretion. Intravenous infusion should be made over a 1- to 2-hr period. *Intrathecal, adult*, **4** to **8 mg** once a day (use preservative-free preparation); *infants* and *children over 3 mo*, **1** to **2 mg** once a day. *Topical* (*NOTE:* as the sulfate), to eye, **0.05** to **1 mL** of **0.3%** solution every 4 to 8 hr or a small amount of **0.3%** ointment every 6 to 12 hr; *topical*, to skin, as **0.1**% cream or ointment 3 to 4 times a day. Except for enterococcal infections, the urine should be alkalinized in urinary tract infections.

Dosage Forms (as the sulfate)—Cream: 0.1%; Injection: 60 mg/1.5 mL; 4, 20 and 80 mg/2 mL; 400 mg/10 mL; 800 mg/20 mL; 60 mg/ 60 mL; and 100 mg/100 mL; Ointment: 0.1%; Ophthalmic Ointment: 0.3%; Ophthalmic Solution: 0.3%; Intrathecal: 4 mg/2 mL (preservative-free).

Kanamycin Sulfate

D-Streptamine, *O*-3-amino-3-deoxy-α-glucopyranosyl(1→6)-*O*-[6-amino-6-deoxy-α-D-glucopyranosyl(1→4)]-2-deoxy-, sulfate (1:1) (salt); Kantrex (*Apothecon*); (*Various Mfrs*)

[133-92-6; 25389-94-0] $C_{18}H_{36}N_4O_{11}.H_2SO_4$ (582.58); contains kanamycin sulfate equivalent to not less than 75% of kanamycin (583.58) (the antibiotic activity of 750 μg of kanamycin in each mg) and not more than 5% of kanamycin B sulfate on the anhydrous basis.

Preparation—Solely by fermentation using *Streptomyces kanamyceticus*. Review: *Analytical Profiles of Drug Substances*, vol 6, Academic Press, New York, 259–296 1977.

Description—White, crystalline powder; odorless; pK_a 7.2.

Solubility—Freely soluble in water; insoluble in alcohol, acetone, ethyl acetate or benzene.

Uses—Active against gram-netative organisms such as *Klebsiella, Enterobacter, Acinetobacter, Brucelia, E coli, Serratia marcescens* and many strains of *Proteus*. Unfortunately, *Pseudomonas aeruginosa* and *Bacteroides* are resistant. It is also effective against some gram-positive bacteria, especially *Staph pyogenes* and *Staph epidermidis*, most of which strains are inhibited by 1 μg/mL and many others by 2 to 2.5 μg/mL: others, such as streptococci and pneumococci, are not inhibited at levels usually attained in body fluids. However, in combination with a penicillin or cephalosporin it is effective against *Strep faccalis*. It is also effective against mycobacteria in a concentration of 2.5 to 10 μmg/mL. Most sensitive organisms can develop resistance to it. Furthermore, there is almost complete cross-resistance with neomycin and paromomycin. It is used only when there is resistance to safer drugs. It is used in the treatment of *gram-negative septicemias* (particularly in *shock*) serious *urinary tract infections*, gram-negative *bacterial endocarditis, peritonitis, Klebsiella pneumoniae pneumonia, otitis media, sinusitis, osteomyelitis, burn wound infections* and *neonatal meningitis* (especially *E coli*). It is used sometimes in combination with other drugs for use against serious staphylococcal infections and tuberculosis. It is used orally for bowel sterilization in heaptic coma and prior to bowel surgery. The toxicity is that of aminoglycosides in general (see the general statement). About 30% of patients will manifest a hearing deficit and 7% disturbed vestibular function. Ototoxicity is highly probable if the total (cumulative) dose exceeds 10 g. With oral administration, vomiting, diarrhea, steatorrhea and other malabsorption syndromes can occur. Pain occurs at the injection site. Because of its toxicity, it is not used widely, and its status is that of a third-order "back-up" drug. The absorption, distribution and elimination are those of aminoglycosides in general (see the general statement). Intramuscular injection of 1 g yields a plasma concentration of 20 to 35 μg/mL in about 1 hr. Although the half-life is about 2.5 hr in adults, it is 18 hr in premature infants less than 2 days old, and 6 hr in infants 5 to 22 days old. The half-life is prolonged in renal failure, and doses must be adjusted according to creatinine clearance assuming 100% renal elimination.

Dose—(base equivalent): *Oral, adult* for *intestinal infections*. **1 g** 3 times a day for 5 to 7 days: for *preoperative preparation* of the bowel, **1 g** every hr for 4 doses, then **1 g** every 6 hr for 36 to 72 hr; in *hepatic coma*, **2** to **3 g** every 6 hr. *Intramuscular, adult* and *children*. **3.75** mg/kg every 6 hr. **5 mg/kg** every 8 hr, or **7.5 mg/kg** every 12 hr. *Intravenous, adult* and *children*. **3.75 mg/kg** every 6 hr, **5 mg/kg** every 8 hr. or **7.5 mg/kg** every 12 hr for 7 to 10 days. *Intraperitoneal, adults*, **0.5 g** the dose is to be diluted with sterile water to a volume of 20 mL. By any parenteral route, the dose should not exceed 1.5 g/day for up to 5 days. *Inhalation, adults*, **250 mg** every 6 to 12 hr.

Dosage Forms—(as base): Capsules: 500 mg: Injection: 75 and 500 mg/2mL. 1 g/3 mL.

Neomycin Sulfate

Mycifradin Sulfate (*Upjohn*); (*Various Mfrs*)

Neomycin sulfate [1405-10-3]; the sulfate of an antibacterial substance produced by the growth of *Streptomyces fradiae* Waksman (Fam. *Streptomycetaceae*). Potency: equivalent to not less than 600 μg of neomycin/mg, calculated on the dried basis.

Neomycin consists almost entirely of a pair of $C_{23}H_{46}N_6O_{13}$ epimers designated as neomycin B and neomycin C, and the ratio of B to C has been observed to vary widely among different production lots. The total structure and the common names of the component parts of neomycin C are shown below. One g of salt should contain no less than 600 mg of the base.

(Neosamine C) neamine neobiosamine B (2-Desoxy-D-streptamine) (Neosamine C) D-Ribose

Neomycin B

Systematically, it is *O*-2,6-diamino-2,6-dideoxy-α-D-gluco-pyranosyl-(1→3)-*O*-β-D-ribofuranosyl-(1→5)-*O*-[2,6-diamino-2,6-dideoxy-α-D-glucopyranosyl-(1→4)]-2-deoxy-D-streptamine. Neomycin B is identical except that the α-D-glucopyranosyl residue in the neobiosamine moiety is β-L-idopyranosyl.

Description—White to slightly yellow powder or cryodesiccated solid; odorless or practically odorless; hygroscopic; pH (aqueous solution 33 mg/mL) between 5 and 7.5.

Solubility—1 g in about 1 mL water; very slightly soluble in alcohol; practically insoluble in acetone, chloroform or ether.

Uses—Gram-negative bacteria that are sensitive to neomycin are: *E coli, Klebsiella-Enterobacter, Proteus, Pasteurella, Hemophilus, Salmonella, Shigella, N meningitidis, V cholerae* and *Bordetella pertussis; Ps aeruginosa* is usually not sensitive. Sensitive gram-positive organisms are *B anthracis, C diphtheriae, Listeria, Borellia, Leptospira, M tuberculosis, Staph aureus* and *Strep fecalis;* Group A *Strep pyogenes* and *Strep viridans* are resistant. Concentrations of 5 to 10 μg/mL are usually adequate to inhibit susceptible organisms. The antibiotic is used topically in a wide variety of local infections, including *infected dermatoses, burns, wounds, ulcers, impetigo, furunculosis, otitis externa, conjunctivitis* and *sty*, as well as for irrigation of the bladder and urethra during catheterization, as prophylaxis. It mostly is combined with other antibiotics, especially polymyxin B sulfate, bacitracin zinc and gramicidin. It also is incorporated into topical steroid preparations, to control secondary infections in inflammatory disorders; however, evidence indicates that in such preparations, often it fails to control the infections.

Orally, the drug is used to produce intestinal antisepsis prior to large bowel surgery, for the treatment of gastroenteritis caused by toxigenic *E coli* and to suppress ammonia-producing bowel flora in the management of hepatic coma. Orally, it interferes with the absorption of cholesterol and, hence it is used in the treatment of *hypercholesterolemia.* Because of rapid overgrowth of nonsusceptible bacteria, including staphylococci, oral therapy should not be continued for longer than 72 hr; this is not possible for antihyperlipidemic therapy, so a less than maximal dose is used in order to cause less disruption of the enteric floral ecology.

Because it has high toxicity, it is used systematically only in very desperate situations in which the usual antibiotics are ineffective. These are usually septicemias or serious urinary tract or respiratory infections caused by gram-negative bacilli. In some countries it is used as an aerosol in the treatment of respiratory infections.

Although the orally administered drug rarely causes systemic toxic effects, it frequently produces loose stools, nausea, vomiting and malabsorption syndromes. Applied topically, the drug is tolerated well, relatively nonirritating and has a low index of sensitivity. However, contact dermatitis occasionally occurs. Injected parenterally, it causes serious nephrotoxic, ototoxic and neurotoxic effects. The renal injury is usually reversible and is manifested by albumin and granular casts in the urine and an elevation of nonprotein nitrogen in the blood; ototoxicity is mainly auditory and may be additive to that produced by streptomycin. Because of the potential toxicity, parenteral injection and prolonged oral administration are avoided if possible.

About 97% of the orally administered drug is eliminated unchanged in the feces; an oral dose of 3 g produces a peak serum level of only 1 to 4 μg/mL. An intramuscular dose of 1 g produces a peak serum level of 20 μg/mL. Unlike other aminoglycosides, only 50% is excreted unchanged. The half-life is 2 hr.

Dose (base equivalent)—*Oral, adult,* for *preoperative prophylaxis for elective colorectal surgery,* neomycin plus erythromycin base (**1 g** each at 1 pm, 2 pm and 11 pm the day prior to surgery (surgery at 8 am); for *hepatic coma* (as adjunct), *adults,* **4** to **12 g** a day in divided doses for 5 to 6 days, *children,* **50** to **100 mg** a day in divided doses; for *hypercholerolemia,* **350 mg** 4 times a day; *infants and children,* for *bowel sterilization,* **10.3 mg/kg** or **292 mg/m²** every 4 hr for 3 days; for *hepatic encephalopathy,* **437.5 mg** to **1.225 g/m²** every 6 hr for 5 or 6 days. *Topical,* to the skin, as **0.35**% cream or ointment 1 to 3 times a day; to the conjunctiva, as **0.35**% ophthalmic ointment, 1 to 3 times a day.

To calculate doses in terms of the sulfate, multiply by 1.43 (500 mg of the sulfate is equivalent to 350 mg of the base).

Dosage Forms (base equivalent)—Cream: 3.5 mg/g; Ointment: 3.5 mg/g; Ophthalmic Ointment: 3.5 mg/g; Oral Solution: 87.5 mg/5 mL; Sterile Powder, to be reconstituted to 2 mL: 350 mg; Tablets: 350 mg.

Netilmicin Sulfate

D-Streptamine, *O*-3-deoxy-4-*C*-methyl-3-(methylamino)-β-L-arabinopyranosyl-(1→6)-*O*-[2,6-diamino-2,3,4,5-tetradeoxy-α-D-*glycero*-hex-4- enopyranosyl-(1→4)]-2-deoxy-*N*[1]-ethyl-, sulfate (2:5) (salt); Netromycin (*Schering*)

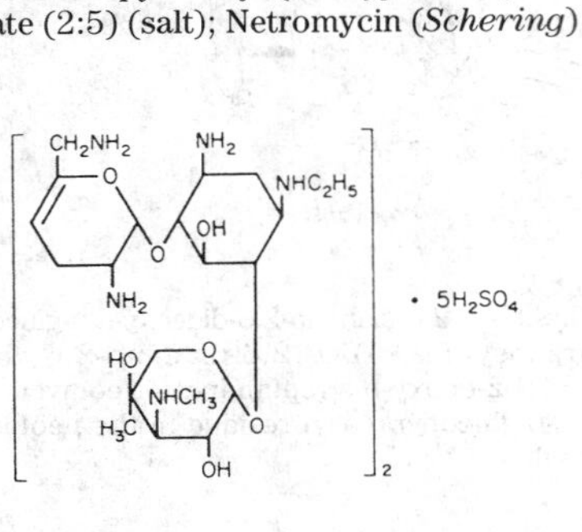

[56391-57-2] $(C_{21}H_{41}N_5O_7)_2.5H_2O$ (1441.54); contains not less than 595 μg of netilmicin base calculated on the dried basis.

Preparation—A semi-synthetic derivative of sisomicin formed by ethylation of the amimo group in the 1-position of the 2-deoxystreptamine ring; see *Chem Commun 206:* 1976.

Description—Off-white powder, p (1 in 25 solution) between 3.5 and 5.5; pKa 8.1.

Solubility—Very soluble in water.

Uses—Has an antibacterial spectrum of activity much like that of gentamicin and tobramycin. However, it is not degraded by certain bacterial enzymes that degrade gentamicin and tobramycin, so that it may be effective at times when there is resistance to gentamicin and tobramycin, especially by *Ecterobacteriaceae.* A large clinical trial found it to be comparable to tobramycin. It does not appear to offer advantages over amikacin. Its toxicity, contraindications and pharmacokinetics are like those of aminoglycosides in general (see the general statement); dose adjustments must be made in renal failure.

Dose—*Intramuscular* or *intravenous infusion, adult,* for serious *systemic infections,* **1.3** to **2.2 mg/kg** every 8 hr or **2** to **3.25 mg/kg** every 12 hr; for serious *urinary tract infections,* **1.5** to **2 mg/kg** every 12 hr. *Infants older than 6 wk* and *children up through 12 yr,* **1.8** to **2.7 mg/kg** every 8 hr or **2.7** to **4 mg** every 12 hr. *Neonates less than 6 wk,* **2** to **3.25 mg/kg** every 12 hr.

Dosage Form—Injection: 20 and 50 mg/2 mL, 150 mg/1.5 mL.

Paromomycin—page 1325.

Streptomycin Sulfate

D-Streptamine, *O*-2-deoxy-2-(methylamino)-α-L-glucopyranosyl-(1→2)-*O*-5-deoxy-3-*C*-formyl-α-L-lyxofuranosyl-(1→4)-*N,N'*-bis(aminoiminomethyl)-, sulfate (2:3) (salt); *(Various Mfrs)*

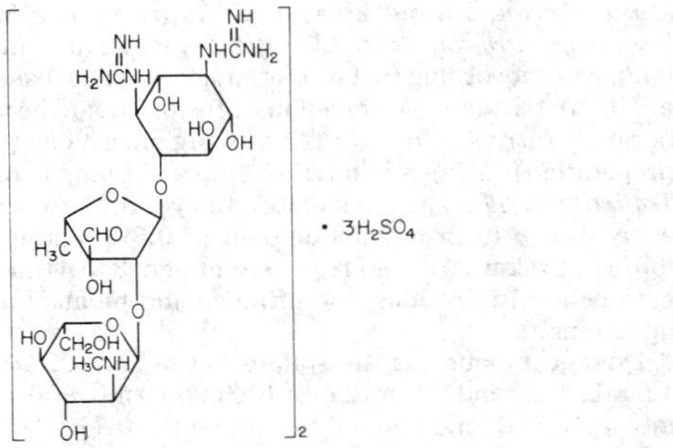

Streptomycin sulfate (2:3) (salt) [3810-74-0] $(C_{21}H_{39}N_7O_{12})_2 \cdot 3H_2SO_4$ (1457.38). Potency: equivalent to 650 to 850 μg of streptomycin $(C_{21}H_{39}N_7O_{12})$/mg.

Streptomycin is an organic base, consisting of *N*-methyl-*l*-glucosamine and streptidine linked through the carbohydrate streptose. The overall structure is portrayed above.

Preparation—Isolated from soil by Waksman and his colleagues of Rutgers University in 1943.

Streptomycin is produced in organic or synthetic media, in surface or submerged cultures of an actinomycete, *Streptomyces griseus,* a mold-like organism with filaments (mycelium) of bacterial thickness.

Commercially, streptomycin is manufactured much like penicillin, microbiologically in tank fermenters with aeration and agitation.

Description—White or practically white powder; odorless or has not more than a faint odor; hygroscopic; but stable toward air and light; pH (1 in 5 solution) between 4.5 and 7.0.

Solubility—Freely soluble in water; very slightly soluble in alcohol; practically insoluble in chloroform.

Uses—Bacteriostatic in low concentrations and bactericidal in high concentrations to a large number of gram-negative and gram-positive bacteria. *Brucella, H ducreyi, Yersinia pestis, Francisella tularensis,* many strains of *M tuberculosis* are sensitive to concentrations that are usually achievable in man. Strains of *E coli, Salmonella, Staph aureus* and *epidermidis, Strep faecalis, pneumoniae, pyogenes* (Group A) and *viridans* and *Yersinia enterocolitica* are variably sensitive.

The only infections in which it alone is the drug of choice are *tularemia* and *bubonic plague.* In combination with a tetracycline it is first choice in the treatment of *brucellosis* and infections caused by *Pseudomonas mallei.* It is an alternate choice drug in the treatment of chancroid, *rat-bite fevers (Spirillum* and *Streptobacillus)* and *tuberculosis;* in tuberculosis, however, it is never used alone, because of the rapidity of development of resistance. Occasionally, it is used as a secondary choice in combination with other drugs in desperate situations, such as gram-negative bacillary bacteremia, meningitis, pneumonia and urinary tract infection.

The toxicity is that of aminoglycosides in general (see the general statement). In addition, malaise and myalgia may occur. Vestibular disturbances are more frequent than loss of hearing.

The absorption, distribution and elimination are those of aminoglycosides in general. An intramuscular dose of 1 g causes a peak plasma concentration of 30 to 48 μg/mL in the adult. Doses must be decreased with impaired renal function.

Dose (base equivalent)—*Intramuscular, young* and *middle-aged adult*, for *tuberculosis*, in combination with one or more of the drugs isoniazid, ethambutol, rifampin or aminosalicylic acid, **1 g** once a day, to be reduced to **1 g** 2 to 3 times/wk, until toxicity or resistance supervenes; *elderly adult*, **0.5** to **0.75 g** once a day; for *tularemia*, **1** to **2 g/day** in 2 or 4 divided doses until the patient has been afebrile for 5 to 7 days (total of about 7 to 10 days); for *plague*, **2** to **4 g/day** in 2 to 4 divided doses until the patient has been afebrile for at least 3 days; for *various fulminating infections* **0.25** to **1 g** every 6 hr *or* **0.5** to **2 g** every 12 hr; *children*, for *tuberculosis*, in combination with other antitubercular drugs, **20** to **40 mg/kg** once a day, not to exceed 1 g/day.

Dosage Forms (base equivalent)—Injection: 5 g/12.5 mL; Sterile powder: 1 and 5 g. 1.25 g of the sulfate is equivalent to 1 g of the base.

Tobramycin

D-Streptamine, *O*-3-amino-3-deoxy-α-D-glucopyranosyl-(1→6)-*O*-[2,6- diamino-2,3,6-trideoxy-α- D-*ribo*-hexopyranosyl-(1→4)]-2-deoxy-, Tobrex (*Alcon*); Nebcin (sulfate) (*Lilly*)

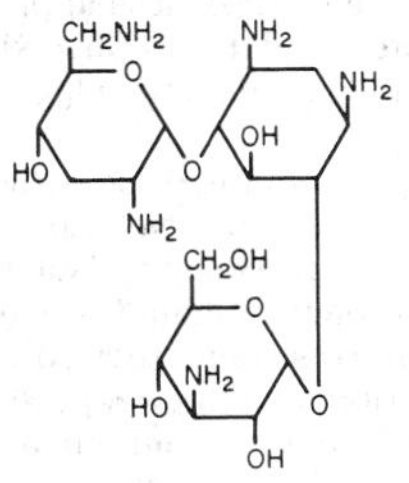

[32986-56-4] $C_{18}H_{37}N_5O_9$ (467.52). Potency: Not less than 900 μg of $C_{18}H_{37}N_5O_9$ per mg, calculated on the anhydrous basis.

Preparation—An antibiotic entity separated from an antibiotic complex produced by *Streptomyces tenebrarius*. In its injection dosage form tobramycin is present as a sulfate.

Description—White or off-white, hygroscopic powder; hygroscopic; pK_a 6.7, 8.3, 9.9.

Solubility—1 g in 1.5 mL water; slightly soluble in alcohol; practically insoluble in chloroform or ether; a 1 in 10 aqueous solution, pH between 9 and 11.

Uses—Bactericidal to most strains of *Klebsiella-Enterobacter-Serratia* organisms in concentrations of 0.75 μg/mL or less, *Staph aureus* in 1 μg/mL and most other gram-negative organisms in 2 μg/mL, except 50% *Proteus* spp and *E coli* in 3 μg/mL and *Pseudomonas* in 5 to 10 μg/mL. Thus, it is generally less active than gentamicin, but it is approximately 4 times as active against *Pseudomonas*. Carbenicillin and certain other penicillins synergize its actions against *Pseudomonas*. Strains with low-level resistance to gentamicin are sensitive to tobramycin, but strains with high-level resistance are not.

Because of its efficacy against *Pseudomonas* infections, it should be used only in the treatment of such infections when they are caused by organisms insensitive not only to gentamicin but other less-toxic antimicrobial drugs as well. In this way, the development of resistant strains is discouraged, and the future value of the drug is not likely to be jeopardized. Despite this precept, the drug is promoted for the treatment of serious infections caused by generally sensitive strains of *Pseudomonas, E coli, Proteus* spp (irrespective of indole character), *Providencia, Klebsiella-Enterobacter-Serratia, Citrobacter* and *Staph aureus*. Although a few staphylococci are susceptible, it is not used for staphylococcal infections, except in combination with penicillin G against identified susceptible strains of *Strep faecalis*.

The toxic effects are those of aminoglycosides in general (see the general statement). Both auditory and vestibular functions may be affected. Plasma concentrations should be monitored and concentrations above 12 μg/mL avoided. Urine should be examined regularly.

The absorption, distribution and elimination is that of aminoglycosides in general (see the general statement). Intramuscular injection of 1 mg/kg will yield a peak plasma concentration of about 4 μg/mL. Elimination is impaired in renal failure.

Dose (base equivalent)—*Intramuscular* or *intravenous infusion, adult*, **0.75** to **1.25 mg/kg** every 6 hr *or* **1** to **1.7 mg/kg** every 8 hr for 7 to 10 days or longer, except up to **5 mg/kg** a day, divided in 3 or 4 equal doses, in life-threatening infections; *neonates up to 1 wk* and *premature infants*, up to **4 mg/kg** of body weight every 12 hr; *older infants* and *children*, **1.5** to **1.9 mg/kg** every 6 hr *or* **2** to **2.5 mg/kg** every 8 hr. In renal failure the dose must be adjusted according to the creatinine clearance, based on 100% excretion.

Dosage Forms (base equivalent; the injection is prepared with the aid of sulfuric acid to solubilize the tobramycin and it exists, therefore, as the sulfate salt)—Injection: 20 and 80 mg/2 mL and 60 mg/1.5 mL. Sterile Powder: 1.2 g.

Aminoglycoside-Containing Combinations

Some examples of aminoglycoside-containing combinations (with content/mL or g provided) are as follows:

Neomycin Sulfate and Polymyxin B Sulfate [Neosporin G.U. Irrigant (*Burroughs Wellcome*)]—40 mg and 200,000 Units, respectively; G.U. irrigant. [Neosporin (*Burroughs Wellcome*); Startol (*Alcon*)]—3.5 and 10,000 Units, respectively; cream, ophthalmic ointment. [Statrol (*Alcon*)]—3.5 mg and 16,250 units, respectively; ophthalmic solution.

Neomycin Sulfate, Polymyxin B Sulfate and Bacitracin Zinc [Neosporin and Neosporin Ophthalmic (*Burroughs Wellcome*); Triple Antibiotic (*Various Mfrs*); Mycitracin Triple Antibiotic and Mycitracin Ophthalmic (*Upjohn*); (*Various Mfrs*)]—3.5 or 5 mg, 5000 Units and 400 or 500 Units, respectively; ointment and ophthalmic ointment.

Neomycin Sulfate, Polymyxin B Sulfate and Gramicidin [AK-Spore (*Akorn*); Neocidin (*Major*), Neosporin Ophthalmic (*Burroughs Wellcome*)]—1.75 mg, 10,000 units and 0.025 mg, respectively; ophthalmic solution.

Macrolides

The macrolides are hydroxylated macrocyclic lactones containing 12 to 20 carbon atoms in the primary ring. There are 37 known members of this class but only erythromycin and its derivatives have been used widely. Two new macrolides, clarithromycin and azithromycin were approved in 1991. These are chemically similiar to the 14-membered-ring maculolide, erythromycin. Clarithromycin is a 6-methoxyerythromycin. Azithromycin is a 15-membered-ring macrolide.

Macrolides bind to the 50s subunit of the bacterial ribosome. The main effect is an inhibition of the translocation step in protein synthesis, so that the synthesis itself is inhibited. The complex has a low-enough affinity constant that some protein synthesis can take place, so that these drugs are mainly bacteriostatic in therapeutic concentrations. Macrolides bind equally to ribosomes from gram-positive and gram-negative bacteria; the much greater effect on gram-positive organisms is the result of greater permeation of the cell membrane. Macrolides do not bind to mammalian ribosomes. The activities and uses of erythromycin-type macrolides are discussed mainly under the prototype, erythromycin.

Azithromycin

Oxa-6-azacyclopentadecan-15-one, 13-[(2,6-dideoxy-3-*C*-methyl-[2*R*-(2*R**,3*S**,4*R**,5*R**,8*R**,10*R**,11*R**,12*S**,13*S**,14*R**)]-3-*O*-methyl-α-L-*ribo*-hexopyranosyl)oxy]-2-ethyl-3,4,10-trihydroxy-3,5,6,8,10,12,14-heptamethyl-11-[[3,4,6-trideoxy-3-(dimethylamino)-β-D-*xylo*-hexopyranosyl]oxy]-, Zithromax (*Pfizer*)

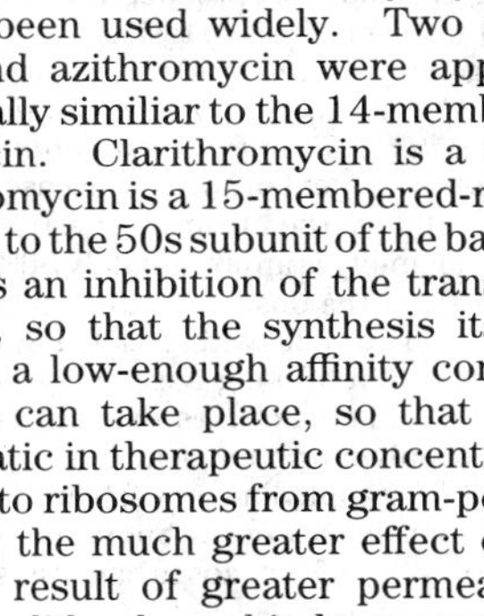

[83905-01-5] $C_{38}H_{72}N_2O_{12}$ (749.00).

Preparation—A semisynthetic macrolide similar to erythromycin A; US pat 4,517,359.

Description—White crystals; melts about 114°.

Uses—A new alternative macrolide to erythromycin that has a similar spectrum of activity. It is active against staphylococci and streptococci but is more active than erythromycin against *Haemophilus influenzae* and some aerobic gram-negative bacilli. Differences have yet to be clinically significant for treatment of any infections. Azithromycin should be taken at least 1 hr before or 2 hr after a meal because food decreases bioavailability. It has a half-life of 68 hr, which is much longer than any other macrolide. Only 6% is recovered from the urine; hepatic metabolism and biliary excretion account for most of its clearance. It is concentrated in phagocytes and fibroblasts. Side effects most frequently reported are diarrhea, nausea and abdominal pain, but these are less than those observed with erythromycin. Azithromycin should not be taken with food or antacids containing aluminum or magnesium.

It currently is being evaluated for treatment of some difficult-to-treat infections in AIDS patients with promising results (eg, disseminated *Mycobacterium* infections, *Toxoplasma* encephalitis and crytosporidiosis).

Dose—*Oral, adult* $\geq$ *16 yr*, **500 mg** on first day followed by **250 mg** a day for a total of **1.5 g;** for nongonococcal urtheritis due to *C trachomatis*, give a single 1-g dose.

Dosage Forms—Capsules: 250 mg.

Clarithromycin

Erythromycin, 6-*O*-methyl; Biaxin (*Abbott*)

[81103-11-9] $C_{38}H_{69}NO_{13}$ (747.96)

For the structure of *Erythromycin base*, see next monograph.

Preparation—US Pat 4,331,802.

Description—Crystals; colorless; melts about 220° with decomposition.

Uses—An alternative to erythromycin for treatment of streptococcal pharyngitis, community-acquired respiratory tract infections, skin and soft tissue infections and acute sinusitis. It is two- to fourfold more active than erythromycin against most streptococci and staphylococci, but organisms resistant to erythromycin are also resistant to clarithromycin. It has moderate activity against *Haemophilus influenzae* and *N gonorrhae*. Also susceptible are *Moraxella catarrhalis, Legionella pneumophilia, Mycoplasma pneumoniae, Chlamydia trachomatis and pneumoniae* and *Borrelia burgdorferi* (agent of Lyme's disease).

Clarithromycin is well absorbed from the gastrointestinal tract with or without food. Bioavailability is approximately 50%. It is metabolized in the liver and 30 to 40% of the dose is recovered in the urine. It has an elimination half-life of 3 to 4 hr with a 250 mg dose every 12 hr but increases to 5 to 7 hr with a 500 mg dose every 12 hr. It is 65 to 70% bound to plasma proteins but penetrates well into tissues and cells, including macrophages and polymorphonuclear leukocytes. It may increase serum concentrations of theophylline or carbamazepine. Diarrhea, nausea, vomiting and dyspepsia may occur but seem to be less frequent than reported with erythromycin. High doses have caused fetal abnormalities in animals.

It currently is being evaluated for treatment of some refractory infections in AIDS patients, with promising results (eg, disseminated *Mycobacterium* infections, *Toxoplasma* encephalitis and crytosporidiosis).

Dose—*Oral, adult,* **250** to **500 mg** every 12 hr.

Dosage Forms—Tablets: 250 and 500 mg.

Erythromycin

Ilotycin (*Lilly*); E-Mycin (*Upjohn*); (*Various Mfrs*)

(3*R**,4*S**,5*S**,6*R**,7*R**,9*R**,11*R**,12*R**,13*S**,14*R**)-4-[(2,6-Di-deoxy-3-*C*-methyl-3-*O*-methyl-α-L-*ribo*-hexopyranosyl)oxy]-14-ethyl-7,12,13-trihydroxy-3,5,7,9,11,13-hexamethyl-6-[[3,4,6-trideoxy-3-(dimethylamino)-β-D-*xylo*-hexopyranosyl]oxy]oxacyclotetradecane-2,10-dione [114-07-8] $C_{37}H_{67}NO_{13}$ (733.94). Potency: not less than 850 μg of $C_{37}H_{67}NO_{13}$/mg, calculated on the anhydrous basis.

Preparation—Elaborated during the growth of a strain of *Streptomyces erythreus.* US Pat 2,823,203.

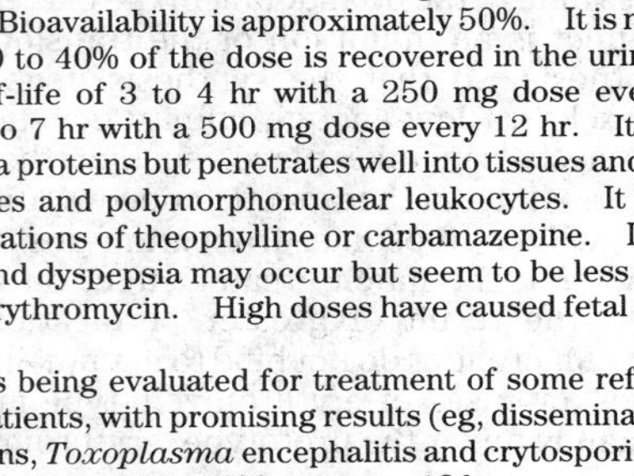

Description—White or slightly yellow crystals or powder; odorless or practically odorless; slightly hygroscopic; pK_a 8.7.

Solubility—1 g in about 1000 mL of water; soluble in alcohol, chloroform or ether.

Uses—A relatively broad spectrum of activity that overlaps the activity of penicillin. It is most effective against gram-positive cocci, such as enterococci, Group A hemolytic streptococci, pneumococci and *Staph aureus. Neisseria meningitidis* and *gonorrhoeae, Listeria, Corynebacterium diphtheria* and *acnes* and some strains of *H influenzae* are also sensitive. Mycoplasma and the agent of Legionnaires' disease are inhibited by low concentrations of the drug. Enterococci are resistant. The drug is equally sensitive against both penicillin-sensitive and penicillin-resistant strains of staphylococci; it is also active against bacteria that have developed resistance to streptomycin. The activity demonstrated by erythromycin against mycoplasma, chlamydia and rickettsia places this drug in the so-called "broad-spectrum" group, although showing low activity against some of the important disease-producing organisms of the gram-negative group. There is no cross-resistance between it and other antibiotics except to other macrolides.

It is the drug of choice in the treatment of infections caused by *Campylobacter jejuni, Chlamydia trachomatis* (pneumonia, urethritis or pelvic inflammation), *Corynebacterium diphtheriae* or *minutissimum, H ducreyi, Bordetella pertussis* (especially the carrier state), *Legionella pneumophila* and *micdadei, Mycoplasma pneumoniae* and *Ureoplasma ureolyticum.* It is one of a number of alternative drugs for the treatment of infections by *Bacillus anthracis, Borrelia burgdorferei, Moraxella catarrhalis, Eikenella corrodens, H influenzae, Mycobacterium fortuitum, Listeria monocytogenes* or *Strep pneumoniae, pyogenes* or *viridans* or *Treponema pallidum.* Although medical authorities do not list it among the choices, it is approved for the treatment of gonorrhea, amebic dysentery and the prophylaxis of neonatal ocular chlamydial and gonococcal conjunctivitis (in which use it is inferior to silver nitrate).

Local infections susceptible to the drug include *impetigo, wound* and *burn infections, infected eczema, acne vulgaris* and *sycosis vulgaris.* Because of the possibility of producing resistant strains of staphylococci, indiscriminate use of erythromycin should be avoided. A large number of staphylococci have acquired resistance to the drug since it was introduced.

Untoward reactions attributable to therapy are uncommon and usually are of little consequence. Nausea, vomiting and, occasionally, diarrhea and stomatitis may occur, particularly with large doses. Serious systemic toxicity has not been observed and there are no absolute contraindications except hypersensitivity; skin eruptions, fever and eosinophilia occasionally occur. Suprainfections, especially of *Candida,* may occur. The drug antagonizes lincomycin and chloramphenicol. Because hepatic dysfunction, with or without jaundice, occurs in some patients receiving oral erythromycin products (especially the estolate), the FDA requires all manufacturers of such products to include in package literature a statement that caution should be exercised in administering the antibiotic to patients with impaired hepatic function.

It is absorbed variably after oral administration. Absorption appears to be of zero reaction order, especially with higher doses. Food interferes with absorption. The antibiotic is destroyed by gastric acid. Peak plasma levels are attained in 1 to 4 hr, following which the concentration declines sharply by the 4th to 6th hr. It is 73% bound to plasma proteins. The volume of distribution is 0.72 mL/g. The plasma half-life is 1.2 to 2 hr, except that it may be up to 5 to 6 hr in renal insufficiency. A single oral dose of 200 to 300 mg usually provides a plasma concentration of 0.6 to 0.8 μg/mL.

The antibiotic does not readily diffuse into cerebrospinal fluid, but attains antibacterial concentrations in peritoneal and pleural fluids. Only 2% of oral and 20% of parenteral erythromycin is excreted in active form by the kidney. Alkalinization favors resorption and thus lowers urine concentration (pK_a = 8.6), but it also increases potency disproportionately, so that the urine should be alkalinized for treatment of urinary tract infections. Alkalinization also broadens the spectrum, so that urinary tract infections caused by gram-negative bacilli respond. The antibiotic is concentrated in the liver and excreted in active form in the bile; the feces of patients given large oral doses contain about 0.5 mg/g. Erythromycin increases the plasma levels of theophylline, caffeine, alfentanil, carbamazepine, cyclosporine, digoxin, warfarin and bilirubin. It interferes with the determination of alanine- and aspartate-aminotransferases and urinary catecholamines.

Dose—*Oral, adult,* **250 mg** every 6 hr, **333 mg** every 8 hr, or **500 mg** every 6 to 12 hr (for *bacterial infections* only). The usual adult oral dose is 250 mg every 6 hr, but the dose may be doubled for more severe infections and infections caused by *Legionella.* In *gonorrhea,* the dose is **500 mg** every 6 hr for 6 or 7 days and in *syphilis* **500 mg** every 6 hr for 14 days except 30 days in late syphilis. In *intestinal amebiasis* (obsolete), **250 mg** every 6 hr or **333 mg** every 8 hr for 10 to 14 days. *Oral, children,* **7.5** to **25 mg/kg** every 6 hr or **15** to **50 mg/kg** every 12 hr for bacterial infections. The dose can be doubled, if necessary. For prophylaxis against streptococci in rheumatic fever and chorea, **250 mg** every 12 hr. *Topical*, to the *skin*, as **1%** ointment 3 or 4 times a day or **1.5** or **2%** solution twice a day and to the *conjunctiva* as a thin strip (about 1 cm) of **0.5%** ointment 1 or more times a day.

Dosage Forms—Enteric-Coated Capsules: 250 mg; Ointment: 10 mg/g; Ophthalmic Ointment: 5 mg/g; Powder: 10, 25 and 100 g; Topical Solution: 1.5 and 2%; Enteric-Coated Tablets: 250, 333 and 500 mg.

Erythromycin Estolate

Ilosone (*Dista*); (*Various Mfrs*)

[3521-62-8] $C_{40}H_{71}NO_{14}.C_{12}H_{26}O_4S$ (1056.39).

Potency: equivalent to not less than 600 μg of erythromycin/mg calculated on the anhydrous basis.

Preparation—Erythromycin is reacted with propionic acid anhydride in acetone solution to form the 2′-propionate ester which then is converted to its hydrochloride. The ester salt then is metathesized with sodium dodecyl sulfate. *J Am Phaarm Assoc 48*:620, 1959.

Description—White, crystalline powder; odorless or practically so; practically tasteless; decomposes about 138°; pK_a 6.9.

Solubility—Practically insoluble in water; 1 g in 20 mL alcohol, 10 mL chloroform or 15 mL acetone.

Uses—The actions and uses are those of *Erythromycin*. The estolate is very insoluble in water, and it is more acid-stable and less affected by presence of food in the stomach than are other erythromycin preparations. About 20% of the estolate is absorbed as the base, and 80% as the ester; the latter undergoes continuing hydrolysis to maintain approximately this ratio. Further hydrolysis at the bacterial-cell level contributes to the activity of the drug. Hepatic dysfunction, with or without jaundice, has occurred in association with its administration, chiefly in adults. The drug is contraindicated in patients with hepatic dysfunction or preexisting liver disease.

Dose—*Oral*, see under *Erythromycin*.

Dosage Forms—Capsules: 125 and 250 mg; Suspension: 100 mg/mL and 125 and 250 mg/5 mL; Tablets: 500 mg; Chewable Tablets: 125 and 250 mg.

Erythromycin Ethylsuccinate

Erythromycin 2′-(ethyl butanedioate); E.E.S. (*Abbott*); (*Various Mfrs*)

Erythromycin 2′-(ethyl succinate) [41342-53-4] $C_{43}H_{75}NO_{16}$ (862.06).

Potency: the equivalent of not less than 765 μg of erythromycin ($C_{37}H_{67}NO_{13}$)/mg, calculated on the anhydrous basis.

Preparation—Erythromycin is esterified at the 2′-position by reacting it with ethyl 3-chloroformylpropionate [$ClCOCH_2CH_2CO_2Et$] in dry acetone in the presence of sodium bicarbonate.

Description—White or slightly yellow, crystalline powder; odorless or practically so; practically tasteless; pK_a 7.1.

Solubility—Very slightly soluble in water; freely soluble in alcohol, chloroform or polyethylene glycol 400.

Uses—Relatively tasteless and, hence, is used in flavored oral "suspensions" for pediatric use. Its actions and uses are essentially those of *Erythromycin*, into which it is converted in the body. In combination with sulfisoxazole, it is approved for use in the treatment of *otitis media* caused by *H influenzae*.

Dose (base equivalent)—*Oral, adults*, for disseminated *gonorrhea*, **800 mg** every 6 hr for 7 days; for *Legionella*, **400 mg** to **1 g** every 6 hr; for *syphilis*, **800 mg** every 6 hr for 15 days in early and 30 days in late syphilis; for *other bacterial infections*, **400 mg** every 6 hr *or* **800 mg** every 12 hr; for *intestinal amebiasis*, **400 mg** every 6 hr for 7 days; for prophylaxis against streptococci in rheumatic fever and chorea, **400 mg** every 12 hr. *Children, see* under *Erythromycin*.

Dosage Forms (base equivalent)—Oral Suspension: 200 and 400 mg/5 mL; Powder for Oral Suspension: 100 mg/2.5 mL and 200 and 400 mg/5 mL; Chewable Tablets: 200 mg; Film-Coated Tablets: 400 mg.

Erythromycin Gluceptate

Erythromycin monoglucoheptonate (salt); Ilotycin Glucoheptonate (*Dista*)

Erythromycin glucoheptonate (1:1) (salt) [304-63-2] $C_{37}H_{67}NO_{13}.C_7H_{14}O_8$ (960.12). Potency: the equivalent of not less than 600 μg of erythromycin ($C_{37}H_{67}NO_{13}$)/mg, calculated on the anhydrous basis.

Preparation—By dissolving erythromycin in an aqueous solution containing the proper amount of glucoheptonic acid and removing the solvent under reduced pressure.

Description—White powder; odorless or practically so; slightly hygroscopic; pH (1 in 20 solution) neutral or slightly acid.

Solubility—Freely soluble in water or alcohol; slightly soluble in chloroform; practically insoluble in ether.

Uses—See *Erythromycin*. This salt is particularly suited for intravenous administration. There may be reversible hearing loss when the intravenous dose exceeds 4 g a day.

Dose (base equivalent)—*Intravenous infusion, adults*, **250** to **500 mg** or **3.75** to **5 mg/kg** every 6 hr, but may be as much as 4 g or more a day, if necessary; *children*, **3.75** to **5 mg/kg** every 6 hr. Intravenous doses should be administered slowly over a period of 20 to 60 min. As soon as the patient's condition indicates an effect on the infection, the erythromycin should be changed to an oral form.

Dosage Form (base equivalent)—Sterile: 250 and 500 mg, and 1 g.

Erythromycin Lactobionate

Erythrocin Lactobionate (*Abbott*); (*Various Mfrs*)

Erythromycin mono(4-*O*-β-D-galactopyranosyl-D-gluconate) (salt) [3847-29-8] $C_{37}H_{67}NO_{13}.C_{12}H_{22}O_{12}$ (1092.23); contains not less then 90% of labeled amount of $C_{37}H_{67}NO_{13}$ (erythromycin).

Preparation—Using lactobionic acid, erythromycin lactobionate (1:1) (salt) is prepared as described above for the glucoheptonate.

Description—White or slightly yellow crystals or powder; faint odor; pH (1 in 20 solution) between 6.5 and 7.5.

Solubility—Freely soluble in water, alcohol; slightly soluble in chloroform; practically insoluble in ether.

Uses—The water solubility of this salt allows it to be given parenterally, either intravenously or intramuscularly. It has the same uses and actions as the base (see *Erythromycin*). Intravenous doses in excess of 4 g a day may cause reversible hearing loss. The parenteral route should be employed only if the patient cannot tolerate the base by the oral route. Once some control of the infection is obtained the preparation should be changed to an oral one if the patient is then able to tolerate it.

Dose (base equivalent)—*Intravenous*, see *Erythromycin Gluceptate*.

Dosage Form (base equivalent)—for Injection: 500 mg and 1 g.

Erythromycin Stearate

Erythromycin octadecanoate (salt); Erythrocin Stearate (*Abbott*); (*Various Mfrs*)

Erythromycin stearate (salt) [643-22-1] $C_{37}H_{67}NO_{13}.C_{18}H_{36}O_2$ (1018.42); the stearic acid salt of erythromycin, with an excess of stearic acid. Potency: equivalent to not less than 550 μg of erythromycin ($C_{37}H_{67}NO_{13}$)/mg, calculated on the anhydrous basis.

Preparation—By reacting erythromycin with the proper quantity of stearic acid in acetone solution and then diluting the solution with water to precipitate the salt.

Description—White or slightly yellow crystals or powder; practically odorless; slightly bitter taste; pH (1% aqueous suspension) between 6.0 and 11.0.

Solubility—Practically insoluble in water; soluble in alcohol, chloroform and ether.

Uses—Actions and uses identical to those of *Erythromycin*. It is insoluble in water and, hence, supposedly is destroyed to a lesser extent in the stomach. It is hydrolyzed in the small intestine and in the tissues to yield erythromycin. It is claimed to give the same blood levels as oral erythromycin, but there is considerable variation, which is partly biological and partly pharmaceutical in cause.

Dose (base equivalent)—*Oral*, same as that of *Erythromycin*.

Dosage Form (base equivalent)—Film-Coated Tablets: 250 and 500 mg.

Spiramycin—see RPS-18, page 1207.

Troleandomycin—see RPS-18, page 1208.

Polypeptides

The polypeptides differ from each other in their mechanism of action and antibacterial spectrum, and grouping them together is only an organizational convenience. Only colistin and polymyxin B have close chemical and antibacterial relatedness.

Bacitracin

Ayfivin; Penitracin; Topitracin; Zutracin; (*Various Mfrs*)

Bacitracin [1405-87-4]; polypeptide produced by the growth of the *licheniformis* group of *Bacillus subtilis* (Fam *Bacillaceae*). It has a potency of not less than 40 USP Units of bacitracin/mg. (The USP Unit of Bacitracin is the bacitracin activity exhibited by the weight of USP Bacitracin Reference Standard indicated on the label of the Standard. The USP unit and that defined by the FDA are equivalent.) Sterile bacitracin has a potency of not less than 50 Units/mg.

Bacitracin is a mixture of at least nine polypeptides, principally bacitracin A, $C_{66}H_{103}N_{17}O_{16}S$ (1411). The structure of bacitracin A has been shown to be

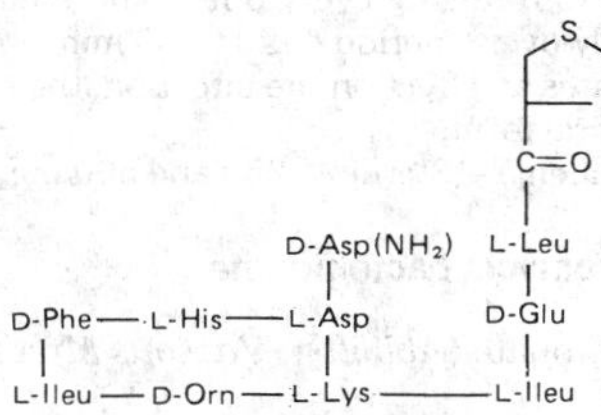

D-Asp(NH₂) — L-Leu; D-Phe — L-His — L-Asp; D-Glu; L-Ileu — D-Orn — L-Lys — L-Ileu

in which the detailed structure at the upper right represents a cyclic condensation moiety derived from cysteine and isoleucine.

Preparation—Several methods for isolation and purification of this antibiotic have been published. For details of certain of these multi-step procedures see US Pats 2,498,165, 2,828,246, and 2,915,432.

Description—White to pale-buff powder; odorless or has a slight odor; hygroscopic; solutions rapidly deteriorate at room temperature; precipitated from its solutions and is inactivated by salts of many of the heavy metals; solutions retain their potency for several weeks if kept in a refrigerator.

Solubility—Freely soluble in water; soluble in alcohol; insoluble in chloroform or ether.

Uses—Effective mainly against gram-positive bacteria. It is limited largely in its use to infections which can be treated by topical application or local infiltration. The high incidence of nephrotoxicity (albuminuria, cylindruria, azotemia, accumulation of drug) which follows its parenteral administration precludes systemic use except in life-endangering staphylococcal infections (pneumonia, empyema) in infants in which other antibiotics have proved to be ineffective or in the treatment of antibiotic-associated (pseudomembranous) enterocolitis caused by *Clostridium difficile.*

It is effective topically in the treatment of the following *cutaneous bacterial infections* where the pathogen is bacitracin-sensitive: impetigo contagiosa, folliculitis, pyoderma, ecthyma, furunculosis, decubitus ulcer, infectious eczematoid dermatitis, scabies and dermatophytosis. The drug is used in the treatment of *ophthalmological conditions* including styes, acute and chronic conjunctivitis, corneal ulcer, keratitis and dacryocystitis. *Infections of the ear, mouth and nasopharynx* such as Vincent's angina, pharyngitis, chronic suppurative otitis media and mastoiditis have been treated successfully with bacitracin. The zinc salt often is preferred for topical therapy and is the form most often incorporated into combinations. It usually is combined with neomycin and polymyxin B sulfate.

Development of bacterial resistance is much less frequent and slower for bacitracin than for penicillin, and for most organisms it is essentially nil. The drug is not inactivated by the metabolic products of mixed infections.

In addition to renal damage, toxic effects of parenteral use include pain, induration and petechiae at the site of injection, skin rash, malaise, anorexia, nausea and vomiting. In a few instances tinnitus and a peculiar taste may be noted. Topical application is usually not irritating and rarely induces allergic reactions.

It is not effective by the oral route. Systemically, the half-life is about 1.5 hr. Approximately 30% is excreted into the urine unchanged.

Dose—*Intramuscular, infants less than 2.5 kg,* **900 units/kg** a day in 2 or 3 divided doses; *infants more than 2.5 kg, up to 1 yr,* **1000 units/kg** a day in 2 or 3 divided doses. *Topical,* to the *conjunctiva,* a thin strip (about 1 cm) of ointment containing 400 or 500 units/g every 3 hr or more frequently; to the skin, ointment containing 500 units/g 3 to 4 times a day. Procaine, 2%, in isotonic sodium chloride solution may be used as a diluent for solutions injected intramuscularly, using a quantity sufficient to provide a bacitracin concentration of 10,000 units/mL. Procaine should not be used in bacitracin solutions injected into cerebral tissue or into spinal fluid. *Oral,* for *antibiotic-associated enterocolitis,* **25,000 units** 4 times a day for 7 to 10 days.

Dosage Forms—*for Injection:* 10,000 and 50,000 units; *Injection:* 50,000 units/20 mL; *Ointment:* 500 units/g; *Ophthalmic Ointment:* 400 and 500 units/g.

Bacitracin Zinc

Bacitracins, zinc complex; (*Various Mfrs*)

Zinc bacitracin [1405-89-6]; the zinc salt of a kind of bacitracin or a mixture of two or more such salts. Potency: not less than 40 Units of bacitracin activity/mg.

Description—White to pale-tan powder; odorless or has a slight odor; hygroscopic.

Solubility—Sparingly soluble in water.

Uses—Incorporated into various ointments used for topical antibiotic therapy (see *Bacitracin*). It is more stable than bacitracin, and the zinc may enhance the activity of the antibiotic. The astringent properties of zinc may reduce inflammation. The zinc also aids wound-healing. It frequently is combined with polymyxin B and/or neomycin.

Dose—*Topical,* as ointment containing 500 units/g 2 or 3 times a day.

Dosage Forms (bacitracin equivalent)—In combination with other antibacterial drugs and/or steroids, 111, 400 and 500 units/g in ointments, and 400 units/g in a topical powder.

Capreomycin Sulfate

Capestat Sulfate (*Lilly*)

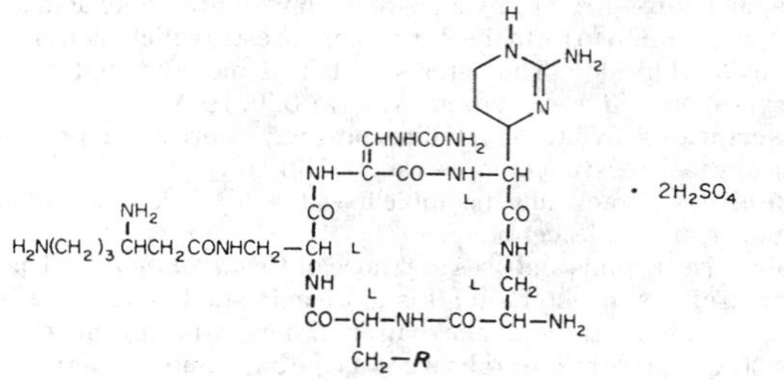

· $2H_2SO_4$

	R	
Capreomycin IA	OH	$C_{25}H_{44}N_{14}O_8$
Capreomycin IB	H	$C_{25}H_{44}N_{14}O_7$

[1405-37-4].

Preparation—An antibiotic produced by *Streptomyces capreolus,* is a mixture of polypeptides, a structure for one of which has been proposed (*Nature 231:* 301, 1971).

Description—White to slightly yellowish white, amorphous powder; essentially odorless; pK_a (in aq DMF) 6.2, 8.2, 10.1 and 13.3; unstable in strong acids or bases; pH (3% solution) 4.5 to 7.5.

Solubility—1 g in 1 mL water; practically insoluble in most organic solvents.

Uses—Possesses antibacterial activity, especially toward acid-fast bacilli, hence used in the treatment of *tuberculosis.* When it is used alone, resistance readily develops. It should be administered only in combination with other antitubercular drugs, such as isoniazid or ethambutol. Capreomycin is a fourth- or fifth-choice drug in tuberculotherapy. It should not be used unless bacteriological sensitivity tests demonstrate its potential usefulness and need. Although it is not chemically related to the aminoglycosides, cross-resistance to kanamycin occurs, and also to viomycin.

As with aminoglycosides, loss of hearing may develop with chronic use; the reported incidence is 11%. Hearing should be tested regularly. Also, as with kanamycin, renal toxicity may occur during treatment; such toxicity includes transient proteinuria, cylindruria and azotemia. Severe renal failure attributable to the drug is rare. Other untoward effects include pain and sterile abscesses at the site of injection, tinnitus, hypokalemia, skin rashes, eosinophilia, leukocytosis, leukopenia and partial neuromuscular blockade that can potentiate that of anesthetics and neuromuscular paralysants.

It is not absorbed after oral administration, so that parenteral administration is required. The half-life is 3 to 6 hr, except longer in renal- insufficiency.

Dose (base equivalent)—*Intramuscular.* **1 g** a day, not to exceed 20 mg/kg a day for 60 to 120 days, then **1 g** 2 or 3 times a wk for 18 to 24 mo. It is always used in combination with other antitubercular drugs.

Dosage Form—Injection: 250 mg.

Colistimethate Sodium

Coly-Mycin M (*Parke-Davis*)

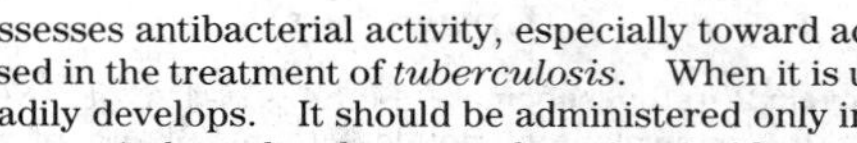

R—C(=O)—Dbu-Thr-Dbu-Dbu-Dbu-DLeu-Leu-Dbu — Dbu-Thr (ring closed through N^γ); N^γ-R′ on the Dbu residues

(Dbu is L-α,γ-diaminobutyric acid; *R* is $CH_3CH_2CH(CH_3)(CH_2)_4$ in the colistin A component and $CH_3CH(CH_3)(CH_2)_4$ in the colistin B component; *R′* is CH_2SO_3Na)

[21236-08-3; 8068-28-8]; contains the pentasodium salt of the penta (methanesulfonic acid) derivative of colistin A, $C_{58}H_{105}N_{16}Na_5O_{28}S_5$;

(1749.81), as the major component, with a small proportion of the pentasodium salt of the same derivative of colistin B, $C_{57}H_{103}N_{16}Na_5O_2S_5$ (1735.78). Potency: the equivalent of not less than 390 μg of colistin base activity/mg.

Preparation—Purified colistin is treated with formaldehyde in aqueous solution, and the resulting colistin-formaldehyde complex (pentamethylolcolistin) is reacted with sodium bisulfite to generate the penta(methanesulfonate).

Description—White to slightly yellow, fine powder; odorless.

Solubility—Freely soluble in water; insoluble in ether.

Uses—Must generate colistin in the body to be effective. Since it is water-soluble, it is a suitable form of colistin for intramuscular injection. By the intravenous route, it has no advantage over polymyxin B sulfate. It has nearly the same antibacterial spectrum as polymyxin B against most gram-negative bacilli, and it also elicits the same renal and neural toxic symptoms. The incidence of nephrotoxicity is about 20%. Like polymyxin B sulfate the drug is especially useful in the treatment of infections caused by *Pseudomonas* and *Serratia* spp. It also may be used to treat serious infections caused by *Ent aerogenes, E coli* and *K pneumoniae.* It is used only when other drugs cannot be used. It is eliminated mainly by renal excretion. It has a plasma half-life of 2 to 4.5 hr. except that it may be 2 to 3 days in severe renal failure. Blood levels should be monitored in renal insufficiency.

Dose (colinstin equivalent)—*Intramuscular* or *intravenous, adults* and *children,* **1.25 mg/kg** 2 to 4 times a day. In *moderate renal insufficiency* (creatinine clearance greater than 20 mL/min), **1.8** to **2.5 mg/kg** every 12 hr; in *severe renal failure* (creatinine clearance 5 to 20 mL/min), **1.25 mg/kg** every 12 hr: with *negligible renal function* (creatinine clearance les sthan 5 mL/min), **0.75 mg/kg** every 12 to 18 hr.

Colistin Sulfate

Colistins Sulfate; Polymyxin E; Coly-Mycin S (*Parke-Davis*)

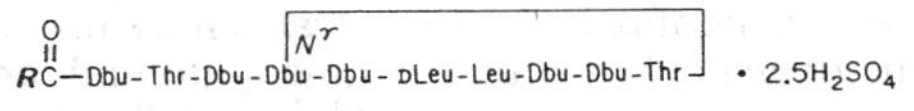

```
  O          ┌Nγ──────────────────────────────┐
  ‖          │                                │
RC—Dbu-Thr-Dbu-Dbu-Dbu-DLeu-Leu-Dbu-Dbu-Thr──┘  • 2.5H2SO4
```

(Dbu is L-α,γ-diaminobutyric acid; *R* is 5-methylheptyl in Colistin A and 5-methylhexyl in Colistin B)

[1264-72-8]. The sulfate salt of an antibacterial substance produced by the growth of *Bacillus polymyxa* var *colistinus.* It consists primarily of colistin A with small amounts of colistin B. Potency: not less than 500 μg of colistin/mg. The colistins are monoacylated decapeptides with seven of the amino acid residues in cyclic union. Colistin B [$C_{52}H_{98}N_{16}O_{13}$ = 1155.45] is a des-homolog of colistin A [$C_{53}H_{100}N_{16}O_{13}$ = 1169.47].

Preparation—Information concerning isolation of colistin from cultures of *Bacillus colistinus* (obtained from Japanese soil), synthesis of colistin A, structure of colistins and probable identity of colistins and polymyxins E is available in reviews by Vogler and Studer (*Experientia 22:* 345, 1966) and in several articles in *Medicanenta 61*(509): 177–234, 1973.

Description—White to slightly yellow, fine powder; odorless; solutions are more stable at an acid pH than at an alkaline pH; the dry powder is stable indefinitely.

Solubility—Freely soluble in water; insolube in acetone or ether.

Uses—The antibacterial spectrum is very similar to that of polymyxin B (this page), but is usually less potent, except against *Klebsiella pneumoniae* and *Serratia marcescens.* It is marketed only for oral administration in the treatment of intestinal infections. It is indicated especially in the treatment in children of acute enteritis caused by *Pseudomonas, Shigella* and *E coli* refractory to other drugs. Resistance rarely occurs. It also is used topically in the treatment of some external ear infections. It has the same toxicity as polymyxin B sulfate (above), but adverse effects by the oral route rarely occur, except in infants. Infants receiving the drug should be examined frequently for impairment of renal function. It is not absorbed by the oral route except in infants, in whom significant blood levels can be obtained by this route of administration. The drug is excreted in the urine. The plasma half-life is about 1.6 to 2.7 hr but it may be 2 to 3 days in severe renal failure.

Dose—*Oral,* **1.67** to **5 mg/kg** 3 times a day; *topical,* to external ear, **0.2 mL** of a **0.3% suspension** with hydrocortisone acetate, neomycin sulfate and thonzonium bromide 3 times a day.

Dosage Form—Powder for Oral Suspension: 300 mg/37 mL (reconstituted).

Daptomycin—see RPS-18, page 1210.

Gramicidin—see RPS-18, page 1210.

Polymyxin B Sulfate

Polymyxin B, sulfate; Aerosporin (*Burroughs Wellcome*); (*Roerig*)

Polymyxin B sulfate [1405-20-5]; the sulfate salt of a substance produced by the growth of *Bacillus polymyxa* (Prazmowski) Migula (Fam *Bacillaceae*). It has a potency of not less than 6000 Units of polymyxin B/mg, calculated on the anhydrous basis.

Preparation—The filtered broth from the fermentation step (see page 1279) is treated with a certified dye and the polymyxin B–dye salt complex thus precipitated is collected by filtration, washed with water and treated with an alcoholic solution of a lower aliphatic amine sulfate. The polymyxin B sulfate thus formed is filtered off, purified and lyophilized.

There are several polymyxins each of which is an *N*-monoacylated decapeptide with seven of the amino acid residues in cyclic union. Polymyxin B is a mixture of polymyxin B_1 ($C_{56}H_{98}N_{16}O_{13}$) and polymyxin B_2 ($C_{55}H_{96}N_{16}O_{13}$) the only difference being in the composition of the *N*-acyl group:

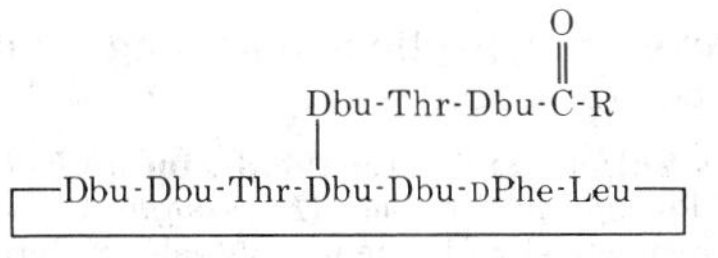

```
                   O
                   ‖
   Dbu-Thr-Dbu-C-R
   |
┌─Dbu-Dbu-Thr-Dbu-Dbu-DPhe-Leu─┐
└──────────────────────────────┘
```

(Dbu = 2,4-diaminobutyric acid)
Polymyxin B_1 R = (+)-5-methylheptyl
Polymyxin B_2 R = 5-methylhexyl

The close relationship between these polymyxins and the colistins (see preceding article) is readily apparent.

Description—White to buff-colored powder; odorless or a faint odor; solutions are slightly acid or are neutral to litmus (pH 5.0 to 7.5); pK_a 8 to 9.

Solubility—Freely soluble in water; slightly soluble in alcohol.

Uses—*In vitro* and *in vivo* antimicrobial spectrum of activity is restricted to gram-negative bacteria, including *Aerobacter, Escherichia, Haemophilus, Klebsiella, Pasteurella, Pseudomonas, Salmonella, Shigella,* most *Vibrio* and *Yersinia;* all strains of *Proteus Providencia* and most of *Serratio marcescens* are unaffected by the antibiotic. Some strains of *Neisseria* and *Brucella* are also resistant. All gram-positive bacteria are resistant. Bacteria initially sensitive to the antibiotic rarely acquire resistance to it.

Systemically, it is indicated only when other drugs cannot be employed. It is used to treat *meningitis* caused by *Ps aeruginosa* and *H influenzae, septicemia* caused by *Ps aeruginosa, Enterobacter aerogenes* and *Kl pneumoniae,* serious *urinary tract* infections caused by *Ps aeruginosa* and other pseudomonal infections. In meningitis, it must be given intrathecally. In systemic therapy it is as effective and no more toxic as colistimethate, despite popular belief to the contrary. The drug also is used topically for the treatment or the prevention and treatment of *external ocular infections* caused by susceptible microorganisms, especially *Ps aeruginosa.* In topical therapy, it often is combined with neomycin, gramicidin and bacitracin. It also is included in glucocorticoid ophthalmologic topical preparations.

It is absorbed readily when injected subcutaneously or intramuscularly. Peak levels are attained within 30 min to 2 hr after injection; the plasma half-life is about 6 hr, but it varies considerably. When the half-life is appreciably longer, the usual doses are cumulative and may lead to toxicity. The drug does not gain access to the cerebrospinal fluid. Gastrointestinal absorption is slow and negligible. The antibiotic is excreted by the kidney; a total of 60% of the administered drug can be recovered from the urine. In renal failure the half-life is longer, and the dose needs to be diminished.

When given parenterally, it adversely can affect the nervous system and the kidney, especially if the total daily dose exceeds 3 mg (30,000 units)/kg. Neurological disturbances are usually subjective and include dizziness, mild weakness and paresthesias of the mouth, face and the extremities. Symptoms are rarely severe when recommended doses are employed; but larger amounts have caused incoordination, ataxia, dysarthria and dyssynergia. Nephrotoxic effects, with damage to the kidney glomerular and tubular epithelium, are manifested by albumin, red blood cells, leukocytes and, occasionally, granular casts in the urine; in severe cases, oliguria and elevated level of serum nonprotein nitrogen are noted. Toxic effects usually clear within 4 days after the last dose of the drug. Substances such as soap, which antagonize cationic surface-active agents, impair the action of the antibiotic.

Dose—*Intramuscular, adult* and *children,* **2.5** to **3 mg/kg** a day in 4 to 6 equally divided doses; *infants* can be given up to **4 mg/kg** a day without adverse effects, and *neonates* and *premature infants* have been given **4.5 mg/kg** a day in serious infections caused by *Ps aeruginosa.*

The intramuscular route is not recommended because of pain at the site of injection. *Intravenous, adults* and *children*, **0.75** to **1.25 mg/kg** every 12 hr; infants with normal renal function may be given up to 4 mg/kg a day. It is imperative to adjust all systemic doses in renal insufficiency. *Topical*, to the *conjunctiva* as a thin strip (about 1 cm) of 0.05, or 0.1% ointment or 1 to 3 drops of 0.1 to 0.163% solution every hour. *Intrathecal*, the following doses are suggested: *children under 2 yr*, 2 mg a day for 3 or 4 days, then 2.5 mg every other day; *children over 2 yr* and *adults*, 5 mg a day for 3 or 4 days, then 5 mg every other day. The intrathecal solution should contain 3 to 5 mg in 1 mL of 0.9% sterile sodium chloride solution. (1 mg represents 10,000 units.)

Dosage Forms—Injection: 50 mg/20 mL; for Injection: 50 mg; Ophthalmic Ointment: 0.5 and 1 mg/g; Sterile Powder for Ophthalmic Solution: 50 mg, to be reconstituted to 20 to 50 mL. Also marketed in combinations for ophthalmic and topical use. 1 mg equals 10,000 units.

Vancomycin—page 1317.

Polypeptide-Containing Combination

An example of a polypeptide-containing combination (with content provided) is as follows:

Polymyxin B Sulfate and Bacitracin Zinc [AK-Poly-Bac (*Akorn*), Polysporin and Polysporin Ointment (*Burroughs Wellcome*)]—10,000 and 500 units, respectively; ointment, ophthalmic ointment and topical powder.

See also *Aminoglycoside-Containing Combinations*.

Tetracyclines

The tetracyclines are all very much alike with respect to their antimicrobial spectra and the untoward effects they elicit. They differ mainly in their absorption, duration of action and suitability for parenteral administration.

Antimicrobial Actions—The tetracyclines are broad-spectrum antibiotics. They are mainly bacteriostatic. They bind to the bacterial 30s ribosomes and prevent t-RNA from combining with m-RNA. Thus, protein synthesis is inhibited. The drugs have activities against both gram-positive and gram-negative bacteria, mycobacteria, *Mycoplasma*, treponemas, leptospira, rickettsia, actinomycetes, *Coxiella, Chlamydiae* and plasmodia. The susceptible gram-positive bacteria are variable but may include *Staph aureus, Strep pyogenes* and *viridans, pneumoniae* (pneumococcus) and *faecalis* (enterococcus), anaerobic streptococci, *B anthracis, Cl tetani*, and *perfringens*, and *Listeria monocytogenes*. Susceptible gram-negative bacteria include *Enterobacteriaceae* such as, *Esch coli, Salmonella, Shigella* and *Klebsiella, Enterobacter Neisseria* (gonococci and meningococci), *H influenzae, B pertussis, Brucella, Pasteurella, Vibrio cholerae* and *vulnificus, Legionella, Bacteroides* and *Ps pseudomallei, Serratia marcescens* and *Ps mirabilis* are usually resistant but many indole-positive Proteus (*Pr vulgaris, Morganella morganii* and *Prov rettgeri*) are sensitive. *Rickettsia* is very sensitive. The acid-fast *Mycobacterium tuberculosis* is poorly susceptible. *Mycoplasma pneumoniae* and the T-strains are sensitive. They have variable efficacy in the treatment of infections caused by anaerobic bacteria (*Clostridium, Bacteroides*). The tetracyclines do not have a direct action against amebas, but they suppress amebic dysentery by altering the intestinal bacterial flora.

Although resistance to the tetracyclines is not acquired as rapidly as to penicillin, it nevertheless does occur readily. Among the gram-positive bacteria up to 44% of *Strep pyogenes* are resistant and 74% of *Strep faecalis*. The incidence of resistance among hospital strains of *Staph aureus* may run from 30 to 50% but may increase to as high as 75% after several days of treatment. Highly resistant gonococci have become prevalent. However, topical tetracycline is comparable with silver nitrate in the prophylaxis of ophthalmia neonatorum and does not cause chemical conjunctivitis.

Various streptococci and pneumococci also become resistant. The incidence of resistance among various gram-negative bacteria is also very high, especially among the *Enterobacteriaceae*, which in the intestine can pass resistance-controlling genes from one species, even genus, to another (infectious drug resistance). Resistance to one tetracycline usually confers resistance to all others, except that some tetracycline-resistant strains of streptococci and *E coli* may retain sensitivity to minocycline. Cross-resistance between penicillin and tetracyclines or between other classes of antibiotics and tetracyclines is uncommon, except in infectious drug resistance, in which the acquired episome or plasmid contains more than one gene for resistance to other drugs.

Uses—A tetracycline alone is the *drug of choice* in the treatment of *cholera, relapsing fever, granuloma inguinale* and infections caused by *rickettsia, Borrelia, Mycobacterium fortuitum* and *marinum* and *Chlamydia psittaci* and *trachomatis* (except pneumonia and inclusion conjunctivitis). With erythromycin it shares *first-choice* status for the treatment of *Mycoplasma pneumonia* (primary atypical pneumonia). A tetracycline is a component of *first-choice combinations* for the treatment of *brucellosis, glanders* and infections by *Ps pseudomallei*. It is an alternative drug for the treatment of *actinomycosis, anthrax, chancroid, mellioidosis, plague, rat-bite fevers, syphilis, yaws* and infections caused by *Aeromonas hydrophila, Brucella, Campylobacter, Cl tetani, Eikenella corrodens, E coli; Kl pneumoniae, H influenzae, Leptospira, Leptotrichia buccalis, Morganella morganii, Prot vulgaris, Prov rettgeri, Streptobacillis moniliformis, Ureaplasma* and *Yersinia pestis*. Tetracyclines may be used in the treatment of minor *staphylococcal infections*, but other drugs take precedence. However, in the treatment of acne, tetracyclines maintain a favored but challengeable status; if there is inflammation with pustules and cysts, an antibiotic may be indicated. Doxycycline has been shown to prevent travelers' diarrhea caused by enterotoxigenic *E coli*.

In the treatment of *peritonitis*, tetracyclines may be of use, but the incidence of resistance is now quite high among the offending organisms, so that other drugs usually are preferred. When susceptible bacteria are causative, tetracyclines may be used to treat *biliary tract infections*. In *urinary tract infections*, other drugs usually are preferred, unless sensitivity testing especially indicates tetracyclines. However, tetracyclines frequently are used in *nongonococcal urethritis* and in *prostatitis* (often a mycoplasma). In urinary tract infections and urethritis, the urine should be acidified to favor antibacterial action. In the treatment of the meningococcal carrier state, minocycline, but not other tetracyclines, appears to be effective.

In combination with quinine, a tetracycline is an alternative drug for the treatment chloroquine-resistant *Pl falciparum* malaria.

Tetracyclines are used as an alternative to silver nitrate in the prevention of neonatal ocular prophylaxis of chlamydial and gonococcal conjunctivitis, but studies have shown them to be inferior.

Adverse Effects—The tetracyclines cause a number of untoward effects. *Gastrointestinal toxicity* is common with oral use; it is probably the combined effect of local irritation and alteration of the intestinal flora. Manifestations are heartburn, epigastric distress, nausea, vomiting, diarrhea and rare esophageal ulceration in persons with esophageal obstruction or spastic disease. Claims that some tetracyclines cause less gastrointestinal distress have not yet been supported by objective clinical evidence, but it is probable that those that are used in the lower doses cause a lesser incidence of such effects. Some tetracyclines occasionally cause *antibiotic-associated* (peudomembranous) *colitis*. Rare hemolytic anemia has been reported.

The broad-spectrum antibacterial activity of the tetracyclines causes marked alterations in the floral ecology, so that microorganisms formerly held in check overgrow to cause *suprainfections*. This occurs most frequently in the bowel but it also may occur readily in the mouth, lungs, vagina and occasionally elsewhere. The most common suprainfection is candidiasis, but overgrowth from staphylococci, enterococci, *Proteus, Pseudomonas* or *Cl difficile* (cause of antibiotic-associated colitis) occurs. Staphylococcal enteric superinfections are frequently fatal. Staphylococcal enteritis is especially likely to happen to children. The usual effect of an overgrowth in the bowel is diarrhea. However, in debilitated patients or patients with very high numbers of monilia in the gut, the yeast can enter the blood stream and disseminate to various locations.

Various *hypersensitivity* reactions, especially urticaria, asthma or facial edema, occur, but they are uncommon. *Phototoxicity* occurs, to a very high extent with demeclocycline but to a low extent with minocycline and other tetracyclines.

Hepatotoxicity, which is sometimes fatal, occasionally results when the daily dose in adults exceeds 1 g/day, especially if the tetracycline is given intravenously; pregnancy and renal failure predispose to this toxicity. Tetracyclines also may increase the risk of hepatic damage by other hepatotoxic drugs.

Although tetracyclines probably do not affect normal kidney function, they *aggravate preexisting renal insufficiency*, which can lead to extreme azotemia, but without oliguria. Doxycycline appears to be free of this effect. Old preparations that have undergone decomposition on the shelf are serious offenders in causing nephrotoxicity. Tetracyclines also interact with diuretics to cause azotemia. They may promote nephrotoxicity caused by methoxyflurane. Minocycline can cause vestibular toxicity.

Tetracyclines *pigment developing teeth* and reversibly *impair bone growth* through complexation with the bone salts and fixation to matrix proteins. The implication is that tetracyclines should be avoided in children under 6 years, in whom the cosmetically important permanent teeth have not erupted. It also should be avoided in pregnancy.

A rare, reversible *cerebral toxicity* which causes a bulging fontanelle in infants and headache, irritability, vomiting, blurred vision and papilledema in children and adults has been observed in tetracycline-treated patients. There are also rare ocular toxicities, such as transient myopia, diplopia, papilledema and blurred vision.

Intravenous tetracyclines may cause *thrombophlebitis*, caused mainly by the acid required to effect solution. The soluble tetracyclines like rolitetracycline rarely cause this complication. Polyvinylpyrrolidone and phosphate in intravenous preparations lessen the irritant action. Because of the various dangers from intravenous tetracyclines (local, hepatic and renal), administration by this route should be withheld unless the illness is so severe that the necessary dose cannot be tolerated by mouth, the patient is unable to take oral medication or oral therapy is inadequate. Intramuscular injections cause local pain, unless a local anesthetic is included.

Absorption, Distribution and Elimination—The extent of gastrointestinal absorption is 58 to 100%. Doxycycline and minocycline are absorbed the best. Tetracyclines complex with bivalent and trivalent metal ions, so that their absorption is greatly impaired by calcium-, magnesium- and aluminum-containing antacids and by iron preparations. If possible, such drugs should be withheld during tetracycline therapy or at least not administered within 1 hour before or after the tetracycline. Food, especially milk products or other high-calcium foods, also interferes with oral absorption of tetracyclines, although a minimal effect occurs with doxycycline and minocycline. Phosphate appears to improve absorption, in part by removing calcium.

All tetracyclines are bound to plasma proteins, to an extent ranging from 35 to 91%. There is no correlation between protein-binding and volume of distribution or half-life. Volumes of distribution range from 0.14 to 1.79 mL/g. Half-lives vary from 6 to 17 hours in normal persons but 12 to 108 hours in renal failure. Doxycycline and minocycline are longer acting, the most lipophilic and pentrate tissues more efficiently. Therapeutic concentrations of minocycline are achieved in saliva and tears to eradicate the meningococcal carrier state. Renal excretion is the principal mode of elimination, except that minocycline is excreted mostly in the bile and doxycycline is more than 50% metabolized and/or excreted into the colon. The tetracyclines penetrate well into the tissues and body fluids, but penetration into the cerebrospinal fluid is low by the oral route, so that concentrations may be no more than 1/50 to 1/10 of those in the plasma; with intravenous administration, higher levels can be achieved. All tetracyclines are excreted somewhat into the bile and not resorbed completely in the intestine, so that even intravenous doses are capable of altering the bowel flora.

Chlorotetracycline Hydrochloride—see RPS-18, page 1215.

Demeclocycline Hydrochloride

2-Naphthacenecarboxamide, [4*S*-(4α,4aα,5aα,6β,12aα)]-7-chloro-4-(dimethylamino)-1,4,4a,-5,5a,6,11,12a-octahydro-3,6,10,12,12a-pentahydroxy-1,11-dioxo-, monohydrochloride; Declomycin (*Lederle*)

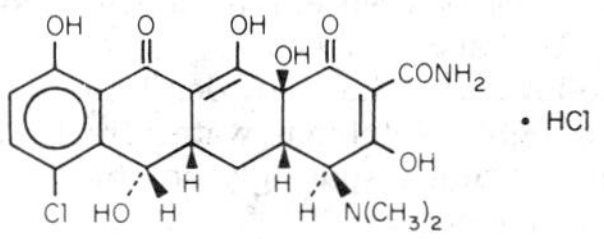

7-Chloro-6-demethyltetracycline Hydrochloride [64-73-3] $C_{21}H_{21}ClN_2O_8.HCl$ (501.32). Potency: not less than 900 μg of $C_{21}H_{21}ClN_2O_8.HCl$/mg, calculated on the anhydrous basis.

Preparation—An appropriate mutant strain of *Streptomyces aureofaciens* is grown in an appropriate liquid nutrient medium under controlled conditions of temperature, pH, and aeration. The harvested broth is acidified and filtered, and the antibiotic is isolated from the filtrate, either by solvent extraction or by chemical precipitation, and converted into the hydrochloride.

Description—Yellow, crystalline powder; odorless; bitter taste; pH (1 in 100 solution) about 2.5; pK_a 3.3, 7.2, 9.3.

Solubility—1 g in about 60 mL water, 200 mL ethanol or 50 mL methanol; sparingly soluble in solutions of alkali hydroxides or carbonates; practically insoluble in chloroform.

Uses—A spectrum of activity similar to other tetracyclines (see the general statement). Its potency *in vitro* against most of the organisms susceptible to the group is equal to that of tetracycline, except that it is twice as potent against *Strep viridans, Klebsiella, Serratia, Ps aeruginosa*, gonococcus and *H influenzae*. It is absorbed better (66%) after oral administration than oxytetracycline but not as well as tetracycline. In plasma it is protein-bound 75 to 91%. Its volume of distribution is 1.8 mL/g. It readily penetrates into body cavities, fluids and cells. Its half-life is about 10 to 17 hr, except up to 60 hr in renal failure. About 42% is eliminated in urine. Because of its slow rate of excretion, its efficacy against urinary tract infections is compromised. In general, it has the same uses as other tetracyclines. However, it has unique usefulness in bone-scanning procedures and in the treatment of inappropriate antidiuretic hormone secretion; the mechanism is not understood; these are considered by some to be the only legitimate uses, since it is too expensive for general tetracycline-appropriate use.

The incidence and type of side effects encountered with this drug are similar to those of other tetracyclines, except that the incidence of gastrointestinal side effects may be lower than with tetracycline, possibly because of the smaller doses used. However, it causes antibiotic-associated colitis more than does tetracycline, and it also can impair renal function or cause diuresis and polyuria. Photodynamic and photosensitivity reactions appear more frequently with the drug. Nonsystemic antacid preparations, milk or food should not be taken with the drug, since these interfere with its gastrointestinal absorption.

Dose—*Oral, adult, antibacterial* and *antiprotozoal*, usually **150 mg** every 6 hr or **300 mg** every 12 hr, but as much as 2.4 g a day may be given, if necessary; for *acne*, initially **300 mg** twice a day until improvement, then a gradual reduction to **75** to **300 mg** a day; for inappropriate *ADH secretion*, **3.25** to **3.75 mg/kg** every 6 hr. *Chidren 8 yr and older, antibacterial* and *antiprotozoal*, **6** to **12 mg/kg** a day, depending on severity, divided into 2 or 4 doses; not recommended for children under 8 yr because of effects on bone and teeth.

Dosage Forms—Capsules: 150 mg; Tablets: 150 and 300 mg.

Doxycycline

2-Naphthacenecarboxamide, [4*S*-(4α,4aα,5α,5aα,6α,12aα)]-4-(dimethylamino)-1,4,4a,5,5a,6,11,12a-octahydro-3,5,10,12,12a-pentahydroxy-6-methyl-1,11-dioxo-, monohydrate; Vibramycin (*Pfizer*); (*Various Mfrs*)

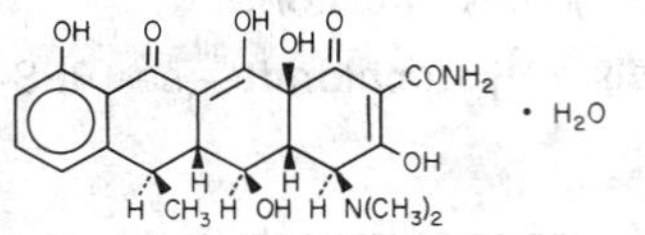

[17086-28-1] $C_{22}H_{24}N_2O_8.H_2O$ (462.46); *anhydrous* [564-25-0] (444.44). Potency: 880 to 980 μg of $C_{22}H_{24}N_2O_8$/mg.

Preparation—6-Deoxy-6-demethyl-6-methylene-5-oxytetracycline (*see Methacycline*) is dissolved or suspended in an inert liquid such as methanol and hydrogenated under the influence of catalytic amounts of noble metals such as rhodium or palladium to give a mixture of the 6α- and 6β-methyl epimers. The desired epimer is then isolated by chromatographic processes. US Pat 3,200,149.

Description—Yellow, crystalline powder; bitter taste; pK_a 3.4, 7.7, 9.7.

Solubility—Very slightly soluble in water; freely soluble in dilute acid or alkali hydroxide solutions; sparingly soluble in alcohol; practically insoluble in chloroform or ether.

Uses—The actions and uses generally are the same as other tetracyclines (see the general statement). Against gram-positive bacteria it is about twice as potent as tetracycline, except that it is up to 10 times as potent against *Strep viridans.* Furthermore, strains of *Strep fecalis* that are resistant to other tetracyclines may be sensitive to the drug. Against gram-negative bacteria it is as potent to twice as potent as tetracycline. It is the drug of first choice for *prophylaxis* of "travelers' diarrhea," commonly caused by enterotoxigenic *E coli.* It is the best of the tetracyclines against anaerobes. It also is efficacious as a chemoprophylactic against leptospirosis.

It is absorbed more completely (90 to 100%) after oral administration than other tetracyclines, and its absorption does not appear to be inhibited by foods. Plasma-protein binding is about 93%. It has a volume of distribution of 0.75 mL/g. It readily penetrates cells, body fluids and cavities. Elimination is about 65% by hepatic metabolism and 35% by biliary/renal excretion. The rate of excretion is slow and the half-life is the longest of the tetracyclines, namely, 12 to 22 hr. The slow rate of excretion means that urine concentrations are lower than with other tetracyclines, which compromises its efficacy in urinary tract infections in which urine concentration is important. Nevertheless, it has been used successfully in the treatment of urinary tract infections, especially those, such as pyelonephritis or prostatitis, in which tissue concentration may be more important than urine concentration. Renal insufficiency has little influence on plasma levels or duration of action.

The toxicity is that of tetracyclines in general, but there is a threefold greater incidence of gastrointestinal effects and more frequent skin rashes than with other tetracyclines. Photosensitization occurs much more frequently than with shorter-acting tetracyclines. Although it complexes calcium to a lesser extent than other tetracyclines, absorption is hindered by calcium-containing as well as by other nonsystemic acids and by iron preparations.

Dose (anhydrous equivalent)—*Oral, adult* and *children over 45 kg, antibacterial* and *antiprotozoal, usually* **100 mg** every 12 hr on the first day followed by either **50** to **100 mg** every 12 hr or **100** to **200 mg** once a day, but up to 300 mg a day may be given; for *prophylaxis of traveller's diarrhea,* **100 mg** once a day for 3 wk. *Children 45 kg or less, initially* 2 doses of **2.2 mg/kg** at 12-hr intervals the first day followed by either **1.1** to **2.2 mg/kg** every 12 hr or **2.2** to **4.4 mg/kg** once a day. Not recommended for children under 8 yr because of effects on bone and teeth.

Dosage Form (anhydrous equivalent)—for Oral Suspension: 25 mg/5 mL (reconstituted, as the monohydrate).

Doxycycline Calcium—see RPS-18, page 1215.

Doxycycline Hyclate

2-Naphthacenecarboxamide, [4*S*-(4α,4aα,5α,5aα,6α,12aα)]-4-(dimethylamino)-1,4,4a,5,5a,6,11,12a-octahydro-3,5,10,12,12a-pentahydroxy-6-methyl-1,11-dioxo-, monohydrochloride, compd with ethanol (2:1), monohydrate; (*Various Mfrs*)

See *Doxycycline* for structure of the parent compound [24390-14-5] $(C_{22}H_{24}N_2O_8.HCl)_2.C_2H_6O.H_2O$ (1025.89). Potency: the equivalent of 800–920 μg of doxycycline/mg.

Preparation—Doxycycline hydrochloride is crystallized from a solution in ethanol containing hydrochloric acid.

Description—Yellow, crystalline powder.

Solubility—1 g in 3 mL water or 60 mL alcohol; soluble in solutions of alkali hydroxides and carbonates; practically insoluble in chloroform and ether.

Uses—See *Doxycycline.*

Dose (base equivalent)—*Oral,* the same as for *Doxycycline. In travenous infusion, adults* and *children over 45 kg, initially* **200 mg** once or **100 mg** twice on the first day followed by **100** to **200 mg** once a day or **50** to **100 mg** twice a day; *children up through 45 kg,* **4.4 mg/kg** once or **2.2 mg/kg** twice on the first day followed by **2.2** to **4.4 mg/kg** once a day or **1.1** to **2.2 mg/kg** twice a day. Not recommended for children under 8 yr because of effects on bone and teeth.

Dosage Forms (base equivalent)—Capsules: 50 and 100 mg; for Injection: 100 and 200 mg; Film-Coated Tablets: 100 mg; tablets 50 and 100 mg.

Meclocycline Sulfosalicylate—see RPS-18, page 1212.

Methacycline Hydrochloride—see RPS-18, page 1213.

Minocycline Hydrochloride

2-Naphthacenecarboxamide, [4*S*-(4α,4aα,5aα,12aα)]-4,7-bis(dimethylamino)-1,4,4a,5,5a,6,11,12a-octahydro-3,10,12,12a-tetrahydroxy-1,11-dioxo-, monohydrochloride; Minocin (*Lederle*)

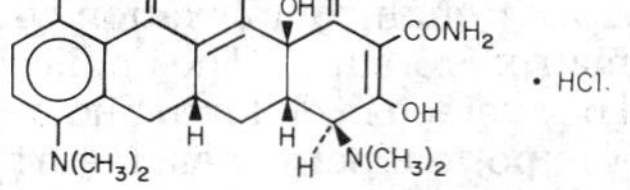

7-Dimethylamino-6-demethyl-6-deoxytetracycline [13614-98-7] $C_{23}H_{27}N_3O_7.HCl$ (493.94). Potency: equivalent to not less than 785 μg of minocycline ($C_{23}H_{27}N_3O_7$)/mg.

Preparation—6-Demethyltetracycline, dissolved in tetrahydrofuran containing methanesulfonic acid, is reacted with dibenzyl azodicarboxylate to form 7-[1,2-bis(carbobenzoxy)hydrazino]-6-demethyltetracycline. Palladium-catalyzed hydrogenation in the presence of formaldehyde yields minocycline which reacts with an equimolar quantity of HCl to form the monohydrochloride. US Pats 3,148,212 and 3,226,436.

Description—Yellow, crystalline powder; odorless; slightly bitter taste; slightly hygroscopic; stable in air when protected from light and moisture (strong light and/or moist air causes it to darken); potency in solution affected primarily due to epimerization; pH (1 in 100 solution) between 3.5 and 4.5; pK_{a1} 2.8; pK_{a2} 5.0; pK_{a3} 7.8; pK_{a4} 9.3.

Solubility—1 g in about 60 mL water and about 70 mL alcohol; soluble in solutions of alkali hydroxides or carbonates; practically insoluble in chloroform or ether.

Uses—The actions and uses are essentially the same as those of the tetracyclines in general (see the general statement). Against most gram-positive organisms it appears to be generally 2 to 4 times as potent as tetracycline, but it shares an equally low potency against *Strep fecalis.* Against *Strep viridans* it is about 8 times as potent. Against gram-negative bacteria it is generally 2 to 4 times as potent as tetracycline. It is especially effective against *Mycobacterium marinum,* and it is now the drug of choice for treating infections caused by that bacterium. It differs from other tetracyclines in that bacterial resistance to the drug is of a lower order and incidence; this is especially true of staphylococci, in which cross-resistance has been reported to be as low as 4%.

The incidence and severity of the usual side effects of tetracyclines, effects like phototoxicity and gastrointestinal upsets, are less than with other tetracyclines. Diarrhea, abdominal pain and flatus are experienced by only 2 to 5% of patients. However, nausea and vomiting are frequent, as the result of ototoxicity and CNS effects. There are also autonomic nervous disorders; dry mouth and cycloplegia occur in 2 to 10% of recipients and caution is advised in persons with glaucoma or males with partial obstruction of the urinary tract. Headache occurs in 33% and myalgia in 12% of patients. Lethargy, fatigue, vertigo, confusion and disorientation occur in about 25% of users. Insomnia occurs in 9%, hot flashes in 8% and tinnitus in 4%. Impairment of hearing and vestibular function can result from use in patients with meningitis, the various manifestations of CNS toxicity and ototoxicity occurring in 50 to 90% of recipients.

It is 90 to 100% absorbed by the oral route. Its absorption is diminished slightly by food and milk and markedly by nonsystemic antacids and iron preparations. It is 70 to 75% protein-bound in plasma. The volume of distribution is 0.14 to 0.7 mL/g. The half-life is 11 to 17 hr. Only

10% is reported to be excreted unchanged, but the half-life has been reported to be greatly prolonged in renal failure.

Dose (minocycline equivalent)—*Oral, adult, antibacterial* and *antiprotozoal*, usually either **200 mg** initially followed by **100 mg** every 12 hr or **100** to **200 mg** initially followed by **50 mg** every 6 hr; in the *meningococcal carrier* state, **100 mg** every 12 hr for 5 days; for infections by *M marinum*, **100 mg** every 12 hr for 6 to 8 wk. *Children 8 yr or older*, initially **4 mg/kg** followed by **2 mg/kg** every 12 hr. Not recommended in children under 8 yr because of effects on bone and teeth. *Intravenous*, same as usual oral dosage.

Dosage Forms (minocycline equivalent)—Capsules: 50 and 100 mg; for Injection: 100 mg (to be reconstituted to 5 mL); Oral Suspension: 50 mg/5 mL; Tablets: 50 and 100 mg.

Oxytetracycline

2-Naphthacenecarboxamide, [4*S*-(4α,4aα,5α,5aα,6β,12aα)]-4-(dimethylamino)-1,4,4a,5,5a,6,11,12a-octahydro-3,5,6,10,12,12a-hexahydroxy-6-methyl-1,11-dioxo-, dihydrate; Terramycin (*Roerig*); (*Various Mfrs*)

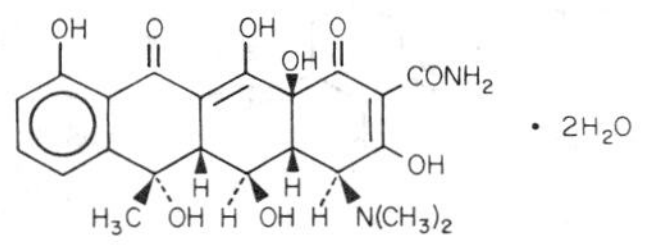

[6153-64-6] $C_{22}H_{24}N_2O_9.2H_2O$ (496.47); *anhydrous* [79-57-2] (460.44). Potency: not less than 832 mg of $C_{22}H_{24}N_2O_9$/mg.

Preparation—By the growth of a selected strain of *Streptomyces rimosus* on a medium consisting of water, proteins and nutrient salts.

Description—Pale yellow to tan, odorless, crystalline powder; stable in air, but exposure to strong sunlight causes it to darken; deteriorates in solutions of pH below 2, and is rapidly destroyed by alkali hydroxide solutions; saturated solution is nearly neutral to litmus, having a pH of about 6.5.

Solubility—1 g in 4150 mL water, 100 mL alcohol, >10,000 mL chloroform, 6250 mL ether; freely soluble in diluted hydrochloric acid or alkaline solutions.

Uses—The actions, toxicity and uses essentially those of tetracyclines in general (see the general statement). The relative susceptibilities of various microorganisms to this drug are virtually the same as for chlortetracycline and tetracycline, with a few exceptions. Bacterial resistance automatically confers resistance to chlortetracycline or tetracycline. This drug also is used in the treatment of intestinal amebiasis; it removes both cysts and motile forms from the intestine and compares favorably with halogenated quinolines. However, all these drugs have been superseded by metronidazole. Approximately 58% of an oral dose is absorbed in the fasting state. It is bound to plasma proteins only about 35%. The volume of distribution is 0.9 to 1.9 mL/g. About 70% is eliminated by renal excretion. The biologic half-life is 6 to 10 hr; it may be 47 to 66 hr in anuria. The gastrointestinal side effects are greater than with other tetracyclines. Food, milk, nonsystemic antacids and iron preparations interfere with oral absorption.

Dose (anhydrous)—*Intramuscular, adult*, **100 mg** every 8 hr, **150 mg** every 12 hr, *or* **250 mg** once a day; up to 500 mg a day may be given, if necessary; *children 8 yr or more*, usually either **5** to **8.3 mg/kg** every 8 hr *or* **7.5** to **12.5 mg/kg** every 12 hr, except that no dose should exceed 250 mg. Not recommended for children under 8 yr because of effects on bone and teeth.

Dosage Form (anhydrous)—*Intramuscular* Injection: 50 and 125 mg/mL (all contain 2% lidocaine).

Oxytetracycline Calcium—see RPS-18, page 1215.

Oxytetracycline Hydrochloride

2-Naphthacenecarboxamide, [4*S*-(4α,4aα,5α,5aα,6β,12aα)]-4-(dimethylamino)-1,4,4a,5,5a,6,11,12a-octahydro-3,5,6,10,12,12a-hexahydroxy-6-methyl-1,11-dioxo-, monohydrochloride; (*Various Mfrs*)

[2058-46-0] $C_{22}H_{24}N_2O_9.HCl$ (496.90). Potency: equivalent to not less than 835 μg of oxytetracycline ($C_{22}H_{24}N_2O_9$)/mg, calculated on the anhydrous basis.

For the structure of the base, see *Oxytetracycline*.

Description—Yellow, crystalline powder; odorless; bitter taste; hygroscopic; decomposes above 180°; exposure to strong sunlight or to temperature above 90° in moist air causes darkening, but no appreciable loss in potency; potency is affected in solutions of pH below 2, and is rapidly destroyed by alkali hydroxide solutions; pH (1% solution) between 2 and 3; pK_a 3.3, 7.3, 9.1.

Solubility—1 g in 2 mL water, but the solution becomes cloudy or turbid due to liberation of oxytetracycline base; 1 g in 35 mL alcohol; less soluble in dehydrated alcohol; insoluble in chloroform or ether.

Uses—See *Oxytetracycline*.

Dose—*Oral, adults*, **250 mg** every 6 hr; *children 8 yr or over*, **6.25** to **12.5 mg/kg** every 6 hr. *Intramuscular*, **adults 250 mg** once every 24 hr or **300 mg** given in divided doses every 8 to 12 hr; *children over 8 yr*, **15** to **25 mg/kg** up to a maximum of 250 mg per single daily injection. Not recommended for children under 8 yr because of effects on teeth and bone. Plasma concentrations should not exceed 15 μg/mL, especially in pregnant women or postpartum women with pyelonephritis. *Topical*, in combination with polymyxin B and/or hydrocortisone, 3% ointment or 0.5% ophthalmic ointment.

Dosage Forms (oxytetracycline equivalent)—Capsules: 250 mg; Injection: 250 and 500 mg.

Tetracycline

2-Naphthacenecarboxamide [4*S*-(4α,4aα,5aα,6β,12aα)]-4-(dimethylamino)-1,4,4a,5,5a,6,11,12a-octahydro-3,6,10,12,12a-pentahydroxy-6-methyl-1,11-dioxo-, (*Various Mfrs*)

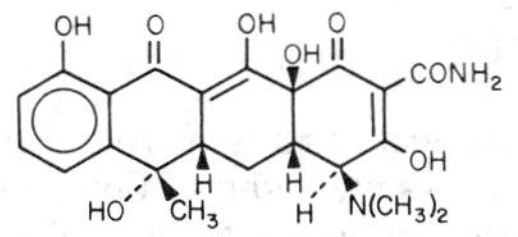

[60-54-8] $C_{22}H_{24}N_2O_8$ (444.44). Potency: equivalent to not less than 975 μg of tetracycline hydrochloride ($C_{22}H_{24}N_2O_8.HCl$)/mg, calculated on the anhydrous basis.

Preparation—By removal of chlorine from chlortetracycline by hydrogenation. Also obtained from a *Streptomyces* species cultured in an appropriate nutrient medium.

Description—Yellow, crystalline powder; odorless; stable in air, but exposure to strong sunlight causes it to darken; potency is affected in solutions of pH below 2, and is destroyed rapidly by alkali hydroxide solutions; more soluble than chlortetracycline and within the physiological and moderately alkaline range of pH is more stable; its solutions darken more rapidly than chlortetracycline but less than oxytetracycline; pH (aqueous suspension, 10 mg/mL) between 3.0 and 7.0; pK_a 3.3, 7.7, 7.9.

Solubility—1 g in about 2500 mL water and about 50 mL alcohol; freely soluble in dilute HCl or alkali hydroxide solutions; practically insoluble in chloroform or ether.

Uses—The antibiotic spectrum, actions, toxicity, absorption, fate and excretion, doses and uses essentially the same as those of the tetracyclines in general (see the general statement). It has been reported to be useful in the treatment of *toxoplasmosis;* it is not known whether this use can be extended to all tetracyclines. The gastrointestinal side effects are less than those from chlortetracycline and oxytetracycline but more than from demeclocycline. About 77% of an oral dose is absorbed. In the plasma 25 to 55% is bound to proteins. The volume of distribution is 1.5 mL/g. About 60% is eliminated by renal excretion. The plasma half-life is 6 to 11 hr in patients with normal renal function; in oliguria it may be as long as 2 to 4 days, and dosage must be adjusted accordingly.

Dose (tetracycline hydrochloride equivalent)—*Oral, adult, systemic infections*, **250** to **500 mg** every 6 hr or **500 mg** to **1 g** every 12 hr; for *acne, initially* **1 g** a day in divided doses, then, after improvement, gradually reduced to **125** to **500 mg** a day; for *gonorrhea*, **500 mg** every 6 hr for 5 days; for *syphilis*, **1.5g** initially then **30** to **40g** in equally divided doses over 10 to 15 days for *late syphilis; children 8 yr* and *older*, **6.25** to **12.5 mg/kg** every 6 hr or **12.5** to **25 mg/kg** every 12 hr. Not recommended for children under 8 yr because of effects on bone and teeth.

Dosage Form (tetracycline hydrochloride equivalent)—Oral Suspension: 125 mg/5 mL.

Tetracycline Hydrochloride

2-Naphthacenecarboxamide, [4*S*-(4α,4aα,5aα,6β,12aα)]-4-(dimethylamino)-1,4,4a,5,5a,6,11,12a-octahydro-3,6,10,12,12a-pentahydroxy-6-methyl-1,11-dioxo-, monohydrochloride (*Various Mfrs*)

[64-75-5] $C_{22}H_{24}N_2O_8.HCl$ (480.90). Potency: not less than 900 μg of $C_{22}H_{24}N_2O_8.HCl$/mg.

For the structure of the base, see *Tetracycline*.

Description—Yellow, crystalline powder; odorless; moderately hygroscopic; stable in air, but exposure to strong sunlight in moist air causes it to darken; potency affected in solutions of pH below 2, and is rapidly destroyed by alkali hydroxide solutions; pH (1 in 100 solution) between 1.8 and 2.8.

Solubility—1 g in 10 mL water or about 100 mL alcohol, the aqueous solution becoming turbid after some time because of hydrolysis; soluble in solutions of alkali hydroxides or carbonates; practically insoluble in chloroform or ether.

Uses—As for *Tetracycline*. Since the hydrochloride is the more soluble form it is used for parenteral administration and in solution for topical use.

Dose—*Oral*, same as for *Tetracycline*. *Intramuscular, adult*, **100 mg** every 8 hr or **150 mg** every 12 hr or **250 mg** once a day; *children 8 yr and over*, **5** to **8.3 mg/kg** every 8 hr or **7.5** to **12.5 mg/ kg** every 12 hr, not to exceed 250 mg a day. *Intravenous, adult*, **250** to **500 mg** once a day; *children 8 yr or older*, **5** to **10 mg/kg** every 12 hr. Not recommended for use in children under 8 yr of age because of effects on bone and teeth. *Topical*, to the *skin* as **3%** ointment once or twice a day or as **0.22%** solution 2 or more times a day; to the conjunctiva as a thin strip (about 1 cm) of **1%** ointment 6 or more times a day or 1 or 2 drops of **1%** suspension into conjunctival sac 2 to 4 times a day.

Dosage Forms—Capsules: 100, 250 and 500 mg; Ophthalmic Ointment: 1%; Topical Ointment: 3%; for Topical Solution: 0.22% (when reconstituted); Ophthalmic Suspension: 1%; Oral Suspension: 125 mg/5 mL; Tablets: 250 and 500 mg.

Fluoroquinolones

Quinolone antibacterial drugs have been in use since 1964, when nalidixic acid was released. Oxolinic acid and cinoxacin were introduced somewhat later. These drugs have limited antibacterial spectra, and resistance to them rapidly develops. Their use is restricted mainly to the treatment of urinary tract infections. The introduction of 6-fluoro and 7-(1-piperazinyl) groups expanded the spectrum, increased potency and appears to have prevented the development of plasmid-mediated resistance. The fluoroquinolones are bacteriostatic at low and bactericidal at high concentrations. They are highly active against most gram-negative pathogens, including *Ps aeruginosa* and the *Enterobacteriaceae*. *Staph aureus* and *epidermidis*, coagulase-negative staphylococci, *Legionella* myobacteria, mycoplasma and chlamydia have intermediate sensitivities. Streptococci are only moderately susceptible to ciprofloxacin and ofloxacin while norfloxacin and enoxacin are even less active. Enterococci require very high concentrations. The drugs inhibit DNA gyrase (topoisomerase II), which results in abnormal linkage between opened DNA and the gyrase. Negative supercoiling (absent in mammalian nuclei) is impaired, so that efficient transcription of DNA into RNA and subsequent protein synthesis is prevented.

Moderate, chromosomal-mediated resistance among strains of *Psuedomonas* occurs clinically in cystic fibrosis patients. Resistance to one fluorolone usually confers resistance to all other quinolones but not to other classes of antimicrobial drugs.

Fluoroquinolones are used to treat upper and lower respiratory infections, gonorrhea, bacterial gastroenteritis, skin and soft tissue infections and both uncomplicated and complicated urinary tract infections, especially those caused by gram-negative bacteria. In general, success is greater against gram-negative than gram-positive infections.

Adverse effects are usually mild and transient. They include gastrointestinal disturbances (nausea, vomiting, diarrhea, dyspepsia, flatulence, constipation, heartburn, abdominal discomfort; 2 to 8%), central nervous symptoms (headache, restlessness, malaise, dizziness, tremor, insomnia, nightmares, depression, paresthesia, visual disturbances, rare hallucinations, phobias, manic excitement, convulsions; 0.5 to 6%), hematologic perturbations (eosinophilia, anemia, elevated erythrocyte sedimentation rate; 1.5 to 5%), mild or moderate rash and/or pruritis (1%), dry mouth, photosensitivity, rare crystalluria and transient arthralgia in a few cystic fibrosis patients. Suprainfections may occur. Some fluoroquinolones prolong the half-life of theophylline; other drug interactions undoubtedly will be discovered. Erosion of cartilage occurs in young animals so the fluoroquinolones are not recommended for use in children under 18 yr or pregnant or nursing women.

Fluoroquinolones are all effective orally but also may be administered parenterally. They have large volumes of distribution and reach therapeutic concentrations in most tissues. They have long half-lives and may be administered only once or twice a day.

Clinically investigated members of this group are ciprofloxacin, enoxacin, lomefloxacin, norfloxacin, ofloxacin and pefloxacin.

Ciprofloxacin Hydrochloride

3-Quinolinecarboxylic acid,
1-cyclopropyl-6-fluoro-1,4-dihydro-4-oxo- 7-(1-piperazinyl)-,
monohydrochloride, monohydrate; Ciloxan (*Alcon*); Cipro (*Miles*)

HN N F N O COOH • HCl • H_2O

[8693-32-0] $C_{17}H_{18}FN_3O_3.HCl.H_2O$ (385.82).

Preparation—From 3-chloro-4-fluoroaniline by condensation with diethyl ethoxymethylenemalonate to form the imine which is thermally cyclized to ethyl 7-chloro-6-fluoro-4-hydroxyquinoline-3-carboxylate. *N*-alkylation with cyclopropyl iodide followed by nucleophilic displacement of the 7-chloro group by *N*-methylpiperazine and hydrolysis of the ester affords the product. *J Med Chem 19:* 1138, 1976.

Description—Pale-yellow crystals; amphoteric; pK_a 6, 8.8.

Solubility—1 g in 25 mL water.

Uses—A fluoroquinolone (see the general statement). It is approved for use in the treatment of *bone* and *joint infections* caused by *Entero cloacae, Ps aeruginosa* and *Serratia marcescens*; *infectious diarrhea* by *Campylobacter jejuni* or *Shigella flexneri* or *sonnei*; *lower respiratory tract infections* by *Entero cloacae, E coli, H influenzae* or *parainfluenzae, Kl pneumoniae, Prot mirabilis, Ps aeruginosa* and *Strep pneumoniae*; *skin infections* by *Citrobacter freundii, Entero cloacae, E coli, Kl pneumoniae, Prot mirabilis* or *vulgaris, Prov stuartii, Ps aeruginosa* or *Staph aureus, epidermidis* or *pyogenes*; and *urinary tract infections* by *Citrobacter diversus* or *freundii, Entero cloacae, E coli, Kl pneumoniae, Morganella morganii, Prot mirabilis, Prov rettgeri, Ps aeruginosa, Serratia marcescens, Staph epidermidis* or *Strep faecalis*. It is a second-choice drug in all of the above. It is the drug of choice for the treatment of infections by *Campylobacter jejuni*. In addition, it is an unlabeled but authoritatively alternative drug for the treatment of gonorrhea and salmonella and yersinia infections.

The adverse effects are those of fluoroquinolones in general. The overall, obviously drug-related incidence is 7.3%. Discontinuation is required in about 3.5% of cases.

The oral bioavailability is about 70 to 80%. A dose of 0.5 g yields a plasma concentration 12 hr after administration of about 0.2 μg/mL. Urinary excretion accounts for the elimination of 40 to 50% of an oral dose. Twenty to 35% is eliminated in the feces. There is hepatic biotransformation of four known metabolites, which accounts for 15% of a dose. The half-life is about 4 hr.

Dose (Base equivalent)—*Oral or intravenous, adults, bone* and *joint, respiratory tract* and *skin* infections or *infectious diarrhea*, **500 mg** every 12 hr; *severe* or *complicated* infections, **750 mg** every 12 hr; *urinary tract* infections, **250 mg** every 12 hr.

Dosage Form—Tablets: 250, 500 and 750 mg; Injection: 200 and 400 mg.

Enoxacin

1,8-Naphthyridine-3-carboxylic acid,
1-ethyl-6-fluoro-1,4-dihydro-4-oxo-7-(1-piperazinyl);
Penetrex (*Rhone-Poulenc Rorer*)

O F COOH N N N HN C_2H_5

[74011-58-8] $C_{15}H_{17}FN_4O_3$ (320.32).

Preparation—The active 2-chloro group of 2,6-dichloro-3-nitropyridine is nucleophilically displaced by *N*-carbethoxypiperazine; then the 6-chloro atom is displaced with ammonia and the resulting amined acylated to the acetamide. The nitro group is reduced, diazotized and treated with HBF_4 to yield the fluoro derivative. The balance of the synthesis is analogous to that for *ciprofloxacin; J Med Chem 27:* 292, 1984.

Description—White crystals; bitter taste; melts about 222°.

Solubility—1 g in 3330 mL water.

Uses—A limited-spectrum fluoroquinolone with an antibacterial spectrum similar to norfloxacin that can be used orally to treat urinary tract infections or gonorrhea. It is highly active against *N gonorrhea, H influenzae, M cararrhalis, Salmonella, Shigella, Aeromonas, Yersinia, Vibrio, E Coli* and *Camplyobacter*. It is less active than ciprofloxacin and ofloxacin against *Chlamydia trachomatis* and *Staph epidermidis. Group A Streptococci* and *Strep pneumoniae* are generally resistant, and higher concentrations are required to be active against *Pseudomonas aeruginosa* and *Staph aureus*.

Enoxacin is well absorbed orally with a bioavailability of 90%. It is partly metabolized and has a half-life of 3 to 6 hr. Clearance decreases with decreased renal function. It is generally well tolerated and has all the adverse effects common to fluoroquinolones (see the general statement).

Dose—For *uncomplicated gonorrhea,* **400 mg** once; for *urinary tract infections,* **200** to **400 mg** every 12 hr for 7 to 14 days.

Dosage Form—Tablets: 200 and 400 mg.

Lomefloxacin Hydrochloride

3-Quinolinecarboxylic acid, (±)-1-ethyl-6,8-difluoro-1,4-dihydro-7-(3-methyl-1-piperazinyl)-4-oxo-, monohydrochloride; Maxaquin (*Searle*)

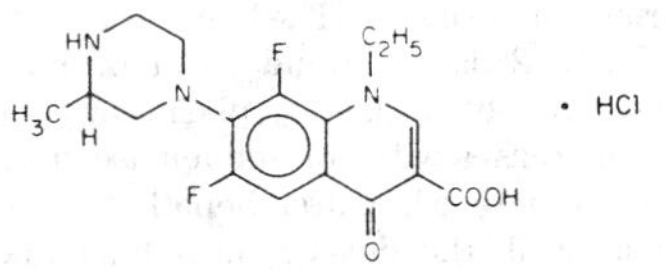

[98079-52-8] $C_{17}H_{19}F_2N_3O_3.HCl$ (387.81).

Preparation—By a method analagous to that for *Enoxacin;* US Pat 4,528,287.

Description—Colorless needles; melts about 295° with decomposition.

Solubility—Soluble in water.

Uses—Another limited-spectrum fluoroquinolone that is similar in antibacterial activity to enoxacin. It is approved only for treatment of urinary tract infections and bronchitis caused by *H influenzae* or *M catarrhalis*. It covers gram-negative organisms frequently associated with urinary tract infections but does not have the activity to cover the same bacterial infections which respond to ciprofloxacin and ofloxacin.

It is absorbed orally almost completely and has a half-life of 7 to 8 hr. About 65% of dose is excreted in the urine unchanged. The adverse effects are similar to the fluoroquinolones (see the general statement)

Dose—**400 mg** once a day for 10 to 14 days; for *preoperative prophylaxis for transurethral surgery,* **400 mg** 2 to 6 hr prior to surgery.

Dosage Form—Tablets: 400 mg

Norfloxacin

3-Quinolinecarboxylic acid,
1-ethyl-6-fluoro-1,4-dihydro-4-oxo-7-(1-piperazinyl)-,
Chibroxin, Noroxin (*MSD*)

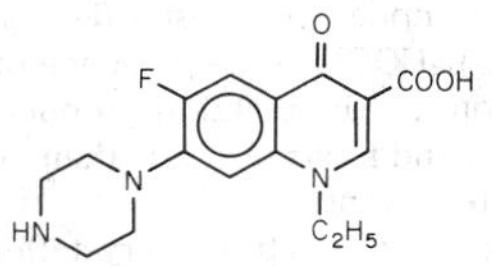

[70458-96-7] $C_{16}H_{18}FN_3O_3$ (319.34).

Preparation—Similar to *Ciprofloxacin,* see *J Med Chem 23:* 1358, 1980.

Description—White to pale-yellow crystalline powder; melts about 221°; hygroscopic and forms a hemihydrate in air; pK_a 6.3, 8.8.

Solubility—Very slightly soluble in water, methanol or alcohol; freely soluble in glacial acetic acid.

Uses—A fluoroquinolone (see the general statement). It is approved for uses in the treatment of *urinary tract infections* caused by *Citrobacter freundii, Entero cloacae, Kl pneumoniae, Morganella morganii, Prot mirabilis* or *vulgaris, Prov rettgeri, Ps aeruginosa, Staph aureus* or *epidermidis* or Group O streptococci. It has been reported to be equal to trimethoprim-sulfamethoxazole or tobramycin and superior to amoxacillin, carbenicillin, ticarcillin, ureidopenicillin, cephalosporins or gentamicin. It also is as effective as spectinomycin in the treatment of penicillin-resistant *gonorrhoea*; a two-dose, single-day regimen suffices in uncomplicated cases. It appears to provide effective *prophylaxis of traveler's diarrhea.*

The adverse effects are those of fluoroquinolones in general. The most frequent are nausea (2.8%), headache (2.7%) and dizziness (1.8%).

Fasting oral bioavailability is 30 to 40%; food decreases absorption. A dose of 400 mg yields a peak plasma concentration of about 1.5 μg/mL. Plasma protein binding is 10 to 15%. Elimination is by renal excretion (67 to 80%), hepatic metabolism (13 to 20%) and biliary secretion. Six metabolites have been identified. The half-life is 3 to 4 hr, except up to 6.5 hr in renal failure. Probenicid prolongs the half-life.

Dose—*Oral, adult, urinary tract infections,* **400 mg** twice a day for 7 to 10 days in uncomplicated and 10 to 21 days in complicated infections. If the creatinine clearance is less than 31 mL/min, the dose is to be given only once a day; for *uncomplicated gonorrhea,* **800 mg** in a single dose.

Dosage Form—Tablets: 400 mg.

Ofloxacin

7H-Pyridol[1,2,3-*de*]-1,4-benzoxazine-6-carboxylic acid, (±)-9-fluoro-2,3-dihydro-3-methyl-10-(4-methyl-1-piperazinyl)-7-oxo-, Floxin (*Ortho*)

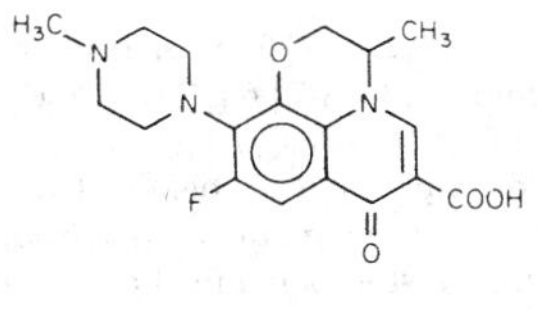

[82419-36-1] $C_{18}H_{20}FN_3O_4$ (361.37). The carbon atom to which the methyl group is attached, in the oxazine ring, is chiral and the clinically used substance is a racemic mixture, whereas the (+) form has twice the activity of the (−) form.

Preparation—By a method analogous to that for *Ciprofloxacin;* US Pat 4,382,892.

Description—Colorless needles; melts about 255° with decomposition; pK_a 7.9.

Solubility—Poorly soluble in water or ethanol.

Uses—A fluroquinolone with an antibacterial spectrum similar to ciprofloxacin, both of which are more active than norfloxacin, enoxacin or lemofloxacin. It is highly active against many bacterial causes of enteritis, including *Salmonella, Shigella, Campylobacter jejuni, Aeromonas, Yersinia, E Coli* and *Vibrio,* but not *C difficile.* It is less active than ciprofloxacin against *Pseudomonas aeruginosa* and, like ciprofloxacin, is much less active than penicillin against streptococci. It has *in vitro* activity against *Legionella pneumophilia, Mycoplasma pneumonia, Chlamydia trachomatis* and *Mycobacterium tuberculosis.* It is approved for treatment of urinary tract, respiratory tract, prostate and skin or soft tissue infections caused by susceptible bacteria. A penicillin or cephalosporin is preferred for known or suspected streptococcal infections.

It is 98% bioavailable upon oral administration and has a serum half-life of 5 to 8 hr. About 70 to 80% of a dose is recovered unchanged in the urine. It has a volume of distribution similar to ciprofloxacin. Adverse effects are the same as other fluoroquinolones (see the general statement).

Dose—*Oral* and *intravenous, adult,* for *urinary tract infections,* **200 mg** every 12 hr for 10 days; for *gonorrhea,* **400 mg** as a single dose, for *Chlamydia,* **300 mg** every 12 hr for 7 days; for *lower respiratory tract infections,* **400 mg** every 12 hr.

Dosage Forms—Tablets: 200, 300 and 400 mg; Injection: 200 and 400 mg.

Miscellaneous Antibiotics

Because of similarities among microorganisms in biosynthetic mechanisms, antibiotics tend to fall into chemical groups. Furthermore, similarities among the target organisms in physiology and metabolism tend to select certain types of molecules as effective antibiotics. Nevertheless, there is species and strain individuality which lends itself to exploitation. Thus, some of the miscellaneous antibiotics are the result of the biosynthetic uniqueness of the generating organism and others of the unique requirements for activity of some specific target organisms.

The similarities in spectrum, mechanism and toxicity of some miscellaneous antibiotics to chemically unrelated drugs are the result of actions at different points in the same general biochemical or physiological function.

Amphotericin B—page 1327.

Candicidin—see RPS-17, page 1226.

Chloramphenicol

Acetamide, [R-(R^*,R^*)]-2,2-dichloro-N-[2-hydroxy-1-(hydroxymethyl)-2-(4-nitrophenyl)ethyl]-,
Chloromycetin (*Parke-Davis*); (*Qualitest*): (*Various Mfrs*)

O_2N–C₆H₄–CH(OH)–CH($NHCOCHCl_2$)–CH_2OH

D-*threo*-(−)-2,2-Dichloro-N-[β-hydroxy-α-(hydroxymethyl)-p-nitrophenethyl]acetamide [56-75-7] $C_{11}H_{12}Cl_2N_2O_5$ (323.13). Potency: not less than 900 μg of $C_{11}H_{12}Cl_2N_2O_5$/mg.

Preparation—Chloramphenicol is believed to be the first naturally occurring compound known to contain a nitro group or to be a derivative of dichloroacetic acid. Its stereochemical configuration is analogous to that of (−)-norpseudoephedrine, and is the only one of the four related stereoisomers that has antibiotic activity.

Chloramphenicol can be obtained from the filtrate of a *Streptomyces venezuelae* culture by extraction with ethyl acetate. If the charcoal extract is rich in chloramphenicol, the latter can be crystallized from the ethyl acetate by diluting with many volumes of kerosene.

Several synthetic methods of preparation are known. One of the better known commences with p-nitroacetophenone and, after converting it into p-nitro-2-aminoacetophenone, proceeds through the following steps: (a) acetylation of the —NH_2 group, (b) reaction with HCHO to introduce the terminal —CH_2OH group, (c) reduction with aluminum isopropoxide to give a mixture of the racemates of the *threo* and *erythro* forms of p-$NO_2PhCH(OH)CH(NH_2)CH_2OH$, (d) isolation of the *threo* racemate and resolution of it using d-camphorsulfonic acid, and (e) condensing the (−) enantiomorph with methyl dichloroacetate.

Description—Fine, white to grayish white or yellowish white, needle-like crystals or elongated plates; odorless; intensely bitter taste; pH (saturated solution) between 4.5 and 7.5; reasonably stable in neutral or moderately acid solutions but rapidly destroyed in alkaline solutions; melts between 149° and 153°; pK_a 5.5.

Solubility—1 g in about 400 mL water; freely soluble in alcohol; slightly soluble in ether or chloroform.

Uses—A wide spectrum of antibacterial activity. The drug is effective in *rickettsial diseases* including epidemic, murine and scrub typhus, Rocky Mountain spotted fever, rickettsial pox and Q fever; *chlamydial diseases* including the psittacosis-lymphogranuloma group and many *bacterial infections* including those caused by *A aerogenes, E coli, K pneumoniae, H pertussis, E typhosa, Brucella, V cholerae*, staphylococci, streptococci, corynebacteria, mycoplasmas, actinomycetes and *T pallidum*. Because of serious toxic reactions, the systemic use of the drug should be limited only to very serious infections that cannot be managed by other drugs. However, it is still used much too promiscuously. It is still the drug of choice for typhoid fever.

It is an alternative drug for the treatment of infections caused by *B fragilis, Brucella, Chlamydia psittaci, Cl perfingens, Francisella tularensis, Fusobacterium, H influenzae* (life-threatening; combined with ampicillin), *Kl pneumoniae, Morganella morganii, N meningitidis, Prot mirabilis, Ps mallei* (with streptomycin), *pseudomallei* (with aminoglycoside) or *cepacia, Rickettsia, Salmonella* (nontyphi) or *Yersinia pestis*. *It should never be used in trivial or mild infections.* It is used topically for superficial conjunctival infections and blepharitis caused by *E coli, H influenzae, Moraxella lacunata, Staph aureus* and *Strep hemolyticus*.

Bone-marrow injury is the major toxic effect. Thrombocytopenia, granulocytopenia and aplastic anemia are the most serious hematopoietic disturbances observed and have resulted in a number of fatalities. Aplastic anemia has occurred even after ophthalmic use. Any patient under treatment must be given a leukocyte and differential count every 2 to 3 days. Bone-marrow depression is more serious in pregnancy and in infants than in other persons. In neonates it may cause the "Gray syndrome," a fatal cyanosis (40% of cases) with symptoms of vomiting, abdominal distention and loose, green stools, owing to the inability of the infant to metabolize the drug in consequence of glucuronyl transferase deficiency. Optic atrophy and blindness occur in a small number of cases, mainly in children on prolonged therapy.

Minor untoward effects such as transient mild euphoria, skin rash and gastrointestinal disturbances (occasional nausea and vomiting, gaseous distention, loose stools and pruritus ani) have been observed; the drug is contraindicated in patients with a history of previous sensitization. Occasional untoward effects include glossitis, stomatitis and pharyngitis. Its use, as with other antibiotics, may result in an overgrowth of microorganisms not susceptible to the drug. It interacts adversely with other drugs that depress bone marrow (antineoplastics, colchicine, gold salts, penicillamine, phenylbutazone). Oral anticoagulants, oral hypoglycemics, phenytoin and perhaps acetaminophen inhibit its metabolism and increase the risk of intoxication; appropriate dose adjustments should be made. Rifampin decreases plasma concentrations.

The drug is absorbed rapidly from the gastrointestinal tract, with a bioavailability of about 90%. Significant serum levels are obtained in 30 min, peak blood concentrations of 10 to 15 μg/mL (after 1-g dose) are reached in about 2 hr, and a therapeutic concentration is maintained for about 6 to 8 hr. Sixty percent of the drug in blood is bound to serum albumin. The volume of distribution is about 0.7 mL/g. From 85 to 95% is biotransformed in the liver. The half-life is 1.5 to 5 hr, except over 24 hr in neonates 1 to 2 days old and 10 hr in infants 10 to 16 days old. Because of considerable variability, plasma levels must be monitored. Also, the clearance increases with continuous use, and dose adjustments are necessary. When there is impaired hepatic function, and sometimes of renal function as well, the dosage must be reduced, according to determined plasma concentrations. It can cross the placental barrier and intoxicate the fetus, so that the drug should be avoided in pregnancy, if possible.

Dose—*Oral, adult, children* and *infants over 2 wk*, usually **12.5 mg/kg** every 6 hr; up to 100 mg/kg a day may be given to adults. *Full-term infants up to 2 wk* and infants with *immature hepatic metabolic function*, **6.25/kg** every 6 hr. *Neonates* (<2 kg) and up to 7 days, **25 mg/kg** once a day; *neonates* (>2 kg) **50 mg/kg** a day in divided doses every 12 hr. The desired plasma concentration is in the range of 5 to 20 μg/mL. *Topical*, as **1%** dermatologic cream 3 or 4 times a day, as **0.5%** otic solution 3 times a day, or as **0.5%** ophthalmic solution or **1%** ophthalmic ointment every 2 to 3 hr for the first 3 days and every 3 to 4 hr thereafter, as required.

Dosage Forms—Capsules: 250 and 500 mg; Cream: 1%; Ophthalmic Ointment: 1%; for Ophthalmic Solution: 25 mg; Ophthalmic Solution: 0.5%; Otic Solution: 0.5%.

Chloramphenicol Palmitate

Hexadecanoic acid, [R-(R^*,R^*)]-2-[(2,2-dichloroacetyl)amino]-3-hydroxy-3-(4-nitrophenyl)propyl ester;
Chloromycetin Palmitate (*Parke-Davis*)

Chloramphenicol α-palmitate [530-43-8] $C_{27}H_{42}Cl_2N_2O_6$ (561.54). Potency: 550 to 595 μg of chloramphenicol ($C_{11}H_{12}Cl_2N_2O_5$)/mg.

Preparation—Chloramphenicol is esterified by treatment with palmitoyl chloride [$CH_3(CH_2)_{14}COCl$] in the presence of pyridine. The crude ester is obtained by pouring the reaction product into a large excess of dilute hydrochloric acid and filtering. It is then purified by recrystallization from an appropriate solvent.

Description—Fine, white, unctuous, crystalline powder; faint odor; bland, mild taste; melts between 87° and 95°.

Solubility—About 1 g in 1000 mL water or 5000 mL petroleum ether; freely soluble in methanol, ethanol and nonpolar solvents.

Uses—The drug is insoluble and hence lacks the bitter flavor of chloramphenicol. It is hydrolyzed in the upper intestinal tract to chloramphenicol. Therefore, its oral uses are those of the parent drug (see *Chloramphenicol*); however, it does not share the topical efficacy of the parent drug. Its toxicity is likewise that of chloramphenicol; it should not be used unless certain severe criteria of indication are met. Since the absorption of the chloramphenicol depends on the hydrolysis of the palmitate ester to chloramphenicol, the blood levels of chloramphenicol rise more slowly after an oral dose than with the parent chloramphenicol and its duration of action is somewhat longer.

Dose—*Oral*, same as for *Chloramphenicol*, expressed as chloramphenicol equivalent.

Dosage Form (chloramphenicol equivalent)—Oral Suspension: 150 mg/5 mL.

Chloramphenicol Sodium Succinate

Butanedioic acid, [*R*-(*R**,*R**)]-mono[2-[(2,2-dichloroacetyl)amino]-3- hydroxy-3-(4-nitrophenyl)propyl]ester, monosodium salt; Chloromycetin Succinate (*Parke-Davis*)

Chloramphenicol α-(sodium succinate) [982-57-0] $C_{15}H_{15}Cl_2N_2NaO_8$ (445.19). Potency: equivalent to 650 to 765 μg of $C_{11}H_{12}Cl_2N_2O_5$ (chloramphenicol)/mg.

Preparation—Chloramphenicol is reacted with an equimolar portion of succinic acid anhydride to yield chloramphenicol hydrogen succinate which, after purification by recrystallization, is neutralized with sodium hydroxide to give the ester-salt.

Description—Light-yellow, crystalline powder.

Solubility—Freely soluble in water or alcohol.

Uses—Useful for parenteral administration by virtue of its high aqueous solubility. Its effectiveness *in vivo* depends on the liberation of the parent compound by hydrolysis, and, therefore, its uses are similar to those of chloramphenicol. Parenteral bioavailability, as chloramphenicol, is more variable (about 70%) with the succinate than with chloramphenicol itself. Also, the volume of distribution (2.1 mL/g) is higher. It may be preferred when oral therapy is not feasible, or when rapid attainment of a high blood level is desired. The toxicity is that of the parent drug; thus, it should not be used unless certain severe criteria of indication are met.

Dose (chloramphenicol equivalent)—*Oral and intravenous, adult,* **12.5 mg/kg** every 6 hr, but up to 100 mg/kg a day in life-threatening infections; *infants 2 wk and older,* **12.5 mg/kg** every 6 hr or **25 mg/kg** every 12 hr; *full-term infants* (<2 kg) **25 mg/kg** once a day or, if >2 kg, given every 12 hr in severe infections, up to 100 mg/kg a day may be given.

Dosage Form—Powder for Injection: 100 mg/1 mL and 1 g/10 mL.

Clindamycin Hydrochloride

L-*threo*-α-D-*galacto*-Octopyranoside, methyl (2*S*-*trans*)-7-chloro-6,7,8-trideoxy-6-[[(1-methyl-4-propyl-2-pyrrolidinyl)carbonyl]-amino]-1-thio-, monohydrochloride; Cleocin Hydrochloride (*Upjohn*); (*Various Mfrs*)

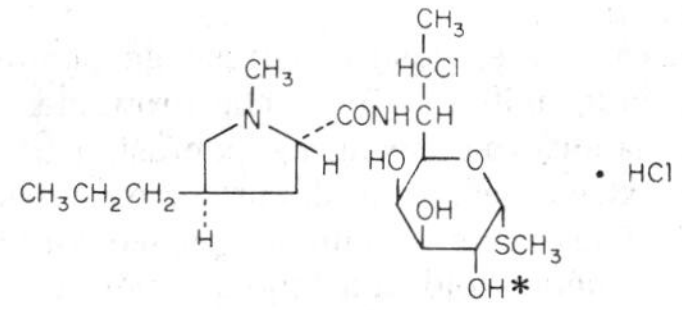

CH_3 HCCl CONHCH $CH_3CH_2CH_2$ HO OH SCH_3 OH* · HCl

(*) Indicates site of esterification to form the palmitate or phosphate derivatives.

[21462-39-5] $C_{18}H_{33}ClN_2O_5S.HCl$ (461.44). Potency: equivalent to not less than 800 μg of clindamycin/mg.

Preparation—*Lincomycin* is treated with a solution of Rydon reagent prepared from triphenylphosphine, acetonitrile, and chlorine. The base is ultimately reacted with HCl. *CA 73:*15185*v*, 1970.

Description—White or practically white, crystalline powder; strong, characteristic taste; odorless or has a faint mercaptan-like odor; stable in air and light; pK_a 7.72; melts about 142°.

Solubility—1 g in 2 mL water or 200 mL ethanol.

Uses—An antibacterial spectrum very much like that of *Lincomycin*, from which it is derived. However, among staphylococci and several streptococci it may be as much as 20 times more potent. It is also more potent against certain gram-negative organisms, but not against gram-negative cocci; with the recommended doses the plasma levels usually are not high enough to be effective against gram-negative bacteria. It is especially useful in the treatment of several infections caused by anaerobes; it is the drug of choice for treatment of gastrointestinal infections caused by *B fragilis* and is one of several alternative drugs for treatment of infections caused by oropharyngeal strains of *B fragilis, Fusobacterium*, anaerobic streptococci and *Cl perfringens* (but not other clostridia). It is important as an alternate drug for treating infections caused by penicillin-resistant *Staph aureus.* It also is used for treatment of respiratory tract infections and pharyngitis or tonsillitis caused by *Strep pyogenes.* It is perhaps the best drug for the topical treatment of *acne vulgaris* (used as the phosphate).

It may cause abdominal pain, nausea, vomiting, diarrhea and loose stools, which may occasionally contain blood and mucus. Incidence of benign diarrhea is about 10 to 20%. Incidence of antibiotic-associated (pseudomembranous) colitis is estimated to be 1:10,000 (by clinical criteria) to 10% (by endoscopy). Allergic rashes and urticaria occur with an incidence of about 10%. Rarely, a Stevens-Johnson-like syndrome occurs. Anaphylaxis also has occurred. Transient neutropenia and eosinophilia occur, and thrombocytopenia and agranulocytosis have been reported.

By the oral route, bioavailability is about 90% with low doses (150 mg) but 23 to 38% with higher doses. The presence of food in the stomach and intestines does not appear to interfere with absorption. In plasma it is 60 to 95% protein-bound. Its volume of distribution is about 0.66 mL/g. It is distributed widely in most tissues, body fluids and bone. However, high enough concentrations are not achieved in CSF to be used to treat meningitis. Most of it is eliminated in the liver, only about 10% being excreted in the urine. The half-life is 2.4 to 3 hr, except 3.5 to 5 hr in anuria and 7 to 14 hr in liver disease. Hepatic failure can be expected to reduce the dose requirement more than renal failure.

Dose (base equivalent)—*Oral, adult,* for *moderately severe infections,* **150** to **300 mg** every 6 hr; for *very severe infections,* **300** to **450 mg** every 6 hr. To avoid esophageal irritation, take each dose with a full glass of water. Treatment of infections caused by anaerobes should be initiated with parenteral clindamycin (clindamycin phosphate), then switched to oral medication when the condition shows improvement.

Dosage Form (clindamycin equivalent)—Capsules: 75, 150 and 300 mg.

Clindamycin Palmitate Hydrochloride

L-*threo*-α-D-*galacto*-Octopyranoside, methyl (2*S*-*trans*)-7-chloro-6,7,8-trideoxy-6-[[(1-methyl-4-propyl-2-pyrrolidinyl)carbonyl]-amino]-1-thio-2-hexadecanoate, monohydrochloride; Cleocin Pediatric (*Upjohn*) (*Various Mfrs*)

[25507-04-4] $C_{34}H_{63}ClN_2O_6S.HCl$ (699.86). Potency: equivalent to not less than 540 μg of clindamycin ($C_{18}H_{33}ClN_2O_5S$)/mg.

Preparation—The 3- and 4-OH groups of clindamycin are protected by condensation with cuminaldehyde and the 2-OH group is then condensed with palmitoyl chloride at the marked hydroxyl group (see structure for *clindamycin hydrochloride*). The protecting group is then removed through appropriate hydrolytic procedure and the clindamycin palmitate is finally reacted with an equimolar quantity of HCl.

Description—White to off-white, amorphous powder; characteristic odor and taste; may form lumps and glass-like crystals when drying; stable in light, heat (up to 50°) and air.

Solubility—1 g in 5 mL water, 3 mL alcohol or 4 mL chloroform; freely soluble in ether.

Uses—Converted to clindamycin in the small intestine. It has the same actions and uses as *Clindamycin Hydrochloride.* The palmitate lacks the bitter taste of clindamycin and is thus suited to use in an oral solution for pediatric use. The absorption time, plasma levels and plasma half-life are identical to those of the hydrochloride; the half-life in young children is about 2 hr.

Dose (clindamycin equivalent)—*Oral, infants 1 mo* and *older* and *children,* **2** to **6.3 mg/kg** every 6 hr or **2.7** to **8.3 mg/kg** every 8 hr. In *children under 10 kg* the dose should be no less than a total of 37.5 mg. Use cautiously in infants less than 1 mo. The palmitate is not usually used in adults.

Dosage Form (clindamycin equivalent)—for Oral Solution: 75 mg/5 mL.

Clindamycin Phosphate

L-*threo*-α-D-*galacto*-Octopyranoside, methyl (2*S*-*trans*)-7-chloro-6,7,8-trideoxy-6-[[(1-methyl-4-propyl-2-pyrrolidinyl)carbonyl]-amino]-1-thio-, 2-(dihydrogen phosphate); Cleocin Phosphate (*Upjohn*) (*Various Mfrs*)

[24729-96-2] $C_{18}H_{34}ClN_2O_8PS$ (504.96). Potency: equivalent to not less than 758 μg of clindamycin/mg.

Preparation—The 3- and 4-OH groups of clindamycin are protected by condensation with cuminaldehyde and the 2-OH* group (refer to the structure of the hydrochloride, p 1209) is then condensed with $POCl_3$. Appropriate hydrolytic procedures finally convert the —$OPOCl_2$ residue to —$OPO(OH)_2$ and remove the protecting group.

Description—White to off-white, crystalline powder; hygroscopic odorless or nearly so; bitter taste; stable in light and air but unstable in temperature of 50° (degrades to free clindamycin); melts with decomposition about 175°.

Solubility—1 g in 2.5 mL water or > 1000 mL alcohol.

Uses—Rapidly hydrolyzed in the plasma to clindamycin. Thus, it has the same actions and uses as *Clindamycin Hydrochloride*, except that the phosphate is given parenterally, which avoids the gastrointestinal side effects of the oral forms of clindamycin. However, the dangers of anaphylaxis are greater. Although the phosphate is promoted for treatment of infections of all grades of severity, it would seem advisable to withhold its use in mild infections, unless the oral forms cannot be tolerated. In infections caused by anaerobes, treatment with clindamycin should be initiated with this derivative given parenterally. This salt also is applied topically in the treatment of acne vulgaris.

Dose—*Intramuscular* or *intravenous, adult, usually* **600** to **1200 mg** a day in 2 to 4 equal doses; up to 2.7 g/day may be given, if necessary; *children over 1 mo,* **20** to **40 mg/kg** in 3 to 4 equal doses; for *life-threatening situations,* **4.8 g** a day have been given IV to adults. *Topical,* to the *skin,* as 1% gel or solution twice a day.

Dosage Forms (clindamycin equivalent)—Gel: 1%; Injection: 300 mg/2 mL and 600 mg/4 mL; Topical Solution: 10 mg/mL.

Cycloserine

(*R*)-3-Isoxazolidinone, 4-amino-, Seromycin (*Lilly*)

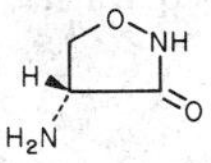

(+)-4-Amino-3-isoxazolidinone [68-41-7] $C_3H_6N_2O_2$ (102.09); a substance produced by the growth of *Streptomyces orchidaceus* or obtained by synthesis. Potency: not less than 900 μg of $C_3H_6N_2O_2$/mg.

Preparation—Cycloserine may be isolated from the fermentation of *Streptomyces orchidaceus* or made synthetically from DL-serine (see RPS-15, page 1146).

Description—White to pale-yellow, crystalline powder; odorless or a faint odor; hygroscopic and deteriorates upon absorbing water; melts about 155° with decomposition.

Solubility—Freely soluble in water.

Uses—Inhibits a wide variety of both gram-positive and gram-negative bacteria and mycobacteria. However, *Pseudomonas, Proteus* and gonococci are resistant. It has been used successfully against stubborn *urinary tract infections* caused by streptococci, staphylococci, *E coli* and *Enterobacter aerogenes.* However, interest mainly centers on its moderate usefulness in the therapy of *tuberculosis* resistant to other drugs; it is a "backup" drug secondary to isoniazid, streptomycin and aminosalicylic acid. It always is combined with other antituberculosis drugs. It should not be used unless other antitubercular drugs have become ineffective or are contraindicated. Resistance to it does develop.

Depending on the dose, toxic effects associated with the CNS occur within the first 2 wk (usually) in a large percentage of patients. These are reversible on discontinuance of therapy. Such effects are headache, vertigo, blurred vision, photosensitivity, anxiety, nightmares, paresis, dysarthria, lethargy, somnolence, depression, confusion, irritability, behavioral changes, psychotic episodes with suicidal tendencies, hyperreflexia, tremors, twitching, ankle clonus and convulsions. CNS toxicity can be controlled by the administration of pyridoxine, anticonvulsants, sedatives and tranquilizing agents. Toxic effects are minimized if blood levels of the drug do not exceed 25 to 30 μg/mL. Skin rashes may occur.

Oral bioavailability is 70 to 90%. It penetrates into all body fluids, cavities and tubercles. The levels in cerebrospinal fluid are 50 to 80% of those in plasma, except 80 to 100% in meningitis. About 70% is eliminated in urine; the half-life is 10 hr but longer in renal failure.

Dose—*Oral, adult* and *children over 10 yr,* **250 mg** every 12 hr; in tuberculosis, after the first 2 wk the dose-interval is cautiously shortened to as short as every 6 hr, according to plasma levels and adverse effects; *children* **10** to **20 mg/kg** a day (maximum of 0.75 to 1 g has been recommended).

Dosage Form—Capsules: 250 mg.

Fusidate Sodium—see RPS-18, page 1219.

Rifampin

Rifamycin, 3-[[(4-methyl-1-piperazinyl)imino]methyl]-, Rifampicin; Rifadin (*Marion Merrell Dow*); Rimactane (*Ciba*)

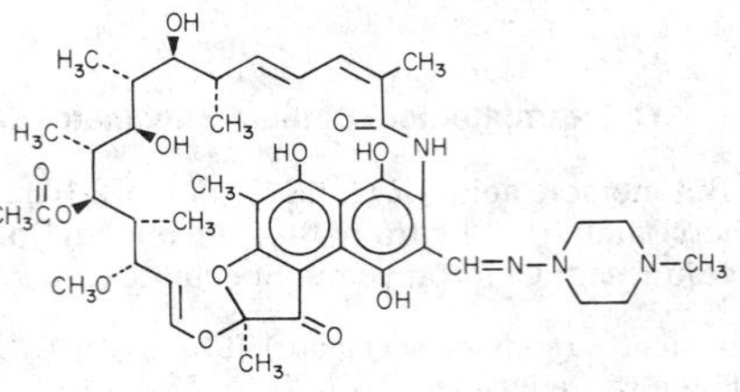

[13292-46-1] $C_{43}H_{58}N_4O_{12}$ (822.95). Potency: not less than 900 μg of $C_{43}H_{58}N_4O_{12}$/mg.

Preparation—Rifamycin SV, which may be prepared by the method of Sensi, *et al* (US Pat 3,313,804), is converted to the 8-carboxaldehyde derivative, known also as 3-formylrifamycin SV, and this is condensed with 1-amino-4-methylpiperazine to form a Schiff base, which is rifampin.

Description—Red-brown, crystalline powder; odorless; unstable in light, heat, air and moisture; melts between 183° and 188° with decomposition; pK_a 1.7, 7.9.

Solubility—1 g in about 762 mL water; freely soluble in chloroform; soluble in ethyl acetate or methanol.

Uses—A broad-spectrum antibiotic effective against most gram-positive bacteria, especially *Staph pyogenes, Strep pyogenes, Strep viridans* and *Strep pneumoniae,* and variably active against gram-negative organisms, especially *H influenzae,* meningococci and gonococci. Both *Mycobacterium tuberculosis* and *Mycobacterium leprae* are very susceptible to the drug. Unfortunately, many bacteria very rapidly acquire resistance to rifampin; this, along with the superiority of other antibiotics against many of the above-cited bacteria and the desire to avoid inadvertent development of resistance of mycobacteria to the drug, is an important reason why the drug has a very limited range of use. Its clinical use is mainly in the treatment of tuberculosis. The rate of development of resistance of the mycobacterium is low. Nevertheless, it always is used in combination with other antitubercular drugs; it may be added to isoniazid and pyrazinamide to make a first-choice combination for treatment of infections caused by *Mycobacterium tuberculosis,* to isoniazid for those caused by *atypical mycobacteria* and to dapsone for *leprosy.* It also appears to be an excellent drug for *prophylaxis of meningococcal* meningitis and pneumonia from *H influenzae Type B and treatment of meningococcal carrier state.*

It may cause heartburn, epigastric distress, gas, cramps, diarrhea, anorexia and nausea and vomiting. Headache, drowsiness and fatigue commonly occur, and inability to concentrate, confusion, muscular weakness, ataxia, pain in the extremities, visual disturbances and generalized numbness are other CNS side effects. Immunological disturbances may occur, such as occasional rheumatoid and lupoid syndromes, allergic rashes, eosinophilia, leukopenia and hemolytic anemia. Thrombocytopenia is frequent and a monthly thrombocyte count is advisable. Avoidance of high doses also helps to obviate thrombocytopenia. Jaundice and other manifestations of hepatotoxicity have occurred during treatment. Where possible, it is wise to avoid using the drug in combination with ethionamide, prothionamide, pyrazinamide or *p*-aminosalicylates, which also can cause hepatic dysfunction. It is teratogenic in laboratory animals and should therefore be withheld in pregnancy.

It induces the hepatic drug-metabolizing enzyme system and accelerates the metabolism of digitoxin, methadone, phenytoin, beta blockers, verapamil, thcophylline, chloramphenicol, oral contraceptives and estrogens, oral anticoagulants, barbiturates, tolbutamide and itself.

It is 100% absorbed after oral administration, but food in the stomach delays absorption of the drug. Bentonite in granules of *p*-aminosalicylic acid also interferes with absorption, and the granules should not be given close to the time of its administration. The drug is distributed widely in the body, even into cerebrospinal fluid. In plasma 98% is protein-bound. The volume of distribution is 0.9 mL/g. About 85% of the drug is eliminated by biotransformation in the liver. An active metabolite is secreted into bile, where it is therapeutically effective. Metabolism is dose-dependent with doses above 300 to 450 mg; with therapeutic doses the serum half-life is 1.5 to 5 hr. Even so, the drug usually is administered at 8- to 12-hr intervals, because absorption is slow enough to sustain effective levels for 8 to 10 hr. Nevertheless, patients who eliminate the drug rapidly probably should be considered for a different schedule. About 1/3 of a dose is excreted in the feces via the bile. Although it does not appear to accumulate in patients with hepatic insufficiency, the hepatic metabolism and the fact that the drug may be hepatotoxic suggest that it should be used cautiously in hepatic dysfunction. The risk of hepatotoxicity is increased when it is used with isoniazid. It imparts a reddish-orange color to urine, stools, sweat, saliva and tears. Soft contact lens may be stained permanently.

Dose—*Oral, adult,* **600 mg** once a day, taken with a glass of water at least 1 hr before a meal or 2 hr after meals against the meningococcal carrier state, only 4 days of use are required; *children,* **10 to 20 mg/kg** once a day. Some authorities recommend 2 or 3 divided doses not to exceed 600 mg a day. The drug always should be used in combination with at least one other antitubercular drug.

Dosage Forms—Capsules: 150 and 300 mg; Capsules (in combination with isoniazid): 300 mg rifampin and 150 mg isoniazid; Powder for Injection: 600 mg.

Spectinomycin Hydrochloride

4*H*-Pyrano[2,3-*b*][1,4]benzodioxin-4-one, [2*R*-(2α,4aβ,5aβ,6β,7β,8β,9α,9aα,10aβ)]-decahydro-4a,7,9-trihydroxy-2-methyl-6,8-bis(methylamino)-, dihydrochloride, pentahydrate; Trobicin (*Upjohn*)

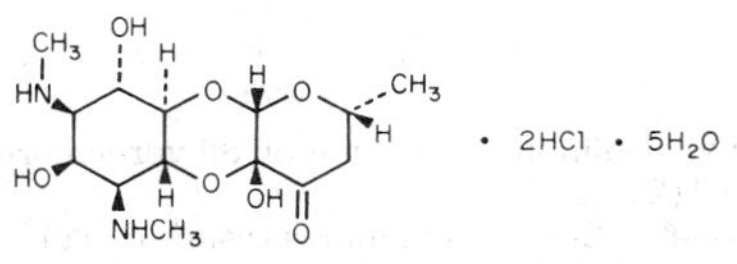

[22189-32-8]; $C_{14}H_{24}N_2O_7.2HCl.5H_2O$ (495.35); *anhydrous* [21736-83-4] (405.27). Potency: equivalent to not less than 603 μg spectinomycin/mg.

Preparation—By growth of the soil microorganism *Streptomyces spectabilis.* Reaction with a double equimolar quantity of HCl yields the hydrochloride. *Antibiot Chemother 11:* 118 and 661, 1961. US Pat 3,234,092.

Description—White, odorless, crystalline powder; slightly bitter taste; stable in light; nonhygroscopic; stable in air at room temperature; pK_a 6.88, 8.84.

Solubility—1 g in about 7 mL water; practically insoluble in alcohol, chloroform or ether.

Uses—A wide-spectrum antibiotic with moderate activity against both gram-positive and gram-negative bacteria. However, it is employed clinically for only one purpose, namely, to treat or prevent acute gonorrhea when the organism is resistant to penicillin, or when the patient is allergic to penicillin. It is not as effective as ceftriaxone. Clinical studies have shown it to be no more efficacious than tetracycline and possibly no better against some strains of gonococcus than ampicillin or erythromycin. Resistance sometimes develops. It is not effective in eradicating pharyngeal gonococcal infections in more than 50% of patients.

Orally, the drug is absorbed poorly and must be given intramuscularly; 2 g will provide a plasma concentration of about 100 μg/mL. The distribution coefficient is 0.12 mL/g. About 75% is excreted into urine unchanged. Plasma half-life is approximately 1 to 3 hr.

Untoward effects caused include frequent pain at the site of injection and infrequent headache, nausea, vomiting, insomnia, chills, fever, mild pruritus and urticaria. It does not eradicate *Treponema* or *Chlamydia trachomatis,* which are common sexually transmitted pathogens.

Dose—*Intramuscular, adult,* as a single injection, usually **2 g**, but **4 g** is used in regions in which partial resistance to the drug is known to occur; *children less than 45 kg,* **40 mg/kg.**

Dosage Form—Injection: 2 and 4 g.

Vancomycin Hydrochloride

Vancomycin, hydrochloride; Lyphocin (*Lyphomed*); Vancocin (*Lilly*); Vancoled (*Lederle*)

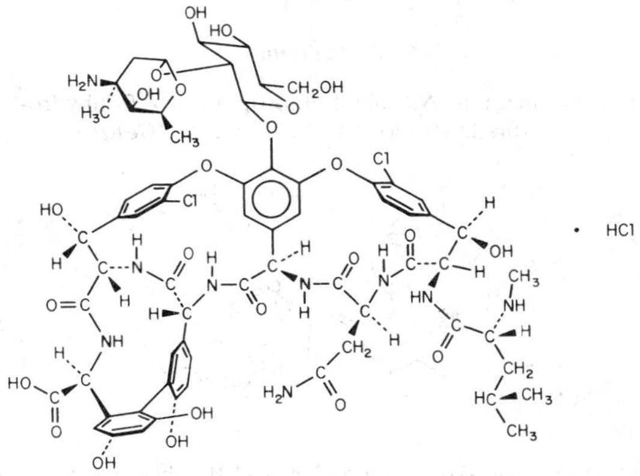

Vancomycin hydrochloride [1404-93-9] is a substance produced by growth of *Streptomyces orientalis* (Fam *Streptomycetaceae).* Potency: equivalent to not less than 900 μg of vancomycin per mg, calculated on the anhydrous basis.

Preparation—Vancomycin is produced by the submerged fermentation process (page 1279). After purification the base is converted to the soluble hydrochloride with HCl. See *Antibiot Ann:*606, 1955–6; US Pat 3,067,099.

Description—Tan to brown, free-flowing powder; odorless; bitter taste.

Solubility—Freely soluble in water; insoluble in ether or chloroform.

Uses—A glycopeptide highly active against gram-positive cocci, neisseria and clostridia. It inhibits synthesis of peptidoglycan in cell-wall formation. It is the drug of choice in the treatment of antibiotic-associated colitis and other infections caused by *Cl difficile.* The rapid emergence of methicillin-resistant staphylococci (especially *Staph* epidermidis) makes this drug valuable in the treatment of severe staphylococcal infections. Development of resistance to vancomycin is rare, and there is no cross-resistance to other antibiotics. Streptococcal (especially Strep *vividans* and *bovis*), enterococcal and pneumococcal infections also are treated with the drug. It is used only in combination with an aminoglycoside in treating enterococcal endocarditis. Because of its toxicity, the drug is held in reserve for serious infections unresponsive to other antibacterial agents or prophylaxis in penicillin-sensitive patients.

It is absorbed poorly from the gastrointestinal tract, so that it may be used orally against staphylococcal and enterococcal enteritis and antibiotic-associated enterocolitis. However, severe enteritis often requires concomitant systemic therapy and hence parenteral administration. In plasma, 55% is protein-bound. It enters the cerebrospinal fluid. The volume of distribution is 0.47 mL/g. The distribution half-life is 0.5 hr. The elimination half-life is 4 to 6 hr in adults and 2 to 3 hr in children. Since the drug is 70% eliminated by excretion in urine, the half-life in anuric patients ranges from 3 to 10 days and doses must be appropriately adjusted. Elimination is accelerated in burn patients, which also requires dose-adjustments.

It is irritating to tissue and may cause thrombophlebitis, or pain at the site of injection and necrosis occurs if extravasated; also chills, fever, occasional urticaria and maculopapular rashes with hypotension (red man's syndrome), nephrotoxicity and ototoxicity and, rarely, thrombocytopenia and neuropathy. The drug is contraindicated in patients taking, or who have recently taken, ototoxic or nephrotoxic drugs, except that it is used in combination with streptomycin for surgical prophylaxis against bacterial endocarditis in penicillin-sensitive patients. Elderly persons should have serial auditory tests and determinations of plasma levels of the drug.

Dose—*Intravenous infusion, adult,* **500 mg** every 6 hr *or* **15 mg/kg** or **1 g** every 12 hr (a total of 3 to 4 g a day have been given in very serious infections); *infants* and *children,* **10 mg/kg** every 6 hr *or* **22 mg/kg** every 12 hr (a total of 60 mg/kg a day have been given in very serious infections). *Oral, adults,* **500 mg** to **2 g** a day in 3 to 4 divided doses for 9 to 10 days or, alternatively, **125 mg** 3 or 4 times a day for *C difficile; children,* **40 mg/kg** a day in divided doses, (do not exceed 2 g a day); *infants and neonates,* **15 mg/kg** initially followed by **10 mg/kg** every 12 hr.

Dosage Forms (vancomycin equivalent)—Capsules: 125 and 250 mg; for Injection: 0.5, 1.5 and 10 g; for Oral Solution: 1 and 10 g.

Miscellaneous Systemic Antibacterial Drugs

Acetohydroxamic acid—see RPS-18, page 1223.

Aminosalicylate Sodium—see RPS-18, page 1221.

Cinoxacin—see RPS 18, page 1223.

Clofazimine

2-Phenazinamine, *N*,5-bis(4-chlorophenyl)-3,5-dihydro-3-[(1-methylethyl)imino]-, Lamprene (*Geigy*)

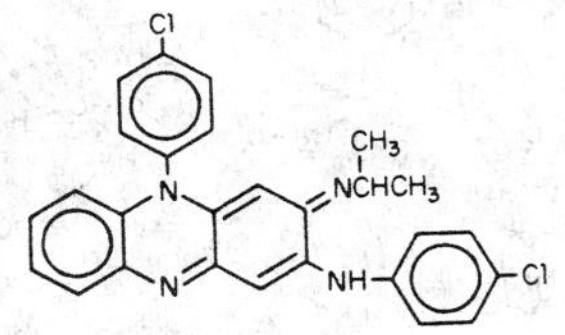

3-(*p*-Chloroanilino)-10-(*p*-chlorophenyl)-2,10-dihydro-2-(isopropylimino)phenazine; [2030-63-9] $C_{27}H_{22}Cl_2N_4$ (473.40).

Preparation—*J Chem Soc:* 859, 1958.

Description—Dark-red crystals; melts about 210°.

Solubility—Practically insoluble in water; soluble in alcohol, acetone, ethyl acetate, chloroform or benzene.

Uses—In combination with other drugs, used for the treatment of *leprosy* and *infections caused by Mycobacterium avium* in AIDS patients. It is not significantly active against other bacteria. It binds to mycobacterial DNA and interferes with growth. It is bactericidal, but as long as 50 days may be required before killing is evident. Nausea, vomiting, diarrhea, abdominal pain and eosinophilic enteritis may occur. Crystalline deposits of drug in the viscera may cause gastrointestinal bleeding and/or obstruction. Antimuscarinic actions cause dry skin and dryness, burning, itching and irritation of the eyes. The drug also causes long-persisting, rufous discoloration of the skin, cornea, conjuctiva and body fluids. The oral-systemic bioavailability is about 50%. The drug has a predilection for adipocytes, reticuloendothelial cells and other macrophages, in which crystals may accumulate. During maintenance, the elimination half-life is about 70 days.

Dose—*Oral, adult,* for *mycobacterial infections,* **50** to **100 mg** a day, in combination with other antileprotic drugs; with recurring leprotic erythema nodosum, up to 300 mg a day may be required. Therapy may continue for 2 mo to a lifetime.

Dosage Form—Capsules: 50 and 100 mg.

Dapsone

Benzenamine 4,4′-sulfonylbis-, DDS; (*Jacobus*)

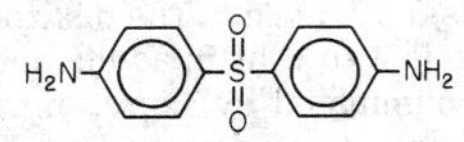

4,4′-Sulfonyldianiline [80-08-0] $C_{12}H_{12}N_2O_2S$ (248.30).

Preparation—Benzene is condensed with sulfuric acid to yield phenyl sulfone [$(C_6H_5)_2SO_2$] which is then nitrated by standard procedures to yield the 4,4′-dinitro derivative. Reduction with tin and HCl or with various other appropriate reductants yields dapsone.

Description—White or creamy white, crystalline powder; odorless; slightly bitter taste; melts between 175° and 181°.

Solubility—Very slightly soluble in water; freely soluble in alcohol; soluble in dilute mineral acids.

Uses—Has an antibacterial spectrum and mechanism of action similar to those of sulfanilamide (see *Sulfonamides*), of which it originally was studied as a congener. Limited success against tuberculosis has been achieved with it, but it is far surpassed by other agents. However, in combination with rifampin, it is the drug of choice in the chemotherapy of *leprosy*. Most of the sulfones used in the treatment of this disease owe both their activity and toxicity to dapsone released from the molecule. For this reason, the drug is the preferred sulfone, since it is cheaper than and equally efficacious to the others. However, resistance is becoming common. Combined with trimethoprim, it is as effective as trimethoprim-sulfametoxazole in the treatment of *Pneumocystis carinii* pneumonia. It is also useful as a suppressant in the treatment of *dermatitis herpetiformis* and *relapsing polychondritis.*

It is absorbed by the oral route. Absorption is more efficient with low than with high doses; 50 mg/day will give a steady-state concentration of 5 to 7 μg/mL, and 100 mg only 7 to 9 μg/mL. It is eliminated in the liver by acetylation. There are slow and fast acetylators among patients. The half-life is 10 to 50 hr, and at least 8 days are required to reach plateau concentrations.

It may cause hemolytic anemia in glucose 6-phosphate dehydrogenase-deficient persons, methemoglobinemia, gastrointestinal upset, headache, nervousness, giddiness, tachycardia, motor neuropathy, blurred vision, paresthesias and pruritus, hematuria, liver damage and jaundice or rash which may become exfoliative. The dermatitis frequently occurs during the 5th week of therapy. Hypermelanosis follows. Lepra reactions (erythema nodosum-like) may occur from a flooding of the body with endotoxins released from killed organisms. Careful initial grading of dose and rest periods avoids much of the toxicity.

Dose—*Oral, adult,* for *leprosy* and *relapsing polychondritis,* **100 mg** or **1.4 mg/kg** once a day up to 200 mg a day; for *dermatitis herpetiformis, initially* **50 mg** a day with gradual increments up to 300 mg a day, if necessary; *children,* for *leprosy* and *dermatitis herpetiformis* **1** to **2** mg/Kg once a day.

Dosage Form—Tablets: 25 and 100 mg.

Ethambutol Hydrochloride

[*R*-(*R**,*R**)]-1-Butanol, 2,2′-(1,2-ethanediyldiimino)bis-, dihydrochloride; Myambutol (*Lederle*)

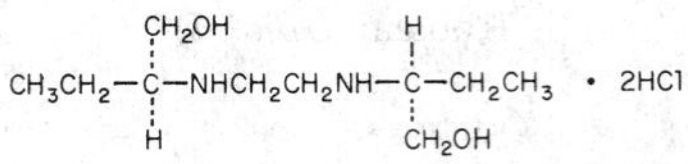

(+)-2,2′-(Ethylenediimino)di-1-butanol dihydrochloride [1070-11-7] $C_{10}H_{24}N_2O_2.2HCl$ (277.23).

Preparation—(±)-2-Aminobutanol is resolved via its tartrate and the (+)-enantiomorph is condensed with 1,2-dichloroethane in an appropriate dehydrochlorinating environment. The ethambutol thus formed is dissolved in a suitable solvent and reacted with HCl. US Pat 3,297,707.

Description—White, crystalline powder; essentially odorless; a bitter taste; stable in light and heat but is hygroscopic when exposed to high relative humidities; melts between 198° and 202°; pK_a 6.3, 9.5.

Solubility—1 g in 1 mL water or 4 mL alcohol; slightly soluble in ether or chloroform.

Uses—A tuberculostatic drug that is effective against tubercle bacilli resistant to isoniazid or streptomycin. It acts only on proliferating cells, apparently by interfering with synthesis of RNA. When used alone in the treatment of tuberculosis, the drug may clear the sputum of mycobacteria within 3 mo in the majority of patients, but bacterial resistance occurs in 35% of cases, and relapses frequently occur. In combination with isoniazid or other tuberculostatic drugs, relapses are uncommon. It should be used as a companion drug to isoniazid. The ethambutol-isoniazid rifampin combinations, are now the most frequently used for patients exposed to drug-resistant organisms.

It occasionally causes optic neuritis, with blurred vision and diminished visual acuity to green light; the effect relates to the duration of use of the drug. Although these effects disappear on discontinuation, the drug should be discontinued at the first indication of a loss in visual acuity. Eye tests should be made before and at monthly intervals after the onset of therapy. Other untoward effects include dermatitis, pruritus, anorexia, nausea, vomiting, abdominal pain, pyrosis, fever, headache, vertigo, malaise, mental confusion, disorientation, hallucinations, paresthesias, elevated serum urate levels (and gout) and abnormal liver function. Multivitamins should be given concurrently. Leukopenia and anaphylaxis are rare occurrences.

The oral bioavailability is 75 to 80%. It is distributed well into most tissues and fluids but poorly in cerebrospinal fluid. The volume of distribution is 1.6 mL/g. Over 80% is eliminated in the urine. The half-life is 3 to 4 hr but up to 8 hr in renal failure.

Dose—*Oral, adult* and *children 13 yr* or *older,* in combination with other tuberculostatic drugs, for *initial treatment,* **15 mg/kg** once a day; for *retreatment* of relapsed cases, **25 mg/kg** once a day for 60 days, then reduced to **15 mg/kg** once a day.

Dosage Form—Film-Coated Tablets: 100 mg and 400 mg.

Ethionamide—see RPS-18, page 1223.

Isoniazid

4-Pyridinecarboxylic acid, hydrazide; Isonicotinylhydrazine; INH; (*Various Mfrs*)

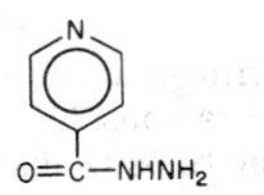

Isonicotinic acid hydrazide [54-85-3] $C_6H_7N_3O$ (137.14).

Preparation—By heating isonicotinic acid or its ethyl ester with anhydrous hydrazine. Isonicotinic acid may be synthesized by various oxidative processes starting with 4-methylpyridine.

Description—Colorless or white crystals, or a white, crystalline powder; odorless; slowly affected by exposure to air and light; solutions are practically neutral to litmus; melts between 170° and 173°; pK_a 1.8, 3.5, 9.5; pH (1 in 100 solution) 5.5 to 6.5.

Solubility—1 g in about 8 mL water and about 50 mL alcohol; slightly soluble in chloroform and ether.

Uses—The most potent and selective of the known *tuberculostatic antibacterial* agents. It is tuberculocidal to growing bacteria and regarded as the most effective agent in the therapy of tuberculosis. The fact that it gains access to all organs and to all body fluids, including cerebrospinal fluid, renders the drug of special value in treating tuberculous meningitis and other extrapulmonary forms of the disease. The drug is never used alone because of the rapid emergence of resistance. Used in combination with other antitubercular drugs, it enhances the clinical response, permits lower doses of the other active agent(s) to be used and retards emergence of resistant tubercle bacilli. It is the central drug around which various combinations are formulated. The first-choice combination contains isoniazid and rifampin, with or without pyrazinamide. It also is used as a *prophylactic*.

Untoward effects are relatively few except in persons who are slow acetylators, when the dose must be lowered. The effects may include restlessness, insomnia, muscle twitching, hyperreflexia, paresthesia and even convulsions, toxic encephalopathy, optic neuritis and atrophy and psychoses. These neurological disorders result from competition of the drug with pyridoxine; pyridoxine administration suppresses the neurological disorders without antagonizing the antitubercular action. Other signs of pyridoxine deficiency may occur. The drug also may cause nausea, vomiting, epigastric distress, agranulocytosis, hemolytic or aplastic anemia, thrombocytopenia, eosinophilia, fever, various rashes and dermatoses and rheumatoid and lupoid syndromes. Hepatitis, with jaundice, is uncommon in patients under 35 yr but occurs in about 2% of recipients over 50 yr, but 10 to 20% will show elevations in SGOT and SGPT. The hepatic, hematological and dermatological effects are probably all allergic.

It is mostly acetylated by the liver; the rate varies considerably. In fast acetylators, the half-life is 1 to 1½ hr; in slow ones, it is 2 to 5 hr. Intramuscular injections cause local irritation.

Dose—*Oral, adult,* for *prophylaxis* or *treatment*, **300 mg** once a day; *infants* and *children*, for *treatment*, **10** to **20 mg/kg** a day, up to 300 to 500 mg of total dose a day, except **30 mg/kg** a day in the 1st week of treatment of tubercular meningitis and for *prophylaxis*, **10 mg/kg** once a day, up to a maximum of 300 mg a day. *Intramuscular, adults,* for *treatment*, **5 mg/kg** once a day, up to 300 mg a day; for *prophylaxis*, **300 mg** once a day; *infants* and *children*, for *treatment*, **10** to **20 mg/kg** up to 300 mg once a day; for *prophylaxis*, **10 mg/kg** up to 300 mg once a day.

Dosage Forms—Injection: 100 mg/mL in 10-mL containers; Powder: 1 lb; Tablets: 50, 100 and 300 mg; syrup: 500 mg/5 mL. For Isoniazid and Rifampin Capsules, see *Rifampin*, page 1317.

Nalidixic Acid—see RPS-18, page 1224.

Nitrofurantoin

2,4-Imidazolidenedione, 1-[[(5-nitro-2-furanyl) methylene]amino]-, Furadantin, Macrodantin (*Procter & Gamble*); (*Various Mfrs*)

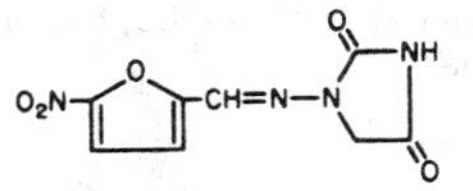

1-[(-5-Nitrofurfurylidene)amino]hydantoin [67-20-9] $C_8H_6N_4O_5$ (238.16).

Caution—It is discolored by alkali and by exposure to light, and is decomposed upon contact with metals other than stainless steel or aluminum.

Preparation—5-Nitro-2-furaldehyde (I) readily undergoes condensation with 1-aminohydantoin (II) to yield nitrofurantoin. I is synthesized by direct nitration of "2-furfural diacetate" [2-furanmethanediol diacetate (III), prepared by the addition reaction between 2-furaldehyde and acetic anhydride] followed by saponification to regenerate the formyl group which, had it not been so protected, would have been oxidized to carboxyl during the nitration. II may be synthesized by effecting the addition of cyanic acid to hydrazinoacetic acid (IV) to produce the 3-carbamoyl derivative (V) which cyclizes by dehydration to II.

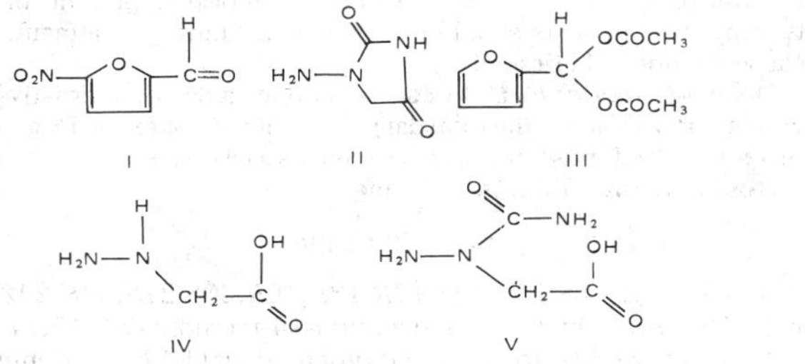

Description—Lemon-yellow crystals or fine powder; odorless; bitter aftertaste; pK_a 7.2.

Solubility—Very slightly soluble in water or alcohol.

Uses—Effective against a majority of urinary tract pathogens, including certain strains of *E coli, Enterobacter, Klebsiella, Proteus* spp, *Staph aureus* and *Strep faecalis*. It is also effective against many staphylococci, clostridia and *B subtilis*. It is indicated for the treatment of infections of the urinary tract caused by the above bacteria: pyelonephritis, cystis and pyelitis. An acid urine favors activity. It is not the drug of first choice in the treatment of any acute infection and it rarely is used. In chronic bacteriuria, it is a second- or third-choice agent. However, as a prophylactic in the prevention of recurrences it is effective, being slightly superior to methenamine mandelate but inferior to sulfamethizole. It is not indicated for treatment of associated perinephric or renal cortical abscesses, prostatitis or other genitourinary tract infections, since in these the blood level is more important than urine concentration. The microcrystalline form is absorbed rapidly and completely; the macrocrystalline form is more slowly and less completely absorbed. About 67% is metabolized in the body, and 33% is excreted into the urine unchanged. The half-life is only 0.3 hr; slow absorption helps to sustain urine levels. Dose adjustment must be made in renal failure. Overall, the side effects are high (10% or more). Nausea, vomiting and diarrhea occur in an appreciable number of patients. Reduction in dosage, or administration with food or milk, lessens the incidence; it is claimed that use of "macrocrystalline" product diminishes the incidence and intensity of gastrointestinal upsets without affecting potency. Absorption is delayed, but bioavailability is not diminished. Gastrointestinal effects also occur in some patients receiving the drug intravenously. Hypersensitivity reactions with dermatological manifestations also occur. Headache, vertigo, drowsiness, malaise, muscular aches, nystagmus and polyneuropathy occasionally occur. Neuropathies appear to be more likely to occur if there is renal insufficiency; they appear to be caused by metabolites. Hemolytic anemia, megaloblastic anemia, granulocytopenia, leukopenia, esoinophilia and maculopapular rashes occur occasionally. It also causes infrequent cholestatic jaundice and hepatocellular damage. Pneumonitis and pulmonary fibrosis can occur, especially in elderly patients. Occasionally, there is transient alopecia. Superinfections may occur. The drug is mutagenic in the Ames test.

Dose—*Oral, adult,* for *treatment*, **50** to **100 mg** or **1.27** to **1.75 mg/kg** every 6 hr; for *prophylaxis*, **50** to **100 mg** or **2 mg/kg** once a day at bed time; *infants* and *children 1 mo* or *over*, **1.25** to **1.75 mg/kg** every 6 hr for 10 to 14 days.

Dosage Forms—Capsules (microcrystals): 50 and 100 mg; Capsules (macrocrystals): 25, 50 and 100 mg; Oral Suspension: 25 mg/5 mL; Tablets: 50 and 100 mg.

Pyrazinamide

Pyrazine carboxamide; (*Lederle*)

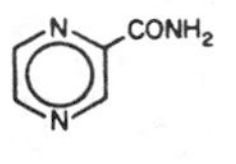

[98-96-4] $C_5H_5N_3O$ (123.11).

Preparation—By thermal decarboxylation of 2,3-pyrazinedicarboxylic acid to form the monocarboxylic acid, which is esterified with methanol and then subjected to controlled ammonolysis; *J Am Chem Soc 74*:3617, 1952.

Description—White to practically white, crystalline powder; sublimes about 60°; melts about 190°; pK_a0.5.

Solubility—1 g in 67 mL water, 75 mL methanol, 175 mL absolute ethanol, 135 mL chloroform, 1000 mL ether or 110 mL alcohol.

Uses—An antituberculosis drug used in initial treatment in combination with isoniazid and rifampin. It generally is administered with isoniazid, which it potentiates. However, it is quite toxic and should be held in reserve until other therapy fails. It may cause fever, anorexia, malaise and hepatic damage, with or without jaundice, and death can occur. All patients intended to be treated with this drug should have prior liver function tests, which tests also must be repeated periodically during therapy. All patients should be hospitalized during treatment. It may cause retention of uric acid.

Dose—*Oral, adult,* **15** to **30 mg/kg** once a day or alternatively **50** to **70 mg/kg** twice a wk; the total daily dose should not exceed 3 g. It is not recommended for use in children except as a last resort.

Dosage form—Tablets: 500 mg.

Rifabutin

(9*S*,12*E*,14*S*,15*R*,16*S*,17*R*,18*R*,19*R*,20*S*,21*S*,22*E*,24*Z*)-6,16,18,20-tetrahydroxyl-1′-isobutyl-14-methoxy-7,9,15,17,19,21,-25-heptamethylspiro[9,4-(epoxypentadeca[1,11,13]trienimino)-2*H*-furo[2′,3′:7,8]naphth[1,2-*d*]imidazole-2,4′-piperidine]-5,10,26-(3*H*, 9*H*)-trione-16-acetate; Mycobutin (*Adria*)

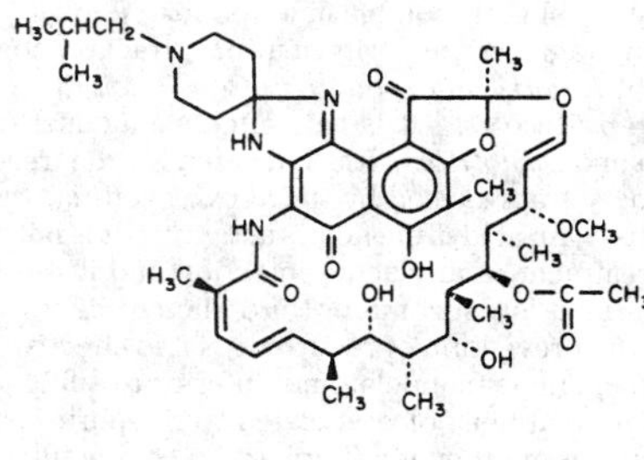

[72559-06-9] $C_{46}H_{62}N_4O_{11}$ (847.02).

Uses—A semisynthetic ansamycin antibiotic that has antimycobacterial activity. It inhibits DNA-dependent RNA polymerase in susceptible strains of bacteria. It is indicated for prevention of disseminated *Mycobacterium avium* complex (MAC) disease in patients with advanced HIV infection.

It should not be administered to patients with active tuberculosis because single agent therapy is likely to lead to development of tuberculosis that is resistant both to rifabutin and rifampin. Adverse reactions primarily may include rash (4%), GI intolerance (3%) and neutropenia (2%). Other reactions may include flu-like syndrome, hepatitis hemolysis, arthralgia, parathesia, aphasia, confusion and nonspecific T wave changes on ECG.

Oral doses are absorbed readily from the GI tract and slowly eliminated with a half-life of 16 to 69 hr. It has a high volume of distribution and good tissue uptake due to its lipophilicity. About 30% of dose is excreted in the feces, and 53% is excreted in urine primarily as metabolites.

Dose—*Oral,* **300 mg** once a day, or for patients with *GI upset,* **150 mg** twice a day with food.

Dosage Form—Capsules: 150 mg.

Trimethoprim

2,4-Pyrimidinediamine, 5-[(3,4,5-trimethoxyphenyl)methyl]-, Proloprim (*Burroughs Wellcome*); Trimpex (*Roche*); (*Various Mfrs*)

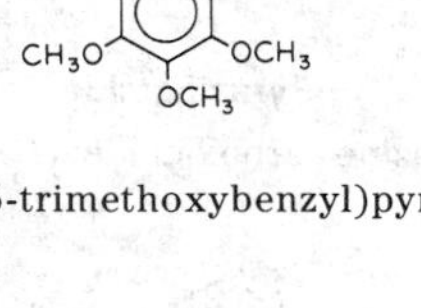

2,4-Diamino-5-(3,4,5-trimethoxybenzyl)pyrimidine [738-70-5] $C_{14}H_{18}$-N_4O_3 (290.32).

Preparation—By interaction of a-(ethoxymethyl)-3,4,5-trimethoxycinnamonitrile and guanidine, the former prepared by condensing 3,4,5-trimethoxybenzaldehyde with β-ethoxypropionitrile. US Pat 3,049,544.

Description—White to cream-colored crystals or crystalline powder; odorless; bitter taste; melts about 199°; pK_a about 6.6.

Solubility—Very slightly soluble in water; 1 g in about 285 mL absolute alcohol or 53 mL chloroform.

Uses—A congener of pyrimethamine and it similarly inhibits dihydrofolate reductase, although it is considerably less potent. It was introduced as an antimalarial drug (mostly against *P falciparum*) and is still used somewhat for that purpose, usually in combination with an appropriate sulfonamide. However, its most important use is as an antibacterial agent. Bacterial dihydrofolate reductases are generally more susceptible than are the plasmodial ones. Therefore, the drug is effective against all bacteria that must synthesize their own folinic acid (leucovorin). This gives it a wide spectrum of activity that includes *Strep pyogenes, viridans* and *pneumoniae, Staph aureus* and *epidermidis, H influenzae, Klebsiella-Enterobacter-Serratia, E coli,* various *Shigella* and *Salmonella, Bordetella pertussis, V cholerae, Pneumocystis carinii, Toxoplasma gondii and Plasmodia.* It is not effective against *Ps aeruginosa* but is against *Ps cepaciae* and *pseudomallei.* Many of these same organisms must also synthesize their own folic acid. Sulfonamides and dapsone block the incorporation of *p*-aminobenzoate into folate, thus inhibiting a crucial biosynthetic step just previous to that where this drug acts. Therefore, the combination of this drug and sulfonamides or dapsone is supposedly more effective than either drug alone, although clinical confirmation of significant synergism is lacking. Nevertheless, it is widely used in combination with sulfamethoxazole. It alone is approved for the same uses as the above combination (see page 1276). It would seem prudent to use the combination for urinary tract infections, even though the cost is greater, but the pharmacokinetics are such that sulfamethoxazole in the present formulation adds little to this drug alone for systemic infections. The combination of dapsone and trimethoprim is used in the treatment of leprosy and infections by *Mycobact avium.*

Mammalian dihydrofolate reductase is about 1:10,000 to 1:50,000 as sensitive to it as the bacterial enzymes, so that there is little interference with folate metabolism in man. The toxicity is low. It includes occasional nausea and vomiting, diarrhea, malaise, immunosuppression and, rarely, rash, leukopenia and thrombocytopenia. It increases bone-marrow suppression and immunosuppression by antineoplastics. It is potentially teratogenic.

By the oral route, it is well absorbed and reaches a peak in 2 to 3 hr. A blood level of 1 to 2 μg/mL in an adult is provided by 160 mg. About 45% is protein-bound in plasma. The volume of distribution is about 1.8 mL/g. The concentration in cerebrospinal fluid reaches 30 to 50% of that in plasma. It is excreted mainly into the urine. The half-life is 9 to 12 hr in normal adults, but may be increased 2- to 3-fold when the creatinine clearance falls below 10 mL/min. It is considerably shorter in infants and children. The drug decreases the renal clearance of procainamide and acecainide. Rifampin accelerates its elimination.

Dose—*Oral, adult* and *children 12 yr* or *over,* for *prophylaxis* of *urinary tract infections,* **100 mg** once a day; for *treatment* of *urinary tract infections,* **100 mg** every 12 hr or **200 mg** once a day for 10 days. Tentative doses: for *chancroid,* 100 mg every 12 hr; *for other infections,* 200 mg every 12 hr. Doses for infants and children under 12 yr probably should be ⅓ to ½ the adult dose.

Dosage Forms—Oral Suspension: 40 mg/5 mL; Tablets: 100 and 200 mg.

Antituberculosis Combinations

Some examples of antituberculosis combinations (with content/capsule or /tablet provided) are as follows:

Isoniazid and Rifampin [Rifamate (*Merrell Dow*)]—150 mg and 300 mg, respectively; capsules; [Rimactane/INH (*Ciba*)]—300 mg each; tablets.

Isoniazid and Pyridoxine Hydrochloride [P-I-N Forte (*Lanette*); Teebaconin and Vitamin B_6 (*CMC*)]—100, 100 or 300 mg and 5, 10 or 30 mg, respectively; tablets.

Antimalarials

Until World War II, malaria was the world's greatest scourge, its steady accumulated toll far exceeding that of the more explosive plague. Even today probably over 125 million people are afflicted, and about 1 million die each year from malaria. Knowledge of mosquito control, insecticides and antimalarials, however, all but have eradicated the disease in the more advanced countries, such as the US; similar strides have been made in certain relatively undeveloped countries, so that malaria now ranks second to tuberculosis in many of these countries.

The export of cinchona from Peru in 1643 allowed the European countries and their colonies some means of suppressing the disease, and the introduction of quinine in the 19th century improved therapy somewhat. However, great advances were not made until the introduction of pamaquine in 1926 and quinacrine (atabrine) in 1930, as the result of screening by I G Farben of over 12,000 candidates. These synthetics did not displace quinine immediately. Only when the supplies of quinine were cut off in World War II did it become imperative to supply synthetic antimalarials to our armed forces in the Pacific and Mediterranean.

The US Office of Scientific Research and Development coordinated a study of about 7000 new, and an equal number of old, synthetic compounds. Not only were the older German compounds "rediscovered," but several new and superior agents (especially amodiaquine, chloroquine, pentaquine and primaquine) resulted. The British counterpart of this program brought forth *chloroguanide*. The continued search in this field has yielded other antimalarials, but the pace recently has been slow. Investigations into the feasability of antimalarial vaccines are in their infancy. Meanwhile, because of the emergence of resistant strains of plasmodia, the effectiveness of several of the "newer" agents is diminishing rapidly, so that not only are new drugs again being sought actively, but combinations of old drugs are in use. In this connection, it is of interest that sulfadoxine or sulfadiazine and tetracycline are being used in combination with quinine and pyrimethamine.

Malaria is caused by several species of the protozoan *Plasmodium*, of which *P vivax* and *P falciparum* are the most common. They all have complex life cycles involving both the anopheles mosquito and the erythrocyte of the human host. In *P vivax*, a persisting tissue phase continues to infect the blood at intervals for many years. Thus, the ideal antimalarial not only should eradicate the microzoan from the blood, (ie, to "suppress" the clinical attack) but from the tissues as well, to effect a "radical cure." The several antimalarials differ in their point of interruption of the cycle of the parasite and in the type of malaria affected.

The 4-aminoquinolines (amodiaquine, chloroquine and hydroxychloroquine) and quinacrine cause similar adverse effects. Gastrointestinal side effects such as nausea, vomiting, diarrhea and sialorrhea are common; they can be diminished by administering the drugs with meals and milk. Oropharyngeal and dermatological side effects may occur, especially during protracted therapy. They include pigmentation of the skin, nailbeds and palate (especially quinacrine), bleaching of hair, pruritus and lichenoid and pleomorphic skin eruptions. They may precipitate severe attacks of psoriasis in patients with that disease. The drugs should not be coadministered with phenylbutazone or gold salts, which have similar dermatotoxicities. There is cross-sensitization among all the 4-aminoquinolines. The drugs may cause neurological disturbances, such as fatigue, lassitude, neuromyopathy, polyneuritis, toxic psychosis and ototoxicity with vertigo and/or decreased auditory sensitivity. The knee and ankle reflexes should be monitored periodically. Ocular disorders, such as corneal opacities, keratopathy and retinopathy (the drugs are concentrated in the retina) occur, especially during long-term treatment. Periodic ophthalmological examinations are advised. The drugs are contraindicated if retinal or visual field disease is present.

The 4-aminoquinolines are concentrated in the liver and may cause hepatotoxicity, and they may precipitate attacks of porphyria; they must be used cautiously in persons with liver disease or who are under medication with other potentially hepatotoxic drugs (gold salts, erythromycin estolate, indomethacin, phenylbutazone, certain anabolic steroids, etc). Hematological disorders occasionally caused by the 4-aminoquinolines include leukopenia, pancytopenia and agranulocytosis; periodic white-blood-cell counts are necessary. The drugs may depress the electrocardiographic T-wave. They pass the placental barrier and can cause cochleovestibular paresis in the fetus; they should be withheld in pregnancy, although chloroquine has been given safely in low doses for chemoprophylaxis.

Chloroguanamide Hydrochloride—see RPS-18, page 1227.

Chloroquine Hydrochloride

1,4-Pentanediamine, N^4-(7-chloro-4-quinolinyl)-N^1,N^1-diethyl-, dihydrochloride; Aralen Hydrochloride (*Winthrop*)

Cl, N, · HCl, HN—CH(CH$_2$)$_3$N(C$_2$H$_5$)$_2$, CH$_3$

7-Chloro-4-[[4-(diethylamino)-1-methylbutyl]amino]quinoline dihydrochloride [3545-67-3]; a sterile solution of chloroquine in water for injection prepared with the aid of hydrochloric acid. It contains, in each mL, 47.5–52.5 mg of $C_{18}H_{26}ClN_3.2HCl$ (392.80).

Preparation—The base is prepared by heating a mixture of 4,7-dichloroquinoline and *N*,*N*-diethylpentyl amine.

Description—White powder; melts about 88°; pK_a 8.4, 10.8.

Solubility—Freely soluble in water.

Uses—Actions and uses are those of *Chloroquine Phosphate*, except that the hydrochloride lends itself better to solutions for intramuscular injection. The intramuscular route may be indicated in patients who cannot tolerate oral chloroquine or in cerebral malaria, in which a very rapid response is desired. The toxicity is like that of the phosphate (see below), even to the occurrence of gastrointestinal complaints; in addition, respiratory depression, hypotension or shock may occur consequent to too-rapid a rate of injection or after an overdose.

Dose—*Intramuscular, adult*, for *malaria*, **200** to **250 mg**, to be repeated in 6 hr, if necessary, but not to exceed 1 g in the first 24 hr; for *extraintestinal amebiasis*, **200** to **250 mg** once a day for 10 to 12 days. *Children*, for *malaria*, **6.25 mg/kg** and no more, to be repeated in 6 hr, if necessary, but not to exceed 12 mg/kg in any 24-hr period; for *extraintestinal amebiasis*, **7.5 mg/kg** a day for 10 to 12 days.

Dosage Form—Injection: 250 mg/5 mL, equivalent to 200 mg/5 mL of chloroquine base.

Chloroquine Phosphate

1,4-Pentanediamine, N^4-(7-chloro-4-quinolinyl)-N^1,N^1-diethyl-, phosphate (1:2); Aralen Phosphate (*Winthrop*); (*Various Mfrs*)

7-Chloro-4-[[4-(diethylamino)-1-methylbutyl]amino]quinoline phosphate (1:2) [50-63-5] $C_{18}H_{26}ClN_3.2H_3PO_4$ (515.87).

For the structure of the base, see *Chloroquine Hydrochloride*.

Preparation—By addition of concentrated phosphoric acid to a hot ethanolic solution of chloroquine base.

Description—White, crystalline powder; odorless; bitter taste; slowly discolors on exposure to light; pH (aqueous solution) about 4.5; 193 to 195° (usual form) or 210 to 215° (other polymorphic form); pK_{a1} 7; pK_{a2} 9.2.

Solubility—Freely soluble in water; practically insoluble in alcohol, chloroform or ether.

Uses—An antimalarial drug that causes dysfunction of the acid phagosomes in plasmodia and also in human leukocytes and macrophages. It is used both for control of acute attacks of *vivax malaria* and for suppression against all plasmodia except chloroquine-resistant *P falciparum*. The drug is neither a prophylactic nor a radical curative agent in vivax malaria. In regions where *P falciparum* is generally sensitive to chloroquine, it is markedly effective in terminating acute attacks of nonresistant *falciparum malaria* and usually bring about complete cure in this type of malaria. However, in some regions a high incidence of resistance (up to 90%) exists, so that other drugs, such as quinine or quinidine, alone or in combination with pyrimethamine, sulfadiazine or tetracycline, may have preference. Resistant strains of *P vivax* also occur.

It is the drug of choice for the oral treatment of all malaria except that caused by resistant *P falciparum*; the hydrochloride is second to quinine or quinidine for parenteral treatment.

Although not useful in intestinal amebiasis, it is an effective agent in the treatment of extraintestinal amebiasis, especially *amebic hepatitis*. It is not used alone but rather in combination with dihydroemetine or emetine. The combination is only the treatment of second choice, behind metronidazole-diiodohydroxyquin. Since chloroquine is well tolerated, it has been recommended that it be employed routinely even in cases of amebiasis without demonstrable hepatic involvement. Like quinacrine, it also may be of value in chronic discoid *lupus erythematosus* and *rheumatoid arthritis*. It is quite effective in the treatment of *photoallergic* reactions.

The adverse effects are those of the 4-aminoquinolines (see the general statement). The incidence is low, except for the gastrointestinal side effects of the oral forms.

The drug is absorbed almost completely from the gastrointestinal tract and usually is administered orally. It (as the hydrochloride) is given intramuscularly when necessary to resort to parenteral administration. Tissues bind the drug, although not quite to the same degree of quinacrine. It is degraded in tissues to unknown products. The drug is slowly excreted in the urine with an initial half-life of 1 wk, changing to 17 days after 4 wk, then ultimately becoming months.

Dose—*Oral, adults,* for *malaria,* as a *suppressive,* **500 mg** (equivalent to 300 mg base) once a wk for 2 wk before exposure, and continue for 4 wk after leaving endemic area: for *therapy,* initially **1 g** followed by **500 mg** in 6 to 8 hr, then **500 mg** once a day on the 2nd and 3rd days; for *extraintestinal amebiasis,* **250 mg** 4 times a day for 2 days followed by **250 mg** twice a day for at least 2 or 3 wk; for *lupus erythematosus,* **250 mg** twice a day for 2 wk then once a day thereafter; to suppress *photoeruptions,* **250 mg** twice a day for 2 wk then once a day; for *rheumatoid arthritis,* **250 mg** once a day, to be increased to as much as 750 mg a day, if necessary. *Children,* for *malaria,* as a *suppressive,* **8.3 mg/kg,** not to exceed 500 mg, once a week, and for *therapy,* initially **16.7 mg/kg,** not to exceed 1 g, then **8.3 mg/kg,** not to exceed 500 mg, 6, 24 and 48 hr later; for *extraintestinal amebiasis,* **10 mg/kg,** not to exceed 600 mg, every day for 3 wk. Suppressive treatment should begin 2 wk in advance of entering into a malarious region and continue for 8 wk after departure; rapid loading for suppression can be achieved by giving the two weekly doses in a single day, 6 hr apart.

Dosage Form—Tablets: 250 and 500 mg, equivalent to 150 and 300 mg, respectively, of chloroquine base.

Dapsone—page 1318.

Hydroxychloroquine Sulfate—see RPS-18, page 1227.

Mefloquine Hydrochloride

4-Quinolinemethanol, (R^*, S^*)-(±)-α-2-piperidinyl-2,8-bis(trifluoromethyl)-, hydrochloride; Lariam (*Roche*)

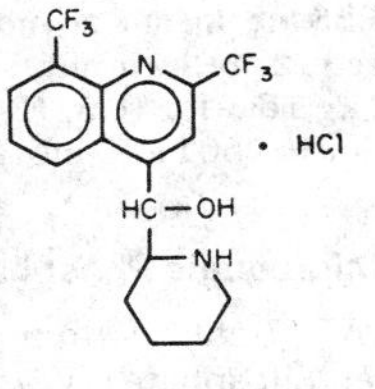

[51773-92-3] $C_{17}H_{16}F_6N_2O.HCl$ (414.78).

Preparation—*J Med Chem, 14:*926, 1971.

Description—White powder; bitter taste; melts about 260° with decomposition; the secondary alcohol group is chiral, but the racemate is used clinically; pK_a 8.6.

Solubility—1 g in 6 mL water or 250 mL alcohol.

Uses—Can eliminate fever and parasitemia and cause a radical cure in infections caused by *Pl falciparum* and can suppress infections caused by *Pl vivax:* with *Pl vivax,* infections usually recur at a later time. Its mechanism is unknown. Resistance develops rapidly, and the WHO is investigating combinations to delay resistance, it is absorbed well orally. In plasma, it is extensively bound to plasma proteins and is concentrated in the liver and lungs. It is eliminated mainly in the feces, mostly after biliary secretion. The half-life is about 13 to 24 days.

Dose—**12.50 mg** as single dose, *prophylaxis* **250 mg** once a wk for 4 wk, then **250 mg** every other wk; *children,* reduced dosage recommended for *suppression* of infections by *Pl vivax,* 250 mg a week.

Dosage Form—Tablets: 250 mg.

Primaquine Phosphate

1,4-Pentanediamine, N^4-(6-methoxy-8-quinolinyl)-, phosphate (1:2); (*Winthrop*)

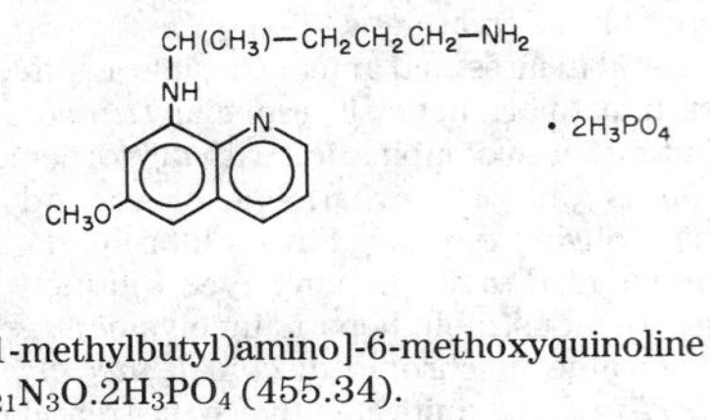

8-[(4-Amino-1-methylbutyl)amino]-6-methoxyquinoline phosphate (1:2) [63-45-6] $C_{15}H_{21}N_3O.2H_3PO_4$ (455.34).

Preparation—2-Chloropentylamine is condensed with 8-amino-6-methoxyquinoline and the resulting primaquine base is reacted with a double molar quantity of phosphoric acid.

Description—Orange-red, crystalline powder; odorless; bitter taste; solutions are acid to litmus; melts about 200°.

Solubility—1 g in about 15 mL water; insoluble in chloroform or ether.

Uses—An antimalarial which is very important for the *radical cure* (ie, prevention of relapse) *of relapsing vivax* or *ovale malaria;* it is not employed for suppressive therapy or for control of the acute clinical attacks of the disease. It often is administered in combination with chloroquine. The incidence of serious untoward effects is low. In Caucasians, therapeutic doses are tolerated adequately. Mild to moderate abdominal cramps and occasional epigastric distress, dizziness and weakness occur in some individuals. Administration of the drug with milk, food or antacids lessens these effects; however, aluminum-containing antacids interfere with absorption. Mild hemolytic anemia, cyanosis (methemoglobinemia) and leukocytosis also may be observed. At higher dose levels these symptoms are accentuated, and leukopenia may be noted. Toxicity is not increased by concurrent administration of quinine or chloroquine, which are often given concurrently. However, quinacrine greatly enhances the toxicity of primaquine and must not be given at the same time. Impairment of liver function has not been noted, even in patients with infectious hepatitis. Persons with tendencies toward granulocytopenia (eg, lupus erythematosus or rheumatoid diseases) should not take it because the blood dyscrasia may be precipitated. Other hemolyzing drugs should not be administered concurrently.

Untoward effects in non-Caucasians are similar, but the incidence and degree of anemia and intravascular hemolysis are greater. A daily dose of 15 mg of the base can be administered safely for 14 days to both Caucasian and non-Caucasian adults without special medical supervision. Larger doses are too toxic for those non-Caucasians and other persons whose erythrocytes are deficient in glucose 6-phosphate dehydrogenase, but usually can be administered to Caucasian subjects, who should be supervised carefully. A sudden darkening of the urine, leukocytosis or severe skin reaction are indicators of hemolysis, and the drug must be discontinued immediately. Bone-marrow depressant drugs (eg, antineoplastics, colchicine, gold salts, penicillamine, phenylbutazone, hydroxyphenylbutazone or quinacrine) given concurrently can cause excessive bone-marrow depression.

Dose—*Oral, adult,* **26.3 mg** once a day for 2 wk, except **52.6 mg** against resistant organisms; to eliminate gametocytes of *Pl falciparum,* **78.9 mg** as a single dose; *infants* and *children,* **667 μg** (0.67 mg)/**kg** once a day for 2 wk.

Dosage Form—Tablets: 26.3 mg, equivalent to 15 mg of primaquine base.

Pyrimethamine

2,4-Pyrimidinediamine, 5-(4-chlorophenyl)-6-ethyl-, Daraprim (*Burroughs Wellcome*)

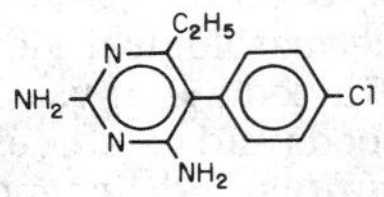

2,4-Diamino-5-(*p*-chlorophenyl)-6-ethylpyrimidine [58-14-0] $C_{12}H_{13}ClN_4$ (248.71).

Preparation—Ethyl propionate is condensed with *p*-chlorophenylacetonitrile in the presence of sodium methylate. The resulting α-propionyl-*p*-chlorophenylacetonitrile is reacted with isoamyl alcohol to form the hemiacetal which undergoes dehydration to α-(*p*-chlorophenyl)-β-ethyl-β-isoamyloxylacrylonitrile (I). I is reacted with guanidine whereupon cyclization occurs due to (*a*) the liberation of isoamyl alcohol by condensation involving the imino hydrogen of guanidine and the isoamyloxy group of I, and (*b*) an addition reaction involving an amino group of guanidine and the nitrile group of I.

Description—White, crystalline powder; odorless; melting range 238° to 242°; pK_a 7.3.

Solubility—Practically insoluble in water; 1 g in about 200 mL alcohol or 125 mL chloroform.

Uses—Inhibits dihydrofolate reductase in plasmodia; thus the developing parasite cannot synthesize and use nucleic acid precursors needed for growth. Its action in preventing the development of the erythrocytic phase of the parasite is slow, so that it is of little value in suppression of acute attacks, except as an adjunct to quinine; rather it is used mainly as a suppressive prophylactic for the prevention of clinical attacks by *P falciparum* in regions where the organism is resistant to chloroquine, in which use it is combined with sulfadoxine. It also renders the parasites incapable of sporulating in the mosquito, so that the life cycle of the parasite is broken. In some regions, treatment with the drug is successful in up to 90% of cases; addition of quinine increases the success rate to about 95%. Combination of the drug and trisulfapyrimidines is the treatment of choice for *toxoplasmosis*.

The toxicity is low. Anorexia and vomiting are common with large doses. Skin rashes are rare. In high doses it may cause megaloblastic anemia and, less commonly, leukopenia, thrombocytopenia and pancytopenia as the result of antagonism of folic acid. Atrophic pharyngitis and esophagitis occasionally results. CNS signs of folate deficiency may occur. Because of the intensive dose regimen for toxoplasmosis, semiweekly blood-cell and platelet counts should be made. The hematopoietic toxicity can be reversed by leucovorin. The antifolate actions are damaging to the fetus, so that the drug should be avoided in pregnancy, if possible, or be coadministered with leucovorin.

Dose—*Oral, adult, antimalarial,* for *prophylaxis* or *suppression* of chloroquine-resistant *P falciparum* malaria, in combination with sulfadoxine, **25 mg** once a week and for *treatment* of uncomplicated attacks, in combination with quinine and sulfadiazine, **25 mg** a day for **2** days; for *toxoplasmosis*, in combination with trisulfapyrimidines, *initially* **50** to **100 mg** once a day for 2 days then **25 mg** once a day. *Infants* and *children, antimalarial,* for *prophylaxis* or *suppression* of chloroquine-resistant *P falciparum* malaria, in combination with sulfadoxine, *4* to *10 yr*, **12.5 mg** once a wk; *<4 yr*, **6.25 mg** once a wk (not to exceed adult dose) and for *treatment* of uncomplicated attack, in combination with quinine and sulfadiazine, 25 mg a day for 2 days; for *toxoplasmosis*, in combination with trisulfapyrimidines, *initially* **1 mg/kg** twice a day for 2 to 4 days then **0.5 mg/kg** twice a day.

Dosage Form—Tablets: 25 mg.

Quinacrine Hydrochloride

1.4-Pentanediamine, N^4-(6-chloro-2-methoxy-9-acridinyl)-N^1,N^1-diethyl-, dihydrochloride, dihydrate-, Atabrine Hydrochloride (*Winthrop*)

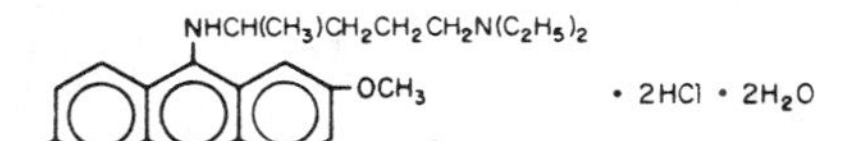

$NHCH(CH_3)CH_2CH_2CH_2N(C_2H_5)_2$; OCH_3 ; Cl ; N ; $\cdot$ 2HCl $\cdot$ $2H_2O$

6-Chloro-9-[[4-(diethylamino)-1-methylbutyl]amino]-2-methoxyacridine dihydrochloride dihydrate, [6151-30-0] $C_{23}H_{30}ClN_3O.2HCl.2H_2O$ (508.91).

Preparation—2,4-Dichlorobenzoic acid is condensed in alkaline solution with *p*-anisidine, and the product, on treatment with phosphorus oxychloride, is cyclized to methoxydichloroacridine. This is heated with 2-amino-5-(diethylamino)pentane in phenol solution and the reaction mixture is added to acetone containing hydrochloric acid. Quinacrine is precipitated as the dihydrochloride while the phenol is held in solution by the acetone.

Description—Bright-yellow, crystalline powder; odorless; bitter; pH (1 in 100 solution) about 4.5; melts about 250° with decomposition.

Solubility—1 g in about 35 mL water; soluble in alcohol; almost insoluble in chloroform.

Uses—Now generally considered an alternative choice for giardiasis for patients who do not tolerate metronidazole. It is obsolete in the treatment of malaria. A small percentage of patients treated with it exhibit untoward effects. These are essentially the same as those caused by the 4-aminoquinolines (see the general statement), of which quinacrine can be considered to be an analog. The gastrointestinal irritancy is higher than with the 4-aminoquinolines, and it is common to give sodium bicarbonate concomitantly. Children do not tolerate it well, and patients with psoriasis should not receive quinacrine because it may exacerbate the condition. Toxic psychosis has been reported in 1.5% of adults who take it. It is absorbed readily from the gastrointestinal tract and from intramuscular and intracavitary sites of injection. It is excreted very slowly in the urine and accumulates in tissue on chronic administration. It usually is administered orally; each dose is given with water after a meal. If the oral route cannot be employed, intramuscular injection is preferred over the intravenous injection.

Dose—*Oral, adult, antimalarial,* as a *suppressive*, **100 mg** once a day for 1 to 3 mo, and for *therapy, initially* **200 mg** every 6 hr for 5 doses followed by **100mg** 3 times a day for 6 days; for *giardiasis*, **100 mg** after meals 3 times a day for 5 to 7 days. Doses for *infants* and *children* and outdated antihelminthic uses and doses, see package literature, *Drug Facts and Comparisons*, the *USP DI* or *The Medical Letter Handbook of Antimicrobial Therapy*.

Dosage Form—Tablets: 100 mg.

Quinidine Gluconate—see page 961.

Quinine Dihydrochloride—see RPS-18, page 1228.

Quinine Sulfate

(8α,9*R*)-Cinchonan-9-ol, 6′-methoxy-, sulfate (2:1) (salt), dihydrate (*Various Mfrs*)

Quinine sulfate (2:1) (salt) dihydrate [6119-70-6] $(C_{20}H_{24}N_2O_2)_2.H_2SO_4.2H_2O$ (782.95); *anhydrous* [804-63-7] (746.92); the sulfate of an alkaloid obtained from the bark of *Cinchona officinalis Linné* (*C ledgeriana* Moens) (Fam *Rubiaceae*) or other species of *Cinchona*. Contains not more than 10.0% of dihydroquinine.

For the structural formula of quinine see page 402.

Preparation—The crude sulfate, obtained when quinine is isolated from the bark of *Cinchona* sp, is recrystallized once or twice from hot water slightly acidified with sulfuric acid.

Description—White, fine, needle-like crystals; usually lusterless, making a light and readily compressible mass; odorless; persistent, very bitter taste; when exposed to light, it acquires a brown tint; kK_a 4.1, 8.5.

Solubility—1 g in about 500 mL water, 120 mL alcohol, 35 mL water at 100° or about 10 mL alcohol at 80°; slightly soluble in chloroform or ether.

Uses—The original antimalarial drug. It only affects the erythrocytic form of the plasmodia and hence is used only as a suppressive in the management of acute attacks of *vivax, malariae* or *ovale malaria*. It may cure up to 50% of infections caused by *falciparum* plasmodia, but some strains are resistant. The drug may be combined with pyrimethamine and a sulfonamide, but it appears to be antagonized by chloroquine. The quinine-pyrimethamine-sulfadiazine (or sulfadoxine) combination is presently the treatment of choice for infections caused by chloroquine-resistant *P falciparum;* an alternative is quinine with tetracycline. In severe infections, intravenous dihydrochloride or quinidine gluconate is the drug of choice. The combination, clindamycin-quinine, is the treatment of choice for *babesiosis*.

It has an effect to suppress neuromuscular transmission. In the symptomatic treatment of a rare myopathy known as *myotonia congenita*, or Thomsen's disease, it exerts a neuromuscular depressant action. It occasionally benefits patients with *spasmodic torticollis* (torsion spasm) and also persons with *nocturnal leg cramps*. It is a frequent constituent of bitter *tonics* and *stomachic* preparations.

A syndrome of toxic effects known as "cinchonism," follows the repeated use of full therapeutic doses. Mild cinchonism is characterized by tinnitus, headache, nausea and slight disturbance of vision. In severe cinchonism the skin is hot and flushed, rashes are frequent and the CNS is involved; headache, fever, vomiting, apprehension, excitement, confusion, delirium and syncope are common. The emesis is due to a central action of the drug as well as to its local irritant action on the intestinal mucosa. In a few cases, renal damage, photosensitivity and hypoprothrombinemia may occur. Agranulocytosis has been observed rarely. Transient ventricular tachycardia is noted in rare instances after massive acute overdosage. Although it generally exerts vasodilator actions, retinal vasoconstriction, leading to loss of vision, has been described; these effects mostly have followed rapid intravenous injections or large overdoses.

It is absorbed readily from the gastrointestinal tract. It is only moderately concentrated in tissues and undergoes degradation particularly in the liver. The drug and its degradation products are excreted rapidly in the urine and for this reason the drug must be given every 6 hr in order to maintain relatively constant plasma levels. The half-life is 5 to 16 hr. An alkaline urine prolongs the half-life. See the *USP DI* for the various pharmacokinetic drug interactions.

The drug is given after meals to minimize gastric irritation. Intramuscular and subcutaneous injections are painful and frequently are followed by local tissue injury. The intravenous route is used rarely and only in emergencies.

Dose—*Oral, adult, antimalarial,* for *infections by chloroquine-resistant Pl falciparum* (in combination with pyrimethamine plus sulfadiazine, sulfadoxine plus pyrimethamine or tetracycline), **650 mg,** every 8 hr for 5 to 7 days, depending upon the adjunct drugs in combination (see the *USP DI*); for *other malarial infections*, **600 mg,** 5 to 7 days every 8 hr for 5 to 7 days; for *babesiosis* (in combination with clindamycin), **650 mg**

3 times a day for 7 days; for *myotonia,* **300** to **600 mg** every 8 or 12 hr; for *nocturnal leg cramps,* **260** to **300 mg** at bedtime and also after the evening meal, if necessary. *Children, antimalarial,* **8.3 mg/kg** every 8 hr for at least 3 days.

Dosage Forms—Capsules: 65, 130, 195, 200, 260, 300 and 325 mg; Tablets: 162.5 and 325 mg.

Sulfadiazine—page 1275.

Sulfadoxine—page 1275.

Antimalarial-Containing Combinations

Examples of antimalarial-containing combinations (with content/capsule or /tablet provided) are as follows:

Chloroquine Phosphate and Primaquine Phosphate [Aralen Phosphate with Primaquine Phosphate (*Winthrop-Breon*)]—500 mg and 79 mg, respectively; tablets.

Pyrimethamine and Sulfadoxine [Fansidar (*Roche*)]—25 mg and 500 mg, respectively; tablets.

Amebicides

The incidence of amebiasis in the US has been estimated to be prevalent in homosexuals to the extent of 25 to 32% of this population. Most infections are essentially asymptomatic, but the number of severe infections is still large.

Amebic infections generally remain confined to the intestines, where they may give rise to dysentery, but in an appreciable fraction of cases the amebae may locate elsewhere, especially in the liver. The chemotherapy of amebiasis thus must provide drugs to treat both the intestinal and extraintestinal forms of the disease. In addition, the ideal amebicide also is capable of eliminating amebic cysts from the intestine. No safe drug exists that will eradicate all of motile forms, cysts and extraintestinal amebas, but judicious combined therapy can eliminate the parasite from all sites. Metronidazole acts on amebae within the lumen and wall of the intestine as well as other organs. Diloxanide, iodoquinol and paromomycin are oral luminal amebicides. Emetine and chloroquine are tissue amebicides.

Dehydroemetine Dihydrochloride—see RPS-18, page 1228.

Diloxamide Furoate—see RPS-18, page 1230.

Emetine Hydrochloride

Emetan, 6′,7′,10,11-tetramethoxy-, dihydrochloride; (*Lilly*)

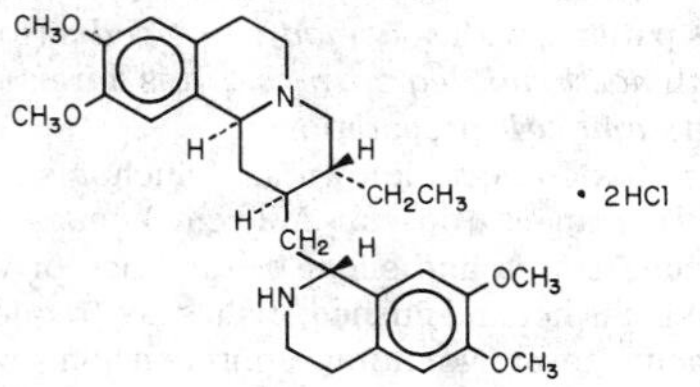

[316-42-7] $C_{29}H_{40}N_2O_4.2HCl$ (553.57); the hydrochloride of an alkaloid obtained from ipecac, or prepared by methylation of cephaeline, or prepared synthetically.

Description—White or very slightly yellowish, crystalline powder; odorless; affected by light; pK_a 7.4, 8.3.

Solubility—1 g in 8 mL water or 12 mL alcohol.

Uses—Eradicates *Entameba histolytica* from both intestinal and extraintestinal sites. It is an alternative drug for *severe intestinal amebiasis* or *amebic hepatitis;* it ranks only as an alternative when other drugs fail. It is concentrated in the liver, hence its value in amebic hepatitis; it is also of considerable value in the treatment of amebic abscesses in other locations. Occasionally, the drug may be life-saving. It rapidly relieves symptoms of intestinal amebiasis by destroying motile amebas, but the percentage of cures is below 15%, since cysts are affected little; other agents are not only safer but superior. It may be used initially to control quickly severe intestinal amebiasis; the drug then is followed by treatment with other agents. It has no place in the therapy of mild ambulatory or chronic cases.

The incidence of toxic effects is very high, both by local and systemic administration. Thus, the IV route is contraindicated. Large doses produce acute lesions in the heart, liver, kidney and intestines, and the dose is now restricted. Nevertheless, deaths still sometimes occur, often because of repeated courses of treatment at close intervals; the drug has a probable half-life on the order of weeks to months. Diarrhea, nausea and vomiting are frequent, as are also skeletal muscle weakness, stiffness and aching. Sensory disturbances also occur. By far the most important toxic effects are cardiovascular; they include hypotension, precordial pain, dyspnea, tachycardia and long-persisting electrocardiographic changes; electrocardiographic and blood-pressure recordings at daily intervals are necessary. It is contraindicated in patients with organic disease of the heart or kidney, unless there is no therapeutic alternative, in pregnancy, and when there has been a previous course of therapy within 6 wk.

A course of the drug should not continue for more than 5 days. The patient should be kept in bed, and carefully watched for toxic effects. Do not give the drug IV. Dehydroemetine is available in US but only from the CDC.

Dose—*Intramuscular, adult* and *children,* **1 mg/kg** (up to maximum of 65 mg) a day, in 1 or 2 doses in adults and always in 2 divided doses in children.

Dosage Form—Injection: 65 mg/1 mL.

Iodoquinol

8-Quinolinol, 5,7-diiodo-, Diiodohydroxyquinoline; Diodohydroxyquin; Yodoxin (*Glenwood*)

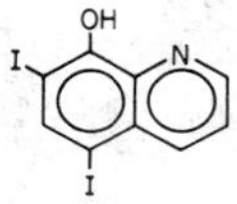

[83-73-8] $C_9H_5I_2NO$ (396.95).

Preparation—8-Quinolinol is iodinated by treatment with iodine monochloride or with a solution of iodine in potassium iodide.

Description—Light yellowish to tan, microcrystalline powder; wetted by water with difficulty; odorless or nearly so; stable in air; melts about 210° with decomposition.

Solubility—Practically insoluble in water; sparingly soluble in alcohol or ether.

Uses—The drug of choice for the treatment of asymptomatic intestinal amebiasis (cyst carrier state) caused by *Entameba histolytica.* In symptomatic intestinal disease, it follows initial treatment with metronidazole or dehydroemetine. In hepatic abscess, it follows metronidazole or emetine. Bed rest is not required. It is the drug of choice in the treatment of infections caused by *Dientameba fragilis.* It is a second-choice drug in the treatment of balantidial dysentery.

It has caused subacute myelo-optic neuropathy when doses larger than recommended for amebiasis were given for three weeks, so long term therapy should be avoided. Iodine toxicoderma, chills, fever, mild to severe dermatitis, irritation, abdominal discomfort, diarrhea and headache occur. The drug may cause goiter. It also can interfere with certain thyroid tests, and protein-bound iodine may remain elevated for as long as 6 mo after termination of a course of treatment. Systemic toxicity can result from topical, especially intravaginal, application. Because of gastrointestinal irritation, it should be taken after meals.

Dose—*Oral, adult,* **630** to **650 mg** 3 times a day after meals for 20 days; *children,* **13.3 mg/kg** (maximum, 650 mg/dose), not to exceed 195 mg a day, 3 times a day for 20 days. Do not exceed 1.95 g in 24 hr.

Dosage Forms—Tablets: 210 and 650 mg; Powder: 25 g.

Metronidazole—page 1325.

Paromomycin Sulfate

D-Streptamine, O-2-amino-2-deoxy-α-D-glucopyranosyl-(1→4)-O-[O-2,6-diamino-2,6-dideoxy-β-L-idopyranosyl-1(1→3)-β-D-ribofuranosyl-(1→5)]-2-deoxy, sulfate (salt); Humatin (*Parke-Davis*)

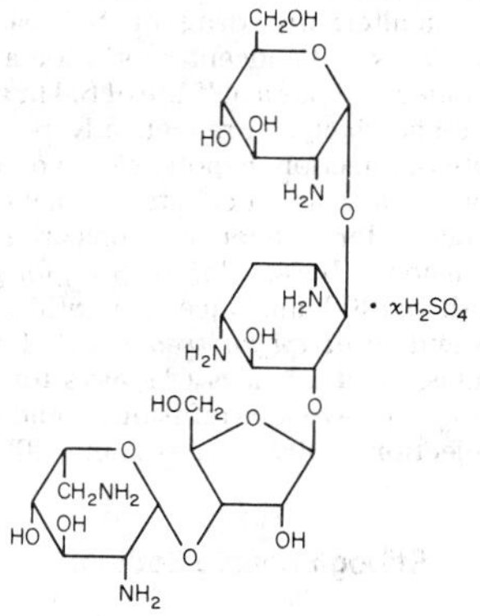

[1263-89-4]; [7542-37-2; 59-04-1 (paramomycin)] $C_{23}H_{45}N_5O_{14}.xH_2SO_4$; the sulfate of an antibiotic substance or substances produced by the growth of *Streptomyces rimosus* var *paromomycinus*, or a mixture of two or more such salts. Potency: equivalent to not less than 675 µg of paromomycin ($C_{23}H_{45}N_5O_{14}$) per mg, calculated on the anhydrous basis.

Preparation—Paromomycin is isolated from fermentation broths by ion-exchange adsorption.

Description—Off-white to light-yellow, amorphous powder; odorless or practically so; very hygroscopic.

Solubility—1 g in < 1 mL water; > 10,000 mL alcohol, chloroform or ether.

Uses—Effective against most clinically significant gram-negative bacteria, especially various species of *Shigella* and *Salmonella* and strains of *E coli*. It is not effective against *Ps aeruginosa*. Among the gram-positive organisms, only staphylococci are sufficiently sensitive to be of clinical significance. It has been used to treat gastroenteritis or bacterial dysentery caused by these organisms, but resistance develops rapidly, the relapse rate is high and other antibiotics are more successful. It also has been used to reduce the bacterial content of the intestine prior to surgery on the bowel or to rid the bowel of nitrogen-forming bacteria in patients with hepatic coma.

Its principal and approved use (US) is in the treatment of asymptomatic intestinal *amebiasis*, for which it is an alternative drug. It alters the ecology of the intestinal flora in such a way that growth of intestinal amebas is discouraged and it also helps to prevent secondary infections that may follow or facilitate amebic invasion of the intestinal walls. It is of no value in treating hepatic or other extraintestinal abscesses. It also is used to treat infections caused by *Dientamoeba fragilis*. It is an obsolete drug for the treatment of tapeworm infestations.

It often causes gastrointestinal hypermotility, nausea, diarrhea and abdominal cramps, which generally appear on the 2nd or 3rd day of treatment and when the daily dose exceeds 2 g. Occasionally, the drug may cause headache, vertigo, vomiting, abdominal pain or skin rash. Overgrowth of enteric staphylococci and other pathogenic bacteria rarely occurs, but may if treatment is prolonged. Malabsorption syndromes have not been reported. There is mutual cross-resistance to kanamycin and neomycin, and often to streptomycin. Although it is absorbed poorly from the gut, there is potential nephrotoxicity, especially in the presence of renal disease.

Dose (base equivalent)—*Oral*, for *intestinal amebiasis* and *Dientamoeba infections*, *adult* and *children*, **25** to **35 mg/kg** a day, in 3 divided doses with meals, for 5 to 10 days; for *hepatic coma*, *adults*, **4 g** a day in divided doses for 5 or 6 days.

Dosage Form (base equivalent)—Capsules: 250 mg.

Miscellaneous Antiprotozoal Drugs

Among the protozoal infections that are endemic to the US are trichomoniasis, amebiasis, giardiasis and malaria. Other protozoal infections, uncommon in the US, nevertheless constitute serious public health and agricultural problems within the possessions and elsewhere. The amebicides and antimalarials are useful in the treatment of a number of other protozoal infections. The antimalarials and amebicides have been treated in separate sections above. Consequently, the drugs listed below are a miscellaneous group of compounds.

Amodiaquine Hydrochloride—RPS-17, page 1217.

Antimony Potassium Tartrate—page 1338.

Atovaquone

Mepron (*Burroughs Wellcome*)

Uses—An analog of ubiquinone with antiprotozoal activity against *Pneumocystis carinii*, *Plasmodium spp* and *Toxplasma gondii*. Its mechanism of action is not fully elucidated but antiprotozoal activity may be explained by an ability to inhibit selectively mitchondrial electron transport that results in inhibition of *de novo* pyrimidine synthesis.

It is highly lipophilic with low aqueous solubility. Bioavailability is increased significantly with food, but especially by fat. It has a half-life of 2.9 days and is believed to be excreted in the bile and to undergo enterohepatic cycling with almost all of the drug eliminated in the feces. It is highly protein bound (> 99.9%).

It is indicated for acute oral treatment of mild to moderate *Pneumocystis carinii* pneumonia (PCP) in patients who are intolerant to trimethoprim-sulfamethoxazole. It has not been evaluated adequately as a chronic suppressive agent to prevent PCP in patients at high risk for it.

Adverse effects in one study of 203 patients have included rash (23%), nausea (21%), diarrhea (19%), headache (16%), vomiting (14%), fever (14%), insomnia (10%), asthenia (8%), pruritus (5%), oral monilial (5%), abdominal pain (4%), constipation (3%) and dizziness (3%).

Dose—*Adult*, **750 mg** administered with food 3 times a day for 21 days.

Dosage Form—Tablets: 250 mg.

Eflornithine Hydrochloride—see RPS-18, page 1231.

Iodoquinol—page 1324.

Meglumine Antimoniate—see RPS-18, page 1231.

Melarsoprol—see RPS-18, page 1231.

Metronidazole

1*H*-Imidazole-1-ethanol, 2-methyl-5-nitro-, Flagyl (*Searle*); (*Various Mfrs*)

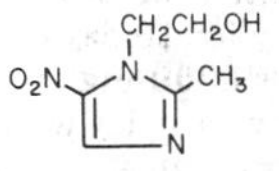

2-Methyl-5-nitroimidazole-1-ethanol [443-48-1] $C_6H_9N_3O_3$ (171.16).

Preparation—2-Methyl-5-nitroimidazole is condensed with ethylene chlorohydrin by heating with a large excess of the chlorohydrin. After removing the surplus chlorohydrin, the residue is extracted with water and the extract is alkalinized and extracted with chloroform. Evaporation of the chloroform yields crude metronidazole which is recrystallized from ethyl acetate. US Pat 2,944,061.

Description—White to pale-yellow, crystals or crystalline powder; odorless; stable in air, but darkens on exposure to light; melts between 159° and 163°; pK_a 2.62.

Solubility—Sparingly soluble in water, alcohol or chloroform; slightly soluble in ether.

Uses—Bactericidal to anaerobic and microaerophilic microorganisms, including *Bacteroides*, *Clostridium* species, *Endolimax nana*, *Entameba histolytica*, *Fusobacterium vincentii*, *Gardnerella vaginalis*, *Giardia lamblia*, *Peptococcus*, *Peptostreptococcus* and *Trichomonas vaginalis*. These organisms reduce the nitro group and generate metabolites that inhibit DNA synthesis. It long has been the drug of choice for the treatment of *trichomoniasis* and more recently in combination with iodoquinol for the treatment of *symptomatic amebiasis* (except in brain). Because it is absorbed well orally, concentrations in the lower bowel sometimes are not high enough to eradicate amebas, so that it is *combined* *with iodoquinol* to make a first-choice combination. It is also the drug of choice for the treatment of *Dracunculus* (guinea worm) *infestations.* It is the alternative drug to treat *giardiasis* (although some authorities consider it the drug of first choice), *balantidiasis, blastocystitis* and infections by *Entameba polecki.* It is used widely for the *treatment* and *prophylaxis of infections caused by anerobic bacteria;* it is a drug of choice against gastrointestinal strains of *Bacteroides fragilis* and vaginal infections by *Gardnerella vaginalis.* It has been used successfully in the treatment of antibiotic-associated pseudomembranous colitis, for which it may be given orally or intravenously. It also has been reported to be of value in Crohn's disease. The drug sensitizes hypoxic tumor cells to radiation and has been employed as an adjunct to radiation therapy.

The most common untoward effects are nausea, diarrhea, anorexia, epigastric distress and abdominal cramps. Unpleasant taste, vomiting, furry tongue and stomatitis are fairly frequent. Urticaria, pruritus, flushing, dysuria, cystitis, dry mouth, dry vulva and vagina, feeling of pelvic pressure, vaginal burning, rash, vertigo, headache, numbness, paresthesias and insomnia occur occasionally. Incoordination and ataxia are rare. Sudden overgrowth of monilia sometimes occurs. The urine sometimes turns a dark color. During treatment the patient should refrain from drinking alcoholic beverages, since the drug has a mild effect similar to *Disulfiram* (page 1167). Neutropenia occurs, so that a blood count should be made, especially before a second course of the drug. In patients with blood dyscrasias great care must be exercised. It should not be used in patients with diseases of the CNS. The drug has been found to be carcinogenic in mice and rats, and mutagenic. Substances mutagenic in the Ames test have been found in the urine of recipients. It has been used in pregnancy without consequence, but it is advisable to withhold it during pregnancy, if possible.

It is usually about 80% absorbed by the oral route, but in some patients absorption is low. Bowel surgery decreases presystemic elimination. Feces contain 6 to 20% of an oral dose. Although metabolism is performed by target anaerobes and microaerophiles, the principal route of elimination is hepatic oxidation and glucuronidation. About 20% of unchanged drug and all of the hepatic metabolites are excreted into the urine. The half-life is about 6 to 12 hr. The drug inhibits the oxidation of warfarin.

Dose—*Intravenous infusion, adults,* for *amebiasis,* **500** to **750 mg** every 8 hr for 5 to 7 days; for *anaerobic infections, treatment, initially* **15 mg/kg**, then **7.5 mg/kg** every 6 hr for at least 7 days; for *perioperative prophylaxis of anaerobic infections* from intestinal surgery, **15 mg/kg** 1 hr before surgery and **7.5 mg/kg** at 6 hr and again at 12 hr. *Oral, adults,* for *antiprotozoal, amebiasis* or *balantidiasis,* **500** to **750 mg** 3 times a day for 5 to 10 days in amebiasis and 5 or 10 days in balantidiasis; for *giardiasis,* **2 g** once a day for 3 days *or* **250** to **500 mg** 3 times a day for 5 to 7 days; for *trichomoniasis,* **2 g** as a single dose or two equally divided doses or **250 mg** 3 times a day for 7 days; *antibacterial,* for *anaerobic infections,* **7.5 mg/kg**, not to exceed 1 g, every 6 hr for at least 7 days; for *burn wound infections, inflammatory bowel disease* or *antibiotic-associated diarrhea* or *enterocolitis,* **500 mg** every 6 hr, except 6 to 8 hr in antibiotic-associated disease; for *Gardnerella vaginitis,* **500 mg** twice a day for 7 days; *antihelminthic,* for *dracunculiasis,* **250 mg** 3 times a day for 10 days; *infants* and *children, antiprotozoal,* for *amebiasis,* **11.6** to **16.7 mg/kg** 3 times a day for 10 days; for *giardiasis* or *trichomoniasis,* **5 mg/kg** 3 times a day for 5 to 7 days in giardiasis and 7 days in trichomoniasis; *antihelminthic,* for *dracunculiasis,* **8.3 mg/kg**, not to exceed 250 mg, 3 times a day for 10 days. *Topical, intravaginal,* as 1 application of a **10%** cream or 1 **500-mg** vaginal suppository or tablet high in the vaginal vault, once or twice a day with the cream and once a day, at bedtime, with the suppository or tablet.

Dosage Forms—Vaginal Cream (Canada): 10%; Injection (buffered with phosphate and citrate to pH of about 6): 500 mg/100 mL. Each 100 mL contains 1.4 mEq of sodium. for Injection: 500 mg; Vaginal Suppositories (Canada): 500 mg; Tablets: 250 and 500 mg; Vaginal Tablets (Canada): 500 mg. Topical dosage forms containing 100,000 units of nystatin/unit dose are available in Canada; Gel: 0.75%.

Metronidazole Hydrochloride—see RPS-18, page 1231.

Nifurtimox—see RPS-18, page 1231.

Ornidazole—see RPS-18, page 1231.

Pentamidine Isethionate

4,4′-(Pentamethylenedioxy)dibenzamidine, bis(2-hydroxyethanesulfonate; Pentam 300, NebuPent (*Lyphomed*)

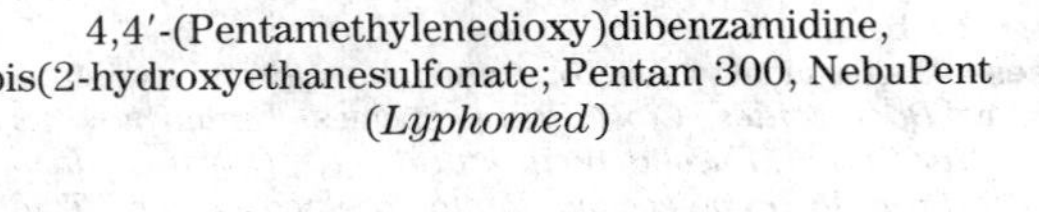

$$H_2N(HN{=})C-C_6H_4-OCH_2(CH_2)_3CH_2O-C_6H_4-C({=}NH)NH_2 \cdot 2\,HOCH_2CH_2SO_3H$$

[140-64-7] $C_{19}H_{24}N_4O_2.2C_2H_6O_4S$ (592.68).

Preparation—*J Chem Soc:* 103, 1942

Description—Crystals; hygroscopic; melts about 180°.

Solubility— Soluble in water; slightly soluble in alcohol; insoluble in ether or chloroform; pK_a 11.4 (base).

Uses—The alternate drug to suramin for treatment of the hemolymphatic stage of African sleeping sickness (trypanosomiasis) caused by *T brucci gambiense* and *T brucei rhodesiense.* It is the alternate drug for the treatment and the drug of choice for prophylaxis of infections caused by *Pneumocystis carinii*; some reports indicate an efficacy equal to that of trimethoprim-sulfamethoxazole and comparable toxicity in patients with AIDS. It is also an alternative drug for the treatment of *kala azar* and *visceral leishmaniasis.* It concentrates in some organs and is eliminated mainly by the kidney. It has a half-life of 6.4 hr and 9.4 hr after 1 IM or IV administration, respectively. Frequent adverse effects include pain and swelling at the site of injection, hypotension, vomiting, blood dyscrasias and renal damage. Occasional effects are diabetes, hypoglycemia, shock and liver damage. Herxheimer reactions are rare. Too-rapid injection causes hypotension. *Dose: Inhalation, for prophylaxis,* 30 or 50 mg twice a month or 300 mg once a month. *Intramuscular* or *intravenous, adults* and *children for treatment,* 4 mg/kg a day for 10 days for trypanosomiasis and 14 days (21 days for AIDS patients) for *Pneumocystis carinii.* Intravenous infusion should last for at least 1 hr.

Dosage Form—Injection: 300 mg, Aerosol: 300 mg.

Stibogluconate Sodium

Gluconic acid, diester with antimonic acid ($H_8Sb_2O_9$), trisodium salt, monohydrate; Pentostam

D-Gluconic acid, cyclic 3,4,5-Sb:3′,4′,5′-Sb′-ester with antimonic acid ($H_8Sb_2O_9$), trisodium salt, nonahydrate [16037-91-5] $C_{12}H_{17}Na_3O_{17}Sb_2.9H_2O$ (907.86); *anhydrous* (745.73). *Note:* Although recorded in the literature, this composition is not in complete agreement with the manufacturer's analytical data.

Description—Amorphous powder; colorless; odorless.

Solubility—Very soluble in water; insoluble in alcohol or ether.

Uses—The drug of choice for the treatment of all forms of *leishmaniasis.* Some of the pentavalent antimony is reduced to trivalent antimony in the body. It is not known whether the active form is the pentavalent or trivalent form.

It has a low toxicity; vomiting and coughing are uncommon. Late in a course of treatment, muscle and joint pains occasionally occur. Bradycardia and electrocardiographic changes are infrequent. Hypersensitivity reactions, such as various rashes, facial edema, hypotension (even rare anaphylaxis), hemolytic anemia, hepatitis, etc, can occur after several doses, but such occurrences are not common. Headache, syncope and abdominal pain also occasionally occur. Liver function may be depressed. Locally, the drug is tolerated fairly well, but pain and other evidences of local toxicity can occur. Dimercaprol will diminish the toxic effects and arrest the development of allergy. It is contraindicated when hepatitis, nephritis or myocarditis are present.

Dose (antimony equivalent)—*Intramuscular* or *intravenous, adult,* **600 mg** a day for 6 to 10 days; *children,* **10 mg/kg** a day for 6 to 10 days. It may be necessary to repeat the course 2 or 3 times, with 10-day rest intervals in between courses. With debilitated persons, it may be advisable to give the drug every other day. In oriental sore, the lesion may be infiltrated around the edges with the equivalent of 200 mg of antimony. In the US this drug is available only from the CDC Drug Service, Centers for Disease Control, Atlanta, GA 30333.

Sulfadoxine—page 1275.

Suramin Sodium

1,3,5-Naphthalenetrisulfonic acid, 8,8′-[carbonylbis[imino-3,1-phenylenecarbonylimino(4-methyl-3,1-phenylene)carbonylimino]]-bis-, hexasodium salt; (*Various Mfrs*)

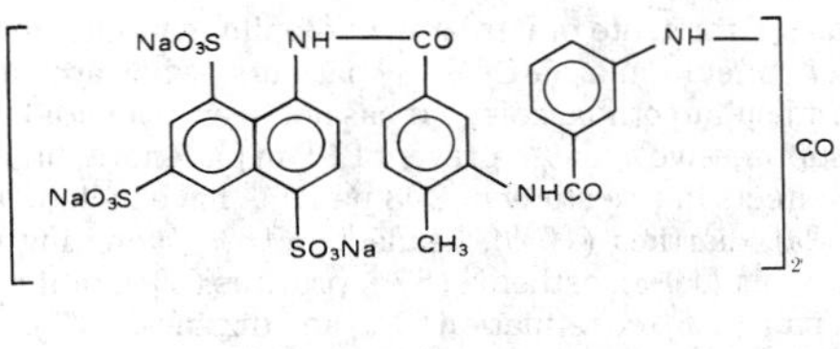

[Structure: NaO3S, NH—CO, NH—, NaO3S, NHCO, CO, SO3Na, CH3; bracketed, subscript 2]

Hexasodium 8,8′-[ureylenebis[*m*-phenylenecarbonylimino(4-methyl-*m*-phenylene)carbonylimino]]di-1,3,5-naphthalenetrisulfonate [129-46-4] $C_{51}H_{34}N_6Na_6O_{23}S_6$ (1429.15).

Preparation—8-Amino-1,3,5-naphthalenetrisulfonic acid is condensed with *m*-nitro-*p*-toluoyl chloride in the presence of sodium acetate. The resulting nitro compound is reduced, and the amino derivative is condensed with *m*-nitrobenzoyl chloride; the product is reduced to the corresponding amino compound which is then reacted with carbonyl chloride in the ratio of two moles of the former to one of the latter. The suramin acid thus obtained is neutralized with NaOH to produce the sodium salt.

Description—White or slightly pink powder; odorless; slightly bitter taste; very hygroscopic and affected by light; pH (1 in 100 solution) between 5.5 and 7.

Solubility—Soluble in water; slightly soluble in alcohol; insoluble in ether or chloroform.

Uses—One of the few nonmetallic compounds effective in the treatment and prophylaxis of *trypanosomiasis* caused by *T rhodesiense*, *T hippicum* and *T gambiense*. If it is used early, it can be used alone, but if there is CNS involvement, arsenicals also must be used. *T cruzi* (agent of Chagas' disease) does not respond. It is also an alternative drug for the treatment of *onchocerciasis*. It also has been employed effectively in the treatment of *pemphigus*. It has moderate antiviral activity, and it is a desperation drug for use against AIDS; however, trials in the US have been suspended.

In some patients, the drug may cause nausea and vomiting, shock and loss of consciousness immediately after injection. Later, sensory disturbances (photophobia, paresthesias, etc) keratopathy, papular eruptions and palpebral edema may occur. Still later, albuminuria, hematuria and casts may occur. Hemolytic anemia and agranulocytosis are rare but possible. It is irritating upon intramuscular injection.

It is not absorbed from the gastrointestinal tract. After intravenous injection, the blood level falls in three phases: rapidly for a few hours, more slowly for several days then very slowly, such that the blood concentration may persist for up to 3 mo. It binds to plasma protein. It does not penetrate the CNS. It is concentrated in the kidney.

Dose—*Intravenous, adult,* for *prophylaxis*, **1 g** by slow infusion every 3 mo; for *active trypanosomiasis*, **1 g** on days 1, 3, 7, 14 and 21; *children;* **20 mg/kg** on days 1, 3, 7, 14 and 21. Initially, try 200 mg to test for sensitivity before giving the full dose. A second course of therapy should not be repeated until 3 mo after the end of the 1st course. For *onchocerciasis, adults,* **1 g** a wk for 7 to 10 wk.

Dosage Form—for Injection: 1 g of sterile powder. In the US this drug is available only from the CDC Drug Service, Centers for Disease Control, Atlanta GA 30333.

Trimetrexate—page 1262.

Tryparasamide—see RPS-18, page 1232.

Antifungal Drugs

The fungi comprise five widely differing classes of primitive flora, including the bacteria; the variations in cell physiology and biochemistry are extreme among fungi. Thus, antifungal agents include a wide variety of chemical types of rather narrow antifungal spectrum. Broad-spectrum antifungal agents in general are toxic and are irritants, as expected from the prerequisite nonselectivity; however, many of these have limited absorption through the epidermis and so may be employed in dermatological preparations. Not all antifungal agents are fungicidal; many are only fungistatic, and certain topical antifungal drugs may owe their efficacy to a keratolytic action that causes a sloughing of the stratum corneum with its entrained fungi.

Aminacrine Hydrochloride—see RPS-18, page 1170.

Amphotericin B

(*Lyphomed*); Fungizone (*Squibb*)

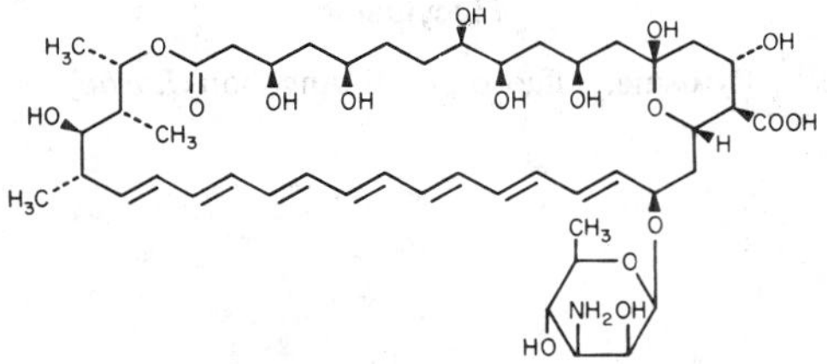

[1*R*-(1*R**,3*S**,5*R**,6*R**,9*R**,11*R**,15*S**,16*R**,17*R**,18*S**,19*E*,21*E*,23*E*,25*E*,27*E*,29*E*,31*E*,33*R**,35*S*,36*S**,37*S**)]-33-[(3-Amino-3,6-dideoxy-β-D-mannopyranosyl)oxy]-1,3,5,6,9,11,17,37-octahydroxy-15,16,18-trimethyl-13-oxo-14,39-dioxabicyclo[33.3.1]nonatriaconta-19,21,23,25,27,29,31-heptaene-36-carboxylic acid [1397-89-3] $C_{47}H_{73}NO_{17}$(924.09); a substance produced by the growth of *Streptomyces nodosus*. Potency: not less than 750 μg of amphotericin B/mg.

Preparation—By the growth of selected strains of *Streptomyces nodosus* in an appropriate medium under controlled conditions of temperature, pH, and aeration. After extracting from the medium, the crude product is purified by treatment with various solvents at controlled acidity.

Description—Yellow to orange powder; odorless or practically so; pK_a (acid) 5.7, (amine) 10.0.

Solubility—Insoluble in water, anhydrous alcohol or ether; aqueous solubility can be increased to about 50 mg/mL by complexation with sodium desoxycholate.

Uses—The widest spectrum of antifungal activity of any systemic antifungal drug. By the intravenous route it is an extremely useful drug for therapy of *systemic fungous diseases*, especially coccidiomycosis, cryptococcosis, systemic moniliasis, histoplasmosis, aspergillosis, rhodotorulosis, sporotrichosis, phycomycosis (mucormycosis) and North American blastomycosis. It also is used topically in the treatment of *superficial monilial infections* and by nasal spray in the prophylaxis of aspergillosis in immunocompromised patients. It is not effective against viruses, protozoa or bacteria. However, it is effective against some species of *Leishmania (L braziliensis* and *mexicana*), for which it is the drug of second choice. Acquired resistance to the drug has not been observed.

It is absorbed very poorly from the gastrointestinal tract. It is highly bound predominantly to β-lipoproteins and is excreted slowly by the kidneys but neither renal failure nor hemodialysis has a consistent effect on plasma levels. The initial half-life is 24 hr which is followed by a terminal half-life of about 15 days.

It may induce chills and fever, nausea and vomiting, diarrhea, abdominal "cramps," hemorrhagic gastroenteritis, dyspepsia, headache, vertigo, pain in the vein injected, thrombophlebitis, muscle and joint pains, anemia, purpura, hypertension, hypotension, cardiac arrest, ventricular fibrillation, skin rashes, hypokalemia, hypomagnesemia, renal damage, blood dyscrasias, loss of hearing and other untoward effects. It has been reported to cause pulmonary deterioration when given with blood products in granulocytopenia. When given intrathecally it may cause grand mal convulsions, radiculitis, arachnoiditis, paralysis of the extremities, urinary retention and other difficulties. Because of the potential seriousness of its toxic effects, intravenous use should be primarily for patients with progressive, potentially fatal infections, and the patient always should be hospitalized during a course of therapy and renal function should be monitored. Hypokalemia may favor digitalis toxicity and sensitize to neuromuscular blocking drugs.

Dose—*Intravenous infusion, adult,* after a test dose of 1 mg to assess tolerance, *initially* **250 μg/kg** a day, increased by daily increments of 5 to 10 mg, if tolerated, up to a maximum of **1 mg/kg** a day or alternate-day doses of **1.5 mg/kg**. *Intrathecal, adults,* **100 μg** *initially* every 48 to 72 hr, with gradual increments up to a single-dose maximum of **500 μg**. *Topical,* as 3% cream, lotion or ointment, apply 2 to 4 times a day.

Dosage Forms—For Injection: 50 mg; Cream: 3%; Lotion: 3%; Ointment: 3%.

Anthralin—page 874.

Benzoic Acid—see RPS-18, page 1235.

Benzoic and Salicylic Acid Ointment—see RPS-18, page 1235.

Butoconazole—see RPS-18, page 1235.

Butylparaben—see RPS-18, page 1170.

Calcium Undecylenate—see RPS-18, page 1235.

Ciclopirox Olamine—see RPS-18, page 1236.

Clioquinol—see RPS-18, page 1236.

Clotrimazole

1*H*-Imidazole, 1-[(2-chlorophenyl)diphenylmethyl]-, Gyne-Lotrimin, Lotrimin (*Schering*); Mycelex, Mycelex-G (*Miles*)

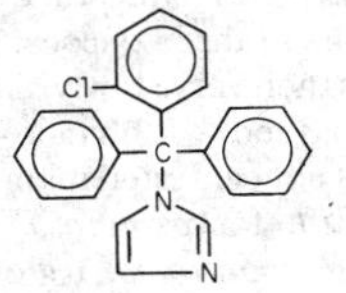

1-(*o*-Chloro-α,α-diphenylbenzyl)imidazole [23593-75-1] $C_{22}H_{17}ClN_2$ (344.84).

Preparation—From the reaction between imidazole and 2-chlorotriphenylmethyl chloride using trimethylamine as a proton receptor.

Description—White, to pale-yellow, crystalline powder; melts about 147° with decomposition weakly basic; hydrolyses on heating with aqueous acid.

Solubility—Slightly soluble in water; soluble in alcohol or chloroform; slightly soluble in ether.

Uses—A broad-spectrum antifungal agent that inhibits growth of pathogenic dermatophytes, yeasts and *Pityrosporon obiculare* (*Malassezia furfur*). It exhibits fungicidal activity *in vitro* against isolates of *Trichophyton rubrum, T mentagrophytes, Epidermophyton floccosum, Microsporum canis* and *Candida albicans*. It shares with econazole and miconazole first-choice status for topical treatment of *tinea pedis, tinea cruris* and *tinea corporis* due to any of the aforementioned organisms, *candidiasis* due to *Candida albicans* and *tinea versicolor* due to Pityrosporon obiculare *Malassezia furfur* as well as for local treatment of *vulvovaginal candidiasis*. It is effective for the topical treatment of *oropharyngeal candidiasis*. In Europe the drug also is used systemically; however, most clinical studies indicate that used orally the drug has limited efficacy yet considerable CNS toxicity.

Adverse effects from topical use include erythema; stinging, blistering and peeling of the skin; pruritus and urticaria. Swallowed (investigational) troches may evoke colic, epigastric pain, nausea, vomiting and diarrhea.

Dose—*Intravaginally*, **5 g** of **1%** cream or one **100-mg** tablet daily, preferably at bedtime, for 7 consecutive days; two 100-mg tablets intravaginally for 3 nights. *Oral, adult* and *children over 4 yr*, **10 mg**, as a troche, slowly dissolved in the mouth 5 times a day for at least 14 days. *Topically*, to the skin, as 1% cream or solution twice a day, morning and evening.

Dosage Forms—Cream: 1%; Vaginal Cream: 1% (one applicatorful contains 5 g of cream); Topical Solution: 1%; Vaginal Tablets: 100 and 500 mg; Troches: 10 mg.

Econazole Nitrate

1*H*-Imidazole, (±)-1-[2-[(4-chlorophenyl)methoxy]-2-(2,4-dichlorophenyl)ethyl]-, mononitrate, Spectrazole (*Ortho*)

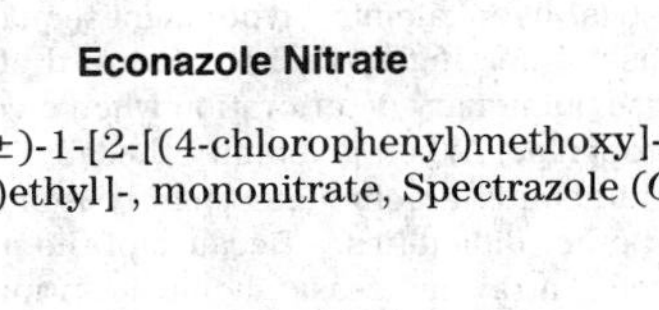

(±)-1-[2,4-Dichloro-β-[(*p*-chlorobenzyl)oxy]phenethyl]imidazole mononitrate [68797-31-9] C_{18}-H_{15}-Cl_3-N_2-O.HNO_3 (440.70).

Preparation—2,4-Dichloroacetophenone is further chlorinated to the phenacyl chloride and this compound treated with imidazole with loss of HCl to yield 1-(1*H*)-(2,4-dichlorophenacyl)imidazole (I). Reduction of the ketone group of I with sodium borohydride forms the secondary alcohol (II). With sodium hydride, the alcoholate of II is produced, which on reaction with *p*-chlorobenzyl chloride produces econazole base. See *J Med Chem 12:* 784, 1969.

Description—White crystals; melts about 162° pK_a 6.6.

Solubility—Very slightly soluble in water or most organic solvents.

Uses—Antifungal activity against the dermatophytes (*Epidermophyton floccosum, Microsporon auduoni, canis* and *gypseum, and Trichophyton rubrum, mentagrophytes* and *tonsurans*), *Pityrosporon obiculare (Malasserzia furfur)* and *Candida albicans*. It is employed in the treatment of *cutaneous Candidiasis*, and *tineas corporis, cruris, pedis* and *versicolor (pityriasis versicolor)*. Its efficacy is comparable to that of miconazole or clotrimazole. It readily penetrates into the stratum corneum, where effective concentrations persist for up to several days. In about 3% of recipients, local erythemia, burning sensation, stinging and itching occur.

Dose—*Topical* to the *skin*, as a **1%** cream twice a day, except only once a day for pityriasis versicolor and 3 times a day for tinea barbae or capitus or paronychia. Treatment should be maintained for at least 2 wk for pityriasis versicolor, tinea corporis, tinea cruris and candidiasis, and 1 mo for tinea pedis.

Fluconazole

1*H*-1,2,4-Triazole-1-ethanol, α-(2,4-difluorophenyl)-α-(1*H*-1,2,4-triazolylmethyl), Diflucan (*Roerig*)

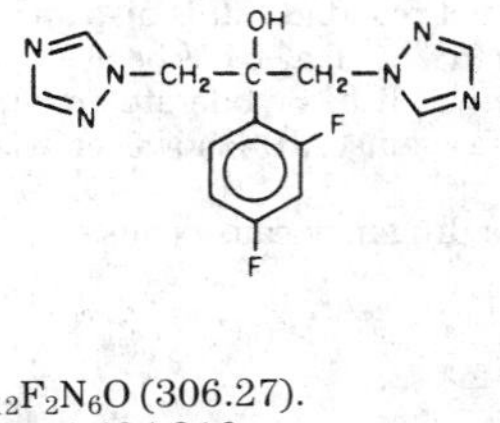

[86386-73-4] $C_{13}H_{12}F_2N_6O$ (306.27).

Preparation—US Pat 4,404,216.

Description—White crystals; melts about 139°.

Uses—A highly selective inhibitor of fungal cytochrome P-450 and sterol C-14 α-demethylation that results in inhibition of ergosterol synthesis. It is a broad-spectrum bistriazole antifungal agent that is primarily fungistatic with activity against *Cryptococcus neoformans* and *Candida* spp. In common with other azole antifungal drugs, most fungi are more susceptible *in vivo*. It is approved for systemic candidiasis, oropharyngeal and esophageal candidiasis and cryptococcal meningitis.

The bioavailability of oral fluconazole is over 90% compared with IV administration. The volume of distribution is 0.8 g/L and reaches concentrations in the CSF that are 80% of that in serum of patients with meningitis. Plasma protein binding is 11% and fluconazole is cleared primarily by renal excretion with 80% of the dose unchanged and 11% as metabolites in the urine. The plasma half-life is about 30 hr. Fluconazole may alter cytochrome P450 pathways of metabolism of several drugs including phenytoin, cyclosporine, warfarin and sulfonylureas.

The most common adverse effects of fluconazole are nausea, vomiting, bloating and abdominal discomfort. Elevated hepatic aminotransferase activity and allergic rashes may occur.

Dose—*Adult, oropharyngeal candidiasis*, **200 mg** the first day followed by 100 mg once a day for a minimum of 2 to 3 wk; *systemic candidiasis* and *cryptococcal meningitis*, **400 mg** the first day followed by **200 mg** once a day for a minimum of 4 wk up to 10 to 12 wk.

Dosage Forms—Tablets: 50,100 and 200 mg; Injection: 200 mg/100 mL and 400 mg/200 mL.

Flucytosine

Cytosine, 5-fluoro-, 5-FC; Ancobon (*Roche*)

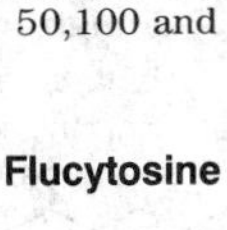

[2022-85-7] $C_4H_4FN_3O$ (129.09).

Preparation—5-Fluorouracil (page 1251) is reacted with $POCl_3$ to form 2,4-dichloro-5-fluoropyrimidine which is reacted with NH_3 to produce 2-chloro-4-amino-5-fluoropyrimidine. Heating the latter in concentrated HCl yields flucytosine. US Pat 3,368,938.

Description—White to off-white, crystalline powder; odorless or has a slight odor; melts about 295° with decomposition; stable in light; nonhygroscopic; stable for at least 3 months at 45°; pK_a 2.9, 10.7.

Solubility—1 g in about 83 mL water or about 12 mL 0.1 *N* HCl; slightly soluble in alcohol; practically insoluble in chloroform or ether.

Uses—Converted in the fungus to 5-fluorouracil which is incorporated into RNA, where it interferes with normal protein synthesis. Certain fungal organisms are more sensitive to interference from the drug than are human cells, so that the drug is useful in the treatment of some fungal infections. Most clinical isolates of *Cryptococcus* and 40 to 92% of *Candida* are sensitive to the drug. It is the drug of choice to treat *chromomycosis* and of second choice to treat *systemic candidiasis*. It may be combined with amphotericin B for first-choice treatment of *aspergillosis* or *cryptococcosis*, especially with meningitis. It also may be used effectively to treat candidiasis of the urinary tract. Since resistance to the drug can develop, not only should sensitivity tests precede therapy but they should be conducted also throughout the course of treatment.

Some patients may be given as much as 5 g a day without toxic effects, and the drug also has been given for as long as 820 days without untoward effects. Nausea, vomiting, diarrhea and rash rather commonly are caused by the drug. There have been a few cases of intestinal perforation. Bone-marrow depression, manifested by anemia, leukopenia and thrombocytopenia, occur in about 10% of patients; there have been a few fatalities. It should not be used with antineoplastics or immunosuppressants. Sedation, confusion, hallucinations, headache and vertigo occur infrequently. Mild azotemia and an increase in liver enzymes in the plasma are rather common effects, but hepatic necrosis seems to be a rare effect. Serum concentrations are monitored if renal function is impaired. Monitor hepatic function and hematopoietic system during therapy. Nausea can be lessened if the several capsules in a dose are taken separately at 10- to 15-min intervals. Nephrotoxicity from concurrently administered amphotericin B will increase the plasma levels and hence the toxicity of it.

About 90% is absorbed orally. It is distributed well among all the tissues, including the CNS. About 80 to 90% is excreted unchanged in the urine with a half-life 0.5 to 1 hr, except 4 to 6 hr in renal failure. The dose needs to be adjusted if renal function is abnormal. If there is any reason to suspect a decrease in renal sufficiency, function tests should be made at the outset.

Dose—*Oral, adult, infants* and *children*, **12.5** to **37.5 mg/kg** (or 375 to 563 mg/m^2 for infants and children) every 6 hr. The duration of treatment varies from a few days to months.

Dosage Form—Capsules: 250 and 500 mg.

Formaldehyde Solution—see RPS-18, page 1171.

Gentian Violet—see RPS-18, page 1171.

Griseofulvin

Spiro[benzofuran-2(3*H*),1′-[2]cyclohexene]-3,4′-dione, 7-chloro-2′,4,6-trimethoxy-6′-methyl-, (1′*S-trans*)-, (*Various Mfrs*)

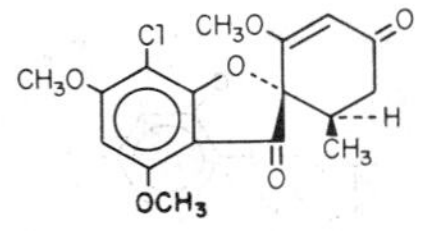

[126-07-8] $C_{17}H_{17}ClO_6$ (352.77); a substance produced by the growth of *Penicillium griseofulvum* or by other means. It has a potency equivalent to not less than 900 μg of $C_{17}H_{17}ClO_6$/mg.

Preparation—By the submerged process using selected strains of *Penicillium patulum*.

Description—White to creamy white, powder, in which particles of the order of 4 μm in diameter predominate; odorless.

Solubility—Soluble in chloroform; sparingly soluble in alcohol; very slightly soluble in water.

Uses—An effective agent in the treatment of superficial fungus infections. It is fungistatic and not fungicidal. Administered systemically, the drug is highly effective in the management of *tinea capitis, tinea corporis, tinea unguium* (onychomycosis) and the chronic form of *tinea pedis* caused by the dermatophytes, *Microsporon, Trichophyton* and *Epidermophyton*. It may also be dramatically effective against *favus*. Infections caused by *T rubrum* may respond, but relapses are frequent. Part of the reason for relapses is that some of the fungi, at least, grow in dead and dying squamous epithelial cells and their keratin residues. Since it does not kill but only arrests reproduction of the organism, it is necessary to continue medication long enough for the entire epidermis to be shed and replaced in order to remove reinfecting organisms. When there is hyperkeratosis, the time for desquamation may be long. It is deposited in the keratin precursor cells and is carried outwards into the epidermis as normal skin growth proceeds. This also makes for a long latency from the time medication is begun until evidence of improvement occurs. Because it disrupts microtubules it has anti-inflammatory properties and has been used successfully in the management of cutaneous inflammatory conditions and several polyarthritic syndromes.

Serious untoward reactions are infrequent, but skin eruptions, leukopenia, granulocytopenia and allergic reactions such as serum sickness or angioneurotic edema are among the serious side effects reported. It is recommended that the drug be reserved for use in infections not amenable to conventional topical measures and for those in which the causative organism has been shown to be susceptible to its effect. It also may cause nausea, vomiting, epigastric distress and diarrhea; these often may be avoided by giving the drug with or shortly following a meal. Headache is also relatively frequent. Infrequently, phototoxicity, proteinuria, lassitude and fatigue occur and, rarely, there is mental confusion and motor incoordination. It is advisable to monitor kidney, blood and liver functions. Ingestion of alcohol during treatment with the drug causes tachycardia and flushing.

The oral bioavailability depends upon particle size; the smaller the crystal size, the more complete the absorption. The percent absorbed from the microsize preparations is 25 to 70%; from the ultramicrosize preparations it is almost complete. Absorption is greater if the drug is administered with a high-fat meal. The principal route of elimination may be transepidermal loss, although a considerable hepatic metabolism and biliary secretion probably also occur. The amount of unchanged drug in the urine is relatively small. The half-life is 24 to 36 hr. It induces the hepatic microsomal system, and the metabolism of warfarin, mexiletine and oral contraceptives is increased, thus necessitating dosage adjustments. Phenobarbital decreases plasma levels of the drug, but it is not clear whether the action is through hepatic enzyme induction or an influence on absorption via alterations in bile acid secretion.

Dose—*Oral, adult,* for *tinea capitis corporis* or *cruris, microcrystalline* form, **500 mg** a day in a single dose or divided doses, or *ultramicrocrystalline* form, **330** to **375 mg** a day in a single dose or divided doses; for *tinea pedia* or *unguium, microcrystalline* form, **1 g** a day in divided doses, or *ultramicrocrystalline* form, **600** to **750 mg** a day in divided doses. *Children, microcrystalline* form, **11 mg/kg**; *or, 14 to 23 kg,* **125** to **250 mg** a day; *over 23 kg,* **250** to **500 mg** a day; *ultramicrocrystalline* form, **5.5** to **7.3 mg/kg** a day; or, *14 to 23 kg,* **82.5** to **165 mg** a day; *over 23 kg,* **165** to **330 mg** a day.

Dosage Forms—*Microsize:* Capsules: 125 and 250 mg; Oral Suspension: 125 mg/5 mL; Tablets: 250 and 500 mg. *Ultramicrosize:* Tablets: 125, 165, 250 and 300 mg.

Haloprogin

Benzene, 1,2,4-trichloro-5-[(3-iodo-2-propynyl)oxy]-, ing of Halotex (*Westwood*)

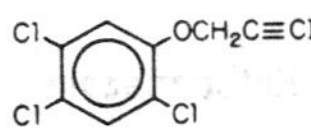

[777-11-7] $C_9H_4Cl_3IO$ (361.39).

Preparation—*CA 58*: 14635g, 1963.

Description—White or pale-yellow, crystalline powder; melts about 114°; decomposes at 190°.

Solubility—Very slightly soluble in water; soluble in alcohol.

Uses—Fungicidal to various species of *Candida, Epidermophyton, Malassezia, Microsporon,* and *Trichophyton*. It is employed topically in the treatment of *tinea pedis* (athlete's foot), *tinea cruris, tinea corporis, tinea manuum* and *tinea versicolor*. In the treatment of athlete's foot, the cure rate is about 80%. It also has been used to treat *cutaneous candidiasis*, for which it has about the same efficacy as nystatin. It has a low order of toxicity. Deliberate attempts to induce contact dermatitis and phototoxicity have been unsuccessful. However, irritation, burning sensation, pruritus, vesiculation, increased maceration and so-called "sensitization" occasionally occur during treatment, especially if occlusive footwear is worn; the apparent sensitization is possibly a response to debris and endotoxins from killed fungi, such as often occurs with other effective antifungal drugs. These reactions give the appearance of the exacerbation of the infection, but mycological examinations show the fungal population to be decreasing. It is absorbed poorly from the skin. That which is absorbed is converted to trichlorophenol. There have been no reports of systemic intoxication from topical application. One 4-yr-old child was treated with 12.1 kg of a 1% preparation over a period of 3 yr without evidences of systemic effects.

Dose—*Topical,* to the *skin, adult, infants* and *children,* as **1%** cream or solution twice a day for 2 to 4 wk.

Dosage Forms—Cream: 1%; Topical Solution: 1%.

Ichthammol—page 875.

Iodine—page 1134.

Itraconazole

3*H*-1,2,4-Triazol-3-one, (±)-4-[4-[4-[4-[[2-(2,4-dichlorophenyl)-2-(1*H*-1,2,4-triazol-1-ylmethyl)-1,3-dioxolan-4-yl]methoxy]-phenyl]-1-piperazinyl]phenyl]-2,4-dihydro-2-(1-methylpropyl)-, Sporanox (*Janssen*)

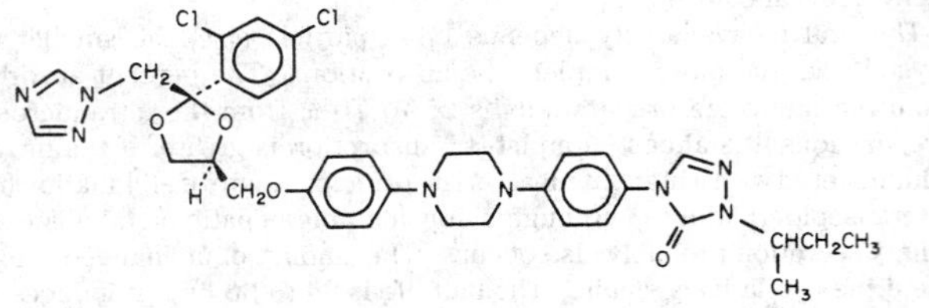

[84625-61-6] $C_{35}H_{38}Cl_2N_8O_4$ (705.65)

Preparation—*J Med Chem, 27:*894, 1984; The racemate is used clinically.

Description—White crystals; melts about 166°; pK_a about 3.5.

Solubility—1 g in 10,000 mL water or 1000 mL of alcohol; more soluble in acidulated polyethylene glycols.

Uses—A triazole antifungal agent with a mechanism of action and broad spectrum similar to fluconazole. It also inhibits chitin synthesis in both yeast-budding and hyphal growth of fungi. It is used to treat fungal infections in immunocompromised and nonimmunocompromised patients with cryptococcosis, blastomycosis, histoplasmosis and aspergillosis. Unlabelled uses include superficial mycoses, systemic mycoses and subcutameous mycoses.

Bioavailability is 55% and food enhances oral absorption. It is 99.8% protein bound and is eliminated in urine and bile after extensive hepatic metabolism. The half-life is 20 to 30 hr. Negligible levels reach CSF.

Adverse effects include nausea, epigastric pain, edema and hypokalemia. Reversible alterations in liver function have been reported in a few cases. Some interactions with drugs metabolized by P450 pathways have been observed in some patients.

Dose—*Oral, adult,* **200 mg** once a day with food, increase by **100-mg** increments if needed to maximum of **400 mg** a day for a minimum of 3 mo. Doses >**200 mg** a day should be in two divided doses. For *life-threatening infections,* a loading dose of **200 mg** 3 times a day for the first 3 days.

Dosage Form—Capsules: 200 mg.

Ketoconazole

Piperazine, *cis*-1-acetyl-4-[4-[[2-(2,4-dichlorophenyl)-2-(1*H*-imidazol- 1-ylmethyl)-1,3-dioxolan-4-yl]methoxy]phenyl]-, Nizarol (*Janssen*)

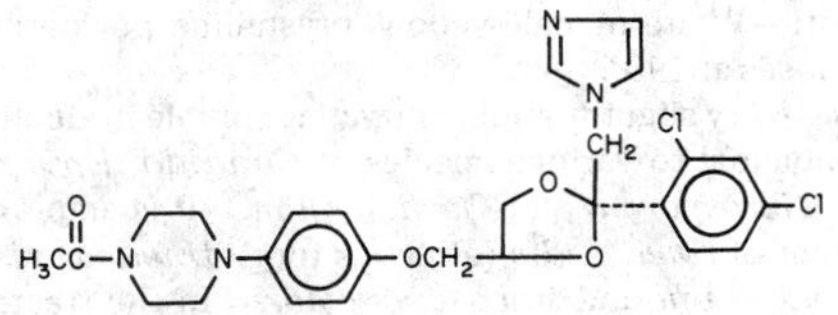

[65277-42-1] $C_{26}H_{28}Cl_2N_4O_4$ (531.44).

Preparation—*J Med Chem 22:* 1003, 1979.

Description—White crystals melts about 146°.

Uses—Blocks the fungal synthesis of ergosterol, which is essential to the integrity of the cell membranes of nearly all the pathogenic fungi. Consequently, it has a broad spectrum of antifungal activity, which includes *Blastomyces dermatitidis, Candida spp, Chromomyces, Coccidioides immitis,* dermatophytes, *Histoplasma capsulatum* and *Paracoccidioides braseliensis* and *Pseudallescheria boydii. Aspergillus, Cryptococcus neoformans* and *Sporothrix schenckii* are affected moderately but *Mucor* is not. It or amphotericin B is the drug of choice for the treatment of *blastomycosis, coccidiodosis, histoplasmosis* and *paracoccidiodosis.* It shares first-choice status with miconazole for the treatment of infections by *Pseudallescheria boydii.* It is an alternative drug for candidiasis and *chromoblastomycosis.* Successful treatment sometimes requires months.

Nausea and vomiting are the most frequent (*ca* 3 to 10%) side effects; these can be avoided by taking the drug with food. Pruritis is the next most frequent (1.5%) and abdominal cramps, third (1.2%). Other effects are pruritus, sleepiness, headache, diarrhea, photophobia, fever, thrombocytopenia, gynecomastia, impotence and oligospermia (from low testosterone levels). Hepatitis is rare (1:12,000). A disulfiram-like reaction to alcohol occurs. Most adverse effects are transient and all are reversible, except that three cases of liver necrosis have been fatal. Monitoring of liver function is mandatory. In rats, it is teratogenic; thus, it should not be used during pregnancy. It inhibits certain cytochrome P-450 enzymes; plasma levels of cyclosporine, estradiol, hydrocortisone, methylprednisolone, rifampin and theophylline can be increased. Cimetidine inhibits and rifampin induces the metabolism of the drug. Ketoconazole inhibits steroid C17-20 lyase and thus decreases the biosynthesis of adrenalcorticoids, androgens and estrogens. This is the basis of its uses to treat *Cushing's syndrome, precocious puberty* and *prostatic carcinoma.*

It is absorbed well by the oral route. A dose of 2 g with a meal will cause a peak plasma level of about 3.5 μg/mL, but up to 50 μg/mL have been reported. In plasma, 95 to 99% is protein-bound. The principal route of elimination is hepatic metabolism and biliary secretion of the metabolites, less than 4% being renal excretion. There are a number of metabolites. Enterohepatic circulation complicates the pharmacokinetics. During the first 10 hr (alpha-phase), the half-life is 1.4 to 3.3 hr; thereafter (beta-phase), it is 6 to 10 hr.

Dose—*Oral, adult* for *vulvovaginal candidiasis* or *tinea versicolor,* **200 mg** once a day for 3 to 5 days in candidiasis and 5 to 10 days in tinea; for *paronychia, fungal cystitis, urinary tract mycoses* or *mild to moderate systemic mycoses,* **200** to **400 mg** once a day; for fungal pneumonia or *septicemia,* **400 mg** to 1 g once a day, not to exceed 1 g a day; for *Cushing's syndrome,* **600 mg** to **1 g** once a day; for *prostatic carcinoma,* **400 mg** 3 times a day, not to exceed 1.2 g a day; *children over 2 yr,* for *mycoses,* **3.3** to **6.6 mg/kg** a day. *Topical,* as **2%** cream, once a day for *candidiasis* or *tinea corporis, cruris* or *versicolor* and 2 or 3 times a day for *paronychia* or *tinea barbis, capitis* or *pedis.*

Dosage Forms—Cream: 2%; Shampoo: 29%; Oral Suspension: 100 mg/5 mL; Tablets: 200 mg.

Mercuric Oxide, Yellow—see RPS-18, page 1172.

Mercury, Ammoniated—see RPS-18, page 1172.

Miconazole

1*H*-Imidazole, 1-[2-(2,4-dichlorophenyl)-2-[(2,4-dichlorophenyl)methoxy]ethyl]-, Micatin (*Ortho*); Monistat (*Janssen*)

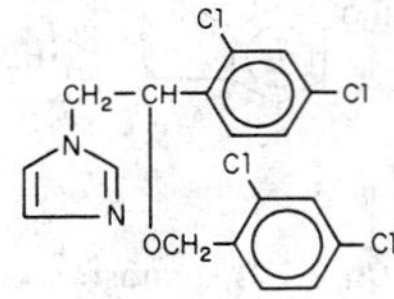

1-[2,4-Dichloro-β-[(2,4-dichlorobenzyl)oxy]phenethyl]imidazole [22916-47-8] $C_{18}H_{14}Cl_4N_2O$ (416.12).

Preparation—2,4-Dichlorophenacyl bromide is used to alkylate imidazole followed by reduction of the ketone group to a secondary alcohol which is converted to the alkoxide. Williamson alkylation with α,*p*,-dichlorotoluene yields the product. *J Med Chem 12:* 784, 1969.

Uses—Fungicidal to various species of *Aspergillus, Blastomyces, Candida, Cladosporium, Coccidioides, Epidermophyton, Histoplasma, Madurella, Pityrosporon (Malassezia), Microsporon, Paracoccidioides, Phialophora, Pseudallescheria* and *Trichophyton.* It also has activity against gram-positive bacteria. It inhibits ergosterol synthesis, which disrupts fungal cell membranes. Sulfonamides enhance the antifungal action in *Candida.* The drug readily penetrates into the stratum corneum and remains there in high concentration for as long as 4 days, which probably contributes to its efficacy against the dermatophytoses. In *tinea pedis* (athlete's foot) a mycological cure rate of 96% has been reported with the nitrate salt, which considerably exceeds that of any other drugs except clotrimazole and econazole. Comparable efficacy has been reported in use against *tinea versicolor,* ringworm, onychomycosis and *cutaneous candidiasis.*

Topically, for *vulvovaginal candidiasis,* the reported cure rate varies from 80 to 95%, considerably superior to that with nystatin (65%) and amphotericin B (75%). Often pruritus is relieved after a single application. It is also effective against some vaginal infections caused by *T glabratus.* The free base is useful in the topical treatment of various ophthalmic mycoses. The base has been used successfully in the systemic treatment of several deep or systemic mycoses, especially those of *candidiasis* and *cryptococcosis.* It is the drug of first choice for the treatment of *allescheriosis* (petriellidiosis) and second choice for *coccidiomycosis.* It is

Table 6—Antifungals for Superficial Mycoses

Drug official name	Trade name(s)	Route	Use: Dermato-phytes	Use: Candida
Allylamine				
Naftifine	Naftin	Topical		x
Imidazoles				
Butaconazole	Femstat	Intravaginal		x
Clotrimazole	Lotromin, Mycelex	Topical, oral	x	x
	Spectazole	Topical	x	x
Econazole				
Ketoconazole	Nizoral	Oral, topical	x	x
Miconazole	Monistat	Topical, intra-vaginal	x	x
Oxiconazole	Oxistat	Topical	x	x
Sulconazole	Exelderm	Topical	x	
Triazole				
Terconazole	Terzol	Intravaginal		x
Polyene antibiotics				
Amphotericin B	Fungizone			x
Mystatin	Mycostatin, Nilstat, Oustain	Oral, intra-vaginal, topical		x
Miscellaneous				
Ciclopirox	Loprox	Toical	x	x
Clioquinol	Vioform	Topical	x	x
Griseofulvin	Various	Oral	x	x
Haloprogin	Halotex	Topical	x	x
Pyrithione zinc	Various	Topical	x	x
Selenium Sulfide	Exsel, Selsun	Topical	x	
Tolnaftate	Aftate, Tinactin, Zeasorb-AF	Topical	x	
Undecylenic acid	Desenex	Topical	x	

also useful against *paracoccidioidomycosis.* Systemic use against minor, self-limiting infections, should be avoided.

Burning, itching and maceration sometimes occur after application of the nitrate to the skin, as happens frequently with effective antifungal drugs; the effect, at least in part, seems to result from irritating debris released from killed organisms. Intravaginally, burning, itching, pelvic discomfort, urticaria and headache occur in 6 to 7% of users, especially during the first few days of treatment. Experimental and clinical studies suggest that the drug is safe for use in pregnancy, but systemic use during pregnancy should probably be avoided, if possible.

Orally, it appears to be tolerated well, but nausea, vomiting and diarrhea occur; no evidence of renal or hepatic toxicity has been observed. Intravenous administration may cause phlebitis, hypercholesterolemia and hypertriglyceridemia (caused by the vehicle), hyponatremia (from ADH secretion), nausea, vomiting, diarrhea, anorexia and infrequent allergic and immune reactions, such as fever, chills, pruritus, rashes, thrombocytopenia, anaphylaxis and anemia. Wheezing and tachypnea and sinoatrial and ventricular tachycardias occur, which can be avoided by slower rates of infusion. Intrathecally, it may cause some meningeal irritation, but the route appears to be safe.

From topical sites, only trace amounts of the drug appear in the blood or urine. Slightly less than 50% of an oral dose is absorbed. In plasma, about 93% is bound to proteins. Less than 1% of an oral dose appears unchanged in urine. The drug manifests three-compartment pharmacokinetics. The terminal (elimination, β) half-life is about 1 day. Systemically, it inhibits the metabolism of warfarin.

Dose—*Intravenous infusion, adults,* for *candidiasis,* **200** to **600 mg** every 8 hr for 1 to over 20 wk; for *coccidiomycosis,* **600 mg** to **1.2 g** every 8 hr for 3 to over 20 wk; for *cryptococcosis,* **400** to **800 mg** every 8 hr for 3 to over 12 wk; for *paracoccidioidomycosis,* **66.7** to **400 mg** every 8 hr for 2 to over 16 wk; for *pseudoallescheriosis,* **200 mg** to **1 g** 3 times a day for 5 to over 20 wk. *Children 1 yr* or *over,* **20** to **40 mg/kg** a day, up to a maximum of 15 mg/kg/dose. *Intrathecal,* **20 mg** every 3 to 7 days. *Bladder irrigation,* **200 mg,** as a diluted injection.

Dosage Form—Injection: 200 mg/10 mL, solubilized with a polyethylene glycol and lactic acid, in water for injection.

Miconazole Nitrate

Monistat (*Ortho*)

[22832-87-7] $C_{18}H_{14}Cl_4N_2O.HNO_3$ (479.15).

Description—White, crystalline powder; melts at 170°.

Solubility—Very slightly soluble in water.

Uses—Actions, uses and side effects discussed under *Miconazole* (above).

Dose—*Topical,* to the *skin* as a **2%** cream, lotion or spray twice a day, except only once a day for *tinea versicolor,* and to the *vagina* as a **2%** cream or **100** or **200 mg** as a suppository once a day at bedtime for 3 or 7 days.

Dosage Forms—Cream: 2%; Vaginal Cream: 2%; Lotion: 2%; Powder: 2%; Spray: 2%; Vaginal Suppository: 100 and 200 mg.

Naftifine Hydrochloride—see RPS-18, page 1236.

Natamycin—see RPS-18, page 1236.

Nystatin

(*Various Mfrs*)

Nystatin [1400-61-9] is a substance produced by the growth of *Streptomyces noursei* Brown, *et al* (Fam *Streptomycetaceae*). It contains not less than 4400 Units of nystatin activity/mg. Nystatin is a mixture of 4 different tetraenes, nystatin A, (principally) and nystatin A_2, A_3 and polyfungin B. Nystatin A_1 [34786-70-4] $C_{47}H_{75}NO_{17}$ is closely related to *Amphotericin B.* Each is a macrocyclic lactone containing a ketal ring, an *all-trans* tetraene system and a mycosamine (3-amino-3-deoxyrhamnose) moiety.

Description—Yellow to light-tan hygroscopic powder; odor suggestive of cereals; hygroscopic; affected by long exposure to light, heat or air; pK_a 4.5, 8.64; gradually decomposes above 160° without melting.

Solubility—(mg/mL, at about 30°) Water, 4; alcohol 1.2; methanol 11.2; chloroform, 0.48; or ethylene glycol, 8.75.

Uses—Active *in vitro* against a number of yeasts and molds, but its clinical usefulness is limited to the treatment of *candidiasis.* The antibiotic is absorbed poorly from the gastrointestinal tract; consequently it is not effective against systemic infections, but is effective against *intestinal candidiasis.* It may prevent emergence of candidal suprainfections resulting from oral therapy with broad-spectrum antibiotics, although such suprainfections are so infrequent that routine "prophylactic" use of nystatin is not worthwhile. It does *not* prevent diarrhea from oral broad-spectrum antibiotics. It has been employed with variable success in the treatment of oral "thrush" (moniliasis). It is used alone to treat vulvovaginal candidiasis. For use on the skin, it may be combined with neomycin, gramicidin and triamcinolone acetonide. It is not the drug of first or second choice in any use. It is relatively nontoxic, but nausea, vomiting and diarrhea may occur with oral therapy.

Dose—*Oral, adult,* **500,000** to **1,000,000 units** 3 times a day; *older infants,* **200,000 units** (4 times a day; *premature or underweight infants,* **100,000 units** 4 times a day. *Oropharyngeal,* **200,000** or **400,000 units** as a lozenge 4 or 5 times a day. *Topical, to the skin, adults and children,* to the affected area 2 or 3 times a day as a cream, ointment or powder containing **100,000 units/g** with or without other agents; *intravaginal,* **100,000** to **200,000 units** high into the vagina once or twice a day.

Dosage Forms—Cream, Ointment or Topical Powder: 100,000 units/g; Lozenges: 200,000 units; Oral Suspension: 100,000 units/mL; Tablets: 500,000 units. Vaginal Tablets: 100,000 units.

Potassium Iodide—page 976.

Potassium Permanganate—see RPS-18, page 1173.

Propylparaben—see RPS-18, page 1173.

Resorcinol—see RPS-16, page 1107.

Resorcinol Monoacetate—see RPS-16, page 1107.

Salicylic Acid—page 879.
Sodium Benzoate—see RPS-18, page 1173.
Sodium Hypochlorite Solution—page 1271.
Sodium Propionate—see RPS-18, page 1236.
Sulconazole Nitrate—see RPS-18, page 1236.
Terconazole—see RPS-18, page 1237.
Tolnaftate—see RPS-18, page 1237.
Triacetin—see RPS-18, page 1237.
Undecylenic Acid—see RPS-18, page 1237.
Zinc Undecylenate—see RPS-18, page 1237.

Antiviral Drugs

Effective, safe, antiviral drugs have been slow to be developed, partly because of insufficient knowledge about viral biochemistry and partly because viruses commandeer part of the host genetic and biochemical apparatus to replicate within the host cell. Many viral targets of chemotherapeutic agents belong to the host or are so similar as to also come under attack. However, recent research on viral molecular biology has described various viral structures in great detail and in relationship to the host cell. With a better understanding of the virion and its control over the host cell, some unique structures suggest themselves as targets and more selective drugs are conceivable.

A virion first attaches to a binding site (receptor) on the exterior surface of the cell membrane. These "docking" sites mostly are well-described molecules, such as the Class I or II histocompatability molecule, CD3 receptor CR2 of lymphocytes, hepatic receptors for polymeric albumin or IgA, CD4 (T4) molecular or IgM receptor of the T lymphocyte epidermal growth factor receptor and even acteylcholine and β-adrenoreceptors. Possible intervention at this stage takes the form of ligating the receptor with an analog of the viral binding aminoacid sequence or inactivating the binding sequence of the virus with an analog of the receptor group. In the case of peptide-T, this has provided a safe but only somewhat effective drug. Nevertheless, this is a most promising approach. Another approach at the receptor locus is one in which a toxin is attached to a receptor ligand or the toxin-ligated receptor itself used as an agent lethal to the infected cell; rCD4-ricin A chain complex kills cells infected by human immunodeficiency virus (HIV) and probably will receive clinical trials.

Receptor activation leads to endocytosis and uncoating of the virion. Details of this step require more elaboration, but this also is a step that probably can be attacked safely. Successful intervention has been achieved thus far only with influenza A virus (amantadine and rimantidine).

Once the viral RNA, DNA and enzymes are free within the cell, selectivity is harder to achieve. However, viral DNA polymerase and retroviral reverse-transcriptase are sufficiently different from the host enzymes that they are possible to attack without severe damage to the host. Some infected cells may be destroyed by the drug, but most infected cells are destined for destruction by the virus, anyway. Various analogs of nucleosides or nucleotides are intended to intervene at this stage in viral replication. However, most of the nucleoside analogs also have varying degrees of adverse effects on uninfected cells. Whether or not highly selective drugs of this class can be developed is uncertain.

The expression of viral genes probably will come to be suppressed by agents designed to attack viral proteins that function to activate genes. The control protein of the HIV is presently under intense study.

The synthesis of the late proteins and assembly of new virions probably will provide loci for selective intervention, but, at present, little progress has been made. However, inhibitors of viral enzymes that trim sugar moieties from new viral glycopeptides are presently under investigation. A key to selective intervention in the budding stage has yet to be discovered. Lastly, virus-infected cells acquire distinct surface properties that make them susceptible to immune attack by macrophages activated by muramyl tripeptides or other ligands on liposomes.

Many antiseptics and astringents are virucidal and may be used for purposes of disinfection of virus-contaminated objects or substances. Also, β-propiolactone and certain other substances are employed specifically to destroy the virus of serum hepatitis that may contaminate human blood products.

Acyclovir

6*H*-Purin-6-one,
2-amino-1,9-dihydro-9-[(2-hydroxyethoxy)methyl]-,
Zovirax (*Burroughs Wellcome*)

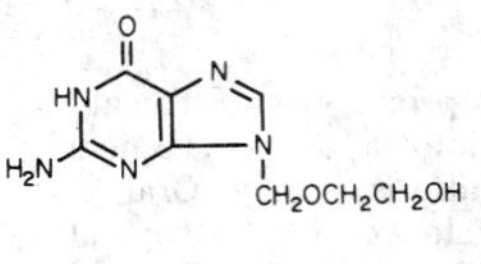

O
HN N
H₂N N N
CH₂OCH₂CH₂OH

9-[(2-Hydroxyethoxy)methyl]guanine [59277-89-3] $C_8H_{11}N_5O_3$ (225.21).

Preparation—Guanine is alkylated with 2-(chloromethoxy)ethyl benzoate and the resulting ester hydrolyzed to the product; See Ger Pat 2,539,963.

Uses—Activity against *Herpes simplex* viruses (HSV) 1 and 2, varicella-zoster, Epstein-Barr viruses and cytomegalovirus. Inside an infected cell, it is changed into the triphosphate, which then is incorporated into DNA; this terminates elongation of the DNA and prevents viral replication. The sodium salt is approved in the US for the oral treatment of recurrent mucosal and cutaneous infections caused by HSV-1 and HSV-2 in immunocompromised adults and children and for severe initial herpes genitalis infections in immunocompetent patients. It decreases but does not completely prevent recurrences or influence the long-term natural history of the disease. However, the drug has been employed effectively in the treatment of HSV encephalitis (drug of choice) and neonatal infections and in the treatment of chicken pox, cytomegalovirus and varicella-zoster infections. Resistant but less virulent strains of HSV have developed during treatment. The drug also is approved for the topical treatment of nonfulminating HSV-1 and HSV-2 infection (except in the eye), but it is only moderately effective, especially against genital herpes in women. It does not eradicate latent herpes. It is somewhat unpredictable as a topical prophylactic against recurrent infections by HSV-1 and HSV-2. Resistance of herpes simplex and cytomegaloviruses occurs and is a source of concern.

The most frequent adverse effect of systemic treatment is irritation at the site of injection (9%). The drug may crystallize in the urine, cause hematuria and impair renal function if fluid intake is inadequate, glomerular filtration rate is low, the dosage-interval is too short or the drug is given as a bolus. Metabolic encephalopathy (1%) with hallucinations, confusion, tremors and seizures, bone-marrow depression and alterations in hepatic function also may result from parenteral therapy. Untoward effects from oral administration are more frequent with long-term than with short-term therapy. In the short term, there may be nausea and vomiting (2.7%), headache (0.6%), diarrhea, dizziness, fatigue, skin rash, sore throat (all 0.3%), anorexia, edema, lymphadenopathy (especially inguinal) and leg pain. In the long term there may be headache (1.9%), diarrhea (2.4%), nausea and vomiting (2.7%), arthralgia, vertigo (both 3.6%), insomnia, fatigue, irritability, depression, rash, acne, alopecia, fever, palpitations, sore throat, muscle cramps and lymphadenopathy. The drug is mutagenic and should be avoided in pregnancy, if possible. Topically, adverse effects occur in about 30% of recipients and consist of local stinging, burning or pain (28%), itching (4%), vulvitis (0.3%) and rash (0.3%).

Infusions of 5 mg/kg at 8-hr intervals at steady-state achieve peak plasma concentrations of 5.5 to 13.8 μg/mL and trough concentrations of 0.7 to 1.0 μg/mL. In plasma, only 9 to 33% is protein-bound. Renal excretion after IV and oral use accounts for 62 to 91% and 9 to 20%, respectively. The half-life is about 2.5 hr but may be as long as 19.5 hr in renal failure.

Dose—*Oral, adult,* for *initial infection* or *intermittent treatment,* **200 mg** every 4 hr while awake (ie, 5 times a day) for 10 days in initial and 5 days in intermittent treatment; for *chronic suppression of recurrent infections,* **400 mg** twice a day for up to 12 mo or alternatively **200 mg** 3 times a day to **200 mg** 5 times a day. *Topical,* to the affected skin or mucous membranes (not conjunctival) every 3 hr, except during sleep, for 7 days.

Dosage Forms—Capsules: 200 mg; Ointment: 5% in a polyethylene glycol base; Tablets: 800 mg; Suspension: 200 mg/5 mL.

Acyclovir Sodium

Uses—See *Acyclovir* (above). The sodium salt is used for intravenous administration.

Dose (acyclovir equivalent)—*Intravenous infusion, adult,* and *children over 12 yr,* for *herpes genitalis, initial infection,* **5 mg/kg** every 8 hr for 5 days; for *disseminated herpes zoster* or *HSV-1* or *HSV-2 mucocutaneous infections* in immunocompromised patients, **5** to **10 mg/kg** every 8 hr for 7 to 10 days; *infants* and *children up to 12 yr,* for *initial infection,* **250 mg/m²** every 8 hr for 5 days; for *HSV-1* or *HSV-2 mucocutaneous infections* in immunocompromised patients, administered for 7 days. Each infusion should last at least 1 hr.

Dosage Form—Powder for injection: 500 mg/10 mL and 1 g/20 mL (reconstituted).

Amantidine Hydrochloride

Tricyclo[3.3.1.1^{3,7}]decan-1-amine, hydrochloride; Symmetrel (*Du Pont*); Symadine (*Reid-Powell*); (*Various Mfrs*)

1-Adamantanamine hydrochloride [665-66-7] $C_{10}H_{17}N.HCl$ (187.71)

Preparation—Adamantane is halogenated with chlorine or bromine in the presence of $AlCl_3$ at the bridgehead carbon atom to yield a very reactive tertiary halide, incapable of dehydrohalogenation. Therefore, even with a weak base, such as CH_3CN, it undergoes an S_N1 reaction to the acetamido derivative. Hydrolysis affords the product, which is converted to the salt. *J Med Chem 6:* 760 (1963).

Description—White crystals; decompose over 360°; pK_a 10.4, (amino group).

Solubility—1 g in 3 mL water or 5 mL alcohol.

Uses—A narrow-spectrum antiviral active against all influenzae A virus strains, some C virus strains, but not effective against B strains. It is approved for chemoprophylaxis and treatment of respiratory tract illness caused by influenzae A virus strains, when immunization is contraindicated or not feasible. It is indicated especially for high-risk patients because of underlying disease (eg, cardiovascular, pulmonary, metabolic, neuromuscular or immunodeficiency disease), close-household or hospital-ward contacts of index cases, immunocompromised patients and health-care and community-services personnel.

Amantidine is well tolerated by most patients but CNS side effects are most common and include difficulty in thinking, confusion, lightheadedness, hallucinations, anxiety and insomnia. These side effects are reversible upon discontinuation of the drug. More severe adverse effects such as mental depression and psychoses may occur with doses exceeding 200 mg daily. Less common side effects include anorexia, nausea, vomiting and orthostatic hypotension. The peripheral and central effects of anticholinergic drugs are increased by concomitant use of amantidine.

Oral absorption is rapid and complete. It is not metabolized and 90% of the dose is excreted unchanged in the urine. The half-life is about 20hr and it reaches levels in the cerebral spinal fluid that are 60% of the plasma concentration. The dose must be reduced with renal insufficiency and in the elderly who have decreased renal function.

Dose—*Oral, adult,* **200 mg** a day as a single dose or **100 mg** twice a day; *children, 9* to *12 yr,* **2** to **4 mg/lb** a day (4.4 to 8.8 mg/kg a day); *children 1* to *9 yr,* once a day or divided twice a day, not to exceed 150 mg a day.

Dosage Forms—Capsules: 100 mg; Syrup: 50 mg/5 mL.

Cytarabine—page 1247.

Didanosine

Inosine, 2′,3′-dideoxy-, ddI; Videx (*Bristol-Myers Squibb*)

[69655-05-6] $C_{10}H_{12}N_4O_3$ (236.23).

Preparation—*Nucleosides Nucleotides 7:* 147, 1988.

Description—White solid; melts 160 to 163°.

Uses—A nucleoside analog that is incorporated into retroviral DNA contributing to chain termination and inhibition of viral replication. The active metabolite, dideoxyadenosine triphosphate, is a reverse transcriptase inhibitor that is active against the human immunodeficiency virus (HIV) infected T cell and monocyte/macrophage cell cultures.

The approved indication is treatment of adult and pediatric patients with advanced HIV infection who have received prolonged prior zidovudine therapy or who have demonstrated intolerance or significant clinical or immunological deterioration during zidovudine therapy.

The major clinical toxicities of didanosine are pancreatitis (9%) and peripheral neuropathy (34%). Several other adverse effects are observed frequently including diarrhea (34%), asthenia (25%), insomnia (25%), nausea and vomiting (25%), rash/pruritus (24%), abdominal pain (21%), CNS depression (19%), constipation (16%), stomatitis (14%), myalgia (13%), arthritis (11%), taste loss/perversion (10%), pain (10%), dry mouth (9%), alopecia (8%) and dizziness (7%).

The clinical trial results are limited but the average bioavailability of didanosine is reported to be 33% ± 14% after a single dose. The elimination half-life is 1.6 hr and renal clearance is about 50%. There is no evidence of accumulation after either IV or oral dosing.

Dose—*Oral, adult, 75 kg,* **300** to **375 mg;** *50* to *74 kg,* **200** to **250 mg;** *35* to *49 kg, 125* to *167 mg,* every 12 hr; *Children,* **100mg/m²** a day in two equal doses every 12 hr.

Dosage Forms—Chewable/Dispersable Buffered Tablets: 25, 50, 100 and 150 mg; Buffered Powder for Oral Solution: 100, 167, 250 and 375 mg; Pediatric Powder for Oral Solution: 2 and 4 g.

Foscarnet Sodium

Phosphinecarboxylic acid, dihydroxy-, oxide, trisodium salt; Foscavir (*Astra*)

$(NaO)_2P(O)COONa$

Phosphonoformic acid, trisodium salt [63585-09-1] CNa_3O_5P (191.95).

Preparation—*Ber 57B:* 1023, 1924.

Description—White crystals (usually as the hexahydrate); melts above 250°; pK_a 7.27, 3.41, 0.49.

Solubility: Very soluble in water; insoluble in alcohol.

Uses—An antiviral agent that acts at the pyrophosphate-binding site and inhibits viral DNA polymerases and reverse transcriptases at concentrations that do not affect cellular DNA polymerases. It does not require activation (phosphorylation) by a kinase. All known herpes viruses are inhibited *in vitro* including cytomegalovirus (CMV), herpes simplex 1 and 2 (HSV-1, HSV-2), human herpes virus 6 (HHV-6), Epstein-Barr virus (EBV) and varicella zoster virus (VZV). The only approved indication is the treatment of CMV retinitis in patients with AIDS.

The major toxicity is renal impairment which occurs in 33% of all patients, so everyone receiving it should be monitored for renal function. The other frequent adverse reactions include fever (65%), nausea (47%), anemia (33%), diarrhea (30%), vomiting or headache (26%) and seizures (10%). Electrolyte abnormalities must be monitored because of the propensity of foscarnet to chelate divalent cations.

The drug is only administered by controlled IV infusion to decrease the incidence of toxicity as a result of excessive plasma levels. Approximately 80 to 90% of IV foscarnet is excreted unchanged in the urine. Plasma half-life of foscarnet increases as renal function is impaired, but initial half-lives of 2 to 8 hr have been reported for patients with 24-hr creatinine clearance of 44 to 90 mL/min. Measurements of urinary excretion are required to detect the longer terminal half-life which is assumed to represent release of foscarnet from bone. The safety and efficacy of foscarnet in children has not been studied because it is deposited in teeth and bone, and deposition is greater in young and growing animals. Development of tooth enamel is adversely affected in animals studies.

Dose—*Adult, intravenous infusion, for induction:* **60 mg/kg** at a constant rate over a minimum of 1 hr every 5 hr for 2 to 3 wk depending on clinical response; *for maintenance,* **90 to 120 mg/kg** a day (individualized for renal function) given as IV infusion over 2 hr.

Dosage Form—Injection: 24 mg.

Ganciclovir Sodium

6*H*-Purin-6-one, 2-amino-1,9-dihydro-9-[[2-hydroxyl-1-(hydroxymethyl)ethoxy]-methyl]-, Cytovene *(Syntex)*

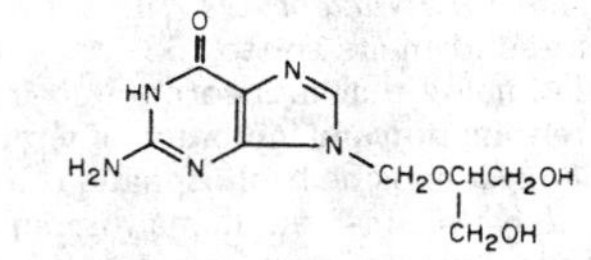

9-[[2-Hydroxyl-1-(hydroxymethyl)ethoxy]methyl]guanine [*82410-32-0*] $C_9H_{13}N_5O_4$ (255.23).

Preparation—US Pat 4,355,032; *J Med Chem 26:* 759, 1983.

Description—White powder.

Solubility—1 g in 250 mL water.

Uses—An antiviral drug active against cytomegalovirus (CMV), herpes simples virus-1 and -2 (HSV-1, HSV-2), Epstein-Barr virus and viricella zoster virus. It is approved for treatment of CMV retinitis in immunocompromised patients, including those with AIDS and prevention of CMV disease in transplant patients at risk for CMV disease. Upon entry into host cells, CMV induce kinases that phosphorylate ganciclovir to its active triphosphate form which is believed to inhibit viral DNA synthesis by competitive inhibitiion of viral DNA, resulting in termination of viral DNA elongation.

The major clinical toxicities of ganciclovir include granulocytopenia (40%) and thrombocytopenia (20%). In animal studies it is carcinogenic, teratogenic and causes aspermatogenesis. Other adverse effects that have led to its withdrawal or interrupted its use in clinical trials are headache (17%), confusion (6%), abnormal thoughts or dreams, ataxia, dizziness, nervousness, parasthesia, psychosis, somnolence, tremor, arrhythmia, hypertension, rash, pruritus, alopecia, urticaria, nausea, vomiting, anorexia, diarrhea, abdominal pain, sepsis, fever, chills, edema, malaise and dyspnea. Retinal detachment has occurred before and after initial treatment of CMV retinitis, so ophthalmological evaluations are advised. Renal toxicity may occur in heart allograft recipients, so renal function should be monitored during therapy.

Ganciclivor is given by IV infusion. Phlebitis and pain at site of injection occur. The high pH (11) of solution may result in severe tissue irritation if given SC or IM. It is eliminated unmetabolized by renal excretion which accounts for 90% of the administered dose. The plasma half-life with normal renal function is about 3 hr but is increased to more than 10 hr with severe renal impairment. There is limited evidence to suggest that ganciclovir crosses the blood brain barrier in adequate concentrations.

Dose—*Adult, CMV retinitis treatment,* induction treatment is **5 mg/kg** (given IV at a constant rate of 1 hr) every 12 hr for 14 to 21 days, followed by **5 mg/kg** over 1 hr once a day 7 days a wk or **6 mg/kg** once a day 5 days a wk.

Dosage Form—Powder for Injection: 500 mg.

Idoxuridine

Uridine, 2′-deoxy-5-iodo-, IDU; Herplex (*Allergan*); Stoxil (*SmithKline Beecham*)

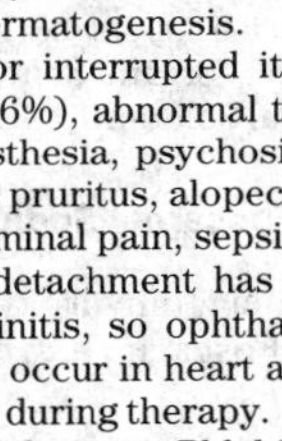

2′-Deoxy-5-iodouridine [54-42-2] $C_9H_{11}IN_2O_5$ (354.10).

Preparation—By refluxing a solution of deoxuridine in aqueous mineral acid in the presence of iodine. Brit Pat 1,024,156. For the preparation of deoxuridine, see *J Chem Soc 1958:* 3035.

Description—White, crystalline powder; practically odorless; turns black 171°; pH (0.1% aqueous solution) about 6; a 0.1% solution in distilled water and preserved with 1:50,000 thimerosal is stable at room temperature for over a year; pK_a 8.25.

Solubility—Slightly soluble in water or alcohol; practically insoluble in chloroform or ether; 1g in 2.5 mL DMSO.

Uses—An antimetabolite of thymidine. It also is incorporated into desoxyribonucleic acid in lieu of thymidine, thus interfering with normal nuclear functions. It is incorporated faster into the DNA of cancer cells than normal cells. It was first studied as an antineoplastic drug. However, its *antiviral* activity has received the greater clinical scrutiny. At present its use is limited to the topical therapy of *herpes simplex, vaccinia keratitis* or *keratoconjunctivitis of the eye;* the dendritic type responds readily, but the stromal type does not respond unless adrenal steroids are given concurrently. Anterior uveitis and adenovirus conjunctivitis have been reported to respond to the drug. Herpetic lesions of the genitalia and skin do not respond. The drug has been given intravenously in successful treatment of herpetic encephalitis.

Local treatment to the eye occasionally may cause reversible epithelial edema and corneal stippling, inflammation, stinging, itching or photophobia. Allergic reactions are rare. It may interfere with the healing of deep lesions of the cornea. When applied to the cornea, it does not produce systemic toxicity. When given systemically, it may cause depression of bone marrow and alopecia, especially if a total of more than 20 g is given.

The ointment does not require as frequent administration as the solution and, hence, is especially advantageous for use at night. The principal metabolite is 5-iodouracil and thymidine; the half-life of the parent drug is less than 5 min.

Dose—*Topical,* to the conjunctiva, as a **0.5%** ointment 5 instillations daily during the day and just before bedtime, or **one** drop of a **0.1%** solution every hr during the day and every 2 hr at night. This schedule is continued until the lesions no longer stain with fluorescein; thereafter, the intervals between applications may be doubled. In herpes simplex keratitis (only), the solution may be applied at 4-hr intervals if at each application 1 drop is instilled every minute for 5 min; continue for 3 to 5 days after healing appears complete.

Dosage Form—Ophthalmic Ointment: 0.5%; Ophthalmic Solution: 0.1%.

Interferons—pages 1252, 1253 and 1262.
Methisazone—see RPS-18, page 1240.

Ribavirin

1*H*-1,2,4-Triazole-3-carboxamide, 1-β-D-ribofuranosyl-, Virazole (*ICN*)

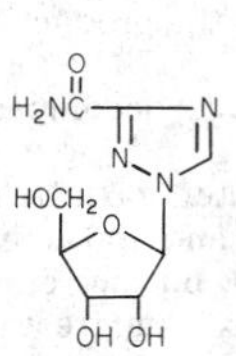

Tribavirin; [36791-04-5] $C_8H_{12}N_4O_5$ (244.21).

Preparation—*J Med Chem 15:* 1150, 1972.

Description—Colorless, crystalline powder existing in two polymorphic forms: melts about 167° (from aqueous ethanol) and melts about 175° (from ethanol)

Solubility—142 mg/mL in water at 25°; slightly soluble in alcohol.

Uses—A nucleoside analog with significant activity against influenza B, respiratory syncytial virus (RSV) and herpes simplex virus. It also has lesser activity against a wide variety of other viruses, such as those of herpes, varicella, Lassa fever, infectious hepatitis, dengue fever, measles and AIDS. It is converted to metabolites that inhibit the 5′ capping of viral mRNA, so that ultimately viral protein synthesis of both DNA and RNA viruses are affected. It is approved for use only in the treatment of *severe upper respiratory infections caused by RSV* in infants and children. If the duration of the infection is judged to be less than that of a full course of treatment, the drug is contraindicated. It has been used successfully as an aerosol in the treatment of influenza A and B. Varying success has been achieved against infectious hepatitis, measles, Lassa fever and Asian hemorrhagic fever.

Intravenous or oral doses of more than 1 g a day suppress erythropoiesis, characterized mostly by normocytic anemia and reticulocytosis. The effect is reversible. There is also occasional hypotension, cardiac arrest or digitalis intoxication. Adverse effects of the inhalation aerosol include occasional rash and conjunctivitis. In chronic obstructive pulmonary disease, pulmonary function often deteriorates. It antagonizes the effect of zidovudine on human immunodeficiency virus replication. It is contraindicated in pregnancy and during breast-feeding.

Systemic absorption occurs after aerosol administration but bioavailability is unknown. It is highly accumulated in erythrocytes but is not bound to plasma proteins. In the cells, the drug is degraded by deribosylation and amide hydrolysis and the product is mono-, di- and triphosphorylated. The triphosphate is thought to be the active metabolite. It is formed more in lung and liver than in other tissues, hence the drug is most effective against infections in these organs. It does not pass the blood-brain barrier. Drug and known metabolites are excreted in the urine (50%) and feces (15%). The plasma half-life is 9.5 hr while the half-life in erythrocytes is about 40 days.

Dose—*Inhalation, infants and children,* **190 μg/L** of air for 12 to 18 hr a day for 3 to 7 days. See the package literature, *PDR, Facts and Comparisons* or the *USP DI* for details of preparation and administration.

Dosage Form—Powder for Aerosol: 6 g/100 mL (reconstituted).

Rifampin—page 1316.

Suramin Sodium—page 1326.

Trifluridine

Thymidine, α,α,α-trifluoro-, Viroptic (*Burroughs Wellcome*)

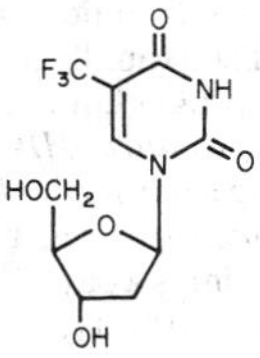

2′-Deoxy-5-(trifluoromethyl)uridine [70-00-8] $C_{10}H_{11}F_3N_2O_5$ (296.20).

Preparation—*J Amer Chem Soc 84:* 3597, 1962.

Description—White crystals; melts about 188°.

Uses—An analog of thymidine which not only inhibits thymidylic phosphorylase and specific DNA polymerases which are involved in the incorporation of thymidine into DNA but also is incorporated itself into viral DNA. It inhibits viral and cellular DNA synthesis but its antiviral actions are not completely known. It is active against *Herpes simplex* viruses (HSV) 1 and 2 and some vaccinia virus. It also has antineoplastic activity. In the US, it is approved for use only in the topical treatment of *herpetic epithelial keratitis* or *keratoconjunctivitis.*

Nearly 5% of recipients experience transient mild stinging or burning of the conjunctiva and sclera and 3% palpebral edema after instillation into the conjunctival sac. Less frequently, there may be irritation, hyperemia, stromal edema, keratitis sicca, epithelial keratopathy, punctate keratopathy and hypersensitivity. There is a rare cross-sensitivity to idoxuridine. It is mutagenic, but its oncogenic potential is unknown. Overdosage by ocular instillation is unlikely because any excess solution is expelled quickly from the conjunctival sac. Reversible bone marrow suppression may occur with IV doses of 15 to 30 mg/kg a day.

Dose—*Topical,* to the *conjunctiva, adults* and *children,* **1 drop** of a **1%** solution every 2 hr during waketime; after re-epithelialization, the dose interval may be lengthened to 4 hr, application continuing for 7 days longer.

Dosage Form—Ophthalmic Solution: 1%.

Vidarabine

9*H*-Purin-6-amine, 9-β-D-arabinofuranosyl-, monohydrate; Adenine Arabinoside; Vira-A (*Parke-Davis*)

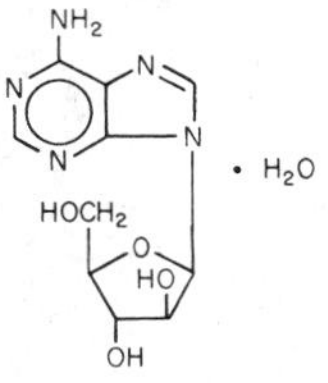

[24356-66-9] $C_{10}H_{13}N_5O_4.H_2O$ (285.26); *anhydrous* [5536-17-4] (267.24). Potency: not less than 845 μg and not more than 985 μg of $C_{10}H_{13}N_5O_4$/mg.

Preparation—Production of vidarabine by culturing a strain of *Streptomyces antibioticus* is described in British Pat 1,159,290 (*CA 71:* 79757z, 1969). Several methods of synthesis have been published. In one of these 2,3,5-tri-*O*-benzyl-β-D-arabinofuranose, readily preparable from D-arabinose, is converted to 2,3,5-tri-*O*-benzyl-D-arabinofuranosyl chloride, which is condensed with *N*-benzoyladenine; subsequent removal of the protecting groups yields vidarabine. *J Org Chem 28:* 3004, 1963.

Description—White to off-white powder; melts about 257°.

Solubility—Very slightly soluble in water; more soluble in alkaline solutions.

Uses—Active against *Herpes simplex* viruses, Types 1 and 2, varicella-zoster, vaccinia virus and cytomegalovirus. In cells, it and its hypoxanthine metabolite are phosphorylated; the several phosphorylated metabolites inhibit the viral DNA polymerase and viral-induced ribonucleotide reductase. It is indicated for topical treatment of superficial *herpetic keratitis* and *keratoconjunctivitis,* especially if idoxuridine has proved to be ineffective or cannot be tolerated. Its efficacy is approximately equal to that of idoxuridine. It is not effective against nonherpetic infections. It also is indicated for the systemic treatment of *herpes simplex virus encephalitis,* and it has been shown to decrease mortality in this disease. It is the least toxic antiviral drug for the purpose. If the drug is started within the first 3 days of herpes zoster, it is effective in reducing complications. No data are available to support efficacy against CMV or vaccinia virus.

Topically, to the eye, adverse effects include a blurring of vision (from chemosis, typical of ophthalmic ointments), and burning, irritation, pain, photophobia, punctal occlusion and sensitization. These effects are less severe than with idoxuridine. By the intravenous route, nausea and other gastrointestinal disturbances are common. Weakness, tremor, dizziness, ataxia and confusion have been reported but may have been disease-related; however, probably drug-related neurological deterioration, coma and death have occurred in renal transplant patients. Decreases in hemoglobin and white-cell and platelet counts have been observed, but severe bone-marrow depression or renal and hepatic toxicities have not occurred. The blood-cell counts should be monitored during treatment. It is oncogenic and mutagenic in mice and rats.

In the body, it is deaminated to the hypoxanthine analog (Ara-HX). The half-life of vidarabine is about 1 hr and that of Ara-HX, 3.3 hr. Ara-HX penetrates into cerebrospinal fluid and is the primary active agent in viral encephalitis. The CSF/plasma ratio is about 1:3. Ara-HX is eliminated primarily by renal excretion, and dose adjustments are required in renal failure. Topically, only small amounts are absorbed from the conjunctiva and too little through the normal cornea to be useful in treating herpetic uveitis, but penetrance through the infected cornea appears to be greater.

Dose (as monohydrate)—*Topical,* to the *conjunctiva* as a thin strip (about 1.25 cm) of **3%** ointment 5 times a day at 3-hour intervals until re-epithelialization, then with decreased frequency, such as twice a day for at least 7 more days. *Intravenous,* by infusion, **15 mg/kg** a day for 10 days; infusion should be made over a 12- to 24-hr period.

Dosage Forms (as monohydrate)—Injection: 1 g/5 mL; Ophthalmic Ointment: 3%.

Zalcitabine

Cytidine, 2′,3′-dideoxy-, ddC; Hivid (*Roche*)

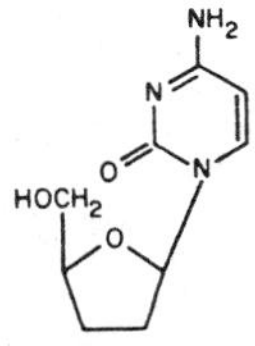

[7481-89-2] $C_9H_{13}N_3O_3$ (211.22).

Preparation—*Chem Pharm Bull 22:* 128, 1974.

Description—White crystals; melts about 216°.

Uses—Antiviral activity against human immunodeficiency virus (HIV) is mediated by its conversion within infected cells to the active nucleoside triphosphate metabolite which inhibits HIV reverse transcriptase and viral DNA synthesis. It is approved for combination therapy with zidovudine in advanced HIV infection (CD4 cell count $\leq 300/mm^3$) who have demonstrated significant clinical or immunological deterioration. This indication is based on two small studies done without a concurrent control group taking the currently recommended dose of zidovudine (100 mg every 4 hr).

The major clinical toxicities of zalcitabine are peripheral neuropathy (17 to 31%) and pancreatitis (< 1%). It may exacerbate hepatic dysfunction and a greater risk of toxicity may occur in patients with renal impairment. Infrequent cases of esophageal ulcers have been attributed to zalcitabine therapy. Other adverse effects include oral ulcers, nausea, dysphagia, anorexia, abdominal pain, vomiting, diarrhea, rash, pruritis, headache, dizziness, myalgia, arthralgia, fatigue, pharyngitis, fever, rigors, chest pain and weight decrease. The mean oral bioavailability is > 80%, but food decreases the extent and rate of absorption. Renal excretion is the major route of excretion with little if any degree of hepatic matabolism. The half-life is 1 to 3 hr but impaired renal function prolongs elimination.

Dose—*Oral, adult,* **0.75 mg** concomitantly with **200 mg** zidovudine every 8 hr.

Dosage Forms—Tablets: 0.375 and 0.75 mg.

Zidovudine

Thymidine, 3′-azido-3′-deoxy-, AZT; Retrovir
(Burroughs Wellcome)

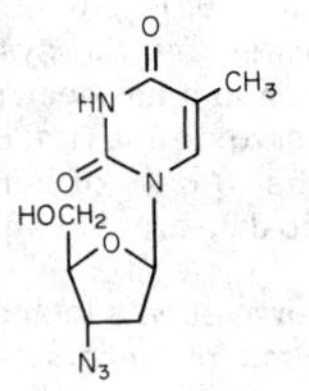

Azidothymidine; [30516-87-1] $C_{10}H_{13}N_5O_4$ (267.24).

Preparatioon—*Tetrahedron Letters 29:* 5349, 1988.

Description—White needles; from petroleum ether melts about 110°; from water, melts about 121°; pK_a 9.68.

Solubility—1 g in 40 mL water or 15 mL alcohol.

Uses—Incorporated into retroviral DNA by reverse-transcriptase to make a nonsense sequence that terminates DNA chain synthesis. The reverse-transcriptase is 100 times more susceptible to the drug than mammalian DNA polymerase. It has activity against human immunodeficiency virus; consequently, it is used for the treatment of AIDS and AIDS-related complex (ARC). It increases the survival and improves the quality of life of patients with complications, such as severe weight loss, fever, pneumocystosis, herpes zoster, herpes or thrush. Because it crosses the blood-brain barrier, it has a favorable effect on the neurological symptoms of AIDS. During prolonged therapy resistance may occur. Cost and toxicity have precluded testing to determine whether earlier treatment prolongs life. In the US, it has been approved for use only if there is evidence of impaired immunity such as pneumocystosis or a CD4 (T4 helper/inducer) lymphocyte count of less than 500/mm^5.

It causes severe anemia from bone-marrow depression in patients with AIDS; 25% of infected persons without AIDS develop anemia. It causes granulocytopenia and/or thrombocytopenia in about 5% of AIDS patients. However, it may increase platelet count if the count is depressed as the result of the disease. Nausea (46%), headaches (42%), gastrointestinal pain (20%), rash (17%), fever (16%), diarrhea (12%), anorexia (11%), myalgia (8%), somnolence (8%), malaise (8%), vomiting, dizziness, paresthesias (each 6%), insomnia, dyspnea, sweating (all 5%) and macrocytosis occur. Polymyositis sometimes occurs. It is weakly mutagenic and should be withheld in pregnancy, if possible. *In vitro* antagonism of AZT inhibition of HIV-1 by ribovarin has been demonstrated, so those agents should not be used simultaneously. Drugs that inhibit hepatic glucuronidation, such as acetaminophen, aspirin, indomethacin, probenecid, pyrimethamine and trimethoprim decrease elimination and increase toxicity.

Oral bioavailability is 52 to 75%. Plasma protein-binding is 34 to 38%. Doses of 3 to 5.4 mg/kg every 4 hr yield mean plasma concentrations of about 0.16 μg/mL. Cerebrospinal fluid levels are nearly the same as in plasma. The drug is metabolized rapidly in the liver with a half-life of 0.8 to 1.9 hr. Only 14% of intact drug is eliminated in urine.

Dose—*Oral, adult, asymptomatic HIV infection, initially* **100mg** every 4 hr while awake (500 mg a day), after 1 mo, dose may be reduced to 100 mg every 4 hr; *intravenous infusion,* **1** to **2 mg/kg** infused over 1 hr every 4 hr around the clock (6 times a day).

Dosage Forms—Capsules: 100 mg; Syrup 50 mg/5 mL; Injection: 200 mg/20mL.

CHAPTER 77

Parasiticides

H Steve White, PhD
Research Associate Professor of Pharmacology & Toxicology
College of Pharmacy
University of Utah
Salt Lake City, UT 84112

Parasitic infections are now a worldwide problem. Increased travel, use of immunosuppressants and the spread of AIDS has led to a greater prevalence of parasitic infections (*Med Lett Drugs Ther 34:* 17, 1992). Consequently, the subject is an important part of pharmacology. In its broadest aspects, it includes the problem of eradication of all organisms that live within or upon man. However, the discussion in this chapter will be limited to the anthelmintics and those agents which are applied directly to the skin of the human host in the treatment of pediculosis and scabies. The antimalarials, *amebicides* and fungicides are discussed in Chapter 76.

Anthelmintics

The term anthelmintic frequently is restricted to drugs acting locally to expel parasites from the gastrointestinal tract. However, there are several types of worms which penetrate other tissues; drugs which act on these parasitic infections are also known as anthelmintics. Furthermore, drugs that kill worms are referred to commonly as vermicides; those that affect the worm in such a manner that peristaltic activity or catharsis expels it from the intestinal tract are referred to as vermifuges. This arbitrary division serves no useful purpose since many anthelmintics manifest both actions, according to the dose employed. Therefore, the anthelmintics are defined more properly as drugs used to combat any type of helminthiasis.

The worm parasites of man belong to two phyla: *Nemathelminthes* (roundworms) and *Platyhelminthes* (flat worms).

The roundworms include the hookworm, roundworm, whipworm, pinworm, *Strongyloides stercoralis, Trichinella spiralis* and *Wuchereria bancrofti.*

There are two common varieties of hookworm: *Necator americanus,* the American variety, and *Ancylostoma duodenale,* the European variety. They are cylindrical worms, 1 to 2 cm long, with two pairs of hooks near the mouth. They attach themselves to the mucosa of the duodenum and derive their nourishment by sucking blood from the surrounding blood vessels.

The common roundworm, *Ascaris lumbricoides,* is the most prevalent of human helminths. It may be 7 to 23 cm in length, 3 to 6 mm in diameter, grayish to reddish in color and inhabits the upper part of the small intestine; therefore, it is vomited up occasionally.

The whipworm, *Trichuris trichiura,* is about 5 cm long and resembles a whip; it inhabits the cecum principally, but is found also in the lower part of the ileum and the appendix.

The pinworm or threadworm, *Enterobius vermicularis,* is 1.5 to 3 mm long and inhabits the small intestine, cecum and colon.

Strongyloides stercoralis is only about 2 mm long. It inhabits the duodenum chiefly, but may be found in the stomach, biliary passages, pancreatic ducts and various parts of the intestinal tract.

Infection with *Trichinella spiralis* causes trichinosis, a condition which results from eating incompletely cooked pork infested with the larvae of the worm. When such meat is eaten, the cysts dissolve, the parasites mature and a new crop of larvae develop which penetrate the intestinal mucosa and eventually lodge in the muscles. The most important filarial worm is *Wuchereria bancrofti,* which is transmitted by the bite of the mosquito. Symptoms result from the blocking of the lymphatic ducts with the adult worms.

The flatworms are of two types: segmented (cestodes) and nonsegmented (trematodes). The cestodes include the tapeworms and the trematodes include the flukes.

Four common varieties of parasitic tapeworms are found in man; *Taenia saginata* (beef tapeworm), *Taenia solium (pork tapeworm), Diphyllobothrium latum* (fish tapeworm) and *Hymenolepis nana (*dwarf tapeworm). Except for the dwarf tapeworm, they are from 2 to 10 m in length and may contain 3000 to 4000 segments, each segment being capable of producing hundreds of eggs. The dwarf tapeworm is only 6 to 12 mm in length, but consists of 150 to 200 segments. The larval stage of all tapeworms is spent in the muscles of the intermediate host, and human infection occurs through eating imperfectly cooked meat and fish.

Three varieties of blood fluke inhabit the blood stream of man causing schistosomiasis: *S haematobium, S mansoni, S mekongi* and *S japonicum.* These parasites cause epigastric distress, abdominal pain, anorexia, diarrhea with blood and mucus in the stools, enlarged and tender liver, pyrexia and ascites. The intermediate host is either a fresh water snail or a fresh water mollusk. Transmission is by way of contaminated water.

Parasitic worms are harmful to the human host for a number of reasons. They deprive the host of food, injure organs or obstruct ducts, may elaborate substances toxic to the host and may provide a portal of entry for other organisms. It is desirable, therefore, to eradicate the parasites as soon as they have been discovered. Nevertheless, the need for treatment must be weighed carefully against the toxicity of the drug; the mere presence of a parasite does not necessarily demand that it must be treated.

Proper choice of the anthelmintic is important, as most drugs are more effective against some species than others, and virtually all antiparasitic drugs induce some adverse effects. The drug selected should offer the best combination of effectiveness and relative safety. There is an excellent review (*Med Lett Drugs Ther 34:* 17, 1992) of the choice of drugs for parasitic infections.

Many of the newer drugs require little or no change in the patient's normal routine. When the patient has a tapeworm infestation, a thorough examination of the stools produced by the second purgation is necessary. Unless the head of the worm has been expelled and identified, the worm will regenerate. Usually three specimens of stools are examined one week after administration of the anthelmintic. If ova or parasites are still present, the treatment should be repeated. All drugs which are poisonous to the worms are also poisonous to the patient. Therefore, the recommended methods of treatment for each drug should be followed carefully and the patient watched closely for the appearance of any untoward drug effects.

Antimony Potassium Tartrate

Antimonate (2-), bis[μ[2,3-dihydroxybutanedioato(4-)-O^1,O^2,O^3,O^4]]-di-, dipotassium, trihydrate, stereoisomer

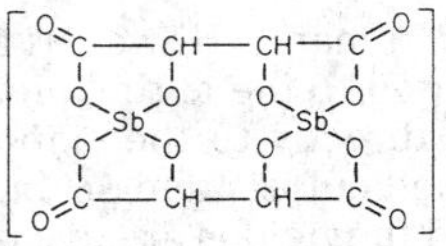

$2K^+ \cdot 3H_2O$

Tartar Emetic [28300-74-5] $C_8H_4K_2Sb_2O_{12} \cdot 3H_2O$ (667.85); anhydrous [11071-15-1] (613.81).

Preparation—By dissolving a mixture of 10 parts of potassium bitartrate with 8 parts of antimony trioxide [Sb_2O_3] in 75 parts of boiling water, filtering the solution while hot and allowing it to crystallize.

Description and Solubility—Colorless, odorless, transparent crystals or a white powder; the crystals effloresce upon exposure to air; solutions are acid to litmus.

Solubility—1 g dissolves in 12 mL water, about 15 mL glycerin or about 3 mL boiling water; insoluble in alcohol.

Incompatibilities—*Mineral acids,* when added to aqueous solutions of antimony potassium tartrate, precipitate basic salts of antimony, with possibly some potassium bitartrate. *Alkali hydroxides* and *carbonates* of sufficient concentration precipitate antimony trioxide. Precipitation is retarded by citrates, tartrates, glycerin or sugar. Many metallic salts form insoluble tartrates. Addition of *alcohol* to an aqueous solution may cause precipitation. An insoluble tannate is formed with *tannic acid.*

Uses—Formerly used for infections caused by *Schistosoma japonicum.* It is also an *emetic,* chiefly by virtue of its irritant action on the gastrointestinal mucosa. Subemetic doses produce an *expectorant* action due to reflex stimulation of the salivary and bronchial glands. Toxic effects induced by antimony potassium tartrate frequently include painful local inflammation, coughing and vomiting when intravenous injection is rapid, muscle and joint stiffness and bradycardia. Occasional adverse effects include colic, diarrhea, rash, pruritus and myocardial damage. Rarely, liver damage, hemolytic anemia, renal damage, shock and sudden death are encountered.

Dose—Usual, intravenous, as a **0.5** to **1% solution,** *initial,* **40 mg,** repeated every 2 days, each dose increased by 20 mg until 140 mg is reached, then **140 mg** every other day for a total course-of-treatment dose of **2 g.**

Bithionol

2,2′-Thiobis(4,6-dichlorophenol); Actamer (*Monsanto*)

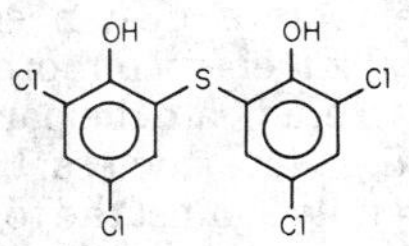

[97-18-7] $C_{12}H_6Cl_4O_2S$ (356.05).

Preparation—By reaction of 2,4-dichlorophenol and sulfur chloride.

Description—White or off-white, crystalline powder; melts at 188°.

Solubility—Practically insoluble in water; freely soluble in alcohol or ether; soluble in solutions of alkali hydroxides.

Uses—The drug of choice for infections caused by *Fasciola hepatica* (sheep liver fluke) and, alternative drug for those caused by *Paragonimus westermani* (lung fluke). Untoward reactions are frequent and include photosensitivity skin reactions, vomiting, diarrhea, abdominal pain and urticaria.

Dose—*Usual, adult, oral,* **30** to **50 mg/kg** on alternate days for 10 to 15 doses. *Pediatric,* as for adults.

Dosage Form—Available from the Parasitic Disease Drug Service, Centers for Disease Control, Atlanta, GA 30333.

Diethylcarbamazine Citrate

1-Piperazinecarboxamide, *N,N*-diethyl-4-methyl-, 2-hydroxy-1,2,3-propanetricarboxylate; Hetrazan (*Lederle*)

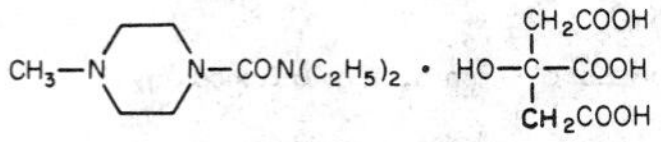

$CH_3-N\langle\rangle N-CON(C_2H_5)_2 \cdot HO-C(CH_2COOH)_2-COOH$

N,N-Diethyl-4-methyl-1-piperazinecarboxamide citrate (1:1) [1642-54-2] $C_{10}H_{21}N_3O.C_6H_8O_7$ (391.42).

Preparation—By acylating piperazine with diethylcarbamoyl chloride, and then methylating at the N^4-position by treatment with formaldehyde and formic acid. Treatment of the purified base with an equimolar portion of citric acid yields the official citrate.

Description—White, crystalline powder; odorless, or has a slight odor; slightly hygroscopic; melts between 134° and 139°.

Solubility—Very soluble in water; sparingly soluble in alcohol; practically insoluble in acetone, chloroform or ether.

Uses—The drug of choice for treating filariasis infections (*Wuchereria bancrofti, Brugia malayi, Mansonella ozzardi, Loa loa* and *tropical eosinophilia).* In adequate dosage it clears the blood rapidly of the microfilariae and appears to be curative. The drug should be administered with special caution in *Loa loa,* because it can provoke an encephalopathy. Antihistamines or corticosteroids may be required to control the allergic reactions due to the disintegration of microfilariae. Untoward reactions are frequent but not serious; they include severe allergic or febrile reactions, due to the filarial infection, and gastrointestinal disturbances. Rarely, encephalopathy and loss of vision are encountered.

Dose—*Usual,* **2 mg/kg** 3 times a day for 10 to 30 days. In *Wuchereria bancrofti* and *Acanthocheilonema perstans (Loa loa)* **50 mg,** day 1; **50 mg,** 3 times, day 2; **50 mg,** 3 times, day 3; **6 to 9 mg/kg** a day in divided doses, day 4 through day 21; **2 mg/kg** 3 times a day. In *Tropical eosinophilia,* **6 mg/kg** in 3 divided doses for 21 days.

Dosage Forms—Syrup: 120 mg/5 mL; Tablets: 50 mg. (*Note*: Available only from the manufacturer.)

Emetine Hydrochloride—page 1324.
Gentian Violet—see RPS-18, page 1171.

Ivermectin

Mectizan (*MSD*)

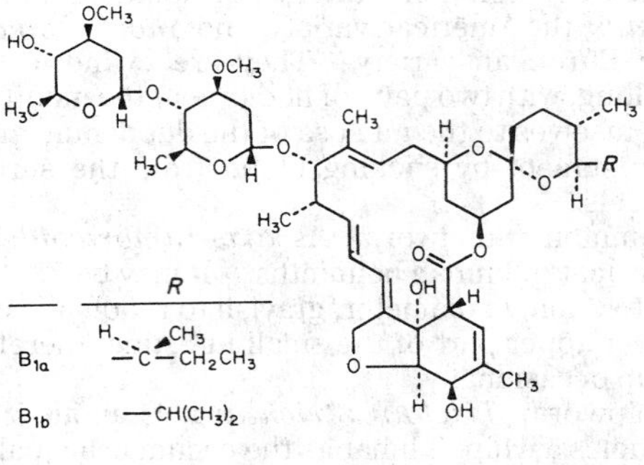

R	
B_{1a}	$-CH(CH_3)CH_2CH_3$
B_{1b}	$-CH(CH_3)_2$

[70288-86-7], [70161-11-4], [70209-81-3]

Preparation—A mixture of components B_{1a} and B_{1b} of ivermectin (in approximately 4:1 ratio. See *J Med Chem 23:* 2377, 1982.

Description—Off-white powder.

Solubility—Practically insoluble in water or alcohol; soluble in methyl ethyl ketone, propylene glycol or polyethylene glycol.

Uses—The anthelmintic of choice for *Onchorcerca volvulus.* It also may be effective against *Mansonella ozzardi.* Invermectin can, on occasion, in onchorarias is result in a Mazzotti-type reaction which may include fever, pruritus, tender lymphnodes, headache and joint/bone pain. It rarely will cause hypotension.

Dose—*Usual, oral, adult* and *children,* 150 μg/kg as a single dose; repeat every 6 to 12 months.

Dosage Form—Available from the Drug Service, Centers for Disease Control, Atlanta, GA 30333.

Mebendazole

Carbamic acid, (5-benzoyl-1*H*-benzimidazol-2-yl)-, methyl ester; Vermox (*Janssen*)

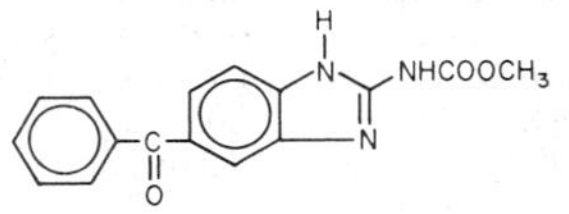

Methyl 5-benzoyl-2-benzimidazolecarbamate [31431-39-7] $C_{16}H_{13}N_3O_3$ (295.30).

Preparation—Synthesis of mebendazole and related anthelmintic benzimidazolecarbamates is described in German Pat 2,029,637 (corresponding to US Pat 3,657,267). See *CA 74:*100047s, 1971.

Description—White to slightly yellow powder; melts at about 290°.

Solubility—Practically insoluble in water, alcohol, ether or chloroform.

Uses—The anthelmintic of choice in hookworm (*Ancylostoma duodenale, Necator americanus*), pinworm (*Enterobius vermicularis*), roundworm (*Ascaris lumbricoides*) and whipworm (*Trichuris trichiura*) in guinea worm (*Dracunculus medinensis*), filariasis (*Mansonella perstans*), and an alternative drug for *Visceral Larva Migrans.* Mebendazole also is used as an adjunct to steroids for the treatment of Trichinosis (*Trichinella spiralis*). It blocks the glucose uptake by susceptible helminths, thereby depleting glycogen stored within the parasite. The glycogen depletion results in a decreased formation of adenosine triphosphate (ATP); the latter is required for survival and reproduction of the helminth. Side effects are usually mild and transient; abdominal pain and diarrhea have occurred in cases of massive infection and expulsion of worms. Leukopenia is rare but has been reported. The drug is contraindicated in pregnancy and in persons who have shown hypersensitivity to it.

Dose—*Usual, adults* and *children, oral,* for control of *pinworm infestation,* **100 mg** administered once; for other infestations, **100 mg,** morning and evening, for 3 consecutive days. If necessary, a second course of treatment may be given in 3 weeks. Tablets may be chewed, swallowed or crushed and mixed with food. The drug has not been studied adequately in children under 2 yr and bene-fit/risk should be considered before use in children of this age.

Dosage Form—Chewable: Tablets, 100 mg.

Metronidazole—page 1325.

Metrifonate—see RPS-18, page 1243.

Niclosamide

Benzamide, 5-chloro-*N*-(2-chloro-4-nitrophenyl)-2-hydroxy-, Niclocide (*Miles*)

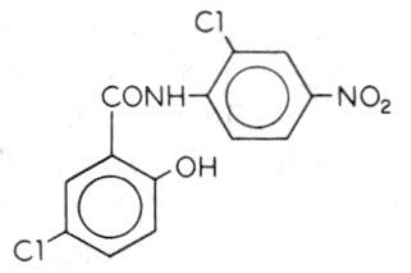

2′,5-Dichloro-4′-nitrosalicylanilide [50-65-7] $C_{13}H_8Cl_2N_2O_4$ (327.12).

Preparation—PCl_3 is slowly introduced into a boiling xylene solution containing 5-chlorosalicylic acid and 2-chloro-4-nitroaniline in equimolar ratio and the heating continued for 3 hr. Crystals of niclosamide separate on cooling and are recrystallized from ethanol. US Pat. 3,079,297.

Description—Pale yellow crystals; melting range, 225° to 230°.

Solubility—Practically insoluble in water; sparingly soluble in alcohol, chloroform or ether.

Uses—One of the anthelmintics of first choice in the treatment of beef tapeworm (*Taenia saginata*), fish tapeworm (*Diphyllobothrium latum*) and pork tapeworm (*Taenia solium*); an alternate drug of choice for dwarf tapeworm (*Hymenolepis nana*) infections. It inhibits phosphorylation in the mitochondria of cestodes. Both *in vitro* and *in vivo*, the scolex and proximal segments are killed on contact with the drug. The loosened scolex may be digested in the intestine; hence, it may be impossible to identify the scolex in the feces. Untoward effects occur only occasionally; nausea and abdominal pain have been reported most frequently.

Dose—*Usual, oral; adult,* a single dose of 4 tablets (**2 g**) chewed thoroughly. *Pediatric,* 11 to 34 kg, a single dose of 2 tablets (**1 g**); >34 kg, a single dose of 3 tablets (**1.5 g**). For dwarf tapeworm infection, the drug should be taken for 6 to 7 days. The patient should omit breakfast but may eat 2 hr after the last dose. The tablets should be chewed thoroughly and then washed down with water.

Dosage Form—Tablets: 500 mg.

Niridazole—see RPS-18, page 1244.

Oxamniquine

6-Quinolinemethanol, 1,2,3,4-tetrahydro-2-[[(1-methylethyl)amino]methyl]-7-nitro-, Vansil (*Pfizer*).

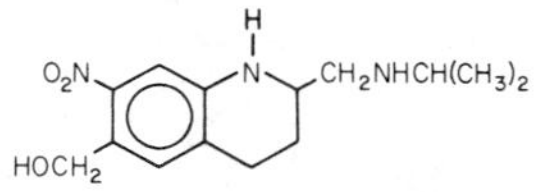

[21738-42-1] $C_{14}H_{21}N_3O_3$ (279.34).

Preparation—From 6-methoxymethylquinaldinic acid to form the acyl chloride, which with diethylamine yields the amide. Reduction of the amide with lithium aluminum hydride and Raney nickel produces the diethylaminomethyl derivative. Nitration of the latter compound in the 7-position followed by demethylation of the 6-position yields oxamniquine (US Pat. 3,821,228).

Description—A light, orange, crystalline powder melting about 151°.

Solubility—Soluble in 3300 in water; soluble in acetone, chloroform or methanol.

Uses—An alternate drug for infection caused by *Schistosoma mansoni,* including the acute and chronic phase with hepatosplenic involvement. It significantly reduces the egg load of *S mansoni.* Contraindicated in pregnancy. Adverse effects observed include occasional headache, fever, dizziness, somnolence, nausea, diarrhea, rash, insomnia and ECG changes. Convulsions and neuropsychiatric disturbances also have been observed, but are rare.

Dose—*Schistosoma mansoni, adults,* **15 mg/kg,** once; *children,* **20 mg/kg** in 2 divided doses for 1 day.

Dosage Form—Capsules: 250 mg.

Piperazine

(Various Mfrs)

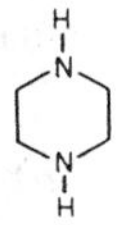

[110-85-0] $C_4H_{10}N_2$ (86.14).

Preparation— By catalytic deamination of diethylenetriamine and of ethylenediamine. US Pat 2,267,686.

Description—White to slightly off-white lumps or flakes having an ammoniacal odor; melts between 109° and 113°; boils between 145° and 146°; in water it crystallizes with $6H_2O$ in colorless crystals called *piperazine hydrate,* melting at 44° and boiling between 125° and 130°. Soluble in water or alcohol; insoluble in ether. Incompatible with salts of heavy metals, alkaloidal salts or with acetanilid, phenacetin or nitrites.

Uses—Piperazine and several of its salts—the *adipate, calcium edetate, citrate, phosphate* and *tartrate*—have been used as anthelmintics for treatment of roundworm and pinworm infections. When administered orally, therapeutic doses have little or no pharmacological effects on the host. Adverse effects are transient, usually mild and disappear when the drug is discontinued. Occasionally, patients may complain of nausea, vomiting, mild diarrhea, abdominal cramps, headache and dizziness. More serious adverse effects such as seizures and respiratory depression are rare and occur after large doses. Piperazine should be used with caution in patients with severe malnutrition oranemia. It is contraindicated in patients with impaired renal or hepatic function or seizure disorders and in those patients who are hypersensitive to piperazine. Piperazine has been used in pregnant women; without adverse effects; however, its safe use in pregnancy has not been established clearly.

Dose—*Enterobiasis, adult and children,* **65 mg/kg** (maximum 2.5 g) daily for 7 consecutive days. Alternatively, adults may be given a single dose of 2 g daily and children 19/m^2 daily for 7 days. In severe enterobiasis, treatment may be reported after 1 wk. *Ascariasis, adult,* **3** to **5 g** once daily and *children,* 75 mg/kg (up to 3.5 g) once daily for 2 consecutive days. Alternatively, *children* may be given **2 g/m^2** daily for 2 days.
Dosage Forms—Tablets: 250 mg (of piperazine hexahydrate); Solution: 500 mg (of piperazine hexahydrate) per 5 mL.

Piperazine Citrate—see RPS-18, page 1244.

Praziquantel

4*H*-Pyrazino[2,1-*a*]isoquinolin-4-one, 2-(cyclohexylcarbonyl)-1,2,3,6,7,11b-hexahydro-, Biltricide (*Miles*)

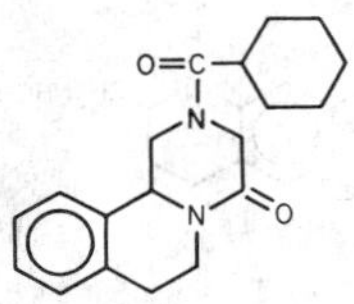

[55268] $C_{19}H_{24}N_2O_2$ (312.41).
Preparation—Aminomethyltetrahydroisoquinoline, cyclohexanecarbonyl chloride, acetonitrile and aqueous hydrochloric acid are refluxed in the presence of pyridine to first form the cyclohexanecarbamoylmethyl derivative which cyclizes to form the product (US Pat 4,001,411).
Description—A hygroscopic solid with a bitter taste, melting about 137°.
Solubility—Freely soluble in chloroform; soluble in ethanol; very slightly soluble in water.
Uses—The drug of choice for infections caused by *Schistosoma japonicum, S mekongi, S haematobium* and *S mansoni.* It is also an investigational drug of choice for tapeworm infestations and numerous fluke infections. It increases the permeability of the worm's cell membrane to calcium ions; this causes massive contraction and paralysis of its musculature and disintegration of its tegumental layer. Adverse effects include sedation, abdominal discomfort, fever, sweating, nausea, eosinophilia, headache and dizziness.
Dose—*Usual, adult or children, S Haematobium, S mansoni, S japonicum,* and *S mekongi,* **40** to **60 mg/kg** 3 times in 1 day; flukes, **75 mg/kg** 3 times a day for 1 to 2 days.
Dosage Form—Tablets: 60 mg.

Pyrantel Pamoate

Pyrimidine, (*E*)-1,4,5,6-tetrahydro-1-methyl-2-[2-(2-thienyl)ethenyl]-, compd with 4,4′-methylenebis[3-hydroxy-2-naphthalenecarboxylic acid] (1:1); Antiminth (*Roerig*); Combatrin (*Pfizer*)

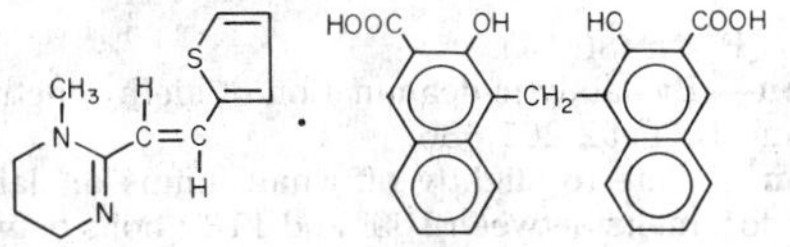

[22204-24-6] $C_{11}H_{14}N_2S.C_{23}H_{16}O_6$ (594.68).
Preparation—Thiophene is converted to 2-thiophenecarboxaldehyde (I) via a Vilsmeier-Haack reaction. *N*-Methyl-1,3-propanediamine is condensed with acetonitrile to yield 1,4,5,6-tetrahydro-1,2-dimethylpyrimidine which is then coupled with I in the presence of methyl formate to yield pyrantel (base). The pyrantel is isolated as the tartrate and metathesized with a soluble alkali-metal pamoate.
Description—Yellow to tan powder that is tasteless and free of characteristic odor; decomposes slowly in light; nonhygroscopic in air under ordinary conditions; relatively stable in heat; melts with decomposition between 247° and 261°.
Solubility—Insoluble in water; very slightly soluble in alcohol.
Uses—One of the anthelmintics of choice in the treatment of *ascariasis* (common roundworm infection) and *enterobiasis* (pinworm) infection. It is also an investigational drug for the treatment of hookworm, moniliformis and trichostrongylus infections. Side effects occur only occasionally and are relatively mild; gastrointestinal disturbances, headache, dizziness, rash and fever have been reported.
Dose—*Usual, oral, children* and *adults,* **11 mg** pyrantel base/**kg,** with a maximum of 1 g, as a single dose repeated in 2 weeks. Members of the family of patients with pinworm infestations also should be treated to prevent recurrence.
Dose Form—Oral Suspension: 50 mg pyrantel base/mL.

Quinacrine Hydrochloride—page 1323.

Suramin Sodium—page 1326.

Thiabendazole

1*H*-Benzimidazole, 2-(4-thiazolyl)-, Mintezol (*MSD*); Thibenzole (*Merck*)

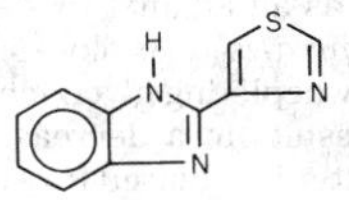

2-(4-Thiazolyl)benzimidazole [148-79-8] $C_{10}H_7N_3S$ (201.25).
Preparation—Ethyl pyruvate is brominated and the resulting 2-bromo ester is reacted with thioformamide whereby cyclization occurs with formation of ethyl 4-thiazolecarboxylate. This ester is saponified and condensed with *o*-phenylenediamine to introduce the benzimidazole moiety. US Pat 3,017,415.
Description—White to practically white, odorless or practically odorless, tasteless powder; stable in light and nonhygroscopic; melts between 296° and 303°; pK_a 4.7.
Solubility—Practically insoluble in water; slightly soluble in acetone or alcohol; very slightly soluble in chloroform or ether.
Uses—The anthelmintic of choice in *Strongyloides stercoralis,* cutaneous larva migrans (creeping eruption), *Angiostrongylus costaricensis. It also is recommended as an alternate drug in the treatment of Capillaris philippensis* and *Dracunculus medinensis* (guinea worm) infections, and visceral larva migrans. No special diet or purgation is needed with this drug. Side effects usually include nausea, vomiting, vertigo, headache and weakness. Leukopenia, crystalluria, rash, disturbance of color vision and hallucinations also have been reported. In rare instances, shock, tinnitus and Stevens-Johnson syndrome have been observed. Since from ⅓ to ½ of patients usually are incapacitated for several hours after receiving the drug, it should be given on days when the patient does not have to go to school or work. Patients on the drug should be cautioned not to engage in activities requiring mental alertness.
Dose—*Usual, oral, adults* and *children,* **25 mg/kg** twice daily after meals; the daily dose should not exceed 3 g. For *Strongyloides stercoralis* infections, this dosage is given 2 days; for severe visceral larva migrans, the dosage is continued for 5 days. For cutaneous larva migrans (creeping eruption), it is applied topically or administered orally in the above dosage for 2 to 5 days. For *Capillaris philippensis* **25 mg/kg** is given each day for 30 days.
Dosage Forms—Oral Suspension: 500 mg/5 mL; Chewable Tablets, 500 mg.

Pediculicides and Scabicides

Pediculicides are compounds effective in the treatment of pediculosis. Pediculosis in man is caused by three species of sucking lice known as *Pediculus humanus* variety *capitis, the head louse, Pediculus humanus* variety *corporis,* the body louse and *Phthirius pubis,* the crab louse. These parasitic, wingless insects thrive where personal hygiene is neglected. The eggs (nits) of the body louse are attached to the fibers of clothing while those of the other two species are attached to hairs by a chitin-like cement. Cutting the hair short or shaving the area is helpful in destroying the eggs. The period of development from egg to adult is about 2 to 4 weeks. To be effective completely, an antipedicular agent must kill both parasites and eggs. Should the latter fail to be destroyed, repeated applications of the agent may be necessary to destroy the newly hatched lice.

Scabicides are compounds that are effective against *Sarcoptes scabiei*, the animal parasite that causes scabies in man. The parasite, a mite, thrives where personal hygiene is neglected. After copulation takes place on the surface of the skin, the female mite excavates a sinuous inward-sloping burrow in the corneous layer of the skin. The eggs are laid in the burrow and, after hatching, the larvae and nymphs may exit. In order to eradicate this infestation, an antiscabious agent must kill both parasites and eggs. If the eggs are not destroyed, repeated applications of the antiscabious agent may be necessary. The life cycle from egg to adult parasite is from 8 to 15 days. Sulfur ointment has been a time-honored scabicide. Except for alternate use in scabies (*Sarcoptes scabies*), it now has been replaced by more effective agents.

Since many agents possess both antipedicular and antiscabious properties, the pediculicides and scabicides are listed together.

Benzyl Benzoate—see RPS-18, page 1246.

Benzyl Benzoate Lotion—see RPS-18, page 1246.

Chlorophenothane—see RPS-18, page 1247.

Crotamiton

2-Butenamide, *N*-ethyl-*N*-(2-methylphenyl)-, Eurax (*Westwood)*

$CH_3CH{=}CHCONCH_2CH_3$ (on 2-methylphenyl, CH_3)

N-Ethyl-*o*-crotonotoluidide [483-63-6] $C_{13}H_{17}NO$ (203.28).

Preparation—By condensation of a crotonyl halide, ester, salt or a derivative thereof with *N*-ethyl-*o*-toluidine.

Description—Colorless to slightly yellowish oil; faint amine-like odor.

Solubility—Practically insoluble in water; miscible with alcohol.

Uses—A scabicidal and antipruritic agent, effective in eradicating scabies infestations and useful for symptomatic treatment of pruritic skin. Allergic sensitivity or primary irritation reactions may occur in some patients. It should not be applied to acutely inflamed skin, raw, weeping surfaces or in the eyes or mouth.

Dose—In *scabies*, thoroughly massage into the skin of the entire body, from the chin down, a **10%** cream or lotion; a second application 24 hr later is advised to assure complete eradication of mites. A cleansing bath should be taken 48 hr after the last application. In *pruritus* the cream is massaged gently into affected areas until absorbed; repeated as needed.

Dosage Form—Cream: 10%; Lotion 10%.

Lindane

Cyclohexane, (1α,2α,3β,4α,5α,6β)-1,2,3,4,5,6-hexachloro-, Gamma Benzene Hexachloride; Gammexane; BHC; 666; Kwell (*Reed & Carnrick*)

γ-1,2,3,4,5,6-Hexachlorocyclohexane [58-89-9] $C_6H_6Cl_6$ (290.83).

Gamma benzene hexachloride, as this compound was formerly officially called, is one of the nine theoretical stereoisomeric forms of 1, 2,-3,4,5,6-hexachlorocyclohexane. It has been shown to have the conformation

and, in terms of equatorial-axial notation, becomes 1*e*,2*e*,3*e*,4*a*,5*a*,6*a*-hexachlorocyclohexane.

Preparation—By the chlorination of benzene in the presence of light. The reaction product is a mixture of stereoisomers containing from 10 to 15% of the insecticidally active gamma isomer which may be separated by solvent extraction processes.

Description—White, crystalline powder; slight, musty odor.

Solubility—Practically insoluble in water; slightly soluble in ethylene glycol; 1 g in 20 mL dehydrated alcohol, 3.5 mL chloroform or 40 mL ether.

Uses—Widely used as an ectoparasiticide and ovicide. It is an alternative drug for the treatment of *Sarcoptes scabiei* (scabies), *Pediculosis capitis* (head lice) and *Phthirus pubis* (crab lice). As a *scabicide*, it is employed in a 1% concentration in a vanishing cream or lotion. The mixture is applied in a thin layer over the entire cutaneous surface from the neck down. One ounce usually is sufficient for an adult. Leave it on for at least 12 hr; remove it by thorough washing. One application is usually curative; retreatment is indicated only if living mites can be demonstrated. The shampoo is used for the treatment of *Pediculosis pubis* and *capitis*. Approximately 1 oz (for short hair) and 2 oz (for long hair) is worked thoroughly into the hair and allowed to remain in place for 4 min; small quantities of water are added then until a lather forms; the hair is rinsed thoroughly, toweled briskly and any nits removed with nit comb or tweezers.

Adverse effects include occasional eczematous skin rash and conjunctivitis; rarely, convulsions and aplastic anemia have been observed.

Dose—*Topical*, **1%** in cream, lotion or shampoo once or twice a week.

Dosage Forms—Cream: 1%/57 g and 1 lb; Lotion: 1%/60 mL, pt and gal; Shampoo: 1%/60 mL, pt and gal.

Malathion—page 1357.

Permethrin

3-(2,2-Dichloroethenyl)-2,2-dimethylcyclopropanecarboxylic acid, (3-phenoxyphenyl)methyl ester; Nix (*Burroughs Wellcome*); Elimite (*Allergan Herbert*)

[52645-53-1] $C_{21}H_{20}Cl_2O_3$ (391.29).

Preparation—See *Pestic Sci 5:* 791, 1974.

Description—Colorless crystals melting about 35° to a viscous, pale orange-brown liquid. Of the 4 theoretically possible isomers which exist it is a mixture of the two active isomers, 1*R-cis*/1*R-trans* (ca 1:3).

Solubility—Practically insoluble in water; soluble in nonpolar organic solvents.

Uses—The drug of choice for the treatment of Sarcoptes scabiei (scabies) and *Pediculus humanus, Pediculus capitis* and *Phthirus pubis.* It acts on the para-site's nerve-cell membranes to disrupt the sodium channel current. A single application is highly effective in patients with scabies and head lice. Residual persistence is detectable on the hair for at least 10 days following a single application. Adverse effects include burning, stinging, numbness, increased pruritus, pain, edema, erythema and rash. Since there have been no adequate well-controlled studies in pregnant women, it should not be used in pregnancy unless clearly needed. For similar reasons it should not be given to nursing mothers. Safety and efficacy in children under 2 yr has not been established.

Dose—*Adult and children*: *Scabies*, a **5%** permathrin cream is massaged into the skin from the head to toes and removed 8 to 14 hr later with a bath or shower. *Head lice* (*Pediculus capitis*), 1% liquid is used after the hair has been washed with shampoo, rinsed with water and towel dried. Apply a sufficient amount to saturate the hair and scalp. Allow it to remain on the hair for 10 min and thoroughly rinse off with water.

Dosage Form—Liquid: 1% in 60 mL. Cream: 5% in 60 g.

Precipitated Sulfur

Precipitated Sulphur; Lac Sulfuris; Milk of Sulfur

Sulfur [7704-34-9] S (32.06).

Preparation—To a slurry of 1 part of lime and 10 parts of water, 2 parts of sublimed sulfur are added, thoroughly mixed and the mixture boiled with frequent agitation until all of the sulfur is dissolved:

$$12S + 3Ca(OH)_2 \rightarrow 2CaS_5 + CaS_2O_3 + 3H_2O$$

After cooling, the clear liquid is decanted through a filter, and a slight excess of HCl, calculated from the quantity of lime used, is added to the filtrate. The acid decomposes the calcium pentasulfide and the thiosulfate with the precipitation of sulfur:

$$2CaS_5 + CaS_2O_3 + 6HCl \rightarrow 3CaCl_2 + 12S + 3H_2O$$

Description—Very fine, pale yellow, amorphous or microcrystalline powder; odorless and tasteless.

Solubility—Practically insoluble in water; very slightly soluble in alcohol; slightly soluble in olive oil. Distinguished from other forms of sulfur by more rapid solubility in carbon disulfide: on shaking 1 g of precipitated sulfur with 5 mL carbon disulfide, it should dissolve quickly except for a small amount of insoluble matter usually present.

Incompatibilities—Sufficiently hydrophobic that it sometimes causes trouble in lotions, where it tends to float on the surface. Among substances which have been shown to promote the wetting of sulfur, and thus aid its dispersion, are triethanolamine oleate and benzoin tincture. Trituration of the sulfur with a few drops of alcohol, glycerin or a dilute solution of a wetting agent is also of some service.

Uses—An active parasiticide; a 10% sulfur paste or ointment is used as an alternative treatment for *Sarcoptes scabiei* (mites). Sulfur also is actively *keratolytic* and, in the form of full-strength ointment or in combination with other keratolytic agents such as salicylic acid, it is used in the treatment of skin disorders such as *psoriasis, seborrhea, eczema-dermatitis* and *lupus erythematosus.* The percentage of sulfur in an ointment should be reduced in the event that a patient's skin shows intolerance. Prolonged use of sulfur may result in a characteristic dermatitis venenata.

Dose—*Topical, as a* **10%** ointment every night for 3 nights.

Sulfur Ointment USP contains 10% of S.

Pyrethrins with Piperonyl Butoxide

RID (*Leeming*); A-200 Pyrinate (*Norcliff Thayer*); (*Various Mfrs*)

Preparation—Pyrethrins are the insecticidal extracts of the pyrethrum flower and are usually synthesized from pyrethrolone [(*Z*)(+)-4-hydroxy-3-methyl-2-(2,4-pentadienyl)-2-cyclopentene-1-one,$C_{11}H_{14}O$] and chrysanthemic acid [2,2-dimethyl-3-(2-methyl-1-propenyl)cyclo-propanecarboxylic acid, $C_{10}H_{17}O_2$] to yield a mixture of pyrethrins I and II. Piperonyl butoxide, [5-[[2-(2-butoxyethoxy)ethoxy]methyl]-6-propyl-1,3-benzodioxazole, $C_{19}H_{30}O_5$] has a synergistic effect on pyrethrins and rotenone, another floral insecticide.

Use—This combination (pyrethrins 0.3%, piperonyl butoxide 3.0%) is an alternative treatment for *Pediculosis humanis, P capitis, and Phthirus pubis.* It is contraindicated in individuals sensitive to the ingredients or ragweed, harmful if swallowed or inhaled and may be irritating to the eyes and mucous membranes. Discontinue use and notify a physician if irritation or skin rash occurs.

Dose—Apply topically only once; it may be necessary to apply a second time 5 to 7 days later to kill hatching progeny.

Dosage Form—Liquid: 60 and 120 mL; Shampoo: 60 and 120 mL; Gel: 30 g.

CHAPTER 78

Pesticides

Ara H Der Marderosian, PhD
Professor of Pharmacognosy & Research Professor of Medicinal Chemistry
Philadelphia College of Pharmacy and Science
Philadelphia, PA 19104

Pesticides may be defined simply as chemical agents used to control pests. In its broadest sense it includes insecticides, rodenticides, fungicides and herbicides. These substances represent big business, with the US once being the largest producer in the world.

Worldwide the annual sales of traditional pesticides is more than $7 billion with more than 95% being synthetic chemicals.

The pesticide usage in the US during the early 1990s has been relatively stable at about 1.1 billion pounds of active ingredient. The agricultural share of pesticide usage is reported to have stabilized at about 75% of the total as it increased steadily throughout the 1960s and 1970s, mainly due to the increased use of herbicides in crop production. Another important recent trend is seen where growth in the use of pesticides has been diminished because of lower application rates due to the introduction of more potent and effective pesticides, more efficiency in their use and lower farm commodity prices.

The overall volume of pesticides used for nonagricultural purposes in this country has been relatively stable in recent years at about 275 million pounds of active ingredient. This translates to some 1.1 pounds per person (the average for 250 million people). However, considering all usage, including agricultural, US pesticide usage comes out to a little more than four pounds per person (4.3 pounds in 1991).

In 1990, the office of pesticide programs of EPA completed a pesticide industry sales and usage market estimate and a national survey of home and garden usage of pesticides. Some of the highlights of the report include

US pesticide user's purchases account for one-third of the world market.

Annual US pesticide-user expenditures totaled about $8.3 billion in 1991 and $8 billion in 1990.

Herbicides are currently the leading types of pesticides (both in volume and user expenditures).

There are about 20,000 pesticide programs registered under the Federal Pesticide Law.

Total US pesticide usage in 1991 was really 2.2 billion pounds of active ingredient (counting wood preservatives, disinfectants and sulfur).

Farmer's expenditure on pesticides equal about 4.7% of total farm production expenditures.

Total pesticide research and development expenditures represent about 16% of pesticide expenditures by the user community.

Net usage of conventional pesticides of about 1.1 billion pounds derives from US production of 1.3 billion, imports of 0.2 billion and exports of 0.4 billion pounds of active ingredient of conventional pesticides.

Significant numbers of firms/individuals are involved in the production/distribution of pesticides (*viz,* 120 leading producers, 2200 formulators, 7300 producing establishments and 17,200 distributors).

The use of pesticides occurs on more than 900,000 farms and in at least 69 million households.

The two most widely used pesticides by volume are the herbicides *atrazine* and *alachlor.*

There were 12 new active ingredients registered as pesticides under FIFRA in 1991 (up from eight in 1990).

Acknowledgment is made of helpful comments and suggestions by Drs M Lee, R Taylor and D MacIver and information provided by Susan Lawrence, Chief, Public Response and Program Resources Branch Field Operations Div, Office of Pesticide Programs, US Environmental Protection Agency.

There are about 1.3 million certified pesticide applicators in the US of which nearly 1 million are for agriculture, and the remainder are 0.3 million certified applicators. Eighty-five percent of all households have at least one pesticide in storage in or around the home.

The specific results of the National Home and Garden survey revealed that

In households without children under five years old, about 75% had at least one pesticide stored less than four feet off the ground and not locked in a cabinet (ie, within reach of children).

In homes with children under five years of age, about 47% stored at least one pesticide within reach of children. Overall, an estimated 85% of all households have at least one pesticide in storage and around the home.

Most families have between one and five pesticide products stored, and slightly over 27% of single family households have over six products stored.

Some 76% of all households used pesticides in their homes themselves, while about 20% hired a commercial applicator to treat such pests as roaches, fleas or ants (termites are not included in these estimates).

Less than 25% could recall receiving written notification about the pesticides used in their home or any safety precautions to follow.

About 15% of households had pesticides applied in or around their homes by someone outside the household. Only half of these people recall receiving written information regarding the pesticides used and safety precautions to be followed.

In the households which dispose of concentrated pesticides, 67% use regular trash, 16% use special collections and 17% give it away, pour it down the toilet or sink, on the street, in the gutter or sewer or on the ground.

Some 44% of all households identified at least one insect that was considered a major problem.

Some 25% of all households were treated for cockroaches in 1990. It appears that cockroaches are the most common pest problem for households living in multifamily dwellings. For households in single family dwellings, ants are the most common problem.

The most difficult pest to control was identified as fleas.

One of the most interesting reports on this scientific random sampling was an amazing response rate of 85 percent. The executive summaries of this 400 page National Home and Garden Pesticide Use Survey are available and may be obtained from the Communications Branch of EPA's Pesticide Programs (Telephone: 703-305-5017).

Pharmacies throughout the US stock a myriad of consumer pesticide products used for these purposes. This represents an important area in which pharmacists can exercise their knowledge and skills, particularly for proper use, handling and disposal of pesticides.

As of June 1993, the EPA (Prevention, Pesticides and Toxic Substances [H-7508W]; report #738-R-93-009, June 1993) published the Status of Pesticides in Registration and Special Review (Rainbow report) which contains a general management directory, a chemical review manager directory and a general information section which covers purpose, timing, comments, additional information and electronic access.

Chapter 2 is entitled *Special Review* and is organized so that the first section explains the special review process including the criteria which EPA uses to initiate a special review, the steps it takes to conduct a Special Review and the risk-reduction alternatives to the conventional Special Review process.

The following section gives an "At a Glance" summary of the dates when Special Review decision documents were published in the *Federal Register.*

The third section provides a comprehensive reference list of all chemicals which have been or are currently in the Special Review program. The various chemicals are listed in alphabetical order.

The final section lists the chemicals in identical sequence and additionally, gives the details of Special Review criteria met or exceeded as well as the outcomes of the reviews. The entire report is 377 pages long and lists almost 1500 compounds.

Further, the EPA lists numerous solvents, surfactants, stabilizers and similar substances. Various economic, political and toxicological considerations which crop up routinely in the pesticide business preclude any more accurate figures within a given year.

For those who question the use of pesticides at all it is important to know something about what damage pests can do on a worldwide basis. First it should be understood that plants are the world's major source of food. These plants are susceptible to between 80,000 to 100,000 diseases caused by everything from viruses to bacteria, fungi, algae and even other higher plants. Food plants have to compete with some 30,000 different species of weeds worldwide, of which at least 1800 species are capable of causing serious economic losses. Various higher organisms like nematodes and insects also devastate crops routinely around the world.

It has been estimated that about one-third of the food crops of the world is destroyed by these various pests at various stages, *viz*, growth, harvest and storage. The rates of destruction often are higher in less developed nations. The Food and Agriculture Organization (FAO) estimates that one-half of cotton production in developing countries would be lost to pests without the use of pesticides. Even in the US crop devastation due to pests is estimated to be about 30% ($20 billion annually) even though pesticides are used widely here. Several studies have shown that this country could not survive as a nation without pesticides. Without herbicides alone, at least 10 to 12% of the US population would be working on our farms instead of the current 3%.

Another important consideration of recent origin is the concept of minimum or reduced tillage. In this relatively new farming practice herbicides help promote savings of energy and soil conservation by reducing plowing and cultivation drastically. Now, farmers till only enough to plant new crops. Previous crop debris and weeds are left on the soil and insects and weeds are controlled chemically rather than mechanically through unnecessary plowing. This method of control requires some 80% less energy.

There have been many who have argued for the return of what is called "organic" farming. Generally, organic farmers prefer to avoid the use of synthetic chemical products at all. They prefer naturally occurring chemicals such as rock phosphate and limestone and the manure of domestic animals. Also, leguminous plants are used as a nitrogen source as well as other plants which contain natural pesticidal compounds. While these are laudable practices, they generally result in higher prices because of the costs of these less available materials and the higher costs involved in the more labor-intensive practices of organic farming. In addition, more land with lower yielding capability would have to be farmed to make up for the lower efficiency of organic farming.

From a scientific point of view all natural materials are not necessarily organic and organic substances are not necessarily natural. All things on earth are made up of chemicals, and plants do not really differentiate between what is made by man or nature. However, organic farming practices are sensible for the smaller farmer who wishes to avoid excess use of unnecessary chemicals and does not mind the use of extra labor practices to save money on materials.

According to a study by the new Natural Resources Defense Council entitled "Harvest of Hope," alternative farming techniques could reduce pesticide applications between 25 and 80% on nine crops grown in California and Iowa. The study showed that over 580 million pounds of pesticide-active ingredients were sold in California in 1987, and 57 million pounds of herbicide per year were used by Iowa farmers.

The study further stated that many ill effects have resulted from use of all of these including pesticide contamination of the food supply, farm worker illness, ecosystem degradation and water pollution. The council study calls on the Federal Government to redirect its agricultural research to make development of alternative farming systems a priority and to adopt alternative farming systems, including crop rotations, without incurring financial penalties. In addition, it promotes the concept that Federal and State Governments should levy fees on fertilizers and pesticides to help finance alternative agricultural research. At the same time that alternative ways of controlling pests are being sought, there are efforts to develop new chemicals with greater specificity to a particular pest and less toxicity to nontarget species. Proponents claim that having different chemical pesticides on hand with varying mechanisms of action allow for rotation of these in order to limit development of resistance.

The first of this type developed is *imidacloprid* (Bayer AG) which has already been introduced in France, Spain, Japan and South America. The EPA will soon allow its sale in the US. It has shown good results in controlling most sucking insects, including aphids and whiteflies, but it is less effective against chewing insects (worms, caterpiller larvae and butterflies).

Imidacloprid works to bind to one type of receptor for the neurotransmitter, acetylcholine, causing the nerves of an insect to fire uncontrollably, leading to muscle paralysis and death. Other new and specific chemical pesticides include *fipronil* (Rhone-Poulenc) and *pyrrole* (American Cyanamid).

Perhaps the major reason for use of pesticides has been the long world history of mass destruction of crops by disease and insects. One constantly is reminded that it would not take long to return to a primitive agriculture status by the numerous reports of crop devastation and disease which appear in various underdeveloped countries. Some of the relatively recent examples of pest effects include the destruction of 3 million tons of wheat by stem rust in western Canada in 1954; the continuous problem of arthropod-borne encephalitides which caused an average of 205 human cases in the US annually between 1964 and 1973; and the reduction of the annual death rate of malaria through the use of pesticides (down from 6 million in 1939 to 2.5 million in 1965 to less than 1 million today). There are at least two dozen common diseases (encephalitis, typhus, anthrax, dysentery, etc), still of concern to man, which are transmitted by a myriad of insects, ticks or mites.

As with all substances used by modern man, pesticides offer a risk-benefit ratio which must be assessed for each application. A modern concerned society should always advocate very specific, carefully planned usage of pesticides, well-integrated with other control practices. This approach has become quite popular today and is referred to as Integrated Pest Management (IPM). It consists of determining a workable combination of the best parts of all possible control procedures and applying them to a specific problem. The concept is to keep pests at a controllable level within the confines of sound ecological principles so that economic injury to plants or man is avoided. Overall, while mistakes have been made (eg, DDT), pesticides have contributed significantly to the increased productivity of the US farmer.

In 1981, each American farmer produced enough food and fiber for 78 people as opposed to only 14 people in 1950. Currently, at least one-third of today's crops are saved through the use of pesticide chemicals in agriculture. On the world scale it is widely known that current food supplies are inadequate. Estimates are given that at least 56% of the population of the world is undernourished with the situation in some countries being much worse. With world population continuing to explode (4.4 billion in 1980; 5.4 billion in 1990) there is little doubt that agriculture needs all the help it can get.

Comparisons between foreign and US farmers is enlightening. The Asian farmer produces about 19,964 kg of food a year, the Russian farmer 14,973 kg, the European farmer 15,880 kg, while the American farmer produces 170,145 kg. This makes it easy to understand why the US can grow 48% of the world's corn and 63% of the world's soybeans with only 2% of the population involved in agriculture. Viewed from the point of view of health alone, millions of humans around the world are killed or made sick annually from a myriad of insect-borne diseases. The overall worldwide losses from insects, weeds, rats and diseases is estimated to be in the vicinity of $90 billion annually. Without pesticides the world population could not exist.

Pesticides and Law

In the US, numerous federal laws protect the user of pesticides as well as the consumers. Many of these laws are quite old and have been amended from time to time for obvious reasons. Since they are all complex and change with time a brief summary is presented here so the pharmacist will be aware of who is responsible for which laws and what the current status of pesticide registration is.

The Federal Insecticide, Fungicide and Rodenticide Act (FIFRA) as amended (EPA, Oct 1988) is administered by the EPA. These new amendments require a substantial acceleration of the reregistration process for previously registered (licensed) pesticides and authorize the collection of fees to support reregistration activities. This law also changes EPA's responsibilities and funding requirements for the storage and disposal of suspended and cancelled pesticides and the indemnification of holders of remaining stocks of such canceled pesticides. Hence, under FIFRA, all pesticides have to be registered with EPA before they may be sold or distributed in commerce in the US.

This agency establishes an overall risk/benefit standard for pesticide registration, requiring that pesticides show efficacy when employed according to label instructions, and should show no unreasonable risk of adverse effects on human health or the environment. Laws require that EPA take into account the economic, social and environmental costs and benefits of pesticide uses.

Because FIFRA was originally enacted in 1947, there has been developed since, literally thousands of pesticides registered for use. However, over time, the standards of use obviously have changed and evolved in tandem with general advances in science and public policy. Specifically, for example, test-data requirements for pesticides have become increasingly stringent in the light of modern advances in analytical chemistry and toxicology. So now, more than ever, companies which hold pesticide registrations are responsible for providing all test data needed to satisfy EPA's registration requirements. To be sure all of these things are done, FIFRA requires the review and *reregistration* of all existing pesticides. Obviously, this has shown to be an enormous undertaking. Several factors have impeded this process, including inadequate resources and the sheer magnitude of the process.

Of the estimated 600 pesticide-active ingredients which require reregistration under FIFRA, the EPA has issued Registration Standards for a little over 185.

To further understand the complexity, note that this requires a comprehensive review of all the available data needed for full registration, and the Agency's current regulatory position on the pesticide. Thus, FIFRA authorizes the EPA to cancel the registration of any pesticide if test data shows that it causes unreasonable adverse effects on human health or even the environment. In order to prevent an imminent hazard, the EPA can take action to suspend the registration of a pesticide.

Up until these more recent 1988 amendments, the EPA was required under older FIFRA rules to accept certain suspended and canceled pesticides for appropriate disposal at government expense. Additionally, there was even an indemnification provision which required EPA to reimburse holders of such suspended and canceled pesticides for financial losses suffered, up to the cost of the pesticide.

It obviously is impossible to provide all the details of the 1988 amendments, but it should be understood that there are several requirements for reregistration with very tight schedules and deadlines. These include five phases which involve

The publishing of lists of pesticide-active ingredients.
The identification of missing and inadequate scientific studies.
The summarization and reformating of key existing studies to facilitate EPA review.
The requirement of EPA to complete its review in a timely manner.
Either the reregistration or the application of other appropriate regulatory action.

A fee structure also has been defined by the FIFRA regulations which is expected to cost about $250 million over the nine years of the 5-phase process. It is estimated that $110 to 120 million of these costs will come from a continuation of the current level of EPA's budget for reregistration activities. The rest of the monies will be derived from the pesticide industry through two types of fees, including a reregistration fee for each active ingredient, plus an annual fee for registration maintenance to be paid for each registered product.

Registrants will be required to pay reregistration fees totalling $150,000 for each active ingredient intended for use on major food or animal feed crops. For the most part, an initial payment of $50,000 is due during Phase 2, and the balance in Phase 3. In those cases where the pesticides are not intended for major food or feed uses, registrants will have to pay a fee of not more than $150,000 and not less than $50,000. Active ingredient fees will be apportioned among registrants of each ingredient based on market share.

The regulations also cover storage and disposal of suspended or canceled pesticides, indemnity (or disposal) payments and various miscellaneous provisions, including penalties, unlawful acts, records and inspection, unregistered pesticides, use of a scientific advisory panel and congressional review.

In May 1992, the EPA issued another update entitled "Pesticide Reregistration" (#700-K92-004) in the form of a 16-page booklet. It further defines

The registration standards program. The status of the accelerated reregistration program.
The List A pesticides (those 194 active ingredient cases or those 350 individual active ingredients, for which EPA had issued Registration Standards prior to December 24, 1988). The List B, C and D Pesticides (List B contain less significant food-use pesticides, outdoor nonfood uses, indoor uses; List C contains antimicrobials, including disinfectants and wood preservatives; List D contains other outdoor and indoor uses, antimicrobials, microbial pesticides.

Overall, by April 1992, EPA had completed Reregistration Eligibility Documents (RED) for eight List A cases, and had begun reregistering products containing active ingredients in several of these cases. At least another 144 of the original 194 List A cases remain supported for reregistration (*viz*, their registrants had provided sufficient required data and had paid the requisite fees), and were either awaiting data or in review. Some forty-two cases had become unsupported or canceled.

In regard to the original Lists B, C and D published in 1989, many of these pesticides were unsupported for reregistration and therefore canceled. By 1992, EPA had completed REDs for six List D cases, but only 261 of the 418 List B, C and D cases were still supported for reregistration. By the end of Phase 4 (as they did at the end of Phase 2 and 3), the EPA will provide public notice for the unsupported uses in case anyone wishes to support them through reregistration.

As can be garnered from all of this data on the EPA's current pesticide reregistration process, it is apparent that it simply will not be possible to complete the process until well beyond the year 2000. Pharmacists who wish to determine the status of any particular pesticide should contact their local or national EPA offices. They will provide answers on the status of individual pesticides but cannot give the general status of any category of pesticides.

Readers are advised to write or call the Special Review and Reregistration Division (H-7508W), Office of Pesticide Programs, US EPA, Washington, DC 20460; telephone: 703-308-8000.

For similar reasons it has not been possible to provide the exact status of every pesticide mentioned in this chapter. For completeness, however, the long-standing status and general properties of many *classically* used pesticides has been retained.

The Environmental Protection Agency Responsibilities

Interpret its laws and implement its provisions.

Has established, by regulation, ten categories of certification for commercial applicators. These include: (1) agricultural pest control (plant and animal); (2) forest pest control; (3) ornamental and turf pest control; (4) seed treatment; (5) aquatic pest control; (6) right-of-way pest control; (7) industrial, institutional, structural and health-related pest control; (8) public health pest control; (9) regulatory pest control and (10) demonstration and research pest control.

Set general standards of knowledge for all categories of certified commercial applicators of pesticides. In each state, the certification is carried out by an appropriate regulatory agency, usually the state department of agriculture. Pesticide applicators are trained through the various cooperative extension services of the state.

State Regulation

Since these vary considerably for each state there is little room to include them in this chapter. For the most part, these laws are similar to the federal regulations. Reference is made to local state agricultural agencies for specific information.

Pesticides and the Law

At the international level, the World Health Organization (WHO) and the Food and Agriculture Organization (FAO) of the United Nations continue to press for wider use of certain pesticides to help raise the level of efficiency in agriculture. Recent WHO literature relates international concern on safe use of pesticides and pesticide residues in food.

Interest in pesticides extends beyond their use simply to increase crop yields, specifically in their use in the control of pests as vectors of disease. For example, it is well known that insects such as chiggers, itch mites and ticks transport disease to man directly or via foodstuffs, and that mosquitoes, tsetse flies, rat fleas and others are capable of directly injecting disease organisms into his blood stream. Pest control also enters into areas where livestock must be protected against predatory animals such as coyotes, wolves and bobcats.

It should be stated at the outset that the various pesticides discussed in this chapter are subject to numerous constraints under new and continually changing rulings. For this reason it is suggested that reference be made directly to the EPA for definitive information on specific pesticides and their registered uses. Each state also publishes its own set of pesticide recommendations.

While it is difficult to classify all pesticides chemically or biologically it will be useful to list some of the major categories with a few examples in each class:

Insecticides

Stomach poison or protective insecticides—Chlorinated hydrocarbons (methoxychlor, chlordane); miscellaneous (carbaryl).

Contact insecticides—Botanicals (nicotine sulfate, pyrethrum, rotenone); organic phosphorus compounds (parathion, malathion); miscellaneous (carbaryl).

Fumigants—Gaseous materials used in tightly closed spaces such as warehouses, ship holds, mills, grain elevators, boxcars, vaults and in the soil; these include methyl bromide, and paradichlorobenzene.

Acaricides (Miticides)

Phosphate insecticides, tetradifon.

Fungicides

Construed under FEPCA (1972) as those chemicals and formulations used to control fungi and bacteria on living and nonliving plants and plant parts, as well as on or in all materials and surfaces but *excluding* all uses on living humans or animals and all uses on or in processed foods, beverages or pharmaceuticals. A *localized fungicide* is dodine; examples of *complete fungicides* are benomyl and thiabendazole.

Nematicides

Construed under FEPCA (1972) as those chemicals and formulations used to control nematodes (roundworms) inhabiting soil and water that are associated with damage to plants or plant parts. A *postplanting nematicides* is VC-13; *systemic nematicides* are aldicarb and demeton.

Herbicides

Selective—Dalapon, siduron, 2,4-D.

Nonselective—bromacil.

Contact—Cacodylic acid, paraquat, DNBP.

Translocated—2,4-DB; MCPA.

Plant Regulators

All preparations intended to alter the behavior or products of plants through physiological action, such as gibberellic acid, maleic hydrazide.

Defoliants and Desiccants

Preparations intended to cause leaves or foliage of plants to drop prematurely, and usually are used to aid harvesting of certain crops as cotton. Endothall, arsenic acid and sodium chlorate are in this class.

Rodenticides

Strychnine, zinc phosphide, warfarin, chlorophacinone.

Sex Pheromones

Chemical substances produced and released by one sex of an insect (usually the female) that elicit a sexual response in an individual of the opposite sex. *cis*-7,8-Epoxy-2-methyloctadecane (Disparlure) is a gypsy moth lure.

Juvenile Hormones (Insect Growth Regulators)

A relatively new type of pest control agent that regulates insect growth. Isopropyl-11-methoxy-3,7,11-trimethyldodeca-2,4-dienoate (generic name, methoprene; brand name Altosid) is used to arrest mosquito development at the pupal stage.

Attractants

These are insect sexual pheromones which are used to attract specific pests to traps where they may be destroyed. Examples include boll weevil sex attractant and muscalure (Z-9-tricosene) a sex and aggregation pheromone for the common fly (*Musca domestica*).

Many of the chemical names given to pesticides are contractions of longer systematic nomenclature that usually serve as nonproprietary names. As with drugs, many proprietary names are featured. Many pesticides are put into proprietary formulations which include the active ingredients often coupled with some adjuvant such as abscission agents, acidifying agents, buffering agents, antifoaming agents, antitranspirants, colors and dyes, compatibility agents, crop oil concentrates, surfactants, deposition agents, dispersants, drift control agents, foam-markers, gustatory/ feeding stimulants, harvest aids, spreaders, penetrants, wetting agents, stickers, extenders, adhesive agents and suspension and gelling agents.

According to the major purpose for which pesticides are used, they may be classified in the following way:

Acaricides—Control ticks or mites.
Algicides—Destroy algae and other aquatic vegetation.
Antiseptics—Protect objects from damage by microorganisms.
Arboricides—Defoliate and/or destroy trees or shrubby vegetation.
Bactericides—Control bacterial infection in plants.
Fungicides—Control fungal infection in plants.
Herbicides—Control weeds or undesirable species of plants.
Insecticides—Control harmful insects. Several specific terms named for the insect group have been coined; eg, aphicide—agents which control aphids.
Larvicides—Control larval stages of insects.
Limacides or **Molluscicides**—Control mollusks, including gastropods.
Nematicides—Control round worms (nematodes).
Predacides—Control predatory mammals or birds.
Zoocides—Control rodents (rodenticides).

General Suggestions to Pharmacists

The pharmacy is a logical source to obtain pesticide and pest-control information. However, if the pharmacist desires to handle pesticides and build a permanent patronage, he should acquaint himself with the common pest problems, with chemicals recommended and how such materials should be used. In particular, the pharmacist should be acquainted with the classification of pesticides since he will be handling and selling the "general use" type and not the "restricted use" group.

The pharmacist also should keep abreast of new laws which will influence the ways in which chemicals may be used legally. Particular attention should be placed on becoming familiar with the FEPCA discussed above and the Pesticide Chemicals Amendment to the Food, Drug and Cosmetic Act dealing with the safety determination needed on the residue of pesticides on raw agricultural commodities. This amendment is commonly known as the "Miller Bill" and was passed in 1954.

The pharmacist also should study the Chemical Additives Amendment to that same Act passed in 1958 and fully effective in 1960. An annual updating of federal and state pesticide legislation may be obtained through the most recent edition of the *Farm Chemicals Handbook*, 1994, published by Meister Publishing Co, 37733 Euclid Ave, Willoughby OH 44094. This reference features a buyer's guide, application equipment, fertilizer, trade names and dictionary and a pesticide dictionary. Particularly noteworthy in this edition is description of crop chemicals, toxicity class, handling and storage cautions. The current regulatory file is an important new supplement and incorporates information on regulatory action at both the federal and state level in the US affecting pesticides. Further information is included on the Endangered Species Act, Superfund Amendment and Reauthorization Act (SARA), the OSHA Hazard Communication Standard and California's Proposition 65.

For further information on pesticides one can refer to the EPA's *Pesticide Fact Handbook* Vols 1 and 2 published by Noyes Data Corp, Mill Rd, Park Ridge NJ 07656, in 1988 and 1990 respectively. This text provides 130 Pesticide Fact Sheets issued by EPA and announced in the *Federal Register* through December 1990. These Pesticide Fact Sheets include a description of the chemical use patterns and formulations, scientific findings, a summary of the Agency's regulatory position/rationale and a summary of major data gaps. These Fact Sheets in Vols 1 and 2 cover more than 980 tradenamed pesticides.

The entomologist and plant physiologist of the state agricultural experiment station, and the county agent of the state's cooperative extension service, should be consulted for identification of insects and up-to-date information about plant diseases. Publications on weed, insect and plant disease control may be obtained from the state experiment station. Also, the Office of Information, US Department of Agriculture, Washington DC, supplies on request a publications list from which those needed for a personal reference library may be selected for ordering. To learn about applicator certification, contact the local state department of agriculture.

Meetings of insecticide dealers, held annually in many states, also can be important sources of knowledge of new developments in the field of insecticides. Information about the scheduling of such meetings may be obtained from the local county agricultural agent. Each year the cooperative extension service in each state publishes recommendations on pesticides.

Since there are many dependable sources of pesticides, the pharmacist generally will find it advantageous to stock packaged materials for his sales. To aid in contacting wholesalers, the guide known as ENTOMA, prepared and distributed by the Entomological Society of America, 4603 Calvert Rd, College Park MD 20740, is invaluable.

Guidance on methods of rodent and predatory animal control may be obtained from the US Fish and Wildlife Service, Department of the Interior, Washington DC.

Authority for promulgating regulations establishing tolerances for pesticide chemicals in or on raw agricultural commodities, or exempting any pesticide chemical from the necessity of such a tolerance, is vested in the administrator of EPA according to the Miller Amendment (Sec 408) of the Federal Food, Drug and Cosmetic Act. It should be emphasized that both FEPCA and state laws require that pesticides be used according to label directions. Failure to do so can result in civil and criminal penalties.

Since garden insecticides are of fair importance in suburban areas, the pharmacist should be aware of the numerous inexpensive publications that are available from the Superintendent of Documents, US Government Printing Office, Washington DC 20402. These include discussion of such topics as diseases and pests of garden and ornamental plants.

Finally, it has been noted that pharmacists frequently are consulted on venereal diseases, which have increased dramatically in recent years. Beyond the usual recommendation to consult a physician, the pharmacist may be of direct service in recommending agents for body lice infestation.

Control of Insects

Insects may be controlled through proper application of chemicals by means of suitable techniques.

Classification of Insect Control Chemicals

Insect control chemicals may be classified as insecticides, fumigants, repellants and attractants.

Insecticides—Insecticides often are classified according to the type of action that results in destruction of the insect. Three broad categories, namely *stomach poisons, contact insecticides* and *fumigants*, are recognized generally. Among older insecticides such classification was rather distinct. However, with the new synthetic organic compounds, a single material often produces insecticidal action in several ways. Certain materials often are selected and used, however, in such a manner as to accomplish control primarily by stomach, contact or fumigating action.

Stomach Poisons—For control of insects by this method it usually is necessary to apply the insecticide to the food that they consume. Stomach poisons are used widely to control leaf-feeding insects or other pests of plants that will result in consumption of the surface-contaminated material. Stomach poisons also are used in specially prepared baits for controlling a variety of insects. With the rapid advances in employing systemic insecticides it is now feasible to destroy by stomach action certain insects which feed on plant juices or blood and tissues of animals, which in the past were considered vulnerable only to contact insecticides.

Systemic insecticides are those chemicals which move in plants and animals from one location where applied to an other location where the insect may be feeding. Some of the more widely used systemic insecticides include *O,O*-diethyl *O* (and *S*)-[2-(ethylthio)ethyl]phosphorothioates), *Meta Systox R* and *dimethoate*, (*O,O*-dimethyl *S*-methylcarbamoylmethylphosphorodithioate). Stomach poisons include a variety of organic *arsenicals, fluosilicates, rotenone*, various *chlorinated hydrocarbons* and the *organic phosphates* and *carbamates*.

Contact Insecticides—Most of the insecticides in use today depend largely on contact action to destroy insects. *Pyrethrum, rotenone, oil emulsions, nicotine* and *soaps* have been used for this purpose for many years. The *chlorinated hydrocarbon* insecticides (BHC, chlordane), the *organic phosphates* (parathion, TEPP, malathion, etc) and the *carbamates* (eg, carbaryl (Sevin)) have been employed extensively for many years but many of these will soon be unavailable for lack of reregistration or because of cancellation. Some now have restricted use for specific purposes as stated in the EPA suspended and cancelled pesticide list of May 1977. Contact insecticides are employed against chewing as well as sucking insects.

Often insecticides appear on the market with added compounds called synergists, which may enhance the effects of the insecticides considerably. Some, like piperonyl butoxide, help block metabolic degradation of the insecticide by the insect.

Fumigants—Fumigants are gases or vapors used for the control of insects, usually in enclosed spaces. The fumigants include *ethylene dichloride, carbon tetrachloride, methyl bromide, chloropicrin* and many others. A number of the *chlorinated hydrocarbon* and *organic phosphorus* insecticides have sufficiently high vapor toxicity to cause marked fumigating action against insects particularly in enclosed spaces and in soils, but many of these, like lindane, have been cancelled for use in vaporizers.

Repellants—A variety of insect control chemicals possess repellant action. *Citronella* and *creosote* are examples of older materials. *Ethohexadiol* and *diethyltoluamide* are examples of materials more recently developed. Such materials often cause insects to avoid contact with treated surfaces. Repellancy in a strict sense might vary greatly as to mode of action. Some insecticides, such as pyrethrum, have little or no repellent action except on contact. However, the action of *pyrethrum* is so rapid that the spraying of animals may cause flies and mosquitoes to leave after alighting and before biting.

Attractants—The use of attractants to lure insects to poisons or traps has been employed as a means of control for many years. The attractants employed are usually favorite foods for the particular insect involved, such as *molasses, sugar* or *milk* for houseflies, sugar or *grease* for ants, *bran* for cutworms, *bananas* for cockroaches, decaying *meats* for blowflies and protein hydrolysate materials for tropical fruit flies such as the Mediterranean fruit fly. In some cases specific chemicals prove highly attractive. Notable examples are *methyl eugenol* for attracting males of the oriental fruitfly, a serious pest of fruits in some tropical areas, and many synthetic substitutes like 10-dodecadienol, the codling moth sex attractant and *cis*-7,8-epoxy-2-methyloctadecane *(Disparlure)*, the gypsy moth sex attractant.

A new trap for Japanese beetles, now on the market, combines a controlled release strip containing a furanone sex attractant and a eugenol odor attractant.

Qualifications of Suppliers of Insecticides

Mere stocking of insecticides is not enough to establish a professionally recognized and economically successful enterprise as a supplier of insecticides, for three basic services must be provided in addition to physical supplies. These services, principally of information, are

Recognition of the type of insect causing the damage, either from examination of the insect or the injury it produces.

Recommendation of a remedy, based on knowledge of the action of various insecticides or other insect-control chemicals and of the life history, habits and structure of the insect responsible.

Familiarity with methods of application of the remedy, for which the user is largely responsible but who may need instruction in such methods.

Pharmacists will find the following specific information useful in developing the aforementioned services:

An understanding of the relative importance of different insects and the relation of the cost of treatment to the increase in value resulting therefrom to the product injured is necessary. Not infrequently, the cost will exceed the damage that might be done. If the value of the product is small, the insect may not cause appreciable loss even though it may be conspicuously evident. Again, the damage may have been done before its recognition and the delayed treatment will not affect the insect or aid in preventing the damage.

A knowledge of the life, history and habits of the common insects is desirable, as all insect control methods are based on a knowledge of these things.

The ability to recognize the common insects is a great aid as it is the first step in providing suitable control. The county agents, federal entomologists and the members of the staff of the respective state agricultural experiment stations are usually available to aid in the identification of insect pests.

A knowledge of how insecticides kill, of the relation of types of mouth parts to the kind of insecticide to use and when and how the material should be applied is useful.

A knowledge of the usual insect problems of a community will enable the supplier to carry in stock the insecticides likely to be needed. This will eliminate surplus stocks and will provide the materials which so often fill emergency needs.

A knowledge of the toxicity of an insecticide to warm-blooded animals, persistence of residues on plants or in animal tissues, hazard of the materials to bees or fish and wildlife is important in order that advice can be given on precautions which should be taken in the use of certain chemicals. A wide variety of chemicals is in use today. They vary in their toxicity and hazards to different organisms. The degree of danger is governed not only by the inherent toxicity to higher animals and beneficial organisms in a lower category but also by the manner of use and extent of exposure. A highly toxic material properly applied in small amounts may be less hazardous than a material low in toxicity which is applied in larger amounts. The variety of insect control chemicals is clearly apparent by mentioning some of the materials in wide use today. They include some organic arsenicals, nicotine compounds, a few chlorinated hydrocarbon insecticides (methoxychlor, lindane) and the insecticides grouped under the name *organic phosphates*, which at present includes *parathion, malathion, dipterex, diazinon, dursban, imidan* and the newer carbamates, which include *Sevin (carbaryl*, 1-naphthyl-*N*-methylcarbamate) and others. Several pamphlets are available from EPA that deal with pesticide disposal, pesticide dust-avoidance respirators and diagnosis and treatment of poisoning by pesticides. These should be kept on hand for reference by pharmacists providing poison control information on pesticides.

It is important to follow the recommendations for each locality. An insecticide effective in one region may not be in others.

It is essential to understand the labels on trade-named preparations and follow the directions very carefully.

A knowledge of the essentials of a good insecticide, its effect on insects and its availability and cost, is important.

Those manufacturing and offering preparations such as insecticides, rodenticides, etc, for sale on the open market, must familiarize themselves with the various regulations of the individual states where the products are being manufactured or are to be sold. If such products are shipped in interstate commerce, these preparations also must comply with the various federal regulations, especially the FEPCA of 1972 and subsequent EPA amendments.

Many states require dealers in pesticides to be licensed. Some require the dealer to pass a written test to obtain the license. The test usually focuses on pesticide laws and regulations.

Mouth Parts and Relation to Insect Control—In general, pests have two kinds of mouth parts: chewing and sucking. An understanding of the mouth parts and how they relate to the use of different chemical insecticides often will aid in recommending a satisfactory insecticide treatment.

Chewing insects include the *grasshoppers, cockroaches, crickets, bird lice, beetles, slugs* and *caterpillars*. Such insects have mandibles or jaws that enable them to cut off and take into their stomachs solid tissue. Consequently, an insecticide can be used that kills when taken into the stomach with food eaten by the insect. Most of the newer insecticides, however, are active both as contact and as stomach poisons.

Sucking insects include *plant bugs, leafhoppers, scale insects, aphids, fleas, mosquitoes, flies* and *sucking lice* on animals. Such an insect punctures the plant or animal but does not take any of the surface tissue into its stomach; consequently, stomach poisons that have no contact action will be ineffective when applied to the surface. During recent years, however, a variety of compounds have been found that are absorbed through the roots, stems or leaves and transported to various parts of the plant where the chemical is available to sucking or chewing insects that feed inside or on the plant or fruit. This class of compounds is referred to as systemics. Insecticides having systemic action offer great promise for controlling insects, and a number of such compounds now are being employed on both plants and animals.

Plants that have been attacked by chewing pests frequently are recognized by the appearance of the eaten areas. Some plant feeders eat the entire tissue, as do *potato beetles;* others eat holes in leaves, as do *flea beetles;* while some chewing insects skeletonize the leaves, as do *slugs* and the *Mexican bean beetle*.

Sucking insects injure plants in different ways and it is often difficult to determine the kind of insect responsible for the damage unless specimens are available. Sucking insects or mites may remove the sap and cause the plant to "stand still," wilt or drop its foliage; or they may deform the plant, causing the leaves or shoots to curl and become deformed. Some sucking insects, such as the *potato leafhopper*, the *tarnished plant bug* and *plant lice* (*aphids*) inject toxic secretions at the time of feeding, causing the death of plant cells while others, such as *plant lice, leafhoppers* and *striped cucumber beetles, may injure plants directly by feeding as well as through the transmission of plant diseases. Sucking insects also may affect animals by removing the blood, injecting toxic secretions, causing swelling and irritation or carrying disease organisms.*

Life History and Habits of Insects—In general, there are two types of metamorphosis or development among insects: incomplete and complete. Those with incomplete metamorphosis, such as aphids, grasshoppers, plant bugs and scale insects, have only three stages in development: the *egg* or *embryo*, the *nymph* and the *adult* or *imago*. Insects with complete metamorphosis, such as beetles, butterflies, moths, flies, bees, ants and wasps, have four stages in development. In this type, the larva hatching from the egg has no resemblance to the adult, there being also an intermediate resting stage known as the *pupa*, during which remarkable changes in structure take place.

The interrelation of insects, where they hibernate, when they are actively feeding, where they lay their eggs, natural enemies which feed on destructive pests, etc, all have an important bearing on controls. The ant is essential to the life of the corn root aphid and cultural practices which eliminate the ant likewise will eliminate the aphid; the fact that anopheles mosquitoes often rest in homes and other sheltered areas explains the great success of residual sprays such as malathion and baytex for controlling malaria which such mosquitoes transmit; a knowledge of the preferred oviposition sites for grasshoppers permits surveys of egg abundance or abundance of newly hatched nymphs to forecast impending outbreaks of grasshoppers.

Methods of Insect Control

For convenience, insect controls can be grouped as follows.

Natural Controls—Those that are usually present and that normally tend to hold insects in check.

Natural Enemies—Parasitic and predacious insects. Every insect is more or less hindered in its increase by other insects as well as by predacious birds, mammals and other animal life. Although insect-eating birds and certain mammals are important, the insect parasites, predators and insect diseases are usually the most important factors in natural insect control. In fact, it is probable that outbreaks of insects, such as the army worm, often are due not so much to favorable conditions for the pests as to unfavorable conditions for the insect parasites and predators which normally hold them in check. The use of a specific insecticide against a major pest on a crop might lead to a serious outbreak of a secondary pest because of the destruction of natural enemies which normally keep it in check, particularly if the pesticide chosen were largely ineffective against the secondary pest. Such an upset in the balance between destructive and useful insects is a problem of increasing concern in developing insect control chemicals.

Weather and Topographic Influences—Summer and winter temperatures, rainfall, soil and atmospheric humidity plus all similar natural factors have their effect on insects and their hosts. No definite statement can be made concerning the effect of these factors on all insects. A severe winter may be harmful to some insects such as those which winter in an exposed condition; on the other hand, such conditions may have little effect on insects which are well-protected. Similarly, a severe winter may weaken trees and make them more susceptible to insect attack, or it may kill the fruit buds and deprive fruit-infesting insects of their food. However, it should be remembered that insects have a high reproductive capacity and the seasonal conditions, especially spring and early summer conditions, may aid insects in becoming destructively abundant even though they pass the winter few in numbers. On the other hand, an insect overwintering in large numbers may not be important the following season if the weather is not favorable for increase. In tropical, temperate and frigid climates there are to be found insect pests peculiar to these areas due to their adaptation to prevailing weather and topographic influences. Topographic features, such as mountain ranges, act as rather effective barriers to insect migration. However, the great increase in the amount and speed of national and international travel and commerce during the last few decades has provided greater opportunities for hitchhiking insect species to overcome such barriers.

Artificial Controls—Those that are scientific developments of man.

Farm Practices—Many of our most effective aids to insect control are those called farm practices. These include rotations, cultivation, time of planting, time of harvesting, sanitation, good seed, good fertility, good planting conditions and drainage. In general, it may be said that the practices recognized as the best garden, agronomic, orchard, greenhouse or other farm practices, are likewise the best for holding insects in check. Certain insect problems are intensified, however, because of changes in practices such as irrigation, prolonged fruiting periods, etc. It generally is recognized, for example, that supplemental irrigation, increased use of fertilizers and the planting of higher-yielding varieties of cotton have increased the boll weevil problem.

Mechanical Devices—Aside from devices for applying insecticides, there are mechanical devices of value in fighting insect pests. The house screens, fly swatters, insect-proof packages for cereals and other contrivances may be included in this classification.

Insecticides—An insecticide may include any material used for the purpose of killing insects or of protecting crops, animals or other property against insect attack. Insect repellants, fumigants and attractants are considered insecticides in a broad sense. It is important to note that some insecticides may destroy only certain insect pests and are not effective against all insects.

Parasiticides—These substances kill animal parasites such as itch mites, ticks, etc.

Sterilizing Agents—The release of large numbers of insects treated by radioisotopes or chemicals to interfere with reproduction has produced high degrees of control of native populations with whom the sterilized individuals mate, particularly where the insect may mate only one time. Intensive research to extend this insect control concept is underway.

Bioinsecticides—In the 1920s, entomologists experimenting with moths and butterflies found that there were natural chemicals internal to the insects which controlled their development. The release of these natural chemicals was controlled by the brain. These findings encouraged the development of so-called insect growth regulator (IGR) pesticides. Further work in the 1970s showed that synthetic analogs could react similarly. For example, methoprene can prevent adult moth emergence from pupae. Thus, insect larvae grow larger and molt repeatedly and never pupate into reproductive adults and eventually die. Because these IGRs are unique to insects and their relatives, they are very specific in their toxicity and are among the safest pesticides known. It has been found to be useful in many areas eg, it can have an effective life of up to 4 years in controlling stored product pests like beetles in tobacco.

Miscellaneous Controls—

Some of the other natural insecticides are those of botanical origin. These include pyrethrins, nicotine and rotenone. They work mainly as nerve-type poisons. Pyrethrins are the most common botanical insecticides and are extracted from the flower heads of a chysanthemum relative grown mainly in South America and Africa. The pyrethrins have been synthesized and many derivatives with specific advantages (last longer) have been used in recent years.

Some of the inorganic pesticides act in a natural manner due to their desiccant or drying properties. They include boric acid, silica gel or sulfur.

Another approach of a natural nature has been the use of microbials. These kill by causing a fatal disease in insects via specifically introduced bacteria or viruses. Among the two most common microbials in use today are *Bacillus thuringiensis*, which kills only larvae (caterpillars) of butterflies and moths, and *B popillae*, which kills the grubs of Japanese bettles. *B thuringiensis* var *israelensis* is a newly developed variety which affects mosquito larvae. While microbials act slowly they are very specific and only attack certain groups of insects. Microbials, therefore, are generally quite safe to use because they will not harm people, pets or nontargeted organisms.

For a more complete list of the biocontrol agents, please refer to the list provided in the Farm Chemicals Handbook (1994) referenced above. They list over 500 different biologically derived pest-control agents. These include semiochemicals (pheromones, allomones, kairomones), plant regulators, hormones and enzymes, either naturally occurring or identical to a natural product, which attract, retard, destroy or otherwise exert a pesticidal activity.

The microbial agents include viruses, bacteria, fungi and protozoa. Beneficial biological control agents include predators, parasites and weed-feeding invertebrates, living organisms used for controlling the population or biological activities of another life form considered to be a pest. The EPA refers to all of these as *birational pesticides.* This list also includes traps and lures.

Application of Insecticides

How Insecticides Kill—An understanding of how insecticides affect insects will assist in explaining methods and timing of applications.

Stomach poisons kill by being taken into the stomach where they are acted upon by the digestive juices, absorbed through the stomach walls and assimilated by the blood. Details of the mode of action that leads to the death of the insect are not too well-known, even for our most common insecticides. However, much information is being obtained on the general nature of toxic action.

Contact insecticides kill by direct or indirect contact with the insect. Sometimes the insecticide may penetrate directly through the body integument; in other cases it causes oxidation and suffocates the insect, dissolves the insect covering or may prevent settling of the young, as in scale insects, when lime-sulfur has been used. Some contact insecticides are effective only when applied in the presence of the insect, a fact that explains the necessity of the proper timing of applications as well as the importance of directing the spray or dust to the insect itself. Other contact insecticides of the residual type may persist on the treated surfaces where insects rest, such as barn walls, leaves of plants, etc, and kill pests that contact the insecticide deposit.

An important contact insecticide is amorphous silica gel. It has an adsorbing action on the wax coating or cuticle of insects, preventing entrance and exit of water, which leads ultimately to dehydration and death (eg, Dri Die and Drione).

Fumigants can be applied only in enclosed spaces. Fumigants surround the insect and, being in a gaseous state, readily enter the breathing pores of the insect and kill much, as do all volatile insecticides. The systemic insecticides like the phosphates are taken up by the plants. These kill insects, which in turn can cause a residual phosphate problem.

Essentials of a Good Insecticide—There are certain important factors that have a definite bearing on the practicability of insecticides.

Insecticidal or killing properties.
Effect on the plant or animal or environment being treated under varying conditions.
Physical properties, such as color, odor, staining properties, adhesiveness, spreading properties, stability under varying seasonal and storage conditions, reaction with other insecticides or with fungicides, consistency and cost of preparing suitable formulations.
Availability.
Cost.
Safety in the hands of the user.
Safety and palatability of the food products exposed to the insecticide.
Ease of application.
Flammability or explosive character.

All of these factors must be kept in mind by those interested in insect control by the use of insecticides, whether researcher, manufacturer, dealer or user.

Insecticide Formulations—Most of the contact and stomach insecticides cannot be used for insect control as manufactured. They must be compounded in forms that will permit the user to apply them directly or in a manner that requires simple mixing with water or some other diluent before application. Many insect repellants, however, are applied to the skin or clothing without being formulated. The fumigants also are used without special preparation before use.

Insecticides generally are employed in three ways—as dusts, sprays or baits.

Dust Preparations—Prepared dusts ready for use may contain from 1 to 20% of the active insecticide in a carrier such as talc, bentonite or pyrophyllite. When the insecticide compound is a crystalline material, it usually has to be ground to a fine state so that the finished product will flow readily from the dusting equipment and disperse readily. In dusts made from insecticide chemicals that are liquid, such as chlordane or parathion, the concentration of the active material seldom can exceed 5% and still have good dusting qualities. Special conditioning agents may be necessary and special equipment might be required to make a satisfactory dust product. For this reason the ultimate user is seldom in position to make his own insecticidal dusts from the manufactured insecticide chemical. Dusts are used mainly for home purposes.

Insecticide dusts are used for controlling pests on agricultural crops, in homes, on man or on animals.

In some instances where it is desired to limit the drift of dust particles and prevent particles from adhering to vegetation, dry preparations are prepared so the particles are about the size of sugar granules. Such preparations, called *granular insecticides,* are used for treating soils for soil-inhabiting pests and certain other pests such as the European cornborer where the granules collect in whorls or leaf axilla and destroy the young larvae before they bore into the stalk. They also are employed to some extent for controlling mosquito larvae, sand-fly larvae and other insects affecting man. In general, however, dusts and granular insecticides are not used as extensively as are sprays.

Spray Preparations—Insecticidal sprays are formulated in three ways—as solutions, emulsions or suspensions.

In preparing *solutions* the material may be dissolved in a suitable solvent such as crude or refined kerosene. The solutions are then ready for use. Many insecticide preparations containing pyrethrum, malathion, chlordane, lindane, methoxychlor, etc, for household use are distributed in solution form ready for application. Ultralow-volume (ULV) spraying by airplanes makes use of some of these.

When employed as *emulsions,* the chemical is dissolved in a solvent in combination with an emulsifying agent. It is usually highly concentrated. Such a concentrate is intended for dilution with water before use. Emulsion concentrates, for example, may contain 40 to 50% *carbaryl,* 45 to 50% xylene and 10% of an oil-soluble emulsifying agent. Depending on the intended use, this concentrate is added to water at rates varying from 1 part of concentrate to 4 or as much as 100 parts of water. Emulsion sprays are used widely in the agricultural field for controlling both plant and animal pests and for controlling household and industrial pests.

Suspensions are prepared in dry form similar to dusts but contain a wetting agent which makes it possible to prepare suspensions in water. These preparations in concentrate form usually are called wettable powders. These may contain from 15 to 75% of the active ingredient depending on the insecticide formulated.

Wettable powder concentrates (25 to 85%) are added to water for application at concentrations ranging from about 0.1 to 2.5% of the active ingredient. Wettable powder sprays are used on crops, livestock and as barn sprays. Such sprays are particularly useful for application to plants that might be sensitive to the oils employed for emulsions or solutions.

Bait Preparation—Many of the active ingredients have been formulated into insect baits. Baygon bait, is an effective example. In very restrictive areas, Amdro (amidinohydrazone) has been packaged as a bait inside a self-contained stick-on bait station. These can be effective in restaurant kitchen ceilings and similar areas.

Other Insecticide Preparations—Insecticides are employed in several other ways. Heat can be used to produce vapors or smokes for dispensing insecticides. This method also can be employed for treating greenhouses with insecticides for controlling insects and mites.

One of the most widely used methods of dispensing insecticides is the aerosol form. The *aerosol bomb* developed just prior to and during World War II, and employed by the military services, has gained general favor by civilians. Millions of the aerosol "bombs," now referred to as "pressure packs," are sold annually for dispensing insecticides in homes and industrial establishments for controlling flies, mosquitoes and other household pests. Pyrethrum, allethrin, organic thiocyanates and methoxychlor in various formulations are used most frequently as the insecticides. The insecticides are dissolved in a liquefied gas, such as butane or propane, plus a suitable solvent under pressure in the container. Producers are substituting the fluorocarbon propellents with hydrocarbons (butane or propane) because of concerns about the effect of fluorocarbons on the ozone layer in the atmosphere. When applied, the gas volatilizes instantly, leaving the insecticide and nonvolatile solvent suspended in the air as minute droplets that contact the insects present. Aerosols also are employed for applying insecticides in greenhouses.

The liquefied gas propellent also is used to apply "wet aerosols" or so-called "self-propelled" sprays. The water droplets here are larger than those usually obtained with aerosol propellants. The amount of nonvolatile solvent is increased so that the droplets are larger and will readily wet the surface treated. Such wet aerosol sprays are used for applying insect repellants to the skin or clothing or for applying insecticides as residual sprays for controlling various household insects.

The development of systemic insecticides for controlling plant and animal pests has led to other special methods of use. For control of cattle grubs in cattle, boluses containing the insecticide are administered orally. In using plant systemics the treatment of soils prior to planting with a slurry of the insecticides or insecticide granules is one of the methods of use.

Insecticidal strips of polymer impregnated with DDVP (*Vapona*) emit vapors for long periods of time. In areas of little human or animal activity these can be effective. Mosquito "coils," which are burned to release pesticides, are also important control measures. Fly traps are still available and catch these insects by sticky material (flypaper) or by attracting them into a device which resembles an inverted funnel from which they are unable to emerge.

Equipment for Applying Insecticides—Often, failure to obtain satisfactory results with insecticide preparations is due to improper equipment for their application. A knowledge of the type of equipment to employ is therefore important to the supplier of insecticides. Equipment might vary from small hand sprayers, or even paint brushes for use in homes, to large power sprayers for treating livestock, field crops, fruit or large shade trees. Use of airplanes and helicopters for insecticide dispersal is increasing steadily. The manufacturers of equipment, also county agents, entomologists and agricultural engineers with state and federal governments, as well as suppliers of insecticides, are in a position to give advice on insect control equipment to the potential user.

Control of Household Pests and Insects Attacking Man

The pharmacist often is asked to provide materials or advise on the control of insects, ticks and mites affecting man or those that are pests in homes or industrial establishments. Suggestions for the control of such arthropods are presented below.

General Considerations

The most important measure to follow in minimizing insect problems in the home or on the person is to practice *sanitation* and *good housekeeping*. Many of the pests in homes and industrial establishments, including mice, rats, cockroaches, ants and silverfish, depend on exposed foods or scraps of food for their existence. Cleanliness, therefore, will go a long way toward reducing the insect problem within homes, restaurants and other buildings. Pantry pests, such as grain moths and weevils of various kinds develop in flour, corn meal, dog biscuits and many other food products. An open container of oatmeal or dog biscuits hidden away in a pantry for several months can produce hundreds of moths or other pests that may continue to emerge over a period of weeks or months. Obviously, the simplest and best solution for such a problem is to destroy the source of the infestation rather than to use insecticides repeatedly.

A homeowner might be alarmed, and rightly so, when an infestation of fleas is detected in his home. In most modern dwellings the odds are great that the source of the fleas is the cat or dog which has not had proper care. The householder can minimize the danger of flying pests such as mosquitoes and flies getting into the premises by maintaining screen doors and windows in proper condition and by closing any openings into the home. Poorly cared-for garbage containers can be responsible for serious fly problems by attracting adult flies and by providing places for fly breeding. A few tin cans or tire casings that catch rainwater can provide the moisture essential for mosquito breeding on the premises.

Among the four general control measures for the prevention of insect and mite damage without chemicals are physical-control measures, mechanical methods, cultural-control procedures and biological methods. Physical control measures simply involve direct action by hand, such as removal of insect nests or egg masses. Mechanical-control methods involve use of equipment specifically designed to control insects, as applying sticky bands around tree trunks to trap tent caterpillars, frequent hosing of foliage to prevent red spider mites and mealybugs from taking hold. Cultural-control methods are based on knowledge of the life history and habit pattern of insects and controlling these in various ways, like cultivating the soil when many insects are in the pupal stage, breeding insect-resistant plants or interplanting. Interplanting marigolds, which discourage nematode growth, with tomatoes is an example. Use of the praying mantis, which devours insects, is an example of biological control.

It is recognized, however, that in spite of proper precautions, every home owner is likely to be faced with insect problems that must be solved by applying insect-control chemicals. In some cases, however, the solution is not simple. It may require knowledge of the habits of the pest, a thorough survey of the problem and know-how to control the pest involved. Often, it is not practical for the owner to attempt to do the job himself. In such circumstances the services of a licensed pest control operator (listed in the yellow pages of telephone directories) should be sought. The National Pest Control Association is in a position to advise on qualified pest-control firms in almost every city. County agents and entomologists in state experiment stations, and with the Federal Government, are prepared to give advice and furnish publications which will be helpful in many cases.

For insect control in living quarters, in food-handling establishments and on the person, the factor of safety in handling and applying toxic chemicals must be considered fully. Fortunately, a number of efficient insecticides have low levels of hazard to man and animals, although no insecticide can be considered completely harmless. The petroleum oil solvent most commonly used as the carrier in household sprays is in itself sufficiently hazardous to cause toxic effects if the operator is careless in use and permits overexposure to it.

Foods and food utensils should not be left uncovered while insecticides are being used. All food preparation surfaces, utensils and food serving areas should be cleaned thoroughly before the next use to avoid contamination by pesticide residues. Care is needed in handling and applying pesticides to avoid excessive inhalation or skin contact. All poisons should be stored so that they are inaccessible to children and unauthorized people or where they cannot be mistaken for food. It also must be kept in mind that many preparations containing petroleum oil are flammable or the vapors are explosive.

While stressing necessary precautions, it must be kept in mind that the proper use of insecticides should not be discouraged. Many pests in and around homes are capable of transmitting diseases, and experience has shown that the disease hazard may be far greater than that of the chemicals needed to control the insects responsible for propagating an epidemic.

Ants—Several species of ants are pests in the home or around the premises. In the past, poison baits of various kinds containing *arsenicals*, *thallium* or other poisons were used to destroy them. The use of thallium sulfate is no longer permitted as ant poison or for any other use around the home due to its excessive toxicity. Such methods are still effective under certain conditions but the use of newer sprays or dusts provides more effective and more rapid results.

Efforts should be made to locate the colony and destroy it if possible, although inside buildings the colony often cannot be found or may be inaccessible for treatment. The use of dusts and suitable sprays applied to the point of runoff on runways and other surfaces where ants have been seen, and along baseboards, borders of floors, window frames, doorsills and similar places usually will give satisfactory control, although follow-up treatments may be necessary. In general, the procedure for poisoning ants is similar to that for controlling roaches.

For ant control on lawns or in gardens, the best procedure is to locate the ant colony and apply Baygon, Dursban, Ficam or one of the other pyrethrin derivatives. Baygon, a carbamate insecticide, and Dursban, an organic phosphate insecticide, have become popular for this use. These currently are formulated at higher concentrations for use by professional applicators only. The material may be applied with a sprinkling can, sprayer or any other convenient method being sure to follow product labels, particularly those allowed for lawn use only. A concentration of 0.25% of these insecticides is suggested for treating individual mounds. The amount to apply varies with the size of the colony. A quart may be sufficient for small colonies and up to 3 gal may be necessary for large fire ant colonies a foot high and 2 to 3 feet in diameter at the base. The surface of the mound or soil should be disturbed by raking and the material poured on and around the nest.

Children and pets should not be permitted to play on the lawns until the area has been watered or rained on and allowed to dry. It is advised that the insecticide be washed off vegetation, into the ground, by sprinkling; this will not reduce the efficacy of the treatment.

Chlordane solution use has been suspended except for subsurface termite control and specific cases of fire ant and beetle control.

Chlorpyrifos (*Dursban*), and synergized pyrethrum sprays, may be employed for ant control in homes, but the use of lindane in vaporizers has been cancelled.

Bedbugs—The bedbug is controlled effectively by spraying thoroughly the bed frame, springs, edges and ticking of mattresses with 1 to 3% malathion by a professional applicator. Cracks, crevices and surfaces behind objects near a wall also should be treated. Bedbugs stay well hidden in such places. Spraying the bed and other hiding places to the point of running off of the solution will provide long-lasting control. The treated mattress should be aired well before use.

Chiggers—Chiggers or red bugs cause severe annoyance to many people. These mites are most common in southern and midwestern areas. Some individuals are particularly susceptible to chigger bites, especially if they have not previously been exposed to them.

The insect repellants dimethyl phthalate, dimethyl carbate, diethyltoluamide, 2-ethyl-1,3-hexanediol and benzyl benzoate, when applied to clothing, are excellent in preventing attack by chiggers. Permettrin aerosols for clothing treatment are also important. The repellants may be applied by hand to socks, inside cuffs of trousers and sleeves and the edges of any other openings in the clothing. Additional application of the repellant to the skin on the legs and forearms and base of neck will increase the probability of complete protection. Chiggers seldom attack the exposed portion of the body and are killed or repelled while crawling over treated clothing or exposed skin.

Clothing may be made repellant by light spraying, by drawing the mouth of the bottle along the parts of cloth to be treated (cuffs, fly, etc) or by complete impregnation of the cloth.

Although the repellants are highly effective in providing protection against chigger attack, persons often become exposed in areas where they do not expect chiggers to be present. After chiggers attack, there is no known treatment of the bites that will destroy the toxic substance which causes the irritation, although certain local anesthetics such as benzocaine will provide relief for several hours. A thorough, soapy bath as soon as chigger irritation is noted, which may be within a few hours after exposure, will reveal those attached and thus allow for removal and subsequent reduction of irritation.

Cockroaches—The German, American and brown-banded are the most common cockroach species found in homes and industrial establishments. Although the efficacy of different insecticides varies with the species, those in common use can be employed effectively in most instances. The German roach accounts for 98% of the problem in the US.

Most aerosol formulas contain pyrethrum, allethrin or resmethrin. Although intended primarily for flying insects, the aerosols can be used fairly effectively for roach control if applied in considerable amounts directly into the hiding places or released in high concentration in closed rooms. A thorough spray or dust treatment is considered more effective and longer-lasting. Many purchasers of aerosols expect roach control in the home by a light treatment. Such treatment, although satisfactory for flies, mosquitoes and similar pests, is inadequate for good roach control.

Boric acid and borax in finely powdered form, applied to hiding places and runways, are used for roach control, although they are less effective and slower to produce results than most other insecticides. The materials also are used in tablet form mixed with food baits which the roaches must eat. When well-distributed in office buildings or rooms where there is little food for roaches, they often provide satisfactory control.

Dursban (chlorpyrifos) sprays and dusts are widely used insecticides for roach control. The sprays, either oil-base or prepared from an emulsifiable concentrate, should contain about 2% and dusts about 5% of the insecticide as described on the label. During the day, roaches usually remain well hidden in cracks, crevices and behind objects. It is important to know where the roaches hide and where they run. The coarse, wet insecticide sprays are applied into these runways and hiding places. A few puffs of a mist spray will not provide satisfactory control. A paint brush may be used to apply the solution instead of a sprayer, if label directions allow it. A dust should be blown directly into hiding places and placed along runways. Dursban [*O,O*-diethyl-*O*-(3,5,6-trichloro-2-pyridyl)phosphorothionate] may be recommended as a first-use agent. *Ficam* (2,2-dimethyl-1,3-benzodioxol-4-yl) or *bendiocarb* (generic name) also is useful and is popular as a highly effective broad-spectrum carbamate insecticide for control of at least six species of cockroach.

Pyrethrum sprays or dusts usually will provide satisfactory roach control. It is necessary, however, to treat with pyrethrum often to obtain and maintain control. The use of synergists with this insecticide has made it more effective.

When chlorinated hydrocarbon resistance is encountered in roaches, malathion as a 1 to 2% spray has proved to be an effective substitute. Diazinon [*O,O*-diethyl-*O*-(2-isopropyl-4-methyl-6-pyrimidinyl)phosphorothioate] also has proved useful where roach resistance has been a problem. The residual life of malathion is generally less than that obtained with methoxychlor prior to the appearance of insecticide-resistant strains.

Fleas—Fleas often are pests in homes and even in lawns in some areas. Infestations usually are associated with the presence of cats, dogs, rats or other animals. To prevent recurrence of fleas, the source of the trouble should be treated. For dogs, powders containing 1% lindane, pyrethrum or rotenone are used per label directions. For cats, only rotenone or pyrethrum insecticides are recommended, because these animals are very susceptible to the toxic effects of chlorinated hydrocarbons. If the source of the fleas is rats, the host animals should be eliminated by following suitable rodent-control measures. Actual flea control in homes is usually not difficult. Bedding where dogs sleep should be removed and the area thoroughly cleaned. Ordinary household sprays containing pyrethrum also may be used although several repeat treatments may be required. Certain volatile organophosphate insecticides are the active ingredients of "flea collars" for dogs and cats. A new insect growth regulator, methoprene, is giving effective indoor flea control. This agent interferes with the life cycle of insects undergoing complete metamorphosis.

Finally, attention must be given to the pesticide label precautions. Some dogs and many cats are allergic to collars. Malathion as well as Sevin (carbaryl) are excellent materials for the control of fleas in the home or in infested yards.

Flies—For most homes or industrial establishments flies can be eliminated by using ordinary household sprays or aerosols. The most common ones consist of deodorized kerosene, about 0.1% pyrethrins or allethrin and 0.75% of a synergist such as piperonyl butoxide or sulfoxide. Many variations in percentages of such insecticides are included in different formulations. Aerosol formulas often contain from 0.25 to 0.6% pyrethrins or allethrin, 0.8 to 1% of a synergist and from 1 to 2% methoxychlor. The method of using the sprays or aerosols generally is known and usually well-described on the labels.

If flies are a serious problem on the premises, other methods of control must be followed. During recent years the use of poison baits has become more widespread. Dry sugar containing 1% Bayer L 13/59, malathion or Diazinon sprinkled around the premises where flies congregate has given good control. The use of these materials in sweetened liquid bait (syrup in sugar) sprinkled in such places also has been used with good success.

Malathion and Diazinon sprays used as residual treatments outdoors around homes, in livestock buildings (including inside dairy barns) and similar places have come into use. When used according to label directions, these materials often provide good fly control up to several weeks after application. Fly traps (paper) and mechanical devices for trapping are still available and popular.

Itch Mite—Many preparations have been employed for controlling the itch mite, or *scabies*. One of the most successful was the NBIN emulsion employed for head-louse control. It is important that all portions of the body be treated, and that a bath be delayed for about 12 hours after treatment. A second treatment may be needed after 1 week although one thorough treatment will usually eliminate the infestation.

Lice—Three kinds of lice attack man: the *body louse*, *head louse* and *crab (pubic) louse*. In the US head louse and pubic louse infestations are more common than those of the body louse.

Body louse infestations can be controlled by regular changes of clothing and sterilization of all wearing apparel and bedding. When the use of insecticides is indicated, a thorough dusting of the clothing with 1% lindane dust is recommended, according to label directions. The Department of Defense and the World Health Organization are considering the adoption of a 1% malathion dust if final toxicological clearance is obtained. This substitute treatment if approved will provide a highly efficient material for louse control. Synergized pyrethrum dusts are also highly effective for body louse control. Later investigations showed that the synergists piperonyl butoxide is equally as effective as the *n*-butyl undecylenamide. It also has been found that allethrin is about as effective as pyrethrins in such formulations. The material most commonly used today for head and body lice treatment is synergized pyrethrum (eg, the OTC product RID).

Head louse infestations are controlled readily with benzyl benzoate followed by a thorough shampoo the next morning. Weekly treatments may be needed. Since eggs are not destroyed easily, treatments should be repeated. One treatment applied to the hair on the head before bedtime will kill all motile stages of the lice, which may be brushed or washed out of the hair in the morning.

Crab louse infestations are controlled effectively with any of the preparations discussed under *head louse*. It is important that all hairy portions of the body be treated.

Mosquitoes—Mosquitoes which occasionally enter homes can be killed easily with the type of space sprays and aerosols discussed in connection with fly control. Mosquitoes often breed in areas several miles from the places where they are serious nuisances. Community mosquito control programs are the only real solution to this problem. The problem of achieving satisfactory mosquito control in a community is usually so complex and extensive that the help and advice of specialists are necessary.

Persons exposed to mosquitoes, biting gnats and flies outdoors in connection with work or recreation can obtain relief by applying skin repellants. The most common individual repellants available on the market are diethyltoluamide, dimethyl phthalate, ethohexadiol (Rutgers 612), dimethyl carbate and Indalone. Various combinations of these also are available. All of these materials used as directed on container labels will provide transient relief from insect attack.

In some circumstances treatment of the exposed skin alone is inadequate because the mosquitoes also may bite through clothing. The application of repellants to clothing by impregnation, by light spraying or by hand will prevent the attack. The same repellant materials intended for skin application may be used. Most of the repellants are plasticizers. They should not be applied to rayons and similar synthetic clothing. Repellents such as dimethyl phthalate (DIMP) are good plasticizers but diethylmethyltoluamide (DEET) is a poor or very weak plasticizer.

Moths and Carpet Beetles—Every home owner is likely to encounter damage due to clothes moths or carpet beetles, often called "buffalo" moths. The damage caused by these insects to woolens and other items such as furs, materials made of animal hair or feathers is very great.

For many years the fumigants, naphthalene and paradichlorobenzene, were the chief means of control. It takes a high concentration of vapor to kill clothes moths or carpet beetles, however. Many pounds of these fumigants are needed to eliminate infestations in closets that are not tight or where the doors are opened too often to permit sufficient concentration of vapor. In using these fumigants add crystals, flakes or balls at the rate of 1 lb/100 ft^3 and make closets tight by sealing cracks and edges of doors. Since the gas is considerably heavier than air, the fumigant should be placed high in the closet. For protecting clothing, furs, etc in trunks and other storage spaces for long periods, about 1 lb for an average-size trunk is sufficient.

In stuffed furniture it is often difficult to get the insecticide to the infestation. Fumigation in vaults by companies prepared to do such work may be necessary. The use of methoxychlor and lindane sprays as contact insecticides and as residual sprays were used in controlling moth infestations in homes but are being phased out or already unavailable. All of these materials will kill the different stages on contact. Methoxychlor is not highly effective as a residual deposit, however, for killing carpet beetles which crawl over treated surfaces. Lindane is superior for this purpose.

As a surface spray or dust to eliminate general infestations in a home, Dycarb (bendiocarb), Dursban, diazinon or resmethrin are effective; the spray or dust being applied to the edges of rugs, floor area between rug and wall and baseboards. In closets, the floors, corners, walls, etc should be treated. Also behind pictures, radiators and other hard-to- clean places. The entire rug may be sprayed with methoxychlor. Lindane is not recommended for general treatment in homes because of possible excessive vapors or skin contact that might be hazardous. Limited spot treatment is advocated for these materials. Other materials, such as fluoride solutions, are also satisfactory for treatment of rugs and similar items. Directions on the label should be followed at all times.

Moth infestations are destroyed and woolen items effectively protected against subsequent infestations by treating with paradichlorobenzene, naphthalene or DDVP (dichlorvos).

Silverfish—For the control of silverfish, use carefully applied residual insecticide sprays and dusts such as bendiocarb, diazinon, propoxur and silica gel. Silverfish may be found in many places in the home—basement, attic, around books and behind wall paper. They feed on the starchy material used as glues or for sizing paper.

Ticks—Ticks are serious pests in some areas. If the infested areas must be used, it is possible to kill the ticks by following the procedures suggested for area chigger control. Protection of individuals from tick attack, however, is fairly effective if clothing is thoroughly impregnated with certain repellants. Emulsions of dimethyl phthalate and diethyltoluamide may be used for such treatment.

Insecticides, Fumigants and Repellants

The number of insecticides and repellants currently in use has increased greatly during the past 30 years. New synthetic compounds have come into use for many pests for which practical chemical control methods were unknown, and in some cases have largely replaced certain inorganic compounds and insecticides of plant origin. However, some of the more recently developed chemicals are being replaced by even newer materials because of development of resistance by various insects to insecticides. This is a problem of major significance in insect control. The housefly, for example, became resistant to DDT and other chlorinated hydrocarbon insecticides within 5 to 10 years after they came into extensive use. Organic phosphorus insecticides were developed as substitutes but within a few years evidence of resistance to them became apparent. A wide variety of insects affecting man, livestock, fruits, vegetables and cotton are resistant to one or more of the newer insecticides. Currently, the resistant strains still are restricted generally to certain localities. However, authorities in insect control generally are agreed that such local resistance problems are likely to become more widespread with continued use of the materials. The use of piperonyl butoxide as a mixed-function oxidase inhibitor and an inducer of cytochrome P450 has led to the reduction of resistance to many insecticides by many insects.

The more widely employed insect control chemicals and their areas of use will be discussed briefly. The extensive literature on the many insecticides may be consulted for further details and the US Dept of Agriculture, state experiment stations, the US Public Health Service and manufacturers of specific insecticides are prepared to provide more detailed information. The EPA should be consulted for the latest information about a particular pesticide since its status may change at any time. A chart for emergency treatment of acute pesticide poisoning is available from the US Navy Disease Vector Ecology and Control Center, Jacksonville, FL 32212.

Common Insecticides

Allethrin (*dl*-2-allyl-4-hydroxy-3-methyl-2-cyclopenten-1-one esterified with a mixture of *cis* and *trans dl*-chrysanthemum monocarboxylic acids)—This synthetic pyrethrin-like compounds has been developed as the result of basic studies on the complex composition of the active principles in pyrethrum insecticides. It has many of the desirable features of pyrethrum—high insecticidal activity with low toxicity to warm-blooded animals. In general, allethrin is effective against the same insects as pyrethrum. For some species such as the *housefly* and the *body louse* it is equally as effective, but against others it is less effective than pyrethrum. At present it can be produced commercially at a cost somewhat lower than the cost of the pyrethrins (principal active ingredients in pyrethrum). This advantage in practical use is offset, however, due to the fact that the insecticidal activity of allethrin is not increased to the same degree as the pyrethrins when combined with synergists available at present.

The development of allethrin is of great significance however. It is now used in household sprays and aerosols as a substitute for pyrethrins or to supplement the pyrethrins. The Dept of Defense uses the insecticide in sprays and aerosols supplied to troops. Research has shown that allethrin is highly efficient for the control of lice affecting man. The availability of allethrin assures a supply of a pyrethrum-like insecticide in the event our source of supply of pyrethrum is cut off or greatly reduced as during World War II.

Arsenicals—The arsenicals, including *Paris green* (an acetoarsenite of copper), *lead arsenate, calcium arsenate, calcium arsenite* and *sodium arsenite,* are among the older insecticides. Arsenicals are still employed to a limited extent as dusts and sprays for controlling a variety of *chewing insects,* for use as dips for *ticks* and other livestock pests, in poison baits for *fly* control or for controlling *cutworms* and as larvicides for *Anopheles mosquitoes.* Due to the development and availability of many new insecticides equally as effective and often less hazardous to plants and animals the arsenicals have been largely replaced by other insecticides. Some use is seen in herbicides, wood preservatives and plant dessicants though not widespread. In the suspended and cancelled list of the EPA (May 1978) and Oct 1979, arsenic trioxide in excess of 1.5% and sodium arsenite in excess of 2.0% are listed as unacceptable for home use. The following statements must appear prominently on labels: "Do not use or store in or around the home" and "Do not allow domestic animals to graze treated area." Organic arsenicals are at present of the most pesticidal interest because of their value as selective herbicides, e.g., cacodylic acid, DSMA, etc.

Fluorine Compounds—*Sodium fluoride,* one of several fluorine compounds, has served a useful purpose for controlling *roaches* and *silverfish* in homes and industrial establishments, but it is not much used today. In the suspended and cancelled list of the EPA (May 1978), sodium fluoride is cancelled for home use if the product contains more than 40% of this compound. Sodium fluoroacetate has been cancelled for use in mammalian predator control; the label should have instructons for predator use blocked out. The Jan 1985 Suspended and Cancelled List of EPA lists only fluoroacetamide which is allowed for use only inside of sewers against the Norway and roof rat by a certified applicator. Sulfuryl fluoride is still used as a restricted use pesticide due to its inhalation hazards.

Lime-Sulfur (Calcium polysulfides)—Originally used as a *sheep dip* for the control of *mites* and *ticks,* lime-sulfur in liquid and dry form is now better known as a dormant spray for the control of *scale insects* and as a summer spray for the control of certain *plant diseases.* For the methods of using the lime-sulfur liquid concentrate, follow the recommendations on the container. It generally is used to control Apple scab and powdery skin irritation mildews.

Nicotine—This, the volatile liquid alkaloid of tobacco (*Nicotiana tabacum*), is a powerful insecticide; however, it is highly toxic to the nervous system of man and other animals. Nicotine extracts usually are obtained from the stems and refuse parts of tobacco. It is available in two forms, namely, free nicotine and nicotine sulfate. The latter is available mainly as a 40% aqueous solution. For the common garden sprays to control *aphids* (*plant lice*) and similar insects, the nicotine sulfate is the form commonly used although dusts containing nicotine sulfate are also available. It kills a wide range of both chewing and sucking insects. Soap or saponin (obtainable from Merck & Co) should always be used with nicotine sulfate unless combined with an alkaline solution such as Bordeaux mixture or lime-sulfur. This is needed to release the nicotine, which is the active killing agent.

It is effective as a destructive agent for *plant lice* and also serves as an efficient stomach poison for some pests. It is water-soluble, but should be kept in tightly stoppered containers as it decomposes very quickly. Nicotine, as used, does not injure the most delicate foliage. It generally is considered to be most effective as a contact insecticide when used during the warm part of the day.

Free nicotine was used for fumigating greenhouses.

It has lost much of its popularity in recent years, due to the introduction of new, synthetic chemicals having improved effectiveness and equal or greater safety. It is no longer produced in the US.

Oil Sprays—Oils made from petroleum are among the insecticides that have been used for many years, chiefly as contact insecticides for *scale insects* and *mites* attacking plants. They are very important today. Oils will destroy other insects however, including *aphids, thrips, leafhoppers* and *eggs* of certain *Lepidopterous* spp.

There are two classes of oils used as insecticides: the *dormant oils* and *summer oils.* The dormant oils are applied to more hardy trees during the dormant period. The summer oils are used on fruit and vegetable crops during the growing season. The chief differences between the two types are the degree of refinement and their heaviness or viscosity, which determine in part the degree of phytotoxicity. The oils are applied as emulsions which permit dilution with water and more uniform distribution on the plants. The concentration of oil in the finished spray for citrus usually ranges from 1.66 to 2.0%. Small amounts of insecticides such as parathion added to the oil sprays increases their efficacy against various insects.

Pyrethrum—Pyrethrum flowers, the first widely used insecticide, possess unusually fast contact action against many insects causing paralysis in a few minutes. Their low mammalian toxicity and rapid toxic action against many pests are features that are not present in the newer materials.

The active substances, pyrethrins I and II, occur in the oleoresin secretion of certain floral parts (achenes) of the closed or partially open flowers. A maximum of about 1.4% of pyrethrins has been adopted by the foremost manufacturers of pyrethrum insecticides.

Formerly, pyrethrum insecticides were prepared as dusts by using the finely ground flowers or were prepared and used as liquids by extracting the active ingredients from the flowers with special fractions of light petroleum oil, preferably odorless kerosene. Today, manufacturers extract and concentrate the active ingredients in products containing about 20% pyrethrins. This concentrate is used to prepare the various preparations employed by the public including dusts, petroleum oil solutions, emulsion concentrates, wettable powders and aerosol formulations.

Pyrethrum still is used as an ingredient in most household sprays and aerosols chiefly for its *knockdown* effects against insects. It also is used in dusts and liquid preparations for controlling a variety of garden pests and *fleas, lice* and *ticks* on pets.

The continued prominent place of pyrethrum as an insecticide has been maintained chiefly because of the development of chemicals which, when combined with pyrethrum, have the remarkable property of increasing the insecticidal activity of the insecticide even though the material added alone has little or no insecticidal properties. This cooperative potentiation is known as *synergism.*

These compounds include piperonyl butoxide, sulfoxide and others and are called "synergists." The development of these synergists has increased the range of activity of pyrethrins and at the same time permits reduction in the cost of formulas containing it.

"Synergized" pyrethrum combinations, although not so long-lasting as the chlorinated hydrocarbon insecticides, are used chiefly in household sprays and aerosols for *flies, mosquitoes* and other *household pests,* in liquid and dust preparations for controlling *external parasites* on pets, as sprays for flies on dairy cattle, and as dusts and sprays for controlling certain *vegetable pests.* Synergized pyrethrum powders and liquids were employed extensively for a time in controlling *lice* attacking man during World War II. Some newer preparations include Pyrefume, Pyrellin, Pyrenone, Pyrexcel and Pyrocide. Most of these contain pyrethrins in varying concentrations and other materials such as piperonyl butoxide, rotenone, or ryania. Many pyrethroid synthetics have been found effective and now are registered for use. These include newer allethrin derivatives, resmethrin products and *S*-bioallethrin.

Rotenone—This is a useful botanical insecticide and represents the chief chemical constituent of derris (*D elliptica* and *D chinensis*) and cubé roots (species of *Lonchocarpus*) and other sources. Rotenone ($C_{23}H_{22}O_6$) is commercially available as such or in the form of derris and cubé roots, sold with assayed rotenone content, usually 5%.

It is classified incorrectly as a nontoxic insecticide. It can cause skin irritation. Its use for louse control on humans is not recommended since irritation often is produced, especially in the groin region. On internal administration in moderately large doses, especially in the presence of fatty foods, it is very toxic to higher animals. In general, however, rotenone insecticides are considered low in hazard. The relatively small amounts applied and rapid loss of toxic action results in minor residues on food crops. Rotenone is used mainly to kill unwanted fish in a pond prior to restocking.

Its paralyzing action on insects is slower than that of pyrethrum but more certain, with usually no recoveries. As a dry, crystalline powder, it is odorless and relatively stable. It is soluble in alcohol, oils, chloroform and carbon tetrachloride (used in the extraction from the crude drug and its quantitative determination). It is slightly soluble in water, but aqueous sprays, particularly in the presence of alkaline soaps, quickly deteriorate and must be prepared fresh before use.

Its dusts at concentrations ranging from 0.75 to 1.0% still are used to control pests such as the *Mexican bean beetle, cabbage worms, leaf hoppers* and other insects attacking a variety of vegetables. It is especially useful for application to vegetables near the time for harvest when certain of the effective newer insecticides cannot be used because of potentially excessive residues.

It also is used for controlling insect parasites of animals. It is effective for controlling *cattle grubs,* and is employed also for *lice, fleas* and *ticks* on pets and livestock.

Sulfur is used widely in insecticide preparations. It formerly was used for controlling such insects as *plant mites, fleahoppers* on cotton, *lice* on livestock and *chiggers.* The new insecticides available today are far more efficient than sulfur for most insects. However, it is still one of the more effective insecticides for certain species of plant mites. Sulfur also is used in combination with many other insecticide dusts as a diluent. It serves a useful purpose in such combinations in controlling or preventing a buildup of mites and for the control of *plant diseases.* It is employed as a spray made from wettable sulfur or is used in wettable powder preparations containing other insecticides.

Other Materials—A number of other insecticides that have been used as pesticides, but for limited purposes, include *pentachlorophenol* (C_6Cl_5OH), widely used as a wood preservative to control termites, other wood infesting insects and wood rots (it is under investigation for dioxin contamination and the health ramifications of this contaminant); *Ryania,* a plant product containing alkaloids, used to some extent for controlling corn borers and codling moths on apples, and *sabadilla,* another plant product, which is effective for controlling squash bugs, lygus bugs and harlequin bugs.

Also of interest in the biopesticide group are the *avermectins.* These are macrocyclic lactones isolated from the soil organism *Streptomyces avermitilis.* One product is available under the trade name Affirm (MSD). It is available as a 0.011% insecticidal bait or as a granular powder for application on turf, lawns or other noncrop, wide outdoor areas (not allowed on pastures, rangeland or croplands). It also is used to treat guinea worm and other parasitic organisms.

Another interesting modern pesticide of biological origin is *neem.* This is a general name given the plant and its products. It is a subtropical shade tree (*Azadirachta indica*) native to the arid regions of India, Pakistan and parts of Africa. Its most important constituent is a limonoid compound named azadirachtin. The tree has been known for centuries as being free of insects, disease and nematodes. All parts of the tree, especially the seeds, are resistant. The bark, leaves and fruit have been used in traditional medicinal remedies and various extracts have been long used as insect repellents and antifeedants in Asia. Recently, Margosan-O, a neem formulation, has been approved by the EPA (1985) for limited use as a pesticide on nonfood crops.

In June 1993 the Clinton administration announced an effort to encourage farmers to reduce their use of pesticides. This was partly due to a National Academy of Sciences report which said that pesticides may have a greater effect on children and that studies should be expanded to determine the possible dangers to children who may consume more pesticides relative to their body weight.

Leaders in biotechnology are expanding efforts to circumvent the use of pesticides and hope to replace 10 to 20% of the current chemical pesticides in use. Already, biotechnology is being used to develop squash plants which are immune to a killer virus by activating the plant's natural defenses. In a similar way, hybrid corn, using genes from rare species, may allow for resistance to corn borer worm.

Opponents are concerned that biotechnology raises ethical questions about tinkering with nature. Of course, this approach will take time and money to see if it will be successful. Until then, the older advice of shopping for fresh vegetables frequently, serving a variety of fruits and washing and peeling vegetables should be continued to minimize pesticide residue consumption.

Chlorinated Hydrocarbon Insecticides

The advances in insect control since about 1940 have been phenomenal because of the development and extensive use of a variety of chemical compounds broadly classified as synthetic chlorinated hydrocarbons. The use of this class of insecticides began with DDT, which was employed first in Switzerland, but within a decade a number of new similar insecticides of comparable, or in some instances greater, insecticidal activity came into use. These materials, although effective against similar pests in many instances, vary in their usefulness for controlling insects. Insect species vary in their susceptibility to the different compounds. In addition, a factor of great significance that limits the practical use of many insecticides is the hazard associated with their use. Some of the insecticides possess long residual action—which may be of great advantage in controlling certain pests—but which is an objectionable feature when applied to food plants consumed by man and animals. Some of the materials are stored in fat or are excreted in milk of animals when the residues are consumed on forage treated for insect control or when the insecticides are applied to the animals for controlling pests. Such residues of some insecticides may persist for months while others are eliminated within a few days or weeks.

Because of the residue problem, DDT use was canceled, and aldrin and dieldrin have been cancelled for all uses except subsurface ground insertion for termite control, dipping of nonfood roots and tops and mothproofing by manufacturing processes in a closed system.

Obviously, it is not possible in this chapter to discuss in detail the many uses for the various chlorinated hydrocarbon insecticides. The formulation to use, amount to apply, method and time of application, precautions that must be observed in avoiding harmful residues on the harvested crop and many other aspects must be considered. Only a brief discussion of the more important compounds in this class and their areas of use follows.

Lindane is used in household sprays and dusts on livestock and other animals and for controlling some *pests on fruits and vegetables.* When *lice* resistant to 10% DDT powder appeared in Korea the Department of Defense substituted a 1% lindane dust for controlling this insect attacking man.

The acute oral toxicity of lindane to animals is somewhat higher than DDT, but when absorbed through the skin it is more toxic than DDT. Lindane possesses high insecticidal activity in vapor form. This property has resulted in certain restricted use for the compound in devices that generate vapors with the aid of heat. In the Jan 1985 EPA List of Suspended, Canceled and Restricted Pesticides, lindane has been canceled for use in vaporizers, canceled for indoor use in smoke fumigation devices and a host of new restrictions developed for limited use on commercial and homeowner ornamentals, hardwood logs and lumber, dog dips, moth sprays, seed treatments, flea collars, etc.

Chlordane [*Velsicol* 1068, CD-68, *Octachlor, Octa-Klor*; 1,2,4,5,-6,7,8,8-octachloro-2,3,3a,4,7,7a-hexahydro-4,7-methanoindene]—This insecticide, developed in the US, is a viscous amber-colored liquid, nearly odorless. It is readily soluble in a wide variety of solvents.

As of Oct 1979, the EPA lists chlordane as suspended for all uses except subsurface ground insertion for termite control, dipping of roots or tops of nonfood plants, in federal/state quarantine programs for the Japanese beetle and imported fire ant, control of blackvine weevil on Japanese yew in Michigan, control of Texas Harvester ant in Oklahoma, control of white-fringed beetle attacking food crops in eight southwestern states of the US, control of soil insects attacking Florida citrus root weevils, control of strawberry root pests by preplant treatments and control of white grubs in Michigan. Other specific uses still are allowed but it is being phased out completely. See the Jan 1985 EPA list. In the US only, the emulsifiable formulation concentrate of chlordane alone or in combination with heptachlor is used for subterranean termite control applications.

DDT [dichlorodiphenyltrichloroethane; 1,1,1-trichloro-2,2-bis(*p*-chlorophenyl)ethane]—This crystalline substance is practically odorless, with low vapor pressure and high toxic action to a wide range of insects. One of its chief uses was in the field of medical entomology, particularly for controlling *mosquito larvae* and *adults, flies, body lice, bedbugs* and *fleas.* It also was used extensively for controlling pests of livestock, farm crops, forest and shade trees and stored products. Due to its persistence and ubiquitous nature, and its accumulation and storage in various members of the food chain, with possible deleterious results, its use in the US was cancelled in 1972. Emergency use is permitted only with EPA approval (see introduction). The Oct 1979 EPA list classifies DDT as canceled except for use by the US Public Health Service and other health service officials for control of vector diseases, for the US Dept of Agriculture or the military for health quarantine, in drugs for controlling body lice (to be dispensed by a physician), and in the formulation of prescription drugs for controlling body lice. These restrictions are continued by the EPA (1985 List, above). All uses, except emergency public health uses and a very few other uses permitted on a case basis, have been canceled as of January 1, 1973.

Ethyl 4,4-Dichlorobenzilate [Chlorobenzilate]—This is an effective ascaricide-miticide, marketed as *Ascaraben* for the use on citrus only, and only with specified restrictions (Jan 1985).

Heptachlor [1,4,5,6,7,8,8-heptachloro-3a,4,7,7a-tetrahydro-4,7-methanoindene]—A crystalline compound chemically related to chlordane, highly active against a wide range of insects. Most registered products containing heptachlor have been canceled.

Methoxychlor [1,1,1-trichloro-2,2-*bis*(*p*-methoxyphenyl)ethane]—This insecticide has chemical and physical properties similar to those of DDT. The chief advantage of this over other chlorinated hydrocarbon insecticides is its low hazard to animals. It is satisfactory for controlling *flies* and other *household pests,* including *clothes moths* and *flies* and *lice* on livestock, *Mexican bean beetles* and a variety of other insects attacking fruit, vegetable and forage crops. It is available in 25 to 50% concentration in various application forms.

Methoxychlor is one of the few chlorinated hydrocarbon insecticides that is not readily stored in animal fat or excreted in milk when consumed as residues on forage crops. For this reason it is used for controlling various insects on livestock feeds and forage. It also was used as a spray for controlling flies and lice on dairy cows but is no longer used thus because small amounts of the insecticide occur in milk.

Toxaphene—This substance is a reproducible mixture of 175 or more polychloro derivatives of camphene produced by chlorination of the latter to a content of 67 to 69% chlorine, representing the empirical formula $C_{10}H_{10}Cl_8$. It is a yellow, waxy solid, practically insoluble in water. This product has had most of its uses suspended by the EPA except for scabies control on cattle and sheep and minor use for army worm, cutworm, grasshopper and mealybug control.

Miticides

A variety of synthetic organic insecticides are used for controlling mites on plants, in addition to older insecticides such as sulfur and the organic phosphates discussed in the next section. Among the compounds used are *Ovex* (*p*-chlorophenyl *p*-chlorobenzenesulfonate), and *Kelthane* (1,1-bis(*p*-chlorophenyl)-2,2,2-trichloroethanol), used extensively on fruits and vegetables. These miticides may be used as dusts or sprays, and they often are combined with other insecticide applications or in insecticide-fungicide formulations.

Organic Phosphorus Compounds

A large variety of organic compounds of phosphorus possess high insecticidal activity. They often are referred to as organophosphorus compounds. Some of these compounds also have unusually high potency as miticides, and many are also extremely toxic to man and other warm-blooded animals because of their action as irreversible inhibitors of cholinesterase.

A number of human fatalities in the US and other parts of the world have occurred as a result of exposure to phosphate insecticides and many other persons have suffered ill effects. It is important, therefore, that the more toxic of these insecticides be handled with extreme caution and strictly in accordance with recommendations outlined by the manufacturer and federal and state agencies.

The reputation of the organic phosphorus insecticides is such that, to the uninformed, most compounds in this class are regarded as being dangerous to use. This is a misconception. The mammalian toxicity of some of the compounds is of a low order, and they can be handled with no more danger than that associated with the use of a number of the synthetic chlorinated hydrocarbon insecticides which are employed without serious toxic reactions.

The organophosphorus compounds will control a wide range of pests and disease carriers. Certain of these compounds possess systemic action, a characteristic that offers great promise for controlling important insect pests of crops as well as livestock.

The organic phosphorus insecticides are used extensively, in many instances replacing in part, at least, some of the chlorinated hydrocarbons and older insecticides such as rotenone. This trend is due to several factors. Resistance to the chlorinated hydrocarbons by a number of pests has necessitated substitute materials possessing a different mode of insecticidal action. Several of the organic phosphorus compounds do not accumulate in meat and milk as readily as do certain chlorinated hydrocarbon insecticides when consumed as residues on forage crops.

The phosphorus insecticides have not been in use as long as the older materials and relatively few insects have become resistant to them. There is no assurance, however, that many pests will not in time become resistant to the phosphorus materials. A number of species of mites on plants became resistant within a few years, and, as already mentioned, the house fly also has developed resistance to certain organic phosphorus compounds. There is some evidence, however, that in some insect species, resistance to the phosphorus insecticides does not develop to the high level of the chlorinated hydrocarbons.

Organic phosphorus insecticides generally destroy a wide range of insect species. Consequently, their use often kills many parasites, predators and pollinating insects, as well as the destructive pests.

The more widely used organic phosphorus insecticides are described briefly, and some of their more important uses are given.

Ciodrin [3-hydroxycrotonic acid α-methylbenzyl ester dimethyl phosphate; Crotoxyphos]—An insecticide for control of animal parasites and for premises use.

Diazinon [*O,O*-diethyl *O*-(2-isopropyl-4-methyl-6-pyrimidinyl)-phosphorothioate; Spectracide *Knox Out*]—An amber-colored liquid with a somewhat objectionable odor in its technical form; it is an excellent insecticide. It is less toxic than parathion but more so than malathion to warm-blooded animals. It is highly toxic to flies as a contact and residual spray as well as a stomach poison and is in use for controlling these insects both as sprays and in poison baits. It also is effective against aphids, mites, leafhoppers, the codling moth, fruitflies, cabbage worms, mosquitoes, roaches and other insects. Some resistant strains of houseflies have been reported. It also is used as a bait to control scavenger yellowjackets in 11 contiguous western states.

Dibrom (1,2-dibromo-2,2-dichloroethyl dimethylphosphate; Naled)—A broad-spectrum insecticide for both plant protection and premises use. Not approved for use in grain bins.

Dipterex [*O,O*-dimethyl 2,2,2-trichloro-1-hydroxyethylphosphonate; *trichlorofon*]—A white, crystalline solid; soluble in water. The material also known as Bayer L 13/59 is used in poison baits for controlling flies and for controlling many different species of insects. Its toxicity to warm-blooded animals is reported to be of a low order.

EPN [*O*-ethyl *O-p*-nitrophenyl phenylphosphonothioate; Velsicol]—An amber liquid, effective against a wide range of pests, including aphids, mites, scale insects, the European corn borer, mosquito larvae, boll weevil, pink bollworm, codling moth, plum curculio and others. It is slightly less toxic to warm-blooded animals than parathion but merits the same degree of extreme caution in its use. In 1985, the EPA listed a host of specific cancellations and new hazard warnings for it.

Guthion [*O,O*-dimethyl *S*-(4-oxo-3*H*-1,2,3-benzotriazine-3-methyl) phosphorodithionate; *azinphosmethyl*]—A compound, also known as Bayer 17147; it is a crystalline material relatively insoluble in water.

It has a wide spectrum of activity as a contact insecticide for the control of insect pests. It is generally more persistent on plants than other commonly used organophosphorus insecticides. The material is employed as a dust or spray. Although the toxicity of Guthion is somewhat lower than that of parathion, it is in the class of highly toxic materials and must be handled with extreme caution. It is finding wide use for controlling cotton insects, particularly the boll weevil, which has become resistant to chlorinated hydrocarbon insecticides. It is also highly effective for the control of fruit pests such as the plum curculio, codling moth, stink bugs, aphids and mites. This has proven useful in integrated fruit pest control. Some or all applications may be classified by EPA as RUPs.

Malathion—This phosphorus compound, *S*-(1,2-dicarbethoxyethyl)-*O,O*-dimethyldithiophosphate, as produced commercially, is a light-amber liquid, having a sulfur-like odor. It is relatively low in toxicity to most warm-blooded animals and is active against a wide range of insects, although in general it is less effective than parathion or TEPP. The much lower toxicity to warm-blooded animals and rapid loss of residues on plants make it an acceptable insecticide for many uses.

It is used extensively for controlling insects on vegetables, fruits and cereal and forage crops as well as for controlling insects affecting man and animals. The residues disappear in a few days to two weeks, thus permitting application near the harvest period. The compound is available commercially as emulsifiable concentrates, wettable powders, dusts and for ultra-low-volume spraying. In the US Malathion ULV concentrate is the only grade registered for use on stored grain, recommended for use inside homes and accepted for use on humans. Over 25 commercial products are marketed in the US which contain this ingredient.

Methyl Parathion—Closely related to parathion with insecticidal and toxic properties somewhat similar to it. It is employed for controlling mites, aphids, thrips and other insects, including such pests as the boll weevil. Some or all applications now classified by EPA as RUPs.

Phorate [*O,O*-diethyl *S*-(ethylthio)methyl phosphorodithioate; Thimet]—A liquid material with an objectionable odor. It is relatively insoluble in water. It is one of the more toxic of the organophosphorus insecticides and must be handled with extreme caution. It is primarily systemic in action and is absorbed readily by the roots of plants when applied to the seeds or when added to the soil. It has had limited use for controlling aphids, spider mites, thrips, leafhoppers and certain other insects on cotton and sugar beets. It is now classed as an RUP by EPA.

Phosdrin [1-methoxycarbonyl-1-propen-2-yl dimethyl phosphate; Mevinphos]—A contact and systemic insecticide-acaricide with broad range of use on vegetable, fruit, field and forage crops. It is a liquid material, miscible with water and quite volatile. Its toxicity is high, and it must be employed with extreme caution such as that required for parathion.

It destroys insects both as a contact and stomach poison. The residue disappears rather rapidly from treated plants which makes it particularly desirable for controlling pests on crops near the harvest time. It is useful for controlling such pests as aphids, mites, flea beetles, cutworms and army worms. It is now classed as an RUP by EPA.

Phosphamidon [2-chloro-2-diethylcarbamoyl-1-methylvinyl dimethyl phosphate]—An organic phosphate, a water-miscible oil, used as a systemic insecticide, with strong stomach action, in small grains, cotton and other field crops.

Carbamate Insecticides

Carbamate insecticides, like the organic phosphorus insecticides, inhibit insect cholinesterases. Their mode of action is sufficiently different, however, for them to be considered a separate class of insecticides. The carbamates of interest as insecticides include

Carbaryl [1-naphthyl *N*-methylcarbamate; *Sevin*]
Carbaryl, occurring as crystals slightly soluble in water, is highly effective against a wide range of insects, including the codling moth, Mexican bean beetle, cabbage worms, gypsy moth, boll weevil and pink bollworm. It is not highly effective against most insects of medical importance or against mites affecting plants. Although the carbamate insecticides are considered to be of moderate to low toxicity to higher animals, carbaryl is highly toxic to the honey bee. It has the greatest range of controlled pests of any insecticide; vegetables, fruits, field crops, ornamentals and pets. It is classed as a broad-spectrum insecticide.

Newer Methods of Insect Control

Extensive research continues on new methods of insect control that reduce or avoid the dangers of toxic insecticide residues. Three experimental procedures that illustrate how such control may be achieved are

1. The use of irradiation to destroy the breeding capacity of the insect. Certain insects breed only once, and when the female of such a species is mated with a sterile mate, that female will not produce fertile eggs. Advantage has been taken of this biological fact in controlling the screw worm—a serious pest of cattle in the southern US. In this operation males are irradiated with controlled doses of radioactive cobalt and then are released in tremendous numbers in the areas to be protected. Preliminary results have been so promising that this procedure is being considered for use against other species of insects with the same biological characteristics.
2. Distribution of the spores of organisms which are pathogenic for certain insect species only. A strain of spores, *Bacillus thuringiensis, Berliner*, var *Kurstaki* has been shown to have value in controlling a small number of insect species and is now commercially available as Bactur, Thuricide and others. The toxin is referred to as deltaendotoxin. Another is *Bacillus popilliae dutky* available in *Doom* and *Japidemic*, also referred to as Milky Spore Powder.
3. The use of certain of the silica aerogels which act on soft-bodied insects by desiccation. Since the silica aerogels are exceedingly low in toxicity to humans, residues may be insignificant.

Pheromones are potentially important for monitoring insect populations. They are chemical substances produced and released by one sex of an insect (usually the female) that elicit a sexual response in an individual of the opposite sex. The specificity of pheromones makes them valuable for detecting and estimating insect populations before an infestation can enlarge or spread. There are at least 90 different pheromones currently available, eg, the boll weevil (*Granlure*), codling moth (*Codlelure*), house fly (*Muscalure*), Mediterranean fruit fly (*Trimedlure*), etc.

Insect population suppression also can be achieved by using large numbers of attractant-bated traps (mass-trapping), by disruption of normal communication between sexes ("confusion technique") and by using a mixture of pheromone and a chemical sterilant.

Fumigants

Fumigants have and still are being used extensively for controlling a wide range of insects. Homes, industrial establishments, ships and other structures may be fumigated to control household or structural pests. Large amounts of fumigants are employed to control pests in grains and woolens, in soil and in living plants or plant products such as nursery stock, fruits and vegetables.

The most common fumigants and their uses are discussed briefly below.

Aluminum Phosphide—A pelletized source of phosphine plus fire retardant. It presently is used widely in grain fumigation. It is available as *Phostoxin*, Al-Phos, Celphine and others.

Carbon Disulfide [CS_2]—This is one of the older fumigants. A colorless to slightly yellow liquid with a disagreeable odor. The vapor is heavy (about 2.6 times that of air). Its chief disadvantage is its extreme explosiveness. It also is toxic to animals and lengthy exposure must be avoided. It is not registered for use in fumigating stored beans, cowpeas or peas.

To reduce its flammability, it is combined with carbon tetrachloride, usually in the ratio of 1 part carbon disulfide to 4 parts carbon tetrachloride. It most often is used for *treatment of grains in storage bins.* It has limited use in emulsion form for controlling *soil-infesting insects.*

Carbon Tetrachloride [CCl_4]—This is a liquid with a heavy vapor (five times that of air). This fumigant alone does not have extensive use because it does not possess a high degree of fumigating action to most insects. It is, however, used in combination with other fumigants, because the vapor is nonflammable; its use with such fumigants as carbon disulfide and ethylene dichloride reduces the fire hazard. It is employed also in combination with methyl bromide or ethylene dibromide to aid in the distribution of the vapor. Combinations of this with other fumigants are employed most extensively in *grain fumigation. Caution: It can be toxic on inhalation.* It is no longer allowed for home use and is not registered for use in fumigating dry beans, peanuts or peas.

Chloropicrin, Trichloronitromethane [CCl_3NO_2]—A colorless liquid which causes intense irritation of the eyes and throat and induces vomiting. It is used chiefly as a *soil fumigant.* It may be injected in the soil in combination with xylene, carbon tetrachloride or ethylene dichloride to help distribute the gas. It also is used in combination with certain other fumigants for *treating stored products* by sprinkling or spraying the infested materials. Since the gas is only slowly volatilized thorough airing after use is required. Several products are on the market, eg, *Acquinite.* It is now classed as an RUP by the EPA.

D-D Mixture—This is a mixture of 1,3-dichloropropene and 1,2-dichloropropene. It is a dark colored liquid having a sharp disagreeable odor. The material is flammable and is highly toxic to humans. The chief use of the mixture is for *soil fumigation* to control *nematodes,* etc. It is toxic to most plants and therefore is applied to the soil several weeks before planting the crop. Some products containing this are on the EPA RUP list.

Methyl Bromide [CH_3Br]—A colorless and usually odorless gas at ordinary temperatures approximately three times as heavy as air. The gas is nonflammable and sometimes is used as a fire extinguisher. It is highly toxic to humans and the absence of odor and slow toxic action are characteristics which increase its hazard. It is among the most widely used fumigants. It destroys a wide range of *pests.* It is not highly toxic to most plants and leaves no objectionable odor in food. Since the chemical is a gas at ordinary temperatures, it is applied from containers into which it has been compressed as a liquid. It readily vaporizes at temperatures ordinarily encountered in fumigating. It usually is formulated with a small amount of chloropicrin to recognize the presence of this colorless and odorless gas.

Some important uses are for *fumigating warehouses, ships, railroad cars, residences, grains, living plants* shipped under quarantine regulations, *tobacco* and many other products. The fumigant also is used to destroy *soil pests.* During World War II it was used successfully to *fumigate clothing of refugees and prisoners of war* to control *body lice.* Currently, all applications are classified by the EPA as RUPs. Only the registrant is authorized to refill cylinders.

Insect Repellents

Repellents are substances used to protect humans, animals and plants from insects by making the hosts objectionable or unattractive by disguising the characteristic odor of the hosts.

During World War II troops on many fronts in tropical and semitropical regions employed repellants effectively in the preventive campaign to keep away mosquitoes and other annoying and disease-carrying insect pests. The problem here was to use compounds that not only had effective staying and nonirritating properties when applied to the skin of man and animals, but also were without pronounced and penetrating odors that would give the enemy information about patroling or combat activities and locations of hideouts, etc. During and since World War II more than 10,000 chemicals were tested for use as insect repellents.

Perhaps the best all-purpose repellent developed since World War II is *diethyltoluamide,* which in various tests has been shown to be the most effective agent against a wide variety of insects.

Repellants, single- or multi-ingredient, generally are compounded in solution, emulsion, cream or semisolid stick application forms. Most will provide relief from attack from mosquitoes, biting flies and gnats for periods of 30 minutes to 2 hours or longer.

The volatile oils of citronella, cedarwood, eucalyptus, pennyroyal, bergamot, cassia, clove, wintergreen and lavender are, to some degree, repellent to mosquitoes and other annoying insects but are not nearly as effective as the aforementioned chemicals.

Individuals who are allergic or sensitive to repellants may show various skin reactions, such as burning, itching and swelling. Most repellents cause smarting when applied to broken skin or mucous membranes, hence care should be exercised when applying them around the eyes or other sensitive areas.

A brief chemical and physical description of the principal repellents follows.

Avitrol [4-Aminopyridine]—An avi-repellent. It controls several species of birds, eg, blackbirds, crows, gulls, pigeons, sparrows, starlings and other birds in and around structures and agriculture (field corn, sunflowers, etc). The odor causes the birds to signal vocal and physical distress which acts as an area repellent to the flock.

***n*-Butyl phthalate** [1,2-benzenedicarboxylic acid dibutyl ester; $C_{16}H_{22}O_4$]—An oily liquid used as an insect repellent for impregnation of clothing.

***n*-Butylacetanilide** [BAA; $C_{12}H_{17}NO$]—A clothing impregnant repellent for ticks and chiggers.

Di-*n*-butyl succinate [$C_{12}H_{22}O_4$; Tabatrex]—A liquid insect repellent against ants, cockroaches and flies used in buildings only. This is not registered for use on livestock or in dairy barns or milk rooms.

Diethyltoluamide [*N,N*-diethyl-*m*-toluamide; *N,N*-diethyl-3-methylbenzamide; (*Delphene,* Deet); $C_{12}H_{27}NO$]—A colorless liquid with a faint, pleasant odor; practically insoluble in water, miscible with alcohol. This is a repellent for mosquitoes, biting flies, gnats, chiggers, ticks, fleas and certain other biting insects. Safe for use on human skin.

Ethohexadiol [2-ethyl-1,3-hexanediol; Rutgers 612; $C_8H_{18}O_2$]—A colorless, oily liquid, odorless or with a slight odor; 1 mL dissolves in about 50 mL of water; miscible with alcohol. A common insect repellent used by humans.

Hinder—Ammonium soaps of higher fatty acids. It is used as a deer and rabbit repellent by odor from fruit trees, vegetables, field crops, ornamentals, etc. It is a viscous, brownish, aqueous solution with an ammonia odor.

Hot Sauce Animal Repellent—Contains capsaicin, the active irritant principle from hot peppers. It is used on ornamental trees and shrubs, fruit trees and nursery stock to repel deer, rabbits and mice.

Methiocarb [3,5-Dimethyl-4-(methylthio)phenyl methylcarbamate]—A nonsystemic insecticide, ascaricide, molluscicide and bird repellent. It is registered in several US states for bird repellency on blueberries.

Methyl Nonyl Ketone [MGK]—A dog and cat repellent. It is used as a training aid for pets, and to prevent damage by stray animals to ornamental plantings.

Thiram [Bis(dimethylthiocarbamoyl)disulfide]—A fungicide, seed protectant and animal repellent.

Control of Rodents

The following compounds are employed commonly to control rodents. They are dangerous and must be handled with caution. Many of the modern rodenticids are now packaged in "bait stations" to minimize larger-animal and human poisonings.

Bromadiolone [3-[3-(4′-bromo[1,1′-biphenyl]-4-yl)-3-hydroxy-1-phenylpropyl]-4-hydroxy-2H-1-benzopyran-2-one]—A yellowish powder, rather insoluble and used in baits or tracking powder for rodent control. It is used in official establishments operating under the Federal meat, poultry, shell egg grading and egg products inspection program. Some applications classed by the EPA as RUPs.

Brodifacoum—A complex benzopyranone derivative. It is an off-white powder. It is an anticoagulant rodenticide, available in pellets and bait blocks. Single feeding causes death.

Chlorophacinone (*Rozol*)—An indandione derivative. It is a white, crystalline material made in grain bait, water bait, paraffin blocks and tracking powder. It has the same uses as above.

Diphenadione [Diphacinone; 2-diphenylacetyl-1,3-indandione]—The most toxic of the anticoagulants in use at present. While other chemicals in this class usually are used, in bait, at a concentration of 0.025%, this is effective in 0.005% concentration.

Pindone [Pival; 2-pivaloyl-1,3-indandione]—This anticoagulant rodenticide resembles warfarin in its action and methods of use. It is available in concentrates, solutions and prepared baits, which must be used as directed.

Red Squill [*Dethdiet, Rodine*]—Because of its relative safety for humans, pets and domestic animals, properly standardized red squill powders and extracts generally were recommended poisons for rats. Red squill contains scilliroside, a cardiac glycoside and strong emetic which causes humans and most species of domestic animals to void the poison promptly. Its specific toxicity is due to the inability of rats to vomit. This allows the absorption of the toxicant. Other animals do vomit, allowing them to survive accidental poisoning. Red squill has never been more than a mediocre rodenticide and is used little in the US today.

Valone (*PMP;* 2-isovaleryl-1,3-indandione)—An anticoagulant used to formulate rat and mouse poisons.

Viruses—Rat viruses are not registered for use in the US at present. Governmental agencies responsible for protecting human and animal health have recommended against the general sale of bacterial cultures for pest mammal control.

Warfarin [*WARF-42, Compound 42;* 3-(α-acetonylbenzyl)-4-hydroxycoumarin]—A chemical relative of dicumarol; it acts by causing a loss of clotting power of the blood, and the animals die of exhaustion from multiple hemorrhages. The product was the first successful anticoagulant rodenticide and was unique in that it had to be eaten repeatedly to cause death. For rats, the feeding time is usually from 3 to 10 days, and for mice a much longer period of daily feeding is needed. Fantastically low percentages of the poison in food are effective, and food baits now on the market contain 0.025 to 0.05%, and concentrates for making solutions of the sodium salt of warfarin containing 0.005% of warfarin equivalent are available. At these levels rats and mice do not detect the material in the baits and will continue to come back to eat or drink until too weak to do so.

Warfarin itself is a highly toxic poison, but the fact that it is needed at such low concentrations in baits and that these must be eaten repeatedly to cause symptoms makes it less likely to injure pets and children than certain other poisons. It has had a good record of safety and is considered one of the less dangerous rat and mouse control materials.

Several other coumarin derivatives are available; eg, 3-(1-furyl-3-acetylethyl)-4-hydroxycoumarin, known by the nonproprietary name coumafuryl and marketed under several tradenames (eg, *Fumarin, Fumasol, Krumkil, Lurat* and *Rat-A-Way*). This was developed and produced by Amchem.

Zinc Phosphide [Zn_3P_2]—A phosphorus preparation which has found a definite place in a specialized rodent control problem in the US. It is blended with a diluent to permit its easier use as a dusting powder over cut apples in the preparation of a highly effective orchard mouse bait. Just enough of the perishable bait is made to supply an afternoon's work, and it is placed by uncovering mouse tunnels and making a bait spot of two or three apple sections placed directly in the runway. This is repeated at several points in the trails around each orchard tree, and when properly done is quite effective. The same zinc phosphide blend can be used on other types of food bait for domestic rat or mouse control. It is dangerous to animals other than rats or mice, and should be handled carefully. Some or all applications of several products containing this (*Gopha-Rid* or *Ridall-Zinc*) are classed by the EPA as RUPs.

Control of Fungi and Bacteria

Fungicides are chemical compounds used to prevent or retard the deleterious action of a varied group of plants called fungi, which for the most part are microscopic, devoid of green coloring matter and reproduce by spores.

Fungi are present throughout the world. They attack other living and dead plants, animals, human beings and such diversified inanimate objects as foodstuffs, cloth, paper, lumber, paint, plastic coverings and leather, to mention only a few of the substances affected.

Some fungicide materials also are toxic to bacteria but in general the term is limited to those materials used for protection against fungi. For many years fungicides have been used extensively in agriculture for the protection of crops.

The prevalence of fungi fluctuates with environmental conditions. Early historical and religious writings contain references to the blasting, blighting, rusting or mildewing of the crops. From the dawn of civilization to the present there has been a constant battle between the agriculturist on one hand and the fungi on the other, with the environmental conditions swinging the balance to one side and then to the other. Prior to 1853 losses resulting from the attacks of fungi were accepted as inevitable since the true cause was not understood. However, in that year Anton de Bary established the parasitism of the fungi associated with the rust and smut diseases. This discovery, establishing the science of plant pathology, has been followed by an increasing number of investigations into the cause of plant diseases and by the development of a wide variety of materials used for the control of these diseases.

Fundamental Requirements of a Fungicide—These materials may be applied in either liquid or powder form. The process of applying substances in liquid form is termed spraying; that of applying them in powder form, dusting.

Irrespective of the method of application a fungicide, to be entirely satisfactory, must be

Capable of destroying, controlling or preventing the growth of the fungus.
Relatively noninjurious to the host plant.
Easy to apply.
Easy to prepare.
Reasonable in cost.

Types of Fungicidal Action—Fungicidal materials are of varied composition and their exact mode of action against specific organisms is beyond the scope of this discussion. In general, however, all materials fall into two general categories; *protective* and *eradicative*.

In the *protective type* the material does not necessarily kill the fungus spores but does prevent their germination. The various forms of elemental *sulfur* used as spray or dust are protective in their action against the spores of the apple scab fungus (*Venturia inaequalis*) and are used widely by commercial orchardists to prevent numerous infections from developing on the apple leaves and fruit. However, the same materials used against certain rust fungi are definitely eradicative in their action upon the rust spores. This diverse effect on different fungi is but one example of the complexity of the problem.

In the *eradicative type* the material kills the fungus and in this way stops the disease either before or soon after initial infection has occurred. The complex *calcium polysulfides* or newer agents like the Captan, Thiram or Benlate preparations, for example, have a definite eradicative effect on the apple scab fungus. Unfortunately, most of the eradicative materials are rather caustic in their action, and they can be used only under certain conditions since they are apt to produce injury often more serious in consequence than the disease they are being used to combat. However, whenever it is possible to use an eradicative type of fungicide without incurring serious injury to the plant, this procedure should be adopted as it is productive of the most satisfactory control results.

Commonly Used Fungicides

It is realized that the pharmacist is not expected to have the detailed knowledge of a technically trained plant pathologist regarding the use of fungicide materials. However, he is asked frequently for advice and he should familiarize himself with directions on pesticide labels and recognize the importance of having his patrons understand and follow the directions; also, he should use the services of state or county extension pathologists when label information is insufficient to deal with specific problems that might arise.

The following list of commonly used materials should enable him to answer intelligently the majority of questions with which he is confronted. Requests for information concerning large-scale usage of fungicides should be referred to the state agricultural experiment station, to the USDA or to the EPA.

Afugan (Pyrazophos)—A systemic fungicide used for powdery mildew on apple, cereals, cucumber, grape, melon, ornamentals, pumpkin, squash, strawberry and watermelon.

Benomyl [Methyl 1-(butylcarbamoyl)-2-benzimidazolecarbamate]—A carbamate type of fungicide of broad spectrum with both protective and curative qualities. It shows local systemic activity within the leaf system and from soil applications where the root system stays within the treated zone. It is registered for use on roses, other ornamentals, turf, stone fruits, melons, beans, cucumbers, grapes, pome fruits and peanuts. The LD50 of a rat oral dose is over 10,000 mg/kg. Avoid contamination of food supplies.

Bioquin I—see *Copper 8-Quinolinolate.*

Botran—This trade name and others (*DCNA, Allisan*) refer to *2,6-dichloro-4-nitroaniline,* which was developed in England. This substituted amine is formulated as a yellow, wettable powder used for spraying (75%) and for dipping (50%); it also is used as dust. It generally is used as a soil and foliar fungicide to control *Sclerotinia* mold, *Monilinia* rot, *Rhizopus* rot, *Sclerotium* and *Botrytus* mold, including storage or transit on vegetables, fruits and ornamentals. It is almost nontoxic to rats but phytotoxic to strawberries, wilted leaf lettuce, asters, petunias and some other greenhouse plants, and to some germinating seeds and annual seedlings. It is persistent on leaf surfaces for 1 to 2 weeks and involves low hazard generally.

Caution—Avoid inhalation of dust and spray mist; occasional cases of contact dermatitis have been reported.

Calcium Hypochlorite [Chloride of lime; bleaching powder]—The activity of this compound as a general disinfectant is based on its ability to release chlorine. Various forms of this are used to sanitize swimming pools. It has fungicidal and bactericidal properties.

Captan [*N*-trichloromethylthio-4-cyclohexene-1,2-dicarboximide]—An organic fungicide used at the rate of 1 to 2 lb/100 gal of water for control of diseases of fruits, vegetables and ornamental plants. It is excellent for summer spraying of apple trees. It is used extensively on fruits and vegetables and on field and ornamental crops. Do not use with lime or other strong alkali. It is classed as a protectant-eradicant fungicide.

Copper 8-Quinolinolate—An organic copper compound (sold under the trade name *Bioquin I*) is used for the control of alternaria blight, botrytis blight and powdery mildew on carnations, chrysanthemums and roses. It also has some industrial fungicide use. It generally is recommended to be used at the rate of 1 lb/100 gal of water. *Zinc* and *magnesium compounds* of similar composition also have been tested as well as *8-hydroxyquinoline sulfate, 8-quinolinol benzoate* and *8-quinolinol.*

Copper Sulfate—In addition to being the principal ingredient of Bordeaux mixture, it is the essential component of many commercial copper fungicides. It is a fungicide and algicide.

Difolatan [(*Chevron; Captafol*); cis-*N*-[(1,1,2,2-tetrachloroethyl)-thio]-4-cyclohexene-1,2-dicarboximide]—This sulfenimide is a solid of low toxicity which is insoluble in water. It is formulated as an 80% wettable powder and a 7.5% dust. It generally is used as a fungicidal protectant-eradicant particularly for the control of early and late blight on potatoes. It also is used extensively on fruits, melons, tomatoes, onions. It is slightly toxic to rats, fish and birds. Foliage of some roses may be injured with this fungicide. It is persistent on plant surfaces for 7 to 10 days. No hazard occurs in its use. It is not compatible with strongly alkaline materials. It should not be used in combination with or closely following oil sprays. One product, *Haipen* is used as a wood preservative.

Diphenyl (biphenyl)—Used as a preservative for citrus in storage and transit. It is used by impregnating citrus fruit wraps.

Dithane M 22—See *Maneb.*

Dithane M 45 [*Mancozeb*]—A zinc ion and manganese ethylene bisdithiocarbamate compound. It is a broad-spectrum fungicide used on vegetables, fruits, turf and ornamentals for leafspot, early and late blight, crown rot, damping off, anthracnose and others. It is one of the most commonly used vegetable fungicides.

Dithane Z 78—See *Zineb.*

Dodine [(*Am Cyanamid*); *N*-dodecylguanidine acetate; *Cyprex, Melprex, Doquadine*]—A fairly stable fungicide formulated as a 65% wettable powder and a protectant and eradicant fungicide, particularly for apple and pecan scab, cherry leaf spot, sycamore anthracnose and other tree diseases. It may cause foliage or fruit injury, particularly if applied at freezing or near-freezing temperatures. *Caution*—It may produce eye and skin irritation. If exposed, flush eyes for at least 15 minutes.

Dyrene [2,4-dichloro-6-(*o*-chloroanilino)-*s*-triazone, anilazine, *Kemate* (*Chemagro*)]—A foliar fungicide for the control of turf diseases, some vegetable diseases, berries and gladiolus. It may be phytotoxic to some fruit and ornamentals and potentially hazardous to animals. It can cause skin irritation.

Ferbam—An iron organic compound, *ferric dimethyldithiocarbamate,* used extensively as a substitute for sulfur and copper compounds in the control of fungus diseases of fruit trees. It is employed as a specific for the control of the apple cedar rust. In the Pacific Northwest it is used instead of sulfur for the control of pear scab since it does not russet the fruit. Likewise, it is used for the control of the fungi causing apple scab, apple blotch and bitter rot since it reduces the risk of spray injury and at the same time gives satisfactory control of these fungi.

It also is used for the control of tomato anthracnose, and is especially effective for the control of anthracnose leaf blight, downy mildew and fruit rot of cucumbers and melons. It causes less leaf injury than copper compounds on tomatoes, cucumbers and melons.

Caution—Ferbam is a flammable material and must not be mixed near an open flame. In mixing sprays the operator should avoid inhaling it.

Ferric Dimethyldithiocarbamate—See *Ferbam.*

Folpet [(*Stauffer*); (*N*-trichloromethylthio)phthalimide; *Phaltan,* Rose and Garden Fungicide (*Ortho; Stauffer*)]—Generally as a protectant–eradicant fungicide for fruit, vegetables, ornamentals and turf. It is especially good for black spot of rose. It is slightly more phytotoxic than captan. It is not recommended for apples before the 4th cover spray, it may burn grape leaves in hot, dry seasons and also may injure sweet cherry leaves and snapdragons severely. It has a low health hazard. Concentrated solutions may cause skin irritation. Its use is limited to the western states.

Krenite—(*Sodium Dinitro-ortho-cresylate.*)—A plant-growth regulator which stops treated plants from refoliating during the next growing season. It is classed as a brush control agent.

Lime-Sulfur Solution—A widely used spray material consisting of approximately 30% *calcium polysulfides* prepared by heating sulfur and lime together with appropriate quantities of water.

Lime-sulfur solution has proved specially effective for the control of the apple scab fungus, and has been used widely for the control of many other plant diseases. The water dilution for use during the growing season varies from 1 gal of the concentrate for 50 gal of spray to 1 gal for 100 gal. Used at a concentration of 12 gal for 100 gal of spray during the winter months, it has been used for a long time on peach trees for the combined control of San Jose scale and the leaf curl fungus.

Since the calcium polysulfides are likely to produce spray injury, it is being replaced by less injurious forms of sulfur and various organic materials in large-scale commercial spraying operations. It also has miticidal activity. It has been supplanted largely by newer synthetic fungicides with a milder action on plants.

Maneb [manganese ethylenebisdithiocarbamate; *Manzate, Dithane M-22, Chem-Neb, MEB,* etc]—The manganese salt of dithiocarbamic acid is used at the rate of 1 to 2 lb/100 gal of water for the control of potato, tomato, celery, carrots and onion diseases. It also has been used to control grape black rot and is used on many fruits and vegetables. It is currently an important fungicide.

Mercaptobenzothiazole [*Niacides*]—Used on apples as a plant fungicide by pesticide formulators in their products.

Nabam [Disodium ethylenebis[dithiocarbamate]—For industrial applications only; not for food crops. It is an algicide in rice.

Pentachloronitrobenzene [*PCNB, Terraclor, Brassicol*]—A nitrobenzene compound as a soil fungicide effective against many soil pathogens which attack vegetables, turf and ornamentals. It also is used as foliar spray on young lettuce, cabbage and cauliflower as well as on fruit trees.

Polyramcombi—This is a mixture of 5.2 parts by weight (83.9%) of ammoniates of [ethylenebis(dithiocarbamato)] zinc with 1 part by weight (16.1%) ethylenebis[dithioarbamic acid], bimolecular and trimolecular cyclic anhydrosulfides and disulfides. These dithiocarbamates are solids and are insoluble in most common solvents. They decompose under strongly basic or acidic conditions. It is available as an 80% wettable powder and several dusts. Moisture can cause deterioration. It generally is used as blight control on potatoes and tomatoes. It can control apple scab, cedar apple rust, sooty blotch and fly speck and also is used on ornamentals. It is also useful on certain other vegetables and some field crops. It has no known phytotoxicity and is persistent on plant surfaces for 10 to 14 days. This agent is compatible with chlorinated hydrocarbons, coppers, sulfurs and phosphates, except parathion oil sprays. Karathane or Diazinon should be added just before use. It is safer than lead arsenate on apples. It has low hazard potential, however some applications are classified by EPA or RUPs.

Sodium *o*-Phenylphenate [*o*-phenylphenol; *Dowicide A*]—Used on a variety of fruits and vegetables to increase storage life.

Sulfur—For a long time one of the standard fungicide materials and still used widely to control a wide variety of plant diseases. It is sold as a dry powder ground to varying degrees of fineness, as a paste, or fused with clay (bentonite) and subsequently ground. Many special brands are available and each manufacturer claims special virtues for his particular product. They all depend for their effectiveness on its inherent toxic property in affecting the growth processes of various fungi. The directions on the packages will be a guide to their use. It is one of the cheapest fungicide materials and probably will continue to be used extensively as spray or dust for many years to come.

Combined with lime and water and heated for a considerable period, it forms complex *polysulfides*. This reaction product called *lime-sulfur* has been described in a preceding paragraph. If it is added to slaking stone lime and the only heat supplied is that of the stone lime combining with water, another type of spray called *self-boiled lime-sulfur* results. Properly prepared self-boiled lime-sulfur has a very low calcium polysulfide content and produces very little injury; it can be used with safety on peaches during the growing season whereas lime-sulfur used at that time would cause excessive injury to the trees.

Tersan—[1,4-dichloro-2,5-dimethoxybenzene; *Chloroneb, Demosan*]—Used in systemic seed treatment, in-furrow soil treatment and turf diseases.

Yellow Cuprous Oxide—This material, containing 47% of metallic copper, is sold under the trade name *Yellow Cuprocide* and may be used as a spray or dust. Used at the rate of 1½ lb/100 gal it is effective against celery blight, Alternaria blight of tomato, early and late blights of potato, anthracnose, downy mildew and other leaf diseases of cucurbits and is recommended for a variety of vegetable crops wherever a copper spray is needed.

Zinc Dimethyldithiocarbamate—See *Ziram*.

Zinc Ethylenebisdithiocarbamate—See *Zineb*.

Zineb [*Zinc ethylenebisdithiocarbamate*]—Exceptionally effective in the control of potato and tomato late blight in Florida. It has not been much superior to copper compounds in the more northern tomato-growing sections. It is less injurious to the tomato and potato plants than copper compounds, a factor of considerable importance in the South where numerous spray applications are required during the long growing season.

It also has been used on cucumbers, muskmelons and watermelons for downy mildew and anthracnose control, especially in Florida. The lack of injury on these plants is a specially valuable feature of this compound, since cucumbers and melons are extremely susceptible to copper injury. For the same reason this compound has proved of value for the control of cabbage and cauliflower diseases and also has many uses on fruits. It sometimes is used to control fire blight on apple and pear trees. It also has been applied as a dust containing 8 to 10% of the fungicide.

Ziram—[*Zinc dimethyldithiocarbamate*]—A white powder and does not leave an objectionable residue. It has found extensive use in the control of vegetable diseases (celery leaf blight, downy mildew of cucurbits, bean anthracnose, cabbage downy mildew and squash black rot). It also has been used for peach brown rot control, but is apt to produce leaf injury and fruit russet when used on applies, sour cherries, pears and several other fruits. It is not an effective material for the control of potato or tomato late blight.

Relatively crude, denatured forms of streptomycin and oxytetracycline are being used to control many bacterial diseases of plants. Cycloheximide, under the name ActiDione, is used to control cherry leaf spot and dollar spot of turf.

Antibiotics

Streptomycin—Marketed as the sulfate or nitrate under the trade names *Agrimycin 17, AG-Strep* and *Phytomycin* by Pfizer, Merck and Olin Mathieson, respectively. It is formulated as a dry, wettable powder (sulfate) and liquid (nitrate). Its salts are very soluble in water. It has general use as an antibacterial against fire blight of applies and pears and similar infections on ornamentals including woody and herbaceous plants. It is persistent on plant surfaces for up to 4 months, but is considered of low general toxicity. It can produce allergenic reactions such as rashes, conjunctivitis and bronochial asthma. This agent should not be applied following Bordeaux mixture and it is incompatible with lime sulfur, pyrethrane and aldrin.

Other animal and plant diseases can be controlled with aureomycin, terramycin and phytoactin.

Control of Weeds and Plants

Between 1987 and 1992 herbicides exhibited a growth of about 5.3% per year to $3.47 billion in sales, aided by many technological advances. Corn and soybean growers will remain the two largest markets. High-activity compounds based on new chemistry have been developed which permit significantly lower application rates, employing new modes of action and lower environmental hazards.

Many herbicides are used for weed control, and others are being evaluated experimentally to determine their usefulness. Only those of current general interest and usefulness are described below.

Available information on the degree of toxicity of herbicides is listed in the descriptions of chemicals used for weed control. The symbol LD50 (lethal dose that kills 50% of the experimental animals) precedes each number that indicates relative oral toxicity. For example, the single acute oral dose for calcium cyanamide, LD50 = 1400 mg/kg, indicates a relatively low oral toxicity. The larger the LD50 number, the less poisonous the herbicide.

All LD values listed in this guide are based on a single dose of material orally administered to animals, followed by observation of the treated animals for a definite period of time. However, these findings do not indicate the possible hazards that may arise from skin contact or inhalation of the substance or substances indicated. Likewise, these data do not accurately predict the toxicity of a formulation which may differ according to the solvent or diluent employed.

Herbicides are materials used mainly for the control of weeds and are used in five general ways.

Preplanting, which means that the herbicides are applied after the soil has been prepared, but before seeding of the desired plant.

Preemergence or contract, which means that nonresidual dosages of herbicide are used after seeding but before emergence of the crop seedlings.

Preemergence or residual, which means that the herbicide is applied at the time of seedling or just prior to crop emergence so that it kills weed seeds and germinating seedlings.

Postemergence, which refers to herbicide application after emergence of a crop.

Sterilant or nonselective, which means that sufficient herbicide is used to effect a complete kill of all treated plant life.

There are at least 15 major classes of herbicides in use today. These include the following.

Inorganic Herbicides

The major examples in this class are ammonium sulfamate, copper sulfate and sodium arsenite.

Copper Sulfate (Pentahydrate) [Basicap (*Griffin Corp*)]—A blue, water-soluble crystalline material, widely used as a fungicide. However, it is used also as a herbicide specifically for the control of algae & pond weeds in impounded potable waters. It also is used in irrigation water conveyance systems, root control in sewers and in rice patties to control algae. *Signal Word:* Danger. *Toxicity Class:* I. *Toxicity:* Acute oral LD50, 470 mg/kg. 1 mg/m^3 for all copper dusts or mists. Toxic to fish. *Antidote/Treatment:* See a physician. May be corrosive to mucous membranes, eyes, skin and gastrointestinal tract if swallowed. For oral poisoning, give two glasses of milk of magnesia, water or milk to dilute the chemical, then induce vomiting. This should be repeated until vomitus is clear. *Handling and Storage Cautions:* Avoid direct contact. Do not use excessive amounts in ponds, streams or lakes as a herbicide. Protective equipment and clothing should be worn during handling. *Formulation:* Numerous crystal forms and sizes, solutions and powders are available from several manufacturers.

Sodium Arsenite [*Chem Pels C, Penite*]—Once commonly used as fungicide, herbicide and insecticide. Because of its extreme toxicity and solubility in soil moisture and hence the possibility of contaminating water supplies, it is not used now for many purposes formerly common practice. All other uses have been banned by the EPA. *Toxicity Class:* I. *Toxicity:* Acute oral LD50 (mammalian), 10 to 50 mg/kg. It is highly toxic.

Petroleum Oils (*90-Par, Volck oils, White Oils, refined grades*)

These long have been used as insecticides, insecticide solvents and insecticide adjuvants to increase their efficacy. Some are used as herbicides by themselves. They are applied as contact herbicides, being used for general or selective weed control. Petroleum products used as herbicides include Stoddart solvent (petroleum distillate between gasoline and kerosene, known also as mineral spirits) and diesel oil.

These should be used with caution and are placed in Toxicity Class III. Various physical and chemical properties of the oils are important in determining their final use, eg, sulfonation percentage (indicates degree of refinement), volability, density, viscosity, etc.

Organic Arsenicals

This group includes monosodium methanearsonate (MSMA), disodium methanearsonate (DSMA) and cacodylic acid.

Monosodium Methanearsonate (MSMA) [*Ansar, Arsonate Liquid, Broadside*]—A white, crystalline solid (mp, 132–139°C). It is a herbicide used for postemergent control of Johnsongrass and other grassy weeds along the banks of ditches, storage yards, rights-of-way and other noncrop locations; preplant in cotton; bearing citrus (except in Florida); nonbearing orchards; and for crabgrass and certain broadleaf control in turf and as a tree killer. *Toxicity Class:* III; it should be used with caution. *Toxicity:* Acute oral LD50 (rat), 700 mg/kg; Arsonate Liquid (51% MSMA); acute oral LD50 (rat) 1738 mg/kg; acute dermal LD50 (rabbit) 2500 mg/kg; acute inhalation LD50 (rat) 20 mg/L. It is midly irritating to skin and eyes (rabbit). *Antidote/Treatment:* If swallowed, induce vomiting; drink lots of water.

Disodium Methanearsonate (DSMA)—Marketed under a variety of trade names (eg, *Ansor DSMA Liquid, Arsinyl, Crab-E-Rad*) and is used as a selective postemergence herbicide for cotton, as a directed spray on weeds such as Johnsongrass, cocklebur, dallisgrass, watergrass, nutgrass and goosegrass, particularly in noncrop areas. *Toxicity and Caution:* Similar to *MSMA*.

Cacodylic Acid [Hydroxydimethylarsine oxide; dimethylarsinic acid; *Bolate, Dilic, Phytar 560,* etc]—A nonselective herbicide, cotton defoliant and silvicide (tree killer) for forestry use. *Toxicity Class:* III; use with caution. *Toxicity:* Acute oral LD50 (rat), 700 mg/kg. It also is used in a number of combination products.

Phenoxy-Aliphatic Acids

This group incudes many so-called plant hormones & related substances such as *2,4-D, 2,4,5-T, 2,4-DB, MCPA* and *Silvex.*

2,4-D [(2,4-dichlorophenoxy) acetic acid; *Acme Amine 4, Hedonal, Transamine, Weed-B-Gon,* etc]—Selective herbicide whose application is for grasses, wheat, barley, oats, sorghum, corn, sugarcane, rice (Philippines) and noncrop areas for postemergent control of weeds such as Canada thistle, dandelion, annual mustards, ragweed and lambs-quarters. Certain formulations are registered for pine release, water hyacinth control and prevention of seed formation, and others for control of wild radish and other broadleaf weeds in cereals. For specific cautions, see the labels of different formulations. The dimethylamine salt form: *Toxicity Class:* I (eyes); EC: III (oral). *Toxicity:* Acute LD50 (rat), 375 mg/kg, 700 mg/kg (isopropyl); 666 to 805 mg/kg (sodium salts). At the usual application rates (usually quite dilute), it has no adverse effect on soil microorganisms. Since this compound is active at low concentrations, spray equipment contaminated with it must be cleaned scrupulously before use for any other material. Avoid contamination in irrigation water. When using its preparations, plastic gloves, goggles, aprons and dust masks are recommended. There are hundreds of commercial formulations and combinations of this agent on the market.

Substituted Amines

The substitute amine herbicides include propanil, naptalam, alachlor and cypromid.

Propanil [BSI, ISO, WSSA, BAY30130 (*Bayer*), Prop Job (*Drexel*), *N*-(3,4-dichlorophenyl)propionamide]—A postemergence, contact-type herbicide with no residual effect against numerous grasses and broadleaved weeds in rice.

Naptalam [ISO, WSSA, ACP 322 (*Ancrack*), sodium 2-[(1-naphthalenylamino)carbonyl]benzoate]—Herbicide for numerous broadleaf weeds on cucurbits and nursery stock.

Alachlor [ANSI, BSI, ISO, WSSA, Chimichlor (*Diachem S.P.A.*), 2-chloro-2′,6′-diethyl-*N*-(methoxy-methyl)acetanilide]—A pre-emergence herbicide used to control most annual grasses and certain broadleaf weeds in corn, dry beans, peanuts, and soybeans. Leaves no carryovers residue in soil.

Cypromid [3′,4′-dichlorocyclopropanecarboxanclide]—herbicide.

Nitroanilines

These herbicides include benefin and triflaralin.

Benefin [Benfluralin, *N*-Butyl-*N*-ethyl-α,α,α,-trifluoro-2,6-dinitro-*p*-toluidine; *Balan, Pel-Tech, Quilan,* etc]—Selective preemergence herbicides to control annual grasses and broadleaf weeds in seeded alfalfa, direct seeded lettuce, peanuts, tobacco and for established turf. It may be applied and soil incorporated as much as 10 weeks prior to planting; however, it will not control established weeds. The caution signal word varies with the formulation used. *Toxicity:* Acute oral LD50 (rat): over 10,000 mg/kg. The pure compound is a yellow-orange, crystalline solid which is readily soluble in organic solvents. It has a flashpoint of 25.5°C (78°F). These characteristics dictate caution in handling & storage. It should not be frozen, nor stored above 4.5°C (40°F), particularly near heat or open flame. It is corrosive and has caused severe eye irritation in lab animals. Certain individuals may show skin-sensitization reactions to it. It can be harmful if swallowed, inhaled or absorbed through the skin. In the case of contact, the eyes & skin should be flushed immediately with plenty of water. Protective clothing is recommended during usage. Several formulations and combination products are marketed.

Substituted Ureas

These herbicides include diuron, monuron, linuron, noria, chloroxuron and baturon.

Diuron [3-(3,4-Dichlorophenyl)-1,1-dimethyl-urea; *N*′-(3,4-dichlorophenyl)-*N,N*-dimethylurea; *Cekiuron, Dailon, Unidron,* etc]—Used at low rates as a selective herbicide to control germinating broadleaf, grass weeds in numerous crops such as sugarcane, pineapple, alfalfa, grapes, cotton and peppermint. At higher rates of application it can be used as a general week killer. As a soil sterilant, it is more persistent and preferred over monuron on lighter soil and/or in areas of heavy rainfall. *Toxicity Class:* III. *Toxicity:* Acute oral LD50 (rat), 3400 mg/kg. *Handling and Storage Cautions:* Similar to other herbicides. It is used commonly as a flowable, wettable powder in formulations and numerous combination products exist.

Carbamates

These include propham, chloropropham, barban and terbutol.

Propham [Isopropyl carbanilate; IPC, Ban-Hoc (*Shellstar*), Premalox (*May & Baker,* etc]—Used primarily as a preemergence and postemergence herbicide. It prevents cell division and acts on meristematic tissue. Major uses include control of weeds in alfalfa, ladino clover, flax, lettuce, safflower, lentils, peas and on fallow land. *Toxicity Class:* III. *Toxicity:* generally low toxicity to wildlife and fish; acute oral LD50 (rat), 5000 mg/kg. It is available in flowable suspensions, wettable powders and in various combination products.

Thiocarbamates

These include pebulate, diallate and EPTC (S-Ethyl dipropylthiocarbamate; Alirox)

Pebulate [*S*-Propyl butylethylthiocarbamate; R-2061 (*Stauffer*)]—A preplant selective herbicide for the control of both grassy and broadleaf weeds. It has been used for selective weed control in sugar beets, tobacco and tomatoes. The signal word is *caution.* *Toxicity Class:* III. *Toxicity:* Acute of LD50 (rat), 921 to 1900 mg/kg; acute dermal LD50 (rabbit) >4640 mg/kg. Formulations include emulsifiable concentrate (6 lb/gal), and granules (10%).

Heterocyclic Nitrogen Compounds

These herbicides include amitrole, pyrazon and picloram.

Amitrole [1*H*-1,2,4-triazol-3-amine; *ANSI, BSI, ISO, WSSA, Amerol, AT-90, Diurol, Herbizole, Simazol*]—Used mainly as a nonselective systemic herbicide for control of annual grasses, broadleaf weeds, perennial broadleaf weeds, poison ivy and certain aquatic weeds in marshes and drainage ditches. Some or all applications may be classified by the EPA as RUPs. It is restricted to noncropland use. The signal word is caution. *Toxicity Class:* III. *Toxicity:* Acute oral LD50 (male albino rat), up to 10,000 mg/kg caused no death nor symptoms of systemic activity. It has an indefinite self-life and should be stored at room temperature. It is available in liquid and solid powder formulations as well as pressurized-container products. Numerous combination products are also available.

Triazines

These herbicides include atrazine, simazine, propazine, prometone and cyanazine.

Atrazine [2-Chloro-4-ethylamino-6-isopropylamino-1,3,5 triazine; ATREX®, *Ciba-Geigy*, etc]—A selective herbicide used in season-long weed control in corn, sorghum and certain other crops. It also is used at higher rates of application for nonselective weed control in noncropped areas. One product (*Crisazina*) is used for pre- and early postemergent weed control on African oil palm, bananas, citrus groves, coffee, corn, pineapples, sorghum and sugarcane. One registration note on *Bellater* [cyanazine, atrazine (*Shell*) lists a use for maize outside the US. *Toxicity Class:* III. *Toxicity:* Acute oral LD50 (rat), 1780 mg/kg. It is listed as harmful if swallowed and contact with eyes and skin should be avoided. Another caution listing states "do not contaminate food, feed or water supplies with the product." The shelf-life is given as 3 years under environmental conditions, provided that the product is stored in its unopened and undamaged original containers, in shaded, possibly well-aired, fresh and dry storehouse conditions and kept away from sources of heat, free flames or spark-generating equipment. Formulations include dry, flowable powders, flowable liquids and wettable powders. Numerous combination products are on the market.

Uracils

These herbicides are bromacil and terbacil.

Bromacil [5-Bromo-3-sec-butyl-6-methyluracil; Borea, Bromax (*Hopkins Agri*), etc]—A weed & brush herbicide in noncrop areas, especially for perennial grasses. It also has been used in selective weed control in pineapple and citrus growing. The dry formulations are water-soluble. *Toxicity Class:* III (dry); II (liquid). *Toxicity:* Acute oral LD50 (rat), 5200 mg/kg. *Handling and Storage Cautions:* there are several due to its irritant & combustible qualities. Protective clothing is advised for proper handling. The formulations include granular powder, liquid, water-soluble liquid and wettable powder. Several combination products are available, particularly with various contact and hormone weed killers.

Aliphatic acids

These herbicides include *dalapon* and *TCA* (trichloroacetic acid).

Dalapon [2,2-Dichloropropionic acid; Basfapon, Ded-Weed, Revenge (*Hopkins*), Unipon, etc]—A selective herbicide and growth regulator used for quackgrass, bermudagrass and other perennial and annual grasses as well as cattails and rushes. This herbicide is used commonly as a preplant treatment to control established perennial grasses in cropland, noncropland areas and irrigation ditch banks in 17 western states. It acts by being translocated to the roots of most species where it acts as a growth regulator. *Toxicity Class:* II. *Toxicity:* Acute oral LD50 (female rats), 970 mg/kg (tech a.i.); 7570 mg/kg (sodium salt). The acid is not used directly and commercial products usually contain 85% of the sodium salt or mixed sodium and magnesium salts. *Handling and Storage Cautions:* There are several, including the avoidance of skin and eye contact because of irritancy and the avoidance of contamination of water, food or feed through storage or disposal. It is formulated mainly as a water-soluble powder and in several combination products.

Arylaliphatic Acids

The herbicides which belong to this class include *dicamba*, *fenac*, *2,3,6-TBA* (trichlorobenzoic acid), *DCPA* (Dacthal; dimethyl tetrachloroterephthalate) and *chloramben*.

Dicamba [2-Methoxy-3,6-dichlorobenzoic acid; 3,6-dichloro-o-anisic acid]—An herbicide. *Toxicity Class:* II. *Toxicity:* Acute oral LD50 (rat), 1707 mg/kg; acute dermal LD50 (rabbit), 2000 mg/kg. Formulations of a flowable liquid potassium product (Marksman) and the dimethylamine salt (4 lb/gal) are available. Several combination products are marketed.

Phenol Derivatives

These herbicides include DNOC and dinoseb.

DNOC [4,6-Dinitro-*o*-cresol; 2-methyl-4,6-dinitrophenol]; *Chemsect, Nitrador, Sinox, Trifrina*]—Insecticide, fungicide, herbicide and defoliant properties. It has use as a dormant spray for killing insect eggs and in apple scab control. The triethanolamine salt has promise as a complete dormant apple spray for light infestations of mite and aphid eggs, as well as other pests. The sodium salt has been used as a weed killer and on apple and peach trees to thin fruit. The signal word is *Danger. Caution. Very phytotoxic. Toxicity Class:* III; I. *Toxicity:* Acute oral LD50 (rat), 20 to 50 mg/kg. It should be stored in cool, well-ventilated areas away from heat and foodstuffs. Formulations include the ammonium salt (50%), flakes (98 to 100% free acid) and a flowable, wettable powder.

Substituted Nitriles

These herbicides include dihlobenil and bromoxynil.

Dichlobenil [2,6-Dichlorobenzonitrile; *Casoron, Decabane, Norosac, Prefix D*, etc]—For selective weed controls in cranberry bogs, ornamentals, nurseries, fruit orchards, vineyards, forest plantations, public green areas and for total weed control (industrial sites, railway lines, etc under asphalt). It also is used to control aquatic weeds in nonflowing water. It has been recommended for selective weed control in woody perennial crops, and for total weed control on industrial sites, car parks, roadsides, railways and related areas. *Toxicity Class:* III. *Toxicity:* Acute oral LD50 (rat), 3160 mg/kg; acute dermal LD50 (rabbit), 1350 mg/kg. It is toxic to germinating seeds. It should not be stored with propagative structures such as seeds, bulbs, tubers, nursery stock etc, or with food or feed products. It is available as granules and wettable powder and in severe combinations.

Bipyridyliums

These herbicides include diquat and paraquat.

Paraquat [1,1′-Dimethyl-4,4′-bipyridinium ion (present as the dichloride salt); *Actor, Herboxone, Weedol*, etc]—A contact herbicide used in the desiccation of seed crops and for noncrop & industrial weed control in bearing and nonbearing fruit orchards, shade trees and ornamentals. Other uses include defoliation and desiccation of cotton, a harvest aid in soybeans, sugarcane, sunflowers, for pasture renovation and for eradication of weeds in coffee plantations and similar situations. Some or all applications may be classified by the EPA as an RUP. The signal words are *danger* and *poison*. *Toxicity Class:* I. *Toxicity:* Acute oral LD50 (rat), 150 mg ion/kg. It can kill if swallowed. Use only with protective clothing and wash thoroughly after using. Various formulations include soluble dichloride concentrate (2 lb/ion/gal in the US), and various liquid & granular forms. Several combination products are available.

Miscellaneous Herbicides

Several herbicides in this miscellaneous group include endothall and bensulide.

Endothall [7-Oxabicyclo [2.2.1] heptane-2,3-dicarboxylic acid]; *Accelerate*, etc]—A pre- and postemergence herbicide, defoliant, desiccant, aquatic algricide and growth regulator. *Toxicity Class:* I. *Toxicity:* Acute oral LD50 (rat), 51 mg/kg.

Bensulide [*S*-(0,0-Diisopropyl phosphoro-dithioate) ester of *N*-(2-mercaptoethyl)benzenesulfonamide; *Bensumec, Exporsan, Prefar*, etc]—For preemergence control of annual grasses, crop use in carrots, cucumbers, peppers and tomatoes, among others. *Toxicity Class:* III. *Toxicity:* Acute oral LD50 (rat), 271 to 1470 mg/kg. Various formulations and combination products exist.

Plant Regulators

A plant-growth regulator is a preparation which, in minute amounts, alters the behavior of ornamental or crop plants, or the products thereof, through physiological (hormone) action rather than physical action. It may act to accelerate or retard growth, prolong or break a dormant condition, promote rooting or in other ways. A classification of plant-growth regulators usually includes auxins—2,4-D, MCPB, BNOA; Gibberillins; cytokinins—kinetin; ethylene generators—ethylene ethephon; inhibitors—benzoic acid, MH; and retardants—A-Rest, Atrinal.

Gibberellic acid is used extensively on seeds to aid in uniform germination and growth and on grapes to increase size. 2-Methyl-4-chlorophenoxyacetic acid (MCPA) and a number of related chemicals are used to thin blossoms, stop the premature drop of fruits or vegetables before harvest, increase the uniformity of ripening and for a wide variety of other purposes. For example, when applied properly, 2,4-D will increase the red color in potatoes, and other chemicals will produce pineapples of more uniform shape than untreated ones. This field of chemical usage is expanding and appears to have a future limited only by the necessity to prove that the uses will be safe, from both the toxicological and nutritional viewpoints. Also, 2,4-D is used on tomatoes to cause all fruits to ripen at the same time for machine harvesting. According to the EPA list of May 1978, products containing 2,4-D for use on grains must include the following label statement: "Do not forage or graze treated grain fields within 2 weeks after treatment with 2,4-D."

The identification of vegetable-growth inhibitors may yield improved storage methods for crops. Growth inhibitors for onions and cabbage have been identified but further studies are necessary to determine their ultimate value. Other growth regulators of potential value include

Ethrel (2-chloroethylphosphonic acid), which functions by releasing ethylene in plant tissues; it can increase appearance of fruit on pineapple with rates of 1 to 4 lb/acre.

Captan (*N*-(trichloromethylthio)-4-cyclohexene-1,2-dicarboximide) is registered for use in increasing the fruit set of both oranges and tangelos at the relatively high rate of 5 lb/acre.

Ripenthol, which contains *endothall* (7-oxabicyclo[2.2.1]heptane-2,3-dicarboxylic acid), can delay sucrose breakdown in mature sugarcane, giving planters a longer harvest period; this has increased yields of sugar in sugarcane up to 25%.

Desiccants and Defoliants

Desiccants and defoliants become increasingly important as mechancial harvesting gains popularity. In the same way that removal of weeds by use of herbicides just before the combines are put into the fields to harvest wheat will prevent clogging of the machines with weed debris, the removal of cotton leaves by chemical treatment aids mechanical harvesting of cotton and other leafy crops. Arsenic acid, pentachlorophenol and more complex chemicals such as *S,S,S*-tributylphosphorotrithionate and *S,S,S*-tributylphosphorotrithioite, and others are being used for this purpose. Requests for information concerning developments in this field should be addressed to the USDA, state experiment stations, or manufacturers of specific products. Questions on the legal status of pesticides should be sent to Director, Pesticides Regulation Division, Environmental Protection Agency (EPA), Washington, DC 20460.

Bibliography

Biological effects of pesticides in mammalian systems. *Ann NY Acad Sci 160* (art 1): 1, 1969.

Melnikov NN: *Chemistry of Pesticides*, Springer-Verlag, New York, 1971.

De Ong ER *et al:* *Insect Disease and Weed Control*, Chem Pub, New York, 1972.

Stevens-White R, ed: *Pesticides in the Environment*, vol 1, part 1, Dekker, New York, 1071; vol 1, part 2, 1971.

Djerassi C *et al:* Insect control of the future: operational and policy aspects. *Science 186:* 596, 1974.

Klingman GC, Ashton FM, Noordhoff LJ: *Weed Science: Principles and Practices*, Wiley, New York, 1975.

Edwards CA: *Persistent Pesticides in the Environment*, Chem Rubber Press, Cleveland OH, 1970.

Brooks GT: *Chlorinated Insecticides*, vol I, *Technology and Application*, Chem Rubber Press, Cleveland OH, 1974; vol II, *Biological and Environmental Aspects*, 1975.

Street JC, ed: *Pesticide Symposia* (Toxicology), Halos and Assoc, Miami, 1970.

Matsumura F, ed: *Environmental Toxicology of Pesticides*, Academic, New York, 1972.

Eto M: *Organophosphorus Pesticides: Organic and Biological Chemistry*, Chem Rubber Press, Cleveland OH, 1974.

Jacbson M: *Pesticides of the Future*, Dekker, New York, 1975.

Morgan DP: *Recognition and Management of Pesticide Poisonings*, EPA-540/9-80, Washington DC, Jan 182, 3rd ed.

EPA Pesticide Reregistration. (700-K92-004). May 1992.

EPA Status of Pesticides in Reregistration and Special Review. (738-R-93-009), June 1993.

EPA Pesticides Industry Sales and Usage 1990 and 1991 Market Estimates. (H-7503Q), Fall 1992.

EPA Suspended and Cancelled Pesticides, 3rd rev, EPA, Office of Public Awareness (A-107), Washington DC, Jan 1985.

Farm Chemicals Handbook, 8th ed, Meister Publ, Willoughby OH, 1994

Ware GW: *Pesticides. Theory and Application*, WH Freeman, San Francisco, 1983.

Wiswesser WJ, ed: *Pesticide Index*, 5th ed, Entomol Soc Am, College Park MD 1976.

Hassall K: *The Chemistry of Pesticides*, Verlag Chemie, Deerfield Beach FL, 1982.

Herbicide Handbook, 5th ed, Weed Sci Soc Am, Champaign IL, 1983.

Sherma J: Pesticides. *Anal Chem 59:* 18R, 1987.

Storck WJ: Pesticides growth slow. *Chem Eng News (Nov 16)*: 35, 1987.

Citizens Guide to Pesticides, EPA, Office of Pesticide Programs, Washington DC, Sep 1987.

The Federal Insecticide, Fungicide, and Rodenticide Act (as amended), EPA, Washington DC, 540/09-89-012, Oct. 1988

Regulating Pesticides in Food, Natl Acad Press, Washington DC, 1987.

40 CFR 150–189 (as of July 1, 1987), Protection of Environment, USGPO, 1987.

Pesticide Fact Handbook (EPA regulatory status of 550 tradenamed pesticides), Noyes Data Corp, Park Ridge NJ, 1988.

Pesticide Fact Handbook, Vol 2. (EPA regulatory status of 430 tradenamed pesticides), Noyes Data Corp., Park Ridge, NJ, 1990.

CHAPTER 79

Diagnostic Drugs and Reagents

Jan N Bair, PhD
Professor of Hospital Pharmacy
College of Pharmacy
Associate Administrator for Professional Services
and Director of Pharmacy Services
University of Utah Hospital
University of Utah
Salt Lake City, Utah 84132

The classic studies of Abed and Rowntree in 1909 demonstrated that parenterally administered phenoltetrachlorophthalein was excreted only in the bile while phenolsulfonphthalein was excreted almost exclusively in the urine. These findings were adopted promptly by Rowntree and his associates as a means of testing liver and kidney function.

Diagnostic methods have become increasingly complex and frequently involve the use of inorganic or organic chemicals that must meet all approval criteria as drugs. These chemicals, or more appropriately drugs, may be used *in vitro*, eg, reagent strips for blood or urine tests, or *in vivo*, eg, thyroid stimulating hormone, as a thyroid function test. A number of radioactive substances have been introduced to measure organic function and these are discussed in Chapter 51.

Although some drugs employed as diagnostic agents are innocuous and very specific in their action, others possess pharmacological activity and/or undesirable side effects. Indeed, no *in vivo* diagnostic test or drug is completely devoid of risk. Sudden death from an anaphylactic reaction has followed the intravenous injection of such relatively inert substances as dehydrocholic acid. Alarming pharmacological responses have been observed to follow the use of more active agents, such as the iodine-containing compounds. Iodism can follow the use of diagnostic agents with a high iodine content, eg, X-ray contrast media. Electrolyte imbalances and cardiovascular reactions can occur as the result of the release of high concentrations of cations, eg, calcium, potassium and sodium. Other untoward effects include mild transient symptoms such as restlessness, sensations of warmth, sneezing, perspiration, salivation, flushing, pressure in the upper abdomen, dizziness, nausea, vomiting, chills, fever, headache, pallor and tremors. Rarely, swollen eyelids, laryngospasm, respiratory difficulties, hypotension, cardiac reactions and cyanosis have been reported.

Hypersensitivity reactions may occur. In rare instances, despite the most careful sensitivity testing, anaphylactoid reactions also may occur. In addition, renal function tests may be altered and renal failure may occur. Moreover, these drugs should be administered with extreme caution to patients known or suspected to have pheochromocytoma. These materials have been shown to promote the phenomenon of sickling in individuals who are homozygous for sickle cell disease. Iodine-containing contrast agents may alter the results of thyroid function tests; such tests, if indicated, should be performed prior to the administration of the contrast agent.

These agents should be used with extreme caution in patients with a positive history of bronchial asthma or allergy, a family history of allergy or a previous reaction or hypersensitivity to a contrast agent, those with combined renal and hepatic disease, severe hypertension or congestive heart failure. The safe use of iodinated drugs during pregnancy has not been established; therefore, these agents should be used in pregnant patients only when, in the judgment of the physician, such use is deemed essential to the welfare of the patient. In general, infant nursing should not be continued following administration of any of these iodinated substances. Therefore, it generally is agreed that the clinician should evaluate carefully the need for every test and should reserve *in vivo* diagnostic drugs for those situations where effective management of the patient depends on their use. In addition, appropriate facilities should be available for coping with situations that may arise as a result of the procedure, as well as for emergency treatment of severe reactions to the agent itself. During intravascular administration of a radiographic contrast agent, competent personnel and emergency facilities should be available, and these should be accessible for 30 to 60 minutes after the procedure, since severe delayed reactions have been known to occur.

There are a great many radiographic contrast agents, and estimates indicate in excess of ten million intravascular injections per year in the US.[1] The absolute quantity of iodine, placed in the path of the X-rays, determines the degree of opacity achieved by the contrast agent and, therefore, the ultimate value of the test result. The radiographic contrast agents can be divided into two general categories; high-osmolality contrast agents (HOCA), which are also known as "conventional agents" or "ionic agents," and the newer, low-osmolality contrast agents (LOCA), approved for use in the US in 1985, which often are called "nonionic agents". References to the ionic or nonionic status of these groups does not always hold true since the latter group contains one low-osmolality ionic dimer, ioxaglate meglumine sodium.[2]

Typical representatives of the HOCA group are diatrizoate, iothalamate and metrizoate salts which are ionic and develop a very high osmotic pressure, as much as eight times, when compared to normal human plasma. Representatives of the LOCA group are iohexol, iopamidol and ioversol, which are nonionic and develop an osmotic pressure roughly twice that of plasma. An additional consideration of the LOCA group is that their cost is approximately 10 to 20 times that of the HOCA group of products, which can have a significant impact on the cost of health care.

There are several categories of procedures wherein radiopaque contrast media are used. A detailed discussion of these procedures is beyond the scope of this chapter. Some of the more common procedures are listed below.

Peripheral angiography, cerebral angiography, computed tomography (CT), coronary angiography ventriculography, excretory urography (intravenous pyelography) and myelography (the low-osmolality nonionic contrast media are the accepted standards of practice).

This chapter includes most of the currently available diagnostic drugs and chemicals. They are listed alphabetically by the category of test functionality, eg, gallbladder function. Many drugs are referenced to the section of this text wherein their major pharmacological actions are described. The use of some of these drugs for diagnostic tests actually may be incidental to their primary pharmacological purpose.

Many test reagents, in the form of tablets or strips, are listed under the name of the agent for which the test is indicated, eg, Acetone, Albumin, etc. These tests are primarily qualitative color reactions that indicate the presence or absence, and occasionally an approximate level of presence, of the agent indicated. They are used as *in vitro* diagnostic aids by a patient at home as well as the physician in the office. Detailed characteristics and specific uses may be found in the manufacturer's package insert.

Acetone (see also *Ketone Bodies,* page 524)

Acetest Reagent (*Ames*) tablets for urine or blood test.
Chemstrip K (*Boehringer Mannheim*) reagent papers for urine test.
Ketostix Strips (*Ames*) reagent strips for urine test.

Adrenocortical Insufficiency

Corticotropin (Acthar, Cortophin-Zinc)—see page 1060.
Cosyntropin (Cortrosyn-Organon)—see page 1061.

Albumin (see also *Protein,* page 524)

Albustix Strips (*Ames*) reagent strips for urine test.

Amyloidosis

Congo Red

1-Naphthalenesulfonic acid, 3,3′-[[1,1′-biphenyl]-4,4′-diylbis(azo)]bis[4-amino-, disodium salt; Direct Red

Colour Index Direct red 28 disodium salt; CI no 22120 [573-58-0] C_{32}-H_{22}-$N_6Na_2O_6S_2$ (696.67).

Preparation—Benzidine is doubly diazotized and coupled with 4-amino-1-naphthalenesulfonic acid. The resulting bisazo acid is then converted to the disodium salt.

Description—Dark-red or reddish brown powder; odorless; decomposes on exposure to acid fumes; solutions have a pH of 8 to 9.5.

Solubility—1 g in about 30 mL water; slightly soluble in alcohol; practically insoluble in ether.

Uses—In a wide variety of diagnostic tests. However, it is recognized only for its use in the detection of *amyloidosis.* As much as 80% of an injected dose can be retained by the abnormal amyloid deposit. Thus, the dye will disappear more rapidly from the blood of affected patients than it does from the normal individual. In amyloid growths in the liver, no dye appears in the urine; in amyloid growths in the kidneys, substantial amounts appear in the urine. The drug should be injected slowly to prevent thrombosis. Except for rare idiosyncratic reactions which may cause death, the drug is relatively free from toxic effects.

Dose—*Intravenous,* **100** to **200 mg** as a **1%** solution in water for injection.

Dosage Form—Injection: 1%.

Bacteriuria

Microstix-3 Strips (*Ames*) test for nitrite in urine and for bacterial growth.
Uricult (*Med Technol*) urine culture test to detect bacteriuria and identify uropathogens.
Isocult for Bacteriuria (*SmithKline Diagnostics*) culture test for bacteriuria

Bilirubin (see also *Bilirubin,* page 525)

Ictotest Tablets (*Ames*) reagent for urine test

Blood Urea Nitrogen

Azostix Srips (*Ames*) reagent strips for blood test

Blood Volume Determination

The estimation of blood volume is important in detecting impending shock and as a guide to the amount of plasma or other fluids to be used in order to avoid inadequate or excessive dosage.

Evans Blue

1,3-Naphthalenedisulfonic acid, 6,6′-[(3,3′-dimethyl[1,1′-biphenyl]-4,4′-diyl)-bis(azo)]bis[4-amino-5-hydroxy]-, tetrasodium salt

Colour Index: direct blue 53 tetrasodium salt; CI no 23860 [314-13-6] $C_{34}H_{24}N_6Na_4O_{14}S_4$ (960.79).

Preparation—By diazotizing *o*-tolidine and coupling the resulting diazonium compound with 1-amino-8-naphthol-2,4-disulfonic acid.

Description—Green, bluish green or brown powder; odorless; the dried product is hygroscopic; exhibits a maximum absorbance at about 610 nm.

Solubility—Very soluble in water; very slightly soluble in alcohol; practically insoluble in benzene, carbon tetrachloride, ether or chloroform.

Uses—A *diagnostic agent* employed in *blood volume estimation.* A known quantity of the dye is injected into the blood stream. It combines firmly with plasma protein and remains within the intravascular compartment. After allowing time for thorough mixing (10 to 15 min), the withdrawal of a sample of blood and determination of the concentration of the dye in the sample enables the clinician to calculate the volume of blood in the patient. No adverse effects—either acute or chronic—have been reported. Massive doses stain the sclerae and skin but disappear over a period of several weeks.

Dose—*Usual, intravenous,* **2** to **4 mL** of injection containing 4.52 mg of dried Evans Blue/mL.

Dosage Form—Injection: 22.6 mg/5 mL.

Bronchial Airway Hyperactivity

Methacholine Chloride

1-Propanaminium, 2-(acetyloxy)-*N,N,N*-trimethyl-, chloride; Provocholine (*Roche*)

$$\left[CH_3COOCH(CH_3)CH_2N^+(CH_3)_3 \right] Cl^-$$

[62-51-1] $C_8H_{18}ClNO_2$ (195.69).

Preparation—Chloroacetone and trimethylamine are reacted to form β-methyl-*N,N,N*-trimethylacetonyl ammonium chloride which is reduced catalytically to the secondary alcohol and esterified with acetic anhydride.

Description—Deliquescent crystals, melts about 171°, after thorough drying; faint putrescent odor.

Solubility—Freely soluble in water, alcohol or chloroform.

Uses—A parasympathomimetic (cholinergic) agent for the *diagnosis of bronchial airway hyperactivity* in subjects who do not display symptoms of asthma. Asthmatics are significantly more sensitive to inhaled methacholine chloride than are healthy subjects. The difference in response provides the pharmacological basis for this diagnostic test. It should not be used in patients with epilepsy, cardiovascular, peptic ulcer or thyroid disease; likewise, it is contraindicated in patients with urinary tract obstruction. Adverse effects *after inhalation* include headache, throat irritation, lightheadedness and itching; those after *oral administration* include nausea, vomiting, hypotension, fainting and transient complete heart block. Patients should be informed of the possibility of these adverse effects and instructed how to manage such symptoms. The safety of the test during pregnancy and lactation, and in children under 5 yr, has not been established.

Dose—*Inhalation,* **0.025** to **25 mg/mL** administered by nebulizer during 5 breaths.

Dosage Form—Powder (for reconstitution of solution for inhalation): 100 mg in 5-mL vials.

Candida

Isocult for Candida (*SmithKline Diagnostics*) culture test for vaginal surface sample.

Coccidiomycosis Skin Test Antigen (see page 1432)

Coccidiodin.

Chlamydia Trachomatis

Chlamydiazyme (*Abbott*) solid-phase enzyme immunoassay

MicroTrak Chlamydia Trachomatis direct specimen test (*Syva*) slide test

Dental Plaque

Erythrosine Sodium

Spiro[isobenzofuran-1(3*H*),9′-[9*H*]xanthen]-3-one, 3′,6′-dihydroxy- 2′,4′,5′,7′-tetraiodo-, disodium salt; Trace (*Lorvic*)

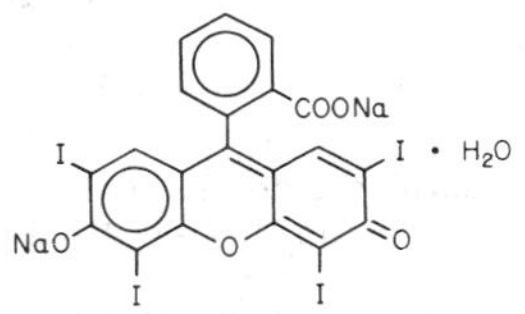

2′,4′,5′,7′-Tetraiodofluorescein disodium salt monohydrate *Colour Index:* Food Red 14; CI no 45430 [49746-10-3] (897.88); *anhydrous* [568-63-8 or 16423-68-0] $C_{20}H_6I_4Na_2O_5$ (879.86); a dye consisting principally of erythrosine sodium, with smaller amounts of lower iodinated fluoresceins; contains not less than 87% of erythrosine sodium.

Preparation—Fluorescein is dissolved in NaOH solution and treated with iodine in KI solution.

Description—Red or brownish red powder; odorless; dissolves in water to form a bluish red solution that shows no fluorescence in ordinary light.

Solubility—Soluble in water, glycerin or propylene glycol; sparingly soluble in alcohol; insoluble in fats or oils.

Uses—A *dental disclosing agent* used to identify areas of plaque on the teeth. When the solution is applied topically to the teeth or the tablets chewed, areas of plaque to be removed are colored red. The identified plaque is removed and the test repeated as necessary.

Dose—For *external use,* apply **solution** *topically* to the teeth or chew **1 tablet** thoroughly. Following use, rinse the mouth with water (*Do not swallow*).

Dosage Forms—Solution: 2%; Tablets: 3.5 and 8.5 mg.

Diabetes Mellitus

Many products are available to test the blood or urine for glucose content. Many additional products are available that will test for more than one single entity in the blood or urine (see also *Glucose* (reducing substances) page 524).

Copper Sulfate Reduction Method for Urine Testing—

Clinitest tablets (*Ames*).

Glucose Oxidase Reagents for Urine Testing—

Chemstrip uG Strips (*Boehringer Mannheim*).

Clinistix Strips (*Ames*).

Diastix Strips (*Ames*).

Tes-Tape (*Lilly*).

Testing Blood for Glucose Content—

Chemstrip bg Strips (*Boehringer Mannheim*).

Dextrostix Reagent Strips (*Ames*).

Diascan-S Reagent Strips (*Home Diagnostics*).

Glucostix Strips (*Ames*).

Tracer bG Reagent Strips (*Boehringer Mannheim*).

Visidex II Reagent Strips (*Ames*).

Testing for Glucose and Other Contents of the Urine

Bili-Labstix (*Ames*) tests for glucose, protein, pH, blood, ketones and bilirubin.

Chemstrip 2 GP (*Boehringer Mannheim*) tests for both glucose and protein.

Chemstrip 2 LN (*Boehringer Mannheim*) tests for nitrite and leukocytes.

Chemstrip 4 THE OB (*Boehringer Mannheim*) tests for glucose, protein, blood and leukocytes.

Chemstrip 6 (*Boehringer Mannheim*) tests for glucose, protein, pH, blood, ketones and leukocytes.

Chemstrip 7 (*Boehringer Mannheim*) tests for glucose, protein, pH, blood, ketones, bilirubin and leukocytes.

Chemstrip 8 (*Boehringer Mannheim*) tests for glucose, protein, pH, blood, ketones, bilirubin, urobilinogen and leukocytes.

Chemstrip 9 (*Boehringer Mannheim*) provides for the same nine tests as *Chemstrip 10 with SG,* except that it does not test for specific gravity.

Chemstrip 10 with SG (*Boehringer Mannheim*) tests for glucose, protein, pH, blood, ketones, bilirubin, urobilinogen, nitrite, leukocytes, and specific gravity.

Chemstrip uGK (*Boehringer Mannheim*) broad range tests for glucose and ketones.

Combistix (*Ames*) tests for glucose, protein and pH.

Glucose & Ketone Urine Test (*Major*) tests for glucose and ketones.

Hema-Combistix (*Ames*) tests for glucose, protein, pH and blood.

Keto-Diastix (*Ames*) tests for glucose and ketones.

Labstix (*Ames*) tests for glucose, protein, Ph, blood and ketones.

Multistix (*Ames*) tests for glucose, protein, pH, blood, ketones, bilirubin and urobilinogen.

Multistix SG (*Ames*) provides for the same tests as Multistix (above) with the addition of specific gravity.

Multistix 2 (*Ames*) tests for nitrite and luekocytes.

Multistix 7 (*Ames*) tests for glucose, protein, pH, blood, ketones, nitrite and leukocytes.

Multistix 8 SG (*Ames*) provides for the same tests as Multistix 7 (above) with the addition of specific gravity.

Multistix 9 (*Ames*) provides for the same nine tests as does *Chemstrip 9* (above).

Multistix 9 SG (*Ames*) tests for glucose, protein, pH, blood, ketones, bilirubin, nitrite and leukocytes, plus specific gravity.

Multistix 10 SG (*Ames*) provides for the same tests as Multistix 9 SG (above) with the addition of urobilinogen.

N-Multistix (*Ames*) tests for glucose, protein, pH, blood, ketones, bilirubin, urobilinogen and nitrite.

N-Multistix SG (*Ames*) provides for the same tests as *N-Multistix* (above) with the addition of specific gravity.

Uristix (*Ames*) tests for both glucose and protein.

Uristix 4 (*Ames*) tests for glucose, protein, nitrite and leukocytes.

Drug-Hypersensitivity

Benzylpenicilloyl Polylysine

Pre-Pen (*Kremers Urban*)

Penicilloyl polylysine [53608-77-8].

Preparation—From penicillenic acid and polylysine. See *J Exp Med 115:* 803, 1962.

Uses—A *skin test antigen* used to assess the risk of hypersensitivity reactions prior to the administration of penicillin G to adults who have a history of sensitivity to penicillin. It appears to be more sensitive than penicillin G skin tests in detecting penicillin hypersensitivity. This test is of particular value in patients with life-threatening infections for which penicillins are the drugs of choice; those testing positive can be desensitized prior to starting therapy. Adverse effects include an occasional local inflammatory response, pruritis, erythema, wheal, urticaria and/or edema. Rarely, these reactions may become generalized with or without some angioneurotic edema, urticaria, dyspnea, hypotension and/or bronchospasm. Its safe use during pregnancy has not been established.

Dose—*Scratch test:* a small drop is placed on a nonbleeding scratch 3 to 5 mm in length on the inner volar surface of the forearm and gently rubbed with an applicator or toothpick. *Intradermal test:* a tuberculin syringe (26- to 30-gauge, 1/8- to 5/8-in needle) is used to inject under the surface of the skin sufficient of the test substance to raise the smallest perceptable bleb; a like amount of 0.9% sodium chloride is injected as a control at least 1.5 in from the test site. A negative response consists of no increase in the size of the original bleb and/or no greater reaction than that at the control site.

Dosage Form—Injection: 6×10^{-5} *M* of benzylpenicilloyl.

Gallbladder Function, Cholecystography and Choleangiography

Ceruletide Diethylamine

Caerulin compound with *N*-ethylethaneamine; Tymtran (*Adria*)

[71247-25-1] $C_{58}H_{73}N_{13}O_{21}S_2 . xC_4H_{11}N$.

Preparation—The free acid has been isolated from the skin of the Australian tree toad, *Hyla caerulea*, as described in *Experientia 23:* 700, 1967. The salt is formed on treatment with diethylamine.

Description—Off-white hygroscopic powder

Solubility—Soluble in dimethylformamide and dimethyl sulfoxide; insoluble in ether or acetone.

Uses—As an aid in oral *cholecystokinetic cholecystography* whenever contraction of the gallbladder would facilitate diagnostic visualization, particularly when the gallbladder is opacified or in any way obscured. This drug is qualitatively identical to cholecystokinin. It contracts the gallbladder, stimulates pancreatic exocrine and gastric secretion, delays gastric emptying, inhibits motility of the proximal duodenum and stimulates motility of the distal duodenum, jejunum, ileum and to a lesser extent, the colon. Gallbladder contraction is evident 10 min after intramuscular injection and contraction exceeding 40% occurs within 15 to 20 min. Adverse reactions are usually mild and of brief duration. Abdominal pain or cramps and nausea occur in about 10% of patients. Other systemic effects include eructation, regurgitation, weakness, flushing, dizziness, hypotension, diarrhea, sweating, an urge to defecate and urinate, hiccoughs and gas. Its safe use in pregnant women, lactating mothers and children has not been established.

Dose—Intramuscular, **0.3 μg/kg.**

Dosage Form—Injection: 40 μg (20 μg/mL) in 2-mL ampuls.

Cholecystokinin

CCK (*Pharmacia*)

Pancreozymin [9011-97-6]. A polypeptide isolated from the mucosa of the intestine which induces contraction and emptying of the gall bladder. Porcine cholecystokinin contains 33 peptide residues; the *C*-terminal peptide is identical to cerulitide (*Eur J Biochem 6:* 156, 1968).

Preparation—Both the *C*-terminal dodecapeptide and the *N*-terminal hexapeptide have been synthesized: see *J Org Chem 37:* 2303, 1972.

Uses: As adjunctive therapy in *cholecystography*, preoperative and secondary *cholangiography*, and X-ray studies of the small bowel. Adverse effects are rare. If the drug is given too rapidly, flushing may occur. See Ceruletide Diethylamine, above.

Dose—Intravenous: 1 to 75 IDU (see package insert).

Dosage Form—Powder for Injection: 75 Ivy Dog Units/vial.

Iocetamic Acid

Propanoic acid, 3-[acetyl(3-amino-2,4,6-triiodophenyl)amino]-2-methyl-, Cholebrine (*Mallinckrodt*)

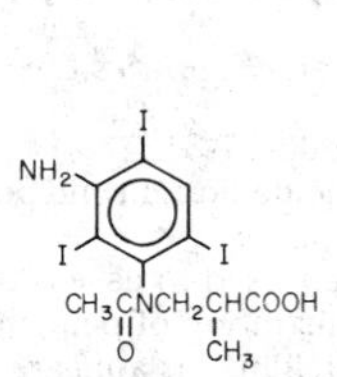

A mixture of two diastereoisomers (A and B). *N*-Acetyl-*N*-(3-amino-2,4,6-triiodophenyl)-2-methyl-β-alanine [16034-77-8] $C_{12}H_{13}I_3N_2O_3$ (613.96).

Preparation—*m*-Nitroaniline is heated with methacrylic acid and the resulting *N*-(3-nitrophenyl)-2-methyl-β-alanine is *N*-acetylated with a mixture of acetic anhydride and acetic acid. After reducing the NO_2 to NH_2 with the aid of Raney nickel, iodination is effected with $NaICl_2$.

Description—White to creamy white powder; odorless or has a faint acetic acid odor; unstable in light; melts between 190 and 222° (isomer A at about 232°, isomer B at about 201°); pK_a (isomer A) 4.25; pK_a (isomer B) 4.10.

Solubility—Insoluble in water; slightly soluble in alcohol, acetone or chloroform; very slightly soluble in ether or benzene.

Uses—An oral *cholecystographic* agent indicated for the radiographic visualization of the gall bladder. It is absorbed rapidly following oral administration, conjugated with glucuronic acid in the liver, secreted into the bile as radiopaque glucuronide and concentrated in the functioning gallbladder. Contraction of the gall bladder also may provide visualization of the biliary ducts. Contraindications, warnings, precautions and adverse reactions are similar to other iodinated diagnostic agents.

Dose—*Usual, oral, adult,* **3 g** (4 tablets) or **4.5 g** (6 tablets) as a single dose. Cholecystography is performed in 10 to 15 hr.

Dosage Form—Tablets: 750 mg.

Iodipamide Meglumine

Benzoic acid, 3,3′-[(1,6-dioxo-1,6-hexanediyl)diimino]bis[2,4,6-triiodo-, compd. with 1-deoxy-1-(methylamino)-D-glucitol (1:2); Cholografin Meglumine, Renovue-Dip and Renovue-65 (*Squibb*)

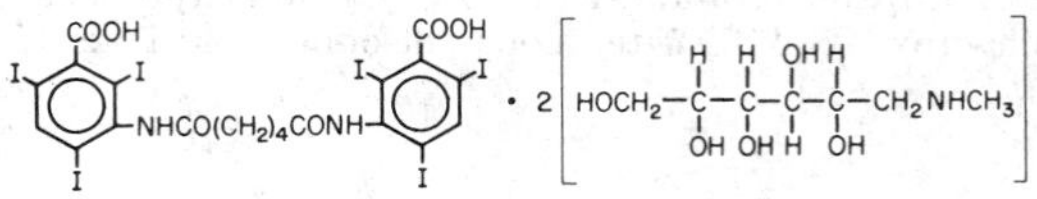

1-Deoxy-1-(methylamino)-D-glucitol 3,3′-(adipoyldiimino)-bis- [2,4,6-triiodobenzoate] (2:1) (salt) [3521-84-4] $C_{20}H_{14}I_6N_2O_6 . 2C_7H_{17}NO_5$ (1530.20).

Preparation—Iodipamide is reacted with a double equimolar quantity of methylglucamine (meglumine), using sufficient water for injection to produce a solution of the required concentration.

Description—Clear, colorless to pale yellow, slightly viscous liquid.

Uses—For *intravenous cholangiography* and *cholecystography* as follows: visualization of the gallbladder and biliary ducts in the differential diagnosis of acute abdominal conditions, visualization of the biliary ducts especially in patients with symptoms after cholecystectomy and visualization of the gallbladder in patients unable to take oral contrast media or to absorb media from the gastrointestinal tract. The contrast medium appears in the bile within 10 to 15 min after injection and the biliary ducts are visualized within 25 min; the gallbladder begins to fill within 1 hr, maximum filling occurring in 2 to 2.5 hr. Adverse reactions and contraindications are similar to those common to iodine-containing compounds.

Dose—*Usual, intravenous, adult,* **100 mL** of 10.3% solution by slow intravenous infusion over 30 to 45 min.; **4.5 mL/kg** by intravenous infusion over 10 min, but not to exceed 300 mL; **20 mL** of 52% solution administered over 10 min.; **0.8 mL/kg** of 65% solution (not to exceed 50 mL) within 1 or 2 min. *Children, less than 6 mo,* **5 mL** of 65%; *6 to 12 mo,* **8 mL**; *1 to 2 yr,* **10 mL**; *3 to 5 yr,* **12 mL**; *6 to 7 yr,* **15 mL**; *8 to 10 yr,* **18 mL**; *11 to 12 yr,* **20 mL**; *over 12 yr,* **0.8 mL/kg**; *maximum dose,* **50 mL.**

Dosage Form—Injection: 10.3, 24, 52 and 65% solution.

Iopanoic Acid

Benzenepropanoic acid, 3-amino-α-ethyl-2,4,6-triiodo-, Telepaque (*Winthrop*)

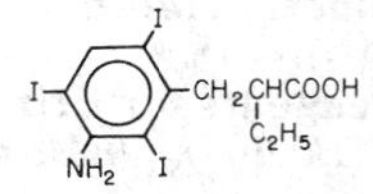

3-Amino-α-ethyl-2,4,6-triiodohydrocinnamic acid [96-83-3] $C_{11}H_{12}I_3NO_2$ (570.93).

Preparation—A mixture of *m*-nitrobenzaldehyde, butyric anhydride and sodium butyrate is heated in xylene to effect a Perkin condensation yielding *m*-nitro-α-ethylcinnamic acid. The acid is reduced with hydrogen in the presence of Raney nickel. The resulting *m*-amino-α-ethylhydrocinnamic acid is iodinated with iodine monochloride in acetic acid solution.

Description—Cream-colored powder; tasteless or nearly so; faint characteristic odor; affected by light; melts with decomposition between 152 and 158°.

Solubility—Insoluble in water; soluble in alcohol, chloroform or ether; soluble in solutions of alkali hydroxides or carbonates.

Uses—Orally, as a *radiopaque medium* in *cholecystography* and *cholangiography*. It is absorbed promptly from the gastrointestinal tract, concentrated in the gallbladder, and subsequently excreted, approximately two-thirds through the gastrointestinal tract and one-third through the kidneys. About 50% of an administered dose is excreted within 24 hr and the remainder in about 5 days. It is relatively free from undesirable reactions and has low toxicity. Occasionally, nausea and diarrhea and, rarely, dysuria have followed its administration. A mild stinging sensation during urination may occur. Hypersensitivity reactions involving the skin, mucous membranes, and a systemic serum sickness-type reaction have been reported. It is contraindicated in patients with acute nephritis and uremia, since it is eliminated by the kidneys. It should not be administered when disorders of the gastrointestinal tract exist which prevent absorption of the medium.

The usual regimen is to give the patient a fat-free evening meal following which it is administered approximately 14 hr before the time scheduled for roentgenography. Immediately after the roentgen examination, the patient is given a high-fat meal and additional exposures are made in order to evaluate the contraction of the gallbladder and to visualize the patency of the extrahepatic ducts. When the latter structures are of particular interest, its dose may be increased to 5 or 6 g.

Dose—**3** to **6 g;** *usual,* **3 g.**

Dosage Form—Tablets: 500 mg, in envelopes of 6 tablets.

Ipodate Calcium

Benzenepropanoic acid, 3-[[(dimethylamino)methylene]amino]-2,4,6- triiodo-, calcium salt; Oragrafin Calcium (*Squibb*)

$$\left[I_3C_6H(CH_2CH_2COO^-)(N{=}CHN(CH_3)_2) \right]_2 Ca$$

Calcium 3-[[(dimethylamino)methylene]amino]-2,4,6-triiodohydrocinnamate [1151-11-7] $C_{24}H_{24}CaI_6N_4O_4$ (1233.99).

Preparation—By precipitation using aqueous solutions of sodium ipodate and calcium chloride. The crude precipitate is recrystallized from a suitable solvent, such as aqueous dimethylformamide. The preparation of *Ipodate Sodium* is described in the next monograph.

Description—White to off-white, fine crystalline powder; odorless and has a chalky, very bitter taste; it should be stored at room temperature in a tightly closed container protected from light; melts at 300° with decomposition.

Solubility—1 g in 1700 mL water or 2.6 mL chloroform; slightly soluble in alcohol.

Uses—A water-insoluble substance that contains 61.7% iodine and is used as a contrast medium for *cholecystography*. It also may be used for *cholangiography*, but is not the drug of choice. The agent is absorbed rapidly from the gastrointestinal tract and excreted in the bile in sufficient quantity to outline the biliary ducts within 30 min after administration; optimal opacification of the ducts occurs 1 to 3 hr after ingestion. Maximal visualization of the gallbladder occurs 10 hr after administration of the salt. Untoward effects reported include abdominal cramping, diarrhea, nausea, vomiting, dysuria, urticaria, headache, heartburn and epigastric pain. Although rare, hypotension and circulatory collapse have been reported. The drug is contraindicated in patients with severe renal disease and in patients known to be allergic to iodine. It also interferes with thyroid function tests based on uptake of radioactive iodine by the gland.

Dose—*Usual,* **3** to **6 g** as a single dose given 10 to 12 hr before the examination.

Dosage Form—Granules for Oral Suspension: 3 g.

Ipodate Sodium

Benzenepropanoic acid, 3-[[(dimethylamino)methylene]amino]-2,4,6-triiodo-, sodium salt; Oragrafin Sodium (*Squibb*)

$$I_3C_6H(CH_2CH_2COONa)(N{=}CHN(CH_3)_2)$$

Sodium 3-[[(dimethylamino)methylene]amino]-2,4,6-triiodohy- drocinnamate [1221-56-3] $C_{12}H_{12}I_3N_2NaO_2$ (619.94).

Preparation—3-Amino-2,4,6-triiodohydrocinnamic acid is condensed with *N,N*-dimethylformamide with the aid of iodomethanesulfonyl chloride to produce 3-[[(dimethylamino)methylene]-amino]-2,4,6-triiodohydrocinnamic acid. Neutralization of the acid with sodium hydroxide yields the sodium salt (*Chem Ber 93:* 2347, 1960).

Description—White to off-white, crystalline powder; odorless; it should be stored at room temperature in a tightly closed container protected from light; melts between 303° and 304° with decomposition.

Solubility—1 g in 1 mL water or 2 mL alcohol; very slightly soluble in chloroform.

Uses—A radiopaque medium for *cholecystography* and *cholangiography*. Except that this drug is somewhat less rapidly absorbed from the gastrointestinal tract, is soluble in water and contains slightly less iodine (61.4%), its actions, uses, onset and duration of effects and contraindications are similar to those for *Ipodate Calcium*.

Dose—**3** to **6 g;** *usual,* **3 g** given 12 hr before examination.

Dosage Form—Capsules: 500 mg.

Sincalide

Caerulein, 1-de(5-oxo-L-proline)-2-de-L-glutamide-5-L-methionine; Kinevac (*Squibb*)

```
  SO3H
   |
Asp-Tyr-Met-Gly-Trp-Met-Asp-Phe—NH2
 1   2   3   4   5   6   7   8
```

[25126-32-3] $C_{49}H_{62}N_{10}O_{16}S_3$ (1143.27).

Sincalide is the synthetic C-terminal octapeptide of cholecystokinin.

Description—White, lyophilized powder.

Solubility—Very slightly soluble in water; practically insoluble in alcohol.

Uses—A synthetic fragment of cholecystokinin reported to be at least five times more active than the physiological hormone that stimulates contraction of the gallbladder and increases intestinal motility. It is used to obtain a *specimen of gallbladder bile,* in conjunction with secretin to *stimulate pancreatic secretion* for analysis, and for *postevacuation cholecystography* in cases where the physician wishes to avoid the usual fatty meal. Untoward reactions include mild, transient, abdominal discomfort and an urge to defecate, and occasional dizziness, flushing and nausea. Its safety in pregnant women or for children has not been established.

Dose—*Usual, adult, intravenous,* for *contraction of gallbladder,* **0.02 μg/kg** injected over a period of 30 to 60 sec; if satisfactory contraction does not occur in 15 min, a 2nd dose, **0.04 μg/kg,** may be administered. For the *secretin-sincalide* test, **0.25 unit/kg** of secretin infused over a period of 60 min, followed in 30 min with **0.02 μg/kg** of this drug administered over a 30-min period.

Dosage Form—Powder for Injection: 5 μg/vial.

Tyropanoate Sodium

Benzenepropanoic acid, α-ethyl-2,4,6-triiodo-3-[(1-oxobutyl)amino]-, monosodium salt; Bilopaque Sodium (*Sterling*)

$$I_3C_6H(CH_2CH(C_2H_5)COONa)(NHCOCH_2CH_2CH_3)$$

Sodium 3-butyramido-α-ethyl-2,4,6-triiodohydrocinnamate [7246-21-1] $C_{15}H_{17}I_3NNaO_3$ (663.01).

Preparation—Iopanoic acid is reacted with butyric anhydride in the presence of H_2SO_4 as a catalyst. The reaction product is converted to the sodium salt with NaOH, and purified by recrystallization from a solvent such as isopropyl alcohol.

Description—Off-white powder; odolress; hygroscopic; bitter taste; decomposes on heating.

Solubility—Soluble in water or alcohol; very slightly soluble in acetone or ether.

Uses—An oral radiopaque agent used in *cholecystography*. Optimal visualization occurs in 10 to 12 hr after oral administration. The drug is contraindicated in patients with advanced hepatorenal disease, severe impairment of renal function, or severe gastrointestinal disease which prevents absorption. Common side effects include nausea, vomiting, abdominal cramps or discomfort. Other allergic responses characteristic of iodine-containing compounds have been observed. It is not recommended for use in children under 12 yr. Although no teratogenic effects have been observed in animals, the safe use of this agent in pregnant women has not been established.

Dose—*Usual, oral, adult* **3 g** administered with water in a single dose. For best results, drug administration is preceded by a diet containing some fat in order to empty the gallbladder. The meal immediately prior to drug administration should be fat-free. If no visualization occurs, the dose is repeated the next day.

Dosage Form—Capsules: 750 mg.

Gastric Function

In some clinical situations it is important to know if the stomach is capable of secreting hydrochloric acid. Proof of the absence of hydrochloric acid in the stomach is essential to the diagnosis of pernicious anemia and, in some circumstances, offers presumptive evidence of gastric cancer. On the other hand, the presence of hydrochloric acid contributes to the diagnosis of peptic ulcer and peptic esophagitis, which conversely can be excluded virtually by the demonstration of true achlorhydria.

Because the volume of acid secreted by the normal stomach covers the entire range of volume encountered in disease and because there is no sharp line of demarcation in the secretory capacity of the stomach variously diseased, the quantity of acid secreted even in response to a controlled stimulus is seldom of any diagnostic importance. Therefore, it is usually important only to establish the presence or absence of free hydrochloric acid in the stomach. The gastric stimulants included in this section and those listed below are frequently of value for this purpose.

Alcohol—page 1404.

Caffeine—page 1231.

Caffeine and Sodium Benzoate—page 1233.

Histamine Phosphate—page 1222.

Pentagastrin

L-Phenylalaninamide, *N*-[(1,1-dimethylethoxy)carbonyl]-β-alanyl-L-tryptophyl-L-methionyl-L-α-aspartyl-, Peptavlon (*Ayerst*)

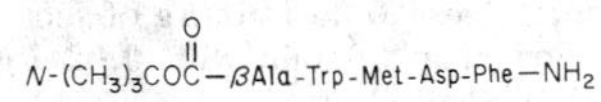

$N\text{-}(CH_3)_3COC(=O)-\beta Ala\text{-}Trp\text{-}Met\text{-}Asp\text{-}Phe-NH_2$

N-Carboxy-β-alanyl-L-tryptophyl-L-methionyl-L-aspartylphenyl-L-alaninamide, *N-tert*-butyl ester [5534-95-2] $C_{37}H_{49}N_7O_9S$ (767.90).

Description—Fine colorless needles; melts about 230° with decomposition.

Solubility—Soluble in dimethyl sulfoxide or dimethylformamide; slightly soluble in alcohol or dilute solutions of ammonia; practically insoluble in water, ether or benzene.

Uses—A diagnostic agent used to evaluate gastric acid secretory function. It is useful in testing for *anacidity* in patients with suspected pernicious anemia, atrophic gastritis or gastric carcinoma; for *hypersecretion* in patients with possible duodenal ulcer or postoperative stomal ulcer; for the diagnosis of Zollinger-Ellison tumor and for determining the adequacy of acid reducing operations for peptic ulcer. Acid secretion is increased within 10 min after a subcutaneous injection and reaches a peak in most patients within 20 to 30 min. Duration is usually between 60 and 80 min. Plasma half-life is reported to be less than 1 min. Excessive doses may inhibit gastric acid secretion. It is contraindicated in patients hypersensitive to the drug. Likewise, it should be used with caution in patients with pancreatic, hepatic or biliary disease. Adverse reactions include abdominal pain, nausea, vomiting, flushing, tachycardia, dizziness, faintness, lightheadedness, drowsiness, blurred vision and headache. Its use in pregnant women and children has not been studied.

Dose—*Usual, subcutaneous, adult:* **6 μg/kg.**

Dosage Form—Injection: 0.25 mg (250 μg)/mL in 2-mL ampuls.

Histoplasmosis Skin Test Antigen (page 1432).

Intestinal Function

Previous to the introduction of barium sulfate as a contrast medium in 1910, insoluble bismuth salts were used in roentgen examination of the gastrointestinal tract. Bismuth subcarbonate was preferred over the subnitrate because of its lower toxicity. In modern medical practice, barium sulfate has replaced the bismuth salts because it is completely innocuous even when taken in very large doses and it is inexpensive. Since the soluble barium salts are highly toxic, it is recommended that when barium sulfate is prescribed, the title should be written out in full.

Barium Sulfate

Sulfuric acid, barium salt (1:1); Synthetic or Artificial Barytes (*Various Mfrs*)

Barium sulfate (1:1) [7727-43-7] $BaSO_4$ (233.39).

Caution—When Barium Sulfate is prescribed, the title always should be written out in full to avoid confusion with the poisonous barium sulfide or barium sulfite.

Preparation—Barium sulfate precipitates when an aqueous solution containing barium ion is mixed with a solution containing sulfate ion. It also can be obtained by suitable purification of native barium sulfate.

Description—Fine, white, bulky powder, free from grittiness; odorless; tasteless; its suspension in water is neutral to litmus paper.

Solubility—Practically insoluble in water, solutions of acids or alkalies or organic solvents.

Uses—Medicinally used in roentgenography for the purpose of making the intestinal tract opaque to the X-ray so that it may be photographed. As the amount required is large, 60 to 250 g (2 to 8 oz), and as soluble salts of barium are extremely poisonous, it is highly important to be sure that the sulfate dispensed is of USP quality. When preparing barium sulfate mixtures for X-ray diagnosis, they should be strained through gauze or mixed well with food, otherwise lumps of the salt may give false indication of an ulcer niche. The following suggestions are offered if specific directions are not given by the attending physician:

For the Roentgen-Ray Examination of the Stomach—The evening before the examination, the patient receives 30 mL of castor oil or other suitable cathartic. In the morning an ordinary portion of wheat-meal porridge, with which 60 g of barium sulfate has been mixed well, together with a little sugar and cream, is administered by mouth. The patient is then directed to abstain from further food. The examination is made 6 hr later.

For the Roentgen-Ray Examination of the Colon—An enema containing barium sulfate and one or more suitable dispersing and/ or suspending agents is warmed to body temperature and injected into the rectum from a height of from 3 to 6 ft (90 to 180 cm). The examination is made with a fluoroscope while the injection is passing into the rectum.

Suspensions of barium sulfate can be very constipating; impaction has occurred after such use.

Dose—*Usual, oral,* **60** to **450 g** in suitable suspension; *usual, rectal,* **150** to **750 g** in suitable suspension.

Dosage Form—for Suspension: a dry mixture containing not less than 90.0% $BaSO_4$, with one or more suitable dispersing and/or suspending agents and that may contain suitable colors, flavors, fluidizing agents and preservatives; in bulk or single-dose powder and disposable, prefilled cups or enema kits.

Xylose

D-Xylose; Xylo-Pfan (*Adria*)

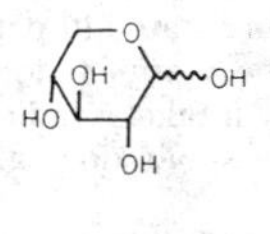

β-D-Xylopyranose [2460-44-8] $C_5H_{10}O_5$ (150.13).

Preparation—Prepared from corn cobs by distilling with 8% sulfuric acid; *J Amer Chem Soc 41:* 1002, 1919.

Description—White, monoclinic prisms or needles melting about 144°; very sweet taste; pK_a 12.14.

Solubility—1 g in 0.8 mL water; soluble in hot alcohol or pyridine.

Uses—The dextrorotatory form of this 5-carbon monosaccharide (Wood Sugar) used for evaluating *intestinal absorption* in both adults and children. Malabsorption may occur in any disease which affects the small bowel directly or indirectly, including such conditions as celiac sprue, tropical sprue, lymphoma, small bowel ischemia, blind loop syndrome, short bowel syndrome, Whipple's gastroenteritis, amyloid disease of the gut, Crohn's disease, radiation enteritis, cow's milk protein intolerance (post-challenge) and certain parasitic diseases such as giardiasis, coccidiosis and ascariasis.

In patients with signs and symptoms of malabsorption, the xylose absorption test may aid in providing an index of the degrees of impairment and the extent of therapy. Both blood and urine samples may be collected and these results may be considered together, for an individual patient, to provide a stricter definition of abnormalities. There are no know contra-indications to the use of xylose for the evaluation of intestinal absorption.

Dose—*For the urine test,* **25 g** is dissolved in 200 to 300 ml water, and the selected dose of 5 g or 25 g is administered orally in a single dose. Additional water intake during the first 2 hr will assure adequate urine flow for collection. *For the blood test,* **25 g** is dissolved in 100 to 200 ml water, and the selected dose of 5 g or 25 g is administered orally in a single dose. Patients must fast for a minimum of 8 hr prior to the test.

Dosage Form—Powder (oral administration only): 25 g.

Kidney Function

The rate of excretion of a number of drugs in the urine has been proposed as a means of measuring the functional capacity of the kidney. Glomerular filtration rate can be measured by the renal plasma clearance of inulin, thiosulfate, mannitol or endogenous creatinine. The inulin clearance is thought to be most reliable since mannitol is subject to some tubular reabsorption, thiosulfate to some tubular excretion and reabsorption and endogenous creatinine to some tubular excretion. Effective renal plasma flow and tubular functional capacity can be measured by the use of sodium aminohippurate and iodohippurate. Because of the greater accuracy and facility of chemical methods for the determination of the compound, sodium amminohippurate is considered the drug of choice. Although the excretion of phenolsulfonphthalein is accomplished by the same mechanisms as the excretion of sodium aminohippurate, its plasma clearance averages about two-thirds of the effective renal plasma flow and its toxicity prevents its use for the determination of functioning tubular capacity.

Aminohippurate Sodium

Glycine, *N*-(4-aminobenzoyl)-, monosodium salt; (*MSD*)

$H_2N-C_6H_4-CONHCH_2COONa$

Monosodium *p*-aminohippurate [94-16-6] $C_9H_9N_2NaO_3$ (216.17).

Preparation—*p*-Aminohippuric acid is prepared from *p*-nitrobenzoyl chloride and glycine and the nitro group reduced with Sn and HCl. The sodium salt of the acid is formed with NaOH and adjusting the pH of the resulting solution to 7 to 7.2 with citric acid. In preparing the injection, the salt is not isolated from the solution.

Uses—To estimate the *effective renal plasma flow* (ERPF) and to measure the functional capacity of the *renal tubular secretory mechanism.* After intravenous administration, the drug is distributed throughout the extracellular space. It is excreted mainly by proximal tubular secretion, although some glomerular secretion occurs. The half-life in patients with normal renal function is 24 min. Approximately 90% of the drug represented in plasma concentrations of 10 to 20 μg/mL is extracted from the renal circulation during a single passage through the kidneys; this results in urinary concentrations of 4 to 8 mg/mL. Normal values for *ERPF* are 675 + 150 mL/min for men and 595 + 125 mL/min for women. The maximum capacity of the proximal tubule cells to secrete PAH is reached at plasma levels of 400 to 600 μg/mL. The average normal values of *maximum tubular secretory capacity* are 80 to 90 mg/min for both men and women. Conditions that impair renal excretion include cardiac failure, primary vascular disease and most primary renal diseases.

Adverse reactions include nausea, vomiting, cramps and vasomotor disturbances. These tests are contraindicated in patients on drugs, such as diuretics, penicillin, probenecid or salicylates, which share the same tubular excretory mechanisms and agents such as procaine, sulfonamides and thiosulfones which interfere with the colorimetric analytical procedures. Safety and effectiveness during pregnancy, in nursing mothers and in children have not been established. Specialized references should be consulted for analysis procedures.

Dose—*Usual, adults, ERPF, intravenous, initially* **6** to **10 mg/ kg** followed by an *infusion dose* of **10** to **24 mg/min.** *Tubular secretory capacity:* see package insert.

Dosage Form—Injection (intravenous use only): 200 mg/mL in 10-mL ampuls.

Indigotindisulfonate Sodium

1*H*-Indole-5-sulfonic acid, 2-(1,3-dihydro-3-oxo-5-sulfo-2*H*-indol-2-ylidene)-2,3-dihydro-3-oxo-, disodium salt;
Soluble Indigo Blue; Indigo Carmine (*HW & D*)

Disodium 3,3′-dioxo[$\Delta^{2,2'}$-biindoline]-5,5′-disulfonate; Colour Index: Food Blue 1; CI no 73015 [860-22-0] $C_{16}H_8N_2Na_2O_8S_2$ (466.35).

Preparation—Anthranilic acid is treated with chloroacetic acid to form phenylglycine-*o*-carboxylic acid. The latter is fused with KOH or NaOH and the resulting indoxylacetic acid loses carbon dioxide to form *indoxyl,* which is oxidized by air to *indigo blue.* Indigo carmine is prepared from indigo blue by sulfonating with H_2SO_4 and neutralizing the SO_3H groups with sodium carbonate.

Description—Dusky, purplish blue powder or blue granules with a coppery luster; affected by light; solutions have a blue or bluish purple color.

Solubility—1 g in about 100 mL water; slightly soluble in alcohol; practically insoluble in most other organic solvents.

Uses—Originally, to measure kidney function, but excretion of the dye does not correlate well with renal failure. Currently used to localize ureteral orifices during cystoscopy and ureteral catheterization, and as a marker dye to identify severed ureters and fistulous communications. It is cleared rapidly from the circulation after intravenous injections; half-life is 4.5 min; approximately 10% is excreted by the kidney within 1 hr. Patients with a history of allergy should be tested for sensitivity before the drug is given. It also is employed as a *reagent,* as a *stain* for microscopic specimens and as a *dye.*

Dose—*Usual, intravenous,* **40 mg;** *usual, intramuscular,* **50** to **100 mg.**

Dosage Form—Injection: 40 mg/5 mL.

Inulin

(*Am Critical Care*)

Inulin [9005-80-5] $C_6H_{11}O_5(C_6H_{10}O_5)_nOH$. A substance, occurring in some plants of the *Compositae* family, closely allied to starch except that it is a levulan rather than a dextran. It differs from starch in the following particulars: it is colored yellow by iodine, does not gelatinize with water and is not found in plants in the form of granules having concentric layers. When hydrolyzed with acid, fructose is produced.

Preparation—Isolated from various *Compositae* members, eg, Inula, Taraxacum, Pyrethrum, Lappa, etc.

Uses—It is filtered only by the glomeruli and is neither secreted nor reabsorbed by the tubules. Therefore, it is used as a *diagnostic agent for evaluation of glomerular filtration.* It is considered the most sensitive and accurate method for the measurement of the glomerular filtration rate. Usually, the patient is hydrated with 1000 mL of water followed by 200 mL every 30 min until the test is completed; 2 hr following the first intake of water, a control blood sample is taken, the drug is administered intravenously and the exact time noted; 1 hr later the bladder is emptied, the urine discarded, the time noted, a blood sample taken and the time once more noted. Urine and blood samples are then collected hourly for 2 hr. The samples are analyzed for this drug. Appropriate calculations then are made. Although considerable variation occurs, normal clearance values are 130 ± 20 mL/min in the male and 120 ± 15 mL/min in the female. Untoward reactions are infrequent and usually mild.

Dose—*Usual, intravenous,* **10 g** dissolved in 100 mL of sodium chloride injection and injected at the rate of 10 mL/min.

Dosage Form—Injection: 100 mg/mL in 50-mL vials.

Iodohippurate Sodium I-131—page 858.

Mannitol—page 1041.

Phenolsulfonphthalein

Phenol Red; P.S.P.; Sulfonphthal; (*Various Mfrs*)

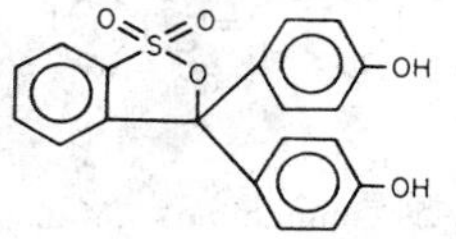

[143-74-8] $C_{19}H_{14}O_5S$ (354.38).

Preparation—By fusing the anhydride of *o*-sulfobenzoic acid with phenol. The *o*-sulfobenzoic anhydride may be obtained by heating the acid with phosphorus pentoxide.

Description—Crystalline powder; varies in color from bright to dark red; stable in air.

Solubility—1 g in about 1300 mL water, about 350 mL alcohol or about 500 mL acetone; almost insoluble in chloroform or ether; freely soluble in solutions of alkali hydroxides or their carbonates.

Uses—A *diagnostic aid* used for determining *kidney function.* When injected intramuscularly or intravenously, it begins to be excreted in patients with normal kidneys in from 5 to 10 min. In patients with deficient renal function, the first appearance of its secretion is delayed. In normal cases, after intramuscular injection, almost the total amount (from 60 to 80%) is excreted within 2 hr. Failure to excrete nearly the full amount within 2 hr indicates a deficient functional activity and the degree of this functional deficiency may be estimated by the proportionate amount excreted within 2 hr.

The average normal eliminations after intravenous administration are from 35 to 45% in 15 min, from 50 to 65% in 30 min and from 65 to 80% in the first hour. From 20 to 30 min before the test, the patient is given 300 to 400 mL of water to insure free urinary excretion: otherwise, delayed appearance may be due to lack of excretion.

Under aseptic precautions a catheter is introduced and the bladder is emptied completely, or the patient is allowed to empty it voluntarily. The time is noted, and 1 mL of a solution of phenosulfonphthalein containing 6 mg/mL is administered intramuscularly into the lumbar muscles, or intravenously, by means of a graduated syringe. Care must be taken that all of the solutions is injected. The urine is allowed to drain into a test tube containing a drop of 25% NaOH solution, and the time of apperance of the first faint pinkish tinge is noted. In patients having no urinary obstruction, the catheter is withdrawn at the time of appearance of the drug in the urine.

If injection is made *intramuscularly,* the patient is instructed to void into a receptacle at the end of 1 hr and 10 min, and into a second receptacle at the end of the second hour. If injection is made *intravenously,* the patient is instructed to void into a receptacle at the end of 15 or 30 min or 1 hr. The urine collected is made alkaline with a 25% solution of NaOH and then diluted to 1 L; a small filtered portion is taken to compare with the standard used for all estimations. Comparison is made in a colorimeter devised for this purpose.

Dose—*Usual, intramuscular* or *intravenous,* 6 mg.

Dosage Form—Injection: 6 mg/1 mL.

Liver Function

Unfortunately, available methods for estimating the extent of liver damage by various measurements of decreased liver function are still comparatively unsatisfactory. The liver itself has such a large reserve of functional capacity that most methods of determining decreased function do not reveal such a state until 70 to 90% of the liver cells have been damaged. The liver function test most commonly used involves the intravenous injection of indocyanine green, an agent *not* taken up by any organ other than the liver. Moreover, it is relatively nontoxic, can be analyzed in low concentrations, not metabolized and has a plasma-disappearance rate-curve which is nearly exponential.

Indocyanine Green

1*H*-Benz[*e*]indolium, 2-[7-[1,3-dihydro-1,1-dimethyl-3-(4-sulfobutyl)- 2*H*-benz[*e*]indol-2-ylidene]-1,3,5-heptatrienyl]-1,1-dimethyl-3-(4- sulfobutyl)-, hydroxide, inner salt, sodium salt; Cardio-Green (*HW & D*)

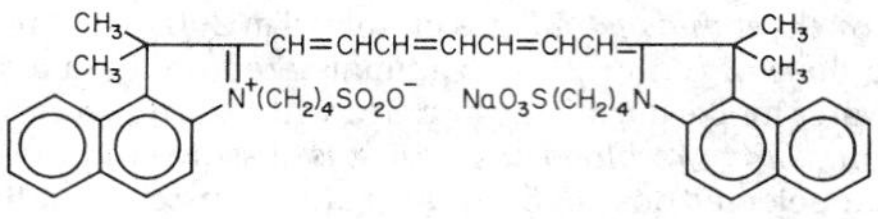

[3599-32-4] $C_{43}H_{47}N_2NaO_6S_2$ (774.96).

Preparation—By reacting 1,1,2-trimethyl-3-(4-sulfobutyl)-1*H*-benz[*e*]indolium hydroxide inner salt (I) with a bis(Schiff base) derived from glutaconic aldehyde. The starting indolium compound I is prepared by heating 1,1,2-trimethyl-1*H*-benz[*e*]indole with 4-hydroxy-1-butanesulfonic acid δ-sultone. Details for preparing these tricarbocyanine dyes are provided in US Pats 2,251,286 and 2,895,955.

Description—Dark green, blue-green, olive brown, dark blue or black powder; odorless or with a slight odor; solutions are deep emerald-green in color; pH (1 in 200 solution) about 6; unstable in solution.

Solubility—Soluble in water or methanol; practically insoluble in most other organic solvents.

Uses—To determine *cardiac output, hepatic function* and *liver blood flow.* It also has been used to measure *plasma volume* and *regional blood flow* in various organs including the kidneys, eyes and lungs. Following intravenous injection, the distribution volume is relatively constant among individuals and approximates that of plasma volume, because tissue binding is negligible and the fraction of unbound drug in blood is very small. Indeed, it is so highly bound to plasma proteins, particularly alpha lipoproteins, that it does not distribute extravascularly and its clearance is not limited by binding. The intrinsic clearance of bound and unbound drug is high, hepatic extraction ratios in man vary from 50 to 80%. It is not metabolized, but is eliminated entirely by active uptake into hepatic parenchymal cells. It then is transported to bile and once excreted in the small intestine is not reabsorbed; consequently, it imparts a green color to the stool. The elimination half-life in healthy adults ranges from 2.2 to 3 min. These properties, together with low toxicity and easy measurement in plasma, have made it a commonly used indicator for the measurement of liver blood flow.

For hepatic function studies, the calculated amount of the diagnostic agent is injected into an arm vein. Twenty minutes after injection, 6 mL of venous blood is withdrawn from the opposite arm. After coagulation and centrifugation, the clear serum is read in a photometer at 800 to 810 nm. A dye retention of less than 4% is found in healthy subjects. Failure to remove the dye, as indicated by serum levels in excess of 4%, is indicative of impaired hepatic function. It contains a small amount of sodium iodide; thus, it should be used with caution in patients allergic to iodides and radioactive iodine uptake studies should not be performed for at least 1 wk following its use. Since probenecid has been shown in dogs to affect hepatic uptake, this possibility should be kept in mind. Its safe use in pregnancy has not been established.

Dose—*Usual, adult, intravenous, cardiac output determination, via cardiac catheter,* **5 mg** in **1 mL;** *children,* **2.5 mL** in **1 mL;** *infants,* **1.25 mg** in **1 mL.** *Hepatic function determination,* **0.5 mg/kg.** *Ophthalmic angiography,* **40 mg** in **2 mL.**

Dosage Form—Sterile: 25- and 50-mg-vials; with two 10-mL ampuls of water for injection.

Sodium Benzoate—see RPS-18, page 1173.

Lymphatic System

Isosulfan Blue

Ethanaminium, *N*-[4-[[4-(diethylamino)-phenyl] (2,5-disulfophenyl)methylene]-2,5-cyclohexadien-1-ylidene]-*N*-ethyl-, hydroxide, inner salt, sodium salt; Lymphazurin (*Hirsch*)

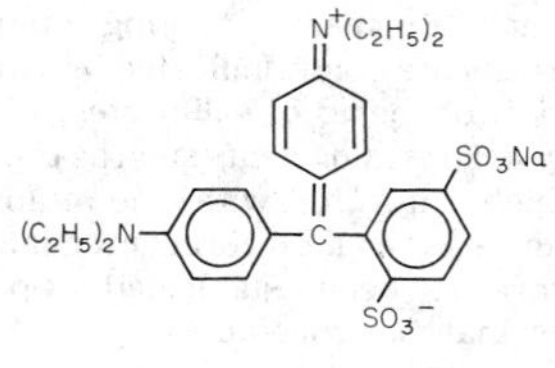

Colour Index: Sulphan Blue; CI no 42045 (often confused with Patent Blue V, CI no 42051) [68238-36-8] $C_{27}H_{31}N_2NaO_6S_2$ (566.66).

Preparation—By condensation of 4-formylbenzene-1,3-disulfonic acid and *N,N*-diethylaniline. See *Colour Index v4*, 1971.

Description—Violet powder; aqueous solutions are blue and the color is stable over a wide range of pH if protected from light.

Solubility—Soluble in water (1 in 20); partially soluble in alcohol.

Uses—An adjunct to lymphography for visualization of the lymphatic system draining the area in which injected. It has no known pharmacological action. Absorption studies in rats indicate that following a single 1-mL subcutaneous injection of a 1% solution, 34% is absorbed in 30 min and 69% and 100% in 1 and 24 hr, respectively; 10% is excreted unchanged in the urine in 24 hr and 90% through the biliary system. Allergic-type adverse effects occur in about 1.5% of patients and include localized swelling and pruritus of the hands, abdomen and neck. Edema of the face and glottis, respiratory distress or shock have been reported. These reactions are more likely to occur in patients with a history of hypersensitivity. Its safe use during pregnancy and lactation, as well as in children, has not been established.

Dose—*Usual, adult, subcutaneous,* **0.5 mL** into 3 interdigital spaces of each extremity; *maximum,* **3 mL** (30 mg).

Dosage Form—Injection: 1% (10 mg/mL) in 5-mL vials.

Mumps Skin Test Antigen (see page 1432).

Myasthenia Gravis (see page 676).

Edrophonium Chloride—page 1005.
Neostigmine Methylsulfate—page 1006.

Ophthalmic Diagnostic Aids

Fluorescein Sodium

Spiro[isobenzofuran-1(3*H*),9′-[9*H*]xanthene]-3-one, 3′,6′-dihydroxy-, disodium salt; Soluble Fluorescein; Resorcinolphthalein Sodium; Uranin; Uranine Yellow; (*Various Mfrs*)

NaO … O … O … COONa

Colour Index: Acid Yellow 73; CI no 45350 [518-47-8] $C_{20}H_{10}Na_2O_5$ (376.28).

Preparation—By heating resorcinol with phthalic anhydride at about 200°. After purifying, the phthalein is dissolved in the required amount of sodium hydroxide solution and evaporated to dryness.

Description—Orange-red, odorless powder; hygroscopic; aqueous solution is strongly fluorescent even in extreme dilution; the fluorescence disappears when the solution is made acid, and reappears when the solution is again made alkaline.

Solubility—Freely soluble in water; sparingly soluble in alcohol.

Uses—Either as an ophthalmic strip or as a 2% aqueous solution as an ophthalmic *diagnostic aid.* It is applied topically for the diagnosis of *corneal lesions,* pressure points on the surface of the cornea under contact lenses and the detection of minute *foreign bodies* embedded in the cornea. While a weak solution of it will not stain the normal cornea, ulcers or parts deprived of epithelium and pressure points will become green and remain so for a time; foreign bodies will appear surrounded by a green ring; loss of substance in the conjunctiva is indicated by a yellow hue. It also reveals defects or disease of the endothelium of the cornea, producing a deep coloration of the diseased area. It also is used to outline and demarcate *tumors,* particularly in the central nervous system. It sometimes is used intravenously as a diagnostic aid for various purposes, particularly to determine circulation time (see *Fluorescein Sodium Injection,* below).

In using the drug in the eye, it is particularly important that the preparation be sterile and that no accidental contamination of the solution with *Pseudomonas aeruginosa* take place. A diseased or injured eye is readily infected with this organism that can cause blindness. Being anionic, it is not compatible with preservatives such as benzalkonium chloride or substances known to be effective against *Pseudomonas aeruginosa,* such as polymyxin B sulfate. The solution is best used as a unit-dose package or dispensed from a container which protects the contents from contamination. It is also available as paper strips impregnated with it which are dried, heat-sterilized and packaged in hermetically sealed unit-dose packets. One of these dipped into the lacrimal fluid of the eye to be examined releases enough of the highly soluble drug to permit examination of the eye for lesions or injury.

Dose—*Topical,* **0.1** to **0.3 mL** of a **2%** solution, to the conjunctiva. *Ophthalmic strip,* moistened with sterile water and applied to conjunctiva.

Dosage Forms—Injection (see below); 5 and 10%; Ophthalmic Strips: 0.6, 1 and 9 mg.

Fluorescein Sodium Injection [Fluorescite (*Alcon*); Ful-Glo (*Barnes-Hind*) Funduscein (*Iolab*)]—*Uses:* A diagnostic aid in *ophthalmic angiography* which includes examination of the fundus, evaluation of the iris vasculature, distinction between viable and nonviable tissue, and observation of the aqueous flow. It is useful in the differential diagnosis of malignant and nonmalignant ocular tumors. It also is used to determine *circulation time* and *circulation adequacy.* To determine circulation time, 5 mL of the injection is administered rapidly via the antecubital vein; the lips of the patient are viewed under long-wave ultraviolet light and the time from the injection to the time the lips acquire a greenish yellow hue noted. The circulation time in adults varies from 15 to 20 sec; the circulation time is prolonged in right heart failure and hypothyroidism, shortened in hyperthyroidism and anemia but is essentially normal in bronchial asthma.

Adverse reactions include cardiac arrest, basilar artery ischemia, severe shock and thrombophlebitis at the site of the injection. Transient nausea, vomiting and allergic reactions have been reported in sensitive patients. A strong taste may develop following high dosage. *Dose: Usual, adult, intravenous,* for *determination of circulation time,* 500 to 750 mg as a 10% solution injected rapidly in the antecubital vein; *usual, pediatric, intravenous,* 7.5 mg/kg, as a 5% solution. Have epinephrine 1:1000, an antihistamine and oxygen available.

Sodium Phosphate P32—page 861.

Thyroid Function

Sodium Iodide I-131—page 860.
Sodium Iodide I-123—page 861.
Thyrotropin—page 1059.

Pancreatic Function

Bentiromide

Benzoic acid, (*S*)-4-[[2-(benzoylamino)-3-(4-hydroxyphenyl)-1-oxopropyl]amino]-, Chymex (*Adria*)

HO–C6H4–CH2–C(H)(NH–CO–C6H5)–CONH–C6H4–COOH

[37106-97-1] $C_{23}H_{20}N_2O_5$ (404.42).

Preparation—See *J Med Chem 15:* 1098, 1972.

Description—White crystals; melts about 240°.

Uses—To diagnose exocrine pancreatic insufficiency and to monitor the adequacy of enzyme replacement therapy in patients with exocrine pancreatic insufficiency. Pancreatic chymotrypsin selectively cleaves para-aminobenzoic acid (PABA) from bentiromide following oral administration. PABA is absorbed rapidly under normal gastrointestinal function, conjugated by the liver and excreted in the urine in about 6 hr. If approximately 50% of the PABA content of bentiromide (170 mg in 500 mg) is collected in the 6-hr urine sample, it is indicative of normal exocrine pancreatic function, gastric emptying, intestinal and kidney function.

This test is a simple, noninvasive test and has been shown to produce reliable, reproducible results in the diagnosis of pancreatic insufficiency. Adverse effects are transient and relatively infrequent; diarrhea, headache, flatulence, nausea, vomiting and weakness are the most frequent. Safety and efficacy in children over 6 yr have not been established. The drug should not be used during pregnancy or in nursing mothers unless clearly needed. Drugs and foods that are metabolized to primary arylamines and multiple vitamins should be discontinued at least 3 days prior to the drug's administration.

Dose—*Usual, adults* and *children over 12 yr, oral,* **500 mg;** *children 6 yr and older,* **14 mg/kg** up to a maximum of 500 mg. Immediately following its administration the patient is given 250 mL of water, another 250 mL of water 2 hr after administration and 500 mL of water during the next 4 hr.

Dosage Form—Oral Solution: 500 mg/7.5 mL.

Secretin

Secretin-Kabi (*Pharmacia*)

Secretin [1393-25-5] is a polypeptide hormone, secreted by the duodenal mucosa and to a lesser extent by the upper jejunal mucosa, which stimulates secretion of water and bicarbonate from the pancreas. As isolated from porcine mucosa and purified, the hormone consists of 27 amino acid units from 12 different amino acids and has the molecular formula $C_{122}H_{220}N_{44}O_{41}$; it has been synthesized (Bodanszky *et al, J Am Chem Soc 89*: 685, 6753, 1967). The hormone supplied for diagnostic use is of porcine origin; it is a sterile, refined, freeze-dried powder, stable for 2 yr when stored in its original, unopened vial at 2 to 7°, but unstable in solution.

Uses—In the diagnosis of *pancreatic disorders*, such as pancreatic exocrine disease and gastrinoma (*Zollinger-Ellison syndrome*). Intravenous injection of the hormone in persons with normal pancreatic secretion increases the bicarbonate content and volume of secretion from the pancreas. Reduced secretory volume and diminished bicarbonate concentration are signs of pancreatic insufficiency. Volume reductions are indicative of pancreatic duct obstruction as seen in neoplasms; bicarbonate concentration reductions indicate pancreatic inflammatory disease.

In performing the test a double-lumen tube is passed through the mouth after a 12- to 15-hr fast, under fluoroscopic guidance so that a proper placement of the proximal tube in the gastric antrum and of the distal tube beyond the papilla of Vater is accomplished. Constant suction is applied to both outlets of the tube throughout the test. After a control period of collection of fluid for 10 to 20 min, and skin testing of the patient for sensitivity to secretin to avoid an anaphylactic reaction, a standard dose of 1 Clinical Unit (CU)/kg of the drug is injected intravenously. A 60-min collection period of aspirated secretions, fractioned into 4 periods, the first two at 10- min intervals and the last two at 20-min intervals, provides separate duodenal and stomach specimens that are analyzed for volume variations, bicarbonate concentrations and other constituents.

It is contraindicated in patients with a history of atopic asthma, allergy and those showing a positive skin test. It should be used with great caution, if at all, in patients with acute pancreatitis.

Dose—See above.

Dosage Form—Powder for Injection: 75 CU/vial (10 CU/mL when reconstituted with 7.5 mL of sodium chloride for injection).

Tolbutamide—page 1081.

Parathroid Function

Teriparatide Acetate

L-Phenylalanine, L-valyl-L-seryl-L-α-glutamyl-L-isoleucyl-L-glutaminyl-L-leucyl-L-methionyl-L-histidyl-L-asparaginyl-L-leucylglycyl-L-lysyl-L-histidyl-L-leucyl-L-asparaginyl-L-seryl-L-methionyl-L-α-glutamyl-L-arginyl-L-valyl-L-α-glutamyl-L-tryptophyl-L-leucyl-L-arginyl-L-lysyl-L-leucyl-L-glutaminyl-L-α-aspartyl-L-valyl-L-histidyl-L-asparaginyl-, acetate (salt) hydrate; Parathar (*Rhone-Poulenc Rorer*)

H-Ser–Val–Ser–Glu–Ile–Gln–Leu–Met–His–Asn–Leu–Gly–Lys–His–Leu–Asn–
1 2 3 4 5 6 7 8 9 10 11 12 13 14 15 16

Ser–Met–Glu–Arg–Val–Glu–Trp–Leu–Arg–Lys–Lys–Leu–Gln–Asp–Val–His–Asn–
17 18 19 20 21 22 23 24 25 26 27 28 29 30 31 32 33

Phe–OH • xH_2O • yCH_3COOH
34

[99294-94-7] $C_{181}H_{291}N_{55}O_{51}S_2.xH_2O.yC_2H_4O_2$.

Description—A synthetic polypeptide composed of 34 amino acids.

Uses—It is used to distinguish between *hypocalcemia* due to *hypoparathyroidism and pseudohypoparathyroidism*, but not between these conditions and normal. Adverse effects include nausea, abdominal cramps, urge to defecate and diarrhea. Hypertensive crisis, hypocalcemia convulsions and tingling of the extremities also have been reported. Its safe use during pregnancy and lactation, as well as in children under 3 yr, has not been established. **Dose**—Diagnostic use in patients with hypocalcemia: *adults,* **200 units** infused *intravenously* over a 10-min period; *children, 3 yr and older,* **3 units/kg** (maximum, 200 units).

Dosage Form—Lyophilized Powder for Injection: 200 units in 10-mL vials with a 10-mL vial of diluent.

Pheochromocytoma

Histamine Phosphate—page 1222.
Phentolamine Mesylate—page 1010.

Phenylpyruvic Acid (see also *Phenylpyruvic Acid,* page 524)

Phenistix (*Ames*) reagent strips for urine test to determine phenylketonuria (PKU) in newborn infants.

Pituitary Function

Arginine Hydrochloride—page 1130.

Gonadorelin Hydrochloride

Factrel (*Ayerst*)

5–oxoPro–His–Trp–Ser–Tyr–Gly–Leu–Arg–Pro–Gly–NH_2 • xHCl
1 2 3 4 5 6 7 8 9 10

Leutinizing hormone-releasing factor hydrochloride [51952-41-1] $C_{55}H_{75}N_{17}O.x$HCl (1182.33; free base – the *hydrochloride* may be either the mono- or dihydrochloride or a mixture thereof).

Preparation—Isolated from the hypothalamus of pigs or sheep. The industrial preparation is described in German Pat 2,213,737.

Description—The base is a white to very pale yellowish powder containing not less than 85% of active peptide and not more than 6% acetic acid.

Uses—A diagnostic agent used for evaluating *hypothalamic-pituitary gonadotropic* function. The test should be conducted in the absence of other drugs which directly effect pituitary secretion of the gonadotropins, including preparations that contain androgens, estrogens, progestins or glucocorticoids. Adverse reactions include headache, nausea, lightheadedness, abdominal discomfort and flushing. Localized swelling may occur at the site of injection. Safety for use during pregnancy has not been established.

Dose—*Subcutaneous or intravenous,* **100 µg** (see *latest* package insert).

Dosage Form—Powder for Injection: 100 and 500 µg (as HCl)/ vial (accompanied by 2-mL ampul of 2% benzyl alcohol and water for injection).

Metyrapone

1-Propanone, 2-methyl-1,2-di-3-pyridinyl-,
Metopirone (*Ciba-Geigy*)

[54-36-4] $C_{14}H_{14}N_2O$ (226.28).

Preparation—Methyl 3-pyridyl ketone is reduced electrolytically to the corresponding pinacol, 2,3-bis(3-pyridyl)-2,3-butanediol; heating with a strong inorganic acid results in dehydration of the pinacol with subsequent rearrangement to form metyrapone. US Pat 2,966,493.

Description—White to light-amber, fine, crystalline powder; characteristic odor; darkens on exposure to light.

Solubility—Sparingly soluble in water; soluble in methanol or chloroform; forms water-soluble salts with acids.

Uses—A synthetic compound that has the unique ability to inhibit 11-beta-hydroxylation in the biosynthesis of cortisol, corticosterone and aldosterone. Hence, it is used to test for *hypothalamic-pituitary* function. In the normal individual, metyrapone blocks the enzymatic step that leads to cortisol and corticosterone synthesis, produces an intense stimulation of ACTH secretion and induces a marked increase in urinary excretion of 17-hydroxycorticosteroids. In patients with abnormal pituitary function, the ability to increase ACTH production is lacking and no significant increase in 17-hydroxycorticosteroids is seen. The drug is particularly valuable as a diagnostic aid in patients suspect of hypopituitarism and Cushing's syndrome. It has a $T_{1/2}$ of about 20 to 26 min. Within 2 days following oral administration of 750 mg every 4 hr for 6 doses, approximately 0.5% of the drug is excreted as the reduced metabolite and 37% as glucuronide conjugates of metyrapone.

Untoward effects include anorexia, nausea, abdominal discomfort, diarrhea, dizziness, vertigo, headache, sedation and allergic rash. The drug is contraindicated in patients with adrenal cortical hypofunction. Since several drugs modify the results obtained in the test, the test should be performed in patients receiving no other medication.

Dose—*Usual, adult, oral,* **750 mg** every 4 hr for 6 doses; *pediatric,* **15 mg/kg** every 4 hr for 6 doses.

Dosage Form—Tablets: 250 mg.

Protirelin

L-Prolinamide, 5-oxo-L-propyl-L-histidyl-, TRH, Thypinone (*Abbott*); Relefact-TRH (*Hoechst-Roussel*)

Thyrotropin releasing factor [24305-27-9] $C_{16}H_{22}N_6O_4$ (362.39).

Preparation—Protirelin obtained from most mammals appears to be identical and is apparently not species specific. A review of synthetic methods is found in *Methods Enzymol 37:* 408, 1975.

Solubility—Highly purified material is partially soluble in chloroform and very soluble in methanol.

Uses—An adjunct in the diagnostic assessment of *thyroid function* and *pituitary or hypothalamic dysfunction.* It is a synthetic tripeptide believed to be structurally identical to the naturally occurring thyrotropin-releasing hormone produced by the hypothalamus. Following intravenous administration, the $T_{1/2}$ is approximately 5 min; TSH levels reach a peak in 20 to 30 min and decline slowly over a period of 3 hr to baseline levels. Adverse effects occur in about 50% of patients and include hypertension or hypotension with or without syncope and breast enlargment. Other reactions include nausea, urge to urinate, flushing, lightheadedness, bad taste, abdominal discomfort, headache and dry mouth. It should be used in pregnant women only when clearly indicated.

Dose—*Intravenous, adult,* **500 µg;** *children 6 to 16 yr,* **7 µg/kg,** up to **500 µg;** *infants and children up to 6 yr,* **7 µg/kg.**

Dosage Form—500 µg/mL in 1-mL ampuls.

Roentgenographic Products: Drugs Used As X-Ray Contrast Media

Diatrizoate Meglumine

Benzoic acid, 3,5-bis(acetylamino)-2,4,6-triiodo-, compd with 1-deoxy-1-(methylamino)-D-glucitol (1:1); Cardiografin, Cystografin (*Squibb*); Hypaque Meglumine, Hypaque-Cysto (*Sterling*); Reno-M (*Squibb*); (*Various Mfrs*)

1-Deoxy-1-(methylamino)-L-glucitol 3,5-diacetamido-2,4,6-triiodobenzoate (salt) [131-49-7] $C_7H_{17}NO_5.C_{11}H_9I_3N_2O_4$ (809.13).

Preparation—Diatrizoic acid is reacted with an equimolar quantity of methylglucamine (meglumine), usually in water for injection to produce a solution of the required concentration.

Uses—In different concentrations for many diagnostic tests. The 76% injection is used for adult *angiocardiography* and *thoracic aortography.* On injection into a vessel or into the heart, it is diffused rapidly in the vascular system and excreted by the kidneys. As the contrast medium enters the cardiac chambers, the vessels and aorta, lesions or malformations of the heart and obstructions or anomalies are visualized. The drug should be used with great care in patients known to have multiple myeloma; anuria resulting in progressive uremia, renal failure and eventually death has occurred. Also, it should be used with extreme caution in patients known to have pheochromocytoma, severe hepatic and renal disease, patients who are homozygous for sickle-cell disease and patients known to be sensitive to iodine compounds. Safe use in pregnancy has not been established.

A 76% solution is used for adult *angiocardiography* and *thoracic aortography;* a 60 or 76% solution in *excretion urography, aortography, pediatric angiocardiography* and *peripheral arteriography;* a 60% solution for *excretory urography, cerebral angiography, peripheral arteriography, venography, splenoportography, arthrography* and *discography* and a 30% solution for *retrograde cystourethrography* and *infusion urography,* and enhancement of *computed tomography* of the brain. Adverse reactions, precautions and contraindications are similar to those for other iodinated diagnostic agents.

Dose—As the dosage and concentration of injections of this drug vary greatly with the many diagnostic uses and techniques of administration of the agent, and often with the physical condition and preliminary preparation of the patient, the *latest* package insert should be consulted for adult and pediatric dosages and other information concerning uses.

Dosage Forms—Injection: 30, 60 and 76%; Urogenital Sterile Solution: 18 and 30%.

Diatrizoate Meglumine and Diatrizoate Sodium [Injection]

Angiovist, Gastrovist (*Berlex*); Renovist, Renografin (*Squibb*); MD- Gastroview (*Mallinckrodt*); Hypaque-M (*Winthrop*)

A sterile solution of diatrizoate meglumine and diatrizoate sodium in water for injection, or a sterile solution of diatrizoic acid in water for injection prepared with the aid of NaOH and meglumine. It may contain small amounts of suitable buffers and of edetate calcium disodium or edetate disodium as a stabilizer. When intended for intravascular use, it contains no antimicrobial agents.

Description—Clear, colorless to pale yellow, slightly viscous liquid; may crystallize at room temperature or below.

Uses—Designed to combine the lower toxicity of the meglumine salt with the lower viscosity and higher iodine content of the sodium salt. In appropriate concentrations it is used as a radiopaque medium for *angiocardiography, aortography, angiography, excretion urography, hysterosalpingography, peripheral arteriography* and *venography* and other radiographic procedures. Contraindications, general warnings and adverse effects are similar to those for other iodinated diagnostic agents.

A solution containing 66% of diatrizoate meglumine and 10% of diatrizoate sodium (Gastrografin, *Squibb*) is used as a contrast medium for radiographic examination of the gastrointestinal tract following oral or rectal administration. The preparation is indicated particularly where use of barium is not feasible or is potentially dangerous. It is contraindicated in patients sensitive to salts of diatrizoic acid and should be used with caution in patients sensitive to iodine. The safety of the oral solution in pregnancy has not been established. It is usually tolerated well; occasionally, some diarrhea occurs.

Dose—As the dosage and concentration vary greatly with the many diagnostic uses and techniques of administration of the injection, and often with the physical condition and preliminary preparation of the patient, the *latest* package insert should be consulted for adult and pediatric dosages and other information concerning uses, as well as of the oral solution used for radiographic examination of the gastrointestinal tract.

Dosage Forms—Injection, containing the following percentages of diatrizoate meglumine and diatrizoate sodium, respectively: 28.5/29.1, 34.3/35, 50/25, 52/8, 60/30 and 66/10. Oral or rectal Solution: 66/10.

Diatrizoate Meglumine and Iodipamide Meglumine [Injection]

Sinografin (*Squibb*)

A sterile, aqueous solution of diatrizoate meglumine equivalent to 40% diatrizoic acid and iodipamide meglumine equivalent to 20% iodipamide, containing approximately 38% of bound iodine.

Uses—A radiopaque medium indicated for *hysterosalpingography.* Following intrauterine administration immediate visualization of the uterus and tubes is achieved. Medium spilled into the peritoneal cavity is absorbed within 20 to 60 min. The preparation is contraindicated during pregnancy or in patients with acute pelvic inflammatory disease. The test should not be performed within 30 days following curettage or conization. Otherwise the precautions, adverse effects and contraindications are similar to those for other iodinated diagnostic agents.

Dose—*Usual, uterus,* **3** to **4 mL**; an additional 3 to 4 mL will outline the *fallopian tubes.* Total dose varies from 1.5 to 10 mL.

Dosage Form—Single-Dose Vials: 10 mL.

Diatrizoate Sodium

Benzoic acid, 3,5-bis(acetylamino)-2,4,6-triiodo-, monosodium salt; MD-50 (*Mallinckrodt*); Urovist Sodium 300 (*Berlex*)

[737-31-5] $C_{11}H_8I_3N_2NaO_4$ (635.90).

Preparation—Diatrizoic acid is reacted with an equimolar quantity of NaOH, usually in water for injection to produce a solution of the required concentration.

Uses—A radiopaque agent with uses, profile of toxicity and precautions similar to those for *Diatrizoate Meglumine* and other iodinated diagnostic agents. It contains somewhat more iodine (59.87%) than the meglumine salt (47.01%); consequently, it is somewhat more toxic. Solutions are considerably less viscous than those prepared from diatrizoate meglumine. Also, this drug should not be used in coronary angiography because it is more likely to cause serious cardiac arrhythmias than is the meglumine salt. When administered orally or given as an enema, it is used as a radiopaque medium to outline the upper and lower gastrointestinal tract.

Dosage—As the dosage and concentration of injections, oral solutions and enemas vary considerably with the diagnostic uses and techniques of administration of the agent, the *latest* package insert should be consulted for adult and pediatric dosages and other information concerning uses.

Dosage Forms—Powder (or oral or rectal solution): 600 mg iodine/g; Solution: 41.66% (249 mg of iodine/mL); Injection: 25% (150 mg of iodine/mL) and 50% (300 mg of iodine/mL); Urogenital Solution: 20% (120 mg of iodine/mL).

Diatrizoic Acid

Benzoic acid, 3,5-bis (acetylamino)-2,4,6-triiodo-,

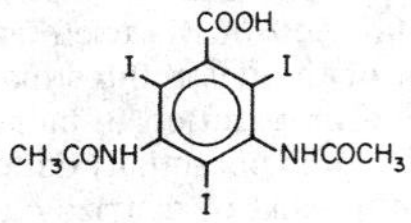

[117-96-4] $C_{11}H_9I_3N_2O_4$ (613.92); *dihydrate* [50978-11-5] (649.95).

Preparation—From benzoic acid by (1) nitration to the 3,5-dinito acid, (2) reduction by means of stannous chloride or other reducing agent to the corresponding diamino acid, (3) iodination with iodine monochloride in acetic acid to the 2,4,6-triiodo derivative or (4) acetylation of the amino groups using acetic anhydride.

Description—White powder; odorless.

Solubility—Very slightly soluble in water or alcohol; soluble in dimethylformamide or alkali hydroxide solutions.

Uses—Radiopaque component of *Diatrizoate Meglumine Injection, Diatrizoate Meglumine and Diatrizoate Sodium Injection, Diatrizoate Sodium Injection* and *Diatrizoate Sodium Oral Solution.*

Ethiodized Oil

Ethiodol (*Savage*)

An iodine addition product of the ethyl ester of the fatty acids of poppyseed oil, containing 35.2–38.9% of organically combined iodine. It is sterile [8008-53-5].

Preparation—By saponifying poppy-seed oil and subjecting the resulting fatty acids to iodination and subsequent esterification with ethanol.

Description—Straw-colored to amber-colored, oily liquid; may have an alliaceous odor.

Solubility—Insoluble in water; soluble in acetone, chloroform or ether.

Uses—A *contrast medium* used in *hysterosalpingography* and *lymphography.* It should not be used in the presence of intrauterine bleeding, pelvic infection or pregnancy. Likewise, it should not be used in patients known to be sensitive to iodine. Except for pulmonary embolism resulting from accidental intravasation of the medium, other side effects, such as transient fever, allergic dermatitis, lipogranuloma formation and delayed wound healing, are rare and of little consequence.

Dose—*Usual, hysterosalpingography, by special injection,* **5 mL** followed by increments of **2 mL** until tubule patency is established or limit of tolerance is reached. *Lymphography, by special injection, lower extremity,* **6** to **8 mL** per extremity, at a rate of 0.1 to 0.2 mL/min; *upper extremity,* **2** to **4 mL** per extremity, at a rate of 0.1 to 0.2 mL/min. *Usual, pediatric, dose, lymphography,* **1 mL** to a maximum of **6 mL.**

Dosage Form—10-mL ampuls.

Iodipamide

Benzoic acid, 3,3′-[(1,6-dioxo-1,6-hexanediyl)diimino] bis[2,4,6-triiodo-, Cholografin (*Squibb*)

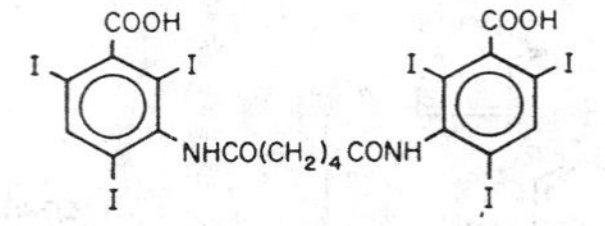

[606-17-7] $C_{20}H_{14}I_6N_2O_6$ (1139.77).

Preparation—From benzoic acid by (1) nitration to 3-nitrobenzoic acid, (2) reduction by means of stannous chloride or other reducing agent to 3-aminobenzoic acid, (3) iodination with iodine monochloride in acetic acid to the 2,4,6-triiodo derivative or (4) acylation of the amino group with adipoyl chloride [$ClCO(CH_2)_4COCl$].

Description—White, crystalline powder; nearly odorless.

Solubility—Very slightly soluble in water, chloroform or ether; slightly soluble in alcohol.

Uses—Radiopaque component of *iodipamide Meglumine Injection.*

Iodamide Meglumine

Benzoic acid, 3-(acetylamino)-5-[(acetylamino)methyl]-2,4,6-triiodo-, compound with 1-deoxy-1-(methylamino)-D-glucitol(1:1); Renovue (*Squibb*)

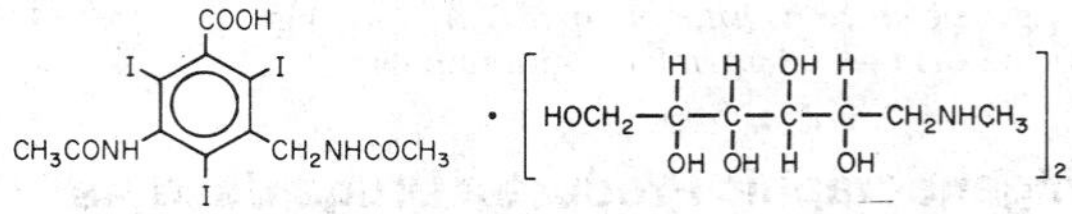

[18656-21-8] $C_{12}H_{11}I_3N_2O_4.C_7H_{16}NO_5$ (823.16).

Preparation—For the synthesis of iodamic acid see *Helv Chim Acta 48:* 259, 1965; this material is converted to the salt in the same fashion as diatrizoate meglumine previously described.

Uses—A diagnostic agent for *excretion urography* administered either by intravenous infusion (Renovue-Dip) or intravenous injection (Renovue-65). Following either intravenous infusion or injection it is rapidly transported to the kidneys and excreted essentially unchanged, principally by glomerular filtration. However, at least one-third of the intravenous dose is secreted by the renal tubules. Thus, it permits visualization of the kidneys and urinary passages through normal physiologic mechanisms of excretion. There are no absolute contraindications to its use. However, urography should be performed with extreme caution in patients with severe hepatic and renal disease, or anuria. Otherwise, the precautions, adverse effects and contraindications are similar to those for other iodinated diagnostic agents.

Dose—*Excretory urography:* by *drip IV infusion,* **4.5 mL/kg** (maximum, **300 mL**), infused over 10-min period; by *intravenous injection,* **0.8 mL/kg** (maximum **50 mL**) injected within 1 to 2 min.

Dosage Forms—IV Infusion: 24% in 300-mL bottles; IV Injection: 65% in 50-mL vials.

Iodized Oil

Iodized Oil Viscous Injection; Lipiodol (*Savage*)

An iodine addition product of vegetable oil or oils, containing 38–42% of organically combined iodine. It is sterile.

Preparation—The methods of preparing iodized oil involve addition of elemental iodine to the unsaturated fatty constituents of a vegetable oil, the resulting oil containing chemically saturated iodoglycerides. The oil most generally used is poppy seed oil.

Description—Thick, viscous, oily liquid; alliaceous odor; oleaginous taste; light to dark-brown in color, and on exposure to air and light it becomes darker due to liberation of iodine; specific gravity about 1.35.

Solubility—Insoluble in water; soluble in ether, chloroform or petroleum benzin; 1 mL of iodized oil should yield a clear solution with 10 mL of solvent hexane.

Uses—Formerly, for visualization of various internal cavities; the stated indications are now restricted to *hysterosalpingography, sialography, visualization of sinus and fistulous tracts* and, with great caution, *bronchography*. Many reports of adverse and toxic effects from use of iodized oils have been published, including deaths from use in bronchography (primarily due to anoxia associated with emphysema or bronchospasm) and in hysterosalpingography (primarily due to cerebral oil embolism). This injection is contraindicated in the presence of active bleeding, in patients with disease in which there is inflammation (pelvic inflammatory disease, pulmonary tuberculosis) and in individuals with known or suspected iodine sensitivity.

Dose—*Usual*, **1** to **30 mL** by special injection, depending on procedure.

Dosage Form—Injection: 1, 5, 10 and 20 mL.

Iohexol

1,3-Benzenedicarboxamide, 5-[acetyl(2,3-dihydroxypropyl)-amino]-*N*,*N'*-bis(2,3-dihydroxypropyl)-2,4,6-triiodo-, Omnipaque (*Winthrop*)

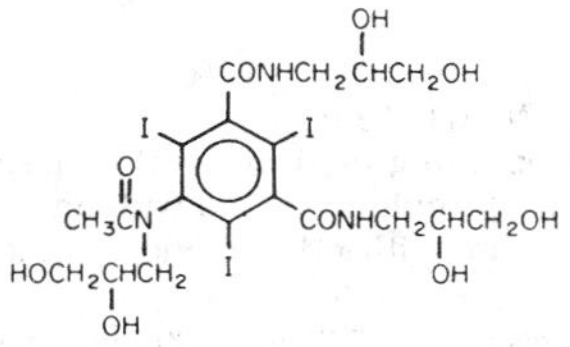

[66108-95-0] $C_{19}H_{26}I_3N_3O_9$ (821.14).

Preparation—US Pat 4,250,113.

Description—White crystals; melts about 176°.

Solubility—Soluble in water to form stable solutions.

Uses—A nonionic, water-soluble radiographic contrast medium used in different concentrations for different tests in both adults and children. Intrathecal doses, used for *myelography* (lumbar, thoracic, cervical, total columnar) and in contrast enhancement for computerized tomography (CT) for *myelography, cisternography*), are absorbed from cerebrospinal fluid into the bloodstream and eliminated by renal excretion. No significant metabolism, deiodination or biotransformation occurs.

Iohexol also may be administered intravascularly, whereupon it is distributed in the extracellular fluid and excreted unchanged by glomerular filtration. Intravascular administration is used in CT imaging of the head and total body as well as for *angiocardiography, arteriography, digital subtraction* and *peripheral angiography* and *excretory urography*.

Iohexol may be injected directly into body cavities as well as used orally for a variety of test procedures, ie, *arthrography, hysterosalpingography, herniography*, etc.

Iohexol should not be administered in the presence of significant local or systemic infection where bacteremia is likely. The concomitant intrathecal administration of corticosteroids is contraindicated. Caution is advised in patients with a history of epilepsy, severe cardiovascular disease, chronic alcoholism or multiple sclerosis.

Drugs which lower seizure threshold, especially phenothiazine derivatives, including those used for their antihistaminic or antinauseant properties, are not recommended for use with iohexol. Others include monoamine oxidase (MAO) inhibitors, tricyclic antidepressants, CNS stimulants, psychoactive drugs described as analeptics, major tranquilizers or antipsychotic drugs. Such medications should be discontinued at least 48 hr prior to myelography, should not be used for the control of nausea or vomiting during or after myelography and should not be resumed for at least 24 hr postprocedure.

Dose—Dosage volume and concentration depends upon the technique employed, the degree and extent of contrast required in the area(s) to be examined and the equipment to be used. See the package insert.

Dosage Forms—Intrathecal Injection: 180, 210, 240 and 300 mg iodine/mL in various sizes of vials and kit combinations. Intravascular/Oral: 140, 210, 240, 300 and 350 mg iodine/mL in various vial and IV bottle sizes. Iohexol solutions must be protected from strong daylight and direct exposure to sunlight and must not be allowed to freeze.

Iopamidol

1,3-Benzenedicarboxamide, (*S*)-*N*,*N'*-bis[2-hydroxy-1-(hydroxymethyl)ethyl]-5-[(2-hydroxy-1-oxopropyl)amino]-2,4,6-triiodo-, Isovue (*Squibb*)

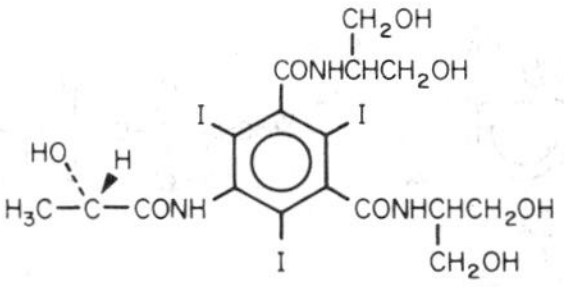

[60166-93-0] $C_{17}H_{22}I_3N_3O_8$ (777.09).

Preparation—See US Pat 4,001,323.

Description—White, odorless crystals; decompose about 300° without melting.

Solubility—Very soluble in water or methanol; soluble in boiling ethanol; practically insoluble in chloroform.

Uses—A nonionic contrast media for intrathecal administration in neuroradiology including *myelography*, (*lumbar, thoracic, cervical, total columnar*), *contrast enhancement of computed tomographic cisternography* and *angiography* throughout the cardiovascular system, including *cerebral* and *peripheral arteriography, coronary arteriography* and *ventriculography*. It is absorbed rapidly into the blood from the cerebrospinal fluid; following intrathecal administration, it appears in the plasma within 1 hr, but does not bind to plasma protein. It is excreted by the kidneys and eliminated within 48 hr. It should be administered with caution in patients with increased intracranial pressure, a history of convulsive disorders, severe cardiovascular disease, chronic alcoholism or multiple sclerosis and in elderly patients. Like other radiopaque diagnostic contrast agents, it is potentially hazardous in patients with multiple myeloma or pheochromocytoma. It should be used during pregnancy only when clearly needed; it should be avoided during delivery and in nursing mothers. Safety and effectiveness in children have not been established.

Dose—*Usual, adult, parenteral*, 46%: **4** to **15 mL**; 61%: **8** to **100 mL**; 76%: **2** to **50 mL**. See the package insert for details.

Dosage Form—Injection: **26%** (13% iodine); **41%** (20% iodine), 20-mL vials; **61%** (30% iodine), 20-, 50- and 100-mL vials; **76%** (37% iodine), 50-, 100-, 150- and 200-mL vials.

Iophendylate

Benzenedecanoic acid, iodo-ι-methyl-, ethyl ester; Pantopaque (*Alcon*)

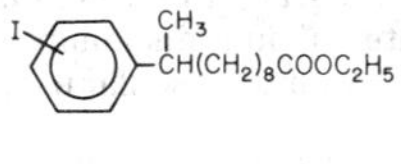

Iophendylate is a mixture of isomers of ethyl iodophenylundeca- noate, consisting chiefly of ethyl 10-(iodophenyl)undecanoate [1320-11-2] $C_{19}H_{29}IO_2$ (416.34).

Preparation—This substance is reported to be manufactured as follows. Benzene is reacted with undecylenic acid forming a mixture of isomers of phenylundecyclic acid. The mixture is iodinated and finally esterified with ethyl alcohol. After decolorization, the desired fraction is separated by distillation.

Description—Colorless to pale yellow, viscous liquid; darkens on long exposure to air; odorless or possesses a faintly ethereal odor; specific gravity between 1.248 and 1.257.

Solubility—Very slightly soluble in water; freely soluble in alcohol, benzene, chloroform or ether.

Uses—A *radiopaque medium* for *myelography*. It is used commonly for visualization of tumors or herniation of the intervertebral disc or other lesions compressing the spinal cord. It is absorbed at a rate of about 1 mL/yr, varying with the condition of the tissues; persistent levels in the body interfere with tracer radioactive iodine. About 80 to 100% can be removed by aspiration from the subarachnoid space following lumbar subarachnoid injection. The incidence of adverse reactions is low.

Note—The use of this agent has mostly been replaced by the low-osmolality nonionic contrast media.

Dose—*Usual, myelography, intrathecal* or *by special injection*, **3** to **12 mL.**

Dosage Form—Injection (sterile iophendylate): 305 mg of iodine/mL.

Iothalamate Meglumine [Injection]

Benzoic acid, 3-(acetylamino)-2,4,6-triiodo-5-[(methylamino)carbonyl]-, compd with 1-deoxy-1-(methylamino)-D-glucitol (1:1); Conray, Cysto-Conray (*Mallinckrodt*)

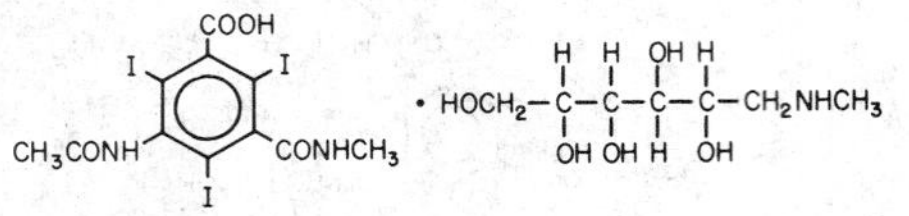

[13087-53-1] $C_{11}H_9I_3N_2O_4.C_7H_{17}NO_5$ (809.13).

Preparation—Iothalamic acid is reacted with an equimolar quantity of methylglucamine (meglumine), using sufficient water for injection to produce a solution of the required concentration.

Uses—A radiopaque media used *parenterally* in a 30, 43 or 60% solution for *urography*, a 30 or 60% solution for *angiography* and *computed tomography*, a 43 or 60% solution for venography, a 43% solution for *pyelography* and *cystourethrography* and a 60% solution for *cholangiography, arteriography, ventriculography* and *arthrography*. It is also available as a 17.2 and 43% *urogenital solution* for *retrograde urography, cystography* and *cystourethrography*. It is contraindicated in patients with a known sensitivity to salts of iothalamic acid and should not be used for urography in patients with anuria. Intravenous urography is hazardous to patients with multiple myeloma; anuria, progressive uremia, renal failure and death have occurred. No form of therapy, including dialysis, has been effective in reversing this effect. It also should be used with extreme caution in patients with pheochromocytoma and individuals homozygous for sickle cell disease. Iodine-containing contrast agents may also alter the result of thyroid-function tests. Adverse effects, precautions and contraindications are similar to those for other iodinated diagnostic agents. Its safety in pregnancy has not been established.

Dose—As the dosage and concentration vary considerably with the diagnostic uses and techniques of administration of the injection, the *latest* package insert should be consulted for adult and pediatric dosages and other information concerning uses.

Dosage Forms—Injection: 30%, 43% and 60% (141, 202 and 282 mg iodine/mL); Urogenital Solution: 17.2% and 48% (81 and 202 mg iodine/mL).

Iothalamate Meglumine and Iothalamate Sodium [Injection]

Vascoray (*Mallinckrodt*)

A sterile solution of iothalamic acid in water for injection, prepared with the aid of meglumine and NaOH. It may contain small amounts of suitable buffers and of edetate calcium disodium or edetate disodium as a stabilizer. When intended for intravascular use, it contains no antimicrobial agents.

Description—Clear, colorless to pale yellow, slightly viscous liquid.

Uses—For *intravascular angiocardiography, aortography,* selective *renal arteriography,* selective *coronary arteriography, excretory urography* and *computerized tomography*. Its warnings, contraindications and adverse effects are the same as for other iodinated diagnostic agents.

Dose—As the dosage varies with its diagnostic uses and techniques of administration, the *latest* package insert should be consulted for adult and pediatric dosages and other information concerning uses.

Dosage Form—Injection: 52% iothalamate meglumine and 26% iothalamate sodium.

Iothalamate Sodium [Injection]

Benzoic acid, 3-(acetylamino)-2,4,6-triiodo-5-[(methylamino)carbonyl]-, monosodium salt; Conray 325, Conray 400, Angio-Conray (*Mallinckrodt*)

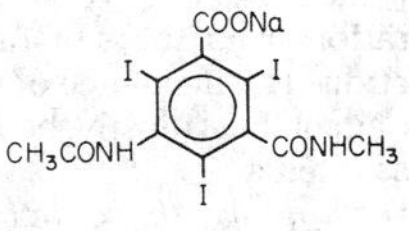

[1225-20-3] $C_{11}H_8I_3N_2NaO_4$ (635.90).

Preparation—Iothalamic acid is reacted with an equimolar quantity of NaOH, using sufficient water for injection to produce a solution of the required concentration.

Uses—For *intravascular angiocardiography, aortography, excretory urography* and enhancement of *computerized tomography*. It is contraindicated in cerebral angiography, and in patients with sensitivity to iothalamic acid. Its adverse effects and precautions are similar to those for other iodinated diagnostic agents.

Dose—As the dosage and concentration vary considerably with the diagnostic uses and techniques of administration, the *latest* package insert should be consulted for adult and pediatric dosages and other information concerning uses.

Dosage Forms—Injection: 54.3, 66.8 and 80% (325, 400 and 480 mg iodine/mL, respectively).

Iothalamic Acid

Benzoic acid, 3-(acetylamino)-2,4,6-triiodo-5-[(methylamino)carbony]-, ing of Vascoray (*Mallinckrodt*)

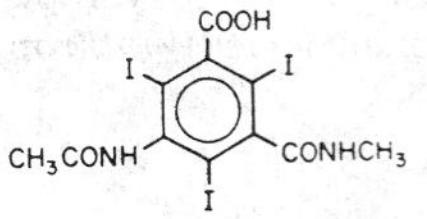

[2276-90-6] $C_{11}H_9I_3N_2O_4$ (613.92).

Preparation—By oxidizing *m*-xylene with potassium permanganate, condensing the resulting isophthalic acid with an equimolar quantity of methylamine and iodinating with iodine monochloride in acetic acid.

Description—White powder; odorless.

Solubility—Slightly soluble in water or alcohol; soluble in solutions of alkali hydroxides.

Uses—Radiopaque component for *Iothalamate Meglumine Injection, Iothalamate Meglumine and Iothalamate Sodium Injection* and *Iothalamate Sodium Injection*.

Ioversol

1,3-Benzenedicarboxamide, *N,N'*-bis(2,3-dihydroxypropyl)-5-[(hydroxyacetyl)-(2-hydroxyethyl)amino]-2,4,6-triiodo-, Optiray (*Mallinckrodt*)

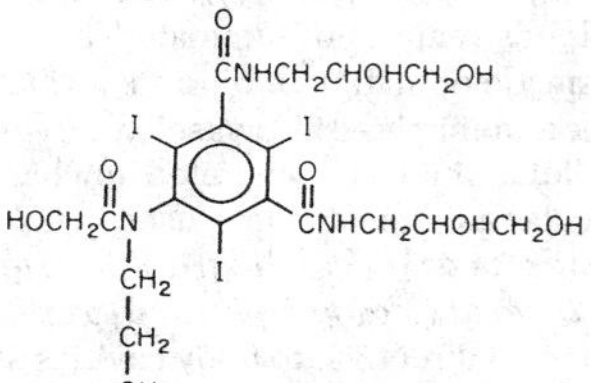

[87771-40-2] $C_{18}H_{24}I_3N_3O_9$ (807.12).

Uses—A nonionic, water-soluble radiographic contrast medium used in different concentrations for different tests in adults. The safety and effectiveness in children have not been established. Intravenous doses are used for *angiography* throughout the cardiovascular system, for contrast-enhanced CT imaging of the head and body, *excretory urography* and *digital subtraction angiography and venography*. One strength is indicated for *intra-arterial digital subtraction angiography (IA-DSA)*. No significant metabolism, deiodination or biotransformation occurs. Ioversol does not bind to serum or plasma proteins to any extent and does not cross the blood-brain barrier. Solutions of ioversol have osmolalities 1.2 to 2.8 times that of plasma and are hypertonic under conditions of use.

Ioversol is distributed rapidly (30 to 90 sec) after IV administration. The pharmacokinetics conform to an open two-compartment model with first-order elimination, eg, a rapid alpha phase for drug distribution and a slower beta phase for drug elimination. The $t_{1/2}$ is 1.5 hr.

Caution must be exercised in patients with severely impaired renal function, combined renal and hepatic disease, severe thyrotoxicosis, myelomatosis or anuria, particularly when large doses are administered. Intravenously administered iodine-containing radiopaque media are potentially hazardous in patients with multiple myeloma or other paraproteinemia, particularly in those with therapeutically resistant anuria. Arterial injection should never be made following the administration of vasopressors since they strongly potentiate neurological effects. In patients known or suspected to have pheochromocytoma, extreme caution should be exercised, blood pressure should be assessed throughout the procedure and measures for treatment of a hypertensive crisis should be available. Patients should be well hydrated prior to and following the administration of ioversol.

Dose—Dosage volume and concentration depends upon the technique employed, the degree and extent of contrast required in the area(s) to be examined and the equipment to be used. See the package insert.

Dosage Forms—Intravenous Injection: 160, 240, 320, and 350 mg/ml of organically bound iodine in various vial, IV bottle and injector syringe sizes. Ioversol solutions must be protected from strong daylight and direct exposure to sunlight and must not be allowed to freeze.

Ioxaglate Meglumine and Ioxaglate Sodium

Hexabrix (*Mallinkrodt*)

COOH CONHCH3 I I I I O O O O HOCH2CH2NHC NHCCH2NHC NCCH3 I I CH3

H H OH H · HOCH2—C—C—C—C—CH2NHCH3 OH OH H OH

A mixture of ioxaglate meglumine 39.3% [[59018-13-2] $C_{24}H_{21}N_5O_9.C_7H_{17}O_5$ (1464.10) and ioxaglate sodium 19.6% ([67992-58-9] $C_{24}H_{20}I_6N_5NaO_8$ (1290.87)]. The structure for the meglumine adduct is depicted above. The other component of Hexabrix is the sodium salt of the benzoic acid moiety of ioxaglate.

Uses—A radiopaque media containing 32% iodine for *urography, arthrography, angiography, angiocardiography, arteriography, aortography, venography, hysterosalpingography* and *computerized tomography*. Its precautions, drug interactions, adverse reactions and clinical procedures are similar to those for other iodine-containing radiopaque agents. Likewise, it should not be used during pregnancy or in nursing mothers.

Dose—*Adults,* **30** to **150 mL**; not to exceed 250 mL total. *Older children,* **30** to **45 mL** in a single dose. *Infants* and *young children,* **1.5 mL/kg** (range, 1 to 2 mL/kg) in a single dose. See package insert for details.

Dosage Form—Injection: 20-, 30- and 50-mL vials; 100- and 200-mL in bottles.

Metrizamide

D-Glucose, 2-[[3-(acetylamino)-5-(acetylmethylamino)-2,4,6-triiodobenzoyl]amino]-2-deoxy-, Amipaque (*Sterling*)

CH2OH O H OH OH HO I NHCOCH3 O NHC I I H3C—N—COCH3

[31112-62-6] $C_{18}H_{22}I_3N_3O_8$ (789.10).

Preparation—The acyl halide of metrizoic acid [3-(acetylamino)-5-(acetylmethylamino)-2,4,6-triiodobenzoic acid] and glucosamine are reacted under conditions whereby the amine portion of the glucosamine is acylated preferentially, in lieu of the hydroxyl groups.

Description—White crystals; melts about 230°.

Solubility—Freely soluble in water; protect aqueous solutions from light.

Uses—A radiopaque agent injected into the subarachnoid space for *lumbar, thoracic, cervical* and *total columnar myelography* and *computerized tomography* of the *intracranial subarachnoid spaces* following spinal subarachnoid injection. In pediatric patients it also is indicated for cisternography and ventriculography. It is absorbed from cerebrospinal fluid into the blood stream. Approximately 60% of the administered dose is excreted unchanged through the kidneys within 48 hr. Following subarachnoid injection conventional radiography will continue to provide good diagnostic contrast for at least 30 min; after 1 hr the degree of diagnostic contrast is not adequate. Metrizamide should not be given to patients known to be hypersensitive to it. The concurrent administration of corticosteroids and metrizamide is contraindicated. Lumbar puncture should not be performed in the presence of significant bacteremic infections. This agent should be used with caution in patients with a history of epilepsy, severe cardiovascular disease, chronic alcoholism or multiple sclerosis. Adverse reactions are similar to those for other iodinated diagnostic agents.

Dose—As the dosage and concentration varies with the diagnostic use and position of the patient, the package insert should be consulted for concentrations and dosage.

Dosage Form—Powder for Injection: 2.5 g in 20-mL vial, 3.75 g in 50-mL vial and 6.75 g in 20-mL vial.

Propyliodone

1(4H)-Pyridineacetic acid, 3,5-diiodo-4-oxo-, propyl ester; Dionosil Oily (*Glaxo*)

I O= N—CH2COOCH2CH2CH3 I

[587-61-1] $C_{10}H_{11}I_2NO_3$ (447.01).

Preparation—4(1*H*)-Pyridone, as the nitrate in aqueous solution, is iodinated with a mixture of sodium iodide and sodium iodate in the presence of sulfuric acid. The 3,5-diiodo-4(1*H*)-pyridone thus formed is isolated and condensed with chloroacetic acid to yield 3,5-diiodo-4-oxo-1(4*H*)-pyridineacetic acid, which is esterified with propyl alcohol.

Description—White, or almost white, crystalline powder; odorless or has a faint odor; melts between 187 and 190°.

Solubility—Practically insoluble in water; soluble in acetone, alcohol or ether.

Uses—A *radiopaque medium* for *bronchographic* use. Direct instillation into the bronchi results in well-defined bronchograms for at least 30 min. It usually is eliminated from the lungs in 7 to 10 days. Because of its toxicity, it should be used only if absolutely essential. It is contraindicated in patients with pulmonary emphysema or bronchiectasis.

Dose—*Usual, bronchography, intratracheal,* **0.75** to **1 mL** of 60% oil suspension, to a maximum of 12 to 18 mL.

Dosage Form—Sterile Oil Suspension: 20 mL of 60% (340 mg of iodine/mL).

Tuberculosis (see page 658).

Tuberculin, Old—page 1433
Tuberculin, Purified Protein Derivative (PPD)—page 1433

References

1. Jacobson PD, Rosenquist CH: *JAMA 260:* 1586, 1988.
2. Lawrence V, Matthai W, Hartmaier S: *Invest Radiol 1992:* 2, 1992.

CHAPTER 80

Pharmaceutical Necessities

William J Reilly, Jr
Manager, Technical Services
Pharmaceutical Division
FMC Corp
Princeton, NJ 08543

Significant changes are underway which could alter the rights of pharmacy practitioners. Extemporaneous compounding is being reviewed carefully by the FDA to ensure that manufacturing operations are not being conducted under the guise of pharmacy-practice rights. Additionally, some serious accidents have resulted from the improper compounding and handling of extemporaneously prepared prescriptions.

This chapter does not address the legalities of compounding by a practitioner, but rather is intended as a reference source which highlights substances of little or no therapeutic value which are useful in the compounding of pharmaceuticals. These substances, referred to as excipients, also are used for the bulk manufacture of pharmaceutical products, but usually for different purposes. The excipients described include antioxidants and preservatives; coloring and flavoring agents; diluents and binders; emulsifying and suspending agents, ointment bases, solvents and miscellaneous agents. A more detailed review of these excipients and their industrial applications can be found in the various chapters of **Part 8** of this text.

Antioxidants and Preservatives

An antioxidant is a substance capable of inhibiting oxidation and that may be added for this purpose to pharmaceutical products subject to deterioration by oxidative processes as, for example, the development of rancidity in oils and fats or the inactivation of some medicinals in the environment of their dosage forms. A preservative is, in the common pharmaceutical sense, a substance that prevents or inhibits microbial growth and may be added to pharmaceutical preparations for this purpose to avoid consequent spoilage of the preparations by microorganisms. Both antioxidants and preservatives have many applications in making medicinal products.

Alcohol—page 1404.

Ascorbyl Palmitate—see RPS-18, page 1286.

Anoxomer—see RPS-18, page 1288.

Benzoic Acid—see RPS-18, page 1235.

Benzalkonium Chloride—page 1264.

Benzethonium Chloride—page 1265.

Benzyl Alcohol—page 1151.

Butylated Hydroxyanisole

Phenol, (1,1-dimethylethyl)-4-methoxy-, Tenox BHA (*Eastman*)

OH, $C(CH_3)_3$, OCH_3

tert-Butyl-4-methoxyphenol [25013-16-5] $C_{11}H_{16}O_2$ (180.25).

Preparation—By an addition interaction of *p*-methoxyphenol and 2-methylpropene. US Pat 2,428,745.

Description—White or slightly yellow, waxy solid having a faint, characteristic odor.

Solubility—Insoluble in water; 1 g in 4 mL alcohol, 2 mL chloroform or 1.2 mL ether.

Uses—An *antioxidant* in cosmetics and pharmaceuticals containing fats and oils.

Butylparaben—see RPS-18 page 1170.

Butylated Hydroxytoluene

Phenol, 2,6-bis(1,1-dimethylethyl)-4-methyl-, Butylated Hydroxytoluene Crystalline (*Diamond-Shamrock*); Tenox BHT (*Eastman*)

OH, $(CH_3)_3C$, $C(CH_3)_3$, CH_3

2,6-Di-*tert*-butyl-*p*-cresol [128-37-0] $C_{15}H_{24}O$ (220.35).

Preparation—By an addition interaction of *p*-cresol and 2-methylpropene. US Pat 2,428,745.

Description—White, tasteless crystals with a mild odor; stable in light or air; melts at 70°.

Solubility—Insoluble in water; 1 g in 4 mL alcohol, 1.1 mL chloroform or 1.1 mL ether.

Uses—An *antioxidant* employed to retard oxidative degradation of oils and fats in various cosmetics and pharmaceuticals.

Cetylpyridinium Chloride—see RPS-18, page 1171.

Chlorobutanol

2-Propanol, 1,1,1-trichloro-2-methyl-, Chlorbutol; Chlorbutanol; Acetone chloroform; Chloretone (*Stauffer*)

$(CCl_3)C(CH_3)_2OH$

1,1,1-Trichloro-2-methyl-2-propanol [57-15-8] $C_4H_7Cl_3O$ (177.46); *hemihydrate* [6001-64-5] (186.46).

Preparation—Chloroform undergoes chemical addition to acetone under the catalytic influence of powdered potassium hydroxide.

Description—Colorless to white crystals, of a characteristic, somewhat camphoraceous odor and taste; anhydrous melts about 95°; hydrous melts about 76°; boils with some decomposition between 165 and 168°.

Solubility—1 g in 125 mL water, 1 mL alcohol or about 10 mL glycerin; freely soluble in chloroform, ether or volatile oils.

Incompatibilities—The anhydrous form must be used in order to prepare a clear solution in liquid petrolatum. It is decomposed by *alkalies; ephedrine* is sufficiently alkaline to cause its breakdown with the formation of ephedrine hydrochloride which will separate from a liquid petrolatum solution. It is only slightly soluble in water, hence alcohol must be used to dissolve the required amount in certain vehicles. A soft mass is produced by trituration with *antipyrine, menthol, phenol* and other substances.

Uses—Topically, as a solution in clove oil as a *dental analgesic.* It has *local anesthetic* potency to a mild degree and has been employed as an anesthetic dusting powder (1 to 5%) or ointment (10%). It has antibacterial and germicidal properties. It is used chiefly as a *preservative* in solutions of epinephrine, posterior pituitary, etc. When administered orally, it has much the same therapeutic use as chloral hydrate. Hence, it has been employed as a sedative and hypnotic. It has been taken orally to allay vomiting due to gastritis.

Dose—*Topical,* as a **25%** solution in clove oil.

Other Dose Information—The oral dose is 300 mg to 1 g, given in tablets or capsules.

Dehydroacetic Acid

Keto form: 2*H*-Pyran-2,4(3*H*)-dione, 3-acetyl-6-methyl-,

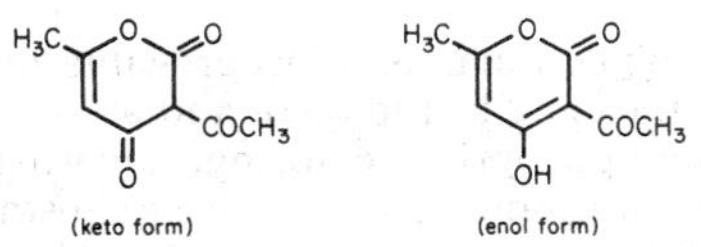

(keto form) (enol form)

Enol form: 3-Acetyl-4-hydroxy-6-methyl-2H-pyran-2-one [520-45-6 (Keto)], [771-03-9 (enol)] $C_8H_8O_4$ (168.15).

Preparation—By fractional distillation of a mixture of ethyl acetoacetate and sodium bicarbonate, maintaining almost total reflux conditions, allowing only ethanol to be removed. The residue is distilled under vacuum. *Org Syn Coll III:* 231, 1955.

Description—White to creamy-white crystalline powder melting about 110° with sublimation.

Solubility—1 g dissolves in 25 g acetone, 18 g benzene, 5 g methanol or 3 g alcohol.

Uses—Preservative.

Ethylenediamine

1,2-Ethanediamine

$H_2NCH_2CH_2NH_2$

Ethylenediamine [107-15-3] $C_2H_8N_2$ (60.10).

Caution—Use care in handling because of its caustic nature and the irritating properties of its vapor.

Note—It is strongly alkaline and may readily absorb carbon dioxide from the air to form a nonvolatile carbonate. Protect it against undue exposure to the atmosphere.

Preparation—By reacting ethylene dichloride with ammonia, then adding NaOH and distilling.

Description—Clear, colorless or only slightly yellow liquid, having an ammonia-like odor and strong alkaline reaction; miscible with water and alcohol; anhydrous boils 116 to 117° and solidifies at about 8°; volatile with steam; a strong base and readily combines with acids to form salts with the evolution of much heat.

Uses—A *pharmaceutical necessity* for *Aminophylline Injection.* It is irritating to skin and mucous membranes. It also may cause sensitization characterized by asthma and allergic dermatitis.

Ethylparaben—see RPS-18, page 1171.
Ethyl Vanillin—page 1386.
Glycerin—pages 1041 and 1405.
Hypophosphorus Acid—page 1410.
Malic Acid BP—see RPS-18, page 1288.
Methylparaben—see RPS-18, page 1171.
Monothioglycerol—see RPS-18, page 1287.
Phenol—page 1412.
Phenylethyl Alcohol—page 1389.
Phenylmercuric Nitrate—page 1270.

Potassium Benzoate

Benzoic acid, potassium salt

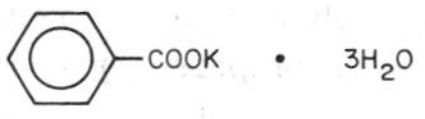

[582-25-2] $C_7H_5KO_2$ (160.21) (anhydrous).

Description—Crystalline powder.

Solubility—Soluble in water or alcohol.

Uses—Preservative.

Potassium Metabisulfite

Dipotassium pyrosulfite

[16731-55-8] $K_2S_2O_5$ (222.31).

Description—White crystals or crystalline powder with an odor of SO_2. Oxidizes in air to the sulfate. May ignite on powdering in a mortar if too much heat develops.

Solubility—Freely soluble in water; insoluble in alcohol.

Uses—Antioxidant.

Potassium Sorbate

2,4-Hexadienoic acid, (*E,E*)-, potassium salt; 2,4-Hexadienoic acid, potassium salt; Potassium 2,4-Hexadienoate

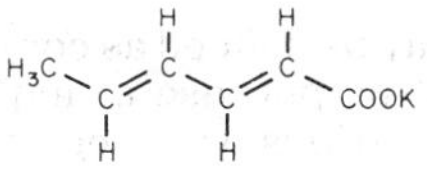

Potassium (*E,E*)-sorbate; potassium sorbate [590-00-1] [24634- 61-5] $C_6H_7KO_2$ (150.22).

Preparation—Sorbic Acid is reacted with an equimolar portion of KOH. The resulting potassium sorbate may be crystallized from aqueous ethanol. US Pat 3,173,948.

Description—White crystals or powder with a characteristic odor; melts about 270° with decomposition.

Solubility—1 g in 4.5 mL water, 35 mL alcohol, > 1000 mL chloroform or > 1000 mL ether.

Uses—A water-soluble salt of sorbic acid used in pharmaceuticals to *inhibit the growth of molds and yeasts.* Its toxicity is low, but it may irritate the skin.

Propyl Gallate BP—see RPS-18, page 1288.
Propylparaben—see RPS-18, page 1171.
Sassafras Oil—page 1392.
Sodium Benzoate—page 1271.

Sodium Bisulfite

Sulfurous acid, monosodium salt; Sodium Hydrogen Sulfite; Sodium Acid Sulfite; Leucogen

Monosodium sulfite [7631-90-5] $NaHSO_3$ and sodium metabisulfite ($Na_2S_2O_5$) in varying proportions; yields 58.5–67.4% of SO_2.

Description—White or yellowish white crystals or granular powder having the odor of sulfur dioxide; unstable in air.

Solubility—1 g in 4 mL water; slightly soluble in alcohol.

Uses—An *antioxidant* and *stabilizing agent.* Epinephrine hydrochloride solutions may be stabilized by the addition of small quantities of the salt. It also is used to help solubilize kidney stones. It is useful for removing permanganate stains and for solubilizing certain dyes and other chemicals (see *Menadione Sodium Bisulfite,* RPS-17, page 1011).

Sodium Metabisulfite

Disulfurous acid, disodium salt

Disodium pyrosulfite [7681-57-4]$Na_2S_2O_5$ (190.10).

Preparation—Formed when sodium bisulfite undergoes thermal dehydration. It also may be prepared by passing sulfur dioxide over sodium carbonate.

Description—White crystals or white to yellowish crystalline powder having an odor of sulfur dioxide; on exposure to air and moisture, it is slowly oxidized to sulfate.

Solubility—1 g in 2 mL water; slightly soluble in alcohol; freely soluble in glycerin.

Uses—A *reducing agent.* It is used in easily oxidized pharmaceuticals, such as epinephrine hydrochloride and phenylephrine hydrochloride injections, to retard oxidation.

Sodium Propionate—see RPS-18, page 1236.

Sorbic Acid

2,4-Hexadienoic acid, (*E,E*)-, 2,4-Hexadienoic acid

(*E,E*)-Sorbic acid; Sorbic acid [22500-92-1] [110-44-1] $C_6H_8O_2$ (112.13).

Preparation—By various processes. Refer to US Pat 2,921,090.

Description—Free-flowing, white, crystalline powder, having a characteristic odor; melts about 133°.

Solubility—1 g in 1000 mL water, 10 mL alcohol, 15 mL chloroform, 30 mL ether or 19 mL propylene glycol.

Uses—A *mold and yeast inhibitor.* It also is used as a fungistatic agent for foods, especially cheeses.

Sulfur Dioxide—see RPS-18, page 1288.

Thimerosal—page 1271.

Coloring, Flavoring and Diluting Agents

The use of properly colored and flavored medicinal substances, although offering no particular therapeutic advantage, is of considerable importance psychologically. A water-clear medicine is not particularly acceptable to most patients, and, in general, is thought to be inert. Many very active medicinal substances are quite unpalatable, and the patient may fail to take the medicine simply because the taste or appearance is objectionable. Disagreeable medication can be made both pleasing to the taste and attractive by careful selection of the appropriate coloring, flavoring and diluting agents. Therefore, judicious use of these substances is important in securing patient cooperation in taking or using the prescribed medication and continued compliance with the prescriber's intent.

Coloring Agents or Colorants

Coloring agents may be defined as compounds employed in pharmacy solely for the purpose of imparting color. They may be classified in various ways, eg, inorganic or organic. For the purpose of this discussion two subdivisions are used: *Natural Coloring Principles* and *Synthetic Coloring Principles.* The members of these groups are used as colors for pharmaceutical preparations, cosmetics, foods and as bacteriological stains and diagnostic agents.

Natural Coloring Principles

Natural coloring principles are obtained from mineral, plant and animal sources. They are used primarily for artistic purposes, as symbolic adornments of natives, as colors for foods, drugs and cosmetics and for other psychological effects.

Mineral colors frequently are termed *pigments* and are used to color lotions, cosmetics and other preparations, usually for external application. Examples are *Red Ferric Oxide* (page 1416) and *Yellow Ferric Oxide* (page 1416), titanium dioxide (page 884) and carbon black.

The term pigment also is applied generically to plant colors by phytochemists. Many plants contain coloring principles that may be extracted and used as colorants, eg, chlorophyll. Anattenes are obtained from annatto seeds and give yellow to orange water-soluble dyes. Natural beta-carotene is a yellow color extracted from carrots and used to color margarine. Alizarin is a reddish-yellow dye obtained from the madder plant. The indigo plant is the source of a blue pigment called indigo. Flavones, such as riboflavin, rutin, hesperidin and quercetin, are yellow pigments. Saffron is a glycoside that gives a yellow color to drugs and foods. Cudbear and red saunders are two other dyes obtained from plants. Most plant colors now have been characterized and synthesized, however, and those with the desirable qualities of stability, fastness and pleasing hue are available commercially as synthetic products.

Animals have been a source of coloring principles from the earliest periods of recorded history. For example, *Tyrian purple,* once a sign of royalty, was prepared by air oxidation of a colorless secretion obtained from the glands of a snail (*Murex brandaris*). This dye now is known to be 6,6′-dibromoindigo, and has been synthesized, but cheaper dyes of the same color are available. Cochineal from the insect *Coccus cacti* contains the bright-red coloring principle *carminic acid,* a derivative of anthraquinone. This dye is no longer used in foods and pharmaceuticals due to *Salmonella* contamination.

Synthetic Coloring Principles

Synthetic coloring principles date from 1856 when WH Perkin accidentally discovered *mauveine,* also known as a *Perkin's purple,* while engaged in unsuccessful attempts to synthesize quinine. He obtained the dye by oxidizing aniline containing *o*- and *p*-toluidines as impurities. Other discoveries of this kind followed soon after, and a major industry grew up in the field of coal-tar chemistry.

The earliest colors were prepared from aniline and for many years all coal-tar dyes were called aniline colors, irrespective of their origin. The coal-tar dyes include more than a dozen well-defined groups among which are *nitroso-dyes, nitro-dyes, azo-dyes, oxazines, thiazines, pyrazolones, xanthenes, indigoids, anthraquinones, acridines, rosanilines, phthaleins, quinolines* and others. These in turn are classified, according to their method of use, as *acid dyes* and *basic dyes,* or *direct dyes* and *mordant dyes.*

Certain structural elements in organic molecules, called *chromophore* groups, give color to the molecules, eg, azo (—N=N—), nitroso (—N=O), nitro ($—NO_2$), azoxy (—N=N—O—), carbonyl (>C=O) and ethylene (>C=C<). Other such combinations augment the chromophore groups, eg, methoxy, hydroxy and amino groups and are known as *auxochromes.*

Stability—Most dyes are relatively unstable chemicals due to their unsaturated structures. They are subject to fading due to light, metals, heat, microorganisms, oxidizing and reducing agents plus strong acids and bases. In tablets, fading may appear as spotting and specking.

Uses—Most synthetic coloring principles are used in coloring fabrics and for various artistic purposes. They also find application as indicators, bacteriological stains, diagnostic aids, reagents in microscopy, etc.

Many coal-tar dyes originally were used in foodstuffs and beverages without careful selection or discrimination between those that were harmless and those that were toxic and without any supervision as to purity or freedom from poisonous constituents derived from their manufacture.

After the passage of the Food and Drugs Act in 1906, the US Department of Agriculture established regulations by which a few colors came to be known as *permitted colors.* Certain of these colors may be used in foods, drugs and cosmetics, but only after certification by the FDA that they meet certain specifications. From this list of permitted colors may be produced, by skillful blending and mixing, other colors that may be used in foods, beverages and pharmaceutical preparations. Blends of certified dyes must be recertified.

The word "permitted" is used in a restricted sense. It does not carry with it the right to use colors for purposes of deception, even though they are "permitted" colors, for all food laws have clauses prohibiting the coloring of foods and beverages in a manner so as to conceal inferiority or to give a false appearance of value.

The certified colors are classified into three groups: FD&C dyes which legally may be used in foods, drugs and cosmetics, D&C dyes which legally may be used in drugs and cosmetics and External D&C dyes which legally may be used only in externally applied drugs and cosmetics. There are specific limits for the pure dye, sulfated ash, ether extractives, soluble and insoluble matter, uncombined intermediates, oxides, chlorides and sulfates. As the use status of these colors is subject to change, the latest regulations of the FDA should be consulted to determine how they may be used—especially since several FD&C dyes formerly widely used have been found to be carcinogenic even when "pure" and, therefore, have been banned from use.

The Coal-Tar Color Regulations specify that the term "externally applied drugs and cosmetics" means drugs and cosmetics which are applied only to external parts of the body and not to the lips or any body surface covered by mucous membrane. No certified dye, regardless of its category, legally may be used in any article which is to be applied to the area of the eye.

Lakes are calcium or aluminum salts of certified dyes extended on a substrate of alumina. They are insoluble in water and organic solvents, hence are used to color powders, pharmaceuticals, foods, hard candies and food packaging.

The application of dyes to pharmaceutical preparations is an art that can be acquired only after an understanding of the characteristics of dyes and knowledge of the composition of the products to be colored has been obtained. Specific rules for the choice or application of dyes to pharmaceutical preparations are difficult to formulate. Each preparation may present unique problems.

Preparations which may be colored include most liquid pharmaceuticals, powders, ointments and emulsions. Some general hints may be offered in connection with solutions and powders, but desired results usually can be obtained only by a series of trials. In general, an inexperienced operator tends to use a much higher concentration of the dye than is necessary, resulting in a dull color. The amount of dye present in any pharmaceutical preparation should be of a concentration high enough to give the desired color and low enough to prevent toxic reactions and permanent staining of fabrics and tissues.

Liquids (Solutions)—The dye concentration in liquid preparations and solutions usually should come within a range of 0.0005% (1 in 200,000) and 0.001% (1 in 100,000), depending upon the depth of color wanted and the thickness of column to be viewed in the container. With some dyes, concentrations as low as 0.0001% (1 in 1,000,000) may have a distinct tinting effect. Dyes are used most conveniently in the form of stock solutions.

Powders—White powders usually require the incorporation of 0.1% (1 in 1000) of a dye to impart a pastel color. The dyes may be incorporated into the powder by dry-blending in a ball mill or, on a small scale, with a mortar and pestle. The dye is incorporated by trituration and geometric dilution. Powders also may be colored evenly by adding a solution of the dye in alcohol or some other volatile solvent having only a slight solvent action on the powder being colored. When this procedure is employed, the solution is added in portions, with thorough mixing after each addition, after which the solvent is allowed to evaporate from the mixture.

Many of the syrups and elixirs used as flavoring and diluting agents are colored. When such agents are used no further coloring matter is necessary. The use of colored flavoring agents is discussed in a subsequent section. However, when it is desired to add color to an otherwise colorless mixture, one of the agents described in the first section may be used.

Incompatibilities—FD&C dyes are mainly anionic (sodium salts), hence are incompatible with cationic substances. Since the concentrations of these substances are generally very low, no precipitate is evident. Polyvalent ions such as calcium, magnesium and aluminum also may form insoluble compounds with dyes. A pH change may cause the color to change. Acids may release the insoluble acid form of the dye.

Caramel —see RPS-18, page 1290.

Flavoring Agents

Flavor

The word flavor refers to a mixed sensation of taste, touch, smell, sight and sound, all of which combine to produce an infinite number of gradations in the perception of a substance. The four primary tastes—*sweet*, *bitter*, *sour* and *saline*—appear to be the result partly of physicochemical and partly of psychological action. Taste buds (Fig 1), located mainly on the tongue, contain very sensitive nerve endings that react, in the presence of moisture, with the flavors in the mouth and as a result of physicochemical activity electrical impulses are produced and transmitted via the seventh, ninth and tenth cranial nerves to the areas of the brain which are devoted to the perception of taste. Some of the taste buds are specialized in their function, giving rise to areas on the tongue which are sensitive to only one type of taste. The brain, however, usually perceives taste as a composite sensation, and accordingly the components of any flavor are not readily discernible. Children have more taste buds than adults, hence are more sensitive to tastes.

Taste partly depends on the ions which are produced in the mouth, but psychologists have demonstrated that sight (color) and sound also play a definite role when certain reflexes

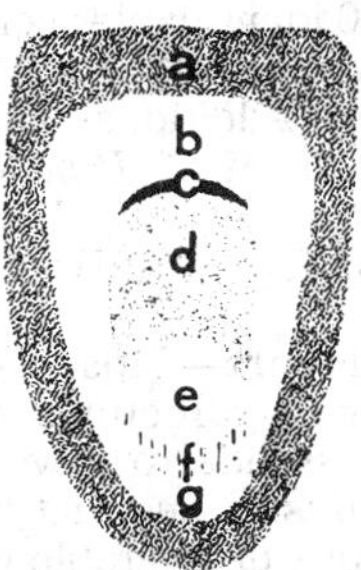

Fig 1. Upper Surface of the tongue. a: Taste receptors for all tastes; b: sweet, salty and sour; c: salty and sour; d: sour only; e: no taste sensation; f: sweet and sour; g: bitter, sweet and sour (adapted from Crocker EC: *Flavor,* McGraw-Hill, New York, 22, 1945).

become conditioned through custom and association of sense perceptions. Thus, in the classic experiments of Pavlov demonstrating "conditioned reflexes," the ringing of a bell or the showing of a circle of light caused the gastric juices of a dog to flow although no food was placed before it, and much of the enjoyment derived from eating celery is due to its crunchy crispness as the fibrovascular bundles are crushed. The effect of color is just as pronounced; oleomargarine is unpalatable to most people when it is uncolored, but once the dye has been incorporated gourmets frequently cannot distinguish it from butter. Color and taste must coincide, eg, cherry flavor is associated with a red color.

A person suffering from a head cold finds his food much less palatable than usual because his sense of smell is impaired, and, if the nostrils are held closed, raw onions taste sweet and it is much easier to ingest castor oil and other nauseating medicines. The volatility of a substance is an important factor that is influenced by the warmth and moisture of the mouth since the more volatile a compound, the more pronounced its odor. The sense of smell detects very minute amounts of material and is usually much more sensitive in detecting the presence of volatile chemicals, but the tongue is able to detect infinitesimal amounts of some vapors if it is protruded from the mouth so that solution of the gases in the saliva may take place. In this manner traces of sulfur dioxide can be detected in the air since it dissolves in the saliva and creates a sour taste.

Flavors described as hot are those that exert a mild counterirritant effect on the mucosa of the mouth, those that are astringent and pucker the mouth contain tannins and acids that produce this effect by reacting with the lining of the mouth and wines possess a bouquet due to the odor of the volatile constituents. Indian turnip (Jack-in-the-pulpit) owes its flavor largely to the stinging sensation caused by the minute acicular crystals of calcium oxalate which penetrate the mucous membrane.

Other physiological and physical factors that also may affect taste are coarseness or grittiness due to small particles, eg, ion-exchange resins. Antidiarrheal preparations have a chalky taste. Menthol imparts a cool taste because it affects the coldness receptors. Mannitol gives a cool sensation when it dissolves because its negative of heat of solution will cause the temperature to drop. For this reason, mannitol often is used as the base for chewable tablets.

There is a definite threshold of taste for every substance, which varies somewhat with the individual and with the environment. The experienced chef tastes his delicacies at the temperature at which they will be served since heat and cold alter the flavor of many preparations. Thus, lemon loses its sour taste entirely at an elevated temperature and other flavors become almost nonvolatile, tasteless and odorless when cooled sufficiently. In addition to the influence of temperature, the sensitivity of each individual must be considered. For example, it has been determined by experiment that the amount of sugar that can just be detected by the average individual is about 7 mg. However, this amount cannot be tasted by some and it is definitely sweet to others.

People are more sensitive to odor than to taste. There are about 10,000 to 30,000 identifiable scents, of which the average person can identify about 4000. Women are more sensitive to odors than men. Additional insights can be obtained by reading Cagan RH, Kare MR: *Biochemistry of Taste and Olfaction*, Academic, NY 1981, and Beidler LM, ed: *Handbook of Sensory Physiology*, vol IV, pts 1 and 2, Springer-Verlag, Berlin 1971.

Preservation of Flavors—Most monographs of official products contain specific directions for storage. Proper methods of storage are essential to prevent deterioration which in many instances results in destruction of odor and taste. Under adverse conditions undesirable changes occur due to one or a combination of the following: enzymatic activity, oxidation, change in moisture content, absorption of odors, activity of microorganisms and effects of heat and light. In certain products some of the changes wrought by these factors are desirable, as when esters are formed due to the activity of enzymes and when blending and mellowing results from the interchange of the radicals of esters (*trans-esterification*).

One method for protecting readily oxidizable substances, such as lemon oil, from deteriorating, and thus preserving their original delicate flavor, is to microencapsulate them by spray-drying. The capsules containing the flavors then are enclosed in various packaged products (eg, powdered gelatins) or tablets which are flavored deliciously when the capsule is disintegrated by mixing and warming with water or saliva.

Correlation of Chemical Structure with Flavor and Odor—The compounds employed as flavors in vehicles vary considerably in their chemical structure, ranging from simple esters (methyl salicylate), alcohols (glycerin) and aldehydes (vanillin) to carbohydrates (honey) and the complex volatile oils (anise oil). Synthetic flavors of almost any desired type are now available. These frequently possess the delicate flavor and aroma of the natural products and also the desirable characteristics of stability, reproducibility and comparatively low cost. Synthetic products such as cinnamaldehyde and benzaldehyde, first officially recognized when several of the essential oils became scarce during World War II, have been used widely.

There is a close relationship between chemical structure and taste. Solubility, the degree of ionization and the type of ions produced in the saliva definitely influence the sensation interpreted by the brain.

Sour taste is caused by hydrogen ions and it is proportional to the hydrogen-ion concentration and the lipid solubility of the compound. It is characteristic of acids, tannins, alum, phenols and lactones. Saltiness is due to simultaneous presence of anions and cations, eg, KBr, NH_4Cl and sodium salicylate. High-molecular-weight salts may have a bitter taste. Sweet taste is due to polyhydroxy compounds, polyhalogenated aliphatic compounds and α-amino acids. Amino and amide groups, especially if the positive effect is balanced by the proximity of a negative group, may produce a sweet taste. Sweetness increases with the number of hydroxy groups, possibly due to increase in solubility. Imides such as saccharin and sulfamates such as cyclamates are intensely sweet. Cyclamates have been removed from the market because they reportedly cause bladder tumors in rats. Free bases such as alkaloids and amides such as amphetamines give bitter tastes. Polyhydroxy compounds with a molecular weight greater than 300, halogenated substances and aliphatic thio compounds also may have bitter tastes. Unsaturation frequently bestows a sharp, biting odor and taste upon compounds.

No precise relationship between chemical structure and odor has been found. There are no primary odors, and odors blend into each other. Polymerization reduces or destroys odor; high valency gives odor and unsaturation enhances odor. A tertiary carbon atom often will give a camphoraceous odor, esters and lactones have a fruity odor and ketones have a pleasant odor. Strong odors often are accompanied by volatility and chemical reactivity.

Selection of Flavors

The proper selection of flavors for disguising nauseating medicines aids in their ingestion. Occasionally, sensitive patients have become nauseated sufficiently to vomit at the thought of having to take disagreeable medication, and it is particularly difficult to persuade children to continue to use and retain distasteful preparations. There is a need to know the allergies and idiosyncrasies of the patient; thus, it is foolish to use a chocolate-flavored vehicle for the patient who dislikes the flavor or who is allergic to it, notwithstanding the fact that this flavor is generally acceptable.

Flavoring Methodology

Each flavoring problem is unique and requires an individual solution. The problem of flavoring is further complicated because flavor and taste depend on individual preferences. In solving flavoring problems the following techniques have been used:

Blending—Fruit flavors blend with sour taste; bitter tastes can be blended with salty, sweet and sour tastes; salt reduces sourness and increases sweetness; chemicals such as vanillin, monosodium glutamate and benzaldehyde are used for blending.

Overshadow—Addition of a flavor whose intensity is longer and stronger than the obvious taste, eg, methyl salicylate, glycyrrhiza and oleoresins.

Physical—Formation of insoluble compounds of the offending drug, eg, sulfonamides; emulsification of oils; effervescence, eg, magnesium citrate solution; high viscosity of fluids to limit contact of drug with the tongue, and mechanical procedures such as coating tablets, are physical methods to reduce flavoring problems.

Chemical—Adsorption of the drug on a substrate, or formation of a complex of the drug with ion-exchange resins or complexing agents.

Physiological—The taste buds may be anesthetized by menthol or mint flavors.

Flavors, as used by the pharmacist in compounding prescriptions, may be divided into four main categories according to the type of taste which is to be masked, as follows:

Salty Taste—Cinnamon syrup has been found to be the best vehicle for ammonium chloride, and other salty drugs such as sodium salicylate and ferric ammonium citrate. In a study of the comparative efficiency of flavoring agents for disguising salty taste, the following additional vehicles were arranged in descending order of usefulness: orange syrup, citric acid syrup, cherry syrup, cocoa syrup, wild cherry syrup, raspberry syrup, glycyrrhiza elixir, aromatic elixir and glycyrrhiza syrup. The last-named is particularly useful as a vehicle for the salines by virtue of its colloidal properties and the sweetness of both glycyrrhizin and sucrose.

Bitter Taste—Cocoa syrup was found to be the best vehicle for disguising the bitter taste of quinine bisulfate, followed, in descending order of usefulness, by raspberry syrup, cocoa syrup, cherry syrup, cinnamon syrup, compound sarsaparilla syrup, citric acid syrup, licorice syrup, aromatic elixir, orange syrup and wild cherry syrup.

Acrid or Sour Taste—Raspberry syrup and other fruit syrups are especially efficient in masking the taste of sour substances such as hydrochloric acid. Acacia syrup and other mucilaginous vehicles are best for disguising the acrid taste of substances, such as capsicum, since they tend to form a colloidal protective coating over the taste buds of the tongue. Tragacanth, unlike acacia, may be used in an alcoholic vehicle.

Oily Taste—Castor oil may be made palatable by emulsifying with an equal volume of aromatic rhubarb syrup or with compound sarsaparilla syrup. Cod liver oil is disguised effectively by adding wintergreen oil or peppermint oil. Lemon, orange and anise or combinations of these are also useful. It is better to mix most of the flavor with the oil before emulsifying it, and then the small remaining quantity can be added after the primary emulsion is formed.

Those flavors that are most pleasing to the majority of people are associated with some stimulant of a physical or physiological nature. This may be a central nervous stimulant such as caffeine, which is the reason so many enjoy tea and coffee as a beverage, or it may be a counterirritant such as one of the spices that produce a "biting" sensation or an agent which "tickles" the throat such as soda water. Sherry owes its sharp flavor to its acetaldehyde content, and some of the volatile oils contain terpenes that are stimulating to the mucous surfaces.

Selection of Vehicles

Too few pharmacists realize the unique opportunity they have in acquainting physicians with a knowledge of how to increase both the palatability and efficacy of their prescribed medicines through the judicious selection of vehicles. Because of the training a pharmacist receives, his knowledge of the characteristics of various pharmaceuticals and therapeutic agents and his technique and skill in preparing elegant preparations are well-developed, so that he is qualified admirably to advise concerning the proper use of vehicles.

A large selection of flavors is available as well as a choice of colors, so that one may prescribe a basic drug for a prolonged period, but by changing the vehicle from time to time, the taste and appearance are so altered that the patient does not tire of the prescription or show other psychological reactions to it.

The statement of the late Dr Bernard Fantus that "the best solvent is the best vehicle" helps to explain the proper use of a flavoring vehicle. For example, a substance that is soluble in alcohol, eg, phenobarbital, will not leave an alcoholic vehicle readily to dissolve in the aqueous saliva.

Waters—These are the simplest of the vehicles and are available with several flavors. They contain no sucrose, a fact to be considered at times, since sucrose under certain circumstances may be undesirable. They are likewise nonalcoholic, another fact which frequently influences vehicle selection.

Elixirs—These have added sweetness that waters lack, and they usually contain alcohol, which imparts an added sharpness to the flavor of certain preparations, making the latter more pleasing to the taste. Elixirs are suitable for alcohol-soluble drugs.

Syrups—These vehicles, like elixirs, offer a wide selection of flavors and colors from which to choose. Their specific value, however, lies particularly in the fact that they are intensely sweet and contain little or no alcohol, a combination which makes them of singular value as masking agents for water-soluble drugs.

Vehicles consisting of a solution of pleasantly flavored volatile oils in syrup or glycerin (1:500) have been employed successfully in producing uniform and stable preparations. These vehicles are prepared by adding 2 mL of the volatile oil, diluted with 6 mL of alcohol, to 500 mL of glycerin or syrup, which has been warmed gently. The solution is added a little at a time with continuous shaking, and then sufficient glycerin or syrup is added to make 1000 mL, and mixed well.

Alcohol solutions of volatile oils are sometimes used as "stock solutions" for flavoring pharmaceuticals.

A listing of substances, most of them official, used as flavors, flavored vehicles or as sweeteners, is given in Table 1. Additional information on flavoring ingredients may be obtained in Furia TE, Bellanca A: *Fenaroli's Handbook of Flavor Ingredients*, Chemical Rubber, Cleveland, 1971.

Acacia Syrup—page 1393.

Anethole—see RPS-18, page 1292.

Anise Oil

Aniseed Oil; Star Anise Oil

The volatile oil distilled with steam from the dried, ripe fruit of *Pimpinella anisum* Linné (Fam *Umbelliferae*) or from the dried, ripe fruit of *Illicium verum* Hooker filius (Fam *Magnoliaceae*).

Note—If solid material has separated, carefully warm the oil until it is completely liquefied, and mix it before using.

Constituents—The official oil varies somewhat in composition, depending upon whether it was obtained from *Pimpinella anisum* or the star anise, *Illicium verum*. *Anethole* is the chief constituent of both oils, occurring to the extent of 80 to 90%. *Methyl chavicol*, an isomer of anethole, and *anisic ketone* [$C_{10}H_{12}O_2$] also are found in both oils, as are small amounts of many other constituents.

Description—Colorless or pale yellow, strongly refractive liquid, having the characteristic odor and taste of anise; specific gravity 0.978 to 0.988; congeals not below 15°.

Solubility—Soluble in 3 volumes of 90% alcohol.

Uses—Extensively as a *flavoring agent*, particularly for licorice candies. It has been given as a *carminative* in a dose of about 0.1 mL.

Aromatic Elixir—page 1394.

Aromatic Elixir, Red—see RPS-15, page 1240.

Table 1—Flavoring Agents

Acacia syrup	Lavender oil
Anethole	Lemon oil
Anise oil	Lemon tincture
Aromatic elixir	Mannitol
Benzaldehyde	Methyl salicylate
Benzaldehyde elixir, compound	Nutmeg oil
Caraway	Orange, bitter, elixir
Caraway oil	Orange, bitter, oil
Cardamom oil	Orange flower oil
Cardamom seed	Orange flower water
Cardamom spirit, compound	Orange oil
Cardamom tincture, compound	Orange peel, bitter
Cherry juice	Orange peel, sweet, tincture
Cherry syrup	Orange spirit, compound
Cinnamon	Orange syrup
Cinnamon oil	Peppermint
Cinnamon water	Peppermint oil
Citric acid	Peppermint spirit
Citric acid syrup	Peppermint water
Clove oil	Phenylethyl alcohol
Cocoa	Raspberry juice
Cocoa syrup	Raspberry syrup
Coriander oil	Rosemary oil
Dextrose	Rose oil
Eriodictyon	Rose water
Eriodictyon fluidextract	Rose water, stronger
Eriodictyon syrup, aromatic	Saccharin
Ethyl acetate	Saccharin calcium
Ethyl vanillin	Saccharin sodium
Fennel oil	Sarsaparilla syrup, compound
Ginger	Sorbitol solution
Ginger fluidextract	Spearmint
Ginger oleoresin	Spearmint oil
Glucose	Sucrose
Glycerin	Syrup
Glycyrrhiza	Thyme oil
Glycyrrhiza elixir	Tolu balsam
Glycyrrhiza extract	Tolu balsam syrup
Glycyrrhiza extract, pure	Vanilla
Glycyrrhiza fluidextract	Vanilla tincture
Glycyrrhiza syrup	Vanillin
Honey	Wild cherry syrup
Iso-Alcoholic elixir	

Benzaldehyde

Artificial Essential Almond Oil

[structure: benzene ring–CHO]

Benzaldehyde [100-52-7] C_7H_6O (106.12).

Preparation—By the interaction of benzal chloride with lime in the resence of water. Benzal chloride is obtained by treating boiling toluene with chlorine.

Description—Colorless, strongly refractive liquid, having an odor resembling that of bitter almond oil, and a burning aromatic taste; affected by light; specific gravity 1.041 to 1.046; boils about 180°, solidifies about −56.5° and on exposure to air it gradually oxidizes to benzoic acid.

Solubility—Dissolves in about 350 volumes of water; miscible with alcohol, ether, chloroform or fixed and volatile oils.

Uses—In place of bitter almond oil for *flavoring* purposes; it is much safer than the latter because it contains no hydrocyanic acid. It also is used extensively in *perfumery* and in the manufacture of dyestuffs and many other organic compounds, such as aniline, acetanilid or mandelic acid.

Compound Benzaldehyde Elixir—*Preparation:* Dissolve benzaldehyde (0.5 mL) and vanillin (1 g) in alcohol (50 mL); add syrup (400 mL), orange flower water (150 mL) and sufficient purified water, in several portions, shaking the mixture thoroughly after each addition, to make the product measure 1000 mL; then filter, if necessary, until the product is clear. *Alcohol Content:* 3 to 5%. *Uses:* A useful vehicle for administering bromides and other salts, especially when a low alcoholic content is desired.

Camphor Water—see RPS-13, page 436.

Caraway—see RPS-18, page 1293.

Caraway Oil—see RPS-18, page 1293.

Cardamom Seed

Cardamom Fruit; Cardamom; Ceylon or Malabar Cardamom

The dried ripe seed of *Elettaria cardamomum* (Linné) Maton (Fam. *Zingiberaceae*).

It should be removed recently from the capsule.

Constituents—A *volatile oil,* the yield of which is 1.3% from Malabar Ceylon Seeds and 2.6% from Mysore-Ceylon Seeds. *Fixed oil* is present to the extent of 10%, also starch, mucilage, etc.

Uses—A *flavor.* For many years it was employed empirically as a *carminative.*

Cardamom Oil—The volatile oil distilled from the seed of *Elettaria cardamomum* (Linné) Maton (Fam *Zingiberaceae*). Varieties of the oil contain *d-α-terpineol* [$C_{10}H_{17}OH$] both free and as the acetate, 5 to 10% *cineol* [$C_{10}H_{18}O$] and *limonene* [$C_{10}H_{16}$]. The Ceylon Oil, however, contains the alcohol 4-*terpineol (4-carbomenthenol)* [$C_{10}H_{17}OH$], the terpenes *terpinene* and *sabinene,* and *acetic* and *formic acids,* probably combined as esters. *Description and Solubility:* Colorless or very pale yellow liquid possessing the aromatic, penetrating and somewhat camphoraceous odor of cardamom, and a persistently pungent, strongly aromatic taste; affected by light; specific gravity 0.917 to 0.947. Miscible with alcohol; dissolves in 5 volumes of 70% alcohol. *Uses:* A *flavor.*

Cardamom Tincture, Compound—see RPS-18, page 1302.

Cherry Juice—see RPS-18, page 1320.

Cherry Syrup—page 1393.

Cinnamon

Saigon Cinnamon; True Cinnamon; Saigon Cassia

The dried bark of *Cinnamomum loureirii* Nees (Fam. *Lauraceae*).

It contains, in each 100 g, not less than 2.5 mL of volatile oil.

Uses—A *flavoring agent.* Formerly, it was used as a carminative.

Cinnamon Oil [Cassia Oil; Oil of Chinese Cinnamon]—The volatile oil distilled with steam from the leaves and twigs of *Cinnamomum cassia* (Nees) Nees ex Blume (Fam *Lauraceae*), rectified by distillation; contains not less than 80%, by volume, of the total aldehydes of cinnamon oil. Cinnamaldehyde is the chief constituent. *Description and Solubility:* Yellowish or brownish liquid, becoming darker and thicker on aging or exposure to the air, and having the characteristic odor and taste of cassia cinnamon; specific gravity 1.045 to 1.063. Soluble in an equal volume of alcohol, 2 volumes of 70% alcohol or an equal volume of glacial acetic acid. *Uses:* A *flavor.* It formerly was used in a dose of 0.1 mL for flatulent colic.

Cocoa —see RPS-18, page 1293.

Cocoa Syrup—page 1393.

Coriander—page 1391.

Coriander Oil—see RPS-18 page 1294.

Denatonium Benzoate—page 1409.

Eriodictyon—see RPS-18, page 1294.

Eriodictyon Fluidextract—see RPS-18, page 1294.

Eriodictyon Syrup, Aromatic—see RPS-18, page 1301.

Ethyl Acetate—see RPS-18, page 1294.

Ethyl Vanillin

Benzaldehyde, 3-ethoxy-4-hydroxy-, Bourbanal; Ethovan; Vanillal; Vanirome

[structure: C_2H_5O, HO–benzene ring–CHO]

3-Ethoxy-4-hydroxybenzaldehyde [121-32-4] $C_9H_{10}O_3$ (166.18).

Preparation—By reacting *o*-ethoxyphenol with formaldehyde and *p*-nitrosodimethylaniline in the presence of aluminum and water.

Description—Fine, white or slightly yellowish crystals; odor and taste similar to vanillin; affected by light; solutions are acid to litmus; melts about 77°.

Solubility—1 g in about 100 mL water at 50°; freely soluble in alcohol, chloroform, ether or solutions of fixed alkali hydroxides.

Uses—A *flavor*, like vanillin, but stronger.

Eucalyptus Oil

The volatile oil distilled with steam from the fresh leaf of *Eucalyptus globulus* Labillardière or of some other species of *Eucalyptus* L'Heritier (Fam *Myrtaceae*). It contains not less than 70% of $C_{10}H_{18}O$ (eucalyptol).

Constituents—The most important constituent is *eucalyptol* (*cineol*). Other compounds include *d*-a-*pinene, globulol, pinocarveol, pinocarvone* and several aldehydes.

Description—Colorless or pale yellow liquid, having a characteristic, aromatic, somewhat camphoraceous odor, and a pungent, spicy, cooling taste; specific gravity 0.905 to 0.925 at 25°.

Solubility—Soluble in 5 volumes of 70% alcohol.

Uses—A *flavoring agent* and an *expectorant* in chronic bronchitis. It also has *bacteriostatic* properties. This oil may be toxic.

Fennel Oil

The volatile oil distilled with steam from the dried ripe fruit of *Foeniculum vulgare* Miller (Fam *Umbelliferae*).

Note—If solid material has separated, carefully warm the oil until it is completely liquefied, and mix it before using.

Constituents—*Anethole* [$C_{10}H_{12}O$] is the chief constituent, occurring to the extent of 50 to 60%. Some of the other constituents are *d*-pinene, phellandrene, dipentene, fenchone, methylchavicol, anisaldehyde and anisic acid.

Description—Colorless or pale yellow liquid, having the characteristic odor and taste of fennel; specific gravity 0.953 to 0.973; congealing temperature is not below 3°.

Solubility—Soluble in 8 volumes of 80% alcohol or in 1 volume of 90% alcohol.

Uses—A flavoring agent. It formerly was employed in a dose of 0.1 mL as a *carminative*.

Glycyrrhiza

Licorice Root; Liquorice Root; Sweetwood; Italian Juice Root; Spanish Juice Root

The dried rhizome and roots of *Glycyrrhiza glabra* Linné, known in commerce as Spanish Licorice, or of *Glycyrrhiza glabra* Linné var *glandulifera* Waldstein et Kitaibel, known in commerce as Russian Licorice, or of other varieties of *Glycyrrhiza glabra* Linné, yielding a yellow and sweet wood (Fam. *Leguminosae*).

Constituents—This well-known root contains 5 to 7% of the sweet principle *glycyrrhizin*, or *glycyrrhizic acid* which is 50 times as sweet as cane sugar. There also is present an oleoresinous substance to which its slight acridity is due. If alcohol or an alkali is used as a menstruum for the root and the preparation not treated to deprive it of acridity, it will have a disagreeable aftertaste. For this reason boiling water is used for its extraction in both the extract and the fluidextract.

Description—The USP/NF provides descriptions of *Unground Spanish and Russian Glycyrrhizas, Histology* and *Powdered Glycyrrhiza*.

Uses—Valuable in pharmacy chiefly for its *sweet flavor*. It is one of the most efficient substances known for masking the taste of bitter substances, like quinine. Acids precipitate the glycyrrhizin and should not be added to mixtures in which glycyrrhiza is intended to mask disagreeable taste. Most of the imported licorice is used by tobacco manufacturers to flavor tobacco. It also is used in making candy.

Pure Glycyrrhiza Extract [Pure Licorice Root Extract]—*Preparation:* Moisten 1000 g of glycyrrhiza, in granular powder, with boiling water, transfer it to a percolator, and percolate with boiling water until the glycyrrhiza is exhausted. Add enough diluted ammonia solution to the percolate to impart a distinctly ammoniacal odor, then boil the liquid under normal atmospheric pressure until it is reduced to a volume of about 1500 mL. Filter the liquid, and immediately evaporate the filtrate until the residue has a pilular consistency. Pure extract of glycyrrhiza differs from the commercial extract in that it is almost completely soluble in aqueous mixtures. The large amount of filler used in the commercial extract to give it firmness renders it unfit to use as a substitute for the pure extract. *Description:* Black, pilular mass having a characteristic, sweet taste. *Uses:* A *flavoring agent*. One of the ingredients in *Aromatic Cascara Sagrada Fluidextract*.

Glycyrrhiza Fluidextract [Licorice Root Fluidextract; Liquid Extract of Liquorice]—*Preparation:* To 1000 g of coarsely ground glycyrrhiza add about 3000 mL of boiling water, mix and allow to macerate in a suitable, covered percolator for 2 hr. Then allow the percolation to proceed at a rate of 1 to 3 mL/min, gradually adding boiling water until the glycyrrhiza is exhausted. Add enough diluted ammonia solution to the percolate to impart a distinctly ammoniacal odor, then boil the liquid actively under normal atmospheric pressure until it is reduced to a volume of about 1500 mL. Filter the liquid, evaporate the filtrate on a steam bath until the residue measures 750 mL, cool, gradually add 250 mL of alcohol and enough water to make the product measure 1000 mL and mix. *Alcohol Content:* 20 to 24%, by volume. *Uses:* A pleasant *flavor* for use in syrups and elixirs to be employed as vehicles and correctives.

Glycyrrhiza Elixir—page 1394.

Glycyrrhiza Syrup—page 1393.

Honey—page 1416.

Hydriodic Acid Syrup—page 1393.

Iso-Alcoholic Elixir—page 1416.

Lavender Oil

Lavender Flowers Oil

The volatile oil distilled with steam from the fresh flowering tops of *Lavandula officinalis* Chaix ex Villars (*Lavandula vera* DeCandolle) (Fam *Labiatae*) or produced synthetically. It contains not less than 35% of esters calculated as $C_{12}H_{20}O_2$ (linalyl acetate).

Constituents—It is a product of considerable importance in perfumery. *Linalyl acetate* is the chief constituent. *Cineol* appears to be a normal constituent of English oils. Other constituents include *amyl alcohol*, *d-borneol* (small amount); *geraniol, lavandulol* ($C_{10}H_{18}O$); *linaloöl; nerol; acetic, butyric, valeric,* and *caproic acids* (as esters); traces of *d-pinene, limonene* (in English oils only) and the sesquiterpene *caryophyllene; ethyl n-amyl ketone;* an aldehyde (probably *valeric aldehyde*) and *coumarin*.

Description—Colorless or yellow liquid, having the characteristic odor and taste of lavender flowers; specific gravity 0.875 to 0.888.

Solubility—1 volume in 4 volumes of 70% alcohol.

Uses—Primarily as a *perfume*. It formerly was used in doses of 0.1 mL as a *carminative*.

Lemon Oil

The volatile oil obtained by expression, without the aid of heat, from the fresh peel of the fruit of *Citrus limon* (Linné) Burmann filius (Fam *Rutaceae*), with or without the previous separation of the pulp and the peel. The total aldehyde content, calculated as citral ($C_{10}H_{16}O$), is 2.2–3.8% for California-type oil, and 3.0–5.5% for Italian-type oil.

Note—Do not use oil that has a terebinthine odor.

Constituents—From the standpoint of odor and flavor, the most noteworthy constituent is the aldehyde *citral*, which is present to the extent of about 4%. About 90% of *d-limonene* is present; small amounts of *l*-α-*pinene*, β-*pinene, camphene*, β-*phellandrene* and γ-terpinene also occur. About 2% of a solid, nonvolatile substance called *citroptene, limettin* or *lemon-camphor*, which is dissolved out of the peel, also is present. In addition, there are traces of several other compounds: α-*terpineol;* the *acetates of linaloöl* and *geraniol; citronellal, octyl* and *nonyl aldehydes;* the sesquiterpenes *bisabolene* and *cadinene* and the ketone *methylheptenone*.

When fresh, the oil has the fragrant odor of lemons. Because of the instability of the terpenes present, the oil readily undergoes deterioration by oxidation, acquiring a terebinthinate odor.

Description—Pale yellow to deep yellow or greenish yellow liquid, with the characteristic odor and taste of the outer part of fresh lemon peel; specific gravity 0.849 to 0.855.

Solubility—In 3 volumes of alcohol; miscible in all proportions with dehydrated alcohol, carbon disulfide or glacial acetic acid.

Uses—A *flavor* in pharmaceutical preparations and in certain candies and foods.

Methyl Salicylate

Benzoic acid, 2-hydroxy-, methyl ester; Gaultheria Oil; Wintergreen Oil; Betula Oil; Sweet Birch Oil; Teaberry Oil; Artificial Wintergreen Oil; Synthetic Wintergreen Oil

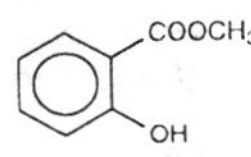

Methyl salicylate [119-36-8] $C_6H_4(OH)COOCH_3$ (152.15); produced synthetically or obtained by maceration and subsequent distillation with

steam from the leaves of *Gaultheria procumbens* Linné (Fam *Ericaceae*) or from the bark of *Betula lenta* Linné (Fam *Betulaceae*).

Note—It must be labeled to indicate whether it was made synthetically or distilled from either of the plants mentioned above.

Preparation—Found naturally in gaultheria and betula oils and in many other plants but the commercial product is usually synthetic, made by esterifying salicylic acid with methyl alcohol in the presence of sulfuric acid and distilling.

Description—Colorless, yellowish or reddish liquid, having the characteristic odor and taste of wintergreen; specific gravity (synthetic), 1.180 to 1.185, (from gaultheria or betula), 1.176 to 1.182; boils between 219 and 224° with some decomposition.

Solubility—Slightly soluble in water; soluble in alcohol or glacial acetic acid.

Uses—A pharmaceutical necessity and *counterirritant* (local analgesic). As a pharmaceutical necessity, it is used to flavor the official *Aromatic Cascara Sagrada Fluidextract*, and it is equal in every respect to wintergreen oil or sweet birch oil. As a counterirritant, it is applied to the skin in the form of a liniment, ointment or cream; care should be exercised since salicylate is absorbed through the skin.

Caution—Because it smells like wintergreen candy, it is ingested frequently by children and has caused many fatalities. *Keep out of the reach of children.*

Dose—*Topical*, in lotions and solutions in **10** to **25%** concentration.

Monosodium Glutamate

Glutamic acid, monosodium salt, monohydrate

[142-47-2] $C_5H_8NNaO_4 \cdot H_2O$ (187.13)

Preparation—From the fermentation of beet sugar or molasses or by hydrolysis of vegetable proteins.

Description—White, crystalline powder. The pentahydrate effloresces in air to form the monohydrate.

Solubility—Very soluble in water; sparingly soluble in alcohol.

Uses—Flavoring agent and perfume.

Nutmeg Oil

Myristica Oil NF XIII; East Indian Nutmeg Oil; West Indian Nutmeg Oil

The volatile oil distilled with steam from the dried kernels of the ripe seeds of *Myristica fragrans* Houttuyn (Fam *Myristicaceae*).

Constituents—It contains about 80% of *d-pinene* and *d-camphene*, 8% of *dipentene*, about 6% of the alcohols *d-borneol*, *geraniol*, *d-linaloöl* and *terpineol*, 4% of *myristicin*, 0.6% of *safrol*, 0.3% of *myristic acid* free and as esters, 0.2% of *eugenol* and *isoeugenol* and traces of the alcohol *terpineol-4*, a citral-like aldehyde and several acids, all present as esters.

Description—Colorless or pale yellow liquid having the characteristic odor and taste of nutmeg; specific gravity (East Indian Oil) 0.880 to 0.910, (West Indian Oil) 0.854 to 0.880.

Solubility—In an equal amount of alcohol; 1 volume of East Indian Oil in 3 volumes of 90% alcohol; 1 volume of West Indian Oil in 4 volumes of 90% alcohol.

Uses—Primarily as a *flavoring agent*. It is used for this purpose in *Aromatic Ammonia Spirit* (page 873). The oil also is employed as a *flavor* in foods, certain alcoholic beverages, dentifrices and tobacco; to some extent, it also is used in perfumery. It *formerly* was used as a *carminative* and *local stimulant* to the gastrointestinal tract in a dose of 0.03 mL. In overdoses, it acts as a narcotic poison. *This oil is very difficult to keep and even if slightly terebinthinate is unfit for flavoring purposes.*

Orange Oil

Sweet Orange Oil

The volatile oil obtained by expression from the fresh peel of the ripe fruit of *Citrus sinensis* (Linné) Osbeck (Fam *Rutaceae*). The total aldehyde content, calculated as decanal ($C_{10}H_{20}O$), is 1.2 to 2.5%.

Note—Do not use oil that has a terebinthine odor.

Constituents—Consists of *d-limonene* to the extent of at least 90%; in the remaining 5 to 10% are the odorous constituents, among which, in samples of American origin, are *n-decylic aldehyde*, *citral*, *d-linaloöl*, *n-nonyl alcohol* and traces of *esters* of *formic*, *acetic*, *caprylic* and *capric* acids.

In addition to most of these compounds, Italian-produced oil contains *d-terpineol*, *terpinolene*, *α-terpinene* and *methyl anthranilate*.

Kept under the usual conditions it is very prone to decompose, and rapidly acquires a terebinthine odor.

Description—Intensely yellow orange or deep orange liquid, which possesses the characteristic odor and taste of the outer part of fresh sweet orange peel; specific gravity 0.842 to 0.846.

Solubility—Miscible with dehydrated alcohol or carbon disulfide; dissolves in an equal volume of glacial acetic acid.

Uses—A *flavoring agent* in elixirs and other preparations.

Orange Flower Oil—see RPS-18, page 1296.

Orange Flower Water—page 1392.

Sweet Orange Peel Tincture

Preparation—From sweet orange peel, which is the outer rind of the nonartificially colored, fresh, ripe fruit of *Citrus sinensis* (Linné) Osbeck (Fam *Rutaceae*), by Process M (page 1522). Macerate 500 g of the sweet orange peel (*Note—Exclude the inner, white portion of the rind*) in 900 mL of alcohol, and complete the preparation with alcohol to make the product measure 1000 mL. Use talc as the filtering medium.

The white portion of the rind must not be used, as the proportion of oil, which is only in the yellow rind, is reduced, and the bitter principle *hesperidin* is introduced.

Alcohol Content—62 to 72%.

Uses—A *flavor*, used in syrups, elixirs and emulsions. This tincture was introduced to provide a delicate orange flavor direct from the fruit instead of depending upon orange oil which so frequently is terebinthinate and unfit for use. The tincture keeps well.

Compound Orange Spirit

Contains, in each 100 mL, 25 to 30 mL of the mixed oils.

Orange Oil	**200 mL**
Lemon Oil	**50 mL**
Coriander Oil	**20 mL**
Anise Oil	**5 mL**
Alcohol, a sufficient quantity,	
To make	**1000 mL**

Mix the oils with sufficient alcohol to make the product measure 1000 mL.

Alcohol Content—65 to 75%.

Uses—A *flavor* for elixirs. An alcoholic solution of this kind permits the uniform introduction of small proportions of oils and also preserves orange and lemon oils from rapid oxidation. These two oils should be bought in small quantities by the pharmacist, since the spirit is made most satisfactorily from oils taken from bottles not previously opened. This will insure that delicacy of flavor which should always be characteristic of elixirs.

Orange Syrup

Syrup of Orange Peel

Contains, in each 100 mL, 450 to 550 mg of citric acid ($C_6H_8O_7$).

Sweet Orange Peel Tincture	**50 mL**
Citric Acid (anhydrous)	**5 g**
Talc	**15 g**
Sucrose	**820 g**
Purified Water, a sufficient quantity,	
To make	**1000 mL**

Triturate the talc with the tincture and citric acid, and gradually add 400 mL of purified water. Then filter, returning the first portions of the filtrate until it becomes clear, and wash the mortar and filter with enough purified water to make the filtrate measure 450 mL. Dissolve the sucrose in this filtrate by agitation, without heating, and add enough purified water to make the product measure 1000 mL. Mix and strain.

Note—*Do not use syrup that has a terebinthine odor or taste or shows other indications of deterioration.*

Alcohol Content—2 to 5%.

Uses—A pleasant, acidic vehicle.

Peppermint

American Mint; Lamb Mint; Brandy Mint

Consists of the dried leaf and flowering top of *Mentha piperita* Linné (Fam *Labiatae*).

Uses—The source of green color for *Peppermint Spirit* (page 902). The odor of fresh peppermint is due to the presence of about 2% of a volatile oil, much of which is lost on drying the leaves in air. It is cultivated widely both in the US and France. It formerly was used as a carminative.

Peppermint Oil—The volatile oil distilled with steam from the fresh overground parts of the flowering plant of *Mentha piperita* Linné (Fam *Labiatae*), rectified by distillation and neither partially nor wholly dementholized. It yields not less than 5% of esters, calculated as menthyl acetate [$C_{12}H_{22}O_2$], and not less than 50% of total menthol [$C_{10}H_{20}O$], free and as esters. *Constituents:* This is one of the most important of the group of volatile oils. The chief constituent is *Menthol* (page 875) which occurs in the levorotatory form; its ester, *menthyl acetate*, is present in a much smaller amount. Other compounds which are present include the ketone *menthone, piperitone, α-pinene, l-limonene, phellandrene, cadinene, menthyl isovalerate, isovaleric aldehyde, acetaldehyde, menthofuran, cineol*, an unidentified *lactone* [$C_{10}H_{16}O_2$] and probably *amyl acetate*.

Description and Solubility—Colorless or pale yellow liquid, having a strong, penetrating odor of peppermint and a pungent taste, followed by a sensation of cold when air is drawn into the mouth; specific gravity 0.896 to 0.908. 1 volume dissolves in 3 volumes of 70% alcohol. *Uses:* A *flavoring agent, carminative, antiseptic* and *local anesthetic*. It also is used extensively as a *flavor* in candy, chewing gum, etc.

Peppermint Spirit—page 902.

Peppermint Water—page 1392.

Phenylethyl Alcohol

Benzeneethanol; 2-Phenylethanol

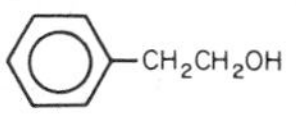

C_6H_5–CH_2CH_2OH

Phenethyl alcohol [60-12-8] $C_8H_{10}O$ (122.17); occurs in a number of essential oils such as those of rose, neroli, hyacinth, carnation and others.

Description—Colorless liquid with a rose-like odor and a sharp, burning taste; solidifies at −27°; specific gravity 1.017 to 1.020.

Solubility—1 g in 60 mL water or < 1 mL alcohol, chloroform or ether; very soluble in fixed oils, glycerin or propylene glycol; slightly soluble in mineral oil.

Uses—Introduced for use as an antibacterial agent in ophthalmic solutions, but it is of limited effectiveness.

It is used in *flavors*, as a *soap perfume* and in the preparation of synthetic oils of rose and similar flower oils. It is also a valuable perfume fixative.

Pine Needle Oil—see RPS-18, page 1297.

Raspberry Syrup—see RPS-18, page 1302.

Rose Oil

Otto of Rose; Attar of Rose

The volatile oil distilled with steam from the fresh flowers of *Rosa gallica* Linné, *Rosa damascena* Miller, *Rosa alba* Linné, *Rosa centifolia* Linné and varieties of these species (Fam *Rosaceae*).

Constituents—From the quantitative standpoint the chief components are the alcohols *geraniol* [$C_{10}H_{18}O$] and *l-citronellol* [$C_{10}H_{20}O$]. The sesquiterpene alcohols *farnesol* and *nerol* occur to the extent of 1% and 5 to 10%, respectively. Together, the four alcohols constitute 70 to 75% of the oil. *Phenylethyl alcohol*, which comprises 1% of the oil, is an important odoriferous constituent. Other compounds present are *linaloöl, eugenol, nonyl aldehyde*, traces of *citral* and two solid hydrocarbons of the paraffin series.

Description and Solubility—A colorless or yellow liquid, which has the characteristic odor and taste of rose; at 25°, a viscous liquid; on gradual cooling it changes to a translucent, crystalline mass, which may be liquefied easily by warming; specific gravity 0.848 to 0.863 at 30° compared with water at 15°; 1 mL mixes with 1 mL of chloroform without turbidity; on the addition of 20 mL of 90% alcohol to this solution, the resulting liquid is neutral or acid to moistened litmus paper and deposits a crystalline residue within 5 min on standing at 20°.

Uses—Principally as a *perfume*. It is recognized officially for its use as an ingredient in *Rose Water Ointment* and cosmetics.

Stronger Rose Water

Triple Rose Water

A saturated solution of the odoriferous principles of the flowers of *Rosa centifolia* Linné (Fam *Rosaceae*), prepared by distilling the fresh flowers with water and separating the excess volatile oil from the clear, water portion of the distillate.

Note—When diluted with an equal volume of purified water, it may be supplied when *Rose Water* is required.

Description—Nearly colorless and clear liquid which possesses the pleasant odor and taste of fresh rose blossoms; must be free from empyreuma, mustiness and fungal growths.

Uses—An ingredient in *Rose Water Ointment*. It sometimes is prepared extemporaneously from concentrates or from rose oil, but such water is not official and rarely compares favorably with the fresh distillate from rose petals.

Saccharin

1,2-Benzisothiazol-3(2*H*)-one, 1,1-dioxide; Gluside; *o*-Benzosulfimide (*Boots; Reisman*) (*Various Mfrs*)

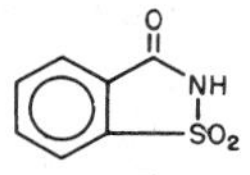

1,2-Benzisothiazolin-3-one 1,1-dioxide [81-07-2] $C_7H_5NO_3S$ (183.18).

Preparation—Toluene is reacted with chlorosulfonic acid to form *o*-toluenesulfonyl chloride, which is converted to the sulfonamide with ammonia. The methyl group then is oxidized with dichromate yielding *o*-sulfamoylbenzoic acid which, when heated, forms the cyclic imide.

Description—White crystals or a white crystalline powder; odorless or has a faint aromatic odor; in dilute solution it is intensely sweet; solutions are acid to litmus; melts between 226 and 230°.

Solubility—1 g in 290 mL water, 31 mL alcohol or 25 mL boiling water; slightly soluble in chloroform or ether; readily dissolved by dilute solution of ammonia, solutions of alkali hydroxides or solutions of alkali carbonates with the evolution of CO_2.

Uses—A sweetening agent in *Aromatic Cascara Sagrada Fluidextract* and highly alcoholic preparations. It is an intensely sweet substance. A 60-mg portion is equivalent in sweetening power to approximately 30 g of sucrose. It is used as a *sweetening agent* in vehicles, canned foods, beverages and in diets for diabetics to replace the sucrose. The relative sweetening power of saccharin is increased by dilution.

Saccharin Calcium

1,2-Benzisothiazol-3(2*H*)-one, 1,1-dioxide, calcium salt, hydrate (2:7) Calcium *o*-Benzosulfimide

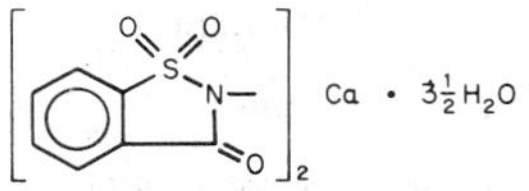

Ca · $3\frac{1}{2}H_2O$

1,2-Benzisothiazolin-3-one 1,1-dioxide calcium salt hydrate (2:7) [6381-91-5] $C_{14}H_8CaN_2O_6S_2.3\frac{1}{2}H_2O$ (467.48); *anhydrous* [6485-34-3] (404.43).

Preparation—Saccharin is reacted with a semimolar quantity of calcium hydroxide in aqueous medium and the resulting solution is concentrated to crystallization.

Description—White crystals or a white, crystalline powder; odorless or has a faint aromatic odor; and an intensely sweet taste even in dilute solutions; in dilute solution it is about 300 times as sweet as sucrose.

Solubility—1 g in 2.6 mL water or 4.7 mL alcohol.

Uses and Dose—See *Saccharin*.

Saccharin Sodium

1,2-Benzisothiazol-3(2*H*)-one, 1,1-dioxide, sodium salt, dihydrate; Soluble Saccharin; Soluble Gluside; Sodium o-Benzosulfimide

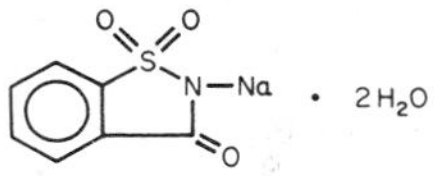

· $2H_2O$

1,2-Benzisothiazolin-3-one 1,1-dioxide sodium salt dihydrate [6155-57-3] $C_7H_4NNaO_3S.2H_2O$ (241.19); *anhydrous* [128-44-9] (205.16).

Preparation—Saccharin is dissolved in an equimolar quantity of aqueous sodium hydroxide and the solution is concentrated to crystallization.

Description—White crystals or a white crystalline powder; odorless or has a faint aromatic odor and an intensely sweet taste even in dilute solutions; in dilute solution it is about 300 times as sweet as sucrose; when in powdered form it usually contains about ⅓ the theoretical amount of water of hydration due to efflorescence.

Solubility—1 g in 1.5 mL water or 50 mL alcohol.

Uses—Same as *Saccharin* but has the advantage of being more soluble in neutral aqueous solutions.

Application—**15** to **60 mg** as necessary.

Dosage Form—Tablets: 15, 30 and 60 mg.

Sarsaparilla Syrup, Compound—see RPS-13, page 445.

Sherry Wine—see page RPS-15, page 1240.

Sorbitol

Sionin; Sorbit; D-Sorbitol; D-Glucitol Sorbo (*EM Labs*)

```
    H  OH H  OH OH H
    |  |  |  |  |  |
HO—C—C—C—C—C—C—OH
    |  |  |  |  |  |
    H  H  OH H  H  H
```

D-Glucitol [50-70-4] $C_6H_{14}O_6$ (182.17); it may contain small amounts of other polyhydric alcohols.

Preparation—Commercially by reduction (hydrogenation) of certain sugars, such as glucose.

Description—White, hygroscopic powder, granules or flakes, having a sweet taste; the usual form melts about 96°.

Solubility—1 g in about 0.45 mL of water; slightly soluble in alcohol, methanol or acetic acid.

Uses—An *osmotic diuretic* given intravenously in 50% (*w/v*) solution to diminish edema, lower cerebrospinal pressure or reduce intraocular pressure in glaucoma. It also is used as a laxative, sweetener, humectant, plasticizer and, in 70% (*w/w*) solution, as a vehicle.

Dose—**50** to **100 mL** of a **50%** solution; *laxative, oral*, **30** to **50 g**.

Sorbitol Solution is a water solution containing, in each 100 g, 69–71 g of total solids consisting essentially of D-sorbitol and a small amount of mannitol and other isomeric polyhydric alcohols. The content of D-sorbitol [$C_6H_8(OH)_6$] in each 100 g is not less than 64 g. *Description:* Clear, colorless, syrupy liquid, having a sweet taste and no characteristic odor; neutral to litmus; specific gravity not less than 1.285; refractive index at 20° 1.455 to 1.465. *Uses:* It is not to be injected. It has been used as a replacement for propylene glycol and glycerin.

Spearmint

Spearmint Leaves; Spearmint Herb; Mint

The dried leaf and flowering top of *Mentha spicata* Linné (*Mentha viridis* Linné) (Common Spearmint) or of *Mentha cardiaca* Gerard ex Baker (Scotch Spearmint) (Fam *Labiatae*).

Fresh spearmint is used in preparing mint sauce and also the well-known mint julep. The volatile oil is the only constituent of importance in this plant; the yield is from ½ to 1%.

Uses—A flavoring agent.

Spearmint Oil is the volatile oil distilled with steam from the fresh over-ground parts of the flowering plant of *Mentha spicata* or of *Mentha cardiaca;* contains not less than 55%, by volume, of $C_{10}H_{14}O$ (carvone = 150.22). The chief odoriferous constituent is the ketone *l-carvone.* American oil also contains *dihydrocarveol acetate* [$CH_3COOC_{10}H_{17}$], *l-limonene* [$C_{10}H_{16}$], a small amount of *phellandrene* [$C_{10}H_{16}$] and traces of *esters of valeric* and *caproic acids.*

Description and Solubility: Colorless, yellow or greenish yellow liquid, having the characteristic odor and taste of spearmint; specific gravity 0.917 to 0.934. Soluble in 1 volume of 80% alcohol, but upon further dilution may become turbid. *Uses:* Primarily as a flavoring agent. It also has been used as a *carminative* in doses of 0.1 mL.

Sucrose

α-D-Glucopyranoside, β-D-fructofuranosyl-, Sugar; Cane Sugar; Beet Sugar

Sucrose [57-50-1] $C_{12}H_{22}O_{11}$ (342.30); a sugar obtained from *Saccharum officinarum* Linné (Fam *Gramineae*), *Beta vulgaris* Linné (Fam *Chenopodiaceae*), and other sources. It contains no added substances.

For the structural formula, see page 384.

Preparation—Commercially from the sugar cane, beet root and sorghum. Originally, sugar cane was the only source, but at present the root of *Beta vulgaris* is used largely in Europe, and to an increasing degree in this country, for making sucrose.

The sugar cane is crushed and the juice amounting to about 80% is expressed with roller mills. The juice after "defecation" with lime and removal of excess of lime by carbonic acid gas, is run into vacuum pans for concentration and the saccharine juice is evaporated in this until it begins to crystallize. After the crystallization is complete, the warm mixture of crystals and syrup is run into centrifuges, in which the crystals of raw sugar are drained and dried. The syrup resulting as a by-product from raw sugar is known as *molasses.* Raw beet sugar is made by a similar process, but is more troublesome to purify than that made from sugar cane.

The refined sugar from either raw cane or beet sugar is prepared by dissolving the raw sugar in water, clarifying, filtering and, finally, decolorizing the solution by passing it through bone-black filters. The water-white solution finally is evaporated under reduced pressure to the crystallizing point and then forced to crystallize in small granules which are collected and drained in a centrifuge.

Description—Colorless or white crystals, crystalline masses or blocks, or a white, crystalline powder; odorless; sweet taste; stable in air; solutions neutral to litmus; melts with decomposition from 160 to 185°; specific gravity of about 1.57; specific rotation at 20° not less than +65.9°; unlike the other official sugars (dextrose, fructose and lactose), it does not reduce Fehling's solution even in hot solutions; also differs from these sugars in that it is darkened and charred by sulfuric acid in the cold; fermentable and, in dilute aqueous solutions, it ferments into alcohol and eventually acetic acid.

Sucrose is hydrolyzed by dilute mineral acids, slowly in the cold, and rapidly on heating into one molecule each of dextrose or levulose. This process is known technically as "inversion" and the product is referred to as "invert sugar"; the term inversion being derived from the change, through the hydrolysis, in the optical rotation from dextro of the sucrose to levo of the hydrolyzed product. The enzyme *invertase* also hydrolyzes sucrose.

Solubility—1 g in 0.5 mL water, 170 mL alcohol or in slightly more than 0.2 mL boiling water; insoluble in chloroform or ether.

Uses—Principally as a pharmaceutical necessity for making syrups and lozenges. It gives viscosity and consistency to fluids.

Intravenous administration of hypertonic solutions has been employed chiefly to initiate *osmotic diuresis.* Such a procedure is not completely safe and renal tubular damage may result, particularly in patients with existing renal pathology. Safer and more effective diuretics are available.

Sugar, Compressible—see RPS-18, page 1298.

Confectioner's Sugar

Sucrose ground together with corn starch to a fine powder; contains 95.0 to 97.0% of sucrose.

Description—Fine, white, odorless powder; sweet taste; stable in air; specific rotation not less than +62.6°.

Solubility—The sucrose portion is soluble in cold water; this is entirely soluble in boiling water.

Uses—A *pharmaceutic aid* as a *tableting excipient* and *sweetening agent.* See also *Sucrose.*

Syrup—page 1393.

Tolu Balsam

Tolu

A balsam obtained from *Myroxylon balsamum* (Linné) Harms (Fam *Leguminosae*).

Constituents—Up to 80% *resin*, about 7% *volatile oil*, 12 to 15% free *cinnamic acid*, 2 to 8% benzoic acid and 0.05% *vanillin.* The volatile oil is composed chiefly of *benzyl benzoate* and *benzyl cinnamate, ethyl benzoate, ethyl cinnamate*, a terpene called *tolene* (possibly identical with *phellandrene*) and the sesquiterpene alcohol *farnesol* also have been reported to be present.

Description—Brown or yellowish brown, plastic solid; transparent in thin layers and brittle when old, dried or exposed to cold temperatures; pleasant, aromatic odor resembling that of vanilla and a mild, aromatic taste.

Solubility—Nearly insoluble in water or solvent hexane; soluble in alcohol, chloroform or ether, sometimes with slight residue or turbidity.

Uses—A *vehicle, flavoring agent* and stimulating *expectorant* as a syrup. It is also an ingredient of *Compound Benzoin Tincture* (page 869).

Tolu Balsam Syrup [Syrup of Tolu; Tolu Syrup]—*Preparation:* Add tolu balsam tincture (50 mL, all at once) to magnesium carbonate (10 g) and sucrose (60 g) in a mortar, and mix intimately. Gradually add purified water (430 mL) with trituration, and filter. Dissolve the remainder of sucrose (760 g) in the clear filtrate with gentle heating, strain the syrup while warm and add purified water (qs) through the strainer to make the product measure 1000 mL. Mix thoroughly. *Note:* May be made also in the following manner: Place the remaining sucrose (760 g) in a suitable percolator, the neck of which nearly is filled with loosely packed cotton, moistened after packing with a few drops of water. Pour the filtrate, obtained as directed in the formula above, upon the sucrose, and regulate the outflow to a steady drip of percolate. When all of the liquid has run through, return portions of the percolate, if necessary, to dissolve all of the sucrose. Then pass enough purified water through the cotton to make the product measure 1000 mL. Mix thoroughly. *Alcohol Content:* 3 to 5%. *Uses:* Chiefly for its agreeable *flavor* in cough syrups. *Dose:* 10 mL.

Tolu Balsam Tincture [Tolu Tincture]—*Preparation:* With tolu balsam (200 g), prepare a tincture by Process M (page 1522), using alcohol as the menstruum. *Alcohol Content:* 77 to 83%. *Uses:* A balsamic preparation employed as an addition to expectorant mixtures; also used in the preparation of *Tolu Balsam Syrup*. *Dose:* 2 mL.

Vanilla

Vanilla Bean

The cured, full-grown, unripe fruit of *Vanilla planifolia* Andrews, often known in commerce as Mexican or Bourbon Vanilla, or of *Vanilla tahitensis* J W Moore, known in commerce as Tahiti Vanilla (Fam *Orchidaceae*); yields not less than 12% of anhydrous extractive soluble in diluted alcohol.

Constituents—Contains a trace of a volatile oil, fixed oil, 4% resin, sugar, *vanillic acid* and about 2.5% *vanillin* (see below). This highest grade of vanilla comes from Madagascar; considerable quantities of the drug also are produced in Mexico.

Uses—A flavor.

Note—Do not use if it has become brittle.

Vanilla Tincture [Extract of Vanilla]—*Preparation:* Add water (200 mL) to comminuted vanilla (cut into small pieces, 100 g) in a suitable covered container, and macerate during 12 hr, preferably in a warm place. Add alcohol (200 mL) to the mixture of vanilla and water, mix well and macerate about 3 days. Transfer the mixture to a percolator containing sucrose (in coarse granules, 200 g), and drain; then pack the drug firmly, and percolate slowly, using diluted alcohol (qs) as the menstruum. If the percolator is packed with an evenly distributed mixture of the comminuted vanilla, sucrose and clean, dry sand, the increased surface area permits more efficient percolation. This tincture is unusual in that it is the only official one in which sucrose is specified as an ingredient. *Alcohol Content:* 38 to 42%. *Uses:* A *flavoring agent*. *See Flavors*, page 1384.

Vanillin

Benzaldehyde, 4-hydroxy-3-methoxy-

4-Hydroxy-3-methoxybenzaldehyde [121-33-5] $C_8H_8O_3$ (152.15).

Preparation—From vanilla, which contains 2 to 3%. It also is found in many other substances, including tissues of certain plants, crude beet sugar, asparagus and even asafetida. Commercially, it is made synthetically. While chemically identical with the product obtained from the "vanilla bean," "flavoring preparations" made from it never equal in flavor the preparation in which vanilla alone is used because vanilla contains other odorous products. It is synthesized by oxidation processes from either coniferin or eugenol, by treating guaiacol with chloroform in the presence of an alkali, and by other methods.

Description—Fine, white to slightly yellow crystals, usually needle-like having an odor and taste suggestive of vanilla; affected by light; solutions are acid to litmus; melts 81 to 83°.

Solubility—1 g in about 100 mL water, about 20 mL glycerin or 20 mL water at 80°; freely soluble in alcohol, chloroform, ether or solutions of the fixed alkali hydroxides.

Incompatibilities—Combines with *glycerin*, forming a compound which is almost insoluble in alcohol. It is decomposed by *alkalies* and is oxidized slowly by the *air*.

Uses—Only as a *flavor*. Solutions of it sometimes are sold as a synthetic substitute for vanilla for flavoring foods but it is inferior in flavor to the real vanilla extract.

Water—page 1392.

Water Purified—page 1392.

Wild Cherry Syrup—page 1393.

Other Flavoring Agents

Anise NF IX [Anise Seed; European Aniseed; Sweet Cumin]—The dried ripe fruit of *Pimpinella anisum* Linné. It contains about 1.75% of volatile oil. *Uses:* A flavor and carminative.

Ceylon Cinnamon—The dried inner bark of the shoots of coppiced trees of *Cinnamomum zeylanicum* Nees (Fam *Lauraceae*); contains, in each 100 g, not less than 0.5 mL volatile oil. *Uses:* A *carminative* and *flavor*.

Clove—The dried flower-bud of *Eugenia caryophyllus* (Sprengel) Bullock et Harrison (Fam *Myrtaceae*). It contains, in each 100 g, not less than 16 mL of clove oil. *Uses:* An *aromatic* in doses of 0.25 g and as a condiment in foods.

Coriander—The dried ripe fruit of *Coriandrum sativum* Linné (Fam *Umbelliferae*); yields not less than 0.25 mL volatile coriander oil/100 g. *Uses:* Seldom used alone, but sometimes is combined with other agents, chiefly as a *flavor*. It also is used as a condiment and flavor in cooking.

Eucalyptol [Cineol; Cajeputol; $C_{10}H_{18}O$ (154.25)]— Obtained from eucalyptus oil and from other sources. Colorless liquid, having a characteristic, aromatic, distinctly camphoraceous odor and a pungent, cooling, spicy taste. 1 volume is soluble in 5 volumes of 60% alcohol; miscible with alcohol, chloroform, ether, glacial acetic acid or fixed or volatile oils; insoluble in water. *Uses:* Primarily as a *flavoring agent*. Locally it is employed for its *antiseptic* effect in inflammations of the nose and throat and in certain skin diseases. It sometimes is used by inhalation in bronchitis.

Fennel [Fennel Seed]—The dried ripe fruit of cultivated varieties of *Foeniculum vulgare* Miller (Fam *Umbelliferae*); contains 4 to 6% of an oxygenated volatile oil and 10% of a fixed oil. *Uses:* A *flavor* and *carminative*.

Ginger NF [Zingiber]—The dried rhizome of *Zingiber officinale* Roscoe (Fam *Zingiberaceae*), known in commerce as Jamaica Ginger, African Ginger and Cochin Ginger. The outer cortical layers often are removed either partially or completely. *Constituents:* A pungent substance, *gingerol;* volatile oil (Jamaica Ginger, about 1%; African Ginger, 2 to 3%), containing the terpenes *d-camphene* and *β-phellandrene* and the sesquiterpene *zingiberene; citral cineol* and *borneol*. *Uses:* A *flavoring agent*. It formerly was employed in a dose of 600 mg as an intestinal stimulant and carminative in colic and in diarrhea.

Ginger Oleoresin—Yields 18 to 35 mL of volatile ginger oil/100 g of oleoresin. *Preparation:* Extract the oleoresin from ginger, in moderately coarse powder, by percolation, using either acetone, alcohol or ether as the menstruum.

Glycyrrhiza Extract [Licorice Root Extract; Licorice]—An extract prepared from the rhizome and roots of species of *Glycyrrhiza* Tournefort ex Linné (Fam *Leguminosae*). *Description:* Brown powder or in flattened, cylindrical rolls or in masses; the rolls or masses have a glossy black color externally, and a brittle, sharp, smooth, conchoidal fracture; the extract has a characteristic and sweet taste which is not more than very slightly acrid. *Uses:* A *flavoring agent*.

Lavender [Lavendula]—The flowers of *Lavandula spica* (*Lavandula officinalis* or *Lavandula vera*); contains a volatile oil with the principal constituent *l*-linalyl acetate. *Uses:* A *perfume*.

Lemon Peel USP XV, BP [Fresh Lemon Peel]—The outer yellow rind of the fresh ripe fruit of *Citrus limon* (Linné) Burmann filius (Fam *Rutaceae*); contains a volatile oil and hesperidin. *Uses:* A *flavor*.

Lemon Tincture USP XVIII [Lemon Peel Tincture]—*Preparation:* From lemon peel, which is the outer yellow rind of the fresh, ripe fruit of *Citrus limon* (Linné) Burmann filius (Fam *Rutaceae*), by *Process M* (page 1522), 500 g of the peel being macerated in 900 mL alcohol and the preparation being completed with alcohol to make the product measure 1000 mL. Use talc as the filtering medium. The white portion of the rind must not be used, as the proportion of oil, which is found only in the yellow rind, is reduced and the bitter principle, hesperidin, introduced. *Alcohol Content:* 62 to 72%. *Uses:* A flavor, its fineness of flavor being assured as it comes from the fresh fruit, and being an alcoholic solution it is more stable than the oil.

Myrcia Oil [Bay Oil; Oil of Bay]—The volatile oil distilled from leaves of *Pimenta racemosa* (Miller) J W Moore (Fam *Myrtaceae*); contains the phenolic compounds eugenol and chavicol. *Uses:* In the preparation of bay rum as a *perfume*.

Orange Oil, Bitter—The volatile oil obtained by expression from the fresh peel of the fruit of *Citrus aurantium* Linné (Fam *Rutaceae*); contains primarily *d*-limonene. Pale yellow liquid with a characteristic; aromatic odor of the Seville orange; if it has a terebinthinate odor, it should not be dispensed; refractive index 1.4725 to 1.4755 at 20°. It differs little from *Orange Oil* (page 1388) except for the botanical source. Miscible with anhydrous alcohol and with about 4 volumes alcohol. *Uses:* A *flavor*.

Orange Peel, Bitter [Bitter Orange; Curacao Orange Peel; Bigarade Orange]—The dried rind of the unripe but fully grown fruit of *Citrus aurantium* Linné (Fam *Rutaceae*). *Constituents:* The inner part of the peel from the bitter orange contains a volatile oil and the glycoside *hesperidin* ($C_{28}H_{34}O_{15}$). This, upon hydrolysis in the presence of H_2SO_4, yields *hesperetin* ($C_{16}H_{14}O_6$), *rhamnose* ($C_6H_{12}O_5$), and D-glucose ($C_6H_{12}O_6$). *Uses:* A *flavoring agent*. It has been used as a bitter.

Orange Peel, Sweet USP XV—The fresh, outer rind of the non-artificially colored, ripe fruit of *Citrus sinensis* (Linné) Osbeck (Fam *Rutaceae*); the white, inner portion of the rind is to be excluded. Contains a volatile oil but no hesperidin, since the glycoside occurs in the white portion of the rind. *Uses:* A *flavor*.

Orris [Orris Root; Iris; Florentine Orris]—The peeled and dried rhizome of *Iris germanica* Linné, including its variety *florentina* Dykes (*Iris florentina* Linné), or of *Iris pallida* Lamarck (Fam *Iridaceae*); contains about 0.1 to 0.2% of a volatile oil (orris butter), myristic acid and the ketone irone; irone provides the fragrant odor of orris. *Uses:* A *perfume*.

Pimenta Oil [Pimento Oil; Allspice Oil]—The volatile oil distilled from the fruit of *Pimenta officinalis* Lindley (Fam *Myrtaceae*). *Uses:* A *carminative* and *stimulant* and also as a *condiment* in foods.

Rosemary Oil—The volatile oil distilled with steam from the fresh flowering tops of *Rosmarinus officinalis* Linné (Fam *Labiatae*); yields not less than 1.5% of esters calculated as bornyl acetate ($C_{12}H_{20}O_2$), and not less than 8% of total borneol ($C_{10}H_{18}O$), free and as esters. *Constituents:* The amount of esters, calculated as bornyl acetate, and of total borneol, respectively, varies somewhat with its geographic source. Cineol is present to the extent of about 19–25%, depending on the source. The terpenes *d-* and *l-α-pinene*, *dipentene* and *camphene*, and the ketone *camphor* also occur in this oil. *Description and Solubility:* Colorless or pale yellow liquid, having the characteristic odor of rosemary, and a warm, camphoraceous taste; specific gravity 0.894 to 0.912. Soluble in 1 volume of 90% alcohol, by volume, but upon further dilution may become turbid. *Uses:* A *flavor* and *perfume*, chiefly, in rubefacient liniments such as *Camphor and Soap Liniment*.

Sassafras—The dried bark of the root of *Sassafras albidum* (Nuttall) Nees (Fam *Lauraceae*). *Uses:* Principally because of its high content of volatile oil which serves to disguise the taste of disagreeable substances. An infusion (*sassafras tea*) formerly was used extensively as a home remedy, particularly in the southern states.

Sassafras Oil—The volatile oil distilled with steam from *Sassafras*. *Uses:* A *flavor* by confectioners, particularly in hard candies. Either the oil or safrol is used as a *preservative* in mucilage and library paste, being far superior to methyl salicylate for this purpose. Since the oil is *antiseptic*, it sometimes is employed in conjunction with other agents for local application in diseases of the nose and throat; safrol also is used in this way.

Wild Cherry [Wild Black Cherry Bark]—The carefully dried stem bark of *Prunus serotina* Ehrhart (Fam *Rosaceae*), free of borke and preferably having been collected in autumn. *Constituents:* A glucoside of *d-mandelonitrile* (C_6H_5.CHOH.CN) known as *prunasin* (page 387), the enzyme *emulsin*, tannin, a bitter principle, starch, resin, etc. In the BP and the English literature this drug has been termed "Virginian Prune"—a literal but incorrect translation of the older botanical name, *Prunus virginiana*. *Uses:* A *flavoring agent*, especially in cough preparations. It is an ingredient in *Wild Cherry Syrup*. As with bitter almond, contact with water, in the presence of emulsin, results in the production of benzaldehyde and HCN. All preparations of wild cherry should be made without heat in order to avoid destruction of the enzyme which is responsible for the production of the free active principles.

Diluting Agents

Diluting agents (vehicles or carriers) are indifferent substances which are used as solvents for active medicinals. They are of primary importance for diluting and flavoring drugs which are intended for oral administration, but a few such agents are designed specifically for diluting parenteral injections. The latter group is considered separately.

The expert selection of diluting agents has been an important factor in popularizing the "specialties" of manufacturing pharmacists. Since a large selection of diluting agents is available in a choice of colors and flavors, the prescriber has an opportunity to make his own prescriptions more acceptable to the patient. The best diluting agent is usually the best solvent for the drug. Water-soluble substances, for example, should be flavored and diluted with an aqueous agent and alcohol-soluble drugs with an alcoholic vehicle. Thus, the diluting agents presented herein are divided into three groups on the basis of their physical properties: aqueous, hydroalcoholic and alcoholic.

Aqueous Diluting Agents

Aqueous diluting agents include aromatic waters, syrups and mucilages. Aromatic waters are used as diluting agents for water-soluble substances and salts, but cannot mask the taste of very disagreeable drugs. Some of the more common flavored aqueous agents and the official forms of water are listed below.

Orange Flower Water

Stronger Orange Flower Water; Triple Orange Flower Water

A saturated solution of the odoriferous principles of the flowers of *Citrus aurantium* Linné (Fam. *Rutaceae*), prepared by distilling the fresh flowers with water and separating the excess volatile oil from the clear, water portion of the distillate.

Description—Should be nearly colorless, clear or only faintly opalescent; the odor should be that of the orange blossoms; it must be free from empyreuma, mustiness and fungoid growths.

Uses—A *vehicle flavor* and *perfume* in syrups, elixirs and solutions.

Peppermint Water

A clear, saturated solution of peppermint oil in purified water, prepared by one of the processes described under *Aromatic Waters* (page 1498).

Uses—A *carminative* and *flavored vehicle*.

Dose—15 mL.

Tolu Balsam Syrup—page 1391.

Water

Water [7732-18-5] H_2O (18.02).

Drinking water, which is subject to EPA regulations with respect to drinking water, and which is delivered by the municipal or other local public system or drawn from a private well or reservoir, is the starting material for all forms of water covered by Pharmacopeial monographs.

Drinking water may be used in the preparation of USP drug substances (eg, in the extraction of certain vegetable drugs and in the manufacture of a few preparations used externally) but not in the preparation of dosage forms, or in the preparation of reagents or test solutions. It is no longer the subject of a separate monograph (in the USP), inasmuch as the cited standards vary from one community to another and generally are beyond the control of private parties or corporations.

Purified Water

Water obtained by distillation, ion-exchange treatment, reverse osmosis or any other suitable process; contains no added substance.

Caution—Do not use this in preparations intended for parenteral administration. For such purposes, use Water for Injection, Bacteriostatic Water for Injection, or Sterile Water for Injection, page 1395.

Preparation—From water complying with EPA regulations with respect to drinking water. A former official process for water, when prepared by distillation, is given below. The pharmacist who is preparing sterile solutions, and must have freshly distilled water of exceptionally high grade, not only free from all bacterial or other microscopic growths but also free from the products of metabolic processes resulting from the growth of such organisms in the water, advantageously may follow this plan. The metabolic products commonly are spoken of as pyrogens and usually consist of complex organic compounds which cause febrile reactions if present in the solvent for parenteral medicinal substances.

Distillation Process

Water	**1000 Vol**
To make	**750 Vol**

Distil the water from a suitable apparatus provided with a block-tin or glass condenser. Collect the first 100 volumes and reject this portion. Then collect 750 volumes and keep the distilled water in glass-stoppered bottles, which have been rinsed with steam or very hot distilled water immediately before being filled. The first 100 volumes are discarded to eliminate foreign volatile substances found in ordinary water and only 750 volumes are collected, since the residue in the still contains concentrated dissolved solids.

Description—Colorless, clear liquid, without odor or taste.
Uses—A *pharmaceutic aid* (vehicle and solvent). It must be used in compounding dosage forms for internal (oral) administration as well as sterile pharmaceuticals applied externally, such as collyria and dermatological preparations, but these must be sterilized before use.
Whenever water is called for in official tests and assays, this must be used.

Syrups Used as Diluting Agents

Syrups are useful as diluting agents for water-soluble drugs and act both as solvents and flavoring agents. The flavored syrups usually consist of simple syrup (85% sucrose in water) containing appropriate flavoring substances. *Glycyrrhiza Syrup* is an excellent vehicle for saline substances because of its colloidal properties, sweet flavor and lingering taste of licorice. *Acacia Syrup* is valuable in disguising the taste of urea. Fruit syrups are especially effective for masking sour tastes. *Aromatic Eriodictyon Syrup* is the diluting agent of choice for masking the bitter taste of alkaloids. *Cocoa Syrup* and *Cherry Syrup* are good general flavoring agents.

Acacia Syrup

Acacia, granular or powdered	**100 g**
Sodium Benzoate	**1 g**
Vanilla Tincture	**5 mL**
Sucrose	**800 g**
Purified Water, a sufficient quantity,	
To make	**1000 mL**

Mix the acacia, sodium benzoate and sucrose; then add 425 mL of purified water, and mix well. Heat the mixture on a steam bath until solution is completed. When cool, remove the scum, add the vanilla tincture and sufficient purified water to make the product measure 1000 mL and strain, if necessary.

Uses—A *flavored vehicle* and *demulcent.*

Cherry Syrup

Syrupus Cerasi

Cherry Juice	**475 mL**
Sucrose	**800 g**
Alcohol	**20 mL**
Purified Water, a sufficient quantity,	
To make	**1000 mL**

Dissolve the sucrose in cherry juice by heating on a steam bath, cool and remove the foam and floating solids. Add the alcohol and sufficient purified water to make 1000 mL, and mix.

Alcohol Content—1 to 2%.
Uses—A pleasantly *flavored vehicle* which is particularly useful in masking the taste of saline and sour drugs.

Citric Acid Syrup USP XVIII—see RPS-18, page 1302.

Cocoa Syrup

Cacao Syrup; Chocolate-flavored Syrup; Chocolate Syrup

Cocoa	**180 g**
Sucrose	**600 g**
Liquid Glucose	**180 g**
Glycerin	**50 mL**
Sodium Chloride	**2 g**
Vanillin	**0.2 g**
Sodium Benzoate	**1 g**
Purified Water, a sufficient quantity,	
To make	**1000 mL**

Mix the sucrose and the cocoa, and to this mixture gradually add a solution of the liquid glucose, glycerin, sodium chloride, vanillin and sodium benzoate in 325 mL of hot purified water. Bring the entire mixture to a boil, and maintain at boiling temperature for 3 min. Allow to cool to room temperature and add sufficient purified water to make the product measure 1000 mL.

Note—Cocoa containing not more than 12% nonvolatile, ether-soluble extractive ("fat") yields a syrup having a minimum tendency to separate. "Breakfast cocoa" contains over 22% "fat."

Uses—A pleasantly *flavored vehicle.*

Aromatic Eriodictyon Syrup—see RPS-18, page 1301.

Raspberry Syrup USP XVIII—see RPS-18, page 1302.

Syrup

Simple Syrup

Sucrose	**850 g**
Purified Water, a sufficient quantity,	
To make	**1000 mL**

May be prepared by using boiling water or, preferably, without heat, by the following process:

Place the sucrose in a suitable percolator the neck of which is nearly filled with loosely packed cotton moistened, after packing, with a few drops of water. Pour carefully about 450 mL of purified water upon the sucrose, and regulate the outflow to a steady drip of percolate. Return the percolate, if necessary, until all of the sucrose has dissolved. Then wash the inside of the percolator and the cotton with sufficient purified water to bring the volume of the percolate to 1000 mL, and mix.

Specific Gravity—Not less than 1.30.
Uses—A *sweet vehicle*, sweetening agent and as the basis for many flavored and medicated syrups.

Other Syrups Used As Diluting Agents

Glycyrrhiza Syrup USP XVIII [Licorice Syrup]—*Preparation:* Add fennel oil (0.05 mL) and anise oil (0.5 mL) to glycyrrhiza fluidextract (250 mL) and agitate until mixed. Then add syrup (qs) to make the product measure 1000 mL, and mix. *Alcohol Content:* 5 to 6%. *Incompatibilities:* The characteristic flavor is destroyed by acids due to a precipitation of the glycyrrhizin. *Uses:* A *flavored vehicle*, especially adapted to the administration of bitter or nauseous substances.

Hydriodic Acid Syrup—Contains, in each 100 mL 1.3 to 1.5 g HI (127.91). *Preparation:* Mix diluted hydriodic acid (140 mL) with purified water (550 mL), and dissolve dextrose (450 g) in this mixture by agitation. Add purified water (qs) to make the product measure 1000 mL, and filter. *Caution: It must not be dispensed if it contains free iodine, as evidenced by a red coloration. Description:* Transparent, colorless, or not more than pale straw-colored, syrupy liquid; odorless and has a sweet, acidulous taste; specific gravity about 1.18; hydriodic acid is decomposed easily in simple aqueous solution (unless protected by hypophosphorous acid) free iodine being liberated, and if taken internally, when in this condition, it is irritating to the alimentary tract. The dextrose used in this syrup should be of the highest grade obtainable. *Incompatibilities:* The reactions of the *acids* (page 1499) as well as those of the water-soluble iodide salts. Oxidizing agents liberate iodine; alkaloids may be precipitated. *Uses:* Traditionally as a *vehicle for expectorant* drugs. Its therapeutic properties are those of the iodides. *Dose: Usual,* 5 mL.

Wild Cherry Syrup USP XVIII—*Preparation:* Pack wild cherry (in coarse powder, 150 g), previously moistened with water (100 mL), in a cylindrical percolator, and add water (qs) to leave a layer of it above the powder. Macerate for 1 hr, then proceed with rapid percolation, using added water, until 400 mL of percolate is collected. Filter the percolate, if necessary, add sucrose (675 g) and dissolve it by agitation, then add glycerin (150 mL), alcohol (20 mL) and water (qs) to make the product measure 1000 mL. Strain if necessary. *It may be made also in the following manner:* The sucrose may be dissolved by placing it in a second percolator as directed for preparing *Syrup*, and allowing the percolate from the wild cherry to flow through it and into a graduated vessel containing the glycerin and alcohol until the total volume measures 1000 mL. *Note:* Heat is avoided, lest the enzyme emulsin be inactivated. If this should happen, the preparation would contain no free HCN, upon which its action as a sedative for coughs mainly depends. For a discussion of the chemistry involved, see *Wild Cherry* (page 1392). *Alcohol Content:* 1 to 2%. *Uses:* Chiefly as a *flavored vehicle* for cough syrups.

Mucilages Used as Diluting Agents

Mucilages are also suitable as diluting agents for water-soluble substances, and are especially useful in stabilizing suspensions and emulsions.

The following mucilage used for this purpose is described under *Emulsifying and Suspending Agents*, page 1395.

Acacia Mucilage—page 1395.

Hydroalcoholic Diluting Agents

Hydroalcoholic diluting agents are suitable for drugs soluble in either water or diluted alcohol. The most important agents in this group are the elixirs. These solutions contain approximately 25% alcohol. *Medicated* elixirs which have therapeutic activity in their own right are not included in this section. Listed below are the common, nonmedicated elixirs which are used purely as diluting agents or solvents for drugs.

Aromatic Elixir

Simple Elixir

Orange Oil	**2.4 mL**
Lemon Oil	**0.6 mL**
Coriander Oil	**0.24 mL**
Anise Oil	**0.06 mL**
Syrup	**375 mL**
Talc	**30 g**
Alcohol,	
Purified Water, each, a sufficient quantity,	
To make	**1000 mL**

Dissolve the oils in alcohol to make 250 mL. To this solution add the syrup in several portions, agitating vigorously after each addition, and afterwards add, in the same manner, the required quantity of purified water. Mix the talc with the liquid, and filter through a filter wetted with diluted alcohol, returning the filtrate until a clear liquid is obtained.

Alcohol Content—21 to 23%.

Uses—A pleasantly *flavored vehicle*, employed in the preparation of many other elixirs. The chief objection to its extensive use is the high alcohol content (about 22%) which at times may counteract the effect of other medicines.

Cardamom Spirit, Compound—see RPS-15, page 1236.

Other Hydroalcoholic Diluting Agents

Glycyrrhiza Elixir [Elixir Adjuvans; Licorice Elixir]—*Preparation:* Mix glycyrrhiza fluidextract (125 mL) and aromatic elixir (875 mL) and filter. *Alcohol Content:* 21 to 23%. *Uses:* A *flavored vehicle*.

Flavored Alcoholic Solutions

Flavored alcoholic solutions, of high alcoholic concentration, are useful as flavors to be added in small quantities to syrups or elixirs. The alcohol content of these solutions is approximately 50%. There are two types of flavored alcoholic solutions: tinctures and spirits. Only nonmedicated tinctures and spirits are used as flavoring agents.

Compound Cardamom Tincture—see RPS-18, page 1302.

Lemon Tincture—page 1391.

Myrcia Spirit, Compound—see RPS-13, page 452.

Orange Spirit, Compound—page 1388.

Orange Peel, Sweet, Tincture—page 1388.

Peppermint Spirit—see RPS-18, page 798.

Diluting Agents for Injections

Injections are liquid preparations, usually solutions or suspensions of drugs, intended to be injected through the skin into the body. Diluting agents used for these preparations may be aqueous or nonaqueous and must meet the requirements for sterility and also of the pyrogen test. Aqueous diluting agents include such preparations as *Sterile Water for Injection* and various sterile, aqueous solutions of electrolytes and/or dextrose. Nonaqueous diluting agents are generally fatty oils of vegetable origin, fatty esters and polyols such as propylene glycol and polyethylene glycol. These agents are used to dissolve or dilute oil-soluble substances and to suspend water-soluble substances when it is desired to decrease the rate of absorption and, hence, prolong the duration of action of the drug substances. Preparations of this type are given intramuscularly. See *Parenteral Preparations*, page 1524.

Corn Oil

Maize Oil

The refined fixed oil obtained from the embryo of *Zea mays* Linné (Fam *Gramineae*).

Preparation—Expressed from the Indian corn embryos or germs separated from the grain in starch manufacture.

Description—Clear, light yellow, oily liquid with a faint characteristic odor and taste; specific gravity 0.914 to 0.921.

Solubility—Slightly soluble in alcohol; miscible with ether, chloroform, benzene or solvent hexane.

Uses—Main official use is as a *solvent* and *vehicle for injections.* It is used as an edible oil substitute for solid fats in the management of hypercholesterolemia. Other uses include making soaps and for burning. It is a semidrying oil and therefore unsuitable for lubricating or mixing paint.

Cottonseed Oil

Cotton Seed Oil; Cotton Oil

The refined fixed oil obtained from the seed of cultivated plants of various varieties of *Gossypium hirsutum* Linné or of other species of *Gossypium* (Fam *Malvaceae*).

Preparation—Cotton seeds contain about 15% oil. The testae of the seeds are first separated, and the kernels are subjected to high pressure in hydraulic presses. The crude oil thus has a bright red to blackish red color. It requires purification before it is suitable for medicinal or food purposes.

Description—Pale yellow, oily liquid with a bland taste; odorless or nearly so; particles of solid fat may separate below 10°; solidifies at about 0° to −5°; specific gravity 0.915 to 0.921.

Solubility—Slightly soluble in alcohol; miscible with ether, chloroform, solvent hexane or carbon disulfide.

Uses—Official as a *solvent* and *vehicle for injections.* It is sometimes taken orally as a mild cathartic in the dose of 30 mL or more. Taken internally, digestible oils retard gastric secretion and motility and increase the caloric intake. It also is used in the manufacture of soaps, oleomargarine, lard substitutes, glycerin, lubricants and cosmetics.

Ethyl Oleate

(*Z*)-9-Octadecenoic acid, ethyl ester

$$\begin{array}{l} HC{-}CH_2(CH_2)_6COOC_2H_5 \\ \;\| \\ HC{-}CH_2(CH_2)_6CH_3 \end{array}$$

Ethyl oleate [111-62-6] $C_{20}H_{38}O_2$ (310.52).

Preparation—Among other ways, by reacting ethanol with oleoyl chloride in the presence of a suitable dehydrochlorinating agent.

Description—Mobile, practically colorless liquid, having an agreeable taste; specific gravity 0.866 to 0.874; acid value not greater than 0.5; iodine value 75 to 85; sterilized by heating at 150° for 1 hr; properties similar to those of almond and arachis oils, but is less viscous and more rapidly absorbed by the tissues; boils about 207°.

Solubility—Does not dissolve in water; miscible with vegetable oils, mineral oil, alcohol or most organic solvents.

Uses—A *vehicle* for certain intramuscular injectable preparations.

Peanut Oil

Arachis Oil; Groundnut Oil; Nut Oil; Earth-Nut Oil

The refined fixed oil obtained from the seed kernels of one or more of the cultivated varieties of *Arachis hypogaea* Linné (Fam *Leguminosae*).

Description—Colorless or pale yellow, oily liquid, with a characteristic nutty odor and a bland taste; specific gravity 0.912 to 0.920.

Solubility—Very slightly soluble in alcohol; miscible with ether, chloroform or carbon disulfide.

Uses—A *solvent* in preparing oil solutions for injection (page 1549). It also is used for making liniments, ointments, plasters and soaps, as a substitute for olive oil.

Sesame Oil

Teel Oil; Benne Oil; Gingili Oil

The refined fixed oil obtained from the seed of one or more cultivated varieties of *Sesamum indicum* Linné (Fam *Pedaliaceae*).

Description—Pale yellow, almost odorless, oily liquid with a bland taste; specific gravity 0.916 to 0.921.

Solubility—Slightly soluble in alcohol; miscible with ether, chloroform, solvent hexane or carbon disulfide.

Uses—A *solvent* and *vehicle* in official injections. It is used much like olive oil both medicinally and for food. It does not readily turn rancid. It also is used in the manufacture of cosmetics, iodized oil, liniments, ointments and oleomargarine.

Water for Injection

Water purified by distillation or by reverse osmosis. It contains no added substance.

Caution—It is intended for use as a solvent for the preparation of parenteral solutions. For parenteral solutions that are prepared under aseptic conditions and are not sterilized by appropriate filtration or in the final container, first render it sterile and thereafter protect it from microbial contamination.

Description—Clear, colorless, odorless liquid.

Uses—*Pharmaceutic aid* (vehicle and solvent).

Bacteriostatic Water for Injection

Sterile water for injection containing one or more suitable antimicrobial agents.

Note—Use it with due regard for the compatibility of the antimicrobial agent or agents it contains with the particular medicinal substance that is to be dissolved or diluted.

Uses—*Sterile vehicle* for parenteral preparations.

Sterile Water for Injection

Water for Parenterals

Water for injection sterilized and suitably packaged. It contains no antimicrobial agent or other added substance.

Description—Clear, colorless, odorless, liquid.

Uses—For the preparation of *all aqueous parenteral solutions*, including those used in *animal assays*. See page 1526 for a detailed discussion.

Sterile Water for Irrigation

Water for injection that has been sterilized and suitably packaged. It contains no antimicrobial agent or other added substance.

Description—Clear, colorless, odorless liquid.

Uses—An *irrigating solution*.

Emulsifying and Suspending Agents

An emulsion is a two-phase system in which one liquid is dispersed in the form of small globules throughout another liquid that is immiscible with the first liquid. Emulsions are formed and stabilized with the help of emulsifying agents, which are surfactants and/or viscosity-producing agents. A suspension is defined as a preparation containing finely divided insoluble material suspended in a liquid medium. The presence of a suspending agent is required to overcome agglomeration of the dispersed particles and to increase the viscosity of the medium so that the particles settle more slowly. Emulsifying and suspending agents are used extensively in the formulation of elegant pharmaceutical preparations for oral, parenteral and external use. For the theoretical and practical aspects of emulsions the interested reader is referred to pages 283 and 1395. More detailed information on the use of suspending agents is given on page 1395.

Acacia

Gum Arabic

The dried gummy exudate from the stems and branches of *Acacia senegal* (Linné) Willdenow or of other related African species of *Acacia* (Fam *Leguminosae*).

Constituents—Principally calcium, magnesium and potassium salts of the polysaccharide *arabic acid*, which on acid hydrolysis yields L-arabinose, L-rhamnose, D-galactose and an aldobionic acid containing D-glucuronic acid and D-galactose.

Description—*Acacia:* Spheroidal tears up to 32 mm in diameter or angular fragments of white to yellowish white color; translucent or somewhat opaque; very brittle; almost odorless; produces a mucilaginous sensation on the tongue. *Flake Acacia:* White to yellowish white, thin flakes. *Powdered Acacia:* White to yellowish white, angular microscopic fragments. *Granular Acacia:* White to pale yellowish white, fine granules. *Spray-dried Acacia:* White to off-white compacted microscopic fragments or whole spheres.

Solubility—Insoluble in alcohol, but almost completely soluble in twice its weight of water at room temperature; the resulting solution flows readily and is acid to litmus.

Incompatibilities—*Alcohol or alcoholic solutions* precipitate acacia as a stringy mass when the alcohol amounts to more than about 35% of the total volume. Solution is effected by dilution with water. The mucilage is destroyed through precipitation of the acacia by *heavy metals*. *Borax* also causes a precipitation which is prevented by glycerin. It contains calcium and, therefore, possesses the incompatibilities of this ion.

It contains a *peroxidase* which acts as an oxidizing agent and produces colored derivatives of *aminopyrine, antipyrine, cresol, guaiacol, phenol, tannin, thymol, vanillin* and other substances. Among the alkaloids affected are *atropine, apomorphine, cocaine, homatropine, hyoscyamine, morphine, physostigmine* and *scopolamine*. A partial destruction of the alkaloid occurs in the reaction. Heating the solution of acacia for a few minutes at 100° destroys the peroxidase and the color reactions are avoided.

Uses—Extensively as a *suspending agent* for insoluble substances in water (page 1515), in the preparation of emulsions (pages 282 and 1509) and for making pills and troches (page 1648).

It is used for its *demulcent* action in inflammations of the throat or stomach.

Its solutions should not be used as a substitute for serum protein in the treatment of *shock* and as a *diuretic* in hypoproteinemic edema, since it produces serious syndromes that may result in death.

Acacia Mucilage [Mucilage of Gum Arabic]—*Preparation:* Place acacia (in small fragments, 350 g) in a graduated bottle having a wide mouth and a capacity not greatly exceeding 1000 mL, wash the drug with cold purified water, allow it to drain and add enough warm purified water, in which benzoic acid (2 g) has been dissolved, to make the product measure 1000 mL. After stoppering, lay the bottle on its side, rotate it occasionally, and when the acacia has dissolved strain the mucilage. *It also may be prepared as follows:* dissolve benzoic acid (2 g) in purified water (400 mL) with the aid of heat, and add the solution to powdered or granular acacia (350 g), in a mortar, triturating until the acacia is dissolved. Then add sufficient purified water to make the product measure 1000 mL, and strain if necessary. This second method is primarily for extemporaneous preparation. *Uses:* A *demulcent* and a *suspending agent*. It also has been employed as an *excipient* in making pills and troches, and as an *emulsifying agent* for cod liver oil and other substances. *Caution—It must be free from mold or any other indication of decomposition.*

Agar

Agar-Agar; Vegetable Gelatin; Gelosa; Chinese or Japanese Gelatin

The dried, hydrophilic, colloidal substance extracted from *Gelidium cartilagineum* (Linné) Gaillon (Fam *Gelidiaceae*), *Gracilaria confervoides* (Linné) Greville (Fam *Sphaerococcaceae*) and related red algae (Class *Rhodophyceae*).

Constituents—Chiefly of the calcium salt of a galactan mono- (acid sulfate).

Description—Usually in bundles of thin, membranous, agglutinated strips or in cut, flaked, or granulated forms; may be weak yellowish orange, yellowish gray to pale yellow or colorless; tough when damp, brittle when dry; odorless or with a slight odor; produces a mucilaginous sensation on the tongue. Also supplied as a white to yellowish white or pale-yellow powder.

Solubility—Insoluble in cold water; soluble in boiling water.

Incompatibilities—Like other gums, it is dehydrated and precipitated from solution by *alcohol*. *Tannic acid* causes precipitation; *electrolytes* cause partial dehydration and decrease in viscosity of sols.

Uses—A relatively ineffective bulk-producing laxative used in a variety of proprietary cathartics. In mineral oil emulsions it acts as a stabilizer.

Dose—4 to **16 g** once or twice a day.

It also is used in culture media for bacteriological work and in the manufacture of ice cream, confectionaries, etc.

Alginic Acid

Alginic acid [9005-32-7] (average equivalent weight 200); a hydrophilic colloidal carbohydrate extracted with dilute alkali from various species of brown seaweeds (*Phaeophyceae*).

Preparation—Precipitates when an aqueous solution of *Sodium Alginate* is treated with mineral acid.

Description—White to yellowish white, fibrous powder; odorless or practically odorless, and tasteless; pH (3 in 100 dispersion in water) 1.5 to 3.5; pK_a (0.1*N* NaCl, 20°) 3.42.

Solubility—Insoluble in water or organic solvents; soluble in alkaline solutions.

Uses—A *pharmaceutic aid* (tablet binder and emulsifying agent). It is used as a sizing agent in the paper and textile industries.

Sodium Alginate

Alginic acid, sodium salt; Algin; Manucol; Norgine; Kelgin (*Kelco*)

Sodium alginate [9005-38-3] (average equivalent weight 220); the purified carbohydrate product extracted from brown seaweeds by the use of dilute alkali. It consists chiefly of the sodium salt of alginic acid, a polyuronic acid composed of beta-D-mannuronic acid residues linked so that the carboxyl group of each unit is free while the aldehyde group is shielded by a glycosidic linkage.

Description—Nearly odorless and tasteless, coarse or fine powder, yellowish white in color.

Solubility—Dissolves in water, forming a viscous, colloidal solution; insoluble in alcohol or in hydroalcoholic solutions in which the alcohol content is greater than about 30% by weight; insoluble in chloroform, ether or acids, when the pH of the solution becomes lower than about 3.

Uses—A *thickening* and *emulsifying agent*. This property makes it useful in a variety of areas. For example, it is used to impart smoothness and body to ice cream and to prevent formation of ice particles.

Bentonite

Wilhinite; Soap Clay; Mineral Soap

Bentonite [1302-78-9]; a native, colloidal, hydrated aluminum silicate.

Occurrence—Bentonite is found in the Midwest of the US and Canada. Originally called *Taylorite* after its discoverer in Wyoming, its name was changed to bentonite after its discovery in the Fort Benton formation of the Upper Cretaceous of Wyoming.

Description—Very fine, odorless powder with a slightly earthy taste, free from grit; the powder is nearly white, but may be a pale buff or cream-colored.

The US Geological Survey has defined bentonite as "a transported stratified clay formed by the alteration of volcanic ash shortly after deposition." Chemically, it is $Al_2O_3.4SiO_2.H_2O$ plus other minerals as impurities. It consists of colloidal crystalline plates, of less than microscopic dimensions in thickness, and of colloidal dimensions in breadth. This fact accounts for the extreme swelling that occurs when it is placed in water, since the water penetrates between an infinite number of plates. A good specimen swells 12 to 14 times its volume.

Solubility—Insoluble in water or acids, but it has the property of adsorbing large quantities of water, swelling to approximately 12 times its original volume, and forming highly viscous thixotropic suspensions or *gels*. This property makes it highly useful in pharmacy. Its gel-forming property is augmented by the addition of small amounts of alkaline substances, such as magnesium oxide. It does not swell in organic solvents.

Incompatibilities—*Acids* and *acid salts* decrease its water-absorbing power and thus cause a breakdown of the magma. Suspensions are most stable at a pH above 7.

Uses—A *protective colloid* for the *stabilization of suspensions*. It also has been used as an emulsifier for oil and as a base for plasters, ointments and similar preparations.

Bentonite Magma—*Preparation:* Sprinkle bentonite (50 g), in portions, on hot purified water (800 g), allowing each portion to become thoroughly wetted without stirring. Allow it to stand with occasional stirring for 24 hr. Stir until a uniform magma is obtained, add purified water to make 1000 g, and mix. The magma may be prepared also by mechanical means such as by use of a blender, as follows: Place purified water (about 500 g) in the blender, and while the machine is running, add bentonite (50 g). Add purified water to make up to about 1000 g or up to the operating capacity of the blender. Blend the mixture for 5 to 10 min, add purified water to make 1000 g, and mix. *Uses:* A *suspending agent* for insoluble medicaments.

Carbomer

Carboxypolymethylene (*Goodrich*)

A synthetic high-molecular-weight cross-linked polymer of acrylic acid; contains 56 to 68% of carboxylic acid (—COOH) groups. The viscosity of a neutralized preparation (2.5 g/500 mL water) is 30,000 to 40,000 centipoises.

Description—White, fluffy powder with a slight characteristic odor; hygroscopic; pH (1 in 100 dispersion) about 3; specific gravity about 1.41.

Solubility (neutralized with alkali hydroxides or amines)—Dissolves in water, alcohol or glycerin.

Uses—A *thickening, suspending, dispersing* and *emulsifying agent* for pharmaceuticals, cosmetics, waxes, paints and other industrial products.

Carrageenan

(*FMC*)

Carrageenan [9000-07-1].

Preparation—The hydrocolloid extracted with water or aqueous alkali from certain red seaweeds of the class *Rhodophyceae*, and separated from the solution by precipitation with alcohol (methanol, ethanol or isopropanol) or by drum-roll drying or freezing.

Constituents—It is a variable mixture of potassium, sodium, calcium, magnesium and ammonium sulfate esters of galactose and 3,6-anhydrogalactose copolymers, the hexoses being alternately linked α-1,3 and β-1,4 in the polymer. The three main types of copolymers present are *kappa*-carrageenan, *iota*-carrageenan and *lambda*-carrageenan, which differ in the composition and manner of linkage of monomeric units and the degree of sulfation (the ester sulfate content for carrageenans varies from 18 to 40%). *Kappa*-carrageenan and *iota*-carrageenan are the gelling fractions; *lambda*-carrageenan is the nongelling fraction. The gelling fractions may be separated from the nongelling fraction by addition of potassium chloride to an aqueous solution of carrageenan. Carrageenan separated by drum-roll drying may contain mono- and di-glycerides or up to 5% of polysorbate 80 used as roll-stripping agents.

Description—Yellow-brown to white, coarse to fine powder; odorless; tasteless, producing a mucilaginous sensation on the tongue.

Solubility—All carrageenans hydrate rapidly in cold water, but only *lambda*-carrageenan and sodium carrageenans dissolve completely. Gelling carrageenans require heating to about 80° for complete solution where potassium and calcium ions are present.

Uses—In the pharmaceutical and food industries as an emulsifying, suspending and gelling agent.

Carboxymethylcellulose Sodium

Carbose D; Carboxymethocel S; CMC; Cellulose Gum (*Aqualon*)

Cellulose, carboxymethyl ether, sodium salt [9004-32-4]; contains 6.5–9.5% of sodium (Na), calculated on the dried basis. It is available in several viscosity types: low, medium, high and extra high.

Description—White to cream-colored powder or granules; the powder is hygroscopic; pH (1 in 100 aqueous solution) about 7.5.

Solubility—Easily dispersed in water to form colloidal solutions; insoluble in alcohol, ether or most other organic solvents.

Uses—*Pharmaceutic aid* (suspending agent, tablet excipient or viscosity-increasing agent). In tablet form it is used as a hydrophilic colloid laxative.

Dose—*Usual, adult, laxative,* **1.5 g** 3 or 4 times a day.

Dosage Form: Tablets: 500 mg.

Powdered Cellulose

(*Degussa*)

Cellulose [9004-34-6] $(C_6H_{10}O_5)_n$; purified, mechanically disintegrated cellulose prepared by processing alpha cellulose obtained as a pulp from fibrous plant materials.

Description—White, odorless substance, consisting of fibrous particles, which may be compressed into self-binding tablets which disintegrate rapidly in water; exists in various grades, exhibiting degrees of fineness ranging from a free-flowing dense powder to a coarse, fluffy, nonflowing material; pH (supernatant liquid of a 10 g/90 mL aqueous suspension after 1 hr) 5 to 7.5.

Solubility—Insoluble in water, dilute acids or nearly all organic solvents; slightly soluble in NaOH solution (1 in 20).

Uses—*Pharmaceutic aid* (tablet diluent, adsorbent or suspending agent).

Cetyl Alcohol—page 1401.

Cholesterol

Cholest-5-en-3-ol, (3β)-, Cholesterin; (*Croda*)

Cholest-5-en-3β-ol [57-88-5] $C_{27}H_{46}O$ (386.66).

For the structural formula, see page 391.

A steroid alcohol widely distributed in the animal organism. In addition to cholesterol and its esters, several closely related steroid alcohols occur in the yolk of eggs, the brain, milk, fish oils, wool fat (10 to 20%), etc. These closely resemble it in properties. One of the methods of commercial production involves extraction of it from the unsaponifiable matter in the spinal cord of cattle, using petroleum benzin. Wool fat also is used as a source.

Description—White or faintly yellow, almost odorless pearly leaflets or granules; usually acquires a yellow to pale tan color on prolonged exposure to light or to elevated temperatures; melts 147 to 150°.

Solubility—Insoluble in water; 1 g slowly dissolves in 100 mL alcohol or about 50 mL dehydrated alcohol; soluble in acetone, hot alcohol, chloroform, dioxane, ether, ethyl acetate, solvent hexane or vegetable oils.

Uses—To enhance incorporation and emulsification of medicinal products in oils or fats. It is a *pharmaceutical necessity* for *Hydrophilic Petrolatum*, in which it enhances water-absorbing capacity. See Chapter 20.

Docusate Sodium—page 900.

Gelatin

White Gelatin; (*Fallek*)

A product obtained by the partial hydrolysis of collagen derived from the skin, white connective tissues and bones of animals. Gelatin derived from an acid-treated precursor is known as Type A and exhibits an isoelectric point between pH 7 and 9, while gelatin derived from an alkali-treated precursor is known as Type B and exhibits an isoelectric point between pH 4.7 and 5.2.

Gelatin for use in the manufacture of capsules in which to dispense medicines, or for the coating of tablets, may be colored with a certified color, may contain not more than 0.15% of sulfur dioxide, may contain a suitable concentration of sodium lauryl sulfate and suitable antimicrobial agents, and may have any suitable gel strength that is designated by Bloom Gelometer number.

Regarding the special gelatin for use in the preparation of emulsions, see *Emulsions* (page 1509).

Description—Sheets, flakes or shreds, or a coarse to fine powder; faintly yellow or amber in color, the color varying in depth according to the particle size; slight, characteristic bouillon-like odor; stable in air when dry, but is subject to microbial decomposition when moist or in solution.

Solubility—Insoluble in cold water, but swells and softens when immersed in it, gradually absorbing from 5 to 10 times its own weight of water; soluble in hot water, acetic acid or hot mixtures of glycerin or water; insoluble in alcohol, chloroform, ether or fixed and volatile oils.

Uses—In pharmacy, to coat pills and form capsules, and as a vehicle for suppositories. It also is recommended as an emulsifying agent. See under *Emulsions* in Chapters 19 and 86, also *Suppositories* (page 1591), and *Absorbable Gelatin Sponge* (page 927). It also has been used as an adjuvant protein food in malnutrition.

Glyceryl Monostearate—page 1402.

Hydroxyethyl Cellulose

Cellulose, 2-hydroxyethyl ether; Cellosize (*Union Carbide*); Natrosol (*Aqualon*)

Cellulose hydroxyethyl ether [9004-62-0].

Preparation—Cellulose is treated with NaOH and then reacted with ethylene oxide.

Description—White, odorless, tasteless, free-flowing powder; softens at about 137°; refractive index (2% solution) about 1.336; pH about 7; solutions are nonionic.

Solubility—Dissolves readily in cold or hot water to give clear, smooth, viscous solutions; partially soluble in acetic acid; insoluble in most organic solvents.

Uses—Resembles carboxymethylcellulose sodium in that it is a cellulose ether, but differs in being nonionic and, hence, its solutions are unaffected by cations. It is used pharmaceutically as a thickener, protective colloid, binder, stabilizer and suspending agent in emulsions, jellies and ointments, lotions, ophthalmic solutions, suppositories and tablets.

Hydroxypropyl Cellulose

Cellulose, 2-hydroxypropyl ether; Klucel (*Aqualon*)

Cellulose hydroxypropyl ether [9004-64-2].

Preparation—After treating with NaOH, cellulose is reacted with propylene oxide at elevated temperature and pressure.

Description—Off-white, odorless, tasteless powder; softens at 130°; burns out completely about 475° in N_2 or O_2; refractive index (2% solution) about 1.337; pH (aqueous solution) 5 to 8.5; solutions are nonionic.

Solubility—Soluble in water below 40° (insoluble above 45°); soluble in many polar organic solvents.

Uses—A broad combination of properties useful in a variety of industries. It is used pharmaceutically as a binder, granulation agent and film-coater in the manufacture of tablets; an alcohol-soluble thickener and suspending agent for elixirs and lotions and a stabilizer for emulsions.

Hydroxypropyl Methylcellulose

Cellulose, 2-hydroxypropyl methyl ether; (*Dow*)

Cellulose hydroxypropyl methyl ether [9004-65-3], available in grades containing 16.5 to 30.0% of methoxy and 4.0 to 32.0% of hydroxypropoxy groups, and thus in viscosity and thermal gelation temperatures of solutions of specified concentration.

Preparation—The appropriate grade of methylcellulose (see below) is treated with NaOH and reacted with propylene oxide at elevated temperature and pressure and for a reaction time sufficient to produce the desired degree of attachment of methyl and hydroxypropyl groups by ether linkages to the anhydroglucose rings of cellulose.

Description—White to slightly off-white, fibrous or granular, free-flowing powder.

Solubility—Swells in water and produces a clear to opalescent, viscous colloidal mixture; undergoes reversible transformation from sol to gel on heating and cooling, respectively. Insoluble in anhydrous alcohol, ether or chloroform.

Uses—A protective colloid that is useful as a dispersing and thickening agent, and in ophthalmic solutions to provide the demulcent action and viscous properties essential for contact-lens use and in "artificial-tear" formulations. See *Hydroxypropyl Methylcellulose Ophthalmic Solution* (page 869).

Lanolin, Anhydrous—page 1401.

Methylcellulose

Cellulose, methyl ether; Methocel (*Dow*)

Cellulose methyl ether [9004-67-5]; a methyl ether of cellulose containing 27.5 to 31.5% of methoxy groups.

Preparation—By the reaction of methyl chloride or of dimethyl sulfate on cellulose dissolved in sodium hydroxide. The cellulose methyl ether so formed is coagulated by adding methanol or other suitable agent and centrifuged. Since cellulose has 3 hydroxyl groups/glucose residue, several methylcelluloses can be made varying, among other properties, in solubility and viscosity. Types useful for pharmaceutical application contain from 1 to 2 methoxy radicals/glucose residue.

Description—White, fibrous powder or granules; aqueous suspensions neutral to litmus; stable to alkalies and dilute acids.

Solubility—Insoluble in ether, alcohol or chloroform; soluble in glacial acetic acid or in a mixture of equal parts of alcohol and chloroform; swells in water, producing a clear to opalescent, viscous colloidal solution; insoluble in hot water and saturated salt solutions; salts of minerals acids and particularly of polybasic acids, phenols and tannins coagulate its solutions, but this can be prevented by the addition of alcohol or of glycol diacetate.

Uses—A synthetic substitute for natural gums that has both pharmaceutic and therapeutic applications. Pharmaceutically, it is used as a *dispersing, thickening, emulsifying, sizing* and *coating agent*. It is an ingredient of many nose drops, eye preparations, burn medications, cosmetics, tooth pastes, liquid dentifrices, hair fixatives, creams and lotions. It functions as a protective colloid for many types of dispersed substances and is an effective stabilizer for oil-in-water emulsions.

Therapeutically, it is used as a *bulk laxative* in the treatment of *chronic constipation*. Taken with 1 or 2 glassesful of water, it forms a colloidal solution in the upper alimentary tract; this solution loses water in the colon, forming a gel that increases the bulk and softness of the stool. The gel is bland, demulcent and nonirritating to the gastrointestinal tract. Once a normal stool develops, the dose should be reduced to a level adequate for maintenance of good function. Although it takes up water from the gastrointestinal tract quite readily, methylcellulose tablets have caused fecal impaction and intestinal obstruction when taken with a limited amount of water. It also is used as a topical ophthalmic protectant, in the form of 0.5 to 1% solution serving as artificial tears or a contact-lens solution applied to the conjunctiva, 0.05 to 0.1 mL at a time, 3 or 4 times a day as needed.

Dose—*Usual*, as laxative, **1 to 1.5 g**, with water, 2 to 4 times a day.

Dosage Forms—Tablets: 500 mg; Ophthalmic Solution: 0.5 and 1%; Syrup: 5.91 g/30 mL.

Octoxynol 9—see RPS-18, page 1307.

Oleyl Alcohol

9-Octadecen-1-ol, (*Z*)-, Aldol 85 (*Sherex*)

$HC-CH_2(CH_2)_7OH$ ‖ $HC-CH_2(CH_2)_6CH_3$

(*Z*)-9-Octadecen-1-ol [143-28-2] $C_{18}H_{36}O$ (268.48); a mixture of unsaturated and saturated high-molecular-weight fatty alcohols consisting chiefly of oleyl alcohol.

Preparation—One method reacts ethyl oleate with absolute ethanol and metallic sodium (*Org Syn Coll III:* 673, 1955).

Description—Clear, colorless to light yellow, oily liquid; faint characteristic odor and bland taste; iodine value between 85 and 90; hydroxyl value between 205 and 215.

Solubility—Soluble in alcohol, ether, isopropyl alcohol or light mineral oil; insoluble in water.

Uses—*A pharmaceutic aid* (emulsifying agent or emollient).

Polyvinyl Alcohol

Ethenol, homopolymer; (*Du Pont*)

$[-CH_2-CH(OH)-]_n$

Vinyl alcohol polymer [9002-89-5] $(C_2H_4O)_n$.

Preparation—Polyvinyl acetate is approximately 88% hydrolyzed in a methanol-methyl acetate solution using either mineral acid or alkali as a catalyst.

Description—White to cream-colored powder or granules; odorless.

Solubility—Freely soluble in water; solution effected more rapidly at somewhat elevated temperatures.

Uses—A *suspending agent* and *emulsifier*, either with or without the aid of a surfactant. It commonly is employed as a lubricant and protectant in various ophthalmic preparations, such as decongestants, artificial tears and contact-lens products (see page 1574).

Povidone

2-Pyrrolidinone, 1-ethenyl-, homopolymer; Polyvinylpyrrolidone; PVP (*ISP; BASF*)

1-Vinyl-2-pyrrolidinone polymer [9003-39-8] $(C_6H_9NO)_n$; a synthetic polymer consisting of linear 1-vinyl-2-pyrrolidinone groups, the degree of polymerization of which results in polymers of various molecular weights. It is produced commercially as a series of products having mean molecular weights ranging from about 10,000 to about 700,000. The viscosity of solutions containing 10% or less is essentially the same as that of water; solutions more concentrated than 10% become more viscous, depending upon the concentration and the molecular weight of the polymer used. It contains 12 to 13% of nitrogen.

Preparation—1,4-Butanediol is dehydrogenated thermally with the aid of copper to γ-butyrolactone, which is then reacted with ammonia to form 2-pyrrolidinone. Addition of the latter to acetylene yields vinylpyrrolidinone (monomer) which is polymerized thermally in the presence of hydrogen peroxide and ammonia.

Description—White to creamy white, odorless powder, hygroscopic; pH (1 in 20 solution) 3 to 7.

Solubility—Soluble in water, alcohol or chloroform; insoluble in ether.

Uses—A *dispersing* and *suspending* agent in pharmaceutical preparations.

Propylene Glycol Monostearate

Octadecanoic acid, monoester with 1,2-propanediol

1,2-Propanediol monostearate [1323-39-3]; a mixture of the propylene glycol mono- and diesters of stearic and palmitic acids. It contains not less than 90% of monoesters of saturated fatty acids, chiefly propylene glycol monostearate ($C_{21}H_{42}O_3$) and propylene glycol monopalmitate ($C_{19}H_{38}O_3$).

Preparation—By reacting propylene glycol with stearoyl chloride in a suitable dehydrochlorinating environment.

Description—White, wax-like solid or white, wax-like beads or flakes; slight, agreeable, fatty odor and taste; congeals not lower than 45°; acid value not more than 2; saponification value 155 to 165; hydroxyl value 150 to 170; iodine value not more than 3.

Solubility—Dissolves in organic solvents such as alcohol, mineral or fixed oils, benzene, ether or acetone; insoluble in water but may be dispersed in hot water with the aid of a small amount of soap or other suitable surface-active agent.

Uses—A *surfactant*. It is particularly useful as a dispersing agent for perfume oils or oil-soluble vitamins in water, and in cosmetic preparations.

Silicon Dioxide, Colloidal—page 1413.

Sodium Lauryl Sulfate

Sulfuric acid monododecyl ester sodium salt; Irium; Duponol C (*Du Pont*); Gardinol WA (*Procter & Gamble*)

Sodium monododecyl sulfate [151-21-3]; a mixture of sodium alkyl sulfates consisting chiefly of sodium lauryl sulfate. The combined content of sodium chloride and sodium sulfate is not more than 8%.

Preparation—The fatty acids of coconut oil, consisting chiefly of lauric acid, are catalytically hydrogenated to form the corresponding alcohols. The latter are then esterified with sulfuric acid (sulfated) and the resulting mixture of alkyl bisulfates (alkylsulfuric acids) is converted into a mixture of sodium salts by reacting with alkali under controlled conditions of pH.

Description—Small, white or light yellow crystals having a slight, characteristic odor.

Solubility—1 g in 10 mL water, forming an opalescent solution.

Incompatibilities—Reacts with *cationic surface-active agents* with loss of activity, even in concentrations too low to cause precipitation. Unlike soaps, it is compatible with dilute acids, and calcium and magnesium ions.

Uses—An emulsifying, detergent and wetting agent in ointments, tooth powders and other pharmaceutical preparations, and in the metal, paper and pigment industries.

Sorbitan Esters

Spans (*Atlas*)

Sorbitan esters (*monolaurate* [1338-39-2]; *monooleate* [1338-43-8]; *monopalmitate* [26266-57-9]; *monostearate* [1338-41-6]; *trioleate* [26266-58-0]; *tristearate* [26658-19-5]).

Preparation—Sorbitol is dehydrated to form a *hexitan* which is then esterified with the desired fatty acid. See *Polysorbates*, page 1403, which are polyethylene glycol ethers of sorbitan fatty acid esters.

Description—*Monolaurate:* Amber, oily liquid; may become hazy or form a precipitate; viscosity about 4250 cps; HLB no 8.6; acid no 7.0 max; saponification no 158 to 170; hydroxyl no 330 to 358. *Monooleate:* Amber liquid; viscosity about 1000 cps; HLB no 4.3; acid no 8.0 max; saponification no 145 to 160; hydroxyl no 193 to 210. *Monopalmitate:* Tan, granular waxy solid; HLB no 6.7; acid no 4 to 7.5; saponification no 140 to 150; hydroxyl no 275 to 305. *Monostearate:* Cream to tan beads; HLB no 4.7; acid no 5 to 10; saponification no 147 to 157; hydroxyl no 235 to 260. *Trioleate:* Amber, oily liquid; viscosity about 200 cps; HLB no 1.8; acid no 15 max; saponification no 170 to 190; hydroxyl no 55 to 70. *Tristearate:* Tan, waxy beads; HLB no 2.1; acid no 12 to 15; saponification no 176 to 188; hydroxyl no 66 to 80.

Solubility—*Monolaurate:* Soluble in methanol or alcohol; dispersible in distilled water and hard water (200 ppm); insoluble in hard water (20,000 ppm). *Monooleate:* Soluble in most mineral or vegetable oils; slightly soluble in ether; dispersible in water; insoluble in acetone. *Monopalmitate:* Dispersible (50°) in distilled water or hard water (200 ppm); soluble in ethyl acetate; insoluble in cold distilled water or hard water (20,000 ppm). *Monostearate:* Soluble (above melting point) in vegetable oils or mineral oil; insoluble in water, alcohol or propylene glycol. *Trioleate:* Soluble in mineral oil, vegetable oils, alcohol or methanol; insoluble in water. *Tristearate:* Soluble in isopropyl alcohol; insoluble in water.

Uses—Nonionic *surfactants* used as *emulsifying agents* in the preparation of water-in-oil emulsions.

Stearic Acid—page 1402.

Stearyl Alcohol

1-Octadecanol [112-92-5] $C_{18}H_{38}O$ (270.50); contains not less than 90% of stearyl alcohol, the remainder consisting chiefly of cetyl alcohol [$C_{16}H_{34}O$ = 242.44].

Preparation—Through the reducing action of lithium aluminum hydride on ethyl stearate.

Description—White, unctuous flakes or granules having a faint, characteristic odor and a bland taste; melts 55 to 60°.

Solubility—Insoluble in water; soluble in alcohol, chloroform, ether or vegetable oils.

Uses—A surface-active agent used to *stabilize emulsions* and increase their ability to retain large quantities of water. See *Hydrophilic Ointment* (page 1402). *Hydrophilic Petrolatum* (page 1401).

Sterculia Gum—see RPS-18, page 788.

Tragacanth

Gum Tragacanth; Hog Gum; Goat's Thorn

The dried gummy exudation from *Astragalus gummifer* Labillardière, or other Asiatic species of *Astragalus* (Fam. *Leguminosae*).

Constituents—60 to 70% bassorin and 30 to 40% soluble gum (*tragacanthin*). The bassorin swells in the presence of water to form a gel and tragacanthin forms a colloidal solution. Bassorin, consisting of complex methoxylated acids, resembles pectin. Tragacanthin yields glucuronic acid and arabinose when hydrolyzed.

Description—Flattened, lamellated, frequently curved fragments or straight or spirally twisted linear pieces 0.5 to 2.5 mm in thickness; white to weak-yellow in color; translucent; horny in texture; odorless; insipid, mucilaginous taste. When powdered, it is white to yellowish white.

Introduced into water, tragacanth absorbs a certain proportion of that liquid, swells very much, and forms a soft adhesive paste, but does not dissolve. If agitated with an excess of water, this paste forms a uniform mixture; but in the course of 1 or 2 days the greater part separates, and is deposited, leaving a portion dissolved in the supernatant fluid. The finest mucilage is obtained from the whole gum or *flake* form. Several days should be allowed for obtaining a uniform mucilage of the maximum gel strength. A common adulterant is *Karaya Gum*, and the USP/NF has introduced tests to detect its presence.

Solubility—Insoluble in alcohol.

Uses—A *suspending agent* in lotions, mixtures and extemporaneous preparations and prescriptions. It is used with emulsifying agents largely to increase consistency and retard creaming. It is sometimes used as a *demulcent* in sore throat, and the jelly-like product formed when the gum is allowed to swell in water serves as a basis for pharmaceutical jellies, eg, *Ephedrine Sulfate Jelly*. It also is used in various confectionery products. In the form of a glycerite, it has been used as a pill excipient.

Tragacanth Mucilage—*Preparation:* Mix glycerin (18 g) with purified water (75 mL) in a tared vessel, heat the mixture to boiling, discontinue the application of heat, add tragacanth (6 g) and benzoic acid (0.2 g) and macerate the mixture during 24 hr, stirring occasionally. Then add enough purified water to make the mixture weigh 100 g, stir actively until of uniform consistency, and strain forcibly through muslin. *Uses:* A suspending agent for insoluble substances in internal mixtures. It is also a *protective* agent.

Xanthan Gum

Keltrol (*Kelco*)

A high-molecular-weight polysaccharide gum produced by a pure-culture fermentation of a carbohydrate with *Xanthomonas campestris*, then purified by recovery with isopropyl alcohol, dried and milled; contains D-glucose and D-mannose as the dominant hexose units, along with D-glucuronic acid, and is prepared as sodium, potassium or calcium salt; yields 4.2 to 5% of carbon dioxide.

Preparation—See above and US Pats 3,433,708 and 3,557,016.

Description—White or cream-colored, tasteless powder with a slight organic odor; powder and solutions stable at 25° or less; does not exhibit polymorphism; aqueous solutions are neutral to litmus.

Solubility—1 g in about 3 mL alcohol; soluble in hot or cold water.

Uses—A hydrophilic colloid to thicken, suspend, emulsify and stabilize water-based systems.

Other Emulsifying and Suspending Agents

Chondrus [Irish Moss; Carrageenan]—The dried sun-bleached plant of *Chondrus crispus* (Linné) Stackhouse (Fam *Gigartinaceae*). *Uses:* Principally, as an emulsifying agent for liquid petrolatum and for cod liver oil. It is also a protective. See also page 1396.

Malt—The partially germinated grain of one or more varieties of *Hordeum vulgare* Linné (Fam *Gramineae*) and contains amylolytic enzymes. Yellowish or amber-colored grains, having a characteristic odor and a sweet taste. The evaporated aqueous extract constitutes malt extract.

Malt Extract—The product obtained by extracting malt, the partially and artificially germinated grain of one or more varieties of *Hordeum vulgare* Linné (Fam *Gramineae*). *Uses:* An infrequently used emulsifying agent.

Ointment Bases

Ointments are semisolid preparations for external application to the body. They should be of such composition that they soften, but not necessarily melt, when applied to the skin. Therapeutically, ointments function as protectives and emollients for the skin, but are used primarily as vehicles or bases for the topical application of medicinal substances. Ointments also may be applied to the eye or eyelids.

Ideally, an ointment base should be compatible with the skin, stable, permanent, smooth and pliable, nonirritating, nonsensitizing, inert and readily able to release its incorporated medication. Since there is no single ointment base which possesses all these characteristics, continued research in this field has resulted in the development of numerous new bases. Indeed, ointment bases have become so numerous as to require classification. Although ointment bases may be grouped in several ways, it is generally agreed that they can be classified best according to composition. Hence, the following four classes are recognized herein: oleaginous, emulsifiable, emulsion bases and water-soluble.

For completeness, substances are included that, although not used alone as ointment bases, contribute some pharmaceutical property to one or more of the various bases.

Oleaginous Ointment Bases and Components

The oleaginous ointment bases include fixed oils of vegetable origin, fats obtained from animals and semisolid hydrocarbons obtained from petroleum. The vegetable oils are used chiefly in ointments to lower the melting point or to soften bases. These oils can be used as a base in themselves when a high percentage of powder is incorporated.

The vegetable oils and the animal fats have two marked disadvantages as ointment bases: their water-absorbing capacity is low and they have a tendency to become rancid. Insofar as vegetable oils are concerned, the second disadvantage can be overcome by hydrogenation, a process which converts many fixed oils into white, semisolid fats or into hard, almost brittle, waxes.

The hydrocarbon bases comprise a group of substances with a wide range of melting points so that any desired consistency and melting point may be prepared with representatives of this group. They are stable, bland, chemically inert and will mix with virtually any chemical substance. Oleaginous bases are excellent emollients.

White Ointment

Ointment USP XI; Simple Ointment

White Wax	**50 g**
White Petrolatum	**950 g**
To make	**1000 g**

Melt the white wax in a suitable dish on a water bath, add the white petrolatum, warm until liquefied, then discontinue the heating, and stir the mixture until it begins to congeal. It is permissible to vary the proportion of wax to obtain a suitable consistency of the ointment under different climatic conditions.

Uses—An emollient and vehicle for other ointments.

Yellow Ointment

Yellow Wax	**50 g**
Petrolatum	**950 g**
To make	**1000 g**

Melt the yellow wax in a suitable dish on a steam bath, add the petrolatum, warm until liquefied, then discontinue the heating, and stir the mixture until it begins to congeal. It is permissible to vary the proportion of wax to obtain a suitable consistency of the ointment under different climatic conditions.

Uses—An emollient and vehicle for other ointments. Both white and yellow ointment are known as "simple ointment." White ointment should be used to prepare white ointments and yellow ointments should be used to prepare colored ointments when simple ointment is prescribed.

Cetyl Esters Wax

"Synthetic Spermaceti"

A mixture consisting primarily of esters of saturated fatty alcohols (C_{14} to C_{18}) and saturated fatty acids (C_{14} to C_{18}). It has a saponification value of 109 to 120 and an acid value of not more than 5.

Description—White to off-white, somewhat translucent flakes; crystalline structure and pearly luster when caked; faint odor and a bland, mild taste; free from rancidity; specific gravity 0.820 to 0.840 at 50°; iodine value not more than 1; melts 43 to 47°.

Solubility—Insoluble in water; practically insoluble in cold alcohol; soluble in boiling alcohol, ether, chloroform or fixed and volatile oils; slightly soluble in cold solvent hexane.

Uses—A replacement for spermaceti used to give consistency and texture to ointments, eg, *Cold Cream* and *Rose Water Ointment*.

Oleic Acid

(*Z*)-9-Octadecenoic acid; Oleinic Acid; Elaic Acid

$$\begin{array}{l} HC-CH_2(CH_2)_6COOH \\ \| \\ HC-CH_2(CH_2)_6CH_3 \end{array}$$

Oleic acid [112-80-1] obtained from tallow and other fats, and consists chiefly of (*Z*)-9-octadecenoic acid (282.47). Oleic acid used in preparations for internal administration is derived from edible sources.

It usually contains variable amounts of the other fatty acids present in tallow such as linolenic and stearic acids.

Preparation—Obtained as a by-product in the manufacture of the solid stearic and palmitic acids used in the manufacture of candles, stearates and other products. The crude oleic acid is known as "red oil," the stearic and palmitic acids being separated by cooling.

Description—Colorless to pale yellow, oily liquid; lard-like odor and taste; specific gravity 0.889 to 0.895; congeals at a temperature not above 10°; pure acid solidifies at 4°; at atmospheric pressure it decomposes when heated at 80 to 100°; on exposure to air it gradually absorbs oxygen, darkens and develops a rancid odor.

Solubility—Practically insoluble in water; miscible with alcohol, chloroform, ether, benzene or fixed and volatile oils.

Incompatibilities—Reacts with *alkalies* to form soaps. *Heavy metals* and *calcium salts* form insoluble oleates. *Iodine solutions* are decolorized by formation of the iodine addition compound of the acid. It is oxidized to various derivatives by *nitric acid, potassium permanganate* and other agents.

Uses—Classified as an emulsion adjunct, which reacts with alkalis to form soaps that function as emulsifying agents; it is used for this purpose in such preparations as *Benzyl Benzoate Lotion* and *Green Soap*. It also is used to prepare oleate salts of bases.

Olive Oil—see RPS-18, page 1309.

Paraffin

Paraffin Wax, Hard Paraffin

A purified mixture of solid hydrocarbons obtained from petroleum.

Description—Colorless or white, more or less translucent mass with a crystalline structure; slightly greasy to the touch; odorless and tasteless; congeals 47 to 65°.

Solubility—Freely soluble in chloroform, ether, volatile oils or most warm fixed oils; slightly soluble in dehydrated alcohol; insoluble in water or alcohol.

Uses—Mainly, to increase the consistency of some ointments.

Petrolatum

Yellow Soft Paraffin; Amber Petrolatum; Yellow Petrolatum; Petroleum Jelly; Paraffin Jelly

A purified mixture of semisolid hydrocarbons obtained from petroleum. It may contain a suitable stabilizer.

Preparation—The "residuums," as they are termed technically, which are obtained by the distillation of petroleum, are purified by melting, usually treating with sulfuric acid and then percolating through recently burned bone black or adsorptive clays; this removes the odor and modifies the color. Selective solvents are also sometimes employed to extract impurities.

It has been found that the extent of purification required to produce *Petrolatum* and *Light Mineral Oil* of official quality removes antioxidants that are naturally present, and the purified product subsequently has a tendency to oxidize and develop an offensive odor. This is prevented by the addition of a minute quantity of α-tocopherol, or other suitable antioxidant, as is now permissible.

Description—Unctuous mass of yellowish to light amber color; not more than a slight fluorescence after being melted; transparent in thin layers; free or nearly free from odor and taste; specific gravity 0.815 to 0.880 at 60°; melts between 38 and 60°.

Solubility—Insoluble in water; almost insoluble in cold or hot alcohol or in cold dehydrated alcohol; freely soluble in benzene, carbon disulfide, chloroform or turpentine oil; soluble in ether, solvent hexane or in most fixed and volatile oils, the degree of solubility in these solvents varying with the composition of the petrolatum.

Uses—A base for ointments. It is highly occlusive and therefore a good emollient but it may not release some drugs readily.

White Petrolatum

White Petroleum Jelly; White Soft Paraffin

A purified mixture of semisolid hydrocarbons obtained from petroleum, and wholly or nearly decolorized. It may contain a suitable stabilizer.

Preparation—In the same manner as petrolatum, the purification treatment being continued until the product is practically free from yellow color.

Description—White or faintly yellowish, unctuous mass; transparent in thin layers, even after cooling to 0°; specific gravity 0.815 to 0.880 at 60°; melts 38 to 60°.

Solubility—Similar to that described under *Petrolatum*.

Uses—Similar to yellow petrolatum but often is preferred because of its freedom from color. It is employed as a protective, a base for ointments and cerates and to form the basis for burn dressings. See *Petrolatum Gauze* (page 867).

Spermaceti—see RPS-18, page 1310.

Starch Glycerite—see RPS-18, page 1310.

White Wax—see RPS-18, page 1310.

Yellow Wax—see RPS-18, page 1311.

Absorbent Ointment Bases

The term absorbent is used here to denote the water-absorbing or emulsifying properties of these bases and not to describe their action on the skin. These bases, sometimes called *emulsifiable ointment bases*, are generally anhydrous substances which have the property of absorbing (emulsify ing) considerable quantities of water and still retaining their ointment-like consistency. Preparations of this type do not contain water as a component of their basic formula, but if water is incorporated, when and as desired, a W/O emulsion results. The following official products fall into this category.

Hydroxystearin Sulfate—see RPS-18, page 1311.

Anhydrous Lanolin

Wool Fat USP XVI; Refined Wool Fat

Lanolin that contains not more than 0.25% of water.

Constituents—Contains the sterols *cholesterol* [$C_{27}H_{45}OH$] and *oxycholesterol*, as well as triterpene and aliphatic alcohols. About 7% of the alcohols are found in the free state, the remainder occurring as esters of the following fatty acids: *carnaubic, cerotic, lanoceric, lanopalmitic, myristic* and *palmitic*. Some of these are found free. The emulsifying and emollient actions of lanolin are due to the alcohols that are found in the unsaponifiable fraction when lanolin is treated with alkali. Constituting approximately one-half of this fraction and known as *lanolin alcohols*, the latter is comprised of *cholesterol* (30%), *lanosterol* (25%), *cholestanol* (*dihydrocholesterol*) (3%), *agnosterol* (2%) and various other alcohols (40%).

Preparation—By purifying the fatty matter (*suint*) obtained from the wool of the sheep. This natural wool fat contains about 30% of free fatty acids and fatty acid esters of *cholesterol* and other higher alcohols. The cholesterol compounds are the important constituents and, to secure these in a purified form, many processes have been devised. In one of these the crude wool fat is treated with weak alkali, the saponified fats and emulsions centrifuged to secure the aqueous soap solution, from which, on standing, a layer of partially purified wool fat separates. This product is further purified by treating it with calcium chloride and then dehydrated by fusion with unslaked lime. It is finally extracted with acetone and the solvent subsequently separated by distillation. This differs from lanolin in that the former contains practically no water.

Description—Yellow, tenacious, unctuous mass; slight, characteristic odor; melts between 36 and 42°.

Solubility—Insoluble in water, but mixes without separation with about twice its weight of water; sparingly soluble in cold alcohol; more soluble in hot alcohol; freely soluble in ether or chloroform.

Uses—An ingredient of ointments, especially when an aqueous liquid is to be incorporated. It gives a distinctive quality to the ointment, increasing absorption of active ingredients and maintaining a uniform consistency for the ointment under most climatic conditions. However, it has been omitted from many ointments on the recommendation of dermatologists who have found that many patients are allergic to this animal wax.

Hydrophilic Petrolatum

Cholesterol	**30 g**
Stearyl Alcohol	**30 g**
White Wax	**80 g**
White Petrolatum	**860 g**
To make	**1000 g**

Melt the stearyl alcohol, white wax, and white petrolatum together on a steam bath, then add the cholesterol, and stir until it completely dissolves. Remove from the bath, and stir until the mixture congeals.

Uses—A *protective* and *water-absorbable ointment base*. It will absorb a large amount of water from aqueous solutions of medicating substances, forming a W/O type of emulsion. See *Ointments* (page 1585).

Emulsion Ointment Bases and Components

Emulsion ointment bases are actually semisolid emulsions. These preparations can be divided into two groups on the basis of emulsion type: emulsion ointment base water- in-oil (W/O) type and emulsion ointment base oil-in-water (O/W) type. Bases of both types will permit the incorporation of some additional amounts of water without reducing the consistency of the base below that of a soft cream. However, only O/W emulsion ointment bases can be removed readily from the skin and clothing with water. W/O emulsions are better emollients and protectants than are O/W emulsions. W/O emulsions can be diluted with oils.

Cetyl Alcohol

Cetostearyl Alcohol; "Palmityl" Alcohol; Aldol 52 (*Sherex*)

$CH_3(CH_2)_{14}CH_2OH$

1-Hexadecanol [124-29-8] $C_{16}H_{34}O$ (242.44); a mixture of not less than 90% of cetyl alcohol, the remainder chiefly stearyl alcohol.

Preparation—By catalytic hydrogenation of palmitic acid, or saponification of spermaceti, which contains cetyl palmitate.

Description—Unctuous, white flakes, granules, cubes or castings; faint characteristic odor and a bland, mild taste; melts 45 to 50°; not less than 90% distils between 316 and 336°.

Solubility—Insoluble in water; soluble in alcohol, chloroform, ether or vegetable oils.

Uses—Similar to *Stearyl Alcohol* (page 1399). It also imparts a smooth texture to the skin and is used widely in cosmetic creams and lotions.

Cold Cream

Petrolatum Rose Water Ointment USP XVI

Cetyl Esters Wax	**125 g**
White Wax	**120 g**
Mineral Oil	**560 g**
Sodium Borate	**5 g**
Purified Water	**190 mL**
To make about	**1000 g**

Reduce the cetyl esters wax and the white wax to small pieces, melt them on a steam bath with the mineral oil and continue heating until the temperature of the mixture reaches 70°. Dissolve the sodium borate in the purified water, warmed to 70° and gradually add the warm solution to the melted mixture, stirring rapidly and continuously until it has congealed.

If the ointment has been chilled, warm it slightly before attempting to incorporate other ingredients (see USP for allowable variations).

Uses—Useful as an emollient, cleansing cream and ointment base. It resembles *Rose Water Ointment*, differing only in that mineral oil is used in place of almond oil and omitting the fragrance. This change produces an ointment base which is not subject to rancidity like one containing a vegetable oil. This is a W/O emulsion.

Glyceryl Monostearate

Octadecanoic acid, monoester with 1,2,3-propanetriol

Monostearin [31566-31-1]; a mixture chiefly of variable proportions of glyceryl monostearate [$C_3H_5(OH)_2C_{18}H_{35}O_2$ = 358.56] and glyceryl monopalmitate [$C_3H_5(OH)_2C_{16}H_{31}O_2$ = 330.51].

Preparation—Among other ways, by reacting glycerin with commercial stearoyl chloride.

Description—White, wax-like solid or occurs in the form of white, wax-like beads, or flakes; slight, agreeable, fatty odor and taste; does not melt below 55°; affected by light.

Solubility—Insoluble in water, but may be dispersed in hot water with the aid of a small amount of soap or other suitable surface-active agent; dissolves in hot organic solvents such as alcohol, mineral or fixed oils, benzene, ether or acetone.

Uses—A thickening and emulsifying agent for ointments. See *Ointments* (page 1585).

Hydrophilic Ointment

Methylparaben	**0.25 g**
Propylparaben	**0.15 g**
Sodium Lauryl Sulfate	**10 g**
Propylene Glycol	**120 g**
Stearyl Alcohol	**250 g**
White Petrolatum	**250 g**
Purified Water	**370 g**
To make about	**1000 g**

Melt the stearyl alcohol and the white petrolatum on a steam bath, and warm to about 75°. Add the other ingredients, previously dissolved in the water and warmed to 75°, and stir the mixture until it congeals.

Uses—A *water-removable ointment base* for the so-called "washable" ointments. This is an O/W emulsion.

Lanolin

Hydrous Wool Fat

The purified, fat-like substance from the wool of sheep, *Ovis aries* Linné (Fam *Bovidae)*; contains 25 to 30% water.

Description—Yellowish white, ointment-like mass, having a slight, characteristic odor; when heated on a steam bath it separates into an upper oily and a lower water layer; when the water is evaporated a residue of *Lanolin* remains which is transparent when melted.

Solubility—Insoluble in water; soluble in chloroform or ether with separation of its water of hydration.

Uses—Largely as a vehicle for ointments, for which it is admirably adapted, on account of its compatibility with skin lipids. It emulsifies aqueous liquids. Lanolin is a W/O emulsion.

Rose Water Ointment

Cold Cream; Galen's Cerate

Cetyl Esters Wax	**125 g**
White Wax	**120 g**
Almond Oil	**560 g**
Sodium Borate	**5 g**
Stronger Rose Water	**25 mL**
Purified Water	**165 mL**
Rose Oil	**0.2 mL**
To make about	**1000 g**

Reduce the cetyl esters wax and the white wax to small pieces, melt them on a steam bath, add the almond oil and continue heating until the temperature of the mixture reaches 70°. Dissolve the sodium borate in the purifed water and stronger rose water, warmed to 70°, and gradually add the warm solution to the melted mixture, stirring rapidly and continuously until it has cooled to about 45°. Incorporate the rose oil.

It must be free from rancidity. If the ointment has been chilled, warm it slightly before attempting to incorporate other ingredients (see USP for allowable variations).

History—Originated by Galen, the famous Roman physician-pharmacist of the 1st century AD, was known for many centuries by the name of *Unguentum* or *Ceratum Refrigerans.* It has changed but little in proportions or method of preparation throughout many centuries.

Uses—An *emollient* and *ointment base.* It is a W/O emulsion.

Stearic Acid

Octadecanoic acid; Cetylacetic Acid; Stearophanic Acid

Stearic acid [57-11-4]; a mixture of stearic acid [$C_{18}H_{36}O_2$ = 284.48] and palmitic acid [$C_{16}H_{32}O_2$ = 256.43], which together constitute not less than 90.0% of the total content. The content of each is not less than 40.0% of the total.

Purified Stearic Acid USP is a mixture of the same acids which together constitute not less than 96.0% of the total content, and the content of $C_{18}H_{36}O_2$ is not less than 90.0% of the total.

Preparation—From edible fats and oils (see exception below) by boiling them with soda lye, separating the glycerin and decomposing the resulting soap with sulfuric or hydrochloric acid. The stearic acid subsequently is separated from any oleic acid by cold expression. It also is prepared by the hydrogenation and subsequent saponification of *olein.* It may be purified by recrystallization from alcohol.

Description—Hard, white or faintly yellowish somewhat glossy and crystalline solid, or a white or yellowish white powder; an odor and taste suggestive of tallow; melts about 55.5° and should not congeal at a temperature below 54°; the purified acid melts at 69 to 70° and congeals between 66 and 69°; slowly volatilizes between 90 and 100°.

Solubility—Practically insoluble in water; 1 g in about 20 mL alcohol, 2 mL chloroform, 3 mL ether, 25 mL acetone or 6 mL carbon tetrachloride; freely soluble in carbon disulfide; also soluble in amyl acetate, benzene or toluene.

Incompatibilities—Insoluble stearates are formed with many *metals.* Ointment bases made with stearic acid may show evidence of drying out or lumpiness due to such a reaction when *zinc* or *calcium* salts are compounded therein.

Uses—In the preparation of sodium stearate which is the solidifying agent for the official glycerin suppositories, in enteric tablet coating, ointments and for many other commercial products, such as toilet creams, vanishing creams, solidified alcohol, etc. (When labeled solely for external use, it is exempt from the requirement that it be prepared from edible fats and oils.)

Wool Alcohols BP—see RPS-18, page 1312.

Water-Soluble Ointment Bases and Components

Included in this section are bases prepared from the higher ethylene glycol polymers (PEG). These polymers are marketed under the trademark of Carbowax. The polymers have a wide range in molecular weight. Those with molecular weights ranging from 200 to 700 are liquids; those above 1000 are wax-like solids. The polymers are water-soluble, nonvolatile and unctuous agents. They do not hydrolyze or deteriorate and will not support mold growth. These properties account for their wide use in washable ointments. Mixtures of PEG are used to give bases of various consistency, such as very soft to hard bases for suppositories.

Glycol Ethers and Derivatives

This special class of ethers is of considerable importance in pharmaceutical technology. Both mono- and polyfunctional compounds are represented in the group. The simplest member is ethylene oxide [$\overline{CH_2CH_2O}$], the internal or cyclic ether of the simplest glycol, ethylene glycol [$HOCH_2CH_2OH$]. External mono- and diethers of ethylene glycol [$ROCH_2CH_2OH$ and $ROCH_2CH_2OR'$] are well-known due largely to research done by Union Carbide.

Preparation—In the presence of NaOH at temperatures of the order of 120° to 135° and under a total pressure of about 4 atmospheres, ethylene oxide reacts with ethylene glycol to form compounds having the general formula $HOCH_2(CH_2OCH_2)_nCH_2OH$, commonly referred to as condensation polymers and termed polyethylene (or polyoxyethylene) glycols. Other glycols besides ethylene glycol function in similar capacity, and the commercial generic term adopted for the entire group is polyalkylene (or polyoxyalkylene) glycols.

Nomenclature—It is to be noted that these condensation polymers are bifunctional; ie, they contain both ether and alcohol linkages. The compound wherein $n = 1$ is the commercially important diethylene glycol [$HOCH_2CH_2OCH_2CH_2OH$], and its internal ether is the familiar dioxane [$\overline{CH_2CH_2OCH_2CH_2O}$]. The mono- and diethers derived from diethylene glycol have the formulas $ROCH_2CH_2OCH_2CH_2OH$ and $ROCH_2CH_2OCH_2CH_2OR'$. The former commonly are termed "*Carbitols*" and the latter "*Cellosolves*," registered trademarks belonging to Union Carbide.

Polyethylene glycols are differentiated in commercial nomenclature by adding a number to the name which represents the average molecular weight. Thus, polyethylene glycol 400 has an average molecular weight of about 400 (measured values for commercial samples range between 380 and 420) corresponding to a value of n for this particular polymer of approximately 8. Polymers have been produced in which the value of n runs into the hundreds. Up to n = approximately 15, the compounds are liquids at room temperature, viscosity and boiling point increasing with increasing molecular weight. Higher polymers are waxy solids and are termed commercially *Carbowaxes* (another Union Carbide trademark).

It should be observed that the presence of the two terminal hydroxyl groups in the polyalkylene glycols makes possible the formation of both ether and ester derivatives, several of which are marketed products.

Uses—Because of their vapor pressure, solubility, solvent power, hygroscopicity, viscosity and lubricating characteristics, the polyalkylene glycols or their derivatives function in many applications as effective replacements for glycerin and water-insoluble oils. They find considerable use as plasticizers, lubricants, conditioners and finishing agents for processing textiles and rubber. They also are important as emulsifying agents and as dispersants for such diverse substances as dyes, oils, resins, insecticides and various types of pharmaceuticals. In addition, they are employed frequently as ingredients in ointment bases and in a variety of cosmetic preparations.

Polyethylene Glycols

Poly(oxy-1,2-ethanediyl), α-hydro-ω-hydroxy-, Carbowaxes (*Union Carbide*); Atpeg (*Zeneca*)

$$H—[OCH_2CH_2—]_nOH$$

Polyethylene glycols [25322-68-3].

Preparation—Ethylene glycol is reacted with ethylene oxide in the presence of NaOH at temperatures in the range of 120° to 135° under pressure of about 4 atm.

Description—*Polyethylene glycols 200, 300, 400* and *600* are clear, viscous liquids at room temperature. *Polyethylene glycols 900, 1000, 1450, 3350, 4500* and *8000* are white, waxy solids. The glycols do not hydrolyze or deteriorate under typical conditions. As their molecular weight increases, their water solubility, vapor pressure, hygroscopicity and solubility in organic solvents decrease; at the same time, freezing or melting range, specific gravity, flash point and viscosity increase. If these compounds ignite, small fires should be extinguished with carbon dioxide or dry-chemical extinguishers and large fires with "alcohol"-type foam extinguishers.

Solubility—All members of this class dissolve in water to form clear solutions and are soluble in many organic solvents.

Uses—These possess a wide range of solubilities and compatibilities, which make them useful in pharmaceutical and cosmetic preparations. Their blandness renders them highly acceptable for hair dressings, hand lotions, sun-tan creams, leg lotions, shaving creams and skin creams (eg, a peroxide ointment which is stable may be prepared using these compounds, while oil-type bases inactivate the peroxide). Their use in washable ointments is discussed under *Ointments* (page 1585). They also are used in making suppositories, hormone creams, etc. See *Polyethylene Glycol Ointment* (below) and *Glycol Ethers* (above). The liquid polyethylene glycol 400 and the solid polyethylene glycol 3350, used in the proportion specified (or a permissible variation thereof) in the official Polyethylene Glycol Ointment, provide a water-soluble ointment base used in the formulation of many dermatological preparations. The solid, waxy, water-soluble glycols often are used to increase the viscosity of liquid polyethylene glycols and to stiffen ointment and suppository bases. In addition, they are used to compensate for the melting point-lowering effect of other agents, ie, chloral hydrate, etc, on such bases.

Polyethylene Glycol Ointment USP—*Preparation:* Heat polyethylene glycol 3350 (400 g) and polyethylene glycol 400 (600 g) on a water bath to 65°. Allow to cool, and stir until congealed. If a firmer preparation is desired, replace up to 100 g of polyethylene glycol 400 with an equal amount of polyethylene glycol 3350. If 6 to 25% of an aqueous solution is to be incorporated in this ointment, replace 50 g of polyethylene glycol 3350 by 50 g of stearyl alcohol. *Uses:* A water-soluble ointment base.

Polyoxyl 40 Stearate

Poly(oxy-1,2-ethanediyl), α-hydro-ω-hydroxy-, octadecanoate; Myrj (*Zeneca*)

$$RCOO(C_2H_4O)_nH$$

($RCOO$ is the stearate moiety; n is approximately **40**)

Polyethylene glycol monostearate [9004-99-3]; a mixture of monostearate and distearate esters of mixed polyoxyethylene diols and corresponding free glycols, the average polymer length being equivalent to about 40 oxyethylene units. *Polyoxyethylene 50 Stearate* is a similar mixture in which the average polymer length is equivalent to about 50 oxyethylene units.

Preparation—One method consists of heating the corresponding polyethylene glycol with an equimolar portion of stearic acid.

Description—White to light-tan waxy solid; odorless or has a faint fat-like odor; congeals between 37 and 47°.

Solubility—Soluble in water, alcohol, ether or acetone; insoluble in mineral or vegetable oils.

Uses—Contains ester and alcohol functions that impart both lyophilic and hydrophilic characteristics to make it useful as a surfactant and emulsifier. It is an ingredient of some water-soluble ointment and cream bases.

Polysorbates

Sorbitan esters, poly(oxy-1,2-ethanediyl) derivs, Tweens (*Zeneca*)

$HO(C_2H_4O)_w$ ... $(OC_2H_4)_xOH$; H; $C(OC_2H_4)_yOH$; $H_2C(OC_2H_4)_zR$

[Sum of $w, x, y,$ and z is 20; R is $(C_{11}H_{23})COO$]

Sorbitan esters, polyoxyethylene derivatives; fatty acid esters of sorbitol and its anhydrides copolymerized with a varying number of moles of ethylene oxide. The NF recognizes: *Polysorbate 20 (structure given above)*, a laurate ester; *Polysorbate 40*, a palmitate ester; *Polysorbate 60*, a mixture of stearate and palmitate esters; and *Polysorbate 80*, an oleate ester.

Preparation—These important nonionic surfactants (page 239) are prepared starting with sorbitol by (1) elimination of water- forming sorbitan (a cyclic sorbitol anhydride); (2) partial esterification of the sorbitan with a fatty acid such as oleic or stearic acid yielding a hexitan ester known commercially as a *Span* and (3) chemical addition of ethylene oxide yielding a *Tween* (the polyoxyethylene derivative).

Description—*Polysorbate 80:* Lemon- to amber-colored, oily liquid; faint, characteristic odor; warm, somewhat bitter taste; specific gravity 1.07 to 1.09; pH (1:20 aqueous solution) 6 to 8.

Solubility—*Polysorbate 80:* Very soluble in water, producing an odorless and nearly colorless solution; soluble in alcohol, cottonseed oil, corn oil, ethyl acetate, methanol or toluene; insoluble in mineral oil.

Uses—Because of their hydrophilic and lyophilic characteristics, these nonionic surfactants are very useful as emulsifying agents forming O/W emulsions in pharmaceuticals, cosmetics and other types of products. Polysorbate 80 is an ingredient in *Coal Tar Ointment* and *Solution.* See *Glycol Ethers* (page 1403).

Other Water-Soluble Ointment Base Component

Polyethylene Glycol 400 Monostearate USP XVI—An ether, alcohol and ester. Semitransparent, whitish, odorless or nearly odorless mass; melts from 30 to 34°. Freely soluble in carbon tetrachloride, chloroform, ether or petroleum benzin; slightly soluble in alcohol; insoluble in water. *Uses:* A nonionic surface-active agent in the preparation of creams, lotions, ointments and similar pharmaceutical preparations, which are readily soluble in water.

Pharmaceutical Solvents

The remarkable growth of the solvent industry is attested by the more than 300 solvents now being produced on an industrial scale. Chemically, these include a great variety of organic compounds, ranging from hydrocarbons through alcohols, esters, ethers and acids to nitroparaffins. Their main applications are in industry and the synthesis of organic chemicals. Comparatively few, however, are used as solvents in pharmacy, because of their toxicity, volatility, instability and/or flammability. Those commonly used as pharmaceutical solvents are described in this section.

Acetone

2-Propanone; Dimethyl Ketone

CH_3COCH_3

Acetone [67-64-1] C_3H_6O (58.08).

Caution—It is very flammable. Do not use where it may be ignited.

Preparation—Formerly obtained exclusively from the destructive distillation of wood. The distillate, consisting principally of methanol, acetic acid and acetone was neutralized with lime and the acetone was separated from the methyl alcohol by fractional distillation. Additional quantities were obtained by pyrolysis of the calcium acetate formed in the neutralization of the distillate.

It now is obtained largely as a by-product of the butyl alcohol industry. This alcohol is formed in the fermentation of carbohydrates such as corn starch, molasses, etc, by the action of the bacterium *Clostridium acetobutylicum* (Weizmann fermentation) and it is always one of the products formed in the process. It also is obtained by the catalytic oxidation of isopropyl alcohol, which is prepared from propylene resulting from the "cracking" of crude petroleum.

Description—Transparent, colorless, mobile, volatile, flammable liquid with a characteristic odor; specific gravity not more than 0.789; distils between 55.5 and 57°; congeals about −95°; aqueous solution neutral to litmus.

Solubility—Miscible with water, alcohol, ether, chloroform or most volatile oils.

Uses—An *antiseptic* in concentrations above 80%. In combination with alcohol it is used as an antiseptic *cleansing* solution. It is employed as a menstruum in the preparation of oleoresins in place of ether. It is used as a *solvent* for dissolving fatty bodies, resins, pyroxylin, mercurials, etc, and also in the manufacture of many organic compounds such as chloroform, chlorobutanol and ascorbic acid.

Alcohol

Ethanol; Spiritus Vini Rectificatus; S. V. R.; Spirit of Wine; Methylcarbinol

Ethyl alcohol [64-17-5]; contains 92.3 to 93.8%, by weight (94.9 to 96.0%, by volume), at 15.56° (60°F) of C_2H_5OH (46.07).

Preparation—Has been made for centuries by fermentation of certain carbohydrates in the presence of *zymase,* an enzyme present in yeast cells. Usable carbohydrate-containing materials include molasses, sugar cane, fruit juices, corn, barley, wheat, potato, wood and waste sulfite liquors. As yeast is capable of fermenting only D-glucose, D-fructose, D-mannose and D-galactose it is essential that more complex carbohydrates, such as starch, be converted to one or more of these simple sugars before they can be fermented. This is accomplished variously, commonly by enzyme- or acid-catalyzed hydrolysis.

The net reaction that occurs when a hexose, glucose for example, is fermented to alcohol may be represented as

$$C_6H_{12}O_6 \rightarrow 2C_2H_5OH + 2CO_2$$

but the mechanism of the process is very complex. The fermented liquid, containing about 15% of alcohol, is distilled to obtain a distillate containing 94.9% of C_2H_5OH, by volume. To produce *absolute alcohol,* the 95% product is dehydrated by various processes.

It may be produced also by hydration of ethylene, abundant supplies of which are available from natural and coke oven gases, from waste gases of the petroleum industry and other sources. In another synthesis acetylene is hydrated catalytically to acetaldehyde, which then is hydrogenated catalytically to ethyl alcohol.

Description—Transparent, colorless, mobile, volatile liquid; slight but characteristic odor; burning taste; boils at 78° but volatilizes even at a low temperature, and is flammable; when pure, it is neutral towards all indicators; specific gravity at 15.56° (the US Government standard temperature for Alcohol) not above 0.816, indicating not less than 92.3% of C_2H_5OH by weight or 94.9% by volume.

Solubility—Miscible with water, acetone, chloroform, ether or many other organic solvents.

Incompatibilities—This and preparations containing a high percentage of alcohol will precipitate many inorganic salts from an aqueous solution. *Acacia* generally is precipitated from a hydroalcoholic medium when the alcohol content is greater than about 35%.

Strong *oxidizing agents* such as *chlorine, nitric acid, permanganate* or *chromate* in acid solution react, in some cases violently, with it to produce oxidation products.

Alkalies cause a darkening in color due to the small amount of aldehyde usually present in it.

Uses—In pharmacy principally for its solvent powers (page 204). It also is used as the starting point in the manufacture of many important compounds, like ether, chloroform, etc. It also is used as a fuel, chiefly in the denatured form.

It is a CNS depressant. Consequently, it occasionally has been administered intravenously for preoperative and postoperative sedation in patients in whom other measures are ineffective or contraindicated. The dose employed is 1 to 1.5 mL/kg. Its intravenous use is a specialized procedure and should be employed only by one experienced in the technique of such use.

It is used widely and abused by lay persons as a sedative. It has, however, no medically approved use for this purpose. Moreover, alcohol potentiates the CNS effects of numerous sedative and depressant drugs. Hence, it should not be used by patients taking certain prescription drugs or OTC medications (see page 1822).

Externally, it has a number of medical uses. It is a solvent for the toxicodendrol causing *ivy poisoning,* and should be used to wash the skin thoroughly soon after contact. In a concentration of 25% it is employed for bathing the skin for the purpose of *cooling* and *reducing fevers.* In high concentrations it is a *rubefacient* and an ingredient of many liniments. In a concentration of 50% it is used to prevent sweating in *astringent* and *anhidrotic* lotions. It also is employed to cleanse and harden the skin and is helpful in preventing *bedsores* in bedridden patients. In a concentration of 60 to 90% it is germicidal. At optimum concentration (70% by weight) it is a good *antiseptic* for the skin (*local anti-infective*) and also for instruments. It also is used as a *solvent* to cleanse the skin splashed with phenol. High concentrations of it often are injected into nerves and ganglia for the *relief of pain,* accomplishing this by causing nerve degeneration.

Denatured Alcohol

An act of Congress June 7, 1906, authorizes the withdrawal of alcohol from bond without the payment of internal revenue tax, for the purpose of denaturation and use in the arts and industries. This is ethyl alcohol to which have been added such denaturing materials as to render the alcohol unfit for use as an intoxicating beverage. It is divided into two classes, namely, *completely denatured alcohol* and *specially denatured alcohol,* prepared in accordance with approved formulas prescribed in Federal Industrial Alcohol Regulations 3.

Information regarding the use of alcohol and permit requirements may be obtained from the Regional Director, Bureau of Alcohol, Tobacco and

Firearms, in any of the following offices: Cincinnati, OH; Philadelphia, PA; Chicago, IL; New York, NY; Atlanta, GA; Dallas, TX and San Francisco, CA. Federal regulation provides that completely and specially denatured alcohols may be purchased by properly qualified persons from duly established denaturing plants or bonded dealers. No permit is required for the purchase and use of completely denatured alcohol unless the purchaser intends to recover the alcohol.

Completely Denatured Alcohol—This term applies to ethyl alcohol to which has been added materials (methyl isobutyl ketone, pyronate, gasoline, acetaldol, kerosene, etc) of such nature that the products may be sold and used within certain limitations without permit and bond.

Specially Denatured Alcohol—This alcohol is intended for use in a greater number of specified arts and industries than completely denatured alcohol and the character of the denaturant or denaturants used is such that specially denatured alcohol may be sold, possessed and used only by those persons or firms that hold basic permits and are covered by bond.

Formulas for products using specially denatured alcohol must be approved prior to use by the Regional Director, Bureau of Alcohol, Tobacco and Firearms in any of the regional offices listed above.

Uses—Approximately 50 specially denatured alcohol formulas containing combinations of more than 90 different denaturants are available to fill the needs of qualified users. Large amounts of specially denaturated alcohols are used as raw materials in the production of acetaldehyde, synthetic rubber, vinegar and ethyl chloride as well as in the manufacture of proprietary solvents and cleaning solutions. Ether and chloroform can be made from suitably denatured alcohols and formulas for the manufacture of Iodine Tincture, Green Soap Tincture and Rubbing Alcohol are set forth in the regulations.

Specially denatured alcohols also are used as solvents for surface coatings, plastics, inks, toilet preparations and external pharmaceuticals. Large quantities are used in the processing of such food and drug products as pectin, vitamins, hormones, antibiotics, alkaloids and blood products. Other uses include supplemental motor fuel, rocket and jet fuel, antifreeze solutions, refrigerants and cutting oils. Few products are manufactured today that do not require the use of alcohol at some stage of production. Specially denatured alcohol may not be used in the manufacture of foods or internal medicines where any of the alcohol remains in the finished product.

Diluted Alcohol

Diluted Ethanol

A mixture of alcohol and water containing 41.0 to 42.0%, by weight (48.4 to 49.5%, by volume), at 15.56°, of C_2H_5OH (46.07).

Preparation—

Alcohol	**500 mL**
Purified Water	**500 mL**

Measure the alcohol and the purified water separately at the same temperature, and mix. If the water and the alcohol and the resulting mixture are measured at 25°, the volume of the mixture will be about 970 mL.

When equal volumes of alcohol and water are mixed together, a rise in temperature and a contraction of about 3% in volume take place. In small operations the contraction generally is disregarded; in larger operations it is very important. If 50 gal of official alcohol are mixed with 50 gal of water, the product will not be 100 gal of diluted alcohol, but only 96¼ gal, a contraction of 3¾ gal. US *Proof Spirit* differs from this and is stronger; it contains 50%, by volume, of absolute alcohol at 15.56° (60°F). This corresponds to 42.5% by weight, and has a specific gravity of 0.9341 at the same temperature. If spirits have a specific gravity lower than that of "proof spirit" (0.9341), they are said to be "*above proof*"; if greater, "*below proof*."

It also may be prepared from the following:

Alcohol	**408 g**
Purified Water	**500 g**

Rules for Dilution—The following rules are applied when making an alcohol of any required lower percentage from an alcohol of any given higher percentage:

I. By Volume—Designate the volume percentage of the stronger alcohol by *V*, and that of the weaker alcohol by *v*.

Rule—Mix *v* volumes of the stronger alcohol with purified water to make *V* volumes of product. Allow the mixture to stand until full contraction has taken place, and until it has cooled, then make up the deficiency in the *V* volumes by adding more purified water.

Example—An alcohol of 30% by volume is to be made from an alcohol of 94.9% by volume.—Take 30 volumes of the 94.9% alcohol, and add enough purified water to produce 94.9 volumes at room temperature.

II. By Weight—Designate the weight-percentage of the stronger alcohol by *W*, and that of the weaker alcohol by *w*.

Rule—Mix *w* parts by weight of the stronger alcohol with purified water to make *W* parts by weight of product.

Example—An alcohol of 50% by weight is to be made from an alcohol of 92.3% by weight.—Take 50 parts by weight of the 92.3% alcohol, and add enough purified water to produce 92.3 parts by weight.

Description—As for *Alcohol*, except its specific gravity is 0.935 to 0.937 at 15.56°, indicating that the strength of C_2H_5OH corresponds to that given in the official definition.

Uses—A menstruum in making tinctures, fluidextracts, extracts, etc. Its properties already have been described fully in connection with the various preparations. Its value consists not only in its *antiseptic* properties, but also in its possessing the *solvent* powers of both water and alcohol. See *Alcohol*.

Nonbeverage Alcohol

This is tax-paid alcohol or distilled spirits used in the manufacture, by approved formula, of such medicines, medicinal preparations, food products, flavors or flavoring extracts as are unfit for beverage purposes. Internal Revenue Service Regulations provide that qualified holders of Special Tax Stamps who use tax paid alcohol or distilled spirits in the types of products listed above, may file a claim for *alcohol tax drawback* or refund of a considerable part of the tax paid.

Amylene Hydrate—see RPS-18, page 1316.

Chloroform—page 1409.

Coconut Oil—see RPS-18, page 1317.

Ether—see RPS-18, page 1041.

Ethyl Acetate—see RPS-18, page 1294.

Glycerin

1,2,3-Propanetriol; Glycerol

$$HOCH_2CH(OH)CH_2OH$$

Glycerol [56-81-5] $C_3H_8O_3$ (92.09).

Chemically, it is the simplest trihydric alcohol. It is worthy of special note because the two terminal alcohol groups are primary, whereas the middle one is secondary. Thus this becomes the first polyhydric alcohol which can yield both an aldose (*glyceraldehyde*) and a ketose (*dihydroxyacetone*).

Preparation—

1. By saponification of fats and oils in the manufacture of soap.
2. By hydrolysis of fats and oils through pressure and superheated steam.
3. By fermentation of beet sugar molasses in the presence of large amounts of sodium sulfite. Under these conditions a reaction takes place expressed as

$$\underset{\text{Glucose}}{C_6H_{12}O_6} \rightarrow \underset{\text{Glycerin}}{C_3H_5(OH)_3} + \underset{\text{Acetaldehyde}}{CH_3CHO} + CO_2$$

4. Glycerin is now prepared in large quantities from propylene, a petroleum product. This hydrocarbon is chlorinated at about 400° to form allyl chloride, which is converted to allyl alcohol. Treatment of the unsaturated alcohol with hypochlorous acid [HOCl] yields the chlorohydrin derivative. Extraction of HCl with soda lime yields 2,3-epoxypropanol which undergoes hydration to glycerin.

Description—Clear, colorless, syrupy liquid with a sweet taste and not more than a slight, characteristic odor, which is neither harsh nor disagreeable; when exposed to moist air it absorbs water and also such gases as H_2S and SO_2; solutions are neutral; specific gravity not below 1.249 (not less than 95% $C_3H_5(OH)_3$); boils at about 290° under 1 atm, with decomposition, but can be distilled intact in a vacuum.

Solubility—Miscible with water, alcohol or methanol; 1 g in about 12 mL ethyl acetate or about 15 mL acetone; insoluble in chloroform, ether or fixed and volatile oils.

Incompatibilities—An explosion may occur if it is triturated with strong *oxidizing agents* such as *chromium trioxide, potassium chlorate* or *potassium permanganate*. In dilute solutions the reactions proceed at a slower rate forming several oxidation products. Iron is an occasional contaminant of it and may be the cause of a darkening in color in mixtures containing *phenols, salicylates, tannin,* etc.

With *boric acid* or *sodium borate*, it forms a complex, generally spoken of as glyceroboric acid, which is a much stronger acid than boric acid.

Uses—One of the most valuable products known to pharmacy by virtue of its *solvent* property. It is useful as a *humectant* in keeping substances moist, owing to its hygroscopicity. Its agreeable taste and high viscosity adapt it for many purposes. Some modern ice collars and ice bags contain it and water hermetically sealed within vulcanized rubber bags. The latter are sterilized by dipping in a germicidal solution and are stored in the refrigerator until needed. It also has some therapeutic uses. In pure anhydrous form, it is used in the eye to reduce corneal edema and to facilitate ophthalmoscopic examination. It is used orally as an evacuant and, in 50 to 75% solution, as a systemic osmotic agent.

Isopropyl Alcohol—page 1267.

Methyl Alcohol

Methanol; Wood Alcohol

CH_3OH

Methanol [67-56-1] CH_4O (32.04).

Caution—It is poisonous.

Preparation—By the catalytic reduction of carbon monoxide or carbon dioxide with hydrogen. A zinc oxide-chromium oxide catalyst is used commonly.

Description—Clear, colorless liquid; characteristic odor; flammable; specific gravity not more than 0.790; distils within a range of 1° between 63.5 and 65.7°.

Solubility—Miscible with water, alcohol, ether, benzene or most other organic solvents.

Uses—*A pharmaceutic aid* (solvent). It is toxic. Ingestion may result in blindness; vapors also may cause toxic reactions.

Methyl Isobutyl Ketone

2-Pentanone, 4-methyl-,

$(CH_3)_2CHCH_2COCH_3$

[108-10-1]; contains not less than 99% of $C_6H_{12}O$ (100.16).

Description—Transparent, colorless, mobile, volatile liquid; faint, ketonic and camphoraceous odor, distils between 114 and 117°.

Solubility—Slightly soluble in water; miscible with alcohol, ether or benzene.

Uses—A *denaturant* for rubbing alcohol and also a *solvent* for gums, resins, nitrocellulose, etc. It may be irritating to the eyes and mucous membranes, and, in high concentrations, narcotic.

Monoethanolamine

Ethanol, 2-amino-, Ethanolamine; Ethylolamine

$HOCH_2CH_2NH_2$

[141-43-5] C_2H_7NO (61.08).

Preparation—This alkanolamine is prepared conveniently by treating ethylene oxide with ammonia.

Description—Clear, colorless, moderately viscous liquid; distinctly ammoniacal odor; affected by light; specific gravity 1.013 to 1.016; distils between 167 and 173°.

Solubility—Miscible in all proportions with water, acetone, alcohol, glycerin or chloroform; immiscible with ether, solvent hexane or fixed oils; dissolves many essential oils.

Uses—A *solvent* for fats, oils and many other substances, it is a pharmaceutical necessity for *Thimerosal Solution* (page 1271). It combines with fatty acids to form soaps which find application in various types of emulsions such as lotions, creams, etc.

Petroleum Benzin—see RPS-18, page 1317.

Propylene Glycol

$CH_3CH(OH)CH_2OH$

1,2-Propanediol [57-55-6] $C_3H_8O_2$ (76.10).

Preparation—Propylene is converted successively to its chlorohydrin (with HOCl), epoxide (with Na_2CO_3) and glycol (with water in presence of protons).

Description—Clear, colorless, viscous and practically odorless liquid; slightly acrid taste; specific gravity 1.035 to 1.037; completely distils between 184 and 189°; absorbs moisture from moist air.

Solubility—Miscible with water, alcohol, acetone or chloroform; soluble in ether; dissolves many volatile oils; immiscible with fixed oils.

Uses—A *solvent, preservative* and *humectant.* See *Hydrophilic Ointment* (page 1402).

Trolamine

Ethanol, 2,2′,2″-nitrilotris-, Triethanolamine

2,2′,2″-Nitrilotriethanol [102-71-6] $N(C_2H_4OH)_3$ (149.19); a mixture of alkanolamines consisting largely of triethanolamine, containing some diethanolamine [$NH(C_2H_4OH)_2$ = 105.14] and monoethanolamine [$NH_2C_2H_4OH$ = 61.08].

Preparation—Along with some mono- and diethanolamine, by the action of ammonia on ethylene oxide.

Description—Colorless to pale yellow, viscous, hygroscopic liquid; slight odor of ammonia; aqueous solution is very alkaline; melts about 21°; specific gravity 1.120 to 1.128; a strong base and readily combines even with weak acids to form salts.

Solubility—Miscible with water or alcohol; soluble in chloroform; slightly soluble in ether or benzene.

Uses—In combination with a fatty acid, eg, oleic acid (see *Benzyl Benzoate Lotion,* page 1519), as an *emulsifier.* See *Monoethanolamine.*

Water—page 1392.

Other Pharmaceutical Solvents

Alcohol, Dehydrated, BP, PhI [Dehydrated Ethanol; Absolute Alcohol]—Transparent, colorless, mobile, volatile liquid; characteristic odor; burning taste; specific gravity not more than 0.798 at 15.56°; hygroscopic, flammable and boils about 78°C. Miscible with water, ether or chloroform. *Uses:* A pharmaceutical solvent; also used by injection for relief of pain (see *Alcohol,* page 1404).

Miscellaneous Pharmaceutical Necessities

The agents listed in this section comprise a heterogeneous group of substances with both pharmaceutical and industrial applications. Pharmaceutically, some of these agents are used as diluents, enteric coatings, excipients, filtering agents and as ingredients in products considered in other chapters. Industrially, some of these agents are used in various chemical processes, in the synthesis of other chemicals and in the manufacture of fertilizers, explosives, etc.

Acetic Acid

Acetic acid; a solution containing 36 to 37%, by weight, of $C_2H_4O_2$ (60.05).

Preparation—By diluting with distilled water an acid of higher concentration, such as the 80% product, or more commonly glacial acetic acid, using 350 mL of the latter for the preparation of each 1000 mL of acetic acid.

Description—Clear, colorless liquid, having a strong characteristic odor and a sharply acid taste; specific gravity about 1.045; congeals about −14°; acid to litmus.

Solubility—Miscible with water, alcohol or glycerin.

Uses—In pharmacy as a *solvent* and *menstruum,* and for making diluted acetic acid. It also is used as a starting point in the manufacture of many other organic compounds, eg, acetates, acetanilid, sulfonamides, etc. It is official primarily as a *pharmaceutic necessity* for the preparation of *Aluminum Subacetate Solution* (RPS-17, page 778).

Diluted Acetic Acid

Dilute Acetic Acid

A solution containing, in each 100 mL, 5.7 to 6.3 g of $C_2H_4O_2$.

Preparation—

Acetic Acid	**158 mL**
Purified Water, a sufficient quantity,	
To make	**1000 mL**

Mix the ingredients.

Note—This acid also may be prepared by diluting 58 mL of glacial acetic acid with sufficient purified water to make 1000 mL.

Description—Essentially the same properties, solubility, purity and identification reactions as *Acetic Acid,* but its specific gravity is about 1.008 and it congeals about −2°.

Uses—*Bactericidal* to many types of microorganisms and occasionally is used in 1% solution for surgical dressings of the skin. A 1% solution is *spermatocidal.* It also is used in vaginal douches for the management of *Trichomonas, Candida* and *Hemophilus* infections.

Glacial Acetic Acid

Concentrated Acetic Acid; Crystallizable Acetic Acid; Ethanolic Acid; Vinegar Acid

CH_3COOH

Glacial acetic acid [64-19-7] $C_2H_4O_2$ (60.05).

Preparation—This acid is termed "glacial" because of its solid, glassy appearance when congealed. In one process it is produced by distillation of weaker acids to which has been added a water-entraining substance such as ethylene dichloride. In this method, referred to as "azeotropic distillation," the ethylene dichloride distils out with the water before the acid distils over, thereby effecting concentration of the latter.

In another process the aqueous acid is mixed with triethanol-amine and heated. The acid combines with the triethanolamine to form a triethanolamine acetate. The water is driven off first; then, at a higher temperature, the triethanolamine compound decomposes to yield this acid.

A greater part of the acid now available is made synthetically from acetylene. When acetylene is passed into this acid containing a metallic catalyst such as mercuric oxide, ethylidene diacetate is produced which yields, upon heating, acetic anhydride and acetaldehyde. Hydration of the former and air oxidation of the latter yield this acid.

Description—Clear, colorless liquid; pungent, characteristic odor; when well-diluted with water, it has an acid taste; boils about 118°; congeals at a temperature not lower than 15.6°, corresponding to a minimum of 99.4% of CH_3COOH; specific gravity about 1.05.

Solubility—Miscible with water, alcohol, acetone, ether or glycerin; insoluble in carbon tetrachloride or chloroform.

Uses—A *caustic* and *vesicant* when applied externally and is often sold under various disguises as a *corn solvent.* It is an excellent *solvent* for fixed and volatile oils and many other organic compounds. It is used primarily as an *acidifying agent.*

Almond Oil—RPS-16, page 720.

Aluminum

Aluminim Al (26.98); the free metal in the form of finely divided powder. It may contain oleic acid or stearic acid as a lubricant. It contains not less than 95% of Al, and not more than 5% of *Acid-insoluble substances,* including any added fatty acid.

Description—Very fine, free-flowing, silvery powder free from gritty or discolored particles.

Solubility—Insoluble in water or alcohol; soluble in hydrochloric and sulfuric acids or in solutions of fixed alkali hydroxides.

Uses—A *protective.* An ingredient in *Aluminum Paste* (RPS-14, page 772).

Aluminum Monostearate

Aluminum, dihydroxy(octadecanoato-*O*-)-,

Dihydroxy(stearato)aluminum [7047-84-9]; a compound of aluminum with a mixture of solid organic acids obtained from fats, and consists chiefly of variable proportions of aluminum monostearate and aluminum monopalmitate. It contains the equivalent of 14.5 to 16.5% of Al_2O_3 (101.96).

Preparation—By interaction of a hydroalcoholic solution of potassium stearate with an aqueous solution of potassium alum, the precipitate being purified to remove free stearic acid and some aluminum distearate simultaneously produced.

Description—Fine, white to yellowish white, bulky powder; faint, characteristic odor.

Solubility—Insoluble in water, alcohol or ether.

Uses—A *pharmaceutical necessity* used in the preparation of *Sterile Procaine Penicillin G with Aluminum Stearate Suspension* (see RPS-18, page 1288).

Strong Ammonia Solution

Stronger Ammonia Water; Stronger Ammonium Hydroxide Solution; Spirit of Hartshorn

Ammonia [1336-21-6]; a solution of NH_3 (17.03), containing 27.0 to 31.0% (*w/w*) of NH_3. Upon exposure to air it loses ammonia rapidly.

Caution—Use care in handling it because of the caustic nature of the Solution and the irritating properties of its vapor. Cool the container well before opening, and cover the closure with a cloth or similar material while opening. Do not taste it, and avoid inhalation of its vapor.

Preparation—Ammonia is obtained commercially chiefly by synthesis from its constituent elements, nitrogen and hydrogen, combined under high pressure and at high temperature in the presence of a catalyst.

Description—Colorless, transparent liquid; exceedingly pungent, characteristic odor; even when well-diluted it is strongly alkaline to litmus; specific gravity about 0.90.

Solubility—Miscible with alcohol.

Uses—Only for chemical and pharmaceutical purposes. It is used primarily in making ammonia water by dilution and as a chemical reagent. It is too strong for internal administration. It is an ingredient in *Aromatic Ammonia Spirit* (page 873).

Bismuth Subnitrate

Basic Bismuth Nitrate; Bismuth Oxynitrate; Spanish White; Bismuth Paint; Bismuthyl Nitrate

Bismuth hydroxide nitrate oxide [1304-85-4] $Bi_5O(OH)_9(NO_3)_4$ (1461.99); a basic salt which, dried at 105° for 2 hr, yields upon ignition not less than 79% of Bi_2O_3 (465.96).

Preparation—A solution of bismuth nitrate is added to boiling water to produce the subnitrate by hydrolysis.

Description—White, slightly hygroscopic powder; suspension in distilled water is faintly acid to litmus (pH about 5).

Solubility—Practically insoluble in water or organic solvents; dissolves readily in an excess of hydrochloric or nitric acid.

Incompatibilities—Slowly hydrolyzed in *water* with liberation of nitric acid; thus, it possesses the incompatibilities of the acid. *Reducing agents* darken it with the production of metallic bismuth.

Uses—A *pharmaceutical necessity* in the preparation of milk of bismuth. It also is used as an *astringent, adsorbent* and *protective;* however, its value as a protective is questionable. This agent, like other insoluble bismuth salts, is used topically in lotions and ointments.

Barium Hydroxide Lime—see RPS-18, page 1318.

Boric Acid

Boric acid (H_3BO_3); Boracic Acid; Orthoboric Acid

Boric acid [10043-35-3] H_3BO_3 (61.83).

Preparation—Lagoons of the volcanic districts of Tuscany formerly furnished the greater part of this acid and borax of commerce. Borax is now found native in California and some of the other western states; calcium and magnesium borates are found there also. It is produced from native borax, or from the other borates, by reacting with hydrochloric or sulfuric acid.

Description—Colorless scales of a somewhat pearly luster, or crystals, but more commonly a white powder slightly unctuous to the touch; odorless and stable in the air; volatilizes with steam.

Solubility—1 g in 18 mL water, 18 mL alcohol, 4 mL glycerin, 4 mL boiling water or 6 mL boiling alcohol.

Uses—A buffer, and it is this use that is recognized officially. It is a very weak *germicide* (*local anti-infective*). Its nonirritating properties make its solutions suitable for application to such delicate structures as the cornea of the eye. Aqueous solutions are employed as an eye wash, mouth wash and for irrigation of the bladder. A 2.2% solution is isotonic with lacrimal fluid. Solutions, even if they are made isotonic, will hemolyze red blood cells. It also is employed as a dusting powder, when diluted with some inert material. It can be absorbed through irritated skin, eg, infants with diaper rash.

Although it is not absorbed significantly from intact skin, it is absorbed from damaged skin and fatal poisoning, particularly in infants, has occurred with topical application to burns, denuded areas, granulation tissue and serous cavities. *Serious poisoning can result from oral ingestion* of as little as 5 g. Symptoms of poisoning are nausea, vomiting, abdominal pain, diarrhea, headache and visual disturbance. Toxic alopecia has been reported from the chronic ingestion of a mouth wash containing it. The kidney may be injured and death may result. Its use as a preservative in beverages and foods is prohibited by national and state legislation. *There is always present the danger of confusing it with dextrose when compounding milk formulas for infants. Fatal accidents have occurred.* For this reason boric acid in bulk is colored, so that it cannot be confused with dextrose.

It is used to prevent discoloration of physostigmine solutions.

Dose—*Topically,* as required.

Calcium Hydroxide

Slaked Lime; Calcium Hydrate

Calcium hydroxide [1305-62-0] $Ca(OH)_2$ (74.09).

Preparation—By reacting freshly prepared calcium oxide with water.

Description—White powder; alkaline, slightly bitter taste; absorbs carbon dioxide from the air forming calcium carbonate; solutions exhibit a strong alkaline reaction.

Solubility—1 g in 630 mL water or 1300 mL boiling water; soluble in glycerin or syrup; insoluble in alcohol; the solubility in water is decreased by the presence of fixed alkali hydroxides.

Uses—In the preparation of *Calcium Hydroxide Solution.*

Calcium Hydroxide Topical Solution

Calcium Hydroxide Solution; Lime Water

A solution containing, in each 100 mL, not less than 140 mg of $Ca(OH)_2$ (74.09).

Note—The solubility of calcium hydroxide varies with the temperature at which the solution is stored, being about 170 mg/100 mL at 15°, and less at a higher temperature. The official concentration is based upon a temperature of 25°.

Preparation—

Calcium Hydroxide	**3 g**
Purified Water	**1000 mL**

Add the calcium hydroxide to 1000 mL of cool, purified water, and agitate the mixture vigorously and repeatedly during 1 hr. Allow the excess of calcium hydroxide to settle. Dispense only the clear, supernatant liquid.

The undissolved portion of the mixture is not suitable for preparing additional quantities of the solution.

The object of keeping lime water over undissolved calcium hydroxide is to insure a saturated solution.

Description—Clear, colorless liquid; alkaline taste; strong alkaline reaction; absorbs carbon dioxide from the air, a film of calcium carbonate forming on the surface of the liquid; when heated, it becomes turbid, owing to the separation of calcium hydroxide, which is less soluble in hot than in cold water.

Uses—Too dilute to be effective as a gastric antacid. It is employed *topically* as a *protective* in various types of lotions. In some lotion formulations it is used with olive oil or oleic acid to form calcium oleate that functions as an emulsifying agent. The USP classes it as an *astringent.*

Dose—*Topically,* in astringent solutions and lotions as required (see *Calamine Lotion,* page 872).

Calcium Pantothenate, Racemic—page 1125.

Calcium Stearate

Octadecanoic acid, calcium salt

Calcium stearate [1592-23-0]; a compound of calcium with a mixture of solid organic acids obtained from fats and consists chiefly of variable proportions of stearic and palmitic acids [calcium stearate, $C_{36}H_{70}CaO_4$ = 607.03; calcium palmitate, $C_{32}H_{62}CaO_4$ = 550.92]; contains the equivalent of 9 to 10.5% of CaO (calcium oxide).

Preparation—By precipitation from interaction of solutions of calcium chloride and the sodium salts of the mixed fatty acids (stearic and palmitic).

Description—Fine, white to yellowish white, bulky powder; slight, characteristic odor; unctuous and free from grittiness.

Solubility—Insoluble in water, alcohol or ether.

Uses—A *lubricant* in the manufacture of compressed tablets. It also is used as a conditioning agent in food and pharmaceutical products. Its virtually nontoxic nature and unctuous properties makes it ideal for these purposes.

Calcium Sulfate

Sulfuric acid, calcium salt (1:1); Gypsum; Terra Alba

Calcium sulfate (1:1) [7778-18-9] $CaSO_4$ (136.14); *dihydrate* [10101-41-4] (172.17).

Preparation—From natural sources or by precipitation from interaction of solutions of calcium chloride and a soluble sulfate.

Description—Fine, white to slightly yellow-white, odorless powder.

Solubility—Dissolves in diluted HCl; slightly soluble in water.

Uses—A *diluent* in the manufacture of compressed tablets. It is sufficiently inert that few undesirable reactions occur in tablets made with this substance. It also is used for making plaster casts and supports.

Carnauba Wax

Obtained from the leaves of *Copernicia cerifera* Mart (Fam *Palmae).*

Preparation—Consists chiefly of *myricyl cerotate* with smaller quantities of *myricyl alcohol, ceryl alcohol* and *cerotic acid.* It is obtained by treating the leaf buds and leaves of *Copernicia cerifera,* the so-called *Brazilian Wax Palm,* with hot water.

Description—Light-brown to pale-yellow, moderately coarse powder; characteristic bland odor; free from rancidity; specific gravity about 0.99; melts about 84°.

Solubility—Insoluble in water; freely soluble in warm benzene; soluble in warm chloroform or toluene; slightly soluble in boiling alcohol.

Uses—A pharmaceutic aid used as a *polishing agent* in the manufacture of coated tablets.

Microcrystalline Cellulose

Cellulose [9004-34-6]; purified, partially depolymerized cellulose prepared by treating alpha cellulose, obtained as a pulp from fibrous plant material, with mineral acids.

Preparation—Cellulose is subjected to the hydrolytic action of 2.5 *N* HCl at the boiling temperature of about 105° for 15 min, whereby amorphous cellulosic material is removed and aggregates of crystalline cellulose are formed. These are collected by filtration, washed with water and aqueous ammonia and disintegrated into small fragments, often termed cellulose crystallites, by vigorous mechanical means such as a blendor. US Pat 3,141,875.

Description—Fine, white, odorless, crystalline powder; consists of free-flowing, nonfibrous particles.

Solubility—Insoluble in water, dilute acids or most organic solvents; slightly soluble in NaOH solution (1 in 20).

Uses—A tablet diluent and disintegrant. It can be compressed into self-binding tablets which disintegrate rapidly when placed in water.

Microcrystalline Cellulose and Sodium Carboxymethylcellulose—A colloid-forming, attrited mixture of microcrystalline cellulose and sodium carboxymethylcellulose. *Description and Solubility:* Tasteless, odorless, white to off-white, coarse to fine powder; pH (dispersion) 6 to 8; swells in water, producing, when dispersed, a white, opaque dispersion or gel. Insoluble in organic solvents or dilute acids. *Uses:* Pharmaceutic aid (suspending agent). *Grades Available* (amounts of sodium carboxymethylcellulose producing viscosities in the concentrations designated): 8.5%, 120 cps in 2.1% solution; 11%, 120 cps in 1.2% solution; 11%, 65 cps in 1.2% solution.

Powdered Cellulose—page 1397.

Cellulose Acetate Phthalate

Cellulose, acetate, 1,2-benzenedicarboxylate

Cellulose acetate phthalate [9004-38-0]; a reaction product of the phthalic anhydride and a partial acetate ester of cellulose. When dried at 105° for 2 hr, it contains 19 to 23.5% of acetyl (C_2H_3O) groups and 30 to 36.0% of phthalyl (*o*-carboxybenzoyl, $C_8H_5O_3$) groups.

Preparation—Cellulose is esterified by treatment with acetic and phthalic acid anhydrides.

Description—Free-flowing, white powder; may have a slight odor of acetic acid.

Solubility—Insoluble in water or alcohol; soluble in acetone or dioxane.

Uses—An *enteric tablet-coating material.* Coatings of this substance disintegrate due to the hydrolytic effect of the intestinal esterases, even when the intestinal contents are acid. *In vitro* studies indicate that cellulose acetate phthalate will withstand the action of artificial gastric juices for long periods of time, but will disintegrate readily in artificial intestinal juices.

Cherry Juice—see RPS-18, page 1320.

Carbon Tetrachloride

Methane, tetrachloro-, Tetrachloromethane

Carbon tetrachloride [56-23-5] CCl_4 (153.82).

Preparation—One method consists of catalytic chlorination of carbon disulfide.

Description—Clear, colorless liquid; characteristic odor resembling that of chloroform; specific gravity 1.588 to 1.590; boils about 77°.

Solubility—Soluble in about 2000 volumes water; miscible with alcohol, acetone, ether, chloroform or benzene.

Uses—Officially recognized as a *pharmaceutical necessity* (solvent). Formerly it was used as a cheap *anthelmintic* for the treatment of *hookworm* infections but it causes severe injury to the liver if absorbed.

Chloroform

Methane, trichloro-,

Trichloromethane [67-66-3] $CHCl_3$ (119.38); contains 99 to 99.5% of $CHCl_3$, the remainder consisting of alcohol.

Caution—Care should be taken not to vaporize it in the presence of a flame, because of the production of harmful gases (hydrogen chloride and phosgene).

Preparation—Made by the reduction of carbon tetrachloride with water and iron and by the controlled chlorination of methane.

The pure compound readily decomposes on keeping, particularly if exposed to moisture and sunlight, resulting in formation of phosgene (carbonyl chloride [$COCl_2$]) and other products. The presence of a small amount of alcohol greatly retards or prevents this decomposition; hence, the requirement that it contain 0.5 to 1% of alcohol. The alcohol combines with any phosgene forming ethyl carbonate, which is nontoxic.

Description—Clear, colorless, mobile liquid; characteristic, ethereal odor; burning, sweet taste; not flammable but its heated vapors burn with a green flame; affected by light and moisture; specific gravity 1.474 to 1.478, indicating 99 to 99.5% of $CHCl_3$; boils about 61°; not affected by acids, but is decomposed by alkali hydroxide into alkali chloride and sodium formate.

Solubility—Soluble in 210 volumes of water; miscible with alcohol, ether, benzene, solvent hexane, acetone or fixed and volatile oils.

Uses—An obsolete *inhalation anesthetic.* Although it possesses advantages of nonflammability and great potency, it rarely is used due to the serious toxic effects it produces on the heart and liver. Internally, it has been used, in small doses, as a *carminative.* Externally, it is an *irritant* and when used in liniments it may produce blisters.

It is categorized as a pharmaceutic aid. It is used as a *preservative* during the aqueous percolation of vegetable drugs to prevent bacterial decomposition in the process of manufacture. In most instances it is evaporated before the product is finished. It is an excellent solvent for alkaloids and many other organic chemicals and is used in the manufacture of these products and in chemical analyses.

Citric Acid

1,2,3-Propanetricarboxylic acid, 2-hydroxy-,

CH_2COOH
HOCCOOH
CH_2COOH

Citric acid [77-92-9] $C_6H_8O_7$ (192.12); *monohydrate* [5949-29-1] (210.14).

Preparation—Found in many plants. It formerly was obtained solely from the juice of limes and lemons and from pineapple wastes. Since about 1925 the acid has been produced largely by fermentation of sucrose solution, including molasses, by fungi belonging to the *Aspergillus niger* group, theoretically according to the following reaction

$$\underset{\text{Sucrose}}{C_{12}H_{22}O_{11}} + \underset{\text{Oxygen}}{3O_2} \rightarrow \underset{\text{Citric Acid}}{2H_3C_6H_5O_7} + \underset{\text{Water}}{3H_2O}$$

but in practice there are deviations from this stoichiometric relationship.

Description—Colorless, translucent crystals, or a white, granular to fine crystalline powder; odorless; strongly acid taste; the hydrous form effloresces in moderately dry air, but is slightly deliquescent in moist air; loses its water of crystallization at about 50°; dilute aqueous solutions are subject to molding (fermentation), oxalic acid being one of the fermentation products.

Solubility—1 g in 0.5 mL water, 2 mL alcohol or about 30 mL ether; freely soluble in methanol.

Uses—In the preparation of *Anticoagulant Citrate Dextrose Solution, Anticoagulant Citrate Phosphate Dextrose Solution, Citric Acid Syrup* and *effervescent salts.* It also has been used to dissolve urinary bladder calculi, and as a mild astringent.

Cocoa Butter

Cacao Butter; Theobroma Oil; Oil of Theobroma

The fat obtained from the roasted seed of *Theobroma cacao* Linné (Fam *Sterculiaceae).*

Preparation—By grinding the kernels of the "chocolate bean" and expressing the oil in powerful, horizontal hydraulic presses. The yield is about 40%. It also has been prepared by dissolving the oil from the unroasted beans by the use of a volatile solvent.

Constituents—Chemically, it is a mixture of stearin, palmitin, olein, laurin, linolein and traces of other glycerides.

Description—Yellowish, white solid; faint, agreeable odor; bland (if obtained by extraction) or chocolate-like (if obtained by pressing) taste; usually brittle below 25°; specific gravity 0.858 to 0.864 at 100°/25°; refractive index 1.454 to 1.458 at 40°.

Solubility—Slightly soluble in alcohol; soluble in boiling dehydrated alcohol; freely soluble in ether or chloroform.

Uses—Valuable in pharmacy for making suppositories by virtue of its low fusing point and its property of becoming solid at a temperature just below the melting point. See *Suppositories* (page 1591). In addition to this use, it is an excellent emollient application to the skin when inflamed; it also is used in various skin creams, especially the so-called "*skin foods.*" It also is used in massage.

Titanium Dioxide—page 884.

Denatonium Benzoate

Benzenemethanaminium *N*-[2-[(2,6-dimethylphenyl)amino]-2-oxoethyl]-*N*,*N*-diethyl-, benzoate;

Benzyldiethyl [(2,6-xylylcarbamoyl)methyl]ammonium benzoate [3734-33-6] $C_{28}H_{34}N_2O_3$ (446.59).

Preparation—2-(Diethylamino)-2′,6′-xylidide is quaternized by reaction with benzyl chloride. The quaternary chloride is then treated with methanolic potassium hydroxide to form the quaternary base which, after filtering off the KCl, is reacted with benzoic acid. The starting xylidide may be prepared by condensing 2,6- xylidine with chloroacetyl chloride and condensing the resulting chloroacetoxylidide with diethylamine. US Pat 3,080,327.

Description—White, odorless, crystalline powder; an intensely bitter taste; melts about 168°.

Solubility—1 g in 20 mL water, 2.4 mL alcohol, 2.9 mL chloroform or 5000 mL ether.

Uses—A *denaturant* for ethyl alcohol.

Dextrin

British Gum; Starch Gum; Leiocom

Dextrin [9004-53-9] $(C_6H_{10}O_5)_n$.

Preparation—By the incomplete hydrolysis of starch with dilute acid, or by heating dry starch.

Description—White or yellow, amorphous powder (*white:* practically odorless; *yellow:* characteristic odor); dextrorotatory; $[\alpha]_D^{20}$ generally above 200°; does not reduce Fehling's solution; gives a reddish color with iodine.

Solubility—Soluble in 3 parts of boiling water, forming a gummy solution; less soluble in cold water.

Uses—An *excipient* and *emulsifier.*

Dextrose

Anhydrous Dextrose; Dextrose Monohydrate; Glucose; D(+)-Glucose; α-D(+)-Glucopyranose; Medicinal Glucose; Purified Glucose; Grape Sugar; Bread Sugar; Cerelose; Starch Sugar; Corn Sugar

D-Glucose monohydrate [5996-10-1] $C_6H_{12}O_6.H_2O$ (198.17); *anhydrous* [50-99-7] (180.16). A sugar usually obtained by the hydrolysis of starch. For the structure, see page 384.

Preparation—See *Liquid Glucose* (page 1410).

Description—Colorless crystals or a white, crystalline or granular powder; odorless; sweet taste; specific rotation (anhydrous) +52.5 to +53°; anhydrous dextrose melts at 146°; dextrose slowly reduces alkaline cupric tartrate TS in the cold and rapidly on heating, producing a red precipitate of cuprous oxide (difference from *sucrose*).

Solubility—1 g in 1 mL of water or 100 mL of alcohol; more soluble in boiling water or boiling alcohol.

Uses—See *Dextrose Injection* (page 916). It also is used, instead of lactose, as a supplement to milk for infant feeding.

Dichlorodifluoromethane

Methane, dichlorodifluoro-,

CCl_2F_2

Dichlorodifluoromethane [75-71-8] CCl_2F_2 (120.91).

Preparation—Carbon tetrachloride is reacted with antimony trifluoride in the presence of antimony pentafluoride.

Description—Clear, colorless gas; faint, ethereal odor; vapor pressure at 25° about 4883 torr.

Uses—A *propellant* (No 12, see page 1678).

Dichlorotetrafluoroethane

Ethane, 1,2-dichloro-1,1,2,2-tetrafluoro-,

$CClF_2CClF_2$

1,2-Dichlorotetrafluoroethane [76-14-2] $C_2Cl_2F_4$ (170.92).

Preparation—By reacting 1,1,2-trichloro-1,2,2-trifluoroethane with antimony trifluorodichloride [SbF_3Cl_2], whereupon one of the 1-chlorine atoms is replaced by fluorine. The starting trichlorofluoroethane may be prepared from hexachloroethane by treatment with SbF_3Cl_2 (Henne AL: *Org Reactions II:* 65, 1944).

Description—Clear, colorless gas; faint, ethereal odor; vapor pressure at 25° about 1620 torr; usually contains 6 to 10% of its isomer, $CFCl_2$—CF_3.

Uses—A *propellant* (No 114 and 114a, see page 1678).

Edetic Acid

Glycine, *N,N'*-1,2-ethanediylbis[*N*-(carboxymethyl)-,

$(HOOCCH_2)_2NCH_2CH_2N(CH_2COOH)_2$

(Ethylenedinitrilo)tetraacetic acid [60-00-4] $C_{10}H_{16}N_2O_8$ (292.24).

Preparation—Ethylenediamine is condensed with sodium monochloroacetate with the aid of sodium carbonate. An aqueous solution of the reactants is heated to about 90° for 10 hr, then cooled and acidified with HCl whereupon the acid precipitates. US Pat 2,130,505.

Description—White, crystalline powder; melts with decomposition above 220°.

Solubility—Very slightly soluble in water; soluble in solutions of alkali hydroxides.

Uses—A *pharmaceutic aid* (metal complexing agent). The acid, rather than any salt, is the form most potent in removing calcium from solution. It may be added to shed blood to prevent clotting. It also is used in pharmaceutical analysis and the removal or inactivation of unwanted ions in solution. Salts of the acid are known as edetates. See *Edetate Calcium Disodium* (page 935) and *Edetate Disodium* (page 935).

Ethylcellulose

Cellulose ethyl ether [9004-57-3]; an ethyl ether of cellulose containing 44 to 51% of ethoxy groups. The *medium-type* viscosity grade contains less than 46.5% ethoxy groups; the *standard-type* viscosity grade contains 46.5% or more ethoxy groups.

Preparation—By the same general procedure described on page 1306 for *Methylcellulose* except that ethyl chloride or ethyl sulfate is employed as the alkylating agent. The 45 to 50% of ethoxy groups in the official ethylcellulose corresponds to from 2.25 to 2.61 ethoxy groups/$C_6H_{10}O_5$ unit, thus representing from 75 to 87% of the maximum theoretical ethoxylation, which is 3 ethoxy groups/$C_6H_{10}O_5$ unit.

Description—Free-flowing, white to light tan powder; forms films that have a refractive index of about 1.47; aqueous suspensions are neutral to litmus.

Solubility—The medium-type is freely soluble in tetrahydrofuran, methyl acetate, chloroform or mixtures of aromatic hydrocarbons with alcohol; the standard-type is freely soluble in alcohol, methanol, toluene, chloroform or ethyl acetate; both types are insoluble in water, glycerin or propylene glycol.

Uses—A *pharmaceutic aid* as a tablet binder and for film-coating tablets and drug particles.

Gelatin—page 1397.

Liquid Glucose

Glucose; Starch Syrup; Corn Syrup

A product obtained by the incomplete hydrolysis of starch. It consists chiefly of dextrose [D(+)-glucose, $C_6H_{12}O_6$ = 180.16] dextrins, maltose and water.

Preparation—Commercially by the action of very weak H_2SO_4 or HCl on starch.

One of the processes for its manufacture is as follows: The starch, usually from corn, is mixed with 5 times its weight of water containing less than 1% of HCl, the mixture is heated to about 45° and then transferred to a suitable reaction vessel into which steam is passed under pressure until the temperature reaches 120°. The temperature is maintained at this point for about 1 hr, or until tests show complete disappearance of starch. The mass is then heated to volatilize most of the hydrochloric acid, sodium carbonate or calcium carbonate is added to neutralize the remaining traces of acid, the liquid is filtered, then decolorized in charcoal or bone-black filters, as is done in sugar refining and finally concentrated in vacuum to the desired consistency.

When made by the above process, it contains about 30 to 40% of dextrose mixed with about an equal proportion of dextrin, together with small amounts of other carbohydrates, notably maltose. By varying the conditions of hydrolysis, the relative proportions of the sugars also vary.

If the crystallizable dextrose is desired, the conversion temperature is higher and the time of conversion longer. The term "glucose," as customarily used in the chemical or pharmaceutical literature, usually refers to dextrose, the crystallizable product.

The name "grape sugar" sometimes is applied to the solid commercial form of dextrose because the principal sugar of the grape is dextrose, although the fruit has never been used as a source of the commercial supply.

Description—Colorless or yellowish, thick, syrupy liquid; odorless, or nearly so; sweet taste; differs from sucrose in that it readily reduces hot alkaline cupric tartrate TS, producing a red precipitate of cuprous oxide.

Solubility—Miscible with water; sparingly soluble in alcohol.

Uses—As an ingredient of *Cocoa Syrup* (page 1393), as a tablet binder and coating agent, and as a diluent in pilular extracts; it has replaced glycerin in many pharmaceutical preparations. It is sometimes given *per rectum* as a *food* in cases where feeding by stomach is impossible. It should not be used in the place of dextrose for intravenous injection.

Hydrochloric Acid

Chlorhydric Acid; Muriatic Acid; Spirit of Salt

Hydrochloric acid [7647-01-0] HCl (36.46); contains 36.5 to 38.0%, by weight, of HCl.

Preparation—By the interaction of NaCl and H_2SO_4 or by combining chlorine with hydrogen. It is obtained as a byproduct in the manufacture of sodium carbonate from NaCl by the Leblanc process in which common salt is decomposed with H_2SO_4. HCl is also a byproduct in the electrolytic production of NaOH from NaCl.

Description—Colorless, fuming liquid; pungent odor; fumes and odor disappear when it is diluted with 2 volumes of water; strongly acid to litmus even when highly diluted; specific gravity about 1.18.

Solubility—Miscible with water or alcohol.

Uses—Officially classified as a pharmaceutic aid that is used as an acidifying agent. It is used in preparing *Diluted Hydrochloric Acid* (see RPS-18, page 783).

Hypophosphorous Acid

Phosphinic acid

Hypophosphorous acid [6303-21-5] HPH_2O_2 (66.00); contains 30 to 32% by weight, of H_3PO_2.

Preparation—By reacting barium or calcium hypophosphite with sulfuric acid or by treating sodium hypophosphite with an ion-exchange resin.

Description—Colorless or slightly yellow, odorless liquid; solution is acid to litmus even when highly diluted; specific gravity about 1.13.

Solubility—Miscible with water or alcohol.

Incompatibilities—Oxidized on exposure to air and by nearly all *oxidizing agents. Mercury, silver* and *bismuth salts* are reduced partially to the metallic state as evidenced by a darkening in color. *Ferric compounds* are changed to ferrous.

Uses—An *antioxidant* in pharmaceutical preparations.

Isopropyl Myristate

Tetradecanoic acid, 1-methylethyl ester

$CH_3(CH_2)_{12}COOCH(CH_3)_2$

Isopropyl myristate [110-27-0] $C_{17}H_{34}O_2$ (270.45).

Preparation—By reacting myristoyl chloride with 2-propanol with the aid of a suitable dehydrochlorinating agent.

Description—Liquid of low viscosity; practically colorless and odorless; congeals about 5° and decomposes at 208°; withstands oxidation and does not become rancid readily.

Solubility—Soluble in alcohol, acetone, chloroform, ethyl acetate, toluene, mineral oil, castor oil or cottonseed oil; practically insoluble in water, glycerin or propylene glycol; dissolves many waxes, cholesterol or lanolin.

Uses—*Pharmaceutic aid* used in cosmetics and topical medicinal preparations as an emollient, lubricant and to enhance absorption through the skin.

Kaolin—page 907.

Lactic Acid

Propanoic acid, 2-hydroxy-, 2-Hydroxypropionic Acid; Propanoloic Acid; Milk Acid

$CH_3CH(OH)COOH$

Lactic acid [50-21-5] $C_3H_6O_3$ (90.08); a mixture of lactic acid and lactic acid lactate ($C_6H_{10}O_5$) equivalent to a total of 85 to 90%, by weight, of $C_3H_6O_3$.

Discovered by Scheele in 1780, it is the acid formed in the souring of milk, hence the name *lactic*, from the Latin name for milk. It results from the decomposition of the lactose (milk sugar) in milk.

Preparation—A solution of glucose or of starch previously hydrolyzed with diluted sulfuric acid is inoculated, after the addition of suitable nitrogen compounds and mineral salts, with *Bacillus lactis*. Calcium carbonate is added to neutralize the lactic acid as soon as it is formed, otherwise the fermentation stops when the amount of acid exceeds 0.5%. When fermentation is complete, as indicated by failure of the liquid to give a test for glucose, the solution is filtered, concentrated and allowed to stand. The calcium lactate that crystallizes is decomposed with dilute sulfuric acid and filtered with charcoal. The lactic acid in the filtrate is extracted with ethyl or isopropyl ether, the ether is distilled off and the aqueous solution of the acid concentrated under reduced pressure.

Description—Colorless or yellowish, nearly odorless, syrupy liquid; acid to litmus; absorbs water on exposure to moist air; when a dilute solution is concentrated to above 50%, lactic acid lactate begins to form; in the official acid the latter amounts to about 12 to 15%; specific gravity about 1.20; decomposes when distilled under normal pressure but may be distilled without decomposition under reduced pressure.

Solubility—Miscible with water, alcohol or ether; insoluble in chloroform.

Uses—In the preparation of *Sodium Lactate Injection* (page 933). It also is used in babies' milk formulas, as an acidulant in food preparations, and in 1 to 2% concentration in some spermatocidal jellies. A 10% solution is used as a bactericidal agent on the skin of neonates. It is corrosive to tissues on prolonged contact. A 16.7% solution in flexible collodion is used to remove warts and small cutaneous tumors.

Lactose

D-Glucose, 4-*O*-β-D-galactopyranosyl-, Milk Sugar

Lactose [63-42-3] $C_{12}H_{22}O_{11}$ (342.30); *monohydrate* [10039-26-6] (360.31); a sugar obtained from milk.

For the structural formula, see page 385.

Preparation—From skim milk, to which is added diluted HCl to precipitate the casein. After removal of the casein by filtration, the reaction of the whey is adjusted to a pH of about 6.2 by addition of lime and the remaining albuminous matter is coagulated by heating; this is filtered out and the liquid set aside to crystallize. Animal charcoal is used to decolorize the solution in a manner similar to that used in purifying sucrose.

Another form of lactose, known as β-lactose, also is available on the market. It differs in that the D-glucose moiety is β instead of α. It is reported that this variety is sweeter and more soluble than ordinary lactose and for that reason is preferable in pharmaceutical manufacturing where lactose is used. Chemically, β-lactose does not appear to differ from ordinary α-lactose. It is manufactured in the same way as α-lactose up to the point of crystallization, then the solution is heated to a temperature above 93.5°, this being the temperature at which the α form is converted to the β variety. The β form occurs only as an anhydrous sugar whereas the α variety may be obtained either in the anhydrous form or as a monohydrate.

Description—White or creamy white, hard, crystalline masses or powder; odorless; faintly sweet taste; stable in air, but readily absorbs odors; pH (1 in 10 solution) 4.0 to 6.5; specific rotation +54.8 to +55.5°.

Solubility—1 g in 5 mL water or 2.6 mL boiling water; very slightly soluble in alcohol; insoluble in chloroform or ether.

Uses—A *diluent* largely used in medicine and pharmacy. It is generally an ingredient of the medium used in penicillin production. It is used extensively as an addition to milk for infant feeding.

Magnesium Chloride

Magnesium chloride hexahydrate [7791-18-6] $MgCl_2.6H_2O$ (203.30); *anhydrous* [7786-30-3] (95.21).

Preparation—By treating magnesite or other suitable magnesium minerals with HCl.

Description—Colorless, odorless, deliquescent flakes or crystals, which lose water when heated to 100° and loose HCl when heated to 110°; pH (1 in 20 solution in carbon dioxide-free water) 4.5 to 7.

Solubility—Very soluble in water; freely soluble in alcohol.

Uses—*Electrolyte replenisher; pharmaceutical necessity* for hemodialysis and peritoneal dialysis fluids.

Magnesium Stearate

Octadecanoic acid, magnesium salt

Magnesium stearate [557-04-0]. A compound of magnesium with a mixture of solid organic acids obtained from fats, and consists chiefly of variable proportions of magnesium stearate and magnesium palmitate. It contains the equivalent of 6.8 to 8.0% of MgO (40.30).

Description—Fine, white, bulky powder; faint, characteristic odor; unctuous, adheres readily to the skin and free from grittiness.

Solubility—Insoluble in water, alcohol or ether.

Uses—A *pharmaceutical necessity (lubricant)* in the manufacture of compressed tablets.

Meglumine

D-Glucitol, 1-deoxy-1-(methylamino)-,

```
         H  H  OH H
         |  |  |  |
HOCH2—C—C—C—C—CH2NHCH3
         |  |  |  |
         OH OH H  OH
```

1-Deoxy-1-(methylamino)-D-glucitol [6284-40-8] $C_7H_{17}NO_5$ (195.21).

Preparation—By treating glucose with hydrogen and methylamine under pressure and in the presence of Raney nickel.

Description—White to faintly yellowish white, odorless crystals or powder; melts about 130°.

Solubility—Freely soluble in water; sparingly soluble in alcohol.

Uses—In forming salts of certain pharmaceuticals, surface-active agents and dyes. See *Diatrizoate Meglumine Injections* (page 1375), *Iodipamide Meglumine Injection* (page 1368) and *Iothalamate Meglumine Injection* (page 1378).

Light Mineral Oil

Light Liquid Petrolatum NF XII; Light Liquid Paraffin; Light White Mineral Oil

A mixture of liquid hydrocarbons obtained from petroleum. It may contain a suitable stabilizer.

Description—Colorless, transparent, oily liquid, free, or nearly free, from fluorescence; odorless and tasteless when cold, and develops not more than a faint odor of petroleum when heated; specific gravity 0.818 to 0.880; kinematic viscosity not more than 33.5 centistokes at 40°.

Solubility—Insoluble in water or alcohol; miscible with most fixed oils, but not with castor oil; soluble in volatile oils.

Uses—Officially recognized as a *vehicle*. Once it was used widely as a vehicle for nose and throat medications; such uses are now considered dangerous because of the possibility of lipoid pneumonia. It sometimes is used to cleanse dry and inflamed skin areas and to facilitate removal of dermatological preparations from the skin. It should never be used for internal administration because of "leakage." See *Mineral Oil* (page 889).

Nitric Acid

Nitric acid [7697-37-2] HNO_3 (63.01); contains about 70%, by weight, of HNO_3.

Preparation—May be prepared by treatment of sodium nitrate (Chile saltpeter) with sulfuric acid, but usually produced by catalytic oxidation of ammonia.

Description—Highly corrosive fuming liquid; characteristic, highly irritating odor; stains animal tissues yellow; boils about 120°; specific gravity about 1.41.

Solubility—Miscible with water.

Uses—*Pharmaceutic aid* (acidifying agent).

Nitrogen

Nitrogen [7727-37-9] N_2 (28.01); contains not less than 99%, by volume, of N_2.

Preparation—By the fractional distillation of liquified air.

Uses—A diluent for medicinal gases. Pharmaceutically, is employed to replace air in the containers of substances which would be affected adversely by air oxidation. Examples include its use with fixed oils, certain vitamin preparations and a variety of injectable products. It also is used as a propellant.

Persic Oil—see RPS-18, page 1323.

Phenol

Carbolic Acid

C_6H_5OH

Phenol [108-95-2] C_6H_6O (94.11).

Preparation—For many years made only by distilling crude carbolic acid from coal tar and separating and purifying the distillate by repeated crystallizations, it now is prepared synthetically.

A more recent process uses chlorobenzene as the starting point in the manufacture. The chlorobenzene is produced in a vapor phase reaction, with benzene, HCl and oxygen over a copper catalyst, followed by hydrolysis with steam to yield HCl and phenol (which is recovered).

Description—Colorless to light pink, interlaced, or separate, needle-shaped crystals, or a white or light pink, crystalline mass; characteristic odor; when undiluted, it whitens and cauterizes the skin and mucous membranes; when gently heated, phenol melts, forming a highly refractive liquid; liquefied by the addition of 10% of water; vapor is flammable; gradually darkens on exposure to light and air; specific gravity 1.07; boils at 182°; congeals not lower than 39°.

Solubility—1 g in 15 mL water; very soluble in alcohol, glycerin, chloroform, ether or fixed and volatile oils; sparingly soluble in mineral oil.

Incompatibilities—Produces a liquid or soft mass when triturated with *camphor, menthol, acetanilid, acetophenetidin, aminopyrine, antipyrine, ethyl aminobenzoate, methenamine, phenyl salicylate, resorcinol, terpin hydrate, thymol* and several other substances including some *alkaloids*. It also softens *cocoa butter* in suppository mixtures.

It is soluble in about 15 parts of water; stronger solutions may be obtained by using as much glycerin as phenol. Only the crystallized form is soluble in fixed oils and liquid petroleum, the liquefied form is not all soluble due to its content of water. *Albumin* and *gelatin* are precipitated by it. *Collodion* is coagulated by the precipitation of pyroxylin. Traces of *iron* in various chemicals such as *alum, borax*, etc, may produce a green color.

Uses—A *caustic, disinfectant, topical anesthetic* and pharmaceutical necessity as a *preservative* for injections, etc. At one time widely used as a germicide and still the standard against which other antiseptics are compared, it has few legitimate uses in modern medicine. Nevertheless, it is still used in several proprietary antiseptic mouthwashes, hemorrhoidal preparations and burn remedies. In full strength, a few drops of the liquefied form may be used to cauterize small wounds, dog bites, snake bites, etc. It commonly is employed as an *antipruritic*, either in the form of phenolated calamine lotion (1%), phenol ointment (2%) or a simple aqueous solution (0.5 to 1%). It has been used for sclerosing hemorrhoids, but more effective and safer drugs are available. A 5% solution in glycerin is used in simple earache. Crude carbolic acid is an effective, economical agent for disinfecting excrement. It is of some therapeutic value as a *fungicide*, but more effective and less toxic agents are available. If accidentally spilled, it should be removed promptly from the skin by swabbing with alcohol.

Liquefied Phenol [Liquefied Carbolic Acid is phenol maintained in a liquid condition by the presence of 10.0% of water. It contains not less than 89.0%, by weight, of C_6H_6O. *Note—When it is to be mixed with a fixed oil, mineral oil or white petrolatum, use the crystalline Phenol, not Liquefied Phenol. Preparation:* Melt phenol (a convenient quantity) by placing the unstoppered container in a steam bath and applying heat gradually. Transfer the liquid to a tared vessel, weigh, add 1 g of purified water for each 9 g of phenol, and mix thoroughly. *Description:* Colorless liquid, which may develop a red tint upon exposure to air and light; characteristic, somewhat aromatic odor; when undiluted it cauterizes and whitens the skin and mucous membranes; specific gravity about 1.065; when it is subjected to distillation, the boiling temperature does not rise above 182°, which is the boiling temperature of phenol; partially solidifies at about 15°. *Solubility:* Miscible with alcohol, ether or glycerin; a mixture of liquefied phenol and an equal volume of glycerin is miscible with water. *Uses:* A formulation which facilitates the dispensing of concentrated phenol. Its therapeutic uses are described above under *Phenol*. It is a *pharmaceutical necessity for Phenolated Calamine Lotion* (page 872).

Phenyl Salicylate—see RPS-15, page 1269.

Phosphoric Acid

Orthophosphoric Acid; Syrupy Phosphoric Acid; Concentrated Phosphoric Acid

Phosphoric acid [7664-38-2] H_3PO_4 (98.00); contains 85 to 88%, by weight, of H_3PO_4.

Preparation—Phosphorus is converted to phosphorus pentoxide [P_2O_5] by exposing it to a current of warm air, then the P_2O_5 is treated with water to form phosphoric acid. The conversion of the phosphorus to the pentoxide takes place while the phosphorus, distilling from the phosphorus manufacturing operation, is in the vapor state.

Description—Colorless, odorless liquid of a syrupy consistency; specific gravity about 1.71.

Solubility—Miscible with water or alcohol, with the evolution of heat.

Uses—To make the diluted acid and as a weak acid in various pharmaceutical preparations. Industrially, it is used in dental cements and in beverages as an acidulant.

Diluted Phosphoric Acid [Dilute Phosphoric Acid] contains, in each 100 mL, 9.5 to 10.5 g of H_3PO_4 (98.00). *Preparation:* Mix phosphoric acid (69 mL) and purified water (qs) to make 1000 mL. *Description and Solubility:* Clear, colorless, odorless liquid; specific gravity about 1.057. Miscible with water or alcohol. *Uses:* A *pharmaceutical necessity*. It also has been employed in *lead poisoning* and in other conditions in which it is desired to administer large amounts of phosphate and at the same time produce a mild acidosis. It has been given in the dose of 60 mL a day (5 mL/hour) under carefully controlled conditions.

Potassium Metaphosphate

Metaphosphoric acid (HPO_3), potassium salt

Potassium metaphosphate [7790-53-6] KPO_3 (118.07); a straight-chain polyphosphate, having a high degree of polymerization; contains the equivalent of 59 to 61% of P_2O_5.

Preparation—By thermal dehydration of monopotassium phosphate (KH_2PO_4).

Description—White, odorless powder.

Solubility—Insoluble in water; soluble in dilute solutions of sodium salts.

Uses—*Pharmaceutic aid* (buffering agent).

Monobasic Potassium Phosphate

Phosphoric acid, monopotassium salt; Potassium Biphosphate; Potassium Acid Phosphate; Potassium Dihydrogen Phosphate; Sørensen's Potassium Phosphate

Monopotassium phosphate [7778-77-0] KH_2PO_4 (136.09).

Preparation—H_3PO_4 is reacted with an equimolar quantity of KOH and the solution is evaporated to crystallization.

Description—Colorless crystals or a white, granular or crystalline powder; odorless and stable in air; pH (1 in 100 solution) about 4.5.

Solubility—Freely soluble in water; practically insoluble in alcohol.

Uses—A component of various buffer solutions. Medicinally, it has been used as a urinary acidifier.

Pumice

Pumex

A substance of volcanic origin, consisting chiefly of complex silicates of aluminum, potassium and sodium.

Description—Very light, hard rough, porous, grayish masses or a gritty, grayish powder of several grades of fineness; odorless, tasteless and stable in the air.

Three powders are available:

Pumice Flour or *Superfine Pumice*—Not less than 97% passes through a No 200 standard mesh sieve.

Fine Pumice—Not less than 95% passes through a No 150 standard mesh sieve, and not more than 75% passes through a No 200 standard mesh sieve.

Coarse Pumice—Not less than 95% passes through a No 60 standard mesh sieve, and not more than 5% passes through a No 200 standard mesh sieve.

Solubility—Insoluble in water and is not attacked by acids or alkali hydroxide solutions.

Uses—A *filtering* and *distributing medium* for pharmaceutical preparations. Because of its grittiness the powdered form is used in certain types of soaps and cleaning powders and also as a *dental abrasive.*

Pyroxylin

Cellulose, nitrate; Soluble Guncotton

Pyroxylin [9004-70-0]; a product obtained by the action of a mixture of nitric and sulfuric acids on cotton, and consists chiefly of cellulose tetranitrate [$(C_{12}H_{16}N_4O_{18})_n$].

Note—The commercially available form is moistened with about 30% of alcohol or other suitable solvent. The alcohol or solvent must be allowed to evaporate to yield the dried substance described in the Pharmacopeia.

Preparation—Shönbein, in 1846, found that nitric acid acts on cotton and produces a soluble compound. It subsequently was proved that this substance belongs to a series of closely related nitrates in which the nitric acid radical replaces the hydroxyl of the cellulose formula. This usually is indicated by taking the double empirical formula for cellulose $C_{12}H_{20}O_{10}$ and indicating replacement of four of the OH groups thus

$$\underset{\textbf{Cellulose}}{C_{12}H_{20}O_{10}} + 4HNO_3 \rightarrow \underset{\textbf{Cellulose Tetranitrate}}{C_{12}H_{16}O_6(NO_3)_4} + 4H_2O$$

The compound used in preparing collodion is a varying mixture of the di-, tri-, tetra- and pentanitrates, but is mainly tetranitrate. The hexanitrate is the true explosive guncotton, and is insoluble in ether, alcohol, acetone or water.

Description—Light yellow, matted mass of filaments, resembling raw cotton in appearance, but harsh to the touch; *exceedingly flammable* burning, when unconfined, very rapidly and with a luminous flame; when kept in well-closed bottles and exposed to light, it is decomposed with the evolution of nitrous vapors, leaving a carbonaceous residue.

Solubility—Insoluble in water; dissolves slowly but completely in 25 parts of a mixture of 3 volumes of ether and 1 volume of alcohol; soluble in acetone or glacial acetic acid and precipitated from these solutions by water.

Uses—A *pharmaceutical necessity* for *Collodion* (RPS-16, page 717).

Rosin

Resina; Colophony; Georgia Pine Rosin; Yellow Pine Rosin

A solid resin obtained from *Pinus palustris* Miller, and from other species of *Pinus* Linné (Fam *Pinaceae*).

Constituents—American rosin contains *sylvic acid* [$C_{20}H_{30}O_2$], α-, β- and γ-*abietic acids* [$C_{20}H_{30}O_2$], γ-*pinic acid* (from which α- and β-pinic acids are gradually formed) and *resene*. Some authorities also include *pimaric acid* [$C_{30}H_{20}O_2$] as a constituent. French rosin is called *galipot*.

Description—Sharply angular, translucent, amber-colored fragments, frequently covered with a yellow dust; fracture brittle at ordinary temperatures, shiny and shallow-conchoidal; odor and taste are slightly terebinthinate; easily fusible and burns with a dense, yellowish smoke, specific gravity 1.07 to 1.09.

Solubility—Insoluble in water; soluble in alcohol, ether, benzene, glacial acetic acid, chloroform, carbon disulfide, dilute solutions of sodium hydroxide and potassium hydroxide or some volatile and fixed oils.

Uses—A pharmaceutical necessity for *Zinc-Eugenol Cement* (see RPS-18, page 1328). Formerly, and to some extent still, used as a component of plasters, cerates and ointments, to which it adds adhesive qualities.

Purified Siliceous Earth

Purified Kieselguhr; Purified Infusorial Earth; Diatomaceous Earth; Diatomite

A form of silica [SiO_2] [7631-86-9] consisting of the frustules and fragments of diatoms, purified by boiling with acid, washing and calcining.

Occurrence and Preparation—Large deposits of this substance are found in Virginia, Maryland, Nevada, Oregon and California, usually in the form of masses of rocks, hundreds of feet in thickness. Under the microscope it is seen to consist largely of the minute siliceous frustules of diatoms. It must be purified carefully in a manner similar to that directed for *Talc* (page 1415), and thoroughly calcined. The latter treatment destroys the bacteria which are present in large quantities in the native earth.

Description—Very fine, white, light-gray or pale-buff mixture of amorphous powder and lesser amounts of crystalline polymorphs, including quartz and cristobalite; gritty, readily absorbs moisture and retains about four times its weight of water without becoming fluid.

Solubility—Insoluble in water, acids or dilute solutions of alkali hydroxides.

Uses—Introduced into the USP as a distributing and *filtering medium* for aromatic waters; also suitable for filtration of elixirs. Like talc, it does not absorb active constituents.

Sarsparilla—see RPS-18, page 1329.

Colloidal Silicon Dioxide

Silica [7631-86-9] SiO_2 (60.08); a submicroscopic fumed silica prepared by the vapor-phase hydrolysis of a silicon compound.

Description—Light, white, nongritty powder of extremely fine particle size (about 15 nm).

Solubility—Insoluble in water or acids (except hydrofluoric); dissolved by hot solutions of alkali hydroxides.

Uses—A *tablet moisture adsorber, glidant* and as a *suspending* and *thickening agent* in pharmaceutical preparations.

Soda Lime

A mixture of calcium hydroxide and sodium or potassium hydroxide or both.

It may contain an indicator that is inert toward anesthetic gases such as ether, cyclopropane and nitrous oxide, and that changes color when the soda lime no longer can absorb carbon dioxide.

Description—White or grayish white granules; if an indicator is added, it may have a color; absorbs carbon dioxide and water on exposure to air.

Uses—Neither a therapeutic nor a pharmaceutical agent. It is a *reagent for the absorption of carbon dioxide* in anesthesia machines, oxygen therapy and metabolic tests. Because of the importance of the proper quality for these purposes it has been made official and standardized.

Sodium Borate

Sodium Tetraborate; Sodium Pyroborate; Sodium Biborate

Borax [1303-96-4] $Na_2B_4O_7.10H_2O$ (381.37); anhydrous [1330-43-4] $Na_2B_4O_7$ (201.22).

Preparation—Found in immense quantities in California as a crystalline deposit. The earth, which is strongly impregnated with borax, is lixiviated; the solution is evaporated and crystallized.

Calcium borate, or *cotton balls*, also occurs in the borax deposits of California, and sodium borate is obtained from it by double decomposition with sodium carbonate.

Description—Colorless, transparent crystals, or a white, crystalline powder; odorless; the crystals often are coated with white powder due to efflorescence; solution alkaline to litmus and phenolphthalein; pH about 9.5.

Solubility—1 g in 16 mL water, 1 mL glycerin or 1 mL boiling water; insoluble in alcohol.

Incompatibilities—Precipitates many *metals* as insoluble borates. In aqueous solution it is alkaline and precipitates *aluminum salts* as aluminum hydroxide, *iron salts* as a basic borate and ferric hydroxide and *zinc sulfate* as zinc borate and a basic salt. *Alkaloids* are precipitated from solutions of their salts. Approximately equal weights of *glycerin* and boric acid react to produce a decidedly acid derivative generally called glyceroboric acid. Thus, the addition of glycerin to a mixture containing it overcomes incompatibilities arising from an alkaline reaction.

Uses—As a pharmaceutical necessity, it is used as an alkalizing agent and as a buffer for alkaline solutions. Its alkalizing properties provide the basis for its use in denture adhesives and its buffering action for its use in eyewash formulations.

Sodium Carbonate

Carbonic acid, disodium salt, monohydrate; Monohydrated Sodium Carbonate USP XVII

Disodium carbonate monohydrate [5968-11-6] $Na_2CO_3.H_2O$ (124.00); *anhydrous* [497-19-8] (105.99).

Preparation—The initial process for its manufacture was devised by Leblanc, a French apothecary, in 1784, and consists of two steps: first, the conversion of common salt [NaCl] into sodium sulfate by heating it with sulfuric acid and, second, the decomposition of the sulfate by calcium carbonate (limestone) and charcoal (coal) at a high temperature to yield this salt and calcium sulfide. The carbonate then is leached out with water.

It currently is prepared by the electrolysis of sodium chloride, whereby sodium and chlorine are produced, the former reacting with water to produce sodium hydroxide and this solution treated with carbon dioxide to produce the salt. The process is used most extensively in localities where electric power is very cheap.

The monohydrated form is made by crystallizing a concentrated solution of this salt at a temperature above 35° (95°F), and stirring the liquid so as to produce small crystals. It contains about 15% of water of crystallization.

Soda ash is a term designating a commercial quality of the anhydrous salt. Its annual production is very large, and it has a wide variety of applications, among which are the manufacture of glass, soap and sodium salts; it also is used for washing fabrics.

Washing soda, or *sal soda*, is the salt with 10 molecules of water. It is in the form of colorless crystals which rapidly effloresce in the air.

Description—Colorless crystals or a white, crystalline powder; stable in air under ordinary conditions; when exposed to dry air above 50° it effloresces, and at 100° becomes anhydrous; decomposed by weak acids forming the salt of the acid and liberating carbon dioxide; aqueous solution alkaline to indicators (pH about 11.5).

Solubility—1 g in 3 mL water or 1.8 mL boiling water; insoluble in alcohol.

Incompatibilities—*Acids, acid salts* and *acidic preparations* cause its decomposition. Most *metals* are precipitated as carbonates, hydroxides or basic salts. *Alkaloids* are precipitated from solutions of their salts.

Uses—Occasionally, for dermatitides topically as a lotion; it has been used as a mouthwash and a vaginal douche. It is used in the preparation of the sodium salts of many acids. The USP recognizes it as a pharmaceutic aid used as an alkalizing agent.

Sodium Hydroxide

Caustic Soda, Soda Lye

Sodium hydroxide [1310-73-2] NaOH (40.00); includes not more than 3% of Na_2CO_3 (105.99).

Caution—Exercise great care in handling it, as it rapidly destroys tissues.

Preparation—By treating sodium carbonate with milk of lime, or by the electrolysis of a solution of sodium chloride as explained under *Potassium Hydroxide* (page 877). It now is produced largely by the latter process. See also *Sodium Carbonate*, above.

Description—White, or nearly white, fused masses, small pellets, flakes, sticks and other forms; hard and brittle and shows a crystalline fracture; exposed to the air, it rapidly absorbs carbon dioxide and moisture; melts at about 318°; specific gravity 2.13; when dissolved in water or alcohol, or when its solution is treated with an acid, much heat is generated; aqueous solutions, even when highly diluted, are strongly alkaline.

Solubility—1 g in 1 mL water; freely soluble in alcohol or glycerin.

Incompatibilities—Exposed to air, it absorbs *carbon dioxide* and is converted to sodium carbonate. With *fats* and *fatty acids* it forms soluble soaps; with *resins* it forms insoluble soaps. See *Potassium Hydroxide* (page 877).

Uses—Too alkaline to be of medicinal value but occasionally used in veterinary practice as a caustic. It is used extensively in pharmaceutical processes as an alkalizing agent and is generally preferred to potassium hydroxide because it is less deliquescent, and less expensive; in addition, less of it is required since 40 parts of it are equivalent to 56 parts of KOH. It is a pharmaceutical necessity in the preparation of *Glycerin Suppositories* (see RPS-18, page 785).

Sodium Stearate

Octadecanoic acid, sodium salt

Sodium stearate [822-16-2] $C_{18}H_{35}NaO_2$ (306.47) consists chiefly of sodium stearate and sodium palmitate [$C_{16}H_{31}NaO_2$ = 278.41).

Preparation—Stearic acid is reacted with an equimolar portion of NaOH.

Description—Fine, white powder, soapy to the touch; usually has a slight, tallow-like odor; affected by light; solutions are alkaline to phenolphthalein TS.

Solubility—Slowly soluble in cold water or cold alcohol; readily soluble in hot water or hot alcohol.

Uses—Officially, a pharmaceutic aid used as an emulsifying and stiffening agent. It is an ingredient of glycerin suppositories. In dermatological practice it has been used topically in sycosis and other skin diseases.

Starch

Corn Starch; Wheat Starch; Potato Starch

Starch [9005-25-8]; consists of the granules separated from the mature grain of corn [*Zea mays* Linné (Fam *Gramineae*)] or of wheat [*Triticum aestivum* Linné] (Fam *Gramineae*), or from tubers of the potato [*Solanum tuberosum* Linné (Fam *Solanaceae*)].

Preparation—In making starch from corn, the germ is separated mechanically and the cells softened to permit escape of the starch granules. This generally is done by permitting it to become sour and decomposed, stopping the fermentation before the starch is affected. On the small scale, it may be made from wheat flour by making a stiff ball of dough and kneading it while a small stream of water trickles upon it. It is carried off with the water, while the *gluten* remains as a soft, elastic mass; the latter may be purified and used for various purposes to which gluten is applicable. Commercially, its quality largely depends on the purity of the water used in its manufacture. It may be made from potatoes by first grating them, and then washing the soft mass upon a sieve, which separates the cellular substances and permits the starch granules to be carried through. It then must be washed thoroughly by decantation, and the quality of this starch also depends largely on the purity of the water that is used in washing it.

Description—Irregular, angular, white masses or fine powder; odorless; slight, characteristic taste. *Corn starch:* Polygonal, rounded or spheroidal granules up to about 35 μm in diameter which usually have a circular or several-rayed central cleft. *Wheat starch:* Simple lenticular granules 20 to 50 μm in diameter and spherical granules 5 to 10 μm in diameter; striations faintly marked and concentric. *Potato starch:* Simple granules, irregularly ovoid or spherical, 30 to 100 μm in diameter, and subspherical granules 10 to 35 μm in diameter; striations well-marked and concentric.

Solubility—Insoluble in cold water or alcohol; when it is boiled with about 20 times its weight of hot water for a few minutes and then cooled, a translucent, whitish jelly results; aqueous suspension neutral to litmus.

Uses—Has absorbent and demulcent properties. It is used as a dusting powder and in various dermatological preparations; also as a pharmaceutic aid (filler, binder and disintegrant). *Note—Starches obtained from different botanical sources may not have identical properties with respect to their use for specific pharmaceutical purposes, eg, as a tablet-disintegrating agent. Therefore, types should not be interchanged unless performance equivalency has been ascertained.*

Under the title *Pregelatinized Starch* the NF recognizes starch that has been processed chemically or mechanically to rupture all or part of the granules in the presence of water, and subsequently dried. Some types may be modified to render them compressible and flowable.

Storax

Liquid Storax; Styrax; Sweet Gum; Prepared Storax

A balsam obtained from the trunk of *Liquidambar orientalis* Miller, known in commerce as Levant Storax, or of *Liquidambar styraciflua* Linné, known in commerce as American Storax (Fam *Hamamelidaceae*).

Constituents—The following occur in both varieties: *styracin* (*cinnamyl cinnamate*), *styrol* (*phenylethylene*, C_8H_8), α- and β-*storesin* (the cinnamic acid ester of an alcohol called *storesinol*), *phenylpropyl cinnamate*, free *cinnamic acid* and *vanillin*. In addition to these, Levant storax contains *ethyl cinnamate*, *benzyl cinnamate*, free *storesinol*, *isocinnamic acid*, *ethylvanillin*, *styrogenin* and *styrocamphene*. This variety yields from 0.5 to 1% of *volatile oil;* from this have been isolated *styrocamphene*, *vanillin*, the cinnamic acid esters of *ethyl*, *phenylpropyl*, *benzyl* and *cinnamyl alcohols*, *naphthalene* and *styrol*.

The American variety contains, in addition to the aforementioned substances common to both varieties, *styaresin* (the cinnamic acid ester of the alcohol *styresinol*, an isomer of storesinol) and *styresinolic acid*. It yields up to 7% of a dextrorotatory volatile oil, the composition of which has not been investigated completely; styrol and traces of vanillin have been isolated from it.

Description—Semiliquid, grayish to grayish brown, sticky, opaque mass, depositing on standing a heavy dark brown layer (Levant storax); or a semisolid, sometimes a solid mass, softened by gently warming (American storax); transparent in thin layers; characteristic odor and taste; more dense than water.

Solubility—Insoluble in water, but soluble, usually incompletely, in an equal weight of warm alcohol; soluble in acetone, carbon disulfide or ether, some insoluble residue usually remaining.

Uses—An *expectorant* but is used chiefly as a local remedy, especially in combination with benzoin; eg, it is an ingredient of *Compound Benzoin Tincture* (page 869). It may be used, like benzoin, to protect fatty substances from rancidity.

Sucrose Octaacetate

α-D-Glucopyranoside, 1,3,4,6-tetra-*O*-acetyl-β-D-fructofuranosyl-, tetraacetate

(Ac is $CH_3C(=O)-$)

Sucrose octaacetate [126-14-7] $C_{28}H_{38}O_{19}$ (678.60).

Preparation—Sucrose is subjected to exhaustive acetylation by reaction with acetic anhydride in the presence of a suitable condensing agent such as pyridine.

Description—White, practically odorless powder; intensely bitter taste; hygroscopic; melts not lower than 78°.

Solubility—1 g in 1100 mL water, 11 mL alcohol, 0.3 mL acetone or 0.6 mL benzene; very soluble in methanol or chloroform; soluble in ether.

Uses—A *denaturant* for alcohol.

Sulfurated Potash

Thiosulfuric acid, dipotassium salt, mixt. with potassium sulfide ($K_2(S_x)$); Liver of Sulfur

Dipotassium thiosulfate mixture with potassium sulfide (K_2S_x) [39365-88-3]; a mixture composed chiefly of potassium polysulfides and potassium thiosulfate. It contains not less than 12.8% of S (sulfur) in combination as sulfide.

Preparation—By thoroughly mixing 1 part of sublimed sulfur with 2 parts of potassium carbonate and gradually heating the mixture in a covered iron crucible until the mass ceases to swell and is melted completely. It then is poured on a stone or glass slab and, when cold, broken into pieces and preserved in tightly closed bottles. When the heat is regulated properly during its production, the reaction is represented approximately by

$$3K_2CO_3 + 8S \rightarrow 2K_2S_3 + K_2S_2O_3 + 3CO_2$$

As this product rapidly deteriorates on exposure to moisture, oxygen and carbon dioxide, it is important that it be prepared recently to produce satisfactory preparations.

Description—Irregular pieces, liver-brown when freshly prepared, changing to a greenish yellow; decomposes upon exposure to air; an odor of hydrogen sulfide and a bitter, acrid, alkaline taste; even weak acids cause the liberation of H_2S from sulfurated potash; 1 in 10 solution light brown in color and alkaline to litmus.

Solubility—1 g in about 2 mL water, usually leaving a slight residue; alcohol dissolves only the sulfides.

Uses—Extensively in dermatological practice, especially in the official *White Lotion* or *Lotio Alba* (page 873). It is used as an opacifier.

The equation for the reaction of the potassium trisulfide in preparing the lotion is

$$ZnSO_4 + K_2S_3 \rightarrow \underline{ZnS} + 2\underline{S} + K_2SO_4$$

Talc

Talcum; Purified Talc; French Chalk; Soapstone; Steatite

A native, hydrous magnesium silicate, sometimes containing a small proportion of aluminum silicate.

Occurrence and Preparation—The native form, called *soapstone* or *French chalk*, is found in various parts of the world. An excellent quality is obtained from deposits in North Carolina. Deposits of a high grade, conforming to the USP requirements, also are found in Manchuria. The native form usually is accompanied by variable amounts of mineral substances. These are separated from it by mechanical means, such as flotation or elutriation. It then is powdered finely, treated with boiling dilute HCl, washed well and dried.

Description—Very fine, white, or grayish white crystalline powder; unctuous to the touch, adhering readily to the skin, and free from grittiness.

Uses—Officially, as a dusting powder and pharmaceutic aid; in both categories it has many specific uses. Its medicinal use as a dusting powder depends on its desiccant and lubricant effects. When perfumed, and sometimes medicated, it is used extensively for toilet purposes under the name *talcum powder;* for such use it should be in the form of an impalpable powder. When used as a filtration medium for clarifying liquids a coarser powder is preferred to minimize passage through the pores of the filter paper; for this purpose it may be used for all classes of preparations with no danger of adsorption or retention of active principles. It is used as a lubricant in the manufacture of tablets, and as a dusting powder when making handmade suppositories. Although it is used as a lubricant for putting on and removing rubber gloves, it should not be used on surgical gloves because even small amounts deposited in organs or healing wounds may cause granuloma formation.

Tartaric Acid

Butanedioic acid, [*R*-(*R**,*R**)] 2,3-dihydroxy-,

COOH
H—C—OH
HO—C—H
COOH

L-(+)-Tartaric acid [87-69-4] $C_4H_6O_6$ (150.09).

Preparation—From *argol*, the crude cream of tartar (potassium bitartrate) deposited on the sides of wine casks during the fermentation of grapes, by conversion to calcium tartrate which is hydrolyzed to tartaric acid and calcium sulfate.

Description—Large, colorless or translucent crystals, or a white granular to fine crystalline powder; odorless; acid taste; stable in the air; solutions acid to litmus; dextrorotatory.

Solubility—1 g in 0.8 mL water, 0.5 mL boiling water, 3 mL alcohol or 250 mL ether; freely soluble in methanol.

Uses—Chiefly, as the acid ingredient of preparations in which it is neutralized by a bicarbonate, as in effervescent salts, and the free acid is completely absent or present only in small amounts in the finished product. It also is used as a buffering agent.

Trichloromonofluoromethane

Methane, trichlorofluoro-,

$CFCl_3$

Trichlorofluoromethane [75-69-4] CCl_3F (137.37).

Preparation—Carbon tetrachloride is reacted with antimony trifluoride in the presence of a small quantity of antimony pentachloride. The reaction produces a mixture of CCl_3F and CCl_2F_2 which is readily separable by fractional distillation.

Description—Clear, colorless gas; faint, ethereal odor; vapor pressure at 25° is about 796 torr; boils about 24°.

Solubility—Practically insoluble in water; soluble in alcohol, ether or other organic solvents.

Uses—A *propellant* (No 11, see page 1696).

Tyloxapol

Phenol, 4-(1,1,3,3-tetramethylbutyl)-, polymer with formaldehyde and oxirane; (*Various Mfrs*)

[*R* is $CH_2CH_2O(CH_2CH_2O)_mCH_2CH_2OH$; *m* is 6 to 8; *n* is not more than 5]

p-(1,1,3,3-Tetramethylbutyl)phenol polymer with ethylene oxide and formaldehyde [25301-02-4].

Preparation—*p*-(1,1,3,3-Tetramethylbutyl)phenol and formaldehyde are condensed by heating in the presence of an acidic catalyst and the polymeric phenol thus obtained is reacted with ethylene oxide at elevated temperature under pressure in the presence of NaOH. US Pat. 2,454,541.

Description—Amber, viscous liquid; may show a slight turbidity; slight aromatic odor; specific gravity about 1.072; stable at sterilization temperature and in the presence of acids, bases and salts; oxidized by metals; pH (5% aqueous solution) 4 to 7.

Solubility—Slowly but freely soluble in water; soluble in many organic solvents, including acetic acid, benzene, carbon tetrachloride, carbon disulfide, chloroform or toluene.

Uses—A nonionic detergent that depresses both surface tension and interfacial tension. It also is used in contact-lens-cleaner formulations.

Zinc-Eugenol Cement—see RPS-18, page 1328.

Iso-Alcoholic Elixir

Iso-Elixir

Low-Alcoholic Elixir	
High-Alcoholic Elixir	of each a calculated volume

Mix the ingredients.

Low-Alcoholic Elixir

Compound Orange Spirit	**10 mL**
Alcohol	**100 mL**
Glycerin	**200 mL**
Sucrose	**320 g**
Purified Water, a sufficient quantity,	
To make	**1000 mL**

Alcohol Content—8 to 10%.

High-Alcoholic Elixir

Compound Orange Spirit	**4 mL**
Saccharin	**3 g**
Glycerin	**200 mL**
Alcohol, a sufficient quantity,	
To make	**1000 mL**

Alcohol Content—73 to 78%.

Uses—Intended as a general *vehicle* for various medicaments that require solvents of different alcohol strengths. When it is specified in a prescription, the proportion of its two ingredients to be used is that which will produce a solution of the required alcohol strength.

The alcohol strength of the elixir to be used with a single liquid galenical in a prescription is approximately the same as that of the galenical. When galenicals of different alcohol strengths are used in the same prescription, the elixir to be used is to be of such alcohol strength as to secure the best solution possible. This generally will be found to be the average of the alcohol strengths of the several ingredients.

For nonextractive substances, the lowest alcohol strength of the elixir that will yield a perfect solution should be chosen.

Other Miscellaneous Pharmaceutical Necessities

Bucrylate [Propenoic acid, 2-cyano-, 2-methylpropyl ester; Isobutyl 2-cyanoacrylate [1069-55-2] $C_8H_{11}NO_2$ (153.18); (*Ethicon*)]—*Preparation:* One method reacts isobutyl 2-chloroacrylate with sodium cyanide. *Uses:* Surgical aid (tissue adhesive).

Ceresin [Ozokerite; Earth Wax; Cerosin; Mineral Wax; Fossil Wax]—A hard, white odorless solid resembling spermaceti when purified, occurring naturally in deposits in the Carpathian Mountains, especially in Galicia. It is a mixture of natural complex paraffin hydrocarbons. Melts between 61 and 78°; specific gravity 0.91 to 0.92; stable toward oxidizing agents. Soluble in 30% alcohol, benzene, chloroform, petroleum, benzin or hot oils. *Uses:* Substitute for beeswax; in dentistry, for impression waxes.

Ethylenediamine Hydrate BP, PhI [$H_2NCH_2CH_2NH_2.H_2O$]—Clear, colorless or slightly yellow liquid with an ammoniacal odor and characteristic alkaline taste; solidifies on cooling to a crystalline mass (mp 10°); boils 118 to 119°; specific gravity about 0.96; hygroscopic and absorbs CO_2 from the air; aqueous solutions alkaline to litmus. Miscible with water or alcohol; soluble in 130 parts of chloroform; slightly soluble in benzene or ether. *Uses:* In the manufacture of aminophylline and in the preparation of aminophylline injections. See *Ethylenediamine* (page 1381).

Ferric Oxide, Red—Contains not less than 90% Fe_2O_3. It is made by heating native ferric oxide or hydroxide at a temperature which will yield a product of the desired color. The color is governed by the temperature and time of heating, the presence and kind of other metals and the particle size of the oxide. A dark-colored oxide is favored by prolonged heating at high temperature and the presence of manganese. A light-colored oxide is favored by the presence of aluminum and by finer particle size. *Uses:* Imparting color to neocalamine and cosmetics.

Ferric Oxide, Yellow—Contains not less than 97.5% Fe_2O_3. It is prepared by heating ferrous hydroxide or ferrous carbonate in air at a low temperature. *Uses:* As for *Red Ferric Oxide* (above).

Honey NF XII [Mel; Clarified Honey; Strained Honey]—The saccharine secretion deposited in the honeycomb by the bee, *Apis mellifera* Linné (Fam *Apidae*). It must be free from foreign substances such as parts of insects, leaves, etc, but may contain pollen grains. *History:* Honey is one of the oldest of food and medicinal products. During the 16th and 17th centuries it was recommended as a cure for almost everything. *Constituents: Invert sugar* (62 to 83%), *sucrose* (0 to 8%) and *dextrin* (0.26 to 7%). *Description:* Thick, syrupy liquid of a light yellowish to reddish brown color; translucent when fresh, but frequently becomes opaque and granular through crystallization of dextrose; characteristic odor and a sweet, faintly acrid taste. *Uses:* A sweetening agent and pharmaceutic necessity.

Hydriodic Acid, Diluted—Contains, in each 100 mL 9.5 to 10.5 g of HI (127.91), and 600 mg to 1 g of HPH_2O_2 (66.00). The latter is added to prevent the formation of free iodine. *Caution: Diluted Hydriodic Acid must not be dispensed or used in the preparation of other products if they contain free iodine. Preparation:* On a large scale, by the interaction of iodine and hydrogen sulfide. *Description* and *Solubility*: Colorless or not more than pale-yellow, odorless liquid; specific gravity about 1.1. Miscible with water or alcohol. *Uses:* In *Hydriodic Acid Syrup* (page 1393). The latter has been used as an expectorant. It also is used in the manufacture of inorganic iodides and disinfectants. The 57% acid also is used for analytical purposes, such as methoxyl determinations.

Lime [Calx; Calcium Oxide; Quicklime; Burnt Lime; Calx Usta; CaO (56.08)]—*Preparation:* By calcining *limestone* (a native calcium carbonate) in kilns with strong heat. *Description and Solubility:* Hard, white or grayish white masses or granules, or a white or grayish white powder; odorless; solution strongly alkaline. 1 g is soluble in about 840 mL water and 1740 mL boiling water; soluble in glycerin or syrup; insoluble in alcohol. *Uses:* In making mortar, whitewash, and various chemicals and products. It is an ingredient in *Sulfurated Lime Solution* (RPS-16, page 1187). In the USP, calcium hydroxide has replaced it, as it is more stable and more readily available of a quality suitable for medicinal use than the lime usually obtainable. Unless protected from air, lime soon becomes unfit for use, due to the action of carbon dioxide and moisture in the air. See *Calcium Hydroxide* (page 1408).

Peach Oil—An oil resembling almond oil obtained from *Persica vulgaris* (Fam *Rosaceae*). See *Persic Oil* (RPS-18, page 1323).

Polacrilin Potassium [Methacrylic acid polymer with divinylbenzene, potassium salt [39394-76-5]; Amberlite IRP-88 (*Rohm & Haas*)]—Prepared by polymerizing methacrylic acid with divinylbenzene and the resulting resin is neutralized with KOH. Dry, buff-colored, odorless, tasteless, free-flowing powder; stable in light, air, and heat; insoluble in water. *Uses: Pharmaceutic aid* (tablet disintegrant).

Poloxalene [Glycols, polymers, polyethylene-polypropylene [9003-11-6]—Polypropylene glycol is reacted with ethylene oxide. *Uses: Pharmaceutic aid* (surfactant).

Raspberry Juice—The liquid expressed from the fresh ripe fruit of *Rubus idaeus* Linné or of *Rubus strigosus* Michaux (Fam *Rosaceae*); contains not less than 1.5% of acids calculated as citric acid. *Preparation:* Express the juice from the washed, well-drained, fresh, ripe, red raspberries. Dissolve 0.1% of benzoic acid in the expressed juice and allow it to stand at room temperature (possibly for several days) until a small portion of the filtered juice produces a clear solution when mixed with ½ of its volume of alcohol, the solution remaining clear for not less than 30 min. Strain the juice from the mixture or filter it, if necessary. *Description:* Clear liquid with an aromatic, characteristic odor and a characteristic, sour taste; the freshly prepared juice is red to reddish orange; affected by light. *Uses:* In the preparation of *Raspberry Syrup* (see RPS-18, page 1302), a *flavored vehicle.*

Sodium Glutamate [Sodium Acid Glutamate [142-47-2] $HOOCCH(NH_2)CH_2CH_2COONa$]—White or nearly white, crystalline powder. Very soluble in water; sparingly soluble in alcohol. *Uses:* Imparts a meat flavor to foods.

Sodium Thioglycollate [Sodium Mercaptoacetate; $HSCH_2COONa$]—Hygroscopic crystals which discolor on exposure to air or iron. Freely soluble in water; slightly soluble in alcohol. *Uses:* Reducing agent in Fluid Thioglycollate Medium for sterility testing.

Suet, Prepared [Mutton Suet]—Internal fat of the abdomen of the sheep, *Ovis aries* (Fam *Bovidae*), purified by melting and straining. White, solid fat with a slight, characteristic odor and taste when fresh; melts between 45° and 50° and congeals between 37° and 40°; must be preserved in a cool place in tight containers. *Uses:* In ointments and cerates.

Urea [Carbamide [57-13-6] $CO(NH_2)_2$(60.06)]—A product of protein metabolism; prepared by hydrolysis of cyanamide or from carbon dioxide by ammonolysis. Colorless to white crystals or white, crystalline powder; almost odorless but may develop a slight odor of ammonia in presence of moisture; melts 132 to 135°. 1 g dissolves in 1.5 mL of water or 10 mL of alcohol; practically insoluble in chloroform or ether. *Uses:* A protein denaturant that promotes hydration of keratin and mild keratolysis in dry and hyperkeratotic skin. It is used in 2 to 20% concentrations in various dry-skin creams.

CHAPTER 81

Immunizing Agents and Diagnostic Skin Antigens

Frank Roia, PhD
Professor of Biology
Philadelphia College of Pharmacy and Science
Philadelphia, PA 19104

The Food and Drug Administration (FDA) refers to immunizing agents as *biologics (biologicals, biological products)*; whereas the Advisory Committee on Immunization Practices (ACIP) refers to immunizing agents as *immunobiologics.* The term *biologic* will be used in this discussion. In its broadest meaning, a biologic refers to something produced from a living source and thus would include hormones, vitamins, antibiotics, enzymes and so forth. However, according to the *Code of Federal Regulations (CFR)*, a biological product is any virus, therapeutic serum, toxin, antitoxin or analogous product applicable to the prevention, treatment or cure of diseases or injuries of man. These preparations are primarily designed to develop a type of immunity or are concerned with immunity. *Immunity*, in the most general sense, may be defined simply as natural or acquired resistance to disease.

Providing immunity by using a biologic is referred to as *immunization.* The term vaccination, as it often is used, refers to the administration of a biologic such as a vaccine for active immunity (see following discussion) without any consideration as to whether or not it confers resistance. ACIP, in its statements of recommendation, uses the two terms interchangeably when referring to active immunization. ACIP, however, points out that whichever term is used, one should not equate automatically the administration of a biologic with the development of adequate immunity because of a variety of specific factors which might interfere with the immune response.

Types of Immunity

Before discussing biologics, it is important to have an understanding of the different types of immunity. Fig 1 illustrates the main categories into which the various kinds of natural and acquired immunity may be classified.

The following discussion is an overview of Fig 1 and is in no way intended to be a comprehensive treatment.

Natural Immunity

Species Immunity—It is well-known that humans are resistant to a variety of infections common in lower animals including canine distemper, hog cholera and cattle plague. In a similar manner lower animals exhibit a *nonsusceptibility* to certain human infections such as gonorrhea, measles, bacillary dysentery and smallpox. In fact, an important reason for the eradication of smallpox (the last naturally occurring case recorded was in Somalia in 1977) was that man was the only host and there were no lower animals to serve as reservoirs for the infection. On the other hand, there are some ninety diseases, such as tuberculosis, anthrax, ornithosis and rabies which occur in both man and lower animals alike.

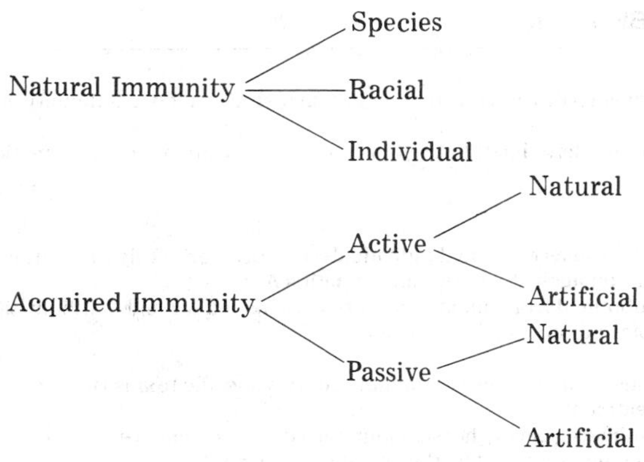

Natural Immunity — Species / Racial / Individual

Acquired Immunity — Active (Natural / Artificial) / Passive (Natural / Artificial)

Fig 1.

Not all factors involved in species immunity are known, but in part, it is determined by the anatomy and physiology of the particular animal species. There is evidence, for example, that certain microorganisms are able to penetrate the epithelial barrier, or other tissue barriers, of one species and not another. It also has been shown that certain species are resistant to specific infections because they possess *natural antibodies* which, as far as is known, are present without obvious external stimuli.

Racial Immunity—Certain races are more resistant or susceptible to specific diseases (eg, yellow fever or tuberculosis).

Like species immunity, the factors which determine racial immunity are not all known. Some, like resistance to malaria, have some physiological basis in that resistance is highest in persons carrying the sickle cell trait. Racial immunity should not be confused with "environmental immunity," which may be the result of resistance to infection among individuals in a given community due to the degree of acquired immunity and to such factors as nutrition, fatigue and genetic constitution (Chapter 44).

Individual Immunity—Individuals in good health are endowed with a high level of natural immunity without having had an opportunity to generate specific antibodies as a result of a previous infection (Chapter 44). General good health also implies healthy body tissues, skin and mucous membranes (all important bacterial barriers), leukocytes in plentiful supply, properly active etc. Also involved in individual resistance is the kind and quality of the resident bacterial flora in the large intestine, in the upper respiratory tract, including the oral cavity and in other parts of the body. Undoubtedly, the resident flora play a part in resisting invasion by other species of microorganisms capable of producing infection. Similarly, the gastric juice, as a result of acidic properties, is bactericidal to a marked degree and capable of destroying many species of harmful bacteria and viruses which may be ingested during eating and drinking. In addition, the intestinal enzymes help to set up a valuable secondary defense mechanism. Another important consideration in individual immunity is the as yet undefined role of immune response genes (Chapter 44).

Active Acquired Immunity

Active acquired immunity occurs when the stimulus is an immunogen which elicits an immune response (Chapter 44). Thus, the host (human or lower animal) is "actively" involved in the production of protecting antibodies (immunoglobulins).

Active acquired immunity may be acquired in one of two general ways: natural or artificial.

Naturally Acquired Active Immunity—This occurs when the introduction of a *virulent immunogen* results in a disease state in its recognizable clinical presentation. However, in some individuals, either because of increased host resistance, moderate exposure to the immunogen or decreased virulence of the immunogen, the disease may be so mild that it never reaches the clinical stage (*subclinical infection*). Immunoglobulins, however, may be produced in sufficient amount to protect the individual from possible future infections by the same species of microorganism. Infections such as polio and rubella, for example, often occur subclinically and are detected, along with protective antibodies to a variety of other infections, in routine immunological studies of individuals who never have had a clinically recognizable case of the disease in question.

It must be kept in mind that the degree of immunity possessed is the determining factor in successful resistance against future exposures. It is known that a level of immunity can be entirely effective against a moderate contact with a given pathogen, yet become ineffective in the event of exposure to an overwhelming dose of the same organism.

The outcome of any infection, therefore, is determined not only by the degree of acquired immunity but also by several complex interreacting factors including the virulence of the invading microorganism, the level of resistance offered by body tissues and cells and by the general level of health in the host.

Artificially Acquired Active Immunity—This involves the use of *avirulent immunogens* in the form of biologics such as *vaccines* and *toxoids* (Table 1). Vaccines and toxoids contain immunogens that are modified so as to be incapable of producing the disease state, yet at the same time modified so slightly that when introduced into the body will elicit the production of specific protective immunoglobulins against the disease.

The duration of active acquired immunity, both natural and artificial, is variable. In some cases it is rather brief but protection usually lasts many years and, in some diseases, for life. For most vaccines and toxoids secondary stimuli or *boosters* are required at periodic intervals of months to years if the acquired immunity is to be maintained.

Passive Acquired Immunity

In passive acquired immunity, the immunoglobulins are produced in another individual (human or lower animal). Thus immunity is acquired by the introduction of these immunoglobulins into the host who is not involved in their production. Passive acquired immunity, like active acquired immunity, may be classified as natural or artificial.

Naturally Acquired Passive Immunity—This occurs by placental transmission of immunoglobulin G (IgG) from mother to fetus (Chapter 44). The infant may have passive immunity for the first four to six months of life to diphtheria, tetanus, measles, mumps and other infections because of the transfer of these immunoglobulins.

Artificially Acquired Passive Immunity—Several biologics (Table 1) are involved in providing immunoglobulins including antitoxins' immune globulin and hyperimmune sera derived from human plasma. In this category also would be placed antivenins used for the treatment of the bites of poisonous snakes and spiders.

Biologics for passive immunity are limited to temporary prophylaxis of susceptible individuals, for example during an epidemic, and to supplying immediate immunoglobulins for the treatment of infections and toxicities.

The immunity provided by these means is not long-lasting, and such immunoglobulins leave the body tissues and fluids of the host within a comparatively short time (usually 1 or 2 weeks). Thus, the administration of diphtheria antitoxin to a susceptible patient exposed to diphtheria will offer protection during the critical period when resistance is needed most urgently, but will not be permanent because the injected immunoglobulins will be utilized either by binding to the pathogen as needed or metabolized by the body if not needed for immunological purposes.

Hypersensitivity to Biologics

Certain biological components can cause hypersensitive (allergic) reactions ranging from mild local symptoms to severe systemic anaphylaxis (eg, hives, swelling of the mouth and throat, difficulty in breathing, hypotension or shock). These reactions primarily are associated with three general types of biologics.

1. *Antisera or Antitoxins of animal origin (usually equine).*
2. *Viral vaccines grown in embryonic egg.*
3. *Biologics (mainly viral vaccines) with antibiotics.*

Antisera or Antitoxins of Animal Origin

Antivenins and antitoxins such as botulism and diphtheria are prepared from horse sera which are proteinaceous and foreign to the recipient and thus may be immunogenic in their own right.

Before the administration of any product containing horse serum, it is customary for the physician to inquire into the history of the patient to determine whether or not equine antisera may have been given some time earlier. It also is important to ascertain whether the patient has a history of asthma or any allergy and particularly whether the patient suffers distress when in proximity to horses. Patients with such a history may develop serious systemic reactions.

Sensitiveness can be determined readily by an intracutaneous skin test or the less commonly used conjunctival test using small quantities of a dilution of the product to be administered. In fact the manufacturers' package inserts recommend that all

Table 1—Types of Biologics

Biologics for Active Immunity

- *Vaccine*—a suspension of attenuated (live) or inactivated (killed) microorganisms or fractions thereof administered to induce immunity and thus prevent infectious disease.
- *Toxoid*—a modified bacterial toxin (exotoxin) that has been rendered nontoxic (detoxified) but retains the ability to stimulate the formation of antitoxin and thus prevent bacterial toxicities.

Biologics for Passive Immunity

- Human Immune Sera (Homologous Sera)
  - *Immune Globulin*—a solution containing immunoglobulins from the pooled plasmas of normal individuals. It is used primarily for routine maintenance of certain immunodeficient persons and for passive immunization against measles and hepatitis A.
  - *Hyperimmune Serum* (Specific Immune Globulin)—a special preparation obtained from human donor pools selected for high antibody titer against a specific disease, eg, hepatitis B immune globulin (HBIG) and rabies immune globulin (RIG).
- Animal Immune Sera (Heterologous Sera)
  - *Antitoxin*—a solution of immunoglobulins derived from the plasma of animals (usually a horse) immunized with specific toxins (toxoids) eg, botulism and diphtheria used to achieve passive immunity or to effect a treatment.
  - *Antivenin*—a preparation of immunoglobulins derived from the plasma of animals (usually horses) immunized with specific venoms, eg, rattlesnakes, coral snake and black widow spider, used to neutralize the venoms produced by the specific organisms.

patients regardless of history be tested before the injection of the biologic. If the patient is sensitive, positive reactions will occur within 30 minutes. In the case of the skin test a positive reaction is a wheal with a hyperaemic areola and in the conjunctival test it is lacrimation and conjunctivitis.

A negative sensitivity test usually is considered reliable but does not preclude entirely the possibility of the occurrence of systemic reactions. If the sensitivity test is positive, the biologic still may be administered to the patient but with *extreme* caution. This is accomplished by following a *desensitization* schedule which involves a series of injections, beginning with a very small dose of diluted antitoxin given *subcutaneously* and increased at 15- to 20-minute intervals until the biologic eventually is given undiluted *intramuscularly* and the required therapeutic dose has been administered. The various manufacturers' package inserts may vary somewhat and therefore should be consulted before using a specific product.

It should be noted that it is exceedingly dangerous to readminister any animal antiserum of the same animal origin. In such cases serious systemic reactions are a real possibility.

Fortunately there currently is little need for use of immunizing agents from animal sera. With proper utilization of diphtheria toxoid for active immunization, the use of antitoxin can be avoided. Only lifesaving antisera such as botulism antitoxin and the antivenins must be used occasionally.

Viral Vaccines Grown in Embryonic Egg

Vaccines propagated in embryonic egg (or cell cultures of chick embryo) may cause hypersensitivity reactions, including anaphylaxis, especially when there is a substantial amount of egg protein in the final product, as is the case with yellow fever vaccine. This vaccine, therefore, should not be administered to an individual with a proved sensitivity to egg or chicken embryo protein. If there is any question, an intracutaneous sensitivity skin test should be performed. The vaccine is contraindicated if the sensitivity test is positive.

Measles, mumps and influenza vaccines also are propagated in egg or cell cultures of chick embryo but can be given safely to individuals sensitive to chicken protein provided that the allergies are not manifested by anaphylactic symptoms. Influenza vaccines, both whole and split, are purified highly during preparation and have been reported only rarely to be associated with hypersensitivity reactions.

Screening persons by a history of ability to eat eggs without adverse effects usually is sufficient to identify those individuals at possible risk from receiving measles, mumps or influenza vaccines. The vaccines should not be given to those individuals who have demonstrated anaphylactic hypersensitivity.

Biologics with Antibiotics

Viral vaccines, such as rubella, that are propagated on human tissue culture essentially are devoid of any potential hypersensitivity related to host tissue but they may contain trace amounts of antibiotics, eg neomycin, to which patients occasionally may be hypersensitive. However, except for anaphylactic reactions to neomycin or streptomycin, viral vaccines are not contraindicated for persons with allergies to penicillin and other antibiotics. Patients also very rarely may be hypersensitive to other additives such as stabilizers and preservatives in biologics, eg thimerosal, a common preservative of many biologics.

Health personnel administering these biologics should review carefully the information provided with the package insert before deciding whether a person with a known hypersensitivity to such ingredients be administered the biologic.

Note: No currently recommended biologic contains penicillin or its derivatives.

Other Reactions

All biologics can cause a variety of local and systemic adverse reactions which appear to be toxic rather than hypersensitive. These reactions range from frequent minor local reactions such as redness, tenderness and induration surrounding the injection site to systemic manifestations including malaise, generalized aches and pains and fever. In extremely rare situations there have been severe, systemic illness, such as paralysis associated with oral polio vaccine.

Generally, the risk of serious reaction is far outweighed by the lifesaving benefits derived by prudent use of these agents. The relative balance of benefits and risks may change as diseases are brought under control or eradicated. This is best exemplified by smallpox vaccination. Since smallpox has been eradicated the very small risk from receiving smallpox vaccine now exceeds the risk of smallpox itself. Thus, smallpox vaccination is limited to civilian laboratory personnel directly involved with smallpox or closely related orthopox viruses and to certain categories of military personnel.

The vaccines for cholera, plague and typhoid fever frequently are associated with local and systemic adverse effects. It is not possible to discuss these specific reactions here; however, it should be noted that some of the recommendations for their use are based upon minimizing potential adverse reactions.

Even the pertussis vaccine component of DTP (diphtheria and tetanus toxoids and pertussis vaccine) has been responsible for serious systemic reactions including collapse or shock, persistent screaming episodes, temperatures of 105° or greater, convulsions and encephalopathy including severe alterations in consciousness with generalized or focal neurological signs. For these reasons the ACIP recommends that further use of pertussis vaccine-containing preparations is contraindicated if any of these adverse reactions occur. The vaccine also is contraindicated in the presence of a neurological condition characterized by changing developmental or neurological findings, regardless of whether a definitive diagnosis has been made. However, in spite of these and other contraindications, the vaccine still is recommended for normal infants and those with resolved and corrected neurological conditions including well-controlled seizures, because the benefits of pertussis immunization continue to outweigh its risks.

The National Childhood Vaccine Injury Act of 1986 (NCVIA)

NCVIA, which became effective on March 21, 1988, has two objectives:

To avoid future "crises" that may interrupt the National Immunization Program.

To provide financial compensation for those patients who suffer vaccine-related injuries.

In order to meet these two goals, the Act requires that health-care providers who administer any vaccine containing measles, mumps, rubella, poliomyelitis, diphtheria, tetanus or pertussis antigens maintain permanent vaccination records, including type of biologic administered; date of administration; manufacturer and lot number; name, address and title of person administering the vaccine; and the patient's occupation, life style and history of vaccine-preventable illnesses. Ideally, the permanent record also should contain information on all other vaccines and toxoids adminstered.

The Act requires that certain specified occurrences of adverse reactions be reported in detail to the Vaccine Adverse Event Reporting System (VAERS) in order to expand knowledge of such reactions. The Act also requires that a surcharge be placed on these biologics in order to establish a fund to compensate victims.

Contraindications

In general, there are two situations in which some biologics may be contraindicated: pregnancy and altered immunocompetence.

Pregnancy—Although very little data is available on the safety of vaccines and toxoids during pregnancy, the administration of any inactivated vaccine or toxoid usually is delayed until the second or third trimester, whenever possible, to minimize concern about potential teratogenicity. The administration of live Bacille Calmette-Guerin (BCG) vaccine and live virus vaccines should not be given to pregnant women or to those likely to become pregnant within 3 months because of a theoretical risk to the developing fetus.

Altered Immunocompetence—BCG, live oral typhoid vaccine or live virus vaccines should not be given to persons who are immunocompromised, eg, those with immune deficiency diseases, leukemia, lymphoma or generalized malignancy or persons immunocompromised from therapy with radiation, corticosteroids or other agents. Severe complications have resulted from immunization with live vaccines as a result of enhanced viral replication and bacterial growth in persons with altered immunocompetence.

Note—There are several conditions as outlined in ACIP recommendations that are not contraindicated to vaccination. Some of the more common conditions that are not considered contraindications are soreness, redness or swelling in the immediate vicinity of the vaccination site or a temperature <105°F as a result of a previous dose of DTP; mild acute illness with low grade fever or mild diarrheal illness in an otherwise well child; current antimicrobial therapy; convalescent phase of illnesses; prematurity; pregnancy of mother or other household contact; recent exposure to an infectious disease; breastfeeding; history of nonspecific allergies or relatives with allergies; allergies to penicillin or any other antibiotic, except anaphylactic reactions to neomycin or streptomycin; allergies to duck meat or duck feathers; family history of convulsions in persons considered for pertussis or measles vaccination; family history of sudden infant death syndrome in children considered for DTP vaccination; and family history of an adverse event, unrelated to immunosuppression, following vaccination.

Routine Immunization of HIV-Infected Persons

HIV-infected infants, children and adults are associated with increased risk of complications from infectious disease, and it is important that they be protected. Although the effectiveness of biologics given to immunocompromised patients may be limited, the minimal adverse reactions and possible benefits outweight the substantial risk of disease.

As previously indicated, the use of live bacterial and virus vaccines is contraindicated in persons with altered immunocompetence. However, several inactivated biologics are recommended by ACIP for the routine vaccination of known HIV asymptomatic or symptomatic persons. These are: diphtheria and tetanus toxoids and pertussis vaccine adsorbed (pediatric) or tetanus and diphtheria toxoids, adsorbed (for adult use); inactivated polio vaccine; *Haemophilus influenzae* type b conjugate vaccine and pneumococcal vaccine. In addition, influenza vaccine is recommended for symptomatic HIV-infected persons and should be considered for known asymptomatic carriers, whereas measles, mumps and rubella vaccine is recommended routinely for known asymptomatic individuals and should be considered for those that are symptomatic.

In the event that a susceptible individual is exposed to an infectious agent, the various human hyperimmune globulins should be considered for those diseases that are preventable by the use of immune globulins.

Federal Control of Biologics

The production and distribution of biologics is regulated by the Center for Biologics Evaluation and Research (CBER), of the FDA. The Center develops standards for safety, potency and purity and conducts research on the development, manufacture and testing of biologics. The Center also reviews data for licensing of biologics and their manufacturers and conducts periodic inspections of the manufacturing sites.

Care in Dispensing

In dispensing biologics, the pharmacist is dealing with preparations mostly intended for injection subcutaneously, intramuscularly, intravenously or by some other parenteral route. It is, therefore, of paramount importance that the sterility and potency of the preparations be maintained until they actually are injected. Sterility is assured by the processes used in manufacturing, and no product is released until repeated tests have shown it to be safe in this respect.

The pharmacist contributes to the maintenance of the potency of the product and insures safety to the patient by observing specified requirements. The label should be examined carefully for specific instructions as to the temperature at which the product should be stored, the expiration date and other essential information pertaining not only to the product but also to the particular lot. All products must be dispensed in the unopened containers in which they were placed by the manufacturer. Freezing temperatures should be avoided, unless otherwise directed on the labeling. The risk of damage from freezing may be greatest for the aqueous diluents frequently packaged with biologics.

Sources of Information

The information presented in this chapter is derived primarily from the following:

Morbidity and Mortality Weekly Report (MMWR)—This report is published weekly by the Centers for Disease Control (CDC) and contains reports on specific disease activity, policy statements and the regular and special recommendations of the Advisory Committee of Immunization Practices (ACIP) on biologics, including (a) *Update on Adult Immunization* Vol 40/No. RR-12, 11/15/91 and (b) *General Recommendations on Immunization*, Vol 43/No. RR-1, 1/28/94.

Manufacturers' Package Inserts—In addition to the type of information discussed in this chapter, the package insert contains data on contraindications, warnings, precautions, adverse reactions, clinical pharmacology, storage requirements, references, etc.

United States Pharmacopeia—This compendium contains the official monographs for some of the biologics described in this chapter. These monographs cover aspects of identity, purity, potency, packaging and storage that are of particular interest to pharmacists and physicians responsible for purchase, storage and use of biologics.

Code of Federal Regulations (CFR)—Title 21, Chapter 1, Subchapter F- Biologics, Parts 600–680, 1993 contains federal regulations (as administered by the CBER) pertaining to licensing, good manufacturing practices, general biologic standards and additional standards on specific biologics.

Biologics for Active Immunization

Bacterial Vaccines

Preparation—The organisms are grown in suitable broth medium under controlled conditions of temperature, pH, oxygen tension and so forth. Whenever possible the medium consists of chemically defined ingredients to reduce the potential for hypersensitivity reactions of the finished product. The incubation period is usually 24 hours but may be extended to 48 to 72 hours or longer for slower growing bacteria.

Following a suitable amount of growth, the culture then is processed in two main steps:

1. If the vaccine is killed, the organisms are *inactivated* with formaldehyde or phenol. Typhoid fever vaccine is inactivated with heat and phenol or heat and acetone.
2. The organisms then are separated from the medium by means of centrifugation and resuspended in sterile saline or sterile water for injection.

The cells may be purified further by several methods including additional centrifugation and/or dialysis.

In the preparation of anthrax and pertussis acellular vaccines, the cultures are filtered and the filtrates, not the organisms, are processed further and used as the source of the immunogens.

Product Form—In cholera, pertussis (whole-cell) plague and typhoid fever (inactivated) vaccines, the resuspended cells are standardized (see *Strength*) and the final vaccine is in the form of a suspension of cells. Anthrax vaccine, as mentioned, is a liquid filtrate and the filtrate is adsorbed onto aluminum hydroxide. Aluminum hydroxide is an *adjuvant* which is used to enhance the immune response. For the preparation of BCG vaccine, the purified living cells are lyophilized (freeze-dried) and the vaccine is reconstituted as directed with a diluent before use. Live oral typhoid vaccine is also a lyophilized product, but the living lyophilized cells are in the form of an enteric-coated capsule.

Meningococcal, pneumococcal and haemophilus b conjugate vaccines are prepared by processing further the suspended cells in a series of steps including, lyses and differential centrifugation in order to extract the polysaccharide capsular immunogens. The pneumococcal vaccine contains a mixture of polysaccharide immunogens in a liquid form; whereas the meningococcal vaccine is a lyophilized product.

Haemophilus b conjugate vaccine is either a solution or lyophilized product of the purified capsular polysaccharide covalently bound to diphtheria toxoid protein or the meningococcal protein to produce an enhanced antibody response and an immunologic memory.

The final vaccine product may contain a single immunogen (*monovalent*), eg, typhoid fever vaccine, or it may contain multiple immunogens (*polyvalent*, *trivalent*, etc) to elicit immunity against the same disease state, eg, cholera vaccine (has two serotypes of the cholera vibrio).

In addition the product may be in the form of a mixed vaccine or a mixed biologic. A *mixed vaccine* such as measles, mumps and rubella vaccines (MMR) is a single product with three viral immunogens for three different disease states. A *mixed biologic*, on the other hand, has a combination of a vaccine(s) and toxoid(s) in the same preparation, eg, DTP.

Strength—The strength of a bacterial vaccine may be expressed in terms of total

Organisms (or colony-forming units, as with BCG vaccine). When the total number of organisms is used to designate strength, the potency of that number of organisms usually is verified by an animal protection test as compared to a US Reference Vaccine for that organism. For example, the number of vaccine organisms, when injected into a specified laboratory animal, should stimulate enough antibodies to protect the animal from a specific challenge with the corresponding pathogenic organism.

Protective units. For some vaccines the strength is expressed directly as protective units per mL or dose rather than a specified number of organisms. Pertussis vaccine, for example, contains four protective units. One protective unit of pertussis vaccine is the amount of vaccine needed to protect a mouse against a lethal intracerebral challenge with *Bordetella pertussis.*

Micrograms of immunogen found in each mL or in each dose of vaccine. The strength of a vaccine composed of extracts of cellular components is expressed in μg of immunogen per mL or per dose. For example, meningococcal vaccine contains 50 μg of polysaccharide immunogen in each 0.5 mL dose, an amount which, when injected into no less than 25 volunteers, will show a four fold or greater rise in antibody titer in not less than 90% of the volunteers.

It is important to note that the strengths of these vaccines (and other biologics), regardless of how they are expressed, are correlated with the dosage schedule and are based upon theoretical considerations, experimental trials and clinical experience.

Anthrax Vaccine Adsorbed

A sterile, slightly opaque liquid derived from a microaerophilic culture of an avirulent, nonencapsulated strain of *Bacillus anthracis.* A sterile filtrate of the culture is obtained and the filtrate then is adsorbed on sterile aluminum hydroxide. The potency is determined by a guinea pig protection test compared to a US Reference Anthrax Vaccine. Formaldehyde in a final concentration not to exceed 0.02% and benzethonium chloride (0.0025%) are added as preservatives.

Uses—Recommended for active immunization of individuals who may come in contact with animal products such as hides, hair or bones which come from endemic areas and may be contaminated with *Bacillus anthracis* spores; and for individuals engaged in diagnostic or investigational activities which may bring them into contact with *B anthracis* spores. It also is recommended for high-risk persons such as veterinarians and others handling potentially infected animals. Routine immunization is not recommended for the general population since risk of exposure to anthrax infection is slight.

Dose—*Subcutaneous,* **3 injections** of **0.5 mL** 2 wk apart, followed by **3 more 0.5-mL doses** 6, 12 and 18 mo after the initial injection.

Booster—**0.5 mL** at 1-yr intervals.

Dosage Form—Injection: 5 mL.

BCG Vaccine

Tice BCG (*Organon*)

A lyophilized living culture of the Tice strain of the bacillus Calmette-Guérin strain of *Mycobacterium bovis.* Each 2-mL ampule contains 1 to 8 × 10^8 colony forming units (CFU) of Tice BCG which is equivalent to approximately 50-mg wet-weight. The product contains no preservatives.

Uses—*Percutaneous:* Strongly recommended for tuberculin-negative infants and children who are at high risk of prolonged and intimate exposure to (1) Persons with persistently untreated and/or ineffectively treated infectious pulmonary tuberculosis, and who cannot be removed from the source of infection nor be placed on long-term preventive therapy. (2) Persons with tuberculosis caused by isoniazid or rifampin-resistant bacilli. Also for tuberculin-negative infants and children living in groups with an excessive rate of new infections (exceeding 1% per year) for whom the usual surveillance and treatment programs are not operationally feasible. Such groups would include those who do not have regular access to modern health care; those who consider modern health care socially or culturally unacceptable or groups who have demonstrated an inability to use existing health-care facilities effectively. *Intravesical:* indicated under certain situations for the primary or secondary treatment of carcinoma *in situ* of the bladder in the absence of associated invasive cancer.

Dose—*Percutaneous for immunization against tuberculosis,* **0.2** to **0.3 mL** of reconstituted vaccine administered with a sterile multipuncture disc; *infants less than 1 mo,* reduced by 1/2 by using 2 mL of sterile water for injection (rather than 1 mL) when reconstituting. A tuberculin test (5TU) should be conducted 2 to 3 months after vaccination. If the test is negative, the vaccination should be repeated. Vaccinated infants who remain tuberculin negative to 5 TU should receive a full dose after 1 yr of age if the above high risk indications persist. *Intravesical for carcinoma of the bladder,* **1 ampule** suspended in 50 mL of preservative-free saline instilled weekly for 6 wk and repeated once if necessary, followed by monthly intravesical instillations for at least 6 to 12 mo. The vaccine should be refrigerated, protected from light and used within 2 hr following reconstitution. Any remaining product should be discarded and preferably incinerated or treated with a strong disinfectant, eg, a strong hypochlorite solution.

Booster—*Percutaneous, for immunization against tuberculosis*—Protection from tuberculosis by BCG vaccination is only relative and is not permanent or entirely predictable. If the tuberculin test again becomes negative and the risk of infection continues, then a booster shot may need to be given.

Dosage Form—Injection: 2 mL.

Cholera Vaccine

A sterile, whitish suspension of equal parts of phenol killed Ogawa and Inaba serotypes of *Vibrio cholerae.* These strains are selected for high immunogenic efficiency. Each mL contains not more than 4 × 10^9 (8 units) of each serotype based on a mouse protection test compared to a US Reference Cholera Vaccine for each respective serotype. Phenol (0.5%) is added as a preservative.

Uses—Has limited usefulness, protects only about 50% of those immunized for a period of 3 to 6 mo and does not prevent transmission of the disease. In addition, the risk of cholera to travelers is very low and the spread of the disease can be controlled effectively by surveillance and treatment. Therefore, cholera vaccination generally is not recommended for travelers; however, some countries require that travelers arriving from epidemic or endemic areas have evidence of receiving a single dose within 6 mo of entry.

Dose—*Subcutaneous* or *intramuscular*, **2 injections** of **0.5 mL**, 1 wk to 1 mo or more apart. For dosage schedules for children 10 yr and younger and for intradermal administration, see the package insert.

Booster—0.5 mL reinforcing dose repeated every 6 mo in areas where cholera is epidemic or endemic (adult booster).

Dosage Form—Injection: 1.5 and 20 mL.

Haemophilus b Conjugate Vaccine

HibTITER (*Lederle*); OmniHIB (*SmithKline Beecham*); Pedvax HIB (*MSD*); ProHIBiT (*Connaught*)

ProHIBiT and HibTITER are sterile, colorless solutions prepared from the purified capsular polysaccharide, a polymer of ribose, ribitol and phosphate (PRP) of the Eagen *Haemophilus influenzae* type b strain covalently bound to diphtheria toxoid or protein. Each 0.5 mL of ProHIBiT contains 25 μg of purified capsular polysaccharide and 18 μg of diphtheria toxoid protein. Each 0.5 mL of HibTITER contains 10 μg of purified saccharide and approximately 25 μg of CRM_{197} protein (nontoxic variant of diphtheria toxin.)

OmniHIB is a lyophilized product prepared from the high-molecular-weight capsular polysaccharide from *H influenzae* type B strain 1482 covalently bound to tetanus toxoid. When reconstituted, each 0.5 mL dose contains 10 μg of purified capsular polysaccharide and 24 μg of tetanus toxoid.

Pedvax HIB is a lyophilized product prepared from the purified capsular polysaccharide of the Ross strain of *H influenzae* type B covalently bound to an outer membrane protein complex (OMPC) of the B11 strain of *Neisseria meningitidis* serogroup B. When reconstituted, each 0.5-mL dose contains 15 μg of purified capsular polysaccharide and 250 μg of meningococcal protein. As a result of the conjugation to the diphtheria, tetanus or meningococcal protein, the polysaccharide is postulated to be presented as a T- dependent immunogen which results in both an enhanced antibody response and immunologic memory.

Note—Diphtheria toxoid or protein, tetanus toxoid and meningococcal protein should not be considered as immunizing agents against diphtheria, tetanus or meningococcal disease.

Thimerosal (1:10,000 or 1:20,000) is added as a preservative.

Uses—ProHIBiT—Indicated for routine active immunization of children 15 mo to 5 yr against invasive disease caused by *H influenzae* type b. HibTITER, OmniHIB and Pedvax HIB—licensed for routine immunization starting at 2 to 6 mo.

Note—HibTITER is available in combination with Triimmunol [diphtheria and tetanus toxoids and whole-cell pertussis vaccine (DTP)] as Tetramune, formulated for use in vaccinating children against diphtheria, tetanus, pertussis and HiB disease. The dose is 4 injections given at 2, 4, 6 and 15 mo. A booster of DTP or DTaP is given between 4 and 6 yr.

Dose—*Intramuscular*, ProHIBiT, **1 injection** of **0.5 mL;** HibTITER and OmniHIB, **3 injections** of **0.5 mL** given 2 mo apart; Pedvax HIB, **2 injections** of **0.5 mL** given 2 mo apart. For dosage schedules of HibTITER, OmniHIB and Pedvax HIB starting after 6 mo, see package inserts.

Booster—ProHIBiT, not required; HibTITER and OmniHIB, at 15 mo; Pedvax HIB, at 12 mo if primary series is given at 2 to 6 mo, at 15 mo if primary series is given after 6 mo.

Dosage Form—Injection: 0.5, 2.5 and 5 mL. Pedvax HIB-single dose with vial of aluminum hydroxide diluent.

Haemophilus b Polysaccharide Vaccine—see RPS-18, page 1393.

Meningococcal Polysaccharide Vaccine Groups A, C, Y and W-135 Combined

Menomune-A/C/Y/W-135 (*Connaught*)

A sterile, lyophilized extract of the group-specific polysaccharide immunogens from *Neisseria meningitidis*. After reconstitution as directed, each 0.5-mL dose contains 50 μg of each polysaccharide immunogen for each of Groups A, C, Y and W-135. Potency is based on a gel-permeation chromatography determination and on immunization of not less than 25 healthy adult human subjects, in whom the antibody titers of the sera from no less than 90% of the subjects show a fourfold or greater rise after immunization. After reconstitution the vaccine contains thimerosal (1:10,000) as a preservative.

Uses—Primarily for active immunization of persons 2 yr and older at risk in epidemic or highly endemic areas. For more detailed information on use, see the package insert.

Dose—*Subcutaneous*, **1 injection** of **0.5 mL** of reconstituted vaccine. Any unused reconstituted vaccine should be stored at 2 to 8° and discarded within 5 days.

Booster—May be indicated for high-risk individuals, particularly children who received their immunization before 4 yr. These children, if they remain at high risk, should be considered for a booster after 2 or 3 yr. The need for boosters for older children and adults has not been determined.

Dosage Form—Injection: 10-dose; 50-dose *for jet injector use only.*

Pertussis Vaccine

A sterile, whitish suspension of a formalin killed strain of Phase I *Bordetella pertussis*. Each 0.5-mL dose contains 4 protective units of pertussis vaccine based on a mouse protection test compared to a US Reference Pertussis Vaccine. Thimerosal (1:10,000) is added as a preservative.

Uses—Available in the multiple immunogen form of Diphtheria and Tetanus Toxoids and Pertussis Vaccine Adsorbed (DTP) which is recommended for active immunization of infants and children 6 wk through 6 yr against diphtheria, tetanus and pertussis simultaneously. Injections should be completed no later than the age of 6 yr.

Note—(1) *Pertussis Vaccine is not recommended for immunizing persons 7 yr and older because the severity of adverse reactions to pertussis vaccine increases with age, whereas the severity of pertussis infection decreases.* (2) *See Other Reactions earlier in this chapter for contraindications and adverse reactions.*

Dose—*Intramuscular*, **3 injections** of **0.5 mL** given 4 to 8 wk apart followed by a fourth reinforcing dose of **0.5 mL** 6 to 12 mo after the third dose. Primary immunization cannot be considered complete without the fourth reinforcing dose being given since this dose is an integral part of the basic immunizing course.

Booster—0.5 mL between 4 and 6 yr (prior to entering kindergarten or elementary school).

Dosage Form (For DTP)—Injection: 5 and 7.5 mL.

Pertussis Vaccine Acellular

A sterile preparation isolated from culture fluids of Phase I *Bordetella pertussis*. Two forms are available.

The Connaught product is purified to isolate the antigenic components by using salt precipitation, ultracentrifugation and ultrafiltration. The antigenic components—filamentous hemagglutinin (FHA) and pertussis toxin (PT)—are combined to obtain a 1:1 ratio and then treated with formaldehyde to inactivate the PT. Each dose of the final vaccine contains 23.4 μg each of protein of FHA and PT.

The Lederle vaccine is purified using ammonium sulfate fractionation and sucrose density gradient centrifugation. Each dose of the final product contains approximately 40 μg (but not more than 60 μg) of pertussis antigen detoxified with formaldehyde, with approximately 86% of this protein being FHA and 8% as PT.

The potency of both vaccines is evaluated using an ELISA system to measure antibody response to PT and FHA in immunized mice. Both vaccines are preserved with 1:10,000 thimerosal.

Uses—Available in the multiple immunogen form of Diphtheria and Tetanus Toxoids and Acelular Pertussis Vaccine Adsorbed (DTaP), which is licensed only for use as the fourth and fifth doses of the DTP series among children 15 mo through 6 yr who have previously received 3 or 4 doses of whole-cell DTP. Acellular pertussis vaccine substantially reduces local reactions, fever and other common systemic events that occur often with whole-cell pertussis preparations. (See *Other Reactions* earlier in this chapter for contraindications and adverse reactions.)

Data is not available on the use of DTaP in children for whom whole-cell pertussis DTP vaccine is contraindicated; thus, Diphtheria and Tetanus Toxoids Adsorbed (for Pediatric Use) should be used for each of the remaining doses in these instances. Efficiency data for acellular pertussis vaccine in infants also is not available; thus, DTaP is not recommended for use in children below the age of 15 mo. There are also questions as to whether protection which is induced using acellular pertussis vaccines is equivalent to that of whole-cell preparations. Therefore, it is recommended that whole-cell pertussis vaccines be continued for the initial 3-dose vaccination series until acellular vaccines have demonstrated essentially equivalent or higher efficacy.

Dose—*Intramuscular*, **0.5 mL** given at 15 mo as the fourth primary dose, 6 to 12 mo after the third dose of DTP.

Booster—0.5 mL between 4 and 6 yr prior to entering kindergarten or elementary school (not necessary if fourth primary dose given after fourth birthday).

Dosage Form (for DTaP)—Injection: 5 and 7.5 mL.

Pertussis Vaccine Adsorbed

A sterile, whitish suspension of formalin-killed *Bordetella pertussis* which has been adsorbed by the addition of aluminum phosphate. Each 0.5-mL dose contains 4 protective units of pertussis vaccine based on a mouse protection test compared to a US Reference Pertussis Vaccine. Thimerosal (1:10,000) is added as a preservative.

Uses—Available in the multiple immunogen form of Diphtheria and Tetanus Toxoids and Pertussis Vaccine Adsorbed (DTP) and as a single-antigen product. The single-antigen product is indicated for active immunization of children (older than 6 wk) against pertussis especially when the commonly used DTP causes untoward reaction or is contraindicated.

Note—(1) *Pertussis Vaccine Adsorbed is not recommended for immunizing persons 7 yr and older because the severity of adverse reactions to pertussis vaccine increases with age, whereas the severity of pertussis infection decreases.* (2) *See Other Reactions earlier in this chapter for contraindications and adverse reactions.*

Dose—*Intramuscular*, **3 injections** of **0.5 mL** given 4 to 8 wk apart followed by a fourth reinforcing dose of **0.5 mL** 1 yr later. Primary immunization cannot be considered complete without the fourth reinforcing dose being given since this dose is an integral part of the basic immunizing course.

Booster—0.5 mL between 4 and 6 yr (prior to entering kindergarten or elementary school).

Dosage Form—Injection: 5 mL.

Plague Vaccine

A sterile, whitish suspension of formaldehyde-killed *Yersinia pestis*. Each mL contains 1.8 to 2.2 × 10^9 organisms based on a mouse protection test compared to a US Reference Plague Vaccine. Phenol (0.5%) is added as a preservative.

Uses—For active immunization of persons at particularly high risk to plague including persons engaged in laboratory and field work involving *Y pestis* organisms and those involved in natural disasters or in situations when regular sanitary practices are interrupted. Routine vaccination is not necessary for travelers in countries where cases have been reported particularly if travel is limited to urban areas. For more detailed information, see the package insert.

Dose—*Intramuscular, adults and children over 10 yr*, **2 injections** of **1.0 mL** followed by **0.2 mL** 1 to 3 mo later. A third injection of **0.2 mL** 3 to 6 mo after the second injection is recommended strongly. For children less than 10 yr, see the package insert.

Booster—1 injection (0.1 to 0.2 mL) every 6 mo for individuals remaining in a known plague area. The smaller dose should be approached as the total number of such injections increases.

Dosage Form—Injection: 20 mL.

Pneumococcal Vaccine Polyvalent

Pneumovax 23 (*MSD*); Pnu-Imune 23 (*Lederle*)

A sterile, colorless liquid consisting of a mixture of purified capsular polysaccharide immunogens from 23 types of *Streptococcus pneumoniae*. For specific capsular immunogens, see the package insert. The capsular immunogens from each bacterial type are purified separately and then pooled so that each dose of vaccine contains 25 μg of each polysaccharide immunogen. The preservative used is phenol (0.25%) or thimerosal (1:10,000).

Uses—Indicated for persons over 2 yr for selective immunization against infections caused by the 23 most prevalent types of pneumococci responsible for approximately 90% of serious pneumococcal disease in the US and the rest of the world. Examples of persons for whom the vaccine is intended include (1) those with chronic illnesses in which there is an increased risk of experiencing more severe pneumococcal disease, such as alcoholism or coexisting diseases including diabetes mellitus, and functional impairment of cardiorespiratory, hepatic and renal systems; (2) those who have anatomical asplenia or who have splenic dysfunction due to sickle cell disease or other causes; (3) those 65 yr or older; (4) those about to undergo immunosuppressive therapy and those with asymptomatic or symptomatic human immunodeficiency virus infection.

Dose—*Subcutaneous* or *intramuscular*, **1 injection** of **0.5 mL.**

Booster—Not recommended routinely.

Dosage Form—Injection: 0.5 and 2.5 mL.

Typhoid Vaccine

A sterile, milky suspension of phenol and heat killed *Salmonella typhi* (Ty-2 strain). The vaccine contains not more than 1,000 million organisms per mL based on a potency of 8 units per mL determined by the mouse protection test compared to a US Reference Typhoid Vaccine. Phenol (0.5%) is added as a preservative.

Uses—Indicated for active immunization against typhoid fever in selective situations including expected intimate exposure to a known typhoid carrier; foreign travel to areas where typhoid fever is endemic; and workers in microbiology laboratories with expected frequent contact with *S. typhi*. The vaccine is estimated to be 70% or more effective in preventing typhoid fever depending in part on the degree of exposure.

Dose—*Subcutaneous, adults* and *children over 10 yr*, **2 injections** of **0.5 mL** at least 4 wk apart. For children less than 10 yr, **2 injections** of **0.25 mL** at least 4 wk apart.

Booster—Under conditions of continued or repeated exposure, a single booster injection of **0.5 mL** or **0.25 mL** (according to age) every 3 yr.

Dosage Form—Injection: 5, 10 and 20 mL.

Typhoid Vaccine Live Oral Ty21a

Vivotif Berna Vaccine (*Berna*)

An enteric-coated capsule containing live-attenuated Ty21a strain of *Salmonello typhi* grown under controlled conditions and lyophilized. Each capsule contains 2 to 6 × 10^9 colony forming units (CFU) of viable *S typhi* Ty21a and 5 to 50 × 10^9 bacterial cells of nonviable *S typhi* Ty21a.

Uses—See *Typhoid Vaccine*.

Note—It is recommended that the vaccine not be given to children under 6 yr.

Dose—*Oral*, a four-dose series, **1 capsule** on days 1, 3, 5 and 7, taken with cool liquid approximately 1 hr before a meal.

Booster—A 4-dose series every 5 yr.

Note—An optimal booster schedule has not been determined and the booster recommendation may change as more data become available on the duration of protection.

Dosage Form—Capsules: single foil blister with 4 capsules.

Other Bacterial Vaccines

Bacterial Antigen Made from Staphylococcus*

Staphage Lysate (SPL) (*Delmont*)

A preparation of lysed cultures of *Staphylococcus aureus*, serologic Types I and III. Indicated for the treatment of either staphylococcal infections or polymicrobial infections with a staphylococcal component.

BCG Vaccine for Percutaneous Use—see RPS-18, page 1394.

Francisella Tularensis Vaccine, Live

Tularemia Vaccine

A live lyophilized IND distributed by the military for high-risk personnel.

Mixed Respiratory Vaccine*

MRV (*Hollister-Stier Miles*)

A killed vaccine containing *Staphylococcus aureus*, *Streptococcus (viridans* and non hemolytic), *Streptococcus pneumoniae*, *Branhamella (Neisseria) catarrhalis*, *Klebsiella pneumoniae* and *Haemophilus influenzae*. Used in the hopes of favorably altering the course of the inflammatory process in recurrent and chronic infections of the respiratory tract and occasionally of the skin.

Q-Fever Vaccine, Inactivated

An inactivated lyophilized IND distributed by the military.

Typhoid Vaccine, Acetone Inactivated, Dried

A sterile lyophilized product distributed by the military.

Note— In the preparation of hepatitus B vaccine recombinant, the gene for hepatitis B surface antigen (HBsAg), is cloned into the *yeast Saccharomyces cerevisiae*.

---

* *Based on a review by the Panel on Bacterial Vaccines and Bacterial Antigens with no US Standard of Potency and other information, the FDA has directed that further investigation be considered before these two products* (Bacterial Antigen made from Staphylococcus and Mixed Respiratory Vaccine) *are determined fully effective for the labeled indication*(s).

Viral Vaccines

Preparation—Viruses are intracellular obligate parasites that cannot be grown on inanimate media used for cultivating bacteria and must be propagated on one of several types of *animate media* including

Embryonic egg—influenza and yellow fever viruses.
Cell cultures of chick embryo—measles and mumps viruses.
Human diploid cell culture—rubella and rabies (rabies vaccine) viruses.
Monkey cell culture—polio and rabies (viruses rabies vaccine adsorbed).
Skin of living calves—smallpox virus.
Intact mice—Japanese encephalitis virus

Following growth, various techniques including disintegration, column filtration, differential centrifugation and so forth, are used to separate the virus from its host cell or in the case of hepatitis B the surface antigen from yeast cells. The purification steps reduce the incidence of possible hypersensitivity due to the animate media or host cells, especially embryonic egg.

Influenza vaccine may remain as the *whole virion* or be further processed chemically and split into subunit particles (subvirion vaccine). Hepatitis B recombinant also is a subunit vaccine (since only the surface antigen is present) and is processed with aluminum hydroxide as an adjuvant for prolonged stimulation of antibodies. Rabies vaccine (adsorbed) is adsorbed to aluminum phosphate which may also serve as an adjuvant.

Some viral vaccines are living and have the advantage of being able to continue to multiply in the body of the immunized individual; thus exerting a prolonged and increasingly strong stimulation to the host to produce antibodies. Other viral vaccines (hepatitis B, recombinant, influenza, Japanese encephalitis and polio for injection) are inactivated with formaldehyde; whereas the vaccines for rabies and one formulation for influenza are inactivated with beta-propiolactone (BPL).

Product Form—Many viral vaccines occur as a lyophilized (freeze-dried) final product that must be reconstituted before injection with the diluent provided. Inactivated vaccines like hepatitis B, influenza, poliovirus and rabies (adsorbed) occur as suspensions for injection; whereas living polio vaccine is in a liquid drop form for oral use.

As with bacterial vaccines, the final viral vaccine product may contain a single immunogen (monovalent), eg, measles vaccine or it may contain multiple immunogens (polyvalent, trivalent, etc) to elicit immunity against the same disease state, eg, trivalent influenza vaccine and trivalent polio vaccines. In addition there is the mixed vaccine (measles, mumps and rubella) which is a single product with three immunogens for three different disease states.

Strength—The strength of a viral vaccine is expressed most commonly in terms of

Tissue culture infectious doses ($TCID_{50}$), which is the quantity of virus estimated to infect 50% of inoculated cultures. Rubella vaccine, for example, contains 1000 $TCID_{50}$, or 1,000 times the amount of virus present in one tissue culture infectious dose.

μg of immunogen present—hepatitis B recombinant and influenza vaccines.

International units—rabies vaccine, based on mouse potency tests.

Plaque-forming units (PFU)—yellow fever vaccine.

D antigen units—poliovirus vaccine inactivated, determined by single radial immunodiffusion.

Hepatitis B Vaccine—see RPS-18, page 1395.

Hepatitis B Vaccine (Recombinant)

Engerix-B (*SmithKline Beecham*); Recombivax HB (*MSD*)

A sterile, slightly opaque, white suspension of formaldehyde-inactivated hepatitis B surface antigen (HBsAg) produced in yeast. The gene for the adw subtype of HBsAg is cloned into the yeast *Saccharomyces cerevisiae*. The HBsAg is then harvested from the fermentation cultures of the recombinant strain, purified and adsorbed onto aluminum hydroxide. Thimerosal (1:20,000) is added as a preservative. The HBsAg dosage concentration of individual products varies with the specific recommended use as follows: Recombivax HB (RHB), 10 μg per mL—for adults 20 yr and older; Recombivax HB Dialysis Formulation (DF), 40 μg per mL—for adult predialysis and dialysis patients; Engerix-B, 20 μg per mL—for individuals older than 10 yr and Engerix-B, 10 μg per 0.5 mL—for children (including neonates) 10 yr and under.

Uses—Recommended for immunization against infection caused by all known subtypes of hepatitis B virus in persons who are or will be at increased risk of infection with hepatitis B. These higher risk groups include health-care personnel, dialysis patients, morticians, embalmers, immigrants from areas of high hepatitis B virus endemicity, homosexually active males, users of illicit injectable drugs, prisoners and clients in institutions for the mentally retarded. For more detailed information, see the package insert.

Dose—*Intramuscular*, **3 injections** of **0.25**, **0.5** or **1 mL** (depending upon age and product) with the second and third injections given 1 mo and 6 mo after the first dose. For more complete dosage schedules, see the package insert.

Booster—The duration of the protective effect is approximately 9 yr; however, the need for a booster(s) is not defined yet. A booster may be considered in predialysis/dialysis patients whose anti-HBs level is less than 10 mIU/mL, 1 to 2 mo after the third dose.

Dosage Form—Injection: 0.5, 1 and 3 mL.

Influenza Virus Vaccine

Influenza Virus Vaccine, Trivalent, types A and B; Flu-Immune (*Lederle*); Fluogen (*Parke-Davis*); Flu Shield (*Wyeth*); Fluzone (*Connaught*)

A sterile, slightly opalescent suspension of the formaldehyde or beta-propiolactone (BPL) inactivated influenza virus types A and B which are harvested from allantoic fluids of chicken embryos infected with the specific influenza virus. The virus may be used whole (whole virion vaccine) or may be in the form of a split virus (subvirion or surface antigen vaccine) prepared by chemical disruption (ethyl ether, glycol p-isooctylphenyl ether or tri(n)butylphosphate and polysorbate 80). There are several methods employed for concentrating and purifying the virus including: column chromatography, ultracentrifugation, zonal centrifugation and continuous flow centrifugation. For more detailed information, see the package insert.

The vaccine is standardized each year according to USPHS requirements; eg, each 0.5 mL dose of the vaccine recommended for the 1994–1995 influenza season contained not less than 15 μg of hemagglutinin each of A/Texas/36/91-like (H1N1), A/Shangdong/9/93-like (H_3N_2) and B/Panama/45/90-like viruses. *Note*—Because of immunogenic variation (drift), the immunogenic characteristics of influenza vaccine may vary from year to year. Thimerosal (1:10,000) is added as a preservative.

Uses—Indicated only for immunization against those strains of viruses from which the vaccine is prepared or against closely related strains. Annual routine immunization is recommended for any persons 6 mo or older, who because of age or an underlying medical condition, is at increased risk of adverse consequences from influenza infection. Health-care workers and others (including household members) in close contact with high-risk persons also should be vaccinated. Groups at greatest risk include (1) adults and children with chronic disorders of the pulmonary or cardiovascular systems requiring regular medical followup or hospitalization during the preceding year, including children with asthma; (2) persons 65 yr and older and (3) residents of nursing homes and other chronic-care facilities housing patients of any age with chronic medical conditions. For other persons at increased risk and other target groups, see the package insert.

Dose—*Intramuscular*, **1** injection of **0.5 mL.** See package inserts for dosage for persons under 13 yr.

Note—because the split vaccine has been shown to be less reactogenic than whole-virus vaccines, particularly in the younger age groups, it is recommended that only the subvirion vaccine be given to those persons under 13 yr.

Booster—A single yearly dose for high-risk individuals.

Dosage Forms—Injection: 0.5 and 5 mL; 25 mL *for jet injector use.*

Japanese Encephalitis Virus Vaccine Inactivated

JE Vaccine; JE-VAX (*Connaught*)

A sterile lyophilized vaccine prepared by harvesting the infected brains of mice intracerebrally inoculated with the Nakayama-NIH strain of the Japanese encephalitis (JE) virus. The harvest is homogenized, centrifuged and inactivated with formaldehyde and then further purified by ultracentrifugation. Thimerosal (0.007%) is added as a preservative. The potency is determined by measuring neutralizing antibodies in a plaque-neutralization assay performed on sera from mice immunized with either the test vaccine or the JE reference vaccine. The potency of the test vaccine must be no less than that of the reference vaccine.

Uses—Recommended for active immunization against JE in persons 1 yr and older who plan to reside or travel more than 1 mo in areas where JE is endemic or epidemic. It is not recommended for all persons traveling to or residing in Asia. For more specific considerations in determining the feasibility of immunization, see the package insert.

Dose—*Subcutaneous, 3 yr and older,* three, **1.0-mL** of reconstituted vaccine on days 0, 7 and 30; *1 to 3 yr,* **0.5 mL.**

Booster—Since the full duration of protection is unknown, definitive recommendations can not be given. However, booster doses may be administered after 2 yr.

Dosage Form—Injection: Single- and 10-dose.

Measles Virus Vaccine Live

Measles Virus Vaccine Live, Attenuated; Attenuvax (*MSD*)

A bacterially sterile, lyophilized preparation of a more attenuated line of live measles virus derived from Enders' attenuated Edmonston strain prepared in cell cultures of chick embryo at low temperature. When reconstituted as directed each 0.5 mL dose of vaccine contains not less than the equivalent of 1,000 $TCID_{50}$ of the US Reference Measles Virus. The reconstituted vaccine is clear yellow and each dose contains approximately 25 μg of neomycin.

Uses—Recommended for active immunization against measles (rubeola) in persons 15 mo or older, especially with the commonly used mixed vaccine form of Measles, Mumps and Rubella Virus Vaccine. Live (MMR) causes untoward reaction or is contraindicated.

In certain populations, eg, groups in which natural measles infections may occur in a significant proportion of infants before 15 mo, infants less than 12 mo may be vaccinated, but should be revaccinated after reaching 15 mo. For further information on vaccination of infants under 15 mo, see the package insert.

Persons born in 1956 or earlier are likely to have been infected naturally and generally need not be immunized. However, all persons born after 1956 are considered susceptible and should be vaccinated if there are no contraindications. This includes persons who may be immune to measles but lack adequate documentation, eg, physician-diagnosed measles, laboratory evidence of measles immunity or adequate immunization with live measles vaccine on or after the first birthday. The vaccine may provide some protection if given within 72 hr after exposure to natural measles. However, better protection may be provided if the vaccine is given a few days before exposure.

Dose—*Subcutaneous,* **1, 0.5 mL** injection of reconstituted vaccine. Any unused reconstituted vaccine should be stored at 2 to 8° and discarded within 8 hr.

Booster—1, 0.5-mL injection. ACIP recommends revaccination at 4 to 6 yr (at entry into kindergarten or first grade), whereas the American Academy of Pediatrics (AAP) recommends routine revaccination at entry to middle school or junior high school. It also should be noted that some state and local health agencies have their own mandates as to the specific age for revaccination.

Dosage Form—Injection: Single-dose; 10- and 50-dose (available only to government agencies/institutions).

Mumps Virus Vaccine Live

Mumpvax (*MSD*)

A bacterially sterile, lyophilized preparation of the Jeryl Lynn (B level) strain of live mumps virus grown in cell cultures of chick embryo. When reconstituted as directed each 0.5 mL dose of vaccine contains not less than the equivalent of 20,000 $TCID_{50}$ of the US Reference Mumps Virus. The reconstituted vaccine is clear yellow and each dose contains approximately 25 μg of neomycin.

Uses—Recommended for active immunization against mumps in persons 12 mo or older especially with the commonly used mixed vaccine form of Measles, Mumps and Rubella Virus Vaccine Live (MMR) causes untoward reaction or is contraindicated or when it is advantageous to begin immunization against mumps before 15 mo (the recommended starting age for MMR). Most adults are likely to have been infected naturally and generally may be considered immune, even if they did not have clinically recognizable disease. The vaccine will not offer protection after exposure to natural mumps.

Dose—*Subcutaneous,* **1, 0.5 mL** injection of reconstituted vaccine. Any unused reconstituted vaccine should be stored at 2 to 8° and discarded within 8 hr.

Booster—Given as MMR (see **Booster** for Measles Virus Vaccine Live).

Note.—Recent studies show that a substantial number of mumps cases have occurred among individuals with histories of prior vaccination.

Dosage Form—Injection: Single-dose; 10- and 50-dose (available only to government agencies/institutions).

Poliovirus Vaccine Inactivated

Inactivated Polio Vaccine (IPV), Poliomyelitis Vaccine, Salk Polio Vaccine; IPOL (*Connaught*)

A sterile, colorless and clear suspension of three types of poliovirus, Type 1 (Mahoney), Type 2 (MEF-1) and Type 3 (Saukett). The virus strains are grown separately in monkey kidney cell cultures, concentrated, purified and inactivated with formaldehyde. The vaccine is formulated to contain 40, 8 and 32 D Antigen units per dose, determined by single radial immunodiffusion and compared to reference preparations of types 1, 2 and 3, respectively. Formaldehyde (0.02%) and 2-phenoxyethanol (0.5%) are added as preservatives.

Uses—For persons under 18 yr Poliovirus Vaccine Inactivated (IPV) has been replaced largely by Poliovirus Vaccine Live Oral (OPV) in the US. IPV is used for adult immunization because there is less risk of vaccine-associated paralysis than with OPV for adults. IPV likewise is safer to administer to immune-deficient persons. Current recommendations of the Immunization Practices Advisory Committee (ACIP), however, indicate that routine primary polio vaccination of adults (18 yr or older) residing in the US is not necessary. For more details, see the package insert.

Dose—*Subcutaneous,* **2 injections** of **0.5 mL** 8 wk apart, followed by a third dose of **0.5 mL** at least 6 and preferably 12 mo after the second dose.

Booster—Children receiving the initial three doses in early childhood should be given a booster dose of **0.5 mL** before entering school. If the third dose of the primary series is administered on or after the fourth birthday, a fourth (booster) dose is not required at school entry. The need for routine additional doses is not known at this time. When revaccinating certain high-risk adults, an interval of 5 yr is recommended; see the package insert for more details.

Dosage Form—Injection: 0.5 mL.

Poliovirus Vaccine Live Oral Trivalent

Oral Polio Vaccine (OPV); Trivalent Oral Polio Vaccine (TOPV), Sabin Vaccine; Orimune (*Lederle*)

A mixture of three types of live, attenuated polioviruses which have been propagated separately in monkey kidney cell culture. The potency is expressed in terms of the amount of virus contained in the recommended dose as $TCID_{50}$. Each dose contains infectivity titers of $10^{5.4}$ to $10^{6.4}$ for Type 1, $10^{4.5}$ to $10^{5.5}$ for Type 2, and $10^{5.2}$ to $10^{6.2}$ for Type 3. The vaccine is free from any known microbial agent other than the attenuated polioviruses listed. Each 0.5-mL dose contains less than 25 μg of each of the antibiotics, streptomycin and neomycin. The usual color of the vaccine is pink and clear because of the phenol red pH indicator. However, some containers of vaccine shipped in ice may exhibit a yellow color due to very low temperature or the possible absorption of carbon dioxide. The color (red-pink-yellow) of the vaccine prior to use has no effect on the virus or efficacy of the vaccine.

Uses—Indicated for active immunization against infections of poliomyelitis caused by Poliovirus Types 1, 2 and 3 in infants starting at 6 to 12 wk and all unimmunized children and adolescents up to 18 yr. Poliovirus Vaccine Live Oral (OPV) is considered by the Advisory Committee on Immunization Practices to be the vaccine of choice for primary immunization of children. Because of the potential risk of developing vaccine-associated paralysis with OPV in adults, adults 18 yr and older should be administered Poliovirus Vaccine Inactivated; however, it is recommended that routine primary polio vaccination of adults (18 yr or older) residing in the US is not necessary. For further information, see the package insert.

Dose—*Oral,* **3 doses** 6 to 8 wk apart (third dose should be administered at 6 mo of age).

Booster—Oral dose upon entering elementary school. This booster is not required if the third primary dose was received on or after the fourth birthday.

Dosage Form—Oral Liquid: 10- and 50-dose (each dose in a disposable pipette).

Rabies Vaccine

Rabies Vaccine Human Diploid Cell (HDCV); Imovax Rabies (*Connaught*); Imovax Rabies ID (*Connaught*)

A sterile lyophilized preparation of the Wistar rabies virus strain PM-1503-3M grown on human diploid cell cultures and inactivated with beta-propiolactone (BPL). Two vaccines, one for intramuscular use and one for intradermal use, are available. When reconstituted as directed, the vaccine for intramuscular use contains at least 2.5 International Units (IU) of rabies antigen in each 1-ml dose. An IU is established by tests in parallel with the Standard Rabies Vaccine in the NIH mouse potency test as required by the Center for Biologics Evaluation and Research. The intramuscular vaccine also contains less than 150 μg of neomycin sulfate and 20 μg of phenol red indicator per dose. The vaccine for intradermal use contains at least 0.25 IU of rabies antigen and less than 22 μg of neomycin sulfate and 3 μg of phenol red indicator per each 0.1-ml dose.

Uses—Both vaccines indicated for active immunization in pre-exposure situations for high-risk groups such as veterinarians, animal handlers, researchers and other similar personnel working in laboratories, hospitals etc. whose pursuits bring them in contact with potentially rabid animals or with the handling of rabies virus or potentially contaminated material. The intramuscular vaccine also is recommended for post-exposure treatment of animal bites with a potential risk of rabies. For more detailed information on both pre-exposure immunization and the rationale of post-exposure treatment with the intramuscular vaccine, see the package inserts.

Dose—*Intramuscular, pre-exposure:* **3 injections** of **1 mL** of reconstituted vaccine on each of days 0, 7 and 21 or 28; *postexposure:* **5** injections of **1 mL** of reconstituted vaccine on each of days 0, 3, 7, 14 and 28 in conjunction with Rabies Immune Globulin (RIG) on day 0. This dosage schedule is recommended by the CDC. For WHO recommendations and further information, see package insert. *Intradermal, preexposure only:* **3** injections of **0.1 mL** of reconstituted vaccine on days 0, 7 and 21 or 28. Both reconstituted vaccines should be used immediately.

Booster—Both vaccines given selectively every 2 yr to persons with continuing risk of exposure, or titers are checked every 2 yr, and if the titer is inadequate a booster is given. Persons working with the live virus in research laboratories or vaccine production facilities should have rabies antibody titers checked every 6 mo and boosters given as needed. For further information see package insert.

Dosage Form—Injection: Single-dose.

Rabies Vaccine Adsorbed

RVA

A sterile, slightly pink, clarified suspension of the CVS Kissling/MDPH strain of rabies virus grown on a diploid cell line derived from fetal rhesus lung cells, inactivated with beta-propiolactone (BPL) and adsorbed to aluminum phosphate. Each 1-mL dose contains 0.01% thimerosal as a preservative and 2.5 IU or more or rabies antigen. See *Rabies Vaccine* (HDCV). This product differs from HDCV in that a different virus strain, cell-line culture and concentration process are used. RVA also differs in that it is a liquid rather than being lyophilized because it is adsorbed on aluminum phosphate (which also may serve as an adjuvant).

Uses—Indicated for both pre-exposure situations for high-risk individuals and postexposure treatment. See *Rabies Vaccine* (HDCV).

Dose—*Intramuscular* only. See *Rabies Vaccine* (HDCV).

Booster—See *Rabies Vaccine* (HDCV).

Dosage Form—Injection: 1.0 mL.

Rubella Virus Vaccine Live

Meruvax$_{II}$ (*MSD*)

A bacterially sterile, lyophilized preparation of the Wistar Institute RA 27/3 strain of live attenuated rubella virus propagated in human diploid cell culture. When reconstituted each 0.5 mL dose contains not less than the equivalent of 1000 $TCID_{50}$ of the US Reference Rubella Virus. The reconstituted vaccine is clear yellow and each 0.5-mL dose contains approximately 25 μg of neomycin.

Uses—Indicated for active immunization against rubella (German measles) in children from 12 mo to puberty especially when the commonly used mixed vaccine form of Measles, Mumps and Rubella Virus Vaccine, Live (MMR) causes untoward reaction or is contraindicated or when it is advantageous to begin immunization against rubella before 15 mo of age (the recommended starting age for MMR). Increased emphasis should be placed on immunizing susceptible non-pregnant adolescent and adult females of childbearing age to protect against subsequently acquiring rubella infection during pregnancy, which in turn prevents infection of the fetus and consequent congenital rubella injury. Vaccination of adolescent and adult males in high-risk groups, eg, college and military bases, may be useful in preventing or controlling outbreaks. For more detailed information on usage, see the package insert.

Dose—*Subcutaneous,* **1, 0.5-mL** injection of reconstituted vaccine. Any unused reconstituted vaccine should be stored at 2 to 8° and discarded within 8 hr.

Booster—Given as MMR (see **Booster** for Measles Virus Vaccine Live Attenuated.) Rubella vaccine failure has not been a major problem. However, there are substantial potential consequences of rubella vaccine failure (ie, congenital rubella syndrome). Thus, a booster of MMR should provide an additional safeguard.

Dosage Form—Injection: Single-dose; 10- and 50-dose (available only to government agencies/institutions).

Yellow Fever Vaccine

YF-Vax (*Connaught*)

A bacterially sterile, lyophilized preparation of the live 17D strain of yellow fever virus prepared in chicken embryos. When reconstituted as directed the vaccine appears slightly opalescent and light orange in color. Each 0.5 mL dose contains not less than 5.04 $\log_{10}$ PFU. There is no preservative added.

Uses—For active immunization of all travelers 9 mo and older planning a trip to areas of South America and Africa where yellow fever infection is reported officially. Children under 9 mo and pregnant women should not be vaccinated unless they live in or are traveling to a high-risk area requiring a certificate of vaccination against yellow fever. However, infants less than 4 mo should not receive yellow fever vaccine because of the risk of encephalitis. For more detailed information on usage, see the package insert. Yellow Fever Vaccine is supplied in the US to designated authorized Yellow Fever Vaccination Centers only. The location of the nearest Centers may be obtained from the CDC.

Dose—*Subcutaneous,* **1 injection** of **0.5 mL** of reconstituted vaccine. Any unused reconstituted vaccine must be sterilized and discarded within 60 min.

Booster—Every 10 yr.

Dosage Form—Injection: 1-, 5- and 20-dose volume; 100 dose for *jet injector use only.* The 20-dose vial may be administered with needle and syringe or jet injector use.

Mixed Vaccines

There are three commonly used mixed viral vaccines that contain multiple immunogens for different viral infections. These combinations provide a broad immunization coverage with a reduced number of injections.

Measles, Mumps and Rubella Virus Vaccine Live

MMR Vaccine; M-M-R$_{II}$ (*MSD*)

A bacterially sterile, lyophilized preparation of a combination of Measles Virus Vaccine Live, Attenuated; Mumps Virus Vaccine Live and Rubella Virus Vaccine Live. The three viruses are mixed before being lyophilized. When reconstituted as directed each 0.5-mL dose contains not less than the equivalent of 1000 $TCID_{50}$ of the US Reference Measles Virus; 20,000 $TCID_{50}$ of the US Reference Mumps Virus; and 1000 $TCID_{50}$ of the US Reference Rubella Virus. The reconstituted vaccine is clear yellow and each 0.5-mL dose contains approximately 25 μg of neomycin.

Uses—Indicated for simultaneous active immunization against measles (rubeola), mumps and rubella (German measles) in persons 15 mo or older. For other recommendations see the package insert.

Dose—*Subcutaneous,* **1 injection** of **0.5 mL** of reconstituted vaccine. Any unused reconstituted vaccine should be stored at 2 to 8° and discarded within 8 hr.

Booster—**1 injection** of **0.5 mL.** ACIP recommends routine revaccination at 4 to 6 yr (at entry to kindergarten or first grade),whereas AAP recommends routine vaccination at entry to middle school or junior high school. It should also be noted that some state and local healthy agencies have their own mandates as to the specific age for revaccination.

Dosage Form—Injection: Single-dose volume; 10-dose (available only to government agencies/institutions).

Measles and Rubella Virus Vaccine Live

MR Vaccine; M-R-Vax$_{II}$ (*MSD*)

A bacterially sterile, lyophilized preparation of a combination of Measles Virus Vaccine Live, Attenuated, and Rubella Virus Vaccine Live. The two viruses are mixed before being lyophilized. When reconstituted as directed each 0.5-mL dose contains not less than the equivalent of 1000 $TCID_{50}$ of the US Reference Measles Virus and 1000 $TCID_{50}$ of the US

Reference Rubella Virus. The reconstituted vaccine is clear-yellow and each 0.5-mL dose contains approximately 25 μg of neomycin.

Uses—Indicated for simultaneous active immunization against measles (rubeola) and rubella (German measles) in persons 15 mo or older. For other recommendations, see the package insert.

Dose—*Subcutaneous*, **1 injection** of **0.5 mL** of reconstituted vaccine. Any unused reconstituted vaccine should be stored at 2 to 8° and discarded within 8 hr.

Booster—See *Measles Mumps and Rubella Virus Vaccine Live.*

Dosage Form—Injection: Single-dose volume; 10- and 50-dose (available only to government agencies/institutions).

Rubella and Mumps Virus Vaccine Live

RM Vaccine; Biavax$_{II}$ (*MSD*)

A bacterially sterile, lyophilized preparation of a combination of Rubella Virus Vaccine Live and Mumps Virus Vaccine Live. The two viruses are mixed before being lyophilized. When reconstituted as directed each 0.5-mL dose contains not less than the equivalent of 1000 $TCID_{50}$ of the US Reference Rubella Virus and 20,000 $TCID_{50}$ of the US Reference Mumps Virus. The reconstituted vaccine is clear yellow and each 0.5-mL dose contains approximately 25 μg of neomycin.

Uses—Indicated for simultaneous active immunization against rubella (German measles) and mumps in persons 12 mo or older. For other recommendations, see the package insert.

Dose—*Subcutaneous*, **1 injection** of **0.5 mL** of reconstituted vaccine. Any unused reconstituted vaccine should be stored at 2 to 8° and discarded within 8 hr.

Booster—Usually given as MMR. See *Measles Mumps and Rubella Virus Vaccine Live.*

Note—Recent studies show that a substantial number of mumps cases have occurred among individuals with histories of prior vaccination. Rubella vaccine failure has not been a major problem. However, there are substantial potential consequences of rubella vaccine failure (ie, congenital rubella syndrome). Thus, a booster should provide an additional safeguard.

Dosage Form—Injection: Single-dose.

Other Viral Vaccines

Adenovirus Vaccine Live Oral Type 4

An oral tablet formulation indicated for immunization of military populations in which epidemic respiratory disease due to adenovirus, Type 4, has been shown likely to occur.

Adenovirus Vaccine Live Oral Type 7

An oral tablet formulation indicated for immunization of military populations in which epidemic respiratory disease due to adenovirus, Type 7, has been shown likely to occur.

Eastern Equine Encephalitis Vaccine, Inactivated

An inactivated lyophilized Investigational New Drug (IND) distributed by the military.

Hepatitis A Vaccine

Havrix (*SmithKline Beecham*)

An inactivated IND for active immunization against hepatitis A.

Smallpox Vaccine

Dryvax (*Wyeth*)

A lyophilized preparation of the live vaccinia virus grown on calf lymph and distributed by the CDC. Production of smallpox vaccine for general use was discontinued in 1982 and in May, 1983 distribution of the vaccine to civilians was discontinued. Smallpox vaccination of civilians now is indicated only for laboratory workers directly involved with smallpox or closely related orthopox viruses. In addition, smallpox vaccine is currently not being given routinely to military recruits.

Varicella Vaccine

A live attenuated IND intended for active immunization against varicella (chicken pox) in immunocompromised and healthy children.

Venezuelan Equine Encephalitis Vaccine, Inactivated

An inactivated lyophilized IND distributed by the military.

Western Equine Encephalitis Vaccine, Inactivated

An inactivated lyophilized IND distributed by the military.

Toxoids

Preparation—Bacteria are propagated in a similar manner as for a bacterial vaccine, and after the required growth is attained, the culture is filtered through a sterilizing membrane filter. The filtrate containing the toxin (exotoxin) then is processed usually as

A concentrated salt solution is added to precipitate the toxin from the filtrate.
The precipitated toxin is washed and purified by dialysis.
The toxin is detoxified with formaldehyde.

The detoxified toxin (toxoid) may be *plain* or may contain an *adjuvant* such as alum, aluminum hydroxide or aluminum phosphate. These adjuvants are insoluble materials which act to keep the immunogens (toxoids) in tissue for longer periods and thus cause a prolonged immunoglobulin stimulation.

Product Form—As with both bacterial and viral vaccines, the final preparation may contain single, multiple or mixed immunogens. If the toxoid is adsorbed, it is in the form of a liquid suspension and if plain, a slightly cloudy solution.

Strength—The strength of a toxoid is expressed in terms of flocculating (Lf) units. A flocculating unit is the smallest amount of toxin which flocculates most rapidly one unit of standard antitoxin in a series of mixtures containing fixed amounts of antitoxin and varying amounts of toxin.

Diphtheria Toxoid Adsorbed

A sterile, white or slightly gray suspension of purified diphtheria toxoid (formaldehyde-treated toxin of *Corynebacterium diphtheriae*) either adsorbed onto aluminum phosphate or precipitated with alum. Each 0.5-mL dose of the pediatric formulations (see *Uses*) contains between 6.6 and 12.5 Lf Units of diphtheria toxoid. The adult formulation (see *Uses*) contains not more than 2 Lf Units of diphtheria toxoid per each 0.5-mL dose. Thimerosal (1:10,000) is added as a preservative.

Uses—Not currently available as a single-antigen product. It is adminstered commonly as Tetanus and Diphtheria Toxoids Adsorbed for Adult Use and as one of the following mixed toxoids and biologics for pediatric use: Diphtheria and Tetanus Toxoids Adsorbed (for Pediatric Use); Diphtheria and Tetanus Toxoids and Pertussis Vaccine Adsorbed (DTP); Diphtheria and Tetanus Toxoids and Acellular Pertussis Vaccine Adsorbed; and the mixed biologic containing DTP and Haemophilus b Conjugate Vaccine.

Dose—*Intramuscular;* see individual mixed toxoids and mixed biologics.

Booster—0.5 mL every 10 yr. For adults and children 7 yr and older, Tetanus and Diphtheria Toxoids Adsorbed (Td) For Adult Use is recommended.

Dosage Form—See individual mixed toxoids and biologics containing diphtheria toxoid.

Tetanus Toxoid

Tetanus Toxoid Fluid; Tetanus Toxoid Plain

A clear, or slightly turbid sterile solution of fluid tetanus toxoid (formaldehyde treated toxin of *Clostridium tetani*). Products of different manufacturers may vary in potency from 4 to 5 Lf Units per 0.5-mL dose. Thimerosal (1:10,000) is added as a preservative.

Uses—May be used for active immunization against tetanus. However, Tetanus Toxoid Adsorbed is preferred for all basic immunizing and recall reactions because of more persistent antitoxin titer induction.

Dose—*Intramuscular* or *subcutaneous*, **3 injections** of **0.5 mL** 4 to 8 wk apart, followed by a fourth, reinforcing dose of **0.5 mL** 6 to 12 mo later. Primary immunization cannot be considered complete without the fourth reinforcing dose being given since this dose is an integral part of the basic immunizing course.

Booster—0.5 mL every 10 yr. For additional information on wound management, see the package insert.

Dosage Form—Injection: 0.5 and 7.5 mL.

Tetanus Toxoid Adsorbed

Te Anatoxal (*Berna*)

A sterile, white or whitish gray suspension of purified tetanus toxoid (formaldehyde treated toxin of *Clostridium tetani*) alum precipitated or adsorbed onto aluminum phosphate. Products of different manufacturers may vary in potency from 5 to 10 Lf Units per 0.5-mL dose. Thimerosal (1:10,000) is added as a preservative.

Uses—For active immunization against tetanus in children and adults. It commonly is administered for routine prophylaxis in the form of Diphtheria and Tetanus Toxoids and Pertussis Vaccine Adsorbed (DTP) to children under 7 yr or as Tetanus and Diphtheria Toxoids Adsorbed (Td) For Adult Use for adults and children 7 yr and older. Tetanus Toxoid Adsorbed or Tetanus Toxoid (Fluid) usually is administered to patients at the time of injury for recall, but it can be used for boosters and establishing immunization at all ages.

Dose—*Intramuscular*, **2 injections** of **0.5 mL** 4 to 8 wk apart, followed by a third, reinforcing dose of **0.5 mL** 6 to 12 mo later.

Booster—0.5 mL every 10 yr. For additional information on wound management, see the package insert.

Dosage Form—Injection: 0.5 and 5 mL.

Mixed Toxoids and Mixed Biologics

A mixed toxoid such as Tetanus and Diphtheria Toxoids Adsorbed (Td) For Adult Use contains two or more toxoids in a single preparation for active immunization of *different toxicities*.

A mixed biologic such as Diphtheria and Tetanus Toxoids and Pertussis Vaccine Adsorbed (DTP) has *toxoids and vaccines* in a single dose form for active immunization of different *toxicities and infections*.

These two types of biologics differ from *polyvalent* products which are used for different strains of the same toxicity or infection, eg, Botulism Antitoxin Trivalent (for passive immunization) and Pneumococcal Vaccine Polyvalent.

Mixed toxoids and biologics have the obvious advantage of providing broad immunization coverage with a reduced number of injections.

Diphtheria and Tetanus Toxoids Adsorbed (For Pediatric Use)

DT

A sterile, white or slightly gray suspension of purified diphtheria and tetanus toxoids alum precipitated or adsorbed onto aluminum phosphate. Products of different manufacturers may vary in potency from 6.6 to 12.5 Lf Units of diphtheria toxoid and from 5 to 7.5 Lf Units of tetanus toxoid per 0.5-mL dose. Thimerosal (1:10,000) is added as a preservative.

Uses—Recommended for active immunization against diphtheria and tetanus in infants and children 6 wk through 6 yr of age when it is unadvisable or contraindicated to give the preferred Diphtheria and Tetanus Toxoids and Pertussis Vaccine Adsorbed (DTP).

Note—DT is not recommended for immunizing persons on or after their seventh birthday due to the increased possibility of severe reactions attributed to the pediatric levels of diphtheria toxoid.

Dose—*Intramuscular*, children less than 1 yr, **3 injections** of **0.5 mL** 4 to 8 wk apart followed by a fourth, reinforcing dose of **0.5 mL** 6 to 12 mo later. For children 1 yr and older, **2** injections of **0.5 mL** 4 to 8 wk apart, followed by a third, reinforcing dose of **0.5 mL** 6 to 12 mo later. Primary immunization cannot be considered complete without the reinforcing dose being given since this dose is an integral part of the basic immunizing course.

Booster—0.5 mL at 4 to 6 yr preferably prior to entrance into kindergarten or elementary school. If last dose of primary immunizing series was administered after the fourth birthday, a booster prior to school entry is not considered necessary. Over age 6, Tetanus and Diphtheria Toxoids Adsorbed (Td) For Adult Use is recommended every 10 yr.

Dosage Form—Injection: 0.5 and 5 mL.

Tetanus and Diphtheria Toxoids Adsorbed For Adult Use

Td

A sterile, white or slightly gray suspension of purified diphtheria and tetanus toxoids alum precipitated or adsorbed onto aluminum phosphate. Each 0.5 mL contains not more than 2 Lf Units of diphtheria toxoid and from 2 to 5 Lf Units of tetanus toxoid depending upon the manufacturer. Thimerosal (1:30,000 to 1:10,000) is added as a preservative.

Uses—For active immunization of adults and children 7 yr and older. The small amount of diphtheria toxoid in the product minimizes sensitivity reactions. Td is not recommended for immunizing persons less than 7 yr.

Dose—*Intramuscular*, **2 injections** of **0.5 mL** 4 to 8 wk apart, followed by a third, reinforcing dose of **0.5 mL** 6 to 12 mo later. Primary immunization cannot be considered complete without the third reinforcing dose being given since this dose is an integral part of the basic immunizing course.

Booster—0.5 mL every 10 yr. For additional information on wound management, see the package insert.

Dosage Forms—Injection: 0.5 and 5 mL; 30 mL *for jet injector use only*.

Diphtheria and Tetanus Toxoids and Acellular Pertussis Vaccine Adsorbed

DTaP; Acel-Imune (*Lederle*); Tripedia (*Connaught*)

A sterile white suspension of purified diphtheria and tetanus toxoids and acellular pertussis vaccine. The Tripedia formulation has the diphtheria and tetatnus toxoids in the adsorbed form (alum precipitated) combined with nonadsorbed pertussis vaccine. The Acel-Imune product has all three components (diphtheria and tetanus toxoids, and pertussis vaccine) combined, diluted in phosphate buffered saline and adsorbed to aluminum. Each 0.5-mL dose contains from 6.7 to 7.5 Lf Units of diphtheria toxoid, 5 Lf Units of tetanus toxoid and approximately 40 μg (but not more than 60 μg) of pertussis antigen. Thimerosal (1:10,000) is added as a preservative.

Uses—Licensed only for use as the fourth and fifth doses of the DTP series among children 15 mo through 6 yr who previously have received 3 or 4 doses of whole-cell DTP. DTaP substantially reduces local reactions, fever and other common systemic events that often occur with whole-cell DTP. (See *Other Reactions* earlier in this chapter for contraindications and adverse reactions.) However, data is not available on the use of DTaP in children for whom whole-cell pertussis DTP vaccine is contraindicated, and thus DT should be used for each of the remaining doses in these instances. Efficacy data for the acellular pertussis vaccine in infants is also not available, and thus DTaP is not recommended for use in children below the age of 15 mo. There are also questions as to whether protection which is induced using acellular pertussis vaccines is equivalent to that of whole-cell pertussis preparations. Therefore, it is recommended that whole-cell pertussis vaccines be continued for the initial 3-dose vaccination series until acellular vaccines have demonstrated essentially equivalent or higher efficacy.

Dose—*Intramuscular*, **0.5 mL** given at 15 mo as the fourth primary dose, 6 to 12 mo after the third dose of DTP.

Booster—0.5 mL between 4 and 6 yr prior to entering kindergarten or elementary school (not necessary if fourth primary dose given after fourth birthday).

Dosage Form—Injection: 5 and 7.5 mL.

Diphtheria and Tetanus Toxoids and Pertussis Vaccine Adsorbed (For Pediatric Use)

DTP; Tri-immunol (*Lederle*)

A sterile, whitish suspension of purified diphtheria and tetanus toxoids alum precipitated or aluminum phosphate adsorbed and Phase 1 pertussis vaccine. The pertussis component varies with the manufacturer and may or may not be adsorbed. Each 0.5-mL dose contains from 6.7 to 12.5 Lf Units of diphtheria toxoid, approximately 5 Lf Units of tetanus toxoid and 4 protective units of pertussis vaccine. Thimerosal (1:10,000) is added as a preservative.

Uses—For active immunization of infants and children through 6 yr against diphtheria, tetanus and pertussis simultaneously. Injections should be started at 6 wk to 2 mo and completed no later than the age of 6 yr.

Dose—*Intramuscular*, **3 injections** of **0.5 mL** 4 to 8 wk apart, followed by a fourth, reinforcing dose of **0.5 mL** 1 yr later. Primary immunization cannot be considered complete without the fourth reinforcing dose being given since this dose is an integral part of the basic immunizing course.

Note: 0.5 mL DTaP may be given as the fourth reinforcing dose.

Booster—For children between 4 and 6 yr (preferably prior to entrance into kindergarten or elementary school), **0.5 mL.**

Note—0.5 mL DTaP may be given as the booster.

For persons 7 yr and older, Tetanus and Diphtheria Toxoids Adsorbed (Td) For Adult Use is recommended every 10 yr. DTP is not used after 6 yr because of the increased possibility of severe reactions, most often attributed to the pediatric levels of diphtheria toxoid, and moreover, because the incidence, severity and fatality of pertussis decrease with age.

Note: See *Other Reactions* earlier in this chapter for contraindications and adverse reactions of Pertussis Vaccine.

Dosage Form—Injection: 5 and 7.5 mL.

Diphtheria and Tetanus Toxoids and Pertussis Vaccine Adsorbed and Haemophilus b Conjugate Vaccine

Tetramune (*Lederle*)

A sterile, while suspension of a combination of diphtheria and tetanus toxoids adsorbed on aluminum phosphate and Phase 1 pertussis vaccine (DTP, Tri-Immunol) mixed with a conjugate of oligosaccharides of the capsular antigen of *Haemophilus influenzae* type b and diphtheria CRM_{197} protein (Haemophilus b Conjugate Vaccine, HibTITER). Each 0.5-mL dose is formulated to contain 12.5 Lf Units of diphtheria toxoid, 5 Lf Units of tetanus toxoid, 10 μg of purified Haemophilus b saccharide and an estimated 4 protective units of pertussis vaccine. Thimerosal is added as a preservative to the combination vaccine to a final concentration of 1:10,000.

Uses—Indicated for the active immunization of children 2 mo to 5 yr for protection against diphtheria, tetanus, pertussis and Haemophilus b disease when indications for immunization with DTP vaccine and Haemophilus b Conjugate Vaccine coincide. Typically, this is at 2, 4, 6 and 15 mo. See the package insert for additional information pertaining to children who have recovered from culture-confirmed pertussis and those who have experienced invasive Haemophilus b disease.

Dose—*Intramuscular*, **3 injections** of **0.5 mL** approximately 2 mo apart beginning at 2 mo, followed by a fourth **0.5-mL** dose at approximately 15 mo.

Note—Children 15 to 18 mo may receive DTaP plus a Haemophilus B conjugate vaccine as separate injections.

Booster—*Intramuscular*, **0.5 mL** of DTP or DTaP at 4 to 6 yr. Haemophilus B conjugate component is not given as a booster.

Dosage Form—Injection: 5 mL.

Other Toxoids

Botulinum Toxoid Pentavalent (ABCDE)

An Investigational New Drug (IND) available from CDC for nonemergency, high laboratory risk immunization.

Biologics for Passive Immunization

Human Immune Sera (Homologous Sera)

Human immune sera or homologous sera include immune globulin and hyperimmune sera (including $Rh_0(D)$ immune globulin) for specific diseases (Table 1).

An homologous serum has less potential for hypersensitivity reactions and a longer half-life than does the more foreign heterologous serum of animal origin. The half-life of an homologous serum such as tetanus immune globulin (TIG) is approximately 26 to 30 days and that for a corresponding heterologous serum is approximately 7 days. Thus not only does TIG have less potential for hypersensitivity reactions but it can be administered in a smaller dose, since it is capable of remaining in the body longer.

The source of homologous sera is the pooled plasma [free of hepatitis B antigen and antibodies to human immunodeficiency virus (HIV)] of adult donors either from the general population (for immune globulin) or from hyperimmunized donors (for immune globulins for specific diseases). The plasma then is precipitated fractionally, usually with cold ethanol, under rigorous controls of pH and ionic strength. Different manufacturers may modify the precipitation procedure to increase the yield.

The precipitated immunoglobulins are purified further and the finished biologic is a solution usually containing not less than 15% and not more than 18% protein. Hepatitis B, $Rh_0(D)$ and varicella-zoster immune globulins contain not less than 10% protein.

Most immune sera are intended for *intramuscular* use only and should not be given *intravenously*. However, two products, immune globulin intravenous (which contains 3 to 12% protein) and cytomegalovirus immune globulin are intended for intravenous use.

Immune Globulin (Human)

Immune Serum Globulin Human, "Gamma" Globulin, IG; Gammar (*Armour*)

A sterile, transparent or slightly opalescent and colorless, nonpyrogenic solution of immunoglobulins, primarily immunoglobulin G (IgG). *Note: the term "gamma" globulin is a misnomer, as some of the immunoglobulins present are beta globulins.* The product is prepared by cold alcohol fractionation of pooled plasma. It contains 16.5% ± 1.5% protein and meets the potency requirements of certain antibodies as determined by the FDA. Thimerosal (1:10,000) is added as a preservative.

Note—The product is prepared from human plasma that was nonreactive when tested for hepatitis B surface antigen and for antibodies to human immunodeficiency virus (HIV).

Uses—Recommended for (1) Passive prevention of hepatitis A when given before or soon after exposure (not more than 2 wk) to hepatitis A. *Note—not indicated in persons with clinical manifestation.* (2) Passive prevention or modification of measles (rubeola) in a susceptible individual (particularly household contacts under 1 yr, for whom the risk of complications is highest) exposed fewer than 6 days previously. *Note—Measles vaccine should not be given at the same time. If a child is older than 12 mo and has received IG, he/she should be given measles vaccine about 3 mo later when the measles antibody titer will have disappeared.* (3) Possible prevention of serious infections in patients with immunoglobulin deficiencies. (4) Use when Varicella-Zoster Immune Globulin is indicated but not available. (5) Possible benefit in lessening the likelihood of infection and fetal damage in women exposed to rubella in early pregnancy and who will not consider a therapeutic abortion.

Note—Routine use of IG for prophylaxis of rubella in early pregnancy is of dubious value and cannot be justified.

Dose—*Intramuscular* only. For doses and frequency of administration for various uses and other essential information, see the package insert.

Dosage Form—Injection: 2 and 10 mL.

Hepatitis B Immune Globulin (Human)

H-Big (*Abbott*); Hep-B Gammagee (*MSD*); HyperHep (*Miles*)

A sterile, slightly amber, nonpyrogenic solution consisting of immunoglobulin prepared by cold alcohol fractionation of blood plasma of human donors who have high titers of antibodies against hepatitis B surface antigen (anti-HBs). Each vial contains anti-HBs antibody equivalent to or exceeding the potency (217 IU/mL) of anti-HBs in a US Reference Hepatitis B Immune Globulin. Thimerosal (1:10,000) is added as a preservative.

Note—The product is prepared from human plasma that was nonreactive when tested for hepatitis B surface antigen and antibodies to human immunodeficiency virus (HIV).

Uses—Indicated for postexposure passive immunization following either parenteral exposure, direct mucous membrane contact, sexual exposure or oral ingestion involving HBsAg-positive materials such as blood, plasma or serum. The product also is recommended for passive immunization of infants born to HBsAg-positive mothers. Hepatitis B Immune Globulin may be given either preceding or concomitant with Hepatitis B Vaccine to provide a more rapid achievement of protective levels of hepatitis B antibody.

Dose—*Intramuscular, adult*, **0.06 mL/kg** (usually 3 to 5 mL), preferably administered within 24 hr of exposure concomitantly with Hepatitis B

Vaccine (Recombinant). The second and third doses of vaccine are given 1 and 6 mo after. For dosage for newborns, see the package insert.

Dosage Form—Injection: 0.5, 1 and 5 mL.

Rabies Immune Globulin (Human)

Hyperab (*Miles*); Imogam Rabies (*Connaught*)

A sterile, transparent or slightly opalescent, nearly colorless nonpyrogenic solution of antirabies immunoglobulins derived from cold fractionation of the blood plasma of individuals hyperimmunized with rabies vaccine. Each mL contains 150 International Units (IU) based on the US Standard Rabies Immune Globulin and using the CVS Virus Challenge by neutralization test in mice or tissue culture. The US unit of potency is equivalent to the International Unit for rabies antibody. Thimerosal (1:10,000) is added as a preservative.

Note—The product is prepared from human plasma that was found nonreactive when tested for hepatitis B surface antigen and antibodies to human immunodeficiency virus (HIV).

Uses—Used in conjunction with Rabies Vaccine and indicated for individuals suspected of exposure to rabies, particularly severe exposure, with the exception of persons who have been immunized previously with rabies vaccine and have confirmed adequate antibody titers. For more complete information, see the package insert.

Dose—*Intramuscular,* **20 IU/kg** (0.133 mL/kg) at the time of administration of the first vaccine dose. If possible up to half the dose should be used to *infiltrate* the wound and the rest administered *intramuscularly*, preferably in the gluteal or deltoid region.

Dosage Form—Injection: 2 mL (pediatric, 300IU); 10 mL (adults, 1500IU).

Rh_0(D) Immune Globulin (Human)

Gamulin Rh and Mini-Gamulin Rh (*Armour*); Rho Gam and MICRho GAM (*Ortho*); HypRho-D Full-Dose and Mini-Dose (*Miles*)

A sterile, transparent or slightly opalescent and practically clear, nonpyrogenic solution of immunoglobulins derived from human blood plasma containing antibody to the erythrocyte factor Rh_0(D). The Rh_0(D) antibody level in each single *full* dose vial is equal to or greater than that of the Center For Biologics Evaluation and Research Reference Rh_0(D) Immune Globulin (Human). This dose (approximately 300 μg) has been shown to inhibit effectively the immunizing potential of up to 15 mL of Rh-positive packed red blood cells. The *mini* or *micro* dosage form contains approximately 1/6 the quantity of Rh_0(D) antibody. Thimerosal (0.03 to 0.01%) is added as a preservative.

Note—The product is prepared from human plasma that was not reactive when tested for hepatitis B surface antigen and antibodies to human immunodeficiency virus (HIV).

Uses—The 300-μg dose is indicated (1) whenever it is known or suspected that fetal red blood cells have entered the circulation of an Rh-negative mother unless the fetus or the father can be shown conclusively to be Rh-negative and (2) for any Rh-negative female or childbearing age who receives any Rh-positive red blood cells or component such as platelets or granulocytes prepared from Rh-positive blood.

Note—If the product is administered antepartum (at 28 wk gestation), it is essential that the mother receive another dose of Rh_0(D) Immune Globulin after delivery of an Rh-positive infant. The 150-μg dose is indicated for an Rh-negative woman following spontaneous or induced abortion or termination of ectopic pregnancy up to and including 12 wk gestation, unless the father is conclusively shown to be Rh-negative. Administration of Rh_0(D) immune globulin within 72 hr reduces the incidence of Rh isoimmunization from 12 to 13% to 1 to 2%, thus offering protection to the next infant if born Rh_0(D) positive.

Dose—*Intramuscular,* **1 vial** or **syringe.** (For transfusion accidents, the number of vials or syringes needed depends on the volume transfused. For more complete information, see the package insert).

Dosage Form—Injection: Single-dose.

Tetanus Immune Globulin (Human)

TIG
Hyper-Tet (*Miles*)

A sterile, transparent or slightly opalescent and practically clear, nonpyrogenic solution of immunoglobulins derived from the cold ethanol fractionation of blood plasma of adult human donors who have been immunized with tetanus toxoid. Each container has not less than 250 antitoxin units based on the US Standard Tetanus Antitoxin and the US Control Tetanus Test Toxin tested in guinea pigs. Thimerosal (1:10,000) is added as a preservative.

Note—The product is prepared from human plasma that was not reactive when tested for hepatitis B surface antigen and antibodies to human immunodeficiency virus (HIV).

Uses—Administered with tetanus toxoid as soon as possible after tetanus-prone injuries to provide immediate passive immunization against tetanus toxin in patients whose immunization is incomplete (have received less than three doses of tetanus toxoid) or uncertain. It also is used in the regimen of treatment of clinical tetanus although the evidence of effectiveness is limited.

Dose—*Intramuscular, prophylactic,* **250 units** in conjunction with Td (adults) or DTP or DT (children less than 7 yr). *Intramuscular, therapeutic,* **500 units to 6,000 units** in combination with other accepted clinical and nursing procedures; however, the optimum therapeutic dose has not yet been established and no claim can be made for the therapeutic effectiveness of the recommended dose.

Dosage Form—Injection: 250 units.

Varicella-Zoster Immune Globulin (Human)

VZIG

A sterile, 10.0 to 18.0% solution of immunoglobulins (primarily IgG) derived from the blood plasmas of adult human volunteers selected for high titers of varicella-zoster antibodies. Each dose contains 125 units of antibody to varicella-zoster virus. Thimerosal (1:10,000) is added as a preservative.

Note—The product is prepared from human plasma that was nonreactive when tested for hepatitis B surface antigen and antibodies to human immunodeficiency virus (HIV).

Uses—For passive immunization of susceptible high-risk individuals following exposure to varicella (chicken pox). High-risk groups include immunocompromised children, newborns of mothers with varicella shortly before or after delivery, premature infants, immunocompromised adults and normal susceptible adults (evaluated on an individual basis) and may also include susceptible high-risk infants less than 1 yr.

Dose—*Intramuscular,* **1 to 5 vials** depending upon body weight. For more detailed information, see the package insert. The proposed dosage, if given within 96 hr after exposure, was found to be effective in modifying significantly the expected severity of chickenpox and reducing the observed frequency of death, pneumonia and encephalitis to less than 25% of the expected rate without treatment.

Its value given after 96 hr of exposure is uncertain and there is no evidence that it can modify an established varicella infection. For more information, see the package insert.

Dosage Form—Injection: Single-dose, 2.5 mL or less. Distributed outside of Massachusetts by the American National Red Cross. Distributed within Massachusetts by The MAPH Biologic Labs.

Other Human Immune Sera

Bacterial Polysaccharide Immune Globulin (Human)

An Investigational New Drug (IND) derived from human plasma from volunteers immunized with 14-valent pneumococcal vaccine, meningococcal vaccine (serogroups A, C, Y and W-135) and *Haemophilus influenzae* type b vaccine. Indicated for prevention of infections caused by pneumococcus, meningococcus and *H influenzae* type b in patients who are at especially high risk of developing such infections.

Cytomegalovirus Immune Globulin (Human) For Intravenous Use

Indicated for the attenuation of primary cytomegalovirus (CMV) disease associated with kidney transplantation. Specifically, the product is indicated for kidney transplant recipients who are seronegative for CMV and who receive a kidney from a CMV seropositive donor.

Immune Globulin Intravenous Human IGIV

Gamimune N(*Miles*); Gammagard (*Baxter*) Sandoglobulin (*Sandoz*)

Contains less protein (3 to 6%) than Immune Globulin for Intramuscular use which has 16.5 ± 1.5%. Gamimune N, 10% consists of 9% to 11% protein. IGIV is indicated in the treatment of primary immunodeficiency states in which severe impairment of antibody forming capacity has been shown, such as congenital agammaglobulinemias, common variable immunodeficiency, Wiskott-Aldrich syndrome and severe combined immunodeficiencies. It is preferable to Immune Globulin (for intramuscular use) in treating patients who require an immediate and high increase in the intravascular immunoglobulin level. For more detailed information, see the package insert.

Respiratory Syncytial Virus Immune Globulin (Human)

An Investigational New Drug (IND) for the passive prevention of respiratory syncytial virus infections in children (less than 2 yr) with congenital heart disease.

Vaccinia Immune Globulin (Human)

Available from the CDC for prevention or modification of smallpox and possible treatment of complications to smallpox vaccine. It is of limited value since the eradication of naturally occurring smallpox and thus the limited use of the vaccine.

Western Equine Encephalitis (WEE) Immune Globulin

An Investigational New Drug (IND) distributed by the military.

Animal Immune Sera (Heterologous Sera)

Animal immune sera or heterologous sera include antitoxins and antivenins (Table 1).

These preparations are obtained from the plasma of horses that have been immunized against the specific immunogen (toxin or venom). The refining and concentration of the immunoglobulins from the plasma may vary with the manufacturer and the particular biologic. In general, plasma is separated into fractions which are immunologically active (immunoglobulins) and immunologically inactive (albumins and clotting factors) by fractional precipitation using ammonium sulfate. The immunologically active fraction then is digested briefly with pepsin to remove the complement-activating component of the molecules and also render them less immunogenic. The immunologically active component then is recovered by dialysis and fractional precipitation or centrifugation.

The finished biologic is either in the form of a solution or, if an antivenin, lyophilized.

As previously indicated, these products have potential for hypersensitivity reactions and the precautions mentioned previously should be followed.

Antitoxins (Equine)

Botulism Antitoxin (Equine)

Botulism Antitoxin Trivalent (Equine)

A sterile, transparent or slightly opalescent, nearly colorless, non- pyrogenic solution containing refined and concentrated immunoglobulins, obtained from the blood of healthy horses that have been immunized against the toxins produced by Type A, Type B and Type E strains of *Clostridium botulinum*. Each vial contains 7500 International Units (IU) of Type A, 5500 IU of Type B, and 8500 IU of Type E. The potency is determined with the US Standard Botulism Antitoxin of relevant type, tested by neutralizing activity in mice of the corresponding US Control Botulism Test Toxin. The product contains phenol (0.4%) as a preservative.

Uses—Indicated for the passive prevention and treatment of botulism known or suspected to be produced by *Clostridium botulinum*, Types A, B or E. The antitoxin will only neutralize circulating toxin and will not counteract the effect of toxin already bound to receptor cells in tissue, hence it will not be effective unless administered before extensive binding of toxin has occurred.

Dose—*Warning: Before the administration of any product containing horse protein, appropriate measures including a sensitivity test with suitable controls should be taken in an effort to detect the presence of dangerous sensitivity. For more details, see the package insert.*

Prophylactic, intramuscular, **1/5 to 1 vial** depending upon the amount of food eaten. A second injection of **1 vial** may be given in 12 to 24 hr if any signs and symptoms of botulism appear. *Therapeutic, intravenous* and *intramuscular,* **1 vial** *intravenously* diluted 1:10 followed by **1 vial** *intramuscularly* (to provide reservoir of antitoxin). Further doses may be indicated in 2 to 4 hr if signs and symptoms worsen.

Dosage Form—Injection: Vial containing not less than 7500 IU of Type A, 5500 IU of Type B and 8500 IU of Type E. (Distributed by the CDC.)

Diphtheria Antitoxin (Equine)

A sterile, transparent or slightly opalescent, nearly colorless, nonpyrogenic solution containing refined and concentrated immunoglobulins obtained from the blood of healthy horses that have been immunized against diphtheria toxin or toxoid (produced by *Corynebacterium diphtheriae*). It has a potency of not less than 500 antitoxin units per mL based on the US Standard Diphtheria Antitoxin, and a diphtheria test toxin, tested in guinea pigs. The preparation contains tricresol (0.4%) as a preservative.

Uses—Indicated for passive prevention and treatment of diphtheria. Prevention should be given to contacts intimately exposed and not immunized previously with toxoid.

Dose—*Warning: Before the administration of any product containing horse protein, appropriate measures including a sensitivity test with suitable controls should be taken in an effort to detect the presence of dangerous sensitivity. For more details, see the package insert.*

Prophylactic, intramuscular, **10,000 units** (varies with exposure, etc). For more details, see the package insert. *Therapeutic, intramuscular* or *intravenous,* **20,000 to 120,000** depending upon severity (administered all at one time). For more details, see the package insert.

Note—The incidence of serum sickness with prophylactic doses is generally below 10%; with therapeutic dosage a higher incidence should be anticipated, depending upon the amount administered.

Dosage Form—Injection: 20,000 units. (Distributed by the CDC.)

Tetanus Antitoxin (Equine)—see RPS-18, page 1402.

Antirabies Serum—see RPS-18, page 1402.

Antivenins (Equine)

Antivenin (*Crotalidae*) Polyvalent (Equine)

A sterile, nonpyrogenic, lyophilized preparation containing refined and concentrated immunoglobulins obtained from the blood of healthy horses immunized with the venoms of the following four species of crotalids (pit vipers): *Crotalus adamanteus* (eastern diamond rattlesnake), *C atrox* (western diamond rattlesnake), *C durissus terrificus* (tropical rattlesnake, Cascabel) and *Bothrops atrox* ("Fer-de-lance"). The potency is determined by a mouse protection test. Phenol (0.25%) and thimerosal (0.005%) are added as preservatives to the lyophilized preparation and phenylmercuric nitrate (0.001%) is added as a preservative to the diluent (Bacteriostatic Water for Injection, USP).

Uses—Indicated only for the treatment of envenomation caused by the bites of the four pit vipers mentioned above and for other pit vipers native to North, Central and South America including copperheads, cottonmouth moccasins and others as described in the package insert.

Dose—*Warning: Before the administration of any product containing horse protein, appropriate measures including a sensitivity test with suitable controls should be taken in an effort to detect the presence of dangerous sensitivity. For more details, see the package insert.*

Intravenous (preferred), *initially* **20** to **150 mL** (2 to 15 vials) or more of a 1:1 to 1:10 dilution of reconstituted Antivenin depending upon an estimate of the severity of the envenomation. The administration of additional Antivenin is based upon the clinical response to the initial dose and continuing assessment of the severity of poisoning. For complete information, see the package insert.

Dosage Form—Injection: A vial of lyophilized serum and a 10-mL vial of diluent.

Antivenin (*Latrodectus Mactans*) (Equine)

Black Widow Spider Antivenin

A sterile, nonpyrogenic lyophilized product containing immunoglobulins obtained from the blood of horses immunized with the venom of the black widow spider (*Latrodectus mactans*). Each vial contains not less than 6000 Antivenin units based on a mouse protection test. One unit of Antivenin will neutralize one average mouse lethal dose of black widow spider venom when the Antivenin and the venom are injected simultaneously. Thimerosal (1:10,000) is added as a preservative.

Uses—Indicated only for the treatment of symptoms due to bites by the black widow spider.

Dose—*Warning: Before the administration of any product containing horse protein, appropriate measures including a sensitivity test with suitable controls should be taken in an effort to detect the presence of dangerous sensitivity. For more details, see the package insert.*

Intramuscular, **1 vial** of reconstituted Antivenin. A second dose may be necessary in some cases. *Intravenous,* for severe cases, or when the patient is under 12 yr, or in shock, **1 vial** of reconstituted Antivenin in 10 to 50 mL of saline solution over a 15-min period.

Dosage Form—Injection: A vial of lyophilized serum and a 2.5-mL vial of sterile diluent. (A 1-mL vial of normal horse serum (1:10 dilution) also is supplied for sensitivity testing.)

Antivenin (*Micrurus Fulvius*) Equine

North American Coral Snake Antivenin

A sterile, non-pyrogenic, lyophilized preparation containing refined and concentrated immunoglobulins obtained by fractionating blood from healthy horses immunized with the venom of eastern coral snake (*Micrurus fulvius fulvius*). Each 10 mL of the reconstituted product will neutralize approximately 250 mouse LD_{50} (lethal doses) or approximately 2 mg of *M fulvius fulvius* venom. Phenol (0.25%) and thimerosal (0.005%) are added as preservatives prior to lyophilization. Phenylmercuric nitrate (1:100,000) is added to the diluent as a preservative.

Uses—Indicated only for the neutralization of the venom of North American coral snake and the venom of *M fulvius tenere* (Texas coral snake). It will not neutralize the venom of *Micruroides euryxanthus* (Arizona or Sonoran coral snake).

Dose—*Warning: Before the administration of any product containing horse protein, appropriate measures including a sensitivity test with suitable controls should be taken in an effort to detect the presence of dangerous sensitivity. For more details, see the package insert.*

Intravenous infusion, **3** to **5 vials** of reconstituted product administered as directed in the package insert. Some patients may require administration of the contents of **10** or more vials if the entire venom load were delivered by the bite(s).

Dosage Form—Injection: A vial of lyophilized serum and a 10-mL vial of diluent.

Diagnostic Skin Antigens

In certain instances antigens may be used as *in vivo* diagnostic aids when injected intradermally into the patient. Most diagnostic skin tests are based upon a hypersensitivity reaction. A positive reaction in these tests indicates sensitivity to the antigen and therefore, the presence of antibodies due either to a present or past infection with the particular organism.

Hypersensitivity skin tests also may be used for the assessment of immunocompetency in individuals with possible cell-mediated immune deficiency diseases (see *Mumps Skin Test Antigen* and *Other Diagnostic Skin Biologics*).

The number of diagnostic skin biologics is relatively small. Several of them were removed from the market as a result of the study made by the FDA Panel on Review of Skin Test Antigens whose principle conclusions and recommendations were reported in the FDA *Drug Bull,* Mar–Apr, 1978.

Coccidioidin

Spherulin (*Berkeley*)

A clear, sterile filtrate prepared from spherules of *Coccidioides immitis,* grown in liquid synthetic medium. The product may be either in the form of the usual skin-test strength or the high skin-test strength. The usual skin-test strength is tested in known positive subjects and is prepared to be bioequivalent in potency to the US Reference Standard Coccidioidin 1:100. The high-test strength (1:10 dilution) is to be used only on persons who are negative to the usual skin-test strength. Thimerosal (1:10,000) is added as a preservative.

Uses—Used as an aid in the diagnosis of coccidioidomycosis and in the differentiation of this disease from sarcoidosis, histoplasmosis and other mycotic and bacterial infections.

Dose—*Intradermal,* **0.1 mL**.

Interpretation—A positive reaction consists of the development of induration measuring 5 mm or more in diameter. Erythema in the absence of induration is considered negative. Readings should always be made at both 24 and 48 hr. A positive skin test is indicative of a present or past infection with *C immitis.* A negative reaction may indicate either that the patient has never been sensitized or has lost sensitivity.

Dosage Form—Injection: 1 mL (usual skin-test strength 1:100) and 0.5 mL (high skin-test strength 1:10).

Histoplasmin

Histolyn-Cyl (*Berkeley*)

A sterile, colorless solution containing standardized culture filtrates of *Histoplasma capsulatum* (yeast or mycelial phase) grown on liquid synthetic medium. The product is standardized to be clinically equivalent in potency to the US Reference Standard Histoplasmin H-42, 1:100. Phenol (0.4 or 0.5%) is added as a preservative.

Uses—Used to detect delayed hypersensitivity to *H capsulatum* and is employed as an aid in the diagnosis of histoplasmosis. It also may be helpful in the differentiation of histoplasmosis from coccidioidomycosis, sarcoidosis and other mycotic or bacterial infections. However, many authorities consider the skin test of little diagnostic or prognostic value except in cases of disseminated disease, in which absence of reactivity denotes anergy, or in very early infections, in which the test also may be negative. In addition, the skin test may evoke a false rise in the complement fixation titer for histoplasmosis. For other possible uses, see the package insert.

Dose—*Intradermal,* **0.1 mL**.

Interpretation—The reaction should be described and measured in terms of mms of induration and degree of reaction from slight induration to vesiculation and necrosis. In many studies reported in the literature a positive reaction is considered to be an induration of 5 mm or greater. A positive reaction may be indicative of a past infection or a mild, subacute or chronic infection with *H capsulatum* or related organisms such as *Blastomyces* or *Coccidioides* species. The reaction should be read 48 to 72 hr after injection. For further information on interpretation, see the package insert.

Dosage Form—Injection: 1 and 1.3 mL.

Mumps Skin Test Antigen

MSTA (*Connaught*)

A sterile, slightly opalescent suspension of formaldehyde-inactivated mumps virus prepared from the extraembryonic fluid of mumps virus-infected chicken embryo, and concentrated and purified by differential centrifugation. Each mL of the skin test antigen contains at least 40 complement-fixing units. Thimerosal (1:10,000) is added as a preservative.

Uses—Indicated when the detection of a delayed hypersensitivity reaction is desired. Most of the population (except for the very young) have had contact or infection with mumps virus and therefore usually demonstrate a delayed hypersensitivity reaction to mumps skin-test antigen if an adequate cellular immune system exists.

Note—Mumps Skin Test Antigen is neither recommended for immunization, diagnosis or treatment of mumps, nor for the diagnosis of immunity to mumps.

Dose—*Intradermal,* **0.1 mL**.

Interpretation—A positive reaction (delayed hypersensitivity to the antigen) is indicated by an induration with a mean diameter (i.e., the longest width plus the longest length, divided by 2) of 5 mm or more. A negative reaction (if the test dose has been given correctly) usually indicates either anergy or nonsensitivity. Pseudopositive reactions may develop in persons sensitive to egg protein. Readings should be made in 48 to 72 hr.

Dosage Form—Injection: 1 mL (10 tests).

Tuberculin, Old

Old Tuberculin; OT; Mono-Vacc Test (*Connaught*); Tine Test (*Lederle*)

A sterile solution derived from the concentrated soluble products of *Mycobacterium tuberculosis.* Old tuberculin is a culture filtrate that has been standardized by clinical evaluation in human subjects to give reactions equivalent to or more potent than 5 TU [US (International) tuberculin units] of standard old tuberculin administered intradermally in the Mantoux test. No preservative is added.

Uses—Indicated for use with multiple-puncture devices as a screening test for the detection of tuberculin sensitivity in high-risk children including American Indian and native Alaskan children; children living in neighborhoods where the case-rate is higher than the national average; children from or whose parents have immigrated from Asia, Africa, the Middle East, Latin America or the Caribbean; and children in households with one or more cases of tuberculosis. For other groups, including persons infected with the human immunodeficiency virus, recommended to be screened for tuberculosis and tuberculosis infection, see the package insert.

Note—Annual testing of low-risk groups (from areas of low prevalence) is not indicated.

Dose—*Intradermal*, multiple-puncture technique, **5 TU.**

Interpretation—The Mono-Vacc Test is read after 48 to 96 hr and a positive reaction is determined by a palpable induration (even 1 to 2 mm). A negative reaction is indicated by a complete absence of induration. Since this test is a screening procedure and diagnostic aid, all positive reactions should be confirmed by a Mantoux test [see *Tuberculin (PPD)*] and possibly other diagnostic test procedures such as a chest X-ray and microbiological examination of sputa and other specimens. The Tine Test is read at 48 to 72 hr and a positive reaction is determined by vesiculation (and management of the patient is the same as that for one classified as positive to the Mantoux test) or an induration 2 mm or greater (may be considered positive but further diagnostic procedures as described above must be considered). A negative test is an induration less that 2 mm and requires no further testing unless the person is a contact of a patient with tuberculosis or there is clinical evidence suggestive of the disease. A significant tuberculin reaction in either test indicates the presence of infection but does not signify disease.

Dosage Forms—Injection: Individual disposable units with 4 stainless-steel prongs or tines (Tine Test) in containers of 25, 100 or 250 individual tests; individual disposable units with a 8-point plastic scarifier (Mono-Vacc Test) in boxes of 25 tests.

Tuberculin (Purified Protein Derivative)

PPD; Aplisol, Aplitest (*Parke-Davis*); PPD Tine Test (*Lederle*); Tubersol (*Connaught*)

A sterile solution derived from a further purified protein fraction of culture filtrates obtained from a human strain of *Mycobacterium tuberculosis* grown on a protein-free synthetic medium. It is standardized with the US Standard Tuberculin, PPD and the potency is tested by comparison with the corresponding US Standard Tuberculin on sensitized guinea pigs. Phenol (0.28% to 0.5%) is used as a preservative, or the product is sterilized with ethylene oxide and no preservative is added.

Uses—Indicated for use with multiple-puncture devices as a mass-screening test for the detection of tuberculin sensitivity in high-risk children as indicated under Tuberculin, Old. PPD also is used in the more sensitive intradermal Mantoux test which is recommended as the standard tuberculin test.

Dose—*Intradermal*, multiple-puncture screening technique, the equivalent of **5 tuberculin units** (TU).

Intradermal, Mantoux test, customary initial dose, **0.1 mL** containing the equivalent of **5 TU.** There are two other strengths available: 1 TU per 0.1 mL and 250 TU per 0.1 mL. The 1-TU dose is recommended as the initial dose for individuals suspected of being highly sensitized, since larger initial doses may result in severe skin reactions. The 250-TU strength is used exclusively for testing individuals who fail to react to a previous injection of either 1 TU and/or 5 TU and *under no circumstances should be used for the initial injection.*

Note—The American Lung Association recommends 5TU as the standard tuberculin test and regards other dosages as having no demonstrable usefulness in ordinary practice.

Interpretation—Both the multiple-puncture and Mantoux tests should be read within 48 to 72 hr of administration.

In the multiple-puncture technique a positive reaction is either vesiculation or a palpable induration of 2 mm or greater. If vesiculation is present the management of the patient is the same as that for one classified as positive to the Mantoux test. However, with a positive induration, further diagnostic procedures must be considered, including confirmation with a Mantoux test. A negative test (induration less than 2 mm) requires no further retesting unless the person is a contact of a patient with tuberculosis or there is clinical evidence suggestive of the disease.

In the Mantoux test only induration is considered in interpreting a positive reaction. A positive test (an induration measuring 10 mm or more) indicates hypersensitivity and is interpreted as positive for past or present infection with *M tuberculosis.* An induration measuring 5 to 9 mm indicates a doubtful reaction and should be repeated in a different site. In the case of known contacts, an induration of 5 to 9 mm should be interpreted as positive. A negative reaction (an induration of less than 5 mm) indicates lack of sensitivity and tuberculosis infection is highly unlikely.

Dosage Forms—Injection: Individual disposable units for multiple-puncture screening tests in multidose packets containing from 25 to 100 tests. PPD for the Mantoux test: 5 TU (10 and 50 test vials), 1 TU and 250 TU (10 test vials).

Other Diagnostic Skin Biologics

Skin Test Antigens for Cellular Hypersensitivity

Multitest CMI (*Connaught*)

An 8-test applicator system consisting of Tetanus Toxoid Antigen, Diphtheria Toxoid Antigen, Streptococcus Antigen, Tuberculin, Old, Glycerin Negative Control, Candida Antigen, Trichophyton Antigen and Proteus Antigen.

This is used to screen for the detection of anergy (nonresponsiveness to antigens) by means of delayed hypersensitivity skin testing and to assess the immunocompetence of patients who may be at high risk.

CHAPTER 82

Allergenic Extracts

H Richard Shough, PhD
Associate Dean and Professor
University of Oklahoma, Health Sciences Center
College of Pharmacy
Oklahoma City, OK 73190

Allergenic extracts comprise a large group of products that are unique compared to other biologicals and conventional pharmaceuticals. A specific license is required for their manufacture and they are available mainly from specialty companies. In spite of more than 75 years of clinical use for the diagnosis and treatment of allergy, allergenic extracts are relatively crude drugs by contemporary standards. Their composition is heterogeneous and ill-defined, their mechanism of action is understood poorly and to date there are no totally reliable standards of potency. Allergenic extracts are administered (or dispensed) primarily in the allergist's office and, with few exceptions, these drugs do not enter conventional pharmaceutical distribution systems.

Common allergies are estimated to affect routinely 10 to 20% of the population and allergenic extracts, despite their shortcomings, are mainstays in the control of these diseases. Every pharmacist should have a fundamental understanding of allergenic extracts and some clinical, institutional and industrial specialists require expertise. In recent years allergy research has intensified but an unfortunately small number of pharmaceutical scientists have entered the field.

Because of the complexity and large number of allergenic extracts only the fundamental terminology, principles, properties and types of products are included in this chapter. The reader desiring detailed information on allergy and allergenic extracts may consult the *Bibliography*. More information on the products as well as specialty supplies and services employed in allergy is also available from the manufacturers. The *Panel on Review of Allergenic Extracts—Final Reports* (March 1981 and December 1983) are excellent reviews and the FDA has established an *Allergenic Products Advisory Committee* for continuing examination of these products.

Allergy

Allergy (*hypersensitivity)* may be defined as an *untoward immunological reaction* to an immunogen called the *allergen.* The phenomenon is not a simple cause-effect relationship, however, for exposure to an allergen results in disease only in a small portion of the population. The occurrence of allergic disease is determined by the characteristics of the individual as well as those of the allergen and even the conditions of exposure. Disease occurs only in those previously *sensitized* by exposure to the allergen and the ability to become sensitized is, at least sometimes, genetically determined (see *Atopy*). Sensitization also may vary with the age of the individual, nature of the allergen, route and degree of exposure and many other factors.

The immunological processes involved in allergy result in tissue damage but otherwise do not differ fundamentally from those seen in the normal immune response (Chapter 44). Allergy can be divided into four types on the basis of the immune effectors, mediators and cells involved in the reaction (Table 1[1]). While this classification is not totally reflective of the clinical situation, it is a very useful frame of reference providing one recognizes its limitations (eg, similar manifestations by different mechanisms).

Most of the common allergies to environmental allergens involve mainly the Type I immediate reactions. It is for this group that sensitivity testing and immunotherapy with allergenic extracts is most useful. Type II and III reactions are more prominent in autoimmune and alloimmune diseases (Chapter 44) and are not as important in the present context. Common *contactant allergens* (eg, poison ivy) produce dermatitis by the cellular-mediated Type IV processes and the *patch-testing materials* described later are used to detect this type of sensitivity.

Atopy

The term atopy was coined by allergists early in the century to describe a set of common allergies which appeared to correlate well with positive skin tests to specific allergens. The meaning of the term has changed somewhat over the years and today atopy generally implies an *inherited tendency* to develop these common allergies. The *atopic diseases* include allergic rhinitis (*hay fever*), allergic asthma, allergic urticaria (*hives*) and atopic eczema (*atopic dermatitis*).

The atopic individual frequently has a family history of allergy and typically is allergic to multiple allergens. Serum IgE usually is elevated and the diseases appear to involve mainly the Type I mechanism. The regulation of IgE synthesis appears to be different from that of other immunoglobulins and it has been suggested that atopy may involve a deficiency of IgE-specific *suppressor* cells. *HLA associations* (Chapter 44) have been described for several ragweed and grass pollen allergens and the ability to develop specific allergies may, in some cases, be inherited through *immune response (Ir) genes* for specific allergens.

Atopic individuals may be more prone to develop immediate-type hypersensitivities to certain drugs (eg, penicillins) but this point is controversial. It is important that pharmacists recognize atopic patients and have as much information as possible on their specific allergies in the patient profiles.

Allergens

Allergens are the inciting agents of allergy. It is common to speak of substances such as pollens, danders, dusts, etc, as *allergens* when, in fact, the true allergens comprise only a small part of these materials.

The chemical identity of most allergens is unknown, but the tools of molecular biology are being employed for both the elucidation of structure and synthesis of recombinant allergens. Baldo has reviewed the structural characteristics of both environmental and drug allergens.[2]

Most known allergens are *proteins* or *glycoproteins* and do not appear to differ much from other immunogens except perhaps being somewhat smaller (mol wt 10,000–70,000). Most allergenic substances contain multiple allergens which vary in their allergenic potency, ie, "major" and "minor" allergens. Allergens from related sources often are similar chemically and *cross-allergenic.* The number and diversity

Table 1—Mechanisms and Manifestations of Allergy[a]

	Type I	Type II	Type III	Type IV
Name(s)	Immediate Reagin-mediated	Cytotoxic	Immune complex Arthus type	Delayed: Cellular-mediated Tuberculin-type
Immujne effectors	IgE	IgG; IgM	IgG (IgM)	Effector T cells
Cells involved in inflammation	Mast cells Basophils	Macrophages (cell-mediated lysis) or	Neutrophils	Macrophages Lymphocytes
Mediators	Histamine Leukotrienes	Complement (C′-mediated lysis)	Lysosomal enzymes	Lymphokines
Time of onset in sensitized individuals	0–30 min	Immediate but may not be apparent for some time	2–24 hr	6–24 hr
Manifestations	Rhinitis Urticaria Angiodema Asthma Anaphylaxis	Hemolytic anemia Neutropenia Thrombocytopenia	Serum sickness Vasculitis Glomerulonephritis Extrinsic alveolitis	Contact dermatitis Allergy of many infections

[a] Based on classification of Coombs and Gell.[1]

of potential allergens in the environment is great which provides a major complication in the control of allergy.

A variety of low-molecular-weight chemicals may serve as *allergenic haptens* (partial immunogens) and induce allergy after combining covalently with a suitable protein carrier. While this is an important process in *drug allergy*, most common environmental allergens appear to be complete immunogens. A notable exception is the case of common *allergic contact dermatitis* caused by a variety of plants, drugs, clothing additives and other substances. The plants most responsible for contact dermatitis in North America belong to the Anacardiaceae family, primarily the genus *Toxicodendron* (*Rhus*), and include poison ivy, oak and sumac. The allergenic components of these plants, called *urushiols*, are found in the oleoresin fraction and are derivatives of pentadecylcatechol or heptadecylcatechol. Many plants of the Compositae family, which includes the ragweeds, also cause contact dermatitis and the allergens have been identified as sesquiterpenoid lactones.

The chemical differences between the common *atopic* and *contactant allergens* are of significance in the preparation of allergenic extracts. The plant oleoresins containing the contactants usually are removed during the defatting process and are not present in the aqueous allergenic extracts. The ether-soluble fraction, on the other hand, can be used for the preparation of patch-testing materials.

Diagnosis of Allergy

The diagnosis of an allergic disease requires first the determination of allergic etiology and second the identification of the specific allergen(s).

Physical diagnosis, while important, is not sufficient to establish allergic etiology since the symptoms of allergic diseases can result from other causes. Important in this respect are the *intrinsic* (nonallergic) diseases of asthma, rhinitis and urticaria which must be distinguished from the *extrinsic* (allergic) diseases. This distinction between allergy and intrinsic diseases is not always clear and some clinical conditions likely involve both. It is important, however, since a number of *drug idiosyncrasies* are associated with intrinsic disease and may be mistaken for allergy.

A *detailed history* is one of the most important steps both in determining whether the condition is an allergy as well as suggesting possible allergens. This should include consideration of the patient's symptoms in relation to familial, seasonal, home environment, occupational, medication and related personal factors.

Clinical laboratory tests are assuming greater importance in the diagnosis of allergy. Diagnostic testing services are available to measure total serum IgE and immunogen-specific IgE for many allergens. These tests can be used in conjunction with sensitivity tests and in those with dermographia, very young patients or others where skin testing may be unreliable. Determination of IgG, IgA and IgM may be helpful in differentiating various autoimmune, infectious or other diseases that may mimic allergies. These and related tests also may be used to monitor immunotherapy.

Sensitivity testing with allergenic extracts is still the principal method of determining specific allergic etiology.

Sensitivity Testing

Sensitivity testing with allergenic extracts has been used since the early part of the century for the diagnosis of allergy. A variety of different test methods may be employed but all involve the administration of a small amount of allergen to the patient who is observed for reactions suggestive of allergy. While simple in principle, both the administration and interpretation of sensitivity tests require a great deal of expertise and should be conducted only by qualified individuals. Also, since sensitivity testing is an expensive, discomforting and time-consuming procedure, it is impractical to test the patient for all possible allergens. A careful history provides the main basis for selection of the specific tests to be performed.

Intradermal Tests—These are the most sensitive of the direct skin tests and are accomplished by injecting allergenic extracts directly into the skin on the volar surface of the lower or upper arm. The back, which may be used in scratch testing, should not be used because of the difficulty in dealing with systemic reactions. Multiple extracts can be tested at one time using sites 2 to 3 inches apart and marked with an appropriate code. The tests are inspected after 15 minutes or again at 30 minutes if the characteristic *wheal and flare reactions* are not developed fully. The tests are graded from 0 to 4+ depending upon the size of the wheal, although the specific grading systems vary extensively.

Generalized allergic reactions are relatively uncommon, but a rubber tourniquet and epinephrine (1:1000) should always be available when tests are performed.

Histamine controls are used to eliminate false-negative reactions by confirming the wheal/flare reaction of the skin and quality of the technique. *Diluent controls* are used to detect the rare dermographic individual that gives positive tests to the skin trauma. Although a single concentration of allergenic extract often is used for testing, more information can be obtained by a *threshold dilution titration* using a 10-fold dilution series.

Prick or Scratch Tests—These tests are simpler and somewhat safer than intradermal tests. They also are less sensitive which some feel is an advantage that provides better correlation with clinical allergy. Many allergists employ a combination of the two methods, using the scratch tests for preliminary screening purposes. The skin is abraded with a sharp needle (prick test) or scarifier (scratch test) either before or after application of one drop of allergenic extract. Much more concentrated extracts are employed since these tests require up to 1000-fold higher concentration to elicit an equivalent reaction to the intradermal test. The test sites, grading of reactions and precautions are similar to those for the intradermal tests.

Other types of sensitivity tests such as *challenge tests* and *passive transfer tests* are employed rarely and are described in earlier editions of *Remington's Pharmaceutical Sciences.*

Patch Testing—This is presently the only routine method for demonstrating allergic contact dermatitis. The procedure usually involves application of the test substance to a piece of cloth or soft paper placed on the outer arm or upper back, covered with an impermeable substance and taped in place. After 24 to 48 hr the patch is removed and the test site examined for presence of the characteristic rash. The specific test procedures used over the years have varied considerably and only recently has there been an attempt to standardize patch testing. The monograph of Marks and DeLeo[3] is an excellent introduction to patch testing and includes a description of each of the twenty allergens included in the American Academy of Dermatology standard tray.

Effect of Drugs on Tests—Antihistamines (H_1-antagonists, Chapter 73) and other drugs with antihistaminic activity such as the tricyclic antidepressants (TCA) suppress the immediate skin-test reactions. Long-acting agents such as astemizole may suppress the reaction for as long as six weeks. H_2-antagonists do not appear to suppress the immediate skin-test reactions alone but may act synergistically with the H_1-antagonists. Oral and parenteral β_2-adrenergic agonists have been reported to decrease the allergen induced wheal, and potent topical corticosteroids may suppress skin reactivity locally. Inhaled β_2-adrenergic agonists, methylxanthines and cromolyn do not interfere with skin testing. Oral corticosteroids have little effect on immediate skin tests but may suppress the cellular-mediated reactions in patch-testing. A task force[4] of the National Institute of Allergy and Infectious Diseases recommends avoiding TCA, chlorpromazine and hydroxyzine at least 5 days before testing, and the short-acting antihistamines should be discontinued for at least 24 hours. Beta-blocking agents can increase the immediate skin test reaction significantly and patients on these drugs may be less responsive to the beta-agonists needed to treat a systemic reaction to an allergenic extract. The optimal time for skin testing is when the patient has recently taken no drugs which may potentially interfere, and in all cases it is important to administer a positive control (ie, histamine).

Treatment of Allergy

The types, causes and contributing factors of allergy are numerous. Therapy is thus complex and variable but can be divided into three main types.

Environmental controls are designed to eliminate or at least minimize exposure to the allergen.[5] The avoidance of an allergen is relatively simple and effective in some instances but most allergens cannot be eliminated totally from the environment. However, minimizing exposure to the allergen nearly always enhances the effectiveness of other measures.

Symptomatic drug therapy is required in the control of most common allergies. The many drugs used for this purpose include the antihistamines (Chapter 73), corticosteroids (Chapter 64) and sympathomimetics (Chapter 57).

Specific *immunotherapy* may be employed for certain allergies as described below.

Immunotherapy

The immunotherapy of allergy is accomplished by administration of gradually increasing doses of allergen over a period of months or years with the anticipation of the patient developing increasing tolerance to the allergen. This is called commonly *desensitization* or *hyposensitization* but these terms tend to imply unconfirmed mechanisms and may be confused with other clinical procedures. For example, in some special cases of penicillin or horse-serum allergy the patient may be desensitized by administering the allergen in sufficient speed and quantity to neutralize effectively the IgE present.

The precise mechanism of immunotherapy still is unknown but a variety of both humoral and cellular immunological changes have been observed over the course of allergen administration.[6] Clinical improvement in some patients correlates well with the level of IgG *blocking antibodies*, which act presumably by binding the allergen and preventing its interaction with the mast cell-bound IgE. The *in vitro* evaluation of antibodies both prior to and during immunotherapy is becoming more common. The AREST Allergy Management System (*Iatric*) is a mail service that includes diagnostic assays of total IgE and allergen-specific IgE, preparation of therapeutic extracts and monitoring of IgG during immunotherapy. The FAST System (*BioWhittaker*) provides clinicians with all of the necessary materials for IgE screening and IgG monitoring in their offices. The *in vitro* methods still are limited by the lack of complete understanding of the mechanisms of both allergic disease and immunotherapy. However, the rapidly expanding knowledge of fundamental immunological mechanisms is clearly leading to better diagnostic, therapeutic and monitoring agents and procedures.

The efficacy of immunotherapy is difficult to judge. There have been many controlled clinical trials but most of these have considered allergic rhinitis and asthma caused by common aeroallergens (eg, ragweed pollens, common grass and tree pollens). Immunotherapy commonly is recommended and is considered to be effective for these conditions when properly employed. The treatment of hay fever and asthma due to other aeroallergens (eg, molds) is also fairly common but based mainly upon experience with the common allergens.

Immunotherapy rarely is recommended for food allergies which are best treated by elimination diets or for dander allergies except in rare instances where avoidance is impossible (eg, veterinarians). It is recommended commonly for the serious stinging-insect allergy and the purified venom extracts are most effective for this purpose. Information on the use of immunotherapy for other allergic diseases is either scanty or contradictory (eg, atopic dermatitis).

Three main techniques are used for the immunotherapy of allergic rhinitis and asthma due to the common aeroallergens.

Coseasonal therapy generally is not recommended but may be employed when the patient first is seen during the allergy season.

Preseasonal treatment is used in some instances and consists of administering the allergen for 3 to 6 months prior to the allergy season at 4- to 7-day intervals.

Perennial treatment is considered by most to provide maximum therapeutic benefit.

Typically, the allergenic extract is administered once or twice a week by subcutaneous injection in the upper arm; intradermal injections often result in severe local reactions, intramuscular injections are painful and intravenous injections may result in serious systemic reactions. The dose is increased gradually up to maximum tolerated levels and the frequency of maintenance doses may sometimes be reduced to every 2 to 4 weeks with amelioration of symptoms. The optimum duration of therapy is variable but usually continues until the patient is symptom-free for 1 year. The average course of therapy may require 3 to 5 years. Success often is relative but some patients remain free of symptoms for extended periods. In others there is sufficient reduction of symptoms that symptomatic therapy alone can be employed but some patients require resumption of immunotherapy.

Immunotherapy is not without risk.[7] Most patients develop some swelling and redness at the injection site but reactions that persist for more than 24 hours are a signal to proceed cautiously. Particularly uncomfortable local reactions may be treated with oral antihistamines and cold compresses. The possibility of serious generalized allergic reactions always is present. Patients should remain in the physician's office for at least 20 minutes after each course of immunotherapy or longer if they are in one of the following high-risk groups: unstable asthma, seasonal exacerbation, high degree of hypersensitivity, receiving beta-blockers or *rush immunotherapy* (ie, more rapid dose escalation than with conventional therapy). During pregnancy there is no evidence of major adverse effects of allergenic extracts on the fetus but uterine contractions may occur as part of a generalized allergic reaction. It generally is recommended that immunotherapy not be started during pregnancy and that slight reduction of the maintenance dose be considered for those who become pregnant during therapy.

Immunotherapy should not be continued indefinitely in the absence of clinical improvement. Treatment failures may result from improper selection of allergens, development of new sensitivities, improper use of environmental controls and various problems associated with the allergenic extracts. The characteristics of these products are discussed in the next section.

Allergenic Extracts

Allergenic extracts are concentrated solutions or suspensions of allergens used for the diagnosis and treatment of allergic diseases. Most are injectable products administered in the physician's office and for many years they were prepared by the individual users. Commercial extracts have gradually replaced extemporaneous preparation as a number of small specialty companies began marketing allergenic extracts several decades ago. In recent years many of the familiar names in allergy products have disappeared with the merger into larger pharmaceutical companies, and today several of the manufacturers of allergenic extracts are multinational corporations. Because of the great number of allergenic extracts on the market only the general characteristics of the products are described here. Additional information on these and related products may be obtained from the licensed manufacturers listed in Table 2.[8]

Federal Licensure

The manufacture of allergenic extracts intended for interstate sale, export or import must be carried out in laboratories that have been licensed as required by Section 351 of the Public Health Services Act (see *Federal Control of Biological Products*, Chapter 81). The provisions of this Act do not prohibit compounding of allergenics dispensed on a prescription when dispensing and patient-use are within the state of origin of the prescription order.

Types

Allergenic extracts usually are designated as being *aqueous* or *glycerinated* products. Normal saline or similar isotonic electrolyte solution is the diluent for the former while the latter contain 50% glycerin in the diluent. The preparations normally are buffered to pH 8 and contain phenol (0.4%) as a preservative.

Diagnostic mixtures are available commercially and since many patients have multiple allergies *custom treatment mixtures* are employed commonly. The formulation of these requires a great deal of expertise and should be done only under the direction of the attending physician. Six or seven allergen sources (less according to some) is the maximum that should be included in any therapeutic mixture and it is recommended that allergens to which a patient particularly is sensitive be administered separately.

Scratch-testing extracts are glycerinated products supplied in 1- to 5- mL dropper vials. They are relatively concentrated solutions, usually in strengths of 1:5 to 1:20, depending on the allergen (see *Standardization*, below).

Intradermal-test extracts are aqueous solutions supplied in 1- to 5- mL multiple dose vials and are more dilute (1:500 to 1:5000).

Therapeutic extracts, both aqueous and glycerinated, are supplied in multiple-dose vials in a variety of sizes (5 to 100 mL) and dilutions (1:10 to 1:100). Since these extracts are diluted before use, most companies provide a variety of *dilution vials* which contain a volume of diluent that facilitates preparation of 10-fold dilutions.

Standard and custom *diagnostic and therapeutic sets and mixtures* also are available as are a variety of auxiliary supplies used in allergy practice.

Autogenous extracts sometimes are prepared from allergenic substances collected from the individual patient's environment.

Adjuvant extracts of several types have been used for many years but only *alum-adsorbed* extracts are available commercially. *Standardized extracts* have been compared to FDA-approved reference standards and have potency expressed in *allergy units* (see *Standardization* below).

There are several *investigational products* which show promise for improving the diagnosis and therapy of allergic disease. These include formalin-treated *allergoids*, along with the glutaraldehyde-polymerized and urea-treated allergens described above (see *Immunotherapy*). Furthermore, improvement in all allergenic extracts may be expected to result from the rapid progress being made in the use of better source materials (eg, venom extracts), identification of specific protein allergens (eg, short ragweed antigen E, cat allergen 1) and methods of standardization (see below).

Table 2—Licensed Manufacturers of Allergenic Extracts[8]

Manufacturer
ALK Laboratories, Inc.
Allergy Laboratories, Inc.
Allergy Laboratories of Ohio, Inc.
Allermed Laboratories, Inc.
Antigen Laboratories, Inc.
Center Laboratories Div, EM Industries, Inc[a]
Greer Laboratories, Inc
Iatric Corp
Meridian Bio-Medical, Inc
Miles Inc[a]
Nelco Laboratories, Inc
Pharmacia A/B

[a] Aqueous and alum precipitated extracts.

Preparation

The preparation of allergenic extracts involves the same general procedures and precautions employed with all parenteral products (Chapter 87). In addition to the usual aseptic procedures the extraction process should be carried out in a cold room. The extracts are thermolabile and must be sterilized by filtration (Chapter 84), and sterility tests for both aerobic and anaerobic microorganisms must be performed on the finished product. Toxicity testing usually is performed in guinea pigs and recommended particularly for autogenous extracts where unknown toxic constituents may be present. Recent concerns for possible mycotoxin contaminants in mold extracts or from mold contamination of other substances have resulted in more intensive efforts to detect and eliminate these toxins. The general procedures used for the preparation of other extractives (Chapter 86) are employed and only those unique for allergenic extracts are included below.

Materials—The allergenic substances to be extracted are obtained mainly from commercial suppliers and only the most reliable sources should be used. For example, pollens are obtained from botanical supply houses that specialize in pollen collection. Samples must be identified properly, free of other pollens and contain no more than 1% of extraneous foreign matter. Prompt and proper dehydration is important to prevent alteration of the allergens and microbial contamination. In spite of these, and other precautions, one can expect lot-to-lot variation in the allergenicity of pollens due to climatic, geographical and other factors. Such variation in the original allergenic substances is largely uncontrollable at present and is unquestionably a major source of the variation ultimately seen in the final products.

Grinding—The material to be extracted must be ground or subdivided in order to effect efficient extraction of the allergens. Household blenders or small plant mills can be used for dried materials, while juicers or food grinders can be used for those containing much moisture. Materials such as hairs, feathers and textiles should be divided finely with shears.

Defatting—Many allergenic substances, including all pollens, should be defatted before final extraction. Ether and petroleum ether are used most commonly for this purpose but alcohols occasionally may be included in the menstruum. Defatting provides a clearer final extract and also removes irritants found in large amounts in some substances, eg, coffee, tea, cocoa, cottonseed, pepper, mustard, ginger. The extract obtained in the defatting process may be used in the preparation of some patch-testing substances.

Extraction—The extraction procedures in current use are based upon the assumption that allergens are water-soluble proteins or glycoproteins although the identity of only a few is known. Extraction is carried out normally for 24 to 72 hours in a cold room using sterile, pyrogen-free buffered saline, Coca's solution or similar aqueous menstruum of pH 8.

Buffered Saline

Sodium chloride	5	g
Monobasic potassium phosphate	0.36	g
Dibasic sodium phosphate, anhydrous	7	g
Phenol crystals	4	g
Water for Injection USP, to make	1000	mL

Coca's Solution

Sodium chloride	5	g
Phenol crystals	5	g
Sodium bicarbonate	2.5	g
Water for Injection USP, to make	1000	mL

After extraction the mixture is clarified by coarse filtration. Some extracts are dialyzed against saline or running tap water to remove irritants or coloring agents. Most pollens require no dialysis but some substances (eg, house dust, mustard, potato, spinach, beets) give nearly universally positive reactions unless dialyzed. Concentration of the extract, where required, may be achieved by a number of methods but care should be taken not to alter the allergens. The processed extract is sterilized by filtration, usually through a cellulose-membrane filter. Prefilters usually are required but asbestos should not be used since it may adsorb some immunogens and may be carcinogenic.

Freeze-dried pollen extracts are prepared essentially as described above except that water rather than electrolyte solution is used as the extracting medium. The lyophilized products are reconstituted with buffered saline at time of use.

Standardization—Most allergenic extracts carry the statement "*No US Standard of Potency.*" Although the first *standardized* allergenic extract was licensed in 1982 and there has been much progress realized in this area, there are still no completely satisfactory means of assaying allergenic extracts and expressing their potency.

The two most common measures of allergenic potency are by *weight/volume* (*w/v*) and the *protein nitrogen unit* (PNU) (Table 3[9]). *Weight/volume* is the weight of allergenic substance extracted per volume of extracting fluid. For example, a 1:50 extract is prepared by extracting 1 g of substance with 50 mL of solvent and decimal dilutions of this extract provide 1:500, 1:5000, etc concentrations. The *protein nitrogen units* also are listed often along with the *w/v* concentration on commercial products and 1 mg of protein nitrogen equals 100,000 PNU. The allergenic protein is virtually always a small and variable part of the total protein, and neither the PNU nor weight/volume standards correlate consistently with each other or clinical potency.

Table 3—Units of Potency for Allergenic Extracts[9]

Unit	Description	Used
Weight/volume (*w/v*)	Allergen (*g*) per volume (mL) of extracting fluid	Worldwide
Protein Nitrogen Unit (PNU)	1 mg proteiin N = 100,000 PNU	Worldwide
Allergy Unit (AU)	Skin testing to endpoint	US
Biological Unit (BU)	Skin testing relative to histamine	Europe

Three general methods are used to estimate potency better in the preparation of *standardized allergenic extracts*.[9]

Specific allergens in an extract are compared to those in the reference standard by immunoelectrophoresis.

Two systems of *bioassay* (Chapter 30) based upon skin testing in patients sensitive to the particular extract are used presently to establish the potency of a reference standard. The *Nordic system* is used in Europe and potency is expressed in *biological units* (BU). The *American system* adopted by the FDA expresses potency in terms of *allergy units* (AU).

Radioallergosorbent-inhibition (RAST-inhibition) tests are used widely to evaluate allergenic extracts. RAST-inhibition (not skin testing) is the main method of comparing the different batches of standardized allergenic extracts with reference standards.

Standard extracts (see Tables 4–9) represent a major improvement in allergenic extracts and, in general, probably are more potent than the conventional extracts. However, a standardized extract can be either more or less potent than the corresponding *w/v* extract and the two should never be used interchangeably. The same general principles of administration apply to both standardized and conventional extracts.

Because allergenic extracts are not standardized completely the appropriate dosage for immunotherapy must be determined clinically. The initial dilution of extract, starting dose and progression of dosage must be determined carefully on the basis of the patient's history and sensitivity tests. Because dilute extracts tend to lose activity more rapidly, the first dose from a more concentrated vial generally should be the same or less than the previous dose. Also, it is common to reduce the dose whenever a new lot of extract is started and then build the dose back to the maintenance level over a period of several weeks.

Stability and Storage

Allergenic extracts tend to show reduced potency within a matter of weeks or months after their preparation, but there have been few detailed studies on the stability of these products. Both high temperatures and freezing usually have deleterious effects, and the latter may cause agglomeration of adjuvant extracts. Some extracts also contain proteolytic enzymes and these may contribute to decomposition of the allergens. Both glycerinated and lyophilized products are more stable than aqueous extracts. Very dilute extracts tend to lose potency by adsorption to the surfaces of containers and syringes and thus usually are prepared close to the time of use. Several studies have shown that the inclusion of Tween 80, Tween 20 or human serum albumin reduces adsorption but a more-complete investigation of this problem is required. The adjuvant extracts should not be diluted with either phosphate buffered saline or Coca's solution since these may cause partial release of allergen; normal saline containing 0.4% phenol is a satisfactory diluent. The adjuvant extracts may be mixed with one another but should not be mixed with other types of extracts.

All allergenic extracts should be refrigerated at 2 to 8° and freezing should be avoided. The expiration date for aqueous extracts is usually 18 months, while for glycerinated scratch-test and bulk extracts it is usually 3 years. Lyophilized products have an expiration date of 4 years or 18 months after reconstitution, so long as the time falls within the original 4 years. Care must be exercised in changing to new lots or different dilutions of extracts because of possible variations in potency. It generally is recommended that quantities of extract sufficient to last the patient for 1 year be prepared to avoid frequent changes in extracts.

Role of the Pharmacist

Few pharmacists are called on today to prepare allergenic extracts or to dispense prescriptions for these products. Some pharmacies, particularly in hospitals, may stock allergenic extracts and related supplies for allergists. Actually, the training of a pharmacist is suited uniquely to many of the services required in the allergy clinic, and it is unfortunate that more pharmacists have not become involved in this area.[10]

In a few institutions allergenic extracts are provided by the pharmacist on a prescription order. Some patients require only a single extract but even in these cases appropriate dilutions must be prepared. More frequently, patients are allergic to multiple allergens and extract mixtures are required. The basic techniques and facilities required for this service are essentially the same as those used in a typical IV-additive program but the pharmacist should have some additional training and experience in handling allergenic extracts.[10]

In addition to assuming responsibility for the preparation and control of allergenic extracts,[10] the pharmacist also may provide a variety of patient-oriented services in the allergy clinic.[11] These services include obtaining patient histories, performing allergy testing procedures and patient consultation.

Common allergic diseases are found in 10 to 20% of the population and patients with these ailments obtain a variety of drugs and medical supplies from community pharmacies. Thus, there are many opportunities for pharmacists to be of service to the allergy patient in traditional practice sites as well as the allergy clinic. To accomplish this effectively, pharmacists must have a fundamental understanding of allergy and the products used in the control of allergic diseases.

Products

This section contains a summary of the principal allergenic extracts available today. It is impractical to provide an individual monograph for each product and they have been grouped according to the type of allergenic substance (eg, pollens or dusts). This classification is not perfect but was chosen in part because the extracts are listed this way in manufacturers' literature. It also is found to have some merit when considering both the product characteristics and clinical allergy. These are described briefly for each group with emphasis on the following: clinical significance of the allergen group, most-common offenders of the group and general usefulness and limitations of the extracts.

The lists of allergenic extracts are intended to be reasonably comprehensive but there have been some intentional omissions. Only one name—usually the common one—is given for each extract, while in practice a number of both common and scientific names may be used. Similarly, individual extracts usually are derived from a single species of plant, animal or microorganism but only the genus is given in the list; however, extracts of most of the common allergenic species are commercially available. Extracts containing allergens from more than one source are designated as *mixtures* and, while many are commercially available, only a few are listed. Not all manufacturers produce all of the extracts, and it should be recognized that different companies may employ significantly different source materials and processes in preparing products of the same name.

Most of the products listed are provided as *diagnostic extracts* for both scratch and intradermal testing, but *therapeutic extracts* may or may not be routinely available. Similarly, the availability of both lyophilized and adjuvant products is limited. Many of the extracts also are available in diagnostic *test sets.* These are not listed but include various regional, pollen, food, mold, pediatric, titration and other test sets. Manufacturing services for *custom therapeutic mixtures* and *autogenous* extracts are also available. The individual manufacturers should be contacted for more specific information on their products and services.

FDA Panel on Review of Allergenic Extracts

The *Panel on Review of Allergenic Extracts* (Dec 1981) evaluated, on a generic basis, about 1670 products for safety and efficacy and recommended classification into one of the following categories:

Category I: Safe, effective and not misbranded
Category II: Unsafe, ineffective or misbranded
Category III: Insufficient data for classification

Only a small number of products could be placed in Category I, and the vast majority (about 1300) of products were classified in Category IIIA. These are extracts of materials known or highly suspected to be allergenic but for which there is little published data to establish efficacy. Category III was abolished by legal action against the FDA, and all products in this category must be reclassified into either Category I or II. Several hundred products have been placed in Categories II and IIIB since the review began, and nearly all have been removed from the market. A complete review of the Category III extracts is not expected to be complete until 1995.

The Panel has been replaced by the *Allergenic Products Advisory Committee* and summary minutes of their deliberations are available from the FDA. The reader should consult the Panel Reports and Committee minutes for a detailed review of the safety and efficacy of these products for diagnosis and immunotherapy.

Pollen Extracts

Pollens are the most common cause of the atopic diseases and, in fact, hay fever is sometimes called "pollinosis." Pollens are produced only by seed-bearing plants and not by algae, fungi, mosses or ferns. Not all pollens are of equal clinical significance for there is variation in both allergenicity and degree of exposure. Allergy usually results from *anemophilous* (wind-borne) rather than *entomophilous* (insect-borne) pollens. Conifers such as the pines are copious pollen producers but the pollens, with few exceptions, are hypoallergenic.

Pollen allergy is largely a problem of *temperate climates.* In arctic and alpine regions where summers are short, plants generally reproduce vegetatively (asexually) and most subarctic plants are conifers. In the tropics there tends to be a proliferation of species with a small number of individual plants so that exposure to a specific pollen is minimized. Anemophilous plants also tend to be less common in regions of extremely high humidity.

Seasonal and geographical variation is more pronounced with pollen allergy than other types. Pollen seasons vary with both the plant and locale but the following generalizations can be made: trees from late winter to spring, grasses from spring to early summer and weeds from late summer to fall. Pollen allergy is a significant problem in most parts of this country, but the allergens vary somewhat with the region and are determined best by consulting one of the published guides. Perhaps 100 of the approximately 300 pollens represented in commercial extracts are fairly common offenders.

Allergenic extracts prepared from some of the common pollens (eg, ragweed, several grass and tree) have been among the most widely studied. Controlled studies generally have shown these products to be reliable for both diagnosis and, in several cases, for therapy when properly prepared and employed. Many of the products listed have not been studied extensively but their reliability often is assumed based on extrapolation of the data on the common pollens. (Table 4).

Dust Extracts

House dust is probably the most common nonpollen inhalant allergen. The allergens in house dust are not related to the inorganic dirt from outside but to the products of aging and decomposition of materials around the home. Whether there is a specific dust-associated allergen is not known for sure, but dust contains mold spores, feathers, hairs, food, cleaning-agent residues, danders, etc, and the composition may vary considerably with the source. The dust for commercial extracts usually is obtained from house-cleaning or rug-cleaning firms and is pooled to obtain some homogeneity.

Table 4—Pollen Extracts

	Trees	
Acacia	Elderberry	Orange
Alder, grey[a]	**Elm, American**[a]	Osage orange
Almond	Eucalyptus	Palo verde
Apple	Fir	Peach
Apricot	Hackberry	Pear
Arbor vitae	Hazelnut	Pecan
Ash	Hemlock	Pepper tree
Aspen	Hickory	Pine
Bayberry	Hop-hornbeam	Plum
Beech	Ironwood	Poplar
Birch, spring[a]	Juniper	Privet
Birch, white[a]	Locust	Redwood
Bottle brush	Maple	Russian olive
Box elder[a]	Melaleuca	Spruce
Carob tree	Mesquite	Sweet gum
Cedar	Mock orange	Sycamore
Cherry	Mulberry	Tamarack
Chestnut	**Oak, white**[a]	Tree of heaven
Cottonwood	Olive	Walnut
Cypress		Willow
	Grasses	
Bahia	Corn	**Redtop**[a]
Barley	**Fescue, meadow**[a]	**Rye grass, perennial**[a]
Beach	Grama	Salt
Bent	Johnson	Sorghum
Bermuda grass[a]	**June grass**[a]	Sudan
Bluegrass, Kentucky[a]	Koeler's	**Sweet vernal grass**[a]
Brome	Oats	**Timothy grass**[a]
Bunch	**Orchard grass**[a]	Velvetgrass
Canarygrass	Quack	Wheat
Chess		Wheatgrass
	Weeds and garden plants	
Alfalfa	Fireweed	Poppy
Amaranth	Gladiolus	Povertyweed
Aster	Goldenrod	Quailbush
Balsam root	Greasewood	**Ragweed, giant**[a]
Bassia	Hemp	**Ragweed, short**[a]
Beach bur	Honeysuckle	**Ragweed, western**[a]
Broomweed	Hops	Rose
Burrow brush	Iodine Bush	**Russian thistle**[a]
Careless weed	Jerusalem oak	Sagebrush
Castor bean	Kochia	Saltbrush
Chamise	**Lamb's quarters**[a]	Scale
Clover	Lily	Scotch broom
Cocklebur	Marigold	Sea blight
Coreopsis	Marshelder	Sheep sorrel
Cosmos	Mexican tea	Snapdragon
Daffodil	**Mugwort**[a]	Sugar beet
Dahlia	Mustard	Sunflower
Daisy	Nettle	Western waterhemp
Dandelion	Pickleweed	Winter fat
Dock	Pigweed	Wormseed
Dog fennel	**Plantain, English**[a]	Wormwood

[a] *Standardized extract* for which FDA reference standard is available.

Most attention has been focused on the *dust mite* and standardized extracts of *Dermatophagoides* spp are now available. The dust mite appears to be distributed virtually universally and usually is found in furnishings stuffed with vegetable fibers (eg, cotton) used by humans. While many feel that mite allergens are responsible for most dust allergy, this is not a complete explanation of the phenomenon. Some individuals are allergic to dust but not the dust mite as it is not found in some dusts.

House-dust sensitivity differs from pollen allergy in several respects and is suspected particularly when the patient's history includes one or more of the following factors: perennial symptoms that worsen when the patient remains indoors, increased nocturnal symptoms, increased symptoms when performing household chores and increased symptoms associated with turning on heating or air conditioning systems.

House dust is a ubiquitous allergen and its total elimination is virtually impossible. However, it is important that the patient maintain as *dust-free environment*[5] as possible, particularly in the bedroom. Instructions for the preparation of dust-free rooms and products to minimize the circulation of dust (Allergex, *Miles*) and kill mites (Acarosan, *Fisons*) are available.

Allergy to house dust is probably the most common immediate hypersensitivity observed in clinical sensitivity testing. House-dust extracts (Table 5) have been investigated extensively and in some study groups 75% or more of allergic patients have shown positive reactions. However, significant numbers of nonallergic individuals also show positive reactions and it is indeed difficult to evaluate the efficacy of these heterogeneous products. The standardized dust mite extracts are more reliable products for both the diagnosis and immunotherapy of house-dust allergy. However, it is still important to effect stringent environmental controls[5] prior to attempting immunotherapy.

Relatively little information is available on other dust extracts. These are generally less-common allergens and many are associated with occupational allergies. Some of these may also be involved in the *extrinsic allergic alveolitis* described under *Fungal Extracts.*

Fungal Extracts

The fungi are a large group of organisms that may be involved in many types of diseases, including intoxications, infections and allergy. Most fungi are saprophytes and compared to bacteria are relatively uncommon causes of infectious disease. *Mycotoxins* are of great concern in several areas of health including as possible contaminants of allergic extracts. A number of fungi have been implicated increasingly as important causes of several types of allergic disease.

Molds are one of the major causes of nonpollen atopic allergies. Asthma and rhinitis, as well as various cutaneous reactions, can be precipitated by inhalation of mold spores or mycelial fragments in sensitive individuals. Fungi are ubiquitous and may be found in the home on textiles, leather goods, upholstered furniture, food and plants. Damp, warm places such as basements and closets tend to favor mold growth, which is often encountered as common "mildew," which most often is *Aspergillus* or *Penicillium* spp. Fungal allergy resulting from indoor exposure tends to be perennial; that from outdoor exposure shows more distinctive seasonal and geographical patterns but these are less pronounced than in pollen allergy. Fungal allergy is also more likely to be associated with an occupation or hobby.

Sensitivity testing for fungal allergens appears to be generally reliable. It also is useful at times to identify the specific fungi in the patient's environment and fungal identification services are available. Therapy should include efforts to create a *mold-free environment* but this is difficult to accomplish completely. Several studies indicate that immunotherapy may be of value for some patients. One problem is that the allergenic extracts are prepared variously from mycelium, medium or both and too little is known about the fungal allergens to know the most-appropriate method of preparation.

Fungi, along with a variety of organic dusts, have been found to be important causes of another respiratory allergy, *extrinsic allergic alveolitis* (hypersensitivity pneumonitis). Many names related to either the allergen or affected individuals have been applied to this condition; eg, farmer's lung,

Table 5—Dust Extracts

	House dusts	
House	Mattress	Upholstery
	Dust mites	
D farniae[a]	**D pteronyssinus**[a]	**Mite mix**[a]
	Other dusts[b]	
Cedar and red cedar	Cotton gin	Oak
Grain, elevator	Padauk	Wood dusts

[a] *Standardized extract* for which FDA reference standard is available.
[b] See also Table 7.

mushroom-workers disease, wood-dust asthma, etc. The disease shows no relationship to atopy but usually can be related to recent high-level exposures to the offending inhalant. Extrinsic allergic alveolitis appears to result from the formation of IgG immune complexes in the lung (Type III reaction) but may involve cellular-mediated (Type IV) reactions. Diagnosis is based mainly on a detailed personal history but the demonstration of specific *precipitins* in the serum of the patient provides supporting evidence. Commercial tests and testing services are available for this purpose. Both Type III and IV allergies may provide cutaneous reactions on allergen challenge, but they differ in time-course and type from the immediate skin-test reactions. The products listed in Table 6 are not useful in the diagnosis of extrinsic allergic alveolitis; effective therapy depends mainly on avoidance of the allergen.

Miscellaneous Inhalant Extracts

Atopic allergies may be caused by a variety of inhalant allergens other than pollens, dusts and molds. The epidermals from domestic animals (cat, dog, horse) are the best-known, but the variety of inhalant allergens is remarkable. Exposure of an average individual to some of the substances listed below might appear unlikely but this is not necessarily the case. Probably few people recognize that orris root is a common component of cosmetics, including many dusting powders; that camel hair may be found in imported textiles and rugs; that the plant gums acacia, karaya and tragacanth are present in hundreds of food, cosmetic and drug products and that pyrethrum is an active constituent of many household insecticides. Many of these substances are also ingestant (see *Food Extracts*) and contactant (see *Patch-Testing Materials*) as well as inhalant allergens.

Sensitivity testing with many of the extracts listed in Table 7 is fairly common but based largely on experience with common aeroallergen extracts. Little information is available on the use of most of these products for immunotherapy. Several cat allergens have been characterized and standardized extracts are available. Avoidance of the allergen remains the preferred method of control and usually can be achieved, although at times only with great effort.

Insect Allergy

Insect allergy is a term rather loosely applied to describe allergy from both insects and arthropods such as spiders and mites. Allergy may result from inhalation of body emanations but most often occurs following a sting or bite.

Allergy to stinging insects of the order *Hymenoptera* is of greatest clinical significance and has been studied most widely. The honeybee is the most common offender but the bumblebee, wasp, hornet and yellow jacket also may cause reactions. *Hymenoptera* sensitivity is estimated to result in 40 deaths annually in this country and the incidence of serious allergy is estimated at 1 to 10:100,000. Allergy with few exceptions involves Type I reactions and may be manifest as urticaria, angioedema, asthma or systemic anaphylaxis. Death usually results from cardiovascular collapse and/or respiratory failure and typically occurs within *1 hour* following the sting.

Serious reactions may occur in individuals without a history of sensitization but they are more common in those who have previously exhibited a systemic reaction following a sting. It is of the utmost importance that sensitive individuals be aware of their problem and understand preventive measures and emergency procedures. *Emergency kits* are available for the treatment of *hymenoptera* sensitivity in the field. These and the services that can be rendered by the community pharmacist are discussed by Sadik and Delafuente.[12]

Diagnosis of insect allergy usually is self-evident but problems may arise in identifying the insect. *Cross-sensitivity* among *hymenoptera* is common but by no means absolute and species-specific allergens are important.

Sensitivity testing and immunotherapy commonly are recommended and employed for allergy to the stinging insects. The venom extracts (Table 8) have been shown to be highly effective when properly employed. These products are *standardized* somewhat differently than the other standardized extracts. The venoms are assayed for several known components (ie, hyaluronidase, antigen 5, phospholipase A), as well as total protein nitrogen. The quantity and potency of the products are expressed in μg rather than allergy units.

Fire-ant allergy is being reported with increasing frequency. The fire ant has now spread over 13 Southern states and is particularly a problem along the Gulf coast. It is a member of the *hymenoptera* and causes similar allergic reactions but its allergens appear to differ considerably from those of other stinging insects. Skin-testing with whole-body extracts appears to be reliable for the determination of sensitivity and early reports on immunotherapy are encouraging.

Table 6—Fungal Extracts

Alternaria	Fusarium	Phoma
Aspergillus	Gelasinospora	Pullularia
Botrytis	Geotrichum	Rhizopus
Candida	Gliocladium	Rhodotorula
Cephalosporium	Helminthosporium	Rusts
Cephalothecium	Hormodendrum	Saccharomyces
Chaetomium	Microsporium	Smuts
Cladosporium	Mucor	Spondylocladium
Cryptococcus	Mycogone	Stemphylium
Curvularia	Nigraspora	Trichoderma
Epicoccum	Paecilomyces	Trichophyton
Epidermophyton	Penicillium	Verticillium

Table 7—Miscellaneous Inhalant Extracts

	Mammalian epidermals	
Camel	Dog	Horse
Cat hair[a]	Gerbil	Mohair
Cat pelt[a]	Goat	Monkey
Chinchilla	Guinea pig	Mouse
Cow	Hamster	Rabbit
Deer	Hog	Wool (sheep)
	Feathers	
Canary	Duck	Pigeon
Chicken	Goose	Turkey
	Parakeet	
	Miscellaneous inhalants	
Acacia	Hemp fiber	Lycopodium
Algae	Henna	Orris root
Castor bean	Flaxseed	Pyrethrum
Cotton linters	Guar gum	Silk, raw
Cottonseed	Jute	Sisal
Derris root	Karaya gum	Tobacco leaf
Fern spores	Kapok	Tragacanth
Grain dusts	Leather	Wood dusts

[a] *Standardized extract* for which FDA reference standard is available.

Table 8—Insect Extracts[a]

	Stinging insect—whole body	
Ant, black	Ant, carptenter	Ant, fire
Ant, red	Ant mix (black/red)	
	Stinging insect—venom protein	
Honey bee[a]	**Wasp**[a]	**White-faced hornet**[a]
Yellow hornet[a]	**Yellow jacket**[a]	**Mixed vespid**[a]
	Inhalant allergy to insects	
Aphid	Deerfly	**Mites, dust**[a]
Black fly	Fruit fly	Mosquito
Butterfly	Honey bee, whole body	Moth
Caddis fly	Horse fly	Mushroom fly
Cicada/locust	House fly	Screwworm fly
Cricket	Leafhopper	Sow bugs
Cockroach	May fly	Spider
Daphnia	Mexican bean weevil	Water flea

[a] *Standardized extracts* (See text, page 1438).

Allergic reactions have been attributed to many *biting insects* including the mosquito, chigger, flea, louse, bedbug, kissing bug and many flies. The majority of the reactions have been localized, with both the immediate- and delayed-types reported. The pathogenesis of most of these sensitivities remains to be verified but, since many appear to be cellular-mediated Type IV reactions, it is not surprising that the limited information on sensitivity testing and immunotherapy is contradictory.

Allergic rhinitis and asthma can develop after *inhalation* of scales, hairs or other emanations of various insects. This is analogous to the allergy seen with common inhalants but most often is seen in individuals who by reason of occupation or hobby are exposed to large numbers of insects. The caddis fly, mayfly and aphid occur in large numbers in some locales and have been implicated most frequently. Allergenic extracts for a number of these have proven to be effective for skin-test diagnosis and may be of value for immunotherapy (see Table 8).

Food Extracts

Various food products are the most common *ingestant allergens.* Food allergy may seem simple but, in fact, is an extremely complex clinical entity. One problem stems from the tendency of many to attribute virtually any gastrointestinal disturbance of unknown etiology to "food allergy." Gastrointestinal disturbance may arise from many causes, including enzyme deficiencies (lactose intolerance), intoxications, infections and others. Also, food allergy may and often is manifest outside the GI tract. The indiscriminate use of the term "food allergy" is to be condemned strongly.

Food allergy may be responsible for an amazing array of symptoms including rhinitis, urticaria, asthma, GI disturbances and headache. Rarely, systemic anaphylaxis may occur and there are reports of fatal reactions. Most of these have been in highly atopic individuals with serious asthma, atopic dermatitis and/or rhinitis. Patients with these conditions may be more at risk for serious reactions and/or less responsive to therapy. Strongly allergic individuals should be trained in the use of epinephrine and carry *emergency kits* to deal with inadvertent exposures.

Relatively few foods are responsible for the majority of reactions—peanuts, milk, nuts, fish, shellfish, eggs and soy are the most common offenders—but many others may cause food allergy.[13] Food allergy may occur at any age but is probably most common in childhood and may be related to an underdeveloped GI system. Patients commonly appear to "outgrow" some food allergy (eg, cow's milk), but this is probably not the case with most foods.

Only a few food allergens have been characterized, but it is possible that many are not present in fresh foods but are the products of food processing or digestion. The diagnosis of food allergy depends heavily upon a detailed history along with the use of carefully designed *elimination* and *challenge test diets.* Skin testing is useful in the hands of experienced clinicians but requires some modified techniques.[13]

The therapy of food allergy is often more difficult than the diagnosis. Elimination of the offending food(s) is about the only effective therapy, but it is often difficult to design a nutritious and palatable diet when multiple and/or common allergens are involved (eg, milk, eggs, peanuts). Immunotherapy is very difficult to assess for reasons noted above and therapeutic food extracts are not used as routinely as those of inhalant allergens.

Food allergy may involve food additives in addition to the natural allergens. Tartrazine dye (FDC Yellow No 5) is perhaps the best-known food (and drug) additive reputed to cause rhinitis, urticaria, asthma and anaphylaxis. In spite of these typically allergic manifestations this appears to be a *pharmacologic response* related to intolerance to aspirin and nonsteroidal anti-inflammatory drugs.

Idiosyncrasy to these compounds is seen mainly in individuals with *intrinsic* rhinitis, asthma or urticaria, rather than in atopics. It also is interesting that these individuals occasionally may be intolerant to *natural salicylates* and *benzoates* which occur in many foods, especially fruits. Under the circumstances it is quite understandable that these idiosyncrasies are mistaken for allergies but the distinction between the two fundamentally different mechanisms has important implications in the control of these reactions.

Of all of the allergies to environmental substances, food allergy is probably the most similar to *drug allergy.*[14] Foods and drugs are the most common *ingestants* and may, in fact, share common allergens (eg, flavoring agents, preservatives or dyes). It is clear that the pharmacist must be concerned with more than simply the patient's drug regimen.

The FDA *Panel on Review of Allergenic Extracts* has recommended that nearly all of the commercially available food extracts, except for most mixtures and processed foods, be classified in Category I for the diagnosis of IgE-mediated allergy but that *all extracts* be placed in Category II for immunotherapy. Because of the large number of extracts, the product list in Table 9 is abbreviated by giving the number of products in several major groups.

Patch-Testing Materials

Contact dermatitis is a term that has been used in two main ways: first, to describe any rash resulting from a substance touching the skin and second, as a synonym for *allergic contact dermatitis.* The latter is used in present context and refers to eczematous lesions resulting from cellular-mediated Type IV reactions analogous to tuberculin sensitivity (Chapter 81). Similar clinical manifestations may occur by other mechanisms: *primary irritant dermatitis,* from direct chemical irritation; *photocontact (phototoxic) dermatitis,* which requires light to generate the irritant; and *photoallergic dermatitis,* which requires light to generate the allergen. These are not necessarily independent, for a number of contact allergens also may be irritants but allergic reactions generally occur with lower concentrations of the offending agent. A variety of other conditions also must be differentiated from contact dermatitis (eg, atopic dermatitis, dermatomycoses), and virtually any disease of the skin may result in increased response to both contact irritants and allergens.

Table 9—Food Extracts[a]

	Animal products	
Beef (3)	Fish (19)	Milk, goat
Chicken (2)	Goat	Pork (3)
Deer	Goose	Rabbit
Duck	Lamb	Shellfish (6)
Egg, chicken (3)	Milk, cow	Turkey
	Plant products	
Apple	Date	Pea
Apricot	Eggplant	Peanut
Arrowroot	Fig	Pear
Artichoke	Grain (12)	Pimento
Asparagus	Grape (6)	Pineapple
Avocado	Greens (11)	Plum
Banana	Gums (5)	Potato (3)
Bean (15)	Hops	Prune
Beet (2)	Lettuce (2)	Pumpkin
Berries (16)	Malt	Radish
Cabbage family (6)	Mango	Rhubarb
Carrot	Melon (2)	Spice/condiment (45)
Celery	Mushroom	Spinach
Cherry (4)	Nuts (11)	Squash (7)
Chocolate	Okra	Tapioca
Citrus fruit (6)	Olive (2)	Tea
Coconut	Onion	Tomato
Coffee	Papaya	Watermelon
Cucumber	Parsnip	Yeast (2)

[a] The number of parentheses represents the approximate number of generic products in each category.

Contact sensitivity is a common problem but the incidence and causes vary in different populations. The overall socioeconomic impact is great for it is a leading cause of *industrial illness.* The American Academy of Dermatology standard-tray allergens are listed in Table 10. These 20 allergens are among the most common causes of allergic contact dermatitis and generally are included in an initial screen for contact sensitivity. Particularly notable are the *drugs and drug additives* which laymen may not recognize as constituents of drug products. The pharmacist should assist the sensitive patient with both drug selection and avoidance.

The likelihood of developing contact sensitivity depends on both the characteristics of the allergen and the individual. Dinitrochlorobenzene (DNCB), for example, will induce sensitivity in nearly everyone and has been used to evaluate the status of cellular-mediated immunity. The oleoresins of poison ivy also are strong sensitizers. However, sensitization, in part, is determined genetically, since about 5% of the population cannot be sensitized to DNCB and others are sensitized easily, even to weak allergens. This susceptibility is not related to atopy although atopic individuals are more likely to show topical sensitization of the immediate type. Also, individuals with atopic dermatitis or other skin conditions may more readily be sensitized and exhibit more pronounced reactions. This should be kept in mind when recommending topical medications.

The diagnosis of contact dermatitis depends mainly on a detailed history and complete physical examination. The area of the body affected is suggestive of the contactant and other factors (eg, light, dermatophytes). The patch test is presently the only practical way to demonstrate contact sensitivity (see *Sensitivity Testing*). The patch test may be used for the following purposes: to verify clinically diagnosed contact sensitivity, to determine the specific allergens including those that may not have been clinically suspected, as a predictive test to determine what the patient can safely tolerate and to exclude contact dermatitis in puzzling clinical situations.

The therapy of contact dermatitis involves most importantly avoidance of the contactant. Cool compresses and topical steroids are the mainstays of therapy but systemic steroids may be employed for serious cases. Other topical medications should be avoided since they may contain irritants or sensitizers.

Several forms of immunotherapy have been used in the treatment of contact dermatitis. *Oral immunotherapy* appears to be effective for the treatment of both poison ivy and poison oak, but there is little information on its efficacy for other conditions. *Parenteral immunotherapy* has been quite controversial. Both forms of therapy have the potential of precipitating serious reactions in highly sensitive individuals. Avoidance of the allergen is definitely the preferred method of control, and immunotherapy should be attempted only in patients with severe allergy when exposure is unavoidable.

The *Panel on Review of Allergenic Extracts* recommended that nearly all available plant oleoresin extracts be classified in Category I for patch-testing. Oral poison ivy and oak extracts also were recommended in Category I for immunotherapy but no other therapeutic extracts were recommended for continued licensing.

Table 10—Standard-Tray Patch-Testing Allergens[a]

Medicaments	*Metals*
Benzocaine	Nickel sulfate
Neomycin sulfate	Potassium dichromate
Preservatives	*Resins*
Quaternium-15	Epoxy
Imidazolidinylurea	*p-tert*-Butylphenolformaldehyde
Formaldehyde	Colophony
Vehicles	*Fragrances*
Lanolin alcohol	Cinnamic aldehyde
Rubber compounds	Balsam of Peru
Thiuram mix	*Miscellaneous*
Mercaptobenzothiazole (MBT)	Ethylenediamine dihydrochloride
Carba mix	*p*-Phenylenediamine
Mercapto mix	
Black rubber *p*-phenylenediamine mix (PPD)	

[a] For a description of the individual American Academy of Dermatology standard-tray allergens, consult Marks and DeLeo.[3]

Veterinary Allergenic Products

Veterinary allergy is an emerging field and pharmacists involved in animal health can expect increasing activity in this area. The general principles of immunology and allergy noted earlier apply for the most part to animals as well. Veterinary pharmaceuticals are controlled by the US Department of Agriculture (USDA), but the products essentially are analogous to the human products described in this chapter. *Greer Laboratories* markets a line of veterinary allergenic extracts and supplies.

Canine Allergic Inhalant Dermatitis is one of the most common and widely studied of the animal allergies. It is a IgE-mediated immediate (Type I) hypersensitivity which is illustrative of the close relationship of animal and human allergy. Canine inhalant dermatitis is a hereditary hypersensitivity to environmental allergens such as pollens (tree, grass, weed), molds, epidermals, house dust, etc. Symptoms may be seasonal or perennial and include primarily *pruritus* with associated scratching, footlicking and face rubbing. Sneezing, rhinitis and conjunctivitis may be present.

Canine inhalant dermatitis usually appears at 1 to 3 years of age and diagnosis is similar to that of human allergies including intradermal skin testing with allergenic extracts. The symptoms respond to corticosteroids. Immunotherapy is claimed to control the disease without steroids in up to 50% of the afflicted animals and to permit steroid dosage reduction in others. Unfortunately about 25% are reported to be unresponsive to immunotherapy. However, the reader is reminded that the evaluation of the safety and effectiveness of veterinary allergenic extracts is subject to problems similar to those of human products.

References

1. Coombs RRA, Gell PGH. In Gell PGH, Coombs RRA, Lachmann PJ, eds: *Clinical Aspects of Immunology.* Blackwell, London, 1975.
2. Baldo BA: *Curr Opin Immunol 3:* 841, 1991.
3. Marks JG, DeLeo VA: *Patch Testing for Contact and Occupational Dermatology.* Mosby Year Book, St Louis, 1992.
4. Bernstein IL, ed: *J Allergy Clin Immunol 82(Suppl)*: 487, 1988.
5. Evans R: *Ibid 90:* 462, 1992.
6. Creticos PS: *Immunol Clin N Am 12:* 13, 1992.
7. Stewart GE, Lockey RF: *J Allergy Clin Immunol 90:* 567, 1992.
8. *Establishments and Products Licensed under Section 351 of the Public Health Services Act,* Publ No (FDA)-91-003, HEW, Washington, DC, 1991.
9. Platts-Mills TAE, Chapman MD: *J Allergy Clin Immunol 87:* 621, 1991.
10. Grabenstein JD: *Hosp Pharm 27:* 145, 1992.
11. Hunter RB, Osterberger DJ: *Am J Hosp Pharm 32:* 392, 1975.
12. Sadik F, Delafuente JC. In *Handbook of Nonprescription Drugs,* 9th ed, APhA, Washington, DC, 945, 1990.
13. Sachs MI, Yunginger JW: *Immunol Allergy Clin of N Am 11:* 743, 1991.
14. VanArsdel PP: *Ibid:* 461, 1991.

Bibliography

Baldo BA: Structural features of allergens large and small with emphasis on recombinant allergens. *Curr Opin Immunol 3:* 841, 1991.

Bernstein IL, ed: Proceedings of the task force on guidelines for standardizing old and new technologies used for the diagnosis and treatment of allergic diseases. *J Allergy Clin Immunol 82(Suppl)*: 487, 1988.

Evans R: Environmental control and immunotherapy for allergic disease. *Ibid 90:* 462, 1991.

FDA (proposed rule) Biological products; allergenic extracts; implementation of efficacy review. *Fed Reg 50:* 3082, 1985.

Grabenstein JD: Allergen extract compounding by pharmacists. *Hosp Pharm 27:* 145, 1992.

Greenberger PA, ed: Immunotherapy of IgE-mediated disorders. *Immunol Allergy Clin N Am 12:* 13, 1992.

Hunter RB, Osterberger DJ: Role of the pharmacist in an allergy clinic. *Am J Hosp Pharm 32:* 392, 1975.

Lockey RF, Bukantz SC: *Allergen Immunotherapy*, Dekker, New York, 1991.

Marks JG, DeLeo, VA: *Patch Testing for Contact and Occupational Dermatology.* Mosby Year Book, St Louis, 1992.

Panel on Review of Allergenic Extracts—Final Report, Publ No PB-81-182115, U.S. Dept of Commerce, NTIS, Springfield, VA, 13 Mar 1981.

Panel on Review of Allergenic Extracts—Category IIIA Reclassification—Final Report, DHHS PHS FDA, Center for Drugs and Biologics, Rockville, MD, Dec 1983.

Platts-Mills TAE, Chapman MD: Allergen standardization. *J Allergy Clin Immunol 87:* 621, 1991.

Sachs MI, Yunginger JW: Food-induced anaphylaxis. *Immunol Allergy Clin N Am 11:* 743, 1991.

Stewart GE, Lockey RF: Systemic reactions from allergen immunotherapy. *J Allergy Clin Immunol 90:* 567, 1992.

Stites DP, Terr AI, eds: *Basic and Clinical Immunology*, Appleton & Lange, Los Altos, CA, 1991.

Turkeltaub, PC: Biological standardization of allergenic extracts. *Curr Concepts Allergy Clin Immunol 17:* 1, 1987.

VanArsdel PP: Drug Allergy. *Immunol Allergy Clin N Am 11:* 461, 1991.

PART 7

Industrial Pharmacy

Joseph B Schwartz PhD
Tice Professor of Pharmaceutics
Philadelphia College of Pharmacy and Science
Philadelphia PA 19104

CHAPTER 83

Preformulation

Galen W Radebaugh, PhD
Director of Pharmaceutics
Parke-Davis Pharmaceutical Research Division
Warner-Lambert Company
Morris Plains, NJ 07950

Louis J Ravin, PhD
Pharmaceutical Consultant
Watertown, CT 06795

The intelligent selection of new potential drug compounds from the discovery process, and their formulation into dosage forms with high and consistent bioavailability, is more important than ever in the pharmaceutical industry. Reasons for this importance include the time and expense required to discover and develop new drugs; the cost of drug substances; more drugs with solubility and bioavailability problems; the advent of highly potent biotechnology-derived proteins and peptides; lot-to-lot changes in the physical-chemical properties of drug substance and multisourcing of drug substance and drug product.

Statistics indicate that the odds of a new compound synthesized in the discovery process becoming a commercially viable drug product is less than 1 in 10,000. The reasons for these poor odds are many and include those of scientific and marketing origins. Included in the reasons is the selection of compounds for development that had unsuitable physical-chemical properties such as instability or insolubility that ultimately led to poor bioavailability or efficacy in human clinical studies. Solutions for these problems often are found in the preformulation process where the physical, chemical and mechanical properties of drug substances are determined.

The stage in the research and development process at which preformulation begins can greatly affect the odds of a new compound becoming a commercially viable drug product. In general, the sooner preformulation data is available, the earlier decisions can be made about the nature of the physical-chemical properties and how these might impact on the development potential of a new drug candidate. For example, when the preformulation scientist works closely with discovery scientists, preformulation data along with biological data can be used to select from a group of compounds, the best compound for future development. It is all too common that new compounds are chosen for development without adequate preformulation data. Hence, problems with stability, solubility and bioavailability occur in the dosage-form development process that could have been prevented or modified had preformulation data been part of the compound selection process.

The bioequivalency of multisource pharmaceutical products continues to receive great attention from practitioners and regulatory authorities alike. It is well documented that the bioavailability of certain drugs is very susceptible to the physical-chemical properties of the drug substance and the process and composition of the formulation. As a result, the efficacy of the formulations can vary dramatically. Even though this does not occur with all drugs, the manner in which the information has been reported by scientists often appears unclear to the practitioner. The information also has been interpreted differently depending on the motivation, viewpoint and attitude of the interpreter.

To optimize the performance of drug products, it is necessary to have a complete understanding of the physical-chemical and mechanical properties of drug substances prior to formulating them into drug products. The development of an optimum formulation is not an easy task, and many factors readily influence formulation properties. Drug substances rarely are administered as pure chemical entities, and are almost always given in a formulation containing excipients. The complexity of the formulation can vary from a simple aqueous solution to a complex controlled-release dosage form containing several polymeric materials. Sometimes the degree of complexity is determined by patent motivation, but more often it is determined by the properties that are expected from or built into the dosage form and by the resulting composition that is required to achieve these qualities.

The high degree of uniformity, physiological availability and therapeutic quality expected of modern medicinal products usually are the result of considerable effort and expertise on the part of the formulating pharmacist. These qualities are attained by careful selection and control of the quality of the various ingredients employed, appropriate manufacturing according to well-defined processes and, most importantly, adequate consideration of the many variables that may influence the composition, stability and utility of the product. In dealing with the formulation of new products it has become necessary to apply the best research methods and tools in order to develop, produce and control the potent, stable and effective dosage forms which make up our modern medical armamentarium.

The pharmaceutical formulator has a need for specialized areas of science in order to acquire and understand scientific information about the drug substance that is necessary to develop an optimum dosage form. The pharmaceutical industry no longer can rely only on past experience or empirical thinking to formulate dosage forms. Industry does not have the time or resources to operate by empirically putting dozens of formulations on a stability-testing schedule and waiting to see which were the most stable. Nor does it have the time or resources to test all these formulations for optimum bioavailability. In short, as much information must be acquired about the drug substance very early in its development. This requires an interdisciplinary approach during the preformulation exercise. Figure 1 shows how the development of a drug requires a multidisciplinary approach involving basic science during the preformulation phase followed by applied science during the development phase.

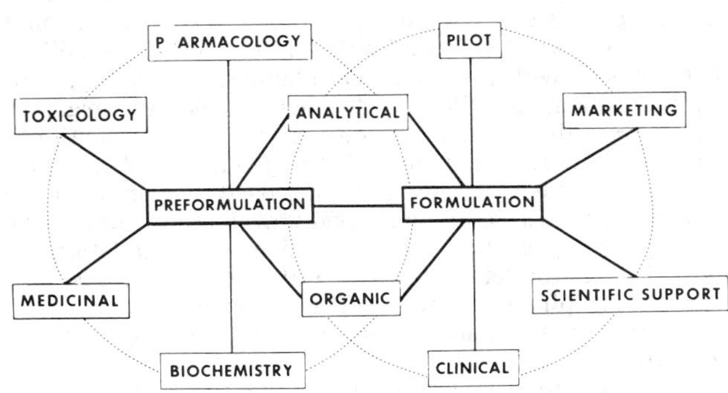

Fig 1. The wheels of product development.

This chapter will discuss the physical-chemical evaluation that takes place during the preformulation stage of development. In addition, consideration will be given to some specialized formulation ingredients that may require discretion in their selection.

Preformulation may be described as a phase of the research and development process where the preformulation scientist characterizes the physical, chemical and mechanical properties of a new drug substance, in order to develop stable, safe and effective dosage forms. Ideally, the preformulation phase begins early in the discovery process such that appropriate physical-chemical data is available to aid in the selection of new chemical entities that enter the development process. At this stage, experiments typically focus on salt selection and its effect on solubility and stability. In all likelihood, the lot sizes synthesized by the medicinal chemist at these early phases are on the order of 200 to 300 mg. Because the synthetic process is likely to change (especially the last step whereby the chemical is crystallized), properties such as crystal size and shape are not critical at this point. It also should be noted that solubility data, in particular, is useful to the pharmacologist and toxicologist in selecting solubilizing vehicles for efficacy and safety studies in animals. Many drug candidates are deemed unefficacious by pharmacology and/or safe by toxicology because of low solubility (and hence low bioavailability) in the dosing vehicles.

The bulk of preformulation work occurs after a new chemical entity and its appropriate salt form have been selected for testing in humans. The initial phase of this work focuses on the filing of an Investigational New Drug Application (INDA) and development of a dosage form for Phase 1 and early Phase 2 clinical studies. Since the odds are less than 1 in 10 that a drug entering Phase 1 clinical trials will proceed to the filing of a New Drug Application (NDA), the Phase 1 dosage form may not warrant the effort to give it the attributes of the market-image dosage form. In today's industrial environment it is imperative to move the drug into human clinical trials as soon as possible in order to determine if the candidate is a potential marketable drug. If the candidate is such a drug, a market-image dosage form can be developed after Phase 1 testing. For example, oral Phase 1 dosage forms are invariably powder-filled, hard-gelatin capsules because they can be easily blinded with respect to color, size and taste. Hence, preformulation studies at this phase of development should be designed to meet the needs of the initial INDA filing. Typical studies would include a pH-stability profile, a pH-solubility profile, studies for polymorphs, partitioning, dissolution behavior, crystal size and shape and compatibility with excipients to be used in the Phase 1 formulation. It should be noted that the lot size of drug substance is increasing at this stage of development, and the last step of the synthetic process may be defined. Therefore it is important to begin to gather historical data on lot-to-lot differences in physical properties, such as crystal habit or polymorphism.

A stability-indicating assay is very important. Typically high-performance liquid chromatography is the analytical method of choice, but development of the assay can take time and depends upon identification of the synthetic impurities and degradation products. In the meantime, thin-layer chromatography can be used to determine if a drug molecule is degrading. It is important for the preformulation scientist to work closely with the analytical chemists who support the synthetic chemists. Pooled effort can accelerate the analytical-methods development process by sharing information on synthetic impurities and degradation products. Accelerated conditions (heat, light, humidity) are used to promote degradation of the drug compound being evaluated. In order to identify and quantitate the mechanism of degradation, the degradation products must be identified and separable in the chromatographic procedure. This information is critical to the formulation scientist in order to stabilize the drug molecule in the dosage form.

During a preformulation study, it is necessary to maintain a high degree of flexibility. Problem areas must be identified early and focused upon. The preformulation scientist can not afford to spend time generating data simply to check off activities on a check-list when the lack of other important data could significantly delay the development of a new drug. For example, selection of a suitable salt or polymorphic form is critical to the toxicology studies. If an unsuitable form is selected without careful preformulation testing, major portions of the toxicology program would have to be repeated. This could delay the overall development program by months or years, depending upon the phase of development in which the unsuitability is identified. Consequently, items such as salt form, hydrate form and polymorphic form are among the first items to be investigated.

When preformulation studies are initiated, the amount of drug substance usually is limited. The first supply of drug substance usually comes from the medicinal chemist where a typical lot size may be less than 1 g. For the remainder of preformulation studies, 25 to 150 g may be available from the chemical-development scientist. The medicinal chemist typically generates preliminary data such as melting point, spectral data and structure of the compound. The direction taken for preformulation is determined by the chemical structure of the new drug and the intended primary dosage forms to be developed. Many areas must be evaluated critically for each new drug substance, and it is essential that problem areas be identified early, otherwise delays could occur later in the development program. Some consequences of inadequate preformulation include possible use of unsatisfactory salt form, poor physical and chemical stability of the new drug substance, toxicological and clinical testing of compounds with marginal activity, increased development costs and increased development time. As preformulation studies progress, data is compiled, analyzed and transferred to scientists in discovery and development. In particular, the formulation scientist uses this information to develop dosage forms.

Physical Properties

Description

Since the pure drug entity is in short supply at the outset of most preliminary evaluations, it is extremely important to note the general appearance, color and odor of the compound. These characteristics provide a basis for comparison with future lots. During the preparation of scale-up lots the chemist usually refines or alters the original chemical synthetic route. This sometimes results in a change in some of the physical properties. When this takes place, comparisons can be made with earlier lots and decisions made regarding solvents for recrystallization.

Taste usually warrants some consideration, especially if the drug is intended for oral use in pediatric dosage forms. In such cases consideration should be given to the preparation of alternate salt forms or possible evaluation of excipients that mask the undesirable taste.

Microscopic Examination

Each lot of drug substance, regardless of size, is examined microscopically and a photomicrograph taken. The microscopic examination gives a gross indication of particle size and characteristic crystal properties. These photomicrographs are useful in determining the consistency of particle size and crystal habit from batch to batch, especially during the early periods of chemical synthesis; if a synthetic step is changed, they also give an indication of any effect the change may have on crystal habit. One must keep in mind that the photomicrograph only gives a qualitative indication of particle size distribution; it always is necessary to do a particle-size analysis for a more accurate picture of the distribution of particles in any particular batch of drug substance.

Particle Size

The uses of pharmaceutical products in a finely divided form are diverse. From knowledge of their particle size, such drugs as griseofulvin, nitrofurantoin, spironolactone, procaine penicillin and phenobarbital have been formulated so as to optimize activity. Other drugs, formulated in suspension or emulsion systems, in inhalation aerosols or in oral dosage forms, may contain finely divided material as an essential component. One of the basic physical properties common to all these finely divided substances is the particle-size distribution, ie, the frequency of occurrence of particles of every size. What is of practical interest usually is not the characteristics of single particles but rather the mean characteristics of a large number of particles. It must be emphasized, however, that knowledge of size characteristics is of no value unless adequate correlation has been established with functional properties of specific interest in the drug formulation. Many investigations demonstrating the significance of particle size are reported in the literature. It has been shown that dissolution rate, absorption rate, content uniformity, color, taste, texture and stability depend to varying degrees on particle size and distribution. In preformulation work it is important that the significance of particle size in relation to formulation be established early. Preliminary physical observations sometimes can detect subtle differences in color. If this can be attributed to differences in particle-size distribution, it is important to define this distribution and recommend that more attention be given to particle size in preparing future batches of drug substance. This effect also is evident when preparing suspensions of poorly soluble materials. One may observe batch-to-batch differences in the color of a suspension which can be related to differences in particle size. Sometimes, when small particles tend to agglomerate, a subtle change in color or texture may be evident.

Sedimentation and flocculation rates in suspensions are in part governed by particle size. In concentrated deflocculated suspensions the larger particles exhibit hindered settling and the smaller particles settle more rapidly. In flocculated suspensions the particles are linked together into flocs which settle according to the size of the floc and porosity of the aggregated mass. Flocculated suspensions are preferred since they have less tendency to cake and are more rapidly dispersible. Thus, it is apparent that the ultimate height, H_u, of sediment as a suspension settles depends on particle size. The ratio H_u/H_o, or the degree of suspendibility as affected by particle size, is valuable information for the formulator in order to prepare a satisfactory dosage form.

The rate of dissolution of small particles usually is faster than that of larger ones because rate of dissolution depends on the specific surface area in contact with the liquid medium. This usually is described by the modified Noyes-Whitney equation for dissolution rate dA/dt

$$\frac{dA}{dt} = KS(C_s - C) \tag{1}$$

where A is the amount of drug in solution, K is the intrinsic dissolution rate constant, S is the surface area, C_s is the concentration of a saturated solution of the drug and C is the drug concentration at time t. The surface area of an object, regardless of shape, varies inversely with its diameter and confirms the above effect of particle size on dissolution rate. Solubility also has been observed to depend on particle size. Hussain demonstrated the power of a related equation, Fick's first law, for predicting the dissolution rates of slightly water-soluble powders.[1] Fick's first law can be written as

$$Q = (ASDt)/h$$

where Q = amount of drug (in grams) dissolved in time t, A = surface area occupied by total weight of the sample, S = solubility of the drug (g/mL) in dissolution media, D = diffusion coefficient of the drug (cm²/sec) and h = thickness of the diffusional layer (cm).

By using experimentally determined values of 9×10^{-6} cm²/sec and 50×10^{-4} cm for D and h, respectively, Hussain showed excellent correlation between dissolution rates calculated theoretically and those determined experimentally. Dittert, *et al*,[2] reported data for an experimental drug, 4-acetamidophenyl 2,2,2-trichloroethyl carbonate, which demonstrated that the dissolution rate and, in turn, bioavailability were affected by particle size. Although the ultimate amount of drug in solution may not be significant with respect to the dose administered, the formulator should be aware of this potential. With poorly soluble drugs it is extremely important to take these factors into account during the design of the dosage form. See also Chapter 34.

Flow properties of drugs can be influenced by particle size, and particle size reduction to extremely small sizes (less than 10 μm) may be inadvisable for some drug substances. Entrapped air adsorbed on the surface of the particles and/or surface electrical charges sometimes impart undesirable properties to the drug. For example, adsorbed air at the drug-particle surface may prevent wetting of the drug by surrounding fluid, and electrically induced agglomeration of fine particles may decrease exposure of the drug surface to surrounding dissolution medium. Such effects act as dissolution rate-limiting steps since they minimize maximum drug surface-liquid contact.

Crystal growth is also a function of particle size. Finer particles tend to dissolve and subsequently recrystallize and adhere to larger particles. This phenomenon is referred to as *Ostwald ripening*. Protective colloid systems can be used to suppress this nucleation. Preformulators can generate information concerning the effectiveness of different colloids that is extremely important to the formulator when he is given the task of preparing a suspension dosage form.

Particle-size reduction may be deleterious for some drug substances. Increasing surface area by milling or other methods may lead to rapid degradation of a compound. Drug substances also may undergo polymorphic transformation during the milling process. The preformulator must always be cognizant of these potential problems, and whenever the decision is made to reduce particle size, the conditions must be controlled and the stability profile evaluated. If a problem does arise, it is the responsibility of the preformulator to note it and attempt to resolve it prior to turning the drug substance over to the formulating pharmacist.

Gastrointestinal absorption of a poorly soluble drug may be affected by the particle-size distribution. If the dissolution rate of the drug is less than the diffusion rate to the site of absorption and the absorption rate itself, then the particle size of the drug is of great importance. Smaller particles should increase dissolution rate and, thus, bring about more rapid gastrointestinal absorption. One of the first observations of this phenomenon was made with sulfadiazine. Blood-level determinations showed that the drug in suspension containing particles 1 to 3 μm in size was absorbed more rapidly and more efficiently than from a suspension containing particles 7 times larger. Maximum blood levels were about 40% higher and occurred 2 hours earlier. Increased bioavailability with particle-size reduction also has been observed with griseofulvin. The extent of absorption of an oral dose increased 2.5 times when the surface area was increased approximately sixfold. Micronized griseofulvin permits a 50% decrease in dosage to obtain a satisfactory clinical response.

On the other hand, it was found that with nitrofurantoin there was an optimal average particle size that minimized side effects without affecting therapeutic response. In fact, a commercial product containing large particles is available. For chloramphenicol, particle size has virtually no effect on total absorption but it significantly affects the rate of appearance of peak blood levels of the drug. After administration of 50-μm particles, as well as 200-μm particles, peak levels occurred in 1 hour; with 400-μm particles peak levels occurred in 2 hours; with 800-μm particles peak levels occurred in 3 hours. All four preparations had the same physiological availability, which implies that the absorption of chloramphenicol occurs uniformly over a major portion of the intestinal tract.

Reduction of particle size also may create adverse responses. For example, fine particles of the prodrug trichloroethyl carbonate were more toxic in mice than regular and coarse particles.[3] Increasing the surface area for water-soluble drugs, and possibly for weakly basic drugs, appears to be of little value. Absorption of weak bases usually is rate-limited by stomach emptying time rather than by dissolution. As previously mentioned, particle size is of importance only when the absorption process is rate-limited by the dissolution rate in gastrointestinal fluids.

The previous discussion considered the effect of particle size of the drug substance and its relationship to formulation. The particle size of the inert ingredients merits some attention. When one is concerned with particle size, all ingredients used in preparing the dosage form should be evaluated and some recommendation regarding their control should be made prior to full-scale development of a dosage form. It is recommended highly that particle size and its distribution be determined, optimized, monitored and controlled when applicable, particularly during early preformulation studies when the decision is made with regard to a suitable dosage form. The more common methods of determining particle size of powders used in the pharmaceutical industry include sieving, microscopy, sedimentation and stream scanning.

Sieving or Screening—Sieving or screening is probably one of the oldest methods of sizing particles and still is used commonly to determine the size distribution of powders in the size range of 325 mesh (44 μm) and greater. These data serve usually as a rough guideline in evaluating raw materials with regard to the need for milling. The basic disadvantages of screen analysis are the large sample size required and the tendency for blinding of the screens due to static charge or mechanical clogging. The advantages include simplicity, low cost and little skill requirement of the operator.

Microscopy—Microscopy is the most universally accepted and direct method of determining particle-size distribution of powders in the subsieve range, but this method is tedious and time-consuming. The preparation of the slide for counting particles is important because the sample must represent the particle-size distribution of the bulk sample. Extreme care must be taken in obtaining a truly representative sample from the bulk chemical. The cone and quartering technique usually gives a satisfactory sample. The sample should be properly suspended, dispersed and mixed thoroughly in a liquid which has a different refractive index from the particles being counted. A representative sample is mounted on a slide having a calibrated grid. For counting, random fields are selected on the slide and the particles are sized and counted. Between 500 and 1000 particles should be counted to make statistical treatment of the data meaningful.

The utility of microscopy has been enhanced greatly by the advent of computerized-image analysis systems. These systems give the operator the ability to observe the particles in the microscopic field, to consider particle-shape factors during measurement, to discriminate between drug and excipient particles and to remove operator bias during microscopic measurement. In addition, the computer provides sophisticated statistical analysis automatically, thereby eliminating manual tabulation and calculations. Computerized-image analysis systems can be validated fully and used on either pure drug substance or drug substance in the presence of excipients.[4]

Sedimentation—Sedimentation techniques utilize the dependence of velocity of fall of particles on their size. Application is made of the Stokes equation (see page 295) which describes a relationship between the rate at which a particle settles in a fluid medium to the size of that particle. Although the equation is based on spherical-shaped particles, it is used widely to determine the weight-size distribution of irregularly shaped particles. Data obtained by this procedure are usually reliable; however, the result may not agree with those obtained by other methods because of the limitations of the shape factor.

The *Andreasen Pipette Method* is used most commonly for sedimentation studies. Exact volumes are withdrawn at prescribed times and at a specified liquid depth. The liquid is evaporated and the residue of powder is weighed. The data are used in the Stokes equation and a weight-size distribution is calculated. Precautions must be observed with this method. Proper dispersion, consistent sampling, temperature control of the suspending medium and concentration should be achieved in order to obtain consistent results.

Stream Scanning—Stream scanning is a technique in which a fluid suspension passes through a sensing zone where the individual particles are electronically sized, counted and tabulated. The great advantage of this technique is that data can be generated in relatively short periods of time with reasonable accuracy. Literally thousands of particles can be counted in seconds and used in determining the size-distribution curve. The data are in a number of particles per class interval and can be expressed mathematically as the arithmetic mean diameter and graphed accordingly. Figure 2 illustrates a plot of typical data obtained for NBS Standard Reference Material No 1003.

The *Coulter Counter* and the *HIAC Counter* are used widely in the field of particle-size analysis in the pharmaceutical industry. They can be used to follow crystal growth in suspensions very effectively. Figure 3 shows the change in particle size with time for an aqueous suspension of Form I of an experimental drug. It appears that the growth of the particles decreases significantly after 6 hours. The photomicrograph shown in Fig 4 depicts the significant increase in particle size after 6 hours. Further treatment of the data as shown in Fig 5 enables one to establish rates of growth for suspended particles. Simply reading off the intercepts at the 1%, 2% or 3% oversize and plotting this increase in diameter with time enables one to calculate the rate of growth of particles in a suspension. This is shown in Fig 6.

Light Scattering—Light-scattering methods are generally fast, inexpensive and induce minimal artifacts. In general, such methods operate by measuring light diffraction from suspended particles without forming an image of the particles onto a detector. A typical unit is the laser diffraction particle sizer (*Malvern*). In it, a liquid dispersion of particles flows through a beam of laser light. Light scattered by the particles and the unscattered remainder are incident onto a receiver lens that forms a diffraction pattern of the scattered

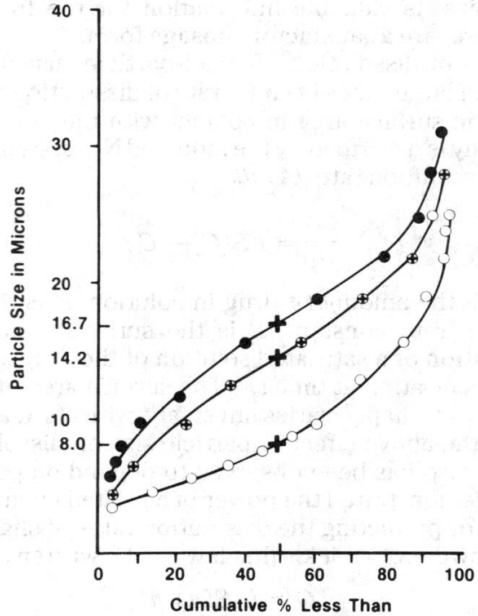

Fig 2. Particle size distribution of NBS glass beads (Standard Reference Material No 1003) expressed in terms of ○ = number of particles; ● = weight of particles; ⊗ = surface area of particles.

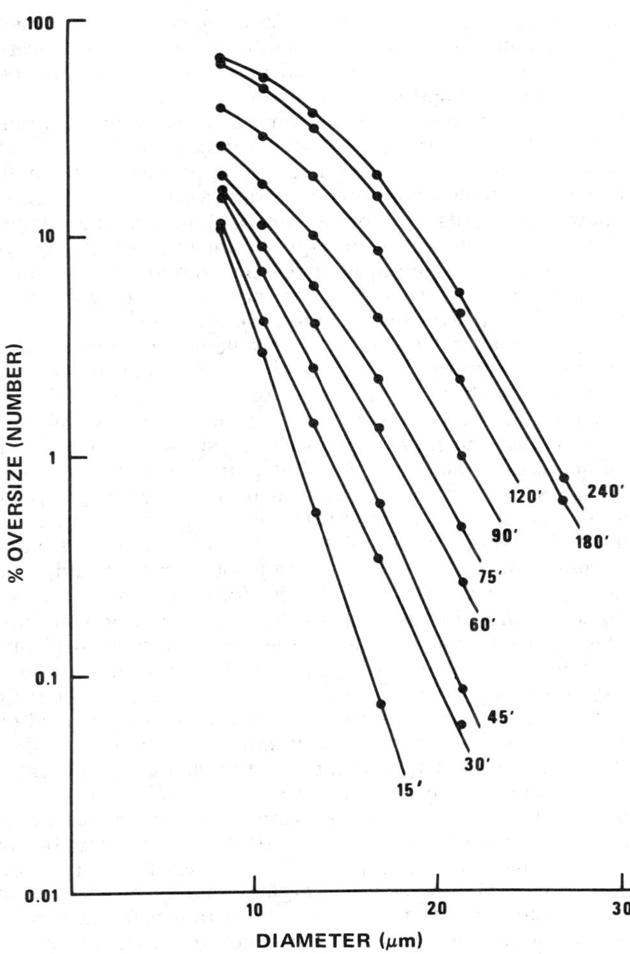

Fig 3. Change in particle size with time for an aqueous suspension of Form I of an experimental drug.

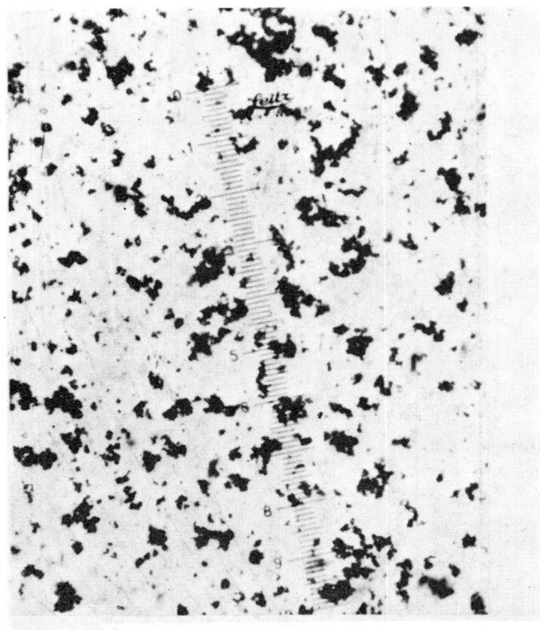

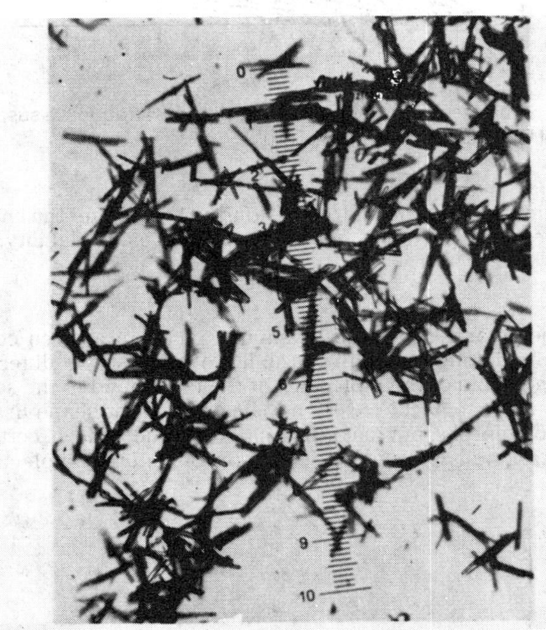

Fig 4. Photomicrographs showing change in crystal size for a suspension of Form I of an experimental drug.

light. The scattered light and unscattered light then are gathered on detectors so the total light power is monitored as it allows the sample volume concentration to be determined. Each particle scatters light at a favored scattering angle that is related to its diameter. The detector provides an electronic output that makes it possible for a computer to deduce the volume-size distribution that gives rise to the observed scattering characteristics. Results may also be transformed to the equivalent surface or number distribution. Refer to Chapters 21 and 33.

Partitioning Effect

If an excess of liquid or solid is added to a mixture of two immiscible liquids, it will distribute itself between the two phases so that each becomes saturated. If the substance is added to the immiscible solvents in an amount insufficient to saturate the solutions, it still will distribute between the two layers in a definite concentration ratio. If C_1 and C_2 are the equilibrium concentrations of the substance in Solvent 1 and Solvent 2, the equilibrium expression becomes

$$\frac{C_1}{C_2} = k \tag{2}$$

The equilibrium constant k is known as the distribution ratio or partition coefficient. Biologically, in order for a pharmacological response to occur, it is necessary that the drug molecule cross a biological membrane. The membrane, consisting of protein and lipid material, acts as a lipophilic barrier to most drugs. The resistance of this barrier to drug transfer is related to the lipophilic nature of the molecule involved. See Chapter 41.

Understanding the partitioning effect and the dissociation constant enables one to estimate the site of absorption of a new chemical entity. If one assumes the stomach to have a pH range of 1.0 to 3.0 and the small intestines to have a pH range from 5 to 8, in most cases acidic drugs (pK_a 3) will be absorbed more rapidly in the stomach while more basic drugs (pK_a 8) will be absorbed more rapidly in the intestinal tract. There are exceptions, however. Some compounds have low

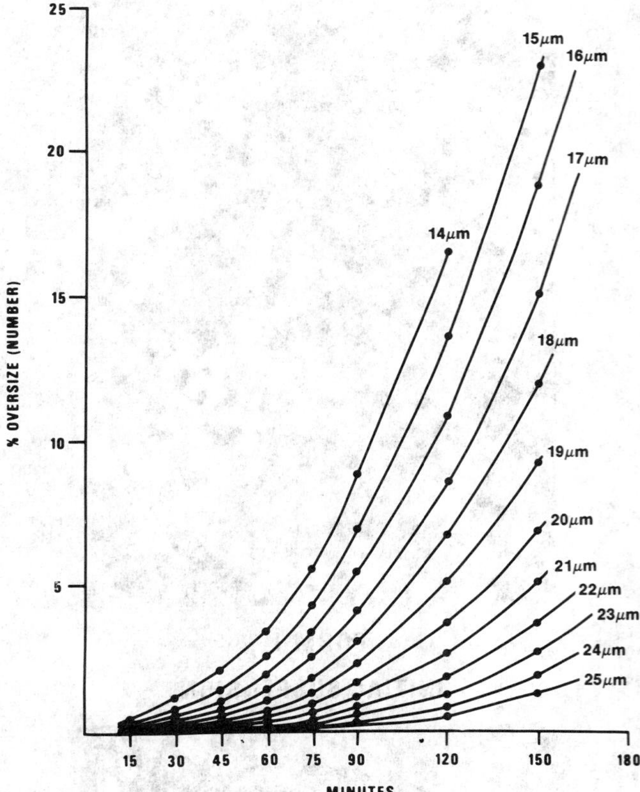

Fig 5. Change in cumulative count with time for an aqueous suspension of Form I of an experimental drug.

partition coefficients and/or are ionized highly over the entire physiological pH range, but still show good bioavailability.

Polymorphism

A polymorph is a solid crystalline phase of a given compound resulting from the possibility of at least two different arrangements of the molecules of the compound in the solid state. The molecule itself may be of different shape in the two polymorphs, but that is not necessary and, indeed, certain changes in shape involve formation of different molecules

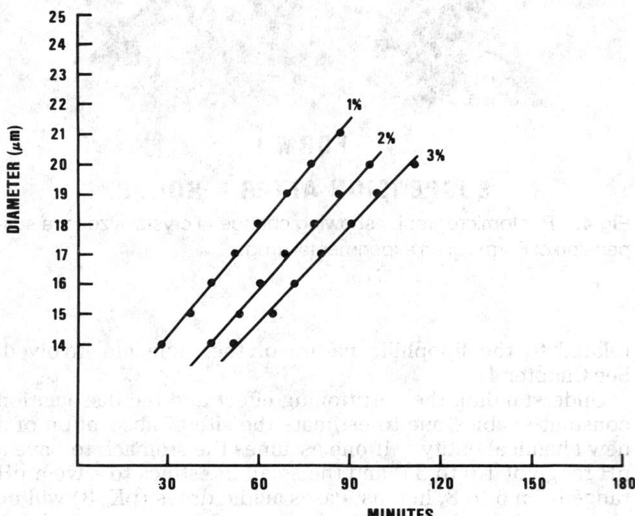

Fig 6. Rate of growth of Form I of experimental drug in aqueous suspension.

and, hence, do not constitute polymorphism. Geometric isomers or tautomers, even though interconvertible and reversibly so, cannot be called polymorphs although they may behave in a confusingly similar manner.

A safe criterion for classification of a system as polymorphic is the following: two polymorphs will be different in crystal structure but identical in the liquid or vapor states. Dynamic isomers will melt at different temperatures, as do polymorphs, but will give melts of different composition. In time, each of these melts changes to an equilibrium mixture of the two isomers with temperature-dependent compositions. Some reported cases of polymorphism are undoubtedly dynamic isomerism, since the two behave quite similarly.

Polymorphism is the ability of any element or compound to crystallize as more than one distinct crystalline species, eg, carbon as a cubic diamond or hexagonal graphite. Different polymorphs of a given compound are, in general, as different in structure and properties as the crystals of two different compounds. Solubility, melting point, density, hardness, crystal shape, optical and electrical properties, vapor pressure, stability, etc all vary with the polymorphic form. In general, it should be possible to obtain different crystalline forms of a drug substance exhibiting polymorphism and, thus, modify the performance properties for that compound. To do so requires a knowledge of the behavior of polymorphs. There are numerous reviews on the subject of polymorphism. In addition, numerous indications of the importance of polymorphism in pharmaceuticals are reported in the literature. Extensive studies of polymorphism have been conducted on steroids, barbiturates, antihistamines and sulfonamides. Preformulation usually includes rigorous studies to determine the presence of polymorphs in new drug substances being prepared for preliminary investigation in test animals. Some of the parameters routinely investigated are the number of polymorphs that exist, relative degree of stability of the various polymorphs, presence of a glassy state, stabilization of metastable forms, temperature stability ranges for each polymorph, solubilities, method of preparation of each form, effect of micronization or tableting and interaction with formulation ingredients.

The initial task of the preformulator is to determine whether or not the drug substance being evaluated exists in more than one crystalline form. The following procedures are usually followed to cause crystallization of a metastable form:[5]

1. Melt completely a small amount of the compound on a slide and observe the solidification between crossed polars. If, after spontaneous freezing, a transformation occurs spontaneously or can be induced by seeding or scratching, the compound probably exists in at least two polymorphic forms. It is essential to prevent nucleation of the stable form by inducing supercooling. Supercooling can be induced by using a small sample size, holding the melt for approximately 30 seconds about 10° above the melting point; carefully setting aside the compound without physical shock before observing it and rapid cooling of the compound.
2. Heat a sample of the compound on a hot stage and observe whether a solid-solid transformation occurs during heating.
3. Sublime a small amount of the compound and attempt to induce a transformation between the sublimate and the original sample by mixing the two in a drop of saturated solution of one of them. If the two are polymorphs, the more stable one will be more insoluble and will grow at the expense of the more soluble metastable form. This process will continue until the metastable form is transformed completely to the stable form. If the samples are not polymorphs, one may dissolve but the other will not grow. If the two are identical forms, nothing will occur.
4. Maintain an excess of the compound in a small amount of solvent held near the melting point of the compound. Isolate the suspended solid. Care should be taken to maintain the temperature during this step. Test the isolated material with an original sample using the procedure outlined in 3, above.
5. Recrystallize the compound from solution by shock-cooling, and observe a portion of the precipitated material suspended in a drop of the mother liquor. The drop then may be seeded with the original compound to check for solution-phase transformation. If the precipitate is a different polymorph, a solution-phase transformation should take place.

Once it has been established that polymorphism occurs, there are procedures which enable the preformulator to prepare the various forms in larger quantities for further evaluation and suitability for incorporation into dosage forms.

Once a compound has been shown to exist in more than one crystalline form, a number of techniques are available to identify the different polymorphic phases present. Each of these techniques could be successful in identifying the phase, but a combination of methods provides a means for isolation and identification of each crystalline modification. In order to confirm the presence of more than one crystalline form of a compound, it is advisable to identify the modifications present by more than one method. Using only one method for confirming the presence of polymorphs sometimes may be misleading.

Microscopy—Optical crystallography is used in the identification of polymorphs. Crystals exist in isotropic and anisotropic forms. When isotropic crystals are examined, the velocity of light is the same in all directions, while anisotropic crystals have two or three different light velocities or refractive indices. This method requires the services of a trained crystallographer. Video recording systems have made it possible to record the events visualized during the heating and cooling stages, thereby providing a permanent record that can be re-examined.

Hot-Stage Methods—The polarizing microscope, fitted with a hot or cold stage, is very useful for investigating polymorphs. An experienced microscopist can tell quickly whether polymorphs exist: the degree of stability of the metastable forms; transition temperatures and melting points; rates of transition under various thermal and physical conditions and whether to pursue polymorphism as a route to an improved dosage form.

X-Ray Powder Diffraction—Crystalline materials in powder form give characteristic X-ray diffraction patterns made up of peaks in certain positions and varying intensities. Each powder pattern of the crystal lattice is characteristic for a given polymorph. This method has the advantage over other identification techniques in that the sample is examined as presented. Some care should be exercised in reducing and maintaining particle-size control. A very small sample size is needed and the method is nondestructive. This method has been used by several investigators in identifying polymorphs in pharmaceuticals.

Infrared Spectroscopy—This procedure is useful in identification of polymorphs. Solid samples must be used since polymorphs of a compound have identical spectra in solution. The technique can be used for both qualitative and quantitative identification.

Thermal Methods—Differential scanning calorimetry and differential thermal analysis have been used extensively to identify polymorphs. In both methods, the heat loss or gain resulting from physical or chemical transitions occurring in a sample is recorded as a function of temperature as the substance is heated at a uniform rate. Enthalpic changes, both endothermic and exothermic, are caused by phase transitions. For example, fusion, sublimation, solid-solid transition and water loss generally produce endothermic effects while crystallization produces exothermic effects. Thermal analysis enables one to calculate the thermodynamic parameters for the systems being evaluated. Heats of fusion can be obtained and the rate of conversion of polymorphs determined.

Dilatometry—Dilatometry measures the change in volume caused by thermal or chemical effects. Ravin and Higuchi[6] used dilatometry to follow the melting behavior of theobroma oil by measuring the specific volume of both rapidly and slowly cooled theobroma oil as a function of increasing temperature. The presence of the metastable form was shown by a contraction in the temperature range of 20 to 24°. This is illustrated in Fig 7. Dilatometry is extremely accurate; however, it is very tedious and time-consuming. It is not used widely.

Proton magnetic resonance, nuclear magnetic resonance and electron microscopy sometimes are used to study polymorphism.

Polymorphs can be classified into one of two types: (1) *enantiotropic*—one polymorphic form can be changed reversibly into another one by varying the temperature or pressure, eg, sulfur and (2) *monotropic*—one polymorphic form is unstable at all temperatures and pressures, eg, glyceryl stearates. At a specified temperature and pressure, only one polymorphic form will be thermodynamically stable. However, other metastable forms may exist under the same conditions. These metastable forms will convert to the stable lattice structures with time. The first indication of the significance of a polymorphic transformation in a pharmaceutical system was noted with novobiocin. The amorphous form of novobiocin was found to be well-absorbed; however, when formulated into a suspension, a reversion of the metastable form to the more stable crystalline form occurred resulting in poor absorption.

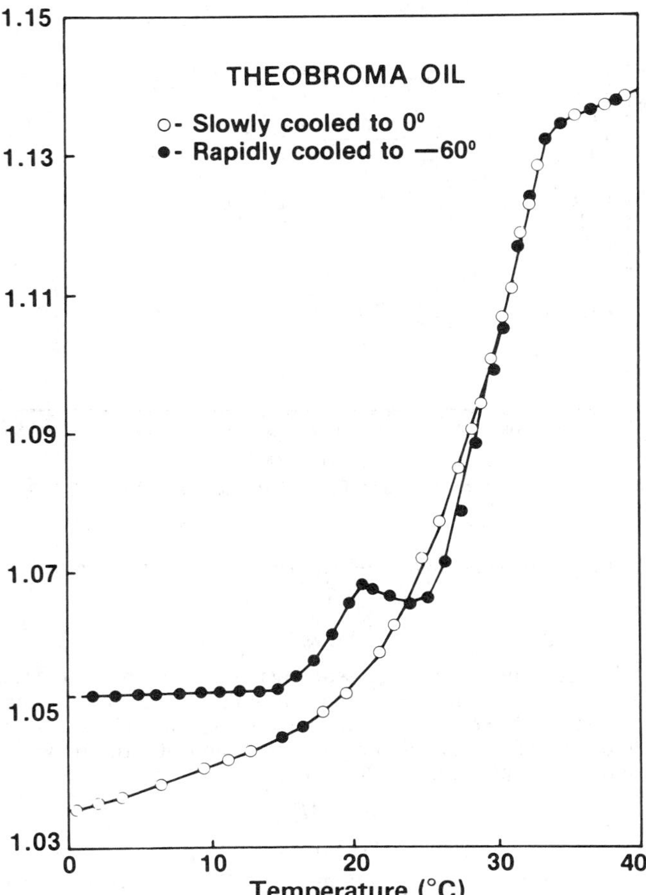

Fig 7. Dilatometric curves: theobroma oil, slowly and rapidly cooled.

After it has been determined that a drug substance does exist in more than one crystalline form, the conditions under which each can be produced should be established. In this manner, proper crystallizing conditions can be maintained from batch to batch to ensure a uniform and acceptable raw material. Recrystallization solvent, rate of crystallization and other factors may cause one crystal form to dominate. During the preliminary investigation to establish these conditions, it is necessary to monitor the forms prepared. For example, during the preliminary work with an indole derivative, differential scanning calorimetry, X-ray analysis and infrared analysis were used to establish that polymorphs were present and that they could be prepared satisfactorily. Figures 8, 9 and 10 show the respective data for this conclusion. When polymorphs are shown to be present, experiments should be designed to determine whether or not the properties differ sufficiently to alter their pharmaceutic or biologic behavior.

Dissolution tests can be used initially to show differences in apparent equilibrium solubilities provided a discriminating solvent system is used. Figure 11 illustrates dissolution data for two polymorphs of an indole derivative which had similar dissolution in the medium used; however, when a more discriminating dissolution medium was used, it was possible to show differences in their dissolution characteristics. This is illustrated in Fig 12. From the data presented for the indole derivative, it was concluded that there would be no appreciable difference in the availability of the two forms if they were to be administered orally in a solid dosage form. Subsequent testing in animals confirmed this. The Nernst equation relates the rate of concentration increase to the

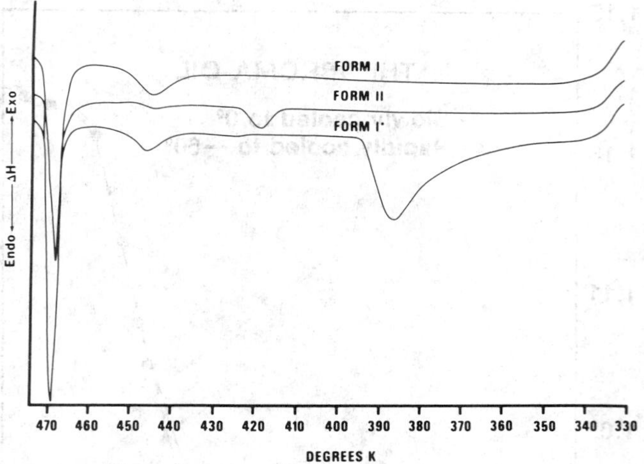

Fig 8. Thermograms for Forms I, I* and II of SK&F 30097.

solubility of a dissolving solid and is commonly written as

$$\frac{dc}{dt} = \frac{AD}{Vh}(C_s - C_t) \tag{3}$$

where A is the area of the dissolving interface of the solid, D is the diffusion coefficient of the solute in the solvent, V is the volume of the solvent, h is the thickness of the diffusion layer and C_s and C_t are concentration of the solute at saturation and at time t, respectively. The equation reduces to

$$\frac{dc}{dt} = \frac{AD}{Vh}C_s \tag{4}$$

for the experimental conditions where $C_s > C_t$. Since D is a property of the solute molecule and the solvent, it is independent of the solid-state form. The experimental conditions can be selected such that A, V and h can be maintained constant in measuring the dissolution rates of different polymorphic forms. The dissolution rate then is directly proportional to C_s, the saturation solubility, and the differences in the solubilities, can be related to their free energies.

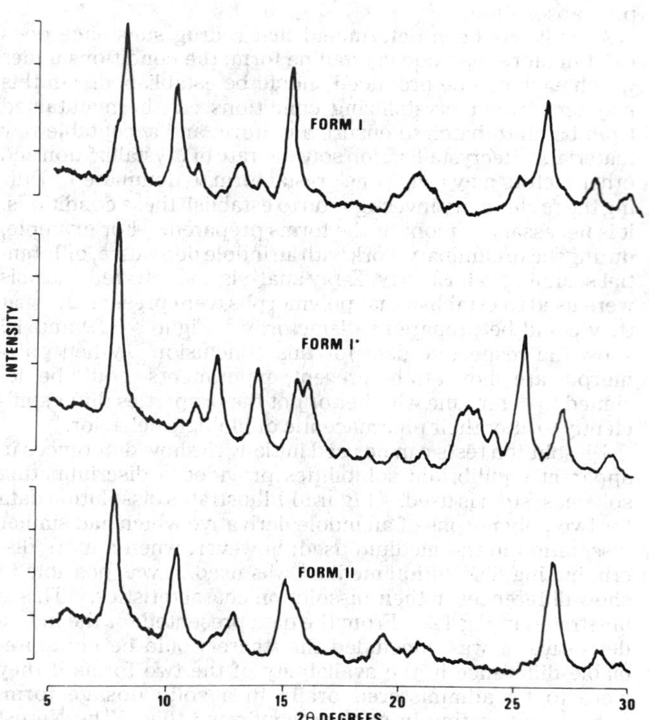

Fig 9. X-Ray diffractograms for Forms I, I* and II of SK&F 30097.

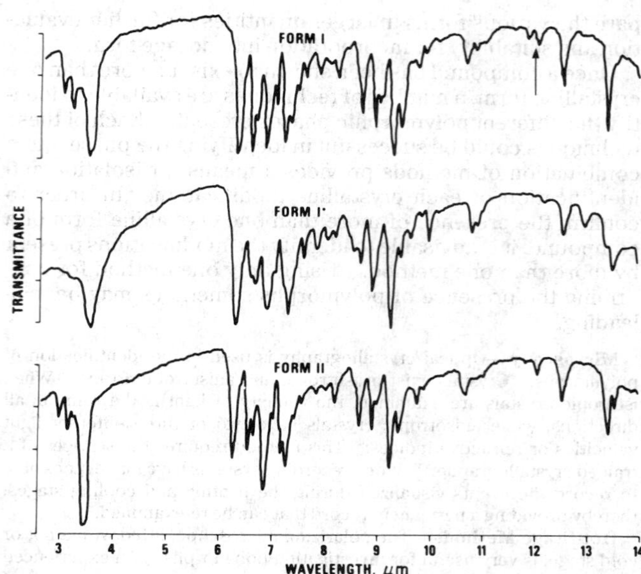

Fig 10. Infrared spectra of Forms I, I* and II of SK&F 30097.

The solubility and dissolution behavior of several polymorphs of chloramphenicol palmitate have been determined. Figures 13 and 14 illustrate the data obtained at several temperatures. It is apparent from the dissolution behavior that the maximum values obtained were good approximations of the solubility of the various forms. Therefore, obtaining data at several temperatures would enable one to calculate the thermodynamic quantities involved in the transition from the metastable to the stable form. A plot of the solubility data as a function of temperature in a typical van't Hoff fashion is

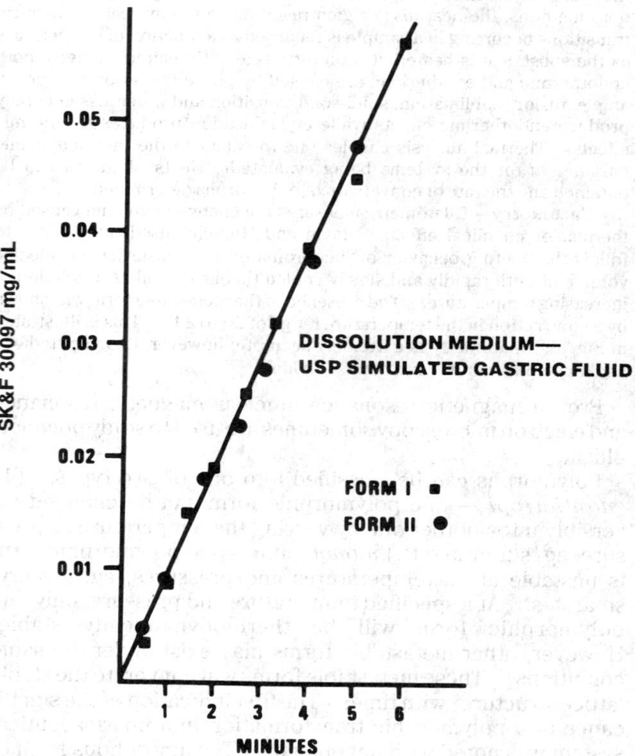

Fig 11. Dissolution behavior of Forms I and II of SK&F 30097 in artificial gastric fluid.

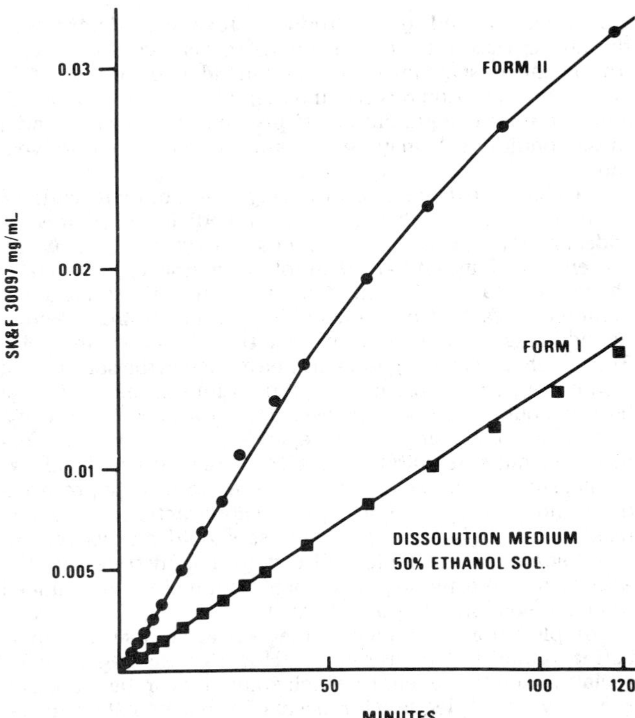

Fig 12. Dissolution behavior of Forms I and II of SK&F 30097 in 50% ethanol solution.

shown in Fig 15. The straight-line relationship enables one to calculate the heats of solution for the various forms and also, by extrapolation, to approximate the transition temperatures for the various forms. These values are shown in Table 1.[7]

At constant temperature and pressure, the free-energy differences between the polymorphs can be calculated by

$$\Delta G_t = RT \ln \frac{C_s \text{ Polymorph A}}{C_s \text{ Polymorph B}} \quad (5)$$

This equation relates the solubility, C_s, of the polymorphic forms at a particular temperature, T, to the free energy differences, ΔG_t. Table 1 also contains the free-energy differences calculated for the polymorphs. The enthalpy changes also can be determined for the various transitions by subtracting the heat of solution derived for the stable form from that of the metastable form. Also, at any particular temperature, T, the entropy for the transition of polymorphs can be evaluated by the following relationship

$$\Delta S_t = \frac{\Delta H_{B \to A} - \Delta G_t}{T} \quad (6)$$

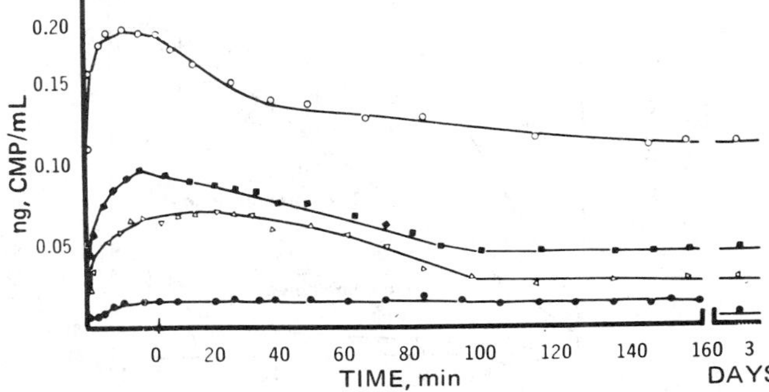

Fig 13. Dissolution curves for Polymorph C of chloramphenicol palmitate in 35% *t*-butyl alcohol and water at 30, 20, 15 and 6°. Key: 30°, ○—○; 20°, ■—■; 15°, △—△; 6°, ●—●.

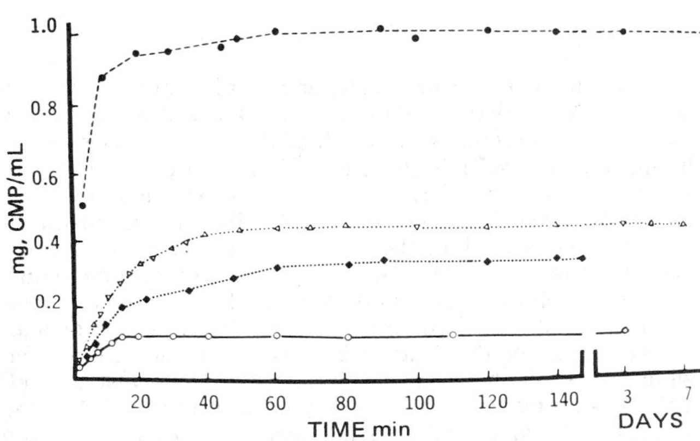

Fig 14. Dissolution curves for Polymorphs A and B of chloramphenicol palmitate in 35% *t*-butyl alcohol and water at 30 and 38°. Key: Polymorph A, 30°, ○—○: Polymorph B, 30°, △—△; Polymorph A, 38°, ◆- - -◆: Polymorph B, 38° ●—●.

The values computed for the transitions also are included in Table 1. At the transition temperature, ΔG_t is equal to zero and the entropy can be calculated, neglecting the free-energy term in Eq 6.

The thermodynamic relationships discussed are based on the assumption that Henry's law is obeyed. Knowledge of these thermodynamic relationships enables the preformulator to select more rationally the more energetic polymorphic form of the drug being investigated for further pharmacological studies and also to have a preliminary assessment of its probable stability.

When a preformulation group inadequately investigates polymorphic drug forms, problems may develop during the development stage. Crystal growth in suspensions resulting in poor uniformity, poor appearance, poor bioavailability, transformation occurring during milling or granulation resulting in changes in the physical and biological characteristics, inadequate pharmacological response and poor chemical stability are typical problems that may become evident.

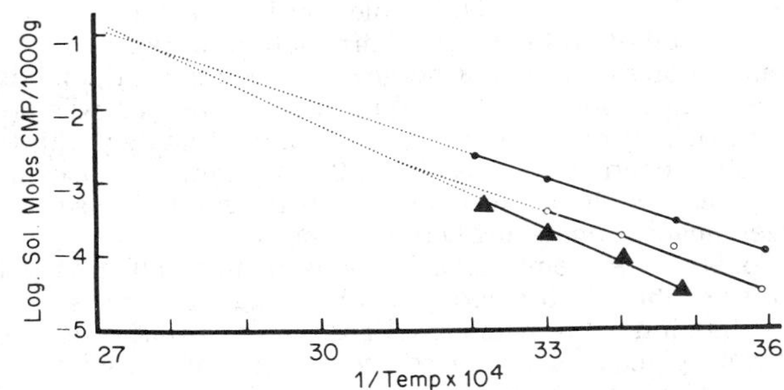

Fig 15. The van't Hoff type plot for Polymorphs A, B, and C of chloramphenicol palmitate. Key: Polymorphs A ▲; B ●—●; and C ○—○.

Table 1—Thermodynamic Values Calculated for Polymorphs *A*, *B* and *C* of Chloramphenicol Palmitate[7]

Polymorph	Transition temp. (°C) to form *A*	Heat of solution, kcal/mole	ΔG_T, cal/mole[a]	ΔS_{303} esu	ΔS_{trans} esu[a]
A	—	21.8	—	—	—
B	88	15.4	−774	−18	−17
C	50	17.2	−465	−13	−14

[a]Calculated for the conversion to Polymorph *A*.

Solubility

In dealing with new drug substances, it is extremely important to know something about their solubility characteristics, especially in aqueous systems since they must possess some limited aqueous solubility to elicit a therapeutic response. In addition, solubility information is critical to developing a discriminating dissolution test method. When a drug substance has an aqueous solubility less than 1 mg/mL in the physiological pH range (1 to 7), a potential bioavailability problem may exist and preformulation studies should be initiated to alleviate the problem. Equilibrium solubility of the drug substance should be determined in a solvent or solvent system which does not have any toxic effects on the test animal. This is done by placing an excess of drug in a vial with the solvent. The vial is agitated at constant temperature and the amount of drug determined periodically by analysis of the supernatant fluid. Equilibrium is not achieved until at least two successive samples have the same result. Experience with solubility determinations would indicate that equilibrium is usually attained by agitating overnight (approximately 24 hours). Solubility determinations can be conducted at several temperatures since the resultant drug products ultimately will be subjected to a wide variation in temperature.

If the solubility of the drug substance is less than the required concentration necessary for the recommended dose, steps must be taken to improve its solubility. The approach taken usually will depend on the chemical nature of the drug substance and the type of drug product desired. If the drug substance is acidic or basic, its solubility can be influenced by pH. Through the application of the Law of Mass Action, the solubility of weakly acidic and basic drug substances can be predicted as a function of pH with a considerable degree of accuracy, using the following equations for the weakly acidic and basic drugs.

Weak Acid *Weak Base*

$$S_t = K_s\left(1 + \frac{K_a}{[H^+]}\right) \qquad S_t = K_s\left(1 + \frac{[H^+]}{K_a}\right) \qquad (7)$$

There are many drug substances for which pH adjustment does not provide an appropriate means for effecting solution. Very weakly acidic or basic drugs may require a pH that could fall outside the accepted tolerable physiological range or may cause stability problems with formulation ingredients. For example, an experimental indole had an equilibrium solubility at pH 1.2 of approximately 50 mg/mL. However, when the pH of this system was increased to approximately 2.0, the solubility decreased to less than 0.1 mg/mL. In cases like this one, or with nonelectrolytes, it is necessary to use some other means of achieving better solubility.

Cosolvent systems have been used quite effectively to achieve solubility for poorly soluble drug substances under investigation. Propylene glycol, glycerin, sorbitol and polyethylene glycols have enjoyed a wide range of success in this area. They have been very useful and generally acceptable for improving solubility. Additional solvents such as glyceryl formal, glycofurol, ethyl carbonate, ethyl lactate and dimethylacetamide have been cited in a review article by Spiegel and Noseworthy;[8] however, it must be emphasized that with the possible exception of dimethylacetamide all of these solvents have not been used in oral products and their acceptability may be doubtful. The number of vehicles readily available to improve solubility is rather limited, yet the frequency of their use is rather high. Solubilizing a new drug substance can improve its availability. For example, when a triazinoindole was administered in a 0.02% solution it showed an equivalent response in antiviral activity to a 2.5% suspension. Information generated early in the preformulation stage can result in a refinement of the dosage regimen and allow for a more accurate estimation of the effective dose.

Cosolvents usually serve a twofold purpose in many pharmaceutical liquid products. They not only effect solution of the drug substance but also improve the solubility of flavoring constituents added to the product. Ideally, in determining the appropriate ratio of cosolvents to achieve the concentration one must achieve, it is recommended to effect solution at the concentration desired and then place the solution at 5° and allow it to equilibrate. If precipitation occurs under these conditions, it may be necessary to alter the cosolvent ratio.

The use of surfactants of various types—nonionic, cationic or anionic—as solubilizing agents for medicinal substances is widespread (see Chapter 19 for illustrations of specific uses). The effect of Triton WR-1339 in solubilizing several steroids is shown in Fig 16.[9] The effect of an anionic, a cationic and a nonionic surfactant on the solubility of an antianginal compound being considered for clinical trials is shown in Fig 17. From such data investigators may be guided in the selection of solubilizing agents for use in preparations to be studied in humans, but it must be emphasized that the acceptability of a particular solubilizing agent depends also on other factors that determine its suitability for the intended use. For example, surfactants are known to interact with some preservatives and thereby decrease preservative action, for which reason the preformulation scientist should always recommend some type of biological test to demonstrate that the activity of the drug substance being studied is not reduced when it is solubilized by a surfactant.

Complexation phenomena sometimes can be used to impart better solubility characteristics. However, the degree of association and the extent to which solubility can be increased generally is not adequate for use in pharmaceutical products. In addition, many complexing agents have physiological activity. The most noteworthy example of the utility of complexation to enhance solubility is the PVP-iodine complex. Hydrotropy sometimes can be used to enhance solubility. High concentrations of urea, salicylates and xanthines have been used successfully on several occasions. Again, the concept is available but the increase in solubility normally observed is not adequate for use in pharmaceutical products.

Salt Formation

Salt-forming agents often are chosen empirically by the pharmaceutical chemist primarily on the basis of the cost of raw materials, ease of recrystallization and percentage yield. Unfortunately, there is no reliable way of predicting the influence of a particular salt species on the behavior of the parent compound in dosage forms. Furthermore, even when many

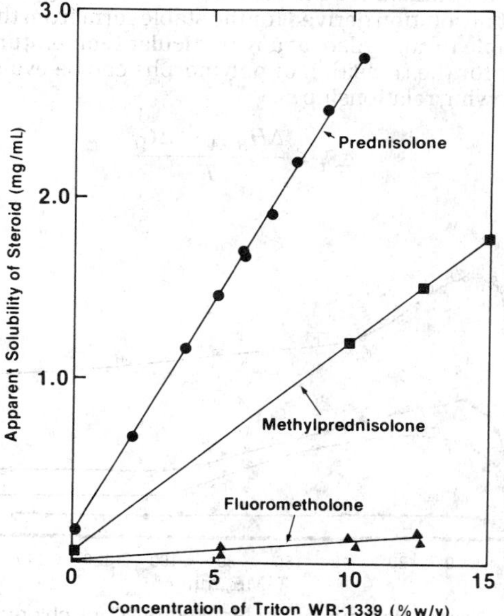

Fig 16. The effect of varying concentrations of Triton WR-1339 in water on the solubility of some anti-inflammatory steroids.[7]

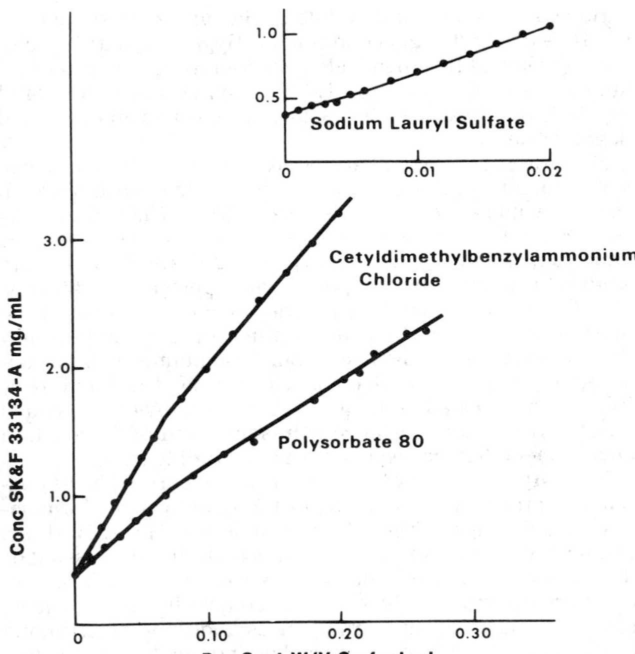

Fig 17. Effect of surfactant concentration on the solubility of SK&F 33134-A.

Table 2—FDA-Approved Commercially Marketed Salts

Anion	Percent[a]	Anion	Percent[a]
Acetate	1.26	Iodide	2.02
Benzenesulfonate	0.25	Isethionate[i]	0.88
Benzoate	0.51	Lactate	0.76
Bicarbonate	0.13	Lactobionate	0.13
Bitartrate	0.63	Malate	0.13
Bromide	4.68	Maleate	3.03
Calcium edetate	0.25	Mandelate	0.38
Camsylate[b]	0.25	Mesylate	2.02
Carbonate	0.38	Methylbromide	0.76
Chloride	4.17	Methylnitrate	0.38
Citrate	3.03	Methylsulfate	0.88
Dihydrochloride	0.51	Mucate	0.13
Edetate	0.25	Napsylate	0.25
Edisylate[c]	0.38	Nitrate	0.64
Estolate[d]	0.13	Pamoate (Embonate)	1.01
Esylate[e]	0.13	Pantothenate	0.25
Fumarate	0.25	Phosphate/diphosphate	3.16
Gluceptate[f]	0.18	Polygalacturonate	0.13
Gluconate	0.51	Salicylate	0.88
Glutamate	0.25	Stearate	0.25
Glycollylarsanilate[g]	0.13	Subacetate	0.38
Hexylresorcinate	0.13	Succinate	0.38
Hydrabamine[h]	0.25	Sulfate	7.46
Hydrobromide	1.90	Tannate	0.88
Hydrochloride	42.98	Tartrate	3.54
Hydroxynaphthoate	0.25	Teoclate[j]	0.13
		Triethiodide	0.13

Cation	Percent[a]	Cation	Percent[a]
Organic:		Metallic:	
Benzathine[k]	0.66	Aluminum	0.66
Chloroprocaine	0.33	Calcium	10.49
Choline	0.33	Lithium	1.64
Diethanolamine	0.98	Magnesium	1.31
Ethylenediamine	0.66	Potassium	10.82
Meglumine[l]	2.29	Sodium	61.97
Procaine	0.66	Zinc	2.95

[a] Percent is based on total number of anionic or cationic salts in use through 1974. [b] Camphorsulfonate. [c] 1,2-Ethanedisulfonate. [d] Lauryl sulfate. [e] Ethanesulfonate. [f] Glucoheptonate. [g] *p*-Glycollamidophenylarsonate. [h] *N,N'*-Di(dehydroabietyl)ethylenediamine. [i] 2-Hydroxyethanesulfonate. [j] 8-Chlorotheophyllinate. [k] *N,N'*-Dibenzylethylenediamine. [l] *N*-Methylglucamine.

salts of the basic compound have been prepared, there are no effective screening techniques which make the selection process of the salt an easier task for the pharmacist. The fundamental considerations which may have some influence on salt selection are physical and chemical stability, hygroscopicity, flowability and solubility.

The number of salt forms available to the chemist is large. Table 2 lists the cations and anions present in FDA-approved commercially marketed salts of pharmaceutical agents.[10] The monoprotic hydrochlorides have been the most frequent choice of the available anionic salt-forming radicals, while sodium has been the most predominant cation. During preformulation evaluation it is extremely important to establish that the particular salt form in question will have properties that will result in a minimum of problems during the development of the dosage forms. Since toxicity studies usually are initiated soon after a compound has been designated for further studies in man, it is important that the salt form selected has been given a critical evaluation to determine whether or not its properties are suitable.

Since physical and chemical stability are vital to any pharmaceutical product, it is imperative that the preformulator evaluate both parameters. A systematic determination of the thermal stability, solution stability (at several pH's) and light-sensitivity of the drug substance provides essential input toward the selection of the most suitable derivative. Studies usually are initiated early to identify problems. Samples of the salts in question usually are placed under exaggerated conditions of heat and light in the presence and absence of moisture and subsequently analyzed to determine the amount of breakdown. In many instances stability-indicating analytical methods may not be available. In these cases it is necessary to resort to thin-layer chromatography to establish a qualitative assessment of stability. At the same time, samples are placed under high-humidity conditions and weighed periodically to determine the degree of hygroscopicity of the compounds. Compounds that have a tendency to adsorb or absorb moisture may present flowability problems during encapsulation.

Solubility characteristics also are evaluated. When a particular salt form has very good solubility (greater than 10%) it sometimes is difficult to prepare a suitable granulation using an aqueous granulating fluid, especially for high doses. Granulations prepared by these methods will not dry satisfactorily or the granulation will not flow uniformly from the hopper, resulting in a large weight variation during the compression stage. A critical evaluation of this type with different salt forms has been proven quite effective in enabling the preformulator to make the selection of the salt form of choice for further development.

Compressibility and Compactibility

Tablets remain a preferred dosage form, and information obtained during preformulation studies on the ability of powdered drugs to be compressed and compacted can be a valuable aid to formulators. Compressibility and compactibility relate directly to tableting performance. Compressibility can be defined as the ability of a powder to decrease in volume under pressure, while compactibility can be defined as the ability of a powder to be compressed into a tablet of a certain strength or hardness. Even though powdered drugs usually are formulated with excipients to modify compression and compaction properties, the properties of the powdered drug alone may be the primary determinant of its ability to be manufactured into a tablet. Significant differences in compression and compaction behavior often can be observed in different lots of the same drug. For example, changes in crystallization or milling procedures may produce differences in behavior.

Compression and compaction most often are evaluated by measuring the tensile strength and hardness of compacts. Tensile strength commonly is measured by diametral compression of round tablets, where the analysis of strength accounts for the dimensions of the tablet.[11] Transverse compression of square compacts between platens narrower than the compact is reported to provide more reproducible results on a wider variety of powders.

Hardness can be defined as the resistance of a solid to local permanent deformation. Deformation hardness tests usually are measured by static impression or dynamic methods. The static method involves the formation of a permanent indentation on a solid surface by a gradual and regularly increasing stress load. Hardness is determined by the load and size of the indentation and is expressed as force per unit area. In dynamic tests, the solid surface is exposed to an abrupt impact such as a swinging pendulum or an indenter allowed to fall under gravity onto the surface. Hardness then is determined from the rebound height of the pendulum or the volume of the resulting indentation.

Hiestand has used adaptations of a compression test and a hardness test to obtain measurements that are used to formulate three dimensionless parameters or indices.[12] The indices are used to characterize the relative tableting performance of individual components or mixtures. The *Strain Index* is the ratio of dynamic indentation hardness to reduced Young's modulus. The *Bonding Index* is the ratio of tensile strength to indentation hardness. The *Brittle Fracture Index* is obtained by comparing the tensile strengths of square compacts with and without a hole at their center. The indices themselves do not measure intrinsic properties of a chemical compound, but rather the traits that influence the tableting performance of a specific lot of chemical. It is necessary to know the magnitude of all three indices to predict the variety of tableting properties that may be incurred. Such information can act as a guide in selecting excipients to overcome problem properties of a drug ingredient.

Chemical Properties

The evaluation of the physical and chemical stability of a new drug substance is an important function of the preformulation group. The initial work should be designed to identify those factors that may result in an alteration of the drug substance under study. The physical pharmacist initially can anticipate the possible type of breakdown that a compound will be subjected to by examination of the chemical structure of the compound. For example, esters and amides are sensitive to hydrolytic degradation while acridanes and catecholamines are sensitive to oxidative degradation. With this preliminary knowledge one may more effectively design studies to identify the problems early. At this point the primary concern is not the pathway or mechanism of degradation. A stability-indicating method of analysis usually is not available early in the preformulation phase. Techniques such as thin-layer chromatography, diffuse reflectance and thermal analysis can be used to provide data to assess preliminary stability. Sometimes, the preliminary evaluation is complicated by the presence of impurities. It is essential that the drug under study be pure before any stability tests are undertaken. The presence of impurities can lead to erroneous conclusions in the preformulation evaluation.

Drug Substance Stability—It is extremely important to determine the stability of the bulk chemical as early as possible. One hardly would expect to prepare stable dosage forms with a chemical substance that was not stable in the pure state. Samples of the chemical are subjected usually to various conditions of light, heat and moisture in the presence and absence of oxygen. The chemical is placed in sealed vials with and without moisture and stored at various elevated temperatures which may vary to some degree from laboratory to laboratory. Light-sensitivity is measured by exposing the surface of the compound to light. Sunlamps are sometimes used to exaggerate light conditions. Hygroscopicity is evaluated by placing the chemical in open petri dishes at relative humidities from 30 to 100%. The samples are monitored regularly for physical changes, moisture pickup and chemical degradation.

Most drug substances are either stable at all conditions, stable under special conditions of handling, unstable with special handling or completely unstable. When drug substances are found to have some stability problems, it may be important to define the pathway of degradation and initiate studies to stabilize the compound with appropriate additives.

At this point, it may be advisable to consider some of the more prominent reactions accounting for instability of new drug substances. Obviously, some compounds will not undergo any appreciable decomposition if kept dry and away from air in a sealed container. It must always be assumed that the new drug substance is in some kind of formulation environment that may lead to instability problems.

Hydrolytic Degradation—Hydrolysis is probably the degradative process encountered most frequently in the formulation of new drugs. It is safe to assume that most new drugs will be exposed to water at some stage during processing or during storage; hence, hydrolysis may occur unless the conditions are optimum. Hydrolysis occurs with esters, amides, salts of weak acids and strong bases and thioesters, among others. A few drug compounds that undergo hydrolytic degradation are procaine, penicillin, aspirin and chlorothiazide.

From a kinetic standpoint, hydrolysis reactions are second-order reactions because the rate is proportional to the concentration of two reactants. However, in aqueous solutions, since water is usually present in excess and at relatively constant concentration, the reactions are treated experimentally as monomolecular or first-order reactions. This simplification permits calculations of the extent of decomposition under precise experimental conditions by less-complicated means. Extrapolation of the exaggerated rates to room temperature makes it possible to establish more expeditiously shelf-life stability of potential new drug products.

The rate of hydrolysis can be affected by temperature and by hydrogen or hydroxyl ion concentration when the hydrolytic process is dependent on pH. Figure 18 shows the pseudo-first-order behavior as a function of pH for carbuterol in aqueous solution at constant ionic strength at 85°. The effect of temperature is illustrated in Fig 19 for carbuterol at pH 4.0 and 10.0 respectively.[13] For solids, the amount of moisture present is minimal. When considering a drug substance that undergoes hydrolytic degradation, studies are designed to establish the conditions of pH and buffer concentration where minimum decomposition occurs. There sometimes is a wide range of pH adjustment which a drug substance can tolerate, and then sometimes the range is narrow. For example, CI-988, a dipeptoid cholecystokinin-B receptor antagonist, was shown to have maximum stability between pH 6.0 and 6.5. The pH-rate stability profile,

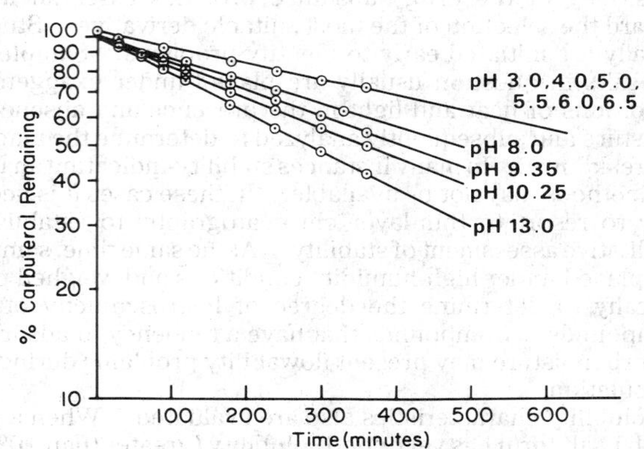

Fig 18. Effect of pH on carbuterol degradation at 85° (μ = 0.5).

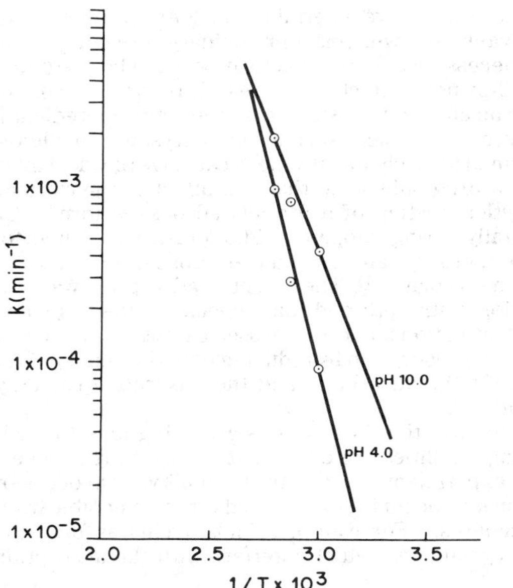

Fig 19. Typical Arrhenius-type plot depicting the temperature dependency of carbuterol hydrolysis at pH 4.0 and 10.0.

which was shown to be independent of salt form, is shown in Fig 20.[14] It is described by two reaction pathways: spontaneous or water-catalyzed degradation of the nonionized form and specific base-catalyzed degradation of the ionized form. A similar pH-rate stability profile, as shown in Fig 21, was found to occur for the lactamization of gabapentin.[15] In aqueous solution, gabapentin undergoes an intramolecular aminolysis to yield a stable, cyclized lactam product over the pH range of 1.4 to 11.1, with maximum stability occuring at pH 6.0. The buffer-independent pH-rate profile was described by two reaction pathways: a specific acid-catalyzed and specific base-catalyzed lactamization of the uncharged species. Another drug substance, carbuterol, hydrolyzed by an intramolecular process showed maximum stability over a wide pH range. Even though these compounds exhibited a wide range of pH for optimum stability in aqueous solution, they could not be formulated and provide products with satisfactory shelf lives without special cosolvent systems and/or special storage conditions. Buffering aqueous solutions to provide a pH for optimum stability can lead to stability problems. Stability sometimes is affected by buffer concen-

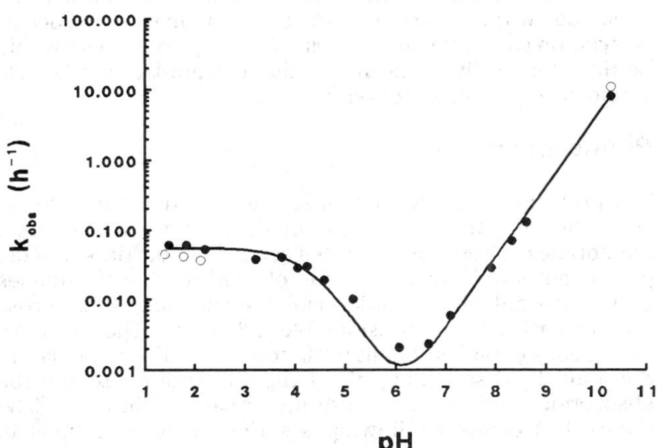

Fig 20. pH-rate profile for the degradation of CI-988 meglumine (○) and CI-988 sodium (●) at 80° and μ = 0.5*M* (with NaCl). The line represents the theoretical profile generated with nonlinear least-squares regression of the experimental data (●).

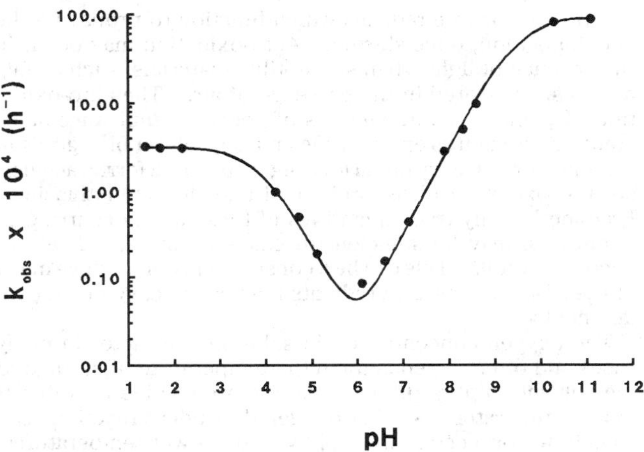

Fig 21. pH-rate profile for the lactamization of gabapentin at 80° and μ = 0.5*M* (with NaCl). The line represents the theoretical profile generated with nonlinear least-squares regression of the experimental data (●).

tration; for example, carbuterol stability was shown to be affected by phosphate buffer concentration.

Another manner in which the preformulation scientist can overcome an instability due to hydrolysis is to recommend the preparation of an insoluble salt form or to prepare a solid dosage form. Insoluble chlorothiazide is stable in neutral aqueous suspensions, but solutions of the sodium salt at relatively high pH decompose rapidly. Frequently, the replacement of water by some other solvent, such as alcohol or the polyhydroxy solvents, reduces the hydrolytic rate of degradation for some systems. Acetylsalicylic acid suspensions containing high concentrations of sorbitol improved stability. Ampicillin also was shown to be more stable when the concentration of alcohol was increased. The formation of molecular complexes with aromatic esters greatly reduces the hydrolytic rate of degradation.

It also has been shown that stability of some compounds may vary depending on whether or not they exist in the micellar or nonmicellar state. For example, a difference in the chemical stability of penicillin exists in the micellar state from that in the monomeric state.

Oxidation—Oxidative degradation is as important as hydrolysis in the preliminary stability evaluation of new-drug substances. Studies should be initiated to establish the oxidative route, then steps should be taken to determine what additives can minimize the degradation. Oxidative degradation is common with many drug compounds. Ascorbic acid, epinephrine, vitamin A, chlorpromazine, isoproterenol, morphine, resorcinol and unsaturated fats and oils are subject to oxidative degradation. The oxidation reaction depends on several factors, including temperature, oxygen concentration in the liquid, impurities present and the concentration of the oxidizable component. The temperature effect in solutions is usually minimal; however, in the dry state it is more pronounced since other factors such as moisture dictate its stability behavior.

Initially, it is important to establish that oxidation is taking place. Solutions of the drug substance in question are exposed to various exaggerated conditions of light and oxygen tension in amber and flint-glass containers. Samples are analyzed for degradation. When it has been established that the oxidative route is the principal pathway for degradation, appropriate additives are used to determine what effect they might have on the stability. Sometimes pH is critical, since a great number of oxidation-reduction processes depend on the concentration of hydrogen or hydroxyl ions. Light usually accelerates degradation, thus the storage of products in dark containers does much to preserve stability. Photochemical changes many times involve the formation of other reactive compounds or free radicals which function to propagate the decomposition, once started. Auto-oxidation may occur in the absence of light when susceptible materials, such as fats and oils, are stored in the presence of air. The auto-oxidation of phenolic compounds is of special significance since compounds such as epinephrine and isoproterenol degrade in this manner. Heavy metal ions, eg, cupric and ferric, accelerate the oxidation of ascorbic acid and the phenothiazines. Frequently, only trace quantities of these ions, occurring as impurities, may be sufficient to cause an increased rate of decomposition. This can be a consistent problem since many of the so-called inert ingredients may have heavy metal contaminants.

The oxygen concentration in solution is a factor in many cases and often depends upon the temperature of storage or the solvent employed. Oxygen is more soluble in water at lower temperatures so that oxygen-dependent reactions can sometimes proceed more rapidly at the lower temperatures. Ascorbic acid is more stable in 90% propylene glycol or in Syrup USP than in water, presumably because of the lower oxygen concentration in these vehicles. Oxidative degradation is an extremely complex process since the overall rate is dependent upon several factors. Preparations sensitive to oxidation are sometimes stabilized by effectively removing the oxygen and by the addition of suitable additives. Nitrogen flushing has been used successfully for this purpose. A wide variety of reducing agents and compounds to sequester metals and inhibit chain reactions has been employed for stabilization, but relatively few are acceptable for parenteral products. Often, it is necessary to combine ingredients and adjust pH to maximize stability. Detailed kinetic studies have been reported for the oxidative decomposition of prednisolone.

The physical pharmacist has a difficult task with oxidative degradation. Initially, experiments must be designed that will encompass many variables. Preparing samples at several concentrations containing antioxidants plus sequestering agents at several pH levels and placing them in flint or amber containers with and without nitrogen is a common procedure. The subsequent evaluation of these limited data is critical. Light-sensitivity studies with several formulations of prochlorperazine resulted in the selection of a stable formula. In a study with idoxuridine it was shown that placing the aqueous solution in an amber container was sufficient to protect the product from oxidative degradation.

Drug Substance–Excipient Interaction—Drug substance–excipient studies are designed to determine a list of excipients that can be used routinely in the final dosage forms. Lactose, sucrose, calcium sulfate, dicalcium phosphate, starch and magnesium stearate are some of the substances routinely tested in combinations. Some basic observations with the drug substance and/or its salt form sometimes can dictate what excipients can be used. For example, one would not consider using sucrose or lactose if the drug substance being considered is a primary amine. This system has the potential for interaction to form a colored compound readily detected by a color change.

Various means have been used for detecting potential interactions and incompatibilities. Diffuse reflectance techniques have been used to detect interactions. This has been done by comparing the spectra obtained initially with those obtained after storage at exaggerated conditions. A shift in absorption has been interpreted as an interaction. Thin-layer chromatography also has been used. When excipients are present it is usually advisable to set a mixture of the excipients at the same conditions as the excipient-drug mixtures. This will give a comparison of the chromatograms of both systems. If any new degradation products are present, the source may be determined more easily.

Mixtures containing at least two levels of drug concentration with excipients are sealed in vials containing 5% water. These vials are stored under exaggerated conditions of light and heat for various time periods. The resultant samples are observed physically and analyzed by an appropriate technique to get a qualitative determination. At this point in the stability evaluation, which is a preliminary screening process, it is not necessary to know exactly how much has degraded. It is an all-or-none effect. The search is for the excipients that have no effect on the stability of the active ingredient.

Even an excipient such as microcrystalline cellulose, often assumed to be chemically inert, can have physical interactions with a drug substance that can affect the performance and analytical testing of a formulated dosage form. CI-977, a centrally acting kappa-opioid agonist, was found to adsorb onto microcrystalline cellulose, croscarmellose and sodium starch glycolate.[16] The extent of adsorption was affected by pH, ionic strength and ionic species. Results showed that divalent cations, and to a lesser extent monovalent cations, inhibited adsorption by reducing both the affinity of the adsorbent for the adsorbate, and the adsorptive capacity of the adsorbent.

When solution interactions are being investigated and no incompatibilities are evident, it is wise to recommend an *in vivo* experiment to evaluate availability. On occasion, interaction may occur in solution that is not detectable with routine procedures. For example, clindamycin was found to interact with cyclamates, which interfere with the absorption of the drug.

Other Changes—Optically active substances may lose their optical activity; eg, through racemization. If the entiomorphic compounds possess different degrees of physiologic action, such changes may result in reduced therapeutic effects. The FDA is constantly adopting stricter guidelines for the development of stereoisomeric drugs.[17,18] Even though stereoisomeric pairs essentially may have the same physical (except for optical rotation) and chemical (except in a chiral environment) properties, they are often readily distinguishable by biological systems. The development of racemic mixtures raises issues of acceptable manufacturing control of synthesis and impurities, adequate pharmacological and toxicological assessment, proper characterization of metabolism and distribution, and appropriate clinical evaluation. Hence, the interconversion from one isomer to another can lead to different pharmacokinetic properties (absorption, distribution, biotransformation and excretion) and quantitatively or qualitatively different pharmacological or toxicological effects. Epinephrine has been shown to undergo racemization under various acidic and basic conditions. Although the potential for this to become evident during a preformulation evaluation is rare, one should always be aware of this possibility. Polymerization is also a remote possibility. Darkening of glucose solution is attributed to polymerization of the breakdown product, 5-(hydroxymethyl)furfural. Isomerization, which is the process involving the change of one structure into another having the same empirical formula but with different properties in one or more respects, also can occur; again, the occurrence is rare. Deamination and decarboxylation can occur sometimes. This type of change would be detected easily since the resultant degradation products would have completely different properties.

Permeability

A preformulation evaluation should include studies to assess the passage of drug molecules across biological membranes. These membranes act as lipid barriers to most drugs and permit the absorption of lipid-soluble substances by passive diffusion. Lipid-insoluble substances can cross the barrier only with considerable difficulty. The pH-partition theory explains the interrelationship of the dissociation constant, lipid solubility, pH at the absorption site and the absorption characteristics of drugs across membranes. The theory has evolved following a series of investigations in laboratory animals and man and is the basis of much of the current understanding of absorption of drugs.

Data obtained from basic physical-chemical studies described earlier may give the preformulation scientist an indication of possible absorption difficulties. Experimental techniques are available that can be used to give a more accurate assessment of absorption problems. An *in vitro* system that has been used extensively consists of an aqueous/organic solvent/aqueous system which has the advantage of being simple, allows for accurate pH control, membrane thickness and other variables. It can be described mathematically in precise terms. However, the interpretation and correlation of data are limited when applied to biologic systems.

Another *in vitro* procedure, the everted sac technique, is a simple and reproducible method for determining the absorption characteristics of drugs. Isolated segments of rat small intestines are everted and filled with a solution of the drug being evaluated, and the passage of drug through the membrane is determined. This technique has been used to measure the permeability of a number of drug substances.[19] It also can evaluate both passive and active transport of drugs. The fact that the preparation has been removed from the animal and its normal blood supply is a distinct disadvantage.

The *in situ* technique developed by Doluisio, *et al*,[20] for the study of membrane permeability appears to overcome the disadvantages of the everted sac technique. Since the intestine is not removed from its blood supply, the results would be expected to be similar to those obtained in intact animals. A disadvantage of the technique is that the procedure does not account for the loss of fluid from the solution by absorption in the intestine. Nonabsorbable markers, such as phenol red, can be added to the drug solution to solve this problem.

The techniques described can give the preformulation scientist an indication of possible absorption problems or suggest that little or no difficulty will be observed in the passage of a particular drug product through the biological membranes. This information, along with eventual studies in man, serves to establish possible *in vitro / in vivo* correlation for dissolution and bioavailability. These data are important in establishing quality-control specifications for the products which will ensure consistent biological performance from subsequent lots.

Proteins and Peptides

Proteins and peptides produced by the commercialization of biotechnology are presenting preformulation scientists with new challenges. In general, protein and peptide drugs are more expensive to produce, more potent and more difficult to analyze than nonprotein and nonpeptide drugs. They frequently are formulated as parenterals instead of oral dosage forms because they are unable to be absorbed from the GI tract, unstable in GI fluids or subject to rapid first-pass metabolism. Degradation of proteins and peptides occurs not only by covalent bond reaction but also by denaturation. The prediction of shelf-life by the Arrhenius equation is usually not applicable.

Degradation by reaction of the covalent bond can be characterized by the following major reactions: hydrolysis, transpeptidation, racemization, oxidation, diketopiperazine formation, disulfide exchange and photodecomposition. Hydrolysis can occur at the peptide linkage (R-NH-CO-R), but it is more stable than the ester linkage (R-O-CO-R) unless cleavage is assisted by a neighboring group. Hence, peptides such as oxytocin and captopril are stable enough for liquid parenteral formulations. Transpeptidation occurs when amino acid residues cyclize back onto the peptide chain and the cyclic intermediate undergoes hydrolysis. Racemization can occur in acidic or alkaline medium, and if proline or glycine occur in the *N*-terminal position, diketopiperazine formation is facilitated. Cysteine, methionine and tryptophan are susceptible to oxidation, and since disulfide exchange is concentration-dependent, oligomers are formed frequently as a result of the creation of disulfide bonds between peptide chains. Photodecomposition of tryptophan residues may lead to discoloration and photoproducts of increased molecular weight.

Degradation via denaturation occurs when the conformational structure of a protein or peptide is altered. Potential factors that can denature a molecule include ionic strength, surface-active agents or processing conditions that subject the molecule to shear or adsorption. Identification of the preferred conformation, and mechanisms by which it can be altered, is critical in formulating the molecule as a stable drug. Hydrogen bonds act to stabilize conformational structure and the presence of water promotes hydrogen bonding. Hence, agents that disrupt the water-protein interaction such as salts and molecules with ionic side chains can promote conformational instability.

The increased size of the protein molecule, as compared to more traditional synthetic organic drug molecules, complicates traditional analytical methods and makes any one method itself inadequate to fully quantitate and characterize the protein. Consequently, an array of analytical methods is required and stability studies are a complex and time-consuming exercise. Usually, characterization of the protein requires probing each structural or functional feature of the molecule. Characterization assays may include amino acid sequence, isoelectric point, molecular size and glycosylation pattern. An electrophoretic technique, sodium dodecyl sulfate polyacrylamide gel electrophoresis (SDS-PAGE), is the most common technique for determination of molecular weight. Gel-permeation chromatography and ultracentrifugation also are used to determine molecular size and size distribution. HPLC chromatographic techniques, such as reversed-phase, ion-exchange and size-exclusion, are being used increasingly to quantitate proteins.

Several methods can be used to study denaturation of proteins. These include thermal analysis, determination of critical micelle concentration, determination of cloud-point, light scattering and fluorescence spectrometry. Thermal analysis with a scanning microcalorimeter is used to measure energies of transition in solution and is useful for determining the effect of stabilizing excipients on proteins in solution. Measurement of the critical micelle concentration also can be used as a tool to study the ability of an excipient to stabilize or disrupt the hydrophobic interactions which promote micellerization. Cloud-point measurements (the temperature, when cooled, at which a solution becomes cloudy) also have been suggested as a tool to study the effects of solvents or excipients on denaturation. Fluorescence spectrometry can be used to measure thermal denaturation by using a fluorescent probe whose fluorescence increases when a protein is denatured.

The ultimate analytical procedure for proteins is the bioassay that evaluates the desired biological activity. Even though bioassays determine the biological activity of the molecule, these tests usually show large assay variability. In addition, they are often unable to distinguish between two similarly acting proteins. Even so, regulatory agencies typically require a bioassay as part of any stability protocol.

Proteins and peptides can be stabilized in many ways, usually employing empirical, rather than theoretical, procedures. For parenteral formulations, excipients are added to enhance stability. Serum albumin, itself a relatively stable protein, is used commonly as a stabilizer for peptides and proteins. It may inhibit surface adsorption and act as a cryoprotectant during lyophilization. Amino acids, such as glutamic or aspartic acid, may chelate metals such as zinc, which may cause aggregation; however, metal ions, such as calcium, are essential to the stability of certain amylases and proteases. Phospholipids and fatty acids also are potential stabilizers. Even though surfactants have a high denaturing effect, they also may inhibit the effects of other denaturants.

Proteins, as opposed to nonprotein drugs, may find a dilute aqueous medium unfavorable. Therefore, one should attempt to create an environment similar to the natural habitat of the specific protein. This environment would be rich in proteins and carbohydrates, low in oxygen and have a high degree of immobilized water. However, as methodologies for studying denaturation and degradation become more defined, the number of excipients needed to stabilize a formulation can be limited selectively.

Formulation Ingredients

Although preliminary screening of commonly used excipients with new-drug substances has become routine in preformulation studies, there are occasions when problems arise because of the interaction with additives such as preservatives, stabilizers, dyes and, possibly, flavors. A discussion of some problems that have risen is in order to make formulators aware that they should be concerned about the potential for interaction whenever another ingredient is added to a formulation.

Preservatives—Each time a liquid or semisolid pharmaceutical dosage form is prepared, it is necessary to include a preservative in the formulation. Such preservatives as sodium benzoate, sorbic acid and the methyl and propyl esters of *p*-hydroxybenzoic acid (parabens) have been used in these systems for many years. There have been reports that the parabens have been inactivated when used in the presence of various surface-active agents and vegetable gums. This loss of activity might be due to the formation of complexes between the preservative and the surfactant. A dialysis technique has been used to demonstrate an interaction between polysorbate 80 and the parabens. This observation becomes critical if the level of preservative added is borderline with respect to the preservative-activity threshold. The desired preservative effect may not be achieved unless an excess of the preservative is added to compensate for that which is complexed. It also has been shown that molecular complexes form when the parabens are mixed with polyethylene glycol, methylcellulose, polyvinylpyrrolidone or gelatin. The degree of binding was less than that observed with polysorbate 80. Sorbic acid also interacts with polysorbates but does not interact with polyethylene glycols. The quaternary ammonium compounds also are bound by polysorbate 80 to reduce their preservative activity. Benzyl alcohol also was shown to be adsorbed by certain types of rubber stoppers. Subsequent work has shown that butyl rubber does not interact with benzyl alcohol.

Antioxidants—During the preformulation evaluation of compounds that are sensitive to oxidation often it is commonplace to test several levels of antioxidant concentrations added to aqueous systems in order to determine the relative effectiveness of the antioxidants. Sodium bisulfite and ascorbic acid are two antioxidants that are used widely in pharmaceutical systems. Sodium bisulfite yields a colorless water-soluble salt when it is oxidized. It will add to double bonds, react with aldehydes and certain ketones and contributes in bisulfite cleavage reactions. Many of the reactions with bisulfite are irreversible, and the resulting sulfonic acids frequently are biologically inactive. Epinephrine has been shown to interact with bisulfite to form a bisulfite addition product. Other sympathomimetic drugs, principally the *ortho-* or *para*-hydroxybenzyl alcohol derivatives, also react with bisulfite in a similar manner. The *meta*-hydroxy alcohol does not react. Sometimes these interactions are reversible as in the case with the adrenocorticosteroid molecules.

Ascorbic acid, on the other hand, is less reactive. However, when mixed with compounds having a primary amine nucleus, there is the tendency for interaction to form a highly colored Schiff base. One must be aware of this possibility when selecting a suitable antioxidant.

Suspending Agents—Occasionally, it will be necessary to consider the use of a suspending agent to prepare some preliminary suspension preparations for stability evaluation prior to starting toxicity testing. The physical pharmacist should be aware of the potential for these additives to react with the drug substance being evaluated. Anionic water-soluble compounds, such as sodium carboxymethylcellulose, alginic acid, carrageenin and other hydrocolloids, although generally considered inert, frequently interact with drug compounds in solution. Carboxymethylcellulose and carrageenin form complexes, or possibly salts, with many medicinal agents including procaine, chlorpromazine, benadryl, quinine, chlorpheniramine, neomycin and kanamycin. In some instances the formation of the complex imparted better stability to the system. When this problem is suspected, it is important to conduct appropriate tests to insure that an interaction does not take place in the system being evaluated.

Dyes—Although preformulation tests usually are conducted long before any consideration of coloring the intended dosage forms, they should not be overlooked. Dyes are chemical in nature and contain reactive sites capable of causing incompatibilities. Several studies have demonstrated that certified dyes do react with drug substances. Sugars, such as dextrose, lactose and sucrose, were found to increase the rate of fading of FD&C Blue #2. Insoluble complexes also were formed when quaternary ammonium compounds were formulated with FD&C Blue #1.

Summary

The preformulation evaluation of new-drug substances has become an integral part of the development process. A thorough understanding of the physical-chemical properties of the new-drug substance under study provides the development pharmacist with data that are essential in designing stable and efficacious dosage forms. Many of the problems discussed and the solutions offered in this chapter resulted from application of scientific training of present-day pharmaceutical scientists. Their diverse skills, creative aptitudes and initiative provide the pharmaceutical industry with the essential ingredients to develop drug products that help maintain the health-care process at its highest level of excellence.

References

1. Hussain A: *J Pharm Sci 61:* 811, 1972.
2. Dittert LW, *et al:* *Ibid 57:* 1146, 1968.
3. Dittert LW, *et al:* *J Pharm Sci 57:* 1269, 1968.
4. Zingerman JP, *et al:* *Int J Pharm 88:* 303, 1992.
5. Haleblain H, McCrone W: *J Pharm Sci 58:* 911, 1969.
6. Ravin LJ, Higuchi T: *J APhA Sci Ed 46:* 732, 1957.
7. Aguiar A, Zelmer JE: *J Pharm Sci 58:* 983, 1969.
8. Spiegel AJ, Noseworthy MM: *Ibid 52:* 917, 1963.
9. Guttman DE, *et al:* *Ibid 50:* 305, 1961.
10. Berge SM, Bighley LD, Monkhouse DC: *Ibid 66:* 1, 1977.
11. Fell J, Newton J: *Ibid 59:* 688, 1970.
12. Hiestand H, Smith D: *Powder Tech 38:* 145, 1984.
13. Ravin LJ, *et al:* *J Pharm Sci 67:* 1523, 1978.
14. Kearney AS, Mehta SC, Radebaugh GW: *Pharm Res 9:* 1092, 1992.
15. Kearney AS, Mehta SC, Radebaugh GW: *Int J Pharm 78:* 25, 1992.
16. Senderoff RI, Mahjour M, Radebaugh GW: *Int J Pharm 83:* 65, 1992.
17. *Fed Reg 57:* 22249, 1992.
18. Stinson SC: *C&E News:* Sep 28, 1992.
19. Kaplan SA, Cotler S: *J Pharm Sci 61:* 1361, 1972.
20. Doluisio JT, *et al:* *Ibid 58:* 1196, 1969.

Bibliography

Carstensen JT: *Pharmaceutics of Solids and Solid Dosage Forms*, Wiley, New York, 1977.

Fiese EF, Hagan TA: Preformulation. In Lachman L, Lieberman HA, Kanig JL, eds: *The Theory and Practice of Industrial Pharmacy*, Lea & Febiger, Philadelphia, Chap 8, 1986.

Leuenberger H, Rohera BD: *Pharm Res 3:* 12, 1986.

Pearlman R, Nguyen TH: Analysis of protein drugs. In Lee VHL, ed: *Peptide and Protein Drug Delivery*, Dekker, New York, Chap 6, 1991.

Wang YJ, Hanson M: *J Parenter Sci Technol 42 (2S)*: S3, 1988.

Wells JI: *Pharmaceutical Preformulation: The Physicochemical Properties of Drug Substances*, Ellis Horwood Ltd, Chichester, England, 1988.

Zito SW, ed: *Pharmaceutical Biotechnology: A Programmed Text*, Technomic Publ, Lancaster, PA, 1992.

CHAPTER 84

Sterilization

Barry Garfinkle, PhD
Martin Henley, PhD
Merck & Co.
West Point, PA 19486

The aim of a sterilization process is to destroy or eliminate microorganisms which are present on or in an object or preparation, to make sure that this has been achieved with an extremely high level of probability and to assure that the object or preparation is free from infection hazards. The currently accepted performance target for a sterilization process is that it provide for a probability of finding a nonsterile unit of less than one in one million. That is, the process (including production, storage, shipment, etc) will provide a *Sterility Assurance Level* (SAL) equal to or better than 10^{-6}.

The variety and amounts of sterile products and their packages required for health care have increased continuously and been modified in recent years. Accordingly, sterilization technologies have adapted to the changing need. Some of these also are brought about by changing requirements and guidelines issued by regulatory or advisory bodies.

Not many years ago, sterility testing of the finished product was the basic means of monitoring the success of a sterilization process. Today, qualification and validation of the equipment and the process carried out in that equipment is considered essential. This stems from the general principles of Total Quality systems. National and international standards that define this system (ISO9000, EN29000, etc) indeed state that ". . .Sterilization is a *special* process because its efficacy cannot be verified by simple inspection and testing on the final product. . . . For this reason, sterilization processes have to be validated before use, the performance monitored routinely and the equipment regularly maintained. . . ."

The purpose of this chapter is to provide a basic understanding of the following sterilization methods currently being used in pharmaceutical technology and the equipment employed to carry out these methods:

Method	*Equipment*
Moist heat sterilization	Saturated steam autoclaves
	Superheated water autoclaves
	Air over steam autoclaves
Dry heat sterilization	Batch sterilizers
	Continuous tunnel sterilizers
Chemical "Cold" sterilization	Ethylene oxide
	Vaporized hydrogen peroxide
	Hydrogen peroxide/steam
	Other gases
Radiation sterilization	Electromagnetic
	Particulate
Filtration	Membranes

Definitions

The following terms, relating to sterilization, should be understood by those carrying out sterilization processes or handling sterile products:

Antiseptic—A substance that arrests or prevents the growth of microorganisms by inhibiting their activity without necessarily destroying them.

Aseptic Processing—Those operations performed between the sterilization of an object or preparation and the final sealing of its package. These operations are, by definition, carried out in the complete absence of microorganisms.

Bactericide—Any agent which destroys microorganisms.

Bacteriostat—Any agent which arrests or retards the growth of microorganisms.

Bioburden—The number of viable microorganisms in or on an object or preparation entering a sterilization step (usually expressed in colony forming units per unit of volume).

Disinfection—A process which decreases the probability of infection by destroying vegetative microorganisms, but not ordinarily bacterial spores. The term usually is applied to the use of chemical agents on inanimate objects.

Germicide—An agent which destroys microorganisms, but not necessarily bacterial spores.

Sterility—The absence of viable microorganisms.

Sterility Assurance Level (SAL)—A term related to the probability of finding a nonsterile unit following a sterilization step. It usually is expressed in terms of the negative power of 10 (ie, one in one million = 10^{-6}).

Sterilization—A process by which all viable microorganisms are removed or destroyed, based on a probability function.

Terminal Sterilization—A process which destroys all viable microorganisms within the final, sealed package.

Validation—The act of verifying that a procedure is capable of producing the intended result under all expected circumstances. This usually is accomplished through appropriate challenge(s).

Viricide—An agent which will destroy viruses.

Sterility as a Total System

It is necessary to reiterate the concept already briefly addressed in the introduction. The task of the technology we are dealing with is to provide the product in sterile conditions to the end user.

It is currently acknowledged that the *quality* of the product must be "built into" the process. This concept is particularly true when one of the essential qualities of the product is sterility.

Accordingly, the above-mentioned task is accomplished with a series of design, production and distribution steps that can be summarized as activities for the selection and routine checking of the following items:

Active constituents, additives, raw materials in general
Water used both as solvent and as washing/rinsing agent
Packaging suitable for the product and for the sterilization process that will be used
Working environment and equipment
Personnel

These procedures clearly have the purpose of providing the sterilization process with a product that has a minimum, definite and consistent bioburden. There are also the following activities:

Selection of the sterilization method that most suits the unit formed by the product and its packaging, and definition of the process variables for obtaining the intended SAL
Selection of the machine that is most suitable for performing the selected method and of the utilities that this machine requires
Qualification and validation of the machine and of the process
Routine checking of the process
Checking of the results of the sterilization process
Proper storage of sterile goods and verification that their sterility is maintained with full reliability throughout the allowed storage period
Delivering, opening and using sterile goods without recontamination.

It also should be noted that, on October 11, 1991, the FDA proposed new regulations for aseptic processing and terminal sterilization. The proposed rules requires manufacturers of sterile products to use terminal sterilization wherever possible. The proposal will affect 21 CFR 211, 314 and 514. Aseptic processing may be used only in those cases where terminal sterilization has significant detrimental effects on the product. This ruling is based on the ability to prove higher SAL's with current terminal sterilization processes, thus reducing the risk of a nonsterile unit reaching the patient.

Contamination

Certain facts about microorganisms must be kept in mind when preparing sterile products. Some microbes (bacteria, molds, etc) multiply in the refrigerator, others at temperatures as high as 60°. Microbes vary in their oxygen requirements from the strict anaerobes that cannot tolerate oxygen to aerobes that demand it. Slightly alkaline growth media will support the multiplication of many microorganisms while others flourish in acidic environments. Some microorganisms have the ability to utilize nitrogen and carbon dioxide from the air and thus can actually multiply in distilled water. In general, however, most pathogenic bacteria have rather selective cultural requirements, with optimum temperatures of 30 to 37° and a pH of 7.0. Contaminating yeasts and molds can develop readily in glucose and other sugar solutions.

Actively growing microbes are, for the most part, vegetative forms with little resistance to heat and disinfectants. However, some forms of bacteria—among them the bacteria that cause anthrax, tetanus and gas gangrene—have the ability to assume a spore state, which is very resistant to heat as well as to many disinfectants. For this reason, an excellent measure of successful sterilization is whether the highly resistant spore forms of nonpathogenic bacteria have been killed.

The nature of expected contamination and the bioburden are important to the pharmacist preparing materials to be sterilized. The raw materials he works with rarely will be sterile and improper storage may increase the microbial content. Because the pharmacist seldom handles all raw materials in a sterile or protected environment, the environmental elements of the manufacturing area (air, surfaces, water, etc) can be expected to contribute to the contamination of a preparation. The container or packaging material may or may not be presterilized and thus may contribute to the total microbial load.

Understanding the nature of contaminants prior to sterilization and application of methods for minimizing such contamination is vital to preparing for successful pharmaceutical sterilization. Examples of such methods include:

Maintenance of a hygienic laboratory.
Frequent disinfection of floors and surfaces.
Minimization of traffic in and out of the area.
Refrigerated storage of raw materials and preparations which support microbial growth.
Use of laminar airflow devices (see page to be referenced) for certain critical operations.
Use of water that is of appropriate USP quality and is free of microbial contamination. It is preferrable to use presterilized water to avoid any possible contamination.

Methods

General

The procedure to be used for sterilizing a drug, a pharmaceutical preparation or a medical device is determined to a large extent by the nature of the product. It is important to remember that the same sterilization technique cannot be applied universally because the unique properties of some materials may result in their destruction or modification. Methods of inactivating microorganisms may be classified as either physical or chemical. Physical methods include moist heat, dry heat and irradiation. Sterile filtration is another process, but it only removes, not inactivates, microorganisms. Chemical methods include the use of either gaseous or liquid sterilants. Guidelines for the use of many types of industrial and hospital sterilization are available.[1–10]

Each sterilization method can be evaluated using experimentally derived values representing the general inactivation rates of the process. For example, a death rate or survival curve for a standardized species can be diagrammed for different sterilization conditions. This is done by plotting the logarithm of surviving organisms against time of exposure to the sterilization method. In most instances, these data show a linear relationship, typical of first-order kinetics and suggest that a constant proportion of a contaminant population is inactivated in any given time interval. Based on such inactivation curves, it is possible to derive values that represent the general inactivation rates of the process. For example, based on such data, it has become common to derive a decimal reduction time or D value, which represents the time under a stated set of sterilization exposure conditions required to reduce a surviving microbial population by a factor of 90%.

D values, or other expressions of sterilization process rates, provide a means of establishing dependable sterilization cycles. Obviously, the initial microbial load on a product to be sterilized becomes an important consideration. Beyond this, however, kinetic data also can be used to provide a statistical basis for the success of sterilization cycles. A simple example will suffice (Fig 1). When the initial microbial contamination level is assumed to be 10^6, and if the D value of the sterilization process is 7 minutes, complete kill is approached by application of 6 D values (42 minutes). However, at this point reliable sterilization would not be assured because a few abnormally resistant members of the population may remain. In this example, by extending the process to include an additional 6 D values, most of the remaining population is inactivated, reducing the probability of one organism surviving to one in one million.

Moist Heat

Essentials of Steam Sterilization Kinetics—Let us suppose a system contaminated by microorganisms (which we assume, for the sake of simplicity, to be pure and homogeneous) is immersed in pressurized saturated steam, at constant temperature; for example a vial containing an aqueous suspension of a certain spore-forming microorganism.

It has been shown experimentally that, under the above conditions, the reaction of thermal degradation of the microorganism obeys the laws of chemical reactions: the rate of reduction of the number of microorganisms present in the system in each moment is proportional to the actual number itself. The proportionality coefficient is typical of the species and conditions of the chosen microorganism.

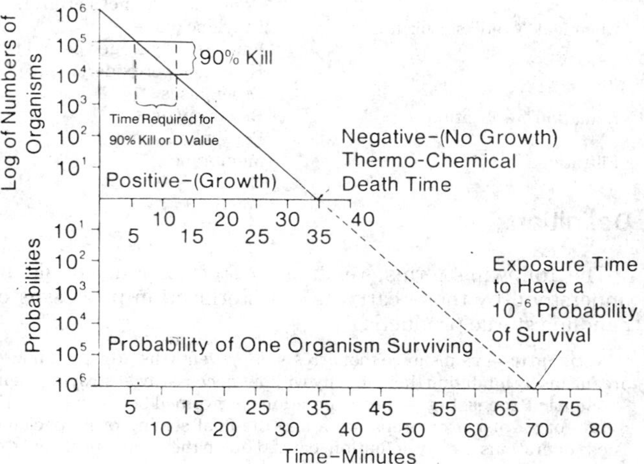

Fig 1. Sterilization model using D values.

The degradation reaction, (the sterilization process) therefore, develops like a first-order chemical reaction in which the reaction rate is proportional, in each moment, only to the amount of microorganisms still to be inactivated. This seems to be obvious for dry sterilization, but less rigorous for steam sterilization, in which the water vapor molecules also seem to take part in the reaction. Actually, this bimolecular reaction is of the first order, since the steam is present in high excess during the entire reaction and its concentration may be regarded as constant.

The most frequently used mathematical expression of the above facts is

$$N = N_0\, 10^{-t/D} \tag{1}$$

where N_0 = initial number of microorganisms, t = elapsed exposure (= sterilization time), N = number of microorganisms after the exposure time t and D = "decimal decay time," defined as the time interval required, at a specified *constant* temperature, to reduce the microbial population being considered by 1/10 (ie, by one logarithmic value, eg, from 100% to 10% or from 10% to 1% of the initial value).

The D value is inversely proportional to the first-order reaction coefficient and is therefore typical of the species and conditions of the chosen microorganism. Depending on the initial hypothesis of exposure at constant temperature, each D value always refers to a specified temperature.

Equation 1 allows one to draw a first very important conclusion: the time required to reduce the microorganism concentration to any preset value is the function of the initial concentration.

The sterilization reaction is therefore neither an "all-or-nothing" process nor a "potential barrier" process as was once thought.

It also is evident immediately that the effect of sterilization at the same constant temperature will be very different depending on the D value of the contaminating microbial species (or on the largest D value in the usual case of mixed contamination). Figure 2 shows that the same reduction ratio for different species is achieved after exposure time proportional to the D value of each species. The graph derives only from Eq 1 and from the definition of D value. The basic hypothesis of the temperature being constant is thoroughly valid.

Sterility Is a "Probable" Effect of Exposure Time—Let us now consider what happens within a batch of units (vials, bottles or others) with an initial constant unit contamination of 100 microorganisms = 10^2. If the D value at 121° is assumed = 1, after 1 minute at 121°, the reduction = to 10^1 = 10 microorganisms is achieved; after another minute, only 10^0 = 1 microorganism is still surviving. After another minute the surviving microbial population would be 10^{-1} = 1/10 microorganism. A contamination of 1/10 must not be understood to mean that each unit contains 1/10 of a microorganism, which is biologically meaningless (in this case the unit probably would be sterile. . .) but that there is a probability of having 1/10 of the units still contaminated within the batch of sterilized units.

In fact, 3 minutes would be the necessary time to reduce the microbial population to a single surviving microorganism if the initial population were ten times larger than the one at issue. This higher initial contamination could be regarded either as a ten times larger number of microorganisms in the same unit, or as the initial contamination of a ten times larger unit.

If the unit is not considered any longer as the single vial or bottle, but as the whole of all the items produced over a period of time, the initial number of microorganisms present in each item has to be multiplied times the number of items produced, and the exposure time to achieve the reduction to the same number of viable microorganisms left in the whole of the items produced, has to be increased correspondingly. The following example will be helpful to focus the matter.

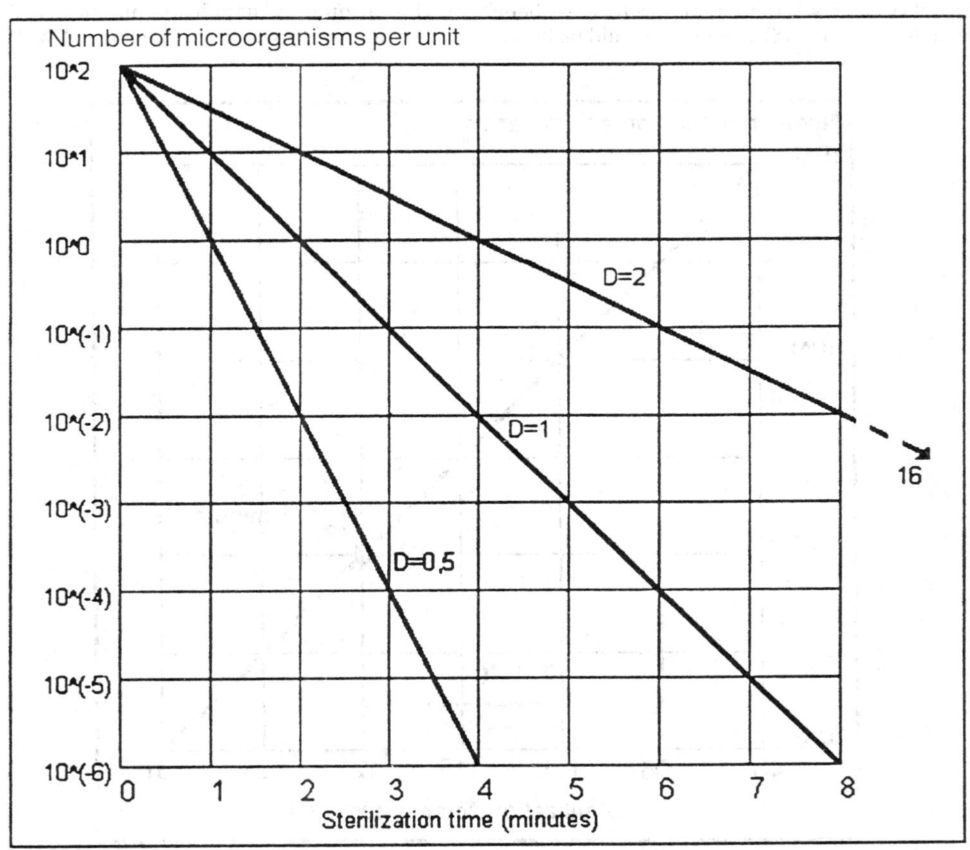

Fig 2. Effect of varying D values on sterilization rate (courtesy, Fedegari Autoclavi).

A new sterile product in ampules has to be manufactured; the number of ampules to be produced over all the life period of the product is expected to be 10^{10}. The maximum number of contaminated ampules deemed to be acceptable is $10^{0} = 1$: this obviously means that the probability of having nonsterile ampules after sterilization must not exceed 10^{-10}. Let us also suppose that the microbial population within each ampule after the filling and the sealing does not exceed 10^{3} microorganisms. These must be destroyed by means of moist heat-terminal sterilization at 121°. The applicable D value is 1 minute. The total number of microorganisms to be destroyed during the life of the product will be

$$10^{10+3} = 10^{13}$$

If this whole microbial population were exposed to moist heat at 121° over a period of 13 minutes, it would be reduced to 10^{-13} times it initial number, ie, to $10^{13\text{-}13} = 10^{0} = 1$. The exposure time of 13 minutes thus would be sufficient (under all the other above hypotheses) to prevent the total number of contaminated ampules from exceeding the value of one.

From the point of view of each single ampule, 13 minutes of exposure would reduce the microbial population to the theoretical value of

$$10^{3-13} = 10^{-10}$$

To interpret this numeric value as the probability of still having one contaminated ampule in ten billion sterilized ampules means that a single ampule will still be contaminated out of a whole lot of 10^{10}. This probability value is defined as PNSU (Probability of Non Sterile Unit).

In recent times the PNSU as a sterility evaluation criterion is being replaced by the SAL (Sterility Assurance Level). The name itself could generate some misunderstanding since a level of assurance commonly is deemed to be good if high, but SAL seems to have been defined in such a way that its numerical value is the same as PNSU. This notwithstanding, it is sometimes calculated as the reciprocal value of PNSU. The SAP (Sterility Assurance Probability) criterion has been proposed as well and SAP seems for the moment to have been granted the same definition of PNSU, even if it would be better understandable if its value approached unity after a satisfactory sterilization.

The above discussion and example lead to the conclusion that the optimum exposure time for a sterilization process must take into account not only the initial microbial population within the single item to be sterilized and the species and conditions of the contaminating microorganism, but also the total number of items expected to be sterilized over the life of the product.

Effect of Temperature Changes—All the above considerations have been developed under the basic assumption that the temperature is kept constant during the entire exposure time. It seems rather obvious that the D value will change as the temperature changes. If the D values experimentally obtained for a given microbial species are plotted on a semilogarithmic chart as the function of the temperature T, a path similar to Fig 3 is obtained.

In this case, it can be seen that D value is 1 minute at 121° (ie, the average value which very often is assumed to be acceptable in the absence of more exact experimental data). It also can be seen that D value varies by a factor of 10 if the temperature varies by 10°.

The z value is defined as the temperature coefficient of microbial destruction, ie, as the number of degrees of temperature which causes a 10-fold variation of D (or, more generally, of the sterilization rate).

The z-values generally oscillate between 6 and 13 for steam sterilization in the range 100 to 130° and z value often is assumed to be equal to 10 in the absence of more precise experimental data.

The fact that D value varies by 10 times for a variation of 10° when z = 10 must not lead to the false assumption that D varies by one time (ie, doubles) for an increase of 1°. Obviously, this is not true.

It is actually a matter of finding the number which yields 10 when raised to the tenth power. This number is 1.24. Therefore, a variation of 1° entails a variation of D value of 24%.

This is quite a significant number, which illustrates the dramatic effects which are generated when the sterilization

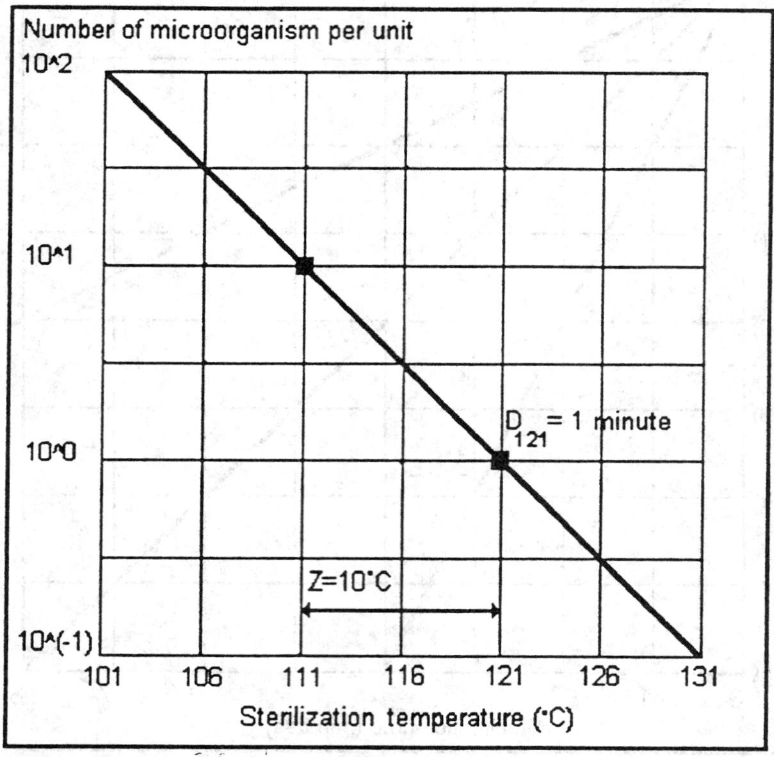

Fig 3. Effect of temperature on microbial destruction (courtesy, Fedegari Autoclavi).

temperature is also only a few degrees lower than the expected value, perhaps only in some areas of the sterilizer load.

It is also useful to remember that the effect of temperature variation decreases considerably as the temperature rises and drops to approximately 1/2 (or even less) for dry sterilization at approximately 200°. Under these condition the z value is about 20 instead of about 10. Therefore, the small temperature differences which can be so dramatic in steam sterilization have much less effect in dry sterilization.

The foregoing refers to average values since the actual D values and z values depend to a large extent on the medium which contains the microorganisms and on their history. At 121° no microorganism has exactly D = 1 and z = 10. However, the combined use of these two parameters in calculating F_0 and PNSU provides ample margins of safety with regard to the microorganisms with which we deal commonly.

F_0 or Equivalent Sterilization Time at 121°—It is of the utmost interest to calculate the lethal effect of the exposure of a microbial population to a variable temperature, T, by relating it to an hypothetical sterilization performed at a constant temperature, T_0, for the time, t_0. If the constant reference temperature is assumed equal to 121.1° (originally 250°F) and the z value equal to 10, the equivalent time is termed F_0.

Thus, F_0 is the equivalent exposure time at 121.1° of the actual exposure time at a variable temperature, calculated for an ideal microorganism with a temperature coefficient of destruction equal to 10.

First introduced in the *Laboratory Manual for Food Canners and Processors* by the National Canners Association in 1968, F_0 has become a common term in pharmaceutical production since the FDA used it extensively in the "Proposed rules" of June 1st, 1976 (21 CFR 212.3) with the following meaning:

> F_0 means the equivalent amount of time, in minutes at 121.1°C or 250°F, which has been delivered to a product by the sterilization process.

For the calculation of it

> A z value of 10°C or 18°F is assumed; the term z value means the slope of the thermal death time curve and may be expressed as the number of degrees . . . required to bring about a tenfold change in the death rate.

In practice, the knowledge of the temperature values as the continuous function of elapsing time is not available, and F_0 is calculated as

$$F_0 = \Delta t \, \Sigma \, 10^{\frac{T-121.1}{z}} \qquad (2)$$

where Δt = time interval between to following measurements of T, T = temperature of the sterilized product at time t and z = temperature coefficient, assumed to be equal to 10.

Saturated Steam

Principles—Sterilization with saturated steam is the method that provides the best combination of flexibility in operation, safe results and low plant and running costs.

The sterilizing medium obviously is pressurized saturated steam and the typical operating temperature is 121° (250°F), but higher or lower temperatures often are used.

The term *dry* saturated steam sometimes is used: it should be made clear that this is an "ideal" condition of steam, and that *moist* saturated steam is used in practice for sterilization. However, the steam must entrain the smallest possible amount of condensate. The "water vapor ratio" of the steam defines the amount of condensate entrained by 100 parts by weight of moist steam; a water vapor ratio of 0.95 means that 100 g of steam consist of 95 g of dry saturated steam plus 5 g of condensate which is, or should be, *at the same temperature as the steam.*

The reliability of sterilization performed with saturated steam is based on three particular characteristics of this medium.

When steam condenses, it releases calories at a *constant temperature* and in a *considerable amount:* 1 kg of pure saturated steam condensing at 121° (turning into water at 121°, thus without cooling) releases as much as 525 kcal.

The temperatures and pressures of saturated steam have a two-way correlation. Once the temperature of the steam is determined, so is its pressure, and vice versa. Saturated steam at 121° inevitably has a pressure of 2.05 abs bar.

This entails two very interesting practical possibilities: (1) a pure saturated steam autoclave can be controlled indifferently according to the temperature parameter or according to the pressure parameter and (2) regardless of the parameter used for control, the second parameter can be used easily to cross-monitor the first one.

One gram molecule of water (18 g, ie, 18 mL in the liquid state) as steam at 121° and 2.05 abs bar occupies a volume of approximately 15 L. This means that when steam condenses at 121° it shrinks in volume by almost 1000 times. Accordingly, additional available steam *spontaneously* reaches the object to be sterilized. The condensate that forms can be removed easily from the autoclave chamber by means of a condensate discharge or, with a more modern technique, by continuous and forced bleeding (as occurs for example in so-called *dynamic steam* sterilizers).

However, three other phenomena must be considered.

In order to perform its microorganism inactivating action (coagulation of cellular proteins), the steam, or more generally the moist heat, must make contact with the microorganisms. This can occur directly or indirectly. For example, it occurs directly when the steam that is present in the autoclave chamber is in direct contact with a surgical instrument. It instead occurs indirectly when moist steam is generated (by heat exchange with the steam present in the chamber) inside a sealed ampul that contains an aqueous solution. However, it is evident that it is not possible to steam-sterilize the inside of an empty closed ampul or the contents of an ampul if they are constituted by an anhydrous oil-based solution.

The air that is initially present in the autoclave chamber and the *incondensables* that possibly are entrained by the steam (generally CO_2) have molecular weights, and thus densities, 1.5 to 2 times higher than steam (under equal temperature/pressure conditions). Therefore, the air must be eliminated initially from the chamber and the steam must not introduce incondensables in the chamber; otherwise, these tend to stratify in the lower portions of the chamber, creating intolerable temperature gradients.

When closed nondeformable containers that contain aqueous solutions are sterilized, the pressures inside them can reach values far above those of the chamber. All air has been removed from the chamber, which in fact only contains steam: accordingly, at 121° the pressure is 2.05 abs bar. The container instead almost always has a head space that contains air (or other gases).

During sterilization, the aqueous solution of the container produces a vapor pressure which is approximately equal to 2.05 abs bar, but this value is increased by the partial pressure of the air of the head space; assuming that its initial value is 1.0 bar, it will increase to approximately 1.3 bar due to heating.

Pressure increases also will occur due to the thermal expansion of the solution (which is not entirely compensated by the expansion of the glass of the container) and because any gases dissolved in the solution may leave it.

Generally, in the conditions described above the total pressure inside the container exceeds by approximately 1.4 bar the pressure in the chamber if the initial head space is, as usually occurs, 10 to 20% of the total volume of the container. This overpressure generally is well tolerated by glass ampules, even those of considerable capacity (20 to 30 mL). However, it becomes hazardous for glass containers fitted with rubber stoppers held in place by a seal (due to the risk of stopper lifting) and intolerable for deformable containers, such as rigid (and even flexible) plastic containers, prefilled syringes or cans. In all these cases, it is necessary or convenient to use the *counterpressure* sterilization methods (described later).

Saturated Steam Autoclaves—

Materials—All autoclaves intended for the pharmaceutical industry are made of Class AISI 316 stainless steel, including valves and piping. See Fig 4. Only the service elements arranged *downstream* of the autoclave (for example the vacuum pump or the condensate discharge) are accepted if they are made of other materials. The service elements *upstream* of the autoclave (eg, heat exchangers or water pumps) also must be made of stainless steel.

Silicone rubber or Teflon and derivatives thereof generally are used for the gaskets (of doors, valves, etc).

Structure—Saturated steam autoclaves generally have a quadrangular, or rarely cylindrical, chamber. The doors are generally quadrangular even if the structure is cylindrical; in

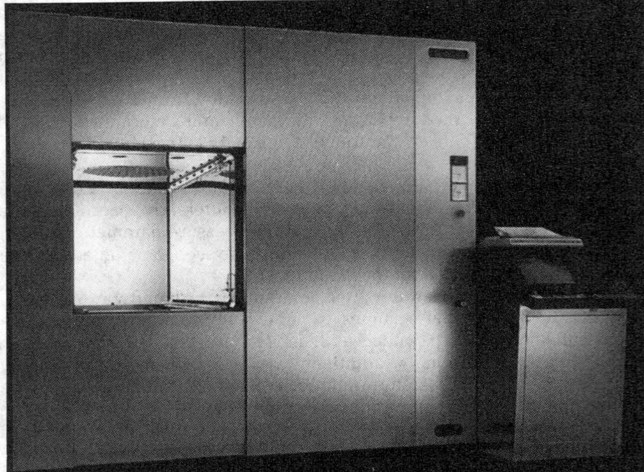

Fig 4. A modern computerized steam autoclave with horizontal sliding door (courtesy, Fedegari Autoclavi).

this case, the doors are inscribed in the circumference. There may be one or two doors: when the autoclave leads to a sterile room, there are always two doors.

Two-door autoclaves often are used when this requirement does not occur but the need is nonetheless felt to separate the loading area, where products *to be sterilized* are placed, from the unloading area, where *already sterilized* products are placed. *This concept applies to all types of sterilizers.*

Doors may be of various kinds. The most common types are

Hinged, manually operated, retained by radial locking bars, with a solid and fixed gasket.

Hinged, semiautomatically operated, retained by means of abutments in which the door engages automatically and with a movable gasket activated by compressed air.

Vertically or laterally sliding, with retention and gaskets as mentioned immediately above.

Saturated steam autoclaves generally are jacketed. There is no room here to discuss the various kinds of jacket and their purposes. However, there are two ways to feed steam into the jacket and into the chamber:

Single Feed—the steam circulates first in the jacket and passes from the jacket into the chamber.

Separate Feed—usually the chamber is fed pure steam and the jacket is fed industrial steam.

Single feed steam has some advantages in terms of control, but separate feed steam is preferred since it provides better assurances of lack of microbiological and particle contamination.

Management Systems—The management systems used on currently manufactured autoclaves are programmable logic controllers (PLCs) or personal computers (PCs) or, sometimes, combinations of PLCs and PCs. This is also true for other kinds of autoclaves and sterilizers, which we will discuss later.

However, a very large number of autoclaves controlled by electropneumatic systems are still in operation and still perform acceptable work. Naturally, the current control systems offer a kind of performance that was undreamed of earlier.

Pressure or temperature control (we mentioned previously that these parameters are interchangeable for a saturated steam autoclave) generally is performed with a proportional-integral-derivative method. Control by temperature is the generally accepted scheme since it is not influenced by trapped air. Sterilization can be time-managed or F_0-managed (with the F_0 being accumulated by heat probes enabled for this function), or time-managed with simultaneous calculation of F_0 for monitoring purposes.

Some management systems offer exceptional flexibility in composing programs and in setting parameters even to operators that have no knowledge of electronic programming. The information provided in real time (on same display device) is extremely detailed; so is the permanent information, which can be produced on paper or stored on various kinds of electronic medium.

Process—

Initial Removal of the Air from the Chamber—The main reason the air must be removed from the autoclave chamber has been pointed out above.

Loads often are made up of porous materials or materials packaged in sterilization paper or in plastic/paper bags, or contained in filter boxes. All these situations require reliable and rapid removal of the air from the load. The so-called *gravity* removal method is considered obsolete. Modern autoclaves have a water-ring vacuum pump that can produce a vacuum of approximately 70 residual mbar in the chamber. Accordingly, only about 10% of the air remains in the chamber. There are essentially two methods for completing air removal:

Pulsed Vacuum—Once the initial vacuum has been reached, the pump is stopped and steam is introduced in the chamber (up to approximately atmospheric pressure), then vacuum is produced again. Three or more of these vacuum/steam pulses are performed.

Dynamic Vacuum—Once the initial vacuum has been reached, the pump continues to run, but at the same time a 5- to 10-minute injection of steam is performed (from the side of the chamber that lies opposite the vacuum drain).

Modern autoclaves are capable of performing either of these methods, chosen according to the load to be processed.

Heating-Sterilization—During heating phases, and much less during the sterilization phase, considerable amounts of condensate form in the chamber. Except for particular instances, this condensate must be removed from the chamber. There are basically two extraction methods:

A condensate trap located at the bottom of the chamber. This is the simplest and cheapest method, but it causes significant pressure drops, and therefore temperature drops, inside the chamber due to the inertia of the condensate trap. Essentially, it discharges not only the condensate but also significant amounts of steam, which cause instantaneous expansion, and thus cooling, of the steam that remains in the chamber.

Dynamic steam. This is the most reliable and elegant system, but is also more expensive. During the heating and sterilization phases, the vacuum pump is kept running and draws from the chamber all the condensate that forms in it through a low-capacity valve. A certain amount of steam is naturally aspirated continuously, and a *dynamic* condition of the steam is thus produced, hence the name of the method.

Autoclaves also are required to have a continuous steam bleed past the controlling sensor in the drain line.

Post-Sterilization Phases—These may be different according to the material to be sterilized and depending on the results to be obtained on the material itself. The most common solutions are

1. **Vacuum and Time-Controlled Vacuum Maintenance**—This method is used to dry and simultaneously cool loads of solid materials, both porous and non-porous. It is performed by restarting the vacuum pump until a preset value (eg, 100 mbar) is reached; the pump then is kept running for a preset time (eg, 20 minutes).

2. **Cooling by Circulating Cold Water in the Jacket**—This method is used to cool containers that are partially filled with solution (eg, culture media) and closed with sleeve (Bellco-type) stoppers. Naturally, with these loads Item 1 is not applicable, since the solution would boil, and Item 3 is dangerous due to possible contaminations. This method is performed by removing the steam present in the chamber through the introduction of compressed sterile air at a pressure that is equal to, or greater than, the sterilization pressure. Then, cold water is circulated in the jacket. The pressurized compressed air in the chamber has two purposes: (1) to prevent the solution from boiling and (2) to improve heat exchange between the load and the jacket.

3. **Cooling by Spraying Water on the Load**—This method generally is used for loads of filled and closed ampuls and plastic intravenous containers. It is performed with deionized water (to avoid salt residues on the ampuls) which is nebulized onto the load by means of a sparger provided in the ceiling of the chamber. Naturally the ampuls, which preferably are arranged in an orderly fashion, must be contained in trays with a perforated bottom. Nebulization of the water causes a rapid con-

densation of the steam that produces a sudden pressure drop in the chamber, whereas the pressure inside the ampuls still remains rather high because the solution cools rather slowly. Ampuls of good quality (even large ones up to approximately 20 mL) tolerate this method adequately. Cooling stops when the solution inside the ampuls has reached the temperature of 70 to 80°. In this manner, the load, removed from the autoclave, still contains enough heat energy to dry spontaneously.

4. **Ampul Tightness with Fast Vacuum**—The pressure stress described in Item 3, above, is produced deliberately and increased by activating the vacuum pump as soon as the sterilization phase ends. The pressure in the chamber quickly drops to values that can reach 150 to 200 mbar (obviously this value can be controlled easily), whereas the pressure inside the closed ampuls initially remains above 3.0 bar. The ΔP thus produced breaks ampuls with "closed defects," ie, thinner regions and tensions in the glass, closed cracks, etc.

Obviously, if the ampuls have "open defects" (ie, holes at the tip or open cracks), the ΔP does not arise or is very small and thus the ampuls rarely break. What happens instead is that the solution in the ampul boils and thus evaporates, reducing the volume of the solution. Unfortunately, this evaporation is very limited. Since it requires a considerable amount of energy, the solution cools very quickly and the boiling ends. One cannot rely on the transmission of heat from the adjacent ampuls or from the jacket, since the chamber is evacuated.

It is evident that in such conditions, solution in the liquid state leaks from the ampuls; at least from the "open defects" that lie *below* the level of the solution. Accordingly, it may be convenient to load the ampuls upside down (i.e. with their tip pointing downward) if it is known that most defects occur at the tip or shoulder of the ampules.

Naturally, the breakage of the ampuls or the leakage of solution soils the load, which must therefore be washed and dried. With appropriate methods it usually is possible to achieve all this in the autoclave itself.

5. **Cooling as in Item 3, but with Air Counterpressure**—In many cases it is not possible or reasonable to subject the load, during cooling, to the pressure stress that arises with the method described in Item 3. In such cases, it is possible to remove the steam present in the chamber by replacing it with sterile compressed air at a pressure which is equal to, or higher than, the sterilization pressure. Only after this has occurred does the cooling water spray described in Item 3 begin. This method only prevents the load from suffering the pressure stress of the cooling phase, whereas the stress of the sterilization phase is unavoidable. Reference is made to the section on "Counterpressure Methods" below for an explanation of this phenomenon and for the autoclaves that allow to avoid it.

6. **Spontaneous Cooling**—In some particular cases it may be necessary to resort to this cooling method, which is the simplest but also obviously requires a very long time. Clearly, at the end of this cooling the autoclave will be in vacuum, and the longer the cooling the deeper the vacuum.

7. **Ampul Tightness Test with Dye Solution Penetration**—This test generally is performed with an aqueous solution of methylene blue. However, it is also possible to use other dyes. This test is effective only on "open defects" of ampuls and is performed as follows:

a. Vacuum in the chamber to approximately 100 to 150 mbar.

b. The chamber is filled with the colored solution until the load is completely covered; the ampuls must of course be contained in appropriate trays that do not allow them to escape, since they tend to float.

c. During this filling operation, the chamber vacuum reached in Item a is maintained continuously by connecting the vacuum pump to the ceiling of the chamber

d. The colored solution is pressurized at 2 to 3 bar and is maintained in this condition for 30 to 60 minutes or more.

e. The colored solution is discharged and recovered.

f. The load is washed several times with spray water.

g. The load is washed by flooding the chamber.

h. The washing water is discharged.

There are alternatives to this method, such as electronic spark discharge inspection which detects leakage of liquid from the ampul by a decrease in resistance across electrodes placed across the ampul.

The vacuum is not maintained continuously while the chamber is being filled with the colored solution.

The vacuum is produced only after filling the chamber with the colored solution.

The vacuum is not produced at all.

This test has in any case the following problems:

It has been demonstrated extensively that with usual values for dye concentration, differential test pressure and test time, tip holes with a diameter of less than 5 to 10 μm allow very small amounts of colored solution to enter. This prevents detection of the coloring of the ampuls during subsequent checking.

The preparation of sterile colored solution for each test entails very high costs.

Recovery and reuse of the colored solution entails keeping it in conditions that prevent microbial proliferation (80°) and subjecting it to sterilizing filtration prior to each test. All these procedures are expensive and complicated. In any case, the solution recovered from each test is contaminated chemically by the broken or defective tested ampuls.

Decolorization/destruction of the solution is very difficult, since methylene blue is very stable; however, good decolorization results have been achieved by using ozone. The use of amber glass ampuls makes detection of the dye difficult.

Sterilizing the Air Introduced in the Chamber—In the previous paragraphs we noted that it is often necessary to introduce air in the chamber, especially in poststerilization phases. This air must be sterile, otherwise it may recontaminate the sterilized load and can, in any case, contaminate the sterile environment if the autoclave is of the two-door type connected to the sterile area.

The air generally is sterilized by filtration using a system that is part of the autoclave. It is thus necessary to

Provide a filtration cartridge with sterilizing porosity.

Allow *in situ* sterilization of the assembled filtration system with an appropriate sterilization program of the autoclave itself.

Ensure that the filtration system and the line for connecting it to the autoclave maintain their sterility between one production sterilization program of the autoclave and the next.

Allow validation of all of the above described procedures.

If one wishes to operate in perfect safety, the filtration system also should be subjected to an integrity test each time it is operated.

Counterpressure Methods

Autoclaves operating with counterpressure are defined as devices able to control, during sterilization, the pressure of the moist sterilizing medium independently of its temperature.

Conventional pure saturated steam autoclaves do not belong to this category. The temperature of the pure saturated steam present in the chamber in fact automatically generates a specific pressure which cannot be modified without modifying the temperature as well. If the temperature of the steam is 121°, its pressure is unavoidably 2.05 bar abs and vice versa, assuming no trapped air.

For many kinds of load it is necessary or convenient to use an autoclave operating with counterpressure.

In order to understand this need, let us see what happens in a conventional autoclave during the sterilization of a rigid container partially filled with an aqueous solution and closed tight. For the sake of simplicity, let us assume that the container is filled with pure water.

A glass bottle is filled partially in standard conditions: 20° and 1.013 bar; the bottle is closed with a rubber stopper and aluminum seal. In the head space there is a total pressure of 1.013 bar, which is actually the sum of two factors: a partial water-vapor pressure which corresponds to the vapor pressure of water at 20°, ie, 0.025 bar, and a partial air pressure of 0.988 bar.

When the bottle is subjected to the sterilization phase at 121°, these two factors change as follows:

	Initial condition		Sterilization condition
Partial water-vapor pressure	0.025	→	2.050 bar (1)
Partial air pressure	0.988	→	1.330 bar (2)
Total pressure in head space	1.013	→	3.380 bar abs

Value 1, 2.050 bar, is obviously the pressure of water vapor at 121° and *corresponds to the pressure which occurs in the autoclave chamber.* Value 2, 1.330 bar, is a theoretical value which is calculated by applying the law of perfect gases to air, ie

$$0.988 \times \frac{121 + 273}{20 + 273} = 1.330$$

Therefore, the total pressure of 3.380 bar abs is also a theoretical value.

There are some reports which demonstrate that the *practical* value is slightly higher than the theoretical one and largely depends on the ratio between the head space and the volume of the filling solution. The practical pressure of the head volume is, on average, higher at 121° by approximately 1.40 bar, with respect to the pressure in the chamber. This is caused by two mechanisms:

The thermal expansion of water is significantly greater than that of glass and increases very rapidly as the temperature rises. The specific volumes of water at the temperatures we are interested in are in fact

Temperature °C	Specific volume mL/g
0	1.0002
4	1.0000 (maximum density)
20	1.0017
120	1.0606

In passing from 20 to 121°, water increases its volume by approximately 6% according to the following ratio:

$$\frac{1.0606}{1.0017} = 1.058$$

This fact must be considered carefully by those who tend to reduce or eliminate the head space in containers and then are surprised to find that such containers explode or warp during sterilization.

Solutions (especially if filtered under gas pressure) contain considerable amounts of dissolved gases which leave the liquid phase as the temperature rises.

The overpressure of approximately 1.40 bar which occurs in the bottle naturally generates a force of approximately 1.4 kg per cm^2 of internal surface of the bottle. A rubber stopper with a diameter of 24 mm is subjected to an expulsion force of approximately 6.3 kg.

These conditions therefore prevent or advise against the use of a pure saturated steam autoclave to sterilize solutions contained in a wide variety of containers. For example

Large-Volume Parenterals (LVP) in glass containers
Small-Volume Parenterals (SVP) in glass vials with rubber stopper
LVP or SVP in plastic containers (flexible, semirigid or rigid plastic)
Prefilled syringes
Jars or similar containers with press-on or screw on closures
Blisters containing various materials, eg, disposable contact lenses.

Two counterpressure methods currently in use are

Superheated water spray method (sometimes named "water cascade process").
Air overstream method (sometimes named "steam + air method").

Superheated Water Spray Autoclaves—A typical functional diagram of this autoclave is shown in the Fig 5. Obviously, different solutions are also possible which, however, do not change the essence of the method.

The chamber generally has a circular crosssection (with quadrangular door(s) inscribed in the circumference) and has a single wall.

At the beginning of the program, after the goods have been loaded, the lower circular sector is filled with purified water. The air contained in the chamber is *not* removed.

The water, drawn by a sanitary-type pump, circulates in a heat exchanger (plate or other sanitary type) which is *indirectly* heated in countercurrent with industrial steam. The water returns then into the upper part of the chamber and is distributed to the load by a system of solid-cone spray nozzles. The uniform redistribution of the water on the lower layers of the load is ensured by appropriate perforated racks which support the load. Side spray bars sometimes are used, even if their actual usefulness is not demonstrated.

The heating of the circulation water, and therefore of the load, is gradual but quite fast; eg, the temperature of 121° is reached in approximately 20 to 30 minutes *inside* 500-mL containers, mainly dependent on the solution and the material and shape of the containers.

The sterilization phase lasts 15 to 20 minutes, and temperature uniformity (in time and space) is excellent: it is well

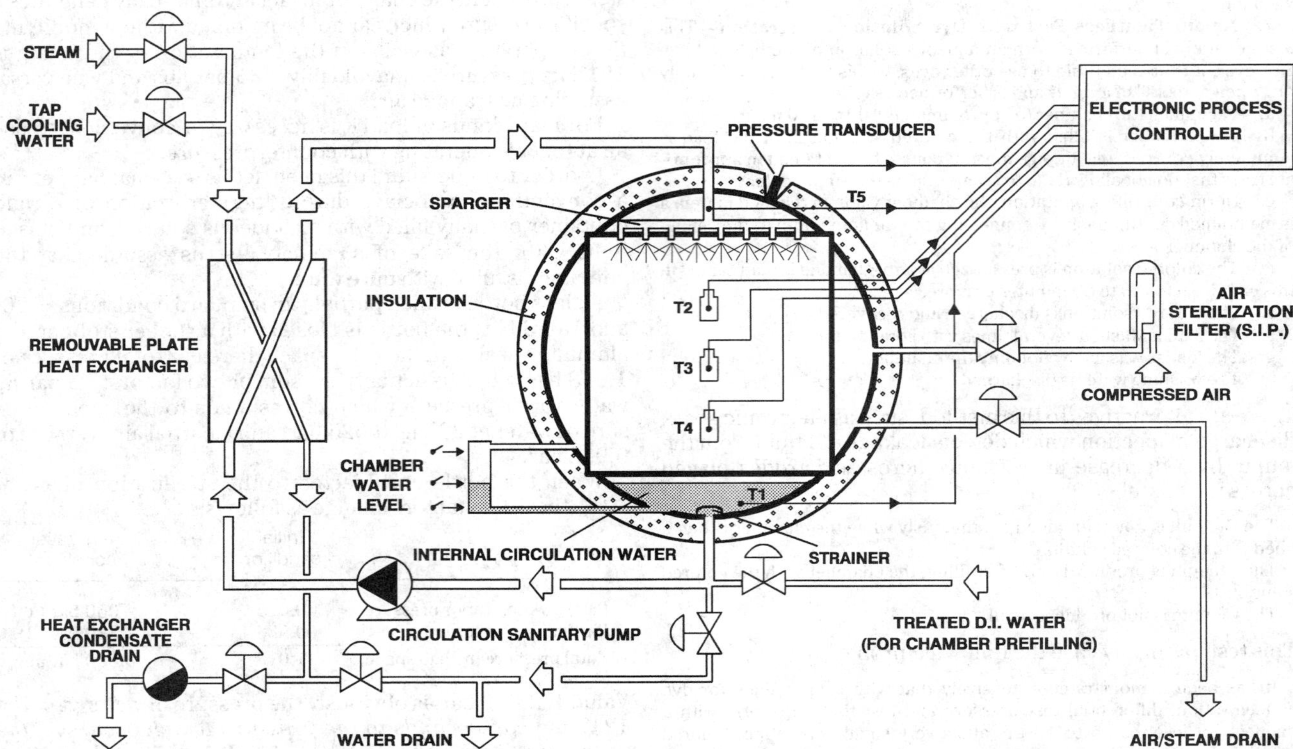

Fig 5. Superheated water-spray autoclave: simplified piping and instrumentation diagram (courtesy, Fedegari Autoclavi).

within the quite narrow limits required by FDA for LVP sterilization, ie, ±0.5°. This allows very small F_0 dispersions and therefore minimum sterilization times.

The cooling phase is performed while the circulation water, now sterile, continues to circulate. However, cold tap water now flows in the plates of the exchanger, where steam was flowing earlier. In less than 15 minutes, the temperature *inside* the 500-mL containers drops to approximately 70°, which is also the ideal temperature for obtaining a rapid and spontaneous drying of the load removed from the autoclave.

During all the phases of the process, an appropriate sterile air counterpressure is maintained inside the chamber to counterbalance the overpressure in the bottles.

There are various methods for controlling this counterpressure in each phase. With computerized management, it is even possible to generate a total pressure (steam + air) inside the chamber which is correlated, in each phase, to the average of the internal temperatures of two or more *witness* containers.

The load suffers no thermal or pressure shock and the differential pressure between containers and chamber can be eliminated or maintained in a direction convenient, in each phase, for the particular type of load. Even highly deformable products (semirigid plastic containers or plastic-aluminum blisters) or products which are particularly sensitive to differential pressures (eg, prefilled syringes) can be treated (from 60 to 127°) without problems.

The autoclaves are obviously highly specialized machines, and as such they have some limitations in application, such as

It is illogical to attempt to dry the load *inside* the autoclave by putting the chamber in vacuum or by circulating warm air.

In the case of materials with concavities directed upward, these concavities will be filled with water at the end of the program: the most obvious solution is to load these materials upside down.

When PVC bags are sterilized, the phenomenon of *blushing*, ie, the whitening of the PVC due to water absorption, usually occurs.

The intensity of this phenomenon and the time required for its disappearance depend on the type of PVC and of plasticizer employed. Blushing does not occur with rigid or semirigid plastic or with polylaminate plastics; it also is reduced considerably with PVC containing special plasticizers.

Air Over Steam Autoclaves—A typical functional diagram of this type of autoclave is shown in Fig 6. Alternatives are also possible in this case. The most important one is the use of horizontal faus placed on a side of the chamber. As in the previous case, the chamber has a circular cross section (with quadrangular door(s) inscribed in the circumference) and has a single wall.

There are two reasons for choosing a circular cross-section for autoclaves operating in counterpressure.

These autoclaves operate at significantly higher pressures than conventional pure saturated steam autoclaves, and generally are not put in vacuum. It is well known that a cylindrical structure withstands internal pressure much better than a quadrangular one.

The circular sectors of the chamber which are not occupied by the load are used to place elements required for the operation of these autoclaves.

The air is *not* removed initially from the chamber. The steam enters directly into the chamber through a sparger which is located in the chamber's lower portion.

The partial air pressure of the mixture can be adjusted during the entire process, similarly to what occurs for the previously described superheated water spray autoclaves.

The fan(s) placed against the ceiling of the chamber and the flow deflectors have the purpose of homogenizing the steam + air mixture which forms inside the chamber.

The task of these fans is very important and demanding. In fact, for equal pressure and temperature conditions, the air is approximately 1.6 times denser than the steam (one only has to consider their respective molecular weights) and would tend to stratify on the bottom, producing intolerable temperature gradients.

The cooling phase consists of feeding air into the chamber (in order to condense and replace all the steam which is present) while maintaining the same sterilization pressure or possibly increasing it. Cold tap water then is fed into the

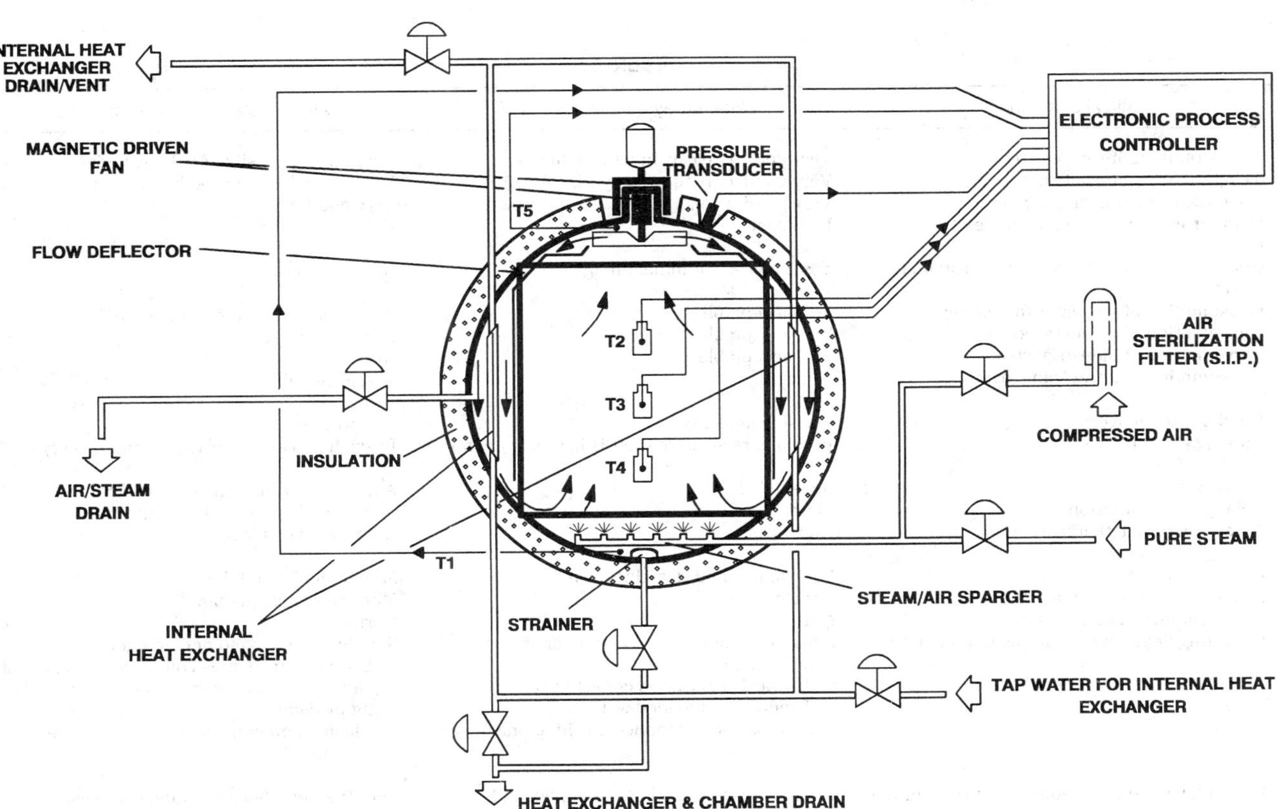

Fig 6. Air over steam autoclave: simplified piping and instrumentation diagram (courtesy, Fedegari Autoclavi).

heat exchangers, which are constituted by batteries of hollow plates located in the two circular sectors of the sides of the chamber (only one plate is shown in the diagram for the sake of simplicity). A tube heat exchanger can be used as an alternative.

The load is thus cooled while constantly maintaining a controlled pressure inside the chamber. However, this cooling comprises two solid-gas heat exchanges (plates → air; air → load) which, as is known, have a very poor efficiency. An attempt is made to improve this exchange by increasing the pressure of the air in the chamber (within the limits allowed by the product and the autoclave) so as to increase its density and therefore its heat-exchange capacity. The fans obviously continue to run during the cooling phase.

Despite these refinements, the cooling phase is definitely longer than the same phase in superheated water spray autoclaves.

A critical mechanical aspect of these autoclaves is the tightness of the fan shaft. This aspect can be solved completely by using magnetic-drive fans.

With steam + air mixture autoclaves, the blushing of PVC bags is less intense than with water spray autoclaves and generally affects essentially the regions where the bag rests on the supporting racks.

Table 1 compares the characteristics of the two kinds of counter pressure autoclaves.

Dry Heat Treatments

Sterilization and Depyrogenation—Dry heat treatments have two targets: microorganisms and their by-products. The aim of sterilization is to destroy the ability of microorganisms to survive and multiply. Depyrogenation seeks to destroy the chemical activity of the by-products: pyrogens or endotoxins (these terms do not mean exactly the same thing, but we will consider them to be synonymous for the sake of simplicity).

Both processes consist of an oxidation which is almost a combustion. However, the temperatures required to achieve depyrogenation are distinctly higher than those needed to obtain sterilization. We can summarize the situation as

If an effective dry heat depyrogenation is performed, sterilization generally is achieved *as well*.

Effective dry heat sterilization can be performed even *without* achieving depyrogenation.

If moist heat sterilization is performed, in normal operating conditions depyrogenation is *not* achieved.

The kinetics of dry heat treatments is not substantially different from that of moist heat sterilization. The values of the algorithms F_T and F_H (analogous to F_0) and those of the parameters D and z, however, are different not only from those of moist heat sterilization but also from each other. Furthermore, the two dry heat treatments are verified biologically with different biochallenges. Accordingly, the two dry heat treatments require different validation approaches.

The materials subjected to dry heat treatments naturally-must be heat-stable: the most common are glass containers for parenterals. Elastomeric compounds generally are unable to tolerate these treatments.

The literature generally mentions the following operating conditions:

Sterilization:	160°—120 to 180 minutes
	170°—90 to 120 minutes
	180°—45 to 60 minutes
Depyrogenation:	230°—60 to 90 minutes
	250°—30 to 60 minutes

However, the current trend is towards using treatments at higher temperatures than those listed.

The sections that follow describe the most common types of equipment used to perform the above-mentioned processes. The following general remarks should be made regarding this equipment:

If the load (bottles/vials/ampuls made of glass or other materials) is wet when it is introduced, a large part of the energy required by the process is used initially to evaporate the water that wets the load, and the process accordingly takes more time.

Table 1.

Critical comparison	Water spray autoclaves = WS	Air over steam autoclaves = AS
Temperature uniformity in time	Very good } easily in ±0.5°C limits	Very good } easily in ±0.5°C limits
Temperature uniformity in space	Very good } requested by FDA for LVP	Very good } requested by FDA for LVP
Total pressure uniformity in time	Very good	Very good
Counterpressure management flexibility	Excellent	Excellent
Consumption of high microbiological quality water	Yes, modest, for initial filling	No
Consumption of tap water for cooling	Yes, acceptable	Yes, approx. 3 times higher than WS
Consumption of compressed air	Yes, acceptable	Yes, acceptable
Consumption of industrial steam	Yes, acceptable	No
Consumption of ultraclean steam	No	Yes, acceptable
Condensate recovery	Possible and easy	Not possible
Cooling water recovery	Possible, recovered water is initially very hot	Possible, recovered water is initially very hot
Autoclave price	Acceptable	Approx. 1.1 times higher than WS
Total process duration	Short	Approx. 1.3 times higher than WS
Autoclave productivity/price	High	Approx. 70% of WS
Operating principle	Very simple and straightforward	More complicated than WS
Mechanical construction	Simple	More complicated than WS
Qualification/validation	Normal	Normal
Operating flexibility according to type of load	Suitable for any kind of container with the following remarks: · Upward concavities collect water · Product is unloaded wet · PVC bags can produce blushing phenomena	Suitable for any kind of container: · Upward concavities collect condensate only · Other kind of container can be unloaded lighly damp · Blushing phenomena of PVC bags are limited
Possibility of combination with pure saturated steam processes	Strongly discouraged: it is complex and expensive and complicates validation	Very frequent, but moderately expensive

The equipment uses large amounts of air which generally is recirculated partially and must be filtered in HEPA filters in order to have, in the critical regions of the equipment, Class 100 environment which is indispensable to obtain a load which is not only sterile and depyrogenated but also has extremely low particulate contamination. This is relatively easy to achieve in the sterilization phases (or regions) in which the *thermal situation* of the filters is stable. It is much less easy to achieve in the heating/cooling phases (or regions), because the changes in temperature entail expansions/contractions of the filters, with consequent release of particles.

Dry Heat Batch Sterilizers—The forced-convection batch sterilizer is a type of dry heat unit widely used in the industry. It uses the principle of convective heat transfer to heat the load. Figure 7 is a schematic diagram of a modern unit. It shows a two-door sterilizer in which the unloading door leads to the sterile area. The two doors are, of course, parallel to the plane of the drawing and are hinged vertically.

The pressure inside the chamber must be controlled continuously so that it is slightly higher than the pressure in the loading area (nonsterile) and slightly lower than the pressure in the unloading area (sterile).

The unit is made entirely of stainless steel; particular care must be placed in selecting the insulating materials and in the methods for applying them. It is in fact important also to avoid the forming of so-called *thermal bridges* that allow dissipation and therefore excessive external temperatures of the sterilizer and *cold spots* in the chamber.

The main features shown in the sketch are

1. Air-circulation fan
2. Water-cooled battery (for the cooling phase)
3. Circulation HEPA filters
4. Launch/recovery bulkheads
5. Trolley and load
6. Discharge duct
7. HEPA filter on the discharge duct to prevent back-flow contamination
8. Variable-speed fan for chamber pressurization (proportionally controlled)
9. Prefilter and HEPA filter on the chamber pressurization loop
10. Electric heater (proportionally controlled)
11. Four flexible Pt100 4-wire RTDs
12. Main control Pt100 4-wire RTD
13. Pressure transducer

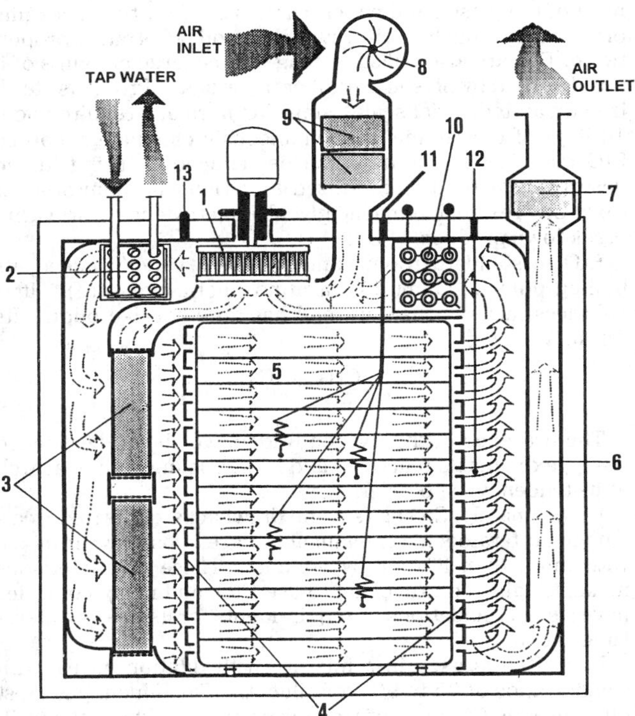

Fig 7. Dry-heat batch sterilizer: simplified diagram (courtesy, Fedegri Autoclavi).

Dry Heat Tunnels—The drying, sterilizing/depyrogenation, and cooling tunnel is the only continuous sterilizing apparatus widely used in the pharmaceutical industry (apart from filters). It basically consists of a horizontally rotating transport belt made of a stainless-steel mesh (some devices must be provided to confine the product on the transport belt without particulate generating friction), installed in a thermally insulated "tunnel" directly connecting an upstream cleaning machine to the downstream sterile area or to "isolated" devices.

Inside the tunnel, the product (most frequently glass vials) is dried, heat-treated either by radiant heat or, as more usual today, by hot air and finally cooled. In both cases the internal part of the tunnel must be pressurized dynamically by ventilation at an intermediate pressure level between the downstream system and the loading room. From a process point of view, higher temperature and shorter exposure time are used than in batch sterilizers. During the last 10 years the practice has changed from 20 minutes at 280° to 3 or 4 minutes at 300° or more. Since a minimum safety margin is required for the duration of exposure, and glass of most types becomes more difficult to handle above 320° and more fragile after such a treatment, it is likely that the trend toward higher temperature values has reached its practical limit.

In IR (infrared radiant heat) tunnels, heat is supplied by resistance-in-glass heaters located above and below the transport belt; prefiltered and HEPA-filtered air is fed into the cooling zone mainly for pressurizing and cooling. This air, countercurrent slowly flowing through the entire tunnel, has also an important drying and preheating effect of the load in the infeed zone. Figure 8 schematically represents an IR tunnel: even if this type of apparatus is no longer widely used, the basic concepts have not been modified in the LF (hot air laminar flow) tunnel, but airflow patterns are a little more complex.

LF tunnels do not radiate heat directly to the product, but heating is provided by circulation of hot filtered air forced onto the product. A circulation fan withdraws the air, leaving the product through heating bars below the transport belt and feeds it again to the inside of the tunnel through HEPA filters suitable for operating at high temperature. Airtightness of the coupling of HEPA filters with tunnel framework is of utmost importance from the point of view of particulate contamination. It must cope with the strong thermal expansion of different materials. Some makeup air is required in the heating zone, and the total number of installed fans may be as high as five, or six if an additional extraction below tunnel outfeed is required in case of high pressure in the sterile room.

Despite the complexity of its airflow, the LF tunnel has the main advantage of quicker heating and consequent shorter process time. This results in reduced size compared with the IR tunnel, since the belt speed cannot be reduced below a certain value. As the name itself declares, the air speed in the LF tunnel is kept around 0.5 m/sec (1.5 ft/sec), aiming to avoid particulate contamination.

The comparison between continuous tunnel and batch oven is favorable to the continuous tunnel from the point of view of handling the product. No batch work is needed after the unpacking of the components and loading of them into the cleaning machine until the final removal of the packaged product from the line after the filling and the following operations.

This can be very important in the case of large-scale production, but the batch oven provides a much easier isolation of the sterile area. In the case of continuous tunnel, there must be a steady flow of air through the open connection from the sterile area to the tunnel. The pressure difference between the two systems must be such that the sterile area always is kept at a higher pressure level than the tunnel. Too big a difference would result in an excessive escape of air to the tunnel, both reducing the pressure in the sterile area and disturbing the laminar air flow and the temperature profile inside the tunnel.

Experience has proved that these problems can be solved satisfactorily only if the design of the air-conditioning system

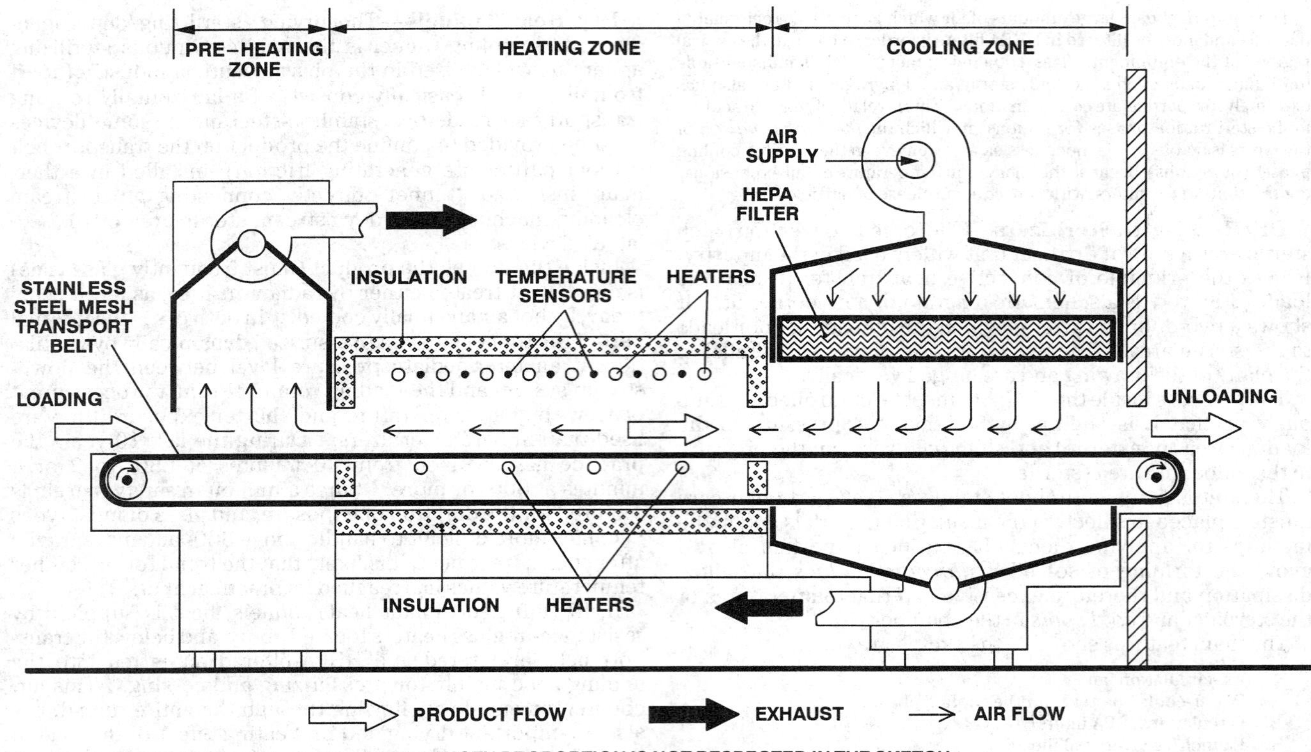

Fig 8. Dry-heat tunnel: simplified diagram (courtesy, Fedegari Autoclavi).

of the sterile area is developed from the very beginning keeping in mind the foreseen installation of a specified tunnel. Baffle systems also aid in maintaining pressure differentials between the aseptic-processing area and the sterilizing tunnel.

Chemical "Cold" Sterilization

Many products do not tolerate the sterilization conditions of moist-heat or dry-heat processes. In such cases it is possible to resort to cold or at least low-temperature sterilization methods performed with chemical means, ie, gases or vapors.

The continuously increasing use of plastic disposable products or components for medical treatments has been made possible by the development of reliable cold sterilization processes.

A variety of gases and vapors have shown germicidal properties: ethylene oxide, propylene oxide, formaldehyde, betapropiolactone, ozone, hydrogen peroxide, peracetic acid, etc. Ethylene oxide (EtO) is currently in widespread use for medical product sterilization. Vaporized hydrogen peroxide and hydrogen peroxide/steam mixtures are being used to sterilize a variety of materials and work surfaces.

Ethylene Oxide—The sterilizing action of EtO is based on an alkylation reaction: it is, accordingly, a truly chemical action rather than a physical one. This chemical reaction must be activated by the presence of water vapor (approximately 60% of RH or relative humidity) and is increased by temperature and EtO concentration.

Process temperature is limited by the characteristics of the product. Generally, it is between 40 and 60°, but it must be remembered that the reaction rate increases by approximately 2.5 times for each 10° increase in temperature. Normally used EtO concentrations range between 400 and 1200 mg/L. It has in fact been demonstrated that beyond 1200 mg/L the consequent increase in the reaction rate is no longer economically convenient.

The EtO must make *direct* contact with the microorganism for the microbe to be inactivated. Any packagings that contain the object to be sterilized must therefore be permeable to air, EtO and any dilution gases (as mentioned later). Generally, it is not possible to use EtO to sterilize liquids, solutions, emulsions, etc. Powders, too, are difficult to treat unless microbial contamination is only on the outside of the granules.

Fortunately, EtO, air and dilution gases easily penetrate most of the plastic and paper barriers used for the packaging of medical products. However, the good penetrating properties of EtO are also a disadvantage, since large amounts of it are absorbed by plastic or rubber materials. Products sterilized on an industrial scale using EtO normally require about 14 days of quarantine to spontaneously eliminate absorbed EtO residuals. This time can be reduced by using forced desorption methods. Sterilized goods must be monitored for toxic EtO residual, ethylene glycol and ethylene chlorhydrin-breakdown products of EtO.

EtO in standard room conditions is a vapor (indeed, its boiling point is about 11° at atmospheric pressure). It is colorless, heavier than air, and has an ether-like odor. Its formula is

$$\underbrace{CH_2\text{—}CH_2}_{O}$$

The presence of the oxygen bridge, which can be opened easily, explains its reactivity and its sterilizing action, as well as its tendency to polymerize.

Unfortunately, EtO has several drawbacks: it is toxic, carcinogenic, teratogenic, inflammable and explosive when mixed with more than 3% air by volume. These characteristics make it highly controversial to use EtO, and many countries have issued regulations or requirements for its use as a sterilizing agent.

EtO often is used in a mixture with dilution gases, with weight ratios of 85 to 90% of diluent. The diluent gas most often used is CO_2; use of freon is shrinking, due to the well-known international restrictions to its use; N_2 is beginning to be used quite often.

These mixtures are considered nonflammable and nonexplosive, and many countries consider them mandatory for use in industrial autoclaves. These countries allow the use of pure EtO in small individual single-use cylinders only for small autoclaves (100 to 200 L). If a 10 to 12% mixture of EtO in CO_2 is used to obtain an acceptable EtO concentration (at least 500 mg/L), it is necessary to work at 3 to 4 absolute bar. Accordingly, one must use an autoclave that can withstand relatively high pressures and is therefore expensive, and the duration of the sterilization process is rather long because of EtO concentration is rather low.

Other countries accept the use (including industrial use) of pure EtO or of inflammable/explosive mixtures with a low percentage of dilution gas (the presence of the dilution gas generally is ascribed to a reduction in the tendency of pure EtO to polymerize). In such circumstances one can operate at less than atmospheric pressures and still reach high EtO concentrations that shorten the sterilization time. It is therefore not necessary to use true autoclaves, but merely sterilizers capable of tolerating the very hard vacuum required for the initial elimination of the air from the chamber and from the load and for the final extraction of the EtO. Obviously, in these circumstances the use of plants constructed with explosion-proof criteria cannot be avoided.

The P/T/t diagrams of EtO sterilization are therefore different, depending on whether one or the other of the above described principles is used. A typical diagram of an overpressure sterilization with a mixture using 10% EtO and 90% CO_2 is shown in Fig 9. The steps are

Load and/or chamber heating
Vacuum
Vacuum hold for leak test
Humidification by steam injection
Penetration of humidity in the load
Loading of EtO mixture
Sterilization
EtO mixture evacuation
Air/vacuum pulses
Vacuum hold
Vacuum breaking

A typical diagram of a subatmospheric sterilization with a mixture using 85% EtO and 15% CO_2 is shown equally in Fig 9. One can see clearly that the phases are substantially the same as in Fig 8; what changes is the sterilization pressure, the EtO concentration and therefore the duration of the sterilization phase.

In performing industrial sterilizations, which accordingly involve large loads, the load is heated and humidified before placing it in the sterilizer, in adequately conditioned rooms. The heating/humidification phases described above in Figs 8 and 9 diagrams therefore are reduced drastically.

The layout of an industrial EtO sterilization plant is shown in Fig 10. Some remarks should be made regarding some of the items of this layout. This unit contains

The EtO or EtO-mixture cylinders.

The automatic devices that connect/disconnect the various cylinders to and from the sterilizer; disconnection of a cylinder (especially for mixture cylinders) often is controlled by its weight reduction, which must accordingly be checked individually.

The heat exchanger that must provide the vaporization calories to the liquid EtO mixture.

The pressure reduction unit that bring the liquid EtO mixture to the vapor state.

Any cylinders of N_2, which is used in the most advanced plants to "wash," after each process, the pipes that have carried EtO.

The EtO that is produced in the desorption chamber is at a very low concentration and it is generally too expensive to eliminate it with a catalytic burner. It is preferred to absorb it on activated-charcoal columns through which the air of the desorption chamber is recirculated.

Obviously, the EtO discharged by the sterilizer (and possibly the EtO arriving from the desorption chamber) must not be discharged into the atmosphere. Catalytic burners generally are used today: they convert the EtO into $CO_2 + H_2O$. These burners must be highly efficient, and their efficiency must be checked systematically, since the laws enforced in the various countries are generally very strict as to the limits of residual EtO. The asterisks (*) in the figure indicate points where continuous monitoring of EtO concentration must be provided.

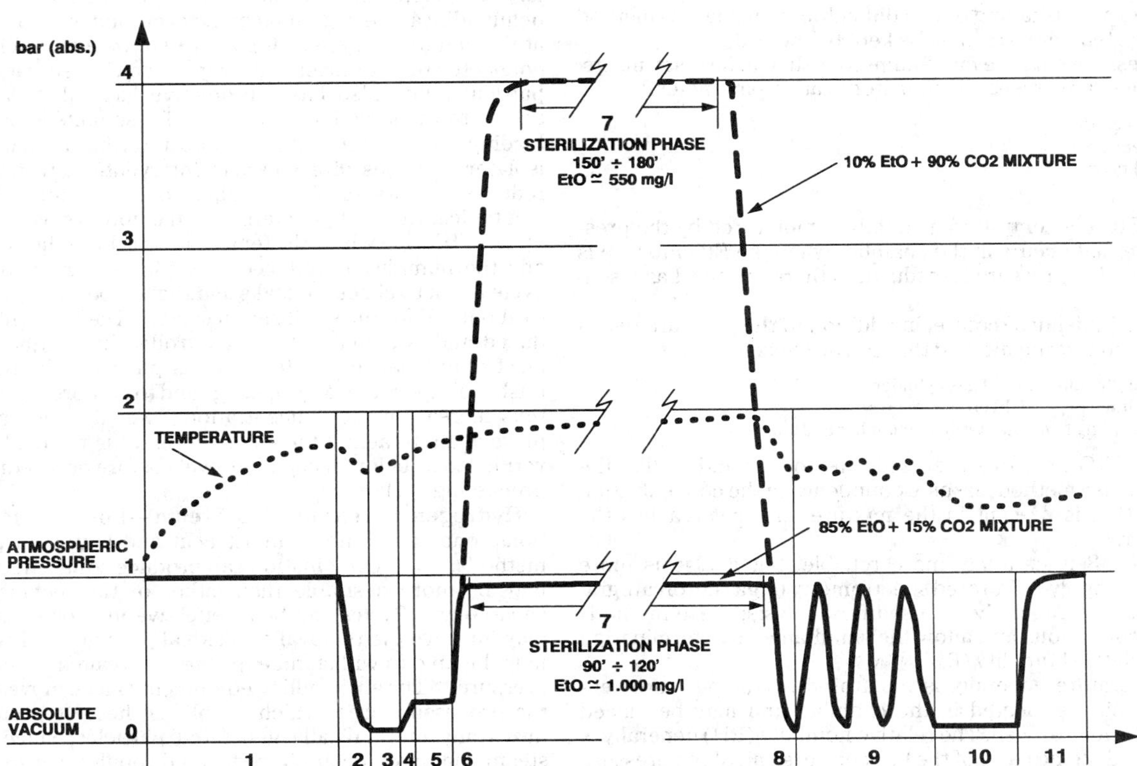

Fig 9. EtO sterilization pressure-time diagram: overpressure and subatmospheric pressure (courtesy, Fedegari Autoclavi).

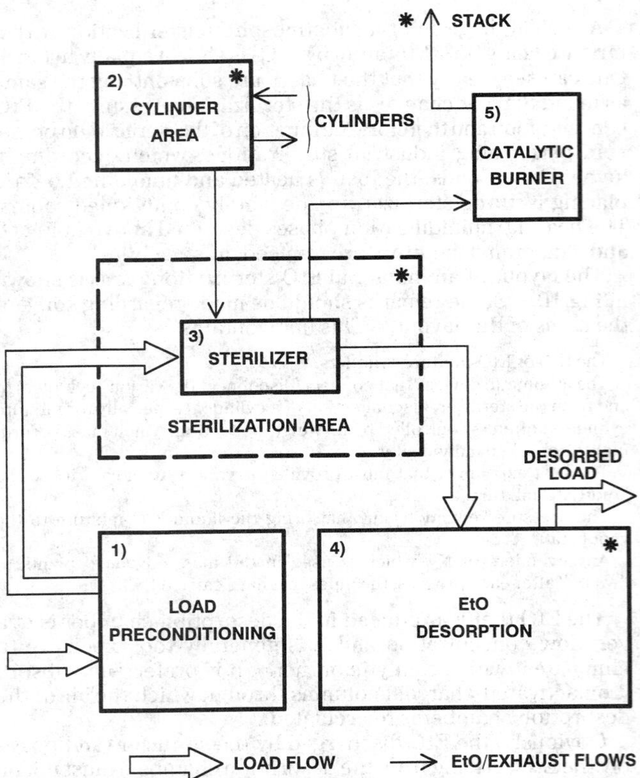

Fig 10. Flow diagram of an EtO sterilization industrial plant (courtesy, Fedegari Autoclavi).

EtO sterilizers generally are made of stainless steel, although there also are machines made of carbon steel coated with epoxy paints. The chamber generally is jacketed in order to circulate thermostat-controlled warm water to maintain the sterilization temperature. Use of water vapor for the same purpose is fading due to difficulties in using this method when the temperature must be kept below 100°.

Process sensors are more numerous than in heat sterilizers, since there are essentially four sterilization parameters:

EtO concentration
Temperature
Humidity or RH
Time

The EtO concentration generally is monitored by the pressure rise that occurs in the chamber when the EtO mixture is introduced; a pressure transducer is therefore used as a sensor.

Many Guidelines require, in addition to the pressure rise, a second monitoring method that can be chosen among

1. Weight difference of gas cylinder
2. Volume of gas delivered
3. Sampling from the sterilizer chamber and analysis

When EtO mixtures are used, Methods 1 and 2, like the pressure rise method, assume confidence in the concentration of EtO that is present in the mixture and that reaches the sterilizer.

Method 3 is certainly more reliable, but it also is more difficult to apply. Infrared spectrometry or gas chromatography methods generally are used for analysis; these methods can be continuous and allow the simultaneous determination of the relative humidity (RH).

Temperature generally is monitored by temperature sensors which are located in the chamber and may be placed inside the load as well. The relative humidity (RH) generally is monitored on the basis of the temperature and of the pressure rise of the steam injection of the humidification phase. This method obviously is not very reliable, and many guidelines recommend also to use a sensor that can determine the RH. Unfortunately, sensors of this kind are generally "poisoned" by the EtO and become unreliable after a few cycles. The solution often used is to keep the sensor inside the chamber during the humidification phases, removing it before introducing the EtO in the chamber.

Finally, it is evident that if the load is preconditioned, the preconditioning temperature/humidity/time also must be monitored.

Hydrogen Peroxide—Hydrogen Peroxide (HP), chemically H_2O_2, is normally a liquid at room temperature. However, it can be vaporized and the resultant gas is an effective sterilant for certain packaged materials and for equipment and enclosures used in processing sterile materials. The most frequent and successful use of HP as a sterilant is for isolators (also known as barriers, locally controlled environments, etc). These units are very sophisticated versions of their ancestors ("glove boxes"), which were used to isolate processes in the past.

Isolators now are used widely for sterility testing, transporting sterilized goods from moist and dry heat units to sterile areas or processing isolators and processing of supplies. HP also is being used to sterilize more sophisticated processing equipment, such as freeze dryers and filling lines, and even may be used to sterilized small clean rooms. High humidity can inhibit the effectiveness of vaporized HP and must therefore be controlled during the exposure of the gas. Figure 11 represents a typical vaporized HP cycle.

While HP is broken down readily to water and oxygen, the effluent gas can represent a safety hazard at higher levels. Just as with EtO, catalytic converters are used to assure that all materials are rendered safe before they are released to the atmosphere. Figure 12 represents a typical installation using vaporized HP to sterilize a freeze dryer and condenser system. VHP DV1000 is a model manufactured by the Am Sterilizer/Finn Aqua Co, who hold many of the patents on the use of this technology.

Systems for larger applications may require fans to aid in uniformly distributing the vaporized HP. In addition, auxiliary air systems may be added to reduce the time required to dehumidify at the beginning of the cycle and to aerate the load at the end of the cycle. Figure 13 shows a transfer isolator connected to a sterilizer and a vaporized HP generator. This particular unit also has a protective half-suit to allow full access to the large internal area. These units allow the unloading of the sterilizer directly into a sterilized isolator. The isolator excludes direct human intervention, which greatly reduces the potential for microbial contamination.

A typical freeze-dryer sterilization involves several vacuum "pulses" during which the temperature is brought to 40 to 60° and the humidity is reduced (dry phase). A vacuum hold cycle is run to check for leaks and the temperature is reduced to about 25° for the sterilization cycle. The sterilant is introduced and is monitored and controlled by weight using an electronic balance. Filtered air is pulsed with sterilant to push the vapors into any deadlegs and to compress the vapors, thus increasing the concentration. Finally, the vacuum is pulse again to aerate the chamber, and the residual vapor is verified to be below acceptable levels before proceeding to the processing cycle.

Hydrogen Peroxide Plus Steam—For certain applications, one can combine moist heat and hydrogen peroxide methods. The combination can produce some effects which may be more desirable than either of the techniques run separately. Cycles can be as effective in shorter times and may improve the removal of residual peroxide. The system must be able to withstand exposure to steam at atmospheric pressure. The air-handling equipment can be moved outside the processing area, which simplifies the system and minimizes any mechanically generated particles, since the air, steam and peroxide are introduced through the same type of HEPA filters used for laminar-flow hoods.

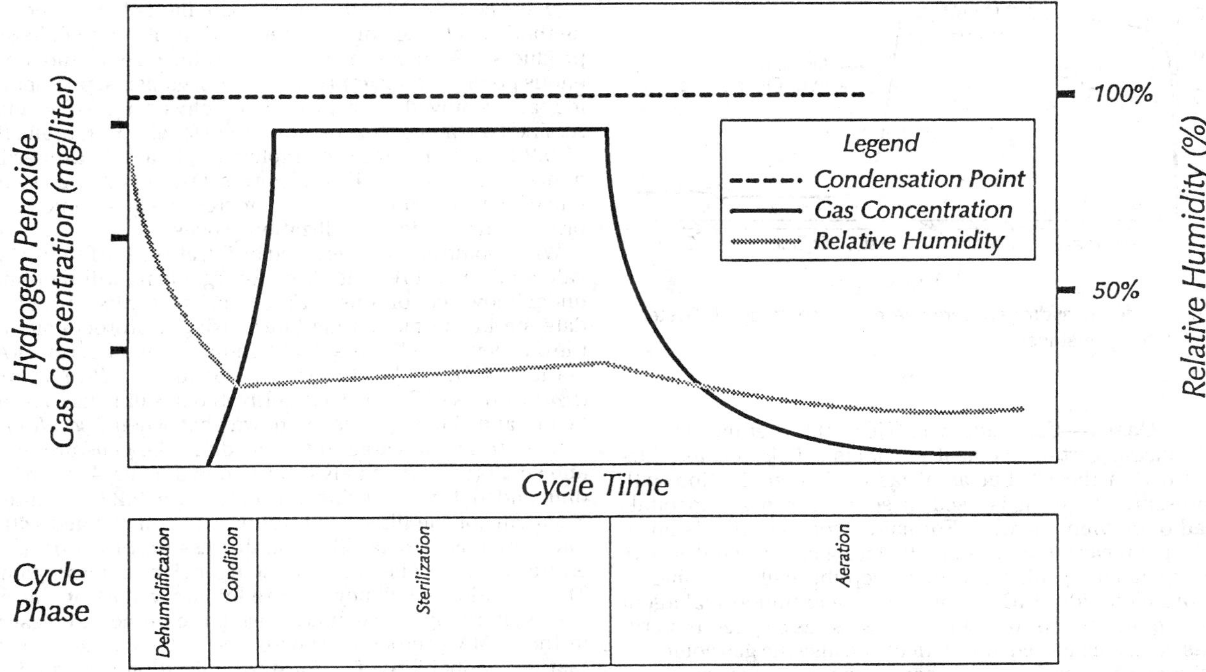

Fig 11. A typical vaporized HP cycle (courtesy, Am Sterilizer/Finn Aqua).

The process is basically as follows:

The process area is raised to about 80° by introducing dry heated air through the HEPA filters. The steam is introduced and surfaces are raised to about 100°. During the steam cycle, hydrogen peroxide is introduced and is carried with the steam. When the cycle has been completed, the steam and peroxide are stopped and the dry heated air is started again. This aids in removal of residual condensate and helps break down the peroxide to water and oxygen. After sufficient heat has been introduced to dry and remove residuals, cool air is introduced to bring the unit to the desired operating temperature.

Since the hydrogen peroxide is mixed intimately with the steam, temperature can be used to monitor the progression of the cycle. However, the heated portions of the cycle must be validated using biological indicators and residual peroxide measurements, to assure their effectiveness in sterilizing and removing residuals to a safe level. Figure 14 diagrams a cycle using steam and hydrogen peroxide to sterilize as a filler in an isolator.

Figure 15 is included to show the synergistic effects of steam and hydrogen peroxide in some sterilization cycles. The challenge organism was *Bacillus stearothermophilis*, which typically is used to validate steam cycles. It should be noted that the kill rate was not only considerably faster, but was accomplished using atmospheric steam. This means that instead of 121° the equipment was only subjected to 100° and was exposed for 15 minutes less to achieve the same reduction in microorganism count.

Fig 12. A typical installation using vaporized HP to sterilize a freeze dryer and condenser (Courtesy, Am Sterilizer/Finn Aqua).

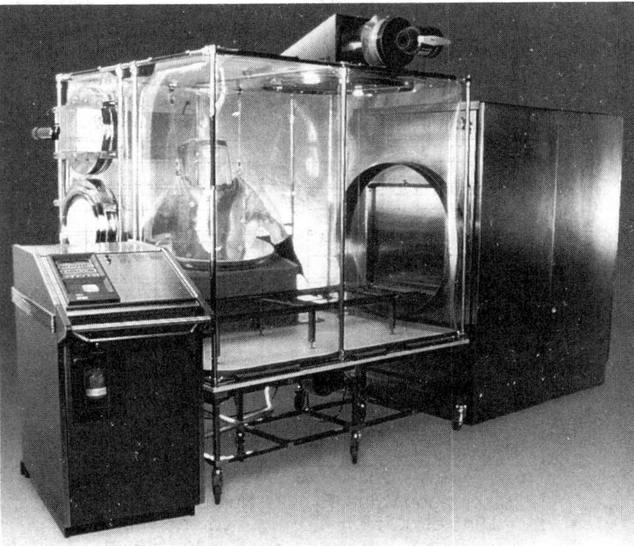

Fig 13. A transfer isolator connected to a sterilizer and a vaporized HP generator (Courtesy, Am Sterilizer/Finn Aqua).

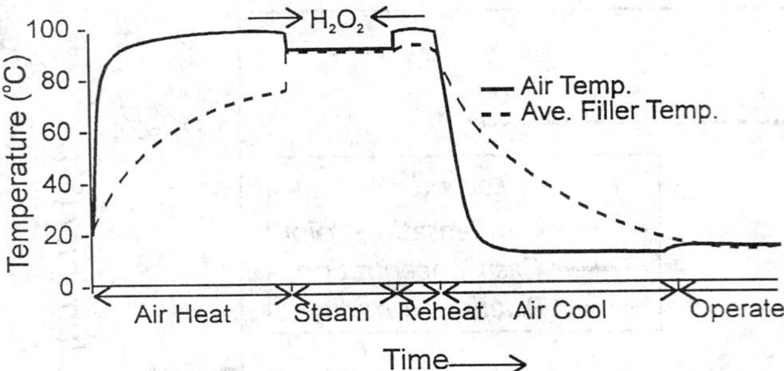

Fig 14. A steam/hydrogen peroxide cycle (courtesy TL Systems and Despatch Industries).

Other Gases—Formaldehyde (HCHO) sometimes is used for sterilizing certain medical products. It is not in widespread use in the US but as a gas or in combination with low-pressure steam, it is used in some European hospitals instead of ethylene oxide. Formaldehyde, a toxic chemical and a human carcinogen, is an alkylating agent and destroys microorganisms by alkylation of susceptible cell components.

Chlorine dioxide (ClO_2) is an effective antimicrobial agent in both liquid and gaseous states. Its use as a gaseous sterilant has been considered impractical because the gas could not be shipped or stored. There have been, however, some recent innovations allowing for *in situ* generation of the gas, which would make possible its future use in a sterilization chamber.[11]

Filtration

Filtration is the removal of particulate matter from a fluid stream. Sterilizing filtration is a process which removes, but does not destroy, microorganisms. Filtration, one of the oldest methods of sterilization, is the method of choice for solutions that are unstable to other types of sterilizing processes.

Pasteur, Chamberland, Seitz and Berkfeld filters have been used in the past to sterilize pharmaceutical products. These types of filters were composed of various materials such as sintered glass, porcelain or fibrous materials (ie, asbestos or cellulose). The filtration mechanism of these depth filters is random adsorption or entrapment in the filter matrix. The disadvantages of these filters are low flow rates, difficulty in cleaning and media migration into the filtrate. Fiber-releasing and asbestos filters now are prohibited by the FDA for the filtration of parenteral products.[12,13]

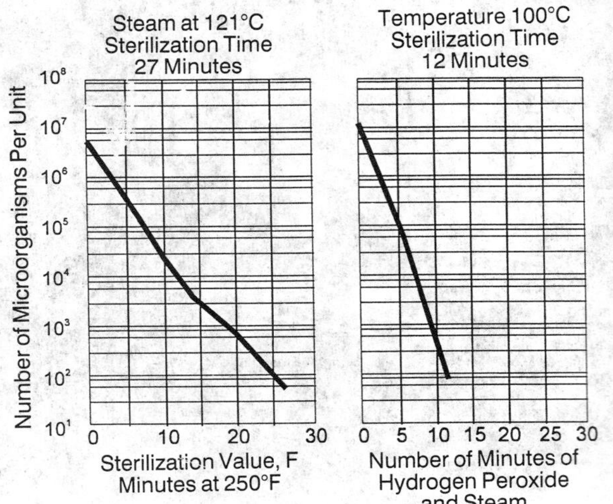

Fig 15. Comparison of steam under pressure with hydrogen peroxide/atmospheric steam mixture (courtesy, TL Systems and Despatch Industries).

Over the past 30 years, membrane filters have become the method of choice for the sterilization of heat-labile sterile products. Membrane filters are thin, strong and homogenous polymeric structures. Microorganisms, present in fluids, are removed by a process of physical sieving and are retained on or near the membrane surface. Membrane filters of 0.22-μm pore size are employed commonly as sterilizing filters. However, 0.45-μm pore size filters are used to remove bacteria from antibiotics or steroids in organic vehicles prior to an aseptic crystallization process.

When solutions are sterilized by filtration, the filters must be validated to assure that all microorganisms will be removed under known conditions. Filter manufacturers normally validate sterilizing membrane filters using a protocol similar to the one developed by the Health Industry Manufacturers Association (HIMA).[14] In this procedure, *Pseudomonas diminuta* (ATTC 19146) is cultivated in saline lactose broth. Leahy and Sullivan[15] have shown that when *Pseudomonas diminuta* is cultivated in this medium the cells are discrete and small (approximately 0.3 μm in diameter)—a range recommended for sterilizing filtration with 0.22-μm filters. Each cm^2 of the filter to be validated is challenged with 10^7 microorganisms at a differential pressure of 30 psig. The entire filtrate is collected and tested for viable microorganisms. The retention efficiency (log reduction value) of the membrane filter may be calculated using the procedure described in the HIMA protocol. Dawson *et al*[16] have demonstrated that the probability of a nonsterile filtration with a properly validated membrane filter is approximately 10^{-6}. Another aspect in filter validation is adsorption of the product by the filter and extractables from the filter and housing.

Once the performance of the membrane filter has been validated, a nondestructive integrity test that has been correlated to the bacterial challenge test (the bubble point or diffusion test) can be used routinely prior to and after a sterilizing filtration to assure that the membrane filter is integral.[17,18] Unique to membrane filtration is the condition that beyond a certain challenge level of microorganisms, the filter will clog. For a typical sterilizing filter this level is 10^9 organisms per cm^2. Initially, membrane filters were available only in disc configuration. Advances in membrane technology have provided filters in stacked-disc, pleated-cartridge and hollow fiber configurations. These advances have provided larger surface areas and higher flow-rate capabilities. Figure 16 is an example of these larger surface area filters.

Membrane filters are manufactured from a variety of polymers; cellulosic esters (MCE), polyvinylidiene fluoride (PVF), polytetrafluoroethylene (PTFE), etc. The type of fluid to be

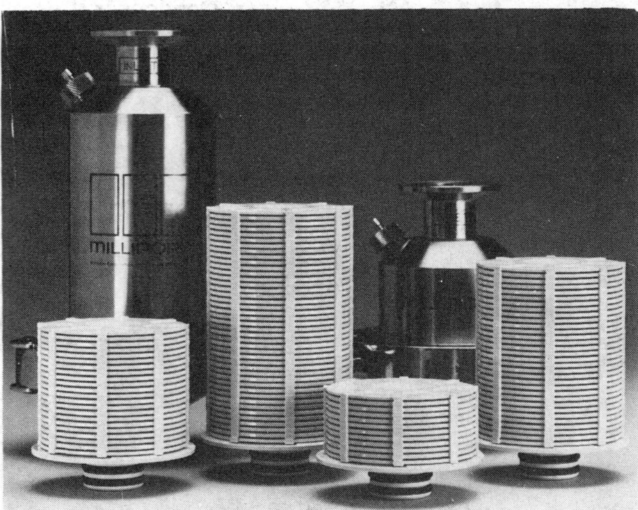

Fig 16. Stacked-disk membrane filters. This new technology allows filter manufacturers to supply filters with large surface area in relatively small packages (courtesy, Millipore). vaporized HP generator (Courtesy, Am Sterilizer/Finn Aqua).

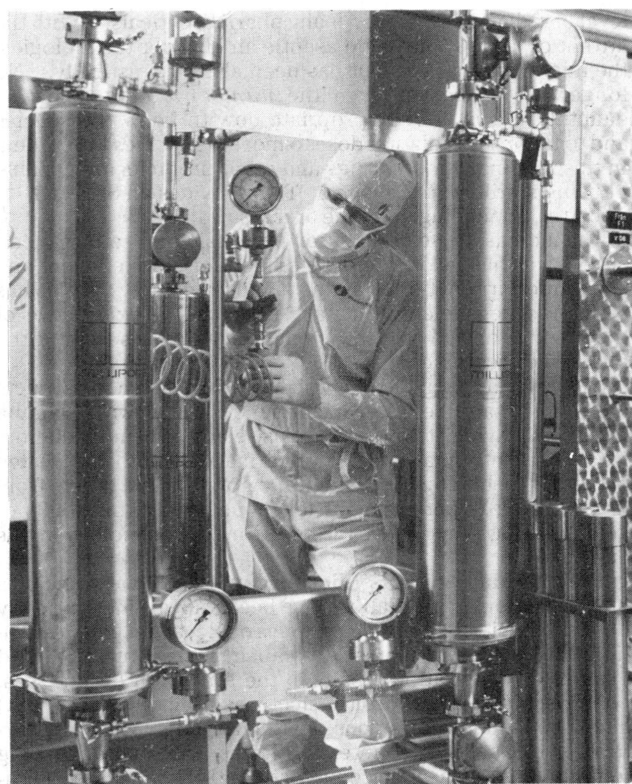

Fig 17. An example of a process filtration system in a pharmaceutical plant (courtesy, Millipore).

sterilized will dictate the polymer to be used. The listing below is intended to serve only as a guide for the selection of membrane filters for a particular application. The filter manufacturer should be consulted before making a final choice.

Fluid	*Polymer*
Aqueous	PVF, MCE
Oil	PVF, MCE
Organic solvents	PVF, PTFE
Aqueous, extreme pH	PVF
Gases	PVF, PTFE

Figure 17 is an example of a sterilizing filtration system commonly used in the pharmaceutical industry.

Positive pressure commonly is used in sterilizing filtrations. It has the following advantages over vacuum; it provides higher flow rates, integrity testing is easier and it avoids a negative pressure on the downstream (sterile) side of the filtrate, thus precluding contamination. Membrane filters are sterilized readily by autoclaving, *in-situ* steaming or by using ethylene oxide.

In addition to their use in the pharmaceutical industry, membrane filters are used in many applications in the hospital pharmacy. The membrane filters commonly used in these applications are small disposable units. Examples of these are shown in Figs 18 and 19. Typical applications for membrane filters in hospital pharmacies include sterilization of intravenous (IV) admixtures and hyperalimentation solutions, sterilization of extemporaneously compounded preparations, sterility testing of admixtures as well as in direct patient care (see Chapter 88).

Radiation Sterilization

The retail or hospital pharmacist probably has little opportunity to use radiation sterilization. However, they should be aware that many of the products sold in stores and used daily in hospitals are sterilized by this technology. Products such as contact lens solutions, bandages, baby bottle nipples and

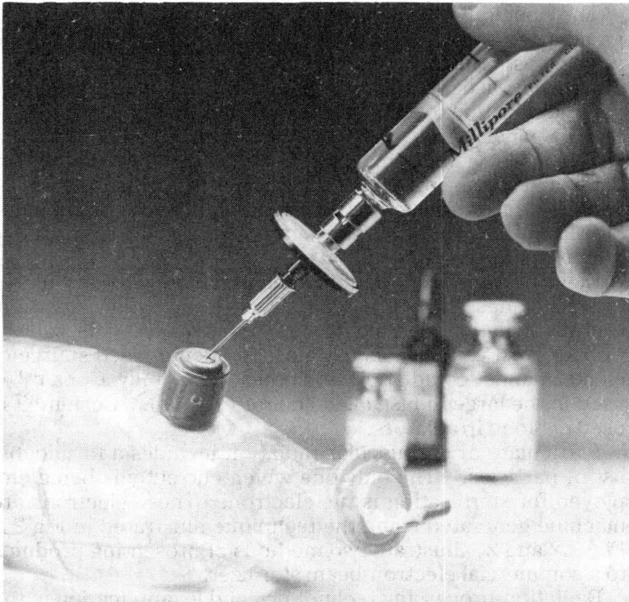

Fig 18. IV additive filtration using a small disposable membrane filter (courtesy, Millipore).

teething rings (the kind containing water/gel) are a few examples of the everyday type of product encountered in a Pharmacy. Several drugs, including some anticancer drugs also are sterilized *terminally* using gamma radiation.

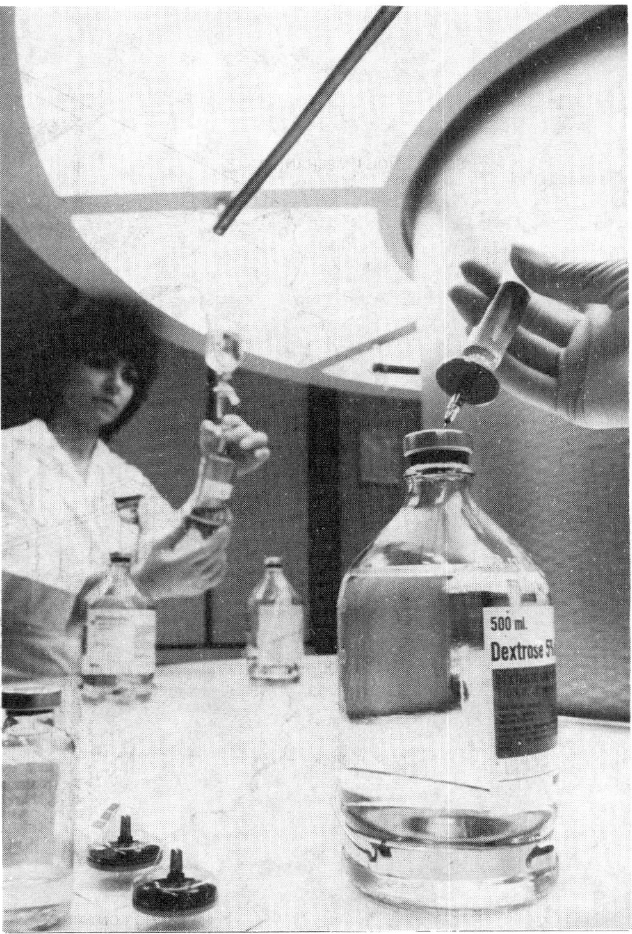

Fig 19. IV additive filtration and sterility testing. Both procedures employ membrane filtration (courtesy, Millipore).

The hospital pharmacist is likely to encounter the use of gamma or X-ray treatment of blood to eliminate white blood cells in host versus graft reactions following transplant surgery. The serum used for tissue cultures is frequently sterilized with gamma radiation to eliminate viruses, viruse-like particles and mycoplasmas.

The pharmaceutical industry historically has relied on steam, dry heat, ethylene oxide gas, filtration and chemical processes to meet sanitization or microbial load reduction requirements. Sterilization by radiation may employ either electromagnetic radiation or particle radiation.

Electromagnetic radiation, comprised of photons of energy, includes ultraviolet, gamma, X- and cosmic radiation. Gamma radiation, emitted from radioactive materials, such as Cobalt^{60} or Cesium^{137}, is the most frequently used source of electromagnetic radiation. Of these two, only Cobalt^{60} is used in the large industrial irradiator (Fig 20). Cesium^{137} is used in blood irradiators.

Particulate or corpuscular radiation includes a formidable list of particles. The only one which currently is being employed for sterilization is the electron. These electrons are machine generated using the technique illustrated in Fig 21; Figs 22 and 23 illustrate two methods of presenting products to a commercial electron-beam sterilizer.

Radiation-processing technology, and its application in the manufacture of pharmaceuticals, is being investigated more actively now than at any other time. This renewed interest is in part due to the development of aseptic and barrier technology, as well as an overall improvement in the environment in which pharmaceuticals are manufactured.

In the past the use of a radiation dose of 25 kGy was required to ensure that all spores had been destroyed, and that a Sterility Assurance Level (SAL) of 10^{-6} was achieved. This level of radiation destroyed many pharmaceuticals. With the advent of clean rooms, and aseptic and barrier technologies, the microbial environment has been altered drastically. No longer are spores or even the *number* of organisms as daunting. It is more appropriate now to know the species and to tailor the radiation dose to meet the *species* bioburden. In this way many more drugs and other products are capable of being sterilized terminally. This provides an SAL of 10^{-6} or better, depending upon the organism.

The increased use of radiation processing to sterilize medical devices has led to the development of more efficient and economical irradiation equipment and processes. It also has generated new scientific data. The positive experience of the medical-device industry should be a "sign post" for the pharmaceuticals industry.

Several pharmaceutical raw materials and finished products are being sanitized/sterilized successfully with gamma radiation. While it is possible to use electron beam radiation, we are presently unaware of any pharmaceuticals being treated using this technology. This should not preclude others from investigating its potential. The unique penetrating ability of gamma radiation provides the edge for this technology in this application.

How Radiation Kills Microorganisms—The principles of sterilization by irradiation have been known since the early 1940s. Basically, charged particles or electromagnetic radiation interact with matter to cause both ionization and excitation. Ionization results in the formation of ion pairs, comprised of ejected orbital electrons (negatively charged) and their counterparts (positively charged). Charged particles such as electrons interact directly with matter causing ionization, whereas electromagnetic radiation causes ionization through various mechanisms that result in the ejection of

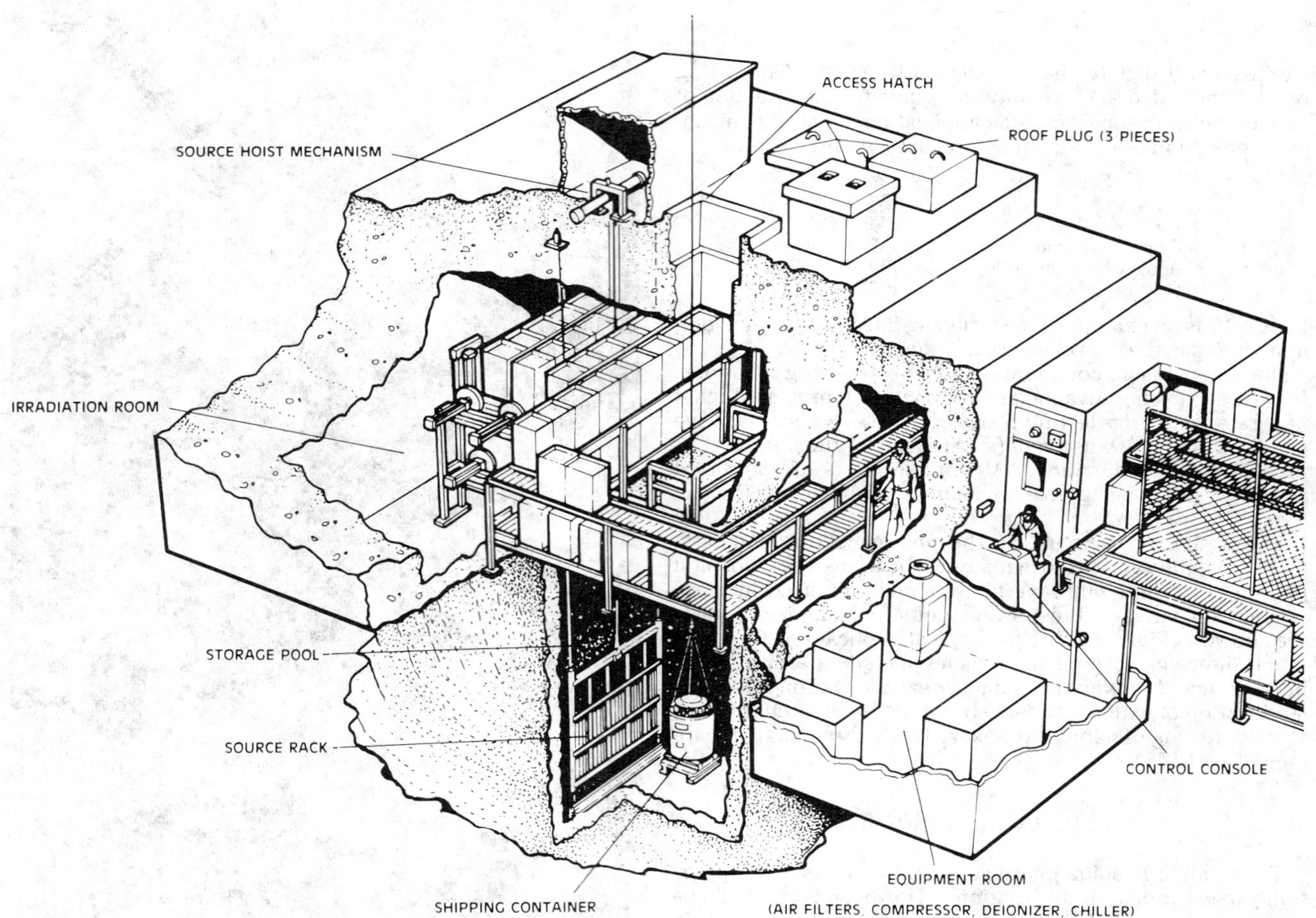

Fig 20. Tote box irradiator: automatic (courtesy, Nordion Intl).

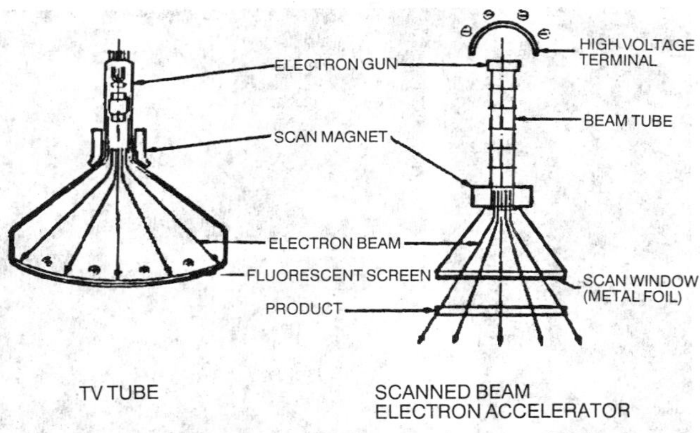

Fig 21. To produce an electron (courtesy, RDI).

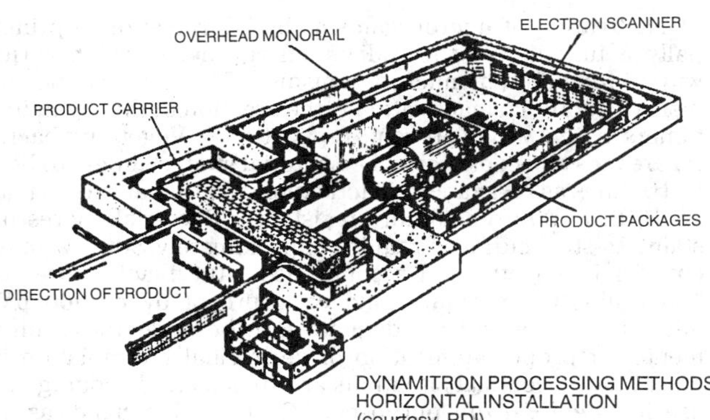

Fig 23. Dynamitron processing methods: horizontal installation (courtesy, RDI).

an orbital electron with a specific amount of energy transferred from the incident gamma ray. These ejected electrons then behave similarly to machine-generated electrons in ionization reactions. Thus, both particle and electromagnetic radiation are considered as ionizing radiation and differ from ultraviolet radiation in this respect.

Ionizing radiation kills or inactivates microorganisms through the interaction of the ion pairs or excitations altering the molecular structure or spatial configuration of *biologically active* macromolecules. In particular, those involved in cell replication are most critical. It can do this in two ways. The first is to deposit energy directly in a bond of the macromolecule. This can cause a rearrangement of its structure, altering or destroying its normal function. The second is to generate free radicals, primarily from the water contained within the cytoplasm. The free radicals thus generated react with the macromolecules to subvert their normal function. In either case the result is the loss of reproductive capability of the microorganism.

The number of organisms inactivated by a given radiation dose is a statistical phenomenon. It depends upon the sensitivity of the biologically active macromolecule(s) to alteration (denaturation), the number of alterations elicited within the cell and the ability of the cell to repair these alterations. Different organisms have different capabilities to withstand or repair such alterations. This sensitivity is referred to as the D_{10} value. The size of the organism, its state of hydration and the presence or absence of radical scavengers all affect the outcome of exposure to ionizing radiation.

The ability of gamma radiation to inactivate microorganisms has been well documented. New documentation relating to viruses, or new strains/reclassifications of microorganisms, is being added continually. The major benefit of using radiation sterilization as the terminal step in the manufacturing process as opposed to autoclaving, or dry-heat methods, is the lack of, or reduction in, product degradation with this technology.

The process has been in use in the medical device industry for over 20 years. Ample evidence as to its efficacy exists in the literature. Materials and processes have been developed to reduce the impact of radiation on the product. It is the intent of this update to present some of the process developments which will facilitate the use of this technology for the terminal sterilization of pharmaceutical products. It also will assist those wishing to improve the microbial quality of raw materials entering the manufacturing process. Clean materials reduce the bioburden impact on a clean room facility.

Sterilization by ionizing radiation requires consideration of the dose (or the amount of radiation that is absorbed by the material), the energy level available (which along with the bulk density of the material will determine the thickness of penetration) and the power output available (which determines the rate at which the dose can be applied).

The unit of absorbed dose is the Gray (Gy), where 1 Gy = 1 J/kg, independent of the nature of the irradiated substance. Sterilization doses, for convenience, usually are expressed in kilogray (Kgy).

Many investigators have studied the relative resistance of microorganisms to sterilization by radiation. The consensus is that vegetative forms are most sensitive, followed by molds, yeasts, viruses and spore-formers. While past practice has been to use 15 to 25 kGy, today the radiation dose is more closely tailored to the bioburden. It is not unusual to use doses as low as 2 to 8 kGy. The use of the AAMI guidelines or the soon-to-be-published ISO Guidelines are highly recommended.

Modern gamma sterilization facilities used by pharmaceutical and medical device firms generally hold up to 4 MCi of Cobalt^{60}. The largest facility holds 12 Mci. Figure 19 shows a schematic of a modern Cobalt^{60} radiosterilization facility.

Two types of electron accelerators are used in sterilization: alternating-current machines with ranges up to 50 kW of power and 5 to 12 meV of energy, and direct-current machines with ranges of 30 to 200 kW and 0.5 to 5 mev. These machines generate electrons at high voltage, accelerate the electrons and spray them on to the product to be sterilized. The greater the machine power (kW), the more electrons can be generated per unit time. The higher the energy (meV), the greater the penetration of the electron into the material to be sterilized.

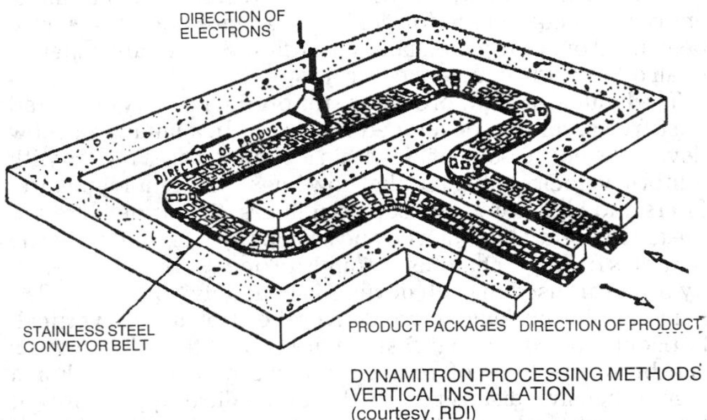

Fig 22. Dynamitron processing methods: vertical installation (courtesy, RDI).

Ultraviolet (UV) Radiation

Artifically produced UV radiation in the region of 253.7 nm has been used as a germicide for many years. While UV radiation often is used in the pharmaceutical industry for the maintenance of aseptic areas and rooms, it is of limited value as a sterilizing agent.

Inactivation of microorganisms by UV radiation is principally a function of the radiant energy dose, which varies widely for different microorganisms. The primary mechanism of microbial inactivation is the creation of the thymidine dimers in DNA which prevents replication. Vegetative bacteria are most susceptible, while bacterial spores appear to be 3 to 10 times as resistant to inactivation and fungal spores may be 100 to 1000 times more resistant. Bacterial spores on stainless-steel surfaces require approximately 800 μw min/cm^2 for inactivation. By comparison, the black spores of Aspergillus niger require and exposure of over 5000 μW min/cm^2. Even with an adequate dose, however, the requirements for proper application of germicidal UV radiation in most pharmaceutical situations are such as to discourage its use for *sterilization* purposes. On the other hand, as an ancillary germicidal agent, UV radiation can be useful.

When using UV radiation, it is very important that lamps be cleaned periodically with alcohol and tested for output: also its use requires that personnel be properly protected; eye protection is particularly important.

The principal disadvantage to the use of germicidal UV radiation is its limited penetration—its 253.7 nm wavelength is screened out by most materials, allowing clumps of organisms, and those protected by dust or debris, to escape the lethal action. The use of UV radiation as a sterilizing agent is not recommended unless the material to be irradiated is very clean and free of crevices that can protect microorganisms. Many organisms are capable of repairing the UV-induced DNA damage using photoreactivation (light repair) and dark repair.

Aseptic Processing

Although not actually a sterilization process, aseptic processing is a technique frequently used in the compounding of prescriptions or commercial products that will not withstand sterilization but in which all of the ingredients are sterile. In such cases, sterility must be maintained by using sterile materials and a controlled working environment. All containers and apparatus used should be sterilized by one of the previously mentioned processes and such work should be conducted only by an operator fully versed in the control of contamination. The use of laminar-airflow devices or barrier technology for aseptic processing is essential.

With the availability of sterile bulk drugs and sterilized syringe parts from manufacturers, the purchase of several pieces of equipment permits pharmacies to produce filled sterile unit-dose syringes with minimum effort. The equipment needs have been described in a paper by Patel *et al.*[19] Figure 24[19] illustrates this system.

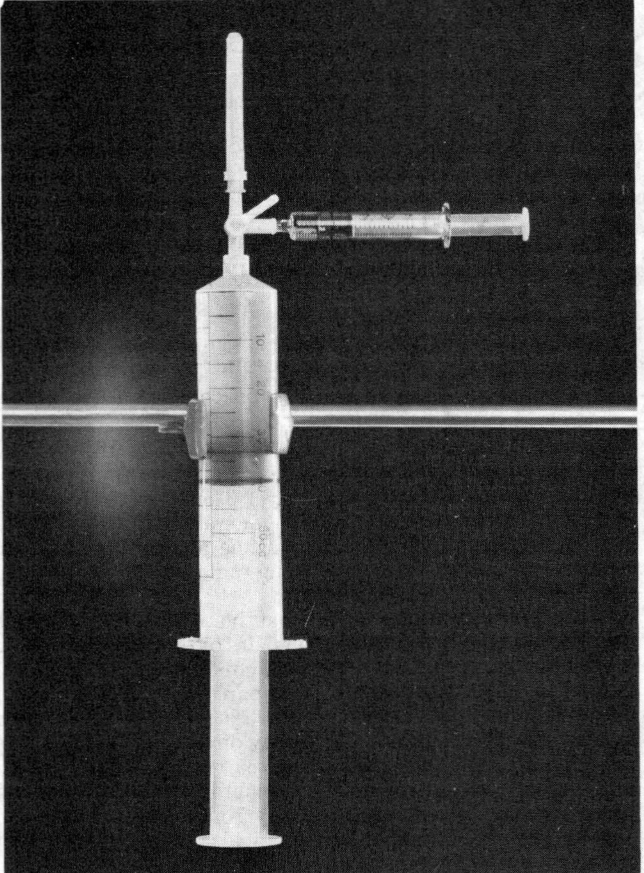

Fig 24. Unit-of-use system for sterile injectable medication.[19]

Packaging

Following exposure of a product to a well-controlled sterilization treatment, the packaging material of the product is expected to maintain sterility until the time of use. Packaging must be durable, provide for permanent-seal integrity and have pore sizes small enough to prevent entry of contaminants. Obviously, the packaging must be compatible with the method of sterilization.

The package design is important if the contents are to be removed without recontamination. Tearing of plastics or paper can be tempered by coatings, and sealed containers should be tested carefully to assure retention of sterility at the time of use.

If sterile material passes through many hands, it is important to provide a tamperproof closure to indicate if the container has been opened inadvertently. These four features—compatibility with sterilization, proven storage protection, ease of opening, tamperproofing—are highly desirable characteristics of medical packaging.

For hospitals and pharmacies, there are a wide variety of woven reusable materials or nonwoven disposable materials which provide acceptable sterile barriers and are offered by major packaging suppliers. These suppliers normally conduct extensive programs to assure the ability of the material to maintain sterility. Both hospitals and industry have guidelines and accepted practices for sterile-product packaging.[5]

A review of the principles of sterile-material packaging by Powell[20] discusses the suitability of packaging materials for various sterilization methods, including resistance to bacteria, types of openings, strength of packaging, testing of packaging and types of packaging. These topics also are discussed in Chapter 85.

Laminar Airflow

Laminar-airflow equipment is essential for proper performance of sterility tests and aseptic filling or assembling operations. These procedures require exact control over the working environment, but while many techniques and different types of equipment for performing these operations have been used over the years, laminar-airflow devices are superior to all other environmental controls.

The laminar-airflow procedure for producing very clean and dust-free areas was developed in 1961. In a laminar-airflow device the entire body of air within a confined area moves with uniform velocity along parallel flow lines. By employing prefilters and high-efficiency bacterial filters, the air delivered to the area essentially is sterile and sweeps all dust and airborne particles from the chamber through an open side. The velocity of the air used in such devices is generally 90 fpm ± 20%. Laminar-airflow devices that deliver the clean air in a vertical, horizontal or curvilinear fashion are available. The devices can be in the form of rooms, cabinets or benches. For a comprehensive discussion of the biomedical application of laminar airflow the reader is referred to Runkle and Phillips.[21]

Each laminar-airflow cabinet or bench should be located in a separate, small, clean room having a filtered air supply.

The selection of the type of cabinet will depend on the operation itself. For most sterility-testing operations, horizontal laminar-airflow units appear to be superior to vertical-flow hoods because the air movement is less likely to wash organisms from the operator's hands or equipment into the sterility test media. Figure 25 shows the sterility testing of syringes in a horizontal laminar airflow hood. Figure 26 shows the design of a typical horizontal, laminar-airflow hood. The major disadvantage of the horizontal laminar-airflow units is that any airborne particulate matter generated in the units is blown directly into the room and against the working personnel. In situations where infectious material is involved, or where one must prevent contamination of the environment with a powder or drug, the use of specifically designed vertical, recirculating laminar-flow units is recommended. Units are available that do an excellent job of providing both product and personnel protection. Such a unit is shown in Fig 27.

To achieve maximum benefit from laminar airflow, it is important first to realize that the filtered airflow does not itself remove microbial contamination from the surface of objects. Thus, to avoid product or test contamination, it is necessary to reduce the microbial load on the outside of materials used in sterility testing. Laminar flow will do an excellent job of maintaining the sterility of an article bathed in the airflow; however, to be accurate, the sterility-testing, or product-assembly procedure must create the least possible turbulence within the unit. Moreover, an awareness of the turbulent air patterns created by the operation is necessary to avoid performing critical operations in turbulent zones. To illustrate how effectively airborne particles are washed from an environment by laminar airflow, Fig 28 shows the distance various-size particles will travel horizontally before falling 5 ft in a cross-flow of air moving at 50 fpm.

Laminar-flow clean benches should supply Class 100 air as defined in Federal Standard 209B.[22] They should be certified to this standard when installed and then tested periodically An air velometer should be used at regular intervals to check the airflow rates across the face of the filter. Smoke tests are useful in visualizing airflow patterns and a particle analyzer can be used to check the quality of the air. The hot dioctyl phthalate (DOP) test generally is employed to check filter efficiency. This standard acceptance test determines the validity of the filter and its seal using DOP smoke (mean particulate diameter of 0.3 μm) and a light-scattering aerosol photometer. The smoke, at a concentration of 80 to 100 mg/L, is introduced to the plenum of the unit and the entire perimeter of the filter face is scanned with the photometer probe at a sampling rate of 1 ft^3/min. A reading of 0.01% of the upstream smoke concentration is considered a leak.

In addition to the routine airflow measurements and filter-efficiency testing, biological testing should be done to monitor the effectiveness of laminar-airflow systems. Microbial air sampling and agar-settling plates are useful in monitoring these environments. Phillips evaluated horizontal laminar-flow hoods by tabulating the number of "false positives" appearing in sterility-test media over a period of time. These results (Table 2) showed very low numbers of "false positives."

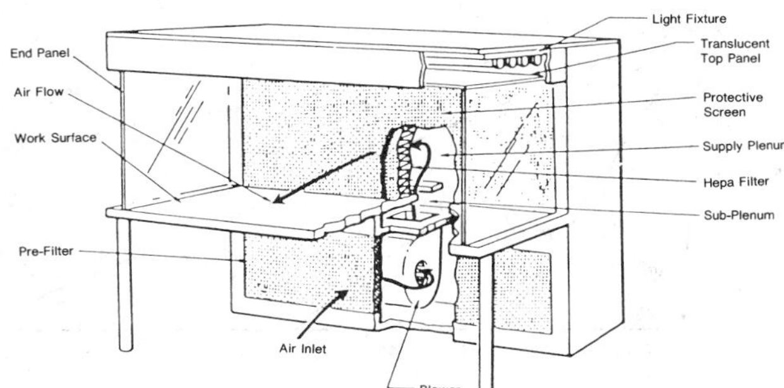

Fig 26. Horizontal laminar-airflow hood.

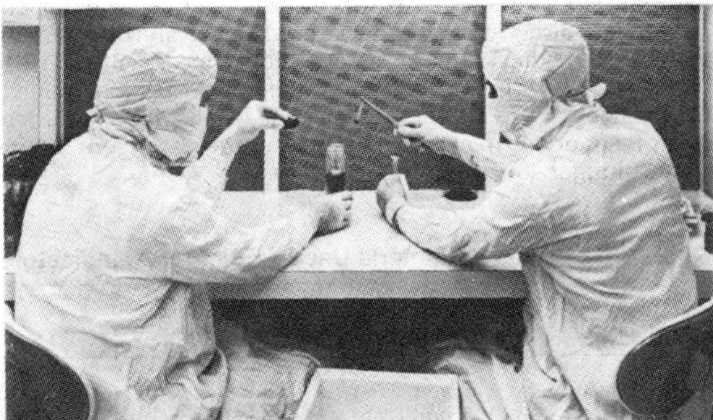

Fig 25. Serility testing of plastic disposable syringes in a horizontal laminar-airflow bench (courtesy, Becton Dickinson & Co).

Testing

After sterilization, there are several techniques for determining mining whether or not the particular lot of material is sterile. The only method for determining sterility with 100% assurance would be to run a total sterility test, ie, to test every item in the lot.

Representative probabilities are shown in Tables 3 and 4 to illustrate more specifically how low levels of contamination in treated lots of medical articles may escape detection by the usual sterility-test procedures. The data are calculated by binomial expansion, employing certain assumed values of percent contamination with large lot sizes (greater than 5000)

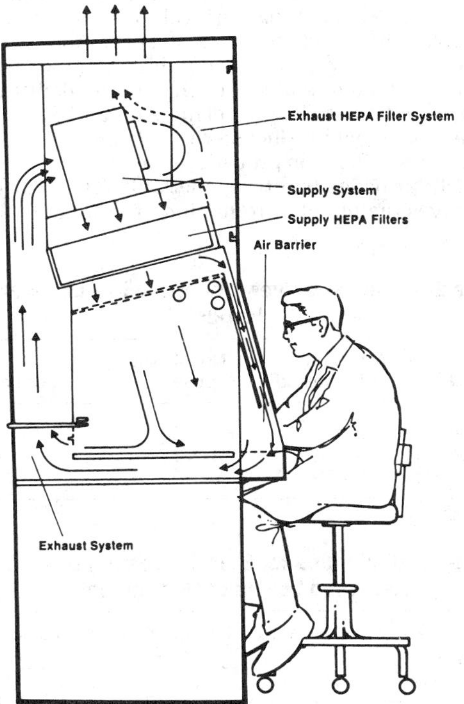

Fig 27. Sketch (*above*) of a biological cabinet with vertical, recirculating laminar-airflow and HEPA-filtered exhaust. HEPA-filtered air is supplied to the work area at 90 fpm ± 20%. Airflow patterns in combination with a high-velocity curtain of air form a barrier at the front access opening which protects both the work and the worker from airborne contamination (courtesy, Bioquest).

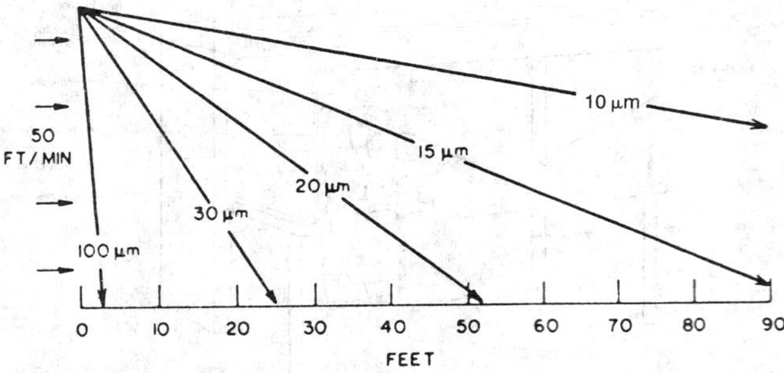

Fig 28. Distance traveled by particles settling from a height of 5 ft.

Table 4—Relationship of Probabilities of Acceptance of Lots of Varying Assumed Degrees of Contamination to Sample Size

Number of samples tested (n)	Probability of no positive growth "True" % contamination of lot					
	0.1	1	5	10	15	20
10	0.99	0.91	0.60	0.35	0.20	0.11
20	0.98	0.82	0.36	0.12	0.04	0.01
50	0.95	0.61	0.08	0.007		
100	0.91	0.37	0.01	0.00		
300	0.74	0.05				
500	0.61	0.01				

and including standard assumptions with regard to the efficiency of recovery media, etc.

In Table 3 the probability data are calculated for lots with various degrees of assumed contamination when 10 random samples per lot are tested. For example, a lot that has one in each 1000 items contaminated (0.1% contamination) could be passed as satisfactory (by showing no positive samples from 10 tested) in 99 tests out of 100. Even at the 10% contamination level, contamination would be detected only two out of three times.

Table 4 shows the difficulty in attempting to improve the reliability of sterility tests by increasing sample size. For contamination levels as low as 0.1%, increasing the sample size from 10 to 100 has a relatively small effect in improving the probability of accepting lots. Even a sample size of 500 would result in erroneously accepting a lot six times out of ten. On the other hand, with a lot contaminated to the extent of 10%, by testing 100 samples the probability of acceptance of the lot would be reduced to a theoretical zero.

The information in Table 4 may be viewed in another way. If, for the probability values shown for each different sample size, the value that approximates the 95% confidence level (P = 0.05) is selected, it is clear that using 20 samples only will discriminate contamination levels of 15% or more. If the 20 tubes show no growth the lot could, of course, be sterile but there would be no way of knowing this from the test. From such a test it could be stated only that it is unlikely that the lot would be contaminated at a level higher than 15%. It is clear from these data that product sterility testing is a poor method of validating sterilization procedures.

The USP provides two basic methods for sterility testing. One involves the direct introduction of product test samples into culture media; the second involves filtering test samples through membrane filters, washing the filters with fluids to remove inhibitory properties and transferring the membrane aseptically to appropriate culture media. Test samples may be sterilized devices that simply are immersed aseptically into the appropriate culture-broth washings of the sterile object with sterile diluent, or dilutions of sterile materials. The USP recommends three aqueous diluting fluids for sterility tests while the Antibiotic Regulations list four; all are nontoxic to microorganisms. In the case of petrolatum-based drugs, a nonaqueous diluting fluid is required.

Many studies have been conducted to find the minimum number of culture media that will provide the greatest sensitivity in detecting contamination. Internationally recognized experts and bodies now recommend the use of two culture media: Soybean-Casein Digest Medium, incubated at 20 to 25°, and Fluid Thioglycollate Medium, incubated at 30 to 35°. The time of incubation specified usually is 7 days for the membrane filtration method and 7 to 14 days for the direct-inoculation method, depending on the method of sterilization. The requirements are described in detail in the USP.

The preferred method of verifying sterility is not by testing sterilized materials but by the use of biological indicators. This is not possible, however, when products are sterilized by filtration and filled aseptically into their final containers, as is the case with such important drugs as antibiotics, insulin or hormones. The indicators generally are highly resistant bacterial spores present in greater numbers than the normal contamination of the product and with equal or greater resistance than normal microbial flora in the products being sterilized. Various properties of commercially available bacterial spores have been recommended for specific methods of sterilization based on unique resistance characteristics. Commonly accepted species of bacteria used for biological indicators are shown in Table 5. Other species can be employed, probably without serious impact on the validity of sterility interpretation, so long as the prime requirements of greater numbers and higher resistance, compared to material contamination characteristics, are maintained.

Included with the materials being sterilized, biological indicators are imbedded on either paper or plastic strips or are inoculated directly onto the material being sterilized. Obviously, the indicator has greater validity in verifying sterility if it is located within product spaces that are the most difficult to sterilize. For example, in the case of a syringe, the location of a paper strip or inoculation of spores between the ribs of the plunger stopper is recommended.

Table 2—False Positives Occurring in a Laminar-Flow Hood[26]

Product	No. of units sterility tested	No. of false positives	% false positives
Syringes	9793	2	0.02
Needles	4676	2	0.04
Misc	306	0	0

Table 3—Probabilities for Sterility Testing of Articles with Assumed Levels of Contamination

"True" % contamination	Probability of designated positives out of 10 samples tested			
	0	1	5	10
0.1	0.990	(Total = 0.010)		
1.0	0.904	0.091		
5.0	0.599	0.315		
10.0	0.349	0.387	0.001	
30.0	0.028	0.121	0.103	
50.0	0.001	0.010	0.246	0.001

Table 5—Species of Bacteria Used as Biological Indicators

Method of sterilization	Bacterial species
Moist heat	*B stearothermophilus*
Dry heat	*B subtilis*
Ethylene oxide	*B stearothermophilus*
Radiation	*B pumilus, B stearothermophilus, B subtilis*

The use of isolators (barrier technology) for processing materials is discussed under *Advanced Aseptic Processing*. The first widespread use of these modern "glove boxes" in the pharmaceutical industry was in sterility testing. As filling speeds became faster, batches became larger. This, coupled with more expensive drug substances, created the need to avoid false-positive sterility tests. Even with laminar-flow hoods becoming widely used, the large number of manipulations carried out by people, created a significant chance for contamination through the testing procedure.

Government standards for SAL basically eliminated the possibility to repeat sterility tests. This means that batches which fail for any reason cannot be released. They are only useful for investigation of potential contamination hazards. Industry in turn needed more assurance that the product was indeed not sterile and the test was valid. This led to the development of more sophisticated isolation units. Figure 29 shows a stainless-steel half-suit system, which is typical of those used in sterility testing. The units can be "docked" to a sterilizer, which eliminates the possibility of contamination during transfer of materials to the test area. The units can be sterilized using vaporized hydrogen peroxide. The exterior of any test materials required to be transferred into the units also can be sterilized in this manner. Validation of these steps allows one to virtually eliminate false-positive test results. Most manufacturers have adopted this technique and have agreed to a policy of essentially no sterility retests. Only where obvious system breakdowns can be shown to have led to failures will a retest be considered.

Advanced Aseptic Processing—Isolator technology also is being used with increasing frequency in the processing of sterile products and associated packaging materials. This is driven by the same need to minimize human intervention and thus increase dramatically the assurance of sterility (SAL). The minimization of people was expanded throughout the 1980s with the advent of more widespread use of form, fill and seal technology. This involved the molding, filling and sealing of plastic bottles, containing sterile products, on-line. The technology was housed in rigid walled areas and product was supplied through filters and sterilized in place, at the last possible area before filling.

While form, fill and seal is a technology on its own, it did lead to the recognition that by updating significantly the older concepts of "glove boxes," one could dramatically affect the sterility assurance of an aseptic process. People contribute the largest percentage of the contamination risk. By minimizing their interaction the probability of nonsterility is greatly reduced.

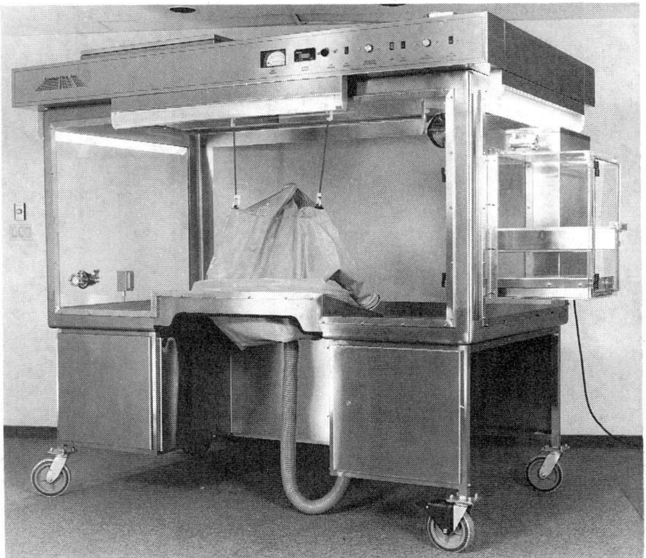

Fig 29. Stainless-steel half-suit isolator (courtesy, Laminar Flow).

Glove boxes were not designed to support modern (and especially more automated) operations. This may explain why they did not become popular as aseptic processing units. It was only when the need for increased assurance drove designers to develop ergonomically designed isolators that the usage began to expand.

More recently, the manufacturers of high-speed processing equipment have begun to redesign their machinery in line with the principles of isolator units. Since the mechanics of these machines have been proved to be very reliable and require very little human intervention, the timing seems to be correct for such modifications. Isolator units are relatively inexpensive also. They have allowed for aseptic processing without the construction of large processing areas, sterile suites or gowning areas. The development of relatively safe sterilization methods, such as vaporized hydrogen peroxide (with or without atmospheric steam) also has allowed the technology to become more viable for widespread use. Prior to this, the use of toxic (and sometimes corrosive) materials was required. This limited their use to more sophisticated operators, who were able to afford the resources required to build and maintain facilities for their use.

Training

It is desirable that personnel involved with sterilization or aseptic processing be instructed in the basic behavior of microorganisms. This would include the differentiation of vegetative, spore-forming and slow-growing life forms such as molds and yeasts. This would allow those being trained in the operations to understand the reasons for many of the restrictions necessary to carry out these processes.

It is imperative that each person involved in these operations be instructed in two main areas.

Safety is the first and foremost area of concentration for a training program. Each of the pieces of equipment and processes described above have unique hazards associated with them. The operators must be made to understand the dangers of steam under pressure and exposure to gaseous sterilants, prior to their neutralization.

The equipment design and installation should undergo safety reviews prior to its general operation. This review for potential hazards must be done by highly trained individuals and should include computer control and piping systems. It is important that the equipment fail (should a failure occur) in a manner which is safe to the operators. Valves should fail in a way to vent pressure to some safe area and/or gases to a relatively safe, unoccupied site.

The second major area of training involves that of gowning for entry into the sterile areas and subsequent performance of aseptic operations. Personnel must be instructed in proper gowning techniques, so that they do not contaminate the exterior of garments and gloves during the process. Gowning areas should be supplied with full length mirrors so that personnel can verify that all areas of their body have been covered fully and properly prior to entering a sterile work area. Recent trends indicate that gowning training be followed by personnel monitoring with contact plates containing growth media. This allows one to verify the effectiveness of the training and, should growth occur, one can use this growth as a training tool to emphasize the importance of careful attention to detail during the gowning process. Since these plates require incubation, one does not allow operators to enter the sterile area until the results of these tests have been collected and reviewed with the candidate.

Continuing with the above approach, those performing aseptic operations require additional training and subsequent verification. This principle of competency-based training (ie, verifying the capabilities of those being trained) is necessary to assure that the operators have developed the skills to carry out these vital operations while minimizing the risk of contamination. Again, it allows for constructive feedback to those who have not yet become fully accomplished in the techniques. It is prudent to reinforce these skills periodically through refresher sessions, and reverification of the skills. It has become standard practice to do unannounced spot-checks of the gloves and gowns of aseptic operators. This practice helps to maintain a level of vigilance, with regard to proper gowning and operating technique.

Acknowledgments

Special thanks to Paul J Haas of Despatch Industries, Dario Pistolesi of Fedegari Autoclavi, Brian Reid of Nordion International and James R. Rickloff of American Sterilizer for supplying significant contributions to the text updates.

References

1. *Medical Device Sterilization Monographs* (Rep Nos 78-4.13 and 78-4.11), Health Ind Manuf Assoc, Washington DC, 1978.
2. Block SS, ed: *Disinfection, Sterilization and Preservation*, 3rd ed, Lea & Febiger, Philadelphia, 1983.
3. *Steam Sterilization and Sterility Assurance, Good Hospital Practice* (AAMI Recommended Practice, ST.1-1980), Assoc Adv Med Instrum, Arlington VA, 1980.
4. *Guideline for Industrial Ethylene Oxide Sterilization of Medical Devices* (AAMI Recommended Practice, OPEO-87), Assoc Adv Med Instrum, Arlington VA, 1987.
5. *In-Hospital Sterility Assurance—Current Perspectives, Aseptic Barrier Evaluation, Sterilizer Processing, Issues in Infection Control and Sterility Assurance* (AAMI Technol Assess Rep No 4-82), Assoc Adv Med Instrum, Arlington VA, 1982.
6. *Hospital Steam Sterilizers* (Am Natl Std, ANSI/AAMI ST8-1982) Assoc Adv Med Instrum, Arlington VA, 1983.
7. *Process Control Guidelines for Gamma Radiation Sterilization of Medical Devices* (AAMI Recommended Practice, RS-3/84), Assoc Adv Med Instrum, Arlington VA, 1984.
8. *Performance Evaluation of Ethylene Oxide Sterilizers—Ethylene Oxide Test Packs, Good Hospital Practice* (AAMI Recommended Practice, EOTP-2.85), Assoc Adv Med Instrum, Arlington VA, 1985.
9. *Biological Indicators for Saturated Steam Sterilization Processes in Health Care Facilities* (Am Natl Std, ANSI/AAMI ST 19-1985), Assoc Adv Med Instrum, Arlington VA, 1986.
10. *Good Hospital Practice: Steam Sterilization Using the Unwrapped Method (Flash Sterilization)* (AAMI Recommended Practice, SSUM-9/85), Assoc Adv Med Instrum, Arlington VA, 1986.
11. Rosenblatt *et al*: *Use of Chlorine Dioxide Gas as a Chemosterilizing Agent*, US Pat 4,504,422 (Scopas Technol Corp), 1985.
12. National Archives: *Fed Reg* 40: 11865, Mar 14, 1975.
13. *21 CFR 211.72.*
14. *Microbiological Evaluation of Filters for Sterilizing Liquids*, No 3, Vol 4, Health Ind Manuf Assoc, Washington DC, 1981.
15. Leahy TJ *et al*: *Pharm Technol 2*: 65, 1978.
16. Dawson FW *et al*: *Nordiska Foreningen for Renlighelsteknik och Rena Rum*, Goteborg, Sweden, 5, 1981.
17. *Test for Determination of Characteristics of Membrane Filters for Use in Aerospace Liquids* (Proposed Tentative Test Method), ASTM, Philadelphia, June 1965.
18. Reti, AR *et al*: *Bull Parenter Drug Assoc 31*: 187, 1977.
19. Patel JA, Curtis EG, Phillips GL: *Amer J Hosp Pharm 29*: 947, 1972.
20. Powell DB: in Phillips GB, Miller WS, eds: *Industrial Sterilization*, Duke Univ Press, Durham NC 79, 1973.
21. Runkle RS, Phillips GB, eds: *Microbial Contamination Control Facilities*, Van Nostrand-Reinhold, New York, 1969.
22. *Clean Room and Work Station Requirements: Controlled Environment* (Fed Std No 209B), USGPO, Washington DC Apr 24, 1973.
23. Lysfjord JP *et al*: *The Potential For Use of Steam at Atmospheric Pressure to Decontaminate or Sterilize Parenteral Filling Lines Incorporating Barrier Isolation Technology*, Spring Mtg of the PDA, Philadelphia, Mar 10, 1993.
24. Edwards LM: *Pharm Eng 13(2)*: 50, 1993.
25. Johnson J: *Vaporized Hydrogen Peroxide Sterilization of Freeze Dryers*, ISPE Annual Mtg, Panama City FL, 1993.

CHAPTER 85

Plastic Packaging Materials

Barrett E Rabinow, PhD
Director, Strategic Development

Theodore J Roseman, PhD
Vice President
Pharmaceutical Sciences Research and Development
Baxter Healthcare Corp
Glendale CA 91203

As defined by the American Society for Testing and Materials (ASTM)

A plastic is a material that contains as an essential ingredient one or more polymeric organic substances of large molecular weight, is solid in its finished state and at some stage in its manufacture or processing into finished articles can be shaped by flow.

The large-molecular-weight organic substance is called a polymer. The use of plastics in the health-care industry has grown at a very rapid rate since the 1960s. This phenomenal growth is due primarily to the wide flexibility in choice of properties offered by plastics. However, because of the wide range of properties of plastics, judicious selection must be made for the intended application.

Prior to the recognition of the potential use of plastics in health-care practice, glass was the predominate material used in the primary packaging of pharmaceutical products. Glass has a definite advantage in being a relatively unreactive and inert substance (although leachable aluminum and glass particles or delamination have posed problems on occasion). As such, it can be used in contact with many critical products, either dry or liquid. It provides excellent protection against water vapor and gas permeation, and it can withstand steam sterilization (autoclaving) without incurring physical distortion. Two definite disadvantages of glass in the field of packaging, however, are its fragility and weight. Due to these negative aspects, coupled with the many positive attributes of plastics, significant inroads for the use of plastic in pharmaceutical packaging have been made. Today, for example, plastics are being used in the following primary packaging areas, where in the 1960s only glass could be considered: syringes, bottles, vials and ampuls.

There are many other significant medical uses which, without the use of plastics, would never have been feasible technically. A few examples include indwelling catheters, prosthetic devices, tracheotomy tubes and flexible containers for intravenous, irrigation and inhalation solutions, as well as for the collection of blood. An additional use for plastics is in secondary container packaging; ie, packaging that is not in direct contact with the product itself. This particular use normally involves plastic films of various types and thicknesses used for tamperproof over-wrapping, whereas the previously mentioned devices normally are fabricated by molding or extrusion of the finished part.

Selection of the appropriate materials for a packaging application should be performed with an understanding of the intended overall design of the package. The requirements should be specified with regard to customer usage, regulatory approval, marketing presentation, manufacturability, sterility and, very importantly, protection of the pharmaceutical product or device during transportation, storage and use. These functional requirements then must be analyzed in terms of the stress requirements they impose on the material, permitting translation of those requirements into material properties. A target material profile is developed by assigning required values of design and performance properties that predict or correlate with the container functions. Likely candidate materials are determined by comparing their properties with the property profile derived from the functional requirements. A prototype is built, and tested via functionally oriented tests such as maintenance of product stability, simulated usage and storage tests, and customer focus groups. Material properties affecting functional performance are now described.

Material Properties

Mechanical Properties

Important mechanical properties in plastic packaging materials are

Tensile strength is the maximum force needed to pull apart a specimen of material, divided by its cross-sectional area. Elongation is the percentage change over original length at breaking point and measures a film's ability to stretch.

Impact strength is a measure of the ability to withstand shock-loading, where a specimen receives a blow from a swinging pendulum, for example. Fracture will occur if the impact force exceeds the limit of elasticity of the material. Glass, for example, has a much lower impact strength than many plastics, although its has appreciable tensile strength.

Tear strength is measured both as the force necessary to initiate a tear and force to propagate a tear. Propagation of tear is undesirable in shipping sacks, but desirable in tear tapes. Orientation of the material can affect results, because the polymer chains can be aligned along a particular direction during manufacturing, thus conferring greater strength in that direction.

Stiffness is the resistance of bending where deflection against a load can be measured.

Flex resistance to the development of pinholing and fracture, when subjected to repeated flexing or creasing, is important in shipping applications. Unsupported aluminum foil, unless it is heavy gauge, is prone to this failure mode.

Coefficient of friction or ***slip*** relates to the ease with which one material will slide over another. Passage of films through packaging machinery requires high slip to prevent binding, and is important in form, fill-seal-operations.

Blocking is the tendency of two adjacent layers of film to stick together. This can create difficulties during manufacturing.

Fatigue resistance, or the ability to withstand the imposition of repetitive short-time stress or deformation without cracking, is relevant in applications involving continual cyclical loading, such as toggle mechanisms, gear teeth of a pump or peristaltic compression of IV tubing.

Creep failure occurs when a plastic is subjected to a constant static load, it deforms quickly and elastically (reversibly) to a predicted strain value and then continues to deform at a slower rate indefinitely. Rupture may eventually occur. Creep is both temperature and time dependent. The design life of the package thus plays a role, because both strength and stiffness may be time related. The loss of torque of a static bottle-closure system over time or deformation of plastic IV tubing under constant compression are examples.

Other properties of plastics may affect their usage in a particular application. For example low temperature, mechanical behavior is important if a plastic is exposed to frozen temperatures during its use, since the impact strength of certain plastics decreases in the frozen state. The density of plastics, which vary between 0.8 to 1.8 g/cm^3 is an important property, since lower density materials will produce more moldings per unit weight. Additionally, the melting point which may extend over a range of temperatures is important for determining processing temperatures, heat sterilizability, ability to hot-fire a product and heat-sealing characteristics.

Optical Properties

Important optical properties in plastic packaging materials are

Light transmission is the ratio of the intensity of a light source measured with the film interposed to the intensity without the film. It gives no indication of image distortion or blurring.

Clarity indicates the degree of distortion of an object seen through the film.

Haze is a measure of milkiness, caused by light scattering by surface imperfections or film inhomogeneities such as crystallites, voids, cross-linked materials and undissolved additives. Haze obscures visibility for product inspection.

Gloss measures specular reflection, or the reflectance of light as a mirror reflects. This parameter indicates the ability to produce a sharp image of any light source, giving rise to a pleasing sparkle of the film.

Electrical Properties

Electrical properties can be important, as for the dissipation of static charge in the operating room. This was previously of greater concern when ether was more widely used as an anesthetic and poured from a bottle, resulting in a potential fire hazard. More importantly, static electricity is a hazard to electronic equipment and devices. In addition, dirt and dust are attracted by static to the surface and increase the chance of contamination.

Physicochemical Properties

Mass Transfer

Many pharmaceutical preparations must be protected adequately from oxygen, water vapor, carbon dioxide and many other permeants. An effervescent tablet requires a barrier to moisture, for example, whereas an oil-based product must be protected from oxygen-induced oxidation. Unlike glass, plastics are permeable. Barrier properties indicate permeability to water vapor, oxygen, carbon dioxide, etc. In addition, components of the product can permeate through the package. Examples include the parabens, flavorants, water vapor and oils. Permeation through a plastic barrier depends on the composition of the plastic, permeation area, thickness of the barrier, partial pressure differential of the permeant across the barrier and time. Permeation through a plastic also can be affected greatly by additives and the crystalline structure of the plastic. Specific additives, primarily plasticizers, can increase the permeation rate greatly. Highly crystalline plastics such as polypropylene generally exhibit low water-permeation rates.

As a guide, the approximate relative permeation rates for water vapor, oxygen and carbon dioxide through the more commonly used plastics in packaging are given in Table 1.[1] The total ingress of gas into a package can be divided into contributions from the separate components, for example, permeation through the lid, bottle, outer protective overpouch and gross leakage through microscopic cracks and pinholes. This analysis can be performed kinetically to verify container integrity or to resolve manufacturing problems.[2]

Table I—Permeability Rates of Selective Plastic Packaging Materials[1]

Plastic	g/100 in²/24 hr/mil @ 37.8°C	cc/100 in²/mil/24 hr/atm @ 25°C	
	Water vapor	Oxygen	Carbon dioxide
Nylon			
Type 6	16–22	2.6	10–12
Type 12	4	34–92	153–336
Polyethylene terephthalate	1.0–1.3	3.0–6.0	15–25
Polyethylene			
Low density	1.0–1.5	500	2700
Medium density	0.7	250–535	1000–2500
High density	0.3	185	580
Polypropylene	0.7	150–240	500–800
Polystyrene	7–10	250–350	900
Vinyl			
Nonplasticized	2–5	4–30	4–30
Plasticized	15–40	600	20–500
Vinyl chloride-acetate copolymer			
Nonplasticized	4	15–20	40–70
Plasticized	5–8	20–150	70–800
Polyvinylidene chloride	0.2–0.6	0.8–6.9	3.8–44
Polycarbonate	11	300	1075

Chemical Attack

Resistance to acids, alkalies, fats, solvents, water and light are important if compatibility with these materials is required. Some plastics are incompatible with plasticizers used with PVC polymers, lipid emulsions, detergents or antiseptic solutions. Iodine-containing liquids permanently stain many polyolefin compounds after a brief exposure. Absorption of the migrating chemical forces the polymer chains apart, swelling the plastic and causes stress cracking. This can occur, as well, from solvents used to solvent-bond plastic components.

Rubber, when exposed to ozone, as from electrostatic dust precipitators, will lose elasticity and become brittle. In this case, chemical reaction of the ozone with the polymer backbone is responsible. Another failure mode involves simply the leaching of components, such as silicone lubricant from rubber syringe plungers, into the contained solution. This increases the particulate burden and can form a visual haze. In some instances pigmentation used in the plastic is attacked chemically and leached by the product.

In the case of plastics used in direct contact with a product—either in dry or liquid form—the length of time that the medication and the container are in contact may determine if problems such as discoloration, leaching and absorption or adsorption of a constituent of the product may arise. It is possible that both the product and the package containing it could change significantly from the time of manufacture. Lack of visual indication of a reaction at the onset of a stability study does not imply that the reaction(s) was not occurring during the early stages of storage.

In certain instances, a specific set of storage parameters must exist before a reaction is initiated. For many drugs, generally the higher the temperature and humidity in the storage area, the more rapid the chemical attack. For many IV solutions in flexible plastic containers, however, shelf-life is limited by water-vapor loss, which is diminished in the presence of high humidity. Other factors that may affect the plastic packaging and product are pH, surface treatment of the plastic, container configuration, type of polymer used, method of package preparation, light transmission and means of assembly or sterilization.[3]

Theory and experiment have been developed sufficiently to permit prediction of the maximal accumulation of leachables in solution without waiting for the results of shelf-life stability studies. This expedites product development and addresses material/solution compatibility concerns. Accumulation of a leachable material from a container into solution can be limited by any of four physical factors:[4]

1. The initial amount of leachable material present in the container material (total available pool, TAP).
2. The solubility limit of the leachable material in the solution phase.
3. The equilibrium partitioning of the leachable component between the container and the solution.
4. The rate of migration of the leachable component from the container into solution.

The TAP, solubility limit and equilibrium partitioning can be evaluated for each identified leachable substance. These characteristics then can be used to identify the process which would limit the accumulation of leachable chemicals. The lowest value found determines the limiting accumulation and identifies the limiting mechanism. The solubility limit, equilibrium partitioning and rate of migration may restrict actual solution accumulation below the total available pool estimate. Kinetic control produces the minimum accumulation estimate, since no matter how fast the rate of migration, a leachable component cannot accumulate in excess of what is thermodynamically available. As an example, the equilibrium solution accumulation of a leachable material, C_e, is given by

$$C_e = (TAP \times W_c)/[(W_c \times E_b) + V_s]$$

where TAP is the μg leachable/g of film, W_c = weight of the container (in grams), V_s is the solution volume (in liters) and E_b is the equilibrium partitioning constant, the ratio of the concentration of solute in the film to that in water, at equilibrium. This can be calculated from the more familiar, and referenced, solvent-solvent partition coefficients.

This methodology also can be used to predict the extent of the reverse process, that of adsorption of solution components (drugs or antimicrobial agents) into the plastic.[5]

Safety Testing

Numerous testing procedures must be followed in order to ensure the safety of use of any plastic. Among these are biological, chemical, physical and pharmacological assessments. A greater degree of safety testing is warranted as the extent of contact of the material with the body increases. Thus, an IV solution container is studied in greater depth than is secondary packaging. Medical devices that are left intact in the human body for prolonged periods of time (vascular grafts, cartilage replacements, pacemakers or prosthetics) are studied most extensively. Their reactivity and degree of safety and toxicity must be determined. In all cases, it is imperative that the plastic, and its processing procedure, provide a nonreactive and nontoxic end product.

The official compendia provide procedures for performing certain biological and physicochemical tests on plastic containers; for details, see the USP. The principles of these tests are described in the following sections.

Biologic Testing Procedures—The official USP biologic procedures are designed to determine the suitability of plastic materials intended for use in fabricating containers or accessories for both parenteral and ophthalmic preparations. The procedures for the former determine the reaction of living animal tissues and normal animals to implanted portions of the plastic or injected extracts prepared from it. Depending on the use of the plastic, other biological tests may be performed, such as pyrogenicity, blood compatibility, antigenicity, suitability for use in cardiovascular devices, embryological reaction and tissue-toxicity testing.

Physiochemical Testing Procedures—Many chemical and physical tests are applied to plastics, the particular ones used depending on the intended applications of the substances. The physicochemical procedures used by the USP are designed to determine the physical and chemical properties of plastics used as containers, based on tests with extracts prepared by heating samples with Water for Injection at 70° for 24 hours. Portions of the extract are used to determine Nonvolatile Residue, Residue on Ignition, Heavy Metals and Buffering Capacity or Reaction, official limits for each of which are specified. Also described is a procedure for determining the light transmission of plastics, with limits for maximum transmission.

The actual product/package should be evaluated under simulated use conditions, including shipping and storage, to assure product integrity throughout its shelf-life. Potential incompatibilities between the primary plastic container and secondary packaging should be addressed to anticipate adulteration of the product. Prolonged exposure to ultraviolet light has been shown to enhance the migration of certain additives which, in turn, can accelerate the aging characteristics of the plastic and decrease the shelf-life of the product. In some instances, incompatibilities that might occur readily can be detected visually; in others, sophisticated extraction techniques must be followed in order to ascertain the effects storage conditions may have had. For this reason, well-planned stability studies need to be established.

Desirable features used for health-care packaging are transparency, thermal stability, physical strength, formability, sealability, biological barrier, radiation resistance and disposability. Usually one cannot find all the desired properties in a single material, but two or more plastics can be combined into a composite packaging material.

Failure Mode Analysis

After development and subsequent distribution of plastic packaged items, functional problems may occur occasionally. Resolution of these problems requires analysis of the causative-failure mode. This involves problem isolation, segregating the problem material to a particular batch, for example, to identify potential causative factors. The failed parts are subjected to mechanical, microscopic and chemical analysis to further determine how they differ from acceptable parts. The analytical techniques chosen are dictated by the observed mode of failure.

Physical tests, such as mechanical, electrical and optical determinations can be performed quickly, and control values exist in the form of manufacturers' specifications, which are readily available. As the problem becomes more precisely focused, more specific, and often elaborate testing, is performed to further isolate the cause. For example, reduced stiffness of a part may be attributable to lowered molecular weight of the plastic. Microscopic analysis is rapid, and a skilled analyst often can identify the problem as a pinhole, improper seal, delamination of a composite material or foreign material acting as a stress fracture initiator.

Chemical analysis of impurities caused bloom or preventing seal formation is often time consuming because of the tiny amounts present, large variety of potential compounds and lack of control information from the supplier. The expense and variety of chemical instrumentation available requires judicious selection of the approach to be used.

Classification

There are over 100 different polymer types available for use which can be classified further into two subcategories. These are identified as *Thermoplastics* and *Thermosets* (thermosetting plastics). Thermoplastics consist of those plastics which normally are rigid at operating temperatures, but can be remelted and reprocessed. Thermosets consist of those plastics which, when subjected to heat, normally will become infusible or insoluble, and as such cannot be remelted.

Additives

Thermoplastics can be modified greatly and their properties enhanced by the addition of specific additives. As chemicals may act synergistically, any two safe additives may have the potential to produce undesirable effects when combined. For these reasons, the Food and Drug Administration (FDA) requires that these blends or combinations be evaluated totally, prior to marketing in product form. Chemical, pharmacological and biological tests should be conducted in order to establish safety. Problems involving additives include migration to the surface of molded parts and leaching into aqueous solutions. Additives used routinely in thermoplastic formulations are

Lubricants are used to assist processing of the plastic during the molding or extrusion operation. A commonly used lubricant in the case of polyethylene is zinc stearate. The quantities employed vary from formulation to formulation.

Stabilizers are used to retard or prevent degradation of the polymer by heat and light, during manufacturing, as well as to improve its aging characteristics. Common stabilizer families include organometallic compounds, fatty acid salts and inorganic oxides.

Plasticizers are used in order to achieve softness and flexibility. They are used commonly in plastic materials such as vinyls, cellulosics and propionates.

Antioxidants are a special type of stabilizer used primarily to assist in retarding oxidation. Combinations of antioxidants with other additives may result in undesirable chemical reactions.

Antistatic agents are used to prevent the buildup of static charges on the plastic surface.

Slip agents are added primarily to polyolefins (polyethylene and polypropylene) in order to reduce the coefficient of friction of the material. These particular chemicals result in antitack and antiblock characteristics in the end product.

Dyes and pigments are added to impart color.

Processing

Besides the addition of additives, the manner in which a plastic is formed into the desired configuration can affect the end properties. It is important that process parameters, such as temperature, pressure and time, be controlled rigidly to ensure batch-to-batch uniformity for plastic objects. If process parameters are not controlled adequately, such deleterious effects on plastic properties as thermal degradation, piece-part stresses and incorrect physical dimensions may result. Process thermal degradation of a plastic can affect the leaching characteristics of the plastic object, its permeation characteristics and its long-term stability during the shelf-life of the pharmaceutical product. Piece-part stresses may be relieved when the pharmaceutical package is subjected to certain environmental conditions resulting in package failure during the shelf-life of the product.

The more common plastic processing methods employed for pharmaceutical packaging components follow.

Injection Molding

Injection molding is an intermittent process, the plastic being heated to a melted or viscous state and then forced into a cavity (mold) at high pressure. The melted material cools in the cavity and solidifies. The mold is then opened and the part removed. A wide range of thermoplastic and several thermosetting materials can be injection-molded. Besides threads on bottle caps, very intricate configurations can be obtained by injection- molding of plastics.

Extrusion

Extrusion is a continuous process, the plastic being heated to a melted or viscous state and forced under pressure through a die, resulting in a configuration of desired shape. The extruded profile is cooled to a solid state, generally by spraying with water, by immersion in water or by using chilled rolls for film material. A wide range of thermoplastic materials can be extruded. Typical extruded profiles used by the pharmaceutical industry are packaging films and medical tubing. Plastic packaging film also is formed by blow extrusion, an extruded tube being blown into a large cylinder and then slit after cooling.

Besides simply imparting a new shape to the molten plastic, the manufacturing process can preferentially orient the molecular chains in a given direction, by stretching the plastic. This in turn affects physical properties such as clarity and impact strength, as the chains are oriented along the load-bearing direction. Crystallites can be formed and oriented to yield increases in strength, albeit at reduction in elongation at break. Barrier properties are improved for polypropylene. Biaxially oriented film has balanced properties if the same extent of stretching is used in each direction. In cast film, orientation in the machine direction is achieved by feeding the film through a series of rolls running at gradually increasing speeds. Rolls are heated sufficiently to bring the film to suitable temperature below the melting point. Transverse orientation is obtained by use of a tenter frame, which has two divergent endless belts fitted with clips. These grip the film so that, as it travels forward, it is drawn transversely at the required draw ratio. Uniaxial orientation is used for high-performance tape.

Blow Molding

The plastic is heated to a melted or viscous state and formed into a hollow cylinder (parison). The parison generally is extruded, but may be injection-molded. If extruded, the parison is cut to the required length and transferred to the blowing cavity (mold). The bottom of the parison is pinched off by the mold and air is blown into the parison, expanding the viscous plastic to the walls of the cavity, thus forming the desired shape of the container. The melted material cools in the cavity and solidifies. The mold is opened and the container removed. Pharmaceutical bottles are blow-molded from a wide range of thermoplastic materials, of which polyethylene and polypropylene are used predominantly.

Solvent Casting

A liquid suspension of rubber is deposited on an endless belt and the solvent is vaporized. The belt carries the rubber material through a heat cabinet to cure it, whereupon the film is stripped off the belt, cooled and wound onto reels.

Compression Molding

Compression molding is used for thermosetting materials and is an intermittent process. The thermosetting material (powder or a tablet preform) is placed into a heated cavity (mold). The material melts and flows to fill the cavity. The mold is held under pressure until the thermosetting material cures, after which the mold is opened and the part removed. As with injection molding, very intricate configurations can be obtained by compression-molding of thermosetting materials.

Types and Uses

The following types of plastics are used commonly in health-care practice; several of their properties and end uses are indicated.

Thermoplastics

The following are used commonly in injection molding, blow molding, extrusion and fabricated sheeting.

Acrylics—This class includes the polymethacrylates, polyacrylates and copolymers of acrylonitrile. There are many variations in this class, mainly concerned with the combinations of methacrylate and acrylate esters, as well as acrylonitrile. These plastics are characterized by clarity and unusual optical properties, low water absorption, good electrical resistivity, excellent weatherability and fair tensile strength. Their heat resistance is low and care should be taken to keep them below temperatures of 200°F, at which they tend to soften. Acrylics find considerable use in a multiplicity of devices employed in today's hospitals and clinics. A specific application is in the adapters used in solution-administration sets and blood-collection sets.

Cellulosics—To be used as a thermoplastic without charring, cellulose must be modified. The range of modification available permits a wide variety of physical characteristics, including toughness, surface gloss, good clarity, good scuff resistance and high gas permeability. To achieve these properties, the cellulosic alcohol groups are esterified with acetate, butyrate and/or propionate. Butyrate and propionate are chosen over acetate for applications requiring low-temperature impact strength and dimensional stability. Extruded butyrate and propionate sheeting have good gage uniformity, surface quality, brilliance and visual effects. Propionate is selected over butyrate and acetate when increases in hardness, tensile strength and stiffness are important. Increased plasticizer level lowers hardness, stiffness and tensile strength but increases impact strength. Combined esters such as cellulose acetate propionate and cellulose acetate butyrate are especially popular for medical applications. This family of cellulosics is used in such articles as tubing and special trays for urological or spinal procedures, membranes in dialyzers and some filters, and IV buret housings.

Nylons—Nylon is the generic designation for a class of polyamides containing repeating amide groups (—CONH—) connected to methylene units (—CH_2—) in the structure of the polymer. They are characterized by good chemical resistance to most solvents and chemicals, with the exception of strong solutions of certain mineral acids, phenolic compounds and strong oxidizers. Nylons can be used in the fabrication of precision parts and adapters for devices and equipment. Aerosol valves, for example, have a low wear requirement which is satisfied by nylon's low friction-bearing surfaces. Nylon also is used in the manufacture of packaging films and laminates, providing clarity and imparting excellent resistance to puncture and abrasion; but, because sterilization survival is not good (it wrinkles during autoclaving and degrades upon irradiation), its success in form/fill/seal food-packaging applications has not made an impact on health-care packaging.

Polyethylene Terephthalate (PET)—PET is prepared from ethylene glycol and either terephthalic acid or the dimethyl ester of terephthalic acid. Its chemical structure is $p\text{-}HO(COC_6H_4COOCH_2CH_2O)_nH$. PET exists in an amorphous state, an oriented and partially crystalline state and a highly crystalline state. Most applications require orientation and/or crystallization in order to take advantage of the dramatically increased strength and improved serviceability at high temperatures that result. PET polymers offer many advantages to the container and packaging field. Among those are its high strength, excellent clarity and low transmission rate to gas and water vapor and sterilizability by all major modes. PET bottles are used for a wide variety of foods and beverages, as well as pharmaceutical containers. Heavier gauge, semirigid, unoriented polyester is used in the manufacture of blister packs.

Polyethylene—The properties of polyethylene vary according to molecular weight and type: low-density or branched and high-density or linear. The linear type is more crystalline, more heat-resistant and stiffer than the low-density or conventional type. Both have low water absorption, excellent electrical resistance, high resistance to most solvents and chemicals and is tasteless and odorless. It, thus, is well-suited to many applications where only moderate to low heat exposure will be encountered. Due to its excellent properties, polyethylene has found widespread application in the pharmaceutical industry and in hospitals. Its use ranges from containers for liquid or dry products, to both laminated and unsupported films for sterile-device packaging and to molded parts for a variety of devices and equipment. Unsupported polyethylene is used for shrink-wrapping, stretch-wrapping, skin-packaging and bags.

The properties of polyethylene vary according to molecular weight and type: low-density (LDPE) or branched and high-density (HDPE) or linear. The length and number of side-chain branches determine the degree of crystallinity and density of this amorphous-crystalline polymer. The linear type is more crystalline, more heat-resistant and stiffer than the low-density or conventional type. As crystallinity and density increase, opacity, stiffness, tensile strength, surface hardness and chemical resistance increase. Silicone oil and surfactants, however, can act as stress-crack agents, leading to cracks forming in stressed areas, as the permeants spread apart the polymeric chains.

With more tightly packed molecules HDPE has better moisture-barrier properties with less elongation (better tensile strength) than LDPE. It is used widely, where rigidity and barrier properties are preferrred, for bottles of solid dosage-form products. However, LDPE is used, where flexibility is required, for squeeze bottles of sprays and drops. Blown-films of LDPE have very low haze and high gloss whereas HDPE films have higher haze, because of crystalline induced light scattering, and are semiglossy. The less crystalline LDPE has a lower melting point with broader melting range than does HDPE and, therefore, is easier to heat-seal. The low melting point, however, negates steam sterilization for LDPE, unlike HDPE.

Polyethylene is used as primary packing film but its use as a sealant, through the application of heat and pressure, is more important. To increase its sealing and adhesion to more polar materials, polyethylene often is modified by comonomers, such as 3 to 5% ethylene-vinyl acetate, acrylic acid, methacrylic and methyl acrylate.

Ethylene-Vinyl Acetate (EVA)—Addition of vinyl acetate comonomer to ethylene reduces polymer crystallinity, improving clarity, low-temperature flexibility and toughness, impact strength, stress-crack and flex-crack resistance, and reduces hardness. Melting and heat-seal temperature are lowered, as are the barrier properties. Increased vinyl acetate concentration also increases polarity, resulting in increased tackiness and adhesion to a variety of substrates. The copolymer also can be cross-linked (chemical bonds form between the polymer chains) by either radiation or addition of organic peroxides. This increases the melting temperature, permitting autoclaving as a sterilization option. Adding vinyl acetate softens the material, resulting in a smoother surface. The copolymer, EVA, is used in tip protectors, where flex resistance is required, and for low-temperature IV bags.

The two main characteristics controlled in the copolymerization of vinyl acetate and ethylene are crystallinity and molecular weight. Molecular weight is controlled by the addition of radical chain-transfer agents. As the molecular weight of EVA increases, so does the melt viscosity, heat-seal strength, toughness, flexibility, stress-crack resistance and hot-tack strength. One of the leachables is acetic acid, resulting from the hydrolysis of the acetate esters.

Polypropylene—Propylene is lighter than polyethylene, yet it is much stiffer and more heat- resistant with the same chemical and electrical resistance properties. This material is available as the highly crystalline, isotactic polypropylene and the higher impact grades of atactic and syndiotactic types. *Isotactic* refers to a plastic with the organic groups (R) being on the same side of the polymer chain. *Syndiotactic* refers to the alternation of organic groups above and below the polymer chain and *atactic* signifies no regular sequences of the groups.

Polypropylenes can be used in almost every application employed for polyethylene. Devices made of this material can be sterilized with steam and ethylene oxide, but not radiation, unless modified polypropylenes are used. Polypropylenes can be modified with polyethylene or rubber to improve their impact resistance. Higher levels of ethylene lower stiffness and improve clarity. Biaxial orientation also will improve its clarity. It is, however, the nonoriented cast copolymer that is most used for health-care packaging. Polypropylene is used widely for solid dosage products. Injection-molded bottles, for example, can be made either with separate lids or with integrally molded lids which exhibit high flexural strength.

The low density of polypropylene offers an economic advantage, as more molds can be made from a given weight of the material. Nucleating agents may be added to speed the rate of crystallization, thus shortening the molding cycle, resulting in more economical manufacturing processes and cheaper products. Because polypropylene is largely chemically resistant, it cannot be solvent-bonded. It can, nevertheless, be heat-bonded. Bonding by use of adhesives requires surface pretreatment using corona, plasma or flame, or chemical etching. It can be made heat sealable by applying a coating of polyvinylidene chloride or ethylene-polypropylene copolymer.

Tyvek (*Du Pont*)—is a spun-bonded polyolefin that appears white, smooth, water repellant and offers high tear strength as well as good porosity for sterilization. However, it is expensive, has poor print quality and its web varies in thickness and density. It usually is not used for autoclaving. Prior to thermal disintegration, it will become translucent, indicating that its properties have been compromised.

Polystyrene (PS)—This polymer is one of the oldest and most widely used plastics. In pharmaceutics and therapeutics it has enjoyed wide use for fabrication of containers and syringes. Polystyrene (PS) has relatively low heat resistance and is attacked by a number of chemical agents, such as phthalate plasticizers in vinyl polymers, resulting in crazing (microcracks). It is available in a clear crystal grade and an increasingly popular rubber-modified impact-resistant grade, in which polystyrene is copolymerized with acrylonitrile and butadiene. The crystal versions craze during most ethylene oxide cycles, but impact grades withstand both gas and radiation sterilization. Polystyrene cannot, however, be autoclaved. While this polymer is inexpensive, the lack of impact strength in the conventional grade, and poor optical properties in impact-modified grades, limit its use in more demanding applications.

Vinyl Plastics—The term vinyl comes from the group, ($CH_2{=}CH$—), which has many derivatives, such as vinyl chloride ($CH_2{=}CHCl$) and vinyl acetate ($CH_2{=}CHOCOCH_3$) and vinylidene chloride ($CH_2{=}CCl_2$, Saran). With this group of vinyl compounds, many polymers are made either as homopolymers of themselves or as copolymers with other vinyl derivatives or other monomeric materials. For example, polyvinylidene chloride resins are, for the most part, copolymers of vinylidene chloride with vinyl chloride, acrylonitrile and acrylate esters.

These are used primarily where high barrier properties to moisture, oxygen and other chemicals are required.

The versatile vinyl plastics are used to prepare materials ranging from soft flexible sheeting to rigid, hard tubing. The great variety of PVC resins, with their wide range of physical properties, had led to the development of many applications of this material in the fields of pharmacy and medicine. It is used in the manufacture of blood bags, examination gloves, IV solution containers and pump tubing. An unplasticized form is used in the fabrication of rigid parts for devices. Because PVC has glass-like clarity and is inexpensive, it makes an appealing blister pack. It finds limited use in packaging devices because it turns brown when exposed to radiation sterilization, is too heat sensitive for steam sterilization and degassing ethylene oxide is too lengthy. However, more than 25% of all plastic-based medical devices used in hospitals are made of PVC, because of its weldability, cost, response to heat and pressure and versatility.[6]

Flexible PVC has excellent impact and flex-crack resistance at room temperature. As the temperature is lowered, the material becomes stiffer, resulting in decreased flex-crack resistance and impact strength. The type and amount of plasticizer determines the temperature at which the failure mode changes from ductile to a brittle failure. For flexible medical applications such as IV bags and tubing, the plasticizer DEHP (Di(2-ethylhexyl)phthalate) is used most often. Because it can leach into solution, the safety of DEHP has been studied extensively throughout the years, and no long-term exposure problems have been identified.[7]

Cyclohexanone can be used to bond PVC to most materials. When bonded to DEHP-noncompatible materials, such as polycarbonate and impact-grade polystyrene, a barrier adhesive must be used.

Polycarbonates—These are formed by condensation of polyphenols such as Bisphenol-A with phosgene. The polymers are transparent thermoplastics (although opacifiers are added for some applications), with high strength and high temperature resistance. Because they are expensive, their use is limited to specialty applications where dimensional stability or high-impact resistance are valued, such as in rigid, transparent, blood oxygenator housings. The polycarbonates have hardness properties similar to those of metals and are being used to replace metals in numerous industrial applications.

Creep-resistance is good over a broad range of temperatures and parts can be molded consistently to tolerances of 0.002 in/in. They can be heat- or solvent-sealed, facilitating fabrication procedures, but this advantage also renders them susceptible to phthalate crazing, when placed in contact with plasticized vinyls.

Ionomer—Is used as an inner ply in laminates, offering good heat-sealing (even when the seal area is contaminated by liquid or powder) over a wide temperature range. Heat-sealing usually can proceed faster than by using alternate materials. Ionomers are clear, semiflexible, tough materials with good abrasion resistance, all of which are features valued in sachet and pouch packs.

Chemically, ionomers are the sodium or zinc salts of ethylene/methacrylic acid polymers. The ionic cross-links occur randomly along the long-chain polymer molecules to produce solid-state properties usually associated with polymers of high molecular weight. Heating ionomers to normal thermoplastic-processing temperatures, however, diminishes these ionic forces, allowing the material to be melt-processed in conventional molding and extrusion equipment. The long-chain semicrystalline hydrocarbon polymer imparts polyolefinic character, chemical inertness, thermal stability and low water-vapor transmission.

Fluoropolymer-Aclar Film (polymonochlorotrifluoroethylene, PCTFE)—Fluoropolymer has extremely low transmission of moisture, is transparent and can be heat-sealed, laminated, printed, thermoformed, metallized and sterilized. Because it is the most expensive plastic used in the pharmaceutical industry, it is employed only where the most demanding barrier properties are required. Laminated Aclar/PVC sheet is used widely in thermoformed blister packs for moisture sensitive solid dosage forms.

Polyurethane foams are formed by polymerization in the presence of a foaming agent and have been used as a replacement for cotton wool in tablet containers.

Thermosets

The following are some of the commonly used compression-molded thermosetting compounds. These plastics are used when good dimensional and temperature stability are required. Parts are fabricated by means of compression-molding techniques. The formaldehyde plastics are obtained by condensation reactions between formaldehyde and substances such as melamine, phenol and urea.

As a family, the formaldehydes have been found to be of most use in the pharmaceutical industry as closures for glass and/or plastic containers. By virtue of high resistance to heat, they are used in specific applications where the molded part requires sterilization by steam.

Melamine Formaldehyde—This family of plastics exhibits good to excellent dimensional stability. When used in the manufacture of closures, high torque strength and good impact strength are obtained. These plastics also exhibit good resistance to oils, grease and many organic solvents.

Phenol Formaldehyde—This type of plastic provides good scratch-resistant parts. It exhibits very low shrinkage, and low water-absorption properties. It is, however, a relatively brittle plastic.

Urea Formaldehyde—This plastic exhibits good dimensional stability as well as good strength properties. Articles produced from this material are highly rigid and provide good resistance to alcohols, oils, grease and some of the weaker acids.

Applications

Composite materials, incorporating several components or plies, are used often to obtain the numerous advantages of multiple materials, all of which are unavailable from just one component. A stable material, forming the bulk of the film is selected, such as PET, which is very popular for flexible packaging, providing dimensional and thermal stability. To this can be added protective coatings, such as barrier materials affording protection from oxygen, water vapor and gasses. Also available are sealant layers permitting the package to be heat-sealed, bonding layers to accommodate printing inks, and to bond the various layers together in multiple-ply extrusions or laminations.

Health-Care Device Packaging is designed to protect medical devices during sterilization and shipping. The material porosity required for steam or ethylene oxide gas sterilization must be considered in conjunction with the need for maintaining a bacterial barrier following sterilization. Some candidate materials must be rejected because they cannot survive the sterilization mode. For example, PVC, unless specially stabilized, turns brown when subjected to radiation sterilization. Polypropylene becomes brittle only months following radiation exposure.

A satisfactory vent bag consist of a porous Tyvek patch incorporated into a 3-mils or thicker LDPE bag. This permits rapid in- and out-gassing of ethylene oxide, minimizing expensive sterilization and hold-storage times. The thickness represents a compromise between cost and performance, because thinner bags tend to tear thus occasioning repacking and resterilizing.

For products requiring better protection than that afforded by a flexible pouch, tray packages can be used. These may be either preformed or formed on-line. The latter uses thermoform/fill/seal machinery which forms a container from a web of flexible material which is unwound from a reel. This is then filled with product and sealed on-line, in one continuous operation. Polyester often is considered for the blister tray, using its thermoforming capability, appearance, toughness and dimensional stability, subsequently sealing it to a Tyvek or paper lid.

Heat-seal coating technology is important to ensure a reliably sterile product. Modified PE often is used for the heat-seal coating. Sealant properties of PE can be modified, depending upon the product requirements, by branching the polymer chain, which decreases its crystallinity and hence density. By decreasing density, the sealing range, elongation, stress-flex resistance, elasticity and impact strength increase. As density increases, the following properties increase: sealing temperature, tensile strength, stiffness, hardness, barrier properties and chemical resistance.

For packaging products high in alcohol content, EMA (ethylene methacrylic acid) copolymers may be used because of their ability to seal despite contact with organic contaminants in the seal area. For bonding to metal foils, PE must be made more hydrophilic. This is accomplished by copolymerizing hydrophobic ethylene with the more hydrophilic EAA (ethylene acrylic acid), EMA or ionomer. Polypropylene also can be modified by the incorporation of random ethylene monomers in the polymer chain. This confers rubbery character to the sealant, increasing impact strength and flexibility.

Blister Packaging involves forming a heat-softened plastic film into or around a deep-drawn pocketed mold to make a plastic tray (thermoforming), filling with a solid dosage-form product and sealing with push-through or peelable covering. The forming film, covering and product must flow at the right rates without sticking. Appropriate heat and pressure must be applied to ensure that permanent sealing will be formed which will protect the product throughout its shelf-life.

Choice of film thickness affects both material costs and barrier properties. Other considerations are machineability, production rates, depth of the blister, wall thickness and uniformity of the blister, and sealing properties. Unplasticized, or rigid, PVC is the most common material for forming film because it is thermoformed easily and has barrier properties which are adequate for many drugs. The typical film thickness of 250 μm (10 mil) can be increased by applying a 25 to 50 μm coating of PVDC (polyvinylidene chloride) which increases the water vapor barrier properties 5- to 10-fold.

For better protection, films are made from PVC and CTFE (chlorotrifluoroethylene, Aclar). Such films are 15-fold less permeable to moisture than is PVC of comparable thickness. Maximal protection from water vapor is provided by biaxially oriented polyamide/aluminum/PVC (nylon-Al-PVC) which gives barrier properties that are immeasurably low. Aluminum makes the material more recyclable. The cost is comparable to PVDC-coated PVC. Other materials such as PP, PS or PET have been tried for blister packs but have not achieved commercial success due to technical difficulties, poor barrier properties or economic issues.

Lidding (covering) material is usually aluminum/paper or preprinted aluminum. A standard 25-μm thickness of aluminum is considered to be pinhole free and represents an optimum combination of cost and product protection. The hardness of the aluminum can be optimized either for facilitating a push-through opening or hindering it, if a child-proof feature is desired. Lidding material is also perforated along the sealed seams to prevent it from being peeled from the formed film in one piece. The lidding material has a printing primer on one side and a heat-sealing lacquer on the other, which faces the product and forming film. A value-added feature is a peel-off-push-through foil, offered by a paper-polyester-aluminum laminate. The paper/PET laminate first is peeled from the aluminum, and then the tablet is pushed through the aluminum.[8]

Strip and sachet packaging are other unit-type packs used for tablets, capsules, powders, etc. Multidose packs for solid dosage forms can be made from PS, PVC, polyester, PP or HDPE. The latter two are preferred for their better barrier properties toward moisture. All can be made child resistant and tamper evident/resistant using innovative closure systems reflecting the versatility of plastic materials.

Intravenous (IV) Solutions—Compared to glass bottles, plastic packaging offers nonbreakability and light weight, affording easier transport and handling. Additionally, flexible packaging permits collapsibility, which provides greater protection from aerial contamination. Also, squeezing the bag with a pressure cuff enables rapid administration of large fluid quantities in emergency situations. This puts a burst-strength requirement on both the material and the quality of the seals.

Because of its transparency, durability, autoclavability and manufacturability at an economical cost PVC has been a material of choice. The realities of shipping require pinhole resistance. This is offered by flexible, high-yield strength materials like plasticized vinyl, rather than stiffer, more brittle materials like unmodified polyolefins. The polar nature of PVC permits rapid radio-frequency sealing of the bag, incorporating the port tubes for an IV administration set and medication sites. A polyolefin overwrap is used as a water-vapor barrier to prevent excessive moisture loss through the plasticized PVC.

Automatic packaging of IV solutions can be accomplished with an aseptic form (blow molding)-fill-seal system for rigid containers or a seal-fill-seal system for flexible containers. The latter requires preformed plastic film which is reel-fed onto a forming manifold, and side-sealed to form a tube, which is then filled. After incorporating fitments and closures, the final seal is made, and the completed container is cut from the web of material. The materials used are primarily polyethylene, polypropylene and polyolefin modified with rubber to increase yield strength for flexible containers. Composite materials may be used, incorporating a heat-seal layer facing the solution, economical bulk layer for strength and polyester outside layer for scuff resistance and glossy appearance.[9]

Sterilization

For plastic medical devices and packaging materials, a number of sterilizing agents have been used, including (1) steam, (2) gas and (3) irradiation (cobalt and electron discharge). Of these agents, steam can be used only on a few polymers due to their inability to withstand heat without distortion. The following commonly used plastic types generally can withstand steam sterilization at temperatures of 121°: polypropylene, high-density polyethylene, polycarbonate, PVC for certain applications and all thermosets.

The most commonly used procedure for sterilizing plastic devices is gas sterilization. Some of the gases available are (1) 100% ethylene oxide, (2) 88%/12% mixtures of Freon and ethylene oxide and (3) 80%/20% or 90%/10% mixtures of carbon dioxide and ethylene oxide.

Gas sterilization cannot be used for containers of aqueous products because side-reaction products such as ethylene glycol and 2-chloroethanol are formed. Ethylene oxide itself is carcinogenic.[7] It also can react with body proteins and certain material leachables to form immunogenic compounds that can elicit hypersensitivity reactions. For this reason, regulatory permissible limits have been established for residual layers of ethylene oxide. To meet these limits, packaged products are degassed prior to shipping or use. Degassing properties depend upon geometry, heat-history, storage conditions, contact with other plastics and type of secondary packages used. Because of this complexity, degassing hold times must be determined for each product.

Irradiation can cause degradation or cross-linking of certain polymers. For example, PVC loses hydrochloric acid upon irradiation, decomposing into unstable fragments which may then cross-link. This dehydrochlorination leads to the formation of conjugated double bonds which impart yellow discoloration to the plastic. As part of the additive package to make PVC more radiation resistant, blue dyes are added to mask the yellow coloration. Radical-chain terminators also are added to minimize chain scission. Certain polymers like polyethylene acquire improved tensile and impact strength because of the cross-linking attendant with radiation. The effect upon composite materials may not necessarily correlate with the properties of the individual components. Thus, the loss of strength of a cellulosic film may not be noticed if the film is supported by polyethylene or foil.

Quality-Control Considerations

The selection and approval of a polymer type (and a specific compound within that type) is as important as the need to check it routinely against the criteria used in its selection. The following basic areas of control and/or procedures are recommended regarding an ongoing quality-control program.

Tissue-cell toxicity testing (or a similar toxicity test) should be conducted in order to provide assurance that the material being used is nontoxic or falls within the toxicity range originally specified.

Characterization analysis should be conducted in order to provide assurances that the proper polymer type is used and that the physical parameters have not been altered, which in turn could affect the function of the product/package. Such techniques as infrared spectrometric analysis, density and melt-flow can assist in providing the necessary assurances.

Any plastic part or package should be inspected routinely on an incoming basis for dimensional and attribute variables against statistically accepted sampling plans such as MIL-STD-105D.

Environmental Considerations

Disposal is a critical issue as the volume of solid waste continues to increase and the capacity of landfill sites dwindles. Hospitals are coming under increasing pressure as communities frown upon incineration and disposal costs escalate. Of the total municipal waste generated, plastic packaging accounts for only 4% by weight. While paper accounts for 50% and glass about 25%, plastics draw much of the concern of environmentalists, because of their persistence (nondegradability) in landfill sites. Additionally, plastics are increasingly displacing conventional packaging materials, and on a volume basis, bulky and resilient plastic bottles constitute more of a problem than their weight percentage would imply. The problem is being addressed from a number of standpoints.

Disposal is a complex issue, involving both economics and regulatory requirements. Often the plastic selection alternatives depend upon many factors, such as the mode of disposal or incineration versus landfill. For example, PVC has come under attack because it forms hydrochloric acid when incinerated, necessitating expensive scrubbing systems to neutralize the acid. Dioxins also may be formed if the incineration system is not optimized. If incineration will not be used to dispose of the medical waste for a given location, however, these objections become irrelevant for the particular case.

In response to their customers, hospital supply manufacturers are reducing the amount of packaging material accompanying their products. Some are working with hospitals to establish successful recycling efforts. This requires convenience of collection, viable reprocessing technology, markets for waste derived products and good economics. The individual plastic resins must first be sorted prior to being reprocessed for relatively undemanding, nonpackaging applications such as fiberfill. Under some circumstances, homogeneous resins, such as the PET in beverage bottles, can be recycled more easily than composite materials, because of this sorting issue. Plastics manufacturers can, however, incorporate scrap into one of the component layers of some composite materials, making such items potentially recyclable. Recycling of PVC infusion containers is hampered by the difficulties involved in separating metal and rubber components, disinfecting and drying the products to render them suitable for processing.[7] Nevertheless, the industry is investing in sorting technology and reclamation capacity to create commercially viable recycling programs.[10]

Summary

Before the selection of a plastic for a packaging application is made, all the functional and safety requirements must be specified. These requirements are restated in terms of engineering and scientific material testing parameters. Candidate materials are reviewed and selected on the basis of the most economic solution that addresses the critical needs. Within each polymer class, properties may be altered to an extent by modifying molecular weight, copolymerizing with other polymers or blending in particular additives. Often, composite materials are used to combine the advantages of the individual components. Proper sterilization procedures, including adequate degassing, must be identified in order to obtain a sterile product that is nontoxic. Once designed, the product/package must demonstrate physical and chemical stability in formal stability studies over the shelf-life of the product. An ongoing quality-assurance program should be designed to ensure that packaging-product requirements are maintained. After use, disposal of the packaging is becoming more of an issue from economic and environmental standpoints. For more specific and in-depth information, consult the *Bibliography*.

References

1. *Modern Plastics Encyclopedia*, vol 64, McGraw-Hill, New York, 554, 1987.
2. Rabinow B, Payton R. Raghavan N: *J Pharm Sci 75:* 808, 1986.
3. Wang YJ, Chien YW: *Sterile Pharmaceutical Packaging: Compatibility and Stability* (Tech Rpt #5), PDA, Philadelphia, 1984.
4. Sanchez IC, Chang SS, Smith LE: *Polymer News 6:* 249, 1980.
5. Jenke DR *et al:* *Int J Pharm 78:* 115, 1992.
6. *Med Device Technol* Jun, 1991.
7. Van Dooren AA: *Pharm Weekbl [Sci] 13(3):* 109, 1991.
8. Reiterer F: *Pharm Technol (Mar):* 74, 1991.
9. Lambert P: *Ibid (Apr):* 48, 1991.
10. *J Vinyl Technol 13(2):* 1991.

Bibliography

Briston JH: *Plastic Films*, 3rd ed, Wiley, New York, 1988.

Brostow W, Corneliussen RD: *Failure of Plastics*, Macmillan, New York, 1986.

Dean DA: "The Packaging of Pharmaceuticals," Int Pkg Conf, CONEX 85 (Oct 22–25, 1985), Beijing, vol 1: China Pkg Technol Assoc, pp 287, 1985.

Dean DA: *Plastics in Pharmaceutical Packaging*, Antony Rowe Ltd, England, 1990.

Finlayson KM: *Plastic Film Technology, High Barrier Plastic Films for Packaging*, vol 1, Technomic Publ Co, Lancaster PA, 1989.

Modern Plastics Encyclopedia, vol 68, McGraw-Hill, New York, 1992.

Wiley Encyclopedia of Packaging Technology, Wiley, New York, 1986.

CHAPTER 86

Solutions, Emulsions, Suspensions and Extracts

J G Nairn, PhD
Professor of Pharmacy
Faculty of Pharmacy
University of Toronto
Toronto, Canada M5S 1A1

The dosage forms described in this chapter may be prepared by dissolving the active ingredient(s) in an aqueous or nonaqueous solvent, by suspending the drug (if it is insoluble in pharmaceutically or therapeutically acceptable solvents) in an appropriate medium or by incorporating the medicinal agent into one of the two phases of an oil and water system. Such solutions, suspensions and emulsions are further defined in subsequent paragraphs but some, with similar properties, are considered elsewhere. These dosage forms are useful for a number of reasons. They can be formulated for different routes of administration: oral use, introduction into body cavities or applied externally. The dose easily can be adjusted by dilution, and the oral liquid form readily can be administered to children or people unable to swallow tablets or capsules. Extracts eliminate the need to isolate the drug in pure form, allow several ingredients to be administered from a single source (eg, pancreatic extract) and permit the preliminary study of drugs from natural sources. Occasionally, solutions of drugs such as potassium chloride are used to minimize adverse effects in the gastrointestinal tract.

The preparation of these dosage forms involves several considerations on the part of the pharmacist: purpose of the drug, internal or external use, concentration of the drug, selection of the liquid vehicle, physical and chemical stability of the drug, preservation of the preparation and use of appropriate excipients such as buffers, solubilizers, suspending agents, emulsifying agents, viscosity controlling agents, colors and flavors. Oral preparations require that consideration be given to improving patient compliance by making an acceptable product; consequently, color, odor and taste must be considered. These organoleptic factors are described in Chapter 80. The viscosity of a product also must be considered in order that it has the proper palatability for an oral preparation and to have the appropriate suspending properties if it is an emulsion or suspension. The theory pertaining to these systems is provided in Chapters 21 and 22. The theory of solutions, which involves solubility, ionization, pH control through the use of buffers and solubilization, is discussed in Chapters 16 and 17. Because of the complexity of some manufactured products, compounding may be carried out with the aid of linear programming models in order to obtain the optimal product. Chapters (87 to 89) should be consulted for information on the preparation and characteristics of those liquid preparations that are intended for ophthalmic or parenteral use.

Much has been written during the past decade about the biopharmaceutical properties of, in particular, the solid dosage forms. In assessing the bioavailability of drugs in tablets and capsules, many researchers first have studied the absorption of drugs administered in solution. Since drugs are absorbed in their dissolved state, frequently it is found that the absorption rate of oral dosage forms decreases in the following order: aqueous solution > aqueous suspension > tablet or capsule. The bioavailability of a medicament, for oral ingestion and absorption, should be such that eventually all of the drug is absorbed as it passes through the gastrointestinal tract, regardless of the dosage form. Some formulation factors which may influence the bioavailability and pharmacokinetics of drugs in solution include concentration of the drug, volume of liquid administered, pH, buffer capacity and viscosity. Emulsions and suspensions are more complex systems and consequently the extent of absorption and pharmacokinetic parameters may be affected by a number of additional formulation factors such as surfactants, type of viscosity agent, particle size and particle-size distribution, polymorphism and solubility of drug in the oil phase. Specific examples are provided in Chapter 19. There are a number of reasons for formulating drugs in forms in which the drug is not in the molecular state. These are improved stability, improved taste, low water solubility, palatability and ease of administration. It becomes apparent, then, that each dosage form will have advantages and disadvantages.

Liquid preparations may be dispensed in one of three ways. The pharmacist may dispense the product in its original container, buy the product in bulk and repackage it at the time a prescription is presented by the patient or compound the solution, suspension or emulsion in the dispensary. Compounding may involve nothing more than mixing marketed products in the manner indicated on the prescription or, in specific instances, may require the incorporation of active ingredients in a logical and pharmaceutically acceptable manner into the aqueous or nonaqueous solvents which will form the bulk of the product.

The pharmacist, in the first instance, depends on the pharmaceutical manufacturer to produce a product that is effective, elegant and stable when stored under reasonably adverse conditions. Most manufacturers attempt to guarantee efficacy by evaluating their products in a scientifically acceptable manner but, in some instances, such efficacy is relative. For example, cough mixtures marketed by two different manufacturers may contain the same active ingredients and it becomes difficult to assess the relative merits of the two products. In such instances the commercial advantage gained by one over the other may be based on product acceptability and preference which includes such factors as color, odor, taste, pourability, uniformity and packaging. Two additional important factors which must be considered in formulations are the stability of active and other ingredients, and the prevention of microbial contamination.

The stability of the active ingredient in the final product is of prime concern to the formulator. In general, drug substances are less stable in aqueous media than in the solid dosage form and it is important, therefore, to properly stabilize and preserve, in particular those solutions, suspensions and emulsions that contain water. Certain simple chemical reactions can occur in these products. These may involve an ingredient-ingredient interaction which implies a poor formulation, a container-product interaction which may alter product pH and thus, for pH-sensitive ingredients, be responsible for the subsequent formation of precipitates or a direct reaction with water, ie, hydrolysis. The stability of pharmaceutical products is discussed in Chapter 38.

The more complicated reactions usually involve oxygen. Vitamins, essential oils and almost all fats and oils can be oxidized. Formulators usually use the word *autoxidation* when the ingredient(s) in the product react with oxygen but without drastic external interference. Such reactions first must be initiated by heat, light (including ultraviolet radiant energy), peroxides or other labile compounds or heavy metals such as copper or iron. This initiation step results in the formation of a free radical (R*) which then reacts with oxygen.

$$R^* + O_2 \rightarrow RO_2^* \text{ (peroxy radical)}$$

$$RO_2^* + RH \rightarrow ROOH + R^*$$

The free radical thus is regenerated and reacts with more oxygen. This propagation step is followed by the termination reactions.

$$RO_2^* + RO_2^* \rightarrow \text{inactive product}$$

$$RO_2^* + R^* \rightarrow \text{inactive product}$$

$$R^* + R^* \rightarrow \text{inactive product}$$

The effect of trace metals can be minimized by using citric acid or EDTA ie, sequestering agents. Antioxidants, however, may retard or delay oxidation by reacting with the free radicals formed in the product. Examples of antioxidants are the propyl, octyl and dodecyl esters of gallic acid, butylated hydroxyanisole (BHA) and the tocopherols or vitamin E. For a more detailed approach to the prevention of oxidative deterioration in pharmaceuticals, the information provided by Connors *et al*[1] should be consulted. A description of many antioxidants is given in Chapter 80.

The problem of drug stability has been well-defined by pharmaceutical scientists, but during the past few years a secondary and, in some respects, more serious problem has confronted the manufacturer of liquid preparations. Such pharmaceutically diverse products as baby lotions and milk of magnesia have been recalled from the market because of microbial contamination. In a survey of retail packages of liquid antacid preparations containing magnesium hydroxide, it was found that 30.5% of the finished bottles were contaminated with *Pseudomonas aeruginosa.* The aerobic plate count ranged from less than 100 to 9,300,000 organisms/g. Kurup and Wan[2] describe many preparations that are not preserved adequately and thus are not able to resist microbial contamination. Other examples could be cited but the range of microorganisms which can contaminate the liquid preparation includes the *Salmonella* sp, *E coli*, certain *Pseudomonas* sp, including *P aeruginosa*, and *Staphylococcus aureus*. Bruch[3] describes the types of microorganisms found in various products and attempts to evaluate the hazards associated with the use of nonsterile pharmaceuticals. Coates[4] in a series of papers describes various interactions which must be considered when preservatives are selected.

The USP recommends that certain classes of products be tested for microbial count and for specified indicator microbial contaminants, eg, natural plant, animal and some mineral products, for freedom from *Salmonella* sp; oral solutions and suspensions, for freedom from *E coli*; articles applied topically, for freedom from *P aeruginosa* and *S aureus* and articles for rectal, urethral or vaginal administration, for yeasts and molds.

Products may become contaminated for a number of reasons.

The raw materials used in the manufacture of solutions, suspensions and emulsions are excellent growth media for bacteria. Water, in particular, must be handled with care but substances such as gums, dispersing agents, surfactants, sugars and flavors can be the carriers of bacteria which ultimately contaminate the product.

Equipment. Bacteria grow well in the nooks and crevices of pharmaceutical equipment (and in the simple equipment used in the dispensary). Such equipment should be cleaned thoroughly prior to use.

Environment and personnel can contribute to product contamination. Hands and hair are the most important carriers of contaminants. General cleanliness thus is vital. Head coverings must be used by those involved in the manufacturing process and face masks should be used by those individuals suffering from colds, coughs, hay fever and other allergic manifestations.

Packaging should be selected so that it will not contaminate the product and also will protect it from the environment.

Finally, consumer use may result in the introduction of microorganisms as a source of contamination, and this is of particular concern if the organism is pathogenic. The consumer should be instructed in the proper technique in order to minimize contamination, and the manufacturer should ensure, through the use of suitable challenge tests, that the product is preserved appropriately and will reduce a severe microbial challenge.

Most factors cited above relate to good manufacturing practice. However, the formulator should add a preservative to the product and decrease the probability of product contamination. If the product contains water, which is an important requirement for microbial growth, it almost is mandatory to include a preservative in the formulation. Nearly all products described in this chapter contain water and, thus, with certain exceptions, eg, aqueous acids, will support microbial growth. Microbes will grow in an aqueous solution, and in the aqueous phase of multiphase systems such as emulsions and suspensions. It must be stressed that the addition of an appropriate preservative in no way replaces good manufacturing practice but merely provides further assurance that the product will retain its pharmaceutically acceptable characteristics until it is used by the patient and for sometime thereafter.

The major criteria that should be considered in selecting a preservative are as follows: it should be effective against a wide spectrum of microorganisms, stable for its shelf life, nontoxic, nonsensitizing, compatible with the ingredients in the dosage form inexpensive and essentially relatively free of taste and odor.

In addition to the above discussion, there are a number of specific factors which should be taken into account when a preservative is selected:

1. The site of use, eg, external, internal or ophthalmic.
2. The pH of the liquid, as it may affect both the ionization of the preservative and its stability.
3. The solvent, as this will affect the solubility of the preservative.
4. Partitioning into the oil phase of an emulsion, thereby reducing the concentration in the aqueous phase where preservative action takes place.
5. Adsorption onto the solid phase of a suspension, thereby reducing the concentration in the aqueous phase.
6. Processing and packaging variables such as heat, order of addition of the ingredients, stirring or container materials.
7. Type of dosage form, eg, solution, emulsion or suspension.

Preservatives[5,6] may be grouped into a number of classes depending upon their molecular structure and only a few will be discussed. The reader should consult Chapter 80 or selected texts in the bibliography for further description.

Alcohols—Ethanol is useful as a preservative when it is used as a solvent; however, it does need a relatively high concentration, somewhat greater than 10%, to be effective. Too high a concentration may result in incompatibilities in suspension and emulsion systems. Propylene glycol also is used as a solvent in oral solutions and topical preparations, and it can function as a preservative in the range of 15 to 30%. It is not volatile like ethanol and is used frequently not only in solutions but also in suspensions and emulsions. Other alcohols used in lower concentrations, about 1%, for preservative action, include chlorobutanol and phenylethyl alcohol.

Acids—Benzoic acid has a low solubility in water, about 0.34% at 25°. The concentration range used for inhibitory action varies from 0.1% to 0.5%. Only the nonionized form is effective and therefore its use is restricted to preparations with a pH below 4.5. Sorbic acid also has a low solubility in water, 0.3% at 30°. Suitable concentrations for preservative action are in the range of 0.05 to 2%. Its preservative action is due to the nonionized form; consequently, it is only effective in acid media. Because of the double bond in its structure, it is subject to oxidation.

Esters—Parabens are esters of *p*-hydroxybenzoic acid and include the methyl, ethyl, propyl and butyl derivatives. The solubility in water decreases as the molecular weight increases from 0.25% for the methyl ester to 0.02% for the butyl ester. These compounds are used widely in pharmaceutical products and are effective and stable over a pH range of 4 to 8. They are employed at concentrations up to about 0.2%. Frequently, two esters are used in combination in the same preparation. This achieves a higher total concentration, and the mixture tends to be active against a wider range of microorganisms. Their activity is reduced in the presence of nonionic surface active agents due to binding. In alkaline solutions, ionization takes place and this reduces their activity; in addition, hydrolytic decomposition of the ester group occurs with a loss of activity.

Quaternary Ammonium Compounds—Benzalkonium chloride is a mixture consisting principally of the homologs $C_{12}H_{25}$ and $C_{14}H_{29}$. This preservative is used at a relatively low concentration, 0.002 to 0.02%, depending on the nature of the pharmaceutical product. This class of compounds has an optimal activity over the pH range of 4 to 10 and is quite stable at room temperature. Because of the cationic nature of this type of preservative, it is incompatible with many anionic compounds such as surfactants and can bind to nonionic surfactants. It is used generally in preparations for external use or those solutions which come in contact with mucous membranes.

It now should be obvious that when the pharmacist dispenses or compounds the various liquid preparations responsibility is assumed along, with the manufacturer, for the maintenance of product stability. The USP includes a section on stability considerations in dispensing, which should be studied in detail. Certain points are self-evident. Stock should be rotated and replaced if expiration dates on the label so indicate. Products should be stored in the manner indicated in the compendium; eg, in a cool place or a tight, light-resistant container. Further, products should be checked for evidence of instability. With respect to solutions, elixirs and syrups, color change, precipitation and evidence of microbial or chemical gas formation are major signs of instability. Emulsions may cream but if they break (ie, there is a separation of an oil phase) the product is considered to be unstable. Sedimentation and caking are primary indications of instability in suspensions. The presence of large particles may mean that excessive crystal growth has occurred.

The USP states that if the product must be repackaged, care and the container specified by the compendium must be used. For example, a suitably opaque plastic container should be used if a light-resistant container is specified. If a product is diluted, or where two products are mixed, the pharmacist should use his or her knowledge to guard against incompatibility and instability. Oral antibiotic preparations constituted into liquid form should never be mixed with other products. If the chemical stability of extemporaneously prepared liquid preparations is unknown, their use should be minimized and every care taken to insure that product characteristics will not change during the time it must be used by the patient.

Because of the number of excipients and additives in these preparations, it is recommended that all the ingredients be listed on the container to reduce the risks which confront hypersensitive patients when these products are administered. Finally, the pharmacist should inform the patient regarding the appropriate use of the product, the proper storage conditions and the time after which it should be discarded.

Solutions

Aqueous Solutions

A solution is a homogeneous mixture that is prepared by dissolving a solid, liquid or gas in another liquid and represents a group of preparations in which the molecules of the solute or dissolved substance are dispersed among those of the solvent. Solutions also may be classified on the basis of physical or chemical properties, method of preparation, use, physical state, number of ingredients and particle size. The narrower definition in this subsection limits the solvent to water and excludes those preparations that are sweet and/or viscid in character and nonaqueous solutions. This section includes, therefore, those pharmaceutical forms that are designated as *Water, Aromatic Waters, Aqueous Acids, Solutions, Douches, Enemas, Gargles, Mouthwashes, Juices, Nasal Solutions, Otic Solutions* and *Irrigation Solutions.*

Water

The major ingredient in most of the dosage forms described herein is water. It is used both as a vehicle and as a solvent for the desired flavoring or medicinal ingredients. Its tastelessness, freedom from irritating qualities and lack of pharmacological activity make it ideal for such purposes. There is, however, a tendency to assume that its purity is constant and that it can be stored, handled and used with a minimum of care. While it is true that municipal supplies must comply with Environmental Protection Agency (EPA) regulations (or comparable regulations in other countries), drinking water *must* be repurified before it can be used in pharmaceuticals. For further information on water, see Chapter 23.

Five of the six solvent waters described in the USP are used in the preparation of parenterals, irrigations or inhalations. *Purified Water* must be used for all other pharmaceutical operations, dosage forms and, as needed, in all USP tests and assays. It must meet rigid specifications for chemical purity. Such water may be prepared by distillation, by use of ion-exchange resins or by reverse osmosis.

A wide variety of commercially available stills are used to produce distilled water. The end use of the product dictates the size of the still and extent of pretreatment of the drinking water introduced into the system. A description of stills is provided in Chapter 87. Such water may be sterile provided the condenser is sterile, but to be called sterile it must be subjected to a satisfactory sterilization process. However, it has been shown that *P aeruginosa* (and other microorganisms) can grow in the distilled water produced in hospitals. The implications of this are obvious. Sterile water may be sterile at the time of production but may lose this characteristic if it is stored improperly. Hickman *et al*,[7] by regrouping the components of conventional distillation equipment, have described a method for the continuous supply of sterile, ultrapure water. Quality-control procedures for monitoring the microbiological quality of water should be performed in the pharmaceutical manufacturer's production facilities.

The major impurities in water are calcium, iron, magnesium, manganese, silica and sodium. The cations usually are combined with the bicarbonate, sulfate or chloride anions. "Hard" waters are those that contain calcium and magnesium cations. Bicarbonates are the major impurity in "alkaline" waters.

Ion-exchange (deionization, demineralization) processes will remove most of the major impurities in water efficiently and economically. A cation exchanger, H_2R, first converts bicarbonates, sulfates and chlorides to their respective acids, eg,

$$\left.\begin{array}{l} CaSO_4 \\ MgSO_4 \\ Na_2SO_4 \end{array}\right| + H_2R \rightarrow \left.\begin{array}{r} Ca \\ Mg \\ Na_2 \end{array}\right| R + H_2SO_4$$

$$\left.\begin{array}{l} Ca(HCO_3)_2 \\ Mg(HCO_3)_2 \\ 2NaHCO_3 \end{array}\right| + H_2R \rightarrow \left.\begin{array}{r} Ca \\ Mg \\ Na_2 \end{array}\right| R + 2H_2CO_3$$

Carbonic acid decomposes to carbon dioxide (which is removed by aeration in the decarbonator) and water.

The anion exchanger may contain either a weakly basic or a strongly basic anion resin. These adsorb sulfuric, hydrochloric and nitric acids. Chemical reactions may involve complete adsorption or an exchange with some other anion.

$$H_2SO_4 + A \rightarrow A \cdot H_2SO_4$$

If the resin contains a hydroxyl group, water is formed during the purification process.

$$H_2SO_4 + 2AOH \rightarrow A_2SO_4 + 2H_2O$$

Weakly dissociated carbonic and silicic acids can be removed only by strongly basic anion resins.

$$H_2SiO_3 + 2AOH \rightarrow A_2SiO_2 + 2H_2O$$

Unit capacity varies with the nature of the installation, but it is possible to process as much as 15,000 gal of water/min.

Deionization processes do not necessarily produce *Purified Water* which will comply with EPA requirements for drinking water. Resin columns retain phosphates and organic debris. Either alone or in combination, these substances can act as growth media for microorganisms. Observations have shown that deionized water containing 90 organisms/mL contained, after 24-hour storage, 10^6 organisms/mL. Columns can be cleaned partially of pseudomonads by recharging, but a 0.25% solution of formaldehyde will destroy most bacteria. The column must be washed thoroughly and checked for the absence of aldehyde (with a Schiffs Reagent) before it can be used to generate deionized water.

Ultraviolet radiant energy (240–280 nm), heat or filtration can be used to limit the growth, kill or remove microorganisms in water. The latter method employs membrane filters and can be used to remove bacteria from heat-labile materials as described under membrane filters in Chapter 84.

The phenomenon of osmosis involves the passage of water from a dilute solution across a semipermeable membrane to a more concentrated solution. Flow of water can be stopped by applying pressure, equal to the osmotic pressure, to the concentrated solution. The flow of water can be reversed by applying a pressure, greater than the osmotic pressure. The process of reverse osmosis utilizes the latter principle; by applying pressure, greater than the osmotic pressure, to the concentrated solution, eg, tap water, pure water may be obtained (see *Reverse Osmosis* in Chapter 37).

Cellulose acetate is used in the manufacture of semipermeable membranes for purifying water by reverse osmosis. This polymer has functional groups that can hydrogen-bond to water or other substances such as alcohol. The water molecules which enter the polymer are transported from one bonding site to the next under pressure. Because of the thin layer of pure water strongly adsorbed at the surface of the membrane, salts, to a large extent, are repelled from the surface, the higher-valent ions being repelled to a greater extent, thus causing a separation of ions from the water. Organic molecules are rejected on the basis of a sieve mechanism related to their size and shape. Small organic molecules, with a molecular weight smaller than approximately 200, will pass through the membrane material. Since there are few organic molecules with a molecular weight of less than 200 in the municipal water supply, reverse osmosis usually is sufficient for the removal of organic material. The pore sizes of the selectively permeable reverse-osmosis membranes are between 5 and 100 A. Viruses and bacteria larger than 100 A are rejected if no imperfections exist in the membrane. The membranes may and do develop openings which permit the passage of microorganisms. Because of the semistatic conditions, bacteria can grow both upstream and downstream of the membrane. Improvements in membranes are being made continually in type and manufacturing process such as the use of polyamide materials. It is expected that the preparation of water with negligible or no bacteria present will be achieved by this process.

The selection of water-treatment equipment depends upon the quality of water to be tested, the quality of water required and the specific pharmaceutical purpose of the water. Frequently, two or more methods are used to produce the water desired, for example, filtration and distillation, or filtration, reverse osmosis and ion exchange.

Aromatic Waters

Aromatic waters, known also as medicated waters, are clear, saturated aqueous solutions of volatile oils or other aromatic or volatile substances. Their odors and tastes are similar to those of the drugs or volatile substances from which they are prepared. They are used principally as flavored or perfumed vehicles. Aromatic Waters may be prepared by distillation or solution of the aromatic substance with or without the use of a dispersing agent such as talc. Peppermint Water USP and Stronger Rose Water USP are examples of aromatic waters.

Other methods have been suggested for preparing aromatic waters based on the use of soluble concentrates or on incorporation of solubilizing agents such as polysorbate 20.

Concentrated waters eg, peppermint, dill, cinnamon and caraway, may be prepared as follows:

Dissolve 20 mL of the volatile oil in 600 mL of 90% ethanol. Add sufficient purified water in successive small portions to produce 1000 mL. Shake vigorously after each addition. Add 50 g of sterilized purified talc, shake occasionally for several hours and filter.

The aromatic water is prepared by diluting the concentrate with 39 times its volume of water.

The chemical composition of many of the volatile oils is known and suitable synthetic substances may be used in preparing pharmaceuticals and cosmetics. Similarly, many synthetic aromatic substances have a characteristic odor; eg, geranyl phenyl acetate has a honey odor. Such substances, either alone or in combination, can be used in nonofficial preparations. Additional information regarding the appropriate preparation of aromatic waters is provided in RPS-18, Chapter 83, and RPS-17, Chapter 84.

The principal difficulty experienced in compounding prescriptions containing aromatic waters is due to a "salting out" action of certain ingredients, such as very soluble salts, on the volatile principle of the aromatic water. A replacement of part of the aromatic water with purified water is permissible when no other function is being served than that of a vehicle.

Preservation—Aromatic waters will deteriorate with time and should, therefore, be made in small quantities and protected from intense light, excessive heat and stored in airtight, light-resistant containers.

Aqueous Acids

The official inorganic acids and certain organic acids, although of minor significance as therapeutic agents, are of great importance in chemical and pharmaceutical manufacturing. This is especially true of acetic, hydrochloric and nitric acids.

Percentage Strengths—Many of the more important inorganic acids are available commercially in the form of concentrated aqueous solutions. The percentage strength varies from one acid to another and depends on the solubility and stability of the solute in water and on the manufacturing process. Thus, the official Hydrochloric Acid contains from 36.5 to 38% by weight of HCl, whereas Nitric Acid contains from 69 to 71% by weight of HNO_3.

Because the strengths of these concentrated acids are stated in terms of % by weight, it is essential that specific gravities also be provided if one is to be able to calculate conveniently the amount of absolute acid contained in a unit volume of the solution as purchased. The mathematical relationship involved is given by the equation $M = V \times S \times F$, where M is the mass in g of absolute acid contained in V mL of solution having a specific gravity S and a fractional percentage strength F. As an example, Hydrochloric Acid containing 36.93% by weight of HCl has a specific gravity of 1.1875. Therefore, the amount of absolute HCl supplied by 100 mL of this solution is given by:

$$M = 100 \times 1.1875 \times 0.3693 = 43.85 \text{ g HCl}$$

Incompatibilities—Although many of the reactions characteristic of acids offer opportunities for incompatibilities, only a few are of sufficient importance to require more than casual mention. Acids and acid salts decompose carbonates with liberation of carbon dioxide and, in a closed container, sufficient pressure may be developed to produce an explosion. Inorganic acids react with salts of organic acids to produce the free organic acid and a salt of the inorganic acid. If insoluble, the organic acid will be precipitated. Thus, salicylic acid and benzoic acid are precipitated from solutions of salicylates and benzoates. Boric acid likewise is precipitated from concentrated solutions of borates. By a similar reaction, certain soluble organic compounds are converted into an insoluble form. Phenobarbital sodium, for example, is converted into phenobarbital which will precipitate in aqueous solution.

The ability of acids to combine with alkaloids and other organic compounds containing a basic nitrogen atom is used in preparing soluble salts of these substances.

It should be borne in mind that certain solutions, syrups, elixirs and other pharmaceutical preparations, may contain free acid, which causes these preparations to exhibit the incompatibilities characteristic of the acid.

Acids also possess the incompatibilities of the anions which they contain and, in the case of organic acids, these are frequently of prime importance. These are discussed under the specific anions.

Diluted Acids—The diluted acids in the USP are aqueous solutions of acids, of a suitable strength (usually 10% *w/v* but Diluted Acetic Acid is 6% *w/v*) for internal administration or for the manufacture of other preparations.

The strengths of the official undiluted acids are expressed as percentages *w/w*, whereas the strengths of the official diluted acids are expressed as percent *w/v*. It, therefore, becomes necessary to consider the specific gravities of the concentrated acids when calculating the volume required to make a given quantity of diluted acid. The following equation will give the number of mL required to make 1000 mL of diluted acid:

$$\frac{\text{Strength of diluted acid} \times 1000}{\text{Strength of undiluted acid} \times \text{sp gr of undiluted acid}}$$

Thus, if one wishes to make 1000 mL of Diluted Hydrochloric Acid USP using Hydrochloric Acid which assays 37.5% HCl (sp gr 1.18), the amount required is

$$\frac{10 \times 1000}{37.5 \times 1.18} = 226 \text{ mL}$$

Diluted Hydrochloric Acid USP has been used in the treatment of achlorhydria. However, it may irritate the mucous membrane of the mouth and attack the enamel of the teeth. The usual dose is 5 mL, well-diluted with water. In the treatment of achlorhydria no attempt is made to administer more than a relief-producing dose.

Solutions

A solution, in the present context, is a liquid preparation that contains one or more soluble chemical substances dissolved in water. The solute usually is nonvolatile. Solutions are used for the specific therapeutic effect of the solute, either internally or externally. Although the emphasis here is on the aqueous solution, certain preparations of this type such as syrups, infusions and decoctions have distinctive characteristics and, therefore, are described later in the chapter.

Solvents, solubility and general methods for the incorporation of a solute in a solvent are discussed in Chapter 16. Solutions are usually bottled automatically with equipment of the type shown in Fig. 1.

Preparation—A specific method of preparation is given in the compendia for most solutions. These procedures fall into three main categories.

Simple Solutions—Solutions of this type are prepared by dissolving the solute in most of the solvent, mixing until dissolved, then adding sufficient solvent to bring the solution up to the proper volume. The solvent may contain other ingredients which stabilize or solubilize the active ingredient. Calcium Hydroxide Topical Solution USP (Lime Water), Sodium Phosphates Oral Solution USP and Strong Iodine Solution USP are examples.

Calcium Hydroxide Topical Solution contains, in each 100 mL, not less than 140 mg of $Ca(OH)_2$. The solution is prepared by agitating vigorously 3 g of calcium hydroxide with 1000 mL of cool, purified water. Excess calcium hydroxide is allowed to settle out and the clear, supernatant liquid dispensed.

An increase in solvent temperature usually implies an increase in solute solubility. This rule does not apply, however, to the solubility of calcium hydroxide in water, which decreases with increasing temperature. The official solution is prepared at 25°.

Solutions containing hydroxides react with the carbon dioxide in the atmosphere.

$$OH^- + CO_2 \rightarrow HCO_3^-$$

$$OH^- + HCO_3^- \rightarrow CO_3^{2-} + H_2O$$

Calcium Hydroxide Topical Solution, therefore, should be preserved in well-filled, tight containers, at a temperature not exceeding 25°.

Strong Iodine Solution contains, in each 100 mL, 4.5–5.5 g of iodine, and 9.5–10.5 g of potassium iodide. It is prepared by dissolving 50 g of iodine in 100 mL of purified water containing 100 g of potassium iodide. Sufficient purified water then is added to make 1000 mL of solution.

One g of iodine dissolves in 2950 mL of water. However, solutions of iodides dissolve large quantities of iodine. Strong Iodine Solution is, therefore, a solution of polyiodides in excess iodide.

$$I^- + nI_2 \rightarrow I^-_{(2n+1)}$$

Doubly charged anions may be found also

$$2I^- + nI_2 \rightarrow I^{2-}_{(2n+2)}$$

Strong Iodine Solution is used in the treatment of iodide deficiency disorders such as endemic goiter.

Several antibiotics (eg, cloxacillin sodium, nafcillin sodium and vancomycin), because they are relatively unstable in aqueous solution, are prepared by manufacturers as dry powders or granules in combination with suitable buffers, colors, diluents, dispersants, flavors and/or preservatives. These preparations, Cloxacillin Sodium for Oral Solution, Nafcillin for Oral Solution and Vancomycin Hydrochloride for Oral Solution meet the requirements of the USP. Upon dispensing to the patient, the pharmacist adds the appropriate amount of water. The products are stable for up to 14 days when refrigerated. This period usually provides sufficient time for the patient to complete the administration of all the medication.

Solution by Chemical Reaction—These solutions are prepared by reacting two or more solutes with each other in a suitable solvent. An example is Aluminum Subacetate Topical Solution USP.

Aluminum sulfate (145 g) is dissolved in 600 mL of cold water. The solution is filtered, and precipitated calcium carbonate (70 g) is added, in several portions, with constant stirring. Acetic acid (160 mL) is added slowly and the mixture set aside for 24 hr. The product is filtered and the magma on the Büchner filter washed with cold water until the total filtrate measures 1000 mL.

The solution contains pentaquohydroxo- and tetraquodihydroxoaluminum (III) acetates and sulfates dissolved in an aqueous medium saturated with calcium sulfate. The solution contains a small amount of acetic acid. It is stabilized by the addition of not more than 0.9% boric acid.

The reactions involved in the preparation of the solution are given below. The hexaquo aluminum cations first are converted to the nonirritating $[Al(H_2O)_5(OH)]^{2+}$ and $[Al(H_2O)_4(OH)_2]^+$ cations.

$$[Al(H_2O)_6]^{3+} + CO_3^{2-} \rightarrow [Al(H_2O)_5(OH)]^{2+} + HCO_3^-$$

$$[Al(H_2O)_6]^{3+} + HCO_3^- \rightarrow [Al(H_2O)_5(OH)]^{2+} + H_2O + CO_2$$

As the concentration of the hexaquo cations decreases, secondary reactions involving carbonate and bicarbonate occur.

$$[Al(H_2O)_5(OH)]^{2+} + CO_3^{2-} \rightarrow [Al(H_2O)_4(OH)_2]^+ + HCO_3^-$$

$$[Al(H_2O)_5(OH)]^{2+} + HCO_3^- \rightarrow [Al(H_2O)_4(OH)_2]^+ + H_2CO_3$$

The pH of the solution now favors the precipitation of dissolved calcium ions as the insoluble sulfate. Acetic acid now is added. The bicarbonate which is formed in the final stages of the procedure is removed as carbon dioxide.

Aluminum Subacetate Topical Solution is used in the preparation of Aluminum Acetate Topical Solution USP (Burow's Solution). The latter solution contains 15 mL of glacial acetic acid, 545 mL of Aluminum Subacetate Topical Solution and sufficient water to make 1000 mL. It is defined as a solution of aluminum acetate in approximately 5%, by weight, of acetic acid in water. It is stabilized by the addition of not more than 0.6% boric acid.

Solution by Extraction—Drugs or pharmaceutical necessities of vegetable or animal origin often are extracted with water or with water containing other substances. Preparations of this type may be classified

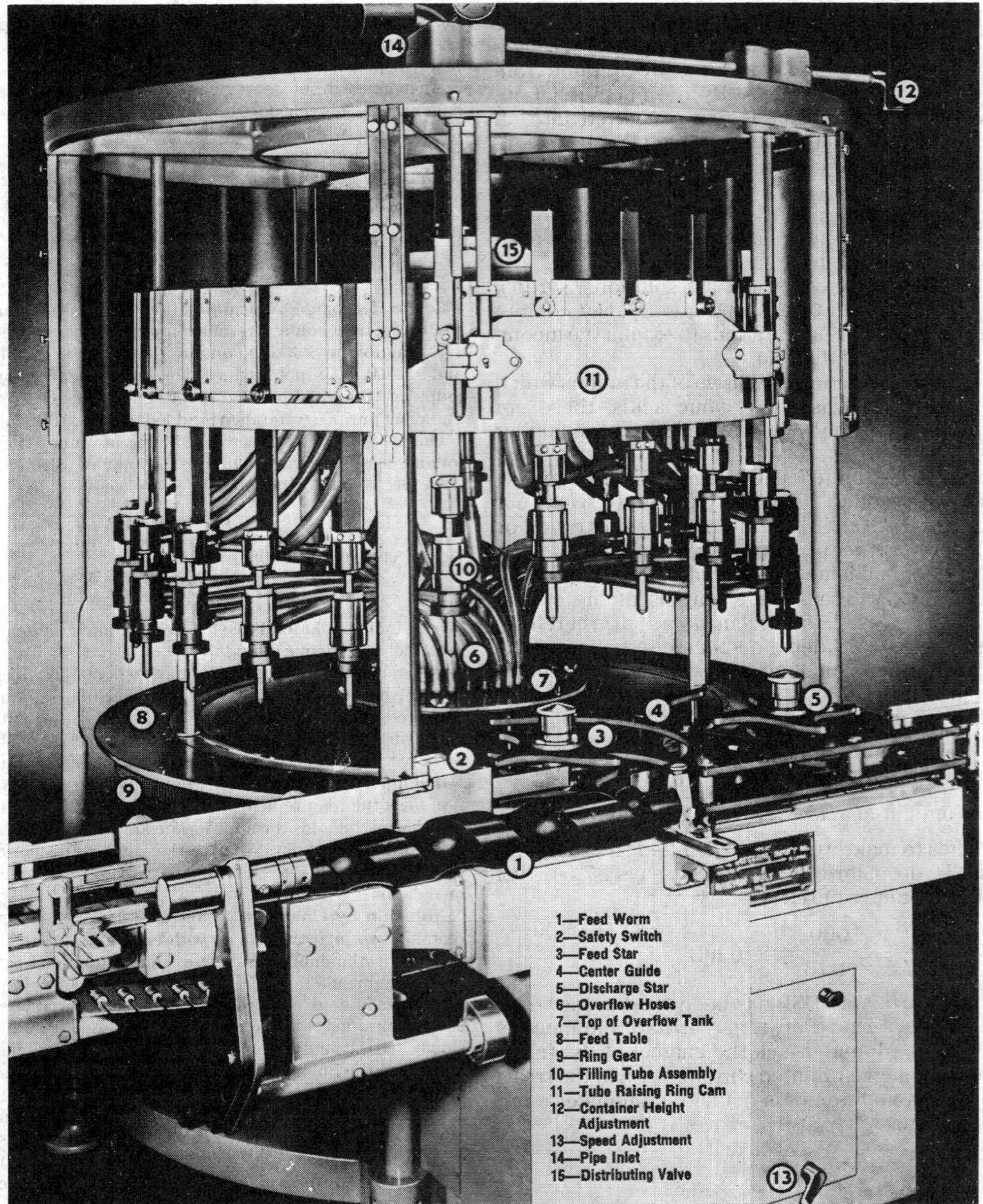

Fig 1. A rotary gravity bottle filler (courtesy, US Bottlers).

as solutions but, more often, are classified as extracts and are described at the end of this chapter.

Douches

A douche is an aqueous solution directed against a part or into a cavity of the body. It functions as a cleansing or antiseptic agent. An *eye douche*, used to remove foreign particles and discharges from the eyes, is directed gently at an oblique angle and allowed to run from the inner to the outer corner of the eye. *Pharyngeal douches* are used to prepare the interior of the throat for an operation and cleanse it in suppurative conditions. Similarly, there are *nasal douches* and *vaginal douches*. Douches usually are directed to the appropriate body part by using bulb syringes (Chapter 107).

Douches most frequently are dispensed in the form of a powder with directions for dissolving in a specified quantity of water (usually warm). However, tablets for preparing solutions are available (eg, Dobell's Solution Tablets) or the solution may be prepared by the pharmacist. If powders or tablets are supplied, they must be free from insoluble material, in order to produce a clear solution. Tablets are produced by the usual processes (see Chapter 92) but any lubricants or diluents used must be readily soluble in water. Boric acid may be used as a lubricant and sodium chloride normally is used as a diluent. Tablets deteriorate on exposure to moist air and should be stored in airtight containers.

Douches are not official as a class of preparations but several substances in the compendia frequently are employed as such in weak solutions, eg, benzalkonium chloride is used in various douches and Compound Sodium Borate Solution NFXI (Dobell's Solution) has been used as a nasal or pharyngeal douche. A sodium bicarbonate vaginal douche has been used to improve the postcoital test.

Vaginal douches are the most common type of douche and are used for cleansing the vagina and hygienic purposes. Liquid concentrates or powders, which may be prepared in bulk or as single-use packages, should be diluted or dissolved in the appropriate amount of warm water prior to use. The ingredients used in vaginal douches include antimicrobial agents such as benzalkonium chloride, the parabens or chlorothymol, anesthetics or antipruritics such as phenol or menthol. Astringents such as zinc sulfate or potassium alum, surface-active agents such as sodium lauryl sulfate and chemicals to alter the pH such as sodium bicarbonate or citric acid also are used.

Enemas

These preparations are rectal injections employed to evacuate the bowel (evacuation enemas), influence the general system by absorption or to affect locally the seat of disease. The latter two are called retention enemas. They may possess anthelmintic, nutritive, sedative or stimulating properties, or they may contain radiopaque substances for roentgenographic examination of the lower bowel.

Sodium chloride, sodium bicarbonate, sodium monohydrogen phosphate and sodium dihydrogen phosphate are used in enemas to evacuate the bowel. These substances may be used alone, in combination with each other or in combination with irritants such as soap. Enema of Soap BPC 1963 is prepared by dissolving 50 g of soft soap in sufficient purified water to make 1000 mL of enema. Sodium Phosphate Enema USP contains 6 g of dibasic sodium phosphate heptahydrate and 16 g of monobasic sodium phosphate monohydrate in each 100 mL. Evacuation enemas usually are given at body temperature in quantities of 1 to 2 pt injected slowly with a syringe.

An official retention enema used for systemic purposes is aminophylline. Retention enemas are to be retained in the intestine and should not be used in larger quantities than 150 mL for an adult. Usually, the volume is considerably smaller, such as a few mL. *Microenema* is a term used to describe these small-volume preparations. Vehicles for retention microenemas have been formulated with small quantities of ethanol and propylene glycol, and no significant difference in irritation, as compared with water, was found. A number of other drugs such as valproic acid, indomethacin and metronidazole have been formulated as microenemas for the purpose of absorption. The absorption of large molecular weight drugs, such as insulin, is under current investigation.

Sulfasalazine rectal enema has been administered for the treatment of ulcerative colitis and may be prepared by dispersing the tablets (1-g strength) in 250 mL water. An enema in the form of a suspension is 5-aminosalicylic acid, 168 g; NaH_2PO_4, 1.6 g; Na_2HPO_4, 17.9 g; NaCl, 36 g; sodium ascorbate, 2 g; tragacanth, 16 g; methylparaben, 8 g; propylparaben, 2 g; propylene glycol, 100 mL; and distilled water to make 4000 mL. It has been prepared by Montgomery *et al*[8] and shown to be stable for 90 days at both room and refrigerator temperatures. Barium sulfate enema contains 120 g of barium sulfate, 100 mL of acacia mucilage and sufficient starch enema to make 500 mL. An enema containing 30 to 50 g of sodium polystyrene sulfonate has been prepared using 100 mL of sorbitol solution.

Starch enema may be used either by itself or as a vehicle for other forms of medication. A thin paste is made by triturating 30 g of powdered starch with 200 mL of cold water. Sufficient boiling water is added to make 1000 mL of enema. The preparation then is reheated to obtain a transparent liquid.

Gargles

Gargles are aqueous solutions frequently containing antiseptics, antibiotics and/or anesthetics used for treating the pharynx and nasopharynx by forcing air from the lungs through the gargle which is held in the throat; subsequently, the gargle is expectorated. Many gargles must be diluted with water prior to use. Although mouthwashes are considered as a separate class of pharmaceuticals, many are used as gargles, either as is, or diluted with water.

A gargle/mouthwash containing the antibiotic tyrothricin has been shown to provide levels of gramicidin, a component of tyrothricin, in saliva when used as a gargle rather than a mouthwash. Higher saliva levels of gramicidin were obtained when a lozenge formulation was employed. Rapid relief of pharyngeal and oral pain was obtained when Cepacaine solution, which contains a topical anesthetic, was used as a gargle.

Potassium Chlorate and Phenol Gargle is official in the PC. It contains potassium chlorate, 30 g, patent blue V (Color Index No 42051) commercial food grade (0.01 g), liquified phenol (15 mL) and water for preparations qs to 1000 mL. It should be diluted with 10 volumes of warm water before use. The product should be labeled so that it cannot be mistaken for preparations intended for internal administration.

A flavored solution containing 7.5% povidone-iodine and 35% alcohol (*Isodine*) is available commercially as a mouthwash or gargle after suitable dilution.

Mouthwashes

A mouthwash can be used for two purposes, therapeutic and cosmetic. Therapeutic rinses or washes can be formulated to reduce plaque, gingivitis, dental caries and stomatitis. Cosmetic mouthwashes may be formulated to reduce bad breath through the use of antimicrobial and/or flavoring agents.

Recent information indicates that mouthwashes are being used as a dosage form for a number of specific problems in the oral cavity; for example, mouthwashes containing a combination of antihistamines, hydrocortisone, nystatin and tetracycline have been prepared from commercially available suspensions, powders, syrups or solutions for the treatment of stomatitis, a painful side effect of cancer therapy. Other drugs include allopurinol, also used for the treatment of stomatitis, pilocarpine for xerostoma (dry mouth), tranexamic acid for the prevention of bleeding after oral surgery, amphotericin B for oral candidiasis, chlorhexidine gluconate for plaque control and hexetidine as an antibactericidal and antifungal agent.

Mouthwashes may be used for a number of other purposes; for example, cetylpyridinum chloride and dibucaine hydrochloride mouthwashes provide satisfactory relief of pain in patients with ulcerative lesions of the mouth, mouthwashes or creams containing carbenoxolone are highly effective dosage forms for the treatment of orofacial herpes simplex infections and undetected oral cancer has been recognized using toluidine blue in the form of a mouth rinse.

Mouthwashes generally contain four groups of excipients as suggested by Tricca.[9]

Alcohols—Alcohol is often present in the range of 10–20%. It enhances the flavor, provides a certain sharpness to the taste, aids in masking the unpleasant taste of active ingredients, functions as a solubilizing agent for some flavoring agents and may function as a preservative. Humectants such as glycerin and sorbitol, may form 5–20% of the mouthwash. These agents increase the viscosity of the preparation and provide a certain *body* or *mouth feel* to the product. They enhance the sweetness of the product and, along with the ethanol, improve the preservative qualities of the product.

Surfactants, usually of the nonionic class such as polyoxyethylene/polyoxypropylene block copolymers or polyoxyethylene derivatives of sorbitol fatty acid esters may be used. The concentration range is 0.1–0.5%. An anionic surfactant occasionally used is sodium lauryl sulfate. Surfactants are used because they aid in the solubilization of flavors and in the removal of debris by providing foaming action. Cationic surfactants such as cetylpyridinium chloride are used for their antimicrobial properties, but these tend to impart a bitter taste.

Flavors are used in conjunction with alcohol and humectants to overcome disagreeable tastes, and at the same time they must be safe to use. The principle flavoring agents are peppermint, spearmint, cinnamon, wintergreen oils, menthol or methyl salicylate. Other flavoring agents may be used singly or in combination.

Coloring agents also are used in these products.

The products of commerce (eg, Cepacol, Listerine, Micrin or Scope) vary widely in composition. Antiseptic Solution and Mouthwash are described in NF XII. The latter wash contains sodium borate, glycerin and potassium bicarbonate. The reactions which take place when these substances are dissolved in water are given below.

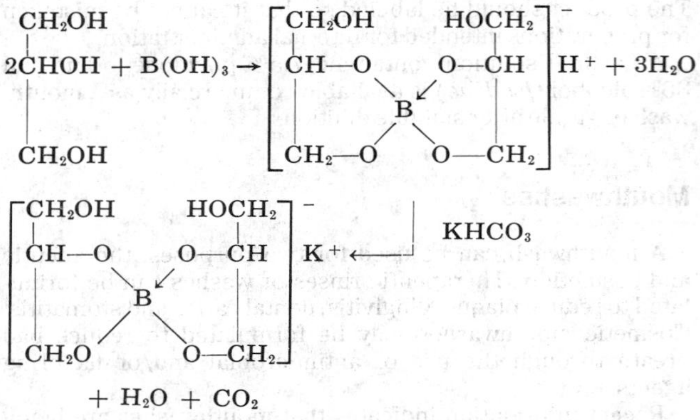

$$2\begin{array}{l}CH_2OH\\ |\\ CHOH\\ |\\ CH_2OH\end{array} + B(OH)_3 \rightarrow \left[\begin{array}{ccc}CH_2OH & & HOCH_2\\ | & & |\\ CH-O & & O-CH\\ & \searrow\ \swarrow & \\ & B & \\ & \diagup\ \diagdown & \\ CH_2-O & & O-CH_2\end{array}\right]^- H^+ + 3H_2O$$

$$\left[\begin{array}{ccc}CH_2OH & & HOCH_2\\ | & & |\\ CH-O & & O-CH\\ & \searrow\ \swarrow & \\ & B & \\ & \diagup\ \diagdown & \\ CH_2O & & O-CH_2\end{array}\right]^- K^+ \leftarrow KHCO_3 \quad + H_2O + CO_2$$

Compound Sodium Chloride Mouthwash and Zinc Sulphate Mouthwash are described in the BP and the PC, respectively. The former wash contains sodium chloride, sodium bicarbonate, concentrated peppermint emulsion and double-strength chloroform water. Extemporaneously compounded preparations include allopurinol at a strength of about 0.1% prepared from tablets in a suspending vehicle of 0.5% methylcellulose sweetened and flavored. Modifications of this preparation have been shown to have considerable stability.

Juices

A juice is prepared from fresh ripe fruit, is aqueous in character and is used in making syrups which are employed as vehicles. The freshly expressed juice is preserved with benzoic acid and allowed to stand at room temperature for several days, until the pectins which naturally are present are destroyed by enzymatic action, as indicated by the filtered juice yielding a clear solution with alcohol. Pectins, if allowed to remain, would cause precipitation in the final syrup.

Cherry Juice (RPS-18 page 1320) is described in the USP XXI and Raspberry Juice in USP XVIII. Concentrated Raspberry Juice PC is prepared from the clarified juice of raspberries. Pectinase is stirred into pulped raspberries and the mixture allowed to stand for 12 hours. The pulp is pressed, the juice clarified and sufficient sucrose added to adjust the weight at 20° to 1.050 to 1.060 g per mL. The juice then is concentrated to one-sixth of its original volume. Sufficient sulfurous acid or sodium metabisulfite is added as a preservative.

Artificial flavors now have replaced many of the natural fruit juices. Although they lack the flavor of the natural juice, they are more stable and easier to incorporate into the final pharmaceutical form. Commercial juices such as orange, apple, grape and mixed vegetables have been used recently to prepare extemporaneous preparations of cholestyramine and nizatidine.

Information on cranberry juice indicates that it may be effective in controlling some urinary tract infections and urolithiosis.

Nasal Solutions

Nasal solutions are usually aqueous solutions designed to be administered to the nasal passages in drops or sprays. While many of the drugs are administered for their local sympathomimetic effect such as Ephedrine Sulfate or Naphazoline Hydrochloride Nasal Solution USP, to reduce nasal congestion, a few other official preparations, Lypressin Nasal Solution USP and Oxytocin Nasal Solution USP, are administered in spray form for their systemic effect for the treatment of diabetes insipidus and *milk letdown* prior to breast feeding, respectively. The current route of administration of peptides and proteins is limited to parenteral injection because of inactivation within the gastrointestinal tract. As a result, there is considerable research on intranasal delivery of these drugs such as analogs of enkephalins or luteinizing hormone releasing hormone and insulin. Other drugs which are absorbed poorly from the GI tract such as gentamicin sulfate, are being administered in the form of nasal solutions, in order to obtain appropriate blood levels.

Nasal solutions are prepared so that they are similar in many respects to nasal secretions, so that normal ciliary action is maintained. Thus, the aqueous nasal solutions usually are isotonic and slightly buffered to maintain a pH of 5.5 to 6.5. In addition, antimicrobial preservatives, similar to those used in ophthalmic preparations, and appropriate drug stabilizers, if required, are included in the formulation.

Commercial nasal preparations, in addition to the drugs listed above also include antibiotics, antihistamines and drugs for asthma prophylaxis.

A formula for Ephedrine Nasal Drops PC is

Ephedrine Hydrochloride	0.5 g
Chlorobutanol	0.5 g
Sodium Chloride	0.5 g
Water for preparations	to 100 mL

Current studies indicate that nasal sprays are deposited mainly in the atrium and cleared slowly into the pharynx with the patient in an upright position. Drops spread more extensively than the spray and three drops cover most of the walls of the nasal cavity, with the patient in a supine position and head tilted back and turned left and right. It is suggested that drop delivery, with appropriate movement by the patient, leads to extensive coverage of the walls of the nasal cavity.

Otic Solutions

These solutions occasionally are referred to as aural preparations. Other otic preparations often include formulations such as suspensions and ointments for topical application in the ear.

The main classes of drugs used for topical administration to the ear include analgesics, eg, benzocaine; antibiotics, eg, neomycin; and anti-inflammatory agents, eg, cortisone. The USP preparations include Antipyrine and Benzocaine Otic Solution. The Neomycin and Polymyxin B Sulfates and Hydrocortisone Otic Solutions contain appropriate buffers and dispersants usually in an aqueous solution. The main solvents used in these preparations include glycerin or water. The viscous glycerin vehicle permits the drug to remain in the ear for a long time. Anhydrous glycerin, being hygroscopic, tends to remove moisture from surrounding tissues, thus reducing swelling. Viscous liquids like glycerin or propylene glycol are used either alone or in combination with a surfactant to aid in the removal of cerumen (ear wax). Sodium Bicarbonate Ear-Drops BP may be used if wax is to be removed from the ear. This preparation contains sodium bicarbonate (5 g), glycerin (30 mL) and purified water (a sufficient quantity to make 100 mL).

In order to provide sufficient time for aqueous preparations to act, it is necessary for the patient to remain on his side for a few minutes so the drops do not run out of the ear. Otic preparations are dispensed in a container which permits the administration of drops.

Irrigation Solutions

These solutions are used to wash or bathe surgical incisions, wounds or body tissues. Because they come in contact with exposed tissue, they must meet stringent requirements for Injections of the USP such as sterility, particulate matter and the requirements of the Pyrogen Test. These products are prepared by dissolving the active ingredient in Water for Injection. They are packaged in single-dose containers, preferably Type I or Type II glass, or suitable plastic containers, and then sterilized. See Chapter 84 for sterilization procedures. A number of irrigations are described in the USP: Acetic Acid Irrigation for bladder irrigation, Dimethyl Sulfoxide Irrigation for relief of internal cystitis, Neomycin and Polymyxin B Sulfates Solution for Irrigation for infection and Sodium Chloride Irrigation for washing wounds.

Extemporaneous formulations frequently are prepared using an isotonic solution of sodium chloride as the solvent. For example, cefazolin or gentamicin in 0.9% sodium chloride are used as anti-infective irrigations, dinoprostone in lactated ringers injection is used by continuous intrauterine irrigation for severe postpartum hemorrhage and 5-fluororacil in 0.9% sodium chloride is employed for bladder irrigation. Alum, either potassium or ammonium, in either sterile water or 0.9% sodium chloride for irrigation has been used for bladder hemorrhage. Amphotericin in sterile water has been used for the treatment of localized infections of the bladder and urinary tract. All the extemporaneous preparations should meet the general requirements noted above for USP irrigations.

Sweet or Other Viscid Aqueous Solutions

Solutions which are sweet or viscid include syrups, honeys, mucilages and jellies. All of these are viscous liquids or semisolids. The basic sweet or viscid substances giving body to these preparations are sugars, polyols or polysaccharides (gums).

Syrups

Syrups are concentrated solutions of sugar such as sucrose in water or other aqueous liquid. When Purified Water alone is used in making the solution of sucrose, the preparation is known as *Syrup*, or *simple syrup*. In addition to sucrose, certain other polyols, such as glycerin or sorbitol, may be added to retard crystallization of sucrose or to increase the solubility of added ingredients. Alcohol often is included as a preservative and also as a solvent for flavors; further resistance to microbial attack can be enhanced by incorporating antimicrobial agents. When the aqueous preparation contains some added-medicinal substance, the syrup is called a *medicated syrup*. A *flavored* syrup is one which usually is not medicated, but which contains various aromatic or pleasantly flavored substances and is intended to be used as a vehicle or flavor for prescriptions, eg, Acacia, Cherry, Cocoa and Orange USP XXI.

Flavored syrups offer unusual opportunities as vehicles in extemporaneous compounding and are accepted readily by both children and adults. Because they contain no, or very little, alcohol they are vehicles of choice for many of the drugs that are prescribed by pediatricians. Their lack of alcohol makes them superior solvents for water-soluble substances. However, sucrose-based medicines continuously administered to children apparently cause an increase in dental caries and gingivitis; consequently, alternate formulations of the drug either unsweetened or sweetened with noncariogenic substances should be considered. A knowledge of the sugar content of liquid medicines is useful for patients who are on a restricted calorie intake; a list has been prepared by Bergen.[10]

Syrups possess remarkable masking properties for bitter or saline drugs. Glycyrrhiza syrup has been recommended for disguising the salty taste of bromides, iodides and chlorides. This has been attributed to its colloidal character and its double sweetness—the immediate sweetness of the sugar and the lingering sweetness of the glycyrrhizin. This syrup is also of value in masking bitterness in preparations containing the B complex vitamins. Acacia Syrup USP XXI (page 1393), because of its colloidal character, is of particular value as a vehicle for masking the disagreeable taste of many medica- ments. Raspberry Syrup BP is one of the most efficient-flavoring agents and is especially useful in masking the taste of bitter drugs. Many factors, however, enter into the choice of a suitable flavoring agent. Literature reports are often contradictory and there appears to be no substitute for the taste panel. The literature on this subject has been reviewed by Meer[11] and this reference and Chapter 80 should be consulted for further information on the flavoring of pharmaceuticals and the preparation of a number of official syrups. A series of papers by Schumacher deals with improving the palatability of bulk-compounded products using flavoring and sweetening agents.[12]

In manufacturing syrups the sucrose must be selected carefully and a purified water, free from foreign substances, and clean vessels and containers must be used. The operation must be conducted with care to avoid contamination, if the products are to be stable.

It is important that the concentration of sucrose approach but not quite reach the saturation point. In dilute solutions sucrose provides an excellent nutrient for molds, yeasts and other microorganisms. In concentrations of 65% by weight or more, the solution will retard the growth of such microorganisms. However, a saturated solution may lead to crystal lization of a part of the sucrose under conditions of changing temperature.

When heat is used in the preparation of syrups, there is almost certain to be an inversion of a slight portion of the sucrose. Sucrose solutions are dextrorotary but, as hydrolysis proceeds, the optical rotation decreases and becomes negative when the reaction is complete. This reaction is termed *inversion* because *invert sugar* (dextrose plus levulose) is formed. The speed of inversion is increased greatly by the presence of acids; the hydrogen ion acts as a catalyst in this hydrolytic reaction. Invert sugar is more readily fermentable than sucrose and tends to be darker in color. Nevertheless, its two reducing sugars are of value in retarding the oxidation of other substances.

Invert Syrup is described in the BP. It is prepared by hydrolyzing sucrose with hydrochloric acid and neutralizing the solution with calcium or sodium carbonate. The sucrose in the 66.7% *w/w* solution must be at least 95% inverted. The monograph states that invert syrup, when mixed in suitable proportions with syrup, prevents the deposition of crystals of sucrose under most conditions of storage.

The levulose formed during inversion is sweeter than sucrose and, therefore, the resulting syrup is sweeter than the original syrup. The relative sweetness of levulose, sucrose and dextrose is in the ratio of 173:100:74. Thus, invert sugar is $1/100\,(173 + 74)\frac{1}{2} = 1.23$ times as sweet as sucrose. The levulose formed during the hydrolysis also is responsible for the darkening of syrup. It is sensitive to heat and darkens readily, particularly in solution. When syrup or sucrose is overheated, it caramelizes. See *Caramel* (RPS-18 page 1290). Occasionally, it is appropriate to use a sugar-free liquid preparation; a list of these has been published.[13]

Preparation—Syrups are prepared in various ways, the choice of the proper method depends on the physical and chemical characteristics of the substances entering into the preparation.

Solution with Heat—This is the usual method of making syrups when the valuable constituent is neither volatile nor injured by heat, and when it is desirable to make the syrup rapidly. The sucrose usually is added to the purified water or aqueous solution and heated until solution is effected, then strained and sufficient purified water added to make the desired weight or volume. If the syrup is made from an infusion, a decoction or an aqueous solution containing organic matter, such as sap from maple trees, it usually is proper to heat the syrup to the boiling point to coagulate albuminous matter; subsequently, this is separated by straining. If the albumin or other impurities were permitted to remain in the syrup, fermentation probably would be induced in warm weather. Saccharometers are very useful in making syrups by the hot process in cases where the proper specific gravity of the finished syrup is known. They may be floated in the syrup while boiling, and thus the exact degree of concentration determined without waiting to cool the syrup and having to heat it again to concentrate it further. When taking a reading of the specific gravity of the hot syrup, allowance must be made for the variation from the official temperature (specific gravities in the USP are taken at 25°).

Excessive heating of syrups at the boiling temperature is undesirable since more or less inversion of the sucrose occurs with an increased tendency to ferment. Syrups cannot be sterilized in an autoclave without some caramelization. This is indicated by a yellowish or brownish color resulting from the formation of caramel by the action of heat upon sucrose.

The formula and procedure given for Acacia Syrup (page 1393) illustrates this method of preparation.

Agitation without Heat—This process is used in those cases where heat would cause the loss of valuable, volatile constituents. In making quantities up to 2000 mL the sucrose should be added to the aqueous solution in a bottle of about twice the size required for the syrup. This permits active agitation and rapid solution. Stoppering the bottle is important, as it prevents contamination and loss during the process. The bottle should be allowed to lie on its side when not being agitated. Glass-lined tanks with mechanical agitators, especially adapted to dissolving of sucrose, are used for making syrups in large quantities.

This method and that previously described are used for the preparation of a wide variety of preparations that are described popularly as syrups. Most cough syrups, for example, contain sucrose and one or more active ingredients. However, the exact composition of such products is not given on the label. Furthermore, some of these products are listed in the USP but no directions are given for their preparation. For example, Guaifenesin Syrup USP (glyceryl guaiacolate syrup) is official but the only known ingredients are guaifenesin (glyceryl guaiacolate) and ethanol (not less than 3% or more than 4%).

The PC, on the other hand, gives a method for the preparation of Codeine Phosphate Syrup. This contains codeine phosphate (5 g), water for preparations (15 mL), chloroform spirit (25 mL) and sufficient syrup to make 1000 mL. It can be used for the relief of cough. Another syrup for this purpose is Codeine Linctus PC. This is really a medicated syrup which possesses demulcent, expectorant or sedative properties. Unlike the syrup, it is colored and flavored. The formula for Codeine Linctus PC is

Codeine Phosphate	3 g
Compound Tartrazine Solution	10 mL
Benzoic Acid Solution	20 mL
Chloroform Spirit	20 mL
Water for Preparations	20 mL
Lemon Syrup	200 mL
Syrup	to 1000 mL

Dissolve the codeine phosphate in the water, add 500 mL of the syrup and mix. Add the other ingredients and sufficient syrup to produce 1000 mL.

For pediatric use, 200 mL of this linctus is diluted with sufficient syrup to make 1000 mL. If sugar is contraindicated in the diet, Diabetic Codeine Linctus can be used:

Codeine Phosphate	3 g
Citric Acid monohydrate	5 g
Lemon Spirit	1 mL
Compound Tartrazine Solution	10 mL
Benzoic Acid Solution	20 mL
Chloroform Spirit	20 mL
Water for Preparations	20 mL
Sorbitol Solution	to 1000 mL

Dissolve the codeine phosphate and the citric acid in the water, add 750 mL of the sorbitol solution and mix. Add the other ingredients and sufficient sorbitol solution to produce 1000 mL.

Sorbitol Solution is the sweetening agent and contains 70% *w/w* of total solids, consisting mainly of D-sorbitol. It has about half the sweetening power of syrup. In the US the FDA has banned the use of chloroform in medicines and cosmetics because of reported carcinogenicity in animals.

Basic formulations can be varied easily to produce the highly advertised articles of commerce. The prescription-only drug (eg, codeine phosphate or methadone) must, of course, be omitted from the formulation but, in certain countries, such as Canada, a decreased quantity of codeine phosphate is permitted in an OTC cough syrup. In addition to the ingredients cited or listed in the official compendia (eg, tolu, squill or ipecacuanha), many cough syrups contain an antihistamine.

Many other active ingredients (eg, ephedrine sulfate, dicyclomine hydrochloride, chloral hydrate or chlorpromazine hydrochloride) are marketed as syrups. Like cough syrups, these preparations are flavored, colored and recommended in those instances where the patient cannot swallow the solid dosage form.

Addition of a Medicating Liquid to Syrup—This method is resorted to in those cases in which fluidextracts, tinctures or other liquids are added to syrup to medicate it. Syrups made in this way usually develop precipitates since alcohol is often an ingredient of the liquids thus used, and the resinous and oily substances dissolved by the alcohol precipitate when mixed with the syrup, producing unsightly preparations. A modification of this process, frequently adopted, consists of mixing the fluidextract or tincture with the water, allowing the mixture to stand to permit the separation of insoluble constituents, filtering and then dissolving the sucrose in the filtrate. It is obvious that this procedure is not permissible when the precipitated ingredients are the valuable medicinal agents.

The formula and procedure given for Aromatic Eriodictyon Syrup USP XXI (RPS-18 page 1301) illustrate this method of preparation.

Percolation—In this procedure, purified water, or an aqueous solution, is permitted to pass slowly through a bed of crystalline sucrose, thus dissolving it and forming a syrup. A cotton pledget is placed in the neck of the percolator and the water or aqueous solution added. By means of a suitable stopcock the flow is regulated so that drops appear in rapid succession. If necessary, a portion of the liquid is recycled through the percolator to dissolve all the sucrose. Finally, sufficient purified water is passed through the cotton to make the required volume.

To be successful in using this process, care in several particulars must be exercised: (1) the percolator used should be cylindrical or semicylindrical and cone-shaped as it nears the lower orifice; (2) a coarse granular sugar must be used, otherwise it will coalesce into a compact mass, which the liquid cannot permeate; (3) the purified cotton must be introduced with care.

If pressed in too tightly, the cotton will stop the process effectually; if inserted too loosely, the liquid will pass through the cotton rapidly and the filtrate will be weak and turbid (from imperfect filtration); it should be inserted completely within the neck of the percolator, since a protruding end, inside the percolator, up through the sucrose, will permit the last portions of water to pass out at the lower orifice without dissolving all the sucrose. For specific directions see *Syrups* (page 1393). The process of percolation is applied on a commercial scale for the making of official syrups as well as those for confectionary use.

Percolation is the preferred method for the preparation of Syrup USP (page 1301). The sucrose, in this instance, is placed in the percolator. However, a slightly modified approach must be used if a drug of vegetable origin is to be incorporated into the syrup. For example, wild cherry bark is first percolated with water; the collection vessel contains sucrose (800 g) and glycerol (50 mL). When the total volume is 1000 mL, the percolate is agitated to produce Wild Cherry Syrup PC.

Reconstitution—In order to improve stability and minimize microbial contamination, dry syrup formulations can be prepared and Purified Water USP added just prior to dispensing or use. Powder mixtures, wholly granulated products and partially granulated products have been investigated for this purpose by Ryder.[14]

The powder mixture preparation requires less equipment and energy to prepare. Chemical stability problems are minimal, since no heat or solvents are used in the process and a low moisture content can be obtained in the final product; unfortunately, powder mixtures are prone to homogeneity problems. In the case of the wholly granulated product all the ingredients are included in the granulation stage. The drug may be incorporated into the dry product before granulation or dissolved or suspended in the granulating fluid. After formation, the granules are dried and then screened to break down oversize particles. The advantages of granulated over powder mixtures include better appearance, better flow, fewer segregation problems and less dust during processing. Partially granulated mixtures are used to gain some of the advantages of granulation without the disadvantages. Usually the drug, and other fine particles, are included at the granulation stage, perhaps with some diluents to improve flow and reduce segregation and dust. Materials selected for mixing with the dried granules would include thermolabile excipients, such as flavors, and free flowing materials, such as sugars.

Preservation—Syrups should be made in quantities which can be consumed within a few months, except in those cases where special facilities can be employed for their preservation; a low temperature is the best method. Concentration without super-saturation is also a condition favorable to preservation. The USP states that syrups may contain preservatives such as glycerin, methylparaben, benzoic acid and sodium benzoate to prevent bacterial and mold growth. Combinations of alkyl esters of *p*-hydroxybenzoic acid are effective inhibitors of yeasts which have been implicated in the contamination of commercial syrups.

The official syrups should be preserved in well-dried bottles, preferably those which have been sterilized. These bottles should not hold more than is likely to be required during 4 to 6 weeks and should be filled completely, stoppered carefully and stored in a cool, dark place.

Syrups Prepared from Juices

Blackberry, pineapple and strawberry syrups may be prepared by following the directions for Raspberry Syrup BP. One volume of the concentrated raspberry juice is diluted with 11 volumes of syrup. Black Current Syrup BP is prepared in a similar manner but also can be prepared from black currants, with certain modifications. The pectin in the juice is destroyed with pectinase. The syrup is prepared by dissolving 700 g of sucrose in 560 mL of clarified juice and may be preserved with sodium metabisulfite. The addition of a dye is permitted, provided it complies with the pertinent government regulations. Cherry Syrup USP XXI is prepared from cherry juice by the addition of alcohol, sucrose and water (page 1393).

Syrups, either as a syrup or as a flavored syrup, are useful for preparing liquid oral dosage forms from not only the pure drug but also injections, capsules or tablets if the pure drug is not readily available. On one hand, if the drug and all the excipients in the preparation, eg, injectables or capsules, are water soluble, a solution will result if a syrup is prepared. On the other hand, if the preparation to be used contains water-insoluble ingredients, as is usually the case with tablets and some capsules, a suspension will be formed. Several of the above preparations have been described in the literature, not only in regard to their formulation but also in regard to stability and bioavailability. Some drugs which have been prepared from either the pure drug or an injectable form include midazolam, atropine, aminocaproic acid, terbutaline, procainamide, chloroquin, propranolol and citrated caffeine. If the appropriate salt of the drug is used, a solution will result. When tablets are used to prepare liquid formulations, a suspension usually is formed because there is usually a nonwater-soluble ingredient used in table preparations. Some formulations prepared from tablets are clonidine hydrochloride, cefuroxime axetil, famotidine, terbutaline sulfate, spironolactone, ranitidine, propranolol and rifampin. The resulting suspensions should have a uniform distribution of particles so that a consistent dose is obtained. If the materials are not distributed uniformly, more appropriate suspending formulations should be considered, which are described later in the chapter. If pharmaceutical preparations contain a liquid such as valproic acid or simethicone, to be incorporated into syrups, which is insoluble in water, an emulsion will form and a uniform product will not result.

Honeys

Honeys are thick liquid preparations somewhat allied to the syrups, differing in that honey, instead of syrup, is used as a base. They are unimportant as a class of preparations today but at one time, before sugar was available and honey was the most common sweetening agent, they were used widely. The BP lists one preparation for coughs containing honey. Squill Oxymel contains squill, water, acetic acid and honey and is prepared by a maceration process.

Honey and sugar pastes are used to a small extent and have been discussed in the pharmaceutical literature for topical application for the treatment of certain types of ulcers and abscesses. Thick and thin sugar pastes containing Caster sugar (very fine granular sugar), icing sugar (additive-free), polyethylene glycol 400 and hydrogen peroxide (in a final concentration of 0.15%) have been prepared and shown to be beneficial in the process of wound healing.

Mucilages

The official mucilages are thick, viscid, adhesive liquids, produced by dispersing gum in water, or by extracting the mucilaginous principles from vegetable substances with water. The mucilages all are prone to decomposition, showing appreciable decrease in viscosity on storage; they should never be made in quantities larger than can be used immediately, unless a preservative is added. Acacia Mucilage NF XII contains benzoic acid and Tragacanth Mucilage BPC (1973) contains alcohol and chloroform water. Chloroform in manufactured products for internal use is banned in some countries.

Acacia Mucilage may be prepared by placing 350 g of acacia in a graduated bottle, washing the drug with cold purified water, allowing it to drain and adding enough warm purified water, in which 2 g of benzoic acid has been dissolved, to make the product measure 1000 mL. The bottle then is stoppered, placed on its side, rotated occasionally and the product strained when the acacia has dissolved.

Tragacanth Mucilage BPC (1973) is prepared by mixing 12.5 g of tragacanth with 25 mL alcohol (90%) in a dry bottle and then quickly adding sufficient chloroform water to 1000 mL and shaking vigorously. The alcohol is used to disperse the gum to prevent agglomeration on addition of the water.

Mucilages are used primarily to aid in suspending insoluble subtances in liquids; their colloidal character and viscosity help prevent immediate sedimentation. Examples include sulfur in lotions, resin in mixtures and oils in emulsions. Both tragacanth and acacia either are partially or completely insoluble in alcohol. Tragacanth is precipitated from solution by alcohol, but acacia, on the other hand, is soluble in diluted alcoholic solutions. A 60% solution of acacia may be prepared with 20% alcohol and a 4% solution of acacia may be prepared even with 50% alcohol.

The viscosity of tragacanth mucilage is reduced by acid, alkali or sodium chloride, particularly if the mucilage is heated. It shows maximum viscosity at pH 5. Acacia is hydrolyzed by dilute mineral acids to arabinose, galactose, aldobionic and galacturonic acids. Its viscosity is low but is maintained over a wide pH range.

Recent research on mucilages includes the preparation of mucilage from plantain and the identification of its sugars, the preparation and suspending properties of cocoa gum, the preparation of glycerin ointments using flaxseed mucilage and the consideration of various gums and mucilages obtained from several Indian plants for pharmaceutical purposes.

Several synthetic mucilage-like substances such as *polyvinyl alcohol*, *methylcellulose*, *carboxymethylcellulose* and related substances, as described in Chapter 80, are used at the appropriate concentration as mucilage substitutes, emulsifying and suspending agents. Methylcellulose (page 1397) is used widely as a bulk laxative since it absorbs water and swells to a hydrogel in the intestine, in much the same manner as *psyllium* or *karaya gum*. Methylcellulose Oral Solution USP is a flavored solution of the agent. It may be prepared by adding slowly the methylcellulose to about one-third the amount of boiling water, with stirring, until it is thoroughly wetted. Cold water then should be added and the wetted material allowed to dissolve while stirring. The viscosity of the solution will depend upon the concentration and the specifications of the methylcellulose. The synthetic gums are non-glycogenetic and may be used in the preparation of diabetic syrups. Several formulas for such syrups, based on sodium carboxymethylcellulose, have been proposed.

Uniformly smooth mucilages sometimes are difficult to prepare due to the uneven wetting of the gums. In general, it is best to use fine gum particles and disperse them with good agitation in a little 95% alcohol or in cold water (except for methylcellulose). The appropriate amount of water then can be added with constant stirring. A review of the chemistry and properties of acacia and other gums has been prepared.[15]

Jellies

Jellies are a class of gels in which the structural coherent matrix contains a high portion of liquid, usually water. They are similar to mucilages, in that they may be prepared from similar gums, but they differ from the latter in having a jelly-like consistency. A whole gum of the best quality, rather than a powdered gum, is desirable in order to obtain a clear preparation of uniform consistency. Tragacanth is the gum used in the preparation of Ephedrine Sulfate Jelly NF XII. While the specific thickening agent in the USP jellies is not indicated, reference usually is made in the monograph to a water-soluble, sterile, viscous base. These preparations also may be formulated with water from acacia, chondrus, gelatin, carboxymethylcellulose, hydroxyethylcellulose and similar substances.

Jellies are used as lubricants for surgical gloves, catheters and rectal thermometers. Lidocaine Hydrochloride Jelly USP is used as a topical anesthetic. Therapeutic vaginal jellies are available and certain jelly-like preparations are used for contraceptive purposes, which often contain surface-active agents to enhance the spermatocidal properties of the jelly. Aromatics, such as methyl salicylate and eucalyptol, often are added to give the preparation a desirable odor.

Jellies are prone to microbial contamination and therefore contain preservatives, eg, methyl *p*-hydroxybenzoate is used as a preservative in a base for medicated jellies. This base contains sodium alginate, glycerin, calcium gluconate and water. The calcium ions cause a cross-linking with sodium alginate to form a gel of firmer consistency. A discussion of gels is provided later in the chapter.

Nonaqueous Solutions

It is difficult to evaluate fairly the importance of nonaqueous solvents in pharmaceutical processes. That they are important in the manufacture of pharmaceuticals is an understatement. However, pharmaceutical preparations, and, in particular, those intended for internal use, rarely contain more than minor quantities of the organic solvents that are common to the manufacturing or analytical operation. For example, industry uses large quantities of chloroform in some operations but the solvent is of only minor importance with respect to the final product. One mL of chloroform dissolves in about 200 mL of water and the solution so formed finds some use as a vehicle (see the section on *Aromatic Waters*). Chloroform has been an ingredient in a number of cough syrups in the past but it has been banned in the US by the FDA in manufactured products intended for internal use. Solvents such as acetone, benzene and petroleum ether must not be ingredients in preparations intended for internal use.

Products of commerce for internal use may contain solvents such as ethanol, glycerin, propylene glycol, certain oils and liquid paraffin. Preparations intended for external use may contain solvents in addition to those just mentioned, namely isopropyl alcohol, polyethylene glycols, various ethers and certain esters. A good example of preparations of this type are the rubefacient rubbing alcohols. Rubbing Alcohol must be manufactured in accordance with the requirements of the Bureau of Alcohol, Tobacco and Firearms, US Treasury Dept, using Formula 23-H denatured alcohol. This mixture contains 8 parts by volume of acetone, 1.5 parts by volume of methyl isobutyl ketone and 100 parts by volume of ethanol. Besides the alcohol in the Rubbing Alcohol, the final product must contain water, sucrose octaacetate or denatonium benzoate and may contain color additives, perfume oils and a suitable stabilizer. The alcohol content, by volume, is not less than 68.5% and not more than 71.5%. The isopropyl alcohol content in Isopropyl Rubbing Alcohol can vary from 68.0% to 72.0% and the finished product may contain color additives, perfume oils and suitable stabilizers.

Although the lines between aqueous and nonaqueous preparations tend to blur in those cases where the solvent is water-soluble, it is possible to categorize a number of products as nonaqueous. This section is, therefore, devoted to groups of nonaqueous solutions; the alcoholic or hydroalcoholic solutions (eg, elixirs and spirits), ethereal solutions (eg, collodions), glycerin solutions (eg, glycerins), oleaginous solutions (eg, liniments, oleovitamins and toothache drops), inhalations and inhalants.

Although the above list is limited, a wide variety of solvents are used in various pharmaceutical preparations. Solvents such as glycerol formal, dimethylacetamide and glycerol dimethylketal have been suggested for some products produced by the industry. However, the toxicity of many of these solvents is not well-established and, for this reason, careful clinical studies should be carried out on the formulated product before it is released to the marketplace.

It is essential that the toxicity of solvents be tested appropriately and approved in order to avoid problems: for example, the tragic loss of life which occurred during 1937 when diethylene glycol was used in an elixir of sulfanilamide. The result of this tragedy was the 1938 Federal Food, Drug and Cosmetic Act, which required that products be tested for both safety and effectiveness.

Collodions

Collodions are liquid preparations containing pyroxylin (a nitrocellulose) in a mixture of ethyl ether and ethanol. They are applied to the skin by means of a soft brush or other suitable applicator and, when the ether and ethanol have evaporated, leave a film of pyroxylin on the surface. The official medicated collodion, Salicylic Acid Collodion USP, contains 10% *w/v* of salicylic acid in Flexible Collodion USP and is used as a keratolytic agent in the treatment of corns and warts. Collodion USP and Flexible Collodion USP are water-repellent protectives for minor cuts and scratches. Collodion is made flexible by the addition of castor oil and camphor. Collodion has been used to reduce or eliminate the side effects of fluorouracil treatment of solar keratoses. Vehicles other than flexible collodion, such as a polyacrylic base, have been used to incorporate salicylic acid for the treatment of warts with less irritation.

Elixirs

Elixirs are clear, pleasantly flavored, sweetened hydroalcoholic liquids intended for oral use. The main ingredients in elixirs are ethanol and water but glycerin, sorbitol, propylene glycol, flavoring agents, preservatives and syrups often are used in the preparation of the final product. Elixirs are more fluid than syrups, due to the use of less viscous ingredients such as alcohol and the minimal use of viscosity-improving agents such as sucrose. They are used as flavors and vehicles such as Aromatic Elixir USP (page 1394) for drug substances and, when such substances are incorporated into the specified solvents, they are classified as medicated elixirs, eg, Dexamethasone Elixir USP and Phenobarbital Elixir USP. Occasionally, certain adverse effects, eg, mucosal erosions, may be eliminated or reduced if the active drug, eg, potassium chloride, is administered in elixir rather than in a solid dosage form.

The distinction between some of the medicated syrups and elixirs is not always clear. For example, Ephedrine Sulfate Syrup USP contains between 20 and 40 mL of alcohol in 1000 mL of product. Ephedrine Elixir BP contains a suitable flavored vehicle and 12% alcohol. Definitions are, sometimes, inconsistent and, in some instances, not too important with respect to the naming of the articles of commerce. To be designated as an elixir, however, the solution must contain alcohol.

The alcoholic content will vary greatly, from elixirs containing only a small quantity to those that contain a considerable portion as a necessary aid to solubility. For example, Aromatic Elixir USP contains 21 to 23% of alcohol; Compound Benzaldehyde Elixir USP, on the other hand, contains 3 to 5%.

Elixirs also may contain glycerin and syrup. These may be added to increase the solubility of the medicinal agent for sweetening purposes or to decrease the pharmacological effects of the alcohol. Some elixirs contain propylene glycol. Claims have been made for this solvent as a satisfactory substitute for both glycerin and alcohol. Sumner,[16] in his paper on terpin hydrate preparations, summarized the advantages and disadvantages of this solvent and suggested several formulations with therapeutic characteristics superior to those of the elixir described in NF XIII.

One of the four formulations described in Sumner's paper is given below:

Terpin Hydrate	6.0 g
Orange Oil	0.1 mL
Benzaldehyde	0.005 mL
Sorbitol Solution USP	10.0 mL
Propylene Glycol	40.0 mL
Alcohol	43.0 mL
Purified Water, a sufficient quantity to make	100.0 mL

Dissolve the terpin hydrate in the propylene glycol and sorbitol solution which have been heated to 50°. Add the oil and the benzaldehyde to the alcohol and mix with the terpin hydrate solution at 25°. Add sufficient purified water to make the product measure 100 mL.

The elixir contains 300 mg of terpin hydrate/5 mL, a minimal quantity of alcohol and flavoring agents which adequately mask the taste of propylene glycol.

Although alcohol is an excellent solvent for some drugs, it does accentuate the saline taste of bromides and similar salts. It often is desirable, therefore, to substitute some other solvent that is more effective in masking such tastes for part of the alcohol in the formula. In general, if taste is a consideration, the formulator is more prone to use a syrup rather than a hydroalcoholic vehicle.

Because only relatively small quantities of ingredients have to be dissolved, elixirs are more readily prepared and manufactured than syrups, which frequently contain considerable amounts of sugar. An elixir may contain both water- and alcohol-soluble ingredients. If such is the case, the following procedure is indicated:

Dissolve the water-soluble ingredients in part of the water. Add and solubilize the sucrose in the aqueous solution. Prepare an alcoholic solution containing the other ingredients. Add the aqueous phase to the alcoholic solution, filter and make to volume with water.

Sucrose increases viscosity and decreases the solubilizing properties of water and so must be added after primary solution has been effected. A high alcoholic content is maintained during preparation by adding the aqueous phase to the alcoholic solution. Elixirs always should be brilliantly clear. They may be strained or filtered and, if necessary, subjected to the clarifying action of purified talc or siliceous earth.

One of the former official elixirs, Iso-Alcoholic Elixir NF XV (RPS-18 page 1328), actually is a combination of two solutions, one containing 8 to 10% alcohol and the other containing 73 to 78%. It is used as a vehicle for various medicaments that require solvents of different alcoholic strengths. For example, the alcoholic strength of the elixir to be used with a single liquid galenical, which is a liquid preparation of vegetable origin, is approximately the same as that of the galenical. When preparations with different alcoholic strengths are em- ployed in the same prescription, the elixir to be used is the one that produces the best solution. This is usually the average of the alcoholic strengths of the several preparations. For nonextractive substances, the lowest alcoholic strength of elixir that will produce a clear solution should be selected.

The formula for High-Alcoholic Elixir is

Compound Orange Spirit	4 mL
Saccharine	3 g
Glycerin	200 mL
Alcohol, a sufficient quantity, to make	1000 mL

This elixir, and many other liquid preparations intended for internal use eg, the diabetic syrups thickened with sodium carboxymethylcellulose or similar substances, contain saccharin as a sweetening agent. In the past, scientists have studied the toxic effects of this sweetening agent and found bladder tumors in rats. However, it is now generally accepted that this does not apply to humans when saccharin is used as a sweetener. Research on another sweetening agent, cyclamate,[17] showed that it could produce cancer in animals and, as a result, this substance was removed from a wide variety of products.

Cyclamates and saccharin have been banned in some countries as ingredients in manufactured products. Much research has been done to find a safe synthetic substitute for sucrose. As a result, aspartame (methyl *N*(-L-α-aspartyl)-L-phenylalaninate), which is about 200 times sweeter than sucrose, is being used now in many commercial preparations as the sweetening agent. It is sparingly soluble in water and is most stable at a pH of 4.3.

Incompatibilities—Since elixirs contain alcohol, incompatibilities of this solvent are an important consideration during formulation. Alcohol precipitates tragacanth, acacia and agar from aqueous solutions. Similarly, it will precipitate many inorganic salts from similar solutions. The implication here is that such substances should be absent from the aqueous phase or present in such concentrations that there is no danger of precipitation on standing.

If an aqueous solution is added to an elixir, a partial precipitation of alcohol-soluble ingredients may occur. This is due to the reduced alcoholic content of the final preparation. Usually, however, the alcoholic content of the mixture is not sufficiently decreased to cause separation. As vehicles for tinctures and fluidextracts, the elixirs generally cause a separation of extractive matter from these products due to a reduction of the alcoholic content.

Many of the incompatibilities between elixirs, and the substances combined with them, are due to the chemical characteristics of the elixir *per se*, or of the ingredients in the final preparation. Thus, certain elixirs are acid in reaction while others may be alkaline and will, therefore, behave accordingly.

Glycerins

Glycerins or glycerites are solutions or mixtures of medicinal substances in not less than 50% by weight of glycerin. Most of the glycerins are extremely viscous and some are of a jelly-like consistency. Few of them are used extensively. Glycerin is a valuable pharmaceutical solvent forming permanent and concentrated solutions not otherwise obtainable.

Glycerin is used as the sole solvent for the preparation of Antipyrine and Benzocaine Otic Solution USP. As noted under *Otic Solutions*, glycerin alone is used to aid in the removal of cerumen. Externol, a commercial product, contains 5% carbamide peroxide (urea hydrogen peroxide) in glycerin, has shown superior qualities in dispersing ear wax. A glycerin base was chosen as the optimum solvent for an otic preparation in a study involving the stability and antimicrobial activity of kanamycin sulfate otic drops.

Glycerins are hygroscopic and should be stored in tightly closed containers.

Inhalations and Inhalants

Inhalations

These preparations are so used or designed that the drug is carried into the respiratory tree of the patient. The vapor or mist reaches the affected area and gives prompt relief from the symptoms of bronchial and nasal congestion. The USP defines Inhalations in the following way:

Inhalations are drugs or solutions or suspensions of one or more drug substances administered by the nasal or oral respiratory route for either a local or systemic effect. Solutions of drug substances in sterile water for inhalation or in sodium chloride inhalation solution may be nebulized by the use of inert gases. Nebulizers are suitable for the administration of inhalation solutions only if they give droplets sufficiently fine and uniform in size so that the mist reaches the bronchioles. Nebulized solutions may be breathed directly from the nebulizer, or the nebulizer may be attached to a plastic face mask, tent or intermittent positive pressure breathing (IPPB) machine.

Another group of products, also known as metered dose inhalers (MDIs) are propellant-driven drug suspensions or solution in liquified-gas propellant with or without a cosolvent and are intended for delivering metered doses of the drug to the respiratory tract. An MDI contains multiple doses, often exceeding several hundred. The most common single-dose volumes delivered are from 25 to 100 μL (also expressed as mg) per actuation.

Examples of MDIs containing drug solutions and suspension in this pharmacopeia are Epinephrine Inhalation Aerosol and Isoproterenol Hydrochloride and Phenylephrine Bitartrate Inhalation Aerosol, respectively.

Powders also may be administered by mechanical devices that require manually produced pressure or a deep inhalation by the patient, eg, Cromolyn Sodium for Inhalation.

As stated in the USP, particle size is of major importance in the administration of this type of preparation. The various mechanical devices that are used in conjunction with inhalations are described in some detail in Chapter 107. It has been reported that the optimum particle size for penetration into the pulmonary cavity is of the order of 0.5 to 7 μm. Fine mists are produced by pressurized aerosols and hence possess basic advantages over the older nebulizers; in addition, metered aerosols deliver more uniform doses. See Chapter 95. A number of inhalations are described in the USP XXI, eg, Epinephrine Inhalation Solution is a solution of Epinephrine in Purified Water prepared with the aid of Hydrochloric Acid, and Isoproterenol Inhalation Solution is a solution of Isoproeterenol Hydrochloride in Purified Water and may contain Sodium Chloride.

The term *inhalations*, defined by the BP, has a different meaning. These are solutions or suspensions of one or more active ingredients which may contain an inert, suspended diffusing agent. They are intended to release volatile constituents for inhalation, either when placed on a pad or when added to hot, but not boiling, water. Benzoin Inhalation BP contains benzoin, storax and alcohol. The vapors from a preparation containing 1 teaspoonful of the tincture and 1 qt of boiling water may be inhaled. The device known as a *vaporizer* may be used with a number of commercially available preparations of this type (see Chapter 107).

Inhalants

The USP defines inhalants as follows:

A special class of inhalations termed "inhalants" consists of drugs or combinations of drugs that, by virtue of their high vapor pressure, can be carried by an air current into the nasal passage where they exert their effect. The container from which the inhalant is administered is known as an inhaler.

Propylhexedrine Inhalant USP and Tuaminoheptane Inhalant USP consist of cylindrical rolls of suitable fibrous material im pregnated with propylhexedrine or tuaminoheptane (as car bonate), usually aromatized, and contained in a suitable inhaler. Propylhexedrine is the active ingredient in the widely used Benzedrex Inhaler. Both of these drugs are vasoconstrictors used to relieve nasal congestion. Inhalers which come in contact with the mouth or nasal passages become contaminated by bacteria, thus, they should be restricted to personal use.

Another inhalant is Amyl Nitrite USP which is very flammable and should not be used where it may be ignited. It is packaged in sealed glass vials in a protective gauze. Upon breaking the vial, the gauze absorbs the drug which is then inhaled for the treatment of anginal pain. See page 953.

Liniments

Liniments are solutions or mixtures of various substances in oil, alcoholic solutions of soap or emulsions and may contain suitable antimicrobial preservatives. They are intended for external application and should be so labeled. They are rubbed onto the affected area and, because of this, were once called *embrocations*.

Liniments usually are applied with friction and rubbing of the skin, the oil or soap base providing for ease of application and massage. Alcoholic liniments are used generally for their rubefacient, counterirritant, mildly astringent and penetrating effects. Such liniments penetrate the skin more readily than do those with an oil base. The oily liniments, therefore, are milder in their action but are more useful when massage is required. Depending on their ingredients, such liniments may function solely as protective coatings. Liniments should not be applied to skin that is bruised or broken.

Many of the marketed "white" liniments are based on the formulation below or variations thereof.

White Liniment BP

Oleic Acid	85 mL
Turpentine Oil	250 mL
Dilute Ammonia Solution	45 mL
Ammonium Chloride	12.5 mL
Purified Water	625 mL

Mix the oleic acid with the turpentine oil. Dilute the dilute ammonia solution with 45 mL of the water, previously warmed, add to the oily solution and shake to form an emulsion. Separately dissolve the ammonium chloride in the remainder of the water, add to the emulsion and mix.

Other liniments contain antipruritics, astringents, emollients or analgesics and are classified on the basis of their active ingredient. An example is:

Compound Calamine Application PC (Compound Calamine Liniment)

Calamine	100 g
Zinc Oxide	50 g
Wool Fat	25 g
Zinc Stearate	25 g
Yellow Soft Paraffin	250 g
Liquid Paraffin	550 g

The powders are triturated to a smooth paste with some of the liquid paraffin (Liquid Petrolatum). The wool fat, zinc stearate and yellow soft paraffin (Petrolatum) are melted, mixed with some of the liquid paraffin, the mixture incorporated with the triturated powders and the rest of the liquid paraffin added with mixing.

Dermatologists prescribe products of this type but only those containing the rubefacients are advertised extensively and used by consumers for treating minor muscular aches and pains. It is essential that these applications be marked clearly for external use only.

Because of the confusion of camphorated oil (camphor liniment) with castor oil, which has resulted in ingestion and, perhaps, to poisoning, camphorated oil has been banned from the market. Camphorated Oil presently is classified as a new drug by the FDA for which a new drug application is required.

Oleovitamins

Oleovitamins are fish-liver oils diluted with edible vegetable oil or solutions of the indicated vitamins or vitamin concentrates (usually vitamin A and D) in fish-liver oil. The definition is broad enough to include a wide variety of marketed products.

Oleovitamin A and D is official; vitamin D may be present as ergocalciferol or cholecalciferol obtained by the activation of ergosterol or 7-dehydrocholesterol or may be obtained from natural sources. Synthetic vitamin A, or a concentrate, may be used to prepare oleovitamin A. The starting material for the concentrate is a fish-liver oil, the active ingredient being isolated by molecular distillation or by a saponification and extraction procedure. The latter procedure is described in detail in the monograph for Concentrated Vitamin A Solution PC.

These vitamins are unstable in the presence of rancid oils and, therefore, these preparations and, in particular, Oleovitamin A, should be stored in small, tight containers, preferably under vacuum or under an atmosphere of an inert gas, protected from light.

Spirits

Spirits, sometimes known as essences, are alcoholic or hydroalcoholic solutions of volatile substances. Like the aromatic waters, the active ingredient in the spirit may be a solid, liquid or gas. The genealogical tree for this class of preparations begins with the distinguished pair of products, Brandy (*Spiritus Vini Vitis*) and Whisky (*Spiritis Frumenti*), and ends with a wide variety of products that comply with the definition given above. Physicians have debated the therapeutic value of the former products and these are no longer official in the compendia.

Some of these spirits are used internally for their medicinal value, a few medicinally by inhalation and a large number as flavoring agents. The latter group provides a convenient and ready means of obtaining the volatile oil in the proper quantity. For example, a spirit or spirit-like preparation may be used in the formulation of aromatic waters or other pharmaceuticals that require a distinctive flavor.

The BP's definition of Spirits is very broad. Some examples are Aromatic Ammonia Spirits BP, which has a different formula from the USP XXI, is used as a flavoring agent, Soap Spirits BP is used instead of a shampoo for scalp disorders and Surgical Spirits BP is used for its astringent action on unbroken skin.

Spirits should be stored in tight, light-resistant containers and in a cool place. This tends to prevent evaporation and volatilization of either the alcohol or the active principle and to limit oxidative changes. Spirits usually contain a high alcohol content and consequently should be kept away from an open flame.

Preparation—There are four classic methods of preparation:

Simple Solution—This is the method by which the majority of spirits are prepared. Aromatic Ammonia Spirit USP is official and a formula and procedure is given in USP XXI, which illustrates this method of preparation.

Aromatic Ammonia Spirit USP XXI

Ammonium Carbonate, in translucent pieces	34 g
Strong Ammonium Solution	36 mL
Lemon Oil	10 mL
Lavender Oil	1 mL
Nutmeg Oil	1 mL
Alcohol	700 mL
Purified Water, a sufficient quantity to make	1000 mL

Dissolve the ammonium carbonate in the strong ammonia solution and 195 mL of purified water by gentle agitation and allow the solution to stand for 12 hours. Dissolve the oils in the alcohol, contained in a graduated bottle or cylinder, and gradually add the ammonium carbonate solution and enough purified water to make the product measure 1000 mL. Set the mixture aside in a cool place for 24 hours, occasionally agitating it, then filter, using a covered funnel.

The spirit is a respiratory stimulant and is administered by inhalation of the vapor as required. It is marketed in suitable tight, light-resistant containers but is also available in a single-dose glass vial wrapped in a soft cotton envelope. The vial is broken easily; the cotton acts as a sponge for the spirit.

Ammonium carbonate is a mixture of ammonium bicarbonate and ammonium carbamate (NH_2COONH_4). The carbamate reacts with water to form the carbonate. An ammonium carbonate solution is, therefore, a solution of ammonium bicarbonate and ammonium carbonate in water. However, it decomposes in water, the decomposition products being ammonia, carbon dioxide and water. The stability of the spirit is improved by the addition of strong ammonia solution. This represses the hydrolysis of ammonium carbonate and, in this way, decreases the loss of dissolved gases.

Solution with Maceration—In this procedure, the leaves of a drug are macerated in purified water to extract water-soluble matter. They are expressed and the moist, macerated leaves are added to a prescribed quantity of alcohol. The volatile oil is added to the filtered liquid. Peppermint Spirit USP is made by this process (RPS-18 page 798). Peppermint Spirit BP differs from the official product in that it is a solution of the volatile oil in ethanol 90% only. The concentration of volatile oil in the final product is about the same but the official preparation possesses a green color.

Chemical Reaction—No official spirits are prepared by this process. Ethyl nitrite is made by the action of sodium nitrite on a mixture of alcohol and sulfuric acid in the cold. This substance then is used to prepare Ethyl Nitrite Spirit (Sweet Spirit of Nitre), a product no longer official and which has been removed from the market.

Distillation—Brandy and Whisky are made by distillation. The latter is derived from the fermented mash of wholly or partially germinated malted cereal grains and the former from the fermented juice of ripe grapes.

Incompatibilities—Spirits are, for the most part, preparations of high alcoholic strength and do not lend themselves well to dilution with aqueous solutions or liquids of low alcoholic content. The addition of such a solution invariably causes separation of some of the material dissolved in the spirit, evidenced by a turbidity which, in time, may disappear as distinct layering occurs. Salts may be precipitated from their aqueous solutions by the addition of spirits due to their lesser solubility in alcoholic liquids.

Some spirits show incompatibilities characteristic of the ingredients they contain. For example, Aromatic Ammonia Spirit cannot be mixed with aqueous preparations containing alkaloids (eg, codeine phosphate). An acid-base reaction (ammonia-phosphate) occurs and, if the alcohol content of the final mixture is too low, codeine will precipitate.

Toothache Drops

Toothache drops are preparations used for temporary relief of toothache by application of a small pledget of cotton saturated with the product into the tooth cavity. Anesthetic compounds include clove oil, eugenol or benzocaine; other ingredients include camphor, creosote, menthol and alcohol. Clove oil, containing a high concentration of eugenol, which is the main constituent, has been considered safe and effective for toothache.

These preparations no longer are recognized officially. Furthermore, dentists do not recommend the use of toothache drops if the patient has ready access to adequate dental services. Some preparations may damage the gums and produce complications more severe than the original toothache. However, many areas do not have adequate dental services and the pharmacist will, of necessity, handle these preparations, and should warn the patient of possible hazards associated with their use.

Toothache Drops NF XI contains 25 g of chlorobutanol in sufficient clove oil to make the product measure 100 mL. Another formulation contains creosote, clove oil, benzocaine and alcohol in a flexible collodion base.

Emulsions

An emulsion is a two-phase system prepared by combining two immiscible liquids, one of which is dispersed uniformly throughout the other and consists of globules that have diameters equal to or greater than those of the largest colloidal particles. The liquid that is dispersed into small droplets is called the dispersed, internal or discontinuous phase. The other liquid is the dispersion medium, external phase or continuous phase.

Most emulsions incorporate an aqueous phase into a nonaqueous phase (or *vice versa*). However, it is possible to prepare emulsions that are basically nonaqueous. For example, investigations of the emulsifying effects of anionic and cationic surfactants on the nonaqueous immiscible system, glycerin and olive oil, have shown that certain amines and three cationic agents produced stable emulsions. This broadening of the basic definition for the term *emulsion* is recognized in the USP.

While the USP definition, given below, is broad enough to encompass nonaqueous systems, emphasis is placed on those emulsions which contain water, as they are by far the most common in pharmacy.

The USP defines emulsions as follows:

Emulsions are two-phase systems in which one liquid is dispersed throughout another liquid in the form of small droplets. Where oil is the dispersed phase and an aqueous solution is the continuous phase, the system is designated as an oil-in-water (O/W) emulsion. Conversely, where water or an aqueous solution is the dispersed phase and oil or oleaginous material is the continuous phase, the system is designated as a water-in-oil (W/O) emulsion.

Applications

When it is necessary to administer oils by the oral route, patient acceptance is enhanced when the oil is prepared in emulsion form. Thus, mineral oil, a laxative, valproic acid an anticonvulsant, oil-soluble vitamins, vegetable oils and preparations for enteral feeding are formulated frequently in an O/W emulsion form to enhance their palatability.

The bioavailability of oils for absorption may be enhanced when the oil is in the form of small droplets. Furthermore, the absorption of some drugs, eg, griseofulvin, sulfonamides and vitamin A, may be enhanced when they are prepared in the form of an O/W emulsion. Emulsion formulations of drugs such as erythromycin and physostigmine salicylate have been considered, in order to improve their stability. Finally, the greatest use of emulsions is for topical preparations. Both O/W and W/O emulsions are used widely, depending upon the effect desired. Emulsion bases of the W/O type tend to be more occlusive and emollient than O/W emulsion bases, which tend to be removed more easily by water. Further information may be found in Chapter 90. The effects of viscosity, surface tension, solubility, particle size, complexation and excipients on the bioavailability of oral suspensions and emulsions have been discussed in detail by Rettig.[17]

Practically, emulsions possess a number of important advantages over other liquid forms. These may be summarized in the following way:

1. In an emulsion, the therapeutic properties and the spreading ability of the constituents are increased.
2. The unpleasant taste or odor of an oil can be masked partially or wholly, by emulsification. Secondary masking techniques are available to the formulator but these must be used with caution. If flavors and sweetening agents are added to the emulsion, only minimal amounts should be used in order to prevent the nausea or gastric distress that results on ingestion of larger quantities of these.
3. The absorption and penetration of medicaments are controlled more easily if they are incorporated into an emulsion.
4. Emulsion action is prolonged and the emollient effect is greater than that observed with comparable preparations.
5. Water is an inexpensive diluent and a good solvent for the many drugs and flavors that are incorporated into an emulsion.

While this section on emulsions focuses primarily on those for oral use and to a lesser degree those for topical application, it should be noted that there are a number of emulsions used parenterally which are described in specialized textbooks on this topic. For example, emulsions of the O/W type are used for intravenous feeding of lipid nutrients. These are used to provide a source of calories and essential fatty acids. These emulsions must meet exacting standards in regard to particle size, safety and stability. Examples of commercial products include Intralipid (*Cutter*) and Liposyn (*Abbott*). Other specialized uses of emulsions include radiopaque emulsions which are used as diagnostic agents for X-ray examination. Other types of emulsions employed parenterally include W/O emulsions of allerginic extracts which are given subcutaneously and radiopaque O/W sustained-release depot preparations given intramuscularly.

Ingredients

The selection of the oil phase for oral preparations depends upon the purpose of the product. For example, mineral oil is used as a laxative and corn oil is used for its nutrient properties. Vegetable oils can be used to dissolve or suspend pharmaceuticals such as oil-soluble vitamins. The selection of the oil phase for topical O/W or W/O preparations is discussed in Chapter 90.

Emulsions are thermodynamically unstable because of the large increase in surface energy due to the combination of interfacial tension and large surface area of the dispersed phase and the different densities of the two phases. As a result, emulsions tend to cream, ie, the less dense phase rises and the more dense phase falls in the container. Subsequently, the droplets can coalesce with a considerable reduction in surface free energy. Consequently, considerable research has been conducted on their preparation and stabilization. The theory of emulsification is described in Chapter 20. In order to prepare suitable emulsions and to have them remain stable for a suitable period of time, a number of excipients are used in their preparation. The most important are those called emulsifying agents, which may be divided into three classes.

1. **Natural Emulsifying Agents**—These substances may be derived from vegetable sources and include acacia, tragacanth, alginates, chrondrus and pectin. While the surface activity of these is low, they achieve their emulsifying power by increasing the viscosity of the aqueous phase, as indicated by White.[18] Examples of emulsifying agents derived from animal sources include gelatin, egg yolk, casein, wool fat, cholesterol and lecithin. Because of the widely different chemical constitution of these compounds, they have a variety of uses, depending upon the specific compound, in both oral and topical preparations. All naturally occurring agents show variations in their emulsifying properties from batch to batch.
2. **Finely Divided Solids**—The compounds most frequently used in pharmacy are the colloidal clays: bentonite (aluminum silicate) and veegum (magnesium aluminum silicate). These compounds are good emulsifiers and tend to be absorbed at the interface, effect an increase in viscosity, generally in the aqueous phase, and usually are used in conjunction with a surfactant to prepare O/W emulsions, but both O/W and W/O preparations can be prepared by adding the clay to the external phase first. They are used frequently for external purposes such as a lotion or cream.
3. **Synthetic Emulsifying Agents**—This group of emulsifying agents is most effective at lowering the interfacial tension between the oil and water phases because the molecule possess both hydrophilic and hydrophobic properties. This property is described by their hydrophilic-lipophilic balance (HLB) number which may vary from 40 for sodium dodecyl sulfate to 1 for oleic acid. Emulsifying agents, sometimes used singly, are preferably a combination of two emulsifying agents, which will give a weighted HLB of 8 to 16 which is satisfactory for O/W emulsions and an HLB 3 to 8 for W/O emulsions. These emulsifying agents are available in different ionic types: anionic, eg, sodium dodecyl sulfate; cationic, eg, benzalkonium chloride; nonionic, eg, polyethylene glycol 400 monostearate and ampholytic, eg, long-chain amino acid derivatives. Many of these agents are described in Chapter 80 and the mechanism of action is discussed in Chapter 20.

In addition to the emulsifying agents, viscosity agents are employed, namely the hydrophilic colloids such as naturally occurring gums, noted above, and partially synthetic polymers such as cellulose derivatives, eg, methylcellulose, hydroxypropylmethylcellulose, sodium carboxymethylcellulose or a number of synthetic polymers that may be used, such as carbomer polymers. These materials are hydrophilic in nature and dissolve or disperse in water to give a viscous solution and function as emulsion stabilizers.

The aqueous phase of the emulsion favors the growth of microorganisms and, because of this, a preservative usually is added to the product. Some of the preservatives that have been used include chlorocresol, chlorobutanol, mercurial preparations, salicylic acid, the esters of *p*-hydroxybenzoic acid, benzoic acid, sodium benzoate or sorbic acid. The preservative should be selected with regard for the ultimate use of the preparation and possible incompatibilities between the preservative and the ingredients in the emulsion, eg, binding between the surface-active agent and the preservative. Low pH values of 5 to 6 and low concentrations of water are characteristics also likely to inhibit microbiological growth in emulsions.

Most emulsions consist of a nonaqueous (or oil or lipid) phase and an aqueous (or water) phase, thus some of the preservative may pass into the oil phase and be removed from the aqueous phase. It is in the aqueous phase that microorganisms tend to grow. As a result, water-soluble preservatives are more effective since the concentration of the unbound preservative in the aqueous phase assumes a great deal of importance in inhibiting the microbial growth. Esters of *p*-hydroxybenzoic acid appear to be the most satisfactory preservatives for emulsions. Many mathematical models have been used to determine the availability of preservatives in emulsified systems. However, because of the number of factors which reduce the effectiveness of the preservative, a final microbiological evaluation of the emulsion must be performed.

While emphasis concerning preservation of emulsions deals with the aqueous phase, microorganisms can reside also in the lipid phase. Consequently, it has been recommended that pairs of preservatives be used to ensure adequate concentration in both phases. Esters of *p*-hydroxybenzoic acid can be used to ensure appropriate concentrations in both phases because of their difference in oil and water solubilities.

The oxidative decomposition of certain excipients in the oil phase in some pharmaceuticals is possible in emulsions, not only because of the usual amount of air dissolved in the liquid, and the possible incorporation of air during the preparation of the product, but also the large interfacial area between the oil and water phase. The selection of the appropriate antioxidant briefly described at the beginning of the chapter depends on such factors as stability, compatibility with the ingredients of the emulsion, toxicity, effectiveness in emulsions, odor, taste and distribution between the two phases. Additional information can be found in appropriate references and in textbooks listed in the *Bibliography*.

Other excipients for the proper formation of emulsions include flavoring agents and fragrances.

Preparation

After the purpose of the emulsions has been determined, ie., oral or topical use, and the type of emulsions, O/W or W/O, and appropriate ingredients selected and the theory of emulsification considered, described in Chapter 21, experimental formulations may be prepared. One method is suggested by Griffin.[19]

1. Group the ingredients on the basis of their solubilities in the aqueous and nonaqueous phases.
2. Determine the type of emulsion required and calculate an approximate HLB (hydrophile-lipophile balance) value.
3. Blend a low HLB emulsifier and a high HLB emulsifier to the calculated value. For experimental formulations, use a higher concentration of emulsifier (eg, 10 to 30% of the oil phase) than that required to produce a satisfactory product. Emulsifiers should, in general, be stable chemically, nontoxic and suitably low in color, odor and taste. The emulsifier is selected on the basis of these characteristics, the type of equipment being used to blend the ingredients and the stability characteristics of the final product. Emulsions should not coalesce at room temperature, when frozen and thawed repeatedly or at elevated temperatures of up to 50°. Mechanical energy input varies with the type of equipment used to prepare the emulsion. The more the energy input, the less the demand on the emulsifier. Both process and formulation variables can affect the stability of an emulsion.
4. Dissolve the oil-soluble ingredients and the emulsifiers in the oil. Heat, if necessary, to approximately 5 to 10° over the melting point of the highest melting ingredient or to a maximum temperature of 70 to 80°.
5. Dissolve the water-soluble ingredients (except acids and salts) in a sufficient quantity of water.
6. Heat the aqueous phase to a temperature which is 3 to 5° higher than that of the oil phase.
7. Add the aqueous phase to the oily phase with suitable agitation.
8. If acids or salts are employed, dissolve them in water and add the solution to the cold emulsion.
9. Examine the emulsion and make adjustments in the formulation if the product is unstable. It may be necessary to add more emulsifier, to change to an emulsifier with a slightly higher or lower HLB value or to use an emulsifier with different chemical characteristics.

The technique of emulsification of pharmaceutical preparations has been described by White.[18] The preparation of an emulsion requires work to reduce the internal phase into small droplets and disperse them throughout the external phase. This can be accomplished by a mortar and pestle or a high-speed emulsifier. The addition of emulsifying agents not only reduces this work but also stabilizes the final emulsion. Emulsions may be prepared by four principle methods.

Addition of Internal Phase to External Phase—This is usually the most satisfactory method for preparing emulsions since there is always an excess of the external phase present which promotes the type of emulsion desired. If the external phase is water and the interal phase is oil, the water-soluble substances are dissolved in the water and the oil- soluble substances mixed thoroughly in the oil. The oil mixture is added in portions to the aqueous preparation with agitation. Sometimes, in order to give a better shearing action during the preparation, all of the water is not mixed with the emulsifying agent until the primary emulsion with the oil is formed; subsequently, the remainder of the water is added. An example using gelatin Type A is given below.

Addition of the External Phase to the Internal Phase—Using an O/W emulsion as an example, the addition of the water (external phase) to the oil (internal phase) will promote the formation of a W/O emulsion due to the preponderance of the oil phase. After further addition of the water, phase inversion to an O/W emulsion should take place. This method especially is useful and successful when hydrophilic agents such as acacia, tragacanth or methylcellulose are first mixed with the oil, effecting dispersion without wetting. Water is added and, eventually, an O/W emulsion is formed. This "dry gum" technique is a rapid method for preparing small quantities of emulsion. The ratio 4 parts of oil, 2 parts of water and 1 part of gum provides maximum shearing action on the oil globules in the mortar. The emulsion then can be diluted and triturated with water to the appropriate concentrations. The preparation of Mineral Oil Emulsion described below is an example.

Mixing Both Phases after Warming Each—This method is used when waxes or other substances which require melting are used. The oil-soluble emulsifying agents, oils and waxes are melted and mixed thoroughly. The water-soluble ingredients dissolved in the water are warmed to a temperature slightly higher than the oil phase. The two phases then are mixed and stirred until cold. For convenience, but not necessity, the aqueous solution is added to the oil mixture. This method frequently is used in the preparation of ointments and creams. An example of an oral preparation containing an insoluble drug is given below.

Alternate Addition of the Two Phases to the Emulsifying Agent—A portion of the oil, if an O/W emulsion is being prepared, is added to all of the oil-soluble emulsifying agents with mixing, then an equal quantity of water containing all the water-soluble emulsifying agents is added with stirring until the emulsion is formed. Further portions of the oil and water are added alternately until the final product is formed. The high concentration of the emulsifying agent in the original emulsion makes the initial emulsification more likely and the high viscosity provides effective shearing action leading to small droplets in the emulsion. This method often is used successfully with soaps.

Examples of some emulsions are given below.

In NF XIII it was suggested that only O/W emulsions are suitable for oral use because these are water-miscible and thus their oiliness is masked. This compendium gave specific directions for the preparation of emulsions using gelatin as an emulsifying agent. These preparations are based on either Type A or Type B gelatin.

Type A gelatin is prepared by acid-treated precursors and is used at a pH of about 3.2. It is incompatible with anionic emulsifying agents such as the vegetable gums. The following formula was recommended.

Gelatin (Type A)	8 g
Tartaric Acid	0.6 g
Flavor as desired	
Alcohol	60 mL
Oil	500 mL
Purified Water, to make	1000 mL

Add the gelatin and the tartaric acid to about 300 mL of purified water, allow to stand for a few minutes, heat until the gelatin is dissolved, then raise the temperature to about 98° and maintain this temperature for about 20 min. Cool to 50°, add the flavor, the alcohol and sufficient purified water to make 500 mL. Add the oil, agitate the mixture thoroughly and pass it through a homogenizer or a colloid mill until the oil is dispersed completely and uniformly.

This emulsion cannot be prepared by trituration or by the use of the usual stirring devices.

Type B gelatin is prepared from alkali-treated precursors and is used at a pH of about 8.0. It may be used with other anionic emulsifying agents but is incompatible with cationic types. If the emulsion contains 50% oil, 5 g of Type B gelatin, 2.5 g of sodium bicarbonate and sufficient tragacanth or agar should be incorporated into the aqueous phase to yield 1000 mL of product of the required viscosity.

An emulsion that may be prepared by the mortar and pestle method is the following Mineral Oil Emulsion USP.

Mineral Oil	500 mL
Acacia, in very fine powder	125 g
Syrup	100 mL
Vanillin	40 mg
Alcohol	60 mL
Purified Water, a sufficient quantity	1000 mL

The mineral oil and acacia are mixed in a dry Wedgwood mortar. Purified water (250 mL) is added and the mixture triturated vigorously until an emulsion is formed. A mixture of the syrup, 50 mL of purified water and the vanillin dissolved in alcohol is added in divided portions with trituration; sufficient purified water is then added to the proper volume, the mixture mixed well and homogenized.

An Oral Emulsion (O/W) Containing an Insoluble Drug[20]

Cottonseed Oil	460.0 g
Sulfadiazine	200.0 g
Sorbitan Monostearate	84.0 g
Polyoxyethylene 20 Sorbitan Monostearate	36.0 g
Sodium Benzoate	2.0 g
Sweetener	qs
Purified Water	1000.0 g
Flavor Oil	qs

The procedure as indicated by Rieger[20] is

1. Heat the first three ingredients to 50° and pass through colloid mill.
2. Add the next four ingredients at 50° to the first three ingredients at 65° and stir while cooling to 45°.
3. Add the flavor oil and continue to stir until room temperature is reached.

Properties

The type of emulsion O/W or W/O depends, to some extent, on the phase-volume ratio. The higher the fraction of one phase, the greater likelihood it will form the external phase. Thus, O/W emulsions are favored if water forms a greater fraction of the volume than the oil phase. However, it is possible for the internal phase of an emulsion to occupy up to 0.74 of the volume of the emulsion and still form a stable product. Emulsifiers with high HLB level values (8 to 16) tend to form an O/W emulsion, while those with low HLB values (3 to 8) tend to form a W/O emulsion.

The consistency of emulsions, as suggested by White,[18] can be increased by increasing the viscosity of the continuous phase, increasing the fractional volume of the internal phase, reducing the particle size of the internal phase, increasing the proportion of the emulsifying agent or adding hydrophobic emulsifying agents to the oil phase of the emulsion.

The physical stability of emulsions may be defined by a number of expressions. The first of these, which is called *creaming*, is the movement of the droplets either upward or downward, depending upon their density. This gives a product which is not homogenous and can lead to a nonuniform dose. Generally, creaming is not a serious problem because a moderate amount of shaking will redisperse the droplets uniformly. The rate of creaming may be decreased by considering the theory of creaming using Stokes law, Chapter 20. This equation relates the rate of creaming to the size of the droplets, the difference in densities and the viscosity of the external phase. Thus, the rate of creaming may be decreased by decreasing the size of the droplets and increasing the viscosity of the external phases, both of which have been discussed above. Minimizing the difference between densities is more difficult to achieve due to a number of practical difficulties.

When the droplets aggregate, they come together and act as a single unit, but do not fuse. As a result of the larger size, they tend to cream faster and further provoke physical instability. Aggregation is to some extent reversible and may be controlled by choosing a somewhat different surfactant system and controlling the electrical potential of the droplets. Coalescence of an emulsion is the fusion of the droplets, leading to a decrease in their numbers and eventually the complete separation of the two phases, yielding an unsatisfactory product which should be reformulated completely (see Chapter 21).

Multiple Emulsions—A recent innovation in emulsion technology is the development of multiple emulsions. The dispersed phase of these emulsions contains even smaller droplets which are miscible with the continuous phase. Thus, the multiple emulsion may be O/W/O where the aqueous phase is between two oil phases, or W/O/W where the internal and external aqueous phases are separated by an oil phase. In these systems both hydrophobic and hydrophilic emulsifiers are used and both have an effect on the yield and stability, as noted by Florence and Whitehill.[21]

It appears that O/W/O emulsions are formed better by lipophilic, nonionic surfactants using gum acacia-emulsified simple systems, while W/O/W multiple emulsions are formed better by nonionic surfactants in a two-stage emulsification procedure. A specific formulation for a W/O/W emulsion may be prepared by forming the primary (W/O) emulsion from isopropyl myristate (47.5%), sorbitan monooleate (2.5%) and distilled water to 100%. This primary emulsion (50%) is added to a polyoxyethylene sorbitan monooleate (2% *w/v*) solution in water as suggested by Florence and Whitehill.[21] Other formulations of multiple emulsions include carboxymethylcellulose sodium, microcrystalline cellulose, sorbitan monooleate and sorbitan trioleate.

While the technique of preparing these emulsions is more complicated, research indicates potential use of these emulsions for prolonged action, taste-masking, more effective dosage forms, improved stability, parenteral preparations, protection against the external environment and enzyme entrapment. These emulsions also may be used to separate two incompatible hydrophilic substances in the inner and outer aqueous phases by the middle oil phase.

Microemulsions—The coarse pharmaceutical macro emulsions appear white and tend to separate on standing. Microemulsions are translucent or transparent, do not separate and have a droplet diameter in the nanometer size range. The microemulsions are not always distinguishable from micellar solutions.

Both O/W and W/O types are possible and may be converted, one to the other, by adding more of the internal phase or by altering the type of emulsifier. As the internal phase is added, the emulsion will pass through a viscoelastic gel stage; with further addition, an emulsion of the opposite type will occur.

The most obvious benefit of microemulsions is their stability, thus providing dose uniformity. Usually, the emulsifier should be 20 to 30% of the weight of the oil used. The W/O systems are prepared by blending the oil and emulsifier with a little heat, if required, and then adding the water. The order of mixing for O/W systems is more flexible. One of the simplest methods is to blend the oil and the emulsifier and pour this into water with a little stirring. In no case can a microemulsion be formed unless there is a match between the oil and emulsifier.

If the emulsifier has been selected properly, microemulsification will occur almost spontaneously, leading to a satisfactory and stable preparation. The details of various preparations and the relationship between microemulsions and micellar solutions have been reviewed by Prince *et al.*[22] Microemulsions containing hydrocortisone have been prepared.

Other authors suggest that the preparation of microemulsions is considerably more difficult than the preparation of coarse suspensions. Rosano *et al*[23] discusses the use of a primary surfactant adsorbed at the interface which influences the curvature of the dispersed phase. The amount of surfactant required may be estimated from the surface area of the droplets and the cross-sectional area of the surfactant molecule. The use of a cosurfactant to form a duplex film has been indicated. The authors also suggest that the order of mixing is important.

General methods are available for testing the instability of emulsions including bulk changes, centrifugal and ultracentrifugal studies, dielectric measurement, surface-area measurement and accelerated-motion studies. Low-shear rheological studies measuring viscoelasticity are suggested as the optimal method of stability testing.

Equipment

The preparation of emulsions requires a certain amount of energy to form the interface between the two phases, and additional work must be done to stir the system to overcome the resistance to flow. In addition, heat often is supplied to the system to melt waxy solids and/or reduce the viscosity of the oil phase. Consequently the preparation of emulsions on a large scale usually requires the expenditure of considerable amounts of energy for heating and mixing. Careful consideration of these processes has led to the development of low-energy emulsification by using an appropriate emulsification temperature and selective heating of the ingredients. This process, described by Lin,[24] involves the preparation of an emulsion concentrate subsequently diluted with the external phase at room temperature.

Because of the variety of oils used, emulsifier agents, phase-volume ratios and the desired physical properties of the product, a wide selection of equipment is available for preparing emulsions and an outline of the main classes of equipment is discussed below. Further information may be obtained from the *Bibliography*.

Special techniques and equipment in certain instances, will produce superior emulsions, including rapid cooling, reduction in particle size or ultrasonic devices. A wide selection of equipment for processing both emulsions and suspensions has been described by Eisberg.[25] A number of improvements have been made to make the various processes more effective and energy-efficient.

The mortar and pestle may be used to prepare small quantities of an emulsion, and it is one of the simplest and least expensive methods. It may be used for most of the different techniques of preparing emulsions. Generally, the final particle size is considerably larger than is achieved by the equipment described below. In addition, it is necessary for the ingredients to have a certain viscosity prior to trituration in order to achieve a satisfactory shear. Satisfactory emulsions of low-viscosity ingredients and small volumes may be prepared using the appropriate equipment described below.

Agitators—Ordinary agitation or shaking may be used to prepare the emulsion. This method frequently is employed by the pharmacist, particularly in the emulsification of easily dispersed, low-viscosity oils. Under certain conditions, intermittent shaking is considerably more effective than ordinary continuous shaking. Continuous shaking tends to break up not only the phase to be dispersed but also the dispersion medium and, in this way, impairs the ease of emulsification. Laboratory shaking devices may be used for small-scale production.

Mechanical Mixers—Emulsions may be prepared by using one of several mixers which are available. Propeller-type mixers which have a propeller attached to a shaft driven by an electric motor are convenient and portable and can be used for both stirring and emulsification. This type operates best in mixtures which have low viscosity, ie, mixtures with a viscosity of glycerin or less. They are also useful for preparing emulsions. A turbine mixer has a number of blades which may be straight or curved, with or without a pitch, mounted on a shaft. The turbine tends to give a greater shear than propellers. The shear can be increased by using diffuser rings which are perforated and surround the turbine so that the liquid from the turbine must pass through holes. The turbines can be used for both low-viscosity mixtures and medium-viscosity liquids, up to that of molasses. The degree of stirring and shear by propeller or turbine mixers depends upon several factors, such as the speed of rotation, pattern of liquid flow, position in the container and baffles in the container as discussed by Fox.[26]

Production-size mixers include high-powered propeller-shaft stirrers immersed in a tank or self-contained units with propeller and paddle systems. The latter usually are constructed so that the contents of the tank either may be heated or cooled during the production process. Baffles often are built into a tank and these increase the efficiency of mixing. Two mixers manufactured by the same company are shown in Figs 2 and 3.

Small electric mixers may be used to prepare emulsions at the prescription counter. They will save time and energy and produce satisfactory emulsions when the emulsifying agent is acacia or agar.

The commercially available *Waring Blendor* disperses efficiently by means of the shearing action of rapidly rotating blades. It transfers large amounts of energy and incorporates air into the emulsion. If an emulsion first is produced by using a blender of this type, the formulator must remember that the emulsion characteristics obtained in the laboratory will not be duplicated necessarily by the production-size equipment.

Colloid Mills—The principle of operation of the colloid mill is the passage of the mixed phases of an emulsion formula between a stator and a high-speed rotor revolving at speeds of 2000 to 18,000 rpm. The clearance between the rotor and the stator is adjustable, usually from 0.001 in upward. The emulsion mixture, in passing between the rotor and stator, is subjected to a tremendous shearing action which effects a fine dispersion of uniform size as indicated by Griffin *et al.*[19] A colloid mill and various rotors are shown in Figs 4 and 5. The operating principle is the same for all, but each manufacturer incorporates specific features which result in changes in oper-

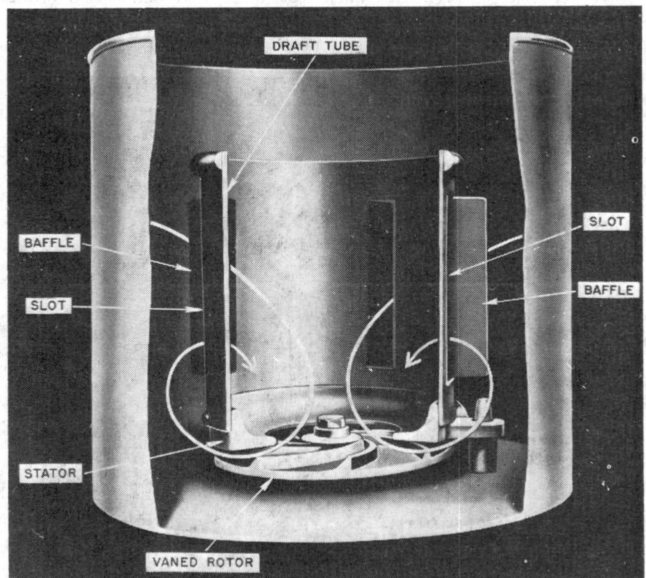

Fig 2. Standard slurry-type dispersall mixer with vaned-rotor "mixing" element and slotted draft-tube circulating element (courtesy, Abbe Eng).

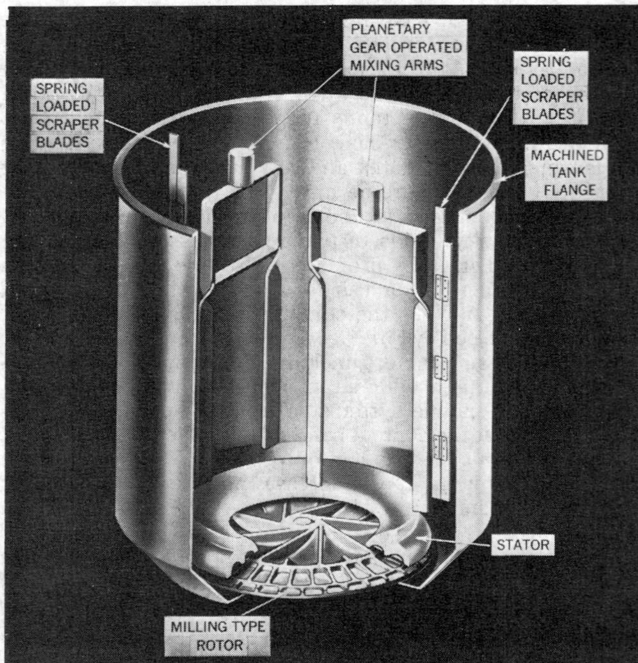

Fig 3. Standard paste-type dispersall mixer with "cupped-rotor" milling element and double-rotating mixing arm circulating element (courtesy, Abbe Eng).

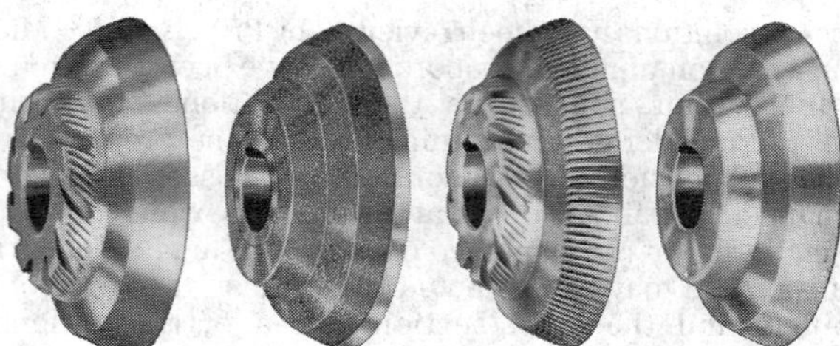

Fig 5. Types of rotors used in colloid mills. These may be smooth (for most emulsions), serrated (for ointments and very viscous products) or of vitrified stone (for the paints and pigment dispersions) (courtesy, Tri-Homo).

ating efficiency. The shearing forces applied in the colloid mill usually result in a temperature increase within the emulsion. It may be necessary, therefore, to cool the equipment when the emulsion is being produced.

Colloid mills are used frequently for the comminution of solids and for the preparation of suspensions, especially suspensions containing solids which are not wetted by the dispersion medium.

Homogenizers—Impeller types of equipment frequently produce a satisfactory emulsion; however, for further reduction in particle size, homogenizers may be employed, as indicated by Scott.[27]

Homogenizers may be used in one of two ways:

1. The ingredients in the emulsion are mixed and then passed through the homogenizer to produce the final product.

2. A coarse emulsion is prepared in some other way and then passed through a homogenizer for the purpose of decreasing the particle size and obtaining a greater degree of uniformity and stability.

The mixed phases or the coarse emulsion are subjected to homogenization and are passed between a finely ground valve and seat under high pressure. This, in effect, produces an atomization which is enhanced by the impact received by the atomized mixture as it strikes the surrounding metal surfaces. They operate at pressures of 1000 to 5000 psi and produce some of the finest dispersions obtainable in an emulsion.

Figure 6 shows the flow through the homogenizing valve, the heart of the high-pressure APV Gaulin homogenizer. The product enters the valve seat at high pressure, flows through the region between the valve and the seat at high velocity with a rapid pressure drop, causing cavitation; subsequently, the mixture hits the impact ring causing further disruption and then is discharged as a homogenized product. It is postulated that circulation and turbulence are responsible mainly for the homogenization that takes place. Different valve assemblies, two stage valve assemblies and equipment with a wide range of capacities are available.

Two-stage homogenizers are constructed so that the emulsion, after treatment in the first valve system, is conducted directly to another where it receives a second treatment. A single homogenization may produce an emulsion which, although its particle size is small, has a tendency to clump or form clusters. Emulsions of this type exhibit increased creaming tendencies. This is corrected by passing the emulsion through the first stage of homogenization at a high pressure (eg, 3000 to 5000 psi) and then through the second stage at a greatly reduced pressure (eg, 1000 psi). This breaks down any clusters formed in the first step.

The Macro Flow-Master *Kom-bi-nator* employs a number of different actions, each of which takes the ingredients a little further along in the process of subdividing droplets, until complete homogenization results. The machine is equipped with a pump which carries the liquid through the various stages of the process. In the first stage, the ingredients are forced between two specially designed rotors (gears) which shoot the liquid in opposite directions in a small chamber and, in this way, are mixed thoroughly. These rotors also set up a swirling action in the next chamber into which the liquid is forced and swirled back and forth in eddies and crosscurrents. The second stage is a pulsing or vibrating action at rapid frequency. The product then leaves this chamber, goes through a small valve opening and is dashed against the wall of

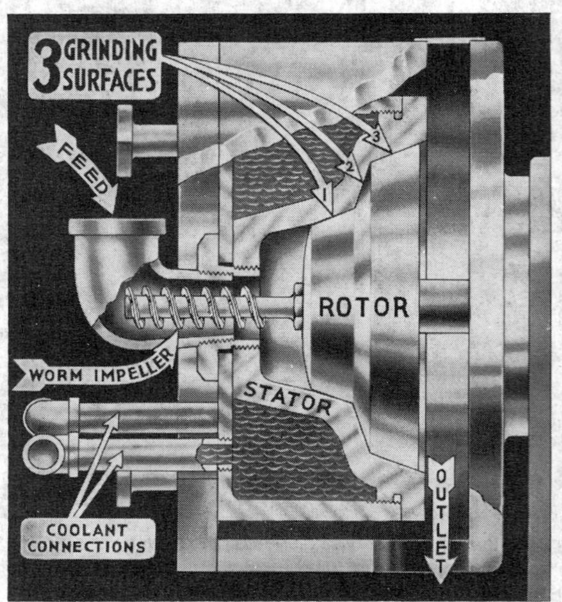

Fig 4. A colloid mill shown in cross section (courtesy, Tri-Homo).

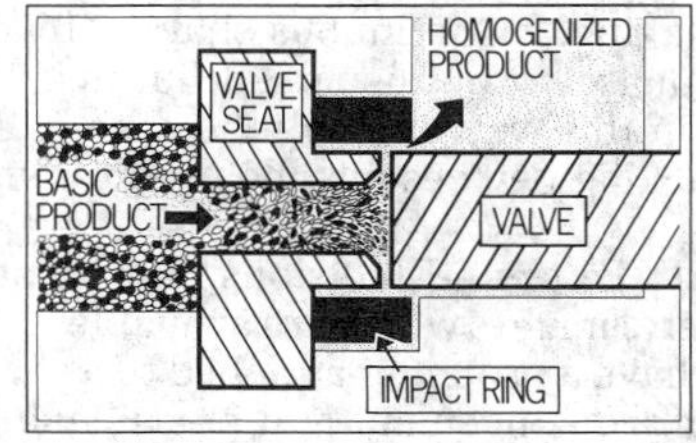

Fig 6. Operation of the homogenizer value assembly (Courtesy APV Gaulin).

the homogenizing chamber. Pressure is applied, but it is not as great as that used in other types of homogenizers. Pressure is controlled accurately by adjusting devices on the front of the machine, and temperature is controlled by passing coolants through the stators.

For small-scale extemporaneous preparation of emulsions, the inexpensive *hand-operated homogenizer* (available from *Central Scientific*) is particularly useful. It is probably the most efficient emulsifying apparatus available to the prescription pharmacist. The two phases, previously mixed in a bottle, are hand pumped through the apparatus. Recirculation of the emulsion through the apparatus will improve its quality.

A homogenizer does not incorporate air into the final product. Air may ruin an emulsion because the emulsifying agent is adsorbed preferentially at the air/water interface, followed by an irreversible precipitation termed *denaturization*. This is particularly prone to occur with protein emulsifying agents.

Homogenization may spoil an emulsion if the concentration of the emulsifying agent in the formulation is less than that required to take care of the increase in surface area produced by the process.

The temperature rise during homogenization is not very large. However, temperature does play an important role in the emulsification process. An increase in temperature will reduce the viscosity and, in certain instances, the interfacial tension between the oil and the water. There are, however, many instances, particularly in the manufacturing of cosmetic creams and ointments, where the ingredients will fail to emulsify properly if they are processed at too high a temperature. Emulsions of this type are processed first at an elevated temperature and then homogenized at a temperature not exceeding 40°.

Homogenizers have been used most frequently with liquid emulsions, but now they may be used with suspensions, as the metal surfaces are formed from wear-resistant alloys which will resist the wear of solid particles contained in suspensions.

Ultrasonic Devices—The preparation of emulsions by the use of ultrasonic vibrations also is possible. An oscillator of high frequency (100 to 500 kHz) is connected to two electrodes between which is placed a piezoelectric quartz plate. The quartz plate and electrodes are immersed in an oil bath and, when the oscillator is operating, high-frequency waves flow through the fluid. Emulsification is accomplished by simply immersing a tube containing the emulsion ingredients into this oil bath. Considerable research has been done on ultrasonic emulsification, particularly with regard to the mechanism of emulsion formation by this method. Limited data indicate that these devices will produce stable emulsions only with liquids of low viscosity. The method is not practical, however, for large-scale production of emulsions.

Commercial products may be prepared using ultrasonics based upon the device known as the Pohlman whistle. In this apparatus, the premixed liquids are forced through a thin orifice and are allowed to impinge upon the free end of a knife-edge bar which is made to vibrate. Ultrasonic waves are produced and areas of compression and rarefaction are formed. Shock waves are produced by the collapse of bubbles which produce a shear effect, thereby producing fine particle sizes as described by Scott.[27]

Suspensions

The physical chemist defines the word "suspension" as a two-phase system consisting of a finely divided solid dispersed in a solid, liquid or gas. The pharmacist accepts this definition and can show that a variety of dosage forms fall within the scope of the preceding statement. There is, however, a reluctance to be all-inclusive, and it is for this reason that the main emphasis is placed on solids dispersed in liquids. In addition, and because there is a need for more specific terminology, the pharmaceutical scientist differentiates between such preparations as suspensions, mixtures, magmas, gels and lotions. In a general sense, each of these preparations represents a suspension, but the state of subdivision of the insoluble solid varies from particles which settle gradually on standing to particles which are colloidal in nature. The lower limit of particle size is approximately 0.1 μm, and it is the preparations containing dispersed solids of this magnitude or greater that are defined pharmaceutically as suspensions.

Suspensions have a number of applications in pharmacy. They are used to supply drugs to the patient in liquid form. Many people have difficulty swallowing solid dosage forms, consequently a liquid preparation has an advantage for these people; in addition, the dose of a liquid form may be adjusted easily to meet the patient's requirements. Thus, if the drug is insoluble or poorly soluble, a suspension may be the most suitable dosage form. If a drug is unstable in an aqueous medium, a different form of the drug, such as an ester or insoluble salt, which does not dissolve in water, may be used in the preparation of a suspension.

In order to improve the stability of an antibiotic such as ampicillin, formulations are made in such a way that the dispersion medium, water, is added upon dispensing to form a satisfactory suspension. Generally, the taste of pharmaceuticals can be improved if they are supplied in suspension form, rather than solutions; thus, chloramphenicol palmitate is used instead of the more soluble form, chloramphenicol. Another way to decrease the solubility of the drug is to replace part of the water with another appropriate liquid such as alcohol or glycerin. Insoluble drugs may be formulated as suspensions for topical use such as calamine lotion.

Other preparations of suspensions, in addition to those noted above, include parenteral preparations, ophthalmic preparations or medicated applications discussed in Chapters 87, 89 and 90, respectively.

Certain authors also include liniments, and the newer sustained-release suspensions, in any discussion of this particular subject. The former preparations now usually are considered as solutions although a number of older liniments were, in fact, suspensions. The sustained-release suspensions represent a very specialized class of preparation and, as such, are discussed in more detail in Chapter 94. Some insoluble drugs also are administered in aerosol form; one example is dexamethasone phosphate suspended in a propellant mixture of fluorochlorocarbons. More detail on aerosols is available in Chapter 95.

Suspension formulation and control is based on the principles outlined in Chapters 20 and 22. Formulation involves more than suspending a solid in a liquid. A knowledge of the behavior of particles in liquids, of suspending agents and of flavors and colors is required to produce a satisfactory suspension.

Well-formulated suspensions should possess certain basic properties. The dispersed phase should settle slowly, if at all, and be redispersed readily on shaking. The particles should not cake on settling and the viscosity should be such that the preparation pours easily. As with all dosage forms, there should be no question as to the chemical stability of the suspension.

Ingredients

The main ingredients in a suspension are the drug and agents to wet the drug, influence flocculation, control viscosity, adjust pH, and the external medium, usually water. In addition, flavoring, sweetening and coloring agents and preservatives are employed.

A *wetting* agent, ie, a suitable surfactant with a HLB value between 7 and 9, is used; although surfactants with higher HLB values are recommended sometimes, eg, certain polysorbates and poloxamers. They are employed at a low concentration (0.05 to 0.5%) to allow the displacement of air from hydrophobic material and permit the liquid, usually water, to surround the particles and provide a proper dispersion. If it is desirable to flocculate the particles, then flocculating agents are employed. Usually low concentrations, less than 1%, of electrolytes such as sodium or potassium chloride are employed to induce flocculation. Water-soluble salts possessing divalent or trivalent ions may be considered if the particles are highly charged.

Viscosity agents such as natural gums, eg, acacia, xanathan and cellulose derivatives such as sodium carboxymethylcellulose and hydroxypropylmethylcellulose, may be used at low concentrations (<0.1%) to function as protective colloids, but at higher concentrations they can then function as viscosity-increasing agents and they decrease the rate of settling of deflocculated particles or provide stability in a flocculated suspension.

The choice of an appropriate viscosity agent depends upon the end-use of the product (external or internal), facilities for preparation and the duration of storage.

Extemporaneous preparations of suspensions for internal use showing good flow and suspending properties are provided by sodium carboxymethylcellulose 2.5%, tragacanth 1.25% and guar gum 0.5%. Avicel RC-591, a coprecipitate of microcrystalline cellulose and sodium carboxymethylcellulose stabilized with hydroxypropylmethylcellulose, has been used as a suspending vehicle for propranolol and orphenadrine hydrochloride dispersions prepared from tablets. It also may serve as a general-purpose suspending agent. Carbopol 934, 0.3% or greater, was a satisfactory suspending agent for sulfamethazine 10%, maintaining a permanent suspension for more than 6 months. Other agents include acacia, methylcellulose or other cellulose derivatives and sodium alginate or tragacanth.

Buffers may be considered if the drug has ionizable groups in order to maintain a low solubility of the drug. Buffers also may be considered to control the ionization of preservatives, ionic viscosity agents or to maintain the pH of the suspensions within a suitable range. The external phase is usually water for oral preparations; however, other polar liquids such as glycerin or alcohol may be considered in order to control solubility, stability and taste. The selection of the external phase is based upon taste, viscosity, density and stability. Nonpolar liquids such as aliphatic hydrocarbons and fatty esters may be considered if the preparation is used for external purposes.

Appropriate preservatives should be incorporated in order to minimize microbiological contamination as discussed previously. The suspension must be acceptable to the patient on the basis of its taste, color and cosmetic qualities (elegance), the latter two factors being of particular importance in preparations intended for external use.

Preparation

The preparation of suspensions involves several steps; the first is to obtain the particles in the proper size range which is in the lower micrometer size. Oral preparations should not feel gritty, topical preparations should feel smooth to the touch and injectables should not produce tissue irritation. Particle size and distribution also should be considered in terms of bioavailability, or alternately, to control the rate of release. Particles of an extremely small size, less than 1 μm will have a higher solubility than larger particles, which may cause problems in regard to dissolution and then the formation of larger particles.

Milling is the term given to the mechanical process of reducing the particle size, which may be accomplished by a number of different types of machines, as described by Parrot.[28] The hammer mill grinds the powders by the impact of rotating hammers and particles which subsequently fall through a screen in a range of 4 to 325 mesh are obtained. A ball mill contains a number of steel balls in a container which revolves, and the balls reduce the particle size to a 20 to 200 mesh by both attrition and impact. A fluid-energy mill produces particles 1 to 30 μm through violent turbulence in high-velocity air. Roller mills have two or more rollers which revolve at different speeds and the particles are reduced to a mesh of 20 to 200 by means of compression and a shearing action.

On a small scale, in a pharmacy, the particles should be wetted thoroughly with a small quantity of water-miscible solvent, such as glycerin or alcohol, which reduces the liquid/air interfacial tension. The suspending agent in the aqueous medium then is added. Alternately, the dry suspending agent can be triturated with the drug particles using a small quantity of glycerin or alcohol and then brought up to volume with the diluent water.

On a large scale, the drug particles are treated with a small portion of water which contains the wetting agent and allowed to stand for several hours in order to release entrapped air. At the same time, the suspending agent should be dissolved or dispersed in the main portion of the external phase and allowed to stand until complete hydration takes place. Subsequently, wetted drug particles should be added slowly to the main portion of the dissolved suspending agent. Other excipients such as electrolytes or buffers should be added in a careful manner to prevent variation in particle charge. The preservatives, flavoring agents and coloring agents are added. After all additions have been made, treatment with homogenizers or ultrasonic devices should be used to reduce the size of agglomerated particles, as described by Nash.[29]

Suspension equipment such as colloid mills or homogenizers normally are used in wet-milling finished suspensions to reduce particle agglomerates and to form a suitable preparation (Figs. 4, 5 and 6).

Quality

The quality of the suspension can be determined in a number of ways, such as photomicroscopy, to determine particle shape, size and flocculation. The Coulter counter can be used to determine the size distribution. Physical stability, ie, the degree of settling or flocculation, may be determined by using cylindrical graduates. Viscosity of the final product and the suspending agent dissolved in the liquid medium may be determined by moisture instruments such as the Brookfield viscometer. Specific-gravity measurements are useful for determining the degree of air entrapped. Of course both microbiological as well as aging tests should be performed to determine the efficiency of the preservative and the appropriateness of the formulation with respect to stability and time.

Suspensions from Tablets

Occasionally, it is necessary to prepare a liquid formulation of a drug in order to meet certain requirements of the patient such as inability to injest a solid dosage form or to prepare a product for a different route of administration or different strength. The pure drug should be used to prepare the dosage form rather than a tablet or a capsule because there is only one ingredient in the product; thus, no consideration has to be given to the excipients in the tablet or capsule. If it is necessary to prepare a liquid dosage form from tablets or capsules, a suspension is formed if either the drug or one of the excipients in the tablets or capsule is insoluble. The solubility of the drug may be determined from the literature; however, the excipients in the tablets or capsules are usually not known.

Insoluble excipients in these dosage forms may include certain disintegrants, lubricants, glidants, colors, diluents and coatings; consequently, although the drug may be soluble in water, many excipients are not. It is preferable to use the contents of capsules, or tablets which are not coated, or if coated, those tablets with a water-soluble coat. In any case, the contents of the capsules or the tablets should be ground finely with a mortar and pestle and then wetted using a little alcohol or glycerin as mentioned above, or with the dispersion medium using the mortar and pestle.

Finally, it may be desirable to use a hand homogenizer to prepare a more suitable product. Some drugs which have been formulated in this manner include clonidine hydrochloride and simple syrup, cefuroxime axetil in an orange syrup vehicle, famotidine in cherry syrup, terbutaline in syrup, prednisone in a tuttifrutti formulation, metoprolol tartrate or spironolactone in a tragacanth-suspending vehicle or propranolol hydrochloride in a simple syrup. Many other examples may be found in current hospital and community pharmacy journals such as the *American Journal of Hospital Pharmacy, Canadian Journal of Hospital Pharmacy, U.S. Pharmacist Drug Development* and *Industrial Pharmacy.* Frequently, stability data and, occasionally, bioavailability and/or taste data are provided.

If the drug is soluble in water, a solution of the drug may be prepared by crushing the tablets in a mortar and pestle, triturating with water, filtering and bringing the solution up to appropriate volume with water or other suitable vehicle if the preparation is for topical application or with a flavored aqueous vehicle if it is for oral use.

If the active ingredient in the tablet or capsule is not stable in an aqueous system, a different method of preparing the suspension is required. The tablet may be crushed and placed in a powder paper and dispensed in the form of individual powders. Each paper contains the active drug in one tablet or an appropriate dose. The powder is placed in a glass of water or suitable liquid, stirred and administered immediately. See Chapter 91 for divided powders.

A general formula to prepare suspensions from crushed tablets is given in Martindale.[30]

Methylcellulose 20	0.75
Parabens	0.1
Purified Water	60.0
Propylene Glycol	2.0
Simple Syrup, to make	100.0

An extemporaneous suspension of cimetidine tablets which retained its potency at 40° over 14 days is:

Cimetidine 300-mg tablets	24 (7.2 g)
Glycerin	10 mL
Simple Syrup, to make	120 mL

The tablets are triturated to a fine powder using a mortar, the mixture is levigated with the glycerin, simple syrup added, mixed well, placed in a blender until smooth and then refrigerated as described by Tortorici.[31]

Satisfactory suspensions have been compounded from diazepam tablets and propranolol hydrochloride tablets, and they possess chemical stability for 60 days and 4 months, respectively, at room temperature or under refrigeration. Frequently, since the drug may be soluble, it is the excipients which are being suspended.

A comprehensive checklist of suspension formulations has been reported in the literature by Scheer.[32]

Gels

Pharmaceutical terminology is, at best, confusing and no two texts will classify gels, jellies magnas, milks and mixtures in the same way. The USP's definition for gels is given below.

Gels (sometimes called Jellies) are semisolid systems consisting of either suspensions made up of small inorganic particles or large organic molecules interpenetrated by a liquid. Where the gel mass consists of a network of small discrete particles, the gel is classified as a two-phase system (eg, *Aluminum Hydroxide Gel*). In a two-phase system, if the particle size of the dispersed phase is relatively large, the gel mass is sometimes referred to as a magma (eg, *Bentonite Magma*). Both gels and magmas may be thixotropic, forming semisolids on standing and becoming liquid on agitation. They should be shaken before use to ensure homogeneity and should be labeled to that effect. (See *Suspensions.*)

Single-phase gels consist of organic macromolecules distributed uniformly throughout a liquid in such a manner that no apparent boundaries exist between the dispersed macromolecules and the liquid. Single-phase gels may be made from synthetic macromolecules (eg, *Carbomer*) or from natural gums (eg, *Tragacanth*). The latter preparations also are called mucilages. Although these gels are commonly aqueous, alcohols and oils may be used as the continuous phase. For example, mineral oil can be combined with a polyethylene resin to form an oleaginous ointment base.

Gels can be used to administer drugs topically or into body cavities (eg, *Phenylephrine Hydrochloride Nasal Jelly*).

The definition in the BP tends to be more restrictive in the sense that the gels are homogenous and are intended to be applied to the skin or certain mucous membranes. Gels may contain auxiliary substances such as antimicrobial preservatives, antioxidants and stabilizers.

Schott[33] has described various aspects of gels. At appropriate concentrations of solute and solvent, gels consisting of two phases, eg, bentonite, are formed because of the attraction between positively charged edges and the negatively charged faces, producing a three-dimensional network penetrated by the liquid phase. In the case of a single-phase system, the gels are formed as a result of secondary valence forces between the polymer molecules due to entanglement of the chains. Permanent gels are formed when three-dimensional polymerization of multifunctional polymers occurs or when there is cross-linking of dissolved polymer molecules by primary valence bonds. These permanent gels are used as matrices for prolonged-release preparations (see Chapter 94) and are not discussed further in this chapter.

Two-phase gels containing bentonite may be used as a base for topical preparations such as plaster and ointment. Another two-phase gel, Aluminum Hydroxide Gel USP is used for its therapeutic properties.

The USP states that

Aluminum Hydroxide Gel is a suspension, each 100 g of which contains the equivalent of not less than 5.5 g and not more than 6.7 g of aluminum hydroxide [$Al(OH)_3$], in the form of amorphous aluminum hydroxide in which there is a partial substitution of carbonate for hydroxide.

The gel itself usually is prepared by the interaction of a soluble aluminum salt, such as a chloride or sulfate, with ammonia solution, sodium carbonate or bicarbonate. The reactions which occur during the preparation are

$$3CO_3^{2-} + 3H_2O \rightarrow 3HCO_3^- + 3OH^-$$

$$[Al(H_2O)_6]^{3+} + 3OH^- \rightarrow [Al[H_2O)_3(OH)_3] + 3H_2O$$

$$2HCO_3^- \rightarrow CO_3^{2-} + H_2O + CO_2$$

The physical and chemical properties of the gel will be affected by the order of addition of reactants, pH of precipitation, temperature of precipitation, concentration of the reactants, the reactants used and the conditions of aging of the precipitated gel.

Aluminum Hydroxide Gel is soluble in acidic (or very strongly basic) media. The mechanism in acidic media is

$$\text{Aluminum Hydoxide Gel} + 3H_2O \rightarrow [Al(H_2O)_3(OH)_3]^0$$

$$[Al(H_2O)_3(OH)_3]^0 + H_3O^+ \rightarrow [Al(H_2O)_4(OH)_2]^+ + H_2O$$

$$[Al(H_2O)_4(OH)_2]^+ + H_3O^+ \rightarrow [Al(H_2O)_5(OH)^{2+} + H_2O$$

$$[Al(H_2O)_5(OH)]^{2+} + H_3O^+ \rightarrow [Al(H_2O)_6]^{3+} + H_2O$$

It is unlikely that the last reaction given proceeds to completion. Since the activity of the gel is controlled by its insolubility (solubility will decrease with an increase in the pH of the gastric media), there is no acid rebound. Further, since a certain quantity of insoluble gel always is available, the neutralizing capability of the gel extends over a considerable period of time.

Aluminum hydroxide gels also may contain peppermint oil, glycerin, sorbitol, sucrose, saccharin and various preservatives. Sorbitol improves the acid-consuming capacity, apparently by inhibiting a secondary polymerization that takes place on aging. In addition, polyols such as mannitol, sorbitol and inositol have been shown to improve the stability of aluminum hydroxide and aluminum hydroxycarbonate gels.

Other two-phase gels of the USP include Aluminum Phosphate Gel and Aluminum Carbonate gels. Some of these products also occur in the dried form and are also called gels.

Single-Phase Gels—The single-phase gels are being used more frequently in pharmacy and cosmetics because of several properties: semisolid state, high degree of clarity, ease of application and ease of removal and use. The gels often provide a faster release of drug substance, independent of the water solubility of the drug, as compared to creams and ointments.

Some recent gel formulations include ophthalmic preparations of pilocarpine, carbachol and betamethasone valerate; topical preparations for burn therapy, anti-inflammatory treatment, musculoskeletal disorders and acne; peptic ulcer treatment with sucralfate gel and bronchoscopy using lidocaine. Cosmetic gels include shower gels, after shave gels and sunscreen gels. The USP lists a number of gels: Sodium Fluoride and Phosphoric Acid Gel for application to the teeth to reduce cavities, Betamethasone Benzoate Gel and Fluocinonide Gel, anti-inflammatory corticosteroids, Tolnaftate Gel, an antifungal agent and Tretinoin Gel for the treatment of acne. Gels may be used as lubricants for catheters, bases for patch testing, sodium chloride gels for electrocardiography.

Gels can be prepared from a number of pharmaceutical agents such as tragacanth 2 to 5%, sodium alginate 2 to 10%, gelatin 2 to 15%, methylcellulose 450 at 3 to 5%, sodium carboxymethylcellulose 2 to 5%, carbomer 0.3 to 5% or polyvinyl alcohols 10 to 20% as noted by Collett.[34] Other gelling agents include methylhydroxyethyl cellulose, polyoxyethylene-polyoxypropylene, hydroxyethylcellulose and gelatin. Gels prepared from nonpolar materials such as magnesium soap-hydrocarbon and hydrocarbons are being investigated. The percentages above indicate the concentration ranges of the gelling agent.

Some fluid gels at or below the lower of the above concentrations can be used as artificial saliva and artificial tears. The lower-percentage preparations, noted above, may be used as lubricants and the higher-percentage preparations as dermatological bases. Some of the gelling agents are available in different grades indicating the viscosity at a definite concentration. In general, high-viscosity grades result in gels at lower concentrations. An example of a gel containing a natural polymer, tragacanth, is:

Ephedrine Sulfate Jelly NF XII

Ephedrine Sulfate	10 g
Tragacanth	10 g
Methyl Salicylate	0.1 g
Eucalyptol	1.0 mL
Pine Needle Oil	0.1 mL
Glycerin	150 g
Purified Water	830 mL

Dissolve the ephedrine sulfate in the purified water and add the glycerin, tragacanth and then the remaining ingredients. Mix well and keep in a closed container for 1 week, stirring occcasionally.

In order to prepare uniform gels, it is necessary to disperse the gelling agent in such a manner that it does not form clumps upon the addition of water. Some techniques include the addition of a small quantity of dispersing agent such as alcohol or glycerin and trituration. Another technique is to sprinkle the gelling agent into a vortex of stirred water. If there are a number of other powders in the preparation, the gelling agent first may be triturated with these powders, followed by the addition of water. Shaking the material in a bottle, mixing in a mortar with a pestle or using a mechanical stirrer also are employed. Specific information on the gelling agents is useful in preparing the gels, as described by Zatz and Kushla.[35]

Gels have been prepared in adhesive form in order to increase the contact time of the active ingredients, such as insulin with the oral and nasal mucosa, leading to a decrease in plasma glucose. This system also has been investigated as a vaginal dosage form for cervical cancer and a topical dosage form for aphthous stomatitis.

Preservatives should be incorporated into the gels, especially those prepared from natural sources. Appropriate preservatives, depending upon use and the gelling agent, include the parabens at about 0.2%, benzoic acid 0.2% (if the product is acidic) and chlorocresol 0.1%.

The preparation of a few gel bases is given below:

Sodium Alginate Gel Base

Sodium Alginate	2–10 g
Glycerin	2–10 g
Methyl Hydroxybenzoate	0.2 g
a soluble calcium salt (calcium or gluconate)	0.5 g
Purified Water, to make	100 mL

The sodium alginate is wetted in a mortar with glycerin, which aids the dispersion. The preservative is dissolved in about 80 mL of water with the aid of heat, allowed to cool and the calcium salt added, which will increase the viscosity of the preparation. This solution is stirred in a high speed stirrer and the sodium alginate-glycerin mixture added slowly while stirring, until the preparation is homogeneous. The preparation should be stored in a tightly sealed container in a wide mouth jar or tube.

Carbomer Jelly

Carbopol 934	2 g
Triethanolamine	1.65 mL
Parabens	0.2 g
Purified Water, to make	100 mL

The parabens are dissolved in 95 mL of water with the aid of heat and allowed to cool. The Carbopol 934, a commercial grade of carbomer, is added in small amounts to the solution using a high speed stirrer and, after a smooth dispersion is obtained, the preparation is allowed to stand permitting entrapped air to separate. Then the gelling agent, triethanolamine, is added, dropwise, stirring with a plastic spatula to avoid entrapping air and the remaining water incorporated. Other concentrations of carbomer can be used to prepare gels, creams or suspensions.

Gels may contract on standing and some of the solvent then is squeezed out. This process is called *syneresis* and will present a problem in the long-term stability of gels. The addition of relatively large quantities of salts may cause a salting-out of polymers, especially those of an ionic nature. The effect of increasing the temperature may cause rigid gels to melt. An example of an exception to this phenomenon is the gelification of methylcellulose which gels as the temperature rises above $\simeq 50°$. This phenomenon is called *thermal gelation*, as described by Schott.[33] In order to minimize water loss from single-phase gels, humectants such as propylene glycol, glycerin or sorbitol are added.

Lotions

Lotions are not defined specifically in the USP, but the BP provides a definition which is broad in nature and indicates that lotions are either liquid or semiliquid preparations which contain one or more active ingredients in an appropriate vehicle. Lotions may contain antimicrobial preservatives and other appropriate excipients such as stabilizers. Lotions are intended to be applied to the unbroken skin without friction. Lotions are usually suspensions of solids in an aqueous medium. A few lotions are, in fact, emulsions or solutions.

Even though lotions usually are applied without friction the insoluble matter should be divided very finely. Particles approaching colloidal dimensions are more soothing to inflamed areas and effective in contact with infected surfaces. A wide variety of ingredients may be added to the preparation to produce better dispersions or to accentuate its cooling, soothing, drying or protective properties. Bentonite is a good example of a suspending agent used in the preparation of lotions. Methylcellulose or sodium carboxymethylcellulose, eg, will localize and hold the active ingredient in contact with the affected site and at the same time be rinsed off easily with water. A formulation containing glycerin will keep the skin moist for a considerable period of time. The drying and cooling effect may be accentuated by adding alcohol to the formula.

Dermatologists frequently prescribe lotions containing anesthetics, antipruritics, antiseptics, astringents, germicides, protectives or screening agents, to be used in treating or preventing various types of skin diseases and dermatitis. Antihistamines, benzocaine, calamine, resorcin, steroids, sulfur, zinc oxide, betamethasone derivatives, salicylic acid, safflower oil, minoxidil and zirconium oxide are ingredients common in unofficial lotions. In many instances the cosmetic aspects of the lotion are of great importance. Many lotions compare badly with cosmetic preparations of a similar nature. The manufacture of fine lotions to meet the specialized needs of the dermatologist provides the pharmacist with an excellent opportunity to demonstrate professional competence. Extensive studies on lotions, as described by Harb,[36] will assist the pharmacist to attain this goal.

Lotions may be prepared by triturating the ingredients to a smooth paste and then adding the remaining liquid phase with trituration. High-speed mixers or colloid mills produce better dispersions and, therefore, are used in the preparation of larger quantities of lotion. Calamine Lotion USP is the classic example of this type of preparation and consists of finely powdered, insoluble solids held in more or less permanent suspension by the presence of suspending agents and/or surface-active agents.

The formula and the method of preparation of Calamine Lotion USP is given

Calamine Lotion

Calamine	80 g
Zinc Oxide	80 g
Glycerin	20 mL
Bentonite Magma	250 mL
Calcium Hydroxide Topical Solution, a sufficient quantity, to make	1000 mL

Dilute the bentonite magma with an equal volume of calcium hydroxide topical solution. Mix the powder intimately with the glycerin and about 100 mL of the diluted magma, triturating until a smooth, uniform paste is formed. Gradually incorporate the remainder of the diluted magma. Finally add enough calcium hydroxide topical solution to make 1000 mL, and shake well.

If a more viscous consistency in the Lotion is desired, the quantity of bentonite magma may be increased to not more than 400 mL.

Many investigators have studied Calamine Lotion and this has led to the publication of many formulations, each possessing certain advantages over the others but none satisfying the collective needs of all dermatologists.

Formulations containing Avicel R (hydrated microcrystalline cellulose, *FMC*) and carboxymethylcellulose settle less than the official preparations.

Calamine Lotion

Calamine	8 g
Zinc Oxide	8 g
Glycerin	2 mL
Avicel R Gel	2 g
Carboxymethylcellulose	2 g
Calcium Hydroxide Solution, a sufficient quantity, to make	100 mL

Mix 45 g of Avicel R with 55 g of water with a suitable electric mixer. This gel is used in the preparation of the calamine lotion. Mix the calamine and the zinc oxide with the glycerin, the gel and the carboxymethylcellulose. Add sufficient calcium hydroxide solution to make the product measure 100 mL.

While most lotions are prepared by trituration, some lotions are formed by chemical interaction in the liquid. White Lotion is an example.

White Lotion

Zinc Sulfate	40 g
Sulfurated Potash	40 g
Purified Water, a sufficient quantity to make	1000 mL

Dissolve the zinc sulfate and the sulfurated potash separately, each in 450 mL of purified water and filter each solution. Add slowly the sulfurated potash solution to the zinc sulfate solution with constant stirring. Then add the required amount of purified water, and mix.

Sulfurated potash is a solid of variable composition but usually is described as $K_2S_3{\cdot}K_2S_2O_3$. The chemical reaction which occurs when sulfurated potash solution is added to the zinc sulfate is

$$ZnSO_4 \cdot 7H_2O + K_2S_3 \cdot K_2S_2O_3 \rightarrow ZnS + S_2 + K_2SO_4 + K_2S_2O_3 + 7H_2O$$

This lotion must be prepared fresh and does not contain a suspending agent. Bentonite Magma has been used in some formulations. Coffman and Huyck[37] include a detailed discussion of the chemistry and the problems involved in the preparation of a suitable product.

An example of a lotion that is an emulsion is Benzyl Benzoate Lotion USP. The formula and method of preparation are as follows:

Benzyl Benzoate	250 mL
Triethanolamine	5 g
Oleic Acid	20 g
Purified Water	750 mL
To make about	1000 mL

Mix the triethanolamine with the oleic acid, add the benzyl benzoate, and mix. Transfer the mixture to a suitable container of about 2000-mL capacity, add 250 mL of purified water, and shake the mixture thoroughly. Finally add the remaining purified water, and again shake thoroughly.

The triethanolamine forms a soap with the oleic acid and functions as the emulsifying agent to form a stable product. This type of emulsifying agent is almost neutral in water and gives a pH of about 8 and thus should not irritate the skin.[6] An example of the wide variety of formulations of benzyl benzoate is provided by Bhargava and Nicolai.[38]

Some lotions are clear solutions as exemplified by Aminobenzoic Acid Lotion BP.

Aminobenzoic Acid	50 g
Glycerol	200 mL
Ethanol 96%	600 mL
Purified Water freshly boiled and cooled, sufficient to produce	1000 mL

Dissolve the aminobenzoic acid in the ethanol 96%, add the glycerol and sufficient purified water to produce 1000 mL and mix. The ethanol is used to dissolve the aminobenzoic acid and provide a cooling effect. The glycerol (glycerin) is used for its emollient effect. Since lotions may be solutions, suspensions or emulsions, the method of preparation is similar to those types of formulations described above.

Several lotions are listed in the USP and contain, for example, antibiotics, steroids, scabicides and sunscreens.

A formula for hydrocortisone lotion is given in the PC.

Hydrocortisone Lotion

Hydrocortisone, in ultrafine powder	10.0 g
Chlorocresol	0.5 g
Self-emulsifying monostearin	40.0 g
Glycerol	63.0 g
Purified water, freshly boiled and cooled to make	1000.0 g

To prepare the base, the chlorocresol is dissolved in 850 mL of water with the aid of gentle heat, the self-emulsifying monostearin is added and the mixture heated to 60° with stirring until completely dispersed. The hydrocortisone is triturated with the glycerol and the trituration is then incorporated, with stirring, into the warm base, allowed to cool while stirring, then add the remainder of the water and mix.

Certain lotions tend to separate or stratify on long standing, and they require a label directing that they be shaken well before each use. All lotions should be labeled "For External Use Only."

Microorganisms may grow in certain lotions if no preservative is included. Care should be taken to avoid contaminating the lotion during preparation, even if a preservative is present.

Magmas and Milks

Magmas and milks are aqueous suspensions of insoluble, inorganic drugs and differ from gels mainly in that the suspended particles are larger. When prepared, they are thick and viscous and, because of this, there is no need to add a suspending agent.

Bentonite Magma USP is prepared by simple hydration. Two procedures are given for the preparation of this product, and these are described in Chapter 80. Dihydroxyaluminum Aminoacetate Magma is the other magma in the USP.

Milk of Magnesia USP is a suspension of magnesium hydroxide containing not less than 80 mg of $Mg(OH)_2$ per mL. The specifications for double strength or triple strength are that these products should contain not less than 160 mg or 240 mg of $Mg(OH)_2$ per mL, respectively. It has an unpleasant, alkaline taste which can be masked with 0.1% citric acid (to reduce alkalinity) and 0.05% of a volatile oil or a blend of volatile oils. Magnesium hydroxide is prepared by the hydration of magnesium oxide.

$$MgO + H_2O \rightarrow Mg(OH)_2$$

Milk of Bismuth USP contains bismuth hydroxide and bismuth subcarbonate in suspension in water. The Magma is prepared by reacting bismuth subnitrate with nitric acid and ammonium carbonate with ammonia solution and then mixing the resulting two solutions.

The following reactions occur during the preparation of the magma.

$$(NH_4)_2CO_3 \rightarrow 2NH_4^+ + CO_3^{2-}$$

$$NH_3 + H_2O \rightarrow NH_4^+ + OH^-$$

$$2BiO^+ + CO_3^{2-} \rightarrow (BiO)_2CO_3$$

$$BiO^+ + OH^- \rightarrow BiO(OH)$$

If the insoluble substance is precipitated fresh by mixing hot, dilute solutions, there is only slight sedimentation on standing. This characteristic of milks or magmas sometimes is enhanced by passing the product through a colloid mill.

For the most part, magmas and milks are intended for internal use, eg, Milk of Magnesia USP and Dihydroxy Aluminum Aminoacetate Magma USP, although Bentonite Magma is used primarily as a suspending agent for insoluble substances for local application and occasionally for internal use. All magmas require a "Shake Well" label. Freezing must be avoided.

Several antimicrobial preservatives have been tested in liquid antacid preparations for their stability and effectiveness, such as benzoic acid, chlorhexidine, methylparaben, propylparaben, sorbic acid, propylene glycol or ethanol. It was found that a combination of methylparaben and sorbic acid was superior to the parabens alone.

Mixtures

The USP does not recognize the term mixture; however, the BP defines the term as

Mixtures are oral liquids containing one or more active ingredients, dissolved, suspended or dispersed in a suitable vehicle. Suspended solids may separate slowly on standing, but are easily redispersed on shaking.

The insoluble substance usually does not make the mixture very viscous, and the particles may be held in suspension by using suitable suspending or thickening agents. This class was introduced originally to secure uniformity in the formulas of certain well-known and largely used preparations. Frequently, the term *mixture* is applied loosely to aqueous preparations of every description. The term *shake mixture* is used often for liquid preparations which contain insoluble ingredients and, therefore, must be shaken before use. The term *suspension* is used to describe a number of similar preparations.

The following is a formula for a mixture in the BP, which is a solution for an extemporaneous preparation.

Ammonium Chloride Mixture

Ammonium Chloride	100 g
Aromatic Ammonia Solution	50 mL
Liquorice Liquid Extract	100 mL
Water for Preparations to	1000 mL

It should be prepared recently.

The following mixture is an example of a suspension and is used for the treatment of diarrhea. The pectin and the tragacanth in Kaolin Mixture with Pectin act as suspending agents. An alternate formula, based on Veegum (*Vanderbilt*) and sodium carboxymethylcellulose, has been proposed by Kalish.[39]

Kaolin Mixture with Pectin

Veegum	0.88 g
Sodium Carboxymethylcellulose	0.22 g
Purified Water	79.12 g
Kaolin	17.50 g
Pectin	0.44 g
Saccharin	0.09 g
Glycerin	1.75 g

Add the Veegum and the sodium carboxymethylcellulose to the water with continuous stirring. Add, with mixing, the kaolin. Mix the pectin, saccharin and glycerin and add to the suspension. A preservative and flavoring agent may be added to the product.

The insoluble material in mixtures must be in a very finely divided state and uniformly distributed throughout the preparation. This is accomplished with colloid mills, special methods of precipitation and suspending agents. There are three main reasons for having the insoluble substances in as fine a state of subdivision as possible.

1. The more nearly the colloidal state is approached by protectives, such as kaolin, magnesium trisilicate or magnesium phosphate, the more active they become as adsorbents and protectives when in contact with inflamed surfaces.
2. Finely divided particles are suspended more readily and settle out much more slowly than large particles, thus enabling the patient to obtain uniform doses of suspended substances. Homogeneous mixtures are desirable especially when administering medication to form an evenly distributed, protective coating on the gastrointestinal tract.
3. The palatability of many preparations is enhanced by the use of colloidal suspending agents.

Mixtures containing suspended material should have a "Shake Well" label affixed to the container in which they are dispensed.

Mixtures, including suspensions, are subject to contamination by microorganisms that remain viable and are a potential health hazard during the period of use of the products. Survival times of organisms depend on the preservative used. A kaolin pediatric mixture that contains benzoic acid kills organisms rapidly, whereas organisms survived for more than a week in a magnesium trisilicate mixture that contained no more than a trace of peppermint oil, as noted by Westwood.[40]

Official Suspensions

The USP places particular emphasis on the term suspension by providing specific definitions for a variety of oral, parenteral and ophthalmic preparations formulated in such a way that an insoluble substance is suspended in a liquid at some stage of the manufacturing or dispensing process. The USP definition begins as follows:

Suspensions are liquid preparations which consist of solid particles dispersed throughout a liquid phase in which the particles are not soluble. Dosage forms officially categorized as Suspensions are designated as such if they are not included in other more specific categories of suspensions, such as Oral Suspensions, Topical Suspensions, etc. (see these other categories). Some suspensions are prepared and ready for use, while others are prepared as solid mixtures intended for constitution just before use with an appropriate vehicle. Such products are designated "for Oral Suspension," etc.

This definition relates the term suspension to milks, magmas and lotions which have been described above.

While there are a number of monographs dealing with suspensions in the USP, neither the definition nor the monographs give specific directions for the preparation of the suspension, although pharmacopeias usually permit the addition of suitable flavoring agents, suspending agents, preservatives and certified color additives. One procedure for the preparation of the commonly used Trisulfapyrimidines Oral Suspension is given below.

Trisulfapyrimidines Oral Suspension

Veegum	1.00 g
Syrup USP	90.60 g
Sodium Citrate	0.78 g
Sulfadiazine	2.54 g
Sulfamerazine	2.54 g
Sulfamethazine	2.54 g

Add the Veegum, slowly and with continuous stirring, to the syrup. Incorporate the sodium citrate into the Veegum-syrup mixture. Premix the sulfa drugs, add to the syrup, stir and homogenize. Add sufficient 5% citric acid to adjust the pH of the product to 5.6. A preservative and a flavoring agent may be added to the product.

Methods of preparation for those formulations which contain several active ingredients and are produced in large quantities tend to be more complex than that given above and are described previously.

Many formulations for suspensions are given in the BP and the PC under *Mixtures*.

A properly prepared suspension has a number of desirable properties:

1. The suspended material should not settle rapidly.
2. Particles that do settle should not form a hard cake and easily should be resuspended uniformly on shaking.
3. The suspension should pour freely from the container.

Insoluble powders that do not disperse evenly throughout the suspending medium, when shaken, should be powdered finely and levigated with a small amount of an agent such as glycerin, alcohol or a portion of the dispersion of the suspending agent. The other ingredients are incorporated and the remainder of the dispersion of the suspending agent is incorporated gradually by trituration to produce the appropriate volume.

Suspensions intended for parenteral or ophthalmic use also are described in the USP. For a discussion of these suspensions, see Chapter 87 and 89.

Extracts

Extraction

Extraction, as the term is used pharmaceutically, involves the separation of medicinally active portions of plant or animal tissues from the inactive or inert components by using selective solvents in standard extraction procedures.

The products so obtained from plants are relatively impure liquids, semisolids or powders intended only for oral or external use. These include classes of preparations known as decoctions, infusions, fluidextracts, tinctures, pilular (semisolid) extracts and powdered extracts. Such preparations popularly have been called galenicals, after Galen, the 2nd century Greek physician. For additional information concerning extraction and extractives, see RPS 15, Chapter 86.

Extraction continues to be of considerable interest in order to obtain improved yields of drugs derived from plant and animal sources. For example, improved extraction of digitalis glycosides has been carried out using a pulsating, perforated, bottom column. Other techniques include ultrasonics, rotary-film evaporators, liquid and supercritical carbon dioxide, hydrodistillation, liquid chromatography, multiple-solvent extraction, countercurrent extraction and gravitation dynamics.

This discussion is concerned primarily with basic extraction procedures for crude drugs to obtain the therapeutically desirable portion and eliminate the inert material by treatment with a selective solvent, known as the menstruum. Extraction differs from solution in that the presence of insoluble matter is implied in the former process. The principal methods of extraction are maceration, percolation, digestion, infusion and decoction. The quality of the finished product can be enhanced by standardizing primary extracts and carrying out analytical assays during production on the raw materials, intermediate products and manufacturing procedures.

The processes of particular importance, insofar as the USP is concerned, are those of maceration and percolation, as described specifically for Belladonna Extract USP and Cascara Sagrada Extract USP. Most pharmacopeias refer to such processes for extraction of active principles from crude drugs. The USP provides general directions for both maceration and percolation under the heading of *Tinctures*.

Maceration—In this process the solid ingredients are placed in a stoppered container with 750 mL of the prescribed solvent and allowed to stand for a period of at least 3 days in a warm place with frequent agitation, until soluble matter is dissolved. The mixture is filtered and, after most of the liquid has drained, the residue on the filter is washed with sufficient quantity of the prescribed solvent or solvent mixture; the filtrates are combined to produce 1000 mL.

Percolation—The ground drug is mixed with the appropriate quantity of the prescribed solvent to make it evenly and uniformly damp. It is allowed to stand for 15 minutes, then transferred to a percolator (a narrow coned-shaped vessel, open at both ends). Sufficient prescribed solvent is added to saturate the drug. The top is placed on the percolator and, when the liquid is about to drip from the apparatus, the lower opening is closed. The drug is allowed to macerate for 24 hours or for the specified time. If no assay is directed, the percolation is allowed to proceed slowly or at the specified rate gradually adding sufficient solvent to produce 1000 mL of solution. If an assay is required, only 950 mL of percolate are collected and mixed and a portion assayed as directed. The rest of the percolate is diluted with the solvent to produce a solution that conforms to the required standard and then mixed.

Digestion—This is a form of maceration in which *gentle heat* is used during the process of extraction. It is used when moderately elevated temperature is not objectionable and the solvent efficiency of the menstruum is increased thereby.

Infusion—An infusion is a dilute solution of the readily soluble constituents of crude drugs. Fresh infusions are prepared by macerating the drugs for a short period of time with either cold or boiling water. US official compendia have not included infusions for some time. An example is Concentrated Compound Gentian Infusion BP 1973.

Decoction—This once-popular process extracts water-soluble and heat-stable constituents from crude drugs by boiling in water for 15 min, cooling, straining and passing sufficient cold water through the drug to produce the required volume.

Extractive Preparations

After a solution of the active constituents of a crude drug is obtained by maceration or percolation, it may be ready for use as a medicinal agent, as with certain tinctures or fluidextracts, or it may be processed further to produce a solid or semisolid extract.

For a discussion of *resins* and *oleoresins* obtained by solvent extraction of plant exudates see Chapter 26, under *Plant Exudates*.

Tinctures—Tinctures are defined in the USP as being alcoholic or hydroalcoholic solutions prepared from vegetable materials or from chemical substances, an example of the latter being Iodine Tincture. Traditionally, tinctures of potent vegetable drugs essentially represent the activity of 10 g of the drug in each 100 mL of tincture, the potency being adjusted following assay. Most other tinctures of vegetable drugs represent the extractive from 20 g of the drug in 100 mL of tincture.

The USP specifically describes two general processes for preparing tinctures, one by percolation designated as Process P, and the other by maceration, as Process M. These utilize the methods described under *Extraction*.

Process P includes a modification so that tinctures that require assay for adjustment to specified potency thus may be tested before dilution to final volume. A tincture prepared by Process P as modified for assayed tinctures is Belladonna Tincture.

Examples of tinctures prepared by Process M are Compound Benzoin Tincture USP and Sweet Orange Peel Tincture USP XXI (the latter contains the extractive from 50 g of sweet orange peel in 100 mL of tincture).

Fluidextracts—The USP defines fluidextracts as being liquid preparations of vegetable drugs, containing alcohol as a solvent or as a preservative, or both, so made that, in general, each mL contains the therapeutic constituents of 1 g of the standard drug that it represents. While the USP states that pharmacopeial fluidextracts are made by percolation, the official compendia previously have described general procedures for three percolation methods used in making fluidextracts.

Process A is a percolation method that can be modified for fluidextracts that must be assayed.

Process E is an alternative for Process A in which percolation is conducted on a column of drug much greater in length than in diameter.

Process D is used for preparing fluidextracts with boiling water as the menstruum, alcohol being added as a preservative to the concentrated percolate; this is the procedure used for preparing Cascara Sagrada Fluidextract USP XXI.

The BP and PC use the designation *Liquid Extracts* for fluidextracts.

Extracts—Extracts are defined in the USP as concentrated preparations of vegetable or animal drugs obtained by removal of the active constituents of the respective drugs with suitable menstrua, evaporation of all or nearly all of the solvent and adjustment of the residual masses or powders to the prescribed standards.

Three forms of extracts were recognized in USP XXI: semiliquids or liquids of syrupy consistency, plastic masses (known as *pilular* or *solid extracts*) and dry powders (known as *powdered extracts*). Extracts, as concentrated forms of the drugs from which they are prepared, are used in a variety of solid or semisolid dosage forms. The USP states that pilular extracts and powdered extracts of any one drug are interchangeable medicinally, but each has its own pharmaceutical advantages. Pilular extracts, so-called because they are of a consistency to be used in pill masses and made into pills and are suited especially for use in ointments and suppositories. Powdered extracts are suited better for incorporation into a dry formulation, as in capsules, powders or tablets. Semiliquid extracts, or extracts of a syrupy consistency, may be used in the manufacture of some pharmaceutical preparations.

Most extracts are prepared by extracting the drug by percolation. The percolate is concentrated, generally by distillation under reduced pressure. The use of heat is avoided where possible because of potential injurious effect on active constituents. Powdered extracts which are made from drugs that contain inactive oily or fatty matter may have to be defatted or prepared from defatted drug. For diluents that may be used to adjust an extract to prescribed standards, see the USP XXI.

Pure Glycyrrhiza Extract USP XXI is an example of a pilular extract; Belladonna Extract USP and Hyoscyamus Extract PC are examples of powdered extracts (the former is prepared also as a pilular extract and the latter as a liquid extract).

References

1. Connors KA, Amidon GL, Kennon L: *Chemical Stability of Pharmaceuticals*, Wiley, New York, 80, 1979.
2. Kurup TRR, Wan LCS: *Pharm J 237:* 761, 1986.
3. Bruch CW: *Drug Cosmet Ind 111(4):* 51, 1972.
4. Coates D: *Mfg Chem Aerosol News 44(6):* 35, *(8):* 41, *(10):* 34, *(12):* 19, 1973; *45(1):* 19, 1974.
5. Reynolds JEF, ed: *Martindale, The Extra Pharmacopoeia*, 30th ed, The Pharmaceutical Press, London, 1132, 1993.
6. *Handbook of Pharmaceutical Excipients*, APhA & Pharmaceutical Society of Great Britain, Washington DC & London, 4, 1986.
7. Hickman K *et al: Science 180:* 15, 1973.
8. Montgomery HA *et al: Am J Hosp Pharm 43:* 118, 1986.
9. Tricca RE: *Drug Cosmet Ind 142(5):* 32, 1988.
10. Bergen A: *Can J Hosp Pharm 30(4):* 109, 1977.
11. Meer T: *Flavoring Pharmaceutical Preparations* (SK&F Selected Pharm Res Refs No 4), SmithKline, Philadelphia, Feb 11, 1957.
12. Schumacher GE: *Am J Hosp Pharm 24:* 588, 713, 1967; *25:* 154, 1968.
13. *Am Drug 175(5):* 24, 1977.
14. Ryder J: *Int J Pharm Technol Prod Mfg 1(1):* 14, 1979.
15. *The Chemistry and Rheology of Water-Soluble Gums and Colloids* (Monograph 24), Society of Chemical Industry, London, 1966.
16. Sumner ED: *JAPhA NS8:* 250, 1968.
17. Rettig H: *Acta Pharm Technol 24:* 143, 1978 through *Int Pharm Abstr 19:* 5096, 1982.
18. White RF: *Pharmaceutical Emulsions and Emulsifying Agents*, 4th ed, Chemist & Druggist, London, 1964.
19. Griffin WC, Lynch MJ, Lathrop LB: *Drug Cosmet Ind 101(4):* 41, *(5):* 52, 1967.
20. Rieger MM. In Lachman L, Lieberman HA, Kanig JL, eds: *The Theory and Practice of Industrial Pharmacy*, 3rd ed, Lea & Febiger, Philadelphia, Chap 17, 1986.
21. Florence AT, Whitehill D: *Int J Pharm 11:* 277, 1982.
22. Prince LM, ed: *Microemulsions: Theory and Practice*, Academic, New York, 1977.
23. Rosano HL *et al: J Soc Cosmet Chem 39:* 201, 1988.
24. Lin TJ: *Ibid 29:* 117, 1978; *35:* 357, 1984.
25. Eisberg N: *Mfg Chem 53(1):* 27, 1982.
26. Fox C. In Breu MM, ed: *Cosmetic Science*, vol 2, Academic, New York, Chap 1, 1980.
27. Scott RR. In Lieberman HA, Rieger MM, Banker GS, eds: *in Pharmaceutical Dosage Forms: Disperse Systems*, vol 2, Dekker, New York, Chap 1, 1989.
28. Parrot EL. In Lachman L, Lieberman HA, Kanig JL, eds: *Theory and Practice of Industrial Pharmacy*, 3rd ed, Lea & Febiger, Philadelphia, Chap 2, 1986.
29. Nash RA. In Lieberman HA, Rieger MM, Banker GS, eds: *Pharmaceutical Dosage Forms: Disperse Systems*, vol 1, Dekker, New York, Chap 5, 1989.
30. Reynolds JEF, ed: *Martindale, The Extra Pharmacopoeia*, 28th ed, Pharmaceutical Press, London, 947, 1982.
31. Tortorici MP: *Am J Hosp Pharm 36:* 22, 1979.
32. Scheer AJ: *Drug Cosmet Ind 128(4):* 40, *(5):* 39, *(6):* 52, 1981.
33. Schott H. In Martin A, Swarbrick J, Cammarata A, eds: *Physical Pharmacy*, Lea & Febiger, Philadelphia, Chap 22, 1983.
34. Collett DM. In Collett DM, Aulton ME, eds: *Pharmaceutical Practice*, Churchill Livingstone, Edinburgh, Chap 14, 1990.
35. Zatz JL, Kushla GP. In Lieberman HA, Rieger MM, Banker GS, eds: *Pharmaceutical Dosage Forms: Disperse Systems*, vol 2, Dekker, New York, Chap 13, 1989.
36. Harb NA: *Cosmet Perfum 89(4):* 67, 1974; Shapiro WB: *Cosmet Toiletries 97(3):* 27, 1982.
37. Coffman HL, Huyck CL: *Am J Hosp Pharm 20:* 132, 1963.
38. Bhargava HN, Nicolai DW. In Lieberman HA, Rieger MM, Banker GS, eds: *Pharmaceutical Dosage Forms: Disperse Systems*, vol 2, Dekker, New York, Chap 7, 1989.
39. Kalish J: *Drug Cosmet Ind 94:* 276, 1964.
40. Westwood N: *Pharm J 208:* 153, 1972.

Bibliography

General

Lieberman HA, Rieger MM, Banker GS, eds: *Pharmaceutical Dosage Forms: Disperse Systems*, vol 1 & 2, Dekker, New York, 1989.

Emulsions

Becher P: *Emulsions: Theory & Practice*, 2nd ed, Reinhold, New York, 1965.

Griffin WC, Lynch MJ, Lathrop LB: *Drug Cosmet Ind 101(4):* 41, *(5):* 52, 1967.

Spalton LM. In White RF, ed: *Pharmaceutical Emulsions and Emulsifying Agents*, 4th ed, Chemist & Druggist, London, 1964.

Equipment

Busse DJ: *Mfg Chem 61(7)*: 39, 1990.
Fox C. In Breuer MM, ed: *Cosmetic Science*, vol 2, Academic, New York, 1980.
Lagman B: *Drug Develop Ind Pharm 14(18)*: 2705, 1988.
Oldshue JY: *Fluid Mixing Technology*, McGraw Hill, New York, 1983.
Rees LH: *Drug Cosmet Ind 101(5)*: 102, 1967.
Scott RR. In Lieberman HA, Rieger MM, Banker GS, eds: *Pharmaceutical Dosage Forms: Disperse Systems*, vol 2, Dekker, New York, 1989.
Washington C: *Mfg Chem 59(3)*: 49, 1988.

Excipient Properties

Handbook of Pharmaceutical Excipients, APhA & Pharmaceutical Society of Great Britain, Washington DC & London, 1986.
Reynolds JEF, ed: *Martindale, The Extra Pharmacopoeia*, 29th ed, Pharmaceutical Press, London, 1989.

Solutions

Ryder J: *Int J Pharm Tech Prod Mfg 1(1)*: 14, 1979.

Suspensions

Plaizier-Vercammen JA, Janssens E: *Labo-Pharma—Probl Tech 32(345, Sep)*: 583, 1984.
Scheer AJ: *Drug Cosmet Ind 128(4)*: 40 *(5)*: 39; *(6)*: 52, 1981.

CHAPTER 87

Parenteral Preparations

Kenneth E Avis, DSc
Emeritus Professor, Pharmaceutics
College of Pharmacy
University of Tennessee, Memphis
The Health Science Center
Memphis, TN 38163

John W. Levchuk, PhD
Adjunct Associate Professor of Pharmaceutics
School of Pharmacy
University of Maryland
Baltimore, MD 21201

The distinctive characteristics of parenteral (Gk, *para enteron*, beside the intestine) dosage forms of drugs will be discussed in this chapter. These dosage forms differ from all other drug dosage forms because of the unique requirements imposed because they are injected directly into body tissue through the primary protective system of the human body, the skin and mucous membranes. Therefore, they must be exceptionally pure and free from physical, chemical and biological contaminants. These requirements place a heavy responsibility on the pharmaceutical industry to practice good manufacturing practices (GMPs) in the manufacture of parenteral dosage forms and upon pharmacists to practice good aseptic practices (GAPs) in dispensing them for administration to patients.

Many of the newer drugs, particularly these derived from the new developments in biotechnology, can only be given parenterally because they are inactivated in the gastrointestinal tract, when given by mouth. Further, the potency and specificity of many of these drugs requires strict control of their administration to the patient. A parenteral route of administration meets both of these critical requirements.

This chapter will begin with a brief review of the historical events contributing to the development of this distinctive dosage form. Consideration will then be given to some of the distinguishing characteristics of these dosage forms and how they are administered to patients. The majority of the remainder of the chapter will discuss the various factors required for the preparation of a pure, safe and effective parenteral product.

History[1]

One of the most significant events in the beginnings of parenteral therapy was the first recorded injection of drugs into the veins of living animals, in about 1657, by the architect Sir Christopher Wren. From such a very crude beginning, the technique for intravenous injection and knowledge of the implications therefore developed slowly during the next century and a half. In 1855 Dr Alexander Wood of Edinburgh described what was probably the first subcutaneous injection of drugs for therapeutic purposes using a true hypodermic syringe.

The latter half of the 19th century brought increasing concern for safety in the administration of parenteral solutions, largely because of the work of Robert Koch and Luis Pasteur. While Charles Chamberland was developing both hot-air and steam sterilization techniques and the first bacteria-retaining filter (made of unglazed porcelain), Stanislaus Limousin was developing a suitable container, the all-glass ampul. In the middle 1920s Dr Florence Seibert provided proof that the disturbing chills and fever which often followed the intravenous injection of drugs was caused by potent products of microbial growth, pyrogens, which could be eliminated from water by distillation and from glassware by heating at elevated temperatures.

Of the technical developments that have contributed to the high quality standards currently achievable in the preparation of parenteral dosage forms, the two that have probably contributed most are the development of HEPA-filtered laminar airflow and the development of membrane microfiltration for solutions. The former made it possible to achieve ultraclean environmental conditions for processing from solutions by filtration both viable and nonviable particles of microbial size and smaller. However, many other developments in recent years have produced an impressive advance in the technology associated with the safe and reliable preparation of parenteral dosage forms. The following list identifies a few of the events which have contributed to that development.

1926—Parenterals were accepted for inclusion in the fifth edition of the *National Formulary*.

1933—The practical application of freeze-drying to clinical materials was accomplished by a team of scientists at the University of Pennsylvania.

1938—The Food, Drug and Cosmetic Act was passed by Congress, establishing the Food and Drug Administration (FDA).

1944—The sterilant ethylene oxide was discovered.

1946—The Parenteral Drug Association was organized.

1961—The concept of laminar airflow was developed by WJ Whitfield.

1962—The FDA was authorized by Congress to establish current good manufacturing practice (CGMP or GMP) regulations.

1965—Total parenteral nutrition (TPN) was developed by SJ Dudrick.

1972—The Limulus Amebocyte Lysate test for pyrogens in parenteral products was developed by JF Cooper.

1974—The concept of validation of processes used in the manufacture of parenteral products was introduced by the FDA.

1977—The principles for clean-in-place (CIP) and steam-in-place (SIP) were introduced.

Early 1980s—Home Health Care emerged as an alternative for patients whose health status permitted release from a hospital to care in the home environment.

1982—Insulin, derived through the new discipline of biotechnology, ushered in the drug class of polypeptides with their inherent stability challenges for parenteral dosage-form development.

1987—Parametric release was accepted by the FDA for selected products terminally sterilized by a validated heat process.

The FDA published *Guideline on Sterile Products Produced by Aseptic Processing*, one of several nonregulatory publications to help industry know what the FDA considers to be acceptable.

Late 1980s—The development of computer capabilities has led to the automation of many process operations and to a revolution in documentation and recordkeeping.

1991—The FDA proposed requiring manufacturers to use a terminal sterilization process when preparing a sterile drug product unless such a process adversely affects the drug product.

Administration

Injections may be classified in six general categories:

1. Solutions ready for injection.
2. Dry, soluble products ready to be combined with a solvent just prior to use.
3. Suspensions ready for injection.
4. Dry, insoluble products ready to be combined with a vehicle just prior to use.
5. Emulsions.
6. Liquid concentrates ready for dilution prior to administration.

These injections may be administered by such routes as intravenous, subcutaneous, intradermal, intramuscular, intra-articular and intrathecal. The nature of the product will determine the particular route of administration that may be employed. Conversely, the desired route of administration will place requirements on the formulation. For example, suspensions would not be administered directly into the blood stream because of the danger of insoluble particles blocking capillaries. Solutions to be administered subcutaneously require strict attention to tonicity adjustment, otherwise irritation of the plentiful supply of nerve endings in this anatomical area would give rise to pronounced pain. Injections intended for intraocular, intraspinal, intracisternal and intrathecal administration require the highest purity standards because of the sensitivity of tissues encountered to irritant and toxic substances.

When compared with other dosage forms, injections possess select advantages. If immediate physiological action is needed from a drug, it usually can be provided by the intravenous injection of an aqueous solution. Modification of the formulation or another route of injection can be used to slow the onset and prolong the action of the drug. The therapeutic response of a drug is controlled more readily by parenteral administration since the irregularities of intestinal absorption are circumvented. Also, since the drug normally is administered by a professionally trained person, it confidently may be expected that the dose was actually and accurately administered. Drugs can be administered parenterally when they cannot be given orally because of the unconscious or uncooperative state of the patient, or because of inactivation or lack of absorption in the intestinal tract. Among the disadvantages of this dosage form are the requirement of asepsis at administration, the risk of tissue toxicity from local irritation, the real or psychological pain factor and the difficulty in correcting an error, should one be made. In the latter situation, unless a direct pharmacological antagonist is immediately available, correction of an error may be impossible. One other disadvantage is that daily or frequent administration poses difficulties, either for the patient to visit a professionally trained person or to learn to inject oneself. However, the advent of home health care as an alternative to extended institutional care has mandated the development of programs for training lay persons to administer these dosage forms.

Parenteral Combinations

During the administration of large-volume parenterals (LVPs), such as 1000-mL of 0.9% sodium chloride solution, it is common practice for a physician to order the addition of a small-volume therapeutic parenteral (SVP), such as an antibiotic, to avoid the discomfort for the patient of a separate injection. While the pharmacist is the most qualified health professional to be responsible to prepare such combinations, as is clearly stated in the Hospital Accreditation Manual of the Joint Commission on Accreditation of Healthcare Organizations,[2] interactions among the combined products can be troublesome even for the pharmacist. In fact, incompatibilities can occur and cause inactivation of one or more ingredients or other undesired reactions. In some instances incompatibilities are visible as precipitation or color change, but in other instances there may be no visible effect.

The many potential combinations present a complex situation even for the pharmacist. To aid in making decisions concerning potential problems, a valuable compilation of relevant data has been assembled by Trissel,[3] and is regularly updated. Further, the advent of computerized data storage and retrieval systems has provided a means to organize and gain rapid access to such information. Further information on this subject may be found in Chapter 88.

As studies have been undertaken and more information has been gained, it has been shown that knowledge of variable factors such as pH and the ionic character of the active constituents aids substantially in understanding and predicting potential incompatibilities. Kinetic studies of reaction rates may be used to describe or predict the extent of degradation. Ultimately, a thorough study should be undertaken of each therapeutic agent in combination with other drugs and IV fluids, not only of generic but of commercial preparations, from the physical, chemical and therapeutic aspects.

Ideally, no parenteral combination should be administered unless it has been studied thoroughly to determine its effect on the therapeutic value and the safety of the combination. However, such an ideal situation may not exist. Nevertheless, it is the responsibility of the pharmacist to be as familiar as possible with the physical, chemical and therapeutic aspects of parenteral combinations and to exercise the best possible judgment as to whether or not the specific combination extemporaneously prescribed is suitable for use in a patient.

General Considerations

An inherent requirement for parenteral preparations is that they be of the very best quality and provide the maximum safety for the patient. Therefore, whether they are prepared from commercially available sterile components, as is usually the case in hospital pharmacies and similar sites, or from nonsterile ingredients in a manufacturing mode, as is the case in the pharmaceutical industry, the persons responsible for their preparation must apply their skills intelligently and diligently. Further, the possession and application of high moral and professional ethics on the part of the persons responsible is the ingredient most vital to achieving the desired quality in the products prepared.

The preparation of parenteral products from sterile components in pharmacies of hospitals and similar sites is discussed further in Chapter 88. In this chapter emphasis will be placed on the preparation of parenteral products from non-sterile components in the highly technologically advanced plants of the pharmaceutical industry, using GMP principles. In the pursuit of GMP, consideration should be given to:

1. Ensure the personnel responsible for assigned duties are capable and qualified to perform them.
2. Ensure that ingredients used in compounding the product have the required identity, quality and purity.
3. Validate critical processes to be sure that the equipment used and the processes followed will ensure that the finished product will have the qualities expected.
4. Maintain a production environment suitable for performing the critical processes required, addressing such matters as orderliness, cleanliness and asepsis.
5. Confirm through adequate quality-control procedures that the finished products have the required potency, purity and quality.
6. Establish through appropriate stability evaluation that the drug products will retain their intended potency, purity and quality until the established expiration date.
7. Ensure that processes are always carried out in accord with established, written procedures.
8. Provide adequate conditions and procedures for the prevention of mixups.
9. Establish adequate procedures, with supporting documentation, for investigating and correcting failures or problems in production or quality control.
10. Provide adequate separation of quality-control responsibilities from those of production to assure independent decision making.

The pursuit of GMP is an ongoing effort which must flex with new technological developments and new understanding of existing principles. Because of the extreme importance of quality in health care of the public, the US Congress has given the responsiblity of regulatory scrutiny over the manufacture and distribution of drug products to the FDA. Therefore, the operations of the pharmaceutical industry are subject to the oversite of the FDA and, with respect to manufacturing practices, to the application of the CGMPs.[4] These regulations are discussed more fully in Chapter 110.

In concert with the pursuit of GMPs, the pharmaceutical industry has shown initiative and innovation in the extensive technological development and improvement in quality, safety and effectiveness of parenteral dosage forms in recent years. Further, outstanding innovative development in drug-delivery systems is occurring. These factors have been additive in providing the public with outstanding parenteral dosage forms of drugs at this time in history.

General Manufacturing Process

The preparation of a parenteral product may be considered to encompass four general areas as follows:

1. Procurement and selection o the components and containers.
2. Production facilities and procedures.
3. Control of quality.
4. Packaging and labeling.

These components of the product to be procured include vehicles, solutes, containers and closures. The steps constituting production include maintaining facilities and equipment, preparing and controlling the environment, cleaning the containers and equipment, preparing the product, filtering the solution, filling containers with the product, sealing the containers and sterilizing the product. The control of quality includes the evaluation of the components, qualification of equipment, validation of processes, determination that the production has been executed within prescribed requirements and performance of necessary evaluative tests on the finished product. The final area of packaging and labeling includes all steps necessary to identify the finished product and enclose it in such manner that it is safely and properly prepared for sale and delivery to the user. The remainder of this chapter will be organized in accord with these four general areas, with emphasis on the first two areas.

Components and Containers

Establishing specifications to ensure the quality of each of the components of an injection is essential. These specifications will be coordinated with the requirements of the specific formulation and will not necessarily be identical for a particular component if used in several different formulations. For example, particle-size control may be necessary for powders used in formulating a suspension but be relatively unimportant for preparing a solution.

The most stringent chemical-purity requirements normally will be encountered with aqueous solutions, particularly if the product is to be sterilized at an elevated temperature where reaction rates will be accelerated greatly. Modification of aqueous vehicles to include a glycol, for example, usually will reduce reaction rates. Dry preparations pose relatively few reaction problems but may require definitive physical specifications for ingredients that must have certain solution or dispersion characteristics when a vehicle is added.

Containers and closures are in prolonged, intimate contact with the product and may release substances into or remove ingredients from the product. Assessment and selection of containers and closures is a necessary part of product formulation to ensure that the product retains its purity, potency and quality during the intimate contact with the container throughout its shelf-life. Administration devices that come in contact with the product should be assessed and selected with the same care as are containers and closures, even though the contact period is usually brief.

Vehicles

Since most liquid injections are quite dilute, the component present in the highest proportion is the vehicle. A vehicle normally has no therapeutic activity and is nontoxic. However, it is of great importance in the formulation since it presents to body tissues the form of the active constituent for absorption. Absorption normally occurs most rapidly and completely when a drug is presented as an aqueous solution. Modification of the vehicle with water-miscible liquids or substitution with water-immiscible liquids normally decreases the rate of absorption. Absorption from a suspension may be affected by such factors as the viscosity of the vehicle, its capacity for wetting the solid particles, the solubility equilibrium produced by the vehicle and the distribution coefficient between the vehicle and aqueous body systems.

The vehicle of greatest importance for parenteral products is water. Water of suitable quality for compounding and rinsing product contact surfaces may be prepared either by distillation or by reverse osmosis, to meet USP specifications for Water for Injection (WFI). Only by these two methods is it possible to separate adequately various liquid, gas and solid contaminating substances from water. These two methods for preparation of WFI will be discussed in this Chapter. It should be noted that there is no unit operation more important and none more costly to install and operate than the one for the preparation of WFI.

Preparation of Water for Injection (WFI)

The source water can be expected to be contaminated with natural suspended mineral and organic substances, dissolved mineral salts, colloidal silicates and industrial chemicals. The degree of contamination will vary with the source and will be markedly different whether obtained from a well or from surface sources, such as a stream or lake. Therefore, this water normally is not of sufficient purity to prepare WFI directly. Hence, the source water usually must be pretreated by one or a combination of the following treatments: chemical softening, filtration, deionization, carbon adsorption or reverse osmosis purification. Space does not permit discussion of these processes here, but the interested reader is referred elsewhere for this information.[5,6]

In general, a conventional still consists of a boiler (evaporator) containing feed water (distilland); a source of heat to vaporize the water in the evaporator; a headspace above the level of distilland with condensing surfaces for refluxing the vapor, thereby returning nonvolatile impurities to the distilland, a means for eliminating volatile impurities before the hot water vapor is condensed; and a condenser for removing the heat of vaporization, thereby converting the water vapor to a liquid distillate.

The specific construction features of a still and the process specifications markedly will affect the quality of distillate obtained from a still. Those required for producing high-purity water, such as WFI, must be considerably more stringent than those required for Purified Water USP. Among the factors that must be considered are:

1. The quality of the feed water will affect the quality of the distillate. Controlling the quality of the feed water is essential for meeting the required specifications for the distillate.
2. The size of the evaporator will affect the efficiency. It should be large enough to provide a low vapor velocity, thus reducing the entrainment of the distilland either as a film on vapor bubbles or as separate droplets.
3. The baffles (condensing surfaces) determine the effectiveness of refluxing. They should be designed to remove efficiently the entrainment at optimal vapor velocity, collecting and returning the heavier droplets contaminated with the distilland.
4. Redissolving volatile impurities in the distillate reduces its purity. Therefore, they should be separated efficiently from the hot water vapor and eliminated by aspirating them to the drain or venting them to the atmosphere.
5. Contamination of the vapor and distillate from the metal parts of the still can occur. Present standards for high-purity stills are that all parts contacted by the vapor or distillate should be constructed of metal coated with pure tin, 304 or 316 stainless steel or chemically resistant glass.

The design features of a still also influence its efficiency of operation, relative freedom from maintenance problems or extent of automatic operation. Stills may be constructed of varying size, rated according to the volume of distillate that can be produced per hour of operation under optimum conditions. Only stills designed to produce high-purity water may be considered for use in the production of WFI.

Conventional commercial stills designed for the production of high-purity water, such as shown in Fig 1, are available from several suppliers (*AMSCO, Barnstead, Corning, Vaponics*).

Compression Distillation—The vapor-compression still, primarily designed for the production of large volumes of high-purity distillate with low consumption of energy and water, is illustrated diagrammatically in Fig 2. To start, the feed water is heated in the evaporator to boiling. The vapor produced in the tubes is separated from the entrained distilland in the separator and conveyed to a compressor which compresses the vapor and raises its temperature to approximately 107°. It then flows to the steam chest where it condenses on the outer surfaces of the tubes containing the distilland; thereby the vapor is condensed and drawn off as a distillate while giving up its heat to bring the distilland in the tubes to the boiling point.

Vapor-compression stills are available in capacities from 50 to 2800 gal/hr (*Aqua-Chem, Barnstead, Meco*).

Multiple-Effect Stills—The multiple-effect still also is designed to conserve energy and water usage. In principle, it is simply a series of single-effect stills running at differing pressures. A series of up to seven effects may be used, with the first effect operated at the highest pressure and the last effect at atmospheric pressure. See a schematic drawing of a multiple-effect still in Fig. 3. Steam from an external source is used in the first effect to generate steam under pressure from feed water; it is used as the power source to drive the second effect. The steam used to drive the second effect condenses as it gives up its heat of vaporization and forms a distillate. This process continues until the last effect when the steam is at atmospheric pressure and must be condensed in a heat exchanger.

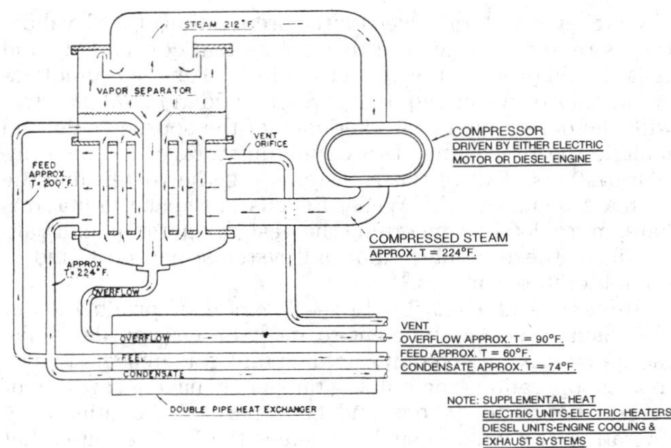

Fig 2. Vapor-compression still.

The capacity of a multiple-effect still can be increased by adding effects. The quantity of the distillate also will be affected by the inlet steam pressure; thus, a 600-gal/hr unit designed to operate at 115 psig steam pressure could be run at approximately 55 psig and would deliver about 400 gal/hr. These stills have no moving parts and operate quietly. They are available in capacities from about 50 to 7000 gal/hr (*AMSCO, Barnstead, Finn-Aqua, Vaponics*).

Reverse Osmosis (RO)—As the name suggests, the natural process of selective permeation of molecules through a semipermeable membrane separating two aqueous solutions of different concentrations is reversed. Pressure, usually between 200 and 400 psig, is applied to overcome osmotic pressure and force pure water to premeate through the membrane. Membranes, usually composed of cellulose esters or polyamides, are selected to provide an efficient rejection of contaminant molecules in raw water. The molecules most difficult to remove are small inorganic ones such as sodium chloride. Passage through two membranes in series is sometimes used to increase the efficiency of removal of these small molecules and to decrease the risk of structural failure of a membrane to remove other contaminants, such as bacteria and pyrogens. For additional information, see *Reverse Osmosis* in Chapter 37 and *Water* in Chapters 80 and 86.

Reverse osmosis systems are available in a range of production sizes. (*AMSCO, Aqua-Chem, Finn-Aqua, Meco, Millipore*, etc).

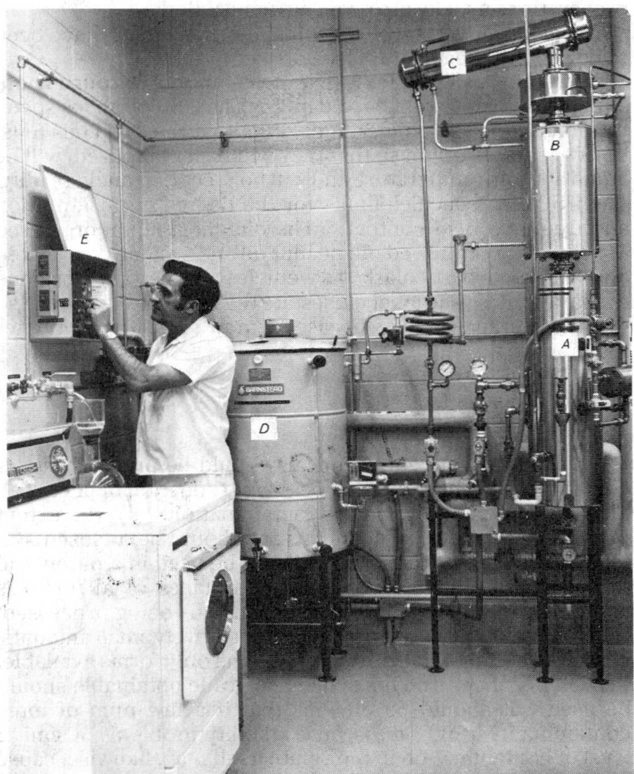

Fig 1. High-purity stilled and sealed water-storage system. *A:* evaporator; *B:* high-purity baffle unit; *C:* condenser; *D:* storage tank with ultraviolet lamp; *E:* control panel (courtesy, Ciba-Geigy).

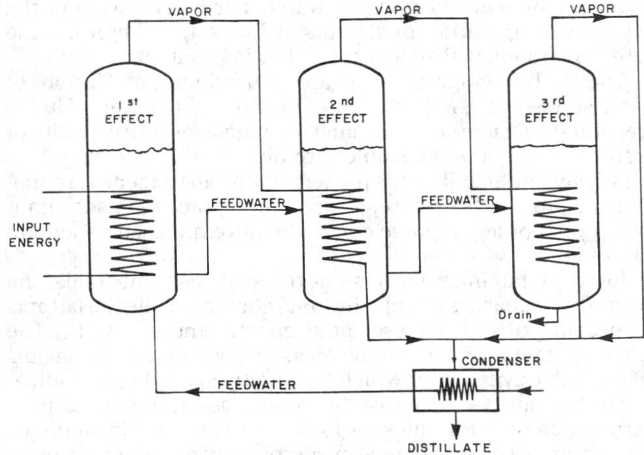

Fig 3. Multiple-effect still. (courtesy, Dekker); taken from Avis KE, Lieberman HA, Lachman L; *Pharmaceutical Dosage Forms: Parenteral Medications,* vol 2, 2nd ed, Dekker, New York, 1993.

Whichever system is used for the preparation of WFI, validation is required to be sure that the system consistently and reliably will produce the chemical, physical and microbiological quality of water required. Such validation should start with the determined characteristics of the source water and include the pretreatment, production, storage and distribution systems. All of these systems together determine the ultimate quality of the WFI. Because of space limitations here, more details concerning the design, operation and validation of these highly important systems may be found in other literature sources.[5,6]

Storage and Distribution—The rate of production of WFI usually is not sufficient to meet processing demands; therefore, it is collected in a holding tank for subsequent use. In large operations the holding tanks may have a capacity of several thousand gallons and be a part of a continuously operating system. In such instances the USP requires that the WFI be held at a temperature too high for microbial growth to occur. Normally, this temperature is a constant 80°.

The USP also permits the WFI to be stored at room temperature, but for a maximum of 24 hours. Under such conditions the WFI usually is collected as a batch for a particular use with any unused water being discarded within 24 hours. Such a system requires frequent sanitization to minimize the risk of viable microorganisms being present. The stainless-steel storage tanks in such systems usually are connected to a welded stainless-steel distribution loop supplying the various use sites with a continuously circulating water supply. The tank is provided with a hydrophobic membrane vent filter capable of excluding bacteria and nonviable particulate matter. Such a vent filter is necessary to permit changes in pressure during filling and emptying. The construction material for the tank and connecting lines is usually electropolished 316L stainless steel with welded pipe. The tanks also may be lined with glass or a coating of pure tin. Such systems are very carefully designed and constructed and often constitute the most costly installation within the plant.

When the water cannot be used at 80°, heat exchangers must be installed to reduce the temperature at the point of use. Bacterial retentive filters should not be installed in such systems because of the risk of bacterial buildup on the filters and the consequential release of pyrogenic substances.

Purity—The USP monographs provide standards of purity for WFI and Sterile Water for Injection (SWFI). A few of these standards require comment.

SWFI must meet the requirements of the USP Sterility Test, but WFI need not since it is to be used in a product which will be sterilized. Both must contain not more than 0.25 Endotoxin units per mL.

The limits for total solids varies in the two monographs. The larger the surface area of the glass container per unit volume of water, the greater the amount of glass constituents that may be leached into the water, particularly during the elevated temperature of steam sterilization. Therefore, the latter treatment will affect the total solids content of SWFI.

The WFL monograph stipulates a maximum of 10 ppm of total solids but SWFI may contain 20 to 40 ppm. This is generally considered to be much too high to assure a quality of water that permits the stable formulation of many drugs. A relatively few metallic ions present often can render a formulation unstable. Therefore, it is common practice to set a limit of 0.1 ppm or less of ionic contaminants expressed as sodium chloride.

Ionic contaminant level is not the same as total solids; the former is a measure of only the ionic content, while the latter is a measure of the undissociated constituents as well. The ionic content of water can be measured very easily by means of a conductivity meter which frequently is used as an indicator of the purity. The results are expressed in one of three terms: as sodium chloride ions, as resistance in ohms or megohms or as conductance in micromhos (or microSiemens). Ohms and mhos have a reciprocal relationship to each other, but they are related to ppm sodium chloride by an experimentally determined curve. The USP is considering introducing a conductivity requirement. To give one point of comparison, 0.1 ppm sodium chloride is equal to approximately 1.01 megohms and 0.99 micromhos. It should be mentioned that conductivity measurements give no direct indication of pyrogen content since pyrogens are undissociated organic compounds.

WFI and SWFI may not contain added substances. Bacteriostatic Water for Injection (BWFI) may contain one or more suitable antimicrobial agents in containers of 30 mL or less. This restriction is designed to prevent the administration of a large quantity of a bacteriostatic agent that probably would be toxic in the accumulated amount of a large volume of solution, even though the concentration was low.

The USP also provides monographs giving the specifications for Sterile Water for Inhalation and Sterile Water for Irrigation. The USP should be consulted for the minor differences between these specifications and those for SWFI.

Types of Vehicles

Aqueous Vehicles—Certain aqueous vehicles are recognized officially because of their valid use in parenterals. Often they are used as isotonic vehicles to which a drug may be added at the time of administration. The additional osmotic effect of the drug may not be enough to produce any discomfort when administered. These vehicles include Sodium Chloride Injection, Ringer's Injection, Dextrose Injection, Dextrose and Sodium Chloride Injection and Lactated Ringer's Injection.

Water-Miscible Vehicles—A number of solvents that are miscible with water have been used as a portion of the vehicle in the formulation of parenterals. These solvents are used primarily to affect the solubility of certain drugs and to reduce hydrolysis. The most important solvents in this group are ethyl alcohol, polyethylene glycol and propylene glycol. Ethyl alcohol is used particularly in the preparation of solutions of cardiac glycosides and the glycols in solutions of barbiturates, certain alkaloids and certain antibiotics. Such preparations usually are given intramuscularly.

These solvents, as well as nonaqueous vehicles, have been reviewed by Spiegel and Noseworthy.[7]

Nonaqueous Vehicles—The most important group of nonaqueous vehicles are the fixed oils. The USP provides specifications for such vehicles, indicating that the fixed oils must be of vegetable origin so that they will be metabolized, will be liquid at room temperature and will not become rancid readily. The USP also specifies limits for the degree of unsaturation and free fatty acid content. The oils most commonly used are corn oil, cottonseed oil, peanut oil and sesame oil. Fixed oils are used particularly as vehicles for certain hormone preparations. The label must state the name of the vehicle so that the user may beware in case of known sensitivity or other reactions to it.

Solutes

Bulk pharmaceutical chemicals should be prepared under conditions designed to preclude the introduction of chemical, physical and microbiological contamination. To the extent possible, the system of manufacture should be a closed system, particularly if the chemical is to be used in a parenteral formulation. Further, the contact surfaces of all process equipment should be inert to the chemicals being processed. Where the chemicals are to be used in relatively small amounts, marketed commercial grades may be the only forms available. In such instances, the best chemical grade obtainable should be used. It should be obvious that if a few ppm of ionic contaminants in WFI may cause stability problems, a similar level of contamination in the solute itself may, likewise, cause stability problems. Metallic catalysis of chemical reactions is one which is encountered frequently.

Other factors to be considered with respect to the quality of solutes include the level of microbial and pyrogenic contamination, solubility characteristics as determined by the chemical or physical form of the compound and freedom from gross dirt.

Added Substances—The USP includes in this category all substances added to a preparation to improve or safeguard its quality. An added substance may:

Effect solubility, as does sodium benzoate in Caffeine and Sodium Benzoate Injection.

Provide patient comfort, as do substances added to make a solution isotonic.

Enhance the chemical stability of a solution, as do antioxidants, inert gases, chelating agents and buffers.

Protect a preparation against the growth of microorganisms. The term "preservative" sometimes is applied only to those substances which prevent the growth of microoganisms in a preparation. However, such limited use is inappropriate, being better used for all substances that act to retard or prevent the chemical, physical or biological degradation of a preparation.

While added substances may prevent a certain reaction from taking place, they may induce others. Not only may visible incompatibilities occur, but hydrolysis, complexation, oxidation and invisible reactions may decompose or otherwise inactivate the therapeutic agent or other added substances. Therefore, added substances must be selected with due consideration and investigation of their effect on the total formulation.

Antimicrobial Agents—The USP states that antimicrobial agents in bacteriostatic or fungistatic concentrations must be added to preparations contained in multiple-dose containers. They must be present in adequate concentration at the time of use to prevent the multiplication of microorganisms inadvertently introduced into the preparation while withdrawing a portion of the contents with a hypodermic needle and syringe. The USP provides a test for *Antimicrobial Preservative Effectiveness* to determine that an antimicrobial substance or combination adequately inhibits the growth of microorganisms in a parenteral product. Because antimicrobials may have inherent toxicity for the patient, the USP prescribes concentration limits for those that are used commonly in parenteral products, as follows:

Phenylmercuric nitrate and thimerosal 0.01%.
Benzethonium chloride and benzalkonium chloride 0.01%.
Phenol or cresol 0.5%.
Chlorobutanol 0.5%.

The above limit is rarely used for phenylmercuric nitrate, most frequently being employed in a concentration of 0.002%. Methyl *p*-hydroxybenzoate 0.18% and propyl *p*-hydroxybenzoate 0.02% in combination, and benzyl alcohol 2% also are used frequently. In oleaginous preparations, no antibacterial agent commonly employed appears to be effective. However, it has been reported that hexylresorcinol 0.5% and phenylmercuric benzoate 0.1% are moderately bactericidal. A few therapeutic compounds have been shown to have antibacterial activity, thus obviating the need for added agents.

Antimicrobial agents must be studied with respect to compatibility with all other components of the formula. In addition, their activity must be evaluated in the total formula. It is not uncommon to find that a particular agent will be effective in one formulation but ineffective in another. This may be due to the effect of various components of the formula on the biological activity or availability of the compound; for example, the binding and inactivation of esters of *p*-hydroxybenzoic acid by macromolecules such as Polysorbate 80 or the reduction of phenylmercuric nitrate by sulfide residues in rubber closures. A physical reaction encountered is that bacteriostatic agents sometimes are removed from solution by rubber closures.

Single-dose containers and pharmacy bulk packs which do not contain antimicrobial agents are expected to be used promptly after opening or to be discarded. Large-volume single-dose containers may not contain an added antimicrobial preservative. Therefore, special care must be exercised in storing such products after the containers have been opened to prepare an admixture, particularly those that can support the growth of microorganisms, such as total parenteral nutrition (TPN) solutions. It should be noted that while refrigeration slows the growth of most microorganisms, it does not prevent their growth.

Buffers are used primarily to stabilize a solution against the chemical degradation that might occur if the pH changes appreciably. Buffer systems employed should normally have as low a buffer capacity as feasible in order not to disturb significantly the body buffer systems when injected. In addition, the buffer range and effect on the activity of the product must be evaluated carefully. The acid salts most frequently employed as buffers are citrates, acetates and phosphates.

Antioxidants are required frequently to preserve products because of the ease with which many drugs are oxidized. Sodium bisulfite 0.1% is used most frequently. The use of sulfites has been reviewed by Schroeter.[8] Acetone sodium bisulfite, sodium formaldehyde sulfoxylate and thiourea also are used sometimes. The sodium salt of ethylenediaminetetraacetic acid has been found to enhance the activity of antioxidants in some cases, apparently by chelating metallic ions that would otherwise catalyze the oxidation reaction.

Displacing the air (oxygen) in and above the solution by purging with an inert gas, such as nitrogen, also can be used as a means to control oxidation of a sensitive drug. Process control is required to be assured that every container is deaerated adequately and uniformly.

Tonicity Agents are used in many parenteral and ophthalmic products to control the tonicity. However, not all preparations need to be isotonic. The agents most commonly used are electrolytes and mono- or disaccharides. This subject is considered much more extensively in Chapter 36.

Pyrogens (Endotoxins)

Pyrogens are products of metabolism of microorganisms. The most potent pyrogenic substances (endotoxins) are constituents of the cell wall of Gram-negative bacteria. Gram-positive bacteria and fungi also produce pyrogens but of lower potency and of different chemical nature. Endotoxins are high-molecular-weight (about 20,000 daltons) lipopolysaccharides. Studies have shown that the lipid portion of the molecule is responsible for the biological activity. Since endotoxins are the most potent pyrogens and Gram-negative bacteria are ubiquitous in the environment, this discussion will focus on endotoxins and the risk of their presence as contaminants in sterile products.

Pyrogens, when present in parenteral drug products and injected into patients, can cause fever, chills, pain in the back and legs, and malaise. While pyrogenic reactions are rarely fatal, they can cause serious discomfort and, in the seriously ill patient, shock-like symptoms that can be fatal. The intensity of the pyrogenic response and its degree of hazard will be affected by the medical condition of the patient, the potency of the pyrogen, the amount of the pyrogen and the route of administration (intrathecal is most hazardous followed by intravenous, intramuscular and subcutaneous). When bacterial (exogenous) pyrogens are introduced into the body, leucocytic phagocytosis is believed to occur and endogenous pyrogen is produced. The endogenous pyrogen then produces the familiar physiological effects. Space will not permit further elaboration of these matters here, but the reader is referred to the work by Pearson[9] if more information is needed.

Control of Pyrogens—Pyrogens are contaminants if present in parenteral drug products, and should not be there. In general, it is impractical, if not impossible, to remove pyrogens once present without adversely affecting the drug product. Therefore, the emphasis should be on the prevention of the introduction or development of pyrogens in all aspects of the compounding and processing of the product.

Pyrogens may enter a preparation through any means that will introduce living or dead microorganisms. However, current technology generally permits the control of such contamination, and the presence of pyrogens in a finished product is indicative of processing under inadequately controlled clean conditions. It also should be noted that time for microbial growth to occur increases the risk for elevated levels of pyrogens. Therefore, compounding and manufacturing processes should be carried out as expeditiously as possible, preferably planning completion of the process, including sterilization, within one work day.

Pyrogens can be destroyed by heating at high temperatures. The recommended procedure for depyrogenation of glassware and equipment is heating at a temperature of 250° for 45 minutes. It has been reported that 650° for 1 minute or 180° for 4 hours likewise will destroy pyrogens. The usual autoclaving cycle will not do so. Heating with strong alkali or oxidizing solutions will destroy pyrogens. It has been claimed that thorough washing with detergent will render glassware pyrogen-free if subsequently rinsed thoroughly with pyrogen-free water. Plastic containers and devices must be protected from pyrogenic contamination during manufacture and storage since known ways to destroy pyrogens will affect the plastic adversely. It has been reported that anion-exchange resins and positively charged membrane filters will remove pyrogens from water. Also, reverse osmosis will eliminate them. However, the most reliable method for their elimination from water is distillation.

A method that has been used for the removal of pyrogens from solutions is adsorption on adsorptive agents. However, since the adsorption phenomenon also may cause selective removal of chemical substances from the solution, this method has limited application. Other in-process methods for their destruction or elimination include selective extraction procedures and careful heating with dilute alkali, dilute acid or mild oxidizing agents. In each instance, the method must be studied thoroughly to be sure it will not have an adverse effect on the constituents of the product. Developments in ultrafiltration now make possible pyrogen separation on a molecular weight basis and the process of tangential flow is making large-scale processing a reality.

Sources of Pyrogens—Through understanding the means by which pyrogens may contaminate parenteral products, their control becomes more achievable. Therefore, it is important to know that water is probably the greatest potential source of pyrogenic contamination, since water is essential for the growth of microorganisms. When microorganisms metabolize, pyrogens will be produced. Therefore, raw water can be expected to be pyrogenic and only when it is appropriately treated to render it free from pyrogens, such as WFI, should it be used for compounding the product or rinsing product contact surfaces such as tubing, mixing vessels and rubber closures. Even when such rinsed equipment and supplies are left wet and improperly exposed to the environment, there is a high risk that they will become pyrogenic. As stated previously, although proper distillation will provide pyrogen-free water, storage conditions must be such that microorganisms are not introduced and subsequent growth is prevented.

Other potential sources of contamination are containers and equipment. Pyrogenic materials adhere strongly to glass and other surfaces. Residues of solutions in used equipment often become bacterial cultures with subsequent pyrogenic contamination. Since drying does not destroy pyrogens, they may remain in equipment for long periods. Adequate washing will reduce and subsequent dry-heat treatment can render contaminated equipment suitable for use. However, all such processes must be validated to assure their effectiveness.

Solutes may be a source of pyrogens. For example, the manufacturing of bulk chemicals may involve the use of pyrogenic water for process steps such as crystallization, precipitation or washing. Bulk drug substances derived from fermentation will almost certainly be heavily pyrogenic. Therefore, all lots of solutes used to prepare parenteral products should be tested to ensure that they will not contribute unacceptable quantities of endotoxin to the finished product.

The manufacturing process must be carried out with great care and as rapidly as possible to minimize the risk of microbial contamination. Preferably, no more product should be prepared than can be processed, completely within one working day, including sterilization.

Containers

Containers are an integral part of the formulation of an injection. No container is totally insoluble or does not in some way affect the liquid it contains, particularly if the liquid is aqueous. Therefore, the selection of a container for a particular injection must be based on a consideration of the composition of the container, as well as of the solution, and the treatment to which it will be subjected.

Table 1 provides a generalized comparison of the three compatibility properties—leaching, permeation and adsorption—of container materials most likely to be involved in the formulation of aqueous parenterals. Further, the integrity of the container/closure system depends upon several characteristics, including container opening finish, closure modulus, durometer and compression set, and aluminum seal application force. These considerations have been reviewed by Morton.[10]

Table 1—Comparative Compatibility Properties of Container Materials

	Leaching		Permeation		Adsorption (selective) extent[a]
	Extent[a]	Potential leachables	Extent[a]	Potential agents	
Glass					
Borosilicate	1	Alkaline earth and heavy metal oxides	0	N/A	2
Soda-lime	5	Alkaline earth and heavy metal oxides	0	N/A	2
Plastic polymers					
Polyethylene					
Low density	2	Plasticizers, antioxidants	5	Gases, water vapor, other molecules	2
High density	1	Antioxidants	3	Gases, water vapor, other molecules	2
PVC	4	HCl, especially plasticizers, antioxidants, other stabilizers	5	Gases, especially water vapor and other molecules	2
Polyolefins	2	Antioxidants	2	Gases, water vapor, other molecules	2
Polypropylene	2	Antioxidants, lubricants	4	Gases, water vapor	1
Rubber polymers					
Natural and related synthetic	5	Heavy metal salts, lubricants, reducing agents	3	Gases, water vapor	3
Butyl	3	Heavy metal salts, lubricants, reducing agents	1	Gases, water vapor	2
Silicone	2	Minimal	5	Gases, water vapor	1

[a] Approximate scale of 1 to 5 with "1" as the lowest.

Plastic

Thermoplastic polymers have been established as packaging materials for sterile preparations such as large-volume parenterals, ophthalmic solutions and, increasingly, for small-volume parenterals. For such use to be acceptable a thorough understanding of the characteristics, potential problems and advantages for use must be developed. A historical review of these factors relative to pharmaceuticals has been prepared by Autian.[11] A recent discussion of polymers for IV solutions has been published by Lambert.[12] Autian stated that three principal problem areas exist in using these materials; namely,

1. Permeation of vapors and other molecules in either direction through the wall of the plastic container.
2. Leaching of constituents from the plastic into the product.
3. Sorption (absorption and/or adsorption) of drug molecules or ions on the plastic material.

Permeation, the most extensive problem, may be troublesome by permitting volatile constituents, water or selected drug molecules to migrate through the wall of the container to the outside and thereby be lost. This problem has been resolved, for example, by the use of an overwrap in the packaging of IV solutions in PVC bags to prevent the loss of water during storage. Reverse permeation also may occur by which oxygen or other molecules may penetrate to the inside of the container and cause oxidative or other degradation of susceptible constituents. Leaching may be a problem when certain constituents in the plastic formulation, such as plasticizers or antioxidants, migrate into the product. Thus, plastic polymer formulations should have as few additives as possible, an objective characteristically achievable for most plastics being used for parenteral packaging. *Sorption* is a problem on a selective basis, that is, sorption of a few drug molecules occurs on select polymers. For example, sorption of insulin, vitamin A acetate and warfarin sodium has been shown to occur on PVC bags and tubing when these drugs were present as additives in IV admixtures. A brief summary of some of these compatibility relationships is given in Table 1.

One of the principle advantages of using plastic packaging materials is that they are not breakable as is glass; also, there is a substantial weight reduction. The flexibility of the low-density polyethylene polymer, for ophthalmic preparations, makes it possible to squeeze the side wall of the container and discharge one or more drops without introducing contamination into the remainder of the product. The flexible bags of polyvinyl chloride or select polyolefins, currently in use for large-volume intravenous fluids, have the added advantage that no air interchange is required; the flexible wall simply collapses as the solution flows out of the bag.

Most plastic materials have the disadvantage that they are not as clear as glass and, therefore, inspection of the contents is impeded. In addition, many of these materials will soften or melt under the conditions of thermal sterilization. However, careful selection of the plastic used and control of the autoclave cycle has made thermal sterilization of some products possible, large-volume parenterals in particular. Ethylene oxide or radiation sterilization may be employed for the empty container with subsequent aseptic filling. However, careful evaluation of the residues from ethylene oxide or its degradation products and their potential toxic effect must be undertaken. Investigation is required concerning potential interactions and other problems that may be encountered when a parenteral product is packaged in plastic. For further details see Chapter 85.

Glass

Glass is employed as the container material of choice for most SVPs. It is composed principally of silicon dioxide with varying amounts of other oxides such as sodium, potassium, calcium, magnesium, aluminum, boron and iron. The basic structural network of glass is formed by the silicon oxide tetrahedron. Boric oxide will enter into this structure, but most of the other oxides do not. The latter are only loosely bound, are present in the network interstices and are relatively free to migrate. These migratory oxides may be leached into a solution in contact with the glass, particularly during the increased reactivity of thermal sterilization. The oxides thus dissolved may hydrolyze to raise the pH of the solution, catalyze reactions or enter into reactions. Additionally, some glass compounds will be attacked by solutions and, in time, dislodge glass flakes into the solution. Such occurrences can be minimized by the proper selection of the glass composition.[13]

Types—The USP has aided in this selection by providing a classification of glass; namely,

Type I, a borosilicate glass.
Type II, a soda-lime treated glass.
Type III, a soda-lime glass.
NP, a soda-lime glass not suitable for containers for parenterals.

Type I glass is composed principally of silicon dioxide and boric oxide, with low levels of the non-network-forming oxides. It is a chemically resistant glass (low leachability) also having a low thermal coefficient of expansion.

Types II and III glass compounds are composed of relatively high proportions of sodium oxide and calcium oxide. This makes the glass chemically less resistant. Both types melt at a lower temperature, are easier to mold into various shapes and have a higher thermal coefficient of expansion than Type I. While there is no one standard formulation for glass among manufacturers of these USP type categories, Type II glass usually has a lower concentration of the migratory oxides than Type III. In addition, Type II has been treated under controlled temperature and humidity conditions with sulfur dioxide to dealkalize the interior surface of the container. While it remains intact, this surface will increase substantially the chemical resistance of the glass. However, repeated exposures to sterilization and alkaline detergents will break down this dealkalized surface and expose the underlying soda-lime compound.

The glass types are determined from the results of two USP tests: the Powdered Glass Test and the Water Attack Test. The latter is used only for Type II glass and is performed on the whole container, because of the dealkalized surface; the former is performed on powdered glass, which exposes internal surfaces of the glass compound. The results are based upon the amount of alkali titrated by 0.02 *N* sulfuric acid after an autoclaving cycle with the glass sample in contact with a high-purity distilled water. Thus, the *Powdered Glass Test* challenges the leaching potential of the interior structure of the glass while the *Water Attack Test* challenges only the intact surface of the container.

Selecting the appropriate glass composition is a critical facet of determining the overall specifications for each parenteral formulation.

In general, Type I glass will be suitable for all products, although sulfur dioxide treatment sometimes is used for a further increase in resistance. Because cost must be considered, one of the other less expensive types may be acceptable. Type II glass may be suitable, for example, for a solution which is buffered, has a pH below 7 or is not reactive with the glass. Type III glass usually will be suitable principally for anhydrous liquids or dry substances. However, some manufacturer-to-manufacturer variation in glass composition should be anticipated within each glass type. Therefore, for highly chemically sensitive parenteral formulations it may be necessary to specify both USP Type and a specific manufacturer.

Physical Characteristics—Some of the physical shapes of glass ampuls and vials are illustrated in Fig 3. Commerically available containers vary in size from 0.5 to 1000 mL. Sizes up to 100 mL may be obtained as ampuls and vials, and larger sizes as bottles. The latter are used mostly for intravenous and irrigating solutions. Smaller sizes are also available as cartridges. Ampuls and cartridges are drawn from glass tubing. The smaller vials may be made by mold-

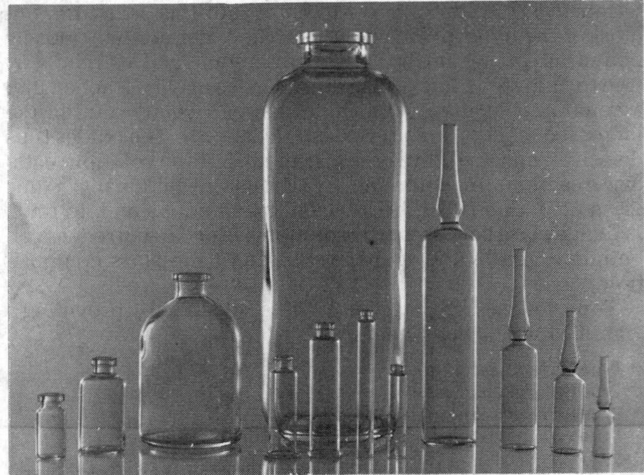

Fig 4. Various types of ampuls and multiple-dose vials for parenterals (courtesy, Kimble).

ing or from tubing. Larger vials and bottles are made only by molding. Containers made by drawing tubing are generally optically clearer and have a thinner wall than molded containers (see Fig 4). Molded containers are uniform in external dimensions, stronger and heavier.

Easy-opening ampuls that permit the user to break off the tip at the neck constriction without the use of a file are weakened at the neck by scoring or applying a ceramic paint having a different coefficient of thermal expansion. An example of a modification of container design to meet a particular need is the double-chambered vial, under the name Univial (*Univial*), designed to contain a freeze-dried product in the lower and solvent in the upper chamber. Other examples are wide-mouth ampuls with flat or rounded bottoms to facilitate filling with dry materials or suspensions, and various modifications of the cartridge for use with disposable dosage units.

Glass containers must be strong enough to withstand the physical shocks of handling and shipping and the pressure differentials that develop, particularly during the autoclave sterilization cycle. They must be able to withstand the thermal shock resulting from large temperature changes during processing, for example, when the hot bottle and contents are exposed to room air at the end of the sterilization cycle. Therefore, a glass having a low coefficient of thermal expansion is necessary. The container also must be transparent to permit inspection of the contents.

Preparations which are light-sensitive must be protected by placing them in amber glass containers or by enclosing flint glass containers in opaque cartons labeled to remain on the container during the period of use. It should be noted that the amber color of the glass is imparted by the incorporation of potentially leachable heavy metals, mostly iron and manganese, which may act as catalysts for oxidative degradation reactions. Silicone coatings sometimes are applied to containers to produce a hydrophobic surface, for example, as a means of reducing the friction of a rubber-tip of a syringe plunger.

The size of single-dose containers is limited to 1000 mL by the USP and multiple-dose containers to 30 mL, unless stated otherwise in a particular monograph. Multiple-dose vials are limited in size to reduce the number of punctures for withdrawing doses and the accompanying risk of contamination of the contents. As the name implies, single-dose containers are opened with aseptic care and the contents used at one time. These may range in size from 1000-mL bottles to 1-mL or less ampuls, vials or syringes. The integrity of the container is destroyed when opened so that the container cannot be closed again.

A multiple-dose container is designed so that more than one dose can be withdrawn at different times, the container maintaining a seal between uses. It should be evident that with

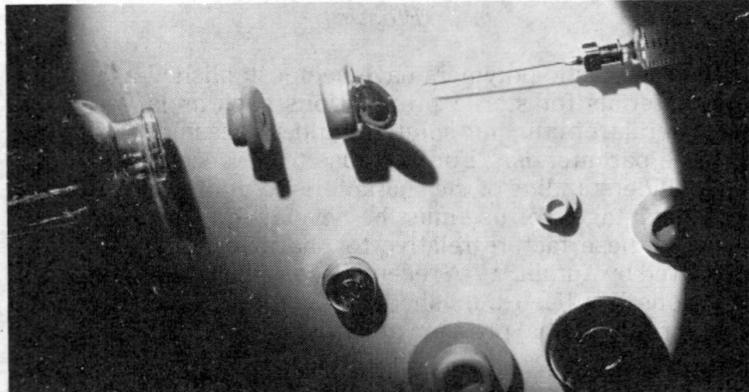

Fig 5. Extended view of scaling components for a multiple-dose vial (courtesy, West).

full aseptic precautions, including sterile syringe and needle for withdrawing the dose and disinfection of the exposed surface of the closure, there is still a substantial risk of introducing contaminating microorganisms and viruses into the contents of the vial. Because of this risk, the USP requires that all multiple-dose vials must contain an antimicrobial agent or be inherently antimicrobial, as determined by the USP *Antimicrobial Preservatives-Effectiveness* tests. There are no comparable antiviral effectiveness tests, nor are antiviral agents available for such use. In spite of the advantagious flexibility of dosage provided by multiple-dose vials, single-dose, disposable container units provide the clear advantage of greater sterility assurance and patient safety.

Rubber Closures

In order to permit introduction of a needle from a hypodermic syringe into a multiple-dose vial and provide for resealing as soon as the needle is withdrawn, each vial is sealed with a rubber closure held in place by an aluminum cap. Figure 5 illustrates how this is done. This principle also is followed for single-dose containers of the cartridge type, except that there is only a single introduction of the needle to make possible the withdrawal or expulsion of the contents.

Rubber closures are composed of multiple ingredients that are plasticized and mixed together at an elevated temperature on milling machines. Subsequently, the plasticized mixture is placed in molds and vulcanized (cured) under high temperature and pressure. During vulcanization the polymer strands are cross-linked by the vulcanizing agent, assisted by the accelerator and activator, so that motion is restricted and the molded closure acquires the elastic, resilient character required for its use. Ingredients not involved in the cross-linking reactions remain dispersed within the compound and,

Table 2—Examples of Ingredients in Rubber Closures

Ingredient	Examples
Elastomer	Natural rubber (latex) Butyl rubber Neoprene
Vulcanizing (curing) agent	Sulfur Peroxides
Accelerator	Zinc dibutyldithiocarbamate
Activator	Zinc oxide Stearic acid
Antioxidant	Dilauryl thiodipropionate
Plasticizer/lubricant	Paraffinic oil Silicone oil
Fillers	Carbon black Clay Barium sulfate
Pigments	Inorganic oxides Carbon black

along with the degree of curing, affect the properties of the finished closure. Examples of rubber-closure ingredients are given in Table 2.

The physical properties to be considered in the selection of a particular formulation include elasticity, hardness, tendency to fragment and permeability to vapor transfer. The elasticity is critical in establishing a seal with the lip and neck of a vial or other opening, and in resealing after withdrawal of a hypodermic needle from a vial closure. The hardness should provide firmness by not excessive resistance to the insertion of a needle through the closure, while minimal fragmentation of pieces of rubber should occur as the hollow shaft of the needle is pushed through the closure. While vapor transfer occurs to some degree with all rubber formulations, appropriate selection of ingredients makes it possible to control the degree of permeability. Physicochemical and toxicological tests for evaluating rubber closures are described in section ⟨381⟩ in the USP.

The ingredients dispersed throughout the rubber compound may be subject to leaching into the product contacting the closure. These ingredients, examples of which are given in Table 2, pose potential compatibility interactions with product ingredients if leached into the product solution, and these effects must be evaluated.[14,15] Further, some ingredients must be evaluated for potential toxicity. In order to reduce the problem of leachables, attempts have been made to coat the product contact surfaces of closures with various polymers, the most successful being Teflon, or to treat the closures in ways considered trade secrets.

The physical shape of some typical closures may be seen in Fig 5. Most of them have a lip and a protruding flange that extends into the neck of the vial or bottle. Many disk closures are being used now, particularly in the high-speed packaging of antibiotics. Slotted closures are used on freeze-dried products to make it possible to insert the closure part way into the neck of the vial during the drying phase of the cycle. Partial insertion provides limited protection from contamination while permitting water vapor to escape from the drying product. The plunger type is used to seal one end of a cartridge. At the time of use, the plunger expels the product by a needle inserted through the closure at the distal end of the cartridge. Intravenous solution closures often have permanent holes for adapters of administration sets; irrigating solution closures usually are designed for pouring.

Production Facilities

A product having components of the best quality quickly may become totally unacceptable if the environment in which it is processed is contaminated or if the manufacturing procedure is not carried out properly. Therefore, the production facilities and the procedure used in processing the product must meet standards adequate for the task. The nearer these standards approach perfection, the better and safer should be the product.

Arrangement of Area

The production area can be considered in terms of five functional areas: the cleanup area, the compounding area, the aseptic area, the quarantine area and the finishing or packaging area. All of these should be designed and constructed for cleaning ease, appropriate environmental control, efficient operation and personnel comfort. The extra requirements for the aseptic area are designed to provide an environment where, for example, an injection may be exposed to the environment for a brief period during subdivision from a bulk container to the individual-dose containers without becoming contaminated. Contaminants such as dust, lint and microorganisms normally are found floating in the air, lying on counters and other surfaces, on clothing and body surfaces of personnel, in the exhaled breath of personnel and deposited on the floor. The design and control of an aseptic area is directed toward so reducing the presence of these contaminants that they are no longer a hazard to aseptic filling. Although the aseptic area must be adjacent to support areas so that an efficient flow of components may be achieved, barriers must be provided to minimize ingress of contaminants to the critical aseptic area. Such barriers may consist of a variety of forms, including sealed walls, manual or automatic doors, airlock pass-throughs, ports of various types or plastic curtains. Figure 6 shows an example of a floor plan in which the two fill rooms and the staging area constitute the walled critical aseptic area, access to which is only by means of pass-through airlocks. Adjacent support areas (rooms) consist of glass preparation, equipment wash, capping, manufacturing (compounding) and various storage areas. Figure 7 shows an adjacent arrangement with the utilization of a through-the-wall port for passage of a filtrate into the critical aseptic filling room.

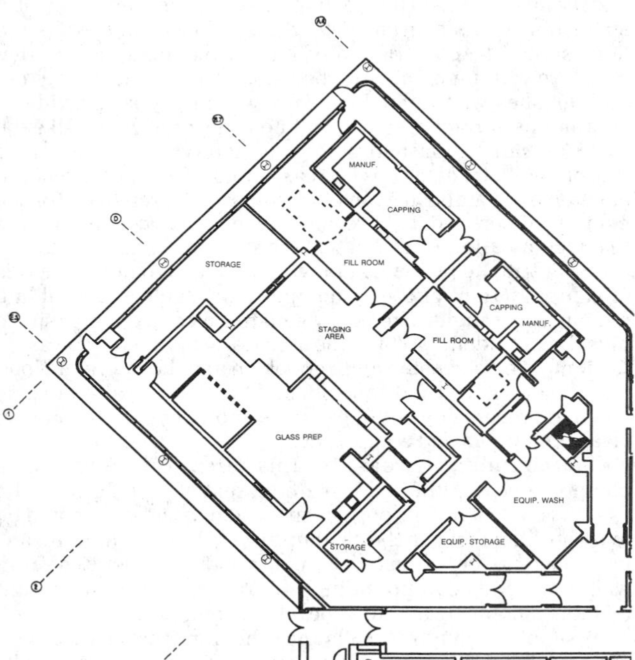

Fig 6. Floor plan of aseptic filling rooms and staging room with adjacent support areas (courtesy, Glaxo).

Flow Plan—In general, the components for a parenteral product flow from the stockroom for released components, either to the compounding area, as for ingredients of the formula, or to the cleanup area, as for containers and equipment. See Fig 8 for a process-flow diagram. After proper processing in these areas, the components flow into the security of the aseptic area for filling of the product in appropriate containers. From there the product passes into the quarantine area where it is held until all necessary tests have been performed. If the product is to be sterilized in its final container, its passage normally is interrupted after leaving the aseptic area for subjection to the sterilization process. After the results from all tests are known and the product has been found to comply with its release specifications, it passes to the finishing area for final labeling and packaging. There sometimes are variations from this flow plan to meet the specific needs of an individual product or to conform to existing facilities. Automated operations convey the components

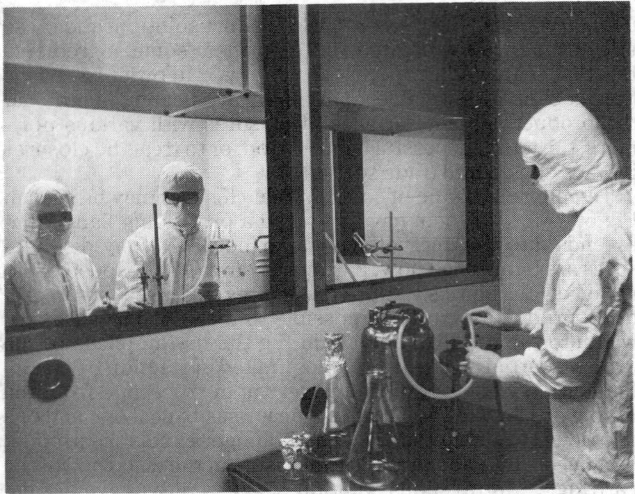

Fig 7. Product filtration from the aseptic staging room through a port into the aseptic filling room (courtesy, The University of Tennessee College of Pharmacy).

from one area to another with little or no handling by operators.

Cleanup Area—The cleanup area is constructed to withstand moisture, steam and detergents. The ceiling, walls and floor should be constructed of impervious materials so that moisture will run off and not be held. One of the "spray-on-tile" finishes with a vinyl or expoxy sealing coat provides a continuous surface free from all holes or crevices. All such surfaces can be washed at regular intervals to keep them thoroughly clean. These areas should be exhausted adequately so that the heat and humidity will be removed for the comfort of personnel. Precautions must be taken to prevent the accumulation of dirt and the growth of microorganisms, especially in the presence of high humidity and heat. In this area preparation for the filling operation, such as assembling equipment, is undertaken. Adequate sink and counter space must be provided. While this area does not need to be aseptic, it must be cleanable and kept clean and the microbial load must be monitored and controlled. Precautions also must be taken to prevent deposit of particles or other contaminants on clean containers and equipment.

Compounding Area—In this area the formula is compounded. Although it is not essential that this area be aseptic, control of microorganisms and particulates should be more stringent than in the cleanup area. For example, means may need to be provided to control dust generated from weighing and compounding operations. Cabinets and counters should, preferably, be constructed of stainless steel. They should fit snugly to walls and other furniture so that there are no catch areas for dirt to accumulate. The ceiling, walls and floor should be constructed similar to those for the cleanup area.

Aseptic Area

This area requires construction features designed for maximum microbial and particulate control. The ceiling, walls and floor must be sealed so that they may be washed and sanitized with a disinfectant, as needed. All counters should be constructed of stainless steel and hung from the wall so that there are no legs to accumulate dirt where they rest on the floor. All light fixtures, utility service lines and ventilation fixtures should be recessed in the walls or ceiling to eliminate ledges, joints and other locations for the accumulation of dust and dirt. As much as possible, tanks containing the compounded product should remain outside the aseptic filling area and the product fed into the area through hose lines. Figure 7 shows such an arrangement. Proper sanitization is required if the tanks must be moved in. Mechanical equipment that is located in the aseptic area should be housed as completely as possible within a stainless-steel cabinet in order to seal the operating parts and their dirt-producing tendencies from the aseptic environment. Mechanical parts that will contact the parenteral product should be demountable so that they can be sterilized.

Personnel entering the aseptic area should enter only through an airlock. They should be attired in sterile coveralls with sterile hats, masks, goggles and foot covers. Movement within the room should be minimal and in-and-out movement rigidly restricted during a filling procedure. The requirements for room preparation and the personnel may be relaxed somewhat if the product is to be sterilized terminally in a sealed container. Some are convinced, however, that it is better to have one standard procedure meeting the most rigid requirements.

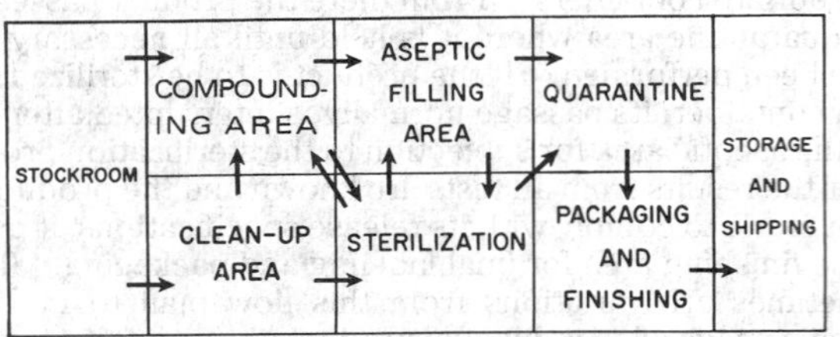

Fig 8. Process-flow diagram.

Air Cleaning

The air in these areas can be one of the greatest sources of contamination. It need not be, however, because several methods are available for providing clean air that is essentially free from dirt particles and microorganisms.

To provide such air, it must be cleaned thoroughly of all contaminants. This may be done by a series of treatments that will vary somewhat from one installation to another. One such series is air from the outside first is passed through a prefilter, usually of glass wool, cloth or shredded plastic, to remove large particles. Then it is treated by passage through an electrostatic precipitator (Suppliers: *Am Air*, *Electro-Air*, *Sturtevant*). Such a unit induces an electrical charge on particles in the air and removes them by attraction to oppositely charged plates. The air then passes through the most efficient cleaning device, a HEPA (high efficiency particulate air) filter having an efficiency of at least 99.97% in removing particles of 0.3 μm and larger, based on the DOP (Dioctyl phthalate) test (Suppliers: *Am Air*, *Cambridge*, *Flanders*).

For personnel comfort, air conditioning and humidity control should be incorporated into the system. Another system, the Kathabar system (*Surface Combustion*), cleans the air of dirt and microorganisms by washing it in an antiseptic solution and, at the same time, controls the humidity. The clean, aseptic air is introduced into the aseptic area and maintained under positive pressure, which prevents outside air from rushing into the aseptic area through cracks, temporarily open doors or other openings.

Laminar-Flow Environments—The required environmental control of aseptic areas has been made possible by the use of laminar airflow enclosures. Laminar airflow provides a total sweep of a confined space because the entire body of air moves with a uniform velocity, usually 90 ft/min, ± 20% along parallel lines, originating through a HEPA filter occupying one entire side of the confined space. Therefore, it bathes the total space with very clean air, sweeping away contaminants.

The arrangement for the direction of airflow can be horizontal (see Fig 9) or vertical (see Fig 10), and may involve a limited area such as a workbench or an entire room.

Figure 10 shows a vial-filling line protected with vertical laminar airflow from ceiling-hung HEPA filters. Plastic curtains are installed to maintain the laminarity of airflow to below the filling line and to circumscribe the critical filling portion of the line. The area outside the curtains can be

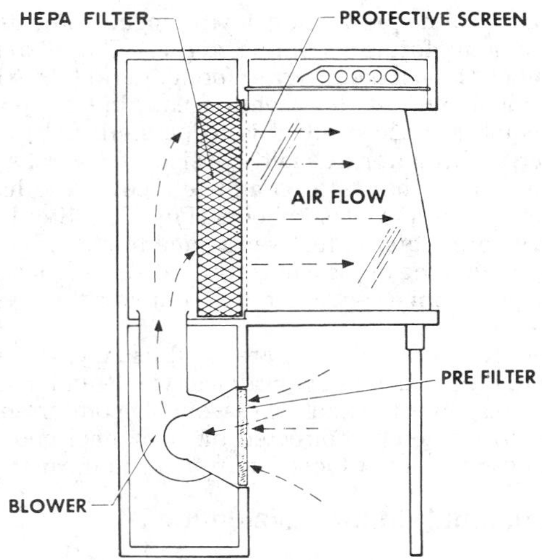

Fig 9. Horizontal laminar-flow workbench (courtesy, adaptation, Sandia).

maintained at a slightly lower level of cleanliness than that inside.

Laminar flow of HEPA-filtered air is capable of meeting the standard for a Class 100 clean room as defined by Federal Standard 209E,[16] which states that such an environment contains no more than 100 particles/ft^3 of 0.5 μm and larger in size. Thus, in Fig 10, the area within the curtains should be a Class 100 environment but the area outside may be Class 10,000 or cleaner, defined on the same basis. Today, it is accepted that critical areas of processing, wherein the product or product contact surfaces may be exposed to the environment, even for a brief period of time, should meet Class 100 clean room standards.

It must be borne in mind that any contamination introduced upstream by equipment, arms of the operator or leaks in the filter will be blown downstream. In the instance of horizontal flow this may be to the critical working site, the face of the operator or across the room. Should the contaminant be, for example, penicillin powder, a biohazard material or viable microorganisms, the danger to the operator is apparent. Further, great care must be exercised to prevent cross-contamination from one operation to another, especially with horizontal laminar air flow. For operations involving such contaminants a vertical system is much more desirable, with the air flowing through perforations in the countertop or through return louvers at floor level, where it can be directed for decontamination. Vertical flow has been recommended for sterility-testing procedures.

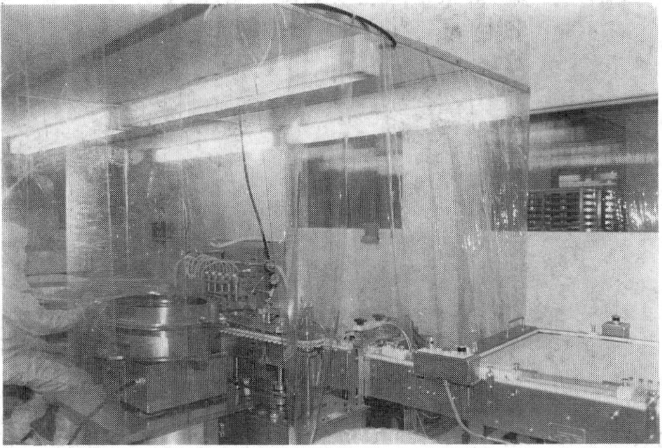

Fig 10. Vial filling line under vertical laminar airflow with critical area enclosed within plastic curtains (courtesy, Merck).

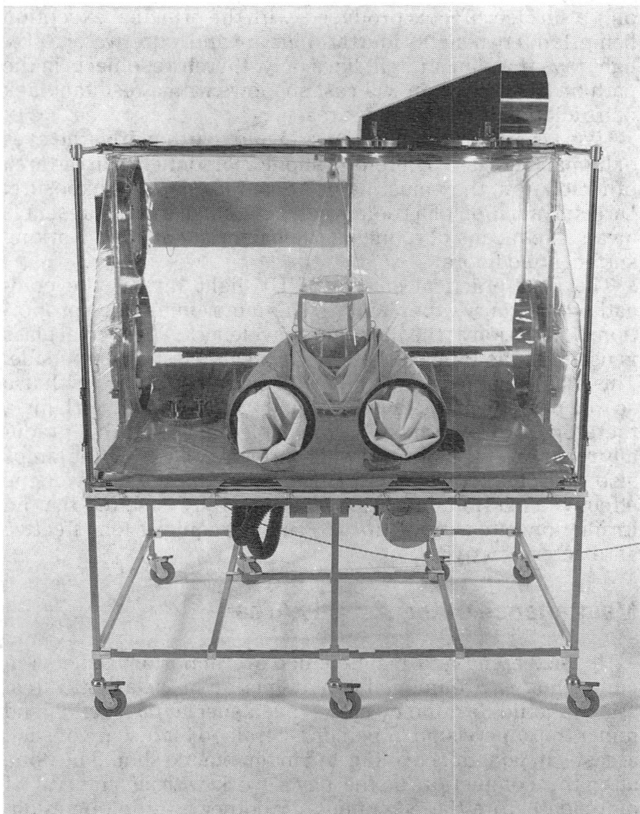

Fig 11. One configuration of an isolator (courtesy, Amsco).

Laminar-flow environments provide well-controlled work areas only if proper precautions are observed. Any reverse air currents or movements exceeding the velocity of the HEPA-filtered airflow may introduce contamination, as may coughing, reaching or other manipulations of operators.

Therefore, laminar-flow work areas should be protected by being located within controlled environments. Personnel should be attired for aseptic processing as described below. All movements and processes should be planned carefully to avoid the introduction of contamination upstream of the critical work area. Checks of the airstream should be performed initially and at regular intervals to be sure no leaks have developed through or around the HEPA filters.

Workbenches and other types of laminar-flow enclosures are available from several commercial sources (Suppliers: *Air Control, Atmos-Tech, Baker, Clean Air, Clestra, EACI/Envirco, Flanders, Laminaire, Liberty, Veco*).

Isolation (barrier) technology is a relatively new approach designed to isolate aseptic operations from personnel. Figure 11 shows the structure of one configuration of an isolator. As can be seen, the operations are performed within transparent, plastic, sealed walls with the operator, in this instance, working through gloves and a half-suit. These isolation work stations are presterilized, usually with peracetic acid or hydrogen peroxide vapor, and sterile supplies are introduced from sterilizing modules through uniquely engineered transfer ports. Results from the use of these units in controlling contamination during sterility testing have reduced false positives to essentially zero. Studies are being undertaken to evaluate these units for aseptic production operations.[17]

Ultraviolet Radiation

Ultraviolet (UV) light rays have an antibacterial action, thereby producing a disinfectant action on directly irradiated surfaces. Since these rays cannot penetrate most materials, only a surface effect is produced, with the principal exception being limited penetration through air and pure water. UV light rays travel in straight lines only; therefore, objects in the path of the light beam will cast shadows with a resultant lack of irradiation in the shadow area.

UV rays are irritating to the skin and, particularly, the eyes of human beings. Therefore, should personnel be in the area of irradiation, they must be protected from direct exposure. Direct irradiation of a room when personnel are not present is a valuable means of reducing the bacterial count on working surfaces and floors.

The best practical source of UV light rays is the cold-cathode mercury vapor lamp. This lamp emits a high proportion of radiation at the 253.7 nm wavelength. A special glass is used for the tube so that the rays will pass to the outside. This glass gradually will change in crystal structure with use so that passage of the rays is gradually reduced. Such lamps, therefore, rarely burn out as do visible-light lamps but gradually reach an emission level which is ineffective. These lamps also must be kept clean, for dust and grease will lower the effective emission drastically. It generally is stated that an irradiation intensity of 20 $\mu w/cm^2$ is required for effective antibacterial activity.

Maintenance of the Aseptic Area

Housekeeping and maintenance are important aspects in controlling environmental contamination in the aseptic area. These should be done by crews given special instruction and under the supervision of personnel trained in the care of such areas. In general, cleaning and maintenance should be done after the completion of the day's work with an interval of quietude before the beginning of another aseptic operation. With the advent of laminar flow of HEPA-filtered air the rigors of cleaning have been reduced since the clean airflow continuously "sweeps" the area clean. All maintenance equipment should be selected for its effectiveness and freedom from lint-producing tendencies and should be reserved for use in aseptic areas only.

Personnel

Personnel selected to work on the preparation of a parenteral product must be neat, orderly and reliable. They should be in good health and free from dermatological conditions that might increase the microbial load. If they show symptoms of a head cold, allergies or similar illness, they should not be permitted in the aseptic area until their recovery is complete. However, a healthy person with the best personal hygiene still will shed large numbers of viable and nonviable particles from body surfaces. This natural phenomenon creates continuing problems when personnel are present in clean rooms, but effective training and proper gowning can reduce, but not eliminate, the problem of particle shedding from personnel.

Aseptic-area operators should be given thorough, formal training in the principles of aseptic processing and the techniques to be employed. Subsequently, the acquired knowledge and skills should be evaluated, to be sure training has been effective, before they are allowed to participate in the preparation of sterile products. Retraining should be performed on a regular schedule to enhance the maintenance of the required level of expertise. An effort should be made to imbue operators with an awareness of the vital role they play in determining the reliability and safety of the final product. This is especially true of supervisors since they should be individuals who not only understand the unique requirements of aseptic procedures but who are able to obtain the full participation of other employees in fulfilling these exacting requirements.

The uniform worn is designed to confine the contaminants discharged from the body of the operator, thereby preventing their entry into the production environment. For use in the aseptic area, uniforms should be sterile. Fresh, sterile uniforms should be used after every break period, or whenever the individual returns to the aseptic area. In some plants this is not required if the product is to be sterilized in its final container. The uniform usually consists of coveralls for both men and women, hoods to completely cover the hair, face masks and Dacron or plastic boots (Fig 12). Sterile rubber gloves also are required for aseptic operations, preceded by thorough scrubbing of the hands with a disinfectant soap. In addition, goggles may be required to complete the coverage of all skin areas.

Dacron or Tyvek uniforms are used usually, are effective barriers to discharged body particles (viable and nonviable), are essentially lint-free and are reasonably comfortable. Air showers are sometimes directed on personnel entering the processing area to blow loose lint from the uniforms.

Environmental Control Evaluation

As evidenced by the above discussion, manufacturers of sterile products use extensive means to control the environment so that these critical products can be prepared free from contamination. Nevertheless, tests should be performed to determine the level of control actually achieved. Normally, the tests consist of counting viable and nonviable particles suspended in the air or settled on surfaces in the workspace. A baseline count, determined by averaging multiple counts when the facility is operating under controlled conditions, is used to establish the optimal test results expected. During the subsequent monitoring program, the test results are followed carefully for high individual counts, a rising trend or other abnormalities. If they exceed selected alert or action levels, a plan of action must be put into operation to determine if or what corrective measures are required.

The tests used generally measure either the particles in a volume of sampled air or the particles that are settling or are present on surfaces. A volume of air measured by an elec-

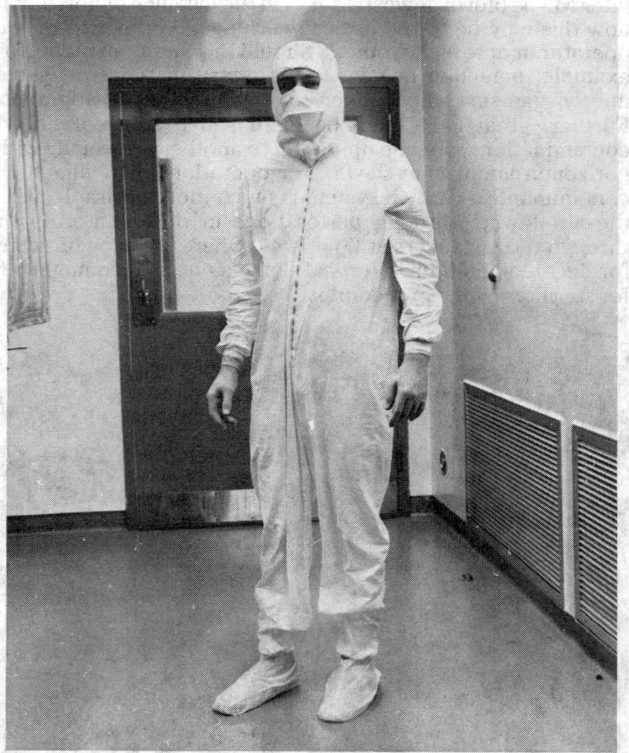

Fig 12. Appropriate uniform for operators entering an aseptic filling room (courtesy, Abbott).

tronic particle counter will detect all particles instantly, but not differentiate between viable and nonviable ones. However, because of the need to control the level of microorganisms in the environment in which sterile products are processed, it also is necessary to detect viable particles. These usually are less in number than nonviable ones and are only detectable as colony forming units (CFUs) after a suitable incubation period at, for example, 30 to 35°C for up to 48 hours.

Locations for sampling should be planned to reveal potential contamination levels which may be critical in the control of the environment. For example, the most critical process step is usually the filling of dispensing containers, a site obviously requiring monitoring. Other examples include the gowning room, high-traffic sites in and out of the filling area, the penetration of conveyor lines through walls and sites near the inlet and exit of the air system.

The size of the sample should be large enough to obtain a meaningful particle count. At sites where the count is expected to be low the size of the sample may need to be increased; for example, in Class 100 areas, Whyte and Niven,[18] suggest that the sample should be at least 30 ft^3 and, probably, much more. They also suggest that settling plates should be exposed in Class 100 areas for an entire fill (up to 7 to 8 hours) rather than the more common 1 hour. However, excessive dehydration of the medium must be avoided, particularly in the path of laminar-flow air.

To measure the total particle content in an air sample, electronic particle counters are available, operating on the principle of the measurement of light-scattered from particles as they pass through the cell of the optical system (Suppliers: *Climet*, *Met One*, *Particle Measuring*, *Royco*). These instruments not only count particles but also provide a size distribution based on the magnitude of the light scattered from the particle.

Several air-sampling devices are used to obtain a count of microorganisms in a measured volume of air. A slit-to-agar (STA) sampler (Suppliers: *Mattson-Garvin*, *New Brunswick*) draws by vacuum a measured volume of air through a narrow opening causing the air to impact on the surface of a slowly rotating nutrient agar plate. Microorganisms adhere to the surface of the agar and grow into visible colonies which are counted as CFUs, since it is not known whether the colonies arise from a single microorganism or a cluster. A centrifugal sampler (Supplier: *Biotest*) pulls air into the sampler by means of a rotating propeller and slings the air by centrifugal action against a peripheral nutrient agar strip. The advantages of this unit are that it can be disinfected easily and is portable so that it can be hand-carried wherever needed. These two methods are used quite widely.

A widely used method for microbiological sampling consists of the exposure of nutrient agar culture plates to the settling of microorganisms from the air. This method is very simple and inexpensive to perform but will detect only those organisms which have settled on the plate; therefore, it does not measure the number of microorganisms in a measured volume of air. Nevertheless, if the conditions of exposure are repeated consistently, a comparison of CFUs at one sampling site from one time to another can be meaningful.

The number of microorganisms on surfaces can be determined with nutrient agar plates having a convex surface (*Rodac Plates*). With these it is possible to roll the raised agar surface over flat or irregular surfaces to be tested. Organisms will be picked up on the agar and will grow during subsequent incubation. This method also can be used to assess the number of microorganisms present on the surface of the uniforms of operators, either as an evaluation of gowning technique immediately after gowning or as a measure of the accumulation of microorganisms during processing. Whenever used, care must be taken to remove any agar residue left on the surface tested.

Further discussion of proposed viable particle test methods and the counts to be accepted will be found in Section ⟨1116⟩ "Microbial Evaluation and Classification of Clean Rooms and Clean Zones" in *Pharm Forum 18:*4048, 1992.

Results from the above tests are very valuable to keep cleaning, production and quality-control personnel apprised of the level of contamination in a given area and, by comparison with baseline counts, will indicate when more extensive cleaning and sanitizing is needed. The results also may serve to detect environmental control defects such as failure in air-cleaning equipment or the presence of personnel who may be disseminating large numbers of bacteria without apparent physical ill effects.

Media Fill—An evaluation which is not strictly an environmental test, but which includes an evaluation of the environment along with the process, the operators and the equipment, is the "media fill." Sterile trypticase soy broth is filled into sterile containers under conditions simulating as closely as possible those characteristics of a filling process for a product. The entire lot, normally at least 3000 units, is then incubated at a suitable temperature, usually 20 to 25°, for at least 14 days and examined for the appearance of growth of microorganisms. If growth occurs, contamination has entered the container(s) during the processing. To pass the test not more than 0.1% of the units may show growth. This evaluation also has been used as a measure of the proficiency of an individual operator. This test is a very stringent evaluation of the efficiency of an aseptic filling process and, by many, is considered to be the most evaluative test available.

Production Procedures

The processes required for preparing sterile products constitute a series of events initiated with the securing of approved raw materials (drugs, excipients, vehicles, etc) and primary packaging components (containers, closures, etc) and ends with the sterile product sealed in its dispensing package. Each step in the process must be controlled very carefully in order that the product will have its required quality. To assure the latter, each process should be validated to be sure that it is accomplishing what it is intended to do. For example, an autoclave sterilization process must be validated by providing data showing that it effectively kills resistant forms of microorganisms; or, a cleaning process for rubber closures should provide evidence that it is cleaning closures to the required level of cleanliness. The validation of processes requires an extensive and intensive effort to be successful, and is an integral part of CGMP requirements.

In the following sections the production procedures used in preparing sterile drug products will be discussed.

Cleaning Containers and Equipment

Containers and equipment coming in contact with parenteral preparations must be cleaned meticulously. It is obvious that if this were not so, all other precautions to prevent contamination of the product would be useless. It also should be obvious that even new, unused containers and equipment will be contaminated with such debris as dust, fibers, chemical films and other materials arising from such sources as the atmosphere, cartons, the manufacturing process and human hands. Much greater contamination must be removed from previously used equipment before it will be suitable for reuse. Equipment should be reserved exclusively for use only with parenteral preparations and, where conditions dictate, only for one product in order to reduce the risk of contamination.

A variety of machines are available for cleaning containers for parenteral products. These vary in complexity from a small rotary rinser (Fig 13) to large automatic washers capable of processing several thousand containers an hour (Fig 14). The selection of the particular type will be determined largely by the physical type of containers, their condition with respect to contamination and the number to be processed in a given period of time.

Characteristics of Machinery—Regardless of the type of cleaning machine selected, certain fundamental characteristics usually are required.

1. The liquid or air treatment must be introduced in such a manner that it will strike the bottom of the inside of the inverted container, spread in all directions and smoothly flow down the walls and out the opening with a sweeping action. The pressure of the jet stream should be such that there is minimal splashing, and the flow should be such that it can leave the container opening without accumulating and producing turbulence inside. Splashing may prevent cleaning all areas, and turbulence may redeposit loosened debris. Therefore, direct introduction of the jet stream within the container with control of its flow is required.
2. The container must receive a concurrent outside rinse.
3. The cycle of treatment should provide for a planned sequence alternating very hot and cool treatments. The final treatment should be an effective rinse with water of a quality equivalent to WFI.
4. All metal parts coming in contact with the containers and with the treatments should be constructed of stainless steel or some other noncorroding and noncontaminating material.

Treatment Cycle—The cycle of treatments to be employed will vary with the condition of the containers to be cleaned. In general, loose dirt can be removed by vigorous rinsing with water. Detergents rarely are used for new containers because of the risk of leaving detergent residues. However, a thermal-shock sequence in the cycle usually is employed to aid, by expansion and contraction, loosening of debris that may be adhering to the container wall. Sometimes only an air rinse is used for new containers, particularly if used for a dry powder. In all instances the final rinse, whether air or WFI, must be ultraclean so that no particulate residues are left by the rinsing agent.

Only new containers are used for parenterals. Improvements have been made in maintaining their cleanliness during shipment from the manufacturer through tight, low-shedding packaging, including plastic blister packs, as can be seen stacked on the right of Fig 14.

Machinery for Containers—The machinery available for cleaning containers embodies the above principles but varies in the mechanics by which it is accomplished. In one approach, the jet tubes are arranged on arms like the spokes of a wheel, which rotate around a center post through which the treatments are introduced. An operator places the unclean containers on the jet tubes as they pass the loading point and removes the clean containers as they complete one rotation. Such a small-scale machine is pictured in Fig 14. A washer capable of cleaning hundreds of containers an hour, shown in Figure 14, uses a row of jet tubes across a conveyor belt. The belt moves the inverted containers past the programmed series of treatments and discharges the clean containers into a sterilizing oven (not shown), which ultimately discharges them through a wall into a clean room for filling. Another type of machine is the rack-loading washer. Stainless-steel racks are designed to fit over the open ends of ampuls or vials as configured in trays of shipping cartons or blister packs. Inverting the trays permits the containers to slide into the racks so that they can be handled by the quantity in the tray, as shown in Fig 15. The clean containers may be transferred directly to the conveyor of a sterilizating tunnel (as shown), or they may be placed in stainless-steel boxes for subsequent dry-heat sterilization and storage. A continuous automated line operation is shown in Figure 16. The vials are fed into the rotary rinser in the foreground, transferred automatically to the covered sterilizing tunnel in the center, conveyed through the wall in the background and discharged through the wall into the filling clean room.

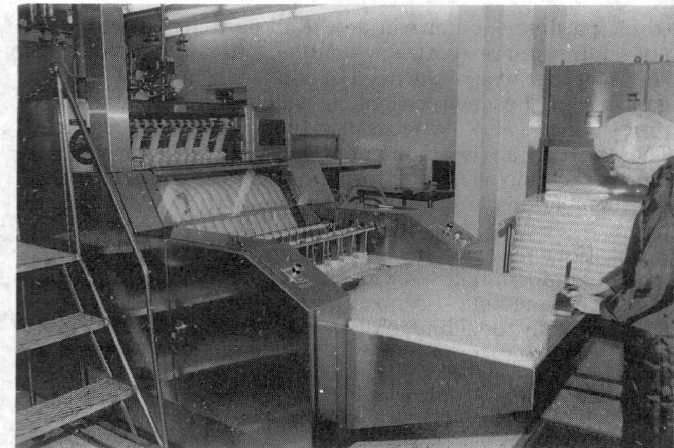

Fig 14. Loading end of large conveyor vial washer that subjects inverted vials to a series of cleaning steps before delivery from the far end of the washer. Note the vials in plastic blister packs at right of operator (courtesy, Merck).

Handling after Cleaning—The wet, clean containers must

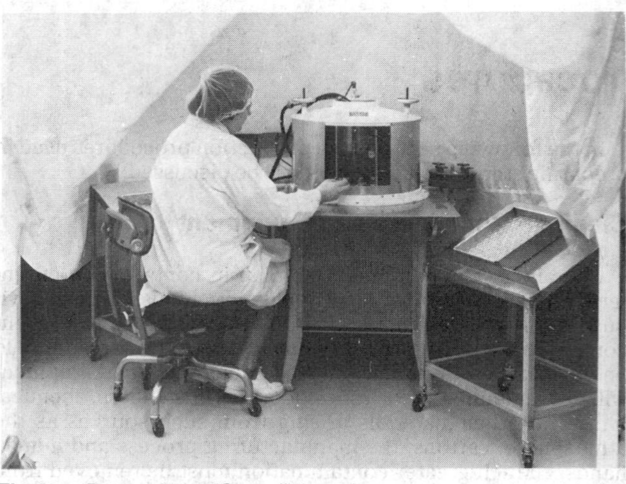

Fig 13. Rotary rinser (Cozzoli) in a clean environment provided by vertical laminar airflow within a curtained enclosure (courtesy, Ciba-Geigy).

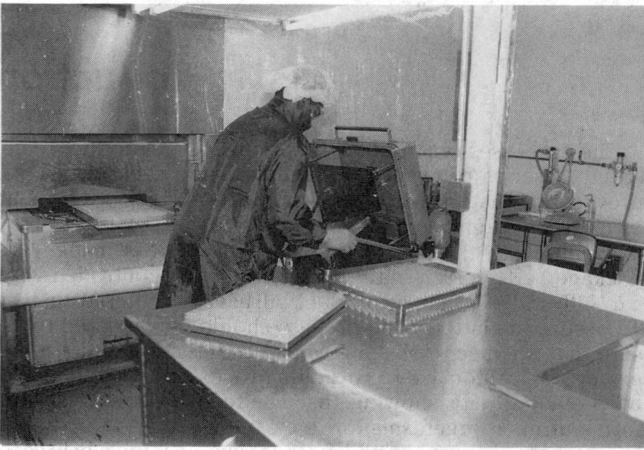

Fig 15. Cleaning vials with rack-loading washer, permitting handling vials by a full rack. After multiple-washing treatments, the racks are placed directly on the conveyor belt of the hot-air sterilizing tunnel (courtesy, Merck).

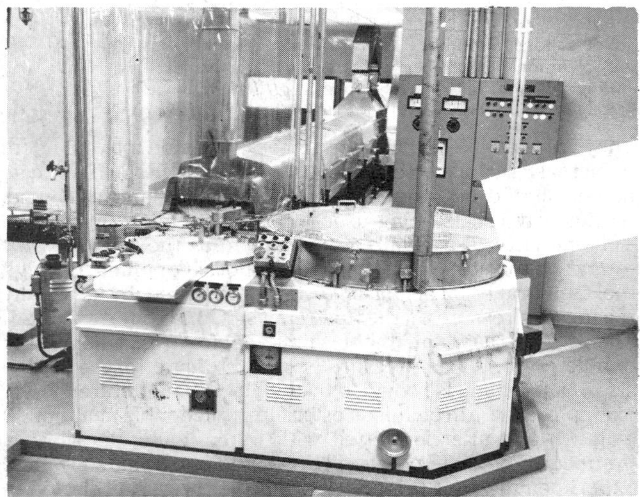

Fig 16. Continuous automatic line operation for vials from a rotary rinser through a sterilizing tunnel with vertical laminar-airflow protection of clean vials (courtesy, Abbott).

be handled in such a way that contamination will not be reintroduced. A wet surface will collect contaminants much more readily than will a dry surface. For this reason wet, rinsed containers must be protected, such as by a laminar flow of clean air until covered, as within a stainless-steel box or within a sterilizing tunnel. Although not clearly visible in each instance, the wet, clean containers in Figs 13–16 were so protected. In addition, microorganisms are more likely to grow in the presence of moisture. Therefore, wet, clean containers should be dry-heat sterilized as soon as possible after washing. Doubling the heating period generally has been considered to be adequate also to destroy pyrogens, but the actual time-temperature conditions required must be validated.

Increases in process rates have necessitated the development of continuous, automated line processing with a minimum of individual handling, still maintaining adequate control of the cleaning and handling of the containers. In Fig 16, the clean, wet containers are protected by filtered laminar-flow air from the rinser through the tunnel and until they are delivered to the filling line.

Closures—Rubber closures are coated with lubricant from the molding operation. In addition, the rough surface and electrostatic attraction tend to hold debris. Also, the surface "bloom" from migrated inorganic constituents of the compound must be removed. The recommended procedure calls for gentle agitation in a hot solution of a mild water softener. The closures are removed from the solution and rinsed several times, or continuously for a prolonged period, with filtered WFI. The rinsing is to be done in a manner which will flush away loosened debris. The wet closures are carefully protected from pick up of environmental contamination, are sterilized, usually by autoclaving, and stored in closed containers until ready for use. This cleaning and sterilizing process must be validated with respect to rendering the closures free from pyrogens. Actually, it is the cleaning and final, thorough rinsing with WFI that must remove pyrogens, since autoclaving does not destroy them. If the closures were immersed during autoclaving, the solution is drained off before storage to reduce hydration of the rubber compound. If the closures must be dry for use, they may be subjected to vacuum drying at a temperature in the vicinity of 100°.

The equipment used for washing large numbers of closures is usually an agitator or horizontal basket-type automatic washing machine. Because of particulate generation from the abrading action of these machines, some heat the closures in kettles in detergent solution and follow with prolonged flush rinsing. The final rinse always should be with low particulate WFI.

Equipment—The details of certain prescribed techniques for cleaning and preparing equipment, as well as of containers and closures, have been presented elsewhere.[19] Here, a few points will be emphasized.

All equipment should be disassembled as much as possible to provide access to internal structures. For thorough cleaning, surfaces should be scrubbed thoroughly with a stiff brush using an effective detergent, paying particular attention to joints, crevices, screw threads and other structures where debris is apt to collect. Exposure to a stream of clean steam will aid in dislodging residues from the walls of stationary tanks, spigots, pipes and similar structures. Thorough rinsing with distilled water should follow the cleaning steps. Large stationary tanks, such as those shown in Fig 17, should be protected as much as possible from contamination after cleaning but should be rinsed thoroughly again with distilled water or WFI prior to reuse.

Because of the inherent variation in the manual cleaning of tanks and other large equipment items, together with the need to validate the process, an automated, usually computer-controlled, system has been developed called "cleaning in place" (CIP).[20] Such an approach involves designing the system, normally of stainless steel, with smooth, rounded internal surfaces and without crevices. That is, for example, with welded rather than threaded connections. The cleaning is accomplished with the scrubbing action of high-pressure spray balls or nozzles delivering hot detergent solution from tanks captive to the system. Thorough rinsing with WFI follows and is accomplished within the same system. The system often is extended to permit sterilizing in place (SIP) as well.[21]

Rubber tubing, rubber gaskets and other rubber parts may be washed in a manner such as described for rubber closures. Thorough rinsing of tubing must be done by passing WFI through it. However, due to the relatively porous nature of rubber compounds and the difficulty in removing all traces of chemicals from previous use, it is considered by some inadvisable to reuse rubber tubing. Rubber tubing must be left wet when preparing for sterilization by autoclaving.

Product Preparation

The basic principles employed in the compounding of the product do not vary from those used routinely by qualified pharmacists. However, selected aspects will be mentioned for emphasis.

A master formula would have been developed and on file. Each batch formula sheet should be prepared from the master and confirmed for accuracy. All measurements of quantities

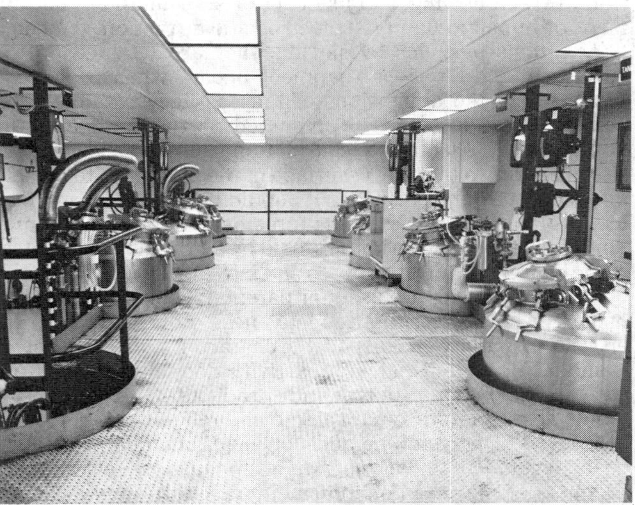

Fig 17. Large stainless-steel tanks for product preparation showing mezzanine access level (courtesy, Abbott).

should be made as accurately as possible and checked by a second qualified person. Frequently, today, the formula documents are generated by a computer and the measurements of quantities of ingredients computer controlled. Although most liquid preparations are dispensed by volume, they are prepared by weight, since weighings can be performed more accurately than volume measurements and no consideration needs to be given to the temperature.

Care must be taken that equipment is not wet enough to significantly dilute the product or, in the case of anhydrous products, to cause a physical incompatibility. The order of mixing of ingredients may affect the product significantly, particularly those of large volume where attaining homogeneity requires considerable mixing time. For example, the adjustment of pH by the addition of an acid, even though diluted, may cause excessive local reduction in the pH of the product so that adverse effects are produced before the acid can be dispersed throughout the entire volume of product.

Parenteral dispersions, including colloids, emulsions and suspensions, provide particular problems. Parenteral emulsions have been reviewed by Singh and Ravin.[22] In addition to the problems of achieving and maintaining proper reduction in particle size under aseptic conditions, the dispersion must be kept in a uniform state of suspension throughout the preparative, transfer and subdividing operations.

The formulation of a stable product is of paramount importance. Certain aspects of this have been mentioned in the discussion of components of the product. Exhaustive coverage of the topic is not possible within the limits of this text, but further coverage is provided in Chapter 83. It should be mentioned here, however, the thermal sterilization of parenteral products increases the possibility of chemical reactions. Such reactions may progress to completion during the period of elevated temperature in the autoclave, or be initiated at this time but continue during subsequent storage. The assurance of attaining product stability requires a high order of pharmaceutical knowledge and responsibility.

Filtration

After a product has been compounded, it must be filtered if it is a solution. The primary objective of filtration is to clarify a solution. A high degree of clarification is termed "polishing" a solution. This term is used when particulate matter down to approximately 2 μm in size is removed. A further step, removing particulate matter down to 0.2 μm in size, would eliminate microorganisms and would accomplish "cold" sterilization. A solution having a high degree of clarity conveys the impression of high quality and purity, desirable characteristics for a parenteral solution.

Filters are thought to function by one or, usually, a combination of the following: (1) sieving or screening, (2) entrapment or impaction and (3) electrostatic attraction. When a filter retains particles by sieving, they are retained on the surface of the filter. Entrapment occurs when a particle, smaller than the dimensions of the passageway (pore), becomes lodged in a turn or impacted on the surface of the passageway. Electrostatic attraction causes particles opposite in charge to that of the surface of the filter pore to be held or adsorbed to the surface. It should be noted that increasing, prolonging or varying the force behind the solution may tend to sweep particles initially held by entrapment or electrostatic charge through the pores and into the filtrate.

Membrane filters are used for parenteral solutions because of their particle-retention effectiveness, nonshedding property, nonreactivity and disposable characteristics. However, it should be noted that nonreactivity does not apply in all cases. For example, polypeptide products may show considerable adsorption through some membrane filters, but those composed of polysulfone and polyvinylidine difluoride have been developed to be essentially nonadsorptive for these products. The most common membranes are composed of

Cellulose ester (Suppliers: *Gelman, Millipore, Sartorius, Schleicher Seitz*).
Nylon (Supplier: *Pall*).
Polysulfone (Supplier: *Gelman*).
Polycarbonate (Supplier: *Nuclepore*).
Polyvinylidene difluoride (Supplier: *Millipore*).
Polytetrafluoroethylene (Teflon) (Supplier: *Millipore*).

They are available as flat membranes or pleated into cylinders to increase surface area and, thus, flow rate. Each filter in its holder should be tested for integrity before and after use, particularly if it is being used to eliminate microorganisms. This integrity test usually is performed as the *bubble-point test*, a test to detect the largest pore, or other opening, through the membrane. The basic test is performed by gradually raising air pressure on the upstream side of a water-wet filter. The pressure at which bubbles first appear downstream is the bubble point. This pressure is characteristic for each pore size of a filter and is provided by the filter manufacturer. For example, a 0.2 μm cellulose ester filter will bubble at about 50 psig. If the filter is wetted with other liquids, such as a product, the bubble point will differ and must be determined experimentally. If the bubble point is lower than the rated pressure, the filter is defective, probably due to a puncture or tear, and should not be used. As the surface area of filters becomes large, diffusion of air through the water-filled pores tends to obscure the bubble point. Therefore, a diffusion, or pressure hold, test has been developed as an integrity test for filters with large surface areas. Particulars are obtainable from the filter manufacturer.

While membrane filters are disposable, and thus discarded after use, the holders must be cleaned thoroughly between uses. Today, clean, sterile, pretested, disposable assemblies for small as well as large volumes of solutions are available commercially. Other characteristics of these filters, important for a full understanding of their use, are given in Chapter 84 and in a review article.[23]

Filling

During the filling of containers with a product, the most stringent requirements must be exercised to prevent contamination, particularly if the product has been sterilized by filtration and will not be sterilized in the final container. Under the latter conditions the process usually is called an "aseptic fill" and is validated with media fills (see page 1537). During the filling operation, the product must be transferred from a bulk container and subdivided into dose containers. This operation exposes the sterile product to the environment, equipment and manipulative technique of the operator until it can be sealed in the dose container. Therefore, this operation is carried out with a minimum exposure time in the aseptic filling area where maximum protection is provided. Additional protection may be provided by filling under a blanket of HEPA-filtered laminar-flow air within the aseptic area.

Normally, the compounded product is in the form of either a liquid or a solid. A liquid is more readily subdivided uniformly and introduced into a container having a narrow mouth than is a solid. Mobile, nonsticking liquids are considerably easier to transfer and subdivide than viscous, sticky liquids, which require heavy-duty machinery for rapid production filling.

Although many devices are available for filling containers with liquids, certain characteristics are fundamental to them all. A means is provided for repetitively forcing a measured volume of the liquid through the orifice of a delivery tube which is introduced into the container. The size of the delivery tube will vary from that of about a 20-gauge hypodermic needle to a tube ½ in. or more in diameter. The size required is determined by the physical characteristics of the liquid, the desired delivery speed and the inside diameter of the neck of the container. The tube must enter the neck and deliver the liquid well into the neck to eliminate spillage, allowing sufficient clearance to permit air to leave the container as the liquid enters. The delivery tube should be as large in diameter as possible in order to reduce the resistance to the flow of the liquid. For smaller volumes of liquids, the delivery usually is obtained from the stroke of the plunger of a syringe, forcing the liquid through a two-way valve providing for alternate filling of the syringe and delivery of mobile liquids. A sliding piston valve would be used for heavy, viscous liquids. Other mechanisms include the turn of an auger in the neck of a funnel or the oscillation of a rubber diaphragm. For large volumes the quantity delivered usually is measured in the container by the level of fill in the container, the force required to transfer the liquid being provided by gravity, a pressure pump or a vacuum pump.

The narrow neck of an ampul limits the clearance possible between the delivery tube and the inside of the neck. Since a drop of liquid normally hangs at the tip of the delivery tube after a delivery, the neck of an ampul will be wet as the delivery tube is withdrawn, unless the drop is retracted. Therefore, filling machines should have a mechanism by which this drop can be drawn back into the lumen of the tube.

Since the liquid will be in intimate contact with the parts of the machine through which it flows, these must be constructed of nonreactive materials such as borosilicate glass or stainless steel. In addition, they should easily be demountable for cleaning and sterilization.

Because of the concern for particulate matter in injectable preparations, a final filter often is inserted in the system between the filler and the delivery tube, as shown in Fig 18. Most frequently this is a membrane filter, having a porosity of approximately 1 μm and treated to have a hydrophobic edge. This is necessary to reduce the risk of rupture of the membrane due to filling pulsations. It should be noted that the insertion of the filter at this point should collect all particulate matter generated during the process. Only that which may be found in inadequately cleaned containers or picked up from exposure to the environment after passage through the final filter potentially remain as contaminants. However, the filter does cushion liquid flow and reduces the efficiency of drop retraction from the end of the delivery tube, sometimes making it difficult to control delivery volume as precisely as would be possible without the filter.

Liquids—The filling of a small number of containers may be accomplished with a hypodermic syringe and needle, the liquid being drawn into the syringe and forced through the needle into the container. A device for providing greater speed of filling is the Cornwall Pipet (*Becton Dickinson*). This has a two-way valve between the syringe and the needle and a means for setting the stroke of the syringe so that the same volume will be delivered each time. Clean, sterile, disposable assemblies (Suppliers: *Burron, Pharmaseal*) operating on the same principle have particular usefulness in hospital pharmacy operations.

Mechanically operated instruments substitute a motor for the operator's hand in the previous devices described. Thereby, a much faster filling rate can be achieved. By careful engineering, the stroke of the syringe can be repeated precisely, and so, once a particular setting has been calibrated to the delivery, high delivery precision is possible. However, the speed of delivery, the expansion of the rubber tubing connecting the valve with the delivery tube and the rapidity of action of the valves can affect the precision of delivery. A filling machine employing a piston valve is shown in Fig 18. Stainless-steel syringes are required with viscous liquids because glass syringes are not strong enough to withstand the high pressures developed during delivery.

When high-speed filling rates are desired but accuracy and precision must be maintained, multiple filling units often are joined together in an electronically coordinated machine, such as shown in Fig 19. When the product is sensitive to metals, a peristaltic-pump filler may be used because the product comes in contact only with silicone rubber tubing. However, there is some sacrifice of filling accuracy.

Most high-speed fillers for large-volume solutions use the bottle as the measuring device, transferring the liquid either by vacuum or positive pressure from the bulk reservoir to the individual unit containers. Therefore, a high accuracy of fill is not achievable.

To insure delivery of the labeled volume to the patient, the USP provides a table of suggested fill volumes to include a slight excess over labeled volume.

Solids—Sterile solids, such as antibiotics, are more difficult to subdivide evenly into containers than are liquids. The rate of flow of solid material is slow and irregular. Even though a container with a larger diameter opening is used to facilitate filling, it is difficult to introduce the solid particles, and the risk of spillage is ever-present. The accuracy of the quantity delivered cannot be controlled as well as with liquids. Because of these factors, the tolerances permitted for the content of such containers must be relatively large. Suggested tolerances can be found in the USP.

Some sterile solids are subdivided into containers by individual weighing. A scoop usually is provided to aid in approximating the quantity required, but the quantity filled into the container finally is weighed on a balance. This is a slow process. When the solid is obtainable in a granular form so that it will flow more freely, other methods of filling may be employed. In general, these involve the measurement and delivery of a volume of the granular material which has been calibrated in terms of the weight desired. In the machine shown in Fig 20 an adjustable cavity in the rim of a wheel is

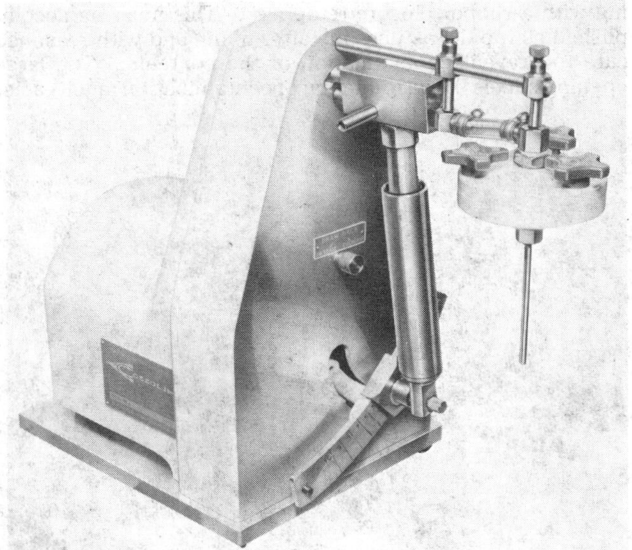

Fig 18. Filling machine employing a piston valve and a stainless-steel syringe (courtesy, Cozzoli).

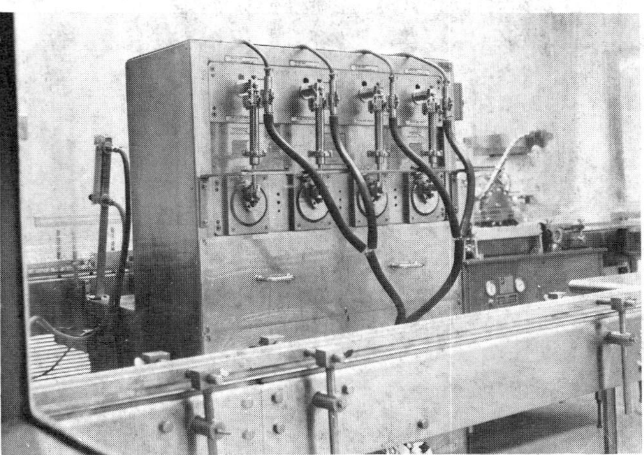

Fig 19. Four-pump liquid filler, with a conveyor line for vials protected by a vertical laminar airflow and plastic curtain; note the automatic stoppering machine on the right within the curtain (courtesy, Abbott).

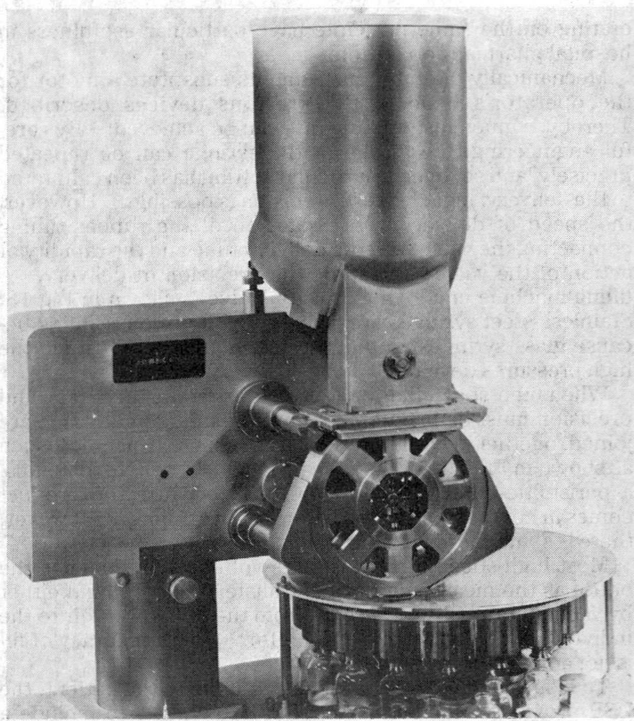

Fig 20. Accofil vacuum powder filler (courtesy, Perry).

filled by vacuum and the contents held by vacuum until the cavity is inverted over the container. The solid material then is discharged into the container by the use of sterile air. Another machine employs an auger in the stem of a funnel at the bottom of a hopper. The granular material is placed in the hopper. By controlling the size of the auger and its rotation, a regulated volume of granular material can be delivered from the funnel stem into the container. Such a machine is shown in Fig 21.

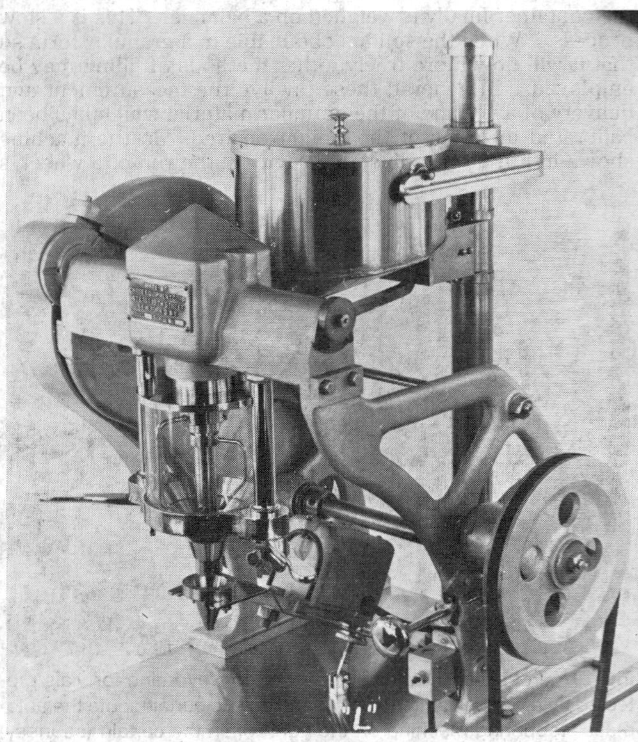

Fig 21. Auger-type powder filler (courtesy, Chase-Logeman).

Sealing

Ampuls—Filled containers should be sealed as soon as possible to prevent the contents from being contaminated by the environment. Ampuls are sealed by melting a portion of the glass neck. Two types of seals are employed normally: tip-seals (bead-seals) or pull-seals.

Tip-seals are made by melting enough glass at the tip of the neck of an ampul to form a bead and close the opening. These can be made rapidly in a high-temperature gas–oxygen flame. To produce a uniform bead, the ampul neck must be heated evenly on all sides. This may be accomplished by means of burners on opposite sides of stationary ampuls or by rotating the ampul in a single flame. Care must be taken to properly adjust the flame temperature and the interval of heating to obtain complete closing of the opening with a bead of glass. Excessive heating will result in the expansion of the gases within the ampul against the soft bead seal and cause a bubble to form. If it bursts, the ampul is no longer sealed; if it does not, the wall of the bubble will be thin and fragile. Insufficient heating will leave an open capillary through the center of the bead. An incompletely sealed ampul is called a "leaker."

Pull-seals are made by heating the neck of the ampul below the tip, leaving enough of the tip for grasping with forceps or other mechanical devices. The ampul is rotated in the flame from a single burner. When the glass has softened, the tip is grasped firmly and pulled quickly away from the body of the ampul, which continues to rotate. The small capillary tube thus formed is twisted closed. Pull-sealing is slower, but the seals are more sure than tip-sealing. Fig 22 shows a machine combining the steps of filling and pull-sealing ampuls.

Powder ampuls or other types having a wide opening must be sealed by pull-sealing. Were these sealed by tip-sealing, the very large bead produced would induce glass strain with subsequent fracture at the juncture of the bead and neck wall. Fracture of the neck of ampuls during sealing also may occur if wetting of the necks occurred at the time of filling. Also, wet necks increase the frequency of bubble formation. If the product in the ampul is organic in nature, wet necks also will result in unsightly carbon deposits from the heat of sealing.

In order to prevent decomposition of a product, it is sometimes necessary to displace the air in the space above the product in the ampul with an inert gas. This is done by introducing a stream of the gas, such as nitrogen or carbon dioxide, during or after filling with the product. Immediately thereafter the ampul is sealed before the gas can diffuse to the outside. This process should be validated to ensure adequate displacement of air by the gas in each container.

Vials and Bottles—These are sealed by closing the opening with a rubber closure (stopper). This must be accomplished as rapidly as possible after filling and with reasoned care to prevent contamination of the contents. The large opening makes the introduction of contamination much easier

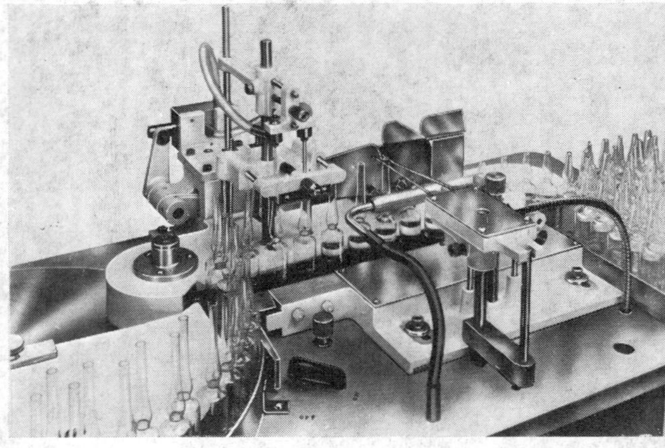

Fig 22. Automatic filling and pull-sealing of ampuls (courtesy, Cozzoli).

than with ampuls. Therefore, a covering should be provided for such containers except for the minimal time required for filling and for the actual introduction of the rubber closure. During the latter critical time the open containers should be protected from the ingress of contamination, preferably with a blanket of HEPA-filtered laminar airflow, as shown in Figs 10 and 19.

The closure must fit the mouth of the container snugly enough so that its elasticity will permit adjustment to slight irregularities in the lip and neck of the container. However, it must not fit so snugly that it is difficult to introduce into the neck of the container. Closures preferably are inserted mechanically using an automated process, especially with high-speed processing. To reduce friction so that the closure may slide more easily through a shute and into the container opening, the closure surfaces often are halogenated or treated with silicone. When the closure is positioned at the insertion site, it is mechanically pushed into the container opening (see Fig 23). When small lots are encountered, manual stoppering with forceps may be used, but such a process poses greater risk of introducing contamination than automated processes.

Rubber closures are held in place by means of aluminum caps. The caps cover the closure and are crimped under the lip of the vial or bottle to hold them in place (see Fig 5). The closure cannot be removed without destroying the aluminum cap; it is tamperproof. Therefore, an intact aluminum cap is proof that the closure has not been removed intentionally or unintentionally. Such confirmation is necessary to assure the integrity of the contents as to sterility and other aspects of quality.

The aluminum caps are so designed that the outer layer of double-layered caps, or the center of single-layered caps, can be removed to expose the center of the rubber closure without disturbing the band which holds the closure in the container. Rubber closures for use with intravenous administration sets often have a permanent hole through the closure. In such cases, a thin rubber disk overlayed with a solid aluminum disk is placed between an inner and outer aluminum cap, thereby providing a seal of the hole through the closure. These are called triple-layered aluminum caps.

Single-layered aluminum caps may be applied by means of a hand crimper known as the Fermpress (Suppliers: *West*, *Wheaton*). Double- or triple-layered caps require greater force for crimping; therefore, heavy-duty mechanical crimpers (see Fig 24) are required (Suppliers: *Bosch*, *Cozzoli*, *Perry*, *West*, *Wheaton*).

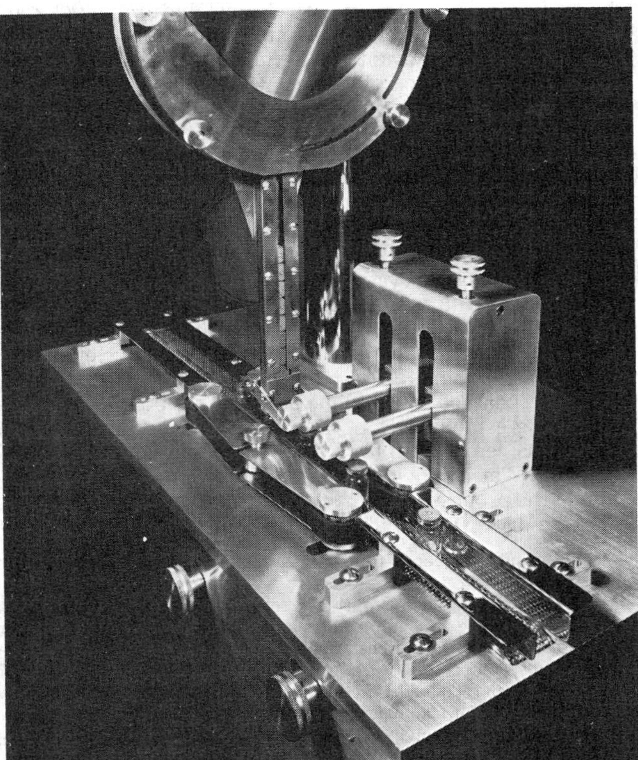

Fig 23. Mechanical device for inserting rubber closures in vials (courtesy, Perry).

Sterilization

Whenever possible, the parenteral product should be sterilized after being sealed in its final container (terminal sterilization) and within as short a time as possible after the filling and sealing have been completed. Since this usually involves a thermal process, due consideration must be given to the effect of the elevated temperature upon the stability of the product. Many products, both pharmaceutical and biological, will be affected adversely by the elevated temperatures required for thermal sterilization. Heat-labile products must, therefore, be sterilized by a nonthermal method, usually by filtration through bacteria-retaining filters. Subsequently, all operations must be carried out in an aseptic manner so that contamination will not be introduced into the filtrate. Colloids, oleaginous solutions, suspensions and emulsions that are thermolabile may require a process in which each component is sterilized separately and the product is formulated and processed under aseptic conditions.

The performance of an aseptic process is difficult and it has been accepted that currently, under the best controlled conditions, a sterility assurance level (SAL) of 10^{-3} is the maximum achievable. On the other hand, technical advances in aseptic processing, including improved automation, use of barrier systems, formulations to include antimicrobial effects and combinations of limited sterilization with aseptic processing, have improved the sterility-assurance levels achievable. Therefore, the successes realized should encourage continued efforts to improve the SAL achievable with aseptic processing. The importance of this is that for many drug solutions aseptic processing is the only method that can be considered for preparing a sterile product.

Nonthermal methods of sterilization, such as irradiation, have been proposed for consideration. However, since there is limited understanding of the molecular transformations that may occur in drug molecules and excipients under exposure to the high-energy levels of the process, extensive research will be required to develop the knowledge needed for an adequate evaluation.

Dry-heat sterilization may be employed for a few dry solids that are not affected adversely by the high temperatures and

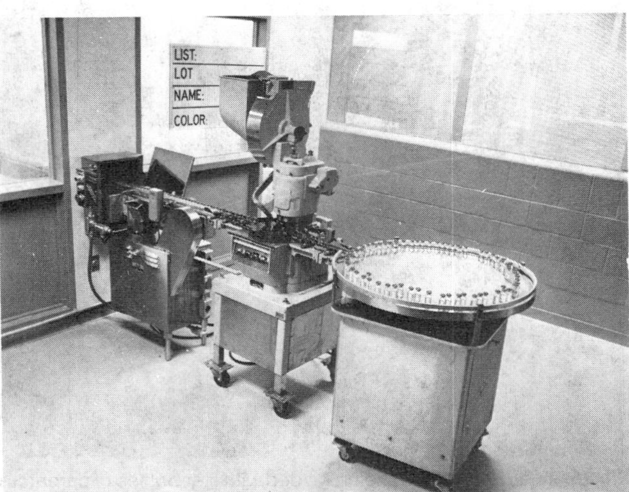

Fig 24. Applying aluminum caps to vials at the end of the process line (courtesy, Abbott).

for the relatively long heating period required. This method is applied most effectively to the sterilization of glassware and metalware. After sterilization, the equipment will be sterile, dry and, if the sterilization period is long enough, pyrogen-free.

Saturated steam under pressure (autoclaving) is the most commonly used and the most effective method for the sterilization of aqueous liquids or substances that can be reached or penetrated by steam. An SAL of 10^{-6} is readily achievable with terminal autoclaving of a thermally stable product. This is a 1000-fold improvement over the currently accepted level for aseptic processing. However, it needs to be noted that for terminal sterilization, as with autoclaving, the SAL is based upon an evaluation of the lethality of the process, ie, of the probable number of viable microorganisms remaining in product units. However, for aseptic processing, the components used have been sterilized by a validated process and the SAL is based upon an evaluation of the probable number of product units that have been contaminated during the process. This difference does not alter the outcome but only the basis for evaluating the probable SAL.

Figure 25 shows liter containers of solution being loaded into an autoclave for sterilization. Since the temperature employed in an autoclave is lower than that for dry-heat sterilization, equipment made of materials such as rubber and polypropylene may be sterilized if the time and temperature are controlled carefully. As mentioned previously, some injections will be affected adversely by the elevated temperature required for autoclaving. For some products, such as Dextrose Injection, the use of an autoclave designed to permit a rapid rise to sterilizing temperature and rapid cooling with water spray after the sterilizing hold-period will make it possible to use this method. It is ineffective in anhydrous conditions, such as within a sealed ampul containing a dry solid or an anhydrous oil. Other products that will not withstand autoclaving temperatures may withstand marginal thermal methods such as tyndallization or inspissation. These methods may be rendered more effective for some injections by the inclusion of a bacteriostatic agent in the product.

It should be obvious that all materials subjected to sterilization must be protected from subsequent contamination to maintain their sterile state. Therefore, they must be wrapped or covered so that microorganisms may not gain access when removed from the autoclave. Equipment and supplies are wrapped most frequently with paper and tied or sealed with special autoclave tape. The wrapping must permit penetration of steam during autoclaving but screen out microorganisms when dry. A double wrapping with lint-free parchment paper designed for such use is probably best. Synthetic fiber cloth such as nylon or Dacron also may be used for the inner wrapping. The openings of equipment subjected to dry-heat sterilization are often covered with silver–aluminum foil or with metal or glass covers. Cellulose wrapping materials are affected adversely by the high temperatures of dry-heat sterilization.

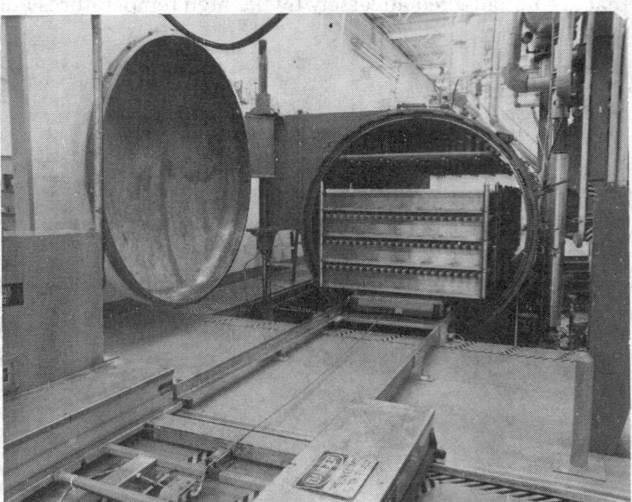

Fig 25. Large autoclave being loaded with liter bottles of parenteral solutions (courtesy, Abbott).

The effectiveness of any sterilization technique must be proved (validated) before it is employed. Since the goal of sterilization is to kill microorganisms, the ideal indicator to prove the effectiveness of the process is a resistant form of an appropriate microorganism, normally resistant spores (a biological indicator or BI). Therefore, during validation of a sterilization process, BIs of known resistance are used and numbers in association with physical-parameter indicators, such as recording thermocouples. Once the lethality of the process is established in association with the physical measurements, the physical measurements can be used for subsequent monitoring of in-use processes without the BIs. Eliminating the use of BIs in direct association with human-use products is appropriate because of the ever-present risk of an undetected, inadvertent contamination of a product or the environment.

The commercial suppliers of BIs have improved the resistance evaluation and lot-to-lot reliability of their products so that the information provided with each lot of BIs is generally reliable and useful in validation procedures.

In addition to the data printout from thermocouples, sometimes other physical indicators are used, such as color-change and melting indicators, to give visual indication that a package or truckload has been subjected to a sterilization process. Such evidence can become a part of the batch record to confirm that sterilization was accomplished.

Further details concerning methods of sterilization and their application will be found in Chapter 84. In addition, the USP provides suggestions concerning the sterilization of injections and related materials.

Freeze-Drying

Freeze-drying (lyophilization) is a process of drying in which water is sublimed from the product after it is frozen.[24] The particular advantages of this process are that biologicals and pharmaceuticals which are relatively unstable in aqueous solution can be processed and filled into dosage containers in the liquid state, taking advantage of the relative ease of processing a liquid. They can be dried without elevated temperatures, thereby eliminating adverse thermal effects, and stored in the dry state in which there are relatively few stability problems.

Further advantages are that these products are often more soluble and/or more rapidly soluble, dispersions are stabilized throughout their shelf life and products subject to degradation by oxidation have enhanced stability because the process is carried out in a vacuum.

However, the increased time and handling required for processing and the cost of the equipment limit the use of this process to those products which significantly have enhanced stability if stored in the dry state.

The fact that ice will sublime at pressures below 3 torr has been a long-established laboratory principle (see Chapter 19). The extensive program for freeze-drying human plasma during World War II provided the impetus for the rapid development of the process.

Freeze-drying essentially consists of

1. Freezing an aqueous product at a temperature below its eutectic temperature.
2. Evacuating the chamber, usually below 0.1 torr (100 μm Hg).
3. Subliming ice on a cold condensing surface at a temperature below that of the product, the condensing surface being within the chamber or in a connecting chamber.
4. Introducing heat to the product under controlled conditions, thereby providing energy for sublimation at a rate designed to keep the product temperature below its eutectic temperature.

Figure 26 shows such a system. The product may be fro-

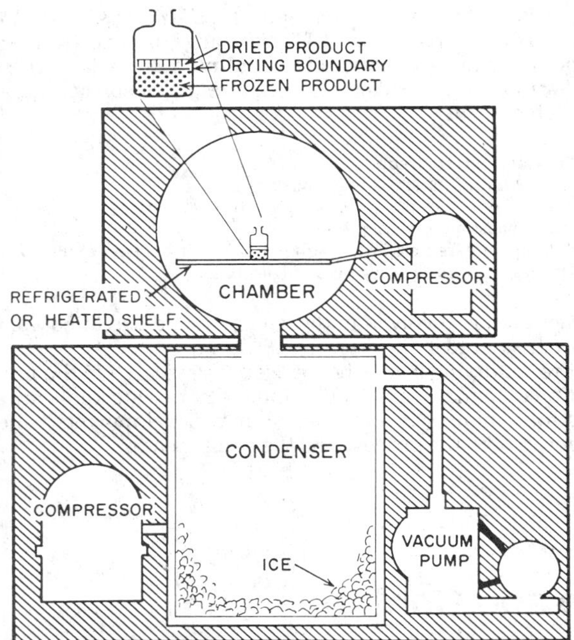

Fig 26. Essential components of a freeze-drying system.

zen on the shelf in the chamber by circulating refrigerant (usually Freon, ammonia or ethylene glycol) from the compressor through pipes within the shelf. After freezing is complete, which may require several hours, the chamber and condenser are evacuated by the vacuum pump, the condenser surface having been chilled previously by circulating refrigerant from the large compressor.

Heat then is introduced from the shelf to the product by electric resistance coils or by circulating hot water, silicone or glycol. The process continues until the product is dry (usually 1% or less moisture), leaving a sponge-like matrix of the solids originally present in the product, the input of heat being controlled so as not to degrade the product.

For most pharmaceuticals and biologicals the liquid product is sterilized by filtration and then filled into the dosage container aseptically. The containers must remain open during the drying process to allow water vapor to escape; therefore, they must be protected from contamination during transfer from the filling area to the freeze-drying chamber, while in the freeze-drying chamber and at the end of the drying process until sealed.

The chambers may be equipped with hydraulic or rubber diaphragm internal-stoppering devices designed to push slotted rubber closures into the vials to be sealed while the chamber is still evacuated, the closures having been partially inserted immediately after filling so that the slots were open to the outside.

If internal stoppering is not available or containers such as ampuls are used, filtered dry air or nitrogen must be introduced to the chamber at the end of the process to establish atmospheric pressure. Then the containers must be removed and sealed under aseptic conditions. If the product is very sensitive to moisture, the environmental humidity also must be controlled until it is sealed.

Factors Affecting the Process Rate—The greater the depth of the product in the container, the longer will be the drying process. Therefore, a product to be frozen by placing the container on a refrigerated shelf (plug freezing) should be filled to a planned, limited depth. If a large volume of solution must be processed, the surface area may be increased and the depth decreased by freezing the solution on a slant or while rotating the container on an angle (shell freezing) in a liquid refrigerant bath, such as dry ice and alcohol.

The actual driving force for the process is the vapor pressure differential between the vapor at the surface where drying of the product is occurring (the drying boundary) and that at the surface of the ice on the condenser. The latter is determined by the temperature of the condenser as modified by the insulating effect of the accumulated ice. The former is determined by a number of factors, including:

1. The rate of heat conduction through the container and the frozen material, both usually relatively poor thermal conductors, to the drying boundary while maintaining all of the product below its eutectic temperature.
2. The impeding effect of the increasing depth of dried, porous product above the drying boundary.
3. The temperature and heat capacity of the shelf itself.

This may be visualized by referring to Fig 26.

The passageways between the product surface and the condenser surface must be wide open and direct for effective operation. Therefore, the condensing surfaces in large freeze-driers are usually in the same chamber as the product. Evacuation of the system is necessary to reduce the impeding effect that collisions with air molecules would have on the passage of water molecules. However, the residual pressure in the system must be greater than the vapor pressure of the ice on the condenser or the ice will be vaporized and pulled into the pump, an event detrimental to most pumps.

The amount of solids in the product, their particle size and their thermal conductance will affect the rate of drying. The more solids present, the more impediment will be provided to the escape of the water vapor. The smaller the particle size, particularly the crystal size of the ice, the faster the drying generally will be. The poorer the thermal conducting properties of the solids in the product, the slower will be the rate of heat transfer through the frozen material to the drying boundary.

The rate of drying is essentially slow, most often requiring 24 hours or longer for completion. The actual time required, the rate of heat input and the product temperatures that may be used must be determined for each product and then reproduced carefully with successive processes.

Factors Affecting Formulation—The active constituent of many pharmaceutical products is present in such a small quantity that if freeze-dried alone its presence would be hard to detect visually. Therefore, excipients often are added to increase the amount of solids.

Some consider it ideal for the dried-product plug to occupy essentially the same volume as that of the original solution. To achieve this, the solids content of the original product must be between approximately 5 and 25%. Among the substances found most useful for this purpose, usually as a combination, are sodium or potassium phosphates, citric acid, tartaric acid, gelatin and carbohydrates such as dextrose, mannitol and dextran.

Each of these substances contributes appearance characteristics of the plug, such as whether dull and spongy or sparkling and crystalline, firm or friable, expanded or shrunken and uniform or striated. Therefore, the formulation of a product to be freeze-dried must include consideration not only of the nature and stability characteristics required during the liquid state, both freshly prepared and when reconstituted before use, but the characteristics desired in the dried plug.

Modifications in the Process and Equipment—In some instances a product may be frozen in a bulk container or in trays rather than in the final container and then handled as a dry solid. This may be desirable when large volumes of a product are processed, but the risk of contamination from the environment is high.

When large quantities of material are processed it may be desirable to use ejection pumps in the equipment system. These draw the vapor into the pump and eject it to the outside, thereby eliminating the need for a condensing surface. Such pumps are expensive and usually practical only in large installations.

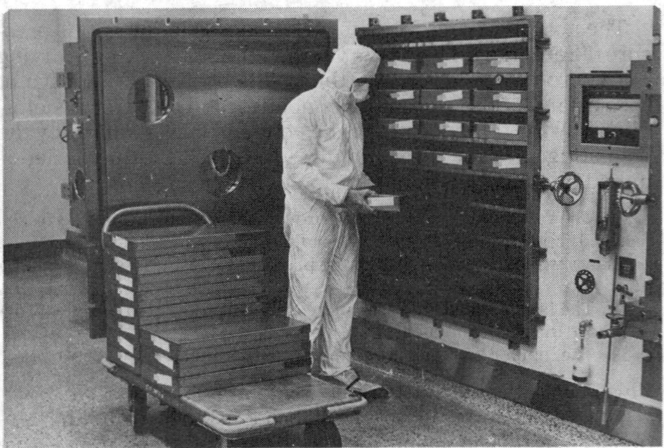

Fig 27. Aseptic loading of freeze-drier (courtesy, Upjohn).

Available freeze-driers (Suppliers: *Edwards, Finn-Aqua, ETS, Hull, NRC, Stokes, Virtis*) range in size from small laboratory units to large industrial models such as the one shown in Fig 27. Their selection requires consideration of such factors as

The tray area required.
The volume of water to be removed.
Whether or not aseptic processing will be involved.
Is internal stoppering required?
Will separate freezers be used for initial freezing of the product.
The degree of automatic operation desired.

Other factors involved in the selection and use of equipment are considered in the literature.[25]

Freeze-drying is now being used for research in the preservation of human tissue and is finding increasing application in the food industry. Progress on new developments is being made in both the process and the equipment.[26]

Quality Assurance and Control

The importance of undertaking every possible means to assure the quality of the finished product cannot be overemphasized. Every component and step of the manufacturing process must be subjected to intense scrutiny to be confident that quality is attained in the finished product. The responsibility for achieving this quality is divided appropriately in concept and practice into Quality Assurance (QA) and Quality Control (QC). QA relates to the studies made and the plans developed for assuring quality of a product prospectively. QC embodies the carrying out of these plans during production and includes all of the tests and evaluations performed to be sure that quality has been achieved in a specific lot of product.

The principles for achieving quality are basically the same for the manufacture of any pharmaceutical. These are discussed in Chapter 39. During the discussion of the preparation of injections, mention was made of numerous quality requirements for components and manufacturing processes. Here, only selected tests characteristically required before a finished product is released will be discussed briefly, including sterility, pyrogen and particulate tests.

Sterility Test

All lots of injections in their final containers must be tested for sterility. The USP prescribes the requirements for this test for official injections. The FDA uses these requirements as a guide for testing unofficial sterile products. The official test has acknowledged limitations in the information that it can provide, particularly those limitations inherent in microbiological procedures. Therefore, it should be noted that this test is not intended as a thoroughly evaluative test for a product subjected to a sterilization method of unknown effectiveness. It is intended primarily as a check test on the probability that a previously validated sterilization procedure has been repeated, or to give assurance of its continued effectiveness. A discussion of sterility testing is given in Chapter 84.

In the event of a sterility-test failure, the immediate issue concerns whether the growth observed came from viable microorganisms in the product (true contamination) or from adventitious contamination during the testing (a false positive). The USP does permit a retest but the position of the FDA is that retest results are only valid if persuasive evidence exists that the cause of the initial sterility-test failure resides in the laboratory. Therefore, a thorough investigation must be launched to support the justification for performing the retest and assessing the validity of the retest results relative to release of the lot of product.

It should be noted that a "lot" with respect to sterility testing is that group of product containers which has been subjected to the same sterilization procedure. For containers of a product which have been sterilized by autoclaving, for example, a lot would constitute those processed in a particular sterilizer cycle. For an aseptic filling operation, a lot would constitute all of those product containers filled during a period when there was no change in the filling assembly or equipment and which is no longer than one working day or shift.

Pyrogen Test

The USP evaluates the presence of pyrogens in parenteral preparations by a qualitative fever response test in rabbits, the Pyrogen Test (Section ⟨151⟩), and by the Bacterial Endotoxins Test (Section ⟨85⟩). These two USP tests are described in Chapter 30. Rabbits are used as test animals in Section ⟨151⟩ because they show a physiological response to pyrogenic substances similar to that by man. While a minimum pyrogenic dose (MPD), the amount just sufficient to cause a positive USP Pyrogen Test response, sometimes may produce uncertain test results, a content equal to a few times the MPD will leave no uncertainty. Therefore, the test is valid and has continued in use since introduced by Seibert in 1923. It should be understood that not all injections may be subjected to the rabbit test since the medicinal agent may have a physiological effect on the test animal such that any fever response would be masked.

The *Bacterial Endotoxins Test* is an *in vitro* test based on the formation of a gel or the development of color in the presence of bacterial endotoxins and the lysate of the amebocytes of the horseshoe crab (*Limulus polyphemus*). The *Limulus Amebocyte Lysate* (LAL) test, as it also is called, is a biochemical test performed in a test tube, and is simpler, more rapid and of greater sensitivity than the rabbit test.[27] Although it detects only the endotoxic pyrogens of gram-negative bacteria, these are the most prominent environmental microbial contaminants likely to invade sterile products. The test also has been automated.[28]

The LAL test is a semiquantitative test. To provide standardization for the test, the USP has established a reference endotoxin against which lots of the lysate are standardized.

Thus, the sensitivity of the lysate is given in terms of endotoxin units (EU). Most USP injections now have been given limits in terms of EUs (eg, Bacteriostatic Sodium Chloride Injection, 1.0 EU/mL) as another measure of the purity of the product.

Particulate Evaluation

Particulate matter in parenteral solutions long has been recognized as unacceptable since the user could be expected to conclude that the presence of visible "dirt" would suggest that the product is of inferior quality. Today, it is recognized that the presence of particles in solution, particularly if injected intravenously, can be harmful. While data defining the extent of risk and the effects produced still are limited, it has been shown that particles of lint, rubber, insoluble chemicals and other foreign matter can produce emboli in the vital organs of animals and man.[29] Further, it has been shown that the development of infusion-phlebitis may be related to the presence of particulate matter in intravenous fluids.[30]

The particle size of particular concern has not been clearly delineated, but it has been suggested that since erythrocytes have a diameter of approximately 4.5 μm, particles of more than 5 μm should be the basis for evaluation. This is a considerably smaller particle than can be seen with the unaided eye; approximately 50 μm is the lower limit unless the Tyndall effect is used whereby particles as small as 10 μm can be seen by the light scattered from them.

The USP specifies that good manufacturing practice requires that each final container of an injection be subjected individually to a visual inspection and that containers in which visible particles can be seen should be discarded. This 100% inspection of a lot of product is designed to prevent the distribution and use of parenterals which contain particulate matter that may be harmful psychologically or organically to the participant. Therefore, all of the product units from a production line currently are being inspected individually by human inspectors under a good light, baffled against reflection into the eye and against a black-and-white background. This inspection is subject to the limitation of the size of particles that can be seen, the variation of visual acuity from inspector to inspector, their emotional state, eye strain, fatigue and other personal factors that will affect what is seen. However, it does provide a means for eliminating the few units which normally contain visible particles. Slow progress has been made on developing equipment for automated inspection of product containers.

Since it is recognized that visual inspection will not detect the presence of particles smaller than approximately 50 μm in size, the USP has established a microscopic test method for identifying particles in large-volume intravenous solutions and has set limits of not more than 50 particles/mL of 10 μm and larger in size and not more than 5 particles/mL of 25 μm and larger in size. This method consists essentially of filtering a measured sample of solution through a membrane filter under ultraclean conditions and then counting the particles on the surface of the filter using oblique light, under a microscope, at both 40x and 100x magnification. These standards are being met readily by the large-volume parenteral solutions currently being manufactured in the US.

More recently the USP established standards for small-volume parenterals to be given intravenously, using an electronic instrument that counts and measures the size of particles by means of a shadow cast by the particle as it passes through a high-intensity light beam (Suppliers: *Climet, HIAC*). The limits prescribed are not more than 10,000 particles/container of $\geq$ 10 μm in size and not more than 1000 particles/container $\geq$ 25 μm in size. These specifications were developed on the premise that as many as five such products may be added to a 1-L bottle of a large-volume parenteral and five products should not contribute more than the overall limits of particles prescribed for a large-volume parenteral. Whether or not these standards are realistic toxicologically has not been established; rather, the objective of the compendium is to establish specification limits that would encourage the preparation of clean parenteral solutions, particularly for those to be given intravenously.

It also should be realized that administration sets and the techniques used in the hospital for preparing and administering intravenous infusion fluid may introduce substantial amounts of particulate matter into an otherwise clean solution. Therefore, the pharmaceutical manufacturer, the administration set manufacturer, the hospital pharmacist, the nurse and the physician must share responsibilities for making sure that the patient receives a clean intravenous injection.

The USP methods for counting and sizing particulate matter in intravenous solutions are not the only methods available for such determinations. A number of electronic particle counters are available that use the light-scattering principle to count particles in a liquid sample (Suppliers: *Climet, Met One, HIAC/Royco*). There also is an instrument available which counts particles and sizes them by measuring the effect on the resistance between two electrodes as the particles pass between them (Supplier: *Coulter*). It is obvious that only the visual inspection can be used for in-line evaluation of every container produced commercially. All of these methods require very stringent ultraclean preparation techniques to assure reasonable accuracy in counting and sizing only the particles in the solution, rather than those that may have been introduced inadvertently during the sample preparation or the testing procedure. Further, these test procedures are destructive and, therefore, can be performed only on samples of the production lot. Further information may be found in a review article.[31]

Leaker Test

Ampuls that have been sealed by fusion must be subjected to a test to determine whether or not a passageway remains to the outside; if so, all or a part of the contents may leak to the outside and spoil the package, or microorganisms or other contaminants may enter. Changes in temperature during storage cause expansion and contraction of the ampul and contents, and will accentuate intechange if a passageway exists, even if microscopic in size.

This test usually is performed by producing a negative pressure within an incompletely sealed ampul while the ampul is entirely submerged in a deeply colored dye solution. Most often, approximately 1% methylene blue solution is employed. The test may be performed by subjecting the ampuls to a vacuum in a vacuum chamber, the ampuls being submerged in a dye bath throughout the process. Another procedure frequently employed is to simply autoclave the ampuls in a dye bath. A modification of this is to remove them from the autoclave while hot and quickly submerge them in a cool bath of dye solution. After carefully rinsing the dye solution from the outside, color from the dye will be visible within a leaker. Leakers, of course, are discarded.

Vials and bottles are not subjected to a leaker test because the sealing material (rubber stopper) is not rigid. Therefore, results from such a test would be meaningless. However, evacuated bottles containing a liquid may be checked for a sharp "click" sound produced when struck with an implement such as a rubber mallet or the ball of the hand. However, assurance of container-closure sealing integrity should be an integral part of product development by developing specifications for the fit of the closure in the neck of the container, the physical characteristics of the closure, the need for lubrication of the closure and the capping pressure.

Safety Test

The National Institutes of Health requires of most biological products routine safety testing in animals. Under the Kefauver-Harris Amendments to the Federal Food, Drug, and Cosmetic Act, most pharmaceutical preparations are now required to be tested for safety. Because it is entirely possible for a parenteral product to pass the routine sterility test, pyrogen test and chemical analyses and still cause unfavorable reactions when injected, a safety test in animals is essential to provide additional assurance that the product does not have unexpected toxic properties. Safety tests in animals are discussed in detail in the USP.

Packaging and Labeling

A full discussion of the packaging of parenteral preparations is beyond the scope of this text. It is essential, of course, that the packaging should provide ample protection for the product against physical damage from shipping, handling and storage as well as protecting light-sensitive materials from ultraviolet radiation. An extensive review of this subject has been published.[32]

Packaging—The USP includes certain requirements for the packaging and storage of injections, as follows:

1. The volume of injection in single-dose containers is defined as that which is specified for parenteral administration at one time and is limited to a volume of 1 L.
2. Parenterals intended for intraspinal, intracisternal or peridural administration are packaged only in single-dose containers.
3. Unless an individual monograph specifies otherwise, no multiple-dose container shall contain a volume of injection more than sufficient to permit the withdrawal and administration of 30 mL.
4. Injections packaged for use as irrigation solutions or for hemofiltration or dialysis or for parenteral nutrition are exampt from the foregoing requirements relating to packaging. Containers for injections packaged for use as hemofiltration or irrigation solutions may be designed to empty rapidly and may contain a volume in excess of 1 L.
5. Injections intended for veterinary use are exempt from the packaging and storage requirements concerning the limitation to single-dose containers and to volume of multiple-dose containers.

Labeling—The labeling of an injection must provide the physician or other user with all of the information needed to assure the safe and proper use of the therapeutic agent. Since all of this information cannot be placed on the immediate container and be legible, it may be provided on accompanying printed matter. General labeling requirements for drugs are discussed in Chapter 110.

A restatement of the labeling definitions and requirements of the USP for Injections is as follows:

The term "labeling" designates all labels and other written, printed or graphic matter upon an immediate container or upon, or in, any package or wrapper in which it is enclosed, with the exception of the outer shipping container. The term "label" designates that part of the labeling upon the immediate container.

The label states the name of the preparation, the percentage content of drug of a liquid preparation, the amount of active ingredient of a dry preparation, the volume of liquid to be added to prepare an injection or suspension from a dry preparation, the route of administration, a statement of storage conditions and an expiration date. Also, the label must indicate the name of the manufacturer or distributor and carry an identifying lot number. The lot number is capable of providing access to the complete manufacturing history of the specific package, including each single manufacturing step.

The container label is so arranged that a sufficient area of the container remains uncovered for its full length or circumference to permit inspection of the contents.

The label must state the name of the vehicle and the proportions of each constituent, if it is a mixture; the names and proportions of all substances added to increase stability or usefulness and the expiration date where required by the individual monograph.

Preparations labeled for use as dialysis, hemofiltration or irrigation solutions must meet the requirements for Injections other than those relating to volume and also must bear on the label statements that they are not intended for intravenous injection.

Injections intended for veterinary use are so labeled.

References

1. Griffenhagen GB: *Bull Parenter Drug Assoc 16(2):* 12, 1962.
2. Joint Commission on Accreditation of Healthcare Organizations, Accreditation Manual for Hospitals, p 107, Chicago, 1992.
3. Trissel LA. *Handbook on Injectable Drugs,* 7th ed, Am Soc Hosp Pharm, Bethesda, MD, 1992.
4. 21 CFR 210, Current Good Manufacturing Practice in manufacturing, processing, packaging or holding of drugs; general, Supt. of Documents, USGPO, Washington DC.
5. *Tech Rep No 4,* Parenteral Drug Association (PDA), Philadelphia, 1983.
6. Brown J *et al: Pharm Eng 11(4):* 15, 1991.
7. Spiegel AJ, Noseworthy MM: *J Pharm Sci 52:* 917, 1963.
8. Schroeter LC: *Ibid 50:* 891, 1961.
9. Pearson FC III: *Pyrogens,* Dekker, New York, 1985.
10. Morton DK: *J Parenter Sci Technol 41:* 145, 1987.
11. Autian J: *Bull Parenter Drug Assoc 22:* 276, 1968.
12. Lambert P: *Pharm Technol 15:* 48, 1991.
13. *Tech Methods Bull No. 3,* PDA, Philadelphia, 1982.
14. *Tech Methods Bull No 1,* PDA, Philadelphia, 1980.
15. *Tech Methods Bull No 2,* PDA, Philadelphia, 1981.
16. Fed Std No 209E, GSA, Washington, DC 20407, Sep. 11, 1992.
17. Davenport SM: *Proc PharmTech Conf,* 92, 1992.
18. Whyte W, Niven L: *J Parenter Sci Technol 40:* 182, 1986.
19. Grimes TL, Fonner DE *et al: Ibid 31:* 179, 1977.
20. Myers T, Chrai S: *J Parenter Sci Technol 35:* 8, 1981.
21. Seiberling DA: *Pharm Eng 6(6):* 30, 1986.
22. Singh M, Ravin LJ: *Ibid 40:* 34, 1986.
23. Levy RV, Souza KS, Neville CB: *Pharm Technol 14:* 160, 1990.
24. *Ann NY Acad Sci 85:* 501–734, 1965.
25. Morgan SL, Spotts MR: *Pharm Technol 3:* 94–101, 114, 1979.
26. Nail SL, Gatlin LA: *J Parenter Sci Technol 39:* 16, 1985.
27. Cooper JF: *Bull Parenter Drug Assoc 29:* 122, 1975.
28. Novitsky TJ, Ryther SS *et al: J Parenter Sci Technol 36:* 11, 1982.
29. Garvan JM, Gunner BW: *Med J Aust 2:* 1, July 4, 1964.
30. Deluca P *et al: Am J Hosp Pharm 32:* 1001, 1975.
31. Borchert SJ, Abe A *et al: J Parenter Sci Technol 40:* 212, 1986.
32. *Tech Report No. 5,* PDA, Philadelphia, 1984.

Bibliography

Akers MJ: *Parenteral Quality Control,* Dekker, New York, 1985.

Avis KE, Levchuk JW. In King RE, ed: *Dispensing of Medication,* 9th ed, Mack Publ Co, Easton PA, Chap 9, 1984.

Avis KE, Lieberman HA, Lachman L, eds: *Pharmaceutical Dosage Forms: Parenteral Medications,* 2nd ed, vol 1, Dekker, New York, 1992.

Ibid, 2nd ed, vol 2, Dekker, New York, 1993.

Ibid, 2nd ed, vol 3, Dekker, New York, 1993.

Avis KE. In Lachman L *et al: The Theory and Practice of Industrial Pharmacy,* 3rd ed, Lea & Febiger, Philadelphia, Chaps 21 & 22, 1986.

Block SS, ed: *Disinfection, Sterilization and Preservation,* 3rd ed, Lea & Febiger, Philadelphia, 1983.

Carleton FJ, Agalloco JP, eds: *Validation of Aseptic Pharmaceutical Processes,* Dekker, New York, 1986.

Gaughran ERL, Kereluk K, eds: *Sterilization of Medical Products,* Johnson & Johnson, New Brunswick NJ, 1977.

Martin EW *et al: Techniques of Medication,* Lippincott, Philadelphia, 1969.

Meltzer TH, ed: *Filtration in the Pharmaceutical Industry,* Dekker, New York, 1987.

Meryman HT, ed: *Cryobiology,* Academic, New York, 1966.

Pearson FC III: *Pyrogens,* Dekker, New York, 1985.

Phillips GB, Miller WS, eds: *Industrial Sterilization,* Duke Univ Press, Durham NC, 1973.

Turco S, King RE: *Sterile Dosage Forms,* 3rd ed, Lea & Febiger, Philadelphia, 1987.

CHAPTER 88

Intravenous Admixtures

Salvatore J Turco, PharmD, FASHP
Professor of Pharmacy
Temple University School of Pharmacy
Philadelphia, PA 19140

It has been estimated that 40% of all drugs administered in hospitals are given in the form of injections and their use is increasing. Part of this increase in parenteral therapy is due to the wider use of intravenous fluids (IV fluids). In the last decade the use of IV fluids has doubled, increasing from 150 million units to 320 million units annually. Not only do IV fluids continue to serve as the means for fluid replacement, electrolyte-balance restoration and supplementary nutrition, but they also are playing major roles as vehicles for administration of other drug substances and in total parenteral nutrition (TPN). Intravenous fluids are finding greater use as the means of administering other drugs because of convenience, the means of reducing the irritation potential of the drugs and the desirability for continuous and intermittent drug therapy. The techniques for providing TPN parenterally have improved steadily in the last decade, and such use is increasing markedly. The use of IV fluids for these purposes requires the compounding of specific intravenous admixtures (parenteral prescriptions) to meet the clinical needs of a given patient. However, the combination of drug substances in an IV fluid can promote parenteral incompatibilities and give rise to conditions not favorable for drug stability. A new area of specialization has been created for hospital pharmacists who can develop the expertise to prepare these solutions—recognizing their compatibility and stability problems and the potential for contamination—and participate in the administration of the solutions. The complex compounding of an order for TPN requires knowledgeable personnel capable of making accurate calculations, compounding and having aseptic technique. The parenteral prescription is becoming increasingly important in hospitals. Centralized admixture programs are now found in 85% of the nation's hospitals having 300 beds or more. Equipment available for administering IV fluids has become more sophisticated, and has made possible increased accuracy of dosage and led to the development of new concepts and methods of nutrition and drug therapy.

Electronic mechanical equipment is now commonplace in hospitals. Its use, as well as its sophistication, continues to increase. Newly designed electronic pumps have been developed for hospital ambulatory use. Multichannel pumps have become available for multiple-drug infusion. Over 500,000 implantable infusion ports have been inserted into patients and 100,000 new patients receive these implantable ports each year in order to accomplish drug therapy. New methods of IV drug delivery systems have been introduced and are constantly evolving. The introduction of patient controlled analgesia (PCA) is commonplace in hospitals. This technology allows the patient with pain to control the degree of analgesia desired.

The growth of TPN in hospitals has been paralleled by home TPN programs. Large numbers of patients conduct parenteral nutrition in the home environment, including those with infectious and neoplastic diseases. More stringent and complete guidelines for the preparation and parenterals in hospitals by pharmacists have been published. These guidelines, promoting sophisticated methods of preparation by the pharmacist, have become recommendations. They are a testament to the importance of parenteral preparation in the institutional setting. Packaging of parenterals in the past five years also has undergone dramatic changes. Prefilled, premixed, prefrozen parenterals are now supplied by the manufacturers. Newly designed plastic mini-bags (*ADD-Vantage* Abbott) have been introduced. Premixed liquids (eg, antibiotics, theophylline, heparin, lidocaine, dopamine) are available from parenteral manufacturers. Multiple-dose containers (*Maxivials*, Lyphomed) have been developed to accommodate new methods of preparation of parenterals by the pharmacist. The pharmaceutical industry has responded to the needs of pharmacists by addressing the packaging, labeling and design requirements necessary to facilitate patient care. The parenteral drug industry continues its efforts to meet higher standards of quality and to assure the availability of sterile and particulate-free products.

Intravenous Fluids

Large-volume injections intended to be administered by intravenous infusion commonly are called IV fluids and are included in the group of sterile products referred to as large-volume parenterals. These consist of single-dose injections having a volume of 100 mL or more and containing no added substances. Intravenous fluids are packaged in containers having a capacity of 100 to 1000 mL. Minitype infusion containers of 250-mL capacity are available with 50- and 100-mL partial fills for solution of drugs when used in the "piggyback" technique (ie, the administration of a second solution through a Y-tube or gum-rubber connection in the administration set of the first intravenous fluid, thus avoiding the need for another injection site). In addition to the IV fluids, this group also includes irrigation solutions and solutions for dialysis.

Intravenous fluids are sterile solutions of simple chemicals such as sugars, amino acids or electrolytes—materials which easily can be carried by the circulatory system and assimilated. Prepared with Water for Injection USP, the solutions are pyrogen-free. Because of the large volumes administered intravenously, the absence of particulate matter assumes a significant role in view of possible biological hazards resulting from insoluble particles. Absence of particulate matter or clarity of IV fluids is as important at the time of administration following their manipulation in the hospital as it is at the time of manufacture of the injection.

Limits for particulate matter occurring in IV fluids, or large-volume injections used for single-dose infusion, are defined in the USP. This represents the first regulatory attempt to define limits for particulate matter in parenterals. Limits also apply to multiple-dose injections, small-volume injections or injections prepared by reconstitution from sterile solids. The USP defines particulate matter as extraneous, mobile, undissolved substances, other than gas bubbles, unintentionally present in parenteral solutions. The total numbers of particles having effective linear dimensions equal to or larger than 10 μm and larger than 25 μm are counted. The IV fluid meets the requirement of the test if it contains not more than 50 particles per mL which are equal to or larger than 10 μm, and not more than 5 particles per mL which are equal to or larger than 25 μm in linear dimension.

Intravenous fluids commonly are used for a number of clinical conditions. These include

- Correction of disturbances in electrolyte balance.
- Correction of disturbances in body fluids (fluid replacement).
- The means of providing basic nutrition.
- The basis for the practice of providing TPN.
- Use as vehicles for other drug substances.

In both of the latter two cases it has become common practice to add other drugs to certain IV fluids to meet the clinical needs of the patient. Using IV fluids as vehicles offers the advantages of convenience, the means of reducing the irritation potential of the drug and a method for continuous drug therapy. However, the practice requires that careful consideration be given to the stability and compatibility of additives present in the IV fluids serving as the vehicle. This approach also demands strict adherence to aseptic techniques in adding the drugs, as well as in the administration of the IV fluids. These procedures are discussed later in the chapter. The IV fluids commonly used for parenterals are shown in Table 1.

Many disease states result in electrolyte depletion and loss. Proper electrolyte concentration and balance in plasma and tissues are critical for proper body function. Electrolyte restoration and balance are achieved most rapidly through administration of IV fluids. Required electrolytes include sodium and chloride ions, which in normal saline more closely approximate the composition of the extracellular fluid than solutions of any other single salt; potassium, the principal intracellular cation of most body tissues and essential for the functioning of the nervous and muscular systems as well as the heart; magnesium, as a nutritional supplement especially in TPN solutions and phosphate ion, important in a variety of biochemical reactions. In addition to the number of standard electrolyte fluids shown in Table 1, a large number of combinations of electrolytes in varying concentrations are available commercially. Some of these electrolyte fluids also contain dextrose.

Dextrose Injection 5% (D5/W) is the most frequently used IV fluid, either for nutrition or fluid replacement. It is isotonic and administered intravenously into a peripheral vein; 1 g of dextrose provides 3.4 cal and 1 L of D5/W supplies 170 cal. The body uses dextrose at a rate of 0.5 g per kg of body weight per hour. More rapid administration can result in glycosuria. Therefore, 1 L of D5/W requires 1½ hours for assimilation. The pH range of D5/W can vary from 3.5 to 6.5. The wide range permitted is due to the free sugar acids present and formed during the sterilization and storage of the injection. To avoid incompatibilities when other drug substances are added to Dextrose Injection, the possible low pH should be considered in using it as a vehicle. More concentrated solutions of dextrose are available and provide in-

Table 1—Fluids Used Commonly for IV Use

Injection	Concentration (%)	pH	Therapeutic use
Alcohol			
with D5/W[a]	5	4.5	Sedative, analgesic, colories
with D5/W in NSS[b]	5		Sedative, analgesic, calories
Amino acid (synthetic)			Fluid and nutrient replenisher
Aminosyn II (*Abbott*)	3.5; 7	5.25	
FreAmine III (*McGaw*)	8.5	6.6	
Travasol (*Baxter*)	3.5; 5.5; 8.5	6.0	
Ammonium chloride	2.14	4.5–6.0	Metabolic alkaloids
Dextran 40			
in NSS	10	5	Priming fluid for extracorporeal circulation
in D5/W	10	4	Priming fluid for extracorporeal circulation
Dextran 70			
in NSS	6	5	Plasma volume expander
in D5/W	6	4	Plasma volume expander
Dextrose (glucose, D5/W)	2.5–50	3.5–6.5	Fluid and nutrient replenisher
Dextrose and sodium chloride	Varying concn of dextrose from 5–20 with varying concn of sodium chloride from 0.22–0.9	3.5–6.5	Fluid, nutrient and electrolyte replenisher
Invert sugar (fructose and dextrose)	5, 10	4.0	Fluid and nutrient replenisher
Lactated Ringer's (Hartmann's)		6.0–7.5	Systemic alkalizer; fluid and electrolyte replenisher
NaCl	0.6		
KCl	0.03		
$CaCl_2$	0.02		
Lactate	0.3		
Mannitol	5	5.0–7.0	Osmotic diuresis
also in combination with	10		
dextrose or sodium	15		
chloride	20		
Multiple electrolyte solutions varying combinations of electrolytes, dextrose, fructose, invert sugar		5.5	Fluid and electrolyte replacement
Ringer's		5.0–7.5	Fluid and electrolyte replenisher
NaCl	0.86		
KCl	0.03		
$CaCl_2$	0.033		
Sodium bicarbonate	5	8	Metabolic acidosis
Sodium chloride	0.45; 0.9; 3; 5	4.5–7.0	Fluid and electrolyte replenisher
Sodium lactate	1/6 *M*	6.3–7.3	Fluid and electrolyte replenisher
Sterile water for injection		5.5	Diluent

[a] 5% Dextrose in water.
[b] Normal saline solution.

creased calorie intake with less fluid volume. Being hypertonic, the more concentrated solutions may be irritating to peripheral veins. Highly concentrated solutions are administered in a larger central vein. Other IV fluids used for intravenous admixtures and providing calories include solutions containing invert sugar. There is some evidence that fructose, unlike dextrose, may be used in diabetic patients; the 10% injection is hypertonic and provides 375 cal per L. Invert sugar consists of equal parts of dextrose and fructose; it is claimed that the presence of fructose promotes more rapid utilization of dextrose.

Intravenous fluids containing crystalline amino acids can provide biologically usable amino acids for protein synthesis (Chapter 65). Protein contributes to tissue growth, wound repair and resistance to infection. The protein requirement for the normal adult is 1 g per kg per day; children and patients under stress require greater amounts. Attempts are made to maintain a positive nitrogen balance, indicating that the protein administered is being utilized properly and not broken down and eliminated through the urine as creatinine and urea, which are normal waste products. In a positive nitrogen balance patients are taking in more nitrogen than they are eliminating. In a negative nitrogen balance there is more nitrogen being eliminated through the urine regularly than is being administered intravenously. This means that tissues are continuing to be torn down and repair is not necessarily taking place. Amino Acid Injection can afford the total body requirements for proteins by the procedure known as TPN (discussed below) or be used for supplemental nutrition by peripheral administration. In addition to the amino acids, these nutritional injections also may contain dextrose, electrolytes, vitamins and insulin. Fat emulsion (*Intralipid*, Kabi Vitrum AB; *Liposyn II*, Abbott and *Travamulsion*, Baxter) sometimes is used concurrently but usually administered at another site. However, new systems such as three-in-one packaging permit mixing of amino acids, carbohydrates and fat in one container for TPN.

Packaging Systems

Containers for intravenous fluids must be designed to maintain solution sterility, clarity (freedom from particulate matter) and nonpyrogenicity from the time of preparation, through storage and during clinical administration. Container closures must be designed to facilitate insertion of administration sets through which the injections are administered, at a regulated flow-rate, into suitable veins. IV fluids are available in glass and plastic containers; the latter may be made from either a flexible or semirigid plastic material. IV fluids are supplied in 1000-mL, 500-mL and 250-mL sizes in addition to 250-mL capacity containers packaged with 50 or 100 mL of D5/W or sodium chloride injection 0.9% for piggyback use in addition to 0.45% sodium chloride and 2.5% dextrose injections. IV fluids in glass containers are packaged under vacuum, which must be dissipated prior to use. For fluid to leave the IV glass container and flow through the administration set, some mechanism is necessary to permit air to enter the container. Current flexible plastic systems do not require air introduction in order to function. Atmospheric pressure pressing on the container forces the fluid to flow.

All glass and plastic containers are single-dose and should be discarded after opening even if not used. Intravenous fluids are packaged with approximately 3% excess fill to allow for removal of air from the administration set and permit the labeled volume to be delivered from the container. The containers are graduated at 20-mL increments on scales that permit the volume in container to be determined either from an upright or inverted position. Glass containers have aluminum and plastic bands for hanging, while plastic containers have eyelet openings or plastic straps for attachment to IV poles.

Fluids for IV use are available from three sources (Abbott, Baxter and McGaw); all provide both glass and plastic containers. The glass-container systems of Baxter and McGaw are similar. The characteristics of current packaging systems are summarized in Table 2.

Table 2—IV Fluid Systems

Source	Container	Characteristics
Baxter	Glass	Vacuum Air tube
Baxter (*Viaflex*)	Plastic	Polyvinyl chloride Flexible Nonvented
McGaw	Glass	Vacuum Air tube
McGaw (*Excell*)	Plastic	Flexible
McGaw (*Accumed*)	Plastic	Polyolefin Semirigid
Abbott	Glass	Vacuum Air filter[a]
Abbott (*Lifecare*)	Plastic	Polyvinyl chloride Flexible Nonvented

[a]Part of administration set.

Administration Sets

Administration sets used to deliver fluids intravenously are sterile, pyrogen-free and disposable. Although these sets are supplied by different manufacturers, each for its own system, they have certain basic components. These usually include a plastic spike to pierce the rubber closure or plastic seal on the IV container, a drip (sight) chamber to trap air and permit adjustment of flow rate and a length (150 to 450 cm) of polyvinyl chloride tubing terminating in a gum-rubber injection port. At the tip of the port is a rigid needle or catheter adapter. An adjustable clamp (screw or roller type) on the tubing pinches the tubing to regulate flow. Since the gum-rubber port is self-sealing, additional medication can be added to the IV system at these ports of entry. Glass containers that have no air tubes require air-inlet filters designed as part of the administration set (Abbott). See Figs 1 to 6.

Administration Procedures

In the administration of IV fluids, the primary IV container provides for fluid replacement, electrolyte replenishment, drug therapy or nutrition; the fluid can be infused over a 4- to 8-hour period. In some cases an IV fluid is infused slowly for the purpose of keeping the vein open (KVO). This will allow additional drugs to be administered when required. The primary IV fluid also can serve as a vehicle for other drugs to be administered, thus becoming an intravenous admixture (IV drip) and results in continuous blood levels of added drugs once the steady state has been reached.

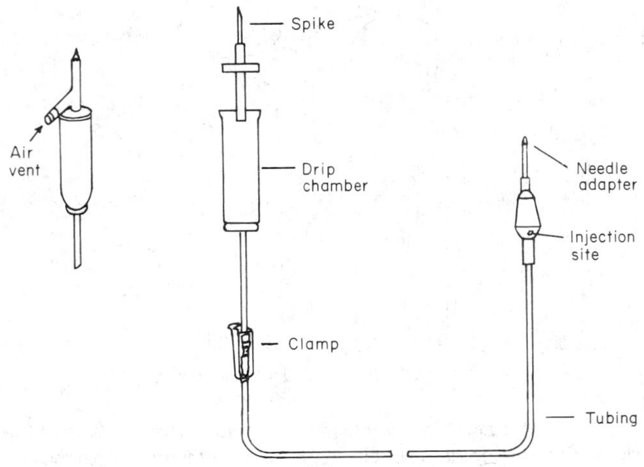

Fig 1. Parts of basic administration sets.

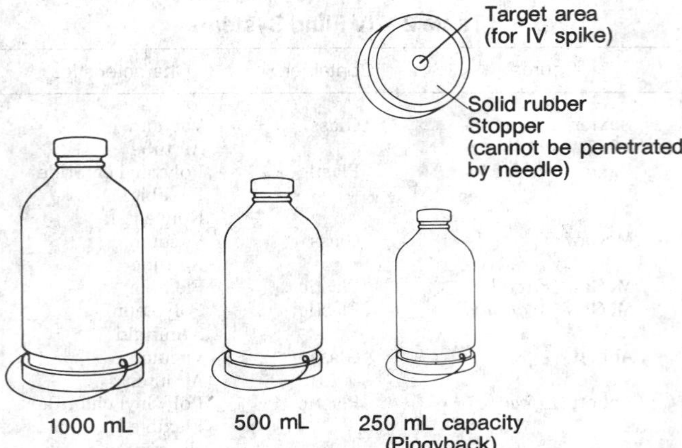

Fig 2. Abbott IV glass container. The air venting is provided through the air filter located in the spike of the administration set. See Fig 1.

The *Accumed* (McGaw) semirigid polyolefin plastic container is being phased out of production in favor of a new non-PVC, non-phthalate flexible container termed *Excell*.

Incinerated PVC products produce hydrogen chloride gas as a toxic pollutant. Diethyl hexyl phthalate (DEHP), a component of PVC containers may leach into the soil in landfills. A number of drugs adsorb on PVC containers, notably nitroglycerin. Some drugs (fat emulsions, blood, taxol) are known to leach DEHP.

The *Excell* container is claimed to eliminate or minimize these problems. The plastic film contains no plasticizers and exhibits no leachability. The solution-contact layer of the container is composed of a rubberized compolymer of ethylene and propylene; which is claimed to be clear, nontoxic and biologically inert. The container is available in 250-mL, 500-mL, and 1-L sizes. Smaller sizes are available in 25, 50 and 100 mL known as PAB containers.

In preparing an IV fluid for administration, the following procedure is used.

The spike adapter of the administration set is inserted into the stopper or seal of the IV container.

The IV fluid is hung on a stand at bedside and air is purged from the administration set by opening the clamp until fluid comes out of needle. The tubing is then clamped off.

The venipuncture is made by member of the IV team, floor nurse or physician.

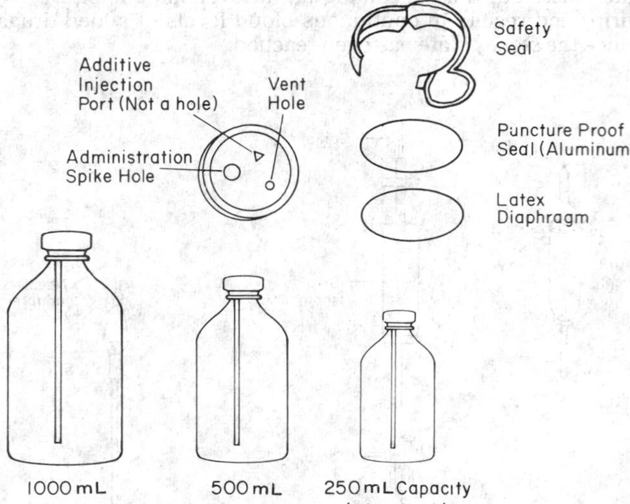

Fig 3. Baxter and McGaw glass containers. The plastic air tube allows the air to enter the bottle as the fluid is infused into the patient. The spike of the administration set is not vented. See Fig 1.

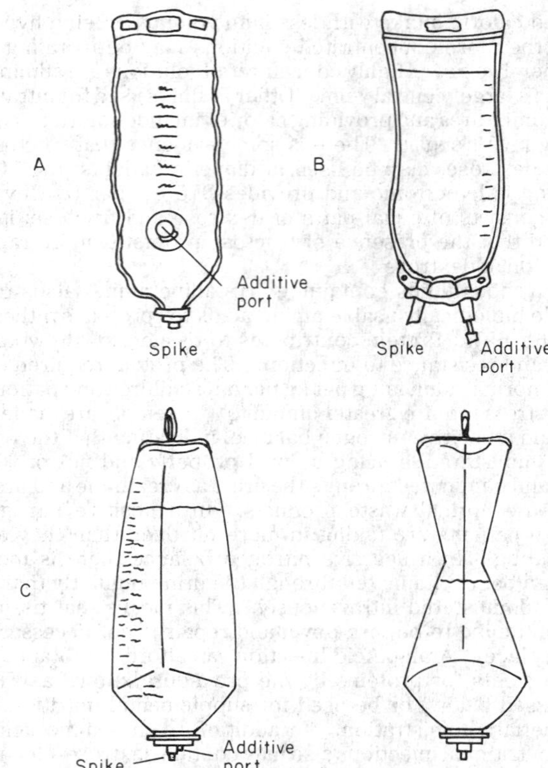

Fig 4. (A) Abbott (*Lifecare*) polyvinyl chloride flexible container; (B) Baxter (*Viaflex*) polyvinyl chloride flexible container. These containers take nonvented administration sets. See Fig 1.

The infusion rate is adjusted by slowly opening and closing the clamp until the desired drop rate, viewed in the drip chamber, is obtained. The usual running time is 4 to 8 hours (usually 125 mL are delivered in 1 hour). Drugs such as heparin, insulin, lidocaine or dopamine may be present in the IV drip. When potent drugs are present, the flow rates will vary depending on the clinical condition of the patient. Sets are calculated to deliver 10, 15, 20, 50 or 60 drops per mL, depending on the manufacturer.

Intermittent administration of an antibiotic and other drugs can be achieved by any of three methods: (1) direct intravenous injection (IV bolus or push), (2) addition of the drug to a predetermined volume of fluid in a volume-control device or (3) use of a second container (minibottle, minibag) with an already hanging IV fluid (piggybacking).

Direct Intravenous Injection—Small volumes (1 to 50 mL) of drugs are injected into the vein over a short period of time (1 to 5 minutes). The injection also can be made through a resealable gum-rubber injection site of an already hanging IV fluid. This method is suitable for a limited number of drugs but too hazardous for most drugs.

Volume-Control Method—Volume-control sets provide a means for intermittent infusion of drug solutions in precise quantities, at controlled rates of flow. These units consist of calibrated, plastic, fluid chambers placed in a direct line under an established primary IV container or more often attached to an independent fluid supply. In either case, the drug to be administered is first reconstituted if it is a sterile solid and injected into the gum-rubber injection port of the volume-control unit. It is then further diluted to 50 to 150 mL with the primary fluid or the separate fluid reservoir. Administration of the total drug-containing solution requires 30 to 60 minutes and produces a peak concentration in the blood followed by a valley if the dosage is discontinued. The following volume-control sets are available commercially: *Soluset*, Abbott; *Buretrol*, Baxter and *Metriset*, McGaw.

The procedure for setting up an intermittent IV infusion with a volume-control set is

Using aseptic technique, the spike of the volume-control set is inserted into the primary IV fluid or a separate fluid container. See Fig 6.

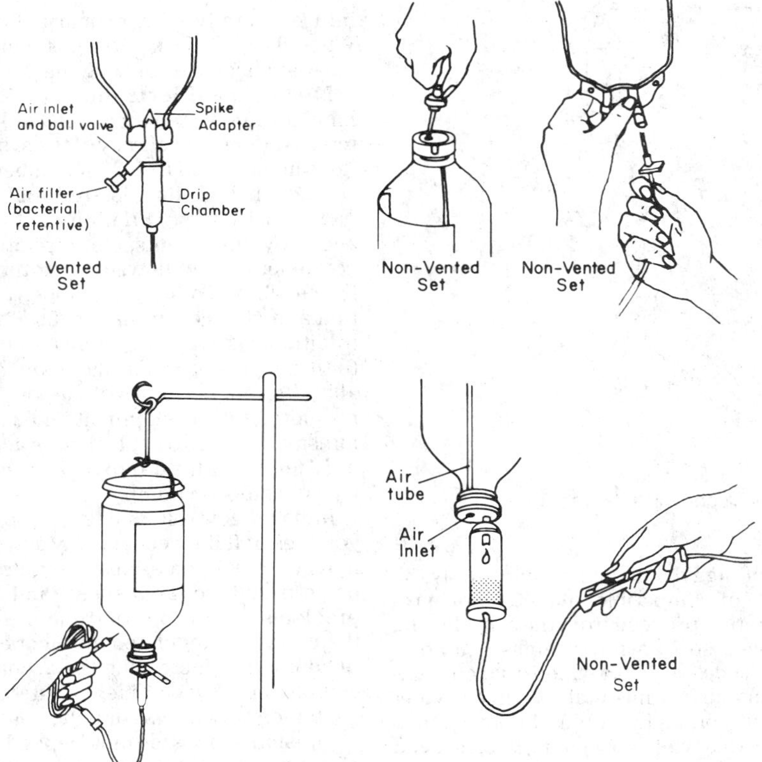

Fig 5. Setting up a primary IV fluid for administration.

Air is purged from tubing of the volume-control set by opening the clamps until fluid comes through.

The clamp is opened above the calibrated chamber and it is filled with 25 to 50 mL fluid from the primary IV container or separate fluid container.

The clamp is closed above the chamber.

The medication is injected through the gum-rubber port of the volume-control unit.

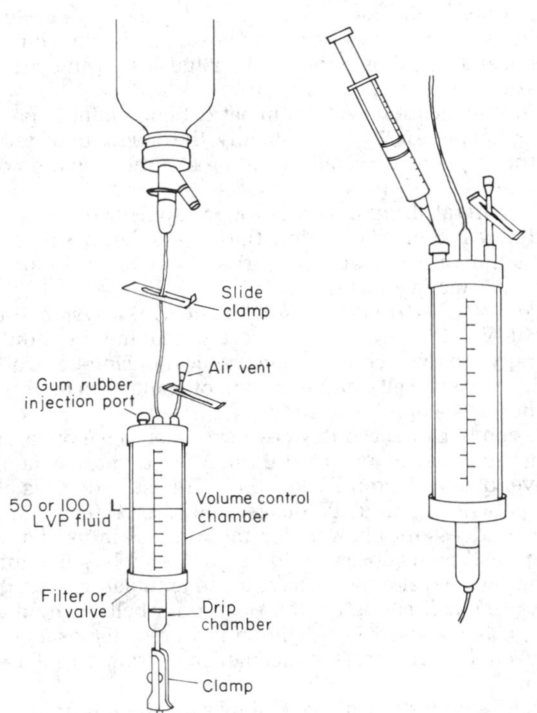

Fig 6. Volume control unit for intermittent administration.

The clamp above the chamber is opened to complete the dilution to the desired volume (50 to 150 mL), then closed.

Flow commences when the clamp below the volume-control unit is opened.

Piggyback Method—The piggyback method (Fig 7) refers to the intermittent IV drip of a second solution, the reconstituted drug, through the venipuncture site of an established primary IV system. With this setup the drug can be thought of as entering the vein on "top" of the primary IV fluid, hence the designation "piggyback." The piggyback technique not only eliminates the need for another venipuncture, but also achieves drug dilution and peak blood levels within a relatively short time span, usually 30 to 60 minutes. Drug dilution helps to reduce irritation, and early high serum levels are an important consideration in serious infection requiring aggressive drug therapy. These advantages have popularized the piggyback method of IV therapy, especially for the intermittent administration of antibiotics. In using the piggyback technique, the secondary unit is purged of air and its needle inserted into a Y-injection site of the primary set or into the injection site at the end of the primary set. The piggyback infusion is then started. Once it is completed, the primary fluid infusion will be restarted. See Fig 7.

Primary IV administration sets are available that have a built-in check valve for use in piggyback administration. When the piggyback is connected to one of these sets and started, the check valve automatically closes off the primary infusion. When the piggyback runs out, the check valve automatically opens, thereby restarting the primary infusion. The check valve works because of pressure differences. To achieve this difference, the primary container is hung lower than the secondary bottle by means of an extension hanger. See Fig 8.

Manufacturers have introduced minibottles prefilled with various antibiotic products; each container is provided with a plastic hanger for direct suspension from an IV pole as the piggyback solution is administered through the resealable gum-rubber injection site or Y-type facility of an existing IV

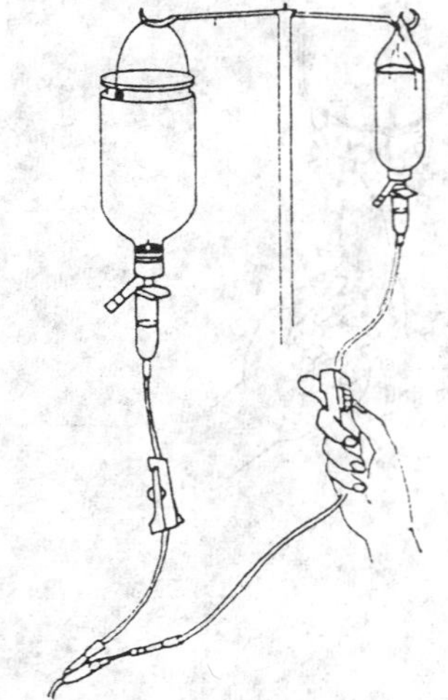

Fig 7. Piggyback administration setup.

system. Reconstitution of piggyback units requires only the addition of a small volume of compatible diluent. Since reconstitution and administration proceed from the same bottle, no drug transfer is involved, so transfer syringes and additional IV containers are not necessary. Prefilled drug containers offer significant advantages to hospitals. Time-saving, less potential for error and contamination and convenience are outstanding qualities of this type of packaging. The need exists in hospitals for these types of innovative packaging to help alleviate the critical nursing shortage and reduce the error potential. It is a significant event that drug manufacturers and intravenous fluid manufacturers have combined efforts to achieve optimal packaging for hospital use.

Partial-fill containers available for piggybacking are 250-mL capacity infusion bottles or bags underfilled with 50 or 100 mL D5/W or normal saline. The drug to be administered first is reconstituted in its original parenteral vial and then added by needle and syringe to the partial-fill container. The needle of the piggyback delivery system is inserted into the Y-site or gum-rubber injection port of a hanging primary infusion set. Flow of the primary intravenous fluid is stopped while the drug solution in the partial-fill container is administered (30 to 60 minutes). After the drug solution has been

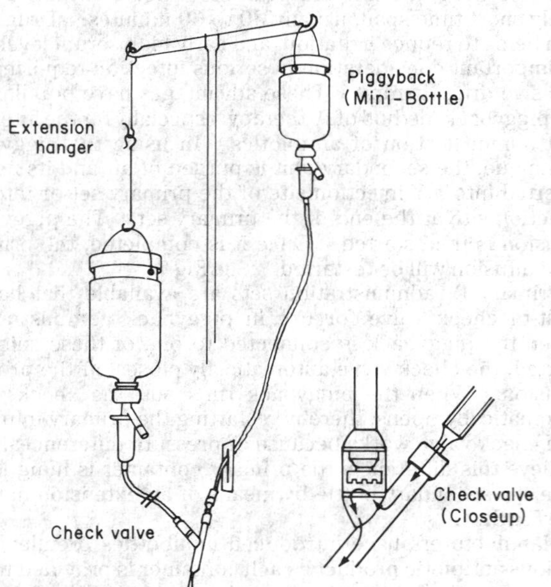

Fig 8. Piggyback administration setup with check valve in primary set.

infused totally, the primary fluid flow is re-established. When the next dose of drug is required, the piggyback procedure is repeated, replacing the prefilled partial-fill container.

Mechanical-Electronic Infusion Devices—Gravity IV administration systems are affected by many variables which tend to alter the accuracy of the system. These include variations in the size of the drip-chamber orifice, the viscosity of the solution being administered, plastic cold flow, clamp slippage, final filters, variations in the patient's blood pressure and body movements, clot formation, pressure changes in IV containers rate of flow, temperature of the IV fluid, changes in the needle and other factors such as kinked tubing, extravasation and changes in the height of the IV container. Flow in traditional gravity IV systems is controlled by manual clamps (either screw or roller clamps) which can provide considerable discrepancies in volume delivery. These factors have promoted the development and use of mechanical-electronic infusion devices to control more accurately the administration of IV fluids. This group of devices includes infusion controllers and infusion pumps.

Infusion controllers count drops electronically or extrude volumes of fluid mechanically and electronically. Having no moving components, controllers are less complex than pumps, being usually less expensive and having fewer maintenance problems. Infusion controllers are gravity-type systems, but the control is regulated automatically rather than manually. In addition to increasing the accuracy of delivery, electronic equipment may be able to detect infiltration of air, empty containers and excess or deficient flow.

Infusion pumps do not depend on gravity to provide the pressure required to infuse the drug. Pressure is provided by an electric pump that propels a syringe, a peristaltic or roller device or a cassette. Most pumps are volumetric in that the delivery is measured in milliliters rather than drops.

The quality of patient care has improved with the use of infusion devices. Flow rates can be maintained, therefore parenteral and enteral nutrition can be conducted safely. In addition, accurate drug therapy can be accomplished with adults and children and "runaways" of IV fluid administration can be eliminated.

Patient-Controlled Analgesia (PCA)—Usually and traditionally the acute or chronic pain experienced by patients in selected diseases are treated initially by oral narcotics and analgesics. However, many clinical situations preclude oral administration. Typically, the unsatisfied pain from disease has been treated by parenteral analgesics given by the IM or SC route.

This medication cycle from patient complaint to pain relief often can be lengthy. Frequently, the dose administered may be too large or too small, resulting in either sedation or poor pain relief. See Fig 10.

Parenteral drugs given IV offer rapid distribution in the body and fast onset of action; the drug undergoes no biotransformation or inactivation and, therefore, allows for more precise dose management.

Patient-Controlled Analgesia (PCA) is a system for delivery of IV or SC narcotics by direct patient intervention. This therapy uses a mechanical, electronic, infusion-control device which permits self-administration of analgesics in proportion to the degree of relief desired.

A number of these devices have been developed and are undergoing development at Bard, Abbott, Pharmacia, Deltec, Travenol and Becton Dickinson. The early devices allowed for patient-triggered IV doses, and later refinement in the microprocessors allowed for tailoring of infusions so that additional bolus doses could be given to a baseline infusion. Additional developments have led to ambulatory PCA devices that are small enough to be worn on a belt. An additional design being used is a balloon-powered disposable device (Travenol) that operates mechanically from an inflated balloon.

In its simplest terms, PCA allows a patient to initiate an IV infusion of a prescribed narcotic analgesic and maintain a

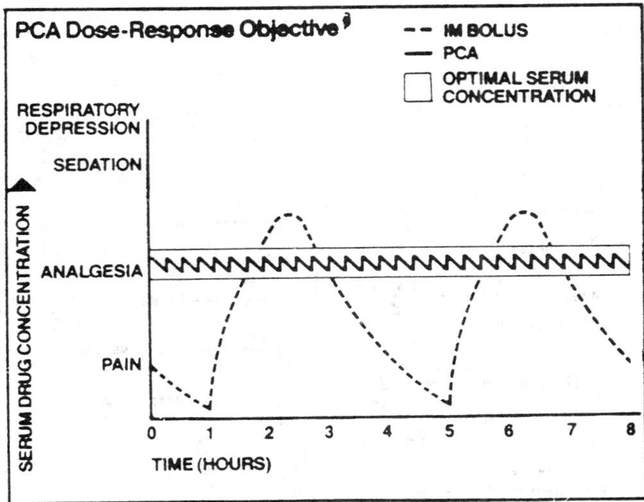

Fig 9. Characteristic pattern comparison of IM bolus serum concentration versus PCA.[3]

self-regulated small amount of incremental doses needed for controlling a variety of pain-associated medical problems.

The success and popularity of PCA is based upon the inadequacy of conventional IM and IV dosing, such as variables that effect absorption and distribution[1] such as conventional nursing practices, inherent procedural delays in securing medication and the ultimate administration to the patient.[2] The perception and sensation of pain in any one patient depends upon individual levels of endorphins and other biochemicals in cerebrospinal fluid.[3]

The last several years have seen the increasing use of infusion devices for epidural or intrathecal administration.

PCA eliminates the peak and valley effects of traditional drug therapy (Fig 9). Epidural or intrathecal therapy of PCA allows a longer duration of drug action.

Kwan[4] reviewed the use of infusion devices for epidural or intrathecal administration.

Final-Filter Devices—Particulate matter in IV fluids and IV admixtures can originate from many sources. It can result from the packaging components of the IV fluid, from admixture incompatibilities, from manipulation in preparing the admixture and even from the administration set itself. Concern for particulate matter led to the design of final-filter devices for attaching to the end of the tubing of the administration set. They afford a final filtration of the IV fluid before it passes through the needle into the vein. The device consists of a plastic chamber containing a membrane or stainless-steel filter having porosities varying from 5 to 0.22 μm. Air lock can be a problem with membrane filters. When wet, membranes with a porosity of 0.22 μm and 0.45 μm are impervious to air at normal pressures and air in the system causes blockage. In order to prevent this, the filter housing must be purged completely of air prior to use. Newer designs have air eliminators. Using final-filter devices increases medication cost but reduces the biological hazards associated with particulate matter.

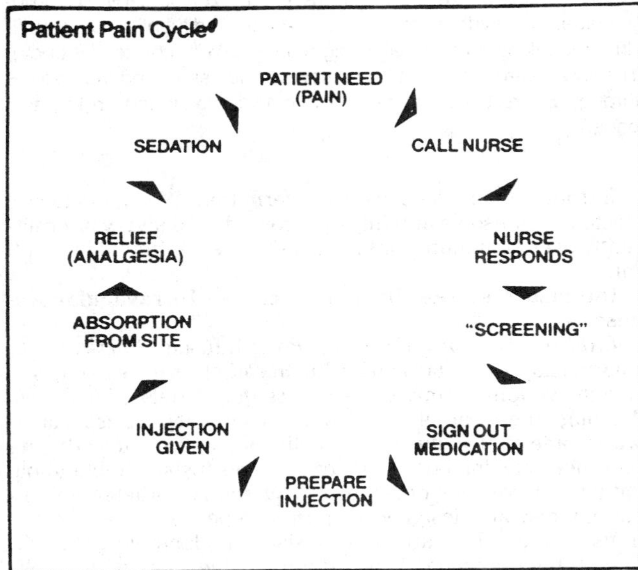

Fig 10. Patient pain cycle—sequence of events.[3]

Although considerable information is available concerning the clinical use of membrane filters in entrapping particulate matter and microorganisms, little information exists describing drug absorption by the filter. Literature on a limited number of drugs and filter materials indicates that drugs administered in low doses might present a problem with drug bonding to the filter.[5] Solutions containing minute dosages of drugs, 5 mg or less, should not be filtered until sufficient data are available to confirm insignificant absorption. Drugs not recommended to be filtered include all parenteral suspensions, blood and blood products, amphotericin B, digitoxin, insulin, intravenous fat emulsions, mithramycin, nitroglycerin and vincristine.

IV Delivery Systems—

Frozen Premixes—Baxter provides delivery to hospitals of frozen drug products packaged in polyvinyl chloride containers. These are stored in a freezer in the hospital's pharmacy, thawed and used when needed. See Fig 11*A*.

Faspak/ADS-100 System—Eli Lilly supplies a non-PVC plastic piggyback container, named Faspak, which contains the dry, powdered form of certain drugs (Keflin, Kefzol, Mandol and ampicillin) which, upon reconstitution with the appropriate diluent, allows direct administration of the diluted drug. This avoids a transferring step that normally takes place when reconstituting a powdered drug. To help in the reconstitution step, a specialized dilution pump named the ADS-100 system is supplied. The package design eliminates the need for transferring between containers after reconstitution, and the Faspak acts as a final delivery container.

Abbott/ADD-Vantage System—Introduced in 1985, the Abbott ADD-Vantage system (Fig 11*B*) has two parts: a plastic IV bag (Abbott) which is filled with solution and a separate glass vial of powder or liquid drug sold by a pharmaceutical manufacturer. The vial is encased by a plastic cover that is removed prior to use. The user locks the vial holding the drug into a chamber at the top of the plastic bag and mixes the drug and solution by externally removing the stopper on the vial.

Nutrimix—A Dual-Compartment container is available from Abbott. This container allows for long-term packaging of amino acids and dextrose mixtures.

IVAC-Cris—The IVAC-Cris (Controlled-Release Infusion System) (Fig 11*F*) is a disposable adapter designed to infuse reconstituted injectable drugs directly from the manufacturer's single-dose vial. The Cris adapter avoids the need to transfer drug doses to piggyback secondary containers and also eliminates the need for a secondary IV set. The adapter has a primary spike that is inserted into the IV fluid container and a secondary spike that receives the drug vial. The vial spike has two fluid paths: one admits IV fluid from the primary container into the vial; the other drains drug solution into the drip chamber of the IV set. A two-position valve allows IV fluid to flow directly from the primary container to the patient or pass through the vial to deliver the drug. A 5 μm in-line filter eliminates particulates.

To operate the Cris adapter, the drug vial first is reconstituted with an appropriate diluent. With the valve dial in the vertical (primary) position, the spike shield is removed and the vial is attached immediately to the Cris spike. The valve dial is then turned toward the vial, directing the flow of primary fluid into the vial of drug solution. The incoming fluid

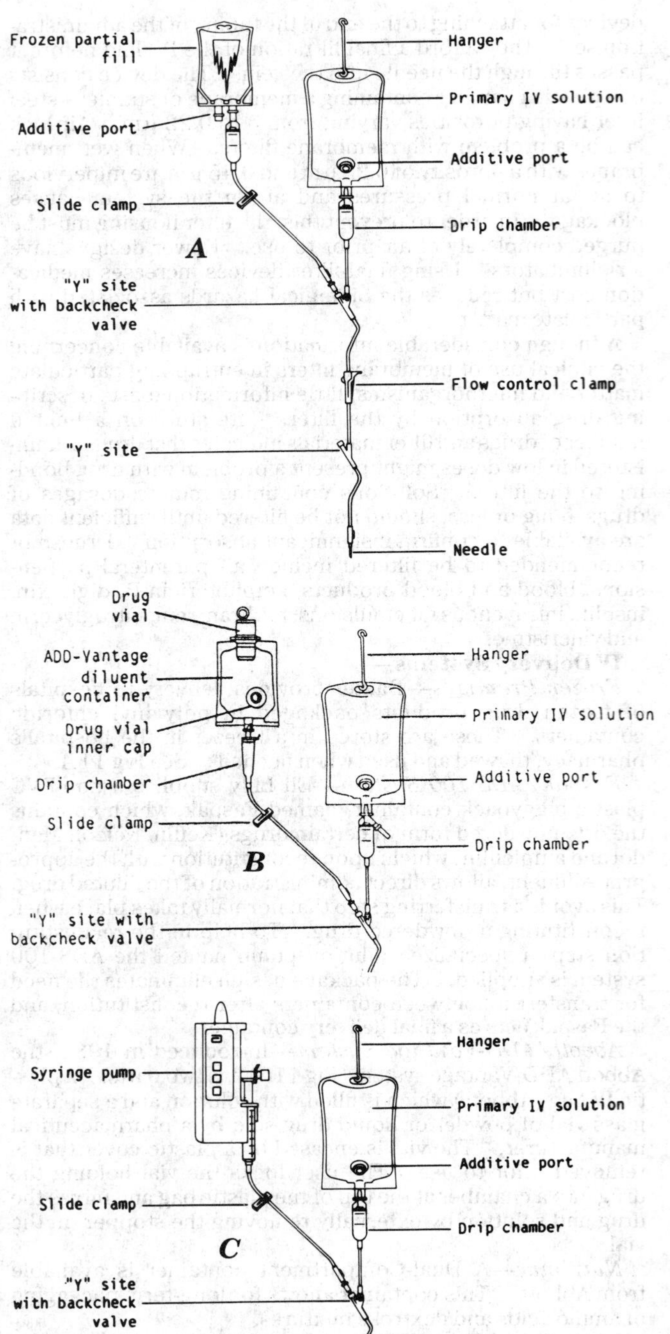

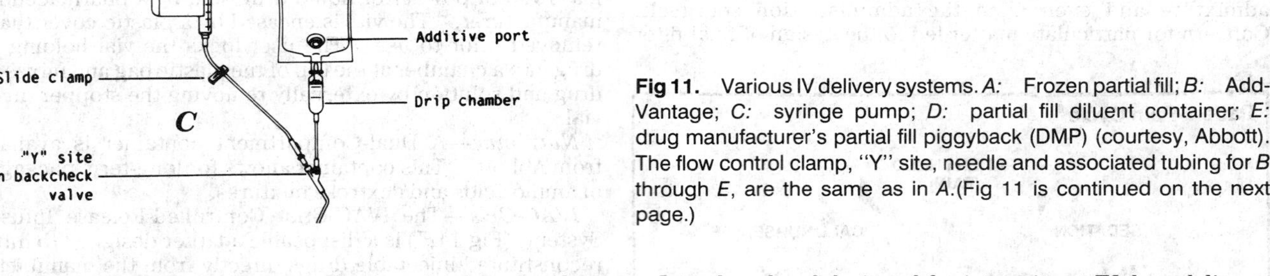

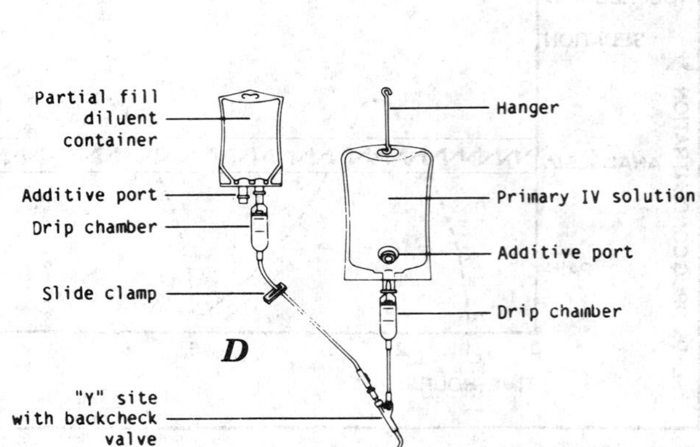

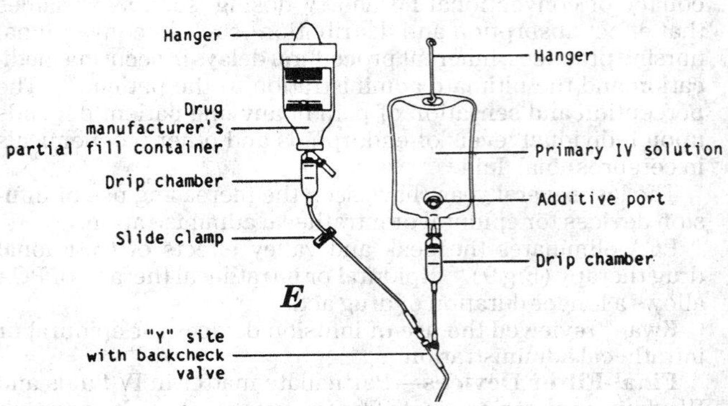

Fig 11. Various IV delivery systems. *A:* Frozen partial fill; *B:* Add-Vantage; *C:* syringe pump; *D:* partial fill diluent container; *E:* drug manufacturer's partial fill piggyback (DMP) (courtesy, Abbott). The flow control clamp, "Y" site, needle and associated tubing for *B* through *E*, are the same as in *A*.(Fig 11 is continued on the next page.)

dilutes and displaces the drug solution into the drip chamber, through the primary set and into the patient. After the dose has been delivered, the vial remains on the spike until the next dose is required. Flow rate can be adjusted using a roller clamp, electronic pump or controller.

Mini-Infuser Pumps for Intermittent IV Drug Delivery—A novel concept in intermittent drug delivery, introduced several years ago, was the Bard-Harvard Mini-Infuser System. This instrument was designed for the administration of antibiotics and other medications delivered intermittently in 40 minutes or less. This battery-generated, lightweight instrument uses standard disposable syringes and microbore disposable extension sets. Different models are available, depending on volume-to-be-delivered selection. This instrument provides accuracy, constant flow, convenience and safety for intermittent drug delivery. See Fig 11*C*.

Introduced and designed for intermittent IV drug delivery, Becton Dickinson's 360 Infusor allows drug delivery intermittently over 60 minutes or less in a volume dilution of up to 60 mL.

Internal Methods Used To Achieve Intravacular Access—

Implantable Ports (*Infuse-A-Port*, Infusaid; *Port-A-Cath*, Pharmacia)—Broviac and Hickman catheters have been used to achieve long-term venous access in a variety of diseases. Although these catheters are widely used, they are associated with some morbidity which includes fracture of catheters entrance site infection and catheters sepsis. Implantable catheters have been developed to overcome catheter complications and are designed to permit repeated access to the infusion site. The catheters consist of implantable-grade silicone tubing connected to a stainless-steel port with a self-

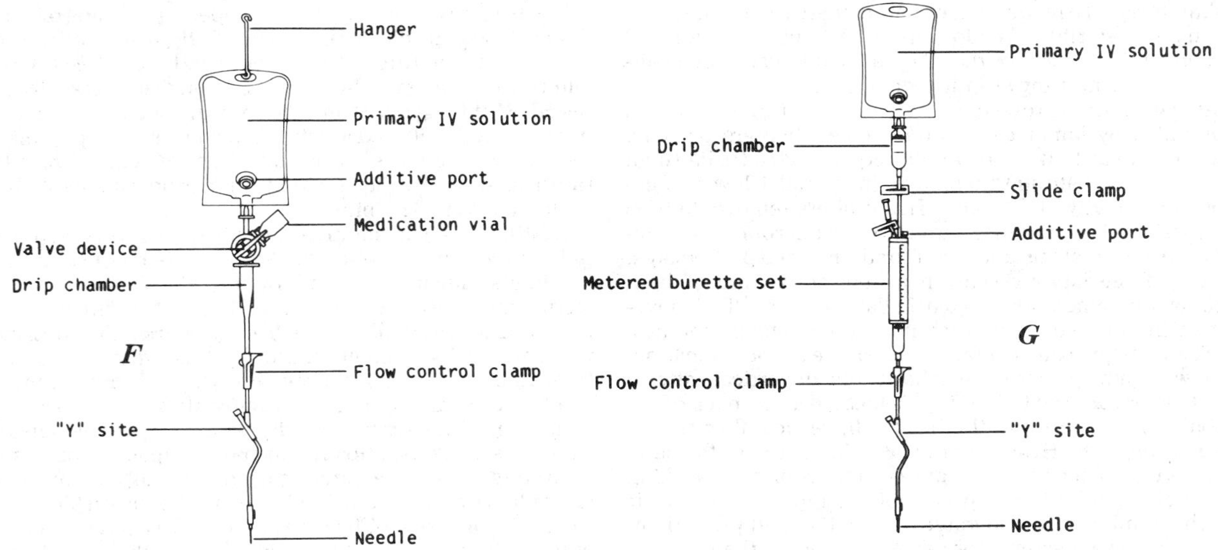

Fig 11 (continued). *F:* Cris infusion; *G:* burette set (courtesy, Abbott).

sealing septum that allows needle access. The delivery catheter can be placed in a vein, cavity, artery or the CNS. The system is accessed with a Huber-point needle through the skin into the self-sealing silicone plug positioned in the center of the portal.

The specialized Huber-point needle is designed with an angle bevel that reduces coring and permits easy entry.

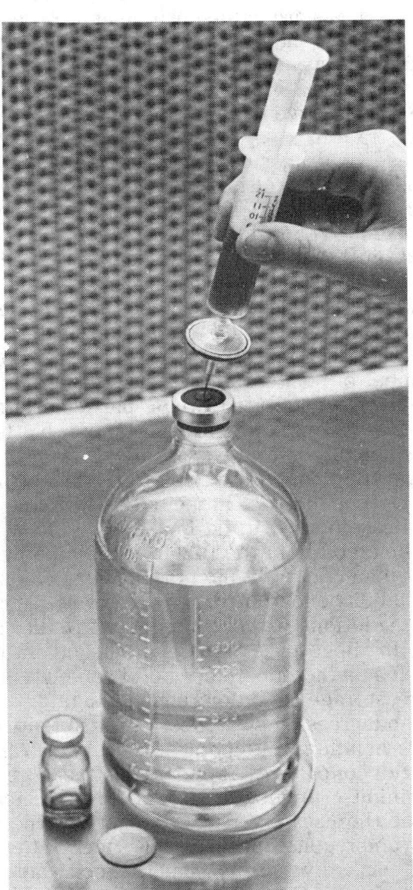

Fig 12. Placing an additive into an IV fluid with filtration through a membrane filter (courtesy, Millipore).

These implantable ports can be used for the injection of IV fluids, total parenteral nutrition, chemotherapy, antibiotics and other drugs.

Some advantages of implantable devices include

The need for a long-term access site to venous, arterial and spinal systems.

An increased dependence on *nonhospital* treatment of chronic disease states.

The direct infusion in a target organ or tumor.

A decrease in infection rates which are seen with percutaneous catheters or repeated spinal taps.

Allowing greater mobility for the patient (a return to normal function).

Implantable Pump (Infusaid)—The Infusaid Implantable Pump was approved for selected drug administration. This pump is the size of a hockey puck and weighs approximately 6½ oz. The construction is titanium, stainless steel and polypropylene. The injection part is constructed of silicone rubber and has a usable life of at least 2000 punctures. Under normal use this device lasts more than 8 years.

The internal power supply uses Freon in equilibrium between the gaseous and liquid states and is *recharged* with each refilling process, thus supplying a power supply for as long as the pump is needed. As the pump is refilled, it compresses the gas back into the liquid state, allowing a fresh supply of energy for the next cycle. The capacity of this pump is 50 mL, which can be administered over a 14-day period. The pump accuracy is stated as over 3%. The cost of one model is approximately $4000.00, not including the surgical implant procedure. The 14-day cycle cannot be altered to any degree.

Model 400 Implantable Drug Delivery System (Infusaid) is designed for long-term therapy in the ambulatory patient. The Model 400 with a 47-mL usable drug volume delivers a precise, continuous flow to a selected organ or site via a soft, nontraumatic, nonthrombogenic silicone rubber catheter. The Model 400 also features an auxiliary *Sideport* septum, completely bypassing the pumping mechanism, for delivery of direct bolus injections to the target site. This allows the clinician easily to supplement the continuous infusion with additional drugs, objectively assess the disease state or monitor catheter location and drug perfusion with the use of radiolabeled microspheres.

Intravenous Admixtures

When one or more sterile products are added to an IV fluid for administration, the resulting combination is known as an

IV admixture. To maintain the characteristics of sterile products, namely sterility, freedom from particulate matter and pyrogens, it is imperative that they be manipulated in a suitable environment using aseptic techniques.

Environment—Proper conditions for aseptic handling can be provided by laminar-flow hoods (see Chapters 84, 87). Within a laminar-flow hood, air filtered through a HEPA (high efficiency particulate air) filter moves in a parallel flow configuration at a velocity of 90 fpm. HEPA filters remove 99.97% of all particles larger than 0.3 μm. Since microbial contaminants present in air usually are found on other particulates, removal of the latter results in a flow of air free of both microbial contaminants and particulate matter. The movement of the filtered air in a laminar-flow configuration at a velocity of 90 fpm can maintain the area free of contamination. The flow of air may be in either a horizontal or vertical pattern. In the former case the HEPA filter is located at the back of the hood and the air flows to the front. In vertical flow the air passes through the HEPA filter located in the top of the cabinet and is exhausted through a grated area around the working surface of the hood. Regardless of the type of laminar air flow, the hood must be operated and maintained properly in order to achieve a satisfactory environment for the preparation of parenteral admixtures.

The hood is situated best in a clean area in which there is little traffic flow past the front of the hood. The inside of the hood is wiped down thoroughly with a suitable disinfectant and allowed to run for at least 30 minutes before starting manipulations. It is important to remember that the laminar-flow hood is not a means of sterilization. It only maintains an area free of microbial contaminants and particulate matter when it has been prepared, maintained and utilized properly by operators having proper aseptic techniques.

Before working in a laminar-flow hood the operator washes his hands thoroughly and scrubs them with a suitable disinfectant. Some laboratories may require gowning and using sterile gloves. Sterile gloves can be an asset but there is always the problem that they can give the operator a false sense of security. Gloved hands can become contaminated as easily as ungloved hands. Additives and IV fluids to be used in the preparation of the admixture, along with suitable syringes, are lined up in the hood in the order they are to be used. The containers must be clean and dust-free. They are inspected for clarity and freedom from cracks. Operators are encouraged to use a lighting device for inspecting IV fluids for particulate matter and cracks. The lighting device should permit the container to be viewed against both a light and a dark background during inspection. If the IV fluid is packaged in plastic containers, pressure is applied to assure that they are sealed properly and do not leak. Some laboratories disinfect the containers prior to placing them in the hood.

In working within the hood the operator works in the center of the hood, with the space between the point of operation and the filter unobstructed. If the flow of air is blocked, the validity of the laminar flow is destroyed. Articles are arranged within the hood in a manner to prevent clean air from washing over dirty objects and contaminating other objects that must remain sterile. The working area must be at least 6 inches from the front edge of the hood. As the operator stands in front of the hood, his body acts as a barrier to the laminar air flow causing it to pass around him and create backflow patterns which can carry room air into the front of the hood.

Laminar-flow hoods must be maintained and evaluated periodically to insure that they are functioning properly. The velocity of air flow can be determined routinely using a velometer. A decrease in the air flow usually indicates a clogged HEPA filter. Some laminar-flow hoods are equipped with pressure gauges indicating pressure in the plenum behind the filter; in these hoods pressure increase also can indicate a clogged filter. Settling plates can be exposed within the hood for given periods of time to determine the presence of microbial contaminants.

The best way to determine the proper functioning of a HEPA filter is to use the dioctyl phthalate (DOP) test using the vapor at room temperature. DOP vapor (particles of ~0.3 μm) is allowed to be taken up by the hood through its intake filter. If the HEPA filter is intact and properly installed, no DOP can be detected in the filtered air stream using a smoke photometer. Certification services are available through commercial laboratories; the HEPA filters within laminar-flow hoods should be evaluated every 6 months.

Additives—The additives are injections packaged in ampuls or vials, or sterile solids; the latter are reconstituted with a suitable diluent before addition to the IV fluid. A fresh, sterile, disposable syringe is used for each additive. Before removing a measured volume from an ampul, the container is wiped with a disinfectant solution. If the ampul is scored, the top can be snapped off; if not scored, an ampul file must be used. A sterile syringe is removed from its protective wrapping. The syringe needle with its cover is separated from the syringe aseptically and may be replaced with a sterile aspirating needle. Aspirating needles usually are made from clear plastic and contain a stainless-steel or nylon filter having a porosity of 5 μm. The filter will remove glass particles and other particulates from the injection as it is drawn up from the ampul into the syringe. The aspirating needle is replaced with the regular needle. The exact volume is calibrated and the injection is ready to be added to the IV fluid (see Fig 12). In the case of additives packaged in multiple-dose vials, the protective cover is removed and the exposed target area of the rubber closure disinfected. A volume of air, equal to the volume of solution to be removed, is drawn up into the syringe and injected into the air space above the injection within the vial. This facilitates withdrawal of the injection. The solution is drawn into the syringe, the exact dose is measured and the injection is ready to be added to the IV fluid.

Certain injections are light-sensitive and protected against photolysis by the container packaging. The manufacturer may use amber glass, individual container wrapping or an amber plastic cover. Many hospital pharmacists use aluminum foil as a protective wrap for light-sensitive drugs during their administration.

In the case of drug substances having poor stability in aqueous solution, the drug is packaged as a sterile solid, either dry-filled or lyophilized. The diluent recommended on the labeling is used to reconstitute the powder; the proper quantity of solution then is removed for addition to the IV fluid. When large volumes of diluent are required for reconstitution, as for Keflin, a sterile needle is placed through the closure to vent the container and facilitate addition of the diluent. In order to increase the efficiency of IV admixture programs, a limited number of hospital pharmacists have found it convenient to freeze reconstituted drugs, particularly antibiotics. The stability of reconstituted drugs is somewhat limited. In some cases stability is limited to only a few hours; in many cases, however, reconstituted solutions can be frozen and thawed at the time of use. In the frozen form the stability of the antibiotic solution can be increased. In a number of instances the stability in the frozen form is known and supplied by the manufacturer. Reports have been published on the frozen stability of certain drugs. However, it is unwise to freeze drug solutions without adequate stability studies for guidance. In those cases where published information is available, close adherence must be observed as to freezing temperature, storage conditions and packaging.

There is an increasing awareness of the potential hazard to pharmacists handling antineoplastic drugs.[6] Although the evidence is not conclusive, it appears that measures should be taken to minimize unnecessary exposure.[7] These precautions include the use of vertical laminar-flow hoods for the preparation and reconstitution of these agents, the wearing of gloves and masks by the personnel, special labeling of the containers to insure their proper handling and disposal and periodic blood studies of personnel involved in preparing admixtures of antineoplastic agents.

The procedure for placing an additive in an IV fluid will vary depending on the type of IV fluid packaging system being used by the hospital. The packaging systems have been described in Table 2.

Abbott Glass Containers (Fig 2)

1. Remove the aluminum tear seal exposing the solid-rubber closure with a target circle in the center.
2. Wipe the closure with suitable disinfectant.
3. Insert the needle of the additive syringe through the target area. The vacuum within the bottle draws in the solution.
4. Gently shake the bottle after each addition.
5. When completed, cover the closure with a plastic protective cap if it is not to be used immediately.

Baxter and McGaw Rigid Glass Containers (Fig 3)

1. Remove the aluminum tear seal and the aluminum disc covering the latex diaphragm.
2. Upon exposing the latex diaphragm, note that the latex cover is drawn in over the openings in the rubber closure.
3. The larger of the two holes receives the administration set, the other is the air vent. The triangle-shaped indentation can serve as the site for injecting the additives as well as the opening for the administration set.
4. Wipe the diaphragm with a suitable disinfectant and pierce the latex cover to place additive into bottle. The vacuum within the bottle will draw additive from the syringe. Do not remove the diaphragm or the vacuum will dissipate. It will be removed at the time of administration prior to the insertion of the administration set.
5. Gently shake the bottle after each additive.
6. When completed, cover the bottle with a plastic additive cap if the administration set is not to be inserted immediately.

Baxter and Abbott Plastic Container (Fig 4)

1. Remove the additive port protective sleeve and rub the gum-rubber plug with a suitable disinfectant.
2. Additives are placed in container by piercing the gum-rubber cover over the additive port.
3. After each addition, milk the container to insure adequate mixing.
4. Containers do not contain a vacuum, but vacuum chambers are available for use in conjunction with the flexible plastic container.
5. Protective additive caps are available if the administration set is not inserted immediately.

McGaw Semirigid Plastic Container (Fig 4)

1. Remove the additive port protective covering and rub the gum-rubber plug with a suitable disinfectant.
2. Additives are placed in containers by piercing the gum-rubber over the additive port.
3. After each addition, shake the container gently to insure adequate mixing.
4. Containers do not contain a vacuum.

Pharmacy Bulk Package—The manufactured bulk package is a sterile container for parenteral use that contains many single doses. These containers are intended for use in admixture programs where large numbers of doses are prepared. It is designed so that the rubber closure is penetrated only one time. It is used in laminar-flow hoods. Pharmacy bulk packages are exempt from the USP requirement that requires multiple-dose containers to have a volume not greater than 30 mL. They also have an exemption in that they are not required to have a bacteriostatic agent. Pharmacy bulk packages have special labeling and storage requirements.

Parenteral Incompatibility—When one or more additives are combined with an IV fluid, their presence together may modify the inherent characteristics of the drug substances present, resulting in a parenteral incompatibility. Parenteral incompatibilities have been divided arbitrarily into three groups: physical, chemical and therapeutic. The latter is the most difficult to observe because the combination results in undesirable antagonistic or synergistic pharmacologic activity. For example, the report that penicillin or cortisone antagonizes the effect of heparin and produces a misleading picture of the anticoagulant effect of heparin represents a therapeutic incompatibility. Physical incompatibilities are observed most easily and can be detected by changes in the appearance of the admixture, such as a change in color, formation of a precipitate or evolution of a gas. Physical incompatibilities frequently can be predicted by knowing the chemical characteristics of the drugs involved. For example, the sodium salts of weak acids, such as phenytoin sodium or phenobarbital sodium, precipitate as free acids when added to intravenous fluids having an acidic pH. Calcium salts precipitate when added to an alkaline medium. Injections that require a special diluent for solubilization, such as diazepam, precipitate when added to aqueous solutions because of their low water solubility.

Decomposition of drug substances resulting from combination of parenteral dosage forms is called a chemical incompatibility, an arbitrary classification since physical incompatibilities also result from chemical changes. Most chemical incompatibilities result from hydrolysis, oxidation, reduction or complexation and can be detected only with a suitable analytic method.

An important factor in causing a parenteral incompatibility is a change in the acid-base environment.[8] The solubility and stability of a drug may vary as the pH of the solution changes. A change in the pH of the solution may be an indication in predicting an incompatibility, especially one involving drug stability, since this is not necessarily apparent physically. The effect of pH on stability is illustrated in the case of penicillin. The antibiotic remains active for 24 hours at pH 6.5, but at pH 3.5 it is destroyed in a short time. Potassium penicillin G contains a citrate buffer and is buffered at pH 6.0 to 6.5 when reconstituted with Sterile Water for Injection, Dextrose Injection or Sodium Chloride Injection. When this reconstituted solution is added to an intravenous fluid such as Dextrose Injection or Sodium Chloride Injection, the normal acid pH of the solution is buffered at pH 6.0 to 6.5, thus assuring the activity of the antibiotic.

While it may be impossible to predict and prevent all parenteral incompatibilities, their occurrence can be minimized. The IV admixture pharmacist should be cognizant of the increasing body of literature concerning parenteral incompatibilities. This includes compatibility guides published by large-volume parenteral manufacturers,[9–11] compatibility studies on individual parenteral products by the manufacturer and published with the product as part of the labeling, the study of the National Coordinating Committee on Large-Volume Parenterals,[12] reference books[13,14] and literature reports of studies with specific parenteral drugs.[15] The pharmacist should encourage the use of as few additives as possible in IV fluids since the number of potential problems increases as the number of additives increases. Physicians should be made aware of possible incompatibilities and the pharmacist can suggest alternate approaches to avoid the difficulties. In some instances, incompatibilities can be avoided by selecting another route of administration for one or more of the drugs involved.

Quality Control—Each hospital should have written procedures covering the handling and storage, use in preparing admixtures, labeling and transportation of IV fluids to the floors. In-use clarity and sterility tests should be devised to assure that IV admixtures retain the characteristics of sterility and freedom from particulate matter. Training and monitoring personnel involved in preparation of IV admixtures should be done on a regular basis.[16] The efforts of the hospital pharmacy should be no less than those of the industry in following Current Good Manufacturing Practice to assure the safety and efficacy of these compounded medications.

Total Parenteral Nutrition

Intravenous administration of calories, nitrogen and other nutrients in sufficient quantities to achieve tissue synthesis and anabolism is called total parenteral nutrition (TPN).[17]

Originally, the term hyperalimentation was used to describe the procedure, but it is being replaced by TPN, the latter being more descriptive for the technique.

The normal caloric requirement for an adult is approximately 2500 per day. If these were to be provided totally by D5/W, approximately 15 L would be required. Each liter contains 50 g dextrose, equivalent to 170 calories. However, it is only possible to administer 3 or 4 L per day without causing fluid overload. To reduce this fluid volume the concentration of dextrose would have to be increased. By increasing the dextrose to 25%, it is possible to administer five times the calories in one-fifth the volume. D25/W is hypertonic and cannot be administered in large amounts into a peripheral vein without sclerosing the vein.

Dudrick developed the technique for administering fluids for TPN by way of the subclavian vein into the superior vena cava where the solution is diluted rapidly by the large volume of blood available, thus minimizing the hypertonicity of the solution. For administration of the TPN fluids, a catheter is inserted and retained in place in the subclavian vein. TPN is indicated in patients who are unable to ingest food due to carcinoma or extensive burns; patients who refuse to eat, as in the case of depressed geriatrics or young patients suffering from anorexia nervosa and surgical patients who should not be fed orally.

The preferred source for calories in TPN fluids is the carbohydrate dextrose. In IV fluid kits commercially available for the preparation of TPN solutions, D50/W is provided. On dilution with amino acid injection, the resulting dextrose concentration is approximately 25%. It is this concentration that is administered.

The source of nitrogen in TPN fluids is crystalline amino acids (*Aminosyn*, Abbott; *FreAmine III*, McGaw; *Travasol*, Travenol). The crystalline amino acid injections contain all the essential and nonessential amino acids in the L-form. For optimum utilization of amino acids and for promoting tissue regeneration, the nitrogen-to-calorie ratio should be 1:150. Calories are needed to provide energy for the metabolism of nitrogen.

Electrolyte requirements vary with the individual patient. The electrolytes present in Amino Acid Injection are given on the label and must be taken into consideration in determining the quantities to be added. Usual electrolyte concentrations are required to fall within the following ranges: sodium, 100–120 mEq; potassium, 80–120 mEq; magnesium, 8–16 mEq; calcium, 5–10 mEq; chloride, 100–120 mEq and phosphate, 40–60 mEq. It is better to keep a 1:1 ratio between sodium and chloride ions. In adding potassium, the acetate salt is preferred to the chloride. If the combination of calcium and phosphate ions exceeds 20 mEq, precipitation occurs.

In addition to the electrolytes, the daily requirement for both water-soluble and fat-soluble vitamins may be added, usually in the form of a multivitamin infusion concentrate. Iron, should be administered separately from the TPN fluids. Trace elements such as zinc, copper, manganese and iodide

Table 3—Typical IV Orders (Parenteral Prescriptions)

Prescription	Comment
1. ℞ NS 1000 mL 125 mL/hr	Sodium Chloride Injection (Normal Saline Solution) 1000 mL, is to be administered at a flow rate of 125 mL per hr. It will require approximately 8 hr.
2. ℞ 1000 D5W + NS + vits 12 hr	Dextrose Injection 5%, 1000 mL, containing 0.9% sodium chloride and container of vitamin B complex with vitamin C is to be administered over a 12-hr period.
3. ℞ 500 D5W + ½NS KVO	Dextrose Injection 5%, 500 mL, containing 0.45% sodium chloride is to be administered at a flow rate to keep the vein open (KVO). The flow rate will be approximately 10 mL per 1 hr.
4. ℞ 1000 cc D5W + ½NS Add 1 amp vits to each + 100 mg thiamine Each to run 6 hr	Dextrose Injection 5%, 1000 mL, containing 0.45% sodium chloride, the contents of one ampul vitamin B complex with vitamin C and sufficient volume of Thiamine Hydrochloride Injection to give 100 mg thiamine, is to be administered over a 6-hr period (approximately 170 mL per hr). Additional orders of the same can be anticipated.
5. ℞ 1000 cc D5W + ½NS + 20 mEq KCl	Dextrose Injection 5%, 1000 mL, is to be provided containing 0.45% sodium chloride and 20 mEq potassium chloride.
6. ℞ 1000 Hyperal + 10 NaCl + 10 KCl + 5 $MgSO_4$ + 10 insulin	One L of the hospital's basic TPN solution is to be provided with the addition of 10 mEq sodium chloride, 10 mEq potassium chloride, 5 mEq magnesium sulfate and 10 units regular zinc insulin.
7. ℞ 1000 cc TPN (FreAmine) + 40 mEq $NaHCO_3$ + 30 mEq KCl + Vits + 5U Reg Insulin to run 80 cc/hr	One L of the basic TPN solution, FreAmine II, is to be provided with the addition of 40 mEq $NaHCO_3$, 30 mEq potassium chloride, the contents of one container vitamin B complex with vitamin C plus 5 units of regular zinc insulin. It is to be administered at the flow rate of 80 mL per hr (approximately 12 hr).
8. ℞ 1000 TPN + 40 mEq NaCl + 10 KCl + 10 Insulin + 10 cal gluconate	One L of the hospital's basic TPN solution is to be provided with the addition of 40 mEq sodium chloride, 10 mEq potassium chloride, 10 units regular zinc insulin and 10 mL Calcium Gluconate Injection.
9. ℞ Keflin 2 g + 100 mL D5W q 6 hr	Cephalothin, 2 g, is reconstituted with Sterile Water for Injection and added to a minibottle containing 100 mL Dextrose Injection 5%. This dose is given every 6 hr using a piggyback technique with a flow rate requiring 30 to 60 min for delivery.
10. ℞ Gentamicin 80 mg IVPB q 8 hr	Gentamicin, 80 mg, is added to a minibottle containing 100 mL Dextrose Injection 5%. This dose is given every 8 hr using the piggyback technique (IVPB) with a flow rate requiring at least 80 min (not less than 1 mg per min).

Table 4—Product Stability

Trade name	Physical form	Shelf-life
Humulin	Liquid solution	2 yr at 2–8°C
Protropin	Lyophilized powder	2 yr at 2–8°C
Humatrope		
Roferon-A	Lyophilized powder	3 yr at 2–8°C
Intron A	Lyophilized powder	2 yr at 2–8°C
Activase	Lyophilized powder	2 yr at 2–30°C
Recombivax-HB	Liquid solution	
Engerix-B	Liquid solution	
Orthoclone	Liquid solution	1 yr at 2–8°C
Epogen	Liquid solution	

are a concern only in long-term cases and can be added when required.

The Parenteral Prescription

The physician writes an admixture order or parenteral prescription on a physician's order form located on the patient's chart. A copy of the order is sent to the pharmacy for compounding. It includes the patient's name, room number, the intravenous fluid wanted, additives and their concentrations, rate of flow, starting time and length of therapy. The order is taken by the technician, nurse or pharmacist to the pharmacy. Orders may be telephoned to the pharmacy; verification with the original order is made on delivery of the admixture. IV orders usually are written for a 24-hour therapy period; the patient's chart is reviewed and new orders are written on a daily basis. The order may be for multiple containers, in which case the containers are numbered consecutively. Unlike the extemporaneously compounded prescription, additives are added without regard to final volume of IV fluid. The prescription is checked for proper dose, compatibility, drug allergies and stability. Additives usually are given an expiration period of 24 hours from the time of preparation. Drugs such as ampicillin may require shorter expiration periods.

The clerical work for the admixture is prepared. This includes typing of the label and the preparation of the profile worksheet. The profile sheet is filed so that the pharmacist will be alerted when subsequent containers are due for preparation. Charging the patient's account can be done from the profile worksheet. The label includes the patient's name, room number, bottle number, preparation date, expiration time and date, intravenous fluid and quantity, additives and quantities, total time for infusion, the milliliters per hour or drops per minute and space for the name of the nurse who hangs the container. The label will be affixed to the container upside down in order that it can be read when hung.

The admixture is prepared by the pharmacist or a supervised technician. In handling sterile products, aseptic techniques as discussed previously must be observed. When completed, a plastic additive cap is affixed before delivery to the floor. The label is applied and checked with the original order. The empty additive containers are checked to confirm the additives present. The admixture is inspected for any color change or particulate matter.

Table 5—Stability after Reconstitution (Lyophilized Products)

Trade name	Shelf-life
Roferon	1 mo at 2–8°C
Intron A	1 mo at 2–8°C
Humatrope	14 days at 2–8°C
Protropin	7 days at 2–8°C
Activase	8 hr at 2–30°C

Table 6—Recombinant Protein Drug

Trade name	Vial strength
Humulin	1000 units
Protropin	5 mg
Humatrope	5 mg
Roferon-A	3 and 18 million units solution
	3 and 18 million units lyo
Intron A	3, 5, 10, 25 and 50 million units
Activase	20, 50 mg
Recombivax HB	5, 10 μg
Engerix-B	20 μg
Orthoclone OKT3	5 μg
Epogen	2, 4 and 10 thousand units

The completed admixture is delivered to the floor. If it is not to be infused immediately (within 1 hour), it is stored under refrigeration; if refrigerated, it must be used within 24 hours. The nurse checks for accuracy of patient's name, drug and concentration, IV fluid, expiration date, time started and clarity. The infusion of admixtures may run ahead or behind schedule, necessitating that the pharmacist modify the preparation of continued orders. Examples of IV orders are shown in Table 3.

Parenterals Derived by Biotechnology

In 1993, 14 biotechnology drugs had been approved for clinical use; 21 were in Phase III clinical studies awaiting approval and over 130 were in various phases of development. The Center for Biologics Evaluation and Review (CBER) had over 3200 INDs under review.

As a result of the stability sensitivities of proteins, the 14 biotechnology pharmaceuticals currently available are all manufactured as parenterals. Many are available as lyophilized parenterals (Table 4). Most have limited shelf-life after reconstitution (Table 5). All are supplied in low dosage, which attest to their potency (Table 6).

For a complete treatment of biotechnology and drugs, see Chapter 49.

References

1. Bennett RL, Griffen WO: *Contemp Surg 23*: 75, 1983.
2. Graves DA et al: *Ann Intern Med 99*: 360, 1983.
3. Bivins BA, Baumann TJ: *Patient Controlled Analgesia (PCA): A Clinical Evaluation of Safety and Efficacy in Hospitalized Trauma/Surgery Patients*, Depts of Surg and Pharm, Henry Ford Hospital, Detroit, Dec, 1984.
4. Kwan JW: *Am J Hosp Pharm 47*: 18, 1990.
5. Turco SJ: *Am J IV Ther. Clin Nutr 9*: 6, 1982.
6. Zimmerman PF, *et al: Am J Hosp Pharm 38*: 1693, 1981.
7. Gallelli JF: *Ibid 39:* 1877, 1982.
8. Newton DW: *Ibid 35:* 1213, 1978.
9. King JC: *Guide to Parenteral Admixtures.* Cutter Laboratories, Berkeley CA, 1987.
10. Shoup LK, Goodwin NH: *Implementation Guide—Centralized Admixture Program*, Travenol Laboratories, Morton Grove IL, 1977.
11. *Good IV Procedures Manual.* Abbott Laboratories, North Chicago IL, 1979.
12. Bergman HD: *Drug Intell Clin Pharm 11*: 345, 1977.
13. Trissel LA: *Parenteral Drug Information Guide*, Am Soc Hosp Pharm, Washington DC, 1974.
14. Trissel LA: *Handbook on Injectable Drugs*, 5th Ed, Am Soc Hosp Pharm, Washington DC, 1992.
15. Kobayashi NH, King JC: *Am J Hosp Pharm 34*: 589, 1977.
16. Sanders SJ *et al: Ibid 35*: 531, 1978.
17. Dudrick SJ, Rhoads JE: *Sci Am 226*: 73, 1972.

Bibliography

General

Am J Hosp Pharm 32: 261, 1975.

Avis, KE, Akers MJ: *Sterile Preparation for the Hospital Pharmacist*, Ann Arbor Sci Publ, Ann Arbor MI, 1981.

Trissel LA: *Handbook on Injectable Drugs*, 5th ed, Am Soc Hosp Pharm, Washington DC, 1992.

Turco SJ, King RE: *Sterile Dosage Forms: Their Preparation and Clinical Applications*, 3rd, Lea & Febiger, Philadelphia, 1987.

PCA

Buchanan C: Development of a Patient Controlled Analgesia Pump System. *Parenterals 4*: 2, 1986.

Graves DA *et al*: Morphine Requirements Using Patient-Controlled Analgesia; Influence of Diurnal Variation and Morbid obesity. *Clin Pharm 2*: 49, 1983.

White PF: Patient Controlled Analgesia: A New Approach to the Management of Postoperative Pain *Semin Anesth 4*: 255, 1985.

Williamson J *et al*: Implementation of an IV Morphine Infusion Program in a Community Hospital *Hosp Pharm 21*: 1098, 1986.

Implantable Systems

Ecoff E *et al:* Implantable Infusion Port, NITA *4:* 406, 1983.

Fulks KD, Kenady DE: Techniques of Chemotherapy Delivery for Cancer Patients, *Hosp Formul 22:* 248, 1987.

Gyves J *et al:* Totally Implanted System for Intravenous Chemotherapy in Patients with Cancer, *Am J Med 73:* 841, 1983.

Kwan JW: Use Of Infusion Devices For Epidural Or Intrathecal Administration Of Spinal Opioids, *Am J Hosp Pharm 47:* 18, 1990.

May GS, Davis C: Percutaneous Catheters and Totally Implantable Access Systems, *J Intraven Nurs 11:* 97, 1988.

McGovern B *et al:* A Totally Implantable Venous Access System for Long Term Chemotherapy In Children, *J Pediatr Surg* 6: 725, 1985

McIntyre KE *et al:* Early Experience with an Implantable Reservoir for Intravenous Chemotherapy, *Ariz Med 42:* 308, 1985.

CHAPTER 89

Ophthalmic Preparations

Gerald Hecht, PhD
Senior Director, Pharmaceutical Sciences
Alcon Laboratories
Fort Worth, TX 76101

Ophthalmic preparations are sterile products essentially free from foreign particles, suitably compounded and packaged for instillation into the eye. Ophthalmic preparations include solutions, suspensions, ointments and solid dosage forms. The solutions and suspensions are, for the most part, aqueous. Ophthalmic ointments usually contain a white petrolatum-mineral oil base.

Ophthalmic preparations can be grouped broadly into two divisions of major significance to the pharmacist. These include single or multidose prescription products and the category described as OTC or over-the-counter ophthalmic products. The latter group has been subjected to a searching review and analysis by a body of experts as a part of the FDA's OTC Drug Review process.

The single dominant factor characteristic of all ophthalmic products is the specification of sterility. Any product intended for use in the eye regardless of form, substance or intent must be sterile. This requirement increases the similarity between ophthalmic and parenteral products, however the physiology of the human eye in many respects imposes more rigid formulation requirements. This will be considered in the following discussion.

Preparations intended for the treatment of eye disorders can be traced to antiquity. Egyptian papyri writings describe eye medications. The Greeks and Romans expanded such uses and gave us the term *collyria*. Collyria refer collectively to materials which were dissolved in water, milk or egg white for use as eyedrops. In the Middle Ages collyria included mydriatic substances to dilate the pupils of milady's eyes for cosmetic purposes, thus the term belladonna or "beautiful lady."

From the time of belladonna collyria, ophthalmic technology progressed at a pharmaceutical snail's pace well into modern times. It was not until after the second World War that the concept of sterility became mandatory for ophthalmic solutions. Prior to World War II and continuing into the 1940s very few ophthalmic preparations were available commercially or were described officially. The USP XIV, official in 1950, included only three ophthalmic preparations and all three were ointments.

Preparations to be used in the eye, either solutions or ointments, invariably were compounded in the community or hospital pharmacy and were intended for immediate (prescription) use. Such preparation and prompt use is reflected in the pharmaceutical literature of the times. The stability of ophthalmic preparations is discussed in terms of days or a few months.

One of the most important attributes of ophthalmic products is the requirement of sterility. Even that, however, is a surprisingly recent event. The USP XV in 1955 was the first official compendium to include a sterility requirement for ophthalmic solutions. The FDA in 1953 adopted the position that a nonsterile ophthalmic solution was adulterated. Sterile ophthalmic products were, of course, available prior to the mid 1950s, however the legal requirement of sterility dates only from 1955.

The sterility requirements for ophthalmic ointments appeared first in the USP XVIII, *Third Supplement* (1972). Prior to that date there was no legal requirement for a sterile ophthalmic ointment. This probably was due to the difficulty (at that time) of testing for sterility in such nonaqueous systems and also for the anticipated difficulties in sterilizing and maintaining sterile conditions during the manufacture and filling of ointments on a large scale.

Anatomy and Physiology of the Eye

The human eye is a challenging subject for topical administration of drugs. The basis of this can be found in the anatomical arrangement of the surface tissues and in the permeability of the cornea. The protective operation of the eyelids and lacrimal system is such that there is rapid removal of material instilled into the eye, unless the material is suitably small in volume and chemically and physiologically compatible with surface tissues. Figures 1[1] and 2[1] include pertinent anatomy of the human eye.

Eyelids—The eyelids serve two purposes: mechanical protection of the globe and creation of an optimum milieu for the cornea. The eyelids are lubricated and kept fluid-filled by secretions of the lacrimal glands and specialized cells residing in the bulbar conjunctiva. The antechamber has the shape of a narrow cleft directly over the front of the eyeball, with pocket-like extensions upward and downward. The pockets are called the superior and inferior fornices (vaults), and the entire space, the cul-de-sac. The elliptical opening between the eyelids is called the palpebral fissure.

Eyeball—The wall of the human eyeball (bulbus, globe) is composed of three concentric layers.

1. The outer fibrous layer.
2. A middle vascular layer—the uvea or uveal tract, consisting of the choroid, the ciliary body and the iris.
3. A nervous layer—the retina.

The outer layer is tough, pliable but only slightly stretchable. In its front portion—the portion facing the outside world—the fine structure of the outer layer is so regular and the water content so carefully adjusted that it acts as a clear transparent window (the cornea). It is devoid of blood vessels. Over the remaining two-thirds the fibrous coat is opaque (the "white" of the eye) and is called the sclera. It contains the microcirculation which nourishes the tissues of this anterior segment and is usually white except when irritated and vessel dilatation occurs.

The eyeball houses an optical apparatus that causes inverted reduced images of the outside world to form on the retina, which is a thin translucent membrane. The optical apparatus consists, in sequence, of the precorneal film, the cornea, the aqueous humor, the pupil, the crystalline lens, the vitreous humor and the retina. The aqueous and vitreous humors are layers of clear fluid or gel-like material interposed between the solid structures. The pupil, a round centric hole in a contractile membranous partition (called the iris), acts as the variable aperture of the system. The crystalline lens is a refractive element with variable power controlled and supported by a muscle incorporated in the ciliary body. The choroid is the metabolic support for the retina.

The optical function of the eye calls for stability of its dimensions, which is provided partly by the fibrous outer coat;

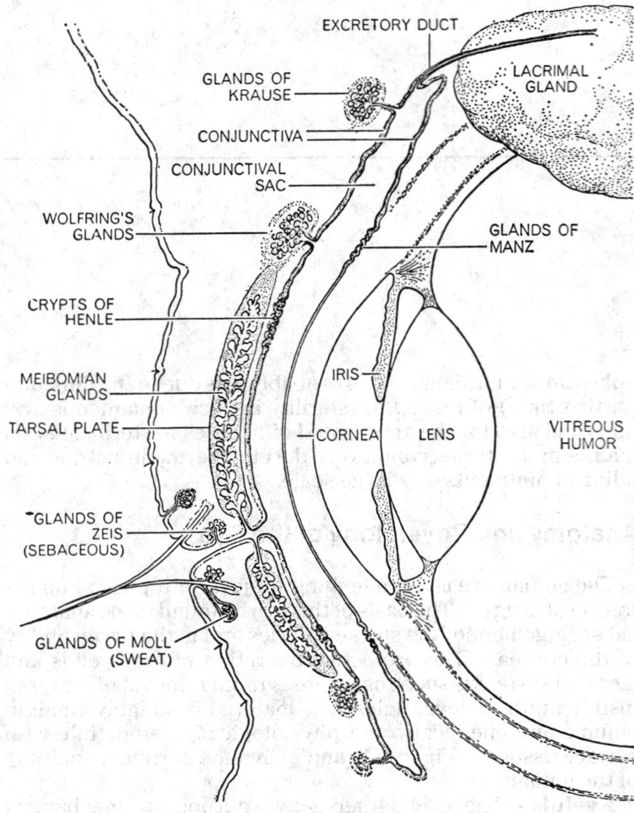

Fig 1. The eye: vertical section.[1]

more effective as a stabilizing factor is the intraocular pressure, which is in excess of the pressure prevailing in the surrounding tissues. This intraocular pressure is the result of a steady production of specific fluid, the aqueous humor, which originates from the ciliary processes and leaves the eye by an intricate system of outflow channels. The resistance encountered during this passage and the rate of aqueous production are the principal factors determining the level of the intraocular pressure. In addition to this hydromechanical function, the aqueous humor acts as a carrier of nutrients, substrates and metabolites for the avascular tissues of the eye.

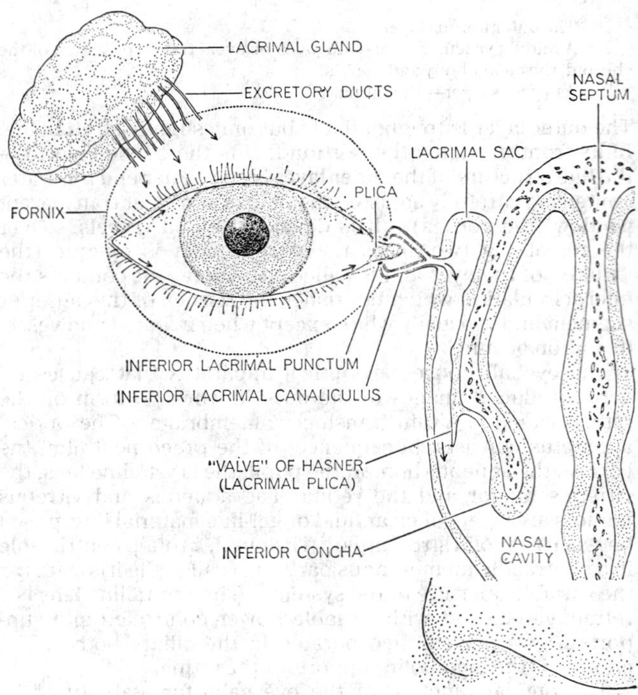

Fig 2. Nasolacrimal duct.[1]

The bones of the skull join to form an approximately pyramid-shaped housing for the eyeball, called the orbit.

Conjunctiva—The conjunctival membrane covers the outer surface of the white portion of the eye and the inner aspect of the eyelids. In most places it is attached loosely and thereby permits free movement of the eyeball. This makes possible subconjunctival injections. Except for the cornea the conjunctiva is the most exposed portion of the eye.

Lacrimal System—The conjunctival and corneal surfaces are covered and lubricated by a film of fluid secreted by the conjunctival and lacrimal glands. The secretion of the lacrimal gland, the tears, is delivered through a number of fine ducts into the conjunctival fornix. The secretion is a clear, watery fluid containing numerous salts, glucose, other organic compounds, approximately 0.7% protein and the enzyme, lysozyme. Small accessory lacrimal glands are situated in the conjunctival fornices. Their secretion suffices for lubrication and cleansing under ordinary conditions and for maintaining a thin fluid film covering the cornea and conjunctiva (the precorneal film). The mucin-protein layer of the film is especially important in maintaining the stability of the film. The main lacrimal gland is called into play only on special occasions. The sebaceous glands of the eyelids secrete an oily fluid which helps to prevent overflowing of tears at the lid margin and reduces evaporation from the exposed surfaces of the eye by spreading over the tear film.

Spontaneous blinking replenishes the fluid film by pushing a thin layer of fluid ahead of the lid margins as they come together. The excess fluid is directed into the lacrimal lake—a small triangular area lying in the angle bound by the innermost portions of the lids. The skin of the eyelids is the thinnest in the body and folds easily, thus permitting rapid opening and closing of the palpebral fissures. The movement of the eyelids includes a narrowing of the palpebral fissures in a zipper-like action from the lateral canthus toward the medial canthus (canthi: the corners where the eyelids meet). This aids the transport or movement of fluid toward the lacrimal lake.

Tears are drained from the lacrimal lake by two small tubes—the lacrimal canaliculi—which lead into the upper part of the nasolacrimal duct, the roomy beginning of which is called the lacrimal sac. The drainage of tears into the nose does not depend merely on gravity. Fluid enters and passes along the lacrimal canaliculi by capillary attraction aided by aspiration caused by contraction of muscle embedded in the eyelids. When the lids close, as in blinking, contraction of the muscle causes dilatation of the upper part of the lacrimal sac and compression of its lower portion. Tears are thus aspirated into the sac, and any which have collected in its lower part are forced down the nasolacrimal duct toward its opening into the nose. As the lids open, the muscle relaxes. The upper part of the sac then collapses and forces fluid into the lower part, which at the same time is released from compression. Thus, the act of blinking exerts a suction-force-pump action in removing tears from the lacrimal lake and emptying them into the nasal cavity. Lacrimation is induced reflexly by stimulation of nerve endings of the cornea or conjunctiva. The reflex is abolished by anesthetization of the surface of the eye and by disorders affecting its nerve components.

The normal cul-de-sac usually is free of pathogenic organisms and often found sterile. The sterility may be due partly to the action of lysozyme in the tears, which normally destroys saprophytic organisms but has little action against pathogens. More effective in producing sterility may be the fact that the secretions, which are normally sterile as they leave the glands, constantly wash the bacteria, dust, etc, down in the nose. In certain diseases the lacrimal gland, like other glandular structures in the body, undergoes involution, with the result that the lacrimal fluid becomes scanty. Furthermore, changes in the conjunctival glands may lead to alteration in the character of the secretion so that quality as well as quantity of tears may be abnormal. This may lead to symptoms of dryness, burning and general discomfort, and may interfere with visual acuity.

Precorneal Film—The cornea must be wet to be an optically adequate surface; when dry, it loses both its regular gloss and its transparency. The precorneal film, part of the tear fluid, provides this important moist surface. Its character depends on the condition of the corneal epithelium. The film, compatible with both aqueous and lipid ophthalmic preparations, is composed of a thin outer lipid layer, a thicker middle aqueous layer and a thin inner mucoid layer. It is renewed during each blink and when blinking is suppressed, either by drugs or by mechanical means, it dries in patches. It seems to be unaffected by the addition of concentrations of up to 2% sodium chloride to conjunctival fluid. A pH below 4 or above 9 causes derangement of the film. The film affects the movement of contact lenses and forms more easily on glass than on plastic prostheses.

Cornea—The cornea, from 0.5 to 1 mm thick, consists mainly of the following structures (from the front backwards):

1. Corneal epithelium.
2. Substantia propria (stroma).
3. Corneal endothelium.

The cornea is transparent to ordinary diffuse light, largely because of a special laminar arrangement of the cells and fibers and because of the absence of blood vessels. Cloudiness of the cornea may be due to any one of several factors including excess pressure in the eyeball as in glaucoma; scar tissue due to injury, infection or deficiency of oxygen or excess hydration such as may occur during the wearing of improperly fitted contact lenses. A wound of the cornea usually heals as an opaque patch which can be a permanent impairment of vision unless it is located in the periphery of the cornea.

The chief refraction of light for the eye occurs at the outer surface of the cornea where the index of refraction changes from that of air (1.00) to that of precorneal substance (1.38). Any alteration in its shape or transparency interferes with the formation of a clear image; therefore, any pathological process, however slight, may interfere seriously with the resolving power or visual acuity of the eye.

The normal cornea possesses no blood vessels except at the corneoscleral junction. The cornea, therefore, must derive its nutrition by diffusion and must have certain permeability characteristics; it also receives nourishment from the fluid circulating through the chambers of the eye and from the air. The fact that the normal cornea is devoid of blood vessels is an important feature in surgical grafting. The corneal nerves do not supply all forms of sensation to the cornea. Pain and cold are well supplied. The pain fibers have a very low threshold, which makes the cornea one of the most sensitive areas on the surface of the body. It now is agreed generally that the cornea possesses a true sense of touch; nerve endings supplying the sensation of heat are lacking.

The corneal epithelium provides an efficient barrier against bacterial invasion. Unless its continuity has been broken by an abrasion (a traumatic opening or defect in the epithelium) pathogenic bacteria, as a rule, cannot gain a foothold. Trauma, therefore, plays an important part in most of the infectious diseases of the cornea which occur exogenously. Any foreign body that either scratches the cornea or lodges and becomes imbedded in the cornea is of serious moment because of the role it may play in permitting pathogenic bacteria to gain a foothold.

A means of detecting abrasions on the corneal surface is afforded by staining the cornea with sodium fluorescein. If there is an abrasion on the epithelium, the underlying layer stains a brilliant green, so that even pinpoint abrasions show up quite clearly. Abrasion may occur during tonometry, that is, during the measurement of ocular tension (pressure) with a tonometer. Care must be used in applying the device to the cornea to avoid abrasion of the cornea. Corneal abrasions sometimes result from wearing contact lenses. Every corneal abrasion is subject to infection.

Bioavailability

Physical Consideration—Under normal conditions the human tear volume averages about 7 μL.[2] The estimated maximum volume of the cul-de-sac is about 30 μL with drainage capacity far exceeding lacrimation rate. The outflow capacity accommodates the sudden large volume resulting from the instillation of an eyedrop. Most commercial eyedrops range from 50 to 75 μL in volume, however, much in excess of 50 μL probably is unable to enter the cul-de-sac.

Within the rabbit cul-de-sac, the drainage rate has been shown to be proportional to the instilled drop volume. Multiple drops administered at intervals produced higher drug concentrations. Ideally, a high concentration of drug in a minimum drop volume is desirable. Patton[3] has shown that approximately equal tear-film concentrations result from the instillation of 5 μL of 1.61×10^{-2} *M* pilocarpine nitrate or from 25 μL of 1.0×10^{-2} *M* solution. The 5 μL contains only 38% as much pilocarpine, yet its bioavailability is greater due to decreased drainage loss.

There is a practical limit or limits to the concept of minimum dosage volume. There is a difficulty in designing and producing a dropper configuration which will deliver small volumes reproducibly. Also, the patient often cannot detect the administration of such a small volume. This sensation or lack of sensation is particularly apparent at the 5.0–7.5-μL dose-volume range.

The concept of dosage-volume drainage and cul-de-sac capacity directly effects the prescribing and administering of separate ophthalmic preparations. The first drug administered may be diluted significantly by the administration of the second. On this basis combination drug products for use in ophthalmology have considerable merit.

Corneal Absorption——Drugs administered by instillation must penetrate the eye and do so primarily through the cornea. Corneal absorption is much more effective than scleral or conjunctival absorption where removal by blood vessels into the general circulation occurs.

Many ophthalmic drugs are weak bases and are applied to the eye as aqueous solutions of their salts. The free base and the salt will be in an equilibrium which will depend on the pH and on the individual characteristics of the drug molecule. To aid in maintaining storage stability and solubility, the medication may be acidic at the moment of instillation but, usually, the neutralizing action of the lacrimal fluid will convert it rapidly to the physiological pH range (approximately pH 7.4), at which there will be enough free base present to begin penetration of the corneal epithelium. Once inside the epithelium the undissociated free base dissociates immediately to a degree. The dissociated moiety then will tend to penetrate the stroma because it is water-soluble. At the junction of the stroma and endothelium the same process that took place at the outer surface of the epithelium must occur again. Finally, the dissociated drug leaves the endothelium for the aqueous humor. Here it can readily diffuse to the iris and the ciliary body, the site of its pharmacological action.

The cornea can be penetrated by ions to a small, but measurable, degree. Under comparable conditions, the permeabilities are similar for all ions of small molecular weight, which suggests that the passage is through extracellular spaces. The diameter of the largest particles which can pass across the cellular layers seems to be in the range 10–25 Å. An instilled drug is subject to protein binding in the tear fluid and metabolic degradation by enzymes such as lysozyme, in addition to the losses by simple overflow and lacrimal drainage.

Since the cornea is a membrane including both hydrophilic and lipophilic layers, most effective penetration is obtained with drugs having both lipid and hydrophilic properties. Highly water soluble drugs penetrate less readily. As an example highly water soluble steroid phosphate esters penetrate the cornea poorly. Better penetration is achieved with the poorly soluble but more lipophilic steroid alcohol; still greater absorption is seen with the steroid acetate form.

In 1976 Lee and Robinson[4] and in 1990, Lee[5] presented a summary of the factors controlling precorneal pilocarpine disposition and pilocarpine bioavailability in the rabbit eye. Combining experimental work and computer simulation the investigators discussed the mechanisms competing with corneal absorption of pilocarpine. Included were solution drainage, drug-induced vasodilation, nonconjunctival loss including uptake by the nictitating membrane, conjunctival absorption, induced lacrimation and normal tear turnover. Subject to experimental conditions the relative effectiveness of the factors involved in precorneal drug removal are drainage ≃ vasodilation > nonconjunctival loss > induced lacrimation ≃ conjunctival absorption > normal tear turnover.

The authors discuss the implications of the mechanisms of precorneal drug loss in the design of ocular drug-delivery systems including the effect of instilled drug volume on aqueous humor concentration and the amount of drug available for systemic absorption. On an absolute basis a smaller volume allows more drug to be absorbed. For a given instilled concentration the opposite is true; however, a smaller volume instilled remains more efficient, ie, the fraction of dose absorbed is greater. Lang[6] discusses the transcorneal route of absorption of a drug into the eye as that route most effective in bringing a given drug to the anterior portion of the eye. This route of absorption is enhanced by the water-lipid gradient found in the cornea. As previously mentioned, the cornea is composed of three general layers: the lipid-rich epithelium, the lipid-poor stroma and the lipid-rich endothelium. Differential studies on the relative lipid contents of these three layers have shown that the corneal epithelium and the corneal endothelium both contain approximately 100 times as much lipid as the corneal stroma. This, coupled with the physiological pH of 7.2 ± 0.2 and its effect on ionizable drug molecules plays the most significant role in corneal penetration.

Ophthalmic ointments generally produce greater bioavailability than the equivalent aqueous solution. Because of the greater contact time drug levels are prolonged and total drug absorption is increased.

Types of Ophthalmic Products

Administration—The instillation of eyedrops remains one of the less precise, yet one of the more accepted means of topical drug delivery. The method of administration is cumbersome at best, particularly for the elderly, patients with poor vision who have difficulty seeing without eyeglasses and patients with other physical handicaps. Perhaps, surprisingly, the majority of patients become quite adept at routine instillation.

The pharmacist should advise each patient to keep the following points in mind to aid in the instillation of eyedrops or ointments:

How to Use Eyedrops

1. Wash hands.
2. With one hand, gently pull lower eyelid down.
3. If dropper is separate, squeeze rubber bulb once while dropper is in bottle to bring liquid into dropper.
4. Holding dropper above eye, drop medicine inside lower lid while looking up; do not touch dropper to eye or fingers.
5. Release lower lid. Try to keep eye open and not blink for at least 30 seconds.
6. If dropper is separate, replace on bottle and tighten cap.

- If dropper is separate, always hold it with tip down.
- Never touch dropper to any surface.
- Never rinse dropper.
- When dropper is at top of bottle, avoid contaminating cap when removed.
- When dropper is a permanent fixture on the bottle, ie, when supplied by a pharmaceutical manufacturer to the pharmacist, the same rules apply to avoid contamination.
- Never use eye drops that have changed color.
- If you have more than one bottle of the same kind of drops, open only one bottle at a time.
- If you are using more than one kind of drop at the same time, wait several minutes before use of other drops.
- It may be helpful in use of the medicine to practice use by positioning yourself in front of a mirror.
- After instillation of drops, do not close eyes tightly and try not to blink more often than usual, as this removes the medicine from the place on the eye where it will be effective.

How to Use Ophthalmic Ointments

1. Wash hands.
2. Remove cap from tube.
3. With one hand, gently pull lower eyelid down.
4. While looking up, squeeze a small amount of ointment (about ¼ to ½ in) inside lower lid. Be careful not to touch tip of tube to eye, eyelid, fingers, etc.
5. Close eye gently and roll eyeball in all directions while eye is closed. Temporary blurring may occur.
6. The closed eyelid may be rubbed very gently by a finger to distribute the drug throughout the fornix.
7. Replace cap on tube.

- Take care to avoid contaminating cap when removed.
- When opening ointment tube for the first time, squeeze out the first ¼″ of ointment and discard as it may be too dry.
- Never touch tip of tube to any surface.
- If you have more than one tube of the same ointment, open only one at a time.
- If you are using more than one kind of ointment at the same time, wait about 10 minutes before use of another ointment.
- To improve flow of ointment, hold tube in hand several minutes to warm before use.
- It may be helpful in use of the ointment to practice use by positioning yourself in front of a mirror.

Ophthalmic Solutions—This is by far the most common means of administering a drug to the eye. The USP describes 59 ophthalmic solutions. By definition, all ingredients are completely in solution, uniformity is not a problem and there is little physical interference with vision. The principal disadvantage of solutions is the relatively brief contact time between the medication and absorbing surfaces. Contact time may be increased to some extent by the inclusion of a viscosity increasing agent such as methylcellulose. Inclusions of this sort are permitted by the USP. A viscosity in the range of 15 to 25 cps is considered optimum for drug retention and visual comfort.

Ophthalmic Suspensions—Suspensions are dispersions of finely divided, relatively insoluble drug substances in an aqueous vehicle containing suitable suspending and dispersing agents. There are 29 listed in the USP. The vehicle is, among other things, a saturated solution of the drug substance. Because of a tendency of particles to be retained in the cul-de-sac, the contact time and duration of action of a suspension probably exceeds that of a solution. The drug is absorbed from solution and the solution concentration is replenished from retained particles. Each of these actions is a function of particle size, with solubility rate being favored by smaller size and retention favored by a larger size; thus, optimum activity should result from an optimum particle size.

For aqueous suspensions the parameters of intrinsic solubility and dissolution rate must be considered. The intrinsic solubility determines the amount of drug actually in solution and available for immediate absorption upon instillation of the dose. As the intrinsic solubility of the drug increases, the concentration of the drug in the saturated solution surrounding the suspended drug particle also increases. For this reason, any comparison of different drugs in suspension systems should include their relative intrinsic solubilities. The observed differences in their biological activities may be ascribed wholly or in part to the differences in this physical parameter. As the drug penetrates the cornea and the initial saturated solution becomes depleted, the particles must dissolve to provide a further supply of the drug. The requirement here is that the particles must undergo significant dissolution within the residence time of the dose in the eye if any benefit is to be gained from their presence in the dosing system.

For a drug whose dissolution rate is rapid, the dissolution requirement may present few problems, but for a slowly soluble substance the dissolution rate becomes critical. If the dissolution rate is not sufficiently rapid to supply significant additional dissolved drug, there is the possibility that the slowly soluble substance in suspension provides no more drug to the aqueous humor than does a more dilute suspension or a saturated solution of the substance in a similar vehicle. Obviously, the particle size of the suspended drug affects the surface area available for dissolution. Particle size also plays an important part in the irritation potential of the dosing system. This consideration is important, as irritation produces excessive tearing and rapid drainage of the instilled dose. It has been recommended that particles be less than 10 μm in size to minimize irritation to the eye. It should be kept in mind, however, that in any suspension system the effects of prolonged storage and changes in storage temperature may cause the smallest particles to dissolve and the largest particles to become larger. In summary, aqueous suspensions should, in general, give a more extended effect than aqueous solutions.

The pharmacist should be aware of two potential difficulties inherent in suspension dosage forms. In the first instance dosage uniformity nearly always requires brisk shaking to distribute the suspended drug. Adequate shaking is a function of the suitability of the suspension formulation but also, and most importantly, patient compliance. Studies have demonstrated that a significant number of patients may not shake the container at all, others may contribute a few trivial shakes. The pharmacist should stress the need of vigorous shaking whenever an ophthalmic suspension is dispensed.

A second and infrequent characteristic of suspensions is the phenomenon of polymorphism or the ability of a substance to exist in several different crystalline forms. A change in crystal structure may occur during storage resulting in an increase (or decrease) in crystal size and alteration in the suspension characteristics causing solubility changes reflected in increased or decreased bioavailability.

The pharmacist should be aware of the procedures used by pharmaceutical manufacturers in the preparation of commercial sterile ophthalmic suspensions and ointments, when called upon to compound such prepations extemporaneously.[7]

Ophthalmic Ointments—Despite disadvantages, ophthalmic ointments remain a popular and frequently prescribed dosage form. There are 58 ophthalmic ointments listed in the USP. Dosage variability probably is greater than with solutions (although probably not with suspensions). Ointments will interfere with vision unless use is limited to bedtime instillation.

Ointments do offer the advantage of longer contact time and greater total drug bioavailability, albeit with slower onset and time to peak absorption. The relationship describing the availability of finely divided solids dispersed in an ointment base was given by Higuchi[8] where the amount of solid (drug) released in unit time is a function of concentration, solubility in the ointment base and diffusivity of the drug in the base.

Special precautions must be taken in the preparation of ophthalmic ointments. They are manufactured from sterilized ingredients under rigidly aseptic conditions and meet the requirements of the official sterility tests. Terminal sterilization of the finished ointment in tubes is accomplished occasionally using a validated dose of gamma radiation. If the specific ingredients used in the formulation do not lend themselves to routine sterilization techniques, other ingredients that meet the sterility requirements described under the official sterility tests, along with aseptic manufacture, may be employed. Ophthalmic ointments must contain a suitable substance or mixture of substances to prevent growth of, or to destroy, microorganisms introduced accidentally when the container is opened during use. The antimicrobial agents currently used are chlorobutanol, the parabens or one of the organic mercurials. The medicinal agent is added to the ointment base either as a solution or as a micronized powder. The finished ointment must be free from large particles. Most ophthalmic ointments are prepared with a base of white petrolatum and mineral oil, often with anhydrous lanolin. Some contain a polyethylene-mineral oil gel. Whichever base is selected, it must be nonirritating to the eye, permit diffusion of the drug throughout the secretions bathing the eye and retain the activity of the medicament for a reasonable period of time under proper storage conditions.

It is obligatory that ophthalmic ointments not contain particulate matter that may be harmful to eye tissues. Hence, in preparing such ointments special precautions must be taken to exclude or to minimize contamination with foreign particulate matter, eg, metal particles fragmented from equipment used in preparing ointments and also to reduce the particle size of the active ingredient(s) to impalpability. The official compendium provides tests designed to limit to a level considered to be unobjectionable the number and size of discrete particles that may occur in ophthalmic ointments. In these tests the extruded contents of 10 tubes of ointment, previously melted in flat-bottom Petri dishes and then allowed to solidify, are scanned under a low-power microscope fitted with a micrometer eyepiece for metal particles 50 μm or larger in any dimension. The requirements are met if the total number of metal particles in all 10 tubes does not exceed 50 and if not more than one tube is found to contain eight such particles.

Testing for sterility of products such as ophthalmic ointments has been facilitated greatly by the use of sterile, bacteria-retaining membranes (those having a nominal porosity of 0.45 or 0.22 μm are used commonly). For ointments soluble in isopropyl myristate (the solvent used in the official test for sterility) a sample of the ointment is dissolved in the sterile test solvent. For ointments insoluble in isopropyl myristate the sample is suspended in a suitable aqueous vehicle that may contain a dispersing agent and tested by the conventional *General Procedure* (see the USP for details).

For a long time the technology available for manufacture of ophthalmic ointments was considered inadequate to produce sterile products; indeed, it was believed by some to be impossible to operate a tube-filling machine so as to maintain sterility even in a sterile room. In recent years technological advances have made it possible to manufacture sterile ophthalmic ointment units. Major improvements have been achieved in the area of filtration technology. Membrane filters have improved the reliability of both sterile filtration procedures and sterility-testing methods. Use of laminar flow of HEPA-filtered air in appropriately designed rooms and hoods has been a major factor in the successful aseptic operation of the roller mill and of devices for filling tubes with ointment. While the ideal method of sterilization is one in which the finished ointment is sterilized in its final container, at present it does not appear feasible to do so by any method with the possible exception of the use of ionizing radiation.

As previously noted, the official compendium directs that ophthalmic ointments be prepared from previously sterilized ingredients, under rigidly aseptic conditions. This is the procedure followed in commercial manufacture as well as in extemporaneous preparation of ophthalmic ointments. In extemporaneous compounding the following information may be helpful: petrolatum vehicles and many medicaments may be sterilized by being heated in a hot air oven and utensils required for compounding may be sterilized by autoclaving. A sterile disposable syringe without a needle may be used to transfer the finished ointment, if it is semifluid, to the presterilized ointment tube, or sterile aluminum foil or powder paper may be used for the same purpose. Probability of microbial contamination may be reduced greatly by carrying out selected steps of the procedure in a laminar-flow hood.

Ocular Inserts—The use of solid dosage forms in the eye actually dates from the *lamellae* of the British Pharmacopeia of the 1940s. These drug-impregnated wafers were designed to dissolve on insertion beneath the eyelid. Other slowly soluble or erodible matrices were investigated from time to time. Each is characterized by a form of enhanced-pulse drug activity. That is, the bioavailability curve of the drug instilled in aqueous solutions was greatly enhanced both in peak absorption and in duration. Drug side effects were enhanced concomitantly as well.

More recently, ocular inserts have been developed in which the drug is delivered based on diffusional mechanisms. Such a device delivers an ophthalmic drug at a constant known rate, minimizing side effects by avoiding excessive absorption peaks. The delivery of pilocarpine by such a device is a well-known commercial product (*Ocusert*, Alza).

Ocular inserts are plagued with some of the same manipulative disadvantages as conventional eyedrops. The insert must be placed in the eye in a manner similar to the insertion of a contact lens. Additionally, the insert, exhausted of its drug content, must be removed from the eye. Such manipulations can be difficult for the elderly patient. Nonetheless, such therapeutic inserts represent a notable scientific contribution to ophthalmic therapy.

Intraocular Solutions—Ophthalmic solutions intended for intraocular use are relatively recent additions to the armamentarium of the ophthalmologist-surgeon. Surgical procedures such as cataract removal require two types of intraocular solutions. During surgery the operating site is rinsed frequently with an irrigating solution. Late in the surgical procedure the surgeon may choose to constrict the iris by the use of a miotic solution such as carbachol or acetylcholine chloride. Drugs such as the latter usually are used in a unit-dose, minimum-volume form. Irrigating solutions, in contrast, may be used over a period of hours during surgery and are available in volumes ranging from 15 to 500 mL.

The formulation of intraocular ophthalmic products presents requirements that differ depending on the type of product. Medicated solutions such as carbachol or acetylcholine are formulated best in relatively simple isotonic vehicles. Preservatives should not be used and buffers should be avoided if possible. The product pH should be adjusted as close to the physiological range as possible. Needless to say, the product should be sterile and particle-free.

Intraocular irrigating solutions present a considerable formulation challenge distinct from the active ingredient solutions described above. Intraocular irrigating solutions are in contact with the delicate internal structures of the eye throughout the course of various surgeries, ie, for time periods measured in hours. The requirements of tonicity, pH, sterility and clarity are obvious; additionally, however, such irrigating solutions require a balanced ionic structure to prevent or minimize deleterious effects on structures such as the corneal endothelium. Edelhauser[9] has shown that isotonic sodium chloride can be toxic to corneal epithelial, endothial, iris and conjunctival cells. The same cells in contrast are unchanged after exposure to Ringer's Solution containing glutathione, bicarbonate and adenosine.

The question of particulate matter in intraocular irrigating solutions is particularly important. In view of the volumes used for irrigations in the surgically opened eye, any particulates could physically block the trabecular meshwork and canals of Schlemm. The latter are vital in the outflow of aqueous humor and help maintain proper intraocular pressure in the intact eye.

Other Modes of Administration

Packs—These sometimes are used to give prolonged contact of the solution with the eye. A cotton pledget is saturated with an ophthalmic solution and this pledget is inserted into the superior or inferior fornix. Packs may be used to produce maximal mydriasis. In this case the cotton pledgets can be, for example, saturated with phenylephrine solution.

Intracameral Injections—Injections may be made directly into the anterior chamber (eg, acetylcholine chloride, alpha-chymotrypsin, carbamylcholine chloride, certain antibiotics and steroids) or directly into the vitreous chamber (eg, amphotericin B, gentamicin sulfate and certain steroids). Injections are not made into the posterior chamber.

Iontophoresis—This procedure keeps the solution in contact with the cornea by means of an eyecup bearing an electrode. Diffusion of the drug (eg, fluorescein sodium, an antibiotic, etc) is effected by difference of electrical potential.

Subconjunctival Injections—Subconjunctival injections (Fig 3[10]) are used frequently to introduce medications which, if applied topically, either do not penetrate into the anterior segment or penetrate too slowly to attain the concentration required. The drug is injected underneath the conjunctiva and probably passes through the sclera and into the eye by simple diffusion. The most common use of subconjunctival injection is for the administration of antibiotics in infections of the anterior segment of the eye. Subconjunctival injections of mydriatrics and cycloplegics also are used to achieve maximal pupillary dilation or relaxation of the ciliary muscle. If the drug is injected underneath the conjunctiva and the underlying Tenon's capsule in the more posterior portion of the eye, effects on the ciliary body, choroid and retina can be obtained.

Retrobulbar Injections—Drugs administered by retrobulbar injection (Fig 1) may enter the globe in essentially the same manner as the medications given subconjunctivally. The orbit is not well-vascularized and the possibility of significant via-blood stream effects from these injections is very remote. In general, such injections are given for the purpose of getting medications (eg, antibiotics, local anesthetics, enzymes with local anesthetics, steroids, vasodilators, etc) into the posterior segment of the globe and to affect the nerves and other structures in that space.

Preparation

The preparation of ophthalmic solutions, suspensions or ointments by the community pharmacist, or even the hospital pharmacist, is becoming less common. The pharmacist may be called upon to prepare a special concentration, particularly of an antibiotic, in the hospital setting. However, the extemporaneous compounding of ophthalmic prescriptions is becoming rare. In those cases where the pharmacist is called upon to compound an ophthalmic preparation extemporaneously, careful documentation, along with physician consultation, is required. Meticulous attention to detail and the use of a detailed, preapproved preparation plan must be in place prior to compounding.[11] In the view of many, the advantages of commercial preparations such as stability, uniformity and sterility outweigh possible disadvantages such as standardization of dosage. A general discussion concerning the preparation of ophthalmic solutions is found in the USP.

Vehicles—Sterile isotonic solutions, properly preserved, are suitable for preparing ophthalmic solutions (see Chapter 36). In most cases, where the concentration of active ingre-

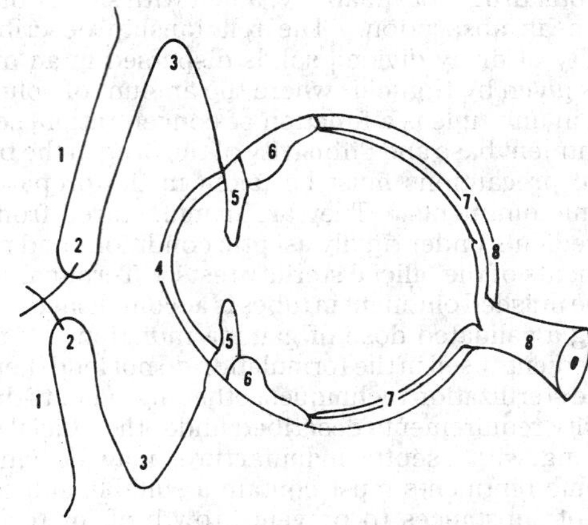

Fig 3. Modes of local therapy in ocular inflammation: *Ointment:* 1–5. *Drops:* 3–5. *Parenteral Injections*— subconjunctival: 4–6; deep subtenons: 6–8; retrobulbar: 8.[10]

dient is low, ie, less than 2.5 to 3.0%, the drug can be dissolved directly in the isotonic vehicle. The finished solutions will be hypertonic somewhat but well within the comfort tolerance of the eye.

Typical stock solutions are as follows:

Isotonic Sodium Chloride Solution

Sodium Chloride USP	0.9 g
Benzalkonium Chloride	1:10,000
Sterile Distilled Water	qs 100 mL

Boric Acid Solution

Boric Acid USP	1.9 g
Benzalkonium Chloride	1:10,000
Sterile Distilled Water	qs 100 mL

Boric acid solution at pH 5 is an appropriate vehicle for the following:

Cocaine	Tetracaine
Neostigmine	Zinc salts
Phenacaine	Piperocaine
Procaine	

Boric acid solution with an antioxidant is useful for oxygen sensitive drugs such as epinephrine, phenylephrine or physostigmine. The following solutions are suggested. Phenylmercuric nitrate replaces benzalkonium chloride as the preservative in the first solution.

Boric Acid	1.9 g
Sodium Sulfite Anhydrous	0.1 g
Phenylmercuric nitrate	1:50,000
Sterile Purified Water	qs 100 mL
Sodium Acid Phosphate (NaH_2PO_4) anhydrous	0.56 g
Disodium Phosphate (Na_2HPO_4) anhydrous	0.284 g
Sodium Chloride	0.5 g
Disodium Edetate	0.1 g
Benzalkonium Chloride	1:10,000
Sterile Purified Water	qs 100 mL

These vehicles are suitable for salts of

Atropine	Homatropine
Ephedrine	Pilocarpine

Sterilization Procedures—Those procedures suited best for the extemporaneous preparation of ophthalmic solutions are:

1. Solutions in Final Container
   a. Place the filtered solution in containers that have been washed and rinsed with distilled water.
   b. Seal dropper bottles with regular screw caps. The dropper assembly should be stapled into a paper envelope.
   c. Sterilize 20 minutes at 15 psi (121°).
   d. Do not assemble until ready to use.
2. Dropper Bottles
   a. Wash container thoroughly and rinse with distilled water.
   b. Loosen caps and place bottles in autoclave.
   c. Autoclave 15 minutes at 15 psi (121°).
   d. Partially cool autoclave.
   e. Remove bottles from autoclave and secure caps.
   f. Store sterilized bottles in a clean, dustproof cabinet.
3. Glassware and Equipment
   a. Wrap adapters (containing filter), syringes, glassware, spatulas, etc, in autoclave paper and secure with masking tape.
   b. Place articles in autoclave and sterilize in the manner described in Section 2 above.
   c. Store in separate cabinet until ready to use.
4. Microbiological Filtration
   a. All equipment and glassware as well as stock solutions should be sterile. The prescription should be dispensed in a sterile container.
   b. Unwrap sterile syringe and draw prepared solution into syringe.
   c. Unwrap sterile adapter containing bacterial filter and attach to syringe. These are available as single-filtration, presterilized disposable units and should be utilized whenever possible.
   d. Force solution through filter directly into sterile container (dropper or plastic *Drop-Tainer* (Alcon) type).
   e. By employing an automatic filling outfit, more than one container of the same prescription can be prepared.
   f. Cap container immediately.

The procedures outlined above should be carried out in a clean area equipped with ultraviolet lighting and preferably in a laminar-flow hood.

Laminar-Flow Principles—A laminar-flow work area is a particularly convenient means of preparing sterile, particulate-free solutions. Laminar flow is defined as air flow in which the total body of air moves with uniform velocity along parallel lines with a minimum of eddies. Laminar flow minimizes the possibility of airborne microbial contamination by providing air free of viable particles and free of practically all inert particulates. Laminar-flow units are available in a variety of shapes and sizes and in two broad categories, horizontal and vertical laminar flow. It should be noted that laminar flow *per se* is not a guarantee of sterility. Correct procedures and sterile techniques remain necessary. See Chapter 84.

General Considerations

A number of requirements must be considered in the preparation of ophthalmic solutions, suspensions or ointments. These include sterility, clarity, buffer, buffer capacity and pH, tonicity, viscosity, stability, comfort, additives, particle size, packaging and preservatives. Many of these requirements are interrelated and must be considered collectively in the preparation of an ophthalmic product. The buffer system must be considered with tonicity and comfort in mind. Stability can be related to the pH, buffer system and packaging. Sterilization must be considered in terms of stability and packaging.

Ophthalmic solutions are formulated to be sterile, isotonic and buffered for stability and comfort. A viscosity-imparting agent may or may not be present. Solutions must be free from foreign particles. Solution pH must be selected for optimum drug stability. The pH then should be maintained by the inclusion of a buffer system of sufficient capacity to maintain pH throughout the extent of the shelf life of the product.

The proper pH, buffer and buffer capacity often represent a compromise between stability of the drug and comfort in the eye, since optimum patient comfort usually is found at the pH of the tear fluid, or about 7.4, while optimum stability for many drugs is generally lower, perhaps as low as 4.0–5.0. Buffer capacity should be sufficient to maintain pH, but minimized to the point where tear fluid can overcome capacity and readjust to pH to 7.4 immediately after instillation in the eye.

Sterilization represents the major requirement of eye products and the method, or methods, employed depend on the active ingredient and product resistance to heat and to the packaging used. More than one means of sterilization may be used. The sterile solution or suspension usually will contain an antimicrobial preservative to deal with inadvertent contamination during use. The preservative should not be relied upon to produce a sterile product and should not be considered as a substitute for sterile techniques and procedures.

Sterilization

Common methods of sterilization include moist heat under pressure (autoclave), dry heat, filtration, gas sterilization and ionizing radiation.

Dangers of Nonsterile Medications—The possibility of serious ocular infection resulting from the use of contaminated ophthalmic solutions has been documented amply in the literature. Such solutions repeatedly have been the cause of corneal ulcers and loss of eyesight. Contaminated solutions have been found in use in physicians' offices, eye clinics and industrial infirmaries, and dispensed on prescription in community and hospital pharmacies. The microbe most frequently found as a contaminant is the *Staphylococcus* group. *Pseudomonas aeruginosa* is a less frequent contaminant and the solution most often found contaminated is that of sodium fluorescein.

Pseudomonas aeruginosa (*B pyocyaneus; Pseudomonas pyocyanea*; Blue pus bacillus)—This is a very dangerous and opportunistic organism that grows well on most culture media and produces both toxins and antibacterial products. The latter tend to kill off other contaminants and allow the *P aeruginosa* to grow in pure culture. This gram-negative bacillus also grows readily in ophthalmic solutions, which may become the source of extremely serious infections of the cornea. It can cause complete loss of sight in 24–48 hours. In concentrations tolerated by tissues of the eye, it seems that all the antimicrobial agents discussed in the following sections may be ineffective against some strains of this organism.

A sterile ophthalmic solution in a multiple-dose container can be contaminated in a number of ways unless precautions are taken. For example, if a dropper bottle is used, the tip of the dropper while out of the bottle can touch the surface of a table or shelf if laid down, or it can touch the eyelid or eyelash of the patient during administration. If the *Drop-Tainer* (Alcon) type of bottle is used, the dropper tip can touch an eyelash, or the cap while removed to permit administration, or its edge may touch a table or finger and that edge can touch the dropper tip as the cap is replaced.

The solution may contain an effective antimicrobial but the next use of the contaminated solution may occur before enough time has elapsed for all of the organisms to be killed, and living organisms can find their way through an abrasion into the corneal stroma. Once in the corneal stroma, any residual traces of antimicrobial agents are neutralized by tissue components and the organisms find an excellent culture medium for rapid growth and dissemination through the cornea and the anterior segment of the eye.

Other Organisms—*Bacillus subtilis* may produce a serious abscess when it infects the vitreous humor. The pathogenic fungus considered of particular importance in eye solutions is *Aspergillus fumigatus*. Other fungi or molds may be harmful by accelerating deterioration of the active drugs.

With regard to viruses, as many as 42 cases of epidemic keratoconjunctivitis were caused by one bottle of virus-contaminated tetracaine solution. Virus contamination is particularly difficult to control because none of the preservatives now available is virucidal. Moreover, viruses are not removable by filtration. However, they are destroyed by autoclaving. The pharmacist and physician have not been made adequately aware of the dangers of transmitting virus infection via contaminated solutions. This is particularly pertinent to the adenoviruses (Types III and VIII) which are now believed to be the causative agents of viral conjunctivitis such as epidemic keratoconjunctivitis.

Methods

Steam under Pressure—Terminal sterilization by autoclaving is an acceptable, effective method of sterilization; however, the solution or suspension components must be sufficiently heat-resistant to survive the procedure. If sterilization is carried out in the final container, the container also must be able to survive the heat and pressure. A recent addition to this technique is the so-called air over steam autoclave. This combination allows pressure adjustments to be made during the autoclave cycle. Pressure manipulations permit the autoclave sterilization of materials which, while heat-resistant, tend to deform (ie, polypropylene containers).

Filtration—The USP states that sterile membrane filtration under aseptic conditions is the preferred method of sterilization. Membrane filtration offers the substantial advantage of room temperature operation with none of the deleterious effects of exposure to heat or sterilizing gas.

Sterilization by filtration does involve the transfer of the finished sterile product into previously sterilized containers using aseptic techniques. The membrane filtration equipment itself usually is sterilized as an assembly by autoclaving.

The application of filtration procedures to the extemporaneous preparation of sterile ophthalmic solutions has been proposed by several workers. Several types of equipment are available for small-scale work, as described in Chapter 37. Particular interest has been shown in the Swinny adapter fitted on a syringe and in the Millipore *Swinnex* disposable filter units. Empty sterile plastic "squeeze" containers and sterile plastic filtration units can be purchased directly from the manufacturers, eg, Wheaton (polyethylene containers) and Millipore (*Swinnex* filter units). They permit extemporaneous preparation of ophthalmic solutions which have a high probability of being sterile if the work is carried out under aseptic conditions. A supplementary device can permit automatic refilling of the syringe. The filter unit must be replaced after use.

Gas—Gas sterilization of heat-sensitive materials may be carried out by exposure to ethylene oxide gas in the presence of moisture. Ethylene oxide gas for sterilization use is available commercially diluted either with carbon dioxide or halogenated hydrocarbons. Ethylene oxide sterilization requires careful consideration of conditions required to effect sterility. Temperature and pressure conditions are quite nominal in contrast to wet or dry heat, however, careful control of exposure time, ethylene oxide concentration and moisture is essential.

Gas sterilization requires the use of specialized but not necessarily elaborate equipment. Gas autoclaves may range from very large walk-in units to small laboratory bench-scale units suitable for small hospitals, laboratories or pharmacies.

In using gas sterilization the possibility of human toxicity must be kept in mind. Care should be taken to restrict exposure to ethylene oxide during the loading, venting and unloading of the sterilizer. Ethylene oxide sterilization produces irritating byproducts which remain as residues in or on the articles sterilized. Residues include ethylene glycol and ethylene chlorohydrin (when in contact with chloride ions) in addition to ethylene oxide itself. To minimize such residues the sterilized articles should be aerated for at least 72 hours, preferably at 40 to 50°.

Ambient aeration time for sterilized polyethylene bottles should be about 48 hours. Ethylene oxide is recommended for the sterilization of solid materials which will not withstand heat sterilization. The FDA has recommended maximum residues in the parts per million range for ethylene oxide, ethylene glycol and ethylene chlorohydrin.

Radiation—Sterilization by exposure to ionizing radiation is an acceptable procedure for components of ophthalmic preparations or indeed for the total product as in certain ophthalmic ointments. Sources of radiation are twofold and include linear electron accelerators and radioisotopes. The linear accelerators produce high-energy electrons with very little penetrating power. Radioisotopes, particularly ^{60}Co, are employed more widely for sterilization. Sterilization by radiation may produce untoward effects such as chemical changes in product components, as well as changes in color or physical characteristics of package components.

Ophthalmic Preparation Characteristics

Clarity—Ophthalmic solutions are by definition free from foreign particles and clarity normally is achieved by filtration. It is, of course, essential that the filtration equipment be clean and well-rinsed so that particulate matter is not contributed to the solution by equipment designed to remove it. Operations performed in clean surroundings, the use of laminar-flow hoods and proper nonshedding garments will contribute collectively to the preparation of brilliantly clear solutions free from foreign particles. In many instances clarity and sterility may be achieved in the same filtration step. It is essential to realize that solution clarity is equally a function of the cleanliness of the intended container and closure. Both container and closure must be thoroughly clean, sterile and nonshedding. That is, the container or closure must not contribute particles to the solution during prolonged contact such as shelf-life storage. This normally is established by thorough stability testing.

Stability—The stability of a drug in solution, ie, an ophthalmic product, depends on the chemical nature of the drug substance, product pH, method of preparation (particularly temperature exposure), solution additives and type of packaging. Until two or three decades ago the stability of ophthalmic solutions was an exceedingly short-term concept; generally, it was the time required for a patient to complete the use of 15 or 30 mL of solution. Now, of course, the stability of ophthalmic products is expressed in terms of years. However, 2- to 3-year stability often is achieved only by virtue of compromise.

Drugs such as pilocarpine and physostigmine are both active and comfortable in the eye at a pH of 6.8; however, at this pH chemical stability (or instability) can be measured in days or months. With either drug, a substantial loss in chemical stability will occur in less than 1 year. On the other hand, at pH 5 both drugs are stable for a period of several years.

In addition to optimal pH, if oxygen sensitivity is a factor, adequate stability may require the inclusion of an antioxidant. Plastic packaging, ie, the low-density polyethylene *Drop-Tainer* (Alcon) that represents a patient convenience, may prove detrimental to stability by permitting oxygen permeation resulting in oxidative decomposition of the drug substance.

The attainment of optimum stability most often imposes a series of compromises on the formulator. The optimum pH may be lower than preferable for product comfort, although this effect may be minimized by adjusting pH with a buffer of minimum capacity. Additives such as chelating agents and antioxidants may be required and convenience packaging may diminish shelf life of the product.

It should be stressed that stability refers to total product stability not just the chemical stability of a single product component. That is an oversimplification. A well-planned stability program will consider and evaluate the chemical stability of the active ingredient, chemical stability of the preservative substance, continuing preservative efficacy against selected test organisms and adequacy of the package as a function of time (ie, does the package protect sterility in addition to various physical measures such as pH, clarity, resuspendability of suspensions and the like). One also must support the thesis that the material on test is representative of all lots of a given product.

Buffer and pH—Ideally, ophthalmic preparations should be formulated at a pH equivalent to the tear fluid value of 7.4. Practically, this seldom is achieved. The large majority of active ingredients used in ophthalmology are salts of weak bases and are most stable at an acid pH. This generally can be extended to suspensions of insoluble corticosteroids. Such suspensions usually are most stable at an acid pH.

Optimum pH adjustment generally requires a compromise on the part of the formulator. The pH selected should be optimum for stability. The buffer system selected should have a capacity adequate to maintain pH within the stability range for the duration of the product shelf life. Buffer capacity is the key in this situation.

It generally is accepted that a low (acid) pH *per se* necessarily will not cause stinging or discomfort on instillation. If the overall pH of the tears, after instillation, reverts rapidly to pH 7.4, discomfort is minimal. On the other hand, if the buffer capacity is sufficient to resist adjustment by tear fluid and the overall eye pH remains acid for an appreciable period of time, then stinging and discomfort may result. Consequently, buffer capacity should be adequate for stability, but minimized so far as possible, to allow the overall pH of the tear fluid to be disrupted only momentarily.

Tonicity—Tonicity refers to the osmotic pressure exerted by salts in aqueous solution. An ophthalmic solution is isotonic with another solution when the magnitudes of the colligative properties of the solutions are equal. An ophthalmic solution is considered isotonic when its tonicity is equal to that of an 0.9% sodium chloride solution.

The calculation of tonicity at one time was stressed rather heavily. The fledging pharmacist was taught in great detail the requirements of and means of achieving exact tonicity, sometimes to the detriment of other factors such as sterility and stability.

In actuality the eye is much more tolerant of tonicity variations than was at one time suggested. The eye usually can tolerate solutions equivalent to a range of 0.5% to 1.8% sodium chloride. Given a choice, isotonicity always is desirable and particularly is important in intraocular solutions. It need not, however, be an overriding concern when total product stability is to be considered.

The tonicity of ophthalmic (and parenteral) solutions has been investigated intensively over the years. These studies have resulted in the accumulation and publication of a large number of sodium chloride equivalents which are useful in calculating tonicity values. See Chapter 36.

Viscosity—The USP permits the use of viscosity-increasing agents to prolong contact time in the eye and thus enhance drug absorption and activity. Substances such as methylcellulose, polyvinyl alcohol and hydroxypropylmethyl cellulose are added frequently to increase viscosity.

Various investigators have studied the effect of increased viscosity on contact time in the eye. In general terms, viscosity increased up to the 15 to 50 cps range significantly improves contact time in the eye. Results tend to plateau beyond the 50-centipose range; higher viscosity values offer no significant advantage and have a tendency to leave a noticeable residue on the lid margins.

Additives—The use of various additives in ophthalmic solutions is permissible, however the choices are few in number. An antioxidant, specifically sodium bisulfite or metabisulfite, is permitted in concentrations up to 0.3%, particularly in solutions containing epinephrine salts. Other antioxidants such as ascorbic acid or acetylcysteine also may be used. The antioxidant acts in this case as a stabilizer to minimize oxidation of epinephrine.

The use of surfactants in ophthalmic preparations is restricted similarly. Nonionic surfactants, that class of such compounds which are least toxic to the ophthalmic tissues, are used in low concentrations particularly in steroid suspensions and as aids in achieving solution clarity. Surfactants may be used rarely as cosolvents to increase solubility.

The use of surfactants, particularly in any significant concentration, should be tempered by recognition of the sorption characteristics of these compounds. Nonionic surfactants, in particular, may react by binding with antimicrobial preservative compounds and inactivate much of the preservative system.

Cationic surfactants are used frequently in ophthalmic solutions but almost invariably as antimicrobial preservatives. Benzalkonium chloride is typical of this class of substances. Concentrations are in the range of 0.005 to 0.02%, with toxicity the limiting factor on the concentration used. Because of its large molecular weight the benzalkonium cation is inactivated easily by macromolecules of opposite charge or by sorption. Despite such limitations, benzalkonium chloride is the preservative used in the large majority of commercial ophthalmic solutions and suspensions.

Packaging

The traditional ophthalmic glass container with accompanying glass dropper has been supplanted almost completely by the low-density polyethylene dropper unit called the *Drop-Tainer* (Alcon). In only a very few instances are glass containers still in use, usually because of stability limitations. Large-volume intraocular solutions of 250 and 500 mL have been packaged in glass, but even these parenteral-type products are beginning to be packaged in specially fabricated polyethylene/polypropylene containers.

One should be ever mindful that plastic packaging, usually low-density polyethylene, is by no means interchangeable with glass. Plastic packaging is permeable to a variety of substances including light and air. The plastic package may contain a variety of extraneous substances such as mold release agents, antioxidants, reaction quenchers and the like, that readily may leach out of the plastic and into the contained solution. Label glues, inks and dyes also may penetrate polyethylene readily. In the opposite sense, volatile materials may permeate from solution into or through plastic containers.

Glass containers remain a convenient package material for extemporaneous preparation of ophthalmic solutions. Type 1 glass should be used. The container should be well-rinsed with sterile distilled water and may be sterilized by autoclaving. Droppers normally are available presterilized and packaged in a convenient blister pack.

Ophthalmic ointments invariably are packaged in metal tubes with an ophthalmic tip. Such tubes are sterilized conveniently by autoclaving or by ethylene oxide. In rare cases of metal reactivity or incompatibility, tubes lined with epoxy or vinyl plastic may be obtained.

Regardless of the form of packaging, some type of tamper-evident feature must be used for consumer protection. The common tamper-evident feature used on most ophthalmic preparations is the moisture- or heat-sensitive shrink band. The band should be identified in such a way that its disruption or absence should constitute a warning that tampering, either accidental or purposeful, has occurred.

The eyecup, an ancillary packaging device, fortunately seems to have gone the way of the community drinking cup. An eyecup should not be used. Its use inevitably will spread or aggravate eye infections. The pharmacist should not fail to discourage such use just as he or she should take the time to instruct the patient in the proper use and care of eye medications. While ophthalmic administration may seem simple enough, it may be a foreign and difficult task for many people. The suggestions and precautions given on page 1566 may be useful in instructing patients.

Antimicrobial Preservatives

The USP states that ophthalmic solutions may be packaged in multiple-dose containers. Each solution must contain a substance or mixture of substances to prevent the growth of, or to destroy, microorganisms introduced accidentally when the container is opened during use. The preservative is not intended to be used as a means of preparing a sterile solution. Appropriate techniques, discussed elsewhere, are to be employed to prepare a sterile solution.

Preservatives are not to be used in solutions intended for intraocular use because of the risk of irritation. Ophthalmic solutions prepared and packaged for a single application, ie, a unit dose, need not contain a preservative because it is not intended for reuse.

The need for proper control of ophthalmic solutions to prevent serious contamination was recognized in the 1930s. The first preservative recommended for use in ophthalmics was chlorobutanol, as an alternative to daily boiling!

The selection of an ophthalmic preservative can be a rather difficult task, in part, because of the relatively small number of suitable candidates. There is, of course, no such thing as an ideal preservative; however, the following criteria may be useful in preservative selection.

1. The agent should have a broad spectrum, and be active against gram-positive and gram-negative organisms as well as fungi. The agent should exert a rapid bactericidal activity particularly against known virulent organisms such as *P aeruginosa* strains.
2. The agent should be stable over a wide range of conditions including autoclaving temperatures and pH range.
3. Compatibility should be established with other preparation components and with package systems.
4. Lack of toxicity and irritation should be established with a reasonable margin of safety.

Preservative substances must be evaluated as a part of the total ophthalmic preparation in the proposed package. Only in this way can the adequacy of the preservative be established. The USP includes a test for preservative effectiveness; additionally, certain manufacturers have developed a panel of test organisms to further challenge and verify preservative activity.

In addition to preservative effectiveness as an immediate measure, its adequacy or stability as a function of time also must be ascertained. This often is done by measuring both chemical stability and preservative effectiveness over a given period of time and under varying conditions.

Many of these test procedures are, of course, not completely pertinent to the preparation of an extemporaneous ophthalmic solution. In such a situation the pharmacist must make selections based upon known conditions and physical and chemical characteristics. In such circumstances it would be prudent to prepare minimum volumes for short-term patient use.

The choice of preservatives suitable for ophthalmic use is surprisingly narrow. The classes of compounds available for such use are described in Table 1.[12] In each case or category there are specific limitations and shortcomings.

Quaternary Ammonium Compounds—Benzalkonium chloride is a typical quaternary ammonium compound and is, by far, the most common preservative used in ophthalmic preparations. Over 65% of commercial ophthalmic prod-

Table 1—Ophthalmic Preservatives[12]

Type	Typical structure	Concentration range	Incompatibilities
Quaternary ammonium compounds	$[R_1—N(R_2)(R_3)—R_1]\ Y^-$	0.004%–0.02% 0.01% most common	Soaps Anionic materials Salicylates Nitrates
Organic mercurials	$SHgC_2H_5$ / $COONa$ (benzene ring)	0.001%–0.01%	Certain halides with phenylmercuric acetate
Parahydroxy benzoates	$COOCH_3$ / OH (benzene ring)	Maximum 0.1%	Adsorption by macromolecules; marginal activity
Chlorobutanol	$CH_3—C(CH_3)(OH)—CCl_3$	0.5%	Stability is pH-dependent; activity concentration is near solubility maximum
Aromatic alcohols	CH_2OH (benzene ring)	0.5%–0.9%	Low solubility in water; marginal activity

ucts are preserved with benzalkonium chloride. Despite this broad use the compound has definite limitations. As a cationic surface-active material of high molecular weight it is not compatible with anionic compounds. It is incompatible with salicylates and nitrates and may be inactivated by high molecular weight nonionic compounds. Conversely, benzalkonium chloride has excellent chemical stability and very good antimicrobial characteristics. Given the alternative it would be preferable to modify a formulation to remove the incompatibility, rather than include a compatible but less effective preservative.

The literature on benzalkonium chloride is somewhat mixed; however, this is not unexpected given the wide variation in test methods and, indeed, the chemical variability of benzalkonium chloride itself. The official substance is defined as a mixture of alkyl benzyldimethylammonium chlorides including all or some of the group ranging from $n\text{-}C_8H_{17}$ through $n\text{-}C_{16}H_{33}$. The $n\text{-}C_{12}H_{25}$ homolog content is not less than 40% on an anhydrous basis.

Reviews[13] of benzalkonium chloride indicate that it is well-suited for use as an ophthalmic preservative. Certain early negative reports have been shown to be quite erroneous; in some cases adverse tissue reactions were attributed to benzalkonium chloride when, in fact, a totally different compound was used as the test material. Although benzalkonium chloride is by far the most common quaternary preservative others occasionally referred to include benzethonium chloride and cetyl pyridinium chloride. All are official compounds. More recently quaternary ammonium compounds have been attached to soluble, reasonably high-molecular-weight polymers. These agents possess good antimicrobial effectiveness with fewer compatibility problems than the official quaternary preservatives. Refer to RPS-14, page 1571 for a summary of quaternary germicides in ophthalmic drugs.

Organic Mercurials—It generally is stated that phenylmercuric nitrate or phenylmercuric acetate, in 0.002% concentration, should be used instead of benzalkonium chloride as a preservative for salicylates and nitrates, and in solutions of salts of physostigmine and epinephrine that contain 0.1% of sodium sulfite. The usual range of concentrations employed is 0.002 to 0.004%. Phenylmercuric borate sometimes is used in place of the nitrate or acetate.

Phenylmercuric nitrate has the advantage, over some other organic mercurials, in not being precipitated at a slightly acid pH. As with other mercurials, it is slow in its bactericidal action, and it also produces sensitization reactions. Phenylmercuric ion is incompatible with halides as it forms precipitates.

The effectiveness of phenylmercuric nitrate against *P aeruginosa* is questionable; it has been found that pseudomonal organisms survive after exposure to a concentration of 0.004% for longer than a week.

Development of iatrogenic mercury deposits in the crystalline lens resulting from use of miotic eye drops containing 0.004% phenylmercuric nitrate, 3 times daily, for periods of 3 to 6 years, has been reported. No impairment of vision was found, but the yellowish brown discoloration of the lens capsule is reported to be permanent.

Thimerosal (*Merthiolate*, Lilly) is an organomercurial with bacteriostatic and antifungal activity and is used as an antimicrobial preservative in concentrations of 0.005 to 0.02%. Its action, as with other mercurials, has been reported to be slow.

Parahydroxybenzoic Acid Esters—Mixtures of methylparaben and propylparaben sometimes are used as ophthalmic antimicrobial preservatives; the concentration of methylparaben is in the range of 0.1 to 0.2%, while that of propylparaben approaches its solubility in water (approximately 0.04%). They are not considered efficient bacteriostatic agents and are slow in their antimicrobial action. Ocular irritation and stinging have been attributed to their use in ophthalmic preparations. In a review of OTC drugs for use in ophthalmology, the FDA expert panel found the parabens unacceptable as ophthalmic solution preservatives.

Substituted Alcohols and Phenols—Chlorobutanol is stated to be effective against both gram-positive and gram-negative organisms, including *P aeruginosa* and some fungi. It broadly is compatible with other ingredients and normally used in a concentration of 0.5%. One of the products of hydrolysis is hydrochloric acid, which causes a decrease in the pH of aqueous solutions. This decomposition occurs rapidly at high temperatures and slowly at room temperature, in unbuffered solutions that were originally neutral or alkaline. Therefore, ophthalmic solutions that contain chlorobutanol should be buffered between pH 5.0 and 5.5. At room temperature it dissolves slowly in water and, although it dissolves more rapidly on heating, loss by vaporization and decomposition is accelerated.

A combination of chlorobutanol and phenylethyl alcohol (0.5% of each) has been reported to be more effective against *P aeruginosa*, *S aureus* and *P vulgaris* than either antimicrobial singly. Also, preliminary solution of the chlorobutanol in phenylethyl alcohol effects solution of the former in water without the use of heat.

Ophthalmic Preparations for OTC Use

A comprehensive review of over-the-counter ophthalmic preparations recently has been completed by an expert panel approved by the FDA. The panel review extended over the period 1973 through 1979. The finding of this panel, in the form of a tentative final monograph, appeared in the *Federal Register*.[14]

In a comprehensive assessment the panel considered the following conditions amenable to OTC drug therapy.

Tear Insufficiency—Rational formulations used to treat tear insufficiency are aqueous solutions containing demulcent agents, tonicity agents and pH and buffering agents. Tear insufficiency includes:

1. Keratoconjunctivitis sicca
2. Sjogren's syndrome
3. Dry eye in the elderly

Corneal Edema—Increased water content in the cornea usually is treated with hypertonic solutions of sodium chloride, either 2 or 5%.

Inflammation and Irritation of the Eye—

1. Presence of loose foreign material in the eye. Commonly treated with an isotonic eyewash properly buffered and preserved.
2. Irritation from airborne pollutants and chlorinated water. Management consists of avoiding the offending allergens and the use of vasoconstrictors, astringents, demulcents and emollients for symptomatic relief.
3. Allergic conjunctivitis. Treatment by topically applied vasoconstrictors and astringents, demulcents, emollients and cold compresses. Only in mild cases, where edema and congestion are slight, is OTC treatment alone adequate.

In providing such OTC medications the pharmacist should take the opportunity to point out that unsupervised use of these products should be limited to 72 hours, when based on self-diagnosis. If the condition persists or worsens at any time, treatment should be discontinued and a physician consulted at once.

Contact Lenses

Contact lenses are optical and/or therapeutic ophthalmic devices divisible into four general categories. The rigid, hydrophobic, so-called hard contact lenses, principally PMMA (polymethyl methacrylate); rigid, semihydrophobic; flexible hydrophilic; flexible hydrophobic and rigid-gas-permeable. Each lens class is accompanied by its support solution products and devices. Solutions used with hard contact lenses are rather conventional compositions, usually regarded as OTC products. Conversely, solutions ancillary to the hydrophilic lenses may be classed as new drugs or devices from a regulatory standpoint. Such preparations require great care and considerable pharmaceutical skill to formulate. Lens materials and support products are further classified and identified in Table 2.

Hard Contact Lens—Some evidence is available to show that contact lenses were visualized by Leonardo da Vinci in

Table 2—Contact Lens Classes, Characteristics and Support Products

Lens type	Chemical classification	Major characteristics	Typical support products
"Hard," rigid, hydrophobic	PMMA (polymethyl methacrylate)	Negligible gas permeability, low water content, medium wettability	Wetting solutions Soaking solutions Cleaning solutions Combination Artificial tears
"Soft," flexible, hydrophilic	HEMA (hydroxyethyl methylmethacrylate)	High water content, low gas permeability, good wettability	Cleaning solutions Disinfection solutions
Flexible hydrophobic	Silicone rubber	Good gas permeability Poor wettability	Wetting solutions Cleaning solutions Soaking solutions
	Silicone vinylpyrollidone	Good gas permeability Good wettability	
Rigid, hydrophilic	CAB (cellulose acetate butyrate)	Good gas permeability Good wettability	Wetting solutions Cleaning solutions Soaking solutions Rewetting solutions

1508 and later, in 1637, by Rene Descartes. In 1827 the British astronomer, Sir John Herschel, described the mathematics of these devices. He speculated on the possibility of filling a glass contact lens with transparent gelatin to correct for corneal irregularities. Not until 1888 was the original concept executed by the artificial eye maker, Albert Muller. He made a glass protective shell for the cornea of a lagophthalmic patient who had carcinoma of the upper lid. The patient wore the device for 20 years, and corneal clarity was maintained. Other cases were reported in Europe of glass shells placed on the eye as corneal protective devices.

Until the latter part of the 1940s almost all contact lenses had a portion resting directly on, or arching over, the cornea with a supporting flange resting beyond the limbus on the sclera. Thus, they were scleral lenses. However, contact lenses without scleral portions (corneal lenses) were in existence at least as early as 1912, when they were being manufactured by Carl Zeiss.

The glass scleral contact lenses that were made from 1888 to 1938 were fitted by a tedious method of trial and error using a fitting set that might contain more than 1000 lenses. The lenses were heavy and adjustments on them by the fitter were impossible. Their life in the eye was short, because the glass was attacked vigorously by lacrimal fluid; in about 6 months the lenses became too rough to wear or to see through. However, they had the advantage that tears readily wet glass. In 1922 Dallos, in Budapest, perfected a molding technique by which a glass shell could be fabricated to approximate closely the curvature of the globe. With the introduction of the methyl methacrylate plastic molded scleral contact lens in 1938 by Obrig and Muller, the feasibility of using plastic for lens fabrication was demonstrated. Although the optical properties of glass are superior to those of plastic, the relative gain in ruggedness and the reduction in weight to one-third that of glass far offset this disadvantage. Not until PMMA became available was a flush-fitting shell possible. The concept was developed by Ridley, in England, in 1954. The protective effect is very useful in various conditions characterized by corneal epithelial fragility and for cosmetic effects.

The "hard" plastic corneal contact lens was introduced by Tuohy in 1948. This was a major development. He specified a lens of smaller diameter that rested within the limbal area of the cornea. The results were poor. Development of a corneal lens was hindered by the fear of traumatizing the cornea with an appliance that fitted directly onto it. The first corneal lens to have any measure of success was developed in the early 1950s by Dickinson, Sohnges and Neill. Its thickness was about 0.2 mm and was considered to be a fairly thick lens. Thinner lenses, about 0.1 mm, were introduced in the early 1960s.

Scleral bifocal lenses were developed initially in 1936 and the corneal type in 1958. Bifocal contact lenses are more difficult to fit, more costly and, in many cases, more uncomfortable than single-vision lenses.

Lens-Care Products

Wetting Solutions—These are preparations designed to furnish an hydrophilic coating over the characteristically hydrophobic surface of PMMA, silicon, acrylate and other rigid lens surfaces. Typically, wetting solutions include an acceptable viscosity-imparting agent, a surfactant and a preservative. The surface-activity and viscosity effect may be obtained from a single compound. Agents commonly used include cellulose derivatives, polyvinyl pyrollidone, polyvinyl alcohol and polyethylene glycol derivatives. Preservatives include those acceptable for ophthalmic use. Such solutions are sterile.

Cleaning Solutions—Cleaning solutions commonly are used to remove surface contaminants—lipids, protein and the like. Cleaning is accomplished by the use of surfactants which preferably are nonionic or amphoteric. Solutions are sterile and properly preserved. Viscosity-imparting agents generally are not included.

Adequate cleaning of hydrophilic lenses is a far more complex and challenging problem than hard-lens cleaning. Because of their permeability characteristics, contaminants penetrate into the lens structure and easily may bind chemically or physically to the HEMA lens material. Contaminants may be surface films or crystals, amorphous aggregates of protein material, cellular debris or insoluble inorganic salts.

Cleaning products generally are specific to the lens material and require FDA approval, with proof of cleaning efficacy and safety. Cleaners are based on surface activity, enzyme action or even abradant action, in which case the abradant material is softer than the lens itself. Adequate cleaning of hydrophilic lens material daily is a necessary prelude to disinfection. Most recently the use of extended-wear lenses has found wide acceptance. Successful use usually depends on the use of an enzyme for cleaning, together with special disinfectants.

Disinfecting Systems—Disinfection of the first hydrophilic lens approved by the FDA was accomplished using a heating device which generated steam from a saline solution. The latter was prepared either by the user or available from the manufacturer. Subsequent to the so-called thermal systems, disinfection solutions were developed which met the requirements necessary for FDA approval. Because of the sorption characteristics of hydrophilic lens materials, many of the accepted ophthalmic preservatives are unsatisfactory for use in soft-lens disinfecting systems, including the ubiquitous benzalkonium chloride. Once again, however, the use of a quaternary disinfectant covalently bonded to a soluble, relatively high-molecular-weight polymer has met with some success.

In addition to possessing satisfactory disinfecting activity, such a preparation must be isotonic, in an acceptable pH range, nonreactive (nonbinding) with lens materials and, over a normal use period, induce or bring about no physical, chemical or optical changes in the lens. It is of course sterile and safe for use in the eye even though direct instillation into the eye is not intended.

Soaking Solutions—Soaking or storage solutions, as the name suggests, are used to store and hydrate hard lenses but, most importantly, to disinfect such lenses. Disinfection should be rapid and as complete as possible making use, once again, of acceptable ophthalmic preservative substances. Soaking solutions typically contain chlorhexidine (gluconate), benzalkonium or quaternary/polymer compounds enhanced by sodium edetate.

Artificial Tears—Solutions intended to rewet hard lenses *in situ* are referred to as rewetting solutions or artificial tears. Such preparations are intended to reinforce the wetting capacity of the normal tear film. Early products of this type tended to be somewhat viscous wetting solutions acceptable for direct installation into the eye. More recent preparations mimic tears more accurately and their viscosity is rather low, thus, user acceptability is improved.

Guidelines for Safety and Efficacy Testing—The FDA periodically issues or updates guidelines describing recommended test procedures for contact lens-care products, other than those used with PMMA lenses and, also, for typical OTC products used with hard lenses. The reader is advised to review the most recent guidelines for appropriate protocols for non-PMMA products.

Tests for OTC (hard) lens products are divided into those appropriate for products intended for direct instillation in the eye and those not so intended. Products intended for direct instillation require multiple-application safety tests in the rabbit eye, preservative efficacy tests and sterility testing, in addition to adequate efficacy tests.

Products not intended for direct instillation require short term evaluation in the rabbit eye and, of course, preservative efficacy and sterility testing.

Soft Contact Lens—In 1960 Wichterle and Lim introduced a new, soft, hydrophilic gel lens synthesized by copolymerization of HEMA with ethylene glycol dimethacrylate (EGDM). Its hydrophilic nature was in marked contrast to the hydrophobic properties of PMMA; its increased permeability to water, oxygen and other constituents of tears having low molecular weight appears to offer metabolic advantages.

Hydrophilic (gel, hydrogel, soft or flexible) lenses are made of polymerized or copolymerized hydrophilic monomers with a cross-linking agent, such as EGDM. The cross-links add stability to the gel lenses and act to decrease the water saturation. The most widely used monomer is HEMA which may be copolymerized with lesser amounts of polyvinylpyrrolidone (PVP), a more hydrophilic polymer. The copolymer acts to increase the hydration level beyond the maximum 40% potential of homogenous poly-HEMA. Gel lenses of even higher water content can be formed by combining a hydrophilic monomer or polymer (usually PVP) with a relatively hydrophobic monomer (usually methyl methacrylate). Lenses of this type are available with as much as 85% water at equilibrium. In addition, these cross-linked polymers cannot be formed by heat or pressure and thus usually are not harmed by boiling in aqueous solution or by autoclaving.

Hydrophilic lenses are elastic and flexible when hydrated, yet brittle when dry. They can absorb and concentrate tear-film constituents as well as environmental pollutants, vapors, cosmetic ingredients, water impurities and antimicrobial preservatives, as well as active ingredients, in ophthalmic preparations. The refractive index for HEMA is 1.43 when hydrated in normal saline; hydrophilic lenses of greater hydration level have a correspondingly lower refractive index. Depending on the amount of cross-linking and the amount and type of additives, the dimensions can be influenced by such factors as pH, tonicity and molecular or ionic species of dissolved substances.

Advantages and Disadvantages of Soft Contact Lenses—Soft contact lenses have the major advantage of wearer comfort and easy adaptability, particularly for the first-time lens wearer. Soft lenses are misplaced or lost less easily and allow an easier transition to eye glasses. The typical vision blurring associated with a transition from hard lenses to eye glasses is absent.

Because of the flexibility of soft contact lenses an accurate fit to the eye is more difficult than is the case with hard lenses. Visual clarity usually is less with soft lenses; indeed, the long-time hard-lens wearer may find visual clarity or acuity of soft lenses unacceptable at first wearing.

Soft lenses require far more care than their hard counterparts. The soft polymers will allow penetration of contaminants deep into the lens body where even simple removal become difficult. Soft lenses may become more or less permanently contaminated by sorption of drug product components, in addition to protein fragments or various other debris.

Even with reasonable care, soft lenses can be expected to have a wearer life substantially shorter than hard lenses. Eye corrective changes requiring refitting and lens replacement may occur well before hard lenses require replacing because of wear.

Despite the obvious practical disparities the popularity of soft contact lenses is immense, and increasing as durability and wearing time are increased. Wearer comfort, easy adaptability and adequacy for most relatively minor visual corrections contribute to soft-lens acceptability and popularity.

Therapeutic Uses

The majority of contact lenses are used for reasons of optical acuity, convenience and/or cosmetic value. However, so far as is known, the first use of such a device, in 1888, was to protect a cornea, and therapeutic usefulness has continued since that time. A major therapeutic advance was made by Ridley, in 1954, using PMMA, at the time that it was replacing glass as the principal material used in making lenses. Currently, there is evidence of contact-lens development of major therapeutic importance in the use of soft lenses in the treatment of very serious pathological conditions. They are of value in several ways, which are interrelated to the extent it is difficult to give an example which illustrates only one point. The several functions can be listed as:

1. As "bandages" (through which one can see) to protect the epithelium of the cornea.
2. While in use as bandages, to permit movement of medicinal fluids through the lens to the eye, as well as under the lens (see below).
3. When so used, to increase the duration of the effect from a given quantity of drug.
4. When so used, to increase the degree of effect from a given amount of drug (see below).

The first two functions have become rather well-established in the past few years; the last two have been of less therapeutic value.

Bullous keratopathy is the most severe form of corneal edema. Its treatment is presented as an example of the first two functions of soft contact lenses. The lens acts basically as a simple bandage, but has the added valuable quality that the ophthalmic solutions, used as drops, can pass through the lenses and act on the eye. The pain of bullous keratopathy usually is relieved dramatically by the use of the lens as a protective shield, as similarly accomplished by the earlier hard scleral lenses. Vision may be improved slightly. The pain results mainly from the lids rubbing on the bullae, rupturing them and exposing corneal nerves. The lenses can be worn fulltime, 24 hours a day for months, except for removal for cleaning. They may need to be cleaned only when protein deposits build up on them. They should be removed and inserted only by a physician. New lenses will be needed as the cornea changes in shape.

Compared with hard lenses, use of the soft lens is much simpler. No moldings of the eye or keratometer readings are needed. The iatrogenic aspects of the hard lens have, to a great extent, been alleviated by the soft lens. Few problems occur on over-wearing the lenses. Usually, no abrasions are found. The eyes are white and usually free of conjunctival infection. As to medicinal agents, because of the concomitant iritis, pupils must be dilated with cycloplegics for the first few days, as by use of atropine. Eyelid hygiene techniques are needed. Antibiotics, such as chloramphenicol drops, are used if secondary infection or blepharitis is present. A 5% hypertonic saline solution may be used to improve vision; the patient can use it as often as it is helpful.

The conditions for which the use of soft lenses is apparently very helpful and well established are

1. Edema
   a. Bullous keratopathy
   b. Aphakic
   c. Secondary to glaucoma
   d. Fuchs' dystrophy
   e. Uveitis, etc
2. Epithelial erosion and defects
   a. Ulcers
   b. Chemical burns
   c. Post-graft
3. Exposure
   a. Neurotropic keratitis
   b. Lid abnormalities
4. Irregular cornea
   a. Scars
   b. Dystrophy
5. Dry eye
   a. Nonprogressive conjunctival cicatrization (Stevens-Johnson syndrome)
   b. Sjögren's syndrome
   c. Trachoma
   d. Pemphigoid

Summary

The progress in ophthalmic pharmaceutics and in lens care pharmaceutics during the last decade must be considered as striking. Very substantial advances have been made in ophthalmic bioavailability and the factors influencing ophthalmic drug absorption. New approaches and new techniques have confirmed (or refuted) many long held tenets of ophthalmic formulation technology. Continuing studies in the general field of ophthalmic pharmaceutics and pharmacokinetics should continue to advance the frontiers of ophthalmic drug therapy and ophthalmic drug delivery.

In the contact-lens and lens-care field one is confronted with a plethora of new lenses and lens polymers. Wearing time has been lengthened substantially, comfort improved and correctable visual defects increased. By the same token the requirements for lens hygiene also have increased. Advances in this broad field also show no signs of abating.

References

1. Botelho SY: *Sci Am 211:* 80, 1964.
2. Shell JW: *Surv Ophthalmol 26:* 207, 1982.
3. Patton TF: *J Pharm Sci 66:* 1058, 1977.
4. Lee VHL, Robinson JR: *Ibid 68:* 673, 1979.
5. Lee VHL, *J Ocul Pharmacol 6(2)*: 157, 1990.
6. Hecht G, *et al*: *Modern Pharmaceutics*, 3rd ed, Dekker, New York, Chap 12.
7. Abshire R, Cash P: *J Parent Sci Technol 40(3)*: 97, 1986.
8. Higuchi T: *J Pharm Sci 50:* 874, 1961.
9. Edelhauser HF, Van Horn DL, Scholtz RO, Hyndiuk RA: *Am J Ophthalmol 81:* 473, 1976.
10. Aronson SD, Elliott JH: *Ocular Inflammation*, Mosby, St Louis, 899, 1972.
11. Reynolds LA: *Am J Hosp Pharm 48*: 2438, 1991.
12. Hoover JE: *Dispensing of Medication*, 8th ed, Mack Publ Co, 237, 1976.
13. Mullen W, Shepherd W, Labovitz J: *Surv Ophthalmol 17:* 469, 1973.
14. *Fed Reg 48(125)*: 29788–29800, June 28, 1983.

Bibliography

Adler FH: *Physiology of the Eye, Clinical Application*, 7th ed, Mosby, St Louis, 1981.

Adler FH: *Textbook of Ophthalmology*, 8th ed, Saunders, Philadelphia, 1969.

Banker GS, Rhodes CT: *Modern Pharmaceutics*, 3rd ed, Dekker, New York, pp 479–564, 1979.

Handbook of Nonprescription Drugs, 7th ed, APhA, Washington DC, 1982, pp 417–450.

Havener WH: *Ocular Pharmacology*, 4th ed, Mosby, St Louis, 1978.

Newell FW: *Ophthalmology—Principles and Concepts*, 4th ed, Mosby, St Louis, 1978.

Stone J, Phillips A: *Contact Lenses*, 2nd ed, Butterworths, Boston, 1980.

Symposium on Contact Lenses, Mosby, St Louis, 1973.

CHAPTER 90

Medicated Applications

Lawrence H Block, PhD
Professor of Pharmaceutics
Duquesne University School of Pharmacy
Pittsburgh, PA 15282

The application of medicinal substances to the skin or various body orifices is a concept doubtless as old as humanity. The papyrus records of ancient Egypt describe a variety of such medications for external use. Galen described the use in Roman times of a forerunner to today's vanishing creams.

Medications are applied in a variety of forms reflecting the ingenuity and scientific imagination of pharmacists through the centuries. New modes of drug delivery have been developed to remedy the shortcomings of earlier vehicles or, more recently, to optimize drug delivery. Conversely, some external medications have fallen into disuse because of changes in the practice of medicine.

Medications are applied to the skin or inserted into body orifices in liquid, semisolid or solid form. Ophthalmics and topical aerosol products will not be discussed in this chapter. Ophthalmic use imposes particle size, viscosity and sterility specifications that require separate, detailed discussion (see Chapter 89). The complexity of pharmaceutical aerosol systems necessitates their inclusion elsewhere (see Chapter 95).

Biopharmaceutic Aspects of the Routes of Administration

Epidermal and Transdermal Drug Delivery

The Skin

The skin often has been referred to as the largest of the body organs: an average adult's skin has a surface area of about 2 m^2. It is probably the heaviest organ of the body. Its accessibility and the opportunity it affords to maintain applied preparations intact for a prolonged time have resulted in its increasing use as a route of drug administration, whether for local, regional or systemic effects.

Anatomically, human skin may be described as a stratified organ with three distinct tissue layers: the epidermis, the dermis and the subcutaneous fat layer (Fig 1).

Epidermis, the outermost skin layer, comprises stratified squamous epithelial cells. Keratinized, flattened remnants of these actively dividing epidermal cells accumulate at the skin surface as a relatively thin region (about 10 μm thick) termed the stratum corneum, or horny layer. The horny layer is itself lamellar with the keratinized cells overlapping one another, linked by intracellular bridges and compressed into about 15 layers. The lipid-rich intercellular space in the stratum corneum is comprised of lamellar matrices with alternating hydrophilic layers and lipophilic bilayers formed during the process of keratinization. The region behaves as a tough but flexible coherent membrane.

The stratum corneum also is markedly hygroscopic—far more so than other keratinous materials such as hair or nails. Immersed in water the isolated stratum corneum swells to about three times its original thickness, absorbing about four to five times its weight in water in the process. The stratum corneum functions as a protective physical and chemical barrier and is only slightly permeable to water. It retards water loss from underlying tissues, minimizes ultraviolet light penetration and limits the entrance of microorganisms, medications and toxic substances from without. The stratum corneum is abraded continuously. Thus, it tends to be thicker in regions more subject to abrasion or the bearing of weight. Its regeneration is provided by rapid cell division in the basal cell layer of the epidermis. Migration or displacement of dividing cells towards the skin surface is accompanied by differentiation of the epidermal cells into layers of flat, laminated plates, as noted above. An acidic film (pH ranging between 4.0 and 6.5, depending on the area tested) made up of emulsified lipids covers the surface of the stratum corneum.

The dermis apparently is a gel structure involving a fibrous protein matrix embedded in an amorphous, colloidal, ground substance. Protein, including collagen and elastin fibers, is oriented approximately parallel to the epidermis. The dermis supports and interacts with the epidermis facilitating its conformation to underlying muscles and bones. Blood vessels, lymphatics and nerves are found within the dermis, though only nerve fibers reach beyond the dermal ridges or papillae into the germinative region of the epidermis. Sweat glands and hair follicles extending from the dermis through the epidermis provide discontinuities in an otherwise uniform integument.

The subcutaneous fat layer serves as a cushion for the dermis and epidermis. Collagenous fibers from the dermis thread between the accumulations of fat cells providing a connection between the superficial skin layers and the subcutaneous layer.

Hair Follicles and Sweat Glands—Human skin is sprinkled liberally with surface openings extending well into the dermis. Hair follicles, together with the sebaceous glands that empty into the follicles, make up the pilosebaceous unit. Apocrine and eccrine sweat glands add to the total.

Pilosebaceous Units—Human hair consists of compacted keratinized cells formed by follicles. Sebaceous glands empty into the follicle sites to form the pilosebaceous unit. The hair follicles are surrounded by sensory nerves; thus, an important function of human hair is sensory. Human hair varies enormously within the same individual, even within the same specific body area. Follicular density varies considerably as well, from values of about 250 follicles per cm^2 for the scalp to 50 per cm^2, or less, for the thigh and other relatively nonhirsute areas. Follicular density is determined genetically, ie, no new follicles are formed after birth. One characteristic human trait is that although most of the body hairs never develop beyond the rudimentary vellus state, the only hairless areas are confined, primarily, to the palmar and plantar surfaces. Individual hairs can vary in microscopic appearance, diameter, cuticle appearance and even presence or absence of medulla.

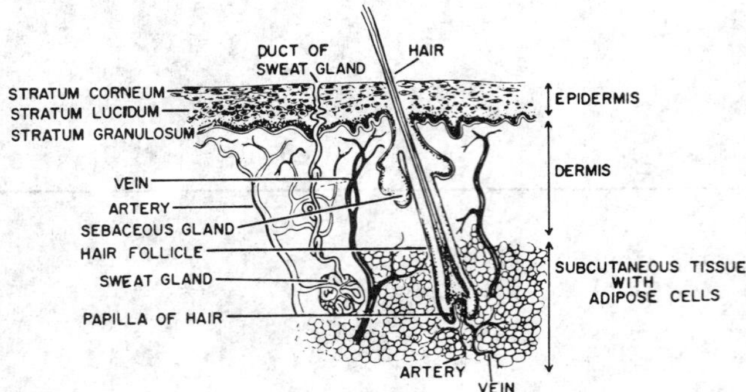

Fig 1. Vertical section of human skin.

Sebaceous glands are similar anatomically and functionally but vary in size and activity according to location. Population in the scalp, face and anogenital areas may vary from 400 to 900/cm^2. Fewer than 100/cm^2 are found in other areas. Sebaceous glands are richly supplied with blood vessels.

Sebaceous cells synthesize and accumulate lipid droplets. This accumulation results in enlarged cells which fragment to form sebum. Sebum is made up of a mixture of lipids, approximately as shown in Table 1.

The sebaceous gland, containing sebum, cell debris and microorganisms such as *Propionibacterium acnes,* is connected to the pilosebaceous canal by a duct of squamous epithelium. When access to the surface is blocked and bacteria multiply, the result is the comedo of acne.

Sebum presumably functions as an emollient, although Kligman once stated it was useless. Montagna suggests that sebum functions as a pheromone to provide the human with a distinctive aroma.

Sweat Glands—Sweat glands are classified as apocrine and eccrine. Apocrine glands are secretory but are not necessarily responsive to thermal stimulation. Such glands do not produce sweat in the normal sense of the word. Apocrine glands, however, often are associated with eccrine sweat glands particularly in the axilla.

Eccrine sweat glands are coiled secretory glands, equipped with a blood supply, extending from the dermis to the epidermal surface. Eccrine sweat glands function to regulate heat exchange in man. As such, they are indispensable to survival.

About 3 million eccrine glands are thought to be distributed over the human body. Distribution varies from less than 100 to more than 300/cm^2. Gland counts after thermal stimulation do not always agree with anatomical counts.

Drug Effects and the Extent of Percutaneous Drug Delivery

Drugs are applied to the skin to elicit one or more of four general effects: an effect on the skin surface, an effect within the stratum corneum, a more deep-seated effect requiring penetration into the epidermis and dermis or a systemic effect resulting from delivery of sufficient drug through the epidermis and the dermis to the vasculature to produce therapeutic systemic concentrations.

Surface Effects—An activity on the skin surface may be in the form of a film, an action against surface microorganisms or a cleansing effect. Film formation on the skin surface may be protective, eg, a zinc oxide cream or a sunscreen. Films may be somewhat occlusive and provide a moisturizing effect by diminishing loss of moisture from the skin surface. In such instances the film or film formation *per se* fulfils the objective of product design. The action of antimicrobials against surface flora requires more than simple delivery to the site. The vehicle must facilitate contact between the surface organisms and the active ingredient. Skin cleansers employ soaps or surfactants to facilitate the removal of superficial soil.

Table 1—Composition of Sebum

Constituents	% w/w
Triglycerides	57.5
Wax Esters	26.0
Squalene	12.0
Cholesterol Esters	3.0
Cholesterol	1.5

Stratum Corneum Effects—Drug effects within the stratum corneum are seen with certain sunscreens; *p*-aminobenzoic acid is an example of a sunscreening agent which both penetrates and is substantive to stratum corneum cells. Skin moisturization takes place within the stratum corneum. Whether it involves the hydration of dry outer cells by surface films or the intercalation of water in the lipid-rich intercellular laminae, the increased moisture results in an apparent softening of the skin. Keratolytic agents, such as salicylic acid, act within the stratum corneum to cause a breakup or sloughing of stratum corneum cell aggregates. This is particularly important in conditions of abnormal stratum corneum such as psoriasis, a disease characterized by thickened scaly plaques.

The stratum corneum also may serve as a *reservoir phase* or depot wherein topically applied drug accumulates due to partitioning into or binding with skin components. This interaction can limit the subsequent migration of the penetrant unless the interaction capacity of the stratum corneum is surpassed by providing excess drug. Examples of drugs which exhibit significant skin interaction include benzocaine, estrogens, scopolamine and corticosteroids.

Epidermal, Dermal, Local and Systemic Effects—The penetration of a drug into the viable epidermis and dermis may be difficult to achieve, as noted above. But, once transepidermal permeation has occurred, the continued diffusion of drug into the dermis is likely to result in drug transfer into the microcirculation of the dermis and then into general circulation. Nonetheless, it is possible to formulate drug delivery systems which provide substantial localized delivery without achieving correspondingly high systemic concentrations. Limited studies in man of topical triethanolamine salicylate, minoxidil and retinoids demonstrate the potential of this approach.

Unwanted systemic effects stemming from the inadvertent transdermal penetration of drugs have been reported for a wide variety of compounds (eg, hexachlorophene, lindane, corticosteroids or *N,N*-diethyl-*m*-toluamide) over the years. With the commercial introduction of transdermal drug delivery systems for scopolamine, nitroglycerin, clonidine, 17β-estradiol, fentanyl, nicotine and testosterone, transdermal penetration is being regarded increasingly as an opportunity rather than a nuisance.

Percutaneous Absorption

Percutaneous absorption involves the transfer of drug from the skin surface into the stratum corneum, under the aegis of a concentration gradient, and its subsequent diffusion through the stratum corneum and underlying epidermis, through the dermis and into the microcirculation. The skin behaves as a passive barrier to diffusing molecules. Evidence for this includes the fact that the impermeability of the skin persists long after the skin has been excised. Furthermore, Fick's Law is obeyed in the vast majority of instances.

Molecular penetration through the various regions of the skin is limited by the diffusional resistances encountered. The total diffusional resistance (R_{skin}) to permeation through the skin has been described by Chien as

$$R_{skin} = R_{sc} + R_e + R_{pd}$$

where R is the diffusional resistance and the subscripts *sc, e and pd* refer to the stratum corneum, epidermis and papillary layer of the dermis, respectively. In addition, resistance to transfer into the microvasculature limits the systemic delivery of drug.

By and large, the greatest resistance to penetration is met in the stratum corneum, ie, diffusion through the stratum corneum tends to be the rate-limiting step in percutaneous absorption.

The role of hair follicles and sweat glands must be considered; however, as a general rule their effect is minimized by the relatively small fractional areas occupied by these appendages. On the other hand, liposomal vehicles and microbead (3 to 10 μm diameter) suspensions appear to accumulate selectively in pilosebaceous and perifollicular areas. In the very early stages of absorption, transit through the appendages may be comparatively large, particularly for lipid-soluble molecules and those whose permeation through the stratum corneum is relatively low.

Rather than characterizing drug transfer into and through the skin in terms of the diffusional resistances encountered, one could define permeation in terms of the *pathways* followed by the diffusing species. Drug permeation through the intact skin of humans involves either an intercellular or transcellular path in the stratum corneum, for the most part, rather than the so-called shunt pathways (transglandular or transfollicular routes).

The conventional wisdom is that, for the most part, lipophilic compounds transfer preferentially into the lipoidal intercellular phase of the stratum corneum, while relatively more hydrophilic compounds transfer into the intracellular domain of the stratum corneum. One should keep in mind that the often-postulated biphasic character of the horny layer—with hydrophilic cells in a lipophilic matrix—is overly simplistic: the hydrophilic cells themselves are enclosed within lipid bilayer membranes, while the lipophilic matrix comprises intercellular lipids which are, in fact, present in lamellar structures which "sandwich in" hydrophilic layers. As Boddé *et al*[1] have suggested, the intercellular pathway is *bicontinuous*, consisting of a nonpolar and a polar diffusion pathway between the corneocytes. The implications for dermatopharmacokinetic modeling are clear.

The stratum corneum can be regarded as a passive diffusion membrane but not an inert system; it often has an affinity for the applied substance. The adsorption isotherm is frequently linear in dilute concentration ranges. The correlation between external and surface concentrations is given in terms of the solvent membrane distribution coefficient K_m. The integrated form of Fick's Law is given as

$$J_s = \frac{K_m D C_s}{\delta}$$

and

$$K_p = \frac{K_m D}{\delta}$$

where K_p is the permeability coefficient, J_s is the steady state flux of solute, C_s is the concentration difference of solute across membrane, δ is the membrane thickness,

$$K_m \text{ is the } \frac{\text{solute sorbed per cc of tissue}}{\text{solute in solution per cc solvent}} = \frac{C_m}{C_s}, \text{ and}$$

D is the average membrane diffusion coefficient for solute.

Permeability experiments have shown that the hydrated stratum corneum has an affinity for both lipophilic and hydrophilic compounds. The bifunctional solubility arises from the *hydrophilic* corneocytes and the lipid-rich lamellar structures in the intercellular space. Thus, attempts to predict permeability constants from oil:water or solvent:water partition coefficients have had limited success.

The effect of regional variation on skin permeability can be marked. It has been suggested that one ought to differentiate between two species of horny layer: the palms and soles (up to 600 μm thick), adapted for weight-bearing and friction; and the body horny layer (~ 10 μm thick), adapted for flexibility, impermeability and sensory discrimination.

Overall, data suggest the following order for diffusion of simple molecules through the skin: plantar < palmar < arms, legs, trunk, dorsum of hand < scrotal and postauricular < axillary < scalp. Electrolytes in solution penetrate the skin poorly. Ionization of a weak electrolyte substantially reduces its permeability, eg, sodium salicylate permeates poorly compared with salicylic acid. The development of iontophoretic devices in recent years may minimize this problem with ionic penetrants. For any specific molecule, the predictability of regional variations in skin permeability continues to elude investigators. This will continue to be true as long as dermatopharmacokinetic models do not adequately reflect the anisotropicity of the skin's composition and structure, its interactions with the drug and the vehicle and the physiologic parameters that affect transfer.

In Vitro and In Vivo Studies

Classically, percutaneous absorption has been studied *in vivo* using radioactively labeled compounds or by *in vitro* techniques using excised human or animal skin. *In vivo* studies in recent years have made use of the skin-stripping method which permits the estimation of the concentration or amount of the penetrating species as a function of depth of the stratum corneum. Layers of the stratum corneum can be removed or stripped successively away by the repeated application and removal of cellulose adhesive tape strips. Skin penetration of *p*-aminobenzoic acid and the effect of additives were studied and evaluated by Lorenzetti through analysis of individual skin strips which provided a profile of skin penetration. Similar experiments have been carried out for a wide range of compounds. Rougier *et al*[2] have championed the use of the skin-stripping method, in conjunction with short-term exposure to the topically applied penetrant, as a predictor of skin permeation.

Clearly, the evaluation of new chemical entities [NCEs] of indeterminate toxicity mandates *in vitro* testing. A diffusion cell frequently used for *in vitro* experiments is shown in Fig 2.[3] In this system the intact skin or the epidermis is treated as a semipermeable membrane separating two fluid media. The transport rate of a particular drug is evaluated by introducing the drug in solution on the stratum corneum side of the "membrane," then measuring penetration by periodic sampling and analysis of the fluid across the skin membrane.

Investigators have recognized that transport across an immersed, fully hydrated stratum corneum may not represent the absorption system or rate observed in *in vivo* studies. Percutaneous absorption across a fully hydrated stratum corneum may be an exaggeration. It may be more representa-

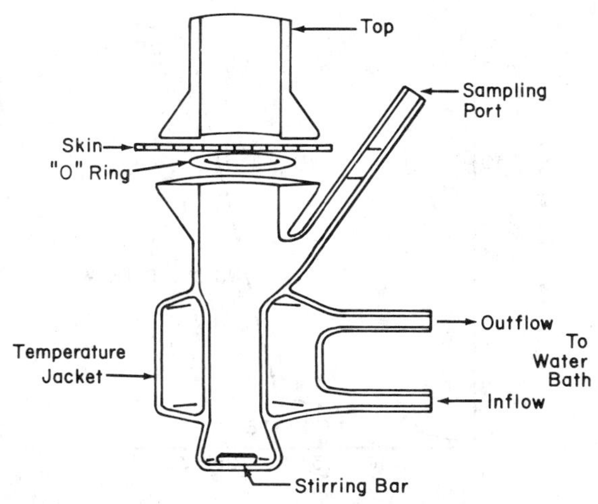

Fig 2. Schematic representation of diffusion cell. Top is open to ambient laboratory environment.[3]

tive of enhanced absorption that is seen after *in vivo* skin is hydrated by occlusive wrapping.

Using separated epidermal skin mounted in diffusion cells, Scheuplein and Ross[4] varied the atmosphere above the skin strip by use of Drierite to simulate dry conditions and wetted paper strips to simulate the effect of occlusion and observed marked reduction in penetration of cortisone under dry conditions but greatly enhanced penetration on humidifying the stratum corneum (see Fig 3).[4]

The studies of Scheuplein and Ross,[4] and of Franz,[3] demonstrate that *in vitro* studies of percutaneous absorption under controlled conditions are relevant to *in vivo* drug penetration. As stated by Franz, "whenever a question is asked requiring only a qualitative or directional answer, the *in vitro* technique appears perfectly adequate."

Relevance of Animal Studies

Any evaluation of a study of percutaneous absorption in animals must take cognizance of species variation. Just as percutaneous absorption in man will vary considerably with skin site, so will absorption in various animal species. Bartek *et al*[5] investigated percutaneous absorption and found a decreasing order of permeability, thus, rabbit > rat > swine > man. They studied the *in vivo* absorption of radioactively labeled haloprogin, *N*-acetylcysteine, testosterone, caffeine and butter yellow; their results with testosterone, shown in Fig 4,[6] illustrate the penetration differences observed with different animal skins.

Subsequently, using a similar *in vivo* technique, Wester and Maibach[7] investigated the percutaneous absorption of benzoic acid, hydrocortisone and testosterone in the rhesus monkey. Radioactively tagged compounds were applied to the ventral surface of the forearm, and absorption was quantified on the basis of radioactivity excreted in the urine for five days following application. The investigators concluded that the percutaneous penetration of these compounds in the rhesus monkey is similar to that in man, and regarded the data as encouraging because of the similarity.

The consensus is that rhesus monkeys and miniature pigs are good *in vivo* models for human percutaneous absorption, while smaller laboratory animals (eg, mouse, rat, rabbit) are not.

It should be stressed again that percutaneous absorption studies in animals, either *in vivo* or *in vitro*, only can be useful approximations of activity in man. The effect of species variation, site variability (about which little is known in animals), skin condition, experimental variables and, of major importance, the vehicle, must be kept in mind.

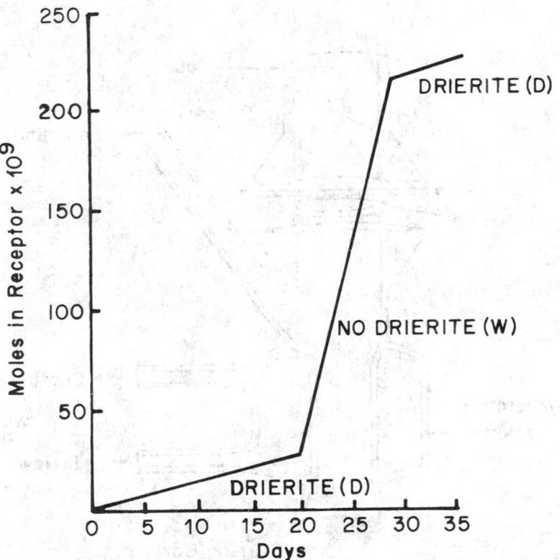

Fig 3. Change in cortisone penetration by alternately drying (D) and humidifying (W) the stratum corneum.[4]

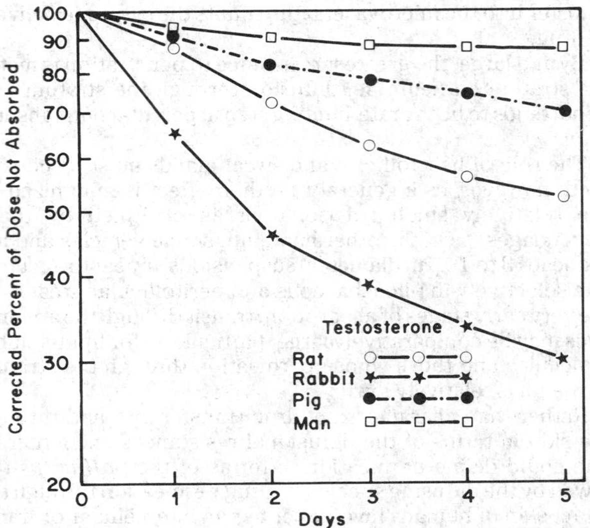

Fig 4. Percutaneous absorption of testosterone in rats, rabbits, swine and man for 5 days after application.[6]

As Bronaugh[8] notes, although human skin is preferable for *in vitro* permeation studies, its availability is limited. Additional constraints apply if one is only willing to use freshly obtained viable human skin from surgical specimens or biopsies as opposed to skin harvested from cadavers.

Concern has been voiced over the notorious variability in barrier properties of excised skin, whether animal or human. Factors responsible for the variability include the source and characteristics of the donor skin (eg, elapsed time from death to harvesting of the skin, age and gender of the donor, health of the skin prior to the donor's death, exposure of the skin to chemicals or mechanical treatment (eg, shaving or clipping prior to harvesting of the skin), etc. The recent development of a *living skin equivalent*—comprising a bilayered system of human dermal fibroblasts in a collagenous matrix upon which human corneocytes have formed a stratified epidermis—offers an alternative, less variable, model for evaluating human skin permeation and biotransformation.

Skin-flap methods represent *in vivo* and *in vitro* techniques for evaluating percutaneous absorption in animals or animal models: the general approach entails the surgical isolation of a skin section of an animal such that the blood supply is singular; this ensures that drug can be collected and assayed in the vascular perfusate as it undergoes absorption from the skin surface. The perfused skin flap can be maintained in the intact animal or mounted in an *in vitro* perfusion system, all the while maintaining its viability.

Animals also have been used to detect contact sensitization, measure antimitotic drug activity, measure phototoxicity and evaluate the comedogenic and comedolytic potential of substances. In each of these test procedures, be it a safety test or assay model, the animal is considered a substitute for man. It is, therefore, important to realize that the animal is not man, even though man is the ultimate test animal. Animal-testing presents the investigator with unique advantages; lack of appreciation of the variables involved can destroy these advantages.

Mershon and Callahan[9] recorded and illustrated the considerations involved in selecting an animal test model. They interpreted the rabbit irritancy data of several investigators, and impressively visualized different possible interpretations of the differing response between rabbit and man.

While the ultimate system for establishing therapeutic efficacy is man, there are specific animal test models that are recognized to be valuable as prehuman-use screens predictive of drug activity in humans. For example, the rat-ear assay and the granuloma-pouch procedure in rats are recognized procedures for the estimation of steroid anti-inflammatory activity.

Lorenzetti[10] tabulated the potency of various topical steroids, comparing the rat-ear-edema assay with potency measured in humans using the vasoconstrictor procedure of Stoughton and McKenzie; the results are given in Table 2.[11] Animal assay models of this kind, particularly the steroid anti-inflammatory assays, are most useful as preliminary activity screens. The simplicity, safety and reproducibility of the vasoconstrictor assay in humans recommend it over any corresponding animal procedure. However, a number of concerns have been raised over the years which need to be addressed, particularly if this bioassay is to be used to assess the bioequivalence of topical corticosteroid formulations. These concerns include the linearity of the vasoconstrictor response-drug concentration relationship and the visual assessment of the blanching or vasoconstrictor response.

As the *in vivo* vasoconstrictor response generally approaches a maximum, one must know whether the microcirculation of the skin has exceeded its capacity to respond linearly to the corticosteroid concentration attained in the skin. It may be that only relatively minimal responses will be elicited by relatively high concentrations. At the other end of the response-dose relationship, what is the minimum dose that will produce a reliable, replicable response? Rather than relying on the somewhat subjective visual evaluation of the response, investigators ought to make use of chromameters to provide objective, quantifiable data.

In Numero Models

In recent years, *in numero* modeling or computer simulation of percutaneous absorption has been advocated as a link between *in vitro* and *in vivo* studies. A number of relatively simplistic dermatopharmacokinetic models have been developed that do provide the formulator with some insight into transdermal drug delivery, in spite of the biological and physicochemical complexity of drug transport into and through the skin. By and large, these models are analogous to the classical pharmacokinetic models which have been employed to assess *in vivo* drug uptake and disposition. Some of the dermatopharmacokinetic models proposed differ from more classically oriented models in that drug transport in the vehicle and in the epidermis, particularly the stratum corneum, is modeled in accordance with Fickian diffusion. Thus, the formulator can anticipate the effect of variables such as the thickness of the applied (vehicle) phase, alterations in drug partitioning between the vehicle and the stratum corneum and the frequency of reapplication on the overall appearance of drug systemically as a function of time following topical application.

Dosage-Form Design

In many (if not most) clinical situations the rate-limiting step is penetration of the drug across the skin barrier, ie, percutaneous penetration through the skin alone. Diffusion of the drug from its vehicle, although dependent on the same diffusion parameters, should not be unknowingly the rate-limiting step in percutaneous absorption. Such a rate limitation or control may, of course, be an objective and the end point of specific drug optimization, but inappropriate formulation can reduce substantially the effectiveness of a topical drug substance.

In the formulation of a vehicle for topical drug application many factors must be considered. Drug stability, specific product use, site of application and product type must be combined in a dosage form which will readily release the drug when placed in contact with the skin. Further, the release characteristics of the vehicle are dependent on the physical-chemical properties of the specific drug substance to be delivered to the skin. A vehicle optimized for delivery of hydrocortisone may be quite inappropriate for delivery of a different steroid.

Higuchi (see *Bibliography*) discussed equations describing the rate of release of solid drugs suspended in ointment bases. Ostrenga *et al*, in a series of publications, discussed the significance of vehicle composition on the percutaneous absorption of fluocinolone acetonide and fluocinolone acetonide 21-acetate (fluocinonide) (see Fig 5).[12] These investigators used propylene glycol/isopropyl myristate partition coefficients, *in vitro* (human) skin penetration and finally *in vivo* vasoconstrictor studies to evaluate formulation variables. They concluded that

> "In general, an efficacious topical gel preparation is one in which (a) the concentration of diffusible drug in the vehicle for a given labeled strength is optimized by ensuring that all of the drug is in solution, (b) the minimum amount of solvent is used to dissolve the drug completely and yet maintain a favorable partition coefficient and (c) the vehicle components affect the permeability of the stratum corneum in a favorable manner."

The effect of propylene glycol concentration on *in vivo* vasoconstrictor activity is illustrated strikingly in Fig 5, taken from Ostrenga, Steinmetz and Poulsen[12]

Experimental work of the kind described by Ostrenga, Steinmetz and Poulson[12] provides a means of optimizing drug release from a vehicle and penetration of the drug into the skin. This is a beginning. The formulator must proceed to develop a total composition in which the drug is stable and causes no irritation to sensitive skin areas. Safety, stability and effective preservative efficacy must be combined with optimum drug delivery in the total formulation.

The work of Flynn, Weiner and others[13] on the physicochemical stability of topical drug delivery systems *postapplication* has facilitated the exploration of additional formula-

Table 2—Relative Potency of Anti-Inflammatory Agents[11]

Compound	Topical anti-inflammatory potency: Rat-ear edema assay	Topical anti-inflammatory potency: Human vasoconstrictor assay
Dexamethasone	73.2 (49.4–110)	10–20
Dexamethasone 21-acetate	117.3 (85.9–106)	10–20
Prednisolone	2.44 (1.54–7.76)	1–2
Prednisolone 21-acetate	5.43 (4.05–7.70)	3
Betamethasone	97.3 (16.7–141)	3–5
Betamethasone 21-acetate	1072.0 (876–1179)	18–33
Fluorometholone	138.3 (57.9–333)	30–40
Fluorometholone acetate	219.5 (9.15–536)	
Fluprednisolone	31.8 (13.3–76.1)	4–6
Fluprednisolone acetate	61.3 (25.6–147)	
Hydrocortisone	1	1

( ) = 95% confidence limits.

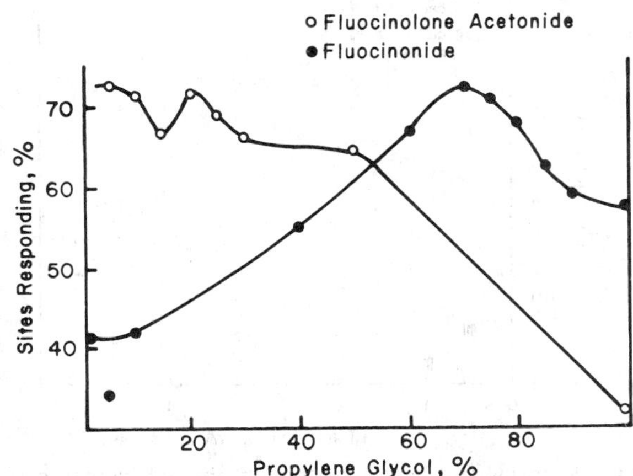

Fig 5. *In vivo* response as a function of vehicle composition (24-hour vasoconstriction).[12]

tion factors which are crucial to the success of topical formulations. Flynn notes that the functionality of topical drug delivery systems stands in stark contrast to those of transdermal drug delivery systems; while both delivery systems are open systems *kinetically* due to the formulation-skin interface, they differ to a considerable extent *thermodynamically* due to the fact that most topical formulations are left open to the air postapplication, while transdermal delivery systems are self-contained *closed* systems.

One study focused on a topical delivery system for minoxidil. The vehicle was 60:20:20 ethanol:propylene glycol:water system, with just enough propylene glycol to maintain 2% minoxidil in solution, following the evaporation of the more volatile ethanol and water. Minoxidil fluxes across human cadaver skin, measured as a function of minoxidil concentration, increased as the initial concentration of drug increased, but only to about 3% (Fig 6[13]). At initial minoxidil concentrations greater than 3%, transport was disproportionately low, relative to initial concentration, due to early precipitation of the drug.

Evaporation and loss of volatile formulation components such as water or ethanol postapplication can be expected to affect topical drug delivery system composition and performance. Flynn *et al*[13] have shown that so-called non-volatile excipients, eg, propylene glycol, evaporate after topical application. Skin permeation by excipients also may occur after application leading to further compositional changes in the applied film on the skin surface. The impact of this evaporative and absorptive loss of adjuvants increases as the volume of the applied formulation is reduced. As Flynn[13] notes, ". . . the momentary compositions, and thus delivery capabilities, of real vehicles are significantly influenced by the amounts applied."

Factors Affecting Drug Absorption

In the foregoing it has been seen that drug-release from its vehicle is a function of concentration, solubility in the vehicle and partition coefficient between the vehicle and the receptor site. Percutaneous absorption of a drug also can be enhanced by the use of occlusive techniques or by the use of so-called penetration enhancers.

Skin Hydration and Temperature—Occluding the skin with wraps or impermeable plastic film such as Saran Wrap prevents the loss of surface water from the skin. Since water is absorbed readily by the protein components of the skin the occlusive wrap causes greatly increased levels of hydration in the stratum corneum. The concomitant swelling of the horny layer ostensibly decreases protein network density and the diffusional path length. Occlusion of the skin surface also increases skin temperature (~2 to 3°) resulting in increased molecular motion and skin permeation.

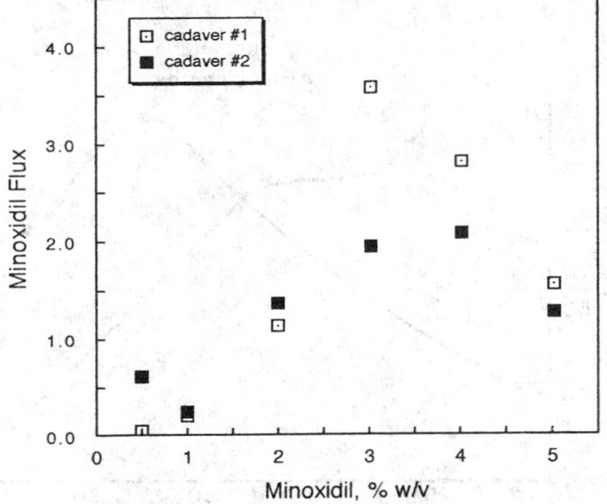

Fig 6. Minoxidil flux (× 10^4 mg/cm^2/h) through human cadaver skin as a function of minoxidil concentration in the topically applied formulation.[13]

Hydrocarbon bases which occlude the skin to a degree will bring about an increase in drug penetration. However, this effect is trivial compared with the effects seen with a true occlusive skin wrap. Occlusive techniques are useful in some clinical situations requiring anti-inflammatory activity and occlusive wrappings are used most commonly with steroids. Since steroid activity can be enhanced so enormously by skin occlusion it is possible to depress adrenal function unknowingly. Early in the 1960s McKenzie demonstrated that penetration of steroid could be increased 100-fold by use of occlusion.

Transdermal delivery systems, with their occlusive backing, can effect increased percutaneous absorption as a result of increased skin temperature and hydration.

In experiments with healthy volunteers wearing transdermal nitroglycerin delivery systems, investigators[14] showed that exposure of the surrounding skin area to localized heating or cooling could cause extensive changes in nitroglycerin bioavailability, presumably due to changes in regional cutaneous blood flow and subsequent systemic uptake (*see below*).

One consequence of occlusion of the skin surface, whether by a transdermal delivery system or a hydrocarbon film, is that an aqueous film may form at the formulation-skin interface. This aqueous film or interphase could result in decreased transfer efficiency, and, in the case of a transdermal delivery system, a loss of adhesion. Accordingly, the suppression of perspiration could enhance vehicle-skin partitioning efficiency and drug permeation.

Penetration Enhancers—This term has been used to describe substances that facilitate absorption through the skin. While most materials have a direct effect on the permeability of the skin, other so-called enhancers (eg polyols, such as glycerin and propylene glycol) appear to augment percutaneous absorption by increasing the thermodynamic activity of the penetrant, thereby increasing the effective escaping tendency and concentration gradient of the diffusing species. Penetration enhancers with a direct effect on skin permeability include solvents, surfactants and miscellaneous chemicals such as urea and *N,N*-diethyl-*m*-toluamide (Table 3).[15,16] The mechanism of action of these enhancers is complex since these substances also may increase penetrant solubility. Nonetheless, the predominant effect of these enhancers on the stratum corneum is either to increase its degree of hydration or disrupt its lipoprotein matrix. In either case, the net result is a decrease in resistance to penetrant diffusion. (The formulator should note that the inclusion of a penetration enhancer in a topical formulation mandates additional testing and evaluation to ensure the absence of enhancer-related adverse effects.)

Foremost among the solvents which affect skin permeability is water. As noted above, water is a factor even for *anhydrous* transdermal delivery systems due to their occlusive nature. Due to its safety and efficacy, water has been described as the ultimate penetration enhancer. Other solvents include the classic enhancer, dimethyl sulfoxide (DMSO), which is of limited utility because of its potential ocular and dermal toxicity, its objectionable taste and odor (a consequence of its absorption and subsequent biotransformation) and the need for concentrations in excess of 70% to promote absorption. Analogs of DMSO such as decylmethyl sulfoxide are used currently in some topical formulations. In contrast with other solvents, laurocapram (1-dodecylazacycloheptan-2-one; Azone) has been shown to function effectively at low concentrations (≤5%). Furthermore, Azone's effect on skin permeability persists long after a single application due apparently to its prolonged retention within the stratum corneum.

Surfactants, long recognized for their ability to alter membrane structure and function, can have a substantial effect on skin permeability.[17] However, given the irritation potential of surfactants applied chronically, their utility as penetration enhancers is limited. Their effect on permeability may be complicated further by surfactant-monomer aggregation to

Table 3—Penetration Enhancers[a]

Solvents	
	Water
	Alcohols
	Methanol
	Ethanol
	2-propanol
	Alkyl methyl sulfoxides
	Dimethyl sulfoxide
	Decylmethyl sulfoxide
	Tetradecylmethyl sulfoxide
	Pyrrolidones
	2-Pyrrolidone
	N-Methyl-2-pyrrolidone
	N-(2-Hydroxyethyl)pyrrolidone
	Laurocapram
	Miscellaneous solvents
	Acetone
	Dimethyl acetamide
	Dimethyl formamide
	Tetrahydrofurfuryl alcohol
Amphiphiles	
	L-α-Amino acids
	Anionic surfactants
	Cationic surfactants
	Amphoteric surfactants
	Nonionic surfactants
	Fatty acids and alcohols
Miscellaneous	
	Clofibric acid amides
	Hexamethylene lauramide
	Proteolytic enzymes
	Terpenes and sesquiterpenes
	α-Bisabolol
	d-Limonene
	Urea
	N,N-Diethyl-*m*-toluamide

[a]Adapted from Refs 15 and 16.

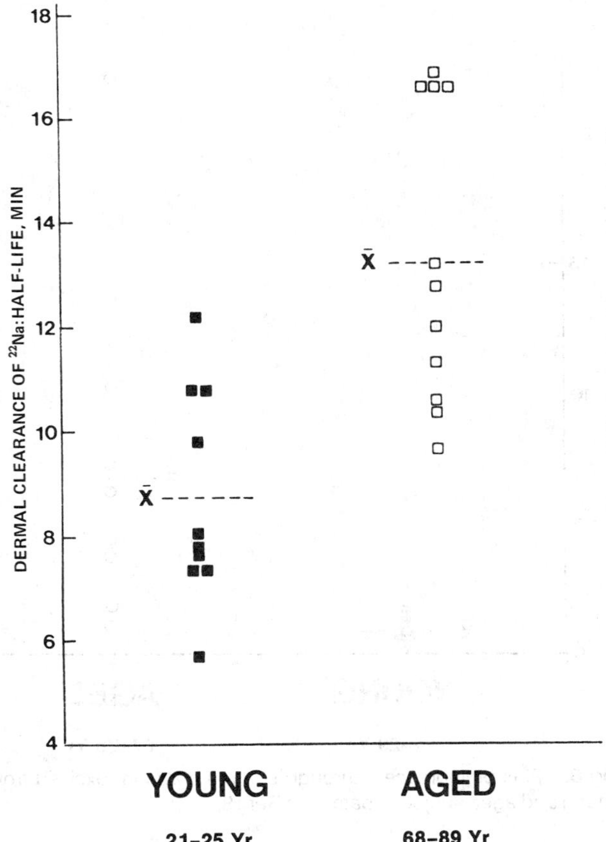

Fig 7. Dermal clearance of ^{22}Na in young and aged subjects after intradermal injection (data from Ref 18).

form micelles and the concomitant solubilization of the permeant. As the impact of surfactants on skin permeability of a penetrant is problematic, the effect of their inclusion in a formulation should be evaluated using appropriate *in vitro* and *in vivo* studies.

Stratum Corneum Barrier Efficacy and Dermal Clearance—Even though *in vitro* studies of percutaneous transport may reflect the resistance of the skin to drug diffusion, there is no way such studies can characterize adequately the transfer of diffusing drug into the microvasculature of the dermis and its subsequent transfer into general circulation.

Christophers and Kligman[18] evaluated the dermal "clearance" of ^{22}Na from the midback skin of volunteers following the intradermal injection of ^{22}Na as normal saline solution. The dermal "clearances," expressed in terms of the half-life for disappearance of radioactivity, are plotted in Fig 7.[18] Similar results were obtained with disappearance of skin fluorescence after intradermal injection of sodium fluorescein. The data are indicative of markedly delayed dermal clearance in the aged. This may reflect, in part, a decrease in older subjects in dermal capillary loop density, a decrease in the rate and/or extent of dermal blood perfusion or an increase in resistance to transfer into the capillaries.

The importance of blood-flow-limited percutaneous absorption was shown by Benowitz *et al*,[19] who documented the effect of the intravenous administration of nicotine, a known cutaneous vasoconstrictor, on the systemic absorption of nicotine administered concurrently in the form of a transdermal delivery system. Plasma nicotine concentrations rose less rapidly and reached a lower peak at a later time than when nicotine was applied transdermally in the absence of the intravenous nicotine infusion. This raises concerns about the potential cutaneous interactions between vasoconstrictors *or* vasodilators *and* topically applied drugs intended for a systemic effect: bioavailability could be increased or diminished as a result! The assessment of the potency of corticosteroids by corticosteroid-induced skin blanching, ie, vasoconstriction, lends credence to this issue.

On the other hand, Christophers and Kligman[18] demonstrated increased *in vitro* skin permeation by sodium fluorescein in the stratum corneum excised from young and old subjects (Fig 8[18]). Thus, the stratum corneum of older subjects may offer less resistance to the penetration of topically applied drugs.

Given the substantial intersubject variations that occur in diffusional resistance and in dermal clearance, it is not surprising that *in vivo* studies of percutaneous absorption often demonstrate marked differences in systemic availability of drugs. Furthermore, the tendency to employ normal, healthy, *young* adults in such studies may not provide data that is indicative of drug permeation through the skin of older subjects or patients.

Roskos, Maibach and Guy[20] made quantitative measurements of the percutaneous absorption of a number of drugs *in vivo* from the urinary excretion profiles of ^{14}C-radiolabeled drugs in young (18 to 40 years) and old (>65 years) subjects: while permeation of hydrocortisone, benzoic acid, aspirin and caffeine was significantly lower in older subjects, testosterone and estradiol absorption was comparable in the two groups. Additional comprehensive studies of percutaneous absorption *as a function of age* continue to be warranted.

Cutaneous Biotransformation—Catabolic enzyme activity in the viable epidermis is substantial. In fact, the viable epidermis is metabolically more active than the dermis. If the topically applied drug is subject to biotransformation during skin permeation, local and systemic bioavailability can be affected markedly. Enzymatic activity in the skin, or for that matter in systemic fluids and tissues, can be taken advantage of to facilitate percutaneous absorption. Sloan and

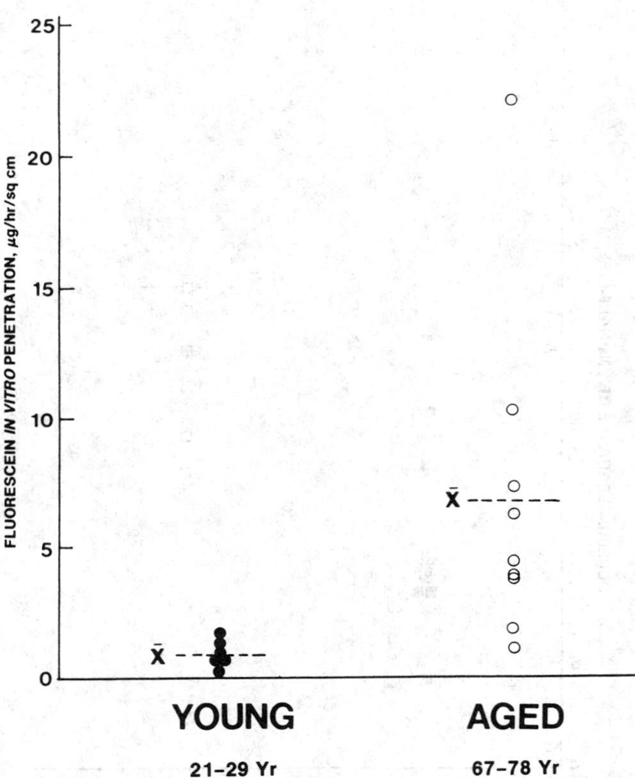

Fig 8. Flux of fluorescein through stratum corneum excised from young and aged subjects (data from Ref 18).

Bodor,[21] for example, synthesized 7-acyloxymethyl derivatives of theophylline which diffuse through the skin far more efficiently than theophylline itself (Fig. 9[21]) but which are biotransformed rapidly to theophylline. Thus, theophylline delivery to systemic circulation can be enhanced substantially.

Further Considerations for Transdermal Drug Delivery

In order for a drug to qualify as a candidate for systemic delivery after topical application, it must satisfy requirements

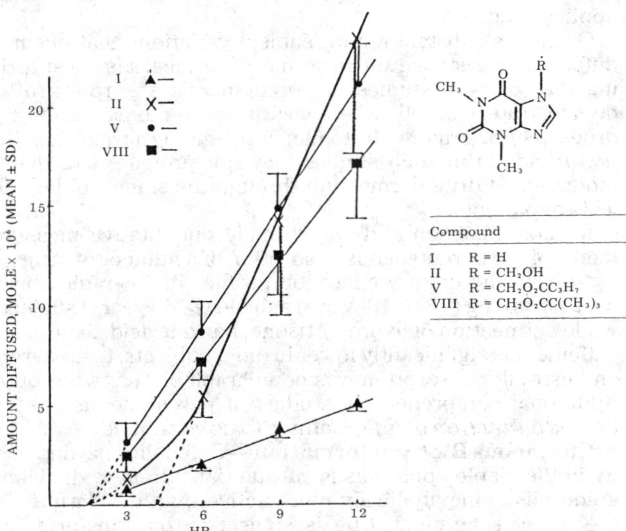

Fig 9. Diffusion of theophylline (I) and its derivatives through hairless mouse skin.[21]

in addition to exhibiting good skin permeation. Successful candidates for transdermal drug delivery should be nonirritating and nonsensitizing to the skin. Since relatively little drug may reach systemic circulation over a relatively long time, drug candidates should be relatively potent drugs. In addition, the limitation to relatively potent drugs can ease problems of formulation since the amount of drug that can be incorporated in the formulation may be limited by physicochemical considerations such as solubility.

Iontophoretic Drug Delivery through the Skin[22,23]—For some poorly absorbed (ionic) compounds, parenteral administration appears to be the only viable option for regional or systemic delivery as chemical penetration enhancers (see Table 3) often do not function well for these compounds. Given the increased risk of adverse reactions associated with the use of such enhancers, the increased evaluation of iontophoretic devices for the enhancement of topical drug delivery has been of great interest. Iontophoretic drug delivery implies the delivery of ionic drugs into the body by means of an electric current. While the stratum corneum forms the principal barrier to electrical conductivity—due, in part, to its lower water content—the skin also acts as a capacitor. Thus, biological tissues such as the skin provide for a reactive electrical circuit. Ionic transport through the skin in the presence of a uniform electric field can be described, in part, in accordance with the Nernst-Planck equation

$$J_i = -D\frac{dC}{dx} + \frac{DzeEC}{kT}$$

where J_i is the flux of ions across the membrane, C is the concentration of ions with valence, z, and electron charge, e, dC/dx is the concentration gradient, E is the electric field, k is Boltzmann's constant and T is the absolute temperature. Thus, the ionic flux is the sum of the fluxes that arise from the concentration gradient and the electric field. Given the complexity of the skin's composition, the thickness of the stratum corneum and the occurrence of electroosmotic effects, the Nernst-Planck equation is only a first approximation of the overall transdermal flux of a solute. Faraday's Law

$$\frac{Q}{t} = \frac{t_j i}{|z|F}$$

further characterizes the iontophoretic flux Q/t in terms of the current i (in amperes) and its duration t (in seconds), the transference number parameter t_j and the Faraday constant F. Additional factors that influence the rate and extent of iontophoretic delivery through the skin include pH and ionic strength of the drug solution.

Although iontophoretic techniques have been shown to increase percutaneous absorption of ionizable or ionic drugs (including lidocaine, salicylates and peptides and proteins such as insulin) markedly, the clinical safety and efficacy of drug delivery systems employing iontophoretic technology have yet to be evaluated fully.

Phonophoretic Drug Delivery—Phonophoresis or sonophoresis is defined as the movement of drug molecules through the skin under the influence of ultrasound. In general, ultrasound frequencies between 20 KHz and 10 MHz at intensities ≤ 3 W/cm^2 have been used with varying degrees of effectiveness,[24] although low-intensity *high*-frequency (10 or 16 MHz) ultrasound has been observed to increase transdermal drug flux and decrease percutaneous diffusional lag times.[25] The precise mechanisms by which ultrasound effects an enhancement of percutaneous absorption remain unclear at this time, although thermal, mechanical and chemical changes all have been suggested.

Ointments

Ointments are semisolid preparations intended for external application to the skin or mucous membranes; usually, but not always, they contain medicinal substances. The types of ointment bases used as vehicles for drugs are selected or designed for optimum delivery of the drugs and also to contribute emolliency or other quasi-medicinal qualities. Ointment properties vary, since they are designed for specific uses, ease of application or extent of application.

The official definition of ointment in its present form was introduced in the USP XV in 1955. The definition is broad and encompasses petrolatum, ie, oleaginous bases, emulsion bases—either water-in-oil (W/O) or oil-in-water (O/W)—and the so-called water-soluble bases.

In unofficial terms, oleaginous bases are described as ointments, but emulsion bases may be termed creams or lotions. Either of these containing large amounts of solids is termed a paste. All of these subclasses are defined officially as ointments.

Pharmaceutical authors have a penchant for defining "ideal" preparations eg, the ideal base, the ideal vehicle and so on. In practice, of course, there is no such thing. An individual cannot be all things to all people; neither can an ointment base be ideal for all drugs, all situations or all skins, for that matter. An ointment base functioning as a drug vehicle should be optimized for a specific drug and, insofar as possible, for specific disease states or skin conditions.

It is, of course, possible to define certain specific requirements for an ointment base to be used for extemporaneous compounding. Such a base should be nonirritating, easily removable, nonstaining, stable, non-pH-dependent and widely compatible with a variety of medicaments. When one adds the stipulation that the base must release the same variety of medicaments, the implausibility of such definitions becomes evident.

Classification and Properties of Ointment Bases

The USP recognizes four general classes of ointment bases, hereunder categorized into five classes for the purpose of indicating more definitively some differences in the principal properties of the bases.

Hydrocarbon Bases (Oleaginous)
Example: White Petrolatum, White Ointment

1. Emollient
2. Occlusive
3. Nonwater-washable
4. Hydrophobic
5. Greasy

Absorption Bases (Anhydrous)
Examples: Hydrophilic Petrolatum; Anhydrous Lanolin

1. Emollient
2. Occlusive
3. Absorb water
4. Anhydrous
5. Greasy

Absorption Bases (W/O Type)
Examples: Lanolin, Cold Cream

1. Emollient
2. Occlusive
3. Contain water
4. Some absorb additional water
5. Greasy

Water-Removable Bases (O/W Type)
Example: Hydrophilic Ointment

1. Water-washable
2. Nongreasy
3. Can be diluted with water
4. Nonocclusive

Water-Soluble Bases
Example: Polyethylene Glycol Ointment

1. Usually anhydrous
2. Water-soluble and washable
3. Nongreasy
4. Nonocclusive
5. Lipid-free

The selection of the optimum vehicle from the classification above may require compromises so often encountered in drug formulation. For example, stability or drug activity might be superior in a hydrocarbon base, however, acceptability is diminished because of the greasy nature of the base. The water-solubility of the polyethylene glycol bases may be attractive, but the glycol(s) may be irritating to traumatized tissue. Drug activity and percutaneous absorption may be superior when using a hydrocarbon base; however, it may be prudent to minimize percutaneous absorption by the use of a less occlusive base.

Ointment Bases

Hydrocarbon Bases

Hydrocarbon bases are usually petrolatum *per se* or petrolatum modified by waxes or liquid petrolatum to change viscosity characteristics. Liquid petrolatum gelled by the addition of a polyethylene resin also is considered a hydrocarbon ointment base, albeit one with unusual viscosity characteristics.

Hydrocarbon ointment bases are classified as oleaginous bases along with bases prepared from vegetable fixed oils or animal fats. Bases of this type include lard, benzoinated lard, olive oil, cottonseed oil and other oils. Such bases are emollient but generally require addition of antioxidants and other preservatives. They are now largely of historic interest.

Petrolatum USP is a tasteless, odorless, unctuous material with a melting range of 38 to 60°; its color ranges from amber to white (when decolorized). Petrolatum often is used externally, without modification or added medication, for its emollient qualities.

Petrolatum used as an ointment base has a high degree of compatibility with a variety of medicaments. Bases of this type are occlusive and nearly anhydrous and thus provide optimum stability for medicaments such as antibiotics. The wide melting range permits some latitude in vehicle selection and the USP permits addition of waxy materials as an aid in minimizing temperature effects.

Hydrocarbon bases, being occlusive, increase skin hydration by reducing the rate of loss of surface water. Bases of this kind may be used solely for such a skin-moisturizing effect, eg, white petroleum jelly as noted above. Skin hydration on the other hand may increase drug activity. Studies have indicated that steroids have increased activity, as measured by vasoconstrictor effects, when applied to the skin in a hydrocarbon vehicle. Stoughton consistently found the same steroid more active when applied in a petrolatum vehicle than when applied in a cream (ie, O/W emulsion) vehicle.

A gelled mineral oil vehicle represents a unique addition to this class of bases comprised of refined natural products. Liquid petrolatum may be gelled by addition of a polyethylene. When approximately 5% of low-density polyethylene is added, the mixture heated and then shock-cooled, a soft unctuous, colorless material resembling white petrolatum is produced. The mass maintains unchanged consistency over a wide temperature range. It neither hardens at low temperatures nor melts at reasonably high temperatures. Its useful working range is between −15° and 60°. Excessive heat, ie, above 90°, will destroy the gel structure.

On the basis of *in vitro* studies, drugs may be released faster from the gelled mineral oil vehicle than from conventional petrolatum. This quicker release has been attributed to easier migration of drug particulates through a vehicle which is essentially a liquid, compared with petrolatum.

Despite the advantages hydrocarbon or oleaginous vehicles provide in terms of stability and emolliency such bases have the considerable disadvantage of greasiness. The greasy or oily material may stain clothing and is difficult to remove. In terms of patient acceptance, hydrocarbon bases, ie, ointments, rank well below emulsion bases such as creams and lotions.

Absorption Bases

Absorption bases are hydrophilic, anhydrous materials or hydrous bases that have the ability to absorb additional water. The former are anhydrous bases which absorb water to become W/O emulsions; the latter are W/O emulsions which have the ability to absorb additional water. The word absorption in this connotation refers only to the ability of the base to absorb water. Both types of base are exemplified by Anhydrous Lanolin and Lanolin. The former is converted to the latter by the addition of 30% water. The latter in turn will absorb additional amounts of water.

Hydrophilic Petrolatum USP is an anhydrous absorption base. The W/O emulsifying property is conferred by the inclusion of cholesterol. This composition is a modification of the original formulation which contained anhydrous lanolin. The lanolin was deleted because of reports of allergy; cholesterol was added. Inclusion of stearyl alcohol and wax add to the physical characteristics, particularly firmness and heat stability.

Hydrophilic Petrolatum USP

Cholesterol	30 g
Stearyl Alcohol	30 g
White Wax	80 g
White Petrolatum	860 g
To make	1000 g

Melt the stearyl alcohol and white wax together on a steam bath, then add the cholesterol and stir until it completely dissolves. Add the white petrolatum and mix. Remove from the bath, and stir until the mixture congeals.

Lanolin is a complex mixture of substances. Its ability to absorb water is probably a characteristic of the material rather than a single component. The chemistry of lanolin has been studied in detail. Such studies have resulted in the introduction of a large variety of lanolin derivatives and separated fractions. Available now are lanolin alcohols, dewaxed lanolins, acetylated lanolins, ethoxylated lanolins, hydrogenated lanolins, lanolin esters and other products. Most of these derivatives have been produced for specific purposes, such as improved emulsification characteristics or to reduce allergic reactivity.

The specific compounds responsible for lanolin allergy remain unknown; however, the greater portion of lanolin allergens reside in the wool wax alcohols fraction. Thus, fractional separation to obtain, for example, the so-called liquid lanolins substantially reduces the incidence of allergic reactions. Given the plethora of lanolin fractions, derivatives, modifications and levels of purity, it is quite possible, even likely, that lanolin-sensitive individuals can tolerate specific lanolin products.

Absorption bases, particularly the emulsion bases, impart excellent emolliency and a degree of occlusiveness on application. The anhydrous types can be used when the presence of water would cause stability problems with specific drug substances, eg, antibiotics. Absorption bases also are greasy when applied and are difficult to remove. Both of these properties are, however, less obvious than with hydrocarbon bases.

Commercially available absorption bases include Aquaphor (*Beiersdorf*) and Polysorb (*Fougera*). Nivea Cream (*Beiersdorf*) is a hydrated emollient base. Absorption bases, either hydrous or anhydrous, are seldom used as vehicles for commercial drug products. The W/O emulsion system is more difficult to deal with than the more conventional O/W systems and there is, of course, reduced patient acceptance because of greasiness.

Water-Removable Bases

Water-washable bases or emulsion bases, commonly referred to as creams, represent the most commonly used type of ointment base. By far the majority of commercial dermatologic drug products are formulated in an emulsion or cream base. Emulsion bases are washable and removed easily from skin or clothing. Emulsion bases can be diluted with water, although such additions are uncommon.

As a result of advances in synthetic cosmetic chemistry the formulator of an emulsion base can be faced with a bewildering variety of selections. Fortunately, the emulsion base can be subdivided into three component parts, designated as the oil phase, the emulsifier and the aqueous phase. The medicinal agent may be included in one of these phases or added to the formed emulsion.

The oil phase, sometimes called the internal phase, is typically made up of petrolatum and/or liquid petrolatum together with one or more of the higher-molecular-weight alcohols, such as cetyl or stearyl alcohol. Stearic acid may be included if the emulsion is to be based on a soap formed *in situ*, eg, triethanolamine stearate. A calculated excess of stearic acid in such a formulation will produce a pearlescent appearance in the finished product.

For drug-delivery vehicles, simplified systems are in order to minimize component interactions, either physical or chemical, and, of course, to minimize cost. Hydrophilic Ointment USP is a typical emulsion base. The composition is as follows:

Hydrophilic Ointment USP

Methylparaben	0.25 g
Propylparaben	0.15 g
Sodium Lauryl Sulfate	10 g
Propylene Glycol	120 g
Stearyl Alcohol	250 g
White Petrolatum	250 g
Purified Water	370 g
To make about	1000 g

Melt the stearyl alcohol and the white petrolatum on a steam bath, and warm to about 75°. Add the other ingredients, previously dissolved in the water and warmed to 75°, and stir the mixture until it congeals.

Stearyl alcohol and petrolatum comprise an oil phase with the proper smoothness and comfort for the skin. Stearyl alcohol also serves as an adjuvant emulsifier. Petrolatum in the oil phase also contributes to the water-holding ability of the overall formulation.

A glance at the cosmetic literature and such volumes as the Cosmetic, Toiletry and Fragrance Association's *International Cosmetic Ingredient Dictionary* impresses one with the enormous number and variety of emulsion-base components, particularly oil-phase components. Many of these substances impart subtle but distinct characteristics to cosmetic emulsion systems. While desirable, many of these characteristics are not really necessary in drug dosage forms and delivery systems.

The aqueous phase of an emulsion base usually, but not always, exceeds the oil phase in volume. The aqueous phase contains the preservative materials, the emulsifier or a part of the emulsifier system and humectant. The last is usually glycerin, propylene glycol or a polyethylene glycol. The humectant normally is included to minimize water loss in the finished composition. Humectants also add to overall physical product acceptability.

The aqueous phase contains the preservative(s) which are included to control microbial growth. Preservatives in emulsion bases usually include one or more of the following: methylparaben and propylparaben, benzyl alcohol, sorbic acid or quaternary ammonium compounds. Propylene glycol insufficient concentration also can function as a preservative. The general subject of preservatives and preservation is discussed elsewhere in this chapter.

The aqueous phase also contains the water-soluble components of the emulsion system, together with any additional stabilizers, antioxidants, buffers, etc that may be necessary for stability, pH control or other considerations associated with aqueous systems.

The emulsifier or emulsifier system in a cream formulation is a major consideration. The emulsifier may be nonionic, anionic, cationic or amphoteric.

Anionic Emulsifiers—Sodium lauryl sulfate, the emulsifier in Hydrophilic Ointment USP, is typical of this class. The active portion of the emulsifier is the anion (lauryl sulfate ion). Similar anionic emulsifiers include soaps such as triethanolamine stearate. Soaps, of course, are alkaline and, hence, incompatible with acids.

Sodium lauryl sulfate and other anionic surfactants of its type are more acid-stable and permit adjustment of the emulsion pH to the desirable acid range of 4.5 to 6.5. As anionic emulsifiers are incompatible with cations, the overall product composition must be kept in mind.

Depending on the chemical type and concentration, anionic surfactants may be irritating in certain situations. It has been reported that percutaneous absorption of certain drugs, notably steroids, may be enhanced by the use of anionic compounds such as sodium lauryl sulfate.

Cationic Emulsifiers—Cationic compounds are highly surface-active but are used infrequently as emulsifiers. The cation portion of the molecule is generally a quaternary ammonium salt including (usually) a fatty acid derivative, eg, dilauryldimethylammonium chloride. Cationics may be irritating to the skin and eyes, and they have a considerable range of incompatibilities, including anionic materials.

Nonionic Emulsifiers—Nonionic emulsifiers show no tendency to ionize in solution. This advantage results in excellent pH and electrolyte compatibility in such emulsions. Nonionic emulsifiers range from lipophilic to hydrophilic. The usual emulsifier system may include both a lipophilic and hydrophilic member to produce a so-called hydrophilic-lipophilic balance (or HLB).

Many nonionic surfactants are the result of condensation of ethylene oxide groups with a long chain hydrophobic compound. The hydrophilic characteristics of the condensation product are controlled by the number of (usually) oxyethylene groups ($—OCH_2CH_2—$). Examples of nonionic surfactants are given in Table 4.[25]

Emulsions containing nonionic emulsifiers usually are prepared by dissolving or dispersing the lipophilic component in the oil phase and the hydrophilic component in the aqueous phase. The two phases then are heated separately and combined as described on page 1509. The nonionic emulsifier content of an emulsion may total as much as 10% of the total weight or volume. Emulsions based on nonionic emulsifiers are generally low in irritation potential, stable and have excellent compatibility characteristics.

Soaps and detergents, ie, emulsifiers, have, overall, a damaging effect on the skin. Both anionic and cationic surfactants can cause damage to the stratum corneum in direct proportion to concentration and duration of contact. Nonionic surfactants appear to have much less effect on the stratum corneum.

After the proper selection of ingredients the emulsion base is formed by heat and agitation. The oil phase is melted and heated to 75° in a container equipped with a variable-speed agitator. The aqueous phase with the emulsifier added is placed in a second container, components are dissolved and the whole heated to 75° or slightly in excess. The aqueous phase then is added slowly with continuous stirring to the oil phase. The first addition should be carried out slowly but continuously with thorough but careful agitation, ie, the emulsion should not be agitated at a rate that incorporates excess air. Progressively slower stirring should be continued during addition of the aqueous phase and until the temperature reaches about 30°. Medicinal agents usually are added after the emulsion has formed and much of the aqueous phase has been added. Drug substances frequently are added as dispersed concentrates in aqueous suspension. Colors and dyes often are added in the same manner as concentrates. Colors sometimes are employed to distinguish different concentrations of the same drug product. Fragrances, if any, are added after the formed emulsion has cooled to about 35°.

Water-Soluble Bases

Soluble ointment bases, as the name implies, are made up of soluble components, or may include gelled aqueous solutions. The latter often are referred to as gels, and in recent years have been formulated specifically to maximize drug availability.

Major components, and in some instances the only components, of water-soluble bases are the polyethylene glycols. These are liquids or waxy solids identified by numbers which are an approximate indication of molecular weight. Polyethylene glycol 400 is a liquid superficially similar to propylene glycol, while polyethylene glycol 4000 is a waxy solid.

Polyethylene glycols have the general chemical formula

$$HOCH_2(CH_2OCH_2)_nCH_2OH$$

They are nonvolatile, water-soluble or water-miscible compounds and chemically inert, varying in molecular weight from several hundred to several thousand. Patch tests have shown that these compounds are innocuous and continuous use has confirmed their lack of irritation.

Polyethylene glycols of interest as vehicles include the 1500, 1600, 4000 and 6000 products, ranging from soft, waxy solids (polyethylene glycol 1500 is similar to petrolatum) to hard waxes. Polyethylene glycol 6000 is a hard wax-like material melting at 58 to 62°; it is nonhygroscopic.

Polyethylene glycols, particularly 1500, can be used as a vehicle *per se;* however, better results often are obtained by using blends of high- and low-molecular-weight glycols, as in Polyethylene Glycol Ointment NF.

Polyethylene Glycol Ointment NF

Polyethylene Glycol 3350	400 g
Polyethylene Glycol 400	600 g

Heat the two ingredients on a water bath to 65°. Allow to cool and stir until congealed. If a firmer preparation is desired, replace up to 100 g of the polyethylene glycol 400 with an equal amount of polyethylene glycol 3350.

Table 4—Nonionic Emulsifiers[25]

Type	Examples
Polyoxyethylene fatty alcohol ethers	Polyoxyethylene lauryl alcohol
Polyoxypropylene fatty alcohol ethers	Propoxylated oleyl alcohol
Polyoxyethylene fatty acid esters	Polyoxyethylene stearate
Polyoxyethylene sorbitan fatty acid esters	Polyoxyethylene sorbitan monostearate
Sorbitan fatty acid esters	Sorbitan monostearate
Polyoxyethylene glycol fatty acid esters	Polyoxyethylene glycol monostearate
Polyol fatty acid esters	Glyceryl monostearate Propylene glycol monostearate
Ethoxylated lanolin derivatives	Ethyoxylated lanolins Ethoxylated cholesterol

Note—If 6 to 25% of an aqueous solution is to be incorporated in polyethylene glycol ointment, replace 50 g of the polyethylene glycol 3350 with an equal amount of stearyl alcohol.

The water-solubility of polyethylene glycol vehicles does not insure availability of drugs contained in the vehicle. As hydrated stratum corneum is an important factor in drug penetration, the use of polyethylene glycol vehicles which are anhydrous and nonocclusive actually may hinder percutaneous absorption due to dehydration of the stratum corneum.

Aqueous gel vehicles containing water, propylene and/or polyethylene glycol, and gelled with a carbomer or a cellulose derivative, also are classed as water-soluble bases. Bases of this kind, sometimes referred to as gels, may be formulated to optimize delivery of a drug, particularly steroids. In such a preparation propylene glycol is used as a steroid solvent as well as an antimicrobial or preservative.

Gelling agents used in these preparations may be nonionic or anionic. Nonionics include cellulose derivatives, such as methylcellulose or hydroxypropyl methylcellulose. These derivatives form gels when dissolved in water but also exhibit the characteristic of reverse solubility. The celluloses are wetted, ie, dispersed in hot water, and then cooled to effect solution. Sodium carboxymethylcellulose is an ionic form of cellulose gelling agent. It is conventionally soluble, and not heat-insoluble.

Carbomers are the USP designation for various polymeric acids which are dispersible but insoluble in water. When the acid dispersion is neutralized with a base a clear, stable gel is formed. Carbomer 934P is physiologically inert and is not a primary irritant or sensitizer. Other carbomers for which monographs appear in the USP include carbomers 910, 940, 941 and 1342.

Another gelling agent is colloidal magnesium aluminum silicate (*Veegum*). It is an inorganic emulsifier and suspending agent, as well as a gelling agent. Veegum dispersions are compatible with alcohols (20 to 30%), acetone and glycols. It frequently is employed as a gel stabilizer, rather than as the sole gelling agent.

Sodium alginate and the propylene glycol ester of alginic acid (*Kelcoloid*) also are satisfactory gelling agents. Sodium alginate is a hydrophilic colloid that functions satisfactorily between pH 4.5 and 10; addition of calcium ions will gel fluid solutions of sodium alginate.

Preparation

Ointment preparation or manufacture depends on the type of vehicle and the quantity to be prepared. The objective is the same, ie, to disperse uniformly throughout the vehicle a finely subdivided or dissolved drug substance(s) (Fig 10). Normally, the drug materials are in finely powdered form before being dispersed in the vehicle.

Incorporation by Levigation

The preparation of small quantities of ointment by the pharmacist, ie, one to several ounces, can be accomplished by using a spatula and an ointment tile (either porcelain or glass). The finely powdered drug material is levigated thoroughly with a small quantity of the base to form a concentrate. The concentrate then is diluted geometrically with the remainder of the base. Such a procedure is useful particularly with petrolatum or oleaginous bases.

If the drug substance is water-soluble it can be dissolved in water and the resulting solution incorporated into the vehicle using a small quantity of lanolin if the base is oleaginous. Generally speaking, an amount of anhydrous lanolin equal in volume to the amount of water used will suffice.

When ointments are made by incorporation in quantities too large to be handled with a tile and spatula, mechanical mixers are used. Hobart mixers, pony mixers and others of the type usually are used for this purpose. The drug substance in finely divided form usually is added slowly or sifted into the vehicle contained in the rotating mixer. When the ointment is uniform, the finished product may be processed through a roller mill to assure complete dispersion and reduce any aggregates.

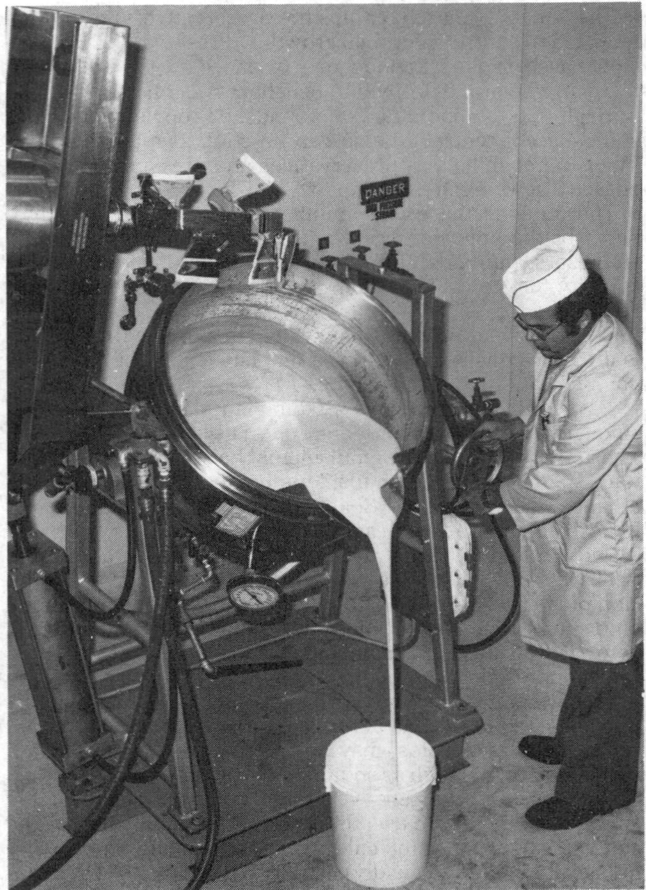

Fig 10. Pilot scale ointment manufacture (courtesy, Alcon).

This procedure may be modified by preparing and milling a concentrate of the drug in a portion of the base. The concentrate then is dispersed in the balance of the vehicle, using a mixer of appropriate size. Occasionally, the base may be melted for easier handling and dispersing. In such cases the drug is dispersed and the base slowly cooled using continuous agitation to maintain dispersion.

Emulsion Products

Medicated creams and lotions are prepared by means of a two-phase heat system. The oil-phase ingredients are combined in a jacketed tank and heated to about 75°. At this temperature the oil-phase ingredients are liquefied and uniform. In a separate tank the aqueous-phase ingredients, including the emulsifier, are heated together to slightly above 75°. The aqueous phase then is added to the oil phase, slowly and with constant agitation. When the emulsion is formed the mixture is allowed to cool, maintaining slow agitation.

At this stage in the process the medicinal ingredients usually are added as a concentrated slurry, which usually has been milled to reduce any particle aggregates. Volatile or aromatic materials generally are added when the finished emulsion has cooled to about 35°. At this point additional water may be added to compensate for any evaporative losses occurring during exposure and transfer at the higher temperatures of emulsion formation.

While the product remains in the tank in bulk, quality-control procedures are performed, ie, for pH, active ingredients, etc. If control results are satisfactory the product is filled into the appropriate containers.

Preservatives in Ointment Bases

Antimicrobial preservative substances are included in ointment formulations to maintain the potency and integrity of product forms and to protect the health and safety of the consumer. The USP addresses this subject in its monograph on Microbiological Attributes of Non-Sterile Pharmaceutical Products. The significance of microorganisms in nonsterile products should be evaluated in terms of the use of the product, the nature of the product and the potential hazard to the user. The USP suggests that products applied topically should be free from *P aeruginosa* and *S aureus*.

The attributes of an ideal preservative system have been defined by various authors as

Effective at relatively low concentrations against a broad spectrum or variety of microorganisms which could cause disease or product deterioration.

Soluble in the required concentration.

Nontoxic and nonsensitizing at in-use concentrations.

Compatible with ingredients of the formulation and package components.

Free from objectionable odors and colors.

Stable over a wide spectrum of conditions.

Inexpensive.

No preservative or preservative system meets these ideal criteria. In fact, preservative substances once considered most acceptable, if not ideal, now have been questioned. Methylparaben and propylparaben, second and third only to water in frequency of use in cosmetic formulations, have been associated with allergic reactions.

Use of parabens as preservatives in topical products began a half-century ago. Animal testing indicated that they virtually are nontoxic and the compounds, usually in combination, became nearly ubiquitous as preservatives in dermatologic and cosmetic products. In 1968 Schorr was among the first in this country to express concern about contact sensitization to parabens. Other investigators have voiced similar concerns.

Topical parabens do not appear to constitute a significant hazard to the public based on their low index of sensitization and low overall toxicity.

Alternative preservation substances available for use in ointment bases, together with comments on possible limitations, are given in Table 5.[26] It is probably sensible to note that, with few exceptions, most of these compounds—in contrast to the parabens—do not have a half-century history of use nor have had extensive patch-testing experiments carried out.

Following selection of preservative candidates and preparation of product prototypes, the efficacy of the preservative system must be evaluated. A variety of methods to accomplish this have been proposed. The organism challenge procedure is currently the most acceptable. In this procedure the test-product formulation is inoculated with specific levels and types of microorganisms. Preservative efficacy is evaluated on the basis of the number of organisms killed or whose growth is inhibited as determined during a specific sampling schedule. Critical to the organism challenge procedure are the selection of challenge microorganisms, the level of organisms in the inoculum, the sampling schedule and data interpretation.

Variations of the organism challenge procedure have usually centered around the selection of organisms, the challenge schedule, use of a rechallenge and standards of effectiveness, ie, cidal activity required rather than static or inhibitory activity.

Table 6 gives the challenge organisms and other criteria used in several preservative challenge procedures.

In addition to efficacy in terms of antimicrobial effects, the preservative system must be assessed in terms of chemical and physical stability as a function of time. This often is done using antimicrobial measurements in addition to chemical analysis.

Safety, Safety Testing and Toxicity

Safety is defined as the condition of being safe from undergoing (or causing) injury. Safety is not absolute but must be taken in the context of conditions of use. Toxicity refers to a specific substance or product and the adverse effect on a system caused by such a substance or product acting for a given period of time at a specific dose level.

Ointment bases may cause irritant or allergic reactions. Allergic reactions are usually to a specific base component. Irritant reactions are more frequent and more important, hence a number of test procedures have been devised to test for irritancy levels, both in the animal and in man. The consequences of species differences and specificity must be included in the evaluation of animal-test results.

Probably the most common irritancy measure is the Draize dermal irritation test in rabbits. In this procedure the test material is applied repeatedly to the clipped skin on the rabbit's back. The test material may be compared with one or more control materials.

End-points are dermal erythema and/or edema. By assigning numerical scores for erythema and edema, mathematical and statistical treatment of results is possible.

In the human, a variety of test procedures are used to measure irritancy, sensitization potential and phototoxicity. Among the most common are the following:

21-Day Cumulative Irritation Study

In this test the test compound is applied daily to the same site on the back or volar forearm. Test materials are applied under occlusive tape and scores are read daily. The test application and scoring is repeated daily for 21 days or until irritation produces a predetermined maximum

Table 5—Topical Preservatives: Benefits and Risks[26]

Preservatives	Limitations relative to use in cosmetic/dermatologic formulations
Quaternary ammonium compounds	a) Inactivated by numerous ingredients including anionics, nonionics and proteins
Organic mercurial compounds	a) Potentially toxic and many sensitize the skin b) Limited use in formulations used near or in the eye
Formaldehyde	a) Volatile compound with an objectionable odor b) Irritating to the skin c) High chemical reactivity
Halogenated phenols hexachlorophene, *p*-chloro-*m*-cresol (PCMC) *p*-chloro-*m*-xylenol (PCMX) dichloro-*m*-xylenol (DCMX)	a) Objectionable odor b) Often inactivated by nonionics, anionics or proteins c) Limited gram-negative antibacterial activity
Sorbic acid potassium sorbate	a) pH-dependent (can be used only in formulations below the pH of 6.5 to 7.0) b) Higher concentrations are oxidized by sunlight resulting in product discoloration c) Limited antibacterial activity
Benzoic acid sodium benzoate	a) pH-dependent (limited to use in formulations with pH of 5.5 or less) b) Replaced by newer antimicrobials because of its limited antimicrobial activity

Table 6—Preservative Effectiveness Test Procedures

	USP	CTFA	FDA
Challenge microorganisms	*S aureus* *E coli* *P aeruginosa* *C albicans* *A niger*	*S aureus* *E coli* *P aeruginosa* *C albicans* *A niger* *P luteum* *B cereus* or *B subtilis* var *globigii*	*S aureus* *E coli* *P aeruginosa* *P putida* *P multivorans* *Klebsiella* *S marcescens* *C albicans* *A niger*
Inoculum level	$1 \times 10^5 - 1 \times 10^6$ Cells/mL or g	1×10^6 Cells/mL or g	$0.8–1.2 \times 10^6$ Cells/mL or g Rechallenge 1–2.0 $\times 10^5$ vegetative cells
Sampling schedule	0, 7, 14, 21, 28 days	0, 1–2, 7, 14, 28 days	Weekly intervals
Standards	Bacteria $<0.1\%$ survival by 14th day. Yeast & molds at or below initial concentration during first 14 days. No increase in organism counts for remainder of 28-day survival	Based on intended use	Vegetative cells $<0.01\%$ survival in 28 days *C albicans* $<1\%$ survival *A niger* $<1\%$ survival Rechallenge 0.1% survival in 28 days

score. Typical erythema scores are

0 = no visible reaction
1 = mild erythema
2 = intense erythema
3 = intense erythema with edema
4 = intense erythema with edema and vesicular erosion.

Usually, 24 subjects are used in this test. Fewer subjects and a shorter application time in days are variants of the test.

Draize-Shelanski Repeat-Insult Patch Test

This test is designed to measure the potential to cause sensitization. The test also provides a measure of irritancy potential. In the usual procedure the test material or a suitable dilution is applied under occlusion to the same site, for 10 alternate-day 24-hour periods. Following a 7-day rest period the test material is applied again to a fresh site for 24 hours. The challenge sites are read on removal of the patch and again 24 hours later. The 0–4 erythema scale is used. A test panel of 100 individuals is common.

Kligman Maximization Test

This test is used to detect the contact sensitizing potential of a product or material. The test material is applied under occlusion to the same site for 48-hour periods. Prior to each exposure the site may be pretreated with a solution of sodium lauryl sulfate under occlusion. Following a 10-day interval the test material again is applied to a different site for 48 hours under occlusion. The challenge site may be treated briefly with a sodium lauryl sulfate solution.

The Maximization test is of shorter duration and makes use of fewer test subjects than the Draize Shelanski test. The use of sodium lauryl sulfate as a pretreatment increases the ability to detect weaker allergens.

These test methods are adequate to detect even weak irritants and weak contact sensitizers. Positive results, however, automatically do not disqualify the use of a substance as unsafe. The actual risk of use depends on concentration, period of use and skin condition. Benzoyl peroxide in tests such as the Draize-Shelanski and Maximization is a potent sensitizer, yet the incidence of sensitization among acne patients is low.

Packaging and Labeling

Ointments usually are packaged in ointment jars or in metal or plastic tubes of a convenient size. Ointment jars are available in one-half to 16-oz sizes; tubes from 3.5-g capacity (often ophthalmic) to 4-oz and on occasion greater capacities.

Ointment Jars—Straight-sided screw cap jars of glass or plastic are available. Clear, amber or opaque glass containers are used, as well as white, opaque, plastic, usually high-density polyethylene, jars. Metal or composition plastic tops are available, with a variety of inner liners to assure a dust- and air-tight closure. Liners are usually paper or plastic laminates or discs glued or otherwise fitted to the closure.

Ointment jars are filled mechanically to somewhat less than capacity to minimize contact between the ointment and the cap or cap-liner. Ointment jars hand-filled by the pharmacist also should be finished to avoid contact between the ointment and cap. This can be accomplished quite readily by skillful use of a flexible spatula. The spatula is forced across the ointment jar while depressed slightly into the ointment. The result is a conical depression that is esthetically acceptable. Much of the same result can be accomplished by depressing the spatula into the center of the filled jar and gradually rotating the jar against the stationary spatula. Small points perhaps, but time well spent to avoid having part of the ointment-jar contents removed inadvertently by the cap when the patient opens the jar.

Ointment Tubes—Ointment tubes made of tin or aluminum, or of an increasing variety of plastic materials, are available. The latter are normally polyethylene, polypropylene or other flexible, heat-sealable plastics. Ointment tubes have obvious advantages over jars; the use of fingers is minimized, as is dust and air contact, and light exposure.

Depending on the expected shelf-life, a number of factors should be considered in selecting an ointment tube. Metal contact and the possibility of metal-ion catalyzed instability must be considered. Conversely, plastic tubes may become stained or discolored by migration of colored materials into the plastic sidewalls of the tube; coal tar in ointment form may cause such discoloration. Tube interactions involving either metal or plastic can be minimized by internal coatings. Such coatings usually are epoxy films that become the primary product contact.

The suitability of ointment containers, either jars or tubes, should be verified by adequate testing prior to use. Compatibility and physical and chemical stability should be established by proper tests before final selection of a jar or tube.

Ointments prepared on prescription can be conveniently filled into a metal ointment tube using the following procedure.

Select an ointment tube of the proper size and remove any lint or dust. Transfer the ointment to a piece of paper of suitable size (use glassine or strong paper). Roll the paper and ointment into a cylinder shape of a diameter slightly less than that of the ointment tube. Insert the rolled paper-ointment cylinder into the ointment tube. The length of the paper cylinder should exceed the tube length. Remove the ointment tube cap and, using a spatula, compress the paper cylinder and tube. Continue compressing the ointment and tube until the ointment appears in the neck-orifice of the open tube. Replace the cap. Using the spatula side as a knife-edge, compress the ointment tube and paper cylinder a reasonable distance from the end of the tube. Holding the spatula firmly in place, draw out the paper cylinder, leaving the ointment within the tube.

The ointment tube selected should be of adequate capacity. After compressing the ointment and paper cylinder into the tube, constrict the tube for cylinder removal at a distance from the end of the tube that will allow at least a double foldover to seal the tube. The fold dimensions are inexact, however, the individual folds on a 1-oz tube are approximately ⅛ to 3/16 in. Ointment tube sealing folds easily can be made by folding the tube over on itself using a spatula blade to flatten the tube and serve as a folding point. Ointment tube clips can be fixed over the tube ends and clamped in place using pliers or a small vise. The sole purpose of folding and clamping is to prevent leakage when routine-use pressure is applied to the tube.

On a larger scale, ointment-tube filling is accomplished using automatic equipment which air-cleans the tubes, fills, folds and crimps the end in one continuous operation (Fig 11). Some equipment will stamp an expiration date onto the crimped surface. In larger-scale manufacturing operations plastic tubes are used with increasing frequency. From a filling standpoint plastic tubes are handled much like metal tubes. The final step, however, is a heat seal with no end foldover.

Labeling Ointment Tubes—Attaching labels to ointment tubes is a minor difficulty compounded by the increasing unsightliness characteristic of many ointment tubes during use. The label increasingly can become obliterated, difficult to read and, frequently, lost. As a general rule the label should be attached to itself, ie, it should completely encircle the tube. It should be attached to the tube, affixed close to the neck end.

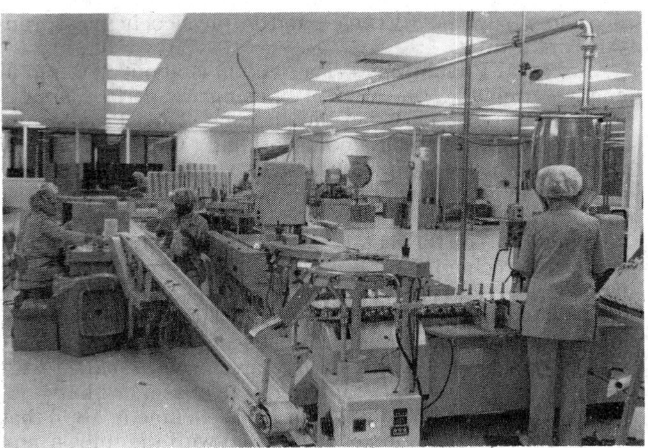

Fig 11. Ointment manufacture and packaging (courtesy, Owen Labs).

Given the usual handling of ointment tubes by the patient, it is good practice to dispense the tube in a vial or hinged pasteboard box of convenient size. The outer container serves to hold and protect the ointment tube as well as to carry the label. The ointment tube is marked with a container prescription number so that both tube and container are identified.

On a manufacturing scale tubes are labeled in a variety of ways. Paper labels may be used, labeling may be silk-screened onto plastic surfaces; expiration dates and code lot numbers may be stamped on as a part of the tube-crimping procedure.

Suppositories

Suppositories are solid dosage forms of various weights and shapes, usually medicated, for insertion into the rectum, vagina or the urethra. After insertion, suppositories soften, melt, disperse or dissolve in the cavity fluids.

The use of suppositories dates from the distant past, this dosage form being referred to in writings of the early Egyptians, Greeks and Romans. Suppositories are suited particularly for administration of drugs to the very young and the very old, a notion first recorded by Hippocrates. Despite the antiquity of this dosage form, little was known about drug absorption or drug activity via suppository administration until recent years.

Types

Rectal Suppositories—The USP describes rectal suppositories for adults as tapered at one or both ends and usually weighing about 2 g each. Infant rectal suppositories usually weigh about one-half that of adult suppositories. Drugs having systemic effects, such as sedatives, tranquilizers and analgesics, are administered by rectal suppository; however, the largest single-use category is probably that of hemorrhoid remedies dispensed over-the-counter. The 2-g weight for adult rectal suppositories is based on use of cocoa butter as the base; when other bases are used the weights may be greater or less than 2 g.

Vaginal Suppositories—The USP describes vaginal suppositories or pessaries, as usually globular or oviform and weighing about 5 g each. Vaginal medications are available in a variety of physical forms, eg, creams, gels or liquids, which depart from the classical concept of suppositories. Vaginal tablets, or inserts prepared by encapsulation in soft gelatin, however, do meet the definition, and represent convenience both of administration and manufacture.

Urethral Suppositories—Urethral suppositories—sometimes referred to as bougies—are not described specifically in the USP, either by weight or dimension. Traditional values, based on use of cocoa butter as base, are as follows for these cylindrical dosage forms: diameter, 5 mm; length, 50 mm female, 125 mm male; weight, 2 g female, 4 g male. Urethral suppositories are an unusual dosage form and seldom are encountered.

Rectal Absorption

Drug absorption for systemic activity generally is limited to rectal administration. As noted previously, the bioavailability of rectally administered drugs is a relatively recent concern. Rectally instilled preparations, whether suppositories, foams or solutions (enemas), tend to be confined to the rectum and sigmoid colon if the volume is less than about 50 mL. Foams tend to dissipate or spread to a lesser extent than solutions, particularly large-volume solutions (~100 to 200 mL). Though large-volume fluid formulations—solutions or enemas—may allow drug to reach the ascending colon, substantial intra- and intersubject variation is evident.[27] Literature information indicates that rectal drug absorption from suppositories can be erratic and may be substantially different from absorption following oral administration. With only a few recent exceptions, suppository studies are based on either *in vivo* or *in vitro* data with few attempts to correlate *in vitro* results with *in vivo* studies.

Major factors affecting the absorption of drugs from suppositories administered rectally are the following: anorectal physiology, suppository vehicle and the physicochemical properties of the drug.

Anorectal Physiology—The rectum is about 150 mm in length, terminating in the anal opening; its surface area is about 200 to 400 cm^2. In the absence of fecal matter the rectum contains a small amount of fluid (1 to 3 mL) of low buffering capacity. Fluid pH is said to be about 7.2; because of the low buffer capacity pH will vary with the pH of the drug product or drug dissolved in it. Böttger *et al.*[28] studied the influence of pH on the rectal absorption of sodium benzoate in man by the technique of rectal lumen perfusion. This study demonstrates that strong buffers in rectal solutions induce a drastic effect on the pH of the boundary layer, an effect that is not seen if unbuffered solutions are used.

Most rectal suppositories today are torpedo-shaped with the apex, or pointed end, tapering to the base, or blunt end, following the recommendation of HS Wellcome in 1893 that rectal suppositories should be inserted with the thicker end foremost so that when the anal sphincter contracts, expulsion is prevented. In the intervening 100 years or so, no study has correlated rectal suppository insertion with anorectal physiology until that of Abd-El-Maeboud *et al*[29] who found that ease of insertion, retention and lack of expulsion were enhanced when the suppository was inserted base or blunt end up. This was ascribed to reversed vermicular contractions of the external anal sphincter, which facilitate movement of the suppository upward into the rectum. The rectal epithelium is lipoidal in character. The lower, middle and upper hemorrhoidal veins surround the rectum. Only the upper vein conveys blood into the portal system, thus drugs absorbed into the lower and middle hemorrhoidal veins will bypass the liver. Absorption and distribution of a drug therefore is modified by its position in the rectum, in the sense that at least a portion of the drug absorbed from the rectum may pass directly into the inferior vena cava, bypassing the liver.

Spreading characteristics of rectal formulations may be affected considerably by intraluminal rectal pressure—due, in part, to the weight of abdominal organs and to respiratory activity—and by periodic contractile activity of the rectal wall.[30]

Suppository Vehicle—The ideal suppository base should meet the following general specifications:

1. The base is nontoxic and nonirritating to mucous membranes.
2. The base is compatible with a variety of drugs.
3. The base melts or dissolves in rectal fluids.
4. The base should be stable on storage; it should not bind or otherwise interfere with release and absorption of drug substances.

Rectal suppository bases can be classified broadly into two types: fatty and water soluble or water miscible. The traditional cocoa butter vehicle is immiscible with aqueous tissue fluids but melts at body temperature. Water-soluble or water-miscible vehicles also have been used. In general, formulators have been reluctant to use glycerinated gelatin as a rectal suppository base because of its relatively slow dissolution. More typical of this class is the polyethylene glycol vehicle. Drug absorption from such dissimilar bases can differ substantially. Lowenthal and Borzelleca[31] investigated the absorption of salicylic acid and sodium salicylate administered to dogs. The drugs were formulated in a cocoa butter base and in a base comprised of polyethylene glycol, synthetic glycerides and a surfactant. Absorption of salicylic acid and sodium salicylate was about equal from the cocoa butter base; how ever, salicylic acid gave higher plasma levels than sodium salicylate when the glycol base was used.

Parrott[32] compared the absorption of salicylates after rectal and oral administration. Using urinary excretion data both aspirin and sodium salicylate were found to be equally bioavailable orally or rectally. Aspirin was released more rapidly from water-miscible suppositories than from the oily type. Conversely, sodium salicylate was released more rapidly from a cocoa butter vehicle.

Based on available data the bioavailability of a drug from a suppository dosage form is dependent on the physicochemical properties of the drug as well as the composition of the base. The drug-dissolution rate and, where appropriate, the partition coefficient between lipid and aqueous phase should be known.

For suppository formulation the relative solubility of the drug in the vehicle is a convenient comparison measure. Lipid-soluble drugs present in low concentration in a cocoa butter base will have little tendency to diffuse into rectal fluids. Drugs that are only slightly soluble in the lipid base will partition readily into the rectal fluid. The partition coefficient between suppository base and rectal fluid thus becomes a useful measure. In water-soluble bases and assuming rapid dissolution, the rate-limiting step in absorption would be transport of the drug through the rectal mucosa.

In the absence of evidence of any substantial carrier-mediated uptake mechanisms, the predominant mechanism of colorectal mucosal permeation appears to involve transcellular passage across cell membranes in accordance with the pH-partition hypothesis. Ease of access to the rectal mucosa has encouraged the evaluation of absorption enhancers. A wide variety of substances have been investigated for their ability to enhance rectal permeability to drugs. Agents such as EDTA have been used to chelate Ca^{2+} and Mg^{2+} in the vicinity of paracellular tight junctions and, thus, alter epithelial permeability. Other promoters of rectal absorption (eg, bile salts and nonsteroidal anti-inflammatory agents, including aspirin, salicylic acid and diclofenac) appear to exert their influence by affecting water influx and efflux rates across the rectal mucosa. Surfactants not only may modify membrane permeability but also enhance wetting or spreading of the base and dissolution of the drug. In any event, it should be evident that, whatever the mechanism, enhancing the *rectal* absorption of drugs—especially those which undergo presystemic elimination—could result in substantially reduced dosage requirements and decreased risk of adverse reactions.

Clearly, the bioavailability of a drug administered rectally depends on the nature of the drug and the composition of the vehicle or base. The physical properties of the drug can be modified to a degree, as can the characteristics of the base selected as the delivery system. Preformulation evaluations of physicochemical properties must then be confirmed by *in vivo* studies in animals and ultimately in the primary primate, man.

***In Vivo* Rectal Absorption Studies**—Dogs are probably the animal of choice in evaluating rectal drug availability. (The pig is a closer physiological match, but size and manageability argue in favor of the dog.) Blood and urine samples can be obtained from the dog and rectal retention can be accomplished with facility. Smaller animals have been used; rabbits, rats and even mice have been employed, but dosing and sampling become progressively more difficult.

Human subjects provide the ultimate measure of drug bioavailability. Subjects are selected on the basis of age, weight and medical history. Subjects usually are required to fast overnight and evacuate the bowel prior to initiation of the study. Fluid volume and food intake usually are standardized in studies of this kind.

Given the difficulty of standardizing pharmacological endpoints the usual measure of rectal drug bioavailability is the concentration of the drug in blood and/or urine as a function of time. A control group using oral drug administration provides a convenient means of comparing oral and rectal drug availability. Such a comparison is meaningful particularly in view of uncertainties and conflicts encountered in the literature. While there is general agreement about drug absorption from the rectum there is less agreement on dosage adequacy and the relationship between oral and rectal dosage. This state of affairs argues in favor of adequate studies to establish proper dosage and verify bioavailability.

Vaginal Absorption

Passive drug absorption via the vaginal mucosa, as with other mucosal tissues, is influenced by absorption site physiology, absorption site pH and the solubility and partitioning characteristics of the drug. The vaginal epithelial surface usually is covered with an aqueous film—emanating from cervical secretions—whose volume, pH and composition vary with age, stage of the menstrual cycle and location. Postmenarche, a vaginal pH gradient is evident with the lowest values (pH ~ 4.0) near the anterior fornix and the highest (pH ~ 5.0) near the cervix.[33]

Following intravaginal administration, some drug absorption from the intact vaginal mucosa is likely, even when the drug is employed for a local effect. In fact, extensive drug absorption can occur from the vagina. For example, Patel *et al*[34] reported that plasma propranolol concentrations following vaginal dosing were significantly higher than those after peroral administration of an equivalent dose; a reflection, in part, of decreased first-pass biotransformation following vaginal absorption. Nonetheless, the notion persists that the vaginal epithelium is relatively impermeable to drugs.

The widespread extemporaneous compounding of progesterone vaginal suppositories,[35,36] as well as the marketing of an intrauterine progesterone drug delivery system [Progestasert, *Alza*] have focused interest on systemic drug absorption following intravaginal administration. However, only limited reports of research on *in vitro* and *in vivo* aspects of vaginal absorption have appeared in the literature to date.

Bases

The USP lists the following as usual suppository bases: cocoa butter, cocoa butter substitutes (primarily, vegetable oils modified by esterification, hydrogenation and/or fractionation), glycerinated gelatin, hydrogenated vegetable oils, mixtures of polyethylene glycols of various molecular weights and fatty acid esters of polyethylene glycol.

Cocoa Butter and other Fatty Bases—Theobroma oil, or cocoa butter, is a naturally occurring triglyceride. About 40% of the fatty acid content is unsaturated. As a natural material there is considerable batch-to-batch variability. A major characteristic of theobroma oil is its polymorphism, ie, its ability to exist in more than one crystal form. While cocoa butter melts quickly at body temperature, it is immiscible with body fluids; this may inhibit the diffusion of fat-soluble drugs to the affected sites. Oleaginous vehicles, such as cocoa butter, seldom are used in vaginal preparations for esthetic reasons: many women consider them messy and prone to leakage.

If, in the preparation of suppositories, the theobroma oil is overheated, ie, heated to about 60°, molded and chilled, the suppositories formed will melt below 30°. The fusion treatment of theobroma oil requires maximum temperatures of 40 to 50° to avoid a change in crystal form and melting point. Theobroma oil, heated to about 60° and cooled rapidly will crystallize in an alpha configuration characterized by a melting point below 30°. The alpha form is metastable and will slowly revert to the beta form with the characteristic melting point approaching 35°. The transition from alpha to beta is slow, taking several days. The use of low heat and slow cooling allows direct crystallization of the more stable beta crystal form.

Certain drugs will depress the melting point of theobroma oil. This involves no polymorphic change although the net effect is similar. Chloral hydrate is the most important of these substances because its rectal hypnotic dose of 0.5 to 1.0 g will cause a substantial melting-point depression. This effect can be countered by addition of a higher melting wax, such as white wax or synthetic spermaceti. The amount to be added must be determined by temperature measurements. The effect of such additives on bioavailability also must be considered.

Various cocoa butter substitutes (hard fat, hydrogenated vegetable oil) are available commercially which offer a number of advantages over cocoa butter such as decreased potential for rancidity and phase transition (melting and solidification) behavior tailored to specific formulation, processing and storage requirements. However, as with cocoa butter, these semisynthetic glyceride mixtures are also subject to polymorphic transformations. Batch-to-batch variations of the physical properties of all of these bases, whether cocoa butter or cocoa butter substitutes, can play havoc with the final products' characteristics. The formulator should ensure that the melting and congealing behavior of these bases and the formulations prepared from them is evaluated thoroughly.

Water-Soluble or Dispersible Bases—Water-miscible suppository bases are of comparatively recent origin. The majority are comprised of polyethylene glycols or glycol-surfactant combinations. Water-miscible suppository bases have the substantial advantage of lack of dependence on a melting point approximating body temperature. Problems of handling, storage and shipping are simplified considerably.

Polymers of ethylene glycol are available as polyethylene glycol polymers (Carbowax, polyglycols) of assorted molecular weights. Suppositories of varying melting points and solubility characteristics can be prepared by blending polyethylene glycols of 1000, 4000 or 6000 molecular weight.

Polyethylene glycol suppositories, while prepared rather easily by molding, cannot be prepared satisfactorily by hand-rolling. The drug-glycol mixture is prepared by melting and then is cooled to just above the melting point before pouring into dry unlubricated molds. Cooling to near the melting point prevents fissuring caused by crystallization and contraction. The USP advises that labels on polyethylene glycol suppositories should instruct patients to moisten the suppository before inserting it.

Water-miscible or water-dispersible suppositories also can be prepared using selected nonionic surfactant materials. Polyoxyl 40 stearate is a white, water-soluble solid melting slightly above body temperature. A polyoxyethylene derivative of sorbitan monostearate is water-insoluble but dispersible. In using surfactant materials the possibility of drug–base interactions must be borne in mind. Interactions caused by macromolecular adsorption may have a significant effect on bioavailability.

Examples of water-miscible suppository bases, devised by Collins, Hohmann and Zopf[37] are

Base 1

Polyethylene glycol 1000	96%
Polyethylene glycol 4000	4%

Base 2

Polyethylene glycol 1000	75%
Polyethylene glycol 4000	25%

Base 1 is low-melting and may require refrigeration; Base 2 is more heat-stable. Each is prepared conveniently by molding techniques.

Water-dispersible bases may include polyoxyethylene sorbitan fatty acid esters. These are either soluble (Tween, Myrj) or water-dispersible (Arlacel), used alone or in combination with other wax or fatty materials. Surfactants in suppositories should be used only with recognition of reports that such materials may either increase or decrease drug absorption.

Hydrogels—In recent years, hydrogels, defined as macromolecular networks that swell but do not dissolve in water, have been advocated as bases for rectal and vaginal drug delivery. The swelling of hydrogels, *ie*, the absorption of water, is a consequence of the presence of hydrophilic functional groups attached to the polymeric network. Cross-links between adjacent macromolecules result in the aqueous insolubility of these hydrogels.

The use of a hydrogel matrix for drug delivery involves the dispersal of the drug in the matrix followed by drying of the system and concomitant immobilization of the drug. When the hydrogel delivery system is placed in an aqueous environment, *eg*, the rectum or the vagina, the hydrogel swells enabling the drug to diffuse out of the macromolecular network. The rate and extent of drug release from these hydrogel matrices depend on the rate of water migration *into* the matrix and the rate of drug diffusion *out of* the swollen matrix.

Hydrogels employed for rectal or vaginal drug administration have been prepared from polymers such as polyvinyl alcohol, hydroxyethyl methacrylate, polyacrylic acid or polyoxyethylene. Although hydrogel-based drug-delivery systems have yet to appear in suppository or insert form commercially, research efforts in this direction are increasing, given their potential for controlled drug delivery, bioadhesion, retention at the site of administration and biocompatibility.

Glycerinated Gelatin—Glycerinated gelatin usually is used as a vehicle for vaginal suppositories. For rectal use a firmer suppository can be obtained by increasing the gelatin content. Glycerinated gelatin suppositories are prepared by dissolving or dispersing the drug substance in enough water to equal 10% of the final suppository weight. Glycerin (70%) is then added and Pharmagel A or B (20%), depending on the drug compatibility requirements. Pharmagel A is acid in reaction, Pharmagel B is alkaline. Glycerinated gelatin suppositories must be formed by molding. The mass cannot be processed by hand-rolling. These suppositories, if not for immediate use, should contain a preservative such as methylparaben and propylparaben.

Preparation

Suppositories are prepared by rolling (hand-shaping), molding (fusion) and cold compression.

Rolled (Hand-Shaped) Suppositories—Hand-shaping suppositories is the oldest and the simplest method of preparing this dosage form. The manipulation requires considerable skill, yet avoids the complications of heat and mold preparation.

The general process can be described as follows:

General Process

Take the prescribed quantity of the medicinal substances and a sufficient quantity of grated theobroma oil. In a mortar reduce the medicating ingredients to a fine powder or, if composed of extracts, soften with diluted alcohol and rub until a smooth paste is formed. The correct amount of grated theobroma oil then is added, and a mass resembling a pill mass is made by thoroughly incorporating the ingredients with a pestle, sometimes with the aid of a small amount of wool fat. When the mass has become plastic under the vigorous kneading of the pestle, it quickly is loosened from the mortar with a spatula, pressed into a roughly shaped mass in the center of the mortar and then transferred with the spatula to a piece of filter paper which is kept between the mass and the hands during the kneading and rolling procedure. By quick, rotary movements of the hands, the mass is rolled to a ball which immediately is placed on a pill tile. A suppository cylinder is formed by rolling the mass on the tile with a flat board, partially aided by the palm of the other hand, if weather conditions permit. The suppository "pipe" frequently will show a tendency to crack in the center, developing a hollow core. This occurs when the mass has not been kneaded and softened sufficiently, with the result that the pressure of the roller board is not carried uniformly throughout the mass but is exerted primarily on the surface. The length of the cylinder usually corresponds to about four spaces on the pill tile for each suppository, thus making the piece, when cut, practically a finished suppository except for the shaping of the point. When the cylinder has been cut into the proper number of pieces with a spatula, the conical shape is given it by rolling one end on the tile with a spatula, or in some cases even by shaping it with the fingers to produce a rounded point.

Compression-Molded (Fused) Suppositories—This method of suppository preparation also avoids heat. The suppository mass, such as a mixture of grated theobroma oil and drug, is forced into a mold under pressure, using a wheel-operated press. The mass is forced into mold openings, pressure is released, the mold removed, opened and replaced. On a large scale cold-compression machines are hydraulically operated, water-jacketed for cooling and screw-fed. Pressure is applied via a piston to compress the mass into mold openings.

Fusion or Melt Molding—In this method the drug is dispersed or dissolved in the melted suppository base. The mixture then is poured into a suppository mold, allowed to cool and the finished suppositories removed by opening the mold. Using this procedure, one to hundreds of suppositories can be made at one time.

Suppository molds are available for the preparation of various types and sizes of suppositories. Molds are made of aluminum alloy, brass or plastic and are available with from six to several hundred cavities.

The method of choice for commercial suppository production (Fig 12) involves the automated filling of molds or preformed shells by a volumetric dosing pump which meters the melt from a jacketed kettle or mixing tank directly into the molds or shells. Strips of preformed shells pass beneath the dosing pump and are filled successively, passed through cooling chambers (to promote solidification), sealed and then packaged. Quality control procedures (eg, weight, fill volume, leakage) are conducted readily "on-line."

An alternative to the melt-and-pour processes described above is that of injection molding, which has been described by Snipes.[38] This process is distinctive in that it makes use of the injection-molding technique developed for the fabrication of plastics. Polyethylene glycols are the excipients of choice in this process with polyethylene oxide, povidone or silicon dioxide added to adjust viscosity or plasticity. Long-chain saturated carboxylic acids also have been added to reduce the hygroscopicity inherent with the use of the polyethylene glycols. Typically, the molten excipient admixture is extruded or injected under pressure into precision-machined multicavity molds followed by the ejection of the molded units from the mold cavities. Advantages claimed for this method include the wide range of shapes and sizes that can be prepared at very high production rates with great precision.

Suppositories usually are formulated on a weight basis so that the medication replaces a portion of the vehicle as a function of specific gravity. If the medicinal substance has a density approximately the same as theobroma oil, it will replace an equal weight of oil. If the medication is heavier, it will replace a proportionally smaller amount of theobroma oil.

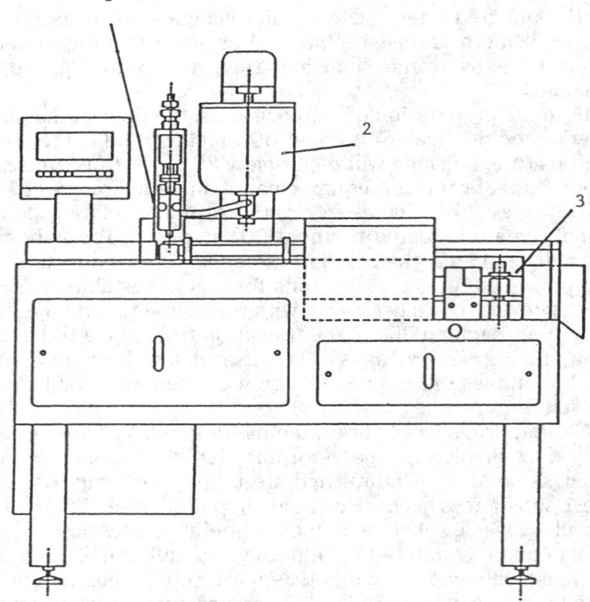

Fig 12. A cross section of the Sarong SpA semiautomatic equipment for the production of suppositories in preformed plastic or foil shells. The fully jacketed piston-type "dosing pump" (1) meters the suppository melt in the jacketed tank (2) into preformed shells which pass direclty beneath injection nozzles. The strips of filled preformed shells continue into a cooling chamber (3) prior to sealing and cartoning.

For instance, tannic acid has a density of 1.6 as compared with cocoa butter (see Table 7[39,40]). If a suppository is to contain 0.1 g tannic acid, then 0.1 g ÷ 1.6 or 0.062 g cocoa butter should be replaced by 0.1 g of drug. If the blank weight of the suppository is 2.0 g, then 2.0 − 0.062 g or 1.938 g cocoa butter is required per suppository. The suppository will actually weigh 1.938 g + 0.1 g or 2.038 g. Table 7 indicates the density factor, or the density as compared with cocoa butter, of many substances used in suppositories.

It always is possible to determine the density of a medicinal substance relative to cocoa butter, if the density factor is not available, by mixing the amount of drug for one or more suppositories with a small quantity of cocoa butter, pouring the mixture into a suppository mold and carefully filling the mold with additional melted cocoa butter. The cooled suppositories are weighed providing data from which a working formula can be calculated as well as the density factor itself.

When using suppository bases other than cocoa butter, such as a polyethylene glycol base, it is necessary to know either the density of the drug relative to the new base or both the densities of the drug and the new base relative to cocoa butter. The density factor for a base other than cocoa butter is simply the ratio of the blank weight of the base and cocoa butter.

For instance, if a suppository is to contain 0.1 g tannic acid in a polyethylene glycol base, then 0.1 g ÷ 1.6 × 1.25 or 0.078 g polyethylene glycol base should be replaced by 0.1 g drug (the polyethylene glycol base is assumed to have a density factor of 1.25). If the blank weight is 1.75 g for the polyethylene glycol base, then 1.75 g − 0.078 g or 1.672 g of base is required per suppository. The final weight will be 1.672 g base + 0.1 g drug or 1.772 g.

Table 7—Density Factors for Cocoa Butter Suppositories[39,40]

Medication	Factor
Acid, boric	1.5
Acid, benzoic	1.5
Acid, gallic	2.0
Acid, salicylic	1.3
Acid, tannic	1.6
Alum	1.7
Aminophylline	1.1
Aminopyrine	1.3
Aspirin	1.3
Barbital	1.2
Belladonna extract	1.3
Bismuth carbonate	4.5
Bismuth salicylate	4.5
Bismuth subgallate	2.7
Bismuth subnitrate	6.0
Castor oil	1.0
Chloral hydrate	1.3
Cocaine hydrochloride	1.3
Digitalis leaf	1.6
Glycerin	1.6
Ichthammol	1.1
Iodoform	4.0
Menthol	0.7
Morphine hydrochloride	1.6
Opium	1.4
Paraffin	1.0
Peruvian, balsam[a]	1.1
Phenobarbital	1.2
Phenol[a]	0.9
Potassium bromide	2.2
Potassium iodide	4.5
Procaine	1.2
Quinine hydrochloride	1.2
Resorcinol	1.4
Sodium bromide	2.3
Spermaceti	1.0
Sulfathiazole	1.6
Tannic acid	1.6
White wax	1.0
Witch hazel fluidextract	1.1
Zinc oxide	4.0
Zinc sulfate	2.8

[a]Density adjusted taking into account white wax in mass.

When the dosage and mold calibration are complete the drug–base mass should be prepared using minimum heat. A water bath or water jacketing usually is used. The melted mass should be stirred constantly but slowly to avoid air entrapment. The mass should be poured into the mold openings slowly. Prelubrication of the mold will depend on the vehicle. Mineral oil is a good lubricant for cocoa butter suppositories. Molds should be dry for polyethylene glycol suppositories.

After pouring into tightly clamped molds the suppositories and mold are allowed to cool thoroughly using refrigeration on a small scale or refrigerated air on a larger scale. After thorough chilling any excess suppository mass should be removed from the mold by scraping, the mold opened and the suppositories removed. It is important to allow cooling time adequate for suppository contraction. This aids in removal and minimizes splitting of the finished suppository.

Packaging and Storage—Suppositories often are packaged in partitioned boxes which hold the suppositories upright. Glycerin and glycerinated gelatin suppositories often are packaged in tightly closed screw-capped glass containers. Though many commercial suppositories are wrapped individually in aluminum foil or PVC-polyethylene, strip-packaging is commonplace.

The most recent innovation in suppository manufacture is the procedure for molding the suppository directly into its primary packaging. In this operation the form into which the suppository mass flows consists of a series of individual molds formed from plastic or foil. After the suppository is poured and cooled the excess is trimmed off and the units are sealed and cut into 3s or 6s as desired. Cooling and final cartoning then can be carried out.

Suppositories with low-melting ingredients are best stored in a cool place. Theobroma oil suppositories, in particular, should be refrigerated.

Other Medicated Applications

Cataplasms (Poultices)

Poultices represent one of the most ancient classes of pharmaceutical preparations. A poultice, or cataplasm, is a soft, moist mass of meal, herbs, seed, etc, usually applied hot in cloth. The consistency is gruel-like, which is probably the origin of the word poultice.

Cataplasms were intended to localize infectious material in the body or to act as counterirritants. The materials tended to be absorptive, which, together with heat accounts for their popular use. None is now official in the USP. The last official product was Kaolin Poultice NF IX.

Pastes

The USP defines pastes as semisolid dosage forms that contain one or more drug substances intended for topical application. Pastes are divided into fatty pastes (eg, Zinc Oxide Paste) and those made from a single-phase aqueous gel (eg, Carboxymethylcellulose Sodium Paste). In the past, pastes have been defined as concentrates of absorptive powders dispersed (usually) in petrolatum or hydrophilic petrolatum. These fatty pastes are stiff to the point of dryness and are reasonably absorptive considering they have a petrolatum base. Pastes often are used in the treatment of oozing lesions where they act to absorb serous secretions. Pastes also are used to restrict the area of treatment by acting as an absorbent and physical dam.

Pastes adhere reasonably well to the skin, and are poorly occlusive. For this reason they are suited for application on and around moist lesions. The heavy consistency of pastes imparts a degree of protection and may, in some instances, make the use of bandages unnecessary. Pastes are less macerating than ointments.

Because of their physical properties pastes easily may be removed from the skin by the use of mineral oil or a vegetable oil. This is particularly true when the underlying or surrounding skin is traumatized easily.

An official paste is the conventional Zinc Oxide Paste; another is Triamcinolone Acetonide Dental Paste, for the specialized use the name implies.

Powders

Powders for external use usually are described as dusting powders. Such powders should have a particle size of not more than 150 μm, ie, less than 100-mesh, to avoid any sensation of grittiness which could irritate traumatized skin. Dusting powders usually contain starch, talc and zinc stearate. Absorbable Dusting Powder USP is comprised of starch treated with epichlorohydrin, with not more than 2.0% magnesium oxide added to maintain the modified starch in impalpable powder form; as it is intended for use as a lubricant for surgical gloves it should be sterilized (by autoclaving) and packaged in sealed paper packets.

The fineness of powders often is expressed in terms of mesh size, with impalpable powders generally in the range of 100- to 200-mesh (149 to 125 mm). Determination of size by mesh analysis becomes increasingly difficult as particle size decreases below 200-mesh.

Dressings

Dressings are external applications resembling ointments usually used as a covering or protection. Petrolatum Gauze is a sterile dressing prepared by adding sterile, molten, white petrolatum to precut sterile gauze in a ratio of 60 g of petrolatum to 20 g of gauze. Topical antibacterials are available in the form of dressings.

Creams

Creams are viscous liquid or semisolid emulsions of either the O/W or W/O type. Pharmaceutical creams are classified as water-removable bases and are described under *Ointments.* In addition to ointment bases, creams include a variety of cosmetic-type preparations. Creams of the O/W type include shaving creams, hand creams and foundation creams; W/O creams include cold creams and emollient creams.

Plasters

Plasters are substances intended for external application made of such materials and of such consistency as to adhere to the skin and attach to a dressing. Plasters are intended to afford protection and support and/or to furnish an occlusive and macerating action and to bring medication into close contact with the skin. Medicated plasters, long used for local or regional drug delivery, are the prototypical transdermal delivery system.

Plasters usually adhere to the skin by means of an adhesive material. The adhesive must bond to the plastic backing and to the skin (or dressing) with proper balance of cohesive strengths. Such a proper balance provides for removal, ie, adhesive breakage at the surface of application thus leaving a clean (skin) surface when the plaster is removed.

Contraceptives

In the context of this chapter contraceptives are considered in the form of creams, jellies or aerosol foams intended for vaginal use to protect against pregnancy. Contraceptive creams and jellies are designed to melt or spread, following insertion, over the vaginal surfaces. These agents act to immobilize spermatozoa.

Creams and jellies for contraceptive use may contain spermicidal agents such as nonoxynol 9 or they may function by a specific pH effect. A pH of 3.5 or less has an appreciable spermicidal effect. It is important to note that a final *in situ* pH of 3.5 or less is required; thus, the dilution effect and pH change brought about by vaginal fluids must be considered. To achieve the proper pH effect and control, buffer systems composed of acid and acid salts such as lactates, acetates and citrates are used frequently. The user must, of course, be assured of the safety, lack of irritancy, acceptability and effectiveness of such products; also, detailed and specific information and instructions should be available to physicians.

References

1. Boddé HE, van den Brink I, Koerten HK, de Haan FHN: *J Contr Rel* 15: 227, 1991.
2. Rougier A, Lotte C. In Shah VP, Maibach HI, eds: *Topical Drug Bioavailability, Bioequivalence, and Penetration,* Plenum Press, New York, 163, 1993.
3. Franz TJ: *J Invest Derm 64:* 191, 1975.
4. Scheuplein RJ, Ross LW: *Ibid 63:* 353, 1974.
5. Bartek MJ, La Bodde JA, Maibach HI: *Ibid 58:* 114, 1972.
6. Maibach HI, ed: *Animal Models in Dermatology,* Churchill Livingstone, Edinburgh, 110, 1975.
7. Wester RC, Maibach HI: *J Invest Derm 67:* 518, 1976.
8. Bronaugh RL. In Kemppainen BW, Reifenrath WG, eds: *Methods for Skin Absorption,* CRC Press, Boca Raton, FL, 61, 1990.
9. Mershon MM, Callahan JF. In Maibach HI, ed: *Animal Models in Dermatology,* Churchill Livingstone, Edinburgh, 36, 1975.
10. Lorenzetti OJ: *Ibid:* 212.
11. Maibach HI, ed: *Ibid:* 221.
12. Ostrenga J, Steinmetz C, Poulsen B: *J Pharm Sci 60:* 1175, 1971.
13. Flynn GL, Weiner ND, *et al: Int J Pharm 55:* 229, 1989.
14. Flynn GL. In Shah VP, Maibach HI, eds.: *Topical Drug Bioavailability, Bioequivalence, and Penetration,* Plenum Press, New York, 369, 1993.
15. Walters KA. In Hadgraft J, Guy RH, eds: *Transdermal Drug Delivery,* Dekker, New York, 197, 1989.
16. Ghosh TK, Banga AK: *Pharm Technol 17(4):* 62, 1993; *17(5):* 68, 1993.
17. Scheuplein RJ, Ross LW: *J Soc Cos Chem 21:* 853, 1970.
18. Christophers E, Kligman AM. In Montagna W, ed: *Advances in the Biology of Skin,* vol 6, Pergamon, Oxford, 163, 1965.
19. Benowitz NL *et al: Clin Pharmacol Ther. 52:* 223, 1992.
20. Roskos KV, Maibach HI, Guy RH: *J Pharmacokin Biopharm 17:* 617, 1989.
21. Sloan KB, Bodor N: *Int J Pharmaceut 12:* 299, 1982.
22. Banga AK, Chien YW: *J Control Rel 7:* 1, 1988.
23. Burnette RR. In Hadgraft J, Guy RH, eds: *Transdermal Drug Delivery,* Dekker, New York, 247, 1989.
24. Ghosh TK, Banga AK: *Pharm Technol 17(3):* 72, 1993.
25. Balsam MS, Sagarin E, eds: *Cosmetics Science and Technology,* 2nd ed, vol 1, Wiley-Interscience, New York, 205, 1972.
26. Lorenzetti OJ, Wernet TC: *Dermatologica 154:* 244, 1977.
27. Wood E, Wilson CG, Hardy JG: *Int J Pharm 25:* 191, 1985.
28. Böttger WM *et al: J Pharmacokin, Biopharm 18:* 1, 1990.
29. Abd-El-Maeboud KH, *et al: Lancet 338:* 798, 1991.
30. Tukker JJ, de Blaey CJ, Charbon GA: *Pharm Res 1:* 173, 1984.
31. Lowenthal W, Borzelleca JF: *J Pharm Sci 54:* 1790, 1965.
32. Parrott EL: *Ibid, 60:* 867, 1971.
33. Benziger DP, Edelson J: *Drug Metab Rev 14:* 137, 1983.
34. Patel LG, Warrington SJ, Pearson RM: *Br Med J 287:* 1247, 1983.
35. Roffe BD, Zimmer RA, Derewicz HJ: *Am J Hosp Pharm. 34:* 1344, 1977.
36. Allen LV, Stiles ML: *US Pharm 13(1):* 16, 1988.
37. Collins AP, Hohmann JR, Zopf LC: *Am Prof Pharm 23*: 231, 1957.
38. Snipes WC: US Pat 5,004,601, Apr 2, 1991.
39. Davis H: *Bentley's Text-Book of Pharmaceutics,* 7th ed, Bailliere, Tindall & Cox, London, 569, 1961.
40. Buchi J: *Pharm Acta Helv 20:* 403, 1940.

Bibliography

Chien YW, ed: *Transdermal Controlled Systemic Medications,* Marcel Dekker, New York, 1987.

Chien YW: *Novel Drug Delivery Systems,* Dekker, New York, 1982.

Flynn GL. In Shah VP, Maibach HI, eds: *Topical Drug Bioavailability, Bioequivalence, and Penetration,* Plenum Press, New York, 369, 1993.

Frost P, Gomez EC, Zaias N: *Recent Advances in Dermatopharmacology*, Spectrum Publ, New York, 1978.
Glas B, deBlaey CJ, eds: *Rectal Therapy*, JR Prous, Barcelona, 1984.
Guy RH, Hadgraft J: In Maibach H, Lowe R, eds: *Models in Dermatology*, vol 2, 5 Karger, Basel, 170, 1985.
Higuchi T: *J Soc Cos Chem 11*: 85, 1960.
Hoover JE, ed: *Dispensing of Medication*, 8th ed, Mack Publ Co, Easton PA, 1976.
International Cosmetic Ingredient Dictionary, 5th ed, The Cosmetic, Toiletry and Fragrance Assoc, Baltimore, 1993.
Kemppanien BW, Reifenrath WG, eds: *Methods for Skin Absorption*, CRC Press, Boca Raton, FL, 1990.
Maibach HI: *Animal Models in Dermatology*, Churchill Livingstone, Edinburgh, 1975.
Mier PD, Cotton DWK: *The Molecular Biology of Skin*, Blackwell, Oxford.
Montagna W, Parrakkal PF: *The Structure and Function of the Skin, 3rd ed, Academic, New York, 1974.*
Marples MJ: *The Ecology of the Human Skin*, Thomas, Springfield IL, 1965.
Scranton AB, Peppas NA: *Adv Drug Del Rev 11:* i, 1993.
Walters KA. In Hadgraft J, Guy RH: *Transdermal Drug Delivery*, Dekker, New York, 197, 1989.
Wester RC, Maibach HI: *Clin Pharmackinet 23:* 253, 1992.

CHAPTER 91

Powders

Robert E O'Connor, PhD
Process Development/Technical Service
RW Johnson Pharmaceutical Research Institute
Raritan, NJ 08869

Edward G Rippie, PhD
Professor of Pharmaceutics
College of Pharmacy, University of Minnesota
Minneapolis, MN 55455

Joseph B Schwartz, PhD
Tice Professor of Pharmaceutics
Director of Industrial Pharmacy Research
Philadelphia College of Pharmacy and Science
Philadelphia, PA 19104

Powders are encountered in almost every aspect of pharmacy, both in industry and in practice. Drugs and other ingredients, when they occur in the solid state in the course of being processed into a dosage form, usually are in a more or less finely divided condition. Frequently, this is a powder whose state of subdivision is critical in determining its behavior both during processing and in the finished dosage form. Apart from their use in the manufacture of tablets, capsules, suspensions, etc, powders also occur as a pharmaceutical dosage form. While the use of powders as a dosage form has declined, the properties and behavior of finely divided solid materials are of considerable importance in pharmacy.

This chapter is intended to provide an introduction to the fundamentals of powder mechanics and the primary means of powder production and handling. The relationships of the principles of powder behavior to powders as dosage forms are discussed.

Production Methods

Molecular Aggregation

Precipitation and Crystallization—These two processes are fundamentally similar and depend on achieving three conditions in succession: a state of supersaturation (super cooling in the case of crystallization from a melt), formation of nuclei and growth of crystals or amorphous particles.

Supersaturation can be achieved by evaporation of solvent from a solution, cooling of the solution if the solute has a positive heat of solution, production of additional solute as a result of a chemical reaction or a change in the solvent medium by addition of various soluble secondary substances. In the absence of seed crystals, significant supersaturation is required to initiate the crystallization process through formation of nuclei. A nucleus is thought to consist of from ten to a few hundred molecules having the spatial arrangement of the crystals that will be grown ultimately from them.

Such small particles are shown by the Kelvin equation to be more soluble than large crystals and, therefore, to require supersaturation, relative to large crystals, for their formation and subsequent growth. It is a gross oversimplification to assume that, for a concentration gradient of a given value, the rate of crystallization is the negative of the rate of dissolution. The latter is generally somewhat greater.

Depending on the conditions of crystallization, it is possible to control or modify the nature of the crystals obtained. When polymorphs exist, careful temperature control and seeding with the desired crystal form are often necessary. The habit or shape of a given crystal form is often highly dependent on impurities in solution, pH, rate of stirring, rate of cooling and the solvent. Very rapid rates of crystallization can result in impurities being included in the crystals by entrapment.

Spray-Drying—Atomization of a solution of one or more solids *via* a nozzle, spinning disk or other device, followed by evaporation of the solvent from the droplets is termed spray-drying. The nature of the powder that results is a function of several variables, including the initial solute concentration, size distribution of droplets produced and rate of solvent removal. The weight of a given particle is determined by the volume of the droplet from which it was derived and by the solute concentration. The particles produced are aggregates of primary particles consisting of crystals and/or amorphous solids, depending on the rate and conditions of solvent removal. This approach to the powdered state provides the opportunity to incorporate multiple solid substances into individual particles at a fixed composition, independent of particle size, and avoiding difficulties that can arise in attempting to obtain a uniform mixture of several powdered ingredients by other procedures.

Particle-Size Reduction

Comminution in its broadest sense is the mechanical process of reducing the size of particles or aggregates. Thus, it embraces a wide variety of operations including cutting, chopping, crushing, grinding, milling, micronizing and trituration, which depend primarily on the type of equipment employed. The selection of equipment in turn is determined by the characteristics of the material, the initial particle size and the degree of size reduction desired. For example, very large particles may require size reduction in stages simply because the equipment required to produce the final product will not accept the initial feed, as in crushing prior to grinding. In the case of vegetable and other fibrous material, size reduction generally must be, at least initially, accomplished by cutting or chopping.

Chemical substances used in pharmaceuticals, in contrast, generally need not be subjected to either crushing or cutting operations prior to reduction to the required particle size. However, these materials do differ considerably in melting point, brittleness, hardness and moisture content, all of which affect the ease of particle-size reduction and dictate the choice of equipment. The heat generated in the mechanical grinding, in particular, presents problems with materials which tend to liquefy or stick together and with the thermolabile products which may degrade unless the heat is dissipated by use of a flowing stream of water or air. The desired particle size, shape and size distribution also must be considered in the selection of grinding or milling equipment. For example, attrition mills tend to produce spheroidal, more free-flowing particles than do impact-type mills, which yield more irregular-shaped particles.

Fracture Mechanics—Reduction of particle size through fracture requires application of mechanical stress to the material to be crushed or ground. Materials respond to stress by yielding, with consequent generation of strain. Depending on the time course of strain as a function of applied stresses, materials can be classified according to their behavior over a continuous spectrum ranging from brittle to plastic. In the case of a totally brittle substance, complete rebound would occur on release of applied stress at stresses up to the yield point, where fracture would occur. In contrast, a totally plastic material would not rebound nor would it fracture. The vast majority of pharmaceutical solids lie somewhere between these extremes and thus possess both elastic and viscous properties. Linear and, to a lesser extent, nonlinear viscoelastic theory has been developed well to account for quantitatively and explain the simultaneous elastic and viscous deformations produced in solids by applied stresses.

The energy expended by comminution ultimately appears as surface energy associated with newly created particle surfaces, internal free energy associated with lattice changes and as heat. Most of the energy expressed as heat is consumed in the viscoelastic deformation of particles, friction and in imparting kinetic energy to particles. Energy is exchanged among these modes and some is, of course, effective in producing fracture. It has been estimated that 1% or less of the total mechanical energy used is associated with newly created surface or with crystal lattice imperfections.

While the grinding process has been described mathematically, the theory of grinding has not been developed to the point where the actual performance of the grinding equipment can be predicted quantitatively. However, three fundamental laws have been advanced:

Kick's Law—The work required to reduce the size of a given quantity of material is constant for the same reduction ratio regardless of the original size of the initial material.

Rittinger's Law—The work used for particulate size reduction is directly proportional to the new surface produced.

Bond's Law—The work used to reduce the particle size is proportional to the square root of the diameter of the particles produced.

In general, however, these laws have been useful only in providing trends and qualitative information on the grinding process. Usually laboratory testing is required to evaluate the performance of particular equipment. A work index, developed from Bond's Law, is a useful way of comparing the efficiency of milling operations.[1] A grindability index, which has been developed for a number of materials, also can be used to evaluate mill performance.[2]

A number of other factors also must be considered in equipment selection. Abrasion or mill wear is an important factor in the grinding of hard materials, particularly in high-speed, close-clearance equipment (eg, hammer mills). In some instances mill wear may be so extensive as to lead to highly contaminated products and excessive maintenance costs that make the milling process uneconomical. Hardness of the material, which often is related to abrasiveness, also must be considered. This usually is measured on the Moh's Scale. Qualitatively, materials from 1 to 3 are considered as soft and from 8 to 10 as hard. Friability (ease of fracture) and fibrousness can be of equal importance in mill selection. Fibrous materials, eg, plant products, require a cutting or chopping action and usually cannot be reduced in size effectively by pressure or impact techniques. A moisture content above about 5% will in most instances also create a problem and can lead to agglomeration or even liquefaction of the milled material. Hydrates often will release their water of hydration under the influence of a high-temperature milling process and thus may require cooling or low-speed processing.

Methods and Equipment—When a narrow particle-size distribution with a minimum of fines is desired, closed-circuit milling is advantageous. This technique combines the milling equipment with some type of classifier (see *Particle-Size Measurement and Classification*). In the simplest arrangement, a screen is used to make the separation, and the oversize particles are returned to the mill on a continuous basis while the particles of the desired size pass through the screen and out of the grinding chamber. Over milling, with its subsequent production of fines, thereby is minimized. Equipment also has been designed to combine the sieving and milling steps into a single operation (see *Centrifugal-Impact Mills and Sieves*).

In order to avoid contamination or deterioration, the equipment used for pharmaceuticals should be fabricated of materials which are chemically and mechanically compatible with the substance being processed. The equipment should be disassembled readily for ease in cleaning to prevent cross-contamination. Dust-free operation, durability, simplified construction and operation and suitable feed and outlet capacities are additional considerations in equipment selection.

While there is no rigid classification of large-scale comminution equipment, it generally is divided into three broad categories based on feed and product size:

1. *Coarse crushers* (eg, jaw, gyratory, roll and impact crushers).
2. *Intermediate grinders* (eg, rotary cutters, disk, hammer, roller and chaser mills).
3. *Fine grinding mills* (eg, ball, rod, hammer, colloid and fluid-energy mills; high-speed mechanical screen and centrifugal classifier).

Machines in the first category are employed ordinarily where the size of the feed material is relatively large, ranging from 1½ to 60″ in diameter. These are used most frequently in the mineral crushing industry and will not be considered further. The machines in the second category are used for feed materials of relatively small size and provide products which fall between 20- and 200-mesh. Those in the third category produce particles, most of which will pass through a 200-mesh sieve, though, often the particle size of the products from fine grinding mills is well into the micron range.

The comminution effect of any given operation can be described mathematically in terms of a matrix whose elements represent the probabilities of transformation of the various-size particles in the feed material to the particle sizes present in the output. The numerical values of the elements in the transition matrix can be determined experimentally and the matrix serves to characterize the mill. Matrices of this type are frequently a function of feed rate and feed particle-size distribution but are useful in predicting mill behavior. Multiplication of the appropriate comminution matrix with the feed-size distribution line-matrix yields the predicted output-size distribution.

Intermediate and Fine Grinding Mills—The various types of comminuting equipment in this class generally employ one of three basic actions or, more commonly, a combination of these actions.

1. *Attrition*—This involves breaking down of the material by a rubbing action between two surfaces. The procedure is particularly applicable to the grinding of fibrous materials where a tearing action is required to reduce the fibers to powder.
2. *Rolling*—This uses a heavy rolling member to crush and pulverize the material. Theoretically, only a rolling-crushing type of action is involved, but in actual practice some slight attrition takes place between the face of the roller and the bed of the mill.
3. *Impact*—This involves the operation of hammers (or bars) at high speeds. These strike the lumps of material and throw them against each other or against the walls of the containing chamber. The impact causes large particles to split apart, the action continuing until small particles of required size are produced. In some instances high-velocity air or centrifugal force may be used to generate high-impact velocities.

Roller Mills in their basic form consist of two rollers revolving in the same direction at different rates of speed. This principle, which provides particle-size reduction mainly through compression (crushing) and shear has been applied to the development of a wide variety of roller mills. Some use multiple smooth rollers or corrugated, ribbed or saw-toothed rollers to provide a cutting action. Most allow adjustment of the gap between rollers to control the particle size of the product. The roller mill is quite versatile and can be used to crush a variety of materials.

An example of a pharmaceutical roller mill is the Crack-U-Lator, in which a series of ribbed rollers are adjusted to reduce sequentially the particle size of the product to produce the desired distribution. The design allows particles which are smaller than the gap between the rollers to pass to the next stage without unnecessary size reduction, thus reducing fines.

Hammer Mills consist of a rotating shaft on which are mounted either rigid or swing hammers (beaters). This unit is enclosed with a chamber containing a grid or removable screen through which the material must pass. On the upper part is the feed hopper. As the material enters the chamber, the rapidly rotating hammers strike against it and break it into smaller fragments. These are swept downward against the screen where they undergo additional "hammering" action until they are reduced to a size small enough to pass through the openings and out. Oversize particles are hurled upward into the chamber where they also undergo further blows by the revolving hammers.

These mills operate at high speed and generally with controlled feed rate. Both impact and attrition provide the grinding action. Particle size is regulated by rotor speed, feed rate, type and number of hammers, clearance between hammers and chamber wall and discharge openings. At a constant screen opening, the speed of the mill and the thickness of the screen will affect the particle size of the milled powder,[3] as shown in Fig 1. The higher the speed, the steeper the approach angle of the particle to the screen hole. Thus, for any screen size opening, the higher the blade speed, the smaller the particle obtained. Increasing the screen thickness will have a similar effect. In general flat-edged blades are most effective for pulverizing, while sharp-edged blades will act to chop or cut fibrous materials.

The FitzMill Comminutor (Fig 2) is an example of this type of mill. It can be used in either the hammer or knife-blade configuration and can be fitted with a wide range of screen sizes to fulfill a variety of milling specifications.

A wide range of particle sizes down to the micron size can be produced by these mills. The particle shape, however, is generally sharper and more irregular than that produced by compression methods. When very fine particles are desired, hammer mills can be operated in conjunction with an air classifier. Under such conditions a narrower particle-size distribution and lower grinding temperatures are obtained. Fine pulverizing of plastic material can be accomplished in these mills by embrittlement with liquid N_2 or CO_2 or by jacketing the grinding chamber.

Centrifugal-Impact Mills and Sieves are useful to minimize the production of fine particles, since their design combines sieving and milling into a single operation. The mill consists of a nonrotating bar or stator which is fixed within a rotating sieve basket. The particles which are smaller than the hole size of the sieve can pass through the mill without comminution; however, the particles or agglomerates larger than the hole size are directed by centrifugal force to impact with the stator. The sieve baskets also can be constructed to have a cutting edge which can aid in particle-size reduction without impact with the stator. The Quick Sieve (Fig 3), Turbo Sieve and CoMill are examples of this type of mill.

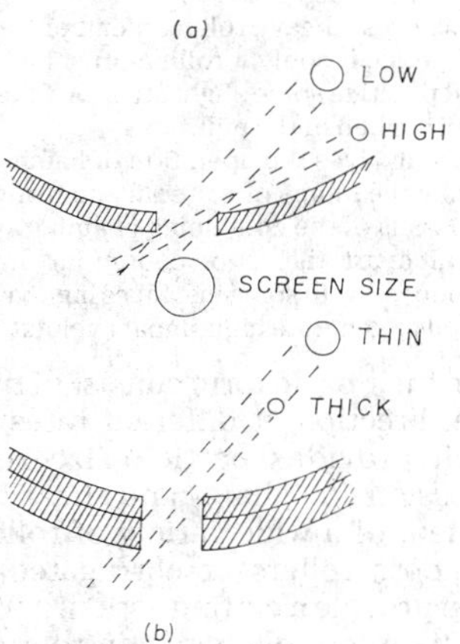

Fig 1. The influence of (*a*) mill speed and (*b*) screen thickness on particle size at a constant screen-opening size.[3]

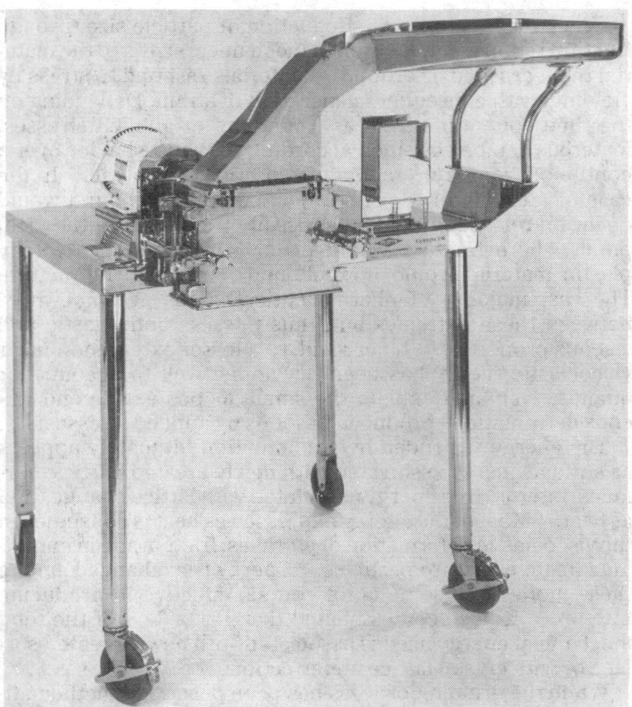

Fig 2. EZ-Clean FitzMill Comminutor (courtesy, Fitzpatrick).

Cutter Mills are useful in reducing the particle size of fibrous material and act by a combined cutting and shearing action. They consist of a horizontal rotor in which are set a series of knives or blades. This rotor turns within a housing into which are set stationary bed knives. The feed is from the top and a perforated plate or screen is set into the bottom of the housing through which the finished product is discharged. The particle size and shape is determined by the plate size, gap between rotor and bed knives and size of the openings. A number of rotor styles are available to provide different particle shapes and sizes, though cutter mills are normally not designed to produce particles finer than 80- to 100-mesh.

Attrition Mills make use of two stone or steel grinding plates, one or both of which revolve to provide grinding mainly through attrition. These mills are most suitable for friable or medium-hard, free-flowing material.

A double-runner attrition mill is an example of a mill which uses two rotating disks revolving in opposite directions. The particle-size reduction is controlled by varying the speed at which the disks revolve, the space between the disks and the size and number of ridges and indentations in the face of the disks. By appropriate combination with a classifier, particle sizes ranging from 10-mesh to 20 μm can be obtained by these attrition mills.

Chaser Mills are so called because two heavy granite stones, or chasers, mounted vertically like wheels and connected by a short horizontal shaft, are made to revolve or *chase* each other upon a granite base surrounded by a curb. Revolution of the chasers produces an upward current of air; this carries over the lighter particles, which fall outside the curb and subsequently are collected as a fine powder.

Pebble or Ball Mills, sometimes called "pot mills" or "jar mills," are operated on the principle of attrition and impact, the grinding being effected by placing the substance in jars or cylindrical vessels, lined with porcelain or a similar hard substance and containing "pebbles" or "balls" of flint, porcelain, steel or stainless steel. These cylindrical vessels revolve hori-

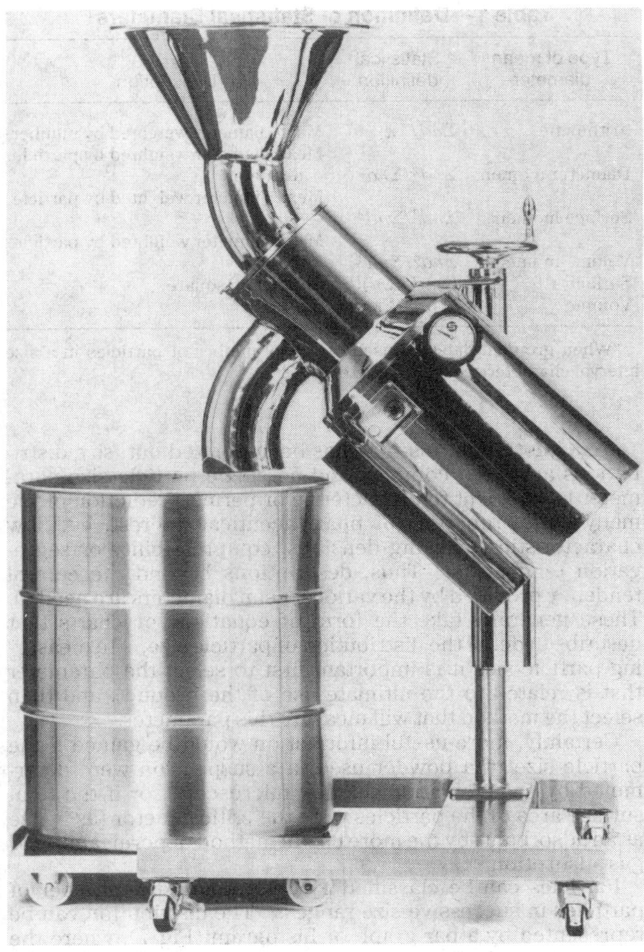

Fig 3. Quick Sieve (courtesy, Glatt Air).

zontally on their long axis and the tumbling of the pebbles or balls over one another and against the sides of the cylinder produces pulverization with a minimum loss of material. Ball-milling is a relatively slow process and generally requires many hours to produce material of suitable fineness. In order to keep the grinding time within reasonable limits, coarse material (> 10-mesh) should be preground before introduction into a ball mill. Fig 4 shows a sectional view of a single jar mill. Rod mills are a modification in which rods about 3 inches shorter than the length of the mill are used in place of balls. This results in a lower production of fines and a somewhat more granular product.

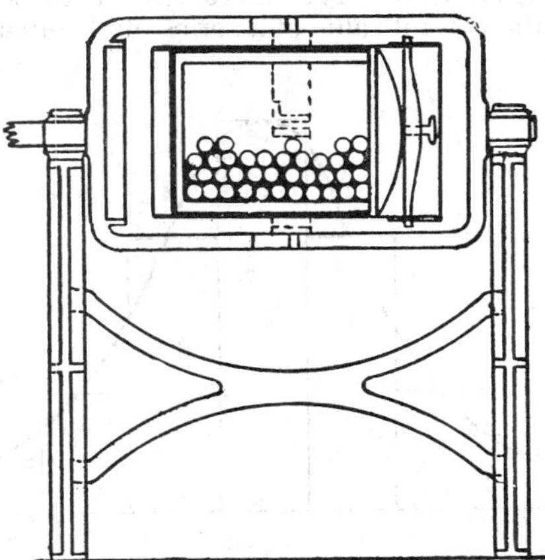

Fig 4. Single jar mill.

Vibrating Ball Mills, which also combine attrition and impact, consist of a mill shell containing a charge of balls similar to rotating ball mills. However, in this case the shell is vibrated at some suitable frequency, rather than rotated. These mills offer the advantage of being free of rotating parts, and thus can be integrated readily into a particle classifying system or other ancillary equipment. Furthermore, there have been several studies which have demonstrated that the vibrating ball mill will grind at rates often as high as 20 to 30 times that of the conventional tumbling mill and offer a higher order of grinding rate and efficiency than other prevailing milling procedures.

Fluid-Energy Mills are used for pulverizing and classifying extremely small particles of many materials. The mills have no moving parts, grinding being achieved by subjecting the solid material to streams of high velocity elastic fluids, usually air, steam or an inert gas. The material to be pulverized is swept into violent turbulence by the sonic and super sonic velocity of the streams. The particles are accelerated to relatively high speeds and when they collide with each other the impact causes violent fracture of the particles.

One type of fluid-energy mill is shown in Fig 5. The elastic grinding fluid is introduced through nozzles in the lower portion of the mill under pressures ranging from 25 to 300 psi. In this way, a rapidly circulating flow of gas is generated in the hollow, doughnut-shaped mill. A Venturi feeder introduces the coarse material into the mill and the particles enter into the jet stream of rapidly moving gas. The raw material is pulverized quickly by mutual impact in the reduction chamber. As the fine particles form they are carried upward in the track. Particles are ground simultaneously and classified in this process. The smaller particles are entrapped by the drag of gas leaving the mill and are carried out to a collecting chamber or bag. Centrifugal force at the top of the chamber stratifies the larger, heavy particles and their greater momentum carries them downward and back to the grinding chamber.

A major advantage of the fluid-energy mill is that the cooling effect of the grinding fluid as it expands in the grinding chamber more than compensates for the moderate heat generated during the grinding process. Another advantage is the rather narrow range of particle sizes produced. When precise control of particle size is an important factor, the fluid-energy mill produces very narrow ranges of particles with minimum effort.

One major disadvantage is the necessity of controlling the feeding of the coarse, raw material into the jet stream. Often, the feeding device becomes clogged by a clump of material,

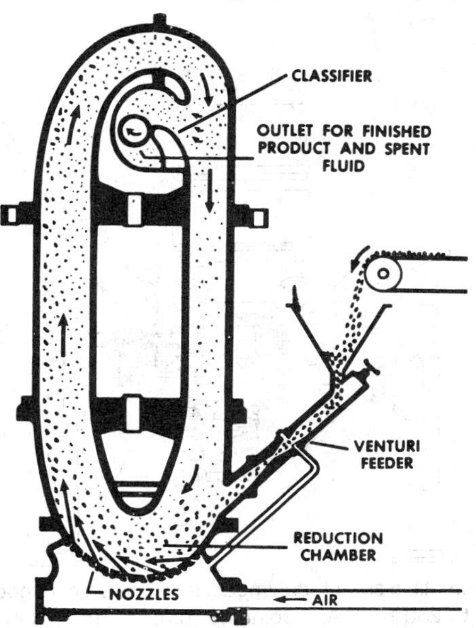

Fig 5. The Jet-O-Mizer fluid energy mill (courtesy, Fluid Energy).

and special feeding devices must be built to produce a uniform rate of feed.

Centrifugal-Impact Pulverizers also have been found to be effective for the reduction of the particle size of a wide variety of materials ranging from very soft, organic chemicals to hard, abrasive minerals. In addition, this type of mill is suited well for the size reduction of heat-sensitive substances. Basically, in these pulverizers, the material is fed into the center of a spinning rotor which applies a high centrifugal force to the particles. The material, thus accelerated, moves toward the impactor set at the periphery of the rotor. On striking these impactors the material is hurled against the outer casing where final reduction is achieved. Processed material is removed from the bottom of the conical discharge hopper (Fig 6). Particle-size reduction in the range of 10- to 325-mesh can be obtained with this type of mill with a minimum of fines.

Particle-Size Measurement and Classification

Size and Distribution

Statistical Parameters—Monodisperse systems of particles of regular shape, such as perfect cubes or spheres, can be described completely by a single parameter, ie, length of a side or diameter. However, when either nonuniform size distributions or anisometric shapes exist, any single parameter is incapable of totally defining the powder. Measurements must be made over the total range of sizes present. Statistical diameters, for example, are useful measures of central size tendency and are computed from some measured property that is a function of size and related to a linear dimension. For irregular particles the assigned size will depend strongly on the method of measurement.

Once a method of assignment of numerical value for the diameter, surface area or other parameter has been established, the average value computed for the parameter is dependent on the weighting given the various sizes. Mean particle diameter is the most important single statistical parameter since, if the proper diameter is chosen, the various other parameters of interest such as specific surface area, number, mean particle weight, etc, often may be calculated. Thus, the choice of the mean diameter to be measured or calculated is based on its intended use. For example, specific surface area, which may control drug dissolution, frequently can be related to the root-mean square diameter. Depending on the method of measurement, various diameters are obtained; these will be discussed later. The particle diameters most commonly used are listed in Table 1.

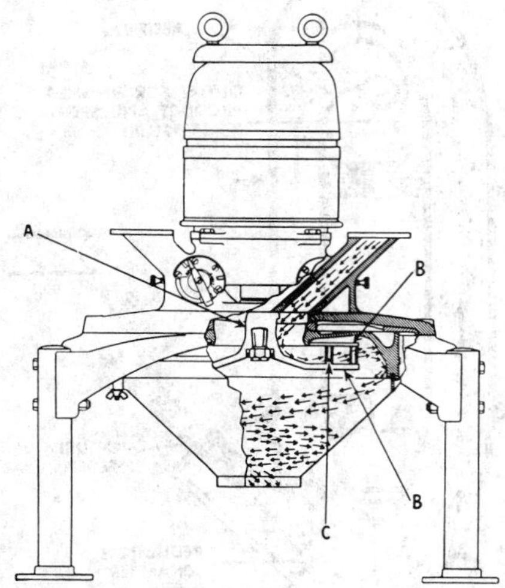

Fig 6. CentriMil, a centrifugal-impact mill, available in models ranging from 2 to 250 hp. A: Spinning roto; B: rotor hub disks; C; impacters (courtesy, Entoleter).

Table 1—Definition of Statistical Diameters[a]

Type of mean diameter	Statistical definition	Description
Arithmetic	$\Sigma nd/\Sigma n$	Mean diameter weighted by number
Diameter moment	$\Sigma nd^2/\Sigma nd$	Mean diameter weighted by particle diameter
Surface moment	$\Sigma nd^3/\Sigma nd^2$	Mean diameter weighted by particle surface
Volume moment	$\Sigma nd^4/\Sigma nd^3$	Mean diameter weighted by particle volume
Surface	$(\Sigma nd^2/\Sigma n)^{1/2}$	Root mean square
Volume	$(\Sigma nd^3/\Sigma n)$	

[a]When grouped data are used, n is the number of particles in a size interval characterized by a diameter, d.

Size Distributions—As has been pointed out, size distributions are often complex and no single particle size parameter is sufficient to characterize or permit prediction of the many bulk properties of pharmaceutical interest, eg, flow characteristics, packing densities, compressibility or segregation tendencies. Thus, descriptions beyond the central tendency provided by the various mean diameters are needed. These generally take the form of equations or charts that describe in detail the distribution of particle size. In measuring particle size it is important first to select the parameter that is related to the ultimate use of the product, and then select the method that will measure this parameter.

Certainly, more-useful information would be gained if the particle size of a powder used in a suspension were determined by sedimentation than by microscopy, or if the total surface area of the particles were the critical factor (as in use as an adsorbant) by the more useful method of permeability or gas adsorption.

Particles can be classified by determining the number of particles in successive size ranges. The distribution can be represented by a bar graph or histogram (Fig 7), where the widths of the bars represent the size range and the heights represent the frequency of occurrence in each range. A smooth curve drawn through the midpoints of the tops of the bars in this case results in a normal probability size-distribution curve. A line drawn through the center of the curve to the abscissa divides the area into two equal parts and represents the mean value. Since a number of other symmetrical distributions could have this same midpoint, a term to describe the scatter about the mean value is needed. Standard deviation (the root-mean square deviation about the mean) serves to define the spread of the curve on either side of the midpoint.

Most particulate material cannot, however, be described by a normal distribution curve. The resultant curves are usually skewed as shown in Fig 8, making mathematical analysis complex. In a skewed size distribution the mean value is affected by very large or very small values. In these cases the median (ie, the central value of a series of observations) is a

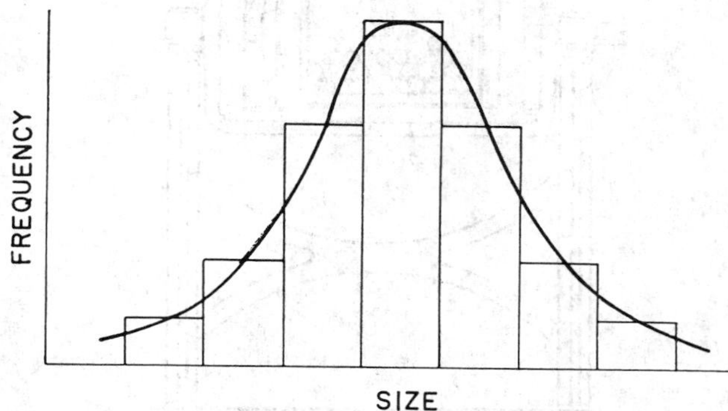

Fig 7. Symmetrical particle-size distribution curve.

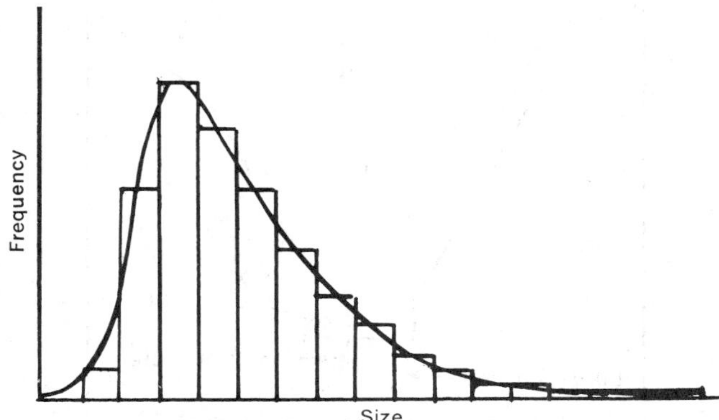

Fig 8. Skewed particle-size distribution curve.

more useful average. In a symmetrical distribution the mean and the median values are the same. Most asymmetrical size distribution curves relating to powders can be converted into symmetrical curves by using the logarithm of the size, ie, Log Normal Distribution curve. The symmetrical shape of the latter curve allows for simplified mathematical analysis.

Cumulative plots are also useful for particle-size distribution analysis. Here the cumulative percent of the particles which are finer (or larger) than a given size is plotted against the size. By use of logarithmic–probability paper the median size (geometric mean) and standard deviation (geometric standard deviation) can be obtained readily by graphical solution. The median is the 50% size and the standard deviation is the slope of the line and equal to the ratio 50% size/15.87% size (Fig 9).

Size Measurement

Frequently, particle-size measurements are made in conjunction with separation of the powder into fractions on the basis of size. Methods that lead primarily to size distribution analysis only are discussed first, followed by methods in which classification by size is a central feature.

The basic processes employed for measurement, classification or fractionation of fine solid particles involve direct and indirect techniques. Direct methods measure the actual dimensions of the particle by use of a calibration scale as in microscopy and sieving. Indirect measurements make use of some characteristic of the particle that can be related to particle size; eg, sedimentation rates, permeability and optical properties.

Microscopy—Microscopic techniques have been classified as one of the most accurate of *direct* methods. Here, particles are sized directly and individually, rather than being grouped statistically by some other means of classification. The linear measurement of particles is made by comparison with a calibrated scale usually incorporated into the microscope. For spherical particles the size is defined by the measurement of the diameter. However, for other-shaped particles some other single size designation is generally used; eg, the diameter of a sphere with the same projected area as the nonspheroidal particle being measured. Other characteristic diameters based on various aspects of the projected particle outline as seen through the microscope also have been reported in the literature to describe non-spheroidal particles.

The method is rather tedious and other limitations are found in the techniques required for preparation of the slides and in the maximum resolution which sets the lower limits of particle size measurement using visible light. White light can resolve particles within the range of 0.2 to 100 μm. This lower limit can be decreased to about 0.1 μm by the use of ultraviolet light and to about 0.01 μm by the use of the ultramicroscope. The electron microscope finds its greatest usefulness in particle-size measurements in the range of 0.2 to 0.001 μm.

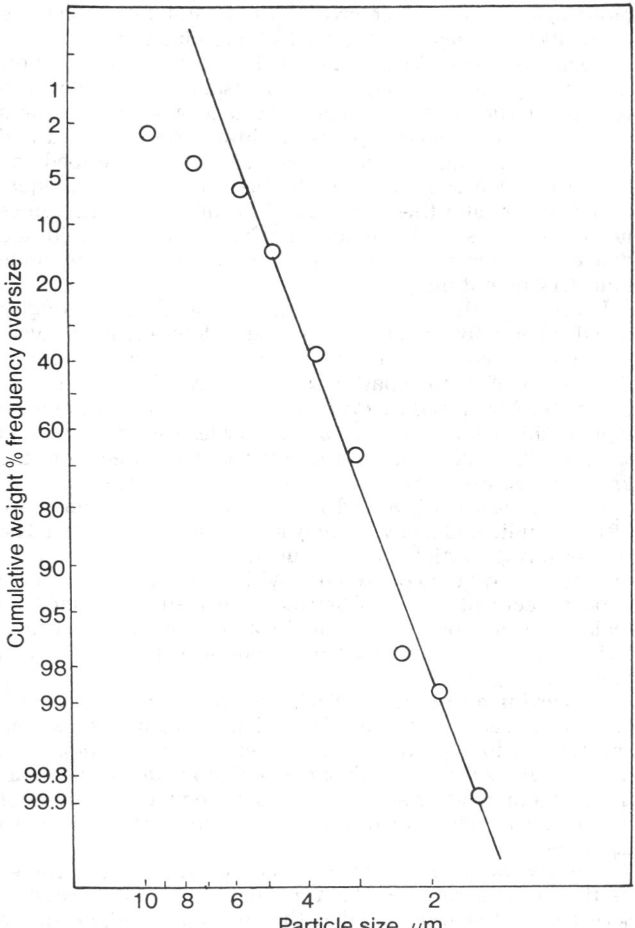

Fig 9. Log-probability plot of particle size versus cumulative weight % frequency oversize.

While microscopic methods for particle size determination are time consuming, tedious, and generally require more skill than some of the other techniques, they offer a number of advantages. They supply information about the shape and thickness that cannot be obtained by other methods and, in addition, supply a permanent record through use of photomicrographs.

A variety of semiautomated procedures have been developed to reduce the fatigue and tedium associated with manual counting of particles. These are represented by instruments such as the Imanco Quantimet 720 and the πMC System (*Millipore*), which scan the powder image in a manner similar to a TV scanner. The signal obtained is analyzed by a pulse-height analyzer and expressed as a particle-size distribution.

Adsorption of Gases—Adsorption of a solute from solution or of a gas at low temperatures onto powdered material serves as a measure of the particle surface area, generally reported as specific surface (area/unit mass). Common adsorption techniques use the adsorption of nitrogen and krypton at low temperatures. The volume of the gas adsorbed by a powdered sample is determined as a function of gas pressure, and an appropriate plot is prepared. The point at which a monomolecular layer of adsorbate occurs is estimated from the discontinuity that shows in the curve. The specific surface area then can be calculated from a knowledge of the volume of gas required to achieve this monolayer, and the area/molecule occupied by the gas, its molecular weight and density. Frequently, more complex expressions such as the Brunauer, Emmett and Teller (BET) equation must be used to describe the surface adsorption of some materials and determine the volume of gas required to produce an adsorbed monolayer. The surface properties of a number of pharmaceuticals have been investigated by this technique.

Permeability—When a gas or liquid is allowed to flow through a powdered material, the resistance to this flow is a function of such factors as specific surface of the powder, area of the bed, pore space, pressure drop across the bed and viscosity of the fluid. This resistance can be described and the specific surface calculated by the Kozeny-Carmen equation, which relates these factors. This method, while it does not provide a size distribution analysis, offers a rapid and convenient means of size estimation that is useful for some industrial operations.

Instruments that measure the rate of flow of a gas through a powder bed under controlled pressure differential are available commercially. The Sub-Sieve Sizer (*Fisher*) permits the reading of average particle size directly. The Blaine Permeameter (produced by *Precision Scientific*) uses the principle of filling the void spaces in a powder with mercury and then weighing it. The void fraction is calculated from the known density of mercury at different temperatures.

The calculations involved in permeability techniques are often complicated and yield only an average size of particles. In measuring particles in the subsieve ranges, rather large deviations may be encountered. With larger mesh sizes, some good agreement is found between the results obtained by techniques employing permeability and microscopy, particularly if the powders are made up of spherical or near-spherical particles.

Impaction and Inertial Techniques—The laws that govern the trajectories of particles in fluid streams are used in several methods of particle-size measurement. Impaction devices are based on the dynamics of deposition of fine particles in a moving air stream when directed past obstacles of defined geometric form, or when forced from a jet device onto a plane surface.

The *cascade impactor*, described by Pilcher *et al*,[4] forces particle laden air at a very high speed and fixed rate through a series of jets (each smaller than the preceding one) onto glass slides; impaction takes place in a series of stages. The velocities of the air stream and the particles suspended in it are increased as they advance through the impactor. As a result, the particles are classified by impaction on the different slides, with the larger particles on the top slides and the smaller ones on the downstream slides. Figure 10 illustrates the principle of the cascade impactor. The exact size of impacted particles on each slide subsequently must be determined. Size analyses may be obtained directly by theoretical treatment or prior calibration of the instrument.

Tillotson[5] described an instrument based on inertial principles similar to those of the cascade impactor. This instrument may be adapted for automatic readout of size distribution by means of light-scattering techniques and electronic counters. The method is claimed to provide complete particle-size distribution data in a few minutes.

Automatic Particle-Size Counters—The Coulter Counter, HIAC Counter and Gelman Automatic Particle Counter represent three examples of automatic counting equipment.

The *Coulter Counter* will determine the particle volume distribution of material suspended in an electrolyte-containing solution. A table of size ranges of several methods compared with the Coulter principle is shown in Fig 11. The principle underlying use of this instrument is described on page 502.

The *HIAC Counter* measures the size distribution of particles suspended in either liquids or gases. The standard models will measure sizes from 2 to 2500 μm at pressures up to 3000 psi. Basically, in this instrument the particles pass a window one-by-one. Each particle as it passes, depending on its size, interrupts some portion of a light beam. This causes an instantaneous reduction in the voltage from a photodetector which is proportional to the size of the particle. Several counting circuits with preset thresholds tally the particles by size.

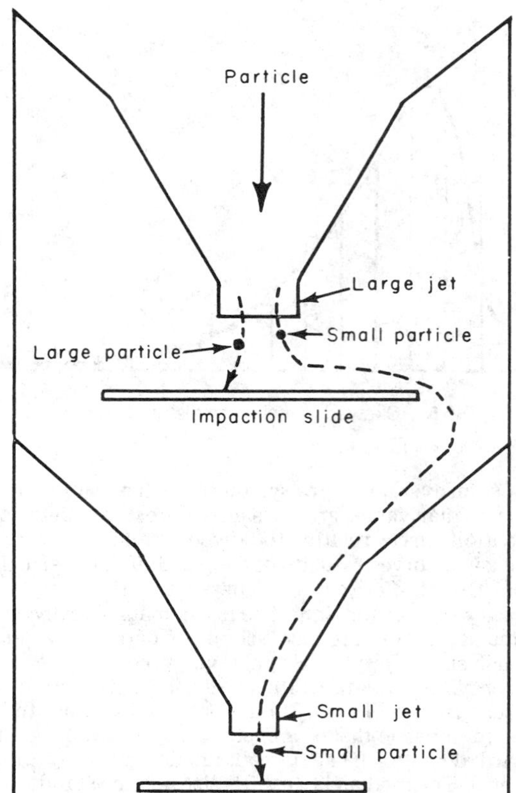

Fig 10. The principle of the cascade impactor.[3]

The *Gelman Counter* uses the principles of light-scattering to count particles in the air in the range of 0.5 μm and larger.

Size Classification

Sieving—This is one of the simplest and probably the most frequently used method for determining particle-size distribution. The technique basically involves size classification followed by the determination of the weight of each fraction.

In this technique, particles of a powder mass are placed on a screen made up of uniform apertures. By the application of some type of motion to the screen, the particles smaller than the apertures are made to pass through. The sieve motion generally is either (1) horizontal, which tends to loosen the packing of the particles in contact with the screen surface, permitting the entrapped subsieve particles to pass through or (2) vertical, which serves to agitate and mix the particles as well as to bring more of the subsieve particles to the screen surface.

One major difficulty associated with this method is the production of screens with uniform apertures, particularly in the very fine mesh sizes. As a result the practical lower limit for woven-wire mesh screens is about 43 μm (325-mesh).

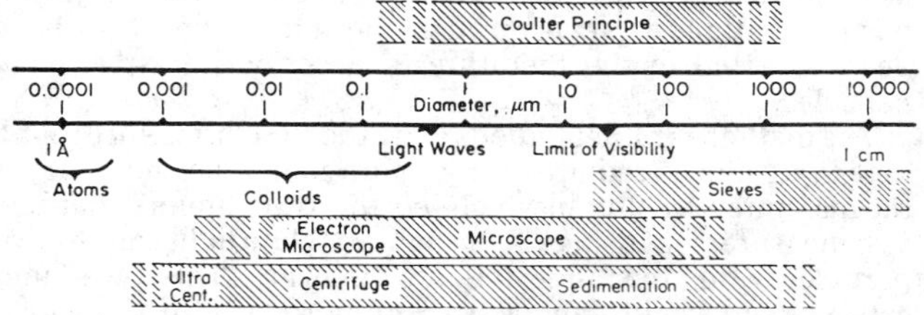

Fig 11. Size range of Coulter method compared with coverage of sieve, sedimentation and microscopic methods, and overlap of electron microscope and centrifuge ranges (courtesy, Coulter).

However, with the introduction of electroformed screens, sieves capable of analyzing particles in the 5-μm range are now available. In addition, "blinding" of the openings by oversized or irregular particles and inefficient presentation of the particles to the screen surface are problems associated with this technique. The use of horizontal and vertical screening motions, airjets, sudden periodic reversal of the sieve motion and continuous cycling all have been used in an attempt to eliminate these problems.

For continuous operations, the screens are attached to mechanical or electromagnetic devices which supply the energy required to shake the particles through the openings in the screen and also prevent accumulation of fines within the openings as this tends to clog them and slow down the operation. The use of an electromagnetic instead of mechanical drive provides a more-gentle sieving action with a resultant decrease in sieve wear, blinding and less machine noise. Sieves may be used either in a sequence of sizes through which the material must pass or singly in the required size.

This apparatus is useful in obtaining size-analysis data under controlled conditions. The sample is placed in the top of the nest of standard sieves arranged in a descending order. The length of time and force of vibration to which the sample is subjected may be preset by variable time and voltage controls. The controlled vibration causes the powder particles to pass through the sieves, each fraction coming to rest in the sieve through which it cannot pass. For the purpose of analysis, the weight of each fraction is determined and the percentage calculated.

The Sonic Sifter (*Allen-Bradley* and *ATM*) is a laboratory sifter that uses sonic oscillation to classify particles. A mechanical pulse action is used to reduce blinding and agglomeration in the subsieve sizes. This combination of sonic and mechanical agitation permits dry sifting down to 5 μm. US Standard Sieves are available for this unit from 3½- to 400-mesh and in precision electroformed mesh sizes from 150 to 5 μm.

Industrial-size mechanical sieves are varied in design and capacity, and include the gyratory, circular rotatory, vibrating, shaking and revolving sifters. In gyratory sifters the motion is in a single horizontal plane, but may vary from circular to reciprocal from the feed to the discharge end. The circular sifter also confines the screen motion to a horizontal plane, but in this case the total motion applied to the sieve is circular. The material enters the top of a gyratory sifter and spreads over the first sieve. Some of the finer particles drop through and are discharged into the "throughs" channel. The remaining powder moves to the next sieve in order, the process is repeated until complete separation is accomplished (Fig 12).

In centrifugal screening, the material is pushed through a spinning vertical wire cloth cylinder. Sharp cuts in particle size can be obtained with this type of equipment. Downward air flow, instead of shaking and tapping, has been used to move the particles through the screen openings; alternating with a reverse air flow serves to prevent "blinding," particularly with fine-mesh sieves.

Wet Screening—The addition of water sometimes is employed to dissolve out any unwanted binders, remove fines or surface contamination, and to reduce surface forces, particularly in micromesh sieves, that oppose the flow of particles through the sieve. Particles that tend to agglomerate or react with oxygen or moisture and thus cannot be dry-sieved often can be handled by wet-sieving. Particles in the 6 to 150-μm range have been classified with good precision using electroformed sieves. Some hydrophobic substances which resist wetting by water may be wet screened by the use of organic liquids such as petroleum ether, acetone or alcohol. Wet-screening may be accomplished by spraying both the screen surface and the material as it is fed onto the screen or by feeding a slurry of material directly onto the screen.

Screening Surfaces—A number of factors must be considered in selecting screening surfaces. Primary consideration is given to the size and shape of the aperture opening, the selection of which is determined by the particle size that is to be separated. Screens commonly used in pharmaceutical processing include *woven wire screens*, *bolting cloth*, *closely spaced bars* and *punched plates*. Punched plates are used for coarse sizing; their holes may be round, oval, square or rectangular. The plates must be sturdy and with stand rough service. Sizes in common use range upward from ¼ in.

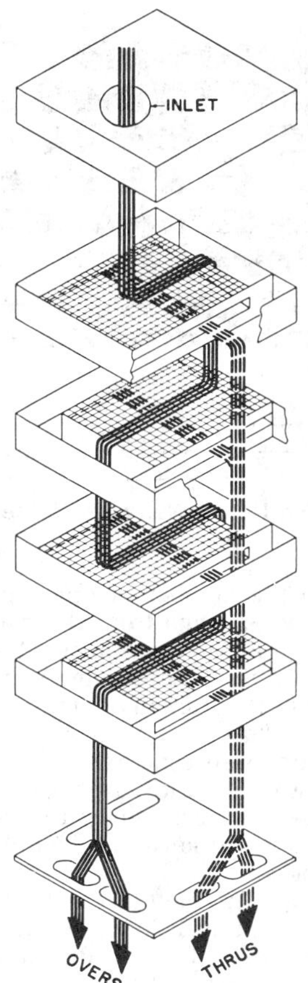

Fig 12. Gyratory sifter (courtesy, Sprout Waldron).

Most screening, however, is accomplished with woven-wire screens ranging in size from those with 400 openings/in to screens with 4-in square openings or larger. There are numerous types of woven wire screens, including plain, twilled and braided weave. An example of the plain and twilled weave is shown in Figs 13 and 14.

In the US, the two common standards are the *Tyler Standard* and *US Standard* sieves. In both these series the sieve

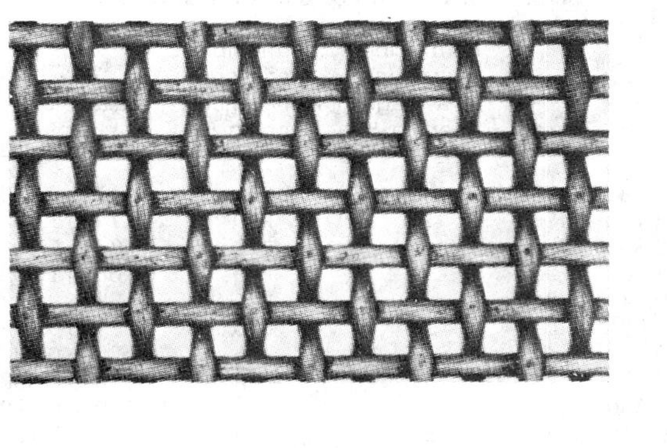

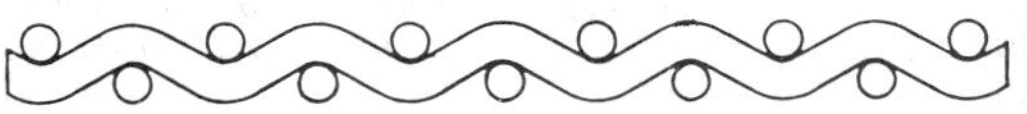

Fig 13. Plain weave screen.

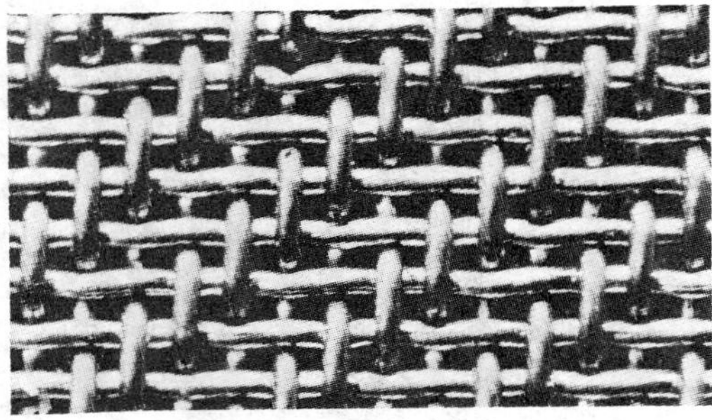

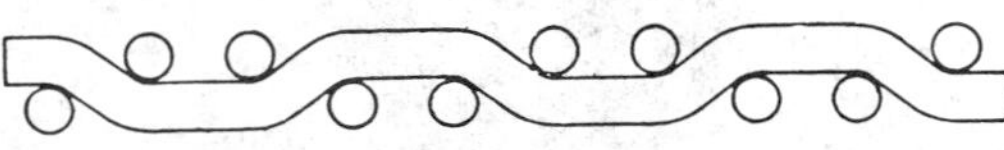

Fig 14. Twilled weave screen.

number refers to the number of openings per linear inch. For most purposes, screens from the two series are interchangeable, though in a few instances the number designations are different. Since these numbers do not define the size of the openings the Bureau of Standards has established specifications for *Standard Sieves*, as given in Table 2. These specifications also establish tolerances for the evenness of weaving, as irregularities from careless weaving might permit much larger particles to pass the sieve than would be indicated. The standard sieves used for pharmaceutical testing are of wire cloth.

Sedimentation—This method employs the settling of particles in a liquid of a relatively low density, under the influence of a gravitational or centrifugal field. In free-settling (ie, no particle–particle interference) the particles are supported by hydraulic forces and their fall can be described by Stokes' law. However, in most real situations particle–particle interference, nonuniformity and turbulence are all present, resulting in more complex settling patterns. The Andreason pipet, which is based on sampling near the bottom of a glass sedimentation chamber, is perhaps the best known of the early instruments. With centrifugation, entrainment of particles in the currents produced by other particles also may interfere with fractionation.

Gravitational settling chambers often are used for large-scale separation of relatively coarse particles in the range of 100 μm. Centrifugal devices are useful for the separation of much smaller particles (5 to 10 μm).

Sedimentation balances are available which provide a means of directly weighing particles at selected time intervals as they fall in a liquid system. For continuous observations, automatic recording balances also are available. A commercially available instrument called a *Micromerograph* uses the principle of sedimentation in an air column. This instrument and others related to it in principle offer more rapid determinations than those which use a liquid medium. There are, however, serious uncertainties in the method which must be taken into consideration. Deviations from Stokes' law and impaction of particles against the inner wall of the settling chamber are sources of possible error.

Table 2—Nominal Dimensions of Standard Sieves

No	Sieve opening, mm	Sieve opening, μm	Permissible variation in average opening, %	Permissible variation in maximum opening, %	Wire diameter, mm
2	9.52	9520	±3	+5	2.11 to 2.59
4	4.76	4760	±3	+10	1.14 to 1.68
8	2.38	2380	±3	+10	0.74 to 1.10
10	2.00	2000	±3	+10	0.68 to 1.00
20	0.84	840	±5	+15	0.38 to 0.55
30	0.59	590	±5	+15	0.29 to 0.42
40	0.42	420	±5	+25	0.23 to 0.33
50	0.297	297	±5	+25	0.170 to 0.253
60	0.250	250	±5	+25	0.149 to 0.220
70	0.210	210	±5	+25	0.130 to 0.187
80	0.177	177	±6	+40	0.114 to 0.154
100	0.149	149	±6	+40	0.096 to 0.125
120	0.125	125	±6	+40	0.079 to 0.103
200	0.074	74	±7	+60	0.045 to 0.061

The Carey and Stairmand *photosedimentometer* photo graphs the tracks of particles as they fall in a dispersion medium. The size determination is derived from the length of the photographic track, which is an indication of the distance traveled by the particles, and the time of exposure of the photograph.

Elutriation—In this process the particles are suspended in a moving fluid, generally water or air. In vertical elutriation at any particular velocity of the fluid, particles of a given size will move upwards with the fluid, while larger particles will settle out under the influence of gravity. In horizontal elutriation a stream of suspended particles is passed over a settling chamber. Particles that leave the stream are collected in the bottom of the chamber. Normally, for all elutriation techniques, both undersize and oversize particles appear in each fraction and recycling is required if a clean cut is desired. By varying the fluid velocities stepwise the sample may be separated into fractions. The amount in each fraction then can be determined and the size limits calculated by the use of the Stokes' equation or measured directly by microscopy. Air elutriation usually will give a sharper fractionation in a shorter time than will water elutriation.

Centrifugal elutriation is basically the same process, except in this case the fluid stream is caused to spin so as to impart a high centrifugal force to the suspended particles. Those particles which are too large to follow the direction of flow separate out on the walls or bottom of the elutriator or cyclone. The finer particles escape with the discharge stream. Separation down to about 0.5 μm can be achieved with some centrifugal classifiers.

The DorrClone (*Dorr-Oliver*) (Fig 15) is an example of a centrifugal-type classifier. The feed enters tangentially into the upper section. Centrifugal forces in the vortex throw the coarser particles to the wall where they collect and then drop down and out of the unit. The fine particles move to the inner spiral of the vortex and are displaced upward and finally out of the top of the unit.

Inertial elutriators, which use an abrupt change in direction of the fluid stream to produce separation, are effective down to about 200-mesh. However, as with other elutriators a clean cut usually cannot be obtained without recycling.

Felvation is a unique process that combines elutriation and sieving along with a varying fluid flow rate and a turbulent fluidized bed to achieve particle separation. The particles are fluidized within the felvation column. By gradually increasing the fluid flow rate the very fine particles are brought up to and then through a sieve surface set into the upper section of the column. These fines are filtered subsequently out of the fluid stream. A further increase in the fluid flow rate causes larger and larger particles to move through the sieve. The final stage is reached when particles just larger than the sieve aperture are elutriated up to the sieve. Because of the way in which the particles are presented to the sieve, very little blinding of the openings occur. Furthermore, since the sieve need only serve as a "go, no go" gauge and not as a supporting surface for the powder, a relatively small sieve surface is required. Thus, the more-uniform but more-expensive electroform sieves, even down to a 10-μm size, can be used in this process.

Miscellaneous Methods—Numerous other methods have been applied to particle-size determination, including X-ray and electron diffraction, ultrasound, flotation and electrostatic, magnetic and dielectrophoretic methods. These techniques either are used principally as research tools or are industrial-scale methods of use outside the pharmaceutical

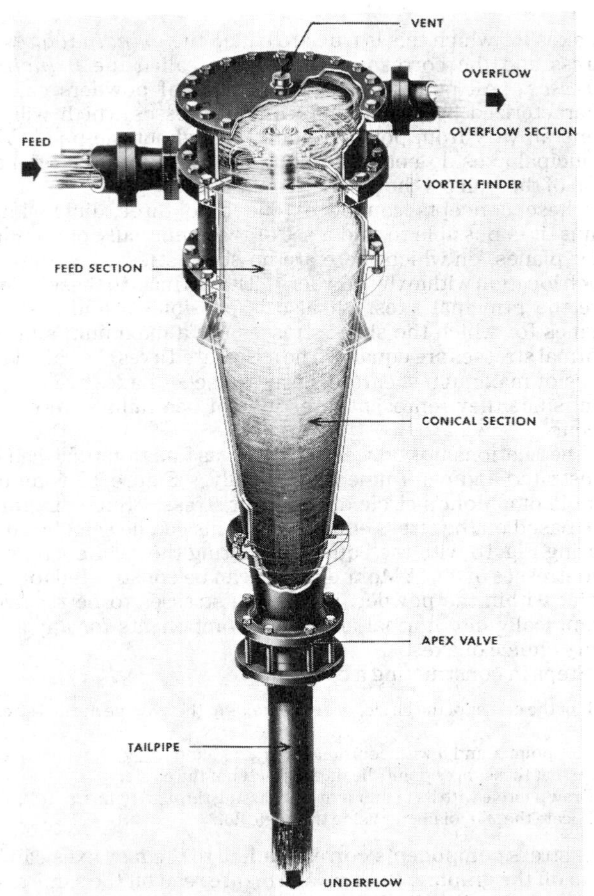

Fig 15. DorrClone, a hydrocentrifugal classifier (courtesy, Dorr-Oliver).

industry. Detailed descriptions of their principles of operation and their applications can be found in the *Bibliography*.

Solids Handling

Packing and Bulk Properties

Bulk Density; Angles of Repose—Systems of particulate solids are the most complex physical systems encountered in pharmacy. No two particles in a powder are identical and the nature of momentum and energy exchange between particles defies description except in the most idealized and approximate terms. Bulk properties of powders are determined in part by the chemical and physical properties of their component solids and in part by the manner in which the various components interact. These interactions in turn frequently depend on the past history of the powder bed as well as on the ambient conditions.

The static properties of a particulate bed depend on particle–particle interactions and, in particular, on the way in which applied stresses are distributed through the bed. The number of contacts between particles and, hence, the average number of interparticulate contact points per particle increases as bed-packing increases. Packing may be expressed in terms of porosity, percent voids or fraction of solids by volume. Packings for regular arrangements of uniform spheres can be calculated and range in fractional solids from 0.53 for cubic to 0.74 for tetrahedral lattices. Powders comprised of irregular-shaped particles in a distribution of sizes can pack to fractional densities approaching unity.

The manner in which stresses are transmitted through a bed and the bed's response to applied stress are reflected in the various angles of friction and repose. The most commonly used of these is the angle of repose which may be determined experimentally by a number of methods, with slightly differing results. The typical method is to pour the powder in a conical heap on a level, flat surface and measure the included angle with the horizontal. Angles of repose range from 23° for smooth uniform glass beads to 64° for granular limestone. Cohesive materials frequently behave in an anomalous manner yielding values in excess of 90°.

The angle of internal friction is a measure of internal stress distributions and is the angle at which an applied stress diverges as it passes through the bed. This angle together with the angle of slide are useful parameters in the design of storage/discharge bins. The latter angle is defined as the least slope at which a powder will slide down an inclined plane surface. Various other angles are in lesser use and will not be discussed here.

Statics—Powders at rest experience stresses that vary with location throughout their volume and arise from pressures exerted by the container as well as from the weight of the bed above. Each point within the bed experiences both normal and shear stresses in general. Normal stresses may be either tensile or compressive. The powder bed will remain motionless and no flow will occur unless the normal and/or the shear strength is exceeded at some point within the bed. In general, the yield strengths, both normal and shear, are functions of the normal and shear stresses at the point of interest and depend upon the orientation of the axes of reference and the nature of the powder itself. It is apparent that to understand powder flow it is necessary to understand the conditions under which bed failure occurs and powder flow is initiated and sustained.

Consider the stresses which are applied to the faces of a small cube that is centered about a point chosen at random within a powder bed. Normal stresses are designated σ_i, where the subscript indicates the axis normal to the face and shear stresses are designated τ_{ij}, where the first subscript indicates the face and the second indicates the direction of the applied force. If the cube has an edge length, l, which is not infinitesimal, and if a stress gradient exists within the region, the corresponding stresses on opposite faces of the cube will not be equal. However, if the cube is made progressively smaller and as l approaches zero, the stress values will converge to those at the point of interest. These forces are illustrated in Fig 16. It can be seen from this diagram that the state of stress at a point can be described by nine stress components.

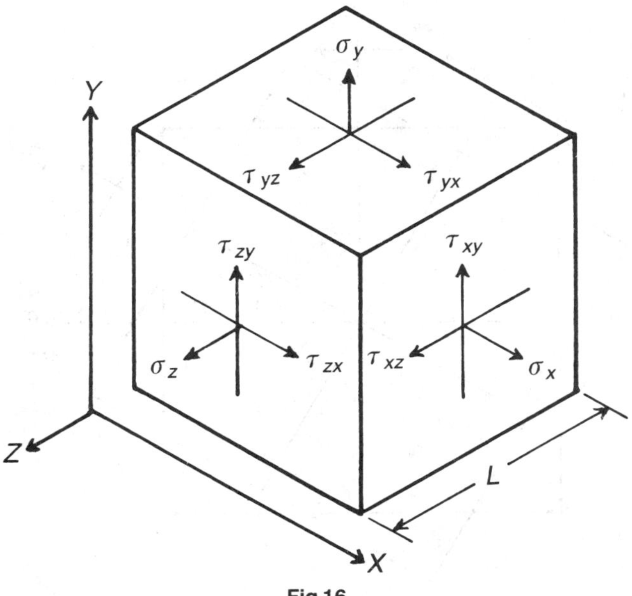

Fig 16.

If the system is in static equilibrium, and is not being accelerated translationally or rotationally, the forces which otherwise would result in movement must be in balance and have the effect of canceling each other. For example, τ_{xy} must equal τ_{yx} if rotation about the z-axis is not to occur. In a similar manner, shear and normal stresses, which would lead to translational movement along any of the three axes, also must balance.

Because the directions of the mutually perpendicular axes in Fig 16 were chosen arbitrarily, any other orientation of the cube corresponding to another set of axes also must result in a balance of forces. However, the distribution of stress among normal and shear components will depend on the particular axes selected. Thus, the stress condition of a powder can be analyzed in terms of the dependence of the normal and shear stresses on the direction chosen for the reference axes. This can be done by a method of analysis devised by Mohr, and can be visualized using a Mohr circle diagram, which permits stresses at any given point within a powder bed to be graphically resolved into normal, σ, and shear, τ, stresses for any arbitrary choice of axes.

For simplicity, assume that stress in the z-direction is not a function of z and that stress gradients exist in the x and y directions only. Stresses then can be analyzed in the xy plane without reference to the z-axis. Fig 17 shows the relationship between stresses relative to two xy coordinate systems at an angle θ to each other. If the condition of stress in the powder remains constant and only the angle θ between the two sets of reference axes is allowed to change, the resolution of stress into normal and shear components will be different for each set of axes and will depend on θ. By means of trigonometry, the relationships between these two sets of stresses is shown to be

$$\sigma_{x'} = \frac{\sigma_x + \sigma_y}{2} + \frac{\sigma_x - \sigma_y}{2}\cos 2\theta + \tau_{xy}\sin 2\theta$$

$$\sigma_{y'} = \frac{\sigma_x + \sigma_y}{2} - \frac{\sigma_x - \sigma_y}{2}\cos 2\theta - \tau_{xy}\sin 2\theta$$

$$\tau_{x'y'} = -\frac{\sigma_x - \sigma_y}{2}\sin 2\theta - \tau_{xy}\cos 2\theta$$

These equations permit the calculation of σ and τ values for any desired set of axes if the values are known for any given set of axes. In particular, if σ is chosen properly, $\tau_{x'y'}$ can be made to vanish and normal stresses only will remain. The set of axes for which this is true are called the *principal axes* of stress and the corresponding σ's are called the *principal stresses*. All points within static beds of powders can be characterized by principal axes and stresses which will, in general, vary from point to point throughout the bed. The principal axes do not correspond necessarily to the orientation of the walls of the powder container.

These concepts can be extended to three dimensions. Thus, it is possible to find a set of three mutually perpendicular planes, on which there are no shear stresses acting, for each location within the powder. The normals to these planes are the principal axes. It also is possible to find a set of planes for which the shear stresses are a maximum and the normal stresses are equal. The associated axes are called the axes of maximum shear. These two sets of axes are important since they represent directions of bed failure were it to occur.

The relationships between strcsses, as functions of θ, can be illustrated and determined graphically. Figure 18 is an example of a Mohr's circle diagram for stress. Such diagrams are based on the stress equations. This can be seen by comparing Fig 18 with the equations, noting the relationships of the stresses of θ. A Mohr diagram can be constructed for any point within the powder, permitting stresses to be resolved graphically into normal and shear components for any arbitrary choice of axes.

Steps in constructing a diagram are

Plot the center of the circle, p, on the σ axis at the average normal stress, $(\sigma_x + \sigma_y)/2$.

Plot point x and y with coordinates (σ_x, τ_{xy}) and (σ_y, τ_{xy}), respectively. Note that these three points lie on a diameter of the circle.

Draw a circle with its center at p and passing through points x and y.

Locate the $x'y'$ diameter using the angle 2θ.

The stress components corresponding to the new axes can be read off the graph. Both $\sigma_{x'}$ and $\sigma_{y'}$ are read off the same axes on the graph since both are normal stresses.

For the particular case in Fig 19, the principal axes lie at an angle of θ^* to the original axes. The axes of maximum shear stress lie at an angle of θ^- from the original axes since the xy line corresponding to maximum shear is perpendicular to the σ axis. Depending on the state of the powder, it is possible to have negative σ values, where the Mohr circle passes to the left of the τ axis.

The application of stress normal to a plane of shear influences the shear stress at which the powder fails. Because of this, a given powder will fail at various combinations of normal and shear stresses. These combinations can be expressed graphically by a line in the σ,τ plane which separates regions on the graph at which the powder either flows or is stable.

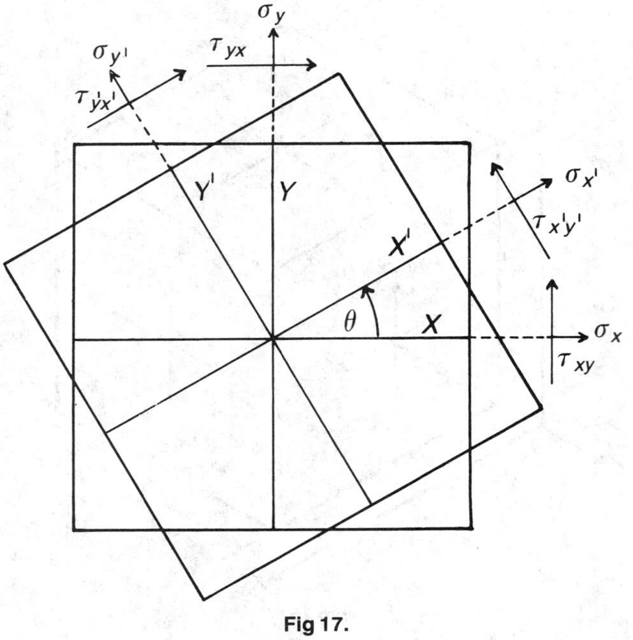

Fig 17.

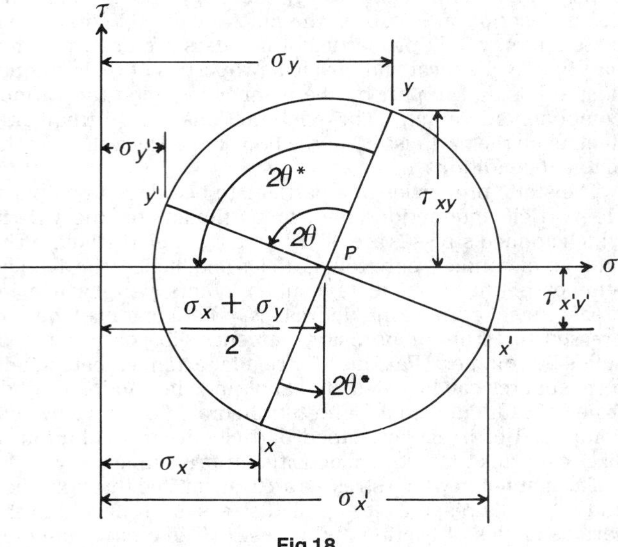

Fig 18.

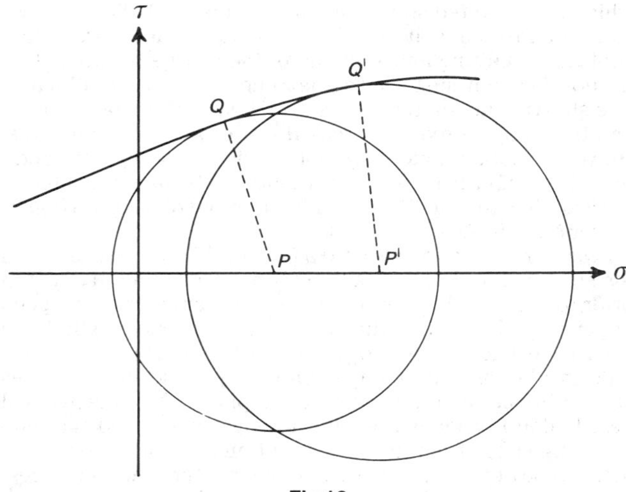

Fig 19.

This is shown in Fig 19 for a typical powder. Various powders will display curves which uniquely define their failure characteristics. Each point on such a curve corresponds to a σ,τ combination at which failure occurs and can be analyzed by constructing a Mohr circle which passes through the point and is centered on the intersection of a line perpendicular to the point, q, and the σ axis. An example is shown in Fig 19.

Bulk Properties—In addition to the angles of repose and friction which reflect bulk behavior, tensile and shear strength and dilatancy are of interest. Tensile strength is measured by forming a powder bed on a roughened and split plate. Half of the plate is laterally movable and the force necessary to rupture the bed by pulling the plate halves apart, minus sliding plate friction corrections, represents the bed tensile strength. Various methods of applying force to the movable plate are used, including tipping the plate from the horizontal and allowing it to react to gravity by rolling on steel balls.

Shear strength is determined from the force necessary to shear horizontally a bed of known cross-section. The Jenike shear cell is typical of those in use. It permits various loads to be applied normal to the plane of shear, whereby a shear failure locus can be determined. With the desired normal load applied, a steadily increasing shearing force is applied until failure occurs. These measurements are the basis for constructing powder-failure curves such as that in Fig 20.

When packed powder beds are deformed, local expansion occurs along the failure planes, barring fracture of the particles themselves. This phenomenon is termed dilatancy and is a direct consequence of the micromechanics of interparticulate movement. For one particle to move past another it is necessary for it to move to the side in order to move forward when the particles are in an "interlocked" arrangement. Such arrangements predominate in packed beds with the consequence that the collective sideways movements in the failure zone produce bed expansion. Room for expansion therefore must be provided when packed beds are forced to flow.

Mixing of Powders

Degree of Homogeneity—Many mathematical expressions have been proposed and used to express the degree of homogeneity of powders comprised of two or more components. For the most part measures of mixture uniformity have been statistical and based on either the standard deviation or variance of the composition from its mean value. It should be recognized that these indices of mixing are scalar quantities and are incapable of uniquely describing the composition profile of a given powder bed. A practical definition of mixing uniformity should be selected to relate as closely as possible to the desired properties of the mix. The manner in which samples are taken (number, size and location of samples) largely determines the validity and interpretation of the derived index.

The standard deviation is presented here as a representative index. It can be estimated solely from a set of n samples. If sample number i has composition x_i, and all samples are of uniform size, the sample standard deviation is defined in the usual way as

$$s = \sqrt{\sum_{i=1}^{n} (x_i - \overline{x})^2/(n - 1)}$$

where $\overline{x}$ is the mean composition estimated from the samples alone.

In sampling a bed, there should be assurance that the bed is sampled uniformly over its entirety. This can be done either by use of a sampling "thief" designed to probe the bed and collect samples at selected points or serially as the powder is discharged from the mixer.

The "scale of scrutiny" at which the powder is examined for uniformity is determined by the sample size. This should be chosen based on the ultimate use of the powder. For a tablet or capsule formulation the appropriate sample size is that of the dosage form.

Two important concepts related to mixing uniformity have been described by Danckwerts as the scale and intensity of segregation. Assuming that zones having uniform but differing compositions exist in a powder bed, the scale of segregation is a function of the size of the zones. The intensity of segregation is in turn a function of the composition differences among zones. Generally, the process of mixing tends to reduce the intensity of segregation while the scale of segregation passes through a minimum.

Mechanisms of Mixing and Segregation—Three primary mechanisms are responsible for mixing:

Convective movement of relatively large portions of the bed.
Shear failure which primarily reduces the scale of segregation.
Diffusive movement of individual particles.

Most efficient mixers operate to induce mixing by all three mechanisms. Thus, mixing can be considered to be a random shuffling-type operation involving both large and small particle groups and even individual particles. However, it should be noted that the use of random motion to achieve random distribution assumes that no other factors influence this distribution. This is rarely if ever the case in practice. Instead, a variety of properties of the powders being mixed influence this approach to complete randomness. Stickiness or slipperiness of particles must be considered, among other factors. As might be expected, the stickier the material, the less readily it mixes and demixes. Electrostatic forces on the particle surface also can produce marked effects on the mixing process, and in fact may produce sufficient particle–particle repulsion to make random mixing impossible.

By enabling particles to undergo movement relative to each other, mixers also provide the conditions necessary for segregation to occur. Any manipulation of a powder bed for purposes of conveying, discharge from a hopper, etc, provides the opportunity for segregation. Thus, many of the so-called mechanisms of segregation are actually conditions under which segregation can happen.

The segregation that occurs in free-flowing solids usually does so as a result of differences in particle size and, to a lesser extent, to differences in particle density and shape. The circumstances leading to segregation can be generalized from a fundamental physical standpoint. The necessary and sufficient conditions for segregation to occur are that (1) various mixture components exhibit mobilities for interparticulate movement which differ and (2) the mixture experience either a field which exerts a directional motive force on the particles or a gradient in a mechanism capable of inducing or modifying interparticulate movement. The combination of these conditions results in asymmetric particle migrations and leads to segregation.

Rates of Mixing and Segregation—Rate expressions analogous to those of chemical kinetics can be derived using any of the various indices of mixing as time dependent variables. When this is done, it usually is found that mixing follows a first-order approach to an equilibrium state of mixedness. More recently, mixing has been described as a stochastic process (by means of stationary and nonstationary Markov chains) in which the probabilities of particle movement from place to place in the bed are determined. When applied to a mixer, this approach is capable of indicating zones of greater and lesser mixing intensity.

Large-Scale Mixing Equipment—The ideal mixer should produce a complete blend rapidly with as gentle as possible a mixing action to avoid product damage. It should be cleaned and discharged easily, be dust-tight and require low maintenance and low power consumption. All of these assets generally are not found in any single piece of equipment, thus requiring some compromise in the selection of a mixer.

Rotating-Shell Mixers—The drum-type, cubical-shaped, double-cone and twin-shell blenders are all examples of this class of mixers. Drum-type blenders with their axis of rotation horizontal to the center of the drum are used quite commonly. These, however, suffer from poor crossflow along the axis. The addition of baffles or inclining the drum on its axis increases crossflow and improves the mixing action. Cubical- and polyhedron-shaped blenders with the rotating axis set at various angles also are available. However, in the latter, because of their flat surfaces, the powder is subjected more to a sliding than a rolling action, a motion which is not conducive to the most efficient mixing.

Double-cone blenders, an important class of rotating-shell or tumbling mixers, were developed in an attempt to overcome some of the shortcomings of the previously discussed mixers. Here, the mixing pattern provides a good crossflow with a rolling rather than a sliding motion. Normally, no baffles are required so that cleaning is simplified. The twin-shell blender is another important tumbling-type blender. It combines the efficiency of the inclined drum-type with the intermixing that occurs when two such mixers combine their flow.

The Cross-Flow blender (*Patterson-Kelley*) (Fig 20) is an example of a twin-shell blender. The uneven length of each shell in this blender provides additional mixing action when the powder bed recombines during each revolution of the blender. The Zig-Zag blender, an extension of the twin-shell blender, provides efficient continuous precision blending.

Fixed-Shell Mixers—The ribbon mixer, one of the oldest mechanical solid–solid blending devices, exemplifies this type of mixer. It consists of a relatively long troughlike shell with a semicircular bottom. The shell is fitted with a shaft on which are mounted spiral ribbons, paddles or helical screws, alone or in combination. These mixing blades produce a continuous cutting and shuffling of the charge by circulating the powder from end to end of the trough as well as rotationally. The shearing action that develops between the moving blade and the trough serves to break down powder agglomerates. However, ribbon mixers are not precision blenders; in addition, they suffer from the disadvantage of being more difficult to clean than the tumbler-type blenders and of having a higher power requirement.

Sigma-Blade and Planetary Paddle Mixers also are used for solid–solid blending, although most generally as a step prior to the introduction of liquids. Mixers with high-speed impeller blades set into the bottom of a vertical or cylindrical shell have been shown to be very efficient blenders. This type, in addition to its ability to produce precise blends, serves also to break down agglomerates rapidly. The mechanical heat buildup produced within the powder mix and the relatively high power requirement are often drawbacks to the use of this type of mixer; however; the shorter time interval necessary to achieve a satisfactory blend may offset these factors.

Vertical Impeller Mixers, which have the advantage of requiring little floor space, employ a screw-type impeller which constantly overturns the batch (Fig 21). The fluidized mixer is a modification of the vertical impeller type. The impeller is replaced by a rapidly moving stream of air fed into the bottom of the shell. The body of the powder is fluidized and mixing is accomplished by circulation and overtumbling in the bed (Fig 22). Generally, when precision solid–solid blend-

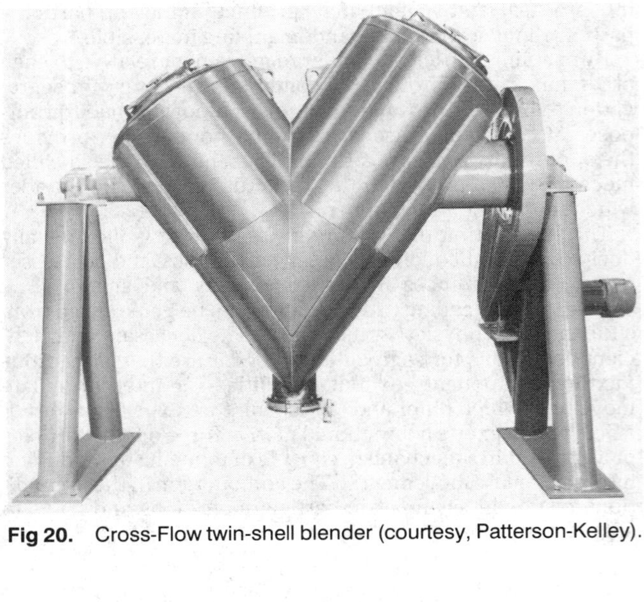

Fig 20. Cross-Flow twin-shell blender (courtesy, Patterson-Kelley).

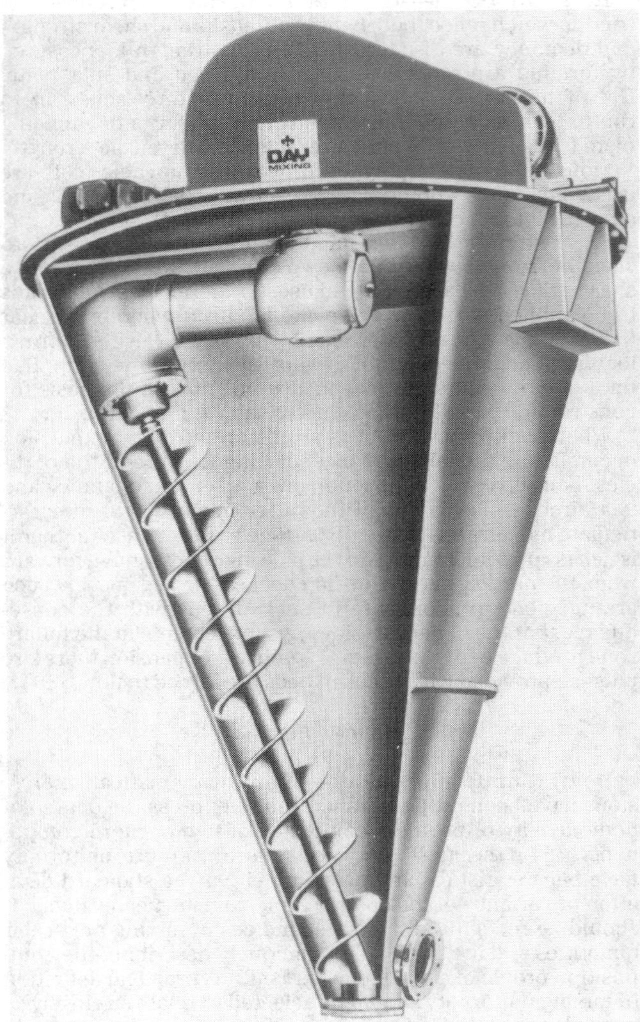

Fig 21. Cutaway view of the Mark II Mixer (courtesy, JH Day).

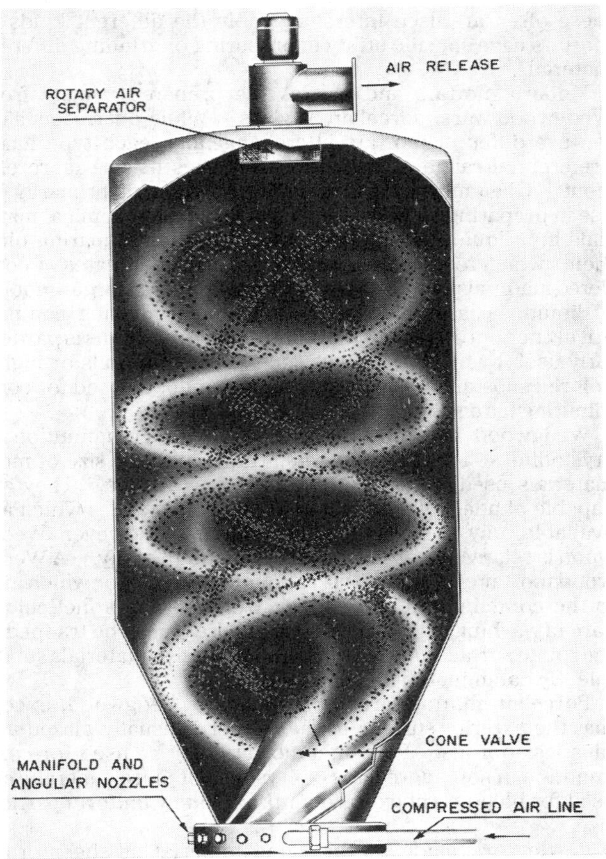

Fig 22. Fluidized air mixer (Courtesy, Sprout, Waldron).

ing is required, the rotating twin-shell or the double-cone-type blenders are recommended.

Motionless Mixers—These are in-line continuous processing devices with no moving parts. They consist of a series of fixed flow-twisting or flow-splitting elements. The Blendex (*Ross & Son*), designed for blending of free-flowing solids, is constructed to operate in a vertical plane. Four pipes interconnect with successive tetrahedral chambers, the number of chambers needed depending on the quality of mix desired. The powders enter the mixer from overhead hoppers and free fall through the mixer and are mixed by what is described as Interfacial Surface Generation. For two input streams entering this mixer the number of layers, L, emerging from each of the successive chambers, C, is $L = 2(4)^C$. Thus for 10 chambers over 2 million layers are generated. This type provides efficient batch or continuous mixing for a wide variety of solids without particle-size reduction or heat generation and essentially no maintenance. Units are available to mix quantities ranging from 100 to 5000 lb/hr.

Small-Scale Mixing Equipment—The pharmacist most generally employs the mortar and pestle for the small-scale mixing usually required for prescription compounding. However, the use of spatulas and sieves also may be used on occasion. The mortar and pestle method combines comminution and mixing in a single operation. Thus, it is particularly useful where some degree of particle-size reduction as well as mixing is required as in the case of mixtures of crystalline material.

The blending of powders with a spatula on a tile or paper, or spatulation, is used sometimes for small quantities of powders often as an auxiliary blending technique or when the compaction produced by the mortar and pestle technique is undesirable. Spatulation is a relatively inefficient method of mixing and is used rarely to prepare a finished dosage form.

Sieving usually is employed as a pre- or post-mixing method to reduce loosely held agglomerates and to increase the overall effectiveness of a blending process. When used alone as a solid–solid blending technique, several passes through the sieve are required to produce a reasonably homogeneous mix.

Storage and Flow

Flow Patterns—Discharge of powders from large-scale mixers, storage bins or machine-feed hoppers primarily generates flow in the form of shear failure, ie, the powder behaves in a manner analogous to a viscous liquid in laminar flow. The analogy ends at that point since conditions are then present in the powder bed conducive to segregation. The overall pattern of discharge from a bin takes the form of either funnel-flow or mass-flow. Bin-design characteristics, which take into account the powder's angles of slide and internal friction and its yield locus in terms of normal and shear stresses, determine which flow pattern will occur.

In funnel flow the powder moves in a column down the center of the bin toward the exit orifice at the bottom. Material surrounding this relatively rapidly moving core remains stationary or is drawn slowly into the core, which is fed primarily from the top where powder moves to the center and then down in the manner of a funnel.

The powder in a mass-flow bin moves downward toward the orifice as a coherent mass. When it reaches the tapered section of the bin leading to the orifice, it is compressed and flows in shear analogous to a plastic mass being compressed. This type of bin is advantageous for use with powders having a strong tendency to segregate.

The rate of discharge from a hopper varies as a function of the cube of the orifice diameter and is nearly independent of the height of the bed. An arch forms over the orifice which in effect is a boundary between material in essentially free fall and material in the closely packed condition of the powder bed. The rate of mass transport across this constantly renewed surface determines the rate of orifice flow. It has been shown that flow can be increased substantially if gas is pumped through the bed and across the orifice in the direction of solids flow. Flow conditioners are also an important means of improving flow and are discussed in Chapter 19.

Pneumatic Transport—This method of transporting powders is of interest since it can be used to mix powders at the same time as they are being conveyed. The method consists of propelling a solids–gas mixture along a conduit *via* a gas pressure drop. The solids are held in suspension by the turbulence of the gas stream. At low-solids concentrations, where the particles are relatively small, the solids are dispersed uniformly over the pipe cross-section. However, at higher solids content or with larger particles some stratification will occur in a horizontal pipe and solids will settle out if the pipe is overloaded.

Gas flow must be turbulent so as to suspend the solids; however, the solids behave as in laminar flow. Slippage between gas and solid occurs, particularly in vertical pipes, with the consequence that gas and solids flow rates are not in proportion to flow-stream composition. Further, smaller and less dense particles flow more rapidly than large and dense material and a chromatographic-like separation occurs. This is not a problem, however, once steady state is achieved. Because of the industrial importance of this process in many fields it has been investigated extensively and a number of useful theoretical and empirical expressions have been derived and may be used to predict conditions necessary for satisfactory pneumatic transport.

Powders as a Dosage Form

Historically, powders represent one of the oldest dosage forms. They are a natural outgrowth of man's attempt to prepare crude drugs and other natural products in a more conveniently administered form. However, with declining use of crude drugs and increasing use of many highly potent compounds, powders as a dosage form have been replaced largely by capsules and tablets.

In certain situations powders possess advantages and thus still represent a portion (although small) of the solid dosage forms currently being employed. These advantages are flexibility in compounding and relatively good chemical stability. The chief disadvantages of powders as a dosage form are they are time-consuming to prepare and they are not suited well for dispensing the many unpleasant-tasting, hygroscopic or deliquescent drugs.

Bulk powders have another serious disadvantage when compared with divided and individually weighed powders—inaccuracy of dose. The dose is influenced by many factors, including size of measuring spoon, density of powder, humidity, degree of settling, fluffiness due to agitation and personal judgment. Not only do patients measure varying amounts of powder when using the same spoon but they often select one differing in size from that specified by their physician.

Extemporaneous Techniques

In both the manufacturing and extemporaneous preparation of powders the general techniques of weighing, measuring, sifting, mixing, etc, as described previously are applied. However, the following procedures should receive special attention.

Use of geometric dilution for the incorporation of small amounts of potent drugs.

Reduction of particle size of all ingredients to the same range to prevent stratification of large and small particles.

Sieving when necessary to achieve mixing or reduction of agglomerates, especially in the preparation of dusting powders or powders into which liquids have been incorporated.

Heavy trituration, when applicable, to reduce the bulkiness of a powder.

Protection against humidity, air oxidation and loss of volatile ingredients.

Powders are prepared most commonly either as divided powders and bulk powders which are mixed with water or other suitable material prior to administration, or as dusting powders which are applied locally. They also may be prepared as dentifrices, products for reconstitution, insufflations, aerosols and other miscellaneous products.

The manually operated procedures usually employed by the pharmacist today are *trituration, pulverization by intervention* and *levigation.*

Trituration—This term refers to the process of reducing substances to fine particles by rubbing them in a mortar with a pestle. The term also designates the process whereby a mixture of fine powders is intimately mixed in a mortar. The circular mixing motion of the pestle on the powders contained in a mortar results in blending them and also breaking up soft aggregates of powders. By means of the application of pressure on the pestle, crushing or grinding also can be effected.

When granular or crystalline materials are to be incorporated into a powdered product, these materials are comminuted individually and then blended together in the mortar.

Pulverization by Intervention—This is the process of reducing the state of subdivision of solids with the aid of an additional material which can be removed easily after the pulverization has been completed. This technique often is applied to substances which are gummy and tend to reagglomerate or which resist grinding. A prime example is camphor which cannot be pulverized easily by trituration because of its gummy properties. However, on the addition of a small amount of alcohol or other volatile solvent, this compound can be reduced readily to a fine powder. Similarly, iodine crystals may be comminuted with the aid of a small quantity of ether. In both instances the solvent is permitted to evaporate and the powdered material is recovered.

Levigation—In this process a paste is first formed by the addition of a suitable nonsolvent to the solid material. Particle-size reduction then is accomplished by rubbing the paste in a mortar with a pestle or on an ointment slab using a spatula. Levigation generally is used by the pharmacist to incorporate solids into dermatological and ophthalmic ointments and suspensions.

The Mortar and Pestle—These are the most frequently used utensils in small-scale comminution. Mortars made of various materials and in diverse shapes are available and while these often are used interchangeably the different kinds of mortars have specific utility in preparing or grinding different materials.

Modern mortars and pestles are prepared usually from Wedgwood ware, porcelain or glass. While pharmacists often use different mortars interchangeably, each type has a preferential range of utility which makes its use more efficient. Glass mortars, for example, are designed primarily for use in preparing solutions and suspensions of chemical materials in a liquid. They also are suitable for preparing ointments which require the reduction of soft aggregates of powdered materials or the incorporation of relatively large amounts of liquid. Glass also has the advantage of being comparatively nonporous and of not staining easily and thus is particularly useful when substances such as flavoring oils or highly colored substances are used. Glass cannot be used for comminuting hard solids.

Wedgwood mortars are suited well for comminution of crystalline solids or for the reduction in particle size of most materials used in modern prescription practice. They are capable of adequately powdering most substances which are available only as crystals or hard lumps. However, Wedgwood is relatively porous and will stain quite easily. A Wedgwood mortar is available with a roughened interior which aids in the comminution process but which requires meticulous care in washing since particles of the drugs may be trapped in the rough surface and cause contamination of materials subsequently comminuted in the mortar.

Porcelain mortars are very similar to Wedgwood, except that the exterior surface of the former is usually glazed and thus less porous. Porcelain mortars may be used for comminution of soft aggregates or crystals but more generally are used for blending powders of approximately uniform particle size.

Pestles are made of the same material as the mortar. Pestles for Wedgwood or porcelain mortars are available with hard rubber or wooden handles screwed into the head of the pestle. Also available are one-piece Wedgwood pestles. Pestles made entirely of porcelain are objectionable, because they are broken easily.

Pestles and mortars should not be interchanged. The efficiency of the grinding or mixing operation depends largely on a maximum contact between the surfaces of the head of the pestle and the interior of the mortar. The pestle should have as much bearing on the interior surface of the mortar as its size will permit. A pestle which does not "fit" the mortar will result in a waste of labor.

Divided Powders

Divided powders (*chartula or chartulae*) are dispensed in the form of individual doses and generally are dispensed in papers, properly folded. They also may be dispensed in metal foil, small heat-sealed plastic bags or other containers.

Dividing Powders—After weighing, comminuting and mixing the ingredients, the powders must be divided accurately into the prescribed number of doses. In order to achieve accuracy consistent with the other steps in the preparation, *each dose should be weighed individually* and transferred to a powder paper. Following completion of this step the powder papers are folded.

Folding Powders—The operations of folding powder papers are illustrated in Fig 23. Care in making the several folds, and experience gained by repetition, are necessary to obtain uniformity when the powders finally are placed in the box for dispensing. Deviation from any of the three main folds will result in powders of varying height being formed, and variations in the folded ends likewise will be noticeable when the powders are placed side by side. A detailed description of folding powder papers is contained in RPS-17, page 1600.

Packaging Divided Powders—Specially manufactured paper and boxes are available for dispensing divided powders.

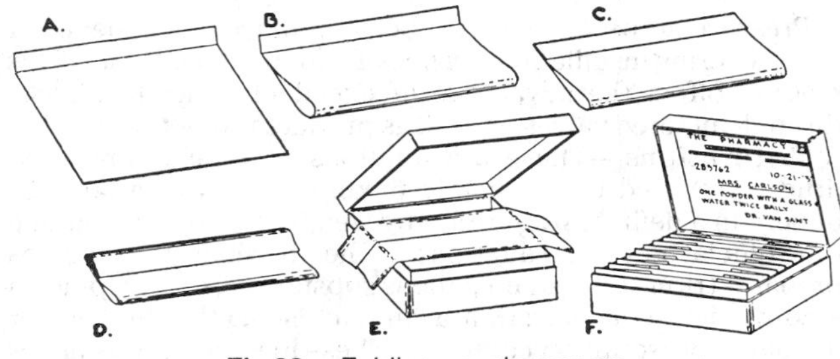

Fig 23. Folding powder papers.

Powder Papers—Four basic types of powder papers are available.

1. Vegetable parchment, a thin semiopaque moisture-resistant paper.
2. White bond, an opaque paper with no moisture-resistant properties.
3. Glassine, a glazed, transparent moisture-resistant paper.
4. Waxed, a transparent waterproof paper.

Hygroscopic and volatile drugs can be protected best by using a waxed paper, double-wrapped with a bond paper to improve the appearance of the completed powder. Parchment and glassine papers offer limited protection for these drugs.

A variety of sizes of powder papers are available. The selection of the proper size depends on the bulk of each dose and the dimensions of the powder box required to hold the number of doses prescribed.

Powder Boxes—Various types of boxes are supplied in several sizes for dispensing divided powders. The hinged-shoulder boxes shown in Fig 23F are the most popular and have the advantage of preventing the switching of lids with the directions for use when several boxes of the same size are in the same home. The prescription label may be pasted directly on top of the lid or inside the lid. In the latter case the name of the pharmacy is lithographed on top of the lid.

Special Problems

The incorporation of volatile substances, eutectic mixtures, liquids and hygroscopic or deliquescent substances into powders presents problems that require special treatment.

Volatile Substances—The loss of camphor, menthol and essential oils by volatilization when incorporated into powders may be prevented or retarded by use of heat-sealed plastic bags or by double wrapping with a waxed or glassine paper inside of a bond paper.

Eutectic Mixtures—Liquids result from the combination of phenol, camphor, menthol, thymol, antipyrine, phenacetin, acetanilid, aspirin, salol and related compounds at ordinary temperatures. These so-called eutectic mixtures may be incorporated into powders by addition of an inert diluent. Magnesium carbonate or light magnesium oxide are used commonly and effective diluents for this purpose, although kaolin, starch, bentonite and other absorbents have been recommended. Silicic acid prevents eutexia with aspirin, phenyl salicylate and other troublesome compounds; incorporation of about 20% silicic acid (particle size, 50 μm) prevented liquefaction even under the compression pressures required to form tablets.

In handling this problem each eutectic compound should be mixed first with a portion of the diluent and gently blended together, preferably with a spatula on a sheet of paper. Generally, an amount of diluent equal to the eutectic compounds is sufficient to prevent liquefaction for about 2 weeks. Deliberate forcing of the formation of the liquid state, by direct trituration, followed by absorption of the moist mass, also will overcome this problem. This technique requires use of more diluent than previously mentioned methods but offers the advantage of extended product stability. Thus, the technique is useful for dispensing a large number of doses that normally would not be consumed over a period of 1 or 2 weeks.

Liquids—In small amounts, liquids may be incorporated into divided powders. Magnesium carbonate, starch or lactose may be added to increase the absorbability of the powders if necessary. When the liquid is a solvent for a nonvolatile heat-stable compound, it may be evaporated gently on a water bath. Lactose may be added during the course of the evaporation to increase the rate of solvent loss by increasing the surface area. Some fluidextracts and tinctures may be treated in this manner, although the use of an equivalent amount of a powdered extract, when available, is a more desirable technique.

Hygroscopic and Deliquescent Substances—Substances that become moist because of affinity for moisture in the air may be prepared as divided powders by adding inert diluents. Double-wrapping is desirable for further protection. Extremely deliquescent compounds cannot be prepared satisfactorily as powders.

Bulk Powders

Bulk powders may be classified as oral powders, dentifrices, douche powders, dusting powders, insufflations and triturations.

Oral Powders—These generally are supplied as *finely divided powders* or *effervescent granules.*

The finely divided powders are intended to be suspended or dissolved in water or mixed with soft foods, eg, applesauce, prior to administration. Antacids and laxative powders frequently are administered in this form.

Effervescent granules contain sodium bicarbonate and either citric acid, tartaric acid or sodium biphosphate in addition to the active ingredients. On solution in water, carbon dioxide is released as a result of the acid–base reaction. The effervescence from the release of the carbon dioxide serves to mask the taste of salty or bitter medications.

Granulation generally is accomplished by producing a moist mass, forcing it through a coarse sieve and drying it in an oven. The moisture necessary for massing the materials is obtained readily by heating them sufficiently to drive off the water of hydration from the uneffloresced citric acid. The completed product must be dispensed in tightly closed glass containers to protect it against the humidity of the air. For a formerly official general formula for preparing effervescent salts see RPS-15, page 1574.

Effervescent powders may be prepared also by adding small amounts of water to the dry salts in order to obtain a workable mass. The mass is dried and ground to yield the powder or granule. Care must be used in this procedure to ensure that the reaction which occurs in the presence of water does not proceed too far before it is stopped by the drying process. Should this happen, the effervescent properties of the product will be destroyed.

Other preparative techniques have been reported for effervescent powders such as a fluidized-bed procedure in which the powders are blended and then suspended in a stream of air in a Wurster chamber. Water is sprayed into the chamber resulting in a slight reaction and an expansion of the particles to form granules ranging in size from 10- to 30-mesh. This approach apparently offers a number of advantages over the older techniques. The extent of reaction and particle size are controlled during the manufacture. A drying oven, trays and even grinding devices are not required. Furthermore, the technique lends itself to a continuous as well as a batch operation.

The heat generated from the blending and mixing operation also has been used to mass the powders by causing the release of the water of hydration from the citric acid. The massed materials can be dried and sieved through a coarse sieve. This technique thus eliminates the need of an external heat source or a granulating solution.

Dentifrices—These may be prepared in the form of a bulk powder, generally containing a soap or detergent, mild abrasive and an anticariogenic agent.

Douche Powders—These products are completely soluble and are intended to be dissolved in water prior to use as antiseptics or cleansing agents for a body cavity. They most commonly are intended for vaginal use, although they may be formulated for nasal, otic or ophthalmic use. Generally, since aromatic oils are included in these powders, they are passed through a No 40 or 60 sieve to eliminate agglomeration and insure complete mixing. Dispensing in wide-mouth glass jars serves to protect against loss of volatile materials and permits easy access by the patient. Bulk-powder boxes may be used for dispensing douche powders, although glass containers are preferred because of the protection afforded by these containers against air and moisture.

Dusting Powders—These are locally applied nontoxic preparations that are intended to have no systemic action. They always should be dispensed in a very fine state of subdivision to enhance effectiveness and minimize irritation. When necessary, they may be micronized or passed through a No 80 or 100 sieve.

Extemporaneously prepared dusting powders should be dispensed in sifter-top packages. Commercial dusting powders are available in sifter-top containers or pressure aerosols. The latter, while generally more expensive than the other containers, offer the advantage of protection from air, moisture and contamination, as well as convenience of application. Foot powders and talcum powders are currently available as pressure aerosols.

Dusting powders are applied to various parts of the body as lubricants, protectives, absorbents, antiseptics, antipruritics, antibromhidrosis agents, astringents and antiperspirants.

While in most cases dusting powders are considered nontoxic, the absorption of boric acid through large areas of abraded skin has caused toxic reactions in infants. Accidental inhalation of zinc stearate powder has led to pulmonary inflammation of the lungs of infants. The pharmacist should be aware of the possible dangers when the patient uses these compounds as well as other externally applied products. See also Chapter 52.

Insufflations—These are finely divided powders introduced into body cavities such as the ears, nose, throat, tooth sockets and vagina. An insufflator (powder blower) usually is employed to administer these products. However, the difficulty in obtaining a uniform dose has restricted their general use.

Specialized equipment has been developed for the administration of micronized powders of relatively potent drugs. The Norisodrine Sulfate Aerohaler Cartridge (*Abbott*) is an example. In the use of this Aerohaler, inhalation by the patient causes a small ball to strike a cartridge containing the drug. The force of the ball shakes the proper amount of the powder free, permitting its inhalation. Another device, the Spinhaler turbo-inhaler (*Fisons*), is a propeller-driven device designed to deposit a mixture of lactose and micronized cromolyn sodium into the lung as an aid in the management of bronchial asthma.

Pressure aerosols also have been employed as a means of administering insufflations, especially for potent drugs. This method offers the advantage of excellent control of dose, through metered valves, as well as product protection.

Triturations—These are dilutions of potent powdered drugs, prepared by intimately mixing them with a suitable diluent in a definite proportion by weight. They were at one time official as 1 to 10 dilutions. The pharmacist sometimes prepares triturations of poisonous substances, eg, atropine, in a convenient concentration using lactose as the diluent, for use at the prescription counter. These medicinal substances are weighed more accurately and conveniently by using this method.

The correct procedure for preparing such triturations or any similar dilution of a potent powder medicament, to insure uniform distribution of the latter, is

Reduce the drug to a moderately fine powder in a mortar.

Add about an equal amount of diluent and mix well by thorough trituration in the mortar.

Successsively add portions of diluent, triturating after each addition, until the entire quantity of diluent has been incorporated.

Under no circumstance should the entire quantity of diluent be added at once to the drug that is to be diluted in the expectation that uniform dispersion of the latter will be more expeditiously achieved on brief trituration of the mixture.

References

1. Parrott EL. In Lachman L *et al: The Theory and Practice of Industrial Pharmacy*, 3rd ed, Lea & Febiger, Philadelphia, 32, 1986.
2. Perry RH *et al: Chemical Engineers' Handbook*, 4th ed, McGraw-Hill, New York, 8–8, 1963.
3. Parrott EL, *loc cit*, 39.
4. Pilcher JM *et al: Proc Chem Spec Mfrs Assoc Ann Mtg:* 66, 1956.
5. Tillotson D: *Aerosol Age 3(5)*:41, 1958.

Bibliography

Irani RR, Callis CF: *Particle Size: Measurement, Interpretation and Application*, Wiley, New York, 1963.

Cadle RD: *Particle Size*, Reinhold, New York, 1965.

Silverman L *et al:* Particle Size Analysis in Industrial Hygiene, Academic, New York, 1971.

Allen T: *Particle Size Measurement*, Chapman & Hall, London, 1968.

Orr C Jr, Dalla Valle JM: *Fine Particle Measurement*, Macmillan, New York, 1959.

Martin AN: *Physical Pharmacy*, 3rd ed, Lea & Febiger, Philadelphia, 1983.

Orr C Jr: *Particulate Technology*, Macmillan, New York, 1966.

Brown RL, Richards JC: *Principles of Powder Mechanics*, Pergamon, Oxford, 1970.

Uhl VW, Gray JW: Mixing, vol II, Academic, New York, 1967.

Stockman JD, Fochtman EG, eds: *Particle Size Analysis*, Ann Arbor Science Pub, Ann Arbor, MI 1977.

Jelinek IZK: *Particle Size Analysis*, Wiley, New York, 1970.

Sterbacek Z, Tausk P: *Mixing in the Chemical Industry*, Pergamon, Oxford, 1965.

DallaValle JM: *Micromeritics*, 2nd ed, Pitman, New York, 1948.

Parfitt GD, Sing KSW: *Characterization of Powder Surfaces*, Academic, London, 1976.

CHAPTER 92

Oral Solid Dosage Forms

Edward Rudnic, PhD
Vice President, Pharmaceutical Research and Development
Pharmavene, Inc.
Gaithersburg, MD 20878

Joseph B Schwartz, PhD
Tice Professor of Pharmaceutics
Philadelphia College of Pharmacy and Science
Philadelphia, PA 19104

Drug substances most frequently are administered orally by means of solid dosage forms such as tablets and capsules. Large-scale production methods used for their preparation, as described later in the chapter, require the presence of other materials in addition to the active ingredients. Additives also may be included in the formulations to facilitate handling, enhance the physical appearance, improve stability and aid in the delivery of the drug to the bloodstream after administration. These supposedly inert ingredients, as well as the production methods employed, have been shown in some cases to influence the absorption or bioavailability of the drug substances.[1] Therefore, care must be taken in the selection and evaluation of additives and preparation methods to ensure that the drug-delivery goals and therapeutic efficacy of the active ingredient will not be diminished.

In a limited number of cases it has been shown that the drug substance's solubility and other physicochemical characteristics have influenced its physiological availability from a solid dosage form. These characteristics include its particle size, whether it is amorphous or crystalline, whether it is solvated or nonsolvated and its polymorphic form. After clinically effective formulations are obtained, such variations among dosage units of a given batch, as well as batch-to-batch differences, should be reduced to a minimum through proper in-process controls and good manufacturing practices. The recognition of the importance of validation both for equipment and processes greatly has enhanced assurance in the reproducibility of formulations. It is in these areas that significant progress has been made with the realization that large-scale production of a satisfactory tablet or capsule depends not only on the availability of a clinically effective formulation but also on the raw materials, facilities, personnel, documentation, validated processes and equipment, packaging and the controls used during and after preparation (Fig 1).

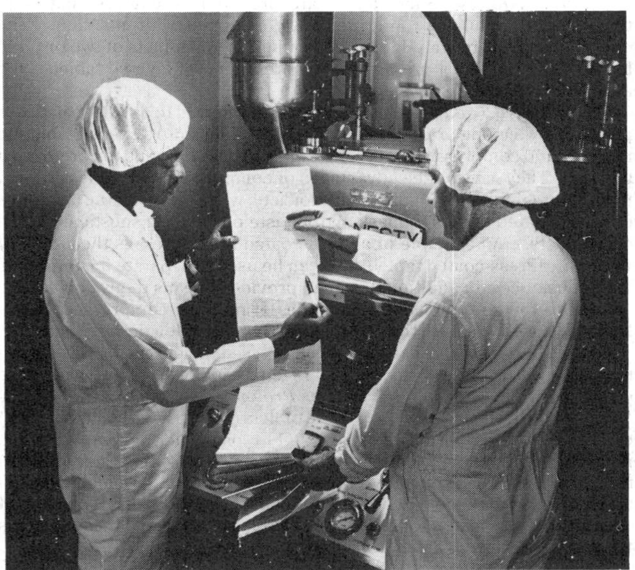

Fig 1. Tablet press operators checking batch record in conformance with Current Good Manufacturing Practices (courtesy, Lilly).

Tablets

Tablets may be defined as solid pharmaceutical dosage forms containing drug substances with or without suitable diluents and prepared either by compression or molding methods. They have been in widespread use since the latter part of the 19th century and their popularity continues. The term *compressed tablet* is believed to have been used first by John Wyeth and Brother of Philadelphia. During this same period, molded tablets were introduced to be used as *hypodermic* tablets for the extemporaneous preparation of solutions for injection. Tablets remain popular as a dosage form because of the advantages afforded both to the manufacturer (eg, simplicity and economy of preparation, stability and convenience in packaging, shipping and dispensing) and the patient (eg, accuracy of dosage, compactness, portability, blandness of taste and ease of administration).

Although the basic mechanical approach for their manufacture has remained the same, tablet technology has undergone great improvement. Efforts are being made continually to understand more clearly the physical characteristics of powder compaction and the factors affecting the availability of the drug substance from the dosage form after oral administration. Tableting equipment continues to improve both as to production speed and the uniformity of tablets compressed. Recent advances in tablet technology have been reviewed.[2–13]

Although tablets frequently are discoid in shape, they also may be round, oval, oblong, cylindrical or triangular. They may differ greatly in size and weight depending on the amount of drug substance present and the intended method of administration. They are divided into two general classes, whether they are made by compression or molding. Compressed tablets usually are prepared by large-scale production methods, while molded tablets generally involve small-scale operations. The various tablet types and abbreviations used in referring to them are listed below.

Compressed Tablets (CT)

These tablets are formed by compression and contain no special coating. They are made from powdered, crystalline or granular materials, alone or in combination with binders, disintegrants, controlled-release polymers, lubricants, diluents and, in many cases, colorants.

Sugar-Coated Tablets (SCT)—These are compressed tablets containing a sugar coating. Such coatings may be colored and are beneficial in covering up drug substances possessing objectionable tastes or odors, and in protecting materials sensitive to oxidation.

Film-Coated Tablets (FCT)—These are compressed tablets which are covered with a thin layer or film of a water-soluble material. A number of polymeric substances with film-forming properties may be used. Film coating imparts the same general characteristics as sugar coating with the added advantage of a greatly reduced time period required for the coating operation.

Enteric-Coated Tablets (ECT)—These are compressed tablets coated with substances that resist solution in gastric fluid but disintegrate in the intestine. Enteric coatings can be used for tablets containing drug substances which are inactivated or destroyed in the stomach, for those which irritate the mucosa or as a means of delayed release of the medication.

Multiple Compressed Tablets (MCT)—These are compressed tablets made by more than one compression cycle.

Layered Tablets—Such tablets are prepared by compressing additional tablet granulation on a previously compressed granulation. The operation may be repeated to produce multilayered tablets of two or three layers. Special tablet presses are required to make layered tablets such as the Versa press (*Stokes/Pennwalt*).

Press-Coated Tablets—Such tablets, also referred to as dry-coated, are prepared by feeding previously compressed tablets into a special tableting machine and compressing another granulation layer around the preformed tablets. They have all the advantages of compressed tablets, ie, slotting, monogramming, speed of disintegration, etc, while retaining the attributes of sugar-coated tablets in masking the taste of the drug substance in the core tablets. An example of a press-coated tablet press is the *Manesty* Drycota. Press-coated tablets also can be used to separate incompatible drug substances; in addition, they can provide a means to give an enteric coating to the core tablets. Both types of multiple-compressed tablets have been used widely in the design of prolonged-action dosage forms.

Controlled-Release Tablets—Compressed tablets can be formulated to release the drug slowly over a prolonged period of time. Hence, these dosage forms have been referred to as *Prolonged-Release* or *Sustained-Release* dosage forms as well. These tablets (as well as capsule versions) can be categorized into three types: (1) those which respond to some physiological condition to release the drug, such as enteric coatings; (2) those that release the drug in a relatively steady, controlled manner and (3) those that combine combinations of mechanisms to release "pulses" of drug, such as repeat-action tablets. The performance of these systems are described in more detail in Chapter 94.

Tablets for Solution—Compressed tablets to be used for preparing solutions or imparting given characteristics to solutions must be labeled to indicate that they are not to be swallowed. Examples of these tablets are Halazone Tablets for Solution and Potassium Permanganate Tablets for Solution.

Effervescent Tablets—In addition to the drug substance, these contain sodium bicarbonate and an organic acid such as tartaric or citric. In the presence of water, these additives react liberating carbon dioxide which acts as a distintegrator and produces effervescence. Except for small quantities of lubricants present, effervescent tablets are soluble.

Compressed Suppositories or Inserts—Occasionally, vaginal suppositories, such as Metronidazole Tablets, are prepared by compression. Tablets for this use usually contain lactose as the diluent. In this case, as well as for any tablet intended for administration other than by swallowing, the label must indicate the manner in which it is to be used.

Buccal and Sublingual Tablets—These are small, flat, oval tablets. Tablets intended for buccal administration by inserting into the buccal pouch may dissolve or erode slowly; therefore, they are formulated and compressed with sufficient pressure to give a hard tablet. Progesterone Tablets may be administered in this way.

Some newer approaches use tablets that melt at body temperatures. The matrix of the tablet is solidified while the drug is in solution. After melting, the drug is automatically in solution and available for absorption, thus eliminating dissolution as a rate-limiting step in the absorption of poorly soluble compounds. Sublingual tablets, such as those containing nitroglycerin, isoproterenol hydrochloride or erythrityl tetranitrate, are placed under the tongue. Sublingual tablets dissolve rapidly and the drug substances are absorbed readily by this form of administration.

Molded Tablets or Tablet Triturates (TT)

Tablet triturates usually are made from moist material using a triturate mold which gives them the shape of cut sections of a cylinder. Such tablets must be completely and rapidly soluble. The problem arising from compression of these tablets is the failure to find a lubricant that is completely water soluble.

Dispensing Tablets (DT)—These tablets provide a convenient quantity of potent drug that can be incorporated readily into powders and liquids, thus circumventing the necessity to weigh small quantities. These tablets are supplied primarily as a convenience for extemporaneous compounding and should never be dispensed as a dosage form.

Hypodermic Tablets (HT)—Hypodermic tablets are soft, readily soluble tablets and originally were used for the preparation of solutions to be injected. Since stable parenteral solutions are now available for most drug substances, there is no justification for the use of hypodermic tablets for injection. Their use in this manner should be discouraged since the resulting solutions are not sterile. Large quantities of these tablets continue to be made, but for oral administration. No hypodermic tablets ever have been recognized by the official compendia.

Compressed Tablets (CT)

In order for medicinal substances, with or without diluents, to be made into solid dosage forms with pressure, using available equipment, it is necessary that the material, either in crystalline or powdered form, possess a number of physical characteristics. These characteristics include the ability to flow freely, cohesiveness and lubrication. The ingredients such as disintegrants designed to break the tablet up in gastrointestinal fluids, and controlled-release polymers designed to slow down drug release, ideally should possess these characteristics, or not interfere with the desirable performance traits of the other excipients. Since most materials have none or only some of these properties, methods of tablet formulation and preparation have been developed to impart these desirable characteristics to the material which is to be compressed into tablets.

The basic mechanical unit in all tablet-compression equipment includes a lower punch which fits into a die from the bottom and an upper punch, having a head of the same shape and dimensions, which enters the die cavity from the top after the tableting material fills the die cavity (see Fig 2). The tablet is formed by pressure applied on the punches and subsequently is ejected from the die. The weight of the tablet is determined by the volume of the material which fills the die cavity. Therefore, the ability of the granulation to flow freely into the die is important in insuring a uniform fill, as well as the continuous movement of the granulation from the source of supply or feed hopper. If the tablet granulation does not possess cohesive properties, the tablet after compression will crumble and fall apart on handling. As the punches must move freely within the die and the tablet must be ejected readily from the punch faces, the material must have a degree of lubrication to minimize friction and allow for the removal of the compressed tablets.

There are three general methods of tablet preparation: the wet-granulation method, the dry-granulation method and di-

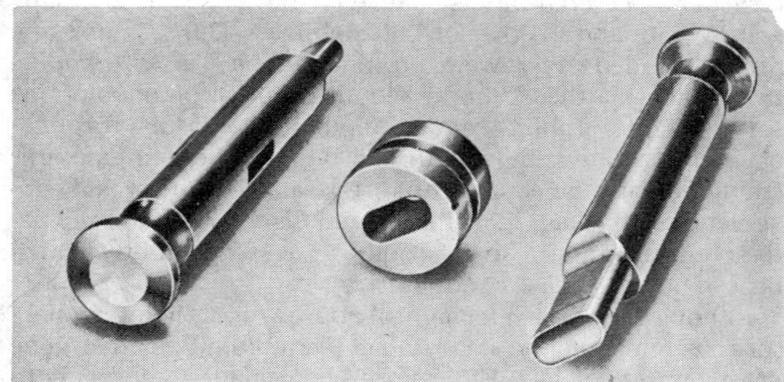

Fig 2. Basic mechanical unit for tabet compression: lower punch, die and upper punch (courtesy, Vector/Colton).

rect compression. The method of preparation and the added ingredients are selected in order to give the tablet formulation the desirable physical characteristics allowing the rapid compression of tablets. After compression, the tablets must have a number of additional attributes such as appearance, hardness, disintegration ability, appropriate dissolution characteristics and uniformity which also are influenced both by the method of preparation and by the added materials present in the formulation. In the preparation of compressed tablets, the formulator also must be cognizant of the effect which the ingredients and methods of preparation may have on the availability of the active ingredients and, hence, the therapeutic efficacy of the dosage form. In response to a request by physicians to change a dicumarol tablet in order that it might be broken more easily, a Canadian company reformulated to make a large tablet with a score. Subsequent use of the tablet, containing the same amount of drug substance as the previous tablet, resulted in complaints that larger-than-usual doses were needed to produce the same therapeutic response. On the other hand, literature reports indicate that the reformulation of a commercial digoxin tablet resulted in a tablet, although containing the same quantity of drug substance, that gave the desired clinical response at half its original dose. Methods and principles that can be used to assess the effects of excipients and additives on drug absorption have been reviewed.[2,14,15] See Chapters 35, 42 and 83.

Tablet Ingredients

In addition to the active or therapeutic ingredient, tablets contain a number of inert materials. The latter are known as additives or *excipients*. They may be classified according to the part they play in the finished tablet. The first group contains those which help to impart satisfactory processing and compression characteristics to the formulation. These include diluents, binders, glidants and lubricants. The second group of added substances helps to give additional desirable physical characteristics to the finished tablet. Included in this group are disintegrants, colors, and in the case of chewable tablets, flavors and sweetening agents, and in the case of controlled-release tablets, polymers or waxes or other solubility-retarding materials.

Although the term *inert* has been applied to these added materials, it is becoming increasingly apparent that there is an important relationship between the properties of the excipients and the dosage forms containing them. Preformulation studies demonstrate their influence on stability, bioavailability and the processes by which the dosage forms are prepared. The need for acquiring more information and use standards for excipients has been recognized in a joint venture of the Academy of Pharmaceutical Sciences and the Council of the Pharmaceutical Society of Great Britain. The result is called the *Handbook of Pharmaceutical Excipients*. This reference now is distributed widely throughout the world.[16]

Diluents

Frequently, the single dose of the active ingredient is small and an inert substance is added to increase the bulk in order to make the tablet a practical size for compression. Compressed tablets of dexamethasone contain 0.75 mg steroid per tablet; hence, it is obvious that another material must be added to make tableting possible. Diluents used for this purpose include dicalcium phosphate, calcium sulfate, lactose, cellulose, kaolin, mannitol, sodium chloride, dry starch and powdered sugar. Certain diluents, such as mannitol, lactose, sorbitol, sucrose and inositol, when present in sufficient quantity, can impart properties to some compressed tablets that permit disintegration in the mouth by chewing. Such tablets commonly are called *chewable tablets*. Upon chewing, properly prepared tablets will disintegrate smoothly at a satisfactory rate, have a pleasant taste and feel and leave no unpleasant aftertaste in the mouth. Diluents used as excipients for direct compression formulas have been subjected to prior processing to give them flowability and compressibility. These are discussed under *Direct Compression*, page 1626.

Most formulators of immediate-release tablets tend to use consistently only one or two diluents selected from the above group in their tablet formulations. Usually, these have been selected on the basis of experience and cost factors. However, in the formulation of new therapeutic agents, the compatibility of the diluents with the drug must be considered, eg, calcium salts used as diluents for the broad-spectrum antibiotic tetracycline have been shown to interfere with the drug's absorption from the gastrointestinal tract. When drug substances have low water solubility, it is recommended that water-soluble diluents be used to avoid possible bioavailability problems. Highly adsorbent substances, eg, bentonite and kaolin, are to be avoided in making tablets of drugs used clinically in small dosage, such as the cardiac glycosides, alkaloids and the synthetic estrogens. These drug substances may be adsorbed after administration. The combination of amine bases with lactose, or amine salts with lactose in the presence of an alkaline lubricant, results in tablets which discolor on aging.

Microcrystalline cellulose (Avicel) usually is used as an excipient in direct-compression formulas. However, its presence in 5 to 15% concentrations in wet granulations has been shown to be beneficial in the granulation and drying processes in minimizing case-hardening of the tablets and in reducing tablet mottling.

Many ingredients are used for several different purposes, even within the same formulation; eg, corn starch can be used in paste form as a binder. When added in drug or suspension form, it is a good disintegrant. Even though these two uses are to achieve opposite goals, some tablet formulas use corn starch in both ways. In some controlled-release formulas, the polymer hydroxypropylmethylcellulose (HPMC) is used both as an aid to prolong the release from the tablet, as well as a film-former in the tablet coating. Therefore, most excipients used in formulating tablets and capsules have many uses, and a thorough understanding of their properties and limitations is necessary in order to use them rationally.

Binders

Agents used to impart cohesive qualities to the powdered material are referred to as binders or granulators. They impart a cohesiveness to the tablet formulation which insures the tablet remaining intact after compression, as well as improving the free-flowing qualities by the formulation of granules of desired hardness and size. Materials commonly used as binders include starch, gelatin and sugars as sucrose, glucose, dextrose, molasses and lactose. Natural and synthetic gums which have been used include acacia, sodium alginate, extract of Irish moss, panwar gum, ghatti gum, mucilage of isapol husks, carboxymethylcellulose, methylcellulose, polyvinylpyrrolidone, Veegum and larch arabogalactan. Other agents which may be considered binders under certain circumstances are polyethylene glycol, ethylcellulose, waxes, water and alcohol.

The quantity of binder used has considerable influence on the characteristics of the compressed tablets. The use of too much binder or too strong a binder will make a hard tablet which will not disintegrate easily and which will cause excessive wear of punches and dies. Differences in binders used for CT Tolbutamide resulted in differences in hypoglycemic effects observed clinically. Materials which have no cohesive qualities of their own will require a stronger binder than those with these qualities. Alcohol and water are not binders in the true sense of the word, but because of their solvent action on some ingredients such as lactose, starch and celluloses, they change the powdered material to granules and the residual moisture retained enables the materials to adhere together when compressed.

Binders are used both as a solution and in a dry form depending on the other ingredients in the formulation and the method of preparation. However, several *pregelatinized* starches available are intended to be added in the dry form so that water alone can be used as the granulating solution. The same amount of binder in solution will be more effective than if it were dispersed in a dry form and moistened with the solvent. By the latter procedure, the binding agent is not as effective in reaching and wetting each of the particles within the mass of powders. Each of the particles in a powder blend has a coating of adsorbed air on its surface, and it is this film which must be penetrated before the powders can be wetted by the binder solution. After wetting, a certain period of time is necessary to dissolve the binder completely and make it completely available for use. Since powders differ with respect to the ease with which they can be wetted, and their rate of solubilization, it is preferable to incorporate the binding agent in solution. By this technique it often is possible to gain effective binding with a lower concentration of binder.

The direct-compression method for preparing tablets (see page 1630) requires a material that not only is free-flowing but also sufficiently cohesive to act as a binder. This use has been described for a number of materials including microcrystalline cellulose, microcrystalline dextrose, amylose and polyvinylpyrrolidone. It has been postulated that microcrystalline cellulose is a special form of cellulose fibril in which the individual crystallites are held together largely by hydrogen bonding. The disintegration of tablets containing the cellulose occurs by breaking the intercrystallite bonds by the disintegrating medium.

Starch Paste—Corn starch is used widely as a binder. The concentration may vary from 10 to 20%. It usually is prepared as it is to be used by dispersing corn starch in sufficient cold purified water to make a 5 to 10% *w/w* suspension and warming in a water bath with continuous stirring until a translucent paste forms. It has been observed that during paste formation, not all of the starch is hydrolyzed. Starch paste then, is not only useful as a binder, but also as a method to incorporate some disintegrant inside the granules.

Gelatin Solution—Gelatin generally is used as a 10 to 20% solution; gelatin solutions should be prepared freshly as needed and used while warm or they will solidify. The gelatin is added to cold purified water and allowed to stand until it is hydrated. It then is warmed in a water bath to dissolve the gelatin, and the solution is made up to the final volume on a weight basis to give the concentration desired.

Cellulosic Solutions—Various cellulosics have been used as binders in solution form. Hydroxypropylmethylcellulose (HPMC) has been used widely in this regard. Typical of a number of cellulosics, HPMC is more soluble in cold water than hot. It also is more dispersable in hot water than cold. Hence, in order to obtain a good, smooth gel that is free from lumps or "fisheyes," it is necessary to add the HPMC in hot, almost boiling water and, under agitation, cool the mixture down as quickly as possible, as low as possible. Other water-soluble cellulosics such as hydroxyethylcellulose (HEC) and hydroxypropylcellulose (HPC) have been used successfully in solution as binders.

Not all cellulosics are soluble in water. Ethylcellulose can be used effectively when dissolved in alcohol, or as a dry binder which then is wetted with alcohol. It is used as a binder for materials that are moisture-sensitive.

Polyvinylpyrrolidone—PVP can be used as an aqueous or alcoholic solution and this versatility has increased its popularity. Concentrations range from 2% and vary considerably.

It will be noted that binder solutions usually are made up to weight rather than volume. This is to enable the formulator to determine the weight of the solids which have been added to the tablet granulation in the binding solution. This becomes part of the total weight of the granulation and must be taken into consideration in determining the weight of the compressed tablet, which will contain the stated amount of the therapeutic agent.

As can be seen by the list of binders in this chapter, most modern binders used in solution are polymeric in form. Because of this, the flow or spreadability of these solutions becomes important when selecting the appropriate granulating equipment. The rheology of polymeric solutions is a fascinating subject in and of itself, and should be considered for these materials.

Lubricants

Lubricants have a number of functions in tablet manufacture. They prevent adhesion of the tablet material to the surface of the dies and punches, reduce interparticle friction, facilitate the ejection of the tablets from the die cavity and may improve the rate of flow of the tablet granulation. Commonly used lubricants include talc, magnesium stearate, calcium stearate, stearic acid, hydrogenated vegetable oils and polyethylene glycol (PEG). Most lubricants, with the exception of talc, are used in concentrations less than 1%. When used alone, talc may require concentrations as high as 5%. Lubricants are in most cases hydrophobic materials. Poor selection or excessive amounts can result in "waterproofing" the tablets, resulting in poor tablet disintegration and/or delayed dissolution of the drug substance.

The addition of the proper lubricant is highly desirable if the material to be tableted tends to stick to the punches and dies. Immediately after compression, most tablets have the tendency to expand and will bind and stick to the side of the die. The choice of the proper lubricant effectively will overcome this.

The method of adding a lubricant to a granulation is important if the material is to perform its function satisfactorily. The lubricant should be divided finely by passing it through a 60- to 100-mesh nylon cloth onto the granulation. In production this is called *bolting* the lubricant. After adding the lubricant, the granulation is tumbled or mixed gently to distribute the lubricant without coating the particles too well or breaking them down to finer particles. Some research has concluded that the order of mixing of lubricants and other excipients can have a profound effect on the performance of the final dosage form. Thus, attention to the mixing process itself is just as important as the selection of lubricant materials.

These process variables can be seen in the prolonged blending of a lubricant in a granulation. Overblending materially can affect the hardness, disintegration time and dissolution performance for the resultant tablets.

The quantity of lubricant varies, being as low as 0.1%, and in some cases as high as 5%. Lubricants have been added to the granulating agents in the form of suspensions or emulsions. This technique serves to reduce the number of operational procedures and thus reduce the processing time.

In selecting a lubricant, proper attention must be given to its compatibility with the drug agent. Perhaps the most widely investigated drug is acetylsalicylic acid. Different talcs varied significantly the stability of aspirin. Talc with a high calcium content and a high loss on ignition was associated with increased aspirin decomposition. From a stability standpoint, the relative acceptability of tablet lubricants for combination with aspirin was found to decrease in the following order: hydrogenated vegetable oil, stearic acid, talc and aluminum stearate.

The primary problem in the preparation of a water-soluble tablet is the selection of a satisfactory lubricant. Soluble lubricants reported to be effective include sodium benzoate, a mixture of sodium benzoate and sodium acetate, sodium chloride, leucine and Carbowax 4000. However, it has been suggested that formulations used to prepare water-soluble tablets may represent a number of compromises between compression efficiency and water solubility. While magnesium stearate is one of the most widely used lubricants, its hydrophobic properties can retard disintegration and dissolution. To overcome these waterproofing characteristics, sodium lauryl sulfate sometimes is included. One compound found to have the lubricating properties of magnesium stearate without its disadvantages is magnesium lauryl sulfate. Its safety for use in pharmaceuticals has not been established.

Glidants

A glidant is a substance which improves the flow characteristics of a powder mixture. These materials always are added in the dry state just prior to compression (ie, during the lubrication step). Colloidal silicon dioxide [Cab-o-sil (*Cabot*)] is the most commonly used glidant and generally is used in low concentrations of 1% or less. Talc (asbestos-free) also is used and may serve the dual purpose as lubricant/glidant.

It is especially important to optimize the order of addition and the mixing process for these materials in order to maximize their effect and to make sure that their influence on the lubricant(s) is minimized.

Disintegrants

A disintegrant is a substance, or a mixture of substances, added to a tablet to facilitate its breakup or disintegration after administration. The active ingredient must be released from the tablet matrix as efficiently as possible to allow for its rapid dissolution. Materials serving as disintegrants have been classified chemically as starches, clays, celluloses, algins, gums and cross-linked polymers.

The oldest and still the most popular disintegrants are corn and potato starch which have been well-dried and powdered. Starch has a great affinity for water and swells when moistened, thus facilitating the rupture of the tablet matrix. However, others have suggested that its disintegrating action in tablets is due to capillary action rather than swelling; the spherical shape of the starch grains increases the porosity of the tablet, thus promoting capillary action. Starch, 5%, is suggested, but if more rapid disintegration is desired, this amount may be increased to 10 or 15%. Although it might be expected that disintegration time would decrease as the percentage of starch in the tablet increased, this does not appear to be the case for tolbutamide tablets. In this instance, there appears to be a critical starch concentration for different granulations of the chemical. When their disintegration effect is desired, starches are added to the powder blends in the dry state.

A group of materials known as *super disintegrants* have gained in popularity as disintegrating agents. The name comes from the low levels (2 to 4%) at which they are completely effective. Croscarmelose, crospovidone and sodium starch glycolate represent examples of a cross-linked cellulose, a cross-linked polymer and a cross-linked starch, respectively.

The development of these disintegrants fostered new theories about the various mechanisms by which disintegrants work. Sodium starch glycolate swells 7- to 12-fold in less than 30 seconds. Croscarmelose swells 4- to 8-fold in less than 10 seconds. The starch swells equally in all three dimensions, while the cellulose swells only in two dimensions, leaving fiber length essentially the same. Since croscarmelose is the more efficient disintegrating agent, it is postulated that the rate, force and extent of swelling play an important role in those disintegrants that work by swelling. Cross-linked PVP swells little, but returns to its original boundaries quickly after compression. Wicking, or capillary action, also is postulated to be a major factor in the ability of cross-linked PVP to function.[17–19]

In addition to the starches, a large variety of materials have been used and are reported to be effective as disintegrants. This group includes Veegum HV, methylcellulose, agar, bentonite, cellulose and wood products, natural sponge, cation-exchange resins, alginic acid, guar gum, citrus pulp and carboxymethylcellulose.[20] Sodium lauryl sulfate in combination with starch also has been demonstrated to be an effective disintegrant. In some cases the apparent effectiveness of surfactants in improving tablet disintegration is postulated as being due to an increase in the rate of wetting.

The disintegrating agent usually is mixed with the active ingredients and diluents prior to granulation. In some cases it may be advantageous to divide the starch into two portions: one part is added to the powdered formula prior to granulation, and the remainder is mixed with the lubricant and added prior to compression. Incorporated in this manner, the starch serves a double purpose; the portion added to the lubricant rapidly breaks down the tablet to granules, and the starch mixed with the active ingredients disintegrates the granules into smaller particles. Veegum has been shown to be more effective as a disintegrator in sulfathiazole tablets when most of the quantity is added after granulation and only a small amount before granulation. Likewise, the montmorillonite clays were found to be good tablet disintegrants when added to prepared granulations as powder. They are much less effective as disintegrants when incorporated within the granules.

Factors other than the presence of disintegrants can affect significantly the disintegration time of compressed tablets. The binder, tablet hardness and the lubricant have been shown to influence the disintegration time. Thus, when the formulator is faced with a problem concerning the disintegration of a compressed tablet, the answer may not lie in the selection and quantity of the disintegrating agent alone.

The evolution of carbon dioxide is also an effective way to cause the disintegration of compressed tablets. Tablets containing a mixture of sodium bicarbonate and an acidulant such as tartaric or citric acid will effervesce when added to water. Sufficient acid is added to produce a neutral or slightly acidic reaction when disintegration in water is rapid and complete. One drawback to the use of the effervescent type of disintegrator is that such tablets must be kept in a dry atmosphere at all times during manufacture, storage and packaging. Soluble, effervescent tablets provide a popular form for dispensing aspirin and noncaloric sweetening agents.

Coloring Agents

Colors in compressed tablets serve functions other than making the dosage form more esthetic in appearance. Color helps the manufacturer to control the product during its preparation, as well as serving as a means of identification to the user. The wide diversity in the use of colors in solid dosage forms makes it possible to use color as an important category in the identification code developed by the AMA to establish the identity of an unknown compressed tablet in situations arising from poisoning.

All colorants used in pharmaceuticals must be approved and certified by the FDA. For several decades colorants have been subjected to rigid toxicity standards and, as a result, a number of colorants have been removed from an approved list of FD&C colors or "delisted." Several have been listed as well. The colorants currently approved in the US are listed in Table 1. Each country has its own list of approved colorants, and formulators must consider this in designing products for the international market.[21]

Any of the approved certified water-soluble FD&C dyes, mixtures of the same or their corresponding lakes may be used to color tablets. A color lake is the combination by adsorption of a water-soluble dye to a hydrous oxide of a heavy metal resulting in an insoluble form of the dye. In some instances multiple dyes are used to give a purposefully heterogeneous coloring in the form of speckling to compressed tablets. The dyes available do not meet all the criteria required for the ideal pharmaceutical colorants. The photosensitivity of several of the commonly used colorants and their lakes has been investigated, as well as the protection afforded by a number of glasses used in packaging tablets.

Another approach for improving the photostability of dyes has been in the use of ultraviolet-absorbing chemicals in the tablet formulations with the dyes. The Di-Pac line (*Am star*) is a series of commercially available colored, direct- compression sugars.

The most common method of adding color to a tablet formulation is to dissolve the dye in the binding solution prior to the granulating process. Another approach is to adsorb the dye

Table 1—Colors Approved for Use in the US in Oral Dosage Forms[a,b]

Color	Other names	Color Index (CI 1971)	Use restriction (US)
FD & C Red 40	Allura red	16035	FDA certification on each lot of dye
D & C Red 33	Acid fuchsin D Naphtalone red B	17200	ADI 0–0.76 mg.
D & C Red 36			ADI 0—1.0 mg
Canthaxanthinin	Food orange 8	40850	None
D & C Red 22	Eosin Y	45380	FDA certification on each lot of dye
D & C Red 28	Phloxine B	45410	FDA certification on each lot of dye
D & C Red 3	Erythrosine	45430	FDA certification on each lot of dye
Cochineal extract	Natural red 4 Carmine	75470	None
Iron oxide—red	—	77491	ADI 0–5 mg elemental iron
FD & C Yellow 6	Sunset yellow FCF Yellow orange 5	15985	None
FD & C Yellow 5	Tartrazine	19140	Label declaration and FDA certification on each lot of dye
D & C Yellow 10	Quinoline yellow WS	47005	FDA certification on each lot of dye
Beta-carotene	—	40800	
Iron oxide—yellow	—	77492	ADI 0–5 mg elemental iron
FD & C Blue 1	Brilliant blue FCF	42090	FDA certification on each lot of dye
FD & C Blue 2	Indigotine Indigo carmine	73015	None
FD & C Green 3	Fast green FCF	42035	FDA certification on each lot of dye
Iron oxide—black	—	77499	ADI 0–5 mg elemental iron
Caramel	Burnt sugar	—	None
Titanium dioxide	—	77891	None

[a] Abbreviations: ADI—Acceptable Daily Intake (per kg body weight)
CI— Color index numbers of 1971 (US)
D & C— Drug and Cosmetic Dyes (US)
FD & C— Food, Drug and Cosmetic Dyes (US)
FDA—Food and Drug Administration (US)

[b] As of February, 1988 and subject to revision.

on starch or calcium sulfate from its aqueous solution; the resultant powder is dried and blended with the other ingredients. If the insoluble lakes are used, they may be blended with the other dry ingredients. Frequently during drying, colors in wet granulations migrate, resulting in an uneven distribution of the color in the granulation. After compression, the tablets will have a mottled appearance due to the uneven distribution of the color. Migration of colors may be reduced by drying the granulation slowly at low temperatures and stirring the granulation while it is drying. The affinity of several water-soluble anionic certified dyes for natural starches has been demonstrated; in these cases this affinity should aid in preventing color migration.

Other additives have been shown to act as dye-migration inhibitors. Tragacanth (1%), acacia (3%), attapulgite (5%) and talc (7%) were effective in inhibiting the migration of FD&C Blue No 1 in lactose. In using dye lakes, the problem of color migration is avoided since the lakes are insoluble. Prevention of mottling can be helped also by the use of lubricants and other additives which have been colored similarly to the granulation prior to their use. The problem of mottling becomes more pronounced as the concentration of the colorants increases. Color mottling is an undesirable characteristic common to many commercial tablets.

Flavoring Agents

In addition to the sweetness which may be afforded by the diluent of the chewable tablet, eg, mannitol or lactose, artificial sweetening agents may be included. Formerly, the cyclamates, either alone or in combination with saccharin, were used widely. With the banning of the cyclamates and the indefinite status of saccharin, new natural sweeteners are being sought. Aspartame (*Searle*), has found applications for pharmaceutical formulations. Sweeteners other than the sugars have the advantage of reducing the bulk volume, considering the quantity of sucrose required to produce the same degree of sweetness. Being present in small quantities, they do not affect markedly the physical characteristics of the tablet granulation.

Powder Compaction

Compressed tablets became a commercially viable and efficient dosage form with the invention of tablet machines. In 1843 William Brockendon, a British inventor, author, artist and watchmaker, received British Patent #9977 for "Shaping Pills, Lozenges, and Black Lead by Pressure in Dies."[22] In over 150 years of tablet manufacture, the basic process has not changed. Surprisingly, improvements have been made only with regards to speed of manufacture and quality control.

The process of compaction has several identifiable phases. As can be seen in Fig 3, when powders undergo compression (a reduction in volume), the first process to occur is a consolidation of the powders. During this consolidation phase, the powder particles adopt a more efficient packing order. The second phase of the compaction process is elastic, or reversible deformation. If the force were to be removed during this phase, the powder would recover completely to the efficiently packed state. For most pharmaceutical powders, this phase is very short in duration, and very difficult to identify on most instrumented tablet presses. The third phase of compaction

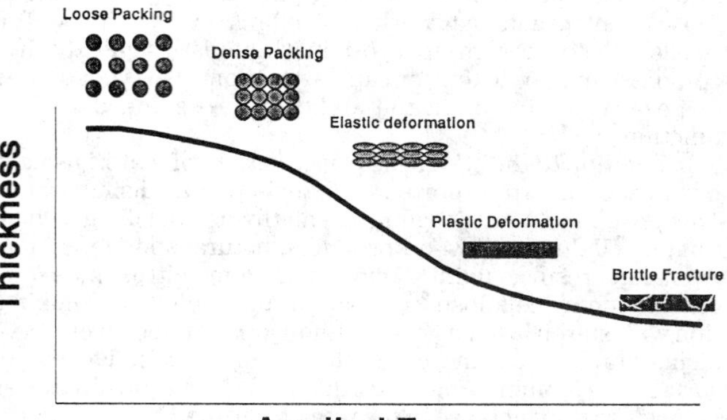

Fig 3. The stages of powder compaction.

is plastic, or irreversible deformation of the powder bed. It is this phase of the compaction process that is the most critical in tablet formation. If too much force is applied to the powder, brittle fracture occurs. If the force was applied to quickly, fracture and debonding during stress relaxation can occur.

In 1950, Stewart reported on the importance of plastic flow, and suggested that if a material has significant plastic flow under compression, it will be more likely to form a compact.[23] David and Augsburger evaluated stress-relaxation data, using the Maxwell model of viscoelastic behavior in an attempt to quantify the rate of plastic deformation of some direct compression excipients.[24] Jones has used the term *contact time* to describe the total time for which a moving punch applies a detectable force to the die contents during the compression and decompression event, excluding ejection.[25]

Rees and Rue evaluated three parameters: stress relation during compaction, effect of contact time on tablet density and rate of application of diametrical compression on tablet deformation.[26]

Jones[25] outlined numerous techniques to evaluate the compactability of powders. Because of the completeness of his review, these parameters are discussed below.

Tablet Strength—Compression Pressure Profile

Most formulators use tablet *hardness*, or tensile strength, as a measure of the cohesiveness of a tablet. With even the simplest of instrumented tablet presses, it is possible to plot tensile strength versus the force applied to the tablet. Figure 4 illustrates such a plot. These plots can be useful in identifying forces which can cause fracture and can lead to a quick, tangible assessment of the compatibility of the formulation. However, there are many limitations to this method, as these plots cannot predict *lamination* or *capping*. In addition, the cohesiveness of a tablet can change upon storage, in either a positive or negative direction.

Tablet Friability

This test is discussed later in the chapter, and there have been many suggestions as to how they should be performed. Many formulators believe this is an important indicator of cohesiveness, but is of limited value in predicting failure in the field.

Changes in Bed Density during Compression

As applied stress (force) increases, elastic and plastic deformation of the particles occurs, which results in plastic flow, and a reduction in inter- and intraparticulate void spaces. This lowers the overall compact density.

For highly cohesive systems, the reduction in void space may yield a compact of sufficient strength for insertion into a capsules shell. However, the inherent cohesiveness for most drugs and excipients is not suitable alone for tablet manufacture.

The Heckel equation is given below; K can be considered to be equal to the reciprocal of the mean yield pressure and A is a function of the original compact volume and is related to the densification and particle rearrangement prior to bonding.

$$\ln\left[\frac{1}{1-D}\right] = KP + A$$

where D is the relative density at pressure P and K and A are constants.

Hersey and Rees[28] have classified Heckel plots into two categories. Figure 5 shows both types of Heckel plots. Type 2 differs from Type 1 in that above a certain pressure a single linear relationship occurs irrespective of the initial bed density. This is independent of particle size and is probable due to fragmentation of particles and their subsequent compaction by plastic deformation. For Type 1 materials, no such fracture occurs, but adjacent particles simply deform plastically.

The pressure at which the plots transition to a linear portion is approximately equal to the minimum pressure required to form a coherent compact.

Changes in Surface Area during Compression

Bulk powders change their state of packing during compaction, and individual particles fracture and/or plastically deform. During this process, the surface area of the powders and the compact in whole, changes. Conventional nitrogen absorption techniques can estimate these changes. Although this can be tedious, these measurements can give a means of examining lamination tendency.

Stress Relaxation

The experimental technique consists of holding the compression process at a point of maximum compression and observing the compression force over various periods of time. By increasing the duration of this period (dwell time), plastic flow is maximized and tablet strength increases.

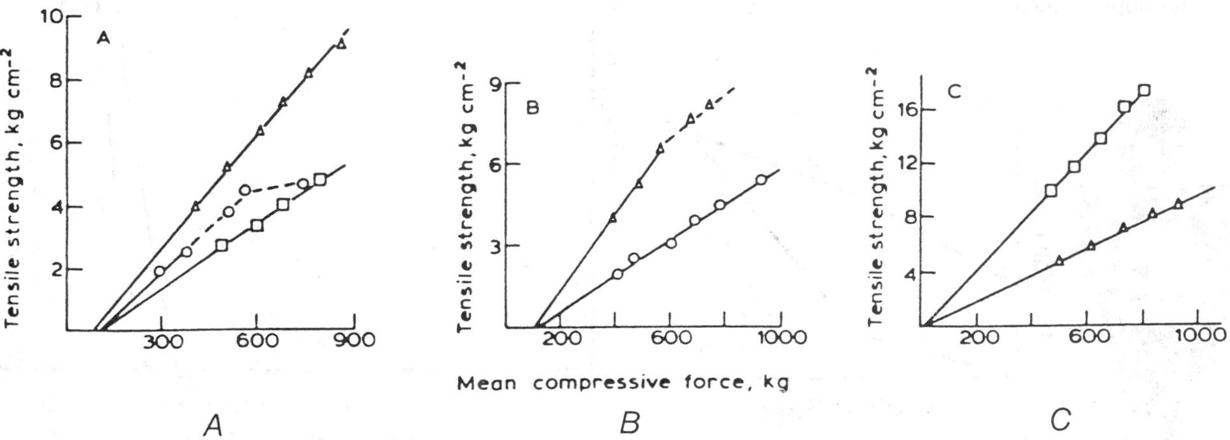

Fig 4. Tensile strength of compacts prepared from different crystal forms. *A:* Barbitone (104–152 μm)—○, Form I; □ Form II; △, Form III. *B:* Sulphathiazole (104–152 μm)—○, Form I; △, Form II. *C:* Aspirin (250–353 μm)—△, Form I; □, Form IV (courtesy, Summers *et al*[27]).

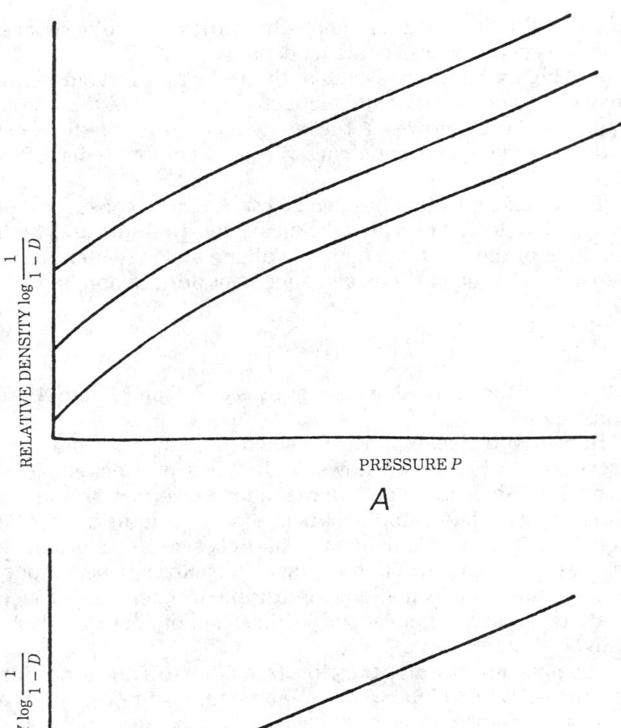

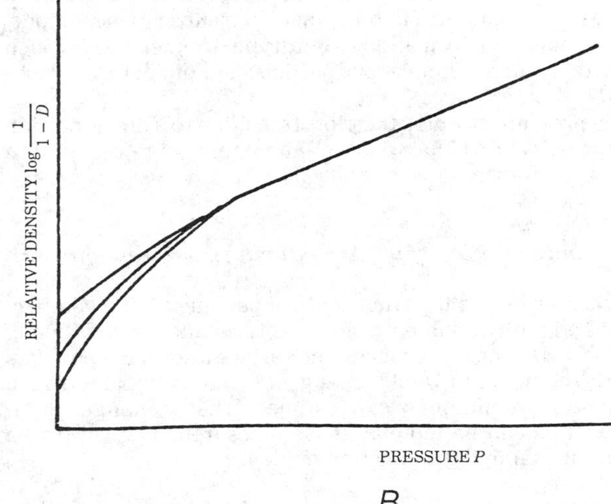

Fig 5. Heckel plots. *A:* Type I; *B:* Type II (courtesy, Jones[29]).

Stress Transmissions during Compression

If the stresses in the upper punch, lower punch and die wall are monitored, as in Fig 6, a general plot can be constructed showing the relationship between these forces. The elastic limit is reached at point *A*. At point *B*, the applied force is released, and the transmitted force on the wall of the die falls rapidly. The upper punch ceases to contact the powder/

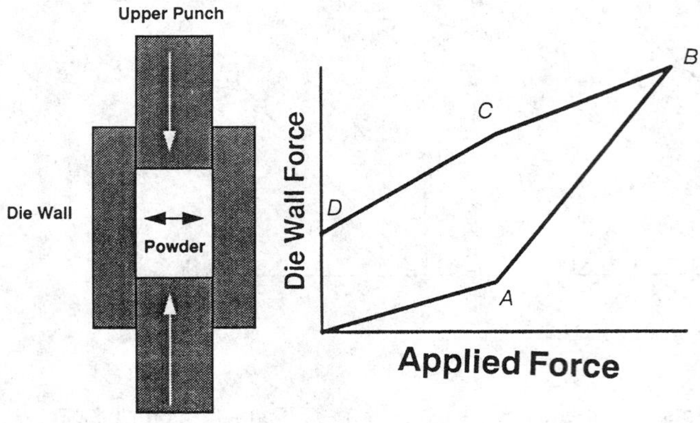

Fig 6. Transmitted stresses during tablet compaction.

compact at point *C*, where the transmitted force falls rapidly to a residual force, point *D*. The force needed to eject the tablet from the die must be greater than the residual force holding it to the sides of the die. Therefore, residual forces tend to be proportional to ejection forces. In addition, these plots can give a good assessment of the elastic component of the compaction process of a powder.

Work and Compaction

Force-displacement (*F-D*) curves are useful in determining the "work" involved in forming a compact. Curves, such as shown in Fig 7,[29] represent the work of the compression process, but all compacts expand somewhat during decompression, and this force is transferred back to the punch. Therefore, by performing a second compression of the compact, the second result can be subtracted from the first for a

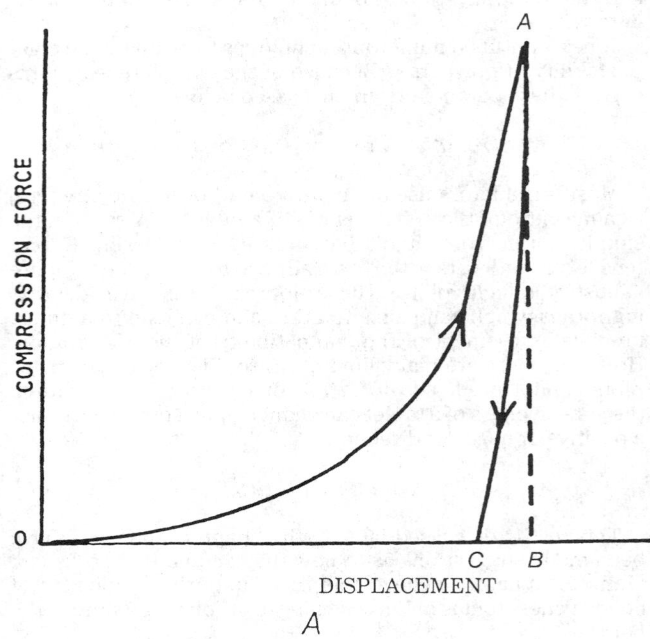

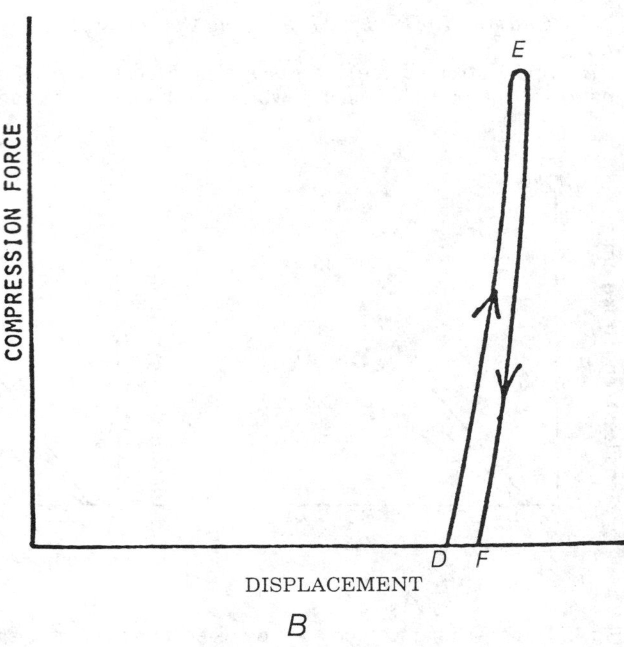

Fig 7. Typical forces. *A:* displacement (*F–D*) curve; *B:* displacement (*F–D*), second compression (courtesy, Jones[29]).

"corrected *F-D* curve." The corrected curve represents the work associated with plastic deformation during powder compaction, as well as a determination of the work of friction of the die wall and the work of elastic deformation.

Granulation Methods

Wet Granulation

The most widely used and most general method of tablet preparation is the wet-granulation method. Its popularity is due to the greater probability that the granulation will meet all the physical requirements for the compression of good tablets. Its chief disadvantages are the number of separate steps involved, as well as the time and labor necessary to carry out the procedure, especially on a large scale. The steps in the wet method are weighing, mixing, granulation, screening the damp mass, drying, dry screening, lubrication and compression. The equipment involved depends on the quantity or size of the batch. The active ingredient, diluent and disintegrant are mixed or blended well. For small batches the ingredients may be mixed in stainless-steel bowls or mortars. Small-scale blending also can be carried out on a large piece of paper by holding the opposite edges and tumbling the material back and forth. The powder blend may be sifted through a screen of suitable fineness to remove or break up lumps. This screening also affords additional mixing. The screen selected always should be of the same type of wire or cloth that will not affect the potency of the ingredients through interaction. For example, the stability of ascorbic acid is affected deleteriously by even small amounts of copper, thus care must be taken to avoid contact with copper or copper-containing alloys.

For larger quantities of powder, the Patterson-Kelley twin-shell blender and the double-cone blender offer a means of precision blending and mixing in short periods of time (Fig 8). Twin-shell blenders are available in many sizes from laboratory models to large production models. Planetary mixers, eg, the Glen mixer and the Hobart mixer, have served this function in the pharmaceutical industry for many years (Fig 9). On a large scale, ribbon blenders also are employed frequently and may be adapted for continuous production procedures. Mass mixers of the sigma-blade type have been used widely in the pharmaceutical industry.

Rapidly increasing in popularity are the high-speed, high-shear mixers such as the Lodige/Littleford, Diosna, Fielder and Baker-Perkins. For these mixers a full range of sizes are available. The processing of granulations in these machines is generally faster than in conventional granulators. However, control over the process is critical, and scale-up issues may become extremely important.[30] Fluid-bed granulation (discussed below) also is gaining wide acceptance in the industry. For both of these types of processing, slight modifications to the following procedures are required.

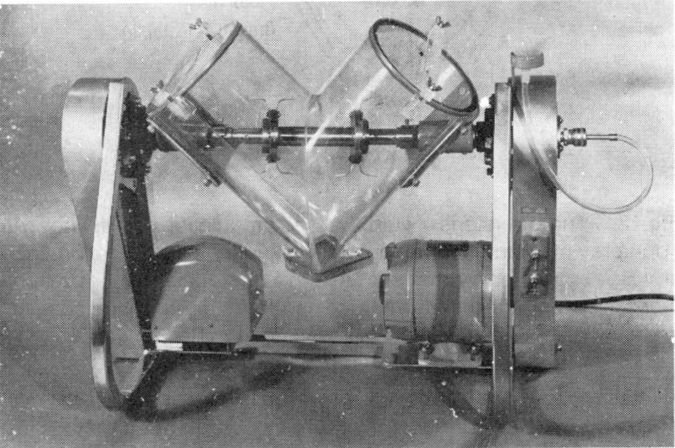

Fig 8. Twin-shell blender for solids or liquid-solids blending (courtesy, Patterson-Kelley).

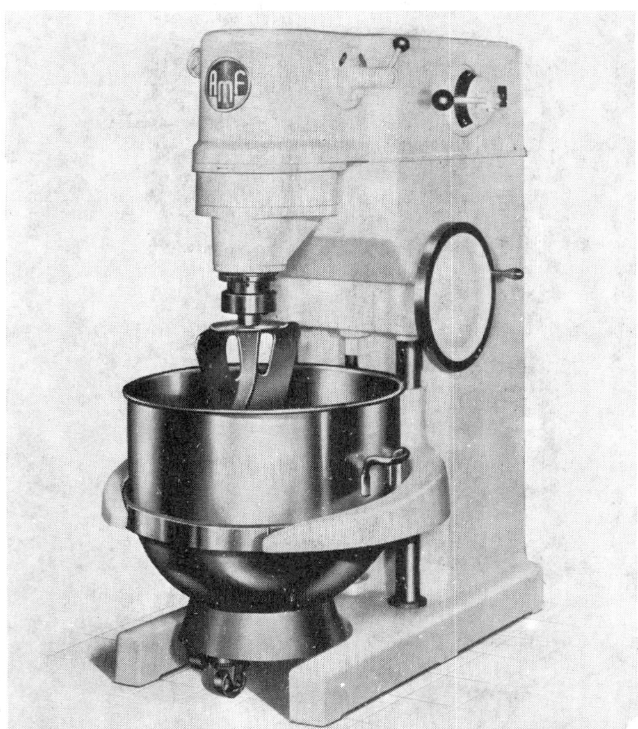

Fig 9. The Glen powder mixer (courtesy, Am Machine).

Solutions of the binding agent are added to the mixed powders with stirring. The powder mass is wetted with the binding solution until the mass has the consistency of damp snow or brown sugar. If the granulation is overwetted, the granules will be hard, requiring considerable pressure to form the tablets, and the resultant tablets may have a mottled appearance. If the powder mixture is not wetted sufficiently, the resulting granules will be too soft, breaking down during lubrication and causing difficulty during compression.

The wet granulation is forced through a 6- or 8-mesh screen. Small batches can be forced through by hand using a manual screen. For larger quantities, one of several comminuting mills suitable for wet screening can be used. These include the Stokes oscillator, Colton rotary granulator, Fitzpatrick comminuting mill or Stokes tornado mill. See Fig 10. In comminuting mills the granulation is forced through the sieving device by rotating hammers, knives or oscillating bars. Most high-speed mixers are equipped with a chopper blade which operates independently of the main mixing blades and can replace the wet milling step, ie, can obviate the need for a separate operation.

For tablet formulations where continuous production is justified, extruders such as the Reitz extructor have been adapted for the wet-granulation process. The extruder consists of a screw mixer with a chamber where the powder is mixed with the binding agent and the wet mass gradually is forced through a perforated screen forming threads of the wet granulation. The granulation then is dried by conventional methods. A semiautomatic continuous process using the Reitz extructor has been described for the preparation of the antacid tablet Gelusil (*Warner-Lambert*).

Moist material from the wet milling step is placed on large sheets of paper on shallow wire trays and placed in drying cabinets with a circulating air current and thermostatic heat control. See Fig 11. While tray drying was the most widely used method of drying tablet granulations in the past, fluid-bed drying is now equally popular. Notable among the newer methods being introduced are the fluid-bed dryers. In drying

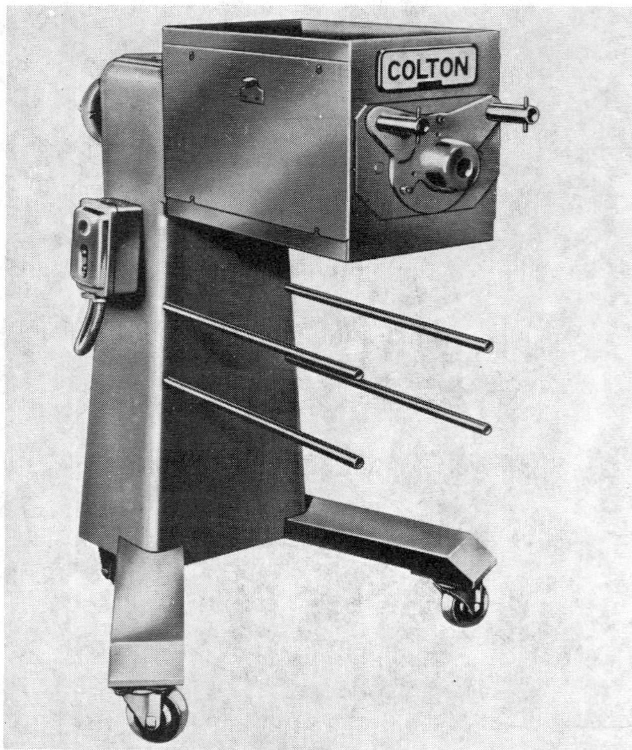

Fig 10. Rotary granulator and sifter (courtesy, Vector/Colton).

tablet granulation by fluidization, the material is suspended and agitated in a warm air stream while the granulation is maintained in motion. Drying tests comparing the fluidized bed and a tray dryer for a number of tablet granulations indicated that the former was 15 times faster than the conventional method of tray drying. In addition to the decreased drying time, the fluidization method is claimed to have other advantages such as better control of drying temperatures, decreased handling costs and the opportunity to blend lubricants and other materials into the dry granulation directly in the fluidized bed. See Fig 12.[31]

The application of radio-frequency drying and infrared drying to tablet granulations has been reported as successful for the majority of granulations tried. These methods readily lend themselves to continuous granulation operations. The study of drying methods for tablet granulations led to the development of the Rovac dryer system by Ciba pharmacists and engineers. The dryer is similar in appearance to the cone blender except for the heating jacket and vacuum connections. By excluding oxygen and using the lower drying temperatures made possible by drying in a vacuum, opportunities for degradation of the ingredients during the drying cycle are minimized. A greater uniformity of residual moisture content is achieved because of the moving bed, controlled temperature and controlled time period of the drying cycle. Particle-size distribution can be controlled by varying the speed of rotation and drying temperature as well as by comminuting the granulation to the desired granule size after drying.

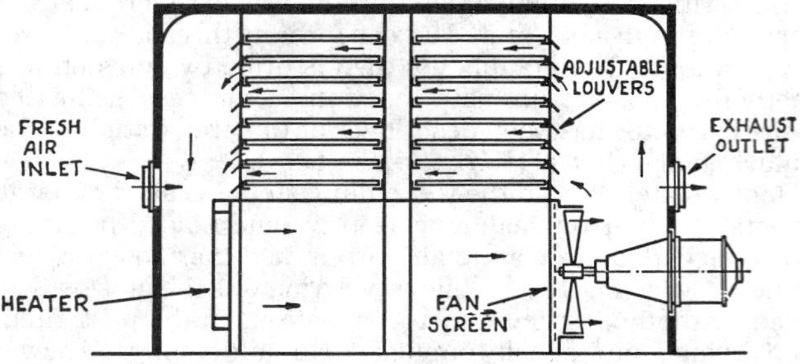

Fig 11. Cross section of tray dryer.

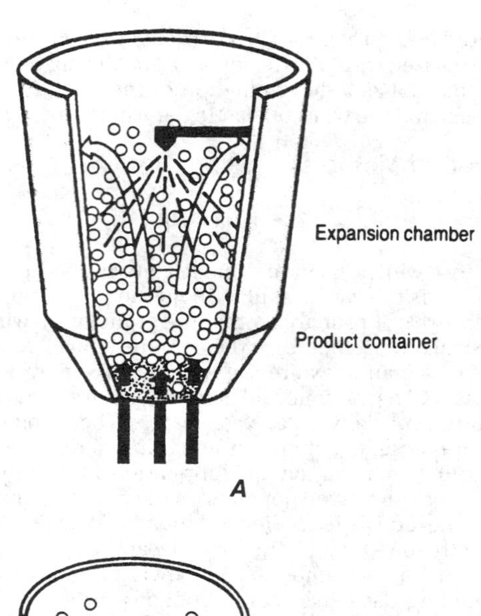

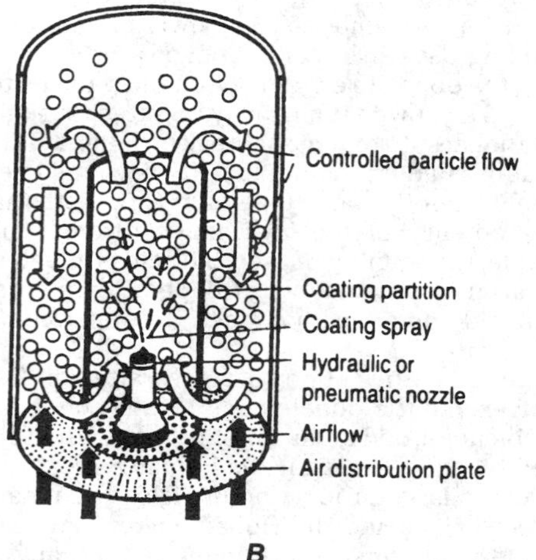

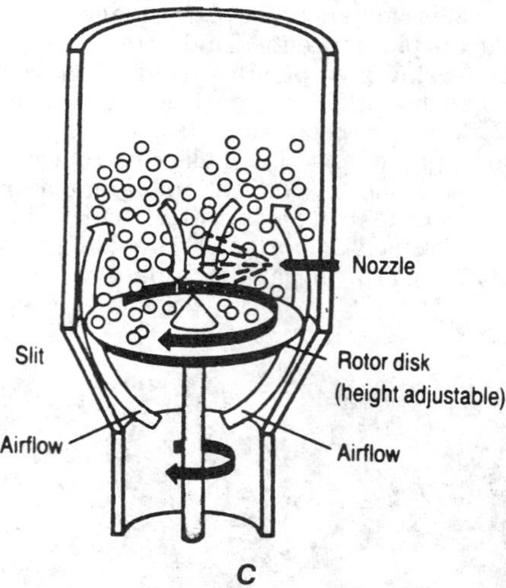

Fig 12. Three versions of fluidized-bed granulation and drying. *A:* Top-spray method used in conventional fluid-bed granulation coaters; *B:* bottom-spray method used in Wurster air-suspension columns; *C:* tangential-spray method used in rotary fluid-bed coaters/granulators (courtesy, Aster Publ, adapted from Ref 31).

In drying granulations it is desirable to maintain a residual amount of moisture in the granulation. This is necessary to maintain the various granulation ingredients such as gums in a hydrated state. Also, the residual moisture contributes to the reduction of the static electric charges on the particles. In the selection of any drying process, an effort is made to obtain a uniform moisture content. In addition to the importance of moisture content of the granulation in its handling during the manufacturing steps, the stability of the products containing moisture-sensitive active ingredients may be related to the moisture content of the products.

Previously it was indicated that water-soluble colorants can migrate toward the surface of the granulation during the drying process, resulting in mottled tablets after compression. This is also true for water-soluble drug substances, resulting in tablets unsatisfactory as to content uniformity. Migration can be reduced by drying the granulation slowly at low temperatures or using a granulation in which the major diluent is present as granules of large particle size. The presence of microcrystalline cellulose in wet granulations also reduces migration tendencies.

After drying, the granulation is reduced in particle size by passing it through a smaller mesh screen. Following dry screening, the granule size tends to be more uniform. For dry granulations the screen size to be selected depends on the diameter of the punch. The following sizes are suggested:

Tablets up to 3/16 inch diam, use 20-mesh
Tablets 7/32 in to 5/16 inch, use 16-mesh
Tablets 11/32 in to 13/32 inch, use 14-mesh
Tablets 7/16 inch and larger, use 12-mesh

For small amounts of granulation, hand screens may be used and the material passed through with the aid of a stainless-steel spatula. With larger quantities, any of the comminuting mills with screens corresponding to those just mentioned may be used. Note that the smaller the tablet, the finer the dry granulation to enable more uniform filling of the die cavity; large granules give an irregular fill to a comparatively small die cavity. With compressed tablets of sodium bicarbonate, lactose and magnesium trisilicate, a relationship has been demonstrated to exist between the particle size of the granulated material and the disintegration time and capping of the resultant tablets. For a sulfathiazole granulation, however, the particle-size distribution did not appear to influence hardness or disintegration.

After dry granulation, the lubricant is added as a fine powder. It usually is screened onto the granulation through 60- or 100-mesh nylon cloth to eliminate small lumps as well as to increase the covering power of the lubricant. As it is desirable for each granule to be covered with the lubricant, the lubricant is blended with the granulation very gently, preferably in a blender using a tumbling action. Gentle action is desired to maintain the uniform granule size resulting from the granulation step. It has been claimed that too much fine powder is not desirable because fine powder may not feed into the die evenly; consequently, variations in weight and density result. Fine powders, commonly designated as *fines*, also blow out around the upper punch and down past the lower punch, making it necessary to clean the machine frequently. Fines, however, at a level of 10 to 20% traditionally are sought by the tablet formulator. The presence of some fines is necessary for the proper filling of the die cavity. Now, even higher concentrations of fines are used successfully in tablet manufacture. Most investigators agree that no general limits exist for the amount of fines that can be present in a granulation but must be determined for each specific formula.

Many formulators once believed (and some still believe) that overblending resulted in an increased amount of fines and, hence, caused air entrapment in the formula. The capping and laminating of tablets associated with overblending lubricants was thought to be caused by these air pockets. Most scientists now recognize that a more plausible explanation has to do with the function of the lubricants themselves. Since the very nature of lubricant tends to make surfaces less susceptible to adhesion, overblending prevents the intergranule bonding that takes place during compaction.

Fluid-Bed Granulation

A new method for granulating evolved from the fluid-bed drying technology described earlier. The concept was to spray a granulating solution onto the suspended particles which then would be dried rapidly in the suspending air. The main benefit from this system is the rapid granulation and drying of a batch. The two main firms that developed this technology are *Glatt* and *Aeromatic*. The design of these systems are basically the same with both companies (see Fig 12). In this method, particles of an inert material, or the active drug, are suspended in a vertical column with a rising air stream; while the particles are suspended, the common granulating materials in solution are sprayed into the column. There is a gradual particle buildup under a controlled set of conditions resulting in a tablet granulation which is ready for compression after the addition of the lubricant. An obvious advantage exists since granulating and drying can take place in a single piece of equipment. It should be noted, however, that many of the mixers discussed previously can be supplied with a steam jacket and vacuum, and can provide the same advantage.

In these systems a granulating solution or solvent is sprayed into or onto the bed of suspended particles. The rate of addition of the binder, temperature in the bed of particles, temperature of the air, volume and moisture of the air all play an important role in the quality and performance of the final product. Many scientists feel that this method is an extension of the wet-granulation method, as it incorporates many of its concepts. However anyone who has developed a formulation in a fluid-bed system knows that the many operating parameters involved make it somewhat more complex.[31] In addition to its use for the preparation of tablet granulations this technique also has been proposed for the coating of solid particles as a means of improving the flow properties of small particles. Researchers have observed that, in general, fluid-bed granulation yields a less dense particle than conventional methods, and this can affect subsequent compression behavior. A large-scale fluid-bed granulation process has been described for Tylenol (*McNeil*). Methods for the preparation of compressed tablets have been reviewed in the literature.[32]

In the *Merck Sharp & Dohme* facility at Elkton, VA, the entire tablet manufacturing process based on a wet-granulation method is computer-controlled. By means of a computer, the system weighs the ingredients, blends, granulates, dries and lubricates to prepare a uniform granulation of specified particle size and particle-size distribution. The computer directs the compression of the material into tablets having exacting specifications for thickness, weight and hardness. After compression, the tablets are coated with a water-based film coating. The computer controls and monitors all flow of material. The plant represents the first totally automated pharmaceutical manufacturing facility. See Fig 13.

Although the Merck facility represents the most fully automated production operation, there are many others throughout the industry which have parts of the operation (such as a coating, compressing or fluid-bed granulation process) operating under a high degree of sophistication and automation. This is the trend for the future. Equipment suppliers work closely with individual pharmaceutical companies in designing specialized and unique systems.

Dry Granulation

When tablet ingredients are sensitive to moisture or are unable to withstand elevated temperatures during drying, and when the tablet ingredients have sufficient inherent binding or cohesive properties, slugging may be used to form granules. This method is referred to as dry granulation, precompression

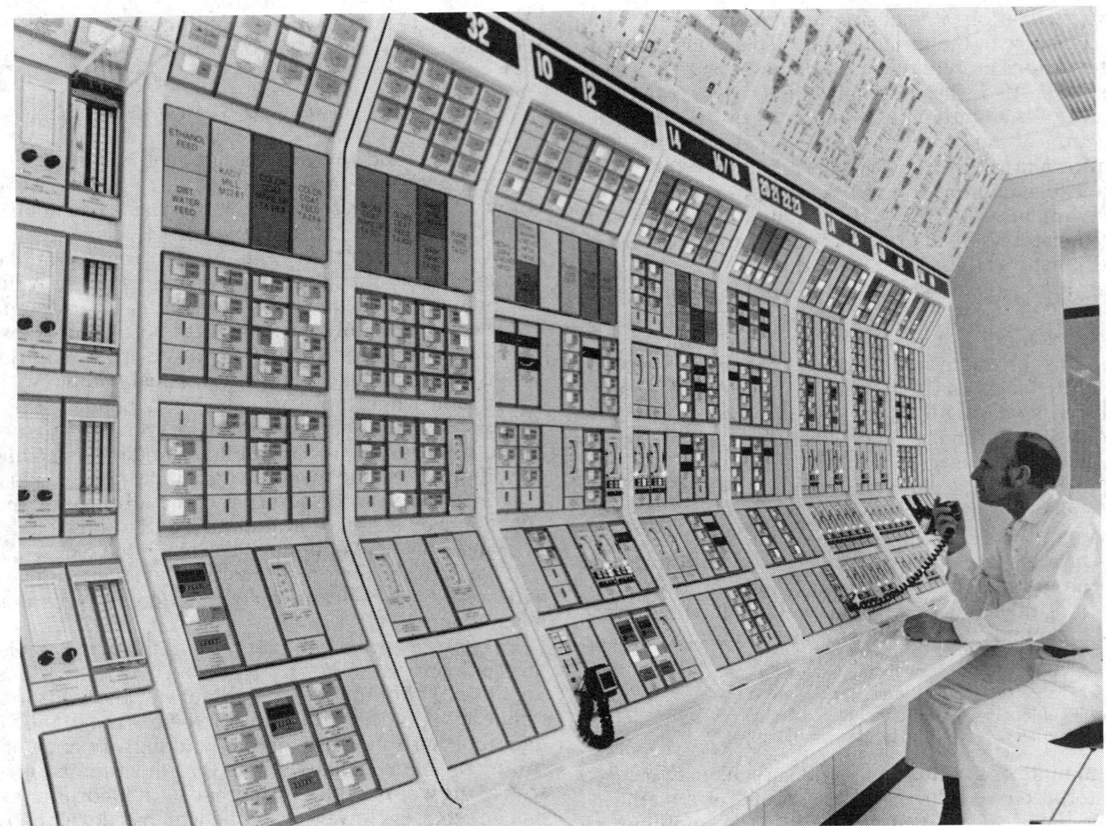

Fig 13. Computer control room for the first large-scale computer-controlled tablet manufacturing facility (courtesy, MSD).

or double-compression. It eliminates a number of steps but still includes weighing, mixing, slugging, dry screening, lubrication and compression. The active ingredient, diluent (if one is required) and part of the lubricant are blended. One of the constituents, either the active ingredient or the diluent, must have cohesive properties. Powdered material contains a considerable amount of air; under pressure this air is expelled and a fairly dense piece is formed. The more time allowed for this air to escape, the better the tablet or slug.

When slugging is used, large tablets are made as slugs because fine powders flow better into large cavities. Also, producing large slugs decreases production time; $\frac{7}{8}$ to 1 in are the most practical sizes for slugs. Sometimes, to obtain the pressure which is desired the slug sizes are reduced to $\frac{3}{4}$ in. The punches should be flat-faced. The compressed slugs are comminuted through the desirable mesh screen either by hand, or for larger quantities through the Fitzpatrick or similar comminuting mill. The lubricant remaining is added to the granulation, blended gently and the material is compressed into tablets. Aspirin is a good example where slugging is satisfactory. Other materials such as aspirin combinations, acetophenetidin, thiamine hydrochloride, ascorbic acid, magnesium hydroxide and other antacid compounds may be treated similarly.

Results comparable to those accomplished by the slugging process also are obtained with compacting mills. In the compaction method the powder to be densified passes between high-pressure rollers which compress the powder and remove the air. The densified material is reduced to a uniform granule size and compressed into tablets after the addition of a lubricant. Excessive pressures which may be required to obtain cohesion of certain materials may result in a prolonged dissolution rate. Compaction mills available include the Chilsonator (*Fitzpatrick*), Roller Compactor (*Vector*) and the Compactor Mill (*Allis-Chalmers*).

Direct Compression

As its name implies, direct compression consists of compressing tablets directly from powdered material without modifying the physical nature of the material itself. Formerly, direct compression as a method of tablet manufacture was reserved for a small group of crystalline chemicals having all the physical characteristics required for the formation of a good tablet. This group includes chemicals such as potassium salts (chlorate, chloride, bromide, iodide, nitrate, permanganate), ammonium chloride and methenamine. These materials possess cohesive and flow properties which make direct compression possible.

Since the pharmaceutical industry constantly is making efforts to increase the efficiency of tableting operations and reduce costs by using the smallest amount of floor space and labor as possible for a given operation, increasing attention is being given to this method of tablet preparation. Approaches being used to make this method more universally applicable include the introduction of formulation additives capable of imparting the characteristics required for compression, and the use of force-feeding devices to improve the flow of powder blends.

For tablets in which the drug itself constitutes a major portion of the total tablet weight, it is necessary that the drug possess those physical characteristics required for the formulation to be compressed directly. Direct compression for tablets containing 25% or less of drug substances frequently can be used by formulating with a suitable diluent which acts as a carrier or vehicle for the drug.[32–34]

Direct-compression vehicles or carriers must have good flow and compressible characteristics. These properties are imparted to them by a preprocessing step such as wet granulation, slugging, spray drying, spheronization or crystallization. These vehicles include processed forms of most of the common diluents including dicalcium phosphate dihydrate, tricalcium phosphate, calcium sulfate, anhydrous lactose, spray-dried lactose, pregelatinized starch, compressible sugar, mannitol and microcrystalline cellulose. These commercially available direct-compression vehicles may contain small quantities of other ingredients (eg, starch) as processing aids. Dicalcium phosphate dihydrate (Di-Tab, *Stauffer*) in its unmilled form has good flow properties and compressibility. It is a white crystalline agglomerate insoluble in water and alcohol. The chemical is odorless, tasteless and nonhygroscopic. Since it has no inherent lubricating or disintegrating properties, other additives must be present to prepare a satisfactory formulation.

Compressible sugar consists mainly of sucrose that is processed to have properties suitable for direct compression. It also may contain small quantities of dextrin, starch or invert sugar. It is a white crystalline powder with a sweet taste and complete water solubility. It requires the incorporation of a suitable lubricant at normal levels for lubricity. The sugar is used widely for chewable vitamin tablets because of its natural sweetness. One commercial source is Di-Pac (*Amstar*) prepared by the cocrystallization of 97% sucrose and 3% dextrins. Some forms of lactose meet the requirements for a direct-compression vehicle. Hydrous lactose does not flow and its use is limited to tablet formulations prepared by the wet granulation method. Both anhydrous lactose and spray-dried lactose have good flowability and compressibility and can be used in direct compression provided a suitable disintegrant and lubricant are present. Mannitol is a popular diluent for chewable tablets due to its pleasant taste and mouthfeel resulting from its negative heat of solution. In its granular form (*ICI Americas*) it has good flow and compressible qualities. It has a low moisture content and is not hygroscopic.

The excipient that has been studied extensively as a direct compression vehicle is microcrystalline cellulose (Avicel, *FMC*). This nonfibrous form of cellulose is obtained by spray-drying washed, acid-treated cellulose and is available in several grades which range in average particle size from 20 to 100 μm. It is water insoluble but the material has the ability to draw fluid into a tablet by capillary action; it swells on contact and thus acts as a disintegrating agent. The material flows well and has a degree of self-lubricating qualities, thus requiring a lower level of lubricant as compared to other excipients.

Forced-flow feeders are mechanical devices available from pharmaceutical equipment manufacturers designed to deaerate light and bulky material. Mechanically, they maintain a steady flow of powder moving into the die cavities under moderate pressure. By increasing the density of the powder, higher uniformity in tablet weights is obtained. See Fig 14.

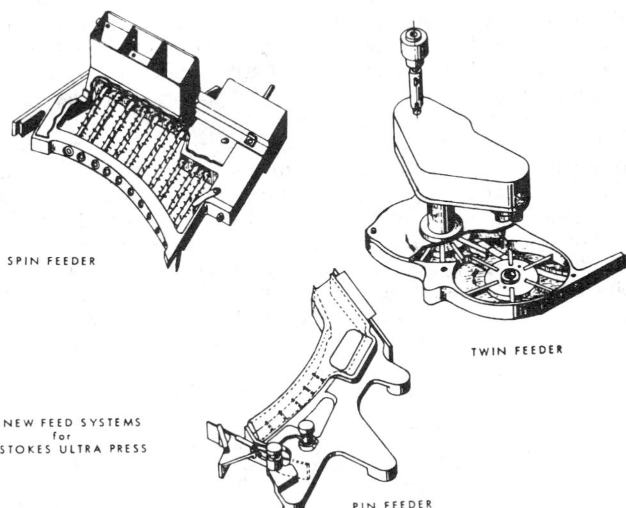

Fig 14. Feeding devices designed to promote flow of granulations for high-speed machines (courtesy, Stokes/Pennwalt).

Recently, many companies have reversed their optimism for some direct-compression systems. Some formulations made by direct compression were not as "forgiving" as were the older wet-granulated products. As raw material variations occurred, especially with the drug, many companies found themselves with poorly compactable formulations. Interest in direct compression also is stimulating basic research on the flowability of powders with and without the presence of additives. Direct compression formulas are included in the formula section found on page 1636.

Related Granulation Processes

Spheronization—Spheronization, a form of pelletization, refers to the formation of spherical particles from wet granulations. Since the particles are round, they have good flow properties when dried. They can be formulated to contain sufficient binder to impart cohesiveness for tableting. Spheronization equipment such as the Marumerizer (*Luwa*) and the CF-Granulator (*Vector*) is commercially available. A wet granulation containing the drug substance, diluent (if required) and binder, is passed first through an extruding machine to form rod-shaped cylindrical segments ranging in diameter from 0.5 to 12 mm. The segment diameter and the size of the final spherical particle depend on the extruder screen size. After extrusion the segments are placed into the Marumerizer where they are shaped into spheres by centrifugal and frictional forces on a rotating plate (see Fig 15). The pellets then are dried by conventional methods, mixed with suitable lubricants and compressed into tablets, or used as capsule-fill material. Microcrystalline cellulose has been shown to be an effective diluent and binder in granulations to be spheronized.[35–38] The advantages of the process include the production of granules, regular in shape, size and surface characteristics; low friability resulting in fewer fines and dust; and the ability to regulate the size of the spheres within a narrow particle-size distribution.

Spheres also can be produced by fluid-bed granulation techniques and by other specialized equipment such as the CF-Granulator (*Vector*). These processes, however, must begin with crystals or nonpareil seeds followed by buildup. Exact results, such as sphere density, are different for the various methods and could be important in product performance. These processes can be run as batches or continuously.

Spray-Drying—A number of tableting additives suitable for direct compression have been prepared by the drying process known as spray-drying. The method consists of bringing together a highly dispersed liquid and a sufficient volume of hot air to produce evaporation and drying of the liquid droplets. The feed liquid may be a solution, slurry, emulsion, gel or paste, provided it is pumpable and capable of being atomized. As shown in Fig 16, the feed is sprayed into a current of warm filtered air. The air supplies the heat for

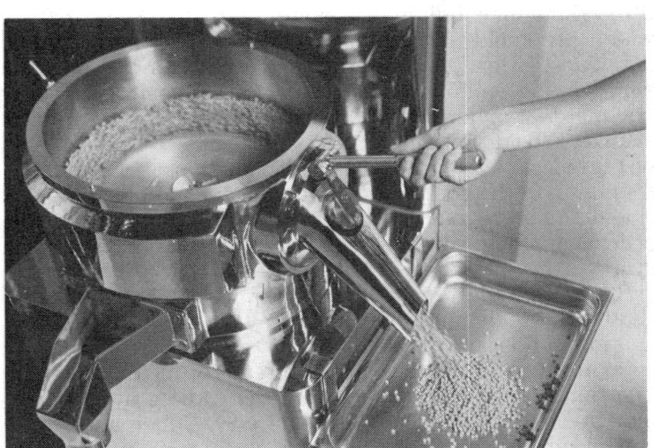

Fig 15. The inside of a QJ-400 Marumerizer (courtesy, Luwa).

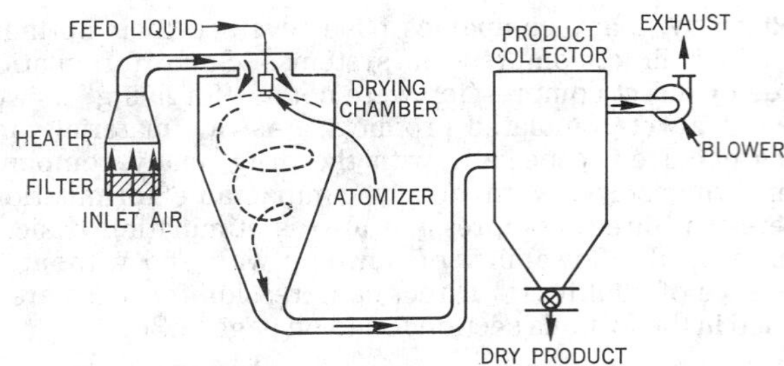

Fig 16. Typical spray-drying system (courtesy, Bowen Eng).

evaporation and conveys the dried product to the collector; the air is then exhausted with the moisture. As the liquid droplets present a large surface area to the warm air, local heat and transfer coefficients are high.

The spray-dried powder particles are homogeneous, approximately spherical in shape, nearly uniform in size and frequently hollow. The latter characteristic results in low bulk density with a rapid rate of solution. Being uniform in size and spherical, the particles possess good flowability. The design and operation of the spray-dryer can vary many characteristics of the final product, such as particle size and size distribution, bulk and particle densities, porosity, moisture content, flowability and friability. Among the spray-dried materials available for direct compression formulas are lactose, mannitol and flour. Another application of the process in tableting is spray-drying the combination of tablet additives as the diluent, disintegrant and binder. The spray-dried material then is blended with the active ingredient or drug, lubricated and compressed directly into tablets.

Since atomization of the feed results in a high surface area, the moisture evaporates rapidly. The evaporation keeps the product cool and as a result the method is applicable for drying heat-sensitive materials. Among heat-sensitive pharmaceuticals successfully spray-dried are the amino acids; antibiotics as aureomycin, bacitracin, penicillin and streptomycin; ascorbic acid; cascara extracts; liver extracts; pepsin and similar enzymes; protein hydrolysates and thiamine.[39]

Frequently, spray-drying is more economical than other processes since it produces a dry powder directly from a liquid and eliminates other processing steps as crystallization, precipitation, filtering or drying, particle-size reduction and particle classifying. By the elimination of these steps, labor, equipment costs, space requirements and possible contamination of the product are reduced. Intrinsic factor concentrate obtained from hog mucosa previously was prepared by *Lederle* using a salt-precipitation process, followed by a freeze-drying. By using spray-drying it was possible to manufacture a high-grade material by a continuous process. The spherical particles of the product facilitated its subsequent blending with vitamin B_{12}. Similar efficiencies have been found in processes producing magnesium trisilicate and dihydroxyaluminum sodium carbonate; both chemicals are used widely in antacid preparations.

Encapsulation of chemicals also can be achieved using spray-drying equipment. The process is useful in coating one material on another in order to protect the interior substance or to control the rate of its release. The substance to be coated can either be liquid or solid, but must be insoluble in a solution of the coating material. The oil-soluble vitamins, A and D, can be coated with a variety of materials such as acacia gum to prevent their deterioration. Flavoring oils and synthetic flavors are coated to give the so-called dry flavors.

Spray-Congealing—Also called spray-chilling, spray-congealing is a technique similar to spray-drying. It consists of melting solids and reducing them to beads or powder by spraying the molten feed into a stream of air or other gas. The same basic equipment is used as with spray-drying although no source of heat is required. Either ambient or cooled air is used depending on the freezing point of the product. For example, monoglycerides and similar materials are spray-congealed with air at 50°F. A closed-loop system with refrigeration cools and recycles the air. Using this process, drugs can be dissolved or suspended in a molten wax and spray-congealed; the resultant material then can be adapted for a prolonged-release form of the drug.

Among the carbohydrates used in compressed tablets, mannitol is the only one which possesses high heat stability. Mannitol melts at 167° and, either alone or in combination with other carbohydrates, can be fused and spray-congealed. Selected drugs have been shown to be soluble in these fused mixtures, and the resultant spray-congealed material possesses excellent flow and compression characteristics.

Tablet Machines

As mentioned previously, the basic mechanical unit in tablet compression involves the operation of two steel punches within a steel die cavity. The tablet is formed by the pressure exerted on the granulation by the punches within the die cavity, or cell. The tablet assumes the size and shape of the punches and die used. See Figs 17 and 18. While round tablets are used more generally, shapes such as oval, capsule-form, square, triangular or other irregular shapes may be used. Likewise, the curvature of the faces of the punches determines the curvature of the tablets. The diameters generally found to be satisfactory and frequently referred to as standard are as follows: 3/16, 7/32, 1/4, 9/32, 5/16, 11/32, 7/16, 1/2, 9/16, 5/8, 11/16 and 3/4 inch. Punch faces with ridges are used for compressed tablets scored for breaking into halves or fourths, although it has been indicated that variation among tablet halves is significantly greater than among intact tablets. However, a patented formulation[40] for a tablet scored to form a groove which is one-third to two-thirds the depth of the total tablet thickness is claimed to give equal parts containing substantially equal amounts of the drug substance. Tablets, engraved or embossed with symbols or initials, require punches with faces embossed or engraved with the corresponding designs. See Figs 19 and 20. The use of the tablet sometimes determines its shape; effervescent tablets are usually large, round and flat, while vitamin tablets frequently are prepared in capsule-shaped forms. Tablets prepared using deep-cup punches appear to be round and when coated take on the appearance of pills. Veterinary tablets often have a bolus shape and are much larger than those used in medical practice.

The quality-control program for punches and dies, frequently referred to as tooling, instituted by large pharmaceutical companies emphasizes the importance of their care in modern pharmaceutical production. To produce physically perfect compressed tablets, an efficient punch-and-die program must be set up. Provisions for inspection of tooling, parameters for cost-per-product determination, product identification and tooling specifications must all be considered. A committee of the Industrial and Pharmaceutical Technology Section of the APhA Academy of Pharmaceutical Sciences has established a set of dimensional specifications and tolerances for standard punches and dies.[41]

Regardless of the size of the tableting operation, the attention which must be given to the proper care of punches and dies should be noted. They must be highly polished and kept free from rust and imperfections. In cases where the material pits or abrades the dies, chromium-plated dies have been used. Dropping the punches on hard surfaces will chip their fine edges. When the punches are in the machine, the upper and lower punches should not be allowed to contact each

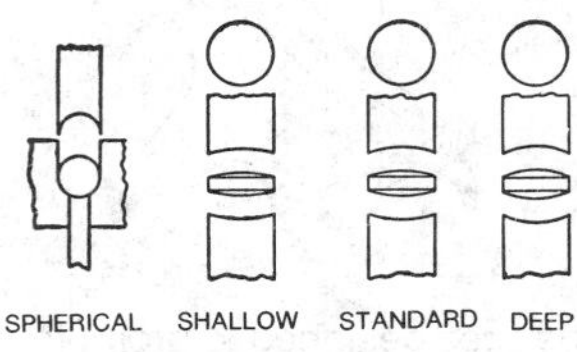

Fig 17. Concave punches.

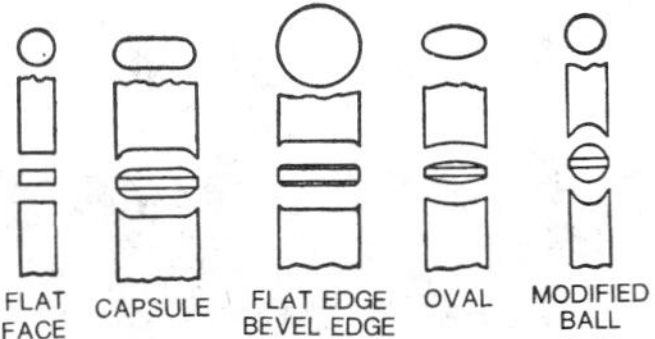

Fig 18. Specially shaped punches.

other. Otherwise, a curling or flattening of the edges will result which is one of the causes of capping. This is especially necessary to observe in the case of deep-cup punches.

When the punches are removed from the machine, they should be washed thoroughly in warm soapy water and dried well with a clean cloth. A coating of grease or oil should be rubbed over all parts of the dies and punches to protect them from the atmosphere. They should be stored carefully in boxes or paper tubes.

Single-Punch Machines

The simplest tableting machines available are those having the single-punch design. A number of models are available as outlined in Table 2. While the majority of these are power-driven, several hand-operated models are available. Compression is accomplished on a single-punch machine as shown in Fig 21. The feed shoe filled with the granulation is positioned over the die cavity which then fills. The feed shoe retracts and scrapes all excess granulation away from the die cavity. The upper punch lowers to compress the granulation within the die cavity. The upper punch retracts and the lower punch rises to eject the tablet. As the feed shoe returns to fill the die cavity, it pushes the compressed tablet from the die platform. The weight of the tablet is determined by the volume of the die cavity; the lower punch is adjustable to increase or decrease the volume of granulation, thus increasing or decreasing the weight of the tablet.

For tablets having diameters larger than ½ inch, sturdier models are required. This is also true for tablets requiring a high degree of hardness as in the case of compressed lozenges.

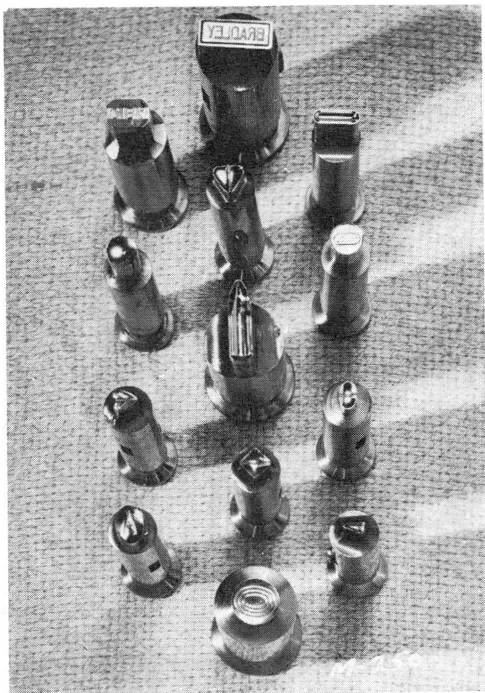

Fig 19. Collection of punches (courtesy, Stokes/Pennwalt).

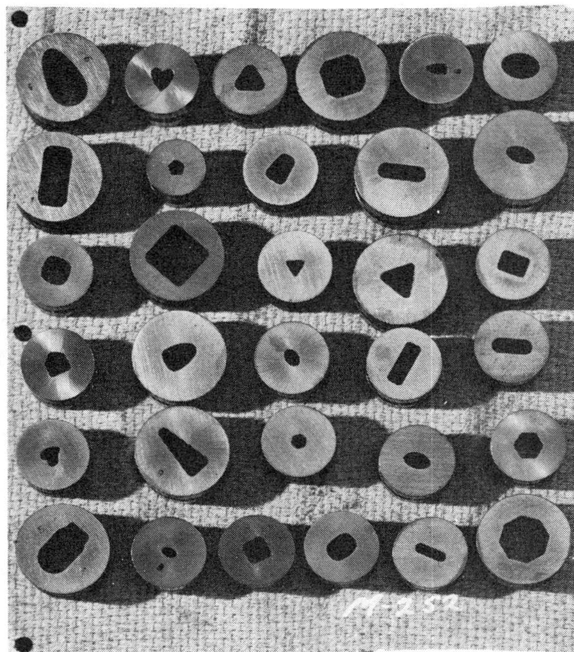

Fig 20. Collection of dies (courtesy, Stokes/Pennwalt).

The heavier models are capable of much higher pressures and are suitable for slugging.

Operation of Single-Punch Machines

In installing punches and dies in a single-punch machine insert the lower punch first by lining up the notched groove on the punch with the lower punch setscrew and slipping it into the smaller bore in the die table; the setscrew is not tightened as yet. The lower punch is differentiated from the upper punch in that it has a collar around the punch head. Slip the die over the punch head so that the notched groove (with the widest area at the top) lines up with the die setscrew. Tighten the lower punch setscrew after seating the lower punch by pressing on the punch with the thumb. Tighten the die setscrew, making certain that the surface of the die is flush with the die table. Insert the upper punch, again lining up the grooved notch with the upper punch setscrew. To be certain that the upper punch is seated securely, turn the machine over by hand with a block of soft wood or wad of cloth between the upper and lower punches. When the punch is seated, tighten the upper punch setscrew. Adjust the pressure so that the upper and lower punches will not come in contact with each other when the machine is turned over. Adjust the lower punch so that it is flush with the die table at the ejection point. Install the feed shoe and hopper.

After adding a small amount of granulation to the hopper, turn the machine over by hand and adjust the pressure until a tablet is formed. Adjust the tablet weight until the desired weight is obtained. The pressure will have to be altered concurrently with the weight adjustments. It should be remembered that as the fill is increased the lower punch moves further away from the upper punch and more pressure will have to be applied to obtain comparable hardness. Conversely, when the fill is decreased, the pressure will have to be decreased. When all the adjust-

Table 2—Single-Punch Tablet Machines

Machine model	Maximum tablet diameter (inches)	Press speed (tablets/min)	Depth of fill (inches)
Stokes-Pennwalt equipment[a]			
511-5	½	40–75	7/16
206-4	1¾	10–40	1 1/16
530-1	2	12–48	1⅝
525-2	3	16–48	2
Manesty equipment (Thomas Eng)			
Hand machine	½	100	7/16
Model F3	⅞	85	11/16
Model 35T[a]	3	36	2¼

[a] Widely used for veterinary boluses.

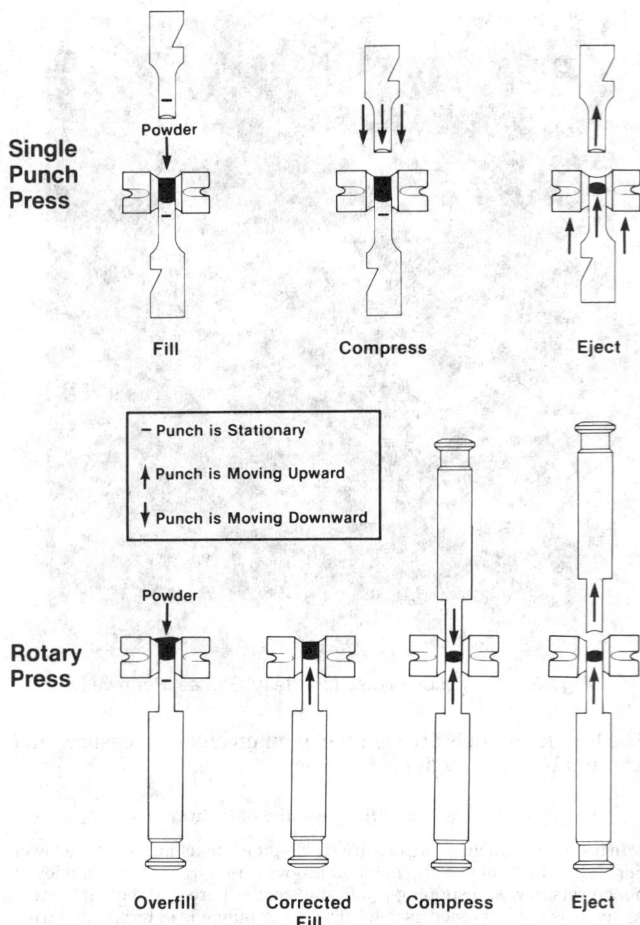

Fig 21. The steps associated with single-punch and rotary tablet machines.

ments have been made, fill the hopper with granulation and turn on the motor. Hardness and weight should be checked immediately and suitable adjustments made if necessary. Periodic checks should be made on the tablet hardness and weight during the running of the batch at 15- to 30-minute intervals.

When the batch has been run off, turn off the power and remove loose dust and granulation with the vacuum cleaner. Release the pressure from the punches. Remove the feed hopper and the feed shoe. Remove the upper punch, the lower punch and the die. Clean all surfaces of the tablet machine and dry well with clean cloth. Cover surfaces with thin coating of grease or oil prior to storage.

As tablets are ejected from the machine after compression, they usually are accompanied with powder and uncompressed granulation. To remove this loose dust, the tablets are passed over a screen, which may be vibrating, and cleaned with a vacuum line.

Rotary Tablet Machines

For increased production, rotary machines offer great advantages. A head carrying a number of sets of punches and dies revolves continuously while the tablet granulation runs from the hopper, through a feed frame and into the dies placed in a large, steel plate revolving under it. This method promotes a uniform fill of the die and therefore an accurate weight for the tablet. Compression takes place as the upper and lower punches pass between a pair of rollers as can be seen in Fig 21. This action produces a slow squeezing effect on the material in the die cavity from the top and bottom and so gives a chance for the entrapped air to escape. The lower punch lifts up and ejects the tablet. Adjustments for tablet weight and hardness can be made without the use of tools

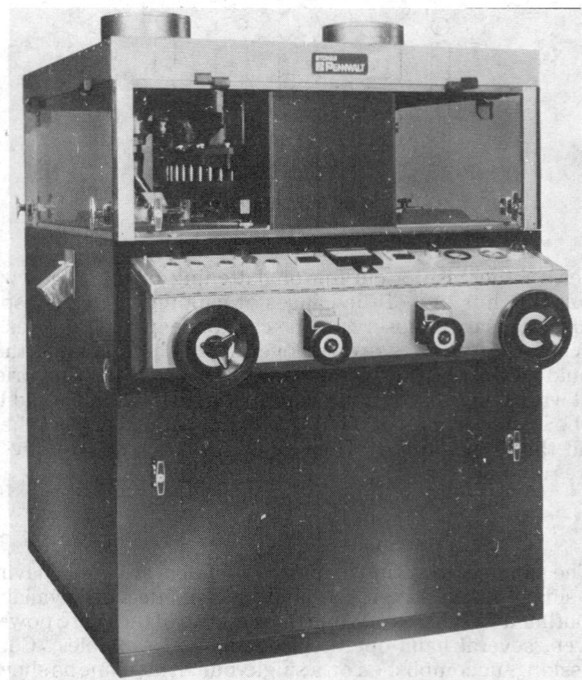

Fig 22. Model 747 High Speed Press, double-sided rotary compacting press designed to produce at speeds over 10,000/min (courtesy, Stokes/Pennwalt).

while the machine is in operation. Figure 23 shows the tooling in a 16-station rotary press in the positions of a complete cycle to produce 1 tablet per set of tooling. One of the factors which contributes to the variation in tablet weight and hardness during compression is the internal flow of the granulation within the feed hopper.

On most rotary machine models there is an excess pressure release which cushions each compression and relieves the machine of all shocks and undue strain. The punches and dies can be removed readily for inspection, cleaning and inserting different sets to produce a great variety of sizes and shapes. Many older presses have been modernized with protective shields to prevent physical injury and to comply with OSHA standards (see Fig 24). It is possible to equip the machine with as few punches and dies as the job requires and thus economize on installation costs. For types of rotary machines available, see Table 3.

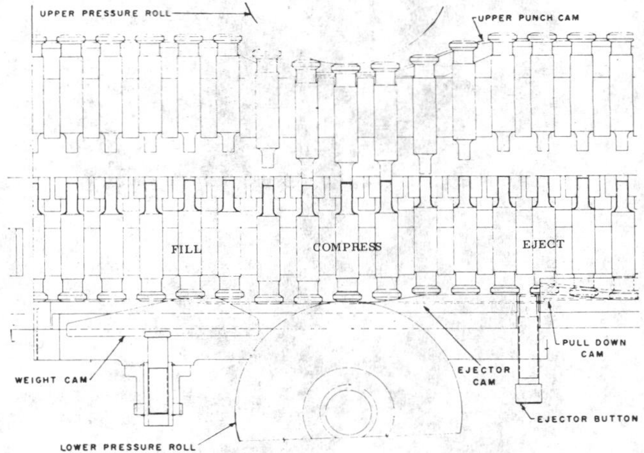

Fig 23. Tooling for a 16-station rotary press showing positions of the cycle required to produce 1 tablet per set of tooling (courtesy, Vector/Colton).

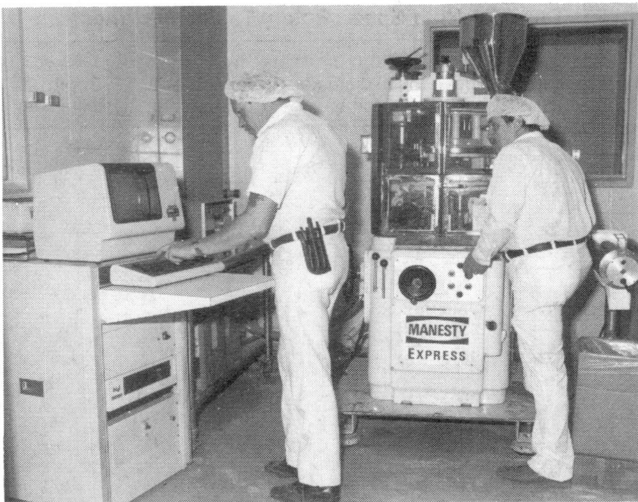

Fig 24. Research technicians use an instrumented tablet press to develop processes at Schering-Plough.

Operation of Rotary Machines

Before inserting punches and dies, make certain that the pressure has been released from the pressure wheel. The die holes should be cleaned thoroughly, making certain that the die seat is completely free of any foreign materials. Back off all die locks and loosely insert dies into the die holes, then tap each die securely into place with a fiber of soft metal rod through the upper punch holes. After all the dies have been tapped into place, tighten each die lockscrew progressively and securely. As each screw is tightened the die is checked to see that it does not project above the die table. Insert the lower punches through the hole made available by removing the punch head. Turn the machine by hand until the punch bore coincides with the plug hole. Insert each lower punch in its place progressively. Insert the upper punches by dropping them into place in the head. Each punch (upper and lower) should be coated with a thin film of mineral oil before inserting them into the machine. Adjust the ejection cam so that the lower punch is flush with the die table at the ejection point.

After insertion of the punches and dies adjust the machine for the tablet weight and hardness. The feed frame should be attached to the machine along with the feed hopper. Add a small amount of the granulation through the hopper and turn over the machine by hand. Increase the pressure by rotating the pressure wheel until a tablet is formed. Check the weight of the tablet and adjust the fill to provide the desired tablet weight. Most likely more than one adjustment of the fill will be necessary before obtaining the acceptable weight. When the fill is decreased, the pressure must be decreased to provide the same hardness in the tablet. Conversely, when the fill is increased, the pressure must be increased to obtain comparable hardness.

Fill the hopper with the granulation and turn on the power. Check tablet weight and hardness immediately after the mechanical operation begins and make suitable adjustments, if necessary. Check these properties routinely and regularly at 15- to 30-minute intervals while the machine is in operation. When the batch has been run, turn off the power. Remove the hopper and feed frame from the machine. Remove loose granulation and dust with a vacuum line. Remove all pressure from the wheel. Remove the punches and dies in the reverse order of that used in setting up the machine. First, remove the upper punches individually, then the lower punches and finally the dies. Wash each punch and die in alcohol and brush with a soft brush to remove adhering material. Dry them with a clean cloth and cover them with a thin coating of grease or oil before storing.

High-Speed Rotary Tablet Machines

The rotary tablet machine has evolved gradually into models capable of compressing tablets at high production rates. See Figs 22, 25 and 26. This has been accomplished by increasing the number of stations, ie, sets of punches and dies, in each revolution of the machine head, improvement in feeding devices, and on some models the installation of dual compression points. In Fig 26, the drawing shows a rotary machine having dual compression points. Rotary machines having dual compression points are referred to as double rotary machines, and those with one compression point, single rotary. In the diagram, half of the tablets are produced 180° from the tablet chute. They travel outside the perimeter and discharge with the second tablet production. While these models are mechanically capable of operating at the production rates shown in Table 3, the actual speed still depends on the physical characteristics of the tablet granulation and the rate which is consistent with compressed tablets having satisfactory physical characteristics. The main difficulty in rapid machine operation is assuring adequate filling of the dies. With rapid filling, dwell time of the die cavity beneath the feed frame is insufficient to ensure the requirements of uniform flow and packing of the dies. Various methods of force-feeding the granulation into the dies have been devised to refill the dies in the very short dwell time permitted on the high-speed machine. These devices are illustrated in Fig 14. Presses with triple compression points (see Table 3) permit the partial compaction of material before final compaction. This provides for the partial deaeration and particle orientation of material before final compression. This helps in the direct compacting of materials and reduces laminating and capping due to entrapped air.

Multilayer Rotary Tablet Machines

The rotary tablet machines also have been developed into models capable of producing multiple-layer tablets; the machines are able to make one-, two- or three-layer tablets [Versa Press (*Stokes/Pennwalt*)]. Stratified tablets offer a number of advantages. Incompatible drugs can be formed into a single tablet by separating the layers containing them with a layer of inert material. It has permitted the formulation of time-delay medication and offers a wide variety of possibilities in developing color combinations which give the products identity.

Originally, the tablets were prepared by a single compression method. The dies were filled with the different granulations in successive layers and the tablet was formed by a single compression stroke. The separation lines of the tablets prepared by this method tended to be irregular. In the machines now available for multilayer production the granulation receives a precompression stroke after the first and second fill, which lightly compacts the granulation and maintains a well-defined surface of separation between each layer. The operator is able to eject either precompressed layer with the machine running at any desired speed for periodic weight and analysis checks.

Other multiple-compression presses can receive previously compressed tablets and compress another granulation around the preformed tablet. An example of a press with this capability is the Manesty Drycota (*Thomas/Manesty*). Pressure coated tablets can be used to separate incompatible drug substances and also to give an enteric coating to the core tablets.

Capping and Splitting of Tablets

The splitting or capping of tablets is one of great concern and annoyance in tablet making. It is quite difficult to detect while the tablets are being processed but can be detected easily by vigorously shaking a few in the cupped hands. A slightly chipped tablet does not necessarily mean that the tablet will cap or split.

There are many factors that may cause a tablet to cap or split:

Excess "fines" or powder which traps air in the tablet mixture.

Deep markings on tablet punches. Many designs or "scores" on punches are too broad and deep. Hairline markings are just as appropriate as deep, heavy markings.

Worn and imperfect punches. Punches should be smooth and buffed. Nicked punches often will cause capping. The development of fine feather edges on tablets indicates wear on punches.

Worn dies. Dies should be replaced or reversed. Dies that are chrome-plated or have tungsten carbide inserts wear longer and give better results than ordinary steel dies.

Too much pressure. By reducing the pressure on the machines the condition may be corrected.

Table 3—Rotary Tablet Machines

Machine model	Tool sets	Maximum tablet diameter (inches)	Press speed (tablets/min)	Depth of fill (inches)
Vector-Colton equipment				
2216	16	5/8	1180	3/4
240	16	7/8	640	13/16
250	12	1 1/4	480	1 1/8
260	25	1 3/16	1450	1 3/8
	31	1	1800	1 3/8
	33	15/16	1910	1 3/8
	43	5/8	2500	1 3/8
270	25	1 3/8	450	2 3/4
Stokes/Pennwalt equipment				
Manesty equipment (Thomas Eng)				
B3B	16	5/8	350–700	11/16
	23	7/16	500–1000	11/16
BB3B	27	5/8	760–1520	11/16
	33	7/16	924–1848	11/16
	35	5/8	1490–2980	11/16
	45	7/16	1913–3826	11/16
D3B	16	1	260–520	13/16
Key equipment				
DC-16	16	15/16	210–510	13/16
BBC	27	5/8	1025–2100	11/16
	35	5/8	1325–2725	11/16
	45	7/16	1700–3500	11/16
Cadpress	37	15/16	850–3500	13/16
	45	5/8	2000–6000	11/16
	55	7/16	2500–7500	11/16
Fette equipment (Raymond Auto)				
		(mm)		(mm)
Perfecta 1000	28	16	2100	18
	33	13	2475	18
Perfecta 2000	29	25	2175	22
	36	16	3600	18
	43	13	4300	18
Courtoy equipment (AC Compact)				
R-100	24	25	285–2260	20
	30	19	356–2850	20
	36	13	550–440	16
Kikusui equipment				
Hercules	18	37	180–540	16
	21	26	210–630	16
	29	25	290–870	16
Virgo	19	16	418–1330	16
	24	11	528–1680	16
Killian equipment				
TX21	21	28	231–1386	20
TX25	25	22	275–2166	20
TX30	30	16	330–3150	20
TX21D	21	25	231–1826	20
TX30A	30	16	330–3150	16
TX40A	40	13	440–4200	16
Korsch equipment				
PH 250/20	20	25	240–1640	22
PH 250/25	25	16	270–2700	18
PH 250/30	30	13	315–3233	18
Elizabeth-Hata equipment				
AP-15-SSU	15	17	300–1050	8–18
AP-18-SSU	18	13	360–1260	8–18
AP-22-SSU	22	11	440–1540	8–18
AP-32-MSU	32	17	640–2240	8–18
AP-38-MSU	38	13	760–2660	8–18
AP-45-MSU	32	11	900–3150	8–18

Unsuitable formula. It may be necessary to change the formula.

Moist and soft granulation. This type of granulation will not flow freely into the dies, thus giving uneven weights and soft or capped tablets.

Poorly machined punches. Uneven punches are detrimental to the tablet machine itself and will not produce tablets of accurate weight. One punch out of alignment may cause one tablet to split or cap on every revolution.

Instrumented Tablet Presses

Compressional and ejectional forces involved in tablet compression can be studied by attaching strain gauges to the punches and other press components involved in compression.

Table 3—High-Speed Rotary Tablet Machines

Machine model	Tool sets	Maximum tablet diameter (inches)	Press speed (tablets/min)	Depth of fill (inches)
Vector-Colton equipment				
2247	33	5/8	3480	3/4
	41	7/16	4300	3/4
	49	7/16	5150	3/4
Magna	66	22/32	10,560	3/4
	74	1/2	11,840	3/4
	90	7/16	14,400	3/4
Stokes/Pennwalt equation				
552-2	35	5/8	800–3200	11/16
328-4	45	3/4	1600–4500	1 3/8
610	65	7/16	3500–10,000	11/16
747	65	7/16	3000–10,000	11/16
	53	5/8	2900–8100	11/16
	41	15/16	2150–6150	11/16
Direct Triple Compression Type				
580-1	45	7/16	525–2100	11/16
580-2	35	5/8	400–1600	11/16
610	65	7/16	3500–10,000	11/16
	53	5/8	2900–8100	11/16
Manesty equipment (Thomas Eng)				
Betapress	16	5/8	600–1500	11/16
	23	7/16	860–2160	11/16
Express	20	1	800–2000	13/16
	25	5/8	1000–2500	11/16
	30	7/16	1200–3000	11/16
Unipress	20	1	970–2420	13/16
	27	5/8	1300–3270	11/16
	34	7/16	1640–4120	11/16
Novapress	37	1	760–3700	13/16
	45	5/8	900–4500	11/16
	61	7/16	1220–6100	11/16
BB3B	35	5/8	1490–2980	11/16
BB4	27	5/8	900–2700	11/16
	35	5/8	1167–3500	11/16
	45	7/16	1500–4500	11/16
Rotapress				
Mark IIA	37	1	710–3550	13/16
	45	5/8	1640–8200	11/16
	61	7/16	2200–11,100	11/16
Mark IV	45	1	2090–6000	13/16
	55	5/8	2550–7330	11/16
	75	7/16	3500–10,000	11/16
Fette tool systems				
		(mm)		(mm)
PT 2080	29	25	435–2900	18
	36	16	540–4100	18
	43	16	645–4900	18
PT 2090IC	22	34	1760	18
	29	25	2900	18
	36	16	4140	18
	43	13	5160	18
	47	11	6110	18
PT 3090IC	37	34	5920	18
	49	25	7840	18
	61	16	9760	18
	73	13	16,748	18
P 3100	37	25	5618	22
	45	16	8100	18
	55	13	9900	18
Courtoy equipment (AC Compact)				
R-200	43	25	750–5833	20
	55	19	916–8500	20
	65	13	1083–10,000	16
Kikusui equipment				
Libra	36	16	900–2520	16
	45	11	1125–3150	16
	49	8	1225–3430	16
Gemini	55	16	2200–7700	16
	67	11	2680–9380	16
	73	8	2920–10,200	16
Elizabeth-Hata equipment				
AP-45-LDU	45	17	1800–6300	8–18
AP-55-LDU	55	13	2200–7700	8–18
AP-65-LDU	65	11	2600–9100	8–18
AP-71-LDU	71	11	2840–9940	8–18
51-XLDU	51	17	2040–7140	8–18
65-XLDU	61	13	2440–8540	8–18

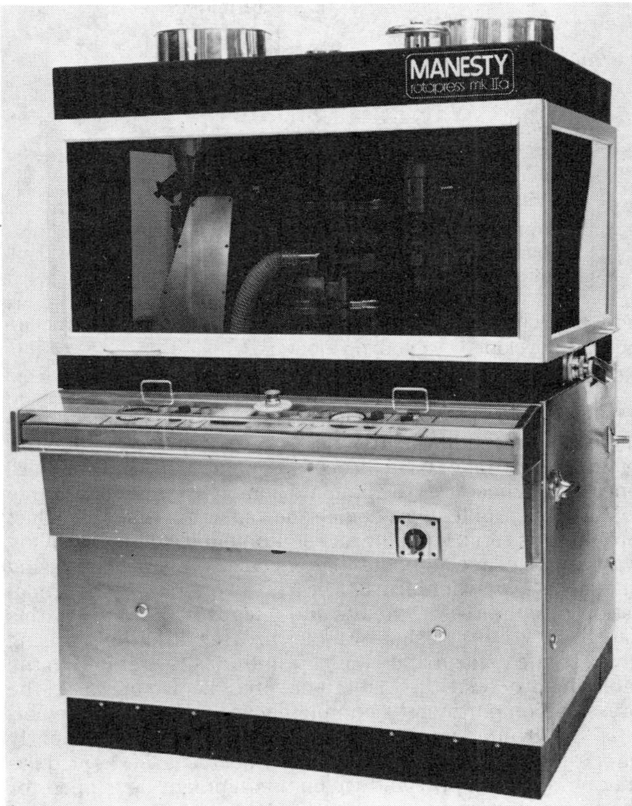

Fig 25. Rotapress Mark IIA: designed for improvements in sound reduction, operator safety, cleanliness and operational convenience; note the control panel on front of machine (courtesy, Thomas/Manesty).

The electrical output of the gauges has been monitored by telemetry or use of a dual beam oscilloscope equipped with camera.[42,43] Instrumentation permits a study of the compaction characteristics of granulations, their flowabilities and the effect of formulation additives, such as lubricants as well as differences in tablet press design, as shown in Figs 29 and 30. Physical characteristics of tablets, such as hardness, friability, disintegration time and dissolution rate, are influenced not only by the nature of the formulation but by the compressional force as well.

As can be seen in Figs 29 and 30, the rate and duration of compaction forces can be quantified. The rate of force application has a profound effect on powder consolidation within the die and, hence, efficiency of packing and powder compaction. The rate of release of force or "decompression" has a direct effect on the ability of the tablet to withstand relaxation. A prominent hypothesis, fostered by Hiestand[44,45]

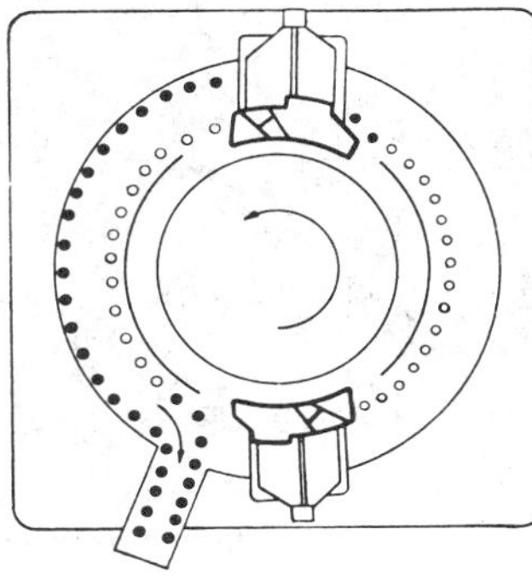

Fig 26. The movement of tablets on die table of a double rotary press (courtesy, Vector/Colton).

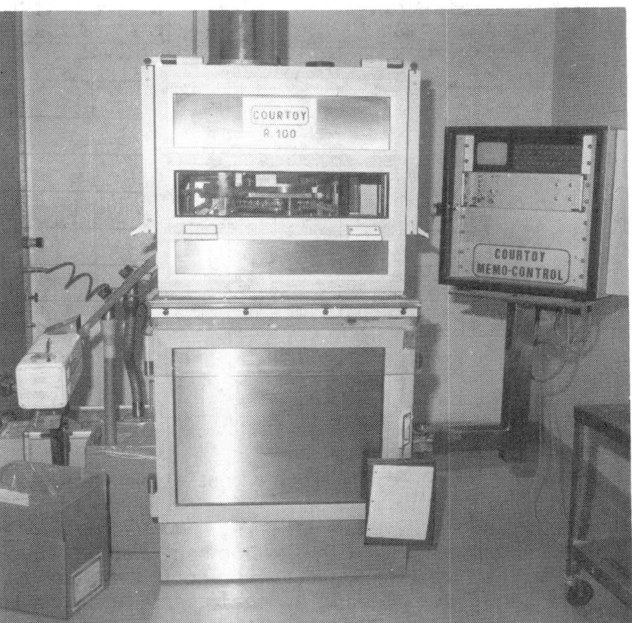

Fig 27. Courtoy R-100 with computer-controlled operation.

and later Luenberger[46] suggested that capping and laminating of tablets is caused by too-rapid stress relaxation or decompression. This explains why slowing a tablet press and using tapered dies is useful in such situations. Most prominent pharmaceutical scientists have embraced this theory and largely have discounted air entrapment as a cause of capping and laminating.

In Fig 30 an interesting set of plots is presented. Walter and Augsburger reported that as compaction force rises, the steel tooling actually compresses in accommodation to the forces applied. The forces used to produce a tablet are considerable, and should be monitored and understood.[47] Therefore, definition of the compressional force and duration of force (dwell time) giving a satisfactory tablet for a formulation provides an in-process control for obtaining both tablet-to-tablet and lot-to-lot uniformity (see Figs 24 and 31).

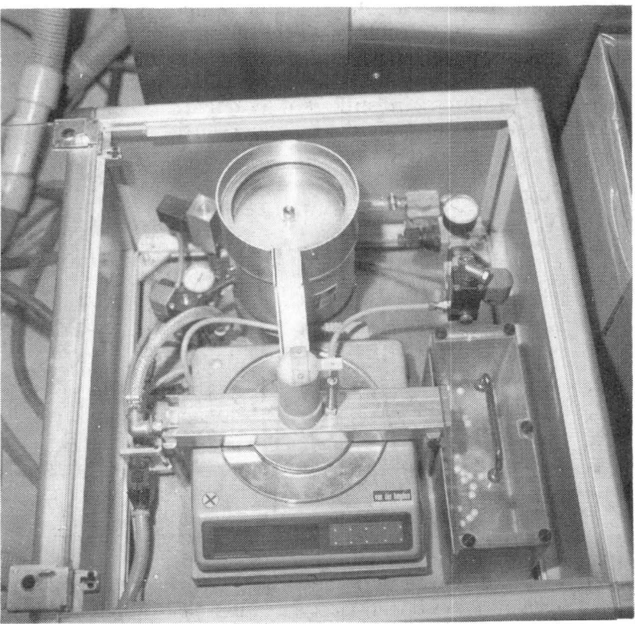

Fig 28. Direct weighing of tablets produced gives actual weight feedback for the controller of the Courtoy R-100 (seen in the bottom left of Fig 27).

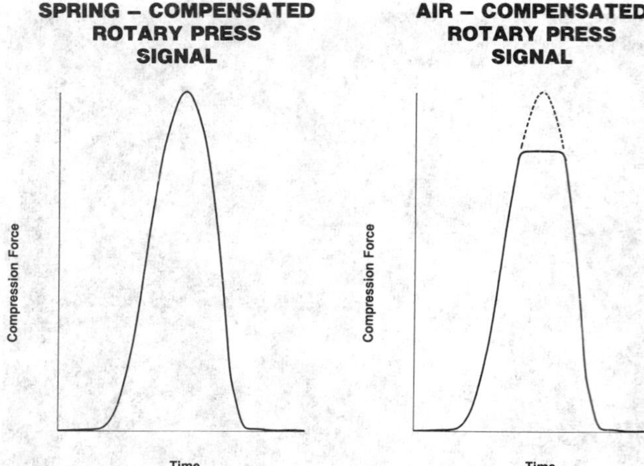

Fig 29. Force-time curves for two types of tablet press.

Instrumentation has led to the development of on-line, automatic, electromechanical tablet weight-control systems capable of continuously monitoring the weights of tablets as they are produced. Units are available commercially [Thomas Tablet Sentinel (*Thomas Eng*); Fette Compression Force Monitor (*Raymond Auto*); Vali-Tab (*Stokes/Pennwalt*)] and are applicable to single or rotary tablet machines. Most commercial presses today can be delivered with some sort of instrumentation attached. When tablet weights vary from preset limits, the monitor automatically will adjust the weight control mechanism to reestablish weights within acceptable limits. If the difficulty continues, the unit will activate an audible warning signal or an optional shut-down relay on the press (see Figs 27 and 28). Most production model tablet presses come equipped with complete instrumentation (optional) and with options for statistical analysis and print out of compression/ejection signals. The techniques and applications of press instrumentation have been reviewed.[48,49]

Contamination Control

While good manufacturing practices used by the pharmaceutical industry for many years have stressed the importance of cleanliness of equipment and facilities for the manufacture of drug products, the penicillin contamination problem resulted in renewed emphasis on this aspect of manufacturing. Penicillin, either as an airborne dust or residual quantities remaining in equipment, is believed to have contaminated unrelated products in sufficient concentrations to cause allergic reactions in individuals, hypersensitive to penicillin,

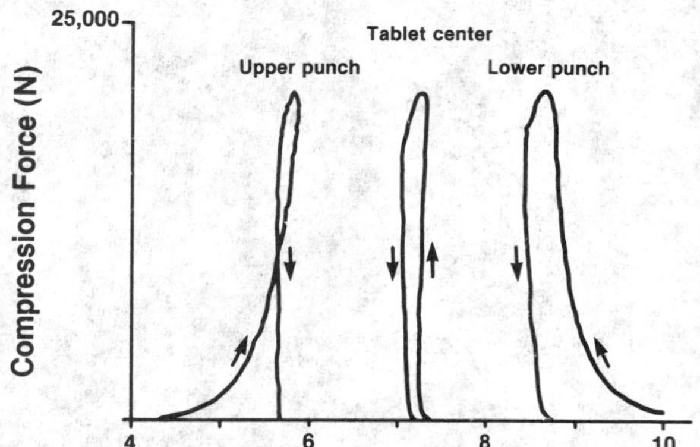

Fig 30. Plot showing the upper and lower punch forces as functions of the position of the punch face within the die. A biaxial force/displacement curve also shown is a plot of the position of the tablet center as a function of the compress ion force.

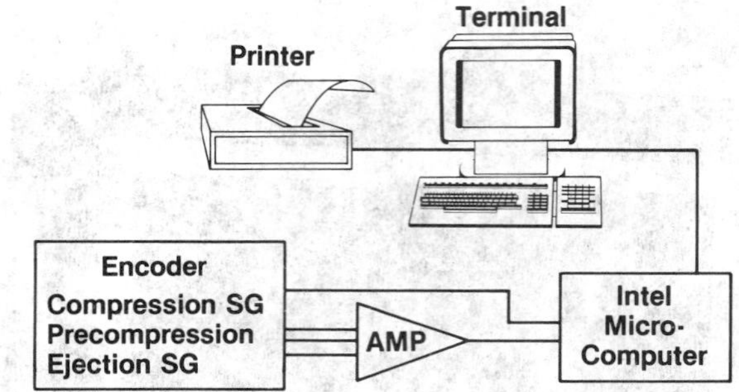

Fig 31. Schematic of an instrumentation system using a microcomputer as developed by Schering-Plough.

who received these products. This resulted in the industry spending millions of dollars to change or modify buildings, manufacturing processes, equipment and standard operating procedures to eliminate penicillin contamination.

With this problem has come renewed emphasis on the dust problem, material handling and equipment cleaning in dealing with drugs, especially potent chemicals. Any process using chemicals in powder form can be a dusty operation; the preparation of compressed tablets and encapsulation falls in this category. In the design of tablet presses attention is being given to the control and elimination of dust generated in the tableting process. In the Perfecta press shown in Fig 32, the pressing compartment is completely sealed off from the outside environment, making cross-contamination nearly impossible. The pressing compartment can be kept dust-free by the air supply and vacuum equipment developed for the machine. It removes airborne dust and granular particles which have not been compressed, thus keeping the circular pressing compartment and the upper and lower punch guides free of dust.

Drug manufacturers have the responsibility to make certain that microorganisms present in finished products are unlikely

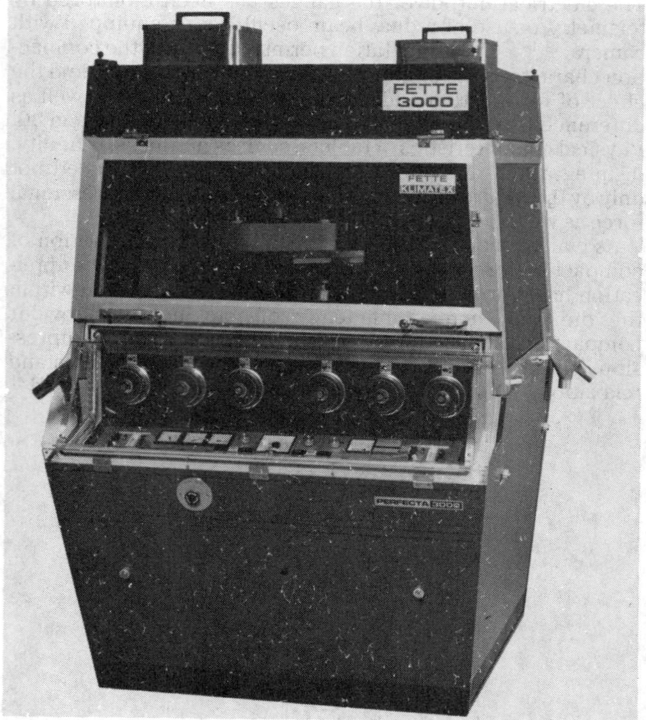

Fig 32. Fette Perfecta 3000 high-speed tablet press with pressing compartment completely sealed off from outside environment making cross contamination impossible (courtesy, Raymond Auto).

to cause harm to the patient and will not be deleterious to the product. An outbreak of *Salmonella* infections in Scandinavian countries was traced to thyroid tablets which had been prepared from contaminated thyroid powder. This concern eventually led to the establishment of microbial limits for raw materials of animal or botanical origin, especially those that readily support microbial growth and are not rendered sterile during subsequent processing. Harmful microorganisms when present in oral products include *Salmonella* spp, *E coli*, certain *Pseudomonas* spp such as *Pseudomonas aeruginosa* and *Staphylococcus aureus*. The compendia have microbial limits on raw materials such as aluminum hydroxide gel, corn starch, thyroid, acacia and gelatin.

These represent examples of the industry's efforts to conform with the intent of current good manufacturing practice as defined by the FDA.

Tablet Formulations

Wet Granulation

CT Acetaminophen, 300 mg

Ingredients	In each	In 10,000
Acetaminophen	300 mg	3000 g
Polyvinylpyrrolidone	22.5 mg	225 g
Lactose	61.75 mg	617.5 g
Alcohol SD3A—200 proof	4.5 mL	45 L
Stearic acid	9 mg	90 g
Talc	13.5 mg	135 g
Corn starch	43.25 mg	432.5 g

Blend acetaminophen, polyvinylpyrrolidone and lactose together; pass through a 40-mesh screen. Add the alcohol slowly and knead well. Screen the wet mass through a 4-mesh screen. Dry the granulation at 50° overnight. Screen the dried granulation through a 20-mesh screen. Bolt the stearic acid, talc and corn starch through a 60-mesh screen prior to mixing by tumbling with the granulation. Compress, using 7/16-inch standard concave punch. 10 tablets should weigh 4.5 g (courtesy, Abbott).

CT Ascorbic Acid USP, 50 mg

Ingredients	In each	In 7000
Ascorbic acid USP (powder No. 80)[a]	55 mg	385 g
Lactose	21 mg	147 g
Starch (potato)	13 mg	91 g
Ethylcellulose N 100 (80–105 cps)	16 mg	112 g
Starch (potato)	7 mg	49 g
Talc	6.5 mg	45.5 g
Calcium stearate (impalpable powder)	1 mg	7 g
Weight of granulation		836.5 g

[a] Includes 10% in excess of claim.

Granulate the first three ingredients with ethylcellulose (5%) dissolved in anhydrous ethyl alcohol adding additional anhydrous alcohol to obtain good, wet granules. Wet-screen through a #8 stainless-steel screen and dry at room temperature in an air-conditioned area. Dry-screen through a #20 stainless-steel screen and incorporate the remaining three ingredients. Mix thoroughly and compress. Use a flat, beveled 1/4-inch punch. 20 tablets should weigh 2.39 g.

Chewable Antacid Tablets

Ingredients	In each	In 10,000
Magnesium trisilicate	500 mg	5000 g
Aluminum hydroxide, dried gel	250 mg	2500 g
Mannitol	300 mg	3000 g
Sodium saccharin	2 mg	20 g
Starch paste, 5%	qs	qs
Oil of peppermint	1 mg	10 g
Magnesium stearate	10 mg	100 g
Corn starch	10 mg	100 g

Mix the magnesium trisilicate and aluminum hydroxide with the mannitol. Dissolve the sodium saccharin in a small quantity of purified water, then combine this with the starch paste. Granulate the powder blend with the starch paste. Dry at 140°F and screen through 16-mesh screen. Add the flavoring oil, magnesium stearate and corn starch; mix well. Age the granulation for at least 24 hours and compress, using a 5/8-inch flat-face bevel-edge punch (courtesy, Atlas).

CT Hexavitamin

Ingredients	In each	In 7000
Ascorbic acid USP (powder)[a]	82.5 mg	577.5 g
Thiamine mononitrate USP (powder)[a]	2.4 mg	16.8 g
Riboflavin[a]	3.3 mg	23.1 g
Nicotinamide USP (powder)[a]	22 mg	154 g
Starch	13.9 mg	97.4 g
Lactose	5.9 mg	41.2 g
Zein	6.4 mg	45 g
Vitamin A acetate:	6250 U	
Vitamin D_2[a] (use Pfizer crystalets medium granules containing 500,000 U vitamin A acetate and50,000 U vitamin D_2/g).	625 U	87.5 g
Magnesium stearate		7.5 g
Weight of granulation		1050 g

[a] Includes the following in excess of claim: ascorbic acid 10%, thiamine mononitrate 20%, riboflavin 10%, nicotinamide 10% and vitamin A acetate–vitamin D_2 crystalets 25%.

Thoroughly mix the first six ingredients and granulate with zein (10% in ethyl alcohol, adding additional alcohol if necessary to obtain good, wet granules). Wet-screen through a #8 stainless-steel screen and dry at 110 to 120°F. Dry-screen through a #20 stainless-steel screen and add the vitamin crystalets. Mix thoroughly, lubricate and compress. 10 tablets should weigh 1.50 g. Coat with syrup.

CT Theobromine–Phenobarbital

Ingredients	In each	In 7000
Theobromine	325 mg	2275 g
Phenobarbital	33 mg	231 g
Starch	39 mg	273 g
Talc	8 mg	56 g
Acacia (powder)	8 mg	56 g
Stearic acid	0.7 mg	4.9 g
Weight of granulation		2895.9 g

Prepare a paste with the acacia and an equal weight of starch. Use this paste for granulating the theobromine and pheno- barbital. Dry and put through a 12-mesh screen, add the remainder of the material, mix thoroughly and compress into tablets, using a 13/32-inch concave punch. 10 tablets should weigh 4.13 g.

Fluid-Bed Granulation

CT Ascorbic Acid USP, 50 mg

Ingredients	In each	In 10,0000
Ascorbic acid USP (powder no 80)[a]	55 mg	550 g
Lactose	21 mg	210 g
Starch (potato)	13 mg	130 g
Ethylcellulose N100 (80-105 cps)	16 mg	160 g
Starch (potato)	7 mg	70 g
Talc	6.5 mg	65 g
Calcium stearate	1 mg	10 g
Weight of granulation		1195.0 g

[a] Includes 10% in excess of claim.

Add the first three ingredients to the granulator. Mix for 5 to 15 minutes or until well mixed. Dissolve the ethylcellulose in anhydrous ethanol and spray this solution, and any additional ethanol, into the fluidized mixture. Cease spraying when good granules are produced. Dry to approximately 3% moisture. Remove the granules and place them in a suitable blender. Sequentially add the remaining three ingredients with mixing steps in between each addition. Compress, using a flat, beveled, ¼-inch punch. 20 tablets should weigh 2.39 g.

Sustained-Release (SR) Procainamide tablets

Ingredients	In each	In 10,000
Procainamide	500 mg	5000 g
HPMC 2208, USP	300 mg	3000 g
Carnauba wax	60 mg	600 g
HPMC 2910, USP	30 mg	300 g
Magnesium stearate	4 mg	40 g
Stearic acid	11 mg	110 g
Talc	5 mg	50 g
Weight of granulation		9100 g

Place the first three ingredients in the granulator and mix for 5 to 15 minutes. Dissolve the HPMC in water (mix in hot water, then cool down) and spray into the fluidized mixture. Dry to approximately 5% moisture. Sequentially add the last three ingredients with mixing steps in between each addition. Compress, using capsule-shaped tooling. 10 tablets should weigh 9.1 g.

Dry Granulation

CT Acetylsalicylic Acid

Ingredients	In each	In 7000
Acetylsalicylic Acid (crystals 20-mesh)	0.325 g	2275 g
Starch		226.8 g
Weight of granulation		2501.8 g

Dry the starch to a moisture content of 10%. Thoroughly mix this with the acetylsalicylic acid. Compress into slugs. Grind the slugs to 14- to 16-mesh size. Recompress into tablets, using a 13/32-inch punch. 10 tablets should weigh 3.575 g.

CT Sodium Phenobarbital

Ingredients	In each	In 7000
Phenobarbital sodium	65 mg	455 g
Lactose (granular, 12-mesh)	26 mg	182 g
Starch	20 mg	140 g
Talc	20 mg	140 g
Magnesium stearate	0.3 mg	2.1 g
Weight of granulation		919.1 g

Mix all the ingredients thoroughly. Compress into slugs. Grind and screen to 14- to 16-mesh granules. Recompress into tablets, using a 9/32-inch concave punch. 10 tablets should weigh 1.3 g.

CT Vitamin B Complex

Ingredients	In each	In 10,000
Thiamine mononitrate[a]	0.733 mg	7.33 g
Riboflavin[a]	0.733 mg	7.33 g
Pyridoxine hydrochloride	0.333 mg	3.33 g
Calcium pantothenate[a]	0.4 mg	4 g
Nicotinamide	5 mg	50 g
Lactose (powder)	75.2 mg	752 g
Starch	21.9 mg	219 g
Talc	20 mg	200 g
Stearic acid (powder)	0.701 mg	7.01 g
Weight of granulation		1250 g

[a] Includes 10% in excess of claim.

Mix all the ingredients thoroughly. Compress into slugs. Grind and screen to 14- to 16-mesh granules. Recompress into tablets, using a ¼-inch concave punch. 10 tablets should weigh 1.25 g.

Sufficient tartaric acid should be used in these tablets to adjust the pH to 4.5.

Direct Compression

APC Tablets

Ingredients	In each	In 10,000
Aspirin (40-mesh crystal)	224 mg	2240 g
Phenacetin	160 mg	1600 g
Caffeine (anhyd USP gran)	32 mg	320 g
Compressible sugar (Di-Pac[a])	93.4 mg	934 g
Sterotex	7.8 mg	78 g
Silica gel (Syloid 244[b])	2.8 mg	28 g

[a] Amstar.
[b] Davison Chem.

Blend ingredients in a twin-shell blender for 15 minutes and compress on a 13/32-inch standard concave punch (courtesy, Amstar).

CT Ascorbic Acid USP, 250 mg

Ingredients	In each	In 10,000
Ascorbic Acid USP (Merck, fine crystals)	255 mg	2550 g
Microcrystalline cellulose[a]	159 mg	1590 g
Stearic acid	9 mg	90 g
Colloidal silica[b]	2 mg	20 g
Weight of granulation		4250 g

[a] Avicel-PH-101.
[b] Cab-O-Sil.

Blend all ingredients in a suitable blender. Compress, using 7/16-inch standard concave punch. 10 tablets should weigh 4.25 g (courtesy, FMC).

Breath Freshener Tablets

Ingredients	In each	In 10,000
Wintergreen oil	0.6 mg	6 g
Menthol	0.85 mg	8.5 g
Peppermint oil	0.3 mg	3 g
Silica gel (Syloid 244[a])	1 mg	10 g
Sodium saccharin	0.3 mg	3 g
Sodium bicarbonate	14 mg	140 g
Mannitol USP (granular)	180.95 mg	1809.5 g
Calcium stearate	2 mg	20 g

[a] Davison Chem.

Mix the flavor oils and menthol until liquid. Adsorb onto the silica gel. Add the remaining ingredients. Blend and compress on 5/16-in flat-face bevel-edge punch to a thickness of 3.1 mm (courtesy, Atlas).

Chewable Antacid Tablets

Ingredients	In each	In 10,000
Aluminum hydroxide and magnesium carbonate, co-dried gel[a]	325 mg	3250 g
Mannitol USP (granular)	675 mg	6750 g
Microcrystalline cellulose[b]	75 mg	750 g
Corn starch	30 mg	300 g
Calcium stearate	22 mg	220 g
Flavor	qs	qs

[a] Reheis F-MA-11.
[b] Avicel.

Blend all ingredients in a suitable blender. Compress, using a 5/8-inch flat-face bevel-edge punch (courtesy, Atlas).

Chewable Multivitamin Tablets

Ingredients	In each	In 10,000
Vitamin A USP (dry, stabilized form)	5000 USP units	50 million units
Vitamin D (dry, stabilized form)	400 USP units	4 million units
Ascorbic Acid USP	60.0 mg	600 g
Thiamine Hydrochloride USP	1 mg	10 g
Riboflavin USP	1.5 mg	15 g
Pyridoxine Hydrochloride USP	1 mg	10 g
Cyanocobalamin USP	2 μg	20 mg
Calcium Pantothenate USP	3 mg	30 g
Niacinamide USP	10 mg	100 g
Mannitol USP (granular)	236.2 mg	2362 g
Corn starch	16.6 mg	166 g
Sodium saccharin	1.1 mg	11 g
Magnesium stearate	6.6 mg	66 g
Talc USP	10 mg	100 g
Flavor	qs	qs

Blend all ingredients in a suitable blender. Compress, using a 3/8-inch flat-face bevel-edge punch (courtesy, Atlas).

CT Ferrous Sulfate

Ingredients	In each	In 7000
Ferrous Sulfate USP (crystalline)	0.325 g	2275 g
Talc		0.975 g
Sterotex		1.95 g
Weight of granulation		2277.93 g

Grind to 12- to 14-mesh, lubricate and compress. Coat immediately to avoid oxidation to the ferric state with 0.410 gr of tolu balsam (dissolved in alcohol) and 0.060 gr of salol and chalk. Use a deep, concave, 11/32-inch punch. 10 tablets should weigh 3.25 g.

CT Methenamine

Ingredients	In each, g	In 7000, g
Methenamine (12- to 14-mesh crystals)	0.325	2275
Weight of granulation		2275

Compress directly, using a 7/16-inch punch. 10 tablets should weigh 3.25 g.

CT Phenobarbital USP, 30 mg

Ingredients	In each	In 10,000
Phenobarbital	30.59 mg	305.9 g
Microcrystalline cellulose[a]	30.59 mg	305.9 g
Spray-dried lactose	69.16 mg	691.6 g
Colloidal silica[b]	1.33 mg	13.3 g
Stearic acid	1.33 mg	13.3 g
Weight of granulation		1330 g

[a] Avicel-PH-101.
[b] QUSO F-22.

Screen the phenobarbital to break up lumps and blend with the microcrystalline cellulose. Add spray-dried lactose and blend. Finally, add the stearic acid and colloidal silica; blend to obtain a homogeneous mixture. Compress, using a 9/32-inch shallow concave punch. 10 tablets should weigh 1.33 g (courtesy, FMC).

Molded Tablets or Tablet Triturates (TT)

Tablet triturates are small, discoid masses of molded powders weighing 30 to 250 mg each. The base consists of lactose, β-lactose, mannitol, dextrose or other rapidly soluble materials. It is desirable in making tablet triturates to prepare a solid dosage form which is rapidly soluble; as the result they are generally softer than compressed tablets.

This type of dosage form is selected for a number of drugs because of its rapidly dissolving characteristic. Nitroglycerin in many concentrations is prepared in tablet triturate form since the molded tablet rapidly dissolves when administered by placing under the tongue. Potent alkaloids and highly toxic drugs used in small doses are prepared as tablet triturates which can serve as dispensing tablets to be used as the source of the drug in compounding other formulations or solutions. Narcotics in the form of hypodermic tablets originally were made as tablet triturates because they rapidly dissolve in sterile water for injection prior to administration. Today with stable injections of narcotics available, there is no longer any justification for their use in this manner. Although many hypodermic tablets currently are made, they are used primarily for oral administration.

Tablet triturates are made by forcing a moistened blend of the drug and diluent into a mold, extruding the formed mass, which is allowed to dry. This method is essentially the same as it was when introduced by Fuller in 1878. Hand molds may vary in size but the method of operation is essentially the same. Molds consist of two plates made from polystyrene plastic, hard rubber, nickel-plated brass or stainless steel. The mold plate contains 50 to 500 carefully polished perforations. The other plate is fitted with a corresponding number of projecting pegs or punches which fit the perforations in the mold plate. The mold plate is placed on a flat surface, the moistened mass is forced into the perforations and the excess is scraped from the top surface. The mold plate is placed over the plate with the corresponding pegs and lowered. As the plates come together, the pegs force the tablet triturates from the molds. They remain on the tops of the pegs until dry and they can be handled (see Fig 33). In some hand molds, as shown in Fig 34, the pegs are forced down onto the plate holding the moist trituration.

Formulation

In developing a formula it is essential that the blank weight of the mold which is to be used is known. To determine this, the weight of the diluent which exactly fills all the openings in the mold is determined by experiment. This amount of diluent is weighed and placed aside. The total amount of the drug required is determined by multiplying the number of perforations in the plate used in the previous experiment by the amount of drug desired in each tablet. The comparative bulk of this medication is compared with that of an equal volume of diluent and that quantity of diluent is removed and weighed. The drug and the remaining diluent are mixed by trituration, and the resulting triturate is moistened and forced into the openings of the mold. If the perforations are not filled completely, more diluent is added, its weight noted and the formula written from the results of the experiments.

It is also permissible in the development of the formula to weigh the quantity of medication needed for the number of tablets represented by the number of perforations in the mold, triturate with a weighed portion (more than ½) of the diluent, moisten the mixture and press it into the perforations of the mold. An additional quantity of the diluent is moistened immediately and also forced into the perforations in the plate until they are filled completely. All excess diluent is removed, the trial tablets are forced from the mold, then triturated until uniform, moistened again, if necessary, and remolded. When these tablets are dried thoroughly and weighed, the difference between their total weight and the weight of medication taken will indicate the amount of diluent required and accordingly supply the formula for future use for that particular tablet triturate.

For proper mixing procedures of the medication with the diluent see Chapter 91.

Preparation

The mixed powders are moistened with a proper mixture of alcohol and water, although other solvents or moistening agents such as acetone, petroleum benzin and various combinations of these may be used in specific cases; the agent of choice depends on the solvent action which it will exert on the powder mixture. Often the moistening agent is 50% alcohol, but this concentration may be increased or decreased depending on the constituents of the formula. Care must be used in adding the solvent mixture to the powder. If too much is used, the mass will be soggy, will require a long time to dry and the finished tablet will be hard and slowly soluble; if the mass is too wet, shrinkage will occur in the molded tablets; finally, a condition known as creeping will be noticed. Creeping is the concentration of the medication on the surface of the tablet caused by capillarity and rapid evaporation of the solvent from the surface. Because molded tablets by their very nature are quite friable, an inaccurate strength in each tablet may result from creeping if powder is lost from the tablet's surface. On the other hand, if an insufficient amount of moistening agent is used, the mass will not have the proper cohesion to make a firm tablet. The correct amount of moistening agent can be determined initially only by experiment.

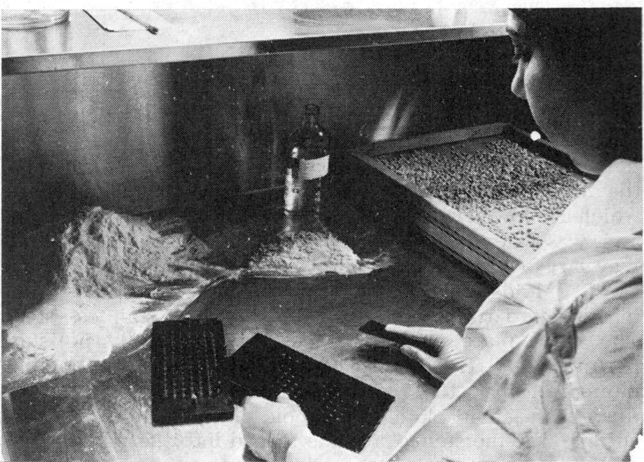

Fig 33. Hand-molding tablet triturates (courtesy, MSD).

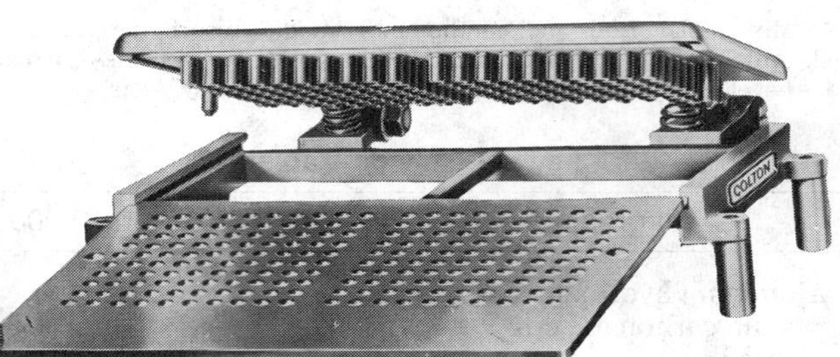

Fig 34. Tablet triturate mold (courtesy, Vector/Colton).

Hand-Molding Tablet Triturates

In preparing hand-molded tablets place the mold plate on a glass plate. The properly moistened material is pressed into the perforations of the mold with a broad spatula exerting uniform pressure over each opening. The excess material is removed by passing the spatula at an oblique angle with strong hand pressure over the mold to give a clean, flat surface. The material thus removed should be placed with the remainder of the unmolded material.

The mold with the filled perforations should be reversed and moved to another clean part of the plate where the pressing operation with the spatula is repeated. It may be necessary to add more material to fill the perforations completely and uniformly. The mold should be allowed to stand in a position so that part of the moistening agent will evaporate equally from both faces. While the first plate is drying, another mold can be prepared. As soon as the second mold has been completed, the first mold should be sufficiently surface-dried so that the pegs will press the tablets from the mold with a minimum of sticking.

To remove the tablets from the mold, place the mold over the peg plate so that the pegs and the perforations are in juxtaposition. The tablets are released from the mold by hand pressure, which forces the pegs through the perforations. The ejected tablets are spread evenly in single layers on silk trays and dried in a clean, dust-free chamber with warm, circulating air. If only a small quantity of tablet triturates is made and no warm-air oven is available, the tablet triturates may be dried to constant weight at room temperature.

Machine-Molding Tablet Triturates

Tablet triturates also can be made using mechanical equipment. The automatic tablet triturate machine illustrated in Fig 35 makes tablet triturates at a rate of 2500/minute. For machine-molding, the powder mass need not be as moist as for plate-molding since the time interval between forming the tablets and pressing them is considerably shorter. The moistened mass passes through the funnel of the hopper to the feed plates below. In this feed plate are four holes having the same diameter as the mouth of the funnel. The material fills one hole at a time and, when filled,

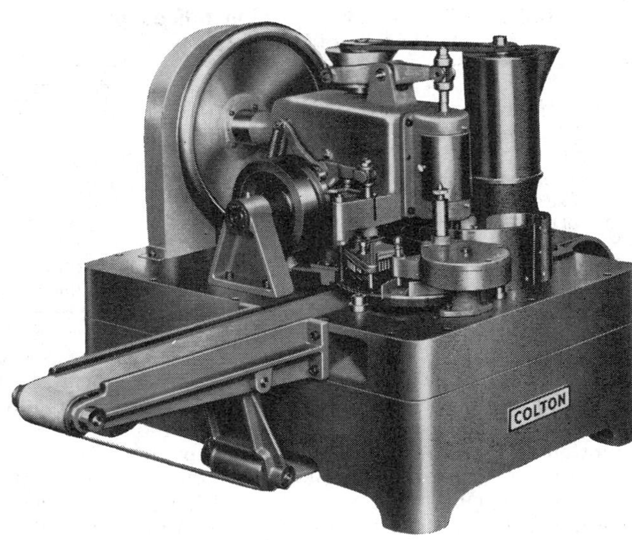

Fig 35. Automatic tablet triturate machine (courtesy, Vector-Colton).

revolves to a position just over the mold plate. When in position the weighted pressure foot lowers and imprisons the powder. At the same time a spreader in the sole of the pressure foot rubs it into the mold cavities and evens it off so that the triturates are smooth on the surface and are of uniform density. When this operation is completed, the mold passes to the next position, where it registers with a nest of punches or pegs which eject the tablets from the mold plate onto a conveyor belt. The conveyor belt sometimes is extended to a length of 8 or 10 feet under a battery of infrared drying lamps to hasten the setting of the tablets for more rapid handling. This method of drying can be used only if the drug is chemically stable to these drying conditions.

Compressed Tablet Triturates

Frequently, tablet triturates are prepared on compression tablet machines using flat-face punches. When solubility and a clear solution are required, water-soluble lubricants must be used to prevent sticking to the punches. The granulations are prepared as directed for ordinary compressed tablets; lactose generally is used as the diluent. Generally, tablet triturates prepared by this method are not as satisfactory as the molded type regarding their solubility and solution characteristics.

Tablet Characteristics

Compressed tablets may be characterized or described by a number of specifications. These include the diameter size, shape, thickness, weight, hardness, disintegration time and dissolution characteristics. The diameter and shape depend on the die and the punches selected for the compression of the tablet. Generally, tablets are discoid in shape, although they may be oval, oblong, round, cylindrical or triangular. Their upper and lower surfaces may be flat, round, concave or convex to various degrees. The concave punches (used to prepare convex tablets) are referred to as shallow, standard and deep cup, depending on the degree of concavity (see Figs 17–20). The tablets may be scored in halves or quadrants to facilitate breaking if a smaller dose is desired. The top or lower surface may be embossed or engraved with a symbol or letters which serve as an additional means of identifying the source of the tablets. These characteristics along with the color of the tablets tend to make them distinctive and identifiable with the active ingredient which they contain.

The remaining specifications assure the manufacturer that the tablets do not vary from one production lot to another. In the case of new tablet formulations their therapeutic efficacy is demonstrated through clinical trials, and it is the manufacturer's aim to reproduce the same tablet with the exact characteristics of the tablets which were used in the clinical evaluation of the dosage form. Therefore, from the control viewpoint these specifications are important for reasons other than physical appearance.

Tablet Hardness

The resistance of the tablet to chipping, abrasion or breakage under conditions of storage, transportation and handling before usage depends on its hardness. In the past, a rule of thumb describes a tablet to be of proper hardness if it is firm enough to break with a sharp snap when it is held between the 2nd and 3rd fingers and using the thumb as the fulcrum, yet doesn't break when it falls on the floor. For obvious reasons and control purposes a number of attempts have been made to quantitate the degree of hardness.

A small and portable hardness tester was manufactured and introduced in the mid-1930s by *Monsanto*. It now is distributed by the Stokes Div (*Pennwalt*) and may be designated as either the Monsanto or Stokes hardness tester. The instrument measures the force required to break the tablet when the force generated by a coil spring is applied diametrically to the tablet. The force is measured in kilograms and when used in production, a hardness of 4 kg is considered to be minimum for a satisfactory tablet.

The Strong-Cobb hardness tester introduced in 1950 also measures the diametrically applied force required to break the tablet. In this instrument the force is produced by a manually operated air pump. As the pressure is increased, a plunger is forced against the tablet placed on anvil. The final breaking point is indicated on a dial calibrated into 30 arbitrary units. The hardness values of the Stokes and Strong-Cobb instruments are not equivalent. Values obtained with the Strong-Cobb tester have been found to be 1.6 times those of the Stokes tester.

Another instrument is the Pfizer hardness tester which operates on the same mechanical principle as ordinary pliers. The force required to break the tablet is recorded on a dial and may be expressed as either kilograms or pounds of force. In an experimental comparison of testers the Pfizer and the Stokes testers were found to check each other fairly well. Again the Strong-Cobb tester was found to give values 1.4 to 1.7 times the absolute values on the other instruments.

The most widely used apparatus to measure tablet hardness or crushing strength is the Schleuniger apparatus, also known as the Heberlein, distributed by *Vector*. This, and other newer electrically operated test equipment, eliminates the operator variability inherent in the measurements described above. Newer equipment is also available with printers to provide a record of test results. See Fig 36.

Manufacturers, such as *Key*, *Van Kel*, *Erweka* and others make similar hardness testers.

Hardness (or more appropriately, crushing strength) determinations are made throughout the tablet runs to determine the need for pressure adjustments on the tableting machine. If the tablet is too hard, it may not disintegrate in the required period of time or meet the dissolution specification; if it is too soft, it will not withstand the handling during subsequent processing such as coating or packaging and shipping operations.

A tablet property related to hardness is *friability*, and the measurement is made by use of the Roche friabilator. Rather than a measure of the force required to crush a tablet, the instrument is designed to evaluate the ability of the tablet to withstand abrasion in packaging, handling and shipping. A number of tablets are weighed and placed in the tumbling apparatus where they are exposed to rolling and repeated

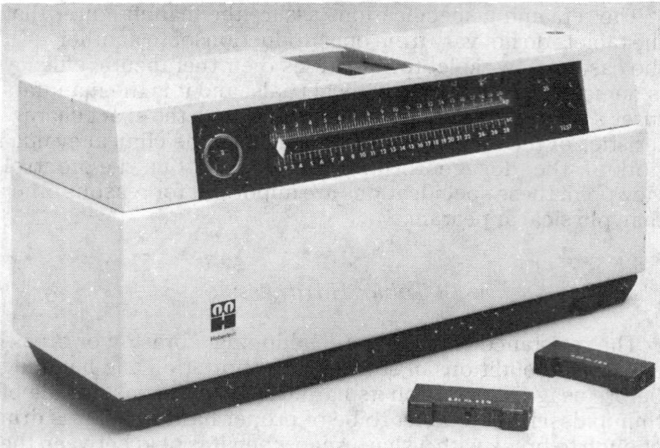

Fig 36. The Schleuniger or Heberlein tablet hardness tester shown with calibration blocks (courtesy, Vector).

shocks resulting from freefalls within the apparatus. After a given number of rotations the tablets are weighed, and the loss in weight indicates the ability of the tablets to withstand this type of wear (Fig 37).

Recent research has proposed that there are at least three measurable hardness parameters that can give a clue to the compatibility and intrinsic strength of powdered materials. These include bonding strength, internal strain and brittleness. Hiestand proposed indeces to quantify these parameters and they are listed in Table 4 for a number of materials.

The higher the bonding index, the stronger a tablet is more likely to be. The higher the strain index, the weaker the tablet. Since the two parameters are opposite in their effect on the tablet, it is possible for a material (such as Avicel) to have a relatively high strain index, but yet have superior compaction properties because of an extraordinary bonding potential. The higher the brittleness index, the more friable the tablet is likely to be. For a more detailed discussion of this subject, the reader is directed to Refs 22, 37, 38.

A similar approach is taken by many manufacturers when they evaluate a new product in the new market package by sending the package to distant points and back using various methods of transportation. This is called a "shipping test." The condition of the product on its return indicates its ability to withstand transportation handling.

Tablet Thickness

The thickness of the tablet from production-run to production-run is controlled carefully. Thickness can vary with no

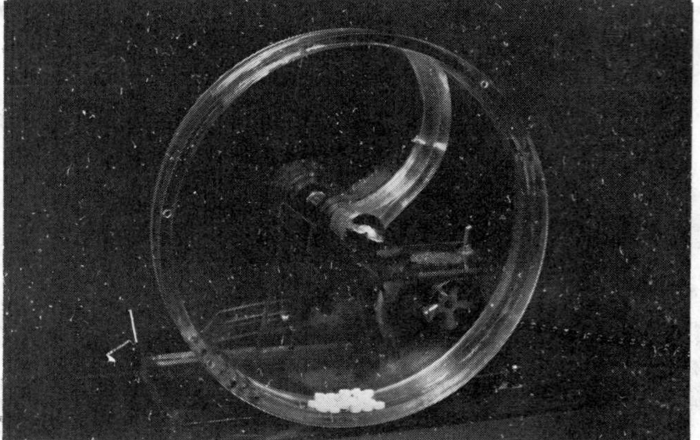

Fig 37. The Roche friabilator (courtesy, Hoffmann-LaRoche).

Table 4—Hiestand Compaction Indices for a Number of Materials

Material	Bonding index	Strain index	Brittleness index
Aspirin	1.5	1.11	0.16
Dicalcium phosphate	1.3	1.13	0.15
Lactose anhydrous	0.8	1.40	0.27
Avicel pH 102	4.3	2.20	0.04
Corn starch	0.4	2.48	0.26
Sucrose NF	1.0	1.45	0.35
Erythromycin dihydrate	1.9	2.13	0.98

change in weight due to difference in the density of the granulation and the pressure applied to the tablets, as well as the speed of tablet compression. Not only is the tablet thickness important in reproducing tablets identical in appearance but also to insure that every production lot will be usable with selected packaging components. If the tablets are thicker than specified, a given number no longer may be contained in the volume of a given size bottle. Tablet thickness also becomes an important characteristic in counting tablets using filling equipment. Some filling equipment utilizes the uniform thickness of the tablets as a counting mechanism. A column containing a known number of tablets is measured for height; filling is accomplished by continually dropping columns of tablets of the same height into bottles. If thickness varies throughout the lot, the result will be variation in count. Other pieces of filling equipment can malfunction due to variation in tablet thickness since tablets above specified thickness may cause wedging of tablets in previously adjusted depths of the counting slots. Tablet thickness is determined with a caliper or thickness gauge which measures the thickness in millimeters. A plus or minus 5% may be allowed, depending on the size of the tablet.

Uniformity of Dosage Forms

Tablet Weight—The volumetric fill of the die cavity determines the weight of the compressed tablet. In setting up the tablet machine the fill is adjusted to give the desired tablet weight. The weight of the tablet is the quantity of the granulation which contains the labeled amount of the therapeutic ingredient. After the tablet machine is in operation the weights of the tablets are checked routinely either manually or electronically to insure that proper-weight tablets are being made. This has become rather routine in most manufacturing operations with newer electronically controlled tablet presses. The USP has provided tolerances for the average weight of uncoated compressed tablets. These are applicable when the tablet contains 50 mg or more of the drug substance or when the latter comprises 50% or more, by weight, of the dosage form. Twenty tablets are weighed individually and the average weight is calculated. The variation from the average weight in the weights of not more than two of the tablets must not differ by more than the percentage listed below; no tablet differs by more than double that percentage. Tablets that are coated are exempt from these requirements but must conform to the test for content uniformity if it is applicable.

Average weight	Percentage difference
130 mg or less	10
More than 130 mg through 324 mg	7.5
More than 324 mg	5

Content Uniformity—In order to ensure that every tablet contains the amount of drug substance intended, with little variation among tablets within a batch, the USP includes the content uniformity test for certain tablets. Due to the increased awareness of physiological availability, the content uniformity test has been extended to monographs on all coated and uncoated tablets and all capsules intended for oral administration where the range of sizes of the dosage form available includes a 50 mg or smaller size, in which case the test is applicable to all sizes (50 mg and larger and smaller) of that tablet or capsule. The official compendia can be consulted for the details of the test. Tablet monographs with a content uniformity requirement do not have a weight variation requirement.

Tablet Disintegration

It is recognized generally that the *in vitro* tablet disintegration test does not necessarily bear a relationship to the *in vivo* action of a solid dosage form. To be absorbed, a drug substance must be in solution and the disintegration test is a measure only of the time required under a given set of conditions for a group of tablets to disintegrate into particles. Generally, this test is useful as a quality-assurance tool for conventional (nonsustained-release) dosage forms. In the present disintegration test the particles are those which will pass through a 10-mesh screen. In a comparison of disintegration times and dissolution rates or initial absorption rates of several brands of aspirin tablets, it was found that the faster absorbed tablets had the longer disintegration time. Regardless of the lack of significance as to *in vivo* action of the tablets, the test provides a means of control in assuring that a given tablet formula is the same as regards disintegration from one production batch to another. The disintegration test is used as a control for tablets intended to be administered by mouth, except where tablets are intended to be chewed before being swallowed or where tablets are designed to release the drug substance over a period of time.

Exact specifications are given for the test apparatus inasmuch as a change in the apparatus can cause a change in the results of the test. The apparatus consists of a basket rack holding six plastic tubes, open at the top and bottom; the bottom of the tubes is covered with 10-mesh screen. See Fig 38. The basket rack is immersed in a bath of suitable liquid, held at 37°, preferably in a 1-L beaker. The rack moves up and down in the fluid at a specified rate. The volume of the fluid is such that on the upward stroke the wire mesh remains at least 2.5 cm below the surface of the fluid and descends to not less than 2.5 cm from the bottom on the downward stroke. Tablets are placed in each of the six cylinders along with a plastic disc over the tablet unless otherwise directed in the monograph. The end-point of the test is indicated when any residue remaining is a soft mass having no palpably soft core. The plastic discs help to force any soft mass which forms through the screen.

For compressed uncoated tablets the testing fluid is usually water at 37°, but in some cases the monographs direct that Simulated Gastric Fluid TS be used. If one or two tablets fail to disintegrate, the test is to be repeated using 12 tablets. Of the 18 tablets then tested, 16 must have disintegrated within the given period of time. The conditions of the test are varied somewhat for coated tablets, buccal tablets and sublingual tablets. Disintegration times are included in the individual tablet monograph. For most uncoated tablets the period is 30 minutes although the time for some uncoated tablets varies greatly from this. For coated tablets up to 2 hours may be required, while for sublingual tablets, such as CT Isoproterenol Hydrochloride, the disintegration time is 3 minutes. For the exact conditions of the test, consult the USP.

Dissolution Test

For certain tablets the monographs direct compliance with limits on dissolution rather than disintegration. Since drug

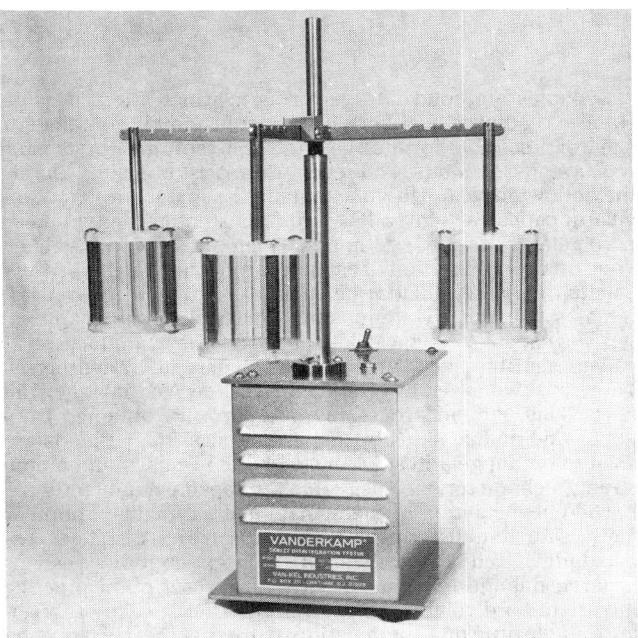

Fig 38. Vanderkamp tablet disintegration tester (courtesy, VanKel).

absorption and physiological availability depend on having the drug substance in the dissolved state, suitable dissolution characteristics are an important property of a satisfactory tablet. Like the disintegration test, the dissolution test for measuring the amount of time required for a given percentage of the drug substance in a tablet to go into solution under a specified set of conditions is an *in vitro* test. It is intended to provide a step towards the evaluation of the physiological availability of the drug substance, but as described currently, it is not designed to measure the safety or efficacy of the tablet being tested. Both the safety and effectiveness of a specific dosage form must be demonstrated initially by means of appropriate *in vivo* studies and clinical evaluation. Like the disintegration test, the dissolution test does provide a means of control in assuring that a given tablet formulation is the same as regards dissolution as the batch of tablets shown initially to be clinically effective. It also provides an *in vitro* control procedure to eliminate variations among production batches. Refer to Chapter 34 for a complete discussion of dissolution testing.

Validation

In this era of increasing regulatory control of the pharmaceutical industry, manufacturing procedures cannot be discussed without the mention of some process validation activity. By way of documentation, product testing and, perhaps, in-process testing as well, the manufacturer can demonstrate that his formula and process perform in the manner expected and that it does so reproducibly.

Although the justification for requiring validation is found in the regulations relating to "Current Good Manufacturing Practices for Finished Pharmaceuticals" as well as other sources, there is still much room for interpretation and the process varies from one company to another. General areas of agreement appear to be that

The validation activity must begin in R&D and continue through product introduction.
Documentation is the key.
In general, three batches represent an adequate sample for validation.

The FDA has rejected historical data or "retrospective validation." They require that new products be validated from beginning to end, a process called "prospective validation."

Capsules

Capsules are solid dosage forms in which the drug substance is enclosed in either a hard or soft, soluble container or shell of a suitable form of gelatin. The soft gelatin capsule was invented by Mothes, a French pharmacist in 1833. During the following year DuBlanc obtained a patent for his soft gelatin capsules. In 1848 Murdock patented the two-piece hard gelatin capsule. Although development work has been done on the preparation of capsules from methylcellulose and calcium alginate, gelatin, because of its unique properties, remains the primary composition material for the manufacture of capsules. The gelatin used in the manufacture of capsules is obtained from collagenous material by hydrolysis. There are two types of gelatin, Type A, derived mainly from pork skins by acid processing, and Type B, obtained from bones and animal skins by alkaline processing. Blends are used to obtain gelatin solutions with the viscosity and bloom strength characteristics desirable for capsule manufacture.[50]

The encapsulation of medicinal agents remains a popular method for administering drugs. Capsules are tasteless, easily administered and easily filled either extemporaneously or in large quantities commercially. In prescription practice the use of hard gelatin capsules permits a choice in prescribing a single drug or a combination of drugs at the exact dosage level considered best for the individual patient. This flexibility is an advantage over tablets. Some patients find it easier to swallow capsules than tablets, therefore preferring to take this form when possible. This preference has prompted pharmaceutical manufacturers to market the product in capsule form even though the product already has been produced in tablet form. While the industry prepares approximately 75% of its solid dosage forms as compressed tablets, 23% as hard gelatin capsules and 2% as soft elastic capsules, market surveys have indicated a consumer preference of 44.2% for soft elastic capsules, 39.6% for tablets and 19.4% for hard gelatin capsules.[51]

Hard Gelatin Capsules

The hard gelatin capsule, also referred to as the dry-filled capsule (DFC), consists of two sections, one slipping over the other, thus completely surrounding the drug formulation. The classic capsule shape is illustrated in Fig 39. These capsules are filled by introducing the powdered material into the longer end or body of the capsule and then slipping on the cap. Hard gelatin capsules are made largely from gelatin, FD&C colorants and sometimes an opacifying agent such as titanium dioxide; the USP permits the gelatin for this purpose to contain 0.15% sulfur dioxide to prevent decomposition during manufacture. Hard gelatin capsules contain 12 to 16% water, but the water content can vary depending on the storage conditions. When the humidity is low, the capsules become brittle; if stored at high humidities, the capsules become flaccid and lose their shape. Storage in high temperature areas also can affect the quality of hard gelatin capsules. Gelatin capsules do not protect hygroscopic materials from atmospheric water vapor as moisture can diffuse through the gelatin wall.

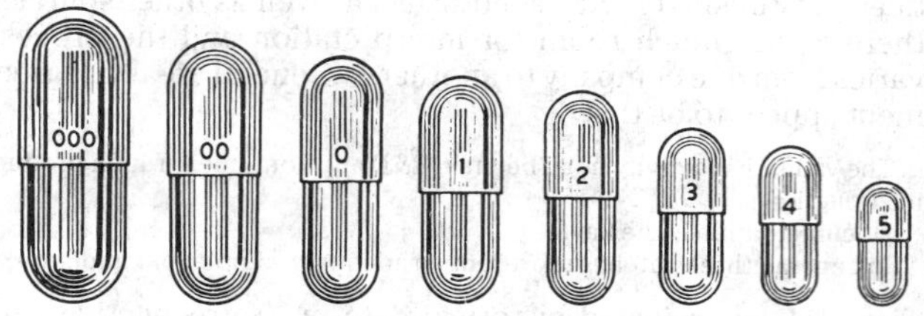

Fig 39. Hard gelatin capsules showing relatives sizes (courtesy, Parke-Davis).

Companies having equipment for preparing empty hard gelatin capsules include *Lilly*, *Parke-Davis*, *Scherer* and *SmithKline*. The latter's production is mainly for its own use; the others are suppliers to the industry. With this equipment stainless-steel pins, set in plates, are dipped into the gelatin solution, which must be maintained at a uniform temperature and an exact degree of fluidity. If the gelatin solution varies in viscosity, it correspondingly will decrease or increase the thickness of the capsule wall. This is important since a slight variation is sufficient to make either a loose or a tight joint. When the pins have been withdrawn from the gelatin solution, they are rotated while being dried in kilns through which a strong blast of filtered air with controlled humidity is forced. Each capsule is stripped, trimmed to uniform length and joined, the entire process being mechanical. Capsule-making equipment is illustrated in Figs 40 and 41. These show the stainless-steel pins being dipped into the gelatin solutions and then being rotated through the drying kiln.

Capsules are supplied in a variety of sizes. The hard, empty capsules (Fig 39) are numbered from 000, the largest size which can be swallowed, to 5, which is the smallest. Larger sizes are available for use in veterinary medicine. The approximate capacity for capsules from 000 to 5 ranges from 600 to 30 mg, although this will vary because of the different densities of powdered drug materials.

Commercially filled capsules have the conventional oblong shape illustrated with the exception of capsule products by *Lilly* and *SmithKline*, which are of distinctive shape. For Lilly products, capsules are used in which the end of the base is tapered to give the capsule a bullet-like shape; products encapsulated in this form are called *Pulvules*. The *SmithKline* capsules differ in that both the ends of the cap and body are angular, rather than round.

After hard gelatin capsules are filled and the cap applied, there are a number of methods used to assure that the capsules will not come apart if subjected to vibration or rough handling, as in high-speed counting and packaging equipment. The capsules can be spot-welded by means of a heated metal pin pressed against the cap, fusing it to the body, or they may be banded with molten gelatin laid around the joint in a strip and dried. Colored gelatin bands around capsules have been used for many years as a trademark by *Parke-Davis* for their line of capsule products, *Kapseals*. Another approach is used in the *Snap-Fit* and *Coni-Snap* capsules. A pair of matched locking rings are formed into the cap and body portions of the capsule. Prior to filling, these capsules are slightly longer than regular capsules of the same size. When

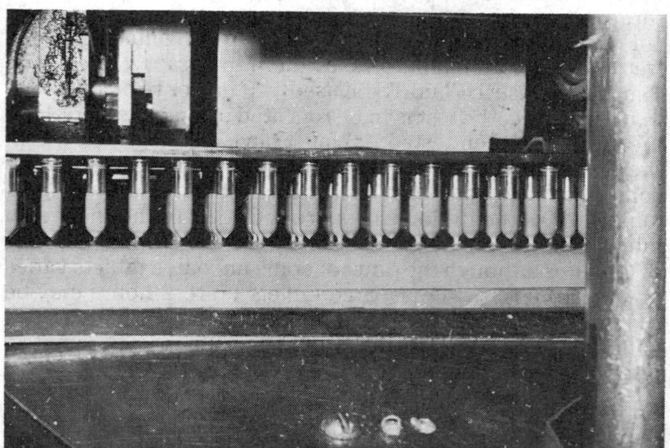

Fig 40. Manufacture of hard gelatin capsules by dipping stainless-steel pins into gelatin solutions (courtesy, Lilly).

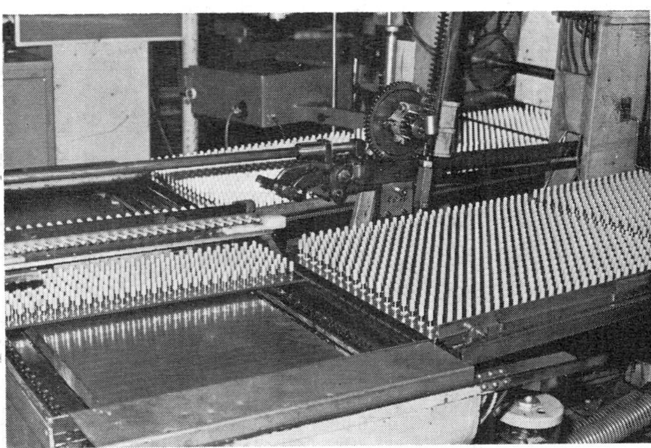

Fig 41. Formed capsules being dried by rotating through a drying kiln (courtesy, Lilly).

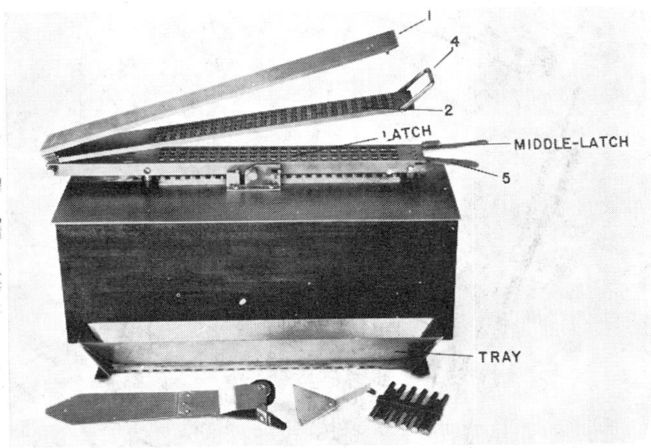

Fig 42. Hand-operated capsule machine (courtesy, Chemi-Pharm).

the locking rings are engaged after filling, their length is equivalent to that of the conventional capsule.

Following several tampering incidents, many pharmaceutical companies now use any number of locking and sealing technologies in order safely to manufacture and distribute these very useful dosage forms. Unfortunately, tamper-resistant packaging has become standard for capsule products.

It is usually necessary for the pharmacist to determine the size of the capsule needed for a given prescription through experimentation. The experienced pharmacist, having calculated the weight of material to be held by a single capsule, often will select the correct size immediately. If the material is powdered, the base of the capsule is filled and the top is replaced. If the material in the capsule proves to be too heavy after weighing, a smaller size must be taken and the test repeated. If the filled capsule is light, it is possible that more can be forced into it by increasing the pressure or, if necessary, some of the material may be placed in the cap. This is not desirable as it tends to decrease the accuracy of subdivision and it is much better to select another size, the base of which will hold exactly the correct quantity. In prescription filling it is wise to check the weight of each filled capsule.

In addition to the transparent, colorless, hard gelatin capsule, capsules are also available in various transparent colors such as pink, green, reddish-brown, blue, yellow and black. If they are used, it is important to note the color as well as the capsule size on the prescription so that in the case of renewal the refilled prescription will duplicate the original. Colored capsules have been used chiefly by manufacturers to give a specialty product a distinctive appearance. Titanium dioxide is added to the gelatin to form white capsules, or to make an opaque, colored capsule. In addition to color contrasts, many commercial products in capsules are given further identification by markings which may be the company's name, a symbol on the outer shell of the capsule or by banding. Some manufacturers mark capsules with special numbers based on a coded system to permit exact identification by the pharmacist or physician.

Extemporaneous Filling Methods

When filling capsules on prescription, the usual procedure is to mix the ingredients by trituration, reducing them to a fine and uniform powder. The principles and methods for the uniform distribution of an active medicinal agent in a powder mixture are discussed in Chapter 91. Granular powders do not pack readily in capsules and crystalline materials, especially those which consist of a mass of filament-like crystals such as the quinine salts, are not fitted easily into capsules unless powdered. Eutectic mixtures that tend to liquefy may be dispensed in capsules if a suitable absorbent such as magnesium carbonate is used. Potent drugs given in small doses usually are mixed with an inert diluent such as lactose before filling into capsules. When incompatible materials are prescribed together, it is sometimes possible to place one in a smaller capsule and then enclose it with the second drug in a larger capsule.

Usually, the powder is placed on paper and flattened with a spatula so that the layer of powder is not greater than about ⅓ the length of the capsule which is being filled. This helps to keep both the hands and capsules clean. The cap is removed from the selected capsule and held in the left hand; the body is pressed repeatedly into the powder until it is filled. The cap is replaced and the capsule is weighed. In filling the capsule the spatula is helpful in pushing the last quantity of the material into the capsule. If each capsule has not been weighed, there is likely to be an excess or a shortage of material when the specified number of capsules have been packed. This condition is adjusted before dispensing the prescription.

A number of manual filling machines and automatic capsule machines are available for increasing the speed of the capsule-filling operation. Figure 42 illustrates a capsule-filling machine which was known formerly as the Sharp & Dohme machine. This equipment is now available through *ChemiPharm*. Many community pharmacists find this a useful piece of apparatus and some pharmaceutical manufacturers use it for small-scale production of specialty items. The machine fills 24 capsules at a time with the possible production of 2000 per day. Entire capsules are placed in the machine by hand; the lower plate carries a clamp which holds the capsule bases and makes it possible to remove and replace the caps mechanically. The plate holding the capsule bases is perforated for three sizes of capsules. The powder is packed in the bases; the degree of accuracy depends on the selection of capsule size and the amount of pressure applied in packing. The hand-operated machine (Model 300, *ChemiPharm*) illustrated in Fig 43 has a production capacity of 2000 capsules per hour. The machine is made for a single capsule size and cannot be changed over for other sizes. A different machine is required for any additional capsule size. Its principle of operation is similar to that of the Sharp & Dohme machine.

Machine Filling Methods

Large-scale filling equipment for capsules operates on the same principle as the manual machines described above, namely the filling of the base of the capsule. Compared with tablets, powders for filling into hard gelatin capsules require the minimum of formulation efforts. The powders usually contain diluents such as lactose, mannitol, calcium carbonate

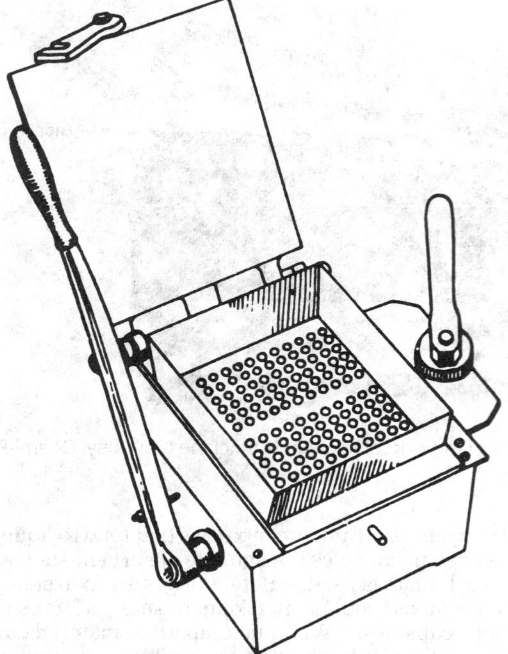

Fig 43. Hand-operated capsule machine, Model 300 (courtesy, ChemiPharm).

or magnesium carbonate. Since the flow of material is of great importance in the rapid and accurate filling of the capsule bodies, lubricants such as the stearates also are used frequently.

Because of the absence of numerous additives and manufacturing processing, the capsule form is used frequently to administer new drug substances for evaluation in initial clinical trials. However, it is now realized that the additives present in the capsule formulation, like the compressed tablet, can influence the release of the drug substance from the capsule. Tablets and capsules of a combination product containing triamterene and hydrochlorothiazide in a 2:1 ratio were compared clinically. The tablet caused approximately twice as much excretion of hydrochlorothiazide and 3 times as much triamterene as the capsule.[52]

Most equipment operates on the principle whereby the base of the capsule is filled and the excess is scraped off. Therefore, the active ingredient is mixed with sufficient volume of a diluent, usually lactose or mannitol, which will give the desired amount of the drug in the capsule when the base is filled with the powder mixture. The manner of operation of the machine can influence the volume of the powder which will be filled into the base of the capsule; therefore, the weights of the capsules must be checked routinely as they are filled. See Table 5.

Semiautomatic capsule-filling machines manufactured by *Parke-Davis* and *Lilly* are illustrated in Figs 44 and 45. The Type 8 capsule-filling machine performs mechanically under the same principle as the hand filling of capsules. This includes separation of the cap from the body, filling the body half and rejoining the cap and body halves.

Empty capsules are taken from the bottom of the capsule hopper into the magazine. The magazine gauge releases one capsule from each tube at the bottom of each stroke of the machine. Leaving the magazine, the capsules drop onto the tracks of the raceway and are pushed forward to the rectifying area with a push blade. The rectifier block descends, turning the capsules in each track, cap up, and drops them into each row of holes in the capsule-holding ring assembly.

As the capsules fall into the holding ring, the cap half has a seat on the counter bore in each hole for the top ring. The

Table 5—Capsule Fill Chart

Capsule Fill Weights (mg) Based on Size and Density

Powder density (g/mL)	Capsule volume (mL)									
	0.95	0.78	0.68	0.54	0.5	0.37	0.3	0.25	0.21	0.13
	Capsule size									
	OO	Oel	O	1el	1	2	3	4el	4	5
0.3	285	234	204	162	150	111	90	75	63	39
0.4	380	312	272	216	200	148	120	100	84	52
0.5	475	390	340	270	250	185	150	125	105	65
0.6	570	468	408	324	300	222	180	150	126	78
0.7	665	546	476	378	350	259	210	175	147	91
0.8	760	624	544	432	400	296	240	200	168	104
0.9	855	702	612	486	450	333	270	225	189	117
1.0	950	780	680	540	500	370	300	250	210	130
1.1	1045	858	748	594	550	407	330	275	231	143
1.2	1140	936	816	648	600	444	360	300	252	156
1.3	1235	1014	884	702	650	481	390	325	273	169
1.4	1330	1092	952	756	700	518	420	350	294	182
1.5	1425	1170	1020	810	750	555	450	375	315	195

body half is pulled by vacuum down into the bottom ring. When all rows in the ring assembly are full, the top ring, filled with caps only, is removed and set aside for later assembly. The body halves now are located in the bottom ring, ready for filling.

The ring holding the body halves is rotated at one of eight speeds on the rotary table. The drug hopper is swung over the rotating ring and the auger forces drug powder into the open body cavities. When the ring has made a complete revolution and the body halves have been filled, the hopper is swung aside. The cap-holding ring is placed over the body-holding ring and the assembly is ready for joining. The capsule-holding ring assembly is placed on the joiner and the joiner plate is swung down into position to hold the capsules in the ring. The peg ring pins are entered in the holes of the body holding ring and tapped in place by the air cylinder pushing the body halves back into the cap halves.

The holding-ring assembly is now pushed by hand back onto the peg ring away from the joiner plate, thus pushing the capsules out of the holding-ring assembly. The joined capsules then fall through the joiner chute into the capsule re-

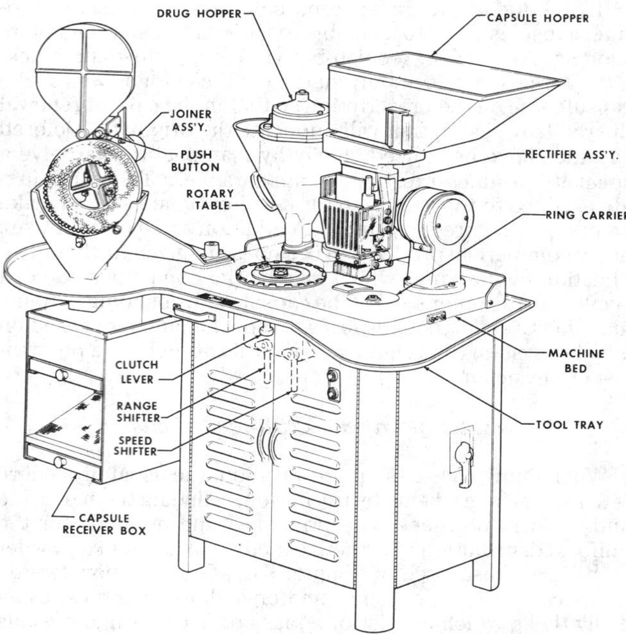

Fig 44. Schematic of Type 8 capsule-filling machine (courtesy, Parke-Davis).

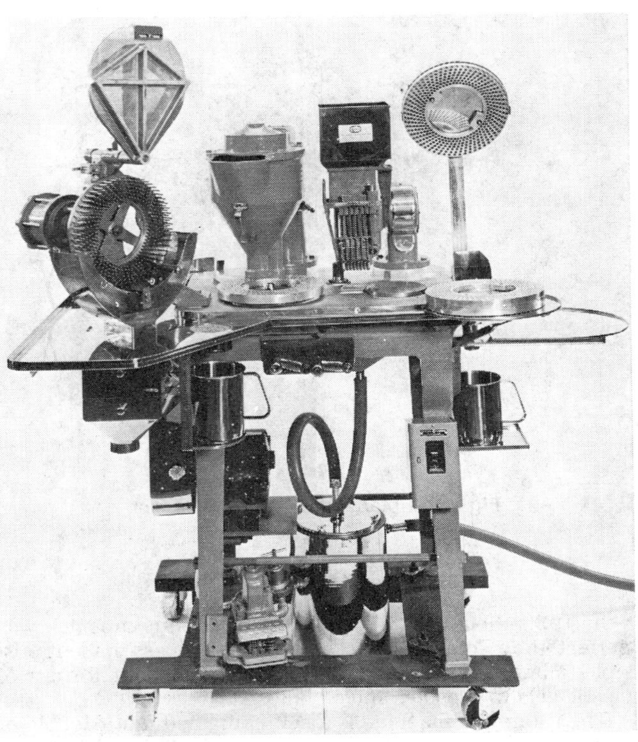

Fig 45. Type 8 capsule-filling machine (courtesy, Lilly).

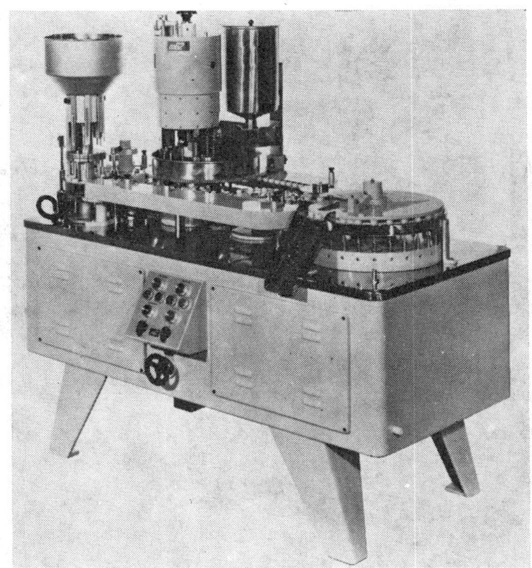

Fig 46. MG-2, automatic capsule-filling machine (courtesy, Supermatic).

ceiver box. The capsule receiver box screens the excess powder from the capsules and delivers them to any convenient container.

Many companies use the Type 8 capsule-filling equipment for small-scale manufacture and clinical supplies for investigational use because of its ease of operation, low cost and extreme flexibility. A Type 8 capsule filling machine will produce approximately 200,000 capsules per day. This, of course, depends upon the operator and the type of material being filled. For this machine, a mathematical model has been developed that describes the effect of selected physical powder properties, as well as mechanical operating conditions on the capsule filling operation. While the Type 8 capsule-filling machine has been in existence for many years, recent modifications have been made to this machine to improve the capsule-filling operations.

There are several pieces of equipment available that are classified as automatic capsule-filling machines. These are automatic in the sense that one operator can handle more than one machine. In this category are the Italian-made Zanasi (*United Machinery*) and MG-2 (*Supermatic*) models plus the West German-made Hoefliger & Karg models (*Bosch*).

Automatic capsule machines are capable of filling either powder or granulated products into hard gelatin capsules. With accessory equipment these machines also can fill pellets or place a tablet into the capsule with the powder or pellets. The capsules are fed at random into a large hopper. They are oriented as required and transferred into holders where the two halves are separated by suction. The top-half and bottom-half of the capsules are each in a separate holder, which at this stage take diverting directions.

A set of filling heads collect the product from the hopper, compresses it into a soft slug and inserts this into the bottom half of the capsule. After filling, each top-half is returned to the corresponding bottom-half. The filled capsules are ejected and an air blast at this point separates possible empty capsules from the filled. The machines can be equipped to handle all sizes of capsules. Depending upon the make and model, speeds from 9000 to 150,000 units per hour can be obtained (see Figs 46–48).

All capsules, whether they have been filled by hand or by machine, will require cleaning. Small quantities of capsules may be wiped individually with cloth. Larger quantities are rotated or shaken with crystalline sodium chloride. The capsules then are rolled on a cloth-covered surface.

Uniformity of Dosage Units

The uniformity of dosage forms can be demonstrated by either of two methods, weight variation or content uniformity. Weight variation may be applied where the product is a liquid-filled soft elastic capsule or where the hard gelatin capsule contains 50 mg or more of a single active ingredient comprising 50% or more, by weight, of the dosage form. See the official compendia for details.

Disintegration tests usually are not required for capsules unless they have been treated to resist solution in gastric fluid (enteric-coated). In this case they must meet the requirements for disintegration of enteric-coated tablets. For certain capsule dosage forms a dissolution requirement is part of

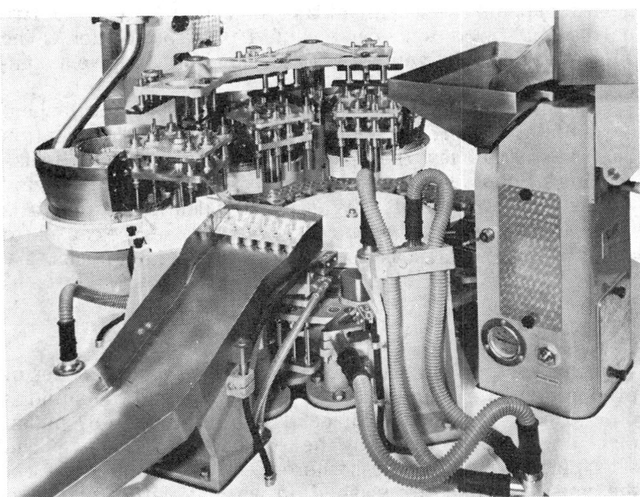

Fig 47. Zanasi automatic filling machine, Model AZ-60. The set of filling heads shown at the left collects the powder from the hopper, compresses it into a soft slug and inserts it into the bottom half of the capsule (courtesy, United Machinery).

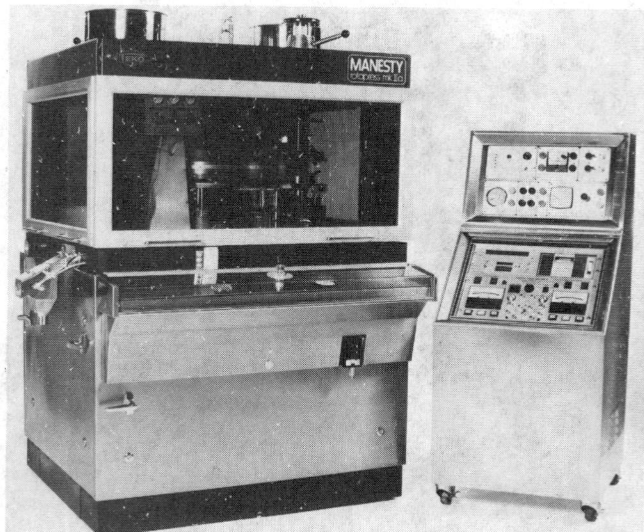

Fig 48. Hoefliger & Karg automatic capsule-filling machine, Model GFK 1200 (courtesy, Amaco).

the monograph. Procedures used are similar to those employed in the case of compressed tablets. (See Chapter 34).

Soft Elastic Capsules

The soft elastic capsule (SEC) is a soft, globular, gelatin shell somewhat thicker than that of hard gelatin capsules. The gelation is plasticized by the addition of glycerin, sorbitol or a similar polyol. The soft gelatin shells may contain a preservative to prevent the growth of fungi. Commonly used preservatives are methyl- and propylparabens and sorbic acid. Where the suspending vehicle or solvent can be an oil, soft gelatin capsules provide a convenient and highly acceptable dosage form. Large-scale production methods generally are required for the preparation and filling of soft gelatin capsules.

Formerly, empty soft gelatin capsules were available to the pharmacist for the extemporaneous compounding of solutions or suspensions in oils. Commercially filled soft gelatin capsules come in a wide choice of sizes and shapes; they may be round, oval, oblong, tube or suppository-shaped. Some sugar-coated tablets are quite similar in appearance to soft gelatin capsules. The essential differences are that the soft gelatin capsule has a seam at the point of closure of the two halves, and the contents can be liquid, paste or powder. The sugar-coated tablet will not have a seam but will have a compressed core.

Oral SEC dosage forms generally are made so that the heat seam of the gelatin shell opens to release its liquid medication into the stomach less than 5 minutes after ingestion. Its use is being studied for those drugs poorly soluble in water having bioavailability problems. When used as suppositories, it is the moisture present in the body cavity that causes the capsule to come apart at its heat-sealed seam and to release its contents.

Plate Process

In this method a set of molds is used. A warm sheet of prepared gelatin is laid over the lower plate and the liquid is poured on it. A second sheet of gelatin is carefully put in place and this is followed by the top plate of the mold. The set is placed under the press where pressure is applied to form the capsules which are washed off with a volatile solvent to remove any traces of oil from the exterior. This process has been adapted and is used for encapsulation by *Upjohn*. The sheets of gelatin may have the same color or different colors.

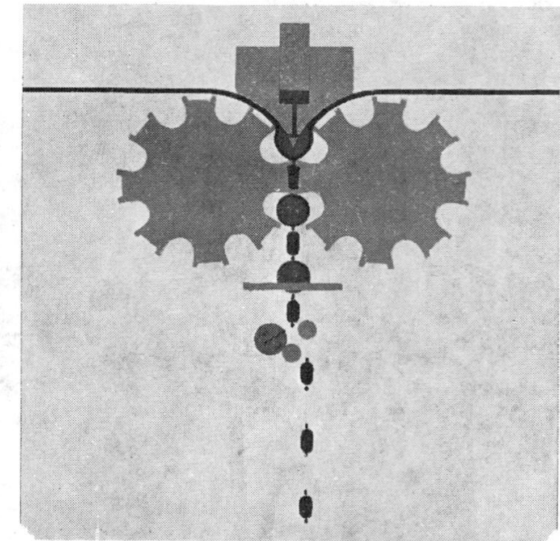

Fig 49. Rotary-die elastic capsule filler.

Rotary-Die Process

In 1933 the rotary-die process for elastic capsules was perfected by Robert P Scherer.[53] This process made it possible to improve the standards of accuracy and uniformity of elastic gelatin capsules and globules.

The rotary-die machine is a self-contained unit capable of continuously and automatically producing finished capsules from a supply of gelatin mass and filling material which may be any liquid, semiliquid or paste that will not dissolve gelatin. Two continuous gelatin ribbons, which the machine forms, are brought into convergence between a pair of revolving dies and an injection wedge. Accurate filling under pressure and sealing of the capsule wall occur as dual and coincident operations; each is delicately timed against the other. Sealing also severs the completed capsule from the net. The principle of operation is shown in Fig 49. See also Fig 50.

By this process the content of each capsule is measured individually by a single stroke of a pump so accurately constructed that plunger travel of 0.025 inch will deliver 1 ♏ (apoth). The Scherer machine contains banks of pumps so arranged that many capsules may be formed and filled simultaneously. All pumps are engineered to extremely small mechanical tolerances and to an extremely high degree of precision and similarity. All operations are controlled on a weight basis by actual periodic checks with a group of analytical balances. Individual net-fill weights of capsules resulting

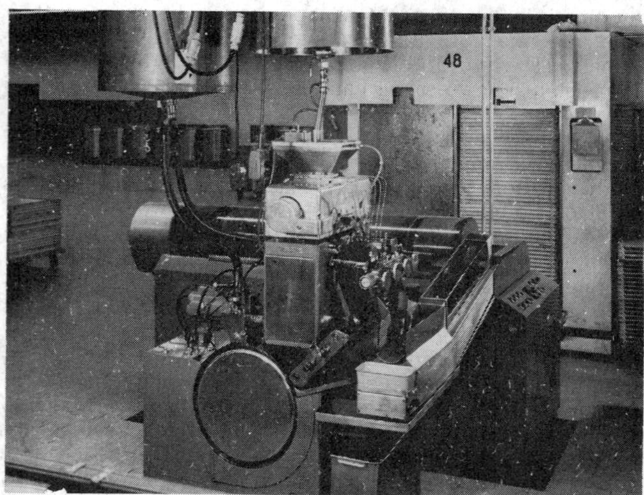

Fig 50. Scherer soft elastic capsule machine (courtesy, Scherer).

from large-scale production vary no more than ±1 to 3% from theory depending upon the materials used.

The rotary-die process makes it possible to encapsulate heavy materials such as ointments and pastes. In this manner solids can be milled with a vehicle and filled into capsules. Where it is desirable to have a high degree of accuracy and a hermetically sealed product, this form of enclosure is suited ideally.

The modern and well-equipped capsule plant is completely air conditioned, a practical necessity for fine capsule production. Its facilities and operations include the availability of carbon dioxide at every exposed point of operation for the protection of oxidizable substances before encapsulation. Special ingredients also have been used in the capsule shell to exclude light wavelengths which are destructive to certain drugs.

Norton Capsule Machine

This machine produces capsules completely automatically by leading two films of gelatin between a set of vertical dies. These dies as they close, open and close are, in effect, a continual vertical plate forming row after row of pockets across the gelatin film. These are filled with medicament and, as they progress through the dies, are sealed, shaped and cut out of the film as capsules which drop into a cooled solvent bath.

Accogel Capsule Machine

Another means of soft gelatin encapsulation uses the Accogel machine and process which were developed in the *Lederle*. The Accogel, or Stern machine, uses a system of rotary dies but is unique in that it is the only machine that successfully can fill dry powder into a soft gelatin capsule. The machine is available to the entire pharmaceutical industry by a lease arrangement and is used in many countries of the world. It is extremely versatile, not only producing capsules with dry powder but also encapsulating liquids and combinations of liquids and powders. By means of an attachment, slugs or compressed tablets may be enclosed in a gelatin film. The capsules can be made in a variety of colors, shapes and sizes.

Microencapsulation

As a technology, microencapsulation is placed in the section on capsules only because of the relationship in terminology to mechanical encapsulation described above. The topic also could have been included in a discussion of coating procedures. Essentially, microencapsulation is a process or technique by which thin coatings can be applied reproducibly to small particles of solids, droplets of liquids or dispersions, thus forming microcapsules. It can be differentiated readily from other coating methods in the size of the particles involved; these range from several tenths of a μm to 5000 μm in size.

A number of microencapsulation processes have been disclosed in the literature.[54] Some are based on chemical processes and involve a chemical or phase change; others are mechanical and require special equipment to produce the physical change in the systems required.

A number of coating materials have been used successfully; examples of these include gelatin, polyvinyl alcohol, ethylcellulose, cellulose acetate phthalate and styrene maleic anhydride. The film thickness can be varied considerably depending on the surface area of the material to be coated and other physical characteristics of the system. The microcapsules may consist of a single particle or clusters of particles. After isolation from the liquid manufacturing vehicle and drying, the material appears as a free-flowing powder. The powder is suitable for formulation as compressed tablets, hard gelatin capsules, suspensions and other dosage forms.

The process provides answers for problems such as masking the taste of bitter drugs, a means of formulating prolonged action dosage forms, a means of separating incompatible materials, a method of protecting chemicals against moisture or oxidation and a means of modifying a material's physical characteristics for ease of handling in formulation and manufacture.

Among the processes applied to pharmaceutical problems is that developed by the National Cash Register Co (NCR). The NCR process is a chemical operation based on phase separation or coacervation techniques. In colloidal chemistry, coacervation refers to the separation of a liquid precipitate, or phase, when solutions of two hydrophilic colloids are mixed under suitable conditions.

The NCR process, using phase separation or coacervation techniques, consists of three steps:

1. Formation of three immiscible phases: a liquid manufacturing phase, a core material phase and a coating material phase.
2. Deposition of the liquid polymer coating on the core material.
3. Rigidizing the coating, usually by thermal, cross-linking or desolvation techniques, to form a microcapsule.

In Step 2, the deposition of the liquid polymer around the core material occurs only if the polymer is absorbed at the interface formed between the core material and the liquid vehicle phase. In many cases physical or chemical changes in the coating polymer solution can be induced so that phase separation (coacervation) of the polymer will occur. Droplets of concentrated polymer solution will form and coalesce to yield a two-phase liquid–liquid system. In cases where the coating material is an immiscible polymer or insoluble liquid polymer, it may be added directly. Also monomers can be dissolved in the liquid vehicle phase and, subsequently, polymerized at the interface.

Equipment required for microencapsulation by this method is relatively simple; it consists mainly of jacketed tanks with variable speed agitators. Figure 51 shows a typical flow diagram of a production installation.

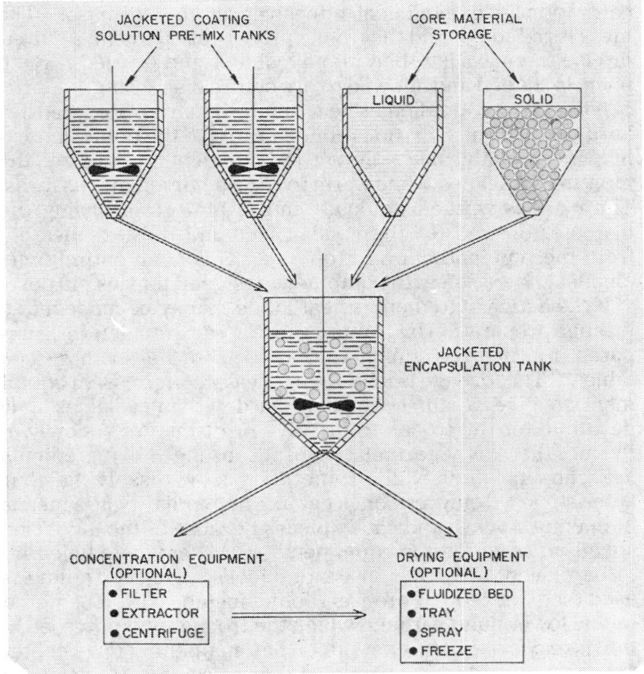

Fig 51. Production installation for the microencapsulation process (courtesy, NCR).

Other Oral Solid Dosage Forms

Pills

Pills are small, round solid dosage forms containing a medicinal agent and are intended for oral administration. Pills were formerly the most extensively used oral dosage form, but they have been replaced largely by compressed tablets and capsules. Substances which are bitter or unpleasant to the taste, if not corrosive or deliquescent, can be administered in this form if the dose is not too large.

Formerly, pills were made extemporaneously by the community pharmacist whose skill at pill-making became an art. However, the few pills which are now used in pharmacy are prepared on a large scale with mechanical equipment. The pill formulas of the NF were introduced largely for the purpose of establishing standards of strength for the well-known and currently used pills. Hexylresorcinol Pills consist of hexylresorcinol crystals covered with a rupture-resistant coating that is dispersible in the digestive tract. It should be noted that the official hexylresorcinol pills are prepared not by traditional methods but by a patented process, the gelatin coating being sufficiently tough that it can not be broken readily, even when chewed. Therefore, the general method for the preparation of pills does not apply to hexylresorcinol pills.

Previous editions of this text should be consulted for methods of pill preparation.

Troches

These forms of oral medication, also known as *lozenges* or *pastilles*, are discoid-shaped solids containing the medicinal agent in a suitably flavored base. The base may be a hard sugar candy, glycerinated gelatin or the combination of sugar with sufficient mucilage to give it form. Troches are placed in the mouth where they slowly dissolve, liberating the active ingredient. The drug involved can be an antiseptic, local anesthetic, antibiotic, antihistaminic, antitussive, analgesic or a decongestant.

Formerly, troches were prepared extemporaneously by the pharmacist. The mass is formed by adding water slowly to a mixture of the powdered drug, powdered sugar and a gum until a pliable mass is formed. Powdered acacia in 7% concentration gives sufficient adhesiveness to the mass. The mass is rolled out and the troche pieces cut out using a cutter, or else the mass is rolled into a cylinder and divided. Each piece is shaped and allowed to dry before dispensing.

If the active ingredient is heat-stable, it may be prepared in a hard candy base. Syrup is concentrated to the point where it becomes a pliable mass, the active ingredient is added and the mixture is kneaded while warm to form a homogeneous mass. The mass is worked gradually into a pipe form having the diameter desired for the candy piece and the lozenges cut from the pipe and allowed to cool. This is an entirely mechanical operation with equipment designed for this purpose.

If the active ingredient is heat-labile, it may be made into a lozenge preparation by compression. The granulation is prepared in a manner similar to that used for any compressed tablet. The lozenge is made using heavy compression equipment to give a tablet which is harder than usual as it is desirable for the troche to dissolve or disintegrate slowly in the mouth. In the formulation of the lozenge the ingredients are chosen which will promote its slow-dissolving char acteristics. Compression is gaining in popularity as a means of making troches and candy pieces because of the increased speeds of compression equipment. In cases where holes are to be placed in troches or candy pieces, core-rod tooling is used (see Fig 52). Core-rod tooling includes a rod centered on the lower punch around which the troche is compressed in the die cavity. The upper punch has an opening in its center for the core rod to enter during compression. It is evident that maximum accuracy is needed to provide alignment as the narrow punches are inserted into the die.

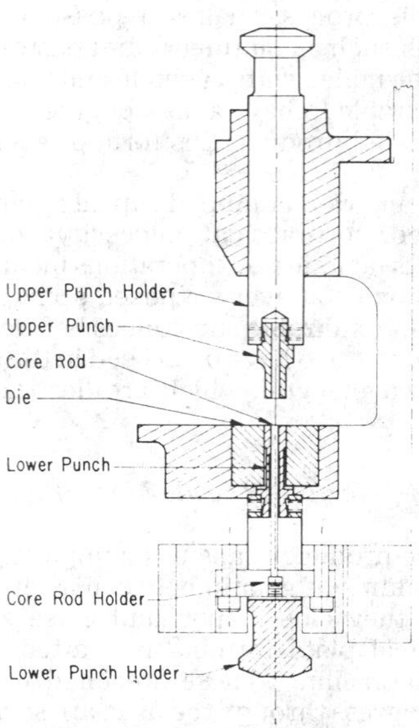

Fig 52. Core-rod tooling for compressing troches or candy pieces with hole in center (courtesy, Vector/Colton).

Cachets

Related to capsules, inasmuch as they provide an edible container for the oral administration of solid drugs, cachets formerly were used in pharmacy. They varied in size from ¾ to ⅛ in in diameter and consisted of two concave pieces of wafer made of flour and water. After one section was filled with the prescribed quantity of the medicinal agent, they were sealed tightly by moistening the margins and pressing them firmly together. When moistened with water, their character was changed entirely; they became soft, elastic and slippery. Hence, they could be swallowed easily by floating them on water.

Pellets

The term pellet is now applied to small, sterile cylinders about 3.2 mm in diameter by 8 mm in length, which are formed by compression from medicated masses.[55] Whenever prolonged and continuous absorption of testosterone, estradiol or desoxycorticosterone is desired, pellets of these potent hormones may be used by implantation.

References

1. Wagner JG: *Fundamentals of Clinical Pharmacokinetics*, Drug Intell Publ, Hamilton, IL, 1975.
2. Benet LZ, Levy G, Ferraiolo BL: *Pharmacokinetics—A Modern View*, Plenum, New York, 1984.
3. Manninen V, Ojala K, Reisell P: *Lancet 2:* 922, 1972.
4. Katchen B, Symchowisz S: *J Pharm Sci 56:* 1108, 1967.
5. Katchen B: *Acta Pharmacol Toxicol 29:* 88, 1971.
6. Hansch C, Dunn, WJ III: *J Pharm Sci 61:* 1, 1972.
7. Flynn GL, Yalkowsky SH and Roseman T: *Ibid 63:* 479, 1974.
8. Lieberman HA, Lachman L, eds: *Pharmaceutical Dosage Forms: Tablets*, vol I, II and III, Dekker, New York, 1980, 1981 and 1982.
9. Evans AJ, Train D: *A Bibliography of the Tableting of Medicinal Substances*, Pharmaceutical Press, London, 1963.
10. Evans AJ: *A Bibliography of the Tableting of Medicinal Substances, Pharmaceutical Press, London, 1964.*
11. Lachman L, *et al: The Theory and Practice of Industrial Pharmacy*, 3rd ed, Lea & Febiger, Philadelphia, 1988.
12. Banker G, Rhodes CT: *Modern Pharmaceutics*, Dekker, New York, 1979.

13. Ansel HC: *Introduction to Pharmaceutical Dosage Forms,* 3rd ed, Lea & Febiger, Philadelphia, 1981.
14. Monkhouse DC, Lach JL: *Can J Pharm Sci 7:* 29, 1972.
15. Blanchard J: *Am J Pharm 150:* 132, 1978.
16. *Handbook of Pharmaceutical Excipients,* APhA/Pharm Soc Great Britian, APhA, Washington, DC 1986.
17. Rudnic EM, Kanig JL, Rhodes CT: *J Pharm Sci, 74:* 647, 1985.
18. Rudnic EM, Rhodes CT, Welch S, Bernardo P: *Drug Dev Ind Pharm 8:* 87, 1982.
19. Kanig JL, Rudnic EM: *Pharm Tech, 8:* 50, 1984.
20. Rudnic EM, Rhodes CT, Bavitz JF, Schwartz JB: *Drug Dev Ind Pharm 7:* 347, 1981.
21. *Capsugel List of Colorants for Oral Drugs,* Capsugel AG, Basel, 1988.
22. Foley VL, Belcastro PF: *Pharm Tech 9:* 110, 1987.
23. Stewart A: *Engineering 169:* 203, 1950.
24. David ST, Augsburger LL: *J Pharm Sci 66:* 155, 1977.
25. Jones TM. In Poldermand J, ed: *Formulation and Preparation of Dosage Forms,* Elsevier, North Holland, 29, 1977.
26. Rees JE, Rue PJ: *J Pharm Pharmacol 30:* 601, 1987.
27. Summers MP, Enever RP, Carless JE: *J Pharm Sci 66:* 1172, 1977.
28. Hersey JA, Rees JE. In Groves MJ, Wyatt-Sargent JL, eds: *Particle Size Analysis,* Soc Anal Chem, London, 1970.
29. Jones TM: *Acta Pharm Tech:* 1978.
30. Chowhan ZT: *Pharm Tech, 12:* 46, 1988.
31. Meht AM: *Ibid 46(Dec)*: 1988.
32. Mendes RW, Roy SB: *Ibid 2(3)*: 35, 1978.
33. Wurster DE: *J APhA Sci Ed 49:* 82, 1960.
34. Mendes RW, Roy SB: *Pharm Tech 2(9)*: 61, 1978.
35. Malinowski HJ, Smith WE: *J Pharm Sci 63:* 285, 1974.
36. Woodruff CW, Nuessle NO: *Ibid 61:* 787, 1972.
37. O'Connor RE, Holinej J, Schwartz JB: *Am J Pharm 156:* 80, 1984.
38. O'Connor RE, Schwartz JB: *Drug Dev Ind Pharm II:* 1837, 1985.
39. Newton JM: *Mfg Chem Aerosol News 37(Apr)*: 33, 1966.
40. US Pat 3,883647, May 13, 1975.
41. *Tableting Specification Manual,* APhA, Washington, DC, 1981.
42. Knoechel EL *et al:* *J Pharm Sci 56:* 116, 1967.
43. Wray PE: *Drug Cosmet Ind 105(3)*: 53, 1969.
44. Hiestand EN and Smith DP: *Powder Tech, 38:* 145, 1984.
45. Hiestand EN, Wells JE, Poet CB, Ochs, J: *J Pharm Sci, 66:* 510, 1977.
46. Luenberger, H: *Int J Pharm, 12:* 41, 1982.
47. Walter JT, Augsburger, LL: *Pharm Tech 10:* 26, 1986.
48. Schwartz JB: *Ibid 5(9)*: 102, 1981.
49. Marshall K: *Ibid 7(3)*: 68, 1983.
50. Jones BE: *Mfg Chem Aerosol News 40(Feb)*: 25, 1969.
51. Delaney R: *Pharm Exec 2(3)*: 34, 1982.
52. Tannenbaum PJ *et al:* *Clin Pharmacol Ther 9:* 598, 1968.
53. Ebert WR: *Pharm Tech 1(10)*: 44, 1977.
54. Madan PL: *Ibid. 2(9)*: 68, 1978.
55. Cox PH, Spanjers F: *Pharm Weekblad 105:* 681, 1970.

CHAPTER 93

Coating of Pharmaceutical Dosage Forms

Stuart C Porter, PhD
Vice President, Research and Development
Colorcon, Inc
West Point, PA 19486

Any introduction to tablet coating must be prefaced by an important question—"Why coat tablets?"—since in many instances, the coating is being applied to a dosage form that already is functionally complete. In attempting to answer this question, if one examines the market, it will become apparent that a significant proportion of pharmaceutical solid dosage forms are coated. The reasons for this range from the esthetic to a desire to control the bioavailability of the drug, and include:

1. Protecting the drug from its surrounding environment (particularly air, moisture and light) with a view to improving stability.
2. Masking of unpleasant taste and odor.
3. Increasing the ease by means of which the product can be ingested by the patient.
4. Improving product identity, from the manufacturing plant, through intermediaries and to the patient.
5. Facilitating handling, particularly in high-speed packaging/filling lines, and automated counters in pharmacies, where the coating minimizes cross-contamination due to dust elimination.
6. Improving product appearance, particularly where there are noticeable visible differences in tablet core ingredients from batch to batch.
7. Reducing the risk of interaction between incompatible components. This would be achieved by using coated forms of one or more of the offending ingredients (particularly active compounds).
8. Improving product mechanical integrity, since coated products generally are more resistant to mishandling (abrasion, attrition, etc).
9. Modifying drug release, as in enteric-coated, repeat-action and sustained-release products.

Evolution of the Coating Process—Tablet coating is perhaps one of the oldest pharmaceutical processes still in existence. Although a great deal has been written about the materials and methods used, the coating process is still often recognized to be more of an art than a science, a factor which may be responsible for many of the problems that can exist. Historically, the literature cites Rhazes (850–932 AD) as being one of the earliest "tablet coaters," having used the mucilage of psyllium seeds to coat pills that had an offending taste. Subsequently, Avicenna[1] was reported to have used gold and silver for pill coating. Since then, there have been many references to the different materials used in "tablet coating." White[2] mentioned the use of finely divided talc in what was at one time popularly known as "pearl coating," while Kremers and Urdang[3] described the introduction of the gelatin coating of pills by Garot in 1838.

An interesting reference[4] reports the use of waxes to coat poison tablets. These waxes, being insoluble in all parts of the gastrointestinal tract, were intended to prevent accidental poisoning (the contents could be utilized by breaking the tablet prior to use).

While earlier coated products were produced by individuals working in pharmacies, particularly when extemporaneous compounding was the order of the day, that responsibility now has been assumed by the pharmaceutical industry. The earliest attempts to apply coatings to pills yielded variable results and usually required the handling of single pills. Such pills would have been mounted on a needle or held with a pair of forceps and literally dipped into the coating fluid, a procedure which would have to be repeated more than once to ensure that the pill was coated completely. Subsequently, the pills were held at the end of a suction tube, dipped and then the process repeated for the other side of the pill. Not surprisingly, these techniques often failed to produce a uniformly coated product.[5]

Initially, the first sugar-coated pills seen in the US were imported from France about 1842;[5] while Warner, a Philadelphia pharmacist, became among the first indigenous manufacturers in 1856.[6]

Pharmaceutical pan-coating processes are based on those used in the candy industry, where techniques were highly evolved, even in the Middle Ages. Today, while most coating pans are fabricated from stainless steel, early pans were made from copper, because drying was effected by means of an externally applied heat source. Current thinking, even with conventional pans, is to dry the coated tablets with a supply of heated air, and remove the moisture and dust-laden air from the vicinity of the pan by means of an air-extraction system.

Pan-coating processes underwent little further change until the late 1940s and early 1950s, with the conventional pan being the mainstay of all coating operations up to that time. However, in the last 20 or 30 years there have been some significant advances made in coating-process technology, mainly as a result of a steady evolution in pan design and its associated ancillary equipment.

Interestingly, in the early years of this development, an entirely new form of technology evolved, that of film coating. Recognizing the deficiencies of the sugar-coating process, advocates of film coating were achieving success by using coating systems involving highly volatile organic solvents. These circumvented the problems associated with the inefficiency in the drying capabilities of conventional equipment, and enabled production quotas to be met with significant reductions in processing times and materials used. The disadvantage of this approach, however, always has been associated with the solvent systems used, which often employed flammable and toxic materials.

The advances that occurred with equipment design, having begun by the development of the Wurster[7] process and continued by the evolution of side-vented pans, have resulted in the gradual emergence of coating processes where drying efficiency can be maximized. Thus, film coating began as a process using inefficient drying equipment, relying on highly volatile coating formulations for success, and evolved into one in which the processing equipment is a major factor in ensuring that rapid drying occurs. Improved drying capabilities have permitted increased use of aqueous film-coating formulations.

Advances in equipment design also have benefited the sugar-coating process, where, because of Current Good Manufacturing Practices (CGMP) and to maintain product uniformity and performance, the trend has been toward using fully automated processes. Nonetheless, film coating tends to dominate as the process of choice for tablet coating.

Pharmaceutical Coating Processes

Basically, there are four major techniques for applying coatings to pharmaceutical solid dosage forms: (1) sugar coating, (2) film coating, (3) microencapsulation and (4) compression coating.

Although it could be argued that the use of mucilage of psyllium seed, gelatin, etc, as already discussed, was an early form of film coating, *sugar coating* is regarded as the oldest method for tablet coating, and involves the deposition from aqueous solution of coatings based predominantly on sucrose as a raw material. The large quantities of coating material that are applied and the inherent skill often required of the operators combine to result in a long and tedious process.

Film coating, the deposition of a thin polymeric film onto the dosage form from solutions that were initially organic-solvent-based, but which now rely more and more on water as the prime solvent, has proven to be a popular alternative to sugar coating.

Microencapsulation is a modified form of film coating, differing only in the size of the particles to be coated and the methods by which this is accomplished. This process is based on either mechanical methods such as pan coating, air-suspension techniques, multiorifice centrifugal techniques and modified spray-drying techniques, or physicochemical ones involving coacervation-phase separation, where the material to be coated is suspended in a solution of the polymer. Phase separation is facilitated by the addition of a nonsolvent, incompatible polymer, inorganic salts or by altering the temperature of the system.

Compression coating incorporates the use of modified tableting machines which allow the compaction of a dry coating around the tablet core produced on the same machine. The main advantage of this type of coating is that it eliminates the use of any solvent, whether aqueous or organic in nature. However, this process is mechanically complex and has not proven popular as a method for coating tablets.

Sugar Coating of Compressed Tablets

While the term "sugar" is somewhat generic, and lends itself to describing various raw materials, sugar coating relies mainly on the use of sucrose. The main reason for this is that, based on the techniques involved, it is probably the only material which has enabled smooth, high-quality coatings to be produced, that are essentially dry and tack-free at the end of the process.

While the popularity of sugar coating has been on the decline, this process still retains some popularity, and many companies have invested in the complete modernization of the process.

In spite of certain inherent difficulties associated with the sugar-coating process, products which have been expertly sugar coated still remain among the most elegant available.

Since sugar coating is a multistep process, where esthetics of the final coated product is an important goal, it has been, and still is in many companies, highly dependent on the use of skilled manpower. For these reasons, the sugar-coating process is often protracted and tedious. However, processing times have been reduced gradually in the last two decades by the adoption of modern techniques and by the introduction of automation.

The sugar-coating process can be subdivided into six main steps: (1) sealing, (2) subcoating, (3) smoothing, (4) color coating, (5) polishing and (6) printing.

Sealing—The sealing coat is applied directly to the tablet core for the purpose of separating the tablet ingredients (primarily the drug) and water (which is a major constituent of the coating formulation) in order to assure good product stability. A secondary function is to strengthen the tablet core. Sealing coats usually consist of alcoholic solutions (approximately 10–30% solids) of resins such as shellac, zein, cellulose acetate phthalate or polyvinyl acetate phthalate. Historically, shellac has proven to be the most popular material although it can cause impaired bioavailability due to a change in resin properties on storage. A solution to this problem has been to use a shellac-based formulation containing a measured quantity of polyvinylpyrrolidone (PVP).[8]

The quantities of material applied as a sealing coat will depend primarily on the tablet and batch size. However, another important factor is tablet porosity, since highly porous tablets will tend to soak up the first application of solution, thus preventing it from spreading uniformly across the surface of every tablet in the batch. Thus, one or more further applications of resin solution may be necessary to ensure that the tablet cores are sealed effectively.

Since most sealing coats develop a degree of tack (stickiness) at some time during the drying process, it is usual to apply a dusting powder to prevent tablets from sticking together or to the pan. A common material used as a dusting powder is asbestos-free talc. Overzealous use of talc may cause problems, firstly, by imparting a high degree of slip to the tablets, thus preventing them from rolling properly in the pan, and secondly, presenting a surface at the beginning of the subcoating stage which is very difficult to wet, resulting in inadequate subcoat buildup, particularly on the edges. If there is a tendency for either of these problems to occur, one solution is to replace part or all of the talc with some other material such as terra alba, which will form a slightly rougher surface. Use of talc now is being frowned upon because of its potential carcinogenicity.

If an enteric-coated product is required, additional quantities of the seal-coat solution are applied. In this situation, however, it is preferable to use synthetic polymers such as polyvinyl acetate phthalate or cellulose acetate phthalate.

Subcoating—Subcoating is a critical operation in the sugar-coating process that can have a marked effect on ultimate tablet quality. Sugar coating is a process which often leads to a 50 to 100% weight increase, and it is at the subcoating stage that most of the buildup occurs.

Historically, subcoating has been achieved by the application of a gum-based solution to the sealed tablet cores, and once this solution has been distributed uniformly throughout the tablet mass, it is followed by a liberal dusting of powder, which serves to reduce tack and facilitate tablet buildup. This procedure of application of gum solution, spreading, dusting and drying is continued until the requisite buildup has been achieved. Thus, the subcoating is a sandwich of alternate layers of gum and powder. Some examples of binder solutions are shown in Table 1 and those of dusting powder formulations in Table 2.

While this approach has proved to be very effective, particularly where there is difficulty in covering edges. If care is not taken, a "lumpy" subcoat will be the result. Also, if the amount of dusting powder applied is not matched to the binding capacity of the gum solution, not only will the ultimate coating be brittle, but also dust will collect in the back of the pan, a factor which may contribute to excessive roughness.

An alternative approach which has proved popular, particularly when used in conjunction with an automated dosing system, is the application of a suspension subcoat formulation.

Table 1—Binder Solution Formulations for Subcoating

	A, % *w/w*	B, % *w/w*
Gelatin	3.3	6.0
Gum acacia (powdered)	8.7	8.0
Sucrose	55.3	45.0
Water	to 100.0	to 100.0

Table 2—Dusting Powder Formulations for Subcoating

	A, % *w/w*	B, % *w/w*
Calcium carbonate	40.0	—
Titanium dioxide	5.0	1.0
Talc (asbestos-free)	25.0	61.0
Sucrose (powdered)	28.0	38.0
Gum acacia (powdered)	2.0	—

In such a formulation the powdered materials responsible for coating buildup have been dispersed in a gum-based solution. A typical formulation is shown in Table 3. This approach allows the solids loading to be matched more closely to the binding capacity of the base solution, and often permits the less-experienced coater to achieve satisfactory results.

Smoothing—Depending on how successfully the subcoat was applied, it may be necessary to smooth out the tablet surface further prior to application of the color coating. Smoothing usually can be accomplished by the application of a simple syrup solution (approximately 60 to 70% sugar solids).

Often, the smoothing syrups contain a low percentage of titanium dioxide (1 to 5%) as an opacifier. This can be particularly useful when the subsequent color-coating formulation uses water-soluble dyes as colorants, since it makes the surface under the color coating more reflective, resulting in a brighter, cleaner final color.

Color Coating—This stage often is the most critical in the successful completion of a sugar-coating process, and involves the multiple application of syrup solutions (60 to 70% sugar solids) containing the requisite coloring matter. The types of coloring materials used can be divided into two categories: dyes or pigments. The distinction between the two simply is one of solubility in the coating fluid. Since water-soluble dyes behave entirely differently than water-insoluble pigments, the application procedure used in the color coating of tablets will depend on the type of colorant chosen.

When used by a skilled artisan, water-soluble dyes produce the most elegant of sugar-coated tablets, since it is possible to obtain a cleaner, brighter final color. However, since water-soluble dyes are migratory colorants (that is to say, moisture that is removed from the coating on drying will cause migration of the colorant, resulting in a nonuniform appearance), great care must be exercised in their use, particularly when dark shades are required. This can be achieved by applying small quantities of colored syrup that are just sufficient to wet the surface of every tablet in the batch, and then allowing the tablets to dry slowly. It is essential that each application is allowed to dry thoroughly before subsequent applications are made, otherwise moisture may become trapped in the coating and may cause the tablets to "sweat" on standing.

The final color obtained may result from up to 60 individual applications of colored syrup. This factor, combined with the need to dry each application slowly and thoroughly, results in very long processing times (eg, assuming 50 applications are made which take between 15 and 30 minutes each, the coloring process can extend over a period of up to 25 hours).

Tablet color coating with pigments, as advocated by Tucker *et al*,[9] can present some significant advantages. First of all, since pigment colors are water-insoluble, they present no problems of migration since the colorant remains where it is deposited. In addition, if the pigment is opaque, or is combined with an opacifier such as titanium dioxide, the desired color can be developed much more rapidly, thus resulting in a thinner color coat. Since each color-syrup application now can be dried more rapidly, fewer applications are required and significant reductions can be made in both processing times and costs.

Table 3—Typical Suspension Subcoating Formulation

	% w/w
Distilled water	25.0
Sucrose	40.0
Calcium carbonate	20.0
Talc (asbestos-free)	12.0
Gum acacia (powdered)	2.0
Titanium dioxide	1.0

Although pigment-based color coatings are by no means foolproof, they will permit more abuse than a dye color-coating approach, and are more amenable for use by less-skilled coaters. Pharmaceutically acceptable pigments can be classified either as inorganic pigments (eg, titanium dioxide, iron oxides) or certified lakes. Certified lakes are produced from water-soluble dyes by means of a process known as "laking," whereby the dye molecule becomes fixed to a suitable insoluble substrate such as aluminum hydroxide.

Certified lakes, particularly when used in conjunction with an opacifier such as titanium dioxide, provide an excellent means of coloring sugar coatings and permit a wide range of shades to be achieved. However, the incorporation of pigments into the syrup solution is not as easy as with water-soluble dyes, since it is necessary to ensure that the pigment is wetted completely and dispersed uniformly. Thus, the use of pigment color concentrates, which are commercially available, is usually beneficial.

Polishing—Sugar-coated tablets need to be polished in order to achieve a final gloss. Polishing is achieved by applying mixtures of waxes (beeswax, carnauba wax, candelila wax or hard paraffin wax) to the tablets in a polishing pan. Such wax mixtures may be applied as powders or as dispersions in various organic solvents.

Printing—In order to identify sugar-coated tablets (in addition to shape, size and color) often it is necessary to print them, either before or after polishing, using pharmaceutical branding inks, by means of the process of *offset rotogravure*.

Sugar-Coating Problems—Various problems may be encountered during the sugar coating of tablets. It must be remembered that any process in which tablets are kept tumbling constantly can present difficulties if the tablets are not strong enough to withstand the applied stress. Tablets which are too soft, or have a tendency to laminate, may break up and the fragments adhere to the surface of otherwise good tablets.

Sugar-coating pans exhibit inherently poor mixing characteristics. If care is not exercised during the application of the various coating fluids, nonuniform distribution of coating material can occur, resulting in an unacceptable range of sizes of finished tablets within the batch.

Overzealous use of dusting powders, particularly during the subcoating stage, may result in a coating being formed in which the quantity of fillers exceeds the binding capacity of the polymer used in the formulation, creating soft coatings or those with increased tendency to crack.

Irregularities in appearance are not uncommon, and occur either as the result of color migration during drying when water-soluble dyes are used, or of "washing back" when overdosing of colored syrups causes the previously dried coating layers to be redissolved. Rough tablet surfaces will produce a "marbled" appearance during polishing, since wax buildup occurs in the small depressions in the tablet surface.

Film Coating of Solid Dosage Forms

Film coating involves the deposition of a thin, but uniform, film onto the surface of the substrate. Unlike sugar coating, the flexibility afforded in film coating allows additional substrates, other than just compressed tablets, to be considered (eg, powder, granules, nonpareils, capsules). Coatings essentially are applied continuously to a moving bed of material, usually by means of a spray technique, although manual application procedures have been used.

Historically, film coating was introduced in the early 1950s in order to combat the shortcomings of the then predominant sugar-coating process. Film coating has proved successful as a result of the many advantages offered, including:

1. Minimal weight increase (typically 2 to 3% of tablet core weight).
2. Significant reduction in processing times.
3. Increased process efficiency and output.
4. Increased flexibility in formulations.
5. Improved resistance to chipping of the coating.

In the early years of film coating, the major process advantages resulted from the greater volatility of the organic solvents used. However, the use of such organic solvents has created many potential problems, including:

1. Flammability hazards.
2. Toxicity hazards.
3. Concerns over environmental pollution.
4. Cost (either relating to minimizing items 1–3, or to the cost of the solvents themselves).

However, since the initial introduction of film coating, significant advances have been made in process technology and equipment design. The emphasis has changed from needing highly volatile organic solvents (to achieve rapid drying), to attaining the same ultimate effect by designing equipment to have more efficient drying characteristics.

Thus, there has been a transition from conventional pans to side-vented pans and fluid-bed equipment, and consequently from the problematic organic solvent-based process to an aqueous one.

Film Coating Raw Materials—The major components in any film-coating formulation consist of a polymer, plasticizer, colorant and solvent (or vehicle).

Ideal properties for the polymer include solubility in a wide range of solvent systems to promote flexibility in formulation, an ability to produce coatings which have suitable mechanical properties and the appropriate solubility in gastrointestinal fluids such that drug bioavailability is not compromised.

Cellulose ethers are the preferred polymers in film coating, particularly hydroxypropyl methylcellulose. Suitable substitutes are hydroxypropyl cellulose, which may produce slightly tackier coatings, and methylcellulose, although this has been reported to retard drug dissolution.[10] Alternatives to the cellulose ethers are certain acrylics, such as methacrylate and methyl methacrylate copolymers.

Most polymers are employed as solutions in either aqueous or organic solvent-based systems. Alternative systems employ aqueous dispersions of water-insoluble polymers (eg ethylcellulose). Such systems usually are combined with aqueous solutions of water-soluble polymer in order to facilitate rapid drug release.

Many of the commonly used polymers are available in a range of molecular-weight grades, a factor which also must be considered in the selection process. Molecular weight may have an important influence on various properties of the coating system and its ultimate performance, such as solution viscosity and mechanical strength and flexibility of the resultant film.

The incorporation of a plasticizer into the formulation improves the flexibility of the coating, reduces the risk of the film cracking and possibly improves adhesion of the film to the substrate. To ensure that these benefits are achieved, the plasticizer must show a high degree of compatibility with the polymer, and be retained permanently in the film, if the properties of the coating are to remain consistent on storage. Examples of typical plasticizers include glycerin, propylene glycol, polyethylene glycols, triacetin, acetylated monoglyceride, citrate esters (eg, triethyl citrate) or phthalate esters (eg, diethyl phthalate).

Colorants usually are used to improve the appearance of the product as well as to facilitate product identification. Additionally, certain physical properties of the coating (eg its performance as a moisture barrier) may be improved. As in the case of sugar coating, colorants can be classified either as water-soluble dyes or insoluble pigments.

The use of water-soluble dyes is precluded with organic solvent-based film coating because of the lack of solubility in the solvent system. Thus, the use of pigments, particularly aluminum lakes, provides the most useful means of coloring film-coating systems. Although it may seem obvious to use water-soluble dyes in aqueous formulations, the use of pigments is preferred, since:

1. They are unlikely to interfere with bioavailability[11] as do some water-soluble dyes.
2. They help to reduce the permeability of the coating to moisture.[12]
3. They serve as bulking agents to increase the overall solids content in the coating dispersion.
4. They tend to be more light stable.

The major solvents used in film coating typically belong to one of these classes: alcohols, ketones, esters, chlorinated hydrocarbons and water. Solvents serve to perform an important function in the film-coating process, since they aid in the application of the coating to the surface of the substrate. Good interaction between solvent and polymer is necessary to ensure that optimal film properties are obtained when the coating dries. This initial interaction between solvent and polymer will yield maximum polymer-chain extension, producing films having the greatest cohesive strength and, thus, the best mechanical properties. An important function of the solvent systems also is to assure a controlled deposition of the polymer onto the surface of the substrate so that a coherent and adherent film coat is obtained.

Although it is very difficult to give typical examples of film-coating formulations, since these will depend on the properties of the materials used, such formulations usually are based on 5 to 15% (w/w) coating solids in the requisite vehicle (with the higher concentration range preferred for aqueous formulations), of which 60 to 70% is polymer, 6 to 7% is plasticizer and 20 to 30% is pigment.

Modified-Release Film Coatings

Film coatings can be applied to pharmaceutical products in order to modify drug release. The USP describes two types of modified-release dosage forms, namely those that are *delayed release* and those that are *extended release*. Delayed-release products often are designed to prevent drug release in the upper part of the gastrointestinal (GI) tract. Film coatings used to prepare this type of dosage form are commonly called *enteric coatings*. Extended-release products are designed to extend drug release over a period of time, a result which can be achieved by the application of a *sustained-* or *controlled-release* film coating.

Enteric Coatings—Enteric coatings are those which remain intact in the stomach, but will dissolve and release the contents of the dosage form once it reaches the small intestine. The purpose of an enteric coating is to delay the release of drugs which are inactivated by the stomach contents, (eg, pancreatin, erythromycin) or may cause nausea or bleeding by irritating the gastric mucosa (eg, aspirin, steroids). In addition, such coatings can be used to give a simple repeat-action effect where additional drug that has been applied over the enteric coat is released in the stomach, while the remainder, being protected by the coating, is released further down the gastrointestinal tract.

The action of enteric coatings results from a difference in composition of the respective gastric and intestinal environments in regard to pH and enzymatic properties. Although there have been repeated attempts to produce coatings which are subject to intestinal enzyme breakdown, this approach is not popular since enzymatic decomposition of the film is rather slow. Thus, most currently used enteric coatings are those which remain undissociated in the low pH environment of the stomach, but readily ionize when the pH rises to about 4 or 5. The most effective enteric polymers are polyacids having a pK_a of 3 to 5. Coatings subject to enzymatic breakdown are being considered now as protective coatings suitable for the colonic delivery of polypeptide drugs.

Historically, the earliest enteric coatings used formalin-treated gelatin, but this was unreliable since the polymerization of gelatin could not be controlled accurately, and often resulted in failure to release the drug, even in the lower intestinal tract. Another early candidate was shellac, but again the main disadvantage resulted from further polymerization that occurred on storage, often resulting in failure to release the active contents. Pharmaceutical formulators now prefer to use synthetic polymers to prepare more effective enteric coatings.

The most extensively used synthetic polymer is cellulose acetate phthalate (CAP) which is capable of functioning effectively as an enteric coating. However, a pH greater than 6 usually is required for solubility and thus a delay in drug release may ensue. It also is relatively permeable to moisture and gastric fluid compared to most enteric polymers. Thus it is susceptible to hydrolytic decomposition where phthalic and acetic acids are split off, resulting in a change in polymeric, and therefore enteric, properties.

Another useful polymer is polyvinyl acetate phthalate (PVAP) which is less permeable to moisture and gastric fluid, more stable to hydrolysis and able to ionize at a lower pH, resulting in earlier release of actives in the duodenum.

Other suitable enteric polymers include hydroxypropyl methylcellulose phthalate (which has properties similar to PVAP); methacrylic acid—methacrylic acid ester copolymers (some of which have a high dissociation constant[13]); cellulose acetate trimellitate (CAT, which has properties similar to CAP); carboxymethyl ethylcellulose (CMEC) and hydroxypropyl methylcellulose acetate succinate (HPMCAS).

Various systems recently have been introduced that allow many of these enteric polymers to be applied as aqueous dispersions, thus facilitating the use of aqueous film-coating technology for the enteric coating of pharmaceutical dosage forms.

Sustained-Release Coatings—The concept of sustained release formulations was developed in order to eliminate the need for multiple dosage regimens, particularly for those drugs requiring reasonably constant blood levels over a long period of time. In addition, it also has been adopted for those drugs which need to be administered in high doses, but where too rapid a release is likely to cause undesirable side effects (eg, the ulceration that occurs when potassium chloride is released rapidly in the gastrointestinal tract).

Formulation methods used to obtain the desired drug availability rate from sustained-action dosage forms include

1. Increasing the particle size of the drug.
2. Embedding the drug in a matrix.
3. Coating the drug or dosage form containing the drug.
4. Forming complexes of the drug with materials such as ion-exchange resins.

Only those methods which involve some form of coating fall within the scope of this chapter.

Materials which have been found suitable for producing sustained-release coatings include

1. Mixtures of waxes (beeswax, carnauba wax, etc) with glyceryl monostearate, stearic acid, palmitic acid, glyceryl monopalmitate and cetyl alcohol. These provide coatings which are dissolved slowly or broken down in the GI tract.
2. Shellac and zein—polymers which remain intact until the pH of gastrointestinal contents becomes less acidic.
3. Ethylcellulose, which provides a membrane around the dosage form and remains intact throughout the gastrointestinal tract. However, it does permit water to permeate the film, dissolve the drug and diffuse out again.
4. Acrylic resins, which behave similarly to ethylcellulose as a diffusion-controlled drug-release coating material.
5. Cellulose acetate (diacetate and triacetate).
6. Silicone elastomers.

As with an enteric coating, many of the synthetic polymers suitable for sustained-release film coating have been prepared as aqueous polymer dispersions (often called latexes or pseudolatexes) that are commercially available and facilitate the use of aqueous film-coating technology for the preparation of extended-release products.[14]

Various methods have been used to prepare sustained-release products using film-coating techniques. Examples include the application of suitable film coatings to

1. Dried granules (either irregular or spheronized).
2. Drug-loaded beads (or nonpareils).
3. Drug crystals.
4. Drug/ion-exchange-resin complexes.
5. Tablets.

In the first four examples, the final coated particles can either be filled into two-piece hard-gelatin capsules or compacted into tablets. Additionally, coated drug/ion-exchange-resin complexes may be dispersed in viscous liquids to create liquid suspensions.

A rather unique application of the film-coated, sustained-release tablet is the elementary osmotic pump. In this device, a tablet core (formulated to contain osmotically active ingredients) is film coated with a semipermeable membrane, which is subsequently "pierced" with a laser to create a delivery orifice. On the ingestion of such a device, the infusion of water generates an osmotic pressure within the coated tablet that "pumps" the drug in solution out through the orifice.

With sustained-release products, one must remain aware constantly of the fact that the final dosage forms typically contain drug loadings that are sufficiently high to cause problems if the entire dose is released quickly. This phenomenon, commonly called "dose-dumping," can be avoided only if:

1. The film coating is mechanically sound and will resist rupture on ingestion of the dosage form.
2. Sufficient coating is applied uniformly across the surface of the material that is to be coated.

Film-Coating Problems

As with sugar coating, difficulties may develop during, or subsequent to, the film-coating process. The tablets being coated may not be sufficiently robust, or may have a tendency to *laminate* while being coated. Since film coats are relatively thin, their ability to hide defects is significantly less than with sugar coating. Hence, tablets which have poor resistance to abrasion (ie, they exhibit high friability characteristics) can be problematic, since the imperfections readily may be apparent after coating. It is very important to identify tablets with suspect properties, whether mechanically or performance related (eg, poor dissolution), prior to a coating process, since subsequent recovery or reworking of tablets may be extremely difficult after a coating has been applied.

Various process-related problems can occur during the application of a film coating. One example is *picking*, which is a consequence of the fluid delivery rate exceeding the drying capacity of the process, causing tablets to stick together and subsequently become broken apart. Another example, *orange peel* or *roughness*, is usually the result of premature drying of atomized droplets of solution, or it may be a consequence of spraying too viscous a coating solution such that effective atomization is difficult.

Mottling, or lack of color uniformity, can result from uneven distribution of color in the coating, a problem often related to the use of soluble dyes in aqueous film coating, when color migration can occur, either by evolution of residual solvent in the film, or by migration of plasticizer in which the colorant may be soluble. The use of pigments in the film-coating process minimizes the incidence of this latter objection considerably. However, uneven color also can result from poor pigment dispersion in the coating solution.

Finally, some major problems occur as the result of internal stress that develops within the film as it dries. One example is *cracking*, which occurs when this stress exceeds the tensile strength of the film. This problem may be compounded by postcompaction stress relaxation (a phenomenon that can occur with certain types of tablet formulations, such as those containing ibuprofen, after ejection from the die), which causes tablets to expand. Another example is *logo-bridging* (ie, bridging of a monogram present in the surface of the tablet core), which occurs when a component of the internal stress is able to overcome the adhesive bonds between the coating and the tablet surface, causing the film to pull away so that legibility of the monogram is lost. An understanding of the properties of the various ingredients used in the film-coating formulation, and how these ingredients interact with one another, can allow the formulator to avoid many of these internal-stress-related problems.[15]

Coating Procedures and Equipment

Coating Pans—Sugar coating historically has involved the ladling of the various coating fluids onto a cascading bed of tablets in a conventional coating pan (Fig 1), fitted with a means of supplying drying air to the tablets and an exhaust to remove moisture and dust-laden air from the pan.

Typically, after the requisite volume of liquid has been applied, an appropriate amount of time is allowed for the tablets to mix and permit the liquid to be dispersed fully throughout the batch. To facilitate the uniform transfer of liquid, the tablets often are "stirred" by hand, or in larger pans, by means of a rake, to overcome mixing problems often associated with "dead spots," an inherent problem associated with the use of conventional pans. Finally, tablets are dried by directing an air supply onto the surface of the tablet bed. Thus, sugar coating is somewhat of a sequential process consisting of consecutive cycles of liquid application, mixing and drying.

During the early history of film coating, the equipment used was adapted essentially from that already employed for sugar coating. Although ladling of coating liquids during the film-coating process has been practiced, usually the liquid is applied using a spray technique. Spray equipment used are essentially of two types:

1. Airless (or hydraulic) spray, where the coating liquid is pumped under pressure to a spray nozzle with a small orifice, and atomization of the liquid occurs as it expands rapidly on emerging from the nozzle. This is analogous to the effect achieved when one places one's finger over the end of a garden hose.
2. Air spray, whereby liquid which is pumped under little or no pressure to the nozzle is atomized by means of a blast of compressed air that makes contact with the stream of liquid as it passes through the nozzle aperture.

Airless-spray techniques typically are used in large-scale film-coating operations for organic solvents, while air-spray techniques are more effective in either a small-scale laboratory set-up or in the currently popular aqueous film-coating operations.

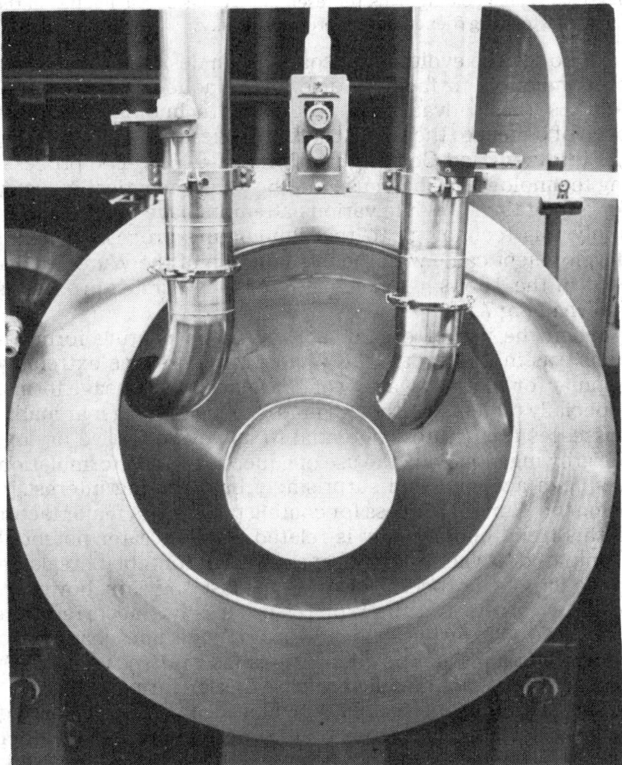

Fig 1. Typical equipment setup for conventional sugar coating.

The use of spray techniques permits the delivery of finely nebulized droplets of a coating solution to the moving tablet mass in such a manner as to ensure uniform coverage while preventing adjacent tablets from sticking together, as the coating solution rapidly dries. Although all the phases that occur during the spray process occur continuously and concurrently, the overall picture can be simplified and represented in the form of several sequential steps, as shown in Fig 2. The spray process can be operated either intermittently or continuously.

In the early years of film coating, the lack of adequate drying conditions inside the coating apparatus, together with the preference for using airless coating techniques (with their inherently higher delivery rates) with organic solvent-based formulations on a production scale, gave rise to the use of an intermittent spray procedure. This procedure allowed excess solvent to be removed during the nonspray part of the cycle, and thus reduced the risk of *picking* and the tendency for tablets to stick together. However, in later years, the improvement in drying capabilities has resulted in a continuous spray procedure being adopted, as this permits a more uniform coating to be developed and results in a shorter, simplified process.

As indicated previously, pan equipment initially was completely conventional in design and, with the exception of the addition of spray-application equipment, was similar to that used in sugar coating. Fortunately, film-coating formulations were based on relatively volatile organic solvents, which enabled acceptable processing times to be achieved in spite of the relative deficiencies of the air-handling systems. Since the equipment rarely represented a completely enclosed system, it did little to minimize the hazards of using organic solvents. Although conventional pans possessed acceptable properties with regard to mixing of the tablet mass in the sugar-coating process (particularly as this could be augmented by manual stirring of the tablets during processing), they were suited poorly to meet the more rigorous demands of the film-coating process, even when some simple form of baffle system was installed. In spite of these inadequacies, the use of conventional pans has persisted.

The introduction of aqueous film coating in recent years has presented the most serious challenge to conventional equipment. Limitations in both drying and mixing capabilities are likely to increase significantly the processing time and risk to product integrity when aqueous processes are used. Fortunately, these problems have been minimized as coating-pan design has evolved and improved.

Although considerable experimentation has taken place with the geometric design of conventional equipment, the most significant change came with the introduction of the Pellegrini coating pan (Fig 3), which is somewhat angular and rotates on a horizontal axis. The geometry of the pan, coupled with the fact that there is an integral baffle system, assures much more uniformity in mixing. Additionally, since the services are introduced through the rear opening, the front can either be left free for inspection purposes or simply closed off to yield

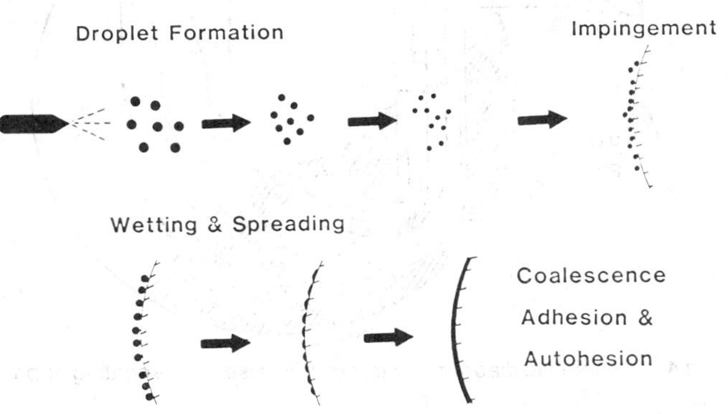

Fig 2. Schematic representation of the film-coating process.

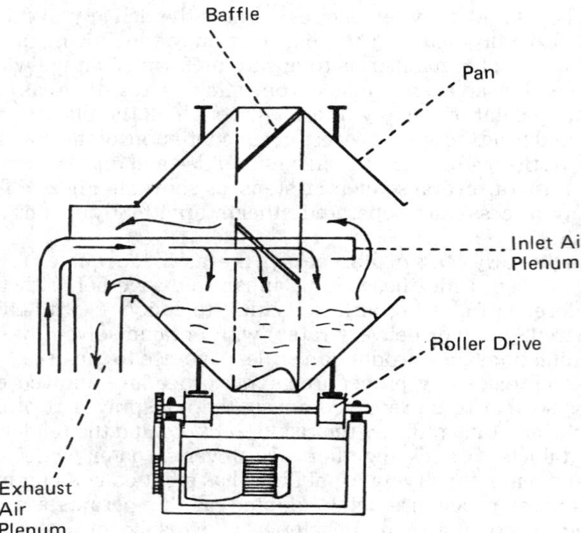

Fig 3. Schematic diagram of a Pellegrini coating pan.

an enclosed coating system. Although drying air is still applied only to the surfaces of the tablet bed, the other advantages derived from the basic overall design ensure that the Pellegrini pan is suitable more for film coating than the conventional equipment previously discussed. Currently, Pellegrini pans are available with capacities ranging from the 10-kg laboratory scale-up to 1000 kg for high-output production.

Considering the relative inefficiencies with equipment in which the majority of drying takes place on the surface of the tablet bed, several attempts have been made to improve air exchange, particularly within the tablet bed. The first to be available on a commercial scale was that developed by Strunck, which, by extending the drying air duct so that it is immersed in the tablet bed, creates a void within the tablet bed from a spraygun located in the opening of the supply air duct (Fig 4). Exhaust air is taken from the pan in a somewhat conventional manner.

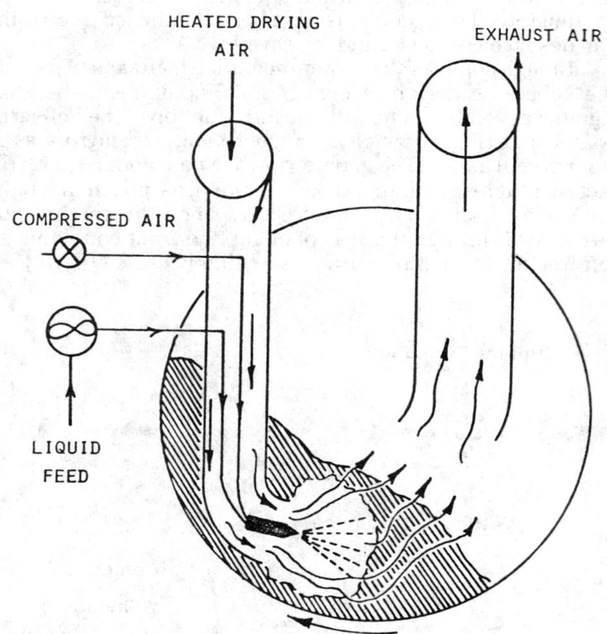

Fig 4. Schematic diagram of Strunck immersed-tube coating apparatus.

A second approach, called the Immersion Sword Process, uses a two-chamber system situated in the bed of tablets, enabling heated air to be introduced directly into the tablet bed through perforated air chambers. After interacting with the cascading bed of tablets, the air is drawn into a perforated exhaust air chamber for venting to the outside. This equipment currently is adaptable to both conventional and Pellegrini-type pans (see Fig 5). An alternative modification to the Pellegrini coating pan is provided by the GS coating system, which also allows drying to take place within the tablet bed. A similar approach is used with the Nicomac coating system.

A major advance in pan-coating technology occurred with the introduction of the side-vented pan concept, an innovation developed by Eli Lilly. Lilly's invention became the Accela-Cota, which is shown in Fig 6. The salient features of this design are

An angular pan (fitted with an integral baffle system) that rotates on a horizontal axis.

A coating system that is completely enclosed.

A perforated pan that allows drying air (that has been introduced into the pan) to be pulled through a cascading bed of tablets while the coating liquid is applied to the tablet surface using a spray-atomization technique.

This pan-coating design drastically improves the drying characteristics of the coating process, a feature which has been a major factor in the successful introduction of aqueous film-coating technology.

Since the introduction of the Accela-Cota, a variety of designs of side-vented coated pans have been introduced by major equipment vendors. A summary of many of these alternative designs is provided in Table 4.

Interesting features of side-vented coating pans in recent years include the fact that

1. Designs have become more complex and now permit multidirectional air flow.
2. Fully-automated, computerized coating processes are becoming commonplace (especially for production-scale coating purposes).
3. Clean-in-place (CIP) systems also are becoming commonplace in order to facilitate compliance with GMPs.
4. Laboratory-scale coating equipment now is being provided with interchangeable coating pans representing batch-size capabilities in the range of 3 to 40 kg (depending on product density).

Although the evolution in coating-pan design has occurred predominately to facilitate use of the aqueous film-coating process, these advances in processing technology also have been of benefit to the sugar-coating process.

Fluidized-Bed Coating Equipment—Fluid-bed processing technology has been used in the pharmaceutical industry for a long time. While various attempts have been made to apply this technology to the film-coating process, a major development came with the introduction of the Wurster concept in the 1950s. A schematic of the Wurster process is shown in Fig 7.

When the use of organic-solvent-based coating formulations was in its heyday, the Wurster process was extremely popular for coating a variety of pharmaceutical dosage forms, especially tablets. Although fluid-bed processing inarguably possesses the greatest potential to achieve effective drying, the growing interest in the use of aqueous coating formulation has been accompanied surprisingly by a waning interest in using the Wurster process for coating tablets. A major factor in this trend undoubtedly is related to the greater potential (compared to when coating pans are used) for tablet breakage in the fluid-bed process. During the last 15 years, however, resurgent interest in the Wurster process has occurred as a result of the growing demand for applying film coatings to pellets, granules and powders (so-called *multiparticulates*) in order to prepare modified-release dosage forms.

The suitability of the fluid-bed process for film coating multiparticulates also has generated interest in processes other than the Wurster for this application. In particular, a modifi-

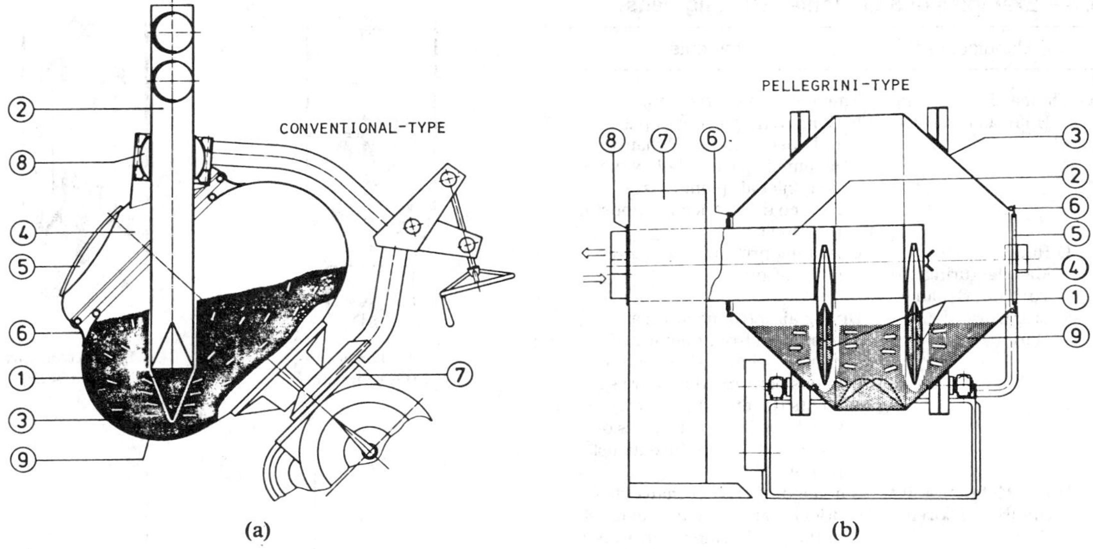

Key: 1. Immersion Sword
2. Coaxial conduit
3. Coating pan
4. Pan cover
5. Clear control cover
6. Silicone seal
7. Stand
8. Coaxial conduit adjustment
9. Coating bed

Fig 5. Schematic diagram of the immersed-sword apparatus for use in either (a) a conventional pan or (b) a Pellegrini pan.

cation of the spray granulation process (often termed the *top-spray coating process*) and a rotary process (often called the *tangential spray process*) have both been used for the film coating of multiparticulates. Schematics for all these processes also are shown in Fig 7.

The three major manufacturers of fluid-bed processing equipment (Glatt Air Techniques, Vector Corporation and Niro-Aeromatic) all have adopted the principle in which a basic processing unit has been designed to accept modular inserts for each of the three fluid-bed coating processes shown

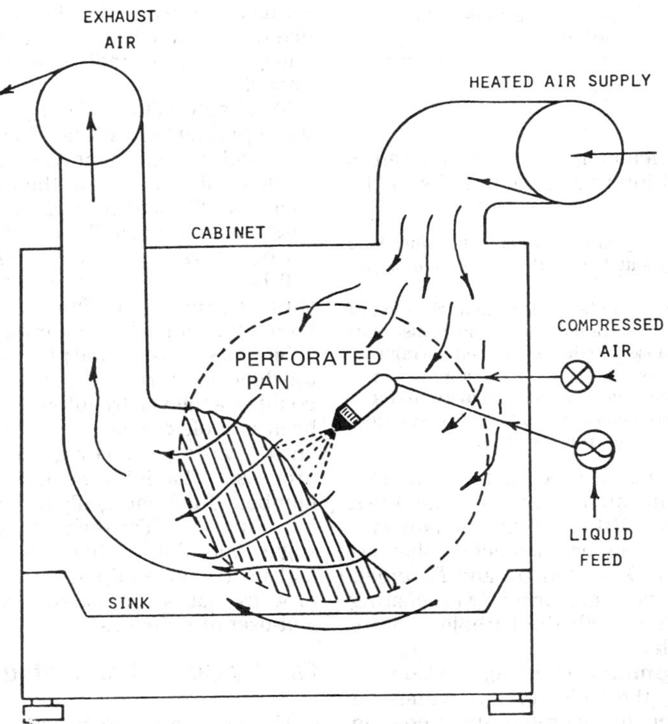

Fig 6. Schematic diagram of a side-vented coating pan (Accela-Cota).

Table 4—Examples of Side-Vented Coating Pans

Pan	Manufacturer	Comments
Accela-Cota	Thomas Engineering Hoffman Estates, IL	The first side-vented pan. Cylindrical portion of pan is fully perforated. Exhaust plenum is located below tablet bed; inlet air plenum is located diametrically opposite (See Fig 6).
Fast Coater	O'Hara Manufacturing Ltd, Toronto, Canada	Operating principle similar to Accela-Cota.
Hi-Coater	Vector Corp. Marion, IA	Drying air introduced via a plenum in front opening of pan. Cylindrical portion of pan is perforated in four segments (located 45° apart) which are linked via ducts on outside of pan to the exhaust plenum.
Driacoater	Driam Metallprodukt GmbH, Eriskirch, Germany	A nonagonal (rather than cylindrical) pan with each segment of the pan having a perforated section. One of the first pans to introduce the multidirectional air-flow concept.
IDA-X	Dumoulin, La Varenne, France	A fully-perforated pan (similar to Accela-Cota). Also uses the multidirectional air-flow concept.
Pro Coater	Glatt Air Techniques, Ramsey, NJ	A fully-perforated pan (similar to Accela-Cota). However, although exhaust plenum is located beneath the tablet bed (8-o'clock position), the inlet on plenum is located in the 4-o'clock position.
Butterfly	Hüttlin, Steinen, Germany	Not a perforated pan. Uses specially engineered slotted openings (at junction of pan-end wall and cylindrical portion of pan) to permit exhausting.
BSC	CMS Ames, IA	A fully perforated pan (similar to Accela-Cota) originally developed for the seed-coating industry.

in Fig 7. Selection of a particular type of insert often is determined by the nature and intended functionality of the coating applied; for example

1. Granulator Top-Spray Process—preferred when a taste-masking coating is being applied; additionally suitable for the application of hot-melt coatings.
2. Wurster, Bottom-Spray Process—preferred for the application of modified-release coatings to a wide variety of multiparticulates; also suitable for drug layering when the drug dose is in the low-to-medium range.
3. Rotor, Tangential-Spray Process—suitable for the application of modified-release film coatings to a wide range of multiparticulate products. Ideal for drug layering when the dose is medium-to-high. Also useful as a spheronizing process for producing spheres from powders.

While the general trend has been to use equipment employing this modular concept, an innovative approach to fluid-bed film coating was introduced by Hüttlin. This company created a design known as the Kugel coater,[16] a machine that has three basic configurations: the *Duo*, *Quattro* and *Turbojet*. The first two configurations are designed primarly for coating granules, pellets and small tablets, while the Turbojet is more suitable for coating regular tablets.

Potential for Totally Automated Coating Systems—During the last few decades, the industry has witnessed a general transition from manually operated sugar-coating procedures, requiring total operator involvement, to film-coating ones in which operator intervention is infrequent.

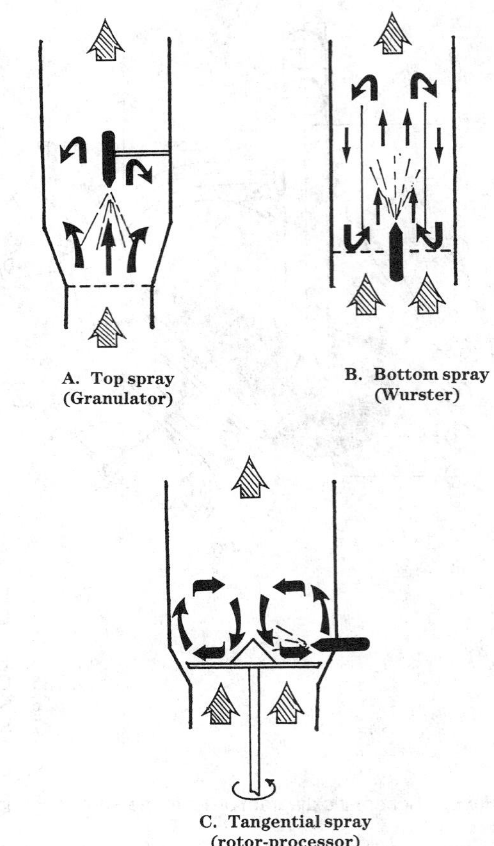

Fig 7. Schematic diagrams for three basic processes used for fluid-bed film coating.

Increasing familiarity with, and understanding of, tablet coating as a unit process, and a desire to ensure compliance with GMPs, ultimately have increased the desire for assuring conformity to design specifications for every batch of product made. Obviously, this is difficult for any process where the idiosyncracies of individual operators can have a significant impact.

Total automation of the process can provide a solution to these problems. Automation involves developing a process where all the important variables and requisite constraints are predetermined. These then can be translated into a form such that ultimate control and monitoring of the various process parameters can be maintained either by a microprocessor or central computer system. However, the system only will be as good as those peripheral devices used to detect various process conditions such as air flow, temperature, humidity, application volumes, delivery rates, etc.

Since a sugar-coating process always has been highly operator-dependent, removal of much of the operator intervention could be achieved by automation. Automation has, however, been complex because of the various sequences that occur and the variety of coating fluids used in a single sugar coating process. That it has been accomplished is evidenced by the number of commercially available systems which have been introduced.[17] The technology for automated control of both sugar- and film-coating processes has become very refined, and most major equipment suppliers are able to offer a coating process that is automated to various degrees (depending on end-user preferences).

Quality Control of Coated Tablets

The most important aspects of coated tablets which must be assessed from a quality-control standpoint are appearance characteristics and drug availability. From the appearance standpoint, coated tablets must be shown to conform, where applicable, to some color standard, otherwise the dispenser and the consumer may assume that differences have occurred from previous lots, signifying a changed or substandard product. In addition, because of the physical abuse that tablets, both in their uncoated and coated forms, receive during the coating process, it is essential to check for defects such as chipped edges, picking, etc, and ensure they do not exceed predetermined limits.

Often, in order to identify the products, coated tablets may be imprinted (particularly with sugar-coated tablets) or bear a monogram (commonly seen with tablets that are film-coated). The clarity and quality of such identifying features must be assessed. The failure of a batch of coated tablets to comply with such preset standards may result in 100% inspection being required or the need for the batch to be reworked.

Batch-to-batch reproducibility for drug availability is of paramount importance, consequently each batch of product should be submitted to some meaningful test such as a dissolution test. Depending on the characteristics of the tablet core to be coated, tablet coatings can modify the drug-release profile, even when not intended (unlike the case of enteric- or controlled-release products). Since this behavior may vary with each batch coated (being dependent, for example, on differences in processing conditions or variability in raw materials used), it is essential that this parameter should be assessed, particularly in products that are typically borderline (refer to Chapter 92).

Stability Testing of Coated Products

The stability-testing program for coated products will vary depending on the dosage form and its composition. Many stability-testing programs are based on studies which have disclosed the conditions a product may encounter prior to end use. Such conditions usually are referred to as normal and include ranges in temperature, humidity, light and handling conditions.

Limits of acceptability are established for each product for qualities such as color, appearance, availability of drug for absorption and drug content. The time over which the product retains specified properties, when tested at normal conditions, may be defined as the *shelf-life*. The container for the product may be designed to improve the shelf-life. For example, if the color in the coating is light-sensitive, the product may be packaged in an amber bottle and/or protected from light by using a paper carton. When the coating is friable, resilient material such as cotton may be incorporated in both the top and bottom of the container, and if the product is affected adversely by moisture, a moisture-resistant closure may be used and/or a desiccant may be placed in the package. The shelf-life of the product is determined in the commercial package tested under normal conditions.

The stability of the product also may be tested under exaggerated conditions. This usually is done for the purpose of accelerating changes so that an extrapolation can be made early, concerning the shelf-life of the product. Although useful, highly exaggerated conditions of storage can supply misleading data for coated dosage forms. Any change in drug release from the dosage form is measured *in vitro*, but an *in vivo* measurement should be used to confirm that drug availability remains within specified limits over its stated shelf-life. This confirmation can be obtained by testing the product initially for *in vivo* availability and then repeating at intervals during storage at normal conditions for its estimated shelf-life (or longer).

Interpretation of stability data for coated, modified-release products should be undertaken with extreme care, since the diffusion characteristics of polymeric films can change significantly under exaggerated temperature conditions. This change may be confounding when trying to predict their diffusion characteristics under more moderate conditions and thus can prove misleading when predicting shelf life.

When elevated-temperature stability studies are conducted on products coated with aqueous polymeric dispersions (latexes or pseudolatexes), the data obtained might be more indicative of morphological changes that have occurred in the film. Such changes may result from partial destruction of the film when coated material adheres together in the container and subsequently is broken apart; additionally, these changes might result from further coalescence of the coating (which can occur when the coating is not coalesced completely during the coating process).

Stability tests usually are conducted on a product at the time of development, during the pilot phase and on representative lots of the commercial product. Stability testing must continue for the commercial product as long as it remains on the market because subtle changes in a manufacturing process and/or a raw material can have an impact on the shelf life of a product.

References

1. Urdang G: *What's New*, 1943, pp 5–14; through *JAPhA 34:* 135, 1945.
2. White RC: *JAPhA 11:* 345, 1922.
3. Kremers E, Urdang G: *History of Pharmacy*, Lippincott, Philadelphia, 20, 319, 1940.
4. Anon: *JAMA 84:* 829, 1920.
5. Wiegand TS: *Am J Pharm 74:* 33, 1902.
6. Warner WR Jr: *Am J Pharm 74:* 32, 1902.
7. Wurster DE: (Wisconsin Alumni Research Foundations) US Pat 2,648,609 (1953).
8. Signorino CA: US Pat 3,738,952 and 3,741,795 (June, 1973).
9. Tucker SJ *et al: JAPhA 47:* 849, 1958.
10. Schwartz JB, Alvino TP: *J Pharm Sci 65:* 572, 1976.
11. Prillig EB: *J Pharm Sci 50:* 1245, 1969.
12. Porter SC: *Pharm Tech 4*, 67, 1980.
13. Delporte JP, Jaminet F: *J Pharm Belg 31:* 38, 1976.
14. Chang RK, Hsiao CH, Robinson JR: *Pharm Tech 11:* 56, 1987.
15. Rowe RC: *J Pharm Pharmacol 33:* 423, 1981.
16. Hütlin H, *Drugs Made in Germany 28:* 147, 1985.
17. Fraade DJ, ed: *Automation of Pharmaceutical Operations*, Pharm Tech Publ, Springfield OR, 1983.

CHAPTER 94

Sustained-Release Drug Delivery Systems

Charles S L Chiao, PhD
Anda SR Pharmaceuticals, Inc
Davie, FL 33314

Joseph R Robinson, PhD
Professor of Pharmacy
School of Pharmacy
University of Wisconsin
Madison, WI 53706

The goal of any drug delivery system is to provide a therapeutic amount of drug to the proper site in the body to achieve promptly, and then maintain, the desired drug concentration. That is, the drug-delivery system should deliver drug at a rate dictated by the needs of the body over the period of treatment. This idealized objective points to the two aspects most important to drug delivery, namely, *spatial placement* and *temporal delivery* of a drug. Spatial placement relates to targeting a drug to a specific organ or tissue, while temporal delivery refers to controlling the rate of drug delivery to the target tissue. An appropriately designed sustained-release drug delivery system can be a major advance toward solving these two problems. It is for this reason that the science and technology responsible for development of sustained-release pharmaceuticals have been and continue to be the focus of a great deal of attention in both industrial and academic laboratories. There currently exist numerous products on the market formulated for both oral and parenteral routes of administration that claim sustained or controlled drug delivery. The bulk of research has been directed at oral dosage forms that satisfy the temporal aspect of drug delivery, but many of the newer approaches under investigation may allow for spatial placement as well. This chapter will define and explain the nature of sustained-release drug therapy, briefly outline relevant physicochemical and biological properties of a drug that affect sustained-release performance and review the more common types of oral and parenteral sustained-release dosage forms. In addition, a brief discussion of some methods currently being used to develop targeted delivery systems will be presented.

Conventional Drug Therapy

To gain an appreciation for the value of sustained drug therapy it is useful to review some fundamental aspects of conventional drug delivery.[1] Consider single dosing of a hypothetical drug that follows a simple one-compartment pharmacokinetic model for disposition. Depending on the route of administration, a conventional dosage form of the drug, eg, a solution, suspension, capsule, tablet, etc, probably will produce a drug blood level versus time profile similar to that shown in Fig 1. The term "drug blood level" refers to the concentration of drug in blood or plasma, but the concentration in any tissue could be plotted on the ordinate. It can be seen from this figure that administration of a drug by either intravenous injection or an extravascular route, eg, orally, intramuscularly or rectally, does not maintain drug blood levels within the therapeutic range for extended periods of time. The short duration of action is due to the inability of conventional dosage forms to control temporal delivery. If an attempt is made to maintain drug blood levels in the therapeutic range for longer periods by, for example, increasing the initial dose of an intravenous injection, as shown by the dotted line in the figure, toxic levels may be produced at early times. This approach obviously is undesirable and unsuitable. An alternate approach is to administer the drug repetitively using a constant dosing interval, as in multiple-dose therapy. This is shown in Fig 2 for the oral route. In this case the drug blood level reached and the time required to reach that level depend on the dose and the dosing interval. There are several potential problems inherent in multiple-dose therapy:

1. If the dosing interval is not appropriate for the biological half-life of the drug, large "peaks" and "valleys" in the drug blood level may result. For example, drugs with short half-lives require frequent dosings to maintain constant therapeutic levels.
2. The drug blood level may not be within the therapeutic range at sufficiently early times, an important consideration for certain disease states.
3. Patient noncompliance with the multiple-dosing regimen can result in failure of this approach.

In many instances, potential problems associated with conventional drug therapy can be overcome. When this is the case, drugs given in conventional dosage forms by multiple-dosing can produce the desired drug blood level for extended periods of time. Frequently, however, these problems are significant enough to make drug therapy with conventional dosage forms less desirable than sustained-release drug therapy. This fact, coupled with the intrinsic inability of conventional dosage forms to achieve spatial placement, is a compelling motive for investigation of sustained-release drug delivery systems. There are numerous potential advantages of sustained-release drug therapy that will be discussed in the next section.

Sustained-Release Drug Therapy

As already mentioned, conventional dosage forms include solutions, suspensions, capsules, tablets, emulsions, aerosols, foams, ointments and suppositories. For this discussion, these dosage forms can be considered to release their active ingredients into an absorption pool immediately. This is illustrated in the following simple kinetic scheme:

$$\text{Dosage Form} \xrightarrow[\text{drug release}]{k_r} \text{Absorption Pool} \xrightarrow[\text{absorption}]{k_a} \text{Target Area} \xrightarrow[\text{elimination}]{k_r}$$

The absorption pool represents a solution of the drug at the site of absorption, and the terms k_r, k_a and k_e are first-order rate constants for drug release, absorption and overall elimination, respectively. Immediate release from a conventional dosage form implies that $k_r >>> k_a$ or, alternatively, that absorption of drug across a biological membrane, such as the intestinal epithelium, is the rate-limiting step in delivery of the drug to its target area. For nonimmediate-release dosage forms, $k_r <<< k_a$, that is, release of drug from the dosage form is the rate-limiting step. This causes the above kinetic scheme to reduce to

$$\text{Dosage Form} \xrightarrow[\text{drug release}]{k_r} \text{Target Area} \xrightarrow[\text{elimination}]{k_e}$$

Essentially, the absorptive phase of the kinetic scheme becomes insignificant compared to the drug release phase. Thus, the effort to develop a nonimmediate-release delivery

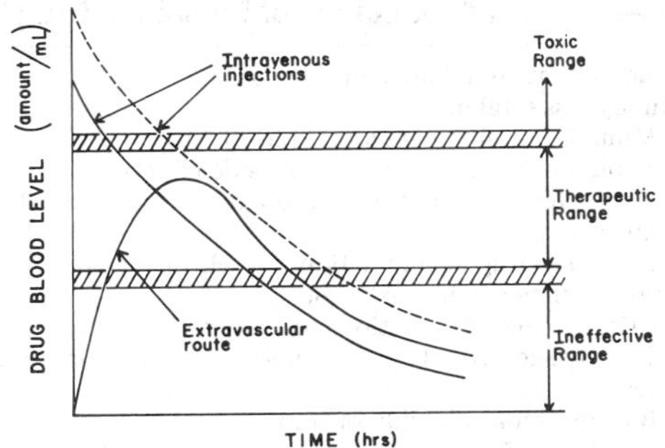

Fig 1. Typical drug blood level versus time profiles for intravenous injections and an extravascular route of administration.

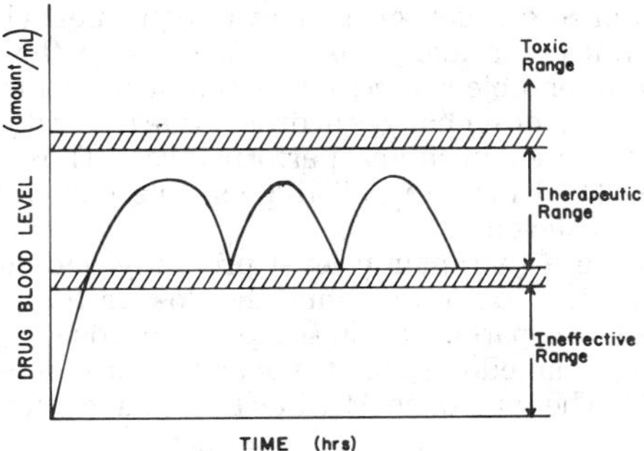

Fig 3. Typical drug blood level versus time profiles for delayed-release drug delivery by a repeat-action dosage form.

system must be directed primarily at altering the release rate by affecting the value of k_r. The many ways in which this has been attempted will be discussed later in this chapter.

Nonimmediate-release delivery systems may be divided conveniently into four categories:

1. Delayed release
2. Sustained release
   a. Controlled release
   b. Prolonged release
3. Site-specific release
4. Receptor release

Delayed-release systems are those that use repetitive, intermittent dosings of a drug from one or more immediate-release units incorporated into a single dosage form. Examples of delayed-release systems include repeat-action tablets and capsules, and enteric-coated tablets where timed release is achieved by a barrier coating. A delayed-release dosage form does not produce or maintain uniform drug blood levels within the therapeutic range, as shown in Fig 3, but, nonetheless, is more effective for patient compliance than conventional dosage forms.

Sustained-release systems include any drug delivery system that achieves slow release of drug over an extended period of time. If the systems can provide some control, whether this be of a temporal or spatial nature, or both, of drug release in the body, or in other words, the system is successful at maintaining constant drug levels in the target tissue or cells, it is considered a *controlled-release* system. If it is unsuccessful at this, but nevertheless prolongs therapeutic blood or tissue level of the drug for an extended period of time, it is considered a *prolonged-release* system. This is illustrated in Fig 4.

Site-specific and *receptor release* refer to targeting of a drug directly to a certain biological location. In the case of site-specific release, the target is adjacent to, or in the diseased organ or tissue; for receptor release, the target is the particular receptor for a drug within an organ or tissue. Both of these systems satisfy the spatial aspect of drug delivery.

Release Rate and Dose Considerations[2]

Although it is not necessary or desirable to maintain a constant level of drug in the blood or target tissue for all therapeutic cases, this is the ideal goal of a sustained-release delivery system. In fact, in some cases optimum therapy is achieved by oscillating, rather than constant, drug levels. An example of this is antibiotic therapy, where the activity of the drug is required only during growth phases of the microorganism. A constant drug level will succeed at curing or controlling the condition, however, and this is true for most forms of therapy.

The objective in designing a sustained-release system is to deliver drug at a rate necessary to achieve and maintain a constant drug blood level. This rate should be analogous to that achieved by continuous intravenous infusion where a drug is provided to the patient at a constant rate just equal to its rate of elimination. This implies that the rate of delivery must be independent of the amount of drug remaining in the dosage form and constant over time. That is, release from the dosage form should follow *zero-order* kinetics, as shown by

$$k_r^0 = \text{Rate In} = \text{Rate Out} = k_e \cdot C_d \cdot V_d \tag{1}$$

where k_r^0 is the zero-order rate constant for drug release (amount/time), k_e is the first-order rate constant for overall drug elimination (time^{-1}), C_d is the desired drug level in the body (amount/volume) and V_d is the volume space in which the drug is distributed. The values of k_e, C_d and V_d needed to calculate k_r^0 are obtained from appropriately designed single-dose pharmacokinetic studies. Equation 1 provides the method to calculate the zero-order release rate constant necessary to maintain a constant drug blood or tissue level for the simplest case where drug is eliminated by first-order kinetics. For many drugs, however, more complex elimination kinetics and other factors affecting their disposition are involved. This in turn affects the nature of the release kinetics necessary to maintain a constant drug blood level. It is important to recognize that while zero-order release may be desirable theo-

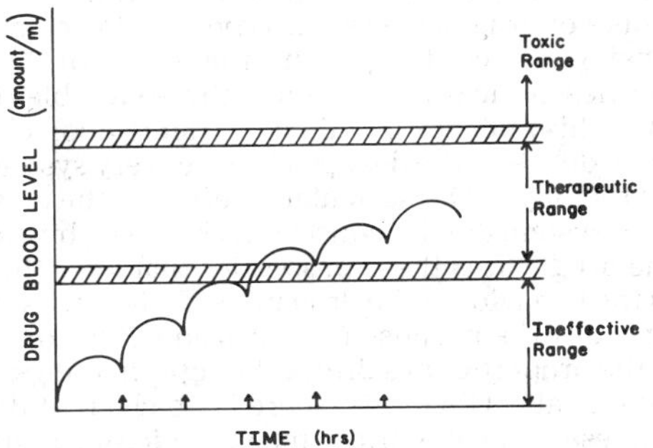

Fig 2. Typical drug blood level versus time profile following oral multiple-dose therapy.

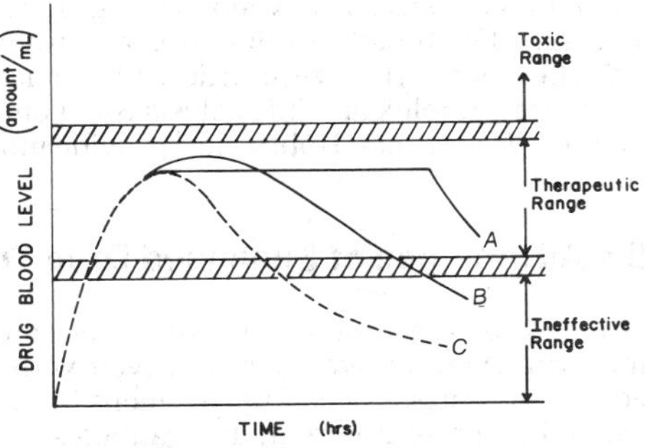

Fig 4. Drug blood level versus time profiles showing the relationship between controlled-release (*A*), prolonged-release (*B*) and conventional-release (*C*) drug delivery.

retically, nonzero-order release may be equivalent clinically to constant release in many cases. Aside from the extent of intra- and intersubject variation is the observation that, for many drugs, modest changes in drug tissue levels do not result in an improvement in clinical performance. Thus, a nonconstant drug level may be indistinguishable clinically from a constant drug level.

To achieve a therapeutic level promptly and sustain the level for a given period of time, the dosage form generally consists of two parts: an initial priming dose, D_i, that releases drug immediately and a maintenance or sustaining dose, D_m. The total dose, W, thus required for the system is

$$W = D_i + D_m \quad (2)$$

For a system where the maintenance dose releases drug by a zero-order process for a specified period of time, the total dose[2] is

$$W = D_i + k_r^0 T_d \quad (3)$$

where k_r^0 is the zero-order rate constant for drug release and T_d is the total time desired for sustained release from one dose. If the maintenance dose begins the release of drug at the time of dosing ($t = 0$), it will add to that which is provided by the initial dose, thus increasing the initial drug level. In this case a correction factor is needed to account for the added drug from the maintenance dose:

$$W = D_i + k_r^0 T_d - k_r^0 T_p \quad (4)$$

The correction factor, $k_r^0 T_p$, is the amount of drug provided during the period from $t = 0$ to the time of the peak drug level, T_p. No correction factor is needed if the dosage form is constructed in such a fashion that the maintenance dose does not begin to release drug until time T_p.

It already has been mentioned that a perfectly invariant drug blood or tissue level versus time profile is the ideal goal of a sustained-release system. The way to achieve this, in the simplest case, is by use of a maintenance dose that releases its drug by zero-order kinetics. However, satisfactory approximations of a constant drug level can be obtained by suitable combinations of the initial dose and a maintenance dose that releases its drug by a first-order process. The total dose for such a system is

$$W = D_i + (k_e C_d / k_r) V_d \quad (5)$$

where k_r is the first-order rate constant for drug release (time^{-1}), and k_e, C_d and V_d are as defined previously. If the maintenance dose begins releasing drug at $t = 0$, a correction factor is required just as it was in the zero-order case. The correct expression in this case is

$$W = D_i + (k_e C_d / k_r) V_d - D_m k_e T_p \quad (6)$$

In order to maintain drug blood levels within the therapeutic range over the entire time course of therapy, most sustained-release drug delivery systems are, like conventional dosage forms, administered as multiple rather than single doses. For an ideal sustained-release system that releases drug by zero-order kinetics, the multiple dosing regimen is analogous to that used for a constant intravenous infusion, as discussed in Chapter 42. For those sustained-release systems having release kinetics other than zero-order, the multiple dosing regimen is more complex and its analysis is beyond the scope of this chapter; Welling and Dobrinska[3] provide more detailed discussion.

Potential Advantages of Sustained Drug Therapy

All sustained-release products share the common goal of improving drug therapy over that achieved with their non-sustained counterparts. This improvement in drug therapy is represented by several potential advantages of the use of sustained-release systems, as shown in Table 1.

Patient compliance has been recognized as a necessary and important component in the success of all self-administered drug therapy. Minimizing or eliminating patient compliance problems is an obvious advantage of sustained-release therapy. Because of the nature of its release kinetics, a sustained-release system should be able to use less total drug over the time course of therapy than a conventional preparation. The advantages of this are a decrease or elimination of both local and systemic side effects, less potentiation or reduction in drug activity with chronic use and minimization of drug accumulation in body tissues with chronic dosing.

Table 1—Potential Advantages of Sustained Drug Therapy

1. Avoid patient compliance problems
2. Employ less total drug
   a. Minimize or eliminate local side effects
   b. Minimize or eliminate systemic side effects
   c. Obtain less potentiation or reduction in drug activity with chronic use
   d. Minimize drug accumulation with chronic dosing
3. Improve efficiency in treatment
   a. Cure or control condition more promptly
   b. Improve control of condition, ie, reduce fluctuation in drug level
   c. Improve bioavailability of some drugs
   d. Make use of special effects, eg, sustained-release aspirin for morning relief of arthritis by dosing before bedtime
4. Economy

Unquestionably the most important reason for sustained-drug therapy is improved efficiency in treatment, ie, optimized therapy. The result of obtaining constant drug blood levels from a sustained-release system is to achieve promptly the desired effect and maintain it for an extended period of time. Reduction or elimination of fluctuations in the drug blood level allows better disease state management. In addition, the method by which sustained release is achieved can improve the bioavailability of some drugs. For example, drugs susceptible to enzymatic inactivation or bacterial decomposition can be protected by encapsulation in polymer systems suitable for sustained release. For drugs that have a "specific window" for absorption, increased bioavailability can be attained by localizing the sustained-release delivery system in certain regions of the gastrointestinal tract. Improved efficiency in treatment also can take the form of a special therapeutic effect not possible with a conventional dosage form (see Table 1).

The last potential advantage listed in Table 1, that of economy, can be examined from two points of view. Although the initial unit cost of most sustained-drug delivery systems usually is greater than that of conventional dosage forms because of the special nature of these products, the average cost of treatment over an extended time period may be less. Economy also may result from a decrease in nursing time/hospitalization, less lost work time, etc.

Drug Properties Relevant to Sustained-Release Formulation

The design of sustained-release delivery systems is subject to several variables of considerable importance. Among these are the route of drug delivery, the type of delivery system, the disease being treated, the patient, the length of therapy and the properties of the drug. Each of these variables are interrelated and this imposes certain constraints upon choices for the route of delivery, the design of the delivery system and the length of therapy. Of particular interest to the scientist designing the system are the constraints imposed by the properties of the drug. It is these properties that have the greatest effect on the behavior of the drug in the delivery system and in the body. For the purpose of discussion, it is convenient to describe the properties of a drug as being either physicochemical or biological. Obviously, there is no clearcut distinction between these two categories since the biological properties of a drug are a function of its physicochemical properties. For purposes of this discussion, however, those attributes that can be determined from *in vitro* experiments will be considered as physicochemical properties. Included as biological properties will be those that result from typical pharmacokinetic studies on the absorption, distribution, metabolism and excretion (ADME) characteristics of a drug and those resulting from pharmacological studies.

Physicochemical Properties

Aqueous Solubility and pK_a—It is well known that in order for a drug to be absorbed it first must dissolve in the aqueous phase surrounding the site of administration and then partition into the absorbing membrane. Two of the most important physicochemical properties of a drug that influence its absorptive behavior are its aqueous solubility and, if it is a weak acid or base (as are most drugs), its pK_a. These properties play an influential role in performance of nonsustained-release products; their role is even greater in sustained-release systems.

The aqueous solubility of a drug influences its dissolution rate, which in turn establishes its concentration in solution and hence the driving force for diffusion across membranes. Dissolution rate is related to aqueous solubility as shown by the Noyes-Whitney equation which, under sink conditions, is

$$dC/dt = k_D A C_s \tag{7}$$

where dC/dt is the dissolution rate, k_D is the dissolution rate constant, A is the total surface area of the drug particles and C_s is the aqueous saturation solubility of the drug. The dissolution rate is constant only if surface area, A, remains constant, but the important point to note is that the initial rate is proportional directly to aqueous solubility C_s. Therefore, the aqueous solubility of a drug can be used as a first approximation of its dissolution rate. Drugs with low aqueous solubility have low dissolution rates and usually suffer oral bioavailability problems.

It will be recalled from Chapter 16 that the aqueous solubility of weak acids and bases is governed by the pK_a of the compound and the pH of the medium. For a weak acid

$$S_t = S_0(1 + K_a/[H^+]) = S_0(1 + 10^{pH-pK_a}) \tag{8}$$

where S_t is the total solubility (both the ionized and unionized forms) of the weak acid, S_0 is the solubility of the unionized form, K_a is the acid dissociation constant and $[H^+]$ is the hydrogen ion concentration of the medium. Equation 8 predicts that the total solubility, S_t, of a weak acid with a given pK_a can be affected by the pH of the medium. Similarly, for a weak base

$$S_t = S_0(1 + [H^+]/K_a) = S_0(1 + 10^{pK_a-pH}) \tag{9}$$

where S_t is the total solubility (both the conjugate acid and free-base forms) of the weak base, S_0 is the solubility of the free-base form and K_a is the acid dissociation constant of the conjugate acid. Analogous to Eq 8, Eq 9 predicts that the total solubility, S_t, of a weak base whose conjugate acid has a given pK_a can be affected by the pH of the medium. Considering the pH-partition hypothesis, the importance of Eqs 8 and 9 relative to drug absorption is evident. The pH-partition hypothesis simply states that the un-ionized form of a drug will be absorbed preferentially, in a passive manner, through membranes. Since weakly acidic drugs will exist in the stomach (pH = 1 to 2) primarily in the un-ionized form, their absorption will be favored from this acidic environment. On the other hand, weakly basic drugs will exist primarily in the ionized form (conjugate acid) at the same site, and their absorption will be poor. In the upper portion of the small intestine, the pH is more alkaline (pH = 5 to 7) and the reverse will be expected for weak acids and bases. The ratio of Eq 8 or 9 written for either the pH of the gastric or intestinal fluid and the pH of blood is indicative of the driving force for absorption based on pH gradient. For example, consider the ratio of the total solubility of the weak acid aspirin in the blood and gastric fluid:

$$R = (1 + 10^{pH_b-pK_a})/(1 + 10^{pH_g-pK_a}) \tag{10}$$

where pH_b is the pH of blood (pH 7.2), pH_g is the pH of the gastric fluid (pH 2) and the pK_a of aspirin is about 3.4. Substituting these values into Eq 10 gives a value for R of $10^{3.8}$ which indicates that aspirin is in a form to be well-absorbed from the stomach. The same calculation for intestinal pH (about 7) yields a ratio close to 1, implying a less-favorable driving force for absorption at that location. Ideally, the release of an ionizable drug from a sustained-release system should be "programmed" in accordance with the variation in pH of the different segments of the gastrointestinal (GI) tract so that the amount of preferentially absorbed species, and thus the plasma level of drug, will be approximately constant throughout the time course of drug action.

In general, extremes in the aqueous solubility of a drug are undesirable for formulation into a sustained-release product. A drug with very low solubility and a slow dissolution rate will exhibit dissolution-limited absorption and yield an inherently sustained blood level. In most instances, formulation of such a drug into a sustained-release system is redundant. Even if a poorly soluble drug was considered as a candidate for formulation into a sustained-release system, a restraint would be placed upon the type of delivery system which could be used. For example, any system relying upon diffusion of drug through a polymer as the rate-limiting step in release would be unsuitable for a poorly soluble drug, since the driving force for diffusion is the concentration of drug in the polymer or solution and this concentration would be low. For a drug with very high solubility and a rapid dissolution rate, it often is quite difficult to decrease its dissolution rate and slow its absorption. Preparing a slightly soluble form of a drug with normally high solubility is, however, one possible method for preparing sustained-release dosage forms. This will be elaborated upon elsewhere in this chapter.

Partition Coefficient—Between the time that a drug is administered and the time it is eliminated from the body, it must diffuse through a variety of biological membranes which act primarily as lipid-like barriers. A major criterion in evaluation of the ability of a drug to penetrate these lipid membranes is its apparent oil/water partition coefficient, defined as

$$K = C_0/C_w \tag{11}$$

where C_0 is the equilibrium concentration of all forms of the drug, eg, ionized and un-ionized, in an organic phase at equilibrium, and C_w is the equilibrium concentration of all forms in an aqueous phase. A frequently used solvent for the organic phase is 1-octanol. Although not always valid, an approximation to the value of K may be obtained by the ratio of the solubility of the drug in 1-octanol to that in water. In general, drugs with extremely large values of K are very oil-soluble and will partition into membranes quite readily. The relationship between tissue permeation and partition coefficient for the drug generally is known as the *Hansch correlation*, discussed in Chapter 28. In general, it describes a parabolic relationship between the logarithm of the activity of a drug or its ability to be absorbed and the logarithm of its partition coefficient for a series of drugs as shown in Fig 5. The explanation for this relationship is that the activity of a drug is a function of its ability to cross membranes and interact with the receptor; as a first approximation, the more effectively a drug crosses membranes, the greater its activity. There is also an optimum partition coefficient for a drug at which it most effectively permeates membranes and thus shows greatest activity. Values of the partition coefficient below this optimum result in decreased lipid solubility, and the drug will remain localized in the first aqueous phase it contacts. Values larger than the optimum result in poorer aqueous solubility, but enhanced lipid solubility and the drug will not partition out of the lipid membrane once it gets in. The value of K at which optimum activity is observed is approximately 1000/1 in 1-octanol/water. Drugs with a partition coefficient that is higher or

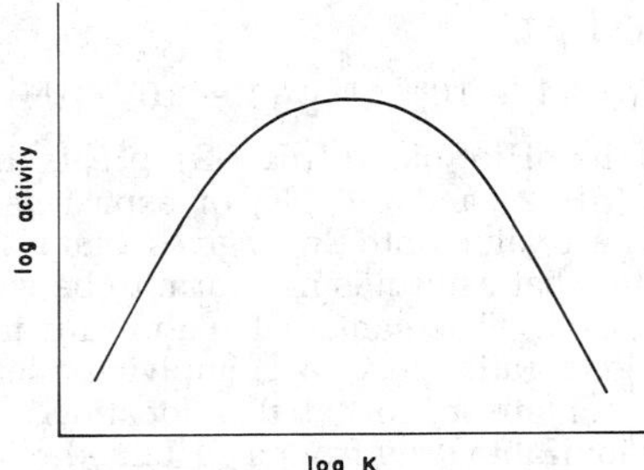

Fig 5. Typical relationship between drug activity and partition coefficient, *K*, generally known as the Hansch correlation.

lower than the optimum are, in general, poorer candidates for formulation into sustained-release dosage forms.

Drug Stability—Of importance for oral dosage forms is the loss of drug through acid hydrolysis and/or metabolism in the GI tract. Since a drug in the solid state undergoes degradation at a much slower rate than a drug in suspension or solution, it would seem possible to improve significantly the relative bioavailability of a drug, which is unstable in the GI tract, by placing it in a slowly available sustained-release form. For those drugs that are unstable in the stomach, the most appropriate sustaining unit would be one that releases its contents only in the intestine. The reverse is the case for those drugs that are unstable in the environment of the intestine; the most appropriate sustaining unit in this case would be one that releases its contents only in the stomach. However, most sustained-release systems currently in use release their contents over the entire length of the GI tract. Thus, drugs with significant stability problems in any particular area of the GI tract are less suitable for formulation into sustained-release systems that deliver their contents uniformly over the length of the GI tract. Delivery systems that remain localized in a certain area of the GI tract eg, bioadhesive drug delivery system, and act as reservoirs for drug release are much more advantageous for drugs that not only suffer from stability problems but have other bioavailability problems as well. Development of this type of system is still in its infancy.

The presence of metabolizing enzymes at the site of absorption is not necessarily a negative factor in sustained-release formulation. Indeed, the prodrug approach to drug delivery takes advantage of the presence of these enzymes to regenerate the parent molecule of an inactive drug derivative. This will be amplified upon below and in Chapter 28.

Protein Binding

Chapters 14 and 43 described the occurrence of drug bind ing to plasma proteins (eg, albumin) and the resulting retention of drug in the vascular space. Distribution of the drug into the extravascular space is governed by the equilibrium process of dissociation of the drug from the protein. The drug–protein complex can serve therefore as a reservoir in the vascular space for sustained drug release to extravascular tissues, but only for those drugs that exhibit a high degree of binding. Thus, the protein binding characteristics of a drug can play a significant role in its therapeutic effect, regardless of the type of dosage form. Extensive binding to plasma proteins will be evidenced by a long half-life of elimination for the drug, and such drugs generally do not require a sustained-release dosage form. However, drugs that exhibit a high degree of binding to plasma proteins also might bind to biopolymers in the GI tract, which could have an influence on sustained-drug delivery.

The main forces of attraction responsible for binding are van der Waals forces, hydrogen bonding and electrostatic forces. In general, charged compounds have a greater tendency to bind a protein than uncharged compounds, due to electrostatic effects. The presence of a hydrophobic moiety on the drug molecule also increases its binding potential. Some drugs that exhibit greater than 95% binding at therapeutic levels are amitriptyline, bishydroxycoumarin, diazepam, diazoxide, dicumarol and novobiocin.

Molecular Size and Diffusivity—As previously discussed, a drug must diffuse through a variety of biological membranes during its time course in the body. In addition to diffusion through these biological membranes, drugs in many sustained-release systems must diffuse through a rate-controlling membrane or matrix. The ability of a drug to diffuse through membranes, its so called diffusivity (diffusion coefficient), is a function of its molecular size (or molecular weight). An important influence upon the value of the diffusivity, D, in polymers is the molecular size (or molecular weight) of the diffusing species. In most polymers, it is possible to relate log D empirically to some function of molecular size, as shown in Eq 12:[4]

$$\log D = -s_v \log v + k_v = -s_M \log M + k_m \quad (12)$$

where v is molecular volume, M is molecular weight and s_v, s_M, k_v and k_m are constants. The value of D thus is related to the size and shape of the cavities as well as size and shape of drugs. Generally, values of the diffusion coefficient for intermediate-molecular-weight drugs, ie, 150 to 400, through flexible polymers range from 10^{-6} to 10^{-9} cm^2/sec, with values on the order of 10^{-8} being most common.[5] A value of approximately 10^{-6} is typical for these drugs through water as the medium. It is of interest to note that the value of D for one gas in another is on the order of 10^{-1} cm^2/sec, and for one liquid through another, 10^{-5} cm^2/sec. For drugs with a molecular weight greater than 500, the diffusion coefficients in many polymers frequently are so small that they are difficult to quantify, ie, less than 10^{-12} cm^2/sec. Thus, high-molecular-weight drugs and/or polymeric drugs should be expected to display very slow-release kinetics in sustained-release devices using diffusion through polymeric membranes or matrices as the releasing mechanism.

Biological Properties

Absorption—The rate, extent and uniformity of absorption of a drug are important factors when considering its formulation into a sustained-release system. Since the rate-limiting step in drug delivery from a sustained-release system is its release from a dosage form, rather than absorption, a rapid rate of absorption of the drug relative to its release is essential if the system is to be successful. As stated previously in discussing terminology, $k_r <<< k_a$. This becomes most critical in the case of oral administration. Assuming that the transit time of a drug through the absorptive area of the GI tract is between 9 and 12 hours, the maximum absorption half-life should be 3 to 4 hours.[6] This corresponds to a minimum absorption rate constant k_a of 0.17 hr^{-1} to 0.23 hr^{-1} necessary for about 80 to 95% absorption over a 9- to 12-hour transit time. For a drug with a very rapid rate of absorption (ie, $k_a \gg 0.23$ hr^{-1}), the above discussion implies that a first-order release-rate constant k_r less than 0.17 hr^{-1} is likely to result in unacceptably poor bioavailability in many patients. Therefore, slowly absorbed drugs will be difficult to formulate into sustained-release systems where the criterion that $k_r <<< k_a$ must be met.

The extent and uniformity of the absorption of a drug, as reflected by its bioavailability and the fraction of the total dose absorbed, may be quite low for a variety of reasons. This usually is not a prohibitive factor in its formulation into a sustained-release system. Some possible reasons for a low extent of absorption are poor water solubility, small partition coefficient, acid hydrolysis and metabolism, or site-specific absorption. The latter reason also is responsible for nonuniformity of absorption. Many of these problems can be overcome by an appropriately designed sustained-release system, as exemplified by the discussion under the potential advantages of sustained drug therapy.

Distribution—For the design of sustained-release systems it is desirable to have as much information as possible regarding drug disposition, but in actual practice decisions usually are based on only a few pharmacokinetic parameters, one of which is the volume of distribution as given in Eq 1. The distribution of a drug into vascular and extravascular spaces in the body is an important factor in its overall elimination kinetics. This, in turn, influences the formulation of that drug into a sustained-release system, primarily by restricting the magnitude of the release rate and the dose size which can be employed.[5] At present, the calculation of these quantities is based primarily on one-compartment pharmacokinetic models as described under terminology. A description of the estimation of these quantities based on multicompartment models is beyond the scope of this chapter. However, the main considerations that need to be dealt with if a two-compartment model is operative will be presented.

Two parameters that are used to describe the distribution characteristics of a drug are its apparent volume of distribution and the ratio of drug concentration in tissue to that in plasma at the steady state, the so-called T/P ratio. The apparent volume of distribution is merely a proportionality constant which relates drug concentration in the blood or plasma to the total amount of drug in the body. The magnitude of the apparent volume of distribution can be used as a guide for additional studies and as a predictor for a drug dosing regimen and hence the need to employ sustained-release system. For drugs which obey a one-compartment model, the apparent volume of distribution is

$$V = \text{dose}/C_0 \qquad (13)$$

where C_0 is the initial drug concentration immediately after an intravenous bolus injection, but before any drug has been eliminated. The application of this equation is based upon the assumption that the distribution of a drug between plasma and tissues takes place instantaneously. This is rarely a good assumption, and it usually is necessary to invoke multi-compartment models to account for the finite time required for the drug to distribute fully throughout the available body space. In the case of a two-compartment model, it has been shown[7] that the best estimate of total volume of drug distribution is given by the apparent volume of distribution at steady state:

$$V_{ss} = (1 + k_{12}/k_{21})V_1 \qquad (14)$$

where V_1 is the volume of the central compartment, k_{12} is the rate constant for distribution of drug from the central to the peripheral compartment and k_{21} is that from the peripheral to the central compartment. As its name implies, V_{ss} relates drug concentration in the blood or plasma at the steady state to the total amount of drug in the body during repetitive dosing or constant-rate infusion. The use of Eq 14 is limited to those instances where a steady-state drug concentration in both compartments has been reached; at any other time, it tends to overestimate or underestimate the total amount of drug in the body.

To avoid the ambiguity inherent in the apparent volume of distribution as an estimator of the amount of drug in the body, the T/P ratio also can be used. If the amount of drug in the central compartment, P, is known, the amount of drug in the peripheral compartment, T, and hence the total amount of drug in the body can be calculated[5] by

$$T/P = k_{12}(k_{21} - \beta) \qquad (15)$$

Here, β is the slow disposition rate constant and k_{12} and k_{21} are as defined previously. The important point to note is that the T/P ratio estimates the relative distribution of drug between compartments, whereas V_{ss} estimates the extent of distribution in the body. Both parameters contribute to an estimation of the distribution characteristics of a drug, but their relative importance in this respect is open to debate.

Metabolism—The metabolic conversion of a drug to another chemical form usually can be considered in the design of a sustained-release system for that drug. As long as the location, rate and extent of metabolism are known and the rate constant(s) for the process(es) are not too large, successful sustained-release products can be developed.

There are two factors associated with the metabolism of some drugs, however, that present problems for their use in sustained-release systems. One is the ability of the drug to induce or inhibit enzyme synthesis; this may result in a fluctuating drug blood level with chronic dosing. The other is a fluctuating drug blood level due to intestinal (or other tissue) metabolism or through a hepatic first-pass effect. Examples of drugs that are subject to intestinal metabolism upon oral dosing are hydralazine, salicylamide, nitroglycerin, isoproterenol, chlorpromazine and levodopa. Examples of drugs that undergo extensive first-pass hepatic metabolism are propoxyphene, nortriptyline, phenacetin, propranolol and lidocaine.

Elimination and Biological Half-Life—The rate of elimination of a drug is described quantitatively by its biological half-life, $t_{1/2}$. The half-life of a drug is related to its apparent volume of distribution V and its systemic clearance:

$$t_{1/2} = 0.693\ V/Cl_s = 0.693\ V\ \text{AUC}/\text{dose} \qquad (16)$$

The systemic clearance, Cl_s, is equal to the ratio of an intravenously administered dose to the total area under the drug blood level versus time curve, AUC. A drug with a short half-life requires frequent dosing and this makes it a desirable candidate for a sustained-release formulation. On the other hand, a drug with a long half-life is dosed at greater time intervals and thus there is less need for a sustained-release system. It is difficult to define precise upper and lower limits for the value of the half-life of a drug that best suits it for sustained-release formulation. In general, however, a drug with a half-life of less than 2 hours probably should not be used, since such systems will require unacceptably large release rates and large doses. At the other extreme, a drug with a half-life of greater than 8 hours also probably should not be used; in most instances, formulation of such a drug into a sustained-release system is unnecessary. Some examples of drugs with half-lives of less than 2 hours are ampicillin, cephalexin, cloxacillin, furosemide, levodopa, penicillin G and propylthiouracil. Examples of those with half-lives of greater than 8 hours are dicumarol, diazepam, digitoxin, digoxin, guanethidine, phenytoin and warfarin.

Side Effects and Safety Considerations—There are very few drugs whose specific therapeutic concentrations are known. Instead, a therapeutic concentration *range* is listed, with increasing toxic effects expected above this range and a falloff in desired therapeutic response observed below the range. For some drugs, the incidence of side effects, in addition to toxicity, is believed to be a function of plasma concentration.[8] As mentioned in the discussion on the potential advantages of sustained drug therapy, a sustained-release system can, at times, minimize side effects for a particular drug by controlling its plasma concentration and using less total drug over the time course of therapy.

The most widely used measure of the margin of safety of a drug is its therapeutic index, TI, discussed in Chapter 41 and defined in the following equation:

$$\text{TI} = \text{TD}_{50}/\text{ED}_{50} \qquad (17)$$

where TD_{50} is the median toxic dose and ED_{50} is the median effective dose. The value of TI varies from as little as unity, where the effective dose is also producing toxic symptoms, to several thousand. For very "potent" drugs, whose therapeutic concentration range is narrow, the value of TI is small. In general, the larger the value of TI, the safer the drug. Drugs with very small values of TI usually are poor candidates for formulation into sustained-release products primarily due to technological limitations of precise control over release rates. A drug is considered to be relatively safe if its *TI* value exceeds 10. Examples of drugs with values of $\text{TI} < 10$ are aprobarbital, digitoxin, phenobarbital and digoxin.

Dose Size—Since a sustained-release system is designed to alleviate repetitive dosing, it naturally will contain a greater amount of drug than a corresponding conventional form. The typical administered dose of a drug in the conventional dosage form will give some indication of the total amount needed in the sustained-release preparation. For those drugs requiring large conventional doses, the volume of the sustained dose may be so large as to be impractical or unacceptable, depending on the route of administration. The same may be true of drugs which require a large release rate from the sustained-release system, eg, drugs with short half-lives. For the oral route the volume of the product is limited by patient acceptance. For the intramuscular, intravenous or subcutaneous routes, the limitation is tolerance of the drug at the injection site. It also should be mentioned that for drugs with a low therapeutic index, incorporation of amounts greater than the TD_{50} potentially may be dangerous if the system fails.

Oral Dosage Forms

For sustained-release systems, the oral route of administration has, by far, received the most attention. This is, in part, because there is more flexibility in dosage-form design for the oral route than there is for the parenteral route. Patient acceptance of the oral route is quite high. It is a relatively safe route of administration, compared to most parenteral routes, and the constraints of sterility and potential damage at the site of administration are minimal. In this section, the more common methods that are used to achieve sustained release of orally administered drugs are discussed.

Diffusion Systems

In these systems, the release rate of drug is determined by its diffusion through a water-insoluble polymer. There are basically two types of diffusion devices: *reservoir devices,* in which a core of drug is surrounded by a polymeric membrane, and *matrix devices,* in which dissolved or dispersed drug is distributed uniformly in an inert polymeric matrix. It should be mentioned that in actual practice many devices which use diffusion also rely upon some degree of dissolution to determine the release rate. Systems using dissolution will be discussed later in this section.

Reservoir Devices—The release of drug from a reservoir device is governed by Fick's first law of diffusion:

$$J = -D\,dC_m/dx \quad (18)$$

where J is the flux of drug across a membrane in the direction of decreasing concentration (amount/area-time), D is the diffusion coefficient of the drug in the membrane (area/time) and dC_m/dx is the change in concentration of drug in the membrane over a distance x. If it is assumed that the drug on either side of the membrane is in equilibrium with the respective surface layer of the membrane, as shown in Fig 6[9], then the concentration just inside the membrane surface can be related to the concentration in the adjacent region by the expressions

$$K = C_{m(0)}/C_{(0)} \text{ at } x = 0 \quad (19)$$

$$K = C_{m(l)}/C_{(l)} \text{ at } x = l \quad (20)$$

where K is a partition coefficient. Assuming that D and K are

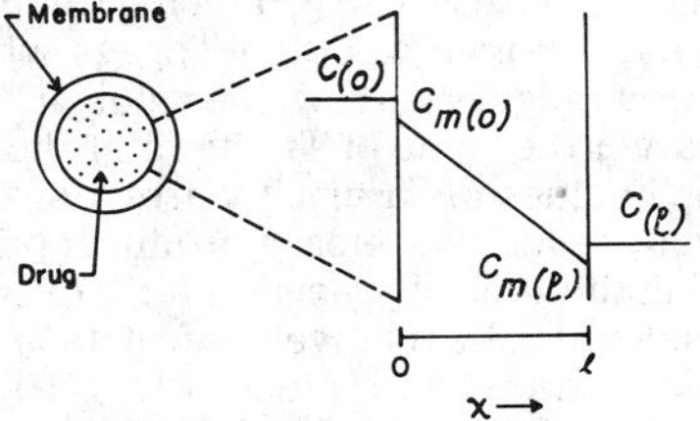

Fig 6. Schematic representation of a reservoir diffusion device. $C_{m(0)}$ and $C_{m(l)}$ represent concentrations of drug at the inside surfaces of the membrane and $C_{(0)}$ and $C_{(l)}$ represent concentrations in the adjacent regions. (Reproduced with permission.[9])

constant, Eq 18 can be integrated to give

$$J = DK\Delta C/l \quad (21)$$

where ΔC is the concentration difference across the membrane.

If the activity of the drug inside the reservoir is maintained constant and the value of K is less than unity, zero-order release can be achieved. This is the case when the drug is present as a solid, ie, its activity is unity. Depending on the shape of the device, the equation describing drug release will vary. Only the simplest geometry, that of a rectangular slab or "sandwich," will be presented here. For the slab geometry, the equation describing release is

$$dM_t/dt = ADK\Delta C/l \quad (22)$$

where M_t is the mass of drug released after time t, dM_t/dt is the steady-state release rate at time t, A is the surface area of the device and D, K and l are as defined previously. Similar equations can be written for cylindrical or spherical geometric devices. In order to obtain a constant drug-release rate, it is necessary to maintain constant area, diffusion path length, concentration and diffusion coefficient. In other words, all of the terms on the right hand side of Eq 22 are held constant. This is often not the case in actual practice because one or more of the above terms will change in the product, thus nonzero-order release is frequently observed.

Common methods used to develop reservoir-type devices include microencapsulation of drug particles and press-coating of tablets containing drug cores. In most cases, particles coated by microencapsulation form a system where the drug is contained in the coating film as well as in the core of the microcapsule. Drug release usually involves a combination of dissolution and diffusion, with dissolution being the process that controls the release rate. If the encapsulating material is selected properly, diffusion will be the controlling process. Microencapsulation is discussed further with reference to systems using dissolution. Some materials used as the membrane barrier coat, alone or in combination, are hardened gelatin, methyl or ethylcelluloses, polyhydroxymethacrylate, hydroxypropylcellulose, polyvinylacetate and various waxes. Examples of some marketed products using an encapsulated reservoir of drug are shown in Table 2. Drug release from these products probably is based primarily on diffusion, but dissolution may be occurring as well.

Matrix Devices—The rate of release of a drug dispersed as a solid in an inert matrix has been described by Higuchi.[10,11] Figure 7 depicts the physical model for a planar slab. In this model, it is assumed that solid drug dissolves from the surface layer of the device first; when this layer becomes exhausted of drug, the next layer begins to be depleted by dissolution and diffusion through the matrix to the external solution. In this fashion, the interface between the region containing dissolved drug and that containing dispersed drug moves into the inte-

Table 2—Reservoir Diffusion Products

Product	Active ingredient(s)	Manufacturer
Plateau CAPS capsules		
Nico-400	Nicotinic acid	Jones
Nitro-Bid	Nitroglycerin	Marion
Cerespan capsules	Papaverine hydrochloride	Rhone-Poulenc Rorer
Histaspan capsules	Chlorpheniramine maleate, phenylephrine hydrochloride, methscopolamine nitrate	Rhone-Poulenc Rorer
Nitrospan capsules	Nitroglycerin	Rhone-Poulenc Rorer
Measurin tablets	Acetylsalicylic acid	Sanofi-Winthrop
Bronkodyl S-R capsules	Theophylline	Sanofi-Winthrop

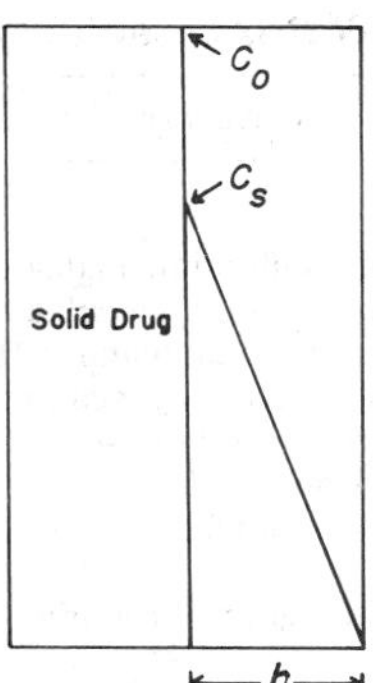

Fig 7. Schematic representation of the physical model used for a planar slab matrix diffusion device.

rior as a front. The assumptions made in deriving the mathematical model are as follows:

1. A pseudo-steady state is maintained during release.
2. The total amount of drug present per unit volume in the matrix, C_0, is substantially greater than the saturation solubility of the drug per unit volume in the matrix, C_s, ie, excess solute is present.
3. The release medium is a perfect sink at all times.
4. Drug particles are much smaller in diameter than the average distance of diffusion.
5. The diffusion coefficient remains constant.
6. No interaction occurs between the drug and the matrix.

Based on Fig 7, the change in amount of drug released per unit area, dM, with a change in the depleted zone thickness, dh, is

$$dM = C_0 dh - (C_s/2)dh \tag{23}$$

where C_0 and C_s are as defined above. However, based on Fick's first law

$$dM = (D_m C_s/h)dt \tag{24}$$

where D_m is the diffusion coefficient in the matrix. If Eqs 23 and 24 are equated, solved for h and that value of h substituted back into the integrated form of Eq 24, an equation for M is obtained:

$$M = [C_s D_m (2C_0 - C_s)t]^{1/2} \tag{25}$$

Similarly, a drug released from a porous or granular matrix is described by

$$M = [D_s C_a(\epsilon/T)(2C_0 - \epsilon C_a)t]^{1/2} \tag{26}$$

where ϵ is porosity of the matrix, T is *tortuosity*, C_a is the solubility of the drug in the release medium and D_s is the diffusion coefficient of drug in the release medium. In this system, drug is leached from the matrix through channels or pores.

For purposes of data treatment, Eqs 25 and 26 are conveniently reduced to

$$M = kt^{1/2} \tag{27}$$

where k is a constant, so that a plot of amount of drug released versus the square root of time should be linear if the release of the drug from the matrix is diffusion-controlled. The release rate of drug from such a device is not zero-order, since it decreases with time but, as previously mentioned, this may be clinically equivalent to constant release for many drugs.

The three major types of materials used in the preparation of matrix devices are insoluble plastics, hydrophilic polymers and fatty compounds. Plastic matrices which have been investigated include methyl acrylate–methyl methacrylate, polyvinyl chloride and polyethylene. The Gradumet tablet (*Abbott*) is an example of a dosage form using a plastic matrix. Hydrophilic polymers include methylcellulose, hydroxypropylmethylcellulose, sodium carboxymethylcellulose and carbopol 934. Fatty compounds include various waxes such as carnauba wax and glyceryl tristearate. An example of a dosage form using a wax matrix is the Lontab tablet (*Ciba*).

The most common method of preparation is to mix the drug with the matrix material and then compress the mixture into tablets. In the case of wax matrices, the drug generally is dispersed in molten wax, which is then congealed, granulated and compressed into cores. In any sustained-release system it is necessary for a portion of the drug to be available immediately as a priming dose, and the remainder to be released in a sustained fashion. This is accomplished in a matrix tablet by placing the priming dose in a coat of the tablet. The coat can be applied by press coating or by conventional pan or air suspension coating. Some marketed matrix diffusion products are listed in Table 3.

Dissolution Systems

As mentioned earlier in the chapter, a drug with a slow dissolution rate will yield an inherently sustained blood level. In principle, then, it would seem possible to prepare sustained-release products by decreasing the dissolution rate of drugs which are highly water-soluble. This can be done by preparing an appropriate salt or derivative, by coating the drug with a slowly soluble material or by incorporating it into a tablet with a slowly soluble carrier. Ideally, the surface area available for dissolution must remain constant in order to achieve a constant release rate. This is, however, difficult to achieve in practice.

The dissolution process can be considered diffusion-layer-controlled, where the rate of diffusion from the solid surface to the bulk solution through an unstirred liquid film is the rate-determining step. In this case the dissolution process at steady state is described by the Noyes-Whitney equation:

$$dC/dt = k_D A(C_s - C) = (D/h)A(C_s - C) \tag{28}$$

where dC/dt is the dissolution rate, k_D is the dissolution rate constant, A is the total surface area, C_s is the saturation solubility of the solid and C is the concentration of solute in the bulk solution. The dissolution-rate constant, k_D, is equal to the diffusion coefficient, D, divided by the thickness of the diffusion layer, h. The above equation predicts a constant dissolution rate if the surface area, diffusion coefficient, diffusion layer thickness and concentration difference are kept constant. However, as dissolution proceeds, all of these parameters may change, especially surface area. For spherical particles, the change in area can be related to the weight of the particle and, under the assumption of sink conditions, Eq 28 becomes the cube-root dissolution equation

$$w_0{}^{1/3} - w^{1/3} = k_D't \tag{29}$$

where k_D' is the cube-root dissolution-rate constant, and w_0 and w are initial weight and weight of the amount remaining at time t, respectively.

Two common formulations relying on dissolution to determine release rate of drug are shown in Fig 8. Most of the products fall into two categories: encapsulated dissolution systems and matrix dissolution systems.

Table 3—Matrix Diffusion Products

Product	Active ingredient(s)	Manufacturer
Gradumet tablets		Abbott
Desoxyn	Methamphetamine HCl	
Fero-Gradumet	Ferrous sulfate	
Fero-Grad-500	Ferrous sulfate, sodium ascorbate	
Tral	Hexocyclium methylsulfate	
Lontab tablets		Ciba
PBZ-SR	Tripelennamine HCl	
Procan SR tablets	Procainamide HCl	Parke-Davis
Choledyl SA tablets	Oxtriphylline	Parke-Davis

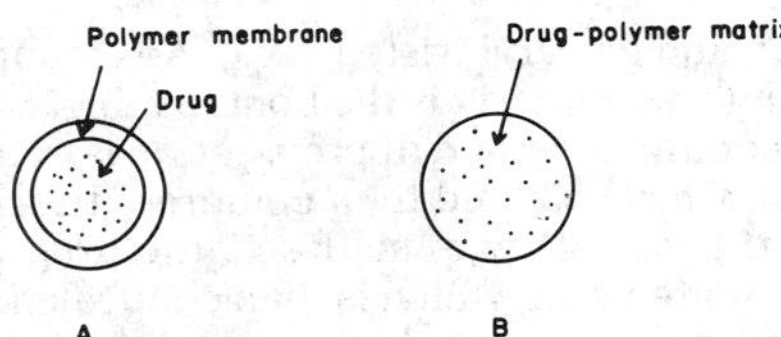

Fig 8. Schematic representation of systems using dissolution. A, encapsulated formulation where drug release is determined by thickness and dissolution rate of the polymer membrane; B, matrix formulation where drug release is determined by dissolution rate of the polymer.

Encapsulated dissolution systems can be prepared either by coating particles or granules of drug with varying thicknesses of slowly soluble polymers or by microencapsulation. Microencapsulation can be accomplished by using phase separation, interfacial polymerization, heat-fusion or the solvent-evaporation method. The coating materials may be selected from a wide variety of natural and synthetic polymers, depending on the drug to be coated and the release characteristics desired. The most commonly used coating materials include gelatin, carnauba wax, shellacs, ethylcellulose, cellulose acetate phthalate or cellulose acetate butyrate. Drug release from microcapsules, is a mass-transport phenomenon; and can be controlled by adjusting the size of microcapsules, thickness of coating materials and the diffusivity of core materials. The coating thickness of microcapsules is normally very thin, and for a given coating-core ratio, it decreases rapidly as the microcapsule size decreases. The thickness can be varied from less than 1 μm to 200 μm by changing the amount of coating material from 3 to 30% of the total weight. If only a few different thicknesses are used, usually three or four, drugs will be released at different, predetermined times to give a delayed release effect, ie, repeat-action. If a spectrum of different thicknesses is employed, a more uniform blood level of the drug can be obtained. Microcapsules commonly are filled into capsules and rarely are tableted as their coatings tend to disrupt during compression. A partial list ing of some marketed sustained-release products relying primarily on encapsulated dissolution are shown in Table 4.

Matrix dissolution devices are prepared by compressing the drug with a slowly soluble polymer carrier into a tablet form. There are two general methods of preparing drug–wax particles: congealing and aqueous dispersion methods. In the congealing method, drug is mixed with a wax material and either spray-congealed or congealed and screened. In the aqueous dispersion method, the drug–wax mixture simply is sprayed or placed in water and the resulting particles are collected. Matrix tablets also are made by direct compression of a mixture of drug, polymer and excipients. Examples of marketed products relying primarily on matrix dissolution are listed in Table 5.

Table 4—Encapsulated Dissolution Products

Product	Active ingredient(s)	Manufacturer
Spansule capsules		SmithKline Beecham
Dexedrine	Dextroamphetamine sulfate	
Hispril	Diphenylpyraline HCl	
Ornade	Phenylpropanolamine HCl, chlorpheniramine maleate	
Thorazine	Chlorpromazine HCl	
Contac capsules	Phenylpropanolamine HCl, chlorpheniramine maleate	SmithKline Beecham
Sequel capsules		Lederle
Artane	Trihexyphenidyl HCl	
Diamox	Acetazolamide	
Ferro-sequels	Ferrous fumarate, docusate sodium	

Table 5—Matrix Dissolution Products

Product	Active ingredient(s)	Manufacturer
Extentab tablets		Robins
Dimetane	Brompheniramine maleate	
Dimetapp	Brompheniramine maleate, phenylpropanolamine HCl	
Donnatal	Phenobarbital, hyoscamine sulfate, atropine sulfate, scopolamine hydrobromide	
Quinidex	Quinidine sulfate	
Timespan tablets		Roche
Mestinon	Pyridostigmine bromide	
Dospan tablets		Lakeside
Tenuate	Diethylpropion HCl	
Chronotab tablets		Schering
Disophrol	Dexbrompheniramine maleate, pseudoephedrine sulfate	
Tempule capsules		Rhone-Poulenc Rorer
Nicobid	Nicotinic acid	
Pentritol	Pentaerythritol tetranitrate	
Repetab tablets		Schering
Chlor-trimeton	Chlorpheniramine maleate	
Demazin	Chlorpheniramine maleate, phenylephrine HCl	
Polaramine	Dexchlorpheniramine maleate	
Trilafon	Perphenazine	

Osmotic Systems

Osmotic pressure can be employed as the driving force to generate a constant release of drug provided a constant osmotic pressure is maintained and a few other features of the physical system are constrained. Consider a tablet consisting of a core of an osmotically active drug, or a core of an osmotically inactive drug, in combination with an osmotically active salt surrounded by a semipermeable membrane containing a small orifice, as shown in Fig 9. The membrane will allow free diffusion of water, but not drug. When the tablet is exposed to water or any fluid in the body, water will flow into the tablet due to osmotic pressure difference and the volume flow rate, dV/dt, of water into the tablet is

$$dV/dt = (kA/h)(\Delta\pi - \Delta P) \tag{30}$$

where k, A and h are the membrane permeability, area and thickness, respectively, $\Delta\pi$ is the osmotic pressure difference and ΔP is the hydrostatic pressure difference. If the orifice is sufficiently large, the hydrostatic pressure difference will be small compared to the osmotic pressure difference, and Eq 30 becomes

$$dV/dt = (kA/h)\Delta\pi \tag{31}$$

Thus, the volume flow rate of water into the tablet is determined by permeability, area and thickness of the membrane. The drug will be pumped out of the tablet through the orifice at a controlled rate, dM/dt, equal to the volume flow rate of water into the tablet multiplied by the drug concentration, C_s:

$$dM/dt = (dV/dt)C_s \tag{32}$$

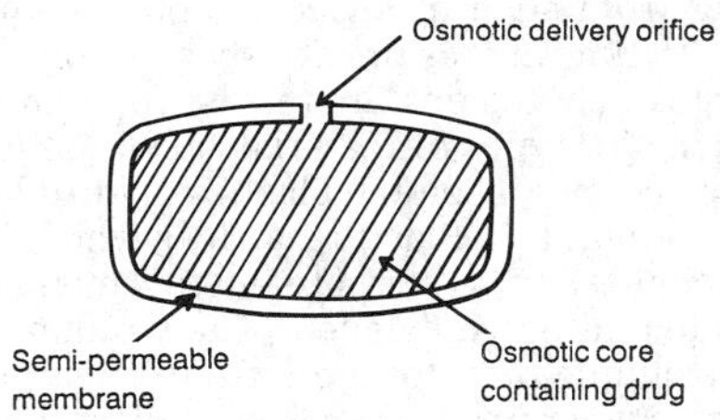

Fig 9. Schematic diagram of an osmotic tablet. (Reproduced with permission.[12])

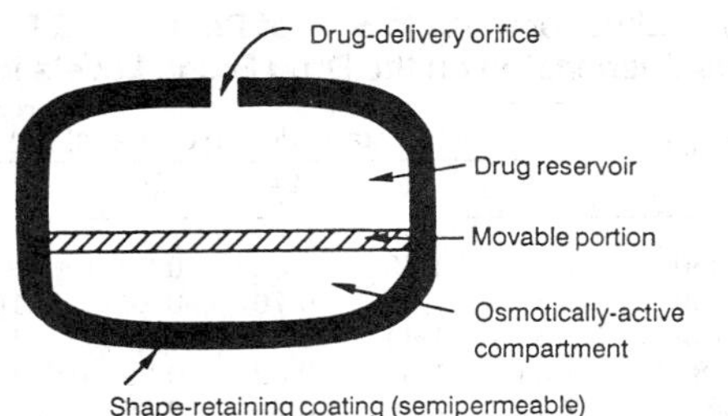

Fig 10. Osmotic pressure-controlled drug-delivery system with two compartments separated by a movable partition.[13]

The release rate will be constant until the concentration of drug inside the tablet falls below saturation.

Several modifications of the osmotic pressure-controlled drug delivery system have been developed. A layer of bioerodible polymer can be applied to the external surface of the semipermeable membrane. A system consists of two compartments separated by a movable partition, as shown in Fig. 10. For a system that does not have an orifice, hydraulic pressure is built up inside as the GI fluid is imbibed until the wall ruptures and the contents are released to the environment.

The advantage of the osmotic system is that it requires only osmotic pressure to be effective and is essentially independent of the environment. The drug release rate can be predetermined precisely regardless of pH change through the GI tract. Some materials used as the semipermeable membrane include polyvinyl alcohol, polyurethane, cellulose acetate, ethylcellulose and polyvinyl chloride. Drugs that have demonstrated successful release rates from an osmotic system *in vivo* after oral dosing are potassium chloride and acetazolamide.

Ion-Exchange Resins

Ion-exchange resins are water-insoluble crosslinked polymers containing salt forming groups in repeating positions on the polymer chain. Drug is bound to the resin by repeated exposure of the resin to the drug in a chromatographic column, or by prolonged contact of the resin with the drug solution. The drug-resin then is washed to remove contaminating ions and dried to form particles or beads. Drug release from the drug–resin complex depends on the ionic environment, ie, pH and electrolyte concentration, within the GI tract as well as properties of the resin.

Drug molecules attached to the resin are released by exchanging with appropriately charged ions in the GI tract, as shown in Fig 11, followed by diffusion of the free drug molecule out of the resin. The rate of diffusion is controlled by the area of diffusion, diffusional pathlength and extent of crosslinking in the resin. A modification of the release rate can be made by coating the drug–resin complex. Further improvement of this ion-exchange type drug delivery system is called the Penn Kinetic system. In this system, the drug-containing resin granules first are treated with an impregnating polymer such as PEG 4000 to retard the rate of swelling in water and further coated with a water-insoluble polymer, such as ethylcellulose, to serve as a rate-limiting barrier to control the drug release.

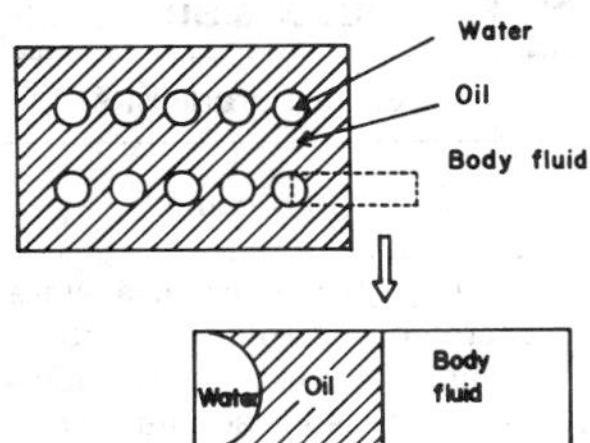

Fig 11. Schematic of drug release from ion-exchange resin.

Most ion-exchange resins currently employed in sustained-release products contain sulfonic acid groups that exchange cationic drugs such as those with an amine functionality. Examples of some of these drugs are amphetamine, phenyl *t*-butylamine (phentermine), phenyltoloxamine and hydrocodone, as shown in Table 6.

Prodrugs

A prodrug is a compound formed by chemical modification of a biologically active compound which will liberate the active compound *in vivo* by enzymatic or hydrolytic cleavage. The primary purpose of employing a prodrug for oral administration is to increase intestinal absorption or to reduce local side effects, such as GI irritation by aspirin. On this basis, one generally does not classify a prodrug as a sustained-release dosage form. However, the ability to bio-reversibly modify the physicochemical properties of a drug allows better intestinal transport properties and hence influences the drug blood level versus time profile. Thus, prodrugs can be used to increase the strategies for sustained release and, in a limited sense, can be sustaining in their own right.

As an example of the use of a prodrug as a sustaining mechanism, consider a water-soluble drug which is modified to a water-insoluble prodrug. The prodrug will have a slower dissolution rate in an aqueous medium than the parent drug and, thus, the appearance of the parent drug in plasma will be slowed. This is observed with theophylline and its prodrug, 7,7′-succinylditheophylline. Alternatively, a water-soluble prodrug of a water-insoluble parent drug can be made to be a substrate for enzymes in the brush border region of the microvilli. The water-soluble prodrug complexes with the enzyme just prior to reaching the membrane surface, is metabolized and its membrane/water partition coefficient increases. The result is an increase in the blood level of the drug. See Chapter 28.

Parenteral Dosage Forms

The most common types of dosage forms used for parenteral sustained-release drug therapy are intramuscular (IM) injections, implants for subcutaneous tissues and various body cavities and transdermal devices. Due to physiological and anatomical constraints, many of the other parenteral routes of administration, eg, intravenous, intra-arterial, intrathecal and intraperitoneal, are not as useful in this regard. The application of the former three types of dosage forms to sustained-release drug delivery will be discussed in this section. The final section is devoted to other parenteral dosage forms being developed for targeted drug delivery.

Intramuscular Injections

Aqueous Solutions—It is conceivable and likely that increased viscosity of the medium not only decreases molecular diffusion but also localizes the injected volume. Thus, the absorptive area is reduced and the rate of drug release is controlled. Examples of thickening agents are methylcellulose, sodium carboxymethylcellulose and polyvinylpyrrolidone.

Complex Formation—The formation of a dissociable complex of a drug with a macromolecule is the same physicochemi-

Table 6—Ion-Exchange Products

Product	Active ingredient(s)	Manufacturer
Biphetamine capsules	Amphetamine, dextroamphetamine	Pennwalt
Tussionex capsules, tablets, suspension	Hydrocodone, chlorpheniramine	Pennwalt
Ionamin capsules	Phentermine	Pennwalt

cal phenomenon which occurs when a drug binds to a plasma protein. In this sense, the drug–macromolecule complex can serve as a reservoir at the site of injection for sustained drug release to the surrounding tissues. The macromolecules used are either biological polymers, such as antibodies and proteins, or synthetic polymers, such as methylcellulose, sodium carboxymethyl-cellulose or polyvinylpyrrolidone. Drug release from the polymer is governed by the degree of association, as given by

$$D + P \overset{K_a}{\rightleftharpoons} DP \tag{33}$$

where D, P and DP represent drug, polymer and complex, respectively, and K_a is the apparent association constant. Only that fraction of the drug which is free, f, can be absorbed:

$$f = \frac{(D)}{(DP) + (D)} = \frac{1}{1 + K_a(P)} \tag{34}$$

where (D), (P) and (DP) are equilibrium concentrations of drug, polymer and complex, respectively. If $K_a(P)$ is much greater than 1, Eq 34 reduces to

$$f = 1/[K_a(P)] \tag{35}$$

The rate of absorption of the drug, $d(C)/dt$, therefore is described by

$$d(C)/dt = k_a f(D_t) = [k_a(D_t)]/[K_a(P)] \tag{36}$$

where (D_t) is the total drug concentration at the absorption site, ie, $(DP) + (D)$, and k_a is the absorption-rate constant. It can be seen from Eq 36 that the rate of absorption can be controlled effectively by the type and concentration of polymer used, assuming that dissociation is instantaneous compared to absorption.

Complexes also can be formed between drugs and small molecules, such as caffeine, rather than macromolecules. The motive behind formation of a drug–small molecule complex is to alter the physicochemical properties of the drug and thus affect changes in its biological disposition. Unlike macromolecular complexes, drug–small molecule complexes are capable of being absorbed. They usually have very small association constants, however, which means that most of the drug is free. This nullifies any advantage gained from alteration of properties upon complexation. If the drug molecule is large, relative to the complexing agent, the association constant will be greater and the complex more stable. This is the approach that has been taken commercially with polypeptide hormones, such as adrenocorticotropic hormone (ACTH) and insulin, and with vitamins such as cyanocobalamin (vitamin B_{12}). The ACTH product, Acthar Gel HP (*Arcum*) consists of an ACTH–zinc tannate complex suspended in a gelatin solution. Tannic acid acts as the complexing agent and gelatin inhibits protein binding of ACTH. With this product, the sustained effect is due to, among other things, a reduction in solubility of the parent drug upon complexation, and not dissociation. In this respect they are much like aqueous suspensions.

Aqueous Suspensions—The rate-limiting step in drug release from an aqueous suspension is dissolution, as given by the Noyes-Whitney equation (Eq 28). The parameters influencing dissolution rate were shown to be surface area (ie, particle size), diffusion coefficient and saturation solubility of the drug. Variation in these parameters for an intramuscular injection is limited by the constraints of stability, occlusion of needles, pain upon injection, minimum effective concentration and other factors. For example, one common approach to decrease dissolution rate is to decrease total surface area by increasing particle size. This generally extends the duration of action of the drug, as illustrated by the data in Table 7.[14] However, increasing the particle size causes an increase in sedimentation rate, as indicated by Stoke's law, resulting in an unstable suspension. In addition, for some drugs there is an upper limit on particle size beyond which therapeutic levels are not attained even though sustained release is achieved.

Table 7—Effect of Particle Size of Penicillin G Procaine in Aqueous Suspension on the Drug Blood Levels in Rabbits[a]

Particle size[b] (μm)	Average drug blood level (hr) 1	4	24	28	48	72
150–250	1.37	1.29	0.82	0.86	0.31	0.12
105–150	1.24	1.50	0.76	0.28	0.16	0.01
58–105	1.54	1.44	0.47	0.25	0.12	—
35–38	1.64	1.51	0.62	0.33	0.15	—
<35	2.40	2.36	0.33	0.16	0.07	—
1–2	2.14	2.22	0.06	0.02	—	—

[a] Compiled from data by Buckwalter and Dickison.[14]
[b] Each aqueous suspension contains 300,000 units/mL of penicillin G procaine with the specified particle-size range.

Another approach to decrease dissolution rate is to decrease the diffusion coefficient by increasing the viscosity of the suspension. For example, injectable nalbuphine HCl suspension containing methylcellulose was found to have prolonged action in dogs compared to a true solution.[15] Recall that the diffusion coefficient is related inversely to viscosity by the Stokes-Einstein relation. An increase in viscosity causes a decrease in sedimentation rate (again by Stoke's law), thus countering the effect of increased particle size. By appropriately varying viscosity and particle size, a stable suspension, that offers sustained release resulting in therapeutic drug blood levels, can be produced.

Probably the most common approach to decrease dissolution rate is to decrease the saturation-solubility of the drug. This is accomplished through the formation of less-soluble salts or prodrug derivatives or by employing polymorphic crystal forms. A typical example of decreasing dissolution rate through salt formation is provided by penicillin G procaine, a sparingly soluble form of penicillin G. Other examples of marketed aqueous suspensions based upon use of less-soluble salts or derivatives of the parent drug are contained in Table 8.

Solubility varies with polymorphic form because different arrangements of molecules in the solid state give rise to different lattice energies. An example of extending duration of action by use of a crystalline polymorph is insulin zinc suspension. Although insulin normally is administered subcutaneously, it is included here merely to illustrate the principle. Insulin precipitates as an insoluble complex in the presence of zinc chloride and, depending on the pH, either an amorphous or crystalline form results. The crystalline form is less soluble than the amorphous form and will result in a longer duration of action than the amorphous form. The two forms can be mixed in various proportions to generate products offering a wide spectrum of duration of action. A list of these products and their reported durations of action is shown in Table 9.[16]

Oil Solutions and Oil Suspensions—In the case of oil solutions the release rate of a drug is determined by partitioning of the drug out of the oil into the surrounding aqueous medium. The partitioning phenomenon is an equilibrium process described by the apparent oil/water partition coefficient given in Eq 11. Only that fractional concentration of

Table 8—Aqueous Suspensions

Product	Active ingredient(s)	Manufacturer
Crysticillin A.S.	Penicillin G procaine	Apothecon
Wycillin	Penicillin G procaine	Wyeth–Ayerst
Depo-Provera	Medroxyprogesterone acetate	Upjohn
Depo-Medrol	Methylprednisolone acetate	Upjohn
Aristospan	Triamcinolone hexacetonide	Lederle
Celeston Soluspan	Betamethasone sodium phosphate, betamethasone acetate	Schering

Table 9—Commercial Insulin Zinc Suspensions and their Reported Durations of Action[a]

Product	Manufacturer	Duration of action (hr)
Semilente Iletin I	Lilly	12–16
Lente Iletin I	Lilly	24
Ultralente Iletin I	Lilly	>36

[a] Compiled from *Physicians' Desk Reference.*[16]

drug in the aqueous phase, f, is available for absorption:

$$f = (1 + \alpha)/(1 + K\alpha) \tag{37}$$

where K is the apparent oil/water partition coefficient and α is the ratio V_0/V_w, the volume of the oil phase to that of the aqueous phase. This equation indicates that the fraction of drug that is available for absorption is controlled by the partition coefficient and the ratio of the volumes of the two phases (α), and that it remains constant so long as α is constant. Since V_w is a physiological parameter, it usually is constant, and therefore the value of α is determined solely by the volume of solution injected, V_0. The rate of drug absorption is described by an equation analogous to Eq 36:

$$d(C)/dt = k_a f(D_t) \tag{38}$$

where (D_t) is the total drug concentration in both phases. The success of an oil solution in achieving sustained release depends on the magnitude of K, which is a function of the drug involved and the oil selected. Only those drugs which are appreciably oil-soluble and have the desired partition characteristics are suitable. Some oils which may be used for intramuscular injection are sesame, olive, arachnis, maize, almond, cottonseed and castor oil. Table 10 contains a partial listing of marketed oil-solution products.

Drug release from oil suspensions combines the principles involved in aqueous suspensions and oil solutions. With the suspended particles acting as a drug reservoir, the drug particles first must dissolve in the oil phase and then partition into the aqueous medium. The concentration of drug in the oil phase remains close to its equilibrium solubility since excess solid is present, unlike an oil solution, but this has no bearing on the fractional concentration in the aqueous phase, as shown in Eq 37. As expected, the duration of action obtained from oil suspensions is longer than that from oil solutions. A list of some marketed oil-suspension products is shown in Table 11.

Emulsions—In the case where dissolved drug makes up the entire oil phase in an O/W emulsion, Higuchi[17] showed that the release rate at steady state can be described by

$$\text{rate} = 4\pi(a_0^2 + 2D\Delta Ct/d)^{1/2}D\Delta C \tag{39}$$

where a_0 is the initial radius of the droplet, D is the diffusion coefficient, ΔC is the concentration difference between the surface of the droplet and the bulk phase, d is the density of the solute and t is time. In the case where the solute makes up only part of the oil phase, appropriate corrections for the distribution coefficient of solute between oil and water phases and partial molal volume of the solute in the droplet must be made.

Table 10—Oil Solutions

Product	Active ingredient(s)	Manufacturer
Prolixin Enanthate	Fluphenazine enanthate in sesame oil	Apothecon
Prolixin Decanoate	Fuphenazine decanoate in sesame oil	Apothecon
Deca-Durabolin	Nandrolone decanoate in sesame oil	Organon
Depo-Testosterone	Testosterone cypionate in cottonseed oil	Upjohn
Ditate-DS	Testosterone enanthate, estradiol valerate in sesame oil	Savage
Delatestryl	Testosterone enanthate in sesame oil	Gynex

Table 11—Oil Suspensions

Product	Active ingredient(s)	Manufacturer
Solganal	Aurothioglucose in sesame oil	Schering

The release rate from W/O emulsions has been treated by Windheuser *et al.*[18] The W/O emulsion is viewed as a uniform dispersion of water droplets containing the drug throughout an external oil phase. Figure 11 depicts a simplified model of the system. Drug release is assumed to proceed via diffusion through the external phase rather than by breaking of the emulsion, and the body fluid acts as a perfect sink. The rate of disappearance of drug from the aqueous phase, $d(C)/dt$, is described by

$$d(C)/dt = -k(C_0)e^{-kt} \tag{40}$$

where (C_0) is the initial concentration in the aqueous phase and k is the rate constant of disappearance of drug from the aqueous phase. The constant k is given by

$$k = ADK/Vl \tag{41}$$

where A is surface area of the droplet, D is the diffusion coefficient of the drug, K is the partition coefficient of the drug between oil and water, V is the volume of the aqueous phase and l is the effective thickness of the oil phase. For a given drug, a fast rate of release is favored by a large K, small droplets (ie, large A for a fixed V) and a phase-volume ratio favoring the oil phase.

If the body fluid is not a perfect sink, an estimate of the fraction of drug in the body fluid can be made using arguments analogous to those for the oil-solution case. Making several simplifying assumptions, an equation identical to Eq 37 is obtained. Based on this argument alone, no apparent advantage is gained by administering a W/O emulsion rather than an oil solution as far as sustained release is concerned. Similar results can be obtained for drug release from O/W emulsions. The development of multiple emulsions for sustained release has gained more attention,[18] although they are more complex than their two-phase counterparts from the standpoint of formulation, stability and drug release. Magnetic emulsions also have been tried as a drug carrier for chemotherapeutic agents.[19]

Implants

Application of biocompatible polymers to the construction of implantable therapeutic systems for achieving a better control of the duration of drug activity and precision of dosing actually started with the discovery of the silicone elastomer. The rate of drug release was found to be controlled by the thickness and surface area of the membrane as well as the polarity of the penetrant. Toward the end of the 1960s, a concentrated effort was made to expand the silicone elastomer-based implantable therapeutic system technology to other biocompatible polymers, in an attempt to control the release of water-soluble molecules. Some of these systems include a microporous membrane made from an ethylene/vinyl acetate copolymer for the ocular delivery of pilocarpine, a biodegradable (lactic/glycolic) copolymer for subcutaneous and intramuscular controlled administration of narcotic antagonists, a bioerodible polysaccharide polymer for the delivery of anti-inflammatory steroids, hydrogel for the subcutaneous controlled administration of estrus synchronizing agents or implantable therapeutic systems activated by osmotic pressure, vapor pressure, magnetism, etc.

The most recent implant systems approved by FDA is the Norplant system (*Wyeth-Ayerst*). The Norplant system kit contains levonorgestrel implants, made of silastic (dimethylsiloxane/methylvinyl siloxane copolymer). The capsules are sealed with silastic adhesive and sterilized. The Norplant system is inserted in a superficial plane beneath the skin of the upper arm. The Norplant system is indicated for the prevention of pregnancy for as long as 5 years and is a reversible contraceptive system. The capsules may be removed at the end of the 5th year. New capsules may be inserted at that time if continuing contraceptive protection is desired.

Controlled Drug Release by Diffusion—In membrane permeation-type controlled drug delivery, the drug is encapsulated within a compartment that is enclosed by a rate-limiting polymeric membrane. The drug reservoir may contain either drug particles or a dispersion (or a solution) of solid drug in a liquid or a solid type dispersing medium. The polymeric membrane may be fabricated from a homogeneous or a heterogeneous nonporous polymeric material or a microporous or semipermeable membrane. The encapsulation of the drug reservoir inside the polymeric membrane may be accomplished by molding, encapsulation, microencapsulation or other techniques.

The drug release (dQ/dt) from this type of implantable therapeutic systems should be constant and defined by

$$\frac{dQ}{dt} = \frac{C_R}{\dfrac{1}{P_m} + \dfrac{1}{P_d}} \tag{42}$$

where C_R is the drug concentration in the reservoir compartment and P_m and P_d are the permeability coefficients of the rate-controlling membrane and of the hydrodynamic diffusion layer existing on the surface of the membrane, respectively. P_m and P_d are defined as

$$P_m = \frac{K_{m/r} D_m}{\delta_m} \tag{43}$$

$$P_d = \frac{K_{a/m} D_a}{\delta_d} \tag{44}$$

where $K_{m/r}$ and $K_{a/m}$ are the partition coefficients for the interfacial partitioning of drug molecules from the reservoir to the membrane and from the membrane to the aqueous diffusion layer, respectively. D_m and D_a are the diffusion coefficients in the membrane and in the aqueous diffusion layer, respectively, and δ_m and δ_a are the thickness of the membrane and of the aqueous diffusion layer, respectively.

Substituting Eq 43 and Eq 44 for P_m and P_d in Eq 42 and then integrating gives

$$\frac{Q}{t} = \frac{K_{m/r} K_{a/m} D_a D_m}{K_{m/r} D_m \delta_d + K_{a/m} D_a \delta_m} \cdot C_R \tag{45}$$

which defines the rate of drug release at the steady-state from a membrane permeation-type controlled drug-delivery device. Examples of this type implantable therapeutic system are Progestasert IUD and Ocusert system.[20]

In matrix diffusion-type controlled drug delivery, the drug reservoir is formed by the homogeneous dispersion of drug particles throughout a lipophilic or hydrophilic polymer matrix. The dispersion of the drug particles in the polymer matrix may be accomplished by blending the drug with a viscous liquid polymer or a semisolid polymer at room temperature, followed by crosslinking of the polymer, or by mixing the drug particles with a melted polymer at an elevated temperature. It also can be fabricated by dissolving the drug particles and/or the polymer in an organic solvent followed by mixing and evaporation of the solvent in a mold at an elevated temperature or under vacuum.

The rate of drug release from this type of delivery device is not constant and is defined by

$$\frac{dQ}{dt} = \left(\frac{AC_p D_p}{2t}\right)^{1/2} \tag{46}$$

where A is the initial drug loading dose dispersed in the polymer matrix and C_p and D_p are the solubility and diffusivity of the drug molecules in the polymer, respectively.Integration of Eq 46 gives

$$\frac{Q}{t^{1/2}} = (2AC_p D_p)^{1/2} \tag{47}$$

which defines the flux of drug release at the steady state from a matrix diffusion type drug delivery device. Examples of this type of implantable therapeutic system are the contraceptive vaginal ring[21] and Compudose implant.[22]

In microreservoir dissolution-controlled drug delivery, the drug reservoir, which is a suspension of drug particles in an aqueous solution of a water-miscible polymer, forms a homogeneous dispersion of a multitude of discrete, unleachable, microscopic drug reservoirs in a polymer matrix. The microdispersion may be generated by using a high-energy-dispersing technique. Release of the drug from this type of drug-delivery device follows either an interfacial partition or a matrix diffusion-controlled process. An example of this type drug delivery device is the Syncro-Mate-C Implant.[20]

Controlled Drug Release by Activation—In osmotic pressure activated drug delivery, the drug reservoir, which is a liquid formulation, is contained within a semipermeable housing. The drug is released in solution form at a controlled, constant rate under an osmotic pressure gradient. An example of this type of drug delivery device is the Alzet osmotic pump.

Infusaid is an example of an implantable infusion pump using vapor pressure activation theory, in which the vapor chamber contains a vaporizable fluid which vaporizes at body temperature and creates a vapor pressure. Under the vapor pressure created, a bellows moves upward and forces the drug to be released. Implantable drug-delivery devices also can be activated by magnetism, ultrasound or hydrolysis.

Implants are typically placed subcutaneously to sustain drug release via various mechanisms. Both nonbiodegradable polymers, such as silicone elastomer (polydimethylsiloxane), and biodegradable polymers, such as poly(caprolactone), poly(lactic acid) or poly(glycolic acid), can be used. An ideal implantable therapeutic system should be biostable, biocompatible, with minimal tissue-implant interactions, nontoxic, noncarcinogenic, removable if required and should release drug at a constant, programmed rate for a predetermined duration of medication.

Transdermal Systems

Among other things, the skin serves as a barrier against penetration of microorganisms, viruses and toxic chemicals, and as a restraint against loss of physiologically vital fluids. A discussion of the fundamentals of percutaneous drug absorption, sometimes referred to as transdermal absorption, can be found in Chapter 90. Investigation of mechanisms of transdermal drug absorption has led to new approaches in using this route for systemic drug delivery. The intensity of interest in the potential biomedical applications of transdermal controlled-drug administration is demonstrated in the increasing research activity in the development of various types of transdermal therapeutic systems for long-term continuous infusion of therapeutic agents, including antihypertensive, antianginal, analgesic, steroidal and contraceptive drugs. Several technologies have been developed to provide rate control over the release and the transdermal permeation of drugs.

Membrane-Moderated Systems—In this system, the drug reservoir is totally encapsulated in a shallow compartment molded from a drug-impermeable backing and a rate-controlling polymeric membrane as shown in Fig 12. The drug molecules may be released only through the rate-controlling polymeric membrane. The rate-limiting membrane can be a microporous or a nonporous polymeric membrane. On the external surface of the membrane, a thin layer of drug-

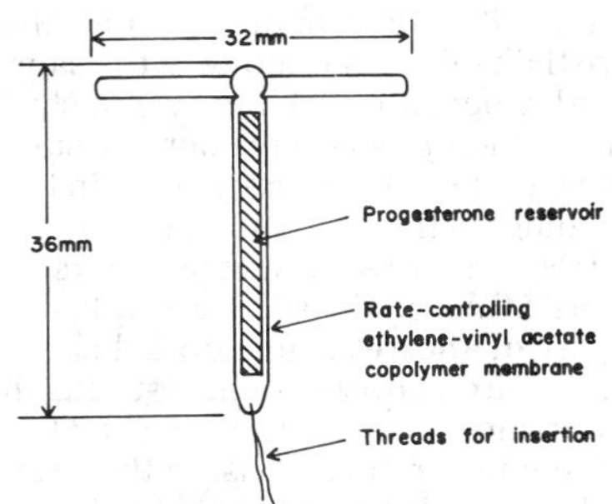

Fig 12. Model of a water-in-oil emulsion. (Reproduced with permission.[1])

compatible, hypoallergenic adhesive polymer, eg, silicone or polyacrylate adhesive, may be applied to achieve an intimate contact of the transdermal system with the skin. The rate of drug release from this type of drug-delivery system can be tailored by varying the polymer composition, permeability coefficient or thickness of the rate-limiting membrane and adhesive. Examples of this type of transdermal therapeutic system are the nitroglycerin-releasing transdermal therapeutic system such as Transderm-Nitro (*Ciba*), scopolamine-releasing transdermal therapeutic system such as Transderm-Scop system (*Ciba*) and clonidine-releasing transdermal therapeutic system such as Catapres transdermal therapeutic system (*Boehringer Ingelheim*). A typical *in vitro* release rate versus time profile from such a system is shown in Fig. 13.

Adhesive Diffusion-Controlled Systems—In this system the drug reservoir is formulated by directly dispersing the drug in an adhesive polymer and then spreading the medicated adhesive, by solvent casting, onto a flat sheet of drug-impermeable backing membrane to form a thin drug-reservoir layer. On the top of the drug-reservoir layer, layers of non-medicated, rate-controlling adhesive polymer of constant thickness are applied to produce an adhesive diffusion-controlled drug-delivery system. Examples of this type of transdermal drug delivery system are the nitroglycerin-releasing transdermal therapeutic system such as the Deponit system (*Pharma-Schwartz*) and isosorbide dinitrate-releasing transdermal therapeutic system such as Frandol tape (*Toaeiyo*).

Matrix Dispersion-Type Systems—In this system, the drug reservoir is formed by homogeneously dispersing the drugs in a hydrophilic or lipophilic polymer matrix, and the medicated polymer then is molded into a medicated disc with a defined surface area and controlled thickness. The disc then is glued onto an occlusive baseplate in a compartment fabricated from a drug-impermeable backing. The adhesive polymer is spread along the circumference to form a strip of adhesive rim around the medicated disc. Example of this type of transdermal drug-delivery system is the nitroglycerin-releasing transdermal therapeutic system such as the Nitro-Dur system (*Key*).

Microreservoir Systems—In this system, the drug reservoir is formed by first suspending the drug particles in an aqueous solution of water-soluble polymer and then dispersing homogeneously in a lipophilic polymer, by high-shear mechanical force, to form a large number of unleachable, microscopic spheres of drug reservoirs. This thermodynamically unstable dispersion is stabilized quickly by immediately crosslinking the polymer *in situ*, which produces a medicated

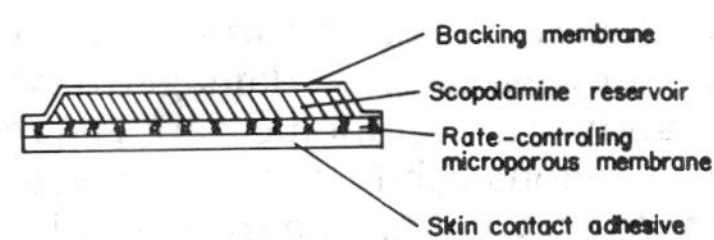

Fig 13. Schematic diagram of a transdermal device for delivery of scopolamine.

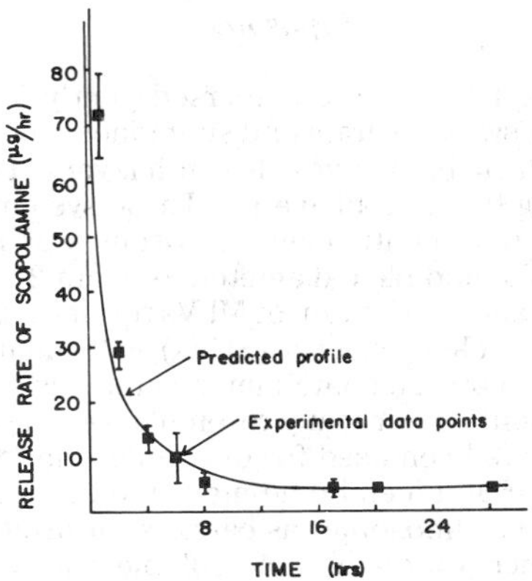

Fig 14. *In-vitro* release rate versus time profile for scopolamine from a transdermal device. (Reproduced with permission.[12])

polymer disk with a constant surface area and a fixed thickness. A transdermal therapeutic system is produced, in which the medicated disc is positioned at the center and surrounded by an adhesive rim. Example of this type of transdermal therapeutic system is the nitroglycerin-releasing system such as the Nitrodisc system (*Searle*).

Targeted Delivery Systems

Nanoparticles

Nanoparticles are one of several types of systems known collectively as colloidal drug delivery systems. Also included in this group are microcapsules, nanocapsules, macromolecular complexes, polymeric beads, microspheres and liposomes. A nanoparticle is a particle containing dispersed drug with a diameter of 200 to 500 nm. The size of a nanoparticle allows it to be administered intravenously via injection, unlike many other colloidal systems which occlude both needles and capillaries. Materials used in the preparation of nanoparticles are sterilizable, nontoxic and biodegradable; examples are albumin, ethylcellulose, casein and gelatin. They usually are prepared by a process similar to the coacervation method of microencapsulation.

There have been two main applications of nanoparticles: as carriers of medical diagnostic agents such as radioisotopic technetium-99m and fluorescein isothiocyanate, and for the delivery of liver flukicides in veterinary medicine. Radioisotopes are used to study the morphology, physiology and blood flow of various organs in the body. The liver commonly is visualized with a technetium-99m/sulfur colloid. Preparation of technetium-99m gelatin nanoparticles, and subsequent intravenous injection into mice, revealed that they are taken up rapidly by the reticuloendothelial system and localized mainly in the liver.[23] The reticuloendothelial system consists of phagocytic cells designed to cleanse the bloodstream of bacteria, viruses, cell debris and other unwanted foreign particles. The behavior of nanoparticles *in vivo* is the same as that exhibited by other colloidal systems of similar size, and points to the possibility of using nanoparticles to target drugs to the liver and phagocytic cells. The use of fluorescein isothiocyanate (FITC) was aimed at determining the availability of surface amino groups on gelatin or albumin nanoparticles. Since FITC is known to bind to amino groups, any such binding on the surface of a nanoparticle would reveal the presence of amino groups and thus their possible use as binding sites for drug molecules as well. Results indicated that free amino groups are, indeed, present on the surface of the nanoparticle.[23] In addition, preliminary work showed that FITC gelatin nanoparticles incubated with tumor cells *in vitro* are taken up by the tumor cells. This observation suggests the possible use of nanoparticles for the targeted delivery of anticancer agents to tumorous tissue.

Liposomes

When phospholipids are dispersed gently in an aqueous medium, they swell, hydrate and spontaneously form multilamellar concentric bilayer vesicles with layers of aqueous media separating the lipid bilayers. These systems commonly are referred to as multilamellar liposomes or multilamellar vesicles (MLVs) and have diameters of from 25 nm to 4 μm. Sonication or solvent dilution of MLVs results in the formation of small unilamellar vesicles (SUVs) with diameters in the range of 300 to 500 Å, containing an aqueous solution in the core. Liposomes bear many resemblances to cellular membranes and have been used for over a decade to study membrane behavior and membrane-mediated processes. It also is possible to use liposomes as carriers for drugs and macromolecules since water- or lipid-soluble substances can be entrapped in the aqueous spaces or within the bilayer itself, respectively. More recent studies have been aimed at investigating the potential of these drug-bearing liposomes for site-specific or receptor release of their active agent.

Phospholipids can form a variety of structures other than liposomes when dispersed in water, depending on the molar ratio of lipid to water. At low ratios the liposome is the preferred structure. Physical characteristics of liposomes depend on pH, ionic strength and the presence of divalent cations. They show low permeability to ionic and polar substances, including many drugs, but at elevated temperatures undergo a phase transition which markedly alters their permeability. The phase transition involves a change from a closely packed, ordered structure, known as the gel state, to a loosely packed, less-ordered structure, known as the fluid state. This occurs at a characteristic phase-transition temperature and results in an increase in permeability to ions, sugars or drugs. In addition to temperature, exposure to proteins can alter the permeability of liposomes. Certain soluble proteins such as cytochrome-C bind, deform and penetrate the bilayer, thereby causing changes in permeability. Cholesterol inhibits this penetration of proteins, apparently by packing the phospholipids more tightly; most liposome formulations used for drug delivery contain cholesterol to help form a more closely packed bilayer system during preparation. Serum high-density lipoproteins cause significant leakage in the membrane, probably due to removal of phospholipid.

The ability to trap solutes varies between different types of liposomes. For example, MLVs are moderately efficient at trapping solutes, but SUVs are extremely inefficient. SUVs offer the advantage of homogeneity and reproducibility in size distribution, however, and a compromise between size and trapping efficiency is offered by large unilamellar vesicles (LUVs). These are prepared by ether evaporation and are three to four times more efficient in terms of trapping water-soluble drug but seem to be somewhat less stable than other types of vesicles. In addition to liposome characteristics, an important determinant in drug entrapment is the physicochemical properties of the drug itself. As mentioned previously, polar drugs are trapped in the aqueous spaces and nonpolar drugs bind to the lipid bilayer of the vesicle. Polar drugs are released when the bilayer is broken, or by permeation but, nonpolar drugs remain affiliated with the bilayer unless it is disrupted by temperature or exposure to lipoproteins. Both types show maximum efflux rates at the phase transition temperature.

Liposomes can interact with cells by four different mechanisms:[24]

1. Endocytosis by phagocytic cells of the reticuloendothelial system such as macrophages and neutrophils.
2. Adsorption to the cell surface either by nonspecific weak hydrophobic or electrostatic forces, or by specific interactions with cell-surface components.
3. Fusion with the plasma cell membrane by insertion of the lipid bilayer of the liposome into the plasma membrane, with simultaneous release of liposomal contents into the cytoplasm.
4. Transfer of liposomal lipids to cellular or subcellular membranes, or *vice versa*, without any association of the liposome contents.

It often is difficult to determine which mechanism is operative and more than one may operate at the same time.

The fate and disposition of intravenously injected liposomes depend on their physical properties, such as size, fluidity and surface charge. They may persist in tissues for hours or days, depending on their composition, and half-lives in the blood range from minutes to several hours. Larger liposomes, such as MLVs and LUVs, are taken up rapidly by phagocytic cells of the reticuloendothelial system, but the physiology of the circulatory system restrains the exit of such large species at most sites. They can exit only in places where large openings or pores exist in the capillary endothelium, such as the sinusoids of the liver or spleen. Thus, these organs are the predominate site of uptake. On the other hand, SUVs show a broader tissue distribution but still are sequestered highly in the liver and spleen. In general, this *in vivo* behavior limits the potential targeting of liposomes to only those organs and tissues accessible to their large size. These include the blood, liver, spleen, bone marrow and lymphoid organs.

Attempts to overcome the limitation on targeting of liposomes have centered around two approaches. One is the use of antibodies, bound to the liposome surface, to direct the antibody and its drug contents to specific antigenic receptors located on a particular cell-type surface. A second approach is to use carbohydrate determinants as recognition sites. Carbohydrate determinants are glycoprotein or glycolipid cell-surface components that play a role in cell–cell recognition, interaction and adhesion. Although the precise mechanism of their action is still unknown, they show potential in directing liposomes to particular cell types by their inclusion in the liposomal membrane. A discussion of the factors influencing targeting of liposomes has been given by Gregoriadis *et al.*[25] Potential therapeutic applications of liposomes include their use in the treatment of malignant tumors, lysosomal storage diseases, intracellular parasites, metal toxicity and diabetes. The liposome acts as the carrier of the active agent used in treatment of these conditions. Most of the applications involve intravenous injection of the liposomal preparation, but other routes of administration are conceivable. For example, liposome-entrapped insulin may offer some degree of protection of drug from gastric degradation and the possibility of GI absorption by endocytosis. Further details of current applications of liposome-entrapped drugs can be found in the literature.[24,25]

Resealed Erythrocytes

When erythrocytes are suspended in a hypotonic medium, they swell to about one and a half times their normal size, and the membrane ruptures resulting in the formation of pores with diameters of 200 to 500 Å. The pores allow equilibration of the intracellular and extracellular solutions. If the ionic strength of the medium then is adjusted to isotonicity and the cells are incubated at 37°, the pores will close and cause the erythrocyte to "reseal." Using this technique with a drug present in the extracellular solution, it is possible to entrap up to 40% of the drug inside the resealed erythrocyte and to use this system for targeted delivery via intravenous injection. The advantages of using resealed erythrocytes as drug carriers are that they are biodegradable, fully biocompatible and nonimmunogenic, exhibit flexibility in circulation time depending on their physicochemical properties, the entrapped drug is shielded from immunologic detection and chemical modification of drug is not required.

The assessment of resealed erythrocytes for use in targeted delivery has been facilitated by studies on the behavior of normal and modified reinfused erythrocytes. In general, normal aging erythrocytes, slightly damaged erythrocytes and those coated lightly with antibodies are sequestered in the spleen after intravenous reinfusion, but heavily damaged or modified erythrocytes are removed from the circulation by the liver.[26] This suggests that resealed erythrocytes can be targeted selectively to either the liver or spleen, depending on their membrane characteristics. In addition to coating with antibodies, removal of portions of cell-surface carbohydrates reduces the circulating half-life. The ability of resealed erythrocytes to deliver drug to the liver or spleen can be viewed as a disadvantage in that other organs and tissues are inaccessible. Thus, the application of this system to targeted delivery has been limited mainly to treatment of lysosomal storage diseases and metal toxicity, where the site of drug action is in the reticuloendothelial system. A more detailed discussion of the application of resealed erythrocytes has been presented by Ihler.[27]

Immunologically Based Systems

As discussed in the section pertaining to intramuscular injections, the formation of dissociable complex of a drug with a macromolecule is a viable method of achieving a sustained-release effect. If the macromolecule used is an antibody, an antigen-specific targeted effect also can be achieved. In addition to complex formation by noncovalent forces, drugs also may be linked covalently to antibodies, provided the activity of both drug and antibody is retained or the activity of drug is recoverable after release.

Most studies of antibody–drug systems have employed covalent conjugation of the drug to the antibody. Chemical crosslinking agents are used commonly to attach a drug to an antibody by reacting with appropriate groups available on both species. Among the crosslinking agents used are carbodiimide, glutaraldehyde, bisazobenzidine, cyanuric chloride, diethylmalonimidate or various mixed anhydrides. The reaction should allow effective control of the antibody–drug conjugate size, and the crosslink must readily be broken by available lysosomal hydrolases within the receptor cell, if drug release is critical to activity.

Certain specificities expressed on tumor cells, referred to as membrane-bound tumor-associated antigens (TAAs), may be exploited for the purpose of targeting antibody–drug conjugates directly at the malignant tumor by various parenteral routes of administration. Since anticancer drugs are indiscriminate to cell type in their action, a targeted delivery system for these drugs would offer a significant improvement in cancer chemotherapy. A wide variety of antineoplastic drugs have been conjugated to tumor-specific antibodies. Three that have received the most attention are chlorambucil, adriamycin and methotrexate. The effectiveness of these systems depends on the nature of the crosslinking agent and the method of reaction. The interested reader is directed to two reviews that discuss the use of antibody–drug conjugates for treatment of tumors.[28,29]

References

1. Lee VHK, Robinson JR, Lee VHL: In Robinson JR, Lee VHL, eds: *Controlled Drug Delivery,* 2nd ed, Marcel Dekker, New York, 3, 1987.
2. Robinson JR, Eriksen SP: *J Pharm Sci 55:* 1254, 1966.
3. Welling PG, Dobrinska MR, in Robinson JR, Lee VHL, eds: *Controlled Drug Delivery,* 2nd ed, Marcel Dekker, New York, 253, 1987.
4. Flynn GL, Yalkowsky SH, Roseman T: *J Pharm Sci 63:* 479, 1974.
5. Burnette RR, in Robinson JR, Lee VHL, eds: *Controlled Drug Delivery,* 2nd ed, Marcel Dekker, New York, 95, 1987.
6. Gibaldi M, Perrier D: *Pharmacokinetics,* 2nd ed, Marcel Dekker, New York, 189, 1982.
7. Riegelman S, Loo JCK, Rowland M: *J Pharm Sci 57:* 128, 1968.
8. Wagner JG: *Am J Pharm 141:* 5, 1969.
9. Park K, Wood RW, Robinson JR, in Langer R, Wise D, eds: *Medical Applications of Controlled Release Technology,* CRC Press, Boca Raton, FL, 171, 1985.
10. Higuchi T: *J Pharm Sci 50:* 874, 1961.
11. Higuchi T: *Ibid 52:* 1145, 1963.
12. Chandrasekaran SK, Benson H, Urquhart J, in Robinson JR, ed: *Sustained and Controlled Release Drug Delivery Systems,* Marcel Dekker, New York, 557, 1978.
13. Hui HW, Robinson JR, Lee VHL: In Robinson JR, Lee VHL, eds: *Controlled Drug Delivery,* 2nd ed, Marcel Dekker, New York, 373, 1987.
14. Buckwalter R, Dickinson J: *JAPhA 47:* 661, 1958.
15. Hussain MA *et al: Drug Dev Ind Pharm 17:* 67, 1991.
16. *Physician's Desk Reference,* 48th ed, Medical Economics, Oradell, NJ 1994.
17. Higuchi WI: *J Pharm Sci 53:* 405, 1964.
18. Windheuser JL, Best ML, Perrin JH: *Bull Parenter Drug Assoc 24:* 286, 1970.
19. Brodin AF, Kavaliunas DR, Frank SG: *Acta Pharm Suec 15:* 1, 1978.
20. Chien YW: In Chien YW, ed: *Novel Drug Delivery Systems,* 2nd ed, Marcel Dekker, New York, 1, 1992.
21. *Ibid:* 43, 1992.
22. Hsieh DST, Smith N, Chien YW: In Meyers WE, Dunn RL, eds: *Proceeding of 11th International Symposium on Controlled Release of Bioactive Materials,* The Controlled Release Society, Chicago, 134, 1984.
23. Oppenheim RC: *J Steroid Biochem 6:* 182, 1975.
24. Juliano RL, Layton D: *Ibid:* 200, 1980.
25. Gregoriadis G *et al:* In Gregoriadis C, Senior J, Trout A, eds: *Targeting of Drugs,* Plenum, New York, 155, 1982.
26. Cooper RA: In William WJ *et al,* eds: *Hematology,* 2nd ed, McGraw-Hill, New York, 216, 1977.
27. Ihler G: In Gregoriadis C, ed: *Drug Carriers in Biology and Medicine,* Academic, London, 129, 1979.
28. Arnon R: In Spreafics F, Arnon R, eds: *Tumor-Associated Antigens and Their Specific Immune Response,* Academic, New York, 287, 1979.
29. O'Neill GJ: In Gregoriadis G, ed: *Drug Carriers in Biology and Medicine,* Academic, London, 23, 1979.

CHAPTER 95

Aerosols

John J Sciarra, PhD
Professor Emeritus and President
Sciarra Laboratories, Inc.
Hicksville, NY 11801

Many therapeutically active ingredients have been administered or applied to the body by means of the aerosol dosage form. This dosage form has been used both orally and topically to dispense a variety of agents such as epinephrine bitartrate and hydrochloride, isoproterenol hydrochloride, albuterol, metaproterenol sulfate, cromolyn sodium, flunisolide, ipratropium bromide, bitolterol mesylate, isoetharine mesylate, beclomethasone dipropionate, dexamethasone sodium phosphate, triamcinolone acetonide, fluinosolide and ergotamine tartrate. Oral aerosols have been used for the symptomatic treatment of asthma as well as for the treatment of migraine headache, while topical aerosols have been used to treat a multitude of dermatological manifestations. From preparations for the treatment of acne to a simple first-aid preparation, aerosols have been accepted readily by both the patient and physician as advantageous dosage forms.

Advantages—One of the main reasons for the rapid and widespread acceptance of the aerosol dosage form for the administration of therapeutically active agents is that it affords many and distinct advantages to the user. These advantages have been described by various investigators and, for metered-dose inhalers, include

Rapid onset of action.
Circumvention of the first-pass effect.
Avoidance of degradation in the gastrointestinal tract.
Lower dosage which will minimize adverse reactions.
Dose titration to individual needs and ideal for prn medication.
Alternate route when therapeutic agent may interact chemically or physically with other medicinals needed concurrently.
Viable alternative when the drug entity exhibits erratic pharmacokinetics upon oral or parenteral administration.

The pressure package is convenient and easy to use. Medication is dispensed in a ready-to-use form at the push of a button. There is generally no need for further handling of the medication. Since the medication is sealed in a tamper-proof pressure container, there is no danger of contamination of the product with foreign materials, and at the same time the contents can be protected from the deleterious effects of both air and moisture. Easily decomposed drugs, such as epinephrine, lend themselves to this type of package. When one considers the danger of contamination of unused topical, ophthalmic, ear, nose and throat preparations, the importance of this advantage is obvious. Sterility is always an important consideration with certain pharmaceutical and medicinal preparations. While initial sterility is generally no problem to the manufacturer, there is concern for the maintenance of the sterility of the package during use as, for example, in ophthalmic preparations. When necessary, the aerosol package can be prepared under sterile conditions and sterility maintained throughout the life of the product. For those products requiring regulation of dosage, a metering valve can be used. An accurately measured dose of therapeutically active drug can be administered quickly and, in the case of drugs for inhalation or nasal application, in the proper particle-size range. When used with topical preparations, indiscriminate use and overuse of the product can be avoided. In addition, when used with expensive products, such as some steriods and antibiotics, savings can be achieved by the user as compared to the use of other topical preparations such as ointments, creams or lotions. The aerosol dosage form allows for the dispensing of the product in the most desirable form; spray, foam or semisolid. Depending on the nature of the product, the characteristics of the spray or foam can be changed to insure the proper and most efficient use of the medication.

Topical aerosol preparations are available as local anesthetics, antiseptics, germicides, first-aid preparations, body rubs, dermatologic products, foot preparations and spray-on protective films. These preparations have met with widespread acceptance, chiefly due to their many advantages over nonaerosol products. In addition to the advantages found in all aerosols, these aerosols possess several distinct advantages of their own.

The irritation produced by the application of an ointment or cream over an abraded area of the skin is reduced and sometimes eliminated by the aerosol. These preparations are more economical since they easily can be applied in a thin layer with no waste by the use of a cotton swab or other applicators. This may result in faster absorption and more efficient use of medications. Since the package is sealed, there is no danger of contamination of the unused portion of the medication. The cooling effect of liquefied-gas aerosols may be desirable in certain skin conditions.

There are many advantages to the administration of medicinal agents by inhalation and nasally. Response to drugs administered by inhalation and nasally is prompt, often very specific and with minimal side effects, faster in onset of activity compared with response to drugs given orally and, with most drugs, approaches intravenous therapy in rapidity of action. Drugs that normally are decomposed in the gastrointestinal tract can be administered safely by inhalation and nasally. The use of the self-pressurized aerosol package makes this type of therapy simple, convenient and acceptable compared to the use of atomizers and nebulizers, which are bulky and require cleaning.

Many drugs, such as insulin and other proteins and the high technology drugs, are being investigated for applications as a nasal aerosol using a metered-dose valve. A uniform particle size can be obtained using a liquified gas propellant, and in the case of aqueous solutions, using a specifically designed pump type valve, and a more recently, a barrier-type system with either a compressed or liquidifed gas.

Definitions—The term "aerosol" is used to denote various systems ranging from those of a colloidal nature to systems consisting of "pressurized packages." Aerosols have been defined as colloidal systems consisting of very finely subdivided liquid or solid particles dispersed in and surrounded by a gas. Originally, the term aerosol referred to liquid or solid particles having a specific size range, but this concept is falling into disuse.

The present-day definition refers to those products which depend upon the power of a liquefied or compressed gas to dispense the active ingredient(s) in a finely dispersed mist, foam or semisolid. Pump systems which also dispense the active ingredient(s) in the form of a finely dispersed mist (although of greater particle size) often are classified as aerosols. These pump systems generally are used to dispense medication intranasally.

An area of development essential to the success of the aerosol package concerned the valve. Various valves were produced that would dispense the product in the form of a fine stream, a fine mist, a coarse spray or solid stream. Especially important are the metered valves that are essential for medicinal aerosols. These valves make it possible to dispense quantities of aerosol ranging from about 25 to 150 μL.

In 1978 the use of certain chlorofluorocarbons was curtailed seriously by the FDA, Environmental Protection Agency and the Consumer Products Safety Commission. These restrictions applied to the use of Propellants 11, 12 and 114. Because of these restrictions, new valve systems and dispensing systems, which allowed greater use of liquefied hydrocarbons and compressed gases, were developed.

Medicinal aerosols are exempted from the ban on propellants 11, 12 and 114. These propellants still can be used for medicinal aerosols taken by inhalation, nasally and orally. While certain pharmaceuticals currently are exempted, such as contraceptive vaginal foams, metered-dose inhalation devices, gauze bandage adhesives and adhesive removers, other drugs used by inhalation and or nasally can be approved upon petition to the FDA for an exemption. At present, propellants 11, 12, and 114 are the only ones acceptable to the FDA for metered-dose inhalers. Several non-CFC propellants have been used with medicinal agents and are currently under clinical study. Possible alternative propellants will be discussed.

Mode of Operation

Liquefied-Gas Systems

Liquefied gases have been used widely as propellants for most aerosol products. These compounds are useful for this purpose since they are gases at room temperature and atmospheric pressure. However, they can be liquefied easily by lowering the temperature (below the boiling point) or by increasing the pressure. The compounds chosen generally have boiling points below 70°F (21°C) and vapor pressures between 13.4 and 135 psia at 70°F (21°C). When a liquefied gas propellant is placed into a sealed container, it immediately separates into a liquid and a vapor phase.

Since these materials are liquefied gases, some of the molecules will leave the liquid state and enter the vapor state. As molecules enter the vapor state, a pressure gradually develops. As the number of molecules in the vapor state increases, the pressure also will increase. An equilibrium soon is attained between the number of molecules changing from a liquid to a vapor and from a vapor to a liquid. The pressure at this point is referred to as the vapor pressure (expressed as psia) and is characteristic for each propellant at any given temperature. The term psig (pounds/square inch gauge) represents the uncorrected gauge pressure and is to be distinguished from psia (pounds per square inch absolute) that is corrected to include atmospheric pressure (0 psig which equals 14.7 psia). This vapor pressure is exerted equally in all directions and is independent of the quantity present.

The pressure exerted against the liquid phase is sufficient to push the latter up a dip tube and against the valve. When the valve is opened, the liquid phase is emitted and comes into contact with the warm air at atmospheric pressure. The liquid propellant immediately reverts to the vapor state since its boiling point is substantially below room temperature. As the contents of the container are expelled, the volume within the container occupied by the vaporized propellant increases causing a temporary fall in pressure. However, as soon as the pressure decreases, a sufficient number of molecules change from the liquid state to the vapor state and restore the original pressure. When a compressed gas is used as the propellant, the relationship is quite different and there is a drop in pressure as the contents are used.

Two-Phase System—This is the simplest of all aerosol systems. It consists of a solution or a suspension of active ingredients in liquid propellant or a mixture of liquid propellant and solvent. Both a liquid and vapor phase are present and, when the valve is depressed, liquid propellant containing dissolved active ingredients and other solvents is released. Depending on the nature of the propellants used, the quantity of propellant present and the valve mechanism, a fine mist or wet spray is produced due to the large expansion of the propellant at room temperature and atmospheric pressure. This system is used to formulate aerosols for inhalation or nasal application.

Fluorocarbon propellants, primarily trichloromonofluoromethane (11), dichlorodifluoro methane (12) and dichlorotetrafluoroethane (114), can be used for oral, nasal and inhalation aerosols provided that an exemption is applied for through the filing of a New Drug Application for all new products and a supplemental application for existing products. All other solution- or suspension-type aerosols must use other fluorocarbon propellants which environmentally are acceptable, a hydrocarbon propellant or a compressed gas. The section dealing with propellants indicates those which are useful for this purpose.

A *space spray* generally contains from 2 to 20% active ingredients and from 80 to 98% propellant. While the pressure of space sprays is in the range of 30 to 40 psig, the particles which are produced are from less than 1 to 50 μm. These particles remain suspended in air for relatively long periods of time. Space insecticides, room deodorants and vaporizer sprays are examples of this type of system.

A *surface-coating spray* (a relatively wet or coarse spray) can be achieved by decreasing the amount of low-boiling propellants and increasing the ratio of active ingredients and solvents. The product concentrate can vary from 20 to 75% and the propellant from 25 to 80%. Particles are produced ranging in size from 50 μm to 200 μm. Products such as hair sprays, residual insecticides, perfumes, colognes, paints, protective coatings and topical sprays are formulated in this manner. The pressure of this system is generally lower than the space spray.

Figure 1 shows a cross section of a typical space or surface-coating aerosol spray.

The propellants widely used for these aerosol systems include those shown in Tables 1 and 2. Combinations of these

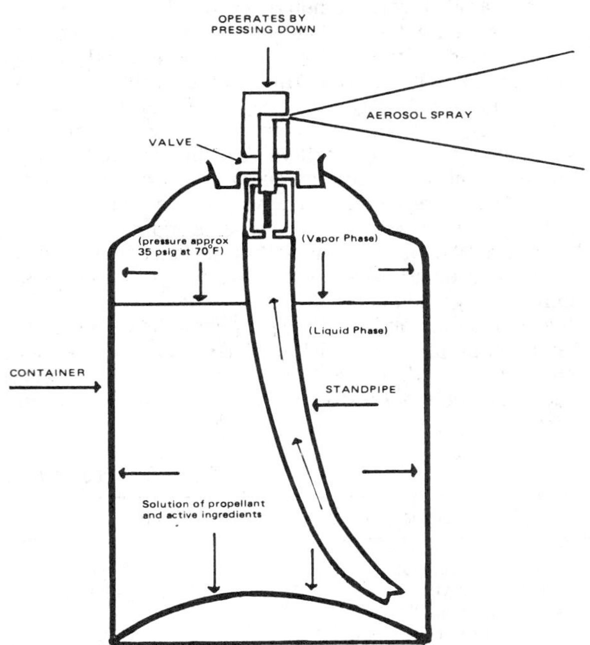

Fig 1. Cross section of a typical space or surface-coating aerosol spray.

Table 1—Properties of Fluorocarbons

Property		Trichloro-monofluoro-methane	Dichloro-difluoro-methane	Dichloro-tetrafluoro-ethane	Difluoro-ethane	Monochloro-diflouro-methane	Monochloro-difluoro-ethane
Molecular formula		CCl_3F	CCl_2F_2	$CClF_2CClF_2$	CH_3CHF_2	$CHClF_2$	CH_3CClF_2
Numerical designation		11	12	114	152a	22	142b
Molecular weight		137.28	120.93	170.93	66.1	86.5	100.5
Boiling point (1 atm)	°F	74.7	−21.6	38.39	−12.0	−41.4	14.4
	°C	23.7	−29.8	3.55	−11.0	−40.8	−9.7
Vapor pressure (psia)	70°F	13.4	84.9	27.6	63.0	−135.7	43.7
	130°F	39.0	196.0	73.5	176.3	355.4	111.7
Liquid density (g/mL)	70°F	1.485	1.325	1.468	0.91	1.21	1.12
	130°C	1.403	1.191	1.360	—	—	—
Solubility in water (weight %)	77°F	0.11	0.028	0.013	< 1.0%	3.0	0.5

propellants are used to achieve the desired results as to spray characteristics. In certain instances the nature of the product will determine the propellant combination. Dispersion or suspension sprays used for metered-dose inhalers are similar to space and surface coating sprays in that they are two-phase systems where the active ingredients are suspended, rather than dissolved, in the liquid phase. At the present time Propellants 12/11, 12/114 and 12/114/11 are used for these inhalation aerosols. Table 3 indicates various trademarks used to identify these propellants.

Three-Phase System—This system is useful in that it allows for a greater use of liquid components not miscible with the propellants. Water is not miscible with liquefied-gas propellants and, in many instances, presents a problem since active ingredients are soluble in water. With the increased emphasis upon the decrease of volatile organic compounds (VOCs) in all products, these systems are finding increased use. These problems have been overcome to a large extent by use of the three-phase system. Depending on the nature of the formulation, one of the following two systems may be employed.

Two-Layer System—In this system the liquid propellant, the vaporized propellant and the aqueous solution of active ingredients make up the three phases. Since the liquid propellant and water are not miscible, the liquid propellant will separate as an immiscible layer. When a hydroalcohol mixture is used, the propellant and hydroalcohol solution will mix and form a single layer. When this propellant is of the fluorocarbon type, being denser than water, it will fall to the bottom of the container. Hydrocarbons, on the other hand, are lighter than water and, when used in this manner, will float on top of the aqueous layer. A typical three-phase aerosol system is shown in Fig 2. A spray is produced by the mechanical action of an exceedingly small-valve orifice through which the liquid and some vaporized propellant is forced by the vapor pressure of the propellant. The vapor layer is replaced continuously by vapors from the liquid layer of propellant.

An important characteristic of this system is that the propellant layer can be adjusted by varying the components so its specific gravity is almost equal to, but does not exceed that of the hydroalcoholic phase. The propellant floats on top of the hydroalcoholic phase and, when shaken, is dispersed easily. When the valve is depressed, sprays are produced of varying characteristics depending on the nature of the formulation.

Figure 2 illustrates a dispenser system which is an example of a water-based system. This system is designed to dispense pressurized products efficiently and economically using relatively small amounts of hydrocarbon or fluorocarbon propellants.

In this system the vapor phase of the propellant and the product enter the mixing chamber in the actuator through separate ducts or channels. The vaporized propellant enters, moving at tremendous velocity, while the product is forced into the actuator by the pressure of the propellant. It is at this point that product and vapor are mixed with violent force, resulting in a uniform, finely dispersed spray. Depending on the configuration of the valve and actuator either a fine dry or a wet spray can be obtained.

Water-based aerosols developed for use in this system would have the advantage that the chilling effect associated with liquefied gas systems is eliminated. Since only vaporized propellant is dispensed, less propellant is required in the container. With greater use of water as a solvent for active ingredients a greater range of products can be developed. Because the use of volatile organic compounds (VOCs) is now being curtailed, water is being used, when possible, as an alternative to some solvents such as alcohol.

Foam System—Foam aerosols, which often are classified separately, consist of three-phase systems wherein the liquid propellant, which normally does not exceed 10% by weight, is emulsified with the propellant. When the valve is depressed, the emulsion is forced through the nozzle and, in the presence of warm air and at atmospheric pressure, the entrapped propellant reverts to a vapor and whips the emulsion into a foam. The use of a dip tube is optional with this type of system and, when present, the container is designed for upright use. For those containers where the dip-tube is omitted, the container must be inverted prior to use. Foam valves have been developed which are applicable to both types of packages. Foam products operate at a pressure of about 40 to 50 psig at 70°F (21°C) and generally contain about 4 to 7% propellant. A typical foam-type aerosol can be seen in Fig 3. Shave creams and shampoos, as well as several topical pharmaceuticals, have been formulated as foam aerosols. Generally, a blend of propane/isobutane is used for foam aerosols. Depending on the formulation, some aerosols use nitrous oxide, carbon dioxide or a mixture of both as the propellant. Con-

Table 2—Properties of Hydrocarbons and Ethers

Property	Propane	Isobutane	n-Butane	Dimethyl ether
Molecular formula	C_3H_8	C_4H_{10}	C_4H_{10}	CH_3OCH_3
Molecular weight	44.1	58.1	58.1	46.1
Boiling point (°F)	−43.7	10.9	31.1	−13
Vapor pressure (psig at 70°F)	110.0	30.4	16.5	63.0
Liquid density (g/mL at 70°F)	0.50	0.56	0.58	0.66
Flash point (°F)	−156	−117	−101	—

Table 3—Trademarks For Propellants

Trademark	Company	Trademark	Company
Freon	Dupont	*Phillips*	Phillips
Dymel	Dupont	*Aeron*	Diversified
Genetron	Allied Signal	*Aeropres (Aeropin)*	Aeropres
		TPI	Technical Propellant,Inc

traceptive foam aerosols are exempt from the ban on fluorocarbons and use 12/114 as the propellant.

Compressed-Gas Aerosols

Aerosols using compressed gases as the propellant are finding increased use. These propellants, especially air, nitrogen and nitrous oxide, are environmentally acceptable. Carbon dioxide also is used. While it is considered to be a *greenhouse* gas, its use has been somewhat curtailed even though its use in aerosols is very small.

Compressed gases are used to dispense the product as a solid stream, wet spray or foam. These aerosol products utilize an inert gas such as nitrogen, carbon dioxide or nitrous oxide as the propellant. The gas is compressed in the container, and it is the expansion of the compressed gas which provides the push or the force necessary to expel the contents from the container. As the contents of the container are expelled, the volume of the gas will increase causing a drop in pressure according to Boyle's law. This enables one to calculate the drop in pressure as the contents of a compressed-gas aerosol are used. Table 4 indicates some of the more important properties of these compressed gases.

Depending upon the nature of the formulation and the type of compressed gas used, the product may be dispensed as a semisolid, foam or spray.

Semisolid Dispensing—The concentrate generally is semisolid in nature and, since the gas is insoluble and immiscible with the concentrate, the product is dispensed in its original form. This system is applicable to the dispensing of dental creams, hair dressings, ointments, creams, cosmetic creams, foods and other products. Compressed-gas aerosols operate at a substantially higher initial pressure of 90 to 100 psig at 70°F (21°C). This pressure is necessary to insure adequate pressure for the dispensing of most of the contents from the container. The amount of product retained in the unit after exhaustion of the pressure varies with the viscosity of the product and loss of pressure due to seepage of gas during storage. Since the concentrate generally is semisolid in nature and the dispensing characteristics depend largely on the viscosity of the product and the pressure within the container, the viscosity of the product concentrate must be adjusted accordingly.

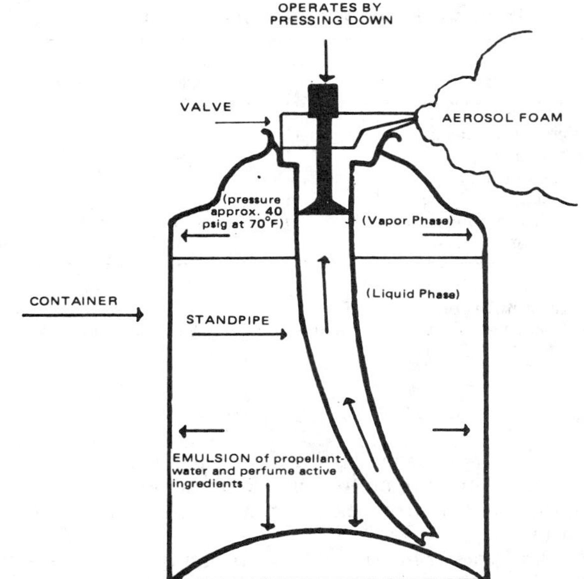

Fig 3. Foam-type aerosol.

Foam Dispensing—Soluble compressed gases such as nitrous oxide and carbon dioxide can be used to produce a foam when used with emulsion products. This system is typical for whipped creams and toppings, and several pharmaceutical and veterinary products. When this system is used, the gas dissolved in the concentrate will be evolved and cause a whipping of the emulsion into a foam. In order to facilitate the formation of a foam this system is shaken prior to use, in order to disperse some of the gas throughout the product concentrate.

Spray Dispensing—This system is similar to a space or surface spray except that a compressed gas is used as the propellant. Since these gases do not possess the dispersing power of the liquefied gases, a mechanical breakup actuator is used. The product is dispensed as a wet spray and is applicable to solutions of medicinal agents in aqueous solvents.

Another application for this type of system is found in the *contact lens saline solutions*. These consist of a normal saline solution packaged in an aluminum aerosol container and pressurized with nitrogen. Since these solutions may come in contact with the eye, they are sterilized using cobalt-60 gamma irradiation.

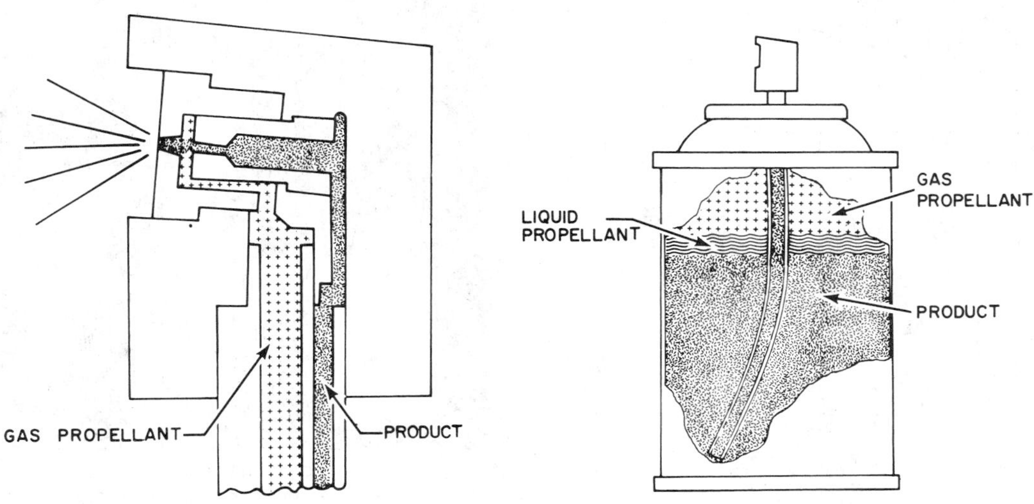

Fig 2. The Aquasol dispenser system (courtesy, Precision Valve).

Table 4—Properties of Compressed Gases

Property	Carbon dioxide	Nitrous oxide	Nitrogen
Molecular formula	CO_2	N_2O	N_2
Molecular weight	44	44	28
Boiling point °F	−109[a]	−127	−320
Vapor pressure, psia, 70°F	852	735	492[b]
Solubility in water,[c] 77°F	0.7	0.5	0.014
Density (gas) g/mL.	1.53	1.53	0.96699

[a]Sublimes
[b]At the critical point (−233°F).
[c]Volume of gas at atmospheric pressure soluble in one volume of water.

Barrier Type Systems

These systems separate the propellant from the product itself. The pressure on the outside of the *barrier* serves to push the contents from the container. The following types are available.

Piston Type—Since it is difficult to empty the contents of a semisolid from an aerosol container completely, a piston-type aerosol system has been developed. This utilizes a polyethylene piston fitted into an aluminum container. The concentrate is placed into the upper portion of the container. The pressure from nitrogen (about 90 to 100 psig), or a liquefied hydrocarbon gas, pushes against the other side of the piston and, when the valve is opened, the product is dispensed. The piston scrapes against the sides of the container and dispenses most of the product concentrate.

The piston-type aerosol system is shown in Fig 4. This system has been used successfully to package cheese spreads, cake decorating icings and ointments. Since the products which use this system are semisolid and viscous, they are dispensed as a lazy stream rather than as a foam or spray. This system is limited to viscous materials since limpid liquids, such as water or alcohol, will pass between the wall of the container and the piston.

Plastic-Bag Type—This system consists of a collapsible plastic bag fitted into a standard, three-piece, tinplate container as shown in Fig 5. The product is placed within the bag and the propellant is added through the bottom of the container. Since the product is placed into a plastic bag, there is no contact between the product and the container wall except for any product which may escape by permeation through the plastic bag.

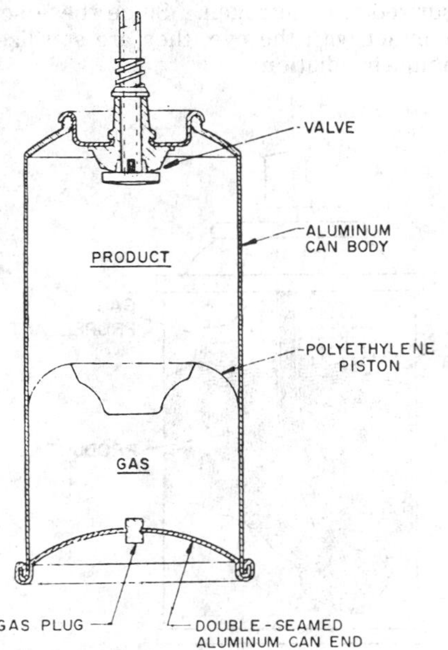

Fig 4. Free-piston aerosol system.

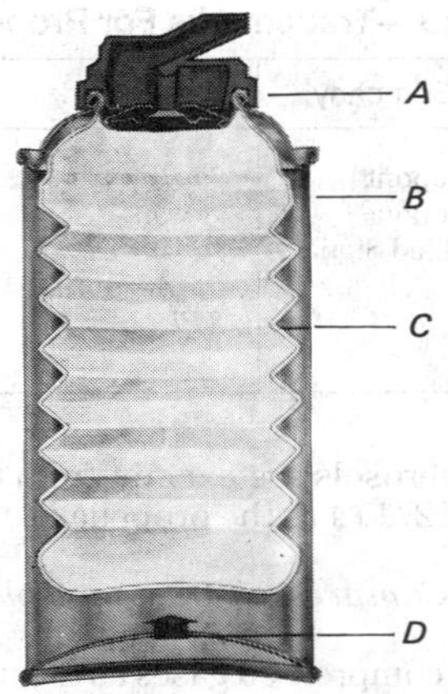

Fig 5. Plastic-bag aerosol system: *A:* valve; *B:* standard three-piece tin-plate container; *C:* plastic bag; *D:* gas filling port.

Limpid liquids, such as water, can be dispensed either as a stream or fine mist depending on the type of valve used, while semisolid substances are dispensed as a stream. In order to prevent the gas from pinching the bag and preventing the dispensing of product, the inner plastic bag is accordion-pleated. This system can be used for a variety of different pharmaceutical and nonpharmaceutical systems, including topical pharmaceutical products as a cream, ointment or gel.

A modification of this system dispenses the product as a gel which will then foam. By dissolving a low-boiling liquid such as isopentane or pentane in the product, a foam will result when the product is placed on the hands and the warmth of the hands will cause vaporization of the solvent. This system, as well as the piston system, is used in post-foaming shave gels.

Can-in-Can Systems—Figure 6 illustrates a system consisting of an aluminum can into which an aluminum thin-walled can has been inserted. This inner can is glued to the outer can and forms a gas-tight seal. Then, the neck of the can is fabricated. The propellant (any acceptable type) is added through a small opening in the bottom of the can which

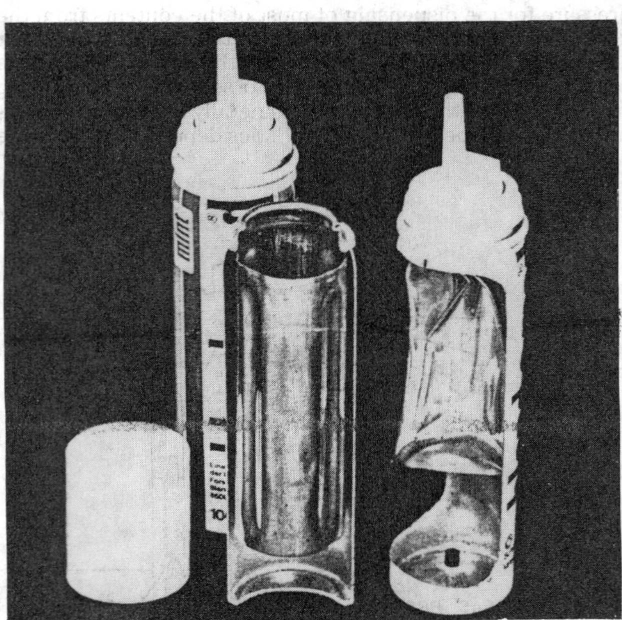

Fig 6. Cross section of the Lechner barrier pack. It consists of a rigid or flexible inner bag which can be evacuated over 95% depending upon the viscosity of the product (courtesy, Lechner GMBH).

is sealed with a rubber plug. A recent addition to this system includes replacement of the inner aluminum pouch with an inner plastic bag made of organic polymers. Sufficient space remains between this bag and the walls and the bottom of the outer container to accommodate sufficient propellant to completely evacuate the product.

Another such system is essentially the same except that the inner aluminum can is supplied separately from the outer can. This allows for insertion of liquified gas prior to adding the inner can (filled with product) and crimping the valve in place. Figure 7 shows this system. Systems illustrated by Figs. 6 and 7 have been suggested for use with a variable-dose valve for dispensing nasal aerosols containing aqueous solutions of insulin.

Other variations of these systems include using a sealed laminate pouch, which is placed into an outer aluminum can. The product is injected into the pouch, and compressed air is added either through a special opening in the valve or by using the under-the-cup method of gassing. Another system includes filling the product into a latex bag which then expands. The energy caused by the *stressed bag* will release the product when the valve is opened.

Propellants

The propellant generally is regarded as the "heart" of the aerosol package. In addition to supplying the necessary force to expel the product, the propellant must also act as a solvent and diluent and has much to do with determining the characteristics of the product as it leaves the container. Various chemical compounds have been used as aerosol propellants.

Compounds useful as propellants can be classified as

- Liquefied gases
  - Fluorinated chlorinated hydrocarbons (halocarbons)
  - Hydrochlorofluorocarbons
  - Hydrochlorocarbons
  - Hydrocarbons
  - Hydrocarbon Ethers
- Compressed gases

Liquefied Gases

The liquefied gas compounds have widespread use as propellants since they are extremely effective in dispersing the active ingredients into a fine mist or foam, depending on the form desired. In addition, they are relatively inert and nontoxic. They have the added advantage that the pressure within the container remains constant. Two types of liquefied gases are used. The fluorinated hydrocarbons find greater use since they are nonflammable as contrasted to the flammable hydrocarbons. The hydrocarbons are advantageous since they are less expensive than fluorocarbons and, generally, are environmentally acceptable.

Chlorofluorocarbons (CFCs) can be used for the following exempted products:

- Metered-dose steroid drugs for nasal inhalation.
- Metered-dose steroid drugs for oral inhalation.
- Metered-dose adrenergic bronchodilator drugs for oral inhalation.
- Contraceptive vaginal foams.
- Metered-dose ergotamine tartrate drug products administered by oral inhalation.
- Certain topical pharmaceutical aerosols containing antibiotics.

These pharmaceutical aerosols include metered-dose inhalers (MDIs) which can be formulated using the chlorofluorocarbons 11, 12, and 114.

Liquefied gases provide a nearly constant pressure during packaging operations and have a large expansion ratio. Several of the fluorinated hydrocarbons have an expansion ratio of about 240, that is, 1 mL of liquefied gas will occupy a volume of approximately 240 mL if allowed to vaporize.

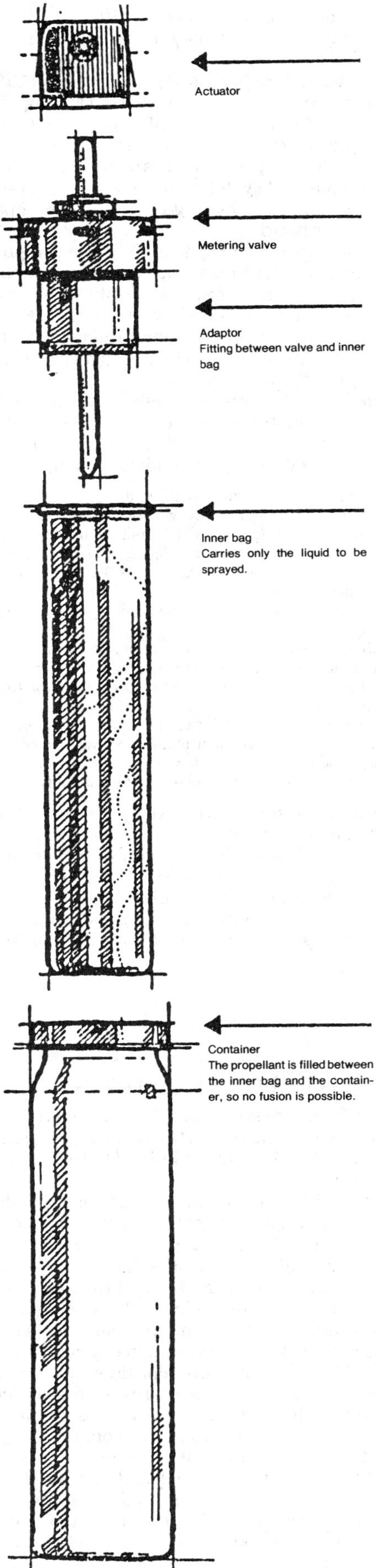

Fig 7. Metered-dose barrier package designed for delivering small quantities of liquids or viscous liquids, creams and ointments.

Dimethyl ether has a value of over 350. On the other hand, compressed gases expand only to the extent of 3 to 10 times the original volume.

Chlorinated-Fluorinated Hydrocarbons (CFCs)—Several of the fluorocarbons have been used as propellants in the past and since 1978 have been of limited use only in specifically exempted metered-dose inhalers and contraceptive vaginal foams. These propellants are derived primarily from methane, ethane and cyclobutane and are prepared by replacing one or more of the hydrogens of these compounds with chlorine and/or fluorine.

The physicochemical properties of these compounds are of prime importance in the formulation and manufacture of aerosol products. The solvent power, stability and reactivity of the propellants must be known and understood. Just as one considers the properties of some of the usually encountered nonaerosol liquids such as ethanol, glycerin or acetone, so should the propellant be considered.

Nomenclature—In order to refer easily to the fluorinated hydrocarbons a relatively simple system of nomenclature was developed some time ago by the refrigeration industry. A numerical designation is used to identify each propellant.

All propellants are designated by three digits. When the first digit is zero, the propellant is designated by two digits.

The first digit is one less than the number of carbon atoms in the compound. Where there are only 2 digits, zero is understood to be this figure and indicates a methane derivative (1 + 0). When this digit is 1, the propellant is an ethane derivative.

The second digit is one more than the number of hydrogen atoms in the compound.

The last digit represents the number of fluorine atoms.

The number of chlorine atoms in the compound is found by subtracting the sum of the fluorine and the hydrogen atoms from the total number of atoms which can be added to saturate the carbon chain.

In the case of isomers, each has the same number and the most symmetric one is indicated by the number alone. As the isomers become more and more asymmetric, the letter a, b, c, etc, follows the number.

For cyclic compounds, a C is used before the number.

The use of this system can be exemplified as follows: Propellant 114 is an ethane derivative, has no hydrogens and contains 4 fluorine atoms. Since 6 atoms are required to saturate the carbon chain, of necessity there must be 2 chlorine atoms. These can be arranged in two different ways; however, since there is no letter following the numerical designation, the symmetrical structure refers to Propellant 114.

```
     F    F              F    F
     |    |              |    |
F—C—C—F        Cl—C—C—F
     |    |              |    |
    Cl   Cl             Cl   F
```

Propellant 114 **Propellant 114a**

Physical Properties—Table 1 shows some of the more useful physicochemical properties of these propellants. Propellants 11, 12 and 114 were admitted to the USP/NF and the British Pharmacopoeia.

From a solubility standpoint, the fluorinated hydrocarbons, which are nonpolar, are miscible with most nonpolar solvents over a wide range of temperature. They also are capable of dissolving many substances. For the most part the propellants are not miscible with water, although the degree of miscibility depends on the individual propellants. A cosolvent such as ethanol, 2-propanol, dimethyl ether or acetone must be used when water is present in order to produce a clear solution. However, when one considers that these propellants are used for metered-dose aerosols, the choice of cosolvent is extremely limited and in many cases, to the use of ethyl alcohol. The alternative is to form an emulsion.

One of the most important physicochemical properties of a propellant is its vapor pressure, which may be defined as the pressure exerted by a liquid in equilibrium with its vapor. When the vapor pressure exceeds atmospheric pressure, boiling and vaporization take place. However, if the vaporized molecules are prevented from leaving the container (by placing the propellant into a sealed container), they will fill the head space and eventually cause an increase in pressure. The pressure developed at equilibrium is the vapor pressure. The vapor pressure of a liquefied gas is independent of the quantity used but is influenced by temperature changes. Assuming ideal behavior for the liquefied gas, the effect of temperature on the vapor pressure can be calculated from

$$\log P = -\frac{\Delta H_{vap}}{2.303\,RT}$$

where P = vapor pressure, ΔH = heat of vaporization, R = gas constant (generally 1.987 cal deg^{-1} mole^{-1}) and T = absolute temperature.

Since

$$\ln P = -\frac{\Delta H_{vap}}{RT} + C$$

a plot of the log P versus $1/T$ should yield a straight line and from this the heat of vaporization may be calculated.

$$\Delta H_{vap}(\text{cal mole}^{-1}) = -(\text{slope})(2.303\,R)$$

These equations can be used to predict the behavior of pure propellants at elevated temperatures. When one considers that an aerosol preparation consists of a propellant and solvents or mixtures of these, the vapor-pressure considerations are somewhat different. By mixing various propellants such as Propellants 11 and 12 or Propellants 12 and 114, a range of vapor pressures is obtained as seen in Fig 8. The vapor pressure of a mixture of propellants may be calculated from Raoult's law, which states that the "vapor pressure of a solution is dependent upon the vapor pressure of the individual components. For ideal solutions, the vapor pressure is equal to the sum of the mole fractions of each component present times the vapor pressure of the pure compound at the desired temperature." Mathematically, this law may be expressed as

$$p_A = \frac{n_A}{n_A + n_B} p_A{}^\circ = N_A p_A{}^\circ$$

where p_A = partial vapor pressure of Component A, $p_A{}^\circ$ = vapor pressure of pure Component A, n_A = moles of Component A, n_B = moles of Component B and N_A = mole fraction of Component A.

$$p_B = \frac{n_B}{n_B + n_A} p_B{}^\circ = N_B p_B{}^\circ$$

The total vapor pressure of the system is obtained by

$$P_{total} = p_A + p_B$$

When the mole fraction of one component is large, the other component has a small mole fraction and, as such, it does not appreciably affect the vapor pressure. This system approaches ideal behavior.

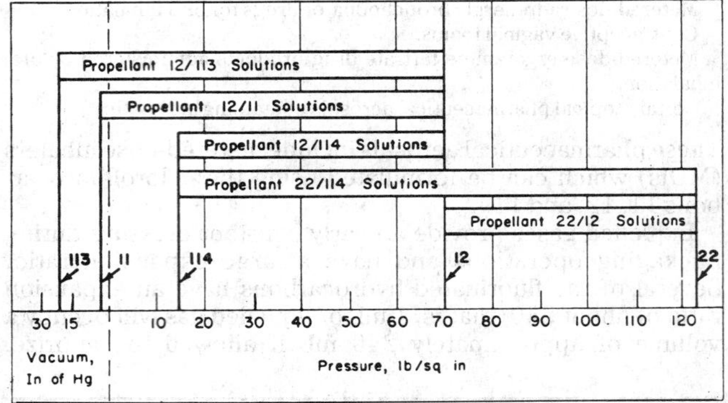

Fig 8. Range of pressures obtainable at 70°F with various propellants.

Where the components are of similar physical and chemical nature, the experimentally determined values and the calculated values are approximately the same. In the case of the fluorinated hydrocarbons, the deviation from ideal behavior is not great and the results are equal approximately or within 5%. Where other solvents are present, such as alcohols or acetone, the vapor pressures can be calculated in a similar manner. However, the vapor pressure of mixtures of these solvents and propellants deviates a great deal from ideal behavior and there is significant difference between the actual and theoretical values. The vapor pressure of many systems consisting of mixtures of various propellants and solvents has been determined. Four factors contribute to any positive deviation.

1. Internal pressure of the two components in the propellant-solvent mixture.
2. Polarity.
3. Length of the hydrocarbon chain or analogous grouping.
4. Association in the liquid phase of either component.

Chemical Properties—The fluorinated hydrocarbons have been used widely as aerosol propellants because they generally are considered to be chemically inert. From the standpoint of formulation, the only chemical property that need be considered is hydrolysis. While addition of fluorine to a carbon atom generally increases stability, a propellant such as trichloromonofluoromethane may undergo hydrolysis with the formation of hydrochloric acid. Propellant 11 is not used with aqueous products as hydrolysis will occur; Propellant 114 generally is used instead. For topical and cosmetic aerosols, hydrochlorocarbons, hydrofluorocarbons or hydrochlorofluorocarbons are used (Propellants 142a, 152b or 22).

Hydrocarbons—Hydrocarbon propellants have replaced fluorocarbons for topical pharmaceutical aerosols. Their low-order toxicity makes them suitable, while their flammability tends to limit their use. With the development of newer types of dispensing valves, the flammability hazard has been reduced considerably. The advantage of hydrocarbons is their greater range of solubility and lower cost compared to fluorinated hydrocarbons. To date they represent a readily available replacement for fluorocarbons as propellants provided that the flammability hazard can be reduced by using various combinations of fluorocarbons, hydrocarbons and a vapor-tap valve.

In addition to having the proper vapor pressure, hydrocarbons have other properties that make them useful as propellants. Their density of less than 1, and their immiscibility with water, make them useful in the formulation of three-phase (two-layer) aerosols. Being lighter than water, the hydrocarbon remains on top of the aqueous layer and serves to push the contents out of the container. Not being halogenated, hydrocarbons generally possess better solubility characteristics than the fluorinated hydrocarbons.

As with fluorocarbons, a range of pressures can be obtained by mixing various hydrocarbons in varying proportions. As the composition of the hydrocarbons is likely to vary somewhat, depending on their source, blending of hydrocarbons must be based on the final pressure desired and not on the basis of a stated proportion of each component, the pressure of which will depend on its purity. Table 5 lists some commonly used blends that are commercially available.

Finally, it should be indicated that the hydrocarbons are characterized further by their extreme chemical stability. They are not subject to hydrolysis, making them useful with water-based aerosols. They will react with the halogens, but only under severe conditions.

Possible Alternative Propellants

Many pharmaceutical aerosols were developed originally using chlorofluorocarbons (CFCs) 11, 12, and 114. These propellants have found widespread use due to their inertness, nonflammability and nontoxicity. Unfortunately, the CFCs have been implicated in depleting the ozone layer, and their use has practically been eliminated, except for a few exempted uses.

Topical pharmaceutical aerosols have been successfully reformulated with Propellants 152a, 142b, 22, dimethyl ether, hydrocarbons and compressed gases. Suitable valves are available which, together with modifications in formulation and propellant blends, produce topical aerosol pharmaceuticals which are satisfactory and acceptable.

Unfortunately, to date, no satisfactory alternative to the use of propellants 11, 12 and 114 for MDIs and nasal aerosols has been found. Several new liquid gas materials have been developed to replace the CFCs as refrigerants, foaming agents and in other nonpharmaceutical uses. Propellant 134a has been developed as a substitute for Propellant 12 in refrigeration. This compound to date has survived many of the short term toxicity studies and shows promise as a substitute for Propellant 12 in MDIs. Another possible replacement for Propellant 12 is Propellant R-227. To date, no suitable replacement has been found for Propellants 11 and 114. Propellant 114 is not essential for use with MDIs, but most of the present suspension formulations require a minimum of Propellant 11. Propellant 11 is used to form a slurry with the active ingredient and dispensing agent. This is impossible to accomplish with Propellants 134a and R-227 (unless these are chilled well below their boiling points and handled as a cold fill).

It also has been noted that many of the currently used dispersing agents are not compatible with these newer materials. The gaskets and sealing compounds used in metered-dose valve present compatability problems to the formulator; however, other gaskets have been developed and found to be satisfactory. Several of the critical properties of these newer suggested propellants are shown in Table 6.

Compressed Gases

The compressed gases such as nitrogen, nitrous oxide and carbon dioxide have been used as aerosol propellants. Depending on the nature of the formulation and the valve design, the product can be dispensed as a fine mist, foam or semisolid. However, unlike the liquefied gases, the com-

Table 5—Commonly Used Hydrocarbon Blends

Designation*	Pressure psig at 70°F	Composition—mole %			
		n-Butane	Propane	*iso*-Butane	Other
A-108	108 ± 4	traces	99	1	traces of ethane
A-31	31 ± 2	3	1	96	
A-17	17 ± 2	98	traces	2	traces of isopentane
A-24	24 ± 2	49.2	0.6	50	0.1 each of *neo*- and *iso*-pentane
A-40	40 ± 2	2	12	86	
A-46	46 ± 2	2	20	78	
A-52	52 ± 2	2	28	70	
A-70	70 ± 2	1	51	48	

[a]Designations used by Phillips Chemical Co, Bartlesville OK.

Table 6—Selected Properties of Possible Alternative Propellants

Property		Trifluoromono-fluoroethane	Heptafluoro-propane
Molecular formula		CF_3CH_2F	CF_3CHFCF_3
Numerical designation		134a	R-227
Molecular weight		102	170
Boiling point (1 atm) °F		−15	—
°C		−27	−17
Vapor pressure (psig)	70°F	71.1	43 (at 20°C)
	130°F	198.7	—
Liquid density (g/mL)	20°C	1.21	1.41

pressed gases possess little, if any, expansion power and will produce a fairly wet spray and foams which are not as stable as liquefied-gas foams. This system has been used for the most part to dispense food products and for nonfoods to dispense the product in its original form as a semisolid. Compressed gases have been used in products such as dental creams, hair preparations, ointments and aqueous antiseptic and germicidal aerosols.

Since compressed gases are used in the gaseous state and not in the liquid state, a higher initial pressure is required, as well as a relatively larger head space than liquefied-gas aerosols. While the pressure of a liquefied-gas aerosol remains constant during use, a drop in pressure is noted during use of a compressed-gas aerosol. This drop in pressure can be calculated by the application of the ideal gas laws.

$$PV = nRT$$

where P = pressure in atmosphere, V = volume in L, n = moles of gas (g/mol wt), R = gas constant (0.08205 L atm deg^{-1} $mole^{-1}$) and T = absolute temperature.

The initial pressure of a compressed-gas aerosol is usually about 90 psig and occupies a volume of about 15 to 25% of the container volume. As the contents of the container are expelled, the volume of head space increases with a corresponding decrease in pressure according to Boyle's law.

The physical and chemical properties of the compressed gases are not as vital to formulation as the properties of the liquefied gases. These gases are, for the most part, chemically inert and do not react with the product concentrate. In the case of nitrogen the gas does not dissolve in the product, whereas nitrous oxide and carbon dioxide are soluble to a certain extent. Table 4 indicates this solubility. Mixtures of nitrous oxide and carbon dioxide have been used as propellants for whipped creams and toppings and also for several veterinary emulsion products. The solubility of carbon dioxide in certain beverage food products is advantageous in that a slight degree of carbonation can be obtained. Since these gases generally are inert and replace the air trapped in the head space, the stability of drugs sometimes is increased.

Containers

Metal

Tin-Plated Steel—In order to produce an aerosol container which was light and relatively inexpensive, tin-plated steel was used for aerosol containers. This resulted in the large scale production of aerosol containers.

For certain products the tin affords sufficient protection so that no further treatment is necessary. Hair lacquers generally can be packaged in this type of container. However, the addition of water and other corrosive ingredients or other substances which will attack tin requires a container having an additional protective coating. This coating is usually organic in nature and may consist of an oleoresin, phenolic, vinyl or epoxy coating. The liner (single or double coat) is added to the container prior to fabrication, that is, it is applied to the flat sheets of tin plate.

Aluminum—Many topical pharmaceutical aerosols use an aluminum container. Aluminum also is preferred for use with most MDIs. These are produced by an impact extrusion process so that the container is seamless. This will give added strength to the container. A variety of different aluminum aerosol containers ranging in size from 10 mL to 45 fl oz is available. While aluminum is less reactive than other metals used in can manufacture, added resistance can be obtained by coating the inside of the container with organic materials such as epoxy, vinyl or phenolic resins.

Glass—For pharmaceuticals and medicinals, glass is preferred due to the absence of incompatibilities, as well as for its esthetic value. The use of glass containers is limited to those products having a lower pressure and lower percentage of propellant. Glass aerosols have found use in packaging of many perfumes, colognes, cosmetics, pharmaceuticals and medicinals. While glass is basically stronger than most metallic containers, a potential hazard is present if, and when, the container is dropped with subsequent breakage. Two types of glass aerosol containers are available. The uncoated glass container has the advantage of decreased cost and high clarity. The contents can be viewed at all times. The plastic-coated glass containers are protected by a plastic coating which prevents the glass from shattering in the event of breakage. In one type the coating is bonded to the glass and becomes an integral part of the container. In another type, the coating fits over the glass container.

Valves

Probably the most basic part of any aerosol or pressurized package is the valve mechanism through which the contents of the package are emitted. Together with the formulation, the valve determines the performance of a pressurized package. The interaction of these two is such that one cannot readily be discussed without reference to the other.

The primary purpose of the valve is to regulate the flow of product from the container. It provides a means of discharging the desired amount when needed and prevents loss at other times. The valve also exerts a major effect on the character of the dispensed product. For example, a product formulated to produce a foam can be dispensed as a spray or as a wet stream by the use of different actuators or push buttons on the valve. The selection of proper propellants also governs whether a foam, spray or wet stream will be produced.

Spray Valves

Since the spray valve is the most common used valve, it will be discussed in detail. Figure 9 illustrates the basic subcomponents used in aerosol valves. A fully assembled valve is shown in Fig. 10.

A small hole of about 0.013 to 0.020" in diameter sometimes is placed in the valve body as seen in Fig 9. This allows for the escape of a small quantity of vaporized propellant along with the product. This gives a greater degree of dispersion to the emitted spray as well as cleaning of the valve orifices following discharge. However, since a greater amount of propellant is used as compared to nonvapor tap systems, care must be exercised during formulation of the product to take this into account. One may also note a change in spray pattern from start to finish due to the change in propellant composition which takes place as the contents are used. Vapor tap valves are used with powder aerosols, water-based aerosols, aerosols containing suspended materials and other agents which would tend to clog the valve. They currently are used with hydrocarbon aerosols since the flame extension of the spray can be reduced substantially through use of a vapor tap valve. This is accomplished by balancing the size of the vapor tap opening and the valve orifice.

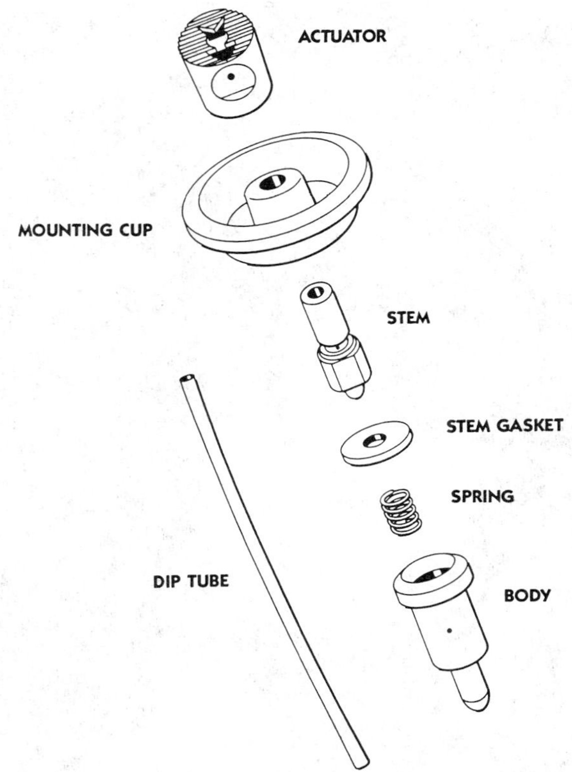

Fig 9. Continuous-spray aerosol valve, showing subcomponents, used for sprays, foams and semisolids (courtesy, Precision Valve).

Foam Valves

Valves for foam or aerated products usually have only one expansion orifice, the one at the seat. Following this is a single expansion chamber which serves as a delivery nozzle or applicator. It is sufficiently large in volume to permit immediate expansion of the pressurized product to form the familiar ball of foam. As demonstrated earlier, the same formulation will be discharged as a solid stream when dispensed with a valve and actuator having small orifices and expansion chambers. Under these latter conditions, the ball of foam will begin to develop where the stream impinges on a surface. This rather interesting performance is utilized in some pressurized surgical soaps on the market.

Because of their large openings, foam valves may lend themselves for use with viscous materials such as syrups, creams and ointments.

After a foam product, such as shaving cream, has been used a small accumulation of foam often will be seen on the end of the actuator. This buildup is not due either to leakage or slow shutoff of the valve, but rather to the expansion of the residual formulation of the actuator. Metered values will be discussed later in this chapter.

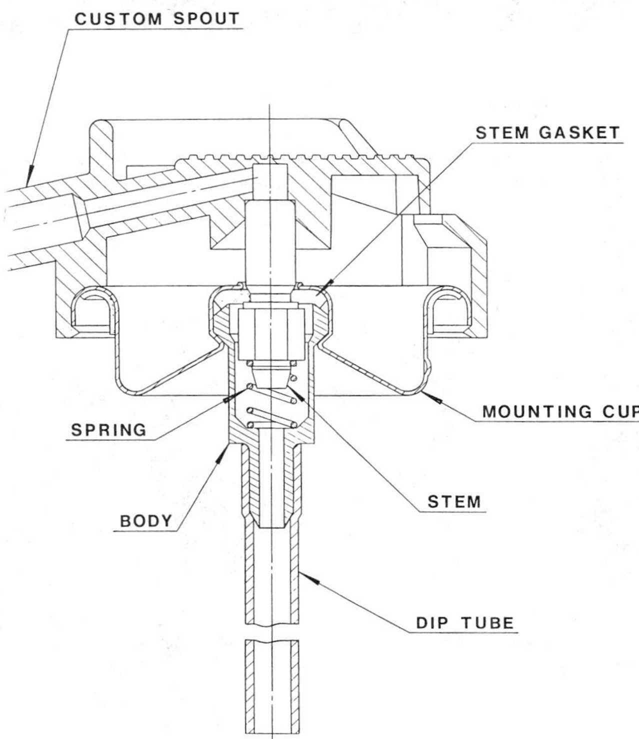

Fig 10. Assembled continuous-spray valve (courtesy, Precision Valve).

Actuators

The actuator provides a rapid and convenient means for releasing the contents from a pressurized container. It provides the additional functional use in allowing the product to be dispensed in the desired form, that is, a fine mist, wet spray, foam or solid stream. Mechanical breakup actuators are used for three-phase or compressed-gas aerosols. In addition, special actuators are available for use with pharmaceutical and medicinal aerosols which allow for the dispensing of products into the mouth, nose, throat, vagina or eye. Several of these actuators and applicators are illustrated in Fig 11.

Dip Tubes

An additional component which should be considered with the valve is the dip tube. The dip tube serves several purposes.

It conveys the liquid from the bottom of the container to the dispensing valve at the top.

It prevents the propellant from escaping without dispensing the contents of the package (when used according to directions).

The dip tube comes into intimate contact with both product and propellant and therefore should be resistant to both physical and chemical attack. Polyethylenes and nylon have been found to possess many desirable properties making them useful for this purpose. However, since the dip tube is stretched to fit tightly on the valve housing, it is possible that on standing the polyethylene or nylon will crack or break down at this point, rendering the product useless since it cannot be dispensed. This has been overcome through the use of specially developed polyethylene or polypropylene compounds.

The tube should extend almost to the bottom of the container. If the tube is too short, all the product will not be dispensed, while a tube touching the bottom of the container will tend to block the passage of liquid. In this connection, most of the materials used for dip tubes tend to elongate when immersed in certain solvents and propellants for long periods of time. This elongation should be anticipated when determining the length of the dip tube.

Packaging

Two methods have been used to package aerosol products. Unlike nonaerosol products, part of the manufacturing of necessity takes place during the filling operation. The propellant and product concentrate must be brought together in such a way as to insure uniformity of product.

Depending on the nature of the product concentrate, the aerosol can be filled by a cold-filling or a pressure-filling process. There are advantages and disadvantages to both

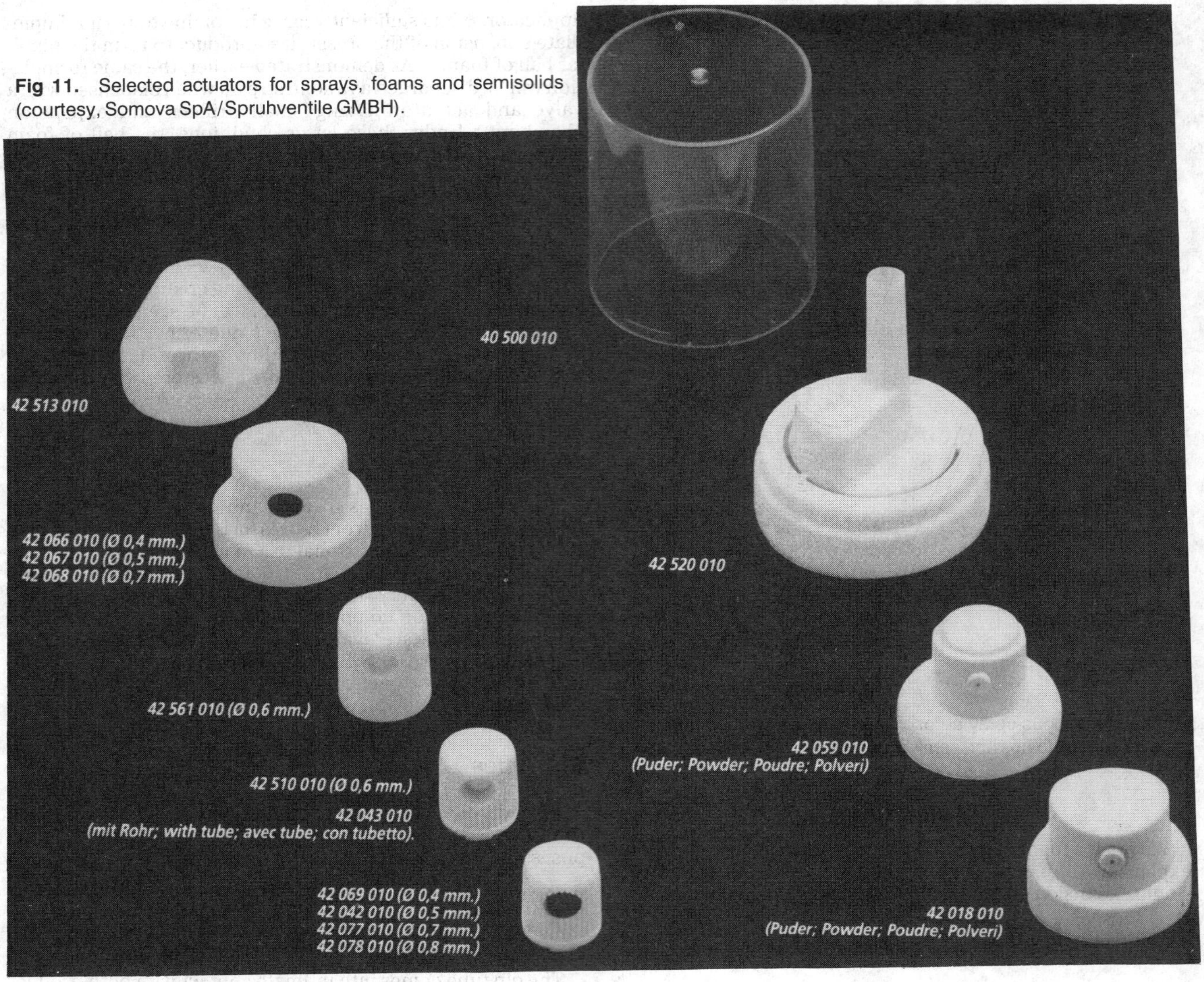

Fig 11. Selected actuators for sprays, foams and semisolids (courtesy, Somova SpA/Spruhventile GMBH).

methods, and there are many factors which must be considered before deciding upon which process to use. Since this is a rather specialized procedure, commercial filling facilities are available. A typical unit used to fill metered-dose inhalers is shown in Fig 12.

Applications

Aerosol technology has been applied to the formulation of products containing therapeutically active ingredients.

A pharmaceutical aerosol may be defined as an aerosol

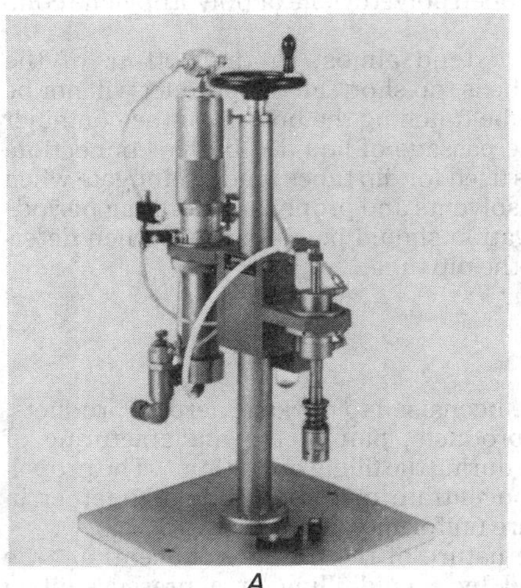

A

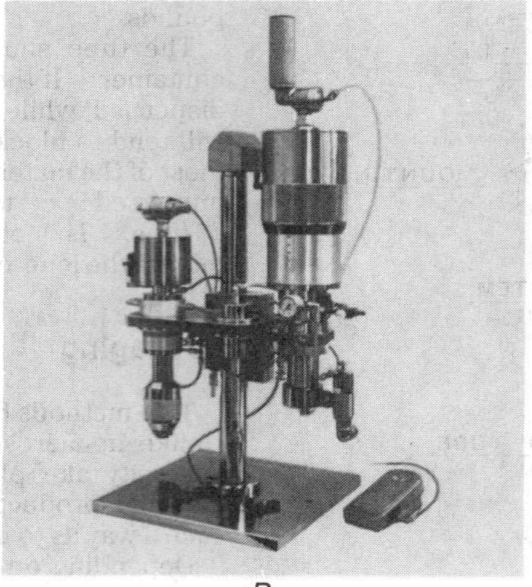

B

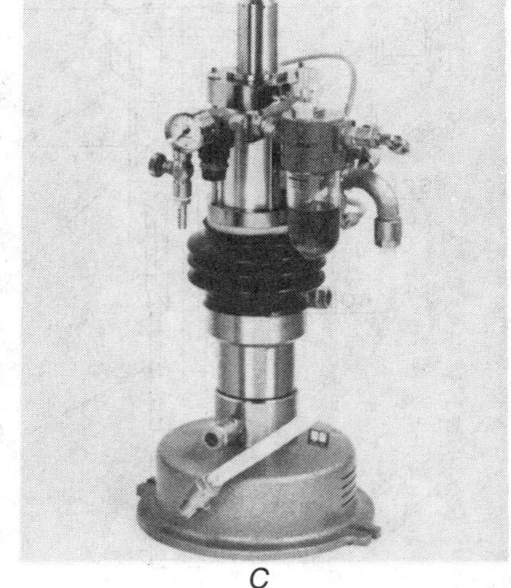

C

Fig 12. Aerosol laboratory and pilot-size filling equipment. *A:* Product filler; *B:* Crimper and pressure filler for propellant; *C:* Propellant pump (courtesy, Pamasol Willi Mader AG).

product containing therapeutically active ingredients dissolved, suspended or emulsified in a propellant or a mixture of solvent and propellant and intended for oral or topical administration or for administration into the nose, eye, ear, rectum or vagina.

Metered-dose inhalers are intended for administration as fine, solid particles or as liquid mists via the respiratory system or nasal passages. They are used for their local action in the nasal areas, throat and lungs, as well as for prompt systemic effect when absorbed from the lungs into the blood stream (inhalation therapy). The particle size must be considerably below 10 μm and, in most instances, should be between 3 and 6 μm for maximum therapeutic response.

According to the USP/NF, "Pharmaceutical aerosols are products that are packaged under pressure and contain therapeutically active ingredients that are released upon activation of an appropriate valve system. They are intended for topical application to the skin as well as local application into the nose (nasal aerosols), mouth (lingual aerosols) or lungs (inhalation aerosols)."

Pharmaceutical Aerosols

Pharmaceuticals may be formulated as aerosols utilizing solutions, suspensions, emulsions, powders and semisolid preparations. Table 7 illustrates the basic formulation of aerosol products for use as a metered-dose inhalant.

Solution Aerosols—These consist of a solution of active ingredients in pure propellant or a mixture of propellant and solvents. The solvent is used to dissolve the active ingredients and/or retard the evaporation of the propellant. Solution aerosols are relatively easy to formulate provided the ingredients are soluble in the propellant. However, the propellants are nonpolar in nature and in most cases are poor solvents for some of the commonly used medicinal ingredients. Through use of a solvent which is miscible with the propellant, one can achieve varying degrees of solubility. There is no limit to the number of solvents which can be used for this purpose except for toxicity considerations. Ethyl alcohol has found the greatest use although some other solvents may be of limited value. For those substances which are insoluble in the propellant or propellant/solvent system, a dispersion or suspension can be produced. In this case the drug must be micronized so that the particles are less than 10 μm in average diameter. While it may be easier to formulate a solution system than a suspension system, the latter generally is preferred since a closer control over the particle size distribution of the droplets dispensed from the solution aerosol may be obtained as well as increased stability.

The usual fluorocarbon substances of Propellants 11, 12 or 114 generally are blended as indicated in Table 7.

For the most part, some of the propellant may be inhaled during use but is exhaled quickly. Propellant 11 is used often when solubility of the drug and solvents presents a problem as it is a better solvent than either Propellant 12 or 114. Additionally, Propellant 11 may be required to prepare a suitable slurry when preparing a dispersion aerosol. Generally the propellant represents upwards of 60 weight-percent of the final formulation and, in most cases, may be as high as 85 to 90%.

Table 7—Metered-Dose Inhalants (Solutions and Suspensions)

Prototype formulation
Solutions
Active ingredient(s)—solubilized
Antioxidants—ascorbic acid
Solvent blends—water, ethanol, glycols
Propellants—12/11, 12/114 or 12 alone
Suspensions
Active ingredient(s)—micronized and suspended
Dispersing agent(s)—sorbitan trioleate, oleyl alcohol, oleic acid, lecithin, etc.
Propellants—12/11, 12/114, 12 or 12/114/11

Propellant 12 may be used alone or in combination as indicated. The proportion of each propellant is varied in order to obtain the desired pressure within the container and the proper particle-size distribution.

Dispersions or Suspensions (Powder Aerosols)—These aerosols are similar to solution aerosols except that the active ingredients are suspended or dispersed throughout the propellant or propellant and solvent phase. This system is useful with antibiotics, steroids and other difficulty soluble compounds. Problems associated with the formulation of this system include agglomeration, caking, particle-size growth and valve clogging. Some of these problems have been overcome through use of lubricants such as isopropyl myristate, light mineral oil or other substances which provide slippage between particles of the compound as well as lubricating component parts of the valve. Surfactants also have been used to disperse the particles. The use of dispersing agents such as sorbitan trioleate, oleyl alcohol, oleic acid, lecithin or corn oil are useful in keeping the suspended particles from agglomerating. Thought also should be given to the particle size as well as the moisture content of the powder. The moisture content should be kept between 100 and 300 ppm or less depending upon the type of product, and the propellants and solvents must be dried by passing them through a drying agent. The particle size for metered-dose inhalants should remain in the micrometer range and should be between 2 and 8 μm with a mass median diameter of between 3 and 6 μm.

Emulsions—An emulsion system is useful for a great variety of products. Since it contains a relatively small amount of propellant (4 to 10%), there is little if any chilling effect. Active ingredients which may be irritating if inhaled can be used as a foam. Depending on the nature of the formulation and the manner in which the product is to be used, the foam is aqueous or nonaqueous and can be stable or quick-breaking.

Emulsions can be dispensed from an aerosol container as a spray, stable foam or quick-breaking foam depending on the type of valve used and the formulation. Two types of emulsions can be formulated for use in an aerosol. A W/O emulsion is one in which the water phase is dispersed throughout the oil phase; an O/W emulsion is one in which the water is the continuous phase.

If the product concentrate is dispersed throughout a propellant, the system behaves similarly to a W/O emulsion. However, since the propellant is in the external phase, the product is dispersed as a wet stream rather than as a foam. When the propellant is in the internal phase (O/W), a foam will be produced. The consistency and stability of the foam can be modified by choice of surfactants and solvents used.

Many water-based aerosols are of the W/O type where the propellant is in the external phase. Stable shave-cream foams, on the other hand, are produced by keeping the propellant in the internal phase.

The stable foam is similar to a shaving-cream formulation into which therapeutically active ingredients are incorporated. The foam is dispensed and rubbed into the skin or affected area. By substituting glycols and glycol derivatives for the water in an emulsion, a nonaqueous foam is obtained. The foam stability can be varied by the choice of surfactant, solvent and propellant. It has been suggested that these foams are applicable to ointment bases, rectal and vaginal medication and burn preparations.

A quick-breaking foam allows for application of medication conveniently and efficiently. In certain instances the product was dispensed as a foam which quickly collapsed. This was useful in covering large areas with no rubbing necessary to disperse the medication. These quick-breaking foams consist of alcohol, surfactant, water and propellant.

Most topical aerosols now use a hydrocarbon propellant. New developments are taking place with valves and barrier packs which allow for greater use of compressed gases for these products. The flammability potential of topical aerosols has been reduced substantially through use of vapor tap valves in which the flame extension can be reduced from over 24″ to less than 18″ and in many instances below 8″. This is accomplished by using a fairly large vapor tap in the valve. The formulator must check to make sure sufficient propellant is present to dispense suitably all of the product. By balancing the vapor tap and dispensing orifices of the valve and by using a capillary dip tube, a satisfactory aerosol system may be formulated.

Semisolid Preparations—These preparations are formulated in the usual manner and depend on nitrogen to push the contents from the package. These systems have been discussed earlier in this chapter.

Container and Valve Components

Pharmaceutical Containers—Various containers have been used for these aerosols. Due to esthetic considerations and excellent compatibility with drugs, glass and aluminum containers have found widespread use in the pharmaceutical industry.

Plastic-coated glass bottles ranging in size from 15 to 30 mL have been employed mainly with metered-dose solution aerosols although there is no technical or scientific rationale for this use other than one can determine the amount of material left in the container by holding the bottle in the path of a strong light. Glass bottles are not recommended for suspension aerosols due to the visibility of the suspensed particles which may present an esthetic problem.

Aluminum is used as the material of construction for most metered-dose aerosols. While aluminum can be used without an internal organic coating for certain aerosol formulations (especially those which contain only active ingredient and propellant) many containers are available which have been anodized. They also may have an internal coating made from an epon- or epoxy-type resin.

Aluminum containers also are made with a 20-mm opening so as to receive the standard metered valves. However, a variety of openings ranging from 15 to 20 mm also are available for special and customized applications. Aluminum containers are manufactured from a "slug" of aluminum and are seamless, therefore, there is virtually no danger of leakage. Figure 13 shows a typical aluminum container used for metered-dose inhalers.

Pharmaceutical Valves—A typical metered-dose aerosol delivery system is illustrated in Fig. 14. Metering valves fitted with a 20-mm ferrule are used with the above containers for all metered-dose inhalation and nasal aerosols.

The metering valve should deliver accurately a measured amount of product and should be reproducible not only for each dose delivered from the same package but from package to package. Two basic types of metering valves are available, one for inverted use and the other for upright use. Generally, valves for upright use contain a thin capillary dip tube and are used with solution type aerosols. On the other

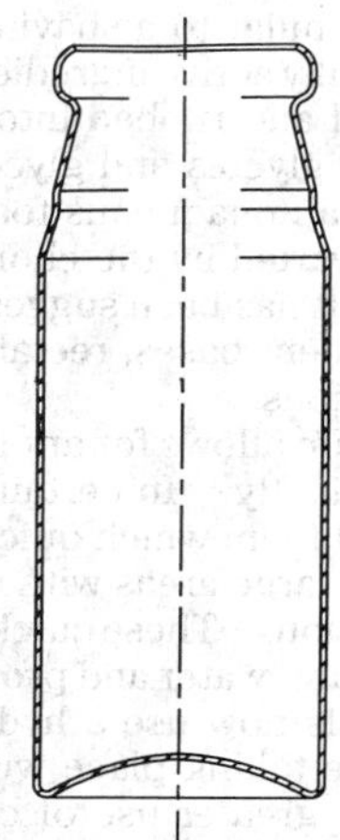

Fig 13. Typical aluminum aerosol container, cut-edge type used with an "O" ring (courtesy, Presspart).

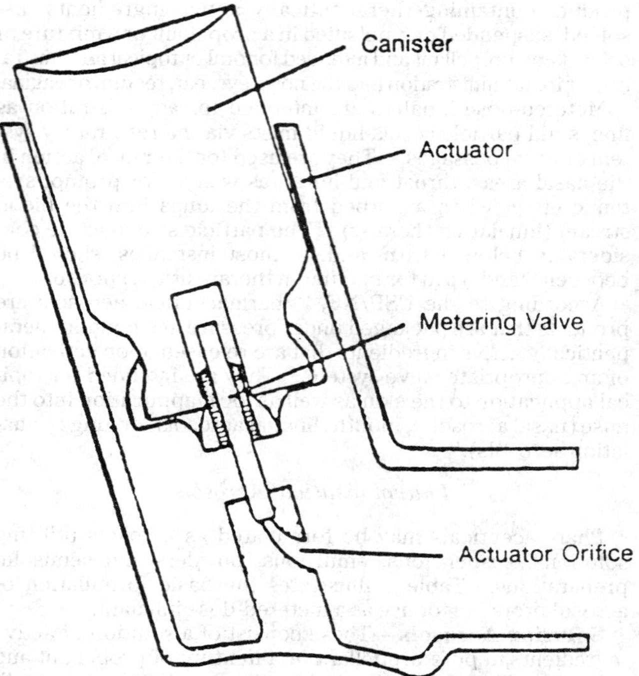

Fig 14. Typical metered-dose aerosol delivery system.

hand, suspension or dispersion aerosols use a valve for inverted use which does not contain a dip tube. Figures 15 and 16 illustrate both types of valves and are typical of those commercially available.

An integral part of these valves is the metering chamber which directly is responsible for the delivery of the desired

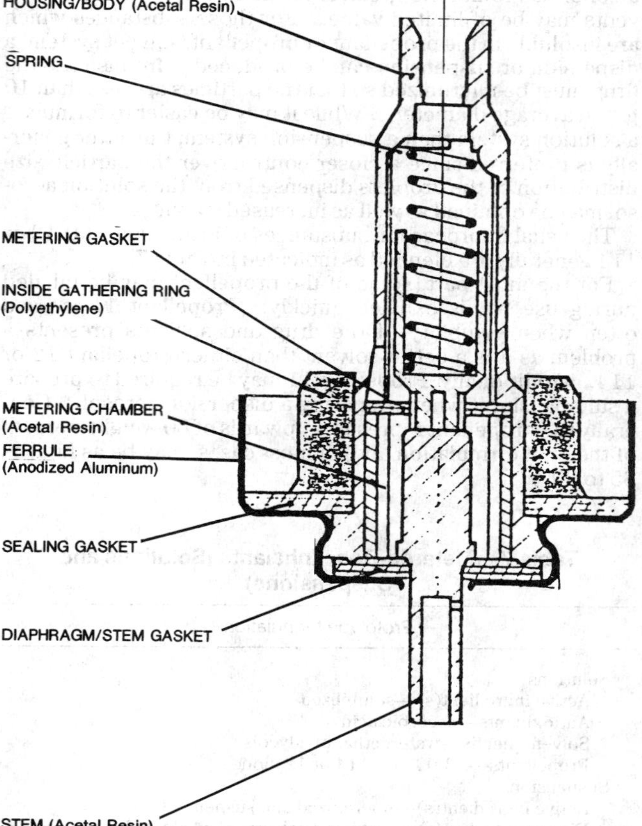

Fig 15. Metering valve—inverted (courtesy, Valois).

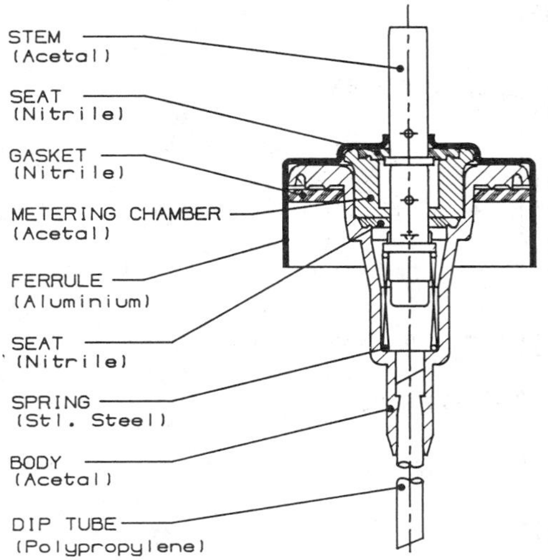

Fig 16. 20-mm metered-dose valve showing the subcomponent parts and metering chamber. It is used in the upright position (courtesy, Bespak).

amount of therapeutic agent. The size of the chamber can be varied so that from about 25 to 150 μL of product can be delivered per actuation. Most of the products commercially available utilize dosages in the range of 50 to 75 μL. The chamber is sealed via the metering and stem gasket. In the actuated position, the stem gasket will allow the contents of the metering chamber to be dispensed while the metering gasket will seal off any additional product from entering the chamber. In this manner the chamber always is filled and ready to deliver the desired amount of therapeutic agent.

These valves should retain their prime charge over fairly long periods of time. However, it is possible for the material in the chamber to return slowly to the main body of product in the event the container is stored upright (for those used in the inverted position). The degree to which this can occur varies with the construction of the valve and the length of time between actuations.

Both types of valves currently are used on commercially available oral inhalation aerosols. During the development stage, the compatibility of the valves should be determined with the exact formulation to be used in order to determine the accuracy of the metered dose developed in regard to doses delivered from the same container of product and from different containers. Additionally, one should ensure that there is no interaction between the various valve subcomponents and the formulation. If distortion or elongation of some of the plastic subcomponents occurs, this may result in leakage, inaccurate dosage and/or decomposition of the active ingredients.

There also have been instances whereby the therapeutic agent was adsorbed or absorbed onto the various plastic components, and a lower than normal dose of the active ingredient was dispensed. For these reasons, one must not only determine the total weight of product dispensed per dose but the actual amount of active ingredient in each dose. Some test procedures use the results obtained by taking 10 doses of material and determining the average amount present in one dose. When possible, and where the analytical procedure permits the detecting of fairly small amounts of active ingredients present per dose, multiple single-dose assays should be performed. Using the average of 10 doses may fail to reveal problems of variations in each of the individual doses dispensed.

Evaluation of Metered-Dose Inhalers and Topical Pharmaceuticals

Various tests have been devised to assure the integrity of the aerosol package. These products are said to be *tamper-proof* since they cannot be opened and closed in the usual manner. Because these products are all under pressure, it is very difficult to add any foreign material to the product once the entire package is assembled. This also makes it rather difficult to obtain suitable samples for an analysis. Special sampling procedures and test methods have been developed and are used to determine the suitability of the product.

Topical pharmaceutical aerosols do not present any special problems other than the sampling procedure. The USP includes several tests under the specific monographs for the topical aerosols. These include delivery rate, leak testing, microbial limit test and assay. While several of these products are dispensed as sprays, no special emphasis or consideration is given to the partial size of the droplets or particles emitted. The spray may be defined as a fine, dry or wet spray.

Metered-dose inhalers require a greater amount of testing since the metered valve, oral adapter and the formulation are collectively responsible for delivering the therapeutically active ingredient to the appropriate site in the respiratory passages. This assumes that the patient will administer the product properly so that both the dose and depth of penetration of the medication can be assured. Unfortunately, this is not always done. Both the physician and the pharmacist can provide a most valuable service to the patient by taking the time to demonstrate the correct use of these inhalers.

Many of the tests required for the evaluation of metered-dose inhalers are similar to those used for other dosage forms. These include description, identification and assay of the active ingredient; microbial limits; moisture content; net weight, degradation products and impurities (if any); extractables and any other tests deemed appropriate for the active ingredient.

Analysis of the metered-dose inhaler also is required in order to determine the amount of drug delivered and its depth of penetration into the respiratory passages, including

Unit Spray Content—This test is described in the USP and determines the average amount of active ingredient delivered through the mouthpiece (oral adapter) per a specified number of actuations (dose taken by patient).

Leakage Rate—This test is also available in the USP and is used to estimate the weight loss over a 1 year period. Since there are several sealing gaskets present in a metered-dose valve, this test determines the integrity of the gaskets as well as the proper crimping of the valve onto the container.

Content Uniformity—This test determines the amount of drug substance delivered per actuation from the mouthpiece of different containers from the same lot.

Number of Doses per Container—This is defined as the number of actuators meeting the *Unit Spray Content* requirements.

Spray Pattern and/or Plume Geometry—This test evaluates the type of spray pattern emitted for the metered-dose inhaler and relates to the characteristics of the metering valve and oral adapter as well as to the formulation.

Valve Delivery—The reproducibility of the amount of product delivered through the valve is evaluated.

It is beyond the scope of this chapter to discuss these tests in greater detail. The reader is referred to the USP. However, particle-size distribution should be covered in greater detail due to its greater importance.

Particle-Size Distribution

Particle-size distribution is probably one of the most important characteristics of a metered-dose inhaler. In order to be effective, the particles emitted from the spray must be below 10 μm and in most cases between 2 and 8 μm in diameter. Several methods are available for the determination of the particle-size distribution for metered-dose inhalers. A common method includes a cascade impactor which depends upon the principle of carrying particles in a stream of air through a series of consecutively smaller jet openings. The heavier and larger diameter particles are impacted on a slide under the larger opening, and as the openings get smaller, the velocity of the stream increases and the next larger particles are deposited on the next slides. Figure 17 illustrates the cascade impactor.

Figure 18 and Table 8 give a typical analysis of a metered-dose inhaler. Other methods include the use of a microscope

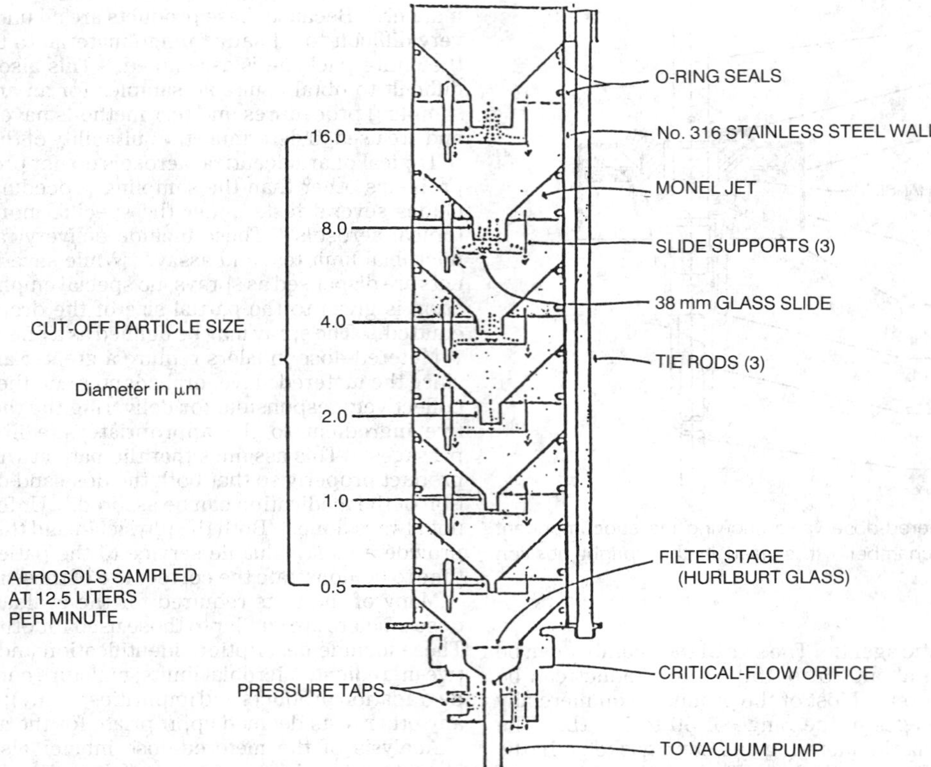

Fig 17. Cascade impactor used for particle-size distribution of metered-dose inhalers.

or instrumentation based on holography and laser beams. The reader is referred to the USP for a more comprehensive review of this subject.

Formulation Factors—Included among formulation factors are the physicochemical characteristics of the active ingredients, the particle size and shape of the formulation, the type and concentration of surface-active agent used and, to some extent, the vapor pressure and the metered volume of propellants. In terms of physicochemical properties, the lipoidal solubility and pulmonary absorption rates of the active ingredient are of utmost importance. Another physicochemical factor governing the biopharmaceutics of a drug is its dissolution characteristics in pulmoanry fluids. Drugs having a rapid dissolution rate in pulmonary fluids predictably produce much more intense and rapid onset of action, having a shorter duration than their less soluble derivatives. Therapeutic agents which exhibit a very poor solubility in pulmonary fluids are to be avoided since they are likely to serve as irritants and precipitate bronchial spasms.

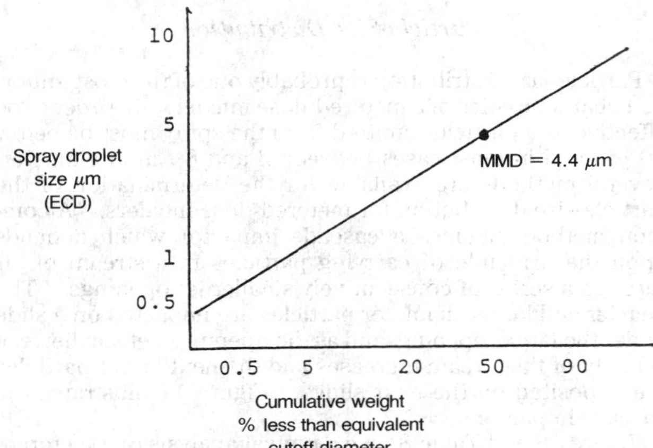

Fig 18. Log probability plot of data from the cascade impactor (MMD: mass median diameter).

The selection of the appropriate surface active agent (required in most pressurized inhalation suspension aerosols) is another important consideration since the surfactant will influence droplet evaporation, particle size and overall hydrophobicity of the particles reaching the respiratory passageways and pulmonary fluids.

The effects of propellant vapor pressure and the metered volume of propellants on drug deposition in the lungs recently have been studied using rather large specialized plastic adapters. Findings in this area have demonstrated that the amount of material deposited in the mouth, tube and actuator (likely sites of material loss) increased as the vapor pressure was decreased and the metered volume increased.

Component Design—Component design, specifically the actuator and adapter, also have been shown to alter the particle size and the penetration and deposition of drugs into the lungs. Numerous studies have demonstrated that a complex set of interactions exist between the actuation type, valve dimensions, distance from actuator and other component variables and that particle size (mass median diameters) could vary up to 40% by altering one or more of the aforementioned components.

One component that has undergone enormous modification in the last few years to improve drug delivery is the adapter. Up to about the mid 1970s, almost all adapters were short and rather simplistic so as to minimize possible hold-up of material in the adapter. The hold-up in the short-stem adapters averages anywhere from 5 to 20%. Recently, however, nu-

Table 8—Cumulative Particle-Size Distribution

Slide no	Particle size (micrometers)	Cumulative particle size Distribution (%)
Filter	less than 0.5	0.55
6	0.5–1	5.35
5	1–2	18.98
4	2–4	61.59
3	4–8	90.20
2	8–16	96.67
1	16–32	100.00

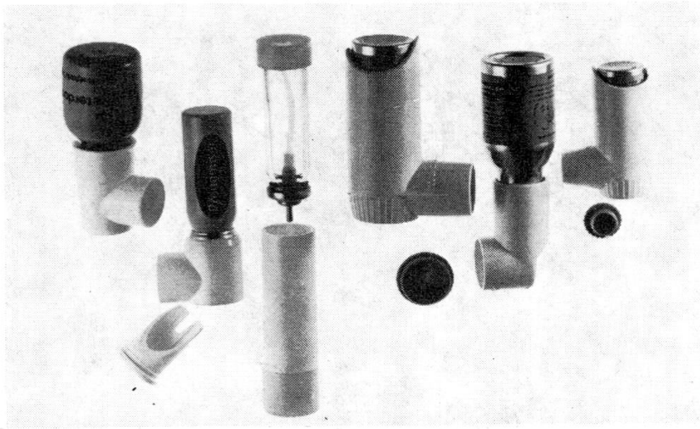

Fig 19. Medicinal aerosols with short oral applicators.

merous customized adapters having specific designs and dimensions have entered the marketplace.

Interest in the larger adapters (often referred to as tube spacers) can be attributed to any one or more of the following reasons. The larger adapter designs permit a complete evaporation of propellant reducing initial droplet velocity and particle size. This reduction of particle size improves depth of drug penetration into the lungs while a lower initial velocity decreases product impaction to the back of the esophagus (whiplash effect), common to short stem adapters. The larger adapter designs also permit a decrease in pressure to drop and increased volume flow which also has been reported to increase penetration of particles into the lungs. It should be pointed out that the larger tube spacers are not without problems. They are inconvenient because of their size, are expensive and somewhat difficult to clean. They also present the manufacturer with the problem of assessing product hold-up in a rather complex device.

Administrative Techniques—The metered inhalation aerosol dosage form, although popular, generally is considered as one of the most complicated drug delivery systems currently marketed by the pharmaceutical industry. It is viewed by many as being only slightly simpler to use than an injectable, since inhalation products often require up to 10 to 15 maneuvers by the patient during use. Failure of the patient to perform correctly any one of these maneuvers may alter significantly the deposition of the drug into the appropriate portion of the lungs.

Differences in the direction of use for each inhalation product are a result of the product formulation and actuator design which the manufacturer deemed most appropriate for the particular product. In light of this, it is not surprising to find patients who require two or more aerosol inhalation products or who are constantly changing their medication (such as the asthmatic patient) occasionally experiencing difficulties in complying with the suggested method of application.

These problems present a unique opportunity for the pharmacist to counsel the patient on the correct use of these inhalers. Several manufacturers will provide placebo inhalers for this purpose. Others will provide video tapes which can be used by the pharmacist and other health professionals to instruct on the correct use if these inhalers. Brown bag and senior citizen programs, health seminars and other similar programs can provide a suitable audience for group presentations. However, the most successful programs are conducted on a one-to-one program in the privacy of the drug store.

Many attempts have been made to overcome these problems and increase the efficacy of this dosage form. A *breath-activated* inhaler has been developed by 3M Pharmaceuticals and is used as an integral part of their pirbuterol acetate inhalation aerosol. They have found that in a study of 70 patients, the use of the breath-activated inhaler increased the

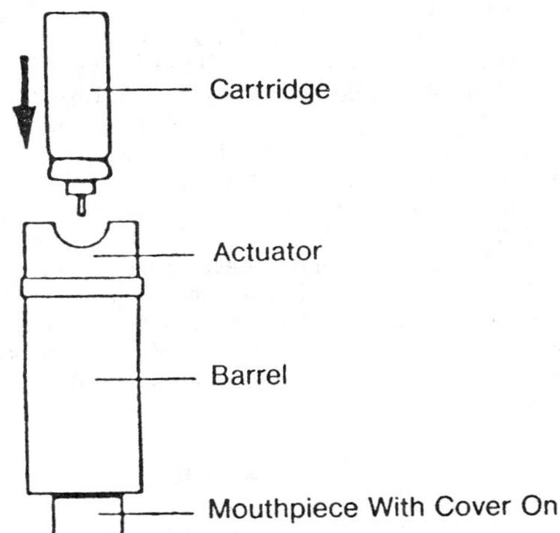

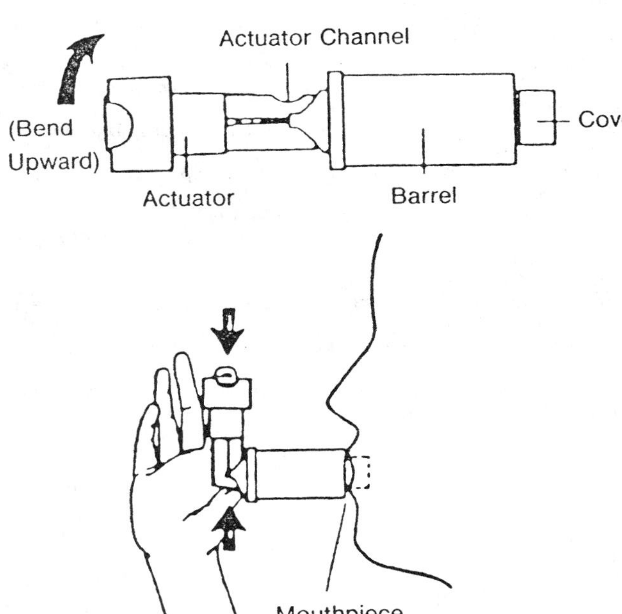

Fig 20. Tube spacer fitted with triamcinolone acetonide metered-dose inhaler (courtesy, Rhone-Poulenc Rorer).

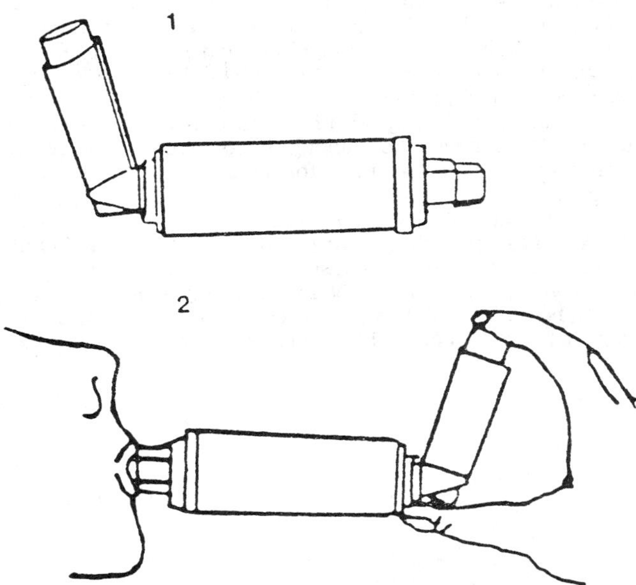

Fig 21. AeroChamber tube spacer (courtesy, Forest).

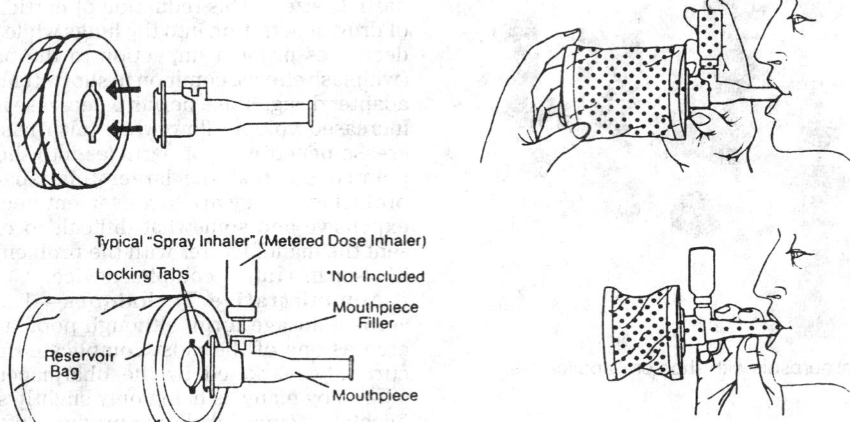

Fig 22. InspirEase unit (courtesy, Schering).

efficient use of these inhalers from 50 to 91%. These patients were given both written and verbal instructions. Reading instructions alone increased the efficiency from 39 to 63%.

Tube spacers also increase the efficiency of drug delivery via metered-dose inhalers. These spacers permit atomization of the delivered dose in a confined chamber or bag, and eliminate the need for the precise synchronization of actuations and deep breathing with inspiration. Triamcinolone acetonide is available as a metered-dose inhaler and is fitted with a tube spacer instead of the conventional short-stem actuators. Figure 19 illustrates several metered-dose aerosols with short stem actuators, while Fig. 20 illustrates the use of a tube spacer. Figs. 21 and 22 show tube spacers which are designed for use with most of the metered-dose aerosols fitted with a short stem. However, the patient must check with their physician before using these spacers since the particle-size distribution of the drug being dispersed through one of these spacers may be substantially different from those emitted from a short-stem actuator. Certainly, the deposition pattern will change and the efficiency of the delivered dose reaching the proper pulmonary airways will be increased.

Newer Developments

At present, there is much interest in developing metered-dose inhalers for a variety of conditions including asthma, emphysema, diabetes, aids, cancer, heart disease and cystic fibrosis. Many of these compounds have been developed using biotechnology processes, and their delivery to the respiratory system via a metered-dose inhaler is an extremely challenging undertaking. With the introduction of newer alternative propellants, the challenge becomes even greater and presents a unique opportunity for the delivery of these compounds.

Generic metered-dose aerosols are not available to the public (except for epinephrine hydrochloride) as yet. Even though albuterol and metaproterenol sulfate have been off-patent for several years, the FDA has not approved any generic metered dose inhalants (MDIs) to date. The development of a bioequivalence guidance by the FDA has been delayed by the lack of information on in vivo testing procedures for nonabsorbing drugs. Anticipating that such guidance will be available, a few generic drug manufacturers have developed these metered-dose aerosols and are awaiting the publication of this guidance in order to conduct a bioequivalence study. Such a guidance became available on January 27, 1994, by the FDA. A *in vivo* test guidance is available for use by manufacturers and the testing required has been covered previously.

With the increased interest by the pharmaceutical manufacturers to develop newer MDIs, the valve and the container suppliers are cooperating with the industry to develop much-needed hardware. A variable-dose valve for use with nasal insulin is currently under development along with different barrier systems, propellants and actuators. These developments will enable the pharmaceutical aerosol team to develop suitable metered-dose delivery systems to meet the high demands of the drugs currently available and those under development.

Bibliography

Anon: *Spray Tech Mark 3(6):* 28, 1993.
Burke GP, Poochikian G, Botstein P: *J Aerosol Med 4:* 265, 1991.
Cutie AJ, Sciarra JJ: *Pharm Times 55(4):* 133, 1989.
Gorman WG, Carroll FA: *Pharm Tech 17(2):* 34, 1993.
Handbook of Pharmaceutical Excipients, APhA/The Pharm Soc of Great Britain, Washington, DC and London, England, 19, 99, 101, 145, 240 and 333, 1986.
Hickey AJ: *Pharmaceutical Inhalation Aerosol Technology*, Dekker, New York, 1992.
Johnsen M: *The Aerosol Handbook*, 2nd ed, Wayne E Darland Co, Caldwell, NJ, 1982.
Mangione RA, Sciarra JJ: *Pharm Times, 57(Jun suppl):* 1, June 1991.
Milosovich SM: *Pharm Tech 16(9):* 82, 1992.
Pharmacopeial Forum 18: (Mar-Apr): 3158, 1992.
Sanders P: *Handbook of Aerosol Technology*, 2nd ed, Robert E Krieger Publ, Malabar, FL, 1987.
Sciarra JJ: *J Pharm Sci 63:* 1815, 1974.
Sciarra JJ, Cutie AJ. In *Industrial Pharmacy*, 3rd ed, Lea Febiger, Philadelphia, 589, 1986.
Sciarra JJ, Cutie AJ. In *Modern Pharmaceutics*, 2nd ed, Dekker, New York, 605, 1990.
Sciarra JJ, Stoller L: *The Science and Technology of Aerosol Packaging*, Wiley, New York, 1974.
USP, 1556, 1689, 1990.

PART 8

Pharmacy Practice

Daniel A Hussar PhD
Remington Professor of Pharmacy
Philadelphia College of Pharmacy and Science
Philadelphia PA 19104

CHAPTER 96

Ambulatory Patient Care

Nicholas G Popovich, PhD
Professor of Pharmacy Practice
School of Pharmacy and Pharmacal Sciences
Purdue University
West Lafayette, IN 47907

Various designations are used to categorize patients: institutionalized, noninstitutionalized, inpatient, outpatient, bedridden and ambulatory.

Strictly speaking, an ambulatory patient is one who is able to walk; that is, one who is not bedridden. Therefore, an ambulatory patient *may* be an inpatient of an institution, such as a hospital or extended-care facility, if he is not confined to bed. However, the term ambulatory patient has become restrictive more in its modern usage simply to mean a noninstitutionalized patient.

The ambulatory patient referred to here is a noninstitutionalized patient who has the responsibility for obtaining his medication, storing it and taking it. He may or may not be an outpatient, depending upon where he receives his treatment. He may even be in a wheelchair and, strictly speaking, not ambulatory, but if he is not institutionalized he will have the same basic responsibility for his medication as a "walking patient."

Whether the patient sees a physician who may prescribe medication or whether he decides to treat himself, the community pharmacist more than likely will come into contact with him. It is important, therefore, for the pharmacist to have an understanding of this patient in order that as a pharmacist and member of the health care team, the best possible health care for the ambulatory patient may be provided through proper use of knowledge and judgment.

The Pharmacist's Responsibility

The pharmacist must play an active role in the proper use of prescription medication by the patient. Indeed, the pharmacist is the learned intermediary in the safe, rational and effective use of medicines. The pharmacist is often the last member of the health-care team to see the patient before he takes the drug without direct medical supervision. In years past, the responsibility of the pharmacist was to ensure the safe and appropriate use of the medication and to answer questions of concern to the patient.

Recently, however, the profession of pharmacy has adopted pharmaceutical care as its mission, and thereby extended the responsibility of the pharmacist.[1] Pharmaceutical care focuses a pharmacist's attitude, behavior, commitment, concern, ethics, functions, knowledge, responsibilities and skills on the provision of a patient's drug therapy. The goal is to achieve optimal outcomes that improve the patient's quality of life. These outcomes may be

Cure of the disease.
Elimination or reduction of symptoms.
Arresting or slowing the disease process.
Prevention of disease.
Diagnosis of disease.
Desired alterations in the physiological processes.

Pharmaceutical care involves pharmacist decisions to avoid, initiate, maintain or discontinue drug therapy, both prescription and nonprescription. Thus, it is practiced in collaboration with patients, physicians, nurses and other health-care providers. In concept, pharmacists are directly responsible to the patient for the cost, quality and results of pharmaceutical care. Since the 1970s there has been active involvement by pharmacists in drug-therapy management for their patients. Research demonstrates that cognitive services provided by pharmacists add value to patient care for both institutionalized and ambulatory patients. This added value includes improvements in patient outcomes and enhanced patient compliance, and reduces health-care costs associated with mismedication problems. In 1990 the US Department of Health and Human Services' Office of the Inspector General summarized the current status of clinical services available in community settings, described barriers that limit the availability of these services and provided recommendations to reduce these barriers and strongly recommended the establishment of strategies to comprehensively deliver pharmaceutical care in the ambulatory setting.[2]

Subsequently, the Omnibus Budget Reconciliation Act of 1990 (OBRA 90) required each state Medicaid Agency to have a Drug Use Review (DUR) program for covered outpatient drugs in effect no later than January 1, 1993. This act also requires pharmacists to provide patient counseling for Medicaid patients. It is hoped that societal and professional pressure will be such to ensure that all patients and not just Medicaid patients will be counseled. OBRA 90 establishes minimum requirements for counseling individuals receiving benefits consistent with applicable state laws and the pharmacist's professional judgment. At a minimum, the pharmacist should discuss

The name and description of the medication.
The dosage form, dosage, route of administration and duration of drug therapy.
Special directions and precautions for preparation, administration and use by the patient.
Common severe side or adverse effects or interactions and therapeutic contraindications that may be encountered, including their avoidance, and the action required if they occur.
Techniques for self-monitoring drug therapy.
Proper storage.
Prescription refill information.
Action to be taken in the event of a missed dose.

To fulfill the intent of OBRA 90, the pharmacist provides certain pharmaceutical services described here which are as important to the health care of the ambulatory patient as those services provided by the other health practitioners.

Proper Use of Medication

The noted philosopher and educator in medicine, Sir William Osler, in 1891, captured the essence of man and medicine when he stated, "the desire to take medicines is perhaps the greatest feature that distinguishes man from animals." Unfortunately, this statement did not capture the mode in which man takes medicine, either correct or incorrect. If the patient complies with the instructions from the physician and pharmacist, there is a strong chance that the therapeutic regimen will be successful. However, if the medication is misused through personal ignorance or inadequate information, it could result in either harm to the patient or ineffective treatment.

It is known that the ambulatory patient does not adhere always to the directions for taking medicine. There are a number of reasons for this and the reader is advised to consult Chapter 103 for a thorough and enlightening discussion of patient compliance. Through the decade of the 1970s, numerous studies have demonstrated that patients widely misuse medications with frequency ranges between 20 and 82%. This wide variation reflects study differences, medication class differences and investigator interpretation of patient misuse of medication. In fact, it is estimated that 90% of all outpatients make mistakes taking their medications; 10% of all hospital admissions in the general population and 25% of all hospital admissions in the elderly are attributed to drug noncompliance.[3] Alternatively, other studies have demonstrated the positive impact of pharmacist intervention to encourage patient compliance. As a health-care provider, the pharmacist is obligated morally and legally and is, perhaps, in the best position to provide patients with adequate, understandable information on the drugs they take or use to maximize the therapeutic outcome and prevent conceivable problems during therapy.

To prevent these problems, the pharmacist must first understand how a patient misuses prescribed medications. Latiolais and Berry[4] compiled a number of ways in which this is accomplished and these are outlined below.

1. Overdosage
   a. Taking more than the prescribed dose at any one administration.
   b. Taking more than the prescribed number of doses in any one day.
   c. Taking a dose, prescribed as needed, at a time other than when needed.
   d. Taking the same medication from two or more different bottles simultaneously.
2. Underdosage
   a. Taking less than the prescribed dose at any one administration.
   b. Omitting one or more doses.
   c. Discontinuing the drug before the prescribed time.
   d. Omitting the dose of a medication, prescribed as needed, when it is needed.
3. Taking a dose at a different time if a time has been specified in the directions.
4. Taking a dose in a form other than that specified in the directions.
5. Using the wrong route of administration.
6. Taking medication that has been discontinued.
7. Taking outdated medications.
8. Taking someone else's medications.
9. Taking two or more medications which are contraindicated therapeutically.
10. Failing to get the prescription filled.
11. Failing to understand how to properly use the administration unit (eg, inhaler).
12. Failing to understand how to properly use or administer the dosage form.

Using the above criteria, they found that 42.8% of the patients sampled were misusing their medications and that 4.4% misused their medicine in such a manner as to pose a serious threat to their health. The types of misuse committed most frequently were overdosage and omission of doses. Overdosage represented 41.3% of the total misused prescriptions. Omitting one or more doses occurred in 23.6% of the misused prescriptions. Another result of this study showed that, of the prescriptions being misused, the patients actually were aware they were misusing about half of them. This apparently deliberate misuse perhaps is more understandable when viewed with respect to the second most frequent reason given by the patients for not following directions: they thought they needed another dose. Another frequent reason was that the patient thought he was cured and stopped taking the drug before the prescribed time. The single most often mentioned reason, occurring fully one-third of the time, was that the patient did not understand the instructions.

It is inconceivable that the patient knowingly would misuse medication in a way that would be injurious to his health. Similarly, with the high cost of health care, it is astounding that patients would not maximize the health care they do receive to gain maximum benefit from their expenditures.

It is estimated that ½ of the 1.8 billion prescriptions dispensed on an annual basis are not taken correctly.[3] As a result, health-care costs increase, there is a lack of work productivity and an alarming reality is that 10% of all hospital admissions are due to patients not taking their medications correctly. It also is estimated that more than 125,000 deaths per year are caused by patient noncompliance with prescribed medications.[3] Thus, an apparent reason for the misuse of medicine may be a lack of knowledge and understanding of the medication and how it is integrated into a treatment regimen for their disease state. For example, it is estimated that of the 14 million Americans with diabetes mellitus, only ½ are under the care of a physician. Historically, the scientific literature documents that patients with this disease administer their insulin in an unacceptable manner, do not follow their diets, exhibit poor foot care and do not test their urine and/or blood correctly.[5] Bad habits and/or a lack of responsibility on the part of the patient play a role, but with this is a professional responsibility to ensure the patient understands how all the components fit into the treatment regimen puzzle.

Unfortunately, many patients have a preconceived notion that all medication will make one free from disease. Many do not realize that medications often are necessary just to maintain one's health at the status quo. This is exemplified vividly by nonsteroidal anti-inflammatory drugs which are intended to provide a level of mobility and relieve the pain, stiffness and swelling of arthritis. These cannot "cure" the underlying disease but attempt to arrest the disease process and the patient must understand this concept.

A further misconception relates to the perception of drug potency. "If one tablet is good, two will be even better," is a philosophy that is fraught with danger. The patient should not be held accountable for a lack of knowledge or understanding of drugs, especially when the most readily available information is found in the lay press and the communications media. The OTC drug industry, comparatively free of restrictions until recent years, has in many instances promoted its products in such a manner that it gives the patient the distinct impression that there are "pills for all ills." Consequently, there is evidence that many people overmedicate themselves and have formed a somewhat distorted or undeserved confidence in all drugs. Pharmacy practice, too, must accept partial responsibility. Some practitioners have bombarded the public with information that "generic medications are cheaper" or "which pharmacy has the lowest prices," rather than promoting the need for proper compliance and selection of health-care providers who, through enhanced professional service, are most cost effective in the long run.

The growing number of published medication guides, directed at the lay person, is a further testimonial to the "drug information gap." But, realistically, it is difficult to write these at a level to be understood by every person. Further complicating the issue is the estimation that 19% of the American population are functionally illiterate, and that about 35% of individuals read below a sixth-grade level.[6] In addition, out of necessity, the scope of some books involves only the most frequently prescribed medications. So what does one do when his medication is not found within the book? This is again an instance where pharmacist guidance can be very useful. For example, the USP-DI Volume II, *Advice for the Patient,* is an excellent text that can be purchased by the patient or made available to the patient in a pharmacy. The pharmacy has permission to photocopy and provide to the patient the information specific to the medicine prescribed.

History documents drug use through the ages and it is interesting that only in the last 25 years has the problem of patient misuse of medication been identified and demonstrated. This evidence has escalated due to better communication technique, better study design, the fact that more people have access to primary health care and the use of potent medication. In 1992 a total of 30 therapeutic agents reached the US market for the first time, one less than the record number of 31 agents marketed in 1991. A large number of these drugs are variations of, or chemically related to, existing drug families/pharmacological classes. Through advances in medicinal chemistry many of these new agents are highly potent, and thus the likelihood that problems may occur is heightened. It is difficult for the medical and the pharmaceutical communities to keep up with the proliferation of new products and rapid therapeutic advancements. Still, however, it is the professional responsibility of the pharmacist to continue to learn about and understand these new chemical entities in the hope of being able to provide necessary and useful information to the patient to ensure that these potent medications are used correctly and to their maximal benefit.

Patient Counseling

It always has been the responsibility of the pharmacist to counsel the patient before dispensing the medication. In reality, however, this did not take place always because of pressure to prepare and dispense prescriptions. It is only after the impetus of the OBRA 90 requirements that make mandatory that which should have been a standard of practice in years past.

During the consultation, the pharmacist should provide him with sufficient information (eg, how to take it, how long to take it, at what times, proper storage, frequently encountered side effects, etc) to ensure that the patient will use the medication safely and appropriately. The amount of information that the pharmacist conceivably could share is awesome.

Indeed, it would be foolhardy to believe that the patient will remember everything. Thus, in addition to verbal information, audiovisual and illustrative materials are beneficial. This would include appropriate materials provided within the package by the drug manufacturer or auxiliary, cautionary labels which can be affixed to the dispensed product. More advanced patient-counseling systems involve advisory leaflets. Some innovative and creative pharmacists have developed these and provide them for their patients to take home. Others have been developed by local and state pharmacy associations and private enterprise. Computer software packages (eg, *Medi-Span Patient Drug Education Database*) allow the pharmacist to prepare, at the time of medication dispensing, product-specific and patient-oriented drug information. It is designed to furnish printed instructions to supplement verbal instructions provided by the pharmacist.

Ask the Pharmacist, Inc. is an innovative drug-information service that employs licensed pharmacists to provide a wide range of drug-information services nationwide on a 24-hour, 365-day basis to individual, group and corporate clients using both 1-800 and 1-900 telephone lines. The advantage of this system for a patient over prerecorded drug information systems is that there is a one-on-one consultation with a licensed pharmacist who can provide individualized information to the patient about prescription and over-the-coutner (OTC) medications. By calling, 1-900-4200-ASK, consumers can secure answers to specific questions about their medication (eg, side effects or drug-drug interactions). A fee of $1.95 is added automatically to the caller's telephone bill. This service can be a valuable backup to reinforce counseling information provided to the patient at the time of dispensing. Or, given individual circumstance if counseling is for some reason not possible at the time of dispensing, the patient may be advised to use this service.

This is a means to help improve compliance and illustrate the service function of the pharmacist. It must be emphasized, however, that this service is not a substitute for active counseling by the pharmacist. The situation for each patient is unique, and the pharmacist must provide relevant information specific to that patient. Then, if necessary, the telephone message service may be used to reinforce what has been imparted to the patient.

Because of illiteracy some patients are unable to read the labels on their prescription medications. No doubt this leads to noncompliance with medications and directions. When one reflects on the plight of these individuals, adult nonreaders have spent the majority of their lives hiding their inability from themselves and others. Thus, the pharmacist must be aware of patient clues that indicate a problem with literacy.[6] For example, the patient may ask the pharmacist to fill out forms for them, bring a friend to help them complete the forms or ask to take the forms home to complete. They may make excuses for not reading printed material, such as "I forgot my glasses," or "I do not have time." In addition, as they pretend to read, a pharmacist might notice that their eyes do not shift from right to left. All of these are clues to a growing and hidden problem that confronts society.

Low-literate patients in need of special help will go unnoticed until the pharmacist can learn to read patients' behavior. Once they are identified, the pharmacist, in a nonthreatening, empathetic and discrete manner, should endeavor to help patients overcome this deficiency to gain the maximum benefit from their drug therapy. One approach would be to use visuals, pictograms or attention-getting graphics (eg, *Pharmex Patient Advisory Leaflets*) or the aforementioned *Ask The Pharmacist, Inc.*, that allow the patient to gain from the instruction. Each situation will differ, however, the patient must perceive that the pharmacist is truly willing to help him with his plight.

The need for pharmacist intervention and counseling about medication cannot be overemphasized. Historically, pharmacists were educated under the influence of the old APhA Code of Ethics, adopted in 1921, which discouraged such a discourse with the patient. The new Code of Ethics adopted in 1969 encouraged counseling with such statements as the pharmacist "should render to each patient the full measure of his ability as an essential health practitioner," and "he should utilize and make available this (his) knowledge as may be required in accordance with his best professional judgment." The pharmacist may be held liable if harm occurs to the patient as a result of the pharmacist's negligence in counseling. For example, if the pharmacist did not warn the patient that the drug may make him drowsy and he harms himself because he was not made aware of this effect, the pharmacist may be held liable. Legislators in at least 19 states (1992) have recognized that there is a void and a potential for problems to surface when people do not have access to useful information about their prescription medications.[7] These states require pharmacist consultation at the time the medication is dispensed for all patients.[7] Further, an additional 22 states have legislation pending that would make it mandatory for pharmacists to counsel all patients.[7] A problem with state laws, however, is that some are nebulous while some are specific and pointedly direct the pharmacist to counsel the patient.

Some pharmacists, in the past, avoided counseling on the premise that it is the responsibility of the physician to provide the information to the patient. The physician does have an obligation to instruct the patient in this regard. However, this environment is not always conducive to counseling. The patient is usually sick, he probably has had to wait a while before seeing the physician and he will experience anticipation, apprehension and even fear while waiting. Coupled with the threat of complex instruments and apparatus that are not understandable to him, unpleasant thoughts may be developed. After examination there either may be a great deal of relief or the worst is anticipated. The patient may be thinking more about what is wrong with him than concentrating on the instructions of the physician. All of these are barriers to a good counseling environment. Indeed, the AMA also has recognized this and has developed for its members advisory leaflets of the most often prescribed medications so that the physician can distribute these to the patient in the hope of encouraging proper medication use. This recognition is convincing evidence that a lack of communication does exist between the physician and the patient.

A majority of pharmacists are not reimbursed for time spent counseling patients about the proper use of prescription medications, advising them on the treatment of minor complaints with the most appropriate nonprescription drug product and monitoring their therapeutic profile. Indeed, many pharmacists believe that the patient is simply unwilling to pay for counseling. However, the body of evidence supports the feeling that clinical pharmacy services, including counseling, add value to patient care by enhancing patient compliance, improving patient outcomes and reducing health-care costs. Consumers are beginning to recognize this, and coupled to this is evidence to support the notion that patients are willing to pay for consultation if they know it is available, its potential benefit and its cost. For example, one enterprising pharmacist in Indiana offers each family who purchases its prescriptions at his pharmacy consultation for a flat annual fee. The cost of the prescription then is based upon the cost to the pharmacy plus a handling charge. The fact remains that pharmacists must "market" their knowledge as a drug expert.

Within the counseling endeavor the pharmacist must remember never to take his impute knowledge to the public. A professional may have the tendency to overlook the fact that things which appear commonplace are not so to others. It must be remembered that, although the pharmacist may be counseling the fifth patient of the day on the proper use of amoxicillin, to that patient it is the first time. The patient needs practical, useful information and the pharmacist should share his knowledge. This affords the pharmacist the opportunity to use his knowledge of drugs and dosage forms and provide services to the patient. The following sections exemplify modes of communication that should be encouraged within the domain of patient consultation.

Removing the Drug from the Package—If, by questioning, it is found that the patient is not familiar with the packaging, the pharmacist should demonstrate how to remove the medicine from the package. In the future, as packaging becomes more sophisticated and tamper-resistant, this will become even more important.

Removing medication from its package may seem to be a simple procedure to the pharmacist, but not always to the patient. Most people think eye drops are administered by using a medicine dropper; seeing a container for eye drops which does not contain a dropper (eg, Drop-tainer) may bewilder the patient. Some people may not understand that the dust cap has to be removed from the aerosol device prior to use. Removing the wrapping from a suppository before insertion is quite obvious to the pharmacist, but not so to some patients; there have been cases of patients who have inserted a wrapped suppository, not realizing that the wrapping must be removed. Opening "safety containers" has presented considerable problems to patients, particularly the arthritic or the elderly.

Administering the Drug—It is important for the pharmacist to tell the patient whether the medicine should be taken by mouth, used in the eye, ear or nose, inserted rectally or vaginally or used externally. It should not be taken for granted that the patient knows how to use the medicine even though it is obvious to the pharmacist. Some parents mistakenly have introduced oral antibiotic drops into the ears of their children because the child was being treated for an ear infection. Some elderly patients have taken transdermal patches orally, as they had no previous experience or advice to the contrary. The pharmacist should insure that the patient understands the details of using the medicine.

Tablets—Consider the most common dosage form, the tablet; then consider how many ways it could be used or administered depending upon the medication and the type of tablet.

1. Place on tongue and swallow with water.
2. Warning: Do not chew.
3. Chew and swallow.
4. Let dissolve in mouth; ie, suck on tablet like a "mint."
5. Place under tongue (sublingual) and let dissolve. Do not swallow.
6. Place between gum and cheek (buccal) and let dissolve. Do not swallow.
7. Dissolve in water and swallow.
8. Dissolve in water and use externally.
9. Moisten with water and insert vaginally or rectally.

The most common method to administer a tablet is to place it on the tongue and to swallow it with water. Most patients understand this method of administration. Some, however, need to be reminded to take the tablet with a glassful of water. This is very important with those drugs that are irritating to the stomach, eg, ferrous sulfate, aspirin, tetracyclines or potassium chloride. Another problem is that some people may assume mistakenly that a tablet must be administered by mouth and proceed to do so.

Another service the pharmacist should provide is to ask the patient if he can swallow a tablet because some people are unable to do so. If a person is unable to swallow a tablet the pharmacist has two options to exercise. The first is to suggest a device that assists in swallowing a tablet (ie, Drink-A-Pill Drinking Glass) or to consult the physician and suggest an equivalent liquid dosage form. If a liquid equivalent is not available a convenient option is to place the tablet in a spoon with some water. After the tablet disintegrates, the contents of the spoon should be swallowed. Some drugs with a disagreeable taste may need to be masked by placing some applesauce, syrup or similar substance on the spoon. Otherwise, the pharmacist should consider preparing extemporaneously a liquid dosage form using a flavored vehicle (eg, cherry syrup). Numerous extemporaneous preparations have appeared in the professional literature in recent years and provide a basis for compounding technique and procedure. However, a main concern is the stability of the drug once it is prepared in liquid form. In some of these instances, pharmaceutical information will be required and the pharmacist should use the telephone number of the manufacturer listed in *Drug Facts and Comparisons*. Severel paperback textbooks on formulations based upon documented and unpublished stability data compiled by pharmaceutical manufacturers and practitioners have been published.

Some tablets must be swallowed in their entirety. These tablets either are enteric-coated or sustained-release. Enteric-coated tablets might contain drugs which are irritating to the stomach or are not stable in gastric fluid. Thus, they are passed through the stomach and ultimate release of the contents in the intestines is preferred. Sustained-release medication is intended to provide medication as the dosage form traverses the gatrointestinal tract. Chewing the tablet unknowingly would alter the release characteristics and may provide the entire effect of the medication at once. This could be hazardous to the patient and at the same time not afford therapeutic coverage for the period of time between doses. Lastly, there are a few tableted medications which have the capability to stain the teeth and mouth. The patient should be told to swallow this type, as well as the aforementioned enteric-coated and sustained-release tablets. See Chapter 94.

Ophthalmic Preparations—The pharmacist should be sure the patient understands how to use these preparations. The use of eye drops can be demonstrated easily by placing a finger below the lower eyelid away from the nose and pulling down. This will form a pocket in the lower lid where the solution should be dropped. For retention in the eye and/or to diminish possible systemic effects of some drugs (eg, timolol maleate), the patient should be told to apply light finger pressure on the lacrimal sac for a minute following administration. Ophthalmic ointments may be used in the eye or on the eyelid depending on the drug and condition of the patient. Therefore, it first should be determined where the ointment should be used. If the ointment is to be used in the eye, pull the lower lid down the same way as when using eyedrops, then squeeze a small amount of ointment inside the lower lid. The eye is then closed and massaged gently. If the ointment is to be used on the eyelid, a thin ribbon of ointment is squeezed from the tube directly onto the eyelid. See Chapter 89.

Inhalations—Currently, medications for inhalation are provided to the patient by a variety of means, from the fine mist of a vaporizer to the powder of cromolyn sodium with a *Spinhaler*. There are now dosage forms for oral and nasal inhalation, and it is obvious that these products will only be effective when properly used. The pharmacist must attempt to educate the patient in the use of these products and provide written instruction, usually found within the product carton. It is difficult to predict what percentage of patients will read or even understand the printed instruction. Thus, the pharmacist must verbally transmit instruction for proper use. Using the oral, metered aerosols as a model the pharmacist should demonstrate how the inhaler is to be assembled, stored and cleaned. The patient should be told if the inhaler requires shaking before use and how to hold it between the index finger and thumb so that the aerosol canister is upside-down. The patient should understand that coordination must be achieved between inhalation (after exhaling as completely as possible) and pressing down the inhaler to release one dose. The patient should be instructed to hold his breath for several seconds, or as long as possible, to gain the maximum benefit from the medication. The patient then is told to remove the inhaler from the mouth and exhale slowly through pursed lips. The pharmacist also should be able to recognize those patients (eg, first-time users, children or the elderly) who typically encounter difficulty when using metered-dose inhalers. Extender devices, some of which are available on prescription only, modify metered-dose inhalers and make them more beneficial for patients who are unable to coordinate drug release and inhalation. The pharmacist should take the initiative to contact the physician in behalf of such a patient and be prepared to suggest such an extender device based upon the patient's circumstances and lifestyle. See Chapter 95 and Chapter 107.

Suppositories—There are several helpful items of information that the pharmacist should relate about the proper use of suppositories. If they must be stored in the refrigerator, they should be allowed to warm to room temperature before insertion. The patient should be advised to rub cocoa butter suppositories gently with the fingers to help melt the surface to provide lubrication for insertion. Glycerinated gelatin or polyethylene glycol suppositories should be moistened with water to enhance lubrication. If the polyethylene glycol suppository formulation does not contain at least 20% water, dipping it in water just prior to insertion prevents moisture from being drawn from rectal tissues after insertion and decreases subsequent irritation. Vaginal inserts (compressed tablets) also should be dipped into water quickly before insertion. This provides lubrication and enhances disintegration. The shape of the suppository determines how it will be inserted. Bullet-shaped rectal suppositories should be inserted pointed-end first. In those instances when the patient is to use one-half of a suppository, the patient should be told to cut the suppository lengthwise with a clean razor blade. See Chapter 90.

Transdermal Systems—In the future there will be many innovative modes of drug delivery by noninvasive means. The advent of this dimension in drug administration is illustrated by the numerous transdermal systems (patches) which are available. Such drugs as nitroglycerin, scopolamine and estradiol are administered in this way. They have the advantage of affording continuous therapy, and in the case of transdermal scopolamine, allow one to enjoy a Caribbean cruise without worry about motion sickness. The duration of use for a patch may vary. For example, for nitroglycerin the patch usually is changed every day, where as with transdermal estradiol it is changed about every 3 days. At the end of that time the patient replaces the old patch with the new. It is incumbent upon the pharmacist to instruct the patient on the proper use of this topical system. The patient should place the adhesive side of the system on a clean, dry, hair-free area of the skin on the trunk of the body, preferably the abdomen. He should be told to rotate the site of application to minimize the possibility of irritation, and the area selected should not be oily, damaged or irritated. The transdermal system should not be applied to the waistline because tight clothing may rub the system off. The patient should be encouraged to apply the system as soon as it is removed from the protective liner and to press it firmly with the palm of the hand for about 10 seconds. It is important to make sure there is good contact, especially around the edges and, in the unlikely event that a patch should fall off, it may be reapplied. If necessary, the patient might have to use a new system but, in either instance, he should continue the original treatment schedule. Although it might seem unimaginable, the patient should be told to replace one patch with another and to discard a patch once it is removed from the skin. Patients should be told that there is enough residual medication (eg, nitroglycerin) in discarded patches that these pose a hazard to children and pets. Thus, these should be disposed of cautiously.

The pharmacist also must ensure that the patient understands about the necessity to wear the patch the entire day or to remove the patch after a set amount of time. For example, starting doses of nitroglycerin between 0.4 and 0.8 mg/hour have shown continued effectiveness for 10 to 12 hours daily for at least 1 month of intermittent administration. Although the minimum nitrate-free interval has not been defined, data show that a nitrate-free interval of 10 to 12 hours is sufficient. Thus, an appropriate dosing schedule would include a daily *patch-on* period of 12 to 14 hours and a *patch-off* period of 10 to 12 hours. Tolerance is a major factor that limits efficacy when the system is used on a continual basis for greater than 12 hours a day. In those instances when the patch is worn overnight, the patient should be told to inspect the patch after awakening. See Chapter 90.

Water—Whenever the directions for the use of a medication refer to water (eg, dissolve in water, mix with water, take with water, etc), the pharmacist should tell the patient how much water to use and in what manner. For example, one laxative product instructs a patient to place a rounded teaspoonful of granules in the mouth and swallow with a glass of water. Another laxative product instructs the patient to add a teaspoon of powder to the liquid before ingesting it. These are points of clarification that are necessary to ensure correct use by the patient.

Timing of the Dose—Interpretation of the directions, "one qid" may be variable between the physician, pharmacist and patient. Conceivable interpretations for this might include the following:

One every 6 hr around the clock (6 am, 12 pm, 6 pm, 12 am).
One every 4 hr while awake (8 am, 12 pm, 4 pm, 8 pm).
One before meals and at bedtime.
One after meals and at bedtime.
One with meals and at bedtime.

The pharmacist must use his biopharmaceutical and pharmacokinetic knowledge of drugs when interpreting the directions and give instructions to the patient to ensure that the drug is maximally effective. If the effectiveness of the drug depends upon a maintained blood level, the patient should be instructed to space out equally through the day appropriate dosing times. If the bioavailability of the drug from oral administration is in doubt when taken with food (eg, antibiotics), it is best to recommend that the drug be taken either 1 hr before or 2 hours after meals. The pharmacist cannot lose sight of the fact that some patients do not eat three meals a day and, thus, if the latter recommendation was made, it would be important to emphasize to the patient that even though a meal may not be eaten, the drug still should be taken. Alternatively, the pharmacist should exercise judgment in those instances where the drug that is administered orally causes stomach distress. In these instances the pharmacist should encourage the patient to take the medication with food or milk to prevent this upset. The pharmacist should never assume that the patient understands completely how to use the medication properly. When the timing of a dose is crucial, the pharmacist should counsel the patient to exercise good judgment.

The pharmacist also should be extremely wary of "as needed" (prn) prescriptions. The patient should be told about the correct use of the product. Probably the foremost example involves pain medication. Exclusive of instances where pain is managed with a specifically scheduled analgesic dosage regimen, eg, cancer therapy, the patient (or family caregiver) should be told to use the medication only as needed for pain relief, and not to prevent subsequent pain. If, however, the pain continues to persist, then the patient should be encouraged to take another dose within the prescribed time indicated on the label, bearing in mind that the drug may not provide immediate pain relief. There likely will be a gap in pain relief if the pain is allowed to return before taking the next dose of medication.

Another example of difficulty with "prn" use entails the tachyphylaxis that develops with the overuse of aerosol in halers to treat asthmatic conditions. A pattern of increasing frequency of refills is a signal to the pharmacist that the patient either is overusing the product or simply does not know how to use it correctly. Pharmacist intervention is a necessity in this instance. Another facet with "prn" medication is that patients may not need the medication for a period of time and thus will have to store it. Adequate instructions should accompany the medication that encourage proper storage. Sometimes, however, "prn" instructions are simply inappropriate, eg, with medications which accumulate in the system for maximum effectiveness, such as the tricyclic antidepressants.

Dosage regimens are established best when consideration is given to the daily routine of the patient. Dosage regimens must be developed to take into account the patient's eating and sleeping habits and work schedule.

Compliance problems with medications increase as the number of medications a person ingests during the day increases. A medication calendar can prove very useful and could be developed almost entirely to the patient's individual needs. The medication calendar should reinforce the correct time to take the medication and afford the opportunity for the patient to mark down that the dose actually was taken. This obviates problems of forgetfulness about whether a dose was taken or missed. Numerous calendars have been developed and an exemplary one is presented (Fig 1). This provides space for writing in *chronic* and *as needed* medications, as well as the administration times within the vertical column. The patient can write in the name and the dosage of the medication (even the prescription number if desired) to be taken at one time. The horizontal column contains the days of the month through day 31. The patient merely checks off the appropriate time slot when a dose of medication has been taken. This helps prevent problems of forgetfulness and avoids unnecessary and dangerous accidental double dosing. Such a calendar can be taped to the refrigerator in the kitchen and encourages the patient to take an active role in the treatment plan by complying with the prescribed medications.

Duration of Use—The pharmacist must ensure that the patient clearly understands the length of time the medication is to be used. Chronic diseases dictate that adequate blood levels of drug be maintained to control the disease process. Thus, emphasis should be toward compliance counseling regarding the medication and periodic revisits with the physician to assess the therapeutic regimen. The pharmacist also must emphasize to the patient that some medications require a lengthy time period to observe the initial effects of the drug (eg, nonsteroidal anti-inflammatory agents, tricyclic antidepressants, etc) and they should exercise patience. At the same time, the pharmacist should provide the patient with a reasonable time period, after which the desired effect may be experienced. After this time, should no effect be observed, the patient should be told to contact his physician.

For acute problems the pharmacist must indicate the length of time the medication should be taken. This is very important with an antibiotic, which must be taken in its entirety over the prescribed time period to cure the infection. Early discontinuation of the medication, because of feeling better, should be discouraged to prevent a relapse of the infection and/or sequelae. The pharmacist must emphasize this fact to the patient because some believe that taking a drug is not good for their body and will only take what they think is necessary. This philosophy particularly is dangerous when dealing with parents of young children who do not want to subject them to more medication than they deem necessary or, simply because of inconvenience, do not elect to continue the medication once the child feels better. Other dosage forms, other than oral, (eg, otic drops, nasal drops, vaginal inserts) might be prescribed for an acute condition. The pharmacist must exercise judgment and instruct the patient on the length of therapy. For example, an infectious otitis externa problem treated with otic drops should be continued for at least 2 to 3 days beyond the time the symptoms have abated. It is not necessary to continue using the otic drops until the medication is exhausted since sufficient material usually is dispensed so that it conceivably could be used for over 20 days. This information should be told to the patient.

Storage—The pharmacist should counsel the patient in the proper storage of the medicine to ensure safety and stability. It is not sufficient to assume the patient will notice, read or even be able to understand an auxiliary label which indicates how to store the medication. Safety is foremost when storing medication, particularly so it is out of the reach of children. Further, medication should be stored in a single area (preferably inside a high cabinet) with external medications separate from internal medications.

Proper storage of the medication also ensures stability of the product. Medications should be stored away from extremes of heat and humidity. Two prime places where medicines should not be stored are in the medicine cabinet of the bathroom and the glove compartment of an automobile or truck. One study demonstrated that temperatures in automobile glove compartments in the northern hemisphere from April to October can range as much as 50° above outdoor temperatures. Thus, medications can be exposed to temperatures in excess of 150° if placed in a glove compartment. Heat and humidity hasten drug degradation and the patient should be told to inspect the medication before using it. Any color change or unusual odor emanating from the product indicates that it may be losing its potency. The patient should be instructed to cap the bottle tightly after use, otherwise environmental humidity could cause stability problems, or the exposure to the atmosphere could promote the evaporation of a liquid vehicle. With topical liquid products (eg, wart removers) this could result in a somewhat more potent and hazardous product due to increased concentration of active ingredients. Further, some products may degrade into toxic products, not merely useless products, eg, tetracyclines.

When a medication is dispensed in its original container and still bears the expiration data on its label (eg, ear drops, eye drops) this should be brought to the attention of the patient so that judgment can be exercised to discard old, outdated medication periodically. Otherwise, medication not used within 1 year after it is obtained should be discarded.

Side Effects—The instructions about a medication should encourage compliance rather than discourage it, and there is no more rapid means to achieve the latter than a hasty, ill-thought presentation by the pharmacist of the side effects that may be encountered with a particular medication. The pharmacist should inform the patient tactfully about side effects that could be encountered. If not so instructed, the patient might discontinue the use of the product with no benefit. The pharmacist only should inform the patient of the most frequently encountered of all the conceivable side effects and provide a mechanism by which to cope with them. For example, metronidazole is used for trichomonal infections, and "may cause headaches in some people. If you experience a headache, do not hesitate to take some aspirin or acetaminophen for it. If this does not help, contact your physician."

The manner in which the patient is told of side effects is crucial. Presentation of the side effect might convince the patient not to take the medication. For example, "Do not drive while taking this medicine; it will make you drowsy." For a person who makes a living traveling, this might dictate against taking the medication at all. Thus, the instruction should be, "this medication may make you drowsy and impair

DAILY MEDS/REASON		DAY																														
		1	2	3	4	5	6	7	8	9	10	11	12	13	14	15	16	17	18	19	20	21	22	23	24	25	26	27	28	29	30	31
Dyazide Caps (Water)	9 AM	X	X		X	X	X	X	X	X	X	X	X	X	X		X	X	X	X	X											
Lanoxin Tabs 0.25mg (Heart)	9 AM	X	X		X	X	X	X	X	X	X	X	X	X	X		X	X	X	X	X											
Somophyllin Liq., 1 tsp (Lungs)	9 AM	X	X	X	X	X	X	X		X	X	X	X	X	X		X	X	X	X	X											
	3 PM	X	X	X	X	X	X	X	X	X		X	X	X	X		X	X	X	X												
	9 PM	X			X	X	X	X	X	X	X	X	X	X	X	X	X	X	X	X	X											
Keflex Caps 250mg (Chest)	6 AM												X	X	X	X	X	X														
	12 PM												X	X		X		X														
	6 PM												X	X	X	X	X															
	12 AM												X	X	X	X	X															
Phenergan Expt., 1 tsp. (Cough)	6 AM												X	X		X		X														
	12 PM												X	X	X	X	X	X	X													
	6 PM												X		X	X	X		X													
	12 AM														X																	
MEDICATIONS ONLY AS NEEDED/REASON																																
Dalmane Caps 15mg (Sleep)	BEDTIME		X			X	X	X				X							X													
Valium Tabs 5mg (Nerves)	BREAKFAST																															
	LUNCH	X				X	X	X			X	X																				
	DINNER					X	X	X			X	X																				

Fig 1. A medication calendar.

your perception. Exercise judgment when doing things that involve your reflexes or alertness. Thus, use caution when you are driving."

Similarly, the patient should be told that some medications cause side effects at first that diminish with continual use, eg, the dizziness or lightheadedness with Catapres TTS should decrease as one adjusts to the medicine. At the same time the patient should be informed if problems persist or get worse they should consult their physician.

Auxiliary labels serve a definite purpose to help inform the patient about prescription medication. These should be used cautiously and explained verbally by the pharmacist when conveying information about side effects or potential drug interactions. For example, one label that is used cautions against excessive exposure to direct sunlight. Unfortunately, without pharmacist explanation, this might be construed to mean avoid going out of doors and keeping the house dark. The word "excessive" is overlooked by the patient, but what does the word mean? Obviously, this label needs interpretation by the pharmacist during counseling. Another label cautions against the concurrent use of alcohol with the medication for fear of an additive depressant effect. Unfortunately, the patient might not read the label or understand that alcohol need not be consumed only from an alcoholic beverage; alcohol is included in a number of liquid medications (eg, cough-cold remedies). Thus, the emphasis should be on good verbal communication with the pharmacist.

Some medications, by virtue of their physical-chemical properties, could cause compliance problems in some patients. Some medications have the ability to change urine color (eg, phenazopyridine), stool color (eg, ferrous sulfate), and saliva, sweat and tear color (eg, rifampin). While these are not side effects, these should be brought to the attention of the patient beforehand to allay any fears encountered when these occur.

Pharmacists also have a professional and legal responsibility to collect information from the patient concerning adverse drug reactions. Both the FDA and pharmaceutical manufacturers have foreseen a need to collect and disseminate this information so that potential problems with a drug can be identified. Protocol restrictions during the clinical trials of a drug may limit its investigation to only certain patient types while excluding others, eg, geriatric patients, children or pregnant women. Thus, reactions which are infrequent may present themselves only after widespread use and the detection of these depends upon the alertness and diligence of the pharmacist and physician.

To report a suspected adverse drug (either prescription or nonprescription) reaction, a pharmacist can complete (to the best extent possible) an *Adverse Reaction Report* (Drugs and Biologics), FDA Form 1639, and submit this directly to the FDA. A copy of this form usually is reproduced on the back cover of the *FDA Medical Bulletin* and also appears within the appendix of Volume I *Drug Information for the Health Care Professional, USP DI.* Alternatively, the pharmacist can telephone (1-800-638-6725) the USP directly to report a suspected adverse drug reaction through its Practitioners' Reporting Network (ie, USP-PRN). The USP shares its information with the FDA, the product manufacturer and the USP Drug Information and Drug Standards Divisions. This alternative is useful because the information received heightens USP awareness about drug reactions that would be beneficial to include within its drug-information monographs. The USP does not reciprocally receive from the FDA adverse drug reaction information which is reported directly to the Agency, so to include the USP *in the loop* serves everyone.

In 1993 the FDA launched MEDWatch, to improve upon the aforementioned voluntary reporting system which for some is difficult to use and that the average health-care professional might be pressed to know what to report, how to report and/or when to report. MEDWatch facilitates the voluntary reporting of serious side effects, defects or other problems in drugs in devices. This was introduced to make the process of adverse drug reporting simpler (only one page required for completion) by encouraging the reporting of only serious effects such as death, life-threatening illness or injury, hospitalization or disability, and complements the USP reporting system which has a broader scope and slightly different focus.

Drug Interactions—The patient should be forewarned about other drugs (eg, legend, nonprescription) that may have the potential to alter the effectiveness of the prescribed medication. Certainly, if there is legend medication within the current profile of the patient that conflicts with a newly prescribed medication, it is the responsibility of the pharmacist to bring it to the attention of the physician. Unfortunately, however, patients perceive nonprescription drugs as entirely safe and do not realize that these have the ability to aggravate their condition or interact with prescription medication. Thus, this discussion also should include instruction to carefully read nonprescription drug labels beforehand and, if in doubt, consult the physician or the pharmacist. It is estimated that well over 1000 drug-drug interactions have been reported in the medical and pharmaceutical literature during the past 25 years. This presents an overwhelming task to the pharmacist to sort out the clinically significant ones from the trivial. Helpful, computerized drug interaction systems are available, many of which are incorporated into the overall pharmacy computer system providing pharmacists with user-friendly and efficient decision support systems. The key, however, is the pharmacist, who after detecting the drug interaction, must assess the risk of the interaction. Assessing the risk of a particular drug interaction requires the knowledge of which factors increase the possibility of adverse effects for each individual interaction. The pharmacist must consider drug-related risk factors and patient-related risk factors, eg, disease of the patient, habits (smoking, alcohol, diet), frequency and type of drug response monitoring and renal/hepatic function.

When the pharmacist takes action to minimize the risk of an interaction, only those drug interactions which are significant clinically (eg, warfarin–aspirin) should be brought to the attention of the patient and alternative means provided to cope with any problems (eg, use of acetaminophen for headache while maintained on warfarin therapy).

This subject also encompasses the ingestion of food concurrent with the oral administration of the medication. When a significant alteration in the bioavailability of a drug or its therapeutic effect occurs with the concurrent administration of foods or liquids (eg, tetracycline with milk) the patient should be warned and provided with a suitable remedy to ensure that he will use the medication. Similarly, if he, by necessity, must ingest food with the medication (eg, phenytoin, propranolol) to avoid gastrointestinal upset, he should be encouraged to maintain this mode of administration whenever possible, to avoid fluctuation in the bioavailability of the drug and, ultimately, the steady-state levels of the drug in the blood. See Chapter 105.

Allergies—Every drug has the potential to effect a hypersensitivity reaction in a patient. However, there are some medications (eg, penicillins, sulfonamides, thiazides, etc) which effect a higher incidence of allergic reactions. When such medications are prescribed, the pharmacist should inquire about the past medication history and any known allergies to any medication. In a tactful manner the patient should be told that the prescribed medication has caused a rash or allergic reaction in some people. Thus, in the event the patient experiences a rash, or an itching and burning of the skin, he should be advised to discontinue the use of the medication and contact the physician.

Refill Information—When presenting the medication to the patient, the pharmacist should indicate verbally whether or not the prescription is refillable, or should be refilled. If the prescription can be refilled, the patient should be informed of this, and told the number of times it may be refilled and the length of time during which the prescription may be refilled. If the prescription is nonrefillable, the patient should be so instructed, so that if he needs additional medication he will know to contact the physician. The pharmacist should not, however, give the patient the impression that there is a need to return to the physician's office only for a new prescription, but to have him contact the physician by telephone, explain the situation and then telephone the pharmacist who in turn can contact the physician for the refill authorization.

Whenever possible, the pharmacist should encourage those patients who take chronic medications to have them refilled on time. Consultation is a time-consuming activity and many pharmacists cannot bring themselves to do it efficiently because they usually are not remunerated for it. One pilot study, however, investigated patient willingness to pay for a community pharmacy-based medication-reminder system.[8] This study blended an initial interview (eg, medication history, counseling session) and followup discussions (ie, return visits to the pharmacy) with a medication-reminder system for a group of patients who were maintained on at least one regularly scheduled cardiovascular medication. These patients received a medication-reminder card in the mail within 3 days after the calculated refill date of the medication was passed. If after 10 days the prescription had not been refilled, the patient was contacted by telephone. The data indicated that nearly 40% of the patients expressed a willingness to pay for the services they received above the cost of the medication. Further, the authors indicated that the reminder system could be maintained in a relatively small amount of time (less than 15 min a day) and effort (clerical and pharmacist) and lent itself nicely to a computer function.

The pharmacist has a responsibility not to refill a nonrefillable prescription without authorization from the physician. In some instances, the physician may have retired from practice, died or designated the prescription as "refill prn." The best rule of thumb for this type is for the pharmacist to refill it only with a frequency consistent with the directions for use, and to check with the prescribing physician after a reasonable amount of time to make certain he wants the patient to continue using the medication. Some states have regulations on the "prn" refill. For example, Texas has taken steps to limit "prn" refills to 1 year, New York allows for one refill only, while Ohio has banned the use of "prn," requiring that it not be interpreted to authorize renewals.

Therapeutic Intent—It is not always advisable for the pharmacist to make reference to the therapeutic use of the medication unless he is absolutely certain of its intended purpose for a particular patient. Often, the pharmacist does not know the diagnosis of the patient, nor the intent of the physician in prescribing a certain drug. Indeed, there are numerous indications for a multitude of drugs which make it difficult to identify the one indication for a specific patient.

In these situations, when confronted by a patient inquiry about the purpose of the medication, the pharmacist should answer a question with a question. A question about the reason the patient consulted a physician and something about their physical health could provide insight for the pharmacist. Careful questioning usually will provide enough information so that the pharmacist can piece together a reasonable answer.

Additional Information—The therapeutic outcome will be successful only if the patient understands the need to comply with his regimen. At the same time, the pharmacist should bring to the attention of the patient other factors which may embellish or enhance the drug therapy. For instance, patients maintained on oral hypoglycemics should be reminded to maintain their caloric intake and be cognizant of their diet; those maintained on daily doses of phenytoin should be advised to exercise good oral hygiene by massaging the gums and brushing the teeth, at least on a daily basis and those with asthmatic conditions can be advised about what may be done to relieve asthmatic attacks before they occur. These are all examples of the use of common sense by the patient and typify the expertise of the pharmacist as a source of information.

Drug Utilization Review (DUR)

Pharmacists always have recognized their responsibility to check the safety of the dosage regimen for each medication dispensed. OBRA 90 now makes mandatory that which should have been a standard of practice for the past several years. In the past this was an easy task, but recently, with the proliferation of many newer, potent medications, this task has become quite formidable. There is no doubt that DUR functions will be enhanced by the use of computer programs. Scanning the profile for therapeutic duplication, over- and underutilization, drug-drug and drug-disease interactions, incorrect dosage or duration of therapy and clinical abuse will be aided considerably by the speed of the computer. However, simple programs cannot interact with the patient in a meaningful way, telephone the prescriber for clarification or judge the severity of the condition and the cooperation of the patient. Each of those judgmental functions will be left to the pharmacist who is educated to do that job.

Checking the safety of a dosage regimen is more complex today because, in addition to higher potency, many drugs can be used for more than one clinical indication, and for nonlabeled uses too. Further, with the diversification of the medical profession into specialty areas, there is a greater chance that patients will consult more than one physician. Thus, the patient of today may be taking a number of drugs, simultaneously, from more than one physician. Very often these physicians will not be aware that their patient is receiving drugs prescribed by other physicians. This is the perfect avenue by which drug interactions occur. In addition, with greater numbers of patients taking medication, there is a greater likelihood of allergic, idiosyncratic or adverse reactions to occur. When these are manifest, it is vital that they be documented to prevent their occurrence in the future. Because of all of these factors it is implicit that the pharmacist be cognizant of each patient as a whole, inclusive of all the medications that the patient may be taking currently when evaluating the safety of a newly prescribed medication or perform DUR. To do this effectively the pharmacist must keep a record of the past medical history of the patient (eg, chronic disease status, allergic/idiosyncratic/adverse reactions) and a medication history. It is inconceivable that the pharmacist could commit to memory the status of each patient and thus the aspect of a patient "profile" or "record" system looms as a necessity for effective ambulatory pharmacy practice. There is no doubt that integrated into this record system is the ability of the pharmacist to monitor the progress with the prescribed therapeutic regimen.

DUR is not new to pharmacy. In fact, another OBRA (OBRA 87) has enhanced the mandate first made in 1974 which virtually created consultant pharmacist services in what then were called nursing homes. Consultant pharmacist services looked much like present DUR, or Drug Regimen Review (DRR) which was once unknown in these facilities. Prior to 1965 the facilities were regulated only by the states, and regulations were few. But with the passage of Medicaid and Medicare laws, the federal agencies became involved. While this review was originally only for skilled facilities, and was at one time the responsibility of either the physicians or nurses, it is now extended to patients in skilled nursing facilities (SNFs), intermediate care facilities (ICFs) and intermediate care facilities for the mentally retarded (ICF-MR). They are also now, appropriately, the exclusive province of the consultant pharmacist.

Medication Profiles

Patient Medication Profiles are synonymous with "Family Prescription Records" or "Patient Medication Cards." Essentially, these systems are a record of information relative to the drug therapy of a patient or an entire family. Ideally, but not too realistically, they also should include OTC drugs/products as well. Prior to the enactment of OBRA 90, the majority of states did not mandate patient profiles, even though pharmacies with commercially developed computer software for prescription processing, as well as some pharmacies with manual systems, already had them. The 1992–1993 *Survey of Pharmacy Law*, published by the National Association of Boards of Pharmacy, lists 16 states which have mandatory patient profiles, two which have rules or laws pending which would mandate them, one with rules under development and 33 which have no such rule.[9] The survey includes information from the District of Columbia and Puerto Rico accounting for the 52 responses. Mandating profiles was only a part of the story. Three states required that the pharmacist consult and examine the profile prior to dispensing.

With the implementation of OBRA 90 much of this became obsolete because Federal legislation mandated that the states pass and implement DUR standards on or before January 1, 1993, as a requirement for participation in Medicaid. Many states have taken the position that if those were to be standard for Medicaid patients, they would extend the requirement to all patients. As part of the process of DUR, the pharmacist is to make a reasonable effort to obtain certain information which forms the basis of the patient medication record. That information includes

Name, address, telephone number, age or date of birth, and gender.
Known drug allergies and adverse reactions.
A list of current medications and relevant devices, either of which may relate to patient's drug therapy.
Known disease states.
Any other information that, in the pharmacist's professional judgment, the pharmacist deems appropriate.
Pharmacist's comments relevant to the individual's drug therapy.

Patient profiles maintained on the pharmacy computer system assist the pharmacist in monitoring the patient and attempting to limit the overlap of medication and drug interactions. Sophistication of computer systems has allowed state-of-the-art clinical screening capabilities for the pharmacist. For example, the Medi-Span Solution is a software implementation tool providing access to Medi-Span's family of DUR databases. The Solution enables drug-drug interaction, drug-allergy, drug-disease contraindication, duplicate therapy, dosage range and duration and compliance screening to be incorporated into a medication order-processing system.

Ideally, patient medication profiles also should include nonprescription drug products/devices. With the movement toward self care, it is conceivable a patient will not be prescribed a prescription drug but asked to purchase a nonprescription one. Patients must be educated about the necessity to share with the pharmacist all medications currently used, including nonprescription ones. Otherwise, the pharmacist would be unable to perform a valid DUR.

The family system of profiling allows all members of the family to be listed within a single profile, which reduces the number of files. This does, however, present a challenge when the pharmacist attempts to monitor the therapy for each patient. Thus, the individual record makes it easier to monitor the patient and is less susceptible to errors of confusion on the part of the pharmacist. This problem is overcome easily by effective computer systems which store a patient record within a family file, but scan only the individual history and medications when necessary.

Purpose—The main purposes of the profile include the documentation of the medication history and the use of medication by the patient (eg, compliance, noncompliance). Further, it provides the basis for retrospective DUR and a data base to facilitate communication and consultation between the pharmacist and other health professionals (eg, drug allergies, idiosyncratic reactions, previous ineffective medication, prevention of potential drug–drug interactions). Computer-based software also provides space for pharmacists to record and document interventions germane to the specific patient.

Essential Information—Historically, there have been a number of different record systems and cards available for the pharmacist. Indeed, because 95% of pharmacies are now computerized, this creates less of a dilemma for the pharmacist. However, pharmacists have been known to design their own cards and have these duplicated, especially when space limitations are real. Aside from the specific patient information mentioned earlier in this section, other essential information on the patient medication profile specific to drug therapy would include

Previous ineffective drug therapy
Prescription number
Date of the prescription
Drug product name
Dosage form of the product
Strength of the product
Quantity dispensed
Name of the prescriber
Identification of the pharmacist

Additional information that can prove useful on the profile are the directions for the medication dispensed, refill information and charge for the medication. Typical family profiles and patient profiles are illustrated in Figs 2 and 3.

The upper left-hand corner contains demographic data of the patient(s). The birth date, not the age of the patient, should be used because it remains constant. When the family system is used, each member must be identified by a key. In Fig 2, the designation (H) is used for the husband, (W) is used for the wife and numbers are used to identify the children.

The upper right-hand portion is reserved for necessary information to prevent the dispensing of contraindicated drugs (ie, clinical conditions/problems, allergies/reactions). Further, space should be allotted for notes (eg, past medication failure, inability to use medication, patient wears contact lens, etc) which provide a complete picture of the patient.

The bottom portion contains relevant information about the dispensed medication.

For those pharmacists still employing handwritten patient profiles, a color dot or symbol system can be used with a profile to identify specific pharmacist concerns; eg, a red dot means to check compliance discrepancy, a green dot to discuss side effects with a particular patient and a red star indicates physician contacted and notation of the prescription face. Further, a color-code system for a certain sequence of the letters in the alphabet is an effective means to overcome the loss of a patient profile. Every practicing pharmacist who has worked with filed records realizes the danger of "lost records"; these are not lost at all, but are merely misfiled. In a pharmacy where there may be well over a thousand profiles, the file may be misplaced in any part of the system. Thus, searching for the file at the time of prescription dispensing is impractical if not impossible. The pharmacist should follow the example of other professions to help identify a misplaced file. Medical records departments are the prime example. For every 100 to 200 files, a different color code is used. A misplaced file becomes very obvious under this system if it is in another color space, or if it is to be found among a very small number of similarly coded files. It also must be mentioned that the likelihood of a person replacing a profile incorrectly is less when the color code does not match. In busy pharmacies when a file is pulled for use, a handy ruler, pencil or tongue depressor usually is placed to mark its spot. The system then resembles a porcupine more than a filing system and when the profile is to be refiled, numerous markers may be confusing and lead to misfiling. An effective color-code system reduces the incidence of misfiled information.

Implementation and Use—The pharmacist must select the medication profile system (family, individual) according to that which best fits his practice. To implement the service the pharmacist must establish a mode to gather and record essential patient information (usually a patient interview). To be effective, the patient medication profile must be used each time a professional service is performed.

The pharmacist must maintain confidentiality of the profile, consistent with the same accorded a prescription. However, the concept of confidentiality is nebulous because the patient is not required to provide the information. The pharmacist usually can divulge information (if in good faith) when it is in the best interest of the patient (eg, contact a physician about his past allergic history). However, the pharmacist should familiarize himself with the state regulations and the state pharmacy laws to be aware of the obligations and responsibilities germane to the dissemination of the information from such a patient profile. Some systems intentionally have the confidential information on the right-side (Fig 2). Thus, information which might be requested for the preparation of income tax or insurance purposes is located on the left side (date, medication order number, physician, charge, etc). Thus, the right-hand side of the card can be covered and a photocopy made of the left-hand portion of the profile.

A key problem with confidentiality occurs when the request for information originates outside of the pharmacy, specifically when the information is requested by an insurance company. Generally, the pharmacist does not know whether the patient is represented by the company. Perhaps there is a history of claims filed for the patient by the pharmacist that gives a clue about the validity of the request. In those in-

FAMILY NAME PUBLIC

ADDRESS 123 W. Columbia

TELEPHONE 555-1212

(H) Nicholas G. 09-30-44
(W) Laura L. 03-04-47
(1) Stanley J. 10-11-72
(2) Gabriel N. 01-04-78
(3) Matthew T. 11-02-79

ALLERGIES/REACTIONS (H) Allergic to Sulfa
(3) Allergic to PCN

CLIN. CONDITIONS/PROBLEMS (W) Glaucoma
(H) Migraine

NOTES: (3) Difficulty swallowing tablets

DATE	RX #	DOCTOR	PT.	DRUG/STRENGTH/AMOUNT	SIG	REF	CHARGE	RPH
1-04-95	224523	Smith	H	100 Inderal 20mg TAB	i qid	5	8.05	NP
1-10-95	225221	Jones	W	10cc Timoptic 0.25%	i ou bid	5	27.60	NP
1-29-95	224523	Smith	H	100 Inderal 20mg TAB	i qid	4	8.05	NP
2-12-95	228461	Cobb	2	30 Amoxicillin 250mg CAP	i tid	4	6.89	NP
2-15-95	231455	Smith	W	24 Dalmane 15mg	1 hs prn	2	12.86	NP
2-15-95	231456	Smith	W	20 Keflex 250mg CAP	1 qid	0	23.50	NP
3-02-95	224523	Smith	H	100 Inderal 20mg TAB	1 qid	3	8.05	NP
3-02-95	233171	Cobb	1	120cc Dimetapp el	5ccq4°	3	6.63	NP
3-04-95	225221	Jones	W	10cc Timoptic 0.25%	i ou bid	4	27.60	NP
4-18-95	238901	Cobb	3	120cc E.E.S. 200/5	5ccq6°	0	8.08	NP
4-18-95	238902	Cobb	3	10cc Cortisporin Sol'n, 2gtts	ear tid	0	20.90	NP
5-22-95	231455	Smith	W	24 Dalmane 15mg	1 hs prn	1	12.86	NP

Fig 2. A family medication record.

stances when there is no obvious relationship or where there is any question, the pharmacist should respect the privacy of the information and not release it without the express permission, either obtained directly from the patient, or from a signed statement of waiver presented by the person requesting the information. Clearly, a telephone request is unacceptable. The patient, for example, could be under investigation for fraud. There could be any number of reasons why the patient would want to know of information requests and have input into the process. The pharmacist cannot make these decisions.

Finally, the pharmacist should familiarize his patients with the profile system and the need to have continual up-to-date information. Thus, patients realize the value of having a current system and a loyalty is fostered between them.

Practice Management—An effective profile system could facilitate additional advantages to the pharmacist that aid in the effective management of his practice. For instance, third-party payment information, generation of tax and insurance receipts and accounting and billing information are just a few examples where the system can be advantageous. Since the first medication profile was introduced into pharmacy prac-

NAME SANTOS, MARIA

ADDRESS 3509 Homewood Dr.
Anywhere, U.S.A.

TELEPHONE 555-1212

BIRTH 06/17/53 SEX M F

CLINICAL CONDITIONS/PROBLEMS
UTI

ALLERGIES/REACTIONS Penicillin

NOTES:

DATE	RX #	DOCTOR	DRUG/STRENGTH/AMOUNT	SIG	REF	CHARGE	RPH
9-27-95	333809	Karberg	Buspar 5mg TAB, #24	i tid		21.69	NP
9-05-95	330536	Karberg	Terazol 3 Cream, 20g	appl hsX3		24.65	NP
8-07-95	325686	Oliver	Feldene 20mg CAP, #10	i qam		23.00	NP
5-31-95	319364	Oliver	Feldene 20mg CAP, #14	i qam		29.69	NP
5-26-95	318874	Pfaff	Cinobac 500mg Pulvule, #10	i q12hr		30.39	NP
8-31-95	318874	Pfaff	Cinobac 500mg Pulvule, #10	i q12hr	1	30.39	NP
5-11-95	317461	Pfaff	Macrodantin 100mg CAP, #28	i qid pc+hs		40.39	NP
3-30-95	313041	Karberg	Terazol 7 0.4% Cream w/appl, 45g	appl hsX7		24.69	NP
3-27-95	312853	Pfaff	Macrodantin 100mg CAP, #40	i qid pc+hs		51.99	NP
3-23-95	312295	Karberg	Buspar 5mg TAB, #24	i tid		20.69	NP
3-23-95	312294	Karberg	Terazol 7 0.4% Cream w/appl, 45g	appl hsX7		24.69	NP
6-15-94	289474	Oliver	Feldene 20mg CAP, #21	i qam	1	41.39	NP

Fig 3. An individual patient medication record.

tice in 1960, there have been numerous discussions concerning the pros and cons of maintaining such a record. The reasons given by pharmacists for not providing this service are it is too time consuming, it costs too much, it increases the pharmacist's liability, this is the physician's responsibility, the patient will not like it and it's an infringement on patient confidentiality. These reasons have been investigated and contested in court with the results in favor of the medication profiles. In addition, good managerial procedures diminish the time-consuming aspect of the profiles. A good example is when a pharmacist deals with one or more members of a family that have different last names. A well-planned and executed cross-reference system negates any problems with these blended families. Further, all pharmacists are required by law to file the original prescription by serial number as received. Finding a "lost number" can be frustrating, both to the pharmacist and the patient. A cross reference to the patient profile is the best mechanism to solve this universal problem. Each time a refill is requested, the pharmacist is required to replace the entire container, if it is a plastic vial, or at least replace the safety closure on a returned glass bottle. It would seem that as more patients become familiar with this practice of replacement, more of them will return for a prescription refill without the original container. Where, then, will the pharmacist retrieve the needed prescription number if there is no patient profile system within the pharmacy? Thus, good business practice dictates the use of a patient profile system. As mentioned earlier a good computer profile system is a valuable management tool for many of these time-consuming problems associated with a manual system.

In the near future, it is possible that with new technology, a patient will be responsible for carrying medical information and prescription and profile information on a *smart card.* One such credit-card size laser recordable card (ie, LaserCard, *Drexler Technol Corp*) holds up to 1600 pages of computerized medical records or 80 medical image scans. This card has been developed to make patients' histories instantly available to physicians and hospitals as a rapid-response diagnostic tool. The company is attempting to develop a pharmacy application which would contain a complete record of a patient's prescriptions.

Once the pharmacy application is in place, rule changes will be necessary regarding the maintenance of the original prescription information. Transfer of information from one pharmacy to another would be facilitated greatly. Out of necessity, the pharmacist filling the prescription would have to update the card. Thus, there finally would be a single accurate source of information about a particular patient and prescription.

Under the current system, it is theoretically possible for an unscrupulous patient to have information on the same prescription in several different pharmacies and receive more drug than the prescriber intended. The pharmacist could enter comments which could include advice, evidence of clinical abuse (if one works, two is better!), documentation as to counseling and other relevant information such as OTC products dispensed, all of which would save time for the next pharmacist serving that patient's pharmaceutical needs. It is easy to see how such a card could aid in treatment of a patient in an emergency. It would be especially helpful if the patient was unresponsive.

Profile Review—As mentioned earlier, to be effective the profile system must be up-to-date and used for the benefit of the patient. Pharmacists must develop their skill and method of reviewing patient profiles to improve monitoring and be of service to the patient.

The importance of profile review in ambulatory pharmacy practice cannot be overstated. Effective monitoring requires a systematic approach by the pharmacist. Presented below is the 10-step method adapted from that developed by Srnka and Self.[10] Each patient, each prescription and each disease state must be considered separately by the pharmacist. Review of patient profiles will illustrate different types of problems varying greatly in significance, urgency and complexity. Thus, the pharmacist must develop a plan of action of what to do and how to do it to effect an appropriate solution to the problem. Often, a solution will involve the coordination of efforts between various individuals (eg, patient, physician). In this context there are three basic options the pharmacist has available:

Dispense the prescription(s) as written.
Do not dispense the prescription(s).
Dispense the prescription(s) after appropriate action has been taken.

The first two are entirely up to the pharmacist; the third involves resolution after consultation with the prescriber. However, before consultation the pharmacist should have a clear grasp of the problem and be able to provide a concise description of the potential problem. Whenever possible, it is helpful if the pharmacist has a literature reference to substantiate the clinical significance. Realistically, however, this is difficult to attain, but the use of a drug-information center might be able to facilitate this. The Medi-Span PAR (*Prior Adverse Reactions*), eg, provides the pharmacist with well-documented advisories and a concise discussion of the primary literature with reference citations. This allows the pharmacist to make a decision about the encountered problem and provide a solution to it (eg, an alternative drug that does not cause the same adverse reaction). Problem resolution depends upon judgment and tact; it is something that is learned only through experience and the willingness to do so by the pharmacist. Through all of this process the pharmacist must keep in mind the patient always is given first priority.[10] A distinct advantage of using computer databases is the periodic updates that are received and can be loaded directly into the program. This has marked advantage over the traditional, print-based library, that for the most part becomes outdated with time.

Srnka and Self[10] suggest the following ten elements to look for on a profile:

History of adverse effects.
Potentially unwarranted/unintended changes in therapeutic regimen.
Potential quantitative misuse (noncompliance, misuse, overuse).
Duplication of medications.
Additive effects from similar medication use.
Inappropriate dosage, route of administration, dosing schedule or dosage form.
Potential current adverse effects.
Drug-drug interactions.
Drug-disease interactions.
Irrational therapeutic regimen.

The authors suggest that the pharmacist have a pocket card with these elements available to aid the review of the patient profile each time he dispenses a prescription. This pocket card provides him with a framework in which to review the profile and, with time, ultimately is committed to memory. For example, when the patient whose profile is illustrated in Fig 93-3 received a prescription for Keflex, there was a possibility he would be allergic to it by virtue of a previous allergy to penicillin (Element 1). It would be important for the pharmacist to advise him tactfully about this possibility. Further, Empirin #3 contains aspirin, a drug which when used with dipyridamole, ie, Persantine, can effect a synergistic antithrombotic effect on small blood vessels and affect clotting time (Element 8). While this situation is not life-threatening it is an example of a situation that must be dealt with by the pharmacist, probably by monitoring the patient's progress while taking the two drugs.

Nonprescription (OTC) Drug Usage

The pharmacist is in a unique position because of his education, training and ready accessibility to the public when it comes to self-medication by the public with OTC drugs. Although the FDA is unsure about the actual number of OTC products, it is estimated to be between 125,000 to 300,000 in number, with sales totalling over $10.9 billion in pharmacies, food stores and mass merchandisers during 1991. The sales of these products will continue to escalate because self-medication continues to increase in importance for two main reasons: (1) the continued sophistication and knowledge of consumers in self-medication and (2) the movement of additional prescription products to OTC status. It is estimated that for every dollar spent on OTC products, two dollars are saved on health-care costs. A void that exists, however, is the unknown impact that patient misadventuring with OTC products costs the health-care system.

At present there is a greater awareness and emphasis on the need for more personal involvement and responsibility for health-care maintenance on the part of the individual. Also, more consumers are beginning to recognize through personal experience and advertising via the media, that the pharmacist is a health-information specialist in this regard.

It is noteworthy to report that the average community pharmacist recommends an OTC product 3888 times per year (324 recommendations per month). As consumer awareness about the pharmacist's knowledge base and skills increases (through, eg, OBRA 90), this will in all likelihood increase pharmacist influence within self-care. Already, the pharmacist has marked influence as evidenced that 97% of 406 respondent pharmacists surveyed indicated that patients always (14%) or usually (83%) purchase the product that the pharmacist recommends. This influence must extend also to patient acceptance of pharmacist advice about safe/effective use of OTC products, and the need for the patient to commit with the pharmacist to share follow-up information to determine the success of the selected self-care regimen.

The second force in this emerging dependence upon OTC drug therapy is the movement of drug products from prescription to nonprescription status. The consuming public now has access to more drugs whose sale in the past was restricted to prescription use only. This movement will continue as a result of the OTC efficacy panel reviews which the FDA initiated in 1972. Predictions indicate that histamine H_2 antagonists, some nonsteroidal anti-inflammatory drugs and nicotine (as the gum/patch) all will be available OTC by the year 2000. The economic impact of these conversions is significant and illustrated by the switch of clotrimazole to OTC status in 1991. The two top-selling products for feminine vaginal yeast infections accounted for over $153 million in sales during 1991.[11] Of the $40 billion dollar drug-therapy expenditure in 1990, approximately $12 billion was spent on OTC drugs. It is estimated that the OTC market segment will grow another $4 to $5 billion by 1996, due in part to numerous additional prescription drugs being switched to OTC status, and because some OTC drugs are drugs-of-choice.

It is interesting to note that pharmacists welcome this movement of drugs from prescription to nonprescription status. While this transfer will continue to have a significant economic impact on pharmacies, the main concern of pharmacists is for patient safety when using these drugs. This area of practice affords the clear opportunity for the pharmacist to use his knowledge and expertise.

A person may not always desire to seek the advice of a physician each time he becomes ill. Correspondingly, the symptoms of the ailment may be minor enough to treat with an OTC product. The decision of the patient concerning which product to purchase usually is based on prior experience with the product, advice received from the pharmacist, neighbor and/or relatives or commercial advertisements by manufacturers. However, the pharmacist is the only expert/specialist in this area of knowledge and should make his particular expertise available to the patient.

In the past the pharmacist often was not consulted about OTC drugs and/or treatments. Two reasons for this were the fact that the pharmacist was too busy and unavailable for consultation or, when available, did not always provide adequate and relevant information. Furthermore, many believe that prior experience with a drug or drug product, or the fact that it is advertised commercially on radio or television, is sufficient for their purpose. Others believe that product labels always are clear and answer consumers' questions and they do not need to be counseled with each purchase.

Studies have demonstrated that some patients have difficulty in physically being capable of reading the information and/or understanding the information which is presented on the OTC product package and label. Many, for example, simply do not understand the meaning of "For therapeutic use only." As a result, in 1990, California enacted a law requiring the pharmaceutical industry to report to the State on the progress made on improvement in readability and clarity of labeling information. Subsequently, the Nonprescription Drug Manufacturers Association developed voluntary industry guidelines that identify specific technical factors that could be addressed to improve the readability of OTC labels. While this is a forward step, these guidelines probably will not be of too much use for those people who experience degenerative eye disorders, most commonly amblyopia (weak eye caused by the destruction of the retinal cones) or be of help to the 20 million people who wear eyeglasses and/or contact lenses that have prescriptions no longer suited to them or an estimated 20 million other people who are in need of some visual correction, but are unaware of this necessity.

It is clear that the pharmacist is in an opportune position to help consumers with their self-care needs and must take an active role to do so.

Consumer trends indicate that the pharmacist slowly is gaining recognition toward providing information to the patient about OTC drugs/products. Consumers seek out pharmacists who provide service. The factors (in descending order of importance) germane to the selection of a pharmacist were:

Discussion of instructions for the use of the product, including effectiveness, side effects and ingredients.
Availability for consultation.
Willingness to offer advice on general health problems.
Friendliness and approachability.

One survey indicated that consumers are so intent on having the personal advice of the pharmacist that even when he was busy a majority of consumers were willing to wait until he was free.

Another study demonstrated that 40% of consumers ask their pharmacist for advice on minor health problems at least once during the year and that people under 50 years seek advice more often than people over 50. This is consistent both with the younger group of people having families about which they are concerned and being more attuned to expect information about their health care. This same study demonstrated that 99% of consumers indicated they would use the product recommended by the pharmacist, and 96% reported they were satisfied with the OTC product recommended by the pharmacist. Further, the FDA supports the concepts of self-medication, but, unfortunately, has not embraced the concept of the pharmacist as the first professional that the patient should consult before using the product. Instead, the FDA has ruled that certain OTC drugs be labeled, "seek the advice of a health professional before using this product." This is unfortunate because "health professional" has a broad definition, sometimes to the exclusion of the pharmacist. However, favorable advertising that suggests that consumers ask their "doctor or pharmacist," helps them identify the valuable counsel the pharmacist has to offer.

Only since the 1960s has a concentrated effort been made to educate the pharmacist to provide accurate and useful advice to the patient seeking symptomatic relief with self-medication. Before that, pharmacy was practiced under the influences and restraints of the APhA Code of Ethics, adopted in 1921, which deemed it unethical for a pharmacist "to prescribe." This was interpreted to mean that a pharmacist recommending an OTC medication would be committing a violation of ethics because he would be "counter-prescribing" (prescribing over the counter). Pharmacists were taught not to provide this service.

Before the adoption of the 1921 Code, and until the 1930s when it began to exert its influence upon the practice of pharmacy, it was common for the patient to seek the advice of a pharmacist for minor ailments and first aid and for the pharmacist to provide this service. Another factor which contributed to isolate the pharmacist from the patient was the increase in prescription volume which occurred in the 1940s.

For a period of about 25 years the pharmacist tended to avoid patient contact. During the 1960s pharmacy was rejuvenated with the promotion and gradual introduction of clinical concepts into the practice of pharmacy. Advising the patient on health matters not only became fashionable but was recognized as a responsibility of the pharmacist, both ethically and legally. The pharmacist was encouraged to question the patient who had decided to self-medicate and either recommend an OTC medication or recommend that the patient seek medical attention. By 1969 the membership of the APhA voted to adopt a new Code of Ethics which held the health and welfare of the patient to be of first consideration for the pharmacist.

Even though the role of the pharmacist has changed, state statutes may not have been updated to reflect this. The pharmacist does walk a very narrow line and quoting the Ohio Revised Code §4731.34 as an example:

"A person is regarded as practicing medicine when he/she prescribes, advises, recommends, administers, or dispenses for compensation any kind, direct or indirect, a drug or medicine for the cure or relief of bodily injury, infirmity, or disease."

This is provided here not to dissuade the pharmacist from performing this valuable service, but to indicate that these statutes do exist. The pharmacist should be familiar with them as they are written and applied. Frequently, these statutes are not applied, but they must be kept in mind when practicing pharmacy.

The above brief historical perspective has been presented in order to explain why the average pharmacist in practice today may not be aware of his responsibility to provide advice to the person who decides to treat himself, and why the pharmacist may have neglected to offer this professional service. A number of pharmacists may have to be educated, or re-educated, on how to counsel the patient who decides upon self-treatment. This is achieved within curriculums of schools and colleges of pharmacy that provide appropriate coursework in the area of OTC drug therapy. Furthermore, continuing-education providers should strive in part to educate these pharmacists who did not have the benefit of a formal course in OTC drug therapy.

Self-medication counseling is a primary-care activity that carries with it a great amount of professional responsibility. Communicating information about OTC products requires the same basic skills used for prescription medication and does not mandate additional specialized training or vast financial expenditures to be done well. In that light, the OTC Drug Review process of the FDA has been a boon to the pharmacist. It has provided him a knowledge base which allows him to make sound decisions on comparative product effectiveness and safety. Although the entire review process is nearing completion, with the panels preparing and submitting final reports, the process has generated substantial scientific research that has produced impressive amounts of new information and data on OTC drugs. At the same time it has placed a burden upon the pharmacist to keep current about new information in this important subject area. A real handicap for the diligent pharmacist is obtaining factual, current information. Few realize that they can contact the National Center for Drug Evaluation and Research, FDA, Rockville, MD 20857, 1-301-295-8000, for appropriate information relative to the review panels.

Usually, it is the patient who looks for assistance and initiates the dialogue when seeking an OTC remedy. Friendliness and courtesy are attributes which facilitate availability and encourage the patient to ask the pharmacist for advice. He may initiate the conversation with several question types such as:

What do you have for diarrhea? (symptom in the form of a question)
What is the best antacid? (product from a specific class of drug)
Do you carry Lotrimin AF Cream? (specific product desired)

Correspondingly, the pharmacist also should recognize that the patient may be deliberating over an awesome number of products in the drug aisle, and offer assistance then or intervene at the time of purchase, when the patient has selected a product that is contraindicated based on his medical history or has a significant potential to cause him harm (eg, corn/callus remover for a diabetic).

When counseling about OTC drugs, there are four basic tenets to follow.

Exercise Active Listening—The patient should be allowed to state the problem completely, and the pharmacist should provide his undivided attention which is necessary to minimize misperception and misunderstanding. The pharmacist then must be able to summarize mentally what the patient has said and provide positive feedback that conveys understanding of the problem, empathy and concern. Using the words of the patient or paraphrasing what he has related indicates understanding the problem. Rewording or having to restate the situation forces the pharmacist to focus on what has been said and indicates that he is processing the information actively and attempting to understand the situation. If the pharmacist can relate to the discomfort of the problem the patient is experiencing, using his own words, it indicates that the pharmacist has exercised a very important component of communication: active listening. This process also facilitates and enhances personal relations between the pharmacist and patient by the demonstration of a true concern.

The initial step in deciding whether or not a complaint or condition is amenable to self therapy involves the identification of the problem that the patient is seeking to treat. Quite often, they provide incomplete or conflicting information, much of which is necessarily subjective. Thus, the pharmacist must exercise the second tenet to the basics of counseling.

Question the Patient Thoroughly—The object is to elicit specific symptoms and determine if self-therapy is appropriate (symptom analysis).

Symptom analysis requires that the pharmacist obtain the following information:

Onset of the problem—When did the symptom(s) start?

Duration of the problem—How long does it last? Is it continual? Does it come and go away at certain times during the day?

Severity—How severe is the problem? Is it getting worse each time?

Description of the symptom—What does it feel like?

Acute versus chronic—Did it occur suddenly? Has it occurred before?

Associated symptoms—Do you have any other symptoms that are occurring?

Exacerbating factors—Does anything make your symptoms worse or seem to cause the problem?

Relieving factors—Has anything you tried previously helped your symptoms?

Previous therapy—Have you tried any products or medications to relieve your symptoms?

The next step in the questioning process is to gather patient-related information. Before an assessment and decision can be made the pharmacist must be cognizant of individual characteristics. The following information should be elicited:

Name—For whom is the request made?

Age—Is the patient an infant, a child, an adult or an elderly person?

Sex—Is the patient male or female? If female, is she pregnant or nursing a baby?

Prior medical history—Are there any other diseases or conditions from which the patient suffers?

Prior drug history—Are there any drugs (ie, prescription/ OTC) that the patient is taking on a daily basis? Do they imbibe social drugs (eg, nicotine, caffeine, alcohol, "recreational" drugs)?

Allergy history—Is the patient allergic to any drugs, environmental agents, etc?

Adverse drug reaction history—Has the patient had any bad experiences or side effects from prior use of any medication?

The pharmacist must ask a sufficient number of questions to identify and assess the problem before a strategy is conceived. Time constraint necessitates keeping the line of questioning direct and to the point. The pharmacist should exercise judgment relative to the pertinence of the question and not probe on the basis of curiosity. With experience, he should develop a style that will gather this information within a period of minutes. If the situation is more complex and time-consuming, the pharmacist can ask the patient to return at a mutually agreeable time, contact him by telephone or refer him directly to a physician.

Interpret Verbal and Nonverbal Communication—Every question asked of the patient should be phrased carefully to facilitate interpretation. The patient should be able to understand that the questions asked come from a genuine interest and desire to be of help. The pharmacist may ask two types of questions:

The open-ended type which are useful to gather information regarding the medical problem. For instance, "can you tell me about the symptoms you have been experiencing?" This question type provides flexibility for patient response and encourages more than a simple yes or no answer.

The second, a direct question, is useful when the information is a specific inquiry, eg, "How long have you noticed the burning sensation in your stomach?"

It is crucial that these questions be asked one at a time, and not in rapid fashion which only results in confusion and frustration for the patient.

Nonverbal communication skills also serve a vital role in this situation. The body posture, facial expression and distance of the patient all provide perception of the patient as a whole. At the same time it is important to be aware of the patient's nonverbal behavior. Physical barriers to communication should be eliminated whenever possible. In fact, anything that impedes the verbal exchange should be eliminated. The pharmacist should make every effort not to talk down to the patient, both verbally (ie, use the vernacular) and physically (the pharmacist and patient should be at the same eye level). These exchanges should be as private and uninterrupted as possible. However, all pharmacies do not have the benefit of a private consultation area or the money to construct one. But privacy can be achieved readily without expense by simply forming a triangle using the patient, the pharmacist and the wall shelf or gondola as sides. This automatically signals others that the consultation is private and not to be interrupted.

Whenever possible the pharmacist physically should assess the patient through observation or inspection. For example, the skin is assessed easily by inspection and palpation. However, the lung requires percussion and auscultation, not easily attainable for the practicing pharmacist. The clear majority of pharmacists obtain physical data (eg, number of comedones per side of the face) exclusively through the use of observation. Further, there are clues to the overall state of health of the patient and these provide insight into the seriousness of the problem. Facial expressions mirror pain and discomfort, pallor and lethargy may be indicative of an infectious process and persistent coughing may be a sign of some systemic illness.

After the pharmacist mentally tabulates all the information (verbal, nonverbal and observed) an assessment must be made to the cause and severity of the condition. These are crucial because it will dictate a particular treatment path.

Assessment of severity will vary among patient complaints. Some problems may be considered severe only when they accumulate to a certain level, such as persistent vomiting or diarrhea in an infant. The longer these persist, the more severe the problem and the greater the potential for referral to a physician. Further, some complaints may be considered severe only when they become symptomatic or the symptoms begin to impair functional activity (eg, bleeding, external hemorrhoids).

Clarify the Facts As Needed—The plan of action that the pharmacist devises is the most important step in the process of self-medication. At this point he has three courses of action from which to select. These are referral, drug therapy or nondrug intervention. Whichever course is chosen the pharmacist must ensure that the patient understands the reasoning behind it and the need to comply.

Before the plan is put into effect, additional information may be necessary to enable a thorough assessment of the problem. This may include the consultation with the parent or guardian of the patient, or communication with the patient's physician. In this latter instance, the pharmacist acts as a direct link between the patient and the physician within the referral process. This communication between physician and pharmacist avoids conflict in the overall management of the patient and alleviates his confusion associated with overlapping responsibilities between the physician and pharmacist. This situation is helpful because it serves several purposes:

It allows for the input of the physician into an evaluation of the problem and determines whether the physician will want to see the patient or deal with the problem over the telephone. In the event that the physician wants to see the patient the pharmacist can provide and share additional information with the physician.

It serves as a method of obtaining additional data on prior medical conditions that need to be clarified to determine if self-therapy is appropriate or acceptable.

Realistically, however, physicians are quite reluctant to give advice on the telephone and to provide service without compensation in the event that the pharmacist cannot handle the question. The pharmacist and the physician may be viewed as "partners" in the health-care system but are not so in the business sense. Thus, communication of this type engenders several questions, eg

Should the pharmacist bill the patient and then respond in compensation to the physician for his service?

Is there a referral fee for the service of the pharmacist when no product is purchased and the patient consults the physician?

Will the physician tire of numerous telephone calls?

The first option is to counsel the self-medicating patient to seek the professional care of a physician. This should be executed in a tactful manner not to alarm or frighten the patient, and at the same time consideration should be given by the pharmacist to the treatment center to which the patient should be directed (ie, emergency, private practice) as well as the urgency. Some conditions dictate immediate attention (eg, persistent epigastric pain with bloody vomitus) whereas others do not (eg, athlete's foot).

When making a decision to recommend physician consultation, the following situations support this:

The symptoms are too severe to be endured by the patient without a definite diagnosis and treatment.

The symptoms are minor but have persisted and do not appear to be due to some easily identifiable cause.

The symptoms are recurring, more frequently, with no recognizable cause.

The pharmacist is in doubt about the condition of the patient.

The misuse of the product by the patient could result in harm to him.

The patient correctly has used (eg, administration, duration) an appropriate OTC product with no positive result.

It is important that the pharmacist emphasize to the patient the need for physician consultation. Sometimes patients listen and then purchase a product anyway. This is frustrating to the pharmacist, but sometimes it cannot be avoided. Conversely, there is a danger that when a pharmacist recommends something to hold the patient over until he can schedule an appointment with a physician, some patients simply will not follow through and make the appointment, particularly if the product seems to work for their condition. However, an earlier mentioned study demonstrated that 9 out of 10 patients will consult a physician when a pharmacist suggests it.

When the pharmacist makes the decision that the patient's condition does not warrant physician intervention, a therapeutic end-point must be identified for the patient and/or the specific condition. This end-point should be attainable and accessible. At this point the pharmacist can either select a drug or nondrug treatment modality. This decision must be based upon patient variables (eg, age, sex, previous medical and/or drug history, life style) in conjunction with drug variables (dosage regimen, side effects, duration of use, comparable effectiveness to other drugs, etc).

There are instances when nondrug treatment measures are indicated. In this instance, the pharmacist will inform the patient to let the condition run its course (eg, canker sores) or recommend ways to help eliminate the problem (eg, humidification of inspired air to relieve the cough and hoarseness associated with laryngitis). There are, however, instances when the pharmacist must recognize that nondrug measures, although appropriate, might not lend themselves to a particular patient. For example, the standard modality to treat diarrhea in an adult is to encourage a liquid diet for a period of time. However, if the patient is diabetic, caloric intake must be maintained. This example is one where pharmacist consultation with the physician is necessary.

When the pharmacist recommends a drug treatment for a condition amenable to self-therapy, he should tell the patient of the condition itself, the monitoring guideposts to bear in mind and the duration of time before the patient should notice the benefit of treatment. Using acne vulgaris as an example, the objective of topical treatment is to control an existing condition, impede acne in the developmental stages and relieve the discomfort (eg, physical, psychological). The patient should be told to note a decrease in the number of lesions that will occur with the continual, daily application of the medication to the entire face and that it may take approximately 2 to 3 weeks before the benefits of the medication are observed. Tied into the discussion should be indices that demonstrate the acne condition may be worsening and require medical attention. Lastly, potential toxicity from the treatment selected should be told to the patient. Using benzoyl peroxide as an example, the acne patient should understand that some skin redness and irritation may develop.

Whenever possible, the pharmacist should follow up with the patient consistent with the concept of pharmaceutical care. To facilitate follow-up the pharmacist should make some notation, perhaps on the patient profile, to document the original problem and reinforce his memory. It is very important, too, that the patient understand the advantage to reporting back to the pharmacist the success of the intervention. If the patient does not seem to be responding to the treatment plan, additional information and data assessment (eg, did he follow instructions correctly and for a reasonable amount of time?) may determine a new course of action. Frequently, this re-evaluation culminates with the referral of the patient to the physician for further treatment. If at all possible the pharmacist should share information attained from the initial and the follow-up evaluation with the physician.

Aside from OTC products the pharmacist also must have a working knowledge of diagnostic aids and tests which are now available to consumers. Since the introduction of the first home pregnancy test in 1977, these do-it-yourself tests have expanded the self-care market and it is estimated that sales of these products will exceed $4 billion by the year 2000. This booming market, represented by an average growth rate of 17%, is attributable to the relatively low cost and reliability of the home tests, as well as their user-friendly nature.

Home pregnancy tests, ovulation prediction tests, fecal occult blood test kits, home blood glucose monitors and blood pressure devices are just a few of the ever-increasing number of in-home diagnostic kits and devices that continue to revolutionize health care within the US. These devices help monitor chronic diseases, decrease unnecessary doctor visits and hospitalizations and, most importantly, actively involve patients in their own health care. With the trend toward preventive medicine, the pharmacist who offers to educate the consumer on the newer diagnostic products that may thwart the leading causes of fatality, eg, colon cancer, diabetes mellitus or high blood pressure, will be in a very opportune professional and economic position. Even though these continue to become more user-friendly, patients encounter problems with the use of these products and do not always follow directions; consequently, the pharmacist will be called upon to problem-solve for the patient and make appropriate recommendations based upon the test result. The patient should understand that these diagnostic kits are intended to be used in close cooperation with health-care professionals who can discuss the test results and their implications.

As a drug informational specialist in the area of OTC products the pharmacist is not displacing the physician when he recommends (or helps the patient select) an OTC product. At least, in this instance, the patient has the benefit of the expertise of the pharmacist, whereas, if the product was purchased in a nonpharmacy outlet there would be no chance for a dialog to occur. In the latter instance there is a great chance for misuse of the product. Given the education of the pharmacist, in conjunction with practical experience, there is no other person who understands the limitations of self-treatment with OTC products and who is in a position to encourage the patient to seek the professional advice of a physician when necessary.

Health Education

A primary concern of the pharmacist should be the welfare of humanity and the relief of human suffering. In fact, one oath contains the passage, "I will use my knowledge and skills to the best of my ability in serving the public and other health professionals." Today, there is little doubt that the continuing "buzz word" in contemporary pharmacy practice is "information"—specifically, consumer health information.

By virtue of the pharmacist's accessibility and familiarity with the community, it is obvious that he can exercise a dynamic impact, which can be translated into not only the triage function but also the dissemination of effective and useful health education. One study revealed that over 90% of those interviewed visited a pharmacy at least once a month and 60%, at least once a week. The hours a pharmacy is open per week greatly exceeds all other health facilities with the possible exception of the hospital emergency room. Although many consumers continue to view the pharmacist as "an invisible man behind a secret counter who delegates responsibility to technicians and clerks to deal directly with the public," this attitude is being changed positively to reflect the pharmacist as a source of health information along with the physician. A vast majority of the public does not hesitate to ask the pharmacist about a health matter and usually he is the first person, other than family or friends, who is consulted.

Frequently, the pharmacist is confronted with a variety of inquiries:

A telephone call from a frantic mother whose child has just swallowed a number of chewable vitamin-iron tablets and wants to know what to do.

A nervous teenage girl who wants to know how to use a home pregnancy kit.

A habitual smoker who is interested in the success rate of the nicotine transdermal patches.

An expectant mother who is afraid for her baby because she may have been exposed to a neighborhood child with German measles.

The situations are endless but typify the need for the pharmacist to be approachable and willing to help.

To answer these people or synthesize a plan of action the pharmacist must maintain professional competence and keep abreast of developments of drugs and disease states. At the same time he should serve as an expeditor to solve patient problems. The familiarity of the pharmacist with the community lends itself to proper referral of patients to other health-care professionals, including providing addresses and telephone numbers. Indeed, the pharmacist is in a position to assess a physician based on personal experience, the types of prescriptions he writes or telephones, patient comments about the care they receive and inquiries about physician follow-up. Beyond health-care assistance the pharmacist also should be able to recommend nonmedical facilities that provide effective care (eg, a shoe store that exercises judgment and care in fitting jogging shoes). Further, pharmacists should know that pharmaceutical companies do offer physicians free drugs for needy patients. While individual manufacturer requirements for assistance may differ, some common requirements include

Eligible patients cannot be covered by Medicaid or a private insurance plan that has prescription-drug coverage.

Physicians must initiate the request on behalf of the patient, and in some instances provide a statement of the patient's financial hardship.

No more that a 3 months' supply is available at one time, although requests may be renewed.

Pharmacists can advise interested patients to seek an alphabetical listing of drugs covered by specific pharmaceutical companies, including information on assistance for AIDS drugs by contacting The Senate Special Committee on Aging, Dirksen Senate Office Building, Room G-31, Washington DC 20510 (1-202-224-5364). Similarly, physicians can be advised to contact the Pharmaceutical Manufacturers' Association, 1100 15th St, NW, Washington, DC 20005 for a directory of manufacturers' assistance programs.

In 1993 there were 100 regional poison control centers in the US (of which 38 were certified centers through the American Association of Poison Control Centers) and every pharmacy should have the telephone numbers and addresses of those in the local area for quick patient referral. Although unintentional poisonings and deaths have dropped dramatically since child-resistant packaging was introduced, tragedies continue to occur among young children. The pharmacist must be able to deal effectively with these emergencies, exercise judgment and be decisive with such inquiries.

Another alarming problem that has surfaced within recent years is child and spouse abuse. This is of concern to all communities, and the pharmacist, by his involvement, can serve in several ways to help alleviate the problem, eg

Be aware of the warning signs of abuse and neglect from the perspective of the child (eg, seems unduly afraid of his parents, shows evidence of repeated skin or other injuries, shows signs of poor overall care) and the parent (eg, makes no attempt to explain the child's most obvious injuries or offers absurd, contradictory explanations, shows a lack of control or fear of losing control). Given the warning signs of child abuse and neglect, the pharmacist gently can coax information from the parent when either taking the initiative to do so or provided the opportunity. A simple conversation may be sufficient encouragement for an abusive parent to admit the need for assistance and guidance. At this point the pharmacist must have the name of an individual at the community abuse center with whom the parent can talk both before and during a crisis. Given uncooperative parents the pharmacist must exercise professional judgment and report the matter to local authorities. The pharmacist, like all citizens, is immune from civil and/or criminal liability when reporting any knowledge or suspicion of child abuse.

By participation with local authorities and professionals in information forums conducted by social workers the pharmacist can provide information to the abusive parent on how drugs, including alcohol, can affect one's behavior, change one's mood, effect depression with long-term use and induce psychotic reactions. When this information is blended with the physician-nurse discussion of physical injury incurred from abuse with teacher awareness of reporting suspicions, it adds immeasurably to the dimension of such a symposium.

The pharmacist also should recognize the need for health education on a broader scale. Many of the health problems encountered by communities can be prevented or alleviated with proper education. But it must be the pharmacist who is willing to share the wealth of knowledge and information he has accrued. All persons are not knowledgable about the extent of the pharmacist's education and thus automatically do not think of him as a source of information. Thus, he must provide the impetus to focus attention toward the capability he has relative to health education. There are several ways he can achieve this.

One method is to make the pharmacy the health center of the community. The willingness to participate in "Poison Prevention Week" or "National Diabetes Month" focuses consumer education toward the pharmacy. Coupled with this is the distribution of pamphlets of public interest on health information for the community. A display of free health literature in the pharmacy demonstrates a commitment to effective health care. There are myriads of pamphlets available on a variety of topics (eg, "Diabetes, Dry Skin and You," "The Professional Treatment of Constipation") from pharmaceutical manufacturers that can be used effectively to promote health care. This encourages inquiries from consumers and, if displayed neatly in the prescription waiting area of the pharmacy, may afford the opportunity to the patient to read health-related information while waiting for a prescription. The pharmacist should make an effort to question pharmaceutical manufacturers' representatives about the availability of such pamphlets for the community. Many times pamphlets are available but, unless requested, they remain confined to the box in which they are contained.

In the event there is an outbreak of a communicable disease (eg, *Pediculosis capitis* at a local elementary school) the pharmacist should obtain and disseminate useful patient-related information; if provided directly at the time of medication purchase or in conjunction with the local school nurse, needless parental worry and confusion is avoided.

The acquired immunodeficiency syndrome (AIDS) crisis continues and ranks as the most significant global health concern of the 1990s. The impact of AIDS on society and on the health-care system is significant, and it is incumbent upon pharmacists to become knowledgeable about this disease process and to identify their role in efforts to stop its spread. Pharmacists can play two major roles in the community HIV disease effort:

1. To actively participate in the provision of care, treatment and information to people afflicted with HIV/AIDS and
2. By virtue of their accessibility, they are in an excellent portion to provide HIV prevention information to consumers and the general public.

The provision of care for HIV and AIDS patients is similar to the treatment of other patients. However, the treatment of these patients is more complex, the disease can be debilitating and the emotional impact upon the patient, the family and health-care providers can be substantial. Aside from normal distributive functions, it is important that the pharmacist provide patient counseling and educational services (eg, treatment options, side effects, transmission information, risk reduction guidelines for sexual activity), emphasize patient compliance (including keeping scheduled medical appointments), provide emotional support and provide referrals to appropriate resources (eg, financial, housing, health-care providers or therapists).

The AIDS patient provides a unique opportunity for pharmacists, and they should interact with the patient in such a way that encourages communication and confidence. It is very important that the patient feel "safe" with the pharmacist. Patients must feel that they are not being judged or scorned because of their disease or sexual orientation. Confidentiality is important to the AIDS patient; protecting it is a particularly important role for the pharmacist. Many patients have legitimate concerns that they may lose their jobs, and/or be alienated from family and friends, if their HIV status becomes known.

Pharmacists should be prepared to listen to a patient's desire to participate in nontraditional therapies. They should be open to discussing with patients the pros and cons of traditional and nontraditional options. It is estimated that health fraud in the US approaches $40 billion on an annual basis. Health fraud knows no bounds and frequently targets certain groups of people, including those with serious illnesses. Products and therapies of quackery waste people's limited financial resources, may offer ineffective or harmful therapy, predispose a patient to harmful adverse effects and even persuade a patient to forego traditional therapy that might be more beneficial. To help patients identify credible clinical trials, pharmacists can encourage them to call the AIDS Clinical Trials Information Service hotline (1-800-874-2572).

A key attribute to being a professional is being accessible to those one serves. In this context the role of the pharmacist is illustrated aptly in the area of family planning. By sharing knowledge and information about oral contraceptive therapy, nonprescription modes of contraception control, prevention of venereal disease, pregnancy testing and by assisting couples dealing with fertility impairment, the pharmacist demonstrates accessibility and increases the awareness of the public that the pharmacy is the place where knowledge and informed advice are available.

Pharmacy school curricula recognize the need for effective oral communication both on an individual patient basis and to larger numbers of assembled people (eg, civic and church groups, clubs, etc) by implementing effective coursework in the undergraduate curriculum. However, if the pharmacist does not accept the challenge and communicate information, then other, less-qualified persons may be asked by the consuming public to fill this informational void. Sometimes pharmacists are fearful of presenting talks or having discussions with interested groups due to a lack of self confidence. At the same time they may feel that they do not have the capability to discuss a topic due to a lack of information.

Recognizing these shortcomings in its past graduates, schools/colleges now have electronic literature-searching programs in their libraries to educate and heighten students' awareness of literature resources. Schools/colleges are commiting toward outcome-based curricula which are anchored toward the development of student oral communication skills, decision-making skills and problem-solving abilities among others. It is hoped that this will encourage greater involvement of the pharmacist in community discussion on health issues. However, one must still deal with the current situation, and pharmacists in practice should look to their local public libraries for information support, or consider contacting either their alma mater or state/local pharmaceutical associations for meaningful information.

It is essential that pharmacists contribute to public informational forums and make the community aware of public-health problems. Information and guidance should not be confined solely to drugs and their use, but also should include health-related issues, eg, sexually-transmitted diseases, hazards of smokeless tobacco, etc. A true concern must center around the casual attitude of the public towards drugs, a concept which, unfortunately, is reinforced through commercial advertising and communication media.

Whenever possible pharmacists must help restore consumer confidence when it has been put in a position of doubt. The classic examples occurred in 1982 and in 1986 with Tylenol-tampering incidents and in 1991 with a Sudafed-tampering incident. Several persons were killed due to the deliberate introduction of cyanide into the capsules on the shelf. Pharmacists responded by displaying posters and informational bulletins that instructed consumers to

Read the label. OTC medicines with tamper-evident packages tell the person on the label what seals and other features he/she should look for.

Inspect the outer packaging. Check for loose, torn, sliced or missing wrappings as well as discolored products and unusual odors.

Inspect the medication once it is opened. Look at it again before taking it. If it looks suspicious, be suspicious.

Never take medications in the dark.

The label should be read and medication inspected at every dose.

The pharmacist must maintain constant surveillance and be willing to allay fears. Unfortunately, there are innovative and creative individuals in the community who may create new problems.

In response to the initial event, the Federal Government passed amendments to its laws (18 USC 65) to provide for tamper-evident and tamper-resistant packaging of OTC products. This amendment (PL 989-127, Oct, 1983) calls for several measures. While the act is complicated, it leaves one the impression that there is not a thing which can be done to a commercial package which is not prohibited, and that is as it should be. The pharmacist must be careful not to inadvertently destroy the tamper-evident or tamper-resistant component of the packaging. To do so may bring the pharmacist under the Act as a violator. Products which have been opened by consumers (often for the purpose of noting how big the tablets are, or for comparing the product to one which is already being used by that individual) renders that particular package unsalable, and it must be removed promptly from the shelf and returned to the supplier.

Most OTC products are covered by the Act. Specifically excluded are insulin, dermatologicals, dentifrices and lozenges. While nothing prevents manufacturers from placing those products into tamper-resistant or tamper-evident packaging, it is not required at this time.

The pharmacist always should remain above reproach in the eye of the public. He should avoid even the appearance of professional impropriety and thereby not create questions of ethics within the mind of the patient. The most important means the pharmacist has in educating society on health matters is the personal contact he has with the public. Whenever possible, he should volunteer health information and encourage people to exercise proper judgment to maintain good health. Some have been very creative and have developed and written patient-oriented newsletters on timely subjects that reinforce the attitude that the pharmacist is both a drug information specialist and health-care educator and provider. Others have achieved this same end by writing health information columns for local newspapers or participating in local media programs to provide health-care information. Professional organizations (eg, NARD) have been helpful, too, through the provision of print-based health information (eg, Pharm/alert) that the pharmacist can use and disseminate for public education.

Finally, by showing a professional interest in and attitude toward the clientele which frequent the pharmacy, the pharmacist makes people feel they are important and that they have someone upon whom they can depend for help. A notable example of this is in ostomy care (see Chapter 104). There are over 1.1 million ostomates in the US with new ones increasing by about 90,000 each year. In the end, though, it is the pharmacist who really benefits by the intangible return of fulfillment and enrichment from using skills and information learned through formal and continuing education and practical experience.

New and Expanded Dimensions

Better care of the public has always been a central goal for the profession of pharmacy. In that context the future direction of the pharmacist in ambulatory care will continue to evolve toward patient-directed services that apply scientific knowledge and clinical skills to the promotion of cost-effective therapy and the prevention and resolution of drug-related needs.

The traditional chain of events in the treatment of the ambulatory patient has been for the physician to make a diagnosis and decide upon a course of treatment. If the treatment required medication the physician wrote or telephoned a prescription to the pharmacist. The three basic functions involved were diagnosing, prescribing and dispensing. The physician diagnosed and prescribed and the pharmacist dispensed. These designations have not been challenged directly but there seems to be a trend developing for the pharmacist to have a greater influence in the prescribing function than he has had in the past.

This trend was initiated when the APhA and consumer groups presented a strong case for the repeal of state anti-substitution laws during the 1970s. Since 1972, all states have repealed laws which prohibited the pharmacist from dispensing a generically equivalent drug product supplied by a different manufacturer than the one prescribed. Gradually, there has been a transition from physician to pharmacist responsibility for selecting the manufacturer of a drug product. In 1992 generic drugs accounted for 14% of all new prescriptions. The use of generic, rather than brandname, drugs offers a significant potential for consumer savings and, when coupled with their availability from a multitude of manufacturing sources, the pharmacist has the opportunity to be a primary decision maker in product selection for a major pharmaceutical segment of more than 500 million new prescriptions written annually within the US. With this opportunity is an accountability, because the pharmacist must exercise ethical and professional responsibility when selecting generic drugs which are of quality and approved for marketing by the FDA. To assist the pharmacist, the FDA recommends generic substitution only among products that it has determined to be therapeutically equivalent. Since 1980 the FDA has published an annual *Approved Drug Products with Therapeutic Equivalence Evaluations*, known synonymously as the "Orange Book." This publication is updated monthly and contains information on more than 8000 approved prescription drugs. Of these, about 6000 are available from more than one manufacturer and, of this number, 80% have been evaluated by the FDA as therapeutically equivalent.

The second critical incident that shaped a future focus of pharmacy practice evolved with the establishment of the American Board of Family Practice in 1969, as the 20th medical specialty. With its establishment the stage was set for the resurrection of the family physician and the concept of personal responsibility for the total health care of the patient, including the selection of appropriate allied health professionals to assist in such care. Inclusion of the clinical pharmacist into the family practice health-care system has gained acceptance on a continual basis, and numerous articles describe this emerging ambulatory role of the pharmacist. Family practice models with clinical pharmacy primary care programs have evolved and have followed one of two paths.

The publicly funded practice model includes programs in the Indian Health Service, the Appalachian Regional Hospitals, family practice residency programs and those within colleges of pharmacy. Their success depends, to an extent, upon the uncertain continuation of government financing.

The private family practice model, which depends upon the more traditional marketing pressures.

Within the model of family practice, the pharmacist works with physicians and other providers to offer clinical skills and practical experience to current and prospective patients. The pharmacist must demonstrate the value of personalized, comprehensive, continuous and convenient services (such as medication history, patient education, dispensing function, patient care functions, etc) provided to patients to ensure the acutely ill get well, the chronically ill gain a better quality of life and the healthy remain healthy.

The success of the pharmacist's role, and acceptance by the physician, depend upon three factors: contributing to better patient care, increasing the quality of the life of the physician by decreasing patient contact time and helping the physician market his services to ensure the financial success of the medical practice. An example is the involvement of the pharmacist with postdiagnostic care of hypertension. The physician selects the patients to be monitored under the hypertension protocol and introduces them to the clinical pharmacist, who explains the protocol, the follow-up appointment schedule, the fee system for services and informs him when to return to see the physician. Ultimately, pharmacist involvement results in better care and fewer procedures which produces overall patient savings which increases the quality of health care at a reduced cost.

Helling proposed an excellent listing of the functions of the Family Practice Clinical Pharmacist.[12] These include

1. Patient medication history.
   a. Drug allergies and sensitivities.
   b. Maintenance prescription medication (current and past).
   c. Nonprescription medication (current and past).
   d. Individual problems associated with the preparation and administration of medication.
   e. Symptoms encountered in past (eg, side effects, drug toxicity, incorrect administration).
2. Patient education
   a. Predictable actions and/or side effects of drugs.
   b. Possible side effects.
   c. Necessity for proper compliance with medication regimens.
   d. Special instructions germane to administration, use and storage of medication.
   e. Specified disease processes relevant to the patient.
   f. Personal hygiene and health maintenance.
   g. Interactions with other prescription and OTC drugs.
   h. Notification of pharmacist or physician if medication problems develop.
3. Patient care
   a. Monitor patient drug therapy.
   b. Therapeutic consultations with physicians and other health professionals.
   c. Audit medication orders: chart review/prescription review.
   d. Participate in nursing home visits.
   e. Pharmacokinetic consulting services.
   f. Coordinate follow-up of laboratory results.
   g. Manage selected acute, self-limiting and chronic disease patients.
   h. Responsible for medication-related inquiries to clinical area.

Clinical pharmacy services will continue to vary in dimension within the framework of pharmacy practice. Some practitioners will participate directly in a number of these activities, while others may participate only from a consulting role (eg, pharmacokinetic consulting service). However, continued escalation of hospital costs and patient charges will encourage the development and implementation of family practice units and off-site clinical areas for routine screening. Studies already have demonstrated the positive impact that pharmacists have had on these ambulatory health-care clinics.

Millis stated that "wise and forceful action to improve education has resulted directly in higher standards of practice with clearly increased benefits to those who receive professional services."[13] The literature supports this comment and is replete with examples of the impact of clinically trained pharmacists on the quality of health care. Furthermore, there is testimony to the impact of the pharmacist within the prescribing role. Already there are settings in which pharmacists prescribe medication in cooperation with other health-care providers and, as the quality of patient care increases, the cost of the care well may be reduced.

In 1981 California Assembly Bill 1868 amended the California Pharmacy Practice Act to allow the pharmacist in a licensed health-care facility (ie, a nursing home) to perform several procedures: adjust the dosage regimen of a patient pursuant to a prescriber order or authorization, order drug-therapy-related laboratory tests and administer drugs and biologicals by parenteral injection pursuant to the orders of the prescriber. These functions, performed under protocol, illustrated the recognition of the pharmacist as a vital member of the health-care team. An outgrowth of this and the California Assembly Bill 717 was California Senate Bill 502 (1985), which authorized a pharmacist to initiate or modify drug therapy in accordance with written guidelines (or protocols) of a licensed health facility. The bill stated that the policies, procedures and education/training requirements must be developed by physicians, pharmacists and nurses, and be approved by the facility's administrator prior to pharmacist participation in this patient-care activity.

Subsequently, the pharmaceutical literature has demonstrated numerous references to the expanding role of pharmacists in a variety of clinical settings. As an example, in one thyroid clinic, a pharmacist can initiate, maintain or modify the drug therapy of a select group of patients under the guidelines of approved protocols.[14] In this clinic, patients treated by the pharmacist include those receiving thyroid-suppression therapy, antithyroid drugs for Graves' disease or thyroid hormone supplementation after surgery or after radioactive iodine therapy. The pharmacist assesses patients, prescribes medications, orders laboratory tests, charts visits and therapeutic plans and educates patients about their conditions. Physicians may refer those noncompliant patients or those desiring additional information also are referred to the pharmacist. Joint therapeutic management between the pharmacist and endocrinologist is necessary when there are major changes in thyroid status.

Prescribing protocols for pharmacists can be found in either the inpatient setting only, or in both inpatient and outpatient, depending upon state law. California, Mississippi, Nevada, South Dakota and Washington have state laws allowing this type of pharmacy practice. California, Mississippi and Nevada limit pharmacist prescribing to inpatient use only; Washington law allows it in both settings. It is important to point out that even in states which do not have existing laws, the trend is to find prescribing protocols in operation using pharmacist expertise.

A positive force in the movement to this practice is that pharmacists must do drug-use evaluation with physicians under the Joint Commission on Accreditation of Healthcare Organizations standards. Thus, it is anticipated that the pharmaceutical literature will continue to evidence references to the expanding role of pharmacists in a variety of settings, eg, hypertension, anticoagulation, thyroid, OB-GYN (birth-control tablets). The important point is that pharmacists are prepared and ready to participate in these protocols that enhance patient outcomes.

In the early 1980s, with the switching of several legend drugs to nonlegend status, an advocacy among certain practitioner groups emerged for the establishment of a third class of drugs. These drugs would be available for OTC sale, but only by or on the advice of a licensed pharmacist. Because the federal Food, Drug and Cosmetic Act (21 USC 301 *et seq*) recognizes only the legend and nonlegend categories, the FDA has maintained that it does not have the authority to establish a "hybrid" category. It also is unlikely that the Congress will amend the law or take other action.

In 1985 Florida found a route to circumvent this dilemma by becoming the first state to grant independent prescribing authority to the pharmacist for a limited number of drugs. A formulary committee established a listing of legend drugs (eg, oral, otic or urinary analgesics, anthelmintics, medicated shampoo with lindane) suitable for pharmacist prescribing as well as dispensing procedures for each drug. While pharmacists were given the right to prescribe, they could elect not to exercise the right, and are not compelled to prescribe.

The Pharmacist Prescribing Law neither insulates the pharmacist from civil liability for prescribing a drug from the approved formulary nor addresses the standard of care to which the pharmacist must adhere.

Experience has demonstrated that this prescribing privilege has been hampered by the fear of lawsuits, dread of red tape and a limited formulary. In fact, many pharmacists indicated that the drugs on the formulary were not worth the trouble to prescribe, and were apt to suggest patient use of more appropriate OTC drugs for their patients.

In 1993 the Pharmacists' Prescriptive Authority Act was passed in New Mexico. It allows a "pharmacist clinician" to prescribe medications using written protocols agreed to by a physician and a pharmacist. The pharmacist clinician is defined as a pharmacist who has received sufficient training as a physician assistant. This act provided the pharmacy board of New Mexico responsibility to develop training requirements and establish rules which are used for guidelines and protocols which pharmacists must follow. Of particular importance, this legislation will allow pharmacists to expand their authority, particularly in long-term care settings and rural areas, where physicians are scarce.

In a similar context, the profession of pharmacy has a unique opportunity to contribute effectively to gerontological care. During the past 40 years the elderly population has increased dramatically. At present about 12% of the population is older than 65 years and, it is estimated that by the year 2025, approximately 20% of the population will be older than 65 years. Thus, community pharmacists can play a vital role in the distribution and maintenance of medical care for the elderly. Indeed, the elderly require the attention of the pharmacist because they may have multiple diseases (most often chronic) for which they may take up to a dozen medications or more. By his unique training, the pharmacist can play a central role in patient assessment, monitoring and coordinating health care and drug distribution in community and extended-health-care facilities. The pharmacist should possess an awareness and a sensitivity to an integrated approach to health care that could help to overcome the more traditional limitations in the health-care model, such as a lack of attention to the social and emotional aspects of care. This recently was demonstrated in a study where the drug use was reduced greatly and chances for early discharge increased when the patient was cared for by a physician/pharmacist teams (versus physician alone) and patients were encouraged to talk about day-to-day concerns with the pharmacist. Pharmacist intervention under the supervision of physicians in this study, effected a decrease in drug use from an average of eight different medications being taken by the patient per month to five, and decreased the amount of tranquilizer use.

Long on the fringes of the health-care system, hospice care is coming into its own. Those pharmacists who dedicate themselves to providing pharmaceutical service to hospice patients have found it personally rewarding and challenging. Hospice care is a team approach to making the terminal cancer patient comfortable for the final days (or months) of life. A majority of hospice care is provided in the home, however, it also is provided in long-term care facilities and hospitals. It is estimated that one in five long-term care facilities offer hospice care.

Pain and symptom control are the cornerstone of pharmacy hospice service. Hospice pharmacists have acquired an unusual latitude in directing patient care. Usually, attending physicians sign standing order lists so that the pharmacist can dispense previously agreed upon medications as the need arises. The array of medications includes laxatives, antidepressants, antianxiety medications and Schedule II narcotics. Those pharmacists in hospice care have learned effective pain control through experience and improvisation. As a result, pharmaceutical service has become a cornerstone in hospice care because the pharmacist has a deep understanding of how to use medications to control pain and to use this knowledge and acquired skills to extend education to other hospice healthcare providers.

One emerging opportunity for pharmacists is the area of home health care. Pharmacy home health care includes all products and services provided by pharmacists to patients or their families outside of the acute-care facility. The emphasis on health-care management is on cost-containment, and prospective payment will pay for hospital services based upon a fixed amount determined according to diagnosis-related groups (DRGs). This implies that a hospital will be reimbursed a fixed fee according to the illness, rather than on the length of stay or the actual cost of treatment. Consequently, there is an incentive for earlier discharge and some patients will be in need, eg, of *intravenous therapy*.

Many pharmacists have responded to this opportunity by working with local discharge planners and home health agencies to arrange for needed "in-home" pharmacy services. Aside from intravenous therapy, a partial listing of home health-care products would include *durable medical equipment* (eg, hospital beds, wheelchairs), *monitoring equipment* (eg, sphygmomanometers, blood glucose meters), *orthotics/prosthetics* (eg, trusses, support hose), *specialized medical equipment* (eg, positive-pressure breathing equipment) and *aids to ambulation* (eg, canes, walkers). As this market has grown, so have the number of suppliers and the sophistication of the equipment. Thus, the enterprising pharmacist who enters this area of practice must be prepared to make a significant commitment of time, effort and money.

An emerging trend in ambulatory practice in future years will be the development of community pharmacy-based therapeutic drug-monitoring (TDM) services.[15,16] This service actively involves pharmacists in analyzing patient blood samples to ensure optimal therapeutic outcomes for their patients. Tailoring medication therapy to the unique needs of the individual patient is an important component of pharmaceutical care. This is particularly true for drugs with known therapeutic serum concentrations (eg, digoxin, theophylline, phenytoin; for drugs with known therapeutic monitoring parameters (eg, insulin/glucose, diuretics/potassium, lovastatin/liver enzymes, warfarin/prothrombin time) and for preventive health measures (eg, assessing and monitoring risk factors related to cholesterol and glucose levels or blood pressure measurements).

An effective patient-monitoring strategy includes therapy assessment (ie, assessing appropriateness of medication therapy), patient compliance evaluation (ie, patient understanding and ownership of the need for medication therapy), documentation (ie, written baseline and outcome goals of therapy, communication with the physician, referral to other appropriate health-care providers) and monitoring/follow up (ie, chronic disease monitoring, drug-therapy monitoring) with patients. To date, the fundamental barrier to implementing TDM is economic, and the traditional pharmacist reimbursement for products dispensed rather than provision of services. Slowly, however, through documentation and positive patient outcome, reimbursement on the basis of cognitive service is gaining acceptance, and research has demonstrated that patients are willing to pay for a TDM service.

Trends indicate that the number of pharmacists practicing "holistic pharmacy" or participating in "holistic health care" will increase in the future. *Holism* is a model of health care that attempts to direct the efforts of health-care providers and patients toward a goal of meeting all the health needs of the individual. From the standpoint of the patient it is a philosophy consistent with pharmaceutical care that maintains that individuals are responsible for themselves and that they have the capacity for self-healing, usually with the cooperative assistance of a health-care provider. This philosophy supports the team concept of providers—physician, nurse, pharmacist and clergyman—with each contributing an integral component of the total health of the patient. There is little doubt that Americans will be handling their health-care problems with more knowledge, confidence and effectiveness in future years. An expanded holistic role for the pharmacist includes the education, screening and monitoring function. High blood pressure intervention is a classic example of how the pharmacist can practice holistic pharmacy, but another is the dynamic movement of men and women toward physical awareness and fitness. It is estimated that over 100 million people exercise on a daily basis, with a notable fitness mode being an activity such as jogging. The pharmacist participates in the holistic role by educating the person to prevent foot problems (eg, proper footwear and attire, running environment, running surface, warmup exercises), screening the patient after an injury has occurred (eg, podiatrist/orthopedist referral, self-medication) and monitoring the person by periodic inquiry, when permissible. Thus, the pharmacist contributes components to the overall health of the individual.

Lastly, health care is concerned with the prevention as well as the treatment of disease. It is more difficult to convince a person what he must do to stay well than it is to convince an individual what he must do to get well once he is sick. When a person is ill he will generally seek help. When he is well he will not, as a rule, seek help to remain well, yet he must take positive steps to maintain good health. He cannot take these steps unless he is aware of them. Even then, he may not take action unless he is educated as to why he must do so and encouraged to take action. Because of his accessibility, professional knowledge and training, the pharmacist is in a premier position to play an important role in maintaining the health of his community by serving as a health educator.

Pharmacists desiring to implement an innovative ambulatory service should first do a needs assessment of the clientele. Questions that need to be answered include

Who are the pharmacy's customers?
What types of patients frequent the pharmacy?
Is there a particular group of patients (eg, hypertensives, diabetics) that lack follow-up?
What is the competition in the locale?
Are there any other considerations (eg, demographics/culture)?

Pharmacists also have to evaluate their own interests and knowledge/skills. It is far easier to implement a service that one is interested in executing.

The goal of implementing an ambulatory service is to create a pharmacy niche. This could be with the elderly, patients with diabetes, animal owners, etc. The advantages of doing so is that it will provide a favorable market position for the pharmacy with less competition and have lower promotional cost. The disadvantage is that the pharmacy might not be able to serve everyone's needs.

Crucial to implementing an ambulatory service is to develop a strategic plan. The pharmacist should outline goals and objectives for the new service. One goal, eg, might be for the pharmacist to become known as a diagnostic test kit/supplies specialist, with an objective to increase the dollar sales of the diagnostic test kits and supplies by 30% during the coming year. To complement the strategic plan, the pharmacist must obtain information and training to provide the service, and coupled with this is the creation of a library of references/patient education materials germane to the service one wishes to offer. Then, the pharmacist must determine space, equipment, personnel and/or financial requirements that will be necessary to implement the service.

Documentation of the value of the service is very important. It is necessary to provide evidence of tangible outcomes and helps to develop a relationship with the prescriber.[17,18] Approaches to documentation may include a consult letter to the prescriber, a detailed consult note, use of a standardized monitoring form and/or a notation on the patient's profile.

When marketing a pharmaceutical service, the pharmacist must think in terms of creating a future that demands access to pharmacist expertise, knowledge and services. To create this image, the pharmacist can participate in health fairs, become a community educational resource and/or become a visible member of the community health-care team. The target groups, of course, become patients, health-care providers and benefits administrators. Marketing options to accomplish this task include brochures, newsletters, personal letters, detailing visits/meetings, signs and advertisements.

Health-Care Delivery Systems

At present, the US is in a period of dramatic change of the patterns of health-care delivery. Social justice dictates equal access to good quality health care for all citizens. Although it has reacted in slow, incremental steps the government has responded in an attempt to provide access to health care for all. The goal is a continuing effort to keep people healthy and out of hospitals, thus containing the high cost of health care.

The major health activities for the US are consolidated with the Department of Health and Human Services (DHHS). One of the components of this department, the Health Care Financing Administration (HCFA), gradually is assuming a greater role in health care, particularly in the financing of health-care services for the elderly, the indigent and the medically indigent. Further, HCFA is charged with the responsibility to administer Medicare and Medicaid (Titles XVIII and XIX).

Historically, the original health-care delivery system was the fee-for-service practice rendered by individual practitioners. A problem with this system is that health-care delivery is fragmented with little or no continuity. Patients consult various physicians and pharmacists, all of whom, after delivering or providing a service to the patient, independently bill the patient for their service. Other fee-for-service practice systems have included group medical practice, prepaid group medical practice and federally funded neighborhood health centers. Quite commonly within these systems, however, no one takes full responsibility for determining the total appropriate level of care and for managing the patient to assure that quality care is supplied.

Health Maintenance Organizations—With the growth in third-party payment for health-care services in the past 20 yr, there has been a trend toward overuse and escalation in costs. This evolved, and was fueled by, government-supported Medicare and Medicaid programs. In response to these high costs, corporate purchasers of health-care services (eg, government, private industry) have initiated strategies to control them. The underlying goal is to manage costs so as to be predictable and controllable while assuring quality. Thus, corporations and health-care coalitions in communities act for large groups of enrolled patients and they have the market power to negotiate with health-care providers, such as Health Maintenance Organizations (HMOs), for services at discounted prices.

At the same time, as corporations were developing strategies to control costs, health-care providers (eg, physician practice groups, aggregates of hospitals, long-term facilities, etc), merged and have become incorporated. Health Maintenance Organizations are examples of incorporated health-care delivery groups, and they have grown rapidly over the past decade. Paraphrasing the official definition, as stated within the Health Maintenance Organization Act of 1973 (Public Law 93-222), an HMO is a private or nonprofit entity which provides basic health-care services to enrollees for a fixed amount on a prepayment basis and provides additional supplemental services for additional payments. It is an organized system of health care that is capable of bringing together the necessary components which a defined population might reasonably require.

There are several types of HMO models:

The staff-model HMO is an organization which typically owns facilities and directly employs physicians. The members of this type of HMO receive health-care service for a prepaid fixed monthly or yearly fee, independent of the actual use of the services.

The group-model HMO contracts directly with rather large, well-established physician groups to provide services to members in return for a capitation fee or a fee-for-service.

The Independent Practice Association (IPA) model is the fastest growing type, in which the HMO contracts individual physicians to provide services on a discounted fee-for-service basis plus profit-sharing.

It is noteworthy to mention that beyond the HMO is the Preferred Provider Organization (PPO). The PPO resembles the IPA, except that the membership may use physicians who are not directly under contract to the organization. However, if a member uses a noncontracting physician, the member will not receive full reimbursement for medical expenses.

A Point of Service (POS) Plan combines the features of HMOs and PPOs. Patients can get care in and out of the network, but there is an in-network gatekeeper who must approve all services. The patient may pay 20 to 50% of the bill for care garnered outside the network.[19]

The concept of the HMO was fostered on the basis of prior prepaid group health plans which date back to the late 1920s, eg, Ross-Loss Group Practice Prepayment Plan, Los Angeles, CA; Community Hospital Association Plan, Elk City, OK. There are some who believe that the HMO system will help this country control runaway health costs by basing health care on prevention as well as treatment.

In 1991 it was estimated that 40.3 million people were cared for by an HMO, and that by the year 2000, every person will be enrolled in some managed care plan.[19] Membership in HMOs continues to increase, and it is estimated that by the year 1994, 53.2 million people will be managed in this environment.

All HMOs have four basic characteristics:

They are organized systems of health care in a specific geographic area, and provide the services of physician and allied health professionals within inpatient and outpatient facilities.

They offer a specified set of comprehensive basic and supplemental health maintenance and treatment services.

Membership is voluntary.

Reimbursement is made through fixed, prenegotiated, periodic payments by, or on behalf of, each person or family unit enrolled in the plan.

The method of paying (capitation payment) for health-care services is the most important characteristic because it dictates the underlying philosophy of this system which is to maintain the health of the individual. If the individual becomes sick, it costs the organization money. If the patient is hospitalized, it costs more money. To keep solvent, the organization must practice preventive medicine. The other alternative is to neglect the patient. Therefore, a review of the quality of patient services is an important element of this system.

Originally, HMOs were funded federally, but this funding was terminated in the early 1980s. Thus, the system has had to develop new sources of income to continue its growth. Business and labor both have a stake in the success of the HMO concept in view of the current economic climate. Thus, the private sector will have to respond and provide increased financial support to the HMO in the future. A key strategy of health-care purchasers to encourage cost-containment is through economic risk-sharing by patients, such as small copayments (typically $2 to $5) per prescription, and by health-care providers, with negotiated rates or fixed-payment schedules (eg, $65 per psychological consultation).

There is no doubt that the development and success of the HMO will have an impact upon pharmacy. Projections which show potential increases in the numbers of HMOs cause corresponding increases in the interest and activity among allied health professionals, and pharmacists are no exception. The most common approaches employed by HMOs to administer drug benefits are through an in-house pharmacy, contracts with community pharmacies or a combination of both. The prescription volume of many independent pharmacies has suffered because members are obligated to have prescriptions dispensed at a specific pharmacy, which has contracted with the HMO to provide this service, or have them dispensed by the HMO pharmacy. Larger staff-model HMOs tend to establish in-house outlets because these can be integrated into existing facilities. Typically, group-model HMOs, IPAs and PPOs do not have their own pharmacies and generally contract the dispensing services.

When an HMO considers implementing pharmacy services it must weigh the convenience and marketing advantages of using a single contractor or multiple-contractor outlets, such as established community pharmacies, against the control over cost afforded by an in-house operation. Alternatively, the independent pharmacist must make an informed decision about whether or not to provide pharmacy services to an HMO. As competition becomes vigorous, managed health-care systems like HMOs will cut premiums and offer new services to attract members. Consequently, these managed health-care systems will press contractor pharmacies for price concessions and place the pharmacy in an unenviable position. If the pharmacy elects not to participate in providing pharmacy services, it may be locked out of a growing prescription market. On the other hand, if it does participate on the basis of price alone, the pharmacy might not be able to generate a profit, even with a large customer base.

The question is whether pharmacists and health-care purchasers can become partners. It is crucial that pharmacists takethe lead to avoid being treated as vendors.[20] Thus, it seems that the best solution to this problem is to win an HMO contract on the basis of an attractive professional service, as well as price. Pharmacy services must be judged or evaluated on patient outcome rather than prescription output.

Purchasers of health care want solutions to meet the health-care needs of their employees. Strandberg, *et al* have proposed ten steps toward becoming a health-care partner.[20] These include

Performing a needs assessment of the potential client's organization. Each organization has a different need and a system must be designed to fit the situation.

Provide assurances that one's managed-care pharmacy plan will offer a true discount. A prospective client will need documented assurance that one's drug distribution system can control costs and that incentives are in place to do so.

Define a management reporting system. One must be capable to provide cost-information summaries in a form that the client can understand.

Define how the on-line network will be funded. Prospective clients are sometimes interested in how the pharmacy on-line computer network is maintained and supported.

Provide for an administrative reporting system. Purchases of health care have needs, e.g., electronic transfer of funds, banking needs and documentation of payments that must be met on a regular basis.

Present a detailed plan, references and program histogram. Demonstrate the length of time that the pharmacy managed-care plan has been in operation and who participates within it.

Describe a well-developed drug use review mechanism. Demonstrate the various aspects of the review system and how it works. Patient confidentiality and how it will be approached is an important facet.

Address antitrust issues. Specifically, does your pharmacy compensation system have any hidden legal problems?

Formulate an overview of the technical and computer system capabilities. Computer systems must be compatible, and some clients may demand paid claims data on computer tape whereas other clients may only request a one-page summary.

Document the quality and background of key management personnel and size of support staff.

Community pharmacies under contract to HMOs dispense prescription drugs to members either for a copayment or at a discount price. The contracted pharmacies then are reimbursed by the system for the balance of the drug price, according to one of several formulas which may be based upon capitation, average wholesale price (AWP), maximum allowable cost (MAC) or actual acquisition cost (AAC), plus a negotiated margin or a flat dispensing fee. Typically, the HMO contract with a pharmacy will call for reimbursement on a *per capita* basis, and claims by individual pharmacies or even a chain of pharmacies usually are subject to audit by the HMO (as with any third party).

Economic incentives to control costs coupled to optimal patient outcomes will become even more important to pharmacists. Focusing on aspects of patient consultation, a recent Schering Report demonstrated that not all pharmacists provide the same degree of pharmaceutical care. Thus, it is possible that those pharmacists who perform a vendor role could be reimbursed at levels less under managed-care incentive programs than those pharmacists who can document cost-savings through pharmaceutical care.[21]

In the past, independent pharmacists were advised by legal counsel that they legally could not join together to bid for third-party business on the basis of price. In fact, antitrust laws basically prohibit combined actions which are in restriction of commerce.

"(P)harmacists cannot act collectively in making a decision whether to participate or not participate in a given third-party program. Moreover, it would be unlawful for a representative to negotiate collectively for a number of individually owned pharmacies with a third-party program administrator over fees to be paid in the program. . . . (A)spects of the decision of whether to participate, which are perfectly lawful when conducted by an individual pharmacy owner acting alone and on his or her own initiative, may not be lawful if done by a group of pharmacy owners." [22]

The reason for this law was the nature of third-party business; bottom-line, dollars and cents price-bidding. Consequently, competitors, that is independent pharmacists, could not agree among themselves on the price to be offered for their services. Multiunit corporations (chain pharmacy operations), however, were regarded by the law as single-entity units for antitrust purposes and thus could take as much of the third-party bid-business as they desired. This created a contradiction in the procompetition philosophy and deprived the bid-market of the effective competition of the independent pharmacist, while allowing the chains to compete among themselves for the market. Guided by recent court decisions (*Maricopa County*, US Supreme Court) and by informal Justice Department Antitrust Division policy changes, it is apparent that independent pharmacists can join together, to form groups such as Pharmacy Service Administrative Organizations (PSAOs and bid for third-party prescription contracts on the basis of price.[23]

A PSAO is a business entity that joins pharmacists together in a legitimate business for the purpose of obtaining new and previously unavailable business through bids and contracts with HMOs, insurance companies and other third parties. The behavior of these groups must have the effect of directly broadening prescription-price competition and also to respond in other ways to meet consumer demands, by improving access to health care.

Experience has demonstrated that on-site pharmacies may have some advantages over their off-site counterparts. For example, rapport and open lines of communication can be developed between the pharmacist and the various providers. Since preventive medication is practiced, patient counseling even before OBRA 90 was dictated with each prescription and continues to necessitate that concise, clear information is provided to the patient. The pharmacist will have access to the entire record of the patient, including prescribed medications, to encourage monitoring and recognition of potential problems with drug therapy. From the standpoint of the management of an on-site pharmacy, volume purchasing, unit-of-use packaging, pharmaceutical manufacturing, drug product selection, development of utilization criteria and a closely controlled formulary system help sustain revenues in excess of expenses and demonstrate the pharmacy as a viable member of the HMO.

Development of an on-site pharmacy takes the innovativeness and creativeness of a skilled pharmacy manager. The HMO pharmacy director should possess good managerial skills and institutional experience. Institutional experience provides a working knowledge of intravenous solution preparation, sterile product preparation and a perspective toward patient monitoring. This person must be clinically adept in identifying both acute and preventive health-care needs of the ambulatory patient and know how to develop and implement pharmacy systems and programs that attain these needs. Good management dictates that this person surround himself with competent and dependable colleagues who can deliver effective, pharmaceutical care. In fact, those pharmacists who practice in on-site situations seem to express a positive feeling toward working within an HMO. It rewards him for service other than providing a product ie, value-added. The ideal attributes of the HMO pharmacist might include the following:

Team-oriented with a commitment toward contributing to and sharing responsibility for patient health care, eg, drug utilization review, monitoring patient drug therapy.

Patient-oriented with a willingness to provide health information, patient counseling and problem-solving abilities that enhance preventive patient care, eg, discharge medication counseling.

Learning-oriented by exhibiting evidence of maintenance of professional competence through continuing education.

An ability and aptitude for drug information retrieval and evaluation, eg, identify drugs of choice, research new drugs and advise on the therapeutic- and cost-effectiveness of a drug.

Good communicative abilities at the patient and the professional level, eg, in-service presentations for physicians and other health professionals.

Management-oriented with responsibilities that include planning, organizing, staffing, directing and controlling functions and activities of the HMO pharmacy and clinical services, eg, preparation, implementation and control of departmental budget.

All of these embody skills which truly are germane to any effective ambulatory pharmacy practice. However, the economic incentive serves as a prompter to the pharmacist to carry out all of these functions on behalf of the patient.

Quebec, Canada, has introduced a unique pharmacist payment program whereby pharmacists are reimbursed by private insurers if they do not dispense or renew a prescription for a clinical reason. Quebec pharmacists receive $5.39 to dispense a prescription, but also receive the same fee for not dispensing a prescription on clinical grounds. Certainly, this seems to be a model for study within the US health-care system, and recognizes that pharmacists can save patients needless medication-related illnesses, which save employers unnecessary costs.

Other Delivery Systems—There is no doubt that drug purchasing by corporate buyers, such as private industry or HMOs, will involve comparisons which include safety, efficacy and cost-effectiveness. Traditional drug distribution is being disrupted and many new forms are being promoted in the marketplace. One example is the emergence of the mail-order pharmacy. It has been predicted that by the end of this century about 10% of patients will secure their medicines by this route. But while mail-order pharmacy offers the advantages of convenience and door-step delivery to the consumer, it has been criticized for a lack of pharmacy services, in that a patient's drug profile will not be reviewed for drug interactions and the patient will not receive counseling at the time of dispensing. However, if the patient does not receive these benefits routinely from the pharmacist in the ambulatory setting, then the incentive for the patient not to use a mail-order pharmacy is lacking, especially if a patient resides in a rural area many miles from the physician and the pharmacy.

There are instances of mail-order pharmacy operations which have provided exemplary pharmacy services. Some have toll-free telephone numbers which allow patients to call in the event questions or problems associated with medicines arise, and some provide patient advisory leaflets for the patient to read when they receive their medicine. Conversely, some mail-order pharmacy operations have been criticized for high-pressure product quotas and volume incentive programs for pharmacists which may engender dispensing mistakes. Other complaints against mail-order pharmacies have included their use of recycled prescription drugs (accepting the return of a prescription drug from one consumer and redispensing it to another), dispensing prescription drugs after the doctor-patient relationship has ended, (eg, the death of the physician), an inability to deliver medicine in a timely manner and the substitution of a generic product for a brandname without first informing the patient. All of these problems have put an increased responsibility upon the individual State Boards of Pharmacy to protect the public interest by developing rules and regulations by which out-of-state mail-order pharmacy firms must abide.

The health-care needs of society are limitless, and society can attempt to provide access to an acceptable quality or minimum level of health care for its members. However, society has limited resources and it must encourage a reduction in health-care costs through the development of health-care systems, like HMOs, that take advantage of the collegiality and strengths of health-care professionals. Another example of the increased access to health care with an attempt to contain cost is the evolving relationship between pharmacy practice and the Visiting Nurse Home Health Service (VNS). Consultant pharmacy services include regular review of VNS patient charts, providing drug parameters for the nurses on chart drug profiles, and notification of the nurses about suspected or potential drug therapy problems. Also, the pharmacists provide in-service programs on drug therapy for the nurses, answer drug information inquiries from the nurses and assist in the resolution of patient therapy problems. Resolution of patient problems may encompass home visitation with nurses, preparation of medication/education sheets and administration schedules, institution of devices for medication setup and/or consultation with the prescribing physician.

The role of the pharmacist has evolved from a product-oriented to a patient-oriented professional. This role modification has been extremely healthy for both patient and pharmacist. It remains now for pharmacy and the health-care industry to ensure that the pharmacist is compensated justly for all of his services. But before this can happen it will be necessary for pharmacy to demonstrate "value-added" to the cost of the prescription. Marketing of the purpose of pharmacy in the health-care morass and of the services provided by the pharmacist is needed to generate an appropriate perceived value among purchasers and users of health-care services. Pharmacists should view themselves as dispensers of therapy and drug effect interpretations as well as of drugs themselves. Service components of pharmacy should be identified clearly to third-party payers and visible to the consumer, so that they know what is available, at what cost and how they may be accessed.

In the future, pharmacy services must be evaluated on patient outcome (ie, pharmaceutical care) rather than the number of prescriptions dispensed, and pharmacy must evolve toward interpretation and patient consultation, related to the use of medication technologies.

References

1. *The Role of the Pharmacist in Comprehensive Medication Use Management. The Delivery of Pharmaceutical Care* (A White Paper), APhA, Washington, DC, Mar 1992.
2. *The Clinical Role of the Community Pharmacist*, Office of the Inspector General, DHHS Washington, DC, Nov 1990.
3. Clepper I: *Drug Topics 136(16)*: 44, 1992.
4. Latiolais CJ, Berry CC: *Drug Intell Clin Pharm 3:* 270, 1969.
5. Rosenstock IM: *Diabetes Care 8(6)*: 610, 1985.
6. Worthen PL, Kwasnik P, Worthen DB. *Pharm Times 59 (6)*: 64, 1993.
7. *1992–1993 Survey of Pharmacy Law*, NABP, Park Ridge, IL, p 48.
8. Brown GH, Kirking DM, Ascione FJ: *Am Pharm NS23:* 325, 1983.
9. *1992–1993 Survey of Pharmacy Law*, NABP, Park Ridge, IL, p 58.
10. Srnka QM, Self TH: *Systematic Medication Profile Review*, 3rd, Am Coll Apothecaries, Alexandria VA, 1991.
11. Gannon K: *Drug Topics 137(2)*: 34, 1993.
12. Helling DK: *Drug Intell Clin Pharm 16:(1)* 35, 1982.
13. Millis JS: *Pharmacists for the Future*, AACP Report of the Study Commission on Pharmacy, Health Administration Press, Ann Arbor, MI, 1975.
14. Dong BJ: *Am J Hosp Pharm 47:* 356, 1990.
15. Knowlton CH, Zarus SA, Voltis O: *Am Pharm NS33(7)*: 57, 1993.
16. Carter BL, Helling DK: *Ann Pharmacother 26:* 701, 1992.
17. Rupp MT: Ibid: 1580, 1992.
18. Banahan BF III, McCaffrey DJ III: *Pharm Times 59(8)*: 29, 1993.
19. Feldman J, Kirway R: *Money* (July), 111 1993.
20. Strandberg LR, Pallari RJ, Fullerton DS: *Am Pharm NS32:* 982, 1992.
21. Glaser M: *Drug Topics 137(12)*: 56, 1993. (DUR and DUE: Managed Competition.)
22. Fink JL III, Siecker BR: *Manager's Guide to Third Party Programs*, Pharm Manage Inst, APhA, Washington, DC, Spring, 1982.
23. Dickinson JG: *US Pharm 11(12)*: 19, 1986.

Bibliography

USP DI Vol I: Drug Information for the Health Care Professional (current edition), USP Convention, Inc, Rockville, MD

USP DI Vol II: Advice for the Patient (current edition), USP Convention, Inc., Rockville, MD

Patient Counseling Handbook, APhA, Washington DC, 1993.

Handbook of Nonprescription Drugs, 10th ed, APhA, Washington DC, 1993.

Geriatric Dosage Handbook, APhA, Washington DC, 1993.

Family Guide to Prescription Drugs, Pharmex, Div of Automatic Business Products, Co., Inc, New Smyrna, FL.

Hansten PD: *Wellcome Trends in Pharmacy 15(2)*: 2, 1993.

Drug Utilization Review. A Systematic Approach to Quality Care, NPC, Reston VA, 1993.

Hager GP: *Wellcome Trends in Pharmacy 15(1)*: 12, 1993.

HIV and AIDS: Issues and Answers for Pharmacists, developed by the Foundation of Pharmacists and Corporate America for AIDS Education, 700 13th St, NW, Washington DC.

Guglielmo BJ, Schweigert BF, Kishi DT: *Am J Hosp Pharm 46:*1366, 1989.

CHAPTER 97

Institutional Patient Care

Harold N Godwin, MS
Professor and Director of Pharmacy
The University of Kansas Medical Center
Kansas City, 66160

Historically, health-care services have been provided primarily through physicians' offices and in hospitals. Thus, pharmaceutical services to patients seen in physicians' offices have been provided through community pharmacies while patients in hospitals normally receive pharmaceutical services through the hospital pharmacy.

The changing nature of health-care delivery has expanded the role of the hospital to include ambulatory-care programs and intermediate-care facilities (such as extended-care facilities and nursing homes). Thus, the term "institutional" care has been coined to reflect this broadened role of the hospital. Concurrently, "institutional" pharmacy also has been coined to coincide with this development. Nonetheless, institutional pharmacy is primarily hospital pharmacy. The term hospital is really the basis for the designation of the term institutional. Institution, as defined in *Webster's Dictionary*, is

> A significant and persistent element (as a practice, a relationship, an organization) in the life of a culture that centers on a fundamental human need, activity, or value, occupies an enduring and cardinal position within a society, and usually is maintained and stabilized through social regulatory agencies.

Certainly, the hospital and its directly related organizational substructures fit the term institution.

As a corollary, the term "organized health care" setting has been used to refer to the wide gamut of organizational subsystems embracing the total health-care delivery system in America. Hospital or institutional pharmacy should not be confused with the provision of pharmaceutical services to all types of organized health-care settings. For example, three physicians practicing in the same office building may have formed a corporation. Thus, they may be referred to properly as a group providing patient-care services in an organized health-care setting, because a corporation is an organized structure. Obviously, providing pharmaceutical services to the patients of these three physicians should not be considered as institutional or hospital pharmacy.

Institutional or hospital pharmacy may be defined as the practice of pharmacy in a hospital setting including its organizationally related facilities or services. It also may be defined as that department or division of the hospital wherein the procurement, storage, compounding, manufacturing, packaging, controlling, assaying, dispensing, distribution and monitoring of medications through drug-therapy management for hospitalized and ambulatory patients are performed by legally qualified, professionally competent pharmacists. In addition to all these traditional functions, the practice of pharmacy in a hospital also includes broad responsibility for the safe and appropriate use of drugs in patients, which includes, among other things, the rational selection, monitoring, dosing and control of the patients overall drug-therapy program. This added dimension requires the application of patient-oriented services superimposed upon the pharmaceutical sciences—to the subject of rational therapeutics. This approach to pharmacy practice has been referred to as "clinical" pharmacy. Thus, clinical pharmacy is simply good, professional, patient-oriented pharmaceutical services. Further, the mission of the pharmacist is to provide pharmaceutical care. Pharmaceutical care is the direct, responsible provision of medication-related care for the purpose of achieving definite outcomes that improve a patient's quality of life.

Such practice is a professional responsibility, not only of institutional or hospital pharmacy but of community pharmacy as well. What then makes the practice of pharmacy in a hospital somewhat different from private or community pharmacy?

Uniqueness of Hospital Pharmacy—A major factor is the organizational structure of a hospital or institution: a formalized pattern of authority, responsibility and coordination which affects every department of the overall health-care team. The administrator implements the policies and philosophies of the governing board, delegates authority and passes on responsibility to department heads to carry out the patient care, teaching, research and public-health objectives of the hospital. Department heads, such as the Director of Pharmacy, are expected to coordinate their services and activities with other department heads; the business and accounting department handles the financial affairs; the building services department provides the essential maintenance, housekeeping and security functions; the human resources department implements personnel policies; the clinical laboratory department performs a multitude of patient laboratory tests and services; dozens of other departments influence and affect the services of all hospital departments. All of these activities interrelate with the hospital pharmacy.

In addition to the traditional physician–pharmacist–patient relationship, which exists in the private practice of medicine and pharmacy, there is a physician–pharmacist–nurse–patient relationship in the hospital. The nurse interjects her professional role in the care of the patient between the traditional physician–pharmacist roles. Thus, the hospital pharmacist must work not only with the physician but also very closely with the nurse.

In addition to the internal forces operating within the hospital there are some external forces which affect, in various ways, the practice of pharmacy in the hospital setting. For example

> Accreditation agencies exert their influence on professional standards of practice as they affect patient care.
>
> Licensing agencies exert legal influences on hospital operations.
>
> The Federal Government imposes standards and regulations on hospitals, such as the "conditions of Participation for Hospitals" under Medicare, third-party (hospitalization insurance) agencies exert their influence on the methods by which hospitals may be reimbursed for services rendered to patients.
>
> Social agencies and governmental welfare agencies influence the services provided to medically indigent and totally indigent patients, and the governing board and public opinion exert their influences over the policies, objectives and philosophies of hospital operation and practice.

Since the hospital is an institution of and for the community, it is influenced heavily by the needs, expectations and demands of the members of that community. These are but a few examples of the socio-medico-economic and organizational forces acting on the practice of pharmacy in the institutional setting. These, among many others, are cogent reasons why hospital pharmacy practice differs significantly from community pharmacy practice.

The hospital pharmacy must be considered as one of the many departments of a hospital and as such it has several basic general functions. These functions have been outlined in a document approved by the American Hospital Association, a "Statement on Functions of a Hospital Department."[1] It reads as follows:

A department carries out its functions according to the philosophy and objectives of the hospital. The philosophy and objectives are established by the governing board. Accordingly, the department head is responsible to the administrator of the hospital. Within the organizational pattern, the functions of the department are:

1. To provide and evaluate service in support of medical care pursuant to the objectives and policies of the hospital.
2. To implement for departmental services the philosophy, objectives, policies and standards of the hospital.
3. To provide and implement a departmental plan of administrative authority which clearly delineates responsibilities and duties of each category of personnel.
4. To participate in the coordination of the functions of the department with the functions of all other departments and services of the hospital.
5. To estimate the requirements for the department and to recommend and implement policies and procedures to maintain an adequate and competent staff.
6. To provide the means and methods by which personnel can work with other groups in interpreting the objectives of the hospital and the department to the patient and community.
7. To develop and maintain an effective system of clinical and/or administrative records and reports.
8. To estimate needs for facilities, supplies and equipment and to implement a system for evaluation, control and maintenance.
9. To participate in and adhere to the financial plan of operation for the hospital.
10. To initiate, utilize and/or participate in studies or research projects designed for the improvement of patient care and the improvement of other administrative and hospital services.
11. To provide and implement a program of continuing education for all personnel.
12. To participate in and/or facilitate all educational programs which include student experiences in the department.
13. To participate in and adhere to the safety program of the hospital.

It is within this framework that the hospital pharmacist practices. The responsibility is to develop a comprehensive pharmaceutical service high in quality, properly coordinated to meet the needs of the numerous diagnostic and therapeutic departments, the nursing service, the medical staff and the hospital as a whole in the interest of providing better patient care.

Hospital pharmacy has developed so significantly in recent years that there is special education and training at the graduate level; it has its own vigorous professional society—The American Society of Hospital Pharmacists (ASHP); it has been developing a useful body of specialized knowledge through its documented literature; it has developed a strong corps of well-qualified career hospital practitioners who have adopted a sound philosophy of professional service and have developed high standards of practice. This professional organization strives to meet the needs of pharmacists practicing in any organized health-care setting. The Society is actively involved in providing continuing-education programs, publications and other services designed to help the institutional practitioner in providing a high level of professional service. The ASHP Practice Standards provide documents that offer a point of reference for use by the pharmacist in evaluating their programs and services.

The setting within which the hospital pharmacist practices requires special education or experience in order to practice with maximum effectiveness. Unlike the pharmacist in community practice, the hospital pharmacist must function within an organization which has additional responsibilities beyond patient care *per se*. These additional responsibilities include education, research and public health.

Hospital pharmacists must concern themselves on a daily basis with professional contacts with other highly specialized and skillfully trained professionals. Pharmacists meet with physician specialists on equal grounds in formal pharmacy and therapeutics committee meetings and in medical patient-care rounds in all matters relating to drug therapy; they meet with the nursing profession constantly in their daily practice; they meet with microbiologists, biochemists and clinical chemists in regard to diagnostic medicine as it relates to drugs; they meet with physicists and radiologists in relation to radioactive pharmaceuticals, diagnostic agents and contrast media; they meet with clinical pharmacologists and research physicians in matters relating to investigational drugs, drug interactions and adverse drug reactions; they meet with specialists who have graduate degrees in medical sociology, medical record librarianships, medical dietetics, methods engineering and hospital administration on a routine basis in the operation of a modern hospital pharmacy.

Hospital pharmacists long recognized the need for additional education and training and developed residency training programs to accomplish these ends. It also was recognized that additional education on a formal basis was desirable. Colleges of pharmacy have recognized the need for providing an educational program for students interested in hospital pharmacy.

Curricula for the professional degree programs (BS and PharmD) include an experiential component in hospital practice. Most of the colleges offer an undergraduate course in hospital pharmacy, while a number of colleges offer a graduate educational program leading to a Master of Science degree in hospital pharmacy. Most of the graduate programs are coordinated so that the student serves a residency in a hospital pharmacy concurrently with his graduate work at the university. These combined programs started in 1947 at the Philadelphia College of Pharmacy and Science and the Jefferson Medical College Hospital, and at the University of Maryland and the Johns Hopkins Hospital; the University of Michigan initiated its combined program in 1948. These combined educational and training programs have contributed much to provide career-minded, well-trained hospital pharmacists. Graduates of such programs have gone into hospitals throughout the country and proved their capabilities through the development of comprehensive pharmaceutical services of broad scope and high quality.

There is a trend toward specialization within hospital pharmacy. Hospital pharmacy residency training programs in years past have trained pharmacists primarily as generalists in pharmacy practice. These 1-year training programs, which follow standardized educational objectives, are surveyed and accredited by the Commission on Credentialing of the ASHP. There is also the need for specialists. Certainly, the drug-information specialty is critical in the development of comprehensive clinical services. There is a need also for a nuclear pharmacy specialist to handle, prepare and formulate new dosage forms, and to conduct research on the large number of diagnostic and therapeutic radioactive pharmaceutical preparations available today. There is the need for a pharmacy administration specialist. There is an expanding need for a variety of clinical pharmacy specialists to assist in the rational selection and use of drug therapy. Some of the clinically trained pharmacists are even further specializing their efforts and expertise in specific areas of drug therapy such as in pediatrics, psychopharmacy, geriatrics, pharmacokinetics, oncology, critical care, nutrition, primary care, adult internal medicine, clinical pharmacokinetics and other specialty areas. Indeed, residency training programs have been developed for most of these specialized areas of practice. In addition, several hospitals or colleges offer fellowship programs to provide the opportunity for 1 to 2 years of research experience in these specialized areas.

Thus, there is a healthy trend developing toward so-called "group practice" in hospital pharmacy, analogous to group medical practice. A number of these specialists in different areas of hospital pharmacy practice make up the team of pharmacists in today's progressive hospital. It is the advancement of this concept that will strengthen the professional role of hospital pharmacists and give them entry to the group of professionals who make up the health-care team.

The Hospital

Hospital pharmacists practice within the framework of an organizational structure called a hospital. In order for them to function effectively, it is essential that they understand thoroughly what a hospital is, how it is organized, what its functions are and how the pharmacy service fits into the overall patient-care program.

Definition—Traditionally, a hospital has been defined in terms of its *form*, that is, its physical makeup and the quantitative nature of its services. This definition is exemplified best by the "registration of hospitals program" of the American Hospital Association. In order to be registered under this program an institution must meet certain requirements which constitute the definition of a hospital. Thus, the program differentiates between a hospital and other institutions such as extended-care facilities, convalescent homes and homes for the aged.

The American Hospital Association has specific definitions for *general* and *special* hospitals in order for these institutions to qualify for the Association's registration program.[2] The AHA's requirements are:

Requirements for Accepting General Hospitals for Registration

1. The institution shall maintain at least six inpatient beds which shall be continuously available for the care of patients who are nonrelated and who stay on the average in excess of 24 hours per admission.
2. The institution shall be constructed, equipped and maintained to ensure the health and safety of patients and to provide uncrowded, sanitary facilities for the treatment of patients.
3. There shall be an identifiable governing authority legally and morally responsible for the conduct of the hospital.
4. There shall be a chief executive to whom the governing authority delegates the continuous responsibility for the operation of the hospital in accordance with established policy.
5. There shall be an organized medical staff of physicians that may include, but shall not be limited to, dentists. The medical staff shall be accountable to the governing authority for maintaining proper standards of medical care, and it shall be governed by bylaws adopted by said staff and approved by the governing authority.
6. Each patient shall be admitted on the authority of a staff member who shall be directly responsible for the patient's diagnosis and treatment. Any graduate of a foreign medical school who is permitted to assume responsibilities for patient care shall possess a valid license to practice medicine, or shall be certified by the Educational Council for Foreign Medical Graduates, or shall have qualified for and have successfully completed an academic year of supervised clinical training under the direction of a medical school approved by the Liaison Committee on Medical Education of the American Medical Association and the Association of American Medical Colleges.
7. Registered nurse supervision and other nursing services are continuous.
8. A current and complete medical record shall be maintained by the institution for each patient and shall be available for reference.
9. Pharmacy service shall be maintained in the institution and shall be supervised by a registered pharmacist.
10. The institution shall provide patients with food service that meets the nutritional and therapeutic requirements; special diets shall also be available.
11. The institution shall maintain diagnostic X-ray service, with facilities and staff for a variety of procedures.
12. The institution shall maintain clinical laboratory service with facilities and staff for a variety of procedures. Anatomical pathology services shall be regularly and conveniently available.
13. The institution shall maintain operating room service with facilities and staff.

Requirements for Accepting Special Hospitals for Registration

1. The institution shall maintain at least six inpatient beds, which shall be continuously available for the care of patients who are nonrelated and who stay on the average in excess of 24 hours per admission.
2. The institution shall be constructed, equipped and maintained to ensure the health and safety of patients and to provide uncrowded, sanitary facilities for the treatment of patients.
3. There shall be an identifiable governing authority legally and morally responsible for the conduct of the hospital.
4. There shall be a chief executive to whom the governing authority delegates the continuous responsibility for the operation of the hospital in accordance with established policy.
5. There shall be an organized medical staff of physicians that may include, but shall not be limited to, dentists. The medical staff shall be accountable to the governing authority for maintaining proper standards of medical care and it shall be governed by bylaws adopted by said staff and approved by the governing authority.
6. Each patient shall be admitted on the authority of a member of the medical staff who shall be directly responsible for the patient's diagnosis and treatment. Any graduate of a foreign medical school who is permitted to assume responsibilities for patient care shall possess a valid license to practice medicine, or shall be certified by the Educational Council for Foreign Medical Graduates, or shall have qualified for and have successfully completed an academic year of supervised clinical training under the direction of a medical school approved by the Liaison Committee on Medical Education of the American Medical Association and the Association of American Medical Colleges.
7. Registered nurse supervision and other nursing services are continuous.
8. A current and complete medical record shall be maintained by the institution for each patient and shall be available for reference.
9. Pharmacy service shall be maintained in the institution and shall be supervised by a registered pharmacist.
10. The institution shall provide patients with food service that meets their nutritional and therapeutic requirements; special diets shall also be available.
11. Such diagnostic and treatment services as may be determined by the Board of Approval of the American Hospital Association to be appropriate for the specified medical conditions for which medical services are provided shall be maintained in the institution, with suitable facilities and staff. If such conditions do not normally require diagnostic X-ray service, laboratory service or operating room service, and if any such services are therefore not maintained in the institution, there shall be written arrangements to make them available to patients requiring them.
12. When the institution provides pregnancy termination services, clinical laboratory services shall include the capability to provide tissue diagnosis.

On the other hand, a hospital may be defined in terms of its broad *purpose* or *mission* instead of its physical form. The contemporary hospital is a community institution which is an instrument of society. It serves as the focal point for the coordination and delivery of patient care to its community. A hospital may be viewed as an organized structure which pools together all the health professions, the diagnostic and therapeutic facilities, equipment and supplies and the physical facilities into a coordinated system for delivering health care to the public.

While the hospital once was considered only as a place where patients were treated, today it is considered as a viable institution which extends its services to the patient wherever he may be located. For example, hospitals provide services to patients within the institution itself (hospitalized patients); in ambulatory-care clinics, emergency rooms and emergency care centers; in physicians' offices at hospitals; in extended-care facilities and nursing homes either affiliated with or owned by the hospital; at home who require home health-care services; at wellness centers and at community or neighborhood health clinics.

Certain other definitions are required for proper understanding of the differences between hospitals and patient-care institutions other than hospitals. In its accreditation program the Joint Commission on Accreditation of Healthcare Organizations (JCAHO) divides long-term care facilities into two categories: a Long-Term Health-Care Facility and a Resident-Care Facility.[3] These facilities are defined as

Long-Term Health-Care Facility—A facility for inpatient care other than a hospital, with an organized medical staff, medical staff equivalent, or medical director and with continuous nursing service under professional nurse direction. It is designed to provide, in addition to the medical care dictated by diagnoses, comprehensive preventive, rehabilitative, social, spiritual and emotional inpatient care to individuals requiring long-term health care and to convalescent patients who have a variety of medical conditions with varying needs.

Resident-Care Facility—A facility providing safe, hygienic living arrangements for residents. Regular and emergency health services are available when needed, and appropriate supportive services, including preventive, rehabilitative, social, spiritual and emotional, are provided on a regular basis.

* * * *

These two broad categories cover the various types of long-term care designated by governmental agencies for licensure, certification and/or reimbursement purposes, including skilled nursing care and intermediate care. Determination of category for accreditation purposes will be made at the time of survey, based on the primary role of the facility. If identifiable roles in both major areas can be determined, accreditation will be considered in both categories.

A *clinic* is a facility or area where ambulatory patients are seen for special study and treatment by a group of physicians practicing together, and where the patient is not confined as in a hospital. The term *clinic* also is used to indicate the outpatient diagnostic facility operated by a hospital and also facilities operated by other agencies for the care of indigent and medically indigent patients. In the past the term clinic usually has been reserved for facilities of a teaching nature where medical students and resident staff offered treatment to patients unable to afford private practitioners. This concept has changed in recent years with the growing trend of physicians to locate their offices in or adjacent to the hospital, and a so-called private outpatient service has been added to the regular clinic facilities. Essentially, these functions now are grouped into a recognized department of ambulatory care at most hospitals.

Development and Expansion—Hospitals had their origin in Indian and Egyptian culture during the 6th century BC. Evolution of the hospital is related to the sociological development of the individual's expansion of interest beyond himself and his family to the welfare of the community. Although early hospitals were really places to remove people from society to protect society, ie, the insane, the incurables and the contagious, other hospitals were developed through religious and divine motives. The temples of the gods in early Greek and Roman civilization were used as hospitals where healing was associated with divine powers, while continued illness or death was associated with a lack of purity. Greek temples were forerunners of the modern hospital in the sense that they provided refuge and treatment for the sick and also provided for the teaching of young medical students. Such temples as the Temple of Aesculapius (Greek god of Medicine) existed in 1134 BC, while the temple at Kos, Greece, was where Hippocrates (born about 460 BC) practiced.

One of the dominant factors in the development and expansion of hospitals was the religious influence. Prior to the Christian Era, hospitals were temples dedicated to the god of medicine in which care of the sick was accompanied by magical, mystical and religious ceremonies. The doctrines of Jesus Christ intensified the emotions and virtues of love, pity and charity. These strong motivating forces toward one's fellow man gave impetus to the expansion of hospitals.

Another major factor in the development and expansion of hospitals devolves from a military influence. Much of the impetus toward medical and surgical progress over the centuries has come from the urgent need for care of the wounded on the battlefield. This was true during the Roman empire; it was also true in the US before, during and after the Civil War. The Civil War, however, focused attention on the inadequacy of hospital construction and also on the lack of nursing care. Lincoln requested Catholic Sisters to care for wounded army personnel because hospital care was so poor. The work done in the army set a pattern for improvement in patient care and combined the military and religious influence on hospital development.

Other factors which have influenced the development and expansion of hospitals were

The Flexner report on medical education (1910) which caused revolutionary developments in medical education *per se* and in medical internship training which helped the development of minimum standards for patient care in hospital surroundings.

The activities of Florence Nightingale during and after the Crimean War which served as the basis for revolutionizing the quality of nursing care in hospitals and for the development of schools of nursing.

The public interest in hospitals through greater dependence and improved confidence in hospital care.

With public dependence and confidence came public support and this support provided the finances for further development, expansion and improvement in hospital facilities. This public interest extended its influence into private hospitalization insurance and government participation in health care through Social Security and other health-related agencies. One of the most significant governmental programs which has affected the development and expansion of hospital facilities in the US was the adoption (in 1946) by the Congress of the Hospital Survey and Construction Act. Commonly known as the Hill–Burton program, this act was passed to provide federal funds for hospital construction on a matching basis with local communities. From 1946 to 1973 hundreds of new hospitals were built while hundreds of other hospitals have undertaken major expansion programs of existing facilities through the availability of government finances through the Hill–Burton Act.

A number of legislative amendments were adopted by the Congress which made funds available for construction and improvement of various health-care facilities, including medical and nursing schools, outpatient facilities, extended-care facilities and specialized diagnostic and therapeutic facilities in hospitals. In addition, the Social Security Amendments of 1965 (Medicare) will have a long-range impact on the development and expansion of hospitals because funds are made available to pay for services of medically indigent patients lacking means to pay hospitals for services rendered.

The National Planning and Resources Development Act was implemented in 1975 creating the development of Health Systems Agencies (HSAs). These agencies have the responsibility of effective health planning and development of health services, manpower and facilities in local areas. Each HSA is responsible for

Improving the health of residents of its health service area.

Increasing the accessibility, acceptability, continuity and quality of services provided.

Restraining increases in the cost of these services.

Preventing unnecessary duplication of health resources.

In 1983, Congress enacted significant changes in the method by which hospitals are reimbursed for medicare patients in an effort to hold down escalating hospital costs. A Prospective Payment System was developed to reimburse hospitals at a specific rate based upon the diagnosis of the patient (diagnosis related groups (DRGs)). This system of payment has influenced the mechanism by which private insurance companies reimburse the hospital or patient for care. This emphasis on cost containment also has prompted a shift from hospital care to ambulatory care for many medical services.

During the early 1990s the public and government promoted efforts for major health-care system reform. The focus issues were universal patient access to a health-care system and the cost of health care. Future restructuring of the system will impact the functions or role of the hospital significantly. The first hospital on the American continent was built by the Spaniards (led by Cortez) in 1524—The Hospital of the Immaculate Conception in Mexico City. In 1663 its name was changed to The Hospital of Jesus of Nazareth and it still exists today. In the American colonies a hospital was built in 1663 on Manhattan Island for sick soldiers. The first incorporated hospital in the US was the Pennsylvania Hospital, established in 1751 through the efforts of Dr Thomas Bond to provide physicians in Philadelphia with a place to treat their private patients. In 1769 New York, with a population of 300,000, had no hospital. Since 1873 the population of the US has more than doubled but the number of hospitals has increased 44 times—from only 149 to approximately 7000.

Beyond the three basic essentials of human existence (food, clothing and shelter), the hospital has become a necessary instrument for providing a fourth basic element of survival—health. The hospital serves as a major instrument through which the health professions are able to provide health care to the people of the community. It is because of the increasing complexity of health care—diagnostic, preventive and therapeutic—that the necessary trained personnel, facilities and equipment are consolidated into what is known as the hospital in order to provide the quality of care the public expects, demands and deserves. Health care has come to be defined as a right for all, rather than a luxury for a few. In the future, hospitals will be an integral part of a health-care system rather than a free-standing entity. They will expand their scope of activity to include ambulatory care, wellness, acute care, emergency care, home-care and long-term care. Indeed, many hospitals will be a part of a larger hospital group much like chain pharmacies.

Classification—Hospitals may be classified in different ways, by

Type of service	Ownership
Length of stay	Bed capacity

Hospitals are classified by *type of service* as either general or special hospitals. A general hospital provides care to patients with any type of illness: medical, surgical, pediatric, psychiatric and maternity. On the other hand, special hospitals are those which restrict the care they provide to special conditions, such as cancer, psychiatric or pediatric cases.

Hospitals are classified by *length of stay* as either short-term or long-term. A short-term hospital is one in which the average length of stay of the patient is less than 30 days. Patients with acute disease conditions and emergency cases usually are hospitalized for less than 30 days. Usually, general hospitals are short-term, since acutely ill patients usually recover in less than 30 days. On the other hand, a long-term hospital is one in which the average length of stay of the patient is 30 days or longer. Such patients have long-term illnesses, such as psychiatric conditions.

Hospitals are classified by *ownership* usually as governmental or nongovernmental. Hospitals falling into these categories of ownership are

Governmental Hospitals	*Nongovernmental Hospitals*
Federal (Armed Forces, Veterans Administration & US Public Health Service)	Nonprofit
	Church related or operated
	Other nonprofit
State	For profit
County	Individual
City (municipal)	Partnership
City-County	Corporation

Hospitals generally are classified by *bed capacity*, according to the following pattern:

Under 50 beds
50–99 beds
100–199 beds
200–299 beds
300–399 beds
400–499 beds
500 beds & over

According to these four general classifications, the approximately 6500 hospitals in the US are 80% nongovernmental, short-term, general or special; roughly half are under 100 beds.

The 6500 hospitals represent approximately 1,500,000 beds, admit about 38 million patients annually and service approximately 400 million outpatient visits per year.

Federal hospitals are owned and operated by various branches of the Federal Government. The US Army, Air Force and Navy hospitals are usually general medical and surgical hospitals, provided to care for military personnel, although there are specialized mental institutions within these groups. The Veterans Administration hospitals provide care for additional specialized groups of our population, and operate general medical and surgical hospitals, and also some mental hospitals.

State hospitals are owned by the state and controlled by a board of control or division of the state government, or a similar organization responsible to state government. They are maintained by state appropriations, and consist mainly of psychiatric hospitals. In some instances, state hospitals are general hospitals affiliated with a university involved in the training of physicians and other professional personnel, often referred to as teaching hospitals.

County hospitals are owned by the county and financed and controlled similarly to state hospitals, only on a county level. They are usually general hospitals caring for the indigent.

City hospitals are owned, financed and controlled by the city government. They are usually general hospitals, caring for the indigent, although there may be a chain of city-owned and operated hospitals as in New York City.

In the nongovernmental hospital group, the majority of institutions are general medical and surgical hospitals, varying only in their control and eligibility for receipt of state funds for charity or indigent patient care. The *proprietary* or *private hospital organized for profit* is usually a corporation composed of physicians, although other businessmen may be involved in the corporate profit-making structure. In recent years, a number of corporations have been formed whereby they own, operate and control large chains of hospitals. There has been a great growth recently of "polycorporate" hospital systems in which one hospital manages several other hospitals or there is a multiple hospital grouping. These multiple hospital arrangements will have an influence upon how health care is delivered.

In the *nonprofit*, nongovernmental grouping of hospitals, some are *church hospitals*, supported financially by fees from paying patients or by contributions from the several religious orders or churches. These hospitals are owned and controlled either by the religious order, or diocese, as in the Catholic churches, or by a separate governing board, as in churches of other denominations.

Community hospitals or private, nonprofit hospitals are owned and operated by members of the community, but with no relationship to the local government. They are financed by fees from patients of the community and surrounding area. The cost of providing medical care for the indigent is a problem for the community hospital and this cost is met through local, state and federal assistance.

Functions—Traditionally, the hospital's basic purpose for existence has been the treatment and care of the sick and injured. In conjunction with this basic function, hospitals have been concerned with teaching, particularly of medical students, ever since the pre-Christian Era of Greek medicine. Research has been another function of the hospital. In modern times a fourth function has been assumed by hospitals, namely, public health (preventive medicine). Thus, the four fundamental functions of hospitals are patient care, teaching, research and public health.

Patient Care—The modern hospital is charged with maintaining and restoring health to the community which it serves. The other three functions are really the handmaidens of patient care since they exist because they contribute either directly or otherwise to the care of the sick and injured. Emergency care of the injured commands prime attention in any hospital—fully as important as the care of the inpatient. Outpatient care also has become an important function of the hospital's responsibility to the community.

Patient care involves the diagnosis and treatment of illness or injury, preventive medicine, rehabilitation, convalescent care, dental care and personalized services.

In providing patient care, hospitals usually have two basic types of accommodations based on the patient's ability to pay: the full-pay or private patient and the partially or totally medical indigent (charity) patient. With the marked increase in prepaid hospitalization insurance (through commercial insurance carriers such as Blue Cross or managed-care contracts such as health maintenance organizations (HMOs)) there has been a great increase in the number of private patients. The Federal Government's involvement with medical care through Medicare and Medicaid expands coverage for a broad population group who previously were partially or totally medical indigents, including nonindigent groups.

Education—This is an important function of the modern hospital whether it is or is not affiliated with a university. Education as a hospital function is of two major forms

1. Education of the medical and allied health professions. This form includes physicians; nurses; medical social service workers; medical record librarians; dietitians; X-ray and laboratory technicians; medical technologists; respiratory, physical and occupational therapists; hospital administrators; pharmacists and others. The hospital's educational program

for these groups includes formal programs (such as medical and nursing schools), in-service training programs for professional personnel such as residencies and on-the-job training programs for nonprofessional personnel. Such educational programs are essential; it is only in a hospital that such concentrated facilities are available to provide the necessary practical learning experience for dealing with the saving of human lives.

2. Education of the patient. This is an important hospital function, the scope of which is seldom realized by the public. It includes providing general education for children confined to long-term hospitalization; special education in the area of rehabilitation—psychiatrically, socially, physically and occupationally; and special education in health care, for example, teaching a diabetic or a cardiac patient to care for his ailment or teaching the colostomy patient who requires a reorientation in caring for his personal needs.

Research—Hospitals carry out research as a vital function for two major purposes: the advancement of medical knowledge against disease and the improvement of hospital services. Both purposes are directed toward the basic aim of better health care for the patient. Examples of research activities in the hospital include devising new diagnostic procedures, conducting laboratory and clinical experiments, developing and perfecting new surgical procedures or techniques and evaluating investigational drugs. Other examples include research to improve administrative procedures for greater efficiency and lower cost to the patient, improvement of accounting procedures for more equitable cost distribution of services, and designing, developing and evaluating new equipment and facilities for improving patient care.

Research in hospitals was performed primarily by medical staffs in the past. However, in recent years there has been a significant increase in research activities in the various hospital departments by other than medical personnel. Nursing, for example, is now engaged in significant research designed to improve patient care. Many drugs are evaluated in hospitalized patients before they are marketed and, thus, the clinical evaluation of investigational drugs presents many opportunities for the hospital pharmacist to participate in research. Pharmacists are involved in many other types of research, such as pharmacokinetic studies involving individualization of drug-dosing in patients, biopharmaceutical studies of drug products and radiopharmaceutical dosage formulations, as well as administrative and professional studies on drug-distribution systems, the effectiveness of clinical roles of pharmacists and drug-utilization review studies.

Public Health—The prime objective of this fourth and relatively new hospital function is to assist the community in reducing the incidence of illness and improve the general health of the population. Examples of public-health activities are: the close working relationships many hospitals have with public-health departments of communicable diseases; the participation in disease detection programs as for tuberculosis, diabetes, hypertension and cancer; the participation in mass public innoculation programs such as against influenza and poliomyelitis and the participation of hospital ambulatory-care departments in teaching better routine hygienic practices, wellness clinics and exercise and fitness programs, as well as ways in which patients should care for themselves when illness strikes. Hospital pharmacists have an opportunity to contribute to this function by providing health-information brochures and services to outpatients and by instructing them on the safe use of drugs and poison-prevention measures.

Standards of Practice—In the US the public is able to determine whether a hospital provides a minimum quality of patient care through its "accreditation" status. The accreditation program is conducted on a national basis, and its purpose is to determine the quality of care rendered to patients. This is achieved through the establishment of minimum standards of quality of patient care and the invitation to all hospitals to meet or surpass these standards by improving their services and facilities.

The accreditation program was carried out by the Joint Commission on Accreditation of Hospitals (JCAH). This name was changed from JCAH to Joint Commission on Accreditation of Healthcare Organizations (JCAHO) in 1988. This change is reflective of the influence this organization has on the standards of health-care delivery. JCAHO sets standards for home-care programs as well as hospitals.

The JCAHO is an independent, voluntary agency, and its actions are not subject to ratification by the organizations represented by its component members. One of its objectives is to make known to the public the names of those hospitals which have invited its scrutiny and have been accredited by it through meeting the minimum standards established for good patient care. The net effect of the program is to enable the public to discriminate between hospitals that are accredited and those that are not.

Accreditation of hospitals began in 1918 when The American College of Surgeons initiated its hospital-standardization program. The purpose was to elevate the quality of surgical care provided in hospitals. The program involved setting up minimum standards of practice for the operating rooms, but it also pointed up the need for similar standards in all departments of the hospital. The first list of approved hospitals, published in 1919, contained 89 approved hospitals out of 692 surveyed. The American College of Surgeons standardization program was taken over by the JCAH in 1953.

During the years the American College of Surgeons carried out the accreditation program, the pharmacy was not included among the essential divisions of the hospital but, rather, was listed as a complementary division. The JCAH continued this classification for several years. However, in 1956, the pharmacy department was included among the essential services of the hospital and thus official recognition was given to the importance of the pharmacy. In 1965 the JCAH amended its standards for medical staff functions by requiring a pharmacy and therapeutics committee. Previously, the JCAH had only considered this committee to be a desirable one rather than an essential committee. A more recent development was the inclusion in the requirement for registration by the American Hospital Association that "Pharmacy service shall be maintained in the institution and shall be supervised by a registered pharmacist."

In the early 1990s JCAHO launched its new direction for the accreditation review process entitled "agenda for change." This new approach now focuses upon quality patient care through outcomes measurements using continuous quality improvement (CQI) techniques. This is in contrast to the previous review system which focused solely upon physical plant, safety procedures and structure and process of patient care.

Another major impetus to the development of standards of practice in hospitals came about with the enactment of the Social Security Amendments of 1965 (Medicare). This law set forth certain conditions which hospitals are required to meet for purposes of participating as providers of services to recipients of federally financed programs. These requirements are published as a manual entitled, *Conditions of Participation—Hospitals* (available from the US Dept of Health and Human Services, Social Security Admin, Washington DC). This manual includes the conditions of participation for the various departments of the hospital, including the pharmacy department. These conditions have played a major role in challenging small hospitals to consider appointing pharmacists to their staffs, providing comprehensive pharmacy services and establishing pharmacy and therapeutics committees.

Organization and Administration—No matter what the type of organization and control of a hospital, there is always a governing body of some sort to which the administrator, director, superintendent, medical director, chief administrative officer or whatever the individual is titled must report. In the case of the federal hospitals, this usually is not a group on a local area level. In state, county and city hospitals the governing body is usually from the political subdivision in which the hospital is located, but need not be so, where persons of special ability are concerned or in cases where political pressure is applied. In the nonprofit, nongovernmental hospital, there is usually a governing board, board of trustees, board of governors or other titled group which assumes overall responsibility for the proper operation of the hospital so adequate service can be rendered to the sick and injured at as low a cost as is compatible with efficiency.

Specifically, the duties of the governing board, performed through the chief administrative officer, are the responsibility for the selection of competent personnel including the medical staff, control of hospital funds and supervision of the physical plant. By reason of certain court decisions the responsibility for injury or other act by a member of the hospital staff on the hospital grounds reverts back to the governing board, although the individual hospital personnel is involved.

The governing body, acting on recommendations of the chief administrative officer, must establish the working hours and conditions, salary schedules and proper checks on personnel. Again, acting on the recommendations of the chief administrative officer, the governing board must establish a schedule of room rates and other charges for hospital inpatient and ambulatory care. The board must devise methods for obtaining endowments and other grants that will supplement income from paying patients and help to balance the hospital budget. The board wisely must invest endowment funds and other grants from which the interest is to be used for operating or other expenses. It must make certain that there is an adequate accounting system and provide for routine audit of the accounts. This board must determine the needs for additional or replacement construction of the physical plant of the hospital and must contract with the most advantageous bidder.

The governing board has its own internal organization, comprised of a president or chairman, vice-chairman, secretary and treasurer. On many boards the chief executive officer of the hospital serves as the secretary. There are usually certain standing committees appointed, such as

The executive committee.

The hospital committee dealing with personnel appointments and especially those of the medical staff, and with other activities of departmental nature.

The finance committee which is concerned with the hospital budget, room rates and other financial matters.

A committee on public relations which is concerned with educating the community on the value of the hospital and with maintaining a desirable relationship with the community.

There may be other committees appointed as the need arises, such as an expansion and development committee where the hospital is concerned with the need for construction of additional hospital beds.

The chief executive officer (CEO) of the hospital is appointed by the governing board and must produce a two-way channel of communication between the board and the hospital staff and personnel insofar as the needs or desires of both are concerned. The CEO is often the secretary of the governing board, and reports to it all essential facts concerning the operation of the hospital and receives from the board all directives it issues. The hospital administrator must have initiative and leadership as well as executive ability in order to carry out his responsibilities. All functions of professional care of the patient must be carried on within budgetary limitations, and there must be interdepartmental cooperation and harmony.

In order for administrators to carry out the overall responsibilities assigned by the governing board, they need assistance. Depending on the size of the hospital there may be one or more associate and several assistant administrators. The administrator also appoints heads of departments. The department heads have the responsibility to operate the departments effectively and properly, within the overall policies and philosophies established by the hospital's governing board.

Among the many departments which make up the modern hospital there are some in which the services involve primarily the *professional care* of the patient while the services of other departments involve mainly the *business management* of the hospital.

Some of the departments which deal with the professional care of the patient (diagnostic or therapeutic) are

Ambulatory Care
Anesthesia
Blood Bank
Central Sterile Supply
Clinical Laboratories
Dental Service
Dietary and Nutrition Service
Electrocardiograph Laboratory
Electroencephalograph Laboratory
Emergency Room
Medical Library
Medical Records
Medical Social Service
Nuclear Medicine
Nursing Service
Occupational Therapy
Pharmacy Service
Physical Medicine
Radiology & X-Ray Therapy
Respiratory Therapy

Departments which deal with the business management or administrative side of the hospital include

Accounting
Admitting
Biomedical Engineering
Business Office
Cafeteria & Coffee Shop
Central Transportation
Credit & Collection
Computer Services
Engineering & Maintenance
Housekeeping
Information Service
Personnel & Payroll
Post Office
Purchase & Store Room
Telephone Switchboard
Volunteer Service

The Medical Staff—The medical staff of a hospital falls in a different category organizationally than the departments listed previously. Physicians are independent agents taking care of their patients, and they use the hospital, its departments, facilities and services to care for these patients. The governing board of the hospital and the community which it represents exercise effective control over the medical staff. Although the governing board neither originates nor implements medical policy, it is responsible for it, and while the board members are not competent to pass judgment on the professional care of the patient they are, as representatives of the ownership of the hospital, liable for dereliction of duties established by law. Thus, the board delegates a portion of its duties and responsibilities to its appointed medical staff to originate medical policy honestly and carry out this policy in good faith. To do this requires that the medical staff be organized to govern itself and appraise its own work, and yet be responsible to the governing board for the details of its work.

In order for a physician to be appointed to the medical staff of a hospital, an application for membership must be made. This application and appropriate credentials are considered by the credentials committee of the medical staff, which determines whether the physician is competent to practice in the claimed specialty. The credentials committee also evaluates the appropriateness of need and the qualifications of the physician to perform certain specialized procedures (eg, cardiac transplant, laser surgery, radiation oncology therapy). The credentials committee, if favorably impressed, makes its recommendation to the medical staff for appointment. Assuming this is approved, the recommendation goes to the governing board for final approval, upon which the physician is designated a member of the medical staff of the hospital for a specified period of time, usually 1 year, subject to renewal.

The organized medical staff of a hospital has certain duties:

Providing professional care to patients of the hospital.
Maintaining its own efficiency.
Self-government.
Participating in the educational program of the hospital.
Auditing its own professional work.
Advising and assisting the administrator and the governing board regarding medical policies.

There are two main types of hospital staffs: *open* and *closed*.

An *open* staff is one in which certain physicians, other than those on the attending or active medical staff, are allowed to use the private-room facilities, providing they comply with all rules and regulations of the institution. These physicians are termed members of the "courtesy" medical staff; the hospital is termed an *open-staff* hospital.

A *closed* staff is one in which all professional services, private and charity, are provided and controlled by the attending or active medical staff. A hospital with this type of staff is termed a *closed-staff* hospital. The closed staff, though it has minor drawbacks, is the more desirable for the average hospital and especially for the teaching hospital, because it allows careful selection of a group of specialists with excellent reputations.

The medical staff consists of the following groups: an honorary staff, a consulting staff, an active staff, an associate staff, a courtesy staff and a resident staff. The *honorary medical staff* is composed of physicians who have been active in the hospital but who are retired, and of those to whom it is desired to do honor because of outstanding contributions. The *consulting medical staff* consists of specialists who are recognized as such by right of passing specialty boards or belonging to the national organization of their specialty, and who serve as consultants to other members of the medical staff when called upon. The *active* or *attending medical staff* is the group primarily concerned with regular patient care. It is the group most actively involved in the hospital. In internal staff government it is the authoritative body. The *associate medical staff* is composed of junior or less-experienced members of the staff. Appointment to this group is the first step toward active or attending staff membership. The *courtesy medical staff* consists of those physicians who desire the privilege of attending private patients but who do not desire active staff membership. The *resident medical staff* is composed of residents, who are full-time employees of the hospital. These persons provide specific services in the care of the patient, for which they receive education and experience.

Financing Hospital Care—The technological developments of our industrialized society and the rapid advances of the medical sciences annually increase the financial burdens of hospitals. Hospitals, in order to provide the best care available, at the insistence of the public, must keep up with these advances by obtaining the newest diagnostic and therapeutic equipment, facilities and products. In addition, the increasing cost of labor is reflected in the increased cost of the personalized services made available in the modern hospital. The cost of hospital care is a direct reflection of these developments. In 1946 the total cost of operating all US hospitals was $1.9 billion; by 1978 it had reached $65.5 billion. By 1992, health-care costs were over $800 billion. This cost is approximately 13% of the Gross National Product (GNP).

Perhaps the most widely used statistic to describe hospital costs is the total expense per patient day. In 1946 the average cost per patient day in hospitals was $5.21; in 1974 it averaged $84; in 1993 it was between $800–$1000. With the trend toward more equitable salaries for hospital personnel, there is every indication that hospital costs will continue to rise dramatically.

For centuries hospitals have struggled with the problem of finances adequate to cover total operating expenses. The fact that, basically, the public does not care to pay for something it does not want has been a major factor in this struggle for financial survival. Individuals resist having to pay hundreds or thousands of dollars for an operation or a long hospital stay which they have not anticipated. At one time hospitals were a place where people went to die; the public cared little about their financial struggles. But, as the hospital developed into a place where people went to get well, the public took a more positive interest in the financial problems. In other words, the public has come to recognize that although it dislikes paying hospital bills it must do so if the hospital is to continue to exist to protect the public health. Over the last few decades the quality of health and the life span have both increased.

Sources of Income—There are several main sources of income for hospitals: patients, government, third-party hospitalization insurance, voluntary contributions, endowment funds and investments.

Since the majority of hospitals in the US are private (nongovernmentally operated), the bulk of income to these institutions is from the patient, either directly or indirectly. Funds may come from the patient directly or they may come through hospitalization insurance (usually referred to as third-party payments). A large segment of the population is covered by hospitalization insurance.

Another third-party principle involves the workmen's compensation regulations in the various states. These vary among the states but essentially each involves the employer taking out an accident insurance policy which will pay for emergency treatment or hospitalization of the employee in case of accident or injury on the job.

Medically indigent patients are those who do not have sufficient income to pay for their own personal health needs. Although some private organizations provide assistance to this group of patients, the bulk of the financial assistance comes from tax funds through local, state and federal agencies. The list of public tax-supported programs for health-care assistance is formidable and becomes complex in determining what department, division or agency of the federal, state, county or city government is involved. In addition, dependents of members of the Armed Forces, members of the Public Health Service and their families and the veterans of foreign wars receive health care through public tax funds.

The Social Security Amendments of 1965 and 1972 extended the benefits for hospitalization, physician's services and outpatient services from the original Social Security Law. A substantial portion of hospital costs is provided under federal auspices. The total percentage of health-care costs covered by third-party reimbursement of some sort approaches 90%.

Other sources of income for hospitals are the voluntary contributions of individuals, corporations, foundations and community fund-raising campaigns. Some of these are direct contributions to the hospitals; others are made available in the form of grants for research; still others are given for major expansion or remodeling programs. Private health-assistance agencies assist individuals who need help by subsidizing the cost of their hospitalization and other health-care needs.

Many hospitals are fortunate in receiving substantial sums for the purpose of setting up endowment trust funds and for use by the hospitals in other ways. In addition, some hospitals receive some income through investments, such as in real estate.

Another category of income sources includes the gift shop, small food-service facility or beauty parlor, many of which are operated by a women's auxiliary on a voluntary basis.

Health Maintenance Organizations—A Health Maintenance Organization (HMO) is a public or private organization which provides comprehensive health services to individuals enrolled with such an organization on a *per capita* prepayment basis. Such comprehensive or "total" health services include minimum emergency care, inpatient hospital and physician care, ambulatory physician care, prescription services and preventive medical services. This type of capitated comprehensive care often is referred to as managed care.

In 1973 Congress passed the "Health Maintenance Organization Act of 1973" (Public Law 93-222) which provided new authority to the Department of Health, Education and Welfare (now Health and Human Services) to develop new HMOs. According to the Act an HMO is an organizational entity which includes four essential attributes:

1. An organized system for providing health care in a geographic area, which entity accepts the responsibility to provide or otherwise assure the delivery of
2. an agreed-upon set of basic and supplemental health maintenance and treatment services to
3. a voluntarily enrolled group of persons
4. and for which services the HMO is reimbursed through a predetermined, fixed, periodic prepayment made by or on behalf of each person or family unit enrolled in the HMO without regard to the amounts of actual services provided.

This legislation authorizes, among many other things, an HMO to "maintain, review and evaluate . . . a drug use profile of its members receiving prescription drugs, evaluate patterns of drug utilization to assure optimum drug therapy and provide for instruction of its members and health professionals in the use of prescription and nonprescription drugs." Thus, opportunities exist for the development of challenging new roles for pharmacy within HMOs in the broad areas of rational drug therapy including diagnostic and curative, as well as preventive, therapy. Many would agree that pharmacy practice within these organized health-care facilities is characteristic of institutional pharmacy practice.

The Hospital Pharmacy

The separation of pharmacy from medicine took place in charitable institutions operated under governmental or ecclesiastic authority. The fact that business interests played no part in the delivery of care to patients in these institutions led to an eventual division of labor in order to improve the quality of care. This division of labor in the physician–apothecary function led to the recognition of pharmacy as a discipline separate from medicine. Since the division occurred in hospitals, the hospital pharmacist was the first recognized practitioner of the profession of pharmacy.

The development of hospital pharmacy in different countries was vitally affected by educational standards and the caliber of its practitioners. Thus, hospital pharmacy as an important professional specialty virtually was neglected in America for almost 168 years, from the time that Jonathan Roberts became the first hospital pharmacist at the Pennsylvania Hospital (Philadelphia) in 1752, to approximately 1920. Others of this period included Charles Rice (1841–1901) of Bellevue Hospital in New York City and Martin I Wilbert (1865–1916) of the German Hospital in Philadelphia.

A National Professional Society—Although the existence of the American hospital covers a span of more than 200 years, only during the past four decades or so have we witnessed the rapid expansion leading to our present vast and complex hospital system. As the movement toward the organization, expansion and growth of the hospital system in the US began to take shape, there also developed a movement toward the organization of hospital pharmacists. As Niemeyer *et al*[4] point out, the critical years for hospital pharmacy were the two decades from 1920 to 1940. The "awakening in the 1920s" came about as a result of a growing realization by hospital pharmacists of the problems, potentialities and importance of their specialty. The "advances in the 1930s" resulted from their determination for organization, recognition and establishment of higher standards of practice.[5]

The activities of hospital pharmacists during this critical period resulted in the formation of The American Society of Hospital Pharmacists (ASHP) in 1942. The development of the Society within the sphere of American pharmacy has been due, in large part, to the adoption of a philosophy of service by hospital pharmacists which places the patient as the focal point for the existence of pharmacy practice.[6] The unity which binds hospital pharmacists through their national professional society stems from their being a goal-oriented group. The common bond among them is the development of higher standards of professional practice and service, *because the patient needs it.* The membership, exceeding 27,000, represents a significant majority of the pharmacists practicing in the institutional setting. Because of this common goal, the ASHP has made significant progress during the first 53 years of its existence.

Despite its relative youth, the ASHP has made significant contributions toward the improvement of hospital pharmacy.

The *American Journal of Hospital Pharmacy* is one of the best professional publications in international pharmaceutical circles. In addition, *Clinical Pharmacy* was published to provide in-depth articles dealing with clinical practice. In 1994 these two significant journals were combined to provide a journal on a semi-monthly basis.

The International Pharmaceutical Abstracts (IPA) was introduced by the ASHP because of the need for such a publication. This abstract service provides extensive coverage of the pharmaceutical literature and now is available for on-line computer searches.

Drug Information (American Hospital Formulary Service) is a comprehensive, unbiased source of current information on drugs provided on a supplemented basis annually. This is a comprehensive reference often used at hospital nursing stations throughout the country. This serves as a basis for the pharmacist to extend his role as pharmaceutical consultant to the medical profession.

In 1964 the *Mirror to Hospital Pharmacy* provided the findings from an exhaustive study of hospital pharmacy in the US. The whole basis for this study was to find out existing practices in hospital pharmacy and determine ways in which to improve the quality and expand the scope of its pharmaceutical service.

Continuing-education programs, known as "Institutes," have served to help the hospital pharmacist keep up with current trends of professional practice. Continuing-education programs such as this are essential for practicing pharmacists to maintain their professional competency.

Maintaining professional competency is one of the greatest challenges of the profession of pharmacy today, indeed the challenge for all health professions. Each year the ASHP conducts two major continuing-education programs on a national basis—the Midyear Clinical Meeting and the Annual Meeting. The Midyear Clinical Meeting has become the world's largest meeting for pharmacy with over 15,000 participants in attendance.

The residency training programs in hospital pharmacy are accredited by the Society and serve as a basis for insuring a high quality of training of future practitioners. In addition to a residency in pharmacy practice with emphasis on pharmaceutical care, specialized residencies in nuclear pharmacy, ambulatory care, pediatric pharmacy, psychiatric pharmacy, geriatric pharmacy, drug information pharmacy practice, oncology pharmacy, primary care, adult internal medicine, clinical pharmacokinetics, critical care, nutrition support and administration serve to provide a means to develop practitioners with specialized skills to meet future practice needs.

The *Minimum Standard for Pharmacies in Institutions* provides a helpful set of principles on which to develop good professional practices within the hospital.

Many other contributions such as computer assisted instruction modules, video tapes and self study modules have been made by the Society and still others are currently under development. Thus, the strengths of a goal-oriented Society are readily apparent in the ASHP's contributions to American hospital pharmacy.

Standards of Practice

The movement to develop standards of practice in the hospital was initiated by the American College of Surgeons during the early 1900s when surgeons recognized the need to standardize and improve on surgical procedures, operating room techniques and medical record-keeping on surgical operations. The College found that to improve the overall care of surgical patients, standards needed to be developed in other departments of the hospital as well as in the operating room. As a result of their initiative, the first Minimum Standard for Pharmacies in Hospitals was presented to the 18th Hospital Standardization Conference of The American College of Surgeons in 1935. In 1942, when The American Society of Hospital Pharmacists was organized, a standing committee on Minimum Standards was appointed for the purpose of maintaining and developing better minimum standards. The original standard of the American College of Surgeons was revised by the ASHP in 1950. This revised Standard was approved by the APhA, American Hospital Association, Catholic Hospital Association and received editorial endorsement by the AMA. The *Minimum Standard for Pharmacies in Hospitals with Guide to Application* has been revised periodically, resulting in the *ASHP Guidelines: Minimum Standard for Pharmacies in Institutions* (available from ASHP, 7272 Wisconsin Avenue, Bethesda MD 20814).

To assist hospital administrators and hospital pharmacists to review their pharmacy service in terms of expected qualitative performance, the JCAHO has continued to revise its standards for a hospital pharmacy. These standards, while not totally inclusive of a broad scope and high-quality pharmaceutical service, do challenge the 6500 hospitals to meet optimum achievable standards of practice in providing a high quality of service.

Another standard of practice relating to institutional pharmacy is the federal requirement imposed under the Social Security Amendments of 1965 (Medicare) and subsequent amendments.

Organization—Within the organizational structure of the hospital, the director of pharmacy, as a department head, reports to the administrator of the hospital on the proper operation and management of the pharmacy. The director of pharmacy formulates and implements departmental administrative and professional policies of the pharmacy subject to the approval of the administrator. The professional and clinical policies relating to hospital-pharmacy practice, which have a direct relationship to the medical staff, are formulated and developed through the pharmacy and therapeutics committee and are subject to administrative approval (see *Pharmacy and Therapeutics Committee*).

The organizational structure of the hospital pharmacy may be as illustrated in Fig 1. This chart attempts to illustrate that coordination and integration of all the technical elements of practice must be implemented effectively into a total pharmaceutical service. For example, there are technical and professional elements of a clinical-pharmacy service. On the other hand, there are clinical components of professional, technical and support services. Likewise, there are educational, technical and clinical implications to the research and supportive components to a pharmacy service. Therefore, one should look at the organizational structure of a modern hospital pharmacy in terms of the overall elements comprising its services rather than viewing it from a clinical versus an operational standpoint. This philosophical approach to the organizational and operational aspects of hospital pharmacy is essential if one is to use effectively all the pharmaceutical sciences which underlie the profession of pharmacy.

A close examination of this organizational chart shows the many ramifications of the practice of pharmacy in today's modern hospital. There follows a comprehensive job description of the pharmacist's responsibilities in general hospital pharmacy activities and in clinical functions and responsibilities.

Pharmacist Responsibilities

I. Inpatient Pharmacist's Responsibilities
   A. Dispensing Area
      1. Insures that established policies and procedures are followed.
      2. Checks for accuracy of doses prepared:
         a. Intravenous admixtures
         b. Unit dose
      3. Provides for proper drug control:
         a. Insures that drugs are stored and dispensed properly (eg, investigational drugs).
         b. Insures that all state and federal drug laws are followed.
      4. Insures that good techniques are used in compounding intravenous admixtures and extemporaneous preparations.
      5. Provides for proper record keeping and billing:
         a. Patient-medication records
         b. Extemporaneous compounding records
         c. Intravenous admixture records and billing
         d. Investigational-drug records
         e. Reports (eg, monthly workload report)

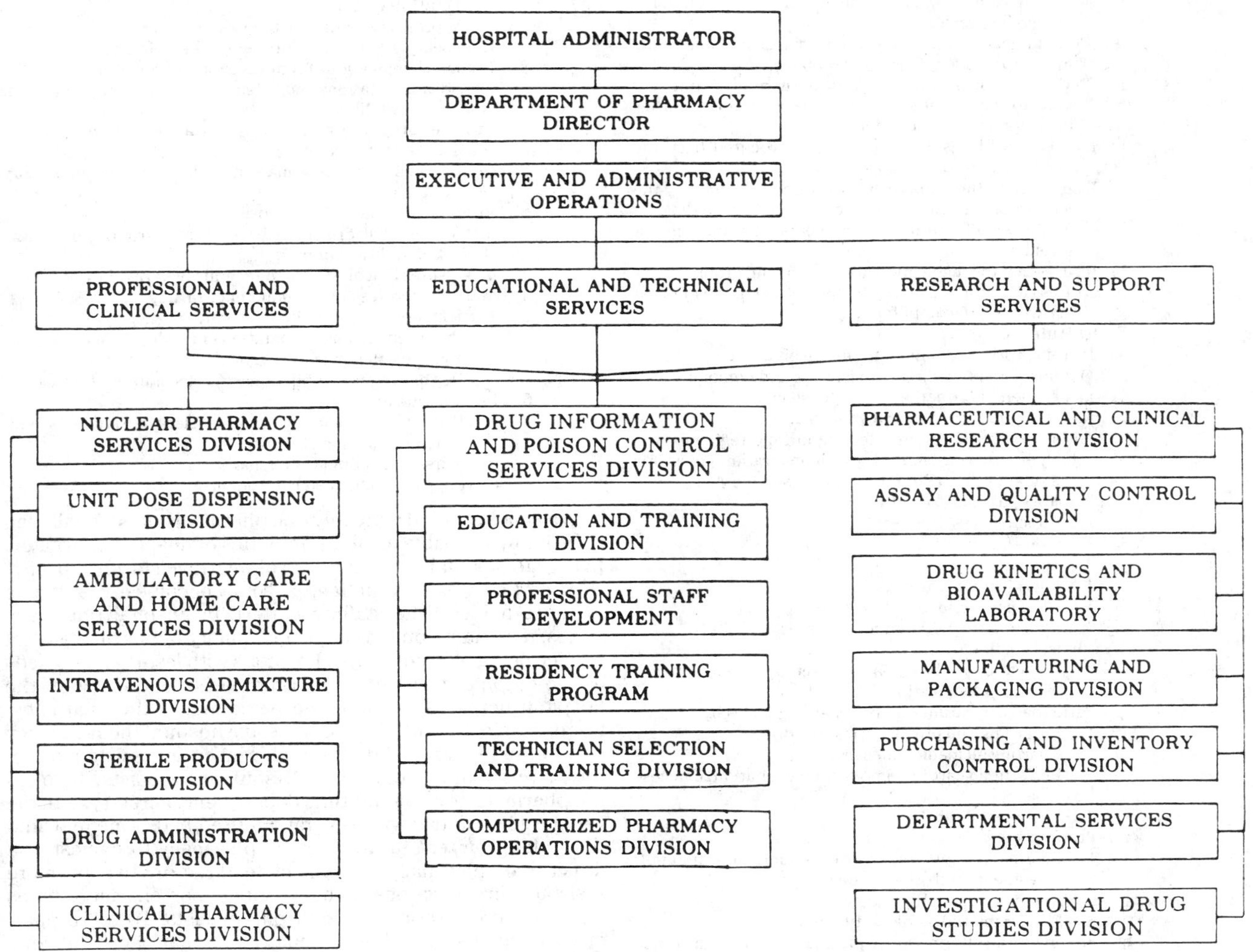

Fig 1. Typical organizational structure of a pharmacy department.

6. Maintains professional competence, particularly in knowledge of drug stability and incompatibilities.
7. Insures that new personnel are trained properly in the policies and procedures of the dispensing area.
8. Coordinates the activities of the area with the available staff to make the best possible use of personnel and resources.
9. Keeps the dispensing area neat and orderly.
10. Communicates with all pharmacy staff regarding new developments in the area and assists in employee evaluations.
11. Provides drug information as necessary to the pharmacy, medical and nursing staff.
12. Coordinates the overall pharmaceutical needs of the patient care areas with the dispensing area (eg delivery schedules).

B. Patient-Care Area
1. Supervision of drug administration.
   a. Reviews and interprets each unit dose and IV admixture medication order to insure that it is entered accurately into the unit-dose or IV-admixture system.
   b. Reviews each patient's drug administration form periodically to insure that all doses are being administered and charted correctly.
      1. Reviews all doses missed, reschedules the doses as necessary and signs all "drugs not given" notices.
      2. Insures that new drug-administration forms are transcribed accurately for continuity of drug therapy and that drug charges are assessed correctly.
   c. Confirms periodically that administered doses are noted correctly on the patient's chart.
   d. Insures that records for administered narcotics are kept correctly and that the physician is informed of all automatic stop orders.
   e. Insures that proper drug-administration techniques are used.
   f. Acts as liaison between the pharmacist and the nursing and medical staff.
   g. Communicates with nurses and physicians concerning medication-administration problems.
   h. Periodically inspects the medication areas on the nursing units to insure that adequate levels of floor-stock drugs and supplies are maintained.
   i. Insures that drugs and supplies are procured from the dispensing area as required.
   j. Insures that other supportive services performed by the department of pharmacy are carried out correctly.
   k. Coordinates all pharmacy services on the nursing-unit level.
   l. Insures that the medication area is neat and orderly.
   m. Insures that proper security is maintained in the medication area to prevent pilferage.
2. Direct Patient Care
   a. Identifies drugs brought into the hospital by patients.
   b. Obtains patient medication histories and communicates all pertinent information to the physician.
   c. Assists in drug-product and entity selection.
   d. Assists the physician in selecting dosage regimens and schedules, then assigns drug-administration times for these schedules. (Pharmacokinetic service.)
   e. Monitors patients' total drug therapy for
      1. Effectiveness/Ineffectiveness
      2. Side effects
      3. Toxicities
      4. Allergic drug reactions
      5. Drug interactions
      6. Appropriate therapeutic outcomes
   f. Counsels patients on
      1. Medications to be self-administered in the hospital
      2. Discharge medications
   g. Participates in cardiopulmonary emergencies by
      1. Procuring and preparing needed drugs
      2. Charting all medications given
      3. Performing cardiopulmonary resuscitation, if necessary
3. General Responsibilities
   a. Provides education to
      1. Pharmacists, pharmacy externs, clerkship students, residents and other students
      2. Nurses and nursing students
      3. Physicians and medical students
   b. Provides drug information to physicians, nurses and other health-care personnel.

II. Ambulatory Pharmacist's Responsibilities
A. Dispensing Area
1. Insures that established policies and procedures are followed.
2. Checks for accuracy in the work of supportive personnel.
3. Insures that proper techniques are used in extemporaneous compounding.
4. Provides for adequate recordkeeping and billing.
   a. Patient medication records
   b. Investigational drug records
   c. Outpatient billing
   d. Reports
   e. Prescription files
5. Maintains professional competence.
6. Insures that new personnel are trained properly in the policies and procedures of the ambulatory pharmacy.
7. Coordinates the activities of the area with the available staff to make the best use of personnel and resources.
8. Keeps the ambulatory pharmacy area neat and orderly at all times.

B. Patient Care Area
1. Inspects periodically the medication areas on the nursing unit to insure an adequate supply of stock drugs and their proper storage.
2. Identifies drugs brought into the clinic by patients.
3. Obtains patient-medication histories and communicates pertinent information to the physician.
4. Assists in drug-product and entity selection.
5. Assists the physician in selecting dosage regimens and schedules.
6. Monitors the patients' total drug therapy for
   a. Effectiveness
   b. Side effects
   c. Toxicities
   d. Allergic drug reactions
   e. Drug interactions
   f. Appropriate patient outcomes
7. Counsels patients on the proper use of their medication.
8. Prepares medications for intravenous administration.
9. Provides medications and/or supplies for patient home care.

C. General Responsibilities
1. Provides drug information as necessary to pharmacy, medical and nursing staffs.
2. Coordinates overall pharmaceutical needs of the ambulatory service area.
3. Provides adequate drug control.
   a. Insures that drugs are handled properly (eg investigational-drug storage).
   b. Insures that all state and federal laws are followed.
4. Maintains professional competence in area.
5. Participates in cardiopulmonary emergencies by
   a. Procurement and preparation of needed drugs
   b. Charting all medications given
   c. Performing cardiopulmonary resuscitation, if necessary
6. Provides in-service education to
   a. Pharmacists, pharmacy externs, clerkship students, residents and other students
   b. Nurses and nursing students
   c. Physicians and medical students

In a small hospital with only one pharmacist it is a challenge to be knowledgeable in all the activities of hospital pharmacy. In a large hospital with a number of pharmacists who specialize in certain areas of practice, each may become expert in one or more fields. The staffing pattern in hospital pharmacy varies, depending on the scope and quality of pharmaceutical service being offered. Most hospitals with less than 100 beds employ a pharmacist on a full-time basis. As the size of the hospital increases, so does the personnel in the pharmacy. For example, in a 300-bed progressive hospital the pharmacy may be staffed with a director of pharmacy, an assistant director of pharmacy, from 7 to 12 staff pharmacists, 5 to 15 nonpharmacists and a full-time department secretary. In the very large hospitals with several hundred beds, one may find the staffing pattern in the hospital pharmacy to consist of a director of pharmacy, an associate director, two or more assistant directors, one or more supervisor pharmacists, as many as 40 to 60 or more staff pharmacists, 10 to 16 pharmacy residents and about as many nonpharmacist helpers, technicians and secretarial personnel as professional personnel. In addition, several clinical pharmacy faculty associated with a college of pharmacy also may be active within the department.

In order to schedule the workload of the department equitably and to insure that all the functions are carried out, various methods are devised, such as work-distribution charts, job descriptions, policy and procedure manuals and functional organizational charts. These and other management aids are used by the director of pharmacy in a large department to insure that all the services and functions are fulfilled adequately.

Facilities—There are great variations in the amount of floor space devoted to the pharmacy in hospitals of the same size and type. Such variations have a direct bearing on the scope of service which can be developed in the pharmacy. A helpful guide for planning hospital pharmacy facilities has been prepared through the cooperative efforts of the Public Health Service and the ASHP.

In the smaller hospital, with one pharmacist, only one room usually is required for the pharmacy, a combination of dispensing, manufacturing, administrative and all other features of a complete pharmaceutical service. When sterile products are to be prepared, there should be a separate room or area for such work. An area of this type is required for reconstituting lyophilized injections, ophthalmic preparations, packaging unit-dose injections into syringes and preparing of intravenous admixtures, all of which must remain sterile.

Hospitals of 200 beds and larger provide the opportunity for departmentalization of pharmacy activities. There should be a separate area for inpatient services and unit-dose dispensing, outpatient service, an office for the chief pharmacist, a compounding, prepacking and labeling room, a storeroom, a sterile products and IV-admixture clean room, a room or area for a departmental computer, a separate area for drug information services and space assigned on various nursing units for unit-dose, drug-administration and clinical-pharmacy services.

As the hospital size advances to 500, 1000 or more beds, so, of course, will the space requirements of pharmaceutical service increase.

Pharmacy and Therapeutics Committee—The relationship between the community pharmacist and the physicians is a direct person-to-person contact. There is a physician–pharmacist–patient relationship which is uncomplicated by organizational lines. On the other hand, the hospital pharmacist is responsible for maintaining proper relationships with from dozens to a few hundred physicians on the medical staff. This is complicated further by the introduction of the nursing profession within the physician–pharmacist–patient relationship. Experience has shown that there is a need for a formal organizational line of communication and liaison between the medical staff and the pharmacy department of a hospital. This was recognized by the American College of Surgeons when it adopted the first *Minimum Standard for Pharmacies in Hospitals* in 1935. The pharmacy and therapeutics also is recognized by the JCAHO committee as an essential committee of the hospital's medical staff.

The ASHP has formulated and adopted a statement embodying the definition, purpose, organization, functions and scope of a pharmacy and therapeutics committee. This statement (Fig 2), is an effective guide in organizing such a committee.

It has been thought by many that the sole purpose of a pharmacy and therapeutics committee was to develop a formulary and operate a formulary system. It can be seen from the preceding statement that there are many important functions of this committee in addition to the formulary system. A hospital's medical staff could have an effective pharmacy and therapeutics committee without having a formulary system. On the other hand, a hospital could not properly operate a formulary system without a pharmacy and therapeutics committee, unless the medical staff served as a "committee of the whole."

During recent years, with the development of the clinical-pharmacy movement, a number of clinical pharmacists on the staff of some departments have developed expertise in specific therapeutic specialty areas. Therefore, it was a logical development that a subcommittee structure could be developed under the pharmacy and therapeutics committee. For example, a cardiologist and a renologist along with a clinical pharmacist who specialized in cardiorenal pharmacology and therapeutics could provide the appropriate expertise to the pharmacy and therapeutics committee in this area of drug therapy. The organizational chart in Fig 3 illustrates a more effective approach for the medical and pharmacy staff to develop and implement a rational drug-therapy program, a subcommittee structure of specialists in defined areas of therapeutics.

In addition, such a structure provides a mechanism for the development of a prospective, on-going and also retrospective, drug-utilization review program in the hospital.

As hospitals enter the era of cost containment and prospective payment systems, the pharmacy and therapeutics committee assumes added responsibility to promote rational and cost effective drug therapy and procedures. Both the clinical pharmacy staff and drug information pharmacist play an ever-increasing role in committee recommendations.

Formulary System—The formulary system and formularies have existed in the US since the days of the American Revolution and in European hospitals for centuries prior to this. The need for hospital formularies becomes increasingly great because of

The increasing number of new drugs being marketed.

The increasing influence of biased advertising and unscientific "scientific" drug literature.

The increasing complexity of untoward effects of the newer more potent drugs.

The highly competitive marketing practices of the pharmaceutical industry.

The public's interest in seeing that the health professions are conscientiously providing the best possible care at the lowest possible cost. This is substantiated by the fact that the federal government requires the establishment of Professional Review Organizations (PROs) whose purpose it is to monitor and control the quality of services rendered to patients. Cost control also is being emphasized by the federal Maximum Allowable Cost (MAC) programs for patients on federally funded programs.

The formulary system—because it has attempted to outline the scientific data on a drug, including its toxicities, untoward side effects and beneficial effects—has been a controversial method of appraising drug therapy. While the pharmaceutical industry promotes the virtues of a trade-named drug, the formulary system evaluates the virtues and defects of that drug in comparison to other trade-named brands with similar therapeutic uses.

In order to outline precisely what the formulary system is, and is not, a *Statement on the Formulary System* was developed and approved by ASHP (Fig 4). This Statement differentiates between the formulary system and the hospital formulary, and lists a number of guiding principles designed to help physicians, pharmacists and administrators to operate a hospital formulary system.

Hospital pharmacists have viewed the hospital formulary system as a means for the pharmacist to assume professional responsibilities in drug-product selection. Essentially, the formulary system provided a mechanism to avoid brand duplication and therapeutic duplication, as well as promoting rational drug therapy. The success of this system is due to "peer review" in a hospital, whereby physicians agree to practice by the policies and procedures established by the committee process.

Many useful reference sources are available to assist pharmacy and therapeutics committees to develop an effective, ongoing rational drug therapy program and formulary system in the hospital. The knowledgeable drug-information specialist and the clinical pharmacist can use these reference sources effectively to encourage the medical staff of the individual hospital to select those drugs its members consider most effective therapeutically, together with the preparations in which they may be administered most effectively. Such reference sources are described in Chapter 106. In addition, these committees have focused increasingly upon the pharmacoeconomics of drug therapy, prompting them to be more selective or restrictive in the use of drugs available for patient care.

ASHP Statement on the Pharmacy and Therapeutics Committee

The multiplicity of drugs available and the complexities surrounding their safe and effective use make it necessary for organized health-care settings to have a sound program for maximizing rational drug use. The pharmacy and therapeutics (P&T) committee, or its equivalent, is the organizational keystone to this program.

The P&T committee evaluates the clinical use of drugs, develops policies for managing drug use and drug administration, and manages the formulary system. This committee is composed of physicians, pharmacists, and other health professionals selected with the guidance of the medical staff. It is a policy-recommending body to the medical staff and the administration of the organization on matters related to the therapeutic use of drugs.

Purposes

The primary purposes of the P&T committee are

1. *Policy Develpment.* The committee formulates policies regarding evaluation, selection, and therapeutic use of drugs and related devices.[a]
2. *Education.* The committee recommends or assists in the formulation of programs designed to meet the needs of the professional staff (physicians, nurses, pharmacists, and other health-care practitioners) for complete current knowledge on matters related to drugs and drug use.

Organization and Operation

While the composition and operation of the P&T committee might vary among specific practice sites, the following generally will apply:

1. The P&T committee should be composed of at least the following voting members: physicians, pharmacists, nurses, administrators, quality-assurance coordinators, and others as appropriate. The size of the committee may vary depending on the scope of services provided by the organization. Committee members should be appointed by a governing unit or authorized official of the organized medical staff.
2. A chairperson from among the physician representatives should be appointed. A pharmacist should be designated as secretary.
3. They should meet regularly, at least six times per year, and more often when necessary.
4. The committee should invite to its meetings persons within or outside the organization who can contribute specialized or unique knowledge, skills, and judgments.
5. An agenda and supplementary materials (including minutes of the previous meeting) should be prepared by the secretary and submitted to committee members in sufficient time before each meeting for them to review the material properly.
6. Minutes of committee meetings should be prepared by the secretary and maintained in the permanent records of the organization.
7. Recommendations of the committee should be presented to the medical staff or its appropriate committee for adoption or recommendation.
8. Liaison with other organizational committees concerned with drug use should be maintained.
9. Actions of the committee should be routinely communicated to the various health-care personnel involved in the care of the patient.
10. The committee should be organized and operated in a manner that ensures the objectivity and credibility of its recommendations. The committee should establish a conflict of interest policy with respect to committee recommendations and actions.
11. In formulating drug use policies for the organization, the committee should be attentive to the content and changes in pertinent guidelines and policies of professional organizations and standards-setting bodies such as the American Society of Hospital Pharmacists, the American Hospital Association, medical and nursing associations, the Joint Commission on Accreditation of Healthcare Organizations, governmental agencies, and others as appropriate.

Functions and Scope

The basic organization of each health-care setting and its medical staff may influence the specific functions and scope of the P&T committee. The following list of committee functions is offered as a guide:

1. To serve in an evaluative, educational, and advisory capacity to the medical staff and organizational administration in all matters pertaining to the use of drugs (including investigational drugs).
2. To develop a formulary of drugs accepted for use in the organization and provide for its constant revision. The selection of items to be included in the formulary should be based on objective evaluation of their relative therapeutic merits, safety, and cost. The committee should minimize duplication of the same basic drug type, drug entity, or drug product.[b]
3. To establish programs and procedures that help ensure safe and effective drug therapy.
4. To establish programs and procedures that help ensure cost-effective drug therapy.
5. To establish or plan suitable educational programs for the organization's professional staff on matters related to drug use.
6. To participate in quality-assurance activities related to distribution, administration, and use of medications.
7. To monitor and evaluate adverse drug (including, but not limited to, biologics and vaccines) reactions in the health-care setting and to make appropriate recommendations to prevent their occurrence.
8. To initiate or direct (or both) drug use evaluation programs and studies, review the results of such activities, and make appropriate recommendations to optimize drug use.
9. To advise the pharmacy department in the implementation of effective drug distribution and control procedures.
10. To disseminate information on its actions and approved recommendations to all organizational healthcare staff.

---

[a] For additional information, see the "ASHP Statement on the Formulary System" (*Am J Hosp Pharm.* 1983; 40:1384–85) and the "ASHP Technical Assistance Bulletin on the Evaluation of Drugs for Formularies" (*Am J Hosp Pharm.* 1988; 45:386–7).

[b] For additional information, see the "ASHP Technical Assistance Bulletin on Drug Formularies" (*Am J Hosp Pharm.* 1991; 48:791–3).

Approved by the ASHP Board of Directories, November 20, 1991, and by the ASHP House of Delegates, June 1, 1992. Revised by the ASHP Council on Professional Affairs. Supersedes previous versions approved by the House of Delegates, May 15, 1978, and June 6, 1984.

Reprinted from the *Am J Hosp Pharm.* 1992; 49:929–30.

Fig 2.

An active pharmacy and therapeutics committee with a well-developed formulary system provides assurance that the medical staff, the pharmacy staff and the administration of the hospital have taken the necessary steps to assure the patient of a rational drug therapy program.

Another significant activity of the pharmacy and therapeutics committee is performing Drug Usage Reviews (DUR) or Drug Usage Evaluations (DUE) studies. The committee, with active involvement by the pharmacy, determines the drugs to be studied, determines the appropriate usage criteria, collects data, evaluates actual usage data against approval criteria and makes recommendations for improvement in appropriate use of the drug studied. Figure 5 illustrates the continuous monitoring of DUE studies by the pharmacy and committee. In addition, the committee is charged by JCAHO to Monitor Adverse Drug Reactions (ADRs) and medication errors as a part of the quality assurance standards of the medical staff.

Purchasing—While the pharmacist may be the actual buyer in a small hospital, the principal function in purchasing is to establish standards and specifications for all drugs, chemicals, diagnostic agents and other preparations used in patients, and pharmaceutical equipment. The pharmacist is responsible for the quality of drugs dispensed to patients. The pharmacy and therapeutics committee serves as a potent force in helping the pharmacist to set up adequate specifications for the purchase of quality pharmaceuticals.

The use of competitive bidding is considered good practice where a drug is used in large amounts and where future continued use seems certain. A quotation request is directed to appropriate manufacturers and the company with the lowest price, and yet with standard quality, usually receives the order for the material, after which the purchase order is prepared.

Many hospitals have adopted the practice of preparing estimates of drug usage for a given period. Thus, manufacturers

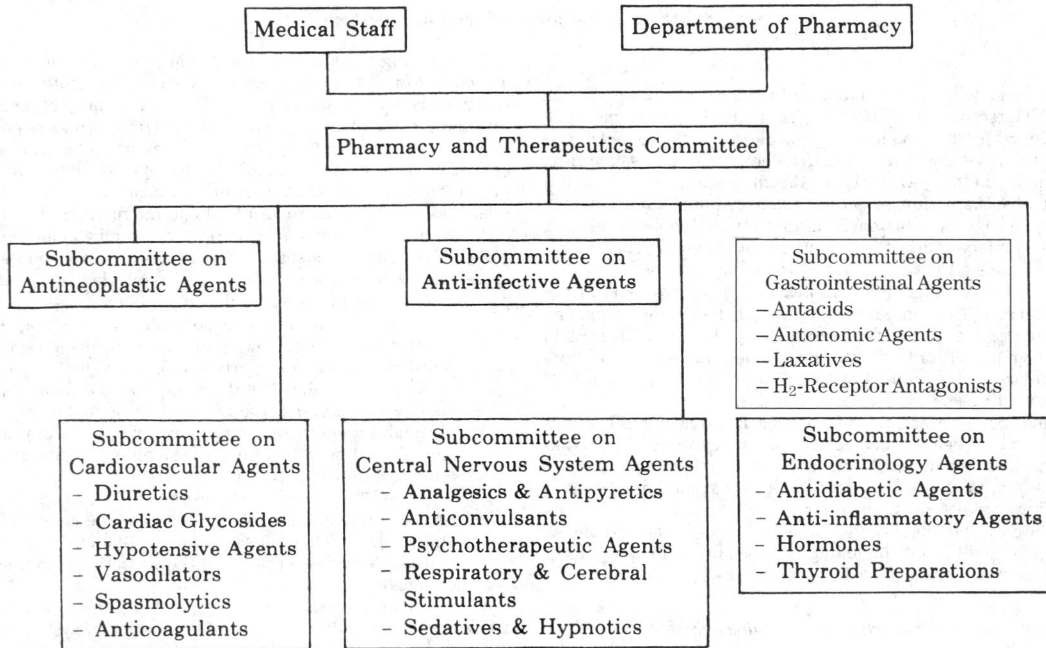

Fig 3. Organization of a pharmacy and therapeutics committee.

are requested to submit their bid quotations on the total quantity of drugs to be used for a 1-year period, or in the case of intravenous solutions, even for a multiple-year period. The stipulation is that the hospital has the option to determine when and how much will be shipped at any time during the contract period.

Upon review of these bids, the hospital pharmacist determines which vendor will receive the contract and a purchase order is sent to the respective manufacturers. Thus, by issuing an annual purchase order to each of the major pharmaceutical manufacturers, the hospital pharmacist eliminates significant amounts of paper work and unnecessary frequent bidding.

A majority of hospital pharmacies now are dispensing all of their contract pharmaceuticals through a single wholesaler, who provides the materials to the hospital for a small percentage fee. This system is known as the *prime-vendor* system and enables the hospital to order all pharmaceuticals from the prime vendor. Thus, multiple purchase orders are eliminated and ordering may be facilitated further using a computer. Most hospitals order electronically on a daily basis. This provides for a minimum inventory at the hospital and provides for an optimum inventory rate. Many departments seek a turnover of stock 10 to 20 times annually. In addition, the prime vendor can provide the hospital with coordinated purchase data and cost-control reports.

Annual inventories should be taken as a check on the theoretical inventory record maintained by either pharmacy or accounting. Various procedures are used to take a drug inventory. Many hospitals are using electronic data processing in inventory value determinations.

In many hospitals it has been observed that trade name duplications abound and clutter the shelves, increasing inventory and decreasing turnover rate and efficiency. The pharmacist should review such inventory periodically and return outmoded and outdated drugs to the manufacturer for credit. In addition, he should bring this matter to the attention of the pharmacy and therapeutics committee since one of its responsibilities is to delete outmoded drugs from the formulary.

Drug-Distribution Systems—The organizational structure of the hospital has placed certain constraints on the manner in which hospitalized patients receive their drugs. These constraints revolve around professional prerogatives and traditions, as well as legal responsibilities, established for medicine, nursing, pharmacy and hospital administration.

Physicians prescribe, pharmacists dispense and, usually, nurses administer drugs. However, in order to have this simple tripartite order executed, many things must take place. The overall drug distribution and utilization process in the hospital involves an infinite number of procedures, personnel, departments, equipment and storage. As an illustration, trace the history of a drug from procurement to administration to the patient.

Before a drug can be purchased, specifications must be prepared. This usually is done through the medical staff and the pharmacist by means of a pharmacy and therapeutics committee. Requisitions outlining the specifications for the drugs selected are prepared and processed in the pharmacy. Drug shipments are received by the receiving department and distributed to the pharmacy where they are checked and stored for future use. Inventory-control procedures must be set up. In the meantime, invoicing for payment must be processed through the accounting department by a coordination of efforts among the pharmacy, purchasing, receiving and business offices.

Physicians must prescribe drugs before they can be administered. Nurses must carry out these medication orders and obtain the necessary drugs from the pharmacy. In the pharmacy the drugs are transferred from the storage area to the dispensing area. There they may have to be prepackaged (for future use), compounded or manufactured and assay and control procedures performed. They must be packaged in proper quantities for use by the nurse to administer to the patient, labeled properly, checked for accuracy and distributed to the nursing unit. Here, the drugs are stored again for continuous use by the patient according to physicians' orders. The nurse prepares the drug for administration, brings it to the patient, returns to the nursing unit and records this information on the patient's record.

In the meantime the pharmacy processes these drug orders for billing purposes and sends these charges to the business office. There, they are posted to the patient's account. Then, through coordination between pharmacy and accounting, data are accumulated on the cost of drugs issued, reduction of drug inventory and income received to offset expenses incurred.

While the mechanics of this operation are taking place, other activities must be completed. Problems must be resolved in the procurement phase regarding overshipments,

ASHP Statement on the Formulary System

Preamble

The care of patients in hospitals and other health-care facilities is often dependent on the effective use of drugs. The multiplicity of drugs available makes it mandatory that a sound program of drug usage be developed within the institution to ensure that patients receive the best possible care.

In the interest of better patient care, the institution should have a program of objective evaluation, selection, and use of medicinal agents in the facility. This program is the basis of appropriate, economical drug therapy. The formulary concept[a] is a method for providing such a program and has been utilized as such for many years.

To be effective, the formulary system must have the approval of the organized medical staff, the concurrence of individual staff members, and the functioning of a properly organized pharmacy and therapeutics (P&T) committee[b] of the medical staff. The basic policies and procedures governing the formulary system should be incorporated in the medical staff bylaws, or in the medical staff rules and regulations.

The P&T committee represents the official organizational line of communication and liaison between the medical and pharmacy staffs. The committee is responsible to the medical staff as a whole, and its recommendations are subject to approval by the organized medical staff, as well as to the normal administrative approval process.

This committee assists in the formulation of broad professional policies relating to drugs in institutions, including their evaluation or appraisal, selection, procurement, storage, distribution, and safe use.

Definition of Formulary and Formulary System

The *formulary* is a continually revised compilation of pharmaceuticals (plus important ancillary information) that reflects the current clinical judgment of the medical staff.[c]

The *formulary system* is a method whereby the medical staff of an institution, working through the P&T committee, evaluates, appraises, and selects from among the numerous available drug entities and drug products those that are considered most useful in patient care. Only those so selected are routinely available from the pharmacy. The formulary system is thus an important tool for assuring the quality of drug use and controlling its cost. The formulary system provides for the procuring, prescribing, dispensing, and administering of drugs under either their nonproprietary or proprietary names in instances where drugs have both names.

Guiding Principles

The following principles will serve as a guide to physicians, pharmacists, nurses, and administrators in hospitals and other facilities utilizing the formulary system:

1. The medical staff shall appoint a multidisciplinary P&T committee and outline its purposes, organization, function, and scope.
2. The formulary system shall be sponsored by the medical staff based on the recommendations of the P&T committee. The medical staff should adapt the principles of the system to the needs of the particular institution.
3. The medical staff shall adopt written policies and procedures governing the formulary system as developed by the P&T committee. Action of the medical staff is subject to the normal adminis trative approval process. These policies and procedures shall afford guidance in the evaluation or appraisal, selection, procurement, storage, distribution, safe use, and other matters relating to drugs, and shall be published in the institution's formulary or other media available to all members of the medical staff.
4. Drugs should be included in the formulary by their nonproprietary names, even though proprietary names may be in common use in the institution. Prescribers should be strongly encouraged to prescribe drugs by their nonproprietary names.
5. Limiting the number of drug entities and drug products routinely available from the pharmacy can produce substantial patient care and (particularly) financial benefits. These benefits are greatly increased through the use of *generic equivalents* (drug products considered to be identical with respect to their active components; eg, two brands of tetracycline hydrochloride capsules) and *therapeutic equivalents* (drug products differing in composition or in their basic drug entity that are considered to have very similar pharmacologic and therapeutic activities; eg, two different antacid products or two different alkylamine antihistamines.) The P&T committee must set forth policies and procedures governing the dispensing of generics and therapeutic equivalents. These policies and procedures should include the following points:
   - That the pharmacist is responsible for selecting, from available generic equivalents, those drugs to be dispensed pursuant to a physician's order for a particular drug product.
   - That the prescriber has the option, at the time of prescribing, to specify the brand or supplier of drug to be dispensed for that particular medication order/prescription. The prescriber's decision should be based on pharmacologic or therapeutic considerations (or both) relative to that patient.
   - That the P&T committee is responsible for determining those drug products and entities (if any) that shall be considered therapeutic equivalents. The conditions and procedures for dispensing a therapeutic alternative in place of the prescribed drug shall be clearly delineated.
6. The institution shall make certain that its medical and nursing staffs are informed about the existence of the formulary system, the procedures governing its operation, and any changes in those procedures. Copies of the formulary must be readily available and accessible at all times.
7. Provision shall be made for the appraisal and use of drugs not included in the formulary, by the medical staff.
8. The pharmacist shall be responsible for specifications as to the quality, quantity, and source of supply of all drugs, chemicals, biologicals, and pharmaceutical preparations used in the diagnosis and treatment of patients. When applicable, such products should meet the standards of the *United States Pharmacopeia*.

Recommendation

A formulary system, based upon these guiding principles, is important in drug therapy in institutions. In the interest of better and more economical patient care, its adoption by medical staffs is strongly recommended.

---

[a] The formulary system is adaptable for use in any type of health-care facility and is not limited to hospitals.

[b] For additional information, see the "ASHP Statement on the Pharmacy and Therapeutics Committee" (*Am J Hosp Pharm 35:* 813, 1978).

[c] For additional information, see the "ASHP Guidelines for Hospital Formularies" (*Am J Hosp Pharm 35:* 326, 1978).

Approved by the ASHP Board of Directors, November 18, 1982, and by the ASHP House of Delegates, June 7, 1983. Developed by the ASHP Council on Clinical Affairs. Supersedes the "ASHP Statement of Guiding Principles on the Operation of the Hospital Formulary System" approved by the Board of Directors, January 10, 1964.

Reprinted from the *Am J Hosp Pharm 40:* 1384, 1983.

Fig 4.

undershipments or other shipping errors; errors in billing may have to be rectified. Outdated or deteriorated drugs may have to be returned to the manufacturer. Further information, such as dosage, toxicity and side effects, may be required from the physician or nurse before the prescription can be filled. Perhaps the staff physician may cancel the resident's medication order and the nurse must return the drug to the pharmacy for credit. Thus, the cycle starts all over again.

How many people are involved in the medication cycle of one drug from the time of its specification to the time it reaches the patient? They include the

Pharmacist and five or more physicians on the pharmacy and therapeutics committee in preparing drug specification.

Pharmacist in selecting the drug to be ordered.

Pharmacy secretary in making out the requisition; the purchasing agent in ordering the drug.

Receiving clerk in accepting shipment.

Delivery clerk from receiving to pharmacy.

Pharmacy stock clerk in checking and storing the drug.

Physician in prescribing the drug; the nurse in processing the drug order.

Pharmacist in preparing and dispensing the drug; the pharmacy delivery clerk in transporting the drug to the nursing unit.

Nursing unit clerk in storing the drug.

Nurse in preparing and administering the drug and in charting the data.

Pharmacy clerk in recording the charge and sending it to the business office.

Account clerk in the receiving and processing of the invoices.

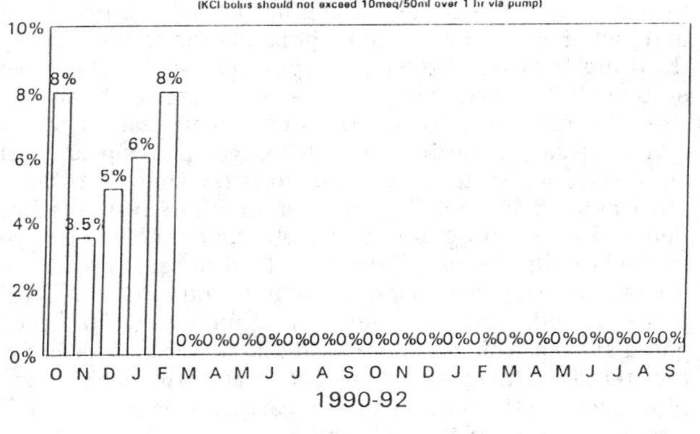

Fig 5.

Business officer in preparing the check for payment.
Posting clerk in posting the charge to the patient's bill.
Credit manager in collecting the bill.

There must be over 20 people involved in some manner or other with one drug order. One can see why the drug distribution system within a hospital is so complex.

Medication is administered to a hospital patient only upon the written order of a physician. Thus, a prescription order originates in the patient's medical record, where the physician writes out all the orders (prescriptions) he wants carried out on or for the patient. Since the patient's medical record remains at the nursing unit, it is essential that some means be utilized to transmit the prescription order from the nursing unit to the pharmacy. These orders are transmitted to the pharmacy usually in one of four ways:

The physician writes the medication order on a separate blank.

The medical record has a duplicate copy so that the pharmacy can obtain a carbon copy of the physician's original medication order.

The physician's order is transcribed by nursing personnel onto an inpatient prescription or requisition form.

The order is transmitted to the pharmacy by the physician inputing the order into a computer terminal. Most hospitals use procedures whereby the pharmacist obtains a direct copy of the physician's medication orders. Some process these orders to the pharmacy by facsimile (FAX) machines in order to expedite order transmission. The transcription method is no longer recognized as an acceptable practice.

The pharmacy department makes drugs available at the nursing unit for patient use usually in one of five ways:

1. Individual prescription medication for each patient.
2. A complete floor-stock system.
3. A combination of 1 and 2.
4. Unit-dose dispensing either centralized in the pharmacy or decentralized at the nursing unit level.
5. A pharmacy-coordinated unit-dose dispensing and drug-administration system.

Systems 1, 2 and 3 are considered poor drug-control methods in comparison to 4 and 5. However, until all hospitals adopt these unit-dose concepts, pharmacists often must operate under these less-desirable systems.

Individual patient medications are compounded and dispensed in the usual manner except that the name and strength of the drug are included on the label. In hospital practice all medications are kept in a nursing unit medication cabinet and are under the custody of the nurse in charge. The nurse or an assistant is responsible for administering the appropriate medication to each patient on the nursing unit. Thus, it is important to know what drug is being administered for it is the nurse's professional responsibility to observe the patient for untoward reactions and report this to the patient's physician. Thus, the patient never sees the prescription container dispensed by the pharmacist to the nursing unit nor has the container in his or her possession. A typical inpatient prescription label would contain the following information:

Mr John Jones		Room 608E
	Tetracycline HCl Capsules, 250 mg	
Quantity #20	Lot #	Exp Date
Doctor's Name	Pharmacist's Name	Data
	THE GENERAL HOSPITAL PHARMACY	

In order to expedite the dispensing of inpatient prescription medication, hospital pharmacists have adopted the practice of prepackaging frequently used drugs in standard dispensing quantities. It is not unusual for a majority of the inpatient prescription medications to be prepackaged. Prepackaging drugs requires accurate procedures, controls and records in order to trace the identity of the drug at all times. Thus, a prepackaging control record form is used for documentation of manufacturer's control numbers, expiration date, pharmacy control number which appears on each prepackaged container label and the pharmacist responsible for the prepackaging operation. In the case of a drug recalled by a manufacturer, the pharmacist easily can trace prepackaged quantities of the drug in question.

Drugs dispensed under a *floor-stock system* are of two classes: free and charge. Free floor stock consists of a predetermined list of medications which are available on every nursing unit of the hospital for use at no specific charge to the patient. Since these drugs are used in large quantities they are prepackaged in standardized containers. Orders usually are received from each nursing unit of the hospital each day of the week. With other systems the pharmacy assumes the responsibility for maintaining the proper inventory of free floor stock drugs on each nursing unit through an automatic floor stock replacement system. Under such a system the nurse is relieved of having to maintain an inventory control, fill out a daily requisition order and return the drug items to the shelves. The pharmacy personnel goes to the nursing unit with an adequate supply of each free floor-stock drug, takes an on-the-spot inventory, brings the inventory to a predetermined level and records the quantities on a preprinted requisition, which lists the drugs in the order in which they are stocked in the drug cabinets. Adequate controls, thus, can be set up on the basis of usage in relation to number of patient days per given interval of time. Some hospitals have adopted electronic data-processing procedures and/or bar-code technology to handle the totaling and cost extension of drugs issued and the preparation of monthly drug usage reports for each nursing unit. Usually these items are inexpensive pharmaceuticals that have a universal patient use (e.g., alcohol, lotion, water for injection, normal saline injection).

Charge floor stock is medication available at each nursing unit of the hospital and for which a charge is made to the patient. Certain medications are required to be used almost immediately after the physician prescribes them, and it is not practical to go to the pharmacy to obtain them in each instance, yet the cost and the volume of usage necessitates a charge to the patient. Such medications are usually injections or other single-dose forms. A common method of handling charge floor-stock drugs is to attach a small removable label, bar-code label or prestamped pharmacy requisition form bearing the name of the drug to the charge floor-stock drug. When the nurse needs the drug she merely removes the label and affixes it to the usual inpatient prescription or requisition slip. This is used then for charging purposes and for replacement of the drug on the nursing unit.

In hospitals where patients pay for their hospitalization—as compared to military or governmental hospitals—the pharmacy often employs a *combination of the individual inpatient prescription system and the floor-stock drug system.* Drugs which are free floor stock are charged against the nursing service and, in the final analysis, the patient does pay for the drugs since the cost is included as a part of the nursing service portion of the daily room and board rate.

Because of the large number and variety of drugs stored on nursing units—including individual patient prescriptions, free and charge floor stock, narcotics and other controlled drugs, investigational drugs and emergency drug tray—it is an important responsibility of the pharmacist to inspect these drugs routinely. Proper storage conditions must be adhered to, dated drugs must be checked, narcotic drugs must be safeguarded and discontinued drugs must be removed from the nursing unit. To insure proper control of a nursing station drug cabinet, the pharmacist prepares a written report to the directors of nursing and of pharmacy. The condition of a nursing-unit medication station may warrant remedial attention by personnel from both departments. In some hospitals, pharmacists are assigned to specific nursing units to coordinate all the drug and drug therapy problems at the nursing-unit level. Rather than simply checking drug-storage conditions, they are developing new roles which brings them closer to the patient-care team.[7]

The most accepted method of dispensing drugs to hospitalized patients, is called *unit-dose dispensing* and has become the standard of practice in the majority of hospitals today. In this system the pharmacist prepares every dose of medication ready for administration, rather than issuing containers of drugs to nursing units where the nurse must prepare the drug for administration. For example, tablets and capsules are labeled for each patient, liquids premeasured, lyophilized injections diluted and measured accurately into sterile syringes, parenteral-drug admixtures added to intravenous solutions prior to use and oral powders and other unusual dosage forms measured and mixed appropriately. Most of these procedures involve pharmaceutical techniques which are properly the pharmacist's responsibility. Hospital pharmacists are studying various methods involving centralized pharmacy versus decentralized pharmacies on the nursing units, using automated systems of communication, information scheduling and retrieval to provide more accurate and effective overall drug distribution and utilization in the hospital.

The unit-dose dispensing concept has changed many of the traditional functions of the hospital pharmacist. For example, the traditional prepackaging system of multiple doses of drugs has been changed to include the use of tablet and capsule strip-packaging, labeling machines and liquid unit-dose packaging equipment. This is necessary since all drugs are not available from the industry in unit-dose packages. The traditional individual inpatient prescription also is eliminated and thereby eliminates prescription-label typing. Free and charge floor-stock drug activities essentially are eliminated. An ASHP national survey of hospital-based pharmaceutical services in 1992 indicated that 90% of all hospitals employed the unit dose dispensing system. This drug distribution system has become the standard of practice.

Unit-dose dispensing lends itself to certain automation procedures, particularly with electronic data processing and computers. On-line computers are used to program patients' total drug-therapy profile, program the times for administering scheduled doses of drugs, maintain records of drugs administered and initiate the drug charges to patients. This eliminates the traditional nurses' drug Kardex (profile), medication ticket and record-of-drug-administered manual system of keeping track of patients' drug-therapy profiles. Thus, the hourly reports of the on-line computer on patients' drug-therapy profiles can be used both by the pharmacy for unit-dose dispensing and by the nurse for drug administration. In fact, automated unit-dose dispensing machines using robotic principles are being used in some locations.[8] The interface with the hospital's computer system can provide a system akin to robotic unit-dose dispensing.

There have been hospitals merging drug dispensing and drug administration into a *coordinated system under pharmacy control.* This makes sense particularly when one considers the fact that when a physician writes a medication order for a hospitalized patient, it is essentially a pharmaceutical order and pharmaceutical orders should be carried out under the supervision of pharmacists. This system was initiated at the Providence Hospital in Seattle.[7] Registered nurses have been employed by the Pharmacy Department and, in conjunction with a unit-dose dispensing system by the pharmacists and technicians, nurses are responsible for administering all the drugs to hospitalized patients. Thus, such a coordinated system effects certain efficiencies and eliminates many steps from the traditional drug-distribution and utilization system.

A pharmacy-coordinated unit-dose dispensing and drug-administration system was initiated at the Ohio State University Hospitals in 1969.[9] This system differs from the Providence Hospital program in that pharmacy technicians were trained to administer the drugs instead of registered nurses. These pharmacy technicians assist in the unit-dose dispensing phase as well as the drug-administration phase of the coordinated system which is controlled and supervised directly by registered pharmacists. Thus, pharmacists work directly with physicians on the nursing unit to carry out pharmacy's mainstream function of the safe and appropriate use of drugs in patients.

A pharmacy-coordinated unit-dose dispensing and drug-administration system requires a complex series of well-integrated procedures in order to administer drugs to patients safely and accurately. A number of studies have shown that uncoordinated drug-distribution systems have a high incidence of medication errors. A two-phase comprehensive study of the pharmacy-coordinated unit-dose dispensing and drug administration-system showed that it reduced significantly the incidence of medication errors in comparison with the other drug-distribution systems in existence.[10]

For effective and efficient functioning, a unit-dose dispensing and drug-administration system should include a *procedural manual* which outlines the stepwise procedures for implementing the myriad tasks and the in-process quality-control checks required for the safe and accurate handling of drugs in the institutional setting in which the system is used.

The General Accounting Office (GAO) studied several distribution systems in its *Study of Health-Care Facilities Construction Costs* (December, 1972), and reported that in addition to safer and better patient care through minimization of medication errors the unit-dose system was to be recommended also because of its favorable life-cycle cost-to-benefit ratio. The JCAHO also recommends the unit-dose distribution system.

Patient Self-Administration of Drugs in Hospitals—Pharmacists generally have considered a unit-dose dispensing system as a panacea for hospital drug problems. However, unit-dose dispensing systems primarily have been "pharmacy-centered" rather than "patient-centered." The new direction in hospital pharmacy is to develop patient-oriented services as the focal point in drug-distribution systems.

The self-administration of drugs by patients in the hospital offers many advantages. It allows the patient to assume more responsibility for his direct care and allows him to learn how to use drugs properly, and to be able to anticipate potential side effects and other drug-created problems. It provides a salient opportunity for the pharmacist to help educate patients on the safe and proper use of drugs and thereby alleviates much time spent by nurses and physicians in this essential pharmaceutical function.

Self-administration of drugs by patients can be implemented effectively on numerous hospital services, such as obstetrics, surgery, medicine, physical medicine and rehabilitation and even in psychiatry.[11,12] Again, a procedural manual should be prepared which outlines the methods used to implement a patient self-administration program as part of a unit-dose distribution system. A self-administration medication program gives the patient possession of his medication and makes the patient responsible for its administration. Both the nurse and pharmacist will make rounds to insure that the patient is using his medication properly.

The self-administration medication program enables the nurse to use her time better. The patient should become more knowledgeable about his medication, thus enhancing proper and safe use of drugs during hospitalization and after discharge.

A nurse-administered medication program places all responsibility for medication administration on the nurse providing the service. This program is used for patients who are not capable of self-administering their medications or for those medications which the patient cannot administer to himself. This is the interacting role which hospital pharmacists have developed under the umbrella term, "clinical pharmacy."

As the pharmaceutical industry develops the unit-dose-packaging concept and as physicians and the FDA continue their drive to provide patients with drugs labeled with the name of the medication in the original manufacturer's package (to insure stability and identity), this virtually will eliminate the count-and-pour and labeling operations in "filling prescriptions." It substantiates the need to use technicians in the physical handling of drugs. It is obvious that this main purpose of the pharmacist must change if he wants to remain a health professional.

There is, however, a challenging professional role which the pharmacist can assume as a member of the health-care team. This role involves the safe and appropriate use of drugs in patients. Taken in a broad context, this implies a high-level role indeed. This is the main purpose for the existence of pharmacy as a health profession. Thus, the concept behind the clinical-pharmacy movement is directed toward the development of this role as the main function of the profession.

Investigational Drugs—The hospital pharmacist is in a strategic position to participate in an evaluation program on investigational drugs because such drugs must be tried in a hospital setting where the necessary laboratory and other medical facilities are available. It is thus a prime responsibility of the pharmacy and therapeutics committee to establish policies and procedures relative to the handling and control of investigational drugs in the hospital. To assist the committees the ASHP developed a statement, entitled *ASHP Guidelines for the Use of Investigational Drugs in Institutions,* embodying basic principles applicable to the safe handling of investigational drugs in the hospital. The ASHP also has provided a manual dealing with pharmacists' responsibilities and opportunities in handling investigational drugs.

There are many problems associated with the use of investigational drugs in the hospital, some of which are

Legal problems may result if a hospital does not exercise due care in the proper handling of investigational drugs in the overall care of the patient.

Nurses, as agents of the hospital, usually are responsible for administering investigational drugs to patients. In performing this act it is essential that sufficient information on the proper dosage, route of administration, possible toxic reactions and side effects, precautions and proper labeling is available to them.

Investigational drugs, as they are made available from the manufacturer to the principal investigator, are not labeled sufficiently in many instances to prevent the possibility of error in their administration to patients.

Because investigational drugs fall in the area of research in contrast to accepted methods of treatment, there are legal implications revolving around the need for written consent by patients.

In the case of double-blind studies it is essential that the person holding the code be readily available 24 hours a day, 7 days a week, in case the patient's condition warrants a breaking of the code.

The legal requirements for proper records on the use of investigational drugs have been delineated by the FDA. In case of a recall because of severe permanent toxicity resulting from an investigational drug, it is essential that records of its use on specific patients in a hospital should be readily available. In cases where the lot number of the drug is a significant factor such records also should be available.

In cases where investigational drugs are used on outpatients it is essential that such drugs be labeled to conform to legal requirements, such as childproof packaging requirements and controlled substances requirements. It should be obvious that information must readily be available to assist physicians in other hospitals who may be required to treat patients suffering from accidental overdosage or toxic symptoms.

It is essential that the supply of an investigational drug is available during the night and weekends as well as when the principal investigator is at the hospital if nurses are to maintain uninterrupted dosage schedules in the best interest of the patient.

Thus, the problems associated with the proper handling of investigational drugs provide ample justification to warrant the establishment of sound policies and procedures governing their use in the hospital. This is a responsibility of the medical staff. The pharmacy and therapeutics committee is a committee of the medical staff and, therefore, should be the responsibility of this committee to formulate policies and procedures relative to the handling of investigational drugs. The hospital pharmacist as a key member of the pharmacy and therapeutics committee makes a real contribution to better patient care and safety by participating in formulating policies and procedures for handling investigational drugs in the hospital. Often, pharmacists serve on The Institutional Review Board (IRB) of a hospital and are involved with the review of all experimentation involving humans. The pharmacist can provide valuable insight on the design, economics and ethics involved in drug studies in human patients.

It is required that physicians obtain written consent from the patient prior to use of an investigational drug.

The hospital pharmacist needs to maintain adequate dispensing records (see Fig 6) for all investigational drugs dispensed.

Many hospital pharmacists are involved clinically with oncology-team members in patient monitoring, drug preparation and administration of investigational drugs. Patient consent and patient information are essential in such activities. Pharmacists often provide specific drug-information cards to patients so that they may understand better their drug regimen and the various side effects or problems to expect (see Fig 7).

A single prescription for a single patient does not raise the question of investigational-drug use. The federal law can be violated by preparing large quantities of drugs which have not been approved for human use by the FDA. To avoid legal violation, a sponsor of a drug investigation must file with the FDA a "Notice of Claimed Investigational Exemption for a New Drug" (IND). Such a form usually is filed by a pharmaceutical manufacturer; however, others may serve as the sponsor, such as a physician, pharmacist, an institution such as a hospital or the hospital-pharmacy department.

An abbreviated form of IND is acceptable to the FDA where a physician wants to study a drug which no manufacturer wants to sponsor. The physician may serve both as sponsor and investigator; or the hospital pharmacy may serve as sponsor and the physician as investigator. Some hospital pharmacy departments serve as sponsors on many abbreviated INDs for special drug dosage forms that are not available commercially. The required forms for the sponsor and investigator plus the new-drug regulations are available from the FDA. Additional information is given in Chapter 48.

Intravenous Admixtures—Health care personnel who are professionally best qualified to prepare intravenous admixtures are hospital pharmacists trained to provide such service. Hospital pharmacists successfully have organized, developed and operated a centralized pharmacy intravenous-admixture service that[13]

Saves nursing time for other professional nursing roles.

Provides a system for screening physical-chemical incompatibilities, and dispensing of stable preparations.

Minimizes pharmaceutical calculation errors.

Reduces the risk of medication error by providing additional checks.[14]

Centralizes responsibility for preparation of parenteral admixtures.

Labels admixtures with rate of infusion as prescribed by the physician and provides a standardized label format.

Provides an aseptic environment for the preparation of admixtures.

Conforms to the standards recommended by the JCAHO.

Conforms to the guidelines established by the National Coordinating Committee on Large-Volume Parenterals.

Provides a mechanism for charging patients for IV therapy and creating revenue.

Insures more effective use of professional personnel in the hospital.

Minimizes the potential for medical-legal liability.

Provides for the preparation of solutions which are not commercially available.

The JCAHO wisely promulgated the concept that the pharmacist should be involved in preparing intravenous admix-

THE UNIVERSITY OF KANSAS MEDICAL CENTER
PHARMACY DEPARTMENT

INVESTIGATIONAL DRUG DISPENSING RECORD

Name and Synonyms ____

Strength and Dosage Form ____

Manufacturer ____

Principal Investigator ____

Date	Patient Name	Case Number	Physician	Rx # or Location	Lot Number	Amount Dispensed	Amount on Hand

Fig 6.

tures. In the Pharmacy Section of its current Standards for Accreditation, the JCAHO frequently refers to the subject of the safe and accurate handling of all drugs, including intravenous admixtures. One especially relevant statement is

> The compounding and admixture of large-volume parenterals should ordinarily be the responsibility of a qualified pharmacist. Individuals who prepare or administer large-volume parenterals should have special training to do so. When any part of the above functions (preparing, sterilizing and labeling parenteral medications and solutions) is performed within the hospital, but not under direct pharmacy supervision, the director of the pharmaceutical service shall be responsible for providing written guidelines and for approving the procedure to assure that all pharmaceutical requirements are met.

In rising to the challenge posed by the JCAHO, it is essential that the pharmacist be involved in preparing intravenous admixtures. A pharmacy-controlled intravenous-admixture service demonstrates that a hospital is fulfilling its responsibilities to patients. The responsibility for preparing intravenous admixtures is actually the same as assumed for the unit-dose distribution system. An intravenous admixture is a unit dose.

Hospital pharmacists need the support of hospital administrators, directors of nursing and medical staffs (through their respective pharmacy and therapeutics committees) in order to develop and operate an effective intravenous admixture service. In establishing such a service it is important that specific guidelines for its operation be formulated.

According to the 1992 ASHP national survey of hospital-based pharmaceutical services, 70% of all hospitals provide a complete IV admixture service. The ASHP has furnished a technical-assistance bulletin regarding pharmacist-prepared sterile products. These guidelines promote greater attention to clean room technology, personnel training and validation, and quality assurance procedures. Specific guidelines for compounding chemotherapy admixtures, are also provided by the ASHP in a technical assistance bulletin. The intravenous-admixture service can serve as a base for other pharmacy services such as chemotherapy compounding, allergy extract preparation and parenteral home-care programs (see also Chapter 88).

Ambulatory-Care Services—As ambulatory-care activities continue to increase within the institutional setting, the hospital pharmacist becomes more and more involved in providing services to these patients. While these pharmacy activities parallel community-pharmacy practice, hospital-pharmacy practitioners have developed many innovative services for the patient. This includes special patient-information brochures, patient-dosing calendars, special packaging, patient-education audiovisual and home-care programs. These activities will continue to increase as more emphasis is placed on ambulatory care as part of the total patient-care program by hospitals.

Clinical Pharmacy—The concept of "clinical or patient-oriented" pharmacy service has gained tremendous acceptance in hospital pharmacy. The hospital environment offers the hospital pharmacist a multitude of opportunities to develop meaningful clinical roles in the safe and rational use of drugs in hospitalized, as well as ambulatory, patients. This chapter does not include a detailed discussion of the hospital pharmacist's clinical roles and responsibilities because they are discussed in Chapters 96, 101, 104 and 105.

It is important to note that significant progress is being made in providing ongoing clinical pharmacy services in hospitals. Various service functions are described in the *ASHP Statement on Clinical Functions in Institutional Practice.* As these roles emerge, various third-party agencies are recognizing the value of the services and specifically are reimbursing the hospital pharmacy department for providing activities not necessarily associated with dispensing a product. Areas of practice in which reimbursement has been made include pharmacokinetic dosing service, patient-education services for home self-administration of growth hormone, total parenteral nutrition solutions service, steroid administration, factor VIII administration, cytarabine administration and injectable analgesics service.

As increased emphasis is being placed on cost containment in hospitals and improved drug-therapy utilization, the clinical pharmacist has been valuable in monitoring patient drug therapy and promoting rational drug therapy. The clinical pharmacist can best carry out the mandates of the pharmacy and therapeutics committee relative to appropriate drug therapy. An evolution of clinical pharmacy practice is occurring in that pharmacists are embracing the concept of pharmaceutical care. In essence the pharmacist is becoming a drug-therapy manager.

The University of Kansas Medical Center

Inpatient Pharmacy

METHOTREXATE

OTHER NAMES: amethopterin, mexate, folex, MTX.

WHAT IS METHOTREXATE?

Methotrexate is a cancer antimetabolite, it interferes with the metabolism of folic acid a compound necessary for the survival of the cell. Methotrexate is S-phase specific, the S-phase is a certain phase the cell goes through during it's life cycle. Methotrexate is used in the treatment of many different cancers. It is used in treatment of solid tumors in adults, which include adenocarcinoma of the breast, lung cancer, squamous cell carcinomas of the head, neck and cervix, and osteogenic sarcoma. Methotrexate is also used to treat malignant lymphoma (nonhodgkins lymphoma and mycosis fungoides), acute lymphoblastic leukemia, choriocarcinoma, and children's solid tumors (rabdomyosarcoma).

WHAT SIDE EFFECTS ARE ASSOCIATED WITH METHOTREXATE?

The possible side effects of methotrexate are:

(1) Bone marrow depression (which clinically causes the patient to become more susceptable to infection.)
(2) Stomatitis (mouth sores)
(3) Diarrhea
(4) Kidney toxicity
(5) Neurologic toxity (behavioral abnormalities, focal sensorimotor signs [example: numbness] and abnormal reflexes)
(6) Possible dermatologic changes (acne and boils)
(7) Alopecia (hair loss)
(8) Weakness, dizziness, and drowsiness.

Your physician should be notified of any of the side effects listed above or any other situation that coincides with the start of the drug.

WHAT PRECAUTIONS SHOULD BE TAKEN WITH THIS MEDICATION?

Notify your physician of any allergies you may have, medications you are currently taking, and if you think you might be pregnant.

SPECIAL INSTRUCTIONS:

(1) Avoid drinking alcohol
(2) Avoid prolonged exposure to the sun and tanning beds
(3) Report any bruising bleeding, black or tarry stools, or blood in your urine to your physician.
(4) Report any fever or sign of infection (cough, chills or weakness) to your physician.
(5) Report any numbness or loss of sensation to your physician.

WHAT IS LEUKOVORIN?

Leukovorin is used in higher dose methotrexate therapy to reverse the toxicity to normal cells. This is often called "leukovorin rescue". The logic behind this treatment is that leukovorin is transported into normal cells and converted into tetrahydrofolic acid (a metabolite necessary for cell survival) while leukovorin is not transported into the cancer cell as fast or not at all.

WHAT ARE THE SIDE EFFECTS OF LEUKOVORIN?

Leukovorin appears to be nontoxic at therapeutic doses. Although thrombocytosis has been reported.

Reviewed by:
Raj Sadasivan, M.D.,Ph.D.
Frank Weinhold. RPh
Virginia Glen Pharm. D.,RPh

Fig 7. Drug-information card for patients.

Future Practice—In reviewing the activities of hospital pharmacy practice one must conclude that no two hospital practices are alike. Hospital-pharmacy practice has made significant strides over the past three decades in changing its practice roles to provide a more patient-oriented pharmacy service. Drug-distribution systems have been improved (unit-dose and IV-admixture services) and patient oriented clinical services have been implemented in large and small hospitals alike. Computerization has increased efficiencies and has provided an improved patient and management database. Practice in hospitals has adjusted to the changing environment of health care. The challenge to the institutional pharmacist and the profession as a whole is to provide pharmaceutical care to all patients by shifting emphasis (not responsibility) from drug distribution to patient care. What the future holds for hospital pharmacy practice in the year 2000 is only speculation.[15] However, with the significant progress in the last few years and the practitioner talent in this area, one can be assured that the role of the hospital pharmacist on the health-care team will be significant and will be directed at meeting the drug-therapy needs of the patient.

References

1. *Hospitals 38 (Jan 1)*: 109, 1964.
2. *Am J Hosp Pharm 32 (9)*: 917, 1975.
3. *The 1992 AHA Guide to the Health Care Field*, Am Hosp Assoc, Chicago IL.
4. Niemeyer GF *et al*: *Bull Am Soc Hosp Pharm 9(4)*: 287, 1962.
5. Spease E, Porter RM: *JAPhA 25*: 65, 1936.
6. *Am J Hosp Pharm 40*: 1384, 1983.
7. Hynniman, C: *Ibid 48*: 524, 1991.
8. Beste D: *Ibid 25(8)*: 396, 1968.
9. Latiolais CJ *et al*: *Ibid 27 (11)*: 886, 1970.
10. Shultz SM *et al*: *Hospitals 47 (Mar 16)*: 106, 1973.
11. Roberts C *et al*: *Drug Intel Clin Pharm 6 (12)*: 408, 1972.
12. Lucarotti RL *et al*: *Am J Hosp Pharm 30 (12)*: 1147, 1973.
13. Shoup LK, Godwin HN: *Implementation Guide for a Centralized Intravenous Admixture Program*, Travenol, 1977.
14. Thur MP *et al*: *Am J Hosp Pharm 29 (4)*: 298, 1972.
15. McConnell WE: *Ibid 40 (8)*: 1315, 1983.

CHAPTER 98

Long-Term Care Facilities

Thomas C Snader, PharmD
Consultant Pharmacist
Sellersville, PA 18960

Long-term health care has become an important issue in the total health care system. There are more long-term facility beds than acute care beds. Future emphasis will be to increase the number of facilities and beds in long-term care, while those of acute care will be reduced.

With advances in the medical sciences and technologies, people are living longer. Prolongation of life expectancy has created a totally new set of problems for the health-care system. There is a rapid rise of chronic disease conditions, with associated social and emotional problems, which require a different approach in their management. Drugs are a key therapeutic modality in the long-term facility care setting.

Health is considered as a microcosm of the broader social system. The growing concern of social obligation and social responsibility in society has advanced the philosophy that health is a right, a right to have access to quality health care without discrimination. The advent of health insurance and government involvement in financing health care has changed the practice and reimbursement of health care services greatly. The assurance of payment for health care services has stimulated utilization of new medical technologies, resulting in higher health care cost and more specialization and subspecialization in medical practice. In addition, most health-care providers are acute-care oriented; they are not equipped and trained to render quality long-term care. Long-term care is more than medical intervention and treatment. It requires a multidisciplinary approach to care as well as an array of psychosocial support and services.

The same forces affecting acute care also have impacted on the growth of long-term care. Long-term care facilities have increased in number and sizes. There are a variety of long-term care facilities, with nursing homes, including skilled-nursing facilities and intermediate-care facilities, among the most common, and an increasing number of alternative-care sites such as board and care. Many patients in these facilities are treated with long-term and multiple drug therapy. With the impact of Diagnosis Related Groups (DRGs) on acute-care settings, there are an increasing number of long-term care admissions requiring high technology pharmacy services. The pharmacist has an important role to play and an opportunity to contribute in the long-term facility care.

Pharmacy services in long-term care facilities are provided primarily by community pharmacist practitioners, who often have little formal institutional-care training. Most of them are self-learners. Government is involved intimately in the financing of long-term facility care, and it is not surprising that it has established numerous regulations and requirements governing the provision of long-term care. The pharmacist has to practice within the established rules and guidelines, but compensation for consultant pharmacist services is reimbursed through the facility, which has created the potential for questionable business arrangements between the pharmacist and the facility, especially where the provider of drugs and the pharmacist consultant are one and the same. And, yet, there is a high level of innovation with emphasis on programs to improve drug utilization and patient care.

Newer standards, eg, OBRA 90 (Omnibus Budget Reconciliation Act of 1990) and impending national health-care reform initiatives require the pharmacist to assume greater responsibility and participation in long-term facility care. In addition to maintaining a safe drug distribution and control system, the pharmacist is asked to apply his knowledge, such as reviewing drug regimens, providing cost containment, participating in patient-care and related committees and developing pharmacy policies and procedures. The new requirements are defined broadly and outcome-oriented. The individual pharmacist has to interpret and apply them according to his own background and experience, assisted by handbooks, Federal Drug Regimen Review Indicators and Interpretive Guidelines for State and Federal Surveyors.

It is impossible to cover the subject of long-term care facilities, pharmacy services in long-term care and geriatric pharmacology and drug therapy, within the context of a single chapter. Therefore, the approach of this chapter is to outline the important issues and topics relating to the provision of pharmacy services in long-term facility care. The emphasis will be addressed to the activities of drug regimen review, development and implementation of pharmacy policies and procedures in long-term care facilities. Also, important principles in geriatric pharmacology and major considerations for monitoring geriatric drug therapy are included.

Historical Background

Long-term care is not and should not be construed as an independent segment of total health care. It is a continuum of acute and episodic care integrated closely with rehabilitative, restorative and supportive care. In order to have a greater appreciation of the mission, role and issues of long-term care facilities, it is necessary to review briefly the major developments in public health and medical technologies which shape current health-care practice.

Since the beginning of time, good health has been considered one of the more important basic needs of man. What separates the human from other mammalian species is man's ability to maintain a state of physical, social, economic and mental well-being.

In ancient times, disease and sickness were considered afflictions of evil spirits and punishment by a god. Those who were sick, weak, poor or aged were deemed social outcasts and undesirable elements of society. The impoverished, aged or elderly who did not have family or relatives to provide for them often were cared for with the sick, the insane, the blind and deaf and other social destitutes, by charitable and religious organizations. The prevailing belief was that institutionalization was an efficient way to manage the dependents of society. The result was a proliferation of public almshouses and church-sponsored institutions whose main services were to provide food, shelter and medical care. They were the prototypes of today's hospitals and long-term care facilities. The principal care providers were the clergy who functioned both as physicians and pharmacists.

Before the middle of the 19th century, communicable and infectious diseases, such as cholera, diphtheria, typhoid, etc, were prevalent in many parts of the world. Little was known about germ theory, public sanitation, personal hygiene and the cause and control of these diseases. The infant mortality rate was high. People did not live long enough to have chronic diseases or become elderly.

During the same period, the Industrial Revolution was fermenting. There was a general public mood favoring more humanism and social reform. Public-health programs were developed and promoted. With the advance of knowledge of bacteriology and immunology, including development of vaccines, the concepts and practices of medical care were altered greatly. Emphasis was placed on prevention and control of epidemic disease. Thus, public-health activities were expanded greatly to include not only disease prevention and improvement of environmental and sanitary conditions, but also the promotion of health and application of social concepts in medical care practice. These public-health measures were responsible mostly for the decrease of infant mortality and the increase in the life span of man.

The 20th century marked the advent of a golden era of medical science and technology. The discovery and development of sulfonamides, penicillin and streptomycin made a spectacular change in the successful management of many common infectious diseases. The isolation and production of insulin revolutionized the treatment and improved the prognosis of patients suffering from diabetes mellitus. Other therapeutic advances in vaccines, antiepileptics, antipsychotics and anesthetics worked wonders in the elimination of some communicable diseases, the management of a substantial number of chronic diseases and also paved the way for surgical innovations. Progress of medical technologies in devices, equipment and procedures resulted in major breakthroughs in the diagnosis and treatment of many diseases. The successes of the medical and scientific technologies have prolonged life and improved its quality. But new problems are emerging, such as the increase of chronic diseases, which require a new approach and different management.

The Right to Health—Interpreted broadly, the right to good health includes a concomitant right to health care. Even though no one can be guaranteed freedom from sickness, the basic concept of the right to health and health care can be construed as society having an obligation to provide its citizens equal access to an acceptable level of health care. Health should not have any racial, sexual, economic or age limitation. Health care should not be a commodity available only to those who are fortunate enough to afford it.

Health as a right is established on the same philosophy as a right to an education and to welfare benefits. Because of the emphasis on individual rights, current social philosophy leans increasingly toward emphasis of social obligation to the individual rather than the individual's obligation to society. Acceptance of health as a right has great implications on the financing and delivery of health-care services as exemplified by the proposal for a national health-care system. Health is only one of the components of our social system. Health as a right has more than moral and philosophical implications; it has political, economic and social ramifications as well. It is especially important to the elderly because, while they account for over 11.6% of the total population, they use between 25 and 30% of the national health-care expenditures and 31% of all prescription drugs.

Impact of Growing Elderly Population

Since the beginning of the 20th century, the elderly population in the US has spiraled precipitously. Actually, there is no specific physical or physiological basis for defining persons 65 years or over as elderly, aged or as senior citizens. Rather, the definition reflects the social, political and legislation perception at the time about aging and life span. The chronological number 65 has been determined as a retirement age, and the beginning of the receipt of social security and other public supported and funded programs. In 1978, Congress enacted legislation abolishing mandatory retirement at 65 to eliminate age discrimination in employment, especially when the life span and productive life of an individual have been greatly extended. In 1900, there were approximately 3 million persons 65 and over, representing 4% of the total population. By 1940 the number had tripled to 9 million or 6.8% of US citizens. In 1965, the year when Medicare and Medicaid were instituted, the elderly were 18.5 million or approximately 9.3% of all people. In 1970 the number of the elderly had more than doubled that of 1940 to over 20 million or 9.9% of total population, and the respective figures for 1980 were 25.5 million and over 11%. Projections of the population of the elderly in the year 2000 and in 2030 are 31 million and 46 million persons, or 12% and 17% of total population, respectively.

With the rapid growth of the elderly population, it is important to identify major characteristics and factors of the elderly in order to meet their social and health-care needs.

The elderly currently celebrating their 65th birthday will, on the average, live an additional 16 years. There are and will be more elderly women than elderly men. The current ratio at ages 65 to 74 is 69 elderly men per 100 elderly women; at 85 years and over it is 44 elderly men per 100 elderly women.

Up to 95% of the elderly live in their homes or with "relatives." More elderly women than men are likely to be living alone. According to the 1970 census, 5% of people 65 years and over were institutionalized and, by 85 years, over 19% were residing in long-term care facilities. The largest number of the elderly live in urban areas. The elderly, as a whole, are more than twice as likely to be poor.

Economic security is probably the number one issue for a large number of elderly because most of the time they are not employed, are on fixed incomes and, thus, are vulnerable to become victims of inflation. Biologically, the elderly are likely to have changes of memory; sensory disturbances in vision, vestibular function and proprioception; loss of muscle strength and decreased joint integrity. They are prone to suffer from falls, incontinence and mental confusion, especially if they are predisposed to infection, toxins, drugs and atherosclerosis. They are more prone to contract chronic diseases.

In terms of patterns of medical-care use, the elderly are two times more vulnerable to hospitalization than those who are under 65. Close to 90% of patients in long-term care facilities are elderly. In 1975, the noninstitutionalized elderly had an average of 6.6 physician visits compared to 5.6 physician visits for persons aged 45 to 65. The elderly as a whole utilize or consume 25% of prescription drugs.

The estimated per capita personal health-care expenditures for the elderly in fiscal 1966 was $445.25, of which 40% was for hospital care, 20% for physician services, 15.4% for nursing home care, 14% for drugs and drug sundries, 3.5% for eye glasses and appliances, 2.9% for dentist service, 2.6% for other professional services and 1.6% for other health services. In fiscal 1971 the *per capita* health-care expenditures had almost doubled to $877.48, with a distribution of hospital care 43%, physician service 16.7%, nursing home care 23.1%, drugs and drug sundries 10%, eye glasses and appliances 2.2%, dentist service 1.9%, other professional services 1.8% and other health services 1.3%. In fiscal 1976 the expenditures ($1521.36) again were almost double those of 1971. Hospital care had a net gain of 2.3% to 45.3%, physician services and nursing home care almost maintained the 1971 levels at 16.8 and 23%, respectively. Drugs and drug sundries were reduced further from 10% in 1971 to 8% in 1976. Eye glasses and appliances and other professional services had reductions from 1.8 to 1.5% and from 2.2 to 1.2%, respectively, while other health services increased from 1.3 to 2.1%. Dental services had increased insignificantly from 1.9 to 2.1%. Within this ten-year interval, the greatest percentage increase in health-care expenditures for the elderly was nursing home care, followed by hospital care. The greatest percentage reduction was for drugs, drug sundries and physician services.

Advent of Health Insurance

The Flexner Report in 1911 not only shaped the trend of today's medical education, but also popularized institutional practice. It was in hospitals that sophisticated knowledge and technologies were available and utilized. The result was a stimulus for proliferation of hospital construction, and the orientation of medical practice was concentrated in acute short-term and highly technological care. Reimbursement for physician services and hospital care was mostly from out-of-pocket and fee-for-service type of payments made by patients. There was no government involvement in financing any aspect of health care.

The depression in the early 1930s posed great financial difficulty for many hospitals. A number of hospitals developed a fixed fee contract for delivery of hospital care to those enrolled in the program. This was the beginning of the voluntary hospital or health insurance. Blue Cross was among the first programs established to assure the health and welfare of hospitals as the primary goal.

Voluntary health insurance had significant impact in the promotion of hospital-based practice by the physicians. It was in the hospital that expensive modern equipment, qualified personnel and appropriate environment were available under one roof. At the time, hospitals were competitive and very protective of their patient population; they were not willing to discharge patients to other types of health-care facilities, even less sophisticated ones. Furthermore, most health insurance policies covered only medical services provided in the hospital setting.

As the elderly population was increasing and there were drastic changes in social and family structure, more of the elderly found themselves living alone and away from their siblings. Those who could not afford single-unit family dwellings, tended to live in residential or boarding homes. With increasing age, health declined and reduced physical capability. They needed general support and assistance in daily living, as well as some basic forms of health-care services. Nurses eventually were hired in these residential institutions and the result was the emergence of the forerunners of nursing homes or long-term care facilities today.

Passage of the Social Security Act in 1935 had great impact on the provision of health care to the elderly. The OASI Program (Old Age Survivors Insurance) which provided monthly payments for the elderly, and the OAA program (Old Age Assistance) which provided financial assistance, participated in and administered by the state for needy elderly, for the first time assured the elderly of some forms of continuous economic support. Both of these programs were considered as cash assistance to the elderly, and not as direct payment for medical care programs. Because of federal support for the elderly, and their need of long-term care, nursing homes and other related facilities, especially those privately operated, were growing in number.

Other federal programs that directly or indirectly contributed to the increase of long-term care facilities were

Hospital and Medical Facilities Construction Program (Hill-Burton) which also provided federal matching funds for constructing and equipping of public or nonprofit-operated long-term care facilities.

The Department of Housing and Urban Development and the Federal Housing Administration also provided mortgage insurance to private lenders to facilitate construction or rehabilitation of qualified proprietary nursing homes, and authority to grant money for loans to nursing homes under the National Housing Act Amendments of 1959.

The Small Business Administration provided commercial loans to privately owned long-term care facilities for construction of new facilities/expansion of new facilities.

The demand and supply of long-term care facilities were stimulated further by the passage of Medicare and Medicaid in 1965. Medicare is a health insurance program and Medicaid is a welfare program through participation and administration by the state. Both programs are designed to meet the medical needs of high-risk groups, the elderly and the poor. Medicare and Medicaid programs are quite similar to the OASI and OAA of the Social Security Act of 1935 except that the former are vendor programs which provide direct payment to providers of health care services. Medicare signifies the beginning of the federal government's involvement in providing health insurance. Because of the provision in both Medicare and Medicaid to pay for care received in long-term care facilities, these programs sparked continued growth of long-term care facilities.

A recent surge of concern over the quality of care given to the institutionalized elderly client has generated broad, sweeping regulations impacting on pharmaceutical services required in long-term care facilities. Included in these regulations are the Medicare Catastrophic Coverage Act of 1988, the 1989 revision of the Health Care Financing Administration's Medicare and Medicaid Requirements for Long Term Care Facilities, the Medicaid Program Conditions for Intermediate Care Facilities for the Mentally Retarded, the Omnibus Budget Reconciliation Act (OBRA) of 1987 and the revision of the Federal Indicators for Surveyor Assessment of the Performance of Drug Regimen Reviews including the surveyor-methodology for detecting medication errors.

Definition of Long-Term Care Facilities

In order to define a long-term care facility and its related institutions, it is important to arrive at a common understanding of what is long-term care. The phrase *long-term care* generally has been accepted by health-care professionals as health care and health-related services provided to individuals who, because of their physical and mental conditions, require medical, nursing or supportive care for a prolonged period of 30 or more days. The Congressional Discursive Dictionary of Health Care defines long-term care as "health and/or personal care services required by persons who are chronically ill, aged, disabled, or retarded, in an institution or at home on a long term basis." The term often is used more narrowly to refer only to long-term institutional care, such as is provided in nursing homes, homes for the retarded and mental hospitals." The APhA publication titled "Pharmaceutical Services in the Long-Term Care Facility" defines a long-term care facility as a facility or unit which is planned, staffed and equipped to accommodate individuals who do not require hospital care but who are in need of a wide range of medical, nursing and related health and social services. Sometimes the term long-term care is used interchangeably with chronic care or care for chronically ill, which describes an impairment of health requiring an extended period of medical supervision. These definitions all equate care for individuals with a prolonged episode of illness, but they also imply the concept of extended care, continuity of care and maintenance care which require a wide range of health and social services other than purely medical care.

Long-term care institutions include, but are not limited to

Nursing homes.
Hospital extended care units.
Psychiatric hospitals.
Chronic disease hospitals, (eg, TB hospitals).
Personal care, shelter care, board and care homes.
Facilities for mentally retarded.
Special facilities for the elderly (eg, geriatric centers or institutes, apartments, communities).
Half-way houses and other special facilities for alcoholics and drug abusers.
Other health and social related institutions (eg, detention centers, special residential facilities for children, jail units).
Hospice-care and respite-care facilities.
Home health care.

For the purpose of this chapter, the discussion on long-term care facilities will focus primarily on the first category, the nursing homes group. These facilities have a great need for quality pharmaceutical services and care, because a very large portion of their patient population is elderly and often has a number of chronic disease conditions treated and maintained by pharmacotherapy. The concept, principles, structure and process of pharmaceutical service and care provided in the nursing home setting are applicable to, or easily modified for, other types of long-term care facilities.

Long-Term Care Facilities (LTCF)

The term *nursing home* has been replaced largely by the broader title, long-term care facility, defined earlier. The services rendered in such facilities are prescribed by, or performed under the supervision of, individuals licensed to provide such services or care in accordance with the laws of the state in which the facility is located. A state-licensed administrator assumes responsibility for facility operations, including the quality of health care rendered to the clients.

The major services provided in the nursing homes as defined by the American Health Care Association are

Nursing Care—Nursing procedures requiring the professional skills of a registered nurse or a licensed practical nurse. These skills include administering medication, injections, catheterizations and similar procedures ordered by the physician. Post-hospital stroke, heart or orthopedic care is available with such related services as physical therapy, occupational therapy, dental services, dietary consultation, laboratory and X-ray services and a pharmaceutical dispensary.

Personal Care—Services such as help in walking, getting in and out of bed, bathing, dressing, eating and the preparation of special diets, as prescribed by a physician.

Residential Care—General supervision in a protective environment, including room and board plus planned programs for the social and spiritual needs of the resident.

The primary goal of a long-term care facility is to preserve the dignity and value of every individual and meet the total emotional, physical, social and spiritual needs of the residents. The professional services and care provided in these settings then should focus on the implementation of this goal with emphasis on rehabilitative, maintenance and psychosocial supports, as well as medical and nursing care. This concept is supported further by the trend toward a social model rather than a medical model of care.

The number of long-term care (LTC) nursing homes seemed to have reached a plateau at 15,362 in 1992, providing 1,665,319 licensed beds. The ratio of beds to those over age 65 rose to 53.3 beds per 1000 from 52.6 in 1991. The average occupancy dropped slightly in 1992 to 94.5% from 94.8% in 1991. The percentage of skilled beds rose from 52.6% in 1991 to 58.9% in 1992 in response to the impact of DRGs on hospitals. There was a shift in nursing-home ownership with 32 of the largest nursing-home chains accounting for 3084 facilities or 20% of the industry and 361,385 licensed beds or 21.7% of the total in 1992. During this time, new nursing-home construction decreased, with 74.1% of all licensed beds and nearly 72% of all nursing homes being 16 years or older. While the facilities aged, Medicare-certified beds increased from 53.6% in 1991 to 58.9% in 1992, supporting the notion of increasing patient acuity.

Fifty-six percent of the residents were covered by Medicaid in 1992, while Medicaid reimbursement supplied 57.5% of the revenue. Average operating costs rose 6.5% in 1992 to $2.6 million. Nursing-home room rates rose 6% to an average of $88 per day for skilled care and 14.7% for intermediate care, to an average of $78 per day. The nursing-home industry employed 1.3 million full-time and 368,000 part-time workers. The average skilled nursing facility with 101 to 150 beds made up ⅓ of total beds. Six states—California, Illinois, New York, Ohio, Pennsylvania and Texas accounted for 38% of all long-term beds and 36% of total nursing homes. Indiana, Iowa, Kansas and Oklahoma had the highest concentrations of beds relative to their population.

Licensed nursing-home beds were distributed among four owner-types in 1992. For-profit facilities accounted for 58% of licensed beds; not-for-profit, 23%; government, 13% and church-related homes, 6%.

Extended-Care Facilities (ECF)

Extended care facility was the term used in the early years of the Medicare program to designate a nursing home which qualified for participation in Medicare. A nursing home has to meet certain requirements in order to be certified as an extended care facility. While nursing homes that provided a lower level of care and qualified for the Medicaid program were called skilled nursing *homes*, only a relatively small number of nursing homes were certified as *extended care facilities*. The concept of extended care, at the time, referred to an extension of care for the original medical condition after hospitalization and not to the duration of long-term facility care required. Medicare covered only up to 100 days of post-hospital extended-care services during any spell of illness. Therefore, the extended-care facility benefit was limited in duration and must follow a hospital stay and be related to the medical condition being treated in the hospital. This remains, even today, as the only federally funded coverage for long-term care under the existing Medicare part A program. Pressure is being exerted to include medication coverage and eventually nursing-home care in the proposed national health-care reform package. If the person exhausted his coverage for extended facility care, he must either finance his own care or resort to seeking eligibility under the Medicaid program. There is an increasing availability of long term care insurance policies but their popularity has been slow in developing. If the person was qualified for Medicaid, his care would be provided in a nursing home that might not be certified or approved by Medicare. In order to establish uniform standards for long-term facility care under Medicare and Medicaid, the term extended-care facility was dropped and replaced by the generic definition of *skilled nursing facility* for both Medicare and Medicaid.

Skilled Nursing Facilities (SNF)

A skilled nursing facility is a nursing home that meets requirements for the conditions for participation in both Medicare and Medicaid programs. Some of the major requirements are

Having a transfer agreement with one or more participating hospitals.

Primarily engaging in providing skilled nursing care and related services.

Having formal policies.

Having a physician, a registered professional nurse or a medical staff responsible for the execution of such policies.

Requiring the health care of every patient to be under the supervision of a physician and providing for having a physician available to furnish necessary medical care in case of an emergency.

Maintaining medical records on all patients.

Providing 24-hour nursing services and having at least one registered professional nurse employed full-time.

Providing appropriate methods and procedures for dispensing and administering drugs and biologicals.

Having, in effect, a utilization review plan.

Meeting licensing standards established by the individual state.

Providing a regular program of independent medical review of the patients in the facility.

Meeting any conditions relating to the health and safety of individuals.

Having the drug regimen of each patient reviewed by the pharmacist at least on a monthly basis.

In addition to providing skilled nursing care, skilled nursing facilities also make available rehabilitative therapy, physical therapy, occupational therapy and other medical services when needed.

Intermediate Care Facilities (ICF)

An intermediate care facility is defined in the Congressional Discursive Dictionary of Health Care as "an institution recognized under the Medicaid program which is licensed under state laws to provide, on a regular basis, health-related care and services to individuals who do not require the degree of care or treatment which a hospital or skilled nursing facility is designed to provide, but who, because of their mental or physical condition, require care and services (above the level of room and board) which can be made available to them only through institutional facilities."

Many long-term care facilities qualify both as a skilled nursing facility and an intermediate care facility, and both types of facilities usually are licensed by the same state agency.

In the recent past, nursing homes were classified as Skilled Nursing Facilities and Intermediate-Care Facilities each having their own regulations and requirements as defined by the level of care required by their clients. Following the recommendations found in the 1987 Omnibus Budget Reconciliation Act (OBRA), the 1989 revision of the Health Care Financing Administration regulations for Skilled and Intermediate

Care Facilities combined regulations, thus applying one set of requirements to both types of facility. Incorporated in this set of regulations are significant additional requirements including

Extending the pharmacist's monthly drug-regimen review to ICF clients.

Assuring resident privacy rights with regard to accommodations, medical treatment, personal care, visits, telephone communications and meetings with resident and family groups.

Assuring proper use of physical restraints and psychoactive drugs including instituting dose reductions, and behavioral intervention programs.

Providing 24-hour licensed nursing services, and services of a registered nurse at least 8 hours a day, 7 days a week, subject to waivers.

Furnishing comprehensive assessments and being subject to civil monetary penalties for falsification of an assessment.

Requiring minimum training of nurse aides, competency-evaluation programs and regular in-service education.

Assuring that the resident's drug regimen is free from unnecessary drugs, significant medication errors or significant medication error rates.

The definition of unnecessary drugs includes drugs

- Given in excessive doses, including duplicate therapy.
- Given for excessive periods of time.
- Given without adequate monitoring.
- Given without adequate indications for use.
- Free of undue adverse consequences, which would indicate the dose should be reduced or the drug discontinued.

Regulation of self-administration of drugs by residents.

Requiring full information prior to institution or alteration of in-care or treatment.

Requiring participation of the competent residents in the development of their plan of care.

Requiring annual independent, external consultant review of the appropriateness of the drug plan of each resident receiving psychopharmacologic drugs.

Any combinations of reasons above.

Specific interpretive guidelines for state surveyors concerning unnecessary drugs were published in April 1992. The specific areas of concern include

Long-Acting Benzodiazepine Drugs—These should not be used in residents of long-term care facilities unless an attempt with a shorter-acting drug has failed.

Even after an attempt with a shorter-acting benzodiazepine drug has failed, a long-acting benzodiazepine should not be used unless

- Evidence exists that other possible reasons for the resident's distress have been considered and ruled out.
- Its use results in maintenance or improvement in the resident's functional status.
- Daily use is less than, or equal to, the listed total *daily* doses in Rev 250 P-140 unless higher doses (as evidenced by resident's response and/or clinical record) are necessary for the maintenance or improvement in the resident's functional status.
- Daily use is less than four continuous months unless an attempt at a *gradual* dose reduction is unsuccessful.

Exceptions:

- When used for neuromuscular syndromes, for withdrawal from short-acting agents, when used in bi-polar disorders, tardive dyskinesia, nocturnal myoclonus or seizure disorders.
- Gradual dosage reduction should be attempted at least twice within one year before determining gradual dose reduction is "clinically contraindicated."

Benzodiazepine or Other Anxiolytic Sedative Drugs—The use of these drugs for purposes other than sleep induction should only occur when

- Evidence exists that other possible reasons for the resident's distress have been considered and ruled out.
- Use results in a maintenance or improvement in the resident's functional status.
- Daily use is less than four continuous months unless an attempt at a gradual dose reduction is unsuccessful.

Use is for one of the following indications as defined by the *Diagnostic and Statistical Manual of Mental Disorders* (3rd edition-revised)

- Generalized anxiety disorder.
- Organic mental syndromes with associated agitated states which are quantitatively and objectively documented and which constitute sources of distress or dysfunction to the resident or represent a danger to the resident or others.
- Panic disorder.
- Symptomatic anxiety.

Drugs used for sleep induction—These drugs should be used only if

- Evidence exists that other possible reasons for insomnia have been ruled out.
- The use of a drug to induce sleep results in the maintenance or improvement of the resident's functional status.
- Daily use of the drug is less than ten continuous days unless an attempt at a gradual dose reduction is unsuccessful.
- The dose of the drug is equal or less than that listed in Rev 250 P-142.

For drugs in this category, a gradual dose reduction should be attempted at least three times within six months before one can conclude that a gradual dose reduction is "clinically contraindicated."

Miscellaneous Sedative Hypnotic/Anxiolytic drugs—These drugs have been deemed inappropriate for use in the elderly including

- Amobarbital
- Butabarbital
- Pentobarbital
- Secobarbital
- Glutethimide
- Meprobamate

Monitoring for Antipsychotic Drug Side Effects—The facility must assure that residents who receive antipsychotic drug therapy receive adequate monitoring for significant side effects of such therapy with emphasis on

- Tardive dyskinesia
- Postural (orthostatic) hypotension
- Cognitive/behavior impairment
- Akathisia
- Parkinsonism.

When antipsychotic drugs are used without monitoring for these side effects, they may be unnecessary drugs because of inadequate monitoring.

Other previously published important guidelines impacting on the use of psychoactive medications include

- The need for an appropriate diagnosis or behavior which causes the resident to become a danger to himself or others, or has a behavior such as continuous crying, screaming, yelling or pacing, if these behaviors cause an impairment in functional capacity.
- A list of symptoms which alone are not sufficient to support the use of antipsychotic drugs.
- Guidelines concerning the use of PRN antipsychotic drugs for dosage reduction or titration. When used PRN to control unexpected harmful behavior, the PRN antipsychotic drug may be used no more than twice in a seven-day period without assessment of the resident and the development of a plan of care to alleviate or reduce the harmful behavior.
- Dosage reduction criteria for antipsychotic drugs require two attempts the first year unless "clinically contraindicated" or for a listed psychiatric condition. Specific documentation criteria are provided in the guidelines for physicians wishing to justify not carrying out a dosage adjustment (Rev 250 P-150).

Intermediate-Care Facilities for the Mentally Retarded (ICF/MR)

The Health Care Financing Administration (HCFA) published its final regulations concerning ICF/MR facilities, effective October 3, 1988. Pharmacy-consultant activities were defined, including a required quarterly drug-regimen review for each client (42 CFR 483.460 (j) (1)). The regulations mandate the following pharmacy-consultant services:

A pharmacist with input from the interdisciplinary team must review the drug regimen of each client at least quarterly.

The pharmacist must report any irregularities in a client's drug regimens to the prescribing physician and to the interdisciplinary team.

The pharmacist must prepare a record of each client's drug regimen review and the facility must maintain that record.

As appropriate, the pharmacist must participate in the development, implementation and review of each client's individual program plan (IPP), either in person, or through a written report to the interdisciplinary team. The IPP identifies the clients needs, as described by the comprehensive functional assessments, and is required to be completed within 30 days of admission.

The perceived positive impact on patient care is typified in the statement by HCFA which accompanied these new regulations ". . . We believe that the proper conduct of these reviews can be assured best by requiring that a pharmacist perform them."

Range and Scope of Resident Care and Services

Long-term care, including both institutional and noninstitutional care, is defined broadly by the Dept of Health and

Human Services as

"Long-term care consists of those services designed to provide diagnostic, preventive, therapeutic, rehabilitative, supportive and maintenance services for individuals of all age groups who have chronic physical and/or mental impairments, in a variety of institutional and noninstitutional health care settings, including the home, with the goal of promoting the optimum level of physical, social, and psychological functioning.

"Provisions of care should be the result of assessment and planning by medical, nursing, social work and therapeutic personnel. The plan of care should be based upon the needs of the individual and family/caretaker who participate in decisions regarding the care plan. Program services and facilities serving the individual requiring long-term care must address the needs of the users of the services. Long-term care programs must focus upon appropriate planning and utilization of resources (medical, social, financial, rehabilitative, and supportive) needed by individuals who have continuing care needs."

Most of the residents cared for in the long-term facility setting are suffering generally from some forms of chronic disease conditions, adjusting to changes in institutional living and experiencing social isolation and individual loneliness. Even though drug therapy is one of the major therapeutic modalities, the residents' needs often are more than medical and physiological, mostly for psychosocial support. Most health professionals are trained technologically and acute-care-oriented, and they are not prepared to care for these patients who need more interpersonal care and contact time from health-care providers.

Because of his easy accessibility and availability to the long-term care facilities, as well as having a vital service role in this setting, the pharmacist can assume a leadership role to improve the quality of care and life in the long-term care facility. Long-term care is broad and diverse and requires the services of a variety of health professionals. The pharmacist must learn to work with other health-care professionals as a true member of a realistic multidisciplinary team. The mission of the pharmacist in the long-term care facility should be more than to provide necessary drugs to patients and assure quality of drug used, but also to participate with other health care providers in rendering necessary psychosocial support to the residents.

Nursing Care and Services

The core of long-term care is nursing care. Nursing service in the long-term care facility accounts for over 90% of all personnel.

The intensity level of nursing care generally is used to classify and define the type of long-term care facilities, such as skilled nursing facilities and intermediate care facilities. The role, as viewed by the nurse in the long-term care facility, is to provide and promote the physical, social, emotional, environmental, recreational, spiritual and rehabilitative aspects of care. The emphasis is directed to preventive, therapeutic and rehabilitative nursing. In addition, the nurse has to coordinate all types and levels of care delivered in the long-term care facility. Because of the chronic nature of the diseases suffered by the long-term facility residents, the infrequent physician contact and the age of the residents, nursing care is the key to the long-term care. The quality of the overall long-term care is related directly to the quality of the nursing care.

Medical Services

In long-term facility care, medical care and services are more than the diagnosing and treatment of diseases. Because of the nature of the illnesses, which are mostly chronic, and the altered physiological states as a result of aging, physicians have to acquire an additional biomedical knowledge base to manage properly the medical problems of the long-term care facility patients. In addition, there are social, psychological and economic needs in this population that may have a higher priority in the view of the individual patient.

The traditional medical practice of most physicians is involved primarily in consultation with individual patients and in advising about treatment of acute episodes of diseases. With the increase in the elderly population and the corresponding rise in chronic diseases, geriatric medicine is being developed and promoted in a number of medical schools. Special geriatric residencies are being established. There is an ongoing debate in the medical community whether geriatric medicine should be taught to all practitioners or established as a specialty in medical practice.

Because of current interest in the care of the elderly, concepts of geriatrics and gerontology have been promoted in the education of many health-care providers. There is general confusion because these terms, *geriatrics* and *gerontology*, have been used interchangeably. Broadly speaking, geriatrics could be considered as a clinical approach to the care and study of the elderly, while gerontology is the basic biological science and psychosocial study and care of the elderly.

The Institute of Medicine, National Academy of Sciences, in its report of a study on "Aging and Medical Education," published in September 1978, includes selected definitions of geriatrics and gerontology:

Geriatrics is the "branch of general medicine concerned with clinical, preventive, remedial, and social aspects of illnesses in the elderly." (British Geriatrics Society.)

Geriatrics is the "clinical side of aging" (Freeman, JT: A Survey of Geriatric Education: Catalogues of US Medical Schools. *J Am Geriatr Soc 19:* 746, 1971).

Gerontology is "a branch of knowledge dealing with aging and the problems of the aged." (*Webster's New Collegiate Dictionary*.)

Gerontology is "the study of aging process—originating in the biological sciences and expanding more recently into the social and behavioral sciences." (DHEW Publication No HRA 74-3117.)

Gerontology denotes "the scientific study of aging in all its aspects—clinical, biological, historical and social" (American Medical Student Association: Curriculum Development in Geriatric Medicine, January 1976).

Thus, physicians who provide long-term facility care, function more than as experts in clinical medicine in the medical evaluation and problem-identification of the institutionalized elderly, but also as an organizer of a multidisciplinary team of clinical and social professionals to plan and deliver continuous and need-oriented therapeutic and psychosocial care. The American Academy of Family Practice recently has incorporated geriatrics as a formal part of the training of family practice physicians. There is also a resurgence of the American Medical Directors Association with special emphasis on the physicians' role in Total Quality Management.

Pharmaceutical Services and Care

Since the beginning of long-term facility care, drugs always have been an indispensable therapeutic modality. Most residents in long-term care facilities are elderly and often are afflicted with a number of chronic disease conditions requiring continuous therapeutic treatment. Drugs are used to eliminate symptoms, reduce suffering, prevent exacerbation and complications of illness, as well as maintain a minimal level of health and enhance the quality of life.

The early phase of pharmaceutical services in long-term care facilities was mostly the provision of medication to individual institutionalized residents. The resident, or the family of the resident, was, and still is, free to select any community pharmacy to provide prescribed medication. As the facility size and number of residents institutionalized increased, it became clear that there was an urgent need for a specific pharmacy designated to be responsible for coordinating and controlling the use of drugs, as well as providing drugs to patients in the facility. Many long-term care facilities were too small to support a pharmacy department of their own, and they negotiated and contracted with specific community pharmacies to provide all pharmaceutical services and needs of the facilities. This marked the advent of the consultant pharmacist in the long-term care setting. The contracted pharmacy was reimbursed for the medications dispensed by submitting bills of services, while the facility usually collected payment from residents or third-party payors including Medicare. In return for providing drugs to the residents in the facility, the contracted pharmacy provider also was required to perform certain services in the facility to assure a safe drug-distribution, storage, administration, control and recording system. Some of these services included in-service training, preparation of policies, procedures and participation in resident-care-related activities.

With the passage of Medicare and Medicaid legislation in the middle 1960s, pharmaceutical services to eligible residents in long-term care facilities were guaranteed under the law. It became very attractive for community pharmacies to expand or specialize their services in the long-term care setting because of assured financial rewards. Whenever government pays for services, there are always strings attached. Specific conditions are spelled out as to how the services should be provided in order to qualify for reimbursement. Long-term care facility pharmacy services have become complicated and complex, and special knowledge and expertise are required to provide pharmacy services in these types of institutions. Most successful long-term care facility pharmacy providers have introduced computer and other technologies in their operations. With the introduction of affordable computers and software packages it has become easier for a newcomer to enter and compete successfully for the delivery of long-term facility care.

The primary source of medications for nursing homes continues to be off-premises pharmacies. The number of nursing homes with in-house pharmacies fell from 6% in 1991 to 5% in 1992. About 11% of the facilities purchased drugs directly through a wholesaler, while 78.7% of nursing homes purchase from provider pharmacies. The largest number of pharmacy providers are community based (41%), with 28% being closed-door community institutional pharmacies. The closed-door pharmacies tend to be large-volume units serving in excess of 2000 residents. Many of the pharmacies serve other than nursing homes including prisons, hospice centers, mental health facilities, alcohol/drug rehabilitation centers, hospitals, home health agencies, HMOs/PPOs and residential-care centers. Many of these pharmacies offer Part B Medicare services, IV admixture programs, durable medical supplies and equipment and consultant pharmacy services.

The typical pharmacy provider dispenses 5000 drug orders per month. Approximately 70% of the pharmacy providers dispense a 30-day supply of medication. Modified unit-dose systems are used by 61% of the pharmacies, 15% use 24-hour unit-dose systems and 24% still use traditional vial systems.

Trends in the future are difficult to predict with accuracy; however, there is an increasing movement toward corporate consolidation of independent providers. The large corporate movements are driven by the reasonable profit margin potential thought to exist in pharmacy. For-profit nursing home chains make up an increasing percentage of these new corporate entities. These changes have resulted in a decrease in the number of pharmacists who remain in control of the pharmacy provider groups. The impact of this change is yet to be realized. In addition to this current trend will come the impact of national health-care reform on the Medicaid programs which comprise the largest single payor. If the state Medicaid programs are turned over to managed health-care providers, there could be dramatic changes including the use of centralized mail-order pharmacies. These changes will impact directly on the consultant pharmacy services which often are provided at below their actual cost to the nursing home client. Separation of provider and consultant pharmacists may become a critical issue in the future. This change in relationship between consultant and provider pharmacists may be fueled further by OBRA Safe Harbor rulings, which could deem underpriced consultant pharmacies to be an illegal inducement to gain Medicaid and Medicare business.

Pharmacist Role and Functions

Needs for Pharmaceutical Care and Services

The profession of pharmacy has a unique body of knowledge and skills to contribute in our health-care system. The pharmacist not only dispenses the appropriate drug product but also has the knowledge to assure safe and rational use of drugs. Early functions of the pharmacist could be grouped into

Assisting in the selection of appropriate drug therapy.

Preparing, compounding and manufacturing drugs for individualized patients.

Dispensing and packaging the prescribed drug products, including proper labeling.

Advising and educating patients on proper use of drugs.

Monitoring the outcome and responses of patients to the effects of drugs, both beneficial and adverse.

Serving as a community resource person on drug and health information.

There is concern among health-care providers over the potential abuse, misuse and inappropriate use of drugs, and the resulting increase in health-care cost and patient suffering. There is need for professionals who are patient-oriented and able to apply and provide drug knowledge to improve drug use in the health care system. Pharmacy colleges have responded by providing clinical training for their undergraduates. This new breed of pharmacists is more clinically and patient-oriented and better prepared to dispense drug knowledge as well as drug products.

Long-term care residents often have a number of chronic disease conditions requiring multiple and continuous drug therapy. Also, they have less frequent physician contact than do patients in acute care facilities. Furthermore, in most long-term care facilities the staffing pattern usually meets only the minimal requirement as stated by law. In addition to having a greater demand for medical care, long-term care residents often have psychosocial and economic needs. A clinically trained and patient-oriented pharmacist will be in an ideal situation to assist and work with other members of the health care team to provide quality long-term facility care.

Federal Requirements in Skilled Nursing Facilities

The Social Security Act Amendment of 1972 (PL 92-603) has established uniform terminology and requirements for long-term care facilities participating under both Medicare and Medicaid programs. Final regulations for skilled nursing facilities were published in the *Fed Reg*, Feb 19, 1974, updated in 1979, 1987 and again in 1992. These regulations outline the conditions, requirements and standards for the provision of pharmaceutical services to long-term care facilities (skilled nursing facilities) qualified for the Medicare and Medicaid programs.

a. *Condition of Participation*—Pharmaceutical Services Paragraph 405.1127 of the regulations outlines the condition for participation of pharmaceutical services and states: "The facility provides routine and emergency drugs and biologicals to its residents, or obtains them under an agreement described in §483.75(h) of this part. The facility may permit unlicensed personnel to administer drugs if state law permits, but only under the general supervision of a licensed nurse. This standard designates the residents facility, rather than the pharmacist, as having responsibility to provide drugs and pharmaceutical services to residents in long-term care facilities. The pharmacists are contracted by the facilities to provide pharmaceutical services. Because pharmacists are reimbursed through the facility, some long-term care facility owners have imposed questionable financial arrangements and requirements on the type of pharmaceutical services provided in the facility. This practice has resulted in "kick-back" scandals and limited development of innovative pharmaceutical services to residents. Examples include free consultant pharmacy services, exorbitant billing discounts, free computer services, forms, telecommunication equipment, medication carts and deep discount supplies.

b. *Procedures*—A facility must provide pharmaceutical services (including procedures that assure the accurate acquiring, receiving, dispensing and administering of all drugs and biologicals) to meet the needs of each resident. The pharmacist (if not a full-time employee) devotes a sufficient number of hours, based upon the needs of the facility, during regularly scheduled visits to carry out these responsibilities. The pharmacist reviews the drug regimen of each resident at least monthly, and reports any irregularities to the attending physician and the director of nursing, and these reports must be acted upon. This provision stipulates the responsibilities of the pharmacist. It differs from the previous concept of a "consultant pharmacist" who does not have direct responsibilities in providing long-term facility care. In addition to spending sufficient time in the facility and making appropriate reports, the pharmacist is required to review the drug regimen of each resident at least monthly. This standard has far-reaching implications and has recognized officially the role of the pharmacist more than as a dispenser of drugs.

OBRA 87 eliminated the differentiation between pharmacy services required for intermediate-care facilities and skilled nursing facilities. At this time, "accuracy" of pharmaceutical services is stressed. Many process-oriented regulations have been replaced by outcome-oriented ones. Drug-labeling requirements are retained with mandatory inclusion of the expiration date. Locked storage requirements and appropriate accessory and cautionary instructions include a permanently affixed compartment for storage of controlled drugs listed in Schedule II of the Comprehensive Drug Abuse Prevention and Control Act of 1976 and other drugs subject to abuse, except when the facility uses single-unit-package drug-distribution systems in which the quantity stored is minimal and missing doses can be detected readily. The Pharmaceutical Services Committee is retained but encouraged to incorporate with the Quality Assessment and Assurance Committee. The revision will remove any obstruction to the individual states permitting unlicensed personnel to administer medications. Monthly drug-regimen reviews were extended to intermediate-care facilities and a response will be required by the appropriate recipient, either the director of nursing or the attending physician. Special emphasis is placed on controlling and reducing the use of psychoactive drugs, especially if chemical restraints are suspected.

c. *Review of Drug Regimens*—The intent of this requirement is to improve drug utilization by reducing adverse drug reactions and interactions, duplication and inappropriate concurrent combination of drugs, and medication errors through the elimination of unnecessary drugs. The pharmacist is asked to deviate from his/her dispensing activities and to apply his/her knowledge in the review of residents' drug regimens. To implement this standard properly, the pharmacist must acquire certain knowledge and skills and undertake some additional activities, such as

1. To develop, obtain and maintain a valid and comprehensive drug data base (drug profile) including pertinent resident information, such as laboratory test results, diagnosis and relevant comments in the resident's medical record.
2. To evaluate the drug data base according to predetermined set of guidelines or standards.
3. To establish monitoring criteria for detecting and preventing potential adverse drug reactions, interactions and iatrogenic disease.
4. To detect medication errors and promote compliance.
5. To assure cost containment and appropriate drug utilization.
6. To eliminate drug abuse and missuse.
7. To educate and inform clients and staff members.
8. To assimilate and communicate significant findings in an objective and concise manner both verbally and in writing.
9. To apply clinical and interpersonal skills.
10. To analyze and report impact of drug reviews on client care.
11. To eliminate all unnecessary medications.

Also, the pharmacist should expand and review his/her knowledge base in geriatric drug therapy.

The costs related to the provision of pharmacist consulting services, such as drug regimen review are recognized by most, if not all, the states. The reimbursement of these services are supposedly reflected in the facility's per diem rate in both Medicaid and Medicare programs. The amount of payment is deemed by many pharmacists as grossly inadequate or non-existent. But this requirement does open the door for the pharmacist to be reimbursed for dispensing knowledge, in addition to dispensing drug products.

For the past few years, the Department of Health and Human Services has proposed specific outcome measures or indicators to assess the performance of pharmacist's review of drug regimens. The consulting pharmacist in addition to providing written records of the monthly drug regimen review activities, would be expected to prepare necessary documentation for the surveyor to apply the proposed indicator measurements. The data most likely to be requested might include

1. The total number of drug regimens reviewed each month (no more than 100 patients should be reviewed in any one day).
2. The average number of prescriptions utilized per patient each month.
3. The total number of drug-related irregularities discovered each month.
4. The number of drug administration errors discovered and reported to nursing staff each month.
5. The average monthly patient census.
6. The monitoring and effectiveness of psychoactive medications.

The general areas that might be addressed by the indicator measurements would include

1. No multiple or duplicative orders for same or similar drugs in the same pharmacological or therapeutic categories (eg, multiple antianxiety agents, antidepressants, antipsychotics, laxatives, multivitamins and sedative-hypnotics).
2. Medication orders on a PRN basis not being given for more than 30 days.
3. Medications being given according to established safe, recommended dosage ranges, especially those requiring reduced dosages in the elderly, such as antianxiety agents, antidepressants, antipsychotics and sedative-hypnotics.
4. Premature changes to higher doses or to other drug agents which require extended periods of time to achieve full therapeutic effects, such as antidepressants, antihypertensives, antipsychotics and some oral hypoglycemics.
5. Drugs requiring periodic or regular laboratory testing (eg, anticoagulants, anticonvulsants, digoxin, diuretics, drugs for anemia, hypoglycemics, thyroid preparations, urinary tract bacterial suppressants and some antirheumatic agents).
6. Monitoring of clinical parameters for efficacy or toxicity of selective drugs such as blood pressures for antihypertensive therapy, daily pulse rate for antiarrhythmics, digoxin and beta blockers.
7. The use of drugs without an appropriate documented supportive diagnosis or symptom.
8. Orders for drugs for which there is a known allergy, as documented in the patient's record.
9. The use of neuroleptics without an acceptable diagnosis or symptom or for nondestructive behavioral disorders.

d. *Control and Accountability*—Regulations stress the importance of control and accountability in the provision of pharmacy services in the long-term care facility. Only approved drugs and biologicals are used in the facility, and are dispensed in compliance with Federal and State laws. Records of receipt and disposition of all controlled drugs are maintained in sufficient detail to enable an accurate reconciliation. The pharmacist determines that drug records are in order and that an account of all controlled drugs is maintained and reconciled.

The pharmacist always has the responsibility for drug control and accountability. Very few long-term care facilities have an in-house or on-site pharmacy department, or employ a full-time pharmacist in the facility. The staffing pattern of many of these facilities is barely adequate to meet minimal requirements of regulation and the staff often lacks the training to assure and implement a good drug control and accountability system. There are publications and reports on congressional hearings describing problems of abuse, misuse and diversion of drugs in long-term care facilities. This statute clearly identifies and emphasizes the role and function of the pharmacist in drug control and accountability.

Specific survey procedures will be applied to determine the presence and rate of medication errors within the facility. The presence of one significant error, as described in the survey process, or a rate of 5% or more of insignificant medication errors will result in a written deficiency. Categories of errors include but are not limited to errors of omission, timing of administration, dose, dosage form and lack of drug authorization. It is incumbent upon the consultant pharmacist to become thoroughly aware of the survey process and to assure facility compliance.

e. *Unit-Dose and Unit per Use System*—The unit-dose system is a medication management technique originally developed and designed for use in acute patient care settings. In the late 1950s and early 1960s, the traditional ward stock system proved to be inadequate to provide safe and accountable drug distribution. In that period many new drugs were introduced into the health care market, resulting in an increase in drug utilization. With the short length of stay and rapid turnover of patients in acute care hospitals, nursing personnel were overwhelmed with the preparation and administration of multitudes of new drugs and dosage forms. Consequently there emerged a growing problem of medication errors. Leaders in hospital pharmacy proposed the unit-dose system as one solution to improve drug distribution and administration in the hospital setting. Since then, the unit-dose system has been accepted and promoted by agencies such as the General Accounting Office of the Congress, and the Joint Commission on the Accreditation of Hospitals as a safe and effective drug distribution and administration system. The objectives of the unit-dose system of drug distribution are

1. To promote safe and effective drug therapy at a reasonable cost.
2. To detect and prevent errors and adverse drug reactions.
3. To promote efficient utilization of health manpower.
4. To minimize drug deterioration, obsolescence, pilferage and abuse.
5. To promote optimum utilization of floor space for medication storage and distribution.
6. To reduce or simplify medication record-keeping requirements.
7. To provide greater drug control through accuracy in medication recordkeeping.

Some of these goals are applicable to long-term care facility settings, while others are not. Long-term care facilities are unique because the drug therapy of most patients is relatively constant and there are few day-to-day changes. Even though the staffing level of nurses in many long-term care facilities is minimal and there is a high turnover rate of staff, the 24 hour pass unit-dose system has not yet been justified to be cost-effective. A modified unit-per-use system may be more logical and easier to adopt. Currently, the reimbursement system under Medicare and Medicaid programs is not inducive for long-term care facilities to venture universally into the 24 hour pass unit-dose system. But everyone will agree that there is need for a safe and efficient medication management system in the long-term care facility. Future implementation of bar-coding technology will reduce dramatically errors, labor costs and facilitate further advancement and integration of drug distribution, administration, recordkeeping, billing, monitoring and information systems.

Important Elements of a Pharmacy Policy and Procedures Manual

Pharmacists, except those involved in institutional care, generally do not ordinarily develop formal and written policies and procedures for the provision of their services. Pharmacy services in the long-term care facility began as an extension of pharmacy practice in the community setting. Whatever policies and procedures existed between pharmacists and management in the facility have been based on common understanding and gentlemen's agreement. As long-term care facilities expand responsibility and scope of services, they demand better organization, management control and accountability of all services, including those of pharmacy. Also, Medicare and Medicaid regulations are requiring more documentation and justification of services reimbursed under these laws. The next unavoidable step was the mandating of written and formal policies and procedures for all long-term care facilities.

A pharmacy policy and procedures manual establishes rules, guidelines and processes which define and govern how pharmacy services are to be delivered. A well-written and designed manual will identify clearly the responsibilities of and relationship between the pharmacist provider and the facility. In general, pharmacists are inadequately trained in management science and the majority are uncomfortable and lack the necessary competency to develop a structured pharmacy policy and procedures manual. Many pharmacists recognize the value of an organized policy and procedures manual, such as

Providing a uniform standard of practice.

Defining specific responsibilities and relationships between provider and facility in the provision of services.

Serving as a teaching guide for in-service training of staff.

Establishing a foundation for planning, developing and reviewing existing and new services.

Serving as a management control and assessment tool.

Providing documentation of services.

A number of excellent continuing-education programs sponsored by national and state pharmaceutical associations and selected universities are designed to assist the pharmacist in the development of a pharmacy policy and procedures manual. One particular manual developed by the American Society of Consultant Pharmacists provides a model workbook for others to adopt, or use to modify and improve their individual manuals. This model-manual workbook offers a systematic approach for the development of a pharmacy policy and procedures manual to meet the specific individual facility needs. Such manuals must include and involve input and participation of other health care providers, such as physicians, nurses and administrators responsible for the delivery of pharmacy and pharmacy-related services. Also, a good manual must meet requirements and conditions for participation established under federal and state laws. Because of tremendous changes occurring externally as well as internally in long-term facility care, the pharmacy policy and procedures should be updated and reviewed periodically, not less than once a year.

Pharmacy policies and procedures can be grouped into two major categories, administration-related and service or operation-related.

Administration-Related Policies and Procedures

This section describes the arrangement between the pharmacist provider and the facility defining the organization and scope of pharmacy services. It should have a signed and dated agreement or contract outlining responsibilities and activities to be performed and, if possible, should state reimbursement or professional fees.

Major topics should include

1. *Those related to the dispensing of drugs and drug products, specifically to*

a. Provide drugs and supplies as required for patients and the facility in accordance with state and federal laws.

b. Furnish and replenish emergency drug supply in acceptable containers and equipment.

c. Label all medications according to state and federal laws.

d. Provide pharmacy services to the facility on a 24-hour day, 7-day week basis.

e. Maintain drug profiles on all active patients.

f. Provide timely delivery of all medications and supplies.

g. Apply prudent buyer concepts to all pharmacy charges.

h. Provide or arrange for pharmacist consultant service.

i. Develop a drug formulary system and product selection policy.

2. *Those related to the dispensing of knowledge:*

a. Review each patient's drug regimen and submit reports at least monthly to the director of nursing and the attending physician.

b. Maintain a log of all visits and activities in the facility.

c. Review at least quarterly the various aspects of the total drug distribution system.

d. Provide complete documentation of all professional review activities in accordance with federal and state laws.

e. Participate as a member of the pharmacy service committee, infection control committee and/or other committees, such as utilization review committee and the patient-care committee.

f. Assist in establishing policies and procedures governing provision of pharmacy services and supplies in the facility.

g. Provide ongoing in-service training for the facility staff at least quarterly.

h. Check emergency drug supply at least monthly.

i. Inspect each nursing station, its related drug storage area and the patient's health record, at least quarterly or more often if the need arises.

j. Make quarterly reports describing problems, solutions, suggestions and improvements to be submitted to the pharmacy services committee.

k. Assist in the destruction of unused controlled substances as prescribed by law.

l. Determine the facility's medication error rate.

m. Report status of staff performance.

n. Assure safe and effective drug usage.

o. Conduct drug-utilization, cost-containment and drug-holiday programs.

p. Document and demonstrate consultant pharmacist's impact on patient care by the use of valid research and study techniques.

Other information that might be included is the number of hours of services, arrangement for on-call or emergency coverage, current pharmacist license number and renewal date and legal provision for such an agreement.

Service-Related or Operation-Related Policies and Procedures

This section covers policies and procedures related to provision of pharmacy services. It describes processes or methods as to how pharmacy services are to be implemented. The following topics should be considered:

1. *Medication Procuring Schedules*

a. A schedule of pharmacy operating hours and drug ordering times should be posted at the nursing station.

b. A drug delivery schedule and log should be kept.

2. *Emergency Medication Services*

a. The 24-hour emergency telephone number of the pharmacist should be posted at the nursing station.

b. A list of emergency medications should be updated periodically.

c. An effective and safe exchange system of emergency medication box or cart to avoid misuse of emergency medications.

3. *Medication Ordering*

a. All medications should be received by authorized personnel.

b. Records for ordering medications from the provider pharmacy should be kept properly.

c. Refills of medications, especially maintenance medications, should be ordered appropriately without interruption of therapy.

d. Direct copies of physician orders should be forwarded to the pharmacy provider within 24 hours.

e. Written copies of all telephone medication orders should be sent promptly to the prescribing physician for signature.

f. Signed copies of telephone orders should be included in the patient's chart.

g. Medication orders should be recapped or rewritten monthly, when appropriate and signed by the physician.

h. Medication orders should be written properly, including the drug name, dose, frequency of administration, route (if other than oral), and if PRN, indication for use.

i. Medication orders in the patient's chart should concur with those in the medication administration sheet.

j. Specific nurses should be authorized to transmit medication orders from the patient's chart to the pharmacy.

k. Special provision should be available for patients who wish to obtain drugs from outside pharmacy providers.

l. Outside pharmacy providers should furnish a drug profile of the patient to the pharmacist consultant every 30 days.

4. *Drug Administration*

a. Administration of routine medications should be recorded properly in the patient's medication record.

b. Administration of PRN medications should be recorded properly in patient's medication record.

c. PRN medications should not be administered on a regular or continuous basis for more than two weeks.

d. All medications should be prepared, dispensed, administered and charted by the same individual.

e. Only licensed personnel should administer medications, except for bedside medications when specifically ordered or when permitted under state regulations.

f. Medications should not be borrowed from one patient and administered to another.

g. "Prepouring" of medications should not be allowed. Medications should be administered as soon as possible, but no more than 2 hours after the doses are poured.

1. Dose not administered, for whatever reason, should be documented in the patient's health record.
2. Drugs ordered "STAT" and not in the emergency drug supply should be available and administered within 1 hour of the time ordered during normal pharmacy hours or within 2 hours if the pharmacy is closed. Anti-infectives, pain medications, antiemetics, antianxiety agents, antidiarrheals should be available and administered within 4 hours.

h. When drugs are removed from the original containers they should be maintained in environments insuring purity and potency up to the time of administration.

i. Procedures and equipment used in drug administration should provide for accurate drug dosage, identification and sanitation.

j. No doses should be charted before administration.

k. There should not be an unusually large amount of doses crushed.

l. The time interval between prescribed doses and actual administration should fall within a range of 2 hours.

m. A procedure for monitoring and recording medication errors should be implemented and adhered to.

5. *Stop Orders*

a. A stop-order policy should be sent to each physician on the staff.

b. A copy of the stop-order policy should be posted in the medicine room.

c. The stop-order procedures should be followed.

d. Stop orders should be in effect for all categories of drugs.

6. *Drug Returns*

a. Drug returns to the pharmacy should be documented in the facility.

7. *Medication Labels*

a. Medication labels should be prepared clearly and properly.

b. Medication labels should not be altered or reused.

c. Non-legend drugs should be labeled properly and stored in original manufacturer's container.

d. The procedure for updating medication labels should be followed.

8. *Storage of Drugs*

a. Test reagents, germicides, disinfectants and other household substances which are considered poisons should be stored separately, away from medications.

b. The utility room or cabinet containing commercial poisons and cleaning supplies should be locked.

c. Medications for external use only should be stored separately, away from medications for internal use.

d. The proper temperature (59–80°F) should be maintained in the medication room or drug cabinet.

e. Medications should be stored in a locked cabinet or room that is not accessible to patients or visitors.

f. Keys to the medicine room or drug cabinet should be under the control of the medicine nurse.

g. Unauthorized personnel should not be permitted to enter or use the drug-storage areas.

h. Drug administration areas should be lighted well.

i. Medication counters in the drug room or drug cabinets should be clean and uncluttered.

j. A metric-apothecary conversion chart should be posted in the medication storage area.

k. Discontinued drug containers should be marked properly, stored and appropriately disposed of.

l. Non-drug items should not be stored in the drug storage area.

m. Medications should be stored in the original containers.

n. Amber or glass bottles or other special containers should be used for certain medications to prevent deterioration.

o. Ophthalmic, otic and nasal medications should be stored separately and away from internal medications.

p. Medications for the same patient should be kept together.

q. There should be no excessive quantities of drugs.

r. There should be no prepackaging of bulk or house drug supplies.

s. The emergency medication box should be stored in an area known to all personnel handling medications.

t. No drugs requiring refrigeration should be in the cabinet of the drug room.

u. The proper temperature (36–46°F) for refrigerator items should be maintained.

v. Only drugs requiring refrigeration should be kept in the refrigerator.

w. Outdated drugs should be removed from the refrigerator.

9. *Emergency Drug Supply*

a. A list of the contents of the emergency medication box should be posted near the telephone at the nursing station and on the outside of the box itself.

b. The emergency medication box should be sealed properly.

c. The emergency medication box drugs should not be expired.

d. Use of any emergency medications should be recorded properly in a log book.

e. Staff physician should be informed in writing regarding use of emergency drug supply.

10. *Drug Disposal*

a. Drugs other than controlled substances under Schedules I, II, III and IV should be destroyed in the facility by the registered nurse in charge of the station and one other licensed nurse or pharmacist.

b. Drug disposal should be documented properly.

c. Discontinued drugs should be identified properly and stored in the medication area.

d. Discontinued drugs not reordered within 90 days should be removed from the cabinet and disposed of.

11. *Discharge Medications*

a. All medications sent with patient on discharge should have been ordered properly by the physician.

b. All medications sent with the patient on discharge should be recorded properly in the patient's health record.

c. All discharge medications should be labeled properly.

12. *"Pass" Medications*

a. All medications sent with the patient on pass should have been ordered properly by the physician.

b. All medications sent with the patient on pass should have been recorded properly in the patient's health record.

c. All medications on pass should be labeled properly.

13. *Controlled Substances*

a. Controlled drugs should not be accessible to nonauthorized personnel.

b. Controlled drugs should be stored in a locked cabinet or drawer separate from non-controlled drugs.

c. Separate records should be maintained for controlled drugs.

d. Controlled drugs and records should be reconciled at least every 24 hours.

e. The procedure for discharge drugs should be followed properly and applied to controlled drugs.

f. Controlled drugs should be destroyed in the presence of a registered pharmacist and a registered nurse employed by the facility.

g. Proper records should be kept for controlled drugs destroyed in the facility.

14. *Bedside Medication*
a. The bedside storage of medications should not be limited if self-administration has been authorized by the physician and facility.
b. The bedside storage of medications should be ordered specifically by the patient's physician and approved by the facility.
c. Medications should be labeled properly.
d. The patient should be instructed properly on the use of bedside medications.
e. Use of bedside medication should be documented properly by the client/resident on a medication administration record.
f. Bedside medication for self-administration must be stored in the resident's room in a locked storage cabinet.

15. *Physician Drug Samples*
a. Physician drug samples should not be used.

16. *Investigational Drugs*
a. The procedure for use of investigational drugs should be strictly adhered to.

17. *Reference Sources and Texts*
a. Each nursing station should have a current edition of *The Physicians' Desk Reference, Facts and Comparisons* and of the *AHFS Drug Information* or equivalent source material.

18. *Equipment and Supplies*
a. The nursing station should have adequate supplies for proper storage and administration of medications.

Considerations in Providing Pharmaceutical Care and Services for the Elderly

In order to review patient drug regimens effectively and serve on committees in a long-term care facility, a pharmacist should understand the nature of the geriatric patient. Physiologic changes that commonly occur with age may render the elderly less able to cope with bodily stresses and may affect drug therapy. Various diseases not only occur more frequently in the elderly but the presentation of the disease may be different from that in younger age groups. Pharmacodynamic and pharmacokinetic profiles of agents may be altered; also, drug toxicity, side effects and interactions appear to be more frequent and more severe in the elderly. Thus, the risk-to-benefit relationship of particular therapeutic choices is altered with age in many cases.

Physiological Variables in the Elderly

Physical Appearance

Most obvious to the pharmacist are physiological changes in the elderly that alter their appearance. Dehydration of vertebral discs and development of kyphosis result in a loss of height of approximately 2 inches between ages 20 and 70, and a change in posture. A decrease in total body weight usually occurs after age 65 and is accompanied by a marked change in the ratio of lean body mass to fat. A 25 to 30% loss of lean body mass results in changes in body contours and more noticeable bony prominences. The lean body mass loss is replaced by increased fat content of the body, primarily in the area of the hips, pelvis and umbilicus. Loss of subcutaneous supportive tissues with age results in thin, dry skin and ecchymoses with minor trauma; simultaneous loss of cells results in atrophy and wrinkling of the skin. The edentulous state, common in the elderly, may result in resorption of the mandible. Hair patterns change as a result of variations in hormonal and cellular activity and there is generalized thinning and a decreased quantity of hair.

Body Composition

Except for changes in lean body mass and fat, other changes in body composition occurring in the elderly are not obvious. Total body water decreases by approximately 25 to 30%, the majority due to intracellular water loss. However, plasma and extracellular fluid volumes also decrease and these changes may affect distribution of drugs in the body. Cell solids, including elements such as potassium, decrease to the same extent as lean body mass. Hypokalemia is common in the elderly, especially with diuretic therapy. Bone mass decreases approximately 1%, with an accompanying loss of calcium. This loss of calcium predisposes the patient to osteoporosis. With loss of lean body mass, an individual's need for energy-producing food is reduced.

Organ Function

Vital to the understanding of the changes in the elderly that may affect drug therapy is the concept of chronologically altered organ function. These changes, which occur in the absence of disease as it is now understood, are thought to result either from decreases in organ cell populations, oxygen consumption and/or blood flow, or a change in the character of organ tissue, such as that which results from a deposition of collagen fibers.

The eyes undergo many changes with age. Arcus senilis, a yellowish white opaque deposition around the periphery of the iris, is found in approximately 40% of the elderly but does not impair vision. The most common change in vision in the elderly is presbyopia which results from a diminished ability of the lens to focus at different distances and requires approximately 90% of the elderly to wear glasses. Senile cataracts, almost always bilateral, result in opacification. Senile macular degeneration may be due to ischemic changes in the retina and may cause blindness in the elderly. With the increased size of the aged lens, the anterior chamber of the eye becomes smaller and the angle between the root of the iris and the corneoscleral posterior surface becomes more acute and should result in increased pressure in the eye. However, resultant glaucoma occurs only in approximately 5% of the elderly due to the decreased production in aqueous humour that occurs after age 50.

Ear-function changes also occur in the elderly with presbycusis, a slow, progressive loss of hearing involving various parts of the hearing system, the most common hearing abnormality. Onset of presbycusis is usually in the seventh decade and results in interference with selectivity of hearing and conversation comprehension.

Many changes occur in the cardiovascular system with age. A decrease in the cardiac output of approximately 40% occurs by age 65. Systemic arterial pressure increases, the systolic increasing to a greater extent than the diastolic. These blood pressure changes often result in hypertrophy of the heart secondary to the increased workload placed on it. Atherosclerosis increases with age with an increased collagen and calcium content of blood vessels and a resultant decreased resilience. The increased atherosclerosis contributes to the increase in blood pressure and *vice versa*. Postural hypotension occurs frequently in the elderly. In one survey of elderly ambulant individuals, 24% showed a postural decrease in systolic blood pressure of 20 torr or more and 5% a decrease of 40 torr or more. This altered compensation by the cardiovascular system for postural change is due to impairment of the baroreceptor reflex. The distribution of peripheral blood flow in the elderly favors coronary, cerebral and skeletal circulations at the expense of visceral, hepatic and renal flow.

The respiratory system also undergoes changes with age. An increased lung collagen content results in loss of elasticity and a resultant decrease in vital and total lung capacities. A progressive increase in the number of alveoli supplied with less than an optimal quantity of pulmonary capillary blood flow occurs. The dimensions of the thoracic cage increase, resulting in hyperinflation. A decrease in the number and activity of cilia as well as decreased efficiency of contraction of the expiratory muscles, which makes coughing more difficult, results in decreased ability to clear mucous secretions.

Renal function decreases with age. The number of functioning nephrons decreases but, because of the large reserve in renal function, this within itself does not pose a major problem. However, coupled with decreased renal blood flow of approximately 50 to 60% by age 70, there is a marked decrease in glomerular filtration rate of between 20 and 50%. This drop in glomerular filtration rate may not be mirrored adequately by the creatinine clearance as 24-hr creatinine excretion decreases by 50% from the 3rd to the 9th decade of life. The serum creatinine is thus not a reliable indicator of changes in creatinine clearance across age groups and in the aged. A normal serum creatinine of 1 mg/dL may correspond to a creatinine clearance of 120 mL/min at age 20 but only 60 mL/min at age 80. Age adjusted nomograms for estimation of creatinine clearance from serum creatinine have been developed. In addition, alterations in respiratory and renal function in the elderly make them less capable of correcting acid-base insults.

Gastrointestinal changes with age include a decrease in peristaltic activity and a diminished defecation reflex. There is also a decrease in intestinal blood flow, a decrease in the volume and acidity of gastric secretions and atrophy and deterioration of the colonic musculature with thinning of the intestinal walls. After age 50, pear-shaped diverticula form which, with poor elimination, can become filled with fecal masses and lead to irritation, infection and diverticulitis. Changes in liver anatomy and function occur late in the aging process. A decrease in liver size is noted after the age of 70. Most liver functions, as measured by plasma bilirubin or plasma enzyme concentrations, remain within normal limits and the reserve capacity of the liver is not compromised severely. A notable exception to this, however, might be drug metabolism enzymes due to the postulated decreased activity of the cytochrome P-450 system and the decreased hepatic blood flow with age.

Endocrine changes noted with time include decreases in glucose tolerance, synthesis and release of insulin and production of thyroid hormone. In addition, there is a change in the anabolic/catabolic ratio of hormones due to a significant decrease in gonadal steroids. Anabolic steroid activity is decreased to 65% with age, while catabolic steroid activity is decreased only 20%. Such changes, in part, account for the osteoporosis seen in the elderly. Loss of calcium is most marked in the postmenopausal female, and resultant fractures may occur spontaneously or with very minor trauma. The activity of the renin-angiotensin-aldosterone system also decreases with age. Also, reduced responsiveness to adrenergic stimuli has been observed in the elderly.

With age, there is a 30% decrease in brain tissue as well as a 30% decrease in nerve conduction velocity. As a result there is a slowing of reflexes and decreased speed of muscle contraction. The central nervous system threshold for excitability and inhibition are reduced, as are perhaps the concentrations of neurotransmitters. Body thermal regulation is impaired. Pain and taste sensations are diminished. In addition, the cardiac conduction system undergoes degeneration.

The immune system responds more slowly and less vigorously in a geriatric patient. Alterations in white blood cell function and reductions in IgG and IgM concentrations have been noted in older individuals.

With all the decreases in organ function occurring over time, the body becomes less able to compensate for stress due to the loss of its reserve capacity. Many of the changes cited predispose the elderly patient to pathologic insults such as infections or fractures which may have devastating results due to the diminished reserve capacity. Drug therapy for these disorders may bear greater risks due to the altered organ function.

Disease Considerations

To perform drug-regimen reviews in any setting, the pharmacist must understand the pathophysiology of disease (see Chapter 40). A detailed review of the numerous diseases that may be found in the elderly is beyond the scope of this chapter. However, for the pharmacist monitoring patients in a long-term care facility, it is important to highlight selected aspects of geriatric diseases.

The symptoms and presentation of a myocardial infarction in the elderly may be very different from those in a younger patient. Classical chest-pain syndromes occur in only approximately one-third of patients with otherwise atypical presentations including acute confusion, severe dyspnea, severe hypotension and vomiting, and weakness being the norm. Bradycardias, Adams-Stokes attacks and cardiac arrhythmias, often asymptomatic, are common. The classical signs and symptoms of congestive heart failure and pulmonary embolism frequently are altered or absent in the elderly and one's index of suspicion must be high.

The management of hypertension in the elderly is a very controversial topic. Patients with diastolic blood pressure greater than 95 torr show mortality rates that increase beyond age 65 for cardiovascular-related death. Thus, classical hypertension is no less a risk factor for those over age 65 and treatment appears effective. Malignant hypertension is rare in the elderly. The bulk of the controversy exists around the management of pure systolic hypertension whose prevalence rises markedly with age. Systolic hypertension has been related to increased morbidity and mortality. The value of treating systolic hypertension in the elderly has been demonstrated. Therefore, the management and investigation of hypertension in the elderly should be carried out but therapy also should be tailored to the individual.

Aged persons with hypertension often manifest diffuse arteriosclerotic disease including the vessels of the head and neck. Treatment of hypertension in such patients may result in sharp reduction in blood pressure associated with syncope, which may lead to injurious falls. In such cases, blood pressure should be reduced gradually with cautious initial dosing. The elderly are more susceptible to complications from diuretics, such as hypokalemia and dehydration, especially when intercurrent illness decreases oral intake. The antihypertensive and central nervous system depressant effects of methyldopa, reserpine and clonidine are greater. Use of beta-blockers often is contraindicated by other concomitant disorders and some investigators report diminished antihypertensive effects in the elderly. Use of reserpine is discouraged in the elderly due to the insidious form of psychic depression which may occur, as is use of guanethidine due to its propensity to cause orthostatic hypotension. The use of calcium channel blockers and angiotensin-converting enzyme inhibitors often are effective and have minimal side effects. It should be recalled that even when diastolic pressure is suitably reduced, a significant systolic elevation may remain. In such cases, a compromise of a slightly higher than desired blood pressure should be accepted.

Peripheral vascular disorders often are seen in the elderly. Peripheral arterial disease is usually unresponsive to vasodilator therapy and, if severe, may lead to gangrene and necessitate amputation. Recent reports indicate that calcium channel blocking agents such as nifedipine may be beneficial medical therapy. Chronic stasis ulcers and deep vein thrombosis also are encountered frequently.

Certain infectious diseases are common and have unique features in the aged. Elderly patients may be predisposed to pneumonias due to decreased immune response, decreased ciliary activity and potential predisposition to aspiration as a result of concomitant strokes, decreased cough reflex and impaired swallowing. The classic picture of lobar pneumonia with abrupt onset of fever and signs of lung consolidation is very much the exception. The elderly patient often has an insidious onset of pneumonia which presents as increasing lassitude, apathy, decreased mobility and, thus, no specific localizing symptoms or signs. Confusion may be the key sign in such cases. The use of pneumococcal vaccine may be of great benefit in the elderly. Influenza, though relatively benign in younger age groups, may cause great morbidity and mortality in the elderly, due to diminished ability to respond to stress. Prophylactic vaccination with influenza vaccine is of great importance in this high-risk group. Incidence of urinary tract infections increases with age in both men and women. Some causes for this include immobility, which may lead to constipation with resultant contamination of the perineum and urethral orifice in the female; increased residual urine volumes secondary to neurogenic bladder or prostatic hypertrophy changes in men; prostatectomy with loss of the antibacterial prostatic substance and use of indwelling catheters. Acute infections should be treated as in the younger patient. Catheters should be avoided where possible; if needed due to incontinence, proper care is vital to limit potential infections. Chronic bacteriuria in the elderly appears to be a relatively benign process which does not lead to renal failure.

Disorders of the gastrointestinal tract commonly seen in the elderly include oral moniliasis, dysphagia, hiatal hernia, achlorhydria, peptic ulcer, diverticulosis, ischemic colitis and cancer of the alimentary tract, the latter being one of the commonest causes of death in the very old. Anemia, weight loss and vague upper abdominal pain are common signs of peptic ulcer disease which warrants vigorous evaluation. One-third of all gastric ulcer deaths occur in the elderly; associated perforation and peritonitis may develop in the absence of classical signs and symptoms. Constipation is not a consequence of old age *per se* but is common in the elderly due to decrease in both mobility and dietary fiber consumption.

Evaluation of mental confusion is very important in the elderly. Though dementia of the Alzheimer type is common, other causes which must be evaluated before this diagnosis is entertained include depression, drug therapy, infections, cerebral hypoxia and metabolic disorders. Cerebral arteriosclerosis often leads to dementia, apraxia and parkinsonism though the latter may be due to other causes. Transient ischemic attacks, drop attacks, strokes and temporal arteritis are common disorders; the drop attacks account for about 20% of fractures of the femur in the aged.

Common bone diseases include osteoporosis, osteomalacia and Paget's disease. The osteomalacia may be due to poor intake of vitamin D coupled with inadequate exposure to sunlight. Postmenopausal estrogen replacement therapy and dietary calcium and fluoride supplementation have been advocated to prevent development of osteoporosis. Fractures are very slow in healing in the aged. Rheumatoid arthritis can start acutely in the elderly or be present in a "burned out" form. However, osteoarthritis, a degenerative joint disease, is much more common. The use of aspirin can produce tinnitus and further compromise high frequency hearing loss in the elderly.

Thyroid disease is not uncommon in old age. Apathetic thyrotoxicosis, a disease of elderly women is characterized by loss of weight, apathy and depression in the absence of clinical signs of thyroid disorder. Diabetes mellitus is common in the elderly. Diabetic ketoacidosis is uncommon but hyperglycemic hyperosmolar, nonketotic coma occasionally develops.

Though red-cell life span and morphology do not change with age, iron deficiency anemia due to blood loss, malabsorption or malnutrition, megaloblastic anemia due to folate and vitamin B_{12} deficiencies and the anemia of chronic disease are common in the elderly.

Urinary and fecal incontinence are frequent maladies in the elderly. Causes for urinary incontinence include: stress incontinence in the female, often associated with age-related changes in the urethra; benign prostatic hypertrophy in the male; fecal impaction with a low-capacity bladder or chronic retention with outflow incontinence; bladder carcinoma; renal calculi; urinary tract infections and impaired neurologic control. Management requires correction of the cause, if possible, with anticholinergic agents occasionally providing some relief. Anticholinergic agents are not without toxicity, especially in the elderly, and should be used carefully. Indwelling catheters should be avoided if possible, but often are required. Fecal incontinence may result from constipation, laxative abuse, drug reactions, diseases of the large bowel and impaired neurologic control of defecation. In both types of incontinence, special patient padding should be used to minimize irritation and effects of moisture on the surrounding skin as this may predispose to decubitus ulcers.

Many geriatric patients require chronic bedrest. Because of their immobility, these patients are more predisposed to complications such as pneumonia, thrombophlebitis, pulmonary embolism, micturition and defecation problems, muscle wasting, stiffness, contractures, accelerated calcium excretion and decubitus ulcers. Decubitus ulcers are localized areas of cellular necrosis commonly called "bed sores" or pressure sores. It has been estimated that approximately one-third of bedridden geriatric patients have pressure sores.

The cause of decubitus ulcers is compression of the skin and subcutaneous tissue severe enough to impair local blood circulation. A pathological sequence of erythema, induration and necrosis results. Bedridden patients are unable to move and thereby remove pressure from a given area. Certain tissues have enhanced pressure on them, such as those which overlie bony prominences (the sacrum, the heels and buttocks) and those under compressing surfaces (chairs, beds, casts, braces, tight dressings and other factors). Poor hygiene, poor nutrition, use of sedating medications, edema, fever and anemia may enhance decubitus ulcer formation. Moisture secondary to excessive perspiration and incontinence may predispose to tissue breakdown. Good nursing care, using special devices (eg, water-support mattresses) to relieve the pressure on certain areas of the patient, is vital to prevent tissue breakdown. Excellent reviews on the prevention and treatment of decubitus ulcers have been published.

Geriatric Pharmacology

The vast majority of studies on drug effects, kinetics and other factors have been carried out in young, healthy volunteers. Little research has been done in the field of geriatric clinical pharmacology to date. Currently, the FDA is assessing the need for additional information about the action of a drug in the elderly patient. The New Drug Application process is likely to be modified to require dosing guidelines for the aged. This field offers great opportunity to the clinical pharmacist investigator. Aspects of what is now known about drug therapy changes with age will be reviewed.

Absorption

The increased pH of the gastrointestinal tract with age could alter drug ionization and solubility, and the decreased blood flow to the gastrointestinal tract could decrease the rate and extent of drug absorption. Likewise, a decreased absorption surface, the decreased physical activity of the elderly as well as the increased incidence of diverticular disease may predispose to problems in drug absorption. However, little research has been done to document such changes. Decreased absorption has been noted for compounds which undergo active transport, such as iron, thiamine, calcium, galactose and glucose. However, acidic drugs undergoing passive diffusion, such as acetaminophen, phenylbutazone and sulfamethizole, have not been shown to have significant changes in the time to peak plasma levels. Basic drugs such as diazepam, levodopa, pentazocine and amitriptyline may undergo gastric absorption and may have decreased absorption as a result of gastric changes. Sustained-release preparations of drugs have not been tested adequately in the geriatric patient and erratic absorption and therapeutic effects may result. Acid-labile compounds, such as potassium penicillin G, may actually reach higher levels in geriatric patients because of increased pH in the gastrointestinal tract. Overall, changes in drug absorption appear to be the least important of age-related changes in pharmacological action.

Distribution

A drug's distribution in the body is determined by its binding characteristics to plasma proteins, red blood cells and other body tissues, the distribution of systemic blood flow and microcirculation and the ability of the drug to pass through various membranes. Serum albumin decreases with age, with a concomitant rise in the globulin-protein fraction. This decrease is more likely the result of disease and immobility, than a function of age *per se;* however, a disturbance in the normal metabolic response to a decreased albumin pool also has been noted. Acidic drugs bind mainly to albumin, and decreases in protein binding as a function of age have been reported with warfarin and phenytoin. The character of protein-binding seems qualitatively the same as in younger individuals. Basic drugs bind primarily to α_1-acid glycoprotein whose concentration is unchanged by age *per se* but is increased as an acute phase reactant in inflammatory disease or myocardial infarction. Concomitant renal disease and drug interactions may further alter drug-binding capacity in the elderly. Unfortunately, most pharmacokinetic studies evaluate total rather than free drug clearance, but free clearance actually determines the steady-state concentration of pharmacologically active unbound drug.

Body fat content increases with age; if a drug is highly lipid-soluble, it may become localized in body fat. Thus, the volume of distribution of drugs such as diazepam, chlorpromazine, barbiturates and glutethimide may be increased in the elderly. Drugs distributed mainly in body water and lean body mass might have higher blood levels in the elderly, particularly if the dose is based on total body weight or surface area; examples are ethanol and lidocaine.

The decrease in cardiac output with age results in a decrease in systemic perfusion but, as noted previously, the reduction of blood flow to various organs is not symmetric; redistribution in favor of cerebral and coronary circulations takes place at the expense of flow to the kidney and liver, which are important organs in drug elimination. Likewise, the ability of a drug to pass through various membranes may ultimately affect its drug action. Increased uptake of morphine in the brain of aged rats may reflect increased permeability of the blood-brain barrier. The amount of local anesthetics needed to produce a desired level of segmental anesthesia after injection into the spinal extradural space has been found to be much less in older patients. This may be explained on the basis of age-related changes in connective tissue and increased permeability of the nerve integuments, resulting in greater drug sensitivity.

Metabolism

Animal studies have shown decreased activity in drug-metabolizing enzymes which has been associated with increases in the serum levels and the intensity and duration of pharmacologic effect of some drugs. Several drugs which undergo hepatic microsomal oxidation have been reported to exhibit reduced clearances in the elderly; these include antipyrine, chlordiazepoxide, diazepam, quinidine, theophylline and nortriptyline. However, conflicting reports make some of this information difficult to interpret; important factors such as cigarette smoking and nutritional status have not been controlled adequately. A significant prolongation of the $t_{1/2}$ of acetanilid versus no age-related increase in the $t_{1/2}$ of isoniazid suggests that liver function does not decline uniformly with age and that while microsomal enzyme pathways may decrease with time, hepatic acetylation may be unaffected. Likewise, the inducibility of drug metabolizing enzymes declines with age. Thus, the effects of aging on the metabolism of a given drug is complex and difficult to predict.

Hepatic blood flow is decreased secondary to the decreased cardiac output with age. Another important component of the metabolizing capacity of the elderly may be their decreased level of activity. Compounds with high hepatic extraction ratios, such as propranolol and indocyanine green, have reduced clearances in the elderly. Fourfold increases in plasma propranolol levels after a single 40-mg dose have been noted in elderly subjects, compared to young individuals.

Excretion

Altered renal function is probably the single most important factor responsible for higher drug levels in an aging population. As noted previously, renal function declines with age; on the average, the decline is approximately 1.5% per year from ages 25 to 65. Also, the serum creatinine level is not a reliable indicator of renal function in the aged. Drugs primarily excreted by the renal route and having a narrow therapeutic index, such as digoxin and the aminoglycoside antibiotics, have been shown to have higher levels in the elderly. The half-life of digoxin has been shown to increase as much as 40% in the elderly, with a decline in creatinine clearance. An important corollary is that many elderly patients are put on digitalis during transient periods of congestive heart failure, secondary to fluid overload and other factors, and then subsequently maintained on digitalis. Studies have shown that such patients can be withdrawn safely from digoxin therapy. Elderly patients also are predisposed to developing alkaline urine. This is due to decreased consumption of protein due to economic factors, with resultant decreased excretion of amino acids, and the catheterizations and other procedures in the elderly which predispose to urinary tract infections with urea-splitting organisms. The end result may be enhanced reabsorption of basic drugs such as the tricyclic antidepressants.

Alteration in Receptor Site Action

Receptor sites for drugs also may be altered in the elderly. A decrease in the number of CNS receptors has been postulated for some drugs. CNS stimulants show decreased activity in the elderly, while CNS depressants show increased activity. Barbiturates may be more likely to cause paradoxical stimulation in the elderly as a result. Atropine's positive chronotropic activity decreases with increasing age, which is thought to be a result of altered receptor site activity. Propranolol reduces the heart rate and cardiac output during exercise, but to a lesser extent in subjects aged 50 to 65 years, than in subjects aged 20 to 35 years. The sympathetic response of the heart elicited by the stimulus of exercise declines with age. Though the reason for this is not clear, reduced numbers of α_2 receptors on platelets and β- receptors on lymphocytes have been demonstrated in the elderly.

Geriatric Predisposition to Adverse Drug Reactions and Interactions

Various factors predispose the elderly to adverse drug reactions and drug interactions. The age-related changes in organ function previously reviewed may alter drug disposition and activity. In this regard, the side effects of digoxin, lidocaine, propranolol, tricyclic antidepressants, benzodiazepines, sedative-hypnotics, antipsychotics, aminoglycoside antibiotics, meperidine, phenytoin and heparin have been noted more frequently in the elderly.

In addition, the elderly suffer from numerous diseases. One autopsy study showed that in 40 patients over 90 years of age, 498 pathological lesions were identified for an average of 12.5 lesions per patient. In many cases, these lesions affected the liver or the kidney and thus had great potential effect on drug elimination. Multiple pathologies may lead to numerous patient complaints. The temptation on the part of the physician is to treat symptomatology with a large number of medications; polypharmacy is very common in the elderly.

As noted previously, patients over age 65 make up 11.6% of the population in the US, but the same group receives 31% of all prescription medications. Patients in long-term facilities account for the majority of such prescription use. The average nursing home patient may receive 5 to 9 medications, while some have been noted to receive as many as 16 medications concomitantly. As a result, medication errors are more common and the number of errors increases with the number and frequency of medication administration.

Thus, it is no wonder drug reactions and medication errors occur more frequently in the elderly; a 10 to 18% incidence of adverse drug reactions has been estimated in institutionalized patients. Drug-related fatalities also have been noted. The incidence of adverse effects has been correlated with age with an increased incidence in the 6th to 8th decade.

As a result of the number of drugs patients receive, the incidence of drug interactions increases. In one study, 49% of nursing home patients had the potential for at least one drug interaction. In another study of 7 nursing homes, 124 of 130 patients had a potential interaction. Chapter 105 reviews drug interactions and the reader is referred to the combinations which are common in the geriatric patient.

As general guidelines, pharmacists should try to insure that the minimal number of drugs and the lowest dosage necessary are being employed by long-term facility care prescribers. The doses the elderly require are often lower than those needed by the younger patient.

CHAPTER 99

The Pharmacist and Public Health

Ara H Der Marderosian, PhD
Professor of Pharmacognosy and Research Professor of Medicinal Chemistry
Philadelphia College of Pharmacy and Science
Philadelphia, PA 19104

Public health and its future during the 1990s has been the subject of concern by many. Breslow[1] pointed out that some have developed a growing perception that the US has lost sight of its public health goals and has allowed the system of public health activities to fall into disarray. Originally public health was established to handle epidemics of acute communicable disease, endemic tuberculosis and very high levels of infant and maternal mortality which were prevalent during the late 1800s and early 1900s. Much of the problem in these times related to lack of sanitation, overcrowding and a general lack of appreciating simple rules of hygiene.

At the beginning there was much support, socially and politically, to address these difficulties. The vast resources of the federal, state and local governments were brought to bear (legislation, regulations, enforcement, nursing, maternal and child care, etc) and by the mid-1900s most of these problems were solved. However, by the 1960s up to now, whole new sets of problems emerged which quickly disabled existing public health resources. These included many unsolvable difficulties of a chronic nature such as cancer epidemics and heart disease, as well as environmental (disposal of toxic wastes) and social problems (care of the elderly, teenage pregnancy and drug abuse). For various reasons this caused many health departments to merge with social welfare agencies with concomitant neglect of public health functions in favor of welfare needs and income maintenance.

Generally, legislators bypassed the public health infrastructure to create new and separate agencies for everything from occupational safety and health to environmental protection and everything in between (water quality, air pollution, etc).

All of this created confusion in the public health community as to its roles and functions. Based on a 1988 report by the Institute of Medicine (IOM) committee entitled *The Future of Public Health*, this was defined as "fulfilling society's interest in assuring conditions in which people can be healthy." Ultimately, the states had to take on this major responsibility with the Federal Government's support, *viz* formulation of objectives, stimulate attention to these, provide financial and technical assistance and adopt interstate health-relevant regulations. However, recent political, economic and social problems have not allowed the public health agencies to gain back their original responsibilities fully.

It is hoped that this will redevelop during the 1990s with at least five major issues needing resolution. These include the functional and structural reconstitution of public health into a coherent pattern instead of a continued drift towards fragmentation, the full national setting of public health objectives with support to achieve the full potential, the shift from disease control to health promotion, the overcoming of long-standing gross inequities (poverty, racism) in health and the full use of accelerating developments in health technology while minimizing the health consequences of industrial advancement.

As time has progressed during the last few decades, it has become more obvious that traditional acute "sickness" services are limited in terms of overall improvement in national health status. This fact has driven all health professionals to the common goal of disease prevention and health promotion or "wellness." Generally, the "clinical" direction of pharmacy has de-emphasized manipulative, product oriented and distributive skills and focused more on "public-health" awareness. Today the pharmacist's attention is directed towards the patient, his environment and his state of general well-being. However, there remains a considerable amount of work to be done in terms of specifically defining and spelling out the role of pharmacy in public health.

Renewed hope appears for major advances in health policy for the US. There continues to be long-cycle theories of social policy as may be seen in the 30-year pattern of Social Security in 1935, Medicare in 1965 and the prospect for action from the 103rd Congress, which may take effect in 1995 for comprehensive health care and public health reform. Certainly, further procrastination will leave many citizens in the US without adequate health coverage and will further burden the economy with its continuing upward spiral of health-care costs.

The current administration has included *Prevention* as one of its primary elements of health policy. The public health community should assure that prevention modalities include both clinical preventive services (community- and office-based) and the population-based public health programs which correspond broadly to the objectives of the HHS *Healthy People 1990* and *Healthy People 2000* reports.

A private/public sector organization, the Partnership for Prevention, the new Advisory Committee to the Director of the Centers for Disease Control and the academic and practice organizations participating in the Council for Linkages between Academia and Public Health Practice all endorsed the concept that private and public payers for medical care also should join to support the *traditional* public health services, strengthened and modified to increase their effectiveness.[2]

The HHS report, *Healthy People 2000* identifies three national health goals which are to increase the span of healthy life, reduce health disparities among Americans and achieve access to preventive services for all Americans. Detailed in the report are 300 specific objectives for health-promotion and disease-prevention programs with quantitative targets to be achieved by the year 2000.

Stoto[3] proposed several new parameters which need to be assessed in public health studies for the future. These include proper assessment, statistical uniformity, specification of individual objectives in surveys, appropriate interpretation of trends, standardization of rates and appropriate health status indicators. Table 1[3] shows proposed health status indicators.

It was not until 1972 and 1973 that Gibson[4] undertook a survey of public-health instruction in colleges of pharmacy and published his findings in the *American Journal of Pharmaceutical Education*. Basically, he found that there was a lack of definition of public health in pharmacy, a lack of perceived relevance to pharmacy, a lack of a text focusing in on the role of pharmacy in public health, a lack of faculty qualified to teach the subject and a lack of sites where students could become involved with public-health projects and personnel. This continues in the 1990s.

By the early 1980s, several authors have continued to promote the importance and need for increased involvement of pharmacists in public health and by the end of this decade considerable progress has been made. This has been summa-

Table 1—Proposed Health Status Indicators[3]

Infants (Under 1 year)
- Deaths: Infant mortality rate (9.1 deaths of infants under 1 year per 1000 live births in 1990)
- Low birth weight: Births of babies weighing less than 2500 g (6.9% of live births)
- Prenatal care: Proportion of infants born to women who received prenatal care in the first trimester of pregnancy (76%)

Children (Ages 1–14)
- Deaths from injury: Death rate for accidents, homicide, and suicide combined (16.6 deaths per 100,000 children ages 1–14)
- Immunization: Proportion of children ages 1–4 reported immunized for measles, rubella, DPT, polio, and mumps (55.3–64.9% for each immunization separately in 1985)
- Toxic exposures: Prevalence of blood lead levels exceeding 15 μg/dL among children ages 6 months through 5 years (15.4 per 100,000 in 1984)

Adolescents/Young Adults (Ages 15–24)
- Deaths from injury: Death rate for accidents, homicide, and suicide combined (75.8 deaths per 100,000 persons ages 15–24)
- Teenage childbearing: Birth rate at ages 15–17 (33.8 live births per 1000 women ages 15–17 in 1988)
- Use of dangerous substances: Proportion of adolescents ages 12–17 who used the following substances in the month
  - Tobacco: (12% in 1990)
  - Alcohol: (25% in 1990)
  - Cocaine: (0.6% in 1990)
- Sexually transmitted diseases: Incidence of gonorrhea (1123 cases reported per 100,000 adolescents ages 15–19 in 1989)

Adults (Ages 25–64)
- Premature chronic disease mortality: Death rate for cancer, heart disease, stroke, and diabetes combined (264.5 deaths per 100,000 persons ages 25–64)
- AIDS/HIV: Incidence of AIDS (16.6 new cases reported per 100,000 persons ages 13 and over in 1990)
- Smoking: Prevalence of cigarette smoking (28.8% of current smokers among persons ages 20 and older)
- Nutrition/physical activity: Prevalence of overweight (21% of persons ages 18 and over with body mass index greater than 27.8 kg/m(2) for men and 27.3 kg/m(2) for women)
- Workplace injury: Incidence of injuries resulting in medical treatment, lost time from work, or restricted work activity (8.1 cases per 100 full-time workers)
- Chronic disease screening:
  - Breast cancer: Proportion of women ages 50 and over who received a clinical breast exam and a mammogram within the preceding year (19%)
  - Serum cholesterol: Proportion of persons ages 18 and over who have ever had their blood cholesterol level checked (59% in 1988)

Older Adults (Ages 65 and over)
- Activity restrictions: Proportion of the noninstitutionalized population age 65 and over with partial or complete limitation of major activity from chronic conditions (22.8% in 1989)
- Disabling injury: Incidence of hip fractures (714 hospital discharges per 100,000 persons age 65 and over in 1988)
- Immunization: Proportion of persons ages 65 and over who receive an influenza vaccination in the preceding 12 months (34%)
- Dental health: Proportion of persons ages 65 and over who have lost all of their natural teeth (36% in 1986)

rized in at least two pertinent articles. One of these is the policy statement (8024 (pp)) of the American Public Health Association which focused on the role of the pharmacist in public health[5] and the other is a booklet edited by Bush, entitled *The Pharmacist Role in Disease Prevention and Health Promotion.* In the former publication there is a statement of the problem (underutilization of the patient-oriented pharmacist), a purpose (the need to maximize the use of existing health-care professionals and facilities) and positions and recommendations (identify current and future roles for pharmacists in public health, provide essential background information about these roles and describe means of implementing or maximizing these functions).

The policy statement provides rather detailed suggestions and identifies the need for "public-health pharmacists," the need for public-health education and role models and the recognition of levels of pharmacist public health activities (eg, micro level, such as speaking to community groups on drug topics and providing hypertension screening, and macro level, such as health planning, evaluation and administration). The mission of public health is defined further as being directed on four fronts including public-health-service delivery, protecting the community against environmental hazards, assisting and reinforcing the community health-care provider system and assisting individuals (consumers) to achieve optimal health status through promoting medical self-help principles.

A particular set of functions for public health and pharmacists'[4] services is given and these include planning for health care for wide geographic areas or communities; managing, administering and evaluating health-care programs, systems and facilities; providing direct-person health-care service (eg, education, maternal and child care, etc) and environmental health; developing and promoting legislation, and deriving regulations pertaining to the public's health; and training health-care workers needed to carry out these functions. While listing these functions, the policy statement does state that, in a few cases, pharmacists have asserted themselves and have established a functional capacity in public health, however, they note that these are exceptions rather than the rule.

In regard to such issues as expenditures for drugs and payment sources, the location and use of health-care facilities and providers, the selection of strategies for health improvement and specific health problems of the community, the policy statement emphasizes that community pharmacists are an underutilized source of factual and anecdotal health data which could assist health planners in these areas.

Health-planning bodies should initiate relationships with local pharmacists to provide epidemiological data on prescribing patterns, patterns of sickness and various socioeconomic factors related to prevalent disease states. Finally, the position paper encourages more exposure of pharmacists to public health in their training and to promote the pursuit of advanced degrees (MPH; DrPH) in schools of public health.

In the latter booklet edited by Bush, the role of the pharmacist in disease prevention and health promotion is taken to the level of actually documenting specific roles in several areas and providing specific articles and cases where pharmacists have shown leadership and significant contributions to the field of community health. This reference provides 12 chapters on the subject including an overall summary. These include an introduction and separate chapters on the role of the pharmacist in general and individual disease prevention and health promotion, community preventive health care, primary care, referral, health education, drug information, toxicology and health planning. The last two chapters cover documentation of pharmacist activities in these areas and competencies required for fulfilling these roles. As an overview coverage of this publication these facts have emerged:

Most pharmacy practitioners are employed in community pharmacies and evidence suggests that they have a significant impact on the health status of the nation's population.

However, the average pharmacist does not participate on a regular basis in community health-promoting activities.

Most of the authors in this publication point to a need to change education and incentive in the direction of public health.

At the managerial or macro level, pharmacists usually are salaried, and they work in private and public institutions, agencies and organizations which focus health care on defined population groups.

The macro-level pharmacist requires a wide breadth and depth of knowledge, usually administrative and organizational skills, eg, health planning, monitoring state medicaid drug programs, providing inservice education, developing health-promotional materials and planning community health campaigns. These require further education.

Currently, it is felt that pharmacy educators should focus on first developing micro-level community practitioners who will interface between fellow pharmacists and community health-planning agencies.

Currently, micro-level pharmacists frequently perform disease-preventing and health-promoting activities which include drug and nutrition counseling, hypertension screening, providing programs on weight control, allergies and proper use of prescribed and OTC medications, referring patients to specific health-care providers and taking drug and medical-problems histories. Some of this is beginning to emerge through federal programs which mandate pharmacists to consult with patients on drug and health matters.

The authors note that community activities, such as speaking to groups on health-related matters, referring patients to community agencies, participating in community based programs on sexually transmitted diseases, mental health, substance abuse, poisoning and cancer signals, are usually not regular activities of practicing pharmacists.

Among the conditions mitigating against pharmacists performing more public-health activities are education, incentives and regulations. However, all of these have improved in recent times.

Even though there are a relatively small number of mostly macro-level pharmacists, their numbers are increasing. Certainly micro-level activities have improved in the past 5 years. While most reimbursement remains product-related, there are trends which make it likely that pharmacists will increase their performance of activities described. These include innovative practice arrangements, drug-information newsletters and pharmacist participation in health fairs.

In a text on pharmacy practice, by Wertheimer and Smith, Bush and Johnson have written a chapter which continued the promotion of the concept of the public-health role of the pharmacist. In addition to the list of public/community activities which have been given above for pharmacists to be involved with, are increased involvement with immunization programs, substance abuse education and monitoring, sexually transmitted disease education, family planning, fluoridation, poison prevention, quackery, disaster preparedness and aversion, environmental protection, work place safety, peer review and health data collection.

Individual patient activities suggested for improvement are increased individual patient education, screening and referral, medication maintenance, compliance counseling, patient monitoring and family counseling. Their chapter concludes with specific suggestions on how the pharmacist generally should approach the responsibility of direct involvement in their patients' public health. Rightly so, they state that participation depends on the pharmacist's "state of mind." There should be a desire to provide these services. The patient's needs must be paramount and the service to be provided a real mission based on commitment.

Straightforward suggestions are given for self-motivated involvement in such existing agencies like the American Cancer Society and the Red Cross. Direct contact with local health departments and promotion of health-related programs based in professional societies such as the American Pharmaceutical Association are advised strongly. The pharmacist is urged strongly to volunteer services, share ideas and knowledge and be available for community health efforts. Initial involvement of a minor nature often leads to greater potential for future mutually beneficial public health endeavors.

While at present, remuneration for such service is difficult to attain directly, it promises to settle in place in future years. They remind pharmacists that the most important income may be "psychic income" and the basic reward of helping others. In this same text, Kilwein also provides information on the pharmacist and public health in a chapter entitled "Selected Readings." Here the author covers similar ground but also gives data on how pharmacists can become aware of sources of health data (Vital Registration System, System of Notifiable Disease Reports, Morbidity and Mortality Weekly Report, National Health Survey, etc) and how epidemiology plays an important part in overall public-health strategies. These references and the updated texts available in public health should continue to serve as guides for pharmacy opportunities in the next decade.

In today's shrunken world, health services must be viewed on all levels, from international to local. In mid-1984, cholera was occurring in 22 countries in the world; its incubation period is 2 to 3 days, and the flight time from anywhere in the world to the US is less than 48 hours. The inference is obvious—the person asking for Kaopectate in the neighborhood pharmacy may be a cholera victim. Insularity is no longer valid in public health—it never was, but today with short travel times and an increasing number of people travelling, it is even more important to be aware of the world picture of health and disease.

Historically speaking, public-health concerns remained dormant until cholera struck England and America in 1832, and the response to the urban environment of flies, filth and feces produced the "Great Sanitary Awakening" of the mid-19th century. The pioneers of this movement were not physicians; they were a lawyer, Edwin Chadwick (1800–1890) in Britain and a bookseller, Lemuel Shattuck (1793–1859), in America. The "Shattuck Report" to the Massachusetts Legislature in 1850 remains to this day the classic document of American public health[6]; many of its recommendations still await promulgation. By 1900, permanent health agencies had replaced *ad hoc* boards of health on a state and local level until, by World War I, an embryonic network of health departments was in existence throughout the US. Public-health programs slowly expanded as funds became available to support them; the unit to administer these programs was the city or county health department with its team of a doctor, a nurse, a sanitarian and a clerk—still the backbone of the local health department.

Prior to World War II, traditional programs formed the bulk of public health work: disposal of sewage, provision of pure water, communicable disease control and the care of mothers and infants, with health education as the main weapon of attack. This changed, however, with the advent of antibiotics and the expanded development of vaccines, both of which reduced the danger of infections. Chronic disease began to assume a major role in morbidity and mortality, and hospital care replaced care in the home. Comparable changes in public health accelerated as federal funding increased, until health departments today are providing an increasing amount of direct patient care in the clinic and in the home. Current inflation has reversed this trend to some extent, but all indications point to a planned, organized medical care service with emphasis on keeping people well, perhaps the forerunner of a true national health service. In 1989 F Mullan, MD, wrote a book entitled *Plagues and Politics* (Basic Book, New York), which explores the politics of public health. He analyzed the way the Public Health Service has responded to political mandates while preserving its medical mission.

With regard to social issues and attitudes about health care into the year 2000 and beyond, there are numerous opposing viewpoints. These have been published in a book entitled, "The Health Crisis, Opposing Viewpoints" by Bonder and Leone. This text is part of a series of books on opposing viewpoints by Greenhaven Press which has covered over 40 topics (eg, abortion, AIDS, Science and Religion). These books include diverse materials taken from well-written sources as well as statements and position papers from a wide range of individuals, organizations and governments. Their basic philosophy is that those who do not completely understand their adversary's point of view do not understand fully their own. In this text there are six chapters and they address the following issues:

Chapter 1—Is There a Health Crisis? (World Health has Worsened, by Joseph D Weissman; World Health Has Improved, by Elizabeth M Whelan; The AIDS Crisis Will Worsen, by William H Masters, Virginia E Johnson and Robert C Kolodny; The AIDS Crisis will Become Less Severe, by Edward N Brandt, Jr; A Critical Thinking Activity: Distinguishing Bias from Reason) and a periodical bibliography is given at the end of this chapter.

In like manner, the other five chapters are structured with opposing viewpoints covered by numerous experts in the field; they address these remaining questions:

Chapter 2—Does Private Industry Make Health Care More Efficient?
Chapter 3—Should Government Provide More Health Care Benefits for the Elderly?
Chapter 4—Are Health Care Costs Too High?
Chapter 5—Is a Holistic Lifestyle Healthier?
Chapter 6—How Can Health Be Improved?

The text ends with an excellent compilation of organizations which are concerned with the issues debated in the book as well as a bibliography of health and public-health books. Anyone involved in public health at any level will want this reference in their library.

In the beginning of the 1990s the world economic problems, coupled with the new world nationalism following the fall of the Soviet Union, created an enormous public health problem worldwide. Public health is at a major crossroad because of the convergence of problems related to social and biological factors, community and individual problems and widespread economic and social policy issues. Generally, public health was always an important indicator of success achieved by society and its governmental institutions. With all the world economic, political, population control and environmental problems, a widespread weakening of public health support has occurred. As a discipline, it is experiencing a severe identity crisis both in organization and accomplishment. In the US both pharmacy and medicine have moved away from teaching public health as an entity. Numerous related disciplines have swallowed up its traditional coverage and diluted its efforts. Hence, public health as a specific area of interest has been relegated to a secondary role in both academia and in applied areas. There has been a vicious cycle between irrelevance and isolation. Frenk[7] addressed the challenges of public health for the 21st century. He proposes an effort to integrate tradition and progress and provides at least seven directions. These include

Research to provide scientifically validated information relevant to the problems of decision-makers at all levels.
Support of continued academic education in public health to promote excellence and broaden university milieu.
Apply the population approach to all related fields of health and integrate levels of analysis through parallel efforts to link disciplines.
Be more open to concepts from the social, biological and behavioral sciences.
To think on an international sphere.
To always look to the future to anticipate problems.
To assume a lasting permanent attitude and concern about the health needs of the population and to learn from them.

In terms of major concerns for the 1990s, a selection of public health literature shows

A wide variety of studies in epidemiology and biostatistics (eg, HIV infection and AIDS in children).
The hantaviruses as etiologic agents of hemorrhagic fever with renal syndrome.
The appropriate amount of physical activity good for health (diet, hormones and cancer).
Environmental and occupational health (eg, health effects of low-level ionizing radiation, occupational health concerns of firefighting, potential adverse health effects from extremely-low-frequency magnetic fields from power lines, worksite drug testing).
Global change, eg, ozone depletion, greenhouse warming and public health (public policy toward municipal solid-waste developmental toxicity).
Public health practice (eg, global immunization, polio eradication from the Western Hemisphere, health issues for college students, mortality of American Indian and Alaska Native infants, the public health practice of tobacco control and lessons learned, the changing epidemiology of asthma morbidity and mortality, mammography use and cost-effectiveness.
Behavioral aspects of health (eg, depression and public health, poverty and cultural diversity challenges for health promotion among the medically underserved, smoking in pregnancy and heterosexual transmission of HIV).
Health services (eg, unnecessary surgery, low preschool immunization coverage in the US, access and cost implications of state limitations on medicaid reimbursement for pharmaceuticals, containing costs while improving quality of care, the insurance gap, retiree health benefits, emergency medical services, aging and national health systems throughout the world).

Epidemiology

Health-care programs must be designed to meet the needs of the communities they serve; to do this, public-health officials must know what these needs are—hence, the importance of disease reporting and investigation, and the knowledge derived from it. This is epidemiology.

The science of epidemiology is the diagnosis of public health, and all pharmacists should have a knowledge of its rudiments. In essence, epidemiology deals with the determinants and occurrence of disease in defined populations and is based on the interaction of the host and his environment, with attention to those particular agents in the environment that are causal factors of the disease in question; a shorter definition is that epidemiology is medical ecology. Originating in the investigation of outbreaks of communicable disease in the nineteenth century, epidemiology is being applied increasingly to those noncommunicable, chronic diseases which are of the most significance in today's aging population—heart disease, cancer and stroke, for example. The alert pharmacist who can apply the basic principles of epidemiology in his or her community will become a significant member of the health team as illustrated by this incident as far back as the 1960s:

"On November 11, 1963, a man went into a pharmacy in New York City and asked the pharmacist for something which would relieve his complaints of fatigue and weakness. These symptoms had bothered him for about a month and had been accompanied by disturbances in vision and swallowing. He also had a dry mouth and a sore throat. He had been seen by several physicians and had received an antibiotic for an 'upper respiratory infection'. The pharmacist questioned him about his eating habits and, on learning that the patient had had some liver paste, suspected botulism. Investigation by the New York City Health Department confirmed the pharmacist's suspicion, thereby adding to the epidemiological picture of botulism which emerged into prominence in 1963. The patient recovered."[4]

This incident illustrates perhaps the most vital application of epidemiological principles by the pharmacist. The public seeks medical advice from pharmacists who quite rightly must refuse to diagnose and treat the patient's illness, but who can be of invaluable help in contributing to the knowledge of disease patterns prevalent in the neighborhood. In another field, the pharmacist can contribute extensively to the reporting of accidental poisoning and is, indeed, an expert to be used in any poison-control program. It is apparent that the pharmacist should fulfill not only the role of referring the patient to a physician but also the position of collaborating epidemiologist with the local health department. It can be said that anyone can practice epidemiology, a statement illustrated by the part played in New York City in 1946 by a pest-control expert in cracking the riddle of rickettsialpox, at that time a completely new disease.[8]

Of recent origin is the specific area of epidemiology referred to as pharmacoepidemiology. This involves the safety or risk assessment of a new drug which starts with its early use and continues with its longer use cycle. It involves generating information about pharmaceutical outcomes and monitoring associated risks, particularly in the postmarketing environment. There are three major parts to these studies which involve a knowledge base, a conceptual framework and an interpretive framework. Using these perspectives a pharmacoepidemiologist can establish surveillance schemes, understand a posed research question, select strategies, apply methodologies and interpret the results of purposeful investigations. Several articles on this topic have appeared in recent issues of *Drug Intelligence and Clinical Pharmacy* by Nelson *et al.*[9] While it is beyond the scope of this chapter to cover this topic in detail, one condensed case report from the Division of Epidemiology and Surveillance (DES) within the Center for Drug Evaluation and Research of the FDA will be illustrative of this risk-assessing function.

Case example: Maprotiline and Seizures

Signal—British Committee on the Safety of Medicines (CMS), FDA-SRS and the medical literature.

Purpose—Although seizures have been reported with the use of most of the antidepressants the signal suggested a higher frequency with maprotiline exposure. The DES was asked whether seizures that occur while on therapy are associated more strongly with maprotiline than with comparable antidepressants.

Data Sources—SRS (Spontaneous Reporting System), NPA (National Prescription Audit), NDIT (National Disease and Therapeutic Index) and the medical literature.

Methods—Standardized event rates were calculated for a comparison of events for maprotiline, amoxapine and trazodone. Seizures in overdose situations were excluded from the analysis.

Results—Seizure events were associated more strongly with maprotiline therapy than with therapy with comparable antidepressants.

Action—Label was modified. A "Dear Doctor" letter was required.

Follow up: Two hypothesis-testing studies using medicaid data were commissioned.

An excellent basic text on *Clinical Epidemiology—The Essentials* by Fletcher *et al* has been published. It covers abnormalities, diagnostic tests and strategies, frequency, risk, prognosis, treatment, chance, rare diseases, cause and a summary.

One of the more remarkable results of epidemiological studies during the last decade has been the revelation that longer life can be achieved by relatively simple measures initiated early in childhood and sustained throughout adulthood. A perfect example is the Report of the Surgeon General[10] who recommended action in 15 different areas. While some are mentioned already in this article, these bear repeating if for nothing else except emphasis of areas in which pharmacists can make major contributions. These areas include family planning, pregnancy and infant care, immunizations, sexually transmissable diseases, control of toxic agents, occupational health and safety, control of accidental injuries, fluoridation of community water supplies, control of infectious agents, smoking cessation, reduction of misuse of alcohol and drugs, improved nutrition, exercise and fitness and stress control. An example of what can be done if enough people get involved has been the remarkable decrease in the number of smokers during the past 5 years. Certainly, the labeling of nicotine as a truly addicting compound in tobacco by the Surgeon General has helped immeasurably in the antismoking campaigns. This has become an idea whose time has come.

Liang *et al*[11] have reviewed the epidemiologically important procedures for regression analysis for correlated data. As is well known, clustered data continue to be increasingly common in public health research for several reasons. The inquiry into earlier risk factors, eg, biomolecular markers of the disease process, has amplified the need for longitudinal studies. This is particularly true in family-related disorders and their genetic roots.

Similarly, the increased relevance of social and behavioral contributions to disease has made multivariate analysis necessary. Simultaneously, increased computing power has made regression analysis more available to public health researchers. Therefore, it is now routine to characterize the nature of the dependence of a response on variable explanations, rather than just questioning whether such a relationship exists. In studies by this group, they focus on generalized linear models, so that the types of outcomes common in public health (eg, continuous measures binary indicators of disease counts, times to events) can be handled in a uniform manner.

Communicable Disease Control

The pattern of twentieth century disease has been shaped by the improvements in medical care, diagnosis, treatment and prevention. The control of infectious diseases, brought about first by the environmental control of food, milk, water and sewage, has resulted in a longer life expectancy and the emergence of the chronic diseases as the main killers in society (Table 2). Heart disease, cancer, stroke and accidents are today's leading causes of death, and there is no readily foreseeable solution to their control as there was with the communicable diseases; there is also, of course, still much to be done in the surveillance and control of infections, although they are no longer lethal in most instances. While serious communicable diseases practically have been eradicated, some like tuberculosis (TB) and syphilis are still common, and certain viral diseases, such as AIDS, have become recognized as very serious.

In the US in 1984 over 20,000 cases of TB were reported. There were also hundreds of thousands of cases of infectious diseases such as hepatitis and salmonellosis. The estimated numbers of sexually transmitted diseases, hospital-acquired infections, influenza and other acute respiratory illnesses were in the millions.

The common cold is the main cause of absenteeism in the US, and there is no prospect of a vaccine in the near, or even distant, future; symptomatic, conservative and common-sense measures remain the best management. The most common infection *reported* is gonorrhea, which has reached epidemic proportions since World War II, but is only one of the many sexually transmitted diseases (STD) rife in society. The pharmacist is in a position to dispel much of the ignorance attached to these diseases.

The classic STDs of syphilis and gonorrhea are similar in their causation but different in their natural history. Both are transmitted by sexual contact, both have causal organisms that disintegrate within seconds outside the human body and both are susceptible to antibiotic treatment; where they differ is in their natural history. Syphilis, fortunately, remains a latent infection in two-thirds of its victims—usually with a low positive response to a serological test for syphilis, in itself a difficult diagnostic problem; the remaining one-third have systemic lesions, mostly in the cardiovascular and central nervous systems. Gonorrhea, on the other hand, manifests itself mainly in local infections in the genitourinary tract with inflammation, and sometimes abscess formation, and scarring (Table 3).

The initial local lesion in syphilis—the hard chancre—rarely will come to the pharmacist's attention but the male urethral discharge produced by "clap" often will require

Table 2—Five Leading Causes of Death in 1900 and 1984 in the US and New Diseases of the 1990s

1990	1984	1990s
1. Pneumonia	1. Diseases of the heart	1. AIDS
2. Tuberculosis	2. Malignant neoplasms	2. Legionnaire's disease
3. Diarrhea, enteritis and ulceration of intestines	3. Cerebrovascular diseases	3. Toxic shock syndrome
4. Diseases of the heart	4. Accidents	4. Lyme disease
5. Intracranial lesions of vascular origin	5. Influenza and pneumonia	

Table 3—Some Common Sexually Transmitted Diseases

	Gonorrhea	Syphilis	Herpes simplex
Causal organism	*Neisseria gonorrhoeae*	*Treponema pallidum*	*Herpes simplex virus*
Incubation period (approx)	6 days	3 weeks	10 days
Initial manifestation	Urethral discharge	Hard chancre (sore)	Blister(s)
Late manifestations	Local	Systemic	None
Diagnosis	Smear	Microscopic & blood	Clinical & viral studies
Treatment	Penicillin	Penicillin	Acyclovir

advice. First, many urethral discharges are not gonorrhea—they are nongonococcal urethritis or prostatitis, and can be caused by many organisms and cured by specific, but different, therapies. Diagnosis by culture and microscopic examination is therefore imperative. A minority of men will have no discharge although infected, in opposition to women in whom 80% will not show the purulent discharge usually associated with gonorrhea. Occasionally, epidemics of STDs occur in both heterosexual and homosexual contacts, and the alert pharmacist often can warn local health officials of this possibility.

Not all genital lesions are sexually transmitted, however, and they range from normal skin or mucous membrane variations to trauma, and local nonsexually transmitted infections or infestations. In all instances, therefore, an accurate diagnosis must be made; this will be made easier when the stigma of the sexual transmission of disease is removed and public education regarding STDs becomes the same as for any other disease.

Again, the pharmacist's role in public education cannot be overemphasized—but it must be by an informed pharmacist who knows the natural history of the sexually transmitted diseases and can therefore judge the efficacy of the advice he offers. It also is ineffective to have a few pamphlets lying in a rack—active distribution to appropriate customers with a few well-chosen words will be more telling. One of the best opportunities for health education is when a customer is waiting for a prescription to be filled and has nothing to do but stand, or sit, and wait.

One STD of current concern is herpes genitalis, which usually is seen as a series of blisters on an inflamed background anywhere in the genital area. In actual fact, the causal virus is associated closely with the cold sore, or oral herpes simplex virus, and treatment is just as ineffective; in itself, herpes genitalis is an unpleasant, innocuous and recurrent nuisance except in those newborn infants infected during delivery—hence, the practice of delivering women with active herpes of the genitals by cesarean section. There also is an unproven association of herpes genitalis and cancer of the cervix which has received undue publicity, although it is prudent at present for women with herpes genitalis to have Pap smears more often than those without—6 months to a year being a reasonable time interval. The use of acyclovir in treating genital herpes has value, but the possibility of a vaccine being produced offers a greater hope for controlling this infection.

The recent spread of acquired immunodeficiency syndrome (AIDS) has catapulted this sexually related disease into critical dimensions. The life-threatening nature of AIDS has caused it to take precedence over all the others in the group. The pharmacist should be involved in educational programs promoting safer sexual practices, particularly where the use of condoms is essential. Already, many pharmacies have prominent displays and ready accessibility of condoms for sale. Certainly, these are important in minimizing barriers to the purchase and use.

From the late 1980s to the early 1990s, the field of STDs has evolved from one with a primary concentration on gonorrhea and syphilis to one of expanded effort addressing a wide spectrum of organisms and syndromes. The emergence of the human immunodeficiency virus (HIV) has accelerated greatly the growth of public concern about STDs and has provided momentum to epidemiologic research in the field.[12] Some have predicted that up to twice as many HIV infections may occur in the 1990s than had occurred during the 1980s.

It should be pointed out one of the "benefits" of the AIDS pandemic is the highlighting of deficiencies in public health and its intrastructures throughout the world. It is hoped the global response to AIDS will reactivate the importance of supporting public health. It should give ministries of health greater visibility and opportunity to provide leadership. It should foster closer collaboration in the governmental and related sectors. There will be increased resources and attention directed to long-neglected areas of health education, prevention of STDs, the blood transfusion industry and research into human behaviors and communication patterns in a variety of cultural settings. AIDS will continue to be one of the greatest public health challenges in this decade. It is felt that it will not be possible to prevent 2 to 3 million AIDS cases projected to occur worldwide over the next decade in individuals infected with HIV before 1990.

The pharmacist also has the opportunity to involve him or herself with sociosexual problems as they relate to public health. There should be an understanding of the subcultures of their patients and how sex and other social behavior varies from one group to another. For example, the subcultures of the promiscuous individual, prostitute, drug abuser, homosexual, etc, must be understood and referred for counsel where appropriate. Patients should be counseled freely and advised on STD-prevention methods, methods for treatment and the necessity for the treatment. In all of this, the personal habits and mores of the pharmacist should be sublimated for the benefit of the patient.

An excellent chapter on sexuality ("The Synthetic Society") may be found in Gable's text on *Psychosocial Pharmacy*. This subject is covered from the viewpoint of how the pharmacist can serve as a major local and readily available consultant in the area. The following chapter in this text deals with the pharmacist as a personal consultant in general sexual and specific female menstrual matters.

Immunization has controlled the childhood infections of measles, mumps, rubella, poliomyelitis, diphtheria and whooping cough. Pharmacists should obtain immunization schedules from health departments and advise parents of the importance of adhering to the times recommended therein. Where mass community clinics are the accepted and best way of bringing immunization to the public, the pharmacist is the obvious person to bear the responsibility of obtaining, storing and preparing the vaccine for administration—this method has been most successful in community immunization programs with oral poliomyelitis vaccine. One other practical aspect of cooperation between the pharmacist and the local health department is an agreement to supply vaccine for immediate or urgent administration, with the understanding that it will be replaced as soon as it can be obtained from the central health-department supply; this has been particularly effective in administering rabies antiserum and vaccine to individual patients where a delay will occur in receiving the vaccine from the state health department. The pharmacist often will have many vaccines in stock for use by private physicians which local health departments need only on an occasional basis and, therefore, do not stock routinely.

The control of communicable disease is based on adequate case finding and the supervision and prophylactic treatment of close contacts.

An indispensable reference book should be in each pharmacy—*The Control of Communicable Diseases in Man*, published by the American Public Health Association and frequently revised (the 1988 edition cost $9.00 and is as good as, or even better than, texts costing many times as much). This publication summarizes, in a concise format, all known communicable diseases, and can be referred to if in doubt about the etiology and control of any disease, from the most common to the rarest exotic importation.

In addition, pharmacists who wish to keep abreast of current communicable disease patterns should subscribe to the *Morbidity and Mortality Weekly Report (MMWR)* of the Centers for Disease Control (CDC) of the US Public Health Service (CDC, Atlanta, GA 30333). This publication is copied by the publishers of the *New England Journal of Medicine* and may be obtained at a considerably reduced cost by subscribing through the Massachusetts Medical Society, PO Box 9120, Waltham MA 02254-9120. The *MMWR* has epidemiologic notes and reports of outbreaks of disease, and current statistics by disease and geographical location at home and abroad, of which all health professionals should keep informed. Most states attempt to develop their own recommended schedule for immunizing children and much confusion exists both among practitioners and parents over this. A sensible schedule recommendation is published periodically by the American Academy of Pediatrics and titled, "Report of the Committee on Infectious Diseases."

Pharmacists more than any professional group will become aware of epidemic infectious diseases in a community. The arrival of an unusual number of people with diarrheal disease for OTC products may be the result of an outbreak of food-borne disease. The monitoring of numbers and types of prescriptions, even in an unscientific way, often suffices to point to an epidemic, and the interested pharmacist can set up a monitoring system of more scientific validity.

Casto[13] in the department of pharmacy at the University of Texas Health Science Center reviewed recent developments in vacines and immunization practices. He notes that dramatic changes have been made in the recommended schedule for immunizations, and for a variety of reasons. These include a greater understanding of risks associated with whole-cell pertussis vaccine, introduction of more immunogenic vaccines to prevent invasive disease caused by *Haemophilus influenzae* type b, a national epidemic of measles that affected many vaccinated individuals and the failure of targeted use of vaccine in high-risk patients to reduce the occurrence of hepatitis B. Generally, new changes in recommended regimens should be expected as new products are developed. However, it seems that good compliance is needed to follow immunization schedules scrupulously so that they will show their greatest effect.

In summary, the role of the pharmacist in the control of communicable diseases consists of an awareness of the natural history of these diseases in both the individual and the community, referral of clients to medical-care facilities where indicated and public education of an informed type at all times. It is possibly in this aspect of community disease control that the pharmacist can play his or her greatest part.

Global Health

Isolationism was a characteristic American trait until World War II, but today the people of the US are only too well aware of the shrunken world beyond their shores. Now, the appearance of an exotic disease in any part of this country is a common event and the pharmacist should have an understanding of the complexity of diseases encountered in international travel. This does not mean, of course, that the pharmacist should be concerned with the differential diagnosis and treatment of schistosomiasis or kala azar, but he or she should know that both of these diseases have been reported by travellers returning to America and thus be aware of the possibility of their occurrence.

One of the most important questions a pharmacist can ask a client who wants advice about a personal disease is that posed by Roman legionnaires to their colleagues—unde venis? (where have you come from?); certainly a routine question in all suspect illnesses should be to ask whether the client has been abroad in the past 2 years.

By international agreement there are today only three diseases to which quarantine regulations apply—cholera, plague and yellow fever (Table 4)—but during the past 15 years, many exotic diseases have been reported by the CDC—schistosomiasis, loiasis, malaria, kala azar, dengue, leishmaniasis, giardiasis, trypanosomiasis and innumerable worm infestations.[7] It is therefore imperative for the pharmacist to ask clients where they have been and ensure that the information elicited is relayed to the physician if medical consultation is sought. The World Health Organization (WHO) is the only official international health organization, and its 156 member nations, apart from reporting disease trends, control many aspects of international health. Its budget for 1982–1983 was $483.3 million. One WHO program is of particular significance to pharmacy—the international standardization of immunological agents such as measles and other vaccines, and toxoids.

Today, the US does not require any immunizations of persons entering the country, wherever they have been or whatever diseases they have been exposed to. Pharmacists can be of invaluable assistance to international travellers in advising them what to take in the way of medications, especially for malaria and traveller's diarrhea, whose ubiquity is evident

Table 4—Global Health

	Quarantinable diseases		
	Cholera	Plague	Yellow fever
Causal organism	*Vibrio cholerae*	*Yersinia pestis*	Yellow fever virus
Incubation period (approx)	2–3 days	2–6 days	3–6 days
Transmission	Fecal-Oral	Flea bite	Mosquito bite
Natural foci	Asia	Worldwide	Central Africa, South America

This Shrunken World and Wanderlust

Americans abroad

1950	1960	1970	1975	1980
676,000	1,634,000	5,260,000	6,354,000	8,163,000

Flying times (hr)

New York to		San Francisco to	
London	New Delhi	Tokyo	Hong Kong
3	14	11	14

from its synonyms of Montezuma's Revenge, the Casablanca Crud, Delhi Belly and even San Franciscitis!

Information on the traveler's "medical chest" is available in several publications and generally will include a broad-spectrum antibiotic, adhesive bandages, remedies for travel sickness, aspirin, thermometer, antibiotic cream, etc. Immunizations must be up-to-date and, again, a CDC publication provides this information in *Health Information for International Travel*. Referral to the local health department may be easier for those pharmacists who have neither the time nor the interest themselves. It is wise, however, for pharmacists to retain some degree of interest in travelers' requirements, if only as a public service. Annually, several of the professional pharmacy journals update travelers' needs in the areas of immunizations and emergency drugs to take along on trips.

Finally, a word about malaria prophylaxis—it is imperative to begin medication 1 week before travel and to continue it for 6 weeks after return from a malarial part of the world if the suppressant (usually chloroquine phosphate) is to be of maximum benefit. A recent increase in strains of *Plasmodia falciparum* resistant to chloroquine phosphate necessitates the addition of other prophylactic drugs such as pyrimethamine–sulfadoxine in some parts of the world.

Disease Prevention

Chronic disease has become the prime target of epidemiological and basic laboratory research. Heart disease recently has shown a slight decrease as a cause of death, the reasons remaining obscure despite claims that it has resulted from a change in diet, more exercise, less smoking and earlier treatment of hypertension—the last reason being the one with most scientific validity. In all probability, the human machine is beginning to adapt to the change in environmental factors which have come into prominence with modern technology—but proof for this, as with causal factors, remains to be seen. Certainly, man has managed to adapt to disease patterns in previous epochs and it would not be unusual to see history repeating itself in the 20th century.

Prevention is of three kinds—primary, secondary and tertiary. Primary prevention is health maintenance—keeping people well. The best example of primary prevention has been discussed already—the control of infections by immunization. Equally important, however, are the many factors of health now generally included under the catchall of "life- style," and there is evidence that following certain health practices leads to longevity, eg, not smoking, limiting alcohol consumption, controlling weight, sleeping 7 to 8 hours a night, being physically active, eating breakfast and not eating between meals have been cited as desirable habits.

In summary, the old saw of "moderation in all things" would seem to be a good dictum to observe. The aim of primary prevention is to modify "lifestyles" to the benefit of the individual and, of course, ultimately to the community—a task easier done on paper than in the flesh. Time will tell whether the current enthusiasm of the newcomers to this popular way of thinking will be justified.

Secondary prevention is the early diagnosis and treatment of an already existing disease and is illustrated best by the use of penicillin in the treatment of streptococcal infections, thereby preventing the occurrence of the much more dangerous rheumatic fever, a disease that "licks the joints but bites the heart." The pharmacist can perform a vital service by advising the patient to see a physician if he has a febrile illness characterized by a sore throat. In no other disease is the old saying that an ounce of prevention is worth a pound of cure more true—although, in this instance, the few cents of prevention by using penicillin is more apropros.

Tertiary prevention is really rehabilitation. Most chronic diseases cannot be cured, but their progress can be retarded with maximum benefit to the patient. Much can be done, for instance, with rheumatoid arthritis to make its victims more comfortable and more productive in their daily lives. It is with this type of disease that the challenge to the pharmacist can be taxed to the utmost in his knowledge, and use, of therapy and resources available to the patient.

Chronic Disease Control

The pharmacist can encourage clients to avail themselves of the few proven techniques in chronic disease prevention. Good living habits never did anyone any harm although their degree of positive protective value is still questionable, and they have been recommended as methods of preventing disease, particularly heart disease. Cancer, however, is not prevented by these measures and, in general, must be dealt with by early diagnosis and treatment; a few techniques such as the Pap smear serve as specific preventive methods but, in general, secondary prevention is the main point of attack. In 1989, the CDC reported that the rate for cancer (second-leading cause of death) is going up. In 1987, the rate was 196.1 deaths for every 100,000 Americans. This is up from 194.7 deaths, the rate for 1986. Cancer killed 447,190 people out of 2.2 million Americans who died in 1987. In economic terms, cancer is the most important health problem in the US. The pharmacist, therefore, should be acquainted with the warning signals of cancer and advise any client who exhibits them to seek medical advice immediately. Local cancer societies will be only too pleased to provide health education literature for professional and public education.

The prevention of strokes is concerned largely with the control of high blood pressure and the revolution in therapy within the past 10 years has probably resulted in the lower death rates from cerebrovascular disease. The pharmacist can, of course, take clients' blood pressure readings, but these may be temporarily high or low, and must, therefore, be followed by at least two more measurements at later dates. As appropriate, local medical societies and heart associations should be consulted as pharmacists become involved in blood pressure screening and monitoring programs. Nevertheless, the pharmacist is in an unique position to advise on and, where indicated, measure clients' blood pressure with the added rider that he or she must also educate them about its normal variations. As the basis of hypertensive therapy is with drugs, the pharmacist should be in the forefront of monitoring their application in his clients, especially in encouraging compliance with prescribed regimens.

As discussed above, pharmacists are becoming more involved in hypertension screening and referral. The death rates for both heart disease and stroke went down from 1986 to 1987 and this was probably due to such well-promoted measures as quitting smoking, controlling high blood pressure, lowering cholesterol intake, increased physical activity and, generally, good overall health consciousness.

The many other chronic diseases all require comparable approaches if they are to be controlled. In the main, secondary and tertiary prevention—that is, early diagnosis and treatment, and rehabilitation—are the main control measures in chronic disease and the pharmacist should be well acquainted with the services that offer diagnosis, treatment and rehabilitation in the community.

The fourth most common cause of death in the US today is accidents. Although there are few specific things that can be done to prevent accidents, such as the use of automobile seat belts, the pharmacist should be the leader in the control of accidental poisoning. In small communities, the pharmacist should be the prime consultant for advice in poisoning cases and should be able to refer the caller to the nearest poison control or information center if unable to deal with the matter personally. In addition, the pharmacist should be the leader in disseminating information about poisoning (eg, in a "Poison Prevention Week" program) and other educational services in the community or neighborhood.

Closely allied to accidental poisoning is deliberate poisoning of the body which is so common today—what is called substance abuse. Drugs, including alcohol, have become an everyday topic of conversation and much misinformation has been distributed about them. Again, the expert knowledge of the pharmacist should be used to good advantage in both an individual and community context. Along with the toxins of self-administered drugs go the many industrial toxins now being encountered with new technology. It is imperative that the pharmacist be aware of the dangers arising from industrial toxins and be alert to their manifestations in clients who seek relief in OTC medicines. Many pharmacists run poison control centers nationally, usually within hospitals in major cities of the US.

In summary, the control of chronic disease can range from the support of proven community programs such as screening clinics for cancer to an alertness for the first signs of disease associated with an occupational hazard. The pharmacist is unique in having a basic understanding of disease processes and in being in daily contact with members of the public on an informal, yet professional, basis. His or her ability, therefore, to intervene in the initial stages of illness in chronic disease is unparalleled and should be avidly seized. Another, and perhaps more significant, area of control is in health education.

Health Education

There is perhaps no aspect of public health more praised than health education although concrete proof of its overall effectiveness is singularly lacking. Certainly no other country in the world pays such lip service to health education from the primary school through college into adulthood but, despite this, many Americans are overweight, smoke too many cigarettes, drink too much alcohol and abuse themselves in many other ways.

There is currently a popular emphasis on changing what are called "life-styles," but how to do this, and whether the result will be beneficial, is still unclear. Take exercise as an example; the current craze for running and jogging is laudable for those who enjoy it, but there is no proof that it achieves its stated object, ie, to improve the circulatory system with subsequent delay of the pathological variations that lead to disease. No doubt those who run derive considerable virtue from their pastime but whether it will do more for them than this is unproven.

The techniques of health education consist of publicizing health data through the local media, whether spoken or written—a process recently entitled health information to distinguish it from the behavior modification which is the objective of health education proper. The use of illustrative material and catchy phrasing is all part of success, but the presentation of advice does not mean that it will be followed—which is the ultimate and only aim of health education.

Many professional pharmacies now participate in patient health education through the use of pamphlets and bulletins freely available on display racks. These cover every medical subject imaginable, including all the major diseases, drug classes, drugs of abuse, drug and food interactions, sexually transmitted diseases, immunizations, family planning, health promotion, fluoridation, poison prevention, quackery, disaster preparedness, environmental protection and work-place safety. Some are general, while others may be prepared by drug companies and are quite specific.

But more than this can be done—the pharmacist actively can promote good health practices by personal example and by reaching out to impart professional information to the public whom he or she serves. The ideal of public service, which is strong at the beginning of a pharmacy student's career, unfortunately becomes dulled by time and the demands of work. If the pharmacist can keep the innate feeling for humans untarnished, much more in the way of health education can be accomplished.

Formal methods of health education have their place in public health, but in the pharmacy the informed direction of members of the public is a much more realistic approach. Certainly, participation of pharmacists in community health education programs must be recommended, but it is in the everyday person-to-person contact with people that the pharmacist serves most effectively. To display pamphlets with health information is admirable but it is substantially better to augment this with verbal instruction. This does not mean that every customer needs counseling, but there are always people who can benefit from a few words of advice on health matters. Too often, the pharmacist remains a figure in a white coat occasionally seen behind and above the service counter.

The keynote of a pharmacist's health-educational service is an informed awareness of the early signs and symptoms of the major diseases of society and a conscientious willingness to pass this information on to those members of the public who require it. Assistance in this matter should be sought from official and voluntary health agencies, remembering that these groups have certain basic differences—of governance, financial support, legal responsibilities and primary aim. In general, official agencies are governed by appointed officials, supported by taxes to provide direct services to the public and somewhat limited by law in what they can do. Voluntary agencies have greater flexibility to experiment with and support new programs, and have no responsibility in law for enforcement (Table 5).

The sequence of events often has been that a philanthropic group forms a voluntary agency which demonstrates a need and, once this has been done, transfers the program to an official agency for direct service purposes. One of the best examples of this succession is in the American Lung Association as it stands in today's health care program—although there has been some blurring of this distinction recently with federal support of all agencies, voluntary and official. Nevertheless, it is important for the pharmacist to understand the basic origins and differences of these agencies if he or she is to work intelligently with them and the public they serve.

Medical Care

The most pressing matter in medical care today is its high cost. The rapid and alarming increase in costs has become a matter of personal and national concern, and it is the federal government's avowed intent to regulate costs by any means at its disposal.

There are three main methods of payment for physician and other health services: direct payment, where the physician is paid directly by the patient, indirect (third-party) payment, where the physician is paid by someone representing the patient (ie, a third party, the patient and the physician being the first and second parties) and salaried payment, where the physician is a salaried member of the government.

In the US today, most medical care is provided through third-party indirect payments, usually of a voluntary insurance nature, but with increasing government participation. The trend in the 1970s and 1980s has been towards the federal provision of more and more dollars for direct patient care—possibly a forerunner of some type of national health program. This will, of course, depend upon the prevailing political climate of the electorate.

The US remains the only country in the world in which a government health service is not a reality, and indications point towards a change within the coming years. Most so-

Table 5—Characteristics of Agencies

	Official	Nonofficial
Basic financing	Taxes	Donations, gifts, fund drives, endowments
Management	Government bureaucracy	Board of trustees or directors
Legal status	Law enforcement	No legal responsibility
Program emphasis	Provision of services	Educational programs
Innovations	Limited by rigidity	Aided by flexibility
Research	Unrestricted	Unrestricted

called health insurance is sickness insurance, ie, payment is made for treating illness, not for keeping people well. The Blue Cross-Blue Shield, and commercial and government insurance, programs provide limited diagnostic and treatment services for most US citizens, either through group or individual premium payments. In addition, the federal programs of Medicare and Medicaid pay for elderly and indigent patients respectively. Uniformity, however, is lacking in many of these programs, with local variation being the rule and not the exception.

Recently, a renewed interest has occurred in prepaid health plans from the standpoint of both preventing disease and curtailing costs. The federal government fostered this interest in the 1970s and 1980s by promoting its version of prepaid medical care through Health Maintenance Organizations (HMOs)—an example now being followed by industry and private enterprise.

The basic principle of a prepaid health plan is that it provides all health services, in or out of hospital, for an annually negotiated premium. The prototype of this method of health care is the Kaiser Permanente program in California.[15] The incentive to keep people well is reflected in the decrease in hospitalization of the prepaid plan members with a consequent increase in money retained by the plan at the end of the fiscal year. Repeated surveys have shown that members of prepaid plans do indeed enter hospitals less often and stay less time when they are admitted. Recently, industries have become interested in prepaid plans and many firms have started plans of their own.

The ultimate decision to be reached in the US today is whether compulsory insurance should replace voluntary insurance, and what proportion of government participation is appropriate to either method. The evolution of health insurance in the US has seen to it that many citizens already have government-financed medical care: the armed forces and their dependents, veterans and those covered by Medicare and Medicaid—and the President of the United States! The major component of government medicine is, however, in two programs—Medicare and Medicaid, which became law in 1965 as Titles XVIII and XIX of the Social Security Act (Table 6).

Medicare is designed to pay for costs of medical care in people who are at least 65 years old. The two parts of the program are designed, in the main, to provide institutional and home care, and medical services wherever the patient may be. Everyone is eligible to participate on reaching the age of 65 and the program is financed and administered by the Federal Government.

Provision for services by all types of health personnel is made, although a monthly premium must be paid by the recipient, and only a percentage of most of the bills will be paid by Medicare. Care in the home is encouraged by paying for skilled nursing visits. Home health services have received much publicity recently, and every indication is that they are becoming an increasingly significant part of health care.

Ill people should be cared for in three, and only three, places—in an institution, in an ambulatory care setting or at home. Anyone requiring 24 hour a day care should be in an institution, usually a hospital or nursing home. The majority of people with disease can, fortunately, be taken care of in an ambulatory care facility—a clinic or office. There is, however, a sizable group of patients who do not need continuous care and yet are unable to walk or ride to an outpatient clinic or office; these people need care in the home. There is a lack of awareness and understanding of the availability and variety of services available for patient care in the home; various estimates have placed from 5 to 25% of patients in hospitals and nursing homes as being able to benefit from home care, which has the advantages of economy and familiarity to the patient. One of the greatest contributions pharmacists can make to cost containment is to become acquainted with the home-health services in the community and promote their use by professional health worker and layman alike.

Table 6—Medicare and Medicaid

	Medicare	Medicaid
Social security act	Title XVIII	Title XIX
Age limit	65 yr or more	None
Eligibility	All if of age	Differs by state
Funding	Federal	Federal and state
Benefits	Uniform	Varies with state
Administration	Federal	State

Medicaid differs from Medicare in that it has no age restriction and is not financed solely by federal funds, each state participating in its support and administration. Medicaid actually has replaced four categorical programs which were operational before 1965—Old Age Assistance, Aid to the Blind, Aid to the Totally and Permanently Disabled and Aid to Dependent Children. In addition, Medicaid is designed to pay for medical care to the "medically needy"—a group of people who cannot afford to pay for medical care although they may or may not be able to pay for other goods and services. States differ in their eligibility requirements, payments and in matters of administration, and pharmacists should obtain information on their state Medicaid program from the appropriate state office.

There has been less talk recently of national health insurance although there almost certainly will be further attempts to introduce some form of this method of care. The form it will take is still debatable—literally debatable—and summaries of proposals may be obtained from government and professional associations. It is unlikely that any drastic change in the current health-care system will ensue unless there is a change in government, which at present leans towards private enterprise and away from government control.

However, this may change with time and prevailing political and economic climate. Much has to do with overall national health expenditures which have risen from $27 billion in 1960 to over $387 billion by 1984. In 1984, the US spent 10.6% of its gross national product on medical care, with hospitals accounting for 41 cents of the health care dollar and physician costs taking 19 cents. For over 25 years, financing programs for medical care (public or private) have served largely to provide financial support for conventional procedures of providing services. The majority of these funds have followed well-established routes into institutional and medical pocketbooks. For the most part, financial programs have rewarded traditional methods and old inefficiencies.

Finally, it should be stated that financing is not the whole problem. Because of the revolution of rising expectations, the consumer has acquired a more informed and expensive taste. These dramatic changes in the health-care market have forced changes in how third-party payments are made. Frequently they are now reimbursed on the basis of a predetermined rate. These and related developments (Diagnostic Related Groups (DRGs) and averaging of payment schedules for all medical procedures) have changed market incentives, prompting both consumers and providers to become more cost-conscious. This has stimulated increased competition among providers to retain their share of the health-care dollars. This has resulted in numerous changes such as surgery centers, free-standing emergency centers, walk-in clinics and numerous prepaid group practice systems and preferred provider organizations. For example, enrollment in HMOs increased over 22% between 1983 and 1984.

Over 2300 ambulatory-care centers are now in existence. Perhaps the most significant change to note here is the emergence of the "for-profit" health-care industry. Figures from 1985 show that at least 20% of all nonfederal hospitals were owned and operated by investor-owned firms. Many experts predict that the health-care system eventually will be dominated by a few large health-care corporations. By the mid-1990s Congress may enact national health insurance to require all employers to provide basic health-care coverage, including drug benefits.

Health Planning

If there is to be a national health insurance program, there must be a national health plan on which it is based. The emphasis on planning for health care is far from new, but it is only within the past 25 years that it has received recognition in this country. The first concerted effort towards planning came with the passage of the federal Comprehensive Health Planning Act (Public Law 89-749) in 1966 which supported national, state and regional planning bodies. Implementation of the act, however, was difficult because of local differences in enthusiasm and in funding, and in 1974 the National Health Planning and Resources Development Act (Public Law 93-641) replaced it.

This legislation already has had a considerable influence on the provision of medical care and was designed to encourage, and indeed enforce, planning for health care at all levels of the nation. Overall, there is a National Health Planning Council appointed by the President which sets the policy through Congress for implementation of local planning in Health Service Areas administered by Health Systems Agencies (HSAs).

The HSAs are the fundamental local units for health planning and they advise, direct and supervise the provision of health services in populations of several hundred thousand people, not necessarily confined by state boundaries. Depending upon their legislative powers, they have the right to review, comment upon and, in many instances, approve or disapprove new health services or changes in existing health services. HSAs deal with *all* health and medical care services, and it is therefore wise for pharmacists to become acquainted with, and active in, their deliberations.

Representation from the pharmacy profession is encouraged, if not required, on the local HSA boards and also on the State Coordinating Councils which act in an advisory capacity in each state. The need for planning to conserve the health resources we have is an obvious move and is echoed by the increasing interest of lay groups in medical care. The HSAs recognize this trend by requiring that a majority of the HSA Board of Directors must be consumers.

Health Services Programs

Health departments in general provide a wide spectrum of services to the public; it must be remembered that the time-honored term for these services is "public health." Too often, public health has the connotation of health care for the poor; in reality, public-health services are supported by taxes and are available to, and should be used by, *all* members of the public.

The local health department is a product of the 20th century. *Ad hoc* local boards of health have existed since the Black Death ravaged Europe in the 14th century, but the first permanent county health department in America was not formed until the early years of the 20th century. The primary aim of public health services at that time was to control communicable disease by enforcing sanitary codes which eliminated contamination of food, water and milk by human excreta. With the advent of immunization, community programs in disease prevention with immunological agents began and, gradually, more personal health services were added to official health agency programs—maternal and child health and crippled children, for example. The chief provider of these services was, and still is, the public-health nurse who, even today in many local areas, is the main and only focus of personal health services in the community. It is a wise pharmacist who is acquainted with the local public-health nurses and the multitude of services they can provide his or her clients.

Most local health departments today are affiliated in varying degree with their state health department. In those states with adequate local coverage, the state health department acts in a consultant capacity but in the more sparsely settled states, and in those with weak local services, direct services often are provided by personnel from the state central office. The state may, in turn, call upon federal health consultants for advice and assistance, but the federal government, in general, cannot encroach on the right of the state to determine its own health policies. Interestingly, all federal health legislation is based on the one phrase in the Preamble to the Constitution which says that the Federal Government has the right to act to "promote the general welfare." It is from these few words that the immense authority of the federal government in health matters is derived.

The state, therefore, has sovereign rights in guarding the health of its inhabitants. Typically, the programs of a local health department are administered by the basic public-health team of a physician, a public-health nurse, a sanitarian and a clerk.

The physician, who usually will have an advanced degree in public health, is responsible for the overall program of the department, with or without the assistance of an administrator.

The public-health nurse provides the bulk of the personal health services, both in clinics and in the home, and spends her time dealing with the care of people ranging from the newborn infant to the aged chronic invalid—her primary concern being to apply the principles of prevention to her patients and to promote health, or to retard the progress of disease where a return to health is not possible.

The sanitarian is responsible for the control of disease by environmental techniques and is following the grand line of the 19th century's "Great Sanitary Awakening" in reviewing the environment in its many intricate interrelationships with society and its constituent members.

The clerk, of course, remains at the center of the health department's activities, and stores, files and retrieves the ever-increasing morass of records required by today's litigious society. Scant justice is accorded to the indispensable clerk and, indeed, to any of the members of the public-health team who perform their work unheralded and unsung in most communities.

Again, pharmacists should become acquainted with their local health department and its wide range of services and avail themselves of these services whenever the need arises.

Maternal and Child Health

The health of the mother and child—maternal and child health as it is generally called—was the first public-health program of the 20th century. Infant and child mortality rates were exceptionally high, largely because of respiratory and diarrheal diseases; many of the latter were propagated by unclean milk, an ideal medium for bacterial proliferation. The first move to combat this disgrace to the nation came in the form of "milk stations" where clean milk was provided to mothers and their children. Gradually, the concept of maternal and child health expanded from this environmental beginning to the formation of programs where direct patient care and advice could be dispensed both in the clinic and at home. No public-health program has proved its worth more than the care of the mother and child. Over the past half century maternal mortality has declined some 45%, while infant mortality has been reduced by about 75%.

The basic idea behind maternal and child health is to shepherd the mother and her child through the time when they are exposed to the greatest risks of disease and death—during pregnancy, the puerperium and the first year of life. The early diagnosis of pregnancy, with informed supervision of its progress through delivery and the immediate postpartum period, constitutes the bulwark of care in maternal and child health programs. The earlier that prenatal care is given, the more beneficial is the effect not only to the mother but also to the child, as the health of the infant is directly influenced by its care *in utero*.

Consequently, the pharmacist who understands the normal course of pregnancy and infancy is at a distinct advantage to one who does not, as he or she can guide the mother in simple matters of hygiene and management of her pregnancy and of her infant. This applies particularly to those women who, through lack of education and other social advantages, have an incomplete understanding of how important it is to have early, professional prenatal care. In addition, the ability of the pharmacist to discuss contraceptive methods intelligently will be a signal service to women in the postpartum phase of their pregnancies or preferably earlier.

Nature has designed the mother to take care of her newborn infant—in many parts of the world she still does this by breast feeding and keeping the baby warm and safe by cuddling it to her body, especially where the climate is tropical. In our society, however, we have produced an artificial environment in which the majority of babies do not receive the food designed for them—that is, their mother's milk. Breast feeding is still the best food for the baby and should be encouraged by the pharmacist whenever possible. One aspect of disease control in the infant, however, which must be supplied by someone other than the mother is protection by immunization, especially in the so-called diseases of childhood. It is paramount that all infants, irrespective of color, creed or income should be immunized with all the toxoids and vaccines available to help them through the dangerous first few years of childhood. Primary immunization should begin at the age of 2 months and is not complete until the fourth dose of triple vaccine (diphtheria, tetanus, pertussis) is given at 18 months with followup at 4 to 6 years for some of these (Table 7).[3]

Other programs which have received much attention in recent years have been family planning, lead poisoning in children, infant and preschool child-health services, services for handicapped children, nutritional education and support for children, if required. Certainly, the economic necessity for mothers to work and the concomitant development of child-care centers has focused interest in all of these.

Vanderpool *et al*[16] reviewed the status of child health in the US and prospects for the 1990s, stating that

> Poverty has become more prevalent among children.
> More children are uninsured for health services than in prior years.
> There has been a serious erosion of the public health system on which poor families depend heavily for health care and related services.
> Single-parent families are increasing in number.
> An increasing percentage of children are living in families of minority background in which poverty often complicates issues related to ethnic differences in child rearing.
> An erosion of the immunization rates achieved earlier in the decade has developed.
> The decline in the infant mortality rate has plateaued.
> AIDS has emerged as a formidable problem among young people.
> Homelessness has come to include children and their parents in increasing numbers.

Population Control

In the realm of maternal and child health, no programs have more significance than those pertaining to population control. Worldwide, the alarming increase in population is the most serious public-health problem. Although in a land of plenty like the US it might seem that population control is of minor significance, the amount of tax dollars required to support unwanted children is immense. Family planning, as population control usually is called in the western countries, consists not only in spacing births by deliberate contraceptive use but also in helping women who cannot conceive to bear children. Although abortion is now legal, it is quite obviously the most unsatisfactory way of determining family size—it is far better to prevent conception than to eliminate its products. Contraceptives are obtained from local pharmacies and it is therefore pharmacists who could be in the front line of family planning.

Health Measurement

In general, the pharmacist has been neglected as a dynamic member of the health team, being relegated, in the eyes of many health professionals, to the role of a dispenser of medicines and other products sold in drug stores. The fact that the pharmacist is the health professional in most frequent

Table 7—Recommended Schedule for Routine Immunization of Infants and Children[a] [3]

Recommended age	Vaccines	Comments
Newborn	HBV	First dose of HBV is administered before hospital discharge.
2 Months	DTP	DTP may be given as early as 6 weeks of age, then at 4–8—week intervals for the first three doses
	OPV	—
	HbCV	HbCV may be given either as HbOC or PRP-OMP
	HBV	Second dose of HBV may be given between 1–2 months
4 Months	DTP	—
	OPV	—
	HbCV	HbCV may be given either as HbOC or PRP-OMP
6 Months	DTP	—
	OPV	Optional dose of OPV, but recommended in high-risk areas
	HbCV	If HbOC was used, recommend another dose at 6 months
	HBV	Third dose of HBV may be given between 6–18 months
	HbCV booster	
12 Months		If PRP-OMP was used previously, recommend a HbCV booster dose given at 12 months as the third dose of PRP-OMP
15 Months	MMR	MMR is usually not given to infants younger than 15 months of age but may be given at 12 months in high-risk areas
	HbCV booster	If HbOC was used previously, recommend another HbCV booster at 15 months, that may be given as PRP-OMP, PRP-D, or HbOC
18 Months	DTP	DTP may be given between 15–18 months, but usually between 6 and 12 months after the third dose, and may be given simultaneously with MMR at 15 months
	OPV	OPV may be given simultaneously with MMR and HbCV at 15 months or any time between 12 and 24 months
4–6 Years (at or before entry to kindergarten or elementary school)	DTP	DTP can be given up to seventh birthday
	OPV	—
	MMR	AAP recommends the administration of the second dose of MMR at 11–12 years of age
14–16 Years	Td	Repeat every 10 years throughout life

[a]Adapted from AAP (Am Acad Pediatrics), 1989; AAP, 1991; AAP, 1992; CDC, 1982; CDC, 1989a; CDC, 1989b; CDC, 1990; & CDC, 1991a. *HBV*, Hepatitis B virus vaccine (refer to Childhood Immunization, Part II, for details); *DTP*, diphtheria toxoid, tetanus toxoid, whole-cell pertussis vaccine; *OPV*, oral poliovirus vaccine; *HbCV*, Hemophilus b conjugate vaccine (three preparations are available [refer to Childhood Immunization, Part II, for details]: PRP-D [ProHIBiT], polyribosylribitol phosphate conjugated to diphtheria toxoid; HbOC [HibTITER], polyribosylribitol phosphate oligosaccharide conjugated with a nontoxic mutant diphtheria toxin; PRP-OMP [PedvaxHIB], polyribosylribitol phosphate conjugated with an outer membrane protein of *N. meningitidis*); *MMR*, measles, mumps, rubella vaccine; *Td*, tetanus toxoid (full dose) and adult strength diphtheria toxoid.

contact with the general public often is forgotten. It is this function as a health educator that makes the pharmacist unique.

As the former Prime Minister of England, Benjamin Disraeli, is reported to have said, "There are three kinds of lies—lies, damned lies and statistics."[17] No pharmacist, however, can ignore statistics, particularly those pertaining to health and disease, however formidable or annoying it may be to wrestle with them. In actual fact, a few basic formulae and their application is all that is necessary—but without them, community health services and practice are meaningless.

All events that are measurable must be related to the population in which they occur—usually known as the population at risk; obviously, to compare the actual number of births in Pittsburgh with those in Podunk is valueless, the difference in population being too great. In other words, the events to be measured must be reduced to a common factor of population—usually, for the sake of convenience, a multiple of ten. This device merely produces a manageable number instead of a fraction, or one preceded by a decimal point. As an example, consider live births. Say that, in 1977 there were 50 births in a population of 1000 people; this means that there were 0.05 births per person—which is ridiculous. By saying that there were 5 births per 100 people, or that the birth rate was 5%, we come up with a workable figure instead of 0.05 births per person. In actual fact, birth rates usually are computed per 1000 of population.

The basic formula for a rate of any type is therefore

$$\text{Rate} = \frac{\text{number of events measured}}{\text{population at risk}} \times k$$

where k is a constant and multiple of ten.

The crude birth rate is what it says—a *crude* measurement of births, as the population at risk includes all the men, women and children in the geographical area of concern—most of whom are incapable of bearing children. A more accurate measurement would be to confine the population at risk to women—a sex-specific rate, but only the women in the child-bearing age group can have babies so a further refinement would be to confine the population at risk to women between the ages of 15 and 44 years—an age/sex-specific rate. This is a much more accurate measurement of births and is known as the fertility rate.

Death rates follow the same pattern as birth rates—ranging from the crude death rate to age and sex-specific rates, the most commonly used as an indicator of health services being the infant death (or mortality) rate. This age-specific rate measures the number of deaths occurring in infants below the age of one year and often is used as an indicator of the effectiveness of a nation's health services, the implication being that the care of the mother and baby reflects the availability and efficiency of medical care. This use is certainly questionable, but it remains the only readily available rate for worldwide comparative purposes.

Earlier in this century the maternal mortality rate—a sex-specific rate—was useful for comparative data but it is now so low in the Western World that it has become useless by dint of the small number of deaths that occur in pregnant women because of better medical care.

Further refinement of rates occurs when particular problems become evident in a community and the measurement of trends becomes necessary. The rise in illegitimacy is a case in point, especially as illegitimate infants have a higher mortality rate than babies born in wedlock. The increase in illegitimate births since World War II has been dramatic, with a proportionally greater rise in white than black populations. The stigma which still attaches to illegitimacy casts some doubt on the validity of the figures but the adverse effect on the infant is apparent. As most of the babies at risk are indigent and, therefore, are cared for by local health departments, it is again imperative for the pharmacist to keep informed of these programs and contribute what he can to them (Table 8).

Kilwein[18] has reviewed several other commonly used rate equations in an article directed to pharmacists. These include crude death rate, age-specific death rate, case fatality rate, incidence rate and prevalence rate. He emphasizes that these are the statistics most frequently used to measure the health status of a community. For example, incident rates show the number of new cases of a disease that occur in a population during a period of time, usually 1 year. Prevalence rates provide the number of new and old cases which are present in a community at a particular point in time. It is obvious that if the pharmacist keeps abreast of local health statistics such as these, he can function as a valuable resource person to researchers conducting epidemiological studies in the community.

Nutrition

For the most part, it is quite rare to encounter severe acute nutritional deficiency such as pellagra, scurvy or beriberi in the US today. However modern public-health studies have shown that a substantial percentage of the population is deficient to some degree in one or more nutrients. Further, there certainly has been developed a distinct relationship between obesity, disease and length of life. For this reason, the pharmacist generally should be aware of normal nutritional requirements and the problem of malnutrition or poor nutrition among his clientele.

The outcry against "fast foods" and "junk foods" has brought nutrition into the public eye as no concerted effort on the part of nutritionists and health educators could have done. In actual fact, many "fast foods" have nutritional value—but generally only if supplemented by the elements commonly missing from their composition. In theory, a hamburger with lettuce, tomato and French fried potatoes contains a balance of protein, fat and carbohydrate which can be beneficial if the food used in their preparation is nutritious to begin with, ie, if

Table 8—Commonly Used Rates

$$\text{Crude birth rate} = \frac{\text{Number of live births}}{\text{Total population}} \times 1{,}000$$

$$\text{Fertility rate} = \frac{\text{Number of live births}}{\text{Total number of women aged 15–44 years}} \times 1{,}000$$

$$\text{Crude death rate} = \frac{\text{Number of deaths}}{\text{Total population}} \times 1{,}000$$

$$\text{Infant mortality rate} = \frac{\text{Number of deaths less than one year of age}}{\text{Number of live births}} \times 1{,}000$$

$$\text{Maternal mortality rate} = \frac{\text{Number of deaths associated with pregnancy}}{\text{Number of live births}} \times 10{,}000$$

$$\text{Illegitimacy ratio} = \frac{\text{Number of illegitimate births}}{\text{Number of live births}} \times 100$$

the hamburger is pure, lean, ground beef and the other foods are of comparable value. In general, however, this type of diet lacks the basic food elements present in fresh fruits and vegetables and, unfortunately, the people to whom "fast foods" appeal seldom bother to obtain these staples.

Fortunately, for the first time, there is sufficient data regarding dietary risk factors for chronic disease to allow for a good opportunity to accelerate the significant health benefits seen in the US population. Generally, these include such simple measures as lower dietary intake of fat (especially saturated fat), using less salt and increasing green and yellow vegetables and whole grain cereals in the diet. For maximum benefit, these measures should be coupled with avoidance of obesity, keeping good physical activity and avoiding alcohol and tobacco.[19]

Allied to nutrition is dental health and most health departments have access to dental services to which medically needy persons should be referred.

Vivian *et al*[20] published an article on the pharmacist's role in the prevention of dental caries. The American Dental Association also published annual pamphlets on the dentist and the pharmacist which cover oral structures and diseases, prevention of caries, OTC and prescription dental drugs and how these professions can work together.

Obesity is the most common form of malnutrition in this country today. Starvation *per se* is almost nonexistent in the Western World but its corollary of fatness is common; one-third of adults, for instance, are calculated to be at least 15 to 20% overweight. Despite this, fashion advertising still emphasizes the skeletal, equine figure of the *haute couture* model as its symbol.

Unless there is some marked glandular disorder in one of the endocrine organs, people become fat by taking in more calories than they are putting out, although there is no doubt that individual metabolic processes enable some people to deal more efficiently than others with this intake–output system. The prevalence of obesity is evident when the best-seller booklists reveal that, year after year, authors are making money from readers desperately trying to be slim; that they don't succeed is also evident by the constant appearance of some new diet fad and book. The correlation of obesity with poor health is well established but, like smoking, it is beyond the power of most fat people to stop eating until some catastrophic event occurs, such as a heart attack, when they dismally will restrict their food intake.

Studies have shown that about 20% of persons over 20 years of age are at least 10% overweight in the US. These are individuals who are at risk and develop diabetes, digestive system diseases, cardiovascular disease and some forms of cancer, later in life. There are, of course, many people who voluntarily lose weight when in good health but the trend in these people is to put it on again within a year or two.

As a practical point, it has been shown that people lose weight better in groups—when they have encouragement, and also competition, from their peers. The proliferation of "health spas" testifies to this dictum. Hence, the pharmacist can acquaint himself with the local organizations aimed at helping men and women (and children) lose weight: Weight Watchers, TOPS (Take Off Pounds Safely) and the many other programs such as those offered by the YMCA and the YWCA. In addition to this, the popular notion that there are magic drugs which will control weight may be dispelled with authority by the pharmacist, nutritional education and guidance offered through the many materials available from voluntary organizations, and local and state health departments.

Thus the pharmacist can make significant contributions in nutrition by advising his patients about basic food needs, helping to correct improper food habits in children, advising on special requirements for nutrients during prenatal and maternal periods in females, suggesting special diet instructions for diabetics and people with food allergies and participating in supporting school lunch programs and food-stamp plans.

Environmental Health

Modern society is suffering physically and emotionally from the technology it has created. The four basic necessities of health—air, water, food and shelter—are all elements of the environment which, in their natural state, have only beneficial effects. To call shelter, whether in the form of personal clothing or housing, an element of nature may seem far-fetched—but the origin of clothes and houses was in skins and wood derived from nature.

Today, society has bent many aspects of nature to its will with harmful results. Air, for instance, now contains noxious substances which are either directly the result of combustion or produced by photochemical change. The classic example of the latter is the famous Los Angeles "smog" (a word first coined from "smoke and fog" in 1905) which results from the interaction of ultraviolet rays in sunshine and unburnt hydrocarbons of automobile engines. The products, when trapped by the thermal inversion engendered by local topography, cause damage to mucous membranes and lungs.

What the long-term danger is from this intermittent pollution we do not yet know; what we do know is that acute episodes of air pollution cause exacerbation of illness and even death in people who already have diseased respiratory and cardiovascular systems. The most famous of these catastrophies was in Donora, PA, in 1948, when there were 20 deaths during a 6-day period of air stagnation. The close correlation of disease with age, and in persons whose heart and lungs were already compromised, became immediately evident during the investigation. Similar major episodes have occurred in Belgium and London, and minor disturbances have been reported in several cities in the US and elsewhere. People with heart or lung disease should stay indoors if air pollution is present or even forecast.

Of more significance than air as a vehicle of disease organisms in this century is food, including milk. Fortunately, pasteurization virtually has eliminated milk as a medium for disease distribution but the same cannot be said for food. Foodborne disease, more commonly but often incorrectly termed food poisoning, is grossly under-reported and the four to five hundred outbreaks comprising some 5 to 10,000 persons per year probably can be multiplied by ten to represent the true magnitude of this common affliction. In most instances the illness produced by contaminated food is mild and of short duration, but more severe diseases such as botulism can occur.

The central packaging and distribution of food and the enormous increase in the number of people eating away from their homes have both contributed to the renewed interest in this minor but distressing group of diseases. Controls extend from the place of food production to the time of consumption and are, in general, simple, effective and inexpensive, particularly in the home—"keep hot food hot and cold food cold" is perhaps the most significant one-liner in the control of foodborne disease. If all food is maintained at temperatures below 45°F or above 140°F, many outbreaks of foodborne disease will be prevented.

Waterborne infectious disease is uncommon today although some 16,000 persons were infected with *Salmonella typhimurium* from a common California water supply.[21] This does not mean, however, that all public water supplies are pure and potable; many complaints about the taste, appearance and physical qualities of locally supplied water have led to a brisk trade in bottled water. In general, the virtues of bottled water have been inflated as most public supplies are bacteriologically safe, even if some may offend a few persons' esthetic senses. Water pollution is, however, a distinct reality and the pharmacist should keep abreast of events in this field.

Housing codes exist in most communities today either in the form of state law or local ordinance. There is no great contribution to be made by pharmacists in this matter except to lend their weight to logical programs for improving housing in their communities.

In summary, the pharmacist's role in environmental health is mainly one of alertness to the conditions prevailing in his community and of working, with others, towards the adequate control of any hazards. This is especially true of air and water pollution which require concerted community action for their control, but pharmacists may play a much more fundamental and personal role in foodborne disease. Often, the first indication of an outbreak of foodborne disease is the unusually large number of people seeking relief from nausea, vomiting and diarrhea, particularly if they are concentrated within a short period of time, a few hours to a day or two. The epidemic pattern of foodborne disease differs completely from the nausea, vomiting and diarrhea of "intestinal flu"—another common complaint, usually seen in the cooler months of the fall and spring.

"Point" epidemics of foodborne disease are dramatic, sudden events with most people becoming sick within 24 to 48 hours. If this type of epidemic results in an increase in across-the-counter sales of antinauseant and antidiarrheal drugs, the local health department should be notified without delay. This action will not only bring about the rapid investigation of the epidemic but also its control—the ultimate object of any epidemiological investigation.

Recent disclosures of the presence of chemical toxins in our environment is disturbing to say the least. "Moderation in all things" has been a wise edict for centuries; this perhaps should be the attitude of the pharmacist whose advice is sought about the need to limit the diet to only those substances pronounced safe. There is well-documented proof of cancer production by ingested materials in animals, but there also is little proof that many of these substances produce human cancer. Certainly host factors must play a significant and vital role in disease of any type—a fact often ignored by the pure environmentalists. Certainly, the community pharmacist should keep abreast of developments pertaining to toxic and carcinogenic substances, but he would do well to maintain a healthy skepticism to the more florid and sweeping statements made today.

Of more real importance are the many diseases resulting from one's occupation, ranging from the classical lead and mercury poisonings of yesteryear to the lung diseases of today. There is no doubt that the workplace may play an immense role in disease occurrence and new occupational hazards emerge every year; one notable example currently in the limelight is asbestos and its relationship to cancer. The pneumoconioses provide another good example of work-related diseases and have been known to occur in miners for hundreds of years in the form of silicosis or "black-lung" disease, but it is only recently that byssinosis or "brown-lung" disease has been demonstrated in textile workers.

All occupations in which the participants are exposed to dust are hazardous to a degree, depending on the size of the dust particles, and their consequent ability to penetrate into the lung substance, combined with their concentration and the length of exposure time in the workers.

Bingham *et al*[22] reviewed the governmental regulation of environmental hazards for the next decade. They provide

Information on the workplace and the future of occupational safety and health regulations.
Hazards of local ambient environments (hazardous and other waste dumps, radioactive waste from weapons production, air emissions and groundwater contamination of unknown magnitude).
The clean air act.
Waste reduction and minimization.
Radioactive waste and weapons production.
Global pollution.
Chlorofluorocarbons and the land ozone layer.
The greenhouse effect and global climate change.
Conserving tropical forest and biological diversity and regulatory initiatives.

They predict that the 1990s will be filled with initiatives to improve environmental health. This will include pollution prevention coupled with remedial efforts. An international cooperation will be needed to address all serious global pollution problems, hopefully with enforceable international agreements. The US likely will follow procedures where workers will be involved in improving their workplace health and safety, *viz*, worker participation, such as that developed in several European countries.

The pharmacist should, therefore, be aware of local occupations and their dangers and be alert to the first symptoms of disease—the case in point being the pneumoconioses, which first become evident in breathlessness occurring on mild exertion.

Again, the emphasis must be on the pharmacist becoming acquainted with the local community and adapting the principles of health and medical care to the particular situations produced therein. The environment is changing constantly—physically, biologically, culturally, socially and economically. The alert citizen, and even more the pharmacist, should cultivate an informed awareness of these changes and adapt his methods of health education, and disease prevention and control, to the changes in each community in which pharmacy services are provided.

The pharmacist's continuing education should include watching the local pattern of society and its diseases, and changing his or her emphasis towards the evolving patterns of disease and its control.

Mental Health

The vast topic of emotional illness and its causation, manifestations and control remains a puzzle to most people, including many health professionals. Even though there are numerous disagreements among professionals about the extent of mental illness in the US, few disagree with the estimate that there are about the same number of beds in this country for the mentally ill as there are for all other ailments combined. At any given time, some have said, approximately 10% of the US population has some form of emotional disorder which requires treatment.

Data in 1986 provided further sobering statistics that an estimated 2.4 million chronically mentally ill individuals have been identified in this country (excluding mental retardation and chronic substance-abuse problem individuals). Out of this number, about half (1.1 million) live at home, some 700,000 are residents of nursing homes, 450,000 live in single rooms or congregate-care facilities and at least 150,000 are found in psychiatric hospitals. The remainder all probably are maintained at home by their families and uncounted numbers may be found among the homeless.

The main trouble with investigating mental disease is that there are few definitive tests on which diagnoses may be based—there is no blood test to measure the occurrence of schizophrenia for instance. In general, pharmacists should be aware of their local community mental health services, especially those catering to ambulatory patients; the timely referral of clients exhibiting bizarre behavior to these facilities may be life-saving, especially in those persons who demonstrate suicidal tendencies.

Suicide is the one manifestation of mental disturbance that can be measured accurately as it results in the death of the person involved. Fortunately, most suicide attempts turn out to be unsuccessful, although this does not negate the importance of prevention whenever possible. The clue to contemplation of suicide may be no more than a solitary phrase expressing disgust with oneself followed by the implication that the best way out is to end it all—comments which should never be ignored. Depression is the forerunner of attempted suicide, and its cardinal symptoms are readily recognizable to the observant layman and even more to a health professional—or they should be.

There is a distinct epidemiology of suicide; it occurs most commonly in older, reasonably well-off men, especially those who are unmarried. Women attempt to commit suicide more often than men but are not as successful in completing the act. The agents used in suicide vary with their availability; in the US firearms figure most prominently, as they are readily available; in England drugs are the main agents because of stringent gun-control laws. With these and other epidemiological facts at his disposal, the pharmacist can be alert to potential suicide victims among clients and should do everything possible to bring aid to them. The "cry for help" which may be offered in the form of overt, or covert, references to worthlessness and to the uselessness of life, should never be neglected.[23] The pharmacist should never be reluctant to ask a client directly whether he or she has ever considered, or is now considering, committing suicide—to contradict one of the many myths which pertain to suicide and its prevention. People who say they will kill themselves often do so, and repeated suicide attempts are not uncommon.

Mechanic[24] reviewed recent developments in mental health and feels that from about 1981–1991 there has been less rhetoric and more appreciation of the tough realities of providing effective community service and care to seriously mentally ill people. There has been more and better understanding of the complexities of finance and organization of service arrangements and their interconnection with housing, welfare, and medical and legal arrangements. Research technology and advanced medications have progressed significantly boding well for the future.

The US currently has a large pool of mental health professionals and facilities. There is also more mental health advocacy. However, there is need to further advance the field. For example, deinstitutionalization has not been complete, freeing mental patients to the streets has contributed a bitter backlash. For the most part the public sector and public welfare, on which many of these mentally ill patients depend, has undergone significant erosion. Many public sector delivery systems are in great disarray and overwhelmed.

The changing demography of the American population has worsened the problem and increased the numbers of seriously mentally ill persons. The federal deficit and public budget pressures have made it difficult to attract enough monies for services in this field. There is need to be more efficient to correct existing fragmentation, duplication and disorganization of the services system and to establish clear priorities so that there is focus on the seriously and persistently mental ill. Lack of insurance and erosion of welfare as well as increases in the numbers of homeless have contributed to the problem.

In summary, if the pharmacist detects what may be a potentially suicidal client, he or she should talk to the client and seek aid from family and professional contacts in the community; the client's plea for help should not be ignored.

Alcoholism and Drug Abuse

The diseases of alcoholism and drug abuse (sometimes lumped together in the phrase "substance abuse") are peculiarly within the purview of the pharmacist. No other disease entities, with the possible exception of poison control, lend themselves more readily to intervention by pharmacists; easy as it may seem to advocate the pharmacy as the central point of control, it is far from having become so. The causal factors in these diseases remain obscure and control measures uncertain.

Alcoholism is estimated to affect many millions of men and women in the US. Society is slowly coming to realize that alcoholism is a biopsychosocial disorder with many causes and many ramifications.

Alcohol and tobacco abuse and drug abuse in general is a worldwide public health problem of enormous dimensions. In the US, between 450,000 and 600,000 premature deaths annually are related to these substances, which represents nearly one-third of all deaths.

One anchor to which the alcoholic may moor himself is Alcoholics Anonymous (AA)—a voluntary organization founded by an alcoholic for alcoholics, with branches for the spouses of alcoholics (Al-Anon) and their children (Alateen). Branches of AA exist in nearly all cities and many smaller towns, and the AA number always is listed in the local telephone directory; willing workers, all of whom were and, still are alcoholics, are ready to help. Apart from AA, various clinics and centers are available through official government agencies such as health and welfare departments, all of which work closely with AA.

The pharmacist will have many opportunities to help individuals who become dependent upon alcohol, although many alcoholics will resist help. This, however, should not be a deterrent, as one victory is worth countless failures. All community agencies, professional and voluntary, should be called into play, including church, voluntary and government groups.

Drug abuse is similar to alcoholism yet different in that it has received more acceptance among younger people—especially marihuana, which has been tried at least once by most teenagers, as has alcohol. The trend to accept the smoking of pot as a normal concomitant of growing up is evident, and the main concern is that hard drugs may follow use of the milder ones. There is still, too, some concern about the long-term effects of marihuana which will not be resolved for many years. Again, the pharmacist is in the unparalleled position of being professionally the most competent member of the community to advise local agencies about drugs and their effects. The knowledge and participation of the pharmacist will add to his or her credit, both professionally and financially, as the contacts and publicity resulting from such interest will be reflected in business returns—a very real, if venal, benefit.

Des Jarlois[25] focused on the AIDS epidemic among injecting drug users (IDUs). His study provides data on

Early epidemiology of HIV infection among IDUs.
Heterosexual and perinatal transmission from IDUs.
Rapid transmission of HIV among IDUs.
Non-AIDS illnesses associated with HIV among IDUs.
Harm-reduction perspective and HIV-prevention programs for IDUs.

In terms of general drug abuse, there are several booklets and pamphlets available through the Drug Enforcement Administration (DEA) and the professional health organizations. One particularly excellent *Resources for Community Action, A Pharmacists Guide to Drug Abuse,* booklet has been produced by the American Council on Marijuana through a grant by ACTION, the Federal volunteer agency, and was published and distributed by McNeil Pharmaceutical Co. The contents include the etiology and health consequences of drug abuse as well as specific coverage of the most commonly abused substances, eg, marijuana, alcohol, cigarettes, cocaine, phencyclidine, the hallicinogens and the sedatives. The back section has an excellent glossary, lists common drugs, symptoms of use and suggested readings and details on how the pharmacist can serve as a community resource for drug-abuse information.

Public Health Research

If the pharmacist evinces a sincere interest in community health programs, there may be opportunities to participate in public health research programs, especially those concerned with drugs and their control. In general, investigation of community disease is based on two methods, known as retrospective and prospective surveys. The retrospective or backward-looking survey is based on past historical data readily obtained by asking questions of the population under investigation.

The prospective or forward-looking method actually observes the events that occur in the population as it progresses through time. Obviously, the retrospective method is inexpensive, takes little time, deals with a stable population and requires a minimum amount of work. Its drawbacks, however, are that it relies on memory, is difficult to conduct with a control group and introduces some observer bias because the surveyor knows what he is looking for. The prospective survey, on the other hand, is the opposite—it may take years to complete, is costly, has to contend with a shifting population and requires a vast amount of work—but it is easy to use with a control group, does not rely on memory and observer

Table 9—Public Health Research Surveys: Advantages (+) and Disadvantages (−)

Type	Time	Cost	Labor	Population stability	Memory	Control	Observer bias
Retrospective (backward)	+	+	+	+	−	−	−
Prospective (forward)	−	−	−	−	+	+	+

bias can be reduced to a minimum or eliminated altogether (Table 9).

The best example of the use of these methods comes from the observation by an Australian ophthalmologist in 1941 that he was seeing an unusually large number of congenital cataracts in infants; investigation revealed that all the women concerned had had rubella (German measles) during their pregnancies—a retrospective discovery. This finding brought about some women obtaining illegal, but medically supervised, abortions when they revealed to their doctors that they had had rubella during their pregnancies and were afraid of having a baby with a congenital deformity.

This practice necessitated a prospective survey to determine what the true incidence of rubella-produced congenital deformities was; pregnant women were observed during their pregnancies and their infants followed after birth to determine whether or not the babies developed congenital deformities. This forward-looking survey revealed that the true incidence was somewhere around 20% instead of the 100% thought to occur at first. Today, of course, with more liberal abortion practices, the question is somewhat academic, but the original work illustrates the principles involved. Practicing pharmacists should offer their services to surveys of these types in investigating disease patterns in their community, particularly in drug therapy and its abuse.

As discussed under *Pharmacoepidemiology*, the clinical pharmacist already has proven valuable in "fine-tuning" drug therapy after marketing medications and the same methodology can be applied in several related areas of community practice. Pharmacists of course, may join the US Public Health Service (USPHS) directly, and information can be obtained by writing the USPHS. Some information on PHS pharmacists is provided in Chapter 6.

Summary

Public-health practice is influenced by the conservatism or liberalism of government and the cultural variations of the people it serves. The trend in the US today is towards private enterprise. Some aspects of health care now resemble those prior to the introduction of medical insurance in the 1930s—but dependence upon the ability to pay a medical bill is sound economy only if charity accepts the burden of the nonpaid bill, and increasing avarice may prevent the "old country doctor" approach being accepted today. The value a society places upon the health of its people has always been regarded as a measure of its humanitarianism. The question being posed today is whether the enormous cost of armament for defense and space exploration is justified at the expense of ill health and disease. How to resolve this dilemma perhaps never will be achieved, but an honest attempt will need more than the superficial platitudes often voiced by politicians.

The pharmacist, as an educated observer, should participate in this debate. In particular, he or she has more contact with the general public and, therefore, more opportunity to influence the well-being than other health professionals. In addition to this role, the pharmacist can offer to be a consultant to, or member of, the many official and voluntary health agencies in the community. Obviously, service as a board member of all the health agencies that exist is impossible, but those to which the most can be contributed can be selected. The pharmacist who is a leader, can lead; if not leading, he can become a useful member of the group in supporting measures that improve the health of the public.

It is hoped that the numerous pleas for pharmacists to "get involved" in public health are heeded and that some of the comments and references present here will be useful to this end.

References

1. Breslow L: *Ann Rev Public Health 11:* 1, 1990.
2. Omenn G: *Ibid* (preface editorial), *14:* V, 1993.
3. Poon, C: *J Pediatr Health Care 6(6):* 370, 1992.
4. Gibson MR: *Am J Pharm Educ 36:* 189, 561, 1972; *37:* 1, 1973.
5. *Am J Public Health 71:* 213, 1981.
6. Shattuck L: *Report of the Sanitary Commission of Massachusetts, 1850* (reprint), Harvard Univ Press, Cambridge, 1948.
7. Frenk J: *Ann Rev Public Health 14:* 469, 1993.
8. Roueche B: *Eleven Blue Men*, Berkley, New York, 1965.
9. Nelson RC: *DICP 22:* 336, 1988.
10. PHS Publ No 79-550 71, DHEW, Washington DC, 1979.
11. Liang K, Zeger SL: *Ann Rev Public Health 14:* 43, 1993.
12. Cates W Jr: *Am J Epiodemiol 131(5):* 749, 1990.
13. Casto DT: *Pharmacotherapy 12:* 94S, 1992.
14. *Morbidity and Mortality Weekly Report* (selected issues, 1968–1983), CDC, Atlanta.
15. Kaiser Foundation medical care program: *Annual Reports, 1960–1983*, Kaiser Center, Oakland CA.
16. Vanderpool N, Richmond J: *Ann Rev Public Health 11:* 185, 1990.
17. Huff D: *How to Lie with Statistics*, Norton, New York, 1954.
18. Kilwein JH: *US Pharm (Mar):*61, 1978.
19. Scrimshaw N: *Ann Rev Public Health 11:* 53, 1990.
20. Vivian AS, Vivian JC, Margolis FJ: *Am Pharm NS21(8):* 25, 1981.
21. *Am J Epidemiol 93:* 33, 1971.
22. Bingham E, Meader W: *Ann Rev Public Health 11:* 419, 1990.
23. Farberow NL, Shneidman ES: *The Cry for Help*, McGraw-Hill, New York, 1961.
24. Mechanic D: *Ann Rev Public Health 12:* 1, 1991.
25. Des Jarlais D: *Ibid 14:* 413, 1993.

Bibliography

Public Health and Preventive Medicine

Bickley HC: *Practical Concepts in Human Disease*, 2nd ed, Williams & Wilkins, Baltimore, 1980.

Grant M: *Handbook of Community Health*, 4th ed, Lea & Febiger, Philadelphia, 1987.

Green: *Community Health*, 6th ed, Mosby Year Book, 1989.

Holland, W *et al*, eds: *Oxford Textbook of Public Health*, Vol I, II, III, Oxford Univ Press, 1991.

Last JM, Maxcy-Rosenau: *Public Health and Preventative Medicine* Appleton & Lange, New York, 1992.

Preventive Medicine USA, Prodist, New York, 1976.

Shindell S, Salloway JS, Oberembt CM: *A Coursebook in Health Care Delivery*, Appleton-Century-Crofts, New York, 1976.

Wilner DM, Walkley RP, O'Neill EJ: *Introduction to Public Health*, 7th ed, Macmillan, New York, 1978.

History

Mullan F: *Plagues and Politics*, Basic Books, New York, 1989.

Rosen G: *A History of Public Health*, MD Publ, New York, 1958.

Rosen G: *Preventive Medicine in the United States, 1900–1975: Trends and Interpretations (Preventive Medicine USA* offprint), Prodist, New York, 1976.

Epidemiology

Bailar J *et al: Assessing Risks to Health: Methodologic Approaches*, Auburn HSE Publ, 1993.

Bres P: *Public Health Action in Emergencies Caused by Epidemics: A Practical Guide*, World Health, 1986.

Fletcher RH *et al: Clinical Epidemiology—The Essentials*, Williams & Wilkins, Baltimore, 1982.

Lilienfeld AM: *Foundations of Epidemiology*, 2nd ed, Oxford Univ Press, New York, 1980.

Mausner JS, Bahn AK: *Epidemiology—An Introductory Text*, Saunders, Philadelphia, 1974.

Public Health and Pharmacy

Bush PJ: *The Pharmacist Role in Disease Prevention and Health Promotion*, ASHP Res Educ Found, Bethesda MD, 1983.

Gable FB: *Psychosocial Pharmacy: The Synthetic Society*, Lea & Febiger, Philadelphia, 1974.

Public Health in the Curricula of Colleges of Pharmacy, AACP, 1965.

Smith MC, Knapp DA: *Pharmacy Drugs and Medical Care*, 2nd ed, Williams & Wilkins, Baltimore, 1976.

Wertheimer AI, Smith MC: *Pharmacy Practice, Social and Behavioral Aspects*, 3rd ed, Williams & Wilkins, Baltimore, 1989.

International Health

Anonymous: *Evaluation of the Strategy for Health for All by the Year 2000*, Vol I, Global Publ, 1992.

Basch PF: *International Health*, Oxford Univ Press, New York, 1978.

Brockington CF: *World Health*, Penguin, Baltimore, 1958.

Graig L: *Health of Nations: An International Perspective on US Health Care Reform*, 2nd ed, Congr Quart, 1993.

Waddell WH, Pierleoni RG, Suter E, eds: *International Health Perspectives*, Springer, New York, 1977.

Occupational Health

Hunter D: *The Diseases of Occupations*, 6th ed, Hodder & Stoughton, London, 1978.

Levy BS and Wegman DH, eds: *Occupational Health*, Little, Brown, Boston, 1983.

Environmental Health

Greenberg M: *Public Health and the Environment*, Guilford Press, New York, 1987.

Karen H: *Handbook of Environmental Health and Safety*. Pergamon Press, New York, 1980.

Purdon PW ed: *Environmental Health*, 2nd ed, Academic, New York, 1980.

Mental Health

Allen RD and Cartier MK: *The Mental Health Almanac*. Garland STPM Press, New York, 1978.

Langsley DG, Berlin IN, and Yarvis RM: *Handbook of Community Mental Health*. Medical Exam Pub, New York, 1981.

Stengel E: *Suicide and Attempted Suicide*, Penguin, Baltimore, 1964.

Suchman E: *Sociology and the Field of Public Health*, Russell Sage Publ, 1963.

Venereal Disease

King A, Nicol C, Rodin P: *Venereal Diseases*, 4th ed, Bailliere Tindall, London, 1980.

Morton RS: *Venereal Diseases*, 2nd ed, Penguin, Baltimore, 1972.

Schofield CBS: *Sexually Transmitted Diseases*, 3rd ed, Churchill, Livingstone, Edinburgh, 1979.

Administration

Curry W, ed: *New Leadership in Health Care Management: The Physician Executive*, Am Coll Phys Execs, 1988.

Hanlon J, Picket GE: *Public Health, Administration and Practice*, 8th ed, Mosby, St Louis, 1984.

Bibliography

Chitty M *et al*: *Federal Information Sources in Health and Medicine: A Selected Annotated Bibliography*, Greenwood Publ, 1988.

La Rocco A, Jones B: A bookshelf in public health, medical care and allied fields. *Bull Med Lib Assoc 60*: 32, 1972.

Opposing Viewpoints

Bender DL, Leone B ser eds. In Szumski B, ed: *The Health Crisis, Opposing Viewpoints*, Greenhaven, San Diego, 1989.

Califano J, Jr: *America's Health Care Revolution: Who Lives? Who Dies? Who Pays?* Random Publ, 1986.

Dental Disease

The Dentist and the Pharmacist, AM Dental Assoc, Chicago, 1985.

Drug Abuse

Resources for Community Action. A Pharmacist's Guide to Drug Abuse, McNeil, Springhouse PA, 1988.

CHAPTER 100

The Patient: Behavioral Determinants

Albert I Wertheimer, PhD
Vice President, Pharmacy Managed Care
First Health Service Corp
Glen Allen VA 23060

Sickness involves more than the biochemical condition portrayed in previous chapters; it is also a social and psychological phenomenon. Perceptions of the state of being sick are taught through socialization, and thus vary among individuals according to social class, ethnicity, attitudes toward health care and availability of services.

Being a patient means yielding responsibility and control of our care to someone else. Someone we may not even know is making decisions having important consequences for an individual and his future. The patient role is an undesirable, unnatural one. The reality, though, is that all of us at one time or another become patients when we, albeit reluctantly, acknowledge that our condition requires care beyond what a layperson might be able to provide.

The pharmacist who wishes to serve his patients to the fullest extent cannot limit his objectives to accurate dispensing. He consciously must address himself to the person in whom the disease process occurs. A totally impersonal approach is not possible in medicine since the pharmacist and the patient react to each other as persons whether they wish to do so or not. Thus, since subjective factors cannot be eliminated, they must be recognized and understood and their therapeutic potentialities used for the patient's benefit.

The personality of the patient is the totality of the characteristic ways the individual deals with internal and external stresses. The signs and symptoms are bound completely with different personality traits and, therefore, true communication is impossible unless the pharmacist is vigilant to this implication.

Illness Behavior

The human psyche is most complex, and many behaviors cannot be predicted with absolute certainty. We can, though, say a few things about the patient. Parsons[1] indicates that we consider a person as ill when he is unable to perform valued tasks. When a sufficient number of tasks cannot be completed so that one's role cannot be fulfilled, that person is regarded generally as too ill to be responsible for the performance of his normal role responsibilities.

Psychosocial factors must be considered to maximize health care outcomes. A patient's past experiences, perceptions, feelings, beliefs, decisions and behaviors can cause a different patient reaction to the same affliction.[2,3]

Illness behavior is a culturally and socially learned response. Much work has demonstrated that members of various ethnic groups react differently to pain and, moreover, react after different threshold levels are reached. With the number of minority groups in the US so rapidly increasing, it is important that the pharmacist be able to differentiate between their accompanying orientation. For instance, Soviet emigres may assume an authoritarian role for the health-care provider, thus hesitating to question medical advice, or even discuss medical issues. A classic study by Zborowski found that the response to similar back pain varied considerably among Italian, Jewish, Irish and Old American (several generations in the US) patients. The Italian and Jewish patients were more expressive regarding their pain than were the Irish and Old American patients. Zborowski further demonstrated that the attitudes toward caretakers differed among these groups; they showed variable levels of confidence, trust, optimism, etc.[4,5] Similar results of differing illness behavior amongst ethnic groups has been demonstrated in recent years, promoting further the necessity for pharmacists to become sensitized to cultural differences. However, the professional must be prudent not to generalize by assuming a patient holds certain attitudes based on an ethnic background.[5] Furthermore, we may expect to find members of different societal subcultures behave rather differently in the face of illness. Most of one's ideas regarding normality, illness and health definitions are developed based on one's views of the immediate world surrounding them. Were everyone in one's peer group to require a hearing aid, the use of such a device soon would be considered normal. What this means, then, is that the practitioner must weigh the response of patients in evaluating their degree of wellness against visible clues of social class, income, occupation and formal education completed.

Countless studies have been performed indicating that views of, reactions to and concern about health and illness vary according to an individual's age, social class, ethnic origin, knowledge about health and medical care, gender and a number of other sociodemographic variables.[6] Additionally, cultural differences play a major role in determining one's illness behavior. Someone from a remote village who has never seen a physician, nurse or pharmacist will seek aid from an elder in the village who might have some medical experience. So, too, would be the expectation if a native American became ill in an area where the power and authority of the medicine man continues and where confidence in his cures and advice endures. There can be little argument that there are links between reaction patterns to pain, illness and physiological response.

Knowing the patient's family is important in understanding him. A person who has had a genuinely caring mother usually has a basic feeling of trust in people that helps in coping with an unpredictable and, at times, unfriendly world. A woman who is inconsistent and emotionally incapable of mothering is apt to send her child out into the world with a wary and hostile attitude. Such children may misinterpret a friendly and helpful gesture as an attempt to hurt or manipulate them.

Siblings usually play an important role in the development of personality. Feelings of jealously toward other patients and the need to win status in the doctor's eyes may be related to childhood sibling rivalries. A positive and loving father, in addition to helping the mother (directly and indirectly) to fulfill her responsibilities to her children, provides goals, standards and conditions that help an individual to orient himself realistically to life. Such an individual, when he ventures from home, is prepared to adjust emotionally and socially to his fellow man.

The pharmacist should consider personality type in order to optimize the interaction between patient and health professional. The manner in which a person reacts to a stressful situation is often amplified by illness due to the patient feeling his/her well-being is threatened, as well as the discomfort of being in an unfamiliar setting. Ten personality types which have been identified are[7]

1. Dependent, demanding patients
2. Orderly, controlling patients
3. Dramatizing, emotional patients
4. Long-suffering, self-sacrificing patients
5. Guarded, suspicious patients
6. Superior and special patients
7. Seclusive, aloof patients
8. Impulsive patients with a tendency to act out
9. Patients with mood swings
10. Patients with chronic memory deficits and a tendency to confusion

Another concept that one must bear in mind is the recognition that an emotional component often has been associated with the etiology of illness or with its development. The vast array of disease states associated with psychosomatic implications should be known and appreciated by the pharmacist. Social scientists even have suggested that the presentation of somatic complaints oftentimes masks an underlying emotional problem which frequently may be the major or compelling reason why the patient has arranged the consultation in the first place.[8,9]

Stress is a variable that has been correlated highly with the use of health services. Yet, both the concept of stress itself as well as the relationship have not been elucidated fully. Even questions dealing with the differential effectiveness of placebos among different patients require greater understanding before definitive or even predictive statements may be made with certainty.

The reactions toward illness also may make illness behavior a candidate as a means to seek secondary advantages. It is acknowledged universally that illness is an acceptable reason for avoiding some role obligations, social responsibilities and expectations.[6] The problems lie in the widely varying definitions of illness and health seen in various locations, institutions and under differing conditions. To be sure, other factors similarly influence illness behavior. These include the patient's self-image with reference to an assessment of vulnerability and problem severity, reaction of family or health-care providers to the problem, demands of family or employment, level of stigmatization of the problem, institutional environment, risks involved in treatment, degree of expected discomfort, expense or disfigurement and confidence in the provider(s) of care.

The pharmacist should have an understanding of patient anxiety, placebo effects, compliance, treatment delay, self-medication, use of home remedies and reticence to seek professional aid.

Parsons suggested that sickness produces a temporary disturbance in an individual's capacity to fulfill his usual roles. This is a conditionally legitimate state, having the effect of insulating the individual from certain types of mutual influence with other persons, and of alienating him from certain norms accepted in the "well" population. The sick person is not held responsible for having incurred his condition, which is by definition undesirable, and, therefore, one is motivated to "get well." Since the patient is incapable of achieving this goal through self-volition, he has an inherent right to receive care, and is, in fact, obligated to seek and accept professional care.

It should be noted that Parson's model of the sick role, while it provides a helpful framework for illness behavior, has been criticized for overlooking important subjective factors of being sick. It also seems to apply most readily to the sickness behavior of the middle-class person who is generally knowledgeable about health and the health-care system. Parson's model also does not apply to patients with mental illness, chronic illness, permanent handicaps and illnesses such as alcoholism and drug abuse.[10,11]

The actual stages of illness and medical care were first delineated by Suchman.[12] He took the concept of illness behavior as proposed by Mechanic and Volkart and arrayed some internal sequences. What we see are five stages of medical events and they are examined along four elements (content, sequence, spacing and variability of behavior). The stages are

Symptom experience
Assumption of the sick-role
Medical-care contact
Dependent-patient role
Recovery or rehabilitation

In the first stage, the decision that something is wrong is made. This is based on recognition of a pain or some other discomfort. It is possible that the individual may elect to do nothing, self-medicate, rest or consult a family member, friend or even decide to visit a physician if the problem worsens.

In the second stage, the decision that one requires professional care is made. One may seek excuse from normal task responsibilities and consult with significant others.

In the third stage, the decision to seek professional medical care is made. A scientific diagnosis and treatment regimen are desired and consulting the physician legitimizes the abrogation of some role responsibilities. The person may ignore the advice and seek another source of aid which is more palatable.

At the onset of the fourth stage, the person truly becomes a patient and accepts transfer of control for his care to the physician. Here, the patient agrees to be placed in another's hands.

At the final stage, a decision is made to relinquish the patient role. Clearly, this is more difficult with some diseases and patients than with others. Now the patient must relearn the full burden of societal responsibilities.

Another system is at work and it oftentimes delivers the would-be patient into the second stage of the Suchman model. This is the Lay Referral System described by Freidson.[13] In this system, one is expected to inquire about a possible medical problem in an ever-widening circle of other individuals. Members of one's nuclear family are queried about the problem, followed by selected persons in the extended family, friends, neighbors, coworkers, etc. In some instances, this search leads to the community pharmacist. The search is terminated when an individual indicates knowledge and/or experience with an identical medical problem and offers sensible-sounding advice.

In some cases, the patient will never recover. It is possible that a permanent impairment will exist or that the patient may even die. Two areas of concern for the pharmacist are seen in these situations. The patient who may have a terminal condition might be seen at home or in a community pharmacy as often as he or she may be found within an institution. Contemporary medical-care practices dictate that a dying patient should be able to return to familiar surroundings, and to be enabled to live one's final time with dignity, eg, the cancer patient might be sent home to be with the family until hospitalization might be required at the very end. The response process to the disclosure of the terminal nature of a disease usually follows a predictable course. The work of Glaser and Kubler-Ross[14] indicates that, after disclosure, the following steps may be seen.

Depression follows disclosure, yet most patients come to terms with the situation and move on to the next stage. Some do not and withdraw from contact with others. Next, the patient either accepts or denies the forthcoming event. Denial may be seen in patients becoming intensely active, emphasizing a future orientation, forcing reciprocal isolation, comparing oneself with other patients or juggling time. Eventually, people overcome the denial stage and accept their fate.

Acceptance may be witnessed in one of two forms. The first—active preparation—involves the patient into becoming philosophical, possibly embracing religion and putting one's social and financial affairs into order. Suicide is a form of active preparation. Here, patients often decide to spare their loved ones protracted grief and expense. Passive preparation for imminent death includes accepting this fate with nonchalance or calm resignation. Accepting the diagnosis but deciding to fight may be seen in this category. A patient may opt for a marginal healer or quack who makes attractive promises.

When the patient defines himself as ill, some of the following sociocultural factors influence how one responds: Socioeconomic Class—It is known that business and professional classes respond to and recover from an illness more so than do persons from blue collar groups. Moreover, persons from lower socio-economic classes and/or who are less educated tend to have greater morbidity, disability and mortality rate in general.

The other problem mentioned earlier that the pharmacist might encounter is that of the permanently impaired patient. Surely, it is obvious to the reader about the possible feelings of an invalid, such as the amputee and others having visible abnormalities. Goffman introduced the study of stigma into the health-care milieu. Stigma refers to something deeply discrediting. Diseases and medical problems may be stigmatized. In such cases, shame and guilt are present. Why do people whisper about mental disorders, cancer, epilepsy or venereal diseases and think nothing about discussing colds, flu, headache, etc, with their friends and co-workers? Why is it that people willingly wear eye glasses, but fight the use of a hearing aid? Is impaired hearing worse than impaired vision? The answer lies in a closer examination of our social mores. Illness has been related closely to religious beliefs. Many persons have believed that illness is a divinely administered punishment and, therefore, have been led to accept the concept that ill persons "might have had it coming." Other stigmatized problems include disfigurement, and this becomes the basis for a problem that the pharmacist might be able to alleviate. Some patients might not be compliant with their medication schedules for fear of having coworkers or others see them swallowing medicine. Others decide not to pursue therapies when they see what visible effects the therapy causes for example, loss of hair from chemotherapy.

Working with Patients—A great deal has been written about the therapeutic relationship between patient and health practitioner. Countless commentators tell us that we must project an image or aura of caring, concern, confidence and competency. It is important to make an assessment of the patient at the outset of an interaction.

The patient is likely to experience greater illness in the same temporal cluster as stress, family problems, personal problems or other traumatic events. Knowledge about the patient's personal life and *understanding of his problems* can be invaluable.

Patient fear/anxiety may be effectively dealt with by the pharmacist. Blood in the stool, breast masses and some central nervous system aberrations can strike fear into patients. The knowledge of a friend or relative's unsuccessful bout with the pathology makes the problem even more acute.

Practitioner-patient relationships have been categorized by Szasz and Hollender.[15] In the active-passive mode the practitioner uses the authority inherent in his role in which the patient does not participate. The guidance-cooperation mode permits the practitioner considerable authority, but the patient is expected to cooperate. In the mutual participation mode the patient is expected to be actively responsible for treatment. The clinician can decide what might be the optimal strategy for each type of patient.

Interviewing the patient is a delicate and important function. Many complaints can be localized in an area of the body. The quality of the discomfort also can be calibrated, with the aid of the patient. The same holds true for the quantity of the perceived stress. The chronology of the problem can be detected with skill and patience. The time of onset, duration and frequency of the disease may be defined sharply. Learning of aggravating or alleviating factors also may be of value. Associated symptoms may be a clue to problems. When the responses to these questions have been considered and evaluated, instructions or advice are forth coming. This communication must be made with due consideration of the person's educational background, intelligence, attitude toward this illness and financial situation.

One can never afford to ignore the possibility of psychophysiological disorders. For example, asthma is thought to be, at least in part, a psychosomatic disease. Classic physicians since Hippocrates saw emotions as playing a crucial role in asthma. The evidence for psychological factors are that, first, most asthmatics state on report and their physicians note a correlation between their episodes and psychological factors, such as fear or anger.

Fifty to 75% of the patients who present gastrointestinal complaints appear to lack a clear pathophysiological basis for their symptoms. The symptom complex presented by such patients variously has been called mucous colitis, spastic colon, functional bowel disorders, nervous diarrhea and, more recently, irritable colon syndrome. In the absence of organic pathology, many physicians ascribe the symptoms to emotional factors. In addition, some gastrointestinal diseases, such as peptic ulcer disease and ulcerative colitis, have a history of being regarded as the result of specific psychological conflicts. In fact, gastrointestinal diseases in general have been regarded as having important psychological components. Sexual dysfunction is another problem which appears to be very much related to psychological factors.

The pharmacist should not joke during the communication process, should not be interrupted for commercial purposes and must be willing to answer questions to explain points two or three times, if necessary, to an agitated and confused patient. False assurances or promises do not benefit anyone and must be avoided.

Dealing with Illness

Defense (or adaptive ego) mechanisms serve as a first line of defense. They may be invoked to keep feelings within bearable limits, restore psychological homeostasis and permit a "time-out" to adjust as well as to deal with unresolvable conflicts. Vaillant's work[16] illuminated this area.

Narcissistic defenses are seen in individuals as adult dreams and fantasies, and in healthy people before the age of five. They alter reality for the user.

Delusional projection of a positive delusion about external reality, usually of a persecutory type. Responsibility for feelings is projected to others.

Denial is seen when one insists that a dead person is still alive, or that a disease is not present, etc, in the face of overwhelming contradictory, comprehendable evidence.

Distortion is a gross reshaping of external reality to suit internal needs. It may include hallucinations, megalomanic beliefs and feelings of delusional superiority or entitlement.

Other immature defenses are seen commonly in healthy juveniles, and in adults with some character and affective disorders. They appear as misbehavior and usually may be corrected by improvements in interpersonal relationships (maturation, or in finding a more mature partner or understanding physician).

Projection is found when a person's emotionally unacceptable feelings unconsciously are rejected and attributed to others.

Schizoid fantasy employs the use of fantasy and withdrawal to avoid a conflict or pleasure. It may be associated with an avoidance of intimacy. Here, the patient may not believe the fantasies or even act them out.

Hypochondriasis is thought of as the transfer of feelings toward others resulting from loneliness, bereavement or unacceptable aggressive impulses into complaints of pain or illness.

Passive-aggressive behavior is aggression expressed indirectly and ineffectively through pouting, negativism, procrastination and illnesses that affect others more than self.

Acting-out is the direct expression of an unconscious wish or impulse in order to avoid being aware of the effect that accompanies it. It may include delinquency, extramarital affairs, exhibitionism, drug use and self-inflicted injury.

Regression is seen as a return to an earlier mode of behavior which was either more successful or pleasant, such as thumb-sucking and baby-talk.

A cogent passage worthy of notation and consideration is one by Coser:[17]

> The sick person who is admitted to the hospital ward frequently is overcome by anxiety to such an extent that he is likely to suffer from a partial blurring of his self-image because of the actual and symbolic threat to his body. His forced passivity, his horizontal pose, the removal of his own clothes and belongings, the fact that doctors and nurses, persons hitherto unknown to him, have full access to his body and the fact that he cannot anticipate what will happen to him—all these factors contribute to a loss of ego identity.

The idea that mind, body and emotions are not separate entities no longer is subject to question. They are so interrelated that it now is recognized that the cause and treatment of a long list of diseases—bronchial asthma, peptic ulcer, colitis, arterial hypertension, migraine headache and many others—are related to the life history and personality of the patient.

Behavioral Science Concepts—Treatment of the total patient has come to be viewed as essential by members of all of the health professions. Failure to use sociodemographic data about a patient permits the existence of bias in predictions made in treatment situations. The application of some behavioral science concepts may aid in the reduction of bias or error in prediction. Moreover, a most-appropriate regimen may be created. For example, instruction of an elderly patient to take one tablet after meals (where we assume three to be normal) may not be effective if the patient eats only one meal a day.

While it probably is unwise for the pharmacist to become involved in behavior modification—a practice which should be left to trained, experienced professionals—he should be aware of techniques and their uses. Natural behaviors include instinct, and *imprinting* (the name for linkages formed between parents and offspring). Through it, only one or two attempts are needed to "learn," and this learning—very heavily preprogrammed behavior—can take place only during a brief period, the critical period in the life of an individual. Learning is a new behavior being acquired, usually through interaction with one's environment.

In classical conditioning, a person who has learned to avoid bees may extend his avoidance to similar insects, such as wasps. In addition, identical elements in a new situation may cause a reactivation of a previously learned response. This occurs in all types of learning. An application of classical conditioning that has gained widespread acceptance is the LaMaze method, which views pain from a Pavlovian view as a response that was unnecessarily conditioned to many stimuli associated with childbirth and, furthermore, as an unconditioned response of lower brain centers that could be inhibited or altered by activity of the higher brain centers (an example of classical "reciprocal inhibition").

In *operant* conditioning, new responses can be acquired and refined. Operant principles may be used to control chronic pain as well as environmental contingencies. This is done by rewarding increases in functioning with praise and by not punishing pain behaviors.

In identification, we see the automatic and largely unconscious process of imitating and copying those who are admired or powerful. It is a continuous process. Persuasion and coercion are practices which can be studied, practiced and learned. We see this with politicians, door-to-door salesmen and others. Such techniques, however, although they produce the desired action or decision, are vulnerable to second thought; hence, they are not particularly effective in inducing changes in ongoing behavior. Peer exploration is another method for changing patterns of preference. Small groups that discuss issues openly can change patterns of interpersonal communication. This has been used successfully for postmyocardial infarct and peptic ulcer patients to modify behaviors.

The pharmacist should understand referral behavior, both to and from medical, as well as nonmedical sources. For example, he should ascertain which patients could be referred to a social worker or psychologist. One must keep in mind that what oftentimes is recommended is a compromise based on the feeling of the recommender as to what is best for the patient, combined with what the patient might accept as a reasonable referral route. It would be pointless to recommend to a patient who has made it clear that he has no faith in physicians that he see a physician. In such a case, it might be wisest to recommend an OTC product or even a self-care book.[18]

Not only is human behavior different among persons in otherwise similar social strata, but differences occur in each of the subcultural groups. For instance, men often behave or react differently than women to the same event or action and we may see these differences in persons with different education, income, etc.

In the Millis Commission Report recommendation number 11 of the 14 recommendations states

> The Study Commission emphasizes that pharmacy is a knowledge system in which *chemical substances and people called patients interact.* Needed and optimally effective drug therapy results only when drugs and those who consume them are understood fully. We suggest that one of the first steps in reviewing the educational program of a college of pharmacy should be weighing the relative emphasis given to the physical and biological sciences against the behavioral and social sciences in the curriculum for the first professional degree.[19]

> Clearly a pharmacist must have ready knowledge about drugs, but he also must have ready knowledge about people, about relationships and communication with them, and about systems and cost service.[20]

The pharmacist is faced with a number of problems beyond the accurate dispensing of the indicated drugs. He is at the end-point where an item of pharmacological activity has been requested. It has been requested by a physician who must be able to handle ignorance and uncertainty. The patient has described the symptoms as best as possible, and the physician understands that these symptoms could be caused by a number of sources. The physician is reminded constantly of his therapeutic inadequacies due to the ever increasing emphasis on postgraduate medical education, pressure from patients in a science worshiping world, specialization accomplishments and the proliferation of medical journals.

The situations which a pharmacist may be expected to face include problems of compliance of prescribed or recommended therapy by patients, the use of the placebo effect, problems in effective communication primarily in the area of patient education and a consideration of the role that a psychological problem can play in symptom development. For instance, about one in four individuals suffer from an affective disorder (such as depression) during their lifetime, and the patient, not recognizing the symptoms, may consult a pharmacist regarding OTC drugs, for example, to address sleeping disturbances. The number of, pervasiveness of and degree to which the symptoms render the patient dysfunctional are good indicators that the patient may be suffering from a psychological illness. Physical symptoms that may indicate the patient is experiencing an illness for which a referral to a specialist would be the most appropriate advice, include fatigue, stomach disorders, sleep disturbances, changes in appetite and/or weight, the ability to concentrate and motor activity.

A placebo drug, one which is not pharmacologically active but may help alleviate a condition because the patient believes it is effective, has been shown to affect a wide variety of biological and disease processes including fever, headache, cough reflex, common cold, insomnia, mood changes, angina pain, postoperative pain, blood-cell count and vasomotor function. Placebo effects are not imaginary and are not necessarily the result of suggestion in the ordinary sense of the term. It is thought that the placebo may result from a patient interaction with health-care personnel or medication and that the patient may be influenced by provider-led expectations.

About one-third of all subjects react to a placebo. A reaction is not merely a matter of mental state, but includes actual physiological responses to an expectation to improve, thus prompting important therapeutic implications for the pharmacist.[21] If there is a failure in therapeutic situations, personnel must consider whether they may have contributed to it through a negative placebo effect.[27]

It is likely that the pharmacist will be involved often with patients who wish to second-guess or question the information offered by a physician. Pharmacists must be careful, as there is always the possibility that a placebo effect was intended or that an unsure diagnosis was made and various therapies are being tried.

Smith[22] provides interesting orientation when he compares the patient to a hunter in almost the same sense as the early pioneers were hunters. The stakes are just as high—survival. There are dangers—economic and medical—since the patient may be taken advantage of by a pharmacist, physician or may be injured by a drug. Many patients are cautious in their hunt and rightly so. Even for prescribed drugs, the patient has the ultimate choice of where to purchase them. These decisions of whether and where are central to the pharmacist-patient relationship and are subject to two kinds of influence: the basic or patient influences and the external or environmental influences. It is proposed that four basic variables control all patient actions: needs, motives, perception and attitudes.

He continues: Patient behavior with regard to pharmacy in general, or to an individual pharmacy, is shaped by individual encounters with the pharmacist and the historical accumulation of such encounters. Whether pharmacist like it or not, this is how the process works.

Roles of Pharmacists

As Dichter has indicated the ideal doctor is gone and community doctors, particularly older ones, were inclined to treat the patient as an illiterate. He writes, "The patient doesn't want to be talked down to—he wants at least to be a knowledgeable participant where his own body is concerned. Pharmacists, being a part of the health system attract a lot of hostility but, to a very large extent, without justification. To better understand the source of the hostility, a number of practical measures could be introduced."

Dichter continues by informing us that the modern patient-consumer has become much more of an individualist. He does not want to be treated as a case or as a number. The pharmacist, accepting this new role, can do a number of things such as inform each patient that there is a complete file maintained about him. Modern patients are antifatalists, and do not accept getting old. They do not want to suffer pains and they tend to plan ahead much more than people used to. This is a good sign, as they are much more health-conscious and prophylactic-conscious. The pharmacist could provide his patients with pamphlets or even prefilled medicine chests for emergencies.

Dichter[30] said

> The modern customer and patient wants to be informed. He unfortunately also has become somewhat more suspicious. In contrast to other countries, in America the prescription filled by the pharmacist is not accompanied by a description of any one of the possible negative side effects. The pharmacist should be on the patient's side. The pharmacist may not want to contradict the physician, but he might advise the patient to ask the physician whether he feels that a low-priced cold remedy would not serve just as well.

Another area where the pharmacist has the opportunity to make major contributions toward the effectiveness and quality of patient care is in patient compliance with therapeutic regimens. Pharmacists are probably in the best position to detect and inform others regarding noncompliance, given their relationship with both patient and physician.[24] Studies indicate a wide variation of noncompliance, but most report that at least one-third of all patients fail to comply with a regimen, and some studies report that more than one-half of all patients are noncompliant.[25] Monitoring and education by the pharmacist can greatly improve patient compliance. Pharmacists should recognize patients who display risk factors that make them more likely to be noncompliant, such as being on a costly regimen, taking drugs that have unpleasant side effects, being on multiple drug therapy or therapy for a chronic condition over an extended period of time.[25]

Both verbal and written instructions should be given and they should be specific and nonambiguous; the label should contain detailed information. The role of the pharmacist does not cease with counseling at the time when the patient receives the prescription. If the pharmacist notes that the patient is not using the drug appropriately (eg, the patient fails to get a refill), the reason for noncompliance should be determined and the situation resolved.[25]

Recent research in patient compliance has shown that a lack of patient understanding is responsible for a significant amount of noncompliance. Merely communicating is not enough; a patient needs to comprehend and recall instructions. Research has shown, eg, that using simple sentences and repetition, categorizing advice, making information concrete and giving reasons for important advice are effective means of communication.[26] The pharmacist also should anticipate potential societal barriers to compliance, such as patient's life-style/schedule or side effects, including those that may not seem significant to the pharmacist. For instance, discussing the issues of skin discoloration, hair loss or foul smells caused by the medication may deter the patient from discontinuing the regimen prematurely.[27]

Ivey *et al*[29] identified ways in which the pharmacist can identify the patient's information needs and thereby control communication, timing and define communication objectives. This information should enable the pharmacist to develop methods of communication and to be able to evaluate the effectiveness of his instructions. Since communications exchanges have centered around the concerns of therapists and patients, it is necessary to know some things about the patient's therapy. The pharmacist should attempt to learn

> The reason or reasons a patient is taking a particular drug.
> Any unpleasant effects produced by the drug that may be self-monitored by the patient.
> Specific instructions on the dosing schedule.
> Interactions with other medications.
> The diet of the patient.
> Instructions for any monitoring tests to be performed by the patient.
> A variety of other information expected by the patient.

Some might argue that health education, preventive medicine and other health services and health educational activities are insufficient and that what is needed, rather, is a health activation or actualization program. It is thought that, in such a program, the patient will come to understand the importance of proper life style, including stress management, diet, use of leisure time and other factors. It was hoped that the patient would be most interested to exercise and take good care of himself. This, then, is what is "wellness." This movement has been transforming the traditionally passive patient into an active, informed and effective participant in health care and health promotion.[29]

Pharmacists should appreciate the potential they hold to influence patient behavior. In a 1991 survey, in which respondents were asked to rank 25 professions in terms of honesty and ethics, pharmacists/druggists ranked first, receiving 60% of either "very high" or "high" ratings; clergy followed closely with 57% of those ratings.[30] Since only a small proportion of people who experience symptoms actually consult a doctor, the pharmacist is often in a position of greater access to the sick person than is the physician. The neighborhood pharmacist often is the only health-care professional who comes into contact with a patient, since 33.6 million people in this country have no health insurance.[31]

There has been an increase in the number of pharmacists over the years. In 1970 there were 55.4 pharmacists per 100,000 people in the US; in 1986 there were 67.1.[33] Furthermore, the role of the pharmacist has broadened, as evidenced by the increase in clinical responsibilities and cognitive services performed by them, and the opportunity for pharmacists to impact patient outcomes positively is definitely growing. With the growth in opportunity comes an increased obligation for the pharmacist to understand the behavioral determinants of patient behavior.

References

1. Parsons T. In Jaco EG, ed: *Patients, Physicians, and Illness*, 3rd ed, Free Press, New York, 112, 1979.
2. Mechanic D: *Soc Psychiatry 1:* 12, 1966.
3. Wertheimer AI, Smith M, eds: *Pharmacy Practice: Social and Behavioral Aspects*, 3rd ed, Williams & Wilkins, Baltimore, 120, 1989.
4. Fincham JE, Wertheimer AI, eds: *Pharmacy and the U.S. Health Care System*, Pharmaceutical Products Press, New York, 365, 1991.
5. Wertheimer AI, Smith M, eds: *Op cit*, 133.
6. Wertheimer AI, Smith M, eds: *Op cit*, 132.
7. Leigh H, Reiser MF: *The Patient*, Plenum, New York, 254–267, 1980.
8. Mechanic D: *Op cit*, 19.
9. Balint M *et al: Treatment or Diagnosis*, Routledge, Chapman & Hall, New York, 1984.
10. Wertheimer AI, Smith M, eds: *Op cit*, 131.
11. Fincham JE, Wertheimer AI, eds: *Op cit*, 337.
12. Suchman EA: *J Health Hum Behav 6:* 2, 1965.
13. Freidson E: *Patient's View of Medical Practice*, Russel Sage Foundation, New York, 146, 1961.
14. Glaser BG: *J Health Hum Behav 6 (Summer):* 83, 1966.
15. Fincham JE, Wertheimer AI, eds: *Op cit*, 332.

16. Bowden CL, Burstein AG, eds: *Psychosocial Basis of Health Care*, 3rd ed, Williams & Wilkins, Baltimore, 27, 1983.
17. Coser RL: *Soc Probl 4:* 3, 1956.
18. Robinson D: *Patients, Practitioners and Medical Care*, Heinemann Books, London, 142, 1973.
19. Millis J, ed: *Pharmacists for the Future: The Report of the Study Commission on Pharmacy*, Health Administration Press, Ann Arbor, 142, 1975.
20. *Ibid*, 126.
21. Leigh H, Reiser MF: *Op cit*, 145.
22. Smith M: *JAPhA NS 17*(12): 761, 1977.
23. Dichter E: *JAPhA NS12(7):* 354, 1972.
24. Fincham JE, Wirtheimer AI, eds: *Op cit*, 401.
25. Wertheimer AI, Smith M, eds: *Op cit*, 185.
26. *Ibid*, 169, 193.
27. Leigh H, Reiser MF: *Op cit*, 305–306.
28. Ivey M *et al: Am J Hosp Pharm 32:* 828, 1975.
29. Wertheimer AI, Smith M, eds: *Op cit*, 420.
30. *Gallup Poll Monthly 308 (May 1):* 29–31, 1991.
31. US Bureau of the Census. *Statistical Abstracts of the United States 1992*, 112th ed, USG PO, Washington, DC, 105, 1992.
32. Kurtz R, Chalfant HP: *The Sociology of Medicine and Illness*, 2nd ed, Allyn & Bacon, Boston, 142, 1991.

Bibliography

Anastasi A: *Psychol Rev 65:* 198, 1958.

Blechman EA: *Handbook of Behavioral Medicine for Women*, Brownell KD, ed, Pergamon NY, 1988.

Brown EL: *Newer Dimensions of Patient Care: Pt. 3, Patients as People*, Russel Sage Foundation, New York, 9, 1964.

Bruhn JG, Phillips BU, Levine PL, eds: *Medical Sociology: An Annotated Bibliography*, 1972–1982, Garland NY, 1985.

Bursztajn H, Feinbloom R, Hamm R, Brodsley A: *Medical Choices—Medical Chances*, Delaconte, New York, 1981.

Cockerham WC: *Medical Sociology*, 3rd ed, Prentice-Hall, Englewood Cliffs NJ, 1986.

Gentry WD, Benson H, DeWolff CJ: *Behavioral Medicine: Work, Stress and Health*, Nijhoff, Boston, 1985.

King NJ, Remenyi A, eds: *Health Care: A Behavioral Approach*, Grune & Stratton, NY, 1986.

Kleinman A: *Patients and Healers in the Context of Culture*, Univ of Calif Press, Berkley, 1980.

Linden W, ed: *Biological Barriers in Behavioral Medicine*, Plenum Press, NY, 1988.

Stone GC, *et al*, eds: *Health Psychology: A Discipline and a Profession*, Univ of Chicago Press, 1987.

Susser M, Watson W, Hopper K, eds: *Sociology in Medicine*, 3rd ed, Oxford Univ Press, NY, 1985.

Talalay P, ed: *Drugs in Our Society*, John Hopkins Press, Baltimore, MD 1964.

Taylor SE, ed: *Health Psychology*, Random House, NY, 1986.

Wertheimer A, Smith M: *A Casebook in Social and Behavioral Pharmacy*, Whitney Books, Cincinnati OH 1987.

Zeiner AR, Bendell D, Walker CE, eds: *Health Psychology: Treatment and Research Issues*, Plenum, New York, 1985.

CHAPTER 101

Patient Communication

Paul L Ranelli, PhD
Assistant Professor of Pharmacy Health Care Administration
University of Florida College of Pharmacy
Gainesville, FL 32610

Pharmacists work in very diverse practice settings—hospitals, community pharmacies, clinics, health maintenance organizations, home health-care organizations, retirement centers and nursing homes. The needs of the patients served in these settings vary greatly: they may have acute or chronic diseases, be ambulatory or bedridden and be under a physician's care or seeking a self-care remedy. Across this spectrum of practice settings and patient types, pharmacists share the role of drug-use expert. To promote rational drug therapy, pharmacists must be able to communicate effectively with patients and other health-care providers.

This chapter provides an overview of the communication process, pharmacists' roles as information givers and information gatherers, aspects of the illness experience that can interfere with professional dialogues and communication techniques pharmacists can incorporate into medication-history interviews and counseling sessions with patients.

Importance of Communication Skills

Pharmacy always has been considered a "people" profession, owing to the large amount of contact pharmacists have with the public, especially in community pharmacies. The profession renewed its commitment to patient-oriented care in 1985 at the American Society of Hospital Pharmacists' Hilton Head consensus development conference on directions for clinical practice in pharmacy. Pharmacists and educators there agreed that it is more important to look at patient-care outcomes—ie, the effect of the intervention of the pharmacist on the health of the patient—rather than just the functions pharmacists perform.

An extension of the patient-oriented care approach is now taking hold within the pharmacy profession, and that initiative is pharmaceutical care. Pharmaceutical care embodies responsibility, outcomes and a patient's quality of life. The concept incorporates many existing ideas about progressive pharmacy practice and brings new meaning to them. It represents an imaginative practice for those who believe the dispensing function alone can no longer support the pharmacy profession at a level it has in the past. Pharmaceutical care is defined by Hepler and Strand (see *Bibliography*) as

> The responsible provision of drug therapy for the purpose of achieving definite outcomes that improve a patient's quality of life.

The pharmacist's role in pharmaceutical care involves identifying, resolving and preventing drug-related problems that come from undertreatment, overtreatment or inappropriate treatment. The practice of pharmaceutical care requires pharmacists to answer the following question: What routine procedure (or system) do you use to monitor your patients' progress toward specific therapeutic outcomes? Only by communicating with patients and other health-care providers can pharmacists provide pharmaceutical care.

Besides the initiatives from within the profession promoting pharmacists' responsibilities for communicating with patients and other health-care professionals, the Federal Government enacted legislation in 1990 requiring pharmacists to offer prospective drug-use review and patient counseling for Medicaid recipients each time a prescription is presented. The requirements outlined within the Omnibus Budget Reconciliation Act of 1990 (OBRA 90), effective in January 1993, are that the pharmacist must offer to discuss with each individual (or caregiver) who presents a prescription the following information:

- Name and description of the medication.
- Dosage form, dose, route of administration and duration of drug therapy.
- Special directions and precautions for preparation, administration and use by the patient.
- Common or severe side effects, adverse effects or interactions and therapeutic contraindications that may be encountered, including ways of avoiding them, and the action required if they occur.
- Techniques for self-monitoring drug therapy.
- Proper storage.
- Prescription refill information.
- Action to be taken in the event of a missed dose.

In addition, the pharmacist must make a reasonable effort to collect, record and maintain the following information about patients receiving Medicaid benefits:

- Patient's name, address, telephone number, date of birth (or age) and gender.
- Patient's individual history where important, including disease state(s), known allergies and drug reactions and a comprehensive list of medications and relevant devices.
- Pharmacist's comments relevant to the individual's drug therapy.

Prospective drug-use review as outlined in OBRA 90 is really about communication, and it challenges pharmacists to interview and counsel patients systematically and to document these activities. It is anticipated that state pharmacy practice acts will expect pharmacists to provide these services for all patients, not just Medicaid recipients.

The responsibilities for medication-history taking and patient counseling as outlined in OBRA 90 should not be new to pharmacists. In fact, the "Standards of Practice for the Profession of Pharmacy," produced jointly by the American Pharmaceutical Association (APhA) and the American Association of Colleges of Pharmacy (AACP) in 1979 list many similar activities that pharmacists should perform:

- Interviews the patient or his/her representative to obtain information for entry into patient record, patient profile or family health record.
- Confirms and further clarifies the patient's understanding of medication dosage, dosage frequency and method of administration.
- Advises patient of potential drug-related or health-related conditions which may develop from the use of the medication for which patient should seek other medical care.
- Consults with patient to identify symptoms properly in order to advise patient for self-medication.

The standards also list other activities pharmacists should perform, all of which illustrate the pervasive need for pharmacists to have good communication skills:

- Refers patient to other health-care providers and/or health resources where indicated.
- Instructs patients in the use of medical or surgical appliances (eg, inhalers, colostomy bags, trusses).
- Advises patients on personal health matters (eg, smoking, drug abuse).
- Participates in appropriate community educational programs relating to health care and drugs (eg, drug abuse, alcoholism, hypertension).

Updated standards are being drafted, and it is anticipated that the pharmacist's role in pharmaceutical care will be reflected in the new standards.

While pharmacy education provides ample opportunities for honing clinical skills, few pharmacists have either a formal background in communication theory or extensive training and practice in communication. As such, some pharmacists may be reluctant to initiate professional dialogues with patients.

Other pharmacists may believe that as licensed professionals they possess all the communication skills necessary for effective practice. They may not realize, however, that there is a difference between credentialed and functional professionals. Credentialed professionals have degrees and certificates indicating they have completed formal training programs and to whom a stamp of approval, such as a license, has been granted. Functional professionals are those persons who possess the necessary skills. Credentialed professionals may not be functional, and *vice versa*.

While pharmacists may become functional communicators through on-the-job experience, that is not always the case. As the saying goes, "Practice makes perfect." But it is also true, especially for pharmacists with bad habits, that "Practice makes permanent." Specific training in patient communication skills in pharmacy school, and periodically thereafter, can provide pharmacists with a good base on which they continually can develop their skills.

The Communication Process

Communication is the sharing of information, ideas, thoughts and feelings. It involves not just the spoken word, but also what is conveyed through inflection, vocal quality, facial expression, body posture and other behavioral responses. As a first step toward communicating more effectively, pharmacists must understand the communication process.

The goal of all communication is understanding. For one person to understand a message composed by another, the receiver must do more than recognize the words used in the message by the sender. The receiver understands the sender if the meaning assigned to the sender's message by the receiver is the same meaning the sender intended. Thus, effective communication occurs only when the meaning of a message is held in common by the participants.

Human nature makes it difficult to attain this point of understanding between two or more people. A major obstacle to effective communication is that people have their own way of making sense of the world. Each person's view of reality is influenced by past life experiences and the current situation. This individualistic perception influences both the way in which a message is sent and the way in which it is received.

When a person wishes to share information with another, the sender must choose how to transmit that message. For instance, the medium of the message can be written, oral, nonverbal or electronic. If the sender decides to transmit the message by the spoken word, the sender must choose words to best convey the intended meaning to the receiver. The choice is aided by the sender's view of reality, feelings at the time and perceptions of the receiver. The process of sending the message is called *encoding*.

Once the information is encoded, the sender loses control of the message. The meaning of the sender's message comes from the *decoding* that occurs at the message's destination, the receiver. The receiver decodes the message based on his view of reality, current feelings and perceptions of the sender. Any response to the message reflects these perceptions and is the result of the receiver's subsequent encoding.

Once receiving a response, the sender can determine if the receiver understood the message. In other words, the response to the message acts as *feedback* to the sender. This gives the sender an opportunity to clarify and correct any misunderstanding.

This sequence of encoding, transmitting and decoding messages continues so long as sender and receiver continue to communicate. Communication usually takes place through multiple nonverbal channels as well. For example, as the words of a message are transmitted, facial expressions, gestures, vocal quality and other nonverbal cues also are sent. These nonverbal signs may modify the intended meaning of a message. A mixed message may result when the intended verbal and nonverbal messages are not understood as meaning similar things.

Information Gatherers and Givers

The interactions of a pharmacist and a patient usually can be categorized as either an information-gathering or information-giving session. Information gathering usually is done during a medication-history interview, which is a conversation with a multifaceted purpose. Pharmacists initiate the interaction to investigate and acquire data about a patient's medication-taking experiences, assess a patient's understanding of past and current medication-taking experiences, assess a patient's motivation for complying with the medication regimen and, possibly, suggest to the prescriber a change in regimens if the information gathered warrants such an action. The direct patient-pharmacist interaction during a medication-history interview frequently provides the pharmacist with an opportunity to begin a professional relationship with the patient.

It is not sufficient for pharmacists to collect information; the information also must be used. Pharmacists incorporate information gathered from medication-history interviews into subsequent counseling—information-giving—sessions. For instance, the pharmacist may learn through a medication-history interview that the patient is not following a prescribed therapeutic regimen. The patient may lack an understanding of the illness, therapy and medication effects, or the patient may lack the motivation to carry out the regimen. Once the compliance problem and its causes are understood, the pharmacist is prepared better to tailor an information-giving session that addresses the patient's specific needs.

In general, the scope of a medication-counseling session includes instruction, motivation and monitoring. Pharmacists should discuss the effects of the prescribed medications, the need to follow medication regimens, special instructions about how and when to take the medication and any unwanted effects and potential drug interactions. As noted earlier in this chapter, OBRA 90 specifically lists the information to be covered for Medicaid patients. Medication-counseling sessions also can serve as a quality-control check for pharmacists. For instance, by showing the patient the product, specifying the directions and stating the product's classification or indication, the pharmacist gives the patient the opportunity to state that the product looks different than before, the directions are different than the prescriber said or he does not have that condition. A further check of the prescription may uncover a dispensing error, or a call to the prescriber may detect a prescribing error—both of which can be corrected before the patient leaves the pharmacy.

A successful counseling session should leave patients trusting that the pharmacist genuinely is interested in their care. Pharmacists should establish and maintain lines of communication so patients feel free to consult them in person or by telephone when questions arise about drugs and drug therapy.

In organized health-care settings, departmental policies generally outline the pharmacists' drug-information responsibilities. A pharmacist usually interviews each patient soon after admittance and records the medication history in the patient's medical record. The counseling session or discharge interview usually occurs the day of discharge, or earlier if more time is needed to ensure the patient's understanding of a complex regimen.

In the community setting, pharmacists should be flexible enough to give or gather information in a variety of situations and environments. Often, the quality of a medication-history interview or a medication-counseling session is hampered by time constraints, a lack of privacy and noise. Pharmacists can overcome these constraints by providing shorter and more frequent patient interactions, making follow-up telephone calls, establishing a private consultation area and making appointments with specific patients, if necessary. Information gleaned from medication-history interviews and counseling sessions should be documented on the patient profile so that all pharmacists working in that setting can use the information when making follow-up consultation and referrals. Indeed, OBRA 90 requires such documentation for Medicaid patients.

It should be noted that the activities of information gathering and information giving are not distinct. In many cases the pharmacist performs both roles interchangeably. For instance, if the patient asks a question during a medication-history interview, the pharmacist usually answers it immediately or at the end of the interview. Similarly, counseling sessions usually begin with some sort of information gathering, such as asking what the prescriber told the patient about the medication or verifying that the patient is not allergic to it.

Many of the communication skills necessary for conducting medication-history interviews also are appropriate for counseling sessions. Here, the focus is on the process of conducting medication-history interviews; Chapter 103 includes information regarding specific ways to improve patient compliance with medication regimens through patient-counseling sessions.

Understanding Illness Experiences

Since a patient's past illness experience or reactions to a present illness contain stressors that may interfere with the communication process, pharmacists need to appreciate and understand these experiences and reactions to communicate effectively in both medication-history interviews and patient-consultation sessions.

For instance, patients may be facing separation from family, loss of important social roles, permanent bodily changes, feelings of helplessness and an uncertain future. For most patients the strain of illness leads to troubling doubts and fears. Patients may knowingly or unknowingly disguise these adaptations, fears and concerns with anger, depression and uncooperative behavior. A skillful pharmacist, aware of both the dynamics of communication and the stressors imposed on patients by an illness, can help patients recognize and cope with these reactions.

Many common fears associated with the illness experience center around the severity of disability and disease. Frequently, patients do not have a clear understanding of what ails them. Aspects of their illness may remain vague and uncertain even after repeated discussions with their physicians. These fears could be abated by more simple explanations, reassurance and positive reinforcement from physicians, pharmacists and other supportive health-care professionals.

Hospitalization can be a terrifying experience, and fear of the unknown can be overwhelming. Sophisticated instruments, electronic monitors, intravenous solutions, laboratory tests, diagnostic machinery, unfamiliar surroundings, strange clothing, a dying patient in the next room, cries of pain and a seriously ill roommate all contribute to an unsettling experience. Because health-care professionals become accustomed to this environment, they may be insensitive to patient fears. By recognizing that patients develop such fears, practitioners can help patients feel more relaxed and remove an important barrier to effective communication.

Patients may fear pain. This should be remembered when talking with patients before a diagnostic or surgical procedure. A patient's anxiety may be so great before a procedure that effective communication virtually is impossible. Practitioners can help relieve the anxiety by offering reassurance and a simple explanation of the procedure.

The fear that arises if a patient faces possible disability must not be underestimated. For instance, patients in serious accidents may have to cope with permanent impairment, and those with heart disease may have to deal with changes in lifestyle. Nurses, physical therapists and other health-care professionals play a vital role in restoring the confidence of patients and helping them adjust to such disabilities.

Patients also may fear death. Even patients without a life-threatening condition may fear death when they are hospitalized if they believe that a hospital is a place where people come to die. Researchers in the area of death and dying have identified five stages of death and the corresponding patterns of patient behavior, beginning with denial and isolation and moving through anger, bargaining, depression and acceptance. By recognizing these stages, health-care professionals can comfort and support a dying patient.

Communicating effectively with dying patients is difficult for both the pharmacist and patient. Sometimes, the professional staff is more uncomfortable talking about death than patients. For example, a community pharmacist may ignore a patient with a terminal illness who is having a prescription refilled simply because the pharmacist feels there is little to say. Being available to listen, however, encourages a patient to express feelings and provides a great source of comfort. Pharmacists should offer reasonable reassurance and accurate statements to strengthen confidence in health-care personnel, hospitals and therapy.

Are there other hindrances to good communication? Absolutely! Patients may be distracted by their disease, its process or their physical state. Patients could be embarrassed, self-conscious, modest or even bored while in the health-care system. The probability of effective communication increases if pharmacists understand that these factors do influence patients.

The way in which an individual reacts is determined partially by characteristics such as age, cultural background, emotional development, education, religious beliefs and previous illness experiences. Observing the adaptive reactions of a patient yields clues toward understanding and, thus, to more effective communication. For example, certain patients fear alienating health-care professionals on whom they depend. This behavior often is reinforced by providers who give positive feedback to "good patients." A patient's fear of alienating providers is not beneficial, however, because it may hinder attempts to detect symptoms. "Noncomplaining" patients need encouragement to express themselves. A genuine interest should be shown by talking with patients and specifically inquiring about their symptoms or other concerns.

Patients who are hostile or uncooperative require patience and understanding. Fears of helplessness and dependency often cause this type of behavior. If these patients become involved in formulating parts of their treatment plan, they may gain a sense of autonomy. For example, if a patient refuses to take medication, the reason should be identified and discussed. Pharmacists should help patients motivate themselves, not scold. They should explain how the medication helps cure the illness or relieve the symptoms, rather than simply talk about generalities on the importance of taking medication. While it is easy to become angry with hostile and uncooperative patients, pharmacists need to understand the reasons for this behavior to attempt effective communication.

Patients may become depressed and withdrawn when an illness strikes, making them reluctant to discuss their illness. Short, frequent conversations with these patients inform them that someone genuinely is interested in them. This eventually may encourage them to talk and discuss their true feelings. Patients should be informed when key staff members are available and when assistance is at hand.

Effective communication with patients, in sum, depends greatly on the degree of empathy demonstrated in the course of conversations. Empathy is the sharing, perception and identification of a patient's beliefs and state of mind without actually sharing those beliefs or having the same experiences. While empathy is essential, it is equally important for health professionals to temper their emotional involvement within the scope of their professional duty. Pharmacists can display an empathic approach by suspending—not surrendering—their own feelings long enough to provide sufficient time to understand the feelings of a patient. Beginning sentences with phrases like, "Boy, you're happy today," "It sounds like you're upset" or "It seems like this really bothers you" help establish an empathic tone by reflecting back on the patient's expression.

Pharmacists can do a great deal to decrease the uncertainties of illness and drug therapy by responding to patient questions, clarifying misconceptions and preparing patients for probable feelings or events. Pharmacists can provide emotional support and appropriate reassurance. A patient's emotional needs require frequent interactions with social support mechanisms. Pharmacists who communicate an empathic point of view are valuable sources of strength to patients coping with an illness.

Preparing for the Interview

How a pharmacist approaches the act of conducting a medication-history interview determines in large measure its success. Interviewers should spend a few moments mentally preparing for the interchange about to occur.

The interviewer should become familiar with the type of questions to ask and issues to pursue. This preparation greatly enhances the experience for both parties and, ultimately, the quality of the interview. As discussed in the previous section, patients may be under stress because of their illness, and pharmacists should be prepared to deal with these reactions to illness.

The interviewer should know as much as possible about the patient before entering the hospital room or approaching the patient in a community pharmacy. This easily is more achievable in a hospital setting where the patient's medical record, as well as other practitioners, can provide valuable background information about the patient. In the community setting, the pharmacist can review the patient's medication record if the patient has been to the pharmacy before. It rarely is possible to know much about a patient before a first pharmacy visit, but supportive personnel can be instructed to prepare a patient profile before the pharmacist begins talking with the patient, so that the pharmacist at least knows the patient's name.

Another issue worth considering before an interview actually begins is the physical state of the patient. Is the patient awake and cooperative, in pain or in distress, lucid or noncommunicative? Was the illness, disease or problem an emergency? A comprehensive interview with a patient who is experiencing acute pain or is semicomatose is difficult and unproductive for both parties.

Knowing the probable diagnosis may help provide a general index of the severity of the disease, the possible diagnostic procedures ahead and the prognosis.

Discovering a patient's social and occupational history are important pieces of the interviewing puzzle. Communication works best using a balanced and understandable vocabulary.

Opening the Interview

Pharmacists begin using verbal and nonverbal skills in the opening segment of the interview. This includes making introductions using the proper names of the patient and interviewer, defining the role of the interviewer, defining and explaining the purpose of the interview, stating the approximate duration of the interview and asking the reason for the patient's visit. The opening should not include specific probes about the physical characteristics of the patient, such as height and weight; background information such as this should be retrieved from other sources or asked later in the interview. A social history, however, may be taken here. This includes inquiring about daily routines, family life, hobbies and whether their medications cause any inconveniences in the workplace or home.

Interviewers properly introduce themselves by making eye contact and greeting the patient by pronouncing clearly both their name and the name of the patient. If help is needed with pronunciation of the patient's name, ask colleagues and the patient to make sure. It is best for the interviewer to begin formally by using the titles Mr, Mrs, Ms or Miss and then to switch to first names if the patient prefers. Some patients may use the interviewer's first name. If this is not acceptable, let the patient know by stating, "I prefer to be called Mr Jones."

The interviewer clearly should identify the purpose of the interview and the role of the interviewer in the situation. For instance, the interviewer could begin by stating, "Hello. My name is Phyllis Smith, and I'm a second-year pharmacy student doing my clerkship at the hospital. I'd like to spend some time talking to you about your medication history."

The interviewer also should explain approximately how long the interview will take and ask for the patient's explanation of the primary medical problem. The latter question gives the interviewer a chance to gather insight into patient concerns before talking about medication. Much of the time the reason for the visit is available from other sources and, in fact, should be acquired before the interview begins, but it is a good idea to hear patients express the reason in their words. Clues to pharmacy-related problems frequently arise using this approach.

Attending to Nonverbal Cues

During medication-history interviews, pharmacists must be observers, self-critics, questioners, listeners and recorders. It is easy to get so involved in these activities that they forget about the nonverbal messages they convey. Pharmacists and patients alike communicate emotions and other information in nonverbal ways. Blank stares, inattentiveness, nervous speech patterns and interruptions are distracting and detrimental to effective communication. Further, staying behind a barrier like a tall counter nonverbally communicates to patients that the pharmacist is unapproachable.

Various definitions of nonverbal phenomena may be found throughout the literature, but the distinction between verbal and nonverbal behavior may represent more of an arbitrary division than a true state of affairs. The verbal and nonverbal aspects of an interaction cannot be separated if one wishes to appreciate fully the nature of the interaction. In the context of interviewing, however, it is necessary to highlight those broad categories of nonverbal cues that communicate information. These categories are eye contact, facilitating movements, gestures or mannerisms and vocal qualities.

Eye Contact—Facial features, as well as facial expressions, are assumed to reveal personality traits. A great deal of information is communicated through head and facial movements, but perhaps the movement of another person's eyes provides more clues than any other facial structure. Therefore, a gaze is a major nonverbal signal to others.

Patients vary in the amount of eye contact that makes them comfortable, so interviewers should take cues from them. The best an interviewer can offer is frequent and attentive eye contact, avoiding blank stares. Eye contact helps assess the meaning that is behind the patient's words and conveys the message, "I'm listening." Thus, eye contact represents an important building block toward establishing patient trust and rapport.

Mannerisms—The study of nonverbal facilitation has led to the marketing of provocative best-sellers that promise readers, "You'll be able to read people like a book." Gestures, vocal qualities, body movement, clothing and hygiene can provide information about interviewers and patients, but ferreting out clues to hidden meanings can be more damaging than helpful to professional relationships.

The interviewer needs to make the patient feel comfortable by enhancing physical and psychological privacy. The interviewer communicates a posture of involvement by facing the patient directly and leaning forward at a slight angle. If the patient is seated or lying down, the interviewer should sit, if possible. This posture of leaning toward the patient is a sign of attentiveness to the patient's needs. Some other examples of nonverbal facilitation are an inclined head, a head nod and hand gestures that suggest understanding or the desire for more information.

Taking notes is appropriate during medication-history interviews so long as it is not the major focus of attention for either interviewer or patient. Excessive writing of notes has disadvantages. It is distracting to patients, impairs interpersonal dynamics and provides a convenient and absorbing escape for interviewers. Novice interviewers should take whatever notes are needed to achieve accuracy during interviews, but they should strive to improve their listening skills by recording only selected information at the moment and then completing the notes immediately after the interview.

Vocal Qualities—Pitch, range, tone, clarity and tempo are vocal qualities. Pitch refers to the frequency level of the voice. Speakers tend to vary pitch according to their learned expressive habits, such that some people vary pitch in a naturally expressive voice that is spontaneous and relatively pleasing, while others speak in a monotone with unvaried pitch. Still others use dramatic and exaggerated pitch changes. Pitch level influences patient attitudes toward interviewers and the content of the message. While monotones generally are disliked by most individuals, exaggerated pitch changes are disliked even more. Speakers with naturally spontaneous voices using neither a wide nor narrow range of pitch tend to be perceived more favorably.

Voice clarity is an important attribute for effective communication. The interviewer must enunciate well and be audible and articulate. To ensure that the patient can hear and comprehend, the interviewer should assess the patient's language and hearing abilities and then change speech patterns, if necessary.

Tempo is the speed of vocal production. Inappropriate silence and delays may irritate patients, while interruptions and cutting off facilitative periods of silence may rush patients and interfere with the smooth flow of conversation.

Fast tempo and frequent pauses often are associated with emotions such as fear or anger. Slow tempo also often is associated with anger, but it can connote sadness, depression or a lack of confidence, as well. A slow tempo with frequent pauses and utterances like "uh," "er" and "um" can indicate uncertainty; perhaps the interviewer is stalling while waiting for the patient's response or while formulating the next question to ask.

Beginning interviewers often express their emotions by talking too fast. Interviewers should keep their rate of speech conversational. A conversational rate of speech does not mean casual, however. The reality is that in professional practice pharmacists cannot afford to be as casual as they otherwise might be in social relationships.

Asking Questions Appropriately

To be good interviewers, pharmacists must be attuned to the types of questions asked, the manner in which questions are asked and the avoidance of repetition. Interviewing is a demanding activity that requires a greater investment of energy than casual conversation, especially if the interviewer is a beginner. The unnecessary repetition of questions often is a sign of interviewer's inattention.

The use of jargon also results from inattentiveness. This is the technical language or the characteristic idiom of a group or groups. Pharmacists and other health-care providers are not immune from using jargon. A sampling includes the terms OTC, po, nocturia, HCTZ, diuretic, hypertension and parenteral. Take OTC, for example. If that term is used in a question aimed at identifying nonprescription drug use, patients may not know that the letters stand for "over-the-counter." Even if they did, they may not understand that it means any medications available in pharmacies and supermarkets that they can buy without a prescription. Interviewers should choose language appropriate to the sophistication of the patient. The unnecessary use of technical terms may increase patient anxiety. If they are necessary, all technical terms should be explained after assessing the patient's understanding.

Open and Closed Questions—The open question is broad and allows the patient sufficient latitude in interpreting and responding to requests for information. An open question asks for information and specifics about the topic in a general way and cannot be answered in one phrase or with a "yes" or a "no." Interviewers often begin a topic or section using open questions since the questions can encourage the patient to discuss a broad range of information, but there can be too much of a good thing. The excessive use of open questions will result in an overly long, rambling, unfocused and inefficient interview.

When starting a section by asking open questions, the interviewer should begin the questions with words or phrases that elicit broad responses rather than words or phrases that restrict responses. For example, questions beginning with terms like "when," "where," "how," "what" and "tell me about" usually result in more information than questions starting with "is," "does," "can," "will" and "are," which usually are used better in follow-up attempts to clarify information.

Open questions beginning with "why" should be used sparingly, as they may imply criticism or result in guesses. The word "why" may have a place in interpersonal communication when the patient sees no threat from the interviewer. Usually, however, the same information can be obtained with other questions using the words "what" or "how." For example, instead of asking, "Why weren't you taking your medicine?" or "Why didn't you come in sooner for a refill?," an interviewer can approach the patient this way: "What tells you it's time for a refill?" or "How do you know it's time for a refill?"

The closed question is narrow and usually limits the patient to a direct and specific answer. Often, closed questions require simple "yes" or "no" answers.

A balance of open and closed questions is the hallmark of an effective, efficient interview. The excessive use of closed questions will result in choppy interviews, reduce the quality and quantity of the information gathered and offer little opportunity to develop a relationship with the patient. Interviewers should use them judiciously to avoid an interrogative approach; however, closed questions are an integral component of an efficient interview. A forced-choice, closed question that asks for a specific bit of information in a word or two can be useful to follow up an open question. An example of a patient response to an open question, followed by several possible closed questions from the interviewer is

Interviewer:	"What problems are you having taking your medication?"
Patient:	"My tablets are hard to swallow."
Closed:	"You said that your tablets are difficult to swallow; are they always difficult to swallow?"
Closed:	"Have you missed any doses?"
Closed:	"Do you have problems swallowing at other times?"

Direct and Indirect Questions—Questions can be categorized as either direct or indirect. Direct questions are to the point. They are outright requests for information, and they may be open or closed.

Indirect questions may not appear to be questions at all. They, too, can be open or closed, but they may not sound like questions. They are implicit and perhaps disguise requests for information. Indirect questions especially come in handy with delicate subjects.

Some examples of direct and indirect questions are

Open direct:	"Tell me about your leg cramps."
Closed direct:	"Are you concerned about your leg cramps?"
Open indirect:	"I'm wondering what you think about your leg cramps."
Open direct:	"What can you tell me about the penicillin you're taking?"
Closed direct:	"Did you finish the penicillin?"
Closed indirect:	"Do you have any penicillin left?"

Loaded and Leading Questions—Loaded and leading questions are forms of closed questions that contain their own answers or imply judgments or both. These types of questions usually are not fruitful for information gathering.

Loaded questions often are emotion-laden and force patients into defensive postures. An example of a loaded question is, "You've never had gonorrhea, have you?"

Leading questions blatantly or subtly steer patients to an answer interviewers anticipate. They put absolute restrictions on how patients may answer the question even though the answer may not be appropriate. Leading questions encourage the patient to give an answer that is simple, avoids the interviewer's disapproval and cuts down the length of the interview. Such questions improperly placed may result in an incomplete, yet seemingly efficient, interview. At times, however, patients need direction, stimulated by a leading question, especially when discussing sensitive areas. An example of a leading question and one possible alternative is

Leading: "Does the medicine make you drowsy?"
Alternative: "How does the medicine make you feel?"

Double or Multiple Questions—Double or multiple questions present patients with two or more inquiries at the same time. They force patients to choose between the questions and respond to one and then the other, if they can remember what the other one was after responding to the first.

Multiple questions, whether presented one right after another or quickly after each answer, trap patients in a barrage of questions and answers that leave patients confused and irritated. What tends to happen is that a question-and-answer pattern is established where patients learn to wait for a question before responding. They adjust to the pattern in such a way that when no questions are posed they remain silent.

An example of a commonly used multiple question in medication-history interviews is

"Are you using medications like aspirin, vitamins, antacids, cough and cold remedies,?"

This has merit if explained properly, but patients may interpret the list as definitive without attempting to think of other nonprescription drugs they take. One way to use this type of question to the interviewer's advantage is to preface it by saying

"I am going to read a list of medicines you can buy in the pharmacy or supermarket without a prescription. Stop me along the way and tell me if you are taking any of them. If the names puzzle you, stop me, and I'll explain them further."

After going through the list, ask whether the patient takes any other nonprescription drugs not mentioned.

Gathering Information and Building Rapport

Accomplished health-care providers recognize and respond to a sense of interpersonal responsibility and are sensitive to how their behavior may affect others. This recognition and sensitivity helps develop positive rapport with patients. Pharmacists should be approachable during interactions, and they should "match" their behavior with true thoughts and feelings, such that the messages communicated are consistent, confident and compatible.

The following points not only help interviewers gather information, but help them build rapport with patients.

Flexibility and Logic—Flexibility is the ability to shift attention on demand, adapting to the total flow of communication. Active listening involves the art of probing for information and analyzing the facts before acting in response. When listening actively, the interviewer's responses to the patient are keener and more insightful, display confidence and are more appropriate than when passively hearing verbal statements. The rapport tends to be reciprocated by the patient, and the relationship tends to be more rewarding.

Logical sequencing is the process of covering groups of related topics in turn, thereby avoiding topic-jumping or asking questions in a random order without any apparent rationale. On occasion it is necessary to follow a patient's lead, even if it does not seem logical. Indeed, patients who are allowed to remember past pharmacy and medical visits in whatever order they choose have recall superior to patients instructed to recall in a temporal order. Logical sequencing permits interviewers to follow patient leads, yet return to the previous sequence without getting lost.

Transitional Phrases and Reinforcers—Transitional statements smoothly shift the interview from one topic to the next. They convey the purpose and importance of the information to be gained. Failure to prepare patients for a shift in topic by a smooth transition may leave them lost, confused and uncooperative. An example of an interviewer's transitional statement is

"You've described your recent medicine-taking experiences; now I'd like to run through the medications you have taken in the last 3 to 6 months."

Simple indications of basic understanding facilitate patient responses. They tell the patient that the interviewer is listening, following along and involved in what is said. Brief statements, such as "Yes," "I see," "Go on," "I understand," "Tell me more about that," "And then" and "Okay" are examples of recognition responses that reinforce. Also, these types of responses indicate encouragement from the interviewer to continue with a verbal communication. Occasionally, it may help to repeat the patient's last word with a rising inflection so that it is a question. For example

Patient: "and then of course every now and then I have a migraine."
Interviewer: "Migraine?"

Since recognition responses can reinforce the speaker, avoid overusing them because of the potential for inadvertently communicating something not intended. It may be hard to believe, but a simple "okay" or "mm-hm" can indicate that the interviewer has made a judgment, even if that is not the case. For example

Patient: "I've been having these leg cramps for awhile."
Interviewer: "Okay."
Patient: "It would be so much better if my legs didn't hurt all the time."
Interviewer: "Mm-hm."
Patient: "A friend of mine said I was lacking vitamins and he gave me some. I've started taking them. Forget that dumb blood pressure drug I take."
Interviewer: "Okay."

Interruptions—Good listeners know how to speak only when the situation calls for it. Waiting patiently and avoiding interruptions (apologize if done so accidentally) may be more beneficial than anything interjected.

Clarification and Verification—Clarification and verification are verbal behaviors that highlight the main topics covered in the interview. Highlighting the main points of one section or the entire interview permits the patient and the interviewer to correct any errors, clear any confusion, confirm information as valid or add new information. For example, the interviewer might say

"Now let me check to make sure I have it. You first noticed the dizziness after your second tablet on the first day, and you stopped taking them on the third day. Okay so far?"

Closing the Interview

Ending a medication-history interview requires attention to many of the skills discussed earlier. The conclusion of an interview should contain a request for additional information which the patient thinks might be helpful, a request for the patient's opinion about the reasons for the problem, a summary of pertinent data along with the opportunity for the patient to make corrections if necessary, an offer to answer any questions now or in the future, a statement of when and where help is available and leave-taking.

Even though summarizing usually is synonymous with closure, it may be necessary, even advantageous, also to summarize at strategic places during the interview. How often to summarize depends on the extensiveness of the medication-history interview, but, as with most anything, too much of a good thing can be damaging. The key point is that an effective summary need not be confined to the closing of the interview.

Information Completeness and Compliance Issues

While the previous sections focused primarily on the process of interviewing, pharmacists cannot be so concerned with the process skills that they neglect to collect accurate drug information and an accurate compliance history. Paying attention to the qualities of completeness and specificity will allow an interviewer to accomplish both tasks.

Although there is not complete consensus about specific questions to ask in a medication-history interview, most authorities expect interviewers to obtain information about prescription and nonprescription medications currently taken by patients. Also, interviewers are expected to gather information about medications taken previously, allergies, problems with adverse effects and possible recreational drug use. In general, the drug information an interviewer gathers should uncover answers to

What medication(s) is (are) being taken?
What is the medication being used for?
Is the medication actually being taken?
How is the medication taken?
How often is the medication taken?
When and with what is the medication taken?
How regularly is the medication taken?
For how long is the medication to be taken?
Is the medication working?
Are there any bothersome effects from the medication?
Does it ever happen that you forget to take the medication?
What happens if you don't take the medication?

Keep in mind that these questions are presented only as a checklist of information to be covered in a medication-history interview. They neither represent the best way to word or ask the question, nor represent an exhaustive list of possibilities.

When a patient answers in nonspecific ways that leave uncertainty regarding the intended message, the interviewer may improve the chance for more complete compliance information by offering a specific response. This does not mean that the interviewer should launch into an interrogation aimed at "just the facts." Complete and specific information can be obtained other than by coldly asking about the particulars of who, what, when, where and how. Simple statements are often sufficient to gain a complete view of compliance, as well as other matters. But, a note of caution should be heeded: Excessive questioning, even with the goal of specificity, tends to establish a pattern where the patient accepts a role of answering, and the interviewer takes the role of asking; if the interviewer does not ask anything about a specific subject, the patient may not offer the sought-after information.

Using a probe will improve specificity, since it urges the patient to say more about a specific topic. It is designed to encourage the respondent to explain or elaborate on something already said. Questions should center on particular streams of events rather than time of occurrence. For example, a patient trying to recall his/her medication history may remember that a specific episode began with a toothache, continued with visits to the dentist and pharmacy and finished with a series of visits to the family physician and the subsequent drug therapy. A probe can be stated in the form of an open statement like, "I'd like you to tell me more about the pain," or by using reflective phrases or words, such as "Really?" and "Why so?" Probes of this type remove the interrogative connotation commonly associated with them. They also present an indirect approach to compliance issues. Barriers to medication compliance may be sensitive areas for patients to talk about, so "soft" probing is a fruitful approach for obtaining specific and complete information.

Patient-Advocates

By communicating with patients and learning about their drug-related problems and concerns, pharmacists are able to serve as patient-advocates in the health-care system. This advocacy approach is forcefully supported by Schulz and Brushwood in their Hastings Center Report (*see Bibliography*). Each pharmacist-patient interaction is different, and the pharmacist determines a plan of action based on an assessment of the situation, including the severity of the problem and the ability of the patient to understand the problem and the available options. For example, in one situation the pharmacist may identify a potential problem in a medication-history interview, point it out to the patient and expect the patient to resolve the problem alone or with the prescriber. In a more serious situation, or when the patient cannot be expected to perform the necessary follow-up, the pharmacist may contact the prescriber about potential problems or concerns on behalf of the patient.

When responding to patient problems and concerns, pharmacists must strive to achieve balance and fulfill their professional duty. The best way to define duty in this context is to offer examples of its opposite. A lack of professional duty by pharmacists either is being so passive toward patient interests such that patient care is compromised, or so active such that the pharmacist shows no regard for the roles of other health-care providers. Teamwork is a treasured commodity worth seeking when patient care is at stake.

Bibliography

Aiken LH, Mechanic D, eds: *Applications of Social Science to Clinical Medicine and Health Policy*, Rutgers Univ Press, New Brunswick NJ, 1986.

American Society of Hospital Pharmacists: Directions for clinical practice in pharmacy: Proceedings of an invitational conference conducted by the ASHP Research and Education Foundation and the ASHP. *Am J Hosp Pharm 42:* 1287–1342, 1985.

Bradburn NM, Rips LJ, Shevell SK: Answering autobiographical questions: the impact of memory and inference on surveys. *Science 36:* 157, 1987.

Coulehan JL, Block MR: *The Medical Interview: A Primer for Students of the Art*, Davis, Philadelphia, 1987.

DiMatteo MR, DiNicola DD: *Achieving Patient Compliance*, Pergamon, New York, 1982.

Friedman HS, DiMatteo MR: *Health Psychology*, Prentice-Hall, Englewood Cliffs NJ, 1989.

Gardner M, Boyce RW, Herrier RN: *Pharmacist-Patient Consultation Program: An Interactive Approach to Verify Patient Understanding* (videotape). USPHS, Indian Health Service/Pfizer, Bethesda MD, 1991.

Hepler CD, Strand LM: Opportunities and responsibilities in pharmaceutical care. *Am J Hosp Pharm 47:* 533, 1990.

Jobe JB, White AA, Kelley CL *et al:* Recall strategies and memory for health-care visits. *Milbank Q 68:* 171, 1990.

Kalman SH, Schlegel JF: Standards of practice for the profession of pharmacy. *Am Pharm NS19:* 133, 1979.

Knapp ML: *Essentials of Nonverbal Communication*, Holt-Rinehart-Winston, New York, 1980.

Meichenbaum D, Turk DC: *Facilitating Treatment Adherence: A Practitioner's Guidebook*, Plenum, New York, 1987.

Metzler K: *Creative Interviewing*, Prentice-Hall, Englewood Cliffs NJ, 1977.

Northouse PG, Northouse LL: *Health Communication: Strategies for Health Professionals*, 2nd ed, Appleton & Lange, Norwalk CT, 1992.

Omnibus Budget Reconciliation Act of 1990, Pub. L. No. 101-508, §4401, 104 Stat. 1388, 1990.

Ranelli PL: The utility of nonverbal communication in the profession of pharmacy. *Soc Sci Med 13A:* 733, 1979.

Ranelli PL, Svarstad BL, Boh L: Factors affecting outcomes of medication-history interviewing by pharmacy students. *Am J Hosp Pharm 46:* 267, 1989.

Ranelli PL: Rediscovering the act of interviewing by pharmacists. *J Clin Pharm Ther 15:* 377, 1990.

Schulz RM, Brushwood DB: The pharmacist's role in patient care. *Hastings Cen Rep 21(1):* 12, 1991.

Stewart CJ, Cash WB Jr: *Interviewing: Principles and Practices*, 5th ed, Wm C Brown, Dubuque IA, 1988.

Tindall WN, Beardsley RS, Kimberlin CL: *Communication Skills in Pharmacy Practice*, 2nd ed, Lea & Febiger, Philadelphia, 1989.

CHAPTER 102

Drug Education

Michael Montagne, PhD
Associate Professor of Social Pharmacy
Massachusetts College of Pharmacy and Allied Health Sciences
Boston, MA 02115

Drug-taking is prevalent in most societies and cultures. Whether the use of a particular drug is for a medical, social, recreational or some other reason, problems often will arise. Preventing drug-use problems is a major concern of most societies and usually is highlighted when specific outbreaks of problems or inappropriate use occur. As pharmacy is the profession to which the control of drugs is attributed, it should be involved intimately with those activities aimed at preventing or reducing drug-use problems. It even could be argued that the pharmaceutical profession should be providing the leadership and directing the research in this area. It is unfortunate that, on the whole, pharmacy has been lacking in its social responsibility for the chemical substances it develops, promotes and dispenses.

Most pharmacists are aware of the important problems which potentially can occur with the appropriate use of prescription medications, such as adverse reactions and drug interactions. Many pharmacists also are knowledgeable about the many potential problems inherent in self-medication with a nonprescription drug, though they probably are less familiar with the use of herbal remedies and homeopathic medications in the same context. However, few pharmacists are aware of the potential problems that can arise with social-recreational drug-taking, or the use of drugs for other nonmedical reasons. The problem of poisoning by a drug has been delegated to poison-control centers and hospital emergency rooms. The individual pharmacist, particularly one working in a community setting, may not feel capable of consulting or educating a particular drug-taker in these problem areas, or may not perceive a need of this type.

Our society, however, is in great need of learning more rational and appropriate uses of all types of drugs, and gaining control over the products of our own technology. The primary importance of drug education is its benefit to the drug user (patient or consumer), by improving the appropriateness of drug-taking behaviors in order to achieve optimal health and well-being. At the center of any educational effort is providing drug information, the strategy with which pharmacists and pharmacy students are most familiar. In today's highly complex, technological world, the availability of current and precise information allows one to understand, to make better choices and to prevent or solve problems.

The individual best suited to assist people in preventing drug-use problems and in achieving optimal, desired experiences from their drug-taking is the pharmacist. The pharmacist is a very accessible source of high-quality information and educational programs and should be concerned with a person's drug-taking behavior, in any context, and with the problems that can arise from such. Whether it be the use of a prescription medicine or an herbal remedy to achieve or maintain a state of health, the use of a drug for its socially oriented effects in a recreational setting or the ingestion of a chemical substance to enhance a religious or aesthetic experience, the perspective presented herein considers the pharmacist to be the leader in efforts to prevent or limit drug-use problems.

In this chapter, the basic principles of drug education are provided with the underlying premise that, for the most part, these principles and strategies are applicable to any type of drug use. While information about, and inherent problems resulting from, specific types of drug-taking might vary from drug to drug, or between reasons for use, the fundamental approach to educating people and effecting changes in drug use is the same. Here, the word "drug" will refer to the use of any substance, other than food, which, by its chemical or physical nature, alters structure or function in a human being, resulting in physiological, behavioral or social changes. This includes all medicinal agents (whether defined legally as prescription or nonprescription), herbal and home remedies, alcohol and caffeine (and other substances that oftentimes are considered to be "food" by consumers, but are used for their pharmacological activity), substances used primarily in a nonmedical context and even poisons.

A number of approaches have been developed for designing drug-information and education programs in medical settings, and many of these are described in other chapters of this book. The majority of the examples in this chapter, therefore, will come from the realm of "drug-abuse" prevention. It should be remembered, however, that these techniques and strategies, and their basic principles, are applicable to educating patients about medicines or providing drug-education programs in any context. It also should be remembered that ideas, strategies and programs developed in the field of patient drug education are applicable to programs on the nonmedical use of drugs, and some examples of this broader view of drug education are provided.

Drug Use and Drug Education

Human beings engage in a great variety of drug-taking behaviors, but one of the most important and rudimentary considerations involves the definition of what constitutes a drug, and which situations or reasons characterize drug-taking. In a 1972 nationwide survey of drug use, adults and youths were asked to indicate which substances they regarded as drugs.[1] Greater than 80% of the respondents regarded substances such as heroin, cocaine, marijuana and psychotherapeutic agents to be drugs. One should realize, however, that a small proportion of the general public (5 to 20%, depending upon the specific drug) did not regard these substances to be drugs. Alcohol and tobacco were regarded as drugs by less than one-third of the respondents. Most of the adolescent respondents (84%) did not consider tobacco to be a drug, though we might expect that if the survey were repeated today, the results would be very different.

The key point is that individuals can hold very different beliefs or perceptions about which chemical substances they regard as being drugs. In fact, this type of survey can be a useful and interesting exercise in a drug-education program. The audience is shown a list of chemical substances and asked to indicate which ones are drugs and which ones are not. Not only can this exercise, and its results, provide the educator with a better idea of the opinions and level of drug knowledge of an individual or group, but it also can be used as a focal point for discussion at that time or subsequent sessions. The belief that certain substances may or may not be drugs is very important in understanding why and how people use such substances, and it should be a primary consideration in the development of any drug-education program.

The nature and extent of certain types of drug-taking varies by drug, availability (or accessibility) and the reason for use. In the medical realm, drug-taking may be initiated by the patient, as in self-medication, or it may be directed by another person, usually a physician, who writes a prescription or suggests it. Studies of self-medication are limited. The research done in this area indicates that self-diagnosis, rather than making contact with the health-care delivery system, occurs in the majority of illness episodes, and that self-medication occurs from 60 to 90% of the time in these situations.

Studies of nonprescription-drug consumption indicate that in general about one-third of a population could be defined as current users of such substances, and that from 25 to 60% of a population may be users of such drugs during any specific period of time.

When a drug is prescribed for a patient, health professionals expect that the drug will be taken precisely as directed. Compliance with medication regimens is another type of drug-taking that is considered to be of major importance in a successful treatment plan. There have been a great number of studies in this area (see Chapter 103 for a thorough review); their results have shown that anywhere from 5 to 90% of patients may be noncompliant in some manner. While there is a wide variation in noncompliance, due to a variety of factors as well as the research design of particular studies, the rate of noncompliance, in general, probably ranges from 33 to 50% in any given population. So in these situations, many patients are *not* taking drugs when they should be.

Drug-taking also occurs in a nonmedical context. While cigarette smoking has declined steadily, with the very important exception of 14- to 25-year-old females, alcohol use has remained about the same over the past few years. The 1991 nationwide survey of drug use by the National Institute on Drug Abuse found that 11% of youths (less than 18 years), 32% of young adults (18 to 25 years) and 28% of adults (26 years or older) were current users of tobacco, while 20% of youths, 64% of young adults and 53% of adults were current users of alcohol.

The nonmedical use of most other types of psychoactive drugs, including marijuana, has declined over the past decade. The exception is the nonmedical use of cocaine, which had increased twofold over the same time period; this, however, is a relative situation, since a very small proportion of the population (in 1991, 1% of youths, 3% of young adults and 2% of adults) currently uses this drug, as compared to other psychoactive agents. Drugs are also the cause of almost one-half of all poisoning episodes (see Chapter 109), a type of drug-taking behavior that is most often unintentional, except in cases of suicide.

It is, perhaps, now obvious that drugs are used appropriately in certain situations for beneficial reasons, that they are not used in some instances when they should be and that they are used inappropriately on many occasions. In all three circumstances, though most often in the last two examples, problems can result from drug use. The prevention or recognition and management of problems resulting from drug use are the main reasons for developing and providing drug-education programs.

Drug education in a medical context has occurred for some time. The earliest health-promotion movement occurred in the late 19th century, and educational activities were an important part of the effort. Patient-counseling always has been a part of the health-professional's role, though the assumption of this role has varied from time to time, especially within pharmacy. Providing drug information or educating patients through verbal interaction have been the principal strategies. Structured educational programs have been developed throughout this century, but it wasn't until after World War II that concerted efforts to develop and implement health-education programs began to occur in public health. In the 1950s and 1960s, a number of attitudinal and behavioral approaches were studied to expand the traditional information-based approach and improve upon the effectiveness of information-only programs. In the 1990s, the behavioral approach has become very popular in health-education programs, and the use of the mass media has increased dramatically.

Early efforts in education about nonmedical drug use consisted of negative portrayals of drugs and moralizing about drug use in the classroom and through the mass media, with very little objective information being presented. Such an approach unfortunately still can be found in many contemporary drug-education programs. These early efforts evolved into the drug-education programs of the late 1960s and early 1970s, which claimed to provide relatively objective information, mostly pharmacological in nature, to children in the health, social science or some other part of a school's curriculum. In most of these cases, the information was provided, but ways of using and incorporating it into one's lifestyle were not presented and discussed. A number of studies in the 1970s found that informational programs in this area aroused the student's curiosity about drugs and increased the likelihood of experimentation with drugs.[2,3]

There came, consequently, a shift in educational programming toward the goal of enhancing social competencies (ie, a person's communication and interpersonal skills, ability to make decisions and to solve problems). The reasoning was that a stable, well-adjusted, socially competent individual surely would have little need for drugs, and in those cases when drugs were used, it only would be socially approved substances in socially accepted and appropriate ways. Such programs usually were quite effective in enhancing these competencies, but the subsequent influence on drug-taking was unknown; indeed, the notion of a causal link is obtuse. It was soon realized, however, that the effectiveness of these programs indicated a general lack of social competency training in the family, schools, religious settings and other places. These programs have value in an educational plan, but mostly when incorporated with drug information, alternatives to drugs, recognition of drug-use problems and other related activities.

In the mid-1970s, in the US, a number of "responsible drug-use" programs were suggested and created, mainly in response to the dominant approach, which implied that a successful drug-education program would result in abstinence from socially disapproved drugs, and of course, a reduction in drug-use problems.[4–6] The "responsible drug-use" movement accepted the notion that people always will want to take chemical substances, and so programs were designed to foster appropriate drug-taking behaviors, rational decision-making in the use of drugs and skills for preventing or recognizing drug-use problems.

Programs employing the responsible drug-use approach ranged from responsible drinking-awareness activities, to drug-overdose first-aid training, to the suggestion that some individuals with alcohol-use problems could reintegrate social drinking into their lives after chemical dependency treatment and counseling. Such programs, however, were not of value to all individuals and groups who engage in drug-taking, and the relative utility and effectiveness of these programs still are not well known.

A few researchers and educators more recently have suggested a rather different approach to drug education and prevention which considers drug-taking as a "natural behavior."[7] In this context, educational programs focus on the need to alter one's state of consciousness in an acceptable way, and to use drugs in a responsible manner consistent with one's lifestyle. The drug-taker is alerted additionally to the importance of values and the influence of societal attitudes in drug-taking. These two notions are extremely important in presenting programs or counseling patients with regard to drug use.

Decisions to use specific chemical substances are based upon the values, attitudes and lifestyles of the user, family and friends, health professionals and society in general. Differences in opinion about and the actual use of many drugs may vary considerably between different individuals and groups.

Tobacco (nicotine) and coffee (caffeine) were considered to be dangerously toxic and addictive substances in earlier times, whereas few people today call either a drug, though renewed interest in combating cigarette smoking has led to the labeling of nicotine as being as addictive as opioids.

In many societies, alcohol is the social drug of choice by adults, while marijuana is the social drug of the young people even though it is socially unaccepted or illegal. In other cultures, alcohol use is forbidden, while marijuana use is socially accepted. As a result of these differences, specific needs for information, education or consultation to resolve problems in drug-taking may not be met; it might be that "what we are now doing in the name of stopping the drug problem *is* the drug problem."[4]

In the 1980s, there was a backlash against these "responsible drug-use" approaches, and a reorientation of prevention efforts from a supply-reduction strategy (ie, preventing or limiting the supply and flow of drugs at the source) to a demand-reduction strategy (ie, preventing or limiting the need, and thus actual use, of drugs in an indigenous population). Thus, the popular contemporary trends are the "Just Say No" campaign and the use of the mass media to inform and educate. The refusal skill technique (eg, "Just Say No" campaign) is an abstinence-based approach, which was developed in the area of smoking-prevention research.

Refusal skills make young people aware of the pressures from peers and the media to use drugs, and through role-playing and other exercises, ways to refuse or avoid drug-taking situations are learned. The use of peers in educational programs also has increased in the 1990s. Much of the effort started in the field of alcohol education as attempts were made to move away from authoritarian-moralistic programs with abstinence as a goal to peer-facilitated strategies based upon the concept of self-discovery, and the fact that alcohol use is socially approved and engendered in most societies, even if it is an illegal activity for certain segments (eg, by age) of the population. Regardless of these trends, "fads" or new approaches in drug-education programming, there are a few basic principles that always should be considered.

Basic Principles of Drug Education

There are a great variety of strategies and techniques that can be used in counseling and educating patients, but before these are considered, the process through which learning takes place is reviewed. The process of learning occurs in three domains or in three different ways (see Fig 1).[8] The basic domain is cognitive, where facts and information are assimilated. A person's knowledge is built through a process of acquiring, understanding, retaining (memory) and reinforcing specific bits of information. The next domain (affective) involves the formation of attitudes such as feelings, beliefs, perceptions, emotions and appreciations. These are constructed through an interactive process, combining knowledge (from the cognitive domain) and real-life experiences during which the person's knowledge is applied and evaluated to see if it fits that reality. The behavioral domain (eg, actions, decision-making, physical abilities) is developed from what the person knows and feels, in conjunction with the nature and requirements of the social environment.

Values may affect all domains of learning. One's viewpoint, ethical orientation or way of life influences drug-taking, and it also influences educators as they develop and provide

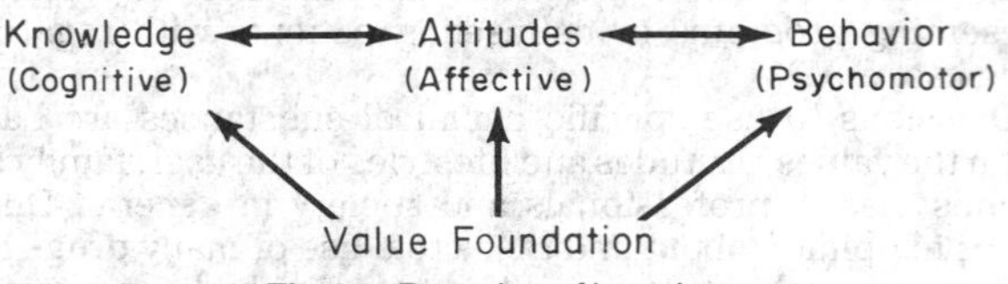

Fig 1. Domains of learning.

programs. The classic philosophical approach is to consider beliefs and decision-making in one of two ways. The deontological approach focuses more on the action or motive behind the decision, while the teleological approach focuses more on the results or consequences of the action or decision. Decisions to give or take drugs can follow the same philosophical lines of thought. In health care, for instance, the outcome or result of therapy usually is more important than the nature of the therapy itself.

In many cases, a vast array of drugs are used to continue the patient's life (the primary "result" of therapy) even when the drugs themselves lead to a variety of negative effects and problems, sometimes worse than the disease itself. Medical and drug research in the past also followed this philosophical approach. The emphasis was on the results of research (ie, finding a drug that would cure a disease), and less on what happened to the patients in the experiment. Contemporary clinical drug trials are much more ethical, but the emphasis on results or the outcome of therapy still remains.

The influence of values also can be seen in the development and provision of drug education programs. As described by Dembo,[9] the two current views or frames of reference in drug prevention and treatment differ in their emphasis on drug use. The positivist view focuses on drug-use problems, and drug education attempts to alter the user's attitudes and behaviors in the direction of total abstinence. The interactionist view stresses the importance of sociocultural and environmental factors leading to drug-taking as a valued activity, and drug education focuses on the development of social sanctions and rituals to prevent or limit dysfunctional drug-taking. It should be obvious that each viewpoint would result in the development of perhaps very different types of drug education programs.

The importance of values in drug-taking and drug education even has been considered as a primary facet in the development of programs. One approach is known as values clarification, which was developed as a strategy to improve an adolescent's general social skills, and which has been adapted to drug-education and prevention programs.[10] The idea behind values clarification is that an individual's beliefs and ability to make decisions are influenced greatly by values. The clearer these values and the process of valuing are, the more self-directed and consistent the individual is in making optimal decisions and choices in life.

The approach of clarifying values focuses on how one chooses a value (eg, freely, from a variety of alternatives and after giving thoughtful consideration to each possible choice), prizes her values (eg, cherishes values and affirms them in public) and acts upon a value (eg, making decisions based upon the value or doing something with the chosen value, and acting upon the value repeatedly in life to form a pattern). The values-clarification strategy has become an important part of some drug-education efforts.

The main problem that educational theorists and researchers have had is in determining what, and how much of what, is learned in one domain influences the learning process in another domain. There is a very dominant notion, based in part on common sense, that the provision of drug information will improve appropriate drug-taking behaviors in most situations (eg, increased compliance, responsible self-medication or decreased social-recreational use). A great variety of research in different areas of drug education suggests that this relationship *does not necessarily* hold true.

Many studies on patient package inserts (PPIs) have found that this form of printed information can lead to reliable gains in drug knowledge, but they seem to have little effect on how patients use a drug. While the patients' knowledge and understanding (cognitive domain) of the drug and drug regimen were improved, their initial decisions regarding drug therapy, their intention of using the drug (attitudinal domain) and their actual compliance with the regimen were not changed greatly. The same also holds in educating people about nonmedical drug use. The relationship between what a person knows about the nonmedical use of drugs, and whether he actually uses drugs in such a way, is not very strong, according to most of the research in this area.[11] This body of research also suggests that the relationship between values and behavior is not very clear and may be quite weak or inconsistent for some individuals or drug-taking situations.

On the other hand, some studies of drug knowledge, attitudes and behaviors in the area of social-recreational drug use have shown a direct link between these three domains in some educational situations. The strongest relationship seems to exist between attitudes and behaviors, but even this appears to be a complex and difficult connection to describe and predict in educational efforts. Interactions with individual patients in practice settings also might show that improving patients' knowledge about their drug therapy, in fact, directly influences their compliance behavior. It is obvious that some things we know do influence our attitudes about them, and what we feel about them will influence how we act toward them.

The relationships illustrated in Fig 1 are assumed to exist, but not necessarily for everyone in all possible situations, and the relationships are shown to occur in either direction. The most important point to realize is that in order to achieve a particular type of effect, the best approach is to focus on the domain of learning where the desired effect or change should occur. Thus, if the goal of the educator's efforts is a more negative attitude toward the use of certain drugs, the educational program should focus its activities more on attitudes, and less on increasing drug knowledge or on discouraging drug-taking. If the goal of the program is to prevent or limit certain types of drug use, the focus should be on building skills and directing behavior away from use, and not so much on increasing drug knowledge or on developing attitudes against drugs and their use.

The key to truly effective drug education may be in individualizing the learning process to the particular needs of the patient or consumer. The pharmacist should become aware of a particular person's situation and be ready to help as needed. Not only is this a part of effective counseling and drug education, but most people indicate that this approach (ie, being considered as a unique human being) is what they desire and expect in interactions with health professionals.

Individualized attention, not surprisingly, is also one of the major factors in a consumer's selection and patronage of a particular pharmacy. In terms of drug education, then, the best way to approach the learning process is to

Assess the person's level of knowledge and provide relevant information in those areas where there is a deficiency.

Counsel the person and encourage positive attitudes toward the appropriate and controlled use of drugs.

Evaluate the person's drug-taking and general health over time to verify appropriate patterns of use and optimal outcomes from use, and to reinforce her positive attitudes and behaviors.

The concepts and principles presented herein apply to people who use a chemical substance for a medical or nonmedical reason in any setting. Many approaches in drug education are based upon social-learning theory, or the concept that individuals learn symbolically through interactions with themselves, others and their environment. In addition, it is important to realize and consider the ways in which people learn. The delineation of educational effects or outcomes is most productive when it is based upon the idea that people learn, and that they act upon what they know, in different ways.

Effects and Outcomes of Drug-Education Programs

The most important concept, which surprisingly often is not stated very explicitly in educational programs, is the behavior or problem that is the target of the educational or prevention effort. This is unfortunately the case with most drug-education programs. There is sometimes a general sense of what should be achieved, but the specific results or outcomes are not clearly delineated. There are a number of different, though not necessarily mutually exclusive, goals for drug-education programs.

An increase in drug knowledge.

A change in attitudes about drugs and their use.

An improvement in social functioning (eg, social competency), which might lead to better decision-making in drug-taking situations.

A change in drug use in general.

A change in the use of specific types of drugs.

A reduction in the occurrence of specific drug-use problems.

Once the overall goals of the program are determined, more specific results and outcomes may be identified and characterized.

This degree of generality appears to occur most often in educational programs on the nonmedical use of drugs. The National Institute on Drug Abuse defines prevention as the process designed to "inhibit or reduce physical, mental, emotional or social impairment which results in or from the abuse of chemical substances."[6] The question of what constitutes "abuse" of a chemical substance usually is not well-defined. This usually results in the adoption of complete abstinence from drug use as the goal of the educational or prevention program. In addition, it becomes difficult to determine at what degree impairment can be defined as occurring; it often results from a dominant social attitude or belief regarding adequate functioning and thus a judgmental definition of when a person is or is not performing up to social standards. Most other definitions of "drug-abuse" prevention are similar in nature and intent, though more recently, the US Government has developed some general goals for the prevention of alcohol and drug misuse that are more quantitative in nature.[12]

What, then, are the effects and outcomes of drug-education programs? The most effective type, in relation to one specific level of learning, addresses drug knowledge. The provision of drug information, and the receipt and understanding of that information, leads to increases at the cognitive level most of the time; patients or consumers show an improvement in their knowledge about drugs, as measured by some cognitive test. This increase in knowledge, however, may not lead to a change in attitudes or behaviors. For instance, the effectiveness of patient package inserts (PPIs) and other programmed medication instruction sheets is variable. Studies of PPIs by the Rand Corp provided a better idea of the use and effectiveness of patient drug information.[13] The principle findings of those studies were that

PPIs are likely to be read widely.

Many patients use PPIs as reference documents.

PPIs lead to reliable gains in drug knowledge.

PPIs seem to have little effect on how patients use a drug.

PPIs do not, in general, lead patients to report more side effects.

PPIs are unlikely to change the frequency with which patients contact their physicians.

Patients find written drug information helpful.

The amount of explanation provided in a PPI makes very little difference in how much information patients understand or remember.

The simplicity with which a PPI is written has little effect on understanding.

Other studies, as well as comprehensive reviews of the literature in this area, have arrived at similar conclusions.[14,15] In a medical context, the provision of drug information often will lead to measurable gains in knowledge about drugs, but corresponding changes in drug-taking (eg, improved compliance or more appropriate self-medication) may not occur, especially if learning also does not take place at the attitudinal or behavioral domain.

Drug-education programs directed at these other domains of learning most often have their impact in those specific domains. The general lack of effectiveness of drug information programs in improving compliance motivated educators to develop other techniques. In the area of compliance, a number of attitudinal and behavioral strategies have been developed (see Chapter 103). For example, health beliefs have been found to influence an individual's decision-making about seeking health care and complying with prescribed therapy. In educational efforts, the Health Belief Model[16] has been used to design specific techniques and strategies, which have been found to be effective in increasing compliance in some patients. Behavioral-modification techniques also have been effective in helping patients to adhere to dieting plans, comply with complex or difficult therapeutic regimens and even stop smoking.

In the area of nonmedical drug education, the informational approach also has been found to have a short-term impact on drug knowledge and very little effect on nonmedical drug use. The interesting and somewhat unfortunate exception is that the provision of information or lecturing solely on the pharmacology of the "drugs of abuse" was found in some studies actually to increase the students' curiosity and their desire to experiment with these substances.[2,3,17] In these studies, drug use increased slightly for a short time after the educational program, and then it fell back to the level measured prior to the educational activity. Early efforts using fear-arousal messages and scare tactics were found to have an immediate effect, when compared to the provision of factual information or discussions of attitudes, but the effect usually lasted for only a short period of time. The consensus of researchers is that fear as a part of punishment is not an effective approach, but positive reinforcement might be effective in some programming efforts.

Some studies formally have evaluated different strategies in "drug-abuse" prevention. In one,[18] a cognitive approach focusing on the provision of drug information, a decision-making approach using role-playing and discussions and a values-clarification program were compared on their effectiveness in preventing or limiting alcohol use. The cognitive approach led to noticeable gains in knowledge about alcohol and its effects, and it was the most positively received of the three. The values-clarification program showed the least amount of change on the outcome measures, though none of the three approaches significantly influenced the use of alcohol in this student population.

In another study,[19] five different approaches were compared and evaluated.

An advocacy program that consisted of information on drugs and alternatives to drug use.

A parent effectiveness approach that focused on communication-skills training for parents.

A peer-group approach that focused on social support and problem-solving exercises.

A social-network approach that was designed to recognize and solve drug-use problems.

A humanistic program that consisted of values-clarification and decision-making exercises.

The peer-group approach and parenting program were the only ones that were effective in actually reducing drug use.

From a meta-analysis of 143 adolescent drug prevention programs, Tobler[20] concluded that of all the different approaches only the peer-counseling programs were effective in producing changes in all three domains of learning and, most importantly, these types of programs were the only ones to prevent or reduce significantly nonmedical drug use in adolescents. Programs using alternatives to drugs were found to be effective in reducing drug use for "high-risk" adolescents. In general, this large-scale analytical review found that multimodality programs were much more effective than programs that used only a single approach or strategy. A review and analysis of 35 drug-education programs, which employed specific-outcome measures, found that the "new generation" of prevention strategies may produce more positive and fewer negative results than did the older drug-information approaches.[21] Even when positive changes were noted in a particular program, those changes were usually small and short-term in effect. Other studies and reviews have arrived at similar conclusions; most educational programs, regardless of the approach or strategy, seem to produce changes in drug knowledge, but few are capable of leading to significant changes in drug-taking behaviors.[22]

Some educators, however, have argued and shown through research that the relationship between knowledge, attitudes and behavior might be a very complex one, and while changes in the cognitive domain can occur quickly, changes in attitudes and behaviors take longer to be internalized by the learner and put into practice in everyday, real-life situations.[23] An interesting variation on the issue of program effectiveness involved a study that assessed changes in teachers' knowledge, attitudes, values-clarification ability and assertiveness skills as a result of a drug-education training program.[24] The results indicated that statistically significant changes had occurred in each area, except for values-clarification ability, as a result of the training program.

Strategies and approaches, that have been developed more recently, have not been shown to be more effective. The refusal-skills approach (eg, "Just Say No" programs) appears to be most effective in smoking prevention, but even then, the impact is short-term in nature. Mass-media approaches to drug education and prevention also have been shown to have a noticeable, short-term effect on drug use, especially in terms of smoking prevention. The use of written drug information, as a supplement to the media content, seems to improve slightly the effectiveness of the mass media.

Drug Education in a Medical Context

The range of audiences for medical drug-education programs can vary from the one-to-one interaction with an individual patient to comprehensive programming for groups of people or whole communities. Drug information and consultation are educational activities which pharmacists have been using for quite some time (see Chapters 7 and 106). Providing information, presenting drug-education programs and consulting with patients and health professionals represent the major prevention effort requiring pharmacy involvement.

Drug-taking in a medical context often is influenced or directed by a health professional. The drug educator should not forget this audience in planning and developing drug-education programs. The primary group is the drug prescriber, mostly physicians. Research has shown that prescribing behaviors are influenced by a variety of factors.

The prescriber's previous education and training, especially when it includes the pharmacology of drugs.

Drug advertising and promotion.

Interactions with colleagues.

Control and regulatory mechanisms in health care.

The demands of patients and society.[25]

These factors should be considered in developing programs to educate physicians and others about drugs and to improve the appropriateness of their prescribing behaviors. Drug- information newsletters and other services, counter-detailing and screening pharmaceutical representatives, in-service seminars and presentations and drug-utilization review with feedback and consultation are the most commonly used approaches to improve drug knowledge and change prescribing practices.

The actual education of patients about their prescribed medications covers a wide range of complex and involved strategies (see Appendix A). At one end of the spectrum, a drug-information sheet (also called a study-instruction sheet), education card or PPI (Patient Package Insert) is given to the patient along with the medication. Information sheets in languages other than English, and in a pictorial formatfor those who cannot read, also have been designed. Programmed instruction sheets, which provide both information and autotutorial learning with reinforcement, also have been developed and used in pharmacy. The value and effectiveness of sheets is variable, with the greatest degree of learning occurring in the cognitive domain.

Written drug information obviously is important, and used by many patients. The best manner to provide such information, however, may not be through mandatory distribution of standardized information, but by individualizing the information to the patient's needs. Supplementing written information with verbal counseling usually increases its effectiveness and utility. The Omnibus Budget Reconciliation Act of 1990 (OBRA 90) regulations will sanction patient counseling and hopefully increase the pharmacist-based counseling of patients. The pharmacist also may help patients' informational needs by being aware of and providing some of the many consumer-oriented drug books now on the market.

Drug information may be obtained from a knowledgeable person (eg, pharmacists and other health professionals or chemical-dependency counselors), a facility (eg, drug-information and poison-control centers, colleges of pharmacy or libraries) or reference materials (eg, articles, textbooks or newsletters). It is all but impossible to have all resources and references for every situation and problem. The amount of drug information that exists is too massive. The best that any pharmacist can expect to have are some key books and people or facilities, which can be used or referred to in difficult situations.

Experience and past research suggests that the vast majority, approximately 85%, of patients' questions and needs can be answered fairly immediately from one's knowledge and experience.[26] The optimal distribution of drug information should be based upon the old adage: the right information, in the right form and amount, to the right person or place at the right time.

Audiovisual materials, and more recently computer-generated video games, have been developed as patient-education tools and as supplements to written and verbal counseling. Programs involving patient education in a small group setting have been developed. These use written and verbal information in a lecture and discussion format. These types of programs have been successful in such diverse areas as dieting, diabetes and epilepsy, and they are now being used to educate patients with glaucoma, hypertension, heart disease and other conditions. These procedures will not be applicable to all situations and settings, especially since they tend to be more time-consuming and costlier.

A newer concept that has emerged recently as an effective learning strategy is social support. Some programs have been designed to include social support in the educational process, and this concept even can be applied to individual counseling situations in health-care settings. The pharmacist and a significant other, such as a spouse, family member or friend, help in motivating the patient toward a positive health behavior by monitoring drug use, noting problems and reinforcing appropriate drug-taking behaviors.

Another moderately new strategy involves the use of behavioral modification to assure appropriate drug use. This problem-solving process employs the observation of behavior, cueing (some type of motivator or reminder to initiate behavior) and rewards to define and modify behavior in a specific way. The patient learns about the medical condition and drug regimen, and then implements a self-management program related to his particular therapy. The patient becomes a partner in the planning of therapy, and consequently feels responsible for following the agreed-upon regimen. These two techniques, social support and behavioral-modification programs, have been found to be quite effective in improving patient compliance with medication regimens.

There is one type of drug-taking behavior for which few educational programs have been developed. Self-medication and related practices involving home remedies have not been well-studied in the past, and consequently, ideas and theories for how to change and improve self-medicating behavior are very limited. Some investigators are working on the application of the Health Belief Model[16] to situations involving self-diagnosis and self-medication. For the most part, educational activities in this area have consisted of drug information, usually in the form of consumer-oriented books on drugs. A perusal of the health and medical sections of local bookstores should give the reader an idea of the range and quality of this information.

Basic principles in the provision of drug information apply to the evaluation and use of these materials as well, before they are suggested or distributed to consumers. In addition to consumer-oriented books and materials, the only other strategies developed in this area are simple, structured educational presentations on self-medication trends, fads and problems, and the use of algorithms or flow charts to assist consumers in their decision-making.[27]

Drug Education in a Nonmedical Context

A great variety of programs have been designed to provide information and education on drug-taking in a nonmedical context (see Appendix A). The classic approach is to provide drug-specific (eg, pharmacology) and drug-related (eg, drug laws or alternatives) information to individuals or groups. The affective or attitudinal approach consists of training in communication skills, values clarification, self- esteem and coping with stress. Informational and affective strategies often are combined in a single program or a series of workshops.

The behavioral approach focuses on the building of skills, such as refusal skills to counter peer pressure, assertiveness, decision-making and problem-solving, or employs behavioral modification techniques to help identify and change inappropriate behaviors. Comprehensive programming involves complex, multisession educational experiences that are designed to have an impact on all domains of learning. Examples of these types of programs include peer-counselor and teacher training, curricular design in school settings, and community-based approaches such as parenting and parent-child interaction workshops and the use of the local mass media.

Research has shown that the best point in a curriculum to begin or to expand "drug-abuse" education programming is around the 6th-grade level.[3] It should be realized, however, that the characteristics of a student population may differ greatly from one school setting to another, thus necessitating the use of a needs assessment survey to determine their level of experience and understanding. Drug-related information (eg, drug laws, alternatives to drugs) also should be presented and discussed as part of any drug education program, particularly if the program goal is abstinence from drug use.

Social competencies are those skills and abilities which promote healthy personal and social functioning. It has been suggested that people who are not socially competent, ie, those with low levels of trust, confidence, self-esteem, identity, directionality and interpersonal skills, are more likely to engage in inappropriate drug use. On the other hand, the socially competent person is more likely to make better decisions about drug use, prevent problems from drug use or recognize such problems and solve them. In fact, the strategy of enhancing social competencies is a major part of Alcoholics/Narcotics Anonymous and related programs.

Well-developed strategies for clarifying values, improving communication and interpersonal skills and encouraging more open discussion of drug-use problems (such as by parents within a family) are available from a number of sources. These techniques are used in mental-health counseling, education and social work for a variety of problem behaviors.

Newer programs involve the learning of coping skills and stress-reduction exercises for the nondrug relief of anxiety and tension, and social-control mechanisms for describing which drugs should be used in what amounts to achieve what effects, reinforcing the use of accepted drugs according to societal values and attitudes and the sanctioning of social relations and settings as appropriate for drug-taking. These types of strategies are probably the ones least familiar to pharmacists, but most of them are relatively easy to learn and apply in an educational program.

The training of gatekeepers and other key people to assist in recognizing drug-use problems and in referring people to appropriate health and social agencies also has been the focus of some educational programs. Gatekeepers are those individuals to whom a person might turn for help in dealing with drug-use problems. Such individuals can be family members, school personnel, religious leaders, local officials, criminal-justice workers, bartenders (with regard to alcohol-use problems), civic organizations and health professionals. Pharmacists perhaps are qualified best to be gatekeepers for individuals with drug-use problems.

Being a gatekeeper essentially means being able to recognize potential or actual drug-use problems, being empathic in understanding the different attitudes or motivations that might have led to the problem and being able to assist the person in solving the problem or making a referral. Such skills are not difficult to learn and actually enhance one's ability to help family, friends, patients and even one's self with all kinds of problems.

Many educational programs for gatekeepers include social-competency skills as a major component of training. Some of these programs can be incorporated into college curricula and continuing-education programs for health professionals. The most important development in this regard has been the formation of peer-counseling programs.

Developing Drug-Education Programs

The provision of drug-education programs occurs to varying degrees, according to the motivations of the pharmacist and the nature of the pharmacy-practice setting. Many factors should be considered in developing a drug-education service: what types of educational programs can be provided and how involved the pharmacist is willing to become, given the constraints of personal knowledge and skills, space, time, manpower, availability of resources and financial considerations. It is good practice to define the exact role one plans to assume as a drug educator, including the specific programs and services to be provided. This provides a framework upon which skills and abilities may be built, and acts as a point of reference from which to work. It also delineates how and what to promote, and makes it clear to patients and consumers what will be offered.

It is very important to recognize that each pharmacist becomes a drug educator to a different degree of involvement. One pharmacist may wish only to provide verbal and written information at his pharmacy, while another may be willing to give structured drug-education presentations before groups of people. Neither should be forced to do more or less. In essence, the type of education recognized by the patients and consumers must be determined, and a personal educational style best suited to meet those needs must be developed (see certain sections of Chapters 96, 99 and 101 for some ideas on this point).

In using any particular educational strategy or program, the pharmacist should be very familiar with its goals and content, the target audience for whom it is intended, its biases and flaws, the results of any evaluation studies performed on it, its known impact on actual use and practical considerations, such as costs, time and manpower requirements, materials and equipment and extra training.

Whether an individual or group effort, drug-education activities require an interactive and structured approach, such as described by the framework illustrated in Fig 2. This general approach is useful when educating individual patients in practice settings or when presenting formal programs before groups of people. The approach basically delineates the important steps one should consider in the conceptualization, development and implementation of any activity intended to educate patients and consumers about drugs.

The first step is the identification or presentation of a specific question, problem or need. This might consist of anything from a patient's noncompliance with prescribed drug therapy to a community's need for comprehensive programming in the area of alcohol use and alcoholism. The problem is identified and defined through interaction with the pharmacist. Once the need has been stated and defined, appropriate strategies can be selected and combined into a specific educational or prevention program. The activity may be as simple as the provision of written and verbal drug information to the patient, or as complex as a multisession

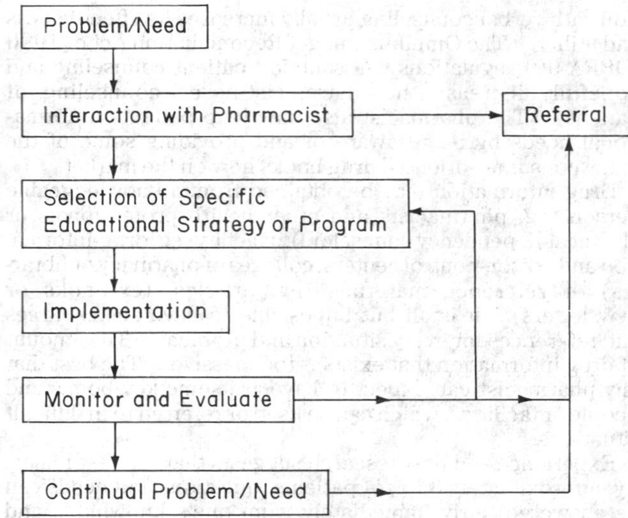

Fig 2. Pharmacist-oriented approach to drug education.

drug-education program involving a variety of strategies. The impact of the activity that has been implemented always should be monitored and evaluated to assure relevance and usefulness in fulfilling the need. In the instance of an ineffective strategy or program, then, the pharmacist can add or drop specific strategies to improve the overall program. If there is a continual need or problem, or if the pharmacist feels that the nature of the stated problem is outside of his area of expertise or comfort, a referral should be made.

A stepwise approach also should be used in developing drug-education programs, but the educator must realize that a list of guidelines (see Table 1) only represents those decisions and activities that should be considered in the planning and developmental stages. These guidelines, and program outlines and curricula from other sources, must never be used in a cookbook fashion, with little or no critical thought about what is being done.

Flexibility in program design and tailoring the program to the individual needs of the audience are most essential for a successful educational endeavor. One procedure for improving the match between the audience's needs and expectations

Table 1—Guidelines for Developing a Drug Education Program

I. Identify Audience and Educational Need or Problem
   1. Receive request for program
   2. Determine need or problem and individual or group at risk.

II. Set Goals and Objectives for the Program
   1. Clarify needs, interests and expectations.
   2. Determine outcomes.
   3. Define specific goals and objectives.
   4. Identify specific topics and content areas based on needs and objectives.
   5. Determine focus and philosophical approach.

III. Develop Resources and Materials
   1. Identify sources of information and gather and evaluate these materials.
   2. Identify key people with expertise.
   3. Prepare new materials.

IV. Select Appropriate Educational Techniques
   1. Choose teaching approach and strategies.
   2. Identify educational setting, time-frame, equipment and other technical needs.

V. Design, Implement and Evaluate the Program
   1. Structure the program format.
   2. Make a complete outline.
   3. Pretest components, content and educational approach.
   4. Implement the program.
   5. Evaluate and refine.

and the educational program's content and approach is to perform a needs assessment. A short questionnaire is prepared to elicit the needs, suggestions and expectations of the target audience, as well as demographic information on the group's characteristics. The results from such a survey then are used to design the content and format of the educational program.

In addition to the program's content and educational materials, there are a few technical matters that need to be considered. The provision of drug-information and education programs always entails the use of time, money and equipment. More complex and involved programs often are more effective in changing drug-taking behaviors, but they also can be more costly and time-consuming. The provider of a drug-education program also must make certain that specific types of equipment (eg, audio-visuals or computers) are available and in good working order for the program. Finally, in most situations, the consent or permission of the audience or their representative, such as in school settings, is necessary prior to the actual implementation of any educational activity.

Developing and providing educational services involves four steps: design, implementation, evaluation and promotion. Each step should be directed by the specific situation. The design of educational services consists of assessing patients' needs, collecting and developing resources and program materials, being trained in their appropriate use and planning their distribution to the target person or audience.

Patient or consumer needs may be determined by recalling past experiences with specific problems, being aware of the mass media and the concerns of consumer-advocacy groups and surveying the local population for current and future needs. Many pharmacists periodically have used patient-need surveys (which simply can consist of a single page of general, open-ended questions soliciting a written response from the person, or a listing of services and programs that the person can check off) to assist them in the design process. They have found that besides being useful for that purpose, it also builds greater trust and loyalty among their patients and gives the pharmacist an idea of what the patients think about the pharmacy and pharmacist in general.

Once the educational services are defined and developed, they can be implemented whenever a need or problem arises. On many occasions, the pharmacist might have to take the initiative, particularly it is perceived there are potential drug-use problems occurring in a person or the community. Most of what is involved in implementation has been described previously. Local and regional resources (eg, drug information and poison-control centers, mental health and chemical-dependency facilities, hospitals, libraries, bookstores and media centers) should be identified beforehand to determine what services or information they can provide, and to know when they are available and how to reach them if necessary.

One should consider evaluating the educational services used to make sure that they are both effective and efficient, and that the information and services provided are understandable and of use in meeting the problem or need. Evaluations can be performed in the same manner as the aforementioned patient-need surveys.

The pharmacist also should consider the promotion of educational programs and services, so that the patients and consumers will become aware of and use them. The promotion of such services is very similar, in concept, to the promotion of any product or service. Detailed descriptions may be found in any reference book on marketing, advertising or business practices. There are many specific techniques which can be used in promotion. Some are free of cost and involve only a small amount of time, while the willingness to spend more time and money will lead to more intricate and diverse promotional schemes. One comprehensive way is through the local mass media. It is not difficult to contact the local town or neighborhood newspaper, local TV/ radio station and local cable networks and ask for a news story, or even request an interview, that would describe the new educational services that will be provided to the community.

If the services are significantly new in nature or potentially beneficial to the community, such as presenting structured drug-education programs, free news stories and public service announcements about these services and their provider could result. Word-of-mouth communication from current users of the services also is important. It is good to end an episode involving counseling and education with the statement, "If you, or anyone else you know, needs further help or information, please don't hesitate to contact me." Advertising in the phonebook and through the media, and placing signs in the pharmacy's window and at key spots around the community also may be effective.

Single-page consumer-oriented drug-information sheets may be produced for distribution. Assistance for the printing of such materials may be obtained from local agencies and businesses as a show of community support. There is also the accepted practice of promoting a new service by informing lay people or community groups about them. Through a process of diffusion, this information will be shared with a larger number of people who come in contact with those who have been informed. In most communities, key people or groups include teachers and counselors at local schools, the Jaycees and Chamber of Commerce, the PTA, women's clubs, consumer groups, governmental agencies, social and welfare organizations, chemical-dependency agencies and other health professionals in the area.

Future Efforts

The nature and focus of most drug-education and prevention programs probably will not change greatly in the near future. A variety of different strategies and techniques have been developed, but what really is needed are more concerted efforts to design and evaluate programs in a rational manner. In a philosophical way, our ability to prevent drug-use problems can be improved in a number of ways. Drugs should not be categorized as being "hard" or "soft," licit or illicit or addictive or nonaddictive, but instead it should be stressed that the use of any chemical substance carries with it a certain potential for the development of problems, depending upon the pattern and setting of use, the reason for use, past experiences with the drug and a variety of additional social and pharmacological factors. Future efforts should focus more on preventing or limiting drug use problems.

Some educators[28] have even argued that a health-promotion, rather than the more traditional disease-prevention, approach should be used. There is also a need to become more cognizant of attitudes, values and motivations in people's drug-taking, especially those that differ from our own, because these factors are most important in recognizing and characterizing the nature and extent of drug use problems. For instance, some educators have argued that it is time to view drug use as a motivated, adaptive behavior that is pursued in the consummation of valued experience, and then to develop strategies and programs based on this notion.[9]

In practical terms, the success of future programs and activities depends upon a clearer and more coordinated effort in using the strategies and techniques that have been developed and tested. Health professionals, the family, schools and communities should combine their efforts and integrate drug education strategies into ongoing activities, instead of just adding them onto irrelevant courses and programs. Affective educational strategies and basic drug information should be combined in educational programs. The various structured and prepackaged materials and techniques should be selected and synthesized into programmatic formats that best meet the needs of the target audience.

It is important to identify individuals or groups at high risk for developing drug-use problems, and to focus educational and prevention efforts on their needs. Finally, a humanistic approach, in which drug-taking is considered to be a natural kind of behavior and in which an awareness of different values is stressed, should be brought into educational programming. Regardless of the degree of involvement, it is time for pharmacists and the pharmaceutical profession to provide more drug-education programs for their patients and all of society.

Acknowledgment

I am very grateful to Victoria Procopion, who assisted in compiling the references, and to the pharmacists and pharmacy students of Kentucky, Massachusetts, Minnesota, New Hampshire and Pennsylvania, who have been involved in the development and use of many ideas, materials and programs described herein.

References

1. *Drug Use in America: Problem in Perspective*, Natl Comm Marijuana Drug Abuse, USGPO, Washington DC, 1973.
2. Tennant FS *et al*: *Pediatrics 52:* 246, 1973.
3. Blum RH: *Drug Education: Results and Recommendations*, Heath, Lexington MA, 1976.
4. Weil A: *The Natural Mind: A New Way of Looking at Drugs and the Higher Consciousness*, rev ed, Houghton-Mifflin, Boston, 1986.
5. Weil A, Rosen W: *Chocolate to Morphine: Understanding Mind-Altering Drugs*, Houghton-Mifflin, Boston, 1983.
6. Kurzman TA: *A Minnesota Primer on the Prevention of Chemical Use Problems*, Dept of Public Welfare, State of Minnesota, St Paul, 1976.
7. Einstein S, ed: *Drugs in Relation to the Drug User*, Pergamon, New York, 1980.
8. Bettinghaus EP: *Prev Med 15:* 475, 1986.
9. Dembo R: *Int J Addict 16:* 1399, 1981.
10. Kirschenbaum H: *Advanced Value Clarification*, Univ Assoc, La Jolla CA, 1977.
11. Goodstadt MS: *Health Educ Monogr 6:* 263, 1978.
12. Segal M *et al*: *Public Health Rep 98:* 426, 1983.
13. Kanouse DE *et al*: *Informing Patients about Drugs*, Rand Corp, Santa Monica CA, 1981.
14. Mullen PD, Green LW: *Measuring Patient Drug Information Transfer: An Assessment of the Literature*, PMA, Washington DC, 1984.
15. Glanz K *et al*: *Med Care 19:* 141, 1981.
16. Becker MH, ed: *The Health Belief Model and Personal Health Behavior*, Slack, Thorofare NJ, 1974.
17. Goodstadt M, ed: *Research on Methods and Programs of Drug Education*, Addict Res Found, Toronto, 1974.
18. Goodstadt MS, Sheppard MA: *J Studies Alcohol 44:* 362, 1983.
19. Sexter J *et al*: *Int J Addict 19:* 79, 1984.
20. Tobler NS: *J Drug Issues 16:* 537, 1986.
21. Schaps E *et al*: *Int J Addict 15:* 657, 1980.
22. *Promising Community Drug Abuse Prevention Programs*, US GAO, Rockville, MD 1991.
23. Gonzalez GM: *J Alcohol Drug Educ 27:* 2, 1982.
24. Sherman RE *et al*: *Ibid 30:* 66, 1984.
25. Hemminki E: *Soc Sci Med 9:* 111, 1975.
26. Montagne M *et al*: *Am J Hosp Pharm 37:* 1211, 1980.
27. Vickery DM, Fries JF: *Take Care of Yourself: A Consumer's Guide to Medical Care*, Addison-Wesley, Reading PA, 1976.
28. Room R: *Public Health Rep 96:* 26, 1981.

Appendix A—Specific Strategies and Programs in Drug Education[a]

Cognitive Programs

Drug-Specific Information

Morris LA: *Communicating Therapeutic Risks*, Springer-Verlag, New York, 1990.
Ray OS, Ksir C: *Drugs, Society and Human Behavior*, 4th ed, Times Mirror, St Louis, 1991.

Drug-Related Information

Corry JM, Cimbolic P: *Drugs: Facts, Alternatives, Decisions*, Wadsworth, Belmont CA, 1985.
Marin P, Cohen AY: *Understanding Drug Use: An Adult's Guide to Drugs and the Young*, Harper & Row, New York, 1971.

Computer-Assisted Instruction

Ellis LBM, Raines JR: *Prev Med 10:* 77, 1981.
Gustafson DH *et al*: *Ann Rev Publ Health 8:* 387, 1987.

Drug Information Services

Montagne M *et al*: *Am J Hosp Pharm 37:* 1211, 1980.
Rolett V, Kinney, J: *How to Start and Run an Alcohol and Other Drug Information Centre: A Guide*, Off Substance Abuse Prev, Rockville MD, 1990.

Affective Programs

Interpersonal Skills

Kurzman TA: *Contemp Drug Probl 3:* 187, 1974.
Meldrum H: *Interpersonal Skills in Pharmaceutical Care*, Haworth, New York, 1994.

Values Clarification

Dembo R: *Int J Addict 16:* 1399, 1981.
Raths LE et al: *Values and Teaching*, Merrill, Columbus OH, 1966.

Social Competencies

Bell C, Battjes R, eds: *Prevention Research: Deterring Drug Abuse among Children and Adolescents*, Natl Inst Drug Abuse, Rockville MD, 1985.
Masters R, Houston J: *Mind Games*, Viking, New York, 1972.

Parenting

Ezetoye S *et al*: *Childhood and Chemical Abuse: Prevention and Intervention*, Haworth, New York, 1986.
Manatt M: *Parents, Peers and Pot II*, Natl Inst Drug Abuse, Rockville MD, 1983.

Coping with Stress

Heit P: *Int J Health Educ 21:* 282, 1978.
Shiffman S, Wills TA, eds: *Coping and Substance Use*, Academic, Orlando FL, 1985.

Behavioral Programs

Refusal Skills and Peer Pressure

Adolescent Peer Pressure: Theory, Correlates, and Program Implications for Drug Abuse Prevention, Natl Inst Drug Abuse, Rockville MD, 1986.
Shore ER, Rivers PC: *J Alcohol Drug Educ 30:* 22, 1985.

Fear-Arousal Messages

Leathar DS *et al*, eds.: *Health Education and the Media II*, Pergamon, New York, 1986.
Smart RG, Fejer D: *J Drug Educ 4:* 225, 1974.

Alternatives to Drugs

Cohen S: *JAMA 238:* 1561, 1977.
Dohner VA: *J Drug Educ 2:* 3, 1972.

Social-Control Mechanisms

Einstein S, ed: *Drugs in Relation to the Drug User*, Pergamon, New York, 1980.
Zinberg NE, Harding WM, eds: *Control Over Intoxicant Use: Pharmacological, Psychological, & Social Considerations*, Human Sciences Press, 1981.

Social Support / Group Activities

Glynn TJ *et al*, eds: *Preventing Adolescent Drug Abuse: Intervention Strategies*, Natl Inst Drug Abuse, Rockville MD, 1983.
Madsen DB: *Int J Addict 14:* 1117, 1979.

Behavioral Modification

Marlatt GA, Nathan PE, eds: *Behavioral Approaches to Alcoholism*, Rutgers Center Alcohol Studies, New Brunswick NJ, 1978.
Serdahely WD: *J Alcohol Drug Educ 29:* 34, 1984.

Decision-Making and Problem-Solving

Goodstadt MS, Sheppard MA: *J Studies Alcohol 44:* 362, 1983.
Koberg D, Bagnall J: *The Universal Traveler: A Soft-Systems Guide to Creativity, Problem-Solving, and the Process of Reaching Goals*, William Kaufmann, Los Altos CA, 1972.

Program Planning

Program Development

Edwards G, Arif A: *Drug Problems in the Sociocultural Context: A Basis for Policies and Programme Planning*, WHO, Geneva, 1980.
Moskowitz JM: *J Stud Alcohol 50:* 54, 1989.

Needs Assessment

Claydon PD, Johnson ME: *J Alcohol Drug Educ 31:* 51, 1985.
World Health Assoc: *Assessment of Public Health and Social Problems with the Use of Psychotropic Drugs,* WHO, Geneva, 1981.

Program Outcomes

Schaps E *et al*: *J Drug Issues 11:* 17, 1981.
Sexter J *et al*: *Int J Addict 19:* 79, 1984.

Program Evaluation

Hawkins JD, Nederhood B: *Handbook for Evaluating Drug and Alcohol Prevention Programs,* Off Substance Abuse Prev, 1987.
Montagne M: *Eval Health Prof 5:* 477, 1982.

Role of the Educator

Dembo R: *Int J Addict 16:* 1399, 1981.
Oshodin OG: *J Alcohol Drug Educ 29:* 1, 1984.

Comprehensive Programming

Mass Media

Flay BR: *J School Health 56:* 401, 1986.
McGuire WJ: *Prev Med 13:* 299, 1984.

Holistic/Integrated Approaches

Nebelkopf E: *J Psychoactive Drugs 13:* 345, 1981.
Winkelman DL, Harbet SC: *J Alcohol Drug Educ 31:* 17, 1985.

School-Based Program

Bangert-Drowns RL: *J Drug Educ 18:* 243, 1988.
Bukoski WJ: *J Child Contemp Soc 18:* 95, 1985.

Community-Based Programs

Giesbrecht N, *et al*, eds: *Research, Action, and the Community: Experiences in the Prevention of Alcohol and Other Drug Problems,* Off Substance Abuse Prev, Rockville MD, 1989.
Johnson CA *et al*: *J Consult Clin Psychol 58:* 447, 1990.

Peer Counseling

Arkin EB, Funkhouser JE: *Communicating about Alcohol and Other Drugs: Strategies for Reaching Populations at Risk,* Off Substance Abuse Prev, Rockville, 1990.
OSAP: *Preventing Adolescent Drug Use: From Theory to Practice,* Off Substance Abuse Prev, Rockville, 1991.

Health-Professional Training

Ewan CE, Waite A: *Int J Addict 17:* 1211, 1982.
Lewis DC *et al*: *JAMA 257:* 2945, 1987.

Gatekeeper Training

Jensen K: *Int J Health Educ 24 (suppl):* 1, 1981.
Schaps E *et al*: *J Alcohol Drug Educ 29:* 35, 1984.

Curricular Guides and Bibliographies

Cornacchia HJ *et al*: *Drugs in the Classroom: A Conceptual Model for School Programs,* 2nd ed, Mosby, St Louis, 1978.
Finn P, O'Gorman PA: *Teaching in Alcohol: Concepts, Methods, and Classroom Activities,* Allyn & Bacon, Boston, 1981.
Prevention Plus II, Off Substance Abuse Prev, Rockville, 1989.
Rodgers T *et al*: *What Works:* Health Promotion Res Center, Palo Alto CA, 1990.

[a]These citations contain specific program descriptions.

CHAPTER 103

Patient Compliance

Daniel A Hussar, PhD
Remington Professor of Pharmacy
Philadelphia College of Pharmacy and Science
Philadelphia, PA 19104

The significant advances that have been made in the understanding of the etiology of many disease states, and the development of many new therapeutic agents, have made it possible to cure or provide symptomatic control of many clinical disorders. However, accompanying the increasing sophistication relative to diagnostic and therapeutic knowledge and skills has been the recognition that, in many circumstances, drugs are not being used in a manner conducive to optimal benefit and safety. In many situations, efforts to maintain or improve health fall short of the goals that are considered attainable and, frequently, the failure to achieve the desired outcomes has been attributable to patient noncompliance or partial compliance.

With regard to the provision of health care the concept of compliance can be viewed broadly, as it relates to instructions concerning diet, exercise, rest, return appointments, etc, in addition to the use of drugs. However, it is in discussions concerning drug therapy that the designation, "patient compliance" is employed most frequently. It is in this context that it will be used in this discussion, and compliance can be defined as the extent to which an individual's behavior coincides with medical or health advice.

Compliance with therapy implies a positive behavior in which the patient is motivated sufficiently to adhere to the prescribed treatment because of a perceived self-benefit and a positive outcome (eg, enhanced daily functioning and well-being). Some have recommended the use of the terms *adherence* or *concordance*, as they may have a less coercive connotation than the designation *compliance;* however, the latter term continues to be the most widely accepted and used.

Problems concerning patient compliance with instructions have been recognized for years and, indeed, Hippocrates once cautioned, "Keep watch also on the fault of patients which often makes them lie about the taking of things prescribed." When the complexity of the patient's illnesses and the actions of potent therapeutic agents are taken into account, the physician, pharmacist and other health professionals easily can become preoccupied with the diagnosis of the disease state as well as the selection and implications of drug therapy and assume that the patient will follow the instructions provided. After all, since the medication is being provided to improve and/or maintain the patient's health, why would the patient not follow instructions? Yet, studies continue to show that a large percentage of patients, for a variety of reasons, do not take their medication according to instructions.

Although some patients make a conscious decision to deviate from the prescribed regimen (ie, *intentional* noncompliance), many intend to take their medication according to instructions and, in some cases, even may be unaware that their use of medication differs from what the prescribed intended.

The term *patient noncompliance* suggests that the patient is at fault for the inappropriate use of medication. Although this is often the case, in a number of situations, the physician and pharmacist have not provided the patient with adequate instructions or have not presented the instructions in a manner that the patient understands them. The most basic questions regarding drug usage must be addressed—Has the patient been provided with adequate instructions? Does the patient understand how the medication is to be taken? Nothing should be taken for granted regarding the patient's understanding of how to use medication, and appropriate steps must be taken to provide patients with the information and counseling necessary to use their medications as effectively and as safely as possible.

Noncompliance

Types

The situations most commonly associated with noncompliance with drug therapy include failure to have the prescription filled or refilled, omission of doses, errors of dosage, incorrect administration, errors in the time of administration and premature discontinuation.

In a survey[1] of consumers, 14% of the respondents indicated that they had obtained prescriptions from their physicians but did not get them filled. The most common explanations for not having the prescriptions filled were that they didn't feel they needed the medication or they didn't want to take it. In the many situations in which infection is associated with fever and local discomfort, patients already may be taking nonprescription medications, such as acetaminophen. The ability of these agents to provide some, if not complete, relief of the symptoms of early infection may lead some patients to conclude that the condition is improving, or better, and that it is not necessary to have the prescription filled.

The omission of doses is one of the most common types of noncompliance and is more likely to occur when a medication is to be administered at frequent intervals and/or for an extended period of time. Errors of dosage include situations in which the amount of an individual dose or frequency of administration is incorrect.

Examples of the incorrect administration of medication include not using the proper technique in using metered-dose inhalers and, in some cases, giving medication by the wrong route of administration. Errors in the time of administration of the drug may include situations in which medication is administered in an inappropriate relationship to meals. Certain drugs—eg, tetracycline, most fluoroquinolones, some erythromycin formulations, didanosine (Videx) and astemizole (Hismanal)—should be administered apart from meals to achieve optimal absorption. The time of day at which a drug is administered also may be important in the use of some medications; eg, diuretics are best administered in the morning.

The premature discontinuation of treatment occurs commonly with the use of antibiotics as well as medications used in the treatment of chronic disorders such as hypertension. An American Association of Retired Persons (AARP) survey of ambulatory elderly found that 33% said they had prematurely discontinued a prescribed medication.[2] Patients must be apprised of the importance of taking the medication in the manner instructed even though their condition may be asymptomatic or, as in the case of infections, the symptoms may have subsided soon after the initiation of therapy.

Studies reflect a wide variation in the degree of noncompliance. Many reports indicate that at least one-third of the patients failed to comply with instructions, and for patients with chronic illnesses on long-term treatment regimens the results suggest a rate of noncompliance of approximately 50%. To provide a better insight into the type and extent of the specific problems identified, the following examples are provided.

One study,[3] which showed that 51% of patients in the outpatient setting were noncompliant for written prescriptions, prompted an investigation of how patients interpret instructions provided on prescription labels. Sixty-seven patients were asked to interpret instructions on each of ten prescription labels and in not one case was a label uniformly interpreted by all patients. Even when the instructions were not felt by the prescriber to be ambiguous, there was frequent misinterpretation with the incidence of interpretive errors ranging from 9 to 64%.

Problems of compliance also have been noted frequently among elderly patients, many of whom have been prescribed complex therapeutic regimens.

In a study[4] conducted in elderly public-housing tenants, noncompliance significantly was associated with taking more than five prescribed medications, an inability to read prescription and auxiliary labels and difficulty opening flip-off-type medication container lids. The challenge of increasing the compliance of elderly patients is the subject of several reviews.[5,6]

Similar challenges have been reported in pediatric patients. In a study of compliance[7] with treatment of acute otitis media in 300 pediatric outpatients, complete compliance in taking prescribed antibiotics was only about 7%. Parents gave fewer than the prescribed number of doses in 36% of cases and therapy was discontinued early in 37%. Other factors contributing to the noncompliance included incorrect labeling and the use of "teaspoons" having widely varying volumes.

Consequences

The importance and scope of the difficulties that result from the failure to use medications in the manner intended has resulted in the National Council on Patient Information and Education designating noncompliance as "America's other drug problem." Others have noted that noncompliance may be the most significant problem that faces medicine today,[8] and that "knowledge of patient compliance is of critical importance in interpreting drug response, whether it be in the individual patient or in a clinical trial.[9] In response to concerns regarding mismedication among elderly patients, including observations that 55% of this patient population is noncompliant, the Office of the Inspector General conducted a study to determine why elderly people fail to follow prescription medication regimens.[10]

"Drugs don't work if people don't take them." This observation made by former Surgeon General C Everett Koop in his keynote address at a symposium on "Improving Medication Compliance,"[11] provides a clear statement of one of the consequences of noncompliance. In many cases noncompliance results in *underutilization* of a drug, thereby depriving the patient of the anticipated therapeutic benefits and possibly resulting in a progressive worsening or other complications of the condition being treated.

Noncompliance also may result in the *overutilization* of a drug. When excessive doses are employed, or when the medication is given more frequently than intended, there is an increased risk of adverse reactions. These problems may develop rather innocently, as in the case where a patient recognizes that he has forgotten a dose of medication and doubles the next dose to make up for it. Some other patients appear to believe that if the one-tablet dose that has been prescribed provides some relief of symptoms, two or three tablets will be even more effective.

The results of several studies suggest that up to 10% of hospital admissions[12] and 23% of nursing home admissions[13] are related to noncompliance. In a recent study of 315 consecutive medical admissions of elderly patients to a community hospital, 28% were medication-related—17% because of adverse reactions and 11% because of noncompliance.[14] In a review of published studies of drug-related hospital admissions, it is noted that eleven reports indicated that 22.7% of adverse drug reaction hospitalizations were induced by noncompliance.[15]

It has been estimated that there are 125,000 deaths and several hundred thousand hospitalizations per year resulting from noncompliance of patients with cardiovascular disease.[16] The deaths attributed to noncompliance have prompted the observation that "noncompliance takes more lives than car accidents and AIDS combined.[17]

Hypertension is the most frequently studied disease with regard to compliance. Although educational and screening programs have significantly reduced the number of individuals who are unaware that they have hypertension, it is estimated that 43% of the nearly 62 million Americans with high blood pressure do not have their condition under control. For those hypertensive patients for whom treatment has been prescribed, numerous studies indicate that fewer than 50% have their blood pressure under effective control and that the major reason for the failure to control hypertension is noncompliance with regimens that would work if administered as intended. Noncompliance is one of the most commonly missed diagnoses, and the manner in which a patient is using his medication should be evaluated before the therapeutic regimen is changed. In one study it is reported that the under-utilization of antihypertensive medications may be associated with hospitalization that could have been prevented if patients had complied with their treatment regimens.[18]

One report[19] has called attention to the hazards of noncompliance with anticonvulsant drug regimens. In examining autopsy records pertaining to 11 cases of unattended, unexpected deaths of epileptic patients, no anticonvulsant drugs were found in four patients and subtherapeutic levels were noted in six others. It is suggested that a number of these deaths may have been preventable had there been better compliance with the instructions for using the medication(s).

Similarly, a leading cause of death in transplant patients, some of whom had waited for years for a donor organ, is the rejection that results from noncompliance in using immunosuppressant medication.[20]

The economic consequences of noncompliance also are alarming. Noncompliance problems among patients with cardiovascular disease have been estimated to represent a loss of 20 million workdays, costing $1.5 billion in earnings, apart from the costs of hospitalization.[16] In 1984 the U.S. Chamber of Commerce estimated that $13 to 15 billion was spent to treat problems arising from noncompliance.[21] The cost of noncompliance and the capacity of improved compliance to reduce health-care expenditures are the subject of a review of a number of studies in which it is observed that "*without exception* the benefits realized from improved compliance outweigh, in some cases far outweigh, the costs of programs designed to improve compliance."[22]

Noncompliance also may take other forms. The problems associated with drug misuse and abuse, whether unintentional or deliberate, are well-recognized. Although usually not thought of in terms of noncompliance, drug-abuse problems sometimes result from excessive use of medications which have been prescribed for existing clinical disorders.

Another implication relates to the storage of drugs that are not used completely during the intended period of treatment. Keeping these drugs may result in their inappropriate use at some later time. Accidental poisonings have resulted, and stockpiled medications have been used to commit suicide.

The recognition that noncompliance is so prevalent has raised questions regarding the attention this variable has received in clinical studies of therapeutic agents. For example, an analysis of the sources and the amount of overt and hidden bias in reports of double-blind studies of nonsteroidal anti-inflammatory drugs published between 1966 and 1985 revealed that only 13% of the studies measured compliance.[23]

The potential changes in therapeutic response resulting from noncompliance dictate that close attention be given to this aspect of the study of the action of therapeutic agents.

Although the consideration of the consequences of noncompliance should focus primarily on the problems that may develop, there also should be an awareness of situations in which some patients may benefit from being noncompliant. Designated by one investigator[24] as *intelligent noncompliance*, it is noted that certain individuals have a rational basis (eg, avoiding adverse effects) for altering the dosage of their medication and that good treatment outcomes are still attained. However, the fact that certain patients may benefit from not adhering to a treatment regimen must not be considered a reason for health professionals being less diligent in detecting noncompliance and initiating the appropriate corrective measures, as any situation in which noncompliance occurs requires careful evaluation.

Detection

Like the diagnosis of medical disorders, detection of noncompliance is a necessary prerequisite for adequate treatment. In addition, like many diseases, compliant or noncompliant behavior is not stable and may change over time, necessitating the regular use of detection methods to measure this behavior as part of the assessment of treatment efficacy.

The ideal detection method would measure compliance at the time and place of the medication-taking (or other treatment) event. Direct observation of the patient would come closest to providing this ideal measure of compliance. However, this method usually is not practical.

Current detection methods include indirect measures, such as self-report, interview, therapeutic outcome, pill count, change in the weight of metered-dose inhaler canisters, medication-refill rate and computerized compliance monitors, and direct measures, such as biological markers, tracer compounds and assay of body fluids. In general, the direct methods of detection have a higher sensitivity and specificity than the indirect methods, making the direct methods more reliable for the assessment of compliance. Still, all of these methods have their limitations. To help overcome limitations of the assessment methods and to provide corroborative information, it is recommended that at least two different detection methods be used to measure compliance.

Indirect Methods—Self-reports and interviews with patients are the most common and simplest methods of attempting to determine compliance with therapy. However, many studies have demonstrated that even the most skilled and highly refined interviewing techniques substantially overestimate medication compliance. In spite of the limitations of interviews, asking carefully constructed questions (eg, "Most people have trouble remembering to take their medicine. Do you have trouble remembering to take yours?")[25] in a nonthreatening manner will be helpful in identifying some noncompliant patients.

Pill counts are another detection method used to measure compliance and frequently are used in clinical drug studies. A patient's adherence to a medication regimen can be assessed by the difference between the number of dosage units initially dispensed and the number remaining in the container on his return visit or during an unscheduled home visit. However, *pill dumping* (ie, attempts by patients to misrepresent their compliance by discarding medication) is common, and several studies have shown that return counts grossly overestimate actual compliance rates.[26,27]

The achievement of treatment goals sometimes has been used as a measure of a patient's compliance. When a particular treatment is associated with a successful outcome (eg, normal blood pressure, glucose level or intraocular pressure), satisfactory compliance with the regimen may be inferred. However, patients may *load-up* on medication or adhere to other treatment regimens (eg, diet) just before their return visit. Such behavior has been called the *toothbrush effect*, after the way people brush their teeth just before seeing a dentist. The toothbrush effect can invalidate almost completely the health-outcome strategy, as well as other detection methods (eg, determination of drug concentrations in body fluid).

Computerized compliance monitors are the most recent and reliable of the indirect-detection methods. The principle of electronic monitoring of compliance was pioneered by Kass *et al.*[28,29] with the development of an electronic eyedrop dispenser and has been adapted to measure compliance with solid dosage forms as well [Medication Event Monitoring System (MEMS) available from Aprex Corp, Fremont, CA]. The system consists of a microprocessor housed in the cap of the medication container. Each time the patient removes the cap, the time and date are recorded. Data are retrieved by connecting the microprocessor unit to a computer. The data not only provide an indication of individual dosing patterns, but also allow correlations with clinical events. Such data might be useful to the clinician in understanding why treatment has not been fully successful. Although the computerized monitors provide no direct information on whether or how much medication was actually taken, their use helps to supplement other methods. For example, in a recent study[30] in which pill counts indicated near-perfect compliance, the monitor in the cap showed that fewer than half of all cap openings occurred at the prescribed interval of 12 ± 2 hours.

Direct Methods—Biological markers and tracer compounds indicate patient compliance over an extended period. For example, measurement of glycosylated hemoglobin in patients with diabetes mellitus gives an objective assessment of metabolic control during the preceding 3-month period. Tracer compounds—small amounts of agents such as phenobarbital and digoxin—can be added to drugs and measured in biological fluids as pharmacological indicators of compliance.[31,32] Both phenobarbital and digoxin have long half-lives and thus have the advantage of indicating compliance for the preceding few weeks rather than days. With either drug, good compliance cannot be simulated by ingesting a few doses immediately before assessment.

Finally, compliance also has been measured through determination of drug concentrations in patients' biological fluids. However, the usefulness of data on drug concentrations in biological fluids is limited because (1) concentrations of drugs are affected by individual differences in absorption, distribution, metabolism and excretion, and low or erratic drug concentrations are not necessarily an indication of noncompliance,[33] (2) drug concentrations do not provide data regarding the timing of doses consumed and (3) brief intake of rapidly cleared drugs before testing can produce results that show adequate drug concentrations, erroneously suggesting regular medication use.

The Noncompliant Patient

Efforts have been made to demonstrate the relationship of noncompliance to a number of variables such as age, education, occupation, socioeconomic status, personality factors, physiological variables and the number, types and severity of illnesses. Although certain patterns have been noted in some studies, the results, in general, have been inconsistent and it continues to be difficult to identify which patients are most likely to be noncompliant.

A distinction has been made between attitudinal and behavioral compliance, since often the attitude and behavior of a patient may be incongruent. For example, a patient fully may intend to take the medication according to instructions but actually not do so because he is forgetful or really does not understand the instructions. On the other hand, some patients may have no intention of complying but nevertheless do so.

Some individuals are intentionally noncompliant. In one study[34] of elderly patients, almost three-quarters of the individuals observed to be noncompliant intentionally did not take their medication(s) according to instructions. The reason most frequently provided was that the patient did not believe the drug was needed in the dosage prescribed by the physician. It was noted that intentional noncompliance was more likely to occur in patients who used two or more pharmacies and two or more physicians.

The recognition that noncompliance may be intentional as well as unintentional underscores the complexity of the challenge to develop strategies to improve compliance. Although considerable progress has been made in recognizing and addressing the problems associated with noncompliance, an observation made in an early discussion[35] of this subject continues to be valid today—"It has not proved possible to identify an uncooperative type. Every patient is a potential defaulter; compliance can never be assumed."

Considerable attention has been directed toward the sociobehavioral determinants of compliance and a number of models based on behavioral principles have been described.[36] A *health-belief model*, which initially was developed[37] to explain preventive health behaviors such as obtaining immunizations and prophylactic dental care, was revised subsequently[38] to apply to compliance with prescribed medical regimens. More recently, a *third-generation* model has been proposed[8] which focuses more specifically on health decisions. This *health-decision model* combines decision analysis, behavioral decision theory and health beliefs to yield a model of health decisions and resultant behavior. The components of this model and the manner in which they are interrelated are outlined in Fig 1.

With respect to the relationship between health beliefs and compliance, if compliance is to be achieved, the patient must believe that

She actually has the illness which has been diagnosed.

The illness could cause severe consequences with regard to her health and daily functioning.

The treatment prescribed will reduce the present or future severity of the condition.

The benefits of the regimen prescribed outweigh the perceived disadvantages and costs of following the recommended action.

In addition, there must be a stimulus to trigger the advocated health behavior, which can be either internal (eg, concern about the disease) or external (eg, interaction with the physician or pharmacist).

Patient education and counseling initiatives should be designed to encourage the beliefs noted above, particularly since many patients believe that "you only need to take medication when you are ill and experience symptoms" and/or "you need to stop taking medication once in awhile or else your body becomes dependent on it or the medication will become less effective."

There are also other "patient factors" which may contribute to noncompliance. Patients who live alone are less likely to comply than those who live with another family member who can take an interest in and/or supervise their therapy. The

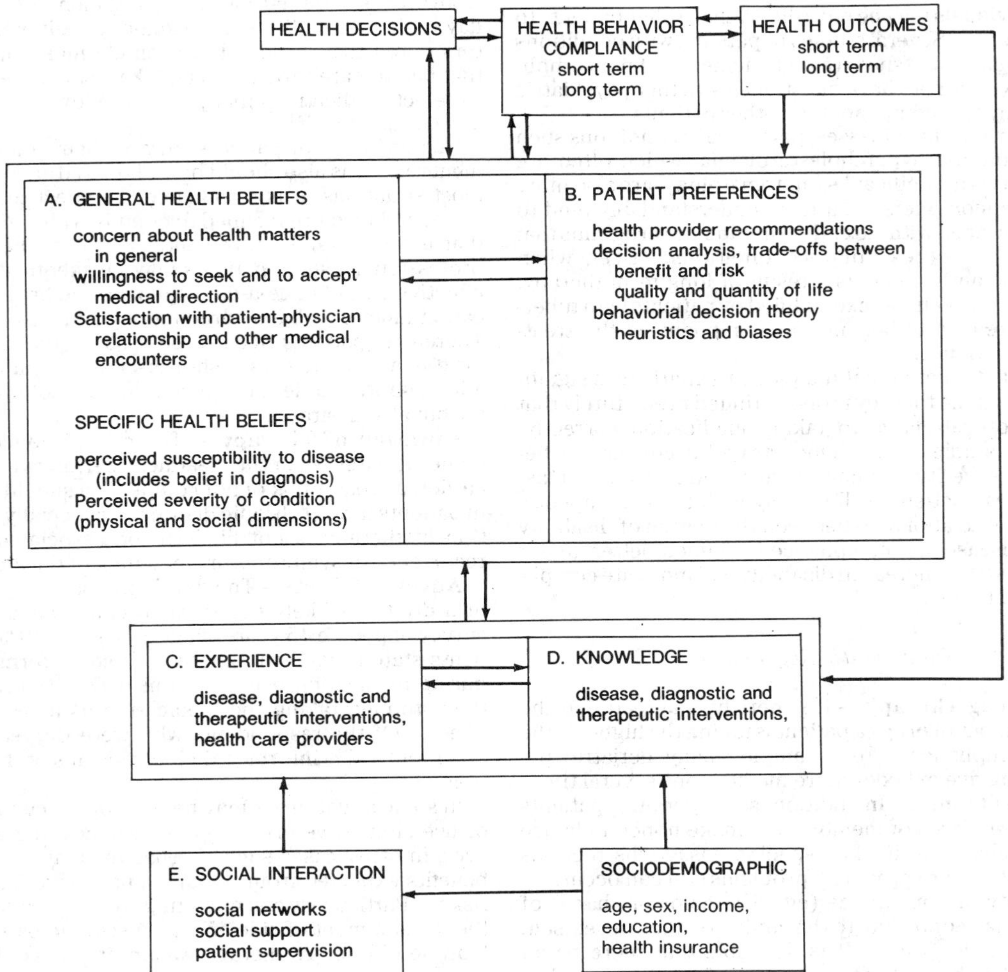

Fig 1. The health-decision model, combining the health-belief model and patient preferences, including decision analysis and behavioral decision theory.[8]

increasing problems of drug abuse and addiction have increased the awareness and concern about becoming dependent on agents that are prescribed for legitimate medical reasons. Although drugs that carry a potential for abuse and development of dependence often are prescribed and used too casually, some patients develop a fear of dependence regarding use of any drug that is to be employed for a prolonged period. To avoid such a possibility or to prove to themselves that they are not dependent, they may interrupt or stop therapy, or use the medication in smaller amounts.

Numerous other factors have been suggested to contribute to patient noncompliance and the most important of these are considered in the following discussion.

Factors Associated with Noncompliance

In addition to the patient factors previously considered, a number of other determinants of patient compliance have been cited. Some of the more important and/or commonly considered factors are discussed below. Although the relationship of some of these factors to the occurrence of noncompliance has not been proven, there should be an awareness of the potential implications in selected patients.

Disease

The nature of the patient's illness may, in some circumstances, contribute to noncompliance. In patients with psychiatric disorders, the ability to cooperate as well as the attitude toward treatment may be compromised by the illness, and these individuals may be more likely than other patients to be noncompliant. Several studies of patients with conditions like schizophrenia have shown a high incidence of noncompliance. However, others have questioned whether psychiatric patients are any less compliant than other patients.

Patients with chronic illnesses, particularly conditions such as hypertension and hypercholesterolemia, which often are not associated with significant symptomatology, are also more likely to be noncompliers. Patients understandably tend to become discouraged with extended therapeutic programs that do not produce "cures" of the conditions. Even when "cures" can be anticipated as a result of long-term therapy, problems still can occur, as exemplified by patients with tuberculosis who frequently become noncompliant as the treatment period continues.

It might be anticipated that if a patient experiences significant symptoms if the therapy is discontinued prematurely that he will be more attentive to taking medication correctly. However, few studies have demonstrated a correlation between disease severity and compliance, and it cannot be assumed that these patients will comply with their therapeutic regimens. The relationship between the degree of disability caused by a disease and compliance is defined better, and it can be expected that increased disability will motivate compliance in most patients.

Therapeutic Regimen

Multiple Drug Therapy— It generally is agreed that the greater the number of drugs a patient is taking the higher is the risk of noncompliance. For example, many geriatric patients are taking five or six or more medications several times a day at different times. In addition, some geriatric patients may experience lapses of memory that make noncompliance even more likely. Even when specific dosage instructions for the medications are provided, problems still can occur.

The similarity of appearance (eg, size, color or shape) of certain drugs may contribute to the confusion that can exist in the use of multiple drugs. It is desirable that there be an awareness of the physical characteristics of the drugs used so that the patient will not be taking, for example, only small white tablets. In one report,[39] serious complications experienced by two patients are described, which were apparently attributable to the patients' confusing digoxin, 0.25 mg, with furosemide, 40 mg, another small white tablet.

The observations in an editorial[40] provide a perspective that is helpful in understanding the challenge for the patient who is to take a number of medications.

> "A common consequence of too many pills is organizational breakdown. Given a regimen of four pills once a day, one pill twice a day, three pills three times daily, and two pills four times daily, compliance suffers. Even the best intentions struggle under such complexity. Day-to-day pill-taking becomes a little like a church dinner, at which no one takes exactly the same foods or the same portions. An assortment of dishes bewilders the senses. Except for the most compulsive patient, a regimen of many pills many times a day breeds more variety than regularity. Reducing pills and reducing intervals helps minimize the randomness of taking drugs. Potluck becomes a balanced diet."

Although combination drug products have certain disadvantages, their use may help improve compliance with therapy since only one tablet need be administered rather than several. Therapy should not be initiated with a combination product but rather with the individual agents. Once the optimal dosages of the individual drugs have been determined, if they correspond to the amounts included in the combination, these products can be used to advantage.

Frequency of Administration—The administration of medication at frequent intervals makes it more likely that the patient's normal routine or work schedule will have to be interrupted to take a dose of medication and in many cases the patient will forget, not want to be inconvenienced or be embarrassed to do so.

In a study in which compliance was observed to improve from 59% on a three-times-a-day regimen to 75% on a twice-a-day regimen to 84% on a once-a-day regimen, the investigators noted that "probably the single most important action that health-care providers can take to improve compliance is to select medications that permit the lowest daily prescribed dose frequency."[41]

The attitudes of patients toward their illnesses and treatment regimens also should be anticipated and addressed. In most situations, it is reasonable to expect that patients will favor, and be more inclined to comply with, a dosage regimen that is simple and convenient. However, like some health professionals, some patients may be skeptical regarding the effectiveness of once-a-day regimens and believe that a medication must be administered more frequently to be effective. Therefore, patients need to be assured that a longer-acting drug is as effective as a shorter-acting medication and that administration at less frequent intervals not only is appropriate but also desirable.

Duration of Therapy— The rate of noncompliance becomes greater when the treatment period is long. As noted earlier, a greater risk of noncompliance should be anticipated in patients having chronic disorders, especially if discontinuation of therapy is not likely to be associated with prompt recurrence of symptoms or worsening of the illness.

Adverse Effects—The development of unpleasant effects of a drug is a likely deterrent to compliance. In an AARP survey of people 45 years of age and older, 40% of the respondents stated they had experienced some form of side effect during medication use.[2] Of this 40%, 50% responded that they stopped taking the medication as a result of the side effect. Of the respondents who were 65 years of age and older, only 47% informed their physicians of the discontinuation.

In some situations it may be possible to change the dosage or use alternative drugs to minimize adverse effects. However, in other cases such alternatives may not exist and the benefits expected from therapy must be weighed against the risks. Particularly disconcerting are those situations in which the development of side effects makes the patient feel worse than he did before therapy was initiated, as often occurs in hypertensive patients.

In a survey[42] of oncologists, over 60% identified noncompliance as a problem. The adverse effects (eg, nausea, vomiting and hair loss) associated with the use of many antineoplastic drugs, are sufficiently distressing to a number of patients that they do not take their medication in the manner intended. The reduction in the quality of life resulting from effects such as severe nausea and vomiting, may be of such importance to some individuals that they do not comply with a regimen which, in some cases, may even offer the hope of being curative.

The ability of certain drugs to cause sexual dysfunction has been cited[43] as a reason for noncompliance by some patients, with the antipsychotic and antihypertensive agents being implicated most frequently.

Even a warning about possible adverse reactions may result in some individuals not complying with instructions. It is inadvisable for patients being treated with sedatives or other agents having a central nervous system depressant effect to consume alcoholic beverages because of the possibility of an excessive depressant response. However, there should be a realistic recognition that some patients, if faced with a mandate not to drink while on drug therapy, will choose not to take their prescribed medication. Although problems of combined alcohol-drug usage are well known, this situation continues to present a challenge of effectively communicating with the patient so that optimal benefit can be achieved at minimal risk.

Patients May be Asymptomatic or Symptoms Subside—It is understandably difficult to convince a patient of the value of drug therapy when the patient has not experienced symptoms prior to initiation of therapy. Such is often the case in the treatment of hypertension, and the lack of previous symptoms coupled with the probable lack of appearance of symptoms if therapy is discontinued contributes to the high rate of noncompliance in these patients.

In other circumstances the patient may feel better after taking the drug and feel that he no longer needs to take it once the symptoms subside. Situations frequently occur where a patient does not complete a full course of antibiotic therapy once he feels that the infection has been controlled. This practice increases the likelihood of a recurrence of the infection, and patients must be advised to take the full course of antibiotic therapy.

Cost of Medication—Noncompliance often occurs with the use of drugs that have a relatively low cost; however, it might be anticipated that patients may be even more reluctant to comply with instructions for the use of more expensive agents. The expense involved has been cited by some patients as the reason for not having prescriptions filled at all, whereas in other cases the medication is taken less frequently than intended or prematurely discontinued because of the cost. Antibiotics are among the higher priced drugs, and some patients may discontinue taking the drug as soon as the symptoms subside and save the balance of the medication for similar problems they or a family member may encounter in the future.

In a discussion regarding health-care plans, one Congressman observed[44] that an older person's decision to skip needed drug therapy due to lack of money "is a true medical catastrophe . . . which is the very thing we want to protect our seniors against." This comment reflects the concern about the general lack of prescription drug coverage for the elderly and the relationship of the cost of therapy to noncompliance in this patient population.

Administration of Medication—Although a patient may fully intend to comply with instructions, he may inadvertently receive the wrong quantity of medication due to incorrect measurement of medication, use of inappropriate measuring devices, or incorrect use of medication-administration devices. In one study[7] of the use of antibiotics in pediatric patients, the volume of 130 "teaspoons" was measured and found to vary from 2 to 9 mL. The inaccuracy of using teaspoons to administer liquid medications is compounded by the possibility of spillage and when the patient is called on to measure a fraction of a teaspoonful. This problem has been long recognized but problems still occur. The importance of providing the patient with measuring cups, oral syringes or calibrated droppers for the use of oral liquids is evident.

Some patients do not use metered-dose aerosol inhalation devices correctly and this could result in inadequate control of the conditions (eg, asthma) for which their use are intended. The provision of oral instruction by the pharmacist has resulted in better patient understanding and performance of the correct steps for inhaler use.[45]

Taste of Medication—Taste problems of medications are encountered most commonly with the use of oral liquids by children. Getting a child to take a dose of medication may be such a difficult task for a parent that doses may be missed or administration of the drug discontinued as soon as the parent sees any sign of improvement. Compliance problems relating to the taste of medication are not limited to children, however. Objections to the taste of liquid potassium chloride preparations often are raised; a number of patients discontinue taking the medication for this reason.

Patient/Health Professional Interaction

The circumstances surrounding the visit of a patient with a physician and pharmacist, and the quality and effectiveness of the interaction of these health professionals with the patient, are major determinants of the patient's under standing of and attitude toward his illness and therapeutic regimen. One of the patient's greatest needs is psychological support provided in a compassionate manner, and it has been observed that patients are more inclined to comply with the instructions of a physician they know well and respect, and from whom they receive information and assurance about their illnesses and medications.

One group of investigators[46] described the patient-physician interaction as a negotiation among two active and equal participants with a strategy which includes the elements of "putting the ill at ease," respect, positive attitude, information, translation, feedback, patient response and negotiation. Respect for the patient and a realistic appraisal of the circumstances of the individual patient are essential if therapeutic goals are to be achieved.

In a discussion of the influence of the patient-physician relationship on compliance, the following observation was made:

> "Our only true influence on the patient is based on the strength of our professional relationship with that patient. And it is this relationship that is central to improving patient compliance with both medication and treatment regimens."[47]

The following factors are among those which could influence compliance adversely if inadequate attention is given to the scope and quality of the interaction with the patient.

Failure to Comprehend the Importance of Therapy—A major reason for noncompliance is that the importance of the drug therapy and the potential consequences if the medication is not used according to instructions have not been impressed upon the patient. Patients usually know relatively little about their illnesses, let alone the therapeutic benefits and problems that could result from drug therapy. Therefore, they establish their own beliefs and expectations with respect to their drug therapy. If the therapy does not meet these expectations they are more likely to become noncompliant. Greater attention to educating the patient regarding his condition, as well as the benefits and limitations of drug therapy, will contribute to better compliance with therapeutic regimens.

Poor Understanding of the Instructions—Prescriptions that state that medication should be taken "as directed" can be the source of misunderstanding as well as serious consequences. Even when instructions are more specific, confusion still may occur and there have been many errors of interpretation of instructions which the prescriber considered to be clear. For example, in interpreting instructions for use of an antibiotic that is to be administered every 6 hours, some patients do not take the medication around the clock for a total of four doses each day as intended, but rather divide the time they are awake into three 6-hour periods and omit the nighttime dose.

Examples of this type point out the confusion that may exist on the part of the patient even when instructions are seemingly clear. However, many prescriptions are written and labeled to indicate how many doses are to be taken each day with no additional clarification as to how the doses are to be scheduled. For example, how should instructions to take one tablet 3 times a day be interpreted? Does this mean every 8 hours, or with meals, or possibly some other schedule? If the drug is to be given with meals or at a specified time before or after meals, it usually is assumed that the patient eats three meals a day. Yet this is not always the case. In one study,[48] patients being treated with antihypertensive medications with instructions to take the medications 3 times a day, were interviewed with respect to the times at which they administered the individual doses of medication. Of 137 patients, only one was administering the medication at regular 8-hour intervals between doses, and 79% of the patients reported taking all three doses within 12 hours, leaving a dosage interval of 12 hours or more.

A patient may be knowledgeable about the dosage and the specific times at which the medication is to be administered but not recognize the importance of *auxiliary* instructions. Some patients have received prescriptions for a tetracycline derivative in a container to which is affixed an auxiliary label with a precaution about exposure to sunlight. However, in the absence of additional explanation, some have concluded that it is the medication that needs to be protected from sunlight (and have placed the container in the refrigerator), and have not recognized that the information applies to an adverse reaction for which *they* are at risk.

In some cases the uncertainty or confusion on the part of the patient is such that medications are given by the wrong route of administration (eg, instilling oral pediatric antibiotic drops into the ear for an ear infection or administering suppositories by the oral route).

A patient being prepared for an electrocardiogram was observed to have 20 transdermal nitroglycerin patches at various locations on his body. Although he had understood the instructions to apply one patch a day, no instruction had been provided regarding their removal.

Although not a complete listing of all factors that result in noncompliance, those discussed give an indication of the difficult challenge of assuring optimal drug therapy.

Improving Compliance

It often is assumed that health professionals recognize the importance of noncompliance and will take the steps necessary to achieve the compliance of their patients with the instructions provided. However, this assumption may not always be valid. In one study,[49] physician compliance with public health recommendations for tuberculosis control was evaluated. The study revealed poor compliance by physicians with recommended policies for the prevention of tuberculosis in health-care workers, thereby raising concerns about the personal risk of tuberculosis for these physicians, as well as questions about how effectively such physicians will promote preventive actions among their patients. In an accompanying editorial,[50] it was noted that "one might wonder how much patient noncompliance is fostered by a less than enthusiastic endorsement by the health-care provider." For strategies to improve compliance to be effective, health professionals must not only believe that noncompliance is an important problem, but also be willing to make a greater commitment to the steps that will help their patients be compliant.

A number of strategies to enhance compliance have been proposed. Inherent in many of the factors considered is the matter of communication of the physician and pharmacist with the patient. This communication is, in many cases, not only incomplete and ineffective, but often there is the impression that physicians and pharmacists are too busy or not interested in talking with the patient. Improving communications must be considered the key to increasing compliance and some of the approaches and recommendations directed toward this goal are reviewed in the following discussion. The pharmacist has a particularly valuable opportunity to encourage compliance since his advice accompanies the actual dispensing of the medication, and he usually is the last health professional to see the patient prior to the time the medication is to be used.

Identification of Risk Factors

All patients should be viewed as potential noncompliers. A first step in efforts to improve compliance should be to recognize individuals who are most likely to be noncompliant, as judged by a consideration of the risk factors noted earlier. These factors should be taken into account in planning the patient's therapy so that the simplest regimen which is, to the extent possible, compatible with the patient's normal activities can be developed.

Development of Treatment Plan

The more complex the treatment regimen, the greater is the risk of noncompliance, and this must be recognized in the development of the treatment plan. The use of longer-acting drugs in a therapeutic class, or dosage forms that are administered less frequently, also may simplify the regimen.

The treatment plan should be individualized based on the patient's needs and, when possible, the patient should be a participant in decisions regarding the therapeutic regimen. The compliant patient sees himself as an active member of the team involved in his care, not as a passive victim of a disease and the health-care system.[51] Involving the patient in the development of the treatment plan will help the patient view the regimen as something that increases his control and options, rather than something that is done to him.

To help reduce inconvenience and forgetfulness, the regimen should be *tailored* so that the doses of medication are administered at times that correspond to regular activities in the patient's daily schedule. When prescriptions are written, the instructions should be as specific as possible. Instructions such as "as directed" or other directions that are subject to misinterpretation should be avoided. Even such seemingly specific instructions as "one tablet 3 times a day" often are misinterpreted, as discussed previously. Where possible, and with a recognition of the patient's normal routine, the specific times of day at which the patient is to take the medication should be indicated.

The APhA and the American Society of Internal Medicine have developed a statement on prescription writing and prescription labeling (Appendix A). Not only do the guidelines provide important information and suggestions, but the statement reflects the type of interdisciplinary cooperation that also must be achieved in practice if patient needs are to be served best.

The prescription can be used as the organizing instrument of instruction. However, "most often the prescription slip simply is handed over as the closing act of the encounter, while the patient or parent is outward bound."[52] The prescription should signal the start of an alliance, and it behooves the physician to emphasize its importance.

Many prescriptions that patients receive from their physicians are never filled. Little progress has been made in detecting and correcting these occurrences, further emphasizing the need for more effective communication and a closer working relationship between physicians and pharmacists.

Patient Education

One of the findings of the report of the Office of the Inspector General is "education is the best way to improve compliance." However, FDA Commissioner David Kessler has expressed concern that "the nation also is facing a communications gap that has serious implications for the public health. This gap extends from what patients want to know about their medicines to what they actually learn from their physicians and pharmacists."[53] He further observes that "physicians . . . need to re-examine the amount of information they give their patients and the way they deliver it. In addition, they need to acknowledge that pharmacists should have a larger role in patient education and advise their patients to expect counseling when they fill their prescriptions."[53]

Many factors influence the effectiveness of educational efforts and a patient's development of compliant behavior. Decisions must be made as to what information should be provided to patients about their illnesses and drug therapy. It must be recognized that when the information is too comprehensive or detailed or is presented inappropriately (eg, a discussion of adverse reactions that alarms the patient), the patient actually may be discouraged from taking the medications. Thus, compliance may be compromised rather than enhanced.

In discussing an illness or drug therapy with a patient, a distinction should be made between "information" and "education." Patients may receive information but not understand it and use it correctly, whereas education implies understanding and behavioral change. Patients should be encouraged to participate in the discussion and, where possible, they should be brought in on the decision-making process.

The goal of patient education is to provide information that the patient is able to understand and use. The anticipated benefits of the therapy should be explained, as should the importance of complying with the provided instructions. Complex terms and unnecessary jargon that can interfere with patient understanding should be avoided.[54] Patients should be asked to repeat the instructions for administering their medications to show that they understand, and they also should be encouraged to ask questions. At the least, the questions noted in Table 1 should be addressed. It is recommended by the National Council on Patient Information and Education (NCPIE) that these questions be discussed each time a patient obtains prescription medication.

Oral Communication/Counseling—Communication between the pharmacist and patient regarding the use of medication can be both oral and written. Although it may be supplemented and reinforced by written instructions, oral communication is the most important component of patient education because it directly involves both the patient and the pharmacist in a two-way exchange and provides the opportunity for the patient to raise questions. For such communication to be most effective it should be conducted in a setting that provides privacy and is free of distractions.

Although most pharmacies do not presently have a separate patient consultation area, this is a desirable goal. Not only will this emphasize to the patient the importance the pharmacist attaches to the information being discussed, but it also will strengthen further the recognition of the pharmacist as one who is contributing to the patient's health care.

In a consumer survey, 59% of respondents said that there is not enough privacy in the pharmacy to speak to the pharmacist confidentially.[55] Most of these respondents, however, did not believe a separate room was necessary to improve privacy, and the majority (71%) believed that a private area at the end of the prescription counter is sufficient.

Medication often is obtained in a manner that does not lend itself to verbal communication. For example, the pharmacist may receive a telephoned prescription from a physician that is to be delivered to the patient's home or picked up at the pharmacy by a relative or friend. In these circumstances, when appropriate, the pharmacist might call the patient to discuss the use of the medication.

Table 1—Patient Questions Regarding Medication[a]

1. What is the name of the medicine, and what is it supposed to do?
2. How much of the medicine should I take, when should I take it and for how long?
3. What foods, beverages and other medicines should I avoid while taking it?
4. What are the possible side effects, and what should I do if they occur?
5. What written material is available about the medicine?

[a]Questions that patients should ask as recommended by the NCPIE.

The effect of pharmacist counseling on patient compliance has been evaluated in a number of studies. In one study,[56] the effect of pharmacist counseling of patients with hypertension was assessed. The results of this study reflect a significant increase in the patients' knowledge of hypertension and its treatment, their compliance with prescribed therapy and the number of patients whose blood pressures were maintained in the normal range.

Other investigators[57] also have demonstrated the value of pharmacist counseling in increasing compliance and further note the contribution the pharmacist makes in the clinic setting in documenting the drug therapy on the medical record and in decreasing the duplication of prescriptions.

A *compliance clinic* has been described[58] in which pharmacists endeavored to improve the compliance of patients referred to the clinic by physicians. Six of the 14 patients seen on a regular basis demonstrated a significant reduction in emergency room visits and eight patients exhibited reduced hospitalizations, as determined by a comparison of pre- and postclinic records. In addition to the therapeutic benefits most patients will experience as a result of improved compliance, there is a considerable cost savings to be achieved as a result of the reduced hospitalization.

Written Communication—The emphasis on verbal communication should not be interpreted to indicate that written communication is not important. Although at the time of the visit to the physician or pharmacist the patient may understand how the medication is to be used, he may not remember later the details relating to administration of the drug. Therefore, specific instructions for use should be placed on the prescription label.

It is also often desirable to provide supplementary written instructions or other information pertaining to the patient's illness or drug therapy, and many pharmacists are now giving patients medication instruction cards or inserts. Information that pertains to the specific medication/formulation being dispensed is preferred to information that applies to a therapeutic class of agents or a general statement that applies to all dosage forms of a particular medication. The provision of supplementary written information appears to be most effective in improving compliance with short-term therapeutic regimens (eg, antibiotic therapy). For drugs used on a long-term basis, written information as a sole intervention has not been shown to be sufficient for improving patient compliance.

As excellent as the labeling and supplemental written instructions may be, they must be viewed as one-way communication unless the patient is permitted to discuss and ask questions about his therapy. Therefore, oral and written communication should be used to complement each other, and both should be viewed as important components of the effort to educate the patient regarding his drug therapy.

Audiovisual Materials—The use of audiovisual aids may be particularly valuable in certain situations because the patient may be better able to visualize the nature of his illness, or how his medication acts or is to be administered (eg, the administration of insulin or sumatriptan, the use of a metered-dose inhaler). An increasing number of health-care professionals have used such aids effectively by making them available for viewing in a patient waiting area or consultation room, and then answering questions the patient may have.

Controlled Therapy—It has been proposed that hospitalized patients be given the responsibility for self-medication prior to discharge. Usually, patients go from a complete dependence on others for the administration of their medication while hospitalized to a situation in which they are given the full responsibility when discharged, often with the assumption that the patient knows about his drugs because he was taking them in the hospital. Similarly, many ambulatory patients who are expected to be responsible for their own treatment, have not been provided with adequate information.

The suggested arrangement would permit the patient to start using the medication on his own before discharge so that health-care professionals can more directly identify problems or situations that might undermine compliance, and answer patient questions.

Special Compliance Programs—In certain situations it is necessary to develop highly structured programs to improve compliance. An example of such a strategy is a behaviorally oriented program that has been developed for teaching medication management skills to patients with schizophrenia (The Medication Management Module, available from UCLA Psychiatric Rehabilitation Consultants, PO Box 6022, Camarillo, CA 93011).[59] Training in medication self-management occurred in four skill areas: (1) obtaining information about the benefits of antipsychotic medication, (2) knowing how to correctly self-administer the medication and evaluate its effects, (3) identifying adverse effects of medication and (4) negotiating medication issues with health-care providers. Training occurred for 3 hours a week for 4 months and 160 (94%) of 170 patients completed the training. This training resulted in important gains in cognitive mastery, skill attainment, skill use and medication compliance. On the average, knowledge about antipsychotic drugs and use of medication management skills increased approximately 50% across the four areas measured. Ratings at 3-month follow-up indicated that patients continued to use the skills that they were taught during training. Medication compliance assessed independently by the patients' psychiatrists and by a designated caregiver indicated that compliance increased significantly, from 63% to 81%.

Special programs for providing information about medication also are needed for sight-impaired and hearing-impaired patients. In a program developed in New York (Herbert Mindlin, Long Island Pharmaceutical Society, personal communication, Feb 26, 1991), participating pharmacies produce prescription labels in Braille for the blind and use a telecommunication device for the deaf (TDD) to communicate with hearing-impaired patients over telephone lines.

Patient Motivation

Many health-care professionals assume that patients who are knowledgeable about their illness and therapeutic regimen are more likely to be compliant. Although this premise is valid for many patients, increased patient knowledge does not necessarily alter patient behavior and compliance. In one study some of the most flagrant noncompliers could identify their drugs by name and correctly recite the instructions for use.[60]

The fact that such observations have been made must not detract from patient education efforts. Indeed, there must be a commitment to further enhance these programs. However, there must be an awareness of the need to motivate the patient to use the knowledge that has been acquired for the purpose of achieving optimum benefit from his therapy.

Information must be provided to patients in a manner that is not coercive, threatening or demeaning. The best-intentioned, most comprehensive educational efforts will not be effective if the patient cannot be motivated to comply with the instructions for taking the medication. In addition to counseling the patient and providing specific written instructions, supplying cues for appropriate behavior (*prompting*) may be of value in motivating the patient to be compliant. Cues may be verbal or nonverbal with examples of the latter including the use of special packaging or reminder systems.

The physician-patient interaction has been characterized as a *negotiation*. This concept has been extended further by the development of *contracts* between patients and health care providers in which the agreed upon treatment goals and responsibilities are outlined.[61] As summarized in a review,[8] contracts offer "a written outline of expected behavior, the involvement of the patient in the decision-making process concerning the regimen and the opportunity to discuss potential problems and solutions with the physician, a formal commitment to the program from the patient, and rewards . . . which create incentives for achieving compliance goals." Although such a structured approach will not be needed with most individuals, it may be effective for patients who have not responded to other initiatives to ensure compliance.

Noncompliance is the greatest challenge in the control of tuberculosis, and the difficulties currently encountered in the management of this infection have prompted one clinician to make the following observations: "Sometimes it takes a little imagination. Give them a cup of coffee. Talk to them. Pay them an honorarium to come in and take the medicine. If the public doesn't want drug-resistant TB, and if bribing people is the way to get them to take their medicine, then I say bribe them."[62]

Compliance Aids

Labeling—The importance of the accuracy and specificity of the information on the label of the prescription container has been noted already. Auxiliary labels which provide additional information regarding the use, precautions and/or storage of the medication also will contribute to the attainment of compliance.

Medication Calendars and Drug Reminder Charts—Various forms, such as medication calendars, have been developed and are designed to assist the patient in self-administering drugs. In addition to their use in helping the patient understand which medication to take and when to take it, the forms on which the patient is to check the appropriate area for each dose of medication he takes, can be evaluated by the pharmacist or physician when the patient returns for more medication or has his next appointment.

Special Medication Containers, Caps and Systems—Several types of medication containers have been developed to help patients organize their medications and to monitor self-administration of the drugs. An example is the 28-compartment MEDISET container (Apothecary Products, Inc, Burnsville, MN). This device contains four compartments for different time periods (eg, morning, noonday, evening, bedtime) for each day of the week.

Specially designed caps for prescription containers also have been developed to facilitate compliance. The Prescript TimeCap (Wheaton Medical Technologies, New Canaan, CT) contains a digital timepiece that displays the time and day on which the last dose of medication was taken. It also sounds an alarm (a beep and a continuous flashing display) when it is time to take the next dose. The use of microelectronic medication monitors (Medication Event Monitoring System) in the caps of prescription containers has been described earlier.

Other sophisticated systems of organizing and monitoring medication use have been developed. CompuMed (CompuMed, Inc., Meeteetse, WY) is a dispensing device that uses cassettes in which the appropriate medications are placed. At the proper time, medication is dispensed automatically into an easily accessed drawer, and audio and visual alarms remind the user that it is time to take his or her medicine.

Although these special prescription containers, caps and systems are not needed by most patients, they may be effective in achieving compliance in patients who forget doses or who are confused by the complexity of the regimen.

Compliance Packaging—The manner in which medication is packaged also has an influence on patient compliance. A *compliance package* has been defined as a prepackaged unit that provides one treatment cycle of the medication to the patient in a ready-to-use package, and a comprehensive review of the use of such packaging as a patient education tool has been published.[63] This type of packaging usually is based on blister packaging using unit-of-use dosing, and designed to serve as a patient-education tool for health professionals and to make it easier for patients to understand and remember to take their medications correctly at home. Specially designed packaging for oral contraceptives was one of the first initiatives of this type and has been valuable in increasing patient understanding of how these agents are to be taken.

Special packages of certain steroids (eg, *Medrol Dosepak*) also have been designed to facilitate the use of steroids in dosage regimens that may be difficult to understand or remember. Some of the other agents that are available in compliance packages include nizatidine (*Axid Convenience Pak*—a 30-day supply of medication in a medication card); and methotrexate (*Rheumatrex Dose Pack*, containing four blister-pack cards each containing three tablets for 1-week's therapy). A special cap (*C Cap Compliance Cap*) has been used for containers of ophthalmic solutions of certain medications [eg, levobunolol] and is designed to help patients remember how many times they have instilled the drops each day. Different caps are available which correspond to the daily number of prescribed doses. For patients who are on once-a-day regimens, another cap is available that is marked with the days of the week.

A possible negative effect of drug packaging on patient compliance is seen with the use of the child-resistant containers. Some patients, particularly the elderly and those with conditions like arthritis and parkinsonism, have difficulty in opening some of these containers and may not persist in their efforts to do so. There also may be difficulty in opening some foil-packed drugs. Pharmacists should be alert to problems of this type and, where appropriate, suggest use of standard containers or caps.

Dosage Forms—New dosage forms of certain drugs also have been developed, in large part as a recognition of problems of noncompliance. For example, the development of longer-acting, controlled-release dosage forms of calcium channel blocking agents has permitted less frequent administration of these agents, which facilitates compliance. The use of transdermal drug-delivery systems permits less frequent administration of the drugs (eg, nitroglycerin, fentanyl) given by this route.

Monitoring Therapy

Self-Monitoring—The patient should be apprised of the importance of monitoring his own treatment regimen and, in some situations, the response parameters. The attention to the responsibility that patients must personally assume also has been considered in consumer publications, as illustrated by an article in *Good Housekeeping* titled, "If your medicine isn't working. . . It may not be the medicine at all. It could be *you!*"[64]

Pharmacist Monitoring—The pharmacist's role in minimizing noncompliance does not end when the prescription is dispensed. The pharmacist is in an excellent position to detect noncompliance pertaining to drugs used in the management of chronic conditions, such as hypertension and diabetes, by being alert to situations in which the frequency of requested refills is not consistent with the directions for use. Pharmacist follow-up with telephoned or mailed refill reminders has been found to increase compliance.[65,66] A computerized system known as Med-Minder (General Computer Corporation, Twinsburg, OH) has been designed to improve compliance by automatically telephoning appropriate patients and delivering a message to have a specific prescription refilled.

One approach in which both health professionals and patients have collaborated effectively in reviewing/monitoring the use of medication has been the *brown bag* program. The Administration on Aging and National Council on Patient Information and Education (NCPIE) have publicized a national *brown bag* program in which older consumers are encouraged to put all their medicines in a bag and take them to their health professional for a personalized medicine review. Pharmacists are encouraged to become involved in this excellent initiative and may obtain additional information by contacting NCPIE at 666 11th St, NW, Ste 810, Washington, DC 20001—Telephone: (202) 347-6711.

Directly Observed Treatment—Even when many of the steps described earlier have been taken, noncompliance may still result. For example, there is great concern about the high rates of treatment failure in patients with tuberculosis and the increasing prevalence of drug-resistant tuberculosis. In one study that used self-administered treatment, 39% of patients were lost from the study with a 6-month antitubercular regimen and 49% with a 9-month regimen.[67] In contrast, in a study that used a 6-month regimen of directly observed treatment (ie, giving patients their medications and seeing that they are swallowed), fewer than 10% of the patients were lost to further treatment.[68] In a commentary advocating the use of directly observed treatment regimens for patients with tuberculosis, it is observed that "we can't afford not to try it."[69]

Conclusion

Considerable time, effort and expense often have gone into the diagnosis of a patient's illness and the development of a treatment program. Yet the goals of therapy will not be reached unless the patient understands and follows the instructions for use of the drugs prescribed. One also cannot help but wonder how often patients have been categorized as treatment failures and have had their therapy changed, possibly to more potent and toxic agents, when the reason for the lack of response or an unanticipated altered response was noncompliance.

Despite the increasing attention directed to the issue of noncompliance, the problem continues to be prevalent. Although not uniformly successful, the approaches taken and suggestions advanced in an effort to improve compliance have contributed substantially to recognition of the problem and provided a valuable base on which to develop modified or new approaches to the problem. Certain approaches that involve a significantly increased commitment of time on the part of health-care professionals may be viewed by some as impractical. Yet can this increased commitment of time compare with the time and money that are currently being wasted as a result of noncompliance?

The improvement of compliance will result in a situation in which all parties benefit. Most importantly the patient benefits from the enhancement of the efficacy and safety of his drug therapy. The pharmacist benefits because there is an increased recognition and respect for the value of the advice and service that he provided. In addition, the pharmacist benefits from the increase in the number of prescriptions filled and refilled. Pharmaceutical manufacturers benefit from the favorable recognition that accompanies the effective and safe use of their drugs as well as from the increased sales resulting from the larger number of prescriptions being filled and refilled. Finally, society and the health-care system benefit as a result of a lesser number of problems associated with noncompliance. Although an increase in compliance will result in more prescriptions being filled and a higher level of expenditures for prescription medications, this increase in costs will be more than offset by a reduction in costs (eg, physician visits, hospitalizations) attributable to problems due to noncompliance.

For too long patients have been deprived of close attention to and monitoring of their drug therapy. An excuse that health-care professionals are too busy to advise patients regarding their drug therapy cannot be accepted; the highest priority must be assigned to taking the steps to ensure that patients will use their medications in the appropriate manner.

References

1. *1985 National Prescription Buyer Survey* (by Market Facts, Inc), Upjohn.
2. Prescription drugs: a survey of consumer use, attitudes and behavior, AARP, Washington, DC, 1984.
3. Mazzullo JM III *et al: JAMA 227:* 929, 1974.
4. Murray MD *et al: DICP 20:*146, 1986.
5. Fedder DO: *Ibid 18:*158, 1984.
6. Bootman JL: *Geriatrics Curriculum Project,* AACP-Health Sciences Consortium Inc, Carrboro, NC, Chap 14, 1984.
7. Mattar ME *et al: J Pediatr* 87:137, 1975.

8. Eraker SA *et al:* *Ann Intern Med 100:*258, 1984.
9. Peck C: *Medic Event Monit Overview 3:*1, 1991.
10. Kusserow RP: Office of the Inspector General, OEI-04-89-89121, Mar 1990.
11. Koop CE: *Proc Symp Nat Pharm Council,* 1, 1984.
12. McKenney JW, Harrison WL: *Am J Hosp Pharm. 33:*792, 1976.
13. Strandberg LR: *Am Health Care Assoc J 10 (7):*20, 1984.
14. Col N *et al:* *Arch Intern Med 150:*841, 1990.
15. Einarson TR: *Ann Pharmacother 27:*832, 1993.
16. Burrell CD, Levy RA: *Proc Symp Nat Pharm Council,* 7, 1984.
17. Advertisement, PRESCRIPT TimeCap Wheaton Medical Technologies.
18. Maronde RF *et al:* *Med Care 27* :1159, 1989.
19. Bowerman DL *et al:* *J Forensic Sci 23:*522, 1978.
20. Rovelli M *et al:* *Transplant Proc 21:*833, 1989.
21. US Chamber of Commerce 1984, as cited in Smith DL: *Patient Compliance: An Educational Mandate,* Norwich Eaton, 12, 1989.
22. Smith M: *Proc Symp Nat Pharm Council,* 35, 1984.
23. Gotzsche PC: *Controlled Clin Trials 10:*31, 1989.
24. Weintraub M: *Contemp Pharm Pract 4:*8, 1981.
25. Sackett DL. In Haynes RB, Taylor DW, Sackett DL, eds: *Compliance in Health Care,* Johns Hopkins Univ Press, Baltimore, 286, 1979.
26. Rudd P *et al:* *Clin Pharmacol Ther 46:*169, 1989.
27. Pullar T *et al:* *Ibid:*163, 1989.
28. Kass MA *et al:* *Am J Ophthalmol 101:*515, 1986.
29. Kass MA *et al:* *Arch Ophthalmol 102:*1550, 1984.
30. Rudd P *et al:* *Clin Pharmacol Ther 48:*676, 1990.
31. Feely M *et al:* *Br J Clin Pharmacol 24:*77, 1987.
32. Maenpaa H *et al:* *Eur Heart J 8(Suppl 1):*31, 1987.
33. Kossoy AF *et al:* *J Allergy Clin Immunol 84:*60, 1989.
34. Cooper JK *et al:* *J Am Geriatr Soc 30:*329, 1982.
35. Porter AMW: *Brit Med J 1:*218, 1969.
36. Svarstad BL: *NARD J (Feb):*75, 1986.
37. Rosenstock IM: *Milbank Mem Fund Q 55(Jul):*94, 1966.
38. Becker MH *et al:* *Med Care 15 (Suppl 5):*27, 1977.
39. Feder R: *N Engl J Med 298:*463, 1978.
40. Kroenke K: *Am J Med 79:*149, 1985.
41. Eisen SA *et al:* *Arch Intern Med 150:*1881, 1990.
42. Hoagland AC *et al:* *Am J Clin Oncol 6:*239, 1983.
43. Aldridge SA: *Clin Pharm 1:*141, 1982.
44. Robinson B: *Drug Topics 131(Feb 16):*37, 1987.
45. DeTullio PL, Corson ME: *Am J Hosp Pharm 44:*1802, 1987.
46. Benarde MA, Mayerson EW: *JAMA 239:*1413, 1978.
47. Sbarbaro JA: *Ann Allergy 64:*325, 1990.
48. Norell SE et al: *Am J Hosp Pharm 41:*1183, 1984.
49. Geiseler PJ, Nelson KE, Cripsen RG: *Am Rev Respir Dis 135:*3, 1987.
50. Miller B, Snider DE: *Ibid:*1, 1987.
51. Schulman BA: *Med Care 17:*267, 1979.
52. Yaffe SJ *et al:* *Drug Ther 7(11):* 64, 1977.
53. Kessler DA: *N Engl J Med 325:*1650, 1991.
54. Korsch BM *et al:* *Pediatrics 42:*855, 1968.
55. Gannon K: *Drug Topics 134 (Jul 9):*13, 1990.
56. McKenney JM *et al:* *Circulation 48:*1104, 1973.
57. Monson R *et al:* *Arch Intern Med 141:*1441, 1981.
58. Cable GL *et al:* *Contemp Pharm Pract 5:*38, 1982.
59. Eckman TA *et al:* *J Clin Psychopharmacol 10:*33, 1990.
60. McKercher PL, Rucker TD: *J APhA NS17:*283, 1977.
61. Dunbar JM, Agros WS: In Ferguson JM, Taylor CB, eds: *Comprehensive Handbook of Behavioral Medicine,* Vol 3. Spectrum, New York, 328, 1980.
62. Reichman L: *Newsweek (Mar 16)* 57, 1992.
63. Smith DL: *Am Pharm NS29(2):*42, 1989.
64. Dawson ML: *Good Housekeeping Apr:* 235, 1991.
65. Garnett WR *et al:* *Am J Hosp Pharm 38:*676, 1981.
66. Simkins CV, Wenzloff NJ: *DICP 20:*799, 1986.
67. Combs DL *et al:* *Ann Intern Med 112:*397, 1990.
68. Cohn, DL *et al:* *Ibid:*407, 1990.
69. Iseman MD *et al:* *N Engl J Med 328:*576, 1993.

Appendix A—Statement on Prescription Writing and Prescription Labeling[a]

Introduction

Historically, the pharmaceutical and medical professions have devoted considerable time and effort to the development and rational utilization of safe and effective drugs for the treatment and prevention of illness. Today, that successful effort continues, helping to achieve the highest standards of health in the world for the American people. But in order to gain maximum benefit from the use of drugs while minimizing their adverse side effects, prescribers and pharmacists must maintain effective communications not only among themselves, but with their patients as well. The directions for drug use and other information which prescribers indicate on prescription orders and which pharmacists transfer to prescription labels are critical to safe and effective drug therapy. In order to assure that this information is conveyed clearly and effectively to patients, the following guidelines have been developed by the American Pharmaceutical Association and the American Society of Internal Medicine.

Guidelines for Prescribers

The following guidelines are recommended for prescribers when writing directions for drug use on their prescription orders.

1. The name and strength of the drug dispensed will be recorded on the prescription label by the pharmacist unless otherwise directed by the prescriber.
2. Whenever possible, specific times of the day for drug administration should be indicated. (For example, *Take one capsule at 8:00 am, 12:00 noon, and 8:00 pm* is preferable to *Take one capsule three times daily.* Likewise, *Take one tablet two hours after meals* is preferable to *Take one tablet after meals.)*
3. The use of potentially confusing abbreviations, ie, *qid, qod, qd,* etc, is discouraged.
4. Vague instructions such as *Take as necessary* or *Take as directed* which are confusing to the patient are to be avoided.
5. If dosing at specific intervals around-the-clock is therapeutically important, this should specifically be stated on the prescription by indicating appropriate times for drug administration.
6. The symptom, indication, or the intended effect for which the drug is being used should be included in the instructions whenever possible. (For example, *Take one tablet at 8:00 am and 8:00 pm for high blood pressure,* or *Take one teaspoonful at 8:00 am, 11:00 am, 3:00 pm, and 6:00 pm for cough.)*
7. The Metric System of weights and measures should be used.
8. The prescription order should indicate whether or not the prescription should be renewed and, if so, the number of times and the period of time such renewal is authorized. Statements such as *Refill prn* or *Refill ad lib* are discouraged.
9. Either single or multi-drug prescription forms may be used when appropriately designed, and pursuant to the desires of local medical and pharmaceutical societies.
10. When institutional prescription blanks are used, the prescriber should print his/her name, telephone number and registration number on the prescription blank.

Guidelines for Pharmacists

1. Pharmacists should include the following information on the prescription label: name, address and telephone number of pharmacy; name of prescriber; name, strength and quantity of drug dispensed (unless otherwise directed by the prescriber); directions for use; prescription number; date on which prescription is dispensed; full name of patient and any other information required by law.
2. Instructions to the patient regarding directions for use of medication should be concise and precise, but readily understandable to the patient. Where the pharmacist feels that the prescription order does not meet these criteria, he should attempt to clarify the order with the prescriber in order to prevent confusion. Verbal reinforcement and/or clarification of instructions should be given to the patient by the pharmacist when appropriate.
3. For those dosage forms where confusion may develop as to how the medication is to be administered (for example, oral drops which may be mistakenly instilled in the ear or suppositories which may be mistakenly administered orally), the pharmacist should clearly indicate the intended route of administration on the prescription label.
4. The pharmacist should include an expiration date on the prescription label when appropriate.
5. Where special storage conditions are required, the pharmacist should indicate appropriate instructions for storage on the prescription label.

Conclusion

Communicating effective dosage instructions to patients clearly and succinctly is a responsibility of both the medical and pharmaceutical professions.

Recent studies documenting the low order of compliance with prescription instructions indicate that poor communication between the medical and pharmaceutical professions and poor comprehension by the public may be causative factors.

The American Pharmaceutical Association and the American Society of Internal Medicine believe that the guidelines as stated above will serve as an initial step toward patients achieving a better understanding of their medication and dosing instructions. The two associations urge state and local societies representing pharmacists and prescribers to appoint joint committees for the purpose of refining these guidelines further as local desires and conditions warrant. The associations believe that such cooperative efforts between the professions are essential to good patient care and that significant progress can be made in other areas by initiating discussions between the two professions concerning common interests and goals.

---

[a]By American Pharmaceutical Association/American Society of Internal Medicine (revised March 1976).

CHAPTER 104

The Prescription

Howard C Ansel, PhD
Professor of Pharmaceutics, College of Pharmacy
The University of Georgia
Athens, GA 30602

A *prescription* is an order for medication issued by a physician, dentist, veterinarian or other properly licensed medical practitioner. Prescriptions designate a specific medication and dosage to be administered to a particular patient at a specified time. Commonly, the prescribed medication also is referred to as the "prescription" by the patient.

The prescription order is a part of the professional relationship between the prescriber, pharmacist and patient. It is the pharmacist's responsibility in this relationship to provide the medication needs of the patient. The pharmacist must be precise, not only in the manual aspects of filling the prescription order, but must provide the patient with the necessary information and guidance to assure the patient's compliance in taking the medication properly. It is also the pharmacist's responsibility to advise the prescriber of drug sensitivities the patient may have, or other medications that the patient may be taking which may alter the effectiveness or safety of the newly and/or previously prescribed medications. To meet these responsibilities it is essential that the pharmacist maintains a high level of practice competence, keeps appropriate records on the health status and medication history of his patients and develops professional working relationships with other health professionals.

Pharmacists must maintain the trust of the prescriber and patient. This includes maintaining confidentiality. The medication being taken by a patient and the nature of his illness is a private matter which must be respected.

There are two broad legal classifications of medications: those which can be obtained only by prescription and those which may be purchased without a prescription. The latter are termed *nonprescription* drugs or *over-the-counter* (OTC) drugs. Medications which may be dispensed legally only upon prescription are referred to as *prescription* drugs or *legend* drugs. The latter term refers to the "legend" that must appear on the label of the product as it is provided to the pharmacist by the manufacturer—"Caution: Federal Law Prohibits Dispensing without Prescription." Occasionally, physicians may issue prescriptions for nonlegend drugs which they desire the patient to receive.

Prescriptions may be written by the prescriber and given to the patient for presentation at the pharmacy, or they may be telephoned or communicated directly to the pharmacist. Prescription orders received verbally should be reduced to proper written form immediately or entered directly into a prescription computer by the pharmacist.

Form of the Prescription Order

Prescriptions usually are written on printed forms that contain blank spaces for the required information. These forms are called *prescription blanks* and are supplied in the form of a pad. Most prescription blanks are imprinted with the name, address, telephone number and other pertinent information of the physician or his practice site; eg, hospital or clinic (Fig 1). The printed information clarifies the prescriber's name when it is signed illegibly, and his address and telephone number facilitates additional professional communication, as may be required.

The Veterans Health Administration provides prescription forms for use only in VA facilities which are printed on security paper and sequentially numbered. The front of the form, printed in gray tone, has check-off blocks to indicate patient status (eg, inpatient) as well as check-off blocks to override the general authority to allow drug substitution and require the product name, strength and quantity to be placed on the label. The back of the form, in white, which must be completed before dispensing an original or refill prescription, provides space to enter the manufacturer and control number of the product, the date dispensed or mailed, the signature or initials of the dispensing pharmacist and any calculations or written notations.

Prescription blanks that are used by the pharmacist in his transposition of verbally received prescriptions commonly are imprinted with the name, address and telephone number of the pharmacy. These blanks also may be used by physicians to write prescriptions when visiting the pharmacy. Specially imprinted prescription blanks are not required legally for prescriptions; any paper or other writing material may be used.

For the purpose of study, the component parts of a prescription are described as follows and identified in Fig 1.

Prescribers office information
Patient information
Date
℞ symbol or *superscription*
Medication prescribed or *inscription*
Dispensing directions to pharmacist or *subscription*
Directions for patient or *signa* (to be placed on label)
Refill, special labeling and/or other instructions
Prescriber's signature and license or DEA number as required

In practice some of the above information (as the patient's address) may be absent when the prescription is received by the pharmacist. In these instances the pharmacist obtains the necessary information from the patient or physician, as is required.

Patient Information—The full name and address of the patient are necessary on the prescription for identification purposes. Names and addresses written illegibly should be clarified on acceptance of the prescription. Incorrect spelling of a patient's name on a prescription label not only might cause concern in the patient's mind as to the correctness of the medication, but also would hamper the desired professional relationship between the pharmacist and patient. Federal law requires that both the full name and address of both the prescriber and the patient be included on prescriptions for certain controlled substances. Controlled substances are drugs which, because of their potential for abuse, are controlled under special regulations by the federal government. The address of the patient is useful for identification purposes as well as for delivery of medication to the patient's home.

Some prescription blanks used by medical specialists, particularly pediatricians, include a space for insertion of the patient's age and/or weight. This information is placed on the prescription by the physician when medication dosage is an important function of age or weight. This information assists the pharmacist in interpreting the prescription, and is

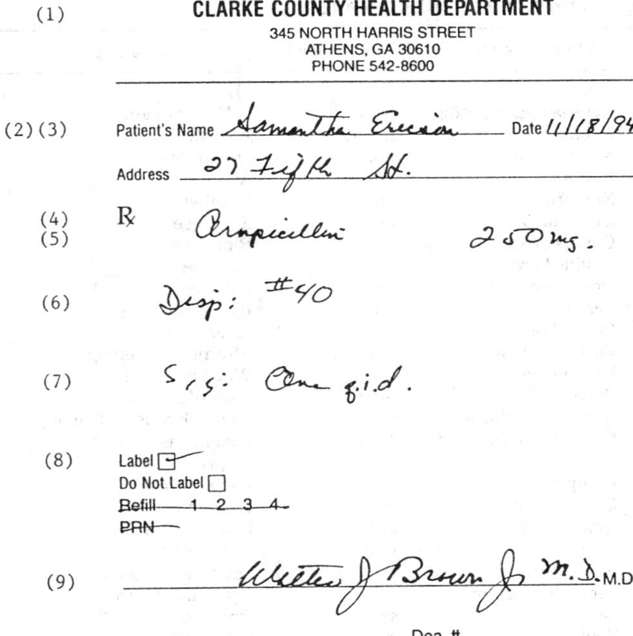

(1) **CLARKE COUNTY HEALTH DEPARTMENT**
345 NORTH HARRIS STREET
ATHENS, GA 30610
PHONE 542-8600

(2) (3) Patient's Name Samantha Ericson Date 4/18/94

Address 27 Fifth St.

(4) ℞
(5) Ampicillin 250 mg.

(6) Disp: #40

(7) Sig: One qid.

(8) Label ☑
Do Not Label ☐
~~Refill 1 2 3 4~~
~~PRN~~

(9) ______ M.D.

Dea. # ______

Fig 1. Example of a physician's prescription showing typical form and content.

particularly useful when a child has the same name as one of his parents.

Date—Prescriptions are dated at the time they are written and also when they are received and filled in the pharmacy. The date is important in establishing the medication record of the patient. An unusual lapse of time between the date a prescription was written and the date it is brought to the pharmacy may be questioned by a pharmacist to determine if the intent of the physician and the needs of the patient can still be met. The date prescribed is also important to a pharmacist in filling prescriptions for controlled substances. The Drug Abuse Control Amendments specify that no prescription order for controlled substances may be dispensed or renewed more than 6 months after the date prescribed.

℞ Symbol or Superscription—The ℞ symbol generally is understood to be a contraction of the Latin verb *recipe*, meaning "take thou" or "you take." Some historians believe this symbol originated from the sign of Jupiter, ♃, employed by the ancients in requesting aid in healing. Gradual distortion through the years has led to the symbol currently used. Today, the symbol is representative of both the prescription and pharmacy itself.

Medication Prescribed or Inscription—This is the body or principal part of the prescription order. It contains the names and quantities of the prescribed ingredients.

Today, the majority of prescriptions are written for medications already prepared or prefabricated into dosage forms by industrial manufacturers. The medications may be prescribed under their trademarked or manufacturer's proprietary name or by their nonproprietary or *generic* names. Pharmacists are required to dispense the trademarked product when prescribed, unless substitution of an equivalent product is permitted by the prescribing physician or by state law. In some instances, the patient must also consent to the drug substitution. Some states require the prescriber to write specific instructions on the prescription to allow or disallow product substitution.

Prescription orders requiring the pharmacist to mix ingredients are termed *compounded* prescriptions. Prescriptions requiring compounding contain the names and quantities of each ingredient required. The names of the ingredients generally are written using the nonproprietary names of the materials, although occasionally proprietary names may be employed. Quantities of ingredients to be used may be indicated in the metric or apothecary system of weights and measures; however, the use of the apothecary system is diminishing. These systems are described in Chapter 9.

In the use of the metric system, the decimal is often replaced by a vertical line that may be imprinted on the prescription blank or drawn by the prescriber. The symbols g or mL often are eliminated, as it is understood that solids are dispensed by weight and liquids by volume.

Dispensing Directions to Pharmacist or Subscription—This part of the prescription consists of directions to the pharmacist for preparing the prescription. With diminished frequency of compounded prescriptions, such directions are likewise less frequent. In a large majority of prescriptions, the subscription serves merely to designate the dosage form (as tablets, capsules, etc) and the number of dosage units to be supplied. Examples of prescription directions to the pharmacist are

M ft caps dtd no xxiv (Mix and make capsules. Dispense 24 such doses).
Ft supp No xii (Make 12 suppositories).
M ft ung (Mix and make an ointment).
Disp tabs No c (Dispense 100 tablets).

Directions for Patient or Signatura—The prescriber indicates the directions for the patient's use of the medication in the portion of the prescription called the *Signatura*. The word, usually abbreviated "Signa" or "Sig" means "mark thou." The directions in the signa commonly are written using abbreviated forms of English or Latin terms or a combination of each. Examples are

Tabs ii q4h (Take two tablets every four hours)
Caps i 4xd pc & hs (Take one capsule four times a day after meals and at bedtime)
Instill gtts ii od (Instill two drops into the right eye)

The directions are transcribed by the pharmacist onto the label of the container of dispensed medication. A list of some prescription abbreviations is presented in Table 1.

It is advisable for the pharmacist to reinforce the directions to the patient upon dispensing the medication since the patient may be uncertain or confused as to the proper method of use. Some pharmacists and physicians provide their patients with written directions outlining the proper use of the medication prescribed. These directions frequently include the best time to take the medication, the importance of adhering to the prescribed dosage schedule, the permitted use of the medication with respect to food, drink and other medications the patient may be taking as well as information about the drug itself. As a requirement of law, certain manufacturers have prepared patient package inserts (PPIs) for specific products for issuance to patients (Fig 2). These present to the patient information regarding the usefulness of the medication as well as its side effects and potential hazards. Other PPIs are available to pharmacists for use in their practices from professional and commercial sources. For example, The United States Pharmacopeial Convention provides patient education leaflets containing supplementary printed instructions on a number of drugs and drug categories to physicians, pharmacists and other health professionals for distribution to patients (Fig 101-3). The information is also available on computer diskette allowing leaflets to be printed in the pharmacy as needed using a compatible computer and standard line printer. Similar microcomputer software programs are available from a number of other sources, designed to generate personalized patient-counseling information for use by the pharmacist in patient education.[1]

In addition to instructions to the patient, many prescribers desire that the name and strength of the prescribed drug be included on the label of the dispensed medication. Precribers indicate this to the pharmacist by including the name and strength of the drug in the signa or by simply writing in the word "label" in the signa. Some prescription blanks have the word "label" printed for circling or checking by the prescribing physician (Fig 1). The practice of including the

Table 1—Examples of Latin and English Prescription Abbreviations

Word or phrase	Abbreviation	Meaning
Ad	Ad	To, up to
Ad libitum	Ad lib	At pleasure, freely
Agita	Agit	Shake, stir
Ampul	amp	Ampul of medication
Ante cibos	ac	Before meals
Ante meridien	am	Before noon, morning
Aqua	aq	Water
Around-the-clock	ATC	A dosing schedule
Auris utrae	au	Each ear
Aurio dextra	ad	Right ear
Aurio læva aurio sinister	al, as	Left ear
Bis in die	bid	Twice a day
Bowel movement	BM	Self explanatory
Blood pressure	BP	Self explanatory
Blood sugar	BS	Self explanatory
Body surface area	BSA	Used in dosage calculation
Capsula	caps	Capsule
Charta	Chart	Paper
Collunarium	collun	A nose wash
Collyrium	collyr	An eye wash
Congestive heart failure	CHF	Self explanatory
Cubic centimeter	cc	A volume approximately equivalent to a milliliter
Cum	c̄	With
Dentur tales doses	dtd	Let such doses be given
Diebus alternis	dieb alt	Every other day
Dilutus	dil	Dilute, diluted
Discontinue	disc or DC	An order to stop a medication or treatment
Dispense	disp	Dispense
Divided	div	Divide
Elixir	elix	A type of liquid dosage form
Emulsum	emuls	Emulsion
Et	. . .	And
Fac, fiat, fiant	F, Ft	Make, let it be made, let them be made
Gastrointestinal	GI	self explanatory
Genitourinary	GU	self explanatory
Gram	g, gm or Gm	Gram
Granum	gr	Grain
Gutta	gtt	A drop
High blood pressure	HBP	self explanatory
Hora	h	An hour
Hora somni	hs	At bedtime
Hypertension	HT	self explanatory
Injectio	inj	An injection
Intravenous	IV or iv	Intravenous injection
Intramuscular	IM	Intramuscular injection
Intradermal	ID	Intradermal injection
Linimentum	lin	Liniment
Liquor	liq	Solution
Microgram	mcg	One-millionth gram
Millequivalent	mEq	one thousandth of a gram equivalent weight
Milligram	mg	One-thousandth gram
Milligrams per kilogram	mg/kg	in dosing; mg of drug per kg of body weight
Milligrams per square meter	mg/m^2	in dosing; mg of drug per sq m of body surface area
Milliliter	ml or mL	One-thousandth liter
Milliosmole	mOsmol	one thousandth of an osmole.
Minimum	m or min	A minim
Misce	m	Mix
Nausea and vomiting	N&V	self explanatory
Nebula	nebul	A spray
Non repetatur	non rep	Do not repeat
Nocte	noct	At night
Numerus	no	Number
Oculo utro	ou	Each eye
Oculus dexter	od	Right eye
Oculus laevus	ol	Left eye
Oculus sinister	os	Left eye
Per os	po	By mouth
Post cibos	pc	After eating
Post meridiem	pm	Afternoon, evening
Pro re nata	prn	When necessary
Pulvis	pulv	A powder
Quantum sufficiat	qs	As much as is sufficient
Quantum sufficiat ad	qs ad	A sufficient quantity to (prepare)
Quaque	q	Each, every
Quaque hora	qh	Every hour
Quater in die	qid	Four times a day
Rectal	Rect	Use rectally
Repetatur	rept	Let it be repeated
Secundum artem	sa	According to art
Semis	ss	One-half
Signa	sig	(You) write
Sine	s̄	Without
Si opus sit	si op sit, sos	If necessary
Solutio	sol	Solution
Solutio saturata	sat sol	Saturated solution
Square meter	sq m, m^2, or M^2	used in calculating dose by body surface area
Statim	stat	Immediately
Subcutaneous	Sub Q or SQ	Subcutaneous injection
Suppositorium	supp	Suppository
Suspension	Susp	Suspension
Syrupus	syr	Syrup
Tabella	tab	Tablet
Ter in die	tid	Three times a day
Tablespoon	tbsp	Tablespoon
Teaspoon	tsp	Teaspoon
Topically	top	(Use) topically
Unguentum	ung	Ointment
Ut dictum	ut dict	As directed
Unus	i, I	One
Duo	ii, II	Two
Tres	iii, III	Three
Quattour	iv, IV	Four
Quinque	v, V	Five
Sex	vi, VI	Six
Septem	vii, VII	Seven
Octo	viii, VIII	Eight
Novem	ix, IX	Nine
Decem	x, X	Ten
Duodecim	XII	Twelve
Quindecim	XV	Fifteen
Viginti	XX	Twenty
Triginta	XXX	Thirty
Quinquaginta	L	Fifty
Centum	C	One hundred
Quingenti	D	Five hundred
Mille	M	One thousand

name of the drug on the medication label is required in some states, and may be excluded only upon the specific direction of the prescriber. The advantages to having the name and strength of the drug identified on the prescription label include the facilitation of communication between the patient and the pharmacist and/or physician and the rapid identification of the medication in times of accidental or purposeful overdose.

The date after which the medication will be subpotent (expiration date) may be placed on the label based on information included on the original manufacturer's package. This precaution is important for certain drugs that rapidly deteriorate and lose their potency. For example, many oral liquid formulations of antibiotics remain stable for only a period of 14 days under refrigeration, and one-half that time when nonrefrigerated following their preparation by the pharmacist. Physicians generally do not specify that expiration dates be noted on the label since they recognize that the pharmacist will provide this information when dispensing such preparations. Statements on auxiliary labels such as "do not use after _ days" or "discard after _ days" serve this purpose. Some state laws require that pharmacists place the expiration

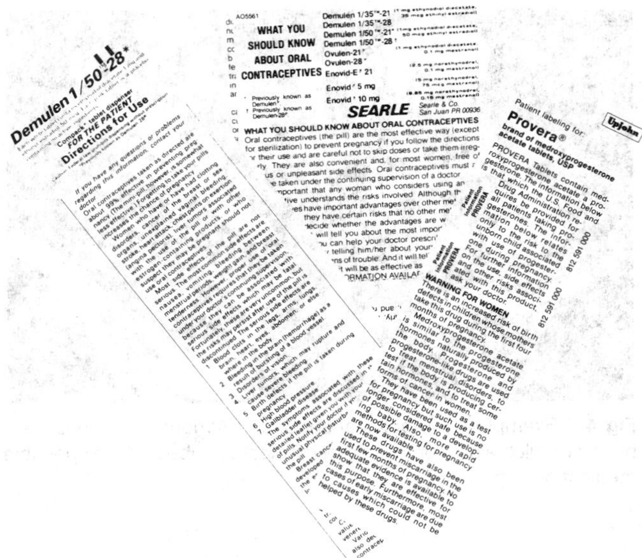

Fig 2. Example of manufacturers' patient package inserts intended to enhance patient understanding of the medication prescribed.

date on the label of all medications dispensed, even those with no special stability problems.

Special Labeling and Other Instructions—The number of authorized refills should be indicated on each prescription by the prescriber. In case no refill information is provided, it is understood that no refills have been authorized. Most prescription blanks include a section where this information may be indicated (see Fig 1). No refills are permitted for Schedule II controlled substances.

Federal law requires that prescriptions for Schedule II controlled substances be validated by the full signature of the prescriber.

Hospital Medication Orders

Medication orders for inpatients in hospitals and other institutions are written by the physician on forms called the "Physician's Order Sheet." The type of form used varies between institutions and even within the institution depending upon the unit rendering the care. Institutional pharmacy practice is discussed in Chapter 97.

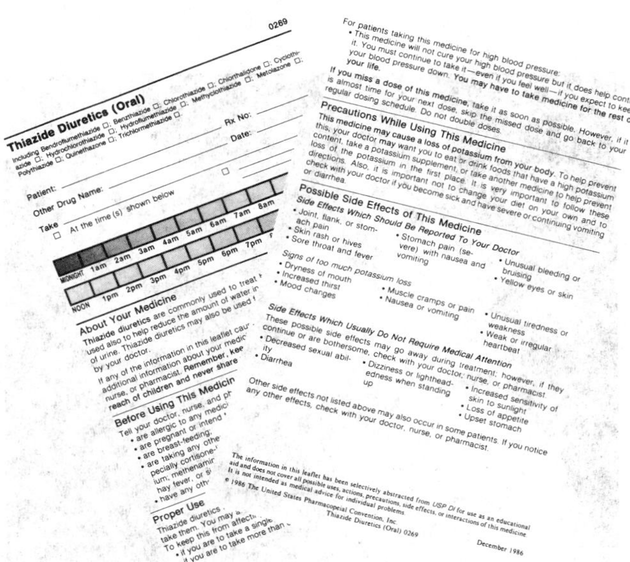

Fig 3. Examples of USP Patient Education Leaflets. The information also is available on computer diskette for use in the pharmacy (courtesy, The USPC).

Reducing Medication Errors

Medication errors, which include inappropriate prescribing, patient noncompliance, dispensing errors and medication administration errors, undermine the purpose of drug therapy and the patient's therapeutic outcomes. Guidelines for the prevention of medication errors have been developed by the Council on Professional Affairs of the American Society of Hospital Pharmacists.[2] Included among the recommendations pertaining to the writing of medication orders are the following:

1. Medication orders should be complete with regard to patient information and drug name and dosage and should be reviewed by the prescriber for accuracy and legibility immediately after writing.
2. Instructions should be written out rather than using nonstandard or ambiguous abbreviations.
3. Vague instructions, as "take as directed" should not be used; instead, more drug-specific instructions should be given.
4. Exact dosage strengths (as "20 milligrams") rather than dosage units (as "one tablet") should be specified.
5. Exact nomenclature for drug names (nonproprietary or proprietary) should be used, rather than fabricated drug-name abbreviations.
6. A leading zero should always precede a decimal expression of less than one (eg, 0.5 mL); conversely, a terminal zero should never be used (eg, 5.0 mL), since failure to note the decimal would result in a tenfold error. When possible avoid the use of decimals (eg, prescribe 500 mg instead of 0.5 g).
7. The word "units" (eg, 10 units of regular insulin) should be spelled out rather than abbreviated with a "U" which could be misinterpreted as a zero (misinterpreted as 100 units rather than the 10 units intended).
8. Use of the metric system should be required.

Processing the Prescription Order

The manner in which a pharmacist processes a prescription order is important in fulfilling his professional responsibilities, and can enhance his image with both the physician and patient. Proper procedures are given below for receiving, reading and checking, numbering and dating, labeling, preparing, packaging, rechecking, delivering and counseling, recording and filing and pricing the prescriptions.

Receiving the Prescription—It is desirable that the patient present the prescription order directly to the pharmacist since this enhances the pharmacist-patient relationship. In situations where this is not practical, the individual receiving the prescription should be trained to accept it in a professional manner and obtain the correct name, address and other pertinent patient information. It is important to determine if the patient's medications are provided through insurance coverage and whether the patient wishes to wait, call back or have the medication delivered. If the pharmacist is unable to receive the prescription order personally, he should be available to provide an estimate of the length of time required to fill the prescription and to price it if requested by the patient. Many pharmacists make it a practice to price prescriptions before dispensing, especially in the case of unusually expensive medication, to avoid subsequent questions concerning the charge.

Reading and Checking the Prescription—The prescription order first should be read completely and carefully; there should be no doubt as to the ingredients or quantities prescribed. From the pharmacy's prescription computer (or other record of the patient's medication history), the pharmacist should determine the compatibility of the newly prescribed medication with other drugs being taken by the patient. Most prescription computer software programs identify possible drug interactions. In addition, references may be used for this purpose, such as *USP Dispensing Information (USP DI)*. Should the probability or likelihood of a drug interaction exist, the pharmacist should consult with the prescriber to determine therapeutic alternatives. The same would apply when a medication is prescribed for a patient with a known drug allergy or sensitivity to the drug prescribed or to other drugs of the same chemical class. If something is illegible or if it appears that an error has been made, the pharmacist should consult another pharmacist or the prescriber. *A pharmacist should never guess at the meaning of an indistinct word or unrecognized abbreviation.* Unfamiliar or unclear abbreviations represent a source of error in interpreting and filling prescriptions.[3] There is no "official" or standard list of prescription abbreviations. Many of them in use are derived from the Latin and generally are recognized (see Table I); however, many others may be simply shorthand creations of the individual prescriber.

Common prescriber abbreviations for drug names include "Pb" for phenobarbital, "MTX" for methotrexate and "ASA" for aspirin. Diseases and conditions also are abbreviated commonly, such as "CHF" for congestive heart failure, "URI" for upper respiratory tract infection and "HBP" for high blood pressure. Other abbreviations, such as "ATC" for around-the-clock and "BM" for bowel movement, also are used in prescription writing.

The use of Latin words, phrases and abbreviations in prescriptions is a carryover from the time that Latin was considered the international language of medicine. Latin was used extensively in writing prescription orders until the early part of the 20th century. Although its use gradually has diminished, it is still used widely, in the form of abbreviations, in the subscription and signa portions of prescriptions.

The pharmacist frequently is confronted in his interpretation of the prescription order with the names of drugs which look alike or sound alike. Examples of such drugs are listed in Table 2.

The pharmacist must take great care and use his broad knowledge of drug products to prevent dispensing errors. A call to the physician, made so as not to alarm the patient, will serve to verify the meaning of a prescription that is unclear and at the same time bolster the professional reputation of the pharmacist as a careful practitioner and valuable member of the health team.

Omissions, such as the failure to specify the desired strength of a medication or its dosage form, should be corrected. In such a case, the pharmacist should never elect to dispense the usual dose or dosage form, but should consult the prescriber. The pharmacist must be familiar with available strengths and dosage forms of prefabricated drug products in order to detect such omissions and provide the physician with the necessary information.

The amount and frequency of a dose must be noted carefully and checked. In determining the safety of the dose of a medicinal agent, the age, weight and condition of the patient, dosage form prescribed, possible influence of other drugs being taken and the frequency of administration all must be considered. A number of guides are available to the pharmacist in evaluating the safety of a prescribed dose. *USP Dispensing Information* provides usual doses and dosage ranges for many drugs in use. Manufacturers' catalogs, file cards and package inserts provide dosage information on their products. References such as *Physicians' Desk Reference*, *AMA Drug Evaluations*, *American Hospital Formulary Service Drug Information*, *Facts and Comparisons* and *Pediatric Dosage Handbook* are useful general sources of such information. In the case of a suspected error in dose, appropriate references should be checked prior to consulting the physician.

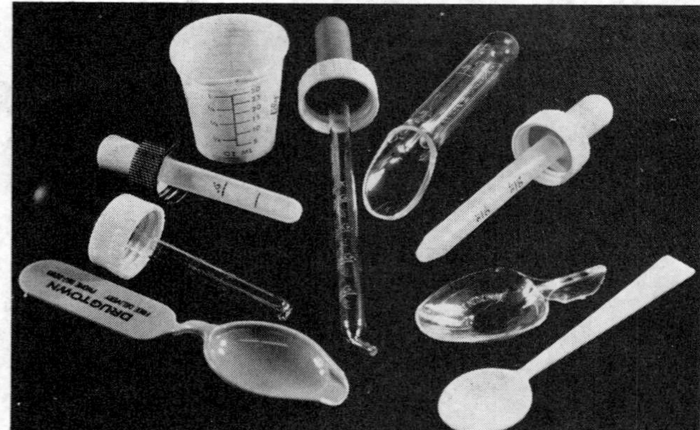

Fig 4. Examples of medicinal spoons of various capacities, calibrated medicine droppers, an oral medication tube and a disposable medication cup.[4]

Measurement of liquid medication may lead to dosage variation due to differences in the capacity of household spoons. The problems associated with teaspoonful dosage have long been recognized. A standard teaspoon has been established by the American National Standards Institute as containing 4.93 ± 0.24 mL. For practical purposes, the standard teaspoonful is considered to be equivalent to 5 mL, although different household teaspoons vary widely in capacity. Thus, 1 fluidounce (29.57 mL) of a medicated liquid is considered to provide approximately six standard teaspoonful doses.

To avoid errors in liquid dosing, pharmacists often dispense calibrated measuring devices with liquid medication. Some of these devices are shown in Figs 4 and 5.

Numbering and Dating—It is a legal requirement to number the prescription order and to place the same number on the label. This serves to identify the bottle or package and to

Table 2—Examples of Look-alike and/or Sound-alike Drug Names

Alupent	Atrovent
Apresoline	Priscoline
Digitoxin	Digoxin
Diphenhydramine	Diphenhydrinate
Doriden	Doxidan
Enalapril	Anafranil
Esimil	Estinyl
Indocin	Lincocin
Isomil	Isordil
Orinase	Ornade
Prednisolone	Prednisone
Prilosec	Prozac
Quinidine	Clonidine
Quinine	Quinidine
Regroton	Hygroton
Xanax	Zantac

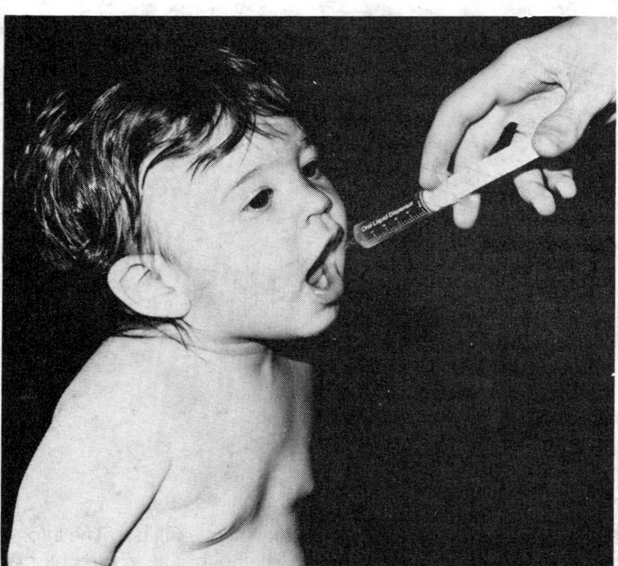

Fig 5. An oral liquid dispenser for the accurate delivery of small doses of liquid medication to infants (courtesy, Baxa Corp).

connect it with the original order for reference or to renew the prescription. Consecutive numbers are assigned by prescription computers or manually by use of numbering machines. These machines can be set to number consecutively in duplicate or triplicate, so that the same number can be stamped clearly and neatly on the prescription order, label and record book as desired.

Dating of the prescription on the date filled is also a legal requirement. This information is important in determining the appropriate refill frequency, patient compliance and as an alternate means of locating the prescription order should the prescription number be lost by the patient. The prescription computer may be employed for these purposes.

Labeling—The prescription label may be typewritten or prepared by computer, using the information entered by the pharmacist or pharmacy assistant. Figure 6 shows a computer-prepared prescription including the label, patient-counseling information and receipt.

A prescription should have an esthetic and professional-appearing label. If the label and the container are not neat and professional in appearance, the patient may conclude that the prescription medication itself also was prepared in a careless manner. This may result in a loss of confidence in the pharmacist or pharmacy.

Since the label is important in the appearance of the finished prescription, a quality label stock should be used. The size of the label used should be in conformance with the size of the prescription container.

The name and address of the pharmacy are required legally to appear on the label; the telephone number also is included commonly. The prescription number, prescriber's name, patient's name, directions for use and the date of dispensing also are required legally; the patient's address and the name and strength of the medication also are included frequently.

The pharmacist should make the directions to the patient for taking the medication as clear and complete as possible. For example, "Take one (1) tablet four (4) times a day before meals and at bedtime" would be preferred to "One 4 times a day."

Some state laws require that the name or initials of the pharmacist dispensing the medication appear on the label. Also, some states require that the name and strength of the medication dispensed appear on the label. Some pharmacists indicate the refill or renewal status of the prescription on the primary label or use an auxiliary label to indicate this information. Occasionally, the manufacturer's lot number for the medication dispensed is entered on the label to aid in rapid identification of medication that might be recalled. Labeling requirements for controlled substances are presented in Chapter 110.

Auxiliary labels are used to emphasize a number of important aspects of the dispensed medication, including its proper

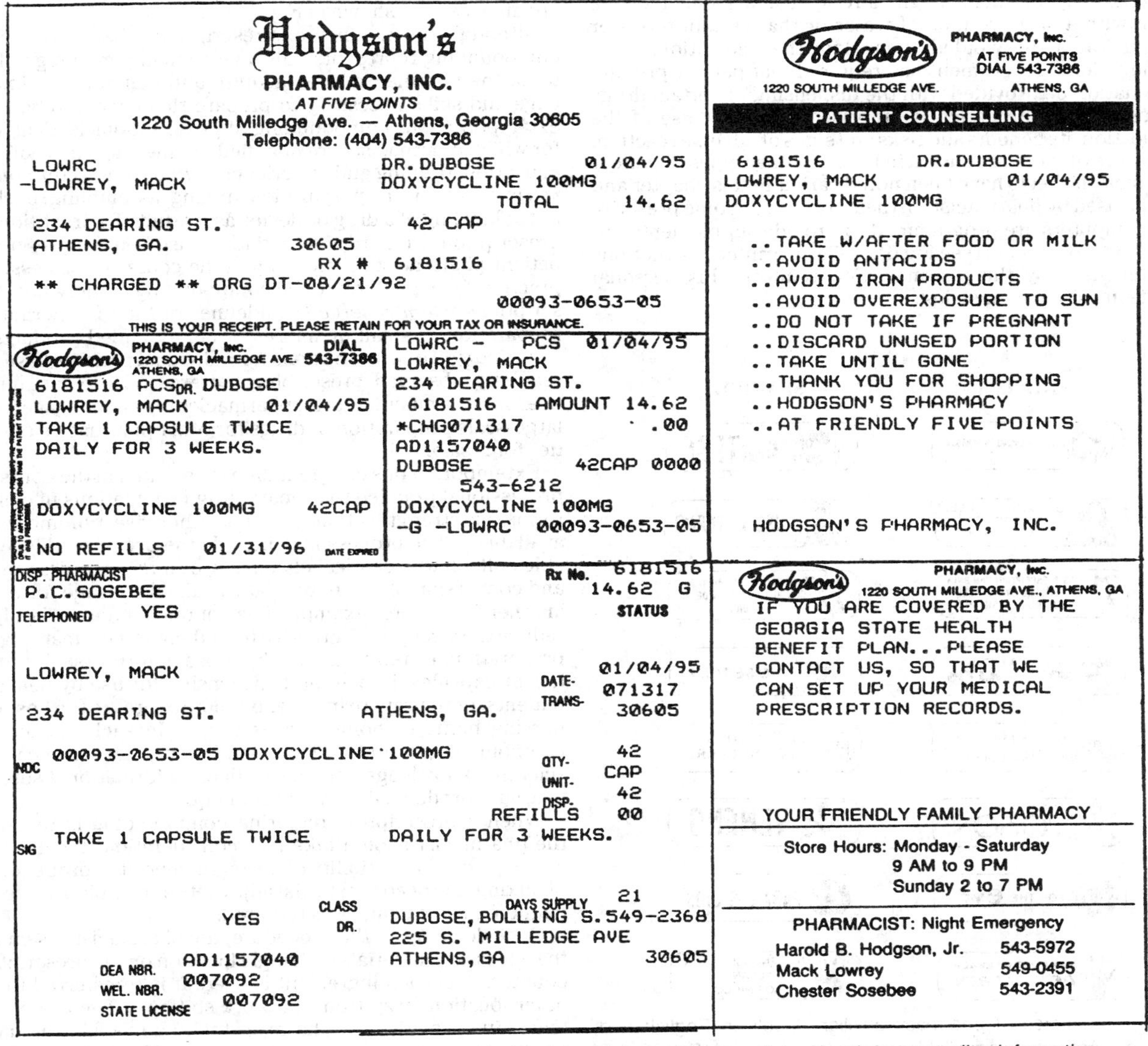

Hodgson's
PHARMACY, INC.
AT FIVE POINTS
1220 South Milledge Ave. — Athens, Georgia 30605
Telephone: (404) 543-7386

LOWRC DR. DUBOSE 01/04/95
-LOWREY, MACK DOXYCYCLINE 100MG
TOTAL 14.62
234 DEARING ST. 42 CAP
ATHENS, GA. 30605
RX # 6181516
** CHARGED ** ORG DT-08/21/92
00093-0653-05
THIS IS YOUR RECEIPT. PLEASE RETAIN FOR YOUR TAX OR INSURANCE.

Hodgson's PHARMACY, Inc. 1220 SOUTH MILLEDGE AVE. ATHENS, GA DIAL 543-7386
6181516 PCS DR. DUBOSE
LOWREY, MACK 01/04/95
TAKE 1 CAPSULE TWICE
DAILY FOR 3 WEEKS.
DOXYCYCLINE 100MG 42CAP
NO REFILLS 01/31/96 DATE EXPIRED

LOWRC - PCS 01/04/95
LOWREY, MACK
234 DEARING ST.
6181516 AMOUNT 14.62
*CHG071317 .00
AD1157040
DUBOSE 42CAP 0000
543-6212
DOXYCYCLINE 100MG
-G -LOWRC 00093-0653-05

DISP. PHARMACIST P.C. SOSEBEE
Rx No. 6181516
14.62 G
STATUS
TELEPHONED YES
LOWREY, MACK
DATE- 01/04/95
TRANS- 071317
234 DEARING ST. ATHENS, GA. 30605
NDC 00093-0653-05 DOXYCYCLINE 100MG
QTY- 42
UNIT- CAP
DISP- 42
REFILLS 00
SIG TAKE 1 CAPSULE TWICE DAILY FOR 3 WEEKS.
DAYS SUPPLY 21
CLASS YES
DR. DUBOSE, BOLLING S. 549-2368
225 S. MILLEDGE AVE
ATHENS, GA 30605
DEA NBR. AD1157040
WEL. NBR. 007092
STATE LICENSE 007092

Hodgson's PHARMACY, Inc.
AT FIVE POINTS
DIAL 543-7386
1220 SOUTH MILLEDGE AVE. ATHENS, GA
PATIENT COUNSELLING
6181516 DR. DUBOSE
LOWREY, MACK 01/04/95
DOXYCYCLINE 100MG
..TAKE W/AFTER FOOD OR MILK
..AVOID ANTACIDS
..AVOID IRON PRODUCTS
..AVOID OVEREXPOSURE TO SUN
..DO NOT TAKE IF PREGNANT
..DISCARD UNUSED PORTION
..TAKE UNTIL GONE
..THANK YOU FOR SHOPPING
..HODGSON'S PHARMACY
..AT FRIENDLY FIVE POINTS
HODGSON'S PHARMACY, INC.

Hodgson's PHARMACY, Inc.
1220 SOUTH MILLEDGE AVE., ATHENS, GA
IF YOU ARE COVERED BY THE
GEORGIA STATE HEALTH
BENEFIT PLAN...PLEASE
CONTACT US, SO THAT WE
CAN SET UP YOUR MEDICAL
PRESCRIPTION RECORDS.

YOUR FRIENDLY FAMILY PHARMACY
Store Hours: Monday - Saturday
9 AM to 9 PM
Sunday 2 to 7 PM

PHARMACIST: Night Emergency
Harold B. Hodgson, Jr. 543-5972
Mack Lowrey 549-0455
Chester Sosebee 543-2391

Fig 6. Example of a computer-prepared prescription record, label, patient receipt and patient-counseling information.

use, handling, storage, refill status and necessary warnings or precautions. A "shake-well" label is indicated for a prescription containing material that may separate on standing, such as mixtures, lotions and emulsions. The use of labels such as "For the Ear," "For the Eye" and "External Use" is recommended because of the added safety they offer, even when the primary directions indicate their proper use. The use of a "poison" label rarely is indicated since it may cause the patient to become unduly alarmed or fearful of using the medication; instead, other precautionary labels may be used to warn that the medication should not be swallowed or used internally or should be kept out of reach of children and others for whom it is not intended.

Auxiliary labels are available in a variety of colors to give them special prominence. They should be placed in a conspicuous spot on the prescription container. Examples of some auxiliary labels in English and Spanish are shown in Fig 7.

In certain circumstances it may be desirable for the pharmacist to supplement the instructions or directions of the prescriber. Some states have passed regulations that recognize that a need may exist for the pharmacist to add to the directions of the prescriber to either clarify or expand his instructions. Such regulations indicate that when, in the judgment of the pharmacist, directions to the patient and/or cautionary messages are necessary, either for clarification or to ensure proper administration of the medication, the pharmacist may add such directions or cautionary messages to those indicated by the prescriber on the original prescription. For example, a pharmacist might advise that a medication be taken with a large volume of water or that certain foods or activities are to be avoided when taking the medication.

The federal government has required that patient product information be provided with the dispensing of certain drugs to ensure that the patient is apprised of proper use of the medication, its benefits and risks and signs of adverse reaction. Examples of these are shown in Fig 2. Other types of patient information sheets have been noted earlier in this chapter and may be used by pharmacists in their practice. Some prescription computers are programmed to provide supplemental instructions to patients (see Fig 6). These printed instructions may be used by the pharmacist to reinforce his personal efforts in patient counseling.

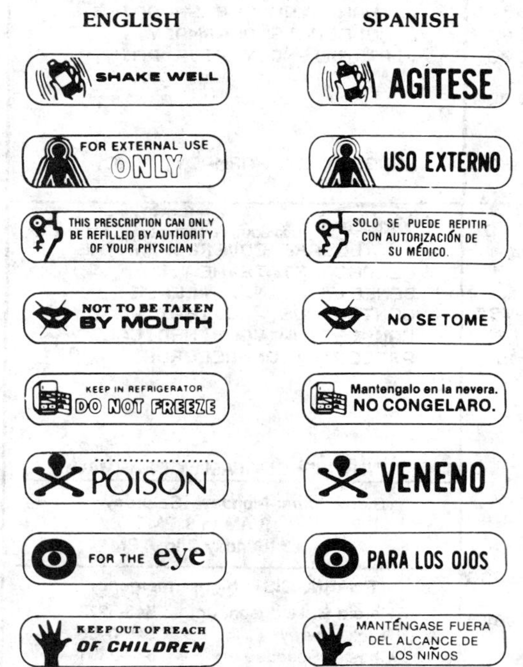

Fig 7. Examples of pharmacy auxiliary labels in English and Spanish. Actual labels available in color (courtesy, PHARMEX).

Preparing the Prescription—After reading and checking the prescription order the pharmacist should decide on the exact procedure to be followed in dispensing or compounding the ingredients.

Most prescriptions call for dispensing medications already prefabricated into dosage forms by pharmaceutical manufacturers. Care must be exercised by the pharmacist in making certain that the product dispensed is of the prescribed dosage, form, strength and number of dosage units. As noted previously, when substitution is permitted, the pharmacist is responsible for the selection of the manufacturer's product to use in filling the prescription. He performs this responsibility on the basis of his knowledge of the quality, effectiveness and cost to the patient of the selected product.

In filling prescriptions with prefabricated products, the pharmacist should check the manufacturer's label, comparing it to the prescription order, before and after filling the order, to make certain of its correctness. Products which show signs of poor manufacture, which look deteriorated or are past the stated expiration date on the label should never be dispensed.

Solid, prefabricated dosage forms generally are counted in the pharmacy using a device such as that shown in Fig 8. Such a device enables the rapid and sanitary counting and transferring of medication from the stock packages to the prescription container. To prevent contamination of tablets and capsules, the counting tray should be wiped clean after each counting, as powder, especially from uncoated tablets, tends to get on the tray. Some pharmacies use automated counting machines. In some practices, unit dose packages are dispensed as shown in Fig 9.

Although the number of prescriptions that now require compounding represents only a very small percentage of the total, the pharmacist must acquire and maintain the knowledge and skills necessary to prepare them accurately. The extemporaneous compounding of prescriptions is an activity for which pharmacists are qualified uniquely by virtue of their education, training and experience. *Pharmacy compounding* is defined as the preparation, mixing, assembling, packaging or labeling of a drug or device as a result of a practitioner's prescription-drug order or initiative based on the prescriber-patient-pharmacist relationship in the course of professional practice.[5] In addition to the compounding of individual prescriptions *when received*, guidelines of the FDA permit the preparation of small quantities of compounded products *in anticipation* of prescriptions for individual patients based on regularly observed prescribing patterns. However, unless licensed as a manufacturer, pharmacies may not engage in the large-scale preparation of drugs for other pharmacies or entities for resale.[6]

Extemporaneous compounding is essential in the course of professional practice to prepare drug formulations in dosage forms or strengths that are not otherwise commercially available. The process may include the use of readily available bulk pharmaceutical chemicals, or it may require the use and conversion of a commercially available dosage form into another form. For example, it is not uncommon to fortify or reduce the strength of an active ingredient in a dermatological preparation, to reformulate adult dosage forms, such as tablets or capsules, into an oral suspension for use by pediatric patients, or to prepare intravenous admixtures in the hospital, nursing home or home-care setting.[7] In each instance of compounding, the pharmacist must apply his technical and scientific knowledge and use available informational sources to assure product efficacy and stability.

When a prescription requiring compounding is received, the pharmacist should take into consideration the chemical and physical compatibility of the ingredients, the proper order of mixing, the need for special adjuvants or techniques and the mathematical calculations required.

Once deciding on the procedure, the pharmacist assembles the necessary materials in a single location on the prescription counter. As each ingredient is used, it is transferred to another location away from the work station. The use of this technique provides the pharmacist with a mechanical check on the introduction of each ingredient. If the pharmacist is

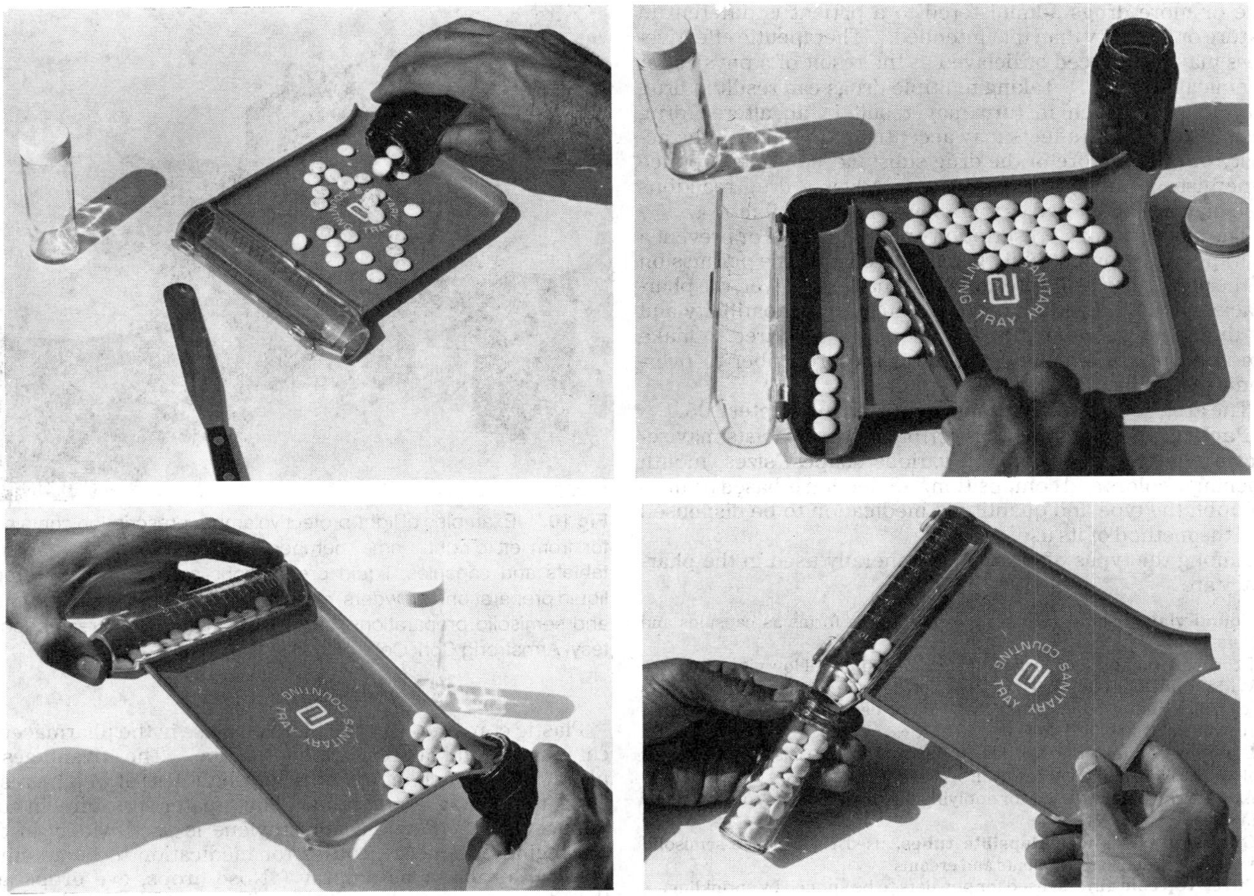

Fig 8. Steps in the hygienic counting of solid dosage units with the Abbott Sanitary Counting Tray: (1) placing units from the stock package onto the tray, (2) counting and transferring the units to the trough, (3) returning the excess units to the stock container and (4) transferring the counted units into the prescription container.

interrupted during the process, there is then no doubt as to which ingredients already have been used. When the pharmacist has finished, all the ingredients are returned to their storage places. Through this process, the pharmacist has the opportunity to read the label of each ingredient three times; once when the container is removed from the storage shelf, again when the contents are weighed and measured and, finally, when the container is returned to the shelf.

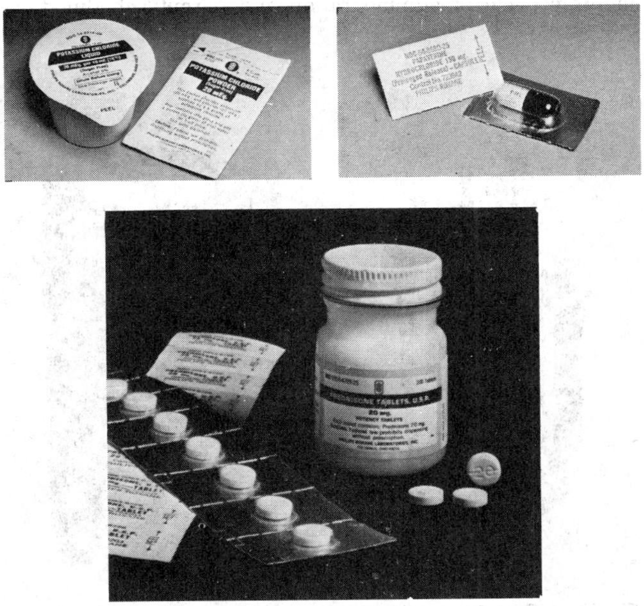

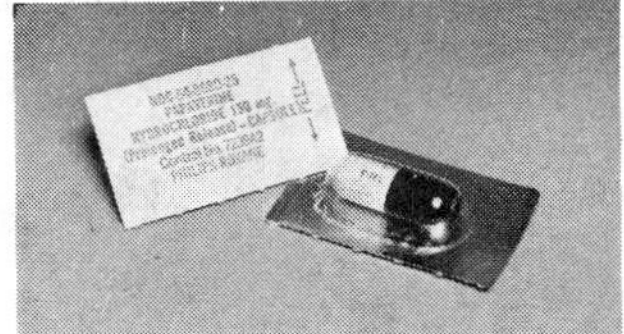

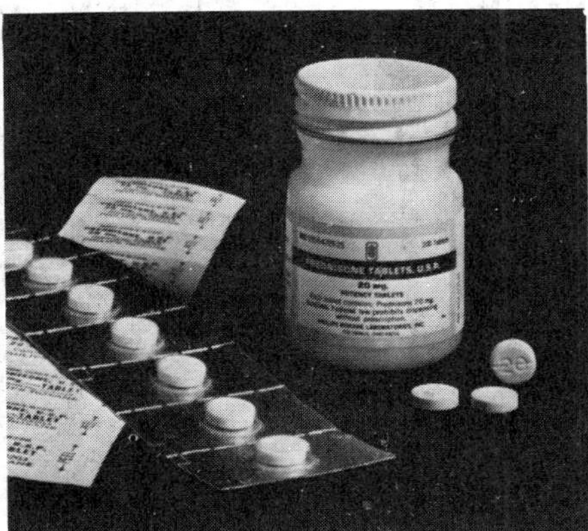

Fig 9. Examples of multiple-unit and single-unit packaging, including patient cup, unit dose of powder, blister packaging of single capsule and strip packaging of tablets (courtesy, Roxane).

Any calculations or compounding information that would be useful in refilling the prescription at a later date should be noted either on the face or back of the prescription order. Adjuvants used, order of mixing, amount of each ingredient, capsule size used, type and size of the container, name and product identification number of the manufacturer, auxiliary labels used, clarification of illegible words or numbers, price charged and any special notations should be recorded. The failure to do this may result in differences in the appearance of the prescription when refilled and possibly create doubt and apprehension in the mind of the patient.

The term *incompatibility* may be applied to prescriptions when certain problems arise during their compounding, dispensing or administration. Incompatibilities are categorized as being physical, chemical or therapeutic. The problems usually develop as a result of using two or more drug substances but problems involving the use of a single drug also may occur.

Physical incompatibility is usually the result of drug insolubility, liquefaction or physical complexation.

Chemical incompatibility may be the result of oxidation-reduction, acid-base, hydrolysis or combination reactions.

The occurrence of physical and chemical incompatibilities generally results in drug deterioration, discoloration, precipitation or other effects which render the product unsatisfactory. These incompatibilities are overcome by the pharmacist through his knowledge of chemistry, physical pharmacy and compounding techniques.

A *therapeutic incompatibility* exists when the response to

one or more drugs administered to a patient is different in nature or intensity than that intended. Therapeutic effectiveness may be reduced or delayed as the result of a physical or chemical reaction. Taking multiple drugs can result in drug interactions, which in turn may result in an altered drug response. These effects may accentuate or diminish the activity of one or more of the drug substances or may produce synergistic or antagonistic effects. Adverse drug reactions also may be considered as therapeutic incompatibilities.

The alteration of a prescription order to correct or prevent a therapeutic incompatibility generally requires the permission of the prescriber. Before contact is made, however, the pharmacist should be certain of the potential incompatibility and its therapeutic significance and should be prepared to make the appropriate recommendation to the prescriber to overcome the problem.

The area of drug interactions is covered in Chapter 105.

Packaging—In filling a prescription, pharmacists may select a container from among various shapes, sizes, mouth openings, colors and composition. Selection is based primarily upon the type and quantity of medication to be dispensed and the method of its use.

Among the types of containers generally used in the pharmacy are

Round vials, used primarily for solid dosage forms as capsules and tablets.

Prescription bottles, used for dispensing liquids of low viscosity.

Wide-mouth bottles, used for bulk powders, large quantities of tablets or capsules and viscous liquids that cannot be poured readily from the narrow-necked standard prescription bottles.

Dropper bottles, used for dispensing ophthalmic, nasal, otic (ear) or oral liquids to be administered by drop.

Applicator bottles, used for applying liquid medication to a wound or skin surface.

Ointment jars and collapsible tubes, used to dispense semisolid dosage forms, such as ointments and creams.

Sifter-top containers, used for powders to be applied by sprinkling.

Hinged-lid or slide boxes, used for dispensing suppositories and powders prepared in packets.

Aerosol containers, used for pharmaceutical aerosol products. They are pressurized systems dispensed by the pharmacist in the original container.

Most of the prescription containers usually are available in colorless or amber-colored glass or plastic. Amber-colored containers are used most widely since they provide maximum protection of their contents against photochemical deterioration. In most instances a container made of good quality amber glass will reduce light transmission sufficiently to protect light-sensitive pharmaceuticals. The containers shown in Fig 10 are examples of such containers. For total light restriction, opaque glass or glass rendered opaque by special coating may be employed. The use of outer wrappings or cartons also may be used to protect light- sensitive pharmaceuticals. Pharmaceutical manufacturers select and use containers which do not affect the composition or stability of their products adversely. Similar types of containers should be used by the pharmacist in dispensing the medication to the patient. FDA regulations require pharmaceutical manufacturers to include in their prescription-product labeling the type of container to be used by the pharmacist when dispensing the prescription drug to preserve its "identity, strength, quality and purity." The regulation does not apply to products intended to be dispensed in the manufacturer's original container.

The closure on a prescription container is as important as the container itself. By law, prescription containers must be moisture-proof and thus the ability of the closure to restrict entrance of moisture into the container is of prime importance. Moisture has a deteriorating effect on many dosage forms, especially capsules, tablets and powders. For example, aspirin tablets will be hydrolyzed in the presence of moisture and broken down into acetic acid and salicylic acid. Many pharmacies use screw-cap glass or tight-fitting closures to reduce moisture penetration (see Fig 11).

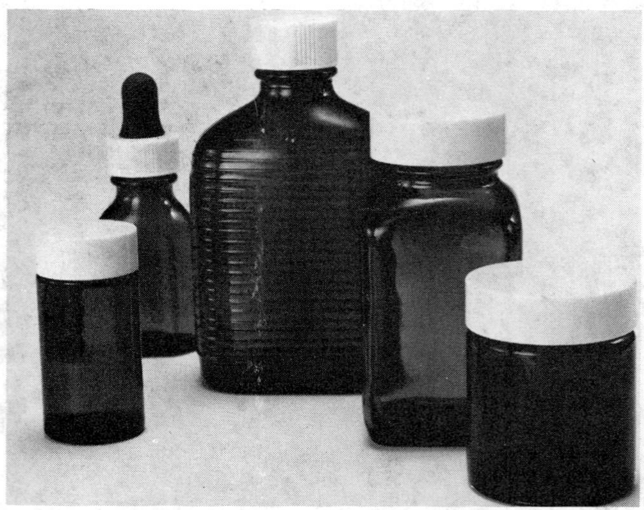

Fig 10. Examples of light-protective amber prescription containers for, from left to right: small numbers of solid dosage forms, such as tablets and capsules; liquid preparations administered by drops; liquid preparations; powders, or large numbers of solid dosage forms and semisolid preparations, such as ointments and creams (courtesy, Armstrong Cork Co).

Plastic containers have widespread use in the pharmaceutical industry and in prescription practice. The advantages of plastic over glass containers include lightness of weight, resistance to breakage upon impact and greater versatility in container design. Flexible polyethylene is used widely in the packaging of squeeze bottles for medication to be administered as drops or as a spray. Nose drops, eye drops and throat sprays, as well as oral medication to be administered dropwise, frequently are packaged and dispensed in these containers. Lotions, medicated shampoos and creams also are packaged conveniently in flexible polyethylene containers. Pliable ointment tubes and flexible plastic containers for intravenous fluids also are used widely.

Rigid polystyrene vials are employed commonly by pharmacists to dispense capsules and tablets. This type of plastic also is used widely in ointment jars and box packages for suppositories. The modern compact-type container used for oral contraceptives, which contain sufficient tablets for a monthly cycle of administration and permit scheduled re-

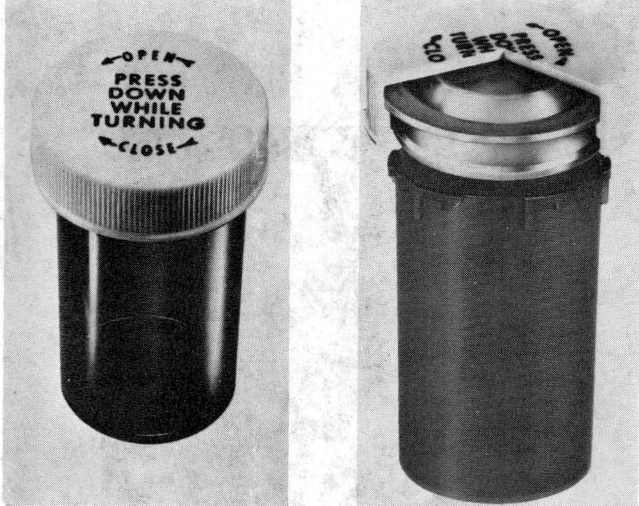

Fig 11. Gross and cutaway views of moisture-tight prescription container (courtesy, Kerr Glass Mfg).

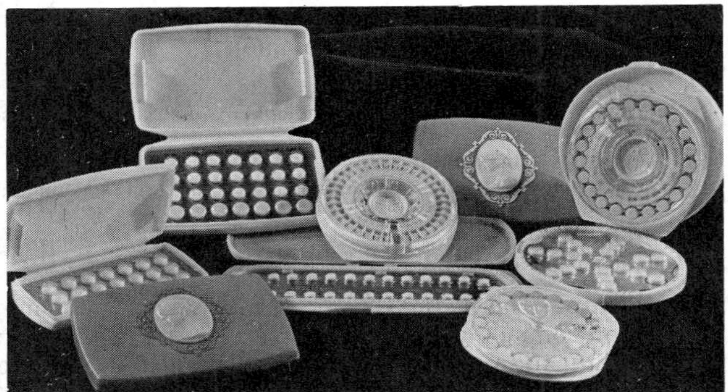

Fig 12. Examples of plastic packaging used for oral contraceptive products.[4]

moval of one tablet at a time, is a prime example of the imaginative packaging possible with plastic. Examples of these containers are shown in Fig 12. These prepackaged containers, as obtained from the manufacturer, are labeled properly by the pharmacist and dispensed in the original container to the patient.

The increased responsibilities of pharmacists in drug distribution and inventory control in hospitals, nursing homes and other patient-care facilities have had an impact on the development of the single-unit drug package, such as the strip-package, blister-package and plastic disposable syringe. These single-unit packages are termed *unit-dose* packages at the time of administration to a specific patient. Examples are shown in Fig 9.

Child-Resistant Containers—The high number of accidental poisonings following ingestion of medication and other household chemicals by children led to the passage of the Poison Prevention Packaging Act in 1970. The initial regulation called for use of "childproof" closures for aspirin products and certain household chemical products shown to have significant potential for causing accidental poisoning in youngsters. As the technical capability in producing effective closures was developed, the regulations were extended to include the use of such safety closures in the packaging of both legend and OTC medications.

The Consumer Product Safety Commission has ruled that manufacturers must place prescription drugs in child-resistant packages if the original package is intended to go directly from the pharmacist to the patient. However, manufacturers need not place drugs in safety packaging if the drugs are intended to be repackaged by pharmacists.

All legend drugs intended for oral use must be dispensed by the pharmacist to the patient in containers having safety closures unless the prescribing physician or the patient specifically requests otherwise. A request for a nonchild-resistant container may be applied to a single prescription or to all of a patient's dispensed medications. The pharmacist should clarify the patient's desires, obtain and file a signed waiver-request and maintain the information in the prescription computer for future reference.[9] There are some exceptions to the overall requirements, such as oral contraceptive packages because of their unique and useful design, and certain cardiac drugs (eg, nitroglycerin) because of the importance to the patient for direct and immediate access to his medication. Exemptions also are permitted in the case of OTC medication for one-package size or specially marked packages to be available to consumers for whom safety closures might be unnecessary or too difficult to manipulate. These consumers include childless persons, arthritic patients and the debilitated. Further, drugs which are used or dispensed in inpatient institutions, such as hospitals, nursing homes and extended-care facilities, need not be dispensed with safety closures unless they are intended for patients who are leaving the confines of the institution. Examples of child-resistant containers are shown in Figs 11 and 13.

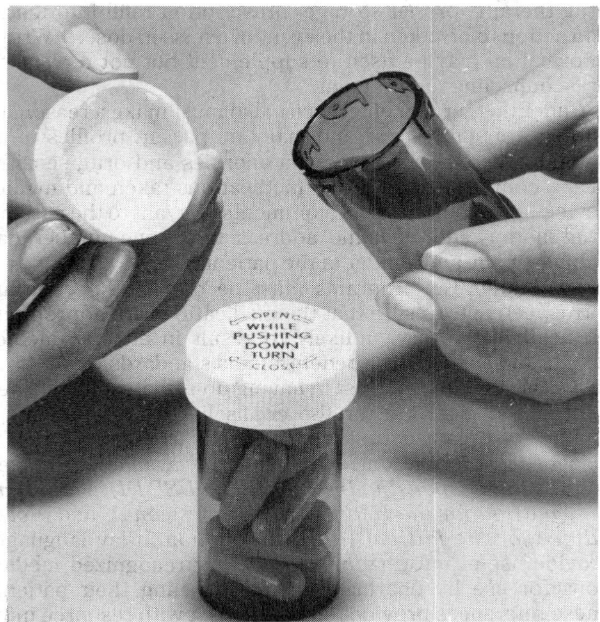

Fig 13. Example of child-resistant safety closure on a prescription container (courtesy, Owens-Brockway).

Rechecking—The importance of this step cannot be overemphasized. Every prescription should be rechecked and the ingredients and amounts used verified by the pharmacist. All details of the label should be rechecked against the prescription order to verify directions, patient's name, prescription number, date and prescriber's name.

Delivering and Patient Counseling—The pharmacist personally should present the prescription medication to the patient (or family member) unless it is to be delivered to the patient's home or workplace. This gives the pharmacist assurance that the patient knows how to use the medication properly. When presenting the medication to the patient, the pharmacist also should call attention to any auxiliary labeling instructions and provide further information regarding the medication as may be desirable. When personal delivery of the prescription is not possible, the pharmacist should make certain that the appropriate instructions are provided to the patient and that he is encouraged to phone should there be any questions.

There is an increased awareness that labeling instructions frequently are inadequate to ensure patient understanding of his medication and his adherence or compliance with recommended instructions. The responsibility that the patient receive specific instructions, precautions and warnings for safe and effective use of prescribed drugs is the shared responsibility of the prescriber and the pharmacist. Reinforcement of the labeled instructions is through verbal communication between the prescriber, pharmacist and patient, or as supplemental printed instructions, as noted previously (see Fig 3).

The Omnibus Budget Reconciliation Act of 1990 (OBRA 90) amended the 1965 Medicaid law and, among other things, required the development of state drug use review (DUR) programs and patient counseling activities by pharmacists. Although the law applies specifically to pharmaceutical care rendered to persons receiving Medicaid benefits, the individual states have developed and adopted similar pharmacy practice standards to apply uniformly to all patients.

The specific requirements of the Act are presented in Chapter 110; however, in brief, pharmacists must offer to discuss with each eligible patient—or caregiver of such individual—who presents a prescription, information on the drug, dosage form, route of administration, any special directions for use, common side effects or interactions and therapeutic contraindications which may apply, techniques for self-monitoring drug therapy, proper storage, prescription refill information and action to be taken in the event of a missed dose. Written information may be used to supplement but not replace the oral counseling requirement.

Under the Act, the pharmacist also must make a reasonable effort to obtain, record and maintain patient profiles of the patient's disease states, known allergies and drug sensitivities, a comprehensive list of medications taken and medical devices used, pharmacists' comments relevant to the patient's drug therapy and the name, address, telephone number, date of birth or age and gender of the patient.

The state DUR programs must be both prospective and retrospective to ensure that the medications are appropriate, medically necessary, unlikely to result in adverse medical results and based upon predetermined standards.

To assist the pharmacist in having up-to-date and pertinent information available for the counseling of his patients, a number of organized and conveniently arranged sources of dispensing information for patients are available. For example, *USP Dispensing Information, (USP DI), Vol I, Drug Information for the Health Care Professional*, and, *Vol II, Advice for the Patient* (drug information in lay language), provide useful information on officially recognized medications for use by pharmacists in counseling their patients. These references provide the pharmacist with resource information including clinical indications and applications, adverse drug reactions, drug interactions, interference with diagnostic tests, known effects on the fetus and newborn, relevant biopharmaceutics and pharmacokinetics, excretion of the drug through breast milk, sugar and/or alcohol content of the medication and other information deemed important.

The prescription medication frequently is placed in specially designed and imprinted prescription bags. Some pharmacists place the patient's name, address, prescription number and price on the package to identify the prescription.

Recording and Filing—A record of the prescriptions dispensed is maintained in the pharmacy through the use of computer and hard copy prescription files.

A variety of prescription file types are available to maintain original prescription orders. Metal or cardboard units, which conveniently store about 1000 prescriptions are common. In using these files, holes are punched in the prescription orders, they then are slipped onto two metal rods firmly attached to the file and placed in a designated compartment in numerical order for safe storage and rapid retrieval.

Suitably partitioned drawers sometimes are used for filing. The partitions may be placed between every 100 or 1000 prescriptions, plainly marked with the numbers of the prescriptions filed in that section. This method permits the removal of a single prescription without preventing ready access to others, as normally occurs when metal rod files are used. Microfilming of prescriptions for purposes of filing and retrieving is an available but little-used method.

Pricing the Prescription—In order for a prescription practice to be successful, the pharmacist must be an effective manager of the financial aspects of his practice. To maintain the types of pharmaceutical services desired by his patients, the pharmacist must make a fair and equitable profit.

Each pharmacy should have a method for pricing prescriptions which is applied consistently by each pharmacist practicing in that pharmacy. The pricing method should be established to ensure the profitable operation of the prescription department. A uniform and consistently applied system is beneficial to the pharmacists and helps to avoid misunderstandings from patrons.

The charge applied to a prescription should cover the costs of the ingredients, including the container and label, the time of the pharmacist and auxiliary personnel involved, the cost of inventory maintenance and other operational costs of the department, as well as providing a reasonable margin of profit on investment.

Although many methods of pricing prescriptions have been used through the years, the most common are

1. *% Markup*
   Cost of ingredients + (cost of ingredients × % markup) = dispensing price.
2. *% Markup + Minimum Fee*
   Cost of ingredients + (cost of ingredients × % markup) + minimum fee = dispensing price.
3. *Professional Fee*
   Cost of ingredients + professional fee = dispensing price.

% Markup—This method and the % markup plus minimum fee method commonly are used in prescription practice. In the straight markup method, the desired percentage markup is taken of the cost of the ingredients and added to the cost of the ingredients to obtain the dispensing price. For example, if the ingredients in a prescription cost the pharmacist $8.00 and he wishes to apply an 80% markup on cost, he would add $6.40 to the cost of the ingredients and arrive at a dispensing price of $14.40. The % markup applied may be varied depending upon the cost of the ingredients, with a lower % markup generally used for prescription items of higher cost and a higher % markup applied for prescription items of a lower cost.

In order to obtain price consistency many multiple-pharmacy operations, such as chain-store pharmacies, provide each pharmacy with a pricing schedule for prescription items. These frequently are provided on microfiche, programmed into the prescription computer or affixed directly to the bulk container of prescription products by chain-store warehouses; the schedules are updated on a regular basis to account for changes in costs of ingredients or in % markup desired.

% Markup Plus Minimum Fee—In this method, a minimum fee is added to the cost of ingredients plus a % markup. The % markup in this method is usually lower than the one used in the method described above. The minimum fee usually is established to recover the combined cost of the container, label, overhead and professional services. This method is applied as follows: if the cost of the prescription ingredients is $8.00, and a 40% markup on cost is applied, the charge to that point would be $11.20. Then, a minimum fee is added and the final dispensing price determined. If, for example, a minimum fee of $4.00 is added, the final prescription price would be $15.20. To achieve the desired profit, the % markup used in this method may be adjusted upward or downward depending upon the minimum fee established.

Professional Fee—This method involves the addition of a specified professional fee to the cost of the ingredients used in filling a prescription. The professional fee includes all the dispensing costs and professional remuneration. A true professional fee is independent of the cost of the ingredients and thus, does not vary from one prescription to another. Some pharmacists use a variable or sliding professional-fee method, whereby the magnitude of the fee is varied somewhat on the cost of the ingredients. By this method, the greater the cost of prescription ingredients, the greater the fee, the rationale being that the cost of inventory maintenance must be recovered in this manner. However, a single fee for all prescriptions is the true basis of the professional-fee method. The fee represents payment for professional service rendered in filling a prescription and is the same without regard to the cost of ingredients.

In practice, the professional fee may vary widely between pharmacies depending on the cost and types of pharmaceutical services rendered (eg, family record systems, delivery service, home health-care needs, etc) and the professional desires of the pharmacist. A pharmacy may determine its professional fee by (1) averaging the amount previously charged, above ingredient cost, for prescriptions dispensed over a specified period of time or (2) using a more exacting cost analysis method in which *all* costs attributed to the prescription department are divided by the prescription volume in determining the actual cost of filling a prescription, with the profit and desired fee then determined. Pharmacies using the professional fee commonly make adjustments for prescriptions requiring compounding to compensate for the extra time, materials and equipment.

Governmental units, such as state human services agencies, and many insurance companies, have adopted the professional-fee method for the reimbursement of pharmacists in filling prescriptions covered under their programs. Such third-party payers negotiate the professional fee to be used with pharmacists interested in participating in the programs. Many of these programs have a "copayment" provision which requires the patient to pay a part of the charge for each prescription he has filled.

After pricing a prescription, pharmacists place the price on the prescription and in the prescription computer for future reference should the prescription later be renewed.

Prescription Refilling—Instructions for refilling a prescription are provided by the prescriber, on the original prescription or by verbal communication. Although prescriptions for noncontrolled substances have no limitation according to federal law as to the number of refills permitted or the date of expiration, state laws may impose such limits. Refilling prescriptions for controlled substances is limited as described later in Chapter 110.

Physicians and pharmacists should work together so that prescriptions are renewed only with the frequency consistent with directions for use and the pharmacist should check with the prescriber after a reasonable time to assure himself that his intent is being met. No prescription should be renewed indefinitely without the patient being reevaluated by the prescriber to assure that the medication as originally prescribed remains the medication of choice.

Renewals should be noted on the reverse side of the prescription order or in the prescription computer with the date, the quantity dispensed, if different from the original, and the name or initials of the pharmacist dispensing the medication. If verbal authorization has been obtained from the prescriber, this should be noted.

The maintenance of accurate records of renewals is not only important to follow federal and state laws, but also is to provide information on the patient's medication history.

Copies of Prescription Orders—These occasionally are requested by the patient or a pharmacist on behalf of the patient. In some instances the intention is to provide information, and in other instances the patient is desirous of having the copy refilled at another pharmacy.

Although the FDA maintains that a copy of a prescription order has no legal status and should not be honored, the agency has opened the door for honoring copies under certain circumstances. The FDA does not object to the exchange of prescription copies between pharmacies for the purpose of renewal, provided that certain safeguards are taken:

The original order is voided and marked to indicate that a copy has been issued, to whom and the date of issuance.

The copy should be so marked and the location and number of original noted.

The copy shows the date of original dispensing, the date of the last renewal and the number of renewals remaining.[8]

This procedure does not apply to Schedule II controlled drugs or if individual states prohibit such a procedure. In instances in which copies of prescriptions are provided by the pharmacist and in which the copy may not be refilled legally, the pharmacist supplying the copy should write "Copy—Not to be Dispensed" or a similar designation across the top. A copy should be made exactly like the original including all pertinent information that a pharmacist might require in dispensing the medication as originally provided. The copy preferably should be written or typed on a preprinted form identifying the pharmacy.

The DEA amended the Code of Federal Regulations in 1981 to permit the transfer of prescription orders between two pharmacies for controlled substance prescriptions which may be renewed lawfully.

The amendment allows for the transfer of an original prescription order for controlled substances listed in Schedules III, IV or V between pharmacies on a *one-time basis only*.

To comply with these regulations, pharmacists first must ascertain if the transfer of a prescription order for renewal dispensing purposes is permissible under state or other applicable law.

When a prescription order is transferred, it must be communicated directly between two licensed pharmacists, and the transferring pharmacist must record the following infor mation:

Write "VOID" on the face of the invalidated prescription order.

On the back of the invalidated prescription order, the name, address and DEA registration number of the pharmacy it was transferred to and the name of the pharmacist who received the information.

The date of transfer and the transferring pharmacist's name.

The pharmacist receiving the transferred prescription order must reduce to writing the following:

The word "transfer" on the face of the transferred prescription order.

All information required on a controlled substance prescription order as it appears on the original prescription order.

Date of issuance of original prescription order.

Original number of renewals authorized on the original prescription order.

The date of the original prescription order.

Number of valid renewals remaining and the date of the last renewal.

Pharmacy's name, address, DEA registration number and original prescription number for which the prescripton order was transferred.

The name of the transferring pharmacist.

The DEA requires that the original and transferred prescription orders must be maintained for a period of 2 years from the date of the last renewal.

Patient Compliance with Prescribed Medication

When a prescriber writes a prescription, he intends the patient to have the prescription filled promptly and to begin using the medication according to directions. Patient adherence or compliance with the prescribed medication schedule has been a source of concern to both the physician and the pharmacist.

Patients may delay unnecessarily the initiation of drug therapy or may wait to see if they "feel better" before having the prescription filled. Some patients discontinue their medication prematurely because they are feeling better and see no particular need to continue taking the medication. Other patients may take excessive doses of the medication believing that they will get better faster, while others take their medication at incorrect intervals or whenever they remember.

On refilling a prescription, a pharmacist generally can determine the compliance of the patient in taking his medication by comparing the dosage units dispensed versus the dosage units apparently taken over the treatment period. Pharmacy computer systems are useful in determining patient compliance.

Specially designed medication containers are useful in assisting a patient to adhere to his medication schedule. These containers have individual compartments for daily medication and generally hold a week's supply (see Fig 14). Containers for oral contraceptive medication, previously discussed and shown in Fig 12, have proven to be effective in patient compliance during the monthly medication cycle. See also Chapter 103.

Pharmacy Computer Systems

The use of computer systems in pharmacy practice is now standard due to the expanded informational needs of the pharmacist, the increased amount of paper work required in the practice, the need for efficiency and the availability of

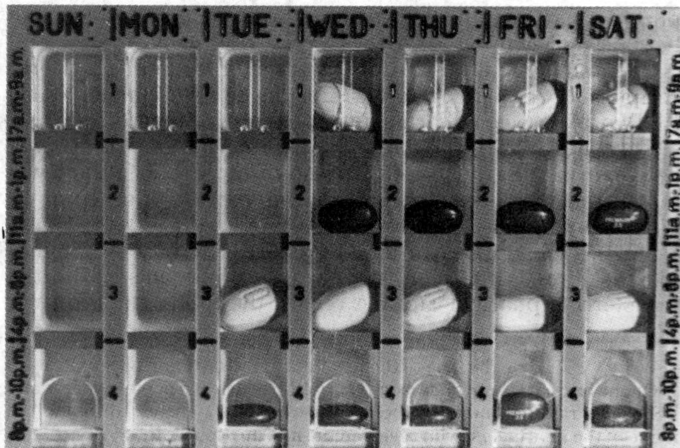

Fig 14. Example of the MEDISET medication container designed to assist patient compliance with prescribed medication schedule (courtesy, Drug Intelligence).

computer technology and expanded data bases to provide the necessary support. (See Fig 15 and also Chapter 11.)

In general, computerized systems in pharmacy are used in three areas: prescription dispensing and associated record maintenance, clinical support and accounting and business management.

Prescription Dispensing and Associated Record Maintenance

Label Preparation—Upon entry of the basic prescription information, the computer produces an error-free label or multiple labels if required.

Prescription Number Assignment—Consecutive numbers are assigned to prescriptions by the computer, and the problem of lost and duplicate numbers virtually is eliminated.

Price Calculations—Prescription computer systems can accommodate multiple pricing methods including: cost plus a professional fee, cost plus % markup or other more complex formulas. The pharmacist specifies the formula desired and the computer calculates the dispensing charge based upon drug-cost information contained in its files.

Receipt Preparation—Prescription computers calculate and store information; thus, it is simple for the computer to prepare a receipt automatically for the patient which may include the amount paid for an individual prescription or for the total prescriptions filled over a given period of time. This information may be important to the patient for insurance or tax purposes.

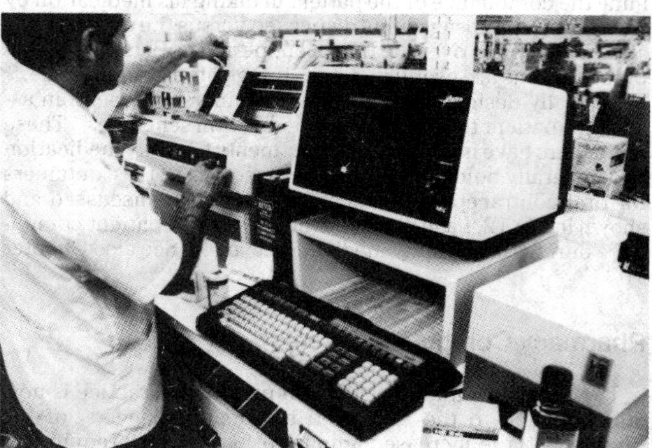

Fig 15. A pharmacist using a prescription computer system in his professional practice (courtesy, General Computer).

Prescription Notation—As a prescription order is processed, the pharmacist typically makes several notations, including: the initials of the dispensing pharmacist, the drug cost and product dispensed and special entries such as "dispensed only one-half at patient request." This information may be retained by the computer and used in renewal processing.

Renewal Processing—The computer-assisted renewal processing of prescriptions is almost automatic. If the computerized records indicate that the prescription renewal is allowable, the computer automatically prepares the new label and receipt, updates the renewal status of the prescription, recalculates the price based on current cost information and adds the entire transaction to the patient's medication profile.

Clinical Support

Patient Medication Profiles—On command, the computer presents on its monitor the most-recent medications that have been dispensed to the individual patient. This information is used by the pharmacist in ascertaining potential drug-drug interactions. Information pertaining to the patient's drug allergies and primary illnesses also permits the pharmacist to assess the drug therapy and dispense only rational and effective medications.

Patient Education Information—Computer-printed information is provided to the patient on the medication dispensed. The information generally includes the proper use of the medication, precautions, possible side effects and a brief description of the purpose of the medication. .

Nursing Home/Consultant Pharmacist Activities—Pharmacists who serve nursing homes as providers or consultants can use computers to prepare physician order sheets, medication administration records, nursing home shipping reports, consultant pharmacist reports, patient medication profiles, patient drug usage and census reports and others.

Drug Utilization Monitoring—By tracking the dispensing dates and quantities dispensed, a pharmacist is able to determine a patient's compliance in taking the prescribed medication properly.

Accounting and Business Management

Business Recordkeeping—The computer may be programmed to provide accounts receivable, payroll, general ledger, accounts payable, third-party claims processing and records, inventory control and ordering, sales analysis functions and daily summary of business.

Prescription Analysis—The computer provides retrievable information on daily, monthly or yearly prescription totals, new versus refilled prescriptions, medication costs per prescription filled and profit per prescription filled.

Drug-Product Defect and Adverse Reaction-Reporting Programs

Monitoring Drug-Product Quality

Monitoring drug-product quality is an important function of the practicing pharmacist. The medications dispensed on prescription and those sold OTC should meet high standards of manufacturing quality to assure safety and efficacy when used properly.

As contained in the *Code of Federal Regulations* (21 CFR 211), manufacturers of pharmaceutical products must comply with FDA standards for *Current Good Manufacturing Practice (CGMP) for Finished Pharmaceuticals* to ensure product quality. A section of these regulations includes provisions for the reporting and handling of drug product complaints. A complaint or concern regarding product quality may arise from a patient or from a health professional and may be communicated directly to the manufacturer or brought to the attention of the FDA. In either case, the information is shared between the agency and manufacturer and each complaint is evaluated to determine whether corrective action is required. Complaints or concerns may relate to any factor of product quality or effectiveness including dosage form integrity, stability, appearance, odor, taste, color, packaging and labeling.

Pharmacists play an important role in the detection and reporting of product defects through participation in the FDA's Medical Products Reporting Program (MedWatch), a voluntary program for the reporting of concerns regarding the quality of distributed prescription and nonprescription drug products. Information provided through this program becomes useful to both the manufacturer and the FDA in maintaining quality standards.[10] Pharmacists may report drug-product quality concerns by telephone or by mail using a form provided for this purpose.

Specific information requested on the FDA MedWatch form includes product name, dosage form, strength and size; National Drug Code Number, if available; lot number and expiration date; name and address of manufacturer and/or distributor/labeler; name, address, and profession of person reporting the suspected product defect; a description of the problem noted or suspected and the date and the signature of the person filing the report. The option is given to the person filing the report to remain anonymous in the subsequent FDA communication to the affected manufacturer or distributor.

Monitoring Adverse Drug Reactions

The FDA has specific requirements for drug manufacturers of investigational and marketed pharmaceutical products to report adverse drug reactions (ADRs) or experiences (ADEs).[11] Pharmacists have the opportunity to participate in reporting such incidents through practices in the institutional and community pharmacy settings. Observations of reactions to investigational drugs generally are observed in the clinical (usually institutional) setting during controlled clinical studies as investigational drugs are evaluated prior to FDA approval for marketing. Reactions to marketed drugs may be observed during any postmarketing clinical studies and through surveillance by health professionals during the course of their practice.

The postmarketing surveillance of pharmaceuticals for adverse reactions is essential in establishing a complete safety profile for marketed drugs. Once marketed, the number and diversity of patients receiving a new drug is far greater than during the controlled clinical trials. Thus, some adverse drug reactions and drug interactions which escape detection during the clinical trials are seen initially after the drug product is marketed.

Pharmacists and other health-care providers who observe *suspect* reactions to drugs are encouraged to report these to the FDA. Serious reactions, observations of events not described in the package insert and reactions to newly marketed products are of particular importance. The FDA provides the MedWatch form for filing a voluntary, or in the case of user-facilities, distributors or manufacturers, a mandatory report. The form includes space for entering patient information; adverse reaction information, including a description of the reaction experience and relevant laboratory tests/data; suspect drug information, such as the drug name, manufacturer, lot number, daily dose, route of administration, dates of administration and duration of administration; concomitant drugs taken and record of administration and name and contact information for the person or manufacturer filing the report. In some institutions in which clinical studies are conducted, computer programs are used to record, monitor and report suspected adverse drug experiences.[12] ADR reports may result in changes in product labeling, warning letters to health-care professionals regarding safe conditions of use, requirements for further clinical/safety studies or, in some instances, withdrawal of the product from the market.[13]

Legal Considerations

All aspects of manufacture, distribution and possession of drugs are controlled by both state and federal laws and regulations. State laws and regulations governing the practice of pharmacy generally are administered by state boards of pharmacy comprised of varying numbers of pharmacy practitioners and in some instances by consumer representation. These boards generally regulate the licensing of pharmacy interns, pharmacists and pharmacies, and enforce rules and regulations pertaining to the legal and ethical practice of pharmacy within the state. State regulations regarding drugs frequently include and extend the federal law. Federal laws are administered by various federal agencies and pertain primarily to products considered to be in interstate commerce.

The laws governing the practice of pharmacy are present ed in Chapter 110.

References

1. Poirier TI, Giudici RA: *Hosp Pharm 27:*408, 1992.
2. *Am J Hosp Pharm 49:*640, 1992.
3. Cohen MR, Davis NM: *Am. Pharm NS32:*112, 1992.
4. Ansel HC: *Introduction to Pharmaceutical Dosage Forms*, 4th ed, Lea & Febiger, Philadelphia, 1985.
5. Resolution 88-4-92, National Association of Boards of Pharmacy.
6. Compliance Guidelines, *Manufacturer, Distribution, and Promotion of Adulterated, Misbranded, or Unapproved New Drugs for Human Use by State-Licensed Pharmacies*, FDA, 1992.
7. Crawford SY, Dombrowski SR: *Am J Hosp Pharm 48:*1205, 1991.
8. *Pharm Pract 13(3):* 18, 1978.
9. *Pharmacy Today*, Dec. 21:3, 1992.
10. Bolger G, Goetsch R: *Amer Pharm NS32:*139, 1992.
11. 21 CFR 312.32; 21 CFR 314.80
12. *Profiles in Hosp Pharm 5:*12, No 3, 1991.
13. Sills JM, Tanner LA, Milstien JB: *Am J Hosp Pharm 43:*2764, 1986.

CHAPTER 105

Drug Interactions

Daniel A Hussar, PhD
Remington Professor of Pharmacy
Philadelphia College of Pharmacy and Science
Philadelphia, PA 19104

Although some drug-related problems develop unexpectedly and can not be predicted, many are related to known pharmacologic actions of the drugs and reasonably can be anticipated. However, as drug therapy becomes more complex and because many patients are being treated with two or more drugs, the ability to predict the magnitude of a specific action of any given drug diminishes. These circumstances point to a need not only for maintenance of complete and current medication records for patients but also for closer monitoring and supervision of drug therapy so that problems can be prevented, or detected at an early stage in their development. The pharmacist is in a unique position to meet these needs, and opportunities exist for greater involvement in and contribution to provision of drug therapy that is both efficacious and safe.

Many drug-related problems are caused by drug interactions. As a basis for this discussion a drug interaction may be considered a situation in which the effects of one drug are altered by prior or concurrent administration of another drug (ie, drug-drug interactions). The concept of drug interaction often is extended to include situations in which

1. Food or certain dietary items influence the activity of a drug (ie, drug-food interactions) or
2. Environmental chemicals or smoking influences the activity of a drug or
3. A drug causes alterations of laboratory test results (ie, drug-laboratory test interactions) or
4. A drug causes undesired effects in patients with certain disease states (ie, drug-disease interactions).

Considerable attention has been focused on the subject of drug interaction in recent years and information pertaining to these occurrences has been widely publicized. Several comprehensive references, such as *Drug Interaction Facts.* (Tatro DS, ed: Facts and Comparisons, St Louis, 1995) and *Drug Interactions and Updates Quarterly* (Hansten PD, Horn JR, eds: Applied Therapeutics, Vancouver, WA, 1995) deal exclusively with this subject, while other references give extensive attention to it. Computer systems that provide for storage and retrieval of drug interaction information also are available.

Problems that may result from drug interactions also have been publicized to the public. In addition to cautions given to patients by physicians and pharmacists, articles on the subject have appeared in many publications widely read by the public. In some of these articles the value of patient medication records kept by the pharmacist has been stressed.

One of the most important consequences of a drug interaction is an excessive response to one or more of the agents being used. For example, a significantly enhanced effect of agents like digoxin and warfarin can result in serious adverse effects. Not as well recognized, but also very important, are those interactions in which drug activity is decreased, resulting in a loss of efficacy. These interactions are especially difficult to detect, since they may be mistaken for therapeutic failure or progression of the disease.

Some drug interactions continue to occur even though they are well documented and recognized. Digoxin and a diuretic often are given concurrently, and rationally so, in treating patients with congestive heart failure. It is well known that most diuretics can cause potassium depletion which, if uncorrected, could become excessive and lead to adverse effects of the digoxin. Yet problems continue to occur as a result of this interaction.

Even with the extensive publicity that drug interactions have received, it is still often difficult to determine their incidence or clinical significance. However, numerous studies have demonstrated that many patients receive multiple drug therapy with agents of recognized potential for interaction. As the number of drugs in a patient's therapeutic regimen increases, the greater is the risk of occurrence of a drug interaction. Although there are only limited data regarding many of the potential drug interactions which have been suggested, considerable progress has been made in defining the level of risk attending the use of a number of combinations of drugs.

Factors Contributing to the Occurrence of Drug Interactions

A number of factors contribute to the occurrence of drug interactions.

Multiple Pharmacological Effects—Most drugs used in current therapy have the capacity to influence many physiologic systems. Therefore, there is an increased possibility that two drugs concomitantly administered will affect some of the same systems. When considering the potential for interactions between drugs there often is a tendency only to be concerned with the primary effects of the drugs involved and to overlook the secondary activities they possess. Combined therapy with a phenothiazine antipsychotic (eg, chlorpromazine), a tricyclic antidepressant (eg, amitriptyline) and an antiparkinson agent (eg, trihexyphenidyl) is employed frequently. Each of these agents has a considerably different primary effect; however, all three possess anticholinergic activity. Even though the anticholinergic effect of any one of the drugs may be slight, the additive effects of the three agents may be significant.

Multiple Prescribers—It is necessary for some individuals to see more than one physician and it is not uncommon for a patient to be seeing one or more specialists in addition to a family physician. Some individuals also are seeing other health professionals (eg, dentists, podiatrists) who may prescribe medication. It frequently is difficult for one prescriber to be aware of all the medications that have been prescribed by others for a particular patient and difficulties could arise from such situations. For example, one physician may prescribe an antihistamine (eg, diphenhydramine) for a patient for whom another physician has prescribed an antianxiety agent, with the possible consequence of an excessive depressant effect.

Even though the patient is seeing different physicians, he

usually will have the prescriptions dispensed by the same pharmacy. Therefore, the pharmacist, by maintaining patient medication records, can play an important role in the detection and prevention of drug-related problems.

Use of Nonprescription Drugs—Many reports of drug interactions have involved the concurrent use of a prescription drug with a nonprescription drug (eg, aspirin, antacids, decongestants). When a physician questions a patient about medications that he is taking, the patient often will neglect to mention the nonprescription medications that he has purchased. Many patients have been taking preparations such as antacids, analgesics and laxatives for such long periods and in such a routine manner that they do not consider them to be drugs. This information often may be missed in questioning a patient and some physicians and pharmacists prefer to utilize a list of symptoms that might ordinarily be treated with nonprescription drugs in trying to obtain this information from the patient.

Interactions also may result from the concurrent use of two or more products available without a prescription. In some situations two nonprescription products promoted for different purposes contain the same active ingredient(s), increasing the risk of an excessive response to these agents. Phenylpropanolamine is used widely as a decongestant, as well as in formulations used as diet aids. Diphenhydramine is included in many products for its antihistaminic action but also is included for its sedative effect in many nonprescription sleep-aid formulations. Patients often are unaware that products they purchase for different conditions may contain the same active ingredients and that they, therefore, are at increased risk of problems with the use of products they might assume to be safe because they do not require a prescription.

Although many individuals will have their prescriptions filled in their local pharmacy, they often purchase nonprescription drugs elsewhere, thus making identification of potential problems extremely difficult for the pharmacist as well as the physician. For this reason, patients should be encouraged to obtain both their prescription and nonprescription medications at a pharmacy. Such advice is justified, however, only when the pharmacist personally supervises the sale of nonprescription medications with which problems may develop.

Patient Noncompliance—For a variety of reasons many patients do not take medication in the manner intended by the prescriber. Some have not received adequate instruction from the prescriber and pharmacist as to how and when to take their medication. In other situations, particularly involving patients who are taking several medications, confusion about the instructions may develop even though the patient may have understood them initially. It is understandable that an older patient who may be taking five or six medications several times a day at different times can be come confused or forget to take his medication, although these occurrences are by no means unique to the geriatric population.

Although the situations involving noncompliance usually would result in a patient not taking enough medication, some circumstances could lead to excessive use of certain medications, thereby increasing the possibility of drug interaction. For example, some patients if they realize they have forgotten a dose of medication, double the next dose to make up for it. Some other patients may act on an assumption that if the one tablet-dose that has been prescribed provides partial, but not complete relief of symptoms, a two-tablet dose will be even more effective.

Drug Abuse—The tendencies of some individuals to abuse or deliberately misuse drugs also may lead to an increased incidence of drug interactions. The barbiturates, opioid analgesics and amphetamines are among the agents most often abused, and the inappropriate use of these drugs can result in a number of problems, including an increased potential for drug interaction.

Many interactions that occur are undetected or unreported. Koch-Weser (*Drug Inform J 6:* 42, 1972) observed that detection of drug interactions by clinicians is inefficient and cited six reasons for existence of this situation. Although initially noted in 1972, many of these observations are just as valid today.

1. In most cases the clinical situation is too complex to allow recognition of an unexpected event in a patient's course as related to his drug therapy.
2. With few exceptions, the intensity of action of drugs in the therapeutic setting cannot be quantitated accurately.

One reason for the many reports of interactions involving anticoagulants, hypoglycemic agents and antihypertensive agents is that there are specific parameters such as prothrombin time, blood glucose concentrations and blood pressure that can be measured and provide a quantitative indication of drug activity. Therefore, any change in these values which may be caused by introducing another drug into therapy can be measured with relative ease. In contrast, when one considers drugs like the antipsychotic agents and analgesics with which it is far more difficult to measure degree of activity, it becomes increasingly difficult to observe and measure the effect of other drugs on their activity.

3. Even when a deficient, excessive or abnormal response to one or both drugs is recognized clearly during concomitant administration, it is attributed usually to factors other than drug interaction.

When an unexpected response to a drug develops, it often is attributed to something other than a drug interaction, such as patient idiosyncrasy in the case of an excessive response, or tolerance in the case of a deficient response.

4. The index of suspicion of most clinicians concerning drug interactions is quite low and many practicing physicians are hardly aware of the phenomenon.
5. Practicing physicians tend to doubt their observations concerning drug interactions unless the same interaction has been reported previously.

Although physicians are now well aware of the occurrence of drug interactions, there are situations in which a drug interaction may be occurring but there are other factors that also could contribute to the altered response noted. Therefore, the physician often accepts a reasonable explanation, albeit incomplete, based on information with which he is familiar, rather than suspecting a possibility that has not been reported previously. Although many interactions that have been reported via case reports have not been confirmed by other observations or additional study, many single-case reports have served as the stimulus for additional study that has resulted in warnings about potentially dangerous interactions.

6. Physicians frequently fail to report drug interactions even when they have unequivocally recognized them.

Several factors, no doubt, contribute to this situation. The time it would take to write up a case report to submit to a journal is a deterrent to many physicians and pharmacists. Also, since drug interactions often represent an undesirable experience for the patient, a health professional often is reluctant to expose himself to possible criticism, or even liability, regarding the therapy. However, it is important that health professionals communicate information that will be useful to others or will help others to avoid the same problems.

Using Drug-Interaction Information

Although there has been considerable progress in identifying drug interactions, a careful analysis of the literature reveals that some of the information is conflicting, incomplete and misleading. Too frequently, the suggested clinical importance of an alleged drug interaction is greatly overstated and publicized.

The use of some of this information unfortunately has led, in some situations, to an undue degree of alarm characterized by some observers as *drug-interaction hysteria* or a *drug-interaction anxiety syndrome*. Caution is needed, therefore, in evaluating and using the information available, because by overreacting to a possible problem, a more difficult situation may result than might have occurred if nothing were done. In some situations patients have been deprived unnecessarily of therapy from which they could benefit as a result of concern about a potential interaction with other medication they are taking. Conversely, some health-care practitioners have found so many of the reports and commentaries regarding drug interactions to be lacking in clinical relevance that their skepticism has precluded adequate attention to those interactions which are clinically important. Recognition of the importance of exercising the appropriate clinical perspective is essential if optimal therapy is to be achieved.

In using the literature on drug interactions and deciding what action is appropriate, a number of factors should be kept in mind.

Interacting Drugs Usually Can Be Used Together—In most cases, two drugs which are known to interact can be administered concurrently so long as adequate precautions are taken (eg, closer monitoring of therapy, dosage adjustments to compensate for the altered response). Although there are some situations in which the use of one drug usually is contraindicated while another is being given, such combinations are not likely to be employed frequently and there may even be exceptions to the contraindication under certain circumstances. In those situations, though, where another agent with similar therapeutic properties and a lesser risk of interacting could be used, such a course of action would be preferable.

Serious reactions have been reported to occur following the concurrent use of a monoamine oxidase inhibitor (eg, tranylcypromine) with a tricyclic antidepressant (eg, amitriptyline), and the literature for most of these products warns that use of such combinations is contraindicated. However, it has been indicated by some that such reactions do not occur commonly and that these combinations, when used under close supervision, may be of benefit in some patients when conventional drug therapy has failed. The fact that these combinations may be used beneficially in some patients does not excuse the pharmacist from his responsibility in checking the therapy with the physician. However, he should be aware that certain circumstances may justify the concomitant use of even "contraindicated" drugs.

Beneficial Interactions—It should be recognized that sometimes a second drug is prescribed deliberately to modify the effects of another. Such an approach might be used in an effort to enhance the effectiveness or to reduce the adverse effects of the primary agent. In these situations the efficacy and/or safety of a drug is increased indicating that interactions are not always harmful as frequently thought, but also can be beneficial.

The ability of probenecid to increase the serum concentrations and prolong the activity of penicillin derivatives has been known for many years, and this interaction has been used to therapeutic advantage in certain infections such as uncomplicated gonorrhea.

An example of a situation in which one drug is given to minimize the undesirable effects of another is seen with the use of an antiparkinson drug with an antipsychotic agent in an effort to reduce the extrapyramidal effects of the latter.

Nature of Reports—Reports and reviews of interactions sometimes attach importance to isolated observations of problems in one patient or a limited number of patients. On several occasions a suspected interaction that was observed in a single patient has been reported in a number of reviews and tables without qualification as to the nature of the report or the possible significance of the interaction. The fact that such an interaction now is included in a number of publications can result in an impression that the problem is well documented and clinically significant.

Depth of Information—Most of the charts and tables of drug interactions do not provide detailed information about specific situations. The mere mention of an increased or decreased effect of one drug in the presence of another is not enough to form a judgment as to the clinical importance and potential severity of the situation. Because of this, most references of this type should be used only to initially screen for possible interactions and more comprehensive reference sources should be consulted for further information.

Current Literature—It is important to review the current literature constantly since new information may change the significance of earlier reports. The existence of conflicting reports regarding some interactions also will become evident as the literature is carefully searched. Although there is no assurance that more recent information is more accurate or pertinent, the date of publication of a particular reference should be noted and, when appropriate, more current references consulted. The importance of having access to the current literature is reflected in the decisions of the publishers of most of the widely used comprehensive drug-interaction references to issue updates at frequent intervals (eg, four times a year).

Recommendations and Therapeutic Alternatives—There is not enough information available on many reported interactions to permit the development of specific guidelines to govern such combination therapy. When such guidelines are presented they can be extremely helpful, and there is an increasing number of such statements in the package inserts for various products. Where possible, the pharmacist should not only identify a potential problem but also be prepared to make a recommendation to the physician and/or patient as to how problems best can be avoided or minimized.

For example, it is known that aspirin may enhance the anticoagulant activity of warfarin. Although many patients taking the two drugs concurrently will not experience a problem, acetaminophen usually would be preferred to aspirin in patients on anticoagulant therapy because it is unlikely to alter the activity of agents such as warfarin. However, before making a recommendation that a patient on anticoagulant therapy use acetaminophen instead of aspirin, there should be an awareness of the purpose for which the aspirin is to be used. Although acetaminophen is comparable to aspirin with regard to analgesic and antipyretic activity, it possesses little anti-inflammatory activity and, unlike aspirin, has not been shown to reduce the risk of problems such as transient ischemic attacks and myocardial infarction. Therefore, it could not be used as an alternative to aspirin in most conditions in which one of these actions is needed.

The use of tetracycline by a patient also taking antacids provides an example of a situation in which a specific recommendation can be made to avoid difficulty. If taken at the same time, the antacid can decrease the absorption and effectiveness of the tetracycline. However, if the two agents are given at least 1 hour apart, difficulty should be avoided.

Viewing Interactions in Perspective—Even after the previously discussed factors have been considered and the data have been analyzed critically, the possibility of interactions developing must be viewed in perspective. Although an altered response appears likely, it might not be clinically significant in many patients. In these situations a patient should not be deprived of needed therapy because of the possibility of an interaction, but such therapy should be monitored closely.

Most health-care practitioners do not have rapid access to a large number of primary literature sources. Therefore, the use of an authoritative and comprehensive reference source such as *Drug Interaction Facts* or *Drug Interactions and Updates Quarterly* is recommended, and these references can be very helpful in identifying potential problems and in making judgments as to their clinical importance and therapeutic alternatives. However, even though certain interactions are well documented, it often is difficult, if not impossible, to predict the severity of an interaction, if indeed it does develop. The many variables which may influence the activity of a drug and its ability to interact with other agents, contribute to the existing uncertainty. Many of these variables pertain to the drugs being used and include dosage, route of administration, time of administration, sequence of administration and duration of therapy, whereas other variables, which are considered in the following discussion, pertain to the patient.

Patient Variables

There are many factors that influence the response to a drug in man. A number of reports have indicated how these factors may predispose a patient to the development of adverse effects to a drug, and it can be anticipated that many of these considerations also apply to the development of drug interactions.

Age—When considering the risk of drug-related problems, age is an important factor. Studies indicate that there is an increased incidence of adverse drug reactions in both young and geriatric patients, and it is reasonable to expect that the occurrence of drug interactions also is highest in these patient groups.

Drug-related problems in young patients are encountered most frequently in newborn infants. Newborn infants do not have fully developed enzyme systems that are involved in the metabolism of certain drugs and they also have immature renal function.

Several factors point to an increased risk of interactions in the elderly. Most elderly patients have at least one chronic illness (eg, hypertension, diabetes) and this is reflected in the prescribing of a larger number of medications for this patient group. The types of diseases more frequently experienced by elderly patients (eg, renal disorders) may contribute to an altered drug response, and there appears to be an increased sensitivity to the action of certain drugs with advancing age. In addition, there may be aging-related changes in the absorption, distribution, metabolism and excretion of certain drugs which increase the possibility of adverse drug reactions and drug interactions. Accordingly, drug therapy in elderly patients must be monitored especially closely.

Genetic Factors—These may be responsible for the development of an unexpected drug response in a particular patient. Isoniazid is metabolized by an acetylation process, the rate of which appears to be under genetic control. Some individuals metabolize isoniazid rapidly, whereas others metabolize it slowly, thus necessitating careful dosage adjustment, as the dose which provides satisfactory concentrations in rapid acetylators may cause toxicity in slow acetylators. For example, isoniazid causes peripheral neuritis in a number of patients and this effect has been noted most frequently in slow acetylators.

It has been observed that isoniazid may inhibit the metabolism of phenytoin, possibly resulting in the development of toxic effects (nystagmus, ataxia, lethargy) of the latter. However, studies have indicated that those patients who developed phenytoin toxicity when also receiving isoniazid were slow acetylators of isoniazid. It is likely that this interaction will be of significance only in patients who metabolize isoniazid at a very slow rate.

Disease States—A number of disease states, other than the one for which a particular drug is being used, may influence patient response to a drug. Impaired renal and hepatic function are the most important conditions that may alter drug activity. However, other disorders also may bring about a change in the activity of a drug. Since many drugs are bound extensively to plasma proteins and only the unbound fraction of the drug is active, a decreased concentration or amount of protein conceivably could change the availability of drugs and, thus, their activity. This possibility must be recognized in patients with conditions that may be associated with hypoalbuminemia.

Renal Function—Renal function is one of the most important determinants of drug activity. The patient's renal status should be known, particularly when drugs that are excreted primarily in an active form by the kidney, are to be used for long periods of time. If there is renal impairment and the usual dose of a drug that is excreted by the kidney is given, there can be an increased and prolonged effect since it is not being excreted at the normal rate. As additional doses are given, serum concentrations will increase, possibly resulting in toxicity. Therefore, a need exists for careful dosage adjustment and particular caution when other potentially interacting drugs are added to the therapeutic regimen.

The alteration of renal excretion as a mechanism by which a number of drug interactions develop is considered later, and the status of the patient's renal function is an obvious determinant of the rate of excretion of the drugs involved and the occurrence of interactions.

Hepatic Function—Many drugs are metabolized in the liver by a number of mechanisms. Therefore, when there is hepatic damage, these drugs may be metabolized at a slower rate and exhibit a prolonged effect. Although each situation should be evaluated to determine whether a reduction in dosage is necessary, it should be recognized that some drugs will be metabolized at the normal rate even though hepatic function is impaired. A number of studies of drug metabolism in patients with liver disease have been conducted. However, the results vary considerably and it is difficult to predict with certainty whether the rate of metabolism will be altered in a given patient.

Many therapeutic agents are metabolized by liver enzymes. If other drugs alter the amount and/or activity of these enzymes, a modified response to the drugs which depend on these enzymes for their metabolism might occur. For example, many agents (eg, barbiturates) are known to stimulate the activity of liver enzymes (enzyme induction). The result would be a more rapid metabolism and excretion of concurrently administered agents which are metabolized by these enzymes. This mechanism of drug interaction is discussed in greater detail later as are the situations in which the action of hepatic enzymes is inhibited.

Alcohol Consumption—Several studies have shown that chronic use of alcoholic beverages may increase the rate of metabolism of drugs such as warfarin, phenytoin and tolbutamide, probably by increasing the activity of liver enzymes. However, in contrast, acute use of alcohol by nonalcoholic individuals may cause an inhibition of hepatic enzymes.

Concurrent use of alcoholic beverages with sedatives and other depressant drugs could result in an excessive depressant response. The fact that the use of such combinations is commonplace cannot be cause for failing to exercise the caution that must be observed if problems are to be averted.

Smoking—A number of investigations have suggested that smoking increases the activity of drug-metabolizing enzymes in the liver with the result that certain therapeutic agents (eg, diazepam, propoxyphene, theophylline, chlorpromazine, amitriptyline) are metabolized more rapidly and their effect is decreased. This response may be more pronounced in young and middle-aged individuals, than in older patients.

Diet—Food often may affect the rate and extent of absorption of drugs from the gastrointestinal tract. For example, many penicillin and tetracycline derivatives should be given at least 1 hour before or 2 hours after meals to achieve optimal absorption.

The type of food may be important with regard to the absorption of concurrently administered drugs. For example, dietary items such as milk and other dairy products that contain calcium may decrease the absorption of tetracycline and fluoroquinolone derivatives by forming a complex with them in the gastrointestinal tract that is absorbed poorly.

Some dietary items, such as certain cheeses and alcoholic beverages, have a relatively high content of the pressor amine tyramine. Tyramine is metabolized by monoamine oxidase, and normally these enzymes in the intestinal wall and liver protect against the pressor actions of amines in foods. However, if these enzymes were to be inhibited by a monoamine oxidase inhibitor, large quantities of unmetabolized tyramine could accumulate which could lead to the development of a severe hypertensive reaction.

Certain dietary items contain an appreciable amount of vitamin K. A change in dietary habits that would significantly alter the intake of these foods could cause problems in patients on anticoagulant therapy.

Diet also may influence urinary pH values. One study has compared the excretion of amphetamine in two groups of patients maintained on different diets. One group was placed on a balanced protein diet that provided an acidic urine (average pH of 5.9) whereas the other group was put on a low-protein diet that provided an alkaline urine (average pH of 7.5). Each group was given a dose of amphetamine and those with the acidic urine excreted 23 to 56% of unchanged amphetamine in the first 8 hours and 5 to 13% in the next 8 hours. In comparison, in those with an alkalinized urine, there was a 2 to 6% excretion in the first 8 hours, followed by an 0.5 to 3% excretion in the next 8 hours.

Environmental Factors—DDT and related materials may increase the activity of liver enzymes and thereby increase the rate of metabolism of other agents. Individuals whose jobs necessitate intensive exposure to these materials should be observed more closely for altered metabolic responses.

Individual Variation—Even after the preceding factors have been considered, wide variations in the response of patients to drugs will be seen that are often difficult to explain. As an example, it has been noted that plasma concentrations of tricyclic antidepressants vary widely among individuals using the same dosage regimen over the same time period. When recognition is taken of the difficulty in predicting the response to many therapeutic agents when they are given alone, the challenge and limitations in endeavoring to anticipate the response with a multiple-drug regimen clearly become apparent.

Mechanisms of Drug Interaction

An understanding of the mechanisms by which drug interactions develop will be valuable in anticipating such situations and dealing with problems that do develop. Although the circumstances surrounding the development of some drug interactions are complex and poorly understood, the mechanisms by which most interactions develop are well documented and relate to the basic processes by which a drug acts and is acted upon in the body.

These mechanisms often are categorized generally as being pharmacokinetic or pharmacodynamic types. *Pharmacokinetic interactions* are those in which one agent (designated by some as the "precipitant drug") alters the absorption, distribution, metabolism or excretion (ADME) of a second agent (the "object drug"), with a resultant change in the plasma concentration of the latter agent. Included among the *pharmacodynamic interactions* are those in which drugs having similar (or opposing) pharmacological effects are administered concurrently and situations in which the sensitivity or responsiveness of the tissues to one drug is altered by another. Pharmacodynamic interactions also have been viewed as situations in which there is a change in drug effect without a change in drug plasma concentration.

Although the pharmacokinetic interactions often present challenging clinical problems which have been publicized widely, the pharmacodynamic interactions are encountered more frequently. It also should be recognized that several mechanisms may be involved in the development of certain interactions.

Pharmacokinetic Interactions

Alteration of Gastrointestinal Absorption

Interactions which involve a change in the absorption of a drug from the gastrointestinal tract may develop through different mechanisms and be of varying clinical importance. In some situations the absorption of the drug may be reduced and its therapeutic activity compromised. In others, absorption may be delayed but the same amount of drug is absorbed eventually. A delay in drug absorption can be undesirable when a rapid effect is needed to relieve acute symptoms, such as pain. The slower absorption rate also may prolong the effects of a drug, and may present difficulty. For example, if the effects of a hypnotic agent are prolonged, the patient may experience excessive residual sedation or "hangover" in the morning. A slower rate of absorption may preclude achievement of effective plasma and tissue concentrations of drugs which are metabolized rapidly and excreted.

Conversely, a delay in drug absorption may not be clinically significant; this is usually the case when a drug is being used on a chronic basis and therapeutic concentrations in the body have already been achieved.

As a general guideline, it is the drugs which are not absorbed completely under "normal" circumstances that are most susceptible to alterations of gastrointestinal absorption.

Alteration of pH

Since many drugs are weak acids or weak bases, the pH of the gastrointestinal contents may influence the extent of absorption. It is recognized that the nonionized form of a drug (the more lipid-soluble form) will be absorbed more readily than the ionized form. Acidic drugs exist primarily in the nonionized form in the upper region of the gastrointestinal tract (having a lower pH). If a drug such as an antacid is ingested, which will raise the pH of the gastrointestinal contents, it is possible that the absorption of such acidic drugs can be delayed and/or inhibited partially.

Although changes in absorption might be predicted for many acidic and basic drugs on a theoretical basis, it would appear that clinically important interactions are likely to occur in only a few situations, and factors other than pH seem to be more important determinants of gastrointestinal absorption.

Aspirin—Antacids—The situation seen with aspirin is an interesting one. As a weak acid it might be anticipated that aspirin would be absorbed primarily from the upper region of the gastrointestinal tract and that antacids would decrease its absorption. Because aspirin produces gastrointestinal side effects in many patients, various efforts including concurrent use of an antacid have been employed to minimize these problems (eg, combination products such as *Bufferin*, *Ascriptin* and *Alka-Seltzer*). Although some studies suggest that absorption of aspirin from buffered products is decreased, other investigations indicate that absorption is not altered or may even be increased. Drugs such as aspirin which are administered orally in solid dosage forms must first dissolve in the gastrointestinal fluids before they can be absorbed. The fact that aspirin dissolves faster in an alkaline medium, even though it is predominantly in the ionized form, is the probable explanation for successful use of aspirin products that also contain antacids.

Ketoconazole—Antacids—An acidic medium is required to achieve dissolution of ketoconazole following oral administration. Therefore, an antacid or a histamine H_2-receptor antagonist (eg, cimetidine, ranitidine) is likely to reduce the dissolution, absorption and effectiveness of the antifungal agent. An antacid should be administered at least 2 hours after ketoconazole; the concurrent use of ketoconazole and a histamine H_2-receptor antagonist is best avoided, and alternative agents having a lesser potential for interaction should be considered.

Bisacodyl—Antacids—A change in the pH of the gastrointestinal contents also may cause another type of problem. For example, oral dosage forms of the laxative bisacodyl are enteric-coated because the drug can be extremely irritating. It has been suggested that this agent should not be given orally within an hour of antacid therapy or ingestion of milk because an increase in the pH of the gastrointestinal contents may cause disintegration of the enteric coating in the stomach, resulting in release of the drug in this area which could cause irritation and vomiting.

Antacids also may alter the gastrointestinal absorption of drugs through other mechanisms and additional examples are considered in the following discussion.

Complexation and Adsorption

Tetracycline—Metals—The interaction between tetracycline derivatives and certain metal ions is well known. Tetracycline can combine with metal ions such as calcium, magnesium, aluminum, iron, bismuth and zinc in the gastrointestinal tract to form complexes which are absorbed poorly. Thus, the simultaneous administration of certain dietary items (eg, milk, containing calcium) or drugs (eg, antacids, iron preparations, products containing calcium salts) with tetracycline could result in a significant decrease in the amount of antibiotic absorbed.

The absorption of doxycycline and minocycline is influenced to a lesser extent by simultaneous ingestion of food or milk and one of these agents may be preferred to tetracycline when gastric irritation occurs or appears likely. However, the concurrent administration of aluminum hydroxide gel will decrease absorption of these analogs, as is seen with other tetracyclines.

When two drugs are recognized as being capable of interacting there is often a tendency to believe that one of them should be discontinued. In the case of the antacid-tetracycline interaction, problems can be avoided by allowing an appropriate interval of time to separate administration of the two agents. This interval should be as long as possible but a minimum period of 1 hour should elapse between administration of the drugs.

The interaction between doxycycline and iron salts calls attention to another factor that must be considered, as the results of one study suggest that the interaction cannot be avoided completely by allowing an interval of 3 hours (or even a longer period) to separate administration of the two drugs. It is noted that a significant amount of doxycycline is transported back to the gastrointestinal tract via the enterohepatic circulation, and the unabsorbed iron still present in the tract prevents reabsorption of the antibiotic.

Fluoroquinolones—Metals—Aluminum- and magnesium- containing antacids, as well as certain dietary items (eg, milk, yogurt), have been reported to reduce markedly the absorption and serum concentrations of fluoroquinolones, probably as a result of the metal ions complexing with the anti-infective agent. Even allowing a long interval to separate the administration of the two drugs may not be sufficient to avoid the interaction, and as long an interval as possible should separate the administration of the fluoroquinolone and metal-containing product. For example, in the product labeling for enoxacin, it is recommended that aluminum- and magnesium-containing antacids, bismuth subsalicylate, sucralfate, products containing iron, and multivitamins containing zinc should not be taken for 8 hours before or 2 hours after enoxacin administration.

Cholestyramine and Colestipol—Other interactions involving complexation might be anticipated when the drugs cholestyramine and colestipol are used. These resinous materials, which are not absorbed from the gastrointestinal tract, bind with bile acids and prevent their reabsorption. In addition to binding with bile acids, cholestyramine and colestipol can bind with drugs that are present in the gastrointestinal tract, and reports suggest that these agents may reduce the absorption of thyroid hormone, warfarin, digoxin and thiazide diuretics. To minimize the possibility of an interaction, the interval between the administration of cholestyramine or colestipol and another drug should be as long as possible.

Two naturally occurring human bile acids, chenodiol and ursodiol, are used in the dissolution of gallstones composed primarily of cholesterol. Because of the affinity of cholestyramine and colestipol for bile acids, the administration of these agents should be separated by as long an interval as possible.

It also should be recognized that prolonged administration of cholestyramine and colestipol can decrease the absorption of fat-soluble vitamins such as vitamin K. This could lead to increased bleeding tendencies in some patients if the vitamin K intake is not increased. When cholestyramine or colestipol is administered to a patient on warfarin therapy, it is understandably difficult to predict the eventual response since, conceivably, the absorption of both the anticoagulant and its antagonist, vitamin K, could be reduced.

Antidiarrheal Agents and Antacids—It has been suggested that since certain antidiarrheal agents (eg, attapulgite) can adsorb toxic substances responsible for causing diarrhea, they also might be capable of adsorbing certain medications that are administered concurrently, resulting in a decrease in their absorption. The occurrence of such interactions has not been evaluated thoroughly. However, since certain antidiarrheal agents and antacids possess this adsorptive potential, the interval between the administration of one of these preparations and another drug should be as long as possible.

Penicillamine—Metals—Aluminum and iron salts have been reported to significantly reduce the absorption of penicillamine, probably through chelation and/or adsorption mechanisms. An interval of at least 2 hours should separate the administration of an antacid or iron salt and penicillamine. Food also will decrease the absorption of penicillanime and the drug should be administered apart from meals.

Alteration of Motility/Rate of Gastric Emptying

Cathartics—A cathartic, by increasing gastrointestinal motility, may increase the rate at which another drug passes through the gastrointestinal tract. This could result in a decreased absorption of certain drugs, particularly those which normally are absorbed slowly and require prolonged contact with the absorbing surface or those which are absorbed only at a particular site along the gastrointestinal tract. Similar problems might be noted with enteric-coated and controlled-release formulations.

Anticholinergics—Anticholinergics, by decreasing gastrointestinal motility, also may influence drug absorption. The effect may be one of decreased absorption, since the reduced peristalsis may retard dissolution, and the slowing of gastric emptying may delay absorption from the small intestine, or increased absorption if a drug is retained for a longer period of time in the area from which it is optimally absorbed.

Metoclopramide and Cisapride—Because metoclopramide and cisapride increase motility of the upper gastrointestinal tract, it should be anticipated that they may influence the absorption of other drugs administered concurrently. For example, it has been suggested that the acceleration of gastric emptying caused by cisapride may potentiate the sedative effects of alcohol and the benzodiazepines.

The Effect of Food

It is known that food can influence the absorption of a number of drugs. In some situations, absorption may be delayed but not reduced, whereas in other circumstances the total amount of drug absorbed may be reduced. The effect of food in influencing drug absorption sometimes is due to its action in slowing gastric emptying. However, food also may affect absorption by binding with drugs, decreasing the access of drugs to sites of absorption, altering the dissolution rate of drugs or altering the pH of the gastrointestinal contents. The drug-administration time schedules used in many hospitals and long-term care facilities may correspond closely to the times at which meals are served. It is important that a specific dosage schedule be established for those drugs that should be administered apart from meals, or with food.

Anti-Infective Agents—Food—The presence of food in the gastrointestinal tract will reduce the absorption of many anti-infective agents. Although there are some exceptions (eg, penicillin V, amoxicillin, doxycycline, minocycline, lomefloxacin), it generally is recommended that the penicillin, tetracycline and fluoroquinolone derivatives, as well as certain other anti-infective agents be given at least 1 hour before meals or 2 hours after meals, to achieve optimum absorption.

Erythromycin stearate formulations should be administered at least 1 hour before meals or 2 hours after a meal, whereas formulations of erythromycin ethylsuccinate and estolate may be given without regard to meals.

The formulations of erythromycin base should be considered on an individual basis because the information for some products indicates they may be given without regard to meals, whereas for other products it is noted that optimum absorption is achieved when given apart from meals.

Food reduces the absorption of the antiviral drug didanosine by as much as 50%, and it is recommended that patients have nothing to eat or drink, except water, for at least 1 hour before and after taking the drug.

The absorption of the antiprotozoal drug atovaquone can be increased significantly (ie, an approximately threefold increase in bioavailability) when the drug is taken with food. Patients must be advised of the importance of administering atovaquone with food because failure to do so may result in an inadequate therapeutic response. In particular, foods with a high fat content (eg, eggs, butter, milk, cheese, pizza, fried foods) significantly enhance the absorption of atovaquone.

Theophylline-Food—It generally has been felt that food does not alter the activity of theophylline significantly when the drug is administered in an immediate-release formulation (ie, those formulations which are not controlled-release). It is likely that many of the controlled-release dosage forms of theophylline also can be given with food without an interaction occurring. However, the extensive discussion that has occurred regarding the influence of food on the absorption of certain of these formulations warrants consideration of these products on an individual basis.

For example, studies with the *Theo-24* formulation indicate that, if the drug is taken less than 1 hour before a high fat-content meal, theophylline absorption and peak serum levels may increase significantly as compared to administration in the fasting state. This response increases the risk of toxicity, and it is recommended that patients receiving large single daily doses (ie, equal to or greater than 900 mg or 13 mg/kg, whichever is less) should avoid eating a high-fat-content breakfast or should take the medication at least 1 hour before eating. If it is anticipated that the patient will not comply with these instructions, a twice-a-day dosing regimen should be used.

Conversely, data indicate that when the *Theo-Dur Sprinkle* formulation is administered with food, the extent of absorption and peak serum concentrations of theophylline are reduced, with as little as 40% of the dose being absorbed following the meal. Therefore, it is advised that this formulation be administered at least 1 hour before or 2 hours after a meal.

Considerable variation is seen among the controlled-release formulations of theophylline with respect to their potential to interact with food. If data are insufficient to assess the potential for a particular theophylline formulation to interact with food, the medication preferably should be administered apart from meals.

It also has been reported that the rate of metabolism of theophylline is increased in individuals consuming large amounts of charcoal-broiled beef, and this has been attributed to the enzyme induction effect of the polycyclic hydrocarbons introduced in this cooking process.

Captopril—Food—The presence of food in the gastrointestinal tract has been reported to reduce the absorption of captopril by 30 to 40%. Although more recent investigations suggest that food is unlikely to alter significantly the effects of captopril, it is advisable to administer the drug 1 hour before meals until this question is resolved. Food does not appear to alter the absorption of most of the other angiotensin converting enzyme inhibitors (eg, enalapril, lisinopril).

Astemizole—Food—The absorption of astemizole is reduced by 60% when taken with meals. The drug should be taken at least 2 hours after a meal and there should be no additional food intake for at least 1 hour after a dose.

Tacrine—Food—Food decreases tacrine bioavailability by as much as 40%, and it is recommended that the drug be administered at least 1 hour before meals. However, gastrointestinal effects commonly are associated with the use of tacrine and, if gastrointestinal upset occurs, the drug may be taken with food to improve tolerability, although a significant reduction in plasma concentrations should be expected.

Alteration of Metabolism in the Gastrointestinal Tract

The absorption of certain agents is influenced by the extent to which they are metabolized in the gastrointestinal tract.

Monoamine Oxidase Inhibitors—Tyramine—There have been reports of serious reactions (hypertensive crisis) occurring in people being treated with a monoamine oxidase (MAO) inhibitor (eg, isocarboxazid, phenelzine, tranylcypromine) following ingestion of certain foods having a high content of pressor substances, such as tyramine.

Tyramine is metabolized by MAO, and normally these enzymes in the intestinal wall and in the liver protect against the pressor actions of amines in foods. However, when these enzymes are inhibited, large quantities of unmetabolized tyramine can accumulate and act to release norepinephrine from adrenergic neurons where greater-than-usual stores of this catecholamine are concentrated as a result of MAO inhibition. Among the foods having the highest tyramine content are aged cheeses (eg, cheddar; in contrast, cottage and cream cheeses contain little or no tyramine and need not be restricted), certain alcoholic beverages (eg, Chianti wine), pickled fish (eg, herring), concentrated yeast extracts and broad-bean pods (also known as fava beans or Italian green beans).

The pharmaceutical companies which market the MAO inhibitors have developed lists of dietary items which patients taking one of these agents should avoid. This information should be provided to and discussed with each patient for whom a MAO inhibitor is prescribed.

Alteration of Gastrointestinal Flora

Changes in the microbial flora of the gastrointestinal tract caused by antibiotics may alter the production or metabolism of certain agents, with a resultant change in the amount of agent being absorbed and available to produce a clinical response.

Anticoagulants—Antibiotics—A number of anti- infective agents have been reported to enhance the effect of concurrently administered anticoagulants. It has been suggested that this effect develops, in part, as a result of interference by the anti-infective agent with production of vitamin K by microorganisms in the gastrointestinal tract. Broad-spectrum antibiotics, such as the tetracyclines, are most likely to cause problems of this type although similar effects also may be seen with other antibiotics. The clinical importance of this mechanism has been questioned, and, if it is a factor, it is likely that problems will occur only in patients who have a low dietary intake of vitamin K.

It is also probable that other mechanisms may be involved in some of these interactions. For example, the increased anticoagulant effect noted when sulfonamides and anticoagulants are given concurrently may be due, in part, to displacement of the anticoagulant from protein-binding sites.

Digoxin—Antibiotics—It is estimated that approximately 10% of patients being treated with digoxin convert a significant portion of the parent compound to inactive reduction metabolites in the gastrointestinal tract. The bacterial flora of the intestine contributes to this metabolic process. Elevated serum digoxin concentrations have been observed in patients receiving erythromycin or tetracycline concurrently, and it is suggested that these antibiotics, by reducing the bacterial flora, decrease the extent to which digoxin is metabolized in the gastrointestinal tract, resulting in the higher serum concentrations of the cardiac glycoside.

Oral Contraceptives—Antibiotics—Several antibiotics (eg, ampicillin) have been suggested to decrease the effectiveness of oral contraceptives. The estrogen component of the contraceptive formulation is conjugated to a large extent in the liver and excreted in the bile. Bacteria in the intestine hydrolyze the conjugated form of the estrogen, permitting the free drug to be reabsorbed and contribute to the serum concentration of the estrogen. Antibiotics, by reducing the bacterial flora, may interrupt the enterohepatic circulation with a resultant reduction in serum estrogen concentrations.

Although questions have been raised regarding the significance of this interaction, it would be desirable for patients to use supplementary contraceptive measures in addition to the oral contraceptive, during cycles in which antibiotics are used.

Malabsorption States

Certain drugs, such as laxatives, colchicine, cholestyramine and colestipol, have been reported to cause malabsorption problems that result in decreased absorption of vitamins and nutrients from the gastrointestinal tract. It should be recognized that these agents may alter absorption of other drugs that are administered simultaneously, and several examples with cholestyramine already have been considered.

Alteration of Distribution

Displacement from Protein Binding Sites

An interaction of this type may occur when two drugs which are capable of binding to proteins are administered concurrently. Although they may bind at different sites on the protein, the binding characteristics of one of the drugs may be altered (noncompetitive displacement). Probably more significant are situations in which two drugs are capable of binding to the same sites on the protein (competitive displacement). Since there are only a limited number of protein binding sites, competition will exist and the drug with the greater affinity for the binding sites will displace the other from plasma or tissue proteins. It is recognized that the protein-bound fraction of a drug in the body is not pharmacologically active. However, an equilibrium exists between bound and unbound fractions, and as the unbound or "free" form of the drug is metabolized and excreted, bound drug is released gradually to maintain the equilibrium and pharmacological response.

The binding of acidic drugs to serum albumin represents the type of drug-protein binding which has been studied most extensively. The binding to albumin is readily reversible and the albumin-drug complex essentially serves as a reservoir that releases more drug as the free drug is metabolized and/or excreted. The importance of the binding of basic drugs (eg, propranolol or lidocaine) to α_1-acid glycoprotein (AAG) also has been recognized. Even small increases in the reactant protein concentration, such as might be associated with infection and inflammation, can result in significant changes in the concentration of free drug.

The risk of an interaction occurring is greatest with drugs that are highly protein-bound (more than 90%) and also have a small apparent volume of distribution. Since only a small fraction of the drug ordinarily would be available in the "free" form, the displacement of even a small percentage of the amount that is bound to proteins could produce a considerable increase in activity.

Warfarin—Phenylbutazone—Both phenylbutazone and warfarin are bound extensively to plasma proteins, in particular to albumin. Phenylbutazone, however, apparently has a greater affinity for the binding sites, resulting in displacement of warfarin and making increased quantities of the "free" drug available. In this situation the activity of the anticoagulant is increased, and risk of hemorrhaging exists. This interaction is highly significant and potentially dangerous and concurrent therapy should be avoided.

The risk of interactions resulting from protein displacement appears to be greatest during the first several days of concurrent therapy. It has been suggested that drugs having the greatest capability of displacing warfarin can increase the anticoagulant response within 24 hours and exhibit maximum potentiation in three to five days. After this period the effect levels off since the drug, as a result of greater amounts being available in the unbound form, also is being metabolized more rapidly and excreted. Therefore, the anticoagulant usually has a shorter half-life when a displacing agent is given concurrently.

In the case of the warfarin-phenylbutazone interaction, it has been noted that the enhancement of anticoagulant activity persisted beyond the time which could be explained by the mechanism of drug displacement alone. Warfarin is a racemic mixture of *R*- and *S*-isomers and subsequent studies have shown that phenylbutazone inhibits the metabolism of the *S*-enantiomer (which is considerably more active than the *R*-enantiomer), resulting in an increased anticoagulant response. This represents a second important mechanism contributing to the occurrence of the interaction and provides the explanation for the continued enhancement of the anticoagulant effect.

Warfarin—Chloral Hydrate—It has been suggested that trichloroacetic acid, a major metabolite of chloral hydrate which is highly bound to protein, can displace warfarin from protein-binding sites, thus increasing the anticoagulant response. Several studies designed to assess the risk of an interaction between chloral hydrate and warfarin have found either no evidence of an interaction or a moderate increase in anticoagulant response. Although the risk of a serious interaction may be low, the possibility cannot be excluded, and it would seem preferable to use an alternate hypnotic agent such as a benzodiazepine, which is not likely to interact.

Methotrexate—Methotrexate is highly bound to plasma proteins, and it has been suggested that agents such as the salicylates may be capable of displacing it from binding sites. Studies also indicate that salicylates may increase the action of methotrexate by inhibiting its renal excretion. Although data pertaining to this interaction are limited, the potential for toxicity with methotrexate dictates extreme caution in any situation in which it is used.

Phenytoin—Valproic acid—Valproic acid has been reported to displace phenytoin from plasma protein binding sites and some studies suggest it also may inhibit the metabolism of phenytoin. In some patients the result may be significantly increased free phenytoin concentrations and the occurrence of adverse reactions, even when the total phenytoin serum concentrations are within what would ordinarily be considered the desired therapeutic range. The evaluation of the potential for these agents to interact is made even more complex by reports that phenytoin may decrease valproic acid plasma concentrations. Combination therapy with these agents should be monitored closely, with dosage adjustments made as needed, in an effort to achieve effective control of the seizure disorders for which they have been prescribed with as low a risk of adverse reactions as possible.

Reduced Albumin Concentrations—Because many drugs are bound extensively to plasma proteins, a decreased concentration or amount of protein theoretically could change the availability of drugs, and thus their activity. Although the type and incidence of clinical problems have not been determined conclusively, several reports suggest that the incidence of adverse effects with certain drugs may be higher in patients with conditions associated with hypoalbuminemia (eg, renal, hepatic and gastrointestinal diseases).

A relationship between prednisone dosage, frequency of side effects and serum albumin concentrations has been shown in one study. When the serum albumin concentration is less than 2.5 g/100 mL, the frequency of prednisone side effects is almost doubled, and this is attributed to an increased concentration of prednisolone, an active metabolite of prednisone.

In another study it was noted that the incidence of adverse reactions to phenytoin was greater in patients with low serum albumin concentrations. It is suggested that the higher incidence of adverse effects in the hypoalbuminemic patients is probably due to increased circulating concentrations of unbound phenytoin.

Protein Binding in Disease States—It has been noted in an increasing number of reports that the response to a particular drug was altered in the presence of a certain pathologic state. Most studies have evaluated the action of drugs in the presence of impaired renal function. In one study the binding of phenytoin to plasma proteins was found to be decreased in patients with poor renal function, this being attributed to a qualitative change in the drug-binding proteins rather than to a decrease in serum albumin or total protein concentrations. Since this results in a greater amount of the drug being available in the "free" or active form, it is likely that favorable clinical responses with phenytoin will be noted at relatively low total plasma concentrations ordinarily considered to be nontoxic. This must be considered when total plasma concentration values of protein-bound drugs are used to establish or monitor dosage regimens.

Stimulation of Metabolism

Many drug interactions have resulted from the ability of one drug to stimulate the metabolism of another, most often by increasing the activity of hepatic enzymes that are involved in the metabolism of numerous therapeutic agents. The increased activity probably is due to enhanced enzyme synthesis, resulting in increased amounts of drug-metabolizing enzymes, an effect frequently referred to as *enzyme induction*. These situations have been documented well with phenobarbital, phenytoin, carbamazepine and rifampin being the agents best recognized as causing enzyme induction.

Drug metabolism most commonly involves oxidation, reduction, hydrolysis and conjugation (eg, with glucuronic acid) reactions. Quantitatively, the most important hepatic enzymes are the mixed-function oxidases (MFO), in particular the cytochrome P-450 enzymes. These enzymes are responsible for the oxidation—often, hydroxylation—of a large number of drugs, such as warfarin and phenytoin.

In most situations, drugs are converted to less active, water-soluble metabolites, and enzyme induction usually will result in an increased metabolism and excretion, and a reduced pharmacologic action of the agent being metabolized by hepatic enzymes. Less frequently, a drug may be converted to a metabolite that is more active than the parent compound and there may be an enhanced response. However, the increased effect may be somewhat offset since the drug will be excreted more rapidly and have a shorter duration of action.

The stimulation of hepatic enzyme activity is not only a factor in the development of drug interactions, but also may be responsible for a drug (eg, carbamazepine) stimulating its own metabolism. With continued use, the half-life of the drug will decrease, possibly resulting in a need to increase the dosage.

Warfarin—Phenobarbital—By causing enzyme induction, phenobarbital can increase the rate of metabolism of warfarin. The result of this interaction is a decreased response to the anticoagulant since it is being metabolized more rapidly and excreted, possibly leading to an increased risk of thrombus formation if the interaction is not recognized. To compensate for this loss of effect, the dose of warfarin would have to be increased until the desired activity was obtained. If the dose of warfarin has been increased to compensate for loss of activity, it will have to be reduced when phenobarbital is discontinued. Otherwise, the readjusted higher dosage that was necessary when phenobarbital was given concurrently may be excessive when it is withdrawn and possibly result in hemorrhaging.

It is probable that all barbiturates have the ability to cause enzyme induction although phenobarbital may be a more potent inducing agent than analogs having a shorter duration of action. Several studies indicate that the effect of barbiturates in decreasing anticoagulant activity is evident within 2 to 5 days, and it is suggested that the administration of a barbiturate for a week or longer is likely to produce this effect in most patients. There have been varying reports as to how rapidly enzyme activity returns to pretreatment levels when the barbiturate is discontinued. However, it is probable that in most situations normal enzyme activity will be restored in 2 to 3 weeks.

Although close monitoring of combined barbiturate-anticoagulant therapy usually will prevent problems from developing, it would seem unwise to expose the patient unnecessarily to the risk of an interaction when therapeutic alternatives are available. The benzodiazepines (eg, diazepam, temazepam) are not likely to interact with anticoagulants and one of these agents might be useful as an alternative to a barbiturate. These alternatives apply to the use of a barbiturate as a sedative-hypnotic. Although some benzodiazepines have been used in certain types of convulsive disorders they would not be adequate alternatives to phenobarbital when the latter is used in the treatment of these conditions.

Oral Contraceptives—Phenobarbital, rifampin and other drugs are known to increase the metabolism of steroid hormones, including estrogens and progestins that are used in oral contraceptive formulations. The high rate of effectiveness of oral contraceptives may suggest that other agents are not likely to reduce their effect significantly. However, there is concern that agents capable of causing enzyme induction indeed may reduce the effectiveness of oral contraceptives. This possibility takes on increased significance in view of the fact that the dosages of the hormones included in these products have been decreased in the interest of minimizing the risk of adverse effects. It is possible that the lower dosages of the hormones used in certain products could be approaching the minimum effective level and that addition of another agent which can reduce their action is sufficient to compromise their effectiveness.

It has been reported that women taking other drugs in addition to an oral contraceptive experience more spotting and breakthrough bleeding. It is suggested that enzyme-inducing agents cause a decrease in hormonal levels which results in withdrawal bleeding and, that when such disturbances occur in women who previously have not experienced such a response with the use of oral contraceptives, the method should be regarded as no longer reliable.

Glucocorticoids—One study of patients with asthma noted increased bronchospasm and pulmonary function deterioration when phenobarbital therapy (120 mg daily in four divided doses) was initiated in three prednisone-dependent patients. Withdrawal of phenobarbital reversed these changes. Other investigations have shown that phenobarbital causes a significant decrease in the half-life of dexamethasone. It is likely that the ability of phenobarbital to increase the rate of metabolism of these steroids is responsible for these effects.

Other studies have shown phenytoin to increase the rate of metabolism of prednisolone and dexamethasone, and similar caution should be exercised when phenytoin or other agents capable of causing enzyme induction are given concurrently with steroid hormones.

Vitamin D—Phenytoin and Phenobarbital—A number of studies have associated disturbances of calcium metabolism and development of rickets and osteomalacia with the use of anticonvulsants such as phenobarbital and phenytoin. Reduced serum calcium concentrations have been noted in a number of patients on long-term anticonvulsant therapy, evidence indicating that this is the result of vitamin D deficiency. Although other factors also may be involved, most reports indicate that anticonvulsants, by causing enzyme induction, increase the rate of metabolism of vitamin D, thereby causing the deficiency.

The possibility of deficiency developing is greater in individuals whose dietary intake of this vitamin is low or borderline. The incidence and severity of the clinical problems are increased with use of multiple-drug regimens and appear to be directly proportional to the total daily dose of anticonvulsant drugs.

Smoking—A number of studies have indicated that the effects of certain drugs may be decreased in individuals who are heavy smokers, presumably due to increased hepatic enzyme activity resulting from the action of polycyclic hydrocarbons which are present in cigarette smoke. Among the drugs whose metabolism is increased and therapeutic activity likely to be reduced are chlorpromazine, diazepam, propoxyphene, theophylline, pentazocine and tricyclic antidepressants. The results of a recent study suggest that the induction of theophylline clearance by phenytoin is additive to that caused by cigarette smoking. In addition to monitoring therapy carefully, with drugs which are metabolized by hepatic enzyme systems in patients who are moderate or heavy smokers, attention also has been called to the need to ascertain the level of smoking when drugs initially are evaluated in clinical trials.

In the examples noted, the effect of smoking is to increase the rate of metabolism of other agents being utilized, and a decreased response to these agents can be anticipated. In contrast, a significant risk of toxicity exists when oral contraceptives are used by women who smoke as it has been noted that smoking markedly increases the risk of serious cardiovascular effects (eg, myocardial infarction), especially in women over 35 years of age.

Charcoal Broiling—When meat is charcoal-broiled, polycyclic hydrocarbons are formed and deposited on the meat. It has been reported that the rate of metabolism of theophylline is increased in individuals consuming large amounts of charcoal-broiled beef. This has been attributed to the enzyme induction effect of the polycyclic hydrocarbons introduced in this cooking process.

Alcohol—Alcohol may either stimulate or inhibit the activity of hepatic enzymes, depending on the circumstances of use. An increased rate of metabolism of tolbutamide, warfarin and phenytoin has been reported in alcoholic patients. This was attributed to increased liver enzyme activity caused by chronic administration of alcohol.

In contrast, acute use of alcohol by nonalcoholic individuals may cause inhibition of hepatic enzymes. This may decrease the rate of metabolism, thereby increasing the effect of other agents administered concurrently, and may be responsible, at least in part, for the enhanced sedation experienced when alcoholic beverages and sedative drugs are taken together by individuals who are not alcoholics. The extent to which the mechanism of enzyme inhibition and central nervous system summation or synergism are involved in this interaction remains to be clarified.

Levodopa—Pyridoxine—Pyridoxine has been shown to antagonize the action of levodopa, presumably by accelerating its decarboxylation to dopamine in the peripheral tissues. Consequently, less levodopa reaches and crosses the blood-brain barrier, with the result that less dopamine is formed in the brain and the therapeutic effect is diminished. The labeling for levodopa formulations notes that pyridoxine, in doses of 10 to 25 mg, rapidly reverses the effect of the antiparkinson drug.

The combination product, *Sinemet*, contains both levodopa and carbidopa, the latter agent acting as an inhibitor of decarboxylase enzymes. When administered with levodopa, carbidopa permits the use of significantly lower doses of the former since it now is metabolized to a lesser extent in the peripheral tissues. The decrease in dosage often is accompanied by a decreased incidence of adverse effects. Since carbidopa does not cross the blood-brain barrier, it will not hinder the conversion of levodopa to dopamine in the brain.

The use of carbidopa with levodopa initially raised questions because of the awareness that agents which are similar chemically to carbidopa can induce pyridoxine deficiency. Therefore, it was anticipated that if such a deficiency did develop, the need to give pyridoxine to overcome the deficiency would result in an antagonism of the effects of levodopa. However, in studies of patients receiving levodopa and carbidopa, the addition of pyridoxine did not result in a reappearance of parkinsonian symptoms; indeed, in some investigations there appeared to be an enhancement of the effect of levodopa.

The apparent explanation for this paradoxical effect of pyridoxine is that carbidopa, which does not enter the brain, blocks the action of pyridoxine in the peripheral tissues, thereby inhibiting the action of decarboxylase enzymes. This permits passage of greater amounts of levodopa to the brain. The pyridoxine that is not blocked enters the brain and activates the decarboxylase enzymes, thereby facilitating the conversion of levodopa to dopamine.

Inhibition of Metabolism

A number of situations have been reported in which one drug has inhibited the metabolism of another, usually resulting in a prolonged and dintensified activity of the latter.

Alcohol—Disulfiram—A well-known example of inhibition of metabolism that has been used to advantage is the use of disulfiram in the treatment of alcoholism. Disulfiram inhibits the activity of aldehyde dehydrogenase, thus inhibiting oxidation of acetaldehyde, an oxidation product of alcohol. This results in accumulation of excessive quantities of acetaldehyde and development of the unpleasant effects characteristic of the disulfiram reaction.

Disulfiram apparently is not a selective inhibitor of aldehyde dehydrogenase but exhibits several inhibitory actions that can result in the development of drug interactions. It has been reported that it can enhance the activity of warfarin and phenytoin, presumably by inhibiting their metabolism.

Alcohol—Cephalosporins—Disulfiram-like reactions have been observed in patients receiving cefamandole, cefmetazole, cefoperazone, cefotetan and moxalactam, following the consumption of alcoholic beverages. The interaction is likely to occur only when the alcohol ingestion follows the administration of the antibiotic and the reaction may be observed as late as 72 hours after the last dose of antibiotic.

The five cephalosporins implicated in these interactions contain a methylthiotetrazole substituent and this structural characteristic is considered to be responsible for these interactions.

Mercaptopurine and Azathioprine—Allopurinol—Allopurinol, by inhibiting the enzyme xanthine oxidase, reduces production of uric acid and is the basis for its use in the treatment of gout. Xanthine oxidase also has an important role in the metabolism of such potentially toxic drugs as mercaptopurine and azathioprine, and when this enzyme is inhibited by allopurinol, the effect of the latter agents can be increased markedly. When allopurinol is given in doses of 300 to 600 mg/day concurrently with either of these drugs, it is advised that the dose of mercaptopurine or azathioprine be reduced to about ⅓ to ¼ the usual dose.

Benzodiazepines—Cimetidine—The inhibition of oxidative metabolic pathways by cimetidine has been demonstrated in a number of investigations, and it should be anticipated that the action of concurrently administered drugs which are metabolized via these pathways will be increased. Cimetidine has been reported to inhibit the metabolism of chlordiazepoxide, diazepam and several other benzodiazepines, and the sedative effect of these agents may be enhanced as a result of the interaction. Particular caution is necessary in elderly patients who may exhibit an increased sensitivity to the depressant effects of the benzodiazepines, even when one of these agents is given alone. The metabolism of lorazepam, oxazepam and temazepam is not likely to be affected, since cimetidine does not alter the glucuronide conjugation of these agents. One of these agents may be preferred when a benzodiazepine is indicated in a patient being treated with cimetidine.

Cimetidine—Because cimetidine is known to inhibit hepatic oxidative enzyme systems, it should be anticipated that the action of other agents which are metabolized extensively via this pathway will be increased. There have been reports of such interactions with carbamazepine, phenytoin, theophylline, warfarin and other agents, and it may be necessary to reduce the dosage of these agents when cimetidine is included in the therapeutic regimen. Although ranitidine also binds to a limited extent to the cytochrome P-450 enzymes involved in the metabolism of these agents, it appears to have a lesser affinity for the enzymes than cimetidine. Consequently, clinically significant interactions are less likely to occur with ranitidine. Studies of the other histamine H_2-receptor antagonists (famotidine and nizatidine) suggest that they are not likely to inhibit oxidative metabolic pathways and to interact with other drugs via this mechanism.

Theophylline—Macrolide Antibiotics—Erythromycin has been reported to increase significantly serum theophylline concentrations by inhibiting its hepatic metabolism. Patients receiving high doses of theophylline or who are otherwise predisposed to theophylline toxicity, should be monitored closely when erythromycin is administered concurrently. It also should be anticipated that clarithromycin and troleandomycin will inhibit the metabolism of theophylline, whereas azithromycin appears unlikely to interact.

Theophylline—Fluoroquinolones—Ciprofloxacin and enoxacin have been reported to markedly increase the plasma concentrations and activity of theophylline, presumably by inhibiting its hepatic metabolism. Norfloxacin and ofloxacin also may increase theophylline concentrations but to a lesser extent than has been reported with ciprofloxacin and enoxacin. Lomefloxacin appears unlikely to interact with theophylline.

Terfenadine and Astemizole anti-infective Agents—There have been rare reports of serious cardiovascular reactions (eg, ventricular arrhythmias) in patients taking terfenadine or astemizole concurrently with ketoconazole or erythromycin. By inhibiting the hepatic metabolism of astemizole and terfenadine (and its active metabolite), these anti-infective agents increase the serum concentrations of the antihistamines and the risk of toxicity. The concurrent use of terfenadine or astemizole with ketoconazole or erythromycin (or the related agents itraconazole, clarithromycin or troleandomycin) should be avoided.

The use of the nonsedating antihistamine loratidine has not been associated with the occurrence of serious cardiovascular reactions, even in a study in which it was used in a dosage that is four times the recommended dosage. Although ketoconazole and erythromycin have been reported to increase the serum concentrations of loratidine, this interaction is probably not of clinical importance because even the higher concentrations of loratidine have not been reported to cause serious adverse reactions.

Monoamine Oxidase Inhibitors—There have been many reports of drug interactions involving use of a monoamine oxidase (MAO) inhibitor with another drug or with certain dietary items. It is likely that MAO inhibitors enhance the effect of drugs like the barbiturates and narcotics by inhibiting hepatic enzyme systems involved in their metabolism. However, other mechanisms are involved in some of the more publicized problems with these compounds and are considered elsewhere in this chapter.

Calcium Channel Blocking Agents—The calcium channel blocking agents (eg, diltiazem, nifedipine or verapamil) have been reported to interact with a number of drugs although the mechanisms through which these interactions occur are not defined well. It has been suggested that verapamil and diltiazem may inhibit the hepatic metabolism of carbamazepine, thereby increasing the activity of the latter agent. Because the calcium channel blocking agents are metabolized themselves in the liver, they may interact with certain drugs because they are competing for the same metabolic pathways.

Propranolol—Food—Observations of an enhanced bioavailability of propranolol and metoprolol in the presence of food, present interesting implications. Both drugs are subject to considerable first-pass metabolism in the liver after oral administration. It is suggested that the transient increase in hepatic blood flow associated with the ingestion of food may reduce hepatic extraction of the drugs and firstpass metabolism, resulting in increased bioavailability. The increase in bioavailability appears to be related to the protein content of the meal and a minimum amount of protein must be present in the meal to induce an effect. In contrast to propranolol and metoprolol, most other beta-adrenergic blocking agents are not metabolized significantly, and it is unlikely that the bioavailability of these agents would be altered appreciably by food.

Alteration of Excretion

Although some therapeutic agents are eliminated via other mechanisms, most drugs and their metabolites are excreted via the kidneys. The most important clinical implications of altering renal excretion involve the use of drugs which are excreted in their unchanged form or in the form of an active metabolite. Thus, substances with pharmacological activity are being reabsorbed or excreted to a greater extent when renal excretion is altered. In contrast, when only inactive metabolites are being excreted, changes in therapeutic activity are less likely to be associated with the use of other drugs which can influence renal excretory pathways.

Alteration of Urinary pH

Alteration of urinary pH can influence the activity of certain drugs. For example, acidifying agents are administered with methenamine to enhance its antibacterial activity. Methenamine must be converted to formaldehyde, which is the active antibacterial substance, and for this conversion to take place so an adequate concentration of formaldehyde is achieved, the urinary pH should be 5.5 or less.

Salicylates—Acidifying and Alkalinizing Agents—A change in urinary pH will influence the ionization of weak acids and weak bases and thus affect the extent to which these agents are reabsorbed and excreted. When a drug is in its nonionized form it will diffuse more readily from urine back into blood. Therefore, for an acidic drug, there will be a larger proportion of drug in the nonionized form in an acid urine than in an alkaline urine—where it will exist primarily as an ionized salt. The result is that from an acid urine more of an acidic drug will diffuse back into the blood and produce a prolonged, and perhaps intensified, activity. In one study it was noted that a salicylate dosage regimen that provided a serum concentration of 20 to 30 μg/mL in a patient when the urinary pH was approximately 6.5, produced serum concentrations that were approximately twice as high when the urinary pH was decreased to 5.5. The risk of a significant interaction is greatest in patients who are taking large doses of salicylates (eg, for arthritis).

The ability of "systemic" antacids such as sodium bicarbonate to increase urinary pH is well-known. Not as well recognized, however, are the circumstances in which "non-systemic" antacids may increase urinary pH. In one study, an aluminum and magnesium hydroxide antacid was administered concomitantly with aspirin to three children with rheumatic fever. In each case the urinary pH was increased, and serum salicylate concentrations decreased by 30 to 70%. The effect of an antacid on urinary pH depends on the kind of antacid, the dose and the pH before antacid administration. In patients on salicylate therapy (especially when the maximum recommended dosage level is approached), the initiation or discontinuation of antacid administration, or switching of antacid products, is cause to monitor serum salicylate concentrations and patient response.

Amphetamines—Alkalinizing Agents—Converse effects will be seen for a basic drug like dextroamphetamine.

In one investigation the excretion of a dose of dextroamphetamine at urinary pH values of approximately 5 and 8 was studied. When the urinary pH was maintained at approximately 5, 54.5% of the dose of dextroamphetamine was excreted within 16 hours, as compared to a 2.9% excretion in the same period when the urinary pH was maintained at approximately 8.

Similar observations have been made with other basic drugs. One report calls attention to the possible development of quinidine toxicity when urine becomes alkaline, since excretion of quinidine was shown to decrease considerably as urinary pH was raised. In another investigation, when the urinary pH was increased to about 8 with sodium bicarbonate, the plasma half-life of pseudoephedrine (*Sudafed*) was approximately double that in normal subjects. When urinary pH in the same subjects was decreased to 5.2, using ammonium chloride, the plasma half-life decreased markedly from control values.

Alteration of Active Transport

Penicillins—Probenecid—A number of organic acids are transported actively from the blood into the tubular urine and vice versa. In some situations these agents interfere with the excretion of each other. It is well-recognized that probenecid can increase serum concentrations and prolong activity of penicillin derivatives by blocking their tubular secretion, and this interaction has been used to therapeutic advantage. Often there will be a twofold to fourfold elevation of serum penicillin concentrations, although the degree to which these concentrations are increased and the duration of activity is prolonged depend on a number of factors.

Probenecid also has been reported to decrease renal excretion of other agents, including methotrexate.

Methotrexate—Nonsteroidal Anti-Inflammatory Drugs—A number of nonsteroidal anti-inflammatory drugs (NSAIDs) have been reported to increase the activity and toxicity of methotrexate. There have been several reports of fatal methotrexate toxicity in patients also receiving ketoprofen, and it has been suggested that ketoprofen inhibited the active renal tubular secretion of methotrexate. However, other mechanisms probably also contribute to an increase in serum methotrexate concentrations. Most of the patients in whom these interactions have been reported were receiving high-dose methotrexate therapy for neoplastic disorders. However, caution also should be exercised in patients receiving lower doses, particularly since there is an increased use of low-dose methotrexate regimens in patients with rheumatoid arthritis who also are taking an NSAID.

Digoxin—Quinidine—A number of reports have noted significantly greater serum digoxin concentrations when quinidine was administered concurrently than when digoxin was given alone. Digoxin is secreted actively in the renal tubules and a primary cause of the quinidine-induced increase in serum digoxin concentrations appears to be a reduction in the renal clearance of digoxin. However, other mechanisms probably are involved also as it has been suggested that quinidine also may reduce the nonrenal clearance of digoxin and reduce the volume of distribution by displacing digoxin from tissue binding sites. In one study, a rise in the serum digoxin concentrations was observed within 2 to 3 days following the addition of quinidine to the regimen. A new plateau was reached in approximately 5 days and, when quinidine was discontinued, an average of 5 days passed before the serum digoxin concentrations returned to the prequinidine concentrations.

Digoxin—Verapamil—Verapamil has been reported to increase serum digoxin concentrations by 50% to 70% during the 1st week in which the agents are administered concurrently, and it usually will be necessary to reduce the dose of the cardiac glycoside. It has been suggested that verapamil may inhibit both the renal tubular secretion and nonrenal elimination of digoxin, resulting in the increase in the serum concentrations of the latter.

Lithium—Nonsteroidal Anti-Inflammatory Drugs—The serum concentrations and incidence of adverse effects of lithium salts have been reported to be increased by the concurrent administration of anti-inflammatory agents such as ibuprofen, indomethacin and piroxicam. It is suggested that the renal clearance of lithium is reduced as a result of the action of these anti-inflammatory agents to inhibit renal prostaglandin synthesis. This interaction probably should be anticipated when any NSAID is administered concurrently with a lithium salt.

Pharmacodynamic Interactions

Although pharmacokinetic interactions often present challenging clinical problems and are publicized widely, pharmacodynamic interactions are the type which occur most frequently.

Drugs Having Opposing Pharmacological Effects

Interactions resulting from the use of two drugs with opposing effects should be among the easiest to detect. However, these sometimes are due to the secondary effects of certain drugs and this, and other factors, may preclude early identification of such situations.

Diuretics—The ability of the thiazides, and certain other diuretics, to elevate blood glucose concentrations is well known. When the diuretic is prescribed for a diabetic patient being treated with insulin or one of the oral hypoglycemic agents, this effect partially may counteract the hypoglycemic action of the antidiabetic drug, necessitating an adjustment in dosage. Similarly, many diuretics may produce a hyperuricemic effect. Therapy in patients with gout should be monitored closely as the hyperuricemic action of a diuretic may necessitate an adjustment in dosage of the agent being used in the treatment of gout.

Drugs Having Similar Pharmacological Effects

An excessive response attributable to the concurrent use of drugs having similar actions is the type of interaction that occurs most often, and these potential problems warrant particular attention.

Central Nervous System Depressants—An excessive central nervous system (CNS) depressant effect, resulting from the concurrent use of two or more drugs exhibiting a depressant action, represents one of the most dangerous drug-related problems. Older patients should be viewed as being especially susceptible to this type of response, and patients experiencing effects such as sedation and dizziness are at increased risk of falls and injuries, such as hip fractures. Patients also must be advised of the risks of operating motor vehicles or machinery. In considering multiple drug regimens, recognition must be taken of the large number of agents (eg, sedative-hypnotics, antipsychotics, tricyclic antidepressants, analgesics and most antihistamines) which can exhibit a depressant effect that will be at least additive to the effect contributed by other drugs. At the minimum, the dosages of the drugs having a depressant effect should be reduced from the "usual" dose, and consideration also should be given as to whether it is necessary to use all the drugs concurrently.

Alcohol—Other Central Nervous System Depressants—The increased CNS depressant effect that is experienced by individuals being treated with depressant drugs when they consume alcoholic beverages is among the best known interactions. However, this interaction also illustrates the difficulties in trying to predict the magnitude of the response that will be experienced by a particular patient as the response will depend on many variables, including the patient's tolerance to alcohol. How then should the patient be instructed when he is to take a depressant medication? Certainly it would be most desirable not to consume alcoholic beverages during the period the medication is being taken. However, there should be a realistic recognition that many patients if faced with a mandate not to drink while on drug therapy, will decide not to take their drug. Every patient should be alerted to the fact that the depressant effect of the drug prescribed may be increased by alcohol. If it is anticipated that the patient would not completely avoid alcoholic beverages, he should be urged to use them in moderation, particularly when therapy is initiated, and cautioned to observe his own tolerance when such combinations are employed. However, the fact that many individuals can take depressant drugs and consume relatively large amounts of alcoholic beverages with no apparent difficulty should not be cause to forget that such combinations have been lethal in some individuals and the cause of injury in others. Thus, there is an important need to caution all patients for whom such drugs are prescribed.

Drugs Having Anticholinergic Activity—Drugs that differ considerably in their primary pharmacological actions may exhibit the same secondary effects. Many patients being treated with antipsychotic agents such as chlorpromazine also are given an antiparkinson agent such as trihexyphenidyl to control the extrapyramidal effects of the former. In addition, a number of patients experience depressive symptoms and a tricyclic antidepressant such as amitriptyline might be added to the therapy. Each of these three agents possesses anticholinergic activity and the additive effect could result in side effects such as dryness of the mouth, blurred vision, urinary retention, constipation and elevation of intraocular pressure.

Even an effect such as dryness of the mouth, which most health professionals would consider as a minor problem, could be troublesome in certain patients. For example, persistent dryness of the mouth could make the use of dentures more difficult and also cause other dental complications. In addition, there may be increased difficulty in chewing and swallowing, an important factor with respect to the problem of malnutrition in many elderly individuals. Dryness of the mouth also may result in other problems as illustrated by a case report of a patient treated with imipramine. The patient experienced persistent dryness of the mouth and when nitroglycerin tablets were administered sublingually for the management of exertional angina, the relief of the symptoms was delayed because of the slower dissolution of the sublingual tablets.

It has been observed that an excessive anticholinergic effect can cause an atropine-like delirium, particularly in geriatric patients. This effect could be misinterpreted as an increase in psychiatric symptoms which might be treated by increasing the dosage of the therapeutic agents that are actually responsible for causing the problem. This example points out the difficulty that often can exist in distinguishing between the symptoms of the condition(s) being treated and the effects of the drug(s) being employed as therapy.

Several studies call attention to other potential problems associated with the use of drugs having anticholinergic activity. In one investigation using volunteers aged 60 to 72, trihexyphenidyl was found to cause substantial memory impairment. In another study of 22 demented nursing-home patients, it was noted that those with high serum anticholinergic concentrations had greater impairment in self-care capacity than patients with low concentrations.

The blurring of vision, which also may be associated with the use of drugs having anticholinergic activity, may be especially distressing for older patients, particularly those whose physical activities may be limited and for whom reading is a favorite activity.

Several reports have described the development of severe hyperpyrexia in patients taking phenothiazine—antiparkinson combinations who were exposed to high environmental temperature and humidity. These investigators call attention to the ability of these combinations to interfere with the thermoregulatory system of the body and recommend that physicians treating patients in hot and humid climates should minimize outdoor exposure of patients receiving high doses of these agents.

Drugs Exhibiting Hypotensive Effects—Certain antihypertensive drugs (eg, prazosin), as well as some other classes of medications (eg, tricyclic antidepressants), can cause orthostatic hypotension, resulting in symptoms such as dizziness, lightheadedness and, in more severe cases, syncope. Older patients are more susceptible to this type of response and the associated risks such as falls and injuries, and appropriate precautions should be exercised whether these agents are given alone or in combination.

Nonsteroidal Anti-Inflammatory Drugs—Several situations exist in which a patient unknowingly may be taking several different products which contain the same NSAID. An arthritic patient whose condition has been managed with ibuprofen obtained via prescription (often at dosage levels at or near the recommended maximum), may purchase an ibuprofen product available without a prescription for pain/discomfort not associated with the arthritis, without recognizing that the two products contain the same drug and that there is an increased risk of adverse effects.

Naproxen and naproxen sodium formulations are marketed under different trade names (*Naprosyn* and *Anaprox*, respectively). The potential exists for one physician to prescribe one formulation for an arthritic disorder and another physician to prescribe the other product for pain and/or inflammation due to another problem (eg, an injury or dental procedures). A patient for whom one of these products is prescribed may purchase a naproxen sodium product available without a prescription without recognizing that the two formulations contain the same active ingredient.

Alteration of Electrolyte Concentrations

Several important drug interactions occur as a result of the ability of certain therapeutic agents to alter the concentration of electrolytes such as potassium and sodium. When these drugs are included in a therapeutic regimen, it is important that electrolyte levels be monitored periodically.

Digoxin—Diuretics—One of the problems associated with the use of most of the commonly employed diuretics (eg, the thiazide derivatives), is that they can cause an excessive loss of potassium. Particular caution is necessary in patients also being treated with digoxin (or other digitalis preparations), many of whom would be candidates for diuretic therapy. If potassium depletion remains uncorrected, the heart may become more sensitive to the effects of the cardiac glycoside and arrhythmia may result.

Although potassium supplementation will be necessary in many individuals being treated with a potassium-depleting diuretic, the initiation of therapy with such a diuretic must not be viewed as a mandate also to provide potassium supplementation. This decision should be based on a consideration of the individual patient situation, and the appropriate parameters should be monitored periodically. It must be recognized that dangers also exist if hyperkalemia occurs as a result of excessive supplementation. This risk of such complications is greatest in patients with diminished renal function.

In addition to the diuretics, other agents also can cause potassium depletion. Prolonged therapy with cathartics and corticosteroids may cause potassium depletion although this is not likely to occur as quickly or to the same extent as with diuretics.

Considerable interest has developed in the clinical implications of magnesium depletion. Concern has been expressed that this condition occurs much more commonly than is recognized and that some clinical problems may continue or worsen despite seemingly adequate electrolyte therapy because magnesium deficiency has not been identified and corrected.

Diuretic therapy may lead to development of magnesium depletion and, as observed when potassium is depleted, the activity of digoxin may be enhanced and possibly result in toxicity. In some patients with digoxin toxicity, low serum-magnesium concentrations may coexist with normal potassium values.

Angiotensin Converting Enzyme Inhibitors—Potassium-sparing Diuretics—The angiotensin converting enzyme (ACE) inhibitors (eg, captopril, enalapril, lisinopril) may cause an elevation of serum potassium concentrations. Potassium-sparing diuretics (amiloride, spironolactone and triamterene) or potassium supplements should be used concurrently only in situations in which hypokalemia is documented, because of the risk of hyperkalemia and associated complications. Salt substitutes containing potassium also should be used with caution.

Lithium—Diuretics—Sodium depletion is known to increase lithium toxicity, for which reason it generally has been recommended that lithium salts should not be used in patients on diuretic therapy or on a sodium-restricted diet. Even protracted sweating or diarrhea can cause sufficient depletion of sodium to result in decreased tolerance to lithium.

The sodium depletion caused by diuretics reduces the renal clearance and increases the activity of lithium. However, it has been noted by some that, if preferable therapeutic alternatives are not available, concurrent therapy need not be contraindicated so long as the interaction is recognized and steps are taken to monitor therapy and adjust dosage.

Interactions at Receptor Sites

Monoamine Oxidase Inhibitors—Sympathomimetic Agents—Monoamine oxidase (MAO) functions to break down catecholamines such as norepinephrine. When the enzyme is inhibited, the levels of norepinephrine within adrenergic neurons increase and a drug that can stimulate its release can bring about an exaggerated response. It is by this mechanism that interactions between MAO inhibitors and indirectly acting sympathomimetic amines (eg, amphetamine) develop. Thus, if amphetamine is administered to a patient whose stores of norepinephrine have been increased by MAO inhibition, he may experience severe headache, hypertension (possibly a hypertensive crisis) and cardiac arrhythmias. The serious consequences associated with these interactions contraindicate use of these agents in combination.

Although most sympathomimetic amines, such as amphetamine, are available only by prescription, others such as ephedrine, phenylephrine and phenylpropanolamine, which also have been reported to interact similarly with MAO inhibitors, are found in many of the popular nonprescription cold and allergy preprations, as well as many of the over-the-counter diet-aid products. It is important that patients being treated with MAO inhibitors avoid using products containing these agents.

MAO Inhibitors—Other Antidepressants—Cautions in the product literature, as well as case reports, warn against concurrent use of an MAO inhibitor with a tricyclic antidepressant (eg, amitriptyline, imipramine) because severe atropine-like reactions, tremors, convulsions, hyperthermia and vascular collapse have been reported to result from such use. It is recommended in the labeling for most of these products that therapy with an MAO inhibitor or a tricyclic antidepressant should not be initiated until at least 7 to 14 days after therapy with the other has been discontinued.

Although the labeling for most MAO inhibitors and tricyclic antidepressants notes that concurrent use is contraindicated, there is controversy as to the degree of risk involved. Several studies of the combined use of these agents have revealed little evidence of interaction and the growing impression that serious interactions are uncommon, coupled with the reports of favorable results with such combinations in selected patients who did not respond to either agent given alone, have led many to conclude that these combinations can be employed cautiously. In patients who are refractory to single antidepressants and who are not candidates for alternative therapeutic approaches, the potential benefits of combination therapy may outweigh the risks. However, such therapy should be undertaken only by those who are thoroughly familiar with the risks involved and under circumstances in which therapy can be monitored closely.

There is only limited data regarding the combined use of fluoxetine and an MAO inhibitor, and it is advised that their combined use be avoided and that at least 14 days elapse between discontinuation of a MAO inhibitor and initiation of treatment with fluoxetine. There have been several reports of deaths of patients in whom therapy with an MAO inhibitor was initiated shortly after discontinuation of fluoxetine. Because of the long half-lives of fluoxetine and its active metabolite, it is recommended that at least 5 weeks should elapse between discontinuation of fluoxetine and initiation of therapy with an MAO inhibitor.

It should be noted that the antineoplastic, procarbazine, and the anti-infective, furazolidone or probably its metabolite, also can inhibit MAO enzymes and warnings applying to the use of other MAO inhibitors should be heeded for these drugs also. With furazolidone, however, it is not likely that enzyme inhibition will occur within the first five days of therapy and usually the course of treatment will be completed within that time.

Guanethidine—Tricyclic Antidepressants—Guanethidine is transported to its site of action within adrenergic neurons by a transport system that also is responsible for uptake of norepinephrine, as well as several indirectly acting sympathomimetic amines such as ephedrine and the amphetamines. Concentration of guanethidine in these neurons is necessary for its hypotensive effect. It appears that tricyclic antidepressants can inhibit uptake of guanethidine into the neuron terminal, thereby preventing its concentration at these sites and reducing its activity. Other studies suggest that antipsychotic agents such as chlorpromazine, haloperidol and thiothixene can act similarly to the tricyclic antidepressants in reducing the antihypertensive effect of these agents.

Although other mechanisms may be involved in the development of drug interactions, the ones cited are the most important. As often stated, more than one mechanism may be responsible for certain interactions; these mechanisms may work in concert or in opposition as determinants of the resulting effect. Still other drug interactions develop by mechanisms yet to be identified.

Even though the discussion of some interactions has raised more questions than have been answered, an awareness of the factors predisposing to the development of drug interactions, as well as the mechanisms by which they occur, will be of value in the identification and prevention of potential problems.

It is evident that significant limitations still exist in trying to predict the results of combination therapy. In the following section, guidelines are provided to minimize the risk of the occurrence of drug interactions.

Reducing the Risk of Drug Interaction

The reduction of the risk of drug interactions is a challenge that embraces a number of considerations. Although they could be applied to drug therapy in general, the following guidelines to reduce and manage drug interactions are offered to assist health professionals having the responsibility of selecting and monitoring therapeutic regimens.

Identify the Patient Risk Factors—Factors such as age, the nature of the patient's medical problems (eg, impaired renal function), dietary habits, smoking and problems like alcoholism will influence the effect of certain drugs and should be considered during the initial patient interview.

Take a Thorough Drug History—An accurate and complete record of both the prescription and nonprescription medications a patient is taking must be obtained. Numerous interactions have resulted from a lack of awareness of prescription medications prescribed by another physician,or nonprescription medications the patient did not consider important enough to mention.

Be Knowledgeable about the Actions of the Drugs Being Used—The knowledge of the properties and the primary and secondary pharmacologic actions of each of the agents used, or being considered for use, is essential if the interaction potential is to be assessed accurately.

Consider Therapeutic Alternatives—In most cases, two drugs that are known to interact can be administered concurrently as long as adequate precautions are taken (eg, closer monitoring of therapy or dosage adjustments to compensate for the altered response). However, in those situations in which another agent with similar therapeutic properties and a lesser risk of interacting is available, it should be used.

Avoid Complex Therapeutic Regimens Where Possible—The number of medications used should be kept to a minimum. In addition, the use of medications or dosage regimens that permit less-frequent administration may help avoid interactions that result from an alteration of absorption (eg, when a drug is administered in close proximity to meals).

Educate the Patient—Patients often know little about their illnesses, let alone the benefits and problems that could result from drug therapy. Individuals who are aware of, and understand, this information can be expected to be in greater compliance with the instructions for administering medications and more attentive to the development of symptoms which could be early indicators of drug-related problems. Patients should be encouraged to ask questions about their therapy and to report any excessive or unexpected responses. There should be no uncertainty on the part of the patient as to how to use his medications in the most effective and safest way.

Monitor Therapy—The risk of drug-related problems warrants close monitoring, not only for the possible occurrence of drug interactions but also for adverse effects occurring with individual agents and noncompliance. Any change in patient behavior should be suspected as being drug-related until that possibility is excluded.

Individualize Therapy—Although the development of a therapeutic regimen that meets the specific needs of individual patients is inherent in many of the above guidelines, the importance of this consideration cannot be emphasized too strongly. Wide variations in the response of patients to the same dose of certain individual drugs is well-recognized. It is difficult to predict the response of many therapeutic agents when they are given alone; the challenge and limitations in anticipating the response with a multiple-drug regimen are even greater. Therefore, priority should be assigned to the needs and clinical response of the individual patient, rather than to the usual dosage recommendations and standard treatment and monitoring guidelines.

The pharmacist will be involved actively in the observance of the guidelines described above. In addition, the need to not only maintain complete and current patient medication records, but also to supervise and monitor drug therapy more closely, places the pharmacist in a strategic position to detect and prevent drug interactions. By observing the preceding guidelines and recommendations, and by strengthening communication with patients and other health professionals, the pharmacist has a valuable opportunity to make a significant contribution toward the further enhancement of the efficacy and safety of drug therapy.

CHAPTER 106

Clinical Drug Literature

Ann B Amerson, PharmD
Professor, College of Pharmacy
University of Kentucky
Lexington, KY 40536-0082

Defining the clinical drug literature is not an easy task. The drug literature is an extensive, heterogenous collection of resources which provides information about drugs. The definition of "clinical" which is most appropriate is "of or pertaining to direct observation and treatment of patients."[1] When this definition is combined with the drug literature as described in Chapter 7, it might be concluded that the clinical drug literature is comprised of primary, secondary and tertiary literature that can be applied to optimize the use of drugs in patients.

This discussion focuses on utilization which requires access, selection and organization. In addition, evaluation becomes a key component in selecting literature and in interpreting and applying the information to patient-care problems.

Opportunities for Utilization

The pharmacist's role as a drug-information provider was a significant focus of the Report of the Study Commission on Pharmacy in 1975.[2] The report stressed that the drug-information needs for both health professionals and consumers were not being met and that the pharmacist was the logical person to fill this gap. While progress in the profession generates opportunities for more active drug-information provision, the full potential has not yet been achieved. The needs and requirements continue to evolve as the profession discusses the concept of pharmaceutical care and addresses the requirements of OBRA 90 (Omnibus Budget Reconciliation Act of 1990).

The opportunities to develop and nurture the role of the drug-information provider exist in almost any practice setting. Different audiences may be involved as the pharmacist in community settings often has more contact with consumers, whereas the pharmacist in the institutional setting may interact more directly with health professionals. Since the publication of the Report of the Study Commission on Pharmacy, the opportunities for pharmacists to be more active drug-information providers have increased. Changes contributing to these opportunities include developments in technology, more health-oriented attitudes by consumers and the evolving education of pharmacists.

Advances in computer technology have enhanced greatly the pharmacist's ability to meet information needs.[3] Computers have improved the efficiency of the distribution operation and recordkeeping. Recent information indicates that about 85% of pharmacies now are computerized for operational needs.[4] This enhances the pharmacist's ability to devote time to other activities. Information retrieval is a second aspect of computer usage that is developing. On-line information systems are becoming widely available for both health professionals and consumers and can be used in practice settings. Journals and texts are available on-line in full-text format. Software focused on specific information areas, such as drug interactions, is available which can be used in conjunction with pharmacy computer systems (eg, *Medicom Micro Plus*-PDS or *Drug Therapy Screening System*-Medi- Span). Information, once available only through printed media, is retrieved quickly and easily using computer technology.

The general public has become increasingly aware of health issues and is more active in seeking information. In addition, information is more available to the public on health issues and drug therapy through newspapers, magazines, radio and television as well as computer systems mentioned previously. Such exposure generates a desire on the part of many individuals to be more knowledgable and thus make inquiries.

The education of pharmacists to handle drug-information inquiries has expanded in many respects with coverage of an increased knowledge base as well as interaction with both health professionals and patients in the educational setting. This should enhance the pharmacist's preparation to meet drug-information needs.

Considerations in Utilization

A key to effective use of clinical drug literature involves a professional commitment by the individual. This ideally develops as a student and continues throughout one's professional life. Aspects of this commitment include a desire to keep informed about new developments, a decision to acquire the resources necessary to do this and a willingness to aid one's health-professional colleagues or patients.

The development of a reference library at the workplace will serve as a foundation for using the clinical drug literature. Such a library, when carefully selected, can provide information for many inquiries. Interestingly, based on surveys conducted several years ago, reference selections by pharmacists were not always adequate in scope to meet the drug-information needs identified by physicians. Areas where physicians indicated needs were information about drugs not commonly used, drug interactions, adverse reactions, specific therapeutic problems, drug costs and availability and poisoning.[5,6] The pharmacist's libraries often were lacking in coverage of most of these areas.[7] Therefore, in approaching resource selection, a needs assessment should be conducted.

The practice site should be considered including the type of facility (community, hospital, nursing home, industry, etc) as well as the type of individuals with which the pharmacist will interact in the practice setting. The types of activities anticipated by the pharmacist in the practice setting also may guide selection. The probable rate-limiting step to acquisition will be the funds available for purchase. Dividing the clinical drug literature into several components assists in evaluation and appropriate selection. Careful selection of the best and most appropriate resources is crucial. Some general guidelines to aid in the selection for each component of the literature will be reviewed. Coupled with the needs assessment, a general framework can be developed for evaluating initial selection of a reference library and potential additions as new sources become available.

Evaluation of Resources

Tertiary Literature—This component involves reference sources characterized by the presentation of information in a condensed and compact form. Two classifications, one by reference type and one by question type, may aid in the initial selection and use for specific questions. A general classification of the references is presented in Table 1. The groups

Table 1—Classification of Drug-Information References

Product-oriented references	
American Drug Index	
Physician's Desk Reference	
Facts and Comparisons	
Handbook of Nonprescription Drugs	
Blue Book	
Red Book	
Drug-oriented references	
General	*Adverse effects*
AHFS Drug Information	Side Effects of Drugs
USP Dispensing Information	Textbook of Adverse Drug Reactions
AMA Drug Evaluations	
Pharmacological Basis of Therapeutics	*Pharmacokinetics*
Martindale's The Extra Pharmacopoeia	Applied Pharmacokinetics
Drug Interactions	*Parenteral Drugs*
Hansten's Drug Interactions	Guide to Parenteral Admixtures
Evaluations of Drug Interactions	Handbook of Injectable Drugs
Drug Interaction Facts	
Therapeutics-oriented references	
Merck Manual	
Conn's Current Therapy	
Current Medical Diagnosis and Treatment	
Current Pediatric Therapy	
Manual of Medical Therapeutics	
Applied Therapeutics: The Clinical Use of Drugs	
Clinical Pharmacy and Therapeutics	
Pharmacotherapy: A Pathophysiologic Basis	
Poisoning information references	
Dreisbach's Handbook of Poisoning	
Clinical Toxicology of Commercial Products	
Dispensing-oriented references	
USP-NF	
Remington's Pharmaceutical Sciences	
Merck Index	

presented are general in nature describing the primary orientation of the reference. This classification is somewhat arbitrary and each reference should be examined to learn its special features and strengths which may make it applicable in other categories. While many references address a number of information needs, no one reference is all-inclusive.

Product-oriented references will be the choice when information on a specific brand-name drug product is required. When information on the generic drug entity is required, drug-oriented references may be the most suitable choice. When information is required on how drugs are used to treat diseases, therapeutics-oriented references are a good choice. Poisoning references are specific for acute or chronic toxicological problems. Dispensing-oriented references are useful particularly for problems related to compounding as well as dispensing. Within each of these categories, a spectrum of references exists which differ in scope and depth. Some provide general information on many aspects related to the drug or product (eg, *Facts and Comparisons* and *Drug Information—American Hospital Formulary Service*) whereas others are focused more on specific content particularly among the drug-oriented references (eg, *Evaluation of Drug Interactions* and *Pediatric Dosage Handbook*). That is why the general classification of references, coupled with a classification of the types of questions received as presented in Table 2

Table 2—Classification of Questions

Identification	Product contents—domestic prescription or OTC, foreign drugs, physical product
Availability	Marketing status—prescription, OTC, investigational
Pharmacokinetics	Absorption, distribution, metabolism, excretion
Dosage	Adult, pediatric, neonatal, geriatric
Interactions	Drug, food, laboratory tests
Adverse reactions / side effects	Untoward effects associated with therapeutic use
Pregnancy / nursing	Teratogenic or other effects on fetus, use when breast feeding
Therapeutic use / efficacy	Drug of choice, relative effectiveness
Stability / compatibility	Injectables, compounding
Toxicity / poisoning	Exposure to chemicals, overdose

more clearly defines the precise needs for drug-information sources. The classification of questions can be modified based on the practice setting. Some examples of crossing the two classifications are as follows: product-oriented references are most useful for answering questions related to identification and availability; pharmacokinetic questions generally are answered best with drug-oriented references and answers for questions involving therapeutic use, particularly the choice of drug, are best found in therapeutics-oriented references. The process described is useful for those beginning to use reference literature as it helps associate specific references with specific information needs. The process becomes second nature for those more experienced in using tertiary literature and allows incorporation of new references into a general framework.

In addition to the informational content, other questions to ask in evaluating initial selection of specific references are

Who are the authors / editors and what are their credentials?—An assessment of the reputation of the individuals who prepare the reference may be in order. Sometimes, colleagues may provide information in addition to the position description of the individuals provided in the reference itself. Determining if the individual(s) has been involved in the preparation of other reference sources or published articles in the topic area of the reference can be helpful.

How recently was the reference published? Are editions published periodically or are supplements provided?—For most text-type references it is important to assess the date of publication. Because of the lag time in the publication process it is reasonable to add 1 year to the date of publication in evaluating the currentness of the information. When multiple editions of a reference are published, a regular schedule for updating may be evident. If the publication of a new edition is imminent, waiting may be the best strategy. More references now provide supplements (eg, *Facts and Comparisons, Drug Information—American Hospital Formulary Service* and *USP Dispensing Information*). The selection of references with this feature generally entails an annual cost but the currentness of the information may be well worth it.

Does the reference have multiple contributors or an editorial panel?—This generally is desirable in that contributors or editorial panel members are recruited because of their expertise in a particular area. On occasion, the cohesiveness of a reference can suffer with multiple contributors due to marked differences in style.

Is the material referenced? If so, what type of references are used and how current are they?—An authoritative reference does not require documentation of its information necessarily (eg, *Facts and Comparisons*). When documented, a careful review of the sources should provide some additional input in the evaluation process. The source references can be reviewed to determine whether they are primary, secondary or tertiary. Primary sources generally are preferred. The currentness of the citations also will indicate how up-to-date the information is.

Does the reference allow easy access?—Will the indexing allow quick retrieval of the information? This feature generally can be determined only with the actual use of the reference. If possible, a wise approach is to try several sample situations where the reference is anticipated to be of benefit.

What is the cost?—Usually, reference purchases will be made within the confines of a budget, either personal or job-related. The anticipated use should justify the expense. Staggering acquisitions should be considered as some involve annual recurring costs while others are purchased every 3 to 5 years.

Secondary Literature—This represents two types of sources: indexing (bibliographic) and abstracting, which serve as guides to primary literature. They represent the most expensive investment of the literature library. Most of these sources are available through on-line retrieval vendors, CD-ROM (compact disc-read only memory) systems and printed versions. Microfiche systems, once popular for several retrieval systems, have been replaced largely by CD-ROM technology.[3,8,9] Microfiche versions allowed significant reduction of the volume of material, but still required the techniques of manual searching. Modern CD-ROM technology provides the system on compact disc at the site of use, allowing the features of on-line retrieval but at a fixed annual cost in contrast to on-line searching. This technology also is finding increased application for several tertiary reference sources for full-text searching.

Several considerations are important in selecting secondary literature sources. These include lag time, coverage of the literature, selectivity of indexing/abstracting and cost.

Lag time refers to when the document was published in the journal versus when it was abstracted or indexed. This time varies among the secondary literature sources and partially may depend on the frequency of updating. Some sources (eg, *Inpharma*, *Reactions*) are published weekly whereas others are published monthly or bimonthly (eg, *Index Medicus* and *deHaen Drugs in Use*). The source with more frequent updating may have less lag time but this should be evaluated carefully for each source.

The number of journals covered by each source is another consideration. This number can vary from a few hundred (eg, *Iowa Drug Information Service*) to thousands (eg, *Index Medicus* and *Excerpta Medica*). This also should be coupled with an examination of whether the source is focused on drugs or whether it is broader in scope. A source focused on drugs may provide the greatest utility but there may be value in selecting a source with broader coverage of topics. The setting where the source will be used may determine which type of source is appropriate.

The form of the system (standard print, microfiche or computerized), should be considered in relation to the needs of the practice site and the needs of the users.

Cost differences exist for sources available in different forms, but such differences should be evaluated carefully, based on number of users and types of information provided.

Primary Literature—Articles appearing in regularly published journals have the greatest diversity and expanse of the three components. It is also the component with which many pharmacy students and practitioners have the least contact. In the more traditional practice, pharmacists may encounter numerous situations with potential for exposure to primary literature; however, this component is generally the least accessible. Technology is changing the potential accessibility, and pharmacists in all types of practices should expect to use primary literature.

One way in which pharmacists are exposed to primary literature presently is personal reading. All pharmacists should be fulfilling a professional commitment to remain up-to-date. One mechanism to accomplish this is by reading journals on a regular basis. Pharmacists also can acquire copies of primary literature from pharmaceutical-company representatives which relate to specific products. Specific drug-information questions often arise at the practice site involving new uses of marketed drugs or recently reported adverse effects, as two examples. The use of primary literature is frequently necessary to answer these questions. Consumer questions, particularly in the situation of media-generated reporting, eg, newspaper, radio or television reports, often are based on studies recently published in major medical journals.

Some criteria to apply in selecting journals for personal use are

What kind of reputation does the journal have?—Several specific points that may be helpful in evaluating a journal's reputation include the duration of publication, the publisher's reputation (an organization or recognized publisher) and colleagues' opinions.

What kind of information is provided?—The educational value and the practicality of information as related to the individual's practice are important. Presentation for ease of use should be considered.

What expert input is there into content?—An editorial board made up of recognized health professionals is a good feature. The use of referees or reviewers of articles submitted for publication is another positive feature that helps to assure that the information presented is authoritative. A journal generally prints such information in the front of each issue.

In most facilities or practice settings, the acquisition of all desirable literature resources will be impossible because of budget limitations. Because the cost of these resources continues to increase, careful selection is necessary. Asking the questions and applying the guidelines will aid in selection of a cost-effective balance of the literature components which will enable the practitioner to function more effectively in the role of a drug-information provider. Accessibility to both secondary and primary literature sources will improve over the next several years, particularly for those practitioners wanting to take advantage of the opportunities.

Evaluating Primary Literature

Many journals have a review process for selecting articles which eventually are published. Some submissions never make it because of lack of overall quality or inappropriate content. One might question why a reader should need to evaluate the literature. With close to 30,000 science serials being published, the volume of primary literature is astounding.[10] In 1979 an estimated two million articles were published, a number which no doubt has increased.[11] With such a large number of journals and articles, the quality is likely to vary regardless of what measures are used. Periodic reviews of the published literature show various kinds of problems with studies even in widely read and respected journals.[12–15] An article classified as a *study* is one which reports the basic elements of experimental design including a statement of purpose, methods, data collection, results and discussion in the evaluation of a drug substance. Therefore, the reader is obligated to make a careful evaluation of studies and determine the applicability of the information to the situation at hand. For efficiency, one approach is to develop a checklist which can be used to determine the positive and negative features of a study. Such a list is included in Table 3. The information is organized by the section of the study where it is anticipated to appear. Others suggest more-detailed evaluation forms.[16]

Identifying the rationale for conducting the study and the specific objectives which are expected to be accomplished is important for both the investigators and the reader. If clearly identifiable in the published study, this information first gives the reader some confidence that the investigators proceeded with a well-defined course. The possibility exists that clear definition happened after the fact; however, for the reader, this information will still help in identifying the anticipated end-points of the study. The rationale for conducting the study may indicate the potential importance of the results in solving some overall controversy or question. The reader should be able to determine if the investigators accomplish the initially established objectives.

The materials and methods section is the most critical part of an article in that it describes how the investigators have conducted the study. If serious flaws occur here the results of the study may be rendered unusable. Table 3 lists four major areas to consider when reviewing this section.

Criteria for patient inclusion or exclusion in the study should define clearly the samples selected. The sample represents the population to which the results will be applicable. The appropriate definition of selection criteria should assure that

Table 3—Checklist for Evaluating Studies

Introduction
- Rationale for conducting study
- Objectives

Materials/methods
- *Patients*
  - Criteria for inclusion
  - Criteria for exclusion
  - Sample size
  - Representation
- *Study design*
  - Controls—type
  - Blinding
  - Randomization
  - Treatment conditions—dosage, compliance
- *Test method*
  - Subjective versus objective
- *Statistical tests*

Results
- *Data presentation*
  - Completeness
  - Dropouts
- *Statistical analysis*
  - Appropriateness

Discussion
- Conclusions

the subjects have the disease which is undergoing treatment. The criteria also will identify such factors as length and severity of disease and age of the sample. The authors also indicate the number of subjects expected to receive treatment. The determination of sample size requires consideration of statistical (Type I and Type II) errors and the anticipated difference between the treatments under study. A detailed discussion of the factors used in determining the sample size is beyond the scope of this discussion. Two references provide further details on this process.[17,18]

Study design is the next portion of the materials and methods section which requires close scrutiny. Controls, blinding and randomization are three key elements to examine. Controls provide a basis for comparison, the most common being groups of subjects who receive placebo or another standard treatment (active control). Subjects also can serve as their own control if they receive more than one dosage regimen under the study conditions. The difference in each subject's performance can be compared on the regimens. Blinding and randomization are two techniques used to reduce bias both on the part of investigators and subjects. Randomization also generally tends to balance treatment groups according to certain prognostic factors, eg, age and length or severity of disease. Incorporation of these three elements are usually indicators of good study design.

The conditions of treatment are particularly important to assess as they often can be sources of bias in the results. The reader should consider the appropriateness of dosage used and treatment duration. The issue of compliance in outpatient studies is always of concern, and efforts to help assure compliance should be evident. If the study employs a crossover design, an appropriate washout period is necessary. Other treatments, whether drug or nondrug, should be standardized.

The tests used to generate the data and thus determine response to the drug require description. Tests used in studies are many and varied, eg, laboratory tests, X-rays, questionnaires and physical assessments. The reader needs to assess whether the test(s) is appropriate and what it actually measures. For example, measuring glucose in the urine is an indication of the control of glucose spillage in a diabetic patient. However, it does not reflect control of the disease process. The tests should be sensitive enough to detect drug action. A certain degree of reliability in the tests is essential so that similar results occur with repeated trials. Variability due to differences in the techniques or interpretation of the investigators is of concern and can become a major problem for tests of a subjective nature. The care taken to establish, explain and standardize the tests is important.

Finally, the investigators should indicate the statistical methods which will be used to analyze the data. If not in the materials and methods section, this information may be reported in the results section as the data are analyzed. Regardless, the investigators should indicate the statistical methods used to allow a review of their appropriateness.

To illustrate why checking for these aspects is important, Der Simonian *et al*[13] evaluated the methods sections of comparative clinical trials in four well-recognized journals. They examined the studies for 11 methodological items which were considered important to study credibility for the reader. The overall means of reporting the 11 methodological items was 56% for the four journals with performance ranging from 46 to 71%. This study simply determined whether the items were present, and not whether the structure was appropriate. However, the absence of many factors indicates potential problems with the studies.

The results section summarizes all the data which is collected during the study. The reader should review the tests for patient assessment as indicated in the materials and methods section to determine that all aspects are reported. The results will be reported in text form and often supplemented with graphs, figures, tables or photographs. Completeness, correctness and agreement with the study goals are three aspects requiring examination. Several questions which require answers are represented by

1. Are results presented on all patients entered into the study? If not, were dropouts identified and explained and how were any results from these subjects analyzed? The text usually indicates such information but, in some cases, the numbers reported in tables are the first indication.
2. Do the text and the data presented in tables, graphs, etc agree?
3. What information actually is presented graphically? Does a close inspection of the graph yield a different perception than the first glance or is it, perhaps, dealing with a single patient? The percent of improvement and percent of patients showing improvement certainly are different parameters but ones which easily could be mistaken for one another.
4. What data are subjected to statistical analysis and what differences are significant statistically versus nonsignificant? In the discussion, differences which are statistically significant generally receive more emphasis than nonsignificant differences. The appropriateness of this emphasis should be determined because nonsignificant differences may be just as important.

A study should be examined for two kinds of statistics: descriptive and inferential.

Descriptive statistics, including such measures as mean, range, variance and standard deviation, give an indication of either the central tendency or the spread of the data. For example, if mean values of diastolic blood pressure ± 1 standard deviation are reported for a sample of 20 patients, a value of 90 ± 16 torr would arouse more concern than a value of 90 ± 5 torr. The first figure indicates a much greater variation in individual values than the second figure, suggesting a less homogeneous sample.

Inferential statistics involve tests applied to data to determine whether a statistically significant difference exists. The test is applied to the "null" hypothesis which indicates that there is no difference. The application of such tests as the t test and chi-square (χ^2) test results in probability values. A probability value equal to or less than 0.05 ($p \leqq 0.05$) is considered generally to indicate a statistically significant difference. The probability value gives an estimate of the risk of making a Type I error (concluding a treatment is effective or different when it is not), which generally is considered more serious than a Type II error (saying there is no difference when one really exists). When the magnitude of the p value is in the range indicated, the risk of a Type I error (α) is low enough that the investigator can conclude that the difference is real and due to the treatment. When an investigator reports no difference between two treatments, the chance that a Type II error (β) has occurred deserves close scrutiny.

In some studies, multiple tests and comparisons may be employed because of the nature of the data reported. When several probability values are reported, careful differentiation of the comparisons being tested and the statistically significant values associated with them is necessary. Values that are not statistically significant must be distinguished from those considered significant. Statistically significant differences should be evaluated for their clinical importance. Refer to Chapter 10 for an in-depth discussion of the statistical treatment of data.

In the discussion of the results, the authors attempt to establish the importance of any observed differences and compare their results with the work of other investigators. Conclusions drawn from the data should conform with the purpose and objectives established at the outset of the study. If conclusions relate to something other than these, the design of the study should be scrutinized closely to see if it provides appropriate data to support such conclusions. If an investigator intends to compare the efficacy of two drugs, the results may indicate no difference in therapeutic effect. However, the investigator concludes that Drug A was more toxic than Drug B because of the number of adverse effects. The methodology should be reevaluated to determine whether appropriate mechanisms were used to assess the adverse effects. Conclusions must conform to the limits of the data and not be extrapolated beyond these limits.

The editorial community continues efforts to improve the overall quality and consistency of the clinical drug literature. A document called *Uniform Requirements for Manuscripts Submitted to Biomedical Journals*, first developed by the International Committee of Medical Journal Editors in 1982, has undergone several revisions with the latest being 1991.[19] Statistical aspects of reporting scientific research are addressed by these guidelines. These are useful not only to those conducting and publishing the research but to readers who evaluate it. Basilar and Mostellar provided a more detailed discussion of many of these points.[20] Numerous journals now use structured abstracts to identify key points for readers.[21] Readers of primary literature must systematically and efficiently evaluate the information presented. Using a checklist, as presented, will aid readers in developing the skills necessary in this area.

General Use of the Literature

Once familiarity develops with the different components of the literature and selections of resources are made, the practitioner then needs a systematic approach for use. Watanabe and Conner[22] described such an approach for handling drug information questions which involved five steps:

1. Classify the question.
2. Obtain background information.
3. Perform a systematic search.
4. Formulate an appropriate response.
5. Follow-up.

Such a process can be adapted for all types of drug-information needs, including specific questions asked of the practitioner, problem solving at the practice site or gathering information for an inservice program. Each step will be reviewed briefly.

Classifying the question involves characterizing it in general terms of the kind noted in Table 2. Combining this classification with a classification of references may aid in selecting the initial sources. Information about the person asking the question should be sought. The second step involves obtaining background information. This includes determining whether the question relates to a specific patient or requires general information. If the question involves a specific patient, information about this individual must be collected, eg, diagnosis, age, renal function and other medications, in order to provide the most appropriate response. In addition, the information collected about the caller must be factored into the situation. Once sufficient background information is obtained, the initial classification may be re-examined. The background information may result in reclassifying the original question.

Performing a systematic search may involve one or more components of the literature. The usual order of search is tertiary, secondary, then primary. Tertiary sources usually are chosen first because of the accessibility and conciseness of the information presented. Secondary literature follows because it aids in quick location of needed citations in the primary literature. The searcher should identify an initial strategy, using one or more of the components of the literature, in seeking the desired information. If this route is not productive, a secondary approach can be identified which provides expanded coverage of the resources. Once appropriate information is obtained, the practitioner should then think about what information needs to be conveyed to provide an adequate response and in what form this should be communicated. In addition, based on the information found, other questions which might arise should be anticipated. Finally, with certain types of questions, a follow-up on the use of the information may be appropriate; poison information being an example.

Conclusion

The opportunities for the pharmacist to fulfill a role as a drug-information provider expand on a daily basis. The clinical drug literature provides the resources to accomplish this role effectively. Strides in technology will aid the pharmacists' accessibility to this literature. The pharmacist must focus on evaluating and carefully selecting from the resources available to optimize the use of this tool in providing pharmaceutical care.

References

1. Morris W (ed): *The American Heritage Dictionary of the English Language*, Houghton Mifflin, Boston; 251, 1980.
2. *Pharmacists for the Future: The Report of the Study Commission on Pharmacy*, Health Admin Press, Ann Arbor; 139, 1975.
3. Dasta JF, Greer ML, Speedie SM: *Ann Pharmacother 26:* 109, 1992.
4. *Fed Reg* 57(212): 49406, Nov 2, 1992.
5. Smith GH, Sorby DL, Sharp LJ: *Am J Hosp Pharm 32:* 19, 1975.
6. Love DS, Hodge NA, Foley WA: *J Fam Pract 10:* 67, 1980.
7. Vrabel RB, Amerson AB: Annual Meeting, APhA, 1975.
8. Wigton RS: *MD Comput 4:* 34, 1987.
9. Wertz RK: *JAMA 256:* 3376, 1986.
10. Okerson A: *Am J Pharm Ed 56:* 407, 1992.
11. Haynes RB, McKibbon KA, Fitzgerald D *et al: Ann Int Med 105:* 149, 1986.
12. Pocock SJ, Hughes MD, Lee RJ: *N Engl J Med 317:* 426, 1987.
13. Der Simonian R, Charette LJ, McPeek B: *Ibid 306:* 1332, 1982.
14. Chalmers TC, Celano P, Sacks HS *et al: Ibid 309:* 1358, 1983.
15. Louis TA, Lavori PW, Bailar JC *et al: Ibid 310:* 24, 1984.
16. Weintraub M: *Drug Ther 12:* 131, 1982.
17. Young MJ, Bresnitz EA, Strom BL: *Ann Int Med 99:* 248, 1983.
18. McLarty JW. *Clin Pharm 7:* 694, 1988.
19. International Committee of Medical Journal Editors: *N Engl J Med 324:* 424, 1991.
20. Basilar JC, Mosteller F: *Ann Int Med 108:* 266, 1988.
21. Haynes RB, Mulrow CD, Huth EJ *et al: Ibid 113:* 69, 1990.
22. Watanabe AS, Conner CS: *Principles of Drug Information Services*, Drug Intell Publ, Hamilton IL; 15, 1978.

CHAPTER 107

Health Accessories

Richard W Knueppel, RPh
President
Knueppel Home Health Care Center
Milwaukee, WI 53222

For too long, many pharmacists treated health accessories as merely a convenience for their prescription patients. Physicians and other health professionals were convinced that the pharmacist had neither the necessary expertise nor equipment and sent their patients elsewhere for such services. In recent years, however, few aspects of professional practice have changed as much or grown as rapidly as the pharmacy's health-accessory department. The specially trained pharmacist is becoming recognized more widely as an expert in this area by other health professionals and can provide a professional and profitable adjunct to the pharmacy's other services.

A comprehensive health-accessory department includes a wide variety of surgical supplies and convalescent aids including wheelchairs, walkers, hospital beds, hydraulic patient lifters, urology and incontinence supplies, ostomy appliances, elastic supports, mastectomy breast forms and orthopedic braces. In addition, many pharmacies specialize in home health-care equipment such as traction devices, blood-glucose monitors, blood-pressure-monitoring devices, suction machines, oxygen and respiratory-therapy equipment, nerve and muscle stimulators, phototherapy lights, apnea monitors and rehabilitation equipment. Some pharmacies may specialize in providing intravenous medications and supplies for enteral or parenteral nutrition.

Even more important than merely providing large varieties of health accessories is the pharmacist's growing involvement in selecting and fitting them and also in instructing the patient in their proper use and maintenance.

To provide these services the pharmacist must acquire new skills and expertise which can be obtained through special courses given by several health-accessory manufacturers, professional associations and some wholesale distributors.

The initial step in selecting the appropriate health accessory is a thorough evaluation of both the patient and the available accessories including

Age	Disability-related factors
Lifestyle	Patient and equipment measurements
Diagnosis	
Prognosis	

Each of these factors should be considered when selecting the most appropriate health accessory for the patient. Also, it is often necessary to verify insurance coverage, including whether particular equipment is mandated by an HMO (see pages 1733 and 1940) and which equipment will be considered for reimbursement by Medicare, Medical Assistance or insurance companies.

Other steps may include consulting with the patient, his physician and his family; preparing a prescription, when applicable, as a recommendation to the physician; selecting the accessory from stock or ordering it from the manufacturer or distributor and checking the accessory to insure that it meets the appropriate specifications. Followup adjustments or modifications also may be necessary.

The author acknowledges the contributions of Barry N Eigen, MBA, Cindy Ciardo, Certified Fitter and Jerry Treptow, Home Medical Equipment Specialist.

Useful forms—eg, certificates of medical necessity (CMNs), disability analysis, measurement, prescription and ordering forms—are usually available from health-accessory manufacturers, insurance companies and government agencies. In fact, some insurance companies and government agencies may mandate the use of their forms.

Wheelchairs

There are literally hundreds of different wheelchairs to serve the patient's different needs. Figure 1 shows one example. The importance of an individualized prescription cannot be overemphasized. A carefully prescribed chair has a prolonged and useful life and promotes the patient's maximal physical independence.

The general loss of body functions in the aged or infirm patient serves as a guide to providing the best chair for his needs. He may have less strength and endurance than a younger or healthier person and, therefore, requires safety and convenience features. This reemphasizes the general rule when fitting any wheelchair: the primary considerations in fitting are the user's physical limitations and lifestyle.

Measurements—Following the disability analysis, the measurements of both the patient and the chair should be considered when preparing a prescription for the proper chair.

The Patient—Ideally, the patient should be sitting when measured, preferably in a chair that allows good body alignment.

Side-to-Side (widest area of hips while sitting)—Important in determining the chair seat width. In order to avoid pressure on the hips or thighs, yet help maintain good seating posture and stability, the chair-seat width should be 2 inches more than the width straight across the hips.

Knee-to-Hip—Critical in determining the actual chair-seat depth. Normally, the seat depth will be approximately 2 to 3 inches less than this measurement in order to provide adequate support, yet avoid pressure behind the knee. If a back panel or back cushion is to be inserted, its thickness must be considered.

Seat-to-Elbow—Serves as an indicator for armrest height. Depending on seating posture, armrest height should provide proper body support. (*Danger signals:* drooping or hunched up shoulders when the patient's elbows are resting on the armrests.) It should be noted that an armrest height 1 inch more than the patient's seat-to-elbow measurement will force the patient's elbows slightly forward, providing a natural brace against forward body slumping, especially when descending ramps.

Floor-to-Knee—Used to determine footrest adjustments from seat level and/or special seat height. The minimum footrest adjustment should be at least 2 inches less than this measurement in order to avoid pressure against the underside of the legs. A good visual guide for proper footrest adjustment (especially when using a standard chair) is to make sure that the tops of the patient's thighs are horizontal and parallel to the floor. To obtain greater-than-standard maximum footrest adjustment, a special seat height must be considered. Sometimes the use of a solid insert seat and/or seat cushion will solve this problem, although it should be remembered that optimum seat height allows the patient to place his feet on the floor without excessive pressure behind the knees.

Seat-to-Armpit—Used to determine back-upholstery height on standard-back chairs. This is important because many patients must be able to put their arms over the back upholstery and hook their elbows under the push handles to achieve leverage when reaching for things.

Other Measurements—May be required for more-involved or custom wheelchairs. Consult manufacturer product literature.

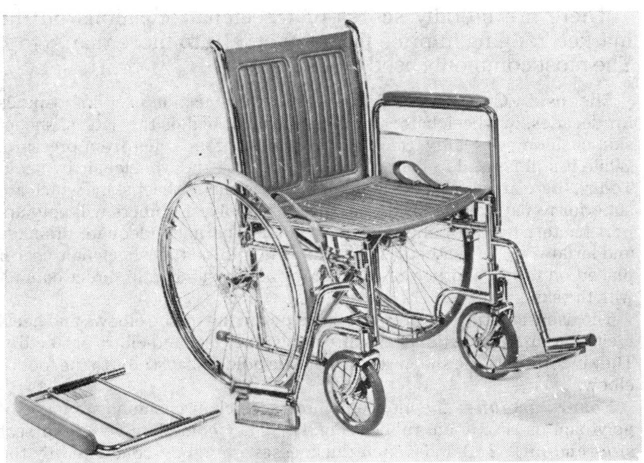

Fig 1. Adult wheelchair with full-length, removable arms and swing-away, detachable footrests (courtesy, Everest & Jennings).

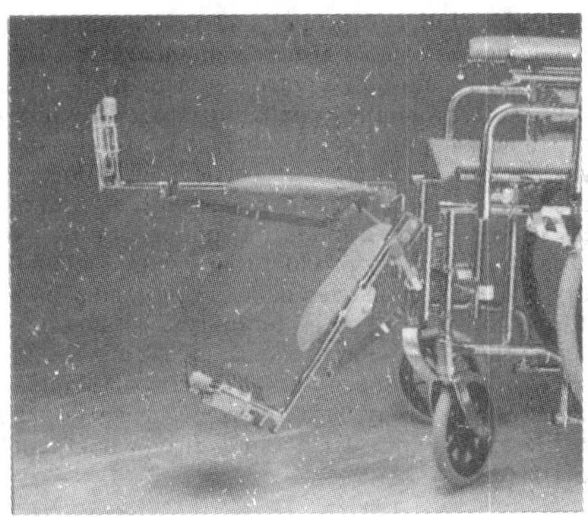

Fig 3. Articulating, elevating leg rest (courtesy, *Invacare*).

The Chair—Certain wheelchair dimensions (Fig 2) are important in preparing an individualized prescription. These are some of the components and measurements which should be considered.

Arms—Full length, nondetachable arms are standard. Desk- or full-length detachable styles are needed if the user must do a lateral transfer. Because detachable arms are offset from the main frame of the wheelchair, they also provide 1½ to 2 inches of additional seat width. Thus, a wheelchair with 18 inches upholstery and detachable arms actually yields 19½ to 20 inches of seat width. Just as this feature widens the seat it also widens the overall width of the wheelchair. If this additional overall width results in an architectural restriction, "wraparound" or "space-saver" arm styles must be considered. They are mounted behind the back uprights instead of between the uprights and the rear wheel. This design allows for the additional seat width and removable convenience, but keeps the overall width to that of a standard-frame wheelchair.

Another consideration of the arm is its height in relation to the seat. Standard arm height is approximately 10 inches. The arm can be manufactured to any specified height; however, a more convenient option is the adjustable-height arm which is available in the detachable styles.

Seat-and-Back-Width—A determination of seat and back width is the most important and fundamental part in selecting the proper wheelchair. A standard adult wheelchair has 18-inch seat and back upholstery. Wheelchairs are typically available in 2-inch increments from 12 to 24 inches. When considering seat width, remember the effect of detachable arms. A wheelchair that is too wide will promote leaning to one side or limit the ability of the user to propel the chair. Too-narrow a wheelchair can result in pressure sores.

Foot Supports—There are two basic types of foot supports: the footrest and the elevating legrest. Both are adjustable in length. To determine which type would be more beneficial to the user, consider the condition of the legs. If there is swelling or infirmity involving the leg or reduced flexion in the knee, elevating legrests might be indicated. A new concept, the articulating elevating leg rest, extends automatically as the leg rest is raised to fit the outstretched leg correctly (Fig 3). In most other cases the simple footrest will suffice. At this point also consider options like removable versus fixed assemblies, quad-release levers, heel-and-toe loops and oversized or nonskid footplates.

Seat Height—The standard seat height is approximately 19 to 20 inches from the floor. Hemi- or low-seat wheelchairs run about 2 inches lower. Seat height is important to those users who propel the wheelchair with one or both feet. A higher seat may be required for users with long legs so the footrest-to-ground clearance will not be less than 1½ to 2-in.

Seat Depth—The standard seat depth is 16 inches. The seat should be deep enough to properly support the thighs without putting pressure on the back of the calf.

Back Height—The standard back height is 16½ inches. A higher back height provides more support for a weak upper body. A lower back height provides less support, but allows for greater freedom of movement. To determine which is best, consider overall physical strength and lifestyle. Try to keep the height of the back to a minimum, high enough to provide adequate support, yet still allow upper-body mobility.

Wheels—Standard wheelchairs use a 24 inch rear wheel with an 8 inch front caster. Hemi wheelchairs have a 22 inch rear wheel. The rear wheel generally is aligned with the back upright. In the case of a reclining or amputee chair the wheels are set back to provide a larger base of support which is needed to prevent tipping backwards.

Note: 1. When taking measurements and adjusting the wheelchair *always* consider the effects of cushions and body positioners if they are to be used.

2. Always fit the wheelchair for the user's present condition. Make some allowances for progressive diseases but never "over prescribe" a wheelchair. Added features add weight and can make the wheelchair cumbersome to its user.

When the pharmacist has completed his measurements and evaluations and actually has the patient sitting in the chair, there are three quick "hand checks" the pharmacist can make.

1. An extended hand should fit between the hip and the skirt guard of the chair.
2. Three or four fingers should fit between the seat upholstery and the back of the calf.
3. Three or four fingers should fit between the top of the back upholstery and the underarm.

This kind of a quick double-check is the type of professional activity which will differentiate a pharmacist as an authority on health accessories.

While most patients will be able to use the manually operated wheelchairs described previously, a growing number will need a battery-powered wheelchair. This will include some quadriplegics and any pa-

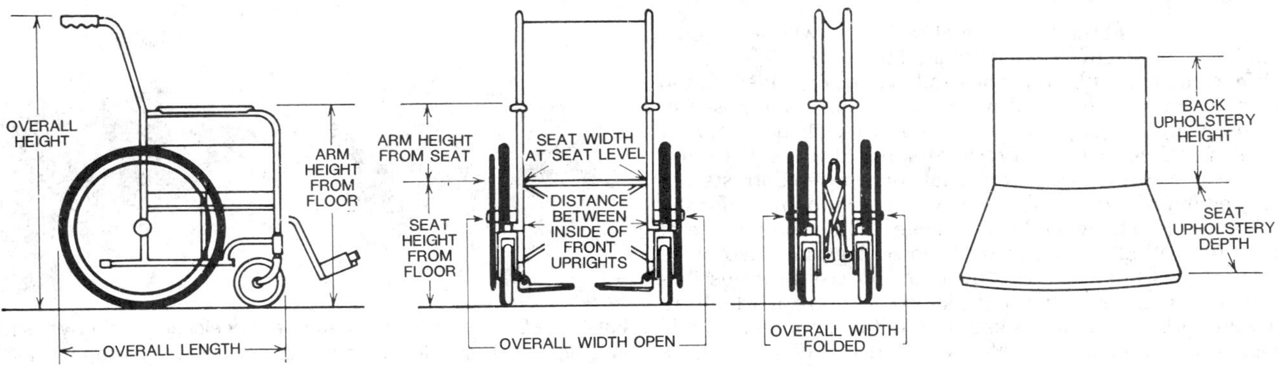

Fig 2. Key to wheelchair dimensions (courtesy, Everest & Jennings).

tients who lack the ability to propel a chair manually. In some cases where the patient has no hand or arm movement a chair can be operated by chin control or a sip-and-puff control, in which the controls may be operated by the patient inhaling or exhaling into a straw-like device.

Since the patient using an electric wheelchair usually spends the major part of his waking hours in his chair, it is especially important that the chair and its accessories be fitted properly to the patient. Manufacturers can provide specialized measuring and fitting guides for power wheelchairs.

One other health-accessory product that can be included in the wheelchair category is the three-wheeled battery-operated scooter. These are often useful for people with limited mobility. A person who can walk a short distance in the home environment may be unable to spend several hours on his feet in a shopping center, or on a trip to a museum or zoo. A battery-operated scooter may be the perfect answer to such a situation, and many health-accessory dealers include three-wheel scooters as part of their product mix.

Cushions and Supplies for Pressure Sores

Many types of cushions are available for a variety of purposes. Some are used to simulate a hospital bed's gatch spring, thus enabling the patient to eat and work in bed in relative comfort, while others are used to bolster the patient's legs to achieve flexion of the lumbar spine during traction. The most important use is to protect the patient from bruises and prevent the occurrence of pressure sores (decubitus ulcers, bed sores).

Pressure sores result from pressure at the thinly covered bony prominences of the body such as the sacrum, tuberosities of the ischium (below the buttocks), heels, elbows, shoulder blades and ears and back of the head in children. When pressure interferes with the normal circulation of capillary blood in the tissues, it can cause localized ulceration and gangrene.

A pressure sore begins as a reddened area which, if left untreated, will develop into an open sore; if not corrected early, surgery may be the only feasible remedy. The best cure is prevention. According to Richard M Meer, Founder and Executive Director of the Center for Tissue Trauma Research and Education (Jensen Beach, FL), "all pressure sores are preventable," a notion which unfortunately is still denied by some health professionals in institutions where pressure sores continue to occur. As health-care consultant to his or her customers, the community pharmacist is in a unique position to facilitate an understanding of pressure sore-prevention techniques which can be used in the home- care environment.

Pressure sores most commonly occur after long-term confinement in either a bed or a wheelchair. In institutions where nursing services are provided or at home where family members are available, the following measures will prevent their occurrence

1. Keep the bed dry and clean.
2. Thoroughly pat dry the skin after baths.
3. To increase circulation, regularly and gently massage the skin.
4. Change the position of the patient in bed as frequently as possible, at least a minimum of every 2 hours.
5. Relieve pressure as soon as the first signs of redness appear.
6. Expose the reddened area to the air and reduce pressure by using commercially available items (ie, cushions) to increase circulation.
7. Maintain proper nutrition.

It has been said that any type of treatment will be of some benefit, because it takes the patient off the sore.

Wheelchairs should never be used over an extended period of time without some kind of seat cushion. The most frequent occurrence of pressure sores in wheelchair users is at the ischial tuberosities. Pressure sores also result from a chair which is too wide, too small or whose footrests are adjusted improperly. Footrests which are too low cause the patient's legs to hang off the front edge of the seat upholstery, thus interrupting circulation to the lower legs, and also cause some patients' knees to come together, increasing the possibility of pressure sores between the knees. Footrests which are too high force the patient's knees up in the air and take body weight off the back of the thighs, resulting in all of the patient's body weight being focused directly on the ischial tuberosities.

There are literally scores of wheelchair cushions on the market, ranging in price from under $10 to more than $450. The most commonly used types are

Sheepskin Cushion (or Pad)—A standard cushion used in hospitals for decades, in wheelchairs and in the hospital bed, is the natural sheepskin cushion. Its fluffy, thick hair provides a good relief from pressure. While it still is used in bed, it is inadequate for the wheelchair by itself. Today, there are several manufacturers of synthetic sheepskins which are superior to natural sheepskin because their polyester fibers will not support bacterial growth and their porous back permits adequate drainage and airflow. The synthetic sheepskin is helpful to the wheelchair user if placed on top of another cushion and works best when in direct contact with the skin.

The usual solution for pressure sores occurring on the elbows and heels is either a large synthetic sheepskin or individual heel-and-elbow protectors. They incorporate the sheepskin in a plastic holder that straps to the foot or elbow.

Foam Cushion—The most common wheelchair cushions are made of polyfoam or latex foam rubber (Fig 4). They come in a variety of seat sizes and in 1, 2, 3 and 4-inch thicknesses. A study conducted by the Rancho Los Amigos Hospital in Downey, CA, compared these and other wheelchair cushions. The study showed that the best for the money was the 3-inch cushion and, further, that dense latex foam rubber was superior to polyfoam. The pharmacist should recommend a cushion with a removable cloth cover that has ties, thus enabling the cushion to be secured to the wheelchair seat back.

Convoluted Foam Cushion—The top surface of this foam cushion consists of rows of cones, giving it an egg-crate appearance. It remains popular in retail stores and many nursing homes, but has yet to be used extensively in the rehabilitation setting.

Coccyx Cushion—This is an effective modification of the foam cushion with its cut-out in one side. It usually comes with a board insert which provides stability in an inherently unstable cushion. This cushion is ideal when pressure sores exist or are anticipated at the base of the patient's spine, and also is used postsurgically for hemorrhoidectomies and patients who have suffered a fracture of the coccyx.

Inflatable Ring Cushion—The wheelchair-size inflatable ring cushion also can be effective providing it neither is underinflated (permitting the patient to bottom out) nor overinflated (making it hard and nonresilient). For most adults a 16-inch cushion with a 4½-inch ID is usually preferred.

Silicone Gel Cushion—The purpose of a silicone gel cushion is to simulate adipose tissue (body fat) and so perfectly distribute body weight that decubitus ulcers will be nearly impossible. While it is an excellent cushion for many patients, it has a drawback in that the loose gel permits some roll and creates a shearing effect damaging to some patients with tendencies toward pressure sores. Less-expensive gel-type cushions are now on the market.

Resin-Filled Cushion—This cushion is considerably lighter than the silicone or water cushions, yet also conforms to the body contours. It does so more slowly, due to its nature, and maintains a "memory" enabling the patient to jostle and move a bit while in his chair without the roll typical of the water and gel cushions. It does have a hard feel to the touch.

Alternating-Pressure Pad—An old standby both in wheelchair cushions and hospital bed mattresses is the alternating pressure pad (APP). The pad is an air mattress arranged in longitudinal tubes and connected to an air pump which alternately inflates and deflates alternate rows of tubes every 60 to 120 seconds. To eliminate counterpressure sometimes created by the smooth long tubes in earlier APP pads, newer configurations include small pillows arranged longitudinally, in lieu of straight tubes. It works on the principle that circulation in the tissues occurs in the absence of pressure. The pad is very effective in preventing and treating pressure sores in hospital beds but is less effective in wheelchairs. The pads, either permanent or the newer disposable type, present problems with respect to punctures and care should be exercised with sharp objects.

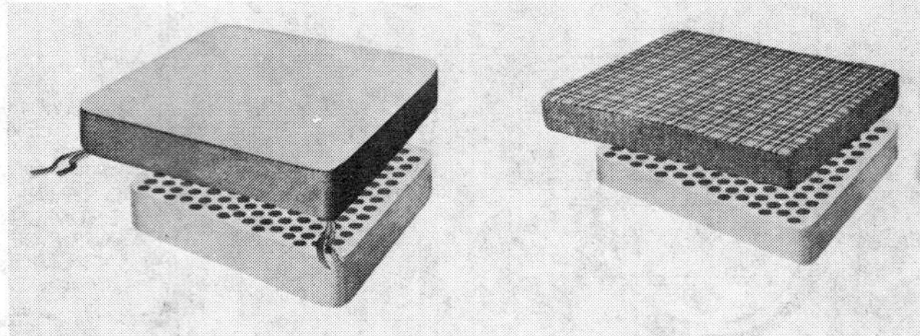

Fig 4. *Left:* 3-inch latex foam-rubber wheelchair cushion with seat ties; *right:* 2-inch latex foam-rubber wheelchair cushion in washable cover (courtesy, Guardian).

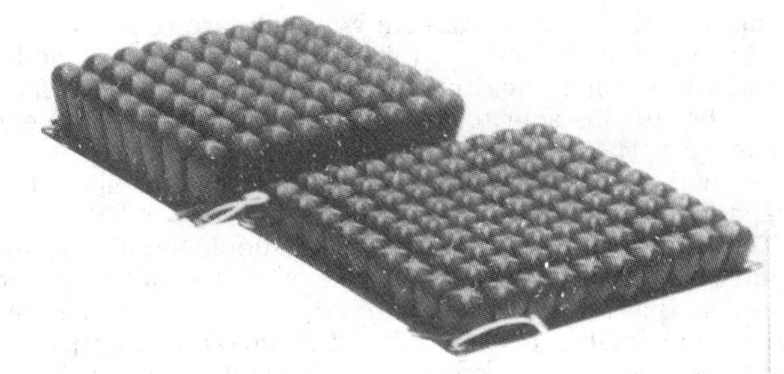

Fig 5. Balloon cushion (courtesy, Roho).

The pad is placed beneath the bottom bed sheet and, with connectors, most machines can operate two pads simultaneously.

Roho Balloon Cushion—Rows of inflatable balloons make up the surface of this cushion. A pressure gauge is used to adjust the pressure of the balloons. Individual balloons can be tied off to achieve an area of zero pressure (Fig 5).

Newer Cushions on the market include cushions which combine decubitus care and body positioning.

A new look at advanced flotation therapy to prevent and manage skin breakdown can be found in the Iris® product line by E R Carpenter. This new technology uses an outer surface produced from Omalux®, a densified, high resiliency foam, and has a dimpled, flat surface for improved flotation. The high-performance foam in the inner core provides optimal support while the Omalux® layers mold to body contours. Together they work to reduce pressure. A tough but supple nylon-taffeta fabric is available to envelop this system which is highly resistant to both moisture and microbial contamination. This system is available as a mattress overlay and as a wheelchair cusion (Fig 6).

All the wheelchair seat cushions described above may be used on the bed, but they usually are inserted in a foam mattress designed to admit the wheelchair seat-size cushion and provide a full level surface.

Canes and Crutches

Canes

Although walking canes are very simple devices, they are misused and misfitted frequently. The problem stems from a lack of basic knowledge as to what a walking cane is supposed to do and how it should be used properly.

A walking cane serves two important functions

Weight Transfer—It provides a means to transfer weight off the weak limb. To accomplish this weight must be put on the cane. If the patient carries the cane on the side of his weak limb and puts 50 lb of weight on it, he transfers 50 lb off his weak limb. The same is true if the cane is carried on the strong side. While the choice of carrying hand has nothing to do with weight transfer, it is crucial for proper balance.

Balance—Good balance in walking is no more than keeping one's center of gravity over the supporting limbs. If you suddenly lift one of your feet off the floor, you would reduce your base of support to one foot, your center of gravity would be outside the base of your support and you would fall. People who walk with legs apart tend to waddle as they must move their centers of gravity from one foot to the other to avoid falling. Fashion models avoid waddling by learning to place one foot directly in front of the other so their centers of gravity move forward rather than side to side.

If the patient carries his cane on the same side as his weak limb, his base of support will be narrow (ie, the distance between the cane tip and his weak limb is small) and he will have to transfer his weight from side to side, increasing the possibility of falling. A narrow base of support makes it difficult for the patient to keep his center of gravity over that base. If he is instructed to carry his walking cane on the side opposite his weak limb, his base of support will be wide and his center of gravity can move primarily forward rather than side to side. He uses the cane together with his weak limb, alternately swinging his strong limb through for the next step.

Again, this kind of instruction in "simple" aids is the type of professional activity which will differentiate a pharmacist as an authority on health accessories.

Unless specifically instructed by the patient's physician or physical therapist to the contrary, always instruct the patient to carry his walking cane on his strong side.

Fitting—A cane should be neither too long nor too short. Each one must be adjusted or cut to fit the patient. Fitting a cane is quite simple. Most schools of physical therapy recommend that a walking cane should fit so that the patient's arm makes a 150 to 160° (from vertical) bend at the elbow; this places the muscle groups in the arm in the best position for firm support. The cane tip should be placed 4 inches in front of the toe at an approximate 45° angle; angle the cane back to the hanging arm and the handle of the cane should be at the crease in the wrist. Then, when the patient lifts his hand up to the cane handle, his elbow will form the desired 20 to 30° bend automatically (Fig 7).

If the patient normally has one shoulder higher than the other, as in cases where the patients has scoliosis (an S-shaped curvature of the spine), no effort should be made to straighten them for the fitting. One cannot measure one side of the patient and then use that measurement for the other side. Each side must be measured separately. His arms should be made to hang normally. If the patient has trouble standing without support, he should be backed up against a wall during the fitting. The back of a chair can be used effectively for support. Rather than measuring at the top of the cane for an indication of where to cut it, turn the cane upside down for the fitting.

These rules apply in the fitting and use of all ambulatory aids including quad canes, forearm crutches, axillary crutches and walkers.

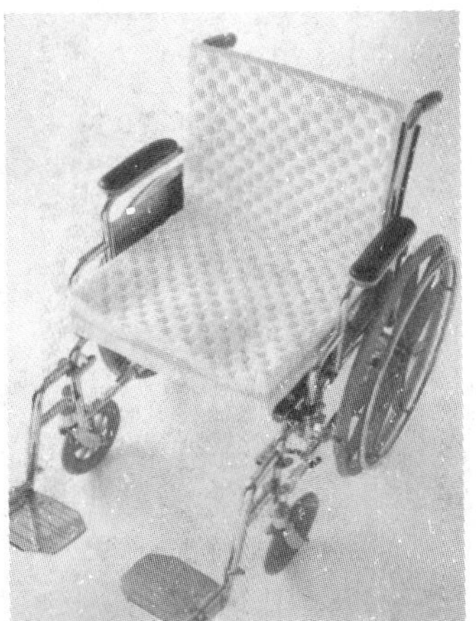

Fig 6. Iris wedge cushion (courtesy, ER Carpenter).

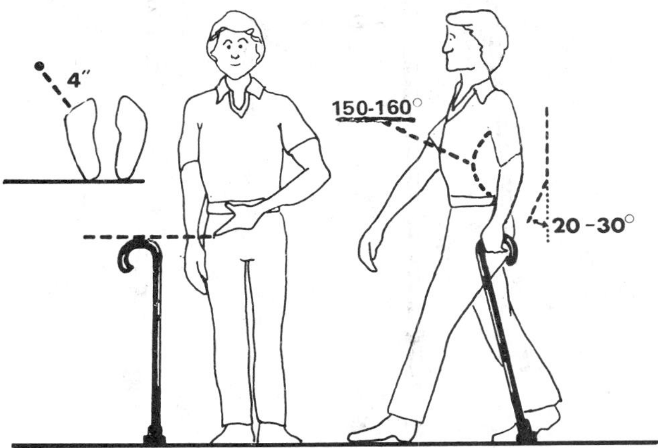

Fig 7. Proper fitting for canes, walkers and crutches.

Walkers

The most common walker in terms of sales and rentals continues to be the adult adjustable walker. A basic inventory of walkers in any pharmacy should include

1. Adult nonfolding adjustable walker
2. Child's adjustable walker
3. Adult folding, adjustable walker
4. Hemiplegic walker
5. Walkane

Proper use is the same for all nonwheeled walkers. The patient is instructed to lift the walker, place it in front of him and walk to it. With this method, the walker is firmly on the floor when the patient is moving. A walker should never be carried by a walking patient; if he is able to do this with relative security, a cane probably would suffice.

A frequent problem encountered is that patients tend to lean into the walker while walking up to it. The danger is that they may lose their balance and push the walker over as it is relatively light. This tendency can be overcome by lengthening the front two legs of the walker by one adjustment making the walker tilt back. This should not be a routine adjustment for all walkers, however; rather, it should be a response to a specific tendency of the patient to lean into the walker.

A folding walker is much more convenient to transport (as in the trunk of a small car) and to use in confined areas or on stairs (Fig 8).

The only safe wheeled walker is one with a braking mechanism, most commonly called a glide brake, that will stop it if the patient trips or loses his balance. The braking mechanism should work when the patient's weight is increased on the normal hand holds.

There are a variety of wheel options available for aluminum walkers: 5 inch rubber wheels, 3 inch rubber wheels, 3 inch rubber swivel wheels and 3 inch plastic wheels. It is recommended that all wheel options be used in conjunction with the glide-brake attachments. Proper application of wheel options should be evaluated by a durable medical equipment technician or physical therapist per individual client's disability and environment for best results.

Yet another ambulatory device being widely prescribed is a rollator walker, technically referred to as a heavy-duty, multibraking system, variable wheel resistant walker. This item is generally of steel construction equipped with 7½ to 8 inch wheels. A hand-brake system is incorporated into this structure with adjustability to control the ambulatory gait of the user. Some units are available with seats for intermittent resting and basket or tray accessories to carry items for daily living needs. Rollator walkers generally are recommended for but are not limited to an individual's need for mobility outside the home environment where a variety of surfaces could be an obstacle to the use of an aluminum-wheeled walker (Fig 9).

As in the case of walking canes, all walkers should be adjusted for each user.

To properly fit a walker, the patient should stand normally against a wall if necessary. The legs of the walker are adjusted so that the top of the handgrips come to the patient's wrist. On raising his hands to the walker handgrips, the patient's elbows will form the proper bend. When it is also necessary to lengthen the front legs of a nonwheeled walker, the wrist-crease length should be accurate for the walker's rear legs. The front legs of the walker will then be 1 to 2 inches longer depending on the extent to which the patient leans into the walker.

In terms of support, a walker can best be compared to the simple cane. While a walker does provide a steadier support for the patient, like the cane, it requires reasonably good arms, wrists and hands.

A patient with a disability or injury involving the hand or wrist making it nonweight-bearing may need a platform attachment which allows the forearm to bear the weight instead of the hand or wrist.

Crutches

Forearm Crutches—Neither walking canes nor walkers provide support to the patient's wrists and elbows. The forearm crutch, however, is designed specifically to provide such support in that it has a vertical member which extends above the wrist and is secured reasonably well to the fleshy part of the forearm by a collar or cuff.

The term forearm crutch is generic. They commonly are referred to as Canadian crutches or Lofstrand crutches. All can be recognized by the collar or cuff which encircles the patient's forearm. The cuff usually is open and the opening either may face the side or front. It is important that the cuff is open so the crutches may be thrown out of the way if the patient falls. The handgrip projects from the main shaft and, unless specifically instructed by the physician or physical therapist to the contrary, the patient should be instructed to hold the handgrip so that it points forward.

If only one crutch is used, it should be used on the side opposite the weak leg. When two crutches are used, the patient should be instructed to step forward with his right leg and his left crutch, followed by his left leg and right crutch and

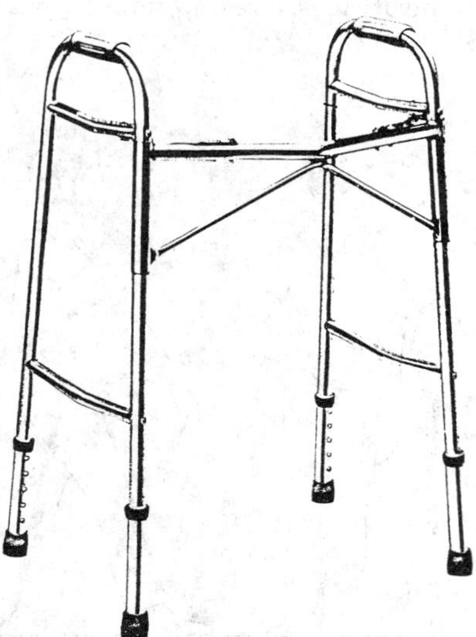

Fig 8. Folding, adjustable walker (courtesy, Guardian).

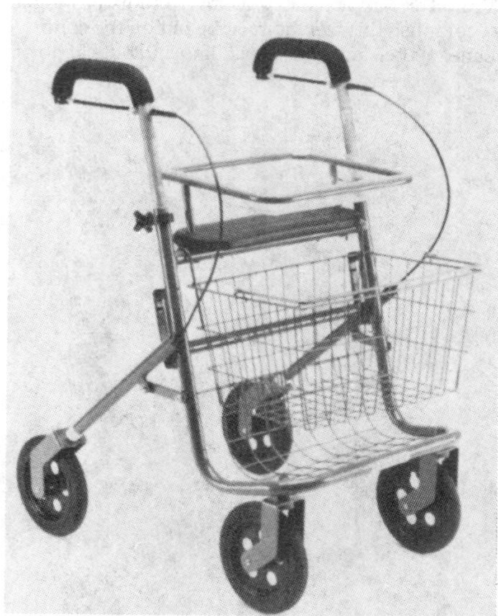

Fig 9. Folding wheeled walker (courtesy, Walker Works).

so on. Commonly known as the two-point gait, it is recommended for persons using forearm crutches unless, of course, the physician or physical therapist suggests a different gait.

In fitting the forearm crutch, the patient should stand normally erect, with arms at his sides. The forearm cuff is flipped back out of the way, and the handgrip is brought to the crease in his wrists by adjusting or cutting the main shaft. The length of the vertical member between the handgrip and the forearm cuff also should be adjusted so that the cuff comes to the middle of the patient's forearm, usually over the fleshiest part. Care should be taken to see that the cuff doesn't interfere with the elbow when it is fully bent. The cuff can be opened or closed by bending and shaping by hand with very little effort. The patient should be shown how to do this as he may want the cuff larger or tighter depending on his clothing.

Axillary Crutches—More common than the forearm crutch is the ordinary wooden or aluminum underarm crutch—the axillary crutch. It provides more support than the forearm crutch because it braces both wrist and elbow.

Adjustable crutches are preferred as they offer better and easier fitting. First, the patient should stand normally erect with arms at his sides. The crutch is placed under the arms with the crutch tip on the floor at a point approximately 6 to 8 inches ahead of his toes and 6 to 8 inches to the side. The main shaft is lengthened or shortened so that the top of the crutch is about 1½ inch (two finger-widths) from the armpit. This fitting should be done with crutch tips and axillary cushions in place on the crutch.

The second step is to adjust the position of the handgrip on the crutch so that it comes to the crease in the wrist. The crutch should be in the same position for this handgrip adjustment as it was during the fitting of its entire length. The arm then is brought out alongside the crutch for the handgrip adjustment.

A flexed elbow is important when using an axillary crutch. If the handgrip is not positioned at the wrist so that the elbow bends when the patient takes hold of the handgrip, the tops of the crutches would push up into his armpits with each swing. But with his elbows bent initially, the crutch tops are safely below the armpits since the patient must straighten his arms on the swing through. When axillary crutches are fitted properly, there is little or no danger of injury to the lymph glands, blood vessels or radial nerves in the armpits which can lead to "crutch paralysis." The primary danger signal is an elevation in the patient's shoulders with each swing through his crutches. When that happens it is clear that the patient's weight is bearing on the crutch tops and not on the handgrips as it should be.

There are several axillary crutch gaits.

The safest, most stable, and most common is the four-point gait. The patient begins by moving his left crutch forward. Next, he moves his right leg forward. His right crutch is then brought up to his right foot and, finally, his left leg is brought up to his left crutch.

The two-point gait, the principal gait used when two canes are employed, also is used commonly with forearm and axillary crutches. Simply, both the left crutch and right leg are brought forward; then the right crutch and left leg are brought forward.

The three-point gait has two variations: the swing-to gait and the swing-through gait. In either form, the patient begins by moving both crutches forward simultaneously. In the swing-to gait, both feet (or one foot for an amputee or when one leg is in a nonweight-bearing cast) are swung to a point between the two crutches. In the swing-through gait, the feet (or foot) are swung through the crutches to a point ahead of the two crutches—it helps to visualize a triangle made by the two crutchtips and foot, and flipping that triangle end-over-end.

Another common crutch gait is the hemiplegic gait. It is nothing more than the use of a single axillary crutch in exactly the same manner as one would use a single cane. The crutch is carried on the strong side and is moved forward together with the weak limb alternating with the good leg.

Accessories

Tips—The most important accessory is the tip which makes contact with the floor. No cane or crutch should ever be sold or rented without a good tip. Safety requires that cane and crutch tips have the following minimum characteristics: they must fit the cane or crutch shaft snugly, have a suction-grip bottom and have a flexible neck so the bottom of the tip will stay in complete contact with the floor when the cane or crutch rocks through a gait. The suction-grip bottom of a crutch or cane tip should be as large as possible—the more rubber in contact with the floor, the less chance of slippage.

Axillary Cushions—These are available in two basic styles—one with a powdery finish and the other without a powdery finish in almost a translucent, amber-colored rubber—and a variety of sizes. Both types adequately protect the underarm from bruises and inhibit slippage of the crutch top from under the arm.

Handgrips—These are more varied in type and style, however, as they are designed for various purposes. The most common kinds are dense foam-rubber sleeves which fit over the standard crutch grip. The split handgrips should be used for nonadjustable crutches only, as they tend to slip around the handgrip. Taping them tightly will secure them somewhat. The nonsplit, often called closed, handgrip is better for the patient, but it requires removal of the crutch's handgrip to put it on.

Other contoured handgrips and "palmgrips" are available. Since the natural palm line is not horizontal, they are designed to alleviate problems such as hand discomfort and wrist soreness associated with the traditional horizontal crutch handgrip.

Commodes

A commode is little more than a portable toilet and yet there are a variety of different types. More than a convenience, a commode can mean the difference between coming home and staying in the hospital. Whenever the patient is unable to ambulate from his bed to the bathroom, or be transported via wheelchair, there is a need for a commode.

Perhaps the most common type is the steel- or aluminum-frame commode with a toilet seat and cover plus a removable plastic pail and cover. It adequately serves its intended purpose although it may look like a commode and be undesirable for that reason. This type comes with either nonadjustable or adjustable legs. The latter is the most desirable since some patients need a rather tall one to aid them both in sitting and getting up more easily. The "Drop-arm" steel commode enables easier lateral transfer to and from the commode seat. Some patients also find this innovation helpful where there is a need to insert suppositories. Depending upon the attitude of the patient and, more often, that of his family, an aluminum folding commode can be removed from view when it is not in use.

The common aluminum- and steel-frame commode uses its uplifted toilet seat cover as a backrest. Commodes are available with padded and nonpadded backs, an upholstered seat and armrests and casters for moving about easily (Fig 10); others are made of wood and resemble furniture—eg, the disguised, Danish Modern commode. Some commodes are designed to be used both in the bedroom and in the bathroom. These are either backless or have a removable back, so as not to interfere with the toilet tank.

Although commodes may be rented in most states, it is unwise to reuse the commode pail; it should be sold to the customer during the first month's rental. It also is helpful to advise the patient's family that a pail filled to one-third with water will be easier to keep clean. Deodorant tablets and drops are also appropriate as an accessory to any commode rental or sale.

It should be mentioned that commodes with wheels should be used with caution.

Bathroom Safety Aids

Safety in the bathroom primarily means safety in the tub or at the toilet. An elevated toilet seat makes it easier for patients to sit or stand and suggests the need for some kind of

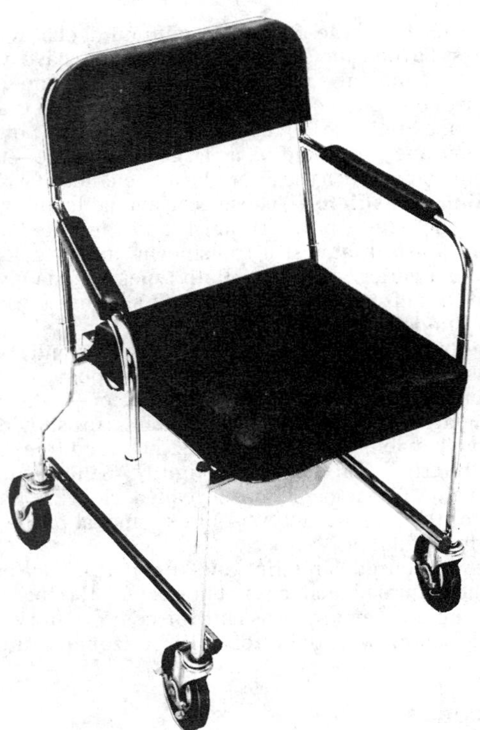

Fig 10. Padded commode on casters with pivot arms (courtesy, Lumex).

toilet guard rail (Fig 11). Attaching-type toilet rails can connect to the bowl with the regular toilet seat bolts. Some attaching types are designed with detachable sides permitting the use of one side only, as well as easier cleaning of the rail in general.

Elevated toilet seats vary considerably with respect to the materials from which they are fabricated, whether or not they have full or partial splash guards, to what extent they are adjustable in height and whether or not they are padded for softness or, like any normal toilet seat, quite hard. The full splash guard may be preferred by many people, but the pharmacist should keep in mind that persons without good legs and body control (paraplegics and quadriplegics, particularly) need the open sides which only the elevated toilet seat with the partial splash guard has in order to administer to their personal cleanliness independently and to insert suppositories without assistance. The least expensive elevated toilet seats are one-piece molded plastic. Combination elevated toilet seats with attached hand rails are available, but may "tip" if equal pressure is not applied to both sides when arising.

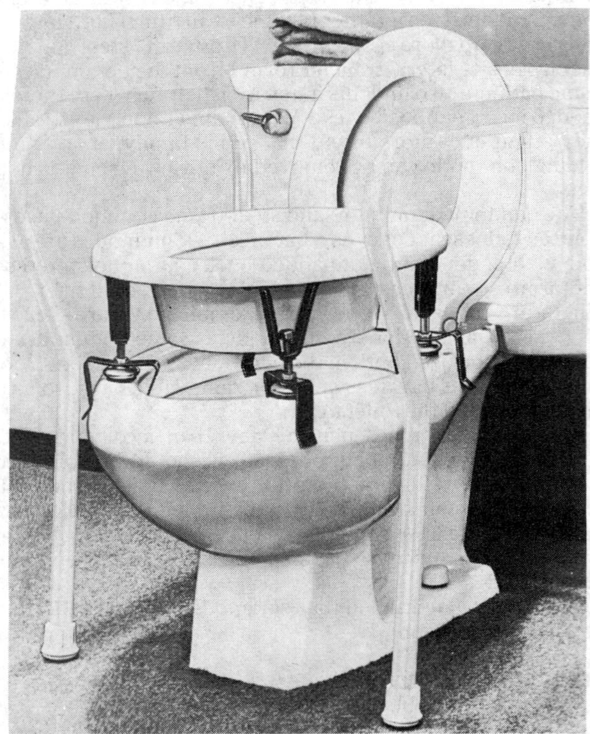

Fig 11. Elevated toilet seat with continuous splash guard (courtesy, Lumex).

Safety aids for the bathtub include adhesive strips and spots for the tub bottom, mats for preventing slips and a variety of tub seats and safety grab bars. Tub seats are either bench types with legs, or seats that straddle the tub sides (Fig 12).

One type of bench has either fixed (standard)- or adjustable-height legs and is available with or without a back. A transfer bench is used with two legs in the tub and two legs on the floor outside the tub. The patient can sit down on that portion of the seat which is outside the tub, swing his legs over the edge of the tub and slide across the bench until the entire body is "inside" the tub. Transfer benches are available with solid seats or with a commode opening to facilitate perineal cleansing. Some models of transfer benches have suction-cup footpieces or clamp on to the side of the tube for security and stability and are available with a plastic or a padded seat for comfort and protection of skin integrity.

Another type of bath seat is powered by either water pressure or a hydraulic pump which actually raises or lowers the height of the seat from the height of the tub side to near the bottom. This seat also can be classified as a bath lift.

Bathtub grab bars range from those which attach to the side of the bathtub to wall-mounted grab bars. Perhaps the most frequently used type is one that extends high enough for a person standing outside the tub to get a firm support before stepping into the tub. Wall grab bars take a variety of shapes, angles and lengths. Finishes of vinyl coating, smooth chrome and a knurled texture for grip security are all available. True grab bars extend from the wall at least 4 to 5 inches, enabling a falling person to slip his forearm behind the bar and hook his elbow over it.

Another important consideration is how the various bars are attached to the wall. Whatever the method, the pharma-

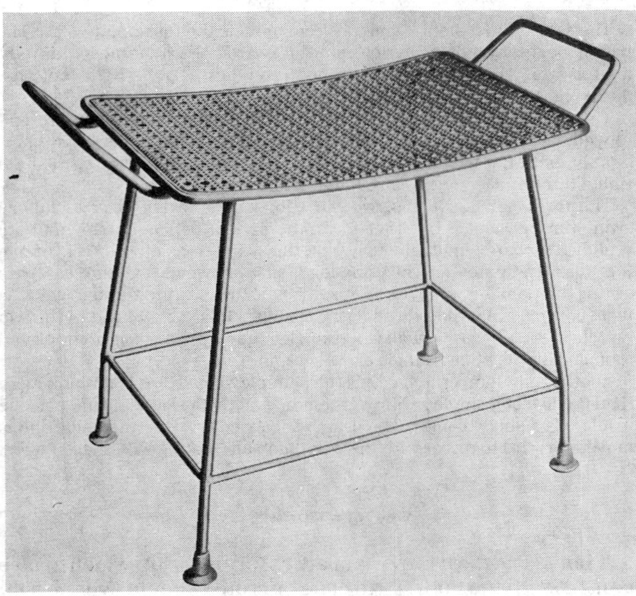

Fig 12. Bath benches (courtesy, Frohock-Stewart).

cist should know how the bars he stocks are mounted best for safety and either be able to instruct the customer in the mounting procedure, provide such service or have someone who will provide installation services on call and also be aware of liability when doing so.

Hospital Beds

The health-accessories department of a pharmacy also may have hospital beds for sale or rental, including manual or electrically-operated beds. The bed either can be fixed or variable height, and its spring should have an adjustable head and foot section that raises the patient's knees as well as permits the feet to be elevated.

The electrically operated bed may be either the 6-way or 4-way type. The height of the 6-way bed is adjustable from the floor, and it has a spring which permits positioning of both the head and foot sections. The 4-way bed can be either fixed height or have a manual crank to adjust the height.

Mattresses—Polyfoam mattresses are excellent for rental purposes, especially with split-spring hospital beds, as one man can handle them easily. An innerspring mattress should be used with an electrically operated bed, or when the heavier mattress is preferred; however, not every innerspring mattress will work well on a hospital bed, since the springs must be hinged in order to have the mattress flex properly when the spring is adjusted. Sometimes the selection of the type of mattress is influenced by the diagnosis or the insurance coverage.

Any mattress used for rental purposes should be covered with a plastic-impregnated mattress ticking and it is well to provide plastic mattress covers. Some states have laws regulating the sanitizing of rental mattresses. The pharmacist should be aware of these as well as the laws in his community.

Bedside Safety Rails—It is recommended to stock three types of bedside safety rails, full-length and half-length rails for use on a hospital bed, and the other for use on any kind of bed normally used in the home. Rails for use with a hospital bed have clamps which attach to the steel parts of the spring. Rails used on home-type beds are attached by connecting rods placed between the regular mattress and box spring. This "any-bed" type of safety rail usually is made of aluminum with cross-members of steel (Fig 13). Hospital bed rails may be constructed of aluminum or steel. Bed rails used on home beds are to provide safety and should not be used as repositioning aids or transfer-assist devices.

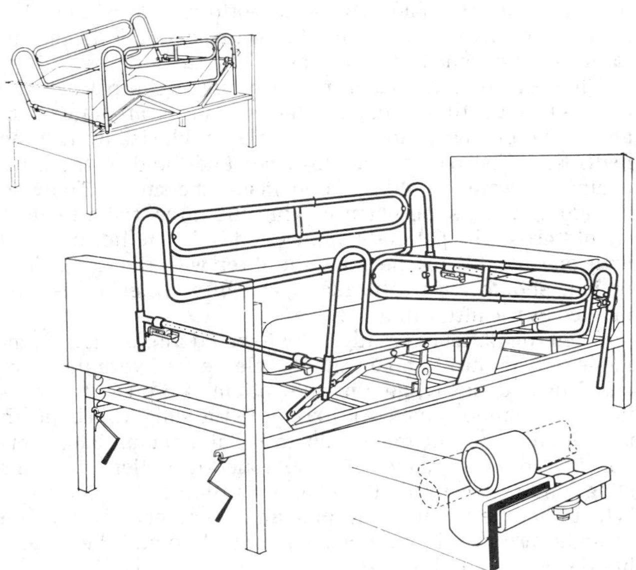

Fig 13. Any-bed model safety rails showing connecting cross bar (courtesy, Edco).

Trapeze Bars—The typical overbed trapeze bar is used by the patient as an assist in sitting up and getting into and out of bed. It usually is made of steel and by means of clamps is attached to the headboard of a hospital bed. A trapeze-bar floor-stand, which enables the trapeze to be used over any bed, is also available (Fig 14).

Trapeze bars are adjustable in height, and some models also provide adjustability in the position of the bar over the bed. A special clamp permits the bar to be swung to various positions and locked for security. A pivoting trapeze bar should never be used with the floor stand, as accidents may occur unless the bar is suspended properly.

Traction

Overdoor traction sets provide for cervical traction at home using any open door for the purpose of mounting the traction pulleys. Weight is applied to the cervical spine by a cord running over the pulleys and attaching to a halter which fits over the patient's head and applies pressure to his mandible and occiput. The weights may be cast-iron traction weights suspended on a traction-weight hanger, or a graduated water-weight bag containing tap water in accordance with the weight-of-water markings on the plastic bag. An additional item in most overdoor traction sets is a metal spreader bar which spreads the top of the head halter in order to avoid pressure against the patient's ears.

Unless specifically instructed by the physician to the contrary, the pharmacist should tell the patient to use the overdoor traction set while sitting in a chair facing the door. When doing so, the patient's head will be pulled toward the front, bending his chin down and flexing his cervical spine. Flexion generally is preferred over hyperextension in any type of traction. If the patient were to sit with his back to the door, as has been illustrated on the covers of overdoor traction sets for many years, his chin would be pulled up and his cervical spine would be hyperextended—usually an undesirable attitude during cervical traction.

The majority of patients who require traction will need it in a flexion posture, the rest needing hyperextension. It may be dangerous to use flexion on patients who require hyperextension.

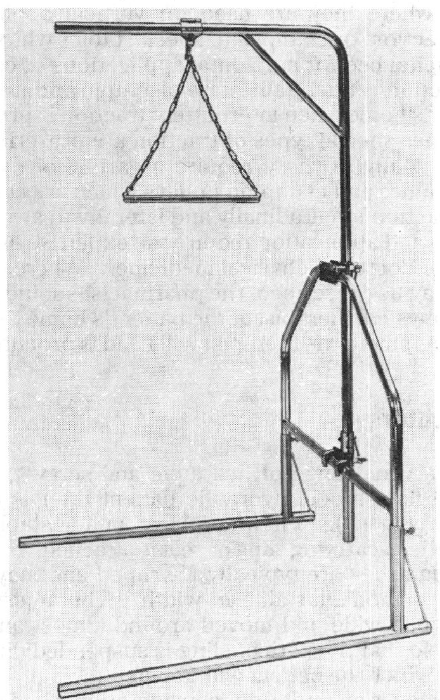

Fig 14. Overbed trapeze bar with floor stand (courtesy, Invacare).

Any traction set—even the ordinary overdoor type—should be sold or rented only on the written prescription of a physician who specifies the frequency of treatment, the length of each treatment, the weight to be applied, whether the traction is to be static or intermittent and special instructions as to positioning of the patient with respect to flexion and hyperextension. It is often necessary for the pharmacist or the patient to call either the physician or the physical therapist to clarify the amount of weight to be used or the length of time of each treatment.

Traction in Bed—While cervical traction may be given either while the patient is sitting in a chair or reclining in bed, pelvic traction is administered at home only when the patient is in prone position. There are two basic types of applied-in-bed traction sets: one is for use with a hospital bed and the other for use with any bed. The any-bed traction device has the typical vertical adjustments and pulleys and is mounted on a floor stand. Buck's extension traction or a mattress clamp set may require a sturdy headboard or footboard as it has no floor stand. Either type is used for both pelvic and cervical traction.

When applying cervical traction to a patient lying in bed, unless specifically instructed by the physician to the contrary, traction pulleys usually are mounted quite high so as to develop flexion of the cervical spine and mildly depress the patient's chin.

When pelvic traction is applied, flexion is also important, and the pulleys should be mounted quite high to produce flexion of the lumbar spine. It also may be helpful to raise the head section of the hospital bed or bolster the ordinary bed with a wedge cushion or mattress elevator. Additionally, the patient's knees should be elevated either with the knee adjustments of the hospital bed spring or ordinary pillows placed under the knees. These recommendations must have the approval of the physician.

A complete traction department also will have pelvic traction belts in a variety of sizes, without which pelvic traction cannot be applied. A universal (one size fits all) belt with velcro fasteners is also available.

An intermittent traction machine that electrically sets pounds of pull, number of seconds of pull and number of seconds of rest during the treatment is available. Some machines also can be set for the length of the entire traction treatment. Intermittent traction machines, used in physical-therapy departments of hospitals, may be attached to wall brackets, where they are used for vertical applications of cervical traction, or clamped to special tables which wheel up to the hospital bed for horizontal applications of cervical and pelvic traction. Such tables are also appropriate for use in the patient's home when intermittent traction is prescribed.

Sometimes special types of traction are prescribed for use at home. Many of these require a variety of over-the-bed fracture frames and clamp-on pulleys which are connected to provide traction longitudinally and laterally to arms and legs; their setup and application require the expertise of a physical therapist or doctor of physical medicine. Where this kind of traction may be prescribed, the pharmacist should arrange to meet the physical therapist at the patient's home to be certain that the equipment the therapist will need is procured.

Patient Lifters

Among a wide range of hydraulic and screw-type patient lifters, the floor-model hydraulic patient lifter is used most commonly (Fig 15). All lifters have an adjustable boom to which a patient-carrying sling or seat is attached. Lifter bases differ though they are typically U-shaped and may be either adjustable or nonadjustable in width. The adjustable base can be spread wide and moved around almost any chair or commode so that the patient sling is suspended directly over the seat to which the patient will transfer.

Sling design is an important consideration when choosing a patient lifter. Slings in all fabrics come as one- or two-piece units, with and without head supports; they also may be had with a commode opening.

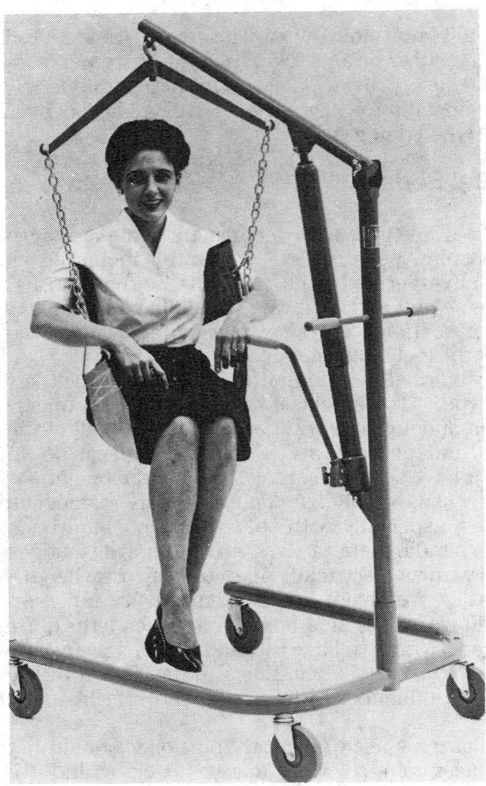

Fig 15. Painted hydraulic patient lifter with nonadjustable base and two-piece canvas patient sling (courtesy, Ted Hoyer & Co).

Positioning the sling under the patient while he is in bed is accomplished in much the same way that bed linens are changed under a patient. He is rolled to his side while half the sling is folded in accordion fashion and tucked up against him. The sling should be so positioned that on rolling him back his spine will rest on the middle of the sling. He is rolled back over the folded portion of the sling and to his other side while the folded part of the sling is unfolded; then he is returned to his back. Attention should be paid to the vertical positioning of the sling also—the bottom edge of the sling should not extend to the middle of the patient's knee, but rather should come just to the knee.

When the sling is placed properly under the patient, the lifter is brought to the bed, the chains or straps are hooked up and the boom raised slowly and gently until he is lifted off the mattress. The patient should never take hold of the lifter chains; his arms should be safely inside the sling. To avoid swinging of the sling when moving the lifter, the attendant should cross the patient's ankles and hold the bottom heel with one hand while he pulls the lifter with the other. The patient should always be facing the lifter when he is suspended by the lifter sling.

When the patient is ready to be lowered into a chair, commode or bed, the attendant should release the hydraulic valve carefully and slowly, guiding the patient into position by his heel. A common mistake is to remove the sling from beneath the patient after transferring him to a chair or commode. It is considerably easier, and safer too, to let the patient sit on his sling, and remove only the chains and lifter from his view. When it's time to pick him up again, the lifter only need be brought into position, the chains hooked up and the patient lifted slowly out of his chair.

A patient lifter with a special type of base must be used for bathtub transfers.

Bedpans

Bedpans, used for the collection of feces, may be round but are predominantly oval and are constructed of plastic, stainless steel, enamelware or porcelain. Single-patient-use plastic bedpans (nonautoclavable) are considerably less expensive than their metal and porcelain counterparts. Plastic, like rubber, also tends to be warmer to the touch and therefore much more comfortable than steel, porcelain or enamelware. There is also available a smaller, sloping and flatter bedpan, called a fracture bedpan, for use, primarily for urine, with immobilized or overweight patients.

It is helpful to the patient for the pharmacist to suggest that, when a hospital bed is available, the back rest and knee section of the gatch spring should be elevated when using the bedpan. The backrest should be elevated substantially while the knee section should be elevated only slightly. When a hospital bed is not available in the patient's home, four or five pillows behind his back will make use of a bedpan much easier.

Accessories for the Bedfast Patient

Special tables and trays for spill-preventing safety and patient comfort are near-essentials in any sickroom (Fig 16). The common overbed table is an ideal accessory whether or not the patient has a hospital bed. Some overbed tables have a center section that can be raised to a slanted position for the support of a book or magazine; others have a vanity tray and mirror which slide out from beneath the tabletop for use by the bedfast patient. Sturdy breakfast trays that straddle the patient's hips while he is in bed, special folding tables and trays with contoured fronts which enable the wheelchair user to get comfortably close and even a special lounge chair with its own adjustable and self-storing table contribute to the nonambulatory patient's comfort and convenience in the sickroom at home.

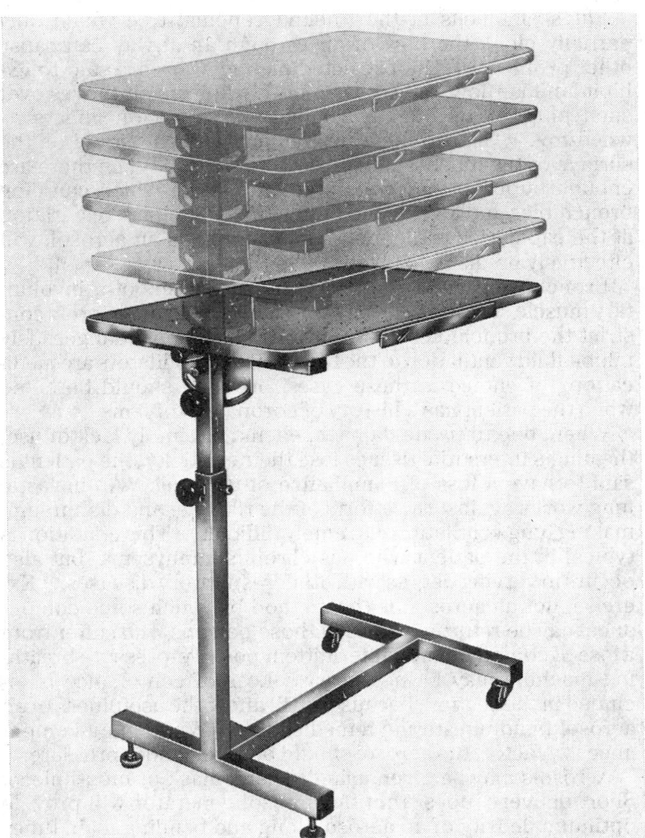

Fig 16. Adjustable overbed table with tilt-top for books or magazines (courtesy, Lumex).

Easy-reachers are devices that enable the bedfast patient to reach out and pick up things normally beyond his reach.

A solid or inflatable plastic shampoo tray facilitates shampooing for patients who cannot leave their beds. The tray fits across the mattress where a pillow normally goes, and is designed to carry shampoo water to a drain at the side of the bed where it may be collected in a plastic bucket. The patient's head rests in the shampoo tray which, though it has quite high sides, has a depression for the back of his neck.

Folding backrests with or without arms, mattress elevators which are placed between an ordinary mattress and the boxspring, wedge-shaped foam cushions, bedboards and footboards with adjustable cushions for the prevention of foot rotation are additional articles for the comfort and convenience of the bedfast patient. When it is necessary to keep bed linens and blankets off the patient's feet and legs, a blanket support, sometimes referred to as a leg or body cradle, is desirable. Holding mitts, built-up forks and swivel spoons, food guards, feeding cups, pencil and cigarette holders and simple drinking straws with accordion hinges that bend without collapsing are some of the devices which make patient home-care effective.

Folding patient-privacy screens are a frequently requested sickroom accessory, especially when the patient will be using a bedside commode.

Finally, a health-accessories department also will stock a modest assortment of safety vests and belts, crib nets and restraints for use by nursing homes and extended-care facilities, as well as by the patient at home.

Respiratory Therapy

Steam Vaporizers—The modern steam inhaler is essentially the same as the now nearly forgotten croup kettle, except that it uses electricity to generate heat and steam. The advantage of this more modern adaptation lies in the attainment of a constant temperature. Also, most forms of this apparatus are equipped with a regulator so that when they run dry, the heating unit shuts off simultaneously. These are easier to handle in the home, especially at night.

The familiar vaporizer provides the conventional hot-steam therapy for the relief of upper respiratory illnesses. Physicians recommend it for colds, sinusitis and similar ailments.

The portable room humidifier, on the other hand, provides a cool mist to compensate for the lack of sufficient moisture in the air in dry, steam-heated rooms, and occasionally for its expectorant effect in liquefying tenacious mucus in the airway. An additional advantage is that, since no heater is used, it is entirely safe for small children.

Vaporizers are used extensively in the home today to humidify bedrooms or chambers where patients suffering from various bronchial conditions may rest. Cool-vapor humidifiers provide effective high-humidity inhalation therapy for respiratory patients, and can be used as well to restore proper humidity to rooms dried out by winter heating.

Aerosol Therapy and Nebulizers—Instruments that generate very fine particles of liquid in a gas of uniform particle size are called nebulizers. Within the container of this apparatus is a small unit that produces atomization inside the flask. The wall of the flask acts as a baffle, removing large droplets from the mist which run down the wall and drop back into the reservoir, and producing a mist of small droplets that penetrate further into the lung. A current of air or oxygen carries the fine mist through the large outlet tube of the nebulizer. The flask of the nebulizer has a mark beyond which fluid should not be added, for atomization will not occur if the level of liquid is higher than the mark.

The nebulizer is not as useful as the plastic-bottle atomizer for applying medication to the nose and pharynx, but because the mist is subdivided very finely, medication can be carried into the deeper parts of the respiratory tract. The nebulizer is especially valuable for diseases of the larynx and trachea as well as various kinds of obstructive airway disease and accompanying conditions which inhibit efficient ventilation.

Within the past decade, the ultrasonic nebulizer (Fig 17) has gained widespread application in respiratory therapy. It produces sound waves by electric current causing vibrations that are used to break up water into aerosol particles. The resulting aerosol is a very dense mist with a water content in excess of 100 mg/L. It is regarded as the most efficient of nebulizers since it is claimed to create better than 90% of its particles within the "effective" range of 0.5 to 3 μm.

The transducer of the ultrasonic nebulizer often is placed in a coupling chamber filled with water. Water helps absorb mechanically produced heat and acts as a transfer medium for sound waves to the nebulizer chamber.

A common use of the term *aerosol* is to describe a nebulized solution consisting of very fine particles carried by a propellent gas under pressure to a site of therapeutic application. The principal purpose of the use of an aerosol in respiratory therapy is the topical administration of medication and/or water or saline solution to the mucosal linings of the tracheobronchial tree (Fig 18). To accomplish this the liquid has to be dispersed as droplets 5 μm or less in diameter. Various medications are used to treat a variety of conditions that accompany respiratory disease. Conditions requiring aerosol therapy, particularly when such therapy can be administered to a patient on a program of home care, include infection, mucosal edema, tenacious secretions, foam buildup, bronchospasms and loss of compliance.

Aerosol therapy provides an efficient means of administering an antibiotic directly to the infection and generally requires a smaller dosage than would be necessary if the drug were given systemically. Infection often is accompanied by one or more of the five other conditions cited above.

Edema of the mucous membrane which lines the interior walls of the tracheobronchial tree seriously may affect ventilation in the alveoli. Any swelling of the linings of the airways, especially in the terminal bronchioles and respiratory bronchioles, may impede severely the flow of air to alveoli, making breathing difficult and reducing the efficiency of oxygen pickup.

When the mucosa becomes edematous the serous fluid it excretes may be profuse and thickened. Cold, dry air or a compressed gas when used without adequate humidification will draw moisture out of the mucus, leaving it sludgelike and tenacious. Such mucus resists movement up the walls of the tracheobronchial tree normally accomplished with efficiency by the cilia throughout the airways and, instead, becomes gradually more viscous and forms mucus plugs which can shut off alveoli and, for that matter, entire airways, depriving whole sections of the lung of oxygen-rich air. Medications that help to loosen these plugs of mucus include wetting agents and a variety of proteolytic enzymes. Distilled water and normal saline solution are also effective in dissolving tenacious secretions.

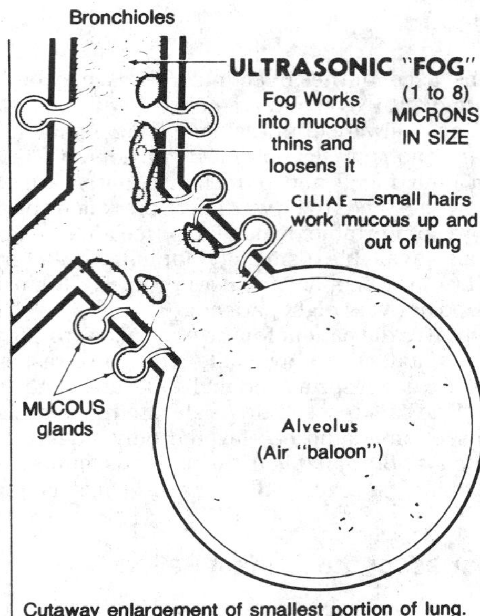

Fig 18. Ultrasonic aerosol is the most efficient at penetrating the terminal bronchioles and alveoli (courtesy, Wisconsin Lung Assoc).

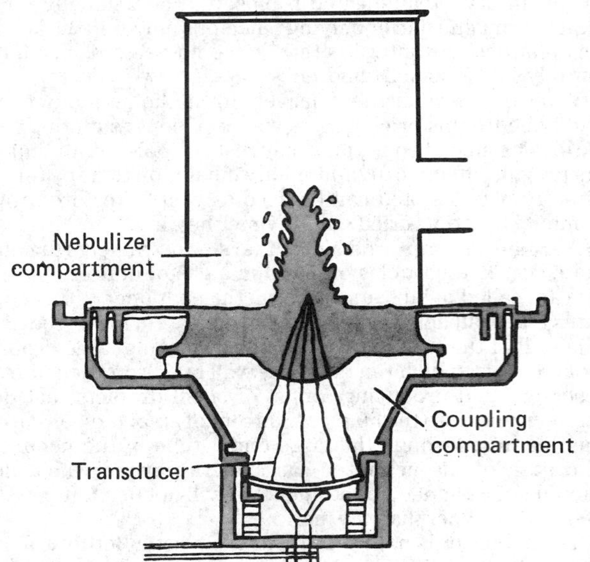

Fig 17. Construction of the ultrasonic nebulizer (from McPherson SP: *Respiratory Therapy Equipment*, Mosby, St Louis, 1981; modified from DeVilbiss).

Plugs of mucus in the tracheobronchial tree which only partially block the flow of air through an airway can cause other problems. Unobstructed passageways are said to exhibit laminar flow, but when smoothly flowing air moves over such plugs it becomes turbulent—a sound one hears as wheezing. The turbulent air then agitates the liquid on the surface of the mucosa and creates bubbles. When there are enough bubbles, they become foam—foam which can clog bronchioles and alveoli and dramatically diminish respiration at the capillaries. Alcohol, administered as an aerosol, will effectively break up foam and clear the airways.

Bronchospasms are contractions of the smooth, involuntary muscle surrounding the bronchioles. They severely constrict the bronchioles and, for obvious reasons, dangerously inhibit fluid ventilation of the lung. Bronchodilators are medications of choice in these cases, but care should be taken when the patient has a history of coronary problems.

When, due to tissue damage, edema or simply lack of use, the lung's interstitial tissues lose their elasticity, the patient is said to have a loss of compliance of the lung. An inelastic lung works against the efforts of the rib cage and diaphragm, making lung ventilation extremely difficult. This condition is typical in the patient who has chronic emphysema, but also occurs in varying degree with other respiratory diseases. Exercise, not an aerosol, is the method by which some compliance may be returned—and in those persons who suffer from a loss of compliance, an intermittent positive-pressure breathing machine may be necessary. Loss of compliance is included in the section, because it will affect the usefulness of an aerosol in administering a medication. Where lung compliance is a factor, the aerosol should be given under pressure.

Aerosols may be given using either a mask or mouthpiece. Short delivery tubes from the aerosol generator will provide optimum density of an aerosol; long and bending main tubes should be avoided as they reduce the concentration of particles in the aerosol which "rain out" on their way to the patient. Warm aerosols tend to carry more moisture into the lung, thereby reducing evaporation from the mucous membrane; they also tend to be more soothing to the patient. If aerosol generators are cleaned scrupulously after each treatment, their effectiveness will be maintained (Fig 19).

Other medicinal and pharmaceutical uses of aerosols are discussed in Chapter 95.

Intermittent Positive Pressure Breathing (IPPB) Machines—These machines for patient treatment at home have been available for many years. IPPB is a technique in which the lungs are inflated actively by means of regulated positive pressure during inspiration. Positive pressure on inspiration enables a patient with chronic obstructive airway disease to inhale deeply when conditions within his lungs make full ventilation impossible on his own. The technique is called intermittent because the positive pressure is cut off when the lung is adequately filled, permitting the patient to exhale without assistance.

IPPB is used to accomplish several things. Pressure is needed in some patients in order to get air into blocked areas of the lungs. In those instances, forcing air into an area of the lung which was blocked previously, or which was not ventilated due to lung tissues having become rigid, allows an aerosol to be delivered to that part of the lung. With air behind a plug of mucus the patient is able to expel the plug by coughing. IPPB therapy may provide a significantly deeper breath than the patient can produce with spontaneous ventilation. Positive pressure also aids in relief of bronchospasms through delivered medication, helps to improve drainage and provides exercise for stiff lung tissues, by far the most important way to return compliance to the lung.

IPPB machines operate using either the force of compressed gas from a cylinder at home or in the hospital or a hospital in-wall system, or, as is the case with most home models, by means of self-contained compression using ordinary room air.

These machines may be either automatic-cycling, manually operated or entirely responsive to the patient's breathing. Machines that operate automatically, beginning and ending each inspiration and expiration regardless of what the patient has in mind, are really respirators designed for unconscious patients and are not well-suited for therapy. While there are some manually operated IPPB machines, the much preferred models are responsive to the patient's breathing.

The latter machines begin the inspiration cycle the instant the patient begins to inhale. The cycling valve responds to the slightest negative pressure and begins the positive flow of air immediately. Machines that have this capability are said to have a "patient-demand" inspiration cycle. These machines also end the inspiration cycle in response to the patient's breathing. The cycling valve reacts to a predetermined positive pressure. On these machines, a pressure gauge is set by adjusting a dial on the front of the machine.

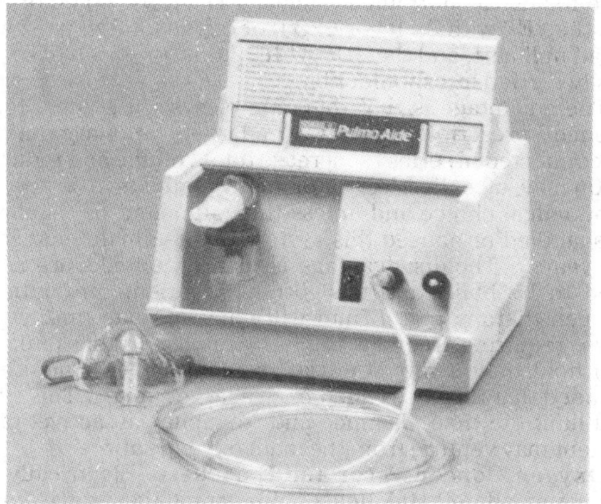

Fig 19. Nebulizer with air compressor (courtesy, DeVilbiss).

Pressure in all IPPB machines is measured in centimeters of water, a uniform standard in all makes and models. Once set, the machine automatically will shut off the flow of air when the patient's pulmonary pressure reaches the preset level. Theoretically, because there is a closed system between the machine's cycling valve and the patient's lung via the main IPPB tube, mouthpiece and trachea, the pressure at the cycling valve is equal to the pressure inside the patient's lung. The cycling pressure then can be set so air will continue to flow into the patient's lung, opening airways and ventilating alveoli in the process, until the preset pressure is reached.

The difficulty frequently encountered with persons just beginning to use an IPPB machine is that they feel uncomfortable having air forced into their lungs, though there is rarely any pain. There is a tendency in these persons to want to stop the flow of air into their lungs. Almost involuntarily, the glottis is closed and the accessory muscles of expiration are brought into action causing back-pressure against the inflow of air and registering an immediate high pressure at the sensitive cycling valve. When that back pressure is equal to the preset cycling pressure in the machine, it does indeed cycle, permitting exhalation. It takes practice and time for most new patients to feel comfortable with an IPPB machine. Part of the responsibility of the pharmacist who sets up such a machine in the patient's home is to guide him in its use and help him get over any initial uneasiness.

During the first few treatments, many patients tend to overdo it, especially soon after they have become used to the machine. Because they may be breathing much deeper than usual while they are using the machine, they easily may become hyperventilated. Oxygen intoxication, as the condition is called sometimes, may leave the patient feeling dizzy. He should be counseled to take his time and, after a couple of breaths on the IPPB machine, alternate with several normal breaths. At signs of dizziness, he should breathe normally until his dizziness disappears. Breathing with an IPPB machine should be a comfortable and relaxing experience.

Among the specifications which the physician will include in his prescription for IPPB therapy at home are

1. The level of positive pressure in centimeters of water, and further instructions as to when, if and to what extent, the pressure should be increased.
2. The duration of each treatment.
3. The number of treatments per day and/or week, and at what times during the day those treatments should be taken.
4. The specific medication or medications for each treatment, including concentration and dosage. If the physician does not want to administer medication with each treatment, he should specify whether the nebulizer should contain distilled water or normal saline solution—an IPPB machine must never be run dry.

On the average, the prescription for IPPB therapy at home requires a pressure setting of between 10 and 20 cm of water pressure and a treatment duration of between 10 and 20 minutes. The number of treatments varies greatly, from 2 to 3 a week, to 3 to 4 times a day. Sometimes the prescription merely suggests "As needed." *Under no circumstances should an intermittent positive pressure breathing machine be rented or sold without a doctor's prescription!*

During equipment setup, the pharmacist should teach the patient how to adjust the pressure dial on the face of the machine and how to read the pressure gauges. IPPB therapy is not without its potential risks, mainly due to overuse. Potential hazards of significant frequency are excessive ventilation, excessive oxygenation, decreased cardiac output, increased intracranial pressure, pneumothorax and hemoptysis. The pharmacist should be aware of these potential hazards and work closely with the respiratory therapist and the physician, following prescription orders precisely. It is generally advisable to type the complete prescription on a gummed label, and paste the label on the face of the machine where the patient can see it.

An IPPB setup is never complete until the pharmacist has reviewed with the patient the details of the doctor's prescription, how the medication is measured and the nebulizer prepared, how the pressure is adjusted, how the gauges are read, how to clean the nebulizer jets and main tube accessories after each treatment and where to reach the pharmacist during and after working hours in the event of an emergency.

Many other types of high-tech respiratory equipment, such as continuous positive airway pressure devices (CPAPs) and ventilators, are available. While these may be a part of the pharmacy's health-accessory department, the actual setup, patient instruction and equipment maintenance usually will be done by a respiratory therapist, who is on call 24 hours a day in case an emergency arises.

Oxygen Therapy—Providing oxygen therapy as an adjunct to a health-accessories department also should be done in conjunction with the services of a respiratory therapist.

Oxygen first became available as a therapeutic gas after the military developed an economical process to distil it in large quantities for use by the pilots and crew of high-altitude aircraft. Prior to this it was not economically feasible to provide oxygen in the quantities required to treat hypoxic patients.

The primary commercial method of manufacturing therapeutic oxygen is by the liquification of air followed by fractional distillation. In this method air is cooled and condensed from a gas into a liquid. As the temperature of the liquid air is increased slowly, the lower boiling points of the nitrogen and inert gases cause them to evaporate out of the solution. The residual liquid oxygen then is stored in its present state in vacuum-insulated vessels or converted under high pressure to the gaseous state in high-pressure steel cylinders.

Supplemental oxygen is used to treat various clinical disorders, both respiratory and nonrespiratory in nature.

Oxygen often is prescribed at a rate of 2 L/min for the relief of arterial hypoxemia and any of its secondary complications. Oxygen also has proved to be therapeutic in treating pulmonary hypertension, polycythemia secondary to hypoxemia, chronic disease states which may be complicated by anemia, cancer, migraine headaches, coronary artery disease, seizure disorders, sickle-cell crisis and sleep apnea.

Some adverse effects and hazards of oxygen therapy include oxygen-induced hypoventilation, absorption atelectasis and oxygen toxicity. Oxygen-induced hypoventilation is probably the greatest potential hazard of oxygen therapy.

In certain clinical situations the respiratory therapy drive that results from carbon dioxide stimulation of the respiratory center is blunted. This phenomenon may be the consequence of a drug overdose such as with a barbiturate or heroin or, more commonly, chronic hypercarbia. Hypoventilation is of particular importance in patients with severe chronic obstructive pulmonary disease (COPD) where carbon dioxide retention and hypoxemia have developed over a long period of time. The respiratory drive of most of these patients results from hypoxic stimulation of the carotid chemoreceptors. Thus, the main stimulation for respiration is hypoxemia. If this hypoxic drive is relieved through the advent of excessive oxygen therapy, hypoventilation may occur and further carbon dioxide retention with possible cessation of ventilation could result.

Absorption atelectasis is the result of collapsed alveoli from a high concentration of oxygen in the inhaled air. Nitrogen, an inert gas which comprises 79% of our atmosphere, maintains the residual volume of space in the alveoli as the oxygen component of inhaled air is diffused through the pulmonary membrane and absorbed into the blood stream. When a high concentration of oxygen is inhaled into the alveoli, the oxygen is absorbed rapidly into the blood, potentially leaving the alveoli empty and collapsed. This is particularly significant in patients with pulmonary disease that involves narrowing or obstructing the airways and a low ventilation-perfusion ratio.

Oxygen toxicity is not a significant hazard until oxygen concentrations are greater than 50% for prolonged periods of time. Oxygen toxicity adversely can affect the pulmonary system, central nervous system, retina and endocrine organs. Pulmonary changes are usually the first to manifest with increased permeability of capillary endothelial cells resulting in alveolar congestion, intraalveolar hemorrhage and fibrinous exudation of the hyaline membrane. Normally, the first symptoms include substernal burning discomfort, cough, paresthesia, nausea and vomiting.

It generally is considered that a prescription of 2 L/min is sufficiently therapeutic without a great increase of risk of the previous hazards.

For the home-care patient on oxygen therapy, there are basically three different types of delivery systems available: the liquid system, compressed gas system and oxygen concentrator. Each has its own distinct advantages and disadvantages. Choosing a system that is most applicable is based on the patient's needs, lifestyle, mobility, convenience, frequency of use and volume of oxygen consumed. Reimbursement criteria set up by Medicare or an HMO also may dictate which type of system is used.

The liquid system is by far the most convenient for patients with an active lifestyle. Oxygen in this system has been compressed and cooled to −184.4° (−300°F). The resulting volume is less than 0.2% of an equivalent amount of oxygen at atmospheric pressure and temperature. The system consists of a large reservoir vessel and a light-weight portable unit. Both are designed to protect the extremely cold contents from heat and to regulate a consistent rate of evaporation from a liquid to a gas for subsequent use by the patient. Most large reservoirs will hold 75 to 100 lb of liquid oxygen and require filling once every week or so. Although considered stationary units, some patients have secured them in vehicles for travel. The portable unit is light enough, at approximately 8 lb when filled, to be transported over the shoulder by its carrying strap. One fill will deliver oxygen at a continuous flow of 2 L/min for approximately 8 hours. The significant advantage of this system is that the portable unit provides the greatest volume and longest continuous-use potential of any portable unit. It also can be refilled or topped off any number of times from the large reservoir vessel. This system affords the patient the greatest mobility and unlimited frequency for excursions outside the home.

The disadvantage of the liquid system is that liquid oxygen is a relatively unstable substance. It does not store well and will waste away through evaporation if not consumed continuously. This is not generally the ideal form of oxygen for patients who use oxygen on an "as needed" basis.

Compressed-gas oxygen systems consist of a basic high-pressure tank and a pressure regulator with an attached flow meter graduated in liters per minute. The most stable and reliable form of oxygen delivery and storage systems, it is most applicable for patients who predominantly are confined to their home with an occasional need for mobility or patients who require oxygen on an "as needed" basis. Compressed oxygen is available in a variety of tank sizes.

The largest, the "H" tank, holds 244 ft^3 or 6900 L of oxygen and is the standard stationary unit of the system. Smaller tanks, some of lightweight aluminum construction, are available for use as portable systems. The most common tanks are the "E" with 22 ft^3 or 622 L of oxygen, often used with a small pull cart, and the "D" with 12.6 ft^3 or 356 L of oxygen, easily carried in a shoulder bag.

The advantage is that this type of system is ideal for "as needed" prescription uses. The large, stationary tanks can be connected in series to increase total volume and reduce the frequency of deliveries. For many patients it is the most economical choice and unless the equipment or regulator is mishandled or abused this system is often maintenance-free for years. The disadvantage is that large tanks are considered to be bulky and unsightly. A patient on continuous oxygen therapy at 2 L/min will consume one tank every 2 days, requiring frequent refills. Small, portable tanks (Fig 20) hold only a few hours of oxygen and it is not recommended that they be refilled from a larger tank. This system will limit the time, distance and frequency an active, mobile patient may venture from the main oxygen source.

Oxygen Concentrator and Enricher—Electrically powered by standard 110-V household current, these devices pump ambient room air through banks of molecular sieves or a

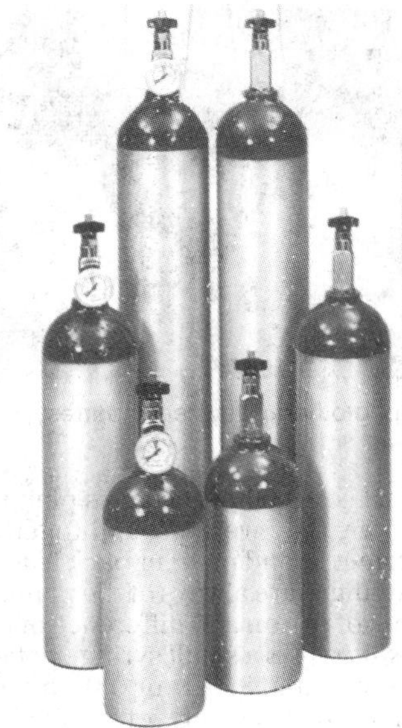

Fig 20. Portable oxygen tanks (courtesy, DeVilbiss).

semipermeable membrane, which then preferentially separates oxygen from nitrogen and delivers approximately 95% oxygen at maximum flows of 3 to 5 L/min. Much improved in efficiency and reliability over the last few years, all concentrators (Fig 21) still require a monthly inspection by a trained technician to verify the percentage of oxygen delivered and perform a scheduled, routine, maintenance program. This type of system never needs refilling and is extremely convenient for the homebound patient. The disadvantage is that the system cannot store any oxygen for portable or emergency use during an electrical outage. Patients should be advised to have a separate source of oxygen, such as a compressed tank, available. It also has the added expense of electricity and produces a certain amount of noise.

Apnea Programs

Sudden infant death syndrome (SIDS) is the number one cause of death in the US for infants under the age of 1 year.

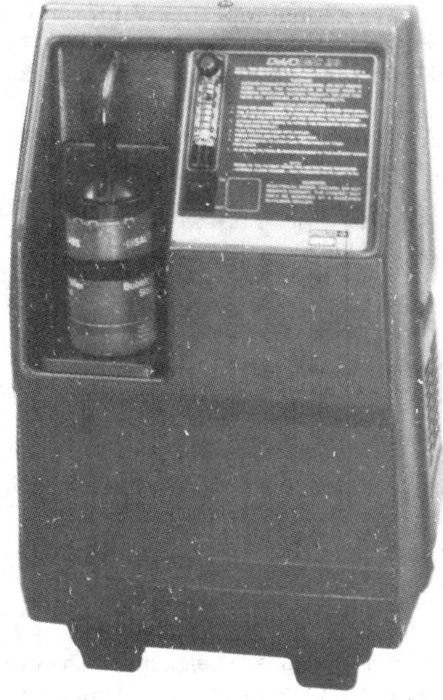

Fig 21. Oxygen concentrator (courtesy, DeVilbiss).

The relationship between SIDS and apnea (a pause in respiration of 15 to 20 seconds or longer) is not exactly clear and is still somewhat controversial. However, a large portion of the pediatric medical community has begun home-monitoring in infants who have experienced episodes of prolonged apnea.

In the last few years a great deal of medical research has been devoted to better understanding the relationship between SIDS and apnea. This has resulted in the publication of a large number of journal articles about apnea and SIDS, the establishment of an annual medical conference on the subject, the startup of numerous hospital-based apnea programs and a general increased awareness in the medical community about the problem.

As the interest in the medical community has increased, so has the number of physicians prescribing home monitors. Apnea programs were once the domain of a select few physicians and hospitals nationwide. Now, most hospitals with a Level II or III nursery have developed their own apnea-monitoring programs, staffed with a team of medical professionals. These programs evaluate infants at risk for apnea and prescribe the use of a home monitor. Typically, a neonatalogist heads up the team and is assisted by nurses and respiratory therapists specializing in the treatment of infants.

The increased interest in SIDS and apnea by the medical community has stimulated tremendous growth in the number of home-health-care dealers offering apnea-monitoring programs. Interest by the medical community is not the only reason for the growth in this area. These programs have become a very lucrative service for many home-health-care dealers. Apnea-monitoring programs have generated a great deal of income and profit for those home-health-care dealers willing to dedicate the resources and time to running a high-quality program.

Pneumograms (Pneumocardiograms)—Apnea monitoring has become much more sophisticated in the last few years. Very-specific and detailed evaluation and screening programs have been established by hospitals to determine which infants will need to go home with an apnea monitor. Once in the home, more follow-up work now is being done. Twelve-hour recordings known as pneumograms now are being performed routinely to evaluate an infant's progress in the home environment. Long-term event recordings are also commonplace for documentation of the types of alarms an infant is having and to determine the proper time for monitor discontinuance.

Pneumograms are two-channel recordings of heart rate (ECG) and respiration. These typically are done in the home for a 12-hour period of time. These recordings then are printed out and analyzed by a physician or technician. The results are used to determine if the infant needs further study at a hospital apnea center or no longer needs to be monitored.

A 12-hour pneumogram is a "snap-shot" recording of one night in an infant's life. The recording may include apnea events in combination with normal activity ("well information") or it may include only "well information." If an infant that previously has had a number of serious problems while being monitored, has an unusual evening during a 12-hour pneumogram, with no events occurring, the physician has a recording that does not reflect accurately an infant's true condition.

An event recorder provides the caregiver long-term information about the events that are causing the monitor to alarm. This provides the physician important documentation about the number and type of events an infant is having over a long period of time. An event recording provides a physician with a more realistic record of an infant's condition. The physician can alter the infant's monitoring program or discontinue monitoring altogether based on the results of the recording.

Event recordings are similar to two-channel pneumograms. They record heart rate and respiration data, but rather than continuously recording this information over a 12-hour period of time, they only record information when the monitor sounds an alarm. An event recording provides the caregiver with information about alarm events occurring in the home.

This information is extremely valuable, particularly when evaluating problem infants or determining when to discontinue monitoring.

Traditionally, home pneumograms are made on small cassette-tape recorders. The recorders and tapes must be delivered to the home the day the recording is scheduled, and the readings printed and analyzed the following day. This takes a lot of valuable time for delivery, pickup and analysis. If a recording is of poor quality and must be repeated, it is even more time-consuming and costly, since dealers are not reimbursed for repeat recordings.

Phototherapy

The treatment of neonatal jaundice (hyperbilirubinemia) often involves the use of a phototherapy light (Fig 22). Phototherapy treatment also may be provided by a fiberoptic system, which consists of an illuminator, a fiberoptic cable and a fiberoptic panel, which can be wrapped around an infant's torso (Fig 23). This may be done in the hospital, or at the doctor's and parent's option, in the home. Home phototherapy costs can be a fraction of the cost of a hospital stay, and the financial resources of the parents or the mandates of an HMO may require home treatment. While the health-accessories pharmacist may stock and set up these units, a nursing service usually will provide the everyday blood-testing required.

Hypodermic Equipment

Syringes are instruments intended for the injection of water or other liquids into the body or its cavities. They are classified according to differences in principle of action into three categories: *plunger syringes*, such as the hypodermic syringes; *bulb syringes*, of which the ear and ulcer syringes are one type and *gravity syringes*, characterized by the fountain syringes.

On the basis of capacity, syringes also may be classified into three groups: *small*, those of 10 mL or less capacity, such as the hypodermic type; *medium*, those from 10 mL to 100 mL in volume, such as ear and ulcer syringes (although some special hypodermic syringes are available in sizes up to 500-mL capacity) and *large*, such as enema or vaginal syringes.

Hypodermic Syringes—These syringes are used to administer medication *subcutaneously* (under the skin) or *intradermally*, *intravenously* (into a vein or artery) or *intramuscularly* (into the muscle).

Parenteral therapy or injection of medication under the skin and through tissues dates from the beginning of the 19th century. The first crude instrument of this type was a needle trocar, developed to deposit morphine in paste form. The principle of introducing medication under the skin, however, became popular in the first half of the 20th century.

Luer Syringes—The inventor of this type of apparatus, Dr Luer, patented his syringe; the letters patent have long since expired but today most hypodermic syringes of this style bear his name. The outstanding feature of the Luer syringe was its ground-glass surfaces. In many instances, the inside of the glass barrel and the outside of the glass plunger were ground individually. Later, they were ground together so that they will provide a perfect fit and prevent back leakage (Fig 24).

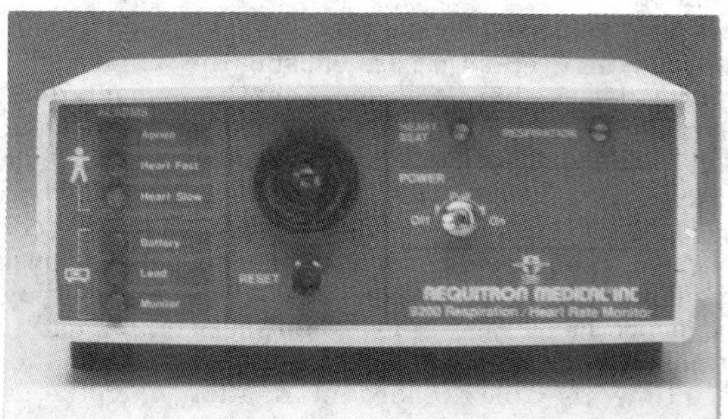

Fig 22. Phototherapy light (courtesy, Aequitron).

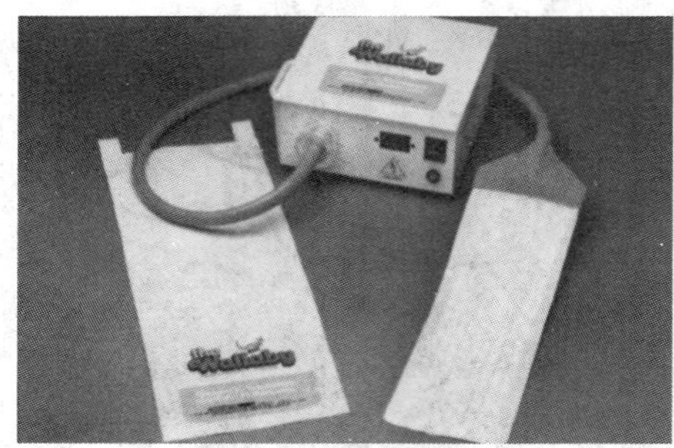

Fig 23. Wallaby phototherapy system (courtesy, Medical Products).

Hypodermic syringes are always of the plunger type, characterized by the type of piston and difference of size or capacity. The *tuberculin syringe* is a small syringe not exceeding 1 mL in capacity, and graduated in 0.1- or 0.01-mL divisions. The *hypodermic syringe* is usually of 2- to 50-mL capacity. There are larger piston syringes, ranging up to 200 mL, for various purposes such as transfusions and in veterinary medicine. Graduations may be in fractions of a mL or in *minims*. Syringes also may be prepared with special graduations, such as *units* of insulin.

To test the efficiency of a hypodermic syringe, close the tip with the finger and attempt to withdraw the plunger. If the plunger and barrel fit perfectly the vacuum created in the cylinder will prevent the withdrawal of the plunger.

Disposable Hypodermic Syringes—Various types of disposable hypodermic syringes, each carrying a single dose of sterile medication, now are supplied as a standard dosage container by many pharmaceutical manufacturers.

Disposable hypodermic syringes—empty, without medication—are available from several sources; some are plastic, others glass. Separate disposable needles, packed sterile in envelopes, are also available.

Hypodermic Needles—Hypodermic needles used with Luer syringes are of metal, and consist of a hub, which locks to the ground-glass tip by friction, and a needle point which varies in diameter and length. Needles also are called *cannulas*. Hypodermic needles may be made of stainless steel, hyperchrome steel, carbon steel, chromium, nickeloid, platinum, platinum-iridium, silver or gold.

Hypodermic needles are characterized by their different points, which have a long, tapering reinforced point and beveled cutting edges of varying degree. A *long-bevel* or *long-taper* needle is used for local anesthesia, aspirating, hypoder-

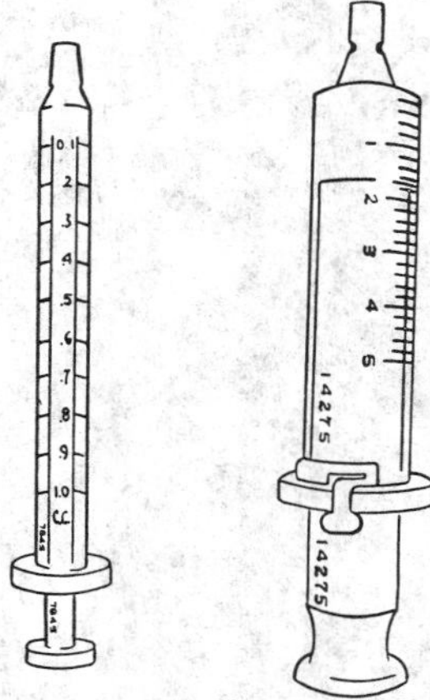

Fig 24. Hypodermic syringes. *Left,* tuberculin or vaccine syringe, graduated in 10ths or 100ths of a mL; *right,* Luer type syringe, of 1- to 50-mL capacity.

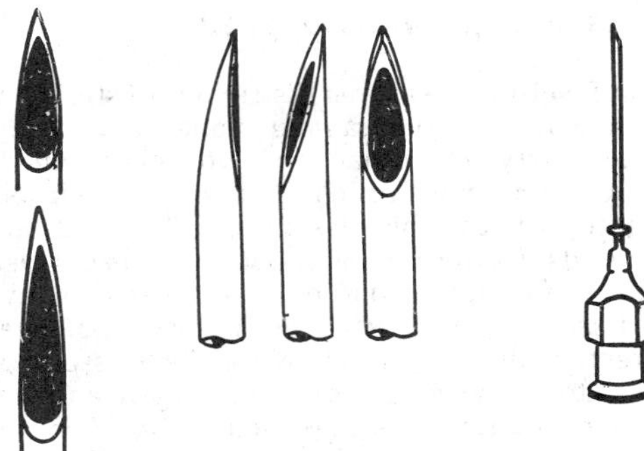

Fig 25. Hypodermic needles. *Left,* short-bevel and long-bevel needle points; *left center,* the Huber point with closed bevel and side opening to avoid producing tissue plugs; *right center,* regular point showing features which insure less cutting, more distention of tissue, reduced trauma, seepage and after-pain; *right,* needle with security button which prevents a broken cannula from becoming lost in the tissues.

moclysis and subcutaneous administration. A *short-bevel* needle is used for intravenous administration, infusions and transfusions. A *special short-bevel* needle is employed for intradermal and spinal administration (Fig 25).

Size—Selection of a size is governed by four factors—safety, rate of flow, comfort of patient and depth of penetration. There are three standard dimensions—length, outside diameter of the cannula and wall thickness. Regular needles are measured for length from where the cannula joins the hub to the tip of the point (hub not included).

The gauge of a needle is measured by the outside diameter of the cannula or needle shaft. The usual range of diameter for needles is from 13-gauge (largest diameter) to 27-gauge. Needles seldom are less than ¼ inch long or longer than 3½ inches.

There are many special needles, designed for a variety of purposes. Various *biopsy* and *bone-marrow transfusion* needles range from 16- to 19-gauge and ½ to 3½ inches long. They are characterized by their heavy shaped hubs.

Needles for *local anesthesia* range from 26-gauge, ½ inch to 20-gauge, 6 inch. *Intravenous, blood transfusion* needles, some with fitted cannulae, range from 19-gauge, 1¼ inch to 15-gauge, 2½ inch.

There are also special needles and cannulae for *abscess, eye, hemorrhoidal, tonsil, laryngeal* and *pneumothorax* use.

These many types of special-purpose hypodermic needles are of varying sizes in diameter and varying lengths. Some of these are shown in Fig 26.

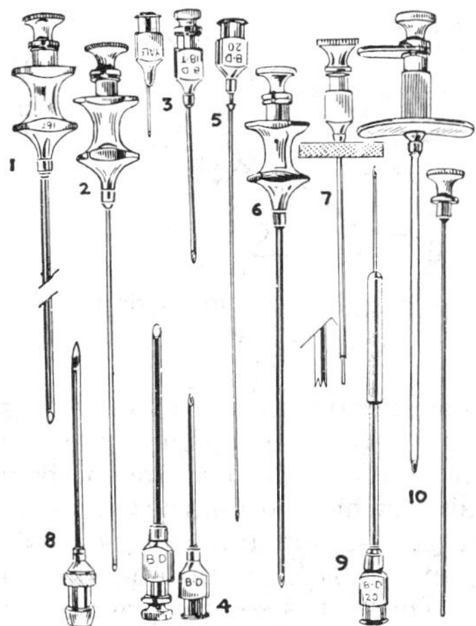

Fig 26. Special hypodermic needles—1: caudal needle; 2: epidural needle for single-shot anesthesia; 3: intravenous anesthesia short-bevel and long needles (with vinyl tubing); 4: blood transfusion needles (with vinyl tubing); 5: short-bevel beaded local anesthesia needles; 6: spinal needle with large spool hub; 7: biopsy needle for bone-marrow aspirations; 8: infusion needle, with female luer slip; 9: hemorrhoidal needle with threaded adjustable gauge to adjust depth of puncture; 10: cerebral angiography needle with thin-walled outer cannula, corrugated shield, and inner cannula (courtesy, Becton-Dickinson).

Bulb Syringes

Bulb syringes frequently are preferred for use where sterility is not necessary or where plunger-type syringes, because of their force, would be dangerous to use. Bulb syringes are of particular value in the nose and ear and for wound and urinary irrigation.

These syringes customarily are known by the name of the part of the body for which they are intended.

Nasal syringes or *nasal aspirators* are soft rubber bulbs of about 1-oz capacity, with an acorn-shaped nasal tip to fit the nostril. The tip may be either glass, plastic or hard rubber. Glass is more popular as the transparency allows visual examination of the mucus removed from the nostril (Fig 27).

Ear syringes and *ulcer syringes* are one-piece molded bulbs of soft, flexible rubber, with long, narrow nozzles and are employed in treating the eye, ear and nose, and for irrigation of any open cavity or ulcer (Fig 28).

If necessary, bulb syringes should be sterilized with germicidal solutions. Prolonged boiling will injure the rubber.

Rectal syringes are customarily of the bulb type, with a long narrow nozzle. They frequently are employed in the administration of enemas to infants. These are the safest and least expensive of syringes requiring minimal maintenance. Such syringes customarily are of 1- to 4-oz capacity. Although many syringes provide hard-rubber or vulcanite tips, the use of hard tips should be discouraged because of occasional injury to the soft tissues from their use (Fig 29).

Vaginal syringes, used for irrigation of the vagina, are 8- to 10-oz capacity bulb syringes with a large vulcanite or rubber spray tube. Pressure on the bulb forces the medicated or irrigating liquid through the tip of the syringe either in a direct stream or with a "whirling" motion. These syringes in white or various colors are provided with rubber sleeve-shaped round or oval shields to prevent leakage when in use. Caps

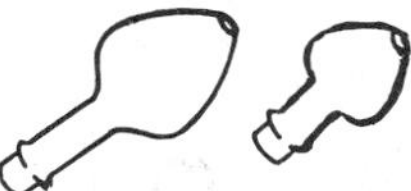

Fig 27. Nasal aspirator tips (either glass or hard rubber).

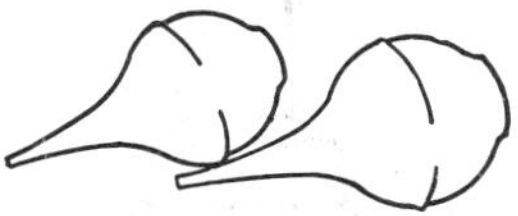

Fig 28. Infant and adult soft-rubber ear and ulcer syringes.

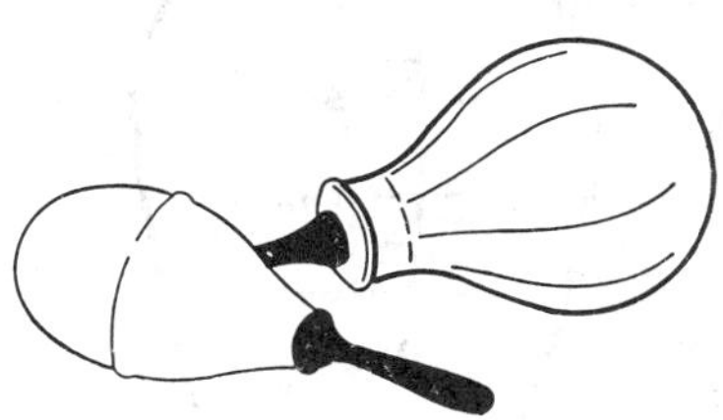

Fig 29. Infant and adult rectal syringes with a soft-rubber bulb and hard tip.

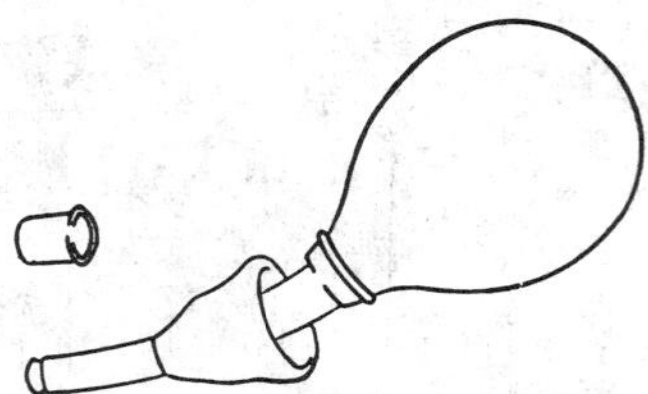

Fig 30. Vaginal syringe.

sealing the nozzles are provided to avoid leakage or loss of the contents before use (Fig 30). One model has a convenient plastic stopper at the bottom of the bulb opening with a removable strainer, which permits mixing of medications.

Enema Syringes—Fountain syringes consist of a reservoir with a capacity of 1 to 3 qt, a 5-ft rubber tube and a vaginal or rectal nozzle. These are used for irrigation with water, salt solution, soap suds or special medications.

Pharmacists should caution users of enema syringes as follows: the "drop" must not exceed 4 ft to prevent excessive gravity pressure, the fluid should be maintained at body temperature to avoid chills or burns and the tube customarily is closed with a mechanical pinchcock. Before using the syringe, the cutoff should be released for a moment until some liquid issues from the nozzle. The user must be certain that no air remains which might be forced from the tube into the body cavity. Hard-rubber nozzles are supplied frequently with enema syringes but, as they may cause damage to the rectum, they preferably are replaced by catheters or tubes of soft rubber with about a $^{3}/_{16}$ inch diameter and 15 inches in length.

Enemas—In simple constipation, whenever evacuation of the lower bowel is indicated, and when proctologic examination or surgery is indicated, an enema customarily is given because of its local, comfortable and safe action in a relatively short period of time.

Enemas should not be used when nausea, vomiting or abdominal pain is present, nor more often than necessary, to avoid dependence. Available as well are plastic, graduated (in ½-oz increments), 4-oz transparent or opaque infant enema syringes which allow accurate filling, mixing and use of the physician's prescribed formulas (Fig 31). Prepared enemas are available for use in simple constipation or whenever evacuation of the lower bowel is indicated, such as in proctologic or sigmoidoscopic examinations; small, disposable units comprising flexible plastic bottles of 6- to 50-mL aqueous or oil solutions, with self-fitted comfortable plastic or rubber tip are available.

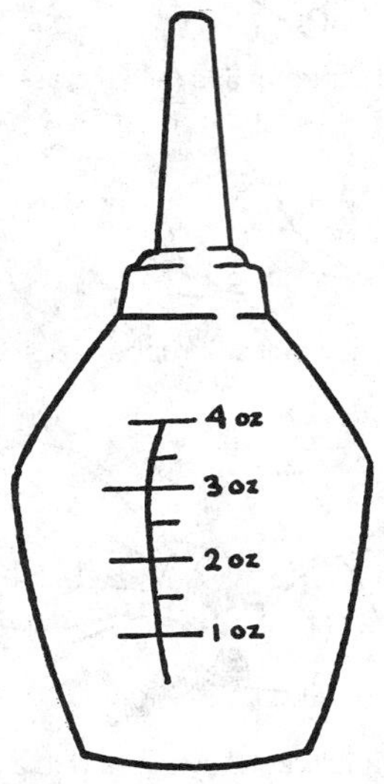

Fig 31. Bulb-type graduated, transparent, infant enema syringe.

Dressings and First-Aid Supplies

The pharmacist is the proper distributor of sterile materials for treating wounds. His training enables him to appreciate the care necessary in their handling and storage, and he often is called upon for advice or instruction as to their use. The following items fall in this class: absorbent cotton, cotton balls and buds, sterile rolls and pads of gauze, elastic bandages, disposable fabric tissues and underpads, eye pads, sponges, tissues and towels, adhesive elastic bandages, aerosol adherent, spray dressings, first-aid kits, scissors, tweezers and applicators. Various types of oxygen and moisture-permeable transparent dressings such as *Tegaderm* or hydroactive dressings such as *Duoderm* serve specialized needs.

The pharmacy with a comprehensive health-accessories department will stock bulk packages of these items for use by nursing homes, visiting nurses services and patients who consume quantities sufficient to warrant their making larger purchases, in addition to the smaller packages for the pharmacy's usual customers.

The Family Medicine Cabinet—There is a place in every home where medicines are kept. The medicine cabinet should either be locked or completely out of the reach of children. Every bottle or box should be labeled clearly. Unused prescription medications, outdated OTC drugs and empty bottles do not belong in the medicine cabinet and should be removed. Some community pharmacists provide folders containing information on first-aid, poison antidotes and simple home medication for use by their customers so that the pharmacy's name is always in view in the medicine cabinet. This also is accomplished by providing a gummed "family prescription record" for the inside of the cabinet door, or an "emergency label" bearing space for entering telephone numbers for the doctor, pharmacy, hospital and fire and police departments, to be attached to the telephone or telephone book.

In addition, the pharmacist should urge that every family car, camper and boat be equipped with an adequate first-aid kit, in addition to a flashlight, flares and a hand fire extinguisher.

Snake-Bite Kits—Anyone in snake, bee or wasp country should carry a snake-bite kit (Fig 32). They usually are available in a compact plastic or metal case containing a tourniquet rubber or other lymph constrictor, antiseptic, razor blade or knife and one or more suction cups or syringes. These are available from Cutter or Becton-Dickinson. Many lives are saved each year by prompt action at the spot where the snake attacks, and relief from the pain and swelling of severe insect stings is also important. Snake bites are medical emergencies that require immediate treatment.

Every hospital pharmacist should have a chart of disaster-unit equipment required for a hospital and all pharmacists should be familiar with the requirements and needs of disaster units.

Hot-Water Bottles—The best instruments for applying dry heat are the hot-water bottle and the electric heating pad. Made of rubber, hot-water bottles may be of the usual 2-qt size, or of the 1-pt capacity in the form of a "face bottle" for neuralgia of the head and for infant conditions. Each hot-water bottle has an opening through which warm water is added and a stopper securely sealed with a washer. It is

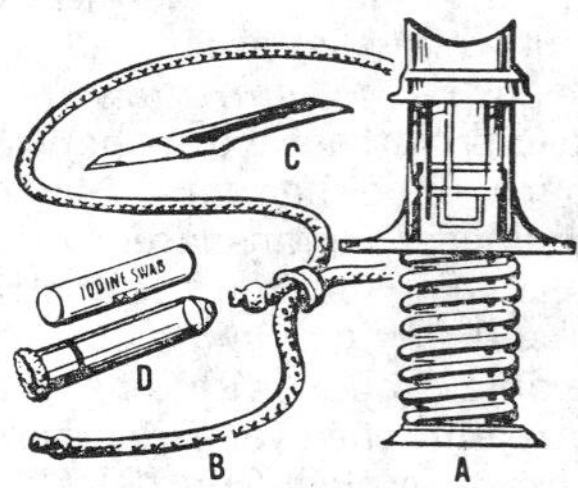

Fig 32. Pocket snake-bite kit contains *A*: suction device, *B*: tourniquet, *C*: incision blade and *D*: antiseptic swab.

more convenient to attach the stopper permanently to the bottle to prevent its loss. Some have screw-stopper attachments, which permit conversion of the bottle into a fountain syringe.

When filling a hot-water bottle, it should be held against the back of the hand or forearm to insure that the temperature is not too high. Bare rubber should never be allowed to come in contact with the skin, or burns may result. Rubber pads, flannelette bags or even a towel wrapped around the hot-water bottle will give adequate passage of heat and comfort and convenience.

After use, the empty hot-water bottle should be hung by the tap at its bottom for thorough draining. Water of boiling temperature, oil, grease, alcohol or turpentine should not be permitted to come in contact with the rubber. When not in use, all rubber devices should be protected from direct light to avoid hardening of the rubber.

Moist-Heat Packs—Various commercial moist-heat packs are now in common use in hospitals and nursing homes, and are also available for use at home. These steam packs appear as compartmented, cloth bean bags when new and are filled with tiny beads. When boiled in water, however, the beads become hydrated and combine into a gelatinous substance which has the unique property of holding its temperature far longer than any other pack—about 30 to 40 minutes.

Moist-heat packs such as these must be wrapped in at least six layers of Turkish towel to prevent burns, and should never be used directly in contact with the skin. They are available in a variety of sizes, including a contoured pack designed specifically for the neck and shoulders. The neck-contour steam pack, as well as others, also have optional terry-cloth covers, lined with foam rubber which takes the place of layers of toweling. Heating units are also available, but the patient at home can prepare a steam pack in an ordinary pot of boiling water. They can be used over and over again without loss of effectiveness if care is taken to avoid dehydration—easily accomplished by wrapping the steam pack in a plastic bag and storing it in the refrigerator. For long-term storage, these packs can be kept in the freezer (again sealed in a plastic bag) to prevent drying out.

Electric Heating Pads—The advantage of the electric heating pad over the hot-water bottle lies in the fact that there is no possibility of leaking or spilling, and the temperature is controlled constantly and indefinitely. Most are wet-proof for wet or dry application, have soft-foam padding and washable flannel covers. Most have adjustable heating elements which permit the temperature to be set at the desired level, and an illuminated temperature-control panel. One of the more popular electric, moist-heating pads is manufactured by Battle Creek under the trade name *Thermophore*. These are controlled by means of a handheld switch which automatically turns the unit off when released, eliminating the possibility of burns due to a patient's falling asleep. The Thermophore heating pad creates moist heat without preboiling or using large amounts of water, hence, its desirability in the home environment. The unit's flannel cover is dipped into water and then wrung dry. Intermittent applications of heat create "fomentation" or intense moist heat. The manufacturer recommends that treatments not exceed 30 minutes in length. All such electrical devices customarily are inspected to insure safe operation; however, short circuits and breakage of the heating element may result from constant use.

Automatic heat bonnets for scalp treatments; heat bandages for sprains, bursitis or arthritis; neck and throat heating pads for stiff neck or whiplash cases; sinus masks for heat therapy of sinus areas; and even thermal massagers are available. The pharmacist always should caution the patient *not* to sleep while using an electric heating pad.

Cold Application—In deep inflammation the effects of external application of either heat or cold are essentially similar, due to reflexes arising from the stimulation of the nerves conducting temperature sensation. Experience has shown that there are some conditions (such as appendicitis) where the application of cold is the more desirable.

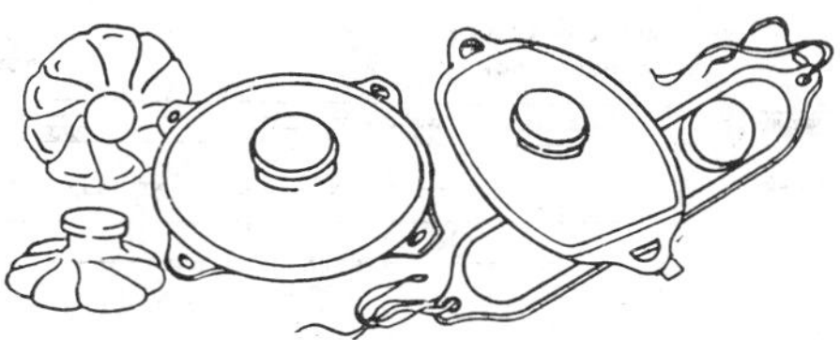

Fig 33. Ice caps and bags. *Left:* mackintosh cloth and rubber collapsible ice cap; *center:* ice bags; *right:* spinal and throat ice bags.

Appliances for local application of cold are reusable cold packs and the familiar ice bag or ice cap (Fig 33). The latter is usually a circular rubber or rubberized mackintosh cloth bag, circular in shape, with a large opening to admit cracked ice. Occasionally thick rubber, similar to that used in hot-water bottles, is employed. Ice caps usually require a cover of some type to protect the skin. The contents of an ice cap are less flaccid than the liquid in hot-water bottles. Therefore, thin-rubber or cloth construction is preferable in order to insure better conformation with the body. The pleated shape common to many ice caps avoids the bulginess and allows the introduction of large amounts of ice.

An adaptation of the ice cap is used for throat inflammation. It is the collar-shaped rubber bag known as a tonsillectomy bag. It fits snugly around the neck, holding the ice on the parts. There are two styles, one with a spring clip and the other tying into place with strings or laces. Ice bags also are made in a long, narrow shape for use around the throat and along the spine.

Cold Packs—Instead of using ice, some hospitals keep their ice bags filled with glycerin or an isopropyl alcohol-water mixture. These *redi-freeze ice packs* are stored in refrigerators until needed and are exchanged for bags which have become warm in use. Thus, cold packs are immediately available at all times, and the liquid contents conform more readily to the contours of the body.

Ice packs of soft rubber or plastic, filled with a nontoxic solution of 10% propylene glycol and water, are available in the usual designs. When stored in the freezing compartment of the refrigerator, the contents freeze to a semisolid or slush which provides greater comfort in use and longer retention of cold temperature than ice cubes. Fitted with tabs and tie-tapes, they are available in throat and body shapes.

In addition, instant hot and cold packs are available which provide a portable modality for heat and cold therapy ideal in situations where refrigeration or heating units are not accessible. To activate the packs, they are struck firmly, which breaks an inner packet containing an activating fluid. This fluid comes into contact with the base chemical and the resulting chemical reaction is either endothermic producing cold, or exothermic producing heat. They maintain heat or cold for about 30 minutes, and then must be discarded.

Thermometers

Hippocrates in 460 BC recognized that abnormal human temperature was a disease symptom. In 1610 AD Sanctorius developed the first clumsy oral thermometer. The thermometer was unreliable until 1714, when Fahrenheit developed the first dependable scale and instrument. It had standard graduations and mercury was used as the heat-measuring liquid. In 1835, two Frenchmen, Becquerel and Breschet, established the mean, or average, temperature of a healthy man as 98.6° on the scale devised by Fahrenheit. A Hollander, Antoon Van Haen, in 1754 developed the first practical clinical thermometer. Thermometers were seldom depended on in medical practice until about 1865, when a Scottish physician named Aitken invented a self-registering thermometer.

Thermometers for Home Use—The types of thermometers usually employed in the home are the *household thermometer* or common type for reading interior or outside air

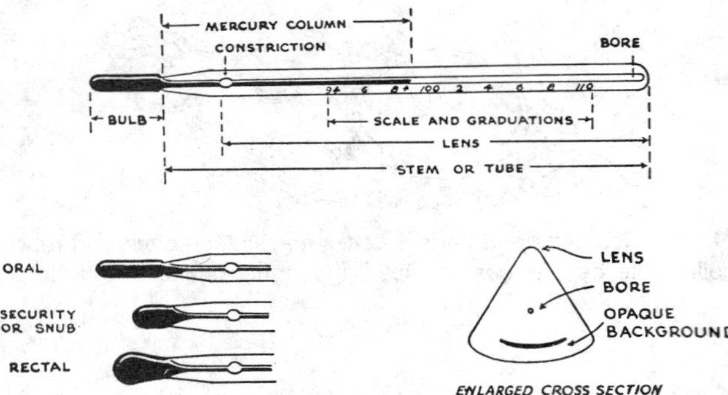

Fig 34. Diagram of thermometer construction.

temperature and *clinical* or *fever thermometers* (Fig 34). The temperature of the atmosphere at the surface of the earth varies more than 200°F, but man's body temperature rarely varies beyond 97° to 104°F, with the portent of danger at either extreme.

The change in temperature of the patient is one of the important symptoms upon which the physician bases his diagnosis and treatment. The instrument employed for body-temperature determination is the *clinical*, or more popularly called, *fever, thermometer.*

An abnormal temperature is nature's warning that something is wrong. A rapid rise or fall and substantial deviations from normal are danger signals. Every home should have a fever thermometer available at all times.

The essential difference between an ordinary thermometer and one designed for determining body temperature is the self-registering feature of the fever thermometer. When the mercury column has risen to the maximum temperature, it remains until shaken back into the reservoir at the bottom of the instrument. This is due to a constriction which acts as a tiny check-valve in the thermometer bore, just above the bulb, and permits passage of the mercury on expansion but does not permit its return on contraction.

Clinical or Fever Thermometers—Three bulb types of fever thermometers are available: (1) the *oral type,* characterized by the slender mercury reservoir, is the most sensitive for mouth use; (2) the *rectal* type has a blunt, strong, pear-shaped bulb for safety and to insure retention in the rectum and (3) a small, sturdy "universal," "security," "snub" or "stubb" type with a short, stubby bulb, for oral or rectal use, and safer for babies or irrational patients (Fig 34).

All fever thermometers have a magnifying-lens front which renders the mercury column visible against an opaque background. Some have a colored line which by reflection helps detect the mercury column, or guidelines which center the eye on the image of the column. Others are flat in shape so that the markings are on the same plane as the mercury when the thermometer is held in normal reading position.

Taking Body Temperature—Fever thermometers should always be sterilized and shaken down below 97°F before taking a reading. For *oral* temperatures, the thermometer should be placed in the mouth with the bulb under the rear edge of the tongue and rotated once or twice to assure complete contact. The transfer of body heat to the thermometer is speeded by then shifting the bulb to the opposite rear edge of the tongue. The lips should be kept closed and the thermometer left in the mouth for at least 3 min. Regardless of length of initial oral exposure, it is always well after the initial reading to return the thermometer to the patient's mouth for another minute, to provide a check or verification of the original reading. Oral temperatures should not be taken for 30 minutes after exercising, smoking, eating or taking hot or cold drinks.

Rectal temperature should be taken only with a rectal or stubby bulb thermometer. The bulb should be lubricated and gently inserted deeply enough to pass the constricting muscle, leaving about half the thermometer exposed. Babies should be held firmly face down, their buttocks separated with one hand and the thermometer held in place with the other. The thermometer should be left in place at least 4 minutes.

A longer time may be necessary for temperature readings if the thermometer is cold or if the patient is anemic or aged, with poor blood circulation. Axillary (under-arm) temperature is not recommended except when all other methods are impossible.

Normal Temperatures—The average normal mouth temperature is 98.6°F but some variations are natural. Healthy persons may have temperatures as much as 1°F above or below the average normal temperature. One's temperature may range from about 97.3°F at 2 to 5 am to about 98°F in the morning and to about 99°F in the late afternoon. One should determine his normal temperature by a series of readings while in good health for comparison as a personal standard when one is ill.

Normal rectal temperatures are usually 1°F higher, or 99.6°F, though the "normal" mark on all types of fever thermometers, including the rectal type, is at 98.6°F.

Basal Temperature Graph—A woman who wishes to become pregnant may increase her chances of conception greatly by having intercourse at the time of ovulation, or she may decrease the chance of contraception by avoiding intercourse then. And one may use her knowledge of the fertile interval for avoidance of conception for some time by natural means, then use it for a planned pregnancy (*natural child spacing*).

Basal temperature graphs are helpful in determining whether and when ovulation occurs. Ovulation is the release of an egg (ovum) from the ovary; it ordinarily occurs only once in each menstrual cycle. Conception can take place only if intercourse takes place at or near this time, during the interval of transition between low- and high-temperature levels.

The basal temperature graph reflects slight body changes taking place during the menstrual cycle; charts for plotting the daily temperatures are available from Schering, Becton-Dickinson and elsewhere. The "basal" *resting* temperature in the first part of the cycle is usually well below normal; in the last 2 weeks or so of the cycle the basal temperature is closer to 98.6°F. Most important, *the shift from the lower to the higher temperature level occurs about the time of ovulation* (Fig 35).

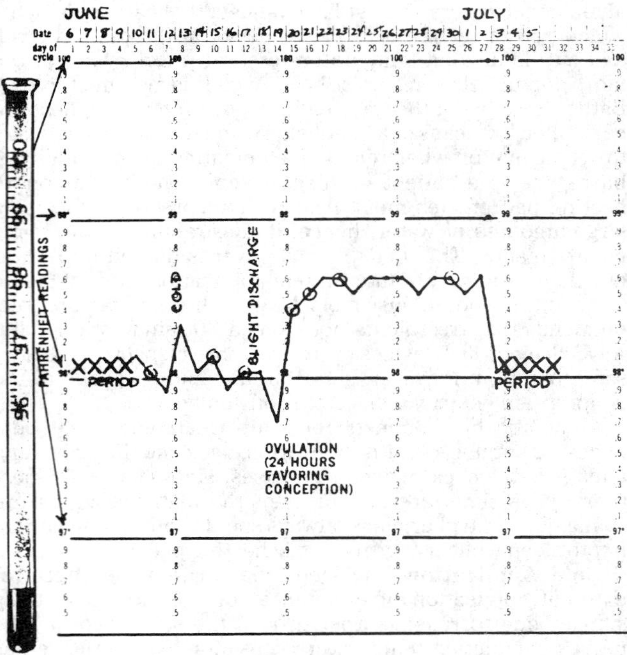

Fig 35. Basal temperature graph for determination of ovulation period in the female.

The variations in the temperature before and after ovulation are slight, often only a few tenths to a half degree, so it is important that the temperature be taken carefully and recorded accurately. Special thermometers are available for this purpose. They record temperatures within the usual range of cyclic variations (from 96 to 100°F only) and are graduated in tenths of a degree and are easier to read than the ordinary fever thermometers, although the latter may be used.

Temperature Comparisons—Throughout the US the Fahrenheit scale still is employed, although the use of the Celcius scale is increasing rapidly in medical circles. Some hospitals and physicians prefer the latter scale, and clinical thermometers graduated in Celcius degrees are available. Normal body temperature on the Celcius scale is 37°. A comparison of temperature equivalents of the two scales, in the range of body temperatures below and above normal, is given in Table 1.

Accuracy—The critical factors in obtaining maximum accuracy are the thermometer must be designed properly, it must be sufficiently accurate to meet each specific requirement and it must be used properly.

In general, the accuracy of fever thermometers is established either by federal standards, or by states, local authorities and sometimes private institutions, usually operating for hospital groups.

Thermometers are offered for sale which exceed the standards, and usually bear specific information on the certificate indicating special accuracy or selection for other factors beyond the minimum requirements. They are valuable for critical temperature use, such as in diagnosis of certain pulmonary diseases and infectious diseases, both surgical and medical, and for basal-temperature studies, now being used widely in the study of human fertility. For ordinary use the CS1-52 *certified thermometer* is entirely adequate.

Reading the Thermometer—Next to accuracy, the most important feature of a fever thermometer is its ease of reading. This is especially true for the inexperienced home user, who will appreciate being shown thermometers with easy-reading features, as offered by many manufacturers. Always demonstrate how to hold the thermometer for reading, which should be done with the back to good light and the instrument held horizontally in the right hand, about 12 in. from the eyes. The bulb should never be held while reading, but the thermometer may be steadied by the left-hand index finger placed behind it. With the markings to the front, the thermometer should be rotated slowly until the mercury is visible.

Care of the Thermometer—After the thermometer has been read and the temperature recorded, it always should be shaken down so that it is ready for use the next time it is needed. In shaking down the mercury column, the thermometer should be grasped firmly between the thumb and the forefinger at the scale end and shaken vigorously by several snaps of the wrist until the reading is below 97°F. This is effective and a good way to describe this method is to liken it to shaking water off the bulb, which the customer can visualize. The thermometer should *never* be held in the fingers while the hand is struck upon a solid surface to jar down the mercury column. Such rough handling is almost certain to cause a breakage or rupture of the constriction, even though it may appear unbroken. If dropped, even though apparently unbroken, the thermometer should be tested before using. Fever thermometers should never be exposed to heat, the sun's rays or a heat unit, or be displayed in a shop window.

Table 1—Temperature Comparison

Fahrenheit	Celcius
96.0°	35.55°
97.0	36.11
97.6	36.36
98.0	36.65
98.6	37.0
99.0	37.22
99.5	37.50
100.0	37.77
101.0	38.33
102.0	38.88
103.0	39.44
104.0	40.0

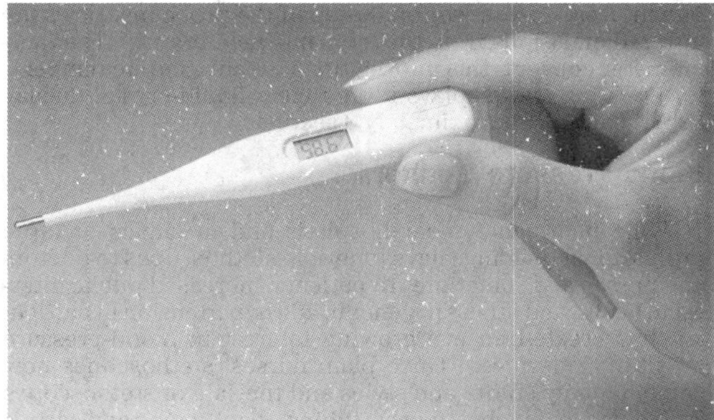

Fig 36. Digital electronic thermometer (courtesy, Omron Healthcare).

Currently there are also available a variety of low-cost, battery-operated electronic fever thermometers, with a visible gauge, that sell for around $5 and up. The most popular is the digital type (Fig 36); however, models with analog indicators are available. This type of thermometer gives precise temperature readings within a minute and are safe to use. Most have a "peak hold" feature so that the maximum temperature attained can be read and use disposable probe covers for sanitation.

A thermometer, designed to make quantitative temperature measurements directly from the surface of the skin, has been developed at the University of Colorado, Craig Rehabilitation Hospital. The instrument is accurate to within one-tenth of a degree when measuring the difference in heat generated by an arthritic joint and that generated by a healthy tissue. Its probe is about 6 inches long and has about a ⅝ inch diameter. Its hollow aluminum barrel holds a spring mechanism—like a ballpoint pen—that permits the user to exert uniform pressure when measuring skin temperatures.

The new tympanic thermometer (Fig 37) can be used on virtually every patient, newborn to elderly. The contoured safety probe of the thermometer is placed snugly into the

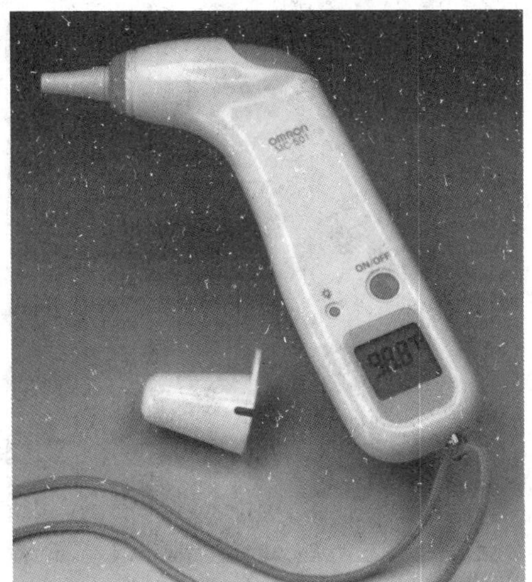

Fig 37. Tympanic thermometer (courtesy, Omron Healthcare).

patient's ear. A sensor on the tip of the probe measures the infrared emissions from the tympanic membrane. The thermometer converts this information into an accurate temperature reading and displays it on a clear liquid-crystal display (LCD) panel in approximately 3 seconds.

Blood-Pressure Monitors

While pharmacies near hospitals and in clinics or large professional buildings have long sold stethoscopes to doctors and nurses and sometimes to patients, increased public interest in health and fitness in general, and hypertension in particular, has created an evergrowing interest in blood-pressure monitoring devices. Once plain nurses' stethoscopes now come in many colors and styles and the sale of stethoscopes and replacement chestpieces, tubing, diaphragms and eartips to nurses not only bring in additional revenue but also introduces nurses to all the other health-related accessories offered by the pharmacy.

Desk-type mercury sphygmomanometers are still used in professionals' offices, but aneroid models are much more popular. Inexpensive self-taking aneroid models can be purchased for home use. More expensive digital models are available and easy to use and some even come with printers. Another digital model takes systolic, diastolic and pulse measurements from the left index finger (Fig 38).

A pharmacist can highlight the blood-pressure monitor department by offering free blood-pressure screening, either on an as-needed basis or specifying a certain morning or afternoon each week. Training in proper techniques for measuring blood pressure may be offered by a local chapter of the American Heart Association.

After taking a subject's blood pressure, the pharmacist, or a properly trained associate, may choose to record the measurement on a folding wallet card (Fig 39). The patient can be advised to return at regular intervals for further readings or encouraged to consult a physician if appropriate. By having the pharmacy name and logo on the opposite side of the folding card, the patient is carrying a reminder of the pharmacy in his wallet. Also, if the patient shows the readings to his physician, the physician may become more aware of the professional level of services provided by the pharmacy.

Blood-Glucose Monitors

A pharmacy can expand its services to diabetic patients by offering blood-glucose monitoring devices and providing training in proper usage. Models are available that are inexpensive and easy to use at home. Ongoing purchases of the test strips and other supplied used with these monitors can provide opportunities for patients to return to the pharmacy on a regular basis.

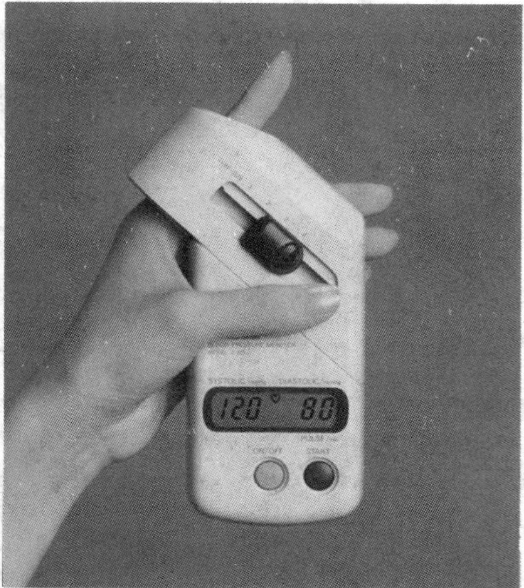

Fig 38. Finger blood-pressure and pulse monitor (courtesy, Omron Healthcare).

Name ______________________

DATE	TIME	BLOOD PRESSURE	INITIALS
		/	
		/	
		/	
		/	
		/	
		/	
		/	
		/	
		/	
		/	
		/	
		/	
		/	
		/	
		/	

Fig 39. Wallet blood-pressure record card.

TENS

Transcutaneous Electrical Nerve Stimulation (TENS) is an electrical method of controlling pain. It is a safe, nonaddictive and noninvasive alternative to drug therapy. A TENS unit delivers mild electrical signals through the skin to the underlying nerves to relieve pain by blocking the pain message before it reaches the brain or by causing the body to release pain-relieving endorphins.

A small battery-powered stimulator generates low intensity electrical impulses to electrodes adhering to the skin. A physician or therapist will set the stimulation parameters. The pharmacist (who has been trained in TENS usage) will instruct the patient in placement of electrodes, use of lead wires to connect the electrodes to the unit, give instructions on adjusting the level of intensity and the treatment schedule, and advise the client on proper skin care.

Vacuum Constriction Devices

A nonsurgical solution to impotence is vacuum constriction therapy. Many men are silent, embarrassed or uneasy about discussing their impotence. Pharmacists can provide the confidential and professional advice essential for the successful use of these devices.

Impotence may result from inadequate blood flow into the penis and/or the inability of blood vessels to retrain the blood flowing into the penis. *Osbon Medical Systems* define therapy as follows: Vacuum constriction involves placing the penis in a patented vacuum cylinder. An erection is achieved by creating a vacuum which generates blood flow into the penis, causing engorgement and rigidity. Similar to the natural erection process, blood flow from the penis then is reduced using a simple retention device. In this manner an erection can be maintained safely and easily for up to 30 minutes (Fig 40).

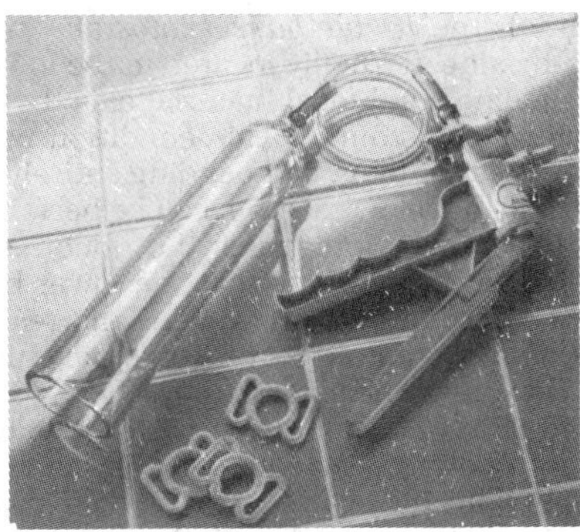

Fig 40. ErecAid vacuum constriction device (courtesy, Osbon Medical Systems).

IV Pharmacy

Historically, parenteral preparations (see Chapter 87) and intravenous admixtures (see Chapter 88) were not a normal component of community pharmacy practice. With increases in both technology and the demand for care in the home, many pharmacies now prepare and dispense these types of pharmaceuticals as well as enteral and parenteral nutrient solutions. The pharmacist in charge is responsible for or supervises the home setup and patient training which is essential for successful home treatment. Different types of infusion pumps to regulate the controlled delivery of these solutions may be supplied by the home-care pharmacist.

Ostomy Appliances and Supplies

Understanding the Ostomy—An ostomy is a surgical procedure whereby parts of the intestinal and/or urinary tract are removed from the patient, the remaining end(s) then are brought to the abdominal wall and a stoma (Gk, mouth), or artificial opening, is constructed surgically through which urine or feces will pass from then on.

It is estimated that more than 50,000 such operations are performed annually in the US, most resulting in the saving of lives. There are approximately a million Americans now living who have had such surgery, and each one of them is buying appliances and supplies on a regular basis.

Since the pharmacist will be called on to offer advice to the ostomy patient as to the kind of appliance that will best serve his needs, and since there are many different kinds of ostomy surgery, each of which has its own special requirements as to the fitting and type of appliance best suited to it, it behooves the pharmacist who wishes to develop a successful ostomy section in his or her health-accessories department to become familiar with every type of surgery and the idiosyncrasies of each.

One could develop three basic classifications of ostomy surgery: those which involve the intestinal tract, those which involve the urinary tract and those which involve both.

Among the surgeries that involve the intestinal tract, there are two types. If the ostomy results from part of the colon being brought to the abdominal wall for the surgical construction of a stoma, the operation is called a *colostomy*. If, on the other hand, the ostomy results from part of the ileum being brought to the abdominal wall for the construction of a stoma, the operation is referred to as an *ileostomy*. The differences in the appearance of these two categories consist primarily in the sizes and locations of their stomas.

Stoma is the name given to the artificial anus on the abdominal wall; it has the appearance of a small bud, normally flush though sometimes protruding up to about ½ inch, and usually pink to bright red, although stomas vary in color and sometimes appear darker. While most stomas do not protrude more than about ½ inch, there are some which may have been constructed so that they protrude an inch or more. But when the pharmacist sees a stoma which protrudes more than 1½ inch he should question the patient as to whether it was that long shortly following his surgery. In cases where the length of the stoma has changed drastically since the surgery, the chances are that it has become distended and the patient should be advised to see his physician for possible corrective surgery to avoid the potentiality of strangulation of the intestine. It also is possible for a stoma to "shrink" back into the body. When it becomes inverted, management can become very difficult, and corrective surgery may be indicated.

Stomas appear red because the surgeon inverts the end of the intestine slightly when he brings it to the outside of the abdominal wall. After suturing the intestine to the abdominal skin, it becomes an integral part of the body wall, and all tissues live normally. The red surface of an ostomy stoma is actually the intestinal capillary bed; it stays red because blood continues to flow through it. As it is also a mucous membrane, it will continue to stay wet.

As most ileostomies result in the entire colon being separated from the small intestine at a point just behind the ileocecal valve (where the ileum joins the cecum), that is usually where the incision is made in the abdominal wall and where the ileum is brought to the outside of the body. The location of the ileocecal valve is near the appendix in the abdomen's lower-right quadrant, and where an ileostomy stoma typically is located. Since the stoma in an ileostomy is constructed from the small intestine, it will be smaller in size than the colostomy stoma, which is made from the colon. However, it is important to note that the location of stomas on the outside of the body cannot be standardized as colostomy on the left side and ileostomy on the right side.

Complications may occur or problems existing unique to the patient obstructing typical stoma placement—eg, a kidney transplant, requiring the surgeon to place the stoma in an unobstructive location. Also, stoma placement may be affected by previous surgical scars, and by the individual patient's body shape. The fecal matter or output indicates what type of surgery was performed.

In a colostomy only part of the colon is removed from the body. The types of colostomies depend upon where the diseased part of the colon is separated from the healthy part of the colon. When only the juncture of the sigmoid colon with the rectum and anus is involved, the surgeon brings the sigmoid colon to the surface of the abdomen and the surgery is termed a *sigmoid colostomy*. When the separation occurs along the length of the descending colon, anywhere between the splenic flexure (the bend where the transverse colon meets the descending colon) and the sigmoid flexure, the operation is called a *descending colostomy*. Accordingly, when the surgeon makes the separation along the length of the transverse colon anywhere between the splenic flexure and the hepatic flexure (where the transverse and ascending colon meet), the surgery is termed a *transverse colostomy; an ascending colostomy* occurs between the hepatic flexure and the cecum. Finally, when the stoma is constructed with that part of the colon called the cecum, the surgery is simply called a *cecostomy*.

These five surgeries, while they are all colostomies, are distinctly different from each other in that different lengths of colon remain in patients having different types of colostomies. Since a primary function of the colon is the removal of water from the feces as it passes through it, it is understandable that the feces produced at a cecostomy stoma will be quite loose and watery while the feces produced at a sigmoid colostomy stoma are generally quite solid. Likewise, the ascending, transverse and descending colostomies produce feces, within the extremes just described, of varying degrees of consistency. The additional fact that all colostomies, because of the reservoir effect of the colon still remaining, can be managed better than ileostomies in which there is no reservoir remaining, has implications for the pharmacist with regard to the types of appliances that are best suited for each type of ostomy.

The implications are that different colostomies in particular, and intestinal ostomies in general, because of differences in fecal products, create nonidentical problems for the patient, ie, not all colostomies can be irrigated successfully, they require different types of appliances and they use different kinds of accessories. There is very little difference in the size of the stomas of each of the five colostomies, but they may be located on the abdominal wall differently. Colostomy stomas which usually are located in the lower-left quadrant of the patient's abdomen tend toward more solid feces, while those usually located in the lower-right quadrant tend toward feces which contain more water and are, therefore, of looser consistency. Most colostomies are performed as the result of cancer of the lower bowel and occur in persons over the age of 60.

When the entire colon must be removed, the surgeon performs an *ileostomy* by separating the colon from the small intestine behind the ileocecal valve. The result is a stoma much smaller than any colostomy stoma, located in the lower-right quadrant and producing fecal material which is always loose and watery. The majority of ileostomies are performed on people between the ages of 18 and 40, and are usually the result of an ulceration of the inner lining of the colon which is called ulcerative colitis.

There are several types of urinary diversions, the most common of which are those in which the patient's bladder must be removed. The preferred surgical procedure brings the two ureters together, implants them in an artificial bladder and enables the patient to have but one stoma to manage and one appliance to wear instead of the usual two.

This operation is frequently referred to as an *ileal bladder*, *ileal conduit* or *urinary diversion*. All three names indicate the same operation, however.

During this operation, the surgeon removes a piece of the healthy small intestine at the ileum, after which he performs a resection of the two ends of the ileum, joining them together again. The missing piece is usually between 6 and 8 inches, and is a relatively insignificant loss to the small intestine, which measures nearly 24 ft in the average adult. One end of the piece of ileum is closed and the other is brought to the outside of the body to become the single stoma. Once the two ureters are implanted in the closed end of the piece of ileum, that piece becomes a conduit for the urine—actually a substitute bladder. Since this conduit or bladder is made from a piece of the ileum, it has gotten the names ileal conduit and ileal bladder.

The stoma has the appearance of an ileostomy stoma and usually is located within the same quadrant, the lower right, but its product is only urine. While most ileostomy stomas are located in the lower half of the lower-right quadrant of the abdomen, most ileal conduit stomas are located in the upper half of the lower-right quadrant. The only way to be sure which ostomy is which is to determine the nature of the waste product.

When the two ureters are severed or cannot be brought forward to the abdominal wall for any reason, the surgeon is forced to bring the ureters to the nearest outside surface—the patient's back. Stomas appearing on the dorsal side or openings through which renal catheters lead directly to the kidneys, indicate an operation called a *nephrostomy*. Persons with bilateral nephrostomies wear two appliances.

Openings directly into the bladder, just above the pubic bone (the symphysis pubis) are the result of a urinary diversion made necessary by involvement of the urethra which normally carries urine from the bladder to the outside. Called *vesicotomies*, these are often temporary operations and are rarely of concern to the pharmacist.

All of the surgeries described above, with the exception of the last, are irreversible and permanent, eg, a patient with an ileostomy will always have an ileostomy. But there are two other ostomies which are temporary and with which the pharmacist should be familiar. One is a modified kind of descending colostomy in which the lower portion of the descending colon, sigmoid colon and rectum are not removed from the patient. After the surgical separation is made, both ends of the colon are brought to the outside and two stomas are constructed, one active and the other inactive.

This operation, the *double-barrel colostomy*, results in two stomas, side-by-side, normally located in the lower-left quadrant and producing solid fecal material exactly like the ordinary descending colostomy. This condition may last from one month to a year or longer, depending entirely on when the surgeon is satisfied that a resection can be performed without further complication. Sometimes the double-barrel colostomy is performed in the hope that the lower bowel can be brought back to normal with treatment and rest. On occasion, a patient with a double-barrel colostomy must return to the hospital for a permanent colostomy.

The second kind of temporary colostomy is called a *loop colostomy*, and is done as an emergency procedure to relieve a bowel impaction and avoid an intestinal rupture. Normally, the patient who has a loop colostomy performed will have his colon repaired and back to normal within a few weeks and before he leaves the hospital. Loop-colostomy appliances are applied during surgery by the physician, and are the only ostomy appliances which are packaged sterile, besides the common postoperative drain. This ostomy gets its name from the fact that, unlike the double-barrel colostomy, the loop colostomy doesn't result in the complete separation of the intestine but, rather, a loop of intestine is brought through an incision and temporarily is secured to the abdominal wall by means of a glass rod which is slipped under the loop and across the incision; the loop then is perforated surgically to relieve the impaction. The wound stays open and the loop remains visible until the perforation in the intestine is closed and the loop is returned to its normal position within the visceral cavity. It is highly unlikely that the pharmacist will ever be called upon to fit a loop-colostomy appliance although he may still want to stock the appliances for use by the hospital.

Choosing the Right Appliance—The various ostomies described above can be grouped into three major categories for the purpose of understanding which kinds of appliances are most appropriate for each.

1. Those ostomies which only produce solid waste at their stomas. They include the sigmoid colostomy, descending colostomy, transverse colostomy, double-barrel colostomy and often the loop colostomy.
2. Those ostomies which only produce urine at their stomas. They include the cutaneous ureterostomy, nephrostomy, vesicotomy and ileal conduit.
3. Those ostomies which, for one reason or another, produce liquid or semisolid fecal matter at their stomas. They include the ileostomy, cecostomy, ascending colostomy and sometimes the loop colostomy.

In real life, neat and perfectly reliable categories such as the ones just described do not exist. People differ, their digestive processes are different and their diets are different. The consistency of the waste matter in any one individual also varies from day to day. Yet these categories are useful generally and, in addition, they point up the fact that an appliance should be chosen primarily for the nature of the waste matter it will have to collect.

Further, the groupings do indicate that among a host of ostomy appliances presently on the market from numerous manufacturers, there are just three basic types, categorized primarily by the nature of the waste material for which they are intended: those designed for pure urine, for semisolids and solid waste matter. Other considerations in choosing the right appliance for each patient include the size of gasket openings which fit around the stoma, method of attaching the appliance around the stoma, patient's financial resources (including what reimbursement limits may be placed either on types, quantities or cost of appliances by government agencies such as Medicare and medical-assistance programs or by HMOs or insurance companies) and activities in which the patient engages at work or at play (Fig 41).

Ostomy Appliances for Solid Wastes—The colostomy appliance, so-called because the majority of colostomies are solid-waste-producing, is the appliance used for most colostomies. There are many types of colostomy appliances on the market, recognizable by larger size gasket openings to accommodate the larger stomas characteristic of all colostomies, and by detachable, throw-away pouches made of thin

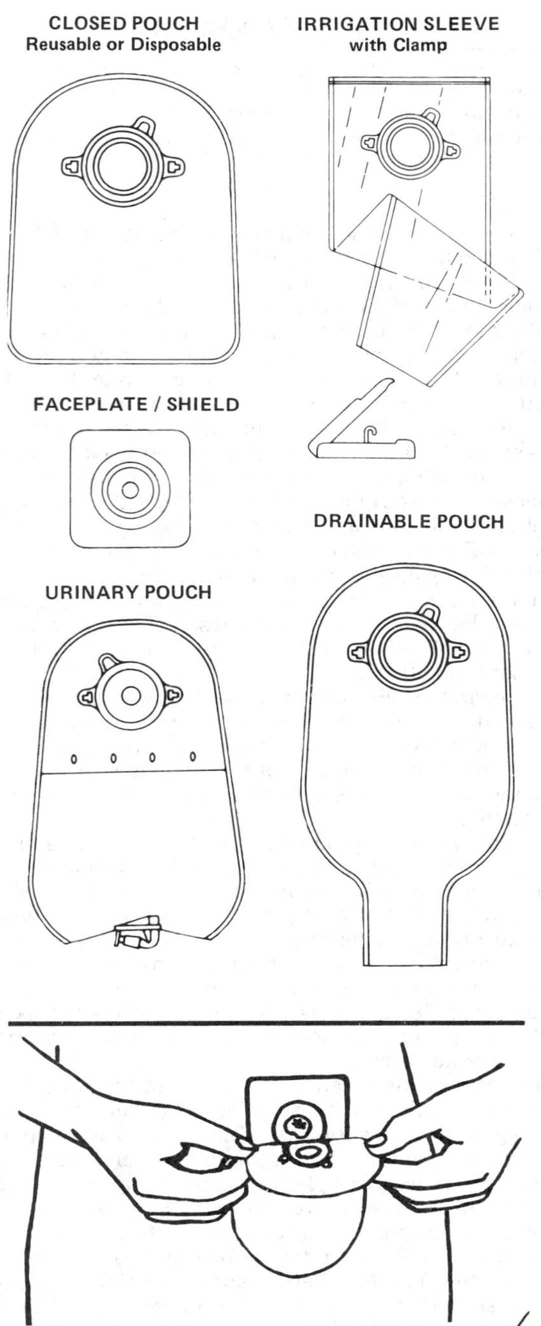

Fig 41. Ostomy appliances (courtesy, Convatec).

polyethylene plastic; most are sealed at their bottoms. However, some colostomates do use open-ended pouches. The fact that these pouches are sealed at the bottom and are disposable indicates the impracticability of bottom drains for solid wastes generally. By and large, colostomy appliances are not the permanent type since those ostomies which produce solid wastes do not cause the problems with skin excoriation typical of the wetter ostomies.

The self-adhesive colostomy appliance is more of a collection bag with adhesive around the stoma opening than it is an appliance. The openings may be cut with scissors to fit the stoma precisely though most manufacturers provide several sizes. The advantages with this type of appliance are that it is light-weight and quite flat against the body so it is less likely to show through clothing. Those colostomates who irrigate regularly find this type of appliance perfect for safety's sake.

Some colostomates are urged by their physicians to irrigate on a regular basis. Irrigation is the process of administering an enema to the colon via the stoma for the purpose of establishing regular, conveniently timed evacuation of the bowel—in other words, to become relatively stool-free. It is necessary just once a day at the most, and may be scheduled in the morning before dressing or in the evening before retiring. It is a highly individual thing and some persons need to irrigate only every other day or two to three times a week. There are some people who have quite irritable bowels and cannot remain stool-free.

After irrigation, the colostomate can expect to have no bowel activity until the next irrigation, except perhaps for slight dripping now and then. Many ostomates, after irrigation, wear only a gauze pad over the stoma for safety and psychological confidence. The pad can be taped over the stoma or secured with a two-way stretch wraparound.

The irrigation process is quite simple and takes between 30 to 45 minutes for completion. The important steps are

The stoma should be dilated with a gloved finger (finger cot) and a bit of lubricating jelly prior to insertion of the irrigator cone.

About one quart of tepid water (some patients add a couple of table spoons of salt) is placed in the irrigating bag—never hung more than head high. About 15 min should be allowed before permitting evacution; after the initial gush it normally takes another 20 to 25 min before the colon is really empty.

Most people close the end of the irrigating sleeve with a rubber band and then shower or shave during this period.

Sometimes drinking a cup of strong black coffee or a glass of ice cold water will start the intestinal peristalsis necessary for complete evacuation.

Irrigation is a technique for accomplishing regularity and security throughout the day, but is only useful in those ostomies which produce solid wastes. Many physicians and enterostomal therapists now are recognizing the importance of diet in gaining control and regularity of bowel movements and irrigation. The question of whether or not a particular colostomy patient should irrigate should be answered only by the physician. Irrigation usually is not advised when the possibility of reconnecting the intestine at a later date exists.

Appliances for Urine and Semisolids—The appliances used for urinary diversions and ileostomies are both similar to the appliances used for colostomies (Fig 41). A notable difference is in the size of the stoma openings (because urostomy and ileostomy stomas are usually much smaller than colostomy stomas). Also, since the discharge from either a urinary diversion or an ileostomy is more liquid than most colostomies, there is more often a need for skin barriers and protectants such as karaya, stomahesive and similar products to maintain a waterproof seal.

The real difference between a urinary appliance and an appliance for semisolids is in their bottoms, however. Where the urinary appliance has a nylon twist-drain plug in the bottom, the "ileostomy" appliance merely narrows down to between 1½ to 2½ inches and is just open. The bottom is closed either by folding and wrapping with a rubber band or folding and securing with a clip. To drain, the clip or rubber band is removed and the bottom of the appliance unfolded.

Different manufacturers make appliances which, although basically similar in design or function, differ with respect to method of securing to the skin. In the past, urinary and ileostomy appliances often were made of rubber and secured to the skin with adhesives. Periodically, these appliances had to be removed, often with the help of an adhesive remover. The appliances then had to be cleaned, dried out and reapplied. Some ostomates still use permanent appliances of this type, but the majority of new ostomates choose the disposable type.

Ostomy Appliance Accessories—Most popular among a host of accessories for ostomy appliances of all kinds are karaya gum powder and karaya gum washers, stomahesive powder and stomahesive and similar barrier pastes. These pastes can be used to fill in irregularities in skin surfaces to protect against leakage.

Varieties of deodorant drops, tablets and sprays are available; some are applied to the outside of the appliance, while others are dropped into the bag prior to applying it. Silicone and benzoin tincture sprays also are used to prepare the skin around the stoma. In addition, racks for drying an appliance after washing, abdominal dressings and cover sponges, gloves and wipes and even zippered, purse-size pouches for supplies are available to make things easier for the ostomate. Some manufacturers now offer new easy-to- apply appliances featuring synthetic materials to reduce skin irritation and prevent leakage.

But perhaps the most helpful things which the pharmacist can provide his customers who have ostomies are suggestions and ideas on how to get along with a minimum of difficulty. Knowledge of these things will come from the ostomates themselves, and it is therefore wise to spend some time asking them questions. It is also important for a pharmacist featuring ostomy-care products to develop a good working relationship with an enterostomal therapist (ET), a nurse specially trained in ostomy care. The ET can advise the pharmacist or the patient when unexpected problems occur. Membership in a local ostomy club or the United Ostomy Association is another way to increase your knowledge of the problems ostomates often encounter.

Urology and Incontinence Supplies

Urinals—These containers are employed to collect urine. They differ in shape according to male or female use. They ordinarily are made of white enamelware or plastic, which is by far the most common, especially for use at home. Plastic urinals come in two basic types: single-patient use or autoclavable.

Catheters—To collect urine from the patient unable to void naturally or where incontinence pants and external catheters are inadequate, indwelling catheters are employed.

The insertion of catheters is a dangerous procedure customarily handled by physicians or trained nurses and orderlies. Serious infections of the bladder and damage to the urethral and bladder tissues may result from improper insertion.

Flexible soft-rubber catheters consist of small rubber tubes with a closed solid tip. At one end is a flaring funnel-shaped opening to facilitate attachment of the catheter to a glass junction or another tube leading to a collection unit. At the inserted end is a wide opening which leads to ths channel through which urine flows to the collection unit. This is referred to as a straight catheter, in contrast to the indwelling catheter, which is designed to remain in the urethra for long periods of time.

The indwelling retention catheter, or Foley catheter as it is commonly known, is characterized by a balloon at its insertion end (Fig. 42). The ballon is designed to secure the catheter tip within the patient's bladder to keep it from slipping or being pulled out. There are two channels which run from the insertion tip to the end of the Foley catheter—one for the passing of urine and the other for the injection of sterile water which inflates the balloon.

Foley catheters are available with either 5- or 30-mL balloons. The 30-mL balloon catheter, which also is known as a hemostatic catheter, is used commonly in nursing homes for patients whose urethras have become dilated or for those patients who have pulled the 5-mL balloon catheter out. A common mistake in filling a balloon catheter is to use too little water. It takes about 10 mL to inflate a 5-mL Foley balloon because nearly 5 mL is held in the filling lumen that runs the length of the catheter. The diameters of the catheter also vary in size. Though their use is limited somewhat, 75-mL balloon retention catheters are also available. The three chief scales used for catheters have been named from their respective countries of origin. They are compared in Table 2. The French scale is employed most commonly (Fig. 43).

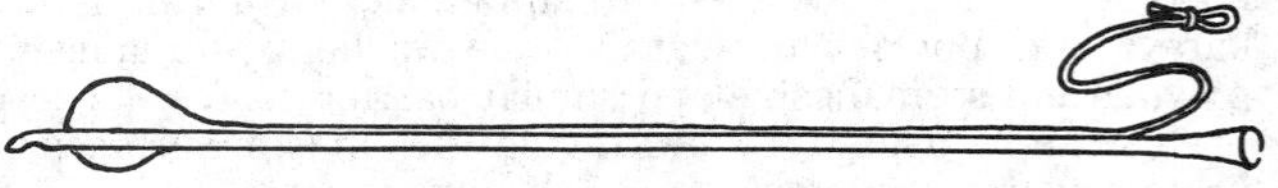

Fig 42. Balloon catheter, for prolonged insertion through the urethra into the bladder.

Table 2—Catheter Scales

French (Nos)	10	12	14	16	18	20	22
American (Nos)	7	8	10	11	12	14	15
English (Nos)	4	5	6	7	9	11	12
Size (inches)	13/100	13/100	18/100	20/100	23/100	26/100	29/100

Other innovations in the urinary catheter include a Foley catheter with its own supply of sterile water for balloon inflation. With these catheters, a valve is released following insertion of the catheter, and the sterile water, which is under pressure, runs up its channel and inflates the balloon. They are especially convenient, as there is no need to prepare a syringe for balloon inflation, but they are considerably more expensive than the typical Foley catheter. Another improvement is the silicone and Teflon coatings on the outside and inside of Foley catheters. Such coatings not only cut down friction during insertion and removal of the catheter, but also inhibit buildup of deposits on catheter walls, thus extending the time between catheter changes. The newest improvement is the all-silicone catheter, now manufactured by Kendall, Bard and others.

The pharmacy also may stock a variety of urine-collection units and catheter administration trays. The bladder-care tray, sometimes called a *cathtray,* is a sterile package containingt the items required during the administration of a Foley catheter, and packed sequentially with those things needed first on top.

Administration trays are also available for catheter irrigation, pulmonary and gastric suction and IV placement.

Male condom catheters and female external catheters are designed to be worn by the patient. They allow mobility and discrete urinary collection without the use of pads or an indwelling catheter. These external types of collection systems are becoming more widely used and are available in a number of different styles. The style selected is usually a matter of personal preference, activity level and size and capacity requirements.

The male condom catheter system consists of two parts: the penile sheath, which resembles a condom with a drainage opening, and a collection bag. The single-use condom catheter may be self-adhesive or attach with an adhesive foam strap. The reuseable style is secured with an adjustable rubber or foam strap worn over the catheter. These are not as secure, but are considerably more cost-effective.

An external collection device for women is also available. According to *Hollister;* their female urinary incontinence system consists of a form-fitting pericup with a urine deflector (a small projection to maintain the position of the device), an external pad and a drain tube which extends from the device and connects to a vented urinary thigh bag.

Both male condom catheters and female urinary collection devices share distinct advantages over other incontinence management methods. Since neither is inserted into the bladder, the incidence of infection is reduced greatly. And since the urine is conveyed to a collection bag the problems of odor and skin breakdown associated with diapers and absorbent pads are minimized.

Urinary Bags—There are two basic types of urinary bags: leg bags and night urinary collection bags. Both can be used with external or indwelling catheter systems.

Leg bags vary in size and capacity and are used by a patient who is ambulatory. The bag is connected to the catheter by a length of plastic or rubber tubing (usually sold separately). The bag itself is worn on the inside of the thigh or lower leg, whichever is most comfortable and least conspicuous. It is secured in place by use of adjustable elastic straps. A common error is to fasten the leg straps so they encircle the bag, thus restricting its volume.

Night urinary collection bags vary in style. The standard is

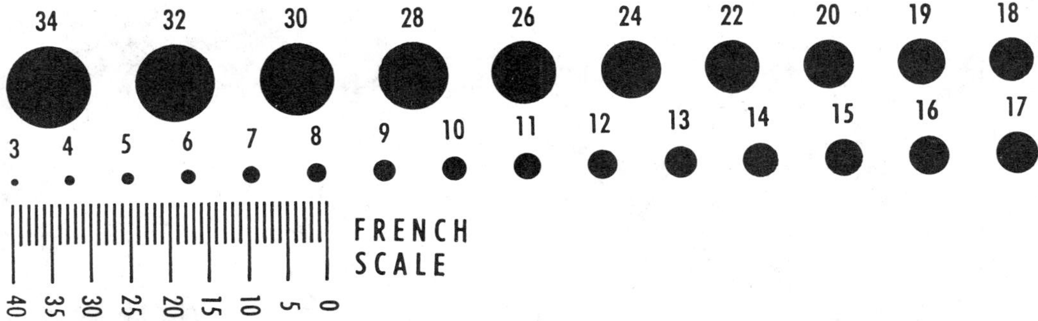

Fig 43. Standard French scale for hospital tubing and catheters as well as rectal and colon, stomach-feeding, suction, urinary drainage and oxygen tubes (courtesy, Becton-Dickinson). To determine the French size if instruments are oval or other shape, use a strip of paper to measure the periphery—then lay on the scale at the left.

a bag that hangs from the side of the bed or the back of the wheelchair. The standard capacity is 2000 mL. Night bags are also available in a cube or a bottle form.

Incontinence Pants—A variety of body-contoured incontinence pants are available for both men and women. Most are of soft, flexible fabric with plastic or rubber coating inside. They are made to remain soft and pliable even after repeated washings. Children's sizes are also available.

Incontinence pants typically are made with elastic tops and legs plus snaps at the sides for ease in putting them on when the patient is bedfast. Newer models consist of an incontinence pouch with waist and leg straps. These briefs are generally more comfortable to wear as they are much less bulky beneath the clothing.

Other products helpful for the incontinent patient include disposable underpads, adult diapers, rubber sheeting, silicone skin sprays and body lotions and deodorants.

Trusses

Hernias and trusses are as old as mankind. The first trusses were nothing more than a rope or strap and a rock. Celsus developed the use of a plate and in medieval times a form of plaster and plate were used. The spring-and-belt-type truss, practically as it is today in principle, was developed by the Netherlands physician Camper in 1785.

True hernias are not the same as ruptures. A true hernia usually is the protrusion of the intestine and its surrounding membrane, the peritoneum, through a natural opening in the abdominal wall, whereas a rupture is such a protrusion through the muscles of the abdomen usually occurring at a point previously weakened. A rupture occurring at the site of a previous surgical incision sometimes is referred to as an incisional hernia. The natural openings in the abdominal musculature through which a true hernia may occur include the umbilical opening; the inguinal openings, through which, in the male, the spermatic cord passes, and in the female, the round ligament passes; and the openings for the femoral arteries (Fig 44).

Abdominal or umbilical hernias are common. Infants in the first year of life show an incidence of 19.6/1000. Between ages 20 and 24, the incidence is lowest, rising to 24.2/1000 in the 70- to 74-year age group.

Of all males afflicted with hernias, 96% suffer from the inguinal type. The corresponding incidence of inguinal hernias among females is just 44.3%. While surgery is becoming the preferred treatment for all hernias, it is not always the best solution for all patients. Some will require trusses in lieu of surgery.

Hernia trusses of all kinds vary from soft-fabric supports to heavier models requiring experienced judgment on the part of the fitter. The type and location of truss pads, and the weight and build of the patient, are important considerations in truss fitting. All trusses must be fitted while the patient is lying down and the hernia is reduced (the protruding intestine has been returned to the abdominal cavity) or the truss itself may cause strangulation.

A well-fitted truss, appropriate to the specific patient and his specific type of hernia, may be tested by having the patient bend, stoop and cough. If the patient can do those things without having a protrusion of the intestine past the truss pad, it is likely that it is fitted properly. Finally, it is important for the pharmacist to teach the patient how to properly put on his truss and test its security while he is in the fitting room, so he can remove it with confidence when he is on his own.

Fitting Schools—The pharmacist who will be in charge of the truss and orthopedic department should attend a fitting school. This may require time and travel, but it basically trains the pharmacist in the anatomy involved, and appliance selection and fitting skills which are absolutely necessary. Several good schools are conducted by surgical-appliance manufacturers and typically run 3 to 5 days. Such programs are given by Camp, OTC, Freeman, Atco and others. Professional organizations such as the National Association of Retail Druggists also conduct information seminars.

No pharmacist or pharmacy employee should attempt any truss or orthopedic fitting involving shaping metal without proper training.

Attendance at one of these schools provides background on the definition, location, varieties, frequency, symptoms, causes, complications and treatment of conditions which could result in the use of these types of surgical appliances:

Orthopedic corsets
Spinal braces
Cervical collars and braces
Knee, ankle and foot orthoses
Traction equipment
Compression hosiery
Trusses
Mastectomy prostheses

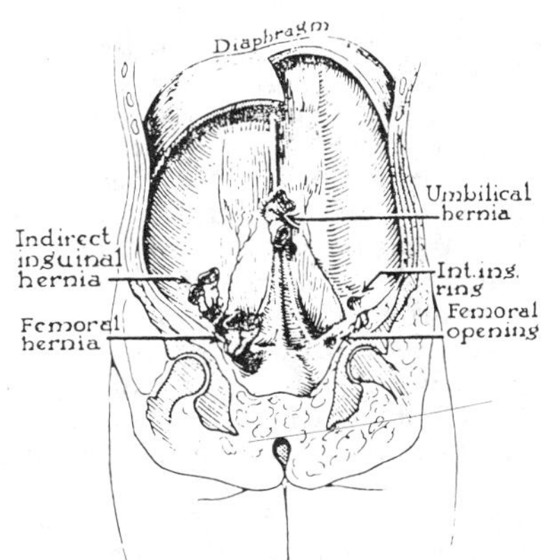

Fig 44. Looking toward the front of the abdominal wall, from within the cavity, showing the five congenitally weak points.

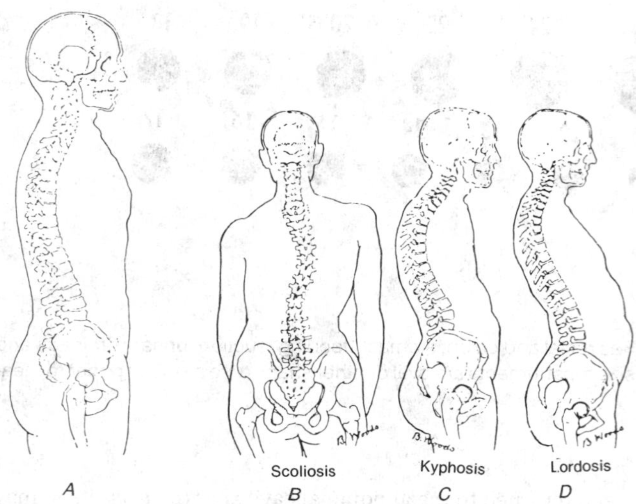

Fig 45. *A:* Curves of the normal spine; *B, C, D:* abnormal curves of the spine.

Reference should be made by the interested pharmacist to literature available from appliance manufacturers.

Orthopedic Supports and Braces

The spinal column can be divided into five major sections:

The cervical spine, consisting of 7 vertebrae, supports the head and is characterized by an anterior curve.

The thoracic spine, consisting of 12 vertebrae to each of which a pair of ribs is attached, is characterized by a posterior curve.

The lumbar spine, consisting of 5 vertebrae and characterized by an anterior curve.

The sacrum, consisting of 5 vertebrae which are joined so tightly as to appear as one bone, is situated beneath the fifth lumbar vertebra and between the two innominate bones of the pelvis forming the sacroiliac joints, and is characterized by a posterior curve.

The coccyx, consisting of 3 to 5 vertebrae immediately beneath the sacrum and continuing its posterior curve (Fig 45*A*).

Apart from the cervical spine, anomalies of the spinal column include lordosis, a hyperextension of the lumbar spine, recognizable as sway-back; kyphosis, a flexion of the lumbar spine and/or hyperextension of the thoracic spine, often appearing as hunch-back and scoliosis, an S-shaped lateral curve of the spine (Fig 45*B*, *C* and *D*). Each of these conditions, in varying degree, often requires use of supportive garments or braces. Sometimes ruptures of the intervertebral discs, the cartilaginous shock-absorbing cushions between separate vertebrae, interfere with the spinal cord or the nerves leading from it. An example is sciatica, in which a ruptured intervertebral disc causes compression or trauma at the base of the sciatic nerve resulting in extreme pain at the back of the thigh and running down the inside of the leg along the course of the sciatic nerve. This condition also may require the use of a spinal garment or brace and, occasionally, the occurrence of spondylolisthesis (the slippage of lower vertebrae usually against the sacrum) will bring the patient to the pharmacy with a prescription for a garment or brace-fitting.

These and other conditions create a need for spinal braces and orthopedic garments to limit motion in the spine and permit healing. While the pharmacist should be knowledgeable about them, he should never diagnose such conditions or prescribe the wearing of an orthopedic appliance. That should be left entirely to the physician. Unhappy consequences can be avoided and the surgical-appliance business strengthened if the pharmacist will adhere to the simple rule of never fitting any brace or support except on the prescription of a physician.

The most commonly prescribed orthopedic back corsets have a back length of from 12 to 15 inches and are made of heavy, cloth material or elastic (Fig 46). They often feature two or four rigid metal stays which the fitter will shape to the physician's order, usually to the contour of the patient's back. Readymade spinal braces often are similar in principle to corsets, but are generally of heavier construction. Braces limit mobility to a greater degree than orthopedic corsets.

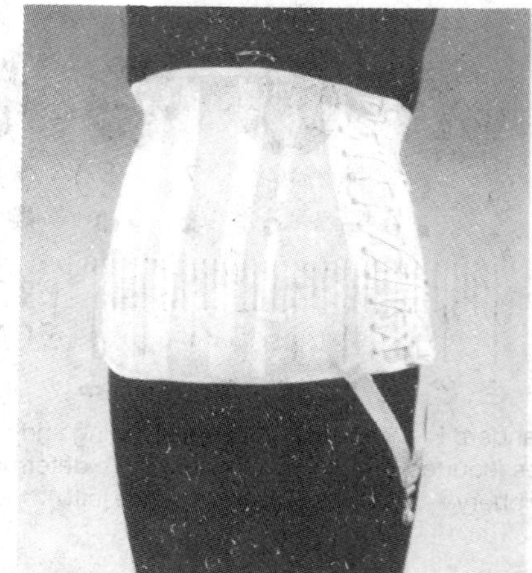

Fig 46. Lumbosacral support (courtesy, Camp).

The procedures for fitting different orthopedic supports and braces are quite involved and are better covered in the week-long schools presented by manufacturers than in a few paragraphs in this text.

Conditions affecting the cervical spine often result in a prescription for a cervical collar or brace. The most popular type is a soft-foam collar with a *velcro* closure. Unless the prescriber specifies flexion or extension, the fitter usually would select a collar that provided support to hold the head in a neutral position. A more rigid plastic collar (Philadelphia type) can be heat-molded to the contours of the patient's neck, chin and shoulders. This type will provide a greater degree of immobilization than a soft collar. Still more immobilization can be obtained by the application of a properly fitted metal cervical brace.

The use of cervical-traction devices also is specified often in the treatment of conditions affecting the cervical spine.

Supports for the knee can vary from a simple pull-on elastic type as found in many pharmacies to 10- or 11 inches long braces with shaped metal hinges and leather straps, to complex braces such as an ACL knee orthosis (Fig 47).

Compression Hosiery—Many types of compression hosiery are available in pharmacy health-accessory departments. Light-weight, fashion-sheer elastic hosiery is very popular,

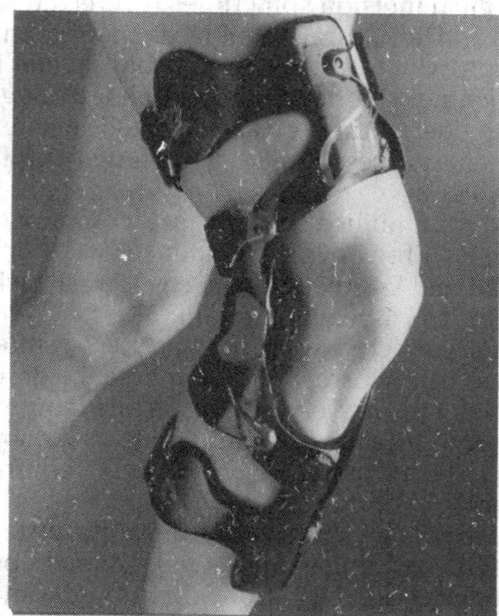

Fig 47. ACL knee orthosis (courtesy, Innovation Sports).

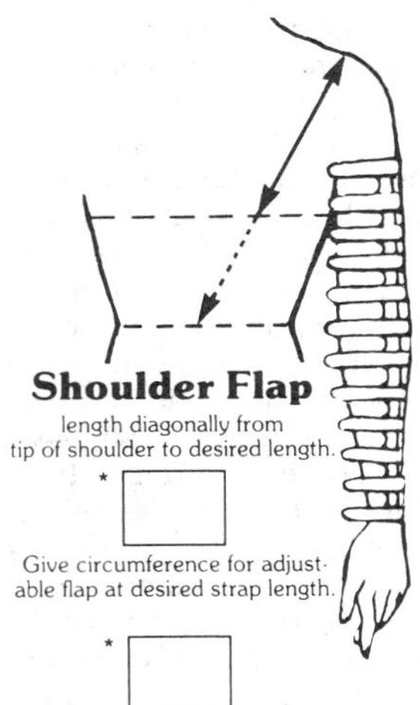

Fig 48. Custom-made elastic support (courtesy, Jobst).

but does not give as much support as heavier, surgical-weight hosiery. For severe or unusual conditions, custom-made elastic supports for arm or leg (such as Jobst, Fig 48) can be ordered. Antiembolism hosiery is intended primarily for bed-fast patients.

Taking the patient into a private fitting room, measuring the limb and then actually applying the hose are the professional activites which will differentiate the qualified health-care-accessories pharmacist from his peers. It should be noted that the best time to measure and fit elastic compression hosiery is early in the morning when the affected limb is likely to be the least distended.

Recent advances in the treatment and management of primary and secondary lymphedema with the use of multicompartmental pneumatic compressors has done much to improve the quality of life for people suffering from lymphedema. Pneumatic compression devices are designed to reduce lymphedema in the extremity by applying pressure sequentially through a multicell pneumatic arm or leg sleeve. The pneumatic sleeve inflates in a distal to proximal direction promoting the flow of lymph fluid through existing lymphatics by exerting pressure on the interstitial tissue. Because the sequential milking pattern is soothing and comfortable, it results in excellent patient compliance (Fig 49).

To maintain the results obtained by home treatments with a multicell compression device, graduated compression hosiery is recommended. The lymphedema garments should be worn during periods of activity to prevent the rapid reaccumulation of lymphatic fluid. Patients should be measured after they have begun their treatments and have achieved some reduction in swelling. Periodic remeasuring is necessary to monitor further reduction.

In some cases, such as severe edema, the physician also may prescribe a special pump and sleeve to reduce the edema prior to applying compression hosiery. Such pumps usually are rented, although sales are not uncommon. Lymphedema pumps, particularly the sequential types, should be rented or sold only by qualified professionals who are very familiar with their uses and contraindications (Fig 49).

Mastectomy Prostheses—The fitting of mastectomy prostheses and bras is often a logical adjunct to an orthopedic corset and compression hosiery section in a pharmacy's health-accessories department. In most cases, it is essential to have a female fitter for this department.

In most cases, breast surgery is the result of breast cancer. Some surgeries, such as a lumpectomy, remove only a portion of the breast. A "simple" mastectomy results in the removal of breast tissue. More-involved surgery results in removal both of breast tissue and additional underlying tissue.

A variety of breast forms is available to fit a woman after each type of surgery, although it is often difficult to fit a woman after a lumpectomy. (Male breast cancer, while rare, does occur.) The breast form is designed not only to help restore a woman's shape, but also to replace the weight lost and restore proper balance (Fig 50).

Although reconstruction is becoming increasingly popular, external breast forms remain a safe alternative. There have been many advances in the technology of manufacturing the forms, resulting in more comfortable, natural-feeling breast prostheses. Although some forms are made with polyester fiberfill or foam, the majority are made with silicone. Conventional silicone forms generally are designed to be worn in conjunction with a specially designed pocketed bra which securely holds the breast form in place.

A new development in silicone breast prostheses allows the form to attach safely and securely directly to the chest wall by means of an adhesive skin support. This new option gives a woman greater freedom for an active lifestyle as well as for fashion flexibility.

The Fitting Room—For such a department, an adequate, private fitting room and stock space nearby are an absolute necessity. The fitting room need be no more than 8 x 8 ft, but should be clean, free of any stock or display and have an inward swinging door to shield the fitting table from view. The fitting room also should be soundproofed to provide privacy and enable the patient to feel comfortable discussing his condition. As many fittings are done with the patient in a horizontal position, a table 72 by 26 and 30 inches high, padded with moistureproof vinyl and a pillow are needed, as well as a chair, coat hooks and clothes hangers, four-legged stool, small dressing table and a full-length mirror. Professional simplicity and cleanliness are exceedingly important. The use of rolled paper on the table is practical and economical. If the pharmacy also has a comprehensive ostomy center, a second chair, so both the patient and the pharmacist can sit, is recommended. As a health-accessories department grows

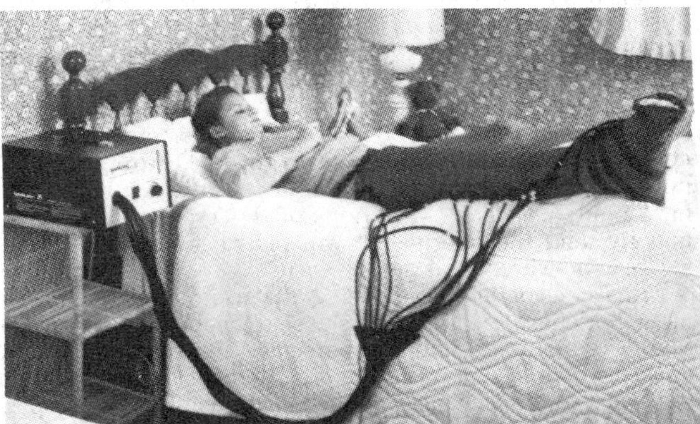

Fig 49. Lymphedema pump (courtesy, Camp).

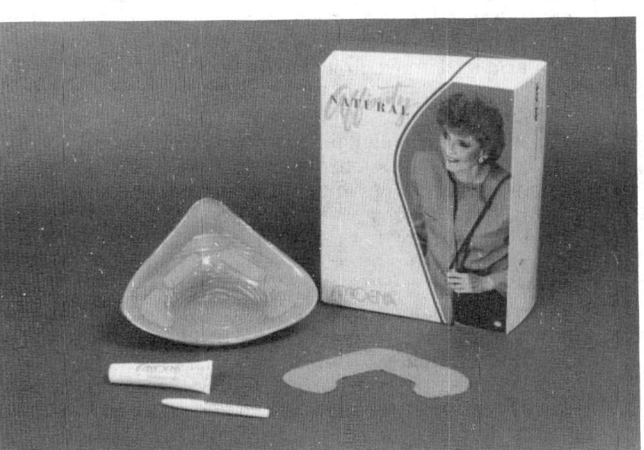

Fig 50. Breast form (courtesy, Amoena).

and prospers, more than one fitting room may be needed. Additional fitting rooms may not all need fitting tables, especially if a large portion of the expected clientele will be for mastectomy or elastic hosiery fittings.

Conveniently near the fitting room should be the orthopedic inventory. It depends on the volume of sales, types and number of physicians prescribing appliances and extent of the pharmacy's promotion. An estimate of the required initial stock space is about 30 to 40 ft^2. Also near the fitting room should be a sink with disposable paper toweling for use by the pharmacist before and after each fitting. Where ostomy fittings are concerned, it is advisable to have such a sink inside the fitting room.

Fitting orthopedic, mastectomy and ostomy appliances is a professional service. While it is advisable to have a trained woman to fit women, with the exception of mastectomies and ostomies, the fitting of both sexes can be done by men or women. Male pharmacists fitting appliances today in a proper environment almost never experience a complaint or unpleasant occurrence with female patients. With the exception of truss-fitting, a female pharmacist should be equally comfortable fitting most surgical appliances on male patients.

Each pharmacy should keep a service record for each patient, with data on physician's instructions, appliances fitted and any reorders.

What to Stock

There are perhaps as many opinions as to which items should be represented within the pharmacy's surgical supplies and convalescent aids department as there are pharmacies, manufacturers and wholesale distributors with experience in this field. Pharmacies differ, one from the other, in a multitude of ways. They face different limitations with regard to the available space within their pharmacies for the establishment of health-accessories departments. Their financial resources are different. The markets they purport to serve are different, both with respect to size and demographics. With regard to their drawing areas, differences exist due to various, specific economic factors reflecting distinctively different kinds of demand:

In an area with a heavy coal-mining industry, the market demand for respiratory therapy equipment might be very high relative to that in a rural farming community.

The extent to which hospital outpatient departments and home-care-oriented health agencies provide the thrust for a viable home health-care market within the community is vastly different from one town to another.

Different pharmacies in different communities face widely divergent forms of competition, both in degree and kind.

All these considerations affect different pharmacies differently. Each pharmacist who contemplates the development of a surgical supplies and convalescent aids department must take these considerations into account when making decisions about what to stock. These are the issues which ultimately determine the optimum variety and depth of in-stock inventory for any given pharmacy.

The pharmacist must first decide which type or types of health accessories he wants to specialize in handling. If he wants to start with durable medical equipment such as canes, crutches, walkers, wheelchairs, commodes and hospital beds, he should contact manufacturers of that type of equipment for advice on which products to stock. The same would be true for ostomy, urological and incontinence supplies. Before opening a department for either orthopedic or mastectomy fitting, it would be necessary to attend a manufacturer's or wholesaler's school to obtain proper instruction. The manufacturer or wholesaler again would be a valuable source of information to assist in selecting those products best suited to an individual pharmacy. Before establishing a comprehensive respiratory-services department, it would be advisable to affiliate with a respiratory therapist who could assist in dealing with manufacturers in selecting the products most suited to a particular market area.

In many pharmacies it is the actual experience of having capital tied up in inventory that does not turn over that has led many owners to the unfortunate practice of choosing a stocking inventory for health-accessories departments solely on the basis of the kind and number of requests received for various types of medical equipment in the past.

Thus begins a vicious circle. The pharmacist has no calls for specialized kinds of wheelchairs, for example; therefore he stocks only four or five basic wheelchair types. Then, when someone comes into the pharmacy for a wheelchair, because of a lack of wheelchair expertise and because more specialized types of wheelchairs are not immediately available, he buys one of the wheelchairs that happens to be in stock. Sometime in the future, if that person visits his physician or physical therapist, he reports, often without realizing it, that the pharmacy was unable to meet his wheel chair needs. The result is that the physician or therapist will not send patients to the pharmacy for further wheelchair fittings.

From then on, the only persons who come to the pharmacy for wheelchairs are those who are either that pharmacy's regular customers or those who are largely uncounseled and self-initiate their visits to the pharmacy. And so, based on his past experience of not having had calls for specialized types of wheelchairs, the pharmacist concludes there is not much demand for them.

Without question, the pharmacist who is interested in developing a successful surgical supplies and convalescent aids department within his pharmacy faces a very serious dilemma. Either he plays it safe, and continues to stock those things for which he knows he will have calls, or he decides to expand his inventory and his expertise in an effort to become relatively sophisticated and, by so doing, runs the risk of raising his operating costs in an industry about which, at the very least, he is uncertain.

What many pharmacists who are involved successfully in providing a comprehensive health-accessories service are finding is that when they give better service with the more specialized kinds of equipment, they also do better with ordinary kinds of equipment. That is because their pharmacies become recognized as *the* places where patients should be sent for a wheelchair, a walker and other kinds of durable medical equipment and surgical supplies. It is also true that an improvement in health-accessories service tends to boost a pharmacy's prescription volume as well.

In preparation for the development of a list of inventory items for a health-accessories department, the pharmacist should formulate guidelines for himself which incorporate those variables discussed previously regarding space available within the pharmacy for such a department, financial resources, etc. It is also helpful to categorize the kinds of equipment and merchandise he might want to stock, and then rank the various articles within each category as to the relative importance of each in meeting the health needs of his community.

One of the very first things the pharmacist must do is to familiarize himself with the industry's manufacturers and become knowledgeable about the products they manufacture. While his local wholesaler may have many of the items he will need in his health-accessories department, he will have to establish direct-buying relationships in order to be able to obtain the scores of things his wholesaler does not stock. He should begin an alphabetical file of manufacturers' catalogs and price lists, and develop an index which cross-references products with their manufacturers. An index of this type will save hours of time and possible embarrassment before his customers as well by enabling him to go quickly to appropriate information when faced with questions for which he doesn't have ready answers. Questions of this type will come frequently, and the pharmacist will realize it as he becomes aware of how broad this field really is.

A final consideration in deciding what to stock are reimbursement guidelines. Pharmacists used to dealing with prescription drug plans will find reimbursement for durable medical equipment much more complex. Medicare mandates that providers submit a bill (assigned or nonassigned) for purchases made by Medicare beneficiaries. Often this results in the pharmacist/provider also billing a second insurance company for the deductibles or co-pays. It is essential that as the pharmacist expands his practice in health-care accessories, he also keeps informed and up-to-date with government-reimbursement mandates, guidelines and procedures. Regional and national pharmacy association meetings are an excellent place to meet with other pharmacists dealing with health-care accessories.

Promotion

The first form of promotion the pharmacist can use is a well-stocked and attractive floor display (see Figs 51 and 52).

Prior to deciding on other kinds of promotion to undertake, the pharmacist first must determine from where the majority of his health-accessories volume is most likely to come. What pharmacists who are involved successfully in comprehensive surgical supplies and convalescent aids departments are finding is that the greatest share of their surgical business is not done with their regular patrons, but with new ones coming to their pharmacies specifically for medical supplies. There is little doubt that the reason most of these new patrons find their way to these pharmacies is that they were sent there by medical and allied health professionals in their own communities.

Referrals for wheelchairs, walkers, ostomy supplies, breathing equipment and other health accessories come from physicians, hospitals, nursing homes and a wide variety of community health professionals, among whom are therapists (physical, occupational, enterostomal, respiratory), nurses, medical social workers, social service directors, home-care coordinators, visiting nurses and trainers in organized athletics. Physicians in most major specialties will make referrals. It is important that each health professional be approached about *products or services relevant to his or her specific discipline.* Organizations in which these and other health professionals can be found include hospitals and nursing homes, visiting nurse associations, private physical therapy associations, state departments of vocational rehabilitation, insurance companies, athletic departments in schools, commercial and manufacturing plants, rehabilitation centers, home-health agencies, clinics and agencies such as the Easter Seal Society, American Cancer Society, Multiple Sclerosis Association, Muscular Dystrophy Foundation, National Paraplegia Foundation, United Cerebral Palsy, United Ostomy Association and many others. These, then, are the people and the organizations at which the pharmacy's principal promotional programs must be aimed. And while promotion to the general public is still very important, it is crucial that the pharmacist develop effective promotional programs aimed at the professional community.

Because it is quite common for many of these "new" patrons to begin to patronize their "new" pharmacy for other health needs, it is not surprising that the very existence of a

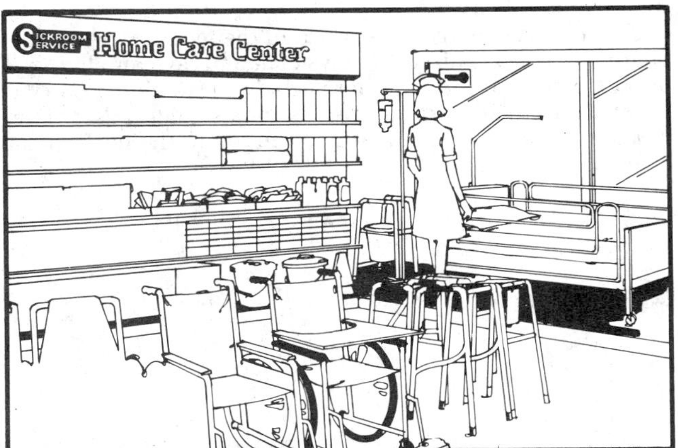

Fig 51. Corner display with window. This arrangement can be extremely beneficial. When placed properly, it is an advertising tool in itself. Its visibility to everyone who walks by, drives past or comes into your store makes this a superb choice.

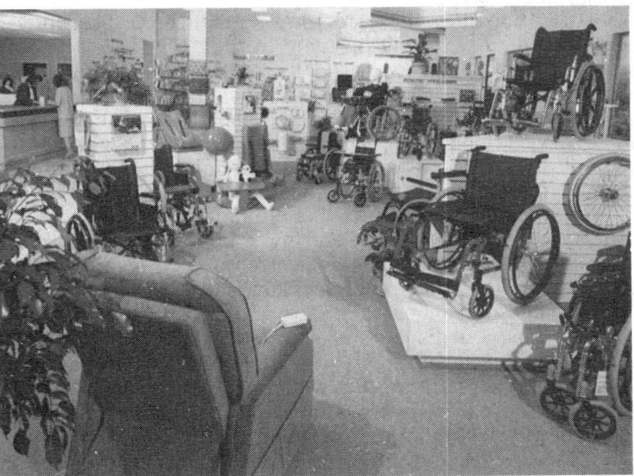

Fig 52. Floor display and wall space. This very common arrangement can be most productive. With the advantage of being able to display all the wheelchairs and walkers open, it gives the consumer a total and comprehensive picture of your home-care department, at once.

comprehensive health-accessories department is regarded by the pharmacies who operate them as an excellent means for promoting the pharmacy as a whole.

Since the largest part of surgical supplies and health accessories volume originates with medical and allied health professionals within the community, the question must be asked: What prompts these professionals to recommend one dealer over another?

Aspects about the retail distribution of medical equipment and supplies, which most concern a community's medical and allied health professionals, are

1. That the supplier have the academic background and practical know-how to recommend the right equipment for each patient need, and be able to show the patient correctly how the equipment should be used.
2. That the supplier not practice medicine, physical therapy, etc, but call on practitioners of these professions for consultation and guidance when appropriate.
3. That the supplier have in stock an adequate inventory, in kind and quantity, to meet the immediate needs of his patients.
4. That the supplier, in addition to having ample stock, have access to wide varieties of medical equipment and supplies from numerous manufacturers, to service the special and unique needs of patients.
5. That the supplier distribute only merchandise of good quality and stand behind what he rents and sells. Many medical professionals are name-brand conscious also.
6. That the supplier have the capability of providing basic maintenance and repair services for what he sells and rents.
7. That the suppliers' equipment be priced competitively in both rentals and sales.
8. That the supplier operate his business in an immaculate, well-organized, efficient and thoroughly professional manner.

Advertising in professional journals, direct-mail campaigns, newspapers and television commercials are all effective and commonly used methods of proclaiming that a pharmacy has the attributes which the professional community expects.

Attending and sponsoring meetings of groups, such as the local ostomy or diabetes assocations, or working with public service groups, such as *Reach to Recovery*, allows the pharmacist to interact with health-care professionals and volunteers who are influential in these areas.

Sending a doctor or other referral source a written "Thank You" for each new referral also helps to remind the doctor of the professional services provided by the pharmacist. Even a simple note stating that a patient was fitted with a particular type of orthopedic support on a certain date as prescribed by the physician may end up in the patient's file where the doctor may see it several times.

One of the most effective ways of promoting a health-accessories department, especially one that features the fitting of orthopedic and mastectomy appliances, is direct physician detailing. Calling on them in their offices is one sure way of promoting your health-accessories department. Even if it is not possible to see the physician each time, contacts with his office personnel, especially a nurse, often can be very effective. Many times the patient will ask the receptionist, while making the next appointment, where they can go for the item just prescribed.

Another effective way to communicate the fact that the pharmacy has the expertise and inventory to meet the community's health-care needs is by a program of regular hospital displays and in-service training classes for the staffs in hospitals and nursing homes.

The "hospital display" is a productive way to meet the physician and have him see the kinds of medical equipment and supplies a pharmacy has available. The hospital display usually runs from about 7:30 am to noon, and is set up in or near the physician's lounge or primary entrance through which they arrive each morning. Permission to set up a display must be obtained well in advance, most often from the hospital administrator, although sometimes from the director of purchasing, the head of central-supply or the manager of the hospital pharmacy. Some hospitals do not allow displays as a general rule, but may permit one to introduce a new service to the community.

There should be plenty of equipment for display, plus a small sign which gives the name of the pharmacy and lists the kinds of articles available. It is also helpful to have business cards and a variety of catalogs handy. Even those physicians who do not stop by to visit will note the availability of a new service and also the variety of equipment supplied. Depending on the size of the hospital, from a half dozen to 70 or more physicians may see the display in the course of the morning—that makes a hospital display worthwhile by any standard.

How better to demonstrate one's expertise in selecting, and when necessary measuring and fitting, health accessories than by providing instruction to groups of health professionals in a hospital or nursing home in the basic principles and proper use of the accessories, particularly those that serve as aids in convalescence or home care of the patient. Thus, for example, the important subject of walking aids—canes, forearm crutches, axillary crutches and walkers—should include a discussion of the physiological factors of ambulation; the selection, measurement and fitting of the devices to provide maximum leverage and comfort and the manner of their use in walking on level areas as well as ascending or descending stairs. Many other subjects can be presented similarly by pharmacists knowledgeable in the use of convalescent aids and other health accessories.

Various equipment manufacturers offer in-service training programs which may be used as a guide to developing training programs for hospitals, nursing homes, visiting nurse associations and schools.

The Future

Increased life expectancy has produced an increase in the number of aged persons and a corresponding increase in the number of ill and infirm persons in this segment of our population. The growing number of aged persons, the trend toward their greater subsidization and the rapid increase in services from home-health-care agencies and hospital-out patient departments portends an ever-increasing number of potential candidates for surgical supplies and convalescent aids in the future. This is also true of many persons who are not aged but still are ill or infirm.

Though nursing homes do care for a substantial number of such patients, more of them want to remain at home and avoid the spiraling costs of institutional care. Hospitals are reluctant to provide services to persons not in need of acute-care facilities, except on an outpatient basis, as it is too costly for both the patient and the hospital. As a result, the trend is to transfer the patient to home care as soon as possible. Encouraged to do so by the principal health-insurance companies such as Blue Cross and by developing home-health-care agencies, the demand for surgical appliances and medical equipment for use in the patient's home is growing daily.

Professional Approach

Not every pharmacist should conclude hastily that he will be successful in this field, regardless of his estimate of the local market, his inventory and his display facilities. Unless the pharmacist is willing to devote time and intelligent effort to the venture, he will fail. He should be interested in helping the aged, the infirm and the sick. His attitude must be professional and his approach to prospective referring physicians and the public must be made on that basis, not on mere availability or price. He must become knowledgeable in the areas of reimbursement and accreditation. Most important, he must have developed the expertise to recommend the right equipment and supplies and instruct his patrons in their proper use.

The pharmacist who seriously is considering developing this specialty will need to expand his reading list of relevant professional journals and periodicals. In addition to the major pharmacy journals, the following publications will broaden his knowledge and perspective concerning convalescent aids and surgical supplies: *Health Industry Today; Ostomy Quarterly; Home Healthcare Business; Medical Products Salesman; Respiratory Therapy; Progress Report, American Physical Therapy Association; American Journal of Occupational Therapy; Homecare* and *HealthWeek.*

The National Association of Retail Druggists (NARD) has created a special division of Home Health Care Pharmacy Services. This division can provide additional information to pharmacists on changes in government programs which affect pharmacists providing home-health-care accessories. A newsletter, the *Home Health Care Pharmacist,* is published monthly. NARD also provides educational programs concerning ostomy, incontinence, wound management, orthotics and prosthetics. A certificate program in orthotics and prosthetics is offered by NARD.

The surgical-supply department of the modern community pharmacy is recognized by physician and layman alike as a proper extension of the pharmacist's professional service. Physicians and allied health professionals quickly assess this new service as an important contribution to the health-team concept.

CHAPTER 108

Surgical Supplies

Barbara Schwartz, PhD
Vice President, New Business Development
Ethicon, Inc
Somerville, NJ 08876

David M Wiseman, PhD
Principal Scientist
Ethicon, Inc
Somerville, NJ 08876

A professional service rendered by many pharmacists consists of supplying surgical instruments, sutures, surgical dressings and other equipment employed by the surgeon prior to, during and after a surgical operation. Some pharmacists, who have obtained the necessary background of information, carry a complete line of such supplies, and even are able to provide operating tables and other heavy equipment.

There are comparatively few such completely equipped pharmacies; the major outlet is through surgical supply houses. Every pharmacist, however, should be familiar with two of the products mentioned above, namely, *Surgical Dressings* and *Sutures*, which are discussed in detail below. The selection of the correct type of surgical dressing or suture is a critical factor in safeguarding the welfare of the patient undergoing surgery. Many items belonging in these categories are handled routinely by the pharmacist and all of these items come within the purview of his professional responsibility.

Surgical Dressings

Definition—*Surgical dressing* is a term applied to a wide range of materials used for the dressing of wounds or injured or diseased tissues. Dressings may serve to

- Provide an environment for moist wound healing. Desiccation of a wound is a major factor in retarding wound healing and increasing scarring. Dressings which prevent desiccation provide an optimal environment for autolysis, cell migration, granulation and re-epithelialization.
- Prevent maceration by permitting evaporation or absorption. In highly exudative wounds, excessive moisture and autolytic enzymes will damage repairing tissue, and will provide a perfect culture medium for microbes.
- Promote hemostasis.
- Protect the wound from further damage (mechanical damage, microbial invasion, dehydration, maceration, chemical damage, alteration in pH).
- Reduce heat loss.
- Control microbial growth (by incorporation of antimicrobial drugs).
- Promote autolysis.
- Promote healing.
- Provide compression, promoting hemostasis and reducing edema.
- Provide support.
- Reduce pain, increase patient comfort and improve functional use of wound site.
- Reduce odor.
- Improve the appearance of the wound site.
- Reduce overall costs associated with wound treatment.

Selection of a Wound Dressing—Dressing selection should be made on the basis of the degree of exudation, presence or likelihood of infection, presence of necrotic tissue and anatomical site. The correct selection of a wound dressing depends not only on the type of wound but on the stage of repair. The use of a wound dressing cannot be considered in isolation, but rather in the context of an integrated wound-care program.

Classification—Functionally, the simplest method of classification uses the terms *primary* and *secondary* dressing. A primary dressing directly contacts the wound. It may provide absorptive capacity and may prevent desiccation, infection and adhesion of the secondary dressing to the wound. A secondary dressing is placed over a primary dressing, providing further protection, absorptive capacity, compression or occlusion. Although some dressings are solely primary or secondary in nature, others have the characteristics of both. The following classification will be made:

- Primary wound dressings
- Primary/secondary wound dressings
- Secondary dressings
  - Absorbents
  - Bandages
  - Adhesive tapes
- Protectives

Within this classification, dressings will be considered on the basis of composition.

Specifications—Surgical dressings and sutures are required to meet specific requirements of the USP for many characteristics. For these specific requirements and the performance of several of the official tests, eg, *Absorbency test* and *Fiber length* of cotton, *Diameter* of sutures and *Tensile strength* of sutures, textile fabrics and films. See the detailed instructions provided in the USP.

Primary Wound Dressings

Plain Gauze has been used as a primary dressing, but will stick to all but clean, incised wounds. Although this property has been used to debride exudative, infected and necrotic wounds, this practice may be painful and is often counterproductive, causing the removal of granulation tissue and new epithelium.

Impregnated Gauze is used to reduce its adherence to wounds. Cotton, rayon or cellulose acetate gauze has been impregnated with a variety of substances such as petroleum or paraffin (Aquaphor, (*Beiersdorf*), Vaseline (*Sherwood*), KY jelly (*Johnson & Johnson*), or petrolatum emulsion (Adaptic, *Johnson & Johnson*). Coatings may wear off, allowing epithelial ingrowth and necessitating a dressing change. A secondary dressing should be used with these dressings to prevent desiccation, provide absorbency and prevent the entrance of pathogens. When used with an appropriate secondary dressing, these dressings may be used in heavily exuding wounds.

Film Dressings (transparent film, occlusive or semiocclusive) are films of polyurethane with acrylic or polyether adhesives. In lightly exuding wounds they permit enough evaporation to promote moist wound healing and prevent maceration. Film dressings exclude bacteria from wounds and permit bathing and observation of the wound. Film dressings will adhere well to intact skin and have a low adherence for wound tissue. They should not be used in infected or heavily exuding wounds. Although some film dressings are permeable to oxygen, this is probably of little consequence to the performance of the dressing.

Film dressings may wrinkle, forming channels for microbial entrance. Difficulty in handling film dressings has been overcome by special design of various application systems. In addition to their use as wound dressings, adhesive films have been used to protect areas vulnerable to pressure, friction or shear ulceration, or for infusion or cannulation sites. Examples of transparent film dressings are Bioclusive (R) Transparent Dressing (*Johnson & Johnson*), Opsite (*Smith & Nephew*) and Tegaderm (*3M*).

Primary/Secondary Wound Dressings

Composite Dressings have primary and secondary components which prevent adherence to the wound with some degree of absorbency. The degree of occlusion provided by these dressings varies. Release (*Johnson & Johnson*) and Telfa (*Kendall*) consist of lightly absorbent rayon or cotton pads sandwiched between porous polyethylene films. Several dressings (Nu-Derm, *Johnson & Johnson*) and Lyofoam A (*Acme United*) comprise polyurethane foams with a film backing.

Hydrogels are complex lattices in which the dispersion medium is trapped rather like water in a *molecular* sponge. The *hydrogel* is typically a crosslinked polymer such as polyvinylpyrrolidone, crosslinked polyethylene oxide gel or polyacrylamide. Hydrogels are nonadherent dressings, which through semipermeable film, allow a high rate of evaporation (and cooling) without compromising wound hydration. This makes them useful in burn treatment. Hydrogels are also very useful in hairy areas where entrapment of hair into the dressing would not be traumatic. Examples of hydrogels are Gel-site (*Baxter*), Clearsite (*NDM*), Geliperm (*Geistlich*), Vigilon (*Bard*) and Nu-Gel TM (*Johnson & Johnson*). The latter is held together with a plastic scrim.

Hydrocolloid Dressings combine the benefits of occlusion and absorbency. Hydrocolloids are dispersions of particles around which water molecules and solvated ions form a shell-like structure. Fluid absorption occurs principally by particle swelling and enlargement of this structure. The *hydrocolloid* mass of these dressings consists of gum-like materials such as guar or karaya, sodium carboxymethylcellulose and pectin, bound by an adhesive such as polyisobutylene.

Hydrocolloid dressings display wet track (adhesion to a wet surface) because of particle swelling. This property facilitates atraumatic removal. The dry tack of hydrocolloid dressings is due to an adhesive such as polyisobutylene, which is inactivated by moisture. The dry tack retained by the dressing around the wound preserves the edge seal. Exudate absorption by most hydrocolloid dressings results in the formation of a yellow/brown gelatinous mass which remains on the wound after dressing removal. This may be irrigated from the wound and should not be confused with pus.

Because hydrocolloids absorb water slowly, they are of little use on acutely exuding wounds. They are, however, very useful for moderately to highly exudative chronic wounds. Examples of hydrocolloid dressings include Duoderm (*Convatec*) and Comfeel Ulcus (*Coloplast*).

Calcium Alginate Dressings—Alginic acid is a naturally occurring polysaccharide derived from brown seaweeds. As the calcium salt, these fibrous nonwoven dressings are highly absorbent and are used on moderately to highly exuding wounds. They may be held in place with gauze tape or a film dressing. They also may be used to pack wounds. Examples of calcium alginate dressings are Sorbsan (*Dow B Hickam*), Algosteril (*Johnson & Johnson*) and Kaltostat (*Calgon Vestal*).

Secondary Wound Dressings

Absorbents

Surgical Cotton—Cotton is the basic surgical absorbent. It is official *Purified Cotton USP*.

Domestic cotton grown in the southern US is suitable for surgical purposes. The domestic cotton plant reaches a height of from 2 to 4 ft. Growing from the seeds is a pod or boll which bursts open upon ripening, exposing a mass of white cotton fibers. Each of these fibers is a minute, hair-like tube, the outer wall being pure cellulose, the opening filled with plant fluids. When the boll bursts open, the fiber collapses into a flat ribbon-like form, twisted and doubled upon itself more than 100 times from end to end.

The raw cotton fiber, mechanically cleaned of dirt and carded into layers, but not otherwise treated, has a limited use for paddings and coverings of unbroken surfaces. This form is supplied under the name of *nonabsorbent cotton*. It also is used frequently as cotton plugs in the bacteriological laboratory because of its nonabsorbency.

Absorbent Cotton is prepared from the raw fiber by a series of processes which remove the natural waxes and all impurities and foreign substances and render the fibers absorbent. It is a practically pure, white cellulose fiber.

Besides the familiar roll form, Purified Cotton may be obtained in various prepared forms such as cotton balls, cotton-tipped applicators, etc.

Absorbent balls made of a uniform surgical viscose-rayon fiber also are available. These absorb fluids faster and retain their shape better than cotton balls.

Nonabsorbent Bleached Cotton, prepared by a modified bleaching process, wherein the water-repellent natural oils and waxes are retained, also is available. This cotton is easily identified by its silky feel. Because it is repellent to water, it does not become matted or inelastic. Consequently, it is well-adapted to packing, padding and cushioning of dressings over traumatized areas and as nonabsorbent backing on sanitary napkins, combines and drainage dressings.

Rayon, or regenerated cellulose, is made from wood or cotton linters. After dissolving it in a mixture of alkali and carbon disulfide, cellulose thread is reprecipitated in an acid-coagulating bath by passage through fine holes in a metal plate. Because plant lignins have been removed, as well as the more circular cross section, rayon fibers are softer and more lustrous than cotton.

Surgical Gauzes—The function of surgical gauze is to provide an absorbent material of sufficient tensile strength for surgical dressings. It is known as *Absorbent Gauze USP*.

In the process of making surgical gauze, the raw cotton fiber is cleaned mechanically and then spun or twisted into a thread, and the thread, in turn, woven into an open-mesh cloth which is gray in appearance and nonabsorbent. It is bleached white and rendered absorbent by much the same processes as those used in the preparation of surgical cotton.

The gauze thus treated is dried by passing a continuous length through a tentering machine. Tenterhooks straighten, stretch and hold it taut as it is dried. When it leaves this apparatus, the dried gauze is cut into lengths, folded, rolled and packaged.

Gauze is classified according to its mesh or number of threads per inch. Some types of surgical dressing require a close-meshed gauze for extra strength and greater protection, while other uses such as primary wound dressings, absorbent secondary dressings and larger dressings to absorb purulent matter or other drainage require softer, more absorbent gauzes, having a more open structure.

Various forms of pads, compresses and dressings are made from surgical gauze, alone or in conjunction with absorbent cotton, tissue paper and other materials.

Filmated Gauze is a folded absorbent gauze with a thin, even film of cotton or rayon distributed over each layer. This filmation fluffs up and gives ample dressing volume, yet costs less than gauze alone of equivalent volume. It possesses quick absorption and unusual softness.

Nonwoven Surgical Sponges—During the past decade, non-woven fabrics have been developed which are suitable alternatives to woven cotton gauze for use in wound cleaning, wound dressing and tissue-handling sponges. These non-woven fabrics depend on dense entanglement of their synthetic fibers (Dacron, Rayon, etc) to provide the fabric with an acceptable tensile strength approaching that of woven cotton gauze. They typically offer greater absorbent capacity than cotton gauze sponges of comparable bulk while generating less lint. Specialty versions of the nonwoven sponges are available prefenestrated for IV tubing or drain-dressing procedures. One manufacturer (*Johnson & Johnson*) provides both a nonwoven sponge for wound dressing (Sof-Wick; very soft texture, very absorbent) and a nonwoven general-purpose cleansing/prep sponge (Nu Gauze; gauze-like texture, more absorbent than gauze).

Antiseptic or *Medicated Surgical Gauze* originated in the Listerian era of surgery, and it is still used to some extent but, with the advent of antibiotics and other therapeutic agents, its popularity is decreasing. Most commonly used is iodoform gauze, which contains 5% iodoform and is used largely as a packing or drainage material. The so-called *Penrose drain*, commonly used for draining surgical wounds, is made by drawing a piece of plain or iodoform gauze through a thin-walled tube of latex and cutting to the desired length.

Selvage-Edge Gauze Strips in widths of ¼ to 2-inch are designed specially and woven for use both as packing strips in surgery of the nose and sinuses, nasal hemostasis, etc, and as drainage wicks in the treatment of boils, abscesses, fistulas and other draining wounds. The ravelproof, selvage edges on both sides eliminate all loose threads. These gauzes are available unmedicated or medicated with 5% iodoform. These strips are obtainable in sterile form packed in sealed glass jars. Nu Gauze Packing Strips are packaged in polystyrene containers.

Gauze Pads or *Sponges* are folded squares of surgical gauze. These are so folded that no cut gauze edges or loose threads are exposed. This prevents loose fibers from entering the wound. The pads are folded such that each size may be unfolded to larger sizes without exposing cut edges or loose threads.

Sterilized packages of these frequently used all-gauze sponges are available in tamperproof packages. Such sterile units particularly are well-suited to the numerous tray sets prepared in hospitals.

X-ray Detectable Gauze Pads are similar to all-gauze pads but contain inserts treated with barium sulfate. They are nontoxic, soft and nonabrasive. They remain permanently detectable because they neither deteriorate in the body nor are they affected by either sterilization or time. Ray-Tec X-Ray Detectable Sponges (*Johnson & Johnson*) contain a nonabrasive vinyl plastic monofilament which gives a characteristic pattern in the X-ray.

Composite absorbent dressings have been developed for specific purposes. They usually consist of layers of absorbent gauze or nonwoven fabric with fillers of cotton, rayon, nonwoven fabric or tissue paper in suitable arrangements. Composite sponges have gauze or nonwoven fabric surfaces with fillers of cotton, rayon, nonwoven fabric or absorbent tissue.

Dressing Combines are designed to provide warmth and protection and to absorb large quantities of fluid that may drain from an incision or wound. Each combine consists of a nonwoven fabric cover enclosing fiber with or without absorbent tissue. They also may incorporate a nonabsorbent layer of cotton, tissue or plastic film to prevent fluid from coming through to soil liners and bedding, though some combined dressings are entirely absorbent.

Laparotomy Sponges, also known as *Abdominal Packs, Tape Pads* or *Packs, Walling-Off Mops, Stitched Pads, Quilted Pads, Gauze Mops,* etc, are used to form a nonabrasive wall that will prevent abdominal or other organs from escaping into the field of operation and to help maintain body temperature during exposure. They are made of four layers of 28- x 24-mesh gauze. The edges are folded in and hemmed. The entire pack is cross-stitched and a looped tape ½-inch wide and 20-inch long is attached to one corner. A desirable feature of one type is an X-ray-detectable insert, so firmly incorporated into the gauze that it cannot become detached. Treated with barium sulfate, the monofilament is nontoxic and, were it to be left inadvertently *in situ*, would cause no more foreign-body reaction than an ordinary dressing.

Sanitary Napkins, intended for special hospital use, otherwise known as *V-Pads, Obstetrical (OB) Pads, Perineal Pads, Maternity Pads,* etc, are used in obstetrical, gynecological or maternity cases. Napkins which have repellent tissue on the side and back surfaces of the napkin usually are preferred because of their greater fluid-holding capacity. Sanitary napkins generally come with two sizes of filler, 3 x 9 or 3 x 11-inch. The napkin cover generally is made from a nonwoven fabric or a nonwoven fabric supported with an open-mesh scrim. Packaged, sterilized napkins are available and used generally to reduce cross-contamination possibilities.

Disposable Cleaners made from various types of nonwoven fabrics are available. They generally offer advantages over paper of wet strength and abrasion resistance, plus having better cleaning ability. Their advantages over cloth are reduced laundry expense and cross-contamination possibilities.

Eye Pads are scientifically shaped to fit comfortably and cover the eye completely thus protecting the eyebrow when taped. These pads are made using nonwoven fabric. Two sides are enclosed to prevent the cotton from escaping and the pad from distorting. Where desired, the pad may be folded and used as a pressure dressing. Eye pads especially are useful in the outpatient clinic of the hospital, the industrial medical department and the physician's office. They are sealed in individual sterile envelopes.

Nursing Pads are designed in a contour shape to fit comfortably under the nursing brassiere or breast binder.

Disposable Underpads are used for incontinent, maternity and other patients with severe drainage. Such pads cost less than the average hospital-made product and provide a neat, clean, easy-to-handle pad that is changed quickly and easily disposed. Disposable briefs are available (*Johnson & Johnson*).

Cotton-Tipped Applicators are used to apply medications or cleanse an area. Machine-made cotton-tipped applicators are uniform in size, resulting in no waste of cotton or medications. The cotton is attached firmly to the stick and may be sterilized readily without affecting the anchorage of the cotton. They are available in 3 or 6 inch lengths.

Bandages

The function of bandages is to hold dressings in place by providing pressure or support. They may be inelastic, elastic or become rigid after shaping for immobilization.

Common Gauze Roller Bandage is listed in the USP as a form in which *Absorbent Gauze* may be provided. It is prepared from *Type I Absorbent Gauze* in various widths and lengths. Each bandage is in one continuous piece, tightly rolled and substantially free from loose threads and ravelings.

Muslin Bandage Rolls are made of heavier unbleached material (56 x 60 mesh). They are supplied in the same widths as the regular gauze bandage. Muslin bandages are very strong and are used wherever gauze bandages do not provide sufficient strength or support. They frequently are used to hold splints or bulky compression dressings in place.

Elastic Bandages are made in several types:

1. **Woven Elastic Bandage** is made of heavy elastic webbing containing rubber threads. Good support and pressure are provided by this type of rubber elastic bandage.
2. **Crepe Bandage** is elastic, but contains no rubber. Its elasticity is due to a special weave that allows it to stretch to practically twice its

length, even after repeated launderings. This elasticity makes it especially serviceable in bandaging varicose veins, sprains, etc, because it conforms closely to the skin or joint surfaces, lies flat and secure, yet allows limited motion and stretches in case of swelling so that circulation is not impaired.

3. **Conforming Bandage** is a new type of readily conforming bandage made from two plies of specially processed, high-quality, 14 x 8 inch cotton gauze folded to the center. This type is much easier to use and apply than ordinary roller bandage since it tends to cling to itself during application, thus preventing slipping. It readily conforms to all body contours without the necessity of "reversing" or twisting. A further advantage is the fact that there can be no rough or frayed edge. Kling Conforming Gauze Bandage (*Johnson & Johnson*) is available in a variety of sizes up to 6 inches wide. This Gauze is used widely to hold dressings or splints firmly in place and occasionally as a primary dressing when sticking to the wound is not a problem. A mercerized cotton Conforming Gauze Bandage clings to itself and thus remains in place better than gauze made of other materials.

4. **High-Bulk Bandage** is made of multiple layers (typically six) of crimped cotton gauze. The high bulk of this bandage type is designed to provide padding protection in wound dressing applications. It also provides the absorbent capacity of a cotton dressing component. One version (Sof-Band High Bulk, *Johnson & Johnson*) is made of mercerized cotton to help the bandage cling to itself, which facilitates application and improves dressing stability.

Triangular Bandages usually are made by cutting a square of bleached muslin diagonally from corner to corner, forming two right triangles of equal size and shape. The length of the base is approximately 54 inches. These bandages were brought into prominence by Esmarch and still bear his name. They are used in first-aid work for head dressings, binders, arm slings and as temporary splints for broken bones.

Orthopedic Bandages are used to provide immobilization and support in the treatment of broken bones and in certain conditions of bones and joints. Plaster of Paris-impregnated gauze has been the standard material for this purpose. More recently introduced are synthetic cast materials made of polyester cotton or fiberglass. Various types of plastic sheets also are offered which can be shaped easily and harden to a rigid form by cooling or chemical reaction. These are useful chiefly for splints and corrective braces.

Individually packaged plaster of Paris bandages and splints are available in a wide variety of sizes. The Specialist brand (*Johnson & Johnson*) is made from specially treated plaster, uniformly spread and firmly bonded to the fabric. This results in a high strength-to-weight ratio in casts made from such bandages. Synthetic casts are applied like plaster of Paris. The Delta-Lite Synthetic Casting System (*Johnson & Johnson*) offers both polyester and fiberglass casting materials. The casts are water-resistant, light weight and durable.

Orthoflex Elastic Plaster Bandages (*Johnson & Johnson*) are plaster of Paris bandages containing elastic threads in the fabric and are intended for specialized prosthetic uses.

Stockinette Bandages are made of stockinette material knitted or woven in tubular form without seams. Surgical stockinette is unbleached. Because it is soft and will stretch readily to conform comfortably to the arm, leg or body, it is used to cover the skin prior to the application of a plaster of Paris or synthetic cast.

Cast Paddings are soft, absorbent, protective paddings, applied like a bandage to the areas affected before application of a cast. They are composed of various fiber constructions which conform and cling, absorb moisture and allow the skin to breathe.

Adhesive Tapes

Surgical adhesive tapes are made in many different forms, varying both in the type of backing and in the formulation of the adhesive mass according to specific needs and requirements. The tapes available today may be divided into two broad categories: those with a rubber-based adhesive and those with an acrylate adhesive. Both types have a variety of uses. Where strength of backing, superior adhesion and economy are required (eg, athletic strapping), rubber adhesives commonly are used. Acrylate adhesives on a variety of backing materials are used widely in surgical dressing applications, where reduced skin trauma is required, as in operative and postoperative procedures; they are supplied in various strength and adhesion levels.

Acrylate Adhesives—Acrylate adhesives on a nonwoven or fabric backing have been accepted widely for use as surgical tapes, owing largely to what may be termed their hypoallergenic nature. Because acrylate adhesives are basically a unipolymeric system, they eliminate the use of a large number of components in rubber-based adhesives. In poly(alkyl- acrylate) adhesives, the desired balance between adhesion, cohesion and flow properties is determined by the choice of monomers and the control of the polymerization reactions. Once the polymer is made, no other formulating or compounding is needed. In addition, the acrylics have an excellent shelf-life because they are not affected readily by heat, light or air, factors which tend to degrade rubber-based adhesives.

Acrylate adhesives combine the proper balance of tack and long-term adhesion. Their molecular structure permits the passage of water vapor so they are nonocclusive, and thus, when coated on a porous backing material, do not cause overhydration in the stratum corneum. Traumatic response to surgical tapes is minimized substantially when tapes are constructed to allow normal skin moisture to pass through adhesive and backing material. With this construction, the moisture content and strength of the horny cell layers remain relatively normal. When a porous tape is removed, the planes of separation develop near the surface of the stratum corneum, in the region of the naturally desquamating cells. This allows for repeated use of tape over the same site with minimal damage to the skin.

Hypoallergenic Surgical Tapes with acrylate adhesive are available with a variety of porous backing materials. Rayon taffeta cloth backing provides a high-strength tape well-suited for affixing heavy dressings. Lighter dressing applications can be accomplished with lower strength, economical paper-backed surgical tapes. A knitted backing tape (Dermiform, *Johnson & Johnson*) provides some of the economies of paper surgical tape with the strength and conformability of a cloth backing. Other tapes feature elastic cloth or foam backing materials for special taping needs.

Rubber-Based Adhesives—A second group of surgical adhesive tapes is the cloth-backed and plastic-backed rubber adhesives. These are used principally where heavy support and a high level of adhesion are required. Modern rubber-based adhesive tape masses consist of varying mixtures of several classes of substances and are composed of an elastomer (para or pale crepe rubber in the case of natural rubber tapes, and synthetic elastomers made from polymers of isobutylene, alkylacrylate or similar materials), one of several types of rosin or modified rosin, antioxidants, plasticizers and fillers and coloring agents to give the tape the desired tint or whiteness.

Adhesive Tape Reactions—While skin reactions formerly were accepted by the medical profession as almost predictable sequelae to the use of adhesive tape, with better understanding of the mechanisms of such reactions and progress in research and technology, the long-sought-for objective of hyporeactivity has, in large degree, been attained.

Because adhesive tape masses historically have consisted of heterogeneous and complex mixtures of organic compounds, it is not surprising that many workers have ascribed adhesive tape reaction to allergy. More recent work, however, has shown that a true allergic response to the modern adhesive tape mass, or to its components, is a factor in only a small proportion of clinical reactions, and that the majority of observed reactions are ascribed properly to other factors, mainly mechanical irritation and, to a lesser degree, chemical irritation. There apparently is no significant difference in reaction between patients with or without a history of allergy, but true specific dermatitis may occur more readily in persons who have manifested some other form of contact dermatitis.

Adverse manifestations produced by adhesive tape are characterized by erythema, edema, papules, vesicles and, in severe cases, desquamation. Itching may be intense, or it may be absent. The reaction may be demonstrated readily by patch-testing, and usually manifests itself early—within 24 to 48 hours. Characteristically, the reaction becomes more severe the longer the tape is left in place and continues to increase in intensity for some time after the tape is removed. This type of reaction is long-lasting and requires days for its complete subsidence.

Two distinct types of irritation can result from the mechanical dynamics of removing tape from the skin. One response—induced vasodilatation—is a relatively nontraumatic, transitory effect in which no actual damage to the skin occurs. A second type—skin stripping—is a traumatic response in which skin is removed with the tape and actual damage to the epidermal layers results. Such mechanical skin removal is possibly the dominant cause of clinical reactions seen with the use of adhesive tape.

Chemical irritation from adhesive tape results when irritating components in the mass or backing of the tape permeate the underlying tissues of the skin. The tape construction can influence the reactivity of such ingredients substantially. For example, many compounds that normally do not penetrate intact stratum corneum can penetrate overhydrated corneum.

When portions of the stratum corneum are removed, the barrier capacity of the skin is damaged substantially. In this situation, any irritating components of the tape have ready access to underlying tissues. These substances then can cause a degree of irritation that is far greater than would be observed on intact skin.

Protectives

Until recently, protectives included only the various impermeable materials intended to be used adjunctively with other dressing components to prevent the loss of moisture or heat from a wound site or to protect clothing or bed liners from wound exudate. Film dressings are excellent devices to protect against infection and dislodgement of vascular cannulae and drainage sites. In addition, they may be used to protect vulnerable areas against pressure sores.

Protectives also are employed to cover wet dressings and hot or cold compresses. In common use as protectives are plastic sheeting and waxed or plastic-coated paper. These prevent the escape of moisture or heat from the dressing or the compress and to protect clothing or bed linens. Rubber sheeting is a rubber-coated cloth, waterproof and flexible, in various lengths and widths for use as a covering for bedding. A so-called "nursery sheeting" is supplied, coated only on one side.

Products for Adhesion Prevention—Adhesions are abnormal connections between organs or tissues that form after trauma, including surgery. They are comprised of fibrovascular scar tissue and complicate all areas of surgery. In gynecological surgery, adhesions may result in infertility and pelvic pain; in intestinal surgery they may result in intestinal obstruction; in cardiac surgery they may render a second sternotomy hazardous and in tendon surgery they will prevent mobility.

Although careful tissue handling and good hemostasis may reduce adhesion formation, there are few proven entities designed for the prevention of adhesions. Interceed Absorbable Adhesion Barrier (Ethicon) is a knitted fabric of oxidized regenerated cellulose which is placed at a site where adhesions are suspected to occur. It swells and gels to form a barrier between two adjacent surfaces, allowing remesothelialization to take place. The fabric then degrades grossly by about 14 days and microscopically by about 28 days. Interceed Barrier is indicated for reducing the incidence of adhesions in pelvic gynecologic surgery.

Operating Room Supplies

Hemostatic Products accelerate hemostasis by providing a thrombogenic surface which promotes platelet aggregation and fibrin polymerization. These include collagen sponges and powder (Instat, *Johnson & Johnson*; Avitene, *Alcon*), gelatin sponge (Gelfoam, *Upjohn*); oxidized cellulose (Oxycel, *Deseret Medical*) and Oxidized Regenerated Cellulose USP (Surgicel, *Johnson & Johnson*). Both oxidized cellulose and oxidized regenerated cellulose are agents whose actions depend on the formation of a coagulum consisting of salts of polyanhydroglucuronic acid and hemoglobin. When applied to a bleeding surface, they swell to form a brown gelatinous mass that is absorbed gradually by the tissues, usually within 7 to 14 days. They are employed in surgery for the control of moderate bleeding where suturing or ligation is impractical or ineffective.

Thrombin (USP) solutions of bovine origin promote hemostasis by catalyzing the conversion of fibrinogen to fibrin. They may be used in conjunction with fibrinogen concentrates prepared from autologous cryoprecipitate or from pooled donor blood.

Disposable Sterile OR and OB Packs are prepared, packaged and sterilized assemblies of diapering and gown units, designed to fulfill the operating and delivery room needs. They eliminate the problems of laundering, storage, assembly and sterilization of muslin drapes and gowns. They introduce many special materials with particular properties of porosity, repellency to water, alcohol, blood and other fluids, abrasion resistance and other desirable attributes.

Double packages of contamination-resistant paper have been developed to permit opening and use without compromising sterility. Retention of sterile characteristics until used, eliminates the need for resterilization.

Face masks for use in the operating room and where contamination must be controlled generally are made of plied, fine-mesh gauze, shaped to cover the nose, mouth and chin. They are laundered and autoclaved. Disposable face masks with special filtration material giving high retention of particulate matter, and designed for more effective fitting, are available from several manufacturers. Surgine Face Mask (*Johnson & Johnson*) claims a 94% filtration efficiency with high user comfort.

Surgical Dressing Monographs

Adhesive Bandage

Adhesive Absorbent Compress; Adhesive Absorbent Gauze.

A compress of four layers of Type I absorbent gauze, or other suitable material, affixed to a film or fabric coated with a pressure-sensitive adhesive substance. It is sterile. The compress may contain a suitable antimicrobial agent and may contain one or more suitable colors. The adhesive surface is protected by a suitable removable covering.

Description—The compress is substantially free from loose threads or ravelings; the adhesive strip may be perforated, and the back may be coated with a water-repellent film.

Gauze Bandage

Type I absorbent gauze; contains no dye or other additives.

Description—One continuous piece, tightly rolled, in various widths and lengths and substantially free from loose threads and ravelings.

Oxidized Cellulose

Absorbable Cellulose; Absorbable Cotton; Cellulosic Acid; Hemo-Pak (*Johnson & Johnson*); Oxycel (*Deseret Medical*)

Sterile gauze or cotton which has been oxidized chemically to make it both hemostatic and absorbable; contains 16–24% of carboxyl (COOH) groups.

Description—In the form of gauze or lint. Is slightly off-white in color, is acid to the taste and has a slight, charred odor.

Solubility—Insoluble in water or acids; soluble in dilute alkalies.

Uses—The value of oxidized cellulose in various surgical procedures is based upon its properties of absorbability when buried in tissues and its remarkable hemostatic effect. Absorption occurs between the second and seventh day following implantation of the dry material, depending on the adequacy of the blood supplied to the area and the degree of chemical degradation of the implanted material. Complete absorption of large amounts of blood-soaked gauze may take 6 weeks or longer and serious surgical complications, and cyst formation has been reported as the result of failure to absorb. Hemostasis depends upon the marked affinity of *cellulosic acid* for hemoglobin. When exposed to blood, either *in vitro* or in surgical conditions, the oxidized gauze or cotton turns very dark brown or black and forms a soft gelatinous mass which readily molds itself to the contours of irregular surfaces and controls surgical hemorrhage by providing an artificially induced clot. Pressure should be exerted on the gauze or cotton for about 2 min in order to facilitate the sealing off of the stomata of the bleeding vessels.

Two factors require emphasis: (1) cellulosic acid does not enter the physiological clotting mechanism *per se* but forms what might be termed an "artificial clot," as described and, therefore, is effective in controlling the bleeding hemophiliac, and (2) the hemostatic action of cellulosic acid is not enhanced by the addition of other hemostatic agents, such as thrombin (which in any case would be destroyed by the pH of the gauze unless some means of neutralization were practicable). The hemostatic effect of either one alone is greater than the combination.

It is useful as a temporary packing for the control of capillary, venous or small arterial *hemorrhage*, but since it inhibits epithelialization, it should be used only for the immediate control of hemorrhage and not as a surface dressing. A purer and more uniform product prepared from oxidized regenerated cellulose has been developed and is available as Surgicel Absorbable Hemostat. This offers many advantages over the older, less-uniform oxidized cellulose derived from cotton and, because of its chemical uniformity, assures dependable performance and overcomes many of the difficulties encountered with the older type of cotton product. The knitted fabric strips do not fragment, may be sutured in place easily if necessary and provide prompt and complete absorption with minimum tissue reaction.

Application—*Topical*, as necessary, to control hemorrhage.

Forms Available—Sterile Pads; Sterile Pledgets; Sterile Strips.

Oxidized Regenerated Cellulose

Surgicel; Surgicel Nu-Knit (*Johnson & Johnson*)

Contains 18–24% of carboxyl groups (COOH), calculated on the dried basis. It is sterile.

Preparation—Cellulose is dissolved and regenerated by a process similar to the manufacture of rayon,which is then oxidized.

Description—Creamy white gauze, lint or woven material.

Solubility—Insoluble in water; soluble in alkali hydroxides.

Uses—Absorbable hemostatic.

Purified Cotton

Gossypium Purificatum; Absorbent Cotton

The hair of the seed of cultivated varieties of *Gossypium hirsutum* Linné or of other species of *Gossypium* (Fam *Malvaceae)*, freed from adhering impurities, deprived of fatty matter, bleached and sterilized in its final container.

Description—White, soft, fine, filament-like hairs appearing under the microscope as hollow, flattened and twisted bands, striate and slightly thickened at the edges; practically odorless and practically tasteless.

Solubility—Insoluble in ordinary solvents; soluble in ammoniated cupric oxide TS.

Dextranomer

Debrisan (*Johnson & Johnson*)

Dextranomer is a three-dimensional cross-linked dextran polymer prepared by interaction of dextran with epichlorohydrin.

Description—White, spherical beads, 0.1 to 0.3 mm in diameter; hydrophilic. Also available, dispersed in polyethylene glycol, as a paste.

Solubility—Insoluble in water or alcohol. Each g absorbs about 4 mL of aqueous fluid, the beads swelling and forming a gel.

Uses—Topically to cleanse secreting lesions such as venous stasis ulcers, decubitus ulcers, infected traumatic and surgical wounds and infected burns. It absorbs the exudates, including the components that tend to impede tissue repair, and thereby retards eschar formation and keeps lesions soft and pliable.

Application—A sufficient amount is applied to cover the cleansed lesion (⅛ to ¼ inch) and a bandage is applied lightly to keep the beads in place. When saturated with exudate the beads become greyish-yellow, and should be removed by irrigation with water, saline solution or other cleansing solution. The dressings usually are changed once or twice a day, but 3 or 4 changes may be required if draining is profuse.

Packaging—Sterile beads, in containers of 60 and 120 g, and in 4-g packets.

Absorbable Dusting Powder

Starch-derivative Dusting Powder

An absorbable powder prepared by processing cornstarch and intended for use as a lubricant for surgical gloves; contains not more than 2% of magnesium oxide.

Description—White, odorless powder; pH (1 in 10 suspension) between 10 and 10.8.

Absorbent Gauze

Carbasus Absorbens; Gauze

Cotton, or a mixture of cotton and not more than 53.0%, by weight, of purified rayon, in the form of a plain woven cloth. If rendered sterile, it is packaged to protect it from contamination.

Description—White cotton cloth of various thread counts and weights; may be supplied in various lengths and widths, and in the form of rolls or folds.

Purified Rayon

A fibrous form of bleached, regenerated cellulose. It may contain not more than 1.25% of titanium dioxide.

Preparation—By the viscose rayon process.

Description—White, lustrous or dull, fine, soft, filamentous fibers, appearing under the microscope as round, oval or slightly flattened, translucent rods, straight or crimped, striate and with serrate cross-sectional edges; practically odorless and practically tasteless.

Solubility—Very soluble in ammoniated cupric oxide TS or dilute H_2SO_4 (3 in 5); insoluble in ordinary solvents.

Uses—Hemostatic.

Adhesive Tape

Sterile Adhesive Tape

Fabric and/or film evenly coated on one side with a pressure- sensitive, adhesive mixture. If rendered sterile, it is protected from contamination by appropriate packaging.

Sutures and Suture Materials

A surgical suture is a strand or fiber used to hold wound edges in apposition during healing, and the process of applying such a strand is called *suturing*. When such material, without a needle, is used to stop bleeding by tying off severed blood vessels, the strand is called a *ligature*, and the process is known as *ligating*. Suture materials, however, have uses beyond those involved in the repair of wounds in that they are often used in reconstructive procedures.

Surgical sutures were first listed in the second supplement of USP XI in a monograph on catgut sutures, which then were designated officially as *Surgical Gut*. USP XII carried a similar monograph on surgical silk. USP XVI contained, in addition to surgical gut, a generalized monograph designed to cover all sutures in addition to catgut, and this is also true of USP XX. USP XXII additionally describes synthetic absorbable sutures.

At one time or another, nearly every form of fibrous material or wire that offered any promise at all has been used as a suture and, indeed, many materials which, by present standards, offer no promise at all, have been evaluated.

Cotton and linen were among the earliest suture materials, but the use of animal intestines and sinews also claims great antiquity. As in many other fields of science, there have been fads, and numerous materials have enjoyed varying favor through the centuries. Frequently, the acceptance of a given suture material depended on its successful use by an eminent surgeon whose authority encouraged emulation and, in many cases, there appeared to be legitimate scientific justification for such use.

Possibly the most important factor in the acceptance of suture materials has been their characteristics in the presence of infection. As knowledge of bacteriology increased and methods of sterilization improved, the earlier disadvantages of certain sutures have been overcome, so that currently a wide variety of surgical suture materials may be sterilized conveniently and effectively.

Among the widely accepted methods for the sterilization of sutures are: autoclave sterilization with free access of water vapor, applicable only for those sutures which are not harmed by this process; dry heat at 310°F; ethylene oxide and irradiation sterilization using either beta or gamma rays. Irradiation sterilization has many advantages over the older methods insofar as commercial production is concerned. The sutures are sterilized in their final sealed packages, eliminating any danger of recontamination. The radiation dose is greater than necessary to kill even the most resistant spore-forming organisms. One great advantage of this method lies in the relative lack of deteriorating effect upon many sutures. Irradiation-sterilized surgical gut is stronger, more pliable and easier to handle than dry-heat-sterilized surgical gut sutures.

Suture materials may be divided into two principal classes: absorbable and nonabsorbable. In the first class are found those materials which are capable of being broken down or digested in animal tissues. Catgut, the classical absorbable suture derived from collagen-rich animal tissue, is proteinaceous in nature and it appears that certain proteolytic enzymes in tissues are responsible for the digestion of catgut and its disappearance from the wound area.

New forms of absorbable sutures based upon synthetic polyesters such as polyglycolic acid, copolymers of lactide and glycolide, polydioxanone and polygluconate have been introduced as alternative absorbable materials.

Absorbable Sutures

Surgical Gut—Catgut probably is still the most widely used suture material and has been of great importance to surgery in general. Its basic constituent is a collagen derived from connective tissue obtained from healthy animals, usually sheep and cattle.

In the older and still widely used method, the catgut is obtained from the submucosal layer of the small intestine of sheep. The intestines from the freshly killed animal are cleaned of their contents and split longitudinally into ribbons. Mechanical processes remove the innermost mucosa and the outer muscularis and serosal layers, essentially leaving only the submucosa. This appears as a thin, strong network consisting chiefly of collagen, whose orientation and strength are increased markedly by subsequent processing. From one to five or six such ribbons are stretched, spun or twisted under tension and dried under tension to form a uniform strand. These strands are polished and cut into appropriate lengths for packaging and sterilization. Intestines from cattle also may be used to prepare catgut but, in this case, it is the serosal layer that is isolated and used.

In another method, collagen sutures are produced from collagen derived from beef tendon. The tendons are suitably treated and dispersed. The dispersed collagen is extruded, precipitated and reconstituted as fine strands which are then twisted, stretched, tanned and otherwise treated to give absorbable sutures with the desired characteristics.

In the US, practically no unsterilized surgical gut is sold, although in certain other countries this is a more common practice.

Diameter and strength requirements for absorbable surgical suture (surgical gut) are specified in the USP, in which will be found descriptions of the suture as well as the apparatus and methods for measuring diameter, tensile strength, sterility and other tests.

Plain and Chromicized Surgical Gut—Two varieties of catgut, as distinguished by their resistance to absorptive action by tissue enzymes, are described in the USP as *Type A*, plain or untreated and *Type C*, medium treatment. The availability of both types reflects the surgeon's requirements for catgut that will retain its tensile strength for varying periods of time, or that will show an increased resistance to the proteolytic substances found in certain body tissues. This is accomplished by the incorporation of chromium salts or other chemicals to prolong its survival in tissues. Such products formerly were designated as 10-, 20- or 40-day catgut, on the assumption that these sutures would remain for such periods in normal tissue. The variations in catgut as a natural product, as well as the variations in patients and in sites of implantations, make such designations qualitative, so that they were replaced by the more general statement of type. While many tests for the expected duration of resistance have been proposed, none is accepted fully as being comparable to digestion in animal tissues, and none has been included in the USP.

Approximately half the surgical gut used in the US has been either chromicized or otherwise treated. Raw catgut is analogous to rawhide, while chromicized catgut is comparable to chrome-tanned leather. The tanning process is applied either to the ribbons before they have been twisted into the strand form or to the finished twisted strand. Treatment in the ribbon form is reported to result in a more uniform deposition of chromium salts throughout the entire cross-section of the suture, while string chromicization sometimes causes the deposition of relatively heavier concentrations of the tanning agent near the periphery of the strand, with less penetration to its center. Deficient tanning of catgut may result in its premature absorption with possible wound disruption, although such incidents now are recognized often as the effects of nutritional or other inadequacies, with resultant weakness of the tissues themselves. Excessive chrome concentration in surgical gut may produce sutures that digest slowly. Since they survive in normal tissues for a long time, they occasionally may extrude through the skin some months following surgery. The mechanism of such extrusion by highly tanned catgut or by nonabsorbable sutures is not clear, although it probably reflects the natural tendency of the body to eliminate or reject foreign material.

Tissue Reaction—Following any surgical incision, there is an outpouring of blood and lymph into and through the wound. These fluids coagulate or clot, forming a network upon which new cells may build. The capillaries in the area dilate, and the blood supply in the vicinity of the wound is increased. Leukocytes in the area also increase in number.

The absorption of surgical gut takes place along with the tissue repair processes. The leukocytes, which appear early in any wound, produce proteolytic enzymes which, among other functions, carry out the digestion of absorbable catgut sutures. After this process is well along, fibroblasts appear and begin to lay down the collagen fibers essential for the increasing strength and healing of the wound. In the first phase of wound healing, the number and character of the debriding cells, together with such secondary effects as swelling, pain and redness constitute "tissue reaction." Chromic catgut elicits a less intense tissue reaction of a leukocytic or exudative type than does the plain variety.

Plain gut is digested by enzymes at a faster rate than chromic gut. The surgeon chooses either plain or chromic gut, depending on the type of tissue involved, the condition of the patient and the estimated healing time of the wound. Small sizes of surgical gut cause less tissue reaction and irritation than large sizes. There is less digestive work for the enzymes to do. For this reason surgeons try never to use a suture that is stronger than the tissue in which it is to be used. The larger sutures merely add to tissue irritation without supplying any needed strength to the wound.

Sterilization and Packaging—Disappointing experiences with many attempts to sterilize gut by chemical means have created widespread distrust of the effectiveness of most chemicals. The exception has been the use of ethylene oxide, which has provided an effective means for sterilizing sutures. The more common methods are dry-heat sterilization (after first dehydrating the catgut) and irradiation sterilization in the final sealed packet.

At one time most surgical gut was produced and labeled as *boilable.* It was packaged in glass tubes with the strands immersed in a water-free high-boiling tubing fluid—usually xylene. The exteriors of the tubes could be sterilized at the hospital by autoclaving—hence, the term *boilable.*

The disadvantage of boilable catgut has been that the drying necessary to permit high-temperature sterilization produces a stiff strand, which is still stiff as removed from the tube, and which requires soaking for several minutes in sterile water before surgeons find it pliable enough to use. This process no longer is used (with isolated exceptions).

The present method of packaging provides sutures ready for use as removed from the packet. The catgut, designated *nonboilable,* is contained in either a foil or plastic packet, immersed in a pliabilizing fluid which generally consists of an alcohol or mixtures of an alcohol with a small percentage of water. The water has a pliabilizing effect, but would ruin the gut if the latter is subjected to high temperatures—therefore, the designation *nonboilable.*

Irradiation and ethylene oxide sterilization techniques, as described in the USP, largely have replaced the older accepted method of dry-heat sterilization. These methods have permitted the development of more convenient packaging innovations which were not practical with the older methods.

For even greater convenience, all foil or plastic packets are now overwrapped in a secondary package. Both the contents and the outside of the inner packet are rendered sterile. By peeling open the overwrap package, the inner packet can be delivered ready for use in a sterile condition on the operating table.

Sterility Testing—Freedom from contamination is the most important property of any suture. Every lot of sutures furnished by reputable manufacturers is subjected to a series of physical and chemical tests, in accordance with prescribed USP sterility test procedures as well as validated sterilization processes. No lot of sutures is released until all of these tests have been passed successfully; hence, the surgeon has developed a justified confidence in the adequacy and sterility of these products. Because of the extraordinary reliability of radiation sterilization, acceptance of product sterility based on validated measurement and control of the radiation process is becoming more widespread.

Operating Room Procedures—Before a scheduled operation, the nurse usually selects the necessary types of sutures designated by the operating surgeon. The required number of overwrapped packages is opened by peeling apart the outer package and flipping or otherwise removing in an aseptic manner the inner sterile packets and placing them on the Mayo stand. The packets are opened by tearing, if foil, and by cutting with sterile scissors, if plastic. Straightening the nonboilable suture is accomplished by a gentle pull. They commonly are used as removed from the packet. Abuse of catgut sutures may lead to their failure in tissues, with possible serious consequences to the patient.

Synthetic Absorbable Sutures—The combination of high tensile strength and absorbability that makes catgut so useful as a suture has been incorporated into synthetic fibers. Polymers derived from condensing the cyclic derivative of glycolic acid (glycolide), mixtures of glycolide and lactide (derived by cyclicizing lactic acid) dioxanone and glycolide with tetramethylene carbonate have been shown to possess properties which make them suitable for many surgical procedures. The first two polyesters mentioned are melt-extruded into multifilament yarns which then are braided into various sizes of sutures. Such braids have high tensile strength and, unlike catgut, must be packaged without fluid and sterilized with ethylene oxide to avoid degradation. The second two polyesters are provided as pliable monofilaments. Synthetic absorbable sutures do not undergo the enzymically mediated absorption process that is well-known for catgut. Rather, the suture is broken down completely by simple hydrolysis as it resides in the tissue. Tissue reaction is minimal since scavenger leukocytes are not involved significantly in the absorption process.

Cargile Membrane—This is a thin sheet of pliable tissue obtained from the appendix ("blind gut") of the steer or ox. It is designed primarily to cover surfaces from which the peritoneum has been removed, especially where a sterile membrane would lessen the formation of adhesions. The membrane is available in sterile sheets of approximately 4 x 6-inches and sometimes is used as a packing or protective sheath. At present, the use of such material is limited.

Fascia Lata—This is obtained from ox fascia and is designed for use as a heavy suture or repair in hernia or similar cases. It usually is attached firmly to a strong structure by means of a nonabsorbable suture. It is supplied in the form of sterile strips approximately ½ inches wide and 8 inches long and also in sheets about 3 x 5 inches.

It should be emphasized, in connection with the above, that catgut strands and ribbons are the only ones which are completely and readily absorbable. The other materials may be absorbed very slowly or may be incorporated in the tissues by invasion of fibroblasts and a kind of replacement process.

Nonabsorbable Sutures

The second principal class of suture consists of natural and synthetic nonabsorbable suture materials which are relatively resistant to attack by normal tissue fluids. Several of these survive, apparently unchanged, for many years in tissue and usually will be found encapsulated in a thin sheath of fibrous tissue. When nonabsorbable sutures are used for skin closure, they usually are removed after the incision or wound has healed to the point where suture support is no longer necessary.

Silk is an important nonabsorbable surgical suture. Selected grades of degummed commercial silk fibers are used, and consist chiefly of the protein fibroin as extruded by the silkworm. Many such fibers are twisted into a single strand of various diameters as specified in the USP, and sold in the natural color or after dyeing. By far the most popular construction is braided silk, in which several twisted yarns are braided into a compact structure favored for its firmness and strength. Most braided silk is dyed and also given a treatment to render it noncapillary. In use as a skin suture this minimizes the rise of tissue fluids to the surface and thus the counterpassage inward of organisms from the surface. Further objectives of such treatments are to impart a degree of stiffness to improve the handling and tying properties, to minimize attachment of tissue cells that would cause pain on removal of the suture and to lubricate the implantation and removal of the silk. When silk, or any other suture, is dyed the USP requires that it be done with a color additive approved by the FDA.

Specifications—The USP describes in the monograph for Nonabsorbable Surgical Suture (which now includes cotton, linen, metallic wire, nylon, rayon, dacron and silk) the respective sizes, diameters and tensile strengths.

Uses—Silk sutures are handled easily, and tolerated well by body tissue, although they may cause significant tissue reaction. In the presence of infection, however, the interstices of silk strands protect organisms from antimicrobial agents and from the body's defense mechanisms, so that chronic sinuses may form which do not heal until the silk is removed or is sloughed by the tissues. Silk, as well as any other nonabsorbable suture, occasionally migrates from the site of implantation and comes to the surface to be extruded months after the operation. In certain sites, the suture knots or ends may serve as centers for the formation of concretions or for other irritating action. Silk usually becomes encapsulated and remains in the tissues for extended periods of time as the protein slowly degrades.

Dermal Silk—These sutures consist of natural twisted silk encased in an insoluble coating of tanned gelatin or other protein. This coating must withstand autoclaving without stripping, and its purpose is to prevent the ingrowth of tissue cells which would interfere with its removal after use as a skin or dermal suture.

Cotton and Linen—Sutures derived from cellulose are among the oldest known but currently are used to a limited extent. These are twisted from fiber staple, have moderately high tensile strength and are stable to heat sterilization. Cotton sutures prepared by suture manufacturers are uniform and have reproducible strength and largely have replaced the household sewing cotton used by many surgeons years ago. These are desirable because of their handling properties and low order of tissue reactivity but are not used widely in critical areas where strength must be maintained for long periods of time because they slowly degrade.

Synthetic Nonabsorbable Sutures

Nylon, the first modern synthetic fiber, came into use as a suture partly as a result of World War II shortages of high-grade silk and partly because of its own merits. It is a synthetic polyamide obtained from the condensation of adipic acid and hexamethylenediamine or from the condensation-polymerization of caprolactam. It is available in the form of monofilaments in the useful range of sizes, as well as in the form of multifilament fibers braided into strands of comparable diameter. It is strong, water-resistant and has come into some use for all suturing or ligating. Monofilament nylon is used as a skin or stay suture or for plastic surgery. Braided nylon more often is buried in tissues and is subject to the same limitations as braided silk in the presence of infection.

Polyester Fiber—Of the numerous multifilament synthetic fibers introduced after the success of nylon, only polyester has been accepted as a suitable braided nonabsorbable suture while polypropylene has enjoyed increasing popularity as a nonabsorbable monofilament suture. Polyester suture is prepared by melt-extruding polyethylene terephthalate into fine filaments which then are braided into various sizes. In general, the tensile strength of polyester braided sutures is superior to that of braided silk and nylon and twisted cotton.

The polyester sutures, in contrast with most other materials except polypropylene and stainless steel, do not lose strength significantly when in contact with water or body fluids. For this reason, they have become a suture of choice when there is a critical need for permanent reinforcement as, for example, in the installation of artificial heart valves. They have the advantage of excellent knot-holding characteristics and are available in the natural color or dyed to enhance visibility in the surgical field.

Recent developments have seen the commercialization of braided polyester fiber sutures coated or impregnated with nontoxic lubricants such as polytetrafluoroethylene or silicone resins. Polybutilate, a lubricant especially designed for polyester suture use, has been derived from a condensation polymer of butanediol and adipic acid. These sutures exhibit the advantage of a smoother surface which gives the suture improved handling properties and permits an easier and more gentle passage through tissue.

Polyolefin Fibers—Of increasing interest in the nonabsorbable suture field is the development of fibers based on polyolefins. Although polyethylene sutures have been available, the use of polypropylene monofilament has increased greatly during recent years. Polypropylene sutures compared to monofilament nylon, tie more secure knots and have a very low order of tissue reactivity. Because of the smoothness of polypropylene sutures, they slip through tissue easily and, because there is no tissue ingrowth, they may be removed easily when necessary. They have found wide application in cardiovascular and other surgical specialties.

A monofilament suture based on polybutylester, reported to have improved pliability, has been introduced. Another new suture, fabricated from expanded polytetrafluoroethylene, has been recommended for use with vascular grafts derived for the same material, as well as in other surgical procedures.

Metallic Sutures

For some years increased attention has been paid to the use of various metal wire sutures and other metallic devices to assist surgical repair.

Silver—Among the older materials which still are used to some extent are silver wire, foil and other forms. Relatively little work has been reported recently on these items. Silver is available readily and is alleged to have some antiseptic action, but in some tissues is definitely irritating. Irritation has been shown by a great many metals and alloys, and now is regarded as a controlling consideration in the choice of substances for implantation in tissues.

Stainless Steel—This ferrous alloy, which so long has been employed usefully in industrial and other applications where resistance to chemical attack is essential, has been used widely in the form of wire sutures, fixation plates, screws and other items. Stainless steel is a rather general term covering a wide variety of materials, and many of the early alloys were attacked by body fluids. The proper selection of stainless steel compositions seems to provide a material essentially inert in tissues and free from the earlier disadvantages. Stainless steel sutures are available both as twisted and monofilament strands and represent the strongest available material. However, they are relatively difficult to use and are employed most commonly in areas where great strength is required, such as in the repair of the sternum after chest surgery.

Surgical Needles

Suture materials may be threaded on eyed needles for suturing. While formerly only eyed needles were available, there is an overwhelming trend to the use of eyeless needles, one or two being attached to each individual strand. One such needle is manufactured with an open channel into which the suture can be placed, and the channel is then swaged around the strand. Another type, known as "seamless," has a very delicate hole drilled in the shank. To prevent pullout, the shank is pressed firmly about the suture. These sutures offer great advantage in minimizing trauma. With an eyed needle an opening in tissue must be made large enough to accommodate the needle and two thicknesses of suture, but with the eyeless needle, the opening need only accommodate the needle, slightly larger than the single suture which follows. This is greatly esteemed in fine surgery such as plastic and ophthalmic work. A wide variety of eyeless needles on catgut and other materials are now available to meet most of the demands of the surgeon. By a recent innovation, it has been possible to control the release of a suture from an eyeless needle by a gentle tug so that the surgeon need not take the time to cut the needle from the suture when it is no longer required.

Vitallium—This metal, which is an alloy of cobalt, chromium and molybdenum, has been applied to many surgical problems in various forms since 1937, although not in the form of sutures or ligatures. The alloy has shown some variability in strength and stiffness and is incapable of much modification at the time of operation, but generally shows negligible tissue reactions. In addition to some use for dentures, surgical forms of vitallium include: fracture plates, screws, bolts, nails and appliances, orbital implants, nasal skeletal supports, tendon rods, tubes for blood vessel anastomosis or bile duct repair and skull plates.

Other Suturing Techniques

Although sutures and ligatures have remained the most effective and popular devices for closing wounds and hemostasis, other techniques are being used with increasing frequency. Surgical stapling devices are available which automatically approximate tissue with rows of steel staples which remain permanently. Such devices exist for closing skin and anastomosing blood vessels as well as for reconstructing other organs such as stomach and intestines. Some surgical staplers are designed to cut tissue before or after the staples are applied.

During the last several years, V-shaped steel, tantalum or titanium clips have been used to clamp small blood vessels and this alternative to ligation is becoming increasingly popular as the application instruments become more convenient and easy to use. Stainless steel clips or staples have been used frequently to coapt skin incisions. More recently, strips of fabric or plastic material coated with a suitable adhesive have been used for the same application.

New approaches to ligating clips are represented by absorbable materials, polydioxanone and lactomer. Ligating clips made from these substances absorb after their function is completed and do not remain in the patient permanently as do metallic clips. Thus, interference with diagnostic imaging techniques such as X-ray and CAT scans is avoided.

With the advent of minimally invasive surgical procedures, the industry faces significant challenges. Several new needles and other devices have been introduced to the market, facilitating the ease with which the surgeon can approximate and suture tissue through a trocar port.

Suture Monograph

Absorbable Surgical Suture

Surgical Catgut; Catgut Suture; Surgical Gut; Sterilized Surgical Catgut BP; Sterilized Surgical Ligature

A sterile strand prepared from collagen derived from healthy mammals or from a synthetic polymer. Its length is not less than 95.0% of that stated on the label. Its diameter and tensile strength correspond to the size designation indicated on the label, within the limits prescribed herein. It is capable of being absorbed by living mammalian tissue, but may be treated to modify its resistance to absorption. It may be modified with respect to body or texture. It may be impregnated or coated with a suitable antimicrobial agent. It may be colored by a color additive approved by the FDA.

Description—Flexible strand varying in treatment, color, size, packaging and resistance to absorption, according to the intended purpose. The collagen suture is either *Type A* Suture or *Type C* Suture. Both types consist of processed strands of collagen, but *Type C* Suture is processed by physical or chemical means so as to provide greater resistance to absorption in living mammalian tissue.

Nonabsorbable Surgical Suture

Surgical Sutures; Surgical Silk; Sterile Surgical Silk

A strand of material that is suitably resistant to the action of living mammalian tissue. Its length is not less than 95.0% of that stated on the label. Its diameter and tensile strength correspond to the size designation indicated on the label, within the limits prescribed herein. It may be nonsterile or sterile. It may be impregnated or coated with a suitable antimicrobial agent.

It may be modified with respect to body or texture, or to reduce capillarity, and may be suitably bleached. It may be colored by a color additive approved by the FDA.

Description—Flexible, monofilament or multifilament, continuous strand, placed in an envelope, tube or other suitable container or wound on a reel or spool. If it is a multifilament strand, the individual filaments may be combined by spinning, twisting, braiding or any combination thereof. Nonabsorbable Surgical Suture is classed and typed as follows: *Class I* Suture is composed of silk or synthetic fibers of monofilament, twisted or braided construction. *Class II* Suture is composed of cotton or linen fibers or coated natural or synthetic fibers where the coating forms a casing of significant thickness but does not contribute appreciably to strength. *Class III* Suture is composed of monofilament or multifilament metal wire.

CHAPTER 109

Poison Control

Anthony R Temple, MD
Executive Director, Medical
McNeil Consumer Products Co
Adjunct Associate Professor, Department of Pediatrics
University of Pennsylvania School of Medicine
Lecturer, Philadelphia College of Pharmacy and Science
Ft Washington, PA 19034

Anthony S Manoguerra, PharmD
Professor of Clinical Pharmacy
School of Pharmacy
University of California San Francisco
San Diego Program
Director, San Diego Regional Poison Center
University of California San Diego Medical Center
San Diego, CA 92103

It is estimated that there are between 5 and 10 million toxic exposures annually in the US. Among children beyond the first year of life, accidents cause more deaths than do the five leading fatal diseases combined. Also among the most common causes of death of preadolescents, adolescents and adults is suicide. Both accidents and suicides frequently involve poisons. Another important cause of morbidity and mortality, especially among the young, is the deliberate abuse of drugs and chemicals for their effects on the central nervous system. Even though the reporting, especially of suicides and abuses, undoubtedly is incomplete, there are known to be over 10,000 deaths in the US each year attributable to poisoning.

In addition to the fatalities due to poisoning, there are staggering numbers of nonfatal cases requiring treatment. The toll in terms of manpower, expense and occupation of medical facilities cannot be estimated, but must be tremendous.

Accidental poisonings should be preventable in most instances. This is especially true of accidental poisonings of young children by drugs and chemicals in the home. This is a problem of great public-health significance, the solution of which will require efforts of individuals in many disciplines. Among these are pharmacists, who can play a key role in preventing or mitigating the consequences of accidental poisonings, especially those due to drugs.

Epidemiology

Effective preventive measures require a knowledge of who and what are involved, how it happened and any predisposing or contributory factors. In order to delineate some of these factors, a description of the experiences of those poison-control centers who report to the National Data Collection System of the American Association of Poison Control Centers (AAPCC) may be instructive. The National Data Collection System of the AAPCC was established in 1983. The data collected by this system constitutes the largest body of data about poisoning exposures in the world. Table 1 summarizes the growth of this System. Starting in 1983 with just over 250,000 reported cases from 16 reporting centers (the largest collection of cases yet reported in the US) representing approximately 11% of the US population, the system grew rapidly over the next 3 years to a point where it recorded over one million cases in 1986. In 1991, 1,837,939 cases were reported from 73 centers representing approximately 80% of the US population.

Table 2 summarizes the pattern of human poisoning exposures by type. Overdose calls made up 98% of all calls, while 1.6% were calls regarding adverse reactions. Poison centers also receive calls that are informational in nature, in which no poisoning victim is involved. The majority of information calls are toxicology or drug-information requests, but also include requests for medical and veterinary information. Of the human poisoning exposure cases, 87.4% were accidental in nature. Suicidal or intentional poisonings made up 7.2%, while poisonings involving drug abuse amounted to 2.5%. Environmental or industrial exposures accounted for 3.4% of the human poisoning exposure cases.

Of the 1,837,939 poisoning cases reported in 1991, 76.3% involved ingestions as the mode of exposure (Table 3). The remainder of exposures were topical, 7.4%, ophthalmic, 6.2%, inhalation, 5.6%, bites and stings, 3.7% and miscellaneous or unknown, 0.9%.

Children 5 years of age and under were involved in 60% of the cases (Table 4). Ages 6 through 19 were involved in 11.3%, while 28.7% involved adults aged 19 and above. In their overall experience, males and females were represented equally.

In terms of the severity of exposures handled by poison-control centers (Table 5), 26.7% had no effect and 22.3% had only a minor effect. Major toxicity was seen in only 0.3%. An additional 34.0% of cases were assessed to have been nontoxic, but the ultimate outcome was not confirmed.

In cases of a poisoning exposure, 71.6% were managed at home or in some non-health-care facility (Table 6). As a general rule, treatment consisted of simple administration of demulcents, dilution, irrigation or emesis. Of the poisoning exposure cases, 25.9% were managed in an emergency-care facility. Less than 0.04% of the cases proved to be fatal.

In the AAPCC data base, the substances most frequently involved in human poisoning exposures were cleaning substances, analgesics, cosmetics, plants, cough and cold preparations, hydrocarbons, bites/envenomations, topicals, foreign bodies, pesticides, foods and sedative/hypnotic/antipsychotics (Table 7). A wide variety of agents made up the remaining cases.

In contrast, the most frequent category of toxic substances involved in reported fatalities was analgesics, followed by antidepressants, stimulants, street drugs, cardiovascular drugs, sedative/hypnotics, gases, fumes, chemicals, alcohols/glycols, asthma therapies, cleaning substances and hydrocarbons (Table 8). Among those categories causing the most fatalities, there is a wide variation in the percent of fatalities with respect to all exposures in that category. At the high end, antidepressant fatalities make up 0.53% of all antidepressant exposures, cardiovascular drugs, 0.35%, and stimulant and street drugs, 0.43%, while analgesic fatalities make up only 0.10% of exposures and cleaning substances, 0.01%.

Of continued importance is therapeutic overdosage, a fact which has important preventive implications for the pharmacist. It is not at all uncommon for a parent who has never been told of the toxic potential of such a commonplace item as aspirin to administer several times the safe dose to a small infant over a period of several days. In fact, such unintentional overdoses are responsible for many of the most serious cases of poisoning.

Particularly tragic are accidental poisonings due to materials which are either outmoded, excessively toxic for their intended use or for which there is only questionable rationale.

Table 1—Growth of the AAPCC National Data Collection System[a]

Year	Number of participating poison centers	Population served (millions)	% of US population served	Human exposures reported
1983	16	43.1	11.0	251,012
1984	47	99.8	42.0	730,224
1985	56	113.6	47.6	900,513
1986	57	132.1	55.0	1,098,894
1987	63	137.5	57.0	1,166,940
1988	64	155.7	63.0	1,368,748
1989	70	182.4	73.0	1,581,540
1990	72	191.7	76.8	1,713,462
1991	73	200.7	80.4	1,837,939

[a] Adapted from Ref 1.

Table 2—Typical Pattern of Human Poison Exposure Cases Reported to AAPCC [a]

Type of poisoning	Number of cases	Total	%	Total
Accidental		1,606,507		87.4
General	1,443,202		78.5	
Misuse	98,373		5.4	
Occupational	36,859		2.0	
Environmental	25,588		1.4	
Unknown	2,485		0.1	
Intentional		194,197		10.6
Suicidal	131,707		7.2	
Abuse	27,581		1.5	
Misuse	18,884		1.0	
Unknown	16,025		0.9	
Adverse Reaction		30,044		1.6
Drug	19,143		1.0	
Food	7,392		0.4	
Other	3,509		0.2	
Unknown		7,191		0.4
Total		1,837,939		100

[a] Adapted from Ref 1.

Table 3—Distribution of Human Poison Exposure Cases by Route of Exposure [a,b]

	Number of cases	%	Number of fatalities	%
Ingestion	1,473,361	76.3	622	75.7
Dermal	143,196	7.4	8	1.0
Ophthalmic	119,027	6.2	2	0.2
Inhalation	107,634	5.6	116	14.1
Bites and stings	72,331	3.7	5	0.6
Parenteral	5,217	0.3	37	4.5
Other/unknown	11,340	0.6	31	3.9

[a] Adapted from Ref 1.
[b] Multiple routes of exposure were observed in many poison exposure victims. Percentage is based upon the total number of exposure routes (1,932,106) for all patients, 822 for fatal cases rather than the total number of human exposures (1,837,939) or fatalities (764).

Also, household chemicals, solvents, cleaners and some pesticides, while valuable to the professional user, are excessively toxic for routine household use. There is little reason for employing highly dangerous inorganic materials such as arsenic, phosphorus or thallium as rodenticides when warfarin practically devoid of acute human toxicity, will do the job.

Influential Factors

A number of factors seem to be important in the consideration of poisoning risk and in poison prevention. The following is a brief discussion of some of those factors.

Table 4—Distribution of Human Poison Exposure Cases by Age of Victim[a]

Age (yr)	% of cases
<1	8.0
1	18.6
2	19.0
3	8.7
4	3.7
5	2.0
6–12	5.6
13–19	5.7
20–29	6.8
30–39	5.8
40–49	3.1
50–59	1.4
60–69	1.1
70–79	0.7
80–89	0.4
90–99	0.1
Unknown adult	9.3
Total	100.0

[a] Adapted from Ref 1.

Table 5—Medical Outcome of Human Exposure Cases[a]

Outcome	Number	%
No effect	490,421	26.7
Minor effect	409,537	22.3
Moderate effect	41,613	2.3
Major effect	5,812	0.3
Death	764	<0.01
Unknown, nontoxic[b]	624,135	34.0
Unknown, potentially toxic[c]	216,726	11.8
Unrelated effect	46,920	2.6
Unknown	2,011	0.1
Total	1,837,939	10.0

[a] Adapted from Ref 1.
[b] No follow-up provided as exposure was assessed as nontoxic.
[c] Patient lost to follow-up. Exposure was assessed as potentially toxic.

Table 6—Management Site of Human Poisoning Exposure Cases[a]

	Number	%
Non-health-facility	1,316,605	71.6
Health-care facility	475,597	25.9
Already there at time of call to poison center	244,544[b]	13.3[b]
Referred by poison center	231,053[b]	12.6[b]
Other/unknown	45,737	2.5
Total	1,837,939	100

[a] Adapted from Ref 1.
[b] These data are not included in the total.

Age—Approximately two-thirds of poisonings occur in children and are accidental, while a majority of the poisonings in adolescents and adults represent suicide attempts. Poisonings do occur in adults from the inadvertent taking of some material other than intended medication or accidental overdosage of proper medication. While such accidents are rather rare, people should nonetheless be cautioned to read labels carefully before taking medications, not to take medications in the dark, not to transfer materials from their original containers, to protect medication labels against destruction and to follow carefully the recommended dosage schedules.

Accidental poisoning is less common beyond 5 or 6 years of age. The most critical age period is between 1 and 3 years, where nearly one-half of poisonings occur. Poisoning is among the most likely reasons to bring a child to the hospital

Table 7—Substances Most Frequently Involved in Human Poison Exposures[a]

	Number	%[b]
Cleaning substances	191,830	10.4
Analgesics	183,013	10.0
Cosmetics	153,424	8.3
Plants	112,564	6.1
Cough and cold preparations	105,185	5.7
Bites/envenomations	76,941	4.2
Pesticides (includes rodenticides)	70,523	3.8
Topicals	69,096	3.8
Antimicrobials	64,805	3.5
Foreign bodies	64,472	3.5
Hydrocarbons	63,536	3.5
Sedatives/hypnotics/antipsychotics	58,450	3.2
Chemicals	53,366	2.9
Alcohols	50,296	2.7
Food poisoning	46,482	2.5
Vitamins	40,883	2.2

[a] Adapted from Ref 1.
[b] Percentages are based on total number of known ingested substances rather than the total number of human exposures cases.
Note: Despite a high frequency of involvement, these substances are not necessarily the most toxic but, rather, often represent only ready availability.

for emergency treatment. The reasons for the high incidence in that age range relate to certain characteristics of child development. During these early years the youngster is inquisitive. By 1 year of age he also usually is able either to creep or walk, yet he is too young to recognize danger. It is to be expected that he will attempt to mouth or ingest any substance left within reach.

No matter how distasteful a product may be, a child still will make an initial attempt to eat or taste it. While pleasant flavoring may be influential in a child's ingesting a larger dose, it has little bearing on the likelihood that he initially will attempt to ingest the material. During the first 2 to 3 years of life, texture is at least as important as flavor in determining acceptability of something to be eaten. Materials that would gag or dissuade an older individual may be ingested readily by the young child. Obviously, even highly caustic substances such as lye are ingested without hesitation by children at this age.

Children less than 1 year old may be given a toxic material by an older sibling. Thus, it is important to keep potentially toxic materials inaccessible not only to very young children but to their older brothers and sisters as well. In addition, children should be educated not to give things to the baby without a parent's permission. Preschool education programs teach children these principles, and they should be a standard part of parenting in every household.

Table 8—Categories with Largest Number of Deaths[a]

Category	No	% of all exposures in category
Analgesics	190	0.104
Antidepressants	188	0.525
Sedative/hypnotics	97	0.166
Stimulants and street drugs	90	0.434
Cardiovascular drugs	87	0.348
Alcohols	72	0.143
Gases and fumes	49	0.188
Asthma therapies	39	0.229
Chemicals	37	0.069
Hydrocarbons	36	0.057
Cleaning substances	26	0.014
Pesticides (includes rodenticides)	18	0.026

[a] Adapted from Ref 1.

It also is of interest that among children older than 3 years of age ingestions may occur as group activities. Occasionally, two or more children will share the material in some form of play, where they might otherwise be unlikely to ingest it by themselves. Again at this age, children are more educable than earlier, so instruction in avoidance of potentially toxic nonfood substances should be given in the home and educational environment.

Some of the supposedly accidental poisonings in teenage and younger children are actually suicide attempts or gestures or attempts at drug abuse. It is important to realize that serious suicide attempts may occur at 9 or 10 years of age. Suicidal attempts or gestures are, of course, quite common among adolescents and in the several years immediately before and after this important transitional stage of life.

"Accident Proneness"—Only a small number of patients treated for poisoning have had a history of having been involved in similar accidents. Thus, while some children may be involved in repetitive episodes, they account for a small percentage of such cases. Nonetheless, a child who has ingested something once, especially if some effort was required in the act, may be at greater future risk and should be treated accordingly. The idea that there are accident-prone children probably is less valid than the fact that there are accident-prone situations and surroundings. Parental education about poison prevention techniques and what to do in case of a poisoning should be considered as part of the routine follow-up in all childhood poisoning episodes.

Location—The vast majority of childhood accidental poisonings occur in the home. Materials which become involved in childhood accidental poisoning usually have been left out after being used, rather than being in their usual place of storage at the time they were taken. The most common areas for poisoning within the home are the kitchen, bathroom and bedroom.

The highest incidence of accidental childhood poisoning is in the late afternoon and around the dinner hour or in the early-morning hours, but poisonings occur with regular consistency during a child's waking hours. Poisonings in the late-morning hours often occur in the kitchen and the substances most frequently involved are common household products such as cleaning agents, polishes and other materials commonly kept in the kitchen. Poisonings that occur in the bedroom may involve cosmetics and, to a lesser extent, medications. Bathroom incidents usually involve either medications or cosmetics. The more often a consumer product is used and stored in the home, the more likely it is involved in an accidental poisoning exposure.

Among cases that occur outside the home, and garage and automobile are common sites of accidental poisoning in young children. Involved most frequently in the automobile are medications left either in the glove compartment or in mother's purse. In the garage, pesticides, petroleum products, cleaning agents and paint products often are stored and thus involved in poisoning. An increasing percentage of cases occurring inside or outside the home involve plants kept for decorative purposes or which are growing either in the yard or wild in the fields. Parents should be reminded that children may be poisoned when they visit the homes of others (especially grandparents) who leave things within reach because they are not accustomed to having children about.

Accessibility—Poison-prevention campaigns often focus on the provision of a locked medicine cabinet. The availability of a safe storage place for medicines is desirable, but this probably would prevent less than one-half the cases of accidental childhood poisoning.

In as many as 75% of the cases, the materials involved in childhood accidental poisoning have been left within reach of a child. In many instances, ingestion occurs when the individual responsible for the care of a child is interrupted during his or her use of the material in question.

People must be instructed not only to provide a storage place for potentially toxic materials, but also to return these materials immediately after use.

The Container—Removal of potentially toxic materials from their original containers is a significant factor in increasing risk of accidental poisoning, especially with certain compounds. The common practice, for example, of storing a small quantity of gasoline or solvents in a soft-drink bottle is especially hazardous, for obvious reasons. Other hazardous materials with which this frequently is done are cleaning solutions, paint products, turpentine and pesticides. Sometimes the container to which they are transferred is a drinking glass or dish. In all such instances, a material may be made to seem more attractive to the child because of resemblance to food or other ingestable items. In addition, transfer of materials from their original containers creates problems of accurate identification if and when poisoning does occur. A similar problem exists when materials, particularly medications, are not identified properly in their original containers. Obviously, all prescription vials should identify accurately the contents on the label.

Supervision—Most children are considered to be under the supervision of one or both parents at the time an accidental poisoning occurs, but usual adult supervision is not adequate to prevent poisoning accidents in young children. This may be due in part because parents underestimate the ability of the child to obtain and ingest a potentially toxic material. A common error is to leave medications on a bedside stand after administering them to a young child, so that the child for whom it was intended or a sibling may ingest the entire contents.

A significant number of childhood poisonings occur when there is a disruption in normal household routine. Times of moving, painting, holidays, visits by friends or relatives or death or illness in the family are occasions when increased caution should be exercised. Other circumstances that invite unsupervised access of children to potentially toxic materials are when items are sent through the mail or after being discarded into a refuse container.

When deteriorated or unwanted materials are to be discarded, the safest procedure for potentially toxic liquids or powders either is to pour them down a drain or flush them down a toilet. With some highly concentrated and highly toxic materials, such as pesticide concentrates, even the amount left remaining in an "empty" bottle may be sufficient to cause serious poisoning. Such containers should be rinsed thoroughly before being discarded and placed carefully in closed refuse containers as far from normal access by children as possible.

Optimal supervision also involves attention to detail in the legitimate use of potentially hazardous materials. As previously noted, drug labels always should be examined carefully to ensure accurate identification before a medication is administered or taken. Self-medication, use of an other individual's medications for the "same problem," and unsupervised self-diagnosis and prescription of a child's treatment by the parents should be encouraged only with appropriate education and potential for consumer understanding.

There is a tendency for many to believe that if a material were significantly hazardous it would not be available for over-the-counter sales, but obviously this is not true. Frequently, parents may overmedicate a child, either because they underestimate the potential hazard or are given inadequate instructions. It is important that physicians who order medications, and pharmacists who dispense them, provide and emphasize specific instructions concerning proper use. The pharmacist can play a key role in this, even if only a minute or two is spent in appropriate patient education.

Although seemingly unlikely, it is not at all uncommon for a patient who has been advised to take or administer "some aspirin every once in a while" to use two or three times the safe dose every few hours for several days or to take concurrent medications containing salicylates until serious intoxication occurs. Instructions on the label are meaningful to the cautious and the concerned, but these are rarely the people who become poisoned. Person-to-person conversation is far more effective and easily can take place at the time a material is prescribed or dispensed.

Treatment

The most important treatment measure for poisoning is prevention. Of course, once a poisoning occurs, it is important to be able to provide highly skilled supportive medical care. It is not sufficient to focus only on simple first-aid measures and antidotal therapy or home remedies.

Actually, there are very few poisons for which there are effective antidotes. Even in those instances where antidotes are available, supportive care is at least as important; indeed, the best antidote in the world is of little value without good supportive care. Most of the home remedies which have been recommended from time to time actually are of little value, and most tend to waste valuable time that could better be devoted to proper treatment under adequate medical supervision.

Unfortunately, many lay publications, including first-aid texts, are outmoded in this respect and continue to recommend all sorts of elaborate but ineffective procedures to be carried out in the home. The same criticism can be leveled at the instructions provided on the many rather complicated antidote lists and first-aid treatment charts that are disseminated for use of the public, often by well-meaning professional organizations.

First-Aid Principles

The cardinal rule for first-aid treatment of poisoning is to remove the poison from contact with the patient (unless such removal is contraindicated) and to obtain further definitive medical care at the earliest possible moment if warranted.

The more simplified one can make any instructions for home treatment, the more likely they are to be followed and the less likely they are to either delay or be substituted for proper care by a physician. Thus, general procedures that can be carried out simply and are applicable almost irrespective of the nature of the poison are to be recommended until medical help can be obtained.

Recommended procedures for lay use in the first-aid treatment of poisoning are outlined in Table 9. The principal elements are knowing what to do before you call someone, obtaining medical advice immediately to determine what to do next and terminating the exposure of the victim by removal of the poison usually through induction of vomiting. In regard to the latter point, it should be noted that induction of vomiting with ipecac syrup is the only really efficacious method of vomiting. Many measures recommended in the past for the induction of vomiting, such as mechanical stimulation of the posterior pharynx or giving mustard water or salt water, are usually not effective and may be dangerous. The most serviceable emetic for first-aid use is ipecac syrup, which is highly effective if used in the doses recommended here. Up to 1 oz can be dispensed without a prescription.

Activated charcoal is a highly effective adsorbent of a large number of poisons and may be just as effective as ipecac-induced vomiting. Most organic and inorganic materials are adsorbed by this material and so its use routinely in cases of poisoning by ingestion is worthwhile. It should be remembered, however, that if activated charcoal is given before ipecac syrup, it will inactivate the latter; consequently, if one is going to both induce vomiting and give activated charcoal, it is advisable to induce vomiting first and then, after the vomiting has subsided, administer the charcoal. Activated charcoal is worthwhile as a nonspecific antidote not only for home use but also for use in hospitals and in poison treatment centers. It is best given as a slurry in water.

In recent years parents have been encouraged to keep ipecac syrup and activated charcoal in homes where there are children of poisoning-prone age. If such items are to be used, it is important that a prominent part of the instruction on

Table 9—First-Aid Treatment for Poisoning

I. DO THESE THINGS BEFORE YOU CALL SOMEONE
  A. Remove poisons from contact with eyes, skin or mouth.
    1. Eyes: Gently wash eyes with plenty of water (or milk) for 10 to 15 minutes with the eyelids held open. Remove contact lenses and again wash the eyes. Do not allow victims to rub their eyes.
    2. Skin: Wash poisons off the skin with large amounts of plain water. Then wash the skin with a detergent if it is possible. Remove and discard all contaminated clothing.
    3. Mouth: Look into victim's mouth and remove all tablets, powder, plants or any other material that you find. Also examine for cuts, burns or any unusual coloring. Wipe out mouth with a cloth and wash thoroughly with water.
  B. Remove victim from contact with poisonous fumes or gases.
    Get the victim into fresh air.
    Loosen all tight-fitting clothing.
    If the victim is not breathing, you should start artificial respiration immediately. Do not stop until the victim is either breathing well or help arrives. Use oxygen if available. Send someone else to call for help.
  C. If a caustic poison has been swallowed, you should dilute it by giving 1 or 2 glassfuls of milk or water.

II. CALL FOR INFORMATION ABOUT WHAT TO DO NEXT:
  A. Call your doctor, or call the poison control center.
    1. Identify yourself and your relationship to the victim.
    2. Describe the victim by name, age and sex.
    3. Have the package or poison in your hand and identify exactly (as best as you can) what the victim took and how much he took.
  B. Call for information even if you are not sure. Keep calm. You have enough time to act, but don't delay unnecessarily.

III. IF YOU ARE INSTRUCTED TO INDUCE VOMITING
  Never induce vomiting until you are instructed to do so.
  A. Have syrup of ipecac available to induce vomiting. Purchase 1 oz of ipecac syrup from your pharmacist. You may do this without a prescription. It will keep stored at room temperature for several years.
  B. To use ipecac syrup:
    In an adult give 2 tablespoonfuls (30 mL), in a child over 1 year give 1 tablespoonful (15 mL), and in a child less than 1 year give 2 teaspoonfuls (10 mL), of ipecac syrup followed by a glass (8 oz) of liquid (water, juices, etc). If patient hasn't vomited within 20 to 30 min, repeat the dose of ipecac syrup and give more water.
  C. Don't waste time trying other ways to make the victim vomit.
    Tickling the back of the throat with your fingers, a spoon, or some other object is not very effective. Do not use salt water. It is potentially dangerous.
  D. Never induce vomiting if the patient:
    Is unconscious.
    Is having convulsions (fits).
    Has swallowed strong caustics or corrosives.
    Has swallowed petroleum products, cleaning fluids, gasoline, lighter fluid, etc., unless specifically instructed to do so.

IV. IF YOU GO TO THE HOSPITAL:
  A. Take with you or send the poison container, poisonous plant, etc.
  B. Take any vomitus you collect.
  A. Don't give substances like coffee, alcohol, stimulants or drugs to the victim.

the label is to call the local poison-control center, an emergency department or a physician before administering either.

Antidotes—It should be emphasized that while activated charcoal is an effective, nonspecific adsorbent of a large number of materials, there is no true "universal antidote." The classic universal antidote which was in use for a long period of time consisted of activated charcoal, tannic acid or magnesium oxide (or, in the home: burnt toast, strong tea or milk of magnesia). It now has been established that the last two constituents have no significant efficacy and may actually impede the one active ingredient, activated charcoal. The long-advocated preparation of burnt toast and strong tea in the home has no merit; the materials do not have significant therapeutic properties.

Because they are not used often, it is important for information to be available readily concerning antidotes, not only so that they can be used properly and at the earliest possible moment, but also so that time is not wasted in searching for nonexistent antidotes. For a few poisons, there are chemical antidotes that react with the poison in the stomach either to inactivate it or to retard its absorption. Such local antidotes are sufficiently innocuous that they can be administered safely.

The most useful antidotes are those available for systemic administration to counteract the effects of poisons which have been absorbed already. Table 10 summarizes the use and administration of antidotes that currently are recommended.

Other Measures—Aside from removal or inactivation of the poison and use of antidotes when available, the treatment of poisoning is supportive. The symptomatic or supportive approach to treatment does not differ significantly from that encountered in other medical problems. Common problems requiring supportive care include coma, respiratory insufficency, convulsions, shock, vomiting, diarrhea, fluid and electrolyte disturbances, cerebral edema, kidney failure and damage to other organs.

Additionally, there are a number of procedures that may be utilized to hasten elimination of a poison. In some instances drugs can be eliminated more rapidly by using diuresis induced by use of pharmacological or osmotic diuretics along with alkalinization of the urine. With poisons that are dialyzable, extracorporeal hemodialysis (use of artificial kidney) is preferred. Sorbent hemoperfusion also is effective with many agents. These procedures are indicated when normal excretory processes fail or prove to be inadequate or when the degree of poisoning portends a fatal outcome unless the level of poison in the body is reduced rapidly.

Centers that are likely to be called on to treat cases of poisoning generally have the necessary supplies and equipment for performance of peritoneal dialysis, hemodialysis and hemoperfusion. If such is not available in a given hospital, the poison center should have information concerning the nearest location of such equipment.

Prevention

A number of preventive measures have been suggested or alluded to previously.

Total prevention through education is an ideal worth striving for. To date, educational programs have eliminated only a portion of the problem. One concern is that educational efforts may be too general, so the public does not know precisely what it should do and has no specific actions to implement. Instruction is most effective when it includes specific directions that can and should be followed. For instance, announcing to parents that they should "keep things out of the reach of small children" helps little until they are told what to keep out of reach.

It is not uncommon in cases of childhood poisoning that parents are not aware that the material was potentially poisonous, or that they took no special precautions because their child had been no problem previously, or they thought the material was inaccessible to the child. Aiming educational efforts at specific actions (see below) has far more chance of being effective. General admonitions about preventing poisoning are much less likely to be effective.

Consonant with the theory of specific instruction is the need to provide specific directions with individual products. This is an important role for the pharmacist. There is a tendency for precautionary labeling to be ignored until after an accident. Labels may be effective in directing individuals to proper treatment, but their preventive value is dependent on the consumer's interest and concern in reading the label in the first place. Person-to-person instruction by the physician or dispensing pharmacist is much more effective.

Limiting the availability of highly toxic materials or directing the consumer to the least toxic material that will serve the intended purpose are of potential value. Outmoded materials that have higher degrees of toxicity should be eliminated as safer substitutes become available. Pharmacists should be in a position to advise about comparative safety as well as efficacy of the products that they dispense or sell.

The Poison Prevention Packaging Act—Enacted in 1970, this legislation (PL 91-601; 16CFR 1700) calls for the packaging of specified potentially hazardous household chemicals and drugs in "safety" containers. The latter include safety-capped vials or bottles, "strip," "blister" or other unit-packaging. Child-resistant packaging must be demonstrated through the use of standardized tests in target-age populations to resist opening by children but not by adults. Such testing demonstrates the particularly effective barrier such packages provide to the poison-prone-age child. Drugs designated thus far as requiring such packaging include, with certain specific exemptions, aspirin-containing preparations, those containing high concentrations of methyl salicylate, prescription drugs, caustics, petroleum distillates, glycols,

Table 10—Summary of Local and Systemic Antidotes

Poison	Local antidote	Systemic antidote
Acetaminophen	Activated charcoal	*N*-acetylcysteine (Mucomyst) initial dose of 140 mg/kg orally in soft drinks, fruit juice, or water; then, 70 mg/kg every 4 hr for 68 hr (17 doses).
Acids, corrosive	Dilute with water or milk	
Alkali, caustic	Dilute with water or milk	
Alkaloids coniine, quinine, strychnine, etc	Activated charcoal	
Anticholinergics	Activated charcoal	Physostigmine, adult: (trial), 2 mg slowly IV, repeat one time, then give 1–4 mg, using lowest effective dose to control life-threatening symptoms; child: (trial) 0.5 mg slowly IV, repeat up to 2 mg max., then give lowest effective dose. (Caution: may cause seizures, asystole, cholinergic crisis).
Anticholinesterases organophosphates neostigmine physostigmine pyridostigmine carbamates	Activated charcoal	Atropine, 2–5 mg (for children under 2 yr, 1 mg or 0.05 mg/kg) IV or IM repeated every 10–30 min until atropinization is evident; then give pralidoxime chloride 25–50 mg/kg (1 g in adults) IV; repeat in 8–12 hr prn.
Antihistamines	(see Anticholinergics)	Atropine as above, but *do not* use pralidoxime
Arsenic	(see Heavy metals)	
Atropine	(see Anticholinergics)	
Belladonna alkaloids	(see Anticholinergics)	
Cadmium	(see Heavy metals)	
Carbon monoxide		100% oxygen by inhalation. Consider hyperbaric oxygen in severe or comatose patients.
Cholinergic compounds	(see Anticholinesterases)	
Copper	(see Heavy metals)	
Cyanide		100% oxygen by inhalation. Consider hyperbaric oxygen in severe or comatose patients. Adult: amyl nitrite inhalation (inhale for 15–30 sec q 60 sec) pending administration of 300 mg sodium nitrite (10 mL of a 3% solution) IV slowly (over 2–4 min); follow immediately with 12.5 g sodium thiosulfate (2.5–5 mL/min of 25% solution) IV slowly (over 10 min) Children: (sodium nitrite should not exceed recommended dose as fatal methemoglobinemia may result). Use the following table as a guide:

Hemoglobin	Initial dose 3% Na nitrite IV	Initial dose 25% Na thiosulfate IV
8g	0.22 mL (6.6 mg/kg)	1.10 mL/kg
10 g	0.27 mL (8.7 mg/kg)	1.35 mL/kg
12 g	0.33 mL (10. mg/kg)	1.65 mL/kg
14 g	0.39 mL (11.6 mg/kg)	1.95 mL/kg

Poison	Local antidote	Systemic antidote
Ethylene glycol	(see Methanol)	
Fluoride	Calcium gluconate or lactate, 150 mg/kg, or milk	Calcium gluconate, 10 mL of 10% solution, given slowly IV until symptoms abate; may be repeated prn.
Gold	(see Heavy metals)	

Table 10—Continued

Poison	Local antidote	Systemic antidote
Heavy metals		BAL (dimercaprol): 3–5 mg/kg/dose deep IM q 4 hr for 2 days, q 4–6 hr for an additional 2 days, then q 4–12 hr for up to 7 additional days
Metal	Usual chelators used	EDTA: 75 mg/kg 24 hr deep IM or slow IV infusion given in 3–6 divided doses for up to 5 days: may be repeated for a second course after a minimum of 2 days; each course should not exceed a total of 500 mg/kg
Arsenic	BAL	
Cadmium	Satisfactory use not demonstrated	
Copper	BAL, penicillamine	
Gold	BAL	
Lead	BAL, EDTA, penicillamine, succimer	
Mercury	BAL, penicillamine	
Silver	Satisfactory use not demonstrated	Penicillamine: 100 mg/kg/day (max 1 g) PO in divided doses for up to 5 days; for long-term therapy do not exceed 40 mg/kg/day
Thallium	Prussian blue	
Hypochlorites	(see Alkali, caustic)	
Iron		Deferoxamine, 20–40 mg/kg IV given as slow drip over 4 hr period not to exceed 15 mg/kg/hr; followed by 20 mg/kg every 4–8 hrs until urine color normal or iron level normal. (Can give 20 mg/kg IM every 4–12 hr if no IV sites available)
Isoniazid	Activated charcoal	Pyridoxine (vitamin B_6) 1 mg/mg of isoniazid ingested in divided doses given slow IV (5–10% concentration in 5% dextrose in water over 30–60 min). If amount of isoniazid is unknown, give 5 g IV over 30 minutes. Use benzodiazepines to control seizures.
Lead	(see Heavy metals)	
Mercury	(see Heavy metals)	
Methanol		Ethanol, loading dose to achieve blood level of 100 mg/dL. Adult: 0.6 g/kg + 7–10 g to be infused IV over 1 hr. Child: 0.6 g/kg + 4–5 g to be infused IV over 1 hr. Maintenance doses should approximate 10 g/hr in adults and 5 g/hr in children, to be adjusted to maintain a blood ethanol level of 100 mg/dL.
Methemoglobinemic agents Nitrites Chlorates Nitrobenzene		Methylene blue, 1–2 mg (0.1–0.2 mL/kg) of a 1% solution IV slowly over 5–10 min if cyanosis is severe (or methemoglobin level is greater than 40%). May be repeated every 4 hr.
Narcotics	Activated charcoal	Naloxone, 0.4–0.8 mg IV, IM or SC. If respiratory depression, give 2 mg. Repeat as necessary.
Nitrites	(see Methemoglobinemic agents)	
Oxalate (hypocalcemic tetany)	Dilute with water or milk, then give calcium glouconate or lactate, 150 mg/kg	Calcium gluconate, 10 mL of 10% solution, given slowly IV until symptoms abate; may be repeated prn
Phenothiazines (neuro-muscular reaction only)		Diphenhydramine, 1–2 mg/kg IM or IV; or benztropine, 1–2 mg IM or IV
Physostigmine	(see Anticholinesterases)	
Silver	(see Heavy metals)	
Thallium	(see Heavy metals)	
Tricyclic antidepressants	(see Anticholinergics)	
Warfarin		Vitamin K_1, 0.5–1.0 mg/kg IV, IM or SC Adults: 10 mg Children: 1–5 mg

For envenomation

Animals	Antivenin[a]
Snake, Crotalidae (all North American rattlers and moccasins)	Antivenin (Crotalidae) Polyvalent (*Wyeth*)
Snake, Coral	Antivenin (Microurus fulvius, monovalent (*Wyeth*)
Spider, Black Widow	Antivenin, Latrodectus mactans (*MSD*)

NOTE: All antisera should be tested for sensitivity to horse serum.
[a] See package insert for dosage and administration.

alcohols, acetaminophen and iron. Additional drugs may be regulated similarly by the time of this publication. For the benefit of the elderly and infirm, the law provides that a single size of regulated products may, at the request of the consumer or prescribing physician, be packaged in conventional containers which are labeled as being intended for households without young children.

While the manufacturer provides the safety packaging for OTC drugs, the pharmacist is responsible for complying with the regulations for prescription products which are repackaged, and plays a key role in implementation of this important poisoning prevention measure. Not only may he be the one to select and employ appropriate packaging for prescription items, but he is in an excellent position to promote effectiveness of the Act. It can succeed only to the extent that purchasing adults accept and use the special packaging. The pharmacist should assure that people are aware of the availability of such packaging for regulated products, that they are instructed as to its importance and proper use and that substitutions of conventional packaging are restricted to legitimate and informed requests. This is particularly important as long as reversible or dual function closures are used, since their comparative safety has yet to be demonstrated.

Poison-Control Centers—The poison-control concept was initiated in Chicago in 1953. Following the impetus of local health officials, pediatricians and other interested physicians, a single center for collecting product data was established. The idea soon caught on and numerous other centers were established. In order to provide a coordinating agency for these centers, the then Bureau of Product Safety in the FDA established the National Clearinghouse for Poison Control Centers. This clearinghouse served as a center for collecting and standardizing product toxicology data and for distributing this data in the form of 5 by 8″ index cards to recognized poison control centers. State health departments were given the responsibility for identifying poison centers within their states. The great interest in poison control eventually resulted in over 580 officially recognized poison-control centers and numerous additional unofficial centers, including drug-information services, bringing the total to well over 600. Unfortunately, many poison centers have had little if any capability for providing sophisticated information or treatment for poisoning, handling as few as one call per week.

From the beginning, studies of poison-control center operation demonstrated a wide variability in the manner by which services were provided. Some centers provide information solely to physicians or health care facilities while others provide information to the public or both. Staffing of poison control centers likewise was quite variable. The staff of a poison center may consist only of full- or part-time clerks, nurses or pharmacists without any direct medical supervision, or they may consist of a full-time clinical toxicologist-medical director and specially trained full-time professional staff, such as clinical pharmacists or nurses. Other centers may include pharmacologists, emergency room physicians, ambulatory pediatricians or other scientifically trained personnel as staff or consultants.

The questions facing the poison-control center movement, now in the 5th decade following its inception, are how best to provide services, how to improve services, how to standardize or monitor services, to whom to provide services and how to organize such services on a regional or national basis. The question of how to organize these services has been resolved to a great degree over these past several years. In the author's view, as well as others, consolidation of manpower and resources into centralized or regional services is crucial. In centralized or regional poison control centers, sophisticated information can be provided both to health professionals and to the public. Treatment facilities are generally an integral part of the regional poison control center, and the staff, particularly the medical staff, can provide the treatment for poisoning victims. In addition, active supervision and even bedside consultation of poisoning cases admitted to other health-care facilities ought to be provided.

There probably should be some 75 to 100 regional programs in the US. A regional poison-control center should be one which, in less densely populated areas, serves a single or multistate region or, in heavily populated areas, serves a portion of a state. Generally, a regional center will be found serving no fewer than 1 million people, but could serve as many as 5 to 10 million people in areas of high population density. A regional center would provide

Comprehensive poison information, both to health professionals and consumers.
Comprehensive poisoning treatment services.
A toll-free communication system.
Access to a full range of analytical toxicological services.
Access to transportation facilities for critically ill patients.
Professional and public education programs.
Collection and dissemination of poisoning experience data.

In essence, these regional centers would be capable of assuming ultimate responsibility for the provision of poisoning consultations and patient care for all poisonings brought to its attention within its region which include the functions mentioned above. The AAPCC has developed standards for regional poison-control centers and provides a process to evaluate a poison center's capabilities and designate centers as "regional poison centers." The types of services and equipment recommended for various types of centers are described in more detail in references noted in the *Bibliography*.

National Poison Prevention Week—Since 1962 the 3rd week of March has been designated National Poison Prevention Week. In addition to giving annual emphasis to the problem of poison control, this week provides an opportunity for concentrated educational efforts directed to the public. Pharmacists can and should play an active role in the activities of this period. Special displays in pharmacies have been one type of effective weapon. Other worthwhile activities have included television or radio messages, special meetings and newspaper articles, all of which can be made more effective by interested pharmacists. By joining forces with the regional or local poison control centers, this week can be used to highlight the year-round educational activities of the center and the community.

Role of the Pharmacist—There is much that the pharmacist can do to help prevent poisoning and improve the treatment thereof. Indeed, it often is the pharmacist of a hospital or medical group who initiates the development of adequate facilities and materials for the treatment of cases.

Undoubtedly, the most important role can be played by the pharmacist in the area of prevention. This role, relative to poison-prevention packaging of prescription drugs, was mentioned above. However, the role of the pharmacist is particularly critical with regard to nonprescription items. With prescription medications there is involvement of a physician who may provide instructions and precautionary advice. However, with OTC materials, the pharmacist is often the only person who is in a position to serve these functions.

The pharmacist can and should provide, explain and amplify directions for proper use of potentially toxic materials, bearing in mind that the concern is not only for the safety of the patient but also for other individuals in the household. Thus, the dispensing of a toxic medication provides an opportunity to warn the buyer about the hazards of leaving the material within reach of children.

In some instances it is desirable to affix warning labels on the products that a pharmacist dispenses or to hand out patient information materials. The dispensing of a drug also provides an opportunity to inquire and give advice about facilities for safe storage. Because of this contact with his patrons the pharmacist can play a personalized role in cautioning about prescription and of commercial products.

The pharmacist can do much to reduce the aforementioned limitations of labeling. While the public often may not read or appreciate precautions on labels, the effectiveness of the latter are increased significantly if they are explained by a pharmacist. He also has a unique role to play in detecting product or labeling defects and an obligation to call to the attention of appropriate manufacturers or regulatory agencies potential labeling or product defects.

As indicated, there has been a tendency in the past for the development of too many small and ineffectual poison centers, the activities of which could be carried out more effectively and efficiently if they were amalgamated with others in the same area. A trend toward centralization and regionalization of poison information and treatment facilities should be encouraged by local pharmacy associations.

Finally, pharmacists can assist greatly in the educational efforts of a community by distributing literature provided by himself or by the local medical or pharmaceutical societies, and by providing space for displays related to poisoning prevention.

Reference

1. Litovitz TL *et al*: 1991 annual report of the American Association of Poison Control Center's National Data Collection System. *Am J Emerg Med 10:* 452–505, 1992.

Bibliography

Ellenhorn MJ, Barcleoux DG: *Medical Toxicology. Diagnosis and Treatment of Human Poisoning.* Elsevier, New York, 1988.

Goldfrank LR *et al*, eds: *Goldfrank's Toxicologic Emergencies*, 3rd ed, Appleton Century Crofts, Norwalk, CT, 1988.

Haddad LM, Winchester JF, eds: *Clinical Management of Poisoning and Drug Overdose*, 2d ed, Saunders, Philadelphia, 1990.

Henretig FM, Cupit GC, Temple AR, Collins M: Toxicologic emergencies. In Fleisher G, Ludwig S, eds: *Textbook of Pediatric Emergency Medicine*, Williams & Wilkins, Baltimore, 1988.

Litovitz TL, Manoguerra AS: Comparison of pediatric poisoning hazards: An analysis of 3.8 million poisoning incidents. *Pediatrics* 89:999, 1992.

Manoguerra AS: The poison information telephone call. In Haddad LM and Winchester JF, eds. *Clinical Management of Poisoning and Drug Overdose*, 2d ed, Saunders, Philadelphia, 1990.

Manoguerra AS: The status of poison control centers in the United States–1989: A report from the American Association of Poison Control Centers. *Vet Human Toxicol 33:*131, 1991.

Manoguerra AS, Temple AR: Observations on the current status of poison control centers in the United States. *Emer Med Clin No Am 2:*185, 1984.

Rumack BH *et al*, eds: *Poisindex*, Micromedex, Denver CO, 1989.

Temple AR: *Ann Rev Pharmacol Toxicol 17:* 215, 1977.

Temple AR: Poison prevention education. *Pediatrics 5:* 964, 1984.

Temple AR: History and present status of American poison control centers. *Vet Human Toxicol 24* (Suppl): 2, 1982.

Temple AR, Mancini RE: Management of poisoning. In Yaffe SJ, ed, *Pediatric Pharmacology*, Grune & Stratton, New York, 1980.

Temple AR, Veltri JC: One year's experience in a regional poison control center. *Clin Toxicol 12:* 277, 1978.

Veltri JC, Temple AR: Telephone management of poisonings using syrup of ipecac. *Ibid 9:* 407, 1976.

CHAPTER 110

Laws Governing Pharmacy

Joseph L Fink III, BS Pharm, JD
Associate Vice Chancellor for Academic Affairs
University of Kentucky
Lexington, KY 40506

Larry M Simonsmeier, BS Pharm, JD
Professor of Pharmacy Law
College of Pharmacy, Washington State University
Pullman, WA 99164

Pharmacists—whether a community practitioner, employed by an institution or employed by a pharmaceutical manufacturer—must be aware of the legal requirements which apply to their daily professional activities. The laws pertaining to the practice of pharmacy may come from different sources, eg, FDA, State Board of Pharmacy, DEA, etc. Moreover, laws may appear in different forms, such as statutes, regulations or court decisions.

There are various types of law. Civil law governs the relationship between individuals within society, whereas criminal law governs the relationship of the individual to society as a whole. Two important subdivisions of civil law are the law of contracts and tort law. The former concerns relationships which the individuals enter into voluntarily, while the latter embodies relationships which exist automatically by virtue of law. Moreover, judicial law is that which results from court decisions, whereas statutes result from action by the legislature. Regulations are promulgated by administrative agencies to enhance enforcement and understanding of statutes. Each type of law is applicable to pharmacists and pharmacy practice.

Laws Governing the Practice of Pharmacy

State Laws

The regulation of the practice of pharmacy is primarily a function of the states and not of the Federal Government. It rests upon the power vested in the state to protect the health, safety and welfare of its citizens.

Like every profession, the practice of pharmacy is a privilege bestowed by the state under the constitutional reservation of "police powers." However, this is a privilege available to a class of persons who satisfy stated minimal qualifications. No one may practice pharmacy without a license, except for those exempted by specification within the act. However, anyone may achieve such licensure by successfully completing the statutory pattern of qualification which the state has established and administered by an agency generally termed a board of pharmacy. In some instances the board of pharmacy is a subagency in that it exists as part of a larger state agency, such as a department of health or licensing.

Once licensure is gained it may not be taken lightly by either the state or the licentiate. The former may suspend, revoke or terminate it after due process and for just cause as set out in the act. At the same time, the state undertakes to protect the public and the licensed pharmacists from practice by unlicensed (hence, unqualified) parties in its jurisdiction.

As to licensed pharmacists, they have gained a profession the practice of which is safeguarded by the federal and state constitutions as a property right. While they must abide by the act to preserve it, must pay fees required to accomplish initial and continuing registration, must satisfy the legal, moral and ethical standards of their peers, as set out in law and regulations, they do have the right to legal redress against any who would seek unjustifiably to deprive them of the benefits and prerogatives of licensure. Pharmacy practice acts specifically must identify the conduct for which sanctions can be imposed.

While pharmacy laws of the different states may vary among themselves, they are in agreement with respect to the fundamental principles, purposes, aims and objectives of pharmaceutical practice.

Pharmacy laws generally provide for

1. The educational and experiential qualifications which pharmacists must meet at the time of examination or registration.
2. The agency, usually known as the State Board of Pharmacy, charged with enforcement and administration of the law.
3. The granting of permits for the conduct of a community pharmacy. In most states permits are issued for 1 year and application must be made for their renewal.
4. Periodic reregistration of pharmacists. In most states, certificates of registration are granted for the period of 1 year.
5. The conditions under which certificates of registration or pharmacy licenses may be canceled or revoked.
6. The prominent display of the certificate of registration in the pharmacy in which the holder is employed.
7. Penalties for violations. Infractions of pharmacy laws are punishable by fines or the revocation or suspension of a license. Some state laws specify that violations of the pharmacy act are punishable as a misdemeanor.
8. Reciprocal registration. A pharmacist licensed by examination in one state may, by conforming to more or less nominal rules, become registered in another state, the latter registration being without full examination.
9. The discretion vested in boards of pharmacy. While the board is authorized to make rules and regulations for the enforcement and administration of the pharmacy law, such rules and regulations must be strictly in accord with the expressed or implied purposes of the law. The board is an administrative, not a legislative, agency. It may not exercise any power or authority not clearly delegated to it.

Every state has a pharmacy practice act which regulates the profession, but there is significant variation in the detail of these acts from state to state. Many of the states' statutes are antiquated, with amendments being added in a haphazard manner. Many of these early acts regulated a profession which primarily was product-oriented and involved in the preparation of dosage forms.

Nuclear pharmacy, clinical pharmacy and drug-product selection are just some of the more recent developments to have an impact upon the regulation of the profession. These developments, along with the need to provide more uniformity among the states, caused the National Association of Boards of Pharmacy to develop a Model State Pharmacy Practice Act. This is intended to provide a greater degree of uniformity but still offer flexibility to the states which adopt it. A number of states are considering either the Act or variations of it.

The NABP's Model State Pharmacy Practice (MSPPA) Act will be reviewed here to afford the reader an example of the overall objectives and purposes of state pharmacy acts. Although the format will be similar to the laws of many states, the pharmacist must be versed in the statutory and regulatory requirements of his own state.

The quoted paragraphs set forth below are taken verbatim either from the MSPPA or from various state pharmacy acts. The source of the quoted paragraph is given in each instance.

Title

The title is an important part of all bills submitted to the legislature. The title must, in a very precise sense, give the purpose of the measure.

"An Act relating to the regulation of the practice of pharmacy, including the sales, use and distribution of drugs and devices at retail; and amending, revising, consolidating and repealing certain laws relating thereto." (*Pennsylvania Pharmacy Act*)

Many acts will also designate a "short title" which is a convenient device by which the legislation may be referred to in a brief, concise manner.

"This Act shall be known as the (name of state) Pharmacy Practice Practice Act." (*MSPPA*)

Declaration of Policy and Purpose

While it is not necessary that a legislative act, such as a state pharmacy law, include a declaration of policy and purpose, such declaration often proves advantageous. It is of aid to the court when the constitutionality of the measure is questioned, and also throws much light upon the meaning of the various provisions of the law. Also, it serves to inform the members of the legislature having the measure under consideration of the objectives sought by the passage of the law.

"The Practice of Pharmacy in the State of ____________ is declared a professional practice affecting the public health, safety and welfare and is subject to regulation and control in the public interest. It is further declared to be a matter of public interest and concern that the Practice of Pharmacy, as defined in this Act, merit and receive the confidence of the public and that only qualified persons be permitted to engage in the Practice of Pharmacy in the State of ____________. This Act shall be liberally construed to carry out these objects and purposes. . . .

"It is the purpose of this Act to promote, preserve and protect the public health, safety and welfare by and through the effective control and regulation of the Practice of Pharmacy; the licensure of pharmacists; the licensure, control, and regulation of all sites or persons, in or out of this State that distribute, manufacture, or sell drugs within this State, and the regulation and control of such other materials as may be used in the diagnosis and treatment of injury, illness and disease." (*MSPPA*)

Definitions

Basic definitions are essential to the clarity, administration and enforcement of any law. The comments to the MSPPA indicate that its writers felt that the definition of the "Practice of Pharmacy" was one of the most important clauses.

Many state statutes have become dated in that they limit the practice of pharmacy to the preparation and distribution of a dosage form. The MSPPA includes very broad language to allow boards of pharmacy to promulgate rules and regulations with considerable flexibility as the profession changes to meet future needs.

The "Practice of Pharmacy" means the interpretation, evaluation, and dispensing of prescription drug orders in the patient's best interest; participation in drug and device selection, drug administration, drug regimen reviews and drug or drug-related research; provision of patient counseling and the provision of those acts or services necessary to provide pharmaceutical care; and the responsibility for: compounding and labeling of drugs and devices (except labeling by a manufacturer, repackager, or distributor of non-prescription drugs and commercially packaged legend drugs and devices), proper and safe storage of drugs and devices and maintenance of proper records for them.

Comments to the MSPPA indicate that the "Practice of Pharmacy" definition, as broadly defined, includes the selection of therapeutic agents in accord with institutional protocols or some other legal authority. The definition also encompasses the concept of consulting with, or providing information to, both the prescriber and the patient regarding drug therapy. Patient counseling and pharmaceutical care are further defined in the model rules.

"Patient Counseling" means the oral communication by the pharmacist of information, as defined in the rules of the Board, to the patient or caregiver, in order to improve therapy by ensuring proper use of drugs and devices.

"Pharmaceutical Care" is the provision of drug therapy and other pharmaceutical patient care services intended to achieve outcomes related to the cure or prevention of a disease, elimination or reduction of a patient's symptoms, or arresting or slowing of a disease process as defined in the Rules of the Board.

Other selected definitions from the MSPPA are

" 'Deliver' or 'Delivery' means the actual, constructive or attempted transfer of a drug or device from one person to another, whether or not for a consideration.

" 'Device' means an instrument, apparatus, implement, machine, contrivance, implant, in vitro reagent or other similar or related article, including any component part or accessory, which is required under federal or state law to be prescribed by a Practitioner and dispensed by a Pharmacist.

" 'Dispense' or 'Dispensing' shall mean the preparation and delivery of a prescription drug pursuant to a lawful order of a Practitioner in a suitable container appropriately labeled for subsequent administration to or use by a patient or other individual entitled to receive the prescription drug.

" 'Drug' means: (i) Articles recognized as drugs in any official compendium or any supplement thereto, designated from time to time by the Board; (ii) Articles intended for use in the diagnosis, cure, mitigation, treatment or prevention of disease in humans or other animals; (iii) Articles (other than food) intended to affect the structure or any function of the body of humans or other animals; and (iv) Articles intended for use as a component of any articles specified in clause (i), (ii) or (iii) of this subsection." (*MSPPA*)

The definitions of a device or a drug are similar to those included in the Federal Food, Drug and Cosmetic Act, but their application often will be different under state law as the board of pharmacy is interested primarily in the dispensing aspects of such drugs or devices.

" 'Manufacture' shall mean the production, preparation, propagation, compounding, conversion, or processing of a Device or a Drug, either directly or indirectly by extraction from substances of natural origin or independently by means of chemical or biological synthesis and includes any packaging or repackaging of the substances or labeling or relabeling of its container, and the promotion and marketing of such Drugs or Devices. Manufacturing also includes the preparation and promotion of commercially available products from bulk compounds for resale by pharmacies, practitioners, or other persons. (*MSPPA*)

It often is difficult to determine what constitutes manufacturing. Such a determination often is necessary for purposes of licensing, inspection and other board procedures. The MSPPA has attempted to clarify the definition of manufacturer by excluding those acts by which a pharmacist prepares a preparation in the course of professional practice.

" 'Person' shall mean an individual, corporation, partnership, association or any other legal entity." (*MSPPA*)

This definition of a person is customary as it provides broad coverage without undue repetition and confusing language throughout the Act.

" 'Pharmacist' shall mean an individual licensed by this State to engage in the Practice of Pharmacy.

" 'Practitioner' shall mean an individual currently licensed, registered, or otherwise authorized by the jurisdiction in which he practices to prescribe and administer drugs in the course of his professional practice." (*MSPPA*)

The various states may include a variety of individuals within the definition of a practitioner, such as a podiatrist. The definition of "Practitioner" anticipates that those persons other than pharmacists who are permitted to prescribe and administer drugs will be specifically authorized in other legislation.

Each state pharmacy practice act, as well as state controlled substances legislation, must be examined carefully to determine the legality of pharmacists filling prescription orders written by prescribers in other states. The majority of the states do not prohibit the dispensing of prescription orders which originate out-of-state, but some states prohibit the dispensing of prescriptions from all out-of-state prescribers except those living in "border states." Pharmacists should consult state statutes carefully and with the board of pharmacy to determine the legal status of prescription orders originating in another state.

" 'Prescription Drug or Legend Drug' shall mean a drug which, under Federal Law is required, prior to being dispensed or delivered, to be labeled with either of the following statements: (1) '*Caution:* Federal law prohibits dispensing without prescription' (2) '*Caution:* Federal law restricts this drug to use by or on the order of a licensed veterinarian'; or a drug which is required by any applicable Federal or State law or regulation to be dispensed on prescription only or is restricted to use by practitioners only.

" 'Non Prescription Drugs' shall mean a drug which may be sold without a prescription and which is labeled for use by the consumer in accordance with the requirements of the laws and rules of this State and the Federal Government." (*MSPPA*)

Board of Pharmacy

"The responsibility for enforcement of the provisions of this Act is hereby vested in the Board of Pharmacy. The Board shall have all of the duties, powers and authority specifically granted by and necessary to the enforcement of this Act, as well as such other duties, powers and authority as it may be granted from time to time by appropriate law.

"The Board of Pharmacy shall consist of (______) members . . . (each) of whom shall be licensed pharmacists who possess the qualifications specified. . . ." (*MSPPA*)

The numerical strength of the board varies greatly, and the number of board members will be determined by each individual state according to its particular requirements. In most states, the total number of board members selected is an odd number. The MSPPA also includes a provision by which states may elect to include public member(s). Many state agencies which are responsible for the protection of the public's health, safety and welfare have included public members to assist in the regulatory process.

"The licensed pharmacist members of the Board of Pharmacy shall at the time of their appointment: (1) Be residents of this State for not less than six (6) months; (2) Be licensed and in good standing to engage in the Practice of Pharmacy in this State; (3) Be actively engaged in the Practice of Pharmacy in this State; (4) Have five (5) years of experience in the Practice of Pharmacy in this State after licensure." (*MSPPA*)

Because one of the duties of the board of pharmacy is to pass upon the fitness of applicants to engage in the practice of pharmacy, it generally is required that the board members shall have been engaged actively in pharmacy practice for a designated period of years. The MSPPA contains very broad language to allow a pharmacist involved in almost any area of practice eligible for appointment.

Appointment and Removal—

"The Governor shall appoint the members of the Board of Pharmacy, in accordance with the other provisions of this Section." (*MSPPA*)

The state pharmacy acts customarily provide for the submittal of a list of nominees by any individual, association or other entity to the governor from which he may select the persons to constitute the board of pharmacy. In most states nominations are recommendations only and are not binding on the governor.

Board of pharmacy members most often serve in staggered terms to provide continuity. Many state provisions prevent a member of the board from serving more than two consecutive full terms. The governor will have the authority to fill any vacancies which might arise and also to remove a member of the board pursuant to specified procedures.

"The Governor may remove a member of the Board, pursuant to the procedures set forth in subsection (b) hereinbelow, upon one or more of the following grounds. (1) The refusal or inability for any reason of a Board Member to perform his duties as a member of the Board in an efficient, responsible and professional manner; (2) The misuse of office by a member of the Board to obtain personal, pecuniary or material gain or advantage for himself or another through such office; (3) The violation by any member of the laws governing the Practice of Pharmacy or the distribution of drugs and/or devices." (*MSPPA*)

Executive Director—

"The Board shall employ a pharmacist to serve as a full-time employee of the Board in the position of Executive Director. The Executive Director shall be responsible for the performance of the regular administrative functions of the Board and such other duties as the Board may direct." (*MSPPA*)

As the board is a functioning agency, it must be organized so as to conform to parliamentary usage. Most states will require that the secretary or executive director of the board be a licensed pharmacist, but in most instances he will not be a voting member of the board. It also is necessary that the executive officer of the board has his duties defined and specific responsibilities fixed insofar as these can be done by the legislative act.

Meetings—

"The Board of Pharmacy shall meet at least once every (______) months to transact its business. The Board shall meet at such additional times as it may determine. Such additional meetings may be called by the President of the Board or by two-thirds (⅔) of the members of the Board. . . . Notice of all meetings of the Board shall be given in the manner and pursuant to requirements prescribed by the State's Administrative Procedures Act. . . . All Board meetings and hearings shall be open to the public. The Board may, in its discretion and according to law, conduct any portion of its meeting in executive session closed to the public." (*MSPPA*)

As a general rule, meetings of a public agency must be open to all parties. The people of the states do not yield their sovereignty to an agency and, thus, the people have the right to be informed of public business. The open meetings statutes of most states do provide exceptions in which public agencies may meet in closed sessions.

Rules and Regulations—

"The Board of Pharmacy shall make, adopt, amend and repeal such rules and regulations as may be deemed necessary by the Board, from time to time, for the proper administration and enforcement of this Act. Such rules and regulations shall be promulgated in accordance with the procedures specified in the Administrative Procedures Act of this State." (*MSPPA*)

It virtually is impossible for the state legislature to detail clearly all the aspects of regulation of the practice of pharmacy. Therefore, administrative agencies are given the power to make rules and regulations which may modify or interpret the legislative mandate. In promulgating rules and regulations, it is vitally important that the board of pharmacy does not exceed its statutory authority. The power to make rules and regulations must not be used to accomplish that which the legislature has not sanctioned specifically. Most states will have adopted some sort of administrative procedure act which will specify the appropriate constitutionally required procedures for rule-making, conduct of hearings and other board functions. It is vital that the board rely upon the provisions of the administrative procedure act so that it can insure that the public, and any affected individuals, are provided due process of law in the promulgation of rules and in the conduct of hearings.

Duties and Powers—The enabling legislation also should set forth the duties and powers of the board. Specifically, the state board of pharmacy has the power to do the following:

"The licensing by examination or by license transfer of applicants who are qualified to engage in the Practice of Pharmacy under the provisions of this Act; The renewal of licenses to engage in the Practice of Pharmacy; The establishment and enforcement of compliance with professional standards and rules of conduct of pharmacists; The determination and issuance of standards for recognition and approval of schools and colleges of pharmacy whose graduates shall be eligible for licensure in this State, and the specification and enforcement of requirements for practical training, including internship; . . . The enforcement of those provisions of this Act relating to the conduct or competence of pharmacists practicing in this State, and the suspension, revocation or restriction of licenses to engage in the Practice of Pharmacy; The licensure and regulation of the training, qualifications and employment of pharmacy interns, and pharmacy technicians. The right to seize any such drugs, devices and other materials found to be detrimental to the public health and welfare; The specifications of minimum professional and technical equipment, environment, supplies and procedures for the compounding and/or dispensing of such medications, drugs, devices and other materials within the Practice of Pharmacy; The control of the purity and quality of such medications, drugs, devices and other materials within the Practice of Pharmacy; The issuance and renewal of licenses of those persons engaged in the manufacture and distribution of drugs . . . . The Board or its authorized representatives shall also have power to investigate and gather evidence concerning alleged violations of the provisions of this Act or of the rules and regulations of the Board." (*MSPPA*)

Licensure

Qualifications—

"To obtain a license to engage in the Practice of Pharmacy, an applicant for licensure by examination shall: (1) Have submitted a written application in the form prescribed by the Board of Pharmacy; (2) Have attained the age of majority; (3) Be of good moral character; . . . (4) Have graduated and received the first professional undergraduate degree from a school or college of pharmacy which has been approved by the Board of Pharmacy; . . . (5) Have completed an internship or other program which has been approved by the Board of Pharmacy, or demonstrated to the Board's satisfaction experience in the Practice of Pharmacy which meets or exceeds the minimum internship requirements of the Board; (6) Have successfully passed an examination given by the Board of Pharmacy; (7) Paid the fees specified by the Board of Pharmacy for examination and issuance of license." (*MSPPA*)

Each state may exercise its police powers by determining the qualifications necessary for an individual to obtain a pharmacy license. It is likely that there will be a substantial degree of similarity among the various state laws regarding qualifications, but each act should be examined by the applicant.

With the increasing trend to lower the age of majority, it is likely that many states will simply require the applicant be 18 years of age. Those individuals who apply for a pharmacy license must be of good moral character. The case law in this area indicates a tremendous variation by the courts as to what constitutes "good moral character." Although it is expected that professional boards will continue to have the authority to inquire as to moral character of the applicant, they must be careful that their inquiry reasonably is related to the protection of the public's health and safety.

One could expect that an applicant for pharmacy licensure must be a graduate of an accredited college of pharmacy. Although the programs of US pharmacy schools are accredited by the American Council on Pharmaceutical Education (ACPE), the board may not delegate the accrediting function to this private organization. The comments to the MSPPA indicate that it is contemplated that boards will accredit those schools with programs whose standards are at least equivalent to the minimum standards required by the ACPE, but it is important that the government agency make its own determinations regarding accreditation, rather than direct reliance upon the private organization.

A requirement that the applicant be a citizen of the US is unconstitutional under existing case law. Such a requirement would deprive non-citizens of the equal protection of the law under the US Constitution.

A variety of internship, externship and clinical clerkship programs have developed in the various states. While the states generally require some sort of internship training, the programs and duration of experience vary among the states. Six-months or 1-year experiences are common. There is an increasing emphasis by the ACPE for colleges of pharmacy to include a substantial portion of the required internship hours within the curriculum of the school.

An examination also is a necessary prerequisite prior to licensure. All but a few states administer the NABPLEX Standard Examination which was developed through the auspices of the National Association of Boards of Pharmacy (NABP). The NABPLEX examination consists of a combined format which determines a candidate's competency to practice through an integrated test, rather than dividing the material into separate subject areas. A national jurisprudence exam also has been introduced, but its use is optional.

Reciprocity—As an alternative to licensure by examination, some applicants also may seek licensure by the reciprocal or license transfer process. Such an applicant must

"Have possessed at the time of initial licensure as a pharmacist all qualifications necessary to have been eligible for licensure at that time in this State; Have engaged in the Practice of Pharmacy for a period of at least one (1) year or have met the internship requirements of this State within the one (1) year period immediately previous to the date of such application; Have presented to the Board proof of initial licensure by examination and proof that such license and any other license or licenses granted to the applicant by any other state or states have not been suspended, revoked, cancelled or otherwise restricted for any reason except non-renewal or the failure to obtain required continuing education credits in any state where the applicant is licensed but not engaged in the Practice of Pharmacy." (*MSPPA*)

At the present time, not all states require 1 year of licensure in order to be eligible to be licensed by reciprocity. However, an applicant will not be eligible for licensure by reciprocity unless the state in which the applicant was licensed initially also grants reciprocal licensure to those from the state wherein the applicant seeks to be registered. At the present time, reciprocity is available from all boards of pharmacy except California and Florida.

The NABP acts as a clearinghouse for the reciprocal process. The applicant provides information to the NABP which in turn verifies these facts relating to licensure and provides that information to the reciprocating state. The reciprocating state reviews the application, and it is highly likely that before it will issue a license it will require the applicant to pass an examination on state laws.

Renewal—In the majority of the states, certificates of licensure expire annually, but may be renewed upon the payment of a specific fee. An increasing number of states require proof that the pharmacist has completed satisfactorily an accredited program of continuing education prior to the issuance of the renewal certificate. It is beneficial if the legislature mandates a continuing-education requirement by statute. The board of pharmacy then may adopt rules and regulations to carry out the objectives and purposes of the statute.

Discipline

As one would expect, the board of pharmacy also is endowed with the power to refuse or revoke the license of those individuals who have failed to exhibit fitness to practice the profession of pharmacy. In order to safeguard the public's health and safety, the board may find it necessary to permanently or temporarily discipline unfit practitioners. The board also has an important role to assist and educate wrongdoers to prevent recurrences of the errant behavior.

The Board of Pharmacy may refuse to issue or renew, or may suspend, revoke or restrict the licenses of any person, pursuant to the procedures set forth in Section 402 herein below, upon one or more of the following grounds: (1) Unprofessional conduct as that term is defined by the rules of the Board; (2) Incapacity of a nature that prevents a pharmacist from engaging in the Practice of Pharmacy with reasonable skill, competence and safety to the public; (3) Being found guilty by a court of competent jurisdiction of one (1) or more of the following: (i) A felony; (ii) Any act involving moral turpitude or gross immorality; or (iii) Violations of the pharmacy or drug laws of this State or rules and regulations of any other state, or of the federal government; (4) Fraud or intentional misrepresentation by a licensee in securing the issuance or renewal of a license; (5)

Engaging or aiding and abetting an individual to engage in the Practice of Pharmacy without a license, or falsely using the title of pharmacist; (6) Being found by the Board to be in violation of any of the provisions of this Act or rules and regulations adopted pursuant to this Act." (*MSPPA*)

Moral turpitude, unprofessional conduct and gross immorality may be terms which defy definition. However, the board of pharmacy must make every attempt to set forth, by rule and regulation, that which is being legislated against. The pharmacist should be able to understand reasonably the type of conduct which is being discouraged. The board of pharmacy will have at its disposal, as per the legislative enactment, the authority to suspend, revoke or restrict the offender's license. In addition, the board may be able to impose a fine for each offense and also may place the offender on probation for a stated period of time. None of these board-imposed penalties would bar a criminal prosecution on behalf of the state for the violations of the Pharmacy Practice Act if the violations were criminal in nature.

Licensing of Facilities

In most states community, as well as institutional, pharmacies may be operated only under permits issued by the board of pharmacy. State law normally will require an annual fee, provisions for inspection of the premises, proper prescription records and the maintenance of certain minimums of equipment or stock. Nonprescription or proprietary medicines usually may be sold in any establishment, and the sale need not be made by licensed pharmacists. However, some states do require such a nonpharmacy outlet to obtain a permit from the state board of pharmacy in order to sell OTC preparations.

The licensure of facilities provides a board with knowledge of all premises involved in the storage, distribution and sale of drugs and devices within the state and those located outside the state which are shipping drugs into the state. These requirements permit a board better to insure against drug diversion from legitimate channels of commerce.

Few states have ownership restrictions on pharmacies. Some states have attempted to legislate against physician-owned pharmacies or any other type of nonpharmacist-owned pharmacies. The US Supreme Court in 1928 held that laws restricting pharmacy ownership only to pharmacists violated the Fourteenth Amendment of the US Constitution. Forty-four years later, the same issue again was raised in the North Dakota courts. The North Dakota Pharmacy Act required that the majority of stock of a pharmacy corporation be owned by registered pharmacists in good standing in North Dakota. The statute was challenged by an out-of-state chain operation, and the case eventually was appealed to the US Supreme Court. The nation's highest court reversed its earlier decision and held that pharmacy-ownership laws were constitutionally sound if such a requirement could be related reasonably to the public's health and welfare. The case was returned to the North Dakota Supreme Court and that court identified seven possible reasons for ownership restrictions:

1. The professional and ethical standards of pharmacy demand the pharmacist's concern for the quantity and quality of stock and equipment. A drug which has deteriorated because of improper storage can be a detriment to public health. A drug not in stock poses a threat to the individual who needs it now. Decisions made in conjunction with the quantity and quality of stock and equipment by nonregistered pharmacist-owners could be detrimental to the public health and welfare.
2. Supervision of hired pharmacists by registered-pharmacist-owners would be in the best interests of public health and safety.
3. Responsibility for improper action could be pinpointed more readily when supervision is in registered pharmacist-owners.
4. The dignity of a profession, and the morale and proficiency of those licensed to engage therein, is enhanced by prohibiting the practitioner from subordinating himself to the direction of untrained supervisors.
5. If control and management is vested in laymen unacquainted with pharmaceutical service, who are untrained and unlicensed, the risk is that social accountability will be subordinated to the profit motive.
6. The term "pharmacy" was intended to identify a particular type of establishment within which a health profession is practiced, and thus was intended to be more than a mere means of making a profit. He who holds the purse strings controls the policy.
7. Doctor-owned pharmacies with built-in conflict-of-interest problems could be restricted.

Although this case cleared the way for state legislatures to develop restrictions on the ownership of pharmacies, there has not been a great deal of momentum in this area. Consumer groups and large national pharmacy corporations have lobbied successfully against such proposals.

Miscellaneous State Provisions

Institutional Pharmacy—The NABP also has developed model rules for institutional pharmacy. These regulations may be applied to facilities such as a hospital, nursing home, psychiatric center, health maintenance organization and others. These regulations include special provisions for the distribution of drugs when the institutional pharmacy is unattended by a licensed pharmacist. The model rules include provisions for night cabinets, emergency kits, investigational drugs, quality assurance and other items which particularly are applicable to the institutional practice of pharmacy.

Nuclear Pharmacy—Nuclear pharmacy, recognized as the first specialty area in the profession, also may have special regulations at the state level. Most regulations make it unlawful for any person to provide radiopharmaceutical services unless under the supervision of a qualified nuclear pharmacist.

"A qualified nuclear pharmacist shall: (a) Be a currently licensed pharmacist in the state; and (b) Be certified as a nuclear pharmacist by the State Board of Pharmacy or by a certification board recognized by the Board of Pharmacy; or (c) Meet the following standards: (1) Meet minimal standards of training for medical uses or radioactive material (cite radiological control agency or NRC licensure guide); (2) Have received a minimum of 200 contact hours of instruction in nuclear pharmacy from a program approved by the Board of Pharmacy; (3) Attain a minimum of 500 hours of clinical nuclear pharmacy training under the supervision of a qualified nuclear pharmacist. (*MSPPA*)

Pharmaceutical Care—The NABP has developed comprehensive model rules to implement the patient-care concepts embodied in the definition of the "practice of pharmacy." The rules provide for the age-old requirements of a prescription-drug order with provisions for the electronic transmittal of the prescription to the pharmacist. The transfer of prescriptions between pharmacies also is addressed in these rules.

The model rules include provisions for drug-product selection, prescription labeling and patient records. These sections provide an important background for the central focus of the pharmaceutical care rules—the requirement for patient counseling and prospective drug review by the pharmacist. Following a review of the patient's records for therapeutic duplication, drug interactions, over or underutilization and a number of other considerations, the pharmacist personally shall initiate discussion with the patient or the patient's caregiver regarding the prescription.

All states that intend to remain in compliance with Federal Medicaid requirements will need to adopt some form of patient counseling. The Omnibus Budget Reconciliation Act (OBRA) of 1990 provides that pharmacists must offer to counsel, in person or by telephone, all Medicaid recipients who receive prescription drugs. The model rules provide a framework for the states to adopt so that the concepts of pharmaceutical care might be extended to all patients, not just those on Medicaid.

Computer Regulations—Computerization has become an important component of the profession as more and more pharmacies keep a wide variety of records on computers. Model rules have been developed by the NABP for states who wish to use them to facilitate the inspection of pharmacies employing computers. These computer systems must have adequate security and systems safeguards to maintain the confidentiality of patients and to prevent unauthorized access or manipulation of patient-profile data.

The computer system must provide for on-line retrieval (via CRT display or hard-copy printout) of original information for those prescription orders which are currently authorized for refilling.

"The computerized system shall have the capability of producing a printout of any prescription-drug order information. The systems should provide a refill-by-refill audit trail for any specified strength and dosage form of any drug. Such an audit trail must be by printout, and include name of the prescribing practitioner, name and location of the patient, quantity dispensed on each refill, date of dispensing of each refill, name or identification code of the dispensing pharmacist and unique identifier of the prescription." *(MSPPA)*

The model rules also provide for special backup procedures when the automated system becomes temporarily inoperative. This auxiliary system must insure that all refills are authorized and that the maximum number of refills is not exceeded, and it must be maintained until the automated system becomes operational. The proposed model rules provide that nothing shall preclude the pharmacist from using professional judgment for the benefit of the patient's health and safety when the computerized system is not working. When the computer returns to operation, all information regarding prescriptions filled and refilled during the inoperative period must be entered into the computer within 96 hours.

Prophylactics—It also is likely that the states will have regulated the sale of prophylactics. Special retail permits often will be required. There is a wide variance among the states as to the type of outlet licensed to sell prophylactics. Statutes which restrict the sale to pharmacies will be found unconstitutional unless the state can support such a limitation. With an increase in the number of cases of AIDS and sexually transmitted diseases being reported, many states are expanding the categories of those who may hold a permit to sell prophylactics to pharmacies, hospitals, family-planning programs, venereal disease prevention and treatment programs and to vending-machine operations. The First Amendment to the US Constitution has been interpreted to permit the advertising and display of prophylactic devices.

Hypodermic Needles and Syringes—Some states permit the sale of hypodermic needles and syringes by the pharmacist on an over-the-counter (OTC) basis. The pharmacist of course must use good professional discretion to insure that the devices are not to be used illegally. Other states will require that these devices be sold only upon a physician's order. This provision has been modified in some states to permit their sale without a prescription order when they are to be used by diabetics, for the administration of adrenalin or for veterinary use. In these latter cases a registry is often required as evidence of the OTC sale.

The Federal Food, Drug and Cosmetic Act

The first attempt by the US government to regulate the quality of drugs occurred during 1848. The government had discovered that adulterated quinine was being supplied for use by American troops in Mexico. In 1906, Congress enacted the first federal statute designed to regulate drug products manufactured domestically.

The Food and Drug Act of 1906 required that drugs marketed in interstate commerce meet their professed minimal standards of strength, purity and quality. This law did not attempt to regulate therapeutic claims for medication. Labeling was first regulated by the Sherley Amendment to the Act, which Congress enacted during 1912. Here the term "misbranded" was used first in drug regulation to refer to fraudulent or false claims of therapeutic effects. A deficiency in this revision was that to establish a violation, the enforcement agency was required to show deliberate fraud.

In 1938 further amendments were made as the result of a firm's marketing a product using diethylene glycol as a vehicle for sulfanilamide. Approximately 40 people were killed by the formulation, so Congress acted to require that a product be shown to be safe before it could be distributed in interstate commerce. However, there was a grandfather clause included in the revision which provided that anything that was on the market prior to enactment of the amendment could continue to be marketed, unless challenged by the FDA.

During the 1940s the FDA began to use internal regulations to establish categories of prescription and nonprescription drugs. The process did not work very well, so in 1951, Senator Hubert Humphrey, a pharmacist from Minnesota, and Congressman Carl Durham, a pharmacist from North Carolina, sponsored legislation to establish clear criteria for such decisions.

In 1962 the Act again was amended to require that drug products, both prescription and nonprescription, be shown to be effective, as well as safe. Once again a grandfather clause was included, covering drugs marketed prior to 1938. However, every product marketed between 1938 and 1962 was now subject to the safety and efficacy requirements. At this time provisions were added to the Act concerning factory inspections and investigational drugs and responsibility for regulating prescription drug advertising was shifted from the Federal Trade Commission to the FDA.

In 1976 the Medical Device Amendments were enacted, representing the first major change in this area since 1938. This amendment substantially increased the regulation of these products.

In 1984 the Drug Price Competition and Patent Term Restoration Act was enacted to facilitate approval of generic versions of established drug products while extending patent protection for pharmaceuticals in certain instances. Due to diversion of medicaments from legitimate channels of distribution, and the resultant risk to patients' health, Congress passed the Prescription Drug Marketing Act of 1987. This latter statute imposed limits on distribution of samples of prescription medications and created strict recordkeeping requirements.

A complete discussion of the provisions of the federal Food, Drug and Cosmetic Act and the regulations promulgated by the FDA for enforcement of the statute likely would be longer than this entire chapter. Consequently, this discussion will focus primarily upon those sections of the Act which are of primary importance to pharmacists. Interested readers may wish to obtain an up-to-date copy of the Act and its effectuating regulations—21 CFR Part 1-end. These may be obtained from the Government Printing Office, Washington DC 20402.

A drug is defined in Section 201(g) of the Act to be an article recognized in the official compendia (*United States Pharmacopeia/National Formulary* or *Homeopathic Pharmacopeia of the United States*), or intended for use in the diagnosis, cure, mitigation, prevention or treatment of disease in man or other animals or intended to alter a bodily function or structure of man or other animal. For purposes of determining the intended use of the drug, reference must be made to the intention of the person labeling the drugs, not the intentions of the purchaser. The same is true in the case of a device, which is an instrument, apparatus, implement or contrivance intended for the same use as a drug. An article may be classified as both a drug and a cosmetic under the Act. Moreover, the distinction between a drug and device under the Act may not be clearcut. For example, is a soft contact lens a drug or a device?

A cosmetic is an item intended to be rubbed, poured, sprinkled or sprayed on, introduced into or otherwise applied to the human body or any part thereof for cleansing, beautifying, promoting attractiveness or altering the appearance. However, the Act specifically excludes soap from the definition of cosmetics. Note that a deodorant would be a cosmetic whereas an antiperspirant may be a drug because it is intended to alter a bodily function.

An important distinction is made in the Act between a label and labeling. A label is a display of written, printed or graphic matter upon the immediate container of the item. Labeling includes the label as well as other written, printed or graphic matter upon the article or any of its containers or wrappers accompanying the item. If information is required to appear on the label, it also must appear on the outside container or wrapper or easily be legible through the container or wrapper. In the case of labeling, it is not necessary that the printed matter directly accompany the item. Literature may be shipped separately and still constitute part of the labeling.

A "new drug" as defined in the Act is one which is not yet generally recognized by medical experts as being safe and effective for the intended use. This might be by virtue of its having a new drug entity as an ingredient, or by having an older chemical ingredient for which a new use, new dosage level or new period of usage is proposed. Sometimes a combination of old drugs in a new dosage form, with claims for use extending beyond those for each ingredient individually, is considered a new drug. Such agents may not be shipped in interstate commerce unless the FDA has approved a New Drug Application (NDA) or Abbreviated New Drug Application (ANDA) for the drug.

However, this provision poses a problem for if the drug cannot be shipped in interstate commerce without being approved by the FDA, how can the drug be tested for safety and efficacy? The Act contains an exemption from the interstate shipment ban for drugs undergoing clinical trials. In order to secure exemption from that provision of the Act, the individual or firm sponsoring the research must apply to the FDA for an exemption by filing an Investigational New Drug (IND) application. Once approved, the drug can be shipped in interstate commerce for testing purposes only. The detailed regulations adopted by the FDA on this topic can be found at 21 CFR 312.

Once the clinical trials have been completed the sponsor may submit an NDA to the FDA. Section 505 of the Act specifies what information must be provided by the sponsor and the basis on which the agency may disapprove the application. At the time of approving the NDA, the FDA determines whether the drug should be available to the public as a nonprescription medication or restricted to prescription-only status. Guidance for this decision can be found in the Durham-Humphrey Amendment of 1951. The applicability of this provision of the Act is restricted to drugs for human use; the standard for restriction of a drug to prescription-only status are

1. The drug is habit-forming.
2. The drug is not safe for self-medication because of its toxicity or other potentiality for harmful effect, or the method of its use or the collateral measures necessary to its use.
3. The drug is a "new drug" which has not been shown to be safe and is restricted to prescription-only distribution by the FDA when it issues the NDA.

The FDA has taken the position that drugs also may be restricted to prescription-only distribution if a layman would not know how to use them properly or because the conditions for which they are used and the diagnostic techniques and collateral therapeutic measures necessary to their use require it. If a drug is to be restricted to prescription-only distribution, the Act requires that its label bear the statement, "Caution—Federal Law Prohibits Dispensing Without Prescription." This phrase is known as the prescription legend and, hence, prescription drugs sometimes are referred to as legend drugs.

Section 301 of the Act sets forth the acts which are prohibited.

1. Introduction or delivery for introduction into interstate commerce of any food, drug, device or cosmetic that is adulterated or misbranded is prohibited.
2. Adulteration or misbranding of any food, drug, device or cosmetic in interstate commerce is violative of the Act.
3. Receipt in interstate commerce of any food, drug, device or cosmetic that is adulterated or misbranded also may subject the individual to the penalties under the Act.

In the landmark case of *United States v Sullivan*, the US Supreme Court stated that under the Act, once something has been in interstate commerce it is considered always to be subject to the interstate jurisdiction of the FDA. Indeed, the Act specifically provides that an article in violation of the Act may be seized at any time while the drug is in interstate commerce or at any time thereafter.

One section of the Act that is of particular interest to pharmacists prohibits alteration, mutilation, destruction, obliteration or removal of the whole or any part of the labeling or the doing of any other act after shipment in interstate commerce which results in the article being adulterated or misbranded. Consequently, the pharmacist may not remove or destroy the label or labeling of a drug product, eg, the package insert.

Refusal to permit entry to an FDA inspector is also a violation of the Act.

The Act is designed to prevent two evils—adulteration and misbranding of products. Adulteration relates to the composition of the product. A drug is deemed to be adulterated if, among other reasons

1. It consists in whole or in part of any filthy, putrid or decomposed substance.
2. It has been prepared, packed or held under insanitary conditions whereby it may have become contaminated with filth or may have been rendered injurious to health.
3. It was manufactured, processed, packed or held under conditions which do not comply with the FDA's current good manufacturing practice (GMP) regulations.
4. Its container is composed of any poisonous or deleterious substance which may render the drug injurious to health.

A drug also will be considered to be adulterated if it purports to meet compendial standards and does not, or if its strength differs from its labeled strength.

Misbranding deals primarily with labeling violations, not the composition of the drug. A drug will be considered to be misbranded if, among other reasons

1. Its labeling is false or misleading in any particular.
2. Its label does not bear the name and address of the manufacturer, packer or distributor as well as an accurate statement of the quantity of the contents.
3. It contains a habit-forming substance specified in the Act or regulations and does not bear the statement "Warning—May Be Habit Forming" directly adjacent to the name of the agent.
4. It does not bear the established name of the agent and, in the case of legend drugs only, the quantity of ingredients.
5. Its labeling does not bear adequate directions for use, unless exempted by FDA, and adequate warnings against use in situations where it may be dangerous to health.
6. It purports to be a drug which meets compendial standards and is not labeled in accordance with compendial standards.
7. Its container is so made, formed or filled as to be misleading.
8. It is an antibiotic or insulin which has not been certified.
9. Its advertising does not meet the standards contained in FDA regulations.
10. It was manufactured or processed in a plant which was not registered with the FDA.
11. Its packaging and labeling are not in conformity with the Poison Prevention Packaging Act of 1970.

Recently, the packaging standards for drug products have been revised. Some drugs must be distributed in containers with "tight" closures and others with "well-closed" caps.

An exemption exists under the Act for the generally applicable labeling requirements when a drug is dispensed pursuant to a prescription. The label of such a drug is required to bear

1. The name and address of the dispenser.
2. The serial number of the prescription and date of its dispensing.
3. The name of the prescriber.
4. The name of the patient, if stated in the prescription.
5. The directions for use and cautionary statements contained in the prescription.

This list in the Act is not intended to be all-inclusive, and the pharmacist may add other truthful information, eg, additional warnings or auxiliary labels bearing messages directed to the patient. It should be emphasized that the requirement that the container "bear" a label has been interpreted to mean that the label be affixed to the *outside* of the container, not inserted *inside* the container.

Also of note is that the labeling and packaging requirements of the Act apply to all who dispense medication, eg, pharmacists, physicians or others.

As noted above, the FDA has the responsibility for enforcement of the federal Food, Drug and Cosmetic Act. Drugs or other articles which violate the Act are subject to seizure by the FDA, and individuals who cause a violation are subject to criminal penalties. Conviction of the first offense under the Act holds the possibility of a fine of up to $1,000 and imprisonment for up to 1 year. Subsequent violations or violations involving an intent to defraud or mislead are punishable by a fine of up to $10,000 and incarceration for up to 3 years for each offense. Note that each act would constitute a separate violation.

Nonprescription Medication—As mentioned above, the Durham-Humphrey Amendment to the Food, Drug and Cosmetic Act embodies the criteria for determining whether a given drug is to be restricted to prescription-only distribution. If a drug does not fall within at least one of those three categories, it is available to the public without a prescription.

Drugs which may be sold legally without a prescription must bear a "7-point label." The elements which must be borne on the label, and the sections of the FDA regulations in which discussion of the requirements can be found, are

1. The name of the product.
2. The name and address of the manufacturer, packer or distributor (21 CFR 201.1).
3. The net contents of the package (21 CFR 201.62).
4. The established name of all active ingredients, and the quantity of certain other ingredients whether active or not, eg, alcohol, potent alkaloids, etc (21 CFR 201.10).
5. The name of any habit-forming drug contained in the preparation (21 CFR 201.10).
6. Cautions and warnings needed for the protection of the user (21 CFR 201.300 et seq).
7. Adequate directions for safe and effective use (21 CFR 201.5).

The most important distinction between nonprescription and prescription medication is based on the availability of "adequate directions for use" under which a layman can use the drug safely and for the purposes for which it is intended.

One issue related to labeling of nonprescription medication is whether a pharmacist must relabel a product which has just been changed from prescription to nonprescription status. The FDA has ruled that former legend drugs which now may be distributed lawfully without a prescription must be relabeled prior to dispensing. The reason for this is that if the drug is still in a package bearing the federal prescription legend, but is lawfully sold without a prescription, the drug is misbranded. Moreover, the labeling requirements which apply to prescription drugs are not the same as those which apply to nonprescription products. Consequently, the former prescription drug probably does not bear all the information required to be on the "7-point label." That, too, would render the drug misbranded. Hence, should a pharmacist wish to distribute a former prescription drug without a prescription, relabeling must occur. The same requirement of relabeling is seen when the pharmacist purchases a large quantity of nonprescription medication and then repackages it in smaller quantities for distribution to the public. All seven points must be included on the label of the repackaged drug.

In 1972 the FDA initiated the Over-the-Counter Drug Review. Nonprescription drugs marketed before 1962 were not required to be shown to be both safe and effective. Rather than review the contents of each of the estimated 100,000 to 500,000 nonprescription products on the market, the agency decided to proceed in a rule-making fashion. The FDA selected panels of experts who reviewed nonprescription drug therapy of 27 categories of drug use, eg, anti- rheumatics, laxatives, antiemetics, etc. When the panel completed its review, it prepared a monograph setting forth the drugs that have been found to be safe and effective for nonprescription use in that area of therapy. Following a period for public comment the monograph was finalized and any product in that therapeutic category which did not meet the standards established in the monograph was subject to FDA sanctions. The FTC is attempting to carry this activity one step further by considering a trade-regulation rule which would prohibit manufacturers or distributors of nonprescription drugs from using any terminology other than that specifically approved in the FDA monograph in its advertising to the public. The OTC Review concluded during the 1980s and it may be several years before the action by the FTC in this area is finalized.

During recent years a number of pharmacy organizations have proposed that a third and fourth class of drug products be established in addition to the currently existing classes of prescription and nonprescription drugs. The third class of drugs would be those which would be available only from a pharmacist and the fourth class of drugs would include those for which a prescription from a licensed prescriber would be required for initiation of therapy but which could be refilled at the professional discretion of the pharmacist.

One additional question which frequently arises is the legal status of refilling a prescription written for a nonprescription medication when no refills have been authorized by the prescriber. The answer turns on the definition of a "prescription" under state law. If it is described as an order for drugs authorized by a licensed practitioner and the statute further states that the pharmacist must have the prescriber's authorization to dispense a prescription, then refilling the prescription probably would not be lawful. Note that this is so even though the patient could merely pick up the same drug from a counter display. On the other hand, if the state statute is phrased differently, then it may be lawful for a pharmacist to refill the prescription because, under the federal scheme of regulation, the drug may be distributed without a prescription.

The Comprehensive Drug Abuse Prevention and Control Act of 1970

The Federal Comprehensive Drug Abuse Prevention and Control Act (Public Law 91-513) became effective on May 1, 1971. Title II of that Act is known as the "Controlled Substances Act" (CSA) and it regulates the manufacture, distribution and dispensing of controlled substances. This law supersedes most previous narcotic and drug-abuse control laws, and places the enforcement of this Act with the Drug Enforcement Administration (DEA), which is part of the US Department of Justice. The DEA has promulgated extensive regulations to implement the Act, and these regulations appear in 21 CFR 1300-end.

The statute provides a "closed" system for virtually every person who legitimately handles controlled substances, other than the ultimate user. Over 500,000 individuals and institutions, such as hospitals, pharmacies, researchers, drug manufacturers and physicians are included in the class of persons subject to direct regulation through registration by the DEA. In addition to replacing or amending the numerous federal laws relating to the control of drugs, the CSA is intended to aid in reducing the widespread diversion of these substances from legitimate channels.

When enacting the CSA Congress no longer relied upon the tax clause of the US Constitution, as had been done in the past. The authority for Congress to enact this legislation was derived from the interstate commerce clause of the Constitution. The power to regulate the health, safety and welfare of the American people has been left primarily within the jurisdiction of the individual states through the "police powers" which were reserved to the states via the Tenth Amendment of the US Constitution. However, Congress determined that the federal control of intrastate incidents of the traffic in controlled substances is essential to the effective control of the interstate incidents of such traffic, and it thereby felt compelled to enter into the regulation of subject matter which previously had been left to the states. It must be remembered that if a provision of state or local law is inconsistent or conflicts with a provision of the CSA, the state or local law must yield to the federal provision. However, if the state or local law augments or strengthens the federal act, the more stringent provision must be followed. In order to provide uniformity with the federal government, the majority of the states have adopted a Uniform Controlled Substances Act.

Important Definitions

The following selected definitions are derived from the CSA or from the DEA regulations. These definitions must be read carefully for their language will affect greatly the use of the words within the Act. The following definitions are those which bear most heavily upon pharmacy practice:

Administer refers to the direct application of a controlled substance to the body of a patient or research subject.

Dispenser means an individual practitioner, an institutional practitioner, pharmacy or pharmacist who dispenses a controlled substance.

Individual practitioner means a physician, dentist, veterinarian or other individual licensed, registered or otherwise permitted, by the US or the jurisdiction in which he practices, to dispense a controlled substance in the course of professional practice, but does not include a pharmacist, a pharmacy or an institutional practitioner.

Institutional practitioner means a hospital or other person (other than an individual) licensed, registered or otherwise permitted, by the US or the jurisdiction in which it practices, to dispense a controlled substance in the course of professional practice, but does not include a pharmacy.

Narcotic drug means any of the following, whether produced directly or indirectly by extraction from substances of vegetable origin, or independently by means of chemical synthesis: (a) opium, coca leaves and opiates; (b) a compound, manufacture, salt, derivative or preparation of opium, coca leaves or opiates; (c) a substance which is chemically identical with any of the substances referred to in a or b.

Person includes any individual, corporation, government or governmental subdivision or agency, business trust, partnership, association or other legal entity.

Pharmacist means any pharmacist licensed by a State to dispense controlled substances, and shall include any other person (eg, pharmacist-intern) authorized by a State to dispense controlled substances under the supervision of a pharmacist licensed by such State.

Prescription means an order for medication which is dispensed to or for an ultimate user but does not include an order for medication which is dispensed for immediate administration to the ultimate user (eg, an order to dispense a drug to a bed patient for immediate administration in a hospital is not a prescription).

Readily retrievable means that certain records are kept by automatic data processing systems or other electronic or mechanized recording systems in such a manner that they can be separated from all other records in a reasonable time and/or records are kept on which certain items are asterisked, redlined or in some other manner visually identifiable apart from other items appearing on the records.

Schedules

The drugs that come under the jurisdiction of the CSA have been categorized according to their potential for abuse and are divided into five schedules. Procedures for controlling a substance under the CSA are set forth in Section 201 of the Act. Proceedings may be initiated by the Department of Health and Human Services (DHHS) by the DEA or by petition of a manufacturer, medical society, pharmaceutical association, public interest group or an individual citizen.

Once the DEA receives a request to control a drug or remove a substance entirely from the schedules, the agency must request the DHHS to conduct a scientific and medical evaluation. The Secretary of the DHHS then consults with the FDA and the other affected agencies regarding recommendations whether the drug or other substance should be controlled or removed from control. The medical and scientific evaluations are binding on the DEA with respect to scientific and medical matters and, if the DHHS recommends that a drug not be controlled, the DEA may not control the substance.

After the DEA receives the DHHS report, it then will proceed to make a final decision. If it has determined to control the drug, a proposal will be published in the *Federal Register* setting forth the proposed schedule and inviting all interested parties to file comments. At this point the affected parties may request a hearing before an administrative law judge. If no hearing is requested, the DEA will evaluate all the comments received and publish a final order in the *Federal Register*.

In reaching a final decision, the DEA is required by the Act to consider a number of factors with respect to each drug proposed to be controlled or removed from the schedules. These include potential for abuse; pharmacological effects; risk to public health; the history, scope, duration and significance of the abuse and the potential for psychic or physiological dependence.

The drugs that come under the jurisdiction of the CSA are divided into five schedules based upon their potential for abuse as follows:

Schedule I

These drugs have a high potential for abuse and no accepted medical use in the US. The three broad categories of substances found in this schedule are the opiates, opium derivatives and hallucinogens. Some examples are heroin, marihuana, LSD, peyote, mescaline, psilocybin, tetrahydrocannabinols (THC) and dihydromorphine and others.

Properly registered persons may use Schedule I substances for research purposes. The FDA has approved the marketing of the THC product, dronabinol (*Marinol*), and the synthetic cannabinoid, nabilone (*Cesamet*), for the treatment of the nausea and vomiting associated with cancer chemotherapy. Both agents have been placed in Schedule II. All other tetrahydrocannabinols and marihuana remain in Schedule I.

Schedule II

These drugs also have a high potential for abuse, but do have a currently accepted medical use in treatment in the US. It has been determined that the abuse of a drug, or other substances included in this schedule, may lead to severe psychological or physical dependence. The broad categories of Schedule II drugs include opiates and opium derivatives, derivatives of coca leaves and certain central nervous system stimulants and depressants. Some examples of Schedule II controlled narcotic substances are opium, morphine, codeine, hydromorphone (*Dilaudid*), methadone (*Dolophine*), pantopon, meperidine (*Demerol*), cocaine, oxycodone (*Percodan*—in combination with aspirin), anileridine (*Leritine*) and oxymorphone (*Numorphan*). Also in Schedule II are amphetamine (*Benzedrine*, *Dexedrine*) and methamphetamine (*Desoxyn*), phenmetrazine (*Preludin*), methylphenidate (*Ritalin*), amobarbital, pentobarbital, secobarbital, etorphine hydrochloride, diphenoxylate and phencyclidine.

The quantity of the substance in a drug product often determines under which schedule it will be controlled. For example, amphetamines and codeine generally are included in Schedule II. However, certain products containing smaller quantities, most often in combination with a noncontrolled substance, are controlled in Schedules III and V.

Schedule III

These drugs have accepted medical use in the US, but they have a lower potential for abuse than Schedule I and II drugs. Schedule III drugs include compounds containing limited quantities of certain narcotic drugs, and nonnarcotic drugs such as derivatives of barbituric acid except those that are listed in another schedule, glutethimide, methyprylon (*Noludar*), nalorphine, benzphetamine, chlorphentermine, clortermine, phendimetrazine and paregoric. Any suppository dosage form containing amobarbital, secobarbital or pentobarbital is in this schedule.

Schedule IV

These drugs have a low potential for abuse relative to those in Schedule III. Abuse of Schedule IV drugs or substances may lead to limited physical dependence or psychological dependence as compared to those included in Schedule III. Schedule IV drugs are generally the long-acting barbiturates, certain hypnotics and the minor tranquilizers. For all practical purposes there are no regulatory differences between Schedule III and IV. Some of the more common drugs found in Schedule IV are barbital, phenobarbital, methylphenobarbital, chloral betaine, chloral hydrate, ethchlorvynol (*Placidyl*), ethinamate (*Valmid*), meprobamate (*Equanil*, *Miltown*), paraldehyde, methohexital, fenfluramine, diethylpropion, phentermine, chlordiazepoxide (*Librium*), diazepam (*Valium*), oxazepam (*Serax*), clorazepate (*Tranxene*), flurazepam (*Dalmane*), clonazepam (*Clonopin*), prazepam (*Verstran*), lorazepam (*Ativan*), mebutamate, propoxyphene (*Darvon*) and pentazocine (*Talwin-NX*).

Schedule V

These drugs have the lowest abuse potential of the controlled substances and consist of preparations containing limited quantities of certain narcotic drugs generally for antitussive and antidiarrheal purposes. As a general rule, Schedule V items are OTC preparations that might be sold without a prescription. There are notable exceptions, and the pharmacist should always check the label to see if the FDA has determined the item to be a prescription-only item. For example, *Lomotil* is a Schedule V item, but it is prescription-only. Paregoric now is restricted to prescription sales and included in Schedule III.

Manufacturers of nonnarcotic substances that may be sold OTC under the terms of the federal Food, Drug and Cosmetic Act may apply to the DEA to have their product excluded from any schedule. Phenobarbital is the most common substance found in those products which are excluded from the scheduling process. One of the prime factors considered in determining whether to exclude a product would be the amount of the controlled substance involved. Once a product is excluded under Section 201 (g)(1) of the CSA it is no longer subject to DEA control. Examples of excluded nonnarcotic OTC products are *Amodrine, Bronkotabs, Primatene P, Tedral* and *Verequad.* However, the pharmacist always should consult state and local laws to determine if these products have been given more restrictive controls.

Schedule V Retail Distribution Restrictions

Controlled substances listed in Schedule V, which are not legend drugs, may be dispensed without a prescription by a pharmacist to a purchaser at retail, provided the following conditions are met:

1. Such dispensing is made only by a pharmacist (which, by definition, also includes a pharmacist intern unless prohibited by state law). However, after the pharmacist has fulfilled his professional and legal responsibilities, the actual cash, credit transaction or delivery may be completed by a nonpharmacist.
2. Not more than 240 mL (8 oz) or 48 solid dosage units of any substance containing opium, or more than 120 mL (4 oz) or 24 solid dosage units of any other controlled substance may be dispensed at retail to the same purchaser in any given 48-hour period without a prescription.
3. The purchaser at retail is at least 18 years of age.
4. The pharmacist requires every retail purchaser of a controlled substance, who is not known to him, to furnish suitable identification (including proof of age where appropriate).
5. A bound record book is maintained which contains the name and address of the purchaser, name and quantity of controlled substance purchased, date of each sale and initials of the selling pharmacist. This record book shall be maintained for a period of 2 years from the date of the last transaction entered in the record book, and it must be made available for inspection and copying by officers of the US, authorized by the Attorney General.
6. Other federal, state or local law does not require a prescription.

The pharmacist must be cautioned that in some states certain, or all, Schedule V substances have been placed on prescription-only status. In these states the more restrictive state law would apply and prohibit the OTC sale of Schedule V items. States may alter any of these restrictions and make them more stringent.

Symbols and Labeling

Each commercial container of controlled substances will have on its label a symbol designating to which schedule it belongs. The symbol for Schedule I through V controlled substances will be as follows:

I or C-I
II or C-II
III or C-III
IV or C-IV
V or C-V.

The symbols will be at least twice as large as the largest letter printed on the label.

There are exceptions to these labeling requirements. In those cases where the commercial container is too small to accommodate the label, only the box and the package insert must contain the "C" symbol.

As a general rule, these symbols are not required on prescription containers dispensed by a pharmacist to a patient in the course of his professional practice, although laws of some states may require such symbols on prescriptions dispensed to extended-care facilities.

Registration

Every person who manufactures, distributes or dispenses any controlled substance or who proposes to engage in the manufacture, distribution or dispensing of any controlled substance shall obtain annually a registration unless exempted. A unique DEA number is assigned to those who must register under the law including manufacturers, distributors, wholesalers and practitioners such as physicians, dentists, veterinarians, scientists, pharmacies, podiatrists and hospitals. There are, however, seven general categories of persons who are exempt from registration under the statute or the regulations, including civil defense officials, law enforcement officials, certain government employees, practitioners affiliated with registered institutions and agents or employees of registrants. It is this latter exemption which permits individual pharmacists not to register with the DEA since such pharmacists serve as agents of the registered pharmacies.

Every pharmacy engaged in distributing or dispensing any controlled substance must register with the DEA. The registration must be renewed every 3 years and a certificate of registration maintained at the registered location and kept available for official inspections. The fee for each 3-year registration or reregistration is $210. If an individual owns and operates more than one pharmacy, each place of business must be registered separately.

Applications for reregistration will be mailed by the DEA to each registered person approximately 60 days before the expiration date of the registration. If a registered pharmacy does not receive such forms within 45 days prior to the expiration date of the registration, it must give notice of such fact and request the reregistration forms by writing to the Drug Enforcement Administration, Registration Section, PO Box 28083, Central Station, Washington, DC 20005.

New Registrations—Pharmacies that seek to become registered for the first time must request a registration application from the DEA (see above address), or from any DEA Field Office. No pharmacy may engage in any activity for which registration is required until its application for registration has been granted and a certificate issued to it by the DEA. However, a pharmacy may not dispense controlled substances if it has not been issued a valid state license, even though the DEA already may have registered the pharmacy and authorized it to obtain controlled substances.

Modifications such as change of address, location or name by existing registrants may be made without going through the new registration process. To make such a modification, the registrant should submit a letter to the DEA requesting it. No fee is required. A registrant also may apply to modify his registration to authorize the handling of additional schedules of controlled substances, but may not modify his registration to transfer it to another party.

Termination—The DEA has the authority under the CSA to suspend or revoke a registration where the registrant has falsified his application, or has been convicted of a felony under the federal or state CSA or has had his state license or registration suspended and no longer is authorized by state law to dispense controlled substances. Except in emergency situations, registrants are assured of a hearing and due process of law prior to suspension or revocation of registration. In addition, the registration of any person terminates if and when such a person dies, ceases legal existence or discontinues business or professional practice.

Distribution

As a general rule a separate DEA registration is required for each activity a registrant wishes to engage in such as manufacturing, distributing, dispensing or conducting research. However, a pharmacy registered to dispense a controlled substance may distribute (without being registered as a distributor) a quantity of controlled substances to a physician, another pharmacy, hospital or nursing home for the purpose of general dispensing by that practitioner provided the following conditions are met:

1. The pharmacy or practitioner to which the controlled substance is being distributed is registered under the Act to dispense that controlled substance.
2. The distribution is recorded as being distributed by the pharmacy and the pharmacist, or practitioner, records the substance being received. The pharmacy distributing a controlled substance must record the name of the substance, the dosage form, the quantity and the name, address and DEA registration number of the pharmacy or practitioner to whom it is distributed as well as the date of distribution.
3. If the substance is listed in Schedule I or II, the transfer must be made on an official DEA order form.
4. The total number of dosage units of controlled substances distributed by a pharmacy may not exceed 5% of all controlled substances dispensed by the pharmacy during the 12-month period in which the pharmacy is registered. If at any time it does exceed 5% the pharmacy is required to register as a distributor as well as being registered as a pharmacy.

As an incident to this distribution, a pharmacist may manufacture (without being registered to manufacture) an aqueous or oleaginous solution or solid dosage form containing a narcotic controlled substance in a proportion not exceeding 20% of the complete solution, compound or mixture.

The regulations also permit a person lawfully in possession of controlled substances to return them to the supplier without registering as a distributor. Registrants would have to use official DEA order forms for the return of Schedule I and II substances to a supplier.

Records and Reports

Every pharmacy handling controlled substances must keep complete and accurate records of all receiving and dispensing transactions which shall be maintained for a period of 2 years. Many states require that the records be kept for as long as 5 years.

All inventories and records of controlled substances in Schedule II must be maintained separately from all other records of the registrant. All inventories and records of controlled substances in Schedules III, IV and V must be maintained separately or must be in such form that they are readily retrievable from the ordinary professional and business records of the pharmacy.

All records pertaining to controlled substances shall be made available for inspection and copying by duly authorized DEA officials.

When a registrant first engages in business, and every 2 years thereafter, he must make a complete and accurate inventory of all stocks of controlled substances on hand. This shall be kept by the registrant for a period of 2 years. Pharmacies are not required to submit a copy of the inventory to the DEA.

Continuing Records—Every pharmacy must maintain, on a current basis, a complete and accurate record of each controlled substance received. Copy 3 of executed DEA order forms retained by the pharmacy, which have been completed as described under the section entitled "Order Forms," will constitute a pharmacy's receiving records for Schedule II controlled substances. Invoices for Schedule III, IV and V controlled substances will be considered as complete receiving records if the actual date of receipt is recorded clearly on the invoices by the pharmacist or other responsible individual.

Filing Prescriptions—Prescription orders for controlled substances must be filed in one of the following three ways:

1. A pharmacy can maintain three separate files—a file for Schedule II drugs dispensed, a file for Schedules III, IV and V drugs dispensed and a file for prescription orders for all other drugs dispensed.
2. A pharmacy can maintain two files—a file for all Schedule II drugs dispensed, and another file for all other drugs dispensed, including those in Schedules III, IV and V. If this method is used, the prescription orders in the file for Schedules III, IV and V must be stamped with the letter "C" in red ink, not less than 1-inch high, in the lower-right corner. This distinctive marking makes the records "readily retrievable" for inspection.
3. A pharmacy can maintain two files—one file for all controlled drugs in all schedules and a second file for all prescription orders for noncontrolled drugs dispensed. If this method is used, the prescription orders for drugs in Schedules III, IV and V in the controlled drug prescription file must be stamped with the red letter "C" not less than 1-inch high in the lower-right corner, as previously mentioned.

In states where the Uniform Narcotic Act (or other state law) requires all narcotic prescription records be kept together, the DEA is of the opinion that a positive conflict exists between federal and state law and, under Section 708 of the CSA, federal requirements prevail.

Inventory

The CSA requires each registrant to make a complete and accurate record of all stocks of controlled substances on hand every 2 years. The biennial inventory date of May 1 may be changed by the registrant to fit his general inventory date, if any, so long as the date is not more than 6 months from the biennial date that otherwise would apply. The actual taking of the inventory should not vary more than 4 days from the biennial inventory date. The inventory record must

1. List the name, address and DEA registration number of the registrant.
2. Indicate the date and time the inventory is taken, ie, opening or closing of business.
3. Be signed by the person or persons responsible for taking the inventory.
4. Be maintained at the location appearing on the registration certificate for at least 2 years.
5. Keep records of Schedule II drugs separate from all other controlled substances.

When taking the inventory of Schedule II controlled substances, an exact count or measure must be made. When taking the inventory of Schedules III, IV and V controlled substances, an estimated count may be made unless the container holds more than 1000 dosage units, in which case an exact count must be made if the container has been opened.

Newly controlled substances—occasionally a drug that has not been controlled previously will be placed in one of the drug schedules or a controlled substance will be moved into a higher or lower schedule. In either case the drug must be inventoried as of the effective date of transfer, and this inventory should be added to the biennial inventory.

Order Forms

The order form system developed by the DEA is a completely closed system of drug distribution. The DEA permits only authorized persons to obtain or distribute Schedule I or II controlled substances and only pursuant to official DEA order forms. The regulations set forth those instances where official order forms are not required to transfer Schedule I or II controlled substances, eg, transfer to a patient pursuant to a written prescription, administration to a patient by a registered practitioner, procurement by civil defense officials or delivery by a common carrier to a warehouse.

A pharmacy desiring official order forms may requisition the appropriate ones from the DEA. Such forms are numbered serially and issued with the name, address and registration number of the pharmacy, the authorized activity and authorized schedules with respect to that pharmacy. Each triplicate form is contained in a book of seven. Up to six books may be ordered at one time unless the pharmacy can show that it needs to exceed this limit. There is no charge for these forms.

The pharmacist must prepare and execute the order form in triplicate using a typewriter, pen or indelible pencil. One must enter the name and address of the supplier from whom the controlled substances are being ordered. Only one supplier may be listed on any one form. There are ten lines in the "item" section of each form. Each of the ten lines must contain a different drug or "item." The number of lines completed must be totaled at the bottom. This is the total number of lines or items and not the total number of commercial containers ordered. The order form must be completed properly and have no material alterations or erasures or a distributor will be obligated to refuse the form, and may elect to do so in other cases as well, if the order form is not completed correctly.

The purchaser must sign his name and date the order form on the day he places the order. If his name is different from the authorized registrant, ie, if he has been given a power of attorney to complete order forms, he also must include the name of the authorized registrant in the signature space. When the form is completed, the purchaser separates the three copies in the following manner: Copies 1 and 2 must be kept intact with the carbon in between them. These are sent in with the registrant's order to his supplier. Copy 3 is retained by the purchaser separately from other records. When the registrant receives the items he must record, on the retained Copy 3, the number of packages and the date such packages were received. A space is provided for this.

Power of Attorney—Any registered pharmacy may authorize one or more individuals, whether or not they are at the registered location of the pharmacy, to obtain and execute order forms on its behalf by executing a power of attorney for each such individual. This must be signed by the same person who signed the most recent application for registration or reregistration and must contain the signature of the individual being authorized to obtain and execute order forms. The power of attorney is not submitted to the DEA but must be retained by the pharmacy with the executed forms. It must be available for inspection together with the order form records. A power of attorney may be revoked at any time by filing a notice of revocation, signed by the individual who signed the most recent application for registration or reregistration and by filing it with the power of attorney being revoked.

Lost or Theft—When unfilled order forms are lost, the pharmacy must execute a new one in triplicate. The pharmacy also must execute a statement containing the serial number and date of the lost form, stating that the drugs in it were never received, and attach a copy of that statement to Copy 3 of the lost form. A copy of that statement also should be attached to Copies 1 and 2 of the newly executed order form.

Whenever any used or unused order forms are stolen or lost, upon discovery, the pharmacy must report this immediately to the Drug Enforcement Administration, Registration Unit, PO Box 28083, Central Station, Washington DC 20005, stating the serial numbers of each form lost or stolen. If an entire book or books of order forms are lost or stolen, and the pharmacist is unable to state the serial numbers, he shall report, in lieu of the serial numbers, the date or approximate date of issuance. Lost or stolen order forms also should be reported to the state board of pharmacy or other state controlled substance agency.

Prescriptions

Who May Issue—In order to issue a prescription an individual practitioner must be both (1) authorized to prescribe controlled substances by the jurisdiction in which he is licensed to practice his profession and (2) either registered or exempted from registration by the DEA.

Purpose of Issue—A prescription for a controlled substance to be effective must be issued for a legitimate medical purpose by a practitioner acting in the usual course of his professional practice. The responsibility for the proper prescribing and dispensing of controlled substances is upon the prescribing practitioner, but a corresponding liability rests with the pharmacist who dispenses the prescription. An order purporting to be a prescription issued not in the usual course of professional treatment, or in legitimate and authorized research, is not a prescription within the meaning and intent of Section 309 of the CSA. The person knowingly dispensing such a purported prescription, as well as the person issuing it, will be subject to the penalties provided for violations of the provisions of law relating to controlled substances.

A prescription by which a practitioner attempts to resupply his office stock or maintain drug-dependent individuals is not a valid prescription and, therefore, is void.

Execution of Prescriptions—All prescriptions for controlled substances shall be dated as of, and signed on, the day when issued and shall bear the full name and address of the patient and the name, address and registration number of the practitioner. A practitioner may sign a prescription in the same manner as he would sign a check or legal document, eg, JH Smith or John H Smith. Where an oral order is not permitted, prescriptions must be executed using a typewriter, ink or an indelible pencil and must be signed manually by the practitioner. The prescription may be prepared by a secretary or agent for the signature of a practitioner, but the prescriber is responsible in case the prescription does not conform, in all essential respects, to the law and regulations.

Prescription orders that are written for controlled substances in Schedule II must be executed using a typewriter, ink or indelible pencil and must be signed by the practitioner issuing such prescription orders. In an emergency, Schedule II drugs may be dispensed upon an oral authorization (see below). Prescription orders for controlled substances in Schedules III, IV or V may be issued either orally or in writing by a practitioner or his authorized agent.

Emergency Dispensing-Schedule II—In the case of a bona fide emergency, as defined by the Secretary of Health and Human Services, a pharmacist may dispense a Schedule II controlled substance upon receiving oral authorization of a prescriber provided that

1. The quantity prescribed and dispensed is limited to the amount adequate to treat the patient during the emergency period. Prescribing or dispensing beyond the emergency period must be pursuant to a written prescription order.
2. The prescription order shall be reduced immediately to writing by the pharmacist and shall contain all information, except for the prescriber's signature.
3. If the prescriber is not known to the pharmacist, he must make a reasonable effort to determine that the oral authorization came from a prescriber, by verifying his telephone number against that listed in the directory and other good-faith efforts to insure his identity.
4. Within 72 hours after authorizing an emergency oral prescription order, the prescriber must cause a written prescription order for the emergency quantity prescribed to be delivered to the dispensing pharmacist. The prescription order shall have written on its face "Authorization for Emergency Dispensing." The written prescription order may be delivered in person or by mail, but if delivered by mail it must be postmarked within the 72-hour period. Upon receipt, the dispensing pharmacist shall attach this prescription order to the oral emergency prescription order which had been reduced to writing earlier. The pharmacist shall notify the nearest office of the DEA, if the prescriber fails to deliver a written prescription order to him. Failure of the pharmacist to do so shall void the authority conferred by the subsection to dispense without a written prescription order of a prescriber.

Definition of Emergency—For the purpose of authorizing an oral prescription order of a controlled substance listed in Schedule II of the Controlled Substances Act, the term "emergency situation" means those situations in which the prescriber determines that

1. Immediate administration of the controlled substance is necessary for the proper treatment of the intended user.
2. No appropriate alternative treatment is available, including administration of a drug which is not a controlled substance under Schedule II of the Act.
3. It is not reasonably possible for the prescriber to provide a written prescription order to be presented to the person dispensing the substance, prior to the dispensing.

Refills and Renewals—No prescription for a Schedule II controlled substance may be refilled, and such prescriptions must be kept in a separate file.

Prescriptions for Schedule III or IV controlled substances may be issued either orally or in writing by a practitioner and may be refilled if so authorized. The prescriptions may not be filled or refilled more than 6 months after the date issued or be refilled more than five times after the date issued. After five refills or after 6 months, the practitioner may renew the prescription. A renewal of any such prescription shall be recorded on a new prescription blank and a new prescription number assigned. Oral prescriptions must be committed to writing and filed by the pharmacist.

Prescriptions for a Schedule V controlled substance may be refilled only as authorized by the prescribing practitioner on the prescription. If no such authorization is given, the prescription may not be refilled. However, if the item may be sold over the counter legally, the burden of determining the propriety of the sale will be upon the pharmacist.

Recording Refills—A pharmacist, after refilling a prescription for any controlled substance in Schedules III, IV or V, must enter on the back of that prescription his initials, the date the prescription was refilled and the amount of drug dispensed. If the pharmacist merely initials and dates the back of the prescription, he shall be deemed to have dispensed a refill for the full face amount of the prescription.

Computerization—A pharmacy is permitted to use a data processing system as an alternative method for the storage and retrieval of prescription refill information for controlled substances in Schedules III and IV.

The computerized system must provide immediate retrieval, (via CRT display or hard-copy printout) of original prescription information for those prescriptions which currently are authorized for refilling. The information which readily must be retrievable must include, but is not limited to, data such as the original prescription number, date of issuance of the prescription by the practitioner, full name and address of the patient, practitioner's name and DEA registration number, name, strength, dosage form, quantity of the controlled substance prescribed, quantity dispensed if different from the quantity prescribed and the total number of refills authorized by the prescriber.

In addition, the system must provide immediate retrieval of the current refill history for Schedule III or IV controlled substance prescriptions that have been authorized for refills during the past 6 months and backup documentation to show that the refill information is correct. The backup documentation must be stored in a separate file at the pharmacy and maintained for a 2-year period from the dispensing date.

Transmittal of Oral Authorization—A practitioner's nurse, or other member of his staff, cannot authorize the renewal of a prescription for a controlled substance that has been refilled five times or is 6-months old. The authority for prescribing controlled substances is vested only with the practitioner, and he cannot delegate this function to anyone else. However, nurses or staff members receiving calls from pharmacies regarding renewals may act as the practitioner's agent and transmit the practitioner's order.

Practitioners' Office Stock—A pharmacist may not dispense a controlled substance on the order of a prescription which is issued by a practitioner and is intended for office use or bag use of the practitioner. Distribution must be made on invoice and/or order form, if required.

Label Requirements—The pharmacist filling a prescription for controlled substances listed in Schedules II, III, IV or V must affix to the package a label showing the pharmacy name and address, serial number and date of initial filling, name of the patient, name of the practitioner issuing the prescription, directions for use and cautionary statements, if any.

The label of any drug listed as a controlled substance in Schedules II, III or IV of the CSA shall, when dispensed to a patient, contain the following warning:

CAUTION: Federal law prohibits the transfer of this drug to any person other than the patient for whom it was prescribed.

Partial Filling-Schedule II—The partial filling of a Schedule II controlled substance prescription is permissible if the pharmacist is unable to supply the full quantity called for in a written or emergency oral prescription. He may supply a portion of the quantity called for provided he makes a notation of the quantity supplied on the face of the written prescription (or written record of the emergency oral prescription). The remaining portion may be filled within 72 hours of the first dispensing; however, if the remaining portion is not, or cannot be filled within the 72-hour period, the pharmacist must notify the prescriber. No further quantity may be supplied beyond the 72 hours except on a new prescription. However, the partial dispensing of a prescription for Schedule II controlled substances beyond the 72-hour limitation is permissible for patients in long-term care facilities.

Partial Filling-Schedule III and IV—Partial filling of prescriptions for controlled substances in Schedules III and IV is permitted if the pharmacist filling or refilling the prescription sets forth the quantity dispensed and his initials on the back of the prescription. In addition, the partial fillings may not exceed the total amount authorized in the prescription and the dispensing of all refills must be within the 6-month limit.

Distribution on Discontinuance or Transfer

Any registrant desiring to discontinue business activities altogether, or with respect to controlled substances (without transferring such business activities to another person), shall return, for cancellation, his certificate of registration and any unexecuted order forms in his possession to the location as per instructions of the DEA Field Office.

Any controlled substances in his possession may be disposed of in accordance with instructions under the section on Drug Security and Disposal.

Any registrant desiring to discontinue business activities altogether, or with respect to controlled substances (by transferring such business activities to another person), shall submit in person or by registered or certified mail, return receipt requested, to the nearest DEA office at least 14 days in advance of the date of the proposed transfer

1. The name, address and registration number of the pharmacy discontinuing business.
2. The name, address and registration number of the person acquiring the pharmacy.
3. Whether the business activities will be continued at the location registered by the person discontinuing business or moved to another location (if the latter, the address of the new location should be listed).
4. The date on which the transfer of controlled substances will occur.

On the day of transfer a complete inventory of all controlled substances being transferred shall be taken in accordance with 21 CFR 1304.11-1304.19. This inventory shall serve as the final inventory of the registrant transferor and the initial inventory for the registrant transferee. A copy of the inventory shall be included in the records of each person. It shall not be necessary to file a copy with the DEA unless requested by the Regional Director. Transfers of any Schedule II substances shall require the use of order forms.

On the day of transfer all records required to be kept by the registrant transferor, with reference to the controlled substances being transferred, shall be transferred to the registrant transferee. Responsibility for the accuracy of records prior to the date of transfer remains with the transferor, but responsibility for custody and maintenance shall be upon the transferee.

Miscellaneous Requirements

Security—Pharmacies must keep Schedules II, III, IV and V controlled substances in a locked cabinet or dispersed throughout the noncontrolled stock in such a manner as to deter theft.

Disposal—A pharmacy wishing to dispose of any excess or undesired stock of controlled substances must contact its nearest DEA Office and request the necessary form (DEA-41). A cover letter from the pharmacy must be attached to the report stating that the controlled substances are not desired and the pharmacy wishes to dispose of them.

Upon the receipt of the letter from the pharmacy, one of four courses of action will be chosen by the DEA; this will be stated in letter form, attached to the original copy of the DEA-41 form and returned to the pharmacy.

The four courses of action are

1. The drugs may be destroyed by two responsible parties employed or acting on behalf of the registrant. This course of action will be used when there are factors which preclude an on-the-site destruction witnessed by DEA personnel, such as the firm's history of compliance and the abuse potential of the drugs involved.
2. The excess or undesired stocks of controlled substances should be forwarded to the appropriate state agency for destruction. In lieu of actual surrender to the state agency, destructions witnessed by state personnel are acceptable.
3. The substances should be held until DEA personnel arrive at a mutually convenient time to witness their destruction. DEA personnel will date and sign the reports or forms after witnessing the destruction.
4. The substances should be forwarded to the DEA Field Office which serves the area in which the registrant is located. Upon receipt of the substances, the DEA Field Office will verify the actual substance submitted. If errors are found, a corrected form must be prepared and the registrant duly notified. The original form will be returned to the registrant.

Drug Theft—Any pharmacy involved in loss of controlled substances must notify the nearest DEA office of the theft or significant loss upon discovery. The pharmacy must make a report regarding the loss or theft by completing DEA-106 form. Such reports shall contain the following information: name and address of firm, DEA registration number, date of theft, local police department notified, type of theft, listing of symbols or cost code used by the pharmacy in marking containers and listing of the controlled substances missing. Such a report should be made in triplicate. The pharmacy should keep the original copy for its records and forward the remaining two copies to the nearest DEA office.

Mailing

Title 39 of the Code of Federal Regulations contains the US Postal Service Regulations regarding nonmailable matter and special mailing rules for various articles and substances. As a general rule, the regulations hold that controlled substances are nonmailable matter and are not to be conveyed in the mail or delivered from any post office. However, controlled substances may be transmitted in the mail between persons registered with the DEA or between persons who are exempted from registration such as military, law enforcement or civil defense personnel in the performance of their official duties. Prescription medicines containing nonnarcotic controlled substances may be mailed from a registered practitioner or dispenser to the ultimate user. Prescription medications containing narcotic drugs may be mailed only by the Veterans Administration medical facilities to certain veterans.

Parcels containing controlled substances must be prepared and packaged for mailing in accordance with the regulations set forth in 39 CFR 124. Regular mail may be used for these parcels.

DEA Inspections

The CSA specifically requires an administrative search warrant for most nonconsentual DEA inspections. Therefore, in order for an agent of the DEA to enter any DEA-registered premise, he must state his purpose and present his credentials. In addition, he must either obtain an informed consent from the registrant, secure an administrative inspection warrant or fit into one of the special exceptions set forth in the statute. The Act recognizes certain exigent circumstances in which an inspection warrant is not required such as the initial registration inspection, inspection of mobile vehicles, emergency situations or dangerous health situations.

Poisons

A poison has been defined as any drug known to the pharmaceutical or medical profession which is liable to be destructive to adult human life if taken in quantities of 60 grains or less. This general definition is helpful in indicating the substances customarily regarded as poisonous, but it is not followed in many of the state poison laws. Regulation of the sale of poisons usually falls within the jurisdiction of the state governments and governmental limits in this area may vary widely from state to state.

State statutes regulating the sale of poisons usually require that the purchaser be of a certain minimum age and that he know, or be informed, that the substance being purchased is a poison. Moreover, the pharmacist frequently has a responsibility to determine that the substance will be used for a lawful purpose. Recordkeeping requirements usually are specified in state statutes. For example, the pharmacist may be required to record the date of sale, name and address of the purchaser, name or initials of the seller, name and quantity of the poison and purpose for which it is intended. Some states require that the purchaser sign the record book to form a receipt and impress upon the purchaser the dangerous nature of the substance. The book in which this information is recorded frequently is referred to as "the Poison Register" and there may be a requirement that the book be used exclusively for recording sales of poisons. Most states specify a time period during which the sales records must be preserved and made available for inspection by appropriate state authorities.

Special labeling requirements for poisons frequently are encountered. The usual minimum requirement is that the container bear the name of the substance, the word "poison" and the name and place of business of the seller. Such state requirements may be supplemented by federal requirements concerning labeling with information about toxicity, cautionary statements and information about treatment.

Poisons are not permitted to be mailed without specific authorization from the US Postal Service.

Poison Prevention Packaging Act

The Poison Prevention Packaging Act was enacted by Congress during 1970 and authorizes the Consumer Product Safety Commission (CPSC) to establish standards for child-resistant packaging. The agency also enforces the statute at the pharmacy level.

Under this statute, federal legend drugs, and some nonprescription medications, are considered to be "hazardous household substances" and, consequently, must be dispensed with a child-resistant closure. However, there are some exceptions to this requirement under the Act.

Most nonprescription medications are not required to be packaged in a child-resistant fashion. However, the CPSC has ordered that aspirin and products containing more than 500 mg of iron per package must be in safety packages. Yet manufacturers of aspirin products may produce one size of a package containing the drug which has a standard closure. Such nonsafety packages are required to bear the warning statement, "This package for households without young children." Other nonprescription products may be added to the list of drugs requiring safety packaging, from time to time, and pharmacists should watch for such developments.

Some prescription drugs are not required to be dispensed in child-resistant packages either. The CPSC has stated that safety packaging is not required for sublingual dosage forms of nitroglycerin as well as sublingual and chewable dosage forms of isosorbide dinitrate in strengths of 5 mg or less. A number of other prescription drugs are being considered for exemption from the requirements of the Act and, while under consideration, child-resistant packaging is not required.

The prescriber may request that a drug, which otherwise would be required to be in a child-resistant package, be dispensed with a standard closure. The patient also has this option under the Act. The legislation does not require any specific fashion for communicating this waiver, ie, it is not required to be in writing. For example, a prescriber transmitting a prescription by telephone could indicate orally that standard packaging is requested. Nonetheless, the pharmacist may desire to have requests by prescribers or patients for noncomplying packaging in writing in order to document the transaction; this could prove to be invaluable in case of an adverse occurrence.

At the outset of the enforcement of this statute, the CPSC took the position that the pharmacist could not advise the patient of the option of standard packaging. This position was taken in furtherance of the agency's view that nonsafety packaging should be the rare exception, not the rule, and a feeling that if pharmacists were to advise patients of their options widely, the Act would be undermined. The APhA challenged this position of the agency and the CPSC now has stated that pharmacists may advise patients of their right to request nonsafety packaging.

Drugs dispensed for use by inpatients, be they in a hospital or a nursing home, probably are not required to be in child-resistant containers because the patients usually do not have access to them.

Manufacturers are not required to use child-resistant closures on stock bottles of medication which are not intended to reach the patient. However, if the packaging provided by the manufacturer is that which will be dispensed to the patient, eg, packages bearing antibiotic powders for reconstitution, safety tops must be used.

Tort Law

Tort law is that subdivision of the civil law which deals with relationships between individuals created by law rather than by the parties themselves. A tort is a private injury or wrong arising from a breach of a duty created by law. It may involve harm to a person, as well as damage to property, caused negligently or intentionally.

Negligent torts are those which arise because the tortfeasor (the person doing the act) breached a duty or level of care expected of him. Intentional torts are those which the actor does purposefully or with an intention of achieving the desired result. A number of miscellaneous torts also will be discussed. These are torts which do not fall clearly into either of the prior categories. Finally, liability of the owner or occupier of land or business premises will be discussed, for there are some special rules applicable in that area.

Negligence

Negligence has been defined as the omission to do something that a reasonable man, guided by those ordinary considerations which ordinarily regulate human affairs, would do, or the doing of something which a reasonable and prudent man would not do. As is obvious from this statement, one can be negligent either by doing or failing to do something. A more direct description is that negligence occurs when a person under a duty to another to use due care breaches that duty, resulting in the other party suffering damages as a direct result of that breach. Using this statement as a point of departure, each element of negligence shall be considered in order.

In the normal situation, the existence of a legal duty will be created by the activities of other persons. The jury will be charged with determining what the fictional reasonable and prudent man mentioned above would have done under the circumstances. To do this, the jurors receive testimony from a number of people to determine what they would have done. The jury then decides what the reasonable and prudent man would have done, and that creates the existence of a legal duty. In the ordinary circumstance, the duty will be created by the actions of laymen. Yet, when the pharmacist is acting within the scope of his professional calling, his performance will be evaluated in light of what his professional peers would have done. Generally, a pharmacist will be held liable for negligence only if he departed from the practice of other reputable practitioners of pharmacy. For the general practitioner of pharmacy, the reference standard to be used is other general practitioners of pharmacy. While there may be individuals within the profession with greater knowledge or skill in a particular area, eg, the detection of drug interactions, the general practitioner of pharmacy will be required to discharge only that amount of skill exhibited by his peers, not the experts.

Nonetheless, this does not mean that the members of a profession can lag unduly in adopting new methods or procedures. A number of courts have ruled that while in the usual case the law will recognize the standard of care established by the members of the trade, industry or profession, the entire group may have lagged in adopting an innovation. In such cases the courts will not be bound by the standards used by the profession, but rather the court will establish the standard of care to be exercised under the circumstance.

The concept of duty is not fixed but constantly evolving and changing. An example of this is the doctrine of the pharmacist's duty to consult with patients about proper drug use. Through a number of cases decided during the past 25 years, various courts have ruled that the pharmacist does have the legal duty to instruct the patient about safe and proper use of medication. This duty is owed to the patient, and should a pharmacist fail to fulfill this responsibility, he may be held answerable in court.

A second requirement for the existence of negligence is damage. The party who is alleging negligence must prove that he suffered legally sufficient damages. Generally, these damages must be substantial, not slight, eg, a temporary skin rash would be insufficient.

The party bringing the suit next must prove that the damages were the direct result of the pharmacist's breach of a legal duty. This may be quite difficult. In some cases it is known that the patient suffered legally cognizable damages, but it cannot be established by a preponderance of the evidence that damages flowed directly from a breach of duty.

The plaintiff has the burden of establishing those first three elements. Once they have been shown in a legally sufficient manner, the pharmacist has a number of defenses which may be available to result in his being held not liable. One such defense may be *contributory negligence.* That is, the rule that a party, which has in some way contributed to his own injury, will not be entitled to recover. In some states the rule is one of comparative negligence. While contributory negligence is a total bar to recovery by the plaintiff, in states which follow the comparative negligence rule the jury engages in an allocation of responsibility and bases the amount of damages awarded on the parties' relative contributions to the injury.

Another defense which the pharmacist has is known as *voluntary assumption of the risk.* This is the doctrine which states that a patient who understands the risk inherent in a transaction or procedure, and who voluntarily gives his informed consent to assume the risk, cannot sue to recover for damages which occur from the defined risk. An unresolved issue is whether presenting a patient with a patient package insert which outlines the potential hazards of a certain medication results in informed consent and, consequently, voluntary assumption of the risk. Generally the procedure required for informed consent is a lengthy discussion covering the alternatives and the relative incidence of the various risks. This point probably will be litigated in the future.

Another defense which may be available to the pharmacist is the *statute of limitations.* The legislature imposes a time limit on filing suits for negligence. Generally, the statute of limitations in this area is 2 years, meaning that the suit must be filed within 2 years of the time of reasonable discovery of the damage. Note, however, that a person may suffer some damage and not be able to discover it until some time long after the incident, as in the diethylstilbestrol cases which are being litigated. In those cases, the injured parties, daughters of women who took the drug during pregnancy, developed precancerous lesions 15 to 20 years after the drug was consumed. The statute of limitations would begin to run at the time of reasonable discovery, not the time when the drug was dispensed.

The issue of liability of the pharmacist for negligence has been raised in conjunction with a number of developments and innovations in pharmacy practice in recent years. A consideration of the application of the above discussion to these developments is in order. Of necessity, a detailed discussion of these areas is impossible in this chapter. The professional literature contains a number of articles which address these issues in detail, and the interested reader may wish to refer to those.

Patient medication records (PMRs) have been adopted widely in pharmacy practice. There are data from some states which indicate that a majority of the pharmacists maintain such records. In such cases, it may be possible for the attorney representing a party injured, due to a pharmacist's failure to detect a drug interaction, to establish that the standard of due care is maintenance and proper use of PMRs. Even without such data it may be possible for the attorney to establish that the pharmacist has a duty to detect potentially serious drug interactions. This well may have become part of the pharmacist's standard of due care just as is detecting other prescribing errors. The PMR probably should be viewed as a tool to assist in discharging the responsibility, but it does not create it. The responsibility has its origins in the activities of other practicing pharmacists.

Even if the majority of pharmacists do not maintain PMRs, the skillful attorney may make the argument that the entire profession has delayed in implementing an innovation.

Some states have mandated, by statute, that the pharmacist maintain PMRs. In such a case, special rules of negligence would apply. The doctrine of negligence *per se* is that where a criminal statute mandates that a certain activity be performed to protect an identifiable group of people from an identifiable type of harm and one does not do it, that fact and the statute may be introduced into evidence at trial to establish the duty and breach of it. This facilitates the case of the plaintiff. Consequently, pharmacists, practicing in states where maintenance and use of PMRs has been dictated by statute, especially should be careful to comply with the law. Note that this rule of negligence *per se* is applicable only in the case where the activity is required by a statute. A regulation of a board of pharmacy, for example, would not suffice to establish the duty in and of itself. Nonetheless, such a regulation could be introduced into evidence to buttress the testimony of pharmacists on this point.

All states have now enacted drug product selection legislation which frees the pharmacist from the restrictions of the antisubstitution laws, enabling him to use his professional judgment in selecting products to be dispensed on certain prescriptions. Naturally, because these statutes give the pharmacist greater responsibility, they increase his potential liability. However, so long as he discharges this responsibility in a prudent fashion, the potential for legal entanglements will be minimal. In some states the government has provided guidance for the pharmacist in the form of a positive formulary, designating those drugs for which interchange is permissible. The FDA also has published such a list. In the case of a pharmacist who selects a product from the formulary for brand interchange, he then should have a fairly good defense based on his reliance on such governmental lists.

There has not been a successful law suit based on negligence in drug product selection. This even more is significant in light of the fact that pharmacists have been selecting extensively the brand of product to be dispensed for years pursuant to prescriptions written using generic terminology.

Pharmacists should not be concerned unduly with their potential liability exposure as they move into new areas of practice. So long as they are competent to assume the new responsibility and perform the task in a diligent fashion, their liability problems should continue to be minimal.

Intentional Torts

The law distinguishes intentional acts from those which are negligent or careless in nature. Intentional wrongs to persons or property involve such torts as assault, battery and false imprisonment. At the onset, it is important to distinguish between a tort and a crime. The same act may give rise, but not necessarily, to both a tort and a crime. The criminal violation will be prosecuted in the name of the state, but the same act also may result in a separate civil lawsuit between the individuals involved. Quite naturally, intentional torts require a showing of the element of intent, but it is not necessary to demonstrate harmful or hostile design.

Assault—An intentional act, other than the mere speaking of words, which places another individual in apprehension of harmful or offensive contact is an assault. The danger must be of an immediate nature and the individual must be aware of the defendant's apparent intent. Bodily contact is not necessary to establish a claim for relief and, thus, damages for an assault alone are likely to be nominal.

Battery—A battery is defined as an intentional act which, directly or indirectly, is the cause of harmful or offensive contact with another's person or something the person is touching. Assault and battery are separate torts but very often will go hand in hand. A person may be liable for battery even though he intended only to play a practical joke or intended to confer a benefit on the other party.

In patient-care settings it is possible for a cause of action based upon battery to arise during unauthorized surgical operations. Assault and battery offenses also may occur when a pharmacist attempts to control the conduct of patrons of the pharmacy. The case law in some states will permit the owner of a place of business, to which the public is invited, to request that individuals who are causing a disturbance leave the premises. Upon noncompliance, the owner may use such force as is necessary to eject the disturber.

A number of defenses exist for the torts of assault and battery. If an individual inflicts an injury in self-defense, he would not be liable if he believes that the other person intended to cause him harm and that the injury could be prevented only by infliction of injury on the other person. However, excessive force is not permissible in the exercise of self-defense.

Some parties are privileged to touch others without fear of claims of assault and battery. Police officers may touch an arrested party without fear as long as reasonable force is used. In some states store owners also are privileged to remove boisterous patrons with reasonable force.

An individual who consents to physical contact may not claim a battery successfully. Consent to physical contact may be expressed or implied in nature. Consent to surgical procedures also will negate an action based upon assault and battery, but the consent obtained from the patient should be an informed consent, ie, the patient must have a sufficient understanding of that to which he is consenting. The use of investigational drugs also will require an informed consent.

False Imprisonment—The unlawful detention of another person for any length of time may result in an action for false imprisonment. The elements of this tort require the intentional confinement of a person so as to deprive him of his liberty to move about. Negligent imprisonment is not actionable as false imprisonment. A confinement does not have to be by means of physical barriers but may be created by threats of physical force.

This tort may pose a real dilemma for the pharmacy owner who has problems with shoplifters. Many states have enacted laws to aid in this situation. These statutes often provide that the owner of a store, or his employee, may detain and question an individual in a reasonable manner to determine whether or not a theft has been committed. The detainment must be for a reasonable time and there must be good cause to believe that the person has committed the act of shoplifting.

An illegal confinement caused by the assertion of legal authority, where there is none, may result in a false arrest situation. Mere words asserting legal authority without acquiescence do not constitute an arrest. The arrestor should have some element of control if the person acted upon does not acquiesce voluntarily. The law does not require the victim to resist the arrest before he has the cause of action for wrongful arrest. In most states an arrest can be made by a police officer or a private party for a crime committed in his presence.

Miscellaneous Torts

Some torts are not pigeon-holed easily into either the negligent or the intentional tort categories. These miscellaneous torts may require some showing of the element of intent, but it is often more subtle in nature than the intentional torts.

Defamation—Defamation is a communication which injures the good name or reputation of another. Defamatory statements which are communicated in a permanent form such as the written word, pictures, statues, etc, are libelous in nature. Communications which are more transient in nature such as the spoken word or a gesture are termed slander.

A defamatory statement, either libel or slander, must be communicated to a third person, ie, one other than the person defamed. The statement will be deemed defamatory if it harms the reputation of another or exposes an individual to scorn, ridicule or contempt.

Because of its historical background, special rules have been developed regarding the showing of actual damages in a case of defamation. Almost any action based upon libel will be able to proceed regardless of whether actual monetary damages have been suffered by the plaintiff. Most courts have held that special harm or actual dollar loss must be shown in cases of slander unless the slander fits into established exceptions.

As is true with the other tort situations, several defenses exist to actions for libel and slander. Truth is always a defense to actions based upon defamation of character. The burden is on the defendant, in a defamation action, to prove that the statement was true.

Certain individuals are said to be privileged to defame, or free from liability for slander or libel. An absolute privilege exists for defamatory remarks made during the course of judicial, legislative or executive proceedings. Many states have enacted statutes which provide immunity from civil lawsuits for pharmacists and other health-care professionals who file charges or present evidence against another member of their profession regarding alleged incompetency or gross misconduct. The immunity often is extended to claims filed with a board of pharmacy or with the regularly constituted review committee of a pharmaceutical society or hospital. In addition, most states also will provide immunity for those individuals, including pharmacists, who are required to report suspected cases of child abuse.

Privilege to defame also may exist in a variety of other situations. Comments made during the course of a business relationship are protected by a qualified privilege which also exists regarding defamatory remarks made about public officials or public figures. However, the defense of qualified or conditional privilege is forfeited if the publication is malicious in nature. Malice means that the defamation was published with improper motive or for an improper purpose.

Pharmacists may subject themselves to litigation for careless remarks made about their patients or other health-care professionals in the community. Oral statements which accuse another of improper conduct of a business or unprofessionalism are slanderous *per se*, and subject the maker to liability without the necessity of showing actual damages. A pharmacist's untrue accusations of unchastity or infidelity or imputation of certain loathsome diseases also could result in litigation based upon slander *per se*.

Right to Privacy—More and more states are recognizing a new tort for the invasion of another's privacy. The oral or written publication of private information about an individual, even if true, may give rise to an action based on invasion of privacy. Information contained in patient medication records or prescriptions is confidential in nature and should be released only on the consent of the patient or pursuant to other statutory authority. The admission of nonessential persons during medical treatment or taking medical photographs without the consent of the patient constitutes an invasion of privacy. The invasion must be objectionable and not too trifling. Truth is not a defense to this type of action nor is the absence of malice.

The right to privacy often conflicts with the state's exercise of its power to protect the public's health, safety and welfare. Certain individuals in the state of New York filed a lawsuit against that state for the inclusion of prescription information in a computerized data bank. The plaintiffs alleged that the inclusion of the names of patients, who receive Schedule II prescription drugs, in a centralized computer file violated their rights to privacy. The case eventually was decided by the US Supreme Court which held that the New York statute did not impair any privacy interest. The court found that the requirement was a reasonable exercise of the state's police powers.

> Disclosures of private medical information to physicians, hospital personnel, insurance companies and public health agencies are often an essential part of modern practice even when the disclosures may reflect unfavorably on the character of the patient. Requiring such disclosures to representatives of the state having responsibility for the health of the community, does not automatically amount to an impermissible invasion of privacy. *Whalen v Roe*, 429 US 589 (1977).

Liability based upon the tortious invasion of privacy should not be confused with the constitutional right of privacy which protects an individual from unconstitutional intrusions by government. The constitutional right of privacy increasingly is being used by courts as the basis for allowing medical decisions to be made, not by health-care professionals, but by the patients themselves. A number of recent cases have relied on this right of privacy doctrine to knock down regulations curbing the use of laetrile by cancer patients. A series of convictions of physicians who have used unapproved drugs or unconventional therapy in such cases have been overturned. These cases show the attempts by courts to balance the possible medical treatment against the right of privacy, but a key element in each of these cases has been the uncertainty of the success of any known therapy or alternative.

Commercial Law

The pharmacist should understand the general principles of the law of contracts in order to realize the responsibility he undertakes when entering a business obligation. The law of commercial paper and advertising has a direct bearing on the day-to-day activities of pharmacists. Questions concerning ownership of prescriptions and application of the federal antitrust laws to the pharmacist's relationships with third-party prescription program administrators may be encountered frequently by pharmacists.

It is impossible in a general treatise of this kind to describe in detail the legal subjects on which the pharmacist should keep posted. All that can be attempted is a general outline.

Because the US is composed of 50 individual jurisdictions, the law may vary from state to state. Nonetheless, it is possible to provide an overview of the law applicable to pharmacists in the operation of their practices. To a certain extent the laws applicable to commercial activities have been rendered uniform in most of the states through enactment of the Uniform Commercial Code (UCC); it was drafted in the early part of this century by a group of noted legal scholars in order to bring some order out of the patchwork quilt of states' laws applicable to business affairs. Enacted nearly intact in almost all states, the UCC has done a great deal to facilitate the flow of commerce among and between the states.

Contract Law

A contract may be defined as a promise or set of promises for the breach of which the law provides a remedy, or the performance of which the law, in some way, recognizes as a duty. Yet, the law requires much more for a contract to result than a mere exchange of promises. Perhaps a more complete definition of a contract is an agreement between legally competent individuals based on genuine assent of the parties and supported by consideration, made for a lawful purpose and in the form required by law, if any. This definition provides a framework for discussion of these elements of a contract.

The agreement between the parties, which forms a basis for the contract, is composed of both an offer and an acceptance. In order for an offer to be legally sufficient the party making it must have the intention of entering into an agreement with the other party. For example, an offer made in jest would not indicate the required contractual intent. Moreover, an invitation to make an offer or an offer to negotiate is not a legally cognizable offer for it, too, lacks contractual intent. Advertisements are not an offer of sale but, rather, an indication of willingness to consider an offer made by the potential purchaser. The offer must be communicated to the other party prior to acceptance for an agreement to result.

An additional requirement for an offer is that it be definite. This means that the offer must be detailed sufficiently to provide a basis for the agreement. Courts will not add an essential element to an offer, agreement or contract. At the time of acceptance the offer must still be viable. An offer may be withdrawn prior to acceptance, in the absence of an option having been granted. An option is a binding promise to keep an offer open for a stated period of time. If an option exists, the person making the offer may not withdraw it until the option period has expired. An offer also may be terminated by rejection or by lapse of a period of time stated in the offer.

Acceptance is assent by the recipient of the offer to the terms of the offer. No particular form of acceptance is required, eg, in writing, unless specified in the offer. However, the acceptance must be absolute and unconditional. Any variation of the terms or conditions in the acceptance will result in rejection of the offer.

The parties entering into a contract must be competent legally to do so. This means that each party must have contractual capacity. Minors generally lack contractual capacity and contracts they enter into are subject to their avoidance. The other party may not be able to enforce the contract against a minor because the contract can be voided by the minor due to his lack of contractual capacity. However, parents may be liable under contract theory for "necessaries" provided to their minor dependents. "Necessaries" are those things relating to the health, education or comfort of the minor. Prescription drugs probably would fall within this category and a pharmacist providing them to a minor would, in all likelihood, be able to collect the reasonable value of the medication from the parents.

Insane persons also may be under a contractual incapacity. If a person is so mentally deranged as not to know that a contract is being made or does not understand the consequences of what he is doing, the contract may be voided on recovering sanity. The same is true of a person who is so intoxicated as to be unaware that he is making a contract.

The requirement of genuineness of assent relates to mistake, misrepresentation, concealment, fraud or exercise of undue influence or duress over one of the parties. Each of these activities has a different effect on the enforceability of the contract, and a full discussion of each is beyond the scope of this discussion. Nonetheless, the pharmacist should be aware that each bears a possibility for interference with the enforceability of the contract.

Consideration is essential for a contract to be enforceable. It may be defined as an act or forbearance, or the promise of either, which is offered by one party to an agreement and accepted by the other as an inducement to the other's act or promise. When you have given consideration you have agreed to do something that you were not bound to do or you have agreed to refrain from doing that which you have the right to do.

Consideration must be provided by both parties to the contract. If only one is providing consideration, no contract results. It is a mere gift and not legally enforceable.

Ordinarily, courts will not inquire into the adequacy of the consideration exchanged by the parties. The fact that the amount of consideration may appear to be small in the eyes of one person does not necessarily mean that the amount is inadequate or inappropriate. Hence, if some consideration is provided, the contract will be enforceable. One sometimes hears of employment contracts for "a dollar-a-year man," as in the case of a wealthy individual working for the government or a charity. Such an employment contract will be enforceable even though the value of a person's services will be much greater than the amount of compensation provided.

In order for a contract to be enforceable it must be made for a lawful purpose, and this must be achieved in a lawful manner. If this were not so, the courts might be placed in the uncomfortable situation of compelling one party to a contract to commit a crime in order to have the contract performed. An example of this doctrine is the rule that contracts of an unlicensed operator cannot be enforced. Hence, one who practices pharmacy without being licensed to do so, not only is likely to be charged with the crime of violating the state pharmacy practice act, but also will be unable to enforce the contracts he made while "practicing" pharmacy, ie, he will be unable to sue to collect for his services.

Contracts for the sale of prohibited articles also are unenforceable. The sale of a federal legend drug without a valid prescription would fall in this category. Contracts which unreasonably restrain trade also are unlawful and, consequently, unenforceable. When a pharmacist sells a pharmacy it is customary for the purchaser to request that the contract contain a "non-competition" clause which bans the seller from owning a pharmacy within certain geographic and time limits. The purpose is to prevent the seller from selling and immediately opening up a pharmacy, attracting all his prior patients. If such a clause is drafted to include too large a geographic area, or for too long a time, it will be unenforceable due to its restraint on trade. However, note that only contracts which "unreasonably" restrain trade are unlawful. Consequently, if the non-competition clause is drafted carefully it will be enforceable.

Most contracts are not required to be in writing to be enforceable. Obviously, though, it is much easier to prove the existence of and enforce one that is written. Each state has a Statute of Frauds which dictates which types of contracts must be in writing to be enforceable. Generally, contracts for creation of an interest in land, which run for more than 1 yr, must be in writing. Those that involve employment for more than 1 year and those which are for sale of goods of a value of $500 or more also must be in writing. Each state may have additional categories, and the minimum limits just mentioned may vary from state to state.

When a contract is breached, the nonbreaching party has the right to bring legal action against the breaching party to recover that sum of money that will place him in the same position as he would have been had the contract been performed. There are a number of types of damages which may be assessed against the breaching party. Nominal damages are awarded when the injured party did not suffer an actual loss. They usually are of minimal magnitude. Compensatory damages are those which are designed to compensate the injured party for his loss. Liquidated damages also may be encountered; these are those for which provision was made in the contract itself by the contracting parties when they entered into the agreement. Liquidated-damage clauses generally will be enforced if the amount specified is not excessive and if the contract is of such a nature that it would be difficult to determine the actual amount of damages.

The UCC addresses a special category of contracts known as "sales." A sale may be defined as a transaction wherein a seller transfers title for personal property to a buyer for a price (consideration). Article 2 of the UCC addresses the law of sales in great detail and, interested readers may wish to refer to that source for information beyond the scope of this discussion.

Of particular interest to pharmacists is the law applicable to warranties in sales transactions. A warranty is an assurance or guarantee, by a seller, that the goods sold are, or will be, as represented. Warranties may be divided into two general categories: express and implied.

Express warranties are those based on an affirmation of fact or promise relating to the goods, whereas an implied warranty is one that exists by virtue of law, not because of an express statement by the seller. Express warranties may be made about almost any attribute of the goods, but the warranties implied by law are more limited in scope. One such implied warranty is the implied warranty of merchantability. It is seen only with sellers who usually deal in goods of that type and means that the goods provided must be fit for the ordinary purposes for which such goods are used.

The implied warranty of fitness for a particular purpose is present when the seller knows the use to which the goods will be put and has reason to know that the buyer is relying on the seller's skill and judgment to select suitable goods for the purpose. These implied warranties automatically are present in a transaction without any action on the part of the seller to place them there. They can be removed from the sale but require a specific type of action.

Goods sold "as is" are sold with no implied warranties. To remove the implied warranty of "merchantability" those specific words must be used, but the disclaimer can be made orally. Removal of the implied warranty of fitness for a particular purpose can be done only by written words, but no special language is required. However, the statement that the warranty is absent must be conspicuous. Naturally, express warranties can be kept out of a transaction merely by not making an express statement about the goods.

The Magnuson-Moss Warranty Act went into effect during 1975 and requires that a firm offering a warranty must state it in simple language and must state clearly what it covers. Under this statute the implied warranty cannot be disclaimed or modified in a written warranty; however, the duration of the implied warranties can be limited. The Act also requires that warranty statements be made available to the public in a form to which they can obtain easy access.

Prescription Ownership

A question arises from time to time regarding ownership of the prescription. When it is issued by the prescriber, the patient gains ownership of the document. When it is transferred to the pharmacist for purposes of dispensing the medication, ownership then passes to the pharmacist, pursuant to the contract between the pharmacist and the patient. However, the patient retains certain rights with regard to the document.

While the document itself is the property of the pharmacist and must be retained by law by him for recordkeeping purposes, the patient has the legal right to refills which the law and the prescriber have authorized. Moreover, the patient may have a right to obtain a copy of the prescription, except in those cases where the giving of a copy is prohibited or limited. For example, in some states copies provided to patients must be marked with a statement indicating that the prescription copy is provided for informational use only and cannot serve as the basis for dispensing medication.

In some situations, such as with prescriptions which are suspected to be forgeries or those which bear the potential for a harmful drug interaction, the pharmacist may wish to retain or deface the document even though he will not be dispensing the medication. He who does so is running the risk that the prescription might be legitimate or that the drug interaction would not result. In such a case he could be sued for any damages which resulted from his action, for he does not own the document. Should the pharmacist receive a prescription which he does not intend to follow, the problem should be handled through communication with either the patient or the prescriber, not by defacing the document which he does not own.

Because the pharmacist owns the prescription records reflecting medication which he has dispensed, they are assets of the pharmacy which may be transferred on the cessation of the practice. Prescription records should be maintained for a minimum of five years, the statute of limitations of the federal Food Drug and Cosmetic Act.

Antitrust and Prescription Insurance Plans

Third-party prescription plans have burgeoned in the US in recent years, and a substantial portion of Americans now have insurance coverage for their medication expenditures. This brief discussion shall center on the legal problems associated with private third-party prescription plans, not those administered by governmental agencies.

In the typical third-party plan, the pharmacy owner receives an offer to participate in the insurance plan and a contract to be signed. This usually provides for reimbursement of the pharmacist's cost in acquiring the drug product dispensed and the addition of a dispensing fee of fixed magnitude. Other provisions may relate to what products are compensable, eg, many plans will not pay for nonprescription medication, or limit quantities which may be dispensed. Provisions also are seen dealing with claims submission, services the pharmacist is required to provide and access to the pharmacist's financial records for purposes of program accountability. Often, the offer to participate in such plans is distributed to many pharmacies in an area in order for the insurer to offer the subscriber maximum flexibility in selecting a pharmacist with whom to deal.

When such offers to participate are disseminated widely, the possibility of the offers being discussed collectively arises. This may run afoul of the Sherman Antitrust Act of 1890, which provides that

> "Every contract, combination . . . or conspiracy, in restraint of trade or commerce among the several States . . . is declared to be illegal."

Thus, collective action by pharmacists to withhold entering into contracts with the insurer because the professional fee is too low or because other provisions of the contract are objectionable may violate this federal statute. Individual penalties may be assessed under this statute.

> "Every person who shall monopolize, or attempt to monopolize, or combine or conspire with any other person or persons, to monopolize any part of the trade or commerce among the several States . . . shall be deemed guilty of a misdemeanor, and, on conviction thereof, shall be punished by fine not exceeding fifty thousand dollars, or by imprisonment not exceeding one year or both."

Applicability of this statute to pharmacy was affirmed in the 1962 case of *United States v Utah Pharmaceutical Association*. In that case the activity which brought federal sanctions was publication of a recommended fee schedule in an attempt to encourage the adoption of a uniform professional fee.

With third-party prescription plans, the activity which may violate the statute is collective action by pharmacists ("combination . . . or conspiracy") to withhold their participation ("restrain trade") in the insurance plan until the contract is worded in terms acceptable to them as a group. While such action is permissible legally, if done by an individual acting alone, collective action toward the same end would not be legally permissible.

In addition to the criminal penalties outlined above, the patients who are injured by such unlawful activity may bring a civil suit to recover damages. Of importance is the fact that in an antitrust claim, the award is for treble damages, ie, the amount of damages is calculated and then multiplied by three to yield the amount the party engaging in the unlawful activity must pay.

Advertising

The regulation of the advertising and promotion of drugs on an interstate commerce basis is a shared commitment of numerous federal agencies, including the Postal Service, Federal Communications Commission, Federal Trade Commission and Food and Drug Administration. The latter two bear the brunt of the responsibility. The FTC is involved actively in the regulation of OTC drug advertising while the FDA exercises its jurisdiction primarily over matters involving the labeling and advertising of prescription drugs. There is, however, considerable overlap between the two agencies because of statutory definitions and by mutual agreement.

In intrastate commerce, analogous controls often exist both in terms of substantive law and enforcement apparatus. However, state limitations imposed primarily by budget give these controls much less effect in comparison to federal activities. The pharmacist, therefore, will be bound primarily by federal restrictions in the area of advertising.

Federal Trade Commission—The FTC derives its authority over advertising in general and drug advertising in particular from the Federal Trade Commission Act. Section 5 of that statute provides

"Unfair methods of competition in commerce and unfair or deceptive acts or practices in commerce are hereby declared unlawful."

In addition, Section 12 makes it unlawful to disseminate a false advertisement for the purpose of inducing, or which is likely to induce, the purchase of food, drugs, devices or cosmetics. The Wheeler-Lea Amendment to the Act defines "false advertising" as follows:

"The term "false advertisement" means an advertisement, other than labeling, which is misleading in a material respect; and in determining whether any advertisement is misleading, there shall be taken into account (among other things) not only representations made or suggested by statement, word, design, device, sound or any combination thereof, but also the extent to which the advertisement fails to reveal facts, material in the light of such representations or material with respect to consequences, which may result from the use of the commodity to which the advertisement relates under the conditions prescribed in said advertisement, or under such conditions as are customary or usual."

Based on the above provision, the FTC has authority to move against not only false advertisements for OTC drug products but also advertisements which operate in an unfair or deceptive way. The Commission can use its powers by either promulgating a Trade Regulation Rule or by issuing a complaint against an advertiser when there is reason to believe that the law has been violated.

In most cases in which a complaint is issued by the FTC, the advertiser is willing to enter into an agreement to cease and desist from the use of the acts and practices being investigated. Such an agreement is for settlement purposes only, and it does not constitute an admission by the advertiser that the law has been violated. The FTC has been successful in obtaining consent agreements from a number of corporations, including those practicing pharmacy, which require all items advertised to be available for sale readily at or below the advertised price. Displays of advertised items must be marked conspicuously by a sign or other means disclosing that the item is "as advertised" or "on sale." In addition, many of the consent orders provide that if the advertised item is unavailable, the consumer may either be given a rain-check or be allowed to purchase a similar product of equal or better quality at or below the advertised price. Phrases such as "regular price" or "manufacturer's suggested list price" and words of similar import should not be used unless they can be documented. Whenever a "free," "2-for-1," "half price sale," "1¢ sale" or similar type of offer is made, all of its terms and conditions to the consumer should be made clear at the outset.

If the parties are unable to agree to a consent order, an FTC complaint will result in a trial before an administrative law judge who will determine if a violation has occurred and, if so, the appropriate remedies. This decision may be appealed by either party to the full Commission sitting as an appellate body. Thereafter, review can be pursued to a US Court of Appeals and possibly to the US Supreme Court. A case involving a well-known mouthwash followed just such a procedure. An administrative law judge ruled that the advertisements for the mouthwash had made claims which were false, misleading and deceptive. Under the administrative ruling, the manufacturer was ordered not only to stop making such claims but also to institute corrective advertising to inform consumers that the product would not help prevent colds or sore throats or lessen their severity. This ruling was upheld by the full Commission and by a federal appeals court, and the US Supreme Court rejected the manufacturer's petition for further review.

In another action, a 1975 FTC complaint alleging false and misleading advertising included a pharmacy retailer as a defendant even though the ads were prepared by the manufacturer's advertising agency. The administrative law judge held that although the retailer did not know whether the ad claims were true or false, it was not relieved of responsibility simply because the ad copy and content were prepared by others. The full FTC bench ruled that the Act does not exempt the seller of a product from investigating the truthfulness of claims set forth over the retailer's own name. The lack of knowledge of the falsity of the ad was found not to be a defense.

Food and Drug Administration—Prior to 1962 the FTC was vested with sole authority for regulating the advertising of drugs. The Kefauver-Harris Amendments of 1962 to the Food, Drug and Cosmetic Act gave the FDA control over prescription drug advertising. Thus, the FDA regulates not only the labeling of prescription drugs but their advertising as well. All advertisements and other descriptive printed matter issued by the manufacturer must include a statement of the established name, quantitative formula and other information such as side effects, contraindications and effectiveness.

The FDA's authority over the regulation of prescription drug advertising extends not only to advertising directed to professionals but also to that presented to the lay public. By regulation, the FDA has determined that any pharmacy which posts or advertises the price of prescription drugs must include the following information: brand name, if any; generic name, if any; the drug's strength, if the product contains a single active ingredient; dosage form and the price charged for a specific quantity of the drug. Optional information such as delivery service, charge account service or senior citizen's discount may be included if such information is not false or misleading. The regulations do not require any pharmacy to post or advertise prescription drug prices, but pharmacies which do so must follow the FDA format.

State Regulation—For some time, many states had pharmacy act provisions or pharmacy board regulations which prohibited prescription drug advertising. Numerous state court decisions had been handed down regarding the permissibility of such prohibitions, but their dictate was anything but clear. In order to obtain an ultimate decision on this controversy, a group of consumers filed suit against the Virginia State Board of Pharmacy alleging a First Amendment right to receive prescription price information. The case of *Virginia State Board of Pharmacy v Virginia Citizens Consumer Council, Inc* eventually reached the US Supreme Court. The court, basing its decision on the First Amendment, held that even speech which primarily is commercial in nature is protected. The consumer should have the freedom to obtain the price information necessary to make a choice regarding prescription drugs. The FTC previously had proposed a Trade Regulation Rule which would preempt and override all state statutes and regulations which prohibited prescription drug advertising, but with the advent of the *Virginia* case the FTC did not feel it was necessary to move further in this area.

A number of states also have maintained restrictions against the advertisement or display of contraceptives. Such a provision of New York law came under judicial attack, and this case also reached the US Supreme Court which relied heavily on its decision in the *Virginia* case in holding that the prohibition of any advertisement or display of contraceptives is unconstitutional. All total bans on the advertising of such products were struck down, but the states would still be allowed to regulate against obscene ads. The case of *Carey v Population Services International* also held that the limiting of retail sales of nonmedical contraceptives by licensed pharmacists only clearly imposed a significant burden upon the right of individuals to use contraceptives. The state of New York could demonstrate no compelling reason for such a limitation and, thus, the Supreme Court found it unconstitutional.

Bibliography

DeMarco CT: *Pharmacy and the Law* 2nd ed, Aspen Systems Corp, Rockville MD, 1984.

Fink III JL, Marquardt KW, Simonsmeier LM: *Pharmacy Law Digest*, Facts & Comparisons, St Louis MO, 1993.

Merrill RA, Hutt PB: *Food and Drug Law: Cases and Materials*, 2nd ed, Foundation Press, Mineola, NY, 1991.

Nielsen JR: *Handbook of Federal Drug Law*, Lea & Febiger, Philadelphia PA, 1986.

Uelman GF, Haddox VG: *Drug Abuse and the Law: Cases, Text and Materials*, West Publ, St Paul MN, 1974.

Wetherbee H, White BD: *Pharmacy Law: Cases and Materials*, West Publ, St Paul MN, 1980.

CHAPTER 111

Community Pharmacy Economics and Management

James W Richards, MBA
Professor of Pharmacy Administration
College of Pharmacy, University of Michigan
Ann Arbor, MI 48109

The economic impact of the health-care industry on our society is difficult to evaluate. It is accepted that advances made by the industry during the past few decades have reduced morbidity and mortality rates which, in turn, have increased productivity and added to the gross domestic product. At the same time, the cost of health care is rising at a faster rate than is the consumer price index for all items, and this cost continues to represent an increasingly larger share of the gross domestic product.

Economics of Health Care

According to the US Health Care Financing Administration, Americans spent $727 billion on personal health care in 1992. Projections based on historical trends indicate that personal health-care expenditures may exceed $1.5 trillion by the year 2000. However, the actual level of future expenditures will be determined by the outcome of current efforts to reform the US health-care system. The increase in expenditures for personal health care is the result of a number of factors, including

Population increases and aging of the population.
Inflation (general and medical).
Increased use of facilities and services.
Increased governmental involvement in health care.
Increased quality of care from new technologies, equipment and drugs.

Further analysis of national health expenditures reveals that a significant portion of personal health costs are paid with public funds. In 1992, governmental outlays represented over 45% of all health-care expenditures. Medicare payments accounted for a major portion of governmental health-care expenditures. However, state Medicaid programs and other social welfare programs also contributed to the public expenditures for health care.

The magnitude of health-care expenditures in the US and the growing governmental involvement as a third-party payer of health-care costs are evidence of society's commitment to providing the best care possible for all citizens. Those involved in the delivery of health care share society's commitment and, therefore, must be concerned with the economics of the delivery system.

The pharmaceutical segment of the health-care industry entails a significant expenditure. In 1992 over $65 billion was spent at the retail level for drugs and drug sundries in the US. The 1992 expenditure for drugs and pharmaceutical services represented 8.9% of the nation's personal health bill.

In view of the level of expenditures for drugs and pharmaceutical services and given the trend of health-care costs, it is apparent that those involved in the delivery of pharmaceutical services must be aware of their responsibility to provide high-quality services in the most economical way. Although some look on third-party payment as a mechanism for solving the high cost of health care, including the drug-cost segment, it should be understood that third-party payment does not reduce the cost. It simply spreads it over a larger population.

Actually, third-party payment may increase the total cost of health care as additional administrative costs and increased use of services are inherent in these programs. It follows that third-party payers, whether governmental or private, have an obligation to their constituents to ensure the delivery of quality services at reasonable prices. In this regard, health professionals find their services under scrutiny by a sophisticated group of agencies representing a large portion of the general public.

In recent years, concern over increasing personal health-care expenditures has led to the development of a variety of alternative delivery systems for prepaid health care. These systems, sometimes referred to as managed-care programs, include Health Maintenance Organizations (HMOs), Preferred Provider Organizations (PPOs) and Administrative Service Organizations (ASOs) sponsored by providers of health care.

The objectives of all of the managed-care programs are to provide quality health services while, at the same time, attempting to reduce the rate of increase of health-care expenditures. The cost-containment objective of managed-care programs has generated increased competition among providers, as only the most cost-effective providers are eligible to participate in some programs.

With the development of managed-care programs, those who provide pharmacy services must consider economic and professional factors, as they make decisions about participation in the programs. Pharmacy owners and managers face the challenge of maintaining the economic viability of their pharmacies as participants in managed-care programs. Participation in such programs often increases administrative expenses for the pharmacy while, at the same time, providing reimbursement which may not be adequate to cover the costs of providing quality pharmacy services.

In response to the move to managed-care programs, a number of pharmacy organizations have formed Pharmacy Services Administrative Organizations (PSAOs) which are attempting to provide an alternative system that balances the public need for cost-effective services with the professional and economic needs of those who provide pharmacy services. For additional information, see Chapter 96.

In the past the cost of health care was given little attention by the providers of health services. It was assumed that the primary obligation of the provider was to ensure the physical well-being of the patient, without regard to cost. It is now apparent that it does little good to develop a level of health care which is unsurpassed in the world if a sizable segment of the population cannot afford to pay for it.

The obligation of health professionals to consider the economic dimensions of health care is now recognized. For example, pharmacy practice laws in all states have been amended to allow pharmacists to practice drug-product selection. These amendments allow the pharmacist, under specified conditions, to choose drug products with due regard for both the physical and the economic well-being of the patient. The drug-product selection amendments are tangible evidence of societal concern with the cost of health care.

The concern of health professionals with the cost of health care now reinforces the efforts of consumer groups, government and others involved in financing health care, to the end of providing the best care for all, regardless of economic status.

According to the Health Insurance Council, comprehensive

health-service planning and delivery should be based upon the following guidelines.

Health services cost money, and good health service costs a good deal of money. Agencies which spend money on behalf of others have a responsibility to get their money's worth for their beneficiaries.

Financing methods for health service should encourage efficient organization and management of the professional personnel and institutions.

Financing methods should distribute the burden of medical care costs in the way which best assures proper care of the entire population.

Health personnel and institutions must be reimbursed in amounts and by methods which permit them to maintain standards and achieve efficiency.

Although these guidelines are intended for the total health-care system, they may be applied to any segment of the system. The guidelines include concepts which are applicable to pharmacy practice. The guidelines suggest that health insurers promote efficient organization and management of personnel and facilities. It follows that pharmacists should promote efficient organization and management. Using carefully developed organizational plans and modern management techniques, pharmacists in community practice can contribute to the efforts being made to contain health-care costs.

The Community Pharmacy

The majority of consumer expenditures for prescription drugs, proprietary medicines and health appliances are channeled through the approximately 60,000 community pharmacies in the US. Although heterogeneous in some respects, as in type of ownership and type of goods and services offered, community pharmacies generally are recognized by the public as the most accessible source of drugs and of information about drugs.

Community pharmacy, as used here, is defined broadly to include all of those establishments that are privately owned and whose function, in varying degrees, is to serve society's need for both drug products and pharmaceutical services. It is difficult to characterize or describe the typical pharmacy because of the great variance among them. They range from the corporately owned chain pharmacy, to the pharmacy department in a supermarket, to the independently owned pharmaceutical center, providing prescription service plus a relatively few lines of health-related products.

According to the operating data submitted to the *Lilly Digest* (Eli Lilly & Co, Indianapolis, IN) by over 1200 community pharmacy owners, the average independent community pharmacy generated sales of $1,021,215 in 1991. These data represent a summary of individual pharmacy operating figures which were supplied voluntarily by pharmacy managers and owners.

It should be noted that the editors of the *Lilly Digest* make no attempt to structure the sample that comprises the data input and, therefore, their citations are subject to the statistical limitations inherent in the collection of unstructured voluntary data. It appears, however, that the figures serve to describe fairly accurately the financial profile of the independent community pharmacy.

The data from the *1992 Lilly Digest* indicate that approximately 75% of the revenues of the pharmacies reporting are derived from prescription medications and services. The average prescription charge in 1991, as reported in the *Digest*, was $22.44, compared with a charge reported 5 years earlier of $14.36. It should be noted that the average prescription charge is not an accurate measure of the price changes for prescription medications. Over a period of years, the types of drugs dispensed have changed with the introduction of new products which usually provide improved drug therapy at a higher cost. In addition, there has been an increase in the number of maintenance drugs prescribed with a corresponding increase in the average number of dosage units per prescription order. Therefore, the average prescription charge in 1991 was for a different mix of prescription products, in larger quantities, than was represented by the average charge in 1986.

Chain Pharmacies—The foregoing discussion dealt mainly with the independent pharmacies which represent about 55% of the community pharmacies in the US. Chain pharmacies also are an important factor in the delivery of pharmaceutical services and products to the public.

There is no consensus on the definition for a chain pharmacy, as there appears to be a question as to what criteria are appropriate for classifying a group of centrally owned pharmacies as chain pharmacies. To some, the matter of central ownership, alone, is sufficient to classify the individual units as chain pharmacies. Another approach is to classify individual units which are owned centrally as chain pharmacies only when there also is centralized organization and management.

The number of centrally owned units also has been used as a method of defining chain pharmacies. However, this criterion does not provide a satisfactory answer to the question, as many multiple-unit pharmacies are owned centrally and yet each unit functions independently from the central ownership. In mode-of-operation these pharmacies are more similar to individually owned community pharmacies. On the other hand, as the number of units under a central ownership increases, at some point there must be some coordination of policies and activities which results in more central management.

Although it is not possible to establish an exact number of units as the point where all units assume the characteristics of a true chain pharmacy operation, it appears that there is some relationship between the number of units owned and the definition of a pharmacy chain. The US Department of Commerce defines a pharmacy chain as those units with prescription departments which are centrally owned by individuals or organizations who own 11 or more units.

The typical chain pharmacy operates from a broader base in the variety of goods offered for sale than does the independent pharmacy. The kinds of goods offered for sale in chain pharmacies are almost limitless, and include durable consumer goods in addition to health-related products.

In this regard it may be somewhat misleading to compare sales in the chain pharmacy with sales in the independent community pharmacy. However, when trends over the past few years are studied, it is apparent that the chain pharmacies also are improving their relative position in such areas as revenues from prescription medications and OTC drugs.

Establishment of a Community Pharmacy

The pharmacist considering the establishment of a new pharmacy should subject the basic decision to an objective analysis which should include a consideration of community needs—does the community really need another facility for pharmaceutical services?

The question may have both a quantitative and a qualitative dimension. Perhaps a given community has a sufficient number of pharmacies and yet none of them is providing the full scope of needed services. If a community need is identified, the analysis should continue in terms of evaluating the various alternatives that are available for satisfying it. Perhaps an existing pharmacy could be purchased and made to provide more-extensive pharmaceutical services, or there may be an opportunity to join with another pharmacist in the ownership of an existing pharmacy and establish a group practice.

Such alternatives provide the opportunity for improving services to the community while promoting the most efficient use of professional personnel and facilities.

If the analysis indicates that a new pharmacy should be established, the pharmacist must consider a number of questions, some of them simultaneously, eg

What is the appropriate legal organization for the enterprise?
What specific location should be chosen?
How may the necessary capital be obtained?

Although each of the foregoing questions is related to the others and cannot be isolated in a practical situation, each will be treated by itself for purposes of this discussion.

Organization

The pharmacist may choose from three widely recognized forms of legal organization for the community pharmacy enterprise. Traditionally, the majority of these have been organized as individual or sole proprietorships, with relatively little governmental control applied to the organizational structure.

In recent years, because of the increase in the joint ownership of pharmacies by two or more individuals, the partnership and corporate forms of organization have become more significant. The partnership, as a form of business organization, enjoys relative independence from governmental control. The corporation, as a creation of the state government, is subject to rather strict governmental regulation. Each form presents advantages that must be weighed against the disadvantages and limitations that become apparent when compared with the alternative forms of organization.

Unincorporated Sole Proprietorships—The business enterprise owned and managed by an unincorporated sole proprietor is not considered in law to be a separate legal entity; rather, the owner and the enterprise are considered as one. It follows that the risk inherent in establishing a business enterprise in this way has implications for the nonbusiness assets of the proprietor.

The unincorporated sole proprietor has unlimited personal liability. Personal assets are available to satisfy business obligations, and business assets may be used to satisfy personal debts. In return for assuming unlimited liability, the sole proprietor enjoys the freedom to conduct the enterprise in any lawful manner he or she deems appropriate.

Except for the required licenses, the sole proprietor may begin or quit operations without legal formality or governmental permission. Some states do require that a statement of ownership be filed with a designated office when the owner's name is not indicated in the name of the enterprise. The sole proprietor receives all profits from the enterprise.

The size or scope of the operation is not necessarily a determining factor in the decision to organize as a sole proprietorship, as opposed to one of the other forms of organization. However, due to the risks involved and the fact that few persons possess all of the abilities and capacities necessary for carrying on a large complex enterprise, the sole proprietorship most often is associated with smaller, less complex, operations.

Historically, the majority of community pharmacists are independent by nature and have chosen this rather informal form of organization. The typical community pharmacy being geographically local and only moderately complex in scope of operation generally succeeds under the unincorporated sole-ownership system.

Partnerships—When the resources of one individual are not sufficient to provide a proper base for establishing a pharmacy, or when the individual does not wish to assume the entire risk associated with the entrepreneurial function, joint ownership may be considered. Partnership arrangements and incorporation are mechanisms that may be used to broaden the financial or talent base for an enterprise and also may serve to spread the risk. The partnership may be described as an association of two or more individuals based on an expressed or implied contract. They combine their resources as co-owners of an enterprise for their mutual profit. This provides a way for the individuals to do jointly what they could not do separately.

As to liability, a partnership may be described as an association of sole proprietors, because at law the partnership is not considered separate from those who compose it. As with the sole proprietorship, each partner is liable for all debts of the partnership, even to the extent of personal assets. Within the scope of partnership activities, each general partner is considered an agent of the other general partners and, as such, each has the right to bind or commit the partnership in business affairs. Because of the mutual-agency concept and the unlimited liability inherent in partnership associations, it is especially important that the full implications of such an arrangement be understood before adopting this form.

Although it is a contractual arrangement, there are relatively few legal restrictions or regulations applied to the partnership association. No expressed governmental consent is required to establish or dissolve a partnership, and the contract may be written or simply based on a handshake, as long as the elements of a valid contract are present. This is not to imply that the partnership should be consummated on the basis of an informal verbal agreement. The contractual relationship between partners should be verified by a written agreement drafted with the assistance of a lawyer.

The close personal relationship among partners tends to foster a disregard for formalized written documents relating to the operation of the partnership. In the interest of producing a smoothly functioning organization and helping to prevent disagreements among the partners, it is most important that a written partnership agreement be prepared at the outset.

Such matters as the investment, duties, responsibilities and division of profits and losses of each partner should be considered and incorporated into the partnership agreement. The agreement not only provides a reference for solving future misunderstanding but also serves to compel the partners, at the inception of the agreement, to consider matters that might otherwise remain hidden until a specific problem arises.

The partnership as a form of business organization provides a mechanism for joint ownership of an enterprise which is relatively free of governmental regulation and which embodies the same flexibility of operation enjoyed by the sole proprietorship. As the partnership is not considered a legal entity, it is not required to pay income taxes on profits; rather, the individual partners are assigned their share of profits and pay income taxes on them as individuals.

When compared to the corporate form of joint ownership, the partnership usually presents an advantage to the co-owners with regard to income tax liability. The partnership has been a popular form of organization for the co-ownership of community pharmacies.

Corporations—Co-ownership also may be effected through a more formal organization known as the corporation, which is a separate legal entity, created by the expressed authority of the state. A properly constituted corporation offers the stockholders the advantage of limited liability for business debts.

In contrast to the sole proprietorship and the partnership, the incorporated business enterprise is considered as a separate entity from the persons who own it. Consequently, in the absence of a statute to the contrary, corporate stockholders are liable only to the extent of their contributions to the capital of the enterprise. As a general rule, creditors of the corporation cannot proceed against the individual stock holders for debts of the corporation.

As a legal entity created by the state, the corporation enjoys continuity of life subject only to the limitation(s) included in its charter. The death or incapacity of a stockholder or the transfer of ownership in no way affects the corporate existence.

The corporation provides a way for individuals to invest in a business venture without placing their personal assets in jeopardy. It also provides a convenient, highly organized mechanism for accumulating a large amount of capital from several individuals in order to establish a business enterprise.

In terms of initial organization, the formation of a corporation is more complex and formal than other types of own ership. Each state has a required procedure to be followed in the creation of a corporation, and once franchised, it is subject to regulation and control by the state.

By definition, the corporation only has those powers and can do those things that are authorized by the state, in contrast to the partnership, which may do any lawful thing agreed to by the partners. The corporation may be dissolved only by or with the expressed consent of the state.

The status of the corporate enterprise as a legal entity

makes it subject to local, state and federal income taxes upon its earnings. When the earnings after corporate income taxes are distributed as dividends, the individual stockholders are required to pay personal income taxes upon them. As a result, the owners of corporations are said to be subject to double taxation, a factor which in many cases has deterred sole proprietorships and partnerships from adopting the corporate form of organization. However, under special conditions the owners of a corporation may avoid double taxation of profits by requesting designation as a Subchapter S corporation under provisions of the US Internal Revenue Code. If Subchapter S status is granted, profits are not subject to corporate income taxes but are passed through to stockholders and taxed as part of their personal income.

In the field of community pharmacy, the majority of chain organizations are corporations. The corporate form provides the protection of limited liability, which is especially important for larger multiunit operations. In addition, a fair number of the larger nonchain pharmacies are also incorporated, although it should be noted that neither size nor scope of operation is necessarily the only determinant in the decision to incorporate.

In establishing a new pharmacy, the prospective owner(s) must decide at the outset which form of organization to follow. The factors of liability, flexibility of operations, governmental regulation, continuity of life and income taxes should be considered in relationship to the scope of the operation and the personal circumstances of the organizers. It is especially important to seek legal counsel in arriving at a decision. For additional information see Chapter 110.

Site Selection

Much has been written on the criteria that should be employed in choosing a specific community as the site for a new pharmacy. Such factors as population in the trading area, distribution of income among the population, type of industry and the competitive climate have been cited as being important.

Sometimes a pharmacy is established in a community because the pharmacist-owner is determined to own a pharmacy in a specific community because of personal factors such as family ties, climate or other appeals of the community. In such cases the decision often is made without regard to the key issue of whether or not the community needs another facility for pharmaceutical services.

If a need is identified in a given town or city, the selection of a specific site will require careful consideration. The degree of success of a community pharmacy may depend on the choice of the location most suitable among those available. In some cases, the choice of a specific site is extremely limited; the pharmacist must choose from what is available rather than that which is most desirable.

The majority of consumers choose the pharmacy they will patronize on the basis of convenience and accessibility, so long as the pharmacy offers adequate service and fair prices. Therefore, the primary emphasis in site selection should be on obtaining a location that is central to the population to be served. The modern pharmacy must provide easy access and adequate parking. The growth of shopping centers may be cited as evidence of the importance of these factors.

As a general rule, shopping centers are located centrally in relation to the neighborhood, community or region they serve, and they provide easy access and adequate free parking. Interestingly, as a general rule, community pharmacies are more successful in neighborhood and community shopping centers than in the larger regional centers. This tends to substantiate the impression that consumers wish to obtain pharmacy services near home.

Although a site in a neighborhood or community shopping center may be considered to be a choice location for a new pharmacy, as a practical matter few independent community pharmacists are able to obtain such locations. Because of the nature of the system used to finance new shopping centers, preference is given by the developers of the centers to large well-established chain pharmacies.

However, it appears that there are other suitable locations for a traditional pharmacy that emphasizes professional services rather than the sale of nonhealth-related merchandise.

The island type of location, where the pharmacy sits by itself on a main traffic artery into a suburb and surrounded by adequate parking facilities, has proved to be attractive to consumers. A location within a large medical clinic also may prove to be valuable, although, because of the tendency of patients to obtain prescription service near home, the clinic location may not be so important as some believe it to be. The selection of a site solely because it is available readily or inexpensively, should be avoided. Usually, a bargain location in terms of rent proves to be a liability rather than an asset in the long run.

The selection of the proper site for a new pharmacy is important especially as it is a decision which the pharmacist may have to live with for 5, 10 or more years, depending on the terms of the lease, if the pharmacy is operated in a rented facility. Whenever possible, advice should be obtained from others regarding site selection. Some wholesale drug firms provide counsel in this regard, or a business consulting firm may be engaged to assist in making an objective evaluation of alternatives.

Capital

Planning and assembling the capital requirements for a new pharmacy are predicated on careful evaluation of projected sales volume, breadth and depth of inventory requirements and estimated operating expenses. The amount of capital required for the operation of a successful pharmacy is a function of its productivity.

Although certain of the assets required represent a fixed core necessary for any pharmacy, regardless of sales volume, beyond these the amount of assets required depends, in large measure, upon the scope of operation and the volume anticipated. As illustrated in Table I, as sales volume increases, investment in inventory, fixtures and other assets also increases.

Other factors also have an impact on capital requirements. For example, the policy of the owner toward offering credit may require more or less working capital. The mix of sales volume also may affect capital requirements. As a general rule, prescription revenues can be generated with a lower inventory investment than revenues from other sources.

The problem of determining capital requirements for a new pharmacy is difficult. Most of the underlying factors are based on conjecture and forecasts regarding the future, for which there is no reliable basis at the outset. However, some judgment must be made as to what assets are required for a specific venture, so that the pharmacist may explore the feasibility of assembling a definite amount of capital.

When making the forecasts and estimates needed to establish the basis from which to estimate capital requirements, a sense of conservatism should prevail. The projected sales volume should be estimated at minimum level; operating expenses, at maximum level. It is usually easier to add new capital if sales exceed expectation than it is to recall committed capital if sales are less than anticipated. When operating expenses are estimated on the high side and planned for accordingly with adequate capital, a margin of safety is provided. If expenses are estimated at a level lower than is actually realized, financial difficulty may be encountered.

The method of estimating the capital requirements for a new pharmacy can be described by example. Assume that a conservative estimate indicates that a new pharmacy can produce $500,000 in sales volume during the first year of operation. The question becomes: What kinds of capital will be necessary to support the estimated volume and in what amounts? These are as follows: cash, inventory, fixtures and equipment. The assumption made here is that the owner will not own the building or land used for the pharmacy. The

Table 1—Balance Sheets for *Lilly Digest* Pharmacies under 5 Years Old: 1991 (Averages per Pharmacy)[a]

	Sales under $400,000	Sales over $600,000
Assets		
Current assets		
Cash	$ 10,395	$ 19,054
Accounts receivable	13,909	45,231
Inventory	51,854	107,586
Total current assets	$ 76,158	$171,871
Fixed assets		
Fixtures and equipment and leasehold improvements (net after reserve for depreciation)	8829	15,355
Other assets		
Prepaid expenses, deposits, etc.	5,416	4,896
Total assets[b]	$ 90,403	$192,122
Liabilities		
Current and accrued liabilities		
Accounts payable	$ 13,623	$ 26,648
Notes payable (within 1 yr)	12,764	12,474
Accrued expenses and other liabilities	3,077	7,137
Total current and accrued liabilities	$ 29,464	$ 46,259
Long-term liabilities		
Notes payable (later than 1 yr)	24,311	52,399
Total liabilities	$ 53,775	$ 98,658
Net Worth	36,628	95,464
Total liabilities and net worth[b]	$ 90,403	$194,122
Net working capital	$ 46,694	$125,612
Sales	$316,679	$760,307
Purchases	$214,548	$547,426
New profit (before taxes)	$ 11,175	$ 39,215

[a] Source: *The Lilly Digest* for 1992.
[b] Excludes land, building, investments and goodwill plus corresponding liabilities.

amount of capital required in each category is related, in varying degrees, to the anticipated sales volume, and may be estimated as follows.

Cash—Sufficient cash is required to pay preopening expenses, operating expenses for a stated period of time and some excess for emergency use. Preopening expenses include license fees, legal fees, utility deposits and advertising. These expenses, with the possible exception of advertising, are fixed relatively for any new pharmacy and are not related to sales volume. They are determined easily and usually total $2,000 to $3,000. The higher figure will be assumed here.

It is considered good practice to start a new business venture with sufficient cash to pay the first 2- to 3-months' operating expenses, on the theory that the first months of operation may be extremely slow. For a new pharmacy, the amount required may be determined by relating estimated monthly sales volume to operating expense statistics, available from such sources as the *Lilly Digest*. Only cash expense items are used in the calculation. Such noncash expenses as depreciation and bad debt losses are not considered.

For a pharmacy in the volume category of this example, the *Lilly Digest* indicates that approximately 25% of sales go to cover cash operating expenses, including a salary for the pharmacy owner. Applying this percentage to 3-month sales of a pharmacy with annual sales of $500,000 gives a figure of $31,250 needed to pay operating expenses for a 3-month period. The total amount of cash required for pre-opening expenses and early operating expenses equals $34,250. In addition, cash will be needed to provide the other kinds of capital described below.

Inventory—The amount of inventory necessary to support a $500,000 sales volume may be determined by referring to data that give averages for cost of goods sold and annual stock-turnover rates. Again referring to the *Lilly Digest*, the cost of goods sold for a pharmacy with sales of $500,000 is about 70%, or $350,000. The average annual stock-turnover rate is given as 5.2 and is determined by dividing the cost of goods sold by average inventory at cost. Knowing the cost of goods sold and the stock-turnover rate, it is possible to estimate the average inventory; in this case it is approximately $67,300.

Fixtures and Equipment—The fixtures and equipment necessary for a new pharmacy also are related to estimated volume. Larger volume means more inventory, which in turn requires more fixtures and equipment to facilitate storage and display. The size of the building to be furnished and the quality of fixtures chosen also will affect the total expended. On occasion, savings may be realized by purchasing good, used fixtures and equipment, usually available at a fraction of the cost of new ones. A reasonable expenditure for these items for a pharmacy properly equipped to generate annual sales of $500,000 would be about $20,000.

Total Investment and Sources of Capital—The total investment required for a new pharmacy with estimated sales per year of $500,000 would be approximately $121,550, broken down as

Cash (for preopening and operating expenses)	$34,250
Inventory	67,300
Fixtures and equipment	20,000
Total investment	$121,550

The total represents the cash value of the assets required to establish the new pharmacy in this example. However, the amount of actual cash needed will be somewhat less than the total amount stated. In most cases, the owner will be able to assemble the required assets by using a combination of equity capital, borrowed capital and credit.

Equity capital consists of the investment of the owner or owners, and comes from personal savings or from other sources that require no security and no commitment as to date of repayment. Relatives may be a source of equity capital, either on a co-ownership basis or simply by providing unsecured, undated loans. It is thought that at least one-half to two-thirds of the total requirement should be equity capital, although many successful pharmacies have been established with lower amounts. The amount of equity capital provided will influence the availability of borrowed capital and the level of credit that may be obtained by the owner.

Commercial lending institutions, such as banks and savings and loan associations, usually require a substantial equity interest in a new business venture before they will consider lending the funds necessary to supplement the owner's contribution. As a general rule, commercial lending institutions should not be depended upon for a significant portion of initial capital needs. Such institutions are limited in the amount of risk they are willing to assume, especially for new ventures.

Trade sources, such as suppliers of fixtures and wholesale drug firms, present the best opportunity for obtaining nonequity capital for the new pharmacy. It is common for wholesalers to supply the opening inventory requirements for a new pharmacy on the basis of approximately 50% of the total cost as a down-payment, with the balance to be paid over an extended period of time, which varies with the individual circumstances. Usually, if the time exceeds 90 to 180 days, the supplier will attach an interest charge to the unpaid balance.

The amount of cash required for inventory may be further reduced by cutting back the level of inventory at the outset and then building it up to the required level as operations continue and sales volume increases. Two cautions should be considered in obtaining any significant amount of capital through the use of trade credit:

The interest factor should be studied; depending upon the rate and the method of calculation, interest charges can be surprisingly high.

The use of credit simply postpones the underlying obligation to some future date or dates. Repayment of credit obligations should be considered in terms of the practical feasibility of meeting the obligations when they are due.

Fixtures and equipment may be obtained by relatively long-term financing through suppliers, or in some cases through finance companies by a mechanism similar to the one used to finance a personal automobile. Underlying this form of financing is a chattel mortgage which places title to the fixtures and equipment in the hands of the lender as security.

The interest charges from this type of financing may be especially significant, often reaching an effective rate of 15% or more annually. Usually a down-payment of one-quarter to one-third of the value of the fixtures is required, with the balance to be paid in installments over as many as 5 years. The scheduled installment payments should be included in long- range financial budgeting and planning.

After the potential sources of capital have been evaluated carefully, it may be necessary to make compromises or adjustments regarding the amounts estimated originally. In some cases the owner will reduce his withdrawals or salary during early operations to reduce the amount of cash needed for operating expenses. Inventories also may be reduced at the outset. In fact, it is considered good practice to hold about 20% of the amount budgeted for inventory in abeyance until the needs of the particular community are identified.

The amount required for fixtures and equipment may be reduced by purchasing some used fixtures and equipment. It also is possible to lease fixtures and equipment, although this may increase the cost of fixtures and equipment over the long term. However, such arrangements also will reduce initial capital requirements. By these means, and through the judicious use of borrowed funds and credit, a new pharmacy may be established with less cash than is indicated by the figure for the total investment.

Management

In general terms, the management function may be described as all those activities involved in the organization and direction of the elements of an economically productive enterprise. Money, material, equipment and people must be brought together in the proper relationships to one another to achieve the objectives and goals that management has identified. Management practices predicated on predetermined goals and objectives provide for more efficient operation and provide a basis for measuring the effectiveness of management activities.

The management activities of the pharmacist too often consist of handling day-to-day problems and crises. Much of the activity labeled management in the typical community pharmacy is actually routine administrative work that can and should be delegated to nonmanagement personnel. Perhaps this point is best illustrated by the axiom "management's job is not to do, but to get others to do."

The traditional approach to community pharmacy management consisting of the *ad hoc* handling of problems as they arise is not consistent with the nature or responsibilities of modern practice. The sum total of all activities in a pharmacy is becoming increasingly complex, due to increased volume of operations and to outside pressures for more efficient delivery of pharmaceutical services and products.

All health workers are being called on to develop a social conscience and assume more responsibility for the economic impact of their activities. Although technological changes may relieve some of the pressure on health-care costs, better management and administrative techniques also can contribute significantly to solving the problem.

The impact of more effective management also may be reflected in improved professional services to the public. For example, a management decision to assign certain record-keeping functions in the prescription department to nonprofessional personnel allows a more economical use of professional staff. At the same time, it provides the pharmacist with more time for consultation with the patient.

The Role of Management

Objectives and Goals—The first role of management for any business enterprise should be to establish the objectives and goals for the organization. Concurrently, management must provide the policies which will serve as the framework for accomplishing the stated objectives. For example, one objective might be an atmosphere of patient orientation, the elements of which would need to be identified. Proper record-keeping procedures, facilities for consultations and patient-oriented personnel, would be prerequisite for carrying out this objective.

Working with predetermined objectives provides the manager with a basis for establishing policy and assists in decision-making. As in the example cited, the objective has implications in the area of personnel policies and practices. Recruitment and selection techniques geared toward obtaining professional and supporting staff who can function effectively in a patient-oriented environment would have to be developed by the manager.

The kinds of objectives to be established by management might be divided into two categories:

1. A set of rather basic, almost philosophical objectives need to be developed; for example, will the pharmacy stress low prices rather than full service?
2. Objectives concerned with more specific operational matters are needed, as meeting a projected sales volume level during a given year.

In either case, it is management's responsibility to provide a sense of direction by setting forth both basic and specific objectives as guidelines for current and future activities.

Objectives lie in the future and, therefore, are subject to adjustments dictated by forces outside the control of management. Management personnel should keep abreast of those technological, economic and social changes that relate to stated organizational objectives. In this regard the role of management in establishing objectives and goals must include a mechanism for continuing re-evaluation and updating of objectives.

Material and Human Resources—The organization of these resources to pursue the objectives of the enterprise represents the second management function. The kinds and amounts of resources required are dictated in large measure by the nature of the objectives. The ability to obtain capital, generally considered to be an entrepreneurial rather than a managerial function, also may influence this management responsibility.

For the typical independent community pharmacy, it neither is possible or practical to divorce acquisition of capital from its application and management. In most cases, the same person is charged with both functions. Assuming that the required inventories, equipment and people can be assembled, it remains for management to provide the organizational structure and the coordination necessary to mold these resources into an efficiently functioning community pharmacy.

Planning and Controlling Operations—Although a major share of the manager's time must be devoted to controlling day-to-day operations, it is important to maintain a balance between the present and the future. Control of current operations far too often becomes the sole function of many managers, who devote little or no time to planning for future operations.

The lack of planning often compounds the problems associated with day-to-day operations, resulting in a situation where the controlling function requires all of the management effort. For example, many managers spend a disproportionate amount of time ordering merchandise and maintaining inventory when, through a properly planned inventory-control program, this routine activity could be delegated to others.

The brief and simplistic description of management functions given here tends to understate their complexity and significance. Management may be considered an art rather than a science. There are few established laws or formulas for solving the problems inherent in conducting an economically productive enterprise. It especially is difficult to make the numerous and varied decisions required in exercising the management functions. Although there have been attempts to quantify these decisions through the use of mathematics and mathematical models, in the last analysis the human element still dominates the decision-making process.

As management decisions are made and implemented by human beings to affect human beings, it is apparent that those who manage need to consider and study the behavioral and social sciences in order to function effectively. For the community pharmacist who performs the dual role of health professional and manager, such a background especially is appropriate.

Essentially, management is an exercise in group dynamics. The manager must be able to organize, direct and control a group of individuals toward the stated objectives of the organization. The manager who is unable to obtain the cooperation of his subordinates or who fails to delegate the responsibility for routine operational matters to others is not functioning effectively.

In the community pharmacy the human dimension of management especially is crucial. The nature of the typical community pharmacy is such that the manager constantly is in close personal contact with his employees, suppliers and patrons.

In such an environment it is difficult to make consistently objective decisions. Further, the dual role of the pharmacist–manager tends to create situations involving conflicts between sound management decisions and professional responsibilities. For example, as a manager, the pharmacist establishes policies regarding the extension of credit to patrons. Yet when a patron with a poor credit rating has an immediate need for prescription medication, the established policies may be waived or adjusted to satisfy the professional obligation of the pharmacist to the patron.

These rather unique characteristics, and the need for the pharmacist–manager to be more flexible than those performing the management function in other types of organizations, should not be construed to minimize the importance of effective management in the community pharmacy. In the current socioeconomic climate, with increasing costs of operation and pressures to reduce the costs of health care, the management function takes on greater, rather than lesser, significance.

The functions of management provide a somewhat theoretical basis for understanding the overall role of management in the continuing operation of an economically viable enterprise. For practical purposes, however, it may be more valuable to examine the role of management as it relates to the various resources and activities which go to comprise the business entity.

In the community pharmacy the following items require effective management: money, inventory, facilities, personnel, credit and risk. Establishing objectives, organization, planning and control apply to each of these items, as well as to the pharmacy as a unit. At this level the objectives will be more specific, and the organization, planning and control more definitive.

Consideration of the management of the specific elements that in total represent the community pharmacy does not imply that each element is managed in isolation. There are many interrelationships among the various elements, and a decision regarding one element often has an impact on one or more of the others. For example, the decision to expand the inventory may have implications to the management of money, facilities, personnel and risk.

Money

To a large extent, the success of a community pharmacy depends on the ability to obtain money from a variety of sources in sufficient quantity to acquire and support the resources necessary for operation. Once the money is obtained it becomes management's function to employ it in the most appropriate way to achieve the objectives of the pharmacy.

In its simplest and most pragmatic form the objective of money management is to maximize the rate of return on investment. Such an objective may appear inconsistent with the responsibilities of professionals engaged in providing health services, yet in the long run the economical use of money is beneficial to society.

In theory, money is in limited supply and demand usually exceeds supply. In the competition for the limited supply, only the most efficient users of money will be able to obtain it. Applying this concept to community pharmacy practice would suggest that only those owners who can manage money effectively, in all its forms, will succeed. In a sense, the foregoing concept simply is a statement of the basis of our economic system, where efficiency is rewarded and inefficiency is not.

In the broad sense money management applies not only to cash but to all those materials and services which are used in the operation of a pharmacy and are purchased with money. Given a limited amount, the manager must make judgments and decisions about the use of the money in terms of the stated objectives.

In this regard conflicts may develop between basic objectives. For example, the objective of maximizing return on investment may conflict with the objective of offering full services, as in the case where a decision must be made regarding the purchase of a delivery vehicle. The money invested for this purpose represents an inefficient use of money for many pharmacies and thus is contrary to the objective of maximizing return on investment. Yet, in order to meet the goal of providing full services to the patrons of the pharmacy, such an investment may be necessary.

The effectiveness of money management may be measured to some extent by the progress made toward meeting noneconomic objectives. For the most part, however, the most meaningful measure of effectiveness is in economic terms, specifically, by the return on investment, which for a pharmacy may be expressed in two ways:

Return on Total Assets—The rate of return on total assets is determined by dividing the total of all assets employed in the pharmacy into the net profit. No distinction is made between owner's equity and borrowed capital in this calculation. This ratio describes the productivity of the total asset investment.

Return on Owner's Equity—The rate of return realized on the owner's investment in the pharmacy is determined by dividing the difference between total assets and total liabilities (owner's equity) into the net profit. This ratio describes how well the funds provided by the owners are being used.

The manager may calculate these rates and compare them with national data to obtain some idea of the effectiveness of the money management policies. Rates below the national averages, such as those reported in the *Lilly Digest*, may indicate too much investment for the level of operation or inefficient management of the pharmacy.

In either event, by using the return on investment concept and analyzing the operation of the pharmacy, the manager is able to identify a problem requiring attention and can take appropriate steps to correct it.

The management of money in terms of both the total commitment of capital and the application of the owner's equity represents only one dimension of the management function in this area. In a narrower sense, money management also is concerned with day-to-day inflow and outflow of cash from operations. The maintenance of balanced cash flow requires the application of the management functions of planning and control.

Budgeting is necessary to assure that sufficient cash will be available to meet such obligations as accounts payable, wages and taxes. To a large extent, cash needs can be anticipated by an analysis of past experiences combined with projections of future operations.

The inflow of cash may be estimated in the same way. Matching cash revenues with cash expenditures is of more than academic significance: both excessive and deficient cash balances may prove to be uneconomical. When more cash is maintained than is necessary for normal operations, the excess represents earning power which is not being used.

For the pharmacy that consistently maintains a balance of

several thousand dollars in its checking account, it may be possible to transfer some of the cash to a savings account or to convert the cash into high-quality marketable securities. In this way, the excess cash will be earning interest or otherwise appreciating and yet still will be available easily for emergency use. A deficient cash position presents some obvious problems, including the possible impairment of the firm's credit rating which may have long-term implications.

One problem associated with an unfavorable cash position is inability to pay bills on time. In many cases this results in a loss of cash discounts. It is a common practice for suppliers to allow a 1 or 2% discount for the payment of invoices within a given time. The usual terms allow the discount to be taken if the amount is paid within 10 days of a specified date; otherwise, the full amount is due in 30 days. The buyer is offered what appears to be a small discount for paying the bill 20 days early. In terms of interest rates, however, the 2% cash discount for paying 20 days early represents an annual interest rate of about 36%.

For the typical pharmacy, cash discounts can amount to thousands of dollars each year. Too often, managers do not recognize the significance of taking advantage of all cash discounts, and consequently they do not devote sufficient thought to alternative courses of action when faced with an unfavorable cash position. It may be possible to borrow money on a short-term basis at a relatively low annual interest in order to take advantage of a 2% cash discount representing an effective annual interest rate of about 36%.

To some extent, the manager is able to control the cash flow in the pharmacy. Although certain obligations such as payrolls and taxes are fixed as to time of payment, the manager may be able to influence other aspects of cash flow. Good management of credit and collection procedures, for example, can increase inflow. Proper scheduling of purchases of inventory can effect a degree of control over the timing of the outflow for such purposes.

The manager makes the decisions regarding acquisition of new fixtures and equipment that requires outflows of cash either in a lump sum or in installments. Depending on future prospects for cash inflow, the manager can decide whether or not to proceed with such acquisitions.

In actual practice, inflow for a given period should be estimated and known fixed obligations for the same period should be deducted. If a balance remains, this represents discretionary cash available for expenditure. If a negative figure results, it is management's responsibility to attempt to increase inflow or decrease outflow in order to achieve a balance. During periods of temporary cash deficiencies, management may be required to obtain additional funds through borrowing. Knowledge of the sources of funds and the cost of such funds is a prerequisite for effective money management.

Inventory

The merchandise inventory represents the largest single asset on the balance sheet for the typical community pharmacy. About 55% of all assets excluding real estate holdings were reported as merchandise inventory for *Lilly Digest* pharmacies in 1991. The extent of this investment plus the fact that the inventory requirements for a given pharmacy are in a constant state of flux forces a need for continuing management attention to this area of operation.

It has been stated that the community pharmacist is the buying agent in the community for health-related products. He must provide the right products in the right quantities at the right time at the right prices to serve the needs of patrons.

Due to varying consumer preferences and geographical differences in prescribing habits of physicians, the management of inventory becomes a highly individualized function in each community pharmacy. Given a limited amount of capital and the responsibility to use the capital economically, the manager must develop systems and policies that will ensure a continuous flow of needed goods while avoiding the problems of excessive inventory levels.

Although the objective of effective inventory management is stated simply here, in practice it represents one of the most challenging responsibilities of management.

In the community pharmacy the management of inventory is complicated by the fact that a major portion of the inventory consists of prescription (legend) drugs. This makes the problem of inventory control in the pharmacy unique in comparison to control in other enterprises which distribute products at the retail level.

The demand for prescription drugs is generated by physicians and other health practitioners rather than by the ultimate consumer. When dealing directly with the consumer, it is easier to manage inventory. Excessive inventory levels can be reduced by special sales and markdowns. These techniques cannot be used to effect reduction in overstock of prescription drugs.

On the other hand, the successful pharmacy depends on maintaining a breadth and depth of prescription drug inventory which is adequate to handle all prescription orders received. Usually, the need for a prescription drug is immediate. The patient cannot wait until it is ordered, to be delivered in a few days. The dilemma of the manager in this situation is apparent: that of providing a continuous supply of products that are characterized by an unpredictable and uncontrollable demand.

The management of other segments of the inventory such as OTC drugs, cosmetics and sundry items, while not subject to the limitations inherent in the prescription drug segment, present no less a problem to the manager. Changing consumer preferences and pressures by suppliers to buy greater quantities and assortments of OTC drugs and nondrug items increase the need for careful attention to this area of management.

Three basic decisions are required for the effective management of inventory: the specific items to be included in the inventory, the quantity of each item required and the best source of supply.

The specific items included in the inventory should be chosen according to the needs of the community. Although there is a core of items common to every pharmacy, a significant portion of the inventory will be dictated by local demand. In this regard the manager must be objective in the selection of goods and ignore those personal preferences that might influence purchasing decisions. For the newly established pharmacy it is important that a portion of the capital budgeted for the initial inventory be held in reserve until the preferences of the local community are identified. As operations continue, the manager constantly will be faced with decisions on additions to the original selection.

Some managers adopt the policy of stocking all new items immediately, as long as the items are related to current merchandise assortments. Other managers adopt the wait-and-see policy, stocking new items only when a local demand is established. Both approaches have advantages and drawbacks.

The wait-and-see manager runs the risk of losing considerable sales volume and, perhaps more importantly, develops a reputation for not having in stock what the patrons desire. On the other hand, the manager who indiscriminately adds all new items to the inventory runs the risk of an overcommitment of capital to inventory, with its serious economic implications. Striking a balance between these two extremes presents a challenge to the manager.

Perhaps as important as the specific items to be included in the inventory is the quantity of each item carried in stock. Assuming that a given item should be stocked, the manager must decide what quantity is necessary. At this point, a number of decisions must be made, based on a consideration of sources of supply, extent of demand and such financial factors as quantity discounts and buying terms.

In most instances the manager may choose from alternative sources of supply. Some manufacturers of prescription drugs and many producers of the other goods distributed through pharmacies will sell directly to the pharmacy. The pharmacist also may obtain inventory needs from indirect sources, such as wholesale drug companies.

Direct sources offer the advantage of lower prices while indirect sources offer the advantage of faster delivery. As a general rule, direct purchasing requires a larger commitment to inventory investment because of minimum order require ments established by the manufacturer and increased delivery time.

Indirect sellers, such as wholesale drug firms, usually do not establish a minimum order level and emphasize rapid and frequent delivery service. The quantity of a given item carried in the pharmacy's stock, therefore, will be influenced, to some degree, by the source of supply.

Quantity-purchase discounts play an important role in decisions regarding inventory levels. As a general rule, the purchase of larger numbers or sizes of the items stocked in the pharmacy will effect a lower cost per item or unit. Such cost savings can be beneficial to both the owner of the pharmacy and to the public being served. It should be noted, however, that cost savings on the purchase of goods in larger quantities can be offset by additional expenses that accrue from excessive inventory levels.

The costs associated with maintaining a merchandise inventory include implicit and explicit interest, obsolescence, deterioration, storage, property taxes and insurance. Generally, these costs increase in direct proportion to the level of inventory.

The capital invested in inventory represents money that could be used in other ways to earn a return. To the extent that such an investment is necessary to generate sales and to earn a profit, it may be said that the investment is economically sound. However, when the investment in inventory exceeds what is actually required for the level of operation realized, the excess represents an uneconomical use of capital.

For example, assume that a pharmacy has $90,000 invested in inventory. The safest alternative use of this capital might be to buy time savings certificates at an effective annual rate of 5%. At this rate, the $90,000 would earn $4,500 per year and it can be said that this inventory investment has an implicit interest cost of $4,500. To the extent that the inventory produces net profit in excess of $4,500 the capital represented is being used economically.

Assume further that it can be shown that the $90,000 inventory could be reduced to $80,000 without adversely affecting sales or net profit. In terms of the safest alternative use of funds, the excess inventory of $10,000 is costing $500 per year in interest that could be earned and added to net profit.

An explicit interest cost also may result from excess inventory levels if the capital tied up in inventory is needed to pay other operational expenses. The pharmacy owner may be forced to borrow money at current interest rates in order to support current activities. To the extent that the need to borrow is caused by excessive inventory investment, the cost of borrowing should be considered as a cost of the excess inventory.

The possibility of obsolescence and deterioration are risks associated with the maintenance of an inventory, and although such risks may result in some unavoidable losses, they are minimized at optimum inventory levels. When the costs of storage, insurance and taxes are added to the interest factors and to the risk of obsolescence and deterioration, the cost of each dollar invested in inventory can be significant. An awareness of the costs associated with inventory investment will prove useful to the manager as he makes decisions regarding the types and quantities of goods to be included in the merchandise inventory.

The effectiveness of inventory management traditionally has been measured by the stock-turnover rate (the annual rate of turnover for the inventory). The rate is calculated using the following formula:

$$\frac{\text{cost of goods sold for the year}}{\text{average inventory at cost}} = \text{stock-turnover rate}$$

This rate denotes the number of times, on the average, that the inventory has been sold and replaced during a given year. It represents the turnover of dollars invested in inventory but tells nothing of the turnover of specific items or units that go to make up the inventory. As presented here, the rate relates to the entire inventory of the pharmacy. However, the same concept may be applied to departments if appropriate data are available.

The stock-turnover rate may be calculated for a specific pharmacy and then compared with national averages such as those reported in the *Lilly Digest*. The average rate reported by the *Lilly Digest* pharmacies for 1991 was 5.8. It generally is assumed that a rate of approximately 5 to 6 times per year is indicative of adequate management of inventory. Rates considerably below this level may indicate an overinvestment in inventory.

It should be noted that pharmacies with rather low sales volumes typically have stock-turnover rates much lower than the average. For these pharmacies, increased sales represent the only real opportunity for improving their position in this area.

The typical community pharmacy with a sales volume near the national average should show an annual stock-turnover rate of at least 5 times/year. If it falls significantly below the average, the management of inventory should be reexamined.

The rate may be improved in two ways. Attempts can be made to increase sales while the inventory level is held constant. Generating more sales with the same inventory increases the rate. In the event it is not possible to increase sales, the alternative is to reduce the inventory level. With constant sales, this will produce a faster rate of turnover.

A combination of the two alternatives, increasing sales while reducing inventory, can have a profound effect on the stock-turnover rate. As a practical matter, the manager may best be able to work toward a reduction of the inventory level as an immediate means of improving the rate. Certain items in the inventory may be returned to suppliers for refunds or credit. Items that cannot be returned may be sold at reduced prices. Most importantly, buying practices should be reviewed with the objective of reducing purchases until a more favorable rate is achieved.

If a stock-turnover rate of 5 is adequate, a rate of 7 or 8 might appear to be excellent. In some cases this is a valid assumption. However, unless the inventory is managed carefully, high rates may cause problems that are as serious as those resulting from low rates. An extremely high rate may be achieved by ultraconservative buying policies. Conservative buying will better the rate for capital invested in inventory, but the improvement may prove to be uneconomical in the long run.

When undue emphasis is placed on maintaining a high stock-turnover rate, quantity discounts may be lost, resulting in an increase in cost of goods sold. As a general rule, a pharmacy can afford to do at least some quantity buying, thus realizing the benefits accruing from quantity discounts. Frequently, buying in small quantities increases the time and effort involved in the buying process. More orders must be submitted and checked in, and more accounting time is required to process several small orders as compared with a few large ones.

Finally, and perhaps most importantly, the manager who attempts to control the inventory level too closely runs the risk of frequently being out of items. The disadvantages of this include a reduced sales volume and accompanying gross margin. Further, a reputation for being out of stock may result in a loss of patrons to other pharmacies where their needs will be met more consistently.

Through good management, however, it is possible to realize an annual stock-turnover rate higher than the accepted norm without creating the problems described here, and many successful pharmacies do this. However, unusually high rates reduce the likelihood of meeting the objective of having on hand the right goods at the right time in the right quantity at the right price.

In the final analysis the key to effective management of merchandise is stock control on a day-to-day basis. The manager is responsible for designing policies, procedures and systems for controlling and maintaining the proper selection and level of goods carried in stock. Proper training of employees in the importance of stock control and proper use of established control systems are the responsibilities of management.

There are a number of formal systems that may be employed to assist in inventory control. Many pharmacies, for example, maintain and control stock by using computer-based reorder systems. Other firms use the perpetual inventory method of stock control.

The pharmacy manager also can effect reasonable control over inventory by implementing a well-organized visual stock-control system. By predetermining the number of units of each item to be carried in stock, based on estimated sales and adequate turnover, the manager can establish minimum and maximum stock levels for each item. The indicated levels for each item are recorded in an inventory-control book or on the shelf where the item is stored. It becomes a simple task for an employee to check the stock on a regularly scheduled basis and to note those items that should be reordered.

There is nothing profound about such a system, but it does formalize an important function and provides a mechanism for the maintenance of inventory levels. Such a system also forces the manager to think in terms of the minimum and maximum stock levels for each item. This in itself effects a degree of control over the total inventory.

Very often, overcommitment of capital to inventory is not apparent until the end of an accounting period, when a physical inventory is made. In many cases the inventory level creeps upward without a corresponding increase in sales. When little attention is given to a comparison of the inflow of goods against the outflow, it is easy to accumulate excessive inventory.

One mechanism that may be used to combat this problem is the buying budget. In its simplest form the buying budget provides a means of dollar control of inventory based upon matching purchases with sales. In a pharmacy, each dollar of sales generally represents about 70 cents in inventory at cost prices. Assuming a balanced inventory level at the outset, about $700 would be required to restore the inventory level after $1,000 worth of goods had been sold at retail.

The buying budget concept is most effective when used to plan purchases in the near future. A budget is determined by estimating sales for a future period, as for the next month, then calculating the amount of new inventory that will be necessary to support the anticipated sales. The resulting figure becomes the buying budget for the period involved.

As purchases of inventory items are made during the period, they are subtracted from the budgeted amount. The balance is termed the open-to-buy allowance for the remainder of the period. Although the budgeted figure represents neither an absolute minimum or maximum, it does provide a guide for management control of the dollars invested in inventory. The real advantage of the buying budget lies in the fact that continuing management attention is directed toward an important operating problem.

Facilities

On the average approximately 15% of the capital required for a typical community pharmacy is invested in fixtures, equipment and leasehold improvements. Charges for housing the pharmacy are second only to wages among the costs of operation. Expressed as a percentage of annual net sales, rent represents about 2.3%.

Overall, the cost of facilities necessary to operate a pharmacy represents a significant portion of total costs. Management of these costs is difficult, especially because they are based on long-term commitments from which there is little opportunity for retreat. Rent, for example, most often is agreed on in advance for a 5- to 10-year period. The lease that establishes the level of rent to be paid is a legal contract which, once agreed to, is enforceable for its term. Fixtures and equipment, once purchased, represent costs that only can be recovered by long-time use.

Management's main role in the effective and economical use of facilities lies in a careful consideration of the original commitment to these assets. In a sense, facilities must be managed in advance.

Rental Agreements—As is the case in most areas of management, decisions regarding the types and amounts of facilities depend in large measure on projections and forecasts of future operations. Basic decisions on the size of the building and quantities of fixtures and equipment are related intimately to anticipated sales volume. The nature of the pharmacy also plays a role in these decisions. An exclusively prescription pharmacy usually requires less space than does a pharmacy that emphasizes general merchandise.

In negotiating the rental agreement the manager must have some notion of anticipated sales and the relationship of rent to sales. Although such information may be useful as a guideline for negotiating with potential landlords, as a general rule landlords refuse to be bound by statistics.

In many cases rental figures for two or more pharmacies are difficult to compare because the services provided by landlords may vary. A pharmacy located in a medical clinic may pay rent considerably in excess of the average figure for a pharmacy doing a similar volume in another location. However, it may be that the rent includes janitorial services, centralized heating, air conditioning or other services normally not provided.

When negotiating a rental agreement or renewing a lease, the manager may be able to get a stabilization of the rental charge as a percentage of sales by obtaining a percentage lease arrangement. This provides that the landlord will receive rent based on a percentage of net sales. Such an arrangement is attractive, especially for a new pharmacy where there is doubt about the level of sales volume that may be realized.

Landlords increasingly are receptive to percentage lease arrangements. In most cases, however, they will insist on a guaranteed minimum rent, with a percentage to be added after a specified sales volume has been realized. If the guaranteed minimum rent is set at a modest figure, this may prove to be advantageous for the pharmacy.

It would be inaccurate to infer that the manager has significant command of the alternatives and terms of the rental agreement. More often than not, the landlord dictates the terms of the lease. Management's main role is to avoid gross errors in judgment, resulting in long-term overcommitments for space and rent.

Fixtures and Equipment—The original commitment for these items should be made only after careful analysis of requirements, and after searching the market for the most economical and suitable fixtures and equipment. The manager has options regarding quantity, quality and sources of supply for these facilities. It is good practice to secure bids from several sources before making the final decision on the purchase of fixtures and equipment. Further, many suppliers will provide counsel and advice.

Once acquired, the problem of proper arrangement of fixtures and equipment requires additional management decisions. For example, should the prescription laboratory be located in the front or the rear of the pharmacy? When located in the front, it is visible from the street and tends to emphasize prescription service to passers-by; when located in the rear it provides a private atmosphere, free from congestion and activity.

Numerous other decisions regarding layout must be made, and the manager is well-advised to make use of the services of experts in store design before making these decisions. Studies have demonstrated that the arrangement of fixtures and proper departmentalization of goods can help increase sales volume, promote employee efficiency and make the pharmacy more pleasant and convenient for patrons. With modern fixtures designed for flexibility, the manager is able to experiment with various arrangements and layouts until the most efficient combination is achieved. Proper management of facilities can play a significant role in efficient and profitable operation.

Personnel

One of the most important aspects of developing an efficiently operating community pharmacy is a well-conceived program of personnel management. The uniquely personal nature of the atmosphere in the typical community pharmacy dictates that the proper selection, training and maintenance of employees be given top priority as management functions. Each employee represents the pharmacy in daily interaction with patrons, physicians and suppliers. Their ability to reflect and to carry out the objectives of the pharmacy may mean the difference between financial success and failure.

In view of the obvious benefits of sound personnel management, it is surprising to observe that many managers look upon good personnel administration as an area for which they have neither the inclination or the time. Deficiencies in this area arise in part from the numerous and diverse responsibilities assumed by most pharmacy managers. Yet, time and attention devoted to personnel management would, in the long run, free more time for other management functions. The properly selected and well-trained employee can assume many duties that otherwise may be the responsibility of the manager.

The nature of retail employment also contributes to the complexity of personnel management in the pharmacy. In general, retail concerns experience significant variations in the demand for employees. Seasonal variations in sales require adjustments in staff needs. Further, retail activity often is concentrated during certain days of the week and certain hours of the day. Under such conditions, it is difficult to manage payroll costs without the extensive use of part-time help.

Due to the extensive use of part-time employees, many of the people employed by retail firms are young people without previous work experience. Quite often they have little understanding of the economic value of the services they are expected to render. Personnel of this type present special problems in training and orientation, not only to a specific job but also to the general obligation of an employee to an employer.

Attracting competent employees is made more difficult by the need to cater to the desires of the public regarding store hours. Modern consumers expect to shop 7 days a week and into the late evening hours. The retail employee, therefore, is expected to work during hours and on days when others in society are free to shop and play.

Other problems associated with obtaining good employees are inherent in the nature of retailing. Retail employees are meeting the public continually, so they must be of at least average intelligence, present a good appearance and have an acceptable personality. Also, wages paid to retail employees ordinarily are well below those paid in other industries.

Selection—Although the nature of retail employment is unique in many respects, the basic principles of personnel management may be applied in the development of a program for selecting, training and maintaining employees for the retail field and specifically for the community pharmacy. Proper selection techniques must be developed to ensure that employees will be compatible with the job to be done and with the objectives of the pharmacy.

A high rate of turnover in a pharmacy often makes the attitude of management towards selecting employees rather casual. Managers rationalize that the employee will not be staying very long, therefore, why worry about selectivity? Further, the manager frequently is faced with the problem of replacing employees on relatively short notice. In such emergencies selectivity often is ignored.

Improper selection of employees has the effect of perpetuating and intensifying the turnover problem, and the employee who is not suited to his job can be detrimental to the operation of the pharmacy. Two general rules should be incorporated into the personnel policies regarding selection.

1. Minimum standards for qualifications of employees should not be allowed to fall below the minimum standards for service established for the pharmacy. To "underhire" for a given position can serve only to undermine the reputation of the pharmacy.
2. "Overhiring" should be avoided; obviously superior people should not be hired for inferior jobs. Such personnel rapidly become discontented and may have an adverse effect on staff morale and efficiency.

Proper selection of personnel for a specific job is predicated on an understanding of the duties and responsibilities involved and on knowledge of the individual characteristics required for efficient performance. The manager should develop a job description and a job specification for each position in the pharmacy.

The job description is a brief summary of the scope of the job, its relationship to other jobs and such details as working hours and pay scales. It also serves to prevent misunderstandings about the nature or duties of a particular job. The job specification sets forth the characteristics and competencies required in the individual who fills the position.

With these materials the manager is in a position to evaluate objectively the candidates who apply for the position. Selection also requires a knowledge of the sources of potential employees. For some jobs, promotion from within the pharmacy staff may be appropriate. In most cases external sources must be used, such as employment agencies, place ment offices of schools and universities or classified newspaper advertising.

A growing source of part-time employees are the co-op work–study programs of many high schools. An availability file should be established in the pharmacy—a record of qualified people who applied for jobs when no openings existed.

The manager should develop an application form to assist in the selection process. Although the application form serves basically to provide information about the applicant, it can serve other purposes as well; eg

It provides a means for observing the applicant's ability to follow simple written instructions.

It serves as a guide in the employment interview. If no openings currently are available, it can go into the availability file.

It serves a practical purpose as a part of the employee's permanent record, and as a source of information for social security and withholding tax reports.

A properly designed application form can serve as an effective screening device for prospective employees. The information supplied on the application form often will indicate that the applicant does not meet the job specifications and, thus, should not be considered further. If the information suggests that the applicant is a good prospect, the selection procedure should continue with an interview.

Often the employment interview is the sole selection procedure used by pharmacy managers, and this is not advisable. At the very least, the references provided by the applicant should be checked thoroughly to substantiate the impressions generated by the interview. The interview, however, is a key step in most selections. It should be conducted in an unhurried manner, in privacy and in a relatively informal atmosphere. Much can be learned about the prospective employee through a properly conducted interview.

The manager also might consider developing some simple tests to be used in the selection process. Testing is used as a selection technique by many larger firms and can be most useful. In the pharmacy, simple arithmetic tests can be used in selecting personnel for sales or clerking positions which may require that the person be able to handle the simple problems involved in making change and computing sales taxes.

It should be noted that all employment policies and procedures must be consistent with applicable federal and state laws governing equal employment opportunity. In general such laws prohibit discrimination in selection and hiring practices.

Orientation and Training—Proper selection needs to be followed by adequate orientation and training of the employee. These can serve to increase productivity and reduce employee turnover. The orientation process should include a give-and-take discussion with the employee on the following questions:

What are the basic philosophies of the pharmacy (toward patrons, other health professionals and employees)?
What hours will the employee be expected to work (evenings, weekends, holidays)?
How long is the lunch hour?
How is overtime handled?
What is the policy regarding coffee breaks?
What are the regulations about smoking?
What are the rules regarding punctuality?
Are uniforms required? If so, who buys them and who pays for laundering?
What are the safety and security regulations?
May this employee answer the telephone? If so what information is he authorized to give?
Can the telephone be used for personal calls?
What is the vacation policy?
What is the policy regarding leave (sick, personal business)?
What are the opportunities and procedures for advancement?
What are the policies on employee purchases and discounts?

These questions are by no means all-inclusive on those matters that might be of concern to both the employer and the employee, but the use of such a list will provide a basis for posing additional specific questions. Although some of the questions may appear to be trivial, these are the kinds of matters that often cause problems between employers and employees.

In an extreme case disagreements over such matters may lead to termination of employment. In other cases, employee resentment may be reflected in attitudes toward and dealings with patrons of the pharmacy and this could be the most serious consequence of such disagreement. If these matters are discussed in advance, misunderstandings may be minimized, to the mutual benefit of both parties.

After a general orientation to the pharmacy the employee needs specific training in the duties and responsibilities of the job. Too often the new pharmacy employee is trained by the sink-or-swim method. The employee simply is put to work and is expected to pick up knowledge on the job. Obviously, such a method of training is inefficient and in the long run costly, although it does offer the advantage of requiring little or no management time or effort.

Even though the typical community pharmacy has neither the staff or the facilities for sophisticated training programs, there are effective, simple, training methods which can be used. The sponsor system of training is the most appropriate for a pharmacy. A new employee is assigned to a capable experienced employee who explains and demonstrates the job in question. The conference method also may be used, by itself or to supplement the sponsor system. Here, the new employee meets privately with the pharmacy manager or a designated employee to discuss the techniques of the job. In either case the management responsibility lies in organizing and structuring the training so that all aspects of the employee's duties are considered.

Compensation—Retaining good employees is one of the most difficult problems faced by the community pharmacy manager. There are many elements in the employment environment that may help in keeping employees, but most important is the compensation plan. Adequate compensation is necessary, not only to retain employees but also to encourage them to work toward the overall goals and objectives of the pharmacy. The basic elements of a sound plan are:

Adequacy—The amount of compensation should be commensurate with the responsibilities of the job. Adequqcy also may be viewed in a legal sense in terms of state and federal minimum wage laws.

Simplicity—Plans that are uncomplicated are understood easily by the employee and have the further advantage of being easy to administer.

Progressiveness—A plan should recognize and reward initiative, productivity and increasing value of the employee to the pharmacy. It should provide incentive for doing a better job. Periodic review of performance and salary should be provided for in the plan.

Patron Protection—The plan should not encourage acts that are detrimental to the best interests of the patrons of the pharmacy. For example, it is inappropriate to offer extra commissions for promoting the sale of OTC drugs. If commissions are paid on these drugs, the employee may be tempted to place personal economic gain ahead of the real needs of the patron.

Traditionally, the compensation plan for pharmacy employees has consisted of an hourly or weekly salary plus the legally required social security contribution by the employer for each employee. Modern personnel management calls for a broader compensation plan in order to compete effectively for the limited number of good employees.

Increasingly, even small pharmacies are offering plans that include not only salary but such fringe benefits as health insurance, life insurance, paid vacation and sick days plus supplemental retirement benefits. When such benefits are provided, the employer should calculate their value in terms of pre-income tax dollars in order to demonstrate to the employee their real economic value.

Credit

The need for credit is apparent especially when health products and services are involved. The need for drugs and pharmaceutical services often is immediate and independent of the cash position of the patient. Further, a charge account statement provides the patient with a mechanism for keeping track of expenditures for drugs for insurance and income tax purposes.

Credit management in the community pharmacy, on occasion, presents a conflict between sound business practice and professional responsibility. Sound business practice may indicate that credit should not be given to a particular patron, while professional responsibility may dictate that credit must be given. It is not possible to develop inflexible credit policies that will solve such problems. However, it is possible to develop policies and procedures that will be effective in a majority of such situations. There are two general areas that require attention in credit management.

Policies and Procedures—Included here are the matters of eligibility, limits on credit, credit terms, maintaining accurate records and identification of credit patrons. Deciding which patrons are eligible for credit is the most troublesome problem for the pharmacy manager.

It is difficult to make a decision without knowing the credit history of the patron. Data on past credit experiences must be obtained and should be checked. The patron can be asked to supply the necessary information and usually will do so. However, verification presents a serious practical problem. Some managers attempt to verify the information personally by contacting each credit reference. Such a procedure is time-consuming and the information received is often incomplete.

A better approach appears to lie in the use of professional credit bureaus. Most localities are now served by such bureaus which, for a fee, will investigate prospective credit customers and supply a report on their ratings. With this information the manager is able to make better decisions and minimize the problems associated with granting credit.

Collection—The best policies can be thwarted by careless collection procedures. The terms of credit granted should be made clear to the grantee at the outset. If the terms are not met, appropriate and prompt action should be taken. The manager is responsible for establishing the guidelines and procedures necessary to ensure prompt payment of credit accounts. Collection policies that result in prompt payment offer a number of advantages.

Prompt payment means rapid turnover of capital invested in accounts receivable and this permits a given level of operations to be supported with less capital. Operating expenses are lower when accounts are paid on time as delinquent accounts cost money in terms of employee time and supplies required for follow-ups.

Finally, there is a definite relationship between the length of time accounts are outstanding and bad debt losses; as a general rule the longer an account is outstanding, the less likely it is to be collected.

Although guidelines and procedures should be established for collecting past-due accounts, rarely is the same procedure appropriate for all such accounts. New accounts, for example, should be handled firmly in order to impress the patron with the importance of prompt payment. Casual handling or lack of follow-up of delinquent new accounts sets a precedent that may be hard to overcome.

For established accounts, more individualized treatment is indicated. Some patrons fail to pay promptly simply out of negligence. Usually a simple reminder will stimulate payment. Others may be willing to pay their debts but for reasons beyond their control are unable to do so. The manager may be able to work out a budget plan for those to help solve their problems.

A small group of patrons may fall into the category of those who simply do not wish to pay. Outside collection agencies or legal action may be the only alternative for this group. In any event, policies and procedures for collection should be included as part of the credit management func tion.

Credit also may be provided to patrons via a variety of credit card systems operated by banks. The credit card system involves the establishment of a line of credit for an individual with a participating bank or group of banks. The individual is issued a credit card which will be honored by participating businesses for goods or services. The participating business then forwards the receipts for sales of goods or services to the bank and receives immediate payment, less a service charge based on the amount of the sale.

The advantages of this system lie in the fact that bad-debt losses are reduced almost to zero and the cost of billing is assumed by the bank. Even though the amount realized from the sales transaction is reduced by the amount of the service charge, some pharmacy owners view the bank credit card system as the answer to problems associated with credit transactions. In fact, many pharmacies use such systems as their only credit program.

As a practical matter, however, many people who require drugs and pharmaceutical services cannot qualify, and some people refuse to participate in the credit card system. As a result, some pharmacies use such systems simply as a supplement to their own charge-account system. In addition, increasing numbers of pharmacies are accepting nationally recognized credit cards.

Most, if not all, community pharmacies today also extend credit for prescription drugs and pharmacy services to private and government third-party programs. In 1993 it was estimated that 45 to 50% of all outpatient prescriptions were paid for, either in full or in part, by third-party programs. As a result a significant portion of the accounts receivable for the typical community pharmacy represents payments due from third-party payors. As a general rule, credit extended to third-party payors involves minimal risk of bad debts losses if services are provided to patients who are eligible for benefits, program requirements are met and accurate claims are submitted. However, the payment cycle from the submission of a claim to receipt of reimbursement varies greatly among third-party payors. Some process claims within 15 to 20 days while others may take a month or more. In order to minimize delays in reimbursement, the pharmacy manager must implement systems which assure the prompt submission of accurately prepared claims to all third-parties. Fortunately, increasing numbers of third-party payors are using electronic systems which provide for on-line processing and adjudication of claims for pharmacy services. The electronic transmission of claims directly from the pharmacy to the third-party payor provides for instant verification of patient eligibility, confirms whether the service provided is a payable benefit and confirms the amount to be paid to the pharmacy provider. Electronic submission of claims also may shorten the payment cycle and reduce the average collection period for accounts receivable from third-party payors.

In order to measure the effectiveness of management control over credit sales, it is useful to calculate the average collection period of customers' accounts receivable. Average daily credit sales are divided into the total of accounts receivable at the end of a period, giving the average collection period for accounts receivable. In theory, this figure should be about 40 days if all accounts are paid on time. Figures in excess of 60 days indicate deficiencies in credit policies and credit management, and call for prompt action.

Risk

As a commercial enterprise, a community pharmacy presents numerous risks in terms of economic gain or loss. Certain of the risks inherent in the operation are speculative in nature. For example, will operations produce a profit or a loss? With this type of risk there is an uncertainty that may work either to the detriment or benefit of the pharmacy owner. Such risks can be managed only indirectly by careful attention to the management of all of the elements comprising the pharmacy. Even then there is no guarantee of success.

Other risks associated with the operation of a pharmacy may be termed pure risks. These involve uncertainty and chance of loss but do not provide a gain directly if the loss is not realized. Tangible destructible property is subject to pure risk; its destruction always is possible but not certain. For example, there is a risk that the merchandise inventory owned by the pharmacy may be destroyed by fire. If a fire occurs a loss surely will be suffered, but if it does not occur no direct increase in value or profit is realized. Pure risk may be controlled or protected against by appropriate direct management action.

Types—The first function of management related to controlling pure risk is to identify and analyze the several perils to which business assets are subject. Some perils are common to all pharmacies while others are unique to specific situations. It is important, therefore, that the analysis of risk be individualized. There are four common categories of perils to be considered.

Actual Loss of Property—All tangible property is subject to being lost. For the pharmacy most such losses are due to dishonesty such as shoplifting, burglary, robbery or embezzlement.

Damage or Destruction of Property—Most tangible property is exposed to possible destruction or damage by fire, the elements, civil commotion and a variety of other causes.

Civil Liability—Every pharmacy is subject to a variety of risks associated with dealing with the public and with employing people. Negligence or breach of responsibility, alleged or proven, can cause financial losses. Injuries to individuals in the pharmacy, malpractice by pharmacists and product liability are examples of these perils.

Contractual Liability—Legal liability beyond that imposed by the law may be assumed in a contractual relationship between a pharmacist and other persons. The lease signed by the pharmacist to obtain the building for the pharmacy is an example of contractual liability.

Risk Management—Each peril identified by the pharmacy manager must be further analyzed to determine the probability of occurrence of an actual loss as follows: the loss must be quantified in terms of its impact on the total assets of the pharmacy and the ability to handle the loss; the manager must decide which of the alternative methods or combination of methods should be utilized to protect against each peril or loss. The three commonly recognized ways to handle risks are

Self-Insurance—This may be used to protect against relatively small losses with a low probability of occurrence. A reserve is established and, in the event such losses occur, they are paid for out of the reserve which is created by systematically setting aside money for this purpose. A major danger is that a large loss may occur before a sufficient reserve has been established. Except for large, multiunit pharmacies, self-insurance is not practical for community pharmacies.

Assumption of Risk—When the probability of loss is low and the loss is of small magnitude, it may be economically advantageous for the owner to assume the risk. For example, when the cost of insuring plate glass against perils other than fire and the elements is compared with the probability of loss from these perils, most owners decide to assume the risk. Assumption of risk differs from self-insurance in that no reserve is established. Obviously, this method of risk management must be used carefully.

Insurance through Others—The majority of pure risks associated with community pharmacy practice are of sufficient magnitude to dictate the placement of risks with other parties such as insurance companies. They offer service to the insured and provide indemnity in the event a loss is suffered. Such firms provide the technical knowledge and the legal experience required to settle losses quickly and efficiently. Often the services of insurance companies are as important as the indemnification they provide, as is the case in liability suits.

Too often the management of risk is considered to be adequate when proper provision has been made to insure indemnification in the event of a loss. A complete-risk management program should include a consideration of loss prevention as well as protection. An attempt to prevent losses can be beneficial in many ways.

Insurance companies are beginning to recognize clients with good records and to reward them by reductions in premiums. A direct cash savings thus is effected by reducing or preventing losses. More importantly, most tangible losses result in other losses that cannot be handled by insurance. For example, when an error is made in dispensing prescription medication and a malpractice suit is brought, the tangible dollar cost of such a suit may be paid by the insurance company.

The intangible loss due to damage to the reputation of the pharmacy can not be alleviated by cash payment. Prevention of such occurrences is the best way to avoid all of the losses involved. Loss prevention, both philosophically and practically, should be an integral part of risk management programs.

The services of an insurance counselor may prove valuable to the manager of a pharmacy in developing a risk management program. The complexities involved in evaluating risks and in understanding the various types of insurance policies and terminology call for expert advice. The insurance counselor generally is the best source of unbiased information.

The insurance counselor usually does not order policies. The counselor's function is to evaluate the risks of a specific individual or firm and to make recommendations regarding the best way to deal with them. The fee for these services is paid by the insured rather than the insurer. Expenditures of money for this service may prove to be extremely economical in the long run.

Insurance—Among the types of coverage required for the community pharmacy are

Fire insurance
Malpractice insurance
General public liability insurance
Products liability insurance
Employer's liability or worker's compensation
Crime insurance
Business interruption insurance

These specific coverages may be acquired separately, or a number of them may be included in a package policy, similar to the well-known homeowner's policy. Package policies have the advantage of offering broader coverage at the same or even at a lower cost than do the individual policies purchased separately. Such policies should be evaluated carefully; the multiple coverage involved may leave gaps in protection that are not apparent until a loss occurs. It often is difficult to know exactly what is covered, and to what extent, under package, "all risks" policies.

Perhaps the most important coverage for the tangible assets of the pharmacy is fire insurance. Although most pharmacies are protected to some degree, often the amount of the fire insurance falls below the actual value of the property.

This is particularly important because most fire insurance policies contain a co-insurance clause. This clause requires that insurance equal to a specified percentage of the value of the property be carried at all times. A common requirement is 80% of the value.

Under co-insurance if, at the time of a loss, the amount of insurance carried is below the required amount, the insured will have to bear part of the loss. For example, if the insurable value of the property owned by a pharmacist is $50,000 and the fire insurance policy has an 80% co-insurance clause, the pharmacist must carry $40,000 worth of insurance on the property. If only $30,000 is carried and a $10,000 loss is suffered, the insurer is required to pay only $7,500. The pharmacist must assume the balance of the loss because only 75% of the required amount of insurance was maintained.

The standard fire insurance policy should be supplemented by an extended coverage endorsement. For a small additional fee this endorsement has the effect of extending protection to cover damage by windstorm, hail, explosion, riot, smoke and from land vehicles and aircraft. It should be noted that usually neither the standard fire insurance policy nor the extended coverage endorsement covers losses of documents, accounts receivable, prescription files or currency.

Several types of liability insurance are becoming increasingly important in modern practice. The pharmacy owner may be required to answer a suit arising out of the negligence or alleged negligence of him or his employees. In addition, the pharmacy is a public facility where there are innumerable opportunities for injury to patrons.

Product liability may arise out of claims of patrons that have suffered injuries from products purchased in the pharmacy. Although the pharmacist may be able to fall back on the manufacturer under the concept of implied warranty, such claims must be answered by the pharmacist. Insurance can provide the financial and legal resources necessary to answer suits of this type.

The owner must obtain coverage of sufficient scope and amounts adequate to protect against liability claims. Without insurance coverage, an unfavorable judgment from one such claim may be sufficient to bankrupt the owner.

Insurance coverage against criminal acts also should be obtained. In addition, the manager is in an excellent position to use loss-prevention as a means of minimizing these risks. Minimizing the amount of cash carried on the premises, installation of burglar alarm systems and carefully observed security measures can greatly reduce losses in this area.

The dishonesty of employees can be controlled best by adequate systems and policies regarding handling of cash and other assets. Shoplifting losses can be reduced by proper surveillance and proper training of employees. As a rule, insurance is not available to cover these losses.

When a pharmacy suffers losses because of fire, or other causes that interrupt operations, the actual loss goes beyond the property that is damaged or destroyed. Profits will be lost while the pharmacy is closed. Certain business expenses continue, even during interrupted operations. Key employees may be forced to seek other employment. Such losses may be covered by business interruption insurance. This is designed to indemnify the owner for lost profits, continuing expenses and salaries of key employees during a reasonable period of interrupted operations.

Life insurance also may have a role in a comprehensive risk-management program for a community pharmacy. If a pharmacist is the sole owner of a pharmacy, insurance on his life can provide funds to take care of the debts of the pharmacy in the event of the owner's death. If the pharmacist is the co-owner of the pharmacy as a partner, arrangements should be made for life insurance on each partner with the other partner(s) named as beneficiaries. The amount of such insurance should be sufficient to pay for each partner's equity in the enterprise.

In the event of the death of a partner, the surviving partner(s) can use the proceeds from the insurance to buy a deceased partner's interest in the pharmacy from the heirs. Such an arrangement reduces the possibility that the enterprise would be dissolved in order to settle the estate of a deceased partner. The premium payments made for part nership life insurance policies are regarded as a business expense.

There are a variety of other risks that may be covered effectively by insurance. Some of these are peculiar to individual circumstances and must be analyzed and managed in terms of the specific pharmacy. Effective management of all the insurable risks associated with modern community pharmacy practice must be combined with effective management of the uninsurable speculative risks inherent in entrepreneurial activity.

Records

For a variety of reasons—some legal, some financial and some professional—the maintenance of records in the pharmacy is becoming increasingly important. The types of records required may be classified as

Records required by law regarding the acquisition and disposition of drugs.

Records regarding patient utilization of drugs.

Records regarding the past and present financial status of the pharmacy.

Management's role in this function is to identify the specific records required, develop systems for keeping them and delegate the responsibility for day-to-day recordkeeping to capable personnel.

Legal Records—According to federal and state law, the pharmacy owner or manager is charged with maintaining accurate up-to-date records on specific classes of drugs and poisons. Under the provisions of the Federal Controlled Substances Act of 1970, the pharmacist is charged with maintaining accurate records related to the acquisition and disposition of certain drugs that are deemed to be subject to possible misuse or abuse. Several states have enacted legislation that requires accurate records on the distribution of poisons and other hazardous substances.

The legal implications of recordkeeping, as it relates to these drugs, are serious. Improperly maintained or incomplete records can bring legal action and penalties. For further details regarding the legal recordkeeping requirements, see Chapter 110.

Patient Records—In recent years many pharmacists have broadened their recordkeeping activities to include patient drug histories. Although the form of patient record varies, the basic idea is to establish a record, usually on a family-unit basis, that will allow the pharmacist to monitor the drug usage of each member of the family. It increasingly is apparent that, because of the kinds and amounts of drugs being taken by the average patient, there is need for a drug history for each individual.

In order to reduce the problems associated with drug interactions and individual idiosyncrasies to drugs, the pharmacist has a professional obligation to maintain records of this type. In addition, these records also may serve economic purposes, as sources of information for insurance claims and for income tax deductions of the patient.

Financial Records—Properly collected and organized accounting data serve a variety of important uses and are of value to the pharmacy owner in the following ways:

Providing the basic tools for efficient management and measuring its effect.

Making sound decisions regarding future cash needs, inventory requirements, personnel matters and expansion of facilities.

Evaluating past operations, controlling current operations and providing information for planning and forecasting.

Analyzing revenues and expenses.

Measuring return on investment.

Providing the required information to potential grantors of credit and loans as well as to federal, state and local governmental agencies regarding income and business taxes.

Helping to ensure a profitable operation.

As a general rule, the manager no longer acts as bookkeeper in the community pharmacy. Considering the complexities of contemporary business and the importance of good financial records, the pharmacist is well-advised to employ experts to assist in the development and maintenance of his accounting system. The experts can help to develop an individualized system that meets the accepted criteria for good financial records: objectivity, conservatism, consistency and comparability.

Financial records should reflect, insofar as is possible, an objective evaluation of the transactions and data on which they are based. Personal opinion and judgment should not be allowed to prevail over an objective analysis of financial data. For example, the cost of fixtures in the pharmacy should be reported in the financial statement on the basis of acquisition cost as evidenced by a bill of sale or an invoice.

The value of these fixtures should not be increased on the statements simply because management feels they are worth more than the original cost because of increasing price levels. Convincing objective evidence of the dollar amounts reported on the financial statement is a prerequisite to maintaining the integrity of such statements.

The general optimism of many owners and managers may be in conflict with the principle of conservatism as it relates to financial records. A moderately conservative approach should be employed in reporting financial data; otherwise, the data may tend to overstate earnings and assets and to understate liabilities. The consequences of overstated earnings include the possibility of excess income tax liability in a given year.

If a choice must be made between understatement or overstatement of income or assets, the principle of conservatism would dictate understatement. This does not imply that earnings or assets should be understated deliberately. However, when estimates or opinions must be used in making decisions regarding financial records, a conservative attitude should prevail. For example, many managers are reluctant to admit that a certain percentage of accounts receivable will prove to be uncollectable.

They are inclined to report accounts receivable in the financial records without a realistic reduction for bad debts. To do this without adjustment based on recognition of the likelihood of some not being collected is to violate the principle of conservatism.

Although there is no hard and fast rule for accounting for financial transactions, it is important that a given enterprise be consistent in its accounting system. This also is linked closely to the final criterion for good financial records: comparability.

There are various methods of recording and reporting financial transactions, and decisions must be made regarding the best method. Once chosen, it should be applied consistently throughout the life of the enterprise so that financial records will be comparable from period to period. For example, there are several ways to allocate depreciation charges to expense. If the policy on depreciation is changed from one period to the next, the net income may be altered significantly. Such a change would have an impact on the comparability of the financial statements for the two periods.

Attention to consistency and comparability should not necessarily rule out all changes in accounting methods. When valid reasons dictate a change in method, it should be made. However, the nature of the change should be indicated clearly on future financial statements.

Comparability of financial records also is important in the broader sense in order to compare records between firms in the same field. It is advantageous to be able to compare the financial statements for the pharmacy with similar statements such as those reported in the *Lilly Digest* and other references. Such comparisons are facilitated if relatively standard accounting systems are used. The manager could instruct his accountant to classify expenses according to the *Lilly Digest* system. He then would be able to analyze the expenses of his pharmacy in relation to national trends and averages.

The day-by-day financial transactions are summarized in the statements prepared at the end of the accounting period. Among the statements most important to those concerned with the financial progress of the pharmacy are the balance sheet and the income statement. Assuming that the underlying data have been treated objectively and conservatively, the balance sheet should represent fairly accurately the financial position of the pharmacy at the end of a given period. It reflects the basic accounting equation:

assets = liabilities + owner's equity

Assets are the items of value owned by the enterprise, listed at cost prices less any allowances for depreciation or doubtful accounts. The liabilities and owner's equity represent the claims against the assets.

The balance sheet is of interest to the owners in terms of the total value of their investment and the value of specific assets that make up the total investment. Managers especially are interested in such items as total merchandise inventory and accounts receivable.

Future management decisions regarding inventory control and credit policies may be influenced by the information included on the balance sheet. Those who are asked to grant credit to the pharmacy will be interested in the current liabilities and the owner's equity, as reported on the balance sheet. A formal detailed balance sheet should be prepared at least once a year. One commonly used format for reporting balance-sheet information for community pharmacies is illustrated in Table 1.

The income statement describes in detail the effects of revenue and expense transactions during a given accounting period. Unlike the balance sheet, which describes the financial position of an enterprise on a given date, the income statement summarizes only those transactions directly related to income production for a specific period of time, usually a year. For most purposes the income statement is used in concert with the balance sheet, each supplementing the other.

The owners of the pharmacy are interested not only in total investment but also in the net profit, which represents return on investment. The manager cannot judge accurately the appropriateness of the level of merchandise inventory reported in the balance sheet without knowing the sales revenue generated by the inventory as reported in the income statement.

The information included in the income statement can be used by the manager to plan for future operations and as a means for controlling current operations. When the information is compared against past years and national averages, trends will be observed and problem areas may be identified. The manager then can make decisions and take actions intended to improve the profitmaking potential of the pharmacy.

Bibliography

Marino FA, Zabloski EJ, Herman CM: *Principles of Pharmaceutical Accounting*, Lea & Febiger, Philadelphia, 1980.

Smith HA: *Principles and Methods of Pharmacy Management*, 3rd ed, Lea & Febiger, Philadelphia, 1986.

Tharp CP, Lecca PJ: *Pharmacy Management for Students and Practitioners*, 2nd ed, Mosby, St Louis, 1979.

Effective Pharmacy Management, 6th ed, Marion Merrell Dow, Kansas City MO, 1990.

The Lilly Digest (ann ed), Eli Lilly & Co, Indianapolis IN.

CHAPTER 112

Pharmacoeconomics

William F McGhan, PharmD, PhD
Professor of Pharmacy, Department of Pharmacy Practice and Pharmacy Administration,
Philadelphia College of Pharmacy & Science,
Philadelphia, PA 19104

Pharmacy practitioners and managers face a multitude of economic challenges. The impact of cost-containment is causing administrators and policy makers in pharmacy to examine closely the costs and benefits of both proposed and existing programs. It is increasingly evident that private employers and public agencies are demanding that health programs be evaluated in terms of clinical and social outcomes related to the costs incurred. Cost-benefit analysis, along with other pharmacoeconomic approaches, is a way to analyze the value of the service to the public, as a supplement to the traditional marketplace value measured by the prices that the patient or patron is willing to pay. As third parties are paying for a higher percentage of prescriptions dispensed, pharmacy managers are beginning to realize that pharmacy services may require further cost-justification in order to thrive in the future.[1,2]

Pharmacy entrepreneurs have established numerous innovative roles for pharmacists, such as home intravenous (IV) therapy, drug-level monitoring, parenteral nutrition management and self-care counseling. The use of valid economic evaluation methods (such as cost-benefit and cost-effectiveness analysis) to measure the value and impact of new services can increase acceptance of such programs by the medical profession, third-party payers and consumers.[3–5]

There is increasing competition among health professionals for the limited dollars and resources available. Within institutions and communities, pharmacists will have to compete increasingly with nursing, medical and other groups for adequate reimbursement and payment.[6,7] Pharmacy must document the cost-benefits of distinct pharmacy services, and must develop priorities for those services to compete successfully within various arenas.

The purpose of this chapter is to present the general concepts related to cost-benefit and cost-effectiveness analysis, and to suggest how these concepts can be applied in justifying, evaluating and improving pharmacy programs and services.

Overview of Cost-Benefit and Other Economic Methods

The intent of this section is to acquaint the reader with some of the methodological issues regarding cost-benefit analysis (CBA) and cost-effectiveness analysis (CEA). Table 1 provides a basic comparison of these two methods, as well as comparing operations analysis, cost-minimization and cost-utility analysis. One can differentiate between the various approaches according to the units used to measure the inputs and outcomes, as shown in Table 1. For example, in operations research, the inputs may be measured in *pharmacy hours* and the output *production* units such as *number of patients monitored.* In general, the outputs in CEA are related in various outcome measures, such as lives saved, life-years added or disability-days prevented. Whereas, CBA is differentiated from CEA through the use of dollars to measure the output of the respective program. Further discussion and examples of these techniques have been presented elsewhere.[1–3,8–16] The evaluation mechanisms delineated may be helpful in demonstrating both the cost-effectiveness and cost-benefit of pharmaceutical services.

Table 1—Comparison of Evaluation Techniques Regarding Inputs and Outputs

Technique	Inputs	Outputs
Classical operations analysis	Units	Units
Cost-effectiveness analysis	Dollars	Natural units
Cost-benefit analysis	Dollars	Dollars
Cost-utility analysis	Dollars	Utiles/preferences
Cost-minimization analysis	Dollars	Assumed equal

Cost-Benefit Analysis

The use of CBA is not a new concept in evaluating health programs. It is a basic tool that can be used to improve the decision-making process in the allocation of funds to health and other programs.[10,17–26] While the overall concept of CBA is simple, many of the methodological considerations require a certain degree of technical expertise in order to apply CBA appropriately.

The concept of CBA evolved from the need to ascertain estimates of the costs and benefits of public investment projects. Expenditures for health care should produce net social benefits for the public. Thus, CBA techniques can be applied to make resource-allocation decisions in the health-care field. Economists have indicated that medical care is both an investment *good* and a consumption *good.* When considered as an investment good, medical care is an investment in human capital.[25–27] As Pigou has pointed out, "the most important investment of all is the investment in health, intelligence, and character of the people."[28] In economic terms, the present value of a person's lifetime productivity generally is considered the appropriate measure of the benefit from investment in human capital.[27–30]

A major function in any pharmacy planning process is the formulation of alternative ways to achieve desired objectives and then choosing between these alternatives. Many times, decisions are made on the basis of intuition and personal judgment. Cost-benefit analysis, by requiring one to state precise definitions and objectives, to identify criteria for judging results and to quantify the results of each alternative, and examination of the effects of assumptions and uncertainties, provides a more solid basis for decision-making.

Although it may not be easy to conduct a full economic evaluation, an important advantage of CBA is that it forces those responsible to quantify input (costs) and output (benefits) as thoroughly as possible rather than to be content with vague qualitative judgments or personal hunches.[29,30]

Cost-benefit analysis consists of identifying all the societal benefits that will accrue from a health program of interest and converting them into equivalent dollars in the year in which they will occur. This stream of benefit-dollars then is discounted to its equivalent present value at the selected interest rate. On the other side of the equation, all costs of the program are identified and allocated to a specific year and, again, the costs are discounted to their present value at the same interest rate. Then, other things being equal, the program with the largest present value of benefits minus costs is the *best* in terms of its economic value.

Ideally, all benefits and costs caused by the program should be included. This presents considerable difficulty—especially on the benefits side of the equation—since many of the benefits are either difficult to measure, difficult to convert to dollars or both. For example, benefits such as improved patient comfort, improved patient satisfaction with the health-care system, improved working conditions for the physician, etc are not only difficult to measure but extremely difficult to convert into dollars.[29–36]

Another problem in CBA is how one determines the proper interest rate for discounting future benefits and costs. Prest and Turvey recommend that the selection of a rate be based on similar projects, followed by sensitivity analysis to determine the effect of a range of discount rates as the final solution.[29] The problem of selecting an appropriate discount rate and other methodological considerations will be discussed in further detail later in the chapter.

Measuring Benefits

The economic benefits of a health program are defined as the reduction in costs realized because of the implementation of that program. The conventional classification of these benefits is threefold: direct, indirect and intangible. As these terms are studied, also realize that programs often have parallel terms on the cost side of the equation, with direct, indirect and intangible costs.[1,2]

Direct Benefits

Direct benefits are defined as that portion of averted costs currently borne that are associated with spending for health services; they represent potential savings in the use of health resources. In other words, direct benefits are estimations of savings on direct costs. Direct costs include those costs incurred prior to diagnosis and hospitalization, during hospitalization, during convalescent care and during continued medical surveillance. Rice suggested that these costs include "expenditures for prevention, detection, treatment, rehabilitation, research, training and capital investments in medical facilities as well as professional services, drugs, medical supplies and nonpersonal health services."[37,38] Most often, direct benefits may be calculated with relatively little difficulty.

Indirect Benefits

Indirect benefits represent the potential savings on indirect costs. Despite extensive treatment in the literature, indirect benefits are difficult to measure. They are the result of the avoidance of earnings and productivity losses which would have been borne without the health program in question. Rice[38] provides a systematic method of measuring indirect benefits. Her estimates include wage and productivity losses resulting from illness, disability and death based on age and sex for major causal categories of morbidity and mortality.

Intangible Benefits

Intangible costs of ill health are difficult, if not impossible, to measure. These costs may be described as the psychic costs of disease such as those incurred from pain, suffering and grief.[38–40]

The measurement of such intangible benefits poses an almost insuperable task. However, Mishan[41] emphasized that an attempt should be made to account for extremely valuable *spillover* effects if at all possible.

Discount Rates

All benefits and costs which occur at different times must be adjusted to reflect comparable values. This is accomplished by converting dollar amounts into present values through the use of an interest rate often referred to as the discount rate. Although most economists agree that discounting should be emphasized, there is much discussion as to the appropriate rate for a given situation. The consequences of choosing a high or a low discount rate are clear: a low discount rate favors projects with benefits accruing in the distant future, while a high rate favors projects with costs in the distant future.[41–45]

One commonly used rate is the current yield rate on long-term government bonds. This seems practical since it represents a riskless long-term alternative use of funds by a tax-free institution and, therefore, appears valid for use by hospitals in evaluating long-term investment proposals.[2,43] Theoretical support can be found in the literature for practically any figure between the pure time-reference (riskless) rate, as low as 4%, and the corporate return on capital, approximately 20%.[44–48]

Cost-benefit methodology is based upon certain assumptions; it is important to have these assumptions clearly in mind before proceeding.[26] The basic assumptions of CBA are

It is possible to separate one service from another service in a sensible way.
There is a possibility of choice between the interventions.
It is possible to estimate the outcomes associated with each service.
It is possible to value these outcomes.
It is possible to estimate the cost of providing each service.
These costs and benefits can be weighed against each other.
We should provide only those services/treatments in which the benefits outweigh the costs.

Using these assumptions, there are several mathematical methods for developing a benefit/cost ratio. All have the same objective, but they differ in the way in which they handle the data mathematically.[49] The most common method is the following calculation:[50]

$$\text{Cost-benefit ratio} = \frac{\sum_{t=1}^{n} [B_t/(1 + r)^t]}{\sum_{t=1}^{n} [C_t/(1 + r)^t]}$$

where B_t = total benefits for time period t, C_t = total costs for time period, t, r = discount rate and n = number of time periods. The decision criterion is

If $B/C > 1$, benefits exceed costs and program is socially valuable.
If $B/C = 1$, benefits equal costs.
If $B/C < 1$, benefits are less than costs; therefore, the program is not socially beneficial.

The major problem with selecting this method is in choosing r, the discount rate, which was discussed earlier.

A second, increasingly more popular equation used in CBA, relates to the logical concept of net present value (NPV) represented in the equation below.[50]

$$\text{Benefit-costs} = \text{NPV} = \sum_{t=1}^{n} [(B_t - C_t)/(1 + r)^t]$$

These equations can be misleading, depending on the potential differences in the magnitude of dollars and time involved when comparing the costs and benefits of competing programs. In Table 2, simplified versions of three different cost-benefit approaches have been presented to illustrate how the decision factors can vary. The third approach presented in the table includes calculation of a *rate of return* on the investment, which is a rearrangements of the above equations to allow calculation of the *interest rate* from an initial program investment over a potential stream of benefits over time. From these various calculation options, one must select which formula is most appropriate in their institution or setting, and

Table 2—Sample Comparison Using Three Different Cost-Benefit Equations

	Costs (t_1)	Benefits (t_1)	Cost-benefit ratio (B/C)	Net present value (B-C)	Internal rate of return $\frac{(B-C)}{C}$
Program A	\$10,000	\$15,000	1.5:1	\$5,000	50%
Program B	\$100,000	\$180,000	1.8:1	\$80,000	80%

perhaps the calculated answers from all three CBA equations should be presented in the report. Many economists recommend the net present value (NPV) approach.

In the example provided in Table 2, Program A might represent a proposal for a medium-size computer in the pharmacy while Program B might represent a large computer system with multiple decentralized terminals. Although Program B has a higher cost-benefit ratio and rate of return, it is an expensive system and the pharmacy may not be able to commit such a substantial amount of funds. Numerous other examples could be considered here which change the results from the various formulas and make it more difficult to select between programs.

It should be emphasized that, for the limited investment streams presented in this example, the calculations have been simplified greatly. The calculations and comparisons become more complex as benefits are accrued at different increments of time and as costs and benefits are discounted properly with the more complete formulas presented earlier.

If a new project involves startup costs, such as a laminar-flow hood for a home IV service, calculations from the above formulas can be considered. If there are extra benefits accrued by an efficient distribution system, the amount of money that must be saved as benefits each year becomes similar to amortizing off a startup loan (SL) over time (t) with interest rate (r) and with extra yearly benefits (BX). Therefore

$$BX = SL[r/1 - (1 + r)^{-t}]$$

Cost-Effectiveness Analysis

Considerations for Cost-Effectiveness Analysis[50–54] are that

The optimal alternative (not necessarily the least costly) for accomplishing an objective should be possible.
At least two alternative interventions should be possible.
It need not be cost-reduction analysis but rather an optimizing process.

In CEA, costs are calculated in dollars but alternative ways then are compared for achieving a specific set of results such as blood pressure or life-expectancy changes. The objective is not just how to use funds most wisely but CEA also includes the constraint that similar output measurements must be achieved in order to compare interventions.[26] Thus, CEA is applied to health matters in situations where the program's inputs can be measured readily in dollars, but the program's outputs are stated more appropriately in terms of the health improvement created (eg, life-years extended). Weinstein and Stason provided an excellent explanation of the use of CEA for the practicing physician as well as for the physician-administrator.[53] Table 3 provides additional comparison points between the CBA and CEA.

Basic mathematical examples of various economic analyses are presented for cost benefit (Table 4), cost-effectiveness (Table 5), cost-utility (Table 6) and cost-minimization (Table 7).

Economic Perspectives

An important consideration in understanding CBA and CEA is that a pharmacy service providing a positive benefit-to-cost ratio may be of benefit to society as a whole but may not be valued in the same way by different segments of society. For example, a drug therapy regimen that reduces the number of patient-days in an acute-care institution is positive from society's point of view but not necessarily from that of the institution's administrator who operates under a fixed level of revenue and who depends upon a fixed number of patient-days to meet expenses. In other words, what is viewed as cost-beneficial to society may be viewed differently by third-party payors, administrators, health providers, governmental agencies or even individual patients. One must determine whose interests are to be measured when identifying outcome criteria for evaluation. From a cost-benefit perspective, one must always consider who pays the costs and who receives the benefits. A proposal justifying a pharmacy program to a hospital administration obviously would want to demonstrate that the benefits to the hospital outweigh the costs to the hospital. Society's perspective should always be discussed in a CBA, CEA report.

Table 3—Comparison of Cost-Benefit with Cost-Effectiveness Analysis

Cost-benefit analysis	Cost-effectiveness analysis
Uses dollar values for output measurement	Does not use dollar values for output measurement
Determines maximum benefit or investment	Determines least cost combination
Assumes limited resources	Assumes adequate resources
Expedites comparisons among several programs	Generally refers to different ways of reaching the same objectives
Less flexible	More flexible
Micro-oriented tool of analysis	Micro-oriented tool of analysis
Maximizes output—not equity or distribution	Maximizes output—not equity or distribution

Quality-of-Life Outcomes and Patient Decisions

Equally significant in pharmacoeconomics and patient-outcomes management is the issue of quality of life.[55,56] Although it is recognized that there are physical, mental and social impairments associated with disease, there is disagreement on how these factors are to be measured. Consequently, the concept of satisfaction with care often is overlooked in cost-effectiveness studies and even in the approval process of the FDA. But pharmacoeconomics and outcomes research considers quality of life an important predictor in creating a full model of survival and improvement.[54–56] Quality of life is related to clinical outcomes as much as drugs, practitioners, settings and types of disease. The question is how to select and use effective instruments (such as listed in Table 8) for measuring quality of life and satisfaction with care in a meaningful way.

Table 4—Cost-Benefit Analysis: Example Applied to Drug Therapy

	Cost of Therapies (\$)	
	Drug A	Drug B
Costs		
Acquisition cost	300	400
Administration	50	0
Monitoring	50	0
Adverse effects	100	0
Subtotal	500	400
Benefits		
Days at work (\$)	1000	1000
Extra months of life (\$)	2000	3000
Subtotal (\$)	3000	4000
Benefit-to-cost ratio	3000/500 = 6:1	4000/400 = 10:1

Table 5—Cost-Effectiveness Analysis: Example Applied to Drug Therapy

	Cost of Therapies ($)	
	Drug A	Drug B
Costs		
Acquisition cost	300	400
Administration	50	0
Monitoring	50	0
Adverse effects	100	0
Subtotal	500	400
Outputs		
Extra years of life	1.5	1.6
Cost-effectiveness ratio	500/1.5	400/1.6
	= $333	= $250
	per extra year of life	

Another important aspect of quality-of-life research is the number of healthy years within life extension. In an average life span of 73 or 74 years, people may have about 11 or 12 dysfunctional years. Therefore, whenever we examine the pharmacoeconomic impact of pharmaceuticals, we should adjust for the quality of life of any extra years of survival so as to reflect whether this increase leads to full, healthy years or includes some dysfunctional adjustments as well. Likewise, if adjustments are not made for comorbidities, the resulting health profile may be skewed. For example, untreated hypertension may escape a quality-of-life measurement because it does not affect daily life overtly. But a myocardial infarction definitely would lessen quality of life. The FDA has been leery of drugs that make patients feel better while life expectancy is reduced. Nevertheless, the patient must be presented with the various probabilities between perfect health and death plus the compromises associated with different treatments and then administer care accordingly.

In order to present these probabilities, though, one must monitor what happens to patients during clinical treatments over a period of time and collect data on patients' utilities. This means that patients should be asked how they feel about their therapy options, which therapies they prefer and how is their quantity and quality of life affected. Pharmaceutical companies have sponsored studies that examine probabilities, utilities and cost-effectiveness and then chart the results over a period of time. Using decision-analysis concepts, researchers can construct a decision tree of what actually happens to the patient from diagnosis to cure. As a result of using such analytical approaches, one can see clearly not only

Table 6—Cost-Utility Analysis: Example Applied to Drug Therapy

	Cost of Therapies ($)	
	Drug A	Drug B
Costs		
Acquisition cost	300	400
Administration	50	0
Monitoring	50	0
Adverse effects	100	0
Subtotal	500	400
Utilities		
Extra years of life	1.5	1.6
Quality of life index	0.33	0.25
QALYs[a]	0.50	0.40
Cost to utility ratio	500/0.5	400/0.4
	= $1000	= $1000
	per extra quality of life year	

[a]QALYs = Quality adjusted life years.

Table 7—Cost-Minimization Analysis: Example Applied to Drug Therapy[a]

	Cost of Therapies ($)	
	Drug A	Drug B
Costs		
Acquisition cost	250	350
Administration	75	0
Monitoring	75	25
Adverse effects	100	25
Subtotal	500	400
Outcomes		
Antibiotic effectiveness	90%	90%
Result = Cost of Drug A > Cost of Drug B		

[a]In cost-minimization, both interventions (drugs) are considered to be equally effective, and in this example, the cost-minimization question is answered by stating that Drug B is $100 less than Drug A.

costs, but also the probability of entering one health state over another.

From all of this computer modeling one also can develop treatment protocols. Each of the branches of the decision tree designates specific treatments for patients at specific health states. In a simplified form, this tree doubles as an educational tool for presenting available therapy options and probable consequences to the patient.[57,58]

Wennberg[58] has been exploring ways to involve patients in this type of decision-making process. One of his recent projects is a computer interactive program on prostate surgery. This program explains to patients the probability of success,

Table 8—Outcomes and Quality-of-Life Measurement Approaches

- Basic-outcomes list
  - Death
  - Disease
  - Disability
  - Discomfort
  - Dissatisfaction
- Major quality-of-life domains
  - Physical status and functional abilities
  - Psychological status and well-being
  - Social interactions
  - Economic status and factors
- Expanded outcomes list
  - Clinical endpoints
    - Symptoms and signs
    - Laboratory values
    - Death
  - Functional parameters
    - Physical (activities)
    - Mental (depression)
    - Social (friends)
    - Role (work)
  - General well-being
    - Pain
    - Energy/fatigue
    - Health perceptions
    - Opportunity (future)
    - Life satisfaction
  - Satisfaction with care
    - Access
    - Convenience
    - Financial coverage
    - Quality
    - General
- Sample of instruments for outcomes measurement
  - Generic instruments—Sickness Impact Profile (SIP), Nottingham, Quality of Well Being (QWB), Medical Outcome Study (MOS)
  - Specific instruments—Pain, Arthritis, Epilepsy, Cancer

what pain might be involved at each step and what the procedure actually entails. After viewing this program with visual graphic depictions of the surgery, many patients changed their decisions about wanting surgery over watchful waiting. This avoidance of a major surgical procedure resulted from a greater focus on quality of life and patient satisfaction. With further evaluation and perhaps modification of the computer program, it also may produce more cost-effective care. Wennberg's work is an application of outcomes research which helped to weigh costs, utilities and quality of life for the patient. This example shows how a concern for patient input and choice can help balance health-care costs.

Discussion

A key impact to which pharmacy needs to give more attention is the idea that the greatest benefit which can be generated for society as a whole is to target and take more responsibility toward decreasing mortality, not just decreased morbidity. Extra years of life for a patient population can be converted to dollars for society, which greatly enhances the benefit-to-cost ratio of a program. More research remains to be done on the potential impact of pharmacists and pharmaceuticals on mortality rate and quality of life. It is expected that the new government reimbursement plans will include incentives to decrease patient mortality rates and improve quality.

Pharmacy practitioners and managers must consider cost-benefit and cost-effectiveness based on the outcomes of the services that pharmacy delivers and the impact that pharmacy services can provide. There are a number of ways that pharmacy can produce positive outcomes. For example, pharmaceutical services can

Decrease morbidity in patient populations.
Increase the percentage of patients in therapeutic control.
Reduce the costs of the treatment by using more efficient modes of therapy.
Reduce the number of physician visits.
Reduce the rate of hospitalization attributable to or affected by the improper use of drugs.
Contribute to better use of health manpower by using computers and technicians.
Decrease the incidence and intensity of iatrogenic disease, such as adverse drug reactions.

Other examples of the types of pharmacy services and their potential benefits and effects include patient education, which improves patient compliance, reduces medication errors, lessens medication misuse and provides efficient use of all personnel. A unit-dose distribution program can improve patient therapy while reducing drug waste and, perhaps, nursing personnel costs.

By monitoring drug therapy in acute-care situations, practitioners can provide early detection of therapy failure or adverse reaction. Admixture programs provide better IV therapy and possibly more efficient use of personnel. Under patient and therapy responsibilities, drug prescribing by pharmacists might be included, which can be highly cost-effective. What is being done in defined patient-care situations is substituting a pharmacists salary for that of a physician, which may be two or even three times greater. Pharmacists can provide a very beneficial service in the areas of patient-discharge interviews and in taking patient histories. Under personnel substitutions, one can look at ways that pharmacists can increase physician productivity and, by using computers and technicians, how the pharmacy salary budget can be allocated best.

In this chapter a general explanation of CBA and CEA has been provided with the intent to help the reader in cost-justification efforts. There are encouraging reports in the literature that demonstrate that pharmacists and pharmaceuticals can produce cost-benefit effects in a number of areas. Still, it must be realized that even though this research is positive, there is a need to continue to develop programs that maximize the benefit-to-cost ratio to society and to institutions.

Even though a pharmacy endeavor can demonstrate a positive ratio of benefit to cost, society or the health-service organizations will ultimately invest their resources in needed programs which have the higher benefit-to-cost ratio. Similarly, the health system must be convinced that beneficial pharmacy services and pharmaceuticals are worth using with modification or even deletion of other less effective programs if necessary. Pharmacy managers must fully understand evaluation tools such as CBA and CEA if their programs are to thrive in the future.[59]

References

1. McGhan WF: *Hosp Formul 28:* 365, 1993.
2. McGhan W, Rowland C, Bootman JL: *Am J Hosp Pharm 35:* 133, 1978.
3. Ray M: *Ibid 36:* 308, 1979.
4. Bootman JL, McGhan WF Schondelmeyer SW: *Drug Intell Clin Pharm 16:* 235, 1982
5. McGhan WF, Lewis NJ: *Clin Ther 3:* 486, 1992.
6. Enright SM: *Am J Hosp Pharm 40:* 835, 1983.
7. Curtiss FR: *Ibid 40:* 586, 1983.
8. Weinstein MC, Statson B: *N Engl J Med 296:* 716, 1977.
9. Shepard DS, Thompson MS: *Pub Health Rep 94:* 535, 1979.
10. Crystal R, Brewster A: *Inquiry 3:* 3, 1966.
11. Acton J: *Law Contemp Probl 40:* 46, 1976.
12. Emlet HE Jr: *Use of Cost-Benefit Analysis in Solutions to National Health Problems,* 1968 Joint Natl Mtg, Op Res Soc Am, San Francisco, May 1–3, 1968.
13. Gellman DD: *Cancer Med Assoc J 4:* 998, 1974.
14. Goldschmidt PG: *Inquiry 13:* 29, 1976.
15. Bootman JL *et al: J Pharm Sci 68:* 267, 1979.
16. Bootman JL *et al: Am J Hosp Pharm 36:* 368, 1979.
17. Strange PV, Sumner AT: *N Engl J Med 298:* 372, 1978.
18. Cretin S: *Health Serv Res 12:* 174, 1977.
19. Mattsson W *et al: Acta Radiol Oncol 18:* 509, 1979.
20. Stason W, Weinstein M: *N Engl J Med 296:* 732, 1977.
21. Estershan RJ Jr *et al: Cancer 37:* 646, 1976.
22. Bryers F, Hawthorne VM: *J Epidemiol Community Health 32:* 171, 1978.
23. Kissick WL: *Cost-Benefit Studies in Health Planning in the U.S.A.,* Health Economics, Copenhagen, 39, 1969.
24. Klarman H: *Int J Health Serv 4:* 325, 1974.
25. Klarman H: *Am J Public Health 57:* 1948, 1967.
26. Smith W: *Public Health Rep 83:* 899, 1968.
27. Mushkin S, d'Accolings F: *Public Health Rep 74:* 338, 1959.
28. Pigou AC: *Socialism Versus Capitalism,* Macmillan, London, 129, 1947.
29. Prest AR, Turvey R: *Econ J 75:* 683, 1965
30. Peters GH: *Cost / Benefit Analysis and Public Expenditures* (Paper 8), Inst Econ Aff, London, 1968.
31. Osteryoung J: *Capital Budgeting: Long-Term Asset Selection,* Grid Inc, Columbus, OH, 1974.
32. Silvers JB, Praholed CK: *Financial Management of Health Institutions,* Spectrum Publ, New York, 1974.
33. Van Horne JC: *Financial Management and Policy,* Prentice-Hall, Englewood Cliffs, NJ, 1974.
34. Torrance G: *A Generalized Cost-Effectiveness Model for Evaluation of Health Programs.* (PhD Dissertation), State Univ of New York at Buffalo, 1971.
35. Klarman H: *J Occup Med Mar:* 172, 1974.
36. Schulbert HC, Sheldon CA, Baker F: *Program Evaluation in the Health Field,* Behavioral Publ, New York, 1969.
37. Rice DP: *Public Health Rep 84:* 91, 1969.
38. Rice DP: *Estimating the Cost of Illness* (Health Econ Ser No 6), USGPO, Washington DC, 1966.
39. Rinehard K, Felsman F, Moody L: *Public Health Rep 85:* 402, 1970.
40. Ridker RG: *Economic Cost of Air Pollution,* Praeger, New York, 1967.
41. Mishan EJ: In Harberger A *et al,* ed: *Benefit / Cost Analysis,* Aldine-Atherton, Chicago, 103, 1971.
42. Packer AH: *Op Res 16:* 227, 1968.
43. Klarman H: *Economics of Health,* Columbia Univ Press, New York, 1965b.

44. Marglin SA: *J Econ 77:* 95, 1963.
45. Baumol WJ: In Haveman R, Margolia J, eds: *Expenditures and Policy Analysis*, Markham, Chicago, 273, 1970.
46. Amadio J, Mueller J, Grey R: In *Public Health Rep*, IL Dept Public Health, Southern Illinois Univ: Carbondale and Jackson County Health Dept, 1976.
47. Joehnk M, McGrail GR, Degal NJ: *Application of a Benefit/Cost Model to Family Practice Nes Denz* (Natl Tech Inf Serv No HRP-0007312), DHEW, Washington DC, 1975.
48. Cohn E: *Public Expenditures Analysis*, Health, Lexington MA, 1972.
49. Ruchlin E, Rogers H: *Economics and Health Care*, Charles C Thomas, Springfield IL, 1973.
50. Mishan EJ: *Cost-Benefit Analysis*, Holt, Rinehart & Winston, New York, 1976.
51. Quade ES: In Goldin T, ed: *Cost/Effectiveness Analysis*, Praeger, New York, 1967.
52. Niskanen WA: *Ibid:* 18.
53. Weinstein MC, Stason B: *N Engl J Med 296:* 716, 1977.
54. Bootman JL, Townsend RB, McGhan WF: *Principles of Pharmacoeconomics*, Harvey Whitney Books, Cincinnati OH, 1991.
55. Ellwood PM: *N Engl J Med 318:* 1549, 1988.
56. MacKeigan LD, Pathak DS: *Am J Hosp Pharm 49:* 236, 1992.
57. Einarson TR, McGhan WF, Bootman JL: *Ibid 42:* 364, 1985.
58. Wennberg JE: *JAMA 258:* 2568, 1987.
59. McGhan WF, Smith MD: *Pharm Bus Spring 4(2):* 6, 1993.

Table of Metric Doses with Approximate Apothecary Equivalents

These ***approximate*** dose equivalents represent the quantities usually prescribed, under identical conditions, by physicians using, respectively, the metric system and the apothecary system of weights and measures. Statements of quantity or strength in the labeling of drug products, when expressed in the metric and apothecary systems, shall utilize ***exact*** equivalents.

When prepared dosage forms such as tablets, capsules, etc, are prescribed in the metric system, the pharmacist may dispense the corresponding ***approximate*** equivalent in the apothecary system and vice versa, as indicated in the following table.

For the conversion of specific quantities in converting pharmaceutical formulas, use the ***exact*** equivalents. For prescription compounding, use the exact equivalents rounded to three significant figures.

Liquid Measure

Metric	Approximate Apothecary Equivalents	Metric	Approximate Apothecary Equivalents	Metric	Approximate Apothecary Equivalents
1000 mL	1 quart	10 mL	2 1/2 fluid drams	0.5 mL	8 minims
750 mL	1 1/2 pints	8 mL	2 fluid drams	0.3 mL	5 minims
500 mL	1 pint	5 mL	1 1/4 fluid drams	0.25 mL	4 minims
250 mL	8 fluid ounces	4 mL	1 fluid dram	0.2 mL	3 minims
200 mL	7 fluid ounces	3 mL	45 minims	0.1 mL	1 1/2 minims
100 mL	3 1/2 fluid ounces	2 mL	30 minims	0.06 mL	1 minim
50 mL	1 3/4 fluid ounces	1 mL	15 minims	0.05 mL	3/4 minim
30 mL	1 fluid ounce	0.75 mL	12 minims	0.03 mL	1/2 minim
15 mL	4 fluid drams	0.6 mL	10 minims		

Weight

Metric	Approximate Apothecary Equivalents	Metric	Approximate Apothecary Equivalents	Metric	Approximate Apothecary Equivalents
30 g	1 ounce	200 mg	3 grains	4 mg	1/15 grain
15 g	4 drams	150 mg	2 1/2 grains	3 mg	1/20 grain
10 g	2 1/2 drams	125 mg	2 grains	2 mg	1/30 grain
7.5 g	2 drams	100 mg	1 1/2 grains	1.5 mg	1/40 grain
6 g	90 grains	75 mg	1 1/4 grains	1.2 mg	1/50 grain
5 g	75 grains	60 mg	1 grain	1 mg	1/60 grain
4 g	60 grains (1 dram)	50 mg	3/4 grain	800 μg	1/80 grain
3 g	45 grains	40 mg	2/3 grain	600 μg	1/100 grain
2 g	30 grains (1/2 dram)	30 mg	1/2 grain	500 μg	1/120 grain
1.5 g	22 grains	25 mg	3/8 grain	400 μg	1/150 grain
1 g	15 grains	20 mg	1/3 grain	300 μg	1/200 grain
750 mg	12 grains	15 mg	1/4 grain	250 μg	1/250 grain
600 mg	10 grains	12 mg	1/5 grain	200 μg	1/300 grain
500 mg	7 1/2 grains	10 mg	1/6 grain	150 μg	1/400 grain
400 mg	6 grains	8 mg	1/8 grain	120 μg	1/500 grain
300 mg	5 grains	6 mg	1/10 grain	100 μg	1/600 grain
250 mg	4 grains	5 mg	1/12 grain		

NOTE: A milliliter (mL) is the approximate equivalent of a cubic centimeter (cc).

PERIODIC CHART

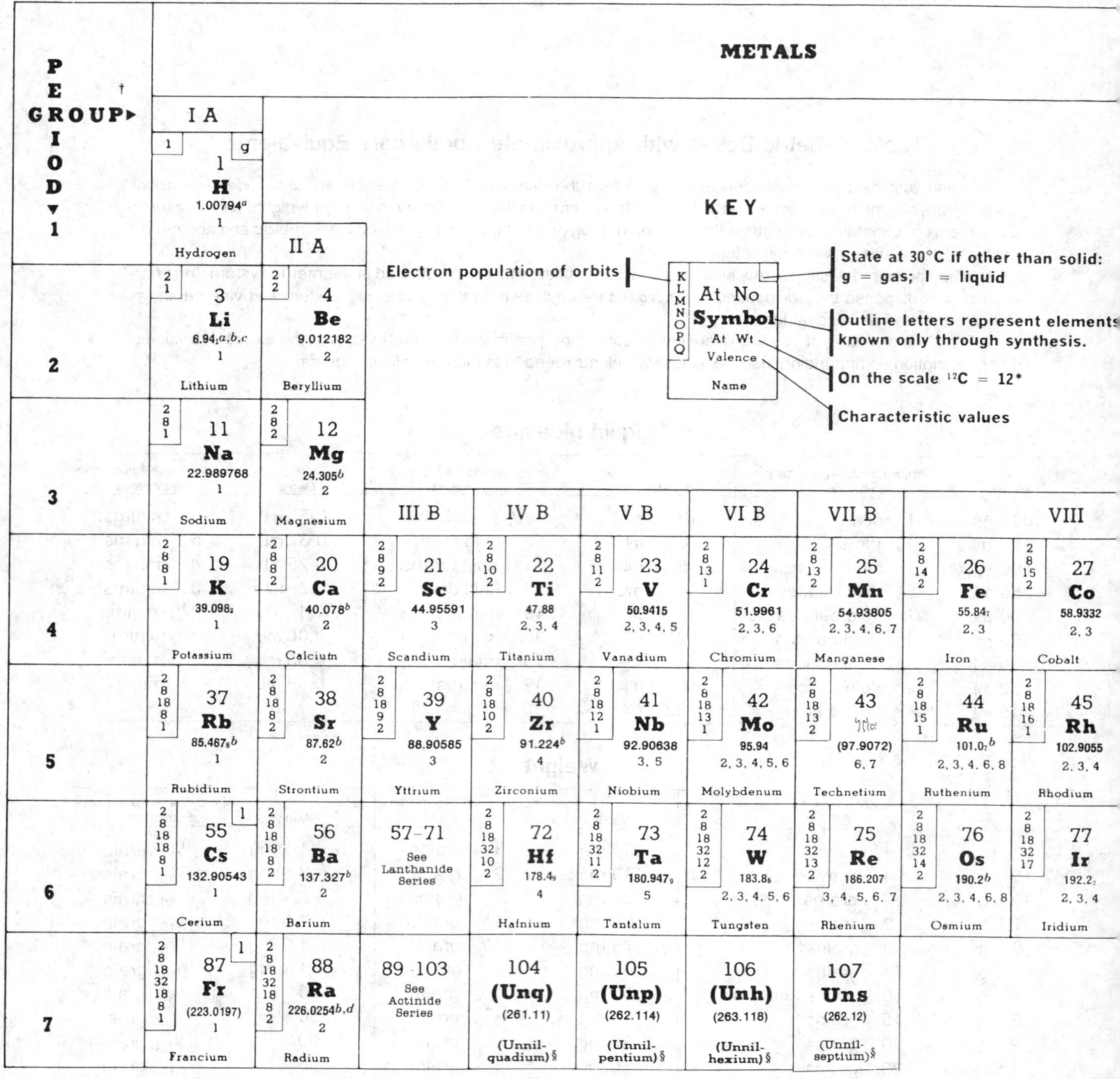

METALS

KEY

PERIOD ▼ † GROUP ▶

PERIOD	IA	IIA	III B	IV B	V B	VI B	VII B	VIII	VIII
1	1 **H** 1.00794[a] 1 Hydrogen (1; g)								
2	3 **Li** 6.94_1[a,b,c] 1 Lithium (2, 1)	4 **Be** 9.012182 2 Beryllium (2, 2)							
3	11 **Na** 22.989768 1 Sodium (2, 8, 1)	12 **Mg** 24.305[b] 2 Magnesium (2, 8, 2)							
4	19 **K** 39.098_3 1 Potassium (2, 8, 8, 1)	20 **Ca** 40.078[b] 2 Calcium (2, 8, 8, 2)	21 **Sc** 44.95591 3 Scandium (2, 8, 9, 2)	22 **Ti** 47.88 2, 3, 4 Titanium (2, 8, 10, 2)	23 **V** 50.9415 2, 3, 4, 5 Vanadium (2, 8, 11, 2)	24 **Cr** 51.9961 2, 3, 6 Chromium (2, 8, 13, 1)	25 **Mn** 54.93805 2, 3, 4, 6, 7 Manganese (2, 8, 13, 2)	26 **Fe** 55.84_7 2, 3 Iron (2, 8, 14, 2)	27 **Co** 58.9332 2, 3 Cobalt (2, 8, 15, 2)
5	37 **Rb** 85.467_8[b] 1 Rubidium (2, 8, 18, 8, 1)	38 **Sr** 87.62[b] 2 Strontium (2, 8, 18, 8, 2)	39 **Y** 88.90585 3 Yttrium (2, 8, 18, 9, 2)	40 **Zr** 91.224[b] 4 Zirconium (2, 8, 18, 10, 2)	41 **Nb** 92.90638 3, 5 Niobium (2, 8, 18, 12, 1)	42 **Mo** 95.94 2, 3, 4, 5, 6 Molybdenum (2, 8, 18, 13, 1)	43 **Tc** (97.9072) 6, 7 Technetium (2, 8, 18, 13, 2)	44 **Ru** 101.0_7[b] 2, 3, 4, 6, 8 Ruthenium (2, 8, 18, 15, 1)	45 **Rh** 102.9055 2, 3, 4 Rhodium (2, 8, 18, 16, 1)
6	55 **Cs** 132.90543 1 Cerium (2, 8, 18, 18, 8, 1; l)	56 **Ba** 137.327[b] 2 Barium (2, 8, 18, 18, 8, 2)	57–71 See Lanthanide Series	72 **Hf** 178.4_9 4 Hafnium (2, 8, 18, 32, 10, 2)	73 **Ta** 180.947_9 5 Tantalum (2, 8, 18, 32, 11, 2)	74 **W** 183.8_5 2, 3, 4, 5, 6 Tungsten (2, 8, 18, 32, 12, 2)	75 **Re** 186.207 3, 4, 5, 6, 7 Rhenium (2, 8, 18, 32, 13, 2)	76 **Os** 190.2[b] 2, 3, 4, 6, 8 Osmium (2, 8, 18, 32, 14, 2)	77 **Ir** 192.2_2 2, 3, 4 Iridium (2, 8, 18, 32, 17)
7	87 **Fr** (223.0197) 1 Francium (2, 8, 18, 32, 18, 8, 1; l)	88 **Ra** 226.0254[b,d] 2 Radium (2, 8, 18, 32, 18, 8, 2)	89–103 See Actinide Series	104 **(Unq)** (261.11) (Unnil-quadium)§	105 **(Unp)** (262.114) (Unnil-pentium)§	106 **(Unh)** (263.118) (Unnil-hexium)§	107 **Uns** (262.12) (Unnil-septium)§		

Lanthanide Series (Rare Earth Elements)	57 **La** 138.905_5[b] 3 Lanthanum (2, 8, 18, 18, 9, 2)	58 **Ce** 140.115[b] 3, 4 Cerium (2, 8, 18, 19, 9, 2)	59 **Pr** 140.90765 3, 4 Praseodymium (2, 8, 18, 20, 9, 2)	60 **Nd** 144.2_4[b] 3 Neodymium (2, 8, 18, 22, 8, 2)	61 **Pm** (144.9127) 3 Promethium (2, 8, 18, 23, 8, 2)	62 **Sm** 150.36 2, 3 Samarium (2, 8, 18, 24, 8, 2)	63 **Eu** 151.965[b] 2, 3 Europium (2, 8, 18, 25, 8, 2)
Actinide Series	89 **Ac** 227.0278[d] 3 Actinium (2, 8, 18, 32, 18, 9, 2)	90 **Th** 232.0381[b,d] 4 Thorium (2, 8, 18, 32, 19, 9, 2)	91 **Pa** 231.0359[d] 5 Protactinium (2, 8, 18, 32, 20, 9, 2)	92 **U** 238.0289[b,c] 3, 4, 5, 6 Uranium (2, 8, 18, 32, 21, 9, 2)	93 **Np** 237.0482[d] 3, 4, 5, 6 Neptunium (2, 8, 18, 32, 22, 9, 2)	94 **Pu** (244.0642) 3, 4, 5, 6 Plutonium (2, 8, 18, 32, 23, 9, 2)	95 **Am** (243.0614) 3, 4, 5, 6 Americium (2, 8, 18, 32, 24, 9, 2)

* Atomic weight is an alternative term for 'relative atomic mass of an element', A_r(E). The IUPAC values given here are scale to $A_r(^{12}C) = 12$ and apply to elements as they exist in materials of terrestrial origin and to certain artificial elements. Whe used with due regard to the footnotes they are considered reliable to ±1 in the last digit or ±3 if that digit is subscript. Val ues in parentheses are for radioactive elements whose atomic weights cannot be quoted precisely without knowledge of th origin of the elements; the value given is the atomic mass number of the isotope of that element of longest known half-life

† Beginning with Group III, authors differ in their presentation of the "A" and "B" groups of elements.

‡ Expected value from theoretical considerations. § Names and symbols provisionally suggested by IUPAC.

OF THE ELEMENTS (Revised 1987)

			NON-METALS					INERT GASES
							VII A	ZERO
							1 g 1 **H** 1.00794[a] −1 Hydrogen	2 g 2 **He** 4.002602[b] 0 Helium
			III A	IV A	V A	VI A		
			2 3 5 **B** 10.811[a,c] 3 Boron	2 4 6 **C** 12.011[a] −4; 2, 4 Carbon	2 5 g 7 **N** 14.00674 −3; 3, 5 Nitrogen	2 6 g 8 **O** 15.999_4[a] −2 Oxygen	2 7 g 9 **F** 18.9984032 −1 Fluorine	2 8 g 10 **Ne** 20.1797[c] 0 Neon
	I B	II B	2 8 3 13 **Al** 26.981539 3 Aluminum	2 8 4 14 **Si** 28.085_5 −4; 4 Silicon	2 8 5 15 **P** 30.973762 −3; 3, 5 Phosphorus	2 8 6 16 **S** 32.066[a] −2; 2, 4, 6 Sulfur	2 8 7 g 17 **Cl** 35.4527 −1; 1, 3, 5, 7 Chlorine	2 8 8 g 18 **Ar** 39.94_8[a,b] 0 Argon
2 8 16 2 28 **Ni** 58.69 2, 3 Nickel	2 8 18 1 29 **Cu** 63.54_6[a] 1, 2 Copper	2 8 18 2 30 **Zn** 65.39 2 Zinc	2 8 18 3 l 31 **Ga** 69.723 3 Gallium	2 8 18 4 32 **Ge** 72.61 4 Germanium	2 8 18 5 33 **As** 74.92159 −3; 3, 5 Arsenic	2 8 18 6 34 **Se** 78.9_6 −2; 4, 6 Selenium	2 8 18 7 l 35 **Br** 79.904 −1; 1, 3, 5, 7 Bromine	2 8 18 8 g 36 **Kr** 83.80[b,c] 0 Krypton
2 8 18 18 46 **Pd** 106.42[b] 2, 4 Palladium	2 8 18 18 1 47 **Ag** 107.868_2[b] 1 Silver	2 8 18 18 2 48 **Cd** 112.411[b] 2 Cadmium	2 8 18 18 3 49 **In** 114.82[b] 3 Indium	2 8 18 18 4 50 **Sn** 118.71 2, 4 Tin	2 8 18 18 5 51 **Sb** 121.7_5 −3; 3, 5 Antimony	2 8 18 18 6 52 **Te** 127.6_0[b] −2; 4, 6 Tellurium	2 8 18 18 7 53 **I** 126.90447 −1; 1, 3, 5, 7 Iodine	2 8 18 18 8 g 54 **Xe** 131.29[b,c] 0 Xenon
2 8 18 32 17 1 78 **Pt** 195.0_8 2, 4 Platinum	2 8 18 32 18 1 79 **Au** 196.96654 1, 3 Gold	2 8 18 32 18 2 l 80 **Hg** 200.5_9 1, 2 Mercury	2 8 18 32 18 3 81 **Tl** 204.3833 1, 3 Thallium	2 8 18 32 18 4 82 **Pb** 207.2[a,b] 2, 4 Lead	2 8 18 32 18 5 83 **Bi** 208.980437 3, 5 Bismuth	2 8 18 32 18 6 84 **Po** (208.9824) 2, 4 Polonium	2 8 18 32 18 7 85 **At** (209.9871) 1, 3, 5, 7‡ Astatine	2 8 18 32 18 8 g 86 **Rn** (222.0176) 0 Radon

2 8 18 25 9 2 64 **Gd** 157.2_5[b] 3 Gadolinium	2 8 18 26 9 2 65 **Tb** 158.92534 3, 4 Terbium	2 8 18 28 8 2 66 **Dy** 162.5_0 3 Dysprosium	2 8 18 29 8 2 67 **Ho** 164.93032 3 Holmium	2 8 18 30 8 2 68 **Er** 167.2_6 3 Erbium	2 8 18 31 8 2 69 **Tm** 168.93421 3 Thulium	2 8 18 32 8 2 70 **Yb** 173.0_4 2, 3 Ytterbium	2 8 18 32 9 2 71 **Lu** 174.96_7 3 Lutetium
2 8 18 32 25 9 2 96 **Cm** (247.0703) 3 Curium	2 8 18 32 26 9 2 97 **Bk** (247.0703) 3, 4 Berkelium	2 8 18 32 27 9 2 98 **Cf** (251.0796) 3 Californium	2 8 18 32 28 9 2 99 **Es** (252.083) 3‡ Einsteinium	2 8 18 32 29 9 2 100 **Fm** (257.0951) 3‡ Fermium	2 8 18 32 30 9 2 101 **Md** (258.10) 3‡ Mendelevium	2 8 18 32 31 9 2 102 **No** (259.1009) 3‡ Nobelium	2 8 18 32 32 9 2 103 **Lr** (262.11) 3‡ Lawrencium

[a] Element for which known variations in isotopic composition in normal terrestrial material prevent a more precise atomic weight being given; A_r(E) values should be applicable to any 'normal' material. [b]Element for which geological specimens are known in which the element has an anomalous isotopic composition, such that the difference between the atomic weight of the element in such specimens and that given in the table may exceed considerably the implied uncertainty. [c]Element for which substantial variations in A_r from the value given can occur in commercially available material because of inadvertent or undisclosed change of isotopic composition. [d]Element for which the value of A_r is that of the radioisotope of longest half-life.

Table of Logarithms

Natural Numbers	0	1	2	3	4	5	6	7	8	9	PP 1	2	3	4	5	6	7	8	9
10	0000	0043	0086	0128	0170	0212	0253	0294	0334	0374	4	8	12	17	21	25	29	33	37
11	0414	0453	0492	0531	0569	0607	0645	0682	0719	0755	4	8	11	15	19	23	26	30	34
12	0792	0828	0864	0899	0934	0969	1004	1038	1072	1106	3	7	10	14	17	21	24	28	31
13	1139	1173	1206	1239	1271	1303	1335	1367	1399	1430	3	6	10	13	16	19	23	26	29
14	1461	1492	1523	1553	1584	1614	1644	1673	1703	1732	3	6	9	12	15	18	21	24	27
15	1761	1790	1818	1847	1875	1903	1931	1959	1987	2014	3	6	8	11	14	17	20	22	25
16	2041	2068	2095	2122	2148	2175	2201	2227	2253	2279	3	5	8	11	13	16	18	21	24
17	2304	2330	2355	2380	2405	2430	2455	2480	2504	2529	2	5	7	10	12	15	17	20	22
18	2553	2577	2601	2625	2648	2672	2695	2718	2742	2765	2	5	7	9	12	14	16	19	21
19	2788	2810	2833	2856	2878	2900	2923	2945	2967	2989	2	4	7	9	11	13	16	18	20
20	3010	3032	3054	3075	3096	3118	3139	3160	3181	3201	2	4	6	8	11	13	15	17	19
21	3222	3243	3263	3284	3304	3324	3345	3365	3385	3404	2	4	6	8	10	12	14	16	18
22	3424	3444	3464	3483	3502	3522	3541	3560	3579	3598	2	4	6	8	10	12	14	15	17
23	3617	3636	3655	3674	3692	3711	3729	3747	3766	3784	2	4	6	7	9	11	13	15	17
24	3802	3820	3838	3856	3874	3892	3909	3927	3945	3962	2	4	5	7	9	11	12	14	16
25	3979	3997	4014	4031	4048	4065	4082	4099	4116	4133	2	3	5	7	9	10	12	14	15
26	4150	4166	4183	4200	4216	4232	4249	4265	4281	4298	2	3	5	7	8	10	11	13	15
27	4314	4330	4346	4362	4378	4393	4409	4425	4440	4456	2	3	5	6	8	9	11	13	14
28	4472	4487	4502	4518	4533	4548	4564	4579	4594	4609	2	3	5	6	8	9	11	12	14
29	4624	4639	4654	4669	4683	4698	4713	4728	4742	4757	1	3	4	6	7	9	10	12	13
30	4771	4786	4800	4814	4829	4843	4857	4871	4886	4900	1	3	4	6	7	9	10	11	13
31	4914	4928	4942	4955	4969	4983	4997	5011	5024	5038	1	3	4	6	7	8	10	11	12
32	5051	5065	5079	5092	5105	5119	5132	5145	5159	5172	1	3	4	5	7	8	9	11	12
33	5185	5198	5211	5224	5237	5250	5263	5276	5289	5302	1	3	4	5	6	8	9	10	12
34	5315	5328	5340	5353	5366	5378	5391	5403	5416	5428	1	3	4	5	6	8	9	10	11
35	5441	5453	5465	5478	5490	5502	5514	5527	5539	5551	1	2	4	5	6	7	9	10	11
36	5563	5575	5587	5599	5611	5623	5635	5647	5658	5670	1	2	4	5	6	7	8	10	11
37	5682	5694	5705	5717	5729	5740	5752	5763	5775	5786	1	2	3	5	6	7	8	9	10
38	5798	5809	5821	5832	5843	5855	5866	5877	5888	5899	1	2	3	5	6	7	8	9	10
39	5911	5922	5933	5944	5955	5966	5977	5988	5999	6010	1	2	3	4	5	7	8	9	10
40	6021	6031	6042	6053	6064	6075	6085	6096	6107	6117	1	2	3	4	5	6	8	9	10
41	6128	6138	6149	6160	6170	6180	6191	6201	6212	6222	1	2	3	4	5	6	7	8	9
42	6232	6243	6253	6263	6274	6284	6294	6304	6314	6325	1	2	3	4	5	6	7	8	9
43	6335	6345	6355	6365	6375	6385	6395	6405	6415	6425	1	2	3	4	5	6	7	8	9
44	6435	6444	6454	6464	6474	6484	6493	6503	6513	6522	1	2	3	4	5	6	7	8	9
45	6532	6542	6551	6561	6571	6580	6590	6599	6609	6618	1	2	3	4	5	6	7	8	9
46	6628	6637	6646	6656	6665	6675	6684	6693	6702	6712	1	2	3	4	5	6	7	7	8
47	6721	6730	6739	6749	6758	6767	6776	6785	6794	6803	1	2	3	4	5	5	6	7	8
48	6812	6821	6830	6839	6848	6857	6866	6875	6884	6893	1	2	3	4	4	5	6	7	8
49	6902	6911	6920	6928	6937	6946	6955	6964	6972	6981	1	2	3	4	4	5	6	7	8
50	6990	6998	7007	7016	7024	7033	7042	7050	7059	7067	1	2	3	3	4	5	6	7	8
51	7076	7084	7093	7101	7110	7118	7126	7135	7143	7152	1	2	3	3	4	5	6	7	8
52	7160	7168	7177	7185	7193	7202	7210	7218	7226	7235	1	2	2	3	4	5	6	7	7
53	7243	7251	7259	7267	7275	7284	7292	7300	7308	7316	1	2	2	3	4	5	6	6	7
54	7324	7332	7340	7348	7356	7364	7372	7380	7388	7396	1	2	2	3	4	5	6	6	7

Natural Numbers	0	1	2	3	4	5	6	7	8	9	PP 1	2	3	4	5	6	7	8	9
55	7404	7412	7419	7427	7435	7443	7451	7459	7466	7474	1	2	2	3	4	5	5	6	7
56	7482	7490	7497	7505	7513	7520	7528	7536	7543	7551	1	2	2	3	4	5	5	6	7
57	7559	7566	7574	7582	7589	7597	7604	7612	7619	7627	1	2	2	3	4	5	5	6	7
58	7634	7642	7649	7657	7664	7672	7679	7686	7694	7701	1	1	2	3	4	4	5	6	7
59	7709	7716	7723	7731	7738	7745	7752	7760	7767	7774	1	1	2	3	4	4	5	6	7
60	7782	7789	7796	7803	7810	7818	7825	7832	7839	7846	1	1	2	3	4	4	5	6	6
61	7853	7860	7868	7875	7882	7889	7896	7903	7910	7917	1	1	2	3	4	4	5	6	6
62	7924	7931	7938	7945	7952	7959	7966	7973	7980	7987	1	1	2	3	3	4	5	6	6
63	7993	8000	8007	8014	8021	8028	8035	8041	8048	8055	1	1	2	3	3	4	5	5	6
64	8062	8069	8075	8082	8089	8096	8102	8109	8116	8122	1	1	2	3	3	4	5	5	6
65	8129	8136	8142	8149	8156	8162	8169	8176	8182	8189	1	1	2	3	3	4	5	5	6
66	8195	8202	8209	8215	8222	8228	8235	8241	8248	8254	1	1	2	3	3	4	5	5	6
67	8261	8267	8274	8280	8287	8293	8299	8306	8312	8319	1	1	2	3	3	4	5	5	6
68	8325	8331	8338	8344	8351	8357	8363	8370	8376	8382	1	1	2	3	3	4	4	5	6
69	8388	8395	8401	8407	8414	8420	8426	8432	8439	8445	1	1	2	2	3	4	4	5	6
70	8451	8457	8463	8470	8476	8482	8488	8494	8500	8506	1	1	2	2	3	4	4	5	6
71	8513	8519	8525	8531	8537	8543	8549	8555	8561	8567	1	1	2	2	3	4	4	5	5
72	8573	8579	8585	8591	8597	8603	8609	8615	8621	8627	1	1	2	2	3	4	4	5	5
73	8633	8639	8645	8651	8657	8663	8669	8675	8681	8686	1	1	2	2	3	4	4	5	5
74	8692	8698	8704	8710	8716	8722	8727	8733	8739	8745	1	1	2	2	3	4	4	5	5
75	8751	8756	8762	8768	8774	8779	8785	8791	8797	8802	1	1	2	2	3	3	4	5	5
76	8808	8814	8820	8825	8831	8837	8842	8848	8854	8859	1	1	2	2	3	3	4	5	5
77	8865	8871	8876	8882	8887	8893	8899	8904	8910	8915	1	1	2	2	3	3	4	4	5
78	8921	8927	8932	8938	8943	8949	8954	8960	8965	8971	1	1	2	2	3	3	4	4	5
79	8976	8982	8987	8993	8998	9004	9009	9015	9020	9026	1	1	2	2	3	3	4	4	5
80	9031	9036	9042	9047	9053	9058	9063	9069	9074	9079	1	1	2	2	3	3	4	4	5
81	9085	9090	9096	9101	9106	9112	9117	9122	9128	9133	1	1	2	2	3	3	4	4	5
82	9138	9143	9149	9154	9159	9165	9170	9175	9180	9186	1	1	2	2	3	3	4	4	5
83	9191	9196	9201	9206	9212	9217	9222	9227	9232	9238	1	1	2	2	3	3	4	4	5
84	9243	9248	9253	9258	9263	9269	9274	9279	9284	9289	1	1	2	2	3	3	4	4	5
85	9294	9299	9304	9309	9315	9320	9325	9330	9335	9340	1	1	2	2	3	3	4	4	5
86	9345	9350	9355	9360	9365	9370	9375	9380	9385	9390	1	1	2	2	3	3	4	4	5
87	9395	9400	9405	9410	9415	9420	9425	9430	9435	9440	0	1	1	2	2	3	3	4	4
88	9445	9450	9455	9460	9465	9469	9474	9479	9484	9489	0	1	1	2	2	3	3	4	4
89	9494	9499	9504	9509	9513	9518	9523	9528	9533	9538	0	1	1	2	2	3	3	4	4
90	9542	9547	9552	9557	9562	9566	9571	9576	9581	9586	0	1	1	2	2	3	3	4	4
91	9590	9595	9600	9605	9609	9614	9619	9624	9628	9633	0	1	1	2	2	3	3	4	4
92	9638	9643	9647	9652	9657	9661	9666	9671	9675	9680	0	1	1	2	2	3	3	4	4
93	9685	9689	9694	9699	9703	9708	9713	9717	9722	9727	0	1	1	2	2	3	3	4	4
94	9731	9736	9741	9745	9750	9754	9759	9763	9768	9773	0	1	1	2	2	3	3	4	4
95	9777	9782	9786	9791	9795	9800	9805	9809	9814	9818	0	1	1	2	2	3	3	4	4
96	9823	9827	9832	9836	9841	9845	9850	9854	9859	9863	0	1	1	2	2	3	3	4	4
97	9868	9872	9877	9881	9886	9890	9894	9899	9903	9908	0	1	1	2	2	3	3	4	4
98	9912	9917	9921	9926	9930	9934	9939	9943	9948	9952	0	1	1	2	2	3	3	4	4
99	9956	9961	9965	9969	9974	9978	9983	9987	9991	9996	0	1	1	2	2	3	3	3	4

Alphabetic Index*

* Main entries in this index will follow in alphabetical order of the entire entry, regardless of spaces or hyphens between words. Indented entries do not alter the alphabetic progression of the principal entry. For example, *Aerosol, propellants* will preceed *Aerosols*, as the main entries are *Aerosol* and *Aerosols*. The indented, subordinate entry does not participate in the alphabetization. However, two or more indented entries under a main heading are arranged in alphabetical order. Prefixes (*n*-, *iso*-, *para*-, etc) and locants (arabic numerals or Greek letters) are disregarded in determining the alphabetical sequence (1-Propanol, β-Blockers), unless spelled out (Dextrocalcium pantothenate). Acronyms are included in the Glossary.

C

D

E

F

G

H

I

J

K

L

M

N

O

P

Q

R

S

T

U

V

W

X

Glossary*

2D-NMR two-dimensional NMR
6-MP 6-mercaptopurine

A

AA atomic absorption
AA Alcoholics Anonymous
AAAD aromatic amino acid decarboxylase
AAC actual acquisition cost
AAC antibiotic-associated colitis
AACP American Association of Clinical Pharmacy
AACP American Association of Colleges of Pharmacy
AAPCC American Association of Poison Control Centers
AAPS American Association of Pharmaceutical Scientists
AARP American Association of Retired Persons
Ab antibody
ABG arterial blood gas
ACCP American College of Clinical Pharmacy
ACE angiotensin converting enzyme
ACIP Advisory Committee on Immunization Practices
ACPE American Council on Pharmaceutical Education
ACS American Chemical Society
ACTH adrenocorticotropic hormone
ADE adverse drug experience
ADH antidiuretic hormone
ADME absorption, distribution, metabolism and elimination
ADP adenosine diphosphate
ADR adverse drug reaction
ADRRS Adverse Drug Reaction Reporting System
AEC Atomic Energy Commission
AEM analytical electron microscopy
AES auger electron spectrometry
AFMS Air Force Medical Service
AFPE American Foundation for Pharmaceutical Education
Ag antigen
AGD agar gel diffusion
AHA American Hospital Association
AHF antihemophilic factor
AHG antihemophilic globulin
AI aortic insufficiency
AIDS acquired immune deficiency syndrome
AJHP American Journal of Hospital Pharmacy
AJPE American Journal of Pharmaceutical Education
ALA aminolevulinic acid
ALS antilymphocyte serum
ALT alanine aminotransferase
ALU arithmetic logic unit
AMA American Medical Association
AMC Air Mobility Command
AML acute myelogenous leukemia
ANA antinuclear antibodies
ANC acid neutralizing capacity
ANDA abbreviated new drug application
ANOVA analysis of variance
AO atomic orbital(s)
APAP acetaminophen
APC antigen-presenting cell(s)
APhA American Pharmaceutical Association
APP alternating pressure pad
APSAC anisoylated plasminogen-streptokinase activator complex
ARDS adult respiratory distress syndrome
ARF acute renal failure
ASCII American Standard Code for Information Interchange
ASHP American Society of Hospital Pharmacists
ASO Administrative Service Organizations
ASPEN American Society for Parenteral and Enteral Nutrition
AST aspartate aminotransferase
ASTM American Society for Testing and Materials
ASV anodic stripping voltammetry
ATN acute tubular necrosis
ATP adenosine triphosphate
ATR attenuated total reflectance
ATTC American Type Culture Collection
AUC area under the concentration-time curve
AV atrioventricular
AWP average wholesale price

B

BAC blood-alcohol concentrations
BAL British antilewisite
BASIC Beginner's Allpurpose Symbolic Instruction Code
BATO boronic acid technetium dioxime
BBB blood-brain barrier
BCA bifunctional chelating agents
BCDSP Boston Collaborative Drug Surveillance Program
BCG Bacille Calmette-Guerin
BCG Boston Consulting Group
BCMS British Committee on the Safety of Medicines
BDZ benzodiazepine
BET Brunauer, Emmett and Teller
BET bacterial endotoxin test
BHA butylated hydroxyanisole
BI biological indicator
BIA bacterial inhibition assay
BIOSIS Biosciences Information Service
BJA basic journal abstracts
BMS between mean squares
BP British Pharmacopeia
BPC British Pharmaceutical Codex
BPL beta-propiolactone
BSA bovine serum albumin
BSP bromosulfonphthalein
BSS between sum-of-squares
BSTFA *N,O*-bistrimethylsilyltrifluoroacetamide
BTMSA *N,O*-bistrimethylsilylacetamide
BUN blood urea nitrogen

C

CA Chemical Abstracts
CAD coronary artery disease
CADD computer aided drug design
CAP cellulose acetate phthalate
CAS Chemical Abstracts Service
CASIA Chemical Abstracts computer-searchable index
CAT computerized axial tomography
CAT cellulose acetate trimellitate
CBA cost-benefit analysis
CBER Center for Biologics Evaluation and Research
CC Current Contents (published by ISI)
CCBs calcium channel blockers
CCD countercurrent distribution
CCRIS Chemical Carcinogenesis Research Information System
CD circular dichroism
CD compact disk
CD4 glycoprotein subset of T4-lymphocytes, thymocytes and macrophages
CDC Centers for Disease Control
CDI compact disk interactive
CE capillary electrophoresis
CEA cost effectiveness analysis
CEO chief executive officer
CEP counter-electrophoresis
CF complement fixation
CFC chlorofluorocarbon
CFR Code of Federal Regulations
CFU colony forming units
CGLP Current Good Laboratory Practice
CGMP Current Good Manufacturing Practice
CGS centimeter-gram-second
CHD coronary heart disease
CHF congestive heart failure
CHRIS Chemical Hazard Response Information System

*Symbols, abbreviations, acronyms, contractions, etc often are used in scientific writing to economize on space and minimize typing fatigue. While most terms are familiar to those working in the field, they may be complete gibberish to the uninitiated. This Glossary includes only those terms found in this book and is not meant to be all-inclusive. It does not define or explain, as in a dictionary. If a term appears to occur only once in a specific chapter, it may not be included herein. No attempt has been made to evaluate the frequency of usage of any particular term so that commonly employed items may appear here, even though the understanding seemingly is universal. Also, it is possible that the same term may not concurrently appear in the Index. This Glossary omits specific page references.

CIMS chemical ionization mass spectrometry
CINAHL Cumulative Index to Nursing and Allied Health Literature
CIP clean-in-place
CK creatine
CK creatine kinase
CLT central limit theorem
CMC critical micelle concentratiom
CMC carboxymethylcellulose
CMI cell mediated immunity
CMN Certificate of Medical Necessity
CMV cytomegalovirus
CNDO complete neglect of differential overlap
CNS central nervous system
CO cardiac output
CoA coenzyme A
COBOL Common Business Oriented Language
COH carboxyhemoglobin
COMPASS Computerized Online Medicaid Pharmaceutical Analysis
COMT catechol-*O*-methyltransferase
COPD chronic obstructive pulmonary disease
CPAP continuous positive airway pressure (devices)
CPK creatinine phosphokinase
CPPDDD calcium pyrophosphate dihydrate deposition disease
CPSC Consumer Product Safety Commission
CPT clinical pharmacology and therapeutics
CPU central processing unit
CQI continuous quality improvement
CRF chronic renal failure
CRF corticotropin-releasing factor
CRT cathode-ray tubes
CSA Controlled Substances Act
CSF cerebrospinal fluid
CSF colony stimulating factors
CSP chiral stationary phases
CSV cathodic stripping voltammetry
CT computerized tomography
CT compressed tablets
CTFE chlorotrifluoroethylene
CTL cytotoxic T lymphocytes
CTZ chemoreceptor trigger zone
CV coefficient of variation
CW continuous wave

D

D5/W dextrose injection 5% in water
DAG diacylglycerol
DCPA dacthal (dimethyl tetrachloroterephthalate)
DDS dapsone
DDVP dichlorvos
DEA Drug Enforcement Administration
DEAE diethylaminoethanol
DEAE diethylaminoethyl (group)
DEHP diethylhexyl phthalate
DES Division of Epidemiology and Surveillance
DET diethyltryptamine
DF degrees of freedom
DFC dry-filled capsule
DHHS Department of Health and Human Services
DHT dihydrotestosterone
DIFT Drug Information Full Text
DIMP dimethyl phthalate
DIP desquamative interstitial
DIP distal interphalangeal
DIS Drug Information Source
DJD degenerative joint disease
DME dropping mercury electrode
DMF dimethylformamide
DMF drug master file
DMSO dimethyl sulfoxide
DMT *N,N*-dimethyltryptamine
DNA deoxyribonucleic acid
DNCB dinitrochlorobenzene
DOD Department of Defense
DOE Department of Energy
DOM dimethoxy-4-methylamphetamine
DOP dioctyl phthalate
DOPA dihydroxyphenylalanine
DOS disk operating system
DPD dihydropyrimidine dehydrogenase
DPM disintegrations per minute
DPS disintegrations per second
DPSV differential pulse stripping voltammetry
DPT dipropyltryptamine
DQRS Drug Quality Reporting System
DRG diagnosis-related groups
DRR Drug Regimen Review
DSC differential scanning calorimetry
DSMA disodium methanearsonate
DT dispensing tablets
DTA differential thermal analysis
DTH delayed-type hypersensitivity
DTP diphtheria & tetanus toxoids & pertussis vaccine
DTPA diethylenetriaminepentaacetic acid
DUE Drug Usage Evaluations
DUR Drug Utilization Review
DVA Department of Veterans Affairs
DVB divinylbenzene
DVT deep venous thrombosis

E

EAA ethylene acrylic acid
EAE experimental allergic encephalomyelitis
EBCDIC Extended Binary Coded Decimal Interchange Code (computer)
ECD electron capture detector
ECF extracellular fluid
ECF extended-care facilities
ECF-A eosinopohil chemotactic factor of anaphylaxis
ECG electrocardiograph (-gram)
ECT enteric-coated tablets
ED end-diastole
ED_{50} median effective dose
EDA electron donor-acceptor
EDRF endothelium-derived relaxing factor
EDS energy dispersive spectrometer
EDTA ethylenediaminetetraacetic acid (edetic acid)
EDV end-diastolic volume
EEG electroencephalograph
EF ejection fraction
EFA esterified forms
EGDM ethylene glycol dimethacrylate
EIA enzyme immunoassays
ELISA enzyme-linked immunosorbent assay
EM electromagnetic
EM erythema multiforme
EMA ethylene methacrylic acid
EMF electromotive force
EMIT enzyme-mediated immunologic technique
EMS error mean square
ENTOMA Entomological Society of America
EPA Environmental Protection Agency
EPMA electron probe microanalysis
EPO erythropoietin
ERM electrochemical relaxation measurement
ERPF effective renal plasma flow
ES end-systole
ESCA electron spectroscopy chemical analysis
ESR erythrocyte sedimentation rate
ESR electron spin resonance
ET enterostomal therapist
EU endotoxin units
EVA ethylene vinyl acetate

F

FAB fast atom bombardment
FAD flavine adenine dinucleotide
FAO Food and Agriculture Organization
FAS fetal alcohol syndrome
FAX facsimile transmission
FCC Food Chemicals Codex
FCT film-coated tablets
FD field description
FD&C Food, Drug and Cosmetic Act
FDA Food and Drug Administration
FDP fibrinogen degradation products
FEF forced expiratory flow
FEV forced expiratory volume
FFT fast Fourier transform (data acquisition)
FHA filamentous hemaglutinin
FID free induction decay
FID flame ionization detector
FIFRA Federal Insecticide, Fungicide and Rodenticide Act
FIR far infrared region
FITC fluorescein isothiocyanate
FNMR Fourier transform NMR
FORTRAN formula translation language (computer)
FPD flame photometric detector
FPIA fluorescence polarization immunoassay
FRC functional residual capacity
FSH follicle-stimulating hormone
FT Fourier transform
FTC Federal Trade Commission
FTIR Fourier transform infrared spectrometry
FTMS Fourier transform mass spectrometry
FUDR floxuridine
FUMP floxuridine monophosphate
FVC forced vital capacity

G

G6P glucose-6-phosphate
G6PD G6P dehydrogenase
Gaba gamma-aminobutyric acid
GAO General Accounting Office
GAP Good Aseptic Practice
GC gas chromatography
GC gonorrhea
GC/MS gas chromatography/mass spectrometry
GDSG Gainesville Drug Study Group
GERD gastroesophageal reflux disease
GFR glomerular filtration rate

GH growth hormone
GHC Group Health Cooperative of Puget Sound
GI gastrointestinal
GLC gas-liquid chromatography
GLDH glutamic dehydrogenases
GLP Good Laboratory Practice
GMP Good Manufacturing Practice
GN glomerulonephritis
GRAS generally regarded as safe
GSC gas-solid chromatography
GSH glutathione

H

HA hepatitis-A
HA hemagglutination
HAA hepatitis associated antigen
HB hepatitis-B
Hb hemoglobin
HbA adult hemoglobin
HbC abnormal Hb with lysine in place of glutamine at position-6
HBDH hydroxybutyric dehydrogenases
HbF fetal hemoglobin
HBIG hepatitis-B immune specific globulin
HbM methemoglobin
HbS sickle hemoglobin
HCFA Health Care Financing Administration
HCG human chorionic gonadotropin
HCN hydrogen cyanide
HDCV rabies vaccine human diploid cell
HDL high density lipoprotein
HDPE high-density polyethylene
HEC hydroxyethylcellulose
HEMA hydroxyethylmethyl methacrylate
HEMA 2-hydroxyethyl methacrylate
HEPA high efficiency particulate air
HETP height equivalent to a theoretical plate
HGF hyperglycemic Factor
HIC hydrophobic interaction chromatography
HIDA Tc-99m labeled analog of iminodiacetic acid
HIMA Health Industry Manufacturers Association
HIV human immunodeficiency virus
HLA human leukocyte antigen
HLB hydrophile-lipophile balance
HMG human menopausal gonadotropin
HMO health maintenance organization
HMPAO hexamethylpropyleneamine oxime
HMPO hexamethylpropylene oxide
HNANB non-A, non-B hepatitis
HOCA high-osmality contrast agents
HP hydrogen peroxide
HPC hydroxypropylcellulose
HPL placental lactogen
HPLC high performance liquid chromatography
HPLC/MS HPLC/mass spectrometry
HPMC hydroxypropylmethylcellulose
HPMCAS hydroxypropyl methylcellulose acetate succinate
HPRS Homeopathic Pharmacopoeia Revision Service
HPUS Homeopathic Pharmacopoeia of the United States
HSA Health Systems Agencies
HSA human serum albumin
HSAB hard and soft acid-base
HSDB Hazardous Substance Databank
HSV-1 herpes simplex virus type-1
HSV-2 herpes simplex virus type-2
HT hypodermic tablets
HVA homovanillic acid
HVL half-value-layer
HWD hot wire detector

I

I/O input/output
IC ion chromatography
ICDH isocitric dehydrogenase
ICF intermediate care facilities
ICF intracellular fluid
ICF-MR intermediate care facilities for the mentally retarded
ICH International Conference on Harmonization
ICP inductively coupled plasmas
ICP-OES inductively coupled plasma optical emission spectrometry
ICR ion-cyclotron resonance
ICSH interstitial cell-stimulating hormone
IDDM insulin-dependent diabetes mellitus
IDP immunodominant peptides
Ig di-immunoglobulin
IgG Ig found in greatest amount in plasma
IgM Ig active against bacteria (gamma M-globulin)
IGR insect growth regulator
IHD ischemic heart disease
IHS Indian Health Service
IND Investigational New Drug
INDA Investigational New Drug Application
INDOR internuclear double resonance
INEPT insensitive nucleus enhancement by polarization transfer
INH isoniazid
INN International Nonproprietary Name
IOM Institute of Medicine
IP intraperitoneal
IP3 1,4,5-inositol triphosphate
IPA Independent Practice Association
IPA International Pharmaceutical Abstracts
IPM integrated pest management
IPP individual program plan
IPPB intermittent positive pressure breathing (machine)
IPV poliovirus vaccine inactivated
IR infrared spectrometry
IRB Institutional Review Board
IRMA immunoradiometric assays
ISA intrinsic sympathomimetic activity
ISCH interstitial cell hormone
ISE ion-specific electrodes
ISF interstitial fluid
ISFET ion-sensitive field effect transistor
ISI Institute for Scientific Information
ISS ion-scattering spectroscopy
IU International Units
IUDs interuterine devices
IUPAC International Union of Pure and Applied Chemistry
IV intravenous
IVF intravascular fluid

J

JCAH Joint Commission on Accreditation of Hospitals
JCAHO Joint Commission on Accreditation of Healthcare Organizations
JE Japanese encephalitis

K

KVO keep vein open

L

LAK lymphokine-activated killer (cells)
LAL *Limulus amebocyte* lysate
LAN local area networks
LAP leucine aminopeptidase
LATS long-acting thyroid stimulator
LCAO linear combination of atomic orbitals
LCD liquid crystal display
LD_{50} median lethal dose
LDH lactic acid dehydrogenase
LDL low density lipoprotein
LDPE low-densitity polyethylene
LED light-emitting diode
LES lower esophageal sphincter
LF laminar flow
LH lutenizing hormone
LISP List Processing Language (computer)
LLC liquid-liquid chromatography
LOCA low-osmolality contrast agents
LRF LH-releasing factor
LSC liquid-solid chromatography
LSD lysergic acid diethylamide
LTCF long-term care facilities
LTH luteotropin hormone
LUV large unilamellar vesicles
LVEDP left ventricular end-diastolic pressure
LVF left ventricular function
LVP large-volume parenterals

M

MAb monoclonal antibodies
MAC maximum allowable cost
MADD Mothers Against Drunk Drivers
MAO monoamine oxidase
MAOI monoamine oxidase inhibitor
MASS magic angle sample spinning
MCA multichannel analyzer
MCE methylcellulosic esters
MCH mean corpuscular hemoglobin
MCHC mean corpuscular hemoglobin concentration
MCPA 2-methyl-4-chlorophenoxyacetic acid
MCT mercury cadmium telluride
MCT multiple compressed tablet
MCT medium-chain triglyceride
MCV mean corpuscular volume
MDH malic dehydrogenase
MDI metered dose inhaler
MDMA 3,4-methylenedioxymethamphetamine
MDP methylenediphosphonate
MDR minimum daily requirements
MEC minimum effective concentration
MEC micellar electrokinetic chromatography
MEDLINE National Library of Medicine medical database
MEMS Medication Event Monitoring System
MES maximal seizures induced by electrical stimulation

MFO mixed-function oxidases
MI mitral insufficiency
MI myocardial infarction
MIA metabolite bacterial inhibition assay
MIBI methoxyisobutylisonitrile
MIF MSH-inhibitory factor
MIL-STD Military Standard (specifications)
MIR multiple internal reflection
MKT mean kinetic temperature
MLVR multilamellar vesicles
MMR measles, mumps and rubella virus vaccine, live
MMWR Morbidity and Mortality Weekly Report
MNOA *N*-methyl-D-aspartate
MNPC medicinal and natural products chemistry
MO molecular orbital(s)
MO-LCAO molecular orbital-linear combination atomic orbitals
MOD maturity-onset diabetes
MPD minimum pyrogenic dose
MPU microprocessor unit [computer]
MQ-NMR multiple quantum NMR technique
MRF MSH-releasing factor
MRI magnetic resonance imaging
MS mean square
MS mass spectrometry
MS mitral stenosis
MS multiple sclerosis
MS/MS mass spectrometry/mass spectrometry
MSD mass spectral detector
MSH melanocyte-stimulating hormone
MSMA monosodium methanearsonate
MSPPA Model State Pharmacy Practice Act
MSUD maple syrup urine disease
MTC minimum toxic concentration

N

NABP National Association of Boards of Pharmacy
NABPLEX National Association of Boards of Pharmacy Licensing Exam
NAD nicotinamide-adenine dinucleotide
NADPH nicotinamide-adenine dinucleotide phosphate
NARD National Association of Retail Druggists
NAS National Academy of the Sciences
NCCLS National Committee for Clinical Laboratory Standards
NCF-A neutrophil chemotactic factor of anaphylaxix
NCPIE National Council on Patient Information & Education
NCVIA National Childhood Vaccine Injury Act of 1986
NDA new drug application
NDIT National Disease and Therapeutic Index
NF National Formulary
NICEM National Information Center for Educational Media
NIDDM noninsulin-dependent diabetes mellitus
NIH National Institutes of Health
NINDS Natl Inst of Neurologic Diseases & Stroke
NIOSH National Institutes of Occupational Therapy and Health
NIR near infrared spectrometry
NK killer T cells and natural killer cells
NLM National Library of Medicine
NMR nuclear magnetic resonance [spectrometry]
NMT not more than (on prescriptions)
NO nitric oxide
NPA National Prescription Audit
NPD nitrogen/phosphorus detector
NPN nonprotein nitrogen compounds
NPV net present value
NRC Nuclear Regulatory Commission
NRC Natl Research Council
NSAID nonsteroidal anti-inflammatory drug
NTD neutral tube defect

O

O/W oil-in-water [emulsion]
O/W/O oil/water/oil [emulsion]
OAA Old Age Assistance
OAM Office of Alternative Medicine
OASI Old Age Survivors Insurance
OBRA 90 Ominbus Budget Reconciliation Act of 1990
ODS octadecylsilyl
OPV poliovirus vaccine live oral
ORD optical rotatory dispersion
OTC over-the-counter

P

P&T pharmacy & therapeutics [committee]
PABA *p*-aminobenzoic acid
PAD premature atrial depolarization
PAF platelet-activating factor
PAGE polyacrylamide gel electrophoresis
PAO peak acid output
PASCAL high-level computer language using English commands
PAW pulmonary arterial wedge
PBE proton-balance equation
PBI protein bound iodine
PBP penicillin-binding proteins
PC Pharmaceutical Codex (11th ed, 1979)
PC personal computer
PCA patient-controlled analgesia
PCP phencyclidine
PCR polymerase chain reaction
PCTFE polymonochlorotrifluoroethylene
PD plasma description
PDD pharmaceutics and drug delivery
PDGF platelet derived growth factor
PE pulmonary embolism
PEG polyethylene glycol
PEMA phenylethylmalonamide
PET polyethylene terephthalate
PET positron emission tomography
PFU plaque-forming units
PFV polyvinylidene fluoride
PHS Public Health Service
PIP proximal interphalangeal
PIT phase inversion temperature
PKU phenylketonuria
PLC programmable logic controller
PMA Pharmaceutical Manufacturers Association
PMMA poly(methyl methacrylate)
PMN polymorphonuclear leukocyte
PMR patient medication record
PND paroxysmal nocturnal dyspnea
PNI psychoneuroimmunology
PNSU probability of non sterile unit
PNU protein nitrogen units
POS point of service
PPDM pharmacodynamics and drug metabolism
PPI patient package insert
PPLO pleuropneumonia-like organisms
PPO preferred provider organization
PPT partial prothrombin time
PRA plasma renin activity
PRO professional review organizations
Pro-UK pro-urokinase
PRP polymer of ribose, ribitol and phosphate
PS polystyrene
PSAO Pharmacy Services Administrative Organization
PSE portal systemic encephalopathy
PSIG pounds per square inch (guage)
PSP phenolsulfonphthalein
PSVT paroxysmal supraventricular tachycardia
PT pertussis toxin
PTFE polytetrafluoroethylene
PTH parathyroid hormone
PTT partial thromboplastin time test
PVAP polyvinyl acetate phthalate
PVC premature ventricular contractions
PVD premature ventricular depolarizations
PVDC polyvinylidene chloride
PVP polyvinylpyrrolidone
PZI protamine zinc insulin

Q

QA quality assurance
QC quality control
QSAR quanitative structure activity relationships

R

R&D research and development
RA rheumatoid arthritis
RAM random access memory
RAS renin-angiotensin system
RAST radioallergosorbent test
RBC red blood cell (erythrocyte)
RCTES Registry of Toxic Effects of Chemical Substances
RDA recommended dietary allowances
RDI US recommended daily allowances
RDW red-cell distribution width
RE reticuloendothelial
RED Registration Eligibility Documents
rem roentgen equivalent man
REM rapid eye movement
RF releasing factor
RFLP restriction fragment length polymorphism
RH releasing hormone
RH relative humidity
RHB Recombivax HB
RIA radioimmunoassay
RIG rabies immune globulin
RISA radioiodinated human serum albumin
RIT radioimmunotherapy
RNA ribonucleic acid

RO	reverse osmosis
ROM	read-only memory
rpm	revolutions per minute
rps	revolutions per second
RPS	Remington's Pharmaceutical Sciences
RRT	relative retention time
RRV	relative retention volume
RSD	relative standard deviation
RSO	Radiation Safety Officer
RTPA	recombinant TPA
RV	residual volume
RVA	rabies vaccine, adsorbed

S

SAL	sterility assurance level
SAP	sterility assurance probability
SARA	Superfund Amendment and Reauthorization Act
SCA	single-channel analyzer
SCE	saturated calomel electrode
SCI	Science Citation Index
SCOT	support-coated open tubular
SCT	sugar-coated tablets
SD	standard deviation
SDH	sorbitol dehydrogenases
SDS	sodium dodecylsulfate
SEAM	Social and Economic Aspects of Medicine
SEC	soft elastic capsule
SFC	supercritical fluid chromatography
SGOT	serum glutamic oxaloacetic transaminase
SHMTADS	Soil and Hazardous Material-Technical Assistance Data System
SIADH	syndrome of inappropriate ADH secretion
SIDS	sudden infant death syndrome
SIMS	secondary ion mass spectrometry
SIP	steam-in-place
SIP	sterilizing in place
SLE	systemic lupus erythematosus
SNF	skilled nursing facilities
SOP	standard operating procedure
SPECT	single photon emission computerized tomography
SRS	Spontaneous Reporting System
SRS-A	slow-reacting substance of anaphylaxis
SS	sum-of-squares
SSBG	specific sex hormone binding globulin
SSD	sudden sniffing death
STA	slit-to-agar
STD	sexually transmitted disease
STH	somatotropin
STP	standard temperature and pressure
STP	serenity, tranquility, peace
SUVs	small unilamellar vesicles
SV	stroke volume
SVP	small-volume parenteral
SWFI	sterile water for injection

T

T3	triiodothyroxine
TAA	tumor-associated antigen
TB	tuberculosis
TBC	thyroxine-binding globulin
TBP	thyroxine-binding proteins
TBPA	thyroxine-binding pre-albumin
TCA	trichloroacetic acid
TCA	tricyclic antidepressants
TCD	thermal conductivity detector
TD_{50}	median toxic dose
TDM	therapeutic drug-monitoring
TEAE	triethylaminoethyl
TEEC	transesophageal echocardiography
TEN	toxic epidermal necrolysis
TENS	transcutaneous electrical nerve stimulation
TETA	tetraethylaminetetraacetic acid
TGA	thermal gravimetric analysis (thermogravimetric analysis)
TGT	thromboplastin generation time test
THC	tetrahydrocannabinol
TIA	transient ischemic attacks
TIG	tetanus immune globulin
TIL	tumor-infiltrating lymprocytes
TLC	total lung capacity
TLC	thin-layer chromatography
TM	transcendental mediatation
TMA	thermomechanical analysis
TMA	3,4,5-trimethoxyamphetamine
TMJ	temporomandibular joint
TMS	tetramethylsilane
TNF	tumor necrosis factor
TOPV	trivalent oral polio vaccine
TPA	tissue plasminogen activator
TPN	total parenteral nutrition
TQM	total quality management
TRH	thyrotropin-releasing hormone
TS	test solution
TSA	tumor-specific antigens
TSD	thermionic specific detector
TSH	thyroid stimulating hormone
TSIM	*N*-trimethylsilylimidazole
TT	tablet triturates
TV	tidal volume

U

UCC	Univorm Commerical Code
ULV	ultralow-volume
URI	upper respiratory [tract] infections
USAN	United States Adopted Name(s)
USDA	US Department of Agriculture
USP	United States Pharmacopoeia
USPC	United States Pharmacopeial Convention
USPDI	USP Dispensing Information
USPHS	US Public Health Service
USRDA	US Recommended Daily Allowance
UTI	urinary tract infections
UV	ultraviolet

V

VA	Veteran's Administration
VAERS	Vaccine Adverse Event Reporting System
VC	vital capacity
VHA	Veterans Health Administration
VIP	vasoactive intestinal polypeptide
VLDL	very low-density lipoproteins
VMA	vanillylmandelic acid
VNS	Visiting Nurse [Home Health] Service
VOC	volatile organic compound
VP	venous pressure
VS	volumetric solution
VWF	von Willebrand factor

W

W/O	water-in-oil [emulsion]
W/O/W	water/oil/water [emulsion]
WBC	white blood cell
WCOT	wall-coated open tubular
WDS	wavelength dispersive spectrometer
WEE	Western Equine Encephalitis
WFI	water for injection
WHO	World Health Organization
WMS	within mean square
WSS	within sum-of-squares

Z

ZE	Zollinger-Ellison
ZSR	zeta sedimentation ratio

Notes

Notes

Notes

Notes

Notes

Notes